Evolve®

YOU'VE JUST PURCHASED
MORE THAN A TEXTBOOK!

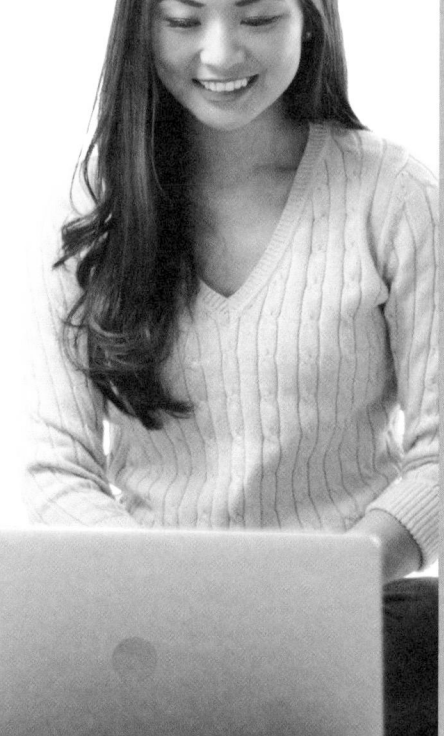

Enhance your learning with Evolve Student Resources.

These online study tools and exercises can help deepen your understanding of textbook content so you can be more prepared for class, perform better on exams, and succeed in your course.

Activate the complete learning experience that comes with each NEW textbook purchase by registering with your scratch-off access code at

http://evolve.elsevier.com/Potter/fundamentals/

If your school uses its own Learning Management System, your resources may be delivered on that platform. Consult with your instructor.

If you rented or purchased a used book and the scratch-off code at right has already been revealed, the code may have been used and cannot be re-used for registration. To purchase a new code to access these valuable study resources, simply follow the link above.

**POTTER
Scratch Gently
to Reveal Code**

REGISTER TODAY!

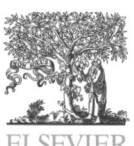

ELSEVIER

2019v1.0

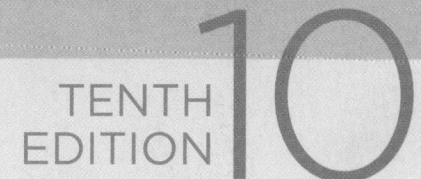

TENTH
EDITION **10**

FUNDAMENTALS of NURSING

Patricia A. Potter, RN, MSN, PhD, FAAN
Formerly, Director of Research
Patient Care Services
Barnes-Jewish Hospital
St. Louis, Missouri

Anne Griffin Perry, RN, MSN, EdD, FAAN
Professor Emerita
School of Nursing
Southern Illinois University Edwardsville
Edwardsville, Illinois

Patricia A. Stockert, RN, BSN, MS, PhD
Formerly, President, College of Nursing
Saint Francis Medical Center College of Nursing
Peoria, Illinois

Amy M. Hall, RN, BSN, MS, PhD, CNE
Professor and Dean
School of Nursing
Franciscan Missionaries of Our Lady University
Baton Rouge, Louisiana

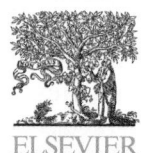

ELSEVIER

Elsevier
3251 Riverport Lane
St. Louis, Missouri 63043

FUNDAMENTALS OF NURSING, TENTH EDITION   ISBN: 978-0-323-67772-1
Copyright © 2021 by Elsevier Inc. All rights reserved.

Notice

Previous editions copyrighted 2017, 2013, 2009, 2005, 2001, 1997, 1993, 1989, 1985.

International Standard Book Number: 978-0-323-67772-1

Director, Traditional Education: Tamara Myers
Senior Content Development Manager: Lisa P. Newton
Senior Content Development Specialist: Tina Kaemmerer
Publishing Services Manager: Julie Eddy
Senior Project Manager: Jodi M. Willard
Design Direction: Maggie Reid
Cover Photo: Gianni Fioretti

Printed in Canada

Last digit is the print number: 9   8   7   6   5   4   3   2

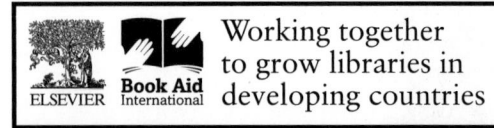

Kimberly Diane Baxter, DNP, APRN, FNP-BC
Associate Dean of Undergraduate Programs
Orvis School of Nursing
University of Nevada, Reno
Reno, Nevada

Sharon Ferguson Beasley, PhD, MSN, RN, CNE
Director
Executive
Accreditation Commission for Education in Nursing (ACEN)
Atlanta, Georgia

Carolyn J. Wright Boon, MSN, BSN
Assistant Professor
Nursing
Saint Francis Medical Center College of Nursing
Peoria, Illinois

Jessica L. Bower, DNP, MSN, RN
Simulation Lab Coordinator
Nursing Department
Pennsylvania College of Technology
Williamsport, Pennsylvania

Karen Britt, DNP, RN-BC, CNE
Associate Professor
Nursing
MCPHS University
Manchester, New Hampshire

Janice C. Colwell, RN, MS, CWOCN, FAAN
Advanced Practice Nurse
Surgery
University of Chicago Medicine
Chicago, Illinois

Sarah Delgado, MSN, RN, ACNP
Clinical Practice Specialist
Practice Excellence
American Association of Critical-Care Nurses
Aliso Viejo, California

Bronwyn Doyle, PhD, RN, CNE
Associate Dean of Undergraduate Nursing
School of Nursing
Franciscan Missionaries of Our Lady University
Baton Rouge, Louisiana

Alice E. Dupler, MSN, JD, RN, CNP, Esq
Professor
Nursing, School of Health Professions
University of Providence
Great Falls, Montana

Jane Fellows, MSN, CWOCN-AP
Wound/Ostomy CNS
Advanced Clinical Practice
Duke University Health System
Durham, North Carolina

Linda Felver, PhD, RN
Associate Professor
School of Nursing
Oregon Health & Science University
Portland, Oregon

Susan Fetzer, BA, BSN, MSN, MBA, PhD
Professor Emeritus
College of Health and Human Services
University of New Hampshire
Durham, New Hampshire;
Director of Research
Patient Care Services
Southern New Hampshire Medical Center
Nashua, New Hampshire

Victoria N. Folse, PhD, APRN, PMHCNS-BC, LCPC
Director and Professor; Caroline F. Rupert Endowed Chair of Nursing
School of Nursing
Illinois Wesleyan University
Bloomington, Illinois

Kay Gaehle, PhD, MSN
Associate Professor
Department of Primary Care and Health Systems Nursing
Southern Illinois University Edwardsville
Edwardsville, Illinois

Lorri A. Graham, DNP-L, RN
Visiting Professor
Nursing
Chamberlain University
Downers Grove, Illinois

Carla Armstead Harmon, PhD (Curriculum & Instruction), MSN, BSN
Associate Professor
School of Nursing
Franciscan Missionaries of Our Lady University
Baton Rouge, Louisiana

Susan Hendricks, EdD, MSN, RN, CNE
Professor and Dean
School of Nursing
Indiana University Kokomo
Kokomo, Indiana

Maureen Hermann, BSN, MSN, DNP, RN
Associate Professor
Nursing
Saint Francis Medical Center College of Nursing
Peoria, Illinois

Tara Hulsey, BSN, MSN, PhD
Vice President and Dean
Nursing
West Virginia University
Morgantown, West Virginia

Lenetra Jefferson, PhD, MSN, BSN, LMT
Nurse Educator
JeffCare
Jefferson Parish Human Services Authority
Metairie, Louisiana;
Contributing Faculty
School of Nursing
Walden University
Minneapolis, Minnesota;, Adjunct Faculty
School of Nursing
Troy University
Troy, Alabama

Noël Marie Kerr, PhD
Associate Professor
School of Nursing
Illinois Wesleyan University
Bloomington, Illinois

Shari Kist, PhD, RN, CNE
Project Supervisor
Missouri Quality Initiate for Nursing Homes
Sinclair School of Nursing
University of Missouri-Columbia
Columbia, Missouri

Mary Koithan, PhD, MSN, BSN
Associate Dean and Anne Furrow Professor
Student and Community Engagement,
College of Nursing
University of Arizona
Tucson, Arizona

Emily McClung, MSN, RN, PhD
Nursing Instructor
Hiram College
Hiram, Ohio

Angela McConachie, FNP, DNP
Associate Professor
Faculty
Goldfarb School of Nursing at Barnes Jewish
　College
St. Louis, Missouri

Emily McKenna, APN, CNS
Illinois Neurological Institute
INI Neurology
OSF St. Francis Medical Center
Peoria, Illinois

Theresa Miller, PhD, MSN, MHA, RN
Associate Professor
Nursing
Saint Francis Medical Center College of Nursing
Peoria, Illinois

Wendy Ostendorf, RN, MS, EdD, CNE
Contributing Faculty
Master of Science in Nursing
Walden University
Minneapolis, Minnesota

Jill Parsons, PhD, RN
Associate Professor
Nursing
MacMurray College
Jacksonville, Illinois

Lynette Savage, BS, BSN, MS, PhD
Associate Professor, Joint Appointment
School of Health Professions
University of Providence
Great Falls, Montana

Angela Renee Starkweather, PhD, ACNP-BC, FAAN
Professor and Associate Dean for Academic
　Affairs
School of Nursing
University of Connecticut
Storrs, Connecticut

Shellye A. Vardaman, PhD
Professor
School of Nursing
Troy University
Troy, Alabama

CONTRIBUTORS TO PREVIOUS EDITIONS

Michelle Aebersold, PhD, RN
Jeanette Adams, PhD, MSN, APRN, CRNI
Paulette M. Archer, RN, EdD
Myra A. Aud, PhD, RN
Katherine N. Ayzengart, MSN, RN
Marjorie Baier, PhD, RN
Sylvia K. Baird, RN, BSN, MM
Karen Balakas, PhD, RN, CNE
Brenda Battle, RN, BSN, MBA
Lois Bentler-Lampe, RN, MS
Janice Boundy, RN, PhD
Anna Brock, PhD, MSN, MEd, BSN
Sheryl Buckner, RN-BC, MS, CNE
Jeri Burger, PhD, RN
Linda Cason, MSN, RN-BC, NE-BC, CNRN
Pamela L. Cherry, RN, BSN, MSN, DNSc
Rhonda W. Comrie, PhD, RN, CNE, AE-C
Maureen F. Cooney, DNP, FNP-BC
Eileen Costantinou, MSN, RN
Cheryl A. Crowe, RN, MS
Ruth M. Curchoe, RN, MSN, CIC
Marinetta DeMoss, RN, MSN
Christine R. Durbin, PhD, JD, RN
Margaret Ecker, RN, MS
Martha Keene Elkin, RN, MS, IBCLC
Antoinette Falker, DNP, RN, CMSRN, CBN, GCNS-BC

Leah W. Frederick, MS, RN CIC
Mimi Hirshberg, RN, MSN
Steve Kilkus, RN, MSN
Judith Ann Kilpatrick, RN, DNSc
Lori Klingman, MSN, RN
Karen Korem, RN-BC, MA
Gayle L. Kruse, RN, ACHPN, GCNS-BC
Anahid Kulwicki, RN, DNS, FAAN
Kristine M. L'Ecuyer, RN, MSN, CCNS
Jerrilee LaMar, PhD, RN, CNE
Joyce Larson, PhD, MS, RN
Kathryn Lever, MSN, WHNP-BC
Ruth Ludwick, BSN, MSN, PhD, RNC
Annette G. Lueckenotte, MS, RN, BC, GNP GCNS
Frank Lyerla, PhD, RN
Deborah Marshall, MSN
Barbara Maxwell, RN, BSN, MS, MSN, CNS
Erin H. McCalley, RN, BSN, MS, CCRN, CCNS
Judith A. McCutchan, RN, ASN, BSN, MSN, PhD
Elaine K. Neel, RN, BSN, MSN
Patricia A. O'Connor, RN, MSN, CNE
Dula Pacquiao, BSN, MA, EdD
Nancy C. Panthofer, RN, MSN
Elaine U. Polan, RNC, BSN, MS

Beverly J. Reynolds, RN, EdD, CNE
Kristine Rose, BSN, MSN
Patsy L. Ruchala, DNSc, RN
Debbie Sanazaro, RN, MSN, GNP
Marilyn Schallom, RN, MSN, CCRN, CCNS
Carrie Sona, RN, MSN, CCRN, ACNS, CCNS
Matthew R. Sorenson, PhD, APN, ANP-C
Marshelle Thobaben, RN, MS, PHN, APNP, FNP
Donna L. Thompson, MSN, CRNP, FNP-BC, CCCN-AP
Jelena Todic, MSW, LCSW
Ann B. Tritak, EdD, MA, BSN, RN
Janis Waite, RN, MSN, EdD
Mary Ann Wehmer, RN, MSN, CNOR
Pamela Becker Weilitz, RN, MSN(R), BC, ANP, M-SCNS
Joan Domigan Wentz, BSN, MSN
Katherine West, BSN, MSEd,CIC
Terry L. Wood, PhD, RN, CNE
Rita Wunderlich, PhD, RN
Valerie Yancey, PhD, RN

**Dr. Colleen Andreoni, DNP, MSN APRN
FNP-BC, ANP-BC, ENP-C**
Clinical Adjunct Faculty
Marcella Niehoff School of Nursing
Loyola University Chicago
Maywood, Illinois;
Nurse Practitioner
Med Express Urgent Care
Naperville, Illinois;
Nurse Practitioner
Emergency Department
Presence St. Joseph's Hospital
Elgin, Illinois

Diane Benefiel, EdD, MSN, RN, CNE
Nursing Faculty
Fresno City College and Fresno Pacific
University
Fresno, California

**Ami A. Bhatt, DNP, MBA, RN, CHPN,
CHCI**
Assistant Professor, Nursing
SUNY Delhi
Delhi, New York

Leigh Ann Bonney, PhD, RN, CCRN, CNE
Associate Professor
Nursing
Saint Francis Medical Center College of
Nursing
Peoria, Illinois

Anna M. Bruch, RN, MSN
Nursing Professor
Illinois Valley Community College
Oglesby, Illinois

**Timothy D. Buchanan, MSN, RN-BC,
CSPHP**
Safe Patient Handling and Mobility Facility
Coordinator
Veterans Affairs Saint Louis Health Care
System (VASTLHCS) and Veterans
Integrated Service Network 15, Point of
Contact
Adjunct Faculty
School of Nursing
Saint Louis University
St. Louis, Missouri

Sheryl Buckner, PhD, RN, ANEF
Assistant Professor
College of Nursing
University of Oklahoma
Oklahoma City, Oklahoma

**Darlene M. Burke, PhD, MS. MA, RN,
CCRN-K, CNE**
Lecturer, Nursing
San Diego State University;
San Diego, California
Associate Faculty
MiraCosta College
Oceanside, California

Pat Callard, MSN, DNP, RN
Associate Professor Emeritus
College of Graduate Nursing
Western University of Health Sciences
Pomona, California

Kim Clevenger, EdD, MSN, RN, BC
Associate Professor of Nursing
Nursing
Morehead State University
Morehead, Kentucky

Tracy D. Colburn, RN, MSN, C-EFM
Associate Professor
Nursing
Lewis and Clark Community College
Godfrey, Illinois

**Barbara A. Coles, RN-BC, PhD, ANCC
Medical-Surgical Certification**
Instructor and Medication Consultant
Nursing
Keiser University and James A. Haley VAMC
Fort Lauderdale, Florida
Tampa, Florida

Pamela Cook, MSN, RN, CNS
Assistant Professor
Nursing Department
Bloomsburg University
Bloomsburg, Pennsylvania

Janie Corbitt, RN, MLS
Nursing Instructor, Retired
LPN, Medical Assisting
Milledgeville, Georgia

Graciela Lopez Cox, MSN, RN
Assistant Professor
Samuel Merritt University
School of Nursing Sacramento Campus
Sacramento, California

Janice M. Crabill, PhD, RN
Associate Professor
Nursing
Northwest Nazarene University
Nampa, Idaho

**Patricia Dettenmeier, PhD(c), DNP,
ANP-BC**
Assistant Professor
Sleep Medicine
Adult Nurse Practitioner
Division of Pulmonary, Critical Care and
Sleep Medicine
SLU Care Physician Group
St. Louis, Missouri

Holly Johanna Diesel, PhD, RN
Associate Professor, Academic Chair,
Accelerated RN to BSN Programs
Nursing
Goldfarb School of Nursing at Barnes-Jewish
College
St. Louis, Missouri

Christine R. Durbin, PhD, JD, RN
Associate Professor and Chair, Primary Care
and Health Systems Department
Primary Care and Health Systems
Southern Illinois University Edwardsville
Edwardsville, Illinois

**Amber Essman, DNP, MSN, APRN,
FNP-BC**
DNP
Nursing
Chamberlain College of Nursing
South University
Cleveland, Ohio

Kelly L. Fisher, PhD, RN, FNAP
Professor and Dean
School of Nursing
Endicott College
Beverly, Massachusetts

Megan D. Frye, RN, MSN
Instructor
Faculty
Saint Francis Medical Center College of
Nursing
Peoria, Illinois

**Linda R. Garner, PhD, RN, PHNA-BC,
CHES**
Associate Professor of Nursing
Department of Nursing
Southeast Missouri State University
Cape Girardeau, Missouri

Joyce Hammer, RN, MSN
Adjunct Nursing Faculty
Nursing
Owens Community College
Toledo, Ohio

Pamela Harvey, RN, ASN, BSN, MSN, BLS
Instructor, LPN Program
North Florida Technical College
Starke, Florida

Nicole M. Heimgartner, DNP, RN, COI
Author and Subject Matter Expert, Elsevier
Nursing Education Consultant, Connect:
    RN2ED
Adjunct Faculty
Mercy College of Ohio
Division of Nursing
Louisville, Kentucky

Dawn Johnson, DNP, RN, Ed
Director of Nursing
Practical Nursing Program
Great Lakes Institute of Technology
Erie, Pennsylvania

Kathleen C. Jones, MSN, RN, CNS
Associate Professor of Nursing
Health Programs
Walters State Community College
Morristown, Tennessee

Vickey Keathley, MSN, RN
Clinical Nurse Educator
School of Nursing ABSN Program
Duke University
Durham, North Carolina

Christina D. Keller, MSN, RN, CHSE
Instructor, Nursing
Radford University Clinical Simulation
    Center
Radford, Virginia

Shari Kist, PhD, RN, CNE
Project Supervisor
Missouri Quality Initiate for Nursing Homes
Sinclair School of Nursing
University of Missouri-Columbia
Columbia, Missouri

Patricia T. Ketcham, RN, MSN
Director of Nursing Laboratories
School of Nursing
Oakland University
Rochester, Michigan

Shannon Lanctot-Shah, RN, MSN, DHSc Dr
Nursing
Selkirk College
Castlegar, British Columbia
Canada

Mollie H. Manning, MSN, RN
Assistant Professor of Nursing
School of Nursing
Arkansas State University
Jonesboro, Arkansas

Angela McConachie, DNP, MSN-FNP, RN
Associate Professor
Family Nurse Practitioner, Cardiology,
    Retail Health
Goldfarb School of Nursing at Barnes-Jewish
    College
St. Louis, Missouri

Janis Longfield McMillan, MSN, RN, CNE
Associate Clinical Professor
School of Nursing
Northern Arizona University
Flagstaff, Arizona

**Katherine Eileen Murphy, RN, MSN, BSN,
    PHN**
Registered Nurse Subject Matter Expert
San Andreas, California

**Kimberly J. Oosterhouse, PhD, RN,
    CCRN-K, CNE**
Assistant Professor
Health Management and Risk Reduction
Marcella Niehoff School of Nursing
Loyola University Chicago
Chicago, Illinois

Rebecca Otten, EdD, RN
Professor Emeritus, Nursing
School of Nursing
California State University, Fullerton
Fullerton, California

**Victoria Plagenz, BSN, MSN, PhD Certified
    Online Instructor**
Associate Professor
Nursing
University of Providence
Great Falls, Montana

**Melissa Anne Radecki, PhD-C, MSN, NEd,
    RN, PCCN-K**
Nursing Instructor
School of Nursing and Health Sciences
Florida Southern College
Lakeland, Florida

Rhonda Ramirez, EdD, FNP-BC
Chair, Family Nurse Practitioner
    Department
Samuel Merritt University
Oakland, California

Cherie R. Rebar, PhD, MBA, RN, COI
Professor of Nursing
School of Nursing
Wittenberg University
Springfield, Ohio

Anita K. Reed, MSN, RN
Department Chair, Community Health
    Practice
Nursing
St. Elizabeth School of Nursing
Lafayette, Indiana

Laura M. Remy, MPH, BSN, RN
Project Manager
School of Health Professions
University of Missouri-Kansas City
Kansas City, Missouri

Scott D. Schaeffer, DC
Professor of Biology
STEM Division
Harford Community College
Bel Air, Maryland

Susan Parnell Scholtz, RN, PhD
Associate Professor of Nursing
Nursing
Moravian College
Bethlehem, Pennsylvania

Lisa J. Scott, DNP, RN
Nursing Faculty
Nursing
Norfolk State University
Norfolk, Virginia

Crystal Slaughter, APN, DNP, CNS
Associate Professor
College of Nursing
Saint Francis Medical Center College of
    Nursing
Peoria, Illinois

Peter D. Smith, BA, MSN, RN
Clinical Education Specialist
ENT/Plastics Reconstruction
Barnes-Jewish Hospital
St. Louis, Missouri

Dr. Mindy Stayner, PhD, RN, CNE
Professor
Nursing
Capella University and Northwest State
    Community College
Minneapolis, Minnesota
Archbold, Ohio

Misty B. Stone, MSN, RN
Assistant Professor
Nursing
The University of North Carolina at
    Pembroke
Pembroke, North Carolina

I wish to dedicate this book to the incredible circle of friends that I call family. Their support, presence, and encouragement are priceless.

You all know who you are. Love you all.

Patricia A. Potter

This book is dedicated to all students who are committed to studying this rewarding but challenging profession.

To all nursing faculty who work tirelessly to provide students with excellent, state-of-the art classroom and clinical experiences.

Finally, to all practicing nurses who welcome students to the clinical practice site and partner with nursing faculty to demonstrate excellence in clinical nursing.

Anne Griffin Perry

During my doctoral education, I was blessed to meet Pat and Anne, who gave me this wonderful opportunity to participate in authoring and editing nursing textbooks. It was an unexpected but wonderful part of my nursing career. Thank you, Pat and Anne, for letting me join your journey of providing nursing students with the best fundamentals nursing textbook! Over the years, I have learned much from both of you and all the wonderful editorial staff at Elsevier. I look forward to continuing the journey with you in the future.

To the nursing students who read this textbook as you start your nursing career, I am glad that we are able to provide you a solid foundation and best evidence to build on as you progress through your nursing programs. You are developing the knowledge and skills necessary to provide safe, competent, patient-centered nursing care. I wish you all the best as you join the wonderful profession of nursing!

And finally, thank you to my husband, Drake, for your patience and support as I spend my time writing and editing. I couldn't have done this without you!

Patricia A. Stockert

To all nurses and nursing faculty, especially those at Franciscan Missionaries of Our Lady University. Your never-ending enthusiasm for nursing is so inspirational and demonstrates the importance of life-long learning to improve patient care every day.

To Patti, Anne, and Pat for your never-ending friendship and support. You push me to be a better person and nurse every day.

To Julia, Tina, Chris, Chuck, Mistie, Blaize, Donna, Jesse, Jenni, Jane, and the rest of the Varsity Sports Running Team for accepting me into your family and showing me the importance of running hard and living easy.

And to Greg. Your love, patience, and support has allowed me to achieve personal and professional goals I never could have imagined.

Amy M. Hall

PREFACE TO THE INSTRUCTOR

The nursing profession is always responding to dynamic change and continual challenges. Today, nurses need a broad knowledge base from which to provide care. More importantly, nurses require the ability to know how to apply best evidence in practice to assure the best outcomes for their patients. The role of the nurse includes assuming the lead in preserving nursing practice and demonstrating its contribution to the health care of our nation. Nurses of tomorrow, therefore, need to become competent clinicians, critical thinkers, patient advocates, clinical decision makers, and patient educators within a broad spectrum of care services.

The tenth edition of *Fundamentals of Nursing* was revised to prepare today's students for the challenges of tomorrow. This textbook is designed for beginning students in all types of professional nursing programs. The comprehensive coverage provides fundamental nursing concepts, skills, and techniques of nursing practice and a firm foundation for more advanced areas of study.

Fundamentals of Nursing provides a contemporary approach to nursing practice, discussing the entire scope of primary, acute, and restorative care. This new edition continues to address a number of key current practice issues, including an emphasis on patient-centered care and evidence-based practice. Evidence-based practice is one of the most important initiatives in health care today. The increased focus on applying current evidence in patient care helps students understand how the latest research findings should guide their clinical decision making. Current evidence is reflected in each chapter's references.

KEY FEATURES

We have carefully developed this tenth edition with the student in mind. We have designed this text to welcome the new student to nursing, communicate our own love for the profession, and promote learning and understanding. Key features of the text include the following:

- Students will appreciate the **clear, engaging writing style.** The narrative actually addresses the reader, making this textbook more of an active instructional tool than a passive reference. Students will find that even complex technical and theoretical concepts are presented in a language that is easy to understand.
- **Comprehensive** coverage and readability of all fundamental nursing content.
- The **attractive, functional design** will appeal to today's visual learner. The clear, readable type and bold headings make the content easy to read and follow. Each special element is consistently color-keyed so students can readily identify important information.
- Hundreds of **large, clear, full-color photographs and drawings** reinforce and clarify key concepts and techniques.
- A **critical thinking model** is incorporated within all clinical chapters, showing how elements of critical thinking, including knowledge, critical thinking attitudes, intellectual and professional standards, and experience, are applied in the nursing process for making clinical decisions.
- The **nursing process** format provides a consistent organizational framework for clinical chapters.
- **Learning aids** to help students identify, review, and apply important content in each chapter include Objectives, Key Terms, Key Points, Clinical Application Questions, and Review Questions.
- **Evolve Resources** lists at the beginning of every chapter detail the electronic resources available for the student.
- **Health promotion and acute and continuing care** are covered to address today's practice in various settings.

- A **health promotion/wellness** thread is used consistently throughout the text.
- **Cultural competence,** care of the **older adult,** and **patient teaching** are stressed throughout chapter narratives, as well as highlighted in special boxes.
- **Procedural Guidelines** boxes provide more streamlined, step-by-step instructions for performing very basic skills.
- **Concept Maps** included in clinical chapters show you the association between multiple nursing diagnoses for a patient with a selected medical diagnosis and the relationship between nursing interventions.
- **Nursing Care Plans** guide students on how to conduct an assessment and analyze the defining characteristics in order to select nursing diagnoses. The plans include NIC and NOC classifications to familiarize students with this important nomenclature. The evaluation sections of the plans show students how to evaluate and then determine the outcomes of care.
- Information related to the **Quality and Safety Education for Nurses (QSEN)** initiative is highlighted by headings that coordinate with the key competencies. Building Competency scenarios in each chapter incorporate one of the six key competencies in QSEN. Answers to these activities can be found online in the Evolve student resources.
- **More than 55 nursing skills** are presented in a clear two-column format, with steps and supporting rationales that are often supported with current evidenced-based research.
- **Delegation Considerations** guide when it is appropriate to delegate tasks to assistive personnel.
- **Unexpected Outcomes and Related Interventions** are highlighted within nursing skills to help students anticipate and appropriately respond to possible problems faced while performing skills.
- **Video Icons** indicate video clips associated with specific skills that are available on the Evolve Student Resources.
- **Printed endpapers** on the inside back cover provide information on locating specific assets in the book, including Skills, Procedure Guidelines, Nursing Care Plans, and Concept Maps.

NEW TO THIS EDITION

- **Reflect Now** boxes interspersed throughout the chapters prompt students to consider a recent clinical experience based on the topic being discussed in the text.
- **Review Questions** have been updated in each chapter, with a minimum of 4 alternate-item type questions. Answers are provided with questions and rationales on Evolve.
- **Evidence-Based Practice** boxes in each chapter have been updated to reflect current research topics and trends.
- A **Reflective Learning** section helps students better understand and think about their clinical and simulation experiences as they progress through their first nursing courses.
- **Teach-back** has been incorporated into the Evaluation section of the Patient Teaching boxes.
- **Chapter 8, Caring for Patients with Chronic Illness,** has been expanded to help prepare students to address the unique health care needs of patients and families who are living with the physical, emotional, social, and economic stressors of chronic illness.

LEARNING SUPPLEMENTS FOR STUDENTS

- The **Evolve Student Resources** are available online at http://evolve.elsevier.com/Potter/fundamentals/ and include the following valuable learning aids organized by chapter:
  - Chapter Review Questions with Answers and Rationales
  - Answers and rationales to Building Competency scenario questions
  - Video clips to highlight common skills
  - Conceptual Care Map (included in each clinical chapter)
  - Case Study with questions
  - Audio Glossary
  - Fluids & Electrolytes Tutorial
  - Printable versions of Chapter Key Points
  - Printable Skills Performance Checklists (included for each skill in the text)
- A thorough *Study Guide* by Geralyn Ochs provides an ideal supplement to help students understand and apply the content of the text. Each chapter includes multiple sections:
  - Preliminary Reading includes a chapter assignment from the text.
  - Case Study with related questions
  - Comprehensive Understanding provides a variety of activities to reinforce the topics and main ideas from the text.
  - Review Questions include multiple-choice, matching, and fill-in-the-blank questions. Answers and rationales are provided in the answer key.
  - Clinical chapters include an Application of Critical Thinking Synthesis Model that expands the case study from the chapter's Care Plan and asks students to develop a step in the synthesis model based on the nurse and patient in the scenario. This helps students learn to apply both content learned and the critical thinking synthesis model.
- The handy *Clinical Companion* complements, rather than abbreviates, the textbook. Content is presented in tabular, list, and outline format that equips your students with a concise, portable guide to all the facts and figures they'll need to know in their early clinical experiences.
- **Virtual Clinical Excursions** is an exciting workbook and video experience that brings learning to life in a virtual hospital setting. The workbook guides students as they care for patients, providing ongoing challenges and learning opportunities. Each lesson in *Virtual Clinical Excursions* complements the textbook content and provides an environment in which students can practice what they are learning. This CD/workbook is available separately or packaged at a special price with the textbook.

TEACHING SUPPLEMENTS FOR INSTRUCTORS

- The **Evolve Instructor Resources** (available online at http://evolve.elsevier.com/Potter/fundamentals) are a comprehensive collection of the most important tools instructors need, including the following:
  - **TEACH for Nurses** ties together every chapter resource you need for the most effective class presentations, with sections dedicated to objectives, teaching focus, nursing curriculum standards (including QSEN, BSN Essentials, and Concepts), instructor chapter resources, student chapter resources, answers to chapter questions, and an in-class case study discussion. Teaching Strategies help you create learning activities you can use to assess students' understanding of the content presented in the textbook. Examples of student activities, online activities, new health promotion–focused activities, and large group activities are provided for more "hands-on" learning.
  - The **Test Bank** contains 1100 questions, with answers coded for NCLEX Client Needs category, nursing process, and cognitive level. The ExamView software allows instructors to create new tests; edit, add, and delete test questions; sort questions by NCLEX category, cognitive level, nursing process step, and question type; and administer/grade online tests.
  - Updated **PowerPoint Presentations** include more than 1500 slides for use in lectures. Art is included within the slides, and progressive case studies include discussion questions and answers.
  - The **Image Collection** contains more than 1150 illustrations from the text for use in lectures.
  - **Simulation Learning System** is an online toolkit that helps instructors and facilitators effectively incorporate medium- to high-fidelity simulation into their nursing curriculum. Detailed patient scenarios promote and enhance the clinical decision-making skills of students at all levels. The system provides detailed instructions for preparation and implementation of the simulation experience, debriefing questions that encourage critical thinking, and learning resources to reinforce student comprehension. Each scenario in *Simulation Learning System* complements the textbook content and helps bridge the gap between lectures and clinicals. This system provides the perfect environment for students to practice what they are learning in the text for a true-to-life, hands-on learning experience.

MULTIMEDIA SUPPLEMENTS FOR INSTRUCTORS AND STUDENTS

- **Nursing Skills Online 4.0** contains 19 modules rich with animations, videos, interactive activities, and exercises to help students prepare for their clinical lab experience. The instructionally designed lessons focus on topics that are difficult to master and pose a high risk to the patient if done incorrectly. Lesson quizzes allow students to check their learning curve and review as needed, and the module exams feed out to an instructor grade book. Modules cover Airway Management, Blood Therapy, Bowel Elimination/Ostomy Care, Cardiac Care, Closed Chest Drainage Systems, Enteral Nutrition, Infection Control, Maintenance of IV Fluid Therapy, IV Fluid Therapy, Administration of Parenteral Medications: Injections, Administration of Parenteral Medications: IV Medications, Administration of Nonparenteral Medications, Safe Medication Preparation, Safety, Specimen Collection, Urinary Catheterization, Caring for Central Vascular Access Devices (CVAD), Vital Signs, and Wound Care. Available alone or packaged with the text.
- **Mosby's Nursing Video Skills: Basic, Intermediate, Advanced, 4th edition** provides 126 skills with overview information covering skill purpose, safety, and delegation guides; equipment lists; preparation procedures; procedure videos with printable step-by-step guidelines; appropriate follow-up care; documentation guidelines; and interactive review questions. Available online, as a student DVD set, or as a networkable DVD set for the institution.

ACKNOWLEDGMENTS

The tenth edition of *Fundamentals of Nursing* is one that we believe continues to prepare the student nurse to practice in the challenging health care environment. Collaboration on this project allows us to be creative, visionary, and thoughtful as to students' learning needs. Each edition is a new adventure for the author team as we to create the very best textbook for beginning nurses. Each of us wishes to acknowledge the professionalism, support, and commitment to detail from the following individuals:

- The editorial and production professionals at Mosby/Elsevier, including:
  - Tamara Myers, Director, Traditional Education, for her vision, organization, professionalism, energy, and support in assisting us to develop a text that offers a state-of-the-art approach to the design, organization, and presentation of *Fundamentals of Nursing*. Her skill is in motivating and supporting a writing team so it can be creative and innovative while retaining the characteristics of a high-quality textbook.
  - Tina Kaemmerer, our Senior Content Development Specialist for *Fundamentals of Nursing*. As a dedicated professional, Tina keeps the writing team organized and focused and performs considerable behind-the-scenes work to ensure accuracy and consistency in how we present content within the textbook. She has limitless energy and is always willing to go the extra mile.
  - Jodi Willard, Senior Project Manager, consistently performs miracles. She is an amazing and accomplished production editor who applies patience, humor, and attention to detail. It is an honor to work with Jodi because of her professionalism and ability to coordinate the multiple aspects of completing a well-designed finished product.
- KJ Filmworks, Hennessey, Oklahoma, for their excellent photography.
- Memorial Hospital East, in Shiloh, Illinois, for granting permission to use its facility for the new photographs.
- To our contributors and clinician and educator reviewers, who share their expertise and knowledge about nursing practice and the trends within health care today, helping us to create informative, accurate, and current information. Their contributions allow us to develop a text that embodies high standards for professional nursing practice through the printed word.
- And special recognition to our professional colleagues at Barnes-Jewish Hospital, Southern Illinois University Edwardsville, Saint Francis Medical Center College of Nursing, and Franciscan Missionaries of Our Lady University.

We believe that *Fundamentals of Nursing*, now in its tenth edition, is a textbook that informs and helps to shape the standards for excellence in nursing practice. Nursing excellence is a goal we all seek, and we are happy to have the opportunity to continue the work we love.

Patricia A. Potter
Anne Griffin Perry
Patricia A. Stockert
Amy M. Hall

CONTENTS

Any updates to this textbook can be found in the Content Updates folder on Evolve at http://evolve.elsevier.com/Potter/fundamentals/.

1

Nursing Today

OBJECTIVES

- Explore the development of professional nursing roles.
- Describe educational programs available for professional registered nurse (RN) education.
- Describe how nursing standards affect nursing care.
- Discuss the roles and career opportunities for professional nurses.
- Discuss the influence of social, historical, political, and economic changes on nursing practices.
- Discuss how advances in nursing science and evidence-based practice improve patient care.

KEY TERMS

Advanced practice registered nurse (APRN), p. 4
American Nurses Association (ANA), p. 2
Caregiver, p. 3
Certified nurse-midwife (CNM), p. 5
Certified registered nurse anesthetist (CRNA), p. 5
Clinical nurse specialist (CNS), p. 4

Code of ethics, p. 3
Continuing education, p. 10
Genomics, p. 9
In-service education, p. 10
International Council of Nurses (ICN), p. 2
Nurse administrator, p. 5
Nurse educator, p. 5
Nurse practitioner (NP), p. 4

Nurse researcher, p. 5
Nursing, p. 2
Patient advocate, p. 3
Professional organization, p. 11
Quality and Safety Education for Nurses (QSEN), p. 8
Registered nurse (RN), p. 10

MEDIA RESOURCES

http://evolve.elsevier.com/Potter/fundamentals/
- Review Questions
- Case Study with Questions

- Audio Glossary
- Content Updates
- Answers to QSEN Activity and Review Questions

Nursing is an art and a science. As an art, you learn to deliver care with compassion, caring, and respect for each patient's dignity and individuality. As a science, nursing practice is based on a body of knowledge and evidence-based practices that are continually changing with new discoveries and innovations. By integrating the art and science of nursing, the quality of care you provide is at the highest standards and benefits patients and their families. Your care reflects your patients' multidimensional needs as well as the needs and values of society and professional standards of care.

Nursing offers personal and professional rewards every day. This chapter presents a contemporary view of the evolution of nursing and nursing practice and the historical, practical, social, and political influences on the discipline of nursing.

NURSING AS A PROFESSION

The patient is the center of your practice. Your patient includes individuals, families, and/or communities. Patients have a wide variety of

health care needs, knowledge, experiences, vulnerabilities, and expectations, but this is what makes nursing both challenging and rewarding. Making a difference in your patients' lives is fulfilling (e.g., helping a young mother learn parenting skills, finding ways for older adults to remain independent in their homes, assisting family caregivers with end-of-life care symptom management).

Nursing is not simply a collection of specific skills, and you are not simply a person trained to perform specific tasks. Nursing is a profession. No one factor absolutely differentiates a job from a profession, but the difference is important in terms of how you practice. To act professionally, use your critical thinking skills to administer quality evidenced-based, patient-centered care in a safe, prudent, and knowledgeable manner. You are responsible and accountable to yourself, your patients, and your peers.

A variety of career opportunities are available in nursing, including clinical practice, education, research, management, administration, and even entrepreneurship. As a student it is important for you to understand the scope of professional nursing practice and how nursing influences the lives of your patients, their families, and their communities.

Health care advocacy groups recognize the importance of the role quality professional nursing has on a nation's health care. One such program was the Robert Wood Johnson Foundation (RWJF) *Future of Nursing: Campaign for Action* (RWJF, 2014a). This program is a multifaceted campaign to transform health care through nursing, and it is a response to the Institute of Medicine (IOM) publication on *The Future of Nursing* (IOM, 2010). A new RWJF (2017) initiative, *Catalysts for Change: Harnessing the power of nurses to build population health in the 21st century*, reinforces the fact that nurses are educated to consider health care issues within a broader context; as a result, nurses identify factors outside health care that affect a person's level of health. These initiatives prepare a professional workforce to meet health promotion, illness prevention, and complex care needs of the population in a changing health care system.

Science and Art of Nursing Practice

Because nursing is both an art and a science, nursing practice requires a blend of current knowledge and practice standards with an insightful and compassionate approach to your patients' health care needs. Your care must reflect the needs and values of society and professional standards of care and performance, meet the needs of each patient, and integrate evidence-based findings to provide the highest level of care.

Clinical expertise takes time and commitment. According to Benner (1984), an expert nurse passes through five levels of proficiency when acquiring and developing generalist or specialized nursing skills (Box 1.1). Expert clinical nursing practice is a commitment to the application of knowledge, ethics, aesthetics, and clinical experience. Your ability to interpret clinical situations and make complex decisions is the foundation for your nursing care and the basis for the advancement of nursing practice and the development of nursing science (Benner et al., 1997, 2010).

Use critical thinking skills to help you gain and interpret scientific knowledge, integrate knowledge from clinical experiences, and become a lifelong learner (Chapter 15). Integrate the competencies of critical thinking in your practice. This includes incorporating knowledge from the basic sciences and nursing, applying knowledge from past and present experiences, applying critical thinking attitudes to a clinical situation, and implementing intellectual and professional standards. When you provide well-thought-out care with compassion and caring, you provide each patient the best of the science and art of nursing care (see Chapter 7).

Scope and Standards of Practice

When giving care, it is essential to provide a specified service according to standards of practice and to follow a code of ethics (ANA, 2015). Professional practice includes knowledge from social and behavioral sciences, biological and physiological sciences, and nursing theories. In addition, nursing practice incorporates ethical and social values, professional autonomy, and a sense of commitment and community (ANA, 2015). The following definition from the American Nurses Association (ANA) illustrates the consistent commitment of nurses to provide care that promotes the well-being of their patients and communities (Fowler, 2015a). Nursing is *the protection, promotion, and optimization of health and abilities; prevention of illness and injury; alleviation of suffering through the diagnosis and treatment of human response; and advocacy in the care of individuals, families, communities, and populations* (ANA, 2015). The International Council of Nurses (ICN, 2018) has another definition: *Nursing encompasses autonomous and collaborative care of individuals of all ages, families, groups, and communities, sick or well, and in all settings. Nursing includes the promotion of health; prevention of illness; and the care of ill, disabled, and dying people.*

BOX 1.1   Benner: From Novice to Expert

- **Novice:** Beginning nursing student or any nurse entering a situation in which there is no previous level of experience (e.g., an experienced operating room nurse chooses to now practice in home health). The learner learns via a specific set of rules or procedures, which are usually stepwise and linear.
- **Advanced Beginner:** A nurse who has had some level of experience with the situation. This experience may be only observational in nature, but the nurse is able to identify meaningful aspects or principles of nursing care.
- **Competent:** A nurse who has been in the same clinical position for 2 to 3 years. This nurse understands the organization and specific care required by the type of patients (e.g., surgical, oncology, or orthopedic patients). He or she is a competent practitioner who is able to anticipate nursing care and establish long-range goals. In this phase the nurse has usually had experience with all types of psychomotor skills required by this specific group of patients.
- **Proficient:** A nurse with more than 2 to 3 years of experience in the same clinical position. This nurse perceives a patient's clinical situation as a whole, is able to assess an entire situation, and can readily transfer knowledge gained from multiple previous experiences to a situation. This nurse focuses on managing care as opposed to managing and performing skills.
- **Expert:** A nurse with diverse experience who has an intuitive grasp of an existing or potential clinical problem. This nurse is able to zero in on the problem and focus on multiple dimensions of the situation. He or she is skilled at identifying both patient-centered problems and problems related to the health care system or perhaps the needs of the novice nurse.

Data from Benner P: *From novice to expert: excellence and power in clinical nursing practice,* Menlo Park, CA, 1984, Addison-Wesley.

BOX 1.2   ANA Standards of Nursing Practice

1. **Assessment:** The registered nurse collects pertinent data and information relative to the healthcare consumer's health or the situation.
2. **Diagnosis:** The registered nurse analyzes the assessment data to determine the actual or potential diagnoses, problems, and issues.
3. **Outcomes Identification:** The registered nurse identifies expected outcomes for a plan individualized to the health care consumer or the situation.
4. **Planning:** The registered nurse develops a plan that prescribes strategies to attain expected, measurable outcomes.
5. **Implementation:** The registered nurse implements the identified plan.
   5a. **Coordination of Care:** The registered nurse coordinates care delivery.
   5b. **Health Teaching and Health Promotion:** The registered nurse employs strategies to promote health and a safe environment.
6. **Evaluation:** The registered nurse evaluates progress toward attainment of outcomes.

Advocacy, promotion of a safe environment, research, participation in shaping health policy and in patient and health systems management, and education are also key nursing roles. Both of these definitions support the prominence and importance that nursing holds in providing safe, patient-centered health care to the global community.

Since 1960 the ANA has defined the scope of nursing and developed Standards of Practice and Standards of Professional Performance (ANA, 2015). It is important that you know and apply these standards in your practice (Box 1.2). Most schools of nursing and practice settings have published copies of the scope and standards of nursing practice.

BOX 1.3   ANA Standards of Professional Performance

1. **Ethics:** The registered nurse practices ethically.
2. **Culturally Congruent Care:** The registered nurse practices in a manner that is congruent with cultural diversity and inclusion principles.
3. **Communication:** The registered nurse communicates effectively in all areas of practice.
4. **Collaboration:** The registered nurse collaborates with health care consumer and other key stakeholders in the conduct of nursing practice.
5. **Leadership:** The registered nurse demonstrates leadership in the professional practice setting and the profession.
6. **Education:** The registered nurse seeks knowledge and competency that reflects current nursing practice and promotes futuristic thinking.
7. **Evidence-Based Practice and Research:** The registered nurse integrates evidence and research findings into practice.
8. **Quality of Practice:** The registered nurse contributes to quality nursing practice.
9. **Professional Practice Evaluation:** The registered nurse evaluates one's own and others' nursing practice.
10. **Resources Utilization:** The registered nurse uses appropriate resources to plan and provide and sustain evidence-based nursing services that are safe, effective, and fiscally responsible.
11. **Environmental Health:** The registered nurse practices in an environmentally safe and healthy manner.

Copyright© American Nurses Association: *Nursing scope and standards of practice*, ed 3, Silver Springs, MD, 2015, The Association. Reprinted with permission. All rights reserved.

The scope and standards of practice guide nurses to make significant and visible contributions that improve the health and well-being of all individuals, communities, and populations (ANA, 2015).

Standards of Professional Nursing Practice. The Standards of Professional Nursing Practice contain authoritative statements of the duties that all registered nurses, regardless of role, population, or specialty, are expected to perform competently (ANA, 2015). The duties are supported by a critical thinking model known as the nursing process: assessment, diagnosis, outcomes identification and planning, implementation, and evaluation (ANA, 2015). The nursing process is the model for clinical decision making and includes all significant actions taken by nurses in providing care to patients (see Unit III).

Standards of Professional Performance. The ANA Standards of Professional Performance (Box 1.3) describe a competent level of behavior in the professional role (ANA, 2015). The standards provide a method to assure patients that they are receiving high-quality care and to ensure that the nurses must know exactly what is necessary to provide nursing care. The standards also are in place to determine whether nursing care meets the standards.

Code of Ethics. The nursing code of ethics is a statement of philosophical ideals of right and wrong that define the principles you will use to provide care to your patients. It is important for you to also incorporate your own values and ethics into your practice. As you incorporate these values, explore what type of nurse you will be and how you will function within the discipline (Fowler, 2015b). Ask yourself how your ethics, values, and practice compare with established standards. The ANA has a number of publications that address ethics and human rights in nursing. *The Code of Ethics for Nurses with Interpretive Statements* is a guide for carrying out nursing

responsibilities and providing quality nursing care; it also outlines the ethical obligations of the profession (Fowler, 2015b). Chapter 22 provides a review of the nursing code of ethics and ethical principles for everyday practice.

Professional Responsibilities and Roles

You are responsible for obtaining and maintaining specific knowledge and skills for a variety of professional roles and responsibilities. Nurses provide care and comfort for patients in all health care settings. Nurses' concern for meeting their patient's needs remains the same whether care focuses on health promotion and illness prevention, disease and symptom management, family support, or end-of-life care.

Autonomy and Accountability. Autonomy is an essential element of professional nursing that involves the initiation of independent nursing interventions without medical orders. Although the nursing profession regulates accountability through nursing audits and standards of practice, you also need to develop a commitment to personal professional accountability. For example, you independently implement coughing and deep-breathing exercises to clear the lungs and promote oxygenation for a patient who recently had major surgery. As you continue to care for this patient, a complication arises. You note that the patient has a fever, and the surgical wound has a yellow-green discharge. You collaborate with other health care professionals to develop the best treatment plan for this patient's surgical wound infection.

With increased autonomy comes greater responsibility and accountability. Accountability means that you are responsible professionally and legally for the type and quality of nursing care provided. You must remain current and competent in nursing and scientific knowledge and in technical skills.

Caregiver. As a caregiver you help patients maintain and regain health, manage disease and symptoms, and attain a maximal level of function and independence through the healing process. You provide evidence-based nursing care to promote healing through both physical and interpersonal skills. Healing involves more than achieving improved physical well-being. You need to support patients by providing measures that restore their emotional, spiritual, and social well-being. As a caregiver you help the patient and family set goals and assist them with meeting these goals with minimal financial cost, time, and energy.

Advocate. As a patient advocate you protect your patient's human and legal rights and provide assistance in asserting these rights if the need arises. As an advocate you act on behalf of your patient and secure your patient's health care rights (Kowalski, 2016). For example, you provide additional information to help a patient decide whether to accept a treatment, or you find an interpreter to help family members communicate their concerns. You sometimes need to defend patients' rights to make health care decisions in a general way by speaking out against policies or actions that put patients in danger or conflict with their rights. Furthermore, advocates ensure that patients' autonomy and self-determination are respected (Gerber, 2018). Patient advocacy is hard and often provides unique emotional challenges to health care providers, especially when caring for patients with terminal or debilitating chronic illnesses (O'Mahoney et al, 2017). As an advocate it is important to be mindful of personal stressors and to identify ways to cope with these stressors (see Chapter 37).

Educator. As an educator you explain concepts and facts about health, describe the reason for routine care activities, demonstrate procedures such as self-care activities, reinforce learning or patient behavior, and evaluate the patient's progress in learning. Some of your patient teaching is unplanned and informal. For example, during a casual conversation you respond to questions about the reason for an intravenous infusion, a health issue such as smoking cessation, or necessary lifestyle changes. Other teaching activities are planned and more formal such as when you teach your patient how to self-administer insulin injections. Assess your patient's and family caregiver's learning styles and needs and develop a teaching plan that includes teaching methods that match your patient's and family's needs (see Chapter 25).

Communicator. An effective communicator is central to the nurse-patient relationship. It allows you to know your patients, including their preferences, strengths, weaknesses, and needs. Quality communication is essential for all nursing roles and activities (see Chapter 24). You routinely communicate with patients and families, other nurses and health care professionals, resource people, and the community. Effective communication strategies are fundamental to providing quality care, coordinating and managing patient care, assisting patients in rehabilitation, advocating for patients, assisting patients and families in decision making, and providing patient education (Christian, 2017).

Manager. Today's health care environment is fast-paced and complex. Nurse managers need to establish an environment for collaborative patient-centered care to provide safe, quality care with positive patient outcomes. A manager coordinates the activities of members of the nursing staff in delivering nursing care and has personnel, policy, and budgetary responsibility for a specific nursing unit or agency. A manager uses appropriate leadership styles to create a nursing environment for patients and staff that reflects the mission and values of the health care organization (see Chapter 21).

Career Development

Innovations in health care, expanding health care systems and practice settings, and the increasing needs of patients have created new nursing roles. Today the majority of nurses practice in hospital settings, followed by community-based care, ambulatory care, home care, and nursing homes/extended care settings.

Nursing provides an opportunity for you to commit to lifelong learning and career development. Because of increasing educational opportunities for nurses, the growth of nursing as a profession, and a greater concern for job enrichment, the nursing profession offers different career opportunities. Your career path is limitless. You will probably switch career roles more than once. Take advantage of the different clinical practice and professional opportunities. Examples of these career opportunities include advanced practice registered nurses (APRNs), nurse researchers, nurse risk managers, quality improvement nurses, consultants, and entrepreneurs.

Provider of Care. Most nurses provide direct patient care in an acute care setting. However, as changes in health care services and reimbursement continue, there will be an increase in direct care activities provided in the home care setting and an increased need for community-based health promotion activities, restorative care, and end-of-life care. Educate your patients and families on how to maintain their health and implement self-care activities. While collaborating with other health care team members, focus your care on returning a patient to his or her home at an optimal functional status.

In the hospital you may choose to practice in a medical-surgical setting or concentrate on a specific area of specialty practice such as pediatrics, critical care, or emergency care. Most specialty care areas require some experience as a medical-surgical nurse and additional

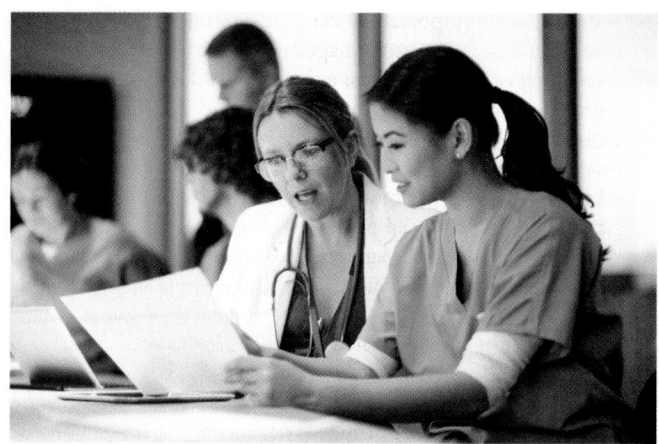

FIG. 1.1 Clinical nurse specialist consults on a complex patient case. (iStock.com/Sturti.)

continuing or in-service education. Many intensive care unit and emergency department nurses are required to have certification in advanced cardiac life support and critical care, emergency nursing, or trauma nursing.

Advanced Practice Registered Nurses. The advanced practice registered nurse (APRN) is the most independently functioning nurse. An APRN has a master's degree or Doctor of Nursing Practice (DNP) degree in nursing; advanced education in pathophysiology, pharmacology, and physical assessment; and certification and expertise in a specialized area of practice (AACN, 2011). In 2008, the APRN Consensus Work Group and the National Council of State Boards of Nursing APRN Advisory Committee developed the Consensus Model for APRN Regulation: Licensure, Accreditation, Certification and Education (APRN, 2008). The Model addresses inconsistent standards in APRN education, regulation, and practice, which had limited APRN mobility from one state to another (Doherty et al., 2018). The consensus model identified that the title of APRN is for nurses with advanced graduate–level knowledge prepared in one of four roles: clinical nurse specialist (CNS), nurse practitioner (NP), certified nurse-midwife (CNM), and certified registered nurse anesthetist (CRNA). The educational preparation for the four roles is in at least one of the following six populations: adult-gerontology, pediatrics, neonatology, women's health/gender related, family/individual across life span, and psychiatric mental health. The Consensus Model, which had an implementation goal of 2015, has not been adopted by all US states and territories, thus requiring nurses to carefully choose their education program (Doherty et al., 2018). APRNs function within their area of practice to plan or improve the quality of nursing care for patients and their families.

Clinical Nurse Specialist. A clinical nurse specialist (CNS) is an APRN who is an expert clinician in a specialized area of practice (Fig. 1.1). The specialty may be identified by a population (e.g., geriatrics), setting (e.g., critical care), disease specialty (e.g., diabetes), type of care (e.g., rehabilitation), or type of problem (e.g., pain) (NACNS, 2018). Clinical nurse specialists provide diagnosis, treatment, and ongoing management of patients in all health care settings. They also provide expertise and support to nurses caring for patients at the bedside, help drive practice changes throughout an organization, and ensure the use of best practices and evidence-based care to achieve the best possible patient outcomes (National Association of Clinical Nurse Specialists, 2019).

Nurse Practitioner. A nurse practitioner (NP) is an APRN who provides comprehensive health care to a group of patients in an inpatient, outpatient, ambulatory care, or community-based setting. This care includes assessment, diagnosis, planning, and treatment; monitoring ongoing health status; evaluation of therapies; and health education. Some NPs provide care to acutely ill patients in hospital settings, including critical care units. Other NPs provide comprehensive care, directly managing the nursing and medical care of patients who are healthy or who have chronic conditions. It is important to review state regulations for advanced practice. Some states require the NP to have a collaborative provider agreement with an agency or physician/physician group to treat a specific group of patients; other states do not.

Certified Nurse-Midwife. A certified nurse-midwife (CNM) is an APRN who is also educated in midwifery and is certified by the American College of Nurse-Midwives (ACNM). The scope of practice of nurse-midwifery has been defined by the ACNM (2011) as encompassing a full range of primary health care services for women from adolescence beyond menopause. These services include primary care; gynecologic and family planning services; preconception care; care during pregnancy, childbirth, and the postpartum period; care of the normal newborn during the first 28 days of life; and treatment of male partners for sexually transmitted infections (ACNM, 2011). The nurse-midwife conducts physical examinations; prescribes medications, including controlled substances and contraceptive methods; admits, manages, and discharges patients; orders and interprets laboratory and diagnostic tests; and orders the use of medical devices.

Certified Registered Nurse Anesthetist. A certified registered nurse anesthetist (CRNA) is an APRN with advanced education from a nurse anesthesia–accredited program. Before applying to a nurse anesthesia program, a nurse must have at least 1 year of critical care or emergency experience. Nurse anesthetists practice both autonomously and in collaboration with a variety of health care providers on the interprofessional team to deliver high-quality, holistic, evidence-based anesthesia and pain care services (American Association of Nurse Anesthetists, 2017). CRNAs practice under the guidance and supervision of an anesthesiologist, a physician with advanced knowledge of surgical anesthesia.

Nurse Educator. A nurse educator works primarily in schools of nursing, staff development departments of health care agencies, and patient education departments. Nurse educators need experience in clinical practice to provide them with practical skills and theoretical knowledge. A faculty member in a nursing program educates students to become professional nurses. Nursing faculty members are responsible for teaching current nursing practice; trends; theory; and necessary skills in classroom, laboratories, and clinical settings. Nursing faculty have graduate degrees such as a master's degree in nursing or an earned doctorate in nursing or related field. Generally, they have a specific clinical, administrative, or research specialty and advanced clinical experience.

Nurse educators in staff development departments of health care institutions provide educational programs for nurses within their institution. These programs include orientation of new personnel, critical care nursing courses, assisting with clinical skill competency, safety training, and instruction about new equipment or procedures. These nursing educators often participate in the development of nursing policies and procedures.

The primary focus of the nurse educator in a patient education department of an agency such as a wound treatment clinic is to teach and coach patients and their families how to self-manage their illness or disability and make positive choices or change their behaviors to promote their health. These nurse educators are usually specialized and hold a certification such as a certified diabetes educator (CDE) or an ostomy care nurse and see only a specific population of patients.

Nurse Administrator. A nurse administrator manages patient care and the delivery of specific nursing services within a health care agency. Nursing administration begins with positions such as clinical care coordinators. Experience and additional education sometimes lead to a middle-management position such as nurse manager of a specific patient care area or house supervisor or to an upper-management position such as an associate director or director of nursing services.

Nurse manager positions usually require at least a baccalaureate degree in nursing, and director and nurse executive positions generally require a master's degree. Chief nurse executive and vice president positions in large health care organizations often require preparation at the doctoral level. Nurse administrators often have advanced degrees such as a master's degree in nursing administration, hospital administration (MHA), public health (MPH), or an MBA.

In today's health care organizations directors have responsibility for more than one nursing unit. They often manage a particular service or product line such as medicine or cardiology. Vice presidents of nursing or chief nurse executives often have responsibilities for all clinical functions within the hospital (e.g., pharmacy, respiratory care, and rehabilitation). This may include all ancillary personnel who provide and support patient care services. The nurse administrator needs to be skilled in business and management and understand all aspects of nursing and patient care. Functions of administrators include budgeting, staffing, strategic planning of programs and services, employee evaluation, and employee development.

Nurse Researcher. The nurse researcher conducts evidence-based practice and research to improve nursing care and further define and expand the scope of nursing practice (see Chapter 5). She or he often works in an academic setting, hospital, or independent professional or community service agency. The preferred educational requirement is a doctoral degree, with at least a master's degree in nursing.

> ### REFLECT NOW
>
> In reviewing the roles and responsibilities of the professional nurse and career options, think about your personal academic and career goals. Design a plan that you can modify as you progress through your academic nursing program.

Nursing Shortage

There is an ongoing shortage of qualified RNs to fill vacant positions (AACN, 2018). This shortage affects all aspects of nursing, including patient care, administration, and nursing education, but it also represents challenges and opportunities for the profession. Many health care dollars are invested in strategies aimed at recruiting and retaining a well-educated, critically thinking, motivated, and dedicated nursing workforce. There is a positive correlation between direct patient care provided by an RN and positive patient outcomes, reduced complication rates, and a more rapid return of the patient to an optimal functional status (Box 1.4) (Giuliano et al., 2016; Aiken, 2013a,b). Research also correlates poor staffing with missed nursing assessments and missed nursing care. In postoperative patients whose status changes rapidly, these missed assessments and care result in poor patient outcomes (Ball et al., 2018).

Professional nursing organizations predict that the number of nurses will continue to diminish (AACN, 2018; Aiken, 2013a). With fewer available nurses, it is important for you to learn to use your patient contact time efficiently and professionally. Time management, therapeutic communication, patient education, and compassionate

BOX 1.4 EVIDENCE-BASED PRACTICE

Impact of Nurse Staffing and Patient Outcomes

PICOT Question: Are patient outcomes improved in hospitals with adequate nursing staffing versus hospitals with lower nursing staffing?

Evidence Summary

There is a growing body of research that shows that nurse staffing affects patient outcomes, patient survival, and the occurrence of adverse events. A secondary data analysis from 661 hospitals showed that there was a significantly lower 30-day readmission rate for patients with heart failure in hospitals that were categorized in the high nurse staffing group, thus reducing health care costs (Giuliano et al., 2016). Patients experiencing an in-hospital cardiac arrest were more likely to survive when there was a decreased patient-to-nurse ratio (McHugh et al., 2016).

Higher nurse staffing was also found to significantly correlate with nursing-sensitive outcomes, such as reduced falls and improved risk assessment for pressure injuries (Burnes Bolton et al., 2017). When there is poor nurse staffing, resulting in larger numbers of patients assigned to a nurse, there is an increase in the occurrence of medication errors, pressure injury formation, and falls with injuries (Cho et al., 2016). Studies demonstrating the positive impact that increased nurse-to-patient ratios have on outcomes provide nursing administrators with evidence to support the hiring of qualified professional nurses.

Application To Nursing Practice

- Consider the nurse-to-patient ratio when looking at a hospital or unit for employment.
- Adequate nursing levels help to improve the nursing work environment (Cho et al., 2016).
- Patient care units in which there is an increased risk for falls due to the patient population or diseases need increased nurse staffing (Burnes Bolton et al., 2017).
- While research supports the economic impact of nurse staffing and improved nursing-sensitive outcomes and other patient outcomes, there needs to be continued research on the impact of nurse staffing ratios (Burnes Bolton, 2017; Giuliano et al., 2016).

implementation of bedside skills are just a few of the essential skills you need. It is important for your patients to leave the health care setting with a positive image of nursing and a feeling that they received quality care. Your patients should never feel that they received rushed or incomplete care. They need to feel that they are important and are involved in decisions and that their needs are met. If a certain aspect of patient care requires 15 minutes of contact, it takes you the same time to deliver organized and compassionate care as it does if you rush through your nursing care.

HISTORICAL INFLUENCES

Nurses have and will always respond to the needs of their patients. In times of war they responded by meeting the needs of the wounded in combat zones and military hospitals in the United States and abroad. When communities face health care crises such as natural disasters, disease outbreaks, or insufficient public health resources, nurses establish community-based immunization and screening programs, treatment clinics, and health promotion activities. Our patients are most vulnerable when they are injured, sick, or dying.

Today nurses are active in determining best practices in a variety of areas such as pressure injury prevention, wound care management, pain control, nutritional management, and care of individuals across the life span. Nurse researchers are leaders in expanding knowledge

in nursing and other health care disciplines. Their work ensures that nurses have the best available evidence to support their practices (see Chapter 5).

Knowledge of the history of the nursing profession increases your ability to understand the social and intellectual origins of the discipline. Although it is not practical to describe all of the historical aspects of professional nursing, some of the more significant nursing leaders and milestones are described in the following paragraphs.

Florence Nightingale

In *Notes on Nursing: What It Is and What It Is Not,* Florence Nightingale established the first nursing philosophy based on health maintenance and restoration (Nightingale, 1860). She saw the role of nursing as having "charge of somebody's health" based on the knowledge of "how to put the body in such a state to be free of disease or to recover from disease" (Nightingale, 1860). During the same year she developed the first organized program for training nurses, the Nightingale Training School for Nurses at St. Thomas' Hospital in London.

Nightingale was the first practicing nurse epidemiologist. Her statistical analyses connected poor sanitation with cholera and dysentery. She volunteered during the Crimean War in 1853 and traveled the battlefield hospitals at night, carrying her lamp; thus, she was known as the "lady with the lamp." The sanitary, nutritional, and basic conditions in the battlefield hospitals were poor, and she was asked to ensure the quality of sanitation facilities. As a result of her actions, the mortality rate at the Barracks Hospital in Scutari, Turkey, reduced from 42.7% to 2.2% in 6 months (Donahue, 2011).

The Civil War To the Beginning of the Twentieth Century

The Civil War (1860–1865) stimulated the growth of nursing in the United States. Clara Barton, founder of the American Red Cross, cared for soldiers on the battlefields, cleansing their wounds, meeting their basic needs, and comforting them at end of life. Dorothea Lynde Dix, Mary Ann Ball (Mother Bickerdyke), and Harriet Tubman also influenced nursing during the Civil War (Donahue, 2011). Dix and Bickerdyke organized hospitals and ambulances, appointed nurses, cared for the wounded soldiers, and oversaw and regulated supplies to the troops. Tubman was active in the Underground Railroad movement and assisted in leading more than 300 slaves to freedom (Donahue, 2011).

The first professionally educated African-American nurse was Mary Mahoney. She was concerned with relationships between cultures and races. As a noted nursing leader, she brought forth an awareness of cultural diversity and respect for the individual, regardless of background, race, color, or religion.

Isabel Hampton Robb helped found the Nurses' Associated Alumnae of the United States and Canada in 1896. This organization became the ANA in 1911. She authored many nursing textbooks and was one of the original founders of the *American Journal of Nursing (Am J Nurs).*

Nursing in hospitals expanded in the late nineteenth century. However, nursing in the community did not increase significantly until 1893, when Lillian Wald and Mary Brewster opened the Henry Street Settlement, which focused on the health needs of poor people who lived in tenements in New York City (Donahue, 2011).

Twentieth Century

In the early twentieth century a movement toward developing a scientific, research-based defined body of nursing knowledge and practice evolved. Nurses began to assume expanded roles. Mary Adelaide Nutting, who became the first nursing professor at Columbia Teachers College in 1906, was instrumental in moving nursing education into universities (Donahue, 2011).

As nursing education developed, nursing practice also expanded, and the Army and Navy Nurse Corps were established. By the 1920s nursing specialization started to develop. The last half of the century saw specialty-nursing organizations such as the American Association of Critical Care Nurses, Association of Operating Room Nurses (AORN), Infusion Nurses Society (INS), and Emergency Nurses Association (ENA) created. In 1990 the ANA established the Center for Ethics and Human Rights, which provides a forum to address the complex ethical and human rights issues confronting nurses and designs activities and programs to increase ethical competence in nurses (Fowler, 2015b).

Twenty-First Century

Today the profession faces multiple challenges. Nurses are revising nursing practice and school curricula to meet the ever-changing needs of society, including an aging population, bioterrorism, emerging infections, and disaster management. Advances in technology and informatics (see Chapter 26), the high-acuity level of care of hospitalized patients, and early discharge from health care institutions require nurses in all settings to have a strong and current knowledge base from which to practice. In addition, nursing and the Robert Wood Johnson Foundation are taking a leadership role in developing standards and policies for end-of-life care through the *Last Acts Campaign* (see Chapter 36). The End-of-Life Nursing Education Consortium (ELNEC), offered collaboratively by the American Association of Colleges of Nursing (AACN) and the City of Hope Medical Center, has brought end-of-life care and practices into nursing curricula and professional continuing education programs for practicing nurses (AACN, 2017).

CONTEMPORARY INFLUENCES

Multiple external forces affect nursing, including the need for nurses' self-care, health care reform and rising health care costs, demographic changes of the population, human rights, and increasing numbers of the medically underserved.

Importance of Nurses' Self-Care

Nursing is a dynamic gratifying career. However, it also has both physical and emotional demands and challenges. You cannot give fully engaged, compassionate care to others when you feel depleted or do not feel cared for yourself. You and your colleagues will have many self-care needs that must be met to function as healthy professionals.

In your educational experience and in your career, you will experience grief and loss. Many times, even before you have a chance to recover from an emotionally draining situation, you will encounter another difficult human story. Nurses in acute care settings frequently witness prolonged, concentrated suffering, leading to feelings of frustration, anger, guilt, sadness, or anxiety (Kelly et al., 2015). Nursing students report feeling initially hesitant and uncomfortable with their first encounters with a dying patient and identify feelings of sadness and anxiety.

Frequent, intense, or prolonged exposure to grief and loss places nurses at risk for developing compassion fatigue. *Compassion fatigue* is a term used to describe a state of burnout and secondary traumatic stress (Potter et al., 2013a). It occurs without warning and often results from giving high levels of energy and compassion over a prolonged period to those who are suffering, often without experiencing improved patient outcomes (Kelly et al., 2015). Secondary traumatic stress is the trauma that health care providers experience when witnessing and caring for others suffering trauma. Examples include an oncology nurse who cares for patients undergoing surgery and chemotherapy over the long term for their cancer or a spouse who witnesses his wife deteriorating over the years from Alzheimer's disease.

Burnout is the condition that occurs when perceived demands outweigh perceived resources (Potter et al., 2013a). It is a state of physical and mental exhaustion that often affects health care providers because of the nature of their work environment. Over time, giving of oneself in often intense caring environments sometimes results in emotional exhaustion, leaving a nurse feeling irritable, restless, and unable to focus and engage with patients (Potter et al., 2013b). This often occurs in situations in which there is a lack of social support, organizational pressures influencing staffing, and the inability of the nurse to practice self-care. Compassion fatigue typically results in feelings of hopelessness, a decrease in the ability to take pleasure from previously enjoyable activities, a state of hypervigilance, and anxiety.

Compassion fatigue negatively impacts the health and wellness of nurses and the quality of care provided to patients. It also affects the organizations as nurses experience changes in job performance and in their personal lives; it can result in nurses' desire to leave the profession or their specialty. In addition, these factors affect patient satisfaction and an agency's ability to maintain a caring, competent staff (Ledoux, 2015).

There is a need for health care agencies to identify early signs of compassion fatigue and to develop interventions to help nurses manage it. Prompt interventions improve nurse retention and job satisfaction rates (Kelly et al., 2015.) Agency-based programs that provide opportunities for nurses to validate their experiences and an opportunity to talk about the challenges of the type of care they give help nurses cope with compassion fatigue and its implication for professional nursing care (Wentzel and Brysiewicz, 2017).

Compassion fatigue may contribute to what is described as *lateral violence* (see Chapter 24). Lateral violence sometimes occurs in nurse-nurse interactions and includes behaviors such as withholding information, making snide remarks, and demonstrating nonverbal expressions of disapproval, such as raising eyebrows or making faces. New graduates and nurses new to a unit are most likely to face problems with lateral or horizontal violence (Sanner-Stiehr and Ward-Smith, 2017).

All nurses require resiliency skills to better manage the stressors that contribute to compassion fatigue and lateral violence. Managing stress and conflict, building connections with colleagues to share difficult stories, and self-care are helpful stress-management techniques in dealing with difficult situations and contribute to safe and effective care (see Chapter 37) (Perez, 2015).

Health Care Reform and Costs

Health care reform affects not only how health care is paid for but also how it is delivered. There is greater emphasis on health promotion, disease prevention, and illness management in the future. More services will be in community-based care settings. However, hospitals will continue to manage the care of very seriously ill patients. As a result, more nurses will be needed to practice in community care centers, patients' homes, schools, and senior centers. This will require nurses to be skilled at assessing for resources, service gaps, and how patients adapt to return to their communities. Nursing needs to respond to such changes by assessing for resources, improving staffing and management models in hospitals, changing nursing education, helping patients adapt to new health care delivery methods, and providing care to safely return patients to their homes.

Skyrocketing health care costs present challenges to the profession, the consumer, and the health care delivery system. As a nurse you are responsible for providing the patient with the best-quality care in an efficient and economically sound manner, including following established protocols, exercising timely well-planned patient discharge from a care setting, and judiciously using supplies and equipment. The challenge is to use health care and patient resources wisely. Chapter 2 summarizes reasons for the rise in health care costs and its implications for nursing.

Demographic Changes

The US Census Bureau (2018) predicts that the 2030s will be a transformative decade, with the population expected to grow at a slower pace, age considerably, and become more racially and ethnically diverse. These changes will require expanded health care resources. The US Census Bureau's 2017 population projections predict that by 2030, all baby boomers will be older than 65 years of age. This will expand the size of the older population so that 1 in every 5 residents will be of retirement age (US Census Bureau, 2018). It is also predicted that by 2044 more than half of the US population will be part of a minority group (Colby et al., 2014). To effectively meet all the health care needs of the expanding minority and aging populations, changes need to occur as to how care is provided, especially in the area of public health. The population is still shifting from rural areas to urban centers, and more people are living with chronic and long-term illness. Not only are outpatient settings expanding, but more and more people want to receive outpatient and community-based care and remain in their homes or community (see Chapters 2 and 3).

Medically Underserved

Unemployment, underemployment and low-paying jobs, mental illness, homelessness, and rising health care costs all contribute to increases in the medically underserved population. Caring for this population is a global challenge; the social, political, economic, and health literacy factors affect both access to care and access to health care–related resources (Kaphingst et al., 2016). In addition, the number of underserved patients who require home-based palliative care services is increasing. This is a group of patients whose physical status does not improve and whose health care needs increase. People with low health literacy are less likely to participate in decision making regarding their care because they do not understand the medical information provided, nor do they understand the consequences of indecision (Seo et al., 2016).

TRENDS IN NURSING

Nursing is a dynamic profession that grows and evolves as society and lifestyles change, as health care priorities and technologies change, and as nurses themselves change. The current philosophies and definitions of nursing have a holistic focus, which addresses the needs of the whole person in all dimensions, in health and illness, and in interaction with the family and community. In addition, there continues to be an increasing awareness for patient safety in all care settings.

Evidence-Based Practice

Today the general public is more informed about their health care needs, the cost of health care, best practices, and the incidence of medical errors within health care institutions. Your current and future practice needs to be based on current evidence, not just according to your education and experiences and the policies and procedures of health care agencies (see Chapter 5). The delivery of and reimbursement for evidence-based nursing care is essential (Melnyk and Gallagher-Ford, 2018). Health care organizations must show their commitment to each health care stakeholder (e.g., patients, insurance companies, and governmental agencies) to reduce health care errors and improve patient safety by implementing evidence-based practices (National Quality Forum, 2010). In addition, many hospitals are achieving Magnet Recognition®, which recognizes excellence in nursing practice (ANCC, n.d.). A component of excellence in practice is quality of care, represented by the implementation of evidence-based practices (see Chapter 2).

Quality and Safety Education for Nurses

The Robert Wood Johnson Foundation sponsored the Quality and Safety Education for Nurses (QSEN) initiative to respond to reports about safety and quality patient care by the Institute of Medicine (IOM) (QSEN Institute, 2018). QSEN addresses the challenge to prepare nurses with the competencies needed to continuously improve the quality of care in their work environments (Table 1.1). The QSEN initiative encompasses the competencies of patient-centered care, teamwork and collaboration, evidence-based practice, quality improvement, safety, and informatics (QSEN Institute, 2018). For each competency there are targeted knowledge, skills, and attitudes (KSAs). The KSAs are elements that were initially developed for prelicensure programs (QSEN Institute, 2018). Now KSAs have been developed for graduate nursing programs (QSEN, 2018; Sherwood and Zomorodi, 2014).

TABLE 1.1	Quality and Safety Education for Nurses
Competency	**Definition With Examples**
Patient-centered care	Recognize the patient or designee as the source of control and full partner in providing compassionate and coordinated care based on respect for patient's preferences, values, and needs. *Examples: Involve family and friends in care. Elicit patient's values and preferences. Provide care with respect for diversity of the human experience.*
Teamwork and collaboration	Function effectively within nursing and interprofessional teams, fostering open communication, mutual respect, and shared decision making to achieve quality patient care. *Examples: Recognize the contributions of other health team members and patient's family members. Discuss effective strategies for communicating and resolving conflict. Participate in designing methods to support effective teamwork.*
Evidence-based practice	Integrate best current evidence with clinical expertise and patient and/or family preferences and values for delivery of optimal health care. *Examples: Demonstrate knowledge of basic scientific methods. Appreciate strengths and weaknesses of scientific bases for practice. Appreciate the importance of regularly reading relevant journals.*
Quality improvement	Use data to monitor the outcomes of care processes and use improvement methods to design and test changes to continuously improve the quality and safety of health care systems. *Examples: Use tools such as flow charts and diagrams to make process of care explicit. Appreciate how unwanted variation in outcomes affects care. Identify gaps between local and best practices.*
Safety	Minimize risk of harm to patients and providers through both system effectiveness and individual performance. *Examples: Examine human factors, basic safety design principles, and commonly used unsafe practices. Value own role in preventing errors.*
Informatics	Use information and technology to communicate, manage knowledge, mitigate error, and support decision making. *Examples: Navigate an electronic health record. Protect confidentiality of protected health information in electronic health records.*

Adapted from QSEN Institute: *QSEN competencies: definitions and pre-licensure KSAs,* 2018, http://qsen.org/competencies/pre-licensure-ksas/. Accessed May 2018.

As you gain experience in clinical practice, you face situations in which your education helps you to make a difference in improving patient care. Whether that difference is to provide evidence for implementing care at the bedside, identify a safety issue, or study patient data to identify trends in outcomes, each of these situations requires competence in patient-centered care, safety, or informatics. Although it is not within the scope of this textbook to present the QSEN initiative in its entirety, subsequent clinical chapters will provide you an opportunity to address how to build competencies in one or more of these areas.

> **QSEN** **Building Competency in Patient-Centered Care** You are caring for Kitty, a 10-year-old with severe delayed development. Kitty, an only child, lives with her parents and goes to a school that is able to meet her needs. Her mom gives her seizure medicine each day, and her seizures are well controlled. Kitty has very little independent function. She needs assistance with all of her activities of daily living (e.g., bathing, toileting, eating, and hygiene). Up to now Kitty's parents have been able to provide all of her care and meet her needs. As a patient advocate, what do you need to know about Kitty's parents goals for her future care? Think about how you can use this information to advocate for Kitty and her parents to achieve these goals.
>
> Answers to QSEN Activities can be found on the Evolve website.

Impact of Emerging Technologies

Emerging technologies have the potential to change nursing practice. These technologies provide more accurate, noninvasive assessment tools; help you to implement evidence-based practices; collect and trend patient outcome data; and use clinical decision support systems. The electronic health record (EHR) is an efficient method for documenting and managing patient health care information (see Chapter 26.) Computerized physician/provider order entry (CPOE) is a critical patient safety initiative (Houston, 2014).

Emerging technologies will assist you to communicate, provide care for, and build relationships with your patients. Telehealth, e-visits, and devices that allow your patient to phone in pertinent health information are examples of technology that open new venues for providing care. Learn how these electronic tools work so that you can teach patients how to use them. Evidence-based practice, clinical decision support systems, and case-based reasoning are all methods to increase information acquisition and distribution.

Technological innovations help family caregivers monitor and manage home environments of older adults, enable older adults to stay in their homes but stay connected to their support systems, and help with decision support and care coordination (Andruszkiewicz and Fike, 2015–2016). Additionally, the availability and use of telehealth and telemedicine functions to provide health care are increasing (NCSBN, 2016).

Genomics

As you use and understand genomics remember to use genomic information in a confidential, ethical, and culturally appropriate manner to help health care providers and patients make informed care decisions (Houston, 2014).

Genetics is the study of inheritance, or the way traits are passed down from one generation to another. Genes carry the instructions for making proteins, which in turn direct the activities of cells and functions of the body that influence traits such as hair and eye color. Genomics is a newer term that describes the study of all the genes in a person and interactions of these genes with one another and with that person's environment (CDC, 2018). Genomic information combined with technology can potentially improve health outcomes, quality,

and safety and reduce health care costs (McCormick and Calzone, 2016). This information allows health care providers to determine how genomic changes contribute to patient conditions and influence treatment decisions (Sharoff, 2016; Miaskowski and Aouizerat, 2012). For example, when a family member has colon cancer before the age of 50, it is likely that other family members are at risk for developing this cancer. Genomics counseling and testing can determine family status. Knowing this information is important for family members who will need a colonoscopy before the age of 50 and repeat colonoscopies more often than the patient who is not at risk. Nurses identify the patients' risk factors through assessment and counsel patients about what this genomic finding means to them personally and to their families.

Public Perception of Nursing

Nursing is a pivotal health care profession. As frontline health care providers, nurses practice in all health care settings and constitute the largest number of health care professionals. They are essential to providing skilled, specialized, knowledgeable care; improving the health status of the public; and ensuring safe, effective quality care (ANA, 2015).

Consumers of health care are more informed than ever; with the Internet consumers have access to more health care and treatment information. For example, *Hospital Compare* is a consumer-oriented website that allows people to select multiple hospitals and directly compare performance measure information on specific diseases such as health attack, heart failure, pneumonia, and surgery (CMS, 2016). This information can help consumers make informed decisions about health care.

Consumers can also access *Hospital Consumer Assessment of Healthcare Providers Systems* (HCAHPS) to obtain information about patients' perspectives on hospital care. Although many hospitals collect information on patient satisfaction, HCAHPS offers a survey that helps consumers obtain valid comparisons about patient perspectives across all hospitals. This information is intended to allow consumers to make "apples to apples" comparisons to support their choice (HCAHPS, 2018).

> **REFLECT NOW**
>
> A nurse is often the first health care professional a patient sees when in the emergency department or following admission to a hospital. Think about the type of impression you want to make in terms of compassion, competency, and professionalism.

Impact of Nursing On Politics and Health Policy

Political power or influence is known as the ability to influence or persuade an individual holding a governmental office to exert the power of that office to effect a desired outcome. Nurses' involvement in politics is receiving greater emphasis in nursing curricula, professional organizations, and health care settings. Professional nursing organizations and state nursing boards employ lobbyists to urge state legislatures and the US Congress to pass legislation that will improve the quality of health care (Mason et al., 2016).

The ANA works for the improvement of health standards and the availability of health care services for all people, fosters high standards of nursing, stimulates and promotes the professional development of nurses, and advances their economic and general welfare. The ANA's purposes are unrestricted by considerations of nationality, race, creed, lifestyle, color, gender, or age.

You can influence policy decisions at all governmental levels. One way to get involved is by participating in local and national efforts

(Mason et al., 2016). This effort is critical to exerting nurses' influence early in the political process. Nurses can help make the future bright by becoming serious students of social needs, activists in influencing policy to meet those needs, and generous contributors of time and money to nursing organizations and to candidates working for universal good health care (Mason et al., 2016).

PROFESSIONAL REGISTERED NURSE EDUCATION

Nursing requires a significant amount of formal education. The issues of standardization of nursing education and entry into practice remain a major controversy. Various prelicensure educational programs are available for individuals intending to be an RN. In addition, graduate nurse education and continuing and in-service education are available for practicing nurses.

Prelicensure

Currently in the United States the most frequent way to become a registered nurse (RN) is through completion of either an associate or baccalaureate degree program. Graduates of both programs are eligible to take the National Council Licensure Examination for Registered Nurses (NCLEX-RN®) to become RNs in the state in which they will practice.

The associate degree program in the United States is a 2-year program that is usually offered by a university or community college. This program focuses on the basic sciences and theoretical and clinical courses related to the practice of nursing.

The baccalaureate degree program usually includes 4 years of study in a college or university. It focuses on the basic sciences; theoretical and clinical courses; and courses in the social sciences, arts, and humanities to support nursing theory. In Canada the degree of Bachelor of Science in Nursing (BScN) or Bachelor in Nursing (BN) is equivalent to the degree of Bachelor of Science in Nursing (BSN) in the United States. The *Essentials of Baccalaureate Education for Professional Nursing* (AACN, 2008) delineates essential knowledge, practice and values, attitudes, personal qualities, and professional behavior for the baccalaureate-prepared nurse and guides faculty on the structure and evaluation of the curriculum. Standards published by nursing program accrediting organizations typically specify core competencies for the professional nurse that should be in the nursing curriculum. In addition, one of the IOM recommendations is that 80% of nurses be prepared with a baccalaureate in nursing by 2020 (IOM, 2010) (see Chapter 2).

Graduate Education

After obtaining a baccalaureate degree in nursing, you can pursue graduate education leading to a master's or doctoral degree in any number of graduate fields, including nursing. A nurse completing a graduate program can receive a master's degree in nursing. The graduate degree provides the advanced clinician with strong skills in nursing science and theory. Graduate education emphasizes advanced knowledge in the basic sciences and research-based clinical practice. A master's degree in nursing is important for the roles of nurse educator and nurse administrator, and it is a minimum requirement for an APRN.

Doctoral Preparation. Professional doctoral programs in nursing (DSN or DNSc) prepare graduates to apply research findings to clinical nursing. Other doctoral programs prepare nurses for more rigorous research and theory development and award the research-oriented Doctor of Philosophy (PhD) in nursing. Recently the AACN recommended the Doctor of Nursing Practice (DNP) as the terminal practice degree and required preparation for all APRNs. The DNP is a practice-focused doctorate. It provides skills in obtaining expanded knowledge through the formulation and interpretations of evidence-based practice.

The need for nurses with doctoral degrees is increasing. Expanding clinical roles and continuing demand for well-educated nursing faculty, nurse administrators, and APRNs in the clinical settings and new areas of nursing specialties such as nursing informatics are just a few reasons for increasing the number of doctoral-prepared nurses.

Continuing and In-Service Education

Nursing is a knowledge-based profession, and clinical decision making and technological expertise are qualities that health care consumers demand and expect. Continuing education updates your knowledge about the latest research and practice developments, helps you to specialize in a particular area of practice, and teaches you new skills and techniques, all of which are crucial factors to improving patient care (Wellings et al., 2017). Continuing education involves educational programs offered by universities, hospitals, state nurses associations, professional nursing organizations, and educational and health care institutions. An example is a program on caring for older adults with dementia offered by a university or a program on safe medication practices offered by a hospital. While many of these programs are on-site as a lecture, seminar, or skills training, there is a growth in virtual learning, especially for those nursing subspecialties, such as oncology, that require continuing nursing education. (das Gracas Silva Matsubara and De Domenico, 2016). Many states require a set number of continuing education hours as part of license renewal. In some cases there are continuing education requirements for specific topics such as bioterrorism and pain management.

In-service education programs are instruction or training provided by a health care agency or institution. An in-service program is held in the institution and is designed to increase the knowledge, skills, and competencies of nurses and other health care professionals employed by the institution. Often in-service programs are focused on new technologies such as how to correctly use the newest safety syringes. Many in-service programs are designed to fulfill required competencies of an organization. For example, a hospital might offer an in-service program on safe principles for administering chemotherapy or a program on cultural sensitivity.

NURSING PRACTICE

You will have an opportunity to practice in a variety of settings, in many roles within those settings, and with caregivers in other related health professions. The ANA standards of practice, standards of performance, and code of ethics for nurses are part of the public recognition of the significance of nursing practice to health care and implications for nursing practice regarding trends in health care. State and provincial nurse practice acts (NPAs) establish specific legal regulations for practice, and professional organizations establish standards of practice as criteria for nursing care.

Nurse Practice Acts

In the United States each State Board of Nursing oversees its NPA. The NPA regulates the scope of nursing practice for the state and protects public health, safety, and welfare. This protection includes protecting the public from unqualified and unsafe nurses. Although each state has its own NPA that defines the scope of nursing practice, most NPAs are similar. The definition of nursing practice published by the ANA is representative of the scope of nursing practice as defined in most states.

During the last decade, many states have revised their NPAs to reflect the growing autonomy of nursing, minimum education requirements, certification requirements, and the expanded roles and scope of practice of APRNs.

Licensure and Certification

Licensure. In the United States all boards of nursing require RN candidates to pass the NCLEX-RN®. Regardless of educational preparation, the examination for RN licensure is the same in every state in the United States. This provides a standardized minimum knowledge base for nurses. Other requirements for licensure such as criminal background checks vary from state to state.

Certification. After passing NCLEX-RN®, a nurse may choose to work toward certification in a specific area of nursing practice. Minimum practice and/or educational requirements are set, based on specific certification. National nursing organizations such as the ANA have many types of certification to enhance your career, such as certification in medical-surgical or geriatric nursing. After passing the initial examination, you maintain your certification by ongoing continuing education and maintaining a set number of hours in clinical or administrative practice.

PROFESSIONAL NURSING ORGANIZATIONS

A professional organization deals with issues of concern to those practicing in the profession. In addition to the educational organizations previously discussed, a variety of specialty nursing organizations exist. For example, some organizations focus on specific areas such as critical care, advanced practice, maternal-child nursing, oncology, and nursing research. These organizations seek to improve the standards of practice, expand nursing roles, and foster the welfare of nurses within the specialty areas. In addition, professional organizations present educational programs and publish journals.

As a student you have the opportunity to take part in organizations such as the National Student Nurses Association (NSNA) in the United States and the Canadian Student Nurses Association (CSNA) in Canada. These organizations consider issues of importance to nursing students such as career development and preparation for licensing. The NSNA often cooperates in activities and programs with the professional organizations.

◼ KEY POINTS

- Nursing responds to the health care needs of society, which are influenced by economic, social, and cultural factors.
- Changes in society, such as health care reform, changing demographic patterns, increases in the medically underserved population, and increased consumerism, affect the practice of nursing.
- Nursing standards provide the guidelines for implementing and evaluating nursing care.
- Advances in nursing's scientific knowledge base and the application of evidence-based practice have improved nursing practice and patient outcomes.
- Nursing education programs must adhere to educational standards established by a nursing education accreditation body.
- A nurse may take multiple professional career paths, such as advanced practice, nurse educator, research, and administration, to advance within the discipline.
- Professional nursing organizations impact educational standards and certifications, specialty practice, consumerism, and patient advocacy.

- Nurses are increasingly aware of the role of politics and its influence on the health care system. As a result, nurses are more aware of the profession's influence on health care policy and practice.

◼ REFLECTIVE LEARNING

- You are on the patient safety committee at your hospital. Your assignment is to identify two resources related to safety. One resource must relate to the individual nurse, and the second must relate to the practice and work environment.
- Thinking back on your recent clinical experiences, which QSEN competencies knowledge, skills, or attitudes did you use while providing care?
- What impact do evidence-based practice and emerging technologies have on quality patient-centered care?

◼ REVIEW QUESTIONS

1. You are preparing a presentation for your classmates regarding the clinical care coordination conference for a patient with terminal cancer. As part of the preparation you have your classmates read the Nursing Code of Ethics for Professional Registered Nurses. Your instructor asks the class why this document is important. Which statement best describes this code?
   1. Improves self–health care
   2. Protects the patient's confidentiality
   3. Ensures identical care to all patients
   4. Defines the principles of right and wrong to provide patient care
2. A nurse is caring for a patient with end-stage lung disease. The patient wants to go home on oxygen and be comfortable. The family wants the patient to have a new surgical procedure. The nurse explains the risk and benefits of the surgery to the family and discusses the patient's wishes with them. The nurse is acting as the patient's:
   1. Educator.
   2. Advocate.
   3. Caregiver.
   4. Communicator.
3. The nurse spends time with a patient and family reviewing a dressing change procedure for the patient's wound. The patient's spouse demonstrates how to change the dressing. The nurse is acting in which professional role?
   1. Educator
   2. Advocate
   3. Caregiver
   4. Communicator
4. The examination for registered nurse (RN) licensure is the same in every state in the United States. This examination:
   1. Guarantees safe nursing care for all patients.
   2. Ensures standard nursing care for all patients.
   3. Provides a minimal standard of knowledge for an RN in practice.
   4. Guarantees standardized education across all prelicensure programs.
5. Contemporary nursing requires that the nurse has knowledge and skills for a variety of professional roles and responsibilities. Which of the following are examples of these roles and responsibilities? (Select all that apply.)
   1. Caregiver
   2. Autonomy
   3. Patient advocate
   4. Health promotion
   5. Genetic counselor

6. Match the advanced practice nurse specialty with the statement about the role.

1. Clinical nurse specialist
2. Nurse anesthetist
3. Nurse practitioner
4. Nurse-midwife

a. Provides independent care, including pregnancy and gynecological services
b. Expert clinician in a specialized area of practice such as adult diabetes care
c. Provides comprehensive care, usually in a primary care setting, directly managing the medical care of patients who are healthy or have chronic conditions
d. Provides care and services under the supervision of an anesthesiologist

7. Health care reform will bring changes in the emphasis of care. Which of these models is expected from health care reform?
   1. Moving from an acute illness to a health promotion, illness prevention model
   2. Moving from an illness prevention to a health promotion model
   3. Moving from hospital-based to community-based care
   4. Moving from an acute illness to a disease management model

8. A nurse meets with the registered dietitian and physical therapist to develop a plan of care that focuses on improving nutrition and mobility for a patient. This is an example of which Quality and Safety in the Education of Nurses (QSEN) competency?
   1. Patient-centered care
   2. Safety
   3. Teamwork and collaboration
   4. Quality improvement

9. A critical care nurse is using a new research-based intervention to correctly position her ventilated patients to reduce pneumonia caused by accumulated respiratory secretions. This is an example of which Quality and Safety in the Education of Nurses (QSEN) competency?
   1. Patient-centered care
   2. Evidence-based practice
   3. Teamwork and collaboration
   4. Quality improvement

10. The nurses on an acute care medical floor notice an increase in pressure injury formation in their patients. A nurse consultant decides to compare two types of treatment. The first is the procedure currently used to assess for pressure injury risk. The second uses a new assessment instrument to identify at-risk patients. Given this information, the nurse consultant exemplifies which career?
    1. Clinical nurse specialist
    2. Nurse administrator
    3. Nurse educator
    4. Nurse researcher

Answers: 1. 4; **2.** 3; **1.** 4; **3.** 5; **1.** 2, 3, 4; **6.** 1b, 2d, 3c, 4a; **7.** 1; **8.** 3; **9.** 2; **10.** 4.

Rationales for Review Questions can be found on the Evolve website.

REFERENCES

Aiken LH: The impact of research on staffing: an interview with Linda Aiken, Part 1, *Nurs Econ* 31(5):216, 2013a.

Aiken LH: The impact of research on staffing: an interview with Linda Aiken, Part 2, *Nurs Econ* 31(5):216, 2013b.

American Association of Colleges of Nursing (AACN): *About ELNEC (website)*, 2017, http://www.aacnnursing-.org/ELNEC/About. Accessed May 2018.

American Association of Colleges of Nursing (AACN): *Essentials of master's education for advanced practice nursing*, Washington, DC, 2011, The Association.

American Association of Colleges of Nursing (AACN): *Nursing shortage, news release*, Washington, DC, 2018, The Association. http://www.aacnnursing.org/News-Information/Nursing-Shortage-Resources/About. Accessed May 2018.

American Association of Colleges of Nursing (AACN): *Essentials of baccalaureate education for professional nursing*, Washington, DC, 2008, The Association.

American Association of Nurse Anesthetists (AANA): Certified Registered Nurse Anesthetist Position Description, 2017, https://www.aana.com/docs/default-source/practice-aana-com-web-documents-(all)/certified-registered-nurse-anesthetist-position-description.pdf?sfvrsn=60649b1_2. Accessed May 20, 2019.

American College of Nurse Midwives (ACMN): Definition of midwifery and scope of practice of certified nurse-midwives and certified midwives, 2011, http://www.midwife.org/Our-Scope-of-Practice. Accessed 20 May 2019.

American Nurses Association (ANA): *Nursing: scope and standards of practice*, ed 3, Silver Spring, MD, 2015, The Association.

American Nurses' Credentialing Center (ANCC): *Magnet Recognition Program* model, n.d, http://www.nursecredentialing.org/Magnet/ProgramOverview/New-Magnet-Model. Accessed May 2018.

APRN Consensus Work Group and the National Council of State Boards of Nursing APRN Advisory Committee: *Consensus model for APRN regulation: licensure, accreditation, certification and education*, 2008, http://www.nursecredentialing.org/Certification/APRNCorner/APRN-FAQ. Accessed May 2018.

Benner P: *From novice to expert: excellence and power in clinical nursing practice*, Menlo Park, CA, 1984, Addison-Wesley.

Benner P, et al.: The social fabric of nursing knowledge, *Am J Nurs* 97(7):16, 1997.

Benner P, et al.: *Educating nurses: a call for radical transformation*, Stanford, CA, 2010, Carnegie Foundation for the Advancement of Teaching.

Centers for Disease Control and Prevention (CDC): *Genomics and diseases*, 2018, https://www.cdc.gov/genomics/disease/genomic_diseases.htm. Accessed May 2018.

Centers for Medicare & Medicaid Services (CMS): *Hospital compare*, updated December 2016, http://www.cms.gov/Medicare/Quality-Initiatives-Patient-Assessment-Instruments/hospitalQualityInits/HospitalCompare.html. Accessed May 2018.

Doherty CL, et al.: The consensus model: What current and future NPs need to know, *American Nurse Today* 13(12), 2018, https://www.americannursetoday.com/consensus-model-nps/. Accessed 20 May 2019.

Donahue MP: *Nursing: the finest art—an illustrated history*, ed 3, St Louis, 2011, Mosby.

Fowler DM: *Guide to nursing's social policy statement: understanding the profession from social contract to social covenant*, Silver Spring, MD, 2015a, American Nurses Publishing.

Fowler DM: *Guide to the Code of Ethics for nurses with interpretive statements: development, interpretation and application*, Silver Spring, MD, 2015b, The Association.

Gerber L: Understanding the nurse's role as a patient advocate, *Nursing* 48(4):55, 2018.

Hospital Consumer Assessment of Healthcare Providers and Systems (HCAHPS): *CAHPS Survey*, May 2018 update, http://www.hcahpsonline.org/. Accessed May 2018.

Houston C: Technology in the health care workplace: benefits, limitations, and challenges. In Houston CJ, editor: *Professional issues in nursing: challenges and opportunities*, ed 3, Philadelphia, 2014, Lippincott Williams & Wilkins.

Institute of Medicine (IOM): *The future of nursing: leading change, advancing health*, Washington DC, 2010, National Academies Press.

International Council of Nurses (ICN): *ICN definition of nursing*, 2018, https://www.icn.ch/nursing-policy/nursing-definitions. Accessed 20 May 2019.

Kowalski K: Professional behavior in nursing, *J Contin Educ Nurs* 47(4):158, 2016.

Mason DJ, et al.: *Policy & politics in nursing and health care*, ed 7, St. Louis, 2016, Elsevier.

McCormick KA, Calzone KA: The impact of genomics on health outcomes, quality, and safety, *Nurs Manage* 47(4):23, 2016.

National Association of Clinical Nurse Specialists (NACNS): *CNS competencies*, 2018, http://nacns.org/professional-resources/practice-and-cns-role/cns-competencies/. Accessed May 2018.

National Council of State Boards of Nursing (NCSBN): A changing environment: 2016 NCSBN environmental scan, *J Nurs Regul* 6(4):4, 2016.

National Quality Forum (NQF): *Safe practices for better healthcare—2010 update: a consensus report*, Washington, DC, 2010, NQF, http://www.qualityforum.org/Publications/2010/04/Safe_Practices_for_Better_Healthcare_-_2010_Update.aspx. Accessed May 2018.

Nightingale F: *Notes on nursing: what it is and what it is not*, London, 1860, Harrison and Sons.

QSEN Institute: *QSEN competencies: definitions and pre-licensure KSAs*, 2018, http://qsen.org/competencies/pre-licensure-ksas/. Accessed May 2018.

Robert Wood Johnson Foundation (RWJF): *Catalysts for change: harnessing the power of nurses to build population health in the 21st century*, 2017, https://www.rwjf.org/en/library/research/2017/09/catalysts-for-change--harnessing-the-power-of-nurses-to-build-population-health.html. Accessed May 2018.

Robert Wood Johnson Foundation (RWJF): *Future of nursing: campaign for action is chalking up successes that will improve patient care*, 2014a, http://www.rwjf.org/en/library/articles-and-news/2014/06/campaign-for-action-is-chalking-up-successes-that-will-improve-p.html. Accessed May 2018.

Sanner-Stiehr E, Ward-Smith P: Lateral violence in nursing: implication and strategies for nurse educators, *J Prof Nurs* 33(2):113, 2017.

Sharoff L: Holistic nursing in the genetic/genomic era, *J Holist Nurs* 34(2):146, 2016.

US Census Bureau: Older people projected to outnumber children for first time in U.S. history, March 13, 2018, Release number CB18-41, https://www.census.gov/newsroom/press-releases/2018/cb18-41-population-projections.html. Accessed 20 May 2019.

RESEARCH REFERENCES

Andruszkiewicz G, Fike K: Emerging technology trends and products: how tech innovations are easing the burden of family caregiving, *Generations* 39(4):64, 2015–2016.

Ball JE, et al.: Post-operative mortality, missed care and nurse staffing in nine countries: a cross-sectional study, *Int J Nurs Stud* 78(10), 2018.

Burnes Bolton L, et al.: Mandated nurse staffing ratios in California: a comparison of staffing and nursing-sensitive outcomes pre- and post regulation, policy, *Polit Nurs Pract* 8(4):238, 2017.

Christian BJ: Translational research—effective communication and teaching strategies for improving the quality of pediatric nursing care for hospitalized children and their families, *J Pediatr Nurs* 34:90, 2017.

Cho E, et al.: The relationships of nurse staffing level and work environment with patient adverse events, *J Nurs Scholarsh* 48(1):74, 2016.

Colby SL, Ortman JM: *Projections of the size and composition of the U.S. population: 2014 to 2060, current population reports, P25-1143*, Washington, DC, 2014, US Census Bureau.

das Gracas Silva Matsubara M, De Domenico EBL: Virtual learning environment in continuing education in nursing in oncology: an experimental study, *J Cancer Educ* 31(4):804, 2016.

Giuliano KK, et al.: The relationship between nurse staffing and 30-day readmission for adults with heart failure, *J Nurs Adm* 46(1):25, 2016.

Kaphingst KA, et al.: Relationships between health literacy and genomics-related knowledge, self-efficacy, perceived importance, and communication in a medically underserved population, *J Health Commun* 21(Suppl 1):58–68, 2016.

Kelly L, et al.: Predictors of compassion fatigue and compassion satisfaction in acute care nurses, *J Nurs Scholarsh* 47:522, 2015.

Ledoux K: Understanding compassion fatigue; understanding compassion, *J Adv Nurs* 71(9):2041, 2015.

McHugh MD, et al.: Better nurse staffing and nurse work environments associated with increased survival of in-hospital cardiac arrest patients, *Med Care* 54(1):74, 2016.

Melnyk BM, Gallagher-Ford L: Outcomes from the first Helene Fuld health trust national institute for evidence-based practice in nursing and health care invitational expert forum, *Worldviews Evid Based Nurs* 15(1):5, 2018.

Miaskowski C, Aouizerat BE: Biomarkers: symptoms, survivorship, and quality of life, *Semin Oncol Nurs* 28(2):129, 2012.

O'Mahony J, et al.: Hospice palliative care volunteers as program and patient/family advocates, *Am J Hosp Palliat Care* 34(9):844, 2017.

Perez GK, et al.: Promoting resiliency among palliative care clinicians: stressors, coping strategies, and training needs, *J Palliat Med* 18(4):332, 2015.

Potter PA, et al.: Developing a systemic program for compassion fatigue, *Nurs Adm Q* 37(4):326, 2013a.

Potter PA, et al.: Evaluation of a compassion fatigue resilience program for oncology nurses, *Oncol Nurs Forum* 40(2):180, 2013b.

Seo J, et al.: Effect of health literacy on decision-making preferences among medically underserved patients, *Med Decis Making* 36(4):550, 2016.

Sherwood G, Zomorodi M: A new mindset for quality and safety: the QSEN competencies redefine nurses' roles in practice, *J Nurs Adm* 44(10):510, 2014.

Wellings CA, et al.: Evaluating continuing nursing education: a qualitative study of intention to change practice and perceived barriers to knowledge translation, *J Nurses Prof Dev* 33(6):281, 2017.

Wentzel D, Brysiewicz P: Integrative review of facility interventions to manage compassion fatigue in oncology nurses, *Oncol Nurs Forum* 44(3):E124, 2017.

2

The Health Care Delivery System

OBJECTIVES

- Describe the six levels of health care.
- Discuss the factors that affect a person's access to health care.
- Explain the concept of "pay for value," used to reward hospitals financially.
- Explain the relationship between levels of health care and levels of prevention.
- Discuss the features of an integrated health care system.
- Discuss the types of settings in which professionals provide various levels of health care.
- Discuss the role of nurses in various health care settings.
- Describe the elements of discharge planning.
- Explain approaches nurses can use to improve patient satisfaction.
- Discuss the nursing implications regarding issues facing the health care system.
- Describe the effects of health disparities on the health of a community.

KEY TERMS

Acute care, p. 17
Adult day care centers, p. 22
Assisted living, p. 22
Diagnosis-related groups (DRGs), p. 23
Discharge planning, p. 18
Extended care facility, p. 20
Health care disparities, p. 27
Health care equity, p. 28
Home care, p. 20
Hospice, p. 22

Inpatient prospective payment system (IPPS), p. 23
Medicaid, p. 20
Medicare, p. 20
Minimum Data Set (MDS), p. 21
Nursing sensitive outcomes, p. 26
Palliative care, p. 22
Patient-centered care, p. 26
Patient Protection and Affordable Care Act, p. 25

Primary health care, p. 16
Rehabilitation, p. 20
Respite care, p. 22
Restorative care, p. 19
Secondary health care, p. 17
Skilled nursing facility, p. 20
Tertiary health care, p. 17

MEDIA RESOURCES

http://evolve.elsevier.com/Potter/fundamentals/
- Review Questions
- Case Study with Questions

- Audio Glossary
- Content Updates
- Answers to QSEN Activity and Review Questions

The US health care system is complex and constantly changing. Over the past decade, efforts focused on reducing the costs of health care while improving access to the health care system and ensuring high-quality outcomes. In 2014, health care expenditures in the United States totaled 17.5% of the gross domestic product, which averaged $9523 per person (Young and Kroth, 2018). A variety of services are available from different disciplines of health professionals, but gaining access to services is often very difficult for those with limited health care insurance. The US Census Bureau reports that 28.1 million people remain uninsured (Himmelstein et al., 2018). There are millions more who have health insurance but do not seek preventive or needed health care because of the high cost of shared expenses (Himmelstein et al., 2018). Patients who are uninsured present a challenge to health care and nursing because they are more likely to skip or delay treatment for acute and chronic illnesses and die prematurely (Young and Kroth, 2018).

You will better succeed in your career if you understand the functioning of the health care system and the roles nurses play. Nursing is a caring discipline. The profession's values are rooted in helping people to regain, maintain, or improve their health; prevent illness; and find comfort and dignity at a time of death.

The practice of nursing is changing. The American Nurses Association (ANA) states: "Nursing promotes the delivery of holistic consumer-centered care and optimal health outcomes throughout the life span and across the health-illness continuum within an environmental context that encompasses culture, ethics, law, politics, economics, access to health care resources and competing priorities" (ANA, 2015). It is critical for nurses to be prepared to face the challenges in the health care system today and to work toward improving access and maintaining quality and safety, while working to lessen health care costs that create a barrier to optimal wellness.

TRADITIONAL LEVEL OF HEALTH CARE

The US health care system has six levels of care for which health care providers offer services: preventive, primary, secondary, tertiary, restorative, and continuing health care. Levels of care describe the scope of services and settings delivered by health care providers to patients in all stages of health and illness. It is important for the nurse to understand how the health care industry organizes and delivers services within these levels of care. Box 2.1 provides examples of the types of services available to patients and families at each level of care.

Each level of care presents different requirements and opportunities for a nurse. For example, in your role within a primary care setting, you will be involved in patient assessment. You will be expected to identify changes in chronic conditions or the development of new acute conditions. You will teach new mothers how to care for their babies or young adults how to use an inhaler. In a continuing care setting, you will apply gerontology nursing principles to help patients adapt to permanent health changes so that they can remain active and engaged.

Levels of care are not the same as levels of prevention (see Chapter 6). Levels of prevention describe the focus of health-related activities in a care setting. These include health promotion and disease prevention (primary prevention), curing of disease (secondary prevention), and reducing complications (tertiary prevention). For example, in a tertiary level of care, such as an intensive care unit, a nurse practices primary prevention by preventing pneumonia through repositioning a patient frequently, secondary prevention by administering antibiotics on time to treat the pneumonia, and tertiary prevention by assessing the patient frequently for signs of antibiotic intolerance.

At every level of care, nurses and other health care providers offer a variety of prevention services. For example, a nurse working in a specialized acute care (secondary/tertiary) hospital setting monitors the recovery of a patient following open heart surgery while also providing health promotion information to the family caregiver concerning diet and exercise.

Health care reform has led to changes unique to each level of care. For example, the health care industry now places greater emphasis on wellness. Thus, the industry directs more resources toward primary and preventive care. Wellness care focuses on the health of populations and their communities rather than simply curing an individual's disease. In wellness care, nurses can help lead communities and health care systems in coordinating resources to better serve their populations. Finding strategies to better address patient needs at all levels of care is critical to improving the functioning of the health care delivery system.

INTEGRATED HEALTH CARE DELIVERY

Integrated health care delivery (IHCD) came about as part of the US health care reform movement in response to the fragmented, costly, and varying quality of health care found in the United States at the time. An integrated health care delivery system is "a network of organizations that provides or arranges to provide a coordinated continuum of services to a defined population and is willing to be held clinically and fiscally accountable for the outcomes and health status of the population served" (Hwang et al., 2013, p.2). IHCDs were developed with a primary focus on improving health care quality and decreasing overall health care costs. The goal of focusing on population health is to decrease health care cost through effective management of patients with chronic health problems. An example of an IHCD is the Accountable Care Organizations that developed in response to health care reform.

There is no single model for an integrated health care system. Basically, two types of integrated health care systems are found: an organizational structure that follows economic imperatives (such as combining financing with all providers, from hospitals, clinics, and physicians to home care and long-term care facilities) and a structure that supports an organized care delivery approach (coordinating care activities and services into seamless functioning) (Hwang et al., 2013).

The Patient-Centered Medical Home model is an example of an integrated health care system. The Patient-Centered Medical Home strengthens the physician-patient relationship with coordinated, goal-oriented, individualized care. In this approach, a patient's primary health care provider is the coordinator/manager who enlists the skills and knowledge of health care professionals from various services. These professionals can include nurses, medical assistants, nutritionists, social workers, pharmacists, hospice care providers, and other caregivers. Members of a Patient-Centered Medical Home care team are linked by information technology, electronic health records and system-best practices to ensure that patients receive care when and where they need it and how they want it. Patient-centeredness is a unifying principle. It describes an ongoing, active partnership with a personal primary care physician or nurse practitioner who leads a team of professionals dedicated to providing proactive, preventive, and chronic care management through all stages of a patient's life (American Academy Family Physicians, 2018).

BOX 2.1 Examples of Health Care Services

Preventive Care
- Adult screenings for blood pressure, cholesterol, tobacco use, and cancer
- Pediatric screenings for hearing, vision, autism, and developmental disorders
- HIV screening for adults at higher risk
- Wellness visits
- Immunizations
- Diet counseling
- Mental health counseling and crisis prevention
- Community legislation (seat belts, car seats for children, bike helmets)

Primary Care (Health Promotion)
- Diagnosis and treatment of common illnesses
- Ongoing management of chronic health problems
- Prenatal care
- Well-baby care
- Family planning
- Patient-centered medical home

Secondary (Acute Care)
- Urgent care; hospital emergency care
- Acute medical-surgical care: ambulatory care, outpatient surgery, hospital
- Radiological procedures

Tertiary Care
- Highly specialized: intensive care, inpatient psychiatric facilities
- Specialty care (such as neurology, cardiology, rheumatology, dermatology, oncology)

Restorative Care
- Rehabilitation programs (such as cardiovascular, pulmonary, orthopedic)
- Sports medicine
- Spinal cord injury programs
- Home care

Continuing Care
- Long-term care: assisted living, nursing centers
- Psychiatric and older-adult day care

Primary and Preventive Health Care Services

Primary health care focuses on improved health outcomes for an entire population. It includes primary care and health education, proper nutrition, maternal/child health care, family planning, immunizations, and control of diseases. The World Health Organization (2018b) holds that 80% to 90% of a person's health care needs in their lifetime can be met with primary care services. Primary health care requires collaboration among health professionals, health care leaders, and community members. In settings in which patients receive preventive and primary care, such as schools, physicians' offices, occupational health clinics, community health centers, and nursing centers, health promotion is a major theme (Table 2.1). Health promotion programs are designed

TABLE 2.1	**Preventive and Primary Care Services**	
Type of Service	**Purpose**	**Available Programs/Services**
School health	Comprehensive programs integrate health promotion principles into a school curriculum. Services emphasize program management, interprofessional collaboration, and community health principles. Research shows a link between the health outcomes of young people and their academic success (CDC, 2015b).	Health education Physical education and physical activity Nutrition environment and services Health services Physical environment Social and emotional climate Counseling, psychological services, and social services Employee wellness Family engagement Community involvement
Occupational health	The workplace is an important setting for delivering comprehensive health-protection, health-promotion and disease/accident-prevention programs. Americans working full time spend an average of more than one-third of their day, 5 days a week at the workplace (CDC, 2015a). The goal is to increase worker productivity, reduce absenteeism, reduce health risks, and reduce the use of expensive medical care.	Environmental surveillance Create company policies that promote healthy behaviors such as a tobacco-free campus policy Work environment: offer healthy foods through vending machines or cafeterias Physical assessment and health screening Health education classes Communicable disease control Counseling
Physicians' offices	Provide primary health care and diagnose and treat acute and chronic illnesses. Practitioners are beginning to focus more on health-promotion practices. Advanced nurse practitioners often partner with a physician in managing a patient population.	Routine physical examination Health screening and risk appraisal Diagnostics Disease management Prevention services: diabetes and osteoporosis screenings, smoking cessation programs, and immunizations Wellness counseling
Nurse-managed clinics	Nurse-managed clinics or centers deliver nursing services with a focus on health promotion and health education, chronic disease assessment and management, and support for self-care and caregivers. Clinics often are associated with a school, college, department of nursing, federally qualified health center, or independent nonprofit health care agency.	Day care Clinical education site for other health care providers in school Prevention services: diabetes screenings, smoking cessation programs, and immunizations Physical exams, cardiovascular checks Health risk appraisal Wellness counseling Employment readiness Acute and chronic care management
Block and parish nursing	Nurses deliver health care services to patients (e.g., older adults or those unable to leave their homes) within their own religious communities. Provides services that are unavailable in traditional health care system.	Running errands/transportation Respite care Counseling Spiritual health: balancing body and mind health to achieve overall wellness
Community centers	Provide comprehensive and cost-effective primary care and supportive services that promote access to health care. Often deliver services to a specific patient population (such as well-baby, mental health, diabetes patients) within underserved communities. Sometimes affiliated with a hospital, medical school, church, or other community organization. The care offered by community centers is culturally appropriate and delivered in languages that many in these communities speak (Center for American Progress, 2018).	Physical assessment and health screening Nutrition education Translation services Dental care Mental health services Care coordination and case management Specialty care (such as orthopedic, cardiac, or podiatric care) Disease management Health education

to lower the overall costs of health care by reducing the incidence of disease, minimizing complications, and thus reducing the need to use more expensive health care resources. In contrast, preventive care is more disease oriented and focused on reducing and controlling risk factors for disease through activities such as immunization and occupational health programs. Chapter 3 provides a more comprehensive discussion of primary health care in the community.

Secondary and Tertiary Care

The traditional reason people use health care services (such as a hospital) is to diagnose and treat illness. When the nature or severity of a condition makes primary care insufficient, secondary and tertiary care may become necessary. The difference between secondary and tertiary care arises from the complexity of a patient's medical needs. Secondary health care is provided by a specialist or agency upon referral by a primary health care provider. It requires more specialized knowledge, skill, or equipment than the primary care physician or nurse practitioner can provide. For example, an individual sees a cardiologist because of increasing shortness of breath with activity.

Tertiary health care is specialized consultative care, usually provided on referral from secondary medical personnel. For example, the cardiac surgeon sees the patient referred from the cardiologist for possible cardiac bypass surgery. However, changes in medical cost reimbursement, improved technology, and less invasive treatments have often made secondary and tertiary care available at the primary care level. For example, more surgeons are performing simple surgeries in outpatient surgical centers or office suites. However, if a patient develops a problem that the surgeon or primary health care provider is not able to treat and/or if intensive nursing care is needed, the patient needs a medical specialist, often resulting in hospitalization. Secondary and tertiary care (also called acute care) typically are expensive, especially if the patient has waited to seek care until after symptoms have developed. Delays in treating or diagnosing chronic illness may cause disability, decreased quality of life, and increased health care costs (Young and Kroth, 2018).

Hospitals. Hospitals provide comprehensive secondary and tertiary health care to patients who are acutely ill. During 2016, over 35 million patients were admitted to American Hospital Association–registered hospitals (AHA, 2018). Even allowing for the fact that some patients are admitted multiple times during a year, a large percentage of the US population receives health care in a hospital each year.

Hospitals vary in the services they offer. Most small rural hospitals offer general inpatient services but have limited emergency and diagnostic services. The exception is critical access hospitals. In comparison, large urban medical centers offer comprehensive, state-of-the-art diagnostic services, trauma and emergency care, surgical intervention, intensive care units (ICUs), inpatient services, and rehabilitation centers. Larger hospitals hire professional staff from a variety of specialties, such as nursing, social service, respiratory therapy, physical and occupational therapy, and speech therapy. Most patients who require these services are having acute episodes of illness. As a nurse, you need to be able to think critically and identify patients' changing problems quickly and accurately. This is challenging when you are assigned multiple patients at one time, depending on your unit. You must be able to deliver an array of nursing interventions safely and effectively and recognize when the needs of your patients no longer match the level of health care where they are receiving treatment. You also must be able to plan and coordinate care with other health care providers quickly and competently.

Hospitals use evidence-based practice guidelines and clinical protocols (see Chapter 5) in the delivery of care to patients. As a nurse,

you need to keep current on evidence-based practices to ensure safe, effective care. As a part of the nursing process, the nurse is expected to continually evaluate patient outcomes.

According to the American Hospital Association (2017), delivering the right care, at the right time, in the right setting is the core mission of hospitals across the country. To fulfill this mission, hospitals fully support quality and safety initiatives. An example of a quality initiative is patient satisfaction. Patient satisfaction is challenging to achieve in a stressful setting, such as an inpatient nursing unit. Patients expect to be treated courteously and respectfully. Patients want to be involved in daily care decisions. Hospitals are adopting models of patient-centered care that focus on care that is responsive to individual patient and family preferences, needs, and values and ensuring that patient values guide clinical decisions (IOM, 2001). In a patient-centered care model nurses engage patients and families early in the decision-making process. As a nurse, you have a key role in learning patient needs and expectations early to form effective therapeutic partnerships. By treating the nurse-patient relationship with respect and dignity, nursing care delivery is improved, which enhances patient satisfaction.

Intensive Care. An ICU or critical care unit is a hospital unit in which patients receive close monitoring and intensive medical care. The status of a patient who is critically ill can change by the minute, so health care providers must have specialized knowledge and skills. ICUs have advanced technologies such as computerized cardiac monitors and high-tech mechanical ventilators. Although many of these devices are on regular nursing units, patients hospitalized within ICUs are monitored and maintained on multiple devices. An ICU is the most expensive health care delivery site because each nurse usually cares for only one or two patients at a time and because of all the treatments and procedures the patients in the ICU require.

Mental Health Facilities. According to the National Alliance on Mental Illness (NAMI) (2018) about 1 in 5 adults in the United States—43.8 million, or 18.5%—experience mental illness in a given year. Perhaps more concerning is the report that only 41% of adults in the United States with a mental health condition received mental health services in the past year (NAMI, 2018). Patients who have emotional and behavioral problems such as depression, mood disorders, violent behavior, and eating disorders require special counseling and treatment in psychiatric facilities. The massive cuts to non-Medicaid state mental health spending in 2011, totaling more than $1.8 billion, resulted in states having to cut vital mental health services for tens of thousands of youth and adults living with the most serious mental illnesses. These services include community- and hospital-based psychiatric care, housing, and access to medications (NAMI, 2011). This reduction of mental health agencies and services continues to have consequences today, such as loss of income due to missed work, high suicide rates, and high education dropout rates (NAMI, 2018). Individuals with serious mental illness are more likely to suffer chronic disease and as a result die on average 25 years earlier than others, largely due to treatable medical conditions (NAMI, 2018).

The psychiatric facilities that do exist are located in hospitals, independent outpatient clinics, and private mental health hospitals. They offer inpatient and outpatient services, depending on the severity of a patient's problem. Patients enter mental health facilities voluntarily or involuntarily. Patients who are hospitalized usually have short stays intended to stabilize them before transfer to outpatient treatment centers. Patients with mental illness receive a comprehensive interprofessional treatment plan that engages patients and their families. Medical, nursing, social work, and activity therapy providers collaborate to develop a plan of care that enables patients to become more functional within their communities. Patients usually receive referrals for follow-up care at clinics or with counselors during discharge from inpatient settings.

Rural Hospitals. Lack of access to health care in rural areas is a serious public health problem. Only about 10% of physicians practice in rural America, while nearly one-fourth of the US population lives in these areas (NRHA, 2018). Rural Americans face a unique combination of factors that create health care disparities that are not found in urban areas, including (1) economic factors (rural Americans are more likely to live below the poverty level), (2) cultural and social differences, (3) lower levels of education, (4) lack of attention to rural problems by legislators, and (5) isolation of living in remote rural areas (NRHA, 2018).

Many rural hospitals have failed economically and closed. To address this problem, the Balanced Budget Act of 1997 changed the designation of some rural hospitals to Critical Access Hospital (CAH) when certain criteria were met (CMS MLN, 2017). A CAH is located in a rural area (35 miles from another hospital) and provides 24-hour emergency care with no more than 25 inpatient beds for temporary care for 96 hours or less to patients needing stabilization before transfer to a larger hospital. Physicians, advanced practice nurses, or physician assistants staff a CAH. The CAH provides inpatient care to acutely ill or injured people before they are transferred to better-equipped health care centers. Basic radiological and laboratory services are also available. To improve care for patients residing in rural areas, rural hospitals are expected to (HealthIT.gov, 2017):

- Improve access to services, including urgent care services, and to meet unmet health needs in isolated rural communities.
- Engage rural communities in developing rural health care systems.
- Develop collaborative delivery systems in rural communities as the hubs of rural health care.
- Create protocols for coordinating care transition by aligning urban health care systems.
- Be the subject matter experts and coordinators for the health care environment of providers, patients, and staff.

Health care reform has enabled urban health care systems to branch out and establish affiliations or mergers with rural hospitals. Rural hospitals and CAH provide a referral base to the larger tertiary care medical centers. Nurses who work in rural hospitals or clinics often function independently without a physician. These nurses must be competent in physical assessment, clinical decision making, and emergency care. Advanced practice nurses (such as nurse practitioners and clinical nurse specialists) use medical protocols and establish collaborative agreements with staff physicians.

Health care payers, such as CMS and private insurers, expect patients who are hospitalized to be treated and discharged within a reasonably predictable time period. Reimbursements are affected by the quality and timeliness of care. Nurses must use resources efficiently and effectively to help patients recover and return home. For example, you may collaborate with members of the interprofessional health care team, such as case managers, advanced practice providers such as nurse practitioners, physical therapists, physicians, and social workers, to plan a quick yet realistic transition to another level of health care. This process is known as *discharge planning.*

Discharge Planning. Discharge planning is a coordinated, interprofessional process that develops a plan for continuing care after a patient leaves a health care agency. Studies have shown that patients tend to be discharged "quicker and sicker" from hospitals. This can result in adverse events during the immediate post-discharge period (Mabire et al., 2013). Such problems include medication prescribing errors, poor communication between hospital and primary care providers, and lack of coordination with community health care services. The focus of discharge planning is to ensure that a patient transitions to the setting in which his or her health care needs can be appropriately met.

According to the Department of Health and Human Services and Centers for Medicare and Medicaid Services (DHHS-CMS) (2017), patients within acute care hospitals have an average length of stay (LOS) of only 2 to 3 days. Thus, *discharge planning with coordination of services must begin the moment a patient is admitted to a hospital.* As a nurse you will play a large role in discharge planning by knowing a patient's plan of care (developed by the interprofessional team) as soon as possible, informing the patient and family of that plan, encouraging their participation, acting on the plan, and evaluating progress (Fig. 2.1). Discharge planning involves these elements (DHHS-CMS, 2017):

- Determining the appropriate post-hospital destination for a patient. A case manager or social worker usually selects this setting based on a patient's health care needs, self-care capacity, insurance, and place of residence.
- Identifying a patient's needs for a smooth and safe transition from the acute care hospital/post–acute care agency to his or her discharge destination. Nurses, therapists (physical, occupational, speech), health care providers, and dietitians usually identify these needs.
- Beginning the process of meeting a patient's needs while the patient is still hospitalized, with approaches such as early mobility protocols, health education, and new medication regimens.

With a well-developed discharge plan, a patient is less likely to have unavoidable complications or unrelated illnesses or injuries and will be able to continue progressing toward the goals of his or her plan of care after discharge (DHHS-CMS, 2017). As a nurse, participate in discharge planning by anticipating and identifying each patient's continuing needs before the actual time of discharge and coordinating efforts to achieve an appropriate discharge plan.

The DHHS-CMS does not require discharge planning for outpatients, including those who present to an emergency department and are not admitted as hospital inpatients. At the same time, hospitals

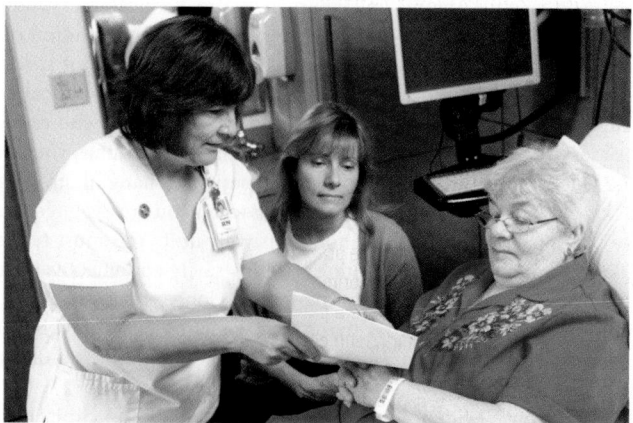

FIG. 2.1 Providing discharge teaching to decrease hospital readmission.

may help some outpatients (such as emergency department or same-day surgery patients) by providing some discharge planning services (DHHS-CMS, 2017). A nurse-driven discharge planning model that includes discharge teaching and follow-up after discharge can help reduce hospital readmission rates (Dizon and Reinking, 2017). Box 2.2 describes models of discharge planning that focus on the patient and his or her family caregiver.

Some patients are more in need of discharge planning because of their health-related risks. For example, some patients have poor health literacy, limited financial resources, or limited family support; others have long-term disabilities or chronic illness, and older adults sometimes have cognitive and/or hearing impairments affecting their attention to discharge instruction. There are also barriers to effective discharge planning, including ineffective communication (health care provider to provider; health care provider to patient), lack of role clarity among health care team members (responsibility and follow-up), and lack of resources (e.g., rehab and nursing home beds) (Okoniewska et al., 2015). You can reduce barriers to discharge planning by clearly communicating about the plan of care with patients, families, and members of the health care team. Change of shift hand-offs and hourly bedside rounds are ways to keep all health care providers and patients informed (Chapter 24). Communicate clearly both verbally and in the entries you make in the electronic health record (EHR) (see Chapter 26). Clarify any role confusion to be sure elements of the plan are completed.

Discharge instructions prepare patients for transition from a hospital to the next level of care (such as home, rehabilitation, or long-term care). Nurses can offer useful and relevant information that will prepare patients and their family caregivers for post-discharge care. To develop discharge instructions, you must understand the proper timing for discharge, engage the patient and family caregiver in the process, and know the health care team's plan of care. Patients cannot learn when they are having pain, nausea, confusion, or other disabling symptoms. Family caregivers can be excellent resources when the patient desires their help. Always involve patients and family caregivers in the decisions about the patient's discharge destination (Mabire et al., 2013).

Provide discharge instruction as early as possible so that you and other health care team members can reinforce the information several times to improve learning. For example, when a patient is receiving care that follows a standard protocol, you can easily anticipate the treatment and the patient's estimated discharge date. When the patient has multiple complications, the plan of care and estimated discharge date might not be clear. Begin to explain discharge instruction as soon as you know the plan of care. The following are required discharge instruction topics (The Joint Commission [TJC], 2016): discharge medications, follow-up care (if needed), list of all medications changed and/or discontinued, dietary needs, and follow-up tests or procedures.

Some patients assume passive roles when they receive instructions. They might be satisfied when a nurse, physician, or therapist rushes through an explanation and finishes by simply inquiring, "Any questions?" This often leads the patient to automatically answer "no." This patient might never have been invited to actively participate in their health care plan. A patient-centered approach does more. The health care provider *invites* the patient to participate: "I want to make sure that I've helped you understand everything you need to know about your illness. Patients usually have questions because their situations can be complicated. Could you tell me what you understand, and then I can help clarify?" The teach-back approach (see Chapter 25) is an excellent way to ensure that a patient understands instructions. Comprehensive discharge instruction ensures that patients know what to do when they get home, how to perform care activities, and what to do when problems develop.

Discharge planning often leads to referrals to other health care providers, especially when specific therapies are planned (such as physical therapy) (see Chapter 18). Some tips for making a successful referral include the following:

- Engage the patient and family caregiver in the referral process, including selecting the care provider. Explain the reason for the referral, the service to be provided, and how the service will be provided.
- Make the referral as soon as possible.
- Give the care provider receiving the referral as much information as possible about the patient. This can avoid unnecessary duplication of assessment (e.g., current vital signs or pain status) and omission of important information.
- The care provider, such as a physical therapist, social worker, dietitian, or radiologist, will make recommendations for the patient's care. Learn these recommendations and incorporate them into the treatment plan as soon as possible.

Restorative Care

Patients recovering from an acute or chronic illness or disability often require additional services to return to their previous level of function or to reach a new level of function limited by their illness or disability. The goals of restorative care are to help individuals regain maximal functional status and to enhance quality of life through promotion of independence and self-care. With the emphasis on early discharge from hospitals, patients usually require some level of restorative care. For example, some patients require ongoing wound care and activity and exercise management until they have recovered enough following surgery to independently resume normal activities of daily living.

BOX 2.2   Discharge Planning Models

Coleman's "Care Transitions Program" (Coleman et al., 2006)

Emphasizes the role of a transition coach in managing/facilitating the discharge of a patient to home or to a rehabilitation center. Model is based on four pillars: (1) medication self-management, (2) patient-centered record, (3) follow-up, and (4) indicators of worsening medical condition. Each pillar has different interventions depending on the stage of the hospitalization.

Naylor's "Transitional Care Model" (Naylor et al., 2009)

Emphasizes comprehensive discharge planning and follow-up for older adults who are chronically ill. Model contains six key components: (1) in-hospital assessment and development of the discharge care plan by a transitional care nurse/advanced practice nurse/gerontological nurse; (2) discharge preparation by an interprofessional care team; (3) patient participation (communication between nursing staff and the patient) regarding the process, the decision making, the discharge planning, and the discharge education; (4) continuity of care and communication among health care providers; (5) predischarge assessment; and (6) postdischarge follow-up.

High-intensity Care Team (GRACE Team Care Model, Indiana University)

The team is headed by *both* a nurse practitioner and a social worker. This team works in tandem to support the primary care physician and, following best practice protocols, to fully address a patient's health conditions. The focus is to help patients manage their health conditions, coordinate their health care, and achieve optimal health (Michigan Care Management Resource Center, 2018). This achieves a patient's goal from the convenience and security of his or her own home (Counsell, 2015).

The intensity of care has increased in restorative care settings because patients leave hospitals earlier. Patients in a home or rehabilitation setting often still receive IV fluids (see Chapter 42), aggressive pain control (see Chapter 44), or enteral nutrition (see Chapter 45). The restorative health care team is interprofessional and includes the patient and family or significant others. In restorative settings nurses recognize that success depends on effective and early collaboration with patients and their families. Patients and families require a clear understanding of goals for physical recovery, the rationale for any physical limitations, and the purpose and potential risks associated with therapies. Patients and families are more likely to follow treatment plans and achieve optimal functioning when they are engaged in their care.

Home Care. Home care is the provision of medically related professional and paraprofessional services and equipment to patients and families in their homes for health maintenance, education, illness prevention, diagnosis and treatment of disease, palliation, and rehabilitation. This care consists of part-time, medically necessary skilled care (nursing, physical therapy, occupational therapy, and speech-language therapy) that is prescribed by a health care provider (CMS, 2016a). A home care service also coordinates the access to and delivery of home health equipment, or durable medical equipment, which is a medical product adapted for home use.

Home care nurses have their own patient caseloads and deliver highly individualized nursing care. They help patients adapt to many permanent or temporary physical limitations so that the patients can assume a daily home routine that is as normal as possible. Home care requires a strong knowledge base in many areas, such as family dynamics (see Chapter 10), cultural competency (see Chapter 9), spiritual values (see Chapter 35), and communication principles (see Chapter 24). Home health nurses must also have expertise in assessment. Nurses who work in Medicare-certified home care agencies conduct patient-specific comprehensive assessments at a patient's start of care, at 60-day follow-ups, at discharge, and before and after an inpatient stay (Research Data Assistance Center [ResDac], 2016). This comprehensive assessment, OASIS (the Outcome and Assessment Information Set), includes a group of standardized core assessment items for an adult home care patient. OASIS forms the basis for measuring patient outcomes for the purposes of outcome-based quality. Data items within OASIS include socio-demographic, environmental, support system, health status, functional status, and health service utilization characteristics of a patient (ResDac, 2016). The OASIS assessment tool was designed to gather the data items needed to measure both outcomes and patient risk factors in the home setting.

Home health care focuses on the goal of helping patients and their family members achieve independence. Home care addresses recovery from and stabilization of illness in the home. In addition, home care identifies problems related to lifestyle, safety, environment, family dynamics, and health care practices in the home. Home care agencies employ skilled and intermittent professional services, such as wound care, administering parenteral and enteral nutrition, administering medications and blood therapy, and home care aide services. These services usually are delivered once or twice a day as often as 7 days a week.

Approved home care agencies usually receive reimbursement for services from governmental programs (such as Medicare and Medicaid in the United States), private insurance, and private payers. The government strictly regulates reimbursement for home care services. An agency cannot simply charge whatever it wants for a service and expect to receive that amount. Governmental programs set the amount of reimbursement for most professional services.

Rehabilitation. The World Health Organization (WHO) defines rehabilitation as the process aimed at enabling people with disabilities to reach and maintain their optimal physical, sensory, intellectual, psychological, and social functional levels. Rehabilitation gives people with disabilities the tools they need to attain independence and self-determination (WHO, 2018a). Patients require rehabilitation after a physical or mental illness, injury, or chemical addiction. Rehabilitation was once offered mostly to patients with illnesses or injury to the nervous or musculoskeletal system, but the expanded scope of services now includes cardiovascular, neurological, musculoskeletal, pulmonary, and mental health rehabilitation programs. The goal of these specialized rehabilitation services is to help patients and families adjust to necessary changes in lifestyle and learn to function with the limitations of their disease. An example is drug rehabilitation centers that help patients become free from drug dependence and return to the community.

Rehabilitation services after acute care include physical, occupational, and speech therapy and social services. Ideally rehabilitation begins the moment a patient enters a health care setting for treatment. For example, some orthopedic programs now have patients perform physical therapy exercises before major joint repair to enhance their recovery after surgery. Initially rehabilitation usually focuses on preventing complications related to an illness or injury, such as promoting early mobility in patients after surgery. As the patient stabilizes, it helps to maximize a patient's functioning and level of independence, often by examining the need for assist devices such as walkers or canes.

Rehabilitation settings include rehabilitation institutions within acute care centers, free-standing outpatient settings, and the home. Patients who have severe disabilities may not be able to carry out the activities of daily living independently. An example would be a patient who has had a stroke or spinal cord injury. These patients may benefit from long-term rehabilitation to reach their maximum potential.

Patients who use rehabilitation services in an outpatient setting receive treatment at appointments during the week but live in their home. Sometimes, specific rehabilitation services are also used in the home to help the patient.

Extended Care Facilities. An extended care facility provides intermediate medical, nursing, or custodial care for patients recovering from acute illness or those with chronic illnesses or disabilities. Extended care facilities include intermediate care and skilled nursing facilities. Some include long-term care and assisted-living facilities. At one point extended care facilities primarily cared for older adults. However, because hospitals discharge their patients sooner, there is a greater need for intermediate care settings for patients of all ages. For example, health care providers transfer a young patient who has experienced a traumatic brain injury resulting from a car accident to an extended care facility for rehabilitative or supportive care until discharge to the home becomes a safe option.

An intermediate care or skilled nursing facility offers skilled care from a licensed nursing staff. This often includes administration of IV fluids, wound care, long-term ventilator management, and physical rehabilitation. Patients receive extensive supportive care until they are able to move back into the community or into residential care. Extended care facilities provide around-the-clock nursing coverage. Nurses who work in a skilled nursing facility need nursing expertise similar to that of nurses working in acute care inpatient settings, along with a background in gerontological nursing principles (see Chapter 14).

Continuing Care

Continuing care describes a variety of health, personal, and social services provided over a prolonged period. These services are for people who are disabled, who were never functionally independent, or who suffer a terminal disease. The need for continuing health care services is growing in the United States. People are living longer, and many of those with continuing health care needs have no immediate family members to care for them. A decline in the number of children families choose to have, the aging of care providers, and the increasing rates of divorce and remarriage complicate this problem.

Continuing care is available within institutional settings (e.g., nursing centers or nursing homes, group homes, and retirement communities), communities (e.g., adult day care and senior centers), or the home (e.g., home care, home-delivered meals, and hospice) (Meiner and Yeager, 2019). Another alternative for the patient who does not need nursing care but needs some assistance to stay independent is elder care services. These services offer companionship, assistance with activities of daily living, and food preparation.

Nursing Centers or Facilities. The language of long-term care is confusing and constantly changing. *Nursing home* was the dominant setting for long-term care (Meiner and Yeager, 2019). With the 1987 Omnibus Budget Reconciliation Act, *nursing facility* became the term for nursing homes and other facilities that provided long-term care. Now *nursing center* is the most appropriate term. A nursing center typically provides 24-hour intermediate and custodial care such as nursing, rehabilitation, dietary, recreational, social, and religious services for residents of any age with chronic or debilitating illnesses. Nursing center services provided by Medicaid-certified nursing homes, offer:

- Skilled nursing
- Rehabilitation
- Long-term care (Medicaid.gov, 2018).

These three services include 24-hour licensed nursing, rehabilitation, medically related social services, pharmaceutical services, dietary services individualized to the needs of each resident, a professionally directed program of activities to meet the interests and needs for the well-being of each resident, emergency dental services, room and bed maintenance services, and routine personal hygiene items and services. A skilled nursing facility must care for its residents in a manner and in an environment that will promote maintenance or enhancement of the quality of life of each resident (Legal Information Institute, 2010).

Most people living in nursing centers are older adults. A nursing center may be a resident's temporary or permanent home with surroundings made as homelike as possible. Residents receive a planned, systematic, and interprofessional approach to care to help them reach and maintain their highest level of function.

Nursing centers must comply with the Omnibus Budget Reconciliation Act of 1987 and its minimum requirements for nursing facilities to receive payment from Medicare and Medicaid. Government regulations require that staff members in nursing centers comprehensively assess each resident and that care planning decisions be made within a prescribed period. A resident's functional ability (such as the ability to perform activities of daily living and instrumental activities of daily living) and long-term physical and psychosocial well-being are the focus.

A nursing facility must complete the Resident Assessment Instrument (RAI) for each resident. The RAI helps nursing facility staff gather definitive information on a resident's strengths and needs, which must then be addressed in an individualized care plan (**CMS, 2015b**). The RAI has three components: the Minimum Data Set (MDS) Version 3.0, the Care Area Assessment (CAA) process, and the RAI Utilization Guidelines (Box 2.3). The components of the RAI yield information about a resident's functional status, strengths, weaknesses, and preferences, as well as offering guidance on further assessment once problems have been identified (CMS, 2015b). The MDS Version

3.0 is an initial overview of a resident's health care needs. It is a preliminary assessment to identify the resident's potential problems, strengths, and preferences. The CAAs are triggered by individual MDS item responses that reveal the need for additional assessment. These item responses identify problems, known as "triggered care areas," which form a critical link between the MDS and decisions about care planning. CAAs enable facilities to identify and use tools that are grounded in current clinical standards of practice, such as evidence-based or expert-endorsed research, clinical practice guidelines, and resources.

The information gathered using the RAI provides a national database for nursing facilities that enables policy makers to better understand the health care needs of the long-term-care population. The MDS and CAAs are a rich resource for nurses in selecting interventions that best meet the health care needs of this growing population.

BOX 2.3 Components of the Resident Assessment Instrument (RAI)

Minimum Data Set (MDS)

A core set of screening, clinical, and functional status elements, including common definitions and coding categories, which forms the foundation of a comprehensive assessment for all residents of nursing homes that are Medicare- or Medicaid-certified. Elements include:

- Resident's background
- Cognitive, communication/hearing, and vision patterns
- Physical functioning and structural problems
- Mood, behavior, and activity pursuit patterns
- Psychosocial well-being
- Bowel and bladder continence
- Disease diagnoses and other health conditions
- Mood and behavior patterns
- Activity pursuit patterns
- Oral/nutritional and dental status
- Skin condition
- Medication use
- Treatments and procedures

Care Area Assessment (CAA) Process

This process is designed to assist the assessor to systematically interpret the information recorded on the MDS. Once a care area has been triggered, nursing home providers use current, evidence-based clinical resources to conduct an assessment of the potential problem and determine a plan of care for it. The CAA process helps the clinician to focus on key issues.

- Care Area Triggers (CATs) are specific resident responses for one or a combination of MDS elements. The triggers identify residents who have or are at risk for developing specific functional problems and require further assessment.
- Care Area Assessment is the further investigation of triggered areas, to determine if the care area triggers require interventions and care planning.
- CAA Summary provides a location for documentation of the care area(s) that have triggered from the MDS and the decisions made during the CAA process regarding whether to proceed to care planning.

Utilization Guidelines

The Utilization Guidelines provide instructions for when and how to use the RAI.

Adapted from Centers for Medicare and Medicaid Services (CMS): Long-Term Care Facility Resident Assessment Instrument 3.0 User's Manual Version 1.13, 2015b. https://www.cms.gov/Medicare/Quality-Initiatives-Patient-Assessment-Instruments/NursingHomeQualityInits/Downloads/MDS-30-RAI-Manual-V113.pdf. Accessed August 2018.

Assisted Living. Assisted living is one of the fastest-growing industries within the United States. There are approximately 30,000 assisted-living facilities that house more than 835,000 people in the United States (NCAL, 2018). Assisted living offers an attractive long-term care setting with an environment more like home and greater resident autonomy. Residents require some assistance with activities of daily living but remain relatively independent within a partially protective setting. A group of residents live together, but each resident has his or her own room and shares dining and social activity areas. Usually people keep all of their personal possessions in their residences.

Assisted-living residences range from hotel-like buildings with hundreds of units to modest group homes that house a handful of seniors. Assisted living provides independence, security, and privacy all at the same time (Touhy and Jett, 2018). These settings promote physical and psychosocial health (Fig. 2.2). Services in an assisted-living center include laundry, assistance with meals and personal care, 24-hour oversight, and housekeeping (NCAL, 2018). Some centers provide assistance with medication administration. Nursing care services are not always directly available, although home care nurses can visit patients in assisted-living residences. Unfortunately, most residents of assisted-living residences pay privately. The national median monthly fee is $3750 for a private unit (NCAL, 2018). With no government fee caps and little regulation, assisted living is not always an option for individuals with limited financial resources.

Respite Care. Caring for family members within the home creates great physical and emotional burdens for adult caregivers. This is especially true when the family member who needs assistance is physically or cognitively limited. The caregiver is usually an adult who not only has the responsibility for providing care to a loved one (such as a spouse, parent, or sibling) but often maintains a full-time job, raises a family, and manages the routines of daily living as well.

Respite care is a service that offers short-term relief by providing a new environment or time to relax for family caregivers who support the ill, disabled, or frail older adult (Alzheimer's Association, 2016). Recommend respite services to the family caregivers of your patient whenever indicated. Respite care can be provided at home by a friend,

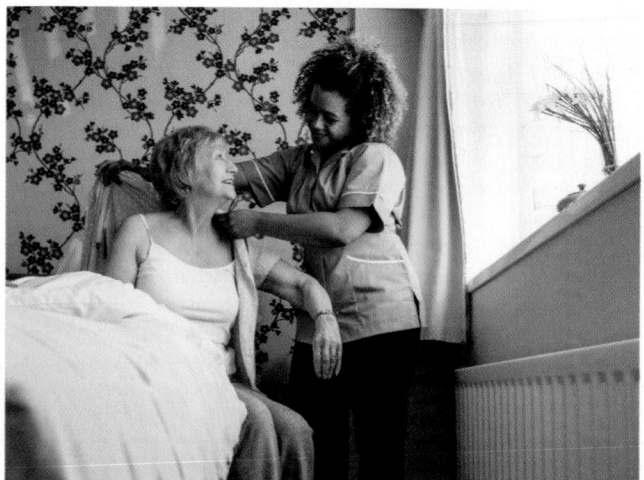

FIG. 2.2 Providing nursing services in assisted-living facilities promotes physical and psychosocial health. (Copyright © DGLimages/iStock/Thinkstock.)

another family member, a volunteer, by a paid service, or in a care setting such as adult day care or a residential center (Alzheimer's Association, 2016). Research has shown that family caregivers must have great trust in the respite care service and that they perceive that the major benefits for the recipients of care are social interaction and meaningful activity, with a resulting improvement in well-being (Stirling, 2014).

Adult Day Care Centers. Adult day care centers provide a variety of health and social services to specific patient populations who live alone or with family in the community. Services offered during the day allow family members to maintain their lifestyles and employment and still provide home care for their relatives (Meiner and Yeager, 2019). Day care centers are associated with a hospital or nursing home or exist as independent centers. Frequently the patients need continuous health care services but not hospitalization (e.g., physical therapy, meals, recreational activities, or counseling) while their families or support people work. Patients who typically use adult day care are physically frail, cognitively impaired, or both and require some supervision but not continuous care (Meiner and Yeager, 2019).

The centers usually operate weekdays during typical business hours and usually charge on a daily basis. Adult day care centers allow patients to retain more independence by living at home, thus potentially reducing the costs of health care by avoiding or delaying an older adult's admission to a nursing center. Nurses working in day care centers provide continuity between care delivered in the home and the center. For example, nurses ensure that patients continue to take prescribed medication and administer specific treatments. Knowledge of community needs and resources is essential in providing adequate patient support (Touhy and Jett, 2018).

Palliative and Hospice Care. Palliative care is a holistic, patient- and family-centered care approach with a goal of improving the quality of life of patients and families who are experiencing problems related to life-threatening illnesses. Palliative care is delivered through the continuum of illness with a focus on early identification and treatment of physical, psychosocial, and spiritual problems; relief of pain and suffering; continuity of care; and helping patients and families make informed decisions (NHPCO, n.d.; Parola et al., 2018). Palliative care can be delivered in any health care setting. Some health care agencies have dedicated palliative care units to care for these patients with complex health problems. Key to palliative care delivery is the nurse-patient and nurse-family relationship. With the patient, the nurse develops a singular relationship, and with the family, a partner, supportive relationship is formed (Parola et al., 2018).

A hospice is a system of family-centered care that allows patients to live with comfort, independence, and dignity while easing the pain of terminal illness. A patient entering into hospice care is in the terminal phase of illness, and the patient, family, and health care provider agree that no further treatment will reverse the disease process. Hospice care is provided in a setting that best meets the needs of each patient and family, such as in a patient's home, in nursing homes, assisted living facilities, freestanding hospices, and hospitals. The focus of hospice care is supportive care, not curative treatment (see Chapter 36). Hospice benefits patients in the terminal phase of any disease, such as cardiomyopathy, multiple sclerosis, acquired immunodeficiency syndrome (AIDS), and cancer. Hospice team members are available 24 hours a day, 7 days a week to answer questions or visit anytime the need for support arises. Team members collaborate to provide care that ensures death with dignity. Services continue without interruption even if a patient's care setting changes. Chapter 36 offers more detail on hospice care.

Palliative and hospice care are similar in that both focus on symptom management and ensuring the patient's comfort. Both care delivery methods are managed by an interprofessional team that works together with the patient's primary health care provider to develop and maintain a patient-directed, individualized plan of care (Pawlow et al., 2018). An essential member of the interprofessional team is the advanced practice registered nurse (APRN). To meet the increasing need for APRNs in palliative and hospice care, integration of core competencies into APRN education, development of clinical education opportunities in palliative and hospice care, and provision of continuing education in palliative and hospice care for practicing APRNs need to occur (Pawlow et al., 2018).

ISSUES IN HEALTH CARE DELIVERY FOR NURSES

The climate in health care today influences both health care professionals and consumers. Because those who provide patient care are the most qualified to make changes in the health care delivery system, you need to participate fully and effectively within all aspects of health care. Health care agencies today are working hard to improve patient experience and engagement while delivering high quality care, improving

outcomes, and controlling cost (Considine, 2018). In today's health care system, the outcomes of patient satisfaction and quality care indicators such as infection rates are tied to health care payments (McCay et al., 2018). As you face issues of how to maintain health care quality while reducing costs, you need to acquire the knowledge, skills, and values necessary to practice competently and effectively. It is also more important than ever to collaborate with other health care professionals to design new approaches for patient care delivery.

Health Care Costs and Quality

It is impossible today to separate two initiatives facing health care institutions: managing costs and achieving high-quality patient care. Health care payers (Table 2.2) (such as Medicare, Medicaid, and private insurers) have been trying to manage and address health care costs for many years. The Social Security Act establishes a system of payment for the operating costs of acute care hospital inpatient stays under Medicare Part A (hospital insurance) based on prospectively set rates (CMS, 2016d). This payment system is referred to as the **inpatient prospective payment system** (IPPS). Under the IPPS, each case is categorized into a **diagnosis-related group** (DRG). Each DRG has a payment weight assigned to it, based on the average resources used to

---

TABLE 2.2 Common Health Care Payers in the United States

Among the current health care payment models, quality is a key component. Most health care cost reimbursement arrangements tie the final payment to the achievement of key quality metrics.

Fee-for-service	• The most traditional health care payment model • Requires patients or payers to reimburse the health care provider for each service performed • No incentive to implement preventive care strategies, prevent hospitalization, or take any other cost-saving measures
Pay-for-coordination	• Coordinates care between the primary care provider and specialists • Coordinating care among multiple providers can help patients and their families manage a unified care plan and can help reduce redundancy in expensive tests and procedures.
Pay for performance (P4P)	• Same as value-based reimbursement • Health care providers are compensated only if they meet certain metrics for quality and efficiency. • Quality benchmark metrics tie physicians' reimbursement directly to quality of care they provide.
Bundled payment or episode-of-care payment	• Reimburses health care providers for specific episodes of care, such as an inpatient hospital stay • Encourages efficiency and quality of care because only a set amount of money will pay for the entire episode of care
Upside shared savings programs (Centers for Medicare and Medicaid Services [CMS] or commercial)	• Provide incentives for providers treating specific patient populations • A percentage of any net savings realized is given to the provider. • Upside-only shared savings is most common with Medicare Shared Savings Program (MSSP) Accountable Care Organizations, but all MSSP participants must move to a downside model after three years.
Downside shared savings programs (CMS or commercial)	• Includes both the gain share potential of an upside model, but also the downside risk of sharing the excess costs of health care delivery between provider and payer • Because providers are taking on greater risk with this model, the upside opportunity potential is larger in most cases than in an all-upside program.
Partial or full capitation	• Patients are assigned a per-member per-month (PMPM) payment based on their age, race, sex, lifestyle, medical history, and benefit design. • Payment rates are tied to expected usage regardless of whether the patient visits more or less. • As with bundled payment models, health care providers have an incentive to help patients avoid expensive procedures and tests in order to maximize their compensation. • Only certain types or categories of services are paid on a capitation basis.

CMS, Centers for Medicare and Medicaid Services; *MSSP*, Medicare Shared Savings Program
Data from American Academy of Pediatrics: Getting paid: alternative payment models, 2019, https://www.aap.org/en-us/professional-resources/practice-transformation/getting-paid/Pages/Payment-Models.aspx. Accessed August 2018; American Hospital Association: Current & emerging payment models, 2019, https://www.aha.org/advocacy/current-and-emerging-payment-models. Accessed August 2018; and Brookings: The beginner's guide to new healthcare payment models, 2014, https://www.brookings.edu/blog/usc-brookings-schaeffer-on-health-policy/2014/07/23/the-beginners-guide-to-new-health-care-payment-models/. Accessed August 2018.

treat Medicare patients in that DRG (CMS, 2016d). Regardless of the amount a hospital spends to care for a patient, the DRG-established payment is the amount the hospital receives. The DRG payment groups are still used, but many payers now demand that evidence-based standards of care be followed to further reduce the cost of health care.

The US Congress created the Centers for Medicare and Medicaid (CMS) Innovation Center to test "innovative payment and service delivery models to reduce program expenditures … while preserving or enhancing the quality of care" for those who receive Medicare, Medicaid, or Children's Health Insurance Program (CHIP) benefits (CMS, 2016b). The Innovation Center supports the following priorities: testing new payment and service delivery models, evaluating results and advancing best practices, and engaging a broad range of stakeholders to develop additional models for testing. One example of an initiative supported by the Innovation Center is the creation of Medicare Accountable Care Organizations (ACOs). The ACOs are groups of doctors, hospitals, and other health care providers who come together voluntarily to give coordinated high-quality care to their Medicare fee-for-service (FFS) beneficiaries and reduce unnecessary costs (CMS, 2016e). As of 2015, 424 ACOs participate in the CMS Shared Savings Program (CMS, 2015a).

The Affordable Care Act ties payment to organizations offering Medicare Advantage plans to the quality ratings of the coverage they offer. If hospitals perform poorly in quality scores, they receive lower payments for services. Quality outcome measures include patient satisfaction and more effective management of care by reducing complications and readmissions and improving care coordination. Examples of reforms that incent or "Pay for Value," designed to build a health care system that better serves the American population (CMS, 2015a), include the following:

- *Hospital Value-Based Purchasing:* This program links a portion of hospitals' Medicare payments (1.5% of base operating DRG payment) for inpatient acute care to their performance in important quality measures. The Hospital Consumer Assessment of Healthcare Providers and Systems (HCAHPS) is the standardized survey instrument and data collection methodology CMS requires for measuring patients' perceptions of hospital care. HCAHPS is a patient satisfaction measure that sets a national standard for collecting or publicly reporting patients' perceptions that enables users to make valid comparisons across all hospitals (HCAHPS, 2018). Research shows that hospitals that have a higher percentage of hospitalists providing care are linking services for improved coordination of care, resulting in higher performance scores (Spaulding et al., 2018).
- *Hospital Readmissions Reduction Program:* This CMS program reduces Medicare payments to hospitals with excess patient readmissions within 30 days of hospital discharge. It is designed to encourage patient safety and care quality. The maximum reduction in payments under the Hospital Readmissions Reduction Program increased in 2015 to 3 percent of base DRG amounts. The conditions that are regulated under this program include heart attack, heart failure, pneumonia, chronic obstructive pulmonary disease, and knee and hip replacements (National Quality Forum, 2018a). Nurses are a vital part of interprofessional teams. These team members collaborate to design treatment and discharge instruction protocols to reduce unnecessary patient readmissions.
- *Bundled Payments for Care Improvements:* Certain health care organizations are testing whether bundled payments (single payment for all services performed to treat a patient) for a specific episode of care (inpatient stays in an acute care hospital) can better coordinate care for Medicare patients and reduce Medicare costs. A bundled payment includes payments for services such as medical, radiological, and therapeutic. This initiative focuses on improving care for specific conditions. Bundling payments for services, such as heart bypass surgery, is one way to encourage doctors and hospitals to better coordinate care during hospitalization and after discharge (CMS, 2015a). Health care institutions enter into payment arrangements that include financial and performance accountability for an episode of care (CMS, 2016c).
- *Hospital Acquired Condition (HAC) Reduction Program.* This program was developed by CMS to encourage hospitals to improve health care quality and patient safety. As a component of this program, hospitals that have a high incidence of HACs, such as pressure injury development, catheter-associated urinary tract infections, central line–associated bloodstream infections, surgical site infections, and *Clostridium difficile* in patients, received reduced or no funding from CMS for the treatment of these HACs (CMS, 2018). This program saves CMS approximately $350 million annually (CMS, 2018). Because of this reduced funding, hospitals have focused quality improvement efforts on reducing and preventing these HACs.

Patient Satisfaction. Patient satisfaction is the responsibility of all health care providers. It is more important than ever because patient satisfaction measures are linked to hospital reimbursement. Patient perceptions of the quality of their health care have been incorporated into quality assessment. As a result, health care organizations have made the patient experience and patient-centered care major components of their health care missions (Cody and Williams-Reed, 2018; Niederhauser and Wolf, 2018). Hospitals now report patient satisfaction scores for patient care units monthly. All health care staff members help identify satisfaction trends and determine ways to improve quality of care. Hospitals and other health care agencies use a variety of instruments to measure patient satisfaction (Al-Abri and Al-Balushi, 2014). Instruments are provided by private vendors. They usually are not published, and their reliability and validity are unclear:

- Public and standardized instruments such as patient satisfaction questionnaires: PSQ-18 and consumer assessment health plans (e.g., HCAHPS). Such instruments have the advantage of good reliability and validity; however, they have a limited scope of survey questions.
- Internally developed instruments that are derived mainly from questions extracted from other instruments

The HCAHPS, developed by the Centers for Medicare and Medicaid Services and the Agency for Healthcare Research and Quality (AHRQ), is a patient satisfaction tool many hospitals use to collect and publicly report data for comparison purposes (HCAHPS, 2018). The HCAHPS survey has 32 questions that ask patients to respond about communication with doctors, communication with nurses, responsiveness of hospital staff, pain management, communication about medicines, discharge information, cleanliness of the hospital environment, quietness of the hospital environment, transition of care, and willingness to recommend the hospital (HCAHPS, 2018). The survey also includes four screening questions and seven demographic items, which are used for adjusting the mix of patients across hospitals and for analytical purposes.

Much research has been conducted to identify the factors that patients perceive affect their satisfaction, including relational communication techniques, hourly rounding (Box 2.4), nurse staffing patterns, and bedside shift report (Cody et al., 2018; Persolja, 2018; Dilts Skaggs et al., 2017). One common factor among the studies is interpersonal skills, especially the courtesy and respect of health care providers. This is in addition to the communication skills of providing explanations and clear information, which are more influential in affecting patient perceptions than other technical skills (George et al., 2018; Pattison et al., 2017).

BOX 2.4   EVIDENCE-BASED PRACTICE

Purposeful Nurse Rounding and Patient Satisfaction

PICOT Question: Does the practice of intentional rounding on a nursing unit improve patient outcomes?

Evidence Summary

Intentional rounding (IR) is a practice that has been adopted by many health care agencies with the goal of improving the patient experience, improving patient satisfaction, ensuring patient safety, and proactively addressing patient concerns or problems (Daniels, 2016; Dilts Skaggs et al., 2018). Typically, IR has a member of the unit's health care team rounding hourly on each patient using an established protocol (Christiansen et al., 2018). Key components to making IR successful are engaging all staff on the unit, holding all workers accountable for the rounding, having an infrastructure and organized approach, and a stable management team monitoring the practice (Daniels, 2016; Flowers et al., 2016). Hourly IR has been found to improve patient satisfaction and patient perception of nurse responsiveness (Bragg et al., 2016; Dilts Skaggs et al., 2018). Studies have also shown that IR reduces the incidence of patient falls and use of the nurse call system because patient problems are addressed proactively (Christiansen et al., 2018). Family members in intensive care units found that IR helped make a connection with staff, provided consistency in communication, and helped prepare families for the future (Cody et al., 2018). Patients also felt that IR helped with the management of their pain (Bragg et al., 2016). Occasionally, patients found IR to be intrusive, but education given by staff on the purpose of the rounding helped patients understand the importance of the practice (Flowers et al., 2016).

Application to Nursing Practice

- Conduct IR on patients as a best practice for your nursing unit.
- Conduct ongoing staff education on the importance of IR to help hard-wire the practice and improve teamwork and compliance (Christiansen et al., 2018; Dilts Skaggs et al., 2018).
- Use a structured approach such as the "12 Step" or "Four Ps" (pain, "potty" (bathroom), positioning, placement of personal items) when rounding (Daniels, 2016).
- Provide education to patients on the practice of IR when orienting patients to the hospital environment and practices (Daniels, 2016; Flowers et al., 2016).
- Participate with the nursing manager to conduct unit audits to monitor compliance of staff with the practice of IR.
- Celebrate successes on your unit such as increased patient satisfaction, decreased incidence of falls, and decreased nurse call system usage.

BOX 2.5   Registered Nurse Competencies

QSEN Competencies

- Patient-Centered Care
- Teamwork and Collaboration
- Evidence-Based Practice (EBP)
- Quality Improvement (QI)
- Safety
- Informatics

Massachusetts Nurse of the Future Nursing Core Competencies

- Patient-Centered Care
- Professionalism
- Leadership
- Systems-Based Practice
- Informatics and Technology
- Communication
- Teamwork and Collaboration
- Safety
- Quality Improvement
- Evidenced-Based Practice (EBP)

Data from Massachusetts Department of Higher Education Nursing Initiative (MDHENI): *Massachusetts Nurse of the Future Nursing Core Competencies© REGISTERED NURSE*, 2016, https://www.mass.edu/nahi/documents/NOFRNCompetencies_updated_March2016.pdf. Accessed August 2018; Quality Safety Education for Nursing (QSEN): *QSEN competencies*, 2018, http://qsen.org/competencies/pre-licensure-ksas/. Accessed August 2018.

percentage of nurses who attain a bachelor's degree to 80% and a doubling in the number of nurses with doctoral degrees. The current nursing workforce falls far short of these recommendations, with only 55% of registered nurses prepared at the baccalaureate or graduate degree level.

- With the passage of the Patient Protection and Affordable Care Act in 2010, more than 32 million Americans are gaining access to health care services, including those provided by RNs and APRNs (AACN, 2017).

The nursing shortage opens great opportunities for every nurse. If you pursue further education and watch trends in health care, you will be able to find employment in any professional position you choose.

Competency

Health care practitioner competencies are an excellent tool for measuring how well a nurse practices nursing and serve as a guide for the development of a professional nursing career. The Quality and Safety Education for Nurses (QSEN) project developed quality and safety competencies for nurses so that they would have the knowledge, skills, and attitudes to meet the challenges in today's health care settings (QSEN, 2018). The Massachusetts Nurse of the Future Nursing Core Competencies were developed by the Massachusetts Department of Higher Education (DHE) and the Massachusetts Organization of Nurse Executives (MONE) to identify knowledge, attitude, and skills for 10 competencies considered essential for the registered nurse for the future (MDHENI, 2016). Box 2.5 shows the QSEN and Massachusetts Nurse of the Future competencies. A consumer of health care expects that the standards of nursing care and practice in any health care setting are appropriate, safe, and effective. Health care organizations ensure quality care by establishing policies, procedures, and protocols that are evidence-based and follow national accrediting standards. Your responsibility is to follow policies and procedures and know the most

Nursing Shortage

The American Association of Colleges of Nursing (AACN) warns of a shortage of registered nurses (RNs) that is expected to intensify as baby boomers age and the need for health care grows (AACN, 2017). The problem is complicated by the fact that nursing schools across the country are struggling to expand their capacity to meet the rising demand for RNs. In addition, aging nurses are retiring from the workforce. The AACN noted important shortage indicators:

- The Bureau of Labor Statistics' (BLS) Employment Projections for 2014-2024 shows RNs among the top occupations in terms of job growth through 2024 (BLS, 2015). The RN workforce is expected to grow 16% (increase of 439,300) by 2024. The Bureau also predicts the need for 649,100 replacement nurses in the workforce, bringing the total number of RN job openings to 1.09 million by 2024.
- The Institute of Medicine's (2010) report, *The Future of Nursing: Leading Change, Advancing Health*, called for an increase in the

current practice standards. Ongoing competency is your responsibility. You are also responsible for obtaining necessary continuing education, following an established code of ethics, and earning certifications in specialty areas.

Patient-Centered Care

In a landmark report, *Crossing the Quality Chasm,* the Institute of Medicine (IOM) defines patient-centered care as "care that is respectful of and responsive to individual patient preferences, needs, and values and (ensures) that patient values guide all clinical decisions" (IOM, 2001). Hospitals across the country have been attempting to implement patient-centered care strategies, specifically delivery of care models (see Chapter 21). Patient-centered care is a component of the total patient experience, which includes all interactions that a patient has in a health care setting. The overall patient experience is influenced by the health care settings' culture and patient perceptions (Wolf, 2017).

Patient-centered care is much more than simply "individualizing" patient care. A critical component of patient-centered care is the nurse, patient, and family caregiver partnering to identify the patient's health care needs within the context of the patient's lifestyle and to coordinate the entire health care team so that patient and family are engaged in the care process and associated decisions. This is a major shift in how care is delivered, empowering the patient and family to participate in the plan of care and engaging patients and families in a dialogue about the patient experience (Niederhauser and Wolf, 2018). The following are the Picker Institute's eight principles of patient-centered care (Oneview, 2015), based on input from patients, families, and health care experts:

1. Respect for patients' values, preferences, and expressed needs
Engage patients in decision making, recognizing that they are individuals with their own unique values and preferences. Treat patients with dignity, respect, and sensitivity to their cultural values and autonomy.

2. Coordination and integration of care
Coordinate care to reduce patients' feelings of vulnerability: coordinate clinical care, coordinate ancillary and support services, and coordinate frontline patient care.

3. Information and education
Improve communication with patients and families.
- Information on clinical status, progress, and prognosis
- Information on processes of care (e.g., discharge, surgery)
- Information to facilitate autonomy, self-care, and health promotion

4. Physical comfort
Provide physical comfort throughout the care experience, including pain management, assistance with activities of daily living needs, and comforting hospital surroundings and environment.

5. Emotional support and alleviation of fear and anxiety
Professional caregivers should pay attention to patients' fear and anxiety, especially:
- Anxiety over physical status, treatment, and prognosis
- Anxiety over the effect of the illness on themselves and family
- Anxiety over the financial impact of illness

6. Involvement of family and friends
Support family and friends in taking a role in the patient's experience. Family dimensions of patient-centered care include:
- Providing accommodations for family and friends
- Involving family and close friends in decision making
- Supporting family members as caregivers
- Recognizing the needs of family and friends

7. Continuity and transition
Offer support and resources so that patients can care for themselves after discharge or receive the assistance they need.

- Provide understandable, detailed information about topics such as medications, physical limitations, and dietary needs.
- Coordinate and plan treatment and services to continue after discharge.
- Provide information about access to clinical, social, physical, and financial support continually.

8. Access to care
Patients need to know they can access care when it is needed, especially ambulatory care.
- Access to hospitals, clinics, and physician offices
- Availability of transportation
- Ease in scheduling appointments
- Availability of appointments when needed
- Accessibility of specialists or specialty services when a referral is made
- Clear instructions provided on when and how to get referrals

> **REFLECT NOW**
>
> After completing your assigned clinical experience, complete a self-assessment evaluating your use of the principles of patient-centered care. Identify areas that you can improve on for your next clinical assignment.

> **QSEN** **Building Competency in Patient-Centered Care** Nathan, a new graduate nurse, is assigned to care for a patient who had surgery yesterday for cancer. The plan is for the patient to be discharged home in 2 days. Identify strategies that Nathan can use to meet his patient's expectations.
>
> Answers to QSEN Activities can be found on the Evolve website.

Magnet Recognition Program®

The American Nurses Credentialing Center (ANCC) established the Magnet Recognition Program® to recognize health care organizations that achieve excellence in nursing practice (ANCC, 2018). Health care organizations that apply for Magnet® status must demonstrate quality patient care, nursing excellence, and innovations in professional practice. The professional work environment needs to allow nurses to practice with a sense of empowerment and autonomy to deliver quality nursing care. The Magnet® Model has five components affected by global issues that are challenging nursing today (ANCC, 2018). The five components are (1) Transformational Leadership, (2) Structural Empowerment, (3) Exemplary Professional Practice, (4) New Knowledge, Innovation, and Improvements, and (5) Empirical Quality Results (Box 2.6). In Magnet® hospitals, the organizational culture is focused on nurse engagement, commitment to quality improvement, clear strategic direction, shared governance, and trust in leadership (Moss et al., 2017; Underwood and Hayne, 2017). Peer review is often used as a mechanism to improve accountability and foster professional growth (Roberts and Cronin, 2017). Magnet® status requires nurses to collect data on specific nursing-sensitive quality indicators or outcomes and compare their outcomes against a national, state, or regional database to demonstrate quality of care.

Nursing-Sensitive Outcomes. Nursing-sensitive outcomes are patient outcomes and nursing workforce characteristics that are directly related to nursing care, such as changes in patients' symptom experiences, functional status, safety, psychological distress, RN job

BOX 2.6 Model and Forces of Magnetism

Magnet® Model Components	Forces of Magnetism
Transformational leadership—A vision for the future and the systems and resources to achieve the vision are created by nursing leaders.	• Quality of nursing leadership • Management style
Structural empowerment—Structures and processes provide an innovative environment in which staff are developed and empowered and professional practice flourishes.	• Organizational structure • Personnel policies and programs • Community and the health organization • Image of nursing • Professional development
Exemplary professional practice—Strong professional practice is established, and accomplishments of the practice are demonstrated.	• Professional models of care • Consultation and resources • Autonomy • Nurses as teachers • Interprofessional relationships
New knowledge, innovations, and improvements—Contributions are made to the profession in the form of new models of care, use of existing knowledge, generation of new knowledge, and contributions to the science of nursing.	• Quality improvement
Empirical quality outcomes—Focus is on structure and processes and demonstration of positive clinical, workforce, and patient and organizational outcomes.	• Quality of care

Adapted from American Nurses Credentialing Center (ANCC): *Magnet Model*, 2018, http://www.nursingworld.org/organizational-programs/magnet/magnet-model/. Accessed August 2018.

satisfaction, total nursing hours per patient day, and costs. As a nurse you assume accountability and responsibility for achieving and accepting the consequences of these outcomes. Measuring and monitoring nursing-sensitive outcomes reveal the interventions that improve patients' outcomes. Nurses and health care agencies use nursing-sensitive outcomes to improve nurses' workloads, enhance patient safety, and develop sound policies related to nursing practice and health care. The American Nurses Association developed the National Database of Nursing Quality Indicators (NDNQI) to measure and evaluate nursing-sensitive outcomes with the purpose of improving patient safety and quality care (Press Ganey, 2018). The NDNQI reports quarterly results on nursing outcomes at the nursing unit level. This provides a database for individual hospitals to compare their performance against nursing performance nationally. The evaluation of patient outcomes and nursing workforce characteristics remains important to nursing and the health care delivery system. Chapter 5 describes approaches for measuring outcomes.

Technology in Health Care

Technological advances continually affect health care organizations and change the ways in which nurses deliver evidence-based care to patients. Emerging technologies that will change how nurses practice include genetics and genomics, less invasive and more accurate tools for diagnosis and treatment, 3-D printing, robotics, biometrics, electronic health records (see Chapter 26), and computerized physician/provider order entry and clinical decision support. Technology makes your work easier in many ways, but it does not replace your judgment. For example, when you manage an IV infusion smart pump, you must monitor the device to ensure that it infuses on schedule and without complications despite its numerous automatic settings. An infusion device infuses at a constant rate, but you must confirm that the rate is calculated correctly. An infusion device sets off an alarm if the infusion slows, making it important for you to respond to the alarm and fix the problem. Technology does not replace a nurse's astute, critical eye and clinical judgment.

Robotics is a form of emerging technology that will greatly impact how nursing is practiced in the future. It is estimated that robotic use will grow due to workforce shortages, a growing elderly population, and a call for higher quality care not subject to human limitations (Huston, 2013; Simshaw et al., 2016). Most robotic applications are limited to food service, medication distribution, infection control, surgery, and even diagnosing patients (Maleski, 2014). However, one area with huge potential for affecting nursing is the use of robots as direct care providers. Maleski (2014) reports that there are daily care robots designed to support older adults and people with disabilities in such activities as preparing and serving meals and in daily care tasks (Simshaw et al., 2016). In addition, exoskeleton-powered robots are used to help patients who are paralyzed stand, with the goal of reducing morbidity and augmenting physical therapy for patients with impaired extremities. The implications for nursing are significant. Nursing must be on the front line in deciding how robotics is utilized in order to advocate for patients and families and to ensure that professional standards of care are delivered.

Telemedicine is a technology that relies on interactive video; it uses medical information gathered and reviewed at one site (such as a hospital, home, clinic, or urgent care center) and transmits treatment recommendations to another site to improve a patient's clinical health status (American Telemedicine Association, 2019). There are a variety of applications and services using two-way video, smartphones, wireless tools, and other forms of telecommunications technology. The benefits of telemedicine include providing services that meet patient demand, increasing access to care, and decreasing cost (American Telemedicine Association, 2019). However, varying federal and state policies on telemedicine use and reimbursement pose an obstacle to wider adoption of this emerging practice (Young and Kroth, 2018).

Nurses need to play a role in evaluating and implementing new technological advances. You use technology to improve the effectiveness of nursing care, enhance safety, and improve patient outcomes. Most important, it is essential for you to remember that the focus of nursing care is not the machine or the technology; it is the patient. Therefore, you need to constantly attend to and connect with your patients and ensure that their dignity and rights are preserved at all levels of care.

Health Care Disparities

Health care disparities are differences in health care outcomes and dimensions of health care, including access, quality, and equity, among population groups (Almgren, 2018; Kneipp et al., 2018). Disparities can be related to many variables, such as race, ethnicity, socioeconomic status, gender, location, or disability (Orgera and Artiga, 2018). Factors such as lack of health insurance, lack of access to care, and poor health outcomes contribute to the disparities for certain groups

BOX 2.7   Social Determinants of Health

- Availability of resources to meet daily needs (such as safe housing, local food markets, pharmacy)
- Access to educational, economic, and job opportunities
- Access to health care services
- Quality of education and job training
- Availability of community-based resources in support of community living and opportunities for recreational and leisure activities
- Transportation options
- Public safety
- Social support
- Social norms and attitudes (such as discrimination, racism, distrust of health care providers)
- Exposure to crime, violence, and social disorder
- Socioeconomic conditions (such as concentrated poverty and stressful conditions that accompany it)
- Residential segregation
- Language/literacy
- Access to mass media and emerging technologies
- Culture

Adapted from *Healthy People 2020: social determinants of health,* 2018, https://www.healthypeople.gov/2020/topics-objectives/topic/social-determinants-of-health. Accessed May 8, 2019.

(Orgera and Artiga, 2018). Social determinants affect health disparities, the differences in the health status of different groups of people. Differences in health status, particularly in a community where the majority have poor health, will affect the productivity and vulnerability of a population. The National Quality Forum (2018b) reports that health care disparities have been linked to the following social determinants: inadequate resources, poor patient-provider communication, a lack of culturally competent care (see Chapter 9), and inadequate access to patient language services, among other factors (Box 2.7). The health care system and the many professionals who serve patients must address these factors and reduce their effect so that all patients receive needed care. One strategy is to establish and support policies that positively influence social and economic conditions and support changes in individual behavior (such as pursuing healthful diets and adhering to medication regimens).

Healthy People 2020 recognizes that health starts in our homes, schools, workplaces, and communities (2018a). One goal of *Healthy People 2020* is to "create social and physical environments that promote good health for all" (Healthy People 2020, 2018a). Another important goal is to achieve **health care equity,** or the highest level of health care for all individuals and populations (Healthy People 2020, 2018b). To achieve health equity, health care disparities and inequalities must be eliminated. Nurses practice in a wide variety of settings that require an awareness of the social determinants of health that contribute to creating health disparities (see Chapter 9). Social determinants of health impact a person's health, overall functioning, and quality of life (Kneipp et al., 2018). Nursing plays a key role in promoting access to health care and in offering appropriate teaching resources to patients and families.

REFLECT NOW

Discuss with your clinical group the social determinants of health impacting the community where you are assigned to complete your clinical experiences. Have these created health disparities in the community?

THE FUTURE OF HEALTH CARE

A discussion of the health care delivery system today is incomplete without discussing the issue of change. The current system is in a constant state of change and reform, making it challenging to try to predict the future (Young and Kroth, 2018). Change is often threatening, but it also opens up opportunities for improvement. The ultimate issue in designing and delivering health care is to ensure the health and welfare of the populations health care institutions serve. Young and Kroth (2018) report that the US health care system is a paradox—extreme successes and technologic advances offset by limited access, high costs, and quality issues. One example of this is the high cost of prescription medications in the United States. Sarnak et al. (2017) reported that the United States had higher prescription drug spending per capita in comparison with nine other high-income countries reviewed. Four factors typically contribute to the spending on prescription drugs for a country. The factors are (1) population numbers and volume of drugs consumed, (2) the amount of drugs used by an individual person, (3) type and mix of drugs prescribed and purchased (e.g., generic drugs versus brand-name drugs), and (4) prices the patient pays at time of purchase (Sarnak et al., 2017). Often patients are uninsured or underinsured and do not have access to necessary services. However, health care organizations are trying to become better prepared to deal with the challenges. Increasingly, they are changing how they provide their services, reducing unnecessary costs, improving access to care, and trying to provide high-quality patient care. Professional nursing is an important player in the future of health care delivery. The solutions necessary to improve the quality of health care depend largely on the active participation of nurses.

▌ KEY POINTS

- Levels of health care describe the scope of services and settings in which health care is delivered to patients in all stages of health and illness.
- The primary level of health care includes medical health care services, health education, nutritional care, maternal/child health care, family planning, and control of diseases.
- Rural Americans' access to health care is affected by economic factors (rural Americans are more likely to live below the poverty level), cultural and social differences, educational shortcomings, lack of recognition of the problem by legislators, and the isolation of living in remote rural areas.
- "Pay for value" ties reimbursement to quality; if hospitals perform poorly in quality scores, they receive lower payments for services. Levels of prevention describe the focus of health-related activities in a care setting. The holistic model of care is used within integrated health care systems and delivers a coordinated continuum of services that supports patients with chronic conditions and improves the health of specific populations.
- Hospitals deliver health care to patients who are acutely ill and need comprehensive specialized secondary and tertiary health care.
- In restorative care settings, nurses know that success depends on their effective and early partnering with patients and their families.
- Discharge planning begins at admission to a health care agency and helps in the transition of a patient's care from one environment to another.

- Barriers to effective discharge planning include ineffective communication, lack of role clarity among health care team members, and lack of resources.
- Nurses promote patient satisfaction through providing patient- and family-centered care and good interpersonal skills, including courtesy, respect, and good communication skills.
- The nursing shortage opens vast opportunities to nurses. Furthering education and following trends in health care open professional options for nurses.
- Social determinants affect health disparities, the differences in the health status of different groups of people in a community. Differences in health status, particularly in a community where the majority have poor health, will affect the productivity and vulnerability of a population.

REFLECTIVE LEARNING

- Investigate whether the clinical unit on which you are assigned displays its patient satisfaction data on the unit. If so, review the data and identify areas that as students you can work on to help improve patient satisfaction. Discuss with your clinical group.
- Select one of the registered nurse competencies identified in Box 2.5. Develop a plan on improving your knowledge, skills, and attitudes for the competency during your upcoming clinical experience.
- Discuss with your clinical group changes in health care that have occurred in the last five years. How have these changes impacted how you practiced nursing today?

REVIEW QUESTIONS

1. Which activity performed by a nurse is related to maintaining competency in nursing practice?
   1. Asking another nurse about how to change the settings on a medication pump
   2. Regularly attending unit staff meetings
   3. Participating as a member of the professional nursing council
   4. Attending a review course in preparation for a certification examination
2. Which of the following are examples of a nurse participating in primary care activities? (Select all that apply.)
   1. Providing prenatal teaching on nutrition to a pregnant woman during the first trimester
   2. Assessing the nutritional status of older adults who come to the community center for lunch
   3. Working with patients in a cardiac rehabilitation program
   4. Providing home wound care to a patient
   5. Teaching a class to parents at the local grade school about the importance of immunizations
3. Which of the following statements is true regarding Magnet® status recognition for a hospital?
   1. Nursing is run by a Magnet manager who makes decisions for the nursing units.
   2. Nurses in Magnet hospitals make all of the decisions on the clinical units.
   3. Magnet is a term that is used to describe hospitals that are able to hire the nurses they need.
   4. Magnet is a special designation for hospitals that achieve excellence in nursing practice.
4. Which of the following nursing activities is provided in a secondary health care environment?
   1. Conducting blood pressure screenings for older adults at the Senior Center
   2. Teaching a patient with chronic obstructive pulmonary disease purse-lipped breathing techniques at an outpatient clinic
   3. Changing the postoperative dressing for a patient on a medical-surgical unit
   4. Doing endotracheal suctioning for a patient on a ventilator in the medical intensive care unit
5. A nurse is providing restorative care to a patient following an extended hospitalization for an acute illness. Which of the following is an appropriate goal for restorative care?
   1. Patient will be able to walk 200 feet without shortness of breath.
   2. Wound will heal without signs of infection.
   3. Patient will express concerns related to return to home.
   4. Patient will identify strategies to improve sleep habits.
6. Which of the following describe characteristics of an integrated health care system? (Select all that apply.)
   1. The focus is holistic.
   2. Participating hospitals follow the same model of health care delivery.
   3. The system coordinates a continuum of services.
   4. The focus of health care providers is finding a cure for patients.
   5. Members of the health care team link electronically to use the EMR to share the patient's health care record.
7. The school nurse has been following a 9-year-old student who has shown behavioral problems in class. The student acts out and does not follow teacher instructions. The nurse plans to meet with the student's family to learn more about social determinants of health that might be affecting the student. Which of the following factors would be appropriate for this type of assessment? (Select all that apply.)
   1. The student's seating placement in the classroom
   2. The level of support parents offer when the student completes homework
   3. The level of violence in the family's neighborhood
   4. The age at which the child first began having behavioral problems
   5. The cultural values about education held by family
8. A nurse is assigned to care for an 82-year-old patient who will be transferred from the hospital to a rehabilitation center. The patient and her husband have selected the rehabilitation center closest to their home. The nurse learns that the patient will be discharged in 3 days and decides to make the referral on the day of discharge. The nurse reviews the recommendations for physical therapy and applies the information to fall prevention strategies in the hospital. What discharge planning action by the nurse has not been addressed correctly?
   1. Patient and family involvement in referral
   2. Timing of referral
   3. Incorporation of referral discipline recommendations into plan of care
   4. Determination of discharge date
9. Which of the following are common barriers to effective discharge planning? (Select all that apply.)
   1. Ineffective communication among providers
   2. Lack of role clarity among health care team members

3. Sufficient number of hospital beds to manage patient volume
4. Patients' long-term disabilities
5. The patient's cultural background

10. A nurse newly hired at a community hospital learns about intentional hourly rounding during orientation. Which of the following are known evidence-based outcomes from intentional rounding? (Select all that apply.)
    1. Reduction in nurse staffing requirements
    2. Improved patient satisfaction
    3. Reduction in patient falls
    4. Increased costs
    5. Reduction in patient call light use

Answers: 1. 4; 2. 1, 2, 5; 3. 4; 4. 3; 5. 1; 6. 1; 7. 2, 3; 8. 2, 9. 1, 2; 10. 2, 3, 5.

Rationales for Review Questions can be found on the Evolve website.

REFERENCES

Almgren G: *Health career politics, policy, and services: a social justice analysis,* New York, 2018, Springer Publishing.

Alzheimer's Association: *Alzheimer's and dementia caregiver center: respite care,* 2018. https://www.alz.org/care/alzheimers-dementia-caregiver-respite.asp. Accessed August 2018.

American Academy Family Physicians: *The medical home,* 2018. https://www.aafp.org/practice-management/transformation/pcmh.html. Accessed August 2018.

American Association of Colleges of Nursing (AACN): *Nursing shortage fact sheet,* 2017. http://www.aacnnursing.org/News-Information/Fact-Sheets/Nursing-Shortage. Accessed August 2018.

American Hospital Association: *Fast facts on US hospitals,* 2018. http://www.aha.org/research/rc/stat-studies/fast-facts.shtml. Accessed August 2018.

American Hospital Association: *Quality and patient safety,* 2017. http://www.aha.org/advocacy-issues/quality/index.shtml. Accessed August 2018.

American Nurses Association (ANA): *Scope and standards of practice,* ed 3, Silver Spring, MD, 2015, American Nurses Association2015.

American Nurses Credentialing Center (ANCC): *Magnet model,* 2018. http://www.nursecredentialing.org/Magnet/ProgramOverview/New-Magnet-Model. Accessed August 2018.

American Telemedicine Association: *Telehealth basics,* 2019. https://www.americantelemed.org/resource/why-telemedicine/. Accessed May 24, 2019.

Bureau of Labor Statistics: *Occupational employment projections to 2024,* 2015. https://www.bls.gov/opub/mlr/2015/article/occupational-employment-projections-to-2024.htm. Accessed August 2018.

Center for American Progress: *The importance of community health centers: engines of economic activity and job creation,* 2018. https://www.americanprogress.org/issues/healthcare/report/2010/08/09/8195/the-importance-of-community-health-centers/. Accessed August 2018.

Centers for Disease Control and Prevention (CDC): *Workplace health promotion: health outcomes measures,* 2015a. http://www.cdc.gov/workplacehealthpromotion/model/evaluation/outcomes.html. Accessed August 2018.

Centers for Disease Control and Prevention (CDC): *Whole school, whole community, whole child (WSCC): a collaborative approach to learning and health,* 2015b. http://www.cdc.gov/healthyschools/wscc/index.htm. Accessed August 2018.

Centers for Medicare and Medicaid Services (CMS): *Better care, smarter spending, healthier people: improving our health care delivery system,* 2015a. https://www.cms.gov/Newsroom/MediaReleaseDatabase/Fact-sheets/2015-Fact-sheets-items/2015-01-26.html. Accessed August 2018.

Centers for Medicare and Medicaid Services (CMS): *Long-term care facility resident assessment instrument 3.0 user's manual version 1.13,* 2015b. https://www.cms.gov/Medicare/Quality-Initiatives-Patient-Assessment-Instruments/NursingHomeQualityInits/Downloads/MDS-30-RAI-Manual-V113.pdf. Accessed August 2018.

Centers for Medicare and Medicaid Services (CMS): *Home Health Quality Initiative,* 2016a. https://www.cms.gov/Medicare/Quality-Initiatives-Patient-Assessment-Instruments/HomeHealthQualityInits/index.html?redirect=/HomeHealthQualityInits/. Accessed August 2018.

Centers for Medicare and Medicaid Services (CMS): *About the CMS Innovation Center,* 2016b. https://innovation.cms.gov/about/index.html. Accessed August 2018.

Centers for Medicare and Medicaid Services (CMS): *Bundled payments for care improvements: general information,* 2016c. https://innovation.cms.gov/initiatives/bundled-payments/. Accessed August 2018.

Centers for Medicare and Medicaid Services (CMS): *Acute inpatient PPS,* 2016d. https://www.cms.gov/Medicare-Fee-for-Service-Payment/AcuteInpatientPPS/index.html?redirect=/acuteinpatientpps/. Accessed August 2018.

Centers for Medicare and Medicaid Services (CMS): *Shared savings programs,* 2016e. https://www.cms.gov/Medicare-Fee-For-Service-Payment/sharedsavingsprogram/index.html. Accessed August 2018.

Center for Medicare and Medicaid Services Medicare Learning Network (CMS MLN): *Critical access hospital,* 2017. https://www.cms.gov/Outreach-and-Education/Medicare-Learning-Network-MLN/MLNProducts/downloads/CritAccessHospfctsht.pdf. Accessed August 2018.

Centers for Medicare and Medicaid Services (CMS): *Hospital-acquired condition (HAC) reduction program,* 2018. https://www.cms.gov/Medicare/Quality-Initiatives-Patient-Assessment-Instruments/Value-Based-Programs/HAC/Hospital-Acquired-Conditions.html. Accessed August 2018.

Considine J: *Better patient experience hinges on improving financial journey,* 2018. https://www.healthmgttech.com/better-patient-experience-hinges-on-improving-financial-journey. Accessed August 2018.

Counsell S: *10 key components of a post-discharge care model,* 2015. http://www.beckershospitalreview.com/quality/10-key-components-of-a-post-discharge-care-model.html. Accessed August 2018.

Department of Health and Human Services Centers for Medicare and Medicaid Services (DHHS-CMS): *Your discharge planning checklist,* 2017. https://www.medicare.gov/pubs/pdf/11376-discharge-planning-checklist.pdf. Accessed August 2018.

George S, et al.: Commit to sit to improve nurse communication, *Crit Care Nurse* 38(2):83, 2018.

HealthIT.gov: *Benefits for critical access hospitals and other small rural hospitals,* 2017. https://www.healthit.gov/topic/health-it-initiatives/benefits-critical-access-hospitals-and-other-small-rural-hospitals. Accessed August 2018.

Healthy People 2020: *Social determinants of health,* 2018a. https://www.healthypeople.gov/2020/topics-objectives/topic/social-determinants-of-health. Accessed August 2018.

Healthy People 2020: *Disparities,* 2018b. https://www.healthypeople.gov/2020/about/foundation-health-measures/Disparities. Accessed August 2018.

Himmelstein DU, et al.: The ongoing U.S. health care crisis: a data update, *Int J Health Serv* 48(2):209, 2018.

Hospital Consumer Assessment of Healthcare Providers and Systems (HCAHPS): *HCAHPS Hospital Survey,* 2018. http://www.hcahpsonline.org. Accessed August 2018.

Huston C: The impact of emerging technology on nursing care: "warp speed ahead," *Online J Issues Nurs* 18(2), 2013.

Institute of Medicine (IOM): *Crossing the quality chasm: a new health system for the 21st century,* Washington DC, 2001, National Academies Press.

Institute of Medicine (IOM): *The future of nursing: leading change, advancing health,* Washington DC, 2010, National Academies Press.

Legal Information Institute: *42 U.S. Code § 1395i-3. Requirements for, and assuring quality of care in, skilled nursing facilities,* 2010. https://www.law.cornell.edu/uscode/text/42/1395i-3. Accessed August 2018.

Maleski DA: *Health care robotics: automated devices to handle tough hospital tasks,* Health Facil Manag, 2014. http://www.hfmmagazine.com/articles/1328-health-care-robotics, Accessed August 2018.

Massachusetts Department of Higher Education Nursing Initiative (MDHENI): *Massachusetts nurse of the future nursing core competencies© registered nurse,* 2016. https://www.mass.edu/nahi/documents/NOFRNCompetencies_updated_March2016.pdf. Accessed August 2018.

Medicaid.gov: *Nursing facilities,* 2018. https://www.medicaid.gov/medicaid/ltss/institutional/nursing/index.html. Accessed August 2018.

Meiner SE, Yeager JJ: *Gerontologic nursing,* ed 6, St Louis, 2019, Mosby.

Michigan Care Management Resource Center: *High intensity care model,* 2018. http://micmrc.org/programs/high-intensity-care-model. Accessed August 2018.

National Alliance on Mental Illness (NAMI): *Mental health by the numbers,* 2018. http://www.nami.org/Learn-More/Mental-Health-By-the-Numbers. Accessed August 2018.

National Alliance on Mental Illness (NAMI): *NAMI describes state mental health cuts in congressional briefing; comprehensive report expected soon,* 2011. https://www.nami.org/Press-Media/Press-Releases/2011/NAMI-Describes-State-Mental-Health-Cuts-in-Congres. Accessed August 2018.

National Center for Assisted Living (NCAL): *Facts and figures,* 2018. https://www.ahcancal.org/ncal/facts/Pages/default.aspx. Accessed August 2018.

National Hospice and Palliative Care Organization: An Explanation of Palliative Care, n.d., https://www.nhpco.org/explanation-palliative-care. Accessed May 24, 2019.

National Quality Forum: *Home vs. Hospital: national efforts to reduce readmissions are helping more patients heal at home,* 2018a. http://www.qualityforum.org/Readmissions_-_Home_vs_Hospitals.aspx. Accessed August 2018.

National Quality Forum: *Disparities*, 2018b. http://ww-w.qualityforum.org/Topics/Disparities.aspx. Accessed August 2018.

National Rural Health Association (NRHA): *About Rural Health Care*, 2018. https://www.ruralhealth-web.org/about-nrha/about-rural-health-care. Accessed August 2018.

Niederhauser V, Wolf J: Patient experience: a call to action for nurse leadership, *Nurs Adm Q* 42(3):211, 2018.

Oneview: *The eight principles of patient-centered care*, 2015. https://www.oneviewhealthcare.com/the-eight-principles-of-patient-centered-care/. Accessed May 24, 2019.

Orgera K, Artiga S: *Disparities in health and health care: five key questions and answers*, Henry J. Kaiser Family Foundation, 2018. https://www.kff.org/disparities-poli-cy/issue-brief/disparities-in-health-and-health-care-five-key-questions-and-answers/. Accessed May 24, 2019.

Press Ganey: *Nursing quality (NDNQI)*, 2018. http://www.pressganey.com/solutions/clinical-quality/nursing-qual-ity. Accessed August 2018.

Quality and Safety Education for Nurses (QSEN): *QSEN competencies*, 2018. http://qsen.org/competencies/pre-li-censure-ksas/. Accessed August 2018.

Research Data Assistance Center: *The home health outcome and assessment information set (OASIS)*, 2016. https://www.resdac.org/cms-data/files/oasis. Accessed August 2018.

Simshaw D, et al.: Regulating healthcare robots: maximiz-ing opportunities while minimizing risks, 2 RICH, JL & TECH 3, 2016. https://scholarship.richmond.edu/jolt/vol22/iss2/1/. Accessed May 24, 2019.

The Joint Commission (TJC): *2016 Comprehensive accredi-tation manual for hospitals*, Oakbrook Terrace, IL, 2016, The Commission.

Touhy TA, Jett K: *Ebersole & Hess' Gerontological nursing & healthy aging*, ed 5, St Louis, 2018, Elsevier.

Wolf JA: Critical considerations for the future of patient experience, *J Healthc Manag* 62(1):9, 2017.

World Health Organization (WHO): *Health topics: reha-bilitation*, 2018a. http://www.who.int/topics/rehabilita-tion/en/. Accessed August 2018.

World Health Organization (WHO): *Primary health care*, 2018b. http://www.who.int/topics/primary_health_care/en/. Accessed August 2018.

Young KM, Kroth PJ: *Sultz & Young's Health care USA: un-derstanding its organization and delivery*, ed 9, Sudbury, 2018, Jones & Bartlett.

RESEARCH REFERENCES

Al-Abri R, Al-Balushi A: Patient satisfaction survey as a tool towards quality improvement, *Oman Med J* 29(1):3–7, 2014.

Bragg L, et al.: How do patients perceive hourly rounding? *Nurs Manage* 47(11):11, 2016.

Christiansen A, et al.: Intentional rounding in acute adult healthcare settings: a systematic mixed-method review, *J Clin Nurs* 27(9/10):1759, 2018.

Cody SE, et al.: Making a connection: family experiences with bedside rounds in the intensive care unit, *Crit Care Nurse* 38(3):18, 2018.

Coleman EA, et al.: The care transitions intervention: re-sults of a randomized controlled trial, *Arch Intern Med* 166(17):1822–1828, 2006.

Daniels JF: Purposeful and timely nursing rounds: a best practice implementation project, *JBI Database System Rev Implement Rep* 14(1):248, 2016.

Dilts Skaggs MK, et al.: Using the evidence-based practice service nursing bundle to increase patient satisfaction, *J Emerg Nurs* 44(1):37, 2018.

Dizon ML, Reinking C: Reducing readmissions: nurse-driven interventions in the transition of care from the hospital, *Worldviews Evid Based Nurs* 14(6):432, 2017.

Flowers K, et al.: Intentional rounding: facilitators, benefits and barriers, *J Clin Nurs* 25(9/10):1346, 2016.

Hwang W, et al.: Effects of integrated delivery system on cost and quality, *Am J Manag Care* 19(5):e175, 2013.

Kneipp SM, et al.: Trends in health disparities, health inequity, and social determinants of health research: a 17-year analysis of NINR, NCI, NHLBI and NIMHD funding, *Nurs Res* 67(3):231, 2018.

Mabire C, et al.: Effectiveness of nursing discharge planning interventions on health-related outcomes in elderly inpatients discharged home: a systematic review protocol, *JBI Database System Rev Implement Rep* 11(8):1–12, 2013.

McCay R, et al.: Nurse leadership style, nurse satisfaction, and patient satisfaction: a systematic review, *J Nurs Care Qual* 33(4):361, 2018.

Moss S, et al.: Creating a culture of success: using the Mag-net Recognition Program* as a framework to engage nurses in an Australian healthcare facility, *J Nurs Adm* 47(2):116, 2017.

Naylor MD, et al.: Translating research into practice: transitional care for older adults, *J Eval Clin Pract* 15(6):1164–1170, 2009.

Okoniewska B, et al.: Barriers to discharge in an acute care medical teaching unit: a qualitative analysis of health providers' perceptions, *J Multidiscip Healthc* 8:83–89, 2015.

Parola V, et al.: Caring in palliative care: a phenomeno-logical study of nurses' lived experiences, *J Hosp Palliat Nurs* 20(2):180, 2018.

Pattison KH, et al.: Patient perceptions of sitting versus standing for nurse leader rounding, *J Nurs Care Qual* 32(1):1, 2017.

Pawlow P, et al.: The hospice and palliative care Advanced Practice Registered Nurse workforce: results of a nation-al study, *J Hosp Palliat Nurs* 20(4):349, 2018.

Persolja M: The effect of nurse staffing patterns on patient satisfaction and needs: a cross-sectional study, *J Nurs Manag* 26(7):858, 2018.

Roberts H, Cronin SN: A descriptive study of nursing peer-review programs in US Magnet* hospitals, *J Nurs Adm* 47(4):226, 2017.

Sarnak DO, et al.: *Paying for prescription drugs around the world: why is the U.S. an outlier?* 2017. https://www.commonwealthfund.org/publications/is-sue-briefs/2017/oct/paying-prescription-drugs-around-world-why-us-outlier. Accessed August 2018.

Spaulding A, et al.: The impact of hospitalists on val-ue-based purchasing program scores, *J Healthc Manag* 63(4):e43, 2018.

Stirling C, et al.: Why carers use adult day respite: a mixed method case study, *BMC Health Serv Res* 14:245, 2014.

Underwood CM, Hayne AN: System-level shared gover-nance structures and processes in healthcare systems with Magnet*-designated hospitals: a descriptive study, *J Nurs Adm* 47(7/8):396, 2017.

3

Community-Based Nursing Practice

OBJECTIVES

- Explain the relationship between public health and community health nursing.
- Differentiate community-oriented nursing from community-based nursing.
- Discuss the role of the community health nurse.
- Discuss the role of the nurse in community-based practice.
- Identify characteristics of patients from vulnerable populations that influence the community-based nurse's approach to care.
- Describe the competencies important for success in community-based nursing practice.
- Describe elements of a community assessment.

KEY TERMS

Community-based nursing, p. 34
Community health nursing, p. 34
Community-oriented nursing, p. 34

Health disparities, p. 34
Incident rates, p. 33
Population, p. 34

Public health nursing, p. 34
Social determinants of health, p. 33
Vulnerable populations, p. 35

MEDIA RESOURCES

Community-based care focuses on health promotion, disease prevention, and restorative care. Patients are often discharged quickly from acute care settings, requiring continued care outside traditional settings. These patients also require preventive care such as immunizations, screenings, lifestyle teaching, and counseling. Health care delivery has changed greatly over the past few decades, resulting in a growing need to provide health care services where people live, work, socialize, and learn. One way to achieve this goal is through a community-based health care model. Community-based health care is a collaborative, patient-centered approach to provide culturally appropriate health care within a community (Centers for Medicare & Medicaid Services [CMS], 2017). A healthy community includes elements that maintain a high quality of life and productivity such as access to health services, preventive care, nutrition, safety, physical activity, oral health, and environmental quality (Office of Disease Prevention and Health Promotion [ODPHP], 2018d). Including interventions that address both mental and physical health is essential for community health programs (CDC, 2016). Nurses directly influence the health and well-being of patients every day and can encourage lifestyle changes within communities (American Nurses Association [ANA], n.d.). As more community health care partnerships develop, nurses are in a strategic position to play an important role in health care delivery and to improve the health of the community.

The focus of health promotion and disease prevention continues to be essential for the holistic practice of professional nursing. Historically, nurses have established and met the public health needs of their patients. Within community health settings, nurses continue to be leaders in assessing, diagnosing, planning, implementing, and evaluating the types of public and community health services needed. Community health nursing and community-based nursing are components of a health care delivery system that improve the health of the general public.

COMMUNITY-BASED HEALTH CARE

Regardless of where you practice nursing, you need to understand the focus of community-based health care. Community-based health care is a model of care that reaches everyone in a community (including the poor and underinsured), focuses on primary rather than institutional or acute care, and provides knowledge about health and health promotion and models of care to the community. Community-based health care occurs outside traditional health care institutions such as hospitals. It provides services to individuals and families within the community for acute and chronic conditions (Stanhope and Lancaster, 2018). Providing care in nontraditional settings such as ambulatory care clinics, community hospice centers, senior centers, parishes, and schools allows those who would not be able to access care in other areas to receive the care they need. Providing necessary care to maintain and restore health decreases vulnerability in at-risk populations.

Today the challenges in community-based health care are numerous. Political policy, social determinants of health, increases in health disparities, and economics all influence public health problems and subsequent health care services. Some of these problems include a lack of adequate health insurance, chronic illnesses (e.g., heart disease and diabetes), substance abuse, an increase in sexually transmitted infections, and underimmunization of infants and children (ODPHP,

2018d). Today's leaders in the health care system must commit to reform and bring attention to health promotion and disease prevention and provide health care services to all communities. Many community health programs are trying to decrease disparity by addressing ways to improve quality of care, access to care, and cost (ODPHP, 2018d).

Achieving Healthy Populations and Communities

The USDHHS Public Health Service designed a program to improve the overall health status of people living in this country. The *Healthy People Initiative* was created to establish ongoing health care goals for the US population (see Chapter 6) to meet the diverse public health needs that exist and to seize opportunities to achieve its goals. Health of the nation is tracked and goals are updated every 10 years based on data gathered during program evaluation and national health trends. *Healthy People* has become a broad-based public engagement initiative, with thousands of citizens helping to shape it at every step along the way. The overall goals of *Healthy People 2020* are to increase life expectancy and quality of life and eliminate health disparities through improved delivery of health care services (ODPHP, 2018a). Improved delivery of health care involves three key components: assessment, development and implementation of public health policies, and improved access to care.

Assessment of health care needs of individuals, families, and communities is the first component. Assessment includes systematic data collection on the population, monitoring the health status of the population, and accessing available information about the health of the community (Stanhope and Lancaster, 2018). Some examples of community assessment include gathering information on incident rates, such as identifying and reporting new infections or diseases, determining adolescent pregnancy rates, and reporting the number of motor vehicle accidents caused by teenage drivers. A comprehensive community assessment informs the development and maintenance of community health programs aimed at infection control, adolescent sex education, or ways to reduce distractions for teen drivers.

The second component of improved health care delivery is policy. Health professionals provide leadership in developing public policies to support the health of the population (Stanhope and Lancaster, 2018). Strong policies are driven by community assessment. For example, assessing the level of lead poisoning in young children often leads to a lead cleanup program to reduce the incidence of lead poisoning. This is the case in Flint, Michigan. Nurses were instrumental as case managers for children exposed to lead but also led public health efforts to lobby for and educate about water filtration and ways to prevent further exposure to lead (Kennedy et al., 2016). Nurses also play an important role in advocating and educating about the nation's opioid epidemic. Nurses can lobby for strict prescription monitoring programs, as well as make referrals and implement evidence-based substance abuse or pain relief treatments to reduce the abuse of opioids (Davis et al., 2015). Identifying evidence-based practices to help people manage chronic illnesses in the home and the community addresses the needs of nurses and their patients (Croft et al., 2018).

The last component of improved health care delivery is access to care. Improved access to care ensures that essential community-wide health services are available and accessible to the entire community (Stanhope and Lancaster, 2018). Insurance coverage, geographic availability of care, and developing relationships with health care providers are essential in establishing access to community-wide health promotion and health maintenance activities (ODPHP, 2018d). Examples include prenatal care programs and programs focusing on disease prevention, health protection, and health promotion. The five-level health services pyramid is an example of how to provide community-based

services within existing health care services in a community (Fig. 3.1). In this population-focused health care services model, the goals of disease prevention, health protection, and health promotion provide a foundation for primary, secondary, and tertiary health care services.

A rural community does not always have a hospital to meet the acute care needs of its citizens. However, the community may have the resources for providing childhood immunizations, flu vaccines, and primary preventive care services and is able to focus on child developmental problems and child safety. For example, a nurse completing a community assessment identifies services available to meet the needs of expectant mothers, reduce teenage smoking, and provide nutritional support for older adults. In addition, the nurse also identifies the health care gaps for the community. Community-based programs provide needed services and are effective in improving the health of the community by ensuring that members of the community are aware of the resources that are available.

Public health services aim at achieving a healthy environment for all individuals. Health care providers apply these principles for individuals, families, and the communities in which they live. Nursing plays a role in all levels of the health services pyramid. By using public health principles, you are better able to understand the types of environments in which patients live and the interventions necessary to help keep them healthy.

Social Determinants of Health

Our health is determined in part by access to social and economic opportunities; the resources and support systems available in our homes, neighborhoods, and communities; the quality of our schooling; the safety of our workplaces; the cleanliness of our water, food, and air; and the nature of our social interactions and relationships.

Health starts in our homes, schools, workplaces, neighborhoods, and communities. We know that taking care of ourselves by eating well and staying active, not smoking, getting the recommended immunizations and screening tests, and seeing a doctor when we are sick all influence our health. However, there are also social determinants of health. Social determinants of health are biological, socioeconomic,

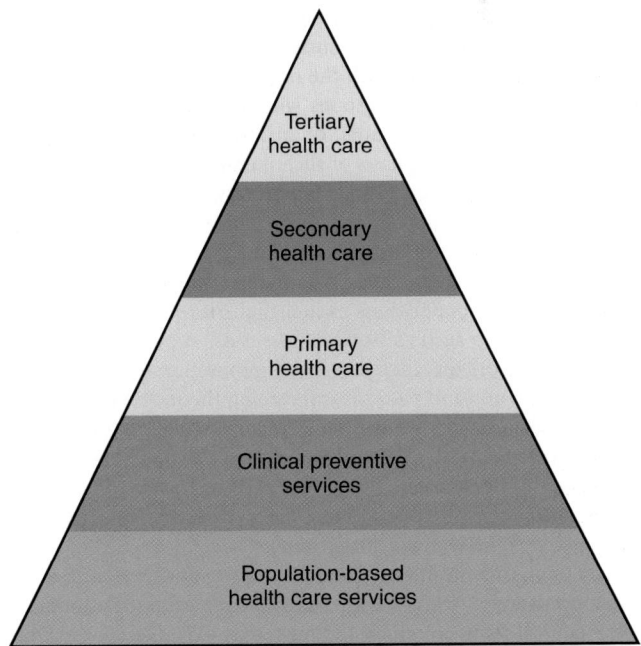

FIG. 3.1 Health services pyramid. (Courtesy US Public Health Service: For a healthy nation: return on investments in public health, Washington DC, 2008, USDHHS.)

psychosocial, behavioral, or social factors that contribute to a person's current state of health (CDC, 2018c). *Healthy People 2020* lists five determinants of health: biology and genetics (sex and age), individual behavior (such as alcohol, injection drug use, unprotected sex, and smoking), social environment (such as discrimination, income, and gender), physical environment (where a person lives or crowding conditions), and health services (such as access to quality health care and having health insurance) (ODPHP, 2018c). Whether these factors affect a single family or the community, they impact the overall health and wellness of that community (see Chapter 2).

Health Disparities

Health disparities negatively affect groups of people who have systematically experienced social or economic obstacles to health. These obstacles stem from characteristics historically linked to discrimination or exclusion such as race or ethnicity, religion, socioeconomic status, gender, mental health, sexual orientation, or geographic location. Other characteristics include cognitive, sensory, or physical disability.

Health disparities are preventable differences in a population's ability to achieve optimal health. Disparity exists if health outcomes vary by population. Populations can be disadvantaged by the burden of disease, injury, violence, or opportunities to achieve optimal health due to social, political, economic, or environmental resources (ODPHP, 2018b). Disparity is multifactorial, including poverty, environmental threats, inadequate access to health care, individual and behavioral factors, and educational inequalities (ODPHP, 2018b).

REFLECT NOW

Consider the community in which your nursing program is located. What are some health disparities that are present within your community?

COMMUNITY-ORIENTED NURSING

Frequently the terms *community health nursing* and *public health nursing* are used interchangeably and fall under the umbrella term *community-oriented nursing*. Community health nursing is nursing practice in the community, with the primary focus on the health care of individuals, families, and groups within the community. The goal is to preserve, protect, promote, or maintain health (Stanhope and Lancaster, 2018). The emphasis of such nursing care is to improve the quality of health and life within a community. Public health nursing is a nursing specialty that requires understanding the needs of a population or a collection of individuals who have one or more personal or environmental characteristics in common (Stanhope and Lancaster, 2018). Examples of populations include high-risk infants, older adults, or an ethnic group such as Native Americans. A public health nurse understands factors that influence health promotion and health maintenance, the trends and patterns influencing the incidence of disease within populations, environmental factors contributing to health and illness, and the political processes that affect public policy. For example, a public health nurse uses data on increased incidence of playground injuries to lobby for a policy to use shock-absorbing material rather than concrete for new public playgrounds.

The community health nurse may also provide direct care services to subpopulations within a community. These subpopulations often have a clinical focus in which the nurse has expertise. For example, a case manager follows older adults recovering from stroke and sees the need for community rehabilitation services, or a nurse practitioner gives immunizations to patients with the objective of managing communicable disease within the community. By focusing on subpopulations, a community health nurse cares for the community and considers an individual or family as only one member of a group at risk. In summary, the focus of community-oriented nursing is on health promotion, disease prevention, and improving quality of life of the population (Stanhope and Lancaster, 2018).

Public health nurses are sometimes required to have a baccalaureate degree in nursing educational preparation and clinical practice in public health nursing. A specialist in public health has a graduate-level education with a focus in the public health sciences (ANA, 2014). Competence as a community health nurse requires the ability to use interventions that include the broad social and political context of the community (Stanhope and Lancaster, 2018). The educational requirements for entry-level nurses practicing in community health nursing roles are not as clear as those for public health nurses. Not all hiring agencies require an advanced degree. However, nurses with a graduate degree in nursing who practice in community settings are considered community health nurse specialists, regardless of their public health experience (Stanhope and Lancaster, 2018).

Nursing Practice in Community Health

Community health nursing practice requires a unique set of skills and knowledge. In the health care delivery system, nurses who become experts in community health practice usually have advanced nursing degrees, yet the baccalaureate-prepared nurse generalist is also able to formulate and apply population-focused assessments and interventions. The expert community health nurse understands the needs of a population or community through experience with individual families or populations, which includes working through their social and health care issues. In this context, critical thinking involves applying knowledge of public health principles, community health nursing, family theory, and communication in finding the best approaches to partner with families.

Successful community health nursing practice involves building relationships with the community and being responsive to changes within the community. For example, when there is an increase in the incidence of grandparents assuming child care responsibilities, a community health nurse becomes an active part of a community by establishing an educational program in cooperation with local schools to assist and support grandparents in this caregiving role. The nurse knows the community members, along with their needs and resources, and works in collaboration with community leaders to establish effective health promotion and disease prevention programs. This requires working with highly resistant systems (e.g., welfare system) and trying to encourage them to be more responsive to the needs of a population. Skills of patient advocacy, communicating people's concerns, and designing new systems in cooperation with existing systems help to make community nursing practice effective.

COMMUNITY-BASED NURSING

Community-based nursing care takes place in community settings such as a home or clinic, where nurses focus on the needs of an individual or family. It involves the safety needs and acute and chronic care of individuals and families, enhances their capacity for self-care, and promotes autonomy in decision making (Stanhope and Lancaster, 2018). Community-based nurses tend to provide illness care within the community setting (Stanhope and Lancaster, 2018). It requires critical thinking and decision making for the individual patient and family—assessing health status, diagnosing health problems, planning care, implementing interventions, and evaluating outcomes of care. Because nurses provide direct care services where patients live, work, and play,

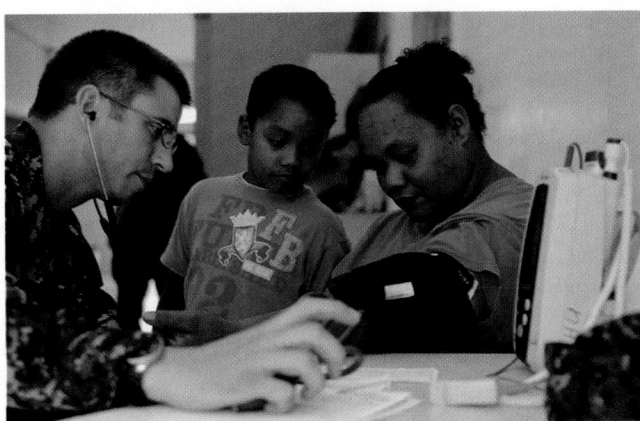

FIG. 3.2 Patient and family receiving care in a community-based care center. (Courtesy Mass Communication Specialist 2nd Class Daniel Viramontes.)

it is important that they place the perspectives of the community members first and foremost when planning care (Stanhope and Lancaster, 2018). This is an example of population-focused care where community is the client.

Community-based nursing centers function as the first level of contact between members of a community and the health care delivery system (Fig. 3.2). Ideally health care services are provided near where patients live, work, and socialize. This approach helps to reduce the cost of health care for the patient and the stress associated with the financial burdens of care. In addition, these centers offer direct access to nurses and comprehensive patient-centered health services and readily incorporate the patient and the patient's family or friends into a plan of care. Community-based nursing centers often care for the most vulnerable of the population (Stanhope and Lancaster, 2018).

With the individual and family as the patients, the context of community-based nursing is family-centered care within the community. This focus requires a strong knowledge base in family theory (see Chapter 10), principles of communication (see Chapter 24), group dynamics, and cultural diversity (see Chapter 9). Nurses partner with their patients and families to enable them to ultimately assume responsibility for their health care decisions.

Vulnerable Populations

Nurses care for patients from diverse cultures and backgrounds and with various health conditions. Changes in the health care delivery system have made high-risk groups the principal patients. For example, you are not likely to visit low-risk mothers and babies. Instead, you are more likely to visit adolescent mothers or mothers with drug addiction. **Vulnerable populations** are groups of patients who are more likely to develop health problems as a result of excess health risks, who are limited in access to health care services, or who depend on others for care. Vulnerable populations include those living in poverty, older adults, the disabled, people who are homeless, immigrants, individuals in abusive relationships, people living with substance abuse, and people with mental illnesses. These vulnerabilities are often associated with the individual's/community's social determinants of health or individual health disparities.

Public and community health nursing and primary care providers share health care responsibility for health promotion, screening, and early detection and disease prevention for vulnerable populations. These patients have intense health care needs that are unmet or ignored or require more care than can be provided in outpatient or hospital settings. Individuals and their families who are vulnerable often belong to more than one of these groups. In addition, health care vulnerability affects all age-groups (Stanhope and Lancaster, 2018).

BOX 3.1 Guidelines for Assessing Members of Vulnerable Population Groups

Setting the Stage
- Create a comfortable, nonthreatening environment.
- Obtain information about a patient's culture so that you understand the practices, beliefs, and values that affect the patient's health care.
- If the patient speaks a different language, use a professional interpreter and observe nonverbal behavior to complete a culturally competent assessment (see Chapter 9).
- Be sensitive to the fact that patients often have priorities other than their health care (e.g., financial, legal, or social issues). Help them with these concerns before beginning a health assessment. If a patient needs financial assistance, consult a social worker. If there are legal issues, provide the patient with a resource. Do not attempt to provide financial or legal advice yourself.

Nursing History of an Individual or Family
- Because you often have only one opportunity to conduct a nursing history, obtain an organized history of all essential information to help an individual or family during that visit.
- Collect data that focus on the specific needs of the vulnerable population with whom you work. However, be flexible so as not to overlook important health information. For example, when with a mother who is an adolescent, obtain a nutritional history on both the mother and baby. Be aware of the developmental needs of the young mother, and listen to her social needs as well.
- Identify both developmental and health care needs. Remember, the goal is to collect enough information to provide family-centered care.
- Identify any risks to the patient's immune system. This is especially important for vulnerable patients who are homeless and sleep in shelters.

Physical Examination and Home Assessment
- Complete a thorough physical and/or home assessment. Only collect data that are relevant to providing care to the patient and family.
- Be alert for signs of physical abuse, substance abuse, or neglect (e.g., inadequately clothed, underweight).
- When assessing a patient's home, observe: Is there adequate water and plumbing? What is the status of the utilities? Are foods and perishables stored properly? Are there signs of insects or vermin? Is the paint peeling? Are the windows and doors adequate? Are there water stains on the ceiling, evidence of a leaky roof? What is the temperature? Is it comfortable? What does the outside environment look like: Are there vacant houses/lots nearby? Is there a busy intersection? What is the crime level?

Modified from Stanhope M, Lancaster J: *Foundations for population health in community/public health nursing*, ed 5, St Louis, 2018, Mosby.

Patients who are vulnerable often come from various cultures, have different beliefs and values, face language and literacy barriers, or have few sources of social support. These diverse needs will be challenging as you care for patients with increasingly complex acute and chronic health conditions. To provide competent care for vulnerable populations, you need to assess these patients accurately (Box 3.1). In addition, you need to evaluate and understand a patient's and family's cultural beliefs, values, and practices to determine their specific needs and the interventions that will be most successful in improving their state of health (see Chapter 9). It is important not to judge or evaluate your patient's beliefs and values about health in terms of your own culture, beliefs, and values. Communication and caring practices are critical in learning a patient's perceptions of his or her problems and then planning health care strategies that will be meaningful, culturally appropriate, and successful.

Barriers to access and use of services often lead to adverse health outcomes for vulnerable populations (ODPHP, 2018b). Because of these poorer outcomes, vulnerable populations have shorter life spans and higher morbidity rates. Members of vulnerable groups frequently have multiple risk factors, resulting in cumulative effects of individual risk factors. It is essential for community-based nurses to assess members of vulnerable populations by considering the multiple stressors that affect their patients' lives. It is also important to learn patients' strengths and resources for coping with stressors. Complete assessment of vulnerable populations enables a community-based nurse to design interventions within the context of the patient's community (Stanhope and Lancaster, 2018).

Immigrant Population. The CDC (2018b) predicts a continued increase in the immigrant population. This continued growth creates many social and health care needs. Social problems involved with immigration sometimes include poverty, acculturation, education, housing, and employment. Some immigrant populations face multiple diverse health issues that cities, counties, and states need to address. These health care needs pose significant legal and policy issues. For some immigrants, access to health care is limited because of language barriers and/or lack of benefits, resources, and transportation. Immigrant populations often have higher rates of hypertension, diabetes mellitus, and infectious diseases; decreased outcomes of care; and shorter life expectancies (Stanhope and Lancaster, 2018).

Frequently patients from immigrant populations practice nontraditional healing practices (see Chapter 9). Although many of these healing practices are effective and complement traditional therapies, it is important that you know how the therapies act physically and understand your patient's health beliefs about these healing practices.

Certain immigrant populations left their homes as a result of oppression, war, or natural disaster. You must be sensitive to these physical and psychological stressors and identify the appropriate resources to help your patients meet their health care needs (Stanhope and Lancaster, 2018).

Effects of Poverty and Homelessness. People who live in poverty are more likely to have more health disparities because they are at a higher risk of living in hazardous environments, working at high-risk jobs, eating less nutritious diets, having multiple stressors in their lives, lacking adequate transportation, and being homeless. Patients who are experiencing homelessness have even fewer resources than people who are poor. They are often jobless, do not have the advantage of a permanent shelter, and must continually cope with finding food and a place to sleep at night. Chronic health problems tend to worsen because of poor nutrition and the inability to store nutritional foods. In addition, people who are experiencing homelessness usually have barriers to accessing health care, causing them to seek health care in emergency departments (American Public Health Association [APHA], 2017).

REFLECT NOW

What health care resources are available to help the homeless and those living in poverty within your community? How can you participate in providing health care to these vulnerable groups?

Patients Who Are Abused. Physical, emotional, and sexual abuse and neglect are major public health problems that often affect older adults, women, and children. Risk factors for abusive relationships include mental health problems, substance abuse, socioeconomic stressors, lack of understanding of child development or parenting skills, and dysfunctional family relationships (CDC, 2018a). For some, risk factors may not be present. When dealing with patients at risk for or who have suffered abuse, it is important to provide protection. Interview a patient you suspect is abused at a time when the patient has privacy and the individual suspected of being the abuser is not present. Patients who are abused may fear retribution if they discuss their problems with a health care provider. Nurses must use therapeutic communication techniques that reinforce that the abuse is not the victim's fault. Nurses are mandatory reporters for abuse involving elders over the age of 65, children under the age of 18, and disabled individuals.

Patients With Mental Illness. Patients with severe mental illness such as schizophrenia or bipolar disorder may experience multiple health and socioeconomic problems. Many patients with severe mental illnesses are homeless or live in poverty and lack the ability to remain employed or to care for themselves on a daily basis (APHA, 2015). Patients who have a mental illness often require medication therapy, counseling, housing, and vocational assistance. In addition, they are at a greater risk for abuse and assault. Patients with mental illnesses are no longer routinely hospitalized in long-term psychiatric institutions. Instead, resources are offered within the community. Although comprehensive service networks may be available in the community, many patients still go untreated or undertreated because of an inability to navigate the health care system (Stanhope and Lancaster, 2018).

Older Adults. The older adult population is increasing, resulting in simultaneous increases in the number of patients suffering from chronic diseases and a greater demand for health care services. Take time to understand what health means to an older adult and which assessment findings to expect; view health promotion in the older adult within a broad context (see Chapter 14). Help older adults and their families understand which steps they need to take to maintain their health and improve their level of function through physical activity (APHA, 2015). Design appropriate community-based interventions that provide an opportunity to improve the lifestyle and quality of life of older adults (Table 3.1).

Competency in Community-Based Nursing

A nurse in community-based practice needs a variety of skills and talents to be successful. In addition to assisting patients with their health care needs and developing relationships within the community, the community-based nurse needs skills in health promotion and disease prevention. Nurses use the nursing process and critical thinking (see Unit III) to ensure individualized nursing care for specific patients and their families. Students' clinical practice in a community-based care setting will probably be in partnership with a community nurse.

Caregiver. First and foremost a nurse is a caregiver (see Chapter 1). In the community setting you manage and care for the health of patients and families in the community. Use a critical thinking approach to apply the nursing process (see Unit III) and ensure appropriate, individualized nursing care for your patients and their families.

Historically, well-baby and child care was integral to community nursing practices. Community child care services are increasing to address changes in the health care delivery system, changing economics, homelessness, and the increased number of people who are medically underinsured. Community nurses are undertaking more complex and expanded child health services for increasingly diverse client populations (ODPHP, 2018e).

In addition, the community nurse must individualize care within the context of a patient's community so that long-term success is more likely. Together with a patient and family you develop a caring

TABLE 3.1 Major Health Problems in Older Adults and Community-Based Nursing Roles and Interventions

Problem	Community-Based Nursing Roles and Interventions
Hypertension	Monitor blood pressure and weight; educate about nutrition and antihypertensive drugs; teach stress management techniques; promote a good balance between rest and activity; establish blood pressure screening programs; assess patient's current lifestyle and promote lifestyle changes; promote dietary modifications by using techniques such as a diet diary.
Cancer	Obtain health history; promote monthly breast self-examinations and recommended screening intervals for Papanicolaou (Pap) smears and mammograms for older women; promote colorectal screening; promote regular physical examinations; encourage smokers to stop smoking; correct misconceptions about processes of aging; provide emotional support and quality of care during diagnostic and treatment procedures.
Arthritis	Educate about management of activities, reducing stress on affected joints, availability of mechanical appliances, and adequate rest; promote stress management; counsel and assist the family to improve communication, role negotiation, and use of community resources.
Visual impairment (e.g., loss of visual acuity, eyelid disorders, opacity of the lens)	Provide support in a well-lighted, glare-free environment; use printed aids with large, well-spaced letters; help adult clean eyeglasses; help make arrangements for vision examinations and obtain necessary prostheses.
Hearing impairment (e.g., presbycusis)	Speak with clarity at a moderate volume and pace, and face audience when performing health teaching; help make arrangements for hearing examination and obtain necessary prostheses; teach how to care for hearing aids.
Cognitive impairment	Provide complete assessment; correct underlying causes of impairment (if possible); provide for a protective environment; promote activities that reinforce reality; help with personal hygiene, nutrition, and hydration; provide emotional support to the family; recommend applicable community resources such as adult day care, home care aides, and homemaker services.
Dementia	Maintain high-level functioning, protection, and safety; encourage human dignity; demonstrate to the primary family caregiver techniques to dress, feed, and toilet adult; provide frequent encouragement and emotional support to caregiver; act as an advocate for patient when dealing with respite care and support groups; protect the patient's rights; provide caregiver support to maintain family members' physical and mental health and to prevent caregiver role strain; maintain family stability; recommend financial services if needed.
Dental problems	Perform oral assessment and refer to dentist as necessary; emphasize regular brushing and flossing, proper nutrition, and dental examinations; encourage patients with dentures to wear and take care of them; calm fears about dentist; help provide access to financial services (if necessary) and dental care resources.
Substance and alcohol abuse	Get drug use history; educate about safe storage, risks for drug, drug-drug, drug-alcohol, and drug-food interactions; give general information about drug (e.g., drug name, purpose, side effects, dosage); instruct adult about presorting techniques (using small containers with one dose of drug that are labeled with specific times to take drug). Counsel adults about substance abuse; promote stress management to avoid need for drugs or alcohol and arrange for and monitor detoxification if appropriate. Provide community resources for substance abuse treatment.
Sexually transmitted infections	Perform a full sexual risk assessment and bring awareness regarding risk factors and susceptibility to human immunodeficiency virus/acquired immunodeficiency syndrome (HIV/AIDS). Educate about safe sexual practices such as abstinence or use of condoms, and refer as necessary for HIV and other infection testing and HPV immunization.

Data from Stanhope M, Lancaster J: *Foundations for population health in community/public health nursing*, ed 5, St Louis, 2018, Mosby; National Prevention, Health Promotion, and Public Health Council: Healthy aging in action: advancing the national prevention strategy, 2016, https://www.cdc.gov/aging/publications/reports.htm. Accessed May 20, 2019; Centers for Disease Control and Prevention (CDC): Health information for older adults, 2018, https://www.cdc.gov/aging/aginginfo/index.htm. Accessed May 20, 2019.

partnership to recognize actual and potential health care needs and identify needed community resources. For example, if a patient is placed on an exercise program, you recommend a safe park or recreational area where the patient can exercise. Competent community-based practice builds healthy communities that are safe and include elements to enable people to achieve and maintain a high quality of life.

> **QSEN Building Competency in Safety** Maria Perez is a 74-year-old widow with heart failure (HF) who has been referred to the Home Care Agency for services. Maria has been admitted to the hospital three times in the past two months. Two admissions were for HF exacerbation and the other was for a fractured wrist after falling in the bathroom. Maria lives alone in a senior housing apartment building that has an elevator. The hospitalist requests a home safety evaluation, along with assessment of medication management. What information does the nurse need to begin this assessment?
>
> Answers to QSEN Activities can be found on the Evolve website.

Case Manager. In community-based practice, case management is an important competency (see Chapter 2). Case managers establish an appropriate plan of care based on assessment of patients and families and coordinate needed resources and services for a patient's well-being across a continuum of care. Generally, a community-based case manager assumes responsibility for the case management of multiple patients. The greatest challenge is to coordinate the activities of multiple providers and payers in different settings throughout a patient's continuum of care. An effective case manager eventually learns the obstacles, limits, and even the opportunities that exist within the community that influence the ability to find solutions for patients' health care needs.

Change Agent. A community-based nurse is also a change agent. This involves identifying and implementing new and more effective approaches to problems. You act as a change agent within a family system or as a mediator for problems within a patient's community. You identify any number of problems (e.g., quality of community child care services, availability of older-adult day care services, or the status of neighborhood violence). As a change agent you empower individuals and their families to creatively solve problems or become instrumental in creating change within a health care agency. For example, if your patient has difficulty keeping regular health care visits, you determine why. Maybe the health clinic is too far and difficult to reach, or perhaps the hours of service are incompatible with a patient's transportation resources. You work with the patient to solve the problem and help identify an alternative site such as a nursing clinic that is closer and has more convenient hours.

To effect change, you gather and analyze facts before you implement programs to help people make changes to improve their health. This requires you to be very familiar with the community itself. Many communities resist change, preferring to provide services in the established manner. Before analyzing facts, it is often necessary to manage conflict among the health care providers, clarify their roles, and clearly identify the needs of the patients. If the community has a history of poor problem solving, you will have to focus on developing problem-solving capabilities (Stanhope and Lancaster, 2018).

Patient Advocate. Patient advocacy is important in community-based practice mainly because of the confusion surrounding access to health care services. Patients often need someone to help them walk through the system and identify where to go for services, how to reach individuals with the appropriate authority, which services to request, and how to follow through with the information they receive. As a patient advocate, you ensure patients have the information necessary to make informed decisions in choosing and using services appropriately. In addition, it is important for you to support and at times defend your patients' decisions.

Collaborator. Community-based nursing practice requires you to be competent in communicating and working with patients, their families, and other members of the health care team. Collaboration, or working in a combined effort with all those involved in care delivery, is necessary to develop a mutually acceptable plan that will achieve common goals (Stanhope and Lancaster, 2018). For example, when your patient is discharged home with terminal cancer, you collaborate with hospice staff, social workers, and pastoral care to initiate a plan to support interprofessional end-of-life care for the patient in the home and support the family. For collaboration to be effective, you need mutual trust and respect for each professional's roles, abilities, and contributions.

Counselor. To be an effective counselor, you need to be aware of a patient's community resources (e.g., mental health clinics, day care services, respite care). A counselor helps patients identify and clarify health problems as well as choose appropriate courses of action to solve those problems. For example, if you are a nurse in an employee-assistance program or a women's shelter, you will often assume the role of counselor with your patients. As a counselor, you are responsible for providing information; listening objectively; and being supportive, caring, and trustworthy. You do not make decisions but rather help your patients reach decisions that are best for them (Stanhope and Lancaster, 2018). Patients and families often require assistance in first identifying and clarifying health problems. For example, a patient who repeatedly reports a problem in following a prescribed diet is unable to afford nutritious foods or has family members who do not support healthy eating habits. You discuss with your patient factors that block or aid problem resolution, identify a range of solutions, and then discuss which solutions are most likely to be successful. You also encourage your patient to make decisions and express your confidence in the choice the patient makes.

Educator. Patient education is often a priority in community-based nursing. Become familiar with community service organizations that offer educational support to a wide range of individuals and patient groups. Prenatal classes, infant care, child safety, and cancer screening are just some of the health education programs provided in a community.

When the goal is to help your patients assume responsibility for their own health care, being an educator takes on greater importance (Stanhope and Lancaster, 2018). Patients and families need to gain skills and knowledge to care for themselves. Assess your patient's learning needs and readiness to learn within the context of the individual, the systems with which the individual interacts (e.g., family, business, and school), and the resources available for support. Adapt your teaching skills so you can instruct a patient within the home setting and make the learning process meaningful. Community-based nursing gives you the opportunity to follow patients over time. Planning for return demonstration of skills, using follow-up phone calls, and referring to community support and self-help groups give you an opportunity to provide continuity of instruction and reinforce important instructional topics and learned behaviors (see Chapter 25).

Epidemiologist. As a community-based nurse, you apply principles of epidemiology, the science dealing with the incidence, distribution, and possible control of diseases and other health problems. Your contacts with families, community groups such as schools and industries, and health care agencies place you in a unique position to initiate epidemiological activities, such as case finding, health teaching, and tracking incident rates of an illness. For example, a cafeteria worker in the local high school is diagnosed with active tuberculosis (TB). As a community health nurse, you help find where the exposure to TB may have occurred, such as within the worker's home, place of employment, or community.

Nurse epidemiologists are responsible for community surveillance (e.g., tracking incidence of elevated lead levels in children and identifying increased fetal and infant mortality rates, increases in adolescent pregnancy, presence of infectious and communicable diseases, and outbreaks of head lice). Nurse epidemiologists protect the level of health of the community, develop sensitivity to changes in the health status of the community, and help identify the cause of these changes.

COMMUNITY ASSESSMENT

When practicing in a community setting, you need to learn how to assess the community at large. Community assessment is the systematic data collection on the population, monitoring the health status of the population, and making information available about the health of the community (Stanhope and Lancaster, 2018). This is the environment in which patients live, work, play, and learn. Without an adequate understanding of that environment, any effort to promote a patient's health and bring about necessary change is unlikely to be successful. The community has three components: structure or locale, the people, and the social systems. To develop a complete community assessment, take a careful look at each of the three components to identify needs for health policy, health programs, and needed health services (Box 3.2).

When assessing the structure or locale, you travel around the neighborhood or community and observe its design, the location of services, and where residents meet. As you assess the physical environment, you look for possible environmental hazards in the air, water, or soil, as well as safety issues, such as abandoned buildings, a lack of sidewalks, or roads that are in poor repair. You obtain the demographics of the population by accessing statistics on the community from reliable websites, a local public health department or public library. You acquire information about existing social systems such as schools or health care agencies by visiting various sites and learning about their services.

Once you have a good understanding of the community, you can perform all individual patient assessments against that background. For example, when assessing a patient's home for safety, you consider the following: Does the patient have secure locks on doors? Are windows

BOX 3.2   Community Assessment

Structure
- Name of community or neighborhood
- Geographical boundaries
- Emergency services
- Water and sanitation
- Housing
- Economic status (e.g., average household income, number of residents on public assistance)
- Transportation
- Safety

Population
- Age distribution
- Sex distribution
- Growth trends
- Density
- Education level
- Predominant ethnic groups
- Predominant religious groups

Social System
- Educational system
- Government
- Communication system
- Welfare system
- Volunteer programs
- Health system

secure and intact? Is lighting along walkways and entryways operational? As you conduct a patient assessment, it is important to know the level of community violence and the resources available when help is necessary. Always assess an individual in the context of the community.

REFLECT NOW

Complete a community assessment in the area surrounding your nursing program. What are the demographics of the population? What social systems exist within the community?

CHANGING PATIENTS' HEALTH

In community-based practice, nurses care for patients from diverse backgrounds and in diverse settings. It is relatively easy over time to become familiar with the available resources within a community practice setting. Likewise, with practice you learn how to identify the unique needs of individual patients. Similarly, you bring together the resources necessary to improve a patient's continuity of care. When you collaborate with your patients and their health care providers, you provide patient-centered care and help reduce duplication of health care services. For example, when caring for a patient with a healing wound, you coordinate wound care services and help the patient and family locate cost-effective dressing materials.

You need to promote and protect a patient's health within the context of the community using an evidence-based practice approach when possible. For example, nurses can help reduce health disparities surrounding childhood obesity in racial/ethnic minority populations through community engagement (Frerichs et al., 2018; Luesse et al., 2018; Subica et al., 2016) (Box 3.3). Frerichs et al. (2018) investigated the effect of an evidence-based community approach to develop strategies to support reducing obesity risk factors among minority groups. Evidence showed that community involvement in collaborative initiatives has a high success rate in reducing obesity among racial/ethnic minority children.

While providing community-based nursing care, it is important to consider how well you understand your patients' lives. You begin by establishing strong, caring relationships with your patients and their families (see Chapter 7). As you gain experience and are accepted by a patient's family, you are able to advise, counsel, and teach effectively and understand what truly makes your patient unique. The day-to-day activities of family life are the variables that influence how you will adapt nursing interventions.

BOX 3.3   EVIDENCE-BASED PRACTICE

Promoting Community Involvement in Reducing Childhood Obesity in Racial/Ethnic Minority Population

PICOT Question: Do community-based interventions decrease childhood obesity rates in diverse populations?

Evidence Summary

Obesity is more prevalent in children from ethnically diverse populations in the United States (Isong et al., 2018). Research has found that there are genetic, epigenetic, biological, social, and environmental risk factors associated with obesity in children (Isong et al., 2018). Current evidence shows links between childhood obesity and ethnicity, lack of physical activity, increased screen time from television and electronics, nutrition, sleep, and socioeconomic status, as well as maternal smoking and breastfeeding (Alexander, 2017; Isong et al., 2018). Childhood obesity has lifelong physical, mental, and social health consequences (Alexander, 2017; Sato et al., 2016).

Evidence shows that early interventions are most successful in decreasing racial/ethnic disparities related to childhood obesity (Isong et al., 2018). Adult perceptions of obesity must align with interventions for success (Alexander, 2017). Evidence shows that when caregivers perceive interventions as useful, children have greater success in adhering to interventions to address obesity (Alexander, 2017). Asking children to adhere to lifestyle changes without adult support and role modeling will not result in positive outcomes (Stanhope and Lancaster, 2018; Trude et al., 2018).

Community involvement is a key element in reducing health disparities (Subica et al., 2018). Community engagement in childhood obesity programs can include community workshops and media resources to gain attendance and community buy-in (Luesse et al., 2018). Collaborative initiatives with community involvement have high success rates in reducing obesity among children, especially those from a variety of racial and ethnic groups (Frerichs et al., 2018). Public policy must ensure that people from underserved communities have access to healthful food choices as well as improved socioenvironmental areas (Stanhope and Lancaster, 2018; Subica et al., 2018). It is important to ensure that families have access to the recommended food to ensure that healthy choices can be followed through on (Frerichs et al., 2018; Luesse et al., 2018). Communities can also help address the socioenvironmental aspects associated with obesity such as underutilized parks (Frerichs et al., 2018). With collaborative community partnerships, childhood obesity in the racial/ethnic minority population can be reduced.

Application to Nursing Practice
- Understand the modifiable risk factors for obesity and design effective interventions targeted at reducing the risk factors (Isong et al., 2018). Interventions need to include both diet and physical activity recommendations (Alexander, 2017). Nutritional information must include information pertaining to both the school and home environments (Luesse et al., 2018). Include culturally and linguistically appropriate interventions and communication, especially when providing care to patients who are from ethnically diverse populations (Luesse et al., 2018).
- Community involvement is a key element in reducing health disparities (Subica et al., 2016). Community engagement in childhood obesity programs can include community workshops and media resources to gain attendance and community buy-in (Luesse et al., 2018).

The time of day a patient goes to work, the availability of the spouse and patient's parents to provide child care, and the family values that shape views about health are just a few examples of the many factors you will consider in community-based practice. Once you acquire a picture of a patient's life, you then design patient-centered interventions to promote health and prevent disease within the community-based practice setting.

KEY POINTS

- The terms *community health nursing* and *public health nursing* are used interchangeably and fall under the umbrella term *community-oriented nursing.*
- The community-oriented nurse's focus is on health promotion, disease prevention, and improving quality of life of the population, while the focus of the community-based nurse is to provide direct illness care to individuals and families within the community setting.
- Vulnerable populations are groups of patients who are more likely to develop health problems as a result of excess health risks, who have limited access to health care services, or who depend on others for care. Individuals living in poverty, older adults, people who are homeless, immigrant populations, individuals in abusive relationships, people with substance abuse disorders, and people with severe mental illnesses are examples of vulnerable populations.
- The community-based nurse needs skills in health promotion, disease prevention, and relationship building to fill the role of caregiver, case manager, change agent, patient advocate, collaborator, counselor, educator, and epidemiologist.
- Community assessment is the systematic collection of data on the population, monitoring of the health status of the population, and making information available about the health of the community. Community assessment includes structure, population, and social system.

REFLECTIVE LEARNING

- What population in the community do you see most frequently in your clinical setting? What are some nursing assessments, skills, or tasks you are able to perform with this population?
- In your clinical setting, what nursing education or community resources do you provide to patients? Do you think the method used to disseminate this information is adequate to meet the patients' needs? Explain your answer.
- Identify key information you learned in your clinical setting that you can take with you in your future nursing practice. How were you inspired to improve your nursing knowledge, practice, and skills by the people you worked with?

REVIEW QUESTIONS

1. Using *Healthy People 2020* as a guide, which of the following would improve delivery of care to a community? (Select all that apply.)
   1. Community assessment
   2. Implementation of public health policies
   3. Home safety assessment
   4. Increased access to care
   5. Determining rates of specific illnesses
2. A community health nurse is working in a clinic with a focus on asthma and allergies. What is the primary focus of the community health nurse in this clinic setting? (Select all that apply.)
   1. Decrease the incidence of asthma attacks in the community
   2. Increase patients' ability to self-manage their asthma
   3. Treat acute asthma in the hospital
   4. Provide asthma education programs for the teachers in the local schools
   5. Provide scheduled immunizations to people who come to the clinic

3. The nurse caring for a refugee community identifies that the children are undervaccinated and the community is unaware of resources. The nurse assesses the community and determines that there is a health clinic within a 5-mile radius. The nurse meets with the community leaders and explains the need for immunizations, the location of the clinic, and the process of accessing health care resources. Which of the following practices is the nurse providing? (Select all that apply.)
   1. Raising awareness about community resources for the children
   2. Teaching the community about health promotion and illness prevention
   3. Promoting autonomy in decision making about health practices
   4. Improving the health care of the community's children
   5. Participating in professional development activities to maintain nursing competency
4. What factor results in vulnerable populations being more likely to develop health problems?
   1. The ability to use available resources to find housing
   2. Adequate transportation to the grocery store and community clinics
   3. Availability of others to help provide care
   4. Limited access to health care services
5. Many older homes in a neighborhood are undergoing a lot of restoration. Lead paint was used to paint the homes when they were built. The community clinic in the neighborhood is initiating a lead screening program. This activity is based on which social determinant of health?
6. A community health nurse conducts a community assessment focused on adolescent health behaviors. The nurse determines that a large number of adolescents smoke. Designing a smoking cessation program at the youth community center is an example of which nursing role?
   1. Educator
   2. Counselor
   3. Collaborator
   4. Case manager
7. A nurse in a community health clinic reviews screening results from students in a local high school during the most recent academic year. The nurse discovers a 10% increase in the number of positive tuberculosis (TB) skin tests when comparing these numbers to the previous year. The nurse contacts the school nurse and the director of the health department. Together they begin to expand their assessment to all students and employees of the school district. The community nurse was acting in which nursing role(s)? (Select all that apply.)
   1. Epidemiologist
   2. Counselor
   3. Collaborator
   4. Case manager
   5. Caregiver
8. A nursing student is giving a presentation to a group of other nursing students about the needs of patients with mental illnesses in the community. Which statement by the student indicates that the nursing professor needs to provide further teaching?
   1. "Many patients with mental illness do not have a permanent home."
   2. "Unemployment is a common problem experienced by people with a mental illness."
   3. "The majority of patients with mental illnesses live in long-term care settings."
   4. "Patients with mental illnesses are often at a higher risk for abuse and assault."

9. The nurse in a new community-based clinic is requested to complete a community assessment. Order the steps for completing this assessment.
   1. Structure or locale
   2. Social systems
   3. Population
10. The public health nurse is working with the county health department on a task force to fully integrate the goals of *Healthy People 2020*. Most of the immigrant population do not have a primary care provider, nor do they participate in health promotion activities; the unemployment rate in the community is 25%. How does the nurse determine which goals need to be included or updated? (Select all that apply.)

1. Assess the health care resources within the community.
2. Assess the existing health care programs offered by the county health department.
3. Compare existing resources and programs with *Healthy People 2020* goals.
4. Initiate new programs to meet *Healthy People 2020* goals.
5. Implement educational sessions in the schools to focus on nutritional needs of the children.

Answers: 1. 1, 2, 4, 5; **2.** 1, 2, 4, 3; **3.** 1, 2, 4, 4; **5.** Physical environment; **6.** 2; **7.** 1, 3; **8.** 1, 3, 2; **9.** 3; **10.** 1, 2, 3.

Rationales for Review Questions can be found on the Evolve website.

REFERENCES

American Nurses Association (ANA): *Public health nursing*, n.d. https://www.nursingworld.org/practice-policy/workforce/public-health-nursing/. Accessed 20 May 2019.

American Nurses Association (ANA): *Standards of public health nursing practice*, ed 2, Washington, DC, 2014, The Association.

American Public Health Association (APHA): *APHA policy statement 201514: building environments and a public health workforce to support physical activity among older adults*, 2015, https://www.apha.org/policies-and-advocacy/public-health-policy-statements/policy-database/2016/01/26/14/18/building-environments-and-a-public-health-workforce-to-support-physical-activity-among-older-adults. Accessed 20 May 2019.

American Public Health Association (APHA): *APHA policy statement 20178: housing and homelessness as a public health issue*, 2017, https://www.apha.org/policies-and-advocacy/public-health-policy-statements/policy-database/2018/01/18/housing-and-homelessness-as-a-public-health-issue. Accessed 20 May 2019.

Centers for Disease Control and Prevention (CDC): *Health-related quality of life*, 2016, https://www.cdc.gov/hrqol/wellbeing.htm. Accessed 20 May 2019.

Centers for Disease Control and Prevention (CDC): *Child abuse and neglect: risk and protective factors*, 2018a, https://www.cdc.gov/violenceprevention/childabuseandneglect/riskprotectivefactors.html. Accessed 20 May 2019.

Centers for Disease Control and Prevention (CDC): *Immigrant and refugee health*, 2018b, https://www.cdc.gov/immigrantrefugeehealth/. Accessed 20 May 2019.

Centers for Disease Control and Prevention (CDC): *Social determinants of health: know what affects health*, 2018c, http://www.cdc.gov/socialdeterminants/faqs/index.htm. Accessed 20 May 2019.

Centers for Medicare and Medicaid Services (CMS): Home- and community-based services, 2017, https://www.cms.gov/Outreach-and-Education/American-Indian-Alaska-Native/AIAN/LTSS-TA-Center/info/hcbs.html. Accessed 20 May 2019.

Croft JB, et al.: Urban-rural county and state differences in chronic obstructive pulmonary disease — United States, 2015, *MMWR* 67(7):205–211, February 23, 2018. https://www.cdc.gov/mmwr/volumes/67/wr/mm6707a1.htm?s_cid=mm6707a1_w/. Accessed 20 May 2019.

Davis CS, et al.: Overdose epidemic, prescription monitoring programs, and public health: a review of state laws, *Am J Public Health* 105(11):e9–e11, 2015.

Kennedy C, et al.: Blood lead levels among children aged <6 years: Flint, Michigan, 2013–2016, *MMWR* 65(25):650–654, July 1, 2016, https://www.cdc.gov/mmwr/volumes/65/wr/mm6525e1.htm?s_cid=mm6525e1_w. Accessed 20 May 2019.

Office of Disease Prevention and Health Promotion (ODPHP): *Healthy People 2020: about healthy people*, 2018a, https://www.healthypeople.gov/2020/About-Healthy-People. Accessed 20 May 2019.

Office of Disease Prevention and Health Promotion (ODPHP): *Healthy People 2020: access to health services*, 2018b, https://www.healthypeople.gov/2020/topics-objectives/topic/Access-to-Health-Services. Accessed 20 May 2019.

Office of Disease Prevention and Health Promotion (ODPHP): *Healthy People 2020: determinants of health*, 2018c, https://www.healthypeople.gov/2020/about/foundation-health-measures/Determinants-of-Health. Accessed 20 May 2019.

Office of Disease Prevention and Health Promotion (ODPHP): *Healthy People 2020: leading health indicators*, 2018d, https://www.healthypeople.gov/2020/Leading-Health-Indicators. Accessed 20 May 2019.

Office of Disease Prevention and Health Promotion (ODPHP): *Healthy People 2020: maternal, infant, and child health*, 2018e, https://www.healthypeople.gov/2020/topics-objectives/topic/maternal-infant-and-child-health. Accessed 20 May 2019.

Stanhope M, Lancaster J: *Foundations for population health in community/public health nursing*, ed 5, St Louis, 2018, Mosby.

RESEARCH REFERENCES

Alexander D, et al.: Do maternal caregiver perceptions of childhood obesity risk factors and obesity complications predict support for prevention initiatives among African Americans, *Matern Child Health J* 21(7):1522–1530, 2017.

Frerichs L, et al.: Development of a systems science curriculum to engage rural African American teens in understanding and addressing childhood obesity prevention, *Health Educ Behav* 45(3):423–434, 2018.

Isong IA, et al.: Racial and ethnic disparities in early childhood obesity, *Pediatrics* 141(1):1–11, 2018.

Luesse HB, et al.: Challenges and facilitators to promoting a healthy food environment and communicating effectively with parents to improve food behaviors of school children, *Matern Child Health J* 22(7):958–967, 2018.

Sato PM, et al.: A youth mentor-led nutritional intervention in urban recreation centers: a promising strategy for childhood obesity prevention in low-income neighborhoods, *Health Educ Res* 31(2):195–206, 2016.

Subica AM, et al.: Communities of color creating healthy environments to combat childhood obesity, *Am J Public Health* 106(1):78–86, 2016.

Trude ACB, et al.: A youth-leader program in Baltimore City recreation centers: lessons learned and applications, *Health Promot Pract* 19(1):75–85, 2018.

4

Theoretical Foundations of Nursing Practice

OBJECTIVES

- Analyze the components of a theory.
- Recognize the evolution of nursing theory.
- Describe types of nursing theories.
- Describe theory-based nursing practice.

- Review selected shared theories from other disciplines.
- Review selected nursing theories
- Understand the use of theories in nursing research.

KEY TERMS

Assumptions, p. 43
Conceptual framework, p. 43
Concepts, p. 43
Content, p. 46
Descriptive theories, p. 45
Domain, p. 43
Environment/situation, p. 44
Feedback, p. 45
Grand theories, p. 44

Health, p. 43
Input, p. 45
Metatheory, p. 42
Middle-range theories, p. 45
Nursing, p. 44
Nursing metaparadigm, p. 43
Nursing theory, p. 43
Output, p. 45
Paradigm, p. 43

Person, p. 43
Phenomenon, p. 43
Practice theories, p. 45
Prescriptive theories, p. 45
Shared theory, p. 45
Theory, p. 42

MEDIA RESOURCES

http://evolve.elsevier.com/Potter/fundamentals/
- Review Questions
- Case Study with Questions

- Audio Glossary
- Content Updates
- Answers to QSEN Activity and Review Questions

Providing patient-centered nursing care is an expectation for all nurses. As you progress through your nursing classes, you will learn to apply knowledge from nursing; social, physical, and biobehavioral sciences; ethics; and health policy. Theory-based nursing practice helps you to design and implement nursing interventions that address individual and family responses to health problems. Some nurses find nursing theory difficult to understand or appreciate. However, as your knowledge about theories improves, you will find that nursing theories help to describe, explain, predict, and/or prescribe nursing care measures.

Common questions nurses have about theory include: What is theory? How are nursing theories created? Why is theory important to the nursing profession? This chapter answers these questions and will help you understand how to use theory in your nursing practice.

Imagine that you are building a house. You need to complete the foundation before you start building the walls. Without a strong foundation, the house will collapse. Such is the case with nursing practice. Theory serves as the foundation for nursing care. Nurses use theory every day but are not always aware of it. For example, when a nurse ensures that a patient's room is free of clutter, excess noise, and soiled linens, the nurse is using Florence Nightingale's environmental theory to promote healing and comfort. A nurse uses Imogene King's theory of goal attainment when encouraging patients to set goals for their recovery. A nurse uses Dorothea Orem's self-care deficit theory when feeding or bathing a patient until the patient is able to do this independently. Even though the term *theory* may sound intimidating, you will find that it is a standard part of everyday nursing practice.

The scientific work used to develop theories expands the scientific knowledge of the profession. Theories offer well-grounded rationales for how and why nurses perform specific interventions and for predicting patient behaviors and outcomes. Expertise in nursing is a result of knowledge and clinical experience. Nursing knowledge improves nursing practice by connecting theory and research. Theory, research, and practice are bound together in a continuous interactive relationship (Fig. 4.1). Nurses develop theories to explain the relationship among variables. Theories may be tested through critical reasoning, description of personal experiences, and use in practice. Throughout this process new information often comes to light that indicates the need to revise a theory, and the cycle repeats (Meleis, 2018). Throughout your nursing career you need to reflect and learn from your experiences to grow professionally and use well-developed theories as a basis for your approach to patient care.

THEORY

What is theory? A theory helps explain an event by defining ideas or concepts, explaining relationships among the concepts, and predicting outcomes (McEwen and Wills, 2019). In the case of nursing, theories are designed to explain a phenomenon such as self-care or caring.

A metatheory is an area of study that looks at the relationships of various components that make up the knowledge of a discipline. These include philosophical, theoretical, and empirical components and provide a broad overview of discipline. Metatheory is used to derive theories and theoretical concepts (Reed and Shearer, 2018).

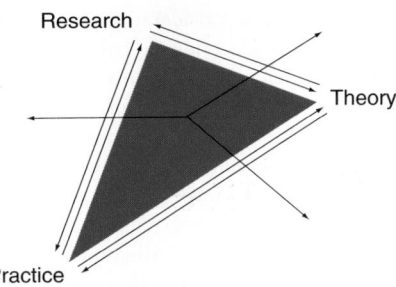

FIG. 4.1 Cyclical relationship among theory, research, and practice. (From LoBiondo-Wood G, Haber J: *Nursing research: methods for critical appraisal for evidence-based practice,* ed 9, St Louis, 2018, Elsevier.)

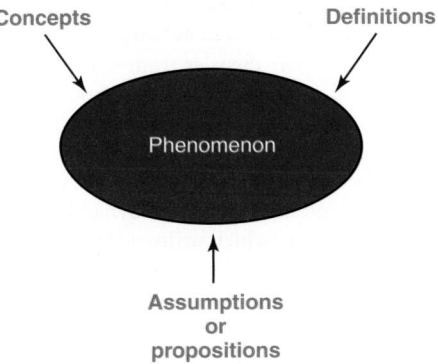

FIG. 4.2 Components of a nursing theory.

A **nursing theory** conceptualizes an aspect of nursing to describe, explain, predict, or prescribe nursing care (Meleis, 2018). Theories offer a perspective for assessing your patients' situations. They also help you organize, analyze, and interpret data. For example, if you use Orem's theory in practice, you assess and interpret data to determine patients' self-care needs, deficits, and abilities in the management of their disease. Orem's theory then guides your development of patient-centered nursing interventions.

Nursing is both a science and an art. The *science* of nursing is based on data obtained from current research, whereas the *art* of nursing stems from a nurse's experience and the unique caring relationship that a nurse develops with a patient (Chinn and Kramer, 2018). A nursing theory helps to identify the focus, means, and goals of practice. Nursing theories enhance communication and accountability for patient care (Meleis, 2018).

Components of a Theory

A theory contains a set of concepts, definitions, and assumptions or propositions that explain a phenomenon. It explains how these elements are uniquely related to the phenomenon (Fig. 4.2). These components provide a foundation of knowledge for nurses to direct and deliver caring nursing practices. Researchers test theories, and as a result they gain a clearer perspective and understanding of all parts of a phenomenon.

Phenomenon. Nursing theories focus on the phenomena of nursing and nursing care. A **phenomenon** is the term, description, or label given to describe an idea or responses about an event, a situation, a process, a group of events, or a group of situations (Meleis, 2018). Phenomena may be temporary or permanent. Examples of phenomena of nursing include caring, self-care, and patient responses to stress.

Concepts. A theory also consists of interrelated concepts that help describe or label phenomena. A concept is a thought or idea of reality that is put into words or phrases to help describe or explain a specific phenomenon (Smith and Liehr, 2018). **Concepts** can be abstract such as emotions or concrete such as physical objects (Chinn and Kramer, 2018). For example, in Meleis and colleagues' theory of transitions, abstract concepts include coping and adapting, while Nightingale described concrete concepts such as physical conditions and health care environments (Meleis, 2018). Theories use concepts to communicate meaning.

Definitions. Theorists use definitions to communicate the general meaning of the concepts of a theory. Definitions may be *theoretical/conceptual* or *operational*. Theoretical or conceptual definitions simply define a particular concept, much like what can be found in a dictionary, based on the theorist's perspective (Meleis, 2018; McEwen and Wills, 2019). Operational definitions state how concepts are measured (Chinn and Kramer, 2018). For example, a nursing concept *conceptually* defines pain as physical discomfort and *operationally* as a patient reporting a score of three or above on a pain scale of zero to ten.

Assumptions. Assumptions are the "taken-for-granted" statements that explain the nature of the concepts, definitions, purpose, relationships, and structure of a theory. Assumptions are accepted as *truths* and are based on values and beliefs (Masters, 2015; Meleis, 2018). For example, Watson's transpersonal caring theory has the assumption that a conscious intention to care promotes healing and wholeness (Alligood, 2018).

The Domain of Nursing

The **domain** is the perspective or territory of a profession or discipline (Meleis, 2018). It provides the subject, central concepts, values and beliefs, phenomena of interest, and central problems of a discipline. The domain of nursing provides both a practical and theoretical aspect of the discipline. It is the knowledge of nursing practice and nursing history, nursing theory, education, and research. The domain of nursing gives nurses a comprehensive perspective that allows you to identify and treat patients' health care needs in all health care settings.

A **paradigm** is a pattern of beliefs used to describe the domain of a discipline. It links the concepts, theories, beliefs, values, and assumptions accepted and applied by the discipline (McEwen and Wills, 2019). The term **conceptual framework** is often used synonymously with paradigm. A conceptual framework provides a way to organize major concepts and visualize the relationship among phenomena. Different frameworks provide alternative ways to view the subject matter of a discipline and represent the perspective of the author. For example, the grand theorists all address similar concepts in their respective theories, but each theorist defines and describes the concepts in a different way based on the theorist's own ideas and experiences (Schmidt and Brown, 2015).

The **nursing metaparadigm** allows nurses to understand and explain what nursing *is*, what nursing *does*, and *why* nurses do what they do (Peterson and Bredow, 2017). The nursing metaparadigm includes the four concepts of person (or human beings), health, environment/situation, and nursing. **Person** is the recipient of nursing care, including individual patients, groups, families, and communities. The person is central to the nursing care you provide. Because each person's needs are often complex, it is important to provide individualized patient-centered care. **Health** has different meanings for each patient, the clinical setting, and the health care profession (see Chapter 6). It is a state of being that people define in relation to their own values, personality, and lifestyle. It is dynamic and continuously changing. Your challenge as a nurse is to provide the best possible care based on a patient's level of health and health care needs at the time of care delivery.

Environment/situation includes all possible conditions affecting patients and the settings where they go for their health care. There is a continuous interaction between a patient and the environment. This interaction has positive and negative effects on a person's level of health and health care needs. Factors in the home, school, workplace, or community all influence the level of these needs. For example, an adolescent girl with type 1 diabetes needs to adapt her treatment plan to adjust for physical activities of school, the demands of a part-time job, and the timing of social events such as her prom.

Nursing includes "care of individuals of all ages, families, groups and communities, sick or well and in all settings. Nursing includes the promotion of health, prevention of illness, and the care of ill, disabled and dying people" (International Council of Nurses, 2018). The scope of nursing is broad. For example, a nurse does not medically diagnose a patient's health condition as heart failure. However, he or she assesses a patient's response to the decrease in activity tolerance as a result of the disease and develops *nursing diagnoses* of fatigue, activity intolerance, and difficulty coping (see Chapter 17). From these nursing diagnoses the nurse creates a patient-centered plan of care for each of the patient's health problems (see Chapter 18). Use critical thinking skills to integrate knowledge, experience, attitudes, and standards into the individualized plan of care for each of your patients (see Chapter 15).

Evolution of Nursing Theory. How are theories created? Nursing theories often build on prior theories. Florence Nightingale is generally regarded as the first nursing theorist; her theory was founded on her belief that nursing could improve a patient's environment to facilitate recovery and prevent complications. In the Nightingale era nurses were taught to observe each patient's condition and report changes to the doctor, thus beginning the status of nursing as subservient to the physician—a sign of the Victorian era in which Nightingale lived (Chinn and Kramer, 2018).

Nursing began to transition from a vocation to a profession in the twentieth century, which prompted American nurses to standardize nursing education in diploma programs and encouraged more nurses to seek academic degrees. The first national gathering of nurses occurred at the World's Fair in Chicago in 1893, and the first edition of the *American Journal of Nursing* (AJN) was published in 1900 (Alligood, 2014). The "curriculum era" of nursing spanned the 1900s to the 1940s. During this period nursing education expanded beyond basic anatomy and physiology courses to include courses in the social sciences, pharmacology, and "nursing arts" that addressed nursing actions, skills, and procedures (Alligood, 2014).

The "research era" encompassed the 1950s, 1960s, and 1970s, during which nurses became increasingly involved in conducting studies and sharing their findings. The earliest research studies had a psychosocial, anthropological, or educational focus. Nurses studied their own attitudes, their relationships with other disciplines, and their functions in work and political settings. In the early years, nursing research did not explore clinical questions based on the medical model of research because the discipline was attempting to show its uniqueness from medicine. At this same time the "graduate education era" began, and early versions of nursing theories were developed that offered more structure to nursing research. The renowned theorists of this time period included Johnson, King, Levine, Neuman, Orem, Rogers, and Roy (Alligood, 2014).

The *theory* era, which included the 1980s and 1990s, significantly contributed to knowledge development, and the nursing metaparadigm was proposed by Fawcett. This era resulted in the publication of several nursing journals, the development of nursing conferences, and the offering of more doctoral programs in nursing (Alligood, 2018).

The twenty-first century is considered the era of *theory utilization*. Today nurses strive to provide evidence-based practice (EBP), which stems from theory, research, and experience. The focus of EBP is safe, comprehensive, individualized, quality health care (see Chapter 5). The original *grand* theories served as springboards for the development of the more modern *middle-range* theories, which, through testing in research studies, provided "evidence" for EBP and promoted the translation of research into practice. Theory use is congruent with current national goals for quality health care (Alligood, 2018).

Nursing theories have changed over time in response to changes in society and the world. The environment of war was a primary factor in developing Nightingale's theory. At the other end of the nursing spectrum, Rogers' introduction of "energy fields" was developed during the 1980s when the advent of the space shuttle program brought an allure of space (Meleis, 2018).

Theorists developed their theories from their own experiences in nursing education and nursing practice and from knowledge gained from the disciplines of philosophy, sociology, psychology, and anthropology. Many nursing theorists revise their theories over time to remain current with health care changes. Such evolution shows that theories are not stagnant; rather they are dynamic and responsive to the changing environment in which we live (McEwen and Wills, 2019).

Types of Theory

The unique theories of a discipline help to distinguish the discipline from other professions. Before the development of nursing theories, nursing was considered a task-oriented occupation that functioned under the direction of the medical profession (McEwen and Wills, 2019). "The primary uses of theory are to provide insights about nursing practice situations and to guide research" and to provide a guideline or explanation of why nurses do what they do (Meleis, 2018, p. 35). Theories have different purposes and are sometimes classified by levels of abstraction (grand vs. middle-range vs. practice theories) or the goals of the theory (descriptive or prescriptive). For example, a descriptive theory describes a phenomenon such as grief or caring and also identifies conditions or factors that predict when a phenomenon may occur but does not guide nursing actions. Prescriptive theory details nursing interventions for a specific phenomenon and the expected outcome of the interventions. Box 4.1 summarizes goals of theoretical nursing models.

Grand theories are abstract, broad in scope, and complex; therefore they require further clarification through research so that they can be applied to nursing practice. A grand theory does not provide guidance for *specific* nursing interventions. Instead it provides the structural framework for general, global ideas about nursing. Grand theories intend to answer the question "What is nursing?" and focus on the *whole* of nursing rather than on a *specific* type of nursing. The

---

BOX 4.1 Goals of Theoretical Nursing Models

- Identify domain and goals of nursing.
- Provide knowledge to improve nursing administration, practice, education, and research.
- Guide research to expand the knowledge base of nursing.
- Identify research techniques and tools used to validate nursing interventions.
- Develop curriculum plans for nursing education.
- Establish criteria for measuring quality of nursing care, education, and research.
- Guide development of a nursing care delivery system.
- Provide systematic structure and rationale for nursing activities.

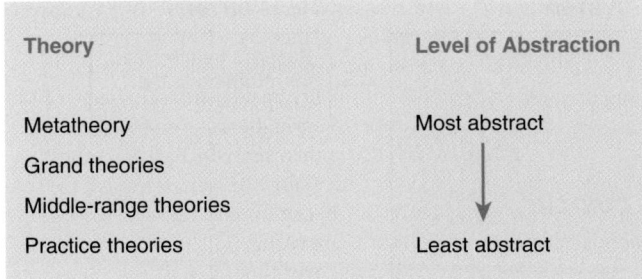

Theory	Level of Abstraction
Metatheory	Most abstract
Grand theories	
Middle-range theories	
Practice theories	Least abstract

FIG. 4.3 Correlation of theory category with level of abstraction. (From McEwen M, Wills EM: *Theoretical basis for nursing*, ed 5, Philadelphia, 2019, Wolters Kluwer Health.)

grand theorists developed their works based on their own experiences and the time in which they were living, which helps to explain why there is so much variation among the theories. Grand theories address the nursing metaparadigm components of person, nursing, health, and environment. For example, in Imogene King's theory of goal attainment, the focus of nursing is the interaction of human beings and the environment with an end goal of health (Meleis, 2018).

Middle-range theories are more limited in scope and less abstract. They address a specific phenomenon and reflect practice (administration, clinical, or teaching). While grand theories take a wide-angled lens perspective to nursing, middle-range theories expand on specific concepts or phenomena in a specific field of nursing such as uncertainty, incontinence, social support, quality of life, and caring (Peterson and Bredow, 2017; Smith and Liehr, 2018). For example, Kolcaba's theory of comfort encourages nurses to meet patients' needs for comfort in physical, psychospiritual, environmental, and sociocultural realms (Schmidt and Brown, 2015). Like many middle-range theories, Kolcaba's theory was based on the works of a grand theorist—in this case, Nightingale. Middle-range theories are also sometimes developed from research, nursing practice, or the theories of other disciplines (McEwen and Wills, 2019).

Practice theories, also known as situation-specific theories, bring theory to the bedside. Narrow in scope and focus, these theories guide the nursing care of a *specific* patient population at a *specific* time (Meleis, 2018). An example of a practice theory is a pain-management protocol for patients recovering from cardiac surgery. Practice theories are less abstract and are often easier to understand and apply than the grand and middle-range theories (Meleis, 2018). Fig. 4.3 demonstrates the level of abstraction for each of the grand, middle-range, and practice theory categories.

Descriptive theories are the first level of theory development. They describe phenomena and identify circumstances in which the phenomena occur (Meleis, 2018). For example, theories of growth and development describe the maturation processes of an individual at various ages (see Chapter 11). Descriptive theories do not direct specific nursing activities or attempt to produce change but rather help to explain patient assessments.

Prescriptive theories address nursing interventions for a phenomenon, guide practice change, and predict the consequences. Nurses use prescriptive theories to anticipate the outcomes of nursing interventions (McEwen and Wills, 2019). Prescriptive theories direct nursing actions toward an explicit goal. Wiedenbach's prescriptive theory of the helping art of nursing conveys the purpose of nursing through three components: to motivate the patient, to facilitate efforts to overcome obstacles, and to develop nursing action based on the immediate situation (Meleis, 2018).

REFLECT NOW

Think about your most recent clinical day.
Consider what type(s) of nursing theories you used when providing care to your patient.

Theory-Based Nursing Practice

Why is theory important to the nursing profession? Nursing knowledge is derived from basic and nursing sciences, experience, aesthetics, nurses' attitudes, and standards of practice. As nursing continues to grow as a practice-oriented profession, new knowledge is needed to prescribe specific interventions to improve patient outcomes. Nursing theories and related concepts continue to evolve. Florence Nightingale spoke with firm conviction about the "nature of nursing as a profession that requires knowledge distinct from medical knowledge" (Nightingale, 1860). The overall goal of nursing knowledge is to explain the practice of nursing as different and distinct from the practice of medicine, psychology, and other health care disciplines. Theory generates nursing knowledge for use in practice, thus supporting EBP (see Chapter 5). The integration of theory into practice leads to coordinated care delivery and therefore serves as the basis for nursing (McEwen and Wills, 2019).

The nursing process is used in clinical settings to determine individual patient needs (see Unit 3). Although the nursing process is central to nursing, it is not a theory. It provides a systematic process for the delivery of nursing care, not the knowledge component of the discipline. However, nurses use theory to provide direction in how to *use* the nursing process. For example, the theory of caring influences what nurses need to assess, how to determine patient needs, how to plan care, how to select individualized nursing interventions, and how to evaluate patient outcomes.

SHARED THEORIES

To practice in today's health care systems, nurses need a strong scientific knowledge base from nursing and other disciplines such as the biomedical, sociological, and behavioral sciences. Shared theory, also known as a *borrowed* or *interdisciplinary* theory, explains a phenomenon specific to the discipline that developed the theory (McEwen and Wills, 2019). For example, Piaget's theory of cognitive development helps to explain how children think, reason, and perceive the world (see Chapter 11). Knowledge and use of this theory help pediatric nurses design appropriate therapeutic play interventions for ill toddlers or school-age children. Knowles' adult learning theory helps a nurse plan and provide appropriate discharge teaching for a patient who is recovering from surgery.

Several nursing theories are based on systems theory. The nursing process is a system (Fig. 4.4). Like all systems, the nursing process has a specific purpose or goal (see Unit 3). The goal of the nursing process is to organize and deliver patient-centered care. As a system the nursing process has the following components: input, output, feedback, and content. Input for the nursing process is the data or information that comes from a patient's assessment. Output is the end product of a system; in the case of the nursing process it is whether the patient's health status improves, declines, or remains stable as a result of nursing care.

Feedback serves to inform a system about how it functions. For example, in the nursing process the outcomes reflect the patient's responses to nursing interventions. The outcomes are part of the feedback system to refine the plan of care. Other forms of feedback in the

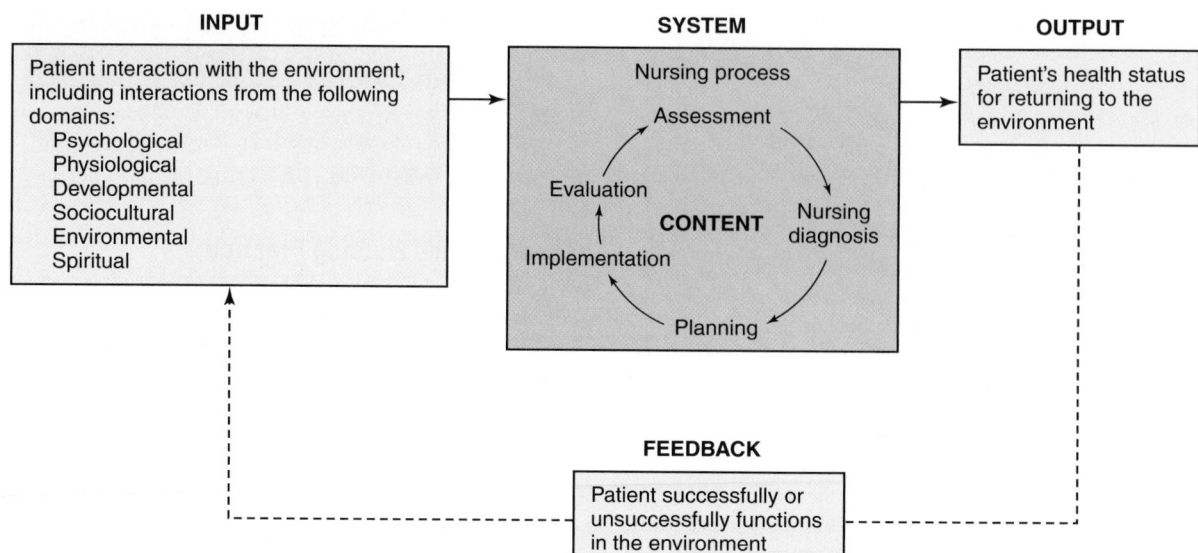

FIG. 4.4 Providing nursing services in assisted-living facilities promotes physical and psychosocial health.

nursing process include responses from family members and consultation from other health care professionals.

The **content** is the product and information obtained from the system. For example, patients with impaired bed mobility have common skin care needs and interventions (e.g., hygiene and scheduled positioning changes) that are very successful in reducing the risk for pressure injuries. Table 4.1 provides an overview of additional select shared theories that are often used in nursing practice.

SELECT NURSING THEORIES

Definitions and theories of nursing can help you understand the practice of nursing. The following sections describe select theories and their concepts. See Table 4.2 for a review of additional grand and middle-range nursing theories.

Nightingale's Environmental Theory

Known as the founder of modern nursing, Florence Nightingale is credited with developing the first nursing theory. The focus of Nightingale's grand theory is a patient's environment, which Nightingale believed nurses should manipulate (e.g., ventilation, light, decreased noise, hygiene, nutrition) so that nature is able to restore a patient to health (McEwen and Wills, 2019). Through observation and data collection, she linked the patient's health status with environmental factors and initiated improved hygiene and sanitary conditions during the Crimean War. Nightingale taught and used the nursing process, noting that "vital observation [assessment] … is not for the sake of piling up miscellaneous information or curious facts, but for the sake of saving life and increasing health and comfort" (Nightingale, 1860).

Peplau's Interpersonal Theory

Hildegard Peplau is considered the mother of psychiatric nursing; the focus of her middle-range theory includes interpersonal relations among a nurse, a patient, and a patient's family and developing the nurse-patient relationship (McEwen and Wills, 2019). According to Peplau, nurses help patients reduce anxiety by converting it into constructive actions (McEwen and Wills, 2019). They develop therapeutic relationships with patients that are respectful, empathetic, and nonjudgmental (Hagerty et al., 2017). The following phases characterize the nurse-patient interpersonal relationship: preorientation (data

gathering), orientation (defining issue), working phase (therapeutic activity), and resolution (termination of relationship). In developing a nurse-patient relationship, the nurse serves as a resource person, counselor, and surrogate. For example, when a patient seeks help, the nurse and patient first discuss the nature of any problems, and the nurse explains the services available. As the nurse-patient relationship develops, the nurse and patient mutually define the problems and potential solutions. When the patient's original needs are resolved, new needs sometimes emerge. This middle-range theory is useful in establishing effective nurse-patient communication when obtaining a nursing history, providing patient education, or counseling patients and their families (see Chapter 24).

Orem's Self-Care Deficit Nursing Theory

Dorothea Orem's Self-Care Deficit Nursing Theory is commonly used in nursing practice (Alligood, 2014). When applying this grand theory, a nurse continually assesses a patient's ability to perform self-care and intervenes as needed to ensure that patients meet physical, psychological, sociological, and developmental needs. According to Orem, people who participate in self-care activities are more likely to improve their health outcomes (Kurtz and Schmidt, 2016; Rustøen et al., 2014). Nursing care becomes necessary when patients are unable to fulfill biological, psychological, developmental, or social needs. Nurses continually assess and determine why patients are unable to meet these needs, identify goals to help them, intervene to help them perform self-care, and evaluate how much self-care they are able to perform. For example, a patient may need a nurse to bathe or feed him or her while acutely ill but, as his or her condition improves, the nurse encourages the patient to begin doing these activities independently.

> ### REFLECT NOW
>
> Consider Orem's Self-Care Deficit Nursing Theory. How can you apply this theory to promote recovery in your patient?

Leininger's Culture Care Theory

As early as the 1950s Madeleine Leininger recognized the need to focus on culture in nursing as she predicted that nursing and health care would

TABLE 4.1 Overview of Select Shared Theories

Theory Categories	Focus	Application To Nursing
Human needs	Need motivates human behavior. Maslow's hierarchy of basic human needs includes five levels of priority (e.g., physiological, safety and security, love and belonging, self-esteem, and self-actualization) (see Fig. 6.3).	Basic physiological and safety needs are usually a patient's first priority, especially when he or she is dependent on others to meet these needs. When a patient has no emergent physical or safety needs, the nurse gives high priority to his or her psychological, sociocultural, developmental, or spiritual needs. Patients entering the health care system generally have unmet needs. A patient in pain after surgery (basic need) is not ready for discharge teaching (higher-level need) until the pain is relieved. The hierarchy of needs is a way to plan for individualized patient care (McEwen and Wills, 2019).
Stress/adaptation	Humans respond to actual or perceived threats by adapting to maintain function and life.	Patients demonstrate a similar pattern of reacting to stress through physiological and psychological responses. Failure to adapt to stress can lead to exhaustion and decline in health. Nurses need to understand the reaction of body and mind to stress and intervene to help patients develop methods of coping/adapting to prevent or manage illness and disease (Masters, 2015).
Developmental	Humans have a common pattern of growth and development.	Human growth and development are orderly, predictive processes that begin with conception and continue through death. Varieties of well-tested theories describe and predict behavior and development at various phases of the life continuum (McEwen and Wills, 2019).
Biomedical	Theory explains causes of disease; principles related to physiology.	Nurses must have knowledge of theories from the fields of biology, medicine, public health, physiology, and pharmacology to provide holistic patient care, promote health, and prevent illness (McEwen and Wills, 2019).
Psychosocial	Theory explains and/or predicts human responses within the physiological, psychological, sociocultural, developmental, and spiritual domains.	Nursing is a diverse discipline that strives to meet holistic needs of patients. Chapter 9 discusses models for understanding cultural diversity and implementing care to meet the diverse needs of the patient. Chapter 10 describes family theory and how to meet the needs of the family when the family is the patient or the caregiver. Chapter 36 discusses several models of grieving and demonstrates how to help patients through loss, death, and grief.
Educational	Theory explains the teaching-learning process by examining behavioral, cognitive, and adult learning principles.	Nurses provide education to patients, families, community groups, and members of the health care team. A basic understanding of arious teaching-learning theories is critical for this aspect of the professional nursing role (Butts and Rich, 2015).
Leadership/management	Theory promotes organization, change, power/empowerment, motivation, conflict management, and decision making.	Nurses often assume leadership positions in the health care realm and as such are expected to effectively manage individuals and groups to promote change and improve quality care and outcomes (McEwen and Wills, 2019).

become more global. She blended her background in anthropology with nursing to form her middle-range theory of cultural care diversity and universality (Alligood, 2014). Human caring varies among cultures in its expressions, processes, and patterns. Social structure factors such as a patient's politics, culture, and traditions are significant forces affecting care and influencing the patient's health and illness patterns. Think about the diversity of patients and their nursing care needs (see Chapter 9). The major concept of Leininger's theory is cultural diversity, and the goal of nursing care is to provide a patient with culturally specific nursing care (Alligood, 2014). To provide care to patients of unique cultures, nurses safely integrate their cultural traditions, values, and beliefs into a plan of care. Leininger's theory recognizes the importance of culture and its influence on everything that involves a patient, including health beliefs, the role of family and community, and dietary practices (Alligood, 2014). For example, some cultures believe that the leader of the community needs to be present during health care decisions. As a result, a health care

team needs to reschedule when rounds occur to include the community leader. In addition, symptom expression also differs among cultures. A person with an Irish background might be stoic and not complain about pain, whereas a person from a Middle Eastern culture might be very vocal about pain. In both cases a nurse needs to skillfully incorporate the patient's cultural practices in assessing his or her level of pain (e.g., asking, "Is the pain getting worse or remaining the same?").

QSEN **Building Competency in Patient-Centered Care** You are caring for a high school student who was in a motor vehicle accident on the way to spring break. She is without her parents. She has not previously been hospitalized and has never been away from home this long. How could you use *Peplau's interpersonal theory* when caring for this patient?

Answers to QSEN Activities can be found on the Evolve website.

TABLE 4.2   Overview of Select Grand and Middle-Range Nursing Theories

Theory Category	Theorist	Focus	Application
Grand theory	Henderson	Principles and practice of nursing	Nurses assist patients with 14 activities (breathing, eating/drinking, elimination, movement/positioning, sleep/rest, clothing, body temperature, hygiene, safety, communication/socialization/play, practice of faith, learning) until patients can meet these needs for themselves or they help patients have a peaceful death (Butts and Rich, 2015; McEwen and Wills, 2019).
	Johnson	Behavioral system	Nurses perceive patients as being more important than their disease; a patient is viewed as a collection of subsystems that form an overall behavioral system focused on meeting basic drives of achievement, affiliation, aggression/protection, dependence, elimination, ingestion, sex, and restoration. The goal of nursing is to help the patient attain/maintain balance, function, and stability in each of the subsystems (Butts and Rich, 2015).
	Neuman	Systems	Nurses view a patient (physical, psychological, sociocultural, developmental, and spiritual) as being an open system that is in constant energy exchange with both internal and external environments. Nurses help a patient (individual, group, family, or community) cope with intrapersonal, interpersonal, and extrapersonal *stressors* that can break through the patient's line of defense and cause illness. The role of nursing is to stabilize a patient or situation, and the focus is on *wellness* and *prevention* of disease (McEwen and Wills, 2019).
	Abdellah	Patient-centered care	Nurses address 21 "nursing problems" to meet patients' physical, psychological, and social needs and should strive to *know* each patient. Nurses use knowledge constructed from previous experiences to determine a general plan of care and then personalize the plan to the patient to provide *patient-centered care*. A nurse also involves a patient's family in the plan of care when appropriate (McEwen and Wills, 2019).
	King	Goal attainment	Nurses view a patient as a unique personal system that is constantly interacting/transacting with other systems (e.g., nurse, family, friends); nurses help patients become active participants in their care by working *with* them to establish goals for attaining, restoring, or maintaining health (Johnson and Webber, 2014; McEwen and Wills, 2019).
	Roy	Adaptation	Nurses help a patient cope with or adapt to changes in physiological, self-concept, role function, and interdependence domains (Masters, 2015).
	Watson	Caring	Caring is a fundamental component of professional nursing practice and is based on 10 *carative factors* (see Chapter 7). The purpose of nursing is to understand the interrelationship among health, illness, and human behavior rather than focus on the disease-cure model. Caring occurs when a nurse and patient engage in a *transpersonal relationship* that facilitates the patient's ability for self-healing (Johnson and Webber, 2014).
	Rogers/Parse/Newman	Unitary beings/human becoming/ expanding consciousness	Nurses view a patient as a unique, dynamic energy field in constant energy exchange with the environment; nursing care focuses on helping a patient use his or her *own* potential to identify and alter personal rhythms/patterns (e.g., eating, breathing, sleeping) to promote and maintain health. Nurses understand that patients are responsible for their own health and that health stems from how patients live their lives in accordance with their own values; the nurse's role is to be truly *present* with the patient and accept his or her view of reality while providing guidance to the patient in making health-related choices in accordance with his or her belief system (Johnson and Webber, 2014; McEwen and Wills, 2019).
Middle-range theory	Benner	Skill acquisition	Nurses progress through five stages of skill acquisition: novice, advanced beginner, competent, proficient, and expert (Butts and Rich, 2015).
	Kolcaba	Comfort	Nurses facilitate health-seeking behaviors in patients by striving to relieve physical, emotional, social, environmental, and/or spiritual distress (McEwen and Wills, 2019).
	Pender	Health promotion	Nurses understand that a patient's personal characteristics, experiences, and beliefs affect his or her motivation for adopting healthy behaviors (see Chapter 6) (McEwen and Wills, 2019).
	American Association of Critical-Care Nurses	Synergy	Matching nurse competencies to patient needs in the critical care environment improves patient outcomes (McEwen and Wills, 2019).
	Meleis, Sawyer, Im, Messias, and Schumacher	Transitions	Patients are more vulnerable during changes in health and illness. Nurses can facilitate healthy *transitions* through the development of nursing interventions specific to each patient. For example, the transition from living at home to a nursing home due to declining health (Alligood, 2018).

LINK BETWEEN THEORY AND KNOWLEDGE DEVELOPMENT IN NURSING

Nursing has its own body of knowledge that is both theoretical and experiential. You acquire theoretical knowledge through "reading, observing, or discussing" concepts (Alligood, 2014, p. 123). Theoretical knowledge stimulates thinking and creates a broad understanding of nursing science and practice. Experiential or clinical knowledge, often called the *art* of nursing, is formed from nurses' clinical experience. Both types of knowledge are needed to provide safe, comprehensive nursing care.

Nursing theories guide nursing practice (McEwen and Wills, 2019). When using theory-based nursing practice, you apply the principles of a theory in delivering nursing interventions. Grand theories help shape and define your practice, middle-range theories continue to advance nursing knowledge through nursing research, and practice theories help you provide specific care for individuals and groups of diverse populations and situations (Peterson and Bredow, 2017).

Relationship Between Nursing Theory and Nursing Research

Research validates, refutes, supports, and/or modifies theory, while theory stimulates nurse scientists to explore significant issues in nursing practice (McEwen and Wills, 2019; Meleis, 2018). The relationship between nursing theory and nursing research builds the scientific knowledge base of nursing, which is then applied to practice. Nurses better understand the appropriate use of a theory to improve patient care as more research is conducted. The relationships between the components of a theory often help identify research questions and determine the overall design of a study. For example, nurse researchers used Peplau's interpersonal theory as the framework for a project to improve communication of a health care team. The aim of the project was to increase health care staff teamwork and communication (Holtmann, 2018). Table 4.3 provides some examples of how theories are used in nursing research. Nurses consider findings from theory-based research to determine whether the theory can be used in practice.

Sometimes research is used to develop new theories (Meleis, 2018). *Theory-generating* research uses logic to explore relationships among phenomena (McEwen and Wills, 2019). In theory-generating research an investigator makes observations (*without* any preconceived ideas) to view a phenomenon in a new way. Middle-range theories are often developed in this manner. For example, the middle-range theory of chronic sorrow stemmed from a researcher's initial observations of cyclic periods of sadness in parents of children with intellectual or developmental disabilities (Vitale and Falco, 2014).

Theory-testing research determines how accurately a theory describes a nursing phenomenon. Testing develops the evidence for describing or predicting patient outcomes. A researcher has *some* preconceived idea as to how patients describe or respond to a phenomenon and generates research questions or hypotheses to test the assumptions of the theory. No one study tests *all* components of a theory; researchers test the theory through a variety of research activities. For example, nurse researchers studied Kolcaba's middle-range nursing theory of comfort in relation to the pain and discomfort experienced by patients with heart disease. The researchers explored the specific intervention of "quiet time" as a comfort measure in this patient population (Krinsky et al., 2014).

Both theory-generating and theory-testing research refine the knowledge base of nursing. In turn, nurses incorporate research-based interventions into theory-based practice (Box 4.2). As research activities continue, not only does the knowledge and science of nursing

TABLE 4.3 Theories Used in Nursing Practice and Research

Theory	Main Concepts Utilized in Research Example	Example of Use in Research
Kolcaba's theory of comfort	Enhanced comfort	The intervention of "quiet time" was studied for possible use with patients experiencing cardiac symptoms (Krinsky et al., 2014).
AACN Synergy Model	Nurse competencies, environmental factors, patient characteristics	Clinical judgment and duration of transport were found to influence patient safety during critical care transport (Swickard et al., 2018).
Mishel's uncertainty in illness theory	Appraisal and management of uncertainty	Study results indicate that young adults with congenital heart disease are at risk for posttraumatic stress disorder (PTSD) and long-term stress due to chronic uncertainty (Moreland and Santacroce, 2018).
Meleis et al.'s transitions theory	Nursing therapeutics (assessment of readiness, preparation for transition, role supplementation), mindfulness	A mindfulness-based transition program was applied to mothers with premature rupture of membranes to measure acceptance of pregnancy, readiness to give birth, maternal attachment, and competency in the role of motherhood (Korukcu and Kukulu, 2017).

AACN, American Association of Critical-Care Nurses.

increase, but patients receive high-quality evidence-based nursing care (see Chapter 5). As an art, nursing relies on knowledge gained from practice and reflection on past experiences. The "expert nurse" translates both the art and science of nursing into the realm of *creative caring*, which takes the extra step of individualizing care to the specific needs of each patient. For example, a nurse provides creative caring when arranging for a patient who is in the hospital to visit with a beloved pet or in finding a way to honor a patient's wish to die at home.

Theory is the foundation of nursing; it defines our unique profession and sets it apart from other disciplines. Theory provides a basis for research and practice and serves as a guide in providing safe, comprehensive, individualized care, which is the hallmark of nursing. As you progress in your nursing education and practice, you will use theory in a variety of ways. Keep in mind that these theories apply not only to patient care but also are useful in communicating with other members of the health care team.

REFLECT NOW

Analyze the nursing program you are enrolled in to determine what theories are reflected in the nursing program and nursing curriculum.

BOX 4.2 EVIDENCE-BASED PRACTICE

Theory-Based Practice in the Management of First-time Parents

PICOT Question: In patients experiencing their first pregnancy, how does application of Meleis' theory of transitions compared to no specific theory application influence a healthy transition to parenthood?

Evidence Summary

The transition to parenthood is a life-changing and often challenging time. Successful transitioning to the role of a parent can be accomplished by gaining confidence, planning for the birth, and developing a strong support system (Barimani et al., 2017; Korukcu and Kukulu, 2017). According to Meleis et al.'s theory of transitions, a transition is required when one's reality is interrupted, causing the need for a change and a new reality to be formed (Vardaman and Mastel-Smith, 2016). Transitions theory can be applied to various types of transitions: developmental, health-illness, situational, and organizational. Nurses can assist expectant parents by providing professional support during the prenatal period. Expectant parents will require information regarding birth plans, feeding routines, maternal and child appointments, and routine testing before birth (Barimani et al., 2017). It is important for the patient to be engaged in all decisions and for the nurse to remain nonjudgmental (Korukcu and Kukulu, 2017). Nursing actions based on Meleis et al.'s theory can assist patients in managing life's transitions (Barimani et al., 2017; Vardaman and Mastel-Smith, 2016).

Application to Nursing Practice

- Ensure that expectant parents are knowledgeable about health care access in the prenatal period (Barimani et al., 2017).
- Help patients identify support groups in the community, allowing expectant parents to share knowledge and emotions with others (Barimani et al., 2017).
- Provide new parent education that covers expectations, coping behaviors, and changes in relationships to facilitate successful transitions (Barimani et al., 2017; Vardaman and Mastel-Smith, 2016).
- Recognize that a first-time parent's level of self-confidence may change during the pregnancy (Barimani et al., 2017; Korukcu and Kukulu, 2017).

KEY POINTS

- The components of a theory provide a foundation for knowledge for nurses to direct and deliver nursing care.
- Theories are dynamic and responsive to the changing environment in which we live.
- The types of nursing theories include grand theories, middle-range theories, practice theories, descriptive and prescriptive theories.
- The integration of theory into practice leads to coordinated care delivery.
- Nurses need a strong scientific knowledge base from nursing and other disciplines, such as the biomedical, sociological, and behavioral sciences.
- Grand and middle-range nursing theories can help you understand the practice of nursing.
- The relationship between theory and research builds the scientific knowledge base of nursing, which is then applied to practice.

REFLECTIVE LEARNING

- Reflect back on a patient you recently were assigned to care for during a clinical or simulation experience. Describe how you did or could have applied Nightingale's environmental theory while you were caring for this patient.
- Reflect back on a patient with a chronic health condition you were recently assigned to care for during a clinical or simulation experience. Explain how you would apply Peplau's interpersonal theory to help this patient prevent complications and promote disease management.
- Reflect on a patient you were assigned to care for in a recent clinical or simulation experience who required total patient care. Describe how you would apply Orem's self-care deficit theory for this patient.

REVIEW QUESTIONS

1. The components of the nursing metaparadigm include:
   1. Person, health, environment, and theory.
   2. Health, theory, concepts, and environment.
   3. Nurses, physicians, health, and patient needs.
   4. Person, health, environment, and nursing.
2. Theory is essential to nursing practice because it: (Select all that apply.)
   1. Contributes to nursing knowledge.
   2. Predicts patient behaviors in situations.
   3. Provides a means of assessing patient vital signs.
   4. Guides nursing practice.
   5. Formulates health care legislation.
   6. Explains relationships between concepts.
3. A nurse ensures that each patient's room is clean; well ventilated; and free from clutter, excessive noise, and extremes in temperature. Which theorist's work is the nurse practicing in this example?
   1. Henderson
   2. Orem
   3. King
   4. Nightingale
4. The nurse is caring for a patient admitted to the neurological unit with the diagnosis of a stroke and right-sided weakness. The nurse assumes responsibility for bathing and feeding the patient until the patient can begin performing these activities. The nurse in this situation is applying the theory developed by:
   1. Johnson.
   2. Orem.
   3. Roy.
   4. Peplau.
5. Match the following types of theory with the appropriate description.

1. Middle-range theory	a. Very abstract; attempts to describe nursing in a global context
2. Shared theory	b. Specific to a particular situation; brings theory to the bedside
3. Grand theory	c. Applies theory from other disciplines to nursing practice
4. Practice theory	d. Addresses a specific phenomenon and reflects practice

6. Match the following descriptions to the appropriate grand theorist.

1. King
2. Henderson
3. Orem
4. Neuman

a. Based on the theory that focuses on *wellness* and *prevention* of disease
b. Based on the belief that people who participate in self-care activities are more likely to improve their health outcomes
c. Based on 14 activities, the belief that the nurse should assist patients with meeting needs until they are able to do so independently
d. Based on the belief that nurses should work with patients to develop goals for care

7. Which of the following statements related to theory-based nursing practice are correct? (Select all that apply.)
   1. Nursing theory differentiates nursing from other disciplines.
   2. Nursing theories are standardized and do not change over time.
   3. Integrating theory into practice promotes coordinated care delivery.
   4. Nursing knowledge is generated by theory.
   5. The theory of nursing process is used in planning patient care.
   6. Evidence-based practice results from theory-testing research.

8. A nurse is caring for a patient who recently lost a leg in a motor vehicle accident. The nurse best assists the patient to cope with this situation by applying which of the following theories?
   1. Roy
   2. Watson
   3. Johnson
   4. Benner

9. Using Maslow's hierarchy of needs, identify the priority for a patient who is experiencing chest pain and difficulty breathing.
   1. Self-actualization
   2. Air, water, and nutrition
   3. Safety
   4. Esteem and self-esteem needs

10. Which of the following categories of shared theories would be most appropriate for a patient who is grieving the loss of a spouse?
    1. Biomedical
    2. Leadership
    3. Psychosocial
    4. Developmental

Answers: 1. 4; **2.** 1, 2, 4, 6; **3.** 4; **4.** 2; **5.** 1d, 2c, 3a, 4b; **6.** 1d, 2c, 3b, 4a; **7.** 1, 3, 4, 6; **8.** 1; **9.** 2; **10.** 3.

Rationales for Review Questions can be found on the Evolve website.

REFERENCES

Alligood MR: *Nursing theory utilization & application*, ed 5, St Louis, 2014, Mosby.

Alligood MR: *Nursing theorists and their work*, ed 9, St Louis, 2018, Elsevier.

Butts JB, Rich KL: *Philosophies and theories for advanced nursing practice*, ed 2, Burlington, MA, 2015, Jones & Bartlett Learning.

Chinn PL, Kramer MK: *Knowledge development in nursing: theory and process*, ed 10, St Louis, 2018, Elsevier.

International Council of Nurses: *Who we are: definition of nursing*, ©2018, International Council of Nurses. https://www.icn.ch/nursing-policy/nursing-definitions. Accessed May 25, 2019.

Johnson BM, Webber PB: *An introduction to theory and reasoning in nursing*, ed 4, Philadelphia, PA, 2014, Lippincott Williams & Wilkins.

Kurtz CP, Schmidt NA: Conceptualizing cognitive-behavioral therapy as a supportive-educative nursing system for patients with insomnia, self-care, *Dependent-Care & Nursing* 22(1):14, 2016.

Masters K: *Nursing theories: a framework for professional practice*, ed 2, Burlington, MA, 2015, Jones & Bartlett Learning.

McEwen M, Wills EM: *Theoretical basis for nursing*, ed 5, Philadelphia, 2019, Wolters Kluwer Health.

Meleis AI: *Theoretical nursing: development & progress*, ed 6, Philadelphia, 2018, Wolters Kluwer.

Nightingale F: *Notes on nursing: what it is and what it is not*, London, 1860, Harrison & Sons.

Peterson SJ, Bredow TS: *Middle range theories: application to nursing research and practice*, ed 4, Philadelphia, 2017, Wolters Kluwer.

Reed PG, Shearer NBC: *Nursing knowledge and theory innovation: advancing the science of practice*, ed 2, New York, 2018, Springer.

Schmidt NA, Brown JM: *Evidence-based practice for nurses: appraisal and application of research*, ed 3, Burlington, MA, 2015, Jones and Bartlett.

Smith MJ, Liehr PR: *Middle range theory for nursing*, ed 4, New York, 2018, Springer.

RESEARCH REFERENCES

Barimani M, et al.: Facilitating and inhibiting factors in transition to parenthood – ways in which health professionals can support parents, *Scand J Caring Sci* 31(3):537, 2017.

Hagerty TA, et al.: Peplau's theory of interpersonal relations: an alternative factor structure for patient experience data? *Nurs Sci Q* 30(2):160, 2017.

Holtmann M: Does the utilization of interactive learning during TeamSTEPPS SBAR, CUS, and debriefing tool sessions increase the perceptions of teamwork and communication in the hospital setting? (Doctoral project), *Retrieved from ProQuest Dissertations & Theses Global*, (Order No. 10792142), 2018.

Korukcu O, Kukulu K: The effect of the mindfulness-based transition to motherhood program in pregnant women with preterm premature rupture of membranes, *Health Care for Women International* 38(7):765, 2017.

Krinsky R, et al.: A practical application of Katharine Kolcaba's comfort theory to cardiac patients, *Appl Nurs Res* 27:147, 2014.

Moreland P, Santacroce SJ: Illness uncertainty and post-traumatic stress in young adults with congenital heart disease, *J Cardiovasc Nurs* 33(4):356, 2018.

Rustøen T, et al.: A randomized clinical trial of the efficacy of a self-care intervention to improve cancer pain management, *Cancer Nurs* 37(1):34, 2014.

Swickard S, et al.: Patient safety events during critical care transport, *Air Med J* 37(4):253, 2018.

Vardaman SA, Mastel-Smith B: The transitions of international nursing students, *Teaching and Learning in Nursing* 11(2):34, 2016.

Vitale SA, Falco C: Children born prematurely: risk of parental chronic sorrow, *J Pediatric Nurs* 29:248, 2014.

5

Evidence-Based Practice

OBJECTIVES

- Discuss the benefits of evidence-based practice.
- Describe the steps of evidence-based practice.
- Develop a PICOT question.
- Explain the levels of evidence available in the literature.
- Discuss how nurses apply evidence in practice.

- Explain how nursing research improves nursing practice.
- Discuss the steps of the research process.
- Explain the relationship among evidence-based practice, research, and performance improvement.

KEY TERMS

Active errors, p. 64
Bias, p. 60
Confidentiality, p. 63
Empirical data, p. 60
Evaluation research, p. 62
Evidence-based practice (EBP), p. 53
Experimental study, p. 61
Generalizability, p. 60
Hypotheses, p. 57

Inductive reasoning, p. 62
Informed consent, p. 63
Latent errors, p. 64
Nursing research, p. 59
Peer-reviewed, p. 55
Performance improvement (PI), p. 63
PICOT question, p. 54
Qualitative nursing research, p. 62
Quantitative nursing research, p. 61

Reliability, p. 60
Research process, p. 62
Sampling error, p. 62
Scientific method, p. 60
Sentinel event, p. 64
Validity, p. 60
Variables, p. 57

MEDIA RESOURCES

http://evolve.elsevier.com/Potter/fundamentals/
- Review Questions
- Case Study with Questions

- Audio Glossary
- Content Updates
- Answers to QSEN Activity and Review Questions

Many nurses practice nursing according to what they learn in nursing school, their experiences in practice, and the policies and procedures of their health care agency. These approaches to practice do not guarantee that nursing practice is always based on up-to-date scientific information. Sometimes it is based on tradition and not on current evidence. Nursing practice is in an "age of accountability," in which nursing care impacts the quality, safety, and cost of health care (Jun et al., 2016; White and Spruce, 2015). People are more informed about their own health and the incidence of medical errors within health care institutions. Health care organizations are required to show their commitment to each health care stakeholder (e.g., patients, insurance companies, governmental agencies) to reduce health care errors and improve safety by putting into place evidence-based safe practices (National Quality Forum, 2018). Nurses and other health care providers can no longer accept and practice the status quo. Nurses need to better understand why certain health care approaches are used, which ones work, and which ones do not. Research priorities identified by nurse administrators include the economic value of nursing, the design of nursing practice and care delivery models, patient safety and outcomes, and creating a healthy practice environment (Scott et al., 2016). Evidence-based practice (EBP) guides nurses and other health care providers in making effective, timely, and appropriate clinical decisions.

Cathy and Tom are two nurses who work in the surgical intensive care unit (ICU). They are members of the interprofessional unit practice committee (UPC) that meets monthly to discuss practice issues on the unit and the quality indicators for their unit. Cathy notes that the monthly quality report shows an increased incidence of central line–associated bloodstream infections (CLABSIs) over each of the past 3 months. Patients with central venous catheters (CVCs) used to deliver fluids and medications are becoming infected, but why? Tom questions whether the problem is related to the type of dressing placed over catheters or the way sites are cleansed before insertion. The occurrence of CLABSIs is considered a "Never Event," meaning that the hospital will not be reimbursed for the care of patients who have this hospital-acquired complication (Centers for Medicare and Medicaid Services, 2015). Thus, it is important for the UPC to find ways to prevent CLABSIs from occurring. The UPC decides to explore these questions as part of its evidence-based practice (EBP) process. The first step is to develop a clinical question to efficiently search the scientific literature. Tom volunteers to do the search with the aid of the hospital librarian. The aim is to determine what evidence is available so that the committee can make an informed decision about standards needed to reduce CLABSIs in their patients.

THE NEED FOR EVIDENCE-BASED PRACTICE

Evidence-based practice (EBP) is a problem-solving approach to clinical practice that combines the deliberate and systematic use of best evidence in combination with a clinician's expertise, patient preferences and values, and available health care resources in making decisions about patient care (Fig. 5.1) (Melnyk and Fineout-Overholt, 2019). Put in simpler terms, EBP addresses a clinical problem by looking for the very best scientific and clinical evidence available for treating or managing the problem and implementing changes in practice. Research shows that EBP enhances the patient experience, decreases cost, empowers clinicians, and improves patient outcomes (Crabtree et al., 2016; Melnyk and Fineout-Overholt, 2019). Use of EBP competencies by nurses and advanced practice nurses further improves the quality and consistency of health care (Melnyk et al., 2017; McNeil, 2016).

Nurses regularly face important clinical decisions when caring for patients (e.g., Why do I use this approach in providing patient care? Is a change needed? Is there a way to improve patient outcomes?). Implementing health care processes or practices that are known to work (evidence based) in a reliable way is a feature of "quality care" and effective timely and appropriate clinical decisions (Peterson et al., 2014). Implementing new knowledge into practice requires a systematic approach that applies evidence to improve clinical educational and administrative practice. EBP is one of the Quality and Safety Education for Nurses' (QSEN) competencies. The overall goal for the QSEN initiative is to prepare nurses in pre-licensure and graduate programs with the knowledge, skills, and attitudes (KSAs) necessary to continuously improve the quality and safety of the health care systems where they work (QSEN, 2018). Following this, Melnyk et al. (2017) developed and validated 12 EBP competencies considered essential for practicing RNs and an additional 11 competencies essential for practicing advanced practice nurses. These EBP competencies are foundational for delivering high-quality care.

There are many sources of evidence. A textbook incorporates evidence into the information, practice guidelines, and procedures it includes. Articles from nursing and health care literature are available on almost any topic involving nursing practice in either journals or on the Internet. Although the scientific basis of nursing practice has grown, some nursing care practices do not have adequate research to guide practice decisions. The challenge is to obtain the very best, most relevant, current, and accurate information when you need it for patient care.

The best scientific evidence comes from well-designed, systematically conducted research studies found in scientific, peer-reviewed journals. Researchers are usually able to conclude whether a new treatment or approach truly makes a difference at the completion of a research study. Unfortunately, much of that evidence never reaches the bedside. While more health care settings have adopted evidence-based practice, there are still nurses who may not have easy access to databases for scientific literature. Instead they often care for patients based on tradition or convenience.

Even when you use the best evidence available, application of the evidence and outcomes differ based on your patients' values, state of health, preferences, concerns, and/or expectations. The correct application of EBP involves ethical and accountable professional nursing practice. As a nurse you use critical thinking skills to determine which evidence is appropriate and related to your patients' clinical situations. For example, a single research article involving adults shows that the use of therapeutic touch is effective in reducing patients' perceptions of abdominal pain after surgery. However, if your patients have cultural beliefs that discourage use of touch, you probably need to search for a different evidence-based therapy that your patients will accept. Using your clinical expertise and considering patients' values and preferences ensure that you apply the evidence available in practice both safely and appropriately.

Steps of Evidence-Based Practice

EBP is a systematic, problem-solving process that facilitates achievement of best practices. Consistently following a step-by-step approach ensures that you obtain the strongest available evidence to apply in

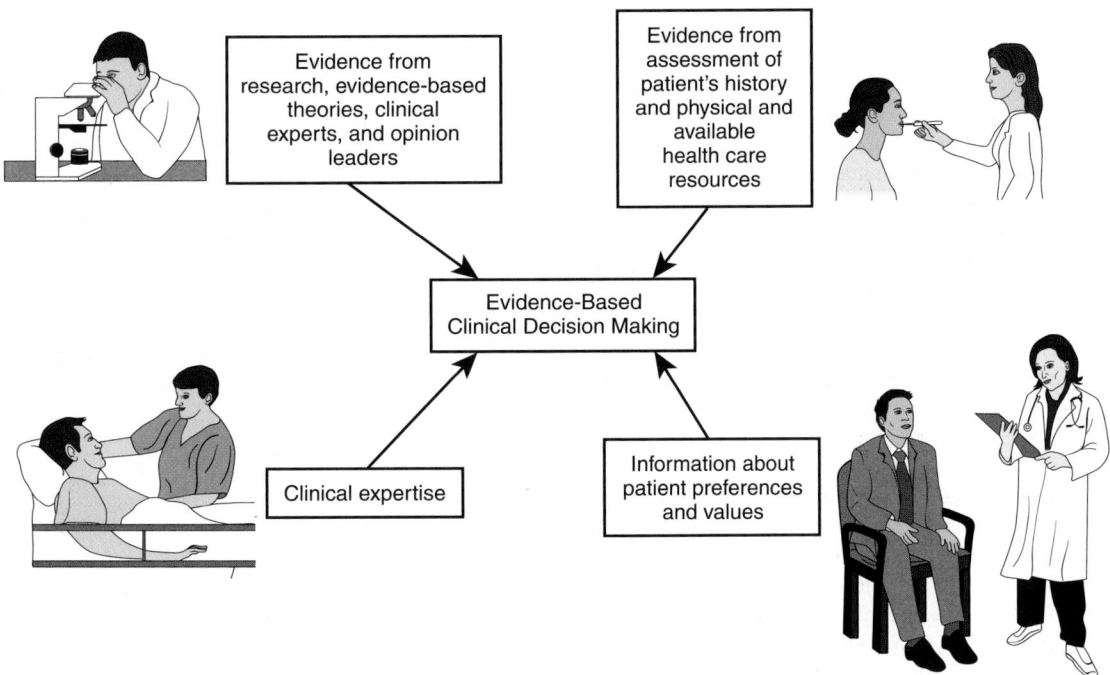

Evidence from research, evidence-based theories, clinical experts, and opinion leaders

Evidence from assessment of patient's history and physical and available health care resources

Evidence-Based Clinical Decision Making

Clinical expertise

Information about patient preferences and values

FIG. 5.1 Model for evidence-based clinical decision making.

patient care. There are seven steps of EBP, which are numbered from zero to six (Melnyk and Fineout-Overholt, 2019):

0. Cultivate a spirit of inquiry within an EBP culture and environment.
1. Ask a clinical question in PICOT format.
2. Search for the most relevant and best evidence.
3. Critically appraise the evidence you gather.
4. Integrate the best evidence with your clinical expertise and patient preferences and values to make the best clinical decision.
5. Evaluate the outcomes of practice changes based on evidence.
6. Communicate the outcomes of EBP decision or changes.

Cultivate a Spirit of Inquiry. Changes in health care are often made slowly because of multiple barriers that often prevent the implementation of EBP. When your care is not evidence based, your patients will sometimes experience poor outcomes. To be an effective change agent and foster optimal patient care, you need to have a never-ending spirit of inquiry. Constantly questioning current practices and believing in the value of EBP lead to the consistent use of EBP in clinical nursing practice. For an institution to be successful at implementing and sustaining EBP changes, there must be a culture that promotes and supports a spirit of inquiry (Melnyk and Fineout-Overholt, 2019).

Health care institutions that promote and support EBP demonstrate a culture in which nurses are encouraged to question practice and identify EBP mentors to mentor other nurses in the process. These institutions have an infrastructure that supports inquiry and provides tools to support EBP, evidence-based policies and procedures, nursing leaders who value EBP, integration of EBP competencies in performance evaluations and clinical ladders, and recognition programs for nurses for their work in EBP (Caramanica and Spiva, 2018; Melnyk et al., 2018a). You need to gain knowledge and skills associated with EBP and maintain a commitment to provide the best care possible to your patients and their families.

Ask a Clinical Question in PICOT Format. Always think about your practice when caring for patients. Question what does not make sense to you and what needs to be clarified. Think about a problem or area of interest that is time consuming, costly, or illogical. These thoughts are part of an ongoing spirit of inquiry into best practice. A problem-focused trigger is one you face while caring for patients or a trend you see on a nursing unit. *For example, Cathy and Tom identified from the quality indicator report that the trend in CLABSIs increased over each of the past 3 months.* Data gathered from a health care setting allows you to examine clinical trends and form questions. Most hospitals keep monthly records on key quality or performance indicators such as medication errors or infection rates. All Magnet®-designated hospitals maintain the National Database of Nursing Quality Improvement (NDNQI). The database has information on falls, pressure injury incidence, and nurse satisfaction. Quality- and risk-management data do not give you evidence for finding a solution to a problem. Rather the data inform you about the nature or severity of problems, which then allows you to form practice questions. Other examples of problem-focused triggers include a patient injury following a fall or a patient who develops a stage III pressure injury following surgery.

A knowledge-focused trigger is a question regarding new information available on a topic. For example, "What current evidence exists to improve pain management in patients with migraine headaches?" Important sources of this type of information are standards and practice guidelines available from national agencies such as the Agency for Healthcare Research and Quality (AHRQ), the American Pain Society (APS), or the American Association of Critical Care Nurses (AACN). Other sources of knowledge-focused triggers include recent research publications and nurse experts within an organization.

Sometimes you use data gathered from a health care setting to examine clinical trends when developing clinical questions. For example, most hospitals keep monthly records on key quality indicators such as medication errors or infection rates. You use quality and risk-management data to help you understand the nature or severity of problems that then allow you to form practice questions. The questions you ask eventually lead you to the evidence for an answer.

After you identify an area of interest, there are two types of questions you may ask: a background question or foreground question. A background question asks general information about a clinical issue and needs to be answered before a searchable and answerable foreground question can be posed (Melnyk and Fineout-Overholt, 2019). For example: What is the best way to reduce wandering in patients with dementia? The question might lead you to a variety of references, some that are even irrelevant, describing approaches for reducing wandering. But background information is often important to help you form a more specific foreground question. A foreground question focuses on specific knowledge that comes from a background question (Melnyk and Fineout-Overholt, 2019). For example, a foreground question might be: In patients with dementia, does the use of stress reduction techniques reduce wandering? Forming a foreground question using a PICOT format is very specific and assists you in finding the right evidence to answer the question with some certainty. When you ask a question and then go to the scientific literature, you do not want to read 100 articles to find the handful that are most helpful. You want to be able to read the best six articles that specifically address your practice question.

Melnyk et al. (2017) suggest using a PICOT format to state a foreground question. Box 5.1 summarizes the five elements of a **PICOT question**. The more focused your question is, the easier it becomes to search for evidence in the scientific literature. *For example, Cathy and Tom first went to the literature with a general background question: "Which factors cause CLABSI in CVCs?" They were quickly frustrated when they found numerous articles about different factors that influence CLABSIs in CVCs. They decide to write two focused PICOT questions: (1) "Does the use of 2% chlorhexidine (I) compared with alcohol (C) for cleansing central catheter insertion sites in hospitalized patients (P) reduce the incidence of CLABSI (O) within 6 months (T)?" (2) "Does the use of sterile barrier techniques during catheter insertion (I) compared with sterile gloving only (C) reduce the incidence of CLABSI (O) in patients who have had surgery (P) during their hospitalization (T)?"*

Proper question formatting allows you to identify key words to use when conducting your literature search. Note that a well-designed EBP question does not have to follow the sequence of P, I, C, O, and

---

BOX 5.1   Developing a PICOT Question

P = Patient population of interest
   Identify patients by age, gender, ethnicity, and disease or health problem.
I = Intervention or area of interest
   Which intervention is worthwhile to use in practice (e.g., a treatment, diagnostic test, prognostic factor)? What area of interest influences a desired outcome (e.g., complementary therapy, motivational interviewing).
C = Comparison intervention or area of interest
   What is the usual standard of care or current intervention used now in practice?
O = Outcome
   What result do you wish to achieve or observe as a result of an intervention (e.g., change in patient behavior, physical finding, or patient perception)?
T = Time
   What amount of time is needed for an intervention to achieve an outcome (e.g., the amount of time needed to change quality of life or patient behavior)?

T. For example, a specific intervention (I), comparison (C), and time (T) are not used in every question. The aim is to ask a question that contains as many of the PICOT elements as possible. For example, here is a meaningful qualitative question that contains only a P and O: How do patients with cystic fibrosis (P) perceive their quality of life (O)? The PICOT format allows you to ask questions that are intervention focused. For questions that are not intervention focused, the meaning of the letter I can be an area of interest instead of an intervention (Melnyk and Fineout-Overholt, 2019). For example, does the use of complementary therapies (I) compared with analgesics (C) lessen pain (O) in patients with osteoarthritis (P)?

The questions you ask using as many elements as possible in a PICOT format help to identify knowledge gaps within a clinical situation. Asking well-thought-out questions allows you to identify evidence needed to guide clinical practice. Remember: Do not be satisfied with clinical routines. Always question and use critical thinking to consider better ways to provide patient care.

Search for the Best Evidence. Once you have a clear and concise PICOT question, you are ready to search for evidence. A variety of sources will provide the evidence needed to answer your question, such as agency policy and procedure manuals, quality improvement data, existing clinical practice guidelines, and journal articles. Do not hesitate to ask for help to find appropriate evidence. Key resources include nursing faculty, librarians, advanced practice nurses, staff educators, risk managers, and infection control nurses.

When using scientific literature for evidence, seek the assistance of a medical librarian who knows the various online databases available to you (Table 5.1). The databases contain large collections of published scientific studies, including peer-reviewed research. A **peer-reviewed** article is reviewed for accuracy, validity, and rigor and approved for publication by experts before it is published. MEDLINE and the Cumulative Index of Nursing and Allied Health Literature (CINAHL) are among the best-known online databases for scientific knowledge in health care (Melnyk and Fineout-Overholt, 2019). Some databases are available through vendors at a cost, some are free of charge, and some offer both options. Students typically have access provided by their schools. One of the more common vendors is OVID, which offers several different databases. Databases are also available on the Internet free of charge. The Cochrane Database of Systematic Reviews is a valuable source of high-quality evidence. It includes the full text of regularly updated systematic reviews and protocols for reviews currently under way. Collaborative review groups prepare and maintain the reviews. The protocols provide the background, objectives, and methods for reviews in progress (Melnyk and Fineout-Overholt, 2019).

Seek the help of a librarian to identify the databases and key words that will provide the best evidence to answer your PICOT question. When conducting a search, you need to enter and manipulate different key words until you get the combination of terms that provides the best articles to help answer your question. It usually takes several searches to find the most appropriate articles. *For example, Cathy and Tom's first PICOT question includes the key words "catheter-associated bloodstream infection," "surgical patients," "chlorhexidine," and "alcohol."* The key words you select often have one meaning to one author and a very different meaning to another. Be patient and persistent and keep trying different words and combinations of words until you find the evidence you need.

Fig. 5.2 represents the hierarchy of evidence. The level of rigor or amount of confidence you can have in the findings of a study decreases as you move down the pyramid. As a nursing student, you cannot be an expert on all aspects of the types of studies conducted. But you can learn enough about the types of studies to help you know which ones have the best scientific evidence. At the top of the pyramid are systematic reviews or meta-analyses, which are state-of-the-art summaries from an individual researcher or panel of experts. Meta-analyses and systematic reviews are the perfect answers to PICOT questions because they rigorously summarize current evidence about a specific topic or intervention.

During either a meta-analysis or a systematic review, a researcher asks a PICOT question, reviews the highest level of evidence available (e.g., randomized controlled trials [RCTs]), summarizes what is currently known about the topic, and reports whether current evidence supports a change in practice or whether further study is needed. The main difference is that in a meta-analysis the researcher uses statistics to show the effect of an intervention on an outcome. In a systematic review, no statistics are used to draw conclusions about the evidence. In the Cochrane Library, all entries include information on meta-analyses and systematic reviews. If you use MEDLINE or CINAHL, enter a text word such as *meta-analysis, systematic reviews,* or *evidence-based medicine* to obtain scientific reviews on your PICOT question.

A randomized controlled trial (RCT) is the highest level of experimental research. In an RCT a researcher tests an intervention (e.g., method for intravenous [IV] site care or patient education) against the usual standard of care. Researchers randomly assign subjects in an experiment to either a control or a treatment group. In other words, all of the subjects have an equal chance to be in either group. The treatment group receives the experimental intervention, and the control group receives the usual standard of care. The researchers measure both groups for the same outcomes and then perform statistical tests to see whether the experimental intervention made a significant difference. When an RCT is completed, the researcher has evidence if the intervention leads to better outcomes than the standard of care.

TABLE 5.1	Searchable Scientific Literature Databases and Sources
Databases	**Sources**
AHRQ	Agency for Healthcare Research and Quality; includes clinical guidelines and evidence summaries http://www.ahrq.gov
CINAHL	Cumulative Index of Nursing and Allied Health Literature; includes studies in nursing, allied health, and biomedicine https://www.ebscohost.com/nursing/products/cinahl-databases/cinahl-complete
MEDLINE	Includes studies in medicine, nursing, dentistry, psychiatry, veterinary medicine, and allied health https://www.nlm.nih.gov/bsd/medline.html
EMBASE	Biomedical and pharmaceutical studies http://www.embase.com
PsycINFO	Psychology and related health care disciplines http://www.apa.org/psycinfo/
Cochrane Database of Systematic Reviews	Full text of regularly updated systematic reviews prepared by the Cochrane Collaboration; includes completed reviews and protocols https://www.cochrane.org/search/site/systematic%20reviews
PubMed	Health science library at the National Library of Medicine; offers free access to journal articles https://www.ncbi.nlm.nih.gov/pubmed/
World Views on Evidence-Based Nursing	Electronic journal containing articles that provide a synthesis of research and an annotated bibliography for selected references

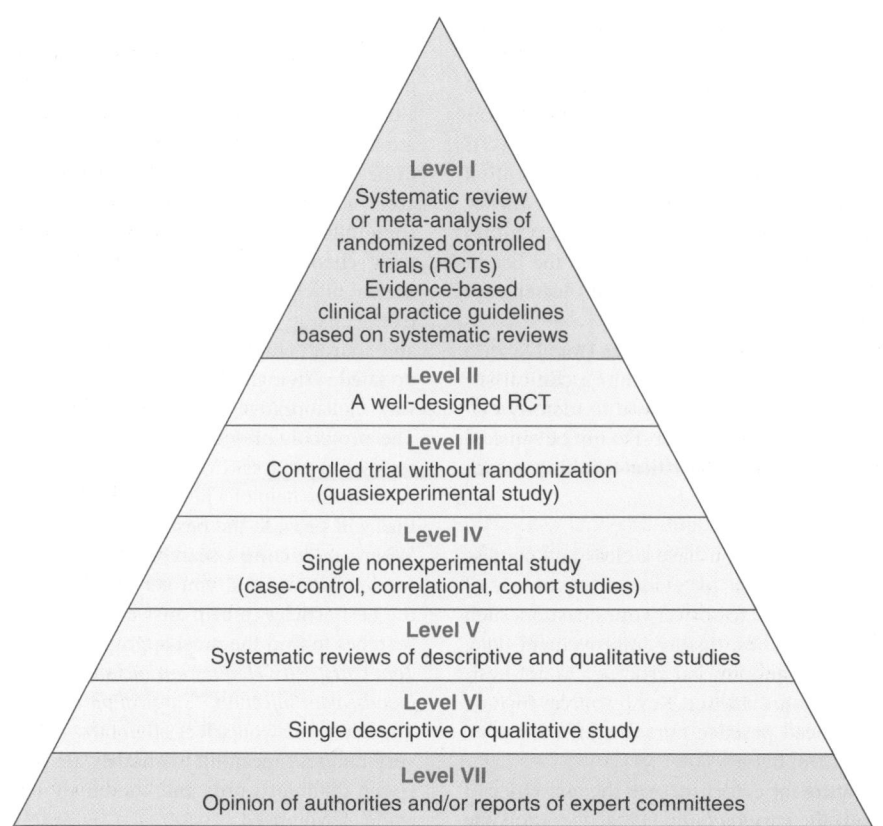

FIG. 5.2 Levels of evidence. (From LoBiondo-Wood G, Haber J: *Nursing research*, ed 9, St Louis, 2018, Elsevier).

A single RCT is not as conclusive as a review of several RCTs on the same question. However, a single RCT that tests the intervention included in your question yields useful evidence. If an RCT is not available on your question, use results from other research studies such as descriptive or qualitative studies to answer your PICOT question. The use of clinical experts may be at the bottom of the evidence pyramid but does not consider clinical experts to be poor sources of evidence. Expert clinicians use evidence frequently as they build their own practice, and they are rich sources of information for clinical problems.

REFLECT NOW

Write a PICOT question related to a situation you encountered during a recent clinical experience. Identify the key words that you would use to search the databases and literature for evidence.

Critically Appraise the Evidence. With the help of the hospital librarian, *Tom searched three databases: PubMed, CINAHL, and the Cochrane Database of Systematic Reviews. He found a systematic review summary on central line dressings from the Cochrane Database. An article from the highly regarded* New England Journal of Medicine *reported on a research study that showed a reduction in CLABSIs after use of a bundling of several interventions (including use of chlorhexidine and barrier precautions). Cathy helped by searching the Centers for Disease Control and Prevention (CDC) website for clinical guidelines on central line catheters. Once they obtained the full text of all articles (not just the abstracts), Cathy and Tom distributed them to members of their UPC for critical review and evaluation.*

Critically reviewing and analyzing the available evidence requires a systematic approach. When evaluating the available evidence, you determine the value, feasibility, and usefulness of evidence for making a practice change (Mitchell and Freise, 2016). There are numerous critical appraisal tools available for nurses to use to evaluate the evidence using a structured format (Buccheri and Sharifi, 2017). Review each source of evidence (article, clinical guideline, expert summary) to determine its value, feasibility, and utility of evidence for making a practice change. This requires you to review each source of evidence carefully to determine its scientific worth and the strength of any study methods (when appropriate), to identify the level of evidence from each source, to summarize your findings, and to determine whether the evidence is conclusive regarding your practice question (Buccheri and Sharifi, 2017). *The ICU UPC committee reviews the articles and clinical guidelines on CLABSIs and decides whether there is convincing evidence for the use of chlorhexidine instead of alcohol in cleansing catheter sites. The team also determines whether the use of barrier precautions during catheter insertion makes a difference in infection rates.*

It takes time to develop skills needed to critique the evidence like an expert. When you read an article, do not put it down and walk away because of the statistics and technical language. To determine its worth to practice, consider:

- What is the level of evidence?
- How well was the study (if research) conducted?
- How useful are the findings to practice?

Know the elements of an article when reviewing each one. Read each article carefully to decide how well the study was conducted. When reading through a scientific study, summarize key elements. Many EBP committees use critical appraisal guides or useful checklists for evaluating studies (Spruce et al., 2016). A guide lists questions about essential elements of research (e.g., purpose, sample size, setting, method of study). It is important to know the elements of scientific articles to decide the value and relevance to your PICOT question (Buccheri and Sharifi, 2017). Evidence-based articles include the following elements:

- *Abstract.* An abstract is a brief summary that quickly tells you if the article is research or clinically based. An abstract summarizes the purpose of the article. It also includes the major themes or findings and the implications for nursing practice.
- *Introduction.* The introduction contains more information about the purpose of the article. There is usually brief supporting evidence as to why the topic is important. Together the abstract and introduction help you decide if you want to continue to read the entire article. You will know if the topic of the article is similar to your PICOT question or related closely enough to provide useful information. If you decide that an article will most likely help answer your question, continue to read the next elements of the article.
- *Literature review or background.* A good author offers a detailed background of the level of science or clinical information about the topic. The literature review offers an argument about what led the author to conduct a study or report on a clinical topic. This section of an article is very valuable. Even if the article itself does not address your PICOT question the way you desire, the literature review may lead you to more useful articles and build your knowledge base in nursing. After reading a literature review, you should have a good idea of how past research led to the researcher's question. *For example, one article Tom found described a study designed to test the effects of aseptic practices on CLABSI. This study reviewed literature that describes the nature of CLABSI and the patients most at risk, the type of factors shown previously in the literature to contribute to CLABSI, and previous interventions used to prevent CLABSI.*
- *Manuscript narrative.* The "middle section," or narrative, of an article differs according to the type of evidence-based article it is (Melnyk and Fineout-Overholt, 2019). A clinical article describes a clinical topic, which often includes a description of a patient population, the nature of a certain disease or health alteration, how patients are affected, and the appropriate nursing therapies. An author sometimes writes a clinical article to explain how to use a therapy or new technology. A research article contains several subsections within the narrative, including the following:
  - *Purpose statement:* Explains the focus or intent of a study. It includes research questions or hypotheses—predictions made about the relationship or differences among study variables (concepts, characteristics, or traits that vary within or among subjects). *An example of a research question is: Does the use of chlorhexidine 2% compared with povidone-iodine reduce CLABSI in patients with CVCs? Within this question the author is studying the variables (independent) of chlorhexidine and povidone-iodine solutions as they affect the outcome (dependent variable) of CLABSI in patients. In contrast, a hypothesis might state: Chlorhexidine 2% for site care reduces the incidence of CLABSI in patients with CVCs.*
  - *Methods or design:* Explains how a research study was organized and conducted to answer the research question or test the hypothesis. This section explains the type of study that was conducted (e.g., RCT, case control study, or qualitative study) and the number of subjects or people who participated in the study. In health care research, subjects often include patients, family members, or health care staff. The methods section is sometimes confusing because it explains details about how the researcher designed the study to obtain the most accurate results possible. Use your faculty member as a resource to help interpret this section.

- *Analysis:* This section explains how the data collected in a study are analyzed. If quantitative data such as physical measurements and scores on surveys are collected, statistical results from the study are explained. Statistics can be confusing. Focus on learning whether the researcher found differences between groups or if an association was found between different variables. For example, if a researcher tests a new fall-prevention strategy, did the strategy reduce falls more so than the standard approach to care? The researcher statistically reports a "p value." The p value (usually set at 0.05) is a probability level that tells you whether the difference between two groups was likely related to the intervention or if it was simply a difference by chance (Lobiondo-Wood and Haber, 2018). When the statistic shows that the value was less than the p value (<0.05), the result was likely the result of the intervention (less than 5% probability caused by chance). If a study involved collection of qualitative information such as audiotaped interviews or open-ended surveys, the analysis describes the major themes from the data. This section helps to determine whether a study was conducted in a way that allows you to trust the results and use them to inform practice (Lobiondo-Wood and Haber, 2018).
- *Results or conclusions:* Clinical and research articles have a summary section. In a clinical article the author explains the clinical implications for the topic presented. In a research article the author details the results of the study and explains whether a hypothesis is supported or how a research question is answered. This section includes a statistical analysis if it is a quantitative research study. A qualitative study summarizes the descriptive themes and ideas that arise from the researcher's analysis of data. Do not let the statistical analysis in an article overwhelm you. Read carefully and ask these questions: Does the researcher describe the results? Were the results significant? An effective author also discusses limitations to a study in this section. The information on limitations is valuable in helping you decide if you want to use the evidence with your patients. Have a faculty member or an expert nurse help you interpret statistical results.
- *Clinical implications:* A research article includes a section that explains whether the findings from the study have clinical implications. The researcher explains the generalizability or how to apply findings in a practice setting for the type of subjects studied.

After you have critically reviewed each article for your PICOT question, combine the findings from all of the articles to determine the state of the evidence. If you used a critical appraisal guide for each article, summarize information in all of the forms into a final evaluation table. As you complete the evaluation table, use critical thinking to consider the scientific rigor or strength of the combined evidence and how well it answers your area of interest. Consider the evidence in light of your patients' concerns, values, preferences, and available health care resources. Your review of articles offers a snapshot conclusion of the combined evidence on your PICOT question. As a new nurse you learn to judge whether to use the evidence for a particular patient or group of patients who usually have complex health care situations (Melnyk and Fineout-Overholt, 2019). Ethically it is important to consider evidence that benefits patients and does no harm.

After appraising all articles, the UPC in the case study focuses on the systematic review, the *research study, and CDC clinical guidelines as offering the most information about the use of chlorhexidine and other interventions for preventing CLABSI. The committee collaborates by discussing their conclusions, reviews the results of the final evaluation table, and applies their clinical expertise. They consider the types of patients they see in the ICU and determine whether the evidence is strong enough for use in practice.*

The systematic review article (evidence level 1) did not address chlorhexidine use but concluded that there was no definitive advantage of transparent IV dressings over gauze for preventing CLABSI. Although Level VII evidence, the clinical guidelines from the CDC contained recommendations categorized on the basis of strength of existing scientific data and applicability. The CDC guidelines reported that research has shown no difference between transparent and gauze dressings in causing bloodstream infection (BSI) and highly recommends use of chlorhexidine for IV site care and the use of sterile barriers during catheter insertion. The cohort study (evidence level IV) showed a significant reduction in CLABSI in ICUs that used a bundle of interventions, including rigorous hand hygiene, chlorhexidine site care, and sterile barriers. The data from all studies were applicable to adult critically ill patients. The committee recommended adopting practice changes to include chlorhexidine site care, sterile barrier precautions for catheter insertion, and reinforcement of strict hand hygiene during all forms of central line site care.

Integrate the Evidence. If you decide that the evidence is strong and applicable to your patients and clinical situation, you begin to identify how to incorporate it into practice. Your first step is simply to apply the research in your plan of care for a patient (see Chapter 18). Use the evidence you find as a rationale for an intervention you plan to try. For instance, you learned about an approach to bathe older adults who are confused and decide to use the technique during your next clinical assignment. If you find that the bathing technique is successful with your own assigned patients, you may begin to work with a group of other students or nurses to revise the policy and procedure for bathing patients or develop a new clinical protocol.

When you work as a part of a hospital committee or task force, sometimes EBP change occurs on a larger scale. Engagement involves bringing all stakeholders (individuals who have an interest or concern in the practice change) together to explain why the evidence-based interventions are important. For example, administrators want to know if the practice change improves patient outcomes and lowers costs. Staff nurses want to know if the practice change improves patient outcomes and how it will affect the way they provide care. Health care providers also want to know how the practice change affects the way they provide care. It is important to consider the setting in which you want to apply the evidence and ask if stakeholders support the change. To integrate evidence into practice, education of all those involved in the practice change must occur. This requires approaches such as teaching seminars, informational newsletters, and ongoing discussions during staff and UPC meetings.

The actual execution of a practice change requires planning, especially if it occurs on a large scale, involving more than one nursing unit or work area. The staff who are implementing a practice change must work closely with those who will be adopting the new practice to anticipate what will be needed to make a change successful. For example, new documentation forms, different types of supplies, or a change in the way information is communicated among disciplines may be needed. It is often best to test a new practice change by conducting a 3-month pilot before implementing on a large scale. A pilot study is a small-scale research study or one that includes a quality or performance improvement (PI) project. The results of the pilot tell you whether the practice change can be implemented easily and whether it results in desired outcomes. Nursing staff buy-in is important to the success of the pilot project and to sustaining the change. Nurses are more likely to use evidence-based practices if they perceive the practices to be useful and relevant and if their work environment is supportive and promotes communication (Jun et al., 2016).

A common approach used for integrating evidence into practice is to incorporate new evidence into policies and procedures (P&Ps). A key feature of a practice environment that supports the use of best evidence is to require clinical practice policies and procedures to be evidence based (Hanrahan et al., 2015; Jun et al., 2016). Many organizations involve staff nurses and research-prepared advanced practice nurses to review scientific articles relevant to P&Ps and make appropriate revisions. P&Ps are important tools for supporting hospital-based nurses in using evidence in their everyday practice and promoting positive patient outcomes (Jun et al., 2016).

After reviewing the evidence on CLABSI, the UPC committee decides to revise the P&P for central catheter insertion and maintenance. Cathy and Tom recommend that the committee conduct in-service sessions to educate all staff about the new P&P. A brief explanation about the change is also placed in the monthly newsletter of the unit. The bundle of interventions (hand hygiene, chlorhexidine use, and full barrier precautions) is implemented after the staff have the opportunity to ask questions about the new protocol in staff meetings. The ICU implements the new P&P with the UPC committee monitoring the monthly reports on CLABSI to determine whether infection rates change. In addition, the UPC audits staff practices to be sure that the new interventions are being followed consistently and that the change in practice is sustained.

Evaluate the Outcomes of the Practice Decision or Change. After applying evidence in your practice, your next step is to evaluate the outcome. How does the intervention work? How effective was the clinical decision for your patient or practice setting? Sometimes your evaluation is as simple as determining whether the expected outcomes you set for an intervention are met (see Chapters 18 and 20). For example, after the use of a transparent IV dressing, does the IV dislodge, or does the patient develop the complication of phlebitis? When using a new approach to preoperative teaching, do patients learn what to expect after surgery?

When an EBP change occurs on a larger scale, an evaluation is more formal. *For example, evidence of factors that reduce the incidence of CLABSI leads the ICU to adopt the new P&P for central line catheter care. To evaluate the procedure, the members of the EBP committee track the outcome of incidence of CLABSI over a course of time before and after the practice change (e.g., 3 to 6 months). Measures from preintervention and postintervention are needed to determine change. In this case the CLABSI measure is collected by the hospital monthly. In addition, the staff collect data to describe both the patients who develop CLABSI and those who do not. This comparative information is valuable in determining the effects of the protocol and whether modifications are necessary.*

When evaluating an EBP change, determine whether the change was effective, whether modifications in the change are needed, or whether the change needs to be discontinued. Events or results that you do not expect may occur. *For example, the changes made in the protocol developed by Cathy and Tom might lead to an increase in CLABSIs. If this is not determined during evaluation, the practice would continue, and patients would suffer.* Never implement a practice change without evaluating its effects.

Communicate the Outcomes of the Evidence-Based Practice Decision. After implementing an EBP change, it is important to communicate the results. If you implement an evidence-based intervention with one patient, you and the patient determine the effectiveness of that intervention. When a practice change occurs on a nursing unit level, the first group to discuss the outcomes of the change is often the clinical staff on that unit. Unit huddles and visual management tools, such as a Gemba board to collect process issues, are effective strategies for communicating EBP changes and practices (Bourgault et al., 2018). To enhance professional development and promote positive patient outcomes beyond the unit level, share the results with various groups of nurses or other care providers such as the nursing practice council, EBP council, or the research council (Carter and Rivera, 2018). Clinicians enjoy and appreciate seeing the results of a practice change. In addition, the practice change will more likely be sustainable and remain in place when staff are able to see the benefits of an EBP change. A good way to share this information on the nursing unit is through a poster presentation to the unit staff.

As a professional nurse it is critical to contribute to the growing knowledge of nursing practice. Nurses often communicate the outcomes of EBP changes during clinical grand rounds and at professional conferences and meetings. Being involved in professional organizations allows them to present EBP changes in scientific abstracts, poster presentations, or even podium presentations.

> **REFLECT NOW**
>
> On your assigned patient care clinical unit, discuss with two nurses the most effective strategies they use to communicate EBP changes to the nursing staff.

Sustain Knowledge Use. Sustaining change in practice as a result of the EBP process is a challenge. Health care institutions are bombarded by change from governmental and accrediting agencies, internal administrative initiatives, and the ongoing demands of delivering safe and effective patient care. When a new practice change is introduced, it is important that it be incorporated into the culture and practice environment of an organization. It is important for health care institutions to use targeted strategies to sustain use of EBP decisions and changes (Box 5.2). Often larger hospitals or health care systems will hire nurse researchers or nurse scientists to manage and further develop the EBP and nursing research programs within the agency (Carter and Rivera, 2018). Mentorship and modeling of EBP by advanced practice nurses facilitate implementation of EBP in clinical settings (Melnyk et al., 2018b). *After the ICU adopts the new P&P for central line catheter care, the committee posts the monthly CLABSI outcome measure on the conference room bulletin board for all staff to see. Members of the UPC conduct occasional audits to be sure that the processes of using chlorhexidine and sterile barriers are being followed by staff members. When the incidence of CLABSI starts to go back up, the UPC committee discusses the results and reviews the causes for each patient situation.* Translating new knowledge into practice requires transformational nursing leadership (see Chapter 21) that provides the resources to develop EBP education for nurses to increase EBP knowledge, such as a toolkit to standardize nursing practices, participation on interprofessional EBP teams, and role modeling of EBP behaviors (Warren et al., 2016a; Warren et al., 2016b)

NURSING RESEARCH

After completing a thorough review and critique of the scientific literature, you might not have enough strong evidence to make a practice change. Instead you may find a gap in knowledge that makes your PICOT question go unanswered. When this happens, the best way to answer your PICOT question is to conduct a research study. At this time in your career you will not be conducting research. However, you may observe nurses performing research within the hospital. It is important for you to understand the process of nursing research and how it generates new knowledge.

Nursing research improves the health and welfare of people who are underserved (NINR, n.d.). **Nursing research** is a way to identify new knowledge, improve professional education and practice, and

---

BOX 5.2 EVIDENCE-BASED PRACTICE

Strategies to Sustain Nurses' Use of Evidence-Based Practice

PICOT Question: Does the use of targeted strategies improve nurses' implementation and sustained use of evidence-based practice (EBP)?

Evidence Summary

Nurses' implementation and sustained use of EBP continues to be a challenge. To be successful in sustaining EBP, health care institutions need to have an implementation plan with targeted strategies (Hanrahan et al., 2015). It is essential that leaders in the institution actively engage in and role model EBP behaviors and provide mentorship to other nurses (Warren et al., 2016b). Nurses who work on units where the leaders have clear vision and use integrated strategies and EBP activities have higher levels of continued use of EBP practices (Caramanica and Spiva, 2018; Fleiszer et al., 2016). Forming a health care agency or unit committee such as a Nursing Clinical Effectiveness Committee or EBP committee within the Shared Governance Councils was found to be an effective targeted strategy to engage nurses in EBP at the unit level (Gallagher-Ford, 2014; McKeever et al., 2016). Nurses are more interested in and willing to adopt innovative practices when they have nursing leaders who provide ongoing communication related to research and EBP (Mortenius et al., 2016). Scholarly mentorships from nursing faculty through academic partnerships or from advanced practice nurses and participation in journal clubs helped nurses develop EBP skills (Carter and Rivera, 2018; Fritz, 2017). EBP fellowship programs increased nurses' EBP knowledge as well as EBP implementation (Friesen et al., 2017; Kim et al., 2017). Visual management tools, such as gemba boards (visual board that includes a method for collecting process issues identified by nurses), and huddles foster an EBP culture (Bourgault et al., 2018). Targeted approaches help nurses engage in EBP in their practices.

Application to Nursing Practice

- Be familiar with the nursing leader's vision as it relates to strategies and activities for EBP in the health care agency (Fleiszer et al., 2016; Melnyk et al., 2018a).
- Form an EBP team or journal club with other nurses to help create a culture of inquiry in your agency (Kitson and Harvey, 2016; Fritz, 2017).
- Watch for strategic communication from leadership about research and EBP educational opportunities and improvements within your agency (Mortenius et al., 2016; Melnyk et al., 2018a).
- Partner with a nursing professor or an advanced practice nurse who can mentor you as you develop your skills in EBP (Carter and Rivera, 2018; Melnyk et al., 2018b).
- As a student, partner with a nurse on the unit to search the literature to answer a practice improvement question and share your findings with the other nurses (Raines, 2016).

---

use nursing and health care resources effectively. Research means to search again or to examine carefully. It is a systematic process that asks and answers questions to generate knowledge. The knowledge provides a scientific basis for nursing practice and validates the effectiveness of nursing interventions. Nursing research improves professional education and practice and helps nurses use resources effectively (e.g., how to best use human resources by determining the best practice mix of nurses and assistive personnel on a nursing unit). The scientific knowledge base of nursing continues to grow, providing evidence that nurses can use to provide safe and effective patient care. Many professional and specialty nursing organizations have agendas for research among their members to advance nursing science.

Translation Research

Translation research focuses on "testing implementation interventions to improve uptake and use of evidence to improve patient outcomes and population health" (Titler, 2018, p. 1). It is also called implementation science. The purpose of studies in translation research is to test implementation strategies to determine which strategies work best to promote use of EBP (Titler, 2018). In testing strategies, translation research helps to uncover which strategies work for whom, in what settings, and why. In conducting translation research, nurses can improve and sustain use of best evidence in practice with the goal of improving patient care, population health, and health outcomes (Titler, 2018). Translation research occurs along a dynamic continuum that moves through five phases—from basic research to application of research findings in a variety of settings. The five phases include:

- Preclinical and animal studies—basic science research
- Phase 1 clinical trials—testing safety and efficacy in a small group of human subjects
- Phase 2 and 3 clinical trials—testing safety and efficacy in a larger group of human subjects and testing for comparison to standard treatment
- Phase 4 clinical trials and outcomes research—translation to practice
- Phase 5 population-level outcomes research—translation to community (Titler, 2018)

Translation research differs from EBP. In translation research, a research study tests the strategies that were used to implement and sustain EBP, whereas EBP focuses on the use of best evidence in practice. Translation research poses a research question and hypothesis. Then a variety of research designs and methods can be used to answer the research question and test the hypothesis (Titler, 2014). Doctorally prepared nurses play a key role in conducting translation research to improve health outcomes (Trautman et al., 2018).

Outcomes Research

In today's health care delivery system, it is more important than ever to understand the results of health care practices. Outcomes research helps patients, health care providers, and those in health care policy make informed decisions based on current evidence (PCORI, 2018). Outcomes research typically focuses on the benefits, risks, costs, and holistic effects of a treatment on patients. For example, researchers are conducting outcomes research when they study the effects of managing Parkinson disease in patients using videoconferencing and telemedicine to increase access to health care.

Care delivery outcomes are the observable or measurable effects of health care interventions (Melnyk and Fineout-Overholt, 2019). Like the expected outcomes you develop in a plan of care (see Chapter 18), a care delivery outcome focuses on the recipients of service (e.g., patient, family, or community) and not the providers (e.g., nurse or physician). For example, an outcome of a diabetes education program is that patients are able to self-administer insulin, not the nurses' success in teaching patients who have diabetes to administer insulin.

Nurses sometimes experience difficulty in clearly defining or selecting measurable outcomes. Components of an outcome include the outcome itself, how it is observed (the indicator), its critical characteristics (how it is measured), and its range of parameters (Melnyk and Fineout-Overholt, 2019). For example, health care facilities commonly identify patient satisfaction as an outcome when introducing new services (e.g., new care delivery model or outpatient clinic). Patient satisfaction is often measured by patients' responses to a satisfaction instrument, which asks patients to rank their satisfaction with different aspects of their experience, such as nursing care, physician care, support services, and the environment. Patients complete the instrument, responding to a scale (parameter) designed to measure their degree of satisfaction (e.g., scale of 1 to 5). The combined score on the instrument yields a measure of patient satisfaction, an outcome that the agency and health care team can track over time.

Nurse-sensitive indicators are outcomes that are directly influenced by nursing practice (Grove and Gray, 2019). Although it is important to research the effects of nursing care on nurse-sensitive indicators, some researchers choose outcomes that do not measure a direct effect of nursing care, such as length of stay, mortality, quality of life, and patient satisfaction. Researchers need to select appropriate outcomes when designing their studies. For example, if a nurse researcher intends to measure the success of a nurse-initiated protocol to manage blood glucose levels in patients who are critically ill, the researcher will not likely measure mortality because it is too broad and susceptible to many factors outside the control of the nurse-initiated protocol (e.g., the selection of medical therapies, the patients' acuity of illness). Instead the nurse researcher will have a better idea of the effects of the protocol by measuring the outcome of patients' blood glucose ranges. The researcher obtains the blood glucose level of patients placed on the protocol and compares them to a desired range that represents good blood glucose control.

Scientific Method

The scientific method is the foundation of research and the most reliable and objective of all methods of gaining knowledge. This method is an objective way to gain and test knowledge. The method guides you in applying research-based evidence in practice and conducting future research. When using research findings to change practice, you need to understand the process used to guide a study. The scientific method is a systematic, step-by-step process. When completed correctly, you know that the study supports the validity, reliability, and generalizability of the data. Thus, you can safely apply the findings of such a study to similar subjects in a different study.

Researchers use the scientific method to understand, explain, predict, or control a nursing phenomenon (Lobiondo-Wood and Haber, 2018). Systematic, orderly procedures reduce the possibility for error. Although this possibility always exists, the scientific method minimizes the chance that a researcher's bias or opinion will influence the results of the study and thus the knowledge gained. Scientific research includes the following characteristics:

- The research identifies the problem area or area of interest to study.
- The steps of planning and conducting a research study are systematic and orderly.
- Researchers try to control external factors that are not being studied but can influence a relationship between the phenomena they are studying. For example, if a nurse is studying the relationship between diet and heart disease, he or she controls other characteristics among subjects, such as stress or smoking history, because they are risk factors for heart disease. Patients on an experimental diet and those on a regular diet would both need to have similar levels of stress and smoking histories to test the true effect of the diet.
- Researchers gather empirical data through the use of observations and assessments and use the data to discover new knowledge.
- The goal is to apply the knowledge gained from a study to a broader group of patients.

Nursing and the Scientific Approach

In the past much of the information used in nursing practice was borrowed from other disciplines, such as biology, physiology, and psychology. Often nurses applied this information to their practice without testing it. For example, nurses use several methods to help patients sleep. Interventions such as giving a patient a back rub, making sure that the bed is clean and comfortable, and preparing the environment

BOX 5.3 Types of Research

- **Historical research:** Studies designed to establish facts and relationships concerning past events. Example: Study examining the societal factors that led to the acceptance of advanced practice nurses by patients.
- **Exploratory research:** Initial study designed to develop or refine the dimensions of phenomena (facts or events) or to develop or refine a hypothesis about the relationships among phenomena. Example: Pilot study testing the benefits of a new exercise program for older adults with dementia.
- **Evaluation research:** Study that tests how well a program, practice, or policy is working. Example: Study measuring the outcomes of an informational campaign designed to improve parents' ability to follow immunization schedules for their children.
- **Descriptive research:** Study that measures characteristics of people, situations, or groups and the frequency with which certain events or characteristics occur. Example: Study to examine RNs' biases toward caring for obese patients.
- **Experimental research:** Study in which the investigator controls the study variable and randomly assigns subjects to different conditions to test the variable. Example: RCT comparing chlorhexidine with Betadine in reducing the incidence of IV-site phlebitis.
- **Correlational research:** Study that explores the interrelationships among variables of interest without any active intervention by the researcher. Example: Study examining the relationship between RNs' educational levels and their satisfaction in the nursing role.

RNs, Registered nurses; *RCT,* randomized controlled trial; *IV,* intravenous.

by dimming the lights are nursing measures that are used frequently and in general are logical, commonsense approaches. However, when these measures are considered in greater depth, questions arise about their applications. For example, are they the best methods to promote sleep? Do different patients in different situations require other interventions to promote sleep?

Research allows you to study nursing questions and problems in greater depth within the context of nursing. Nurses who do not use an evidence-based approach to practice often rely solely on personal experience or the advice of nursing experts. These nurses do not question whether there is an intervention that produces better outcomes. When an intervention is unsuccessful, nurses who do not use EBP will usually use an approach practiced by a colleague or try a different sequence of accepted measures. Even if an intervention discovered with this trial-and-error approach is effective for one or more patients, it is not always appropriate for patients in other settings. Nursing interventions must be tested through research to determine the measures that work best with specific patients.

Nursing research addresses issues important to the discipline of nursing. Some of these issues relate to the profession itself, education of nurses, identification of patient and family needs in specific situations, and issues within the health care delivery system. Once research is completed, it is important to disseminate or communicate the findings. One method of dissemination is through publication of the findings in professional journals. Nursing research uses many methods to study clinical problems (Box 5.3). There are two broad approaches to research: quantitative and qualitative methods.

Quantitative Research. Quantitative nursing research precisely measures and quantifies a study's variables. Two examples of quantitative research are (1) a study dealing with a new pain therapy that quantitatively measures participants' pain severity and (2) a study testing different forms of surgical dressings to measure the extent of wound

healing. Quantitative research is the precise, systematic, objective examination of specific concepts. It focuses on numerical data, statistical analysis, and controls to eliminate bias in findings (Lobiondo-Wood and Haber, 2018). There are many quantitative methods. Some of the more commonly used quantitative methods include experimental, nonexperimental, survey, and evaluation research.

Experimental Research. An RCT is a true experimental study that tightly controls conditions to eliminate bias with the goal of generalizing the results of the study to similar groups of subjects. Researchers test an intervention (e.g., a new drug, therapy, or educational method) against the usual standard of care. They randomly assign subjects to either a control or a treatment group. When an RCT is completed, the researcher hopes to know whether the intervention leads to better outcomes than the standard of care.

Controlled trials without randomization test interventions, but researchers have not randomized the subjects into control (group with no intervention) or treatment groups (group receiving experimental intervention). Thus, there is bias in how the study is conducted. Some findings are distorted because of how the study was designed. A researcher wants to be as certain as possible when testing an intervention that the intervention is the reason for the desired outcomes. In a nonrandomized controlled trial, the way in which subjects fall into the control or treatment group sometimes influences the results. This suggests that the intervention tested was not the only factor affecting the results of the study. Careful critique allows you to determine whether bias was present in a study and what effect, if any, the bias had on the results of the study.

Although RCTs investigate cause and effect and are excellent for testing drug therapies or medical treatments, this approach is not always the best for testing nursing interventions. The nature of nursing care causes nurse researchers to ask questions that are not always answered best by an RCT. For example, nurses help patients with problems such as knowledge deficits and symptom management. When researchers attempt to plan an RCT, ethical issues will often develop if the control group does not receive the new therapeutic intervention. Also, learning to understand how patients experience health problems cannot always be addressed through an RCT. Therefore, nonexperimental descriptive studies are often used in nursing research.

Nonexperimental Research. Nonexperimental descriptive studies describe, explain, or predict phenomena (an observable fact, event, or occurrence). Two examples include (1) a study examining factors that lead to an adolescent's decision to smoke cigarettes, and (2) a study determining factors that lead patients with dementia to fall in a hospital setting.

In a case-control study researchers study one group of subjects with a certain condition (e.g., asthma) at the same time as another group of subjects who do not have the condition. A case-control study determines whether there is an association between one or more predictor variables and the condition (Melnyk and Fineout-Overholt, 2019). For example, is there an association between predictor variables such as family history or environmental exposure to dust and the incidence of asthma? Often a case control study is conducted retrospectively, or after the fact. Researchers look back in time and review available data about the two groups of subjects to understand which variables explain the condition. These studies involve a small number of subjects, creating a risk of bias. Sometimes the subjects in the two groups differ on certain other variables (e.g., amount of stress or history of contact allergies) that also influence the incidence of the condition, more so than the variables being studied, which can make it difficult to interpret the results of the study.

Correlational studies describe the relationship between two variables (e.g., the age of the adolescents and whether the adolescents smoke). The researcher determines whether the two variables are correlated or associated with one another and to what extent.

TABLE 5.2 Comparison of Steps of the Nursing Process With the Research Process

Nursing Process	Research Process
Assessment	Identify area of interest or clinical problem. • Review literature. • Formulate theoretical framework. • Reflect on personal practice and/or discuss clinical issues with experts to better define the problem.
Diagnosis	Develop research question(s)/hypotheses.
Planning	Determine how study will be conducted: • Select research design/methodology. • Identify plan to recruit sample, taking into consideration population, number, and assignment to groups. • Identify study variables: specific interventions (independent variable) and outcomes (dependent variables). • Select data collection methods. • Select approach for measuring outcomes: questionnaires, surveys, physiological measures, interviews, observations. • Formulate plan to analyze data: statistical methods to answer research questions/hypotheses.
Implementation	Conduct the study: • Obtain necessary approvals. • Recruit and enroll subjects. • Implement the study protocol/collect data.
Evaluation	Analyze results of the study: • Continually analyze study methodology. Is study consistently carried out? Are all investigators following study protocol? • Interpret demographics of study population. • Analyze data to answer each research question/hypothesis. • Interpret results, including conclusions, limitations. Use of the findings: • Formulate recommendations for further research. • Determine implications for nursing. • Disseminate the findings: presentations, publications, need for further study, how to apply findings in practice.

Many times researchers use findings from descriptive studies to develop studies that test interventions. For example, if a researcher determines that adolescents 15 years of age and older tend to smoke, he or she might later test whether participation in a program about smoking for older adolescents is effective in helping adolescents stop smoking.

Surveys. Quantitative research often uses surveys to obtain information regarding the frequency, distribution, and interrelation of variables among subjects in the study (Lobiondo-Wood and Haber, 2018). An example is a survey designed to measure nurses' perceptions of physicians' willingness to collaborate in practice. Surveys obtain information about practices, perceptions, education, experience, opinions, and other characteristics of people. The most basic function of a survey is description. Surveys gather a large amount of data to describe the population and the topic of study. It is important in survey research that the population sampled is large enough to keep sampling error at a minimum.

Evaluation Research. Evaluation research is a form of quantitative research that determines how well a program, practice, procedure, or policy is working (Lobiondo-Wood and Haber, 2018). Evaluation research determines why a program (or some components of the program) is successful or unsuccessful. When programs are unsuccessful, evaluation research identifies problems with the program and opportunities for change or barriers to program implementation.

Qualitative Research. Qualitative nursing research studies phenomena that are difficult to quantify or categorize, such as patients' perceptions of illness or quality of life. This research method describes information obtained in a nonnumeric form (e.g., data in the form of transcribed written transcripts from a series of interviews). Qualitative researchers aim to understand patients' experiences with health problems and the contexts in which the experiences occur. Patients tell their stories and share their experiences in these studies. The findings have depth because patients are usually descriptive in what they choose to share. Examples of qualitative studies include (1) patients' perceptions of nurses' caring in a palliative care unit, and (2) the perceptions of stress by family members of critically ill patients.

Qualitative research involves inductive reasoning to develop generalizations or theories from specific observations or interviews (Lobiondo-Wood and Haber, 2018). For example, a nurse extensively interviews cancer survivors and then summarizes the common themes from the interviews to inductively determine the characteristics of cancer survivors' quality of life. Qualitative research involves the discovery and understanding of important behavioral characteristics or phenomena.

There are several different qualitative research methods, including ethnography, phenomenology, and grounded theory. Each is based on a different philosophical or methodological view of how to collect, summarize, and analyze qualitative data.

RESEARCH PROCESS

The research process is an orderly series of steps that allow a researcher to move from asking the research question to finding the answer. Usually the answer to the initial research question leads to new questions and other areas of study. The research process builds knowledge for use in similar situations. For example, a nurse researcher wants to know the best way to provide psychosocial support for patients with breast cancer. The research process ultimately provides knowledge that nurses from a variety of settings will use to provide evidence-based nursing care. Table 5.2 summarizes steps of the research process in comparison to the nursing process (see Unit 3). Initially the researcher identifies an area of inquiry (identifying a problem), which often results from clinical practice. For example, a nurse notices that many surgical patients experience nausea after colon surgery. While speaking with a researcher at a professional nursing conference, the nurse decides to conduct a pilot study on the nursing unit to determine whether chewing peppermint gum following colon surgery prevents patients from having nausea and reduces the incidence of postoperative ileus. The nurse reviews the relevant literature to determine what is known about chewing peppermint gum and its effect on bowel mobility and nausea after abdominal surgery. The nurse notes that although many patients report problems with nausea and return of bowel function, there is limited research on the effects of chewing gum on these two outcomes.

Following identification of the problem and review of the literature, the nurse forms a research team who designs a study with the help of a nurse researcher. The research team includes nurses, gastrointestinal surgeons, and a statistician. The study sample includes all patients who are having elective colon resections. Subjects are excluded if they need to have surgery because of an emergency situation. After obtaining approval from the hospital institutional review board, the research team randomly assigns each subject into one of the two groups (experimental or control), which means subjects have a 50-50 chance of being in each group . The control group receives standard postoperative care. Subjects in the experimental or treatment group get standard postoperative care, and they chew gum for 5 minutes 3 times a day. The research team selects appropriate instruments to measure postoperative nausea and patient assessment data to determine when nurses first hear bowel sounds and when patients first pass flatus and have their first bowel movement after surgery.

Before conducting any study with human subjects, a researcher obtains approvals from the human subjects committee or institutional review board (IRB) of an agency. An IRB includes scientists and laypeople who review all studies conducted in the institution to ensure that ethical principles, including the rights of human subjects, are followed. Informed consent means that research subjects (1) are given full and complete information about the purpose of a study, procedures, data collection, potential harm and benefits, and alternative methods of treatment; (2) are capable of fully understanding the research and the implications of participation; (3) have the power of free choice to voluntarily consent or decline participation in the research; and (4) understand how the researcher maintains confidentiality or anonymity. Confidentiality guarantees that any information a subject provides will not be reported in any manner that identifies the subject and will not be accessible to people outside the research team.

Once the study begins, the nurses on the unit collect data as indicated in the study protocol. Once all data are collected from every patient in the study, the team analyzes the data from the nausea instrument and the chart review about bowel function from the two groups studied. With the help of the statistician, analysis of the results determines whether patients who chewed peppermint gum experienced less nausea and a quicker return of bowel function than the patients who had standard nursing care. The results from this study may advance postoperative nursing care.

Researchers always need to consider study limitations. Limitations are factors that affect study findings, such as a small sample of subjects, a unique setting where the study was conducted, or the failure of the study to include representative cultural groups or age-groups. The research team conducted a pilot study because little data were available about the benefits of chewing gum following abdominal surgery. The sample size included only 20 patients in each group, and it was challenging to collect all the data from the patient charts because of inconsistencies in documentation. Therefore, the results of the study have limited generalizability to other patients who are experiencing abdominal surgery. These limitations help the team decide how to refine or adapt the study for further investigation in the future.

A researcher also addresses the implications for nursing practice. This ultimately helps fellow researchers, clinicians, educators, and administrators apply findings from a study in practice. At the end of the chewing gum study, the research team recommends that patients who have elective colon resections be offered the opportunity to chew peppermint gum following surgery. The surgeons on the unit agreed to the change in practice. The team decides to conduct another study to investigate this intervention with patients who have other types of abdominal surgeries to enhance the generalizability of the results. In addition, the team suggests ways to effectively introduce the use of chewing gum into other surgical units following surgery.

PERFORMANCE IMPROVEMENT

Performance improvement (PI) is a formal approach for the analysis of health care–related processes. It does not involve introduction of new practices, as is the case of EBP, but it can involve review of how interventions within a process function effectively. Health care organizations routinely promote efforts for improving patient care processes and outcomes, particularly with respect to reducing medical errors and enhancing patient safety. PI is the continuous and ongoing effort to achieve measurable improvements in the efficiency, effectiveness, performance, accountability, outcomes, and other indicators of quality services or processes (Green et al., 2018).

Every health care organization gathers and reports data on multiple health outcome measures to determine its quality of care. When findings suggest potential problems, an organization institutes a formal PI initiative. Also, in many cases the trending from PI data reveals problems that lead to EBP projects. PI projects usually occur more quickly than an EBP or research project. An organization analyzes and evaluates current performance data to solve system problems (e.g., supply delivery, appointment scheduling), people problems (e.g., staffing ratios, communication protocols), or clinical problems (e.g., surgical incision infection rates, patient injuries from falls). When interprofessional teams participate in PI activities, they may or may not use research findings to develop strategies; however, an evidenced-based approach is advised when dealing with clinical problems.

Performance Improvement Programs

A well-organized PI program focuses on processes or systems that significantly contribute to outcomes of a specific organization as well as plan on how to sustain measurable improvements over time. Facilities need an organization-wide, systematic approach to ensure that everyone supports a continuous PI philosophy. This begins with the organizational culture, in which all staff members understand their responsibility toward maintaining and improving quality (Connelly, 2018). Typically, in health care many people are involved in single processes of care. For example, medication delivery involves the health care provider who prescribes medications, the secretary who communicates new orders being written, the pharmacist who prepares the dosage, the transporter who delivers medications, and the nurse who prepares and administers the drugs. When an organization identifies a need to improve the medication administration process, all professions involved in medication administration need to be engaged in the PI process. Because most health care processes are interprofessional, all members of the health care team collaborate in PI activities. As a member of the nursing team, you participate in recognizing trends in practice, identifying recurrent problems, and initiating opportunities to improve care.

The PI process begins at the staff level, where all disciplines become involved in identifying quality problems. This requires staff members

TABLE 5.3   Examples of Performance Improvement Models

Performance Improvement Model	Summary Description
1. Balanced scorecard	A multidimensional framework for managing strategy by linking objectives, initiatives, targets, and performance measures across key organization perspectives
2. Root cause analysis (RCA)	A structured method used to analyze serious adverse events. A central tenet of RCA is to identify underlying problems that increase the likelihood of errors while avoiding the trap of focusing on mistakes by individuals.
3. Six Sigma	A disciplined methodology for process improvement that deploys a wide set of tools based on rigorous data analysis to identify sources of variation in performance and ways of reducing them
4. **P**lan-**D**o-**S**tudy-**A**ct (PDSA)	An experiential learning method that involves analyzing a quality problem and testing a change by developing a plan to test the change (Plan), carrying out the test (Do), observing and learning from the consequences (Study), and determining which modifications should be made to the test (Act).

to know the outcomes measured by the organization and the practice standards or guidelines that define quality. Unit PI committees review quality data and the activities or services considered to be most important in providing quality care to patients. One way to identify the greatest opportunity for improving quality is to consider activities that are high volume (greater than 50% of the activity of a unit); high risk (potential for trauma or death); and problem areas for patients, staff, or the institution. For example, on an orthopedic nursing unit hip surgery volume is high, adults over 80 years of age have more postoperative complications, and family members are dissatisfied with patients' pain control. Any one of these factors could become the focus of a PI project.

Another approach to PI is to use The Joint Commission's annual patient safety goals (TJC, 2020), which provide an excellent focus for PI initiatives (see Chapter 27). Sometimes a problem is presented to a committee in the form of a sentinel event, an unexpected occurrence involving death or serious physical or psychological injury of a patient. After a sentinel event, the unit conducts a root cause analysis (RCA). The goal of the RCA is to review all information and identify how the event occurred through identification of active errors (i.e., the acts that personnel perform) and why it occurred through identification and analysis of latent errors (i.e., the organization or steps of the process). Once a committee defines the problem, it applies a formal PI model for exploring and resolving quality concerns. There are several models for PI (Table 5.3). Health care organizations today are changing current organizational culture toward the concept of a "just culture." In a "just culture" the organization values the reporting of errors and is focused on the processes that lead to the error. "Just culture" also values nurses' critical thinking and problem-solving skills and the nurses' work on improving patient care processes (Kennedy, 2016).

PI combined with EBP is the foundation for excellent patient care

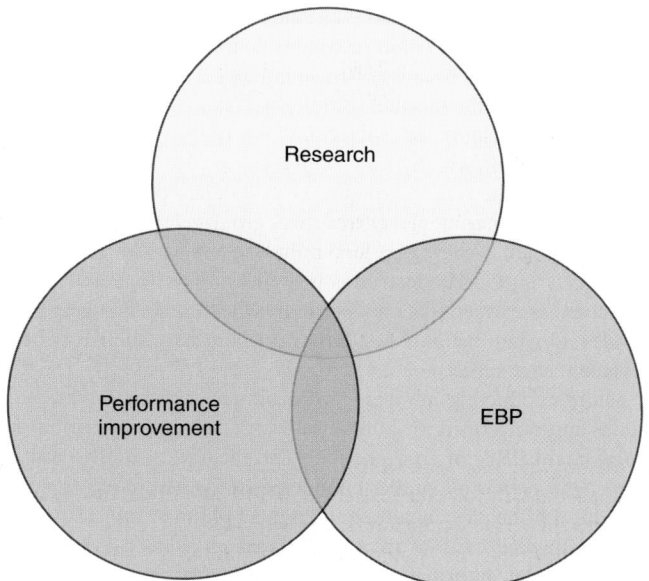

FIG. 5.3 The overlapping relationship among research, evidence-based practice (EBP), and performance improvement.

activities through staff meetings, newsletters, and memos are good communication strategies. Often a PI study reveals information that prompts organization-wide change. An organization must be responsible for responding to the problem with the appropriate resources. Revision of policies and procedures, modification of standards of care, and implementation of new support services are examples of ways an organization responds.

THE RELATIONSHIP BETWEEN EBP, RESEARCH, AND PERFORMANCE IMPROVEMENT

EBP, research, and performance improvement (PI) are closely interrelated (Fig. 5.3) and exist along a continuum of clinical scholarship (Carter et al., 2017). All three processes require you to use the best evidence to provide the highest quality of patient care. As a nurse you are professionally accountable to know the differences and which process to select when facing clinical problems or when you desire to improve patient care. Although you will use all of these in nursing practice, it is important to know the similarities and differences among them (Carter et al., 2017) (Table 5.4). When implementing an EBP project, it is important to first review evidence from appropriate research and PI data. This information helps you better understand the extent of a problem in practice and within your organization. PI data inform you

> **QSEN** **Building Competency in Evidence-Based Practice** The Nursing Practice Council notes that the incidence of falls with injuries has increased on all units in the agency over the past year. When checking its fall prevention protocol, the council notes it was last reviewed 4 years ago. The council knows that falls with injuries are a nursing-sensitive outcome (NDNQI) and established a goal to reduce the incidence of falls in the upcoming year. How should the Nursing Practice Council proceed?
>
> Answers to QSEN Activities can be found on the Evolve website.

and outcomes. Once a PI committee makes an evidence-based practice change, it is important to monitor the results and then communicate the results to staff from all appropriate departments. Practice changes are unlikely to last when PI committees fail to report findings and the results of interventions (Nilsen et al., 2017). Regular discussions of PI

TABLE 5.4 Similarities and Differences Among Evidence-Based Practice, Research, and Performance Improvement

	Evidence-Based Practice	Research	Performance Improvement
Purpose	Use of information from research, professional experts, personal experience, and patient preferences to determine safe and effective nursing interventions with the goal of improving patient outcomes	Systematic inquiry answers questions, solves problems, and contributes to the generalizable knowledge base of nursing; it may or may not improve patient care.	Improves local work processes to improve patient outcomes and efficiency of health systems; results usually not generalizable
Focus	Implementation of evidence already known into practice	New knowledge is generated to find answers for questions that are not known about nursing practice.	Measures effects of practice and/or practice change on specific patient population
Data sources	Multiple research studies, expert opinion, personal experience, patients	Subjects or participants have predefined characteristics that include or exclude them from a study; researcher collects and analyzes data from subjects.	Data from patient records or patients who are in a specific area such as on a patient care unit or admitted to a particular hospital
Who conducts the activity?	Practicing nurses and possibly other members of the health care team	Researchers who may or may not be employed by the health care agency and usually are not a part of the clinical health care team.	Employees of a health care agency such as nurses, physicians, pharmacists
Is activity part of regular clinical practice?	Yes	No	Yes
Is IRB approval needed?	Sometimes	Yes	Sometimes
Funding sources	Internal, from health care agency	Funding is usually external, such as a government grant. However, larger health care organizations often have internal grants available from their foundations.	Internal, from health care agency

IRB, Institutional review board.

about how processes work within an organization and thus offer information about how to make EBP changes. EBP and PI sometimes reveal problems that create opportunities for research.

The following is an example of how the three processes merge to improve nursing practice:

A nursing unit is experiencing a decrease in patient satisfaction with pain management over the last several months. PI data identify factors associated with pain management (e.g., the types of pain medications typically ordered, patient reports of pain relief following administration of pain medications). A thorough analysis of PI data leads a unit-based quality council team of nurses to conduct a literature review and implement the best evidence available to improve their pain-management protocol for the type of patients on the unit. The staff implement a revised pain management protocol and evaluate its results. Despite the implementation of the revised pain-management protocol, patient satisfaction data continue to be lower than desired. Thus, staff decide to conduct a research study to further investigate this clinical problem and improve patient care.

KEY POINTS

- EBP guides nurses and other health care providers in making effective, timely, and appropriate clinical decisions.
- The steps of EBP include cultivate a spirit of inquiry, ask a clinical question in PICOT format, search for the most relevant and best evidence, critically appraise the evidence, integrate the best evidence, evaluate the outcomes of the practice change, and communicate results of the change.
- Using problem- and knowledge-focused triggers to think critically about clinical and operational nursing-unit issues helps you define a PICOT question.

- A focused PICOT question allows you to search for evidence in the scientific literature.
- After appraising the evidence for a PICOT question, if the question is unanswered and there is a gap in knowledge, the research process is the next option for gaining new evidence.
- The research process is an orderly series of six steps that allow the researcher to move from problem identification to finding an answer to the research question.
- The hierarchy of evidence offers a guide to evaluate literature or information and determine whether a source is relevant, valid, and appropriate for use in practice.
- An RCT is the highest level of experimental research.
- Use your clinical expertise and consider patients' values and preference to ensure that you will apply the evidence in practice both safely and appropriately.
- Research is a systematic process that asks and answers questions to generate knowledge and provide a scientific basis for nursing practice.
- The best scientific evidence comes from well-designed, systematically conducted research studies.
- Although EBP, research, and PI are closely related, they are separate processes in nursing practice that all require the use of the best evidence to provide high-quality patient care.

REFLECTIVE LEARNING

- While on the clinical unit, talk to a staff nurse about the PI activities on the nursing unit. Report on the focus of the unit's PI activities to improve patient outcomes.

- Think about the nursing care that you provided to your patients on the clinical unit today. What questions came to your mind about the practices that you were doing? Formulate one of the questions in PICOT format.
- After asking the PICOT question, search the literature and find two or three research studies on the topic. What is the current state of the evidence related to your question?

REVIEW QUESTIONS

1. Match the components of PICO using the question "Does the use of guided imagery compared with standard care decrease the postoperative pain in hospitalized adolescents?"

   _____ (P) Patient/population   A. Adolescents receiving standard care

   _____ (I) Intervention   B. Decreased postoperative pain

   _____ (C) Comparison   C. Hospitalized adolescents

   _____ (O) Outcome   D. Guided imagery

2. Place the steps of the EBP process in the appropriate order.
   1. Critically appraise the evidence you gather.
   2. Ask the clinical question in PICOT format.
   3. Evaluate the outcomes of the practice decision or change.
   4. Search for the most relevant and best evidence.
   5. Cultivate a spirit of inquiry.
   6. Integrate the evidence.
   7. Communicate the outcomes of the EBP change.

3. A nurse is reading a research article discussing a new practice to decrease the incidence of catheter-associated urinary tract infections. One section of the article describes who was studied and how the data were collected to answer the research questions and hypotheses. What section of the research article is currently being read?
   1. The literature review
   2. The data analysis
   3. The methods
   4. The implications for practice

4. A nurse implements an EBP change that teaches patients the importance of taking their diabetes medications correctly and regularly on time using videos streamed on the Internet. The nurse measures the patients' behavioral outcome from the practice change using which type of measurement?
   1. Measuring the patient's weight
   2. Chart auditing teaching sessions
   3. Observing patients viewing the videos
   4. Checking patients' blood sugars

5. A patient in the intensive care unit experiences a sentinel event related to central-line catheter care that resulted in serious injury. What performance improvement model should the unit use to identify errors that led to the sentinel event?
   1. Six Sigma
   2. Root cause analysis
   3. PDSA
   4. Balanced scorecard

6. Which of the following are outcomes measurements? (Select all that apply.)
   1. A nurse teaches a patient how to administer an injection and then observes the patient do a return demonstration.
   2. A nurse implements a new pain-management protocol and checks patients' charts to confirm whether interventions are being provided.
   3. A nursing unit adopts a set of strategies for reducing pressure injuries, and the UPC members use direct observation of the skin to measure incidence of pressure injuries.
   4. A nursing unit implements a new fall-prevention protocol and checks the monthly performance data for incidence of falls on the unit.
   5. A nursing unit implements a patient rounding program, and the charge nurse watches the assistive personnel to see whether hourly rounding is being done on patients.

7. The nurses on a medical unit have seen an increase in the number of pressure injuries developing in their patients. The nurses decide to initiate a performance improvement project using the PDSA model. Which of the following is an example of "Plan" from that model?
   1. Orienting patients to the unit's practice of hourly rounding on patients
   2. Reviewing the incidence of pressure injuries on patients cared for using the protocol
   3. Based on findings from patients who developed injuries, implementing an evidence-based skin care protocol on all units
   4. Meeting with all disciplines to develop a multidisciplinary approach for reducing pressure injuries

8. The nurse is using the QSEN competency of EBP when working with the unit council to initiate a change related to pain management. Which behaviors demonstrate the nurse practicing behaviors associated with EBP? (Select all that apply.)
   1. Initiating plan for self-development as a team member
   2. Reading original research related to pain management
   3. Demonstrating effective use of strategies to reduce risk of harm to self or others
   4. Valuing EBP as critical to the development of pain management guidelines for the unit
   5. Describing to the unit council reliable sources for locating clinical guidelines
   6. Applying technology and information management tools to support safe processes of care

9. Nurses in a community clinic are conducting an EBP project focused on improving the outcomes of children with asthma. The PICO question asked by the nurses is "In school-aged children, does the use of an electronic gaming education module versus educational book improve the usage of inhalers?" In the question, what is the "O"?
   1. School-aged children
   2. Educational book
   3. Use of inhalers
   4. Electronic gaming education

10. During an EBP committee meeting, a nurse discussed two systematic integrative reviews related to the use of prepackaged bath kits versus the standard use of bath basins. What level of evidence is the nurse presenting?
    1. Level I
    2. Level II
    3. Level IV
    4. Level VI

Answers: 1. C, D, A, B; **2.** 5, 2, 4, 1, 6, 3; **7.** 3; **3.** 3; **4.** 4; **5.** 2; **6.** 1, 3, 4; **7.** 4; **8.** 2, 4, 5; **9.** 3; **10.** 1.

Rationales for Review Questions can be found on the Evolve website.

REFERENCES

Carter EJ, et al.: Clarifying the conundrum: evidence-based practice, quality improvement, or research? *J Nurs Adm* 47(5):266, 2017.

Centers for Medicare and Medicaid (CMS): *Hospital acquired conditions*, 2015. https://www.cms.gov/Medicare/Medicare-Fee-for-Service-Payment/HospitalAcqCond/Hospital-Acquired_Conditions.html. Accessed May 21, 2019.

Connelly LM: Overview of quality improvement, *Med Surg Nurs* 27(2):125, 2018.

Crabtree E, et al.: Improving patient care through nursing engagement in evidence-based practice, *Worldviews Evid Based Nurs* 13(2):172, 2016.

Green R, et al.: The CFO's role in accelerating systemwide performance improvement: finance leaders can leverage their operational expertise to serve as catalysts for comprehensive performance improvement: a systematic approach to increasing overall value, *Healthc Financl Manage* 72(6):48, 2018.

Grove SK, Gray JR: *Understanding nursing research: building an evidence-based practice*, ed 7, St. Louis, 2019, Elsevier.

Kennedy B: Team concepts: towards a just culture, *Nurs Management* 47(6):13, 2016.

Lobiondo-Wood G, Haber J: *Nursing research: methods and critical appraisal for evidence-based practice*, ed 9, St Louis, 2018, Elsevier.

McNeil A: Using evidence to structure discharge planning, *Nurs Management* 47(5):22, 2016.

Melnyk BM, et al.: *Implementing the evidence-based practice competencies in healthcare: a practical guide for improving quality, safety, & outcomes*, Indianapolis, IN, 2017, Sigma Theta Tau International.

Melnyk BM, Fineout-Overholt E: *Evidence-based practice in nursing and healthcare: a guide to best practice*, ed 4, Philadelphia, 2019, Lippincott Williams & Wilkins.

Mitchell SA, Freise CR: *Decision rules for summative evaluation of a body of evidence*, 2016. https://www.ons.org/explore-resources/pep/decision-rules-summative-evaluation-body-evidence. Accessed May 19, 2019.

National Institute of Nursing Research (NINR): The National Institute of Nursing Research, n.d., http://www.ninr.nih.gov. Accessed May 20, 2019.

National Quality Forum (NQF): *NQF's strategic direction 2016-2019: lead, prioritize, and collaborate for better healthcare measurement*, 2018. http://www.qualityforum.org/NQF_Strategic_Direction_2016-2019.aspx. Accessed May 20, 2019.

Nilsen P, et al.: Implementation of evidence-based practice from a learning perspective, *Worldviews Evid Based Nurs* 14(3):192, 2017.

Patient-Centered Outcomes Research Institute (PCORI): PCORI, 2018. http://www.pcori.org/. Accessed May 19, 2019.

Peterson M, et al.: Choosing the best evidence to guide clinical practice: application of AACN levels of evidence, *Crit Care Nurse* 34(2):58, 2014.

Quality and Safety Education for Nurses (QSEN) Institute: *QSEN Competencies*, 2018. http://qsen.org/competencies/pre-licensure-ksas/. Accessed July 2018.

Spruce L, et al.: AORN's revised model for evidence appraisal and rating, *AORN J* 103:60, 2016.

The Joint Commission (TJC): *2020 National Patient Safety Goals*, Oakbrook Terrace, IL, 2020, The Commission. http://www.jointcommission.org/en/standards_national-patient-safety-goals/. Accessed January 2, 2020.

Titler MG: Overview of evidence-based practice and translation science, *Nurs Clin N Am* 49(3):269, 2014.

Titler MG: Translation research in practice: an introduction, *Online J Issues in Nurs* 23(2):1, 2018.

Trautman DE, et al.: Advancing scholarship through translational research: the role of PhD and DNP prepared nurses, *Online J Issues in Nurs* 23(2):1, 2018.

RESEARCH REFERENCES

Bourgault AM, et al.: Using Gemba boards to facilitate evidence-based practice in critical care, *Crit Care Nurse* 38(3):e1, 2018.

Buccheri RK, Sharifi C: Critical appraisal tools and reporting guidelines for evidence-based practice, *Worldv Evid-Based Nu* 14(6):463, 2017.

Caramanica L, Spiva L: Exploring nurse manager support of evidence-based practice: clinical nurse perceptions, *JONA* 48(5):272, 2018.

Carter EJ, Rivera RR: Targeted interventions to advance a culture of inquiry at a large multicampus hospital among nurses, *JONA* 48(1):18, 2018.

Fleiszer AR, et al.: Nursing unit leaders' influence on the long-term sustainability of evidence-based practice improvements, *J Nurse Management* 24:309, 2016.

Friesen MA, et al.: Findings from a pilot study: bringing evidence-based practice to the bedside, *Worldviews Evid Based Nurs* 14(1):22, 2017.

Fritz E: Interventions to increase use of evidence-based practice by ambulatory care nurses, *AAACN ViewPoint* 4, 2017, July/August.

Gallagher-Ford L: Leveraging shared governance councils to advance evidence-based practice: the EBP council journey, *Worldviews Evid Based Nurs* 12(1):61, 2014.

Godlock G, et al.: Implementation of an evidence-based patient safety team to prevent falls in inpatient medical units, *Medsurg Nurs* 25(1):17, 2016.

Hanrahan K, et al.: Sacred cow gone to pasture: a systematic evaluation and integration of evidence-based practice, *Worldviews Evid Based Nurs* 12(1):3, 2015.

Jun J, et al.: Barriers and facilitators of nurses' use of clinical practice guidelines: an integrative review, *Int J Nurs Stud* 60(54), 2016.

Kim SC, et al.: Benefits of a regional evidence-based practice fellowship program: a test of the ARCC model, *Worldviews Evid Based Nurs* 14(2):90, 2017.

Kitson AL, Harvey G: Methods to succeed in effective knowledge translation in clinical practice, *J Nurs Scholarsh* 48(3):294, 2016.

McKeever S, et al.: Engaging a nursing workforce in evidence-based practice: introduction of a nursing clinical effectiveness committee, *Worldviews Evid Based Nurs* 13(1):85, 2016.

Melnyk BM, et al.: Outcomes from the first Helene Fuld Health Trust National Institute for evidence-based practice in nursing and healthcare invitational expert forum, *Worldviews Evid Based Nurs* 15(1):5, 2018a.

Melnyk BM, et al.: The first U.S. study on nurses' evidence-based practice competencies indicates major deficits that threaten healthcare quality, safety, and patient outcomes, *Worldviews Evid Based Nurs* 15(1):16, 2018b.

Mortenius H, et al.: Strategic communication intervention to stimulate interest in research and evidence-based practice: a 12-year follow-up study with registered nurses, *Worldviews Evid Based Nurs* 13(1):42, 2016.

Peterson MH, et al.: Choosing the best evidence to guide clinical practice: application of AACN levels of evidence, *Crit Care Nurse* 34(2):58, 2014.

Raines DA: A collaborative strategy to bring evidence into practice, *Worldviews Evid Based Nurs* 13(3):253, 2016.

Scott ES, et al.: Nursing administration research priorities, *JONA* 46(5):238, 2016.

Warren JI, et al.: The strengths and challenges of implementing EBP in healthcare systems, *Worldviews Evid Based Nurs* 13(1):15, 2016a.

Warren JI, et al.: Three-year pre-post analysis of EBP integration in a Magnet-designated community hospital, *Worldviews Evid Based Nurs* 13(1):50, 2016b.

White S, Spruce L: Perioperative nursing leaders implement clinical practice guidelines using the Iowa Model of Evidence-Based Practice 1.3, *AORN J* 102:51, 2015.

6

Health and Wellness

OBJECTIVES

- Explain how *Healthy People* guides public health goals for Americans.
- Discuss how individuals define health.
- Discuss the health belief, health promotion, basic human needs, and holistic health models to understand the relationship between patients' attitudes toward health and health practices.
- Describe variables influencing health, health beliefs, and health practices.

- Describe health promotion, health education, and illness prevention activities.
- Discuss the three levels of prevention.
- Compare and contrast nonmodifiable and modifiable risk factors that threaten health.
- Discuss nursing's role in risk-factor modification and changing health behaviors.
- Describe variables influencing illness behavior.
- Describe the effect of illness on patients and families.

KEY TERMS

Acute illness, p. 76
Chronic illness, p. 76
Health, p. 69
Health Belief Model, p. 69
Health education, p. 73

Health promotion, p. 73
Holistic Health Model, p. 70
Illness, p. 76
Illness behavior, p. 77
Illness prevention, p. 73

Primary prevention, p. 73
Risk factor, p. 74
Secondary prevention, p. 74
Tertiary prevention, p. 74

MEDIA RESOURCES

http://evolve.elsevier.com/Potter/fundamentals/
- Review Questions
- Case Study with Questions

- Audio Glossary
- Content Updates
- Answers to QSEN Activity and Review Questions

Nurses are in a unique position to help individuals, families, communities, and populations become or remain healthy. Because nurses are caregivers, advocates, and educators, they promote health and wellness in all health care settings. Through their knowledge and assessment, nurses identify actual and potential risk factors that predispose an individual or a group to illness. In addition, nurses use strategies to help patients modify those risk factors to prevent illness.

People react in different ways to their own illness or the illness of a family member. Nurses who understand how patients react to illness can help patients and their families maintain or return to the highest level of functioning, which reduces health care costs. Thus, it is important that you help patients make changes to improve their health and wellness.

HEALTHY PEOPLE

The *Healthy People* initiative provides evidence-based, 10-year national objectives for promoting health and preventing disease. *Healthy People* provides a framework to help the United States increase its focus on health promotion and disease prevention (instead of illness care) and encourages cooperation among individuals, communities, and other public, private, and nonprofit organizations to improve health (USDHHS, 2018). Widely cited by the media, in professional journals,

and at health conferences, *Healthy People* emphasizes how the health of communities affects the overall health status of the nation. Because of its interprofessional approach, it has inspired health promotion programs throughout the country since its first publication in 1979.

The current publication, *Healthy People 2020,* was approved in December 2010; it promotes a society in which all people live long, healthy lives. *Healthy People 2020* identifies leading health indicators (LHIs) (e.g., access to health services; injury and violence prevention; maternal, infant, and child health), which are high-priority health issues in the United States. Although the United States has made great progress on the LHIs, it falls behind other developed countries on key measures of health and well-being, including life expectancy, infant mortality, and obesity (USDHHS, 2018). Each month, the HealthyPeople.gov website reports on one or more of the LHIs to explain existing health disparities (USDHHS, 2018).

The Secretary's Advisory Committee on National Health Promotion and Disease Prevention Objectives for 2030 is guiding the development and implementation of *Healthy People 2030*. The framework proposed by *Healthy People 2030* will build on the previous editions of *Healthy People,* promote a holistic approach to health promotion and disease prevention, and help to engage community leaders to act and design policies to improve the health and well-being of all Americans (USDHHS, 2018).

DEFINITION OF HEALTH

The World Health Organization (WHO) defines health as a "state of complete physical, mental, and social well-being, not merely the absence of disease or infirmity" (WHO, 1947, 2018a). Health is a state of being that people define in relation to their own values, personality, and lifestyle. Each person has a personal concept of health. Health is the actualization of inherent and acquired human potential through goal-directed behavior, competent self-care, and satisfying relationships with others (Pender et al., 2015; Murdaugh et al., 2019). People adjust as needed to maintain structural integrity and harmony with the environment.

Individuals' views of health vary among different cultural orientations (Murdaugh et al., 2019). People who are free from disease are not necessarily healthy (Pender, 1996). Health is influenced by a person's values, personality, and lifestyle. People often define their health by the circumstances surrounding their lives rather than by their physical condition. Life conditions can have positive or negative effects on health long before an illness is evident (Murdaugh et al., 2019). Life conditions include socioeconomic variables such as environment, diet, lifestyle practices or choices, and many other physiological and psychological variables.

Individual perceptions and definitions of health are affected by a person's health beliefs and change as a person ages. For example, the definition of health for older people is often influenced by the absence of disease and disability, the maintenance of physical and cognitive functioning, having connections with others, and health practices a person uses regularly (Griffith et al., 2018). Thus, you consider the total person and his or her environment to individualize nursing care and enhance a patient's health.

MODELS OF HEALTH AND ILLNESS

Models help explain complex concepts or ideas, such as health and illness. Models help you understand the relationships between these concepts and a patient's attitudes toward health and health behaviors.

Health beliefs are a person's ideas, convictions, and attitudes about health and illness. They are sometimes based on facts or misinformation, common sense or myths, good or bad experiences, or reality or false expectations. Because health beliefs influence health behavior, they can positively or negatively affect a patient's level of health. Positive health behaviors maintain, attain, or regain health and prevent illness. Common positive health behaviors include immunizations, proper sleep patterns, adequate exercise, stress management, and nutrition. Negative health behaviors include practices that are harmful to health, such as smoking, drug or alcohol abuse, poor diet, and refusing to take necessary medications.

Nurses use several health models to understand patients' unique attitudes and values about health and illness and to provide effective health care. These models allow you to understand and predict patients' health behaviors, including how they use health services and adhere to recommended therapy. Positive health models focus on the individual's strengths, resiliencies, resources, potential, and capabilities rather than on disease or pathology (Murdaugh et al., 2019).

Use these models to individualize plans of care that will be effective in restoring or promoting a patient's health. Remember that each patient has a unique view of health and wellness. A person's individual belief system influences the ability to make lasting changes in health status. Do not make judgments when your patients have views and beliefs that differ from your own.

Health Belief Model

The Health Belief Model (Fig. 6.1) addresses the relationship between a person's beliefs and behaviors (Rosenstoch, 1974; Becker and Maiman, 1975). The first component of this model involves an individual's perception of susceptibility to an illness. For example, a patient whose family history includes one parent and two siblings who have died from a myocardial infarction recognizes the familial link for coronary artery disease and perceives a personal risk of heart disease.

The second component is an individual's perception of the seriousness of the illness. This perception is influenced and modified by demographic and sociopsychological variables, perceived threats of the illness, and cues to action (e.g., mass media campaigns and advice from family, friends, and medical professionals). For example, a patient may not perceive his heart disease to be serious, which may affect the way he takes care of himself.

The third component is the likelihood that a person will take preventive action. This component results from a person's perception of the benefits of and barriers to taking action. Preventive actions include lifestyle changes, increased adherence to medical therapies, or a search for medical advice or treatment. A patient's perception of susceptibility to disease and his or her perception of the seriousness of an illness help to determine the likelihood that the patient will adopt healthy behaviors. This model helps you understand factors influencing patients' perceptions, beliefs, and behaviors to plan care so that you can more effectively help patients maintain or restore health and prevent illness.

Health Promotion Model

The Health Promotion Model (HPM) (Pender, 1982, 1996; Pender et al., 2015; Murdaugh et al., 2019) defines health as a positive, dynamic state, not merely the absence of disease (Fig. 6.2). Health promotion increases a patient's level of well-being. The HPM describes the multidimensional nature of people as they interact within their environment to pursue health (Pender, 1996; Murdaugh et al., 2019). The model focuses on the following three areas: (1) individual characteristics and experiences; (2) behavior-specific knowledge and affect; and (3) behavioral outcomes, in which the patient commits to or changes a behavior. Each person has unique personal characteristics and experiences that affect subsequent actions. The set of variables for behavioral-specific knowledge and affect influence a patient's motivation to change or adopt healthy behaviors. When applying this model, you modify these variables through nursing actions. Health-promoting behaviors result in improved health, enhanced functional ability, and better quality of life at all stages of development (Murdaugh et al., 2019).

Maslow's Hierarchy of Needs

Nurses use Maslow's hierarchy of needs to understand the interrelationships of basic human needs (Fig. 6.3). Basic human needs are necessary for human survival and health (e.g., food, water, safety, and love). Although each person has unique needs, all people share basic human needs, and the extent to which people meet their basic needs is a major factor in determining their level of health.

According to this model, certain human needs are more basic than others, and some needs must be met before other needs (e.g., fulfilling physiological needs before the needs of love and belonging). Self-actualization is the highest expression of one's individual potential and allows for continual self-discovery. Maslow's model considers individual experiences, which are always unique to that individual (Touhy and Jett, 2016).

Maslow's hierarchy provides a basis for nurses to care for patients of all ages in all health settings. However, when applying the model, the focus of care is on a patient's needs rather than on strict adherence to the hierarchy. It is unrealistic to always expect a patient's basic needs to occur in the fixed hierarchical order. In all cases an emergent physiological need takes precedence over a higher-level need. In other situations, a psychological or physical safety need takes priority. For

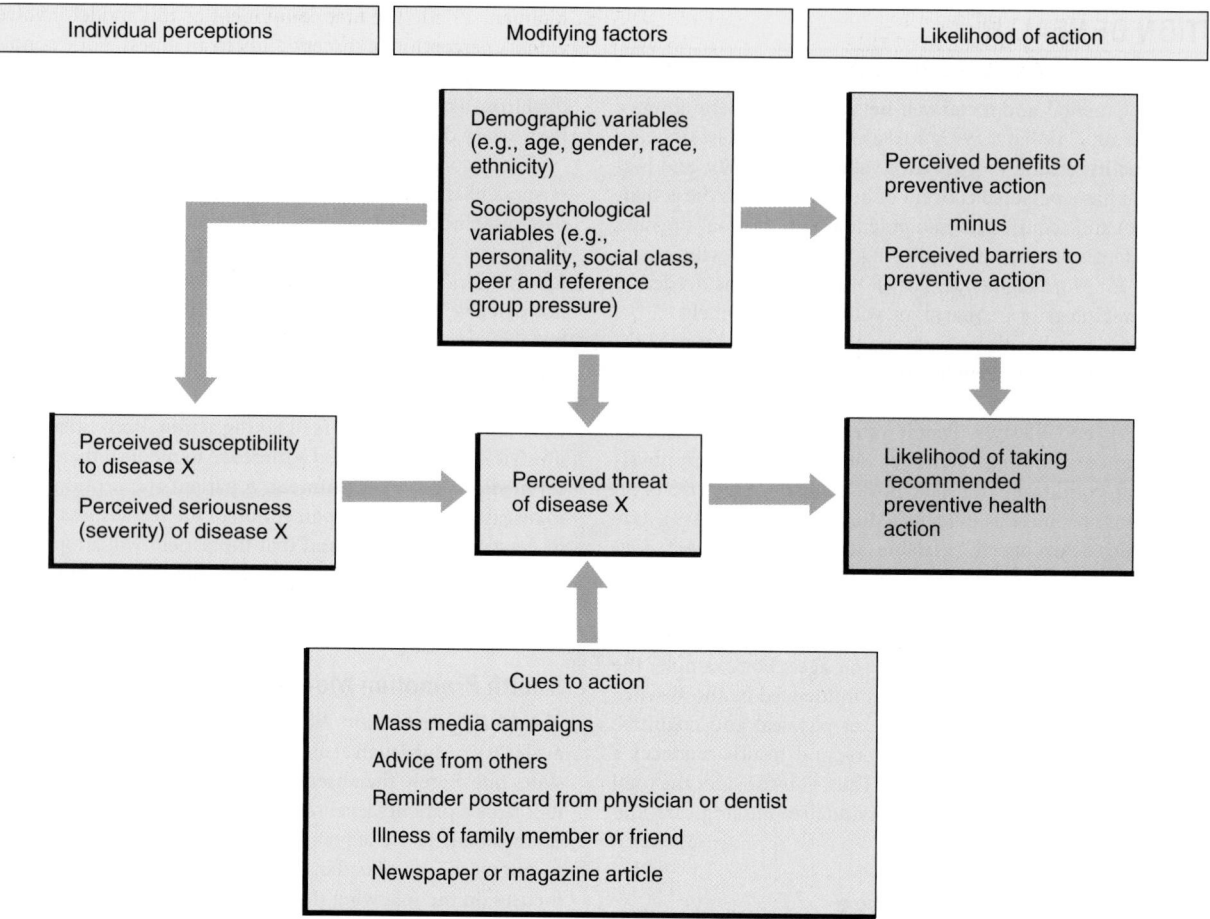

Individual perceptions	Modifying factors	Likelihood of action

FIG. 6.1 Health Belief Model. (Data from Becker M, Maiman L: Sociobehavioral determinants of compliance with health and medical care recommendations, *Med Care* 13[1]:10, 1975.)

example, in a house fire, fear of injury and death takes priority over self-esteem issues. Although you might anticipate a patient who has just had surgery has the strongest need for pain control in the physiological area, if the patient just had a mastectomy, her main need may be in the areas of love, belonging, and self-esteem. It is important not to assume the patient's needs just because other patients reacted in a certain way. Apply Maslow's hierarchy to each patient individually. To provide the most effective care, you need to understand the relationships of different needs and the factors that determine the priorities for each patient.

Holistic Health Model

The relationship between body, mind, and spirit affects a person's health. The Holistic Health Model of nursing promotes a patient's optimal level of health by considering the dynamic interactions among the emotional, spiritual, social, cultural, and physical aspects of an individual's wellness (LaVela et al., 2017). You put your patients at the center of their care and recognize your patients as the ultimate experts concerning their own health. A patient's subjective experience is relevant in maintaining health or assisting in healing. The Holistic Health Model empowers patients to engage in their own recovery and assume some responsibility for health maintenance (Edelman and Kudzma, 2018).

The Holistic Health Model recognizes a person's choices powerfully affect an individual's health. Some of the most widely used holistic interventions include meditation, music therapy, reminiscence, relaxation therapy, therapeutic touch, and guided imagery (see Chapter 32). These holistic strategies, which can be used in all stages of health and illness, are integral in the expanding role of nursing.

Nurses use holistic therapies either alone or in conjunction with conventional medicine. For example, using reminiscence sometimes helps relieve anxiety for older patients dealing with memory loss. Meditation sometimes helps patients cope with the difficult side effects of chemotherapy. Helping your patients understand different holistic therapies allows them to make choices that enhance their health.

VARIABLES INFLUENCING HEALTH AND HEALTH BELIEFS AND PRACTICES

Many variables influence a patient's health beliefs and practices. Internal and external variables influence how a person thinks and acts. Health beliefs usually influence health behaviors or health practices, which positively or negatively affect a patient's level of health. Understanding the effects of these variables allows you to plan and deliver individualized care.

Internal Variables

Internal variables include a person's developmental stage, intellectual background, perception of functioning, and emotional and spiritual factors.

Developmental Stage. A person's perceptions of health, illness, and health behaviors change over time (see Chapter 11). Considering a patient's growth and development stage helps you predict a patient's response to an actual illness or the threat of a future illness. Fear and anxiety are common among ill children, especially if thoughts about illness, hospitalization, or procedures are based on lack of information

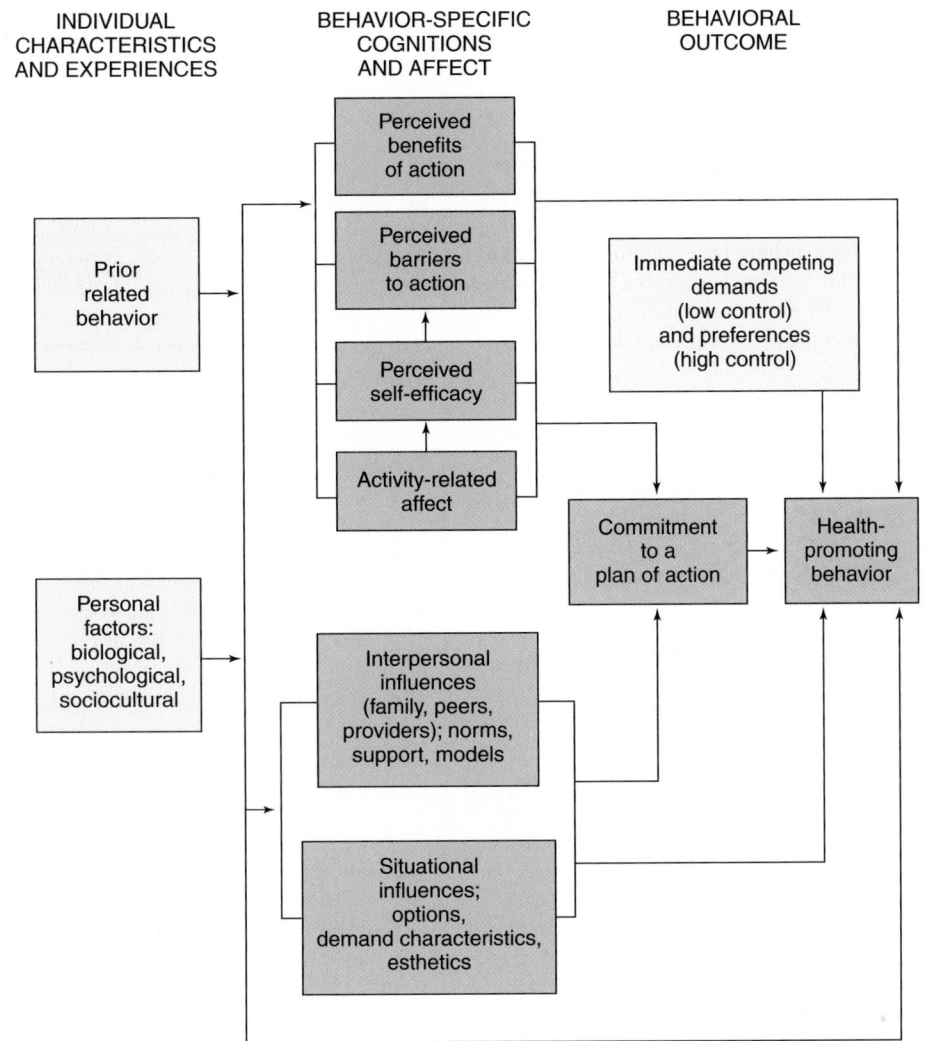

FIG. 6.2 Health Promotion Model (revised). (Redrawn from Maslow AH, Frager RD (Editor), Fadiman J (Editor): *Motivation and personality*, ed 3. ©1987. Reprinted with permission of Ann Kaplan.)

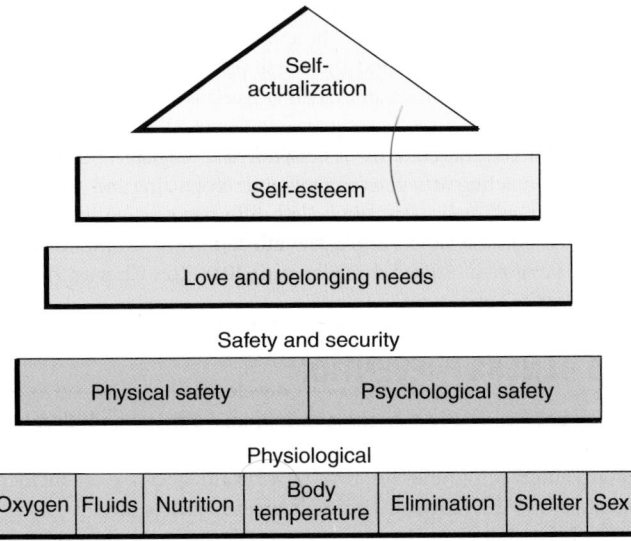

FIG. 6.3 Maslow's hierarchy of needs. (Redrawn from Maslow AH: *Motivation and personality*, ed 3, Upper Saddle River, NJ, 1970, Prentice Hall.)

or lack of clarity of information. Emotional development may also influence personal beliefs about health-related matters. For example, you use different techniques for teaching about the need to be physically active to an adolescent than you use for an adult. A person's developmental stage sometimes differs from his or her chronological age. Adapt your nursing care based on a patient's developmental stage and the ability to participate in self-care.

Intellectual Background. A person's beliefs about health are shaped in part by knowledge or misinformation about body functions and illnesses, educational background, traditions, and past experiences. These variables influence how a patient thinks about health. In addition, cognitive abilities shape the *way* a person thinks, including the ability to understand factors involved in illness and apply knowledge of health and illness to personal health practices. Cognitive abilities also relate to a person's developmental stage. Consider your patient's intellectual background while providing patient teaching (Edelman and Kudzma, 2018).

Perception of Functioning. Perceptions of physical functioning affect people's health beliefs and practices. When you assess a patient's level of health, gather subjective data about the way a patient perceives physical functioning, such as level of fatigue, shortness of breath, or pain. Then obtain objective data about actual functioning such as blood pressure, height measurements, and lung sounds. This information allows you to more successfully plan and implement individualized approaches to improve a person's ability to function (e.g., self-care, mobility).

Emotional Factors. A patient's degree of stress, depression, or fear influences health beliefs and practices. How people handle stress throughout each phase of life influences their reaction to illness. A person who generally is very calm may have little emotional response during illness, whereas another individual may be unable to cope emotionally with the threat of illness and may overreact or deny the presence of symptoms and not take therapeutic action (see Chapter 37).

Spiritual Factors. Spirituality is reflected in how a person lives his or her life, including the values and beliefs exercised, the relationships established with family and friends, and the ability to find hope and meaning in life. Spirituality serves as an integrating theme in people's lives and often provides motivation to participate in health promoting activities (Janssen-Neimeijer et al., 2017; Pilger et al., 2016). Religious practices are one way that people exercise spirituality. Some religions restrict the use of certain forms of medical treatment. For example, persons of the Jehovah Witness faith do not receive blood transfusions. You need to understand patients' spiritual beliefs to incorporate them effectively in nursing care (see Chapter 35).

External Variables

External variables influencing a person's health beliefs and practices include family practices, psychosocial and socioeconomic factors, and cultural background.

Family Role and Practices. The roles and organization of a family influence how each family member defines health and illness and values health practices. Their perceptions of the seriousness of diseases and their history of preventive care behaviors (or lack of them) influence how patients think about health. For example, a child whose parents believe in the importance of eating healthy foods and physical activity may continue to practice these health beliefs, whereas parents who have misconceptions and unhealthy perceptions about diet quality often contribute to eating habits that lead to obesity in their children (Adamo and Brett, 2014; Rausch et al., 2015).

Social Determinants of Health. Health is determined by a person's circumstances and environment. External factors such as where a person lives, the quality of the environment, income, educational level, and relationships with others have a considerable impact on a patient's health. Social determinants of health (SDOH) include a variety of social, commercial, cultural, economic, environmental, and political factors that affect health inequalities. They refer to the conditions in which people are born, grow, live, work, and age (WHO, 2018b). There are five categories of SDOH: economic stability, education, health and health care, social and community context, and neighborhood and built environment (USDHHS, 2018). Examples of SDOH include poverty, food insecurity, access to primary health care, culture, exposure to violence, and access to green spaces (Schroeder et al., 2018).

REFLECT NOW

What is food insecurity, and how does it affect the health of your community?

🌐 BOX 6.1   CULTURAL ASPECTS OF CARE

Cultural Health Beliefs

Cultural beliefs shape patients' views of health, how they treat and prevent illness, and preferences for care. Health beliefs often vary within a cultural group; therefore, it is important to assess the health beliefs of each patient and not stereotype a patient based on cultural background (Abboud et al., 2017; Xu et al., 2016). Cultural health beliefs influence individuals' responses to health and illness such as eye contact, response to pain and pain management, use of touch, perception and treatment of mental illness, and sick role behaviors (Giger, 2017). Recognizing a patient's health beliefs helps you provide culturally competent nursing care that considers the physical, psychological, social, emotional, and spiritual needs of each patient.

Implications for Patient-Centered Care
- Be aware of the effect of culture on a patient's view and understanding of illness (Giger, 2017).
- Understand a patient's traditions, values, and beliefs and how these dimensions may affect a patient's perceptions about illness prevention and treatment (Abboud et al., 2017; Xu et al., 2016).
- Do not stereotype patients based on their culture and do not assume that they will adopt all cultural beliefs and practices (Giger, 2017).
- Recognize your patient's unique cultural perceptions regarding the cause of an illness and attitudes and beliefs about disease prevention when providing patient education about illness and treatment options (Abboud et al., 2017).
- Be aware of your own cultural background and recognize prejudices that lead to stereotyping and discrimination (Geiger, 2017; Smigelski-Theiss et al., 2017).

SDOH, especially those related to economic stability, often affect a patient's level of health by increasing the risk for disease, affecting the ability to find affordable and safe housing, and influencing how or at what point the patient enters the health care system (Schroeder et al., 2018). A person's adherence to a treatment designed to maintain or improve health is also affected by economic status. For example, a patient may give higher priority to food and shelter than to medications, treatments, and food for special diets if the patient has high utility bills, cares for a large family, and has a low income.

Culture, a social and community context, influences a patient's beliefs, values, and customs. It influences the approach to the health care systems, personal health practices, and the nurse-patient relationship. Cultural background also influences an individual's beliefs about causes of illness and remedies or practices to restore health (Box 6.1). If you are not aware of your own cultural patterns of behavior and language, you will have difficulty interacting with your patients and recognizing and understanding your patient's behaviors and beliefs. Effective nursing interventions incorporate cultural factors into a patient's, family's, or community's plan of care (Harris et al., 2016; Schroeder et al., 2018) (see Chapter 9).

HEALTH PROMOTION, WELLNESS, AND ILLNESS PREVENTION

Public health focuses on health promotion, wellness, and illness prevention. Health education, legislation, and policy help individuals, groups, and communities improve their health, decrease the incidence of disease and disability, and improve their quality of life.

Health policies and laws affect all people in a community, state, or country, even if the people affected by the policies or laws are not aware of them. For example, because of the current opioid crisis, all 50 states have passed legislation that facilitates the availability and dispensation of naloxone, especially to certain people, such as first responders and caregivers of people who are addicted to opioids. Most states allow prescribers to order naloxone without examining the patient who needs it to allow qualified individuals the ability to administer naloxone in an emergency (The Network for Public Health Law, n.d.). Other health promotion programs provide guidance in pain management and improve access to substance abuse treatment.

The concepts of health promotion, health education, and illness prevention are closely related and sometimes overlap. All are focused on the future; the differences among them involve motivations and goals. Health promotion helps individuals maintain or enhance their present health. It motivates people to engage in healthy activities such as routine exercise and good nutrition to reach more stable levels of health. Health education includes topics such as physical awareness, stress management, and self-responsibility. Health education helps people develop a greater understanding of their health and how to better manage their health risks. Illness prevention activities such as immunization programs and blood pressure screenings protect people from actual or potential threats to health. They also help people avoid declines in their health or ability to function.

Illnesses, especially chronic illnesses, increase health care costs. Improving self-management and providing preventive services help to reduce health care needs and costs and improve overall health. Taking a holistic approach recognizes that many factors affect a person's health and helps improve well-being in all dimensions (Box 6.2).

Examples of the health topics and objectives as defined by *Healthy People 2020* include physical activity; adolescent health; tobacco use; substance abuse; sexually transmitted diseases; mental health and mental disorders; injury and violence prevention; environmental health, immunization and infectious disease; access to health services; and lesbian, gay, bisexual, and transgender health (USDHHS, 2018). A complete list of topics and objectives is available on the *Healthy People* website (www.healthypeople.gov). These objectives and topics show the importance of health promotion, wellness, and illness prevention and encourage all to participate in the improvement of health.

Some health promotion programs help individuals change their lifestyles by developing more health-oriented habits that affect their overall health. Other programs are aimed at preventing specific health care problems. For example, support groups help people with human immunodeficiency virus (HIV) infection. Exercise programs encourage participants to exercise regularly to reduce their risk of cardiac disease. Stress-reduction programs teach participants to cope with stressors and reduce their risks for multiple illnesses such as infections, gastrointestinal disease, and cardiac disease.

Some health promotion, wellness education, and illness prevention programs are operated by health care agencies; others are operated independently. Many businesses have on-site health promotion activities for employees. Likewise, colleges and community centers offer health promotion and illness prevention programs. These programs often include nurses who provide direct care, act as consultants, or refer patients to them. The goal of these activities is to improve a patient's level of health through preventive health services, environmental protection, and health education.

Health promotion activities are often classified as either passive or active. With passive strategies of health promotion, individuals gain from the activities of others without acting themselves. The fluoridation of municipal drinking water and the fortification of homogenized milk with vitamin D are examples of passive health promotion strategies. With active strategies of health promotion, individuals become personally involved. For example, weight-reduction and smoking-cessation programs require patients to be actively involved in measures to improve their present and future levels of wellness while decreasing the risk of disease.

BOX 6.2 EVIDENCE-BASED PRACTICE

Health Promotion Strategies

PICOT Question: Do holistic approaches effectively promote adult health and assist individuals with lifestyle changes?

Evidence Summary

Nurses use a variety of holistic strategies to improve health promotion in individuals. Holistic strategies focus on a person's body, mind, and spirit and take a person's culture, spirituality, and faith into consideration. Research shows that using culturally appropriate approaches that include a person's faith or provide social support are effective when helping individuals make lifestyle changes (D'Alonzo et al., 2018; Sattin et al., 2016; Schwingel and Gálvez, 2016).

For example, a health promotion program that included spiritual and social support within an African-American faith community was effective in helping people lose weight and maintain weight loss over a 12-month period, thus reducing the risk of developing type 2 diabetes (Sattin et al., 2016). Health promotion programs that use *promotoras*, trained Latino community leaders, to provide evidence-based health promotion interventions and education that is culturally appropriate and includes social support also improve health outcomes. One study found that using *promotoras* who were selected from a church was very effective in improving physical activity, nutrition, and stress management (Schwingel and Gálvez, 2016). Another program trained *promotoras* who were community health workers to improve participants' level of physical activity, aerobic fitness, muscle strength, and flexibility (D'Alonzo et al., 2018)

Application to Nursing Practice

- Use role models from similar cultures when possible to encourage individuals to make health promotion and lifestyle changes (D'Alonzo et al., 2018; Sattin et al., 2016; Schwingel and Gálvez, 2016).
- Provide evidence-based interventions that include a person's faith and provide social support when helping individuals make lifestyle changes (Sattin et al., 2016; Schwingel and Gálvez, 2016).
- Work with churches and other faith-based organizations when implementing community-based health promotion strategies (Sattin et al., 2016; Schwingel and Gálvez, 2016).

Health promotion is a process of helping people gain control of and improve their health and focuses on a wide range of socioeconomic and environmental interventions (WHO, 2018c). An individual takes responsibility for health and wellness by making appropriate lifestyle choices. Lifestyle choices are important because they affect a person's quality of life and well-being. Making positive lifestyle choices and avoiding negative lifestyle choices also play a role in preventing illness. In addition to improving quality of life, preventing illness has an economic impact because it decreases health care costs.

Three Levels of Prevention

Nursing care oriented to health promotion, wellness, and illness prevention is described in terms of health activities on primary, secondary, and tertiary levels (Table 6.1). As a nurse, you will care for patients in all three levels.

Primary Prevention. Primary prevention is true prevention. Its goal is to reduce the incidence of disease. Many primary prevention programs are supported by the government (e.g., federally funded immunization programs). Primary prevention includes health education programs, nutritional programs, and physical fitness activities. It includes all health promotion efforts and wellness education activities that focus on maintaining or improving the general health of

TABLE 6.1 Three Levels of Prevention				
PRIMARY PREVENTION		SECONDARY PREVENTION		TERTIARY PREVENTION
Health Promotion	Specific Protection	Early Diagnosis and Prompt Treatment	Disability Limitations	Restoration and Rehabilitation
Health education Good nutrition based on developmental stage Provision of adequate housing, recreation, and working conditions Marriage counseling, sex education, and genetic screening	Providing immunizations Attention to personal hygiene Use of environmental sanitation Protection from occupational hazards Protection from accidents and carcinogens	Individual and mass screening surveys Focused examinations to cure and prevent diseases, prevent spread of communicable diseases, prevent complications, limit disability, and prevent death	Adequate treatment to stop disease process and prevent further complications Provision of facilities to limit disability and prevent death	Providing retraining and education to return to highest level of functioning Helping people with disabilities find work and accommodating them in the workplace

Modified from Edelman C, Kudzma E: *Health promotion throughout the life span,* ed 9, St Louis, 2018, Mosby.

individuals, families, and communities (Edelman and Kudzma, 2018). Examples of primary prevention include promoting hearing protection in occupational settings and providing education to reduce cardiac disease risk factors.

Secondary Prevention. Secondary prevention focuses on preventing the spread of disease, illness, or infection once it occurs. Activities are directed at diagnosis and prompt intervention, thereby reducing severity and enabling the patient to return to a normal level of health as early as possible (Edelman and Kudzma, 2018). Examples include identifying people who have a new case of a disease or following people who have been exposed to a disease but do not have it yet. It includes screening techniques and treating early stages of disease to limit disability by averting or delaying the consequences of advanced disease. Screening activities may lead to primary prevention intervention. For example, a nurse screens a patient who is obese for diabetes. After gathering more information from the patient, the nurse provides health education about physical activity and preventing hypertension.

Tertiary Prevention. Tertiary prevention occurs when a defect or disability is permanent and irreversible. It involves minimizing the effects of long-term disease or disability by interventions directed at preventing complications and deterioration (Edelman and Kudzma, 2018). Activities are directed at rehabilitation rather than diagnosis and treatment. For example, a patient with a spinal cord injury undergoes rehabilitation to learn how to use a wheelchair and perform activities of daily living independently. Care at this level helps patients achieve as high a level of functioning as possible, despite the limitations caused by illness or impairment.

RISK FACTORS

A risk factor is any attribute, quality, environmental situation, or trait that increases the vulnerability of an individual or group to an illness or accident. An example is risk factors for falls, such as impaired gait, reduced vision, and lower extremity weakness. Risk factors and behaviors, risk factor modification, and behavioral modification are integral components of health promotion, wellness, and illness prevention. Nurses in all areas of practice have opportunities to reduce patients' risk factors to promote health and decrease risks of illness or injury.

Risk factors do not cause diseases or accidents. Instead, they increase the chances that the individual, community, or population will experience a disease or dysfunction. Risk factors play a major role in how you identify a patient's health status. They also often influence health beliefs

BOX 6.3   FOCUS ON OLDER ADULTS

Health Promotion

- Base health promotion for older adults on their common risk factors, chronic health conditions, and health promotion needs, including heart disease, cancer, chronic bronchitis, stroke, diabetes mellitus, dementia, caregiving, and injury prevention (https://www.healthypeople.gov/2020/topics-objectives/topic/older-adults, USDHHS, 2018).
- Consider an older adult's social environment, and strengthen social support to promote health and provide access to resources (Touhy and Jett, 2016).
- Injury prevention is a key strategy to promote and improve health (Touhy and Jett, 2016).
- Promote holistic health promotion programs such as community-based exercise programs and programs that encourage creativity, such as making art or improvisation to improve well-being, decrease social isolation, and increase independence (Cantu and Fleuriet, 2018; Morse et al., 2018; Seo and Chao, 2018).
- Carefully assess each older adult you care for to determine various factors that affect health. Every individual is unique. Current evidence shows factors such as an older adult's social networks, access to transportation, knowledge of local services, mobility, perceptions of age, personal motivation, and perceived confidence in the ability to make effective changes can influence health-promoting behaviors and quality of life (Bardach et al., 2016; Frost et al., 2018; Hong et al., 2018).

and practices if a person is aware of their presence. People can modify some of their risk factors, while other risk factors are unmodifiable.

Nonmodifiable Risk Factors

Nonmodifiable risk factors such as age, gender, genetics, and family history cannot be changed. You use your understanding of nonmodifiable risk factors to select appropriate secondary prevention strategies. For example, a person's age increases the susceptibility to certain illnesses and accidents. Premature infants and neonates are more susceptible to infections. Children are at risk for accidental deaths due to drowning and aspiration. As a person ages, the risk of heart disease and many types of cancers increases. Age risk factors are often closely associated with other risk factors such as family history and personal habits. Educate your patients about the importance of regularly scheduled screenings based on their age. Various professional organizations and federal agencies develop and update recommendations for health screenings, immunizations, and counseling. Box 6.3 discusses ways to support health promotion in older adults.

Sometimes gender affects a person's risk factors. For example, the risk for asthma is higher in boys than girls. However, after puberty, the number of women with asthma becomes more prevalent and severe (Zein and Erzurum, 2015). Men have a higher risk for cardiovascular disease (CVD) than premenopausal women. However, after menopause, the risk for CVD is similar between men and women.

Family history and genetics are other risk factors for some illnesses. Cancers such as breast, ovarian, and colon appear to have a genetic link. These patients can benefit from genetic counseling. A person with a family history of diabetes or CVD is at higher risk for developing these diseases. Sometimes it is difficult to determine if the family link to illness is related to genetics, lifestyle choices, environmental exposure, or a combination of these factors. For example, you are caring for a patient who is obese and develops hypertension. Her parents have hypertension, and her husband smokes. It is difficult for you to determine which risk factor—lifestyle, genetics, or environmental toxins—contributed to her hypertension or whether it was a combination of all of these. In this example, you introduce health promotion strategies targeted at modifiable risk factors for the woman's obesity, such as nutrition counseling and exercise.

Modifiable Risk Factors

Some risk factors such as lifestyle practices and behaviors can be modified. Modifiable risk factors include poor nutrition, overeating, and insufficient rest and sleep. Some risk factors put a person at risk for developing specific diseases. For example, excessive sunbathing increases the risk of skin cancer; smoking increases the risk of lung diseases, including cancer; and a poor diet and being overweight increase the risk of cardiovascular disease.

Examples of modifiable behavioral risk factors that contribute to chronic illnesses include unhealthy diet, physical inactivity, tobacco use, alcohol abuse, poor control of hypertension, and elevated lipid and glucose levels (CDC, 2018). Modifiable risk factors for people who are 10 to 24 years of age include behaviors that lead to unintentional injuries (e.g., texting while driving, driving under the influence of drugs or alcohol, bullying); carrying a weapon; use of tobacco, smokeless tobacco products, alcohol, and other drugs; sexual behaviors leading to unintended pregnancy and sexually transmitted infections; unhealthy diet choices; and physical inactivity (Kann et al., 2018).

Lifestyle behavioral choices are also modifiable. Lifestyle choices can lead to health problems that cause a huge impact on our health care system, our economy, and our communities. Therefore, it is important to understand the effect of lifestyle behaviors on health status. For example, a teenager who makes nutritional choices that lead to obesity will most likely make similar nutritional choices as an adult. Lifestyle choices affect patients throughout the life span. Thus, it is important to understand the relationship between growth and development, lifestyle behaviors, and your patient's health status.

Stress is a lifestyle risk factor if it is severe or prolonged or if the person is unable to cope with life events adequately. Stress threatens both mental health (emotional stress) and physical well-being (physiological stress). Stress also interferes with health promotion activities and the ability to implement needed lifestyle modifications. Some emotional stressors result from life events such as divorce, pregnancy, death of a spouse or family member, and financial instabilities. For example, job-related stressors overtax a person's cognitive skills and decision-making ability, leading to "mental overload" or "burnout" (see Chapters 1 and 37). Stress also threatens physical well-being and is associated with illnesses such as heart disease, cancer, and gastrointestinal disorders (Chiang et al., 2018). Always review life stressors as part of a patient's comprehensive risk factor analysis.

Environment

Where we live and the condition of that area (its air, water, and soil) determine how we live, what we eat, the disease agents to which we are exposed, our state of health, and our ability to adapt. The physical environment in which a person works or lives can increase the likelihood that certain illnesses will occur. For example, some kinds of cancer and other diseases are more likely to develop when industrial workers are exposed to certain chemicals or when people live near toxic waste disposal sites. Environmental exposure rarely occurs at one time, in one location, and from one source because we are constantly interacting with our environment (Edelman and Kudzma, 2018).

RISK-FACTOR IDENTIFICATION AND CHANGING HEALTH BEHAVIORS

You identify your patients' modifiable and unmodifiable risk factors to help them understand what they can modify, control, or even eliminate to promote wellness and prevent illness. Health risk appraisal forms help identify health threats based on the presence of various risk factors (Edelman and Kudzma, 2018). Use data from a health risk appraisal tool to develop educational programs and other community resources if a patient needs to make lifestyle changes and reduce health risks (Murdaugh et al., 2019).

Once you identify a patient's risk factors, you implement appropriate and relevant health education and counseling to help a person change or implement behaviors to maintain or improve health status (Edelman and Kudzma, 2018). Risk-factor modification, health promotion, illness prevention activities, or any program that attempts to change unhealthy lifestyle behaviors is a wellness strategy. Ask patients which changes they perceive they need to make or are willing to make. Patients typically will not change their behaviors unless they see a need and are motivated to change.

Sometimes patients need to stop health-damaging behaviors (e.g., tobacco use or alcohol misuse), while other times patients need to adopt healthy behaviors (e.g., healthy diet or exercise) (Murdaugh et al., 2019). Changing health behavior, especially long-term lifestyle habits, is difficult. Using a health promotion model to identify risky behaviors and implement the change process will help you motivate patients and facilitate health behavior changes (Edelman and Kudzma, 2018). Use evidence-based guidelines and recommendations when helping patients make health behavior changes.

You will be able to help your patients make difficult changes more effectively if you understand the process of change. Current evidence supports that many people go through a series of five stages when they make a change, described by the Transtheoretical Model of Change (Table 6.2) (pro-change Behavior Systems, Inc., 2018; Yusufov et al., 2016). These stages range from no intention to change (precontemplation) to maintaining a changed behavior (maintenance stage) (DiClemente and Prochaska, 1998). Change is not a linear process. People often relapse and cycle through the stages (pro-change Behavior Systems, Inc., 2018). When relapse occurs, a person will return to the contemplation or precontemplation stage before attempting the change again. Help your patients understand that relapse is a learning process; they can apply the lessons learned from relapse to their next attempt to change. It is important to understand what happens at the various stages of the change process to time the implementation of interventions (wellness strategies) adequately and provide appropriate assistance at each stage.

Once an individual identifies a stage of change, the change process facilitates movement through the stages. To be most effective, you choose nursing interventions that match the stage of change. Most behavior-change programs are designed for (and have a chance

TABLE 6.2   Stages of Health Behavior Change

Stage	Definition	Assessment Findings
Precontemplation	No intent to make changes within the next 6 months	Patient is unaware of, not interested in, or underestimates the problem. May be defensive. "There is nothing I really need to change."
Contemplation	Considering a change within the next 6 months	May be ambivalent about the change or is thinking about making a change. "I have a problem that I think I need to work on."
Preparation	Making small changes in preparation for a change in the next month	May have tried to make changes in the past but was unsuccessful. Patient believes that advantages outweigh disadvantages of behavior change. "I started running once, but I didn't keep it up. I think I might try again in a few weeks."
Action	Actively engaged in strategies to change behavior; lasts up to 6 months	Committed to change. Previous habits may become barriers to change. "I am really working hard to stop smoking."
Maintenance stage	Sustained change over time; begins 6 months after action has started and continues indefinitely	Changes integrated into the patient's lifestyle and behaviors adopted to prevent relapse. "I need to avoid people who smoke so I won't be tempted to start smoking again."

of success with) people ready to take action regarding their health behavior problems. Changes are maintained over time only if they are integrated into an individual's overall lifestyle (Box 6.4). Maintaining healthy lifestyles can prevent hospitalizations and potentially lower the cost of health care.

> **QSEN** **Building Competency in Safety** A nurse who works at a health center on a university campus notices that there are many students who smoke. The nurse partners with the local health department to implement a smoking-cessation program on campus. The program is based on the Transtheoretical Model of Change. In applying this model, which strategies does the nurse need to consider?
>
> Answers to QSEN Activities can be found on the Evolve website.

ILLNESS

Illness and disease are different concepts. **Illness** is a state in which a person's physical, emotional, intellectual, social, developmental, or spiritual functioning is diminished or impaired. A person can feel ill in the presence or absence of disease. For example, cancer is a disease. A patient with leukemia continues to function as usual, whereas another patient with breast cancer feels well physically but experiences great spiritual distress. Many patients who have an illness feel healthy. Sometimes illness motivates people to adopt healthy behaviors. Although you need to be knowledgeable about different diseases, you also need to understand illness, which includes the holistic effects of diseases and treatments on your patient's functioning and well-being.

Acute and Chronic Illness

Both acute and chronic illnesses have the potential to affect many dimensions of functioning. An **acute illness** is usually reversible and has a short duration. The symptoms appear abruptly, are intense, and subside after a relatively short period. A **chronic illness** usually lasts more than 6 months, is irreversible, and affects functioning in one or more systems. Patients often fluctuate between maximal functioning and serious health relapses that may be life threatening. A person with a chronic illness is like a person with a disability in that both have varying degrees of functional limitations (Larsen, 2019).

Chronic illnesses and disabilities remain a leading health problem in the United States. Coping and living with a chronic illness is usually complex and overwhelming. Half of the adults in the United

BOX 6.4   PATIENT TEACHING

Lifestyle Changes

Objective
- Patient will reduce health risks related to poor lifestyle habits (e.g., high-fat diet, sedentary lifestyle) through behavior change.

Teaching Strategies
- Practice active listening and establish rapport with the patient.
- Begin with determining information that the patient knows regarding health risks related to poor lifestyle.
- Ask which barriers the patient perceives with the planned lifestyle change.
- Help the patient establish goals for change.
- Collaborate with the patient to establish timelines for modification of eating and exercise lifestyle habits.
- Reinforce the process of change.
- Have patient maintain a log of key behavioral changes (Schneider and Stone, 2016).
- Ensure that educational materials are culturally appropriate (Abboud et al., 2017; Sattin et al., 2016).
- Include family members and significant others to support the lifestyle change (Sattin et al., 2016).

Evaluation
Use the principles of teach-back to evaluate patient/family caregiver learning:
- Ask the patient to repeat back the teaching on reducing risks and lifestyle changes (Dinh et al., 2016).
- Review patient's log to track adherence; ask patient to explain importance of tracking and provide positive reinforcement.
- Ask the patient to discuss success with lifestyle changes (e.g., "How many days did you exercise last week?").

States have one chronic illness, and one in four adults has two or more chronic health problems (CDC, 2018). Many chronic illnesses are related to four modifiable health behaviors: physical inactivity, poor nutrition, tobacco use and secondhand smoke exposure, and excessive alcohol use (CDC, 2018). A major role for nursing is to provide patient education aimed at helping patients manage their illness or disability and to help patients reduce the occurrence or improve the severity of symptoms.

Patients with chronic diseases and their families continually adjust and adapt to their illnesses. How an individual perceives an illness influences the type of coping responses. In response to a chronic illness, an individual develops an illness career. The illness career is flexible and changes in response to changes in health, interactions with health professionals, psychological changes related to grief, and stress related to the illness (Larsen, 2019).

The nature of the illness, either acute or chronic, also affects a patient's illness behavior. Patients with acute illnesses are likely to seek health care and adhere to therapy. On the other hand, a patient with a chronic illness in which symptoms are not cured but only partially relieved may not be motivated to adhere to the therapy plan. Some patients who are chronically ill become less actively involved in their care, experience greater frustration, and adhere less readily to care. Because nurses often spend more time than other health care professionals with chronically ill patients, they are in the unique position of being able to help these patients overcome problems related to illness behavior. A patient's coping skills and his or her locus of control (the degree to which people believe they control what happens to them) are other internal variables that affect the way the patient behaves when ill (see Chapter 37).

Illness Behavior

People who are ill generally act in a way that medical sociologists call illness behavior. People who are ill often adopt cognitive, affective, and behavioral reactions that are influenced by sociocultural and psychological factors. Illness behaviors affect how people monitor their bodies, define and interpret their symptoms, take remedial actions, and use health care resources (Mechanic, 1995). Personal history, social situations, social norms, and past experiences affect illness behaviors (Larsen, 2019). How people react to illness varies widely; illness behavior displayed in sickness is often used to manage life adversities (Mechanic, 1995). In other words, if people perceive themselves to be ill, illness behaviors become coping mechanisms. For example, illness behavior can result in a patient being released from roles, social expectations, or responsibilities.

The nature of the illness also affects a patient's illness behavior. Patients with acute illnesses are likely to seek health care. On the other hand, patients with a chronic illness in which symptoms are only partly relieved may become less actively involved in their care, experience greater frustration, and have difficulty adhering to their treatment plan.

Variables Influencing Illness and Illness Behavior

Many variables influence illness and illness behaviors. Physical stressors such as a poor living environment, work stress, exposure to air pollution, and living in an unsafe environment affect health. Heredity and individual practices such as poor eating habits and not exercising regularly also influence health and health behaviors and illness and illness behaviors. The influences of emotional, intellectual, social, developmental, and spiritual factors often affect the likelihood of seeking health care, adherence to therapy, and health outcomes. Plan individualized care based on an understanding of these variables and behaviors to help patients cope with their illness at various stages. The goal is to promote optimal functioning in all dimensions throughout an illness.

Internal Variables. Internal variables are a patient's perceptions of symptoms and the nature of an illness. A patient's coping skills and his or her locus of control (the degree to which people believe they control what happens to them) are other internal variables that affect the way the patient behaves when ill (see Chapter 37). If patients believe that the symptoms of their illnesses disrupt their normal routine, they are more likely to seek health care assistance than if they do not perceive the symptoms to be disruptive. Patients are also more likely to seek assistance if they believe the symptoms are serious or life threatening.

A patient awakened by crushing chest pain in the middle of the night who sees this symptom as serious and life threatening is motivated to seek assistance. However, such a perception can have the opposite effect. Another patient with the same symptoms fears serious illness, reacts by denying it, and does not seek medical assistance.

External Variables. External variables influencing a patient's illness behavior include the visibility of symptoms, social group, cultural background, economic variables, accessibility of the health care system, and social support. The visibility of the symptoms of an illness affects body image and illness behavior. A patient with a visible symptom (e.g., a high fever) is often more likely to seek assistance than a patient with no visible symptoms (e.g., symptoms associated with ovarian cancer such as fatigue and bloating).

Patients' social groups help them accept or deny the threat of illness. Families, friends, and co-workers all influence patients' illness behaviors. Patients often react positively to social support while practicing positive health behaviors. A person's family and cultural background teach the person how to be healthy, how to recognize illness, and how to be ill. For example, dietary practices, influenced by family and spiritual, religious and cultural beliefs, contribute to illness and disease maintenance (Giger, 2017).

Economic variables are SDOH that influence the way a patient reacts to illness. Financial difficulties often lead to delayed treatment and affect an individual's ability to carry out prescribed treatments and therapies. Patients' access to the health care system is closely related to economic factors. The health care system is a socioeconomic system that patients enter, interact within, and exit. For many patients, entry into the system is complex or confusing. Some patients seek nonemergency medical care in an emergency department because they do not know how to obtain health services in other ways or do not have access to care. The physical proximity of patients to a health care agency often influences how soon they enter the system after deciding to seek care.

Impact of Illness on the Patient and Family

Illness is never an isolated life event. A patient and family deal with changes resulting from illness and treatment. Each patient responds uniquely to illness, requiring you to individualize nursing interventions. The patient and family commonly experience behavioral and emotional changes and changes in roles, body image and self-concept, and family dynamics.

Behavioral and Emotional Changes. People react differently to illness or the threat of illness. Individual behavioral and emotional reactions depend on the nature of an illness, a patient's attitude toward it, the reaction of others to it, and the variables of illness behavior.

Short-term, non–life-threatening illnesses usually require few changes in the functioning of a patient or family. For example, a father who has a cold lacks the energy and patience to spend time in family activities. He becomes irritable and prefers not to interact with his family. This is a behavioral change, but the change is subtle and does not last long. Some may even consider such a change a normal response to illness.

Severe illness, particularly one that is life threatening, leads to more extensive emotional and behavioral changes such as anxiety, shock, denial, anger, and withdrawal. These are common responses to the stress of illness. You develop interventions to help a patient and family cope with and adapt to this stress because the stressor cannot be changed.

Impact on Body Image. Body image is the subjective concept of physical appearance (see Chapter 33). Some illnesses result in changes in physical appearance. Patient and family reactions differ and usually depend on the type of changes (e.g., loss of a limb or an organ), their adaptive capacity, the rate at which changes take place, and the support services available.

When a profound change in body image occurs, such as after a leg amputation or mastectomy, the patient generally adjusts by experiencing phases of the grief process (see Chapter 36). Initially the patient is in shock because of the change or impending change. As the patient and family recognize the reality of the change, they become anxious and often withdraw, refusing to discuss it. Withdrawal is an adaptive coping mechanism that helps the patient adjust. As a patient and family acknowledge the change, they gradually accept the loss. During rehabilitation the patient becomes ready to learn how to adapt to the changed body image.

Impact on Self-Concept. Self-concept is a mental self-image of all aspects of your personality. Self-concept depends in part on body image and roles but also includes other aspects of psychology and spirituality (see Chapters 33 and 35). The effect of illness on the self-concepts of patients and family members is usually more complex and less readily observed than role changes.

Self-concept is important in relationships with other family members. For example, a patient whose self-concept changes (e.g., feeling like a failure) because of illness may no longer meet family expectations, leading to tension or conflict. As a result, family members change their interactions with the patient. While providing care, you observe changes in a patient's self-concept (or in the self-concepts of family members) and develop a care plan to facilitate adjustment to the changes resulting from the illness.

Impact on Family Roles. People have many roles in life, such as wage earner, decision maker, professional, child, sibling, or parent. When an illness occurs, parents and children try to adapt to the major changes that result. Role reversal is common (see Chapter 10). If a parent becomes ill and cannot carry out usual activities, an adult child often assumes many of the parent's responsibilities and in essence becomes a parent to the parent. Such a reversal of the usual situation sometimes leads to stress, conflicting responsibilities for the adult child, or direct conflict over decision making.

An individual and family generally adjust more easily to subtle, short-term changes. In most cases they know that the role change is temporary and will not require a prolonged adjustment. However, long-term changes require an adjustment process similar to the grief process (see Chapter 36). A patient and family often require specific counseling and guidance to help them cope with role changes.

REFLECT NOW

Think about a patient or family member who recently experienced a change in health status. How did this change affect the individual's family?

Impact on Family Dynamics. Family dynamics is the process by which the family functions, makes decisions, gives support to individual members, and copes with everyday changes and challenges. Family dynamics often change because of the effects of illness. For example, a single parent experiences severe injury from a car accident. Her brother assumes some of her roles and responsibilities, such as getting the children to and from school. Although the patient and her brother are very close, the family experiences some tension as roles and responsibilities change. Include the whole family when appropriate to help

patients and their families attain the maximal level of functioning and well-being (see Chapter 10).

CARING FOR YOURSELF

To be able to provide competent, quality, and safe care, nurses need to take care of themselves to ensure they remain healthy. Nurses are particularly susceptible to the development of compassion fatigue, which is a combination of secondary traumatic stress (STS) and burnout (BO) (see Chapter 1). Secondary traumatic stress develops because of the relationships that nurses develop with their patients and families, whereas BO stems from conflicts or nurse job dissatisfaction within the work setting (Kelly and Lefton, 2017). Compassion fatigue frequently affects a nurse's health, often leading to a decline in health, changes in sleep and eating patterns, emotional exhaustion, irritability, restlessness, impaired ability to focus and engage with patients, feelings of hopelessness, inability to take pleasure from activities, and anxiety (Kelly and Lefton, 2017; Henson, 2017). In the workplace the effects of compassion fatigue are often manifested by diminished performance, reduced ability to feel empathy, depersonalization of the patient, poor judgment, chronic absenteeism, high turnover rates, and conflict between nurses (Henson, 2017). It is important for nurses to engage in personal and professional strategies to help combat compassion fatigue and promote resiliency.

Personal strategies focus on health-promoting behaviors and healthy lifestyle choices. To combat STS and BO, you need to eat a nutritious diet, get adequate sleep regularly, engage in regular exercise and relaxation activities, establish a good work-family balance, and engage in regular nonwork activities (Kelly and Lefton, 2017; Mendes, 2017). Other strategies that can help you prevent or deal with STS and BO include developing coping skills, allowing personal time for grieving the loss of patients, and focusing on your spiritual health (Kim and Yeom, 2018). Another strategy is to find a mentor or experienced nurse who understands the stress of the job and can help you identify coping strategies (Doré et al., 2017).

An increasing number of health care institutions and organizations offer educational programs and resources for nurses that are designed to help decrease compassion fatigue and increase resiliency (Kelly and Lefton, 2017). These programs educate nurses about compassion fatigue and its negative effects and provide resources and tools for nurses to use to prevent or cope with STS and BO. For example, participating in debriefing sessions or a compassion fatigue support group allows nurses to identify stressors and work as a group to develop healthy coping strategies (Schmidt and Haglund, 2017; Doré et al., 2017). Health care organizations need to also provide resources for nurses, such as a mental health professional to provide assistance in managing STS and BO.

■ KEY POINTS

- *Healthy People* identifies leading health indicators that are high-priority health issues in the United States.
- Definitions of health vary among individuals based on a person's health beliefs, developmental age, and level of functioning.
- Multiple models of health in which persons are active participants explain relationships among health beliefs, health behaviors, health promotion, and individual well-being.
- Internal variables, such as a person's developmental stage and spirituality, and external factors, such as family roles and SDOH, influence a person's health, health beliefs, and health practices.

- Health promotion activities help maintain or enhance health, health education helps people better understand their health and health risks, and illness prevention activities protect against health threats.
- Primary prevention reduces the incidence of disease, secondary prevention prevents the spread of disease when it occurs, and tertiary prevention minimizes the effects of disease or disability.
- You use your understanding of different types of risk factors to select appropriate secondary prevention strategies for your patients. Nonmodifiable risk factors, such as age and family history, cannot be changed, while modifiable risk factors, such as smoking and activity levels, can be changed.
- Reducing risk factors and improving health usually require a change in health behaviors.
- Illness behaviors are different reactions people have when they become ill. Variables such as perceptions of the illness, the type of illness, and the visibility of symptoms affect a person's illness behaviors.
- Illness has many effects on a patient and family, including changes in behavior and emotions, family roles and dynamics, body image, and self-concept.
- Using personal and professional strategies that focus on caring for self can help to decrease or prevent compassion fatigue.

REFLECTIVE LEARNING

- Understanding a person's risk factors helps you determine appropriate health education and health promotion interventions. Reflect on a patient you recently cared for or someone you know such as a friend or family member. What actual and/or potential health problems does this person have? What risk factors contribute to these health problems? Are the risk factors nonmodifiable or modifiable? What health education or health promotion interventions could you implement to limit the effect of these risk factors?
- Interview a patient or someone you know who is trying to make a health behavior change. What behavior change is the person trying to make? What stage of change is this person currently in based on the Transtheoretical Model of Change (see Table 6.2)? Once this person moves into the maintenance stage, what can you do to help this person prepare for potential relapses?
- Reflect on your own health as well as your beliefs and values. How do you define health? Do you consider yourself healthy? What health behaviors would you like to change or implement right now to improve your health? Develop a plan to make a change in your behavior to improve your health. What barriers might prevent you from implementing your plan? If you implemented this plan, how might your health improve? Remember to consider your health holistically as you reflect on your answers.

REVIEW QUESTIONS

1. A patient discharged a week ago following a stroke is currently participating in rehabilitation sessions provided by nurses, physical therapists, and registered dietitians in an outpatient setting. In what level of prevention is the patient participating?
   1. Primary prevention
   2. Secondary prevention
   3. Tertiary prevention
   4. Transtheoretical prevention

2. Based on the Transtheoretical Model of Change, what is the most appropriate response to a patient who states: "Me, stop smoking? I've been smoking since I was 16!"
   1. "That's fine. Some people who smoke live a long life."
   2. "OK. I want you to decrease the number of cigarettes you smoke by one each day, and I'll see you in 1 month."
   3. "What do you think is the greatest reason why stopping smoking would be challenging for you?"
   4. "I'd like you to attend a smoking-cessation class this week and use nicotine replacement patches as directed."

3. A nurse working on a medical patient care unit states, "I am having trouble sleeping, and I eat nonstop when I get home. All I can think of when I get to work is how I can't wait for my shift to be over. I wish I felt happy again." What are the best responses from the nurse manager? (Select all that apply.)
   1. "I'm sure this is just a phase you are going through. Hang in there. You'll feel better soon."
   2. "I know several nurses who feel this way every now and then. Tell me about the patients you have cared for recently. Did you find it difficult to care for them?"
   3. "You can take diphenhydramine over the counter to help you sleep at night."
   4. "Describe for me what you do with your time when you are not working."
   5. "The hospital just started a group where nurses get together to talk about their feelings. Would you like for me to e-mail the schedule to you?"

4. A patient has been laid off from his construction job and has many unpaid bills. He is going through a divorce from his marriage of 15 years and has been praying daily to help him through this difficult time. He does not have a primary health care provider because he has never really been sick, and his parents never took him to a physician when he was a child. Which external variables influence the patient's health practices? (Select all that apply.)
   1. Difficulty paying his bills
   2. Praying daily
   3. Age of patient (46 years)
   4. Stress from the divorce and the loss of a job
   5. Family practice of not routinely seeing a health care provider

5. A nurse is conducting a home visit with a new mom and her three children. While in the home the nurse weighs each family member and reviews their 3-day food diary. She checks the mom's blood pressure and encourages the mom to take the children for a 15- to 30-minute walk every day. The nurse is addressing which level of need, according to Maslow?
   1. Physiological
   2. Safety and security
   3. Love and belonging
   4. Self-actualization

6. When taking care of patients, a nurse routinely asks whether they take any vitamins or herbal medications, encourages family members to bring in music that the patient likes to help the patient relax, and frequently prays with her patients if that is important to them. The nurse is practicing which model?
   1. Holistic
   2. Health belief
   3. Transtheoretical
   4. Health promotion

7. Using the Transtheoretical Model of Change, order the steps that a patient goes through to make a lifestyle change related to physical activity.

1. The individual recognizes that he is out of shape when his daughter asks him to walk with her after school.
2. Eight months after beginning walking, the individual participates with his wife in a local 5K race.
3. The individual becomes angry when the physician tells him that he needs to increase his activity to lose 30 lb.
4. The individual walks 2 to 3 miles, 5 nights a week, with his wife.
5. The individual visits the local running store to purchase walking shoes and obtain advice on a walking plan.

8. Which of the following are symptoms of secondary traumatic stress and burnout that commonly affect nurses? (Select all that apply.)
   1. Regular participation in a book club
   2. Lack of interest in exercise
   3. Difficulty falling asleep
   4. Lack of desire to go to work
   5. Anxiety while working

9. As part of a faith community nursing program in her church, a nurse is developing a health promotion program on breast self-examination for the women's group. Which statement made by

one of the participants is related to the individual's accurate perception of susceptibility to an illness?
   1. "I have a door hanging tag in my bathroom to remind me to do my breast self-examination monthly."
   2. "Since my mother had breast cancer, I know that I am at increased risk for developing breast cancer."
   3. "Since I am only 25 years of age, the risk of breast cancer for me is very low."
   4. "I participate every year in our local walk/run to raise money for breast cancer research."

10. The nurse assesses the risk factors for coronary artery disease (CAD) in a female patient. Which of these factors are classified as genetic and physiological? (Select all that apply.)
   1. Sedentary lifestyle
   2. Mother died from CAD at age 48
   3. History of hypertension
   4. Eats diet high in sodium
   5. Elevated cholesterol level

Answers: 1. 3; **2.** 3; **3.** 2, 4, 5; **4.** 1, 5; **5.** 1; **6.** 1; **7.** 3, 1, 5, 4; **8.** 2, 3, 4, 5; **9.** 2; **10.** 2, 3, 5.

Rationales for Review Questions can be found on the Evolve website.

REFERENCES

Becker M, Maiman L: Sociobehavioral determinants of compliance with health and medical care recommendations, *Med Care* 13(1):10, 1975.

Centers for Disease Control and Prevention [CDC]: *National center for chronic disease prevention and health promotion*, 2018, https://www.cdc.gov/chronicdisease/. Accessed July 2018.

DiClemente C, Prochaska J: Toward a comprehensive transtheoretical model of change. In Miller WR, Heather N, editors: *Treating addictive behaviors*, New York, 1998, Plenum Press.

Edelman C, Kudzma E: *Health promotion throughout the life span*, ed 9, St Louis, 2018, Mosby.

Giger JN: *Transcultural nursing: assessment and intervention*, ed 7, St Louis, 2017, Mosby.

Harris DA, et al.: Community-based participatory research is needed to address pulmonary health disparities, *Ann Am Thorac Soc* 13(8):1231, 2016.

Henson JS: When compassion is lost, *Medsurg Nurs* 26(2):139, 2017.

Kelly LA, Lefton C: Effect of meaningful recognition on critical care nurses' compassion fatigue, *Am J Crit Care* 26(6):438, 2017.

Larsen PD: *Lubkin's chronic illness: impact and intervention*, ed 10, Boston, 2019, Jones & Bartlett.

Mechanic D: Sociological dimensions of illness behavior, *Soc Sci Med* 41(9):1207, 1995.

Mendes A: How to address compassion fatigue in the community nurse, *Br J Community Nurs* 22(9):458, 2017.

Murdaugh CL, et al.: *Health promotion in nursing practice*, ed 8, New York, 2019, Pearson.

Pender NJ: *Health promotion and nursing practice*, Norwalk, Conn, 1982, Appleton-Century-Crofts.

Pender NJ: *Health promotion and nursing practice*, ed 3, Stamford, C., 1996, Appleton & Lange.

Pender NJ, et al.: *Health promotion in nursing practice*, ed 7, Upper Saddle River, NJ, 2015, Prentice Hall.

pro-change Behavior Systems: *Inc.: the transtheoretical model*, 2018, https://www.prochange.com/transtheoretical-model-of-behavior-change. Accessed July 2018.

Rosenstoch I: Historical origin of the health belief model, *Health Educ Monogr* 2:334, 1974.

Schmidt M, Haglund K: Debrief in emergency departments to improve compassion fatigue and promote resiliency, *J Trauma Nurs* 24(5):317, 2017.

Schroeder K, et al.: Addressing the social determinants of health: a call to action for school nurses, *J Sch Nurs* 34(3):182, 2018.

Smigelski-Theiss R, et al.: Weight bias and psychosocial implications for acute care of patients with obesity, *AACN Adv Crit Care* 28(3):254, 2017.

The Network for Public Health Law: Drug overdose prevention and harm reduction, n.d., https://www.networkforphl.org/resources/topics__resources/drug_overdose_prevention_and_harm_reduction/. Accessed May 20, 2019.

Touhy TA, Jett K: *Ebersole and Hess' toward healthy aging: human needs and nursing response*, ed 9, St Louis, 2016, Mosby.

US Department of Health and Human services [USDHHS]: *HealthyPeople.gov*, 2018, http://www.healthypeople.gov/2020/default.aspx. Accessed May 29, 2018.

World Health Organization Interim Commission [WHO]: Chronicle of WHO, Geneva, 1947, The Organization. [Accessed July 2018].

World Health Organization [WHO]: Constitution of WHO: *principles*, 2018a, http://www.who.int/about/mission/en/. Accessed July 2018.

World Health Organization [WHO]: Social determinants of health, 2018b, http://www.who.int/social_determinants/en/. Accessed July 2018.

World Health Organization [WHO]: Health topics: health promotion, 2018c, http://www.who.int/topics/health_promotion/en/. Accessed July 2018.

Yusufov M, et al.: Baseline predictors of singular action among participants with multiple health behavior risks, *Am J Health Promot* 30(5):365, 2016.

Zein JG, Erzurum SC: Asthma is different in women, *Curr Allergy Asthma Rep* 16(6):28, 2015.

RESEARCH REFERENCES

Abboud S, et al.: Cervical cancer screening among Arab women in the United States: an integrative review, *ONF* 44(1):E20, 2017.

Adamo K, Brett K: Parental perceptions and childhood dietary quality, *Matern Child Health J* 18(4):978, 2014.

Bardach S, et al.: What motivates older adults to improve diet and exercise patterns? *J Community Health* 41(1):22, 2016.

Cantu AG, Fleuriet KJ: "Making the ordinary more extraordinary": exploring creativity as a health promotion practice among older adults in a community-based professionally taught arts program, *J Holistic Nurs* 39(9):123, 2018.

Chiang JJ, et al.: Affective reactivity to daily stress and 20-year mortality risk in adults with chronic illness: findings from the national study of daily experiences, *Health Psychol* 37(2):170, 2018.

D'Alonzo KT, et al.: Outcomes of a culturally tailored partially randomized patient preference controlled trial to increase physical activity among low-income immigrant Latinas, *J Transcult Nurs* 29(4):335, 2018.

Dinh TTH, et al.: The effectiveness of the teach-back method on adherence and self-management in health education for people with chronic disease: a systematic review, *JBI Database Syst Rev Implement Rep* 14(1):210, 2016.

Doré C, et al.: Perspectives on burnout and empowerment among hemodialysis nurses and the current burnout intervention trends: a literature review, *CANNT J* 27(4):16, 2017.

Frost R, et al.: Identifying acceptable components for home-based health promotion services for older people with mid frailty: a qualitative study, *Health Soc Care Community* 26(3):393, 2018.

Griffith D, et al.: "Health is the ability to manage yourself without help": how older African American men define health and successful aging, *J Gerontol B Psychol Sci Soc Sci* 73(2):240, 2018.

Hong M, et al.: Social networks, health promoting behavior and health related quality of life in older Korean adults, *Nurs Health Sci* 20(1):79, 2018.

Janssen-Niemeijer A, et al.: The role of spirituality in lifestyle changing among patients with chronic cardiovascular diseases: a literature review of qualitative studies, *J Religion Health* 56(4):1460, 2017.

Kann L, et al.: Youth risk behavior surveillance—United States, 2017, *MMWR Surveill* 67(No. SS-8):1, 2018. https://www.cdc.gov/mmwr/volumes/67/ss/ss6708a1.htm#suggestedcitation. Accessed July 2018.

Kim HS, Yeom H: The association between spiritual well-being and burnout in intensive care nurses: a descriptive study, *Intensive Crit Care Nurse* 46(92), 2018.

LaVela SL, et al.: Relational empathy and holistic care in persons with spinal cord injuries, *J Spinal Cord Med* 40(1):30, 2017.

Morse LA, et al.: Humor doesn't retire: improvisation as a health-promoting intervention for older adults, *Arch Gerontol Geriatr* 75(1), 2018.

Pilger C, et al.: The relationship of the spiritual and religious dimensions with quality of life and health of patients with chronic kidney disease: an integrative literature review, *Nephrol Nurs J* 43(5):411, 2016.

Rausch JC, et al.: Effect of a school-based intervention on parents' knowledge, attitudes, and behaviors, *Am J Health Educ* 46(1):33, 2015.

Sattin RW, et al.: Community trial of a faith-based lifestyle intervention to prevent diabetes among African Americans, *J Community Health* 41(1):87, 2016.

Schneider S, Stone AA: Ambulatory and diary methods can facilitate the measurement of patient-reported outcomes, *Qual Life Res* 25(3):497, 2016.

Schwingel A, Gálvez P: Divine interventions: faith-based approaches to health promotion programs for Latinos, *J Religion Health* 55(6):1891, 2016.

Seo JY, Chao YY: Effects of exercise interventions on depressive symptoms among community-dwelling older adults in the United States: a systematic review, *J Gerontol Nurs* 44(3):31, 2018.

Xu Y, et al.: Culturally based remedies for initial home treatment of acute musculoskeletal injuries, *Medsurg Nurs* 25(5):360, 2016.

7

Caring in Nursing Practice

OBJECTIVES

- Discuss the role that caring plays in the nurse-patient relationship.
- Compare and contrast theories on caring.
- Discuss the evidence about patients' perceptions of caring.
- Explain how an ethic of care influences nurses' decision making.
- Describe ways to express caring through presence and touch.
- Describe the therapeutic benefit of listening to patients.
- Explain the relationship between knowing a patient and clinical decision making.
- Discuss the relationship of compassion to caring.

KEY TERMS

Caring, p. 82
Comforting, p. 87
Compassion, p. 83

Ethic of care, p. 86
Presence, p. 87
Transcultural, p. 83

Transformative, p. 84

MEDIA RESOURCES

http://evolve.elsevier.com/Potter/fundamentals/
- Review Questions
- Case Study with Questions

- Audio Glossary
- Content Updates
- Answers to QSEN Activity and Review Questions

Nursing is closely related to the core of caring for patients in both illness and health (Theofanidis and Sapountzi-Krepia, 2015). Caring is central to nursing practice, but it is even more important in today's hectic, high-tech health care environment, where productivity and efficiency can interfere with nurses' capacity to be caring, compassionate professionals (Letourneau et al., 2017). The demands, pressure, and time constraints in the health care environment threaten nurses' opportunities to establish therapeutic relationships and interpersonal connections with patients and family caregivers (Percy and Richardson, 2018; Adams, 2016).

It is important to maintain a relationship-centered approach to patient care for all aspects of nursing, whether the care focuses on pain management, teaching self-care, or providing basic hygiene measures. Caring relationships require sincerity, presence, availability, and engagement (Martin, 2015). Despite the challenges in health care, more professional organizations stress the importance of caring in health care and keeping the nurse engaged at a patient's bedside (RWJF, 2014). The American Organization of Nurse Executives (AONE, 2010) describes caring and knowledge as the core of nursing, with caring being a key component of what a nurse brings to a patient experience (Fig. 7.1).

Competent nursing practice values and embraces caring practices and expert knowledge (Benner et al., 2010). Your expertise in caring will come with clinical practice. When you engage patients in a caring and compassionate manner, the therapeutic gain in caring contributes greatly to the health and well-being of your patients. Think about a time when you were ill or experienced a problem requiring health care intervention. Then consider the following two scenarios and select the situation that you believe most successfully demonstrates a sense of caring:

- A nurse enters a patient's room, greets the patient warmly while touching him or her lightly on the shoulder, makes eye contact, sits down for a few minutes and asks about the patient's thoughts and concerns, listens to the patient's story, looks at the intravenous (IV) solution hanging in the room, briefly examines the patient, and then checks the vital sign summary on the bedside computer screen before leaving the room.
- A second nurse enters the patient's room, looks at the IV solution hanging in the room, checks the vital sign summary sheet on the bedside computer screen, and acknowledges the patient but never sits down or touches him or her. The nurse makes eye contact from above while the patient is lying in bed, asks a few brief questions about the patient's symptoms, and leaves.

Both of these scenarios take about the same amount of time but are very different. In times of illness or when a person seeks the professional guidance of a nurse, caring is essential in helping an individual reach positive outcomes.

THEORETICAL VIEWS ON CARING

Caring is a universal phenomenon influencing the ways in which people think, feel, and behave in relation to one another. Since Florence Nightingale, nurses have studied caring from a variety of philosophical and ethical perspectives. Some nursing scholars developed theories on caring because of its importance to nursing practice. This chapter does not detail all of the theories, but it is designed to help you understand how caring enables a nurse to work with all patients in a respectful, therapeutic way.

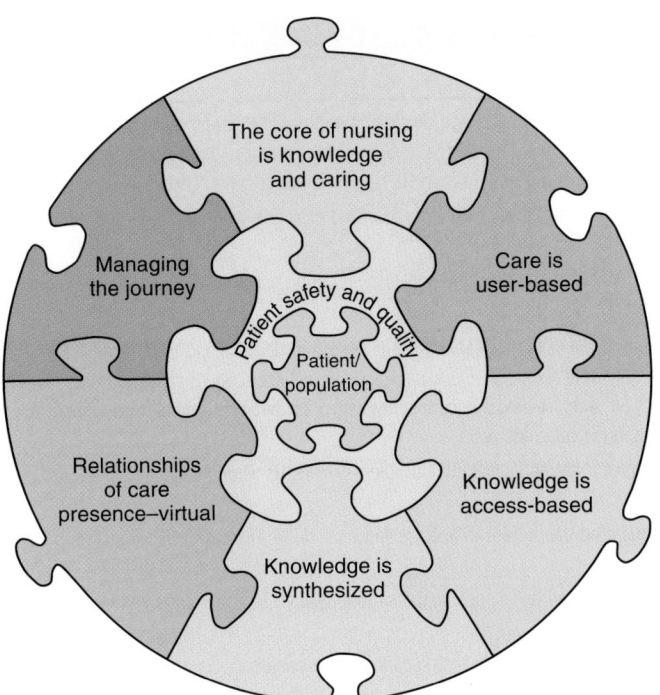

FIG. 7.1 AONE guiding principles for the role of the nurse in future patient care delivery. (Copyright© 2015 by the American Organization of Nurse Executives [AONE]. All rights reserved.)

Caring Is Primary

Dr. Patricia Benner offers nurses a rich, holistic understanding of nursing practice and caring through her research involving the interpretation of expert nurses' stories. After listening to nurses' stories and analyzing their meaning, she described caring as the essence of excellent nursing practice. The stories revealed the nurses' behaviors and decisions that expressed caring. Caring means that people, events, projects, and things matter to people (Benner and Wrubel, 1989; Benner et al., 2010). It is a word for being connected.

Caring underlies a wide range of interactions, from parental love to friendship, from caring for one's work to caring for one's pet, to caring for and about one's patients, and caring for one's self (Hines and Gaughan, 2017). "Caring creates possibility." Personal concern for another person, an event, or a thing provides motivation and direction for people to care. Through caring, nurses help patients recover in the face of illness, give meaning to their illness, and maintain or reestablish connection. Caring and compassion interventions need to be taught and practiced early in nursing education and emphasized in all clinical practice settings (Labraque et al., 2017).

Patients are not all the same. Each person brings a unique background of experiences, values, and cultural perspectives to a health care encounter. Caring is specific and relational for each nurse-patient encounter. As nurses acquire more experience, they typically learn that caring helps them focus on the patients for whom they care (Porter et al., 2014). Caring improves a nurse's ability to know a patient, recognize a patient's problems, and find and implement individualized solutions.

Because illness is the human experience of loss or dysfunction, any treatment or intervention given without consideration of its meaning to an individual is unlikely to be effective. Develop a caring relationship with your patients and listen to their stories to fully understand the meaning and impact of their condition and to provide patient-centered care.

Leininger's Transcultural Caring

Madeleine Leininger (1991) offers a transcultural view of caring. She describes the concept of care as the domain that sets nursing apart from other health care disciplines (see Chapter 4). Care is an essential human need. Care, unlike cure, helps an individual or group improve a human condition. Acts of caring are nurturing and skillful activities, processes, and decisions that help people in empathetic, compassionate, and supportive ways. A caring act depends on the needs, problems, and values of a patient.

Nurses need to understand cultural caring behaviors (Leininger, 1991). Even though human caring is a universal phenomenon, the expressions, processes, and patterns of caring vary among people of different cultures (Box 7.1). Caring is very personal; thus its expression differs for each patient. For caring to be effective, nurses need to learn culturally specific behaviors and words that reflect human caring in different cultures to identify and meet the needs of all patients (see Chapter 9). As nurses we care for patients from certain "subcultures" that have unique needs (e.g., people who are chronically ill, physically disabled, developmentally challenged, or homeless).

Watson's Transpersonal Caring

According to Jean Watson, caring is a central focus of nursing, and it is integral to maintain the ethical and philosophical roots of the profession (Porter et al., 2014; Dey, 2016). Patients and their families expect a high quality of human interaction from nurses; they need conversations with their nurses and caregivers that are meaningful and address their needs (Sitzman, 2017). Unfortunately, many conversations between patients and nurses are brief and disconnected. Many are not really "conversations" but rather simply the nurse reporting information to a patient and family. Watson's theory of caring is a holistic model that supports a nurse's conscious intention to care to promote healing and wholeness (Watson, 2008, 2010). It integrates the human caring processes with healing environments, incorporating the life-generating and life-receiving processes of human caring and healing for nurses and their patients (WCSI, 2018). The theory describes a consciousness that allows nurses to raise new questions about what it means to be a

TABLE 7.1   Watson's 10 Carative Factors

Carative Factor	Example in Practice
Forming a human-altruistic value system	Use loving kindness to extend yourself. Use self-disclosure appropriately to promote a therapeutic alliance with your patient (e.g., share a personal experience in common with your patient such as a child-rearing experience, an illness, or an experience with a parent who needs assistance).
Instilling faith-hope	Provide a connection with the patient that offers purpose and direction when trying to find the meaning of an illness.
Cultivating a sensitivity to one's self and to others	Learn to accept yourself and others for their full potential. A caring nurse matures into becoming a self-actualized nurse.
Developing a helping, trusting, human caring relationship	Learn to develop and sustain helping, trusting, authentic caring relationships through effective communication with your patients.
Promoting and expressing positive and negative feelings	Support and accept your patients' feelings. In connecting with your patients, you show a willingness to take risks in sharing in the relationship.
Using creative problem-solving, caring processes	Apply the nursing process in systematic, scientific problem-solving decision making in providing patient-centered care.
Promoting transpersonal teaching-learning	Learn together while educating the patient to acquire self-care skills. The patient assumes responsibility for learning.
Providing for a supportive, protective, and/or corrective mental, physical, societal, and spiritual environment	Create a healing environment at all levels, physical and nonphysical. This promotes wholeness, beauty, comfort, dignity, and peace.
Meeting human needs	Intentionally help patients meet basic needs with a caring consciousness.
Allowing for existential-phenomenological-spiritual forces	Allow spiritual forces to provide a better understanding of yourself and your patient.

Data from Watson J: *The philosophy and science of caring,* Boulder, CO, 2008, University Press of Colorado.

nurse, to be ill, and to be caring and healing. The transpersonal caring theory rejects the disease orientation to health care and *places care before cure* (Watson, 2008). A nurse who focuses on transpersonal caring looks for deeper sources of inner healing to protect, enhance, and preserve a person's dignity, humanity, wholeness, and inner harmony.

Creating caring-healing environments in the current high-tech health care system is crucial to establishing and maintaining the nurse-patient relationship (Sitzman, 2017). Watson's model emphasizes the nurse-patient caring relationship with the focus on carative behaviors (Table 7.1). A nurse communicates caring-healing to a patient through the nurse's consciousness. This takes place during a single caring moment between nurse and patient when a connection forms. The model is transformative because the relationship influences both the nurse and the patient for better or for worse (Watson, 2008, 2010). Caring-healing consciousness promotes healing. Application of Watson's caring model in practice enhances nurses' caring practices (Box 7.2).

Swanson's Theory of Caring

Kristen Swanson (1991) studied patients and professional caregivers to develop a theory of caring for nursing practice. This theory of caring was developed from three perinatal studies involving interviews with women who miscarried, parents and health care professionals in a newborn intensive care unit, and mothers who were socially at risk and received long-term public health intervention (Swanson, 1999). After analyzing the stories and descriptions of the three groups, Swanson developed a theory of caring, which includes five caring processes (Table 7.2). Swanson (1991) defines caring as a nurturing way of relating to an individual (i.e., when one feels a personal sense of commitment and responsibility). The theory guides nurses in developing useful and effective caring strategies appropriate for multiple age-group and health care settings (Andershed and Olsson, 2009). Caring is a central nursing phenomenon that is not unique to nursing practice; it improves patient satisfaction and outcomes (Ortega Barco and de Rodriguez, 2018). Teaching students and new nurses how to use

Swanson's five caring processes helps new nurses gain confidence when providing patient-centered care (Moffa, 2015).

Summary of Theoretical Views

Caring theories are valuable when assessing patient perceptions of being cared for in a multicultural environment (Suliman et al., 2009). There are common themes among the theoretical view of caring. Porter et al. (2014) support earlier findings and identify these commonalities as human interaction or communication, mutuality, appreciating the uniqueness of individuals, and improving the welfare of patients and families. Caring is relational, and in a health care setting a nurse and patient enter into a relationship that is much more than one person simply doing tasks for another. In a caring relationship a mutual give-and-take develops as nurse and patient begin to know and care for one another (Martin, 2015; Turpin, 2014; Arslan-Ozkan et al., 2013).

Caring is often invisible when a nurse and patient enter a relationship of respect, concern, and support. A nurse's empathy and compassion become a natural part of every patient encounter. However, it is obvious when caring is absent. For example, a nurse who shows disinterest or chooses to avoid a patient's request for help quickly conveys an uncaring attitude. Benner and Wrubel (1989) relate the story of a clinical nurse specialist who learned from a patient what caring is all about: "I felt that I was teaching him a lot, but actually he taught me. One day he said to me (probably after I had delivered some well-meaning technical information about his disease), 'You're doing an OK job, but I can tell that every time you walk in that door you're walking out.'" In this nurse's story the patient perceived that the nurse was simply going through the motions of teaching and showed little caring toward the patient. Patients quickly know when nurses fail to relate to them.

As you gain clinical experience, continue to practice caring, and your patients and their family caregivers will sense your commitment and willingness to enter into a relationship that allows you to understand their experiences of illness (Monsen, et al., 2017). In a study of patients receiving oral chemotherapy, patients noted that it was essential for nurses to develop a partnership and connect with them, to be

BOX 7.2 EVIDENCE-BASED PRACTICE

Enhancing Caring

PICOT Question: Do patient satisfaction scores among adult patients who are hospitalized improve when carative nursing practices are used?

Evidence Summary

Researchers identify a strong, positive relationship between nurse caring behaviors and patient satisfaction. Patients noted that when the nurses listened to their stories and concerns, they felt that their care was individualized and reported greater satisfaction (Brewer and Watson, 2015). Evidence shows that patient and family caregiver satisfaction improves when nurses demonstrate caring behaviors when accommodating patients' specific requests or communicating the reasons why these requests cannot be met immediately (Wyant et al., 2017). Promotion of caring, compassionate, supportive, and therapeutic environments for patients increases patient satisfaction and nurses' job satisfaction (Nightingale et al., 2018). Caring nursing practices also improve patients' functional status, self-efficacy, coping, and self-care (Arslan-Ozkan et al., 2013; Papastavrou et al., 2011). Finally, patient-centered care models emphasize that caring interventions promote patient advocacy and predict patient satisfaction (Compton et al., 2017; Porter et al., 2014).

Application to Nursing Practice

- Use the caring practices of listening, presence, and connectedness to partner with the patient and family through their illness. Use these practices with humility, love, kindness, and compassion (Nightingale et al., 2018; Dobrina et al., 2014).
- Ask patients whether they have questions about their illness, treatment, or home care needs (Compton et al., 2018)
- Knowing the patient enables you to partner with a patient and family to obtain vital health care information, understand the patient's expectations and fears, explore the meaning of the illness to the patient and family caregivers, and identify health care priorities (Compton et al., 2018; Zolnierek, 2014).
- Use every patient interaction to continuously "know" all patients better (Ragan and Kanter, 2017; Zolnierek, 2014).
- Being with and doing for a patient are components of presence, whether it is a dedicated one-on-one interaction or quietly sitting with a patient (Mohammadipour et al., 2017; Yagasaki and Komatsu, 2013). Presence often helps elicit important health care information from a patient and reduces patient fear and anxiety.
- Caring nursing practices also benefit nursing staff by reducing staff turnover, reducing workplace stress, and increasing job satisfaction (Nightingale et al., 2018).

TABLE 7.2 Swanson's Theory of Caring

Caring Process	Definition	Subdimensions
Knowing	Striving to understand an event as it has meaning in the life of the other	Avoiding assumptions Centering on the one cared for Assessing thoroughly Seeking clues to clarify the event Engaging the self or both
Being with	Being emotionally present to the other	Being there Conveying ability Sharing feelings Not burdening
Doing for	Doing for the other as he or she would do for self if it were at all possible	Comforting Anticipating Performing skillfully Protecting Preserving dignity
Enabling	Facilitating the other's passage through life transitions (e.g., birth, death) and unfamiliar events	Informing/explaining Supporting/allowing Focusing Generating alternatives Validating/giving feedback
Maintaining belief	Sustaining faith in the other's capacity to get through an event or transition and face a future with meaning	Believing in/holding in esteem Maintaining a hope-filled attitude Offering realistic optimism "Going the distance"

Data from Swanson KM: Empirical development of a middle-range theory of caring, *Nurs Res*, 40(3):161, 1991.

Knowing the context of a patient's illness helps you choose and individualize patient-centered interventions that will actually help the patient. This approach is more successful than simply selecting interventions on the basis of your patient's symptoms or disease process.

PATIENTS' PERCEPTIONS OF CARING

Theories of caring help nurses understand the behaviors and processes that characterize caring. Researchers have explored nurse caring behaviors as perceived by patients (Table 7.3). Their findings emphasize what patients expect from their caregivers and thus provide useful guidelines for your practice. Patients continue to value nurses' effectiveness in performing tasks; but clearly patients value the affective dimension of nursing care. Caring is a significant part of the art of nursing.

You need to understand patients' perceptions because health care is placing greater emphasis on patient satisfaction (see Chapter 2). Health care consumers can search online for specific information about health care agencies with regard to their ratings by patients in various areas of performance. The Caring Assessment Tool (CAT) was developed to measure caring from a patient's perspective (Duffy et al., 2007). This tool and other caring assessments help you, as a beginning professional, to appreciate the type of behaviors that patients in the hospital identify as caring (Box 7.3). When patients sense that health care providers are sensitive, sympathetic, compassionate, and interested in them as people, they usually become active partners in the plan of care. Suliman et al. (2009) studied the impact of Watson's caring theory as an assessment framework in a multicultural environment. Patients in the study indicated that they did not perceive any

attentive, and be proactive in providing committed patient support (Yagasaki and Komatsu, 2013). Thus, the nurse becomes a coach and partner rather than a detached provider of care.

One aspect of caring is enabling—when a nurse and patient work together to identify alternatives in approaches to care and resources. Consider a nurse working with a patient recently diagnosed with diabetes mellitus. The nurse enables the patient by allowing the patient to modify lifestyle to incorporate diabetes self-management strategies, such as medication administration, exercise, and changes in diet.

Another common theme of caring is understanding the context of a person's life and illness. It is difficult to show caring for another without understanding who the person is and his or her perception of the illness. Ask your patients the following questions to understand their perceptions: How was your illness first recognized? How do you feel about the illness? How does your illness affect what you do each day?

TABLE 7.3   Comparison of Research Studies Exploring Nurse Caring Behaviors (As Perceived by Patients)

Nurses' Caring Behaviors: The Perception of Patients With Cancer At the Time of Discharge After Surgery (Compton et al., 2018)	Learning the Patient's Stories (Ragan and Kanter, 2017)	The Need for a Nursing Presence in Oral Chemotherapy (Yagasaki and Komatsu, 2013)
Used the Caring Assessment Tool (CAT, see Box 7.3) to determine patients' perceptions of nurse caring behaviors at the time of discharge. It was important to patients that nurses appreciated the unique impact of the illness on patient and family caregiver. Patients perceived that the nurses knew what was important to them. Caring behaviors, such as knowing, listening, and presence, contributed to patient satisfaction. Respecting the patient's values, beliefs, and health care choices, such as explaining choices, advocating for resources, and accepting patient decisions, were essential.	Learning and knowing the patient story is an essential element of caring nursing practice. Listening and presence help nurses know patients. Understanding the story establishes a nurse-patient relationship and maintains caring practice. To really hear a patient's story, start by refining listening skills and take the time to "sit and make eye contact" while listening. Knowing the patient and the story is critical to collecting clinical and personal information so that the nurse can better know and understand the patient's health care story and expectations for care, identify and correct missing information, and design patient-centered care.	Nursing presence contributes to knowing the patient. Illness and treatments often cause major changes in a patient's lifestyle. Nursing presence for patients receiving oral chemotherapy is as important as identifying those patients at risk for nonadherence. Nursing presence provides emotional and knowledge-based support for patients who are new to or receiving additional oral chemotherapy.

BOX 7.3   Factors and Items Constituting the Caring Assessment Tool (CAT)

Each item begins with the stem: "Since I have been a patient here, the nurse(s)":

Mutual Problem Solving
- Help me understand how I am thinking.
- Ask me how I think treatment is going.
- Help me explore alternative ways of dealing.
- Ask me what I know.
- Help me figure out questions to ask.

Attentive Reassurance
- Are available.
- Seem interested.
- Support sense of hope.
- Help me believe in self.
- Anticipate my needs.

Human Respect
- Listen to me.
- Accept me.
- Treat me kindly.
- Respect me.
- Pay attention to me.

Encouraging Manner
- Support my beliefs.
- Encourage me to ask questions.
- Help me to see some good.
- Encourage me to go on.
- Help me deal with bad feelings.

Appreciation of Unique Meanings
- Are concerned with how I view things.
- Know what is important to me.
- Acknowledge my inner feelings.
- Show respect for things having meaning.

Healing Environment
- Check up on me.
- Pay attention to me when I am talking.
- Make me feel comfortable.
- Respect my privacy.
- Treat my body carefully.

Affiliation Needs
- Are responsive to my family.
- Talk openly with my family.
- Allow my family to be involved.

Basic Human Needs
- Make sure I get food.
- Help me with routine needs for sleep.
- Help me feel less worried.

Modified from Duffy JR, et al: Dimensions of caring: psychometric evaluation of the Caring Assessment Tool, *Adv Nurs Sci* 30(3):235, 2007.

cultural bias when they perceived nurses to be caring. As institutions strive to improve patient satisfaction, creating an environment of caring is a necessary and worthwhile goal. Patient satisfaction with nursing care is an important factor in a patient's decision to return to a specific health care agency.

As you begin clinical practice, consider how patients perceive caring and the best approaches to provide care. Assess what your patient expects. Build a nurse-patient relationship to learn what is important to your patients. For example, you are caring for a patient who had breast cancer 2 years ago. She needs another breast biopsy and is fearful of the outcome. Instead of giving a lengthy description of why the procedure is necessary, you obtain assistance from an oncology nurse specialist. Knowing your patients helps you select caring approaches that are most appropriate to their needs.

ETHIC OF CARE

Caring is an interaction between the nurse and patient in an atmosphere of mutual respect and trust. In this collaborative environment, the nurse provides encouragement, hope, support, and compassion to help achieve desired outcomes. It is a professional, ethical covenant that nursing has with its public. Caring science provides a disciplinary foundation from which you deliver patient-centered care. Chapter 22 explores the importance of ethics in professional nursing. The term *ethic* refers to the ideals of right and wrong behavior. In any patient encounter a nurse needs to know what behavior is ethically appropriate. Nurses do not make professional decisions based solely on intellectual or analytical principles. Instead, an ethic of care places caring at the center of decision making.

An ethic of care is concerned with relationships between people and with a nurse's character and attitude toward others. Nurses who function from an ethic of care are sensitive to unequal relationships that lead to an abuse of one person's power over another—intentional or otherwise. In health care settings patients and families are often on unequal footing with professionals because of a patient's illness, lack of information, regression caused by pain and suffering, and unfamiliar circumstances. An ethic of care places the nurse as the patient's advocate, solving ethical dilemmas by attending to relationships and giving priority to each patient's unique personhood.

REFLECT NOW

A patient requires a lot of physical and emotional care and is frequently using the nurse call system. The health care providers alternate answering the nurse call system, stating "I just did it" or "It's your turn."
Think about how these comments and actions affect the ethic of care.
How would you convey your thoughts to the health care team?

CARING IN NURSING PRACTICE

It is impossible to determine when a nurse becomes a caring professional. As you deal with health and illness in your practice, you grow in your ability to care and develop caring behaviors. We learn from our patients. Our patients tell us that a simple touch, a simple phrase (e.g., "I'm here"), or a promise to remain at the bedside represent caring and compassion (Engle, 2010).

Caring is one of those human behaviors that we can give and receive. As a nurse it is important to assess both your caring needs and your caring behaviors. Recognize the importance of nurses' self-care (see Chapters 1 and 6). You cannot give fully engaged, compassionate care when you feel depleted. Take time to recognize stressors and reach out to colleagues, family, and friends to help you cope. Use caring behavior to reach out to colleagues to care for them as well (Monsen et al., 2017; Jackson, 2012). Whether you are giving or receiving care, the value of caring in your nursing practice benefits your patients, your colleagues, and your health care agency.

Providing Presence

Nursing practice and patient satisfaction improve when "nursing presence" is part of the health care culture (Mohammadipour et al., 2017; Yagasaki and Komatsu, 2013). Providing presence is a person-to-person encounter conveying a closeness and sense of caring. Presence involves "being there" and "being with." "Being there" is not only a physical presence; it also includes communication and understanding. Nursing presence is the connectedness between a nurse and a patient (Plessis, 2016; Kostovich, 2012).

Presence is an interpersonal process that is characterized by sensitivity, wholism, intimacy, vulnerability, and adaptation to unique circumstances. It results in improved mental well-being for nurses and patients and improved physical well-being in patients. The interpersonal relationship of "being there" requires a nurse to be attentive to the perspectives of the patient and family caregiver. It translates into an actual caring art that affects the healing and well-being of both the nurse and patient (Mohammadipour et al., 2017). Nurses use presence in conjunction with other interventions, such as establishing the nurse-patient relationship, providing comfort measures, providing patient education, and listening (Plessis, 2016). The outcomes of nursing presence include the relief of suffering, a decrease in the sense of isolation and vulnerability, and personal growth.

Establishing presence strengthens your ability to provide effective patient-centered care. Presence is also valuable during patient- and family-centered rounds, during which nurses offer their presence to help patients achieve positive outcomes, diminish the intensity of unwanted feelings, promote reassurance, and guide family caregivers (Sharma et al., 2014; Yagasaki and Komatsu, 2013). As a result, patients often are more satisfied with the nursing care and the health care system in general (Penque and Kearney, 2015).

"Being with" involves a nurse giving of himself or herself, which means being available and at a patient's disposal. If a patient accepts a nurse, the patient will invite the nurse to see, share, and touch his or her vulnerability and suffering. One's human presence never leaves one unaffected (Watson, 2010). The nurse enters the patient's world, and the patient is able to identify feelings and solutions, see new directions, and make choices.

When a nurse establishes presence, eye contact, body language, voice tone, listening, and a positive and encouraging attitude act together to create openness and understanding. Establishing presence enhances a nurse's ability to learn from patients, including their hopes, dreams, need for support, and expectations of care. Learning from a patient strengthens a nurse's ability to provide adequate and appropriate nursing care (Dobrina et al., 2014).

It is especially important to establish presence and caring when patients are experiencing stressful events or situations. Awaiting a physician's report of test results, preparing for an unfamiliar procedure, and planning for a return home after serious illness are just a few examples of events in the course of a person's illness that can create unpredictability and dependency on care providers. A nurse's presence and caring help to calm anxiety and fear related to stressful situations. Giving reassurance and thorough explanations about a procedure, remaining at the patient's side, and coaching the patient through the experience all convey a presence that is invaluable to a patient's well-being.

Touch

Patients face situations that are embarrassing, frightening, and painful. Whatever the feeling or symptom, they look to nurses to provide comfort. The use of touch is one comforting approach that reaches out to patients to communicate concern and support (Hanley et al., 2017).

Touch is relational and leads to a connection between nurse and patient. It involves contact and noncontact touch. Contact touch involves obvious skin-to-skin contact and is referred to as "therapeutic touch" (Hanley et al., 2017). Before implementing touch, be aware of your patient's cultural practices and past experiences. For some people a simple touch on the arm may be perceived as invasive, and for victims of abuse a simple touch may be perceived as a threat. Noncontact touch refers to eye contact. It is difficult to separate the two. Both provide a connectedness between a patient and nurse (Palese et al., 2011; Jackson, 2012).

Nurses use task-oriented touch when performing a task or procedure. The skillful and gentle performance of a nursing procedure conveys security and a sense of competence. An expert nurse learns that any procedure is more effective when it is explained and administered carefully and in consideration of any patient concern. For example, if a patient is anxious about having a procedure such as the insertion of a nasogastric tube, offer comfort through a full explanation of the procedure and what the patient will feel. Then perform the procedure safely, skillfully, and successfully. This is done as you prepare the supplies, position the patient, and gently manipulate and insert the nasogastric tube. Throughout a procedure talk quietly with the patient to provide reassurance and support.

Caring touch is a form of nonverbal communication, which successfully influences a patient's comfort and security, enhances self-esteem, increases confidence of caregivers, and improves mental well-being. You express this in the way you hold a patient's hand, give a back massage, gently position a patient, or participate in a conversation. When using a caring touch, you connect with the patient physically and emotionally.

Protective touch is a form of touch that protects a nurse and/or patient. A patient views it either positively or negatively. The most obvious form of protective touch is in preventing an accident (e.g., holding and bracing a patient to avoid a fall). Protective touch can also protect a nurse emotionally. A nurse withdraws or distances herself or himself from a patient when he or she is unable to tolerate suffering or needs to escape from a situation that is causing tension. When used in this way, protective touch elicits negative feelings in a patient.

Because touch conveys many messages, use it with discretion. Touch itself is a concern when crossing cultural boundaries of either the patient or the nurse (Benner et al., 2010). Patients generally permit task-oriented touch because most individuals give nurses and physicians a license to enter their personal space to provide care (see Box 7.1). Know and understand whether patients accept touch and how they interpret your intentions.

Listening

Listening is necessary for meaningful interactions with patients. It is a planned and deliberate act in which the listener is present and engages the patient in a nonjudgmental and accepting manner. You "take in" what a patient says, interpreting and understanding what the patient is saying, and then give back that understanding to the patient. Listening to the meaning of what a patient says helps create a mutual relationship. True listening leads to knowing and responding to what really matters to a patient and family. Listening, especially when providing end-of-life-care, helps a patient and family caregiver address their concerns and preferences with dignity (Harstade et al., 2018).

Any critical or chronic illness affects all of a patient's life choices and decisions, and sometimes the individual's identity. Being able to tell the story about the illness and its meaning helps a patient break the distress of illness (Borasio and Tamches, 2018; Harstade et al., 2018). The personal concerns that are part of a patient's illness story determine what is at stake for the patient. Caring through listening enables you to become a participant in the patient's life.

To listen effectively you need to silence yourself and listen with an open mind. Remain intentionally silent and concentrate on what the patient has to say. Give patients your full, focused attention as they tell their stories.

When a person chooses to tell his or her story, it involves reaching out to another human being (Borasio and Tamches, 2018). Telling the story implies a relationship that develops only if the clinician exchanges his or her stories as well. Some professionals do not recognize their own need to be known as part of a clinical relationship (Frank, 1998). Unless a professional acknowledges this need, there is no reciprocal relationship, only an interaction.

Through active listening you begin to truly know your patients and what is important to them. Learning to listen to a patient is sometimes difficult. It is easy to become distracted by tasks at hand, colleagues shouting instructions, or other patients waiting to have their needs met. However, the time you take to listen effectively is worthwhile, in both the information gained and the strengthening of the nurse-patient relationship (Engle, 2010). Listening involves paying attention to an individual's words and tone of voice and entering his or her frame of reference (see Chapter 24). By observing the expressions and body language of a patient, you find cues to help the patient explore ways to achieve greater peace.

Knowing the Patient

Knowing the patient is a complex process that occurs over time and within the context of the nurse-patient relationship (Zolnierek, 2014). It is an essential element of nursing practice and is linked to patient satisfaction and successful outcomes of care (Kelley et al., 2013). One of the five caring processes described by Swanson (1991) is knowing the patient. Knowing emerges from a caring relationship between a nurse and a patient, in which the nurse engages in a continuous assessment, striving to understand and interpret the patient's needs across all dimensions (Kelley et al., 2013).

Knowing a patient is at the core of clinical decision making and patient-centered care. Through caring you develop an understanding that helps you to better know the patient as a unique individual and choose the most appropriate and effective nursing therapies (Potter and Savette, 2014). Knowing the patient helps you understand how illness, treatment, or rehabilitation affect the patient and family caregiver (Tyreman, 2015).

Two elements that facilitate knowing are continuity of care and clinical expertise. When patient care is fragmented, nurses have difficulty knowing a patient, compromising patient-centered care (Zolnierek, 2014). Knowing develops over time as a nurse learns the clinical conditions within a specialty and the behaviors and physiological responses of patients. Intimate knowing helps the nurse respond to what really matters to the patient. To know a patient provides the health care team with information to provide patient-focused, team-based interventions that improve patient satisfaction and outcomes (Shippe et al., 2018). Thus, the nurse engages in a caring relationship with the patient that reveals information and cues that facilitate critical thinking and clinical judgments (see Chapter 15).

Factors that contribute to knowing patients include time, continuity of care, teamwork of the nursing staff, trust, and experience. Barriers to knowing a patient are often related to the organizational structure of the organization and economic constraints. Organizational changes that result in decreasing the amount of time that nurses are able to spend with their patients affects nurse-patient relationships. Decreased length of stay also reduces the interactions between nurses and their patients (Zolnierek, 2014).

Many consequences result from not knowing a patient. For example, in the acute care setting, not knowing the patient contributes to risk for falls and actual falls. Patients and their families don't understand the complexities of treatment and their participation in care (Kelley et al., 2013). Finally, patients do not adequately understand their discharge instructions and may administer their home medications or treatments incorrectly. A caring nurse-patient relationship helps you to better know the patient as a unique individual and choose the most appropriate and effective nursing therapies (WCSI, 2018).

A caring relationship coupled with your growing knowledge and experience provides a rich source of meaning when changes in a patient's clinical status occur. Expert nurses develop the ability to detect changes in patients' conditions almost effortlessly (Ragan and Kanter, 2017; Benner et al., 2010). Clinical decision making, perhaps the most important responsibility of a professional nurse, involves various aspects of knowing the patient: responses to therapies, routines and habits, coping resources, physical capacities and endurance, and body typology and characteristics. Experienced nurses know additional facts about their patients such as their experiences, behaviors, feelings, and perceptions (Benner et al., 2010). You will achieve improved patient satisfaction and patient health outcomes when you make clinical decisions accurately in the context of knowing a patient well (Zolnierek, 2014). When you base care on knowing a patient, the patient perceives care as personalized, comforting, supportive, and healing.

The most important thing for a beginning nurse to recognize is that knowing a patient is more than simply gathering data about a patient's clinical signs and condition. Success in knowing a patient is to enter into a caring, social process that also includes interaction with members of the health care team, which results in a deep nurse-patient relationship whereby the patient comes to feel known by the nurse (Ragan and Kanter, 2017; Kelley et al., 2013).

QSEN **Building Competency in Patient-Centered Care** Mrs. Martinez is 72 years of age, has three married sons, and lives in a mother-in-law suite in the home of one son. There are two adult grandchildren who are on their own. Mrs. Martinez's son and daughter-in-law have full-time jobs and are out of the house from 8:00 AM to 6:00 PM each day.

Each summer the other sons and their families visit Mrs. Martinez while the son with whom she lives and his wife go on vacations. Mrs. Martinez's sons and their families spend the holidays together.

Presently she is independent. She takes medication for high blood pressure and an irregular heartbeat. At times these medications make her "light-headed." She also has occasional dizziness from a middle ear problem when she changes position too fast. She is afraid that if she shared this information with her doctor, he'd think that she'd fall and say she must give up her activities. She equates this with losing her independence.

Given the information about her living situation, current level of independence, and symptoms of light-headedness and dizziness, how do you plan and implement patient-centered care?

Answers to QSEN Activities can be found on the Evolve website.

Spiritual Caring

An individual achieves spiritual health after finding a balance between his or her own life values, goals, and belief systems and those of others (see Chapter 35). An individual's beliefs and expectations affect his or her own physical well-being.

Research shows that nurses who develop spiritual caring practices early in their career development are able to identify methods to incorporate these practices into routine care and do not perceive variables such as a lack of sufficient time or patient census as barriers (Ronaldson et al., 2012). Establishing a caring relationship with a patient involves interconnectedness between the nurse and the patient. This interconnectedness is why Watson (2008, 2010) describes the caring relationship in a spiritual sense. Spirituality offers a sense of connectedness: intrapersonally (connected with oneself), interpersonally (connected with others and the environment), and transpersonally (connected with the unseen, God, or a higher power). In a caring relationship the patient and the nurse come to know one another so that both move toward a healing relationship by (Brewer and Watson, 2015; WCSI, 2018):

- Mobilizing hope for the patient and the nurse
- Finding an interpretation or understanding of illness, symptoms, or emotions that is acceptable to the patient
- Assisting the patient in using social, emotional, or spiritual resources
- Recognizing that caring relationships connect us human to human, spirit to spirit

Relieving Symptoms and Suffering

Relieving symptoms such as pain, nausea, and suffering is more than giving pain medications, repositioning a patient, cleaning a wound, or providing end-of-life care (see Chapter 36). Reducing symptoms and suffering requires patient-centered caring actions that give a patient comfort, dignity, respect, and peace and that provide comfort and support measures to the family and friends (Baillie et al., 2018).

Through skillful and accurate assessment of a patient's symptoms, your delivery of patient-centered care will improve a patient's level of comfort. You will use multiple interventions to relieve pain (see Chapter 44), nausea, and fatigue. However, knowing about a patient and the meaning of his or her symptoms guides your care (Baillie et al., 2018). Conveying a quiet, caring presence, touching a patient, or listening helps you to assess and understand the meaning of your patient's discomfort. The caring presence helps you and your patient design goals for symptom relief.

Human suffering is multifaceted, affecting a patient physically, emotionally, socially, and spiritually. It also affects a patient's family caregivers and other family members (Given and Reinhard, 2017). You may find yourself working with a young family whose newborn baby has multiple developmental challenges. Likewise, you may find yourself working with a family providing home care for a parent with dementia. In both of these examples, these families' emotional suffering encompasses anger, guilt, fear, or grief. You cannot fix it, but you can provide comfort through a listening, nonjudgmental caring presence. Patients and their families are comforted by a caring listener.

Family Care

Each person experiences life through relationships with others (see Chapter 10). Thus caring for an individual includes a person's family. As a nurse it is important to know the family and family caregivers as thoroughly as you know a patient (Given and Reinhard, 2017). The family is an important resource (Fig. 7.2). Success with nursing interventions often depends on their willingness to share information about the patient, their acceptance and understanding of therapies, whether the interventions fit with their daily practices, and whether they support and deliver the therapies recommended.

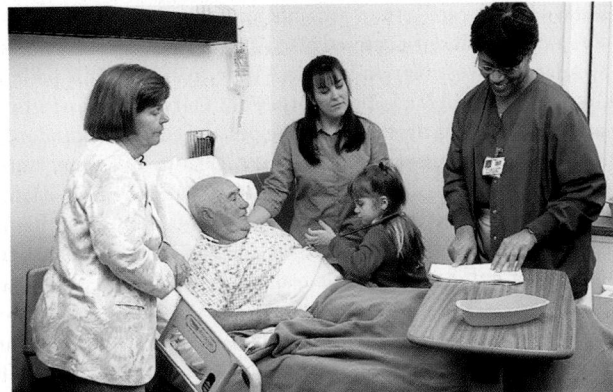

FIG. 7.2 Nurse discusses patient's health care needs with the family.

BOX 7.4 Nurse Caring Behaviors as Perceived by Families

- Providing honest, clear, and accurate information
- Listening to patient and family concerns, complaints, and fears
- Assisting family with implementing advanced directives
- Advocating for patient's care preferences and end-of-life decisions
- Involving family in care and teaching the family how to keep the relative physically comfortable
- Informing the patient and family about the types of nursing services and the people who may enter the personal care area
- Providing comfort (e.g., offering warm blanket, rubbing a patient's back)
- Reading patient passages from religious texts, favorite book, cards, or mail
- Assuring the patient that nursing services will be available
- Helping patients do as much for themselves as possible

Data from Maroon AM: Ethical palliative family nursing care: a new concept of caring for patients and families, *JONA's Healthc Law Ethics Regul* 14(4):115, 2012; Lusk JM, Fater K: A concept analysis of patient-centered care, *Nurs Forum* 48(2):89, 2013.

Families of patients with cancer perceive many nurse caring behaviors to be helpful (Box 7.4). It is critical that a nurse ensures a patient's well-being and safety and helps the family members to be active participants. Although specific to families of patients with cancer, these behaviors offer useful guidelines for developing a caring relationship with all families. Begin a relationship by learning who makes up the patient's family and their roles in the patient's life (Chapter 10). Showing a family that you care for and are concerned about the patient creates an openness that then enables a relationship to form. Caring for the family takes into consideration the context of the patient's illness and the stress it imposes on all members.

REFLECT NOW

Think about a clinical or personal situation in which you needed to provide caring support. Can you identify the caring behaviors you used? Critique your interaction. What was good and helpful? How could you have done better?

THE CHALLENGE OF CARING

The concept of caring motivates people to become nurses. When nurses commit themselves to be caring individuals, they achieve a meaning and purpose in their lives (Benner et al., 2010). Your e). Nurses gain a sense of satisfaction when they know they have made a difference in patients' lives.

Today's health care system presents many challenges for nurses to provide a caring patient-centered plan of care (Percy and Richardson, 2018; Adams, 2016). Nurses have less time to spend with patients, making it much harder to know who they are. Our reliance on technology and cost-effective health care strategies and efforts to standardize and refine work processes all undermine the nature of caring. Nurses are often torn between the human caring model and the task-oriented biomedical model, institutional demands, and time constraints that consume their practice (Letourneau et al., 2017). Too often patients become just a number, with their real needs overlooked or ignored. In addition, nurses deal with multiple stressors (e.g., interdepartmental, technology, paperwork stressors, high patient acuity rates, and multiple patient care interruptions). As a result, nurses are at risk for compassion fatigue and burnout (Mason et al., 2014; Hunsaker et al., 2015).

The American Nurses Association (ANA), National League for Nursing (NLN), American Organization of Nurse Executives (AONE), and American Association of Colleges of Nursing (AACN) recommend strategies to reverse the current nursing shortage (see Chapter 1). A number of these strategies have potential for creating work environments that enable nurses to demonstrate more caring behaviors. In addition, the Robert Wood Johnson Foundation's "Future of Nursing: Campaign for Action" identifies methods to improve both patient care and satisfaction and nurse job satisfaction. This campaign focuses on increasing the amount of time nurses spend with their patients and families. Strategies include greater emphasis on improving the work environment to facilitate more nurse-patient interaction, improving nurse staffing, providing nurses with autonomy over their practice, and promoting increased educational requirements and opportunities (RWJF, 2014).

If health care is to make a positive difference, it must become more compassionate. Nurses play an important role in making care an integral part of health care delivery. This begins when institutions make caring a part of the philosophy and environment of the workplace and incorporate care concepts into standards of nursing care and guidelines for professional conduct.

Finally, during day-to-day practice with patients and families, nurses need to be committed to caring and willing to establish the relationships necessary for personal, competent, compassionate, and meaningful nursing care. "Consistent with the wisdom and vision of Nightingale, nursing is a lifetime journey of caring and healing, seeking to understand and preserve the wholeness of human existence and to offer compassionate, informed knowledgeable human caring ..." (Watson, 2009).

KEY POINTS

- Caring is integral to a nurse's ability to work with people in a respectful and therapeutic manner.
- Theories of caring help explain how caring behaviors are central to a nurse's ability to work with all patients and family caregivers in a respectful and therapeutic way.
- Current evidence emphasizes what patients expect from their caregivers and thus provide useful guidelines for practice.
- An ethic of care is concerned with relationships between people and their values and with a nurse's character and attitude toward others.
- Presence is a person-to-person interaction, conveying closeness and a sense of caring that involves "being there" and "being with" patients or family caregivers.

- Touch includes task-oriented, caring, and protective touch.
- Listening is a therapeutic skill that includes interpreting, understanding, and respecting what a patient or family caregiver is saying and expressing that understanding and respect.
- Knowing the patient is at the core of the process the nurse uses to make clinical decisions about patient-centered care.
- Maintaining compassion in all aspects of nursing care contributes to the health and well-being of patients and can also improve patient and nurse satisfaction.
- Caring involves a mutual give-and-take and is specific and relational for each nurse-patient encounter.

REFLECTIVE LEARNING

- Reflect on a recent clinical experience in which you interviewed the patient and obtained information about his or her current health care problem. How did you prepare to do the interview? Which caring skills did you use? Reflect on the discussion with the patient and determine if you gathered adequate and complete information.
- You enter a patient's room to do a morning assessment and find the patient crying. Think about which caring practices you might use to help this patient.
- Your family member is facing a potentially severe illness; he asks you to come with him to the diagnostic tests and his doctor's visit to discuss the test results. How will understanding how to provide presence and knowing your family member prepare you to support him?

REVIEW QUESTIONS

1. An experienced nurse is explaining the use of touch from a caring perspective. What information does the nurse include in the discussion with the student about touch?
   1. Nurses touch patients only while performing procedures or doing assessments.
   2. Touch is a type of verbal communication.
   3. Nurses use touch only when a patient is in pain.
   4. Touch forms a connection between nurse and patient.
2. Before implementing touch, what does a nurse need to know about touch? (Select all that apply.)
   1. Some cultures may have specific restrictions about non–skill-based touch.
   2. Touch is a type of verbal communication.
   3. Touch can successfully influence a patient's level of comfort.
   4. There is never a problem with using touch at any time.
   5. Touch only reduces physical pain.
3. A young woman comes to a clinic for the first time for a gynecological examination. Which nursing behavior applies Swanson's caring process of "knowing" the patient?
   1. Sharing feelings about the importance of having regular gynecological examinations
   2. Explaining risk factors for cervical cancer
   3. Recognizing that the patient is modest and maintaining her privacy during the examination
   4. Asking the patient what it means to have a vaginal examination
4. A patient is fearful of upcoming surgery and a possible cancer diagnosis. He discusses his love for the Bible with his nurse,

who recommends a favorite Bible verse. Another nurse tells the patient's nurse that there is no place in nursing for spiritual caring. The patient's nurse replies:

1. "You're correct; spiritual care should be left to a pastoral care professional."
2. "You're correct; religion is a personal decision."
3. "Nurses should explain their own religious beliefs to patients."
4. "Spiritual, mind, and body connections can affect health."

5. Which of the following are strategies for creating work environments that support nurse caring interventions? (Select all that apply.)
   1. Increasing technological support
   2. Improving flexibility for scheduling
   3. Providing opportunities to discuss care
   4. Promoting autonomy of practice
   5. Encouraging increased input concerning nursing functions from health care providers

6. A nurse is caring for a patient newly diagnosed with testicular cancer. He asked the nurse to help him find the meaning of cancer by supporting beliefs about life. This is an example of:
   1. Instilling hope and faith.
   2. Forming a human-altruistic value system.
   3. Cultural caring.
   4. Being with.

7. An example of a nurse caring behavior that families of acutely ill patients perceive as important to patients' well-being is:
   1. Making health care decisions for patients.
   2. Having family members provide a patient's total personal hygiene.
   3. Injecting the nurse's perceptions about the level of care provided.
   4. Asking permission before performing a procedure on a patient.

8. A nurse demonstrates caring by helping family members to: (Select all that apply.)
   1. Become active participants in care.
   2. Remove themselves from personal care.
   3. Make health care decisions for the patient.

4. Plan uninterrupted time for family and patient to be together.
5. Discuss their concerns.

9. A hospice nurse sits at the bedside of a male patient in the final stages of cancer. He and his parents made the decision that he would move home and they would help him in the final stages of his disease. The family participates in his care, but lately the nurse has increased the amount of time she spends with the family. Whenever she enters the room or approaches the patient to give care, she touches his shoulder and tells him that she is present. This is an example of what type of touch?
   1. Caring touch
   2. Protective touch
   3. Task-oriented touch
   4. Interpersonal touch

10. Match the following caring behaviors with their definitions.
    1. Knowing
    2. Being with
    3. Doing for
    4. Maintaining belief

    a. Sustaining faith in the other's capacity to get through an event or transition and face a future with meaning
    b. Striving to understand an event as it has meaning in the life of the other
    c. Being emotionally present to the other
    d. Doing for the other as he or she would do for self if it were at all possible

10. 1b, 2c, 3d, 4a.

Answers: 1. 4; **2.** 1,3; **3.** 3,4, 4,5; **2.** 2,3; **4.** 6; **1.** 7; 4,8; 1,4,5; **9.** 1;

Rationales for Review Questions can be found on the Evolve website.

REFERENCES

Adams LY: The conundrum of caring in nursing, *Int J Caring Sci* 9(1):1, 2016.

American Organization of Nurse Executives (AONE): Guiding principles for the role of the nurse in future health care delivery, 2004, 2010, https://www.aonl.org/sites/default/files/aone/role-nurse-future-patient-care.pdf. Accessed May 27, 2019.

Benner P, Wrubel J: *The primacy of caring: stress and coping in health and illness*, Menlo Park, CA, 1989, Addison Wesley.

Benner P, et al.: *Educating nurses: a call for radical transformation*, Stanford, CA, 2010, Carnegie Foundation for the Advancement of Teaching.

Borasio GD, Tamches E: Guest editorial: assessment measures in palliative care: the risk of inflation and the importance of listening to the patient's story, *Palliat Support Care* 12(1), 2018.

Brewer BB, Watson J: Evaluation of authentic human caring professional practices, *JONA* 45(12):622, 2015.

Darnell L, Hickson S: Cultural competent patient-centered nursing care, *Nurs Clin North Am* 50(1):99, 2015.

Engle M: *I'm here: compassionate communication in patient care*, Orlando, FL, 2010, Phillips Press.

Frank AW: Just listening: narrative and deep illness, *Fam Syst Health* 16(3):197, 1998.

Given BA, Reinhard SC: Caregiving at the end of life: the challenges for family caregivers, *Generations J Am Soc Aging* 41(1):50, 2017.

Hanley MA, et al.: A practice-based theory of healing through therapeutic touch, *J Hol Nurs* 35(4):369, 2017.

Jackson C: The interface of caring, self-care, and technology in nursing education and practice, *Holist Nurs Pract* 26(2):69, 2012.

Leininger MM: *Culture care diversity and universality: a theory of nursing*, Pub No 15-2402, New York, 1991, National League for Nursing Press.

Letourneau D, et al.: Humanizing nursing care: an analysis of caring theories through the lens of humanism, *International J Human Caring* 21(1):33, 2017.

Marion L, et al.: Implementing the new ANA standard 8: culturally congruent practice, *Online J Issues Nurs* 22(1):1, 2017.

Markey K, et al.: Understanding nurses' concerns when caring for patients from diverse cultural and ethnic backgrounds, *J Clin Nurs* 27(1/2):e259, 2018.

Martin MB: Caring in nursing professional development, *J Nurses Prof Dev* 31(5):271, 2015.

Mason VM et al.: Compassion fatigue, moral distress, and work engagement in surgical intensive care unit trauma nurses, *Dimens Crit Care Nurs* 33(4):215, 2014.

Moffa C: Caring for novice nurses applying Swanson's Theory of Caring, *Int J Human Caring* 19(1):63, 2015.

Palos GR: Care, compassion, and communication in professional nursing: art, science, or both, *Clin J Oncol Nurs* 18(2):247, 2014.

Penque S, Kearney G: The effect of nursing presence on patient satisfaction, *Nurs Manage* 46(4):38, 2015, 2015.

Percy M, Richardson C: Introducing nursing practice to student nurses: how can we promote care compassion and empathy, *Nurse Educ Pract* 29:200, 2018.

Plessis E: Caring presence in practice: facilitating an appreciative discourse in nursing, *Int Nurs Rev* 63(3):377, 2016.

Potter TM, Savette LA: Ways of knowing: a nurse and physician discuss clinical decisions, actions, and lessons, *Creat Nurs* 20(1):59, 2014.

Ragan SL, Kanter E: Learning the patient's story, *Semin Oncol Nurs* 33(5):467, 2017.

Robert Wood Johnson Foundation (RWJF): *Future of nursing: campaign for action is chalking up successes that will improve patient care*, 2014. http://www.rwjf.org/en/about-rwjf/newsroom/newsroom-content/2014/06/campaign-for-action-is-chalking-up-successes-that-will-improve-p.html. Accessed May 27, 2019.

Sharma A, et al.: A quality improvement initiative to achieve high nursing presence during patient- and family-centered rounds, *Hospital Pediatr* 4(1):1, 2014.

Theofanidis D, Sapountzi-Krepia D: Nursing and caring: an historical overview from ancient Greek tradition to modern times, *Int J Sci* 8(3):791, 2015.

Tyreman S: Trust and truth: uncertainty in health care practices, *J Eval Clin Pract* 21:470, 2015.

Watson Caring Science Institute (WCSI) and International Caritas Consortium: *Caring science theory*, 2018. http://watsoncaringscience.org/about-us/caring-science-definitions-processes-theory/. Accessed May 27, 2019.

Watson J: *The philosophy and science of caring*, Boulder, CO, 2008, University Press of Colorado.

Watson J: Caring science and human caring theory: transforming personal and professional practices of nursing and health care, *J Health Human Serv Adm* 31(4):466, 2009.

Watson J: Caring science and the next decade of holistic healing: transforming self and system from the inside out, *Am Holist Nurses Assoc* 30(2):14, 2010.

RESEARCH REFERENCES

Andershed B, Olsson K: Review of research related to Kristen Swanson's middle-range theory of caring, *Scand J Caring Sci* 23:598, 2009.

Arslan-Ozkan I, et al.: A randomized controlled trial of the effects of nursing care based on Watson's Theory of Human Caring on distress, self-efficacy and adjustment in infertile women, *J Adv Nurs* 70(8):1801, 2013.

Baillie J, et al.: Symptom management, nutrition and hydration at end-of-life: a qualitative exploration of patients', carers' and health professionals' experiences and further research questions, *BMC Palliat Care* 17(1):1, 2018.

Compton EK, et al.: Nurses' caring behaviors: the perception of patients with cancer at the time of discharge after surgery, *Clin J Oncol Nurs* 22(2):169, 2018.

Dey MM: Relationship of hospitalized elders' perceptions of nurse caring behaviors, type of care unit, satisfaction with nursing care, and health outcome of functional status, *Int J Hum Caring* 20(3):134, 2016.

Dobrina R, et al.: An overview of hospice and palliative care nursing models and theories, *Int J Palliat Nurs* 20(2):75, 2014.

Duffy JR, et al.: Dimensions of caring: psychometric evaluation of the caring assessment tool, *Adv Nurs Sci* 30(3):235, 2007.

Harstade CW, et al.: Dignity-conserving care actions in palliative care: an integrative review of Swedish research, *Scand J Caring Sci* 32(1):8, 2018.

Hines MW, Gaughan J: Advanced holistic nursing practice narratives, *J Holist Nurs* 35(4):328, 2017.

Hunsaker S, et al.: Factors that influence the development of compassion fatigue, burnout, and compassion satisfaction in emergency department nurses, *J Nurs Scholarsh* 47(2):186, 2015.

Kelley T, et al.: Information needed to support knowing the patient, *Adv Nurs Sci* 36(4):351, 2013.

Kostovich CT: Development and psychometric assessment of the presence in nursing scale, *Nurs Sci Q* 25(2):167, 2012.

Labraque LJ, et al.: Nursing students' perception of their own caring behaviors: a multi-country study, *Int J Nurs Knowl* 28(4):225, 2017.

Lusk JM, Fater K: A concept analysis of patient-centered care, *Nurs Forum* 48(2):89, 2013.

Mohammadipour F, et al.: An exploratory study on the concept of nursing presence from the perspective of patients admitted to hospitals, *J Clin Nurs* 26(23/24):4313, 2017.

Monsen K, et al.: We can be more caring: a theory for enhancing the experience of being caring as an integral component of prelicensure nursing education, *Int J Hum Caring* 21(1):9, 2017.

Nightingale S, et al.: The impact of emotional intelligence in health care professionals on caring behaviour towards patients in clinical and long-term care settings: findings from an integrative review, *Int J Nurs Stud* 80:106, 2018.

Ortega Barco MA, de Rodriguez LM: Evaluation of the nursing care offered during the parturition process. Controlled clinical trial of an intervention based on Swanson's theory of caring versus conventional care, *Nurs Res Educ* 36(1):e05, 2018.

Palese A, et al.: Surgical patient satisfaction as an outcome of nurses' caring behaviors: a descriptive and correlational study in six European countries, *J Nurs Scholarsh* 43(4):341, 2011.

Papastavrou E, et al.: Nurses' and patients' perceptions of caring behaviours: quantitative systematic review of comparative studies, *J Adv Nurs* 67(6):1191, 2011.

Porter CA, et al.: Nurse caring behaviors following implementation of a relationship centered care professional practice model, *Int J Caring Sci* 7(3):818, 2014.

Ronaldson S, et al.: Spirituality and spiritual caring: nurses' perspectives and practice in palliative and acute care environments, *J Clin Nurs* 21(15):2126, 2012.

Shippe ND, et al.: Effect of a whole-person model of care on patient experience in patients with complex chronic illness in late life, *Am J Hosp Palliat Care* 35(1):104, 2018.

Sitzman K: Evolution of Watson's human caring science in the digital age, *Int J Human Caring* 21(1):46, 2017.

Suliman WA, et al.: Applying Watson's nursing theory to assess patient perceptions of being cared for in a multicultural environment, *J Nurs Res* 17(4):293, 2009.

Swanson KM: Empirical development of a middle-range theory of caring, *Nurs Res* 40(3):161, 1991.

Swanson KM: Effects of caring, measurement, and time on miscarriage impact and women's well-being, *Nurs Res* 48(6):288, 1999.

Turpin RL: State of the science of nursing presence revisited: knowledge for preserving nursing presence capability, *Int J Human Caring* 18(4):14, 2014.

Wyant RA, et al.: Show your stuff and watch your tone: nurses' caring behaviors, *Am J Crit Care* 26(2):111, 2017.

Yagasaki K, Komatsu H: The need for a nursing presence in oral chemotherapy, *Clin J Oncol Nurs* 17(5):512, 2013.

Zolnierek CD: An integrative review of knowing the patient, *J Nurs Scholarsh* 46(1):3, 2014.

Caring for Patients With Chronic Illness

OBJECTIVES

- Describe the characteristics of chronic illness.
- Identify the interaction between genetics and environment as they relate to chronic illness.
- Understand the effects that living with a chronic illness has on patients and their families.
- Explain the components of the Chronic Care Model and the importance of self-management within this model.
- Describe the variation of physical limitations and emotional responses that patients with chronic illnesses frequently experience.
- Explain the role of a nurse in preventing chronic illness through screening, education about healthy lifestyle, and public policy.
- Describe essential components that enhance a patient's ability to self-manage a chronic disease.

KEY TERMS

Adherence, p. 99
Chronic Care Model, p. 98
Chronic disease, p. 93
Chronic illness, p. 93

Incidence, p. 98
Genetic mutation, p. 94
Genetic counseling, p. 94
Multifactorial inheritance, p. 94

Risk behaviors, p. 95
Self-management, p. 101

MEDIA RESOURCES

http://evolve.elsevier.com/Potter/fundamentals/

- Review Questions
- Case Study with Questions

- Audio Glossary
- Content Updates
- Answers to QSEN Activity and Review Questions

Because of advancements in technology and medical treatment, many people are living longer with one or more chronic diseases that affect their daily lives. The increased prevalence of people living longer with multiple complex chronic diseases has greatly affected patients, families, communities, and the health care delivery system. Chronic diseases affect the physical, psychosocial, and economic aspects of a patient and family's life. Changes may occur in a person's interactions and relationships with others as well. Sometimes a disease becomes a person's identity. For example, a patient may be referred to as "the diabetic" or "the cancer patient" instead of a patient living with diabetes or a person diagnosed with cancer.

To care for patients experiencing chronic diseases, you need to understand not only the physical and psychological implications but also the economic impact. In your role in disease prevention, know the risk factors that contribute to the incidence of chronic disease. The Chronic Care Model provides a framework to guide patient care. The roles nurses play in caring for people with chronic diseases include prevention, early detection, and help in identifying effective strategies for patients to manage their chronic illnesses.

THE PREVALENCE AND COSTS OF CHRONIC DISEASE

Although they are separate concepts, the terms chronic disease and chronic illness are often used interchangeably. A chronic disease is a pathophysiologic condition that lasts more than 1 year, requires ongoing medical care, and often limits a person's usual activities of daily living due to symptoms of the disease or self-care activities required to manage the disease (CDC, 2019a). Chronic illness refers to a patient and family's subjective experience of and response to a chronic disease (Meiner and Yeager, 2019).

It is estimated that 60% of all adults in the United States have at least one chronic disease. In addition, 4 out of every 10 adults have two or more chronic conditions (CDC, 2019a). With each additional diagnosed chronic disease, the burden of disease for the individual increases; this translates into additional expenses, such as multiple medications and additional visits to health care providers. Living with two or more chronic diseases often creates the need for patients to make even greater changes to daily activities. Table 8.1 illustrates common chronic diseases listed by body system. Although this is not an exhaustive list, it represents the most common chronic diseases seen in the United States (CDC, 2019a).

The financial burden created by caring for chronic diseases is staggering (Table 8.2). The Centers for Disease Control and Prevention (CDC) (2019b) estimates that 90% of the $3.3 trillion spent on health care in the United States is used to care for people with chronic and mental health diseases. Disease prevention and better symptom management can greatly reduce these costs and potentially save billions of dollars spent yearly on health care (CDC, 2019b). For example, people who have diabetes spend an average of $16,750 per year to manage their disease, which is 2.3 times higher than what people without diabetes spend on their health care (CDC, 2018a). Type 2 diabetes is often preventable or can be managed effectively with lifestyle modifications (e.g., dietary changes, regular exercise).

TABLE 8.1 Examples of Chronic Diseases By Body System

Body System	Disease Examples
Cardiac	Hypertension Heart failure Coronary artery disease
Digestive	Cirrhosis of the liver Ulcerative colitis Obesity
Endocrine	Diabetes mellitus
Pulmonary	Chronic bronchitis Emphysema Asthma Allergies
Musculoskeletal	Arthritis Osteoporosis
Neurologic/psychiatric	Alzheimer's disease Stroke Parkinson's disease Spinal cord injury Systemic lupus Epilepsy Depression Bipolar disorder Multiple sclerosis
Renal	Renal failure
Cancer	Colorectal, breast, cervical, skin, gynecologic
Metabolic	Obesity, metabolic syndrome

TABLE 8.2 Yearly Costs of Chronic Illness Care (2018-2019)

Chronic Disease	Yearly Cost of Medical Care in the United States
Cancer care (NCI, n.d.)	$174 billion
Diabetes (ADA, 2019)	$245 billion
Dementia (AIM, 2019)	$290 billion
Heart disease and stroke (CDC, 2019b)	$199 billion
Obesity (CDC, 2019c)	$147 billion
Arthritis (CDC, 2018b)	$140 billion

REFLECT NOW

What chronic diseases are most prevalent in your community? Which are preventable? What effect would chronic disease prevention have on the health care dollars spent in your community?

MULTIFACTORIAL NATURE OF CHRONIC DISEASE

Numerous factors come into play when describing how individuals develop chronic disease and the symptoms and impairments that result. Each patient presents a unique case for how genetic, environmental, and lifestyle factors collide to create disease. The physical and psychological portraits of patients with the same chronic disease will have commonalities but also important differences that will affect your nursing care. Understanding the interrelationship of the factors contributing to chronic disease better enables you to support patients' illness when they suffer chronic diseases.

Genetic Factors

Autosomal genetic disorders occur when there is a **genetic mutation** or abnormality in inherited genetic material. These genetic mutations cause some inherited chronic diseases. These disorders fall into two categories: autosomal dominant disorders and autosomal recessive disorders. Autosomal dominant disorders such as Huntington's chorea, familial hypercholesterolemia, and neurofibromatosis occur when a person has one parent with the dominant genetic disorder or a new mutation in a gene occurs (NIH, 2019a). Each child born from parents in whom one has the dominant disorder has a 50% risk of having the disorder.

Autosomal recessive disorders such as cystic fibrosis and sickle cell anemia occur most commonly when both parents are carriers of the recessive genetic disorder. Although these parents are carriers of the genetic disease, they do not have the disease. Each child born from two parents who carry a recessive disorder has a 25% risk of having the disease. Both autosomal and recessive genetic disorders account for a small percentage of people with chronic diseases.

Influence of Genetics. Although almost all diseases have a genetic component, most are not the result of a single genetic cause (NIH, 2019b). Multifactorial inheritance, a combination of genetic factors, environmental elements, and lifestyle choices increase the risk for the development of most chronic illnesses (NIH, 2019b; Rappaport, 2016) (Fig. 8.1). Genetic factors are not modifiable. People are born with genetic material from their parents. Simply inheriting a gene mutation for a disease such as diabetes, cancer, or hypertension does not guarantee that a person will develop the disease. **Multifactorial inheritance** explains why a person who carries genetic material for developing a chronic illness may or may not eventually be diagnosed with the disease (NIH, 2019b).

Family History. Identification of a chronic disease occurrence in a family over several generations is the starting point for determining a person's disease risk. In examining a family disease history, important factors to consider include a multigenerational examination for patterns of the same disease, the age of onset of the disease, and generational frequency of the disorder. If a strong disease pattern is identified in a family history, **genetic counseling** may be indicated. Genetic counselors clarify the risk of disease development based on family history, answer questions about the process, recommend screening tests for the disorder if necessary, discuss available genetic testing, and recommend lifestyle changes that may decrease the risk of developing the disease (NIH, 2019c).

Genetic Screening. The science of genetic screening is developing and evolving for chronic diseases. Genetic testing is available for more than 2000 rare and common conditions (NIH, 2018). There are a number of different types of genetic tests, including (1) diagnostic testing (identifies a genetic condition or disease that is making or in the future will make a person ill), (2) predictive and presymptomatic genetic testing (finds genetic variations that increase a person's chance of developing specific diseases), (3) carrier testing (tells people if they "carry" a genetic change that can cause a disease), and (4) prenatal testing (offered during pregnancy to help identify fetuses that have certain diseases) (NIH, 2018). These are just a few examples. Diagnostic testing is available for individuals at high risk for developing certain

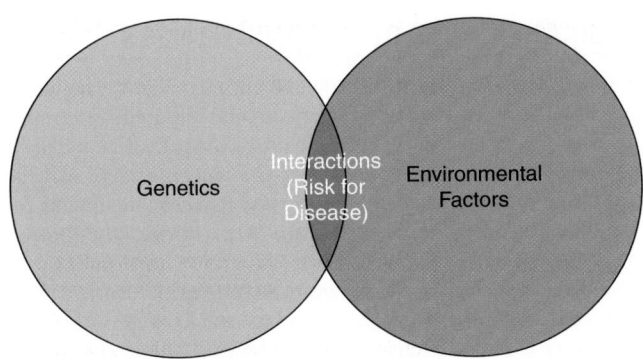

FIG. 8.1 Multifactorial inheritance: interaction of factors promoting chronic disease. (Modified from https://www.genetics.edu.au/publications-and-resources/facts-sheets/fact-sheet-11-environmental-and-genetic-interactions/view. Accessed July 16, 2019.)

breast and colon cancers (HealthyPeople.gov, 2019). Women with a strong family history of breast, ovarian, tubal, or peritoneal cancer may benefit from genetic testing for a *BRCA1* or *BRCA2* mutation (US Preventive Services Task Force, 2013). A positive screen for the *BRCA1* or *BRCA2* genetic mutation indicates the genetic mutation exists in a woman's DNA, placing her at an increased risk for developing one of these cancers. It does not mean that the woman will develop one of these cancers. However, the test results help the woman make informed decisions about her health care and treatment based on scientific data. Knowledge of the presence of a *BRCA1* or *BRCA2* mutation can guide decisions about lifestyle changes, frequency of screening for these cancers, or early preventive therapy such as surgery before cancer develops.

People diagnosed with colon cancer may have an inheritable form of colon cancer called Lynch syndrome (ASCO, 2019). Researchers estimate that 1 in every 300 people carry the gene associated with Lynch syndrome (ASCO, 2019). Because Lynch syndrome is one of the more common hereditary cancer syndromes and because early detection improves survival, genetic screening for this type of colon cancer should be offered to first-degree family members to inform them of the potential risk of developing this cancer. If family members screen positive, more frequent screening for this disease increases the chance of early detection and early treatment to decrease death from this form of colon cancer (ASCO, 2019). Other cancers linked with Lynch syndrome include endometrial, ovarian, small bowel, pancreatic, prostate, urinary tract, liver, kidney, and bile duct cancers. Provide patient education about recommended cancer screenings related to patients diagnosed with Lynch syndrome (Stoffel et al., 2014).

REFLECT NOW

If you have a close relative diagnosed with Lynch syndrome, would you want to have genetic testing? What are the reasons you would want to be tested, and what would prevent you from going for the testing?

Genetic information is also being used to guide care for various chronic diseases, including several types of cancer. Health care providers use testing information to select medications to treat cancer based on how well the medications treated groups of patients with the same cancer type. For some cancers (e.g., lung, colon, melanoma, breast, ovarian), medication choice is often based on the genetic features of a patient's cancer cells (Cleveland Clinic, 2017). Application of knowledge of how genetics impacts people with diseases such as

cancer, diabetes, hypertension, and cardiac disease will continue to be the future focus of research and disease treatment.

Environmental Factors

Ongoing exposure to toxic elements within the environment increases the risk for chronic disease. Public health initiatives are aimed at recognizing individuals' risks, chemical assessment of toxins, exposure reduction and remediation, monitoring, and avoidance (Sears and Genuis, 2012). In the United States the costs of environmental disease in children alone amounted to $76.6 billion in 2008—just from lead poisoning, prenatal mercury exposure, childhood cancer, asthma, intellectual disability, autism, and attention deficit hyperactivity disorder (Sears and Genuis, 2012). However, this estimate is likely low because it does not consider the long-term societal losses for those children who have cognitive impairment such as IQ loss (Grandjean and Bellanger, 2017). Researchers are finding that environmental factors ranging from everyday stress to various chemical agents may alter an individual's DNA. The interaction of environmental toxins and genetic predisposition is likely stronger than genetic risk alone. As a nurse, your role in reducing environmental exposure to toxins involves patient education and risk assessment. Patients are exposed to environmental toxins at home and in the workplace; contaminated water, pesticides, asbestos, mold, heavy metals, and food contamination are a few examples. By identifying exposures and informing individual patients regarding where and how they are being contaminated, you can empower patients to avoid further chemical contamination (Sears and Genuis, 2012).

Lifestyle and Risk Factors

Many risk factors increase the chance that individuals, families, or communities will develop a chronic illness. Some risk factors are modifiable while others are nonmodifiable (see Chapter 6). The most common modifiable risk factors are lifestyle choices or **risk behaviors** that contribute to the development of chronic illness (e.g., smoking cigarettes, exposure to secondhand smoke, poor nutrition, and excessive alcohol consumption) (CDC, 2019a). Lack of physical activity and obesity are associated with heart disease, obesity, diabetes, and some cancers (CDC, 2018c). It is estimated that $117 billion in health care costs are paid yearly due to people who choose a sedentary lifestyle (USDHHS, 2015).

Tobacco Use. Cigarette smoking or extended exposure to secondhand smoke is the leading cause of preventable death in the United States (USDHHS, 2019). Sixteen different types of cancer have been linked to tobacco use, including lung, mouth and throat, bladder, stomach, and liver (Walsberger, 2016). Smoking has also been linked to pulmonary and cardiovascular disease. Although teen smokers are less likely to smoke cigarettes, the use of electronic cigarettes, or e-cigarettes, is on the rise in both middle and high school teens (CDC, 2019d; see Chapter 12). E-cigarettes contain nicotine and other chemicals that negatively affect a person's health (Singh et al., 2016; CDC 2019d). If young people did not start smoking and every smoker stopped smoking, it is estimated that $170 billion could be saved yearly in medical costs (USDHHS, 2014).

Effects of Alcohol. The effects of alcohol on health are directly associated with the pattern, type, and amount of alcohol consumed (WHO, 2019a). Alcohol misuse puts people at increased risk for negative health and social effects. Excessive alcohol use is associated with 1 in 10 deaths in working adults and costs approximately $249 billion yearly in the United States when taking lost productivity, health care expenses, law enforcement, and other costs associated with the criminal justice system into consideration (USDHHS, 2016). Excess consumption of alcohol over a long period of time leads to an increase in chronic disease, including heart disease, liver disease, and several types of cancer.

Nutrition. The rates of chronic diet-related diseases have risen, due in part to changes in lifestyle behaviors. A history of poor eating and physical activity patterns have a cumulative effect and have contributed to significant nutrition-related and physical activity–related health challenges that now face the US population (Health.gov, n.d.). The CDC reports that about half of all adults in the United States have one or more preventable chronic diseases, many of which are related to poor quality eating patterns and physical inactivity. These diseases include cardiovascular disease, high blood pressure, type 2 diabetes, certain cancers, and poor bone health (health.gov, n.d.). Poor nutritional intake is related to a variety of issues, including limited financial resources, poor access to markets selling high-quality foods, limited transportation, and limited understanding of the components of a healthy diet (see Chapter 45). More than two-thirds of adults and nearly one-third of children and youth are overweight or obese, which highlights the enormity of this public health problem (health.gov, n.d.). The educational strategies that you can apply to reduce the health risks from poor nutrition are outlined in Table 8.3.

TABLE 8.3	Strategies for Chronic Disease Prevention
Disease	**Strategy**
Obesity	Increasing physical activity, plus reducing intake of foods high in fat and foods and drinks high in sugars, can prevent unhealthy weight gain.
Type 2 diabetes	Increasing physical activity and maintaining a healthy weight play critical roles in the prevention and treatment of diabetes.
Cardiovascular disease	Reduced intake of saturated and trans fats; sufficient amounts of (omega-3 and omega-6) polyunsaturated fats, fruits, and vegetables; reduced salt intake; physical activity; and controlling weight can reduce the risk of cardiovascular disease.
Cancer	Maintaining a healthy weight will reduce the risk for cancers of the esophagus, colorectum, breast, endometrium, and kidney. Limiting alcohol intake will reduce the risk for cancers of the mouth, throat, esophagus, liver, and breast. Ensuring an adequate intake of fruit and vegetables should further reduce the risk for oral cavity, esophagus, stomach, and colorectal cancer.
Osteoporosis and bone fractures	An adequate intake of calcium (500 mg/day or more) and vitamin D in populations with high osteoporosis rates helps to reduce fracture risk. Sun exposure and physical activity to strengthen bones and muscles also helps to reduce the risk.
Dental disease	Limiting the frequency and amount of sugar consumption and increasing the use of fluoride can prevent tooth decay.

Adapted from World Health Organization: *Diet, nutrition and the prevention of chronic diseases: report of the joint WHO/FAO expert consultation.* WHO Technical Report Series, No. 916 (TRS 916), 2019, https://www.who.int/dietphysicalactivity/publications/trs916/summary/en/. Accessed August 8, 2019.

PHYSICAL EFFECTS OF CHRONIC ILLNESS

The physical effects and limitations of chronic illness vary greatly depending on the disease process and treatments required. Determining patients' individual physical needs and providing patient-centered care are essential. For example, a person who is a cancer survivor may have residual side effects from chemotherapy and radiation treatments such as peripheral neuropathy (Knoerl et al., 2018), cardiac or pulmonary toxicity (Kourie and Klastersky, 2017), or cognitive impairment, called chemo brain, which may last for years (Armstrong, 2016). A person who has emphysema may depend on oxygen and have chronic physical changes such as clubbed fingers or a barrel chest. Other common physical symptoms include malnutrition as a result of difficulty in chewing and digesting food and decreased physical mobility due to poor oxygen reserve.

One person living with heart failure may need to take two medications every day and eat a no-added-salt diet. Another person with heart failure may be dependent on oxygen and confined to home, take continuous IV medications to increase the heart's ability to pump, take eight oral medications per day, and eat a 1-gram sodium diet due to the severity of heart disease. Although these two persons have the same diagnosis, great variations exist regarding their self-care needs.

PSYCHOSOCIAL NEEDS OF PATIENTS WITH CHRONIC ILLNESS

A patient's experience with chronic illness encompasses more than the physical symptoms that result from the effects of the illness on different body systems. The emotional response to living with chronic illness(s) varies even more than a patient's physical response. Emotional responses affect how a person perceives and copes with an illness as well as the person's perceived degree of wellness.

Chronic illness has economic, functional, occupational, psychological, sexual, social, and spiritual effects on patients and families (Chang and Johnson, 2018). Each person with a chronic disease has a unique illness representation (Heid et al., 2018). Illness representations are the responses to bodily and functional changes that occur due to an illness that affect a patient's ability to self-manage an illness (Leventhal et al., 2016). Because every patient has a unique experience with a chronic illness, it is essential to assess patients thoroughly in order to provide patient-centered care.

Psychosocial nursing care for patients with chronic illnesses is very complex and involves many aspects of a patient's life. Patients often have physical and mental illnesses at the same time. Medications used to treat physical illnesses can affect a patient's mental health. Likewise, medications used to treat mental illnesses affect a patient's physical health (Parrish, 2018).

Your role in helping patients manage and cope with the psychosocial effects of a chronic illness depends on your patients' feelings, relationships with others, and ability to access resources. It is essential to develop a therapeutic relationship with patients to help them manage and discuss their feelings about their chronic illnesses.

Depression. Patients who live with chronic illness often experience depression related to frustration, fear about the future, and loss of control over one's life (Lorig et al., 2012). Patients living with chronic illnesses are at a higher risk of experiencing depression when compared with people who are healthy (Parrish, 2018). Patients who experience depression with chronic illness also often express higher levels of pain, fatigue, and social isolation and withdraw from daily activities, which can have an impact on the entire family (Corvin et al., 2017; Parrish, 2018). Depression associated with a chronic illness can be difficult to manage, and it can negatively affect the ability to adhere to a treatment plan (Corvin et al., 2017).

Social Isolation. Social isolation often occurs as an illness or disability becomes more advanced or severe. Some people begin to withdraw as their illnesses become more difficult to manage, have a greater impact on their ability to function, or include symptoms a patient considers to be embarrassing. Managing the symptoms of the chronic illness becomes so overwhelming that the individual chooses to reduce social interactions with others. For some, it is easier to stay at home where the environment is more controllable (Meiner and Yeager, 2019).

For others, friends and family may withdraw from the individual experiencing chronic illness. Friends sometimes become tired of hearing about a patient's chronic illness experience. Physical and psychosocial limitations created by an illness can make friends and family uncomfortable. Some illnesses (e.g., HIV/AIDS, hepatitis) carry a stigma with them, which often leads to social isolation. Regardless of the cause for social isolation, it is essential to carefully assess patients for social isolation and loneliness and ensure that their needs for intimacy are met (Meiner and Yeager, 2019; Garcia-Sanjuan et al., 2018).

Loneliness. A patient's beliefs about treatment benefits often predict the degree of loneliness. People who believe in the treatment and its benefits report less loneliness than those who question the benefits of the treatment (Tuncay et al., 2018). The degree of loneliness a person experiences is negatively related to illness and emotional perception of the chronic disease as well as the person's opinion about the usefulness of the treatment (Tuncay et al., 2018).

People with chronic illness use a variety of personal strengths and strategies to cope with the psychosocial effects of chronic illness (Kristjansdottir, 2018). Internal strengths include being persistent; having a positive outlook; being kind and caring; experiencing positive emotions; being kind toward oneself; reconciling oneself with the situation; and having courage, knowledge, and insight. External strengths include support from family, friends, peers, and health care providers. Self-management strategies include being active, planning and prioritizing, reducing stress, goal setting, and seeking knowledge and help. Encourage patients dealing with chronic illnesses by guiding them to consider personal strengths that can be used to help them cope with the effects of the illness and its related treatment.

QSEN **Building Competency in Patient-Centered Care** Mrs. Jones is a 63-year-old woman who was recently diagnosed with type 2 diabetes mellitus. You are making a home visit to check her progress with the disease. The health record shows that Mrs. Jones is to take an oral tablet twice a day; eat a low carbohydrate, calorie-controlled diet; exercise daily; and check her blood glucose twice a day using a home glucose monitor. You ask Mrs. Jones, "How are you doing?" She responds, "I am so scared and angry. I hate to even say the word 'diabetes'! I can't go out for lunch with my friends anymore. My neighbor has diabetes and just lost both of her legs. I just can't do all of this! What is going to happen to me?" What is the priority issue with Mrs. Jones? What do you plan to discuss with her first?

Answers to QSEN Activities can be found on the Evolve website.

GROWTH AND DEVELOPMENT CONSIDERATIONS

Patients who became chronically ill as children often experience depression and anxiety in adulthood (Secinti et al., 2017). Because the risk for mental health problems in children with chronic illnesses may persist into adulthood, you need to address mental health needs as part of a child's chronic illness treatment plan.

Serious chronic illnesses in children often have a negative effect on school attendance as well as their social engagement with other children, thus putting children with chronic illnesses at greater risk for failing to reach their potential at school (Lum et al., 2017). Some children with chronic illnesses experience poorer relationships with their teachers and are at a higher risk of having to repeat grades and achieving lower levels of educational success (Lum et al., 2017). The siblings of these children often have similar experiences, missing more days of school and experiencing changes in their interactions with their peers and teachers (Gan et al., 2017). Chronic illness also greatly affects children's parents, creating intense psychosocial responses, including chronic sorrow, fatigue, and depression (Coughlin and Sethares, 2017). Ensure that you take a family-centered approach when caring for children and their families affected by chronic illness (see Chapter 10). Be empathetic and compassionate while providing family-centered care. Help children and their families understand that the emotions they are experiencing because of the chronic illness are normal (Coughlin & Sethares, 2017). Involving interprofessional teams helps to ensure that the holistic needs of children and their families affected by chronic illnesses are met (Apple, 2017).

When caring for older adults with chronic illness, the focus of care is often on controlling symptoms, maintaining comfort, and preventing crisis (Meiner & Yeager, 2019). Every older adult patient is unique, and the presence of one or more chronic illnesses creates the need for individualized patient-centered care. Older adults who have chronic illnesses often experience powerlessness and depression because of changes in their body image, changes in their ability to provide self-care, or feelings of loss associated with their illness (Meiner and Yeager, 2019). Having more chronic illnesses is often associated with having more functional limitations and more depressive symptoms (Han, 2018). Older adults who have a negative self-perception of aging often experience more depressive symptoms related to chronic illnesses than those with a positive view of aging (Han, 2018).

Thus you need to assess an older adult patient with chronic illness for depressive symptoms in addition to the patient's perception of aging to provide a foundation for discussing possible coping strategies (Han, 2018). Maximizing functional ability may also improve coping. Consult as needed with members of the interprofessional health care team, such as physical and occupational therapists, to increase a patient's abilities and decrease functional limitations.

FAMILY CAREGIVERS

Advances in disease management have led to more people living longer with chronic illness. As a result, more than 1 in 6 Americans who work either full-time or part-time are providing care for family members or friends with chronic illnesses or disabilities (Family Caregiver Alliance, 2016a). Family caregivers must learn how to perform new tasks and assume new responsibilities that are often time consuming as well as emotionally, psychosocially, and physically draining.

Family caregivers provide a significant amount of direct and indirect patient care for their family members, yet they often fail to address their own personal and health-related concerns (Family Caregiver Alliance, 2016b). They also often receive little help from others, which can lead to anxiety and increased caregiver burden (Moss et al., 2019). Family caregivers report that their personal health worsens over time. Spouses report the largest impact on their health (Family Caregiver Alliance, 2016b). Factors that put the caregiver at greatest risk for poor health outcomes include providing care for more than a year, being 65 years of age or older, providing care for a family member who has significant needs, caring for someone with Alzheimer's disease or other form of dementia, and living with the care recipient (Family Caregiver Alliance, 2016b).

Because chronic illnesses last a long time and their course is often unknown, the uncertainty related to the illness contributes to the stress of the family caregiver. The experience of the family caregiver is related to the characteristics of the chronic illness (Meiner and Yeager, 2019). For example, a family caregiver may report stress when a patient with cognitive changes no longer recognizes family members. Another family caregiver may experience more difficulty coping and managing caregiving when a patient with cancer experiences a relapse and requires more intense care. Ongoing care of a family member with a chronic illness is physically and emotionally draining. When a caregiver is the spouse of the patient, the marital relationship may be greatly affected.

Caring for the family caregiver is essential (see Chapters 7 and 10). Develop a therapeutic relationship with your patients' family caregivers. Assess the physical, psychosocial, and financial effects of the chronic illness on the patient and family caregiver, and ensure that both members of the caregiving dyad have access to appropriate community resources and services, including respite care, social work, and counseling. Provide patient education when needed (see Chapter 25), and include the patient and family caregiver as a part of the interprofessional health care team (Ates et al., 2018).

THE CHRONIC CARE MODEL

The Chronic Care Model provides a framework to guide health care delivery for patients living with chronic illnesses. This model considers the complex nature of factors that affect the care delivery needs of persons with a chronic illness. The Chronic Care Model (Fig. 8.2) illustrates how the community and health care systems interact to influence patient outcomes. The community component focuses on the availability of resources and policies that have the potential to impact health. An effective method to improve preventive health practices includes public policy changes. Examples of these measures include smoke-free legislation, alcohol taxation, or regulations eliminating trans fats in prepared food (Capewell and Capewell, 2018). These policy changes have great potential to enhance preventive health measures and decrease

high-risk behaviors associated with the incidence (or new cases) of chronic disease. You need to be aware of this type of legislation, which focuses on decreasing exposure to health barriers through public policies and legislative changes.

The health care systems component focuses on how providers can best utilize the resources within their system and provide evidence-based care to improve patient outcomes. Using the chronic care model can improve coordination of planned interprofessional care, improve patient follow-up, and educate patients and families on how to manage patient illnesses. There are six essential elements of the Chronic Care Model (Improving Chronic Illness Care, 2006-2019):

1. *Health system*: Needs to constantly attempt to improve the management of chronic illnesses and focus on safety and quality of care.
2. *Delivery system design*: Uses evidence-based care that is patient-centered, preventive in nature, and occurs in a variety of acute, outpatient, and community settings.
3. *Decision support*: Used by health care providers to implement evidence-based guidelines, guide patient education, and encourage patients to participate in their care.
4. *Clinical information systems*: Maintain and share patient health information among providers and patients to ensure effective communication and quality patient care.
5. *Self-management support*: Places the patient in the center of disease management. Self-management support requires providers to collaborate with patients, which ultimately empowers patients to take responsibility for and manage their chronic diseases.
6. *Community*: Help develop partnerships to enhance the effectiveness of chronic disease management programs. Community partnerships between health systems and local, state, and national agencies help fill in the gaps that exist in different services and improve patient care.

Research supports the use of the Chronic Care Model in primary care settings. Kadu and Stolee (2015) reported that barriers and facilitators in implementing this model focused on readiness and climate of the organization, presence of supportive leadership, effective communication, and characteristics and attitudes of the health care providers. When these factors were positively aligned, implementation of the Chronic Care Model in primary care was successful. Reynolds and colleagues (2018)

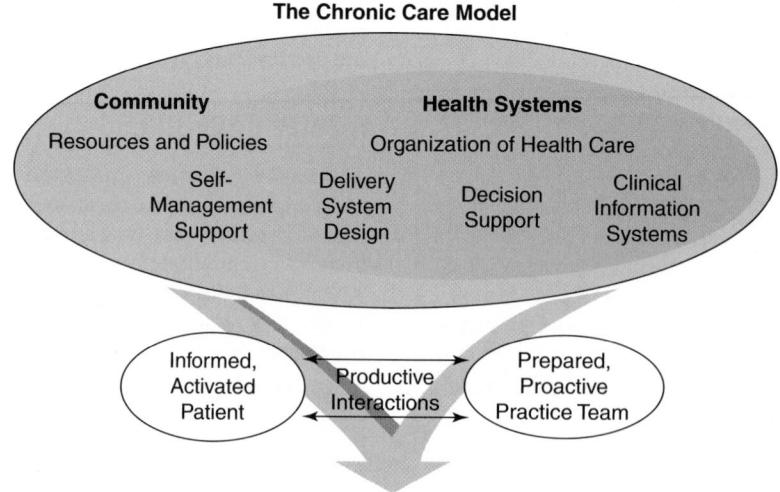

FIG. 8.2 The Chronic Care Model. (© 1996-2018 The MacColl Center. The Improving Chronic Illness Care program is supported by The Robert Wood Johnson Foundation, with direction and technical assistance provided by Group Health's MacColl Center for Health Care Innovation. http://www.improvingchroniccare.org/index.php?p=The_Chronic_Care_Model&s=2. Accessed July 16, 2019.)

identified the primary care chronic disease management interventions most successful in creating positive patient outcomes and disease control. In their systematic review, almost half of the studies demonstrated that *self-management support* was the most effective element from the model for improving patient outcomes, such as improved control of type 2 diabetes and enhancing the quality of life in patients with arthritis and chronic obstructive pulmonary disease (COPD).

IMPLICATIONS FOR NURSING

The excess illness burden of chronic disease and billions of health care dollars could be saved each year if chronic diseases were prevented (CDC, 2019b). Nursing care of patients experiencing chronic illnesses is complex. It is important to promote healthy lifestyles and detect risks for chronic illness early (Fig. 8.3). You first need to thoroughly assess patients to plan appropriate care when the patient has risks for chronic disease or when a chronic disease is diagnosed. Helping patients develop a plan to manage their illness, as well as providing patient education, is essential.

Assessing Patients with Chronic Illnesses

It is important to assess the effect a chronic disease has on your patients. When you collect a nursing history (see Chapters 16 and 30), encourage patients to tell you their stories about their chronic disease and how it affects various aspects of their lives (Tamura-Lis, 2017). The stories your patients tell will provide contextual detail and allow you to better know your patients. As you explore a patient's medical history and treatment, ask open-ended questions such as, "How did that come about?" as opposed to closed-ended questions that require a simple yes or no response (Table 8.4). Let the patient take you on a journey explaining his or her condition. You might ask, "Tell me how your disease most affects you right now" or "What are the biggest problems you are having now?" Encourage your patient to tell you stories that also help you better understand the psychosocial aspects of their illness. Be respectful and caring in your approach to encourage open patient communication (Tamura-Lis, 2017).

Adherence

Wide variation exists from patient to patient regarding adherence to chronic disease management and the effects of treatment on their lives. Adherence depends on the number and type of chronic illnesses, the severity and duration of the chronic illness, and the complexity of a treatment plan. Patients will have different physical symptoms and different pharmacological and nonpharmacological treatments, all of which affect a patient's ability to adhere to a treatment plan. How well a patient with a chronic illness and/or family manages a treatment plan is complex. Assess adherence by asking patients about how they take medications regularly, follow diet plans, or perform routine exercise. Asking patients to keep diaries and then later checking their entries is helpful. Having patients create examples of menu plans is another way to determine if a patient knows how to plan a healthy meal. Family caregivers can also be very helpful in reporting adherence. There are assessment tools available to measure adherence. A standardized self-reported questionnaire, The Adherence in Chronic Diseases Scale (ACDS) assesses the level of adherence to treatment recommendations in chronically ill adults (Kosobucka et al., 2018). The tool was originally developed and validated in patients with coronary artery disease (CAD) (Kubica et al., 2017). The ACDS includes seven questions that focus primarily on how well a patient manages his or her medication regimen.

When patients are unable to adhere to a treatment plan, they often experience increased hospital admissions, poor health outcomes, and increased morbidity and mortality. Nonadherence also greatly increases health care expenses. Current estimates of the annual direct health care costs associated with nonadherence range from $100 billion to $300 billion in the United States (Neiman et al., 2017). Improving adherence is a nursing priority and requires an interprofessional approach (Giddens, 2017; Neiman et al., 2017) (Box 8.1).

Symptom Management

Symptom management is an ongoing problem for many patients with chronic diseases. Explore presenting symptoms as you conduct a physical examination (see Chapter 30) and ask patients to describe the symptoms that are affecting them the most. For example, if a patient is experiencing pain from peripheral neuropathy from cancer treatment, ask whether the pain is affecting the patient's ability to sleep and assess the patient's gait. Explore each symptom that a patient identifies to gain a complete picture of his or her health status. Some patients are reluctant to describe or report their symptoms. Be patient, and when you identify a symptom, explore the extent to which it is currently affecting the patient.

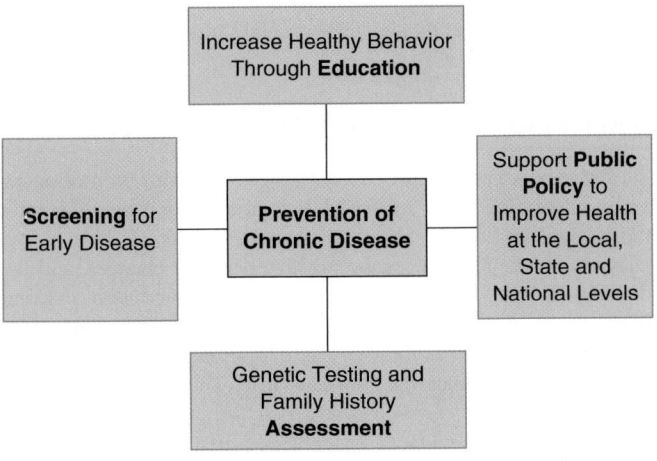

FIG. 8.3 The nurse's role in chronic disease prevention.

TABLE 8.4 Examples of Assessment Questions for Patients Experiencing Chronic Illness	
Category	**Examples of Questions**
Symptoms	Tell me about the symptoms you are experiencing from your illness and its treatment.
	Describe any pain or discomfort you are experiencing.
	Sometimes people with chronic illnesses experience changes in their sleep, appetite, or ability to cope. Describe any changes like these that you are experiencing.
	Tell me about any problems you are having following your treatment plan at home.
Psychosocial problems	How do your family members respond to you now that you have a chronic illness?
	What family members' responses to your chronic illness concern you?
	How has your illness affected the way you see yourself?
	If you have experienced sexual changes because of your illness, which strategies have you tried to make things better? Have these strategies worked?
	Describe any problems you have affording the care your health care provider has prescribed for you.

BOX 8.1   EVIDENCE-BASED PRACTICE

Strategies to Enhance Adherence

PICOT Question: Do interprofessional interventions effectively promote adherence to treatment plans in patients experiencing chronic illness?

Evidence Summary

Chronic diseases require patients and families to make multiple important decisions about their health daily. However, the American health care system does a poor job in supporting self-management of diseases. Patients and providers often express frustration with the approach to chronic disease management, especially due to the many barriers that people who are from underserved populations experience (Stagg et al., 2017).

Current evidence supports the use of interprofessional interventions to enhance adherence to chronic disease management. For example, health care coaches with advanced training in behavioral science that maintain ongoing positive patient relationships have been effective in improving adherence in patients with asthma and COPD (George, 2018). The Patient-Care Medical Home (PCMH) is a patient-care delivery model in which a primary care provider facilitates and coordinates interprofessional patient care to assure that patients receive culturally appropriate care when and where they need it. Patients living with chronic illnesses who used a PCMH recognized by the National Committee for Quality Assurance (NCQA) were better able to adhere to newly prescribed medications for the treatment of their chronic diseases when compared with patients who did not seek their care from a PCMH (Lauffenburger et al., 2017). In addition to interprofessional care, a patient's social support from family and friends is an essential component to patient adherence (Vahedparast et al., 2018).

Application to Nursing Practice

- Carefully assess patients who have difficulty adhering to their treatment plan to determine the factors that are preventing them from being successful. For example, ask: "Are you having difficulty affording your care?" "How many medications do you take on a daily basis and when do you take them?" "Describe the role your family plays in helping you manage your illness" (George, 2018; Vahedparast et al., 2018).
- Assess patients' understanding of their chronic diseases, and provide patient education to help them better manage their chronic illness and adhere to their medications (Yazdanpanah et al., 2019).
- Work with the interprofessional health care team across the continuum of care to enhance adherence to chronic disease treatment. For example, work with pharmacists and a patient's health care providers to ensure that the patient's treatment plan, including the medication regimen, is as simple and cost effective as possible. Make referrals to the health department and home health nurses, and use health information technology such as text messages and electronic health records to ensure continuity of care (Neiman et al., 2017).

Your review of the patient's medical record reveals the type and nature of chronic illness affecting a patient. Focus your physical assessment on the body systems most likely affected to supplement what you learn about symptoms. For example, if a patient tells you he has difficulty breathing, which affects his ability to perform self-care, examine the thorax, assessing lung sounds and degree of excursion.

Tobacco Use

Assess patients to determine their use of tobacco products, including e-cigarettes. Educate patients about the risks related to products of any type that contain nicotine because of the potential to cause disease (WHO, 2019c). Provide education about the benefits of smoking cessation and ways to stop smoking to promote health. Refer patients to resources such as the American Lung Association (www.lung.org), which has online resources for smoking cessation called "Freedom from Smoking Plus." This website provides encouragement and ideas about how to stop smoking, as well as information about why and how to stop.

REFLECT NOW

Go to the World Health Organization website and review global policy suggestions to decrease the use of tobacco (https://www.who.int/health-topics/tobacco). How could you use these guidelines when educating a patient about smoking cessation?

Alcohol Consumption

Assess the amount of alcohol patients drink on a typical day and in a typical week. Suspect alcohol misuse if a patient reports excess daily alcohol consumption (more than 4 drinks for men or more than 3 drinks a day for women) or excess total alcohol consumption (more than 14 drinks a week for men and more than 7 drinks a week for women) (CDC, 2019e). Often patients are reluctant to report the amount of alcohol they drink. The Alcohol Use Disorders Identification Test (AUDIT) is a 10-item screening tool developed by the World Health Organization (WHO) to assess alcohol consumption, drinking behaviors, and alcohol-related problems (Babor et al., 2001). The tool has been tested for its success in identifying patients with drinking problems. Both a clinician-administered version and a self-report version of the AUDIT are available.

In addition to providing information and support, refer patients to resources about alcohol use when appropriate. For example, the CDC (2019e) and National Institute on Alcohol Abuse and Alcoholism (NIAAA, 2016) provide information online on how to calculate alcohol intake and how to stop drinking, as well as available resources if patients have excessive alcohol intake.

Lifestyle

Chronic diseases affect all aspects of a patient's life. Be sure to explore patients' psychological, social, spiritual (see Chapter 35), and sexual (see Chapter 34) needs. If you are unable to identify all your patient's needs on initial assessment, incorporate more detailed assessment questions as you establish rapport and continue to provide care to your patient. Learning how a patient manages care at home is one of the most useful ways to know how an illness affects lifestyle routines. Talk about your patient's daily life and determine the extent to which the chronic illness has affected the patient's ability to perform self-care activities, attend social activities, participate in meals, and obtain adequate sleep. Observe the patient's interactions with family members and friends.

HEALTH PROMOTION AND DISEASE PREVENTION

As a nurse, you need to be actively engaged in health promotion and disease prevention (see Chapter 6). Patient education provides information patients require to understand the effects of their lifestyle behaviors on their health, make positive behavior changes, and lead a healthy lifestyle. Even when patients are diagnosed with a chronic illness, health promotion is important. Understand the nature of a patient's illness as well as the short- and long-term effects of the treatment to guide the topics you choose to teach and the screening interventions you use.

Provide specific evidence-based recommendations focusing on topics such as physical activity, food choices, smoking, and alcohol

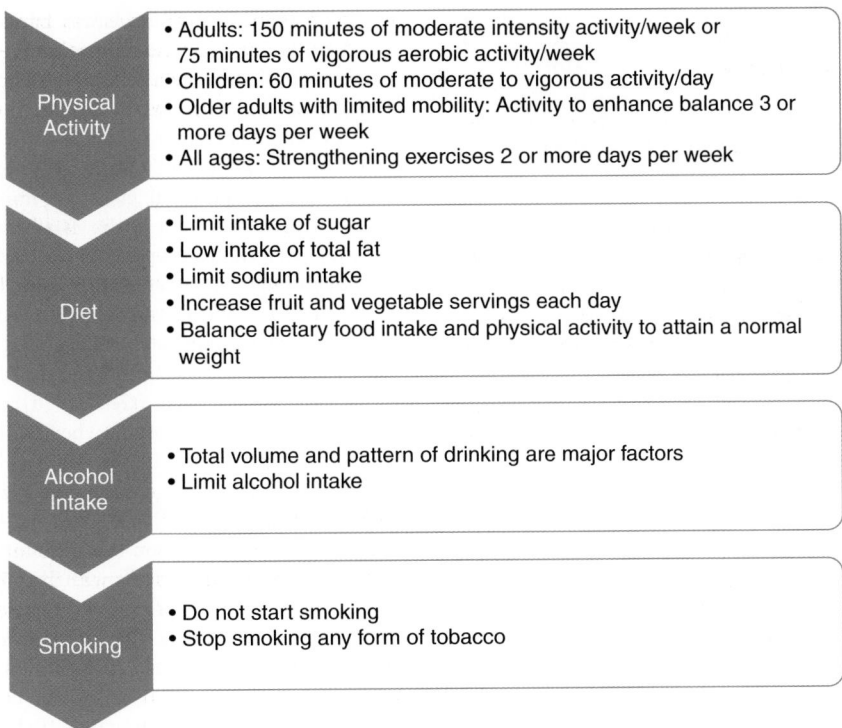

Physical Activity
- Adults: 150 minutes of moderate intensity activity/week or 75 minutes of vigorous aerobic activity/week
- Children: 60 minutes of moderate to vigorous activity/day
- Older adults with limited mobility: Activity to enhance balance 3 or more days per week
- All ages: Strengthening exercises 2 or more days per week

Diet
- Limit intake of sugar
- Low intake of total fat
- Limit sodium intake
- Increase fruit and vegetable servings each day
- Balance dietary food intake and physical activity to attain a normal weight

Alcohol Intake
- Total volume and pattern of drinking are major factors
- Limit alcohol intake

Smoking
- Do not start smoking
- Stop smoking any form of tobacco

FIG. 8.4 World Health Organization recommendations to prevent chronic noncommunicable illnesses. (Source: https://www.who.int/ncds/prevention/en/. Accessed July 13, 2019.)

intake to help patients prevent the development of chronic disease. Use resources such as the World Health Organization's Recommendations to Prevent Chronic Noncommunicable Illnesses (WHO, 2019b) to help you better understand how people can have healthier lives and to guide your interventions (Fig. 8.4).

Use physical activity guidelines for adults, children, and older adults to provide clear activity goals for all age-groups (ODPHP, 2019a; see Chapter 38). Discuss the importance of both the intensity and frequency of exercise. Encourage patients of all age-groups to engage in muscle strengthening 2 to 3 days a week as well. People with chronic diseases need to participate in the same amount of activity and muscle-strengthening as healthy people whenever possible (ODPHP, 2019a). Ensure that these patients consult with their health care provider regarding the types and amounts of activity that are appropriate.

Along with routine exercise, help patients make dietary choices that include an intake of appropriate nutrients to promote health and prevent obesity (see Chapter 45). Healthy food choices, which include a variety of fruits and vegetables, grains, fat-free or low-fat dairy, protein, and oils in an appropriate calorie level, provide balanced nutritional intake (ODPHP, 2019b). Controlling sugar, sodium, fat, and alcohol intake assists in weight control. Refer to evidence-based nutritional guidelines, such as the *Dietary Guidelines for Americans*, available at https://health.gov/dietaryguidelines/, to help guide patient education.

Screening for Diseases

There are a variety of methods to detect disease in its earliest form. When diseases are detected early, treatment can begin, and the consequences of the disease can often be modified. Implement simple screening measures in children, such as blood pressure screening and height and weight screening to gather basic health information. Encourage all patients to have their blood pressure taken regularly. A person with hypertension usually has no symptoms (American Heart Association, 2017). Without routine blood pressure screening, a patient could have

undiagnosed hypertension and without treatment could end up with heart, renal or cardiovascular disease. The earlier high blood pressure is recognized through screening, the earlier treatment can begin and disease can be prevented.

Use health risk assessment data to encourage your patients to have appropriate screenings for diseases such as breast, colon, cervix and prostate cancer. Routine screening at recommended intervals leads to early detection so that if these cancers exist, early treatment with a good prognosis is possible (American Cancer Society, 2019a). Reinforce the need for your patients to routinely participate in these screening processes.

You can also serve as a resource to provide basic information about genetic screening and its benefits based on family history of chronic disease. Genetic counseling is a very specialized area of practice. Refer your patients to reliable sources of information such as the Genetics Home Reference website available at https://ghr.nlm.nih.gov/ (NIH, 2019d) and genetic specialists for expert advice when indicated to ensure that patients receive accurate detailed information about the effect of their genetics on their health.

Patient Education and Chronic Disease Self-Management

Patient education and disease self-management focus on the life changes that a person with a chronic illness must make to live well with his or her illness (Lorig et al., 2003). Living with chronic illnesses requires patients to implement demanding self-care tasks as they learn about their illnesses, how to manage symptoms and emotions, and how to make lifestyle changes to manage their illnesses. Patients are at increased risk of hospitalization or readmission when they are unable to manage their chronic disease at home. Nurses play an instrumental role in patient education to improve home care. When patients are given the tools to manage their illnesses and incorporate healthy behaviors into their daily lives, they usually experience fewer complications and have improved quality of life (CDC, 2018c).

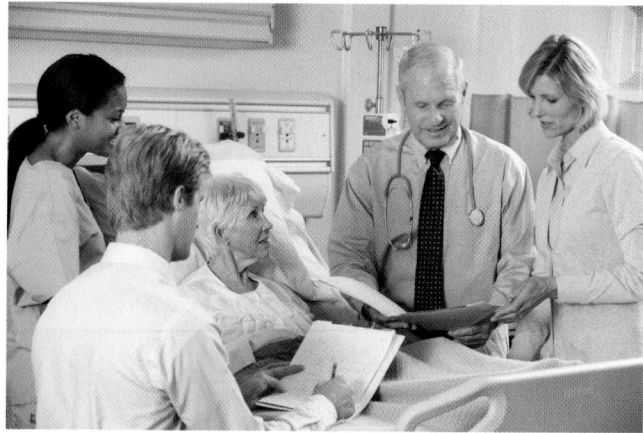

FIG. 8.5 Patients may interact with several members of the health care team. (iStock.com/monkeybusinessimages.)

Provide patient education to help patients understand their illnesses and related treatment. Follow patient education principles (see Chapter 25) to help patients understand their treatment, medications, diet, activity, and what symptoms to report to their health care provider. Emphasize the consequences when treatment plans are not followed. Prepare patients to implement required self-care activities and assist them in making appropriate changes in their behavior. Ensure that patients receive essential information, starting from the time you first meet them. Include family caregivers as appropriate. The AHRQ Health Literacy Universal Precautions Toolkit (2018) provides a variety of evidence-based tools you can implement to help simplify patient communication to reduce miscommunication, make the health care system easier to navigate, and support patients in improving their health.

Ensure that your patients and their caregivers understand the information provided to them. Only 12% of adults in the United States have the health literacy skills required to manage the complex needs related to their health (AHRQ, 2018). Use teach-back to ensure that patients understand this information before discharge from an acute care setting, before leaving an outpatient clinic setting, or at the conclusion of home care visits (AHRQ, 2018).

Include the interprofessional health care team when providing patient education. Members of the interprofessional team include nurses, pharmacists, dietitians, and health care providers (Fig. 8.5). Together, the team explains and reinforces the necessary health behavior changes needed to manage a chronic illness.

Promoting Adherence

Although frequently researched, interventions that promote adherence are not well understood and often do not create changes that are maintained over time (Neiman et al., 2017; Meiner & Yeager, 2019). Many factors affect adherence, including the severity and duration of the illness, the treatment plan, socioeconomic status, patient characteristics (e.g., motivation; personal beliefs about health, illness, and the treatment plan; health literacy; mental health), and characteristics of the health care delivery system (e.g., relationship with health care providers, accessibility) (George, 2018).

One model that supports patients in self-managing their chronic disease is the Five *As* (AHRQ, 2012):

- Assess: Determine a patient's beliefs, behaviors, knowledge.
- Advise: Provide specific information regarding health risks and the benefits of changing behaviors.
- Agree: Collaborate with the patient to set realistic goals.
- Assist: Help the patient identify barriers, strategies, problem-solving skills, and available support.
- Arrange: Determine a follow-up plan such as return visits, phone calls, and text messages.

Your initial assessment provides information about how a patient feels about his or her health, the desire to change behavior (when change is needed), and personal goals for improving health. Motivational interviewing is one strategy that has been found to be very useful in assessing what motivates patients to change. You can advise and assist patients through patient education (see Chapter 25), coaching, providing reminders about treatments (e.g., text messages for taking medications), helping patients establish routines, simplifying treatment plans, being patient advocates, and shared decision making between patients and health care providers (George, 2018; SMRC, 2019). Ongoing follow-up is especially important when your aim long-term is to change patient behavior.

Self-Management Education

Self-management education (SME) programs provide evidence-based interventions to help patients with chronic diseases manage their illness and its related symptoms. The Chronic Disease Self-Management Resource Program (CDSMRP) developed by Kate Lorig is one program that has consistently demonstrated improved patient outcomes for patients and their family caregivers by offering small, highly interactive group workshops that are facilitated by highly trained leaders who have health challenges of their own (SMRC, 2019). Small group participants meet for 2½ hours once a week for 6 weeks in a variety of community settings, such as churches, libraries, clinics, and hospitals. Workshops provide disease-specific information and include the elements of action planning, decision making, and problem solving. Participants identify personal goals and behavioral changes based on their needs and preferences (SMRC, 2019). Current evidence shows that these programs help patients experience improved overall health and use fewer health care resources (Lorig et al., 2016; Cutler et al., 2018).

Refer patients, especially those who are living with multiple chronic diseases, and their caregivers to CDSMRPs whenever possible. Spend time with patients to motivate and promote positive behavioral changes in addition to providing education about disease management. Place your patients at the center of chronic disease management care to enhance patient decision making and motivate change (Cutler, 2018). Providing strategies, such as how to deal with fatigue, pain, isolation, gait training, medication management, and effective communication with family, friends, and health care professionals, helps engage patients in making lifestyle changes for their health (Soderlung, 2018).

Many chronic disease management classes and tools that complement patient information and support provided by CDSMRPs are available (SMRC, 2019). Refer patients to disease-specific websites that offer reliable patient education materials and chronic disease guides to encourage maintaining health through consistent self-management (Table 8.5). For example, if you are caring for patients with heart failure, hypertension, or stroke, you can refer them to the American Heart Association's website (www.heart.org). Some of the free tools provided on this website help you and other health care professionals better understand current evidence-based care and treatment, while other tools are specifically for patients. Patient tools include information on each disease and disease-management principles (e.g., when to seek medical attention, how to monitor blood pressure, and diet information). The American Heart Association's website also provides a digital tracking mechanism with reminders for patients on when to monitor their blood pressure and a self-assessment of heart failure symptoms,

TABLE 8.5 Selected Websites Related to Chronic Illness Management

Chronic Illness(es)	Organization and Website
Heart failure Stroke Hypertension	American Heart Association: www.heart.org
Cancer	American Cancer Society: www.cancer.org
Emphysema Asthma Lung cancer	American Lung Association: www.lung.org
Diabetes	American Diabetes Association: www.diabetes.org

including warning signs that are indicative of deterioration in health and when to seek medical attention.

PUBLIC POLICY

Nurses are responsible to protect the public. Thus, as a nurse, you need to be aware and supportive of legislation that focuses on controlling external environmental factors that contribute to chronic disease development. Your professional nursing responsibility is awareness and support of public policy that decreases disease burden. Review publications and websites from reputable organizations about current policies that promote health, such as the American Cancer Society (2019b). For example, your support of a no-smoking law that prohibits smoking in public spaces, such as restaurants and bars, protects everyone who works and visits these spaces by limiting the exposure to secondhand smoke.

• • •

You will encounter many patients living with chronic illnesses. Use your knowledge and skills to promote health by educating patients about the major risk factors that increase the chance they will develop a chronic illness. Promote health and encourage patients to engage in screenings to detect diseases early to identify potential problems and intervene before permanent damage to health occurs. Helping patients understand how their lifestyle choices affect their health has the potential to decrease occurrence of chronic illness through exercise, healthy food choices, smoking cessation, controlled alcohol intake, and maintaining a healthy weight. Understanding how chronic illnesses affect your patients and their families will help you develop an appropriate patient-centered plan of care to promote optimal patient outcomes.

KEY POINTS

- A chronic disease is a pathophysiologic condition that lasts more than 1 year, requires ongoing medical care, and often limits a person's usual activities of daily living.
- The Chronic Care Model emphasizes the importance of self-management and provides a framework to help members of the health care team understand how community resources and health care systems impact patient outcomes.
- Patients with chronic illnesses must make lifestyle changes and learn to control their illnesses through disease self-management.
- Patients with the same chronic illness often have different symptoms and treatment needs.
- Loneliness and depression may negatively influence a patient's ability to cope with chronic illness.

- Inherited genetics and environmental influences are associated with the onset of chronic illnesses.
- Detecting risk factors for chronic illness before a disease begins provides an opportunity for early intervention to prevent or delay disease onset.
- Teaching healthy lifestyle behaviors provides an opportunity for the nurse to help people identify needed life changes to prevent disease.
- Effective programs that help patients self-manage their chronic diseases provide disease-specific information and help patients make decisions about their care.
- Helping patients understand how to deal with different symptoms related to a chronic disease and its treatment and how to communicate with family, friends, and health care workers assists patients in making lifestyle changes required by their chronic disease.

REFLECTIVE LEARNING

- Consider a patient that you cared for recently in clinical practice. What chronic disease risk factors did this patient have? What focused teaching did you or could you provide to improve the patient's health?
- Assess your patient's or a peer's family history. What patterns of illnesses occur in this family? Based on the family history, what healthy behaviors would prevent the family pattern of illness?
- Evaluate a recent patient's ability to adhere to his or her treatment plan to manage a chronic disease. What factors affected the patient's ability to follow the treatment plan? What interventions may have enhanced the patient's adherence?

REVIEW QUESTIONS

1. A health system upgraded its electronic health record across all its practice settings to enhance patient care and communication among health care providers. This is an example of which component of the Chronic Care Model?
   1. Health systems
   2. Decision support
   3. Clinical information systems
   4. Community
2. A nurse is providing education to a patient with type 2 diabetes. Which characteristics does the nurse include in her teaching to explain why type 2 diabetes is considered a chronic disease? (Select all that apply.)
   1. Type 2 diabetes lasts throughout a person's life.
   2. Genetic mutations drive the treatment for type 2 diabetes.
   3. People with type 2 diabetes have to modify some of their daily activities.
   4. Type 2 diabetes occurs in elderly people.
   5. People with type 2 diabetes require ongoing medical care.
3. Which of the family caregivers listed below will the nurse expect to be most at risk for experiencing poor health outcomes?
   1. A 20-year-old daughter caring for a mother who needs help setting up her medications weekly
   2. The 68-year-old spouse of a patient who is experiencing worsening dementia
   3. A 32-year-old parent of a child who has an ear infection
   4. A married couple who is sharing the caregiving responsibilities for a parent who was recently diagnosed with hypertension and coronary artery disease
4. A school nurse is planning a health fair for children in first, second, and third grade to promote healthy behaviors. The most

appropriate health screening for this age-group would be: (Select all that apply.)

1. Providing information about eating fruits and vegetables
2. Taking the children's blood pressure
3. Recording the children's height and weight on a growth chart
4. Asking the students about their family history of cancer
5. Teaching the students about the risks of secondhand smoke

5. A nurse is providing health promotion information at a health fair for female patients who are diagnosed with cancer. What information should the nurse include? (Select all that apply.)
   1. Recommending that they avoid drinking alcohol to prevent alcohol misuse
   2. Information from the local health department about smoking-cessation classes
   3. The need to avoid physical activity while receiving cancer treatment to lessen fatigue
   4. Strategies to talk with family and friends about the cancer diagnosis and the side effects from their treatment
   5. How nutritional needs may change based on the diagnosis of cancer and its treatment

6. The nurse is caring for a family where there is a strong family history of breast cancer. One of the family members says, "I am afraid of having genetic testing. If it is positive, I know I have cancer." What is the nurse's best response?
   1. "It will help diagnose the cancer early if you have it."
   2. "If the results are positive, it means you have a higher risk for breast cancer, not that you have cancer."
   3. "If it is going to cause you to worry, don't have the screening done."
   4. "I am sure you will be fine. You are a healthy woman."

7. A patient tells the nurse, "My doctor told me to lose weight, exercise, stop smoking, and eat better. I am not sick at all. Why would he tell me that?" The nurse's best response would be:
   1. "Since I was not there to hear the conversation, I am not exactly sure."
   2. "All of these things are behaviors that are good for you and your family. Why not just give it a try?"
   3. "I believe he is trying to get you to think about ways that you can be healthier. All these things help to prevent future health problems."
   4. "Eating a balanced, healthy diet and exercising regularly will help you lose weight. I know stopping smoking is really hard to do."

8. Two nurses are revising a self-management education program to help patients better manage their asthma. What strategies are most important for them to include in the program?
   1. Have patients list the medications they are prescribed to take and describe any problems they are having with their medications.
   2. Create a common set of patient goals that the patients will work toward as a group.
   3. Look for group leaders who are health care providers that are respected by the community.
   4. Provide information on how to balance activities during the day.
   5. Ask patients to discuss how other people in their family react to them now that they have asthma.

9. During a home visit, a patient states, "I am really upset about my heart failure. I can't go out to eat anymore with my friends, I have no energy, and I don't even want to talk on the phone. All I do is focus on how this disease has changed my life and how much time I have left to live." How should the nurse respond? (Select all that apply.)
   1. "Let's talk about going out to lunch. What is making you hesitant about eating with your friends?"
   2. "Tell me about what types of activities you were doing before you knew you had heart failure."
   3. "Eventually you will get used to all of the changes. You are doing OK."
   4. "My mother has heart failure, and she has adjusted to diet, activity, and medication changes."
   5. "How has your heart failure affected your energy level?"

10. A nurse is taking care of a patient who has decided to stop smoking cigarettes. Which online resource would provide evidence-based information about smoking cessation?
    1. The American Lung Association online toolkit for smoking cessation
    2. An online blog led by a nurse for people discussing smoking cessation
    3. A self-help website maintained by a hospital focusing on general wellness behaviors
    4. A CDC website that discusses addictive behavior and risk factors

Answers: 1. 3; **2.** 1, 3, 5; **3.** 2, 4, 2, 3; 5. **4.** 3, 5; **5.** 2, 4, 5; **6.** 2; **7.** 3; **8.** 1, 4, 5; **9.** 1, 2, 5; **10.** 1.

Rationales for Review Questions can be found on the Evolve website.

REFERENCES

Agency for Healthcare Research and Quality (AHRQ): *AHRQ health literacy universal precautions toolkit*, ed 2, 2018. https://www.ahrq.gov/professionals/quality-patient-safety/quality-resources/tools/literacy-toolkit/index.html. Accessed July 13, 2019.

Agency for Healthcare Research and Quality (AHRQ): *Five major steps to intervention (the "5 A's")*, 2012. https://www.ahrq.gov/professionals/clinicians-providers/guidelines-recommendations/tobacco/5steps.html. Accessed June 23, 2019.

Alzheimer's impact Movement (AIM): *Fact sheet*, 2019. http://act.alz.org/site/DocServer/2012_Costs_Fact_Sheet_version_2.pdf?docID=7161. Accessed June 22, 2019.

American Cancer Society: *Help pass laws to defeat cancer*, 2019b. https://www.cancer.org/involved/volunteer/advocate.html. Accessed July 13, 2019.

American Cancer Society: *Stay healthy*, 2019a. https://www.cancer.org/healthy.html. Accessed July 13, 2019.

American Diabetes Association (ADA): *The cost of diabetes*, 2019. http://www.diabetes.org/advocacy/news-events/cost-of-diabetes.html. Accessed June 22, 2019.

American Heart Association: *Why high blood pressure is a "silent killer,"* Dallas, TX, 2017, American Heart Association. https://www.heart.org/en/health-topics/high-blood-pressure/why-high-blood-pressure-is-a-silent-killer. Accessed July 7, 2019.

American Society of Clinical Oncology (ASCO): Lynch syndrome, 2019. https://www.cancer.net/cancer-types/lynch-syndrome. Accessed 22 June 2019.

Armstrong K: Chemobrain: physiological predisposing factors, *Medsurg Nurs* 25(4):215, 2016.

Capewell S, Capewell A: An effectiveness hierarchy of preventive interventions: neglected paradigm or self-evident truth? *J Public Health* 40(2):350, 2018. https://doi.org/10.1093/pubmed/fdx055.

Centers for Disease Control and Prevention (CDC): *How type 2 diabetes affects your workforce*, 2018a. https://www.cdc.gov/diabetes/prevention/how-type2-affects-workforce.htm?CDC_AA_refVal=https%3A%2F%2F. Accessed June 22, 2019.

Centers for Disease Control and Prevention (CDC): *The cost of arthritis in US adults*, 2018b. https://www.cdc.gov/arthritis/data_statistics/cost.htm. Accessed June 22, 2019.

Centers for Disease Control and Prevention (CDC): *Self-management education: learn more. Feel better*, 2018c. https://www.cdc.gov/learnmorefeelbetter/index.htm. Accessed July 13, 2019.

Centers for Disease Control and Prevention (CDC): *National center for chronic disease prevention and health promotion: about chronic diseases.* http://www.cdc.gov/chronicdisease/about/index.htm, 2019a. Accessed June 22, 2019.

Centers for Disease Control and Prevention (CDC): *Health and economic costs of chronic diseases.* https://www.cdc.gov/chronicdisease/about/costs/index.htm, 2019b. Accessed June 22, 2019.

Centers for Disease Control and Prevention (CDC): *Overweight and obesity,* 2019c. https://www.cdc.gov/obesity/index.html. Accessed June 22, 2019.

Centers for Disease Control and Prevention (CDC): *Quick facts on the risks of e-cigarettes for kids, teens, and young adults,* 2019d. https://www.cdc.gov/tobacco/basic_information/e-cigarettes/Quick-Facts-on-the-Risks-of-E-cigarettes-for-Kids-Teens-and-Young-Adults.html. Accessed July 13, 2019.

Centers for Disease Control and Prevention (CDC): *Alcohol and public health,* 2019e. https://www.cdc.gov/alcohol/index.htm. Accessed July 14, 2019.

Chang E, Johnson A: *Living with chronic illness and disability: principles for nursing practice,* ed 3, Chatswood, NSW, 2018, Elsevier Australia.

Cleveland Clinic: *How genetic testing can make your cancer treatment more effective,* 2017. https://health.clevelandclinic.org/how-genetic-testing-can-make-your-cancer-treatment-more-effective/. Accessed July 14, 2019.

Family Caregiver Alliance: *Caregiver statistics: health, technology, and caregiving resources,* 2016b. https://www.caregiver.org/caregiver-statistics-health-technology-and-caregiving-resources. Accessed August 16, 2019.

Family Caregiver Alliance: *Caregiver statistics: work and caregiving,* 2016a. https://www.caregiver.org/caregiver-statistics-work-and-caregiving. Accessed August 16, 2019.

Giddens J: *Concepts for nursing practice,* ed 2, St Louis, 2017, Elsevier.

Grandjean P, Bellanger M: Calculation of the disease burden associated with environmental chemical exposures: application of toxicological information in health economic estimation, *Environ Health* 6(1):123, 2017.

Health.gov: Dietary guidelines for Americans 2015-2020 – Introduction – nutrition and health are closely related, nd https://health.gov/dietaryguidelines/2015/guidelines/introduction/nutrition-and-health-are-closely-related/

HealthyPeople.gov: *Healthy people 2020,* 2019. https://www.healthypeople.gov/. Accessed June 22, 2019.

Improving Chronic Illness Care: *The Chronic Care Model,* 2006-2019. http://www.improvingchroniccare.org/index.php?p=The_Chronic_Care_Model&s=2. Accessed July 7, 2019.

Leventhal H, et al.: Modelling management of chronic illness in everyday life: a common-sense approach, *Psychol Topics* 25(1):18, 2016.

Lorig K, et al.: *Living a healthy life with chronic conditions,* ed 4, Boulder, CO, 2012, Bull Publishing.

Lorig K, et al.: Self-management education: history, definition, outcomes, and mechanisms, *Ann Behav Med* 26(1):1–7, 2003.

Meiner SE, Yeager JJ: *Gerontologic nursing,* ed 6, St Louis, 2019, Elsevier.

Moss K, et al.: Identifying and addressing family caregiver anxiety, *J Hosp Palliat Nurs* 21(1):14, 2019.

National Cancer Institute (NCI): Cancer prevalence and cost of care projections, n.d. , https://costprojections.cancer.gov/. Accessed June 22, 2019.

National Institute on Alcohol Abuse and Alcoholism: *Rethinking drinking: alcohol and your health,* Bethesda, MD, 2016, National Institute of Health Publication No. 15-3770. https://pubs.niaaa.nih.gov/publications/RethinkingDrinking/Rethinking_Drinking.pdf. Accessed July 13, 2019.

National Institutes of Health (NIH): *Genetic testing: how it is used for healthcare,* 2018. https://report.nih.gov/nihfactsheets/ViewFactSheet.aspx?csid=43. Accessed August 8, 2019.

National Institutes of Health (NIH): *What are the different ways in which a genetic condition can be inherited?* 2019a. https://ghr.nlm.nih.gov/primer/inheritance/inheritancepatterns. Accessed June 22, 2019.

National Institutes of Health (NIH): *What are complex or multifactorial disorders?* 2019b. https://ghr.nlm.nih.gov/primer/mutationsanddisorders/complexdisorders, Accessed June 22, 2019.

National Institutes of Health (NIH): *What is a genetic consultation?* 2019c. https://ghr.nlm.nih.gov/primer/consult/consultation. Accessed June 22, 2019.

National Institutes of Health (NIH): *Genetics home reference,* 2019d. https://ghr.nlm.nih.gov/. Accessed July 13, 2019.

Office of Disease Prevention and Health Promotion (ODPHP): *Dietary guidelines,* 2019b. https://health.gov/dietaryguidelines/. Accessed July 14, 2019.

Office of Disease Prevention and Health Promotion (ODPHP): *Physical activity: current guidelines,* 2019a. https://health.gov/paguidelines/second-edition/. Accessed July 14, 2019.

Parrish E: Comorbidity of mental illness and chronic physical illness: a diagnostic and treatment conundrum, *Perspect Psychiatr Care* 54(3):339, 2018.

Sears ME, Genuis SJ: Environmental determinants of chronic disease and medical approaches: recognition, avoidance, supportive therapy, and detoxification, *J Environ Public Health,* 2012, Article ID 356798. https://www.hindawi.com/journals/jeph/2012/356798/.

Self-Management Resource Center (SMRC): *Help your community take charge of its health,* 2019. https://www.selfmanagementresource.com/. Accessed July 13, 2019.

Singh T, et al.: Tobacco use among middle and high school students — United States, 2011–2015, *MMWR* 65(14):361, 2016. https://doi.org/10.15585/mmwr.mm6514a1.

Stoffel EM, et al.: Hereditary colorectal cancer syndromes: American society of clinical Oncology clinical practice guideline endorsement of the familial risk–colorectal cancer: European society for medical Oncology clinical practice guidelines, 2014. https://www.asco.org/practice-guidelines/quality-guidelines/guidelines/gastrointestinal-cancer#/10241. Accessed June 22, 2019.

Tamura-Lis W: Reminiscing — a tool for excellent elder care and improved quality of life, *Urol Nurs* 37(3):151, 2017.

US Department of Health and Human Services (USDHHS): *The health consequences of smoking—50 years of progress: a report of the surgeon general,* 2014. https://www.surgeongeneral.gov/library/reports/50-years-of-progress/full-report.pdf. Accessed June 23, 2019.

US Department of Health and Human Services (USDHHS): *Step it up! the surgeon general's call to action to promote walking and walkable communities,* Washington, DC, 2015, Office of the Surgeon General. https://www.surgeongeneral.gov/library/calls/walking-and-walkable-communities/index.html. Accessed June 23, 2019.

US Department of Health and Human Services (USDHHS): *Facing addiction in America: the surgeon general's report on alcohol, drugs, and health,* 2016. https://www.hhs.gov/surgeongeneral/reports-and-publications/addiction/index.html. Accessed June 23, 2019.

US Department of Health and Human Services (USDHHS): *Tobacco reports and publications,* 2019. https://www.hhs.gov/surgeongeneral/reports-and-publications/tobacco/index.html. Accessed June 23, 2019.

US Preventive Services Task Force: *BRCA-related cancer: risk assessment, genetic counseling, and genetic testing,* 2013. https://www.uspreventiveservicestaskforce.org/Page/Document/UpdateSummaryFinal/brca-related-cancer-risk-assessment-genetic-counseling-and-genetic-testing?ds=1&s=cancer. Accessed June 22, 2019.

Walberger S: Cancer Council: there are 16 cancers that can be caused by smoking. 2016. https://www.cancercouncil.com.au/blog/there-are-16-cancers-that-can-be-caused-by-smoking/. Accessed August 8, 2019.

World Health Organization (WHO): *Alcohol,* 2019a. https://www.who.int/health-topics/alcohol#tab=overview. Accessed July 14, 2019.

World Health Organization (WHO): *Prevention: noncommunicable diseases and their risk factors.* 2019b. http://www.who.int/ncds/prevention/en/. Accessed July 13, 2019.

World Health Organization (WHO): *Tobacco (N Y),* 2019c. https://www.who.int/health-topics/tobacco. Accessed July 14, 2019.

RESEARCH REFERENCES

Apple RW: Children and adolescents coping with chronic illness and disability, *Int J Child Adolesc Health* 10(4):495, 2017.

Ates M, et al.: Educational needs of caregivers of patients hospitalized in a neurology clinic: results of questionnaire, *Int J Caring Sci* 11(2):968, 2018.

Babor TF, et al.: *AUDIT: the alcohol use disorders identification test guidelines for use in primary care,* ed 2, Geneva, 2001, World Health Organization.

Coughlin MB, Sethares KA: Chronic sorrow in parents of children with a chronic illness or disability: an integrative literature review, *J Pediatr Nurs* 37:108, 2017.

Corvin J, et al.: Translating research into practice: employing community-based mixed methods approaches to address chronic disease and depression among Latinos, *J Behav Health Serv Res* 44(4):574, 2017.

Cutler S, et al.: Effectiveness of group self-management interventions for persons with chronic conditions: a systematic review, *Medsurg Nurs* 27(6):359, 2018.

Gan LL, et al.: School experiences of siblings of children with chronic illness: a systematic literature review, *J Pediatr Nurs* 33:23, 2017.

Garcia-Sanjuan S, et al.: Understanding life experiences of people affected by Crohn's disease in Spain. A phenomenological approach, *Scand J Caring Sci* 32(1):354, 2018.

George M: Adherence in asthma and COPD: new strategies for an old problem, *Respir Care* 63(6):818, 2018.

Han J: Chronic illnesses and depressive symptoms among older people: functional limitations as a mediator and self-perceptions of aging as a moderator, *J Aging Health* 30(8):1188, 2018, https://doi.org/10.1177/0898264317711609.

Heid A, et al.: Illness representations of multiple chronic conditions and self-management behaviors in older adults: a pilot study, *Int J Aging Hum Dev* 87(1):90, 2018. https://doi.org/10.1177/0091415018771327.

Kadu MK, Stolee P: Facilitators and barriers of implementing the Chronic Care Model in primary care: a systematic review, *BMC Fam Pract* 16(12), 2015. https://doi.org/10.1186/s12875-014-0219-0.

Knoerl R, et al.: Estimating the frequency, severity, and clustering of SPADE symptoms in chronic painful chemotherapy-induced peripheral neuropathy, *Pain Manag Nurs* 19(4):354, 2018.

Kosobucka A, et al.: Adherence to treatment assessed with the Adherence in Chronic Diseases Scale in patients after myocardial infarction, *Patient Prefer Adherence* 12:333–340, 2018.

Kourie HR, Klastersky JA: Physical long-term side-effects in young adult cancer survivors: germ cell tumors model, *Curr Opin Oncol* 29(4):229, 2017.

Kristjansdottir O, et al.: Personal strengths reported by people with chronic illness: a qualitative study, *Health Expect* 21(4):787, 2018.

Kubica A, et al.: The Adherence in Chronic Diseases Scale: a new tool to monitor implementation of a treatment plan, *Folia Cardiol* 12:19–26, 2017.

Lauffenburger JC, et al.: Association between patient-centered medical homes and adherence to chronic disease medications, *Ann Intern Med* 166:81, 2017.

Lorig K, et al.: Benefits of diabetes self-management for health plan members: a 6-month translation study, *J Med Internet Res* 18(6):1, 2016.

Lum A, et al.: Understanding the school experiences of children and adolescents with serious chronic illness: a systematic meta-review, *Child Care Health Dev* 43(5):645, 2017.

Neiman AB, et al.: CDC grand rounds: improving medication adherence for chronic disease management — innovations and opportunities, *MMWR* 66(45):1248, 2017.

Rappaport S: Genetic factors are not the major causes of chronic diseases, *PLoS One* 11(4):e0154387, 2016. https://www.ncbi.nlm.nih.gov/pmc/articles/PMC4841510/. Accessed 22 June 2019.

Reynolds R, et al.: A systematic review of chronic disease management interventions in primary care, *BMC Fam Pract* 19(1):11, 2018, https://doi.org/10.1186/s12875-017-0682-3.

Secinti E, et al.: Research review: childhood chronic physical illness and adult emotional health: a systematic review and meta-analysis, *J Child Psychol Psychiatry* 58(7):753, 2017, https://doi.org/10.1111/jcpp.12727.

Soderlung PD: Effectiveness of motivational interviewing for improving physical activity self-management for adults with type 2 diabetes: a review, *Chronic Illn* 14(1):54, 2018.

Stagg SJ, et al.: Evaluation of text messaging effects on health goal adherence in the management of participants with chronic disease, *Prof Case Manage* 22(3):126, 2017.

Tuncay F, et al.: Effects of loneliness on illness perception in persons with a chronic disease, *J Clin Nurs* 27(7–8):e1494, 2018. https://doi.org/10.1111/jocn.14273.

Vahedparast H, et al.: The role of social support in adherence to treatment regimens: experiences of patients with chronic diseases, *Medsurg Nurs J* 7(1):e69646, 2018.

Yazdanpanah Y, et al.: Effect of an educational program based on Health Belief Model on medication adherence in elderly patients with hypertension, *Evid Based Care J* 9(1):52, 2019.

9

Cultural Competence

OBJECTIVES

- Explain the concepts of cultural awareness, cultural knowledge, cultural skill, cultural encounter, and cultural desire in the cultural competence model.
- Describe social and cultural influences in health and illness.
- Describe health disparity and the social determinants that affect it.
- Describe the roles that communication and self-examination play in developing cultural competence.

- Explain the approaches to use in conducting a cultural nursing history and physical assessment.
- Describe how teach-back helps a patient with limited health literacy.
- Explain the principles to apply when using an interpreter.

KEY TERMS

Acculturation, p. 111
Assimilation, p. 111
Core measures, p. 111
Culture, p. 107
Cultural assessment, p. 113
Cultural awareness, p. 111
Cultural competence, p. 107
Cultural desire, p. 112
Cultural encounter, p. 112

Cultural knowledge, p. 112
Cultural respect, p. 111
Cultural skill, p. 112
Culturally congruent care, p. 107
Emic world view, p. 108
Ethnic/cultural identity, p. 110
Etic world view, p. 108
Health disparity, p. 108
Health literacy p. 115

Intersectionality, p. 110
Linguistic competence, p. 114
Marginalized groups, p. 109
Oppression, p. 110
Racial identity, p. 110
Social determinants of health, p. 109
Stereotype, p. 108
Unconscious/implicit bias, p. 107

MEDIA RESOURCES

http://evolve.elsevier.com/Potter/fundamentals/
- Review Questions
- Case Study with Questions

- Audio Glossary
- Content Updates
- Answers to QSEN Activity and Review Questions

The term culture refers to the learned and shared beliefs, values, norms, and traditions of a particular group, which guide our thinking, decisions, and actions (Giger, 2017; Leininger and McFarland, 2006). Culture also refers to ways of relating to one another, language and manner of speaking, work and lifestyle practice, social relationships, values, religious beliefs and rituals, and expression of thoughts and emotions (Ball et al., 2019; Giddens, 2017). Culture is a learned behavior, yet it is constantly changing in response to environmental, biological, political, and social influences.

Every one of us has some type of bias that is culturally driven. Such biases can be referred to as an unconscious bias or an implicit bias. Unconscious bias refers to a bias we are unaware of and that happens outside our control, which is influenced by our personal background, cultural environment, and personal experiences. Unconscious bias typically directs one to make quick judgments and assessments of people and situations. An implicit bias is similar; however, we are aware of the bias that is present. We are responsible for implicit bias and must recognize and acknowledge our actions as they impact our behavior, decisions, and patient-centered care provided. One might have a bias toward or against an individual based on his or her culture, such as a bias toward an ethnic group, race, gender, nation, religion, social class, or political party. When you as the nurse hold a bias toward an individual patient or group of patients, it is very difficult to provide patient-centered transcultural care.

Culturally congruent care or transcultural care emphasizes the need to provide care based on an individual's cultural beliefs, practices, and values; therefore, effective communication is a critical skill in culturally competent care and helps you engage a patient and family in respectful, patient-centered dialogue (Hadziabdic et al., 2015). A patient-centered approach to providing transcultural care requires you to address your own implicit bias; be respectful of and responsive to individual patient preferences, needs, and values; and ensure that patient values guide all clinical care decisions (Institute of Medicine [IOM], 2001). This chapter explains the importance of cultural competence and its relationship to patient-centered care. Cultural competence means that professional health care must be culturally sensitive, culturally appropriate, and culturally competent to meet the multifaceted health care needs of each person, family, and community (Spector, 2017). Cultural beliefs, values, and practices are learned from birth, first in the home, then in the church or other places where people congregate, and then in educational and other social settings (Purnell, 2013). This cultural learning applies to both you and your patients. The process of cultural competence in delivering health care services is "a culturally conscious model of care in which a healthcare professional continually strives to achieve the ability and availability to effectively work within the cultural context of a client" (family, individual, or community) (Transcultural C.A.R.E. Associates, 2015). It is a process of becoming culturally competent, not being culturally competent (Transcultural C.A.R.E. Associates, 2015). The goal of delivering cultural care is to utilize research findings to provide culturally specific care that is safe and beneficial to the well-being of the diverse population (McFarland and Wehbe-Alamah, 2015).

The changing demographics of the US population create challenges for the health care system and health care providers. By the year 2060, the percentage of racial and ethnic minority groups in the United States is expected to climb to 32% of the population (US Census Bureau, 2018). The fastest-growing racial ethnic group in the United States is people whose ancestry is from two or more races, and this group is projected to grow by 200% by 2060 (US Census Bureau, 2018). The next fastest-growing is the Asian population, which is projected to double, followed by the Hispanic population (US Census Bureau, 2018). Nearly one in five of the total US population is projected to be foreign born by 2060 (Colby and Ortman, 2015). According to the Administration for Community Living (2017), the population age 60 years and over will increase from 65 million in 2017 to 77 million in 2020 and is projected to reach 94.7 million by the year 2060. The wealth gap between blacks and whites is demonstrated in the fact that blacks lag behind whites in homeownership, household wealth, and median income. These differences remain even when controlling for levels of education (Pew Research Center, 2016). Additionally, the Centers for Disease Control and Prevention (CDC) (2018) reports that studies show adults who self-report the worst health also have the most limited literacy, numeracy, and health literacy skills. A growing body of evidence shows that individuals with the skills and confidence to become actively engaged in their health care have better health outcomes. Although death rates have declined overall in the United States over the past 50 years, people who are poorly educated and people living in poverty still die at a higher rate from the same conditions than people who are better educated and economically advantaged (Ball et al., 2019). These statistics reveal examples of cultural factors that influence the health care system and why issues such as health care resource accessibility, patient adherence to medical therapies, patient satisfaction, and health care outcomes are so difficult to manage.

The Joint Commission (TJC), the National Quality Forum (NQF), and the National Commission on Quality Assurance (NCQA) are a few of the influential organizations that have responded to these complexities in health care by implementing new standards focused on cultural competency, health literacy, and patient-centered and family-centered care. These standards recognize that valuing each patient's unique needs improves the overall safety and quality of a patient's care.

WORLD VIEW

Historical and social realities shape an individual's or group's world view, which determines how people perceive others, how they interact and relate to reality, and how they process information (Walker et al., 2010). World view is a set of assumptions that begins to develop during childhood and guides how one sees, thinks about, experiences, and interprets the world (The Substance Abuse and Mental Health Services Administration [SAMHSA], 2014). It creates a lens through which we view all of life's experiences through our own uniquely tinted view. Our world view evolves during a lifetime process of interacting with family, peers, communities, organizations, media, and institutions (Fig. 9.1). It is important for you to advocate for patients based on their world views. This requires a thorough ongoing assessment, flexibility, and planning in partnership with each patient to ensure that your care is safe, effective, and culturally sensitive.

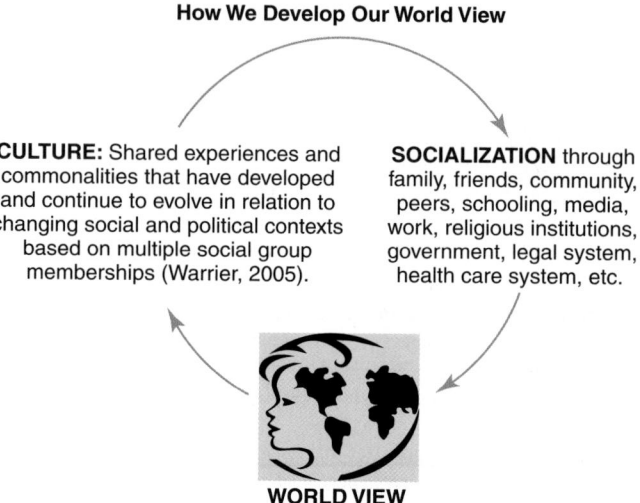

How We Develop Our World View

CULTURE: Shared experiences and commonalities that have developed and continue to evolve in relation to changing social and political contexts based on multiple social group memberships (Warrier, 2005).

SOCIALIZATION through family, friends, community, peers, schooling, media, work, religious institutions, government, legal system, health care system, etc.

WORLD VIEW

FIG. 9.1 How we develop our world view. (Copyright © 2011 Barnes-Jewish Hospital Center for Diversity and Cultural Competence.)

In any intercultural encounter there is an insider perspective (emic world view) and an outsider perspective (etic world view). For example, a Korean woman requests seaweed soup for her first meal after giving birth. This request puzzles her nurse. The nurse has an emic world view of professional postpartum care but is an outsider to the Korean culture. As such, the nurse is not aware of the meal's significance to the patient. Conversely, the Korean patient has an etic world view of American professional postpartum care and assumes that the seaweed soup is available in the hospital because, according to her cultural beliefs, the soup cleanses the blood and promotes healing and lactation (Edelstein, 2011). Conflict arises when health care providers interpret the behaviors of patients through their own world view lens instead of trying to uncover the world view that guides the behavior of their patients.

A **stereotype** is an assumed belief regarding a particular group (Ellis-Fletcher, 2015). It is easy to stereotype various cultural groups after reading general information about their ethnic values, practices, and beliefs. Avoid stereotypes or unwarranted generalizations about any particular group that prevents an inaccurate assessment of an individual's unique characteristics, talents, challenges reflected in the places they live, their socioeconomic circumstances, ethnic heritage, religion, language, abilities, characteristics, and world views (Dayer-Berenson, 2014). Instead, approach each person individually and ask questions to gain a better understanding of a patient's perspective and needs.

HEALTH DISPARITIES

More than a decade ago, a report by the IOM (2001) defined quality health care as health care that is safe, effective, patient centered, timely, efficient, and equitable or fair. Although the US health care system has improved in most of those areas since the IOM report was published, the system still does not emphasize equality of care (Mutha et al., 2012). As a result, many health care disparities remain. *Healthy People 2020* defines a health disparity as "a particular type of health difference that is closely linked with social, economic, and/or environmental disadvantage" (Office of Disease Prevention and Health Promotion [ODPHP], 2016) (Box 9.1). Poor health status, disease risk factors, poor health outcomes, and limited access to health care are types of disparities often interrelated and influenced by the conditions and social context in which people live (CDC, 2013).

BOX 9.1 Examples of Health Disparities Identified by the Centers for Disease Control and Prevention

- Among adults aged 25 years and older in 2011, noncompletion of high school was generally more common among adults who were foreign born than adults born in the United States (CDC, 2013).
- In 2011, 30.3% of US census tracts did not have at least one healthier food retailer (supermarkets, large grocery stores, supercenters and warehouse clubs, or fruit and vegetable specialty stores) within the tract or within a mile of tract boundaries. This represents 83.6 million people, representing approximately 27% of the 2010 continental US population (CDC, 2013).
- Non-Hispanic black adults were at least 50% more likely to die of heart disease or stroke prematurely (i.e., before age 75 years) than their non-Hispanic white counterparts (CDC, 2013).
- Colorectal cancer incidence and mortality increased with advancing age. Incidence and death rates were highest among people aged 75 years and older. Non-Hispanic blacks had higher colorectal cancer incidence and death rates than non-Hispanic whites, Asians/Pacific Islanders, and American Indians/Alaska Natives (CDC, 2013).
- The number of individuals who had colorectal cancer screening (any of the test options) was greater among people aged 65 to 75 years compared with people aged 50 to 64 years among non-Hispanics compared with Hispanics, among people with a disability compared with people with no disability, and among people with health insurance compared with people with no health insurance (CDC, 2013).
- American Indian and Alaska Native adults are twice as likely to be diagnosed with type 2 diabetes mellitus than non-Hispanic whites (CDC, 2016).
- Black and Hispanic children are hospitalized with complications of asthma much more often than are white children (CDC, 2016).

Adapted from Centers for Disease Control and Prevention (CDC): CDC health disparities and inequalities report—United States, 2013, MMWR Morb Mortal Wkly Rep 62(Suppl 3):1, 2013, http://www.cdc.gov/mmwr/pdf/other/su6203.pdf; Centers for Disease Control and Prevention (CDC): CDC selected CDC sponsored interventions—United States, 2016, https://www.cdc.gov/minorityhealth/strategies2016/index.html.

Social determinants of health are the conditions in which people are born, grow, live, work, and age (WHO, 2019). This includes conditions within a health care system. According to the World Health Organization (WHO) (2019), social determinants of health are mostly responsible for health disparities seen with and between countries. Social determinants of health include factors such as age, race, ethnicity, socioeconomic status, access to nutritious food, transportation resources, religion, sexual orientation, age, level of education. literacy level, disability (physical and cognitive), and geographical location (e.g., access to health care) (CDC, 2013). It is important that you understand how patients' cultural factors and their social determinants of health influence their health disparities. You also need to understand the implications this has on how you provide patient-centered care. According to the US Department of Health and Human Services (USDHHS) (n.d.), health care disparities can adversely affect communities, thus identifying a public health concern.

The 2016 National Healthcare Quality and Disparities Report by the Agency for Healthcare Research and Quality (AHRQ) (2017) offers some promise regarding health care access and quality. The report noted that access to health care did not demonstrate significant improvement (2000-2014); however, uninsured rates for Americans decreased from 2010 to 2016. Quality of health care improved overall from 2000 through 2014 to 2015, but the pace of improvement varied. Overall, some disparities were getting smaller from 2000 through 2014-2015, but disparities continue to persist, especially for poor and uninsured populations. People in poor households receive worse care than people in high-income households for almost all quality access measures. Black and Hispanic populations experience worse access to care compared with whites; however, improvements are noted in the number of Americans with a usual source of consistent medical care. The quality of health care improved generally through 2016 based on quality of measures such as patient safety, healthy living, effective treatment, and trends in care coordination (AHRQ, 2017).

In addition to disparity among cultural groups, people who are in **marginalized groups** are more likely to have poor health outcomes and die earlier because of a complex interaction among their individual behaviors, environment of the communities in which they live, the policies and practices of health care and governmental systems, and the clinical care they receive (United Health Foundation, 2015). Examples of marginalized groups include people who are gay, lesbian, bisexual, or transgender; people of color; people who are physically or mentally challenged; and people who are not college educated. Marginalization places or keeps someone in a powerless or an unimportant position within a society or group. Limited access to health care is one social determinant of health that contributes to health disparities. Access to primary care is an important indicator of broader access to health care services. A patient who regularly visits a primary care provider is more likely to receive adequate preventive care than a patient who lacks such access. Nursing intersects with a variety of people from different cultures; therefore, the awareness of marginalization is critical (Hall and Carlson, 2016).

Health care systems and health care providers sometimes contribute significantly to the problem of health care disparities. Disparities have been linked to inadequate resources, poor patient-provider communication, a lack of culturally competent care, and inadequate access to language services (National Quality Forum [NQF], 2018). Populations with a culture that differs from the culture of the health care provider tend to encounter decreased access to care, which leads to poor patient health outcomes (Ingram, 2011). To promote equal treatment for all patients who enter the health care system, we must be deliberate about addressing the impact of health care disparities (NQF, 2018).

Consider this example. *Ms. Millman is a 27-year-old African American. She is overweight and was diagnosed with type 2 diabetes 2 years ago and now requires insulin to control her blood sugar. She became homeless after losing her job and health insurance. She currently lives in housing provided through a neighborhood shelter. Ms. Millman was admitted to the hospital with a blood sugar of 322 mg/dL (her normal targeted range is 80 to 130 mg/dL) and a hemoglobin A1c of 11% (target for Ms. Millman is 7% or less). Hannah, a nursing student, is assigned to care for Ms. Millman. After reading her medical record, Hannah notices that Ms. Millman has come to the emergency department three times during the past 6 months for the same reason. Ms. Millman's previous health care providers documented that she verbalized an understanding of how to manage her diabetes but has difficulty following her treatment plan. Hannah teaches Ms. Millman that it is important to take her insulin as prescribed. She also explains how to make healthy food choices. As Hannah provides patient education, Ms. Millman nods. Hannah gives Ms. Millman a chance to ask questions, but Ms. Millman says she has none.*

In the case study, Ms. Millman has a number of social determinants that affect her health status and ability to manage her diabetes: socioeconomic status (no employment or health insurance, no home, limited financial resources if any), no access to primary care (uses the emergency department), being female, and a questionable literacy problem indicated by her neutral reaction to Hannah's instruction. Hannah needs to consider all these factors to provide Ms. Millman a more culturally competent health care plan.

Intersectionality

Intersectionality is a research and policy model used to study the complexities of people's lives and experiences (Lopez and Gadsden, 2016). The model looks at how being marginalized affects people's health and access to care. It serves to describe the forces, factors, and power structures that shape and influence life. Intersectionality is a way of understanding and analyzing our complex world by looking at the human experience (Lopez and Gadsden, 2016). Each of us is at the intersection of two categories: privilege and oppression. Oppression is a formal and informal system of advantages and disadvantages tied to membership in social groups, reinforced by societal norms, biases, interactions, and beliefs (Goldbach, 2019). Oppression occurs at individual and group experiences. For example, a patient experiencing oppression has limited access to resources, such as health care, housing, education, employment, and legal services. In contrast, a patient experiencing privilege has no difficulty accessing these resources. Individuals who support the theory of intersectionality believe that we must each determine how privileged and how oppressed we are to understand ourselves, the people around us, and the choices we make. Learning about a culture includes becoming familiar with the heritage of the people and understanding how discrimination, prejudice, and oppression can influence beliefs upheld in everyday life (Purnell, 2013). Then as health care providers, we are better able to identify the nature or source of patient's health care problems and how best to find solutions. Social groups affect our daily lives, shape our world view, control our access to resources, and ultimately determine our health outcomes. Whether we live in a disadvantaged community or in a community with access to social power and resources, we all are affected by the system of oppression. Understanding the different levels of oppression and where you stand helps you develop cultural competence (Fig. 9.2).

To apply the intersectionality model to daily nursing practice, think about the following patients who have been diagnosed with type 2 diabetes: a 25-year-old Hispanic woman who is homeless, an 85-year-old African-American retired nurse from rural Alabama, a 32-year-old Latina lesbian executive in San Francisco who is Catholic, and a woman who is an undocumented immigrant from Eastern Europe and has a 3-year-old child with a developmental disability. How may the experiences of each of these women compare with the experiences of other Americans? How do their experiences with the health care system differ? How does age affect their perspective? How would these answers change if you looked at their lives 15 years ago or 35 years ago? These scenarios are likely to draw a wide range of responses. The idea of intersectionality supports a broad view of culture by allowing consideration of a multitude of experiences within the context of power, privilege, and oppression.

RACIAL, ETHNIC, AND CULTURAL IDENTITY

Cultural competence is "a dynamic, fluid, continuous process whereby an individual, system, or health care agency finds meaningful and useful care strategies based on knowledge of the cultural heritage, beliefs, attitudes, and behaviors of those to whom they render care" (Giger, 2017, p. 7). Cultural competence is challenging to achieve, but it begins with one's ongoing development, while gaining an awareness of your own racial, ethnic, and cultural identity. That awareness prepares you to better understand patients within the context of their own racial, ethnic, and cultural identity.

As a nurse, you will counsel and comfort patients to help them better understand their health issues (e.g., medication adherence, ability to follow diet restrictions, knowledge of risk factors) and improve their willingness to partner with you in making important behavioral changes when necessary. Reflect on your own sense of how you identify with race and ethnicity within the context of your family, community, and cultural history (SAMHSA, 2014). Here are two classic definitions. Racial identity is based on one's self-identification with one or more social groups in which a common heritage with a particular racial group is shared (US Census, 2018); ethnic and cultural identity is "the frame in which individuals identify consciously or unconsciously with those with whom they feel a common bond because of similar traditions, behaviors, values, and beliefs" (Chavez & Guido-DiBrito, 1999, p. 41). These definitions help us to understand how individuals negotiate their own and other cultures in life (SAMHSA, 2014). It is important for you to examine your own racial, ethnic, and cultural identity

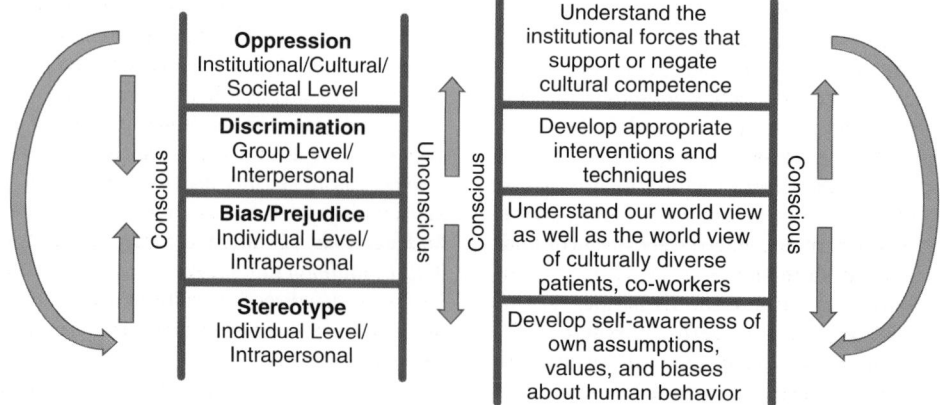

FIG. 9.2 Ladders of oppression and cultural competence. Each level of the ladder of cultural competence offers a response to the ladder of oppression. Because of the extensiveness and complexity of the systems of oppression, individuals and organizations move up and down both ladders simultaneously. (©2011 BJH Center for Diversity and Cultural Competence.)

to better recognize and understand normal and abnormal behavior. If you fail to do this self-examination, you will be more likely to prejudge patients and not accurately assess their health care problems. A self-examination allows you to understand the cultural factors that shape a patient's life experiences, a patient's health care problems, a patient's behavior, and how a patient might perceive those problems, thus supporting the belief that cultural awareness is essential to healing and building trust in the nurse-patient relationship (Conway-Klassen and Maness, 2017; SAMHSA, 2014).

In addition to one's self-examination regarding racial, ethnic, and cultural identities, one must also understand the process of adaptation when transition occurs. The process of acculturation occurs when an individual or group transitions from one culture and develops traits of another culture (Purnell, 2013; Spector, 2017). In this transition, there will be adaptation to the new cultures, traditions, customs, and language. This can lead to stress when the values of the transitioning culture differ from the accepted traits of another. Assimilation is the process in which the individual adapts to the host's cultural values and no longer prefers the components of the origin culture (Frazer, et al., 2017; Spector, 2017).

The National Institutes of Health (2018) has recently coined the term cultural respect, as opposed to cultural competence. Similar to cultural competence, cultural respect is critical to reducing health disparities and improving access to high-quality health care that is respectful and responsive to the needs of the diverse patient. With the growing number of diverse patient populations, the implementation of culturally respectful care is essential and benefits the consumers, stakeholders, and communities, leading to safe and positive health outcomes.

DISEASE AND ILLNESS

People react differently to disease based on their unique cultural perspective. Culture influences our thoughts regarding the way people uniquely define disease and illness. An understanding of the difference between disease and illness allows you to pursue ongoing cultural competence in providing patient care. Illness is the way in which individuals and families react to disease, whereas disease is a malfunctioning of biological or psychological processes. Most health care providers in the United States are primarily educated to treat disease, whereas most individuals seek health care because of their experience with illness. As an example, a patient may have a combination of symptoms that, based on previous experiences with family members and beliefs about illness, the patient believes are untreatable, whereas the patient's physician believes aggressive therapy might offer a cure. Such different perspectives between patients and their health care providers often frustrate patients and providers, fostering a lack of trust, lack of patient adherence to treatment plans, and poor health outcomes. Providing safe, quality care to all patients means taking into consideration both disease and illness (Office of Minority Health [OMH], n.d.).

Culture affects how an individual defines the meaning of illness (see Chapter 6). Some illnesses (e.g., human immunodeficiency virus [HIV], manic depression, cancer, or dementia) are embedded with meaning that is not always based on the physical nature of the condition. Cultural stigma can negatively affect those diagnosed; this can lead to lack of early detection, screening, or diagnosis based on the influence of cultural interpretation and decreased awareness. All illness is socially constructed through the experiences of people—specifically, how individuals come to understand and live with their illnesses (Conrad and Barker, 2010; Shiri et al, 2018). This is particularly true with chronic disease. Patients learn the effects of their diseases and how to adapt to live as normally as possible.

Culture also provides the context in which a person interacts with family members, peers, community members, and institutions (e.g., educational, religious, media, health care, legal). Therefore, culture and life experiences shape a person's world view about health, illness, and health care.

Core Measures

The Centers for Medicare & Medicaid Services (CMS), commercial insurance plans, TJC, Medicare and Medicaid managed-care plans, physician and other care provider organizations, and consumers worked together through the Core Quality Measures Collaborative to identify a set of core measures, which aim to hold health care providers accountable for considering patients' unique cultural perspectives to provide safe quality care (CMS, 2017). The core measures are a set of evidence-based, scientifically researched standards of care (CMS, 2017; TJC, 2018). The core measures are key quality indicators that help health care institutions improve performance, increase accountability, and reduce costs. The measures apply to all patients. The core measures need to be meaningful to patients, consumers, and physicians while reducing variability in outcome measure selection, financial collection burden, and cost (CMS, 2017). All the core measures are consistent with national health priorities and are in the following eight sets (CMS, 2017):

- Accountable care organizations (ACOs), patient-centered medical homes (PCMH), and primary care
- Cardiology
- Gastroenterology
- HIV and hepatitis C
- Medical oncology
- Obstetrics and gynecology
- Orthopedics
- Pediatrics

In addition to improving the standard of care, the core measures are intended to reduce health disparities. When hospitals are held accountable to meet the core quality measures, all patients regardless of cultural and socioeconomic status are to be treated equally because the standard of care applies to all. For example, one obstetrics and gynecology core measure is that women are to receive breast cancer screening (CMS, 2017). In another example, patients who present with heart failure are to receive beta blocker therapy for left ventricular systolic dysfunction (CMS, 2017).

A MODEL OF CULTURAL COMPETENCE

Ongoing development of cultural competence will present as your ability to interact effectively with people from different cultures, identifying the need to be respectful and responsive to the health belief practices or linguistic needs of our diverse population (SAMHSA, 2016). Cultural competence is a self-motivated developmental process that evolves over a lifetime as individuals engage with others and learn from their experiences (SAMHSA, 2016). One must look at cultural competency as a journey, not a destination (Montenery et al., 2013). Campinha-Bacote's model of cultural competency has five interrelated constructs (Transcultural C.A.R.E. Associates, 2015): cultural awareness, cultural knowledge, cultural skill, cultural encounters, and cultural desire. The five constructs provide a framework for you to practice in a culturally competent manner.

- Cultural awareness is the process of conducting a self-examination of one's own biases toward other cultures and the in-depth exploration of one's cultural and professional background. It also involves being aware of the existence of documented racism and other "isms" in health care delivery.

- **Cultural knowledge** is the process in which a health care professional seeks and obtains a sound educational base about culturally diverse groups. In acquiring this knowledge, health care professionals must focus on the integration of three specific issues: health-related beliefs and cultural values, care practices, and disease incidence and prevalence.
- **Cultural skill** is the ability to conduct a cultural assessment of a patient to collect relevant cultural data about a patient's presenting problem, as well as accurately conducting a culturally based physical assessment.
- **Cultural encounter** is a process that encourages health care professionals to directly engage in face-to-face cultural interactions and other types of encounters with patients from culturally diverse backgrounds. A cultural encounter aims to modify a health care provider's existing belief about a cultural group and to prevent possible stereotyping.
- **Cultural desire** is the motivation of a health care professional to "want to" (and not "have to") engage in the process of becoming culturally aware, culturally knowledgeable, and culturally skillful in seeking cultural encounters.

When you provide culturally competent care, you bridge cultural gaps to provide meaningful and supportive care for all patients. Transcultural care is culturally congruent when it fits a person's life patterns, values, and system of meaning. These patterns and meaning are generated by people themselves and not from biased, predetermined criteria. For example, during nursing school you are assigned to care for a female patient who observes Muslim beliefs. You notice the woman's discomfort with several of the male health care providers and you wonder if this discomfort is related to your patient's religious beliefs. While preparing for clinical, you learn that Muslims differ in their adherence to tradition but that modesty is an important Islamic ethic that pertains to interaction between the sexes. Thus you say to the patient, "I know that for many of our Muslim patients, modesty is very important. I want to respect your beliefs; is there some way I can make you more comfortable?" You do not assume that the information will automatically apply to this patient. Instead you combine your knowledge about a cultural group with an attitude of helpfulness and flexibility to provide quality, patient-centered, culturally congruent care. There is great diversity within cultural and racial groups themselves, and knowledge provides a general baseline, which is a great starting point in generating a positive patient outcome based on individual health care needs (Giger, 2017).

CULTURAL AWARENESS AND KNOWLEDGE

Cultural awareness requires a self-examination of one's biases toward other cultures and an in-depth exploration of one's own cultural and professional background (Ingram, 2011; Campinha-Bacote, 2002). Self-examination helps you to understand your own world view of how you perceive and engage patients. Before you begin to assess the cultures, races, and ethnicities of your patients and use this information to improve their care, first examine and understand your own cultural history, racial and ethnic heritage, and cultural values and beliefs (SAMHSA, 2014). Every individual is constructed from a unique cultural background, which can influence an individual's opinions, perceptions, beliefs, biases, or thoughts, thus forming a unique individual identity (Giger, 2017). Nurses who understand themselves and their own cultural groups and perceptions are better equipped to respect patients with diverse belief systems. Being open to understanding a patient's beliefs and forming a partnership is more important than knowing everything about a patient's specific culture (Ball et al., 2019). For example, you are giving discharge instruction to your patient. You

notice the patient is avoiding eye contact, and you perceive this as disrespectful or showing disinterest when, in fact, the patient's lack of eye contact is a sign of respect, as some cultures believe the lack of eye contact when in presence of an authority is expected. Becoming culturally aware is a first step in one's ability to provide positive patient-centered care.

Campinha-Bacote recommends that you begin to gain cultural awareness by not only asking yourself if you hold any biases but also questioning whether there are any "isms" where you work (Transcultural C.A.R.E. Associates, 2015). For example, are there ageism practices in how older adults have their pain treated (e.g., undertreatment)? Be mindful of such practices so that you can adopt care approaches that minimize biases.

Health care providers gain cultural knowledge by taking time to better understand the populations they serve and obtaining specific cultural knowledge as it relates to help seeking, treatment, and recovery (SAMHSA, 2014). Cultural knowledge is learning or becoming educated about the beliefs and values of other cultures and diverse ethnic groups (Campinha-Bacote, 2002). The health care provider must focus on their specific issues: (1) health-related beliefs and cultural values, (2) disease incidence and prevalence, and (3) treatment efficacy (Campinha-Bacote, 2002). Disease incidence and prevalence differ among ethnic groups. Epidemiological data are needed to guide treatment (Campinha-Bacote, 2002). Treatment efficacy is a critical step for providing care to culturally diverse populations.

One's health-related beliefs and cultural values explain how an illness is interpreted by a patient and will guide health care practices delivered throughout patient care. For example, certain cultures believe in the importance of balance and harmony to stay healthy. Aspects of this concept are evident among the beliefs of many Hispanic, Native American, Asian, and Middle Eastern groups (Ball et al., 2019). Box 9.2 summarizes the naturalistic or holistic balance that many people believe they can achieve by using "hot" and "cold" foods and medicines.

BOX 9.2 Balance of "HOT" and "COLD"

Cold Conditions	Hot Treatments	Hot Conditions	Cold Treatments
Cancer	**Foods**	Constipation	**Foods**
Cold, flu	Beef	Diarrhea	Barley water
Earaches	Cereals	Fever	Chicken
Headaches	Chili peppers	Infection	Dairy products
Joint pain	Chocolate	Kidney problems	Fresh vegetables
Menses	Eggs	Rash	Fruits
Pneumonia	Liquor	Sore throat	Honey
Stomach	Onions		**Medicines**
cramps	**Medicines**		**and Herbs**
	and Herbs		Bicarbonate of
	Anise		soda
	Aspirin		Milk of Magnesia
	Castor oil		Sage
	Cinnamon		
	Garlic		
	Ginger root		
	Iron		
	Penicillin		

Adapted from Ball JW, et al: *Seidel's guide to physical examination*, ed 9, St Louis, 2019, Elsevier; and Purnell LD: *Transcultural health care: a culturally competent approach*, ed 4, Philadelphia, 2013, FA Davis.

However, people from different cultures define "hot" and "cold" differently. For example, people who are of Chinese heritage often uphold the philosophical concept of yin (cold) and yang (hot). To restore (treat) a disturbed balance requires the use of opposites (e.g., a "hot" remedy for a "cold" problem and vice versa). If you know about a specific culture's risks for disease, you can focus your nursing history more appropriately during your assessment. If you learn that an individual believes in a "hot" and "cold" balance when choosing certain foods to eat, support your patient's practices, and adapt this information into the patient's dietary plan.

Do not form inappropriate biases or stereotypes when you assess a patient's culture. It is easy to stereotype various cultural groups after reading general information about their ethnic values, practices, and beliefs. Avoid stereotypes or unwarranted generalizations about any particular group that prevents an accurate assessment of an individual's unique characteristics and world view. Instead approach each person individually and ask questions to gain a better understanding of a patient's perspective and needs. Stereotyping occurs in two cognitive phases. In the first phase there is an activation of a stereotype when an individual is categorized into a social group. When this occurs, beliefs and prejudices come to mind about what members of that particular group are like (Ball et al., 2019). Stereotypical views eventually occur without awareness automatically. In the second phase, people use these activated beliefs and feelings when they interact with individuals (Ball et al., 2019). Research shows that health care providers activate these stereotypes or unconscious biases routinely when communicating with and providing care to minority individuals (Dayer-Berenson, 2014). As a result, diagnoses and treatments of patients may be biased even in the absence of the practitioner's intent or awareness.

REFLECT NOW

Consider a patient that you cared for recently. How did the patient's health-related beliefs and cultural values impact the decisions he or she made regarding their health concerns?

Storytelling

One way to begin to understand a patient's cultural perspective is storytelling. Storytelling conveys culture, combining personal experience with the commonalities of all human experiences (Wilson et al., 2015). When you encourage a patient to tell a story or when you tell your own story, you frame important messages in ways that make them memorable for you and your patient. Telling stories engages a nurse and patient in a way that broadens their relational understanding. Use storytelling to explore pertinent health care issues; for example, have patients describe previous surgical experiences, problems with childrearing, or approaches used with self-administration of medications. A story helps identify the real problems affecting a patient's health status and find culturally appropriate ways to intervene (Box 9.3).

World View of Providers and Patients

Health care has its own culture of hierarchies, power, values, beliefs, and practices. Most health care providers educated in Western traditions are immersed in the culture of science and biomedicine through their coursework and professional experience. Consequently, they often have a world view that differs from that of their patients. As a nurse, you need to assume that every patient encounter will be a cross-cultural one.

Patients and all their health care providers bring all their world views into the care process. The iceberg analogy is a tool that helps you visualize

BOX 9.3 EVIDENCE-BASED PRACTICE

Use of Storytelling and Patient Involvement in Health Care.

PICOT Question: Does the use of storytelling compared with standard assessment approaches among adult and pediatric patients affect patient involvement in selecting health care interventions?

Evidence Summary

A patient's ability to understand the complexities of many health issues and to be able to become engaged in decision making requires the ability to discuss and clarify confusing issues. Storytelling allows patients to reflect on their illness experience and create meaning from it (Gucciardi et al., 2016; Hardy and Sumner, 2018). Storytelling enhances self-management of chronic disease (e.g., cancer, diabetes). A recent study involved patients telling stories about their aspirations for the future (Terkildsen and Wittrup, 2015). The shared information allowed clinicians to initiate interventions based on patient experiences of health problems. When patients are able to express their experiences, there is a negotiation with health care providers that leads to a mutual plan of care.

Digital storytelling is also widely used, especially in pediatric patients. Digital storytelling gives children and adolescents with cancer a platform for making sense of and sharing their cancer experience (Wilson et al, 2015). Houston et al. (2011) used DVDs to deliver stories of real patients with hypertension to patients treated for hypertension. Patients with baseline uncontrolled hypertension who watched the storytelling DVDs had a greater reduction in systolic and diastolic blood pressure at 3 months compared with patients watching an attention DVD (a DVD on general health topics unrelated to hypertension). Technology can have a significant impact on providing respect, trust, and justice in patient care (Hardy and Sumner, 2018). The act of telling a story is valuable, allowing a patient to initiate the process of reflection to gain understanding of the self and the disease process (Gucciardi et al., 2016; Hardy & Sumner, 2018).

Application to Nursing Practice

- Create a safe, caring, and nonjudgmental environment when using storytelling (Gucciardi et al., 2016; Hardy and Sumner, 2018).
- Storytelling should be participant-centered; give patients substantial control over when and how to tell a story (Gucciardi et al., 2016).
- Use storytelling to clarify issues when performing a cultural assessment.
- When asking a patient to describe his or her major concerns about a health problem, try to use storytelling to frame the context of those concerns.
- Tell your own stories about patient experiences (respecting confidentiality) to help explain procedures or treatment plans.

the visible and invisible aspects of your own world view (Fig. 9.3). Just as most of an iceberg lies beneath the surface of the water, most aspects of a person's world view lie outside his or her awareness and are invisible to those around the person. For example, a patient who has willingly agreed to be admitted to the hospital for a serious medical condition requiring surgery may refuse the surgery for religious reasons. In the patient's view, she came to the hospital for help to eliminate the pain and infection from her illness. At the same time, she believes that she needs to seek God for a decision that entails removing a body part. The patient's health care provider assumes the patient is in the hospital to receive care for a serious illness and is willing to accept any and all treatments to cure the illness. The patient's deeply held religious beliefs about removing a body part are not obvious by assessing for a religious preference. Thus the nurse needs to conduct a comprehensive cultural assessment to understand how the patient's religious values will affect her willingness to receive care (Box 9.4). These deeply held values reside "underneath the iceberg." The

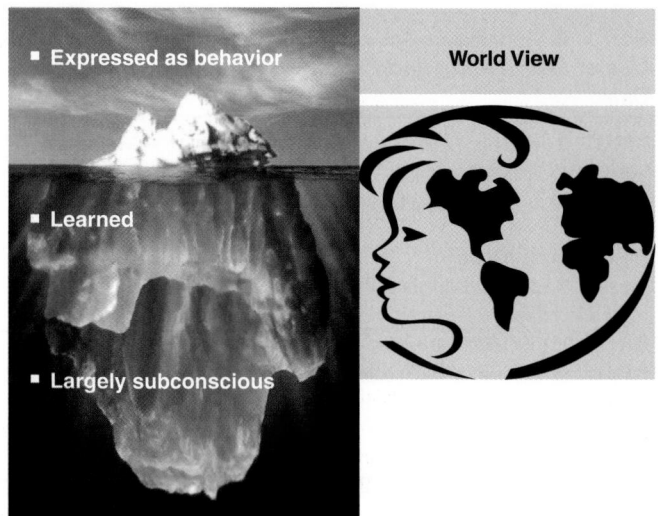

FIG. 9.3 Both nurse and patient act in accordance with their own world views. This model was adapted from Campinha-Bacote et al. (2005) Iceberg Analogy. It incorporates the Kleinman (1980) explanatory model. (Copyright © 2011 Barnes-Jewish Hospital Center for Diversity and Cultural Competence.)

observed behavior (in this case, coming to the hospital) is a visible sign of a person's world view, but the beliefs, attitudes, knowledge, and experiences that guide the behavior are not visible to others. Conflict arises when health care providers interpret the behaviors of patients through their own world view lens instead of trying to uncover the world view that guides the behavior of their patients.

CULTURAL SKILL

Collecting a culturally based nursing history, performing a culturally based physical assessment, and using teach-back with plain language are cultural skills that take practice and require you to apply your cultural awareness and knowledge. The summary of the domains of culture is a framework for the information you might choose to include in a nursing history (Purnell, 2013) (Box 9.5). It takes time to gather a comprehensive culturally based nursing history. If you work in a setting such as home health, school nursing, or a health clinic, you will be able to gather more information with each patient visit. When you are in an acute setting, you must focus your assessment on the domains most relevant to a patient's condition and the impending treatment plan. For example, if you know a patient will require extensive postoperative education, it will be important to assess the patient's and family's language, family roles, and health care practices.

Collecting a Patient History

Begin a patient assessment by being mindful that cultural differences will exist. It is important to grasp exactly what the patient means and know exactly what the patient thinks you mean in words and actions (Ball et al., 2019). Do not make assumptions. Listen carefully, let patients tell their stories, rephrase statements for clarity, and validate any assumptions you make about the patient's condition or health care needs with the patient. As you perform an assessment, the patient may hesitate to offer his or her beliefs and fears, a hesitancy that can be overcome through respectful, nonjudgmental questioning (see Box 9.4). Have a patient help set the agenda for the visit to help you better understand the patient's needs.

A cultural assessment is intrusive and time consuming and requires a trusting relationship between participants. Misunderstandings due

---

BOX 9.4   Cultural Assessment Guide: Aspects of Understanding

Health Beliefs and Practices
- How does the patient define health and illness? How are feelings concerning pain, fatigue, and illness in general expressed?
- Are particular methods used for the treatment of illness?
- What is the attitude toward preventive health measures such as immunizations?
- Are there restrictions imposed by modesty that must be respected (e.g., constraints related to exposure of parts of the body, discussion of sexual health)?
- What are attitudes toward mental illness, pain, chronic disease, being handicapped, and death and dying?
- Is there a person in the family responsible for health-related decisions?
- Does the patient prefer a health professional of the same gender, age, and ethnic and racial background?

Faith-Based Influences and Special Rituals
- Is there a religion or faith to which the patient adheres?
- Is there a significant person to whom the patient looks for guidance?
- What events, rituals, and ceremonies are important within the life cycle of birth, puberty, marriage, and death?

Language and Communication
- What language is spoken in the home?
- How well does the patient understand spoken and written English?
- Are there special signs of demonstrating respect or disrespect?
- Is touch an acceptable form of communication?

Parenting Styles and Family Roles
- Who makes the decisions in the family?
- What is the composition of the family? How many generations are considered to be a single family?
- What is the role of and attitude toward children in the family?
- When do children need to be disciplined or punished, and how is this done?
- Do family members show physical affection toward each other and their children?
- What major events are important to the family, and how do they celebrate?

Sources of Support Beyond the Family
- Are there ethnic organizations that may influence the patient's approach to health care?
- Are there individuals in the patient's social network that influence perception of health and illness?
- Is there a particular cultural group with which the patient identifies?

Dietary Practices
- What does the family like to eat? Does everyone in the family have similar tastes in food?
- Who is responsible for food preparation?
- Are any foods forbidden by the culture, or are some foods a cultural requirement in observance of a rite or ceremony?
- How is food prepared and eaten?
- Are there periods of required fasting?

Adapted from Ball JW, et al: *Seidel's guide to physical examination,* ed 9, St Louis, 2019, Elsevier.

---

to inappropriate communication between a health care provider and the patient are a barrier to accessing health care (Hadziabdic et al., 2015). Misunderstandings occur because of language communication differences between and among participants and differences in interpreting one another's behaviors. **Linguistic competence** is the ability

BOX 9.5   The Twelve Domains of Culture

- Overview, inhabited localities—country of origin and current residence
- Communication—interrelationship of verbal language skills, including dominant language, dialects, touch, contextual use of language, and willingness to share information
- Family roles and organization—defines relationship of insiders and outsiders; includes concepts related to head of household, gender roles, family goals and priorities, and developmental goals of family members
- Workforce issues—type of employment, location, autonomy, language barriers
- Biocultural ecology—skin color, heredity, genetics, drug metabolism
- High-risk behaviors—tobacco, alcohol, recreational drugs, physical activity, safety
- Nutrition—meaning of foods, common foods, deficiencies, rituals, limitations
- Pregnancy and childbearing practices—fertility practices, views toward pregnancy, birthing, postpartum
- Death rituals—bereavement, ceremonies
- Spirituality—religious practices, use of prayer, meaning of life
- Health care practices—focus of health care, traditional practices, responsibility for health, self-medication, pain, sick role, barriers
- Health care providers—perceptions of providers, folk practitioners, gender, and health care status

Adapted from Purnell LD: *Transcultural health care: a culturally competent approach*, ed 4, Philadelphia, 2013, FA Davis.

to communicate effectively and convey information in a manner that is easily understood by diverse audiences. You use transcultural communication skills to interpret a patient's behavior and to behave in a culturally congruent way.

The National Culturally and Linguistically Appropriate Services (CLAS) Standards are intended to advance health equity, improve quality, and help eliminate health care disparities by establishing a blueprint to help individuals and health care organizations implement culturally and linguistically appropriate services (Office of Minority Health [OMH], n.d.). The CLAS standards include standards for communication and language assistance. The standards apply when you care for patients who have limited English proficiency and/or other communication needs. All US health care organizations must meet the following requirements:

- Provide language assistance resources (e.g., trained medical interpreters, qualified translators, telecommunication devices for the deaf) for individuals who have limited English proficiency and/or other communication needs, at no cost to them, to facilitate timely access to all health care and services.
- Inform all individuals of the availability of language assistance services clearly and in their preferred language verbally and in writing.
- Ensure the competence of individuals providing language assistance. Do not use untrained individuals and/or minors as interpreters.
- Provide easy-to-understand print and multimedia materials and signage in the languages commonly used by the populations in the service area.

When you begin a cultural assessment there are some basic questions that can help you explore a patient's culture (Ball et al., 2019):

- What do you call your problem?
- What do you think caused it?
- Why do you think it started when it did?
- What does your sickness do to you?
- How long do you think it will last?

- How different is this problem from the one you had a month ago?
- What is the difference between what we are doing and what you think we should be doing for you?
- Why did you come to us for treatment?
- What benefit do you expect from the treatment?
- How do you typically deal with a problem with your health?

Each question requires an open-ended response, enabling you to gain important details about a patient's perceptions, values, and attitudes. A patient's answer to a question may allow you to explore his or her cultural background more thoroughly.

After realizing that Ms. Millman needs help to better understand the types of foods that are appropriate for a diabetic diet, Hannah refocuses her assessment on some basic questions. How do you think the foods that you eat affect your diabetes? What does diabetes do to you if your blood sugar becomes too high? What benefit will you get from eating healthy foods? Tell me what you eat during a typical day.

Culture influences how feelings are expressed verbally and nonverbally. Verbal and nonverbal communication is an important core of all health care encounters (Hadziabdic et al., 2015). Touch, facial expressions, eye contact, movement, and body posture all have varying significance. The questions in Box 9.4 can help provide further insight to particular situations and help avoid misunderstanding and miscommunication (Ball et al., 2019).

Assessing Health Literacy

Health literacy is the degree to which individuals have the capacity to obtain, process, and understand basic health information and the services needed to make appropriate health decisions (AHRQ, 2015). According to the IOM, 90 million adult Americans have limited health literacy, and 20 million Americans speak poor English and 10 million speak none (NIH, n.d.). Limited health literacy can be a problem for anyone. It is important to understand that even people with good literacy skills find that understanding health care information is a challenge. Patients and family members often do not understand medical vocabulary and the basic concepts in health and medicine, such as how the body works or how to navigate the health care system. During your assessment, be alert for patient behaviors that might reflect a literacy deficit such as having difficulty completing registration forms or health histories, failing to make follow-up appointments, asking few questions during a physical examination, and responding simply "yes" when asked whether explanations are understood. Use health literacy assessment tools to determine the level of a patient's health literacy (AHRQ, 2015). Examples of these tools include:

- The Short Assessment of Health Literacy—Spanish and English (SAHL-S&E) is an instrument consisting of comparable tests in English and Spanish, with good reliability and validity in both languages (Lee et al., 2010).
- The Rapid Estimate of Adult Literacy in Medicine—Short Form (REALM-SF) is a seven-item word recognition test to provide clinicians with a valid quick assessment of patient health literacy (Arozullah et al., 2007). The REALM-SF has been validated and field-tested in diverse research settings.

Assessing a patient's health literacy level is very important in planning appropriate patient education approaches (AHRQ, 2015) (see Chapter 25).

Culturally Based Physical Assessment

When performing a physical assessment, knowledge about a patient directs your physical assessment (see Chapter 30). For example, if you know a patient has diabetes for many years, you focus on the peripheral vascular examination because of the common incidence of circulatory problems in patients with diabetes. If a patient uses an inhaler for asthma, you perform a more detailed assessment of the lungs compared with what you might do for a healthy patient you see during a routine checkup.

Similarly, you learn to anticipate physical findings based on a patient's cultural health practices and distinguish physical characteristics of an ethnic or racial group. There are several ways individuals from one cultural group can differ biologically from members of other cultural groups (Giger, 2017). For example, Mongolian blue spots are a dark pigmented birthmark that may appear shortly after birth on the buttocks, lower back, arms, or legs of dark skin and should not be mistaken for bruising and a signs of abuse. Another example includes the practices of "coining" and "cupping," which are commonly used by some Asian subcultures to release excess force from the body and restore balance (Ball et al., 2019). The practices leave imprints and markings on the skin that can be wrongly interpreted as signs of abuse or disease. Thus it is always important to ask patients about their home remedies and practices. Another example of anticipating findings is to consider sickle cell anemia when blood tests reveal laboratory values that show anemia in a patient of African descent. As you practice and become more knowledgeable of different ethnic groups in your practice, you will more readily recognize physical characteristics of conditions unique to those groups.

Teach-Back and Plain Language

Linguistic competence requires the application of health literacy principles in providing readily available, culturally appropriate oral and written language services to patients and families with limited English proficiency (AHRQ, 2013). The dual challenges of caring for patients with limited health literacy and cultural differences are likely to increase with an expanding, increasingly diverse, and older population. Evidence suggests that health care providers who attend to both issues help reduce medical errors and improve adherence, communication between provider and patient and family, and outcomes of care at both individual and population levels (Lie et al., 2012). Clear communication is essential for effective delivery of quality and safe health care, but most patients experience significant challenges when communicating with their health care providers. Studies show that 40% to 80% of the medical information given to patients during medical office visits is immediately forgotten, and nearly half of the information retained is incorrect (AHRQ, 2018b).

The use of plain language in communicating with patients makes any information you provide easy to read, understand, and use. Plain language is grammatically correct language that includes complete sentence structure and accurate word usage (National Institutes of Health [NIH], n.d.). The Federal Plain Language Guidelines (2011) provide guidance on improving communication through writing. Clear communication is a priority in providing patient care. Written education must be based on specific patient needs. You can find the tips for writing in plain language from the PlainLanguage.gov website: https://www.plainlanguage.gov-/media/FederalPLGuidelines.pdf. Offering patients clear instructions and educational material written in plain language conveys to a learner exactly what to know without using unnecessary words or expressions.

Use the teach-back method following any patient instruction to confirm that you have explained what a patient needs to know in a manner that the patient understands (Fig. 9.4). The teach-back technique is an ongoing process of asking patients for feedback through explanation or demonstration and of presenting information in a new way until you feel confident that you communicated clearly and that your patient fully understands the information presented (Box 9.6). When a family caregiver is the recipient of your instruction, use teach-back to confirm his or her learning. You also use teach-back to identify explanations and communication strategies your patients most commonly understand (AHRQ, 2018a).

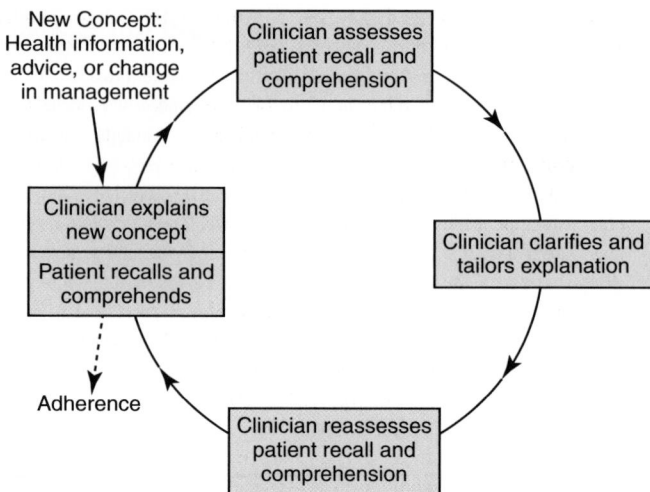

FIG. 9.4 Using the teach-back technique to close the loop. (From the US Health Resources and Services Administration.)

BOX 9.6 PATIENT TEACHING
Medication and Nutritional Adherence

Hannah knows it is important for Ms. Millman to understand her health problems and prescribed treatments. Thus Hannah plans to use teach-back to ensure Ms. Millman understands how to effectively manage her diabetes.

Outcome
At the end of the teaching session, Ms. Millman will be able to:
- Describe how she plans to make healthy food choices at the shelter and neighborhood store.

Teaching Strategies
- Create a shame-free environment by demonstrating a general attitude of helpfulness.
- Use nonmedical language and define in plain language all medical terms.
- Sit instead of stand, and speak slowly.
- Use pictures, models, and written handouts to help Ms. Millman better remember relevant information.
- Have Ms. Millman prepare a meal plan.

Evaluation
Use the principles of teach-back to evaluate patient/family caregiver learning:
- Tell me two strategies that you will use to make healthy food choices when shopping at your neighborhood grocery store.
- We've gone over a lot of information today about changes you plan to make to your diet. In your own words, please review what we talked about. Tell me how you will follow your diet?

When using the teach-back technique, do not ask a patient, "Do you understand?" or "Do you have any questions?" Instead ask open-ended questions to verify a patient's understanding. Some examples include:
- "I've given you a lot of information (e.g., about your insulin) to remember. Please explain it (e.g., how it affects your blood sugar) to me so that I can be sure that I gave you the information you want and need to take good care of yourself."
- "What will you tell your wife (or husband/partner/child) about the changes we made to your medications today?"
- "We've gone over a lot of information today about how you might change your diet, and I want to make sure I explained everything clearly. In your own words, please review what we talked about. How will you follow this diet at home?"

Teach-back is not intended to test a patient but rather to confirm the clarity of your communication (AHRQ, 2018a). Many patients are embarrassed by their inability to sort out health information or instructions. By regarding teach-back as a test of your communication skills, you take responsibility for the success or failure of the interaction and create a shame-free environment for your patients. Following are helpful hints to consider when trying the teach-back method (AHRQ, 2018a).

- Plan your approach. Think about how you will ask your patient to teach back in a shame-free way. Keep in mind that some situations are not appropriate for teach-back.
- Use handouts, pictures, and models to reinforce your teaching.
- "Chunk and check." Do not wait until the end of the visit to initiate teach-back. Chunk out information into small segments and have the patient or family caregiver teach it back. Repeat several times during a visit.
- Clarify and check again. If teach-back uncovers a misunderstanding, explain things again using a different approach. Ask patients to teach-back again until they are able to correctly describe the information in their own words. If they parrot your words back to you, they may not have understood.
- Start slowly and use teach-back consistently. Practice. It will take a little time, but once it is part of your routine, teach-back can be done without awkwardness.
- Use the show-me method. When prescribing new medicines or changing a dose, research shows that even when patients correctly say when and how much medicine they will take, many will make mistakes when asked to demonstrate the dose.
- Clarify. If a patient cannot remember or accurately repeat your instructions, clarify your information, and allow him or her to teach it back again (see Box 9.6).
- Although it takes time to get used to teach-back, studies show that it does not take longer to perform once it becomes a part of your routine (AHRQ, 2018a). *Box 9.6 provides an example of how Hannah used some of these strategies to educate Ms. Millman on how to manage her diet.*

Working With Interpreters

The National CLAS Standards (OMH, n.d.) ensure that qualified translators (written words) and interpreters (verbal words) be provided to patients with limited English proficiency. The CLAS standards require you to notify patients both verbally and in writing of their rights to receive language assistance. If a health care setting does not have timely access to an interpreter, a more feasible option is the use of a telephone service that provides an on-call trained interpreter connected by phone (Juckett and Unger, 2014). Ensure that interpreters are competent in medical terminology and understand issues of confidentiality and impartiality. If available, a cultural broker may be utilized as an interpreter, advocate, or mediator that bridges between the individual or group (Dayer-Berenson, 2014). Do not use a patient's family members to interpret for you or other health care providers. The family member may include his or her own perception or opinion in translation, which can greatly reduce the accuracy of the translated information (Dayer-Berenson, 2014). When you begin a patient interview with an interpreter present, you should speak in the first person ("I" statements), not the third person (e.g., "tell her," "he said"), and speak directly to the patient, as the interpreter functions as an inconspicuous participant for the conversation (Juckett and Unger, 2014). Have the interpreter sit next to or slightly behind the patient. Look at the patient instead of looking at the interpreter and speak in short sentences; then wait for the interpreter to convey them (Juckett and Unger, 2014). Avoid using jargon, acronyms, and jokes; attempts at humor are often lost in interpretation. Ask the patient for feedback and clarification at regular intervals. Be observant of the patient's nonverbal and verbal behaviors. At the end of a conversation thank both the patient and the interpreter.

CULTURAL ENCOUNTER

In every health care setting you will directly interact with patients from culturally diverse backgrounds. This interaction is a cultural encounter, which has two goals (Campinha-Bacote, 2007). One goal is to communicate in a way that generates a wide variety of responses and to send and receive both verbal and nonverbal communication accurately and appropriately in each culturally different context. The second goal is to continuously interact with patients from culturally diverse backgrounds to validate, refine, or modify existing values, beliefs, and practices about a cultural group.

CULTURAL DESIRE

Engaging with people we perceive as "different" from us can be threatening and difficult. It generally takes more effort and patience than engaging with patients who are more similar to us. Cultural desire refers to having the motivation to engage patients so that you understand them from a cultural perspective. It is the pivotal and key construct of cultural competence, for it is a nurse's desire that evokes the entire process of cultural competence (Campinha-Bacote, 2003). Cultural desire involves the concept of caring (see Chapter 7). Establishing a caring relationship with a patient requires you to enter into the patient's world view. Cultural desire includes a genuine passion to be open and flexible with others, to accept differences and build on similarities, and to be willing to learn from others as cultural informants (Campinha-Bacote, 2003).

You will care for patients who display behaviors that may be in direct moral conflict with your own values (e.g., abortion, substance abuse, spouse abuse). For example, you are asked to care for a young male gang member whose beliefs about violence and respect for life are in direct contrast to yours. Yet you care for this patient nonjudgmentally and with respect. Acquiring the willingness to practice cultural desire requires a respect and acceptance of all human beings. The LEARN Model (Campinha-Bacote, 2003) can assist with this process. The mnemonic *LEARN* represents the process of listening, explaining, acknowledging, recommending, and negotiating:

- *Listen* to the patient's perception of the problem. Be nonjudgmental and use encouraging comments, such as "Tell me more" or "I understand what you are saying."
- *Explain* your perception of the problem.
- *Acknowledge* not only the differences between the two perceptions of the problem but also the similarities. Recognize the differences but build on the similarities.
- *Recommendations* must involve the patient.
- *Negotiate* a treatment plan, considering that it is beneficial to incorporate selected aspects of the patient's culture into the plan.

Applying the LEARN mnemonic will help you to reflect at each patient encounter. You recognize that each patient is unique, but you are responsible for understanding what "unique" truly means so that you can engage patients in a patient-centered approach to care.

> **QSEN** **Building Competency in Patient-Centered Care** Mrs. Addelman is 28 years old and 39 weeks pregnant. She has been under medical care since the pregnancy was discovered. At this time, Mrs. Addelman is in labor, and an emergency C-section is needed. She refuses to allow the health care team to prepare her for the C-section until her husband arrives. Her family practices the Muslim faith. What are your concerns related to Mrs. Addelman? What are some steps you, as the nurse, can take to assist?
>
> Answers to QSEN Activities can be found on the Evolve website.

KEY POINTS

- Cultural awareness self-examines the dynamics of personal biases, stereotypes, values, and beliefs related to others different from one's own heritage, while cultural encounter is directly interacting with patients of a diverse population other than one's own.
- Cultural desire is the pivotal and key construct of cultural competence. It is your desire to engage with patients who have cultural differences that evokes the entire process of cultural competence.
- A person's culture and life experiences shape his or her world view about health, illness, and health care.
- Poor health, disease risk factors, poor health outcomes, and limited access to health care are types of preventable health care disparities often interrelated and influenced by the conditions and social context in which people live.
- Disparities in access to quality health care, preventive health care, and health education contribute to poor population health.
- Social determinants of health are defined by conditions in which people are born, grow, live, work, and age.
- Health care systems and providers contribute to the problem of health disparities as a result of inadequate resources, poor patient-provider communication, a lack of culturally competent care, system fragmentation, and inadequate access to language services.
- People who are marginalized are more likely to have poor health outcomes and to die at an early age because of a complex interaction among individual behaviors, public and health policy, cultural factors, and access to and quality of health care.
- Gaining cultural knowledge and conducting a self-examination allows a health care provider to understand the cultural factors that shape a patient's life experiences, a patient's health care problems, a patient's behavior, and how a patient might perceive those problems while building a positive nurse-patient relationship.
- Cultural respect is critical to reducing health disparities and improving access to high-quality health care that is respectful and responsive to the needs of a diverse patient.
- Avoid forming inappropriate biases or stereotypes when assessing a patient's needs. Approach each person individually and ask questions to gain a better understanding of a patient's perspective and needs.
- Ongoing cultural competence and cultural skill are necessary for a nurse to complete a cultural assessment and provide culturally appropriate nursing care for each patient, regardless of the patient's cultural background.
- Knowledge about your patient directs your physical assessment, and the health care provider must learn to anticipate physical findings based on the patient's cultural health practices and the physical characteristics of an ethnic or racial group.
- Teach-back is an ongoing process of asking patients open-ended questions to gather feedback through explanation or demonstration until the health care provider feels confident in the patient's ability to understand and safely apply the new educational content.
- Linguistic competence is the ability to communicate effectively and convey information in a manner that is easily understood by diverse audiences.
- Effective communication is a critical skill in culturally competent care and helps you engage a patient and family in a respectful, patient-centered dialogue. Qualified translators (written words), interpreters (verbal words), and/or the use of a cultural broker (mediator) are options to be utilized to assist with linguistic needs related to effective communication.

REFLECTIVE LEARNING

- Consider a patient that you cared for recently on the clinical unit. How did knowledge of your patient's culture impact your nursing care?
- Discuss some of the social determinants of health that you identified while conducting your assessment of the patient. How have these impacted the health of the patient?
- Review your personal approach to patient education when working with a patient who has a different cultural background from your own. Remember, the teach-back method is a valuable tool for all health care providers to use with each patient. As the health care provider, did you do the following?
  - Use a caring tone of voice and attitude?
  - Display comfortable body language, make eye contact, and sit down at the patient's level?
  - Ask open-ended questions?
  - Take responsibility for making sure the instructions were clear and understood?
  - Use print materials that were reader friendly to support learning?
  - Observe the patient's response to teach-back?

REVIEW QUESTIONS

1. Which of the following is an example of a patient with a health disparity? (Select all that apply.)
   1. A patient who has a homosexual sexual preference
   2. A patient unable to access primary care services
   3. A patient living with a chronic disease
   4. A family who relies on public transportation
   5. A patient who has had a history of smoking for 10 years
2. A 35-year-old woman has Medicaid coverage for herself and two young children. She missed an appointment at the local health clinic to get an annual mammogram because she has no transportation. She gets the annual screening because her mother had breast cancer. Which of the following are social determinants of this woman's health? (Select all that apply.)
   1. Medicaid insurance
   2. Annual screening
   3. Mother's history of breast cancer
   4. Lack of transportation
   5. Woman's age
3. During a nursing assessment a patient displayed several behaviors. Which behavior suggests the patient may have a health literacy problem?
   1. Patient has difficulty completing a registration form at a medical office
   2. Patient asks for written information about a health topic
   3. Patient speaks Spanish as primary language
   4. Patient states unfamiliarity with a newly ordered medicine
4. A nurse desires to communicate with a young woman who is Serbian and who has limited experience with being in a hospital. The nurse has 10 years of experience caring for Serbian women. The patient was admitted for a serious pregnancy complication. Apply the LEARN model and match the nurse's behaviors with each step of the model.

   1. L _____   a. The nurse notes that she has learned that fathers can visit mothers at any time in both Serbia and the United States.

   2. E _____   b. The nurse shares her perception of the woman's experiences as a patient.

   3. A _____   c. The nurse asks the patient how she can maintain bed rest when she returns home.

4. R _____ d. The nurse attends to the patient and listens to her story about hospitals in Serbia.

5. N _____ e. The nurse involves the patient in a discussion of the treatment options for her condition.

5. Health care organizations must provide which of the following based on federal civil rights laws? (Select all that apply.)
   1. Provide language assistance services at all points of contact free of charge.
   2. Provide auxiliary aids and services, such as interpreters, note takers, and computer-aided transcription services.
   3. Use patients' family members to interpret difficult topics.
   4. Ensure that interpreters are competent in medical terminology.
   5. Provide language assistance to all patients who speak limited English or are deaf.

6. A nurse working in a large occupational health clinic knows that many of the workers at her company are marginalized and at risk for poor health outcomes. Which of the following individuals are most likely to be marginalized?
   1. Wives of the employees
   2. The head supervisors of the company
   3. Workers who have a high school education
   4. Workers employed for less than a year at the company

7. A mother is concerned about her child's flulike symptoms. You learn from the health assessment that the mother practices use of "hot" and "cold" foods to treat ailments. Which of the following foods do you expect the mother to use to treat her child?
   1. Chicken
   2. Yogurt
   3. Fresh fruits
   4. Eggs

8. Which explanation provided by the nurse is the most accurate meaning for "providing culturally congruent care"?
   1. It fits the patient's valued life patterns and set of meanings.
   2. It is the same set of values as those of the health care team member providing daily care.
   3. It holds one's own way of life as superior to those of others.
   4. It redirects the patient to a more socially expected set of values.

9. Which statement made by a new graduate nurse about the teach-back technique requires intervention and further instruction by the nurse's preceptor?
   1. "After teaching a patient how to use an inhaler, I need to use the teach-back technique to test my patient's technique."
   2. "The teach-back technique is an ongoing process of asking patients for feedback."
   3. "Using teach-back will help me identify explanations and communication strategies that my patients will most commonly understand."
   4. "Using pictures, drawings, and models can enhance the effectiveness of the teach-back technique."

10. Match the cultural concepts on the left with the correct definitions on the right.
    1. Etic world view _____ a. Factor that shapes how people perceive others and how they relate to reality
    2. World view _____ b. Insider's perspective in an intercultural encounter
    3. Cultural desire _____ c. A policy model that describes factors and power structures that shape and influence life
    4. Intersectionality _____ d. An outsider's perspective in an intercultural encounter
    5. Emic world view _____ e. The motivation of a health care professional to "want to" engage in cultural competency

Answers: 1. 2, 3, 5; **2.** 1, 4, 5; **3.** 1, 4; **4.** 1d, 2b, 3a, 4e, 5c; **5.** 1, 2, 4, 5; **6.** 3; **7.** 4; **8.** 1; **9.** 1; **10.** 1d, 2a, 3e, 4c, 5b.

Rationales for Review Questions can be found on the Evolve website.

REFERENCES

Administration for Community Living: *Projected future growth of older population*, 2017. https://www.acl.gov/index.php/aging-and-disability-in-america/data-and-research/projected-future-growth-of-older-population. Accessed January 2019.

Agency for Healthcare Research and Quality (AHRQ): *What is cultural and linguistic competence*, 2013. http://www.ahrq.gov/professionals/systems/primary-care/cultural-competence-mco/cultcompdef.html. Accessed January 2019.

Agency for Healthcare Research and Quality (AHRQ): *Health literacy measurement tools (revised)*, 2015. http://www.ahrq.gov/professionals/quality-patient-safety/quality-resources/tools/literacy/index.html. Accessed January 2019.

Agency for Healthcare Research and Quality (AHRQ): *2016 National healthcare quality and disparities report*, 2017. https://www.ahrq.gov/sites/default/files/wysiwyg/research/findings/nhqrdr/nhqdr16/final2016qdr-cx.pdf. Accessed January 2019.

Agency for Healthcare Research and Quality (AHRQ): (2018) *Guide to improving patient safety in primary care settings by engaging patients and families*, 2018a. https://www.ahrq.gov/professionals/quality-patient-safety/patient-family-engagement/pfeprimarycare/teachback.html. Accessed January 2019.

Agency for Healthcare Research and Quality (AHRQ): *2015 national healthcare quality and disparities report and 5th Anniversary Update on the national quality Strategy*, 2018b. http://www.ahrq.gov/research/findings/nhqrdr/nhqdr15/index.html. Accessed January 2019.

Ball JW, et al.: *Seidel's guide to physical examination*, ed 9, St Louis, 2019, Elsevier.

Campinha-Bacote J: *The process of cultural competence in the delivery of healthcare services: the journey continues*, ed 5, Cincinnati, OH, 2007, Transcultural C.A.R.E. Associates.

Centers for Disease Control and Prevention (CDC): *CDC health disparities and inequalities report (CHDIR)*, 2013. https://www.cdc.gov/minorityhealth/chdireport.html. Accessed January 2019.

Centers for Disease Control and Prevention (CDC): *Health literacy*, 2018. https://www.cdc.gov/healthliteracy/researchevaluate/evidence-research.html. Accessed January 2019.

Chavez AF, Guido-DiBrito F: *Racial and ethnic identity, new directions for adult and continuing education (84)*, Winter Jossey/Wiley Bass Publishers, 1999.

Colby SL, Ortman JM: *Projections of the size and composition of the U.S. population 2014 to 2060*, US Census Bureau, 2015. https://www.census.gov/content/dam/Census/library/publications/2015/demo/p25-1143.pdf. Accessed January 2019.

Centers for Disease Control and Prevention (CDC): *CDC selected CDC-sponsored interventions – United States*, 2016. https://www.cdc.gov/minorityhealth/strategies2016/index.html. Accessed January 2019.

Centers for Medicare & Medicaid (CMS): *Core measures*, 2017. https://www.cms.gov/Medicare/Quality-Initiatives-Patient-Assessment-Instruments/QualityMeasures/Core-Measures.html. Accessed January 2019.

Dayer-Berenson L: *Cultural competencies for nurses*, ed 2, Burlington, MA, 2014, Jones and Bartlett Learning, LCC.

Edelstein S: *Food, cuisine and cultural competency for culinary, hospitality and healthcare professionals*, Sudbury, MA, 2011, Jones & Bartlett.

Ellis-Fletcher SN: *Cultural sensibility in healthcare: a personal & professional handbook*, Indianapolis, IN, 2015, Sigma Theta Tau International.

Giddens JF: *Concepts for nursing practice*, ed 2, St Louis, 2017, Elsevier, p 2017.

Giger J: *Transcultural nursing*, ed 7, St Louis, 2017, Elsevier.

Goldbach J: *Diversity toolkit: a guide to discussing identity, power, and privilege*, University of California, 2019. https://msw.usc.edu/mswusc-blog/diversity-workshop-guide-to-discussing-identity-power-and-privilege/. Accessed January 2019.

Institute of Medicine (IOM): *Crossing the quality chasm: a new health system for the 21st century*, Washington DC, 2001, National Academy of Sciences, National Academies Press.

Kleinman A: *Patients and healers in the context of culture*, Berkeley, 1980, University of California Press.

Leininger M, McFarland M: *Culture care diversity and universality: a worldwide nursing theory*, ed 2, Sudbury, MA, 2006, Jones and Bartlett.

Lopez N, Gadsden V: Health inequities, social determinants, and intersectionality, *National Academy of Medicine* 2016, 2016. https://nam.edu/wp-content/uploads/2016/12/Health-Inequities-Social-Determinants-and-Intersectionality.pdf. Accessed January 2019.

McFarland MR, Wehbe-Alamah HB: *Leininger's culture care diversity and universality: a worldwide nursing theory*, Burlington, MA, 2015, Jones and Bartlett Learning, LCC.

Mutha S, et al.: *Bringing equity into quality improvement: an overview and opportunities ahead*, San Francisco, 2012, Healthforce Center at UCSF. https://healthforce. ucsf.edu/sites/healthforce.ucsf.edu/files/publication-pdf/6.1%20Part%201%20_Equity%20into%20QI.pdf. Accessed January 2019.

National Institutes of Health (NIH): (n.d.): Clear communication. https://www.nih.gov/institutes-nih/nih-office-director/office-communications-public-liaison/clear-communication. Accessed January 2019.

National Institutes of Health (NIH): *Clear communication: cultural respect*, 2018. https://www.nih.gov/institutes-nih/nih-office-director/office-communications-public-liaison/clear-communication/cultural-respect. Accessed January 2019.

National Quality Forum (NQF): *Disparities*, 2018. http://www.qualityforum.org/Topics/Disparities.aspx. Accessed January 2019.

Office of Minority Health (OMH), US Department of Health and Human Services (USDHHH): (n.d.): National standards for culturally and linguistically appropriate services (CLAS) in health and health care. https://www.thinkculturalhealth.hhs.gov/assets/pdfs/EnhancedNationalCLASStandards.pdf. Accessed January 2019.

Office of Disease Prevention and Health Promotion (ODPHP): Disparities. https://www.healthypeople.gov/2020/about/foundation-health-measures/Disparities, 2016. Accessed January 2019.

Pew Research Center: *5 key takeaways about views of race and inequality in America*, 2016. http://www.pewresearch.org/fact-tank/2016/06/27/key-takeaways-race-and-inequality/. Accessed January 2019.

PlainLanguageGov: *Federal plain language guidelines*, 2011. https://www.plainlanguage.gov/media/FederalPLGuidelines.pdf. Accessed January 2019.

Purnell LD: *Transcultural health care: a culturally competent approach*, ed 4, Philadelphia, PA, 2013, FA Davis.

Spector R: *Cultural diversity in health and illness*, ed 9, Stamford, Ct, 2017, Appleton Lange.

The Joint Commission (TJC): *Measures*, 2018. http://www.jointcommission.org/core_measure_sets.aspx. Accessed January 2019.

The Substance Abuse and Mental Health Services Administration: *Cultural competence*, 2016. https://www.samhsa.gov/section-223/cultural-competency. Accessed July 2019.

The Substance Abuse and Mental Health Services Administration (SAMHSA): *Improving cultural competence. Treatment improvement Protocol (TIP) Series No. 59. HHS Publication No. (SMA) 14-4849*, Rockville, MD, 2014, Substance Abuse and Mental Health Services Administration.

Transcultural C.A.R.E. Associates: *The process of cultural competence in the delivery of healthcare services*, 2015. http://transculturalcare.net/the-process-of-cultural-competence-in-the-delivery-of-healthcare-services/. Accessed January 2019.

United Health Foundation: *America's annual report health rankings*, 2015. http://assets.americashealthrankings.org/app/uploads/2015ahr_annual-v1.pdf. Accessed January 2019.

US Census Bureau: *Demographic turning points for the United States population projection for 2020-2060*, 2018. https://www.census.gov/content/dam/Census/library/publications/2015/demo/p25-1143.pdf. Accessed January 2019.

US Department of Health and Human Services (USDHHS), Office of Minority Health (OMH): (n.d.): Think cultural health: national standards for culturally and linguistically appropriate services (CLAS) in health and health care. https://www.thinkculturalhealth.hhs.gov/assets/pdfs/EnhancedNationalCLASStandards.pdf. Accessed January 2019.

World Health Organization: *Social determinants of health*, 2019. http://www.who.int/social_determinants/sdh_-definition/en/. Accessed January 2019.

RESEARCH REFERENCES

Arozullah AM, et al.: Development and validation of a short-form, rapid estimate of adult literacy in medicine, *Med Care* 45:1026, 2007.

Campinha-Bacote J: The process of cultural competence in the delivery of health care services: a model of care, *J Transcult Nurs* 13:181–184, 2002.

Campinha-Bacote J: Many faces: addressing diversity in health care, *Online J Issues Nurs* 8(1), 2003. www.nursingworld.org/MainMenuCategories/ANAMarketplace/ANAPeriodicals/OJIN/TableofContents/Volume82003/No1Jan2003/AddressingDiversityinHealthcare.aspx, Accessed January 2019.

Conrad P, Barker KK: The social construction of illness: key insights and policy implications, *J Health Soc Behav* S1:S67–S79, 2010.

Conway-Klassen J, Maness L: Critical conversations: cultural awareness, sensitivity, and competency, *Clin Lab Sci* 38(1):34–37, 2017.

Frazer AL, et al.: Acculturation dissonance, acculturation strategy, depressive symptoms, and delinquency in Latina/o adolescents, *Child Youth Care Forum* 46:19–33, 2017.

Gucciardi E, et al.: Designing and delivering facilitated storytelling interventions for chronic disease self-management: a scoping review, *BMS Health Serv Res* 16:249, 2016.

Hadziabdic E, et al.: Boundaries and conditions of interpretation in multilingual and multicultural elderly health care, *BioMed Central Health Services Research* 15:e1–13, 2015.

Hall JM, Carlson K, Marginalization: A revisitation with integration of scholarship on globalization, intersectionality, privilege, microaggressions, and implicit biases, *Adv Nurs Sci* 39(3):200–215, 2016.

Hardy P, Sumner T: *Cultivating compassion: how digital storytelling is transforming health care*, ed 2, Cham, Switzerland, 2018, Palgrave MacMillan/Springer2018.

Houston TK, et al.: Culturally appropriate storytelling to improve blood pressure; a randomized trial, *Ann Intern Med* 154(2):77, 2011.

Ingram R: Using Campinha-Bacote's process of cultural competence model to examine the relationship between health literacy and cultural competency, *J Adv Nurs* 23:695–703, 2011.

Juckett G, Unger K: Appropriate use of medical interpreters, *Am Fam Physician* 90(7):476–480, 2014.

Lee SD, et al.: Short assessment of health literacy—Spanish and English: a comparable test of health literacy for Spanish and English speakers, *Health Serv Res* 45(4):1105–1120, 2010.

Lie D, et al.: What do health literacy and cultural competence have in common? Calling for a collaborative health professional pedagogy, *J Health Commun* 17(3):13–22, 2012.

Montenery S, et al.: Cultural competence in nursing faculty: a journey, not a destination, *J Prof Nurs* 29(6):e51–57, 2013.

Shiri FH, et al.: Explaining the meaning of cancer stigma from the point of view of Iranian stakeholders: a qualitative study, *Int J Cancer Manag* 11(7):e1–8, 2018.

Terkildsen MD, Wittrup I: Negotiating experience in patient involvement: challenges of practicing storytelling in health care conversations, *Tidssfrift for Forskning I Sygdom og Samfund* nr 22:45, 2015.

Walker RL, et al.: Ethnic group differences in reasons for living and the moderating role of cultural worldview, *Cultur Divers Ethnic Minor Psychol* 16(3):e1–15, 2010.

Wilson DK, et al.: *Exploring the role of digital storytelling in pediatric oncology patients' perspectives regarding diagnosis*, Sage Open, 2015. http://sgo.sagepub.com/content/5/1/2158244015572099. Accessed January 2019.

10

Family Dynamics

OBJECTIVES

- Discuss how the term *family* reflects family diversity.
- Examine current trends affecting the American family.
- Discuss the role of families and family members as caregivers.
- Discuss factors that affect family forms and their impact on a family's health.
- Explain how the relationship between family structure and patterns of functioning affects the health of individuals within the family and the family as a whole.
- Compare nursing care that views family as context, family as patient, and family as a system and explain how these different perspectives influence nursing practice.

- Discuss factors that promote or impede family health.
- Use the nursing process to provide for the health care needs of the family.
- Discuss essential aspects of a family assessment.
- Plan family-centered care.
- Create individualized, family-centered interventions to help a family improve its health status.
- Evaluate the effectiveness of family-centered care.

KEY TERMS

Family, p. 122
Family as a system, p. 124
Family as context, p. 124
Family as patient, p. 124
Family caregiving, p. 123

Family diversity, p. 121
Family durability, p. 121
Family dynamics, p. 121
Family forms, p. 122
Family function, p. 124

Hardiness, p. 126
Resiliency, p. 126

MEDIA RESOURCES

http://evolve.elsevier.com/Potter/fundamentals/
- Review Questions
- Case Study with Questions

- Audio Glossary
- Content Updates
- Answers to QSEN Activity and Review Questions

THE FAMILY

Families are very important. They are made up of groups of people who have emotional connections with each other and function as a unit. However, the concept, structure, and function of a family unit continues to change over time. Families face many challenges, including the effects of health and illness, childbearing and childrearing, changes in family structure and dynamics, and caring for older family members. Family characteristics or attributes such as durability, resiliency, and diversity help families adapt to these challenges.

Family durability is a system of support and structure within a family that extends beyond the walls of the household. For example, marriages may end in divorce or death, and remarriage may occur, or children may leave home as adults, but in the end the "family" transcends long periods and inevitable lifestyle changes.

Family resiliency is the ability of a family to cope with expected and unexpected stressors. The family's ability to adapt to role and structural changes, family members' developmental milestones, and crises shows resilience. For example, a family is resilient when the wage earner loses a job and another member of the family takes on that role. A family survives and thrives because of the challenges encountered from stressors.

Family diversity is the uniqueness of each family unit. For example, some families experience marriage and have children in later life. Another family includes parents with young children and grandparents living in the home. Every person within a family unit has specific needs, strengths, and important developmental considerations (see Chapter 11).

As you care for patients and their families, you are responsible for understanding family dynamics, the interactions between family members that are affected by a family's makeup (configuration), structure, function, problem solving, and coping capacity. Use this knowledge to build on a patient's and family's strengths and resources (Duhamel, 2017). The rapidly changing health care delivery system promotes early discharge of patients from acute care settings and even home health visits. Living as a family amid an illness is challenging; family functions, communications, and roles are altered (Kokonya and Fitzsimons, 2018). The goal of family-centered nursing care is to address the comprehensive health care needs of the family as a unit and to advocate, promote, support, and provide for the well-being and health of the patient and individual family members (Coats et al., 2018; Orchard et al., 2017).

Concept of Family

The term *family* suggests a visual image of adults and children living together in a satisfying, harmonious manner (Fig. 10.1). For some this

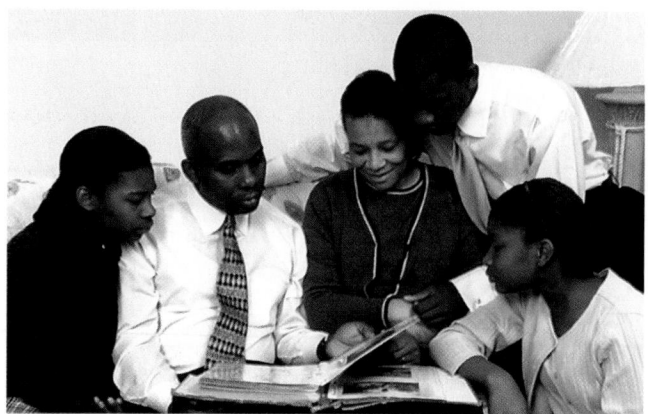

FIG. 10.1 Family celebrations and traditions strengthen the role of the family.

term has the opposite image—a single parent with multiple children living with a grandparent. Families represent more than a set of individuals, and a family is more than a sum of its individual members (Kaakinen et al., 2018). Families are as diverse as the individuals who compose them. Patients have deeply ingrained values about their families that deserve respect.

The specific relationships among patients, families, and health care providers are at the center of patient and family care. Unfortunately, these relationships are often defined and shaped by the beliefs of health care providers and not the needs of patients and family caregivers. As a nurse, you need to assess for and understand how your patients define their families and how they perceive the general state of member relationships. Think of a family as a set of relationships that a patient identifies as family or as a network of individuals who influence one another's lives, whether there are actual biological or legal ties.

Definition: What is a Family?

Defining *family* initially appears to be a simple undertaking. However, different definitions result in heated debates among social scientists who study the dynamics of families and legislators who set the public policies affecting families. The definition of family is significant and affects who is included on health insurance policies, who has access to children's school records, who files joint tax returns, and who is eligible for sick-leave benefits or public assistance programs.

A family is what an individual believes the family to be. It includes a set of interacting individuals who are related through biology or enduring commitments who usually socialize with each other (Kaakinen et al., 2018). For some patients, family includes only people related by marriage, birth, or adoption. To others, aunts, uncles, close friends, and pets are family. Understand that families take many forms and have diverse cultural and ethnic orientations. No two families are alike; each has its own strengths, weaknesses, resources, and challenges. You must care for both the family and the patient. Effective nursing administrators have a clear vision that caring for families is crucial to the mission of their health care agencies and the health of the nation (Orchard et al., 2017).

FAMILY FORMS AND CURRENT TRENDS

Family forms are patterns of people considered by family members to be included in a family (Box 10.1). Although all families have some things in common, each family form has unique problems and strengths. Remain open about who makes up a family to establish a therapeutic relationship with families and to ensure you are aware of a family's resources and concerns.

Families are constantly changing. In some situations, people marry later or delay childbirth. Some choose to have children while others do not have any children. Approximately 50% of people 15 years of age and older are married (US Census Bureau, 2018). However, the number of people living alone is greatly increasing, with approximately 30% of households containing only one person (US Census Bureau, 2018). Calculating divorce rates in the United States is complicated and inaccurate. However, most scholars agree that approximately 40% to 50% of marriages will end in divorce (APA, 2018). Divorce is becoming less common in younger adults but has doubled since the 1990s in adults age 50 and older (Stepler, 2017). Remarriage often results in a blended family with a complex set of relationships among all members.

Marital roles are also more complex as families increasingly have two wage earners. About 70% of mothers with children under 18 years of age are in the workforce, and mothers are the primary or sole earner for about 40% of households (DeWolf, 2017). Balancing employment and family life creates a variety of challenges in terms of child care and household work for both parents.

The number of single-parent families appears to be stabilizing. About 27% of children under the age of 18 live with one parent. Although mothers head most single-parent families, father-only families and the number of children living with other relatives are on the rise (US Census Bureau, 2018).

Although the birth rate for women has dropped 60% since 1991, 6% of all births in the United States occurred in women under 20 years of age in 2015 (Martin et al., 2018; Office of Adolescent Health, 2015). Thus, adolescent pregnancy remains a concern. Most adolescent mothers continue to live with their families. A teenage pregnancy has long-term consequences for the mother. Adolescent mothers are less likely to finish high school and are more likely to require public assistance, live in poverty, and have children with poorer educational, behavioral, and health outcomes (Office of Adolescent Health, 2015). The overwhelming task of being a parent while still being a teenager often severely stresses family relationships and resources. Stressors are also placed on teenage fathers when their partners become pregnant (Hunt, 2015). Teenage fathers usually have poorer support systems and fewer resources to teach them how to parent. Adolescent fatherhood is associated with lower socioeconomic status, lower educational attainment, and incarceration (Lau et al., 2015; Tremblay et al., 2017). Children of teenage fathers are more likely to have low birth weight, live in poverty, and have lower cognitive test scores (Lau et al., 2015). Both adolescent parents often struggle with the normal tasks of development and identity but must accept a parenting role that they are not ready for physically, emotionally, socially, and/or financially.

In 2015 the US Supreme Court issued a groundbreaking ruling that made same-sex marriages constitutional. Since this ruling, the number of same-sex marriages continues to increase, and most same-sex couples who live together (61%) are married (Masci et al., 2017). Individuals in same-sex relationships have become more vocal about their legal rights. Public support for same-sex marriage has grown rapidly over the past 10 years (Masci et al., 2017).

The fastest-growing age-group in America is 65 years of age and over (US Census Bureau, 2017a). In 2016, 49.2 million Americans were 65 years of age or older. This number increased by 33% since 2006 and is expected to almost double to 98 million people in 2060 (ACL, AoA, 2018). This phenomenon, often referred to as the "Graying of America," continues to affect the family life cycle, particularly the "sandwich generation"—composed of the children of older adults. These individuals, who are usually in their middle years, must meet their own needs along with those of their children and their aging family members. This balance of needs often occurs at the expense of their own well-being and resources.

More grandparents are raising their grandchildren (US Census Bureau, 2018). This new parenting responsibility is the result of several societal factors, such as military deployment, unemployment, adolescent pregnancy, substance abuse, and divorce resulting in single parenthood.

Factors Influencing Family Forms

Families face many challenges today, including changing structures and roles related to the changing economic status of society. Some families experience challenges related to chronic illness and aging family members. Family caregiving, poverty, homelessness, and domestic violence create challenges for families.

Family Caregivers. The increases in people living with chronic illnesses or disabilities and in the older adult population have created a greater need for family caregiving (FCA, 2019). Family caregivers are a crucial part of the health care team because they provide most of the physical and emotional care to patients wishing to remain in their homes (FCA, 2016b). In 2015, approximately 43.5 million caregivers provided unpaid caregiving to an adult or child. About 34.2 million caregivers cared for a family member who was 50 years of age or older, and most provided 17 to 22 hours of care per week (FCA, 2016a). More than 1 in 6 Americans who work full- or part-time are family caregivers (FCA, 2016b). Most working family caregivers rearrange their work schedule, decrease their hours, or take an unpaid leave to meet the caregiving needs of their family member (FCA, 2016b). Spouses in their 60s and 70s often are the major caregivers for one another. Older adult caregivers have special needs (Box 10.2).

Caring for a relative who is frail or chronically ill is an ongoing process in which families must continue to redefine their relationships and roles (Hashemi-Ghasemabadi et al., 2016; DePasquale et al., 2018). Family caregiving occurs within the context of a family and requires more than a simple series of tasks. It encompasses multiple cognitive, behavioral, and interpersonal processes. Caregiving activities include finding resources, providing personal care (bathing, feeding, or grooming), monitoring for complications or side effects of an illness or treatment, and providing instrumental activities of daily living (shopping or housekeeping). Family caregivers also provide ongoing emotional support for their loved ones, making decisions about care options, being a

---

BOX 10.2 FOCUS ON OLDER ADULTS

Family Caregiver Concerns

- Families often need help to determine their caregiving roles for the various members of the family (e.g., providing additional financial support, designating someone to obtain groceries and medications, providing hands-on physical care).
- Risk factors related to poor physical health for the caregiving dyad include older age and high school education or lower (Schaffer et al., 2017).
- Risk factors associated with higher emotional distress include younger age, female gender, caring for a spouse, and living with the patient. A caregiver's mental health is often related to the mental health of the patient. (Schaffer et al., 2017).
- Many older adults use spirituality to make end-of-life decisions, cope with life changes, and maintain psychological well-being (Moss et al., 2018; Salamizadeh et al., 2017).
- Social networks and support from close family and friends help to alleviate the stress experienced by caregivers (Newcomb and Hymes, 2017; Kirby et al., 2016).
- Individualized caregiver instruction and support are essential. For example, caregivers who are younger and caring for their spouses often need help in addressing their own and their spouse's psychological distress. Caregivers who are older and less educated may need information about health behaviors and self-care to help them address their physical health (Schaffer et al., 2017).

---

patient advocate, monitoring finances, and maintaining the integrity of the family unit. Whether a husband is caring for his wife or a child is caring for a parent, caregiving is an interactional process. The interpersonal dynamic between family members influences the ultimate quality of caregiving.

Family caregiving can be positive and rewarding, but it can also create caregiver burden and strain. The physical and emotional demands are high. A patient's disease creates changes in the family structure and roles. Family caregivers often do not feel prepared to take on the demands of care for their loved ones. Caregivers have mixed experiences and feelings. For example, they sometimes worry about the patient's illness and how to manage it, experience many life changes and restrictions, need to help the patient cope with illness, and want to show love and affection to the patient despite the burden and anxiety they are feeling (Petruzzo et al., 2017).

Family caregivers are at risk for a variety of physical conditions, ranging from depression, cardiac illness, and eating disorders. In addition, the caregiver often does not consider his or her own health needs as a high priority and misses routine primary care visits, screenings, and dental care (Schaffer et al., 2017).

Poverty. Although the poverty rate in the United States has been falling since 2014, the impact of poverty on families is profound (US Census Bureau, 2017b). Female single-parent families and families with unrelated individuals are especially vulnerable (US Census Bureau, 2017c). Children continue to be the poorest age group in America, with the youngest children and children of color being the poorest (CDF, 2017). Individuals and families who live in poverty are more likely to be uninsured (US Census Bureau, 2017d). Approximately 24 million young adults (18 to 34 years of age) lived in their parents' homes in 2015; about 2.2 million of these adult children were not attending school or working, putting additional economic strains on families (US Census Bureau, 2017e).

Although the Affordable Care Act (ACA) improved access to affordable health insurance, the challenge to access appropriate health care continues, especially for individuals and families who are at or near the poverty level (Martinez and Ward, 2016). When caring for families who live in poverty, be sensitive to their need for independence and help them obtain appropriate financial and health care resources. For example, help a family by providing information about resources within the community to obtain assistance with food, energy bills, dental and health care, and school supplies.

Homelessness. Homelessness is a major public health issue that affects the functioning, health, and well-being of the family and its members (CDF, 2017). Chronic homelessness is experienced by people who need to use homeless shelters for their long-term housing needs. In contrast, people who experience transitional episodic homelessness need shelter for one stay and for a short period of time (National Coalition for the Homeless, 2018). People who are homeless tend to be younger, with a catastrophic event requiring them to seek shelter.

Adults who are homeless face many health risks. They are more likely to have mental and chronic health problems (US Interagency Council on Homelessness, 2018). Exposure to the elements, poor nutritional status and poor access to health care affect the health of people who are homeless. They are also vulnerable to physical and emotional violence, injury, and trauma.

Poverty, domestic violence, reduced government support for families with dependent children, and lack of affordable housing contribute to homelessness in families (National Coalition for the Homeless, 2018). Children of families who are homeless are often in fair or poor health and have higher rates of asthma, ear infections, stomach problems, mental illness, poor dental health, and poor immunization documentation. The emergency department often becomes their only access to health care.

Children who are homeless face barriers such as meeting residency requirements for public schools and inability to obtain previous enrollment records when enrolling into and attending a new school. They often lack adult supervision to help them with homework and school-related issues. As a result, they are more likely to drop out of school, develop risky behaviors, and become unemployable (Barnes et al., 2018; National Alliance to End Homelessness, 2018). Homelessness increases the risk for developing long-term health, psychological, and socioeconomic problems, posing a major challenge for our entire society (Barnes et al., 2018; National Alliance to End Homelessness, 2018) (see Chapter 3).

Domestic Violence. Domestic violence includes not only intimate-partner relationships of spousal, live-in partners and dating relationships but also familial, elder, and child abuse. Emotional, physical, and sexual abuse occurs across all social classes (Futures without Violence, 2018).

Factors associated with family violence are complex and include stress, poverty, social isolation, psychopathology, and learned family behavior. Other factors such as alcohol and drug abuse, pregnancy, sexual orientation, and mental illness increase the incidence of abuse within a family (Futures without Violence, 2018). Although abuse sometimes ends when a person leaves a family environment, negative long-term physical and emotional consequences often linger. One of the consequences includes moving from one abusive situation to another. For example, a child sees marriage as a solution to leave a parents' abusive home and in turn marries a person who continues the abuse in the marriage (Futures without Violence, 2018).

Structure

Structure is based on the ongoing membership of the family and the pattern of relationships, which are often numerous and complex (Kaakinen et al., 2018). Each family has a unique structure and way of functioning. For example, a family member may have relationships with a spouse, child, employer, and work colleagues. Each of these relationships has different demands, roles, and expectations. The multiple relationships and their expectations are often sources for personal and family stress (see Chapter 37).

Structure either enhances or detracts from a family's ability to respond to the expected and unexpected stressors of daily life. Structures that are too rigid or flexible sometimes threaten family functioning. Rigid structures specify who accomplishes different tasks and limit the number of people outside the immediate family allowed to assume these tasks. For example, in one family with a rigid structure, the mother is the only acceptable person to provide emotional support for the children and/or to perform all the household chores. The father is the only acceptable person to provide financial support, maintain the vehicles, do the yard work, and make all the home repairs. A change in the health status of the person responsible for a task places a burden on a rigid family because no other person is available, willing, experienced, or considered acceptable to assume that task. An extremely flexible family structure also presents problems for the family. The absence of stability sometimes prevents other family members from taking action during a crisis or rapid change.

Function

Family function is what a family does, such as how a family interacts to socialize younger family members, cooperates to meet economic needs, and relates to the larger society. Family function involves the processes used by a family to achieve its goals. Some processes include communication among family members, goal setting, conflict resolution, caregiving, nurturing, and the use of internal and external resources. Although family members pursue the family goals at various times during their development, they need emotional and psychosocial support throughout their life span to be successful.

FAMILY NURSING

Family nursing assumes that all people, regardless of age, are members of some type of family form (Fig. 10.2). The goal of family nursing is to help a family and its individual members reach and maintain maximum health throughout and beyond the illness experience. Family nursing is the focus across all practice settings and is important in all health care environments.

There are different approaches for family nursing practice. For the purposes of this chapter, family nursing practice has three levels of approaches: (1) family as context, (2) family as patient, and (3) family as a system. Family as a system includes both relational and transactional concepts. All approaches recognize that patient-centered care

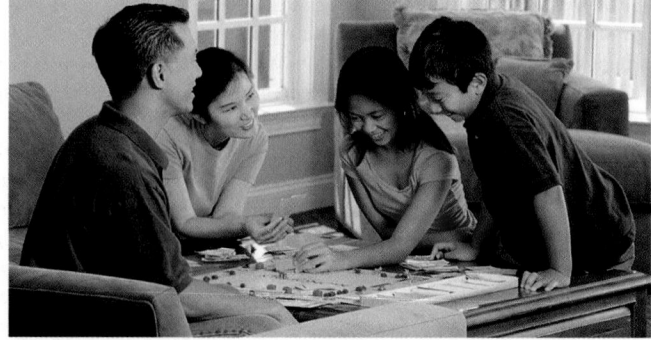

FIG. 10.2 Family recreational activities strengthen family functioning. (Courtesy Bill Branson, National Cancer Institute.)

for one member influences all members and affects family functioning. Families are continually changing. As a result, the need for family support changes over time, and it is important for you to understand that the family is more complex than simply a combination of individual members.

Family As Context

When you view a family as context, the primary focus is on the health and development of an individual member existing within a specific family environment. Although you focus on the health of an individual family member, also assess how much the family provides the individual's basic needs. Needs vary, depending on an individual's developmental level and situation. Consider the family's ability to help your patient meet physical as well as psychological needs when viewing a family as context.

Family As Patient

When you view a family as patient, the family's needs, processes, and relationships (e.g., parenting or family caregiving) are the primary focus of nursing care. Your nursing assessment focuses on family patterns versus characteristics of individual members. Concentrate on patterns and processes that are consistent with reaching and maintaining family and individual health. For example, in the case of family caregiving, determine who the family caregivers are, their different roles, and how they interact to meet a patient's needs. Plan care to meet the patient's and family's changing needs. Dealing with very complex family problems often requires an interprofessional approach. Know the limits of nursing practice, and make referrals when appropriate.

Family As a System

Although you make theoretical and practical distinctions between the family as context and the family as patient, they are not necessarily mutually exclusive. When you care for a family as a system, you are caring for each family member (family as context) and the family unit (family as patient), using all available environmental, social, psychological, and community resources.

The following clinical scenario illustrates three levels of approaches to family care.

You are assisting with end-of-life care for David Daniels, who is 35 years old and is a computer programmer. David and his wife, Lisa, have three school-age children. David expressed a wish to die at home. Lisa is on family leave from her job to help David through this period. Both Lisa and David are only children. David's parents are no longer living, but Lisa's mother is committed to staying with the family to help Lisa and David.

When you view this *family as context,* you focus first on the patient (David) as an individual. You assess and meet David's needs at end-of-life, such as comfort, hygiene, and nutrition, as well as his social and emotional needs. You determine how David is coping with knowing his life is coming to an end and how he perceives it will affect his family. When viewing *the family as patient,* you assess and meet the needs of David's wife and children. Determine to what extent the family's basic needs for normal activity, comfort, and nutrition are being met and whether they have resources for emotional and social support. You determine the family's need for rest (especially the wife) and their stage of coping (the older child shows much anger and fear). You determine the demands placed on David and the family, such as economic survival and well-being of the children. In addition, you continually assess the family's available resources such as time, coping skills, and energy level to support David through the end of life.

When viewing a *family as a system,* you use elements from both the context and patient perspectives and assess the resources available to the family system. Using the knowledge of the family as context, patient, and system, individualize care decisions based on your family assessment and clinical judgment. For example, based on assessment data, you determine that the family is not eating adequately. You also determine that Lisa is experiencing more stress, not sleeping well, and trying to "do it all" regarding her children's school and after-school activities. In addition, Lisa does not want to leave David's bedside when members of their church come to help. You recognize that this family is under enormous stress and that their basic needs such as nutrition, rest, and school activities are not adequately met. As a result, you determine that (1) the family needs help with meals, (2) Lisa needs time to rest, and (3) the family's church is eager to help with David's day-to-day care. Based on these insights, you have a family conference and set up a schedule among Lisa, her mother, and two close church members to provide Lisa with some time away from David's bedside. During the conference, David and Lisa determine when this time will be. Because of the church involvement, members of the church begin to purchase groceries and make all the meals for the family. In addition, other members of the church help with the children's school and after-school activities.

Family and Health

Although American families exist within the same US culture, there are cultural disparities, and individual family members vary greatly in their experiences, beliefs, and values. When a family is victim to low educational preparation, poverty, and decreased social support, these factors compound one another, magnifying their effect on the health and well-being of the family. Economic stability increases a family's access to adequate health care, creates more opportunity for education, increases good nutrition, and decreases stress (CDF, 2017; National Coalition for the Homeless, 2018).

The family is the primary social context in which health promotion and disease prevention take place. A family's beliefs, values, and practices strongly influence the family's structure and function. They also affect family communication patterns, roles, and health-promoting practices. Providing culturally appropriate family-centered interventions and teaching can improve family functioning and self-care (Deek et al., 2016; Srisuk et al., 2017).

Some families do not place a high value on good health. In fact, harmful practices are accepted by some families. For example, some families use high-caloric food intake as an acceptable way to cope with stress. Sometimes a family member gives mixed messages about health. For example, a parent chooses to smoke while telling children that smoking is bad for them. Family environment is crucial because health behavior reinforced in early life has a strong influence on later health practices. In addition, the family environment is a crucial factor in an individual's adjustment to a crisis. Although relationships are strained when confronted with illness, research indicates that when family members receive support from health care professionals, they have the potential to adapt to the stressors and develop coping mechanisms (Phillips and Prezio, 2017).

Attributes of Healthy Families. The family is a dynamic unit; it is exposed to threats, strengths, changes, and challenges. Some families are crisis proof, whereas others are crisis prone. A crisis-proof, or effective, family combines the need for stability with the need for growth and change. This type of family has a flexible structure that allows different family members to complete tasks and accepts help from outside the family system. The structure is flexible enough to allow adaptability but not so flexible that the family lacks cohesiveness and a sense of stability. An effective family controls the environment and influences the immediate environment of home, neighborhood, and school. An ineffective, or crisis-prone, family lacks or believes it lacks control over its environment.

Hardiness and resiliency moderate a family's stress, thus affecting a family's health. Family hardiness is the internal strengths and durability of the family unit. A sense of control over the outcome of life, a view of change as beneficial and growth producing, and an active rather than passive orientation in adapting to stressful events characterize family hardiness (Resilience, Adaptation, and Well-Being, 2016). Resiliency helps individuals and families respond in healthy ways when they experience stressful events. Family resiliency does not develop through evasion of risk but through successful application of protective factors such as family cohesion, self-efficacy, and peer acceptance to engage in adverse situations and emerge from them stronger (Benzies and Mychasiuk, 2009). Resources (e.g., adequate income, education) and techniques (e.g., coping resources) that a family or individuals within the family use to maintain a balance or level of health aid in understanding a family's level of resiliency.

Genetic Factors. Genetic factors reflect a family's heredity or genetic susceptibility to diseases that may or may not result in actual development of a disease. The scope of genomics in nursing care is broad and encompasses risk assessment, risk management, counseling and treatment options, and treatment decisions. Clinical applications of genetic and genomic knowledge for nurses have implications for care of people, families, communities, and populations across the life span (NIH, 2018).

Sometimes identification of genetic factors and genetic counseling help family members decide whether to test for the presence of a disease and/or to have children. Some families choose not to have children; others choose not to know genetic risks and have children; other families choose to know the risk and then determine whether to have children. Some of these diseases (e.g., heart or kidney disease) are manageable. With genetic risks for certain cancers such as some breast cancers, a woman may choose prophylactic bilateral mastectomy to reduce the risk for developing the disease. Families with genetic neurological diseases such as Huntington's disease may choose not to have children. When families know of these risks, they have the opportunity to make informed decisions about their lifestyle and health behaviors, are more vigilant about recognizing changes in their health, and in some cases seek medical intervention earlier.

Living With Acute/Chronic Illnesses or Trauma. Any acute or chronic illness influences an entire family economically, emotionally, socially, and functionally. Illness also affects a family's decision-making and coping resources. Hospitalization of a family member is stressful for the whole family. Hospital environments are foreign, physicians and nurses are strangers, the medical language is difficult to understand or interpret, and family members are often separated from one another.

During an acute illness that requires hospitalization, family members are sometimes left in waiting rooms to receive information about their loved one. Communication among family members may be misunderstood from fear and worry. Previous family conflicts can rise to the surface, whereas others are suppressed. Interprofessional teams often are helpful in meeting the needs of families during acute illnesses.

Chronic illnesses present continuous challenges for families. Frequently family patterns and interactions, roles, social activities, work and household schedules, economic resources, and other family needs and functions must be reorganized around the chronic illness or disability (see Chapter 8).

Trauma is sudden, unplanned, and sometimes life threatening. Family members often struggle to cope with the challenges of a severe life-threatening event. For example, they often deal with stressors associated with a family member hospitalized in an intensive care environment, anxiety, depression, economic burden, and the impact of the trauma on family functioning and decision making (Newcomb and Hymes, 2017). The powerlessness that family members experience makes them very vulnerable and less able to make important decisions about the health of the family.

When implementing a family-centered care model for patients experiencing acute or chronic illnesses or trauma, patients' family members and surrogate decision makers become active partners in decision making and care. Involving family during a hand-off report from one care provider to another, for example, provides an opportunity to involve a patient and family in discussing the present and long-term plan of care (Bigani and Correia, 2018). When possible, patients and family caregivers want to participate in shared decision making about treatment and ongoing disease/symptom management (Sebern et al., 2018). Incorporating a patient's and family's cultural beliefs, values, and communication patterns is essential to provide individualized patient/family-centered care.

In caring for family members, advocate for the patient and family and answer their questions honestly (Newcomb and Hymes, 2017). When you do not know the answer, find someone who does. Ensure that the family knows all the members of the health care team. Provide realistic assurance; giving false hope breaks the nurse-patient trust and affects how the family can adjust to "bad news" (Schultz et al., 2017). When a patient is hospitalized, take time to make sure that the family is comfortable. You can bring them something to eat or drink, give them a blanket, or encourage them to get a meal. Sometimes telling a family that you will stay with their loved one while they are gone is all they need to feel comfortable in leaving.

End-of-Life Care. You will encounter families with a member who is terminally ill. Although people equate terminal illness with cancer, many diseases have terminal aspects (e.g., heart failure, pulmonary and renal diseases, and neuromuscular diseases). Although some family members may be prepared for their loved one's death, their need for information, support, assurance, and presence is great (see Chapter 36). Use presence to develop a therapeutic relationship with a patient and family (see Chapter 7). Also use therapeutic communication to enhance family members' relationships with one another and to promote shared decision making (Brooks et al., 2017). The more you know about your patient's family, how they interact with one another, their strengths, and their weaknesses, the better. Each family approaches and copes with end-of-life decisions differently. Encourage a patient and family to make decisions about care (e.g., pain control or preferred nonpharmacologic comfort measures) and specific therapies. Help a family set up home care if they desire, and make referrals for hospice and other appropriate resources, including grief support (Bickel et al., 2016). Provide information about the dying process and make sure family members know what to do at the time of death. If you are present at the time of death, be sensitive to a family's needs (e.g., provide for privacy and allow sufficient time for saying goodbyes).

FAMILY-CENTERED CARE AND THE NURSING PROCESS

Nurses interact with families in a variety of community-based and clinical settings. Apply the nursing process and use critical thinking to develop and implement family-centered nursing care. The approach to the nursing process is the same whether your focus is family as context, patient, or system. When caring for families, use the same process you use with individual patients, but also incorporate the needs of the family. You use the nursing process to care for an individual within a family (e.g., the family as context) or the entire family (e.g., the family as patient). When initiating the care of families, use these approaches to organize a family approach to the nursing process:

1. Assess all individuals within their family context.
2. Assess the family as patient.
3. Assess the family as a system.

Family Assessment

Using a family-centered approach to assessment allows you to establish a working relationship with a patient and his or her family. A complete assessment provides you a full picture of patient needs as a member of a family and of family needs as well. If your assessment is complete, it ensures that the patient and family needs are correctly identified and that mutual goals and interventions for health care can be established.

Often you will participate in conflict resolution between family members, so each member is able to confront and resolve problems in a healthy way. Ask assessment questions to help the family identify external and internal resources as necessary. For example, who in the family can run errands to get groceries while the patient is unable to drive? Are there members from the church who can come and provide respite care? Ultimately your aim is to help the family reach a point of optimal function, given the family's resources, capacities, and desire to become healthier.

You play an essential role in helping families adjust to acute, chronic, and terminal illness; but first you need to understand the family unit and what a patient's illness means to the family members and family functioning. You also need to understand how the illness affects the family structure and the support the family requires (Kaakinen et al., 2018). Although the family as a whole differs from individual members, the measure of family health is more than a summary of the health of all members. The form, structure, function, and health of the family are areas unique to family assessment. Several culturally sensitive tools and models assess or measure family dynamics (Giddens, 2017). Box 10.3 provides examples of family assessment questions based on the Calgary Family Assessment Model (Shajani and Snell, 2019; Leahey and Wright, 2016).

While completing your assessment, consider knowledge of a patient's illness and its potential impact on the family. Because time is limited in many practice settings, it is critical for you to understand how significant a role the family will play in a patient's recovery. This factor will affect how comprehensive an assessment you conduct. Begin the family assessment by determining a patient's definition of and attitude toward the family. A person's concept of family is highly individualized. The patient's definition will influence how much you are able to incorporate the family into nursing care. When it becomes obvious that family is important for a patient, determine family form and membership by asking who the patient considers family or with whom the patient shares strong emotional feelings. If the patient is unable to express a concept of family, ask with whom he or she lives, spends time, and shares confidences and then ask whether he or she considers them to be family or like family. To further assess the family structure, ask questions that determine the power structure and patterning of roles and tasks (e.g., "Who decides where to go on vacation?" "How are tasks divided in your family?" "Who mows the lawn?" "Who usually prepares the meals?").

Assess family functions such as the ability to provide emotional support for members, the ability to cope with current health problems or situations, and the appropriateness of its goal setting. Also determine

---

BOX 10.3 Family Assessment Questions

Family Structure

Determines members of the family, relationships among family members, and the context of the family

- Who are the members of your family? How are they related to you?
- Who lives with you?
- Has anyone recently moved out of your home?
- Is there anyone who doesn't live with you whom you consider to be family?

Developmental Assessment

Determines how families adapt during predictable and unpredictable changes and difficult times

- What transitions/changes (e.g., recent death, divorce, children leaving/returning home, new births) has your family experienced most recently?
- Are there any members of your family who are having problems (e.g., difficulty in school, acute or chronic illnesses) that are currently affecting your family?
- What aspects of your family do you enjoy the most?
- What plans have you or your family made to care for family members who are in poor health?

Family Functioning

Addresses how individuals behave in relation to one another; includes instrumental aspects, which are routine activities (e.g., making meals, doing laundry), and expressive aspects (e.g., communication, problem solving, roles, influence and power, beliefs)

- Describe a recent problem and how your family resolved it.
- Who is the caregiver for children or older adults?
- What coping strategies does your family use (e.g., exercise, avoidance, overeating, arguing)?
- What are your family beliefs about health/illness, end-of-life care, and advance directives?
- What does your family mean to you?
- How does your family celebrate holidays, birthdays, weddings?
- How do the members of your family manage their health? How do they manage care of a sick family member?
- When someone is ill, who is the caregiver? Is it always the same person?

---

whether the family has sufficient economic resources and whether its social network is extensive enough to provide support.

Cultural Aspects. Always recognize and respect a family's cultural background during your assessment (see Chapter 9). Culture is an important variable when assessing a family because race, ethnicity, language, and norms affect structure, function, health beliefs, values, and the way a family perceives events (Box 10.4). A comprehensive, culturally sensitive family assessment is critical to forming an understanding of family life, current changes in family life, overall goals and expectations, and planning family-centered care.

Forming conclusions about families' needs based on cultural backgrounds requires critical thinking. It is imperative to remember that categorical generalizations are often misleading. Overgeneralizations in terms of racial and ethnic group characteristics do not lead to greater understanding of a culturally diverse family. Culturally different families vary in meaningful and significant ways; however, neglecting to examine similarities leads to inaccurate assumptions and stereotyping (Giger, 2017).

Knowing about a family's culture and the meaning of that culture to a family's structure and functioning, health practices, and family celebrations helps to design family-centered care (see Chapter 9). To

---

⊕ BOX 10.4   CULTURAL ASPECTS OF CARE
Family Nursing

Families have unique perspectives and characteristics, and they have differences in values, beliefs, and philosophies. The cultural heritage of a family or member of the family affects religious, childrearing, and health care practices; recreational activities; and nutritional preferences. Be culturally sensitive and respectful when caring for patients of all cultures. Incorporate individualized cultural preferences into your plan of care so that it is culturally congruent. Design your care to integrate the personal values, life patterns, and beliefs of the patient and family into prescribed therapies.

Implications for Patient-Centered Care

- Focus on the needs of the family, and understand the family's beliefs, values, customs, and roles when designing care (Deek et al., 2016). Perception of events and their impact on the family varies across cultural groups. For example, the care of the grandmother has a great significance to the extended family.
- Family caregiving values, practices, and roles and perceptions of the burden associated with family caregiving vary across cultures (Konerding et al., 2018).
- The family structure sometimes includes multiple generations living together. Intergenerational support and patterns of living arrangements are often related to cultural background (Cohen and Passel, 2018).
- In some cultures, it is a sign of disrespect to place older adults in nursing homes, even when an older adult family member has severe dementia (Giger, 2017).
- Modesty is a strong value among many cultures. Some women bring female family members to health care visits, and a female health care provider must examine the woman.
- In the presence of a critical or terminal illness, some cultures come in groups to pray together with the family at the patient's bedside (Giger, 2017).
- Health beliefs differ among various cultures; these differences affect the decisions of a family and its members about when and where to seek help.

REFLECT NOW

Reflect on a family you know who is currently experiencing a life transition. What questions could you ask to assess their current needs?

Nursing Diagnoses for Families

After assessing a patient's and family's needs and situation, you identify nursing diagnoses. Several positive and negative ICNP* diagnoses can be used when caring for families. Examples of ICNP* nursing diagnoses applicable to family care are:

- *Conflicting Caregiver Attitude*
- *Impaired Family Coping*
- *Risk for Caregiver Stress*
- *Impaired Family Process*
- *Risk for Parent Child Attachment*
- *Family Able to Participate in Care Planning*
- *Family Knowledge of Disease*

Nursing diagnoses that relate to a family often focus on a family's ability to cope with its current situation. Appropriate use of resources helps a family cope with unexpected events that threaten health and stability. Nursing diagnoses often focus on changes in family processes or roles. For example, a man who is married and has four children is in a motor vehicle accident. He sustained multiple fractures to his lower extremities and pelvis and is non–weight-bearing for 6 to 8 weeks after discharge. Thus, he cannot go to work and perform many of the activities (e.g., mowing the lawn, taking the children to school) that he normally performs. His spouse is feeling overwhelmed as she develops a plan to meet all the family's needs, which include her husband's needs for rehabilitation. Based on this data, you determine *Impaired Family Process related to immobility and temporary changes in family roles* is an appropriate nursing diagnosis for this family.

Planning Family-Centered Care

Once you identify pertinent nursing diagnoses, work together with patients and their families to develop plans of care that all members clearly understand and mutually agree to follow. The goals and outcomes you establish need to be concrete and realistic, compatible with the family members' developmental stages (see Chapter 11), and acceptable to family members and their lifestyle.

By offering alternatives for care activities and asking family members for their own ideas and suggestions, you help to include them in the decision making and better meet the patient's needs (Stockwell-Smith et al., 2018). For example, offering options for how to prepare a low-fat diet or how to rearrange the furnishings of a room to accommodate a family member's disability gives a family an opportunity to express their preferences, make choices, and ultimately feel as though they have contributed. Collaborating with other disciplines such as physical therapy and social services increases the likelihood of a comprehensive approach to a family's health care needs, and it ensures better continuity of care. Using other disciplines is particularly important when discharge planning from a health care agency to home or an extended-care facility is necessary.

Implementing Family-Centered Care

You will provide family-centered nursing care in a variety of health care settings, whether you are providing health promotion, acute care, or restorative and continuing care. It is important to develop individualized nursing interventions to meet the needs of your patients and their families.

Health Promotion. Although many people learn health behaviors from their families, the primary focus on health promotion has

---

determine the influence of culture on a family, ask the patient about his or her cultural background. Then ask questions concerning cultural practices. For example, "What type of foods do you eat?" "Who cares for sick family members?" "Have you or anyone in your family been hospitalized?" "Did family members remain at the hospital?" "Do you use any health practices of your culture such as acupuncture or meditation?" "What role do grandparents play in raising your children?"

A comprehensive, culturally sensitive family assessment is critical for you to understand family life, the current changes within it, and a family's overall goals and expectations. These data provide the foundation for family-centered nursing care (Sousza et al., 2017).

Discharge Planning. Discharge planning begins with the initiation of care and includes the family. You are responsible for an accurate assessment of who will provide caregiving and what will be needed for care in the home at the time of discharge. Consider how the patient's physical and/or cognitive limitations will affect daily living activities and the impact this will have on the family. For example, if a patient who is an older adult is discharged to home after surgery and the patient's spouse cannot perform required dressing changes, you need to find out if anyone else in the family or neighborhood is willing and able to do this. If not, you will need to arrange for a home care referral. If the patient also needs exercise and strength training, you consult with the primary health care provider to recommend referral for physical therapy.

traditionally been on individuals. When implementing family nursing, health promotion interventions are designed to improve or maintain the physical, social, emotional, and spiritual well-being of the family unit and its members (Duhamel, 2017). Health promotion behaviors sometimes need to be tied to the developmental stages of the family members (e.g., adequate prenatal care for the childbearing family or adherence to immunization schedules for the childrearing family). Your interventions need to enable individual members and the total family to reach their optimal levels of wellness.

Whether you provide care for the family as context, patient, or system, evidence-based nursing interventions increase family members' ability to provide care, remove barriers to health care, and perform tasks the family is not currently able to do (Box 10.5). Assist a family in problem solving, and express a sense of acceptance and caring by listening carefully to family members' concerns and suggestions.

One of the roles you need to adopt is that of educator (Fig. 10.3). Health education is a process by which a nurse and patient share information (see Chapter 25). Sometimes you recognize family/patient needs for information through direct questioning, but the methods for recognizing these needs are generally subtle. For example, you recognize that a new father is fearful of cleaning his newborn's umbilical cord or that an older-adult woman is not using her cane or walker safely. Respectful communication is necessary. Often you find the subtle needs for information by saying, "I notice you are trying to not touch the umbilical cord. I see that a lot." Or "You use the cane the way I did before I was shown a way to keep from falling or tripping over

it; do you mind if I show you?" When you are confident and skillful instead of coming across as an authority on the subject, your patient's defenses are down, making him or her more willing to listen without feeling embarrassed. You will also recognize patient and family learning needs based on a patient's health condition and physical and mental limitations. Your focus as an educator may be on the family caregiver to prepare that person to manage the skills and processes needed to manage a patient's needs within the home.

REFLECT NOW

Think about a time you provided education to a family to help them manage an illness. How did or could you use the teach-back method to evaluate the effectiveness of your teaching?

One approach for meeting goals and promoting health is the use of family strengths. Families do not always see their strengths. Help families use their strengths to improve their health and meet their goals. Family strengths may include clear communication, adaptability, healthy childrearing practices, and support and nurturing among family members. Other strengths exist in the form of the use of crisis for growth, a commitment to one another and the family unit, a sense of well-being and cohesiveness, and spirituality. Help the family focus on their strengths instead of on problems and weaknesses. For example, point out that a couple's 30-year marriage has endured many crises

BOX 10.5 EVIDENCE-BASED PRACTICE

Caregiving Education for the Family Caregiver

PICOT Question: Do tailored nursing interventions designed for family caregivers reduce caregiver burden and enhance caregiver well-being?

Evidence Summary

When a family member has an acute or chronic illness or experiences a trauma that changes his or her physical or cognitive function, it is often a major life-changing event that affects all family members. The family faces many changes in family dynamics, social interactions, financial commitments, and emotional support systems (Caceres et al., 2016; Newcomb and Hymes, 2017). A patient's physical disabilities and altered mental status affect the family caregiver and other members of the family (Kung, 2015; Weisman de Mamani et al., 2018). As a result, family members report stress and burnout related to the continual demands of the caregiving role (Moriarty et al., 2018). Lower levels of caregiver burden are associated with better mental health in caregivers (Weisman de Mamani et al., 2018). Caregiver coping, especially during hospitalizations, is often influenced by their communication with providers, access to the patient, and the presence of staff helping explain the patient's problems and treatment plan (Newcomb and Hymes, 2017). Providing interventions tailored to the needs of the caregiver reduces caregiver burden and improves caregiver coping and quality of life (Jaffray et al., 2016; Weisman de Mamani et al., 2018).

Application to Nursing Practice

- Teach family caregivers to focus on the present moment using mindfulness-based interventions (e.g., meditation, breathing exercises, guided imagery) to reduce caregiver burden and improve mental health. Current evidence shows mindfulness is often helpful, especially in caregivers for patients with dementia and who are terminally ill (Hicken et al., 2017; Jaffray et al., 2016; Weisman de Mamani et al., 2018).
- Carefully assess the mental health of the caregiver. Encourage caregivers to discuss their feelings about caregiving responsibilities and help shape their perceptions in a way to improve their mental health. For example, if a

caregiver states, "I feel trapped by having to bathe my mother," encourage the caregiver to frame this in a more adaptive way, such as "I now have the opportunity to provide care for someone who used to take care of me" (Weisman de Mamani et al., 2018).
- Encourage family caregivers to remain engaged in a patient's care during hospitalizations (e.g., encourage mobilization, assist with meals, discuss patient education) (Newcomb and Hymes, 2017).
- Teach caregivers for patients living with dementia different ways to cope with and redirect behavioral disturbances associated with dementia to help improve the caregiver's sleep and reduce caregiver burden, distress, and risk for developing depression (Caceres et al., 2016).
- Be aware of and assess for cultural implications of different physical and mental illnesses and their effect on the caregiver. For example, having a mental illness such as schizophrenia is sometimes accompanied by social stigma and isolation in people who are Chinese. Refer caregivers to support groups to encourage them to share their feelings and experiences with others who are in similar situations, and help families communicate effectively with each other to avoid conflict (Kung, 2015).
- Assess the effect (e.g., physical, mental, financial) of a patient's disability on the family. Provide support and patient education targeted to a patient's and family caregiver's needs. For example, some family caregivers of veterans who have posttraumatic stress disorder (PTSD) and/or traumatic brain injury (TBI) experience greater financial issues and depressive symptoms. Providing emotional support and helping families identify financial resources may reduce caregiver burden and improve coping with PTSD and TBI (Moriarty et al., 2018).
- Use telephone- or Internet-assisted technologies based on family caregiver preferences to provide support and patient education when it is difficult for the caregiver to receive effective support due to geographical constraints (e.g., in rural settings) (Hicken et al., 2017).

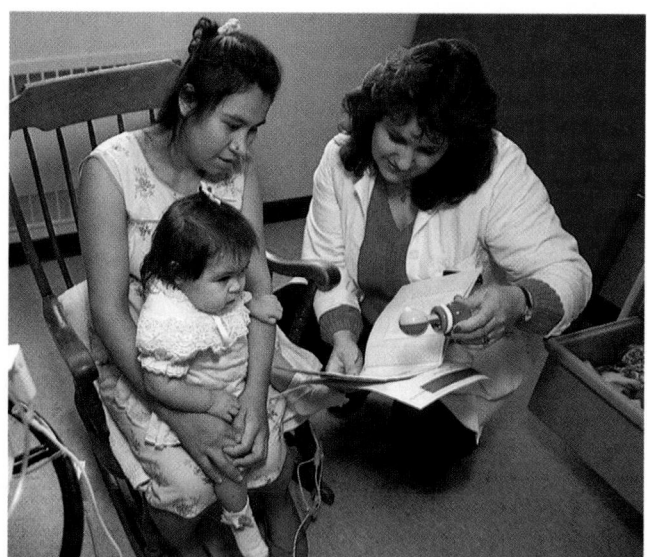

FIG. 10.3 Nurse providing family education. (From Hockenberry MJ, Wilson D, Rodgers CC: *Wong's nursing care of infants and children,* ed 11, St Louis, 2019, Mosby.)

and transitions. Therefore, they are likely to be able to adapt to this latest challenge. Refer families to health promotion programs aimed at enhancing these strengths as needed. For example, some communities have low-cost fitness activities for children and their families that are designed to reduce the risk for obesity (Allar et al., 2017).

Acute Care. The family must be a central focus of nursing care in the acute care setting. It is crucial to emphasize family needs within the context of today's acute health care delivery environment. The complex health care system requires you to be astute, use time wisely, and anticipate the type of interventions needed to support family and patient needs up to and including discharge. The Synergy Model recognizes the importance of the relationship between the nurse and the patient and family to create a healing environment (Fournier, 2017). According to this model, when caring for acutely ill patients and their families, integrate your professional knowledge, skills, experiences, and attitudes to meet the needs of patients and their families. The needs and characteristics of a patient and family drive nursing interventions. When there is synergy between a patient and family and a nurse, optimal patient outcomes result.

Include family caregivers in a patient's care during admission to better prepare them for their role and reduce stress following discharge (Piccenna et al., 2016). Because hospital stays are shortened, it is important to provide education and encourage families to take an active role in caregiving on admission. For example, if you are caring for a patient who will need to go home on multiple medications, including a subcutaneous injection, provide information to the patient and family about the medications and administration of injections throughout the patient's hospital stay.

One growing area in acute care for family caregivers is end-of-life care. You help family members in their caregiving role by allowing them to participate in decision making, ensuring clear communication between the family and the health care team, and supporting a family's resilience (Benzies and Mychasiuk, 2009; Stajduhar et al., 2017). Help family caregivers find home care equipment and community resources and allow them to provide specific aspects of physical care they will need to perform at home. Preparing family members for discharge helps caregiving become a meaningful experience for both caregiver and patient across health care settings.

QSEN **Building Competency in Teamwork and Collaboration** You are caring for the Carlson family. The father, Gary, is a 47-year-old chemical engineer who was diagnosed with amyotrophic lateral sclerosis (Lou Gehrig's disease). He is experiencing a progressive degenerative disease affecting his muscles and is now hospitalized with aspiration pneumonia. He continues to weaken and is preparing to be discharged to home with a hospice consult. His wife, Kathy, is 48 years old and is an information technology specialist. They have two children. Karen is a junior at a local university and lives in the residence hall. Kristen is a high school senior. The family is committed to helping Gary remain at home. Gary has been receiving care from physical therapy, respiratory therapy, the palliative care team, and pastoral care during this hospital stay. What can you do at this time to promote the teamwork and collaboration needed to make the Carlson's transition to home successful?

Answers to QSEN Activities can be found on the Evolve website.

Discharge Planning. Discharge planning with a family is important during the acute care phase of an illness. An open relationship between you and a patient and family leads to a family-centered plan of care at discharge, including coordination of resources in the community and the patient's home (Gaskin, 2018). For example, when a patient who needs home IV antibiotic therapy is discharged, the family caregiver needs to know how to take care of the peripherally inserted central catheter (PICC) line, how to administer the IV antibiotic, how to recognize complications, and when to contact the home health nurse. Be sure the family caregiver is prepared for discharge and knows where to obtain necessary supplies.

Communication. An acute care setting involves multiple health care providers, and therefore clear communication is essential. It is important for the health care team to use communication techniques that are supportive, clear to understand, and consistent and that advocate for a family's expectations (Stajduhar et al., 2017). In addition, clear communication from the health care team helps to clarify medical terminology and enables the family to understand the health care issues, the types of decisions, and potential health care outcomes (see Chapter 24). Use clear plain language when you communicate, and provide professional interpreters if a patient or family does not speak English.

Help the family identify methods to maintain open lines of communication with you and the interprofessional health care team to anticipate your patient's and family members' needs. For example, when caring for a patient with ovarian cancer, how will you use caring practices to help her spouse inform family members about the patient's progress and plan of care? Identify who makes decisions for the family and consistently go to the decision maker. In some situations, the decision maker also needs assistance in developing a method to clearly communicate any decisions. In this electronic age, some families use blogs or social media as a way of providing consistent information. Help the family determine whether this is the best approach for their family needs and structure.

Restorative and Continuing Care. In restorative and continuing care settings, the challenge in family nursing is to maintain patients' functional abilities within the context of the family. This includes having home care nurses help patients remain in their homes following acute injuries or illnesses, surgery, or exacerbation of a chronic illness. It also requires finding ways to better the lives of individuals who are chronically ill or disabled and their families. Work closely with a patient and family to provide well-timed and targeted information, practical guidance, and instructions to help a family caregiver understand the specific care a patient will require in the home (Macleod et al., 2017).

When a patient's functional status changes, make sure that the home environment will accommodate a patient's strengths and limitations. Make a referral to home care. The patient may require other interprofessional care, such as occupational or physical therapy, as well. Clear, concise, and accurate communication with a home care nurse helps to provide continuity of care and facilitates transition from hospital to home. Educate family members about how they can participate in ongoing care and make changes in the home environment to help the patient be as self-sufficient as possible.

Family Caregiving. You help family caregivers by showing them how to perform specific aspects of physical care (e.g., dressing changes), by helping them find home care equipment (e.g., oxygen therapy), and by identifying other community resources (e.g., respite care facilities, rehab centers). Preparing members of the family for care activities and responsibilities helps caregiving become a meaningful experience for both the caregiver and the patient.

When family members become caregivers, their relationship with their significant other often changes. Whenever one individual becomes dependent on another family member for care, significant stress affects both the caregiver and the care recipient (Kaakinen, 2018). Thus, you have a key role in helping the family caregiver and patient develop communication and problem-solving skills to support the relationships needed for successful caregiving (Zhang, 2018).

Without adequate preparation and support from health care providers, caregiving puts the family at risk for serious problems, including a decline in the health of the caregiver and the care receiver, as well as dysfunctional and even abusive relationships (Pickering et al., 2017; Friedman et al., 2017). If your assessment reveals the relationship between potential caregivers and care recipients is not supportive, connect the patient and family with community services to provide the patient's caregiving needs.

You support a family caregiver in many ways. For example, listen to a caregiver's stories and help the caregiver continue to meet the demands of his or her usual lifestyle (e.g., working, raising children). Establish a caregiving schedule that enables all family members to participate, help patients to identify family members who can share the burdens posed by caregiving, and encourage distant relatives to communicate their support. Teach family caregivers to provide physical care for their family member. Recognize that family caregivers also have their own physical and emotional needs. Teach them how to meet their needs (Box 10.6) and set up respite times as appropriate to allow them time to care for themselves (Schaffer et al., 2017).

Connect family caregivers with community resources. National outreach programs such as the Family Caregiver Alliance (https://www.caregiver.org/), The Alzheimer's Association (https://www.alz.org/), and the Caregiver Action Network (https://caregiveraction.org/) provide information and services that can help improve the lives of family caregivers and the care they provide to their loved ones.

Community resources are organizations that can provide needed services or respite care to give the family caregiver time away from the care recipient. Examples of services that are beneficial to families include caregiver support groups, housing and transportation services, food and nutrition services, housecleaning, legal and financial services, home care, hospice, and mental health resources. Before referring a family to a community resource, it is critical that you understand the family's dynamics and their desire for support. Family caregivers sometimes resist help, feeling obligated to be the sole source of support to the care recipient. Be sensitive to family relationships and help caregivers understand the normalcy of caregiving demands. Given the appropriate resources, family caregivers are able to acquire the skills and knowledge necessary to effectively care for their loved ones within the context of the home while maintaining rich and rewarding personal relationships.

BOX 10.6 PATIENT TEACHING

Family Caregiving: Caregiver Role Strain

Objective
- Patient/family will adopt two interventions to reduce caregiver role strain.

Teaching Strategies
- Explain to all family caregivers the signs and symptoms of caregiver role strain such as:
  - Change in caregiver's appetite/weight, sleeping, or leisure activities.
  - Social withdrawal, irritability, anger, or changes in the caregiver's overall level of health.
  - Loss of interest in personal appearance.
- Discuss situations in which caregiver role strain may intensify (e.g., if the patient's health status changes or the patient needs to be hospitalized).
- Describe the importance of having family members set up alternating schedules to give the primary caregiver some rest.
- Provide information about community resources for transportation, respite care, and support groups.
- Offer an opportunity to ask questions and, when possible, provide a phone number for questions and assistance.
- Provide family members with the contact information of the patient's health care provider and instruct them to call if the caregiver has health problems, the caregiver seems overly exhausted, or they observe changes in the caregiver's interactions and attention to normal activities.

Evaluation
Use the principles of teach-back to evaluate patient/family caregiver learning:
- "I want to be sure I explained the effects of being a caregiver so you can recognize when you are under stress. Describe two or three effects that caregiving can have on you."
- "Some families I have cared for have trouble coping with all the responsibilities they have with caring for a family member. Can you explain to me what you are planning to do to help you feel less burdened or overwhelmed?"
- "There may be a time when you are going to need to call your mother's health care provider. Where do you plan on keeping the health care provider's contact information? What situations do you imagine might happen that would require you to call the health care provider?"

Evaluating the Outcomes of Family Care

Through the Patient's and Family's Eyes. It is important to obtain a family's perspective of the nursing care you provided and compare whether it met the family's goals. If your care did not meet the family's expectations, determine what they believe is missing. Consider short-term and long-term goals. Does the family perceive the patient received adequate pain control? Does the family perceive knowing what to do if problems develop at home? Evaluation is continuous and helps you decide when you need to modify your interventions or make referrals to other members of the health care team.

Patient and Family Outcomes. Evaluation is patient- and family-centered. When you care for a family as the context, focus on whether patient and family needs were met. Compare the response of a patient and family with the outcomes you set in the patient's plan of care.

When a family is the patient, your measure of family health becomes more than an evaluation of the health of all family members. You continue to focus on the outcomes you set based on the family-centered nursing diagnoses. For example, you evaluate a family's change in functioning and its satisfaction with the new level of functioning to determine whether a family is achieving its outcomes.

When you are caring for a family as a system, your evaluation focuses on the effects that the interventions had on the entire family, including extended family members. For example, if you are caring for an older adult who is receiving chemotherapy for a new cancer diagnosis, you evaluate how frequent trips to the oncology clinic and the cancer diagnosis affect the patient, the spouse, the children, and the grandchildren.

Evaluation is an ongoing process. Use critical thinking skills and clinical decision making to evaluate a family's response to interventions. Often a patient and/or family does not know how to best deliver care. For example, a family does not think that making dietary changes for a patient who is experiencing anorexia and nausea from chemotherapy is being effective. Evaluate the patient's nutritional status (e.g., laboratory values, weight, skin turgor), and explain to the family which evaluation data show that the dietary changes have been effective. Adjust the patient's diet if indicated.

KEY POINTS

- Families are as diverse as the individuals who compose them. Some family members have different beliefs and traditions, even within the same generation.
- Families face many challenges, including changing structures and roles, especially as the laws, economic status, and demographics of society change.
- Family caregiving is an interactive process that occurs within the context of the relationships among its members. Family caregivers are often spouses who are older adults or adult children trying to work full time and care for aging family members.
- Many factors, including the increased need for family caregivers, poverty, homelessness, and domestic violence, affect family forms and a family's health.
- A family's structure and functioning significantly influence the family's health, health needs, and ability to respond to health problems.
- Your decision to view a family as an important context for an individual family member or to view a family unit as the patient or as a system depends on the situation and the family's needs.
- The family is the primary social context in which health promotion and disease prevention take place. Family members influence one another's health beliefs, practices, and status.
- The concept of family is highly individual; focus the nursing process and nursing care on a patient's attitude and beliefs about family rather than on a traditional definition of family.
- As you provide family-centered care, you continually assess, analyze, and reflect on the changing needs and health care goals of patients and their families.
- The goal of family nursing is to help a family and its individual members reach and maintain maximum health throughout and beyond the illness experience.
- Whether you are caring for a patient with the family as context, patient, or a system, you direct your nursing interventions to increase abilities of family members to function and perform, remove barriers to health care, and do things that the family cannot do for itself.
- Evaluation of nursing care of families is centered on the patient and family. Compare actual responses to care with the outcomes you set in the plan of care, and revise the care plan as needed.

REFLECTIVE LEARNING

- Think about a patient you were assigned to care for recently. Describe the patient's family and its structure. What effect did that structure have on your patient's health?
- Interview a peer about his or her family. How do the beliefs and values of your peer's family affect the family's structure, functioning, health practices, and family celebrations?
- Reflect on a patient you cared for who had a family caregiver. What responsibilities did the family caregiver assume for the patient? Describe how the family caregiver coped with the caregiving role. What stressors related to caregiving did the family caregiver experience?

REVIEW QUESTIONS

1. A family includes a mother, a stepfather, two teenage biological daughters of the mother, and a biological daughter of the father. The father's daughter just moved home following the loss of her job in another city. The family is converting a study into a bedroom and is in the process of distributing household chores. Nursing assessment reveals all members of the family think that their family can adjust to lifestyle changes. This is an example of family:
   1. Diversity.
   2. Durability.
   3. Resiliency.
   4. Configuration.
2. A mother and her two children are homeless and enter a free health care clinic. Which statements most likely describe the effects of homelessness on this family? (Select all that apply.)
   1. The children have stability in their education.
   2. The family members may have symptoms of malnutrition, such as anemia.
   3. The family is at a low risk for experiencing violence.
   4. The children are at higher risk for developing ear infections.
   5. All family members may have mental health issues.
3. A nurse is caring for a 66-year-old patient who lives alone and is receiving chemotherapy and radiation for a new cancer diagnosis. He is unable to care for himself because of severe pain and fatigue. He moves into his 68-year-old brother's home so his brother can help care for him. Which assessment findings indicate that this family caregiving situation will be successful? (Select all that apply.)
   1. Both the patient and his brother attend church together regularly.
   2. The brothers are living together and enjoy eating the same foods.
   3. Other siblings live in the same city and are willing to help.
   4. The patient and his brother have a close network of friends.
   5. The patient has obsessive-compulsive disorder and has difficulty throwing away possessions.
4. A family is facing job loss of the father, who is the major wage earner, and relocation to a new city where there is a new job. The children will have to switch schools, and his wife will have to resign from the job she enjoys. Which of the following contribute to this family's hardiness? (Select all that apply.)
   1. Family meetings
   2. Established family roles
   3. New neighborhood
   4. Willingness to change in time of stress
   5. Passive orientation to life
5. A patient who is newly diagnosed with breast cancer states, "Although I am really scared about what is going to happen to me, I know my family will learn from this experience, and we will be stronger in the end." What term does the nurse use in the patient's

medical record to describe the characteristic displayed in this statement?
1. Resiliency
2. End-of-life care
3. Family functioning
4. Family's culture

6. A hospice nurse is caring for a family that is providing end-of-life care for their grandmother, who has terminal breast cancer. The nurse focuses on symptom management for the grandmother and on helping the family with developing coping skills. This approach is an example of which of the following?
1. Family as context
2. Family as patient
3. Family as a system
4. Family as structure

7. A 7-year-old child was recently diagnosed with asthma. A nurse is providing education to the child and her parents about the treatment and management of asthma and changes they need to make in their home environment to promote her health. Which statement made by the parents requires follow-up by the nurse?
1. "We have made an appointment to talk with the school nurse about the change in our child's health."
2. "We forgot to give our daughter her medications before bedtime, so we made a list of her medications to help us remember."
3. "We have worked out a schedule to check on her before and after school."
4. "We have not been spending time with our parents because we are so busy taking care of our daughter."

8. A family consisting of a grandparent, two adults, and three school-age children just immigrated to the United States. They come to a community wellness center to establish health care. Which of the following questions does the nurse ask to assess the family's function? (Select all that apply.)

1. "What does your family do to keep members healthy?"
2. "How does your family usually make decisions?"
3. "What health services are available in your neighborhood?"
4. "Which rituals or celebrations are important for your family?"
5. "Is there a lot of crime in your neighborhood?"
6. "How many parks are there in your community?"

9. A married couple has three children. The youngest child just graduated from college and is moving to a different city to take a job. The other two children left the home several years ago. Both of their parents are older and are beginning to need help to maintain their home. What assessment questions will help the nurse determine the family's functioning? (Select all that apply).
1. Which transitions or changes in your family are you currently experiencing?
2. Are your children having any problems that are affecting your family right now?
3. Describe a recent family conflict and how your family resolved it.
4. What coping strategies do you typically use as a family?
5. Who is involved in helping care for your parents?

10. During a visit to a family clinic, a nurse teaches a mother about immunizations, the use of car seats, and home safety for an infant and toddler. Which type of nursing interventions are these?
1. Restorative
2. Health promotion
3. Acute care
4. Growth and development

Answers: 1. 3; **2.** 2, 4, 5; **3.** 1, 3, 4; **4.** 1, 2, 4, 5; **5.** 1; **6.** 2; **7.** 4; **8.** 1, 2, 4; **9.** 3, 4, 5; **10.** 2.

Rationales for Review Questions can be found on the Evolve website.

REFERENCES

Administration for Community Living & Administration on Aging (ACL, AoA): *2017 profile of older Americans*, 2018. https://www.acl.gov/sites/default/files/Aging%20and%20Disability%20in%20America/2017OlderAmericansProfile.pdf. Accessed August 2018.

American Psychological Association (APA): *Marriage & divorce*, 2018. http://www.apa.org/topics/divorce/. Accessed August 2018.

Children's Defense Fund (CDF): *The state of America's children® 2017 report*, 2017. http://www.childrensdefense.org/library/state-of-americas-children/. Accessed August 2018.

Cohen D, Passel JS: *A record 64 million Americans live in multigenerational households*, Pew Research Center, 2018. http://www.pewresearch.org/fact-tank/2018/04/05/a-record-64-million-americans-live-in-multigenerational-households/. Accessed August 2018.

DeWolf M: *12 stats about working women*, US Department of Labor Blog, 2017. https://blog.dol.gov/2017/03/01/12-stats-about-working-women. Accessed August 2018.

Duhamel F: Translating knowledge from a family systems approach to clinical practice: insights from knowledge translation research experiences, *J Fam Nurs* 23(4):461, 2017.

Family Caregiver Alliance (FCA): *Caregiver statistics: demographics*, 2016a. https://www.caregiver.org/caregiver-statistics-demographics. Accessed August 2018.

Family Caregiver Alliance (FCA): *Caregiver statistics: work and caregiving*, 2016b. https://www.caregiver.org/caregiver-statistics-work-and-caregiving. Accessed August 2018.

Family Caregiver Alliance (FCA): *National center on caregiving*, 2019. https://www.caregiver.org/. Accessed March 2019.

Fournier AL: Creating a sacred space in the intensive care unit at the end of life, *DCCN* 36(2):110, 2017.

Futures Without Violence: *Futures without violence*, 2018. http://www.futureswithoutviolence.org/. Accessed August 2018.

Giddens JF: *Concepts for nursing practice*, ed 2, St Louis, 2017, Elsevier.

Giger J: *Transcultural nursing assessment and intervention*, ed 7, St Louis, 2017, Mosby.

Kaakinen JR, et al.: *Family health care nursing: theory, practice, and research*, ed 6, Philadelphia, 2018, FA Davis.

Leahey M, Wright L: Application of the Calgary family assessment and intervention models, *J Fam Nurs* 22(4):450, 2016.

Martin JA, et al.: Births: final data for 2016, *Natl Vital Stat Rep* 67(1), 2018. https://www.cdc.gov/nchs/data/nvsr/nvsr67/nvsr67_01.pdf. Accessed August 2018.

Martinez ME, Ward BW: *Health care access and utilization among adults aged 18-64 by poverty level: United States 2013–2015*, National Center for Health Statistics, 2016. https://www.cdc.gov/nchs/products/databriefs/db262.htm. Accessed August 2018.

Masci D: *5 facts about same-sex marriage*, 2017. http://www.pewresearch.org/fact-tank/2017/06/26/same-sex-marriage/. Accessed August 2018.

National Alliance to End Homelessness: *Children and families*, 2018. https://endhomelessness.org/homelessness-in-america/who-experiences-homelessness/children-and-families/. Accessed August 2018.

National Coalition for the homeless: issues, 2018, https://nationalhomeless.org/issues/. Accessed August 2018.

National Institutes of Health (NIH): *What does it mean to have a genetic predisposition to a disease?* 2018. https://ghr.nlm.nih.gov/primer/mutationsanddisorders/predisposition. Accessed August 2018.

Office of Adolescent Health: *Adolescent reproductive health fact sheets*, US Department of Health & Human Services, 2015. https://www.hhs.gov/ash/oah/facts-and-stats/national-and-state-data-sheets/adolescent-reproductive-health. Accessed August 2018.

Orchard CA, et al.: Collaborative leadership, part 2: the role of the nurse leader in interprofessional team-based practice – shifting from task- to collaborative patient-/family-focused care, *Nurs Leadersh* 30(2):26, 2017.

Resilience, adaptation, and well-being: measures, 2016, http://www.mccubbinresilience.org/measures.html. Accessed August 2018.

Shajani Z, Snell D: *Wright & Leahy's Nurses and families: a guide to family assessment and intervention*, ed 7, Philadelphia, 2019, FA Davis.

Stepler R: *Led by baby boomers, divorce rates climb for America's 50+ population*, Pew Research Center, 2017.

http://www.pewresearch.org/fact-tank/2017/03/09/led-by-baby-boomers-divorce-rates-climb-for-americas-50-population/. Accessed August 2018.

US Census Bureau: *The nation's older population is still growing*, Census Bureau reports, 2017a. https://www.census.gov/newsroom/press-releases/2017/cb17-100.html. Accessed August 2018.

US Census Bureau: *Income and poverty in the United States: 2016*, 2017b. https://www.census.gov/library/publications/2017/demo/p60-259.html. Accessed August 2018.

US Census Bureau: Percentage of people in poverty by different poverty measures: 2016, 2017c. https://www.census.gov/content/dam/Census/library/visualizations/2017/demo/p60-261/figure3.pdf. Accessed August 2018.

US Census Bureau: *Health insurance in the United States: 2016 – tables*, 2017d. https://www.census.gov/data/tables/2017/demo/health-insurance/p60-260.html., Accessed August 2018.

US Census Bureau: *The changing economics and demographics of young adulthood: 1975 – 2016*, 2017e. https://www.census.gov/library/publications/2017/demo/p20-579.html. Accessed August 2018.

US Census Bureau: *Families & households tables*, 2018. https://www.census.gov/topics/families/families-and-households/data/tables.html. Accessed August 2018.

US Interagency Council on Homelessness: *Ending family homelessness*, 2018. https://www.usich.gov/goals/families. Accessed August 2018.

RESEARCH REFERENCES

Allar I, et al.: The perceived impact of I am Moving, I am Learning on physical activity and family involvement: a preliminary investigation, *Am J Health Behav* 41(6):683, 2017.

Barnes AJ, et al.: Emotional health among youth experiencing family homelessness, *Pediatrics* 141(4):e20171767, 2018. http://pediatrics.aappublications.org/content/early/2018/03/15/peds.2017-1767. Accessed August 2018.

Benzies B, Mychasiuk R: Fostering family resiliency: a review of the key protective factors, *Child Fam Soc Work* 14:103–114, 2009.

Bickel KE, et al.: An American society of clinical oncology/American academy of hospice and palliative medicine guidance statement, *J Oncol Pract* 12(9):821, 2016.

Bigani DK, Correia AM: On the same page: nurse, patient, and family perceptions of change-of-shift bedside report, *J Pediatr Nurs* 41:84, 2018.

Brooks LA, et al.: Communication and decision-making about end-of-life care in the intensive care unit, *Am J Crit Care* 26(4):336, 2017.

Caceres BA, et al.: Family caregivers of patients with frontotemporal dementia: an integrative review, *Int J Nurs Stud* 55:71, 2016.

Coats H, et al.: Nurses' reflections on benefits and challenges of implementing family-centered care in pediatric intensive care units, *Am J Crit Care* 27(1):52, 2018.

Deek H, et al.: A family-focused intervention for heart failure self-care: conceptual underpinnings of a culturally appropriate intervention, *J Adv Nurs* 72(2):434, 2016.

DePasquale N, et al.: The family time squeeze: perceived family time adequacy buffers work strain in certified nursing assistants with multiple caregiving roles, *Gerontol* 58(3):546, 2018.

Friedman LS, et al.: Physical abuse of elderly adults: victim characteristics and determinants of revictimization, *J Am Geriatr Soc* 65(7):1420, 2017.

Gaskin KL: Patterns of transition experience for parents going home from hospital with their infant after first stage surgery for complex congenital heart disease, *J Pediatr Nurs* 41:e23, 2018.

Hashemi-Ghasemabadi M, et al.: Transition to the new role of caregiving for families of patients with breast cancer: a qualitative descriptive exploratory study, *Support Care Cancer* 24(3):1269, 2016.

Hicken BL, et al.: Supporting caregivers of rural veterans electronically (SCORE), *J Rural Health* 33:305, 2017.

Hunt T, et al.: Family economic stress, quality of paternal relationship, and depressive symptoms among African American adolescent fathers, *J Child Fam Stud* 24(10):3067, 2015.

Jaffray L, et al.: Evaluating the effects of mindfulness-based interventions for informal palliative caregivers: a systematic literature review, *Palliat Med* 30(2):117, 2016.

Kirby S, et al.: Are rural and remote patients, families, and caregiver needs in life-limiting illness different from those of urban dwellers? A narrative synthesis of the evidence, *Aust J Rural Health* 24(5):289, 2016.

Kokonya A, Fitzsimons F: Transition to long-term care: preparing older adults and their families, *Medsurg Nurs* 27(3):143, 2018.

Konerding U, et al.: Investigating burden of informal caregivers in England, Finland and Greece: an analysis with the short form of the Burden Scale for Family Caregivers (BSFC-s), *Aging Ment Health* 22(2):280, 2018.

Kung WW: Culture- and immigration-related stress faced by Chinese American families with a patient having schizophrenia, *J Marital Fam Ther* 42(3):409, 2015.

Lau M, et al.: Clusters of factors identify a high prevalence of pregnancy involvement among US adolescent males, *Matern Child Health J* 19:1713, 2015.

Macleod A, et al.: "There isn't an easy way of finding the help that's available." Barriers and facilitators of service use among dementia family caregivers: a qualitative study, *Int Psychogeriatr* 29(5):765, 2017.

Moriarty J, et al.: Exploration of factors related to depressive symptomatology in family members of military veterans with traumatic brain injury, *J Fam Nurs* 24(2):184, 2018.

Moss KO, et al.: Understanding end-of-life decision-making terminology among African American older adults, *J Gerontol Nurs* 44(2):33, 2018.

Newcomb AB, Hymes RA: Life interrupted: the trauma caregiver experience, *J Trauma Nurs* 24(2):125, 2017.

Petruzzo A, et al.: The lived experience of caregivers of persons with heart failure: a phenomenological study, *Eur J Cardiovasc Nurs* 16(7):638, 2017.

Phillips F, Prezio EA: Wonders & worries: evaluation of a child centered psychosocial intervention for families who have a parent/primary caregiver with cancer, *Psycho-Oncol* 26(7):1006, 2017.

Piccenna L, et al.: The experience of discharge for patients with an acquired brain injury from the inpatient to the community setting: a qualitative review, *Brain Inj* 30(3):241, 2016.

Pickering CEZ, et al.: Identifying elder abuse & neglect among family caregiving dyads: a cross sectional study

of psychometric properties of the QualCare scale, *Int J Nurs Stud* 69:41, 2017.

Salamizadeh A, et al.: The impact of spiritual care education on the self-efficacy of the family caregivers of elderly people with Alzheimer's disease, *Int J Commun Based Nurs Midwifery* 5(3):231, 2017.

Schaffer K, et al.: Mental and physical health correlates among family caregivers of patients with newly-diagnosed incurable cancer: a hierarchical linear regression analysis, *Support Care Cancer* 25(3):965, 2017.

Schultz REC, et al.: Is there hope? Is she there? How families and clinicians experience acute brain injury, *J Palliat Med* 20(2):170, 2017.

Sebern MD: Does an intervention designed to improve self-management, social support and awareness of palliative-care address needs of persons with heart failure, family caregivers and clinicians? *J Clin Nurs* 27(3/4):e643, 2018.

Sousza F, et al.: Calgary family assessment model applied in riverside context, *J Nurs UFPE* 11(12):4798, 2017.

Srisuk N, et al.: Randomized control trial of family-based education for patients with heart failure and their carers, *J Adv Nurs* 73(4):857, 2017.

Stajduhar K, et al.: Bereaved family members' perceptions of the quality of end-of-life care across four types of inpatient care settings, *BMC Palliat Care* 16(1), 2017.

Stockwell-Smith G, et al.: Hospital discharge processes involving older adults living with dementia: an integrated literature review, *J Clin Nurs* 27(5/6):e712, 2018.

Tremblay M, et al.: Fatherhood and delinquency: an examination of risk factors and offending patterns associated with fatherhood status among serious juvenile offenders, *J Child Fam Stud* 26(3):677, 2017.

Weisman de Mamani A, et al.: The interplay among mindfulness, caregiver burden, and mental health in family members of individuals with dementia, *Prof Psychol Res Pract* 49(2):116, 2018.

Zhang Y: Family functioning in the context of an adult family member with illness: a concept analysis, *J Clin Nurs* 27(15/16):3205, 2018.

11

Developmental Theories

OBJECTIVES

- Discuss theoretical underpinnings of growth and development.
- Describe and compare developmental theories.
- Apply developmental theories when planning interventions in the care of patients throughout the life span.

- Discuss nursing implications for the application of developmental principles to patient care.

KEY TERMS

Conventional reasoning, p. 140
Erikson's theory of psychosocial development, p. 137
Freud's psychoanalytical model of personality development, p. 136

Kohlberg's theory of moral development, p. 140
Piaget's theory of cognitive development, p. 138
Postconventional reasoning, p. 140

Temperament, p. 138

MEDIA RESOURCES

http://evolve.elsevier.com/Potter/fundamentals/
- Review Questions
- Case Study with Questions

- Audio Glossary
- Content Updates
- Answers to QSEN Activity and Review Questions

Understanding normal growth and development helps nurses predict, detect, and prevent deviations from patients' expected patterns. Growth encompasses the physical changes that occur from the prenatal period through older adulthood and also demonstrates both advancement and deterioration. Development refers to the biological, cognitive, and socio-emotional changes that begin at conception and continue throughout a lifetime. Development is dynamic and includes progression. However, in some disease processes development is delayed or regresses.

Individuals have unique patterns of growth and development. The ability to progress through each developmental phase influences the overall health of the individual. The success or failure experienced within a phase affects the ability to complete subsequent phases. If individuals have repeated developmental failures, inadequacies sometimes result. However, when an individual experiences repeated successes, health is promoted. For example, a child who does not walk by 20 months demonstrates delayed gross-motor ability that slows exploration and manipulation of the environment. In contrast, a child who walks by 10 months is able to explore and find stimulation in the environment.

When caring for patients, it is important to adopt a life span perspective of human development that takes into account all developmental stages. Traditionally development focused on childhood; however, an understanding of growth and development throughout the life span helps in planning questions for health screenings and health history, health promotion and maintenance, and health education for patients.

DEVELOPMENTAL THEORIES

Developmental theories provide a framework for examining, describing, and appreciating human development. For example, knowledge of

Erikson's psychosocial theory of development helps caregivers understand the importance of supporting the development of basic trust in the infancy stage. Trust establishes the foundation for all future relationships. Developmental theories are also important in helping nurses assess and treat a person's response to an illness. Understanding the specific task or need of each developmental stage guides caregivers in planning appropriate individualized care for patients.

Human development is a dynamic and complex process that cannot be explained by only one theory. This chapter presents biophysical, psychoanalytical/psychosocial, cognitive, and moral developmental theories. Chapters 25 and 35 cover the areas of learning theory for patient teaching and spiritual development.

Biophysical Developmental Theories

Biophysical development is how our physical bodies grow and change. Health care providers compare the changes that occur as a newborn infant grows against established norms. How does the physical body age? What are the triggers that move the body from the physical characteristics of childhood, through adolescence, to the physical changes of adulthood?

Gesell's Theory of Development. Fundamental to Gesell's theory of development is that each child's pattern of growth is unique and this pattern is directed by gene activity (Gesell, 1948). Gesell noted that the pattern of maturation follows a fixed developmental sequence. Sequential development is evident in fetuses, in which there is a specified order of organ system development. Today we know that growth in humans is both cephalocaudal and proximodistal. The cephalocaudal pattern describes the sequence in which growth is fastest at the top (e.g., head and brain develop faster than arm and leg coordination). The proximodistal growth pattern starts at the center of the body and moves toward the extremities (e.g., organ systems in the trunk of the body develop before the arms and legs). Genes direct the sequence of development, but environmental factors also influence development, resulting in developmental changes. For example, genes direct the growth rate in height for an individual, but that growth is only maximized if environmental conditions are adequate. Poor nutrition or chronic disease often affects the growth rate and results in smaller stature, regardless of a person's genetic blueprint. However, adequate nutrition and the absence of disease cannot result in height beyond that determined by heredity.

Psychoanalytical/Psychosocial Theory

Theories of psychoanalytical/psychosocial development describe human development from the perspectives of personality, thinking, and behavior (Table 11.1). Psychoanalytical theory explains development as primarily unconscious and influenced by emotion. Psychoanalytical theorists maintain that these unconscious conflicts influence development through universal stages experienced by all individuals (Berger, 2017).

Sigmund Freud. Freud's psychoanalytical model of personality development states that individuals go through five stages of psychosexual development and that each stage is characterized by sexual pleasure in parts of the body: the mouth, the anus, and the genitals. Freud believed that adult personality is the result of how an individual resolves conflicts between these sources of pleasure and the mandates of reality (Santrock, 2018).

Stage 1: Oral (Birth to 12 to 18 Months). Initially sucking and oral satisfaction are not only vital to life but also extremely pleasurable in their own rights. Late in this stage the infant begins to realize that the mother/parent is something separate from self. Disruption in the physical or emotional availability of the parent (e.g., inadequate bonding or chronic illness) could affect an infant's development.

Stage 2: Anal (12 to 18 Months to 3 Years). The focus of pleasure changes to the anal zone. Children become increasingly aware of the pleasurable sensations of this body region with interest in the products of their effort. Through the toilet-training process the child delays gratification to meet parental and societal expectations.

Stage 3: Phallic or Oedipal (3 to 6 Years). The genital organs are the focus of pleasure during this stage. The boy becomes interested in the penis; the girl becomes aware of the absence of the penis, known as *penis envy*. This is a time of exploration and imagination as a child fantasizes about the parent of the opposite sex as his or her first love interest, known as the *Oedipus* or *Electra complex*. By the end of this stage the child attempts to reduce this conflict by identifying with the parent of the same sex as a way to win recognition and acceptance.

Stage 4: Latency (6 to 12 Years). In this stage Freud believed that children repress and channel sexual urges from the earlier Oedipal stage into productive activities that are socially acceptable. Within the educational and social worlds of the child, there is much to learn and accomplish.

Stage 5: Genital (Puberty Through Adulthood). In this final stage sexual urges reawaken and are directed to an individual outside the family circle. Unresolved prior conflicts surface during adolescence. Once the individual resolves conflicts, he or she is then capable of having a mature adult sexual relationship.

Freud believed that the components of the human personality develop in stages and regulate behavior. These components are the id, the ego, and the superego. The id (i.e., basic instinctual impulses driven to achieve pleasure) is the most primitive part of the personality and originates in the infant. The infant cannot tolerate delay and must have needs met immediately. The ego represents the reality component, mediating conflicts between the environment and the forces of the id. It helps people judge reality accurately, regulate impulses, and make good decisions. Ego is often referred to as one's sense of self. The third component, the superego, performs regulating, restraining, and prohibiting actions. Often referred to as the conscience, the superego is influenced by the standards of outside social forces (e.g., parent or teacher).

TABLE 11.1	Comparison of Major Developmental Theories			
Developmental Stage/Age	**Freud (Psychosexual Development)**	**Erikson (Psychosocial Development)**	**Piaget (Cognitive/ Moral Development)**	**Kohlberg (Development of Moral Reasoning)**
Infancy (birth to 18 months)	Oral stage	Trust vs. mistrust Ability to trust others	Sensorimotor period Progress from reflex activity to simple repetitive actions	
Early childhood/toddler (18 months to 3 years)	Anal stage	Autonomy vs. shame and doubt Self-control and independence	Preoperational period—thinking using symbols Egocentric	Preconventional level Punishment-obedience orientation
Preschool (3-5 years)	Phallic stage	Initiative vs. guilt Highly imaginative	Use of symbols Egocentric	Preconventional level Premoral Instrumental orientation
Middle childhood (6-12 years)	Latent stage	Industry vs. inferiority Engaged in tasks and activities	Concrete operations period Logical thinking	Conventional level Good boy–nice girl orientation
Adolescence (12-19 years)	Genital stage	Identity vs. role confusion Sexual maturity, "Who am I?"	Formal operations period Abstract thinking	Postconventional level Social contract orientation
Young Adult		Intimacy vs. isolation Affiliation vs. love		
Adult		Generativity vs. self-absorption and stagnation		
Old age		Integrity vs. despair		

Some of Freud's critics contend that he based his analysis of personality development on biological determinants and ignored the influence of culture and experience. Others think that Freud's basic assumptions such as the Oedipus complex are not applicable across different cultures. Psychoanalysts today believe that the role of conscious thought is much greater than Freud imagined (Santrock, 2017).

Erik Erikson. Freud had a strong influence on his psychoanalytical followers, including Erik Erikson (1902-1994), who constructed a theory of development that differed from Freud's in one main aspect: Erikson's stages emphasize a person's relationship to family and culture rather than sexual urges (Berger, 2017).

According to Erikson's theory of psychosocial development, individuals need to accomplish a particular task before successfully mastering the stage and progressing to the next one. Each task is framed with opposing conflicts, and tasks once mastered are challenged and tested again during new situations or at times of conflict (Hockenberry et al., 2019).

Trust vs. Mistrust (Birth to 12 to 18 months). Establishing a basic sense of trust is essential for the development of a healthy personality. An infant's successful resolution of this stage requires a consistent caregiver who is available to meet his needs. From this basic trust in parents, an infant is able to trust in herself or himself, in others, and in the world (Hockenberry et al., 2019). The formation of trust results in faith and optimism. A nurse's use of anticipatory guidance helps parents cope with the hospitalization of an infant and the infant's behaviors when discharged to home.

Autonomy vs. Sense of Shame and Doubt (18 Months to 3 Years). By this stage a growing child is more accomplished in some basic self-care activities, including walking, feeding, and toileting. This newfound independence is the result of maturation and imitation. A toddler develops his or her autonomy by making choices. Choices typical for the toddler age-group include activities related to relationships, desires, and playthings. There is also opportunity to learn that parents and society have expectations about these choices. Limiting choices and/or enacting harsh punishment leads to feelings of shame and doubt. A toddler who successfully masters this stage achieves self-control and willpower. The nurse models empathetic guidance that offers support for and understanding of the challenges of this stage. Available choices for the child must be simple in nature and safe.

Initiative vs. Guilt (3 to 6 Years). Children like to pretend and try out new roles. Fantasy and imagination allow them to further explore their environment. Also at this time they are developing their superego, or conscience. Conflicts often occur between a child's desire to explore and the limits placed on his or her behavior. These conflicts sometimes lead to feelings of frustration and guilt. Guilt also occurs if a caregiver's responses are too harsh. Preschoolers learn to maintain a sense of initiative without imposing on the freedoms of others. Successful resolution of this stage results in direction and purpose. Teaching a child impulse control and cooperative behaviors helps a family avoid the risks of altered growth and development. Preschoolers frequently engage in animism, a developmental characteristic that makes them treat dolls or stuffed animals as if they have thoughts and feelings. Play therapy is also instrumental in helping a child successfully deal with the inherent threats related to hospitalization or chronic illness.

REFLECT NOW

You are observing a group of 4- to 5-year-old children in a hospital play group. You notice that some of the children are applying bandages to their stuffed animals. Think about how play activity may help these children cope with hospitalization.

Industry vs. Inferiority (6 to 12 Years). School-age children are eager to apply themselves to learning socially productive skills and tools. They learn to work and play with their peers. They thrive on their accomplishments and praise. Without proper support for learning new skills or if skills are too difficult, they develop a sense of inadequacy and inferiority. Children at this age need to be able to experience real achievement to develop a sense of competency. Erikson believed that an adult's attitudes toward work are traced to successful achievement of this task (Erikson, 1963). During hospitalization it is important for a school-age child to understand the routines and participate, when possible, in his or her treatment. For example, some children enjoy keeping a record of their intake and output.

Identity vs. Role Confusion (Puberty). Dramatic physiological changes associated with sexual maturation mark this stage. There is a marked preoccupation with appearance and body image. This stage, in which identity development begins with the goal of achieving some perspective or direction, answers the question "Who am I?" Acquiring a sense of identity is essential for making adult decisions such as choice of a vocation or marriage partner. Each adolescent moves in his or her unique way into society as an interdependent member. There are also new social demands, opportunities, and conflicts that relate to the emergent identity and separation from family. Erikson held that successful mastery of this stage resulted in devotion and fidelity to others and to their own ideals (Hockenberry et al., 2019).

The adolescent does not consistently perceive vulnerability associated with risk-taking behaviors (Faial et al., 2016). This perceived invulnerability contributes to risk-taking behaviors (Warner, 2018). Nurses have the opportunity to provide education and anticipatory guidance for parents about the changes and challenges and risks to adolescents. When adolescents are hospitalized, help them deal with their illnesses by giving them enough information to help make some decisions about their treatment plan (see Chapter 12).

Intimacy vs. Isolation (Young Adult). Young adults, having developed a sense of identity, deepen their capacity to love others and care for them. They search for meaningful friendships and an intimate relationship with another person. Erikson portrayed intimacy as finding the self and then losing it in another (Santrock, 2017). If the young adult is not able to establish companionship and intimacy, isolation results because he or she fears rejection and disappointment (Berger, 2017). Nurses must understand that during hospitalization a young adult's need for intimacy remains present; thus young adults benefit from the support of their partner or significant other during this time.

Generativity vs. Self-Absorption and Stagnation (Middle Age). Following the development of an intimate relationship, an adult focuses on supporting future generations. The ability to expand one's personal and social involvement is critical to this stage of development. Middle-age adults achieve success in this stage by contributing to future generations through parenthood, teaching, mentoring, and community involvement. Achieving generativity results in caring for others as a basic strength. Inability to play a role in the development of the next generation results in stagnation (Santrock, 2017). Nurses help physically ill adults choose creative ways to foster social development. Middle-age people often find a sense of fulfillment by volunteering in a local school, hospital, or church.

Integrity vs. Despair (Old Age). Many older adults review their lives with a sense of satisfaction, even with their inevitable mistakes. Others see themselves as failures, with their lives marked by despair and regret. Older adults often engage in a retrospective appraisal of their lives. They interpret their lives as a meaningful whole or experience regret because of goals not achieved (Berger, 2017). Because the aging process creates physical and social losses, some adults also suffer loss of status and function (e.g., through retirement or illness). You can enhance feelings of integrity by encouraging older adults to reflect on their meaningful relationships, such as relationships with a higher power, family members, or the community (Touhy & Jett, 2016). These external struggles are met with internal struggles, such as the search for meaning in life. Meeting these challenges creates the potential for growth and the basic strength of wisdom (Fig. 11.1).

Nurses are in positions of influence within their communities to help people feel valued, appreciated, and needed. Erikson stated, "Healthy children will not fear life, if their parents have integrity enough not to fear death" (Erikson, 1963). Although Erikson believed that problems in adult life resulted from unsuccessful resolution of earlier stages, his emphasis on family relationships and culture offers a broad, life span view of development. As a nurse you will use this knowledge of development as you deliver care in any health care setting.

Theories Related to Temperament. Temperament is a behavioral style that affects an individual's emotional interactions with others. Temperamental traits identified in infancy may continue to influence a child's behavior through middle school (Hockenberry et al., 2019). Personality and temperament are often closely linked, and individuals possess some enduring characteristics into adulthood. The individual differences that children display in responding to their environment significantly influence the way others respond to them and their needs. Knowledge of temperament helps parents better understand their child (Hockenberry et al., 2019).

Most children have one of these three broad temperamental traits—easy, slow to warm up, and difficult (Hockenberry et al., 2019):

- *The easy child*—Easygoing and even-tempered. This child is regular and predictable in his or her habits. An easy child is open and adaptable to change and displays a mild to moderately intense mood that is typically positive.
- *The slow-to–warm up child*—Typically displays discomfort when introduced to new situations and needs time to adjust to new environment, authority figures, and expectations. These children respond with tears, somatic complaints, or other maneuvers to avoid the situation (e.g., complaining of a stomachache to avoid going to school).
- *The difficult child*—Highly distracted, active, irritable, and irregular in habits. This child may benefit from "practice" or role playing to be successful with new skills, situations, or environments.

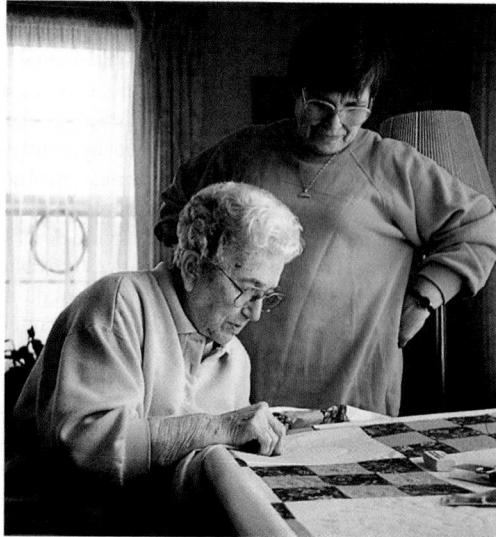

FIG. 11.1 Quilting keeps this older adult active.

Knowledge of temperament and how it impacts the parent-child relationship is critical when providing anticipatory guidance for parents. With the birth of a second child, most parents find that the strategies that worked well with the first child no longer work at all. The nurse individualizes counseling to greatly improve the quality of interactions between parents and children (Hockenberry et al., 2019).

Perspectives on Adult Development

Early studies of development focused only on childhood; however, we now know that although the changes come more slowly, people continue to develop new abilities and adapt to shifting environments.

A life span approach accounts for the multiple life events occurring in adulthood. The contemporary life events approach takes into consideration the variations that occur for each individual. This view considers an individual's personal circumstances (health and family support), how a person views and adjusts to changes, and the current social and historical context in which an individual is living. The increase in life expectancy has made popular the life span approach to development (Santrock, 2018). Life span development is lifelong, multidimensional, multidirectional, and contextual. Development is an interaction of biological, sociocultural, and individual factors (Baltes et al., 2005). Current research on successful aging is much more consistent with a life span approach that emphasizes age-related goals that are relationship oriented and socially oriented to support continued well-being (Nosraty et al., 2015).

Cognitive Developmental Theory

Psychoanalytical/psychosocial theories focus on an individual's unconscious thought and emotions; cognitive theories stress how people learn to think and make sense of their world. As with personality development, cognitive theorists have explored both childhood and adulthood. Some of the theories highlight qualitative changes in thinking; others expand to include social, cultural, and behavioral dimensions.

Jean Piaget. Jean Piaget was most interested in the development of children's intellectual organization: how they think, reason, and perceive the world (Piaget, 1952). Piaget's theory of cognitive development includes four periods that are related to age and demonstrate specific categories of knowing and understanding (see also Chapter 12). He built his theory on years of observing children as they explored, manipulated, and tried to make sense out of the world in which they lived. Piaget believed that individuals move from one stage to the other seeking cognitive equilibrium or a state of mental balance and that they build mental structures to help adapt to the world (Santrock, 2017). Within each of these primary periods of cognitive development are specific stages (see Table 11.1).

Period I: Sensorimotor (Birth to 2 Years). Infants develop a schema or action pattern for dealing with the environment (Box 11.1). These schemas include hitting, looking, grasping, or kicking. Schemas become self-initiated activities (e.g., the infant learning that sucking achieves a pleasing result generalizes the action to suck fingers, blanket, or clothing). Successful achievement leads to greater exploration. During this stage a child learns about himself and his environment through motor and reflex actions. He or she learns that he or she is separate from the environment and that aspects of the environment (e.g., parents or favorite toy) continue to exist even though they cannot always be seen. Piaget termed this understanding that objects continue to exist even when they cannot be seen, heard, or touched *object permanence* and considered it one of the child's most important accomplishments.

Period II: Preoperational (2 to 7 Years). During this time children learn to think with the use of symbols and mental images. They exhibit

BOX 11.1 EVIDENCE-BASED PRACTICE

Applying Developmental Theory to Care of Infants

PICOT Question: In infants who are hospitalized, does parental emotional involvement at bedtime result in improved quality and length of infant sleep?

Evidence Summary

Twenty to thirty percent of infants have difficulty falling asleep and staying asleep (Ball, 2014; Shapiro-Mendoza et al., 2015). Mothers' emotional availability at bedtime has been linked to improved quality of sleep in infants and thought to be associated with infant feelings of safety and security. When mothers are emotionally available, infants are less distressed and sleep more throughout the night (Philbrook & Teti, 2016). In a different study, mothers who did not breastfeed at bedtime noted that increased participation by fathers during the bedtime ritual improved infant sleeping (Tikotzky et al., 2015). It is important that nurses apply developmental theory and recognize the importance of parental engagement in the quality of infant sleep.

Application to Nursing Practice

- Educate parents on how to realign their expectation regarding infant sleeping patterns (Ball, 2014).
- Be aware of the value of involving parents in infant care and feeding, particularly around bedtime (Ball, 2014).
- Help breastfeeding parents set up a bedtime ritual that involves the father (Tikotzky et al., 2015).
- Understand an infant's need for parental involvement in developing a sense of safety and security to enhance quality of sleep.

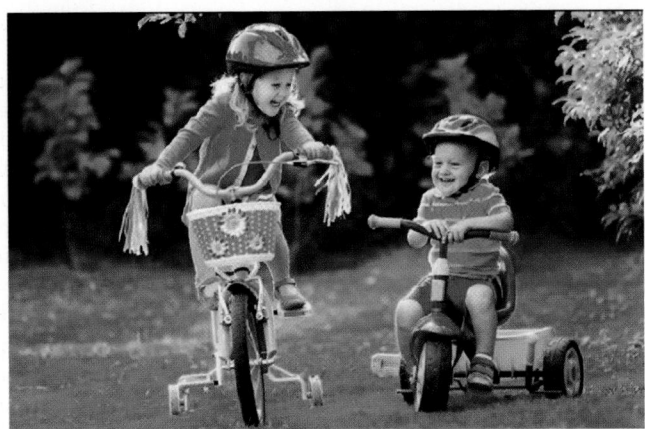

FIG. 11.2 Play is important to a child's development.

by self-consciousness: a belief that their actions and appearance are constantly being scrutinized (an "imaginary audience"), that their thoughts and feelings are unique (the "personal fable"), and that they are invulnerable (Santrock, 2018). These feelings of invulnerability frequently lead to risk-taking behaviors, especially in early adolescence. As adolescents share experiences with peers, they learn that many of their thoughts and feelings are shared by almost everyone, helping them to know that they are not so different. As they mature, their thinking moves to abstract and theoretical subjects. They have the capacity to reason with respect to possibilities.

REFLECT NOW

What nursing actions based on developmental theory could you use to promote an adolescent's emotional well being?

Piaget noted that some aspects of objective performance emerge earlier, and other cognitive abilities can surface later in life. Many adults may not become formal operational thinkers and remain at the concrete stage, and others have cognitive development that goes beyond the stages that Piaget proposed (Santrock, 2018). Assessment of cognitive ability becomes critical as you provide health care teaching to patients and families.

Research in Adult Cognitive Development. Research into cognitive development in adulthood began in the 1970s and continues today. It supports that adults do not always arrive at one answer to a problem but frequently accept several possible solutions. Adults also incorporate emotions, logic, practicality, and flexibility when making decisions. On the basis of these observations, developmentalists proposed a fifth stage of cognitive development termed *postformal thought*. Within this stage adults demonstrate the ability to recognize that answers vary from situation to situation and that solutions need to be sensible. Also within this stage is a struggle with identity and "finding oneself" (Sinnott, 2017).

One of the earliest to develop a theory of adult cognition was William Perry (1913-1998), who studied college students and found that continued cognitive development involved increasing cognitive flexibility. As adolescents were able to move from a position of accepting only one answer to realizing that alternative explanations could be right, depending on one's perspective, there was a significant cognitive change. Adults change how they use knowledge, and the emphasis shifts from attaining knowledge or skills to using knowledge for goal achievement.

"egocentrism" in that they see objects and people from only one point of view, their own. They believe that everyone experiences the world exactly as they do. Early in this stage children demonstrate "animism," in which they personify objects. They believe that inanimate objects have lifelike thought, wishes, and feelings. Their thinking is influenced greatly by fantasy and magical thinking. Children at this stage have difficulty conceptualizing time. Play becomes a primary means by which they foster their cognitive development and learn about the world (Fig. 11.2). Nursing interventions during this period recognize the use of play as the way the child understands the events taking place. Play therapy is a nursing intervention that helps the child work through invasive and intrusive procedures that may occur during hospitalization. In addition, play therapy helps the ill child progress developmentally.

Period III: Concrete Operations (7 to 11 Years). Children now are able to perform mental operations. For example, the child thinks about an action that before was performed physically. Children are now able to describe a process without actually doing it. At this time they are able to coordinate two concrete perspectives in social and scientific thinking, so they are able to appreciate the difference between their perspective and that of a friend. Reversibility is one of the primary characteristics of concrete operational thought. Children can now mentally picture a series of steps and reverse the steps to get back to the starting point. The ability to mentally classify objects according to their quantitative dimensions, known as *seriation,* is achieved. They are able to correctly order or sort objects by length, weight, or other characteristics. Another major accomplishment of this stage is *conservation,* or the ability to see objects or quantities as remaining the same despite a change in their physical appearance (Santrock, 2018).

Period IV: Formal Operations (11 Years to Adulthood). The transition from concrete to formal operational thinking occurs in stages during which there is a prevalence of egocentric thought. This egocentricity leads adolescents to demonstrate feelings and behaviors characterized

Moral Developmental Theory

Moral development refers to the changes in a person's thoughts, emotions, and behaviors that influence beliefs about what is right or wrong. It encompasses both *interpersonal* and *intrapersonal* dimensions as it governs how we interact with others (Santrock, 2018). Although various psychosocial and cognitive theorists address moral development within their respective theories, the theories of Piaget and Kohlberg are more widely known (see Table 11.1).

Kohlberg's Theory of Moral Development. Kohlberg's theory of moral development expands on Piaget's cognitive theory. Kohlberg interviewed children, adolescents, and eventually adults and found that moral reasoning develops in stages. From an examination of responses to a series of moral dilemmas, he identified six stages of moral development under three levels (Kohlberg, 1981). It is important to note that Kohlberg's theory is applicable to age 4 until adulthood. Children younger than 4 do not understand morality.

Level I: Preconventional Reasoning. This is the premoral level, in which there is limited cognitive thinking and an individual's thinking is primarily egocentric. At this stage thinking is mostly based on likes and pleasures. This stage progresses toward having punishment guide behavior. A person's moral reason for acting, the "why," eventually relates to the consequences that the person believes will occur. These consequences come in the form of punishment or reward. It is at this level that children view illness as a punishment for fighting with their siblings or disobeying their parents. Nurses need to be aware of this egocentric thinking and reinforce that the child does not become ill because of wrongdoing.

Stage 1: Punishment and Obedience Orientation. In this first stage a child's response to a moral dilemma is in terms of absolute obedience to authority and rules. A child in this stage reasons, "I must follow the rules; otherwise I will be punished." Avoiding punishment or the unquestioning deference to authority is characteristic motivation to behave. Physical consequences guide right and wrong choices. If the child is caught, it must be wrong; if he or she escapes, it must be right.

Stage 2: Instrumental Relativist Orientation. In this stage the child recognizes that there is more than one right view; a teacher has one view that is different from that of the child's parent. The decision to do something morally right is based on satisfying one's own needs and occasionally the needs of others. The child perceives punishment not as proof of being wrong (as in stage 1) but as something that one wants to avoid. Children at this stage follow their parent's rule about being home in time for supper because they do not want to be confined to their room for the rest of the evening if they are late.

Level II: Conventional Reasoning. At level II, conventional reasoning, the person sees moral reasoning based on his or her own personal internalization of societal and others' expectations. A person wants to fulfill the expectations of the family, group, or nation and also develop a loyalty to and actively maintain, support, and justify the order. Moral decision making at this level moves from "What's in it for me?" to "How will it affect my relationships with others?" Emphasis now is on social rules and a community-centered approach (Berger, 2017). Nurses observe this when family members make end-of-life decisions for their loved ones. Individual members often struggle with this type of moral dilemma. Grief support involves an understanding of the level of moral decision making of each family member (see Chapter 36).

Stage 3: Good Boy–Nice Girl Orientation. The individual wants to win approval and maintain the expectations of one's immediate group. "Being good" is important and defined as having positive motives, showing concern for others, and keeping mutual relationships through trust, loyalty, respect, and gratitude. One earns approval by "being nice." For example, a person in this stage stays after school and does odd jobs to win the teacher's approval.

Stage 4: Society-Maintaining Orientation. During stage 4 individuals expand their focus from a relationship with others to societal concerns. Moral decisions take into account societal perspectives. Right behavior is doing one's duty, showing respect for authority, and maintaining the social order. Adolescents choose not to attend a party where they know beer will be served, not because they are afraid of getting caught but because they know that it is not right.

Level III: Postconventional Reasoning. The person finds a balance between basic human rights and obligations and societal rules and regulations in the level of postconventional reasoning. Individuals move away from moral decisions based on authority or conformity to groups to define their own moral values and principles. Individuals at this stage start to look at what an ideal society would be like. Moral principles and ideals come into prominence at this level (Berger, 2017).

Stage 5: Social Contract Orientation. Having reached stage 5, an individual follows the societal law but recognizes the possibility of changing the law to improve society. The individual also recognizes that different social groups have different values but believes that all rational people would agree on basic rights such as liberty and life. Individuals at this stage make more of an independent effort to determine what society *should* value rather than what the society as a group would value.

Stage 6: Universal Ethical Principle Orientation. Stage 6 defines "right" by the decision of conscience in accord with self-chosen ethical principles. These principles are abstract, like the Golden Rule, and appeal to logical comprehensiveness, universality, and consistency (Kohlberg, 1981). For example, the principle of justice requires the individual to treat everyone in an impartial manner, respecting the basic dignity of all people, and guides the individual to base decisions on an equal respect for all. Civil disobedience is one way to distinguish stage 5 from stage 6. Stage 5 emphasizes the basic rights, the democratic process, and following laws without question; whereas stage 6 defines the principles by which agreements will be most just. For example, a person in stage 5 follows a law, even if it is not fair to a certain racial group. An individual in stage 6 may not follow a law if it does not seem just to the racial group. For example, Martin Luther King believed that although we need laws and democratic processes, people who are committed to justice have an obligation to disobey unjust laws and accept the penalties for disobeying these laws (Crain, 1985).

Kohlberg's Critics. Kohlberg constructed a systemized way of looking at moral development and is recognized as a leader in moral developmental theory. However, critics of his work raise questions about his choice of research subjects. For example, most of Kohlberg's subjects were males raised in Western philosophical traditions. Research attempting to support Kohlberg's theory with individuals raised in the Eastern philosophies found that individuals raised in Eastern philosophies never rose above stages 3 or 4 of Kohlberg's model. To some, these findings suggest that people from Eastern philosophies have not reached higher levels of moral development, which is untrue. Others believe that Kohlberg's research design did not allow a way to measure those raised within a different culture.

Kohlberg has also been criticized for age and gender bias (Zizick et al., 2015). Carol Gilligan criticizes Kohlberg for his gender biases. She believes that he developed his theory on the basis of a justice perspective that focused on the rights of individuals. In contrast, Gilligan's research looked at moral development from a care perspective that viewed people in their interpersonal communications, relationships, and concern for others (Gilligan, 1982; Santrock, 2018). Other researchers have examined Gilligan's theory in studies with children and have not found evidence to support gender differences (Santrock, 2018).

Moral Reasoning and Nursing Practice. Nurses need to recognize their own moral reasoning. Recognizing your own moral developmental level is essential in separating your beliefs from others when helping patients with their moral decision-making process. It is also important to recognize the level of moral and ethical reasoning used by other members of the health care team and its influence on a patient's care plan.

REFLECT NOW

A nurse is caring for a homeless person and believes that all patients deserve the same level of care. The case manager, who is responsible for resource allocation, complains about the amount of resources being expended. What types of moral frustrations is the nurse encountering and how might this impact his or her nursing practice?

Ideally all members of the health care team are on the same level, creating a unified outcome. Research indicates that nurses experience frustration when faced with barriers to doing the right thing rather than confusion over what is the right thing (Rainer et al., 2018).

Developmental theories help nurses use critical thinking skills when asking how and why people respond as they do. From the diverse set of theories included in this chapter, the complexity of human development is evident. No one theory successfully describes all the intricacies of human growth and development. Today's nurse needs to be knowledgeable about several theoretical perspectives when working with patients.

Your assessment of a patient requires a thorough analysis and interpretation of data to form accurate conclusions about his or her developmental needs. Accurate identification of nursing diagnoses relies on your ability to consider developmental theory in data analysis. You compare normal developmental behaviors with those projected by developmental theory. Examples of nursing diagnoses applicable to patients with developmental problems include *impaired development (infant, child, adolescent, adult), risk for delayed growth,* and *risk for disproportionate growth.*

QSEN **Building Competency in Safety** Sam is an 84-year-old patient hospitalized for acute abdominal pain. He does not have any local family and lives in an assisted-housing community. He is confused and disoriented. How would your knowledge of developmental theories guide your nursing care for Sam in ensuring his safety?

Answers to QSEN Activities can be found on the Evolve website.

Growth and development, as supported by a life span perspective, is multidimensional. The theories included are the basis for a meaningful observation of an individual's pattern of growth and development. They are guidelines for understanding important human processes, and they allow nurses to begin to predict human responses and to recognize deviations from the norm.

▮ KEY POINTS

- Development is not limited to childhood and adolescence; people grow and develop throughout the life span.
- Developmental theories are a way to explain and predict human behavior.

- Developmental theory provides a basis through which nurses can assess and understand their patients' cognitive responses and physical capabilities.
- Developmental theories are important guidelines for understanding human processes and assist nurses in predicting human responses and deviations from the norm.
- Developmental tasks are age-related cognitive, social, and physical achievements.

▮ REFLECTIVE LEARNING

- Consider a patient experience you encountered recently and describe how you practiced moral reasoning in providing care.
- How did a patient's developmental stage impact the care you provided during a clinical experience?
- Consider two of your patients and compare their cognitive developmental stages. Describe how you adapted your nursing care.

▮ REVIEW QUESTIONS

1. The nurse is aware that preschoolers often display a developmental characteristic that makes them treat dolls or stuffed animals as if they have thoughts and feelings. This is an example of:
   1. Logical reasoning.
   2. Egocentrism.
   3. Concrete thinking.
   4. Animism.
2. A 9-year-old child has a difficult time making friends at school and being chosen to play on the team. He also has trouble completing his homework and, as a result, receives little positive feedback from his parents or teacher. According to Erikson's theory, failure at this stage of development results in: (Select all that apply.)
   1. Feelings of inadequacy.
   2. A sense of guilt.
   3. A poor sense of self.
   4. Feelings of inferiority.
   5. Mistrust.
3. The nurse teaches parents how to have their children learn impulse control and cooperative behaviors. This would be during which of Erikson's stages of development?
   1. Trust versus mistrust
   2. Initiative versus guilt
   3. Industry versus inferiority
   4. Autonomy versus sense of shame and doubt
4. When Ryan was 3 months old, he had a toy train; when his view of the train was blocked, he did not search for it. Now that he is 9 months old, he looks for it, reflecting the presence of:
   1. Object permanence.
   2. Sensorimotor play.
   3. Schemata.
   4. Magical thinking.
5. When preparing a 4-year-old child for a procedure, which method is developmentally most appropriate for the nurse to use?
   1. Allowing the child to watch another child undergoing the same procedure
   2. Showing the child pictures of what he or she will experience
   3. Talking to the child in simple terms about what will happen
   4. Preparing the child through play with a doll and toy medical equipment

6. A nurse is caring for a man who is recently retired and who appears withdrawn. He says he is "bored with life." The nurse helps this individual find meaning in life by:
   1. Encouraging him to reflect on his relationships with others.
   2. Encouraging relocation to a new city.
   3. Explaining the need to simplify life.
   4. Encouraging him to adopt a new pet.

7. According to Piaget's cognitive theory, a 12-year-old child is most likely to engage in which of the following activities? (Select all that apply.)
   1. Using building blocks to determine how houses are constructed
   2. Writing a story about a clown who wants to leave the circus
   3. Drawing pictures of a family using stick figures
   4. Writing an essay about patriotism
   5. Hanging out with a best friend

8. Elizabeth, who is having unprotected sex with her boyfriend, comments to her friends, "Did you hear about Kathy? You know, she fools around so much; I heard she was pregnant. That would never happen to me!" This is an example of adolescent:
   1. Imaginary audience.
   2. False-belief syndrome.
   3. Personal fable.
   4. Sense of invulnerability.

9. Which of the following are examples of the conventional reasoning form of cognitive development? (Select all that apply.)
   1. A 35-year-old woman is speaking with you about her recent diagnosis of a chronic illness. She is concerned about her treatment options in relation to her ability to continue to care for her family. As she considers the options and alternatives, she incorporates information, her values, and emotions to decide which plan will be the best fit for her.
   2. A young father is considering whether or not to return to school for a graduate degree. He considers the impact the time commitment may have on the needs of his wife and infant son.
   3. A teenage girl is encouraged by her peers to engage in shoplifting. She decides not to join her peers in this activity because she is afraid of getting caught in the act.
   4. A single mother of two children is unhappy with her employer. She has been unable to secure alternate employment but decides to quit her current job.
   5. A young man drives over the speed limit regularly because he thinks he is an excellent driver and will not get into a car accident.

10. Dave reports being happy and satisfied with his life. What do we know about him?
    1. He is in one of the later developmental periods, concerned with reviewing his life.
    2. He is atypical, since most people in any of the developmental stages report significant dissatisfaction with their lives.
    3. He is in one of the earlier developmental periods, concerned with establishing a career and satisfying long-term relationships.
    4. It is difficult to determine Dave's developmental stage since most people report overall satisfaction with their lives in all stages.

Answers: 1. 4; **2.** 1, 4; **3.** 2, 4, 1; **5.** 4; **6.** 1; **7.** 2, 5; **8.** 4; **9.** 1, 2; **10.** 4.

Rationales for Review Questions can be found on the Evolve website.

REFERENCES

Baltes PB, et al.: The psychological science of human aging. In Johnson ML, editor: *The Cambridge handbook of age and aging*, New York, 2005, Cambridge University Press.

Berger KS: *The developing person: through the life span*, ed 10, New York, 2017, Worth.

Crain WC: *Theories of development: concepts and application*, Upper Saddle River, NJ, 1985, Prentice Hall.

Erikson E: *Childhood and society*, New York, 1963, Norton.

Gesell A: *Studies in child development*, New York, 1948, Harper.

Gilligan C: *In a different voice: psychological theory and women's development*, Cambridge, 1982, Harvard University Press.

Hockenberry MJ, Wilson D: *Wong's nursing care of infants and children*, ed 11, St Louis, 2019, Mosby.

Kohlberg L: *The philosophy of moral development: moral stages and the idea of justice*, San Francisco, 1981, Harper & Row.

Piaget J: *The origins of intelligence in children*, New York, 1952, International Universities Press.

Santrock JW: *A topical approach to life span development*, ed 7, New York, 2018, McGraw-Hill.

Santrock JW: *Life span development*, ed 15, New York, 2017, McGraw-Hill.

Touhy TA, Jett K: *Ebersole and Hess' toward healthy aging: human needs and nursing response*, ed 9, St. Louis, 2016, Elsevier.

Zizick B, et al.: *Moral development and citizenship education (9): Kohlberg Revisited*, Rotterdam/Boston/Taipei, 2015, Sense Publishers.

RESEARCH REFERENCES

Ball HL: Reframing what we tell parents about normal infant sleep and how we support them, *Breastfeed Rev* 22(3):11, 2014.

Faial LGM, et al.: Vulnerability in adolescents: a timely area for the practice of health: integrative review, *J Nurs UFPE Online, Recife* 10(9):3473–3482, 2016.

Nosraty L, et al.: Perceptions by the oldest old of successful aging, Vitality 90+ Study, *J Aging Stud* 32:50–58, 2015.

Philbrook L, Teti D: Bidirectional associations between bedtime parenting and infant sleep: parenting quality, parenting practices, and their interaction, *J Fam Psychol* 40(4):431–441, 2016.

Rainer J, et al.: Ethical dilemmas in nursing: an integrative review, *J Clin Nurs* 27(19/20):3446, 2018.

Shapiro-Mendoza CK, et al.: Trends in infant bedding use: National infant sleep position study, 1993-2010, *Pediatrics* 135(1):10, 2015.

Sinnott J: *Identity flexibility in adulthood: perspectives in adult development*, New York, 2017, Springer International Publishing.

Tikotzky L, et al.: Infant sleep development from 3 to 6 months postpartum: links with maternal sleep and paternal involvement, *Monogr Soc Res Child Dev* 80(1):107, 2015.

Warner TD: Adolescent sexual risk taking: the distribution of youth behaviors and perceived peer attitudes across neighborhood contexts, *J Adolesc Health* 62:226, 2018.

12

Conception Through Adolescence

OBJECTIVES

- Describe ways to promote health during pregnancy.
- Discuss common physical and psychosocial changes during the transition of a child from intrauterine to extrauterine life.
- Describe physical changes and growth from conception to adolescence.
- Describe cognitive and psychosocial development from birth to adolescence.
- Explain the role of play in the development of a child.
- Discuss ways in which a nurse is able to help parents meet their children's developmental needs.

KEY TERMS

Adolescence, p. 154
Apgar score, p. 144
Attachment, p. 144
Embryonic stage, p. 143
Fetal stage, p. 143

Fetus, p. 143
Infancy, p. 146
Neonatal period, p. 144
Preembryonic stage, p. 143
Preschool period, p. 151

Puberty, p. 154
School-age period, p. 154
Toddlerhood, p. 149

MEDIA RESOURCES

http://evolve.elsevier.com/Potter/fundamentals/
- Review Questions
- Case Study with Questions

- Audio Glossary
- Content Updates
- Answers to QSEN Activity and Review Questions

STAGES OF GROWTH AND DEVELOPMENT

Human growth and development are continuous and complex processes that are typically divided into stages organized by age-groups. Although this chronological division is somewhat arbitrary, it is based on the timing and sequence of developmental tasks that children accomplish in each stage. This chapter focuses on the physical, psychosocial, and cognitive changes, as well as the health risks and health promotion concerns relevant to each stage of growth and development.

SELECTING A DEVELOPMENTAL FRAMEWORK FOR NURSING

Using a family-centered approach that incorporates knowledge of developmental stages and theories (see Chapter 11) provides a framework to appropriately assess and plan care that meets the needs of the child and family. This approach encourages organized care for the child's current level of functioning to motivate self-direction and health promotion. For example, nurses encourage toddlers to make simple choices and to feed themselves to advance their developing autonomy. Nurses also recognize that adolescents are developing independence and, therefore, that they should feel empowered to participate in decisions regarding their plan of care.

INTRAUTERINE LIFE

From the moment of conception until birth, human development proceeds at a predictable and rapid rate. During gestation, or the prenatal period, the embryo grows from a single cell to a complex, physiological being. All major organ systems develop in utero, with some functioning before birth.

Pregnancy that reaches full term is calculated to last an average of 38 to 40 weeks and is commonly divided into equal phases of 3 months, called *trimesters*. Beginning on the day of fertilization, the first 14 days are referred to as the preembryonic stage, followed by the embryonic stage, which lasts from day 15 until the eighth week. These two stages are then followed by the fetal stage, which lasts from the end of the eighth week until birth (Murray et al., 2019).

The placenta begins development at the third week of the embryonic stage and produces essential hormones that help maintain the pregnancy. The placenta functions as the fetal lungs, kidneys, gastrointestinal tract, and an endocrine organ. Because the placenta is extremely porous, noxious materials such as viruses, chemicals, and drugs also pass from mother to child. These agents are called *teratogens* and can cause abnormal development of structures in the embryo. The effect of teratogens on the fetus depends on the developmental stage in which exposure takes place, individual genetic susceptibility, and the extent of the exposure. The embryonic stage is the most vulnerable since all body organs are formed by the eighth week. Some maternal infections can cross the placental barrier and negatively influence the health of the mother, fetus, or both. It is important to educate women about avoidable sources of teratogens and to help them make healthy lifestyle choices before and during pregnancy.

Health Promotion During Pregnancy

Women who are poorly nourished before pregnancy and who do not consume adequate nutrients and calories during pregnancy may not be able to meet the fetus' nutritional requirements. An increase in weight does not always indicate an increase in nutrients. In addition, the pattern of weight gain is important for tissue growth in a mother and fetus. For women who are at normal weight for height, the recommended weight gain during pregnancy is 25 to 35 pounds (11 to 15 kg) over three trimesters (Murray et al., 2019). As a nurse, you are in a key position to provide women with important nutritional education before conception and throughout pregnancy.

Pregnancy presents a developmental challenge that includes physiological, cognitive, and emotional states that are accompanied by stress and anxiety (see Chapter 13). The expectant woman will soon adopt a parenting role, and relationships within the family will change, whether or not there is a partner involved. Pregnancy can be a period of conflict or support; family dynamics impact fetal development. Parental reactions to pregnancy change throughout the gestational period. Listen carefully to concerns expressed by a mother and her partner, and offer support through each trimester.

The age of a woman sometimes plays a role in fertility, the health of the fetus, and maternal health. As women age, the risk of chromosomal defects and fertility difficulties increases. Pregnant adolescents often seek prenatal care late in the pregnancy or fail to seek prenatal care for a variety of reasons (Murray et al., 2019). Infants of teenage mothers have an increased risk of prematurity and low birth weight (less than 2500 g or 5.5 pounds) (Murray et al., 2019).

Fetal growth and hormonal changes during pregnancy often result in discomfort for the expectant mother. Common concerns expressed include problems such as nausea and vomiting, breast tenderness, urinary frequency, heartburn, constipation, ankle edema, and backache. Always anticipate these discomforts and provide self-care education throughout the pregnancy. Discussing the physiological causes of these discomforts and offering suggestions for safe treatment can be very helpful for expectant mothers and contribute to overall health during pregnancy (Murray et al., 2019).

When assessing a pregnant woman, include questions about the use of complementary and alternative therapies. Some therapies such as herbal supplements can be harmful during pregnancy (Murray et al., 2019). You can promote maternal and fetal health by providing accurate and complete information about health behaviors that support positive outcomes for pregnancy and childbirth.

TRANSITION FROM INTRAUTERINE TO EXTRAUTERINE LIFE

The transition from intrauterine to extrauterine life requires profound physiological changes in the newborn and occurs during the first 24 hours of life. Assessment of the newborn during this period is essential to ensure that the transition is proceeding as expected. Gestational age and development and exposure to depressant drugs before or during labor may influence the adjustment to the external environment.

Physical Changes

An immediate assessment of the newborn's condition to determine the physiological functioning of the major organ systems occurs at birth. The most widely used assessment tool is the Apgar score. Heart rate, respiratory effort, muscle tone, reflex irritability, and color are rated to determine overall status of the newborn. The Apgar assessment generally is conducted at 1 and 5 minutes after birth and is sometimes repeated until the newborn's condition stabilizes. The most extreme physiological change occurs when the newborn leaves the utero circulation and develops independent circulatory and respiratory functioning.

Nursing interventions at birth include maintaining an open airway, stabilizing and maintaining body temperature, and protecting the newborn from infection. The removal of nasopharyngeal and oropharyngeal secretions with suction or a bulb syringe ensures airway patency. Newborns are susceptible to heat loss and cold stress. Because hypothermia increases oxygen needs, it is essential to stabilize and maintain a newborn's body temperature. A healthy newborn may be placed in a radiant warmer, placed directly on the mother's abdomen, or covered in warm blankets with a cap. Preventing infection is a major concern in the care of a newborn, whose immune system is immature. Good handwashing technique is the most important factor in protecting a newborn from infection. You can help prevent infection by instructing parents and visitors to wash their hands before touching the infant.

Psychosocial Changes

After immediate physical evaluation and application of identification bracelets, the nurse promotes early parent-child contact to encourage parent-child attachment. Most healthy newborns are awake and alert for the first hour after birth. This is a good time for parent-child interaction to begin. Close body contact, often including breastfeeding, is a satisfying way for most families to start bonding through eye-to-eye contact and touch. If immediate contact is not possible, incorporate it into the care plan as early as possible, which means bringing the newborn to an ill parent or bringing the parents to an ill or premature child. Attachment is a process that begins during pregnancy and continues for many months after birth (Hockenberry et al., 2019).

NEWBORN

The neonatal period is the first 28 days of life. During this stage the newborn's physical functioning is mostly reflexive, and stabilization of major organ systems is the primary task of the body. Newborn behavior greatly influences interaction among the newborn, the environment, and parents/caregivers. For example, a 2-week-old may smile spontaneously and look at the parent's face, eliciting a positive response from the parent. Alternately, the newborn may cry, which is generally a reflexive response to an unmet need such as hunger, fatigue, or discomfort (Hockenberry et al., 2019). If the newborn is crying when hungry, the nurse may counsel the parents to feed the baby on demand rather than on a rigid schedule. Nurses must use knowledge of growth and development to plan care for the parent and newborn.

Physical Changes

Perform a comprehensive nursing assessment as soon as a newborn's physiological functioning is stable, generally within a few hours after birth. At this time, measure height, weight, head and chest circumference, temperature, pulse, and respirations and observe general appearance, body functions, sensory capabilities, reflexes, and responsiveness. Following a comprehensive physical assessment, assess gestational age and interactions between newborn and parent that indicate successful attachment (Hockenberry et al., 2019).

The average newborn is 6 to 9 pounds (2700 to 4000 g), is 19 to 21 inches (48 to 53 cm) in length, and has a head circumference of 13 to 14 inches (33 to 35 cm). Neonates lose up to 10% of birth weight in the first few days of life, primarily through fluid losses by respiration, urination, defecation, and low fluid intake. They usually regain birth weight by the second week of life, and a gradual pattern of increase in weight, height, and head circumference is evident. Accurate measurement as soon as possible after birth provides a baseline for future comparison (Murray et al., 2019).

Normal physical characteristics of the newborn include the continued presence of lanugo (fine downy hair) on the skin of the back;

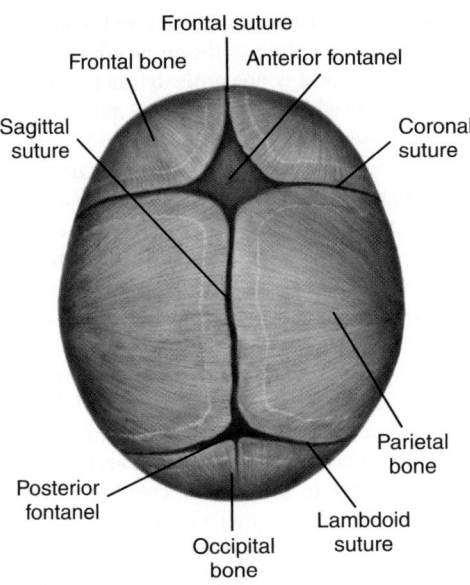

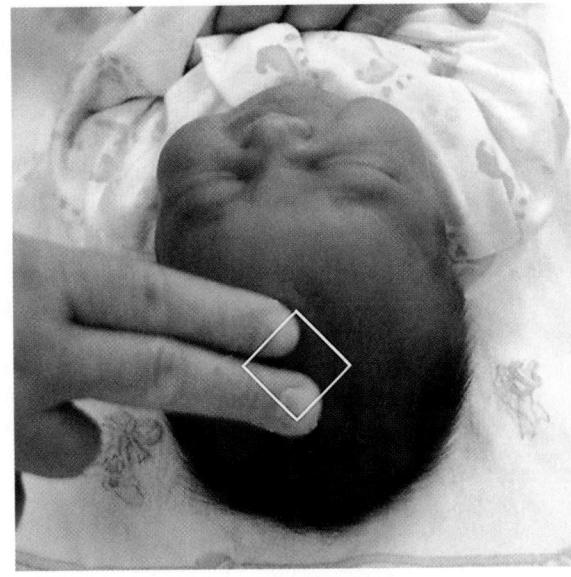

FIG. 12.1 Fontanels and suture lines. (From Hockenberry MJ, et al: *Wong's nursing care of infants and children,* ed 11, St Louis, 2019, Elsevier.)

cyanosis of the hands and feet for the first 24 hours; and a soft, protuberant abdomen. Skin color varies according to racial and genetic heritage and gradually changes during infancy. Molding, or overlapping of the soft skull bones, allows the fetal head to adjust to various diameters of the maternal pelvis and is a common occurrence with vaginal births. The bones readjust within a few days, producing a rounded appearance to the head. The sutures and fontanels are usually palpable at birth. Fig. 12.1 shows the diamond shape of the anterior fontanel and the triangular shape of the posterior fontanel between the unfused bones of the skull. The anterior fontanel usually closes by 12 to 18 months, whereas the posterior fontanel closes by the end of the second or third month.

Assess neurological function by observing the newborn's level of activity, alertness, irritability, and responsiveness to stimuli and the presence and strength of reflexes. Normal reflexes include blinking in response to bright lights, startling in response to sudden loud noises or movement, sucking, rooting, grasping, yawning, coughing, sneezing, swallowing, palmar grasp, plantar grasp, and Babinski. Assessment of these reflexes is vital because the newborn depends largely on reflexes for survival and in response to its environment. Fig. 12.2 shows the tonic neck reflex in the newborn.

Normal behavioral characteristics of the newborn include periods of sucking, crying, sleeping, and activity. Movements are generally sporadic, but they are symmetrical and involve all four extremities. The relatively flexed fetal position of intrauterine life continues as the newborn attempts to maintain an enclosed, secure feeling. Newborns normally watch the caregiver's face, have a nonsocial reflexive smile, and respond to sensory stimuli, particularly the primary caregiver's face, voice, and touch.

Cognitive Changes

Early cognitive development begins with innate behavior, reflexes, and sensory functions. Newborns initiate reflex activities, learn behaviors, and learn their desires. At birth, newborns are able to focus on objects about 8 to 12 inches (20 to 30 cm) from their faces and perceive forms. Newborns respond to human faces, black and white contrasting patterns, and bright colors (Murray et al., 2019). Teach parents about the importance of providing sensory stimulation such as talking to their baby and holding the baby to see the parent's face. This allows

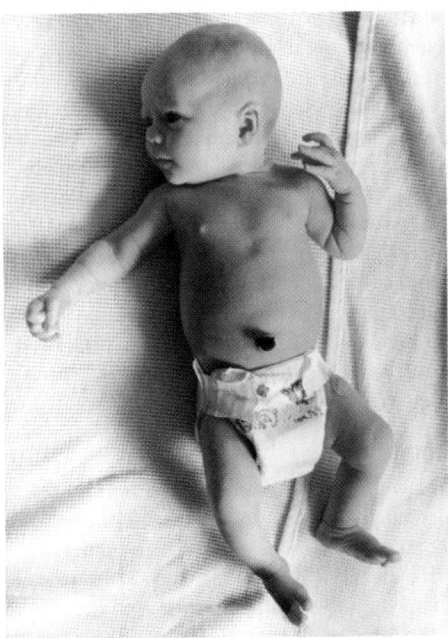

FIG. 12.2 Tonic neck reflex. Newborns assume this position while supine. (From Hockenberry MJ, et al: *Wong's nursing care of infants and children,* ed 11, St Louis, 2019, Elsevier.)

newborns to seek or take in stimuli, thereby enhancing learning and promoting cognitive development.

Crying is a means by which newborns communicate to provide cues to parents. Some babies cry because their diapers are wet or they are hungry or want to be held. Others cry just to make noise or because they need a change in position or activity. The crying may frustrate the parents if they cannot see an apparent cause. With the nurse's help, parents learn to recognize the newborn's cry patterns and take appropriate action when necessary.

Psychosocial Changes

During the first month of life most parents and newborns normally develop a strong bond that grows into a deep attachment. Feeding,

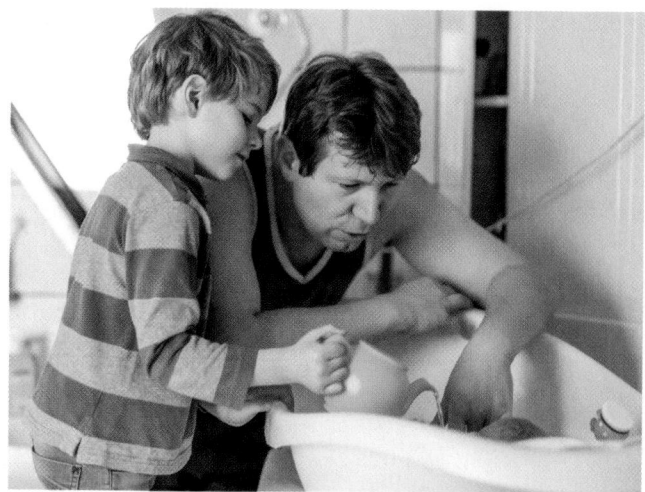

FIG. 12.3 Siblings should be involved in newborn care. (Copyright © romrodinka/iStock/Thinkstock.)

hygiene, and comfort measures consume much of newborns' waking time. These interactions provide a foundation for the formation of deep attachments. Early on, parents can allow siblings to participate in age-appropriate aspects of the newborn's care (Murray et al., 2019). Family involvement helps support growth and development and promotes nurturing (Fig. 12.3).

If parents or children experience health complications after birth, this *may* compromise the attachment process. These newborns' behavioral cues are sometimes weak or absent, and caregiving may be less mutually satisfying. Some tired or ill parents have difficulty interpreting and responding to their newborns. Preterm babies and those born with congenital anomalies are often too weak to be responsive to parental cues and require special supportive nursing care. For example, babies born with heart defects tire easily during feedings. Nurses can support parental attachment by pointing out positive qualities and responses of the newborn and acknowledging how difficult the separation can be for parents and newborn.

Health Promotion

Screening. Newborn screening tests are administered before babies leave the hospital to identify serious or life-threatening conditions before symptoms begin. Results of the screening tests are sent directly to the pediatrician. If a screening test suggests a problem, the baby's physician usually follows up with further testing and may refer the baby to a specialist for treatment if needed. Blood tests help detect inborn errors of metabolism (IEMs). These are genetic disorders caused by the absence or deficiency of a substance, usually an enzyme, essential to cellular metabolism that results in abnormal protein, carbohydrate, or fat metabolism. Although IEMs are rare, neonatal screening is done to detect phenylketonuria (PKU), hypothyroidism, galactosemia, and other diseases to allow appropriate treatment that prevents permanent mental retardation and other health problems.

Studies have indicated that hearing loss is the most common congenital abnormality in newborns. The American Academy of Pediatrics (AAP) recommends universal screening of newborn hearing before discharge or within the first month of life. Early detection of hearing difficulties leads to early treatment and can prevent or decrease developmental delays, especially those related to communication (Murray et al., 2019).

Car Seats. An essential component of discharge teaching is the use of a federally approved car seat for transporting the newborn from the hospital or birthing center to home. Automobile injuries are a leading cause of death in children in the United States. Many of these deaths occur when the child is not properly restrained (Hockenberry et al., 2019). Parents need to learn how to fit the child in the restraint and install the car seat properly. All infants and toddlers should ride in a rear-facing car safety seat until they are 2 years of age or until they reach the highest weight or height allowed by the manufacturer or their car safety seat (AAP, 2018b). Placing an infant in a rear-facing restraint in the front seat of a vehicle is extremely dangerous in any vehicle with a passenger-side air bag. Nurses are responsible for providing education on the use of a car seat before discharge from the hospital.

Sleep and Cribs. In accordance with the recommendations of the AAP (2016c), position infants for sleep on their backs on a firm sleep surface to decrease the risk of sudden infant death syndrome (SIDS). Newborns establish their individual sleep-activity cycle, and parents develop sensitivity to their baby's cues. Co-sleeping or bed sharing (see Chapter 43) is associated with an increased risk for SIDS (AAP, 2016c). Safeguards to reduce the risk for SIDS include proper positioning; removing stuffed animals, soft bedding and crib bumper pads, and pillows; and avoiding overheating the infant. Individuals should avoid smoking during pregnancy and around the infant because it places the infant at greater risk for SIDS (AAP, 2016c). Nurses play an important role in educating parents about safe sleeping for infants.

Federal safety standards now prohibit the manufacture or sale of cribs with drop-side rails and require more durable mattress supports and crib slats (AAP, 2014). New cribs sold in the United States must meet these governmental standards for safety. Unsafe cribs that do not meet the safety standards should be disassembled and thrown away (AAP, 2014). Parents also need to inspect an older crib to make sure the slats are no more than 6 cm (2.4 inches) apart. The crib mattress should fit snugly, and crib toys or mobiles should be attached firmly with no hanging strings or straps. Instruct parents to remove mobiles as soon as the baby is able to reach them (Hockenberry et al., 2019).

INFANT

During **infancy**, the period from 1 month to 1 year of age, rapid physical growth and change occur. This is the only period distinguished by such dramatic physical changes and marked development. Psychosocial developmental advances are aided by the progression from reflexive to more purposeful behavior. Interaction between infants and the environment becomes greater and more meaningful for an infant. During this first year of life, you can easily observe the adaptive potential of infants because changes in growth and development occur so rapidly.

Physical Changes

Steady and proportional growth of an infant is more important than absolute growth values. Charts of normal age- and gender-related growth measurements enable you to compare growth with norms for a child's age. For infants born prematurely, norms will be adjusted based on gestational age. Measurements recorded over time are the best way to monitor growth and identify problems. Size increases rapidly during the first year of life; birth weight doubles in approximately 5 months and triples by 12 months. Height increases an average of 2.5 cm (1 inch) during each of the first 6 months and about 1.2 cm (½ inch) each month until 12 months (Hockenberry et al., 2019).

Throughout the first year, an infant's vision and hearing continue to develop. Patterns of body function also stabilize, as evidenced by predictable sleep, elimination, and feeding routines. Some reflexes that

TABLE 12.1 Gross Motor and Fine Motor Development in Infancy

Age	Gross Motor Skill	Fine Motor Skill
Birth to 1 month	Complete head lag persists Cannot sit upright Primitive reflexes present	Reflexive grasp
2 to 4 months	When prone, lifts head and chest and bears weight on forearms With support, able to sit erect with good head control Can turn from back to side	Holds rattle for short periods but cannot pick it up if dropped Looks at and plays with hands Able to bring objects to mouth
4 to 6 months	Turns from abdomen to back at 5 months and then back to abdomen at 6 months Can support much of own weight when pulled to stand No head lag when pulled to sit	Grasps objects at will and can drop them to pick up another object Pulls feet to mouth to explore Can hold a bottle
6 to 8 months	Sits alone without support Bears full weight on feet and can hold on to furniture while standing	Bangs objects together Transfers objects from hand to hand
8 to 10 months	Scoots or crawls on hands and knees Pulls self to standing position	Picks up small objects Begins to use pincer grasp Shows hand preference
10 to 12 months	Walks holding onto furniture Stands alone, for short periods May attempt first step alone	Can place objects into containers Can turn book pages (more than one page at a time)

Adapted from Hockenberry M, Wilson D: *Wong's nursing care of infants and children*, ed 10, St Louis, 2015, Mosby.

are present in the newborn, such as blinking, yawning, and coughing, remain throughout life, whereas others, such as grasping, rooting, sucking, and the Moro or startle reflex, disappear after several months.

Motor development proceeds in a cephalocaudal (head-to-toe) and proximodistal (central-to-peripheral) pattern, as does myelination of nerves (Hockenberry et al., 2019). Gross-motor skills involve large muscle activities and are usually closely monitored by parents, who easily report recently achieved milestones. Newborns can only momentarily hold their heads up, but by 4 months most infants have no head lag. The same rapid development is evident as infants learn to sit, stand, and walk. Fine-motor skills involve small body movements and are more difficult to achieve than gross-motor skills. Maturation of eye-and-hand coordination occurs over the first 2 years of life as infants move from being able to grasp a rattle briefly at 2 months to drawing an arc with a pencil by 24 months. Development proceeds at a variable pace for each individual but usually follows the same pattern and occurs within the same time frame (Table 12.1).

Cognitive Changes

The complex brain development during the first year is demonstrated by an infant's changing behaviors. As he or she receives stimulation through the developing senses of vision, hearing, and touch, the developing brain interprets the stimuli. Thus, an infant learns by experiencing and manipulating the environment. Developing motor skills and increasing mobility expand an infant's environment and, with developing visual and auditory skills, enhance cognitive development. For these reasons Piaget (1952) named his first stage of cognitive development, which extends until around the third birthday, the sensorimotor period (see Chapter 11). In this stage of cognitive development, infants explore their world through senses. They learn by experimentation and trial and error. They shake and throw things and put things in their mouths. By the age of 7 to 9 months, they begin to realize that things still exist that can no longer be seen. This is known as object permanence and is an important developmental milestone because it demonstrates that their memory is beginning to develop.

Infants need opportunities to develop and use their senses. Assess the appropriateness and adequacy of these opportunities, especially when a child is sick or injured. You must provide alternatives for a child. For example, ill or hospitalized infants sometimes lack the energy to interact with their environment, thereby slowing their cognitive development. Infants need to be stimulated according to their temperament, energy, and age. A nurse may stimulate an infant on tube feeding by offering a pacifier and talking to the child, thereby maximizing development while conserving energy.

Language. Speech is an important aspect of cognition that develops during the first year. Infants proceed from crying, cooing, and laughing to imitating sounds, comprehending the meaning of simple commands, and repeating words with knowledge of their meaning. According to Piaget this demonstrates that an infant is demonstrating some symbolic abilities. By 1 year, infants not only recognize their own names but are also able to say three to five words and understand almost 100 words (Hockenberry et al., 2019). As a nurse, you promote language development by encouraging parents to name objects on which their infant's attention is focused. You also assess the infant's language development to identify developmental delays or potential abnormalities.

Psychosocial Changes

Separation and Individuation. During their first year, infants begin to differentiate themselves from others as separate beings capable of acting on their own. Initially infants are unaware of the boundaries of self; but, through repeated experiences with the environment, they learn where the self ends and the external world begins. As they determine their physical boundaries, they begin to respond to others (Fig. 12.4).

Two- and 3-month-old infants begin to smile responsively rather than reflexively. Similarly they recognize differences in people when their sensory and cognitive capabilities improve. By 8 months most infants are able to differentiate a stranger from a familiar person and respond differently to the two. Close attachment to their primary caregivers, most often parents, usually occurs by this age. Infants seek out these people for support and comfort during times of stress. The ability to distinguish self from others allows infants to interact and socialize more within their environments. For example, by 9 months infants play simple social games such as patty-cake and peek-a-boo. More complex

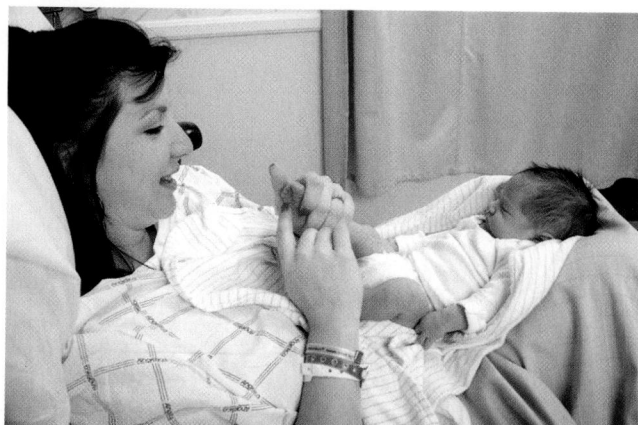

FIG. 12.4 Smiling at and talking to an infant encourage bonding. (From Murray SS, McKinney ES: *Foundations of maternal-newborn and women's health nursing*, ed 6, St Louis, 2014, Saunders.)

interactive games such as hide-and-seek involving objects are possible by age 1.

Erikson (1963) describes the psychosocial developmental crisis for an infant as trust versus mistrust. He explains that the quality of parent-infant interactions determines development of trust or mistrust. The infant learns to trust self, others, and the world through the relationship between the parent and child and the care the child receives (Hockenberry et al., 2019). During infancy a child's temperament or behavioral style becomes apparent and influences the interactions between parent and child. You can help parents understand their child's temperament and determine appropriate childrearing practices.

Assess the availability and appropriateness of experiences contributing to psychosocial development. Hospitalized infants often have difficulty establishing physical boundaries because of repeated bodily intrusions and painful sensations. Limiting these negative experiences and providing pleasurable sensations are interventions that support early psychosocial development. Extended separations from parents complicate the attachment process and increase the number of caregivers with whom the infant must interact. Parents cannot always be present to provide care during hospitalization. When parents are not present, make an attempt to limit the number of different caregivers who have contact with the infant and to follow the parents' directions for care. These interventions foster the infant's continuing development of trust.

Play. Play is important for development of cognitive, social, and motor skills. Much of infant play is solitary and exploratory as infants use their senses to observe and examine their own bodies and objects of interest in their surroundings. Adults facilitate infant learning by planning activities that promote the development of milestones and providing toys that are safe for infants to explore with their mouth and manipulate with their hands such as rattles, wooden blocks, plastic stacking rings, squeezable stuffed animals, and busy boxes.

Health Risks

Injury Prevention. Unintentional injury from all accidents, such as motor vehicle accidents, suffocation, falls, or poisoning, is a major cause of death in children 6 to 12 months old (Kochanek et al., 2017). An understanding of the major developmental accomplishments during this time period allows for injury-prevention planning. As a child achieves gains in motor development and becomes increasingly curious about the environment, constant watchfulness and supervision are critical for injury prevention.

BOX 12.1   Warning Signs of Abuse

- Physical evidence of abuse or neglect over time; this includes previous injuries, emergency department visits
- Conflicting stories about the accident/trauma
- Injury blamed on sibling or another party
- History is not compatible with the pattern or degree of injury
- History inconsistent with the child's developmental age (e.g., a 6-month-old burned by turning on the hot water)
- An initial complaint not associated with the signs and symptoms present (e.g., bringing the child to the clinic for a cold when there is evidence of physical trauma)
- Inappropriate response of the child, especially an older child (e.g., not wanting to be touched, looking at caregiver before answering any questions)
- Previous reports of abuse in the family
- Frequent emergency department or clinic visits at multiple facilities

Adapted from Hockenberry MJ, et al: *Wong's nursing care of infants and children*, ed. 11, St Louis, 2019, Elsevier.

Child Maltreatment. Child maltreatment includes intentional physical abuse or neglect, emotional abuse or neglect, and sexual abuse of children, usually by adults (Hockenberry et al., 2019). More children suffer from neglect than any other type of maltreatment. Children of any age can suffer from maltreatment, but the youngest are the most vulnerable. In addition, many children suffer from more than one type of maltreatment. No one profile fits a victim of maltreatment, and the signs and symptoms vary (Box 12.1).

A combination of signs and symptoms or a pattern of injury should arouse suspicion. By law, nurses are mandated reporters and must report suspected child maltreatment to authorities. Children who are hospitalized for maltreatment have the same developmental needs as other children their age (Hockenberry et al., 2019).

Health Promotion

Nutrition. The quality and quantity of nutrition profoundly influence an infant's growth and development. Many women have already selected a feeding method well before an infant's birth; others will have questions later in the pregnancy. Nurses are in a unique position to help parents select and provide a nutritionally adequate diet for their infant. Understand that factors such as support, culture, role demands, and previous experiences influence feeding methods (Hockenberry et al., 2019).

Breastfeeding is recommended for infant nutrition because breast milk contains the essential nutrients of protein, fats, carbohydrates, and immunoglobulins that bolster the ability to resist infection. Both the AAP and the US Department of Health and Human Services (USDHHS) recommend human milk for the first year of life (Hockenberry et al., 2019). However, if breastfeeding is not possible or if the parent does not desire it, an acceptable alternative is iron-fortified commercially prepared formula. Recent advances in the preparation of infant formula include the addition of nucleotides and long-chain fatty acids, which augment immune function and increase brain development. The use of whole cow's milk, 2% cow's milk, or alternate milk products before the age of 12 months is not recommended. Also, breastfed or formula-fed infants under 4 months of age should not receive supplemental fluids, especially water or juice (Hockenberry et al., 2019).

The average 1-month-old infant consumes approximately 18 to 21 ounces of breast milk or formula per day. This amount increases slightly during the first 6 months and decreases after introducing solid foods. The amount of formula per feeding and the number of feedings vary among infants. The addition of solid foods is not recommended before the age of 6 months because developmentally, infants are not ready for solid food before 6 months. The gastrointestinal tract is not sufficiently mature to handle these complex nutrients, and infants are exposed to food antigens that produce food protein allergies. To identify food sensitivities, one food should be introduced and consumed for approximately 1 week before introducing the next food. This allows for easier identification of which food causes the reaction. The use of fruit juices and nonnutritive drinks such as fruit-flavored drinks or soda should be avoided since these do not provide sufficient and appropriate calories during this period (Hockenberry et al., 2019).

Supplementation. The need for dietary vitamin and mineral supplements depends on an infant's diet. Full-term infants are born with some iron stores. The breastfed infant absorbs adequate iron from breast milk during the first 4 to 6 months of life. After 6 months iron-fortified cereal is generally an adequate supplemental source. Because iron in formula is less readily absorbed than that in breast milk, formula-fed infants need to receive iron-fortified formula throughout the first year.

Fluoride is an essential mineral required for development of healthy teeth. To ensure adequate fluoride ingestion, fluoride is often added to drinking water, toothpaste, and infant formula. Adequate concentrations of fluoride are not available in human milk; however, supplementation in breastfed infants under 6 months of age is generally not needed. In areas where fluoridation of water is inadequate, fluoride supplementation may be indicated. A recent concern is the use of complementary and alternative medical therapies in children that may or may not be safe. Inquire about the use of such products to help the parent determine whether the product is truly safe for the child (Hockenberry et al., 2019).

Immunizations. The widespread use of immunizations has resulted in the dramatic decline of infectious diseases over the past 50 years and therefore is a most important factor in health promotion during childhood. Although most immunizations can be given to people of any age, it is recommended that the administration of the primary series begin soon after birth and be completed during early childhood. Vaccines are among the safest and most reliable drugs used. Minor side effects sometimes occur; however, serious reactions are rare. Parents need instructions regarding the importance of immunizations and common side effects such as low-grade fever and local tenderness. The recommended schedule for immunizations changes as new vaccines are developed and advances are made in the field of immunology. Stay informed of the current policies and direct parents to the primary caregiver for their child's schedule. The AAP maintains the most current schedule on their Internet website (AAP, 2018a). Research documents that infants experience pain with invasive procedures. It is important to be aware of measures such as auditory stimulus or swaddling to reduce or eliminate pain with procedures such as an immunization injection (Azarmnejad et al., 2017; Ho et al., 2016).

Sleep. Sleep patterns vary among infants, with many having their days and nights reversed until 3 to 4 months of age. While young infants may sleep during the day, by 6 months most infants demonstrate nocturnal sleep patterns, sleeping between 9 and 11 hours at night. Most infants take one or two naps a day by the end of the first year. Many parents have concerns regarding their infant's sleep patterns, especially if there is difficulty such as sleep refusal or frequent waking during the night. Carefully assess the individual problem before suggesting interventions to address their concern.

QSEN **Building Competency in Patient-Centered Care** Children rely extensively on their parents and caregivers for their daily needs and health care. Describe how a nurse can best engage in family-centered care that respects the values, preferences, and needs of both the child and the family.

Answers to QSEN Activities can be found on the Evolve website.

TODDLER

Toddlerhood is the period from 12 to 36 months of age during which children enjoy increasing independence bolstered by greater physical mobility and cognitive abilities. Toddlers are increasingly aware of their abilities to control and are pleased with successful efforts with this new skill. This success leads them to repeated attempts to control their environments. Unsuccessful attempts at control result in negative behavior and temper tantrums. These behaviors are most common when parents stop the initial independent action. Parents cite these as the most problematic behaviors during the toddler years and at times express frustration with trying to set consistent and firm limits while simultaneously encouraging independence. Nurses and parents should limit the opportunities for a "no" answer, known as negativism. For example, do not ask the toddler, "Do you want to take your medicine now?" Instead, tell the child that it is time to take medicine, and offer a choice of water or juice to drink with it.

Physical Changes

The average toddler grows 7.5 cm (3 inches) in height, mostly through elongation of the legs, and gains approximately 4 to 6 pounds (1.8 to 2.7 kg) each year (Hockenberry et al., 2019). The rapid development of motor skills allows the child to participate in self-care activities such as feeding, dressing, and toileting. In the beginning the toddler walks in an upright position with a broad stance and gait, protuberant abdomen, and arms out to the sides for balance. Soon the child begins to navigate stairs, using a rail or the wall to maintain balance while progressing upward, placing both feet on the same step before continuing. Success provides courage to attempt the upright mode for descending the stairs in the same manner. Locomotion skills soon include running, jumping, standing on one foot for several seconds, and kicking a ball. Most toddlers ride tricycles and run well by their third birthday.

Fine-motor capabilities progress from spontaneous scribbling to accurately drawing circles and crosses. By 3 years, the child is usually able to stack a small tower of blocks. Toddlers learn to hold crayons with their fingers rather than with their fists and can imitate vertical and horizontal strokes. They are able to manage feeding themselves with a spoon without rotating it and can drink well from a cup without spilling. Toddlers can turn pages of a book one at a time and can easily turn doorknobs (Hockenberry et al., 2019).

Cognitive Changes

Toddlers increase their ability to remember events and begin to put thoughts into words at about 2 years of age. They recognize that they are separate beings from their mothers, but they are unable to assume the view of another. A toddler's reasoning is based on their own experience of an event. They use symbols to represent objects, places, and people. Children demonstrate this function as they imitate the behavior of another that they viewed earlier (e.g., pretend to shave like daddy), pretend that one object is another (e.g., use a finger as a gun), and use language to stand for absent objects (e.g., request bottle).

Language. The 18-month-old child uses approximately 10 words. The 24-month-old child has a vocabulary of up to 300 words and is generally able to speak in two-word sentences, although the ability to understand speech is much greater than the number of words acquired (Hockenberry et al., 2019). According to Piaget, the preoperational stage of development begins in toddlerhood. Children begin to think about things more symbolically as their vocabulary develops (Piaget, 1952). "Who's that?" and "What's that?" are typical questions children ask during this period. Verbal expressions such as "me do it" and "that's mine" demonstrate the 2-year-old child's use of pronouns and desire for independence and control. By 36 months, the child can use simple sentences, follow some grammatical rules, and learn to use five or six new words each day. Parents can facilitate language development best by talking and reading to their children. Reading to children helps expand their vocabulary, knowledge, and imagination. Screen activities such as television, surface pads, or smart phones should not be used to replace parent-child interaction, as it has been shown to delay language development (Canadian Paediatric Society, 2017; Hockenberry et al., 2019).

Psychosocial Changes

According to Erikson (1963) a sense of autonomy emerges during toddlerhood. Children strive for independence by using their developing muscles to do everything for themselves and become the master of their bodily functions. Their strong wills are frequently exhibited in negative behavior when caregivers attempt to direct their actions. Temper tantrums result when parental restrictions frustrate toddlers. Parents need to provide toddlers with graded independence, allowing them to do things that do not result in harm to themselves or others. For example, young toddlers who want to learn to hold their own cups often benefit from two-handled cups with spouts and plastic bibs with pockets to collect the milk that spills during the learning process.

Play. During the preoperational stage of development the child's imagination develops, and children begin to discern the difference between past and future, although they still do not grasp more complex concepts such as cause and effect (Piaget, 1952). Socially, toddlers remain strongly attached to their parents and fear separation from them. In their presence they feel safe, and their curiosity is evident in their exploration of the environment. The child continues to engage in solitary play during toddlerhood but also begins to participate in parallel play, which is playing *beside* rather than *with* another child. Play expands the child's cognitive and psychosocial development. It is always important to consider the safety of a toy and whether the toy supports development of the child.

Health Risks

The newly developed locomotion abilities and insatiable curiosity of toddlers make them at risk for injury. Toddlers need close supervision at all times and particularly when in environments that are not child-proofed (Fig. 12.5).

Poisonings occur frequently because children near 2 years of age are interested in placing any object or substance in their mouths to learn about it. The prudent parent removes or locks up all possible poisons, including plants, cleaning materials, and medications. These parental actions create a safer environment for exploratory behavior. Lead poisoning continues to be a serious health hazard in the United States. Children may ingest or inhale lead, often from chipping of lead-based paint particles in older homes (Hockenberry et al., 2019).

Toddlers' lack of awareness regarding the danger of water and their newly developed walking skills make drowning a major cause of accidental death in this age-group. Limit setting is extremely important for toddlers' safety. Motor vehicle accidents are a significant cause of death in toddlers (Kochanek et al., 2017). Some of these deaths occurred

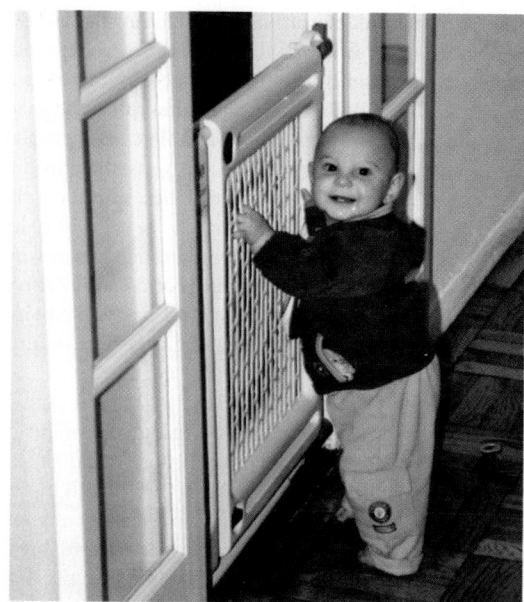

FIG. 12.5 Safety precautions should be provided for toddlers. (Courtesy Elaine Polan, RNC, BSN, MS.)

because children were unrestrained or caregivers failed to use car seat safety guidelines when restraining children (AAP, 2018b; Hockenberry et al., 2019).

Toddlers who become ill and require hospitalization are most stressed by the separation from their parents. Nurses encourage parents to stay with their child as much as possible and actively participate in providing care. Creating an environment that supports parents helps greatly in gaining the trust and cooperation of the toddler. Establishing a trusting relationship with the parents often results in toddler acceptance of treatment.

Health Promotion

Nutrition. Childhood obesity and the associated chronic diseases that result are sources of concern for all health care providers. Children establish lifetime eating habits in early childhood, and there is increased emphasis on food choices. They increasingly meet nutritional needs by eating solid foods. The healthy toddler requires a balanced daily intake of bread and grains, vegetables, fruit, dairy products, and proteins. Because the consumption of more than a quart of milk per day usually decreases a child's appetite for these essential solid foods and results in inadequate iron intake, advise parents to limit milk intake to 2 to 3 cups per day. Children should not be offered low-fat or skim milk until age 2 because they need the fat for satisfactory physical and intellectual growth (Hockenberry et al., 2019).

Mealtime has psychosocial and physical significance. If the parents struggle to control toddlers' dietary intake, problem behavior and conflicts can result. Toddlers often develop "food jags," or the desire to eat one food repeatedly. Rather than becoming disturbed by this behavior, encourage parents to offer a variety of nutritious foods at meals and to provide only nutritious snacks between meals. Serving finger foods to toddlers allows them to eat by themselves and to satisfy their need for independence and control. Small, reasonable servings allow toddlers to eat all of their meals.

Toilet Training. Increased locomotion skills, the ability to undress, and development of sphincter control allow toilet training if a toddler has developed the necessary language and cognitive abilities. Assisting parents in the recognition of the child's patterns and urge to urinate and defecate is crucial in determining a child's readiness. The toddler must also be motivated to hold on to please the parent rather than letting go to please the self to successfully accomplish toilet training (Hockenberry et al., 2019). Remind parents that patience, consistency, and a calm attitude, in addition to the child's readiness, are essential to successful toilet training.

PRESCHOOLERS

The **preschool period** refers to the years between ages 3 and 5. Children refine the mastery of their bodies and eagerly await the beginning of formal education. Many people consider these the most intriguing years of parenting because children are less negative, more accurately share their thoughts, and more effectively interact and communicate. Physical development occurs at a slower pace than cognitive and psychosocial development.

Physical Changes

Several aspects of physical development continue to stabilize in the preschool years. Children have an average annual weight gain of about 4.5 to 6.5 pounds (2 to 3 kg) and grow 6.5 to 9 cm (2.5 to 3.5 inches) per year and stand an average of 110 cm (43.5 inches) tall by their fifth birthday. The elongation of the legs results in more slender-appearing children and little difference exists between the sexes (Hockenberry et al., 2019).

Gross- and fine-motor coordination improves in the preschool years as evidenced by running well, walking up and down steps with ease, and learning to hop. By 5 years they usually skip on alternate feet, jump rope, and begin to skate and swim. Improving fine-motor skills allows intricate manipulations. They learn to copy crosses and squares. Triangles and diamonds are usually mastered between ages 5 and 6 (Hockenberry et al., 2019). Scribbling and drawing help to develop fine-motor skills and the hand-eye coordination needed for the printing of letters and numbers.

Children need opportunities to learn and practice new physical skills. Nursing care of healthy and ill children includes an assessment of the availability of these opportunities. Although children with acute illnesses benefit from rest and exclusion from usual daily activities, children who have chronic conditions or who have been hospitalized for long periods need ongoing exposure to developmental opportunities. The parents and nurses weave these opportunities into the children's daily experiences, depending on their abilities, needs, and energy level.

Cognitive Changes

Preschoolers' cognitive development continues as they accomplish developmental tasks that prepare them for scholastic learning. Much of their development is through imaginative play and interactions with others. Though they begin to recognize others' viewpoints, they remain egocentric in their communication and believe others think as they do. Children have increased social interaction, as is illustrated by the 5-year-old child who offers a bandage to a child with a cut finger.

Preschoolers begin to become aware of cause-and-effect relationships, as illustrated by the statement, "The sun sets because people want to go to bed." Early causal thinking is also evident in preschoolers. For example, if two events are related in time or space, children link them in a causal fashion. For example, the hospitalized child reasons, "I cried last night, and that's why the nurse gave me the shot." As children near age 5, they begin to use or learn to use rules to understand causation. They then begin to reason from the general to the particular. This forms the basis for more formal logical thought. The child now reasons, "I get a shot twice a day, and that's why I got one last night." Children in this stage also believe that inanimate objects have lifelike qualities and are capable of action, as seen through comments such as, "Trees cry when their branches get broken."

Preschoolers' knowledge of the world remains closely linked to concrete (perceived by the senses) experiences. Even their rich fantasy life is grounded in their perception of reality. Preschoolers believe that if a rule is broken, punishment results immediately. During these years they believe that a punishment is automatically connected to an act and do not yet realize that it is socially mediated (Hockenberry et al., 2019).

The greatest fear of this age-group appears to be that of bodily harm. This is evident in children's fear of the dark, animals, thunderstorms, and medical personnel. This fear often interferes with their willingness to allow nursing interventions such as measurement of vital signs. Preschoolers cooperate if they are allowed to help the nurse measure the blood pressure of a parent or to manipulate the nurse's equipment.

Language. Preschoolers' vocabularies continue to increase rapidly; by the age of 5 children have an average of 2100 words that they use to define familiar objects, identify colors, and express their desires and frustrations. They combine four to five words into sentences and use pronouns, prepositions, adjectives, and verbs. Language is more social, and preschoolers often question "Why?" and ask the same question repeatedly until answered. Phonetically similar words such as *die* and *dye* or *wood* and *would* cause confusion in preschool children. Avoid such words when preparing them for procedures and assess comprehension of explanations.

Psychosocial Changes

The world of preschoolers expands beyond the family into the neighborhood where children meet other children and adults. Their curiosity and developing initiative lead to actively exploring the environment, developing new skills, and making new friends. Preschoolers have a surplus of energy that permits them to plan and attempt many activities that are beyond their capabilities, such as pouring milk from a gallon container into their cereal bowls. Guilt arises within children when they overstep the limits of their abilities and think that they have not behaved correctly. Preschoolers also exhibit magical thinking and believe that if they simply think something, it will happen. Children who in anger wished that their sibling were dead experience guilt if that sibling becomes ill. Children need to learn that "wishing" for something to happen does not make it occur. Erikson (1963) recommends that parents help their children strike a healthy balance between initiative and guilt by allowing them to do things on their own while setting firm limits and providing guidance.

Sources of stress for preschoolers can include changes in caregiving arrangements, starting school, the birth of a sibling, parental marital distress, relocation to a new home, or an illness. During these times of stress, preschoolers sometimes revert to bed-wetting or thumb-sucking and want the parents to feed, dress, and hold them. Reassure parents that these are some of the child's normal coping behaviors. Provide experiences that these children are able to master. Such successes help them return to their prior level of independent functioning. As language skills develop, encourage children to talk about their feelings. Play is also an excellent way for preschoolers to vent frustration or anger and is a socially acceptable way to deal with stress.

Play. The play of preschool children becomes more social after the third birthday as it shifts from parallel to associative play. Children playing together engage in similar if not identical activity; however, there is no division of labor or rigid organization or rules. Most 3-year-old children are able to play with one other child in a cooperative manner in which they make something or play designated roles such as mother and baby. By age 4, children play in groups of two or three, and by 5 years the group has a temporary leader for each activity.

During the preoperational stage of growth and development the child begins to engage in make-believe play (Piaget, 1952). Pretend play allows children to learn to understand others' points of view, develop skills in solving social problems, and become more creative. Some children have imaginary playmates. These playmates serve many purposes, are a sign of health, and allow the child to distinguish between reality and fantasy (Hockenberry et al., 2019).

Television (TV), videos, electronic games, and computer programs also help support development and the learning of basic skills. However, these should be only one part of the child's total play activities. The AAP (2016a) advises no more than one hour per day of educational, nonviolent TV programs, which should be viewed by parents or other responsible adults in the home. Limiting TV viewing will provide more time for children to read, engage in physical activity, and socialize with others (Hockenberry et al., 2019).

Health Risks

As fine- and gross-motor skills develop and a child becomes more coordinated with better balance, falls become much less of a problem. Many of the guidelines for injury prevention in the toddler also apply to the preschooler. Children need to learn about safety, and parents need to continue close supervision of activities. Children at this age are great imitators, so parental example is important. For instance, parental use of a helmet while bicycling sets an appropriate example for the preschooler.

Health Promotion

Little research has explored preschoolers' perceptions of their own health. Parental beliefs about health, children's bodily sensations, and their ability to perform usual daily activities help children develop attitudes about their health. Preschoolers are usually quite independent in washing, dressing, and feeding. Alterations in this independence influence their feelings about their own health.

Nutrition. Nutritional requirements for the preschooler vary little from those of the toddler. The average daily intake is 1800 calories. Parents often worry about the amount of food their child is consuming, and this is a relevant concern because of the problem of childhood obesity. However, the quality of the food is more important than quantity in most situations. Preschoolers consume about half of average adult portion sizes. Finicky eating habits are characteristic of the 4-year-old; however, preschoolers engaged in meal preparation are more likely to try new things (Hockenberry et al., 2019).

Sleep. Preschoolers average 12 hours of sleep a night and take infrequent naps. Sleep disturbances are common during these years (Hockenberry et al., 2019). Disturbances range from trouble getting to sleep to nightmares to prolonging bedtime with extensive rituals. Frequently children in this playful age-group have had an overabundance of activity and stimulation. Helping them slow down before bedtime usually results in better sleeping habits.

Vision. Vision screening usually begins in the preschool years and needs to occur at regular intervals. One of the most important tests is to determine the presence of nonbinocular vision or strabismus. Early detection and treatment of strabismus must occur by age 6 to prevent amblyopia (Hockenberry et al., 2019).

REFLECT NOW

Nurses must be careful to recognize their own biases and assumptions when caring for children and families. How can you avoid imposing your beliefs and value system on the families with children that you care for?

SCHOOL-AGE CHILDREN AND ADOLESCENTS

The developmental changes between ages 6 and 18 are diverse and span all areas of growth and development. Children develop, expand, refine, and synchronize physical, psychosocial, cognitive, and moral skills so that the individual is able to become an accepted and productive member of society. The environment in which the individual develops skills also expands and diversifies. Instead of the boundaries of family and close friends, the environment now includes the school, community, and church. With age-specific assessment, you need to review the appropriate developmental expectations for each age-group. You can promote health by helping children and adolescents achieve a necessary developmental balance.

SCHOOL-AGE CHILDREN

During these "middle years" of childhood from age 6 to about age 12, the foundation for adult roles in work, recreation, and social interaction is laid. Puberty marks the end of these middle years and the beginning of adolescence. Children make great developmental strides during these years as they develop competencies in physical, cognitive, and psychosocial skills.

The school or educational experience expands the child's world and is a transition from a life of relatively free play to one of structured play, learning, and work. The school and home influence growth and development, requiring adjustment by the parents and child. The child learns to cope with rules and expectations presented by the school and peers. Parents have to learn to allow their child to make decisions, accept responsibility, and learn from the experiences of life.

Physical Changes

The rate of growth during these early school years is slow and consistent, a relative calm before the growth spurt of adolescence. The school-age child appears slimmer than the preschooler as a result of changes in fat distribution and thickness. Many children double their weight during these middle childhood years, and most girls exceed boys in both height and weight by the end of the school years (Hockenberry et al., 2019).

School-age children become more graceful during the school years because their large-muscle coordination improves and their strength doubles. Most children practice the basic gross-motor skills of running, jumping, balancing, throwing, and catching during play, resulting in refinement of neuromuscular function and skills. Individual differences in the rate of mastering skills and ultimate skill achievement become apparent during their participation in many activities and games.

Fine-motor skills improve, which allows proficiency in a wide range of activities, including handwriting, drawing, and playing. Most 6-year-old children are able to hold a pencil adeptly and print letters and words; by age 12 a child is able to make detailed drawings and write sentences in script. Painting, drawing, playing computer games, and modeling allow children to practice and improve newly refined skills. The improved fine-motor capabilities of children in middle childhood allow them to become very independent in bathing, dressing, and taking care of other personal needs. They develop strong personal preferences in the way these needs are met. Illness and hospitalization threaten children's control in these areas. Therefore, whenever possible, it is important to allow them to participate in care and maintain as much independence as possible. For example, children can help decide the type of fluids and help keep a record of their intake.

As skeletal growth progresses, a child's body appearance and posture change. Earlier the child's posture was stoop shouldered, with slight lordosis and a prominent abdomen. The posture of a school-age child is more erect. The AAP (2016b) recommends screening of scoliosis, the lateral curvature of the spine, in females at age 10 and 12 and in males at age 13 to 14. Early treatment of scoliosis can limit the progression of the curve and the resulting effects.

Eye shape alters because of skeletal growth. This improves visual acuity, and normal adult 20/20 vision is achievable. Screening for vision and hearing problems is easier, and results are more reliable because school-age children more fully understand and cooperate with the test directions. The school nurse typically assesses the growth, visual, and auditory status of school-age children and refers those with possible deviations to a health care provider such as their family practitioner or pediatrician.

Cognitive Changes

According to Piaget, children begin to transition into the concrete-operational stage of growth and development around the age of 7, when they begin to demonstrate logical, more concrete thinking. They become less egocentric and begin to understand that their thoughts and feelings may not be shared by others (Piaget, 1952). Cognitive changes provide the school-age child with the ability to think in a logical manner about the here and now and to understand how one thing relates to another. They are now able to use their developed thinking abilities to experience events without having to act them out (Hockenberry et al., 2019). Their thoughts are no longer dominated by their perceptions; thus their ability to understand the world greatly expands.

School-age children have the ability to concentrate on more than one aspect of a situation. They begin to understand that others do not always see things as they do and even begin to understand another viewpoint. They now have the ability to recognize that the amount or quantity of a substance remains the same even when its shape or appearance changes. For instance, two balls of clay of equal size remain the same amount of clay even when one is flattened and the other remains in the shape of a ball.

The young child is able to separate objects into groups according to shape or color, whereas the school-age child understands that the same element can exist in two classes at the same time. School-age children frequently have collections such as baseball cards or stuffed animals that demonstrate this new cognitive skill. Part of the joy of collecting is the ordering and reordering of items in the collection (Hockenberry et al., 2019).

Language Development. Language growth is rapid during middle childhood. Children improve their use of language and expand their structural knowledge. They become more aware of the rules of syntax, the rules for linking words into phrases and sentences. They also identify generalizations and exceptions to rules. They accept language as a means for representing the world in a subjective manner and realize that words have arbitrary rather than absolute meanings. Children begin to think about language, which enables them to appreciate jokes and riddles. They are not as likely to use a literal interpretation of a word, but rather they reason about its meaning within a context (Hockenberry et al., 2019).

Psychosocial Changes

Erikson (1963) identifies the developmental task for school-age children as industry versus inferiority. During this time children strive to acquire competence and skills necessary for them to function as adults. School-age children who are positively recognized for success feel a sense of worth. Those faced with failure often feel a sense of mediocrity or unworthiness, which sometimes results in withdrawal from school and peers.

School-age children begin to define themselves on the basis of internal more than external characteristics. They begin to define their self-concept and develop self-esteem through ongoing self-evaluation. Interaction with peers allows them to define their own accomplishments in relation to others as they work to develop a positive self-image (Hockenberry et al., 2019).

According to Piaget, school-age children around the age of 11 may begin to enter the fourth and final stage of intellectual development, formal operations. In this stage they begin to ponder abstract relationships. They can formulate hypotheses and consider different possibilities. Piaget believed that this was the final stage of cognitive development and that the continued intellectual development in teenagers and adults depended on the accumulation of knowledge (Piaget, 1952).

Peer Relationships. Group and personal achievements become important to the school-age child. Success is important in physical and cognitive activities. Play involves peers and the pursuit of group goals. Although solitary activities are not eliminated, group play overshadows them. Learning to contribute, collaborate, and work cooperatively toward a common goal becomes a measure of success (Fig. 12.6).

The school-age child prefers same-sex peers. Peer influence becomes quite diverse during this stage of development, and clubs and peer groups become prominent. School-age children often develop "best friends" with whom they share secrets and with whom they look forward to interacting on a daily basis. Group identity increases as the school-age child approaches adolescence.

Sexual Identity. Freud described middle childhood as the latency period because he believed that children of this period had little interest in their sexuality. Children are curious about their sexuality. Children's curiosity about adult magazines or meanings of sexually explicit words is an example of their sexual interest. This is the time for them to have exposure to sex education, including topics about sexual maturation, reproduction, and relationships (Hockenberry et al., 2019).

Stress. Today's children experience more stress than children in earlier generations. Stress comes from parental expectations, peer expectations, the school environment, and violence in the family, school, or community. Some school-age children care for themselves before or after school without adult supervision. Latchkey children sometimes feel increased stress and are at greater risk for injury and unsafe behaviors (Hockenberry et al., 2019). A nurse helps the child cope

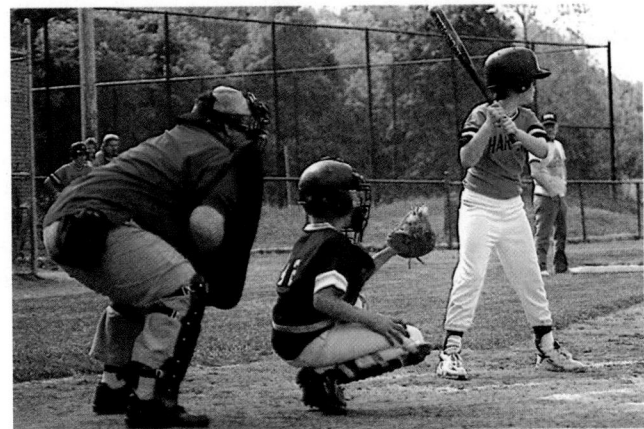

FIG. 12.6 School-age children gain a sense of achievement from working and playing with peers. (From Hockenberry MJ, et al: *Wong's nursing care of infants and children,* ed 11, St Louis, 2019, Elsevier.)

with stress by helping the parents and child identify potential stressors and designing interventions to minimize stress and the child's stress response. Deep-breathing techniques, positive imagery, and progressive relaxation of muscle groups are interventions that most children can learn (see Chapter 37). Include the parent, child, and teacher in the intervention for maximal success.

Health Risks

Accidents and injuries are a major health problem affecting school-age children (Hockenberry et al., 2019). They are exposed to various environments and less supervision, but their developed cognitive and motor skills make them less likely to suffer from unintentional injury. Some school-age children are risk takers and attempt activities that are beyond their abilities. Motor vehicle injuries as a passenger or pedestrian are among the most common in this age-group (CDC, 2018b).

Infections account for the majority of all childhood illnesses. Poverty and the prevalence of illness are highly correlated. Access to primary care is often very limited, and health promotion and preventive health measures are minimal. School nurses play a major role in providing access to meet children's health needs by providing health education and direct care services to children in the school setting.

Health Promotion

Perceptions. During the school-age years identity and self-concept become stronger and more individualized. Perception of wellness is based on readily observable facts such as presence or absence of illness and adequacy of eating or sleeping. Functional ability is the standard by which personal health and the health of others are judged. Children are aware of their body and are modest and sensitive about being exposed. Always provide for privacy when offering explanations of common procedures.

Health Education. Health education during the school-age years is critical to establish behaviors for a healthy adult life. Promotion of good health practices is a nursing responsibility, and effective health education must be developmentally appropriate. Programs directed at health education are frequently organized and conducted in the school. Effective health education teaches children about their bodies and how choices, such as nutrition and routine exercise, impact their health (Hockenberry et al., 2019).

Health Maintenance. Parents need to recognize the importance of annual health maintenance visits for immunizations, screenings, and dental care. When their school-age child reaches 10 years of age, parents need to begin discussions in preparation for upcoming pubertal changes. Topics include introductory information regarding menstruation, sexual intercourse, reproduction, and sexually transmitted infections (STIs). Human papillomavirus (HPV) is a widespread virus that will infect nearly 1 in 4 Americans in their lifetime (AAP, 2018c). For many individuals HPV clears spontaneously, but for others it can cause significant consequences. Females can develop cervical, vaginal, and vulvar cancers and genital warts; and males can develop genital warts. Since it is not possible to determine who will or will not develop disease from the virus, the AAP (2017) recommends routine HPV vaccination for girls and boys, with the first dose given at age 11 to 12. For those who miss this recommended age window, vaccination is still recommended through age 26.

Safety. Because accidents are the leading cause of death and injury in the school-age period, safety is a priority health teaching consideration (Hockenberry et al., 2019). At this age, encourage children to take responsibility for their own safety, such as wearing helmets during bike riding and wearing seat belts when in motor vehicles.

Nutrition. Growth often slows during the school-age period as compared with infancy and adolescence. School-age children are developing eating patterns that are independent of parental supervision. The availability of snacks and fast-food restaurants makes it increasingly difficult for children to make healthy choices. The prevalence of obesity among children 6 to 11 years of age increased from 6.5% in 1980 to 18.4% in 2015 to 2016. In addition, the incidence of adolescents ages 12 to 19 years who were obese increased from 5% to almost 21% during the same period of time (CDC, 2017a). Childhood obesity has become a prominent health problem, resulting in increased risk for hypertension, diabetes, coronary heart disease, fatty liver disease, pulmonary complications such as sleep apnea, musculoskeletal problems, dyslipidemia, and potential for psychological problems (Hockenberry et al., 2019). Nurses promote healthy lifestyle habits, including nutrition and exercise. School-age children need to participate in educational programs that enable them to plan, select, and prepare healthy meals and snacks. These meals and snacks need adequate caloric intake for growth throughout childhood accompanied by activity for continued gross-motor development.

ADOLESCENTS

Adolescence is the period during which the individual makes the transition from childhood to adulthood, usually between ages 13 and 20 years. The term *adolescent* usually refers to psychological maturation of the individual, whereas puberty refers to the point at which reproduction becomes possible. The hormonal changes of puberty result in changes in the appearance of the young person, and cognitive development results in the ability to hypothesize and deal with abstractions. Adjustments and adaptations are necessary to cope with these simultaneous changes and the attempt to establish a mature sense of identity.

Understanding development helps teenagers and parents anticipate and cope with the stresses of adolescence. Nursing activities, particularly education, promote healthy development. These activities occur in a variety of settings and can be developed for the adolescent, parents, or both. For example, a nurse conducts seminars in a high school to provide practical suggestions to a large group of students for solving problems of concern, such as treating acne or making responsible decisions about drugs or alcohol use. Similarly, a group education program for parents about how to cope with teenagers would promote parental understanding of adolescent development.

Physical Changes

Physical changes occur rapidly in adolescence. Sexual maturation occurs with the development of primary and secondary sexual characteristics. The four main physical changes are:
1. Increased growth rate of skeleton, muscle, and viscera
2. Sex-specific changes, such as changes in shoulder and hip width
3. Alteration in distribution of muscle and fat
4. Development of the reproductive system and secondary sex characteristics

Wide variation exists between sexes and within the same sex in the timing of physical changes associated with puberty. Girls generally have prepubescent changes 1 to 2 years before boys do (Hockenberry et al., 2019). The rates of height and weight gain are usually proportional, and the sequence of pubertal growth changes is the same in most individuals.

Hormonal changes within the body create change when the body produces gonadotropin-releasing hormones that stimulate ovarian cells to produce estrogen and testicular cells to produce testosterone. These hormones contribute to the development of secondary sex characteristics, such as hair growth and voice changes, and play an essential role in reproduction. The changing concentrations of these hormones are also linked to acne and body odor. Understanding these hormonal changes enables you to reassure adolescents and educate them about body care needs.

Being like peers is extremely important for adolescents (Fig. 12.7). Any deviation in the timing of their physical changes is extremely difficult for them to accept. It is important to provide emotional support for those undergoing early or delayed puberty. Even adolescents whose physical changes are occurring at the normal times seek confirmation of and reassurance about their normalcy.

Height and weight increases during adolescence, with peak height velocity occurring at about 12 years in girls and at about 14 years in boys. Girls' height increases 5 to 20 cm (2 to 8 inches), and weight increases by 15.5 to 55 pounds (7 to 25 kg). Girls grow less than 2 inches following menarche (the onset of menstruation), reaching their full height by 16 to 17 years of age. Boys' height increases approximately 10 to 30 cm (4 to 12 inches), and weight increases by 15.5 to 66 pounds (7 to 30 kg). Boys continue to grow taller until 18 to 20 years of age (Hockenberry et al., 2019).

Although individual and gender differences exist, growth follows a similar pattern for both sexes. Personal growth curves help nurses assess physical development. However, an individual's sustained progression along the curve is more important than a comparison to the norm.

Cognitive Changes

The adolescent develops the ability to determine and rank possibilities, solve problems, and make decisions through logical operations. The teenager thinks abstractly and deals effectively with hypothetical problems. When confronted with a problem, the adolescent considers an infinite variety of causes and solutions. For the first time the young person moves beyond the physical or concrete properties of a situation and uses reasoning powers to understand the abstract. School-age individuals think about what is, whereas adolescents are able to imagine what might be.

Adolescents are now able to think in terms of the future rather than just current events. These newly developed abilities allow an individual to have more insight and skill in playing video, computer, and board games that require abstract thinking and deductive reasoning about many possible strategies. A teenager even solves problems requiring simultaneous manipulation of several abstract concepts. Development of this ability is important in the pursuit of an identity. For example, newly acquired cognitive skills allow the teenager to define appropriate, effective, and comfortable sex-role behaviors and to consider their impact on peers, family, and society. A higher level of cognitive functioning makes the adolescent receptive to more detailed and diverse

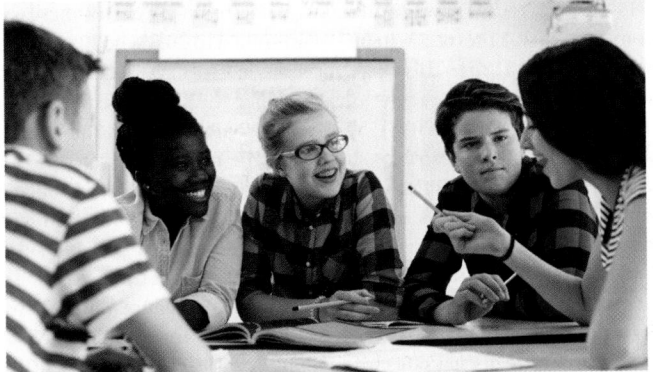

FIG. 12.7 Peer interactions help increase self-esteem during puberty. (Copyright © MachineHeadz/iStock/Thinkstock.)

information about sexuality and sexual behaviors. For example, sex education includes an explanation of physiological sexual changes and birth control measures.

Adolescents also develop the ability to understand how an individual's ideas or actions influence others. Although adolescents have the capability to think as well as an adult, they do not have experiences on which to build. It is common for teenagers to consider their parents too narrow minded or materialistic. At this time adolescents believe that they are unique and the exception, giving rise to their risk-taking behaviors. In other words, they think that they are invincible. For example, an adolescent might believe that he or she is able to drive fast and not have an accident or may argue that e-cigarettes will not impact his or her health.

Language Skills. Language development is fairly complete by adolescence, although vocabulary continues to expand. The primary focus becomes communication skills that an adolescent uses effectively in various situations. Adolescents need to communicate thoughts, feelings, and facts to peers, parents, teachers, and other people of authority. The skills used in these diverse communication situations vary. Adolescents select the people with whom to communicate, decide on the exact message, and choose the way to transmit it. For example, how teenagers tell parents about failing grades is not the same as how they tell friends. Good communication skills are critical for adolescents in overcoming peer pressure and unhealthy behaviors. The following are some hints for communicating with adolescents (Hockenberry et al., 2019):

- Provide privacy and a nonthreatening environment. As adolescents become more autonomous, interviews should be conducted without parents present.
- Ensure confidentiality and explain the limitations of confidentiality, such as disclosure of abuse or suicidal ideations.
- Be nonjudgmental and display genuine interest in the adolescent's perspective.
- Ask open-ended questions (see Chapter 24).
- Start with less sensitive topics and then move to more sensitive issues. Asking questions about sex, drugs, and school opens the channels for further discussion.

Psychosocial Changes

The search for personal identity is the major task of adolescent psychosocial development. Teenagers establish close peer relationships or remain socially isolated. Erikson (1963) sees identity (or role) confusion as the prime danger of this stage and suggests that the cliquish behavior and intolerance of differences seen in adolescent behavior are defenses against identity confusion (Erikson, 1968). Adolescents become more emotionally independent from their parents (Hockenberry et al., 2019). In addition, they develop their own ethical systems based on personal values. They begin to make choices about vocation, future education, and lifestyle. The various components of total identity evolve from these tasks and compose an adult personal identity that is unique to the individual.

Sexual Identity. Physical changes of puberty enhance achievement of sexual identity (see Chapter 34). The physical evidence of maturity encourages the development of masculine and feminine behaviors. Adolescents depend on these physical clues because they want assurance of maleness or femaleness and they do not wish to be different from peers. Also, development of sexual identity involves identification of sexual orientation. By late adolescence, most individuals identify themselves as heterosexual, and a small number identify as bisexual, gay, or lesbian.

Peer Group Identity. Adolescents seek a group identity because they need self-esteem and acceptance. Similarity in dress or speech is common in teenage groups. Peer groups provide the adolescent with a sense of belonging, approval, and the opportunity to learn acceptable behavior. Popularity with opposite-sex and same-sex peers is important. Supportive peer groups can have a positive influence on health choices, while poor peer group selection can lead to poor decision making and negative health outcomes. Nurses should encourage parents to communicate with their adolescents and provide supervision to promote selection of positive peer groups.

Family Identity. Adolescents begin to place more value on peer relationships than on parents. Although financial independence for adolescents is not the norm in American society, many work part-time, using their income to bolster independence. When they cannot have a part-time job because of studies, school-related activities, and other factors, parents can provide allowances for clothing and incidentals, which encourage them to develop decision making and budgeting skills.

Some adolescents and families have more difficulty during these years than others. Adolescents need to make choices, act independently, and experience the consequences of their actions. Nurses help families consider appropriate ways for them to foster the independence of their adolescent while maintaining family structure.

Health Identity. Another component of personal identity is perception of health. This component is of specific interest to health care providers. Healthy adolescents evaluate their own health according to feelings of well-being, ability to function normally, and absence of symptoms (Hockenberry et al., 2019). They also often include health maintenance and health promotion behaviors as important concerns.

Adolescents try new roles, begin to stabilize their identity, and acquire values and behaviors from which their adult lifestyle will evolve. The rapid changes during this period make health promotion programs especially crucial. They are able to identify behaviors such as smoking and substance abuse as threatening to health in general terms but frequently tend to underestimate the effect of the potentially negative consequences of their own actions. Health promotion strategies should focus not only on reducing risk behaviors but also on maximizing protective factors such as coping and adapting (Hockenberry et al., 2019).

Health Risks

Accidents. In the United States, unintentional injury is the leading cause of death in adolescents. Motor vehicle accidents are the most common cause of death (USDHHS, 2018). Adolescents are at particular risk because of lack of driving experience and risk-taking behaviors such as driving too fast, drinking and driving, or riding with someone under the influence (USDHHS, 2014; Hockenberry et al., 2019). The majority of deaths from injury occur in boys. Other frequent causes of accidental death in teenagers are drowning and the use of firearms. Adolescents think that they are invincible, which leads to risk-taking behaviors. The use of alcohol precedes many injuries, and adolescents continue to be both the victims and perpetrators of violence. An objective for *Healthy People 2020* is to reduce the percentage of middle and public high schools that have violent incidents (USDHHS, 2014).

Violence and Homicide. Homicide is the second leading cause of death in adolescents in the United States and is the leading cause of death in African-American teenagers (Hockenberry et al., 2019). Youth Risk Behavior Surveillance System reports that, in 2017, 15.7% of high school students had carried a weapon (e.g., gun, club, or knife) at some point during the preceding 30 days (CDC, 2018c). Teenagers are most likely to be killed by an acquaintance or gang member and most often with a firearm. Because having a gun in the home raises the risk of homicide and suicide for adolescents, include assessment of gun presence in the home and discuss gun safety when counseling families (Hockenberry et al., 2019).

Violence among adolescents has become a national concern. School shootings are increasingly common and contribute to stress in childhood and adolescence. Violence includes physical assaults and fighting, threats and intimidation, sexual harassment or violence, human trafficking (Box 12.2), bullying, or theft. Nurses working with adolescents need to be aware of the potential for school violence and include screening questions when providing health care, regardless of the setting.

REFLECT NOW

School violence and school shootings are on the rise in the United States. Reflect on what you now know about an adolescent's development. How can nurses intervene with this age group to decrease the prevalence of this phenomenon?

Suicide. Suicide is a major leading cause of death in adolescence. A recent survey of high school students in the United States found that 16% of students reported seriously considering suicide, while 8% reported attempting suicide within the past year (CDC, 2017b). Depression and social isolation commonly precede a suicide attempt, but suicide probably results from a combination of several factors. Nurses must be able to identify the factors associated with adolescent depression and suicide risk and precipitating events. Screen for the following changes in behavior:

- Decrease in school performance
- Withdrawal
- Loss of initiative
- Loneliness, sadness, and crying
- Appetite and sleep disturbances
- Verbalization of suicidal thought

If your assessment indicates depression or suicide risk, make immediate referrals to mental health professionals. Guidance helps them focus on the positive aspects of life and strengthen coping abilities.

Substance Abuse. Substance abuse is a concern for all who work with adolescents. Adolescents often believe that mood-altering substances create a sense of well-being or improve level of performance. All adolescents are at risk for experimental or recreational substance use (Hockenberry et al., 2019). The misuse of opioids in high school students has decreased considerably over the past 10 years, while the daily use of marijuana among 12th graders increased from 1.9% in 1992 to 5.9% in 2017 (NIH, 2017).

Tobacco use continues to be a health problem among adolescents. The use of cigarettes by high school students decreased from 15.8% in 2011 to 7.6% in 2017, while the use of electronic cigarettes increased from 1.5% in 2011 to 11.7% in 2017 and spiked to 20.8% in 2018 (CDC, 2018a; CDC, 2018d). This huge increase led to new Food and Drug Administration (FDA) regulations to reduce the sale of electronic cigarettes to youth (FDA, 2018). While electronic cigarettes may be less harmful than cigarettes, they should not be considered safe, as they can harm adolescent brain development and increase the presence of cancer-causing chemicals in the body (CDC, 2018c). In addition, vaping has been associated with serious lung problems likely related to irritation or allergic reactions to contaminants (Shmerling, 2019). The increased use of e-cigarettes and vaping does not reduce the addictive or health effects of nicotine use (CDC, 2018a,d). The long-term effects of nicotine from e-cigarettes and vaping may lead to subsequent frequency of smoking and vaping (Goldenson et al., 2017). Nurses must educate teenagers about smoking cessation and the safety risks associated with smoking and substance and alcohol use.

BOX 12.2   EVIDENCE-BASED PRACTICE

Education Programs to Address Sex Trafficking of Children

PICOT Question: For child and adolescent victims of sex trafficking, will education programs for health care providers and mandatory reporters on the signs and risk factors of sex trafficking victimization improve early identification and intervention?

Evidence Summary

Educational programs on sex trafficking for health care providers are essential to identifying victims and intervening appropriately (Bauer et al, 2019). Sex trafficking of minors is a type of human trafficking involving crimes of a sexual nature committed against children and adolescents. This exploitation may involve prostitution; performing in sexual venues such as strip clubs; survival sex by which a minor performs sex acts for money, food, shelter, or other necessities; pornography; and sex tourism, such as mail-order bride trade or early marriage (Ulibarri, et al., 2017). Because trafficked children do not often disclose that they are victims and there is no uniform data collection system in place to track minor sex trafficking, the prevalence is largely unknown (Bauer et al., 2019; Hartinger-Saunders et al., 2017).

Victims of sex trafficking come from every demographic, but they typically share risk factors that make them vulnerable to exploitation. Common risk factors include history of abuse or neglect, family violence or dysfunction, poverty, substance misuse, mental health issues, runaway/homelessness, and those who identify as lesbian, gay, bisexual, transgender, queer, or questioning (Greenbaum, 2017).

Many sex trafficking victims are "trapped and controlled through assault, threats, false promises, perceived sense of protection, isolation, shaming, and debt" (CDC, 2018e), yet many do not recognize they are being trafficked, do not identify themselves as victims (Perkins and Ruiz, 2017), and may even protect their abuser (Hartinger-Saunders et al., 2017). Common health issues of sex trafficking victims include sexually transmitted infections, HIV/AIDS, pregnancy, physical injury, post-traumatic stress disorder, and depression (Bauer et al., 2019; Greenbaum, 2017).

Application to Nursing Practice

- Develop educational programs that assist health care providers to identify victims of sex trafficking, including how to safely separate the potential victim from the trafficker and knowledge of immediate resources to protect the victim (Bauer et al., 2019).
- Nurses are mandatory reporters and must recognize signs of victimization and know how to intervene (Powell et al., 2017).
- Design "Sex Trafficking Indicator" checklist and educate health care providers on its use (Bauer et al., 2019).
- Use a standardized, evidence-based education program on human trafficking with patient-outcome metrics to educate other health care providers and mandatory reporters to recognize the risk factors and signs of sex traffic victimization (Hartinger-Saunders et al., 2017; Powell et al., 2017).
- Coordinate care and tailor interventions for sex trafficking survivors (Twigg, 2017).
- Lead or participate in research on the best way to educate health care professionals about sex trafficking (Powell et al., 2017).

Eating Disorders. Eating disorders include anorexia nervosa, bulimia nervosa, and binge eating disorder. The highest incidence of eating disorders occurs in 15- to 19-year-olds, so routine nutritional screening should be a part of the health care provided to all adolescents. Areas to include in the assessment are past and present diet history, food records, eating habits, attitudes, health beliefs, and socioeconomic and psychosocial factors (Hockenberry et al., 2019). An important psychosocial factor is assessment of an adolescent's perception of his or her body image and self-esteem or any sources of depression (Laporta-Herrero et al., 2018).

Anorexia nervosa is more common in girls and is a clinical syndrome with both physical and psychosocial components of anxiety and depression. People with anorexia nervosa have an intense fear of gaining weight and refuse to maintain body weight at the minimal normal weight for their age and height. Over time this condition affects both physiological and psychosocial function and impacts quality of life (Carrot et al., 2017).

Bulimia nervosa is most identified with binge eating and behaviors to prevent weight gain. Unlike anorexia, bulimia occurs within a normal weight range; thus it is much more difficult to detect. Behaviors of individuals with eating disorders include self-induced vomiting, misuse of laxatives and other medications, and excessive exercise. It is important to take a thorough dietary history because, if left undetected and untreated, these disorders lead to significant morbidity and mortality (Hockenberry et al., 2019).

Sexually Transmitted Infections. Sexually transmitted infections (STIs) annually affect millions of sexually active adolescents. This high degree of incidence makes it imperative that sexually active adolescents be screened for STIs, even when they have no symptoms. The annual physical examination of a sexually active adolescent includes a thorough sexual history and a careful examination of the genitalia so that STIs are not missed. Be proactive by using the interview process to identify risk factors in the adolescent, and provide education to prevent STIs, including human immunodeficiency virus (HIV) and HPV, and unwanted pregnancies (Hockenberry et al., 2019). As discussed earlier for school-age children, immunization for HPV infection should be considered at this time if not already administered.

Pregnancy. The United States has the highest rate of teenage pregnancy and childbearing annually compared with other industrialized nations (Hockenberry et al., 2019). Adolescent birth rates continue to decline due to improvements in contraceptive use, the use of long-acting reversible contraception, and safe sex practices (Lindberg et al., 2018). However, adolescent pregnancy continues to be a major social challenge. Adolescent pregnancy occurs across socioeconomic classes, in public and private schools, among all ethnic and religious backgrounds, and in all parts of the country. Pregnant teens need special attention to nutrition, health supervision, and psychological support. Adolescent mothers also need help in planning for the future and obtaining competent day care for their infants.

Health Promotion

Health Education. Community and school-based health programs for adolescents focus on health promotion and illness prevention. Nurses need to be sensitive to the emotional cues from adolescents before initiating health teaching to know when the teen is ready to discuss concerns. In addition, discussions with adolescents need to be private and confidential. Adolescents define health in much the same way as adults and look for opportunities to reach their physical, mental, and emotional potential. Large numbers of school-based clinics have been developed and implemented to respond to adolescents' needs. Adolescents are much more likely to use these health care services if they encounter providers who are caring and respectful (Hockenberry et al., 2019).

Nurses play an important role in preventing injuries and accidental deaths. For example, discussing alternatives to substance-impaired driving or riding with someone under the influence of drugs or alcohol prepares them to consider alternatives when such an occasion arises. As a nurse, identify adolescents at risk for abuse, provide education to prevent accidents related to substance abuse, and provide resources to those in need of mental health care.

Minority Adolescents. African-American, Hispanic, Latino, Asian, Native American, and Alaska Native adolescents are the fastest-growing segment in the US population. Minority adolescents experience a greater percentage of health problems and barriers to health care (Hockenberry et al., 2019). Issues of concern for these adolescents living in a high-risk environment include childhood trauma, cyberbullying, death related to violence, unintentional injuries, learning or emotional difficulties, and an increased rate for adolescent pregnancy and STIs (Larson et al., 2017). Poverty is a major factor that negatively affects the lives of many minority adolescents. Limited access to health services is common (Duarte et al., 2018). Nurses are able to make a significant contribution to improving access to appropriate health care for adolescents. With knowledge about various cultures and the means to care for minority adolescents, nurses act as advocates to ensure accessibility of appropriate services.

Gay, Lesbian, and Bisexual Adolescents. Sexual orientation refers to patterns of sexual and emotional attraction to persons of the same gender, opposite gender, or both males and females. While most adolescents identify themselves as heterosexual, many identify themselves as homosexual or bisexual. It is widely known that, although some adolescents participate in same-gender sexual activity, they do not necessarily become homosexual as adults (Hockenberry et al., 2019). Adolescents who believe that they have a homosexual or bisexual orientation often try to keep it hidden to avoid any associated stigma, victimization, or bullying. This increases their vulnerability to depression and suicide. The teens who choose to disclose a homosexual or bisexual orientation become at risk for violence, harassment, and family abuse (Mustanski et al., 2016). If a teen chooses to disclose sexual orientation to you, help the adolescent consider how to discuss with family or friends and to construct a safety plan before telling his or her family or friends in case their response is not supportive (Hockenberry et al., 2019).

KEY POINTS

- Nurses promote the health of pregnant women by addressing nutritional requirements, physical changes, and psychosocial needs.
- At birth, newborns develop independent circulatory and respiratory functioning.
- Promotion of parent-child attachment can begin immediately after birth.
- Physical changes include maturation of organ systems, fine and gross motor development, and physical growth. These changes occur in a regular pattern and are monitored to identify developmental concerns.
- Cognitive and psychosocial development throughout childhood is rapid, and a multitude of factors can foster or hinder a child's development.
- Play provides opportunities for development of cognitive, social, and motor skills. Play evolves from solitary to interactive play throughout childhood.
- Through anticipatory guidance, nurses can prepare parents to reduce their children's health risks and to promote achievement of developmental tasks.

REFLECTIVE LEARNING

- Considering what you know about childhood development, how would your approach to assessment of cognitive function be different if a child were of school age versus an adolescent?
- What anticipatory guidance could you provide for a family you cared for to minimize health risks for their child?
- Family support, including financial and child care assistance, for the adolescent mother significantly increases the likelihood that she

will complete her education and gain skills for the job market. How can you support these goals for an adolescent mother who does not have sufficient family support?

REVIEW QUESTIONS

1. Which of the following should be included in health teaching for a pregnant patient? (Select all that apply.)
   1. Exposure of the fetus to alcohol, drugs, or tobacco can cause abnormal development.
   2. Nutritional needs increase during pregnancy, and eating healthy foods is important.
   3. Complementary and alternative therapies should always be avoided during pregnancy.
   4. Provide education on self-care to reduce common discomforts of pregnancy, such as nausea.
   5. Recommend birthing classes to prepare the mother for the birthing process.

2. A parent has brought her 6-month-old infant in for a well-child check. Which of her statements indicates a need for further teaching?
   1. "I can start giving her whole milk at about 12 months."
   2. "I can continue to breastfeed for another 6 months."
   3. "I can give her plenty of fruit juice to increase her vitamin intake."
   4. "I can start giving her solid food now, introducing one food at a time."

3. A nurse is teaching the mother of a young infant about prevention of sudden infant death syndrome (SIDS). Which of the following statements indicates that the teaching has been effective? (Select all that apply.)
   1. "I'll let the baby sleep in bed with me so I can watch her."
   2. "I'll remove stuffed animals and pillows from the crib."
   3. "I'll place my baby on her back for sleep."
   4. "I'll be sure to keep my baby's room cool."
   5. "I'll keep a crib bumper in the bed to prevent drafts."

4. Sequence the skills in the expected order of gross-motor development in an infant, beginning with the earliest skill.
   1. Can lift head 45 degrees off table, when prone
   2. Pulls self to standing position
   3. Sits upright without support
   4. Rolls from back to abdomen
   5. Rolls from abdomen to back

5. Parents are concerned about their toddler's negativism. To avoid a negative response, which of the following is the best way for a nurse to demonstrate asking the toddler to eat lunch?
   1. Would you like to eat your lunch now?
   2. Would you like to sit at the big table to eat?
   3. When would you like to eat your lunch with your friends?
   4. Would you like apple slices or applesauce with your sandwich?

6. When nurses are communicating with adolescents, they should:
   1. Ask closed-ended questions to get straight answers.
   2. Ask the adolescent to collaborate on plan of care.
   3. Avoid looking for meaning behind adolescents' words or actions.
   4. Avoid discussing sensitive issues such as sex and drugs.

7. You are caring for a 4-year-old child who is hospitalized for an infection. He tells you that he is sick because he was "bad." Which is the most correct interpretation of his comment?
   1. Indicative of maladaptive stress response
   2. Representative of his cognitive development
   3. Suggestive of excessive discipline at home
   4. Indicative of his developing sense of inferiority

8. At a well-child examination, the mother comments that her toddler eats little at mealtime, will sit only briefly at the table, and wants snacks all the time. Which of the following should the nurse recommend? (Select all the apply.)
   1. Provide nutritious snacks for a healthy diet.
   2. Offer rewards for eating at mealtimes.
   3. Avoid snacks so she is hungry at mealtime.
   4. Offer finger foods so she can eat as she walks.
   5. Explain to her why eating at mealtime is important.

9. A 15-year-old patient tells the nurse that she is sexually active. What is the best action by the nurse?
   1. Contact her parents to alert them of her need for birth control.
   2. Explain that having sex is not appropriate for her age-group.
   3. Counsel her on safe sex practices and on minimizing health risks.
   4. Ask her to have her partner come to the clinic for STI testing.

10. A 4-month-old infant has not been feeling well for 2 days. Which number on the image identifies the area of the infant's head where the nurse can assess for dehydration?
    1. 1
    2. 2
    3. 3
    4. 4
    5. 5

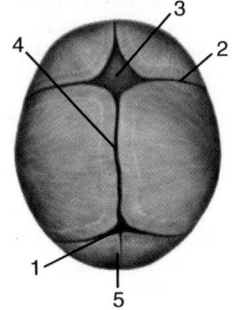

Answers: 1. 1, 2, 4, 5; **2.** 3; **3.** 3, 4; **4.** 1, 5, 4, 3; **5.** 4; **6.** 2; **7.** 2; **8.** 1, 4, 9; **9.** 3; **10.** 3.

Rationales to Review Questions can be found on the Evolve website.

REFERENCES

American Academy of Pediatrics (AAP): *Healthy children: safety and prevention: new crib standards: what parents need to know*, 2014. http://www.healthychildren.org/English/ages-stages/baby/sleep/Pages/New-Crib-Standards-What-Parents-Need-to-Know.aspx. Accessed August 2018.

American Academy of Pediatrics (AAP): Council on communications and Media: Media and young minds, *Pediatrics* 138(5), 2016a. http://pediatrics.aappublications.org/content/138/5/e20162591. Accessed August 2018.

American Academy of Pediatrics (AAP): Screening for Idiopathic scoliosis in adolescents, *Pediatrics* 138(5), 2016b https://doi.org/10.1542/peds.2016-0065. http://pediatrics.aappublications.org/content/early/2016/03/18/peds.2016-0065. Accessed August 2018.

American Academy of Pediatrics (AAP): Task Force on Sudden Infant Death Syndrome: SIDS and other sleep related deaths: Updated 2016 recommendations for a safe infant sleeping environment, *Pediatrics* 138(5), 2016c.

American Academy of Pediatrics (AAP): *HPV vaccine Implementation guidance Updated February 2017*, 2017. https://www.aap.org/en-us/Documents/immunization_hpvimplementationguidance.pdf. Accessed August 2018.

American Academy of Pediatrics (AAP): *Recommended immunization schedule for children and adolescents aged 18 or younger, United States*, 2018a. https://www.aap.org/en-us/Documents/immunization_schedule2018.pdf. Accessed August 2018.

American Academy of Pediatrics (AAP): *Car seats: information for families*, 2018b. https://www.healthychildren.org/English/safety-prevention/on-the-go/Pages/Car-Safety-Seats-Information-for-Families.aspx. Accessed August 2018.

American Academy of Pediatrics (AAP): Why does my son need the HPV vaccine? 2018c. https://www.healthychildren.org/English/tips-tools/ask-the-pediatrician/Pages/why-does-son-need-HPV-vaccine.aspx. Accessed June 2019.

Bauer R, et al.: What health providers should know about human sex trafficking, *MEDSURG Nursing* 28(6):347, 2019.

Centers for Disease Control and Prevention (CDC): *Prevalence of obesity among adults and youth: United States, 2015-2016, NCHS data Brief, No. 288*, 2017a. https://www.cdc.gov/nchs/data/databriefs/db288.pdf. Accessed August 2018.

Centers for Disease Control and Prevention (CDC): *Suicide among youth*, 2017b. https://www.cdc.gov/healthcommunication/toolstemplates/entertainmented/tips/SuicideYouth.html. Accessed August 2018.

Centers for Disease Control and Prevention (CDC): *Youth and tobacco use*, 2018a. https://www.cdc.gov/tobacco/data_statistics/fact_sheets/youth_data/tobacco_use/index.htm. Accessed June 2019.

Centers for Disease Control and Prevention (CDC): *National center for injury prevention and control Web-based injury Statistics Query and reporting system*, 2018b. https://www.cdc.gov/motorvehiclesafety/child_passenger_safety/cps-factsheet.html. Accessed June 2019.

Centers for Disease Control and Prevention (CDC): Youth risk behavior surveillance – United States, 2017, *MMWR (Morb Mortal Wkly Rep)* 67(8), 2018c. https://www.cdc.gov/healthyyouth/data/yrbs/pdf/2017/ss6708.pdf. Accessed June 2019.

Centers for Disease Control and Prevention (CDC): *Electronic cigarettes: what's the bottom line*, 2018d. https://www.cdc.gov/tobacco/basic_information/e-cigarettes/pdfs/Electronic-Cigarettes-Infographic-508.pdf. Accessed June 2019.

Center for Disease Control and Prevention (CDC): *Sex trafficking*, 2018e. https://www.cdc.gov/violenceprevention/sexualviolence/trafficking.html. Accessed June 2019.

Erikson EH: *Childhood and society*, ed 2, New York, 1963, Norton.

Erikson EH: *Identity: youth and crises*, New York, 1968, Norton.

Food and Drug Administration (FDA). FDA statement: statement from FDA Commissioner

Hockenberry M, et al.: *Wong's nursing care of infants and children*, ed 11, St Louis, 2019, Mosby.

Murray SS, et al.: *Foundations of maternal-newborn and women's health nursing*, ed 7, Philadelphia, 2019, Saunders, VitalBook file, Pageburst Online.

National Institutes of Health: *National Institute on Drug Abuse: Monitoring the future 2017 survey results*, 2017. https://www.drugabuse.gov/related-topics/trends-statistics/infographics/monitoring-future-2017-survey-results. Accessed August 2018.

Piaget J: *The origins of intelligence in children*, New York, 1952, International Universities Press.

Shmerling RH: Can vaping damage your lungs? What we do (and don't) know, Harvard Health publishing, 2019. http://www.health.harvard.edu/blog/can-vaping-damage-your-lungs-what-we-do-and-dont-know-2019090417734.

US Department of Health and Human Services (USDHHS): *Health resources and services administration: adolescent health*, 2014. http://healthypeople.gov/2020/topicsobjectives2020/objectiveslist.aspx?topicId=2#16. Accessed March 2015.

US Department of Health and Human Services (USDHHS): National vital statistics reports, vol. 67(No. 5), 26, 2018. https://www.cdc.gov/nchs/data/nvsr/nvsr67/nvsr67_05.pdf. Accessed August 2018.

RESEARCH REFERENCES

Azarmnejad E, et al.: The effectiveness of familiar auditory stimulus on hospitalized neonates' physiologic responses to procedural pain, *Int J Nurs Practr* 23:e12527, 2017.

Canadian Paediatric Society, Digital Health Task Force: Screen time and young children: promoting health and development in a digital world, *Paediatr Child Health* 22(8):461, 2017.

Carrot B, et al.: Are lifetime affective disorders predictive of long-term outcome in severe adolescent anorexia nervosa? *Eur Child Adolesc Psychiatry* 26:969, 2017.

Duarte C, et al.: Correlation of minority status, cyberbullying, and mental health: a cross-sectional study of 1031 adolescents, *J Child Adolesc Trauma* 11(1):39, 2018.

Goldenson NI, et al.: Associations of electronic cigarette nicotine concentration with subsequent cigarette smoking and vaping levels in adolescents, *JAMA Pediatrics* 171(12):1192, 2017.

Greenbaum VJ: Child sex trafficking in the United States: challenges for the healthcare provider, *PLoS Med* 14(11), 2017.

Hartinger-Saunders RM, et al.: Mandated reporters' perceptions of and encounters with domestic minor sex trafficking of adolescent females in the United States, *Am J Orthopsychiatry* 87(3):195, 2017.

Ho LP, et al.: A feasibility and efficacy randomized controlled trial of swaddling for controlling procedural pain in preterm infants, *J Clin Nurs* 25(3/4):472, 2016.

Kochanek KD, et al.: *Mortality in the United States, 2016, NCHS data Brief, no 293*, Hyattsville, MD, 2017, National Center for Health Statistics. https://www.cdc.gov/nchs/data/databriefs/db293.pdf. Accessed August 2018.

Laporta-Herrero I, et al.: Body dissatisfaction in adolescents with eating disorders, *Eat Weight Disord* 23(3):339, 2018.

Larson S, et al.: Chronic childhood trauma, mental health, academic achievement, and school-based health center mental health services, *J School Health* 87(9):675, 2017.

Lindberg LD, et al.: Changing patterns of contraceptive use and the decline in rates of pregnancy and birth among U.S. adolescents 2007-2014, *J Adolescent Health* 63(2):253, 2018.

Mustanski B, et al.: The effects of cumulative victimization on mental health among lesbian, gay bisexual and transgender adolescents and young adults, *Am J Public Health* 106(3):527, 2016.

Perkins EB, Ruiz C: Domestic minor sex trafficking in a rural state: interviews with adjudicated female juveniles, *Child Adolesc Soc Work J* 34(2):171, 2017.

Powell C, et al.: Training US health care professionals on human trafficking: where do we go from here? *Med Educ Online* 22(1), 2017. https://doi.org/10.1080/10872981.2017.1267980.

Twigg NM: Comprehensive care model for sex trafficking survivors, *J Nurs Scholarsh* 49(3):259, 2017, https://doi.org/10.1111/jnu.12285.

Ulibarri MD, et al.: Introduction to special section: research, treatment, and policy regarding trafficking and sexual exploitation of children and adolescents, *J Child Adol Trauma* 10(2):147, 2017, https://doi.org/10.1007/s40653-017-0150-3.

13

Young and Middle Adults

OBJECTIVES

- Discuss developmental theories of young and middle adults.
- List and discuss major life events of young and middle adults and the childbearing family.
- Describe developmental tasks of the young adult, the childbearing family, and the middle adult.
- Discuss the significance of family in the life of the young and middle adult.

- Describe normal physical changes in young and middle adulthood and pregnancy.
- Discuss cognitive and psychosocial changes occurring during the young and middle adult years.
- Describe health concerns of the young adult, the childbearing family, and the middle adult.
- Describe intimate partner violence.

KEY TERMS

Braxton Hicks contractions, p. 167

Climacteric, p. 169

Doula, p. 163

Emerging adulthood, p. 161

Infertility, p. 167

Lactation, p. 167

Menopause, p. 168

Prenatal care, p. 167

Puerperium, p. 163

Sandwich generation, p. 168

MEDIA RESOURCES

http://evolve.elsevier.com/Potter/fundamentals/
- Review Questions
- Case Study with Questions

- Audio Glossary
- Content Updates
- Answers to QSEN Activity and Review Questions

Young and middle adulthood are developmental periods that pose challenges, rewards, and crises. Challenges often include the demands of working and raising families and other crises, such as caring for aging parents or the possibility of job loss in a changing economic environment. Classic works by developmental theorists such as Diekelmann (1976) and Erikson (1963, 1982) attempted to describe the phases of young and middle adulthood and related developmental tasks (see Chapter 11). More recent work has identified an additional phase of development in the young adult: emerging adulthood.

Faced with a societal structure that differs greatly from the norms of 20 or 30 years ago, both men and women are assuming different roles in today's society. Men were traditionally the primary supporters of the family. Today many women pursue careers and contribute significantly to their families' incomes. Women comprise half of the workforce. They are the sole or co-breadwinner in half of American families with children. However, women on average earn less than men in almost every occupation. Women from minority groups and those in lower socioeconomic levels have an even greater wage gap (Institute for Women's Policy Research [IWPR], 2019).

Developmental theories help explain the life events and developmental tasks of the young and middle adult (see Chapter 11). Patients present challenges to nurses who themselves are often young or middle adults coping with the demands of their respective developmental period. Nurses need to recognize the needs of their patients even if they are not experiencing the same challenges and events.

YOUNG ADULTS

Young adulthood is the period between the late teens and the mid to late 30s (Edelman and Kudzma, 2018). In the past several decades, the period of life called emerging adulthood has been identified as lasting from the late teens to mid-twenties (Fioretti et al., 2017). This stage of development is unique from young adulthood and extended adolescence. It is a stage that is much freer from parental control and much more a period of independent exploration compared with adolescence. It differs from young adulthood since most young people in their twenties have not made those transitions historically associated with adult status, especially marriage and parenthood. In this stage young adults are faced with the tasks of identity development, who they want to be, and how to attain their goals (Layland et al., 2018).

It is estimated that in 2017 young adults 20 to 34 years of age made up approximately 22% to 24% of the population (US Census Bureau, 2018). According to the Pew Research Center (2019), today's young adults are history's first "always-connected" generation, with digital technology and social media as major aspects of their lives. They adapt well to new experiences and are more ethnically and racially diverse than previous generations. Young adults increasingly move away from their families of origin, establish career goals, and decide whether to marry or remain single and whether to begin families.

Physical Changes

The young adult usually completes physical growth by the age of 20. An exception to this is the pregnant or lactating woman. The physical, cognitive, and psychosocial changes and the health concerns of the pregnant woman and the childbearing family are extensive.

Young adults are usually quite active, experience severe illnesses less frequently than older age-groups, tend to ignore physical symptoms, and often postpone seeking health care. Physical strength typically peaks, and physical characteristics of young adults begin to change as middle age approaches. Physical changes in weight and muscle mass often occur as a result of diet, exercise, and lifestyle patterns. Assessment findings are generally within normal limits unless an illness is present.

Cognitive Changes

Critical thinking habits increase steadily through the young adult years. Formal and informal educational experiences, general life experiences, and occupational opportunities dramatically increase the individual's conceptual, problem-solving, and motor skills.

Identifying an occupational direction is a major task of young adults. When people know their skills, talents, and personality characteristics, educational preparation and occupational choices are easier and more satisfying. Some young adults pursue postsecondary education to attain their occupational goals. Postsecondary education, which includes vocational training (e.g., carpentry, welding) and earned degrees from colleges or universities (e.g., associate, baccalaureate, and graduate degrees), is often the entry-level educational requirement for many of the fastest-growing occupations in the United States (US Department of Labor, 2019).

An understanding of how adults learn helps nurses develop patient education plans (see Chapter 25). Adults enter the teaching-learning situation with a background of unique life experiences, including illness and injuries. Their adherence to regimens such as medications, treatments, or lifestyle changes such as smoking cessation involves decision-making processes. When determining the amount of information that an individual needs to make decisions about the prescribed course of therapy, consider factors that possibly affect his or her adherence to the regimen, including educational level, lifestyle habits, socioeconomic factors, and motivation and desire to learn.

Because young adults are continually evolving and adjusting to changes in the home, workplace, and social lives, their decision-making processes need to be flexible. The more secure young adults are in their roles, the more flexible and open they are to change. People who are insecure tend to be more rigid in making decisions (Edelman and Kudzma, 2018).

Psychosocial Changes

The emotional health of a young adult is related to the ability to address and resolve personal and social tasks. The young adult is often caught between wanting to prolong some of the freedom of adolescence and assume adult commitments. However, certain trends are relatively predictable. Between the ages of 23 and 28, the person refines self-perception and ability for intimacy. From 29 to 34 the person directs enormous energy toward achievement and mastery of the surrounding world. The years from 35 to 40 are a time of vigorous examination of life goals and relationships. Sometimes as a result of this reexamination people make changes in personal, social, and occupational areas.

Cultural factors such as ethnicity and gender have a sociological and psychological influence in a young adult's life, and these factors pose challenges for nursing care (see Chapter 9). Each person holds individualized definitions of health and illness and the behaviors necessary to stay healthy. Nurses and other health professionals bring with them distinct practices for the prevention and treatment of illness. Knowing too little about a patient's self-perception or beliefs regarding health and illness may create conflict between a nurse and patient.

Changes in the traditional role expectations of both men and women in young adulthood lead to challenges for nursing care. For example, young adults often struggle with balancing job demands, personal relationships, the needs of the family, and socialization (Brough et al., 2018). Thus the struggle to balance these factors is a potential source of stress for the young adult, which may impact coping resources, health promotion behaviors, and level of health (Amnie, 2018).

Health is not merely the absence of disease; it also involves wellness in all human dimensions (see Chapter 6). Through patient education the nurse provides a young adult with access to health promotion resources and appropriate referrals to improve coping and health behaviors. The young adult needs to make decisions concerning career, marriage, and parenthood. Although each person makes these decisions based on individual factors, a nurse needs to understand the general principles involved in these aspects of psychosocial development while assessing the young adult's psychosocial status.

Lifestyle. Family history of cardiovascular, renal, endocrine, or neoplastic disease increases a young adult's risk of illness. In addition, young adults, especially young men, are more likely to participate in some health risk behaviors, such as dangerous driving practices, smoking, substance abuse, overexposure to sun, binge drinking, and increased unprotected sexual activity (Masiero et al., 2018). Your role in health promotion is to identify unique modifiable factors and provide gender and culturally specific patient education and support to reduce unhealthy lifestyle behaviors (Kritsotakis et al., 2016). These lifestyle changes can include diet and exercise modifications, use of seat belts, and reduction in risky sex practices.

A personal lifestyle assessment (see Chapter 6) helps nurses and patients identify habits that increase the risk for cardiac, malignant, pulmonary, renal, or other chronic diseases. The assessment includes general life satisfaction, hobbies, and interests; habits such as diet, sleeping, exercise, sexual habits, and use of caffeine, tobacco, alcohol, and illicit drugs; home conditions and pets; economics, including type of health insurance; occupational environment, including type of work and exposure to hazardous substances; and physical or mental stress. Military records, including dates and geographical area of assignments, may also be useful in assessing the young adult for risk factors. Prolonged stress from lifestyle choices increases wear and tear on the adaptive capacities of the body, and stress-related illnesses, such as ulcers, emotional disorders, and infections, sometimes occur (see Chapter 37).

Career. Successful employment is important in the lives of most men and women. This not only helps to ensure economic security but also leads to fulfillment, friendships, social activities, support, and respect from co-workers.

The average adult under age 35 has an average debt of $67,400 (Renzulli, 2018). The greatest percentage of that debt is educational. The average millennial household owes $14,800 in student loans (Renzulli, 2018). Therefore many young adults choose a two-career family, which has benefits and liabilities. In addition to increasing the family's financial base, the person who works outside the home is able to expand friendships, activities, and interests. However, stress exists in a two-career family as well. These stressors result from a transfer to a new city; increased expenditures of physical, mental, or emotional energy; child care demands; or household needs. When partners share decision making and responsibilities, the stressors related to a two-career family decrease. For example, some families may decide to limit recreational expenses and instead hire someone to do routine housework.

Sexuality. The development of secondary sex characteristics occurs during the adolescent years (see Chapter 12). Physical development is

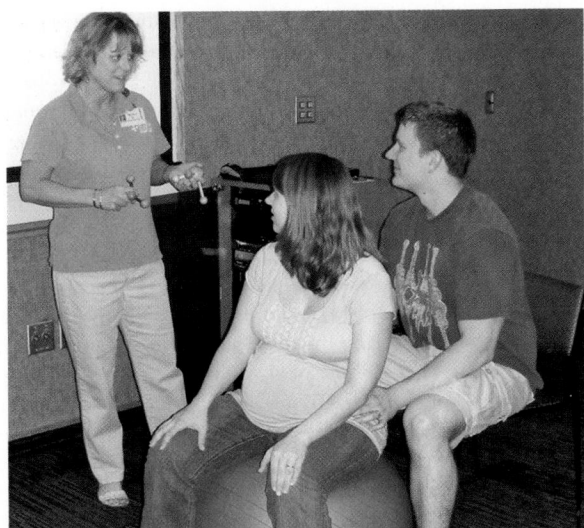

FIG. 13.1 Nurse providing Lamaze class for expectant young adults.

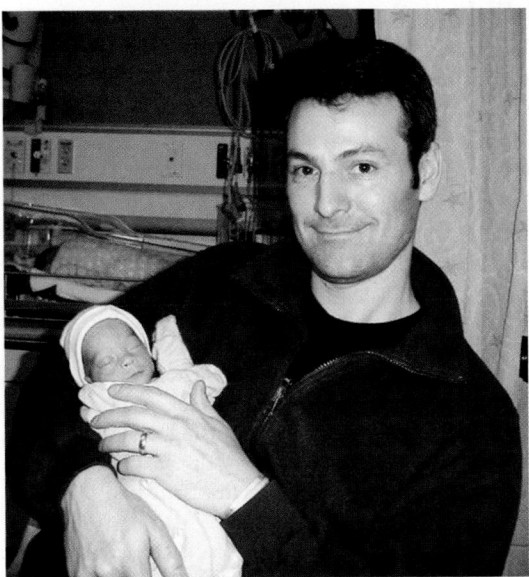

FIG. 13.2 Parent-child nurturing is important in adapting to a newborn. (From Hockenberry MJ, Wilson D: *Wong's nursing care of infants and children*, ed 10, St Louis, 2015, Mosby.)

accompanied by sexual maturation. The young adult usually has emotional maturity to complement the physical ability and therefore is able to develop mature sexual relationships and establish intimacy. Young adults who have failed to achieve the developmental task of personal integration sometimes develop relationships that are superficial and stereotyped (Varcarolis, 2017).

The psychodynamic aspect of sexual activity is as important as the type or frequency of sexual intercourse to young adults (see Chapter 34). To maintain total wellness, encourage young adults to assess their sexual activity and practice safe sex. Assist them to realize that their sexual needs and concerns are normal and may change over time (Shaw and Rogge, 2017). When necessary, help to identify risky sexual behaviors, such as unprotected sex or multiple sexual partners. Ensure that these young adults have adequate sexual health education regarding birth control and the prevention of sexually transmitted infections (STIs).

Childbearing Cycle. Conception, pregnancy, birth, and the **puerperium** are major phases of the childbearing cycle. The changes during these phases are complex. Childbirth education classes can prepare pregnant women, their partners, and other support people to participate in the birthing process (Fig. 13.1). Some health care agencies provide either professional labor support or a lay **doula**, a support person to be present during labor to assist women who have no other source of support. The stress that many women experience after childbirth may have a significant impact on postpartum women's health.

Types of Families. During young adulthood most individuals experience singlehood and the opportunity to be on their own. Those who eventually marry or establish long-term partnerships encounter several changes as they take on new responsibilities. For example, many couples choose to become parents (Fig. 13.2). Some young adults choose alternative lifestyles, and different family forms emerge (see Chapter 10).

Singlehood. The social pressure to get married has changed, and some young adults may choose not to marry until their late 20s or early 30s or not at all. For young adults who remain single, parents and siblings become the nucleus for a family. Some view close friends and associates as "family." One cause for the increased single population is the expanding career opportunities for women. Women

enter the job market with greater career potential and have greater opportunities for financial independence. More single individuals are choosing to live together outside marriage and become parents either biologically or through adoption. Similarly, many married couples choose to separate or divorce if they find their marital situation unsatisfactory.

Parenthood. Knowledge about sexuality and the availability of contraception help people decide when and if to start a family. Sometimes social pressures encourage young adults to have children. Economic considerations frequently enter into the decision-making process because of the expense of childrearing. General health status and age are also considerations in decisions about parenthood.

Alternative Family Structures and Parenting. Changing norms and values about family life in the United States reveal basic shifts in attitudes about family structure (see Chapter 10). The trend toward greater acceptance of cohabitation without marriage is a factor in the greater numbers of infants being born to single women. In addition, approximately 6 million American children and adults have parents who are lesbian, gay, bisexual, transgender, or queer (LGBTQ). Approximately 131,000 same-sex households include children under the age of 18 (Rossi, 2018; Bos et al., 2016). The American Academy of Pediatrics (AAP), in recognizing the needs of gay and lesbian parents and their children, published a policy statement supporting adoption of children and the parenting role by same-sex parents (AAP, 2013). Research demonstrates that there is no difference in child health outcomes between same-sex and different-sex parent households (Bos et al., 2016).

Emotional Health. Young adults need physical and emotional resources and support systems to meet the many challenges, tasks, and responsibilities they face. During psychosocial assessment of young adults, assess for signs of emotional health that support successful maturation in this developmental stage (e.g., satisfaction with personal growth and development, satisfaction with relationships, and attainment of long-term goals related to education, employment, housing, and relationships).

Health Risks

Health risk factors for a young adult originate in the community, lifestyle patterns, and family history. The lifestyle habits that activate the stress response (see Chapter 37) increase the risk of illness. Young adults may have optimistic bias related to specific behaviors, such as smoking and alcohol consumption. When optimistic bias is present, young adults do not perceive that associated health risks for cancer and chronic cardiac and pulmonary diseases will affect their level of health (Masiero et al., 2018). Smoking is a well-documented risk factor for pulmonary, cardiac, and vascular diseases in smokers and the individuals who receive secondhand smoke. Electronic cigarette (e-cigarette) or vaping of substances, such as tobacco or cannabis, has the potential for health risks developing over time due to the inhaled pollutants (Sommerfeld et al., 2018). The nicotine in tobacco is a vasoconstrictor that acts on the coronary arteries, increasing the risk of angina, myocardial infarction, and coronary artery disease. Nicotine also causes peripheral vasoconstriction and leads to vascular problems.

Family History. A family history of a disease sometimes puts a young adult at risk for developing it in the middle- or older-adult years. For example, a young man whose father and paternal grandfather had myocardial infarctions (heart attacks) in their 50s has a risk for a future myocardial infarction. The presence of chronic illnesses such as diabetes mellitus or certain cancers in the family increases the family member's risk of developing the diseases (see Chapter 8). Regular physical examinations and screenings are important since certain conditions such as high blood pressure, high blood sugar, and high cholesterol levels may not have any symptoms in the early stages. In addition, the American Cancer Society (2018) now recommends early routine screening for colorectal cancer and even earlier screening for individuals with a family history of colorectal cancers. Genomic science and resultant technologies identify people at risk for disease through the use of genetic screening. Understanding the role genomics plays in the health of individuals and families enables clinicians to better advise young adults related to current and future health care.

Personal Hygiene Habits. As in all age-groups, some personal hygiene habits in the young adult are risk factors. Sharing eating utensils with a person who has a contagious illness increases the risk of illness. Poor dental hygiene increases the risk of periodontal disease. Individuals avoid gingivitis (inflammation of the gums) and periodontitis (loss of tooth support) through oral hygiene (see Chapter 40).

Violent Death and Injury. Violence is a common cause of mortality and morbidity in the young-adult population (Shane et al., 2018). Factors that predispose individuals to violence, injury, or death include poverty, family breakdown, child abuse and neglect, opioid and other drug use (dealing or illegal use), repeated exposure to violence, and ready access to guns. It is important to perform a thorough psychosocial assessment, including such factors as behavioral patterns, history of physical and substance abuse, education, work history, and social support systems to detect personal and environmental risk factors for violence. Death and injury primarily occur from physical assaults, motor vehicle or other accidents, and suicide attempts in young adults (Shane et al., 2018).

Intimate Partner Violence. Intimate partner violence (IPV), formerly referred to as domestic violence, is a global public health problem. It exists along a continuum from a single episode of violence to ongoing battering. IPV often begins with emotional or mental abuse and may progress to physical or sexual assault. Each year women in the United States experience approximately 4.8 million intimate

partner–related physical assaults and rapes, and men are the victims of approximately 2.9 million intimate partner–related physical assaults (Roberts et al., 2018). Physical injuries from IPV range from minor cuts and bruises to broken bones, internal bleeding, head trauma, and death. IPV is linked to such harmful health behaviors as smoking, alcohol abuse, drug use, and risky sexual activity. Risk factors to look for in an assessment that suggest perpetration of IPV include using drugs or alcohol, especially heavy drinking; unemployment; low self-esteem; gambling; antisocial or borderline personality traits; desire for power and control in relationships; and being a victim of physical or psychological abuse (Roberts et al., 2018; Bonomi et al., 2014). An increased risk of violence occurs during the reproductive years, and a pregnant woman has a greater risk of being a victim of IPV than a nonpregnant woman. Women experiencing IPV may be more likely to delay prenatal care and are at increased risk for multiple poor maternal and infant health outcomes, such as low maternal weight gain, infections, high blood pressure, vaginal bleeding, and delivery of a preterm or low-birth-weight infant (Ferdos et al., 2018).

QSEN **Building Competency in Patient-Centered Care** You are caring for Joan, a 25-year-old patient who has come alone to the clinic because she is experiencing insomnia. Throughout the assessment interview Joan is slightly withdrawn, speaks quietly, and does not make eye contact. She does not work outside the home, and she acknowledges that her relationship with her husband, an engineer who lost his job as a result of downsizing 6 months ago, is "not going well." Physical examination reveals scratches and bruises on Joan's breasts, abdomen, and back. Refer to the CDC's Intimate Partner Violence resource page (https://www.cdc.gov/violenceprevention/intimatepartnerviolence/index.html) to determine which assessment questions, approaches, and tools you can use to determine whether Joan is a victim of IPV. If Joan is experiencing IPV, what resources may help her?

Answers to QSEN Activities can be found on the Evolve website.

Substance Abuse. Substance abuse is a social problem that directly or indirectly contributes to mortality and morbidity in young adults. Substance abuse includes alcohol and drugs. Young adults who are under the influence of substances sometimes are involved in motor vehicle accidents, often resulting in severe injuries, permanent disability, or death to everyone involved in the accident.

Dependence on stimulant or depressant drugs sometimes results in death. Overdose of a stimulant drug ("upper") stresses the cardiovascular and nervous systems to the extent that death occurs. The use of depressants ("downers") leads to an accidental or intentional overdose and death.

There is an ongoing opioid abuse crisis affecting young adults, which often occurs from overuse of opioid prescriptions (Beneitz and Gil-Alegre, 2017). This abuse is the result of the need to take regular and increasing doses of a drug in order to feel good or to avoid feeling bad. The abuse can cause several acute and toxic consequences (Beneitz and Gil-Alegre, 2017). Addiction is an illness that affects the individual, family, and friends; thus it is important to recommend that family and friends participate in the treatment process (Kelly et al., 2017).

Substance abuse can be difficult to diagnose, particularly in its early stages. Nonjudgmental questions about the use of legal drugs (prescribed drugs, tobacco, and alcohol), soft drugs (marijuana), and more problematic drugs (cocaine or heroin) are a routine part of any health assessment. The National Institute on Drug Abuse (NIDA, n.d.) recommends starting a conversation about substance abuse using these questions:

In the past year, how many times have you used the following:

- Alcohol—for men 5 or more in a day; for women 4 or more drinks in a day?
- Tobacco products?
- Prescription drugs for nonmedical reasons?
- Illegal drugs?

If the screening test suggests a patient is at risk, there are online tests available for further assessment, including the NIDA-Modified Alcohol, Smoking, and Substance Involvement Screening Test (NM**ASSIST**). Explain that it is your role as a nurse to convey health recommendations. Recommend quitting before problems (or more problems) develop. Urge patients to talk with their health care providers about the specific medical reasons for quitting (NIDA, n.d.).

Caffeine is a naturally occurring legal stimulant that is readily available in a variety of foods and beverages and in over-the-counter medications such as cold tablets or allergy and analgesic preparations. Caffeine stimulates catecholamine release, which in turn stimulates the central nervous system; it also increases gastric acid secretion, heart rate, and basal metabolic rate. This alters blood pressure, increases diuresis, and relaxes smooth muscle. Consumption of large amounts of caffeine results in restlessness, anxiety, irritability, agitation, muscle tremor, sensory disturbances, heart palpitations, nausea or vomiting, and diarrhea in some individuals.

Human Trafficking. A significant social problem is the number of youth and young adults who run away or are homeless. Many risk becoming involved in illegal and dangerous activities to survive, including human trafficking (Ashe-Goins, 2018). The United Nations Office on Drugs and Crime (2019) defines human trafficking as the recruitment, transport, transfer, harboring, or receipt of a person by threat or use of force for the purpose of exploitation. Nurses in a variety of settings, such as emergency departments, clinics, and public health agencies, are one of the first lines of health professionals who can identify victims of human trafficking and identify safe living and health care and social resources (Egyud et al., 2017). Although human trafficking is often a hidden crime and accurate statistics are difficult to obtain, estimates indicate that over 80% of trafficking victims are female and 50% are children.

Unplanned Pregnancies. Unplanned pregnancies create stress that may result in adverse health outcomes for the mother, infant, and family. Often young adults have educational and career goals that take precedence over family development. Interference with these goals often affects future relationships and parent-child relationships.

The determination of situational factors that affect the progress and outcome of an unplanned pregnancy is important. Exploration of problems such as financial, career, and living accommodations; family support systems; potential parenting disorders; depression; and coping mechanisms is important in assessing the woman with an unplanned pregnancy.

Sexually Transmitted Infections. STIs are a major health problem in young adults. Examples of STIs include syphilis, chlamydia, gonorrhea, genital herpes, human papillomavirus (HPV), and acquired immunodeficiency syndrome (AIDS). STIs have immediate physical effects such as genital discharge, discomfort, and infection. They also lead to chronic disorders, cancer, infertility, or even death. They remain a major public health problem for sexually active people, with almost half of all new infections occurring in men and women younger than 24 years of age (USDHHS, CDC, 2017). Some young adults with STIs also experience intimate partner violence. The US Preventive Services Task Force has relevant recommendations for people with STIs and intimate partner violence. Safe and effective vaccines are available for some STIs. For example, HPV, which can cause several types of cancer, can be prevented through vaccination with Gardasil or Cervarix, both Food and Drug Administration (FDA)–approved vaccines for the prevention of HPV. As young people enter sexual relationships, it is important that health care providers acknowledge the normalcy of these relationships and assess which types of sexual activity young adult patients engage in to determine appropriate screening tests and preventive measures (Gibson, 2016). Also routinely screen for interpersonal violence and refer patients to appropriate community resources.

Environmental or Occupational Factors. A common environmental or occupational risk factor is exposure to work-related hazards or agents that cause diseases and cancer (Table 13.1). Examples include lung diseases, such as silicosis from inhalation of talcum and silicon dust and emphysema from inhalation of smoke. Cancers resulting from occupational exposures may involve the lung, liver, brain, blood, or skin. Include questions regarding occupational exposure to hazardous material as a routine part of your assessment.

Health Concerns

Health Promotion. Some lifestyle choices (e.g., use of tobacco or alcohol, sexual practices) put young adults at risk for illnesses or disabilities

TABLE 13.1 Occupational Hazards/Exposures Associated with Diseases and Cancers		
Job Category	**Occupational Hazard/Exposure**	**Work-Related Condition/Cancer**
Agricultural workers	Pesticides, infectious agents, gases, sunlight	Pesticide poisoning, "farmer's lung," skin cancer
Anesthetists	Anesthetic gases	Reproductive effects, cancer
Automobile workers	Asbestos, plastics, lead, solvents	Asbestosis, dermatitis
Carpenters	Wood dust, wood preservatives, adhesives	Nasopharyngeal cancer, dermatitis
Cement workers	Cement dust, metals	Dermatitis, bronchitis
Dry cleaners	Solvents	Liver disease, dermatitis
Dye workers	Dyestuffs, metals, solvents	Bladder cancer, dermatitis
Glass workers	Heat, solvents, metal powders	Cataracts
Hospital workers	Infectious agents, cleansers, latex gloves, radiation	Infections, latex allergies, unintentional injuries
Insulators	Asbestos, fibrous glass	Asbestosis, lung cancer, mesothelioma
Jackhammer operators	Vibration	Raynaud's phenomenon
Lathe operators	Metal dusts, cutting oils	Lung disease, cancer
Office computer workers	Repetitive wrist motion on computers, eyestrain	Tendinitis, carpal tunnel syndrome, tenosynovitis

during their middle- or older-adult years. Young adults are genetically susceptible to certain chronic diseases such as diabetes mellitus and familial hypercholesterolemia (Huether and McCance, 2017). Making lifestyle changes may prevent these types of diseases in later years. Also encourage adults to perform monthly skin, breast, or male genital self-examination (see Chapter 30). Breast cancer is the most common major cancer among women in the United States, with a steadily increasing incidence. Although the incidence is low in the young adult age-group, every year approximately 1000 women under age 40 die from breast cancer. When breast cancer does develop in young adult women, they face unique challenges (Young Survivors Coalition, 2019):

- The possibility of early menopause and body image concerns and sexual dysfunction
- Potential fertility issues (e.g., the risks associated with pregnancy after diagnosis and treatment)
- Needing to sometimes balance raising small children while enduring treatment and subsequent side effects
- Coping with psychosocial issues (e.g., anxiety, depression).

Your role as patient educator is extremely important in teaching female patients about breast self-examinations (BSEs) and current breast screening recommendations. Prolonged exposure to ultraviolet rays of the sun by adolescents and young adults increases the risk for development of skin cancer later in life. Crohn's disease, a chronic inflammatory disease of the small intestine, most commonly occurs between 15 and 35 years of age. Many young adults have misconceptions regarding transmission and treatment of STIs. Encourage partners to know one another's sexual history and practices. Be alert for STIs when patients come to clinics with complaints of urological or gynecological problems (see Chapter 34). Assess young adults for knowledge and use of safe-sex practices and genital self-examinations.

Psychosocial Health. The psychosocial health concerns of the young adult are often related to job (money and job stability) and family stressors. Stress is valuable because it motivates a patient to change. However, if the stress is prolonged and the patient is unable to adapt to the stressor, health problems develop (see Chapter 37). Some mental health disorders such as depression also begin in this age-group. These conditions may manifest during young adulthood, but symptoms and treatment often continue into middle adulthood and beyond (Varcarolis, 2017).

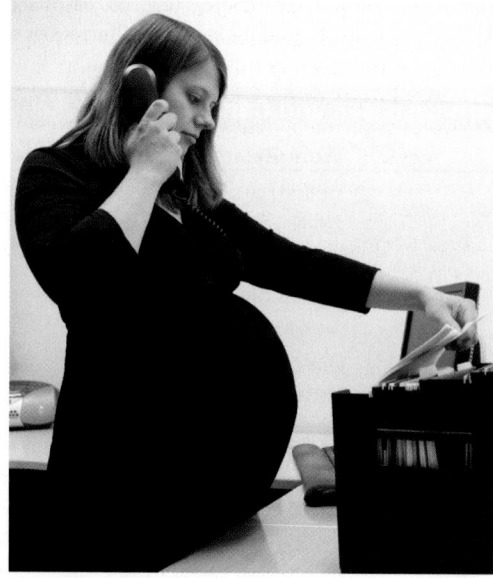

FIG. 13.3 The ability to handle day-to-day challenges at work minimizes stress.

Job Stress. Job stress can occur every day or from time to time. Most young adults are able to handle day-to-day crises (Fig. 13.3). Situational job stress can occur when a new boss enters the workplace, a deadline is approaching, the worker has new or greater numbers of responsibilities, or there is a risk for or actual corporate downsizing. Job stress affects health behaviors, and there is greater use of tobacco and alcohol, poor eating habits, impaired sleeping, and lack of exercise (Wang et al., 2018). Because individuals perceive jobs differently, the types of job stressors, coping strategies, and changes in health behaviors vary from patient to patient (Box 13.1). Your assessment of a young adult includes a description of the usual work performed, changes in job demands, changes in sleep or eating habits, and evidence of an increase in irritability or nervousness.

REFLECT NOW

One of your classmates had a difficult time in yesterday's clinical and is having difficulty participating in the skills lab exercise. During the break she confides that the nurses on the clinical unit don't help her find any equipment, and all she could do last night was think about how "stressful" the clinical site appears to be. Think about what you need to know about how your classmate copes with stress and her health promotion behaviors. How does she prepare for her clinical or skills lab experience?

Family Stress. Because of the multiplicity of changing relationships and structures in the emerging young-adult family, stress is frequently high (see Chapter 10). Situational family stressors occur during events such as births, deaths, illnesses, marriages, and job losses. Stress is often related to a number of variables, including the career paths and job stressors for both partners, and leads to dysfunction in the young-adult family (Padkapayeva et al., 2018). When a patient seeks health care and presents stress-related symptoms, you need to assess for the occurrence of a life-change event.

Each family member has certain predictable roles or jobs. These roles enable a family to function and be an effective part of society. When they change as a result of illness, a situational crisis often occurs. Assess environmental and familial factors, including support systems and coping mechanisms commonly used by family members.

Infertility. According to the American Society for Reproductive Medicine (1996-2019), infertility is the result of a disease (an interruption, cessation, or disorder of body functions, systems, or organs) of the male or female reproductive tract that prevents the conception of a child or the ability to carry a pregnancy to delivery. Infertility evaluation begins after a couple has unprotected intercourse for about 12 months with the failure to conceive. An estimated 10% to 15% of reproductive couples are infertile, and many are young adults. However, approximately half of the couples evaluated and treated in infertility clinics become pregnant. For some infertile couples a nurse is the first resource they identify. Nursing assessment of the infertile couple includes comprehensive histories of both the male and female partners to determine factors that have affected fertility and pertinent physical findings (see Chapter 30).

Obesity. Obesity is a major health problem. Approximately 16% of emerging adults are at risk for significant weight gain, which places them at risk for health problems in later life (Johnson and Annesi, 2018). It is influenced by poor diet, including eating fast food, excessive sugar intake from soft drinks, and increases in portion size, and a steady decline in physical activity (Sahoo et al., 2015). These factors are further complicated by family characteristics, such as parenting style, parents' lifestyles, and environmental factors such as school policies and demographics. Obesity in young adults is further associated with a variety of life events, such as enrolling in college, getting married, and beginning a family (Lanoye et al., 2016). Obesity is linked to the development of conditions such as type 2 diabetes, hypertension, high cholesterol, asthma, and joint problems. In addition, obesity in this age group increases the risk for cancer, morbidity, and mortality (Berger, 2018). Nursing assessment of diet and physical activity of young adults is an important part of data collection

Exercise. People of all ages, both male and female, benefit from regular physical activity (see Chapter 38); however, young many adults spend more time with technology and less time engaged in physical activity. Exercise in young adults is important to prevent or decrease obesity and the development of chronic health conditions such as high blood pressure, diabetes, and specific cancers (Berger, 2018). Conduct a thorough musculoskeletal assessment and exercise history to develop a realistic exercise plan. Encourage regular exercise within the patient's daily schedule.

Pregnant Woman and the Childbearing Family. A developmental task for many young adult couples is the decision to begin a family. Although the physiological changes of pregnancy and childbirth occur only in the woman, cognitive and psychosocial changes and health concerns affect the entire childbearing family, including the baby's father, siblings, and grandparents. Young single-parent families tend to be particularly vulnerable, both economically and socially.

Prenatal Care. Women who are anticipating pregnancy benefit from good health practices before conception, including a balanced diet, folic acid, exercise, dental checkups, prenatal care, avoidance of alcohol, and cessation of smoking once conception occurs.

Prenatal care is the routine examination of the pregnant woman by an obstetrician or advanced practice nurse such as a nurse practitioner or certified nurse-midwife. Prenatal care includes a thorough physical assessment of a pregnant woman during regularly scheduled intervals; provision of information regarding STIs, other vaginal infections, and urinary infections that adversely affect the fetus; and counseling about exercise patterns, diet, and child care. Regular prenatal care addresses health concerns that may arise during the pregnancy.

Physiological Changes. The physiological changes and needs of the pregnant woman vary with each trimester. Be familiar with them, their causes, and implications for nursing. All women experience some physiological changes in the first trimester. For example, they commonly have morning sickness, breast enlargement and tenderness, and fatigue. During the second trimester growth of the uterus and fetus results in some of the physical signs of pregnancy. During the third trimester increases in Braxton Hicks contractions (irregular, short contractions), fatigue, and urinary frequency occur.

Postpartum. Postpartum is a period of approximately 6 weeks after delivery. During this time a woman's body reverts to its prepregnant physical status. Determine the woman's knowledge of and ability to care for both herself and her newborn baby. Assessment of parenting skills and maternal-infant interactions is particularly important. The process of lactation, or breastfeeding, offers many advantages to both the new mother and baby. For the inexperienced mother breastfeeding can be a source of anxiety and frustration. Be alert for signs that the mother needs information and assistance (e.g., the breastfed baby fails to "latch" to the mother's breast or infant weight gain is low).

Needs for Education. The entire childbearing family needs education about pregnancy, labor, delivery, breastfeeding, and integration of the newborn into the family structure.

Psychosocial Changes. Like the physiological changes of pregnancy, psychosocial changes occur at various times during the 9 months of pregnancy and in the puerperium. Table 13.2 summarizes the major categories of psychosocial changes and implications for nursing intervention.

Health Concerns. The pregnant woman and her partner have many health questions. For example, they wonder whether the pregnancy and baby will be normal and whether they have the resources to properly care for the infant. Proper prenatal care has the potential to identify risks and pregnancy problems and meet most of the expectant mother's emotional and physical health needs. For some women, postpartum depression may occur. It is important to educate the mother and family members about common signs, such as overwhelming sadness, mood swings, impaired sleeping, withdrawal, and difficulty bonding with the infant (NIMH, n.d.).

Acute Care

Young adults typically require acute care for accidents, substance abuse, exposure to environmental and occupational hazards, stress-related illnesses, respiratory infections, gastroenteritis, influenza, urinary tract infections, and minor surgery. An acute minor illness causes a disruption in life activities of young adults and can increase stress in an already hectic lifestyle. Lack of insurance or underinsurance, dependency, and limitations posed by treatment regimens also increase frustration. To give them a sense of maintaining control of their health care choices, it is important to keep young adults informed about their health status and involve them in health care decisions.

TABLE 13.2 Major Psychosocial Changes During Pregnancy

Category	Implications for Nursing
Body image	Morning sickness and fatigue contribute to poor body image.
	Increase in breast size sometimes makes the woman feel more feminine and sexually appealing.
	Encourage her to take extra time with hygiene and grooming, trying new hairstyles and makeup.
	Woman begins to "show" during the second trimester and starts to plan maternity wardrobe.
	Woman has general feeling of well-being when she feels the baby move and hears the heartbeat.
	Woman feels big, awkward, and unattractive during third trimester when fetus is growing more rapidly.
Role changes	Both partners think about and have feelings of uncertainty about impending role changes.
	Both partners have feelings of ambivalence about becoming parents and concern about ability to be parents.
Sexuality	Woman needs reassurance that sexual activity will not harm fetus.
	Woman's desire for sexual activity is influenced by body image.
	Woman sometimes desires cuddling and holding rather than sexual intercourse.
Coping mechanisms	Woman needs reassurance that childbirth and child-rearing are natural and positive experiences but are also stressful.
	When indicated, assist her to cope with particular stressors such as finding new housing, preparing the nursery, or participating in childbirth classes.
Stresses during puerperium	Woman returns home from hospital fatigued and unfamiliar with infant care.
	Woman experiences physical discomfort or feelings of anxiety or depression.
	Woman may experience subsequent feelings of guilt, anxiety, or possibly a sense of freedom or relief if she must return to work soon after delivery.

Restorative and Continuing Care

The young adult's need for restorative and continuing care often results from motor vehicle accidents, trauma from violence, or chronic diseases affecting the young adult population, such as multiple sclerosis, rheumatoid arthritis, AIDS, and cancer. In general other chronic illnesses such as hypertension, coronary artery disease, and diabetes may not be recognized until later in life. When present, chronic illness or disability threatens a young adult's independence and results in the need to change personal, family, and career goals. Nursing interventions for the young adult faced with chronic illness or disability may need to focus on problems related to sense of identity, establishing independence, reorganizing intimate relationships, and family structure (see Chapter 8).

MIDDLE ADULTS

The US Census Bureau (2018) reports that approximately 38% of the population are middle-age adults (ages 35 to 64). In middle adulthood an individual makes lasting contributions through involvement with

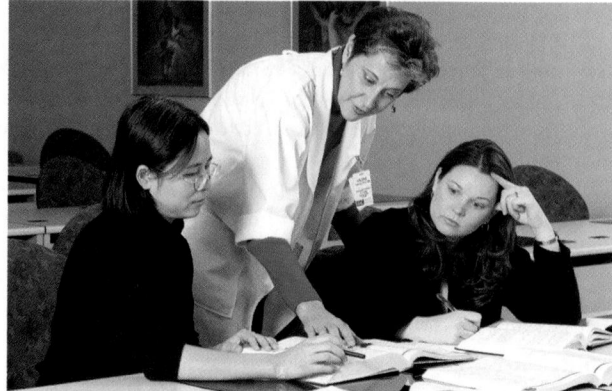

FIG. 13.4 Middle adults enjoy helping young people become productive and responsible adults.

others. During this period personal and career achievements have often already been experienced (see Chapter 11). Many middle adults find joy in helping their children and other young people become productive and responsible adults (Fig. 13.4). They also begin to help aging parents while being responsible for their own children, placing them in the sandwich generation. Using leisure time in satisfying and creative ways is a challenge that, if met satisfactorily, enables middle adults to prepare for retirement.

Men and women need to adjust to inevitable biological changes. As in adolescence, middle adults use considerable energy to adapt self-concept and body image to physiological realities and changes in physical appearance. High self-esteem, a favorable body image, and a positive attitude toward physiological changes occur when middle adults engage in physical exercise, eat balanced diets, obtain adequate sleep, and follow good hygiene practices that promote vigorous, healthy bodies.

Physical Changes

Major physiological changes occur between 40 and 65 years of age. Because of this it is important to assess the middle adult's general health status. A comprehensive assessment offers direction for health promotion recommendations and planning and implementing any acutely needed interventions. The most visible changes during middle adulthood are graying of the hair, wrinkling of the skin, and thickening of the waist. Decreases in hearing and visual acuity are often evident during this period. Often these physiological changes during middle adulthood have an impact on self-concept and body image. Table 13.3 summarizes abnormal findings to consider when conducting a physical examination (see Chapter 30). The most significant physiological changes during middle age are menopause in women and the climacteric in men.

Perimenopause and Menopause. Menstruation and ovulation occur in a cyclical rhythm in women from adolescence into middle adulthood. Perimenopause is the period during which ovarian function declines, resulting in a diminishing number of ova and irregular menstrual cycles; it generally lasts 1 to 3 years. Menopause is the disruption of this cycle, primarily because of the inability of the neurohormonal system to maintain its periodic stimulation of the endocrine system. The ovaries no longer produce estrogen and progesterone, and the blood levels of these hormones drop markedly. Menopause typically occurs between 45 and 60 years of age (see Chapter 34). Approximately 10% of women have no symptoms of menopause other than cessation of menstruation, 70% to 80% are aware of other changes but have no problems, and approximately 10% experience changes severe enough to interfere with activities of daily living.

TABLE 13.3 Abnormal Physical Assessment Findings in the Middle Adult

Body System	Assessment Findings
Integument	Very thin skin Rough, flaky, dry skin Lesions
Scalp and hair	Excessive generalized hair loss or patchy hair loss Excessive scales
Head and neck	Large, thick skull and facial bones Asymmetry in movement of head and/or neck Drooping of one side of the face
Eyes	Reduced peripheral vision Asymmetrical position of the light reflex Drooping of the upper lid (ptosis) Redness or crusting around the eyelids
Ears	Discharge of any kind Reddened, swollen ear canals
Nose, sinuses, and throat	Nasal tenderness Occlusion of nostril Swollen and pale pink or bluish-gray nasal mucosa Sinuses tender to palpation or on percussion Asymmetrical movement or loss of movement of uvula Tonsils red or enlarged
Thorax and lungs	Unequal chest expansion Unequal fremitus, hyperresonance, diminished or absent breath sounds Adventitious lung sounds such as crackles and wheezes
Heart and vascular system	Pulse inequality, weak pulses, bounding pulses, or variations in strength of pulse from beat to beat Bradycardia or tachycardia Hypertension Hypotension
Breasts—female	Recent increase in size of one breast Pigskin-like or orange-peel appearance Redness or painful breasts
Breasts—male	Soft, fatty enlargement of breast tissue
Abdomen	Bruises, areas of local discoloration; purple discoloration; pale, taut skin Generalized abdominal distention Hypoactive, hyperactive, decreased, or absent bowel sounds
Female genitalia	Asymmetrical labia Swelling, pain, or discharge from Bartholin's glands Decreased tone of vaginal musculature Cervical enlargement or projection into the vagina Reddened areas or lesions in the vagina
Male genitalia	Rashes, lesions, or lumps on skin of shaft of penis Discharge from penis Enlarged scrotal sac Bulges that appear at the external inguinal ring or femoral canal when the patient bears down
Musculoskeletal system	Uneven weight bearing Decreased range of joint motion; swollen, red, or enlarged joint; painful joints Decreased strength against resistance
Neurological system	Lethargy Inadequate motor responses Abnormal sensory system responses: inability to smell certain aromas, loss of visual fields, inability to feel and correctly identify facial stimuli, absent gag reflex

Climacteric. The climacteric occurs in men in their late 40s or early 50s (see Chapter 34). Decreased levels of androgens cause climacteric. Throughout this period and thereafter a man is still capable of producing fertile sperm and fathering a child. However, penile erection is less firm, ejaculation is less frequent, and the refractory period is longer.

Cognitive Changes

Changes in the cognitive function of middle adults are rare except with illness or trauma. Some middle adults enter educational or vocational programs to prepare themselves with new skills and information for entering the job market or changing jobs.

Psychosocial Changes

The psychosocial changes in the middle adult involve expected events, such as children moving away from home, and unexpected events, such as separation from a partner or the death of a partner or close friend. You need to assess for major life changes and the impact that the changes have on the middle adult's state of health. Include individual psychosocial factors such as coping mechanisms and sources of social support in your assessment.

In the middle-adult years, as children depart from the household, the family enters the postparental family stage. Time and financial demands on the parents typically decrease, and the couple faces the task of redefining their own relationship. It is during this period that many middle adults take on healthier lifestyles. Assessment of health promotion needs for the middle adult includes regular screening examinations, amount of rest, leisure activities, nutritional intake, and regular exercise. Also assess for the use of tobacco, alcohol, or illicit drugs. Assess the middle adult's social environment, including relationship concerns; communication and relationships with children, grandchildren, and aging parents; and caregiver concerns with parents or an ill spouse.

Career Transition. Career changes occur by choice or as a result of changes in the workplace or society. In recent decades middle adults change occupations more often for a variety of reasons, including limited upward mobility, decreasing availability of jobs, and seeking an occupation that is more challenging. In some cases downsizing, technological advances, or other changes force middle adults to seek new jobs. Such changes, particularly when unanticipated, result in stress that affects health, family relationships, self-concept, and other dimensions.

Sexuality. After the departure of their last child from the home, many couples redefine their relationships and find increased marital and sexual satisfaction. The onset of menopause and the climacteric affect the sexual health of the middle adult. Some women may desire increased sexual activity because pregnancy is no longer possible. Middle-aged men and women are able to engage in satisfying sexual relationships (see Chapter 34 for physical changes).

Other factors influencing sexuality during this period include job stress, diminished health of one or both partners, and effects of some prescription medications. For example, antihypertensive agents have side effects that influence sexual desire or functioning. Antihypertensive medications, diuretics, and beta blockers can cause erectile dysfunction (ED) in men (Burcham and Rosenthal, 2019). Sometimes both partners experience sexual dysfunction caused by stresses related to sexual changes or a conflict between their sexual needs and self-perceptions and social attitudes or expectations.

Family Psychosocial Factors. Psychosocial factors involving the family include the stresses of singlehood, marital changes, transition of the family as children leave home, and the care of aging parents.

Singlehood. Many adults over 35 years of age in the United States have never been married. Many are college-educated people who embrace the philosophy of choice and freedom, delayed marriage, and delayed parenthood. Some middle adults choose to remain single but also opt to become parents either biologically or through adoption. Many single middle adults have no relatives but share a family type of relationship with close friends or work associates. Consequently some single middle adults may feel isolated during traditional "family" holidays such as Thanksgiving or Christmas. In times of illness middle adults who choose to remain single and childless rely on other relatives or friends, increasing caregiving demands of family members who also have other responsibilities. Nursing assessment of single middle adults needs to include a thorough assessment of psychosocial factors, including an individual's definition of family and available support systems.

Marital Changes. Marital changes occurring during middle age include death of a spouse, separation, divorce, and the choice of remarrying or remaining single. A widowed, separated, or divorced patient goes through a period of grief and loss in which it is necessary to adapt to the change in marital status. Normal grieving progresses back and forth through a series of phases, and resolution of grief often takes a year or more. Assess the level of coping of the middle adult to the grief and loss associated with life changes (see Chapter 36).

Family Transitions. The departure of the last child from the home is also a stressor. Many parents welcome freedom from childrearing responsibilities, whereas others feel lonely or without direction. *Empty nest syndrome* is the term used to describe the sadness and loneliness that accompany children leaving home. Eventually parents need to reassess their marriage and try to resolve conflicts and plan for the future. Occasionally this readjustment phase leads to marital conflicts, separation, and divorce (see Chapter 10).

Care of Aging Parents. Increasing life spans in the United States and Canada have led to increased numbers of older adults in the population. Many middle adults find themselves caught between the responsibilities of caring for dependent children and those of caring for aging and ailing parents. Thus they find themselves in the sandwich generation, in which the challenges of caregiving can be stressful. The needs of family caregivers are being given more emphasis in the health care system.

The middle-adult and older-adult parents often have conflicting relationship priorities when the older adult strives to remain independent, such as maintaining his or her own living space or finances. Negotiation and compromise help to define and resolve problems. When meeting family caregivers, take the time to identify the health needs of both groups, and assist the multigenerational family in determining the health and community resources available to them as they make decisions and plans (Liu and Huang, 2018). Evaluate family relationships to determine family members' perceptions of responsibility, willingness and perceived loyalty in relation to caring for older-adult members (Ellington et al., 2018).

REFLECT NOW

You are caring for a middle-age couple who have decided to bring the wife's widowed mother, who has stage 4 metastatic breast cancer, to their home for end-of-life care. In order to help the family unit during the early phase of caregiving, think about information you might need, such as expectations the family may have about caregiving, what resources are available to the family, what other resources they might need, and how the family/couple solves problems.

Health Concerns

Health Promotion and Stress Reduction. Because middle adults experience physiological changes and face certain health realities, their perceptions of health and health behaviors are often important factors in maintaining health. It is important that middle adults maintain regular fitness as they grow older. Routine exercise, 20 to 30 minutes five or six times a week, promotes health (see Chapter 38). For example, there is an association between activity, cardiopulmonary fitness, and long-term health outcomes, especially pertaining to cardiovascular disease (Benck et al., 2018). For women and men with risks for osteoporosis, physical activity several times a week helps to maintain bone health (Tabor et al., 2016).

Stress across the life span is a health concern. Today's complex world makes individuals more prone to stress-related illnesses such as heart attacks and hypertension (see Chapter 37). When adults seek health care, nurses in outpatient and home health settings design targeted, culturally appropriate stress management programs focusing on wellness and guide patients to evaluate health behaviors, lifestyle, and environment (Amnie, 2018; Madva, 2018).

Work with the patient to identify approaches to preventing stressful situations, such as habituation, change avoidance, time blocking, time management, and environmental modification (e.g., adding ramps, removing obstacles). Then help the patient to increase stress resistance (e.g., increase self-esteem, improve assertiveness, redirect goal alternatives, and reorient cognitive appraisal). Finally, help patients learn how to avoid the physiological response to stress. Encourage use of relaxation techniques, imagery, yoga, meditation, and biofeedback to recondition the patient's response to stress (see Chapter 37).

Obesity. Obesity is a growing, expensive health concern for middle adults. It is a complicated, multifactorial disease, with genetic, behavioral, socioeconomic, and environmental origins; obesity reduces quality of life and increases the risk for many serious chronic diseases and premature death (Hruby and Hu, 2015). A *Healthy People 2020* (USDHHS, 2019) goal relates to improvement of health-related quality of life and well-being, including physical well-being. Health consequences of obesity include high blood pressure, high blood cholesterol, type 2 diabetes, coronary heart disease, osteoarthritis, and obstructive sleep apnea. Research shows that the type of diet a patient chooses to follow is not as important as caloric restriction, which is associated with better weight outcomes (Hruby and Hu, 2015).

Forming Positive Health Habits. Positive health habits help maintain optimal function and reduce risk for chronic illnesses. Some habits support health (e.g., exercise and brushing and flossing the teeth each day) or prevent disease. For example, a middle-age woman's health care provider may encourage the patient to take vitamin D and calcium to enhance bone health and prevent osteopenia and osteoporosis (Tai et al., 2015; National Academies of Sciences, 2010).

During assessment obtain data on your patient's health behaviors. Learn what is important to a patient with regard to maintaining his or her health. Then determine which behaviors are positive and negative. Examples of positive health behaviors include regular exercise (see Chapter 38), adherence to healthy dietary habits, avoidance of excess consumption of alcohol, participation in routine screening and diagnostic tests for disease prevention and health promotion (e.g., laboratory screening for serum cholesterol or mammography), and lifestyle changes to reduce stress. Other habits involve risk factors to health (e.g., smoking or eating foods with little or no nutritional value).

BOX 13.2   Barriers to Change

External Barriers
- Lack of facilities
- Lack of resources and materials
- Limited social support
- Lack of motivation
- Poor access to care

Internal Barriers
- Lack of knowledge
- Insufficient skills or motivation to change health habits
- Undefined short- and long-term goals

To help patients form positive health habits, you act as a teacher and facilitator. By providing information about how the body functions and how patients can form and change habits relative to their own goals, patients' levels of knowledge regarding the potential impact of behavior on health are raised (Amnie, 2018). Offer positive reinforcement (such as praise and rewards) for health-directed behaviors and decisions. Such reinforcement increases the likelihood that the behavior will be repeated

Help middle adults consider factors such as avoidance of STIs, prevention of opioid and substance abuse, and accident prevention in relation to decreasing health risks. For example, provide patients with information on STI causes, symptoms, and transmission. Discuss methods of protection during sexual activity with a patient in an open and nonjudgmental manner and reinforce the importance of practicing safe sex (see Chapter 34).

Changing poor health habits is hard; recognize that barriers to change exist (Box 13.2). Help patients recognize and modify unsafe and potential health hazards. You must partner with patients and families to minimize or eliminate these barriers.

Health Literacy. Health literacy is defined as the cognitive and social skills that determine the motivation and ability of individuals to gain access to, understand, and use information in ways that promote and maintain good health (see Chapter 25). Health literacy is essential for a person to take responsibility for his or her own health. Lower health literacy may affect the ability to understand basic written health information or to read a prescription bottle correctly. There is a relationship between health literacy and health promoting behaviors, especially in patients with chronic illnesses, such as diabetes. Therefore, it is important to improve patients' health literacy while providing patient education to enhance health outcomes (Chahardah-Cherik et al, 2018).

People for whom English is a second language are at risk for low health literacy and may be unable to self-manage their health with lifestyle risk-factor modification to prevent the development of chronic diseases (Nierengarten, 2018; Fernandez-Gutierrez et al., 2018). A professional interpreter may be necessary to ensure understanding of health information.

Psychosocial Health

Anxiety. Anxiety is a critical maturational phenomenon related to change, conflict, and perceived control of the environment. Adults often experience anxiety in response to the physiological and psychosocial changes of middle age. Such anxiety motivates an adult to rethink life goals and stimulates productivity. However, for some adults anxiety precipitates psychosomatic illness and preoccupation with death. In this case a middle adult views life as being half or more over and thinks in terms of the time left to live (Varcarolis, 2017).

Clearly, a life-threatening illness, marital transition, loss of a spouse or partner, or job stressor increases the anxiety of a patient and family. Use crisis intervention or stress-management techniques to help a patient adapt to the changes of the middle-adult years (see Chapter 37).

Depression. Depression is a mood disorder that manifests itself in many ways. Although the most frequent age of onset is between ages 14 and 44, it is common among adults in the middle years and has many causes. The risk factors for depression include a family history of depression, being female, being a member of the LGBTQ community, the postpartum period, a lack of social support, chronic illness, and negative stressful life events (Varcarolis, 2017). People with chronic illness or caregivers of family members with chronic and long-term illnesses have a greater level of depression (Madva et al., 2018). Symptoms vary with the individual and may include depressed mood, loss of interest in activities, impaired concentration, or feelings of worthlessness or guilt (Maurer, 2012). Symptoms can also be nonspecific, such as back pain, weight gain or loss, constipation, headaches, or fatigue. The abuse of alcohol or other substances makes depression worse.

Nursing assessment of a middle adult diagnosed with depression will depend on the setting in which you work. A focused data collection regarding individual and family history of depression, mood changes, cognitive changes, behavioral and social changes, and physical changes is ideal. However, there are useful and valid screening tools for depression, including the Patient Health Questionnaire (PHQ)-2, which may rule out, but not definitively diagnose, depression (Whooley et al., 1997). The PHQ-2 contains only two questions, using a Likert scale of 0 to 3: Over the past two weeks, how often have you been bothered by any of the following problems: Little interest or pleasure in doing things; Feeling down, depressed or hopeless. Collect assessment data from both the patient and the patient's family because family data are often particularly important, depending on the level of depression the middle adult is experiencing.

Early-Onset Dementia. Early-onset dementia (EOD), or "presenile dementia," defines all dementia-related conditions before age 65 (Vieria et al., 2013). Depression and anxiety are prominent. As EOD progresses, agitation, apathy, and irritability worsen (Tanaka et al., 2015). EOD has major devastating psychological consequences, affecting people during their productive and leisure years, and also impacts family responsibilities. Patients and families need assistance to maintain independence in decision making and activities (Sakamoto et al., 2017).

Community Health Programs. Community health programs in clinics, self-help groups, and primary care practices offer services to prevent illness, promote health, and detect disease in the early stages. Nurses make valuable contributions to the health of the community by taking an active part in planning screening and teaching programs and support groups for middle adults (see Chapter 3).

Health education programs promote changes in behavior and lifestyle. As a health teacher, offer information that enables patients to make informed decisions about health practices within the context of health promotion. Make sure that educational programs are culturally appropriate (Williams et al., 2018). Changes to more positive health practices during young and middle adulthood lead to fewer or less complicated health problems as an older adult. During health counseling, collaborate with your patient to design a plan of action that addresses his or her health and well-being. Through objective problem solving you can help your patient grow and change (Edelman and Kudzma, 2018).

Acute Care. Acute illnesses and conditions experienced in middle adulthood are similar to those of young adulthood. However, injuries and acute illnesses in middle adulthood require a longer recovery period because of the slowing of healing processes. In addition, they are more likely to become chronic conditions. For middle adults in the sandwich generation, stress levels also increase as they balance responsibilities related to employment, family life, care of children, and care of aging parents while recovering from an injury or acute illness.

Restorative and Continuing Care. Chronic illnesses affect the roles and responsibilities of middle adults. Some results of chronic illness are strained family relationships, modifications in family activities, increased health care tasks, increased financial stress, the need for housing adaptation, social isolation, medical concerns, and grieving. The degree of disability and a patient's perception of both the illness and the disability determine the extent to which lifestyle changes occur. A few examples of the problems experienced by patients who develop debilitating chronic illness during adulthood include role reversal, changes in sexual behavior, and alterations in self-image. Along with the current health status of a middle adult living with a chronic illness, you need to assess the knowledge base of both the patient and family. This assessment includes the medical course of the illness and the prognosis for the patient. You need to determine the coping mechanisms of the patient and family. In addition, you need to assess adherence to treatment and rehabilitation regimens, evaluate the need for community and social services, and make appropriate referrals.

KEY POINTS

- Young and middle adult development involves orderly and sequential changes in characteristics and attitudes and is often related to the natural process of maturation.
- Young adults are in a stable period of normal physical development, which includes changes related to pregnancy.
- Cognitive development continues throughout the young- and middle-adult years.
- Emotional health of young and middle adults is correlated with the ability to address and resolve personal and social problems.
- Pregnant women need to understand physiological changes occurring in each trimester.
- Psychosocial changes and health concerns during pregnancy and the postpartum affect the parents, the siblings, and often the extended family.
- Health concerns of the young adult usually focus on health promotion habits and fertility and pregnancy issues.
- Intimate partner violence, formerly referred to as domestic violence, is a global public health problem. It exists along a continuum from a single episode of violence to ongoing battering.
- Midlife transition begins when a person becomes aware that physiological and psychosocial changes signify passage to another stage in life.
- Cognitive changes in middle age are often related to acute illnesses, early-onset dementia, or physical trauma.
- Psychosocial changes for middle adults often include career transition, sexuality, marital changes, family transition, and care of aging parents.
- Health concerns of middle adults commonly involve stress-related illnesses, health assessment, adoption of positive health habits, and issues with health literacy.

REFLECTIVE LEARNING

- A 24-year-old patient who smokes two packs of cigarettes per day comes to talk with you about quitting smoking. She began smoking when she was 14 years old. She states, "I just can't seem to kick the habit, no matter how hard I try."
    - What information do you need to know to help this patient quit smoking?
    - Which factors will have the greatest impact on health promotion related to smoking cessation in this patient?
- Think about your own health habits. How would you improve them? Select one that you would like to improve. What information would you need to be successful in changing this one habit?
- You have a clinical experience in a community-based clinic. In this clinic there is a young family who is homeless. What are the health risks of the young adult mother in this family?

REVIEW QUESTIONS

1. A nurse is completing an assessment on a 27-year-old female patient. Which questions best assess the psychosocial aspects of this young woman's health? (Select all that apply.)
    1. Do you feel safe in your home and at work?
    2. How many fruits and vegetables do you typically eat every day?
    3. Describe your relationship with your family.
    4. Have you had the vaccine to prevent HPV?
    5. What are your long-term career goals?
2. Which factor affects a middle-age adult's adherence to a treatment plan?
    1. Gender
    2. Lifestyle
    3. Motivation
    4. Family history
3. A 36-year-old patient newly diagnosed with type 1 diabetes shares with you that he is frustrated with the time it takes to prepare meals and monitor his exercise and blood sugar. He also is having trouble understanding his insulin schedule. Which of the following suggestions would be most appropriate? (Select all that apply.)
    1. Provide patient education materials that are easy to read.
    2. Refer this patient to a diabetes support group.
    3. Refer the patient to his endocrinologist.
    4. Suggest that the patient make an appointment with a registered dietitian.
    5. Suggest ways to modify his schedule.
4. Chronic illness (e.g., diabetes mellitus, hypertension, rheumatoid arthritis) may affect a person's roles and responsibilities during middle adulthood. When assessing the health-related knowledge base of both the middle-age patient with a chronic illness and his or her family, the assessment should include which of the following? (Select all that apply.)
    1. Medical course of the illness
    2. Prognosis for the patient
    3. Coping mechanisms of the patient and family
    4. Socioeconomic status
    5. Need for community and social services.
5. A 50-year-old woman has elevated serum cholesterol levels that increase her risk for cardiovascular disease. One method to control this risk factor is to identify the patient's current diet trends and describe dietary changes to reduce the risk. This nursing activity is a form of:

1. Referral.
2. Counseling.
3. Health education.
4. Stress-management techniques.

6. Intimate partner violence (IPV) is linked to which of the following factors? (Select all that apply.)
   1. Alcohol abuse
   2. Marriage
   3. Pregnancy
   4. Unemployment
   5. Drug use

7. Which are examples of positive health habits that may prevent the development of chronic illness later in life? (Select all that apply.)
   1. Routine screening and diagnostic tests
   2. Unprotected sexual activity
   3. Regular exercise
   4. Consistent seat belt use
   5. Excess alcohol consumption

8. A 45-year-old woman who is obese tells a nurse that she wants to lose weight. Which assessment findings may be contributing factors to the woman's obesity? (Select all that apply.)
   1. The woman works in an executive position that is very demanding.
   2. The woman says that she has little time to prepare meals at home and eats out at least four nights a week.
   3. The woman works out at the corporate gym at 5 AM three mornings per week.
   4. The woman says that she tries to eat "low-cholesterol" foods to help lose weight.
   5. The woman says that she vacations annually to reduce stress.

9. A 34-year-old female executive has a job with frequent deadlines. She notes that when the deadlines appear, she tends to eat high-fat, high-carbohydrate foods. She also explains that she gets frequent headaches and stomach pain during these deadlines. After receiving health education from the nurse, the executive decides to try yoga. In this scenario yoga is used as a(n):
   1. Outpatient referral.
   2. Counseling technique.
   3. Health promotion activity.
   4. Stress-management technique.

10. A nurse is completing an assessment on a male patient, age 24. Following the assessment, the nurse notes that his family history is not significant for chronic illnesses, and his physical and laboratory findings are within normal limits. Because of these findings, nursing interventions are directed toward activities related to: (Select all that apply.)
    1. Instructing him to return in 2 years.
    2. Instructing him in secondary prevention.
    3. Instructing him in health promotion activities.
    4. Instructing him about routine screenings.
    5. Instructing him about proper vaccinations.

Answers: 1. 1, 3, 5; 2. 3, 3. 1, 2, 4, 5; 4. 1, 2, 3, 5; 5. 3; 6. 1, 3, 4, 5; 7. 1, 3, 4; 8. 1, 2, 9. 4; 10. 3, 4, 5.

Rationales for Review Questions can be found on the Evolve website.

REFERENCES

American Academy of Pediatrics (AAP): Policy statement: promoting the well-being of children whose parents are gay or lesbian, *Pediatrics* 141(4):827, 2013.

American Cancer Society: *Guideline for colorectal cancer screening*, 2018. https://www.cancer.org/cancer/colon-rectal-cancer/detection-diagnosis-staging/acs-recommendations.html. Accessed July 21, 2019.

American Society for Reproductive Medicine: Infertility, 1996-2019, https://www.asrm.org/topics/topics-index/infertility/. Accessed July 21, 2019.

Ashe-Goins FE: Human trafficking: implications for nurses, *S C Nurse* 25(2):15, 2018.

Berger N: Young adult cancer: influence of the obesity pandemic, *Obesity* 26(4):641, 2018.

Bonomi A, et al.: Intimate partner violence and neighborhood income: a longitudinal analysis, *Violence Against Women* 20(1):42, 2014.

Burcham JR, Rosenthal LD: *Lehne's pharmacology for nursing care*, ed 10, St Louis, 2019, Elsevier.

Conroy J, Tabbenhoff B: Workplace stress: name it, reframe it, tame it, *Virginia Nurses Today* 26(1):6, 2018.

Diekelmann J: The young adult: the choice is health or illness, *Am J Nurs* 76:1276, 1976.

Edelman C, Kudzma EC: *Health promotion throughout the life span*, ed 9, St Louis, 2018, Elsevier.

Ellington L, et al.: Supporting home hospice family caregivers: insights from different perspectives, *Palliat Support Care* 16(2):209, 2018.

Erikson E: *Childhood society*, ed 2, New York, 1963, WW Norton.

Erikson E: *The lifecycle completed: a review*, New York, 1982, WW Norton.

Fernandez-Gutierrez M, et al.: Health literacy interventions for immigrant populations: a systematic review, *Int Nurs Rev* 65(1):54, 2018.

Fioretti C, et al.: The role of this listener on the emotional valence of personal memories in emerging adulthood, *J Adult Dev* 24:252, 2017.

Gibson EJ: *Adolescent and young adult health national resource center: promoting healthy adolescent and young adult sexual and reproductive health*, 2016. http://www.amchp.org/programsandtopics/AdolescentHealth/Documents/Final_SeptemberAYAHCenterNewsletter.pdf. Accessed July 21, 2019.

Huether S, McCance K: *Understanding pathophysiology*, ed 6, St Louis, 2017, Mosby.

Institute for Women's Policy Research (IWPR): *Pay equity and discrimination*, 2019. https://iwpr.org/issue/employment-education-economic-change/pay-equity-discrimination/. Accessed July 21, 2019.

Maurer DM: Screening for depression. *Am Fam Physician* [review], 85(2):139-144, 2012. Review. Erratum in *Am Fam Physician* 87(7):464, 2013.

National Academies of Sciences: *Engineering and Medicine, Health and Medicine division: dietary reference intakes for calcium and vitamin D*, 2010. http://nationalacademies.org/hmd/reports/2010/dietary-reference-intakes-for-calcium-and-vitamin-d.aspx. Accessed July 21, 2019.

The National Institute on Drug Abuse: Talking to patients about their drug use, n.d., https://www.drugabuse.gov/nidamed-medical-health-professionals/about-addiction-performance-project/addiction-performance-project/talking-to-patients-about-their-drug-use. Accessed July 21, 2019.

National Institute of Mental Health: Postpartum depression facts, n.d. https://www.nimh.nih.gov/health/publications/postpartum-depression-facts/index.shtml. Accessed July 21, 2019.

Nierengarten MB: Health literacy: a challenge in diverse populations, 2018, *Contemp Pediatr* 35(1):19, 2018.

Pew Research Center: *Social media fact sheet*, 2019. http://www.pewinternet.org/fact-sheet/social-media/. Accessed July 21, 2019.

Renzulli KA: This is how much debt the average American has now—at every age, *Money*, 2018. http://time.com/money/5233033/average-debt-every-age/. Accessed July 21, 2019.

Rossi N: Commentary on same-sex and different-sex parent households and child health outcomes: additional sources of same-sex parenting stress to consider, *J Dev and Behav Pediatrics* 39(2):180, 2018.

United Nations Office on Drugs and Crime: *Human trafficking FAQs*, 2019. www.unodc.org/unodc/en/human-trafficking/faqs.html. Accessed July 21, 2019.

US Census Bureau: *Annual estimates of the resident population for selected age-groups by sex for the United States, states, counties, and Puerto Rico commonwealth and municipios: April 1, 2010 to July 1, 2017*, 2018. https://factfinder.census.gov/faces/tableservices/jsf/pages/productview.xhtml?pid=PEP_2017_PEPAGESEX&prodType=table. Accessed July 21, 2019.

US Department of Health and Human Services (USDHHS): *Centers for disease control and prevention (CDC): sexually transmitted disease surveillance 2016*, 2017. https://www.cdc.gov/std/stats16/CDC_2016_STDS_Report-for508Web-Sep21_2017_1644.pdf. Accessed July 21, 2019.

US Department of Health and Human Services (USDHHS): *Healthy people 2020*, 2019. www.healthypeople.gov/2020. Accessed July 21, 2019.

US Department of Labor: *Bureau of labor statistics: occupational outlook Handbook*, 2019. www.bls.gov/ooh. Accessed July 20, 2019.

Varcarolis EM: *Essentials of psychiatric mental health nursing*, St Louis, 2017, Elsevier.

Young Survivors Coalition: *Breast cancer in young women: statistics and disparities*, 2019. https://www.youngsurvival.org/learn/about-breast-cancer/statistics. Accessed July 21, 2019.

RESEARCH REFERENCES

Amnie A: An investigation of predictors of self-efficacy to cope with stress and implications for health education practice, *Am J Health Educ* 49(3):155, 2018.

Beneitz MC, Gil-Alegre ME: Opioid addiction: social problems associated and implications of both current and possible future treatments, including polymeric therapeutics for giving up the habit of opioid consumption, *BioMed Res Int* 1, 2017, 5/18/2017.

Benck L, et al.: Association between cardiorespiratory fitness and lung health from young adulthood to middle age, *Am J of Resp and Crit Care Med* 195(9):1236, 2018.

Bos HM, et al.: Same-sex and different-sex parent households and child health outcomes: findings from the national survey of children's health, *J Dev and Behav Pediatrics* 37(3):179, 2016.

Brough P, et al.: Job support, coping, and control: assessment of simultaneous impacts within the occupational stress process, *J Occup Health Psych* 23(2):188, 2018.

Chahardah-Cherik S, et al.: The relationship between health literacy and health promoting behaviors in patient with type 2 diabetes, *Int J Community Based Nurs Midwifery* 6(1):65, 2018.

Egyud A, et al.: Implementation of human trafficking education and treatment algorithm in the emergency department, *J Emerg Nurs* 43(6):526, 2017.

Ferdos J, et al.: Association between intimate partner violence during pregnancy and maternal pregnancy complications among recently delivered women in Bangladesh, *Aggress Behav* 44(3):294, 2018.

Hruby A, Hu FB: The epidemiology of obesity: a big picture, *PharmacoEconomics* 33(7):673–689, 2015. https://www.ncbi.nlm.nih.gov/pmc/articles/PMC4859313/. Accessed July 21, 2019.

Johnson PH, Annesi JJ: Factors related to weight gain/loss among emerging adults with obesity, *Am J Health Behav* 42(3):3, 2018.

Kelly JF, et al.: Coping with the enduring unpredictability of opioid addiction: an investigation of a novel family-focused peer-support organization, *J Subst Abus Treat* 77:193, 2017.

Kritsotakis G, et al.: Gender differences in the prevalence and clustering of multiple health risk behaviors in young adults, *J Adv Nurs* 72(9):2098, 2016.

Lanoye A, et al.: Young adults' attitudes and perceptions of obesity and weight management: implications for treatment development, *Curr Obes Rep* 5(1):14–22, 2016.

Layland EK, et al.: Freedom to explore the self: how emerging adults use leisure to develop identity, *J Positive Psychol* 13(1):78, 2018.

Liu HY, Huang KH: The relationship between family functioning and caregiving appraisal of dementia family caregivers: caregiving self-efficacy as a mediator, *Aging Ment Health* 22(4):558, 2018.

Madva EN: Magnitude and sources of distress in mid-life adults with chronic medical illness: an exploratory mixed-methods analysis, *Psychol Health Med* 23(5):555, 2018.

Masiero M, et al.: Optimistic bias in young adults for cancer, cardiovascular and respiratory diseases: a pilot study on smokers and drinkers, *J Health Psych* 23(5):645, 2018.

Padkapayeva K, et al.: Gender/sex differences in the relationship between psychosocial work exposures and work and life stress, *Ann Work Expo Health* 62(4):416, 2018.

Roberts A, et al.: Gambling and physical intimate partner violence: results from the national Epidemiologic survey on alcohol and related conditions (NESARC), *Am J Addict* 27(1):7, 2018.

Sakamoto, et al.: "I'm still here": Personhood and the early-onset dementia experience, *J Geron Nurs* 43(5):12, 2017.

Sahoo K, et al.: Childhood obesity: causes and consequences, *J Family Med Prim Care* 4(2):187–192, 2015.

Shaw A, Rogge RD: Symbolic meanings of sex in relationships: developing the meanings of sexual behavior inventory, *Psychol Assess* 29(10):1221, 2017.

Shane PD, et al.: Surveillance for violent deaths-national violent death reporting system, 27 states, 2015, *Morbidity and Mortality Weekly Report (MMWR)*, 28(11):67, 2018, 1-12, 2018 https://www.cdc.gov/mmwr/volumes/67/ss/ss6711a1.htm?s_cid=ss6711a1_w. Accessed July 21, 2019.

Sommerfeld D, et al.: Hypersensitivity pneumonitis and acute respiratory distress syndrome from e-cigarette use, *Pediatrics* 164(6):1, 2018.

Tabor E, et al.: The role of physical activity in early adulthood and middle-age on bone health after menopause in epidemiological population from Silesia Osteo Active Study, *Int J Clin Pract* 70:835, 2016.

Tai V, et al.: Calcium intake and bone mineral density: systematic review and meta-analysis, *British J Medicine* 351:h4183, 2015.

Tanaka H, et al.: Relationship between dementia severity and behavioral and psychological symptoms in early-onset Alzheimer's disease, *Psychogeriatrics* 15:242, 2015.

Vieria RT, et al.: Epidemiology of early onset dementia: a review of the literature, *Clin Prac Epidemiol Ment Health* 9:88, 2013.

Wang S, et al.: Job stress in young adults is associated with a range of poorer health behaviors in the childhood determinants of adult health (CDAH) study, *J Occup Environ Med* 60(3):e117, 2018.

Whooley MA, et al.: Case-finding instruments for depression. Two questions are as good as many, *J Gen Intern Med* 12(7):439–445, 1997.

Williams HL, et al.: Do health promotion, behaviors affect levels of job satisfaction and job stress for nurses in an acute care hospital? *J Nurs Adm* 48(6):342, 2018.

14

Older Adults

OBJECTIVES

- Identify common myths and stereotypes about older adults.
- Discuss common developmental tasks of older adults.
- Describe common physiological changes of aging.
- Differentiate among delirium, dementia, and depression.
- Discuss issues related to psychosocial changes of aging.

- Describe the multifaceted aspects of elder mistreatment.
- Describe selected health concerns of older adults.
- Identify nursing interventions related to the physiological, cognitive, and psychosocial changes of aging.

KEY TERMS

Ageism, p. 176

Delirium, p. 181

Dementia, p. 181

Depression, p. 181

Elder mistreatment, p. 190

Gerontological nursing, p. 177

Gerontology, p. 176

Reality orientation, p. 191

Reminiscence, p. 192

Validation therapy, p. 191

MEDIA RESOURCES

http://evolve.elsevier.com/Potter/fundamentals/

- Review Questions
- Case Study with Questions

- Audio Glossary
- Content Updates
- Answers to QSEN Activity and Review Questions

People who are 65 years old are in the lower boundary for "old age" in demographics and social policy within the United States. However, many older adults consider themselves to be "middle age" well into their seventh decade. Chronological age often has little relation to the reality of aging for an older adult. Each person ages in his or her own way. Every older adult is unique. As a nurse you need to approach each person as an individual.

The number of older adults in the United States is growing quickly. In 2016, there were 49.2 million adults over age 65 in the United States, representing 15.2% of the population or one in seven Americans (AOA, 2017). This represents an increase of 33% since 2006. Part of this increase is caused by the increase of the average life span. The aging population is expected to continue to grow to 21.7% of the population by the year 2040. The racial and ethnic diversity of the population over age 65 is also increasing. Between 2014 and 2060, the non-Hispanic white segment of the population is expected to decrease from 78.3% to 54.6% (Population Reference Bureau, 2018). As a nurse, you need to take cultural diversity into account as you care for older adults. The aging of the baby-boom generation and the growth of the population segment over age 85 contribute to the projected increase in the number of older adults. The baby boomers were born between 1946 and 1964. The first baby boomers reached age 65 in 2011. Social and health care programs will need to adapt to meet the needs of this growing segment of the population. The challenge is to gain new knowledge and skills to provide culturally sensitive and linguistically appropriate care (see Chapter 9).

VARIABILITY AMONG OLDER ADULTS

Nursing care of older adults poses special challenges because of variations in their physiological, cognitive, and psychosocial health. Older adults also have a wide range of functional ability. Most older adults are active and involved in their communities. A smaller number have lost the ability to care for themselves, are confused or withdrawn, and/or are unable to make decisions concerning their needs. Most older adults live in noninstitutional settings. In 2017 59% of older adults in noninstitutional settings lived with a spouse/partner (48% of older women, 72% of older men); 28% lived alone (34% of older women, 20% of older men); and only 3.1% of all older adults resided in institutions, primarily nursing homes. As would be expected, the percentage of those living in a nursing home increases with age. Only 1% of the 65 to 74 age-group live in a nursing home, while 9% of those 85 and older do (AOA, 2017).

The physical and psychosocial aspects of aging are closely related. A reduced ability to respond to stress, the experience of multiple losses, and the physical changes associated with normal aging combine to place people at high risk for illness and functional deterioration. Most older adults remain functionally independent despite the increasing prevalence of chronic disease. Nursing assessment provides valuable clues to the effects of a disease or illness on a patient's functional status. Chronic conditions add to the complexity of assessment and care of the older adult. Most older people have at least one chronic condition, and many have multiple conditions. Although the interaction of these physical and psychosocial factors may be serious, do not assume that all older adults have signs, symptoms, or behaviors representing disease and decline or that these are the only factors you need to assess. You also need to identify an older adult's strengths and abilities during the assessment and encourage independence as an integral part of your plan of care (Jett, 2018a).

MYTHS AND STEREOTYPES

Despite ongoing research in the field of gerontology, myths and stereotypes about older adults persist. These include false perceptions about their physical and psychosocial characteristics and lifestyles. When health care providers hold negative stereotypes about aging, their actions often negatively affect the quality of patient care. It is important to correctly assess older adults' functional, physiological, psychosocial, and emotional status.

Some people stereotype older adults as ill, disabled, and physically unattractive. Others believe that older adults are forgetful, confused, rigid, bored, and unfriendly and that they are unable to understand and learn new information. Yet specialists in the field of gerontology view centenarians, the oldest of the old, as having an optimistic outlook on life, good memories, broad social contacts and interests, and tolerance for others. Although changes in vision or hearing and reduced energy and endurance sometimes affect the process of learning, older adults are lifelong learners.

Stereotypes about lifestyles often include mistaken ideas about living arrangements and finances. Misconceptions about financial status range from beliefs that many are affluent to beliefs that many are poor. According to the US Census Bureau, only 9.3% of people over age 65 had incomes below the poverty level. Older women report a significantly lower income than men. Social Security benefits serve as the primary source of income for most older adults (US Census Bureau, 2017).

In a society that values attractiveness, energy, and youth, these myths and stereotypes lead to the undervaluing of older adults. Some people equate worth with productivity; therefore they think that older adults become worthless after they leave the workforce. Others consider their knowledge and experience too outdated to have any current value. These ideas demonstrate ageism, which is discrimination against people because of increasing age, just as people who are racists and sexists discriminate because of skin color and gender. According to experts in the field of gerontology, ageism typically undermines the self-confidence of older adults, limits their access to care, and distorts caregivers' understanding of the uniqueness of each older adult. Nurses should promote a positive perception regarding the aging process when establishing therapeutic relationships and value the experiences of older adults.

Current laws ban age discrimination. The economic and political power of older adults challenges ageist views. Older adults are a significant proportion of the consumer economy. As voters and activists in various issues, they have a major influence in the formation of public policy. Participation of older adults on voting issues adds a unique perspective on social, economic, and technological issues because they have experienced almost a century of developments. Some older adults lived through or were born during the Great Depression of 1929. They also experienced two world wars and wars in Korea, Vietnam, and Iraq and are now experiencing the war on terrorism. They have seen tremendous changes in technology. Changes in health care also impact older adults as the era of the family physician gave way to the age of specialization and managed care. After witnessing the government initiatives establishing the Social Security system, Medicare, and Medicaid, older adults are currently living with the changes imposed by health care reform.

NURSES' ATTITUDES TOWARD OLDER ADULTS

It is important to assess your own attitudes toward older adults, your own aging, and the aging of your family, friends, and patients. Nurses' attitudes come from personal experiences with older adults, education,

employment experiences, and attitudes of co-workers and employing institutions. Given the increasing number of older adults in health care settings, forming positive attitudes toward them and gaining specialized knowledge about aging and the health care needs of older adults are priorities for all nurses. Positive attitudes are based in part on a realistic portrayal of the characteristics and health care needs of older adults. It is critical for you to respect older adults and actively involve them in care decisions and activities. In the past institutional settings such as hospitals and nursing centers often treated older adults as objects rather than independent, dignified people. The time has come for nurses to recognize and address ageism by questioning prevailing negative attitudes and stereotypes and reinforcing the realities of aging as they care for older adults in all settings.

REFLECT NOW

Think about how you feel about caring for older adults. Reflect on positive and negative experiences you have had with older adults and how this may affect your nursing care of older adults.

DEVELOPMENTAL TASKS FOR OLDER ADULTS

Theories of aging are closely linked to the concept of developmental tasks appropriate for distinct stages of life (see Chapter 11). Although no two individuals age in the same way, either biologically or psychosocially, there are common developmental tasks for older adults that are associated with varying degrees of change and loss (Box 14.1). More common changes include alterations in health status, loss of significant others, a decreased sense of usefulness, and decreases in socialization, income, and independent living. How older adults adjust to these changes is individualized. For some, adaptation and adjustment are relatively easy. For others, coping with the changes brought on by aging requires the assistance of family, friends, and health care professionals. Be sensitive to the effect of losses on older adults and their families, and be prepared to offer support.

Older adults need to adjust to the physical changes that accompany aging. The extent and timing of these changes vary by individual, but as body systems age, changes in appearance and functioning occur. These changes are not associated with a disease; they are normal. The presence of disease sometimes alters the timing of the changes or their impact on daily life. The section on physiological changes describes structural and functional changes of aging.

Some older adults, both men and women, find it difficult to accept aging. This is apparent when they understate their ages when asked, adopt younger styles of clothing, or attempt to hide physical evidence of aging with cosmetics. Others deny their aging in ways that are potentially problematic. For example, some older adults deny functional declines and refuse to ask for help with tasks, placing their safety at great risk. Others avoid activities designed for their benefit, such as

---

BOX 14.1 **Developmental Tasks for Older Adults**

- Adjusting to changes in health and physical strength
- Adjusting to retirement and reduced or fixed income
- Adjusting to death of a spouse, children, siblings, friends
- Accepting self as aging person
- Maintaining satisfactory living arrangements
- Redefining relationships with adult children and siblings
- Maintaining quality of life

senior citizens' centers and senior health promotion activities and thus do not receive the benefits these programs offer. Acceptance of personal aging does not mean retreat into inactivity, but it does require a realistic review of strengths and limitations.

Retirement poses challenges, such as adjusting to the loss of the work role and daily interaction with professional colleagues. Some welcome retirement as a time to pursue new interests and hobbies, volunteer in their communities, continue their education, or start new careers. Retirement plans for others include changing residence by moving to a different city or state or to a different type of housing within the same area. Reasons other than retirement also lead to changes of residence. For example, physical impairments sometimes require relocation to a smaller, single-level home or nursing center. A change in living arrangements for the older adult usually requires an extended period of adjustment, during which assistance and support from health care professionals, friends, and family members are necessary.

Many older adults cope with the death of a spouse. In 2017, 33% of all older women were widows, and 11% of older men were widowers (AOA, 2017). They also may need to cope with deaths of adult children and grandchildren and lifelong friends. These deaths represent losses and reminders of personal mortality. Coming to terms with them is often difficult. By helping older adults through the grieving process (Chapter 36), you can help them resolve some of these issues.

Redefining relationships with children continues as older adults experience the challenges of aging. A variety of issues sometimes occur, including control of decision making, dependence, conflict, guilt, and loss. How these issues surface in situations and how they are resolved depend in part on the past relationship between the older adult and his or her adult children. When adult children become their parents' caregivers, they must try to balance the demands of their own children and careers with the many challenges of family caregiving. As adult children and aging parents negotiate the aspects of changing roles, nurses are in the position to act as counselors for the entire family. Helping older adults maintain their quality of life is often a priority. What defines quality of life is unique for each person.

COMMUNITY-BASED AND INSTITUTIONAL HEALTH CARE SERVICES

You will encounter older-adult patients in a wide variety of community and institutional health care settings. Outside of an acute care hospital, nurses care for older adults in clinics, private homes and apartments, retirement communities, adult day care centers, assisted-living residences, and nursing centers (extended care, intermediate care, and skilled nursing facilities). Chapter 2 describes these settings and the services provided in detail.

Sorting through the options for care of older adults can be overwhelming. Nurses and social workers can help older adults and their families by providing information and answering questions as they review care options. Your assistance is especially valuable when patients and families need to make decisions about moving to a nursing center. Some family caregivers consider nursing center placement when in-home care becomes increasingly difficult or when convalescence (recovery) from hospitalization requires more assistance than the family is able to provide. Although the decision to enter a nursing center is never final and a nursing center resident is sometimes discharged to home or another less acute setting, many older adults view the nursing center as their final residence. Results of state and federal inspections of nursing centers are available to the public at the nursing center, online, and at the inspectors' offices. The best way to evaluate the quality of a nursing center is for the patient and family to visit the center and inspect it personally. The Centers for Medicare and Medicaid (CMS, 2018; website http://www.Medicare.gov/NHcompare) provides an excellent resource for you to learn about the quality rating of a nursing center on the basis of health inspections, staffing, and quality measures (Box 14.2). It also offers a nursing center checklist (https://www.medicare.gov/NursingHomeCompare/checklist.pdf).

ASSESSING THE NEEDS OF OLDER ADULTS

Gerontological nursing provides care that addresses mutually established goals for an older adult, his or her family, and health care team members. A comprehensive assessment, including strengths, limitations, and resources, provides a baseline of the older adult's health and functional status. Nursing diagnoses and interventions are selected to either maintain or enhance physical abilities and activity (see Chapter 38) and to create environments for psychosocial and spiritual well-being (see Chapter 35). To complete a thorough assessment, actively engage older adults and provide adequate time, allowing them to share important information about their past and current health. Caring for older adults often requires creative strategies that will maximize the potential of older adults.

Nursing assessment takes into account three key points to ensure an age-specific approach: (1) the interrelation between physical and psychosocial aspects of aging, (2) the effects of disease and disability on functional status, and (3) tailoring the nursing assessment to an older person (Yeager, 2019c). A comprehensive assessment of an older adult takes more time than the assessment of a younger adult because of the longer life and medical history and potential complexity of the history. During the physical examination allow rest periods as needed or conduct the assessment in several sessions if a patient has reduced energy or limited endurance. Review both prescription and over-the-counter medications carefully with each patient.

BOX 14.2 FOCUS ON OLDER ADULTS

Selection of a Nursing Center or Home

An important step in the process of selecting a nursing center is to visit it. A quality nursing home has the following features:

- It is a home, a place where people live. Residents are encouraged to personalize their rooms. Privacy is respected.
- Is Medicare and Medicaid certified.
- Has adequate, qualified staff members who have passed criminal background checks.
- Does not feel like a hospital. However, the nursing center provides quality care. In addition to assistance with basic activities of daily living such as bathing, dressing, eating, oral hygiene, and toileting, staff regularly help residents with social and recreational activities.
- Offers quality food and mealtime choices.
- Welcomes families when they visit the center. Staff always encourage family involvement, whether families wish to provide information, ask questions, participate in care planning, or help with social activities or physical care.
- Is clean. There are no pervasive odors. The environment feels "homelike."
- Provides active communication from staff to patient and family.
- Attends quickly to resident requests. Staff are actively involved with assisting the residents. They focus on the person, not on the task.

Modified from the Centers for Medicare & Medicaid Services (CMS): *Your guide to choosing a nursing home or other long-term care,* Baltimore, MD, 2018, CMS, https://www.medicare.gov/Pubs/pdf/02174-Nursing-Home-Other-Long-Term-Services.pdf. Accessed June 15, 2019.

Sensory changes associated with aging may affect data gathering. Your choice of communication techniques depends on an older adult's visual or hearing impairments. If an older adult is unable to understand your visual or auditory cues, your assessment data will likely be inaccurate or misleading, leading you to incorrectly conclude that the older adult is confused.

When a person has a hearing impairment, move to a quiet area to reduce background noise, face the patient, and speak directly in clear, low-pitched tones. When caring for people with visual impairments, sit or stand at eye level and face them, and always encourage the use of assistive devices such as glasses and hearing aids. Chapter 49 details techniques to use when communicating with older adults who have sensory deficits.

Memory deficits, if present, affect the accuracy and completeness of your assessment. Information contributed by a family member or other caregiver is sometimes necessary to supplement an older adult's recollection of past medical events and information about current self-care habits, medication adherence, allergies, and immunizations. Use tact when involving another person in the assessment interview. The additional person provides supplemental information with the consent of the older adult, but the older adult should remain the primary source of information whenever possible.

During all aspects of an assessment, you are responsible for providing culturally competent care. Your ability to recognize and process your own biases related to ageism, social norms, and racism affects your ability to provide culturally competent care (see Chapter 9). During an assessment, use caution when interpreting signs and symptoms of diseases and laboratory values. Historically, researchers used younger populations to establish these signs and norms. However, the classic signs and symptoms of diseases are sometimes absent, blunted, or atypical in older adults (Jett, 2018a). This is especially true in the cases of bacterial infection, pain, acute myocardial infarction, and heart failure. The masquerading of disease is possibly caused by age-related changes in organ systems and homeostatic mechanisms, progressive loss of physiological and functional reserves, or coexisting acute or chronic conditions. As a result an older adult with a urinary tract infection (UTI) sometimes presents with incontinence, falls, and only a slight elevation of body temperature (within normal limits) instead of having fever, dysuria, frequency, or urgency. Some older adults with pneumonia have tachycardia, tachypnea, and confusion with decreased appetite and functioning, without the more common symptoms of fever and productive cough. Instead of crushing substernal chest pain and diaphoresis, some older adults experience a sudden onset of dyspnea often accompanied by anxiety and confusion when having a myocardial infarction. Variations from the usual norms for laboratory values are sometimes caused by age-related changes in cardiac, pulmonary, renal, and metabolic function.

It is important to recognize early indicators of acute illness in older adults. The Fulmer (2019) SPICES framework (Box 14.3) can be used to guide assessment of an older adult. Box 14.4 provides setting-specific examples of altered presentation of illness. A key principle of providing age-appropriate nursing care is timely detection of these cardinal signs of illness so that early treatment can begin. Mental status changes commonly occur as a result of disease and psychological issues. Some mental changes are often drug related, caused by drug toxicity or adverse drug events.

Falls are complex and often cause life-changing injury. They are sometimes costly, affect functional status, level of independence, and can be a common event for an older adult. You need to investigate every fall carefully to find out whether it was the result of environmental causes or the symptom of a new-onset illness. A fall may be the only symptom in new problems with the cardiac, respiratory, musculoskeletal, neurological, urological, and sensory body systems.

BOX 14.3 SPICES Tool for Overall Assessment of Older Adults

S: Sleep disorders
P: Problems with eating or feeding
I: Incontinence
C: Confusion
E: Evidence of falls
S: Skin breakdown

The nurse should complete further assessment if an older adult demonstrates changes in any of these areas (Fulmer, 2019).

BOX 14.4 Examples of Altered Presentation of Illnesses in Older Adults Occurring in Various Health Care Settings

Hospital
- Confusion is not inevitable. Look for an acute illness, neurological events, new medication, or the presence of risk factors for delirium.
- Many hospitalized older adults have chronic dehydration exacerbated by acute illness (Touhy, 2018e).
- Not all older adults have fevers with infection. Symptoms instead include increased respiratory rate, falls, incontinence, or confusion (Yeager, 2019c).

Nursing Home
- Health care providers often undertreat pain in older adults, especially those with dementia. Look for nonverbal cues of pain presence, such as grimacing or resistance to care (Alderman, 2019).
- Decline in functional ability (even a minor one such as the inability to sit upright in a chair) is a signal of new illness.
- Residents with less muscle mass—both the frail and the obese—are at a much higher risk for toxicity from protein-binding drugs such as phenytoin (Dilantin) and warfarin (Coumadin) (Yeager, 2019b).
- New urinary and/or fecal incontinence is often a sign of the onset of a new illness.

Ambulatory Care
- Fatigue or decreased ability to do usual activities are often signs of anemia, thyroid problems, depression, or neurological or cardiac problems (Yeager, 2019c).
- Severe gastrointestinal problems in older adults do not always present with the same acute symptoms seen in younger patients. Ask about constipation, cramping sensations, and changes in bowel habits.
- Older adults reporting increased dyspnea and confusion, especially those with a cardiac history, need to go to the emergency department because these are the most common manifestations of myocardial infarction in this population (Yeager, 2019c).
- Depression is common among older adults with chronic illnesses. Watch for lack of interest in former activities, significant personal losses, or changes in role or home life.

Home Care
- Investigate all falls, focusing on balance, lower extremity strength, gait, and neurological issues (e.g., loss of sensation).
- Monitor older adults with late-stage heart disease for loss of appetite as an early symptom of impending heart failure (Yeager, 2019c).
- Drug-drug and drug-food interactions in older patients who are seeing more than one provider and taking multiple medications are common. Watch for signs of interactions (Yeager, 2019b).

Dehydration is common in older adults because of decreased oral intake related to a reduced thirst response and less free water as a consequence of a decrease in muscle mass. Additionally, older adults may decrease their intake to avoid additional trips to the bathroom. This is especially true in those with impaired mobility. When vomiting and diarrhea accompany the onset of an acute illness, an older adult is at risk for further dehydration. Decrease in appetite is a common symptom with the onset of pneumonia, heart failure, and UTI.

Loss of functional ability may occur in a subtle fashion over time, or it may occur suddenly, depending on the underlying cause. Thyroid disease, infection, cardiac or pulmonary conditions, metabolic disturbances, and anemia are common causes of functional decline. The nurse is in a position to recognize even subtle changes in the condition of an older adult. You play an essential role in early identification, referral, and treatment of health problems.

Physiological Changes

Perception of well-being defines quality of life. Understanding an older adult's perceptions about health status is essential for accurate assessment and development of clinically relevant interventions. Older adults' concepts of health generally depend on personal perceptions of functional ability. Therefore older adults engaged in activities of daily living (ADLs) usually consider themselves healthy, whereas those who have physical, emotional, or social impairments that limit their activities perceive themselves as ill.

There are common physiological changes associated with normal aging (Table 14.1). These changes are not pathological in themselves, but they can make older adults more vulnerable to common clinical conditions and diseases (Jett, 2018b). Some older adults experience all of these changes, and others experience only a few. The body changes continuously with age, and specific effects on particular older adults depend on health, lifestyle, stressors, and environmental conditions. You need to understand these normal, more common changes to provide appropriate care for older adults and help with adaptation to associated changes.

General Survey. Your general survey begins during the initial nurse-patient encounter and includes a quick but careful head-to-toe

TABLE 14.1 Common Physiological Changes with Aging At a Glance

System	Common Changes
Integumentary	Loss of skin elasticity with fat loss in extremities; pigmentation changes; glandular atrophy (oil, moisture, sweat glands); thinning hair, with hair turning gray-white (facial hair: decreased in men, increased in women); slower nail growth; atrophy of epidermal arterioles
Respiratory	Decreased cough reflex and ciliary activity; increased anterior-posterior chest diameter; increased chest wall rigidity; fewer alveoli, increased airway resistance
Cardiovascular	Thickening of blood vessel walls, narrowing of vessel lumen, loss of vessel elasticity, lower cardiac output, decreased number of heart muscle fibers, decreased elasticity and calcification of heart valves, decreased baroreceptor sensitivity, decreased efficiency of venous valves, increased pulmonary vascular tension, increased systolic blood pressure, decreased peripheral circulation
Gastrointestinal	Periodontal disease; decrease in saliva, gastric secretions, and pancreatic enzymes; smooth-muscle changes with decreased peristalsis and small intestinal motility; gastric atrophy; decreased production of intrinsic factor; increased stomach pH; loss of smooth muscle in the stomach; hemorrhoids; rectal prolapse; and impaired rectal sensation.
Musculoskeletal	Decreased muscle mass and strength, decalcification of bones, degenerative joint changes, dehydration of intervertebral disks, fat tissue increases
Neurological	Degeneration of nerve cells, decrease in neurotransmitters, decrease in rate of conduction of impulses
Sensory	
Eyes	Decreased accommodation to near/far vision (presbyopia), difficulty adjusting to changes from light to dark, yellowing of the lens, altered color perception, increased sensitivity to glare, smaller pupils
Ears	Loss of acuity for high-frequency tones (presbycusis), thickening of tympanic membrane, sclerosis of inner ear, buildup of earwax (cerumen)
Taste	Often diminished; often fewer taste buds
Smell	Often diminished
Touch	Decreased skin receptors
Proprioception	Decreased awareness of body positioning in space
Genitourinary	Fewer nephrons, 50% decrease in renal blood flow by age 80, decreased bladder capacity Male—enlargement of prostate Female—reduced sphincter tone
Reproductive	Male—sperm count diminished, smaller testes, erections less firm and slow to develop Female—decreased estrogen production; degeneration of ovaries; atrophy of vagina, uterus, and breasts; dryness of vaginal mucosa
Endocrine	General—alterations in hormone production with decreased ability to respond to stress Thyroid—diminished secretions Cortisol, glucocorticoids—increased anti-inflammatory hormone Pancreas—increased fibrosis, decreased secretion of enzymes and hormones, decreased sensitivity to insulin
Immune	Thymus decreases in size and volume T-cell function decreases Core temperature elevation is lowered

Modified from Jett K: Biological theories of aging and age-related physiological changes. In Touhy T, Jett K: *Ebersole and Hess' gerontological nursing and healthy aging,* ed 5, St Louis, 2018, Elsevier.

scan of the older adult that you document in a brief description (see Chapter 30). Initial inspection may reveal some universal aging changes (e.g., facial wrinkles, gray hair, loss of body mass in the extremities, an increase of body mass in the trunk). It is also important at this time to observe range of joint motion, grooming, and communication skills.

Integumentary System. With aging, the skin loses resilience and moisture. The epithelial layer thins, and elastic collagen fibers shrink and become rigid. Wrinkles of the face and neck reflect lifelong patterns of muscle activity and facial expressions, the pull of gravity on tissue, and diminished elasticity. Spots and lesions are often present on the skin. Smooth, brown, irregularly shaped spots (age spots or senile lentigo) initially appear on the backs of the hands and on forearms. Small, round, red or brown cherry angiomas occur on the trunk. Seborrheic lesions or keratoses appear as irregular, round or oval, brown, watery lesions. Years of sun exposure contribute to the aging of the skin and lead to premalignant and malignant lesions. You need to rule out these three malignancies related to sun exposure when examining skin lesions: melanoma, basal cell carcinoma, and squamous cell carcinoma (see Chapter 30).

Head and Neck. The facial features of an older adult sometimes become more pronounced from loss of subcutaneous fat and skin elasticity. Facial features may appear asymmetrical because of missing teeth or improperly fitting dentures. In addition, common vocal changes include a rise in pitch and a loss of power and range.

Visual acuity declines with age. This is often the result of retinal damage, reduced pupil size, development of opacities in the lens, or loss of lens elasticity. Presbyopia, a progressive decline in the ability of the eyes to accommodate from near to far vision, is common. More ambient light is necessary for tasks such as reading and other ADLs. Older adults have increased sensitivity to the effects of glare. Pupils are smaller and react slower. Objects do not appear bright, and older adults may have difficulty when moving from bright to dark environments. Changes in color vision and discoloration of the lens make it difficult to distinguish between blues and greens and among pastel shades. Dark colors such as blue and black appear the same. Diseases of the older eye include cataract, macular degeneration (decrease in central vision), diabetic retinopathy (creates visual field loss), and retinal detachment (separation of the retina from surface of the eye, causing increased floaters, flashes of light, and loss of vision). Cataracts, a loss of the transparency of the lens, are a prevalent disorder among older adults. They normally result in blurred vision, sensitivity to glare, and gradual loss of vision. Surgical treatment of cataracts has become a common outpatient procedure that is relatively safe. Chapter 49 outlines nursing interventions for helping patients adapt to their visual changes.

Auditory changes are often subtle. Most of the time older adults ignore the early signs of hearing loss until friends and family members comment on compensatory attempts, such as either turning up the volume on televisions or avoiding social conversations. A common age-related change in auditory acuity is presbycusis. Presbycusis affects the ability to hear high-pitched sounds and conversational speech and is typically bilateral, affecting more men than women. Before the nurse assumes presbycusis, it is necessary to inspect the external auditory canal for the presence of cerumen. Impacted cerumen, a common cause of diminished hearing acuity, is easy to treat.

Salivary secretion is reduced, and taste buds atrophy and lose sensitivity. An older adult is less able to differentiate among salty, sweet, sour, and bitter tastes. The sense of smell also decreases, further reducing taste. Health conditions, treatments, and/or medications often alter taste. It is often a challenge to promote optimal nutrition in an older patient because of the loss of smell and changes in taste.

Thorax and Lungs. Because of changes in the musculoskeletal system, the configuration of the thorax sometimes changes. Respiratory muscle strength begins to decrease, and the anteroposterior diameter of the thorax increases. Vertebral changes caused by osteoporosis lead to dorsal kyphosis, the curvature of the thoracic spine. Calcification of the costal cartilage causes decreased mobility of the ribs. The chest wall gradually becomes stiffer. Lung expansion decreases, and the person is less able to cough deeply. If kyphosis or chronic obstructive lung disease is present, breath sounds become distant. As a result, an older adult is more susceptible to pneumonia and other bacterial or viral infections.

Heart and Vascular System. Decreased contractile strength of the myocardium results in decreased cardiac output. The decrease is significant when an older adult experiences anxiety, excitement, illness, or strenuous activity. The body tries to compensate for decreased cardiac output by increasing the heart rate during exercise. However, after exercising it may take longer for an older adult's heart rate to return to baseline if the person does not regularly exercise or has underlying cardiac disease. Systolic and/or diastolic blood pressures are sometimes abnormally high. Although a common chronic condition, hypertension is not a normal aging change and predisposes older adults to heart failure, stroke, renal failure, coronary heart disease, and peripheral vascular disease.

Peripheral pulses frequently are still palpable but weaker in lower extremities. Older adults sometimes state that their lower extremities are cold, particularly at night. Changes in the peripheral pulses in the upper extremities are less common.

Breasts. As estrogen production diminishes, the milk ducts of the breasts are replaced by fat, making breast tissue less firm. Decreased muscle mass, tone, and elasticity result in smaller breasts in older women. Atrophy of glandular tissue coupled with more fat deposits results in a slightly smaller, less dense, and less nodular breast. Gynecomastia, enlarged breasts in men, is often the result of medication side effects, hormonal changes, or obesity.

Gastrointestinal System and Abdomen. Aging leads to an increase in the amount of fatty tissue in the trunk and abdomen. Because muscle tone and elasticity decrease, the abdomen becomes more protuberant. Gastrointestinal function changes include a slowing of peristalsis and alterations in secretions. An older adult experiences these changes by becoming less tolerant of certain foods and having discomfort from delayed gastric emptying. Alterations in the lower gastrointestinal tract lead to constipation, flatulence, or diarrhea.

Reproductive System. Changes in the structure and function of the reproductive system occur as the result of hormonal alterations. Women experience a reduced responsiveness of the ovaries to pituitary hormones and a resultant decrease in estrogen and progesterone levels. This can cause dryness of the vaginal mucosa, causing irritation and pain with intercourse, and may also cause a decreased libido. Aging men typically experience an erection that is less firm and has a less forceful ejaculation (Jett, 2018a).

Testosterone lessens with age and sometimes leads to a loss of libido. Spermatogenesis begins to decline during the fourth decade and continues into the ninth. However, for both men and women sexual desires, thoughts, and actions continue throughout all decades of life. Less frequent sexual activity often results from illness, death of a sexual partner, or decreased socialization.

Urinary System. Hypertrophy of the prostate gland is frequently seen in older men. This hypertrophy enlarges the gland and places pressure on the neck of the bladder. As a result, urinary retention, frequency, incontinence, and UTIs occur. In addition, prostatic hypertrophy results in difficulty initiating voiding and maintaining a urinary stream and does not always indicate a malignancy. However, when men develop symptoms of prostatic hypertrophy, it is important that this condition is evaluated by a health care provider to differentiate benign prostatic hypertrophy (BPH) from cancer of the prostate. Cancer of the prostate is the second leading cause of cancer death in American men, behind lung cancer. The American Cancer Society estimates that one in nine men will be diagnosed with prostate cancer and 1 in 41 will die (ACS, 2018).

Urinary incontinence is an abnormal and typically embarrassing condition. Older women, particularly those who have had children, experience stress incontinence, an involuntary release of urine that occurs when they cough, laugh, sneeze, or lift an object. This is a result of a weakening of the perineal and bladder muscles. Other types of urinary incontinence are urgency, overflow, functional, and mixed incontinence. The risk factors for urinary incontinence include age, menopause, diabetes, hysterectomy, stroke, and obesity. Men can also experience incontinence but are sometimes reluctant to discuss this with their health care providers because they think that it is a "woman's disease." It is important that male incontinence be evaluated as well.

Musculoskeletal System. With aging, muscle fibers become smaller. Muscle strength diminishes in proportion to the decline in muscle mass. Muscle mass begins to decline when individuals reach their 50s; by the time they reach their 80s, muscle mass is typically 30% to 40% of what is was at the age of 30 (Jett, 2018b). Beginning in the 30s, bone density and bone mass decline in men and women. Older adults who exercise regularly do not lose as much bone and muscle mass or muscle tone as those who are inactive. Osteoporosis is a major public health threat. Fifty-four million Americans have osteoporosis or low bone mass, and approximately one in two women and one in four men over the age of 50 will break a bone because of osteoporosis (National Osteoporosis Foundation, 2018). Postmenopausal women experience a greater rate of bone demineralization than older men. Women who maintain calcium intake throughout life and into menopause have less bone demineralization than women with low calcium intake. Older men with poor nutrition and decreased mobility are also at risk for bone demineralization.

Neurological System. A decrease in the number and size of neurons in the nervous system begins in the middle of the second decade. Neurotransmitters, chemical substances that enhance or inhibit nerve impulse transmission, change with aging as a result of the decrease in neurons. All voluntary reflexes are slower, and individuals often have less of an ability to respond to multiple stimuli. In addition, older adults frequently report alterations in the quality and the quantity of sleep (see Chapter 43), including difficulty falling asleep, difficulty staying asleep, difficulty falling asleep again after waking during the night, waking too early in the morning, and excessive daytime napping. These problems are believed to be caused by age-related changes in the sleep-wake cycle.

Functional Changes

Physical function is a dynamic process. It changes as individuals interact with their environments. Functional status in older adults includes the day-to-day ADLs involving activities within physical, psychological, cognitive, and social domains. A decline in function is often linked to illness or disease and its degree of chronicity. However, ultimately it is the complex relationship among all of these areas that influences an older adult's functional abilities and overall well-being.

Keep in mind that it may be difficult for older adults to accept the changes that occur in all areas of their lives, which in turn have a profound effect on functional status. Some deny the changes and continue to expect the same personal performance, regardless of age. Conversely some overemphasize them and prematurely limit their activities and involvement in life. The fear of becoming dependent is overwhelming for an older adult who is experiencing functional decline as a result of aging. Educate older adults to promote understanding of age-related changes, appropriate lifestyle adjustments, and effective coping. Factors that promote the highest level of function include a healthy, well-balanced diet; paced and appropriate activity; regularly scheduled visits with a health care provider; regular participation in meaningful activities; use of stress-management techniques; and avoidance of alcohol, tobacco, or illicit drugs.

Functional status in older adults refers to the capacity and safe performance of ADLs and instrumental ADLs (IADLs). It is a sensitive indicator of health or illness in the older adult. ADLs (such as bathing, dressing, and toileting) and IADLs (such as the ability to write a check, shop, prepare meals, or make phone calls) are essential to independent living; therefore carefully assess whether an older adult has changed the way he or she completes these tasks. Occupational and physical therapists are your best resources for a comprehensive assessment of functional impairment. A sudden change in function, as evidenced by a decline or change in an older adult's ability to perform any one or a combination of ADLs, is often a sign of either an acute illness (e.g., pneumonia, UTI, or electrolyte imbalance) or worsening of a chronic problem (e.g., diabetes or cardiovascular disease) (Jett, 2018a). An online collection of functional assessment tools used most commonly with older adults is available at the geriatric nursing website of the Hartford Institute for Geriatric Nursing, https://consultgeri.org/. When you identify a decline in a patient's functional status, focus your nursing interventions on maintaining, restoring, and maximizing an older adult's functional status to maintain independence while preserving safety and dignity.

Cognitive Changes

A common misconception about aging is that cognitive impairments are widespread among older adults. Because of this misconception, older adults often fear that they are, or soon will be, cognitively impaired. Younger adults often assume that older adults will become confused and no longer able to handle their affairs. Forgetfulness as an expected consequence of aging is a myth and not a fact or expectation. Some structural and physiological changes within the brain are associated with cognitive impairment. Reduction in the number of brain cells, deposition of lipofuscin and amyloid in cells, and changes in neurotransmitter levels occur in older adults both with and without cognitive impairment. Symptoms of cognitive impairment such as disorientation, loss of language skills, loss of the ability to calculate, and poor judgment *are not* normal aging changes and require you to further assess patients for underlying causes. There are standard assessment forms for determining a patient's mental status, including the Mini-Mental State Exam-2 (MMSE-2), the Mini-Cog, and the Clock Drawing Test (Jett, 2018a).

The three common conditions affecting cognition are delirium, dementia, and depression (Table 14.2). Distinguishing among these three conditions is challenging. A careful and thorough assessment of older adults with cognitive changes to distinguish among them should be completed. Select appropriate nursing interventions that are specific to the cause of the cognitive impairment.

TABLE 14.2   Comparison of Clinical Features of Delirium, Dementia, and Depression

Clinical Feature	Delirium	Dementia	Depression
Onset	Sudden/abrupt; depends on cause	Insidious/slow and often unrecognized	Happens with major life changes; often abrupt but can be gradual
Course	Short, daily fluctuations in symptoms; worse at night, in darkness, and on awakening	Long, no diurnal effects; slow progression over time; some deficits with increased stress	Diurnal effects, typically worse in the morning; situational fluctuations but less than with delirium
Progression	Abrupt	Slow over months and years	Variable; rapid or slow but even
Duration	Hours to less than 1 month; longer if unrecognized and untreated	Months to years	Variable; may be chronic
Consciousness	Reduced/disturbed	Awake	Awake
Alertness	Fluctuates; lethargic or hypervigilant	Generally normal	Normal
Attention	Impaired; fluctuates; inattention	Generally normal	Minimal impairment
Orientation	Generally impaired; severity varies	Generally normal to person but not to place or time	Usually normal
Psychomotor behavior	Variable; hypoactive, hyperactive, or mixed	Normal; some have apraxia	Variable; psychomotor retardation or agitation
Speech	Often incoherent; may call out repeatedly or with the same phrase	Difficulty finding words; perseveration	May be slow
Affect	Variable, but may appear disturbed, frightened	Slowed response; may be labile	Flat

Modified from Touhy T: Care of individuals with neurocognitive disorders. In Touhy T, Jett K: *Ebersole & Hess' gerontological nursing and healthy aging*, ed 5, St Louis, 2018, Elsevier.

Delirium. Delirium, or acute confusional state, is a potentially reversible cognitive impairment that occurs suddenly and worsens at night (Touhy, 2018d). Delirium often has a physiological cause. Physiological causes include electrolyte imbalances, untreated pain, infection, cerebral anoxia, hypoglycemia, medication effects, tumors, subdural hematomas, and cerebrovascular infarction or hemorrhage. A new onset of delirium should trigger the nurse to assess for signs and symptoms of infections such as pneumonia and UTI. Delirium may also be caused by environmental factors such as sensory deprivation or overstimulation, unfamiliar surroundings, or sleep deprivation or psychosocial factors such as emotional distress. Although it occurs in any setting, an older adult in the acute care setting is especially at risk because of predisposing factors (physiological, psychosocial, and environmental) in combination with underlying medical conditions. Between 11% and 42% of hospitalized older adults develop delirium (Touhy, 2018d). Dementia is an additional risk factor that greatly increases the risk for delirium; it is possible for delirium and dementia to occur at the same time. The presence of delirium is a medical emergency and requires prompt assessment and intervention. Nurses are at the bedside 24/7 and in a position to recognize delirium development and report it. The cognitive impairment usually reverses once health care providers identify and treat the cause of delirium.

Dementia. Dementia is a generalized impairment of intellectual functioning that interferes with social and occupational functioning. It is an umbrella term that includes Alzheimer's disease (most common type), Lewy body disease, frontal-temporal dementia, and vascular dementia (Alzheimer's Association, 2018). Cognitive function deterioration leads to a decline in the ability to perform basic ADLs and IADLs. Unlike delirium, dementia is characterized by a gradual, progressive, and irreversible decline in cerebral function (Touhy, 2018d). Because of the similarity between delirium and dementia, you need to assess carefully to rule out the presence of delirium whenever you suspect dementia.

Nursing management of older adults with any form of dementia always considers the safety and physical and psychosocial needs of the older adult and the family. These needs change as the progressive nature of dementia leads to increased cognitive deterioration. To meet the needs of older adults, individualize nursing care to enhance quality of life and maximize functional performance by improving cognition, mood, and behavior. Persons with dementia may exhibit behaviors that may be unsafe, putting them at risk for falls and other injuries. These behaviors are an expression of an unmet need, such as hunger, pain, anxiety, or the need to void or defecate. Therefore, the nurse should consider the meaning behind a person's actions. Nonpharmacological measures should be used first, before administering medications that may be sedating or have other undesirable effects. Box 14.5 lists general nursing principles for the care of older adults with dementia. Support and education about Alzheimer's disease for patients, families, and professionals can be found at the Alzheimer's Association website (www.alz.org).

Depression. Older adults sometimes experience late-life depression, but it is not a normal part of aging. Depression is the most common, yet most undetected and untreated, impairment in older adulthood. It sometimes exists and is exacerbated in patients with other health problems such as stroke, diabetes, dementia, Parkinson's disease, heart disease, cancer, and pain-provoking diseases such as arthritis. Loss of a significant loved one or admission to a nursing center sometimes causes depression. The Geriatric Depression Scale is an easy-to-use screening tool that can be used in conjunction with an interview with the older adult (Jett, 2018a). Clinical depression is treatable. Treatment includes medication, psychotherapy, or a combination of both. Electroconvulsant therapy (ECT) is sometimes used for treatment of resistant depression when medications and psychotherapy do not help. Of special note, suicide attempts in older adults are often successful. Suicide rates in all age-groups are on the rise over the past several years; the age-group of 85 years of age and older has the second highest suicide

BOX 14.5   Dementia Care Practice Recommendations

Person-Centered Care

- Know the person as an individual. Information should include past social and work history, values, interests, and preferences.
- Recognize and accept the person's reality. Do not attempt to reorient the person. Instead, the nurse should recognize that the person's behavior is a form of communication.
- Support opportunities for meaningful interactions. By knowing the person's preferences, interactions are more likely to be effective and meet the needs of the individual. Promote social interaction when possible.
- Nurture authentic, caring relationships. Nurses should focus more on the interaction than the task needing to be accomplished.
- Maintain a supportive community for the person with dementia, the person's family, and staff.

Detection and Diagnosis of Dementia

- Provide information about brain health and related disorders, along with referral to specialists in dementia care.
- Attend to concerns about cognitive changes from family members and other care providers.
- Following a diagnosis of dementia, support and educate the person and family members, including referral to appropriate agencies and support groups.

Person-Centered Assessment and Care Planning

- Ensure that regular ongoing assessments of persons with dementia are conducted. This is an opportunity to support and educate the person, family, and caregivers.
- Involve multiple disciplines when developing a plan of care.
- Regularly evaluate the plan of care for relevance and accuracy.
- Encourage advanced care planning to optimize physical, psychosocial, and fiscal well-being.

Medical Management

- Utilize a holistic approach and manage co-morbidities.
- Encourage nonpharmacological interventions for common behavioral and psychological symptoms.
- Pharmacological measures should be used cautiously and only after attempting nonpharmacological measures. Minimize polypharmacy by decreasing the risk for drug interactions and adverse reactions.

Education and Support of Those Diagnosed With Dementia and Their Families

- Provide education and support early in the disease to better prepare for future events.
- Encourage families and caregivers to work together.
- Educational programming should be culturally sensitive.
- Use technology to reach out to families. Two-way video technology, such as Skype or FaceTime, can be used to enhance family involvement.

Managing Behavioral and Psychological Symptoms of Dementia

- Identify social and environmental triggers of negative behavioral symptoms. Symptoms are individualized responses to the dementia disease process and can vary widely.

- Implement nonpharmacological practices that are tailored to the individual's needs. These include:
  - Sensory practices: aromatherapy, massage, multisensory stimulation, and bright light therapy
  - Psychosocial practices: validation therapy, reminiscence therapy, music therapy, pet therapy, and meaningful activities
  - Structured care protocols (bathing and mouth care)
- Hand in Hand is a training course for direct care providers on safe, effective strategies for caring with persons with dementia. It is available at: https://surveyortraining.cms.hhs.gov/pubs/HandinHand.aspx.

Supporting Activities of Daily Living

- Allow individuals to be involved in their care to the extent of their cognitive abilities, with a focus on preserving self-dignity.
- Provide limited choices with simple instructions.
- Provide dignity and respect in the toileting process by being attuned to cues indicating a need to void/defecate. Toilet continent individuals on a regular basis.
- Support eating nutritious meals and consider food preferences. A quiet homelike atmosphere is conducive to adequate nutritional intake. For some, finger foods may be easier to manipulate than feeding oneself with utensils.
- Monitor and support fluid intake.
- Encourage physical activity. Make sure that the environment is safe for mobility, and promote way-finding with pictures or cues.
- Ensure that assistive devices (hearing aids, glasses, dentures) are functioning and used appropriately.

Recommendations for Staffing

- Provide a thorough orientation that focuses on the care of individuals diagnosed with dementia.
- Provide consistent staff so that the staff member can learn more about the person, as well as the person and their family being able to develop a relationship with staff members.
- Encourage patients, families, and staff to develop and sustain professional, caring relationships.

Providing a Supportive and Therapeutic Environment

- Promote safety, comfort, and dignity.
- Allow for choice for those with dementia to promote safe independence.

Transitions of Care

- Prepare persons living with dementia and their families for common transitions of care by discussing the risks and benefits of a transfer to a new environment (e.g., care facility, hospital).
- Promote timely and effective communication across care settings. Utilizing transfer reports available in the electronic medical record can enhance the quality and timeliness of information sharing.

Modified from Fazio S, et al: Alzheimer's Association dementia care practice recommendations, *Gerontologist* 58(S1):S1–S9, 2018.

rate of all age-groups (American Foundation for Suicide Prevention, 2018). Therefore, suicide prevention considerations for older adults are similar to those for the general population.

Psychosocial Changes

As previously discussed, psychosocial changes occurring during aging involve life transitions and loss. Life transitions, of which loss is a major

component, include retirement and the associated financial changes, changes in roles and relationships, alterations in health and functional ability, changes in one's social network, and relocation.

It is important to assess both the nature of the psychosocial changes that occur in older adults as a result of life transitions and the loss and the adaptations to the changes. During your assessment ask how an older adult feels about self, self in relation to others, and self as one who is aging, and ask which coping methods and skills have been beneficial. Areas to address during the assessment include family, intimate relationships, past and present role changes, finances, housing, social networks, activities, health and wellness, and spirituality. Specific topics related to these areas include retirement, social isolation, sexuality, housing and environment, and death.

Retirement. Many often mistakenly associate retirement with passivity and seclusion. In actuality it is a stage of life characterized by transitions and role changes and may occupy 30 or more years of one's life. This transition requires letting go of certain habits and structure and developing new ones (Touhy, 2018b). The psychosocial stresses of retirement are usually related to role changes with a spouse or within the family and to loss of the work role. Sometimes problems related to social isolation and finances are present. The age of retirement varies; but whether it occurs at age 55, 65, or 75, it is one of the major turning points in life.

Meaningful retirement planning is critical as the population continues to age. Retirement affects more than just the retired. It also affects the spouse, adult children, and even grandchildren. When the spouse is still working, the retired person faces time alone. There may be new expectations of the retired person. For example, a working spouse has new ideas about the amount of housework expected of the retired person. Problems develop when the plans of the retired person conflict with the work responsibilities of the working spouse. The roles of the retiree and the working spouse need clarification. Some adult children expect the retired person to always care for the grandchildren, forgetting that this is a time for the retired person to pursue other personal interests.

Loss of the work role has a major effect on some retired people. When so much of life has revolved around work and the personal relationships at work, the loss of the work role is sometimes devastating. Personal identity is often rooted in the work role, and with retirement individuals need to construct a new identity. They also lose the structure imposed on daily life when they no longer have a work schedule. The social exchanges and interpersonal support that occur in the workplace are lost. In the adjustment to retirement an older adult has to develop a personally meaningful schedule and a supportive social network.

Factors that influence a retired person's satisfaction with life are health status and sufficient income. Positive preretirement expectations also contribute to satisfaction in retirement. You can help the older adult and family prepare for retirement by discussing with them several key areas, including relations with spouse and children; meaningful activities and interests; building social networks; issues related to income; health promotion and maintenance; and long-range planning, including wills and advance directives. This information should be considered part of your psychosocial assessment and provides context for other concerns expressed by the older adult.

Social Isolation. Many older adults experience social isolation. Isolation is sometimes a choice, the result of a desire not to interact with others. Older adults who experience social isolation become vulnerable to its consequences because of the absence of the support of other adults. Impaired sensory function, functional impairment, chronic illness, reduced mobility, and cognitive changes all contribute to reduced interaction with others and often place an older adult at risk for isolation.

Assess patients' potential for social isolation by identifying their social network, access to transportation, and willingness and desire to interact with others. Use your findings to help a lonely older adult rebuild social networks and reverse patterns of isolation. Many communities have outreach programs designed to make contact with isolated older adults. Outreach programs such as daily telephone calls by volunteers or planned social outings also meet socialization needs. A wide range of organizations welcomes older adults as volunteers and provides the opportunity for them to serve while meeting their socialization or other needs. Churches, colleges, community centers, and libraries offer a variety of programs for older adults that increase the opportunity to meet people with similar interests and needs.

Sexuality. All older adults, whether healthy or frail, need to express their need for intimacy and sexual feelings. Sexuality involves love, warmth, sharing, and touching, not just the act of intercourse. It plays an important role in helping the older adult maintain self-esteem. To help an older adult achieve or maintain sexual health, you need to understand the physical changes in a person's sexual response (see Chapter 34). You need to provide privacy for any discussion of sexuality and maintain a nonjudgmental attitude. Open-ended questions should be used to elicit information and concerns related to sex and sexuality. Include information about the prevention of sexually transmitted infections when appropriate. Sexuality and the need to express sexual feelings remain throughout the human life span.

When considering an older adult's need for sexual expression, do not ignore the important need to touch and be touched. Touch is an overt expression with many meanings and is an important part of intimacy (Yeager, 2019a). Touch complements traditional sexual methods or serves as an alternative sexual expression when physical intercourse is not desired or possible. Knowing an older adult's sexual needs allows you to incorporate this information into the nursing care plan. The sexual preferences of older adults are as diverse as those of the younger population. Clearly not all older adults are heterosexual; research is emerging on older adult lesbian, gay, bisexual, and transgender individuals and their health care needs. Nurses often find that they are called on to help other health care professionals understand the sexual needs of older adults. Not all nurses feel comfortable counseling older adults about sexual health and intimacy-related needs. Be prepared to refer older adults to an appropriate professional counselor.

Housing and Environment. Older adults' ability to live independently influences housing choices. However, it is difficult to anticipate what services will be needed by an older adult over the course of several years. For example, a housing unit with only one floor and without exterior steps is a prudent choice for an older adult with severe arthritis who has already had lower-extremity joint replacement surgery and anticipates the need for future operations. A broad range of housing options, with numerous variations, exist. The options may be overwhelming to the older adults and their family.

Aging in place is a concept that is gaining popularity. It is intended to promote successful aging by allowing an older adult to stay in one place while providing the needed supplemental services (National Institute of Health, 2017). Some aging in place initiatives are formal organizations, while others are more loosely organized. Aging in place requires the older adult to anticipate the health and personal services that will be needed and how to access those services, as well as creating a safe physical environment that is accessible in the event of impaired mobility. Some older adults choose to live with family members. Others prefer their own homes or other housing options near their families. Leisure or retirement communities provide older people with living and social opportunities in a one-generation setting. Federally subsidized housing, where available, offers apartments with communal, social, and in some cases food-service arrangements.

The goal of your assessment of a patient's environment is to consider resources that promote safety, independence, and functional ability. Assessment of safety, a major component of an older adult's environment, includes risks within the environment and the older adult's ability to recognize and respond to the risks (see Chapter 27). Bathroom safety is central in an acceptable environment. The bathroom should have:

- Grab bars that can assist with moving and can be reached in case of a potential or actual fall
- Nonslip surfaces on the floor and tub/shower
- Needed supplies in easy reach
- Minimal obstacles (rugs, furniture, equipment)
- Adequate lighting, especially at night

Other considerations include the removal of clutter and throw rugs to decrease the risk of falls. Lighting should be adequate, particularly in walkways and stairs. Water heaters should not be set higher than 120°F. Smoke and carbon monoxide detectors should be installed and batteries changed regularly (Health in Aging, 2019).

Housing and environment can either support or hinder physical and social functioning, enhance or drain energy, and complement or tax existing physical changes such as vision and hearing. For example, furnishings with red, orange, and yellow colors are easiest for older adults to see. Shiny waxed floors may appear to be wet. Ensure that door frames and baseboards are an appropriate color that contrasts with the color of the wall to improve perception of the boundaries of halls and rooms, keeping in mind that older adults often have difficulty distinguishing among pastel shades and between green and blue. Walkways leading to the house need to be flat, even, and in good repair, and stairs need to have a color contrast at the edge of the step so that an older person knows where the stair ends. Glare from highly polished floors, metallic fixtures, or windows is difficult for an older adult to tolerate.

Furniture needs to be comfortable and safe. Older adults need to examine furniture carefully for size, comfort, and function before purchasing it. Furniture should have adequate back support and allow a person to get into and out of the chair or sofa easily and safely. Test dining room chairs for comfort during meals and for height in relation to the table. Many older adults find that armrests on chairs make sitting down and getting up easier. Older adults often prefer to transfer out of a wheelchair to another chair for meals because some styles of wheelchairs do not allow a person to sit close enough to the table to eat comfortably. Raising the table to clear the wheelchair arms brings the table closer to the older adult but makes it too high to eat comfortably. To make getting out of bed easier and safer, ensure that the height of the bed allows an older adult's feet to be flat on the floor when he or she is sitting on the side of the bed.

QSEN Building Competency in Safety Mr. Sousa is an energetic 76-year-old man who is ready for discharge from the hospital. He does not "look" 76, as he appears very fit and states that he is active in social activities and volunteering. He was admitted to the hospital 3 days ago for a right total knee replacement and is doing well after surgery; he now walks with the assistance of one person and is using a walker. He is able to walk to the bathroom and has walked 125 feet in the hallway 3 times today. He will get home health care and home physical therapy rather than going to the hospital rehabilitation unit. He insists on going home because of his dog, Benji, a black Labrador retriever. Mr. Sousa's daughter is going to pick up Benji from the boarding kennel and take him home. Mr. Sousa's wife of 50 years died recently, leaving him alone at home, but he has been getting along well. His daughter lives within 25 miles of his home and will visit him daily. When considering safety for this patient in the home setting, which assessment questions and teaching approaches and resources can you use to enhance his safety in the home environment?

Answers to QSEN Activities can be found on the Evolve website.

Death. Part of one's life history is the experience of loss through the death of relatives and friends (see Chapter 36). This includes the loss of older generations of families and sometimes, sadly, the loss of a child. However, death of a spouse or significant other is the loss that most affects the lives of older people. Do not assume that an older adult is comfortable with death. You play a key role in helping older adults understand and cope with loss.

Current evidence supports that older people have a wide variety of attitudes and beliefs about death but fear of their own death is uncommon. Rather they are concerned with fear of being a burden, experiencing suffering, being alone, and the use of life-prolonging measures (Bub, 2019). The stereotype that the death of an older adult is a blessing does not apply to every older adult. Even as death approaches, many older adults still have unfinished business and are not prepared for it. Families and friends are not always ready to let go of their older significant others. Older adults and family members or friends will often turn to you for assistance. Thus you need knowledge of the grieving process (see Chapter 36), excellent communication skills (see Chapter 24), understanding of legal issues and advance care planning (see Chapter 23), familiarity with community resources, and awareness of one's own feelings, limitations, and strengths as they relate to care of those confronting death.

REFLECT NOW

Reflect on how you would start a conversation with an older adult about end-of-life care, with the intent of determining his or her wishes/goals for care.

ADDRESSING THE HEALTH CONCERNS OF OLDER ADULTS

As the population ages and life expectancy increases, emphasis on health promotion, health maintenance, and disease prevention increases (see Chapter 6). Older adults are becoming more enthusiastic and motivated about healthy lifestyles (AOA, 2017). A number of national programs and projects address preventive practices in the older-adult population. The national initiative *Healthy People 2020* (Office of Disease Prevention and Health Promotion, 2019) has an overarching goal to improve the health, function, and quality of life of older adults. More specifically, *Healthy People 2020* for older adults focuses on:

- Understanding the health services provided to older adults
- Chronic disease management
- Injury prevention
- Caregivers in the home

The challenges of health promotion and disease prevention for older adults are complex and affect health care providers as well. Previous health care experiences, personal motivation, health beliefs, culture, health literacy, and non–health-related factors such as transportation and finances often create barriers for older adults. The interests and desires of older adults should be considered when planning health promotion activities (Campbell et al., 2018). Barriers for health care providers include beliefs and attitudes about which services and programs to provide, their effectiveness and the lack of consistent guidelines, and absence of a coordinated approach. Your role is to focus interventions on maintaining and promoting patients' function and quality of life. You can empower older adults to make their own health care decisions and realize their optimum level of health, function, and quality of life (Davis, 2019). Always be open to recognizing an older adult's concerns so that you can adjust a plan of care accordingly. Although various interventions cross all three levels of care (i.e., health promotion, acute care, and restorative care), some approaches are unique to each level.

Learning Needs

Managing the complexities of chronic disease and the cognitive and sensory changes that may be associated with aging add to the challenges of teaching older adults. As you assess the various physical, cognitive, functional, and psychosocial problems of older adults, it is important to also assess their associated learning needs. For example, during a cognitive and psychosocial assessment, you will gain information that indicates a patient's ability to follow a recommended treatment plan. When assessing a patient's medication history, have the patient describe when he or she takes the medication at home and the dosage. If a patient has slow responses or reaction time when performing physical activities, it is necessary to consider these limitations when teaching new psychomotor skills. During your assessment, carefully consider a patient's learning needs and capability to learn.

Educating Older Adults

Inadequate health literacy disproportionately affects older adults in the United States, causing misunderstanding of health information and subsequent nonadherence, which results in negative outcomes (Cutilli et al., 2018). The World Health Organization (2018) defines health literacy as the ability of individuals to "gain access to, understand and use information in ways which promote and maintain good health" for themselves, their families and their communities. The older adult expects that the patient education delivered is relevant to his or her own situation (Touhy, 2018a). It is important to know how to adapt routine patient education strategies to effectively meet the specific learning needs of older adults (see Box 14.6). When patients do not receive correct and necessary information from an educational session, they may turn to other sources, such as the Internet, relatives, or friends, for information, which may have incomplete or inaccurate information. Thus, nurses have an obligation to provide accurate information in a manner that meets the needs of the older adult.

Health Promotion and Maintenance: Physiological Concerns

The desire and abilities of older adults to participate in health promotion activities vary. Therefore use an individualized approach, taking into account a person's beliefs about the importance of staying healthy and remaining independent. The Federal Interagency Forum on Aging-Related Statistics (2016) reported that in 2014, 22% of older people 65 years and older reported a functional limitation (i.e., difficulty in hearing, vision, cognition, ambulation, self-care, communication), with older women reporting higher levels of functional limitations than men. Difficulties with mobility were the most commonly reported limitation. Some of these disabilities are relatively minor, but others cause people to require assistance to meet important personal needs. The incidence of disability increases with age. Limitations in ADLs limit the ability to live independently. The ADL limitations most often reported include walking, showering and bathing, getting in and out of bed and chair, dressing, toileting, and eating. Healthy Aging in Action (https://www.surgeongeneral.gov/priorities/prevention/about/healthy-aging-in-action-final.pdf) is a resource for promoting healthy aging and improving health and well-being in later life. Evidence-based health promotion programs are highlighted, including community safety and services, walking/physical activity, community engagement, preventive health services, and fall prevention (National Prevention, Health Promotion, and Public Health Council, 2016).

General preventive health measures to recommend to older adults include:

- Regular primary care, dental, vision, and hearing visits (if patient has a hearing aid)
- Participation in recommended screening activities as indicated by age (e.g., blood pressure, mammography, depression, vision and hearing, colonoscopy)
- Immunization for seasonal influenza, tetanus, diphtheria and pertussis, shingles, and pneumococcal disease
- Regular exercise, smoking cessation, and stress management
- Attaining and maintaining target weight
- Eating a low-fat, well-balanced diet or adhering to a specific diet (e.g. diabetic diet, low-sodium diet)
- Moderate alcohol use
- Socialization
- Good handwashing

Those who die from influenza are predominantly older adults. Providers strongly recommend annual immunization of all older adults for influenza, with special emphasis on residents of nursing homes or residential or long-term care facilities.

Other vaccinations, such as pneumonia or shingles, are often recommended. In addition, not all older adults are current with their booster injections, and some never received the primary series of injections. Ask about the current status of all immunizations, provide information about the immunizations, and make arrangements for them to receive immunizations as needed.

Most older adults are interested in their health and are able to take charge of their lives. They want to maintain or improve their health,

---

BOX 14.6   PATIENT TEACHING

Adapting Instruction for Older Adults With Health Literacy Limitations

Objective
- Patient will verbalize an understanding of instructional materials.

Teaching Strategies
- Ensure the patient is ready to learn. Be alert for cues of pain and fatigue.
- Create a comfortable environment (e.g., seating, temperature).
- Allow time to process information and ask questions.
- Adapt teaching materials for culture, language, and health literacy.
- Focus on concrete information and relate to past experiences as appropriate.
- Use printed materials with large black font on either cream or white paper.
- Use clear, concise language; avoid medical terminology.
- Use pictures, demonstrations, videos, and other methods to augment spoken language.

Evaluation
Use the principles of teach-back to evaluate patient/family caregiver learning:
- Tell me the times that you would take your medication.
- Explain three ways that you can improve the safety of your home.
- Show me how you will change the dressing on wound

Modified from Touhy T: Social, psychological, spiritual, and cognitive aspects of aging. In Touhy T, Jett K: *Ebersole and Hess' gerontological nursing and healthy aging*, ed 5, St Louis, 2018, Mosby.

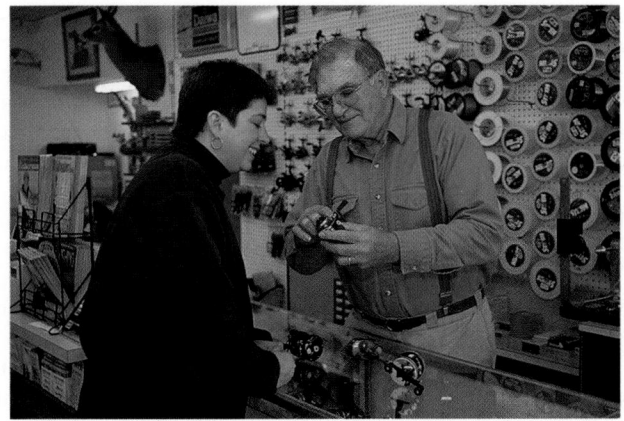

FIG. 14.1 This older adult works part time at a sporting goods store.

remain independent, and prevent disability (Fig. 14.1). Initial screenings establish baseline data to determine wellness, identify health needs, and design health maintenance programs. Following initial screening sessions, share with older adults information on nutrition, exercise, medications, stress management, and safety. You can also provide information on specific conditions such as hypertension, arthritis, and diabetes and self-care procedures such as foot and skin care. By providing information about health promotion and self-care, you significantly improve the health and well-being of older adults.

Heart Disease. Heart disease and cancer are the leading causes of death in older adults (Xu et al., 2018). Common cardiovascular disorders are hypertension and coronary artery disease. Hypertension is a silent killer because older adults, especially African Americans, are often unaware that their blood pressure is elevated (see Chapter 29). The fact that hypertension is common does not make it normal or harmless. Only about half of those diagnosed with hypertension have the condition under control. Treatment is linked to reduced incidence of myocardial infarction, chronic kidney disease, stroke, and heart failure. In coronary artery disease, partial or complete blockage of one or more coronary arteries leads to myocardial ischemia and myocardial infarction. The risk factors for both hypertension and coronary artery disease include smoking, obesity, lack of exercise, and stress. Additional risk factors for coronary artery disease include hypertension, hyperlipidemia, and diabetes mellitus (American Heart Association, 2016).

Nursing interventions for hypertension and coronary artery disease include patient teaching on weight reduction, exercise, dietary changes, limiting salt and fat intake, stress management, and smoking cessation. Additional patient teaching includes information about medication management, blood-pressure monitoring, and the symptoms indicating the need for emergency care.

Cancer. Malignant neoplasms are the second most common cause of death among older adults. Nurses educate older adults about early detection, treatment, and cancer risk factors. Education topics include low-fat diet, smoking cessation, breast self-examination (see Chapter 30), and encouraging all older adults to have recommended annual screening for fecal occult blood. It is also important to educate older adults about the signs of cancer and to encourage prompt reporting of nonhealing skin lesions, unexpected bleeding, change in bowel habits, nagging cough, lump in breast or another part of body, change in a mole, difficulty swallowing, and unexplained weight loss.

Chronic Lung Disease. Chronic lung disease, specifically chronic obstructive pulmonary disease (COPD), is the third leading cause of

death in those 65 and older. More women than men die from COPD (American Lung Association, 2018a). Lung injury from inhalants such as tobacco smoke, exposure to secondhand smoke, and fumes from hair dyes, artificial nail products, and paints can lead to COPD, causing airflow blockage and breathing-related difficulty (American Lung Association, 2018a). Tobacco smoke and exposure to secondhand smoke are key factors in the development and progression of COPD. It is important to provide patients with information about smoking cessation programs. In addition, depending on the severity of a patient's disease, you will teach a patient about proper exercise, how to use inhalers, and techniques for the removal of mucus from the airways (see Chapter 41). Supervised exercise training is a major component of pulmonary rehabilitation programs and is an established safe and effective intervention for improving patients' physical capacity and quality of life (American Lung Association, 2018b).

Stroke (Cerebrovascular Accident). Cerebrovascular accidents (CVAs) are the fourth leading cause of death in the United States and occur as either brain ischemia (inadequate blood supply to areas of brain caused by arterial blockage) or brain hemorrhage (subarachnoid or intercerebral bleeds). Risk factors include hypertension, hyperlipidemia, diabetes mellitus, history of transient ischemic attacks, and family history of cardiovascular disease (American Heart Association, 2018). CVAs often impair a person's functional abilities and lead to loss of independence and nursing home admission. The scope of nursing interventions ranges from teaching older adults about risk-reduction strategies to teaching family caregivers the early warning signs of a stroke and ways to support a patient during recovery and rehabilitation.

Smoking. Cigarette smoking is a risk factor for the four most common causes of death: heart disease, cancer, lung disease, and stroke (American Heart Association, 2016, 2018). Smoking is the most preventable cause of disease and death in the United States. Smoking cessation is a health promotion strategy for older adults just as it is for younger adults. Older smokers still benefit from smoking cessation. In addition to reducing risk, it sometimes stabilizes existing conditions such as COPD and coronary artery disease. Smoking cessation after age 50 reduces the risk of dying prematurely by 50% compared with those who continue to smoke (NCI, 2017). Smoking cessation programs include individual, group, and telephone counseling and the use of nicotine (gum and patch) or non-nicotine medications. If a patient rejects smoking cessation, suggest at least a reduction in smoking. Finally, set a quit or reduction date and a follow-up visit with the older adult to discuss the quit attempt. At follow-up visits, offer encouragement and assistance in modifying the plan as necessary.

Alcohol Abuse. Studies of alcohol abuse in older adults report two patterns: a lifelong pattern of continuous heavy drinking and a pattern of heavy drinking that begins late in life (Lewis et al., 2018). Frequently cited causes of excessive alcohol use include chronic illness, depression, loneliness, and lack of social support.

Alcohol use and late-onset alcohol use disorder (AUD) are often underidentified in older adults. The clues of alcohol abuse in the older adult include stress, role/identity loss, encouragement/approval by friends, multiple chronic health problems, and coexisting dementia or depression (Gibson et al., 2017; Emiliussen et al., 2017). Your suspicion of alcohol abuse increases when there is a history of repeated falls and accidents, social isolation, recurring episodes of memory loss and confusion, failure to meet home and work obligations, a history of skipping meals or medications, and difficulty in managing household tasks and finances. When you suspect that an older adult is abusing alcohol, realize that a variety of treatment options are available. Treatment includes age-specific approaches that acknowledge the stresses experienced by an older adult and encourage involvement in activities that match his or her interests and increase feelings of self-worth. Identifying and treating coexisting depression is also important. The continuum of interventions ranges from simple education about risks to formalized treatment programs that include pharmacotherapy, psychotherapy, and rehabilitation.

Nutrition. Lifelong eating habits and situational factors influence how older adults achieve good nutrition. These habits are based in tradition, cultural habits, and preferences. Religious beliefs influence food choices and preparation. Situational factors affecting nutrition include access to grocery stores, finances, physical and cognitive capability for food preparation, and a place to store food and prepare meals. Older adults' levels of activity and clinical conditions affect their nutritional needs. In addition, conditions such as dementia, poor dentition or ill-fitting dentures, dysphagia, and cardiopulmonary, gastrointestinal, renal, or liver diseases impact nutrition. Healthy nutrition for older adults includes appropriate caloric intake and limited intake of fat, salt, refined sugars, and alcohol. When caring for older adults with dementia and other chronic conditions, routinely monitor weight and food intake; provide small, frequent meals and serve food that is easy to eat such as finger foods (e.g., chicken strips, sandwiches, cut-up vegetables, and fruit), provide assistance with eating, and offer food supplements that the patient likes and are easy to swallow (Brook, 2018). Consult with a registered dietitian when planning nutritional interventions for your patients.

Protein intake is sometimes lower than recommended if older adults have reduced financial resources or limited access to grocery stores. Fat and sodium intake is sometimes higher than usual because of quick and convenient frozen meals or the substitution of fast-food restaurant meals for meals prepared at home. Home-prepared meals that are fried or made with canned goods also are high in fat and sodium. Some use extra salt and sugar while cooking or at the table to compensate for a diminished sense of taste. Home-delivered meals, such as Meals on Wheels, are an excellent source of nutrition for older adults. Newer online ordering and home delivery services can improve access to quality food sources but may require assistance from family members to order appropriately.

Dental Problems. Dental problems with natural teeth and dentures are common in older adults. Dental caries, gingivitis, broken or missing teeth, and ill-fitting or missing dentures affect nutritional adequacy, cause pain, and lead to infection. Weight loss may contribute to ill-fitting dentures. Dentures are a frequent problem because the cost is not covered by Medicare, and dentures tend to be quite expensive. Help prevent dental and gum disease through education about routine dental care (see Chapter 40).

Exercise. Older adults need to maintain physical exercise and activity. The primary benefits of exercise include maintaining and strengthening functional ability and promoting a sense of enhanced well-being and quality of life (Kaushal et al., 2018). Regular daily exercise such as walking builds endurance, increases muscle tone, improves joint flexibility, strengthens bones, reduces stress, and contributes to weight loss. There is some evidence that exercise has some protective effects on cognition and brain health (Tyndall et al., 2018). Other benefits include improved cardiovascular function, increased metabolic rate, increased gastrointestinal transit time, decreased depression, and improved sleep quality. Older adults who participate in group exercise programs, individually tailored balance and strength programs, or

planned walking programs often experience improved mobility, gait, and balance, resulting in fewer falls (CDC, 2015).

Many factors influence an individual's willingness to participate in an exercise program. These include general beliefs about the benefits of exercise, past experience with exercise, personal goals, personality, and any unpleasant sensations associated with exercise. A patient's health care provider should be consulted before initiating an exercise program to be sure there are no medical contraindications. Exercise programs for sedentary older adults who have not been exercising regularly need to begin conservatively and progress slowly. An exercise program should be appropriate to the older adult's physical ability while being enjoyable, increasing the likelihood of maintaining the program.

Developing a habit of routine exercise is not only beneficial for the physiological effects but also improves mood and quality of life and helps to incorporate activity into a person's lifestyle (Kendrick et al., 2018). Walking is one type of exercise many older adults enjoy (Fig. 14.2). Walking and other low-impact exercises such as riding a stationary exercise bicycle or water exercises in a swimming pool protect the musculoskeletal system and joints. Include other exercises in the older adult's daily routine. For example, have an older adult perform arm and leg circles while watching television.

Safety considerations for exercise include wearing supportive shoes and appropriate clothing, drinking water before and after exercising, avoiding outdoor exercise in extreme temperatures, and exercising with a partner. Instruct older adults to stop exercising and seek help if they experience chest pain or tightness, shortness of breath, dizziness or light-headedness, joint pain, or palpitations during exercise.

Falls. There are multiple risks for falls in the older-adult population (see Box 14.7). Falls are a safety concern of many older adults. Falls are the leading cause of fatal injury and are the most common nonfatal trauma-related reason for hospital admission (National Council on Aging, n.d.). When a fall occurs in an older adult, it may lead to other life-changing events such as hip fracture, spine fracture, or head injury and admission to a nursing center. Fall-related injuries are often associated with a person's preexisting medical conditions such as osteoporosis and bleeding tendencies. Hospitalized older adults require extra attention to decrease the risk of falls. Each year about 3 million nonfatal falls among older adults are treated in emergency departments, and more than 800,000 of these patients are hospitalized. The direct

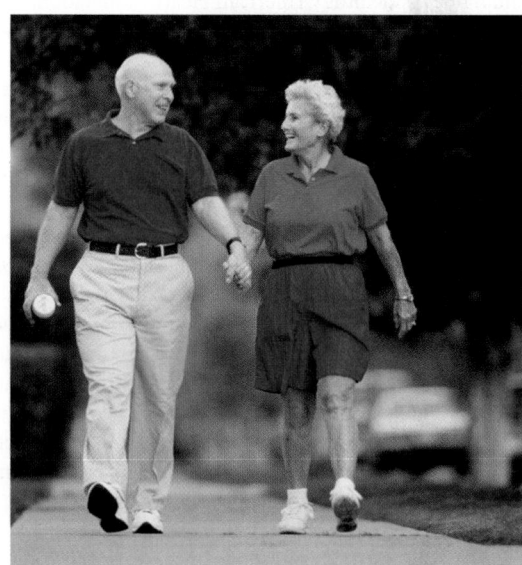

FIG. 14.2 This couple enjoys walking together.

BOX 14.7 Risk Factors for Falls in Older Adults

Intrinsic Factors
- History of a previous fall
- Fear of falling
- Muscle weakness
- Impaired vision
- Postural hypotension
- Problems with balance and gait
- Adverse medication reactions (sedatives, hypnotics, anticonvulsants, opioids)
- Chronic conditions, including arthritis, stroke, incontinence, diabetes, Parkinson's disease, dementia

Extrinsic Factors
- Poor lighting (interior and exterior)
- Lack of handrails on stairs (interior and exterior)
- Poor design of stairwells
- Lack of bathroom grab bars and nonslip surfaces
- Hazards and obstacles (furniture, cords, throw rugs) that contribute to tripping
- Slippery or uneven surfaces
- Improper use of assistive devices
- Inappropriate footwear

medical costs of those falls adjusted for inflation was more than $50 billion (CDC, 2017). Older adults who have fallen will often develop a fear of falling, which in turn often causes them to walk less naturally or to limit their activities, leading to reduced mobility and loss of physical fitness. Routine exercise and activity can help reduce the risk for falls (Roller et al., 2018; Kaushal et al., 2018). See Chapter 38 for a description of fall prevention interventions.

Sensory Impairments. Because of common sensory impairments experienced by older adults, you need to promote existing sensory function and be sure that patients live in safe environments. Whenever you provide care activities, make sure that patients wear assistive devices such as a hearing aid or glasses so that they can fully participate in care. Chapter 49 describes in detail the nursing interventions used to maintain and improve sensory function.

Pain. Pain is a symptom and a sensation of distress, alerting a person that something is wrong. It is prevalent in the older-adult population and may be acute or chronic. The consequences of persistent pain include depression, loss of appetite, sleep difficulties, changes in gait and mobility, and decreased socialization. Many factors influence the management of pain, including cultural influences on the meaning and expression of pain for older adults, fears related to the use of analgesic medications, and the problem of pain assessment with older adults who are cognitively impaired. Nurses caring for older adults have to advocate for appropriate and effective pain management (see Chapter 44). Again, the goal of nursing management of pain in older adults is to maximize and maintain function and improve quality of life.

Medication Use. One of the greatest challenges for older adults is safe medication use. Medication categories such as analgesics, anticoagulants, antidepressants, antihistamines, antihypertensives, sedative-hypnotics, and muscle relaxants create a high likelihood of adverse effects in older adults. They are at risk for adverse medication effects because of age-related changes in the absorption, distribution, metabolism, and

excretion of drugs, collectively referred to as the process of pharmacokinetics (see Chapter 31). Medications sometimes interact with one another, adding to or negating the effect of another drug. Examples of adverse effects include confusion, impaired balance, dizziness, nausea, and vomiting. Because of these effects, some older adults are unwilling to take medications; others do not adhere to the prescribed dosing schedule, or they try to medicate themselves with herbal and over-the-counter medications.

Polypharmacy, the concurrent use of many medications, increases the risk for adverse drug effects (Box 14.8). Although polypharmacy often reflects inappropriate prescribing, the concurrent use of multiple medications is often necessary when an older adult has multiple acute and chronic conditions (Andrew et al., 2018). For example, your patient may be taking one or more medications for hypertension, diabetes, and arthritis. Your role as a nurse is to ensure the greatest therapeutic benefit with the least amount of harm by educating patients about safe medication use. You need to question the efficacy and safety of combinations of prescribed medications by conferring with pharmacists or health care providers. Advocate for the older adult to prevent adverse reactions. Older adults often use over-the-counter or herbal medications. The mix of over-the-counter and herbal medications with prescription medications can create serious adverse reactions.

For some older adults safely managing medications is complex and often becomes overwhelming. This problem is even more complicated when limited health literacy is an issue. Some take their medications incorrectly because they do not understand the administration instructions, thereby complicating your assessment of medication effects and side effects. Medications that need to be taken more than once or twice a day are a concern because a patient may not remember to take them as scheduled. As a nurse you are in a position to help older-adult patients as they carry out this important self-care activity (see Chapter 31).

The cost of prescriptions is often prohibitive. The Medicare Prescription Drug Benefit, Medicare Part D, was created in 2003 as part of the Medicare Modernization Act of 2003. This is not one plan but a designation of many plans that are approved by the Centers for Medicare and Medicaid Services (CMS, n.d.). Although accompanied by a deductible dependent on the number and expense of the medications prescribed, this benefit is of great help to aging adults. In addition, you advocate for patients who need certain medications by working with pharmacies or drug companies to provide the needed medication at less cost. Often a generic medication that will provide the desired effect is available at a reduced cost.

Work collaboratively with older adults and review their medications to ensure safe and appropriate use of all medications, both prescribed and over-the-counter. Teach an older adult the names of all medications that he or she is taking, when and how to take them, and desirable and undesirable effects (Lenander et al., 2018). Pill organizers, bubble packs, and medication calendars help older adults track their doses. Explain how to avoid adverse effects and/or interactions of medications and how to establish and follow an appropriate self-administration pattern. Strategies for reducing the risk for adverse medication effects include reviewing the medications with older adults at each visit, examining for potential interactions with food or other medications, simplifying and individualizing medication regimens, taking every opportunity to inform older adults and their family caregivers about all aspects of medication use, and encouraging older adults to question their health care providers about all prescribed and over-the-counter medications (Van der Linden et al., 2018).

The use of medications to manage confusion should be weighed carefully. Sedatives and tranquilizers sometimes prescribed for older adults who are acutely confused often cause or exacerbate confusion and increase risks for falls or other injuries. Carefully monitor patients

BOX 14.8   EVIDENCE-BASED PRACTICE

Polypharmacy in Older Adults

PICOT Question: Does the use of structured programs to evaluate an older adult's medication regimen decrease the number of potentially inappropriate medications?

Evidence Summary

Polypharmacy is prevalent in older adults due to multiple chronic illnesses and is associated with potentially dangerous outcomes. Health care team members must be alert to potentially harmful medications, as well as adverse reactions and interactions. Studies related to medication management have been conducted in the community, clinics, hospitals, and long-term care facilities. In one study, over half of community-dwelling older adults had questions about their drug regimen, primarily medication side effects and timing (Kovacevic et al., 2017). Additionally, 39.5% reported some sort of practical problem, primarily dosing and remembering instructions that were not written down. Approximately 75% found having a consultation with a pharmacist as beneficial. Another study looked at nursing home residents and older adults receiving home care services (Lenander et al., 2018). The researchers found that 84% of the sample had medication-related problems, including high-risk drugs affecting the nervous, cardiac, and metabolic systems. As a result of the consultation, statistically significant reductions in potentially inappropriate medications and antipsychotics were achieved. A nursing home study compared the number and appropriateness of medications before and after implementing Care by Design, which used an interprofessional team approach and a physician dedicated to each nursing unit (Andrew et al.,2018). While polypharmacy remained high, a statistically significant reduction in polypharmacy was achieved. Additionally, the number of medications identified by the American Geriatric Society's Beers criteria was reduced; however, the reduction was not statistically significant. One hospital study used an interprofessional team to evaluate appropriateness

of medications (Van der Linden et al., 2018). The results demonstrated that the older adults were discharged on fewer medications than they were taking upon admission.

There are two tools to guide appropriate prescribing for older adults. The first tool, the *Beers Criteria for Potentially Inappropriate Medication Use in Older Adults* (American Geriatrics Society, 2015), helps health care providers recognize potentially inappropriate medications. The second, *Screening Tool of Older Person's Prescriptions* and *Screening Tool to Alert Doctors to Right Treatment* (STOPP-START), screens for drug interactions and potentially inappropriate prescribing in older adults (O'Mahony et al., 2015).

Application to Nursing Practice

- Older adults must maintain an accurate listing of all medications being used. Herbal supplements, vitamins, and over-the-counter medications should be included along with prescription medications (Kovacevic et al., 2017).
- If an older adult sees several providers (specialists), there should be one provider that keeps track of the patient's overall medication regimen.
- Older adults can benefit from ongoing education regarding appropriate use of medications and potential adverse effects (Kovacevic et al., 2017).
- The use of a systematic approach to medication reviews has been shown to reduce the number of medications prescribed, including potentially inappropriate medications (Andrew et al., 2018; Lenander et al., 2018).
- The Beers criteria and STOPP-START criteria are two structured tools that provide guidelines for appropriate medication usage (American Geriatric Society, 2015; O'Mahony et al., 2015).
- A number of computer programs and applications can assist with identifying inappropriate medications. These programs are not effective unless the listing of medications is accurate.

---

who receive these medications, taking into account age-related changes in body systems that affect pharmacokinetic activity. When confusion has a physiological cause (such as an infection), health care providers need to treat the cause rather than the confused behavior. When confusion varies by time of day or is related to environmental factors, use creative, nonpharmacological measures such as making the environment more meaningful, providing adequate light, encouraging use of assistive devices, or even calling friends or family members to let older adults hear reassuring voices.

Health Promotion and Maintenance: Psychosocial Health Concerns

Interventions supporting the psychosocial health of older adults resemble those for other age-groups. However, some interventions are more crucial for older adults experiencing social isolation; cognitive impairment; or stresses related to retirement, relocation, or approaching death.

Elder Mistreatment. Elder mistreatment is complex and multifaceted and encompasses a broad range of abuses. It is found across all areas of nursing practice and socioeconomic settings. Elder abuse is defined as an intentional act or failure to act that causes or creates a risk for harm to an older adult (CDC, 2016). Your ability to screen and assess for it is essential to the safety, health, and well-being of the older adult. Types of elder mistreatment include physical abuse, emotional abuse, financial exploitation, sexual abuse, and neglect (intentional and unintentional) (Table 14.3). Although cases remain underreported, data suggest that 10% of older adults in the United States experience some form of elder mistreatment (CDC, 2016). It is also common for

vulnerable older adults to experience a combination of the various types of abuse (Acierno et al., 2018).

Most perpetrators are relative caregivers, making abuse cases more complex to identify because of denial, fear of reporting, and the refusal of community services (Rosen et al., 2018). Higher rates of elder mistreatment occur when there is a greater reliance on the caregiver because of functional and cognitive impairment. Vulnerable older adults may not reach out for help for fear of further retribution, fear of nursing home placement, or because they have become completely isolated from others. They may feel foolish or blame themselves for allowing someone to mistreat them or not want to get caregivers in legal or financial trouble (NIH, 2016).

Elder mistreatment has become the focus of national and international organizations, public and social policy, and research. Established by the US Administration on Aging, the National Center for Elder Abuse (https://ncea.acl.gov/) is a resource center dedicated to the prevention of elder mistreatment. The Elder Justice Act of 2009 is widely regarded as the most comprehensive bill ever passed to address and battle elder mistreatment, providing federal funding to state Adult Protective Services (APS). In most states APS caseworkers are the first responders to reports of abuse, neglect, and exploitation of vulnerable adults. Services include receiving reports of adult abuse, exploitation, or neglect; investigating these reports; case management; monitoring; and evaluation. In addition to casework services, APS arranges medical, social, economic, legal, housing, and law enforcement or other protective emergency or supportive services (National Center on Elder Abuse, n.d.).

You are in a unique position to screen for elder mistreatment and assess for physical and emotional signs of abuse. A necessary part of

TABLE 14.3 Elder Mistreatment: Types, Descriptions, and Examples

Type	Description	Examples
Physical abuse	Occurs when older adults experience illness, pain, or injury as the result of physical force or the threat of physical injury.	Hitting, beating, pushing, slapping, kicking, physical restraint, inappropriate use of drugs, fractures, lacerations, rope burns, untreated injuries
Psychosocial/emotional abuse	Verbal and nonverbal acts that inflict mental pain, anguish, fear, and distress	Insults, threats, humiliation, intimidation, harassment, social isolation, destroying property
Financial abuse	Illegal taking, misuse, or concealment of money, benefits, property, or assets belonging to an elderly person	Check cashing without permission, forging a signature, stealing money or possessions, coercing a signature on legal documents (e.g., will, trust), forcing or improper use of durable power of attorney, unpaid bills, unauthorized credit card use
Sexual abuse	Nonconsensual sexual contact or activity of any kind; coercing an elder to witness sexual behaviors	Unwanted touching, rape, sodomy, forced watching of pornography, coerced nudity, sexually explicit photography
Neglect	Refusal or failure by those responsible to meet basic needs	Refusal or failure to provide basic necessities such as food, water, shelter, hygiene, and medical care

Modified from Centers for Disease Control and Prevention (CDC), National Center for Injury Prevention and Control: *Understanding elder abuse,* 2016, https://www.cdc.gov/violenceprevention/pdf/em-factsheet-a.pdf. Accessed June 15, 2019.

your assessment is completing the interview and assessment privately away from the caregiver. It is definitely a "red flag" if the caregiver refuses to leave the room or area so that you can ask questions confidentially. State laws differ on reporting and investigation of elder mistreatment. However, if you suspect that an older adult is being mistreated, notify your supervisor, who will refer you to the appropriate reporting channels. It is your responsibility to know the reporting provisions of your jurisdiction (Touhy, 2018c).

Therapeutic Communication. Therapeutic communication skills enable you to perceive and respect the older adult's uniqueness and health care expectations. Attentive nurses provide care in a timely fashion, meeting a patient's expressed or unexpressed needs. A caring nurse expresses attitudes of concern, kindness, and compassion. Knowledgeable nurses not only demonstrate procedural competence but also recognize needs and relay information skillfully. Patients accept and respect nurses who meet these expectations and communicate effectively about concern for the older adult's welfare. However, you cannot simply enter an older adult's environment and immediately establish a therapeutic relationship. First, you have to be knowledgeable and skilled in communication techniques (see Chapter 24). Sitting down and engaging an older adult eye to eye goes a long way in establishing a therapeutic relationship.

Touch. Touch is a therapeutic tool that can be used to help comfort older adults. It provides sensory stimulation, induces relaxation, provides physical and emotional comfort, conveys warmth, and communicates interest. It is a powerful physical expression of a relationship. In addition, gentle touch is a technique to use when administering any type of procedure that requires physical contact or repositioning and moving a patient.

Older adults are often deprived of touch when separated from family or friends. An older adult who is isolated, dependent, or ill; who fears death; or who lacks self-esteem has a greater need for touch. You recognize touch deprivation by behaviors as simple as an older adult reaching for the nurse's hand or standing close to the nurse. Unfortunately, older men are sometimes wrongly accused of sexual advances when they reach out to touch others. When you use touch, be aware of cultural variations and individual preferences (see Chapters 7 and 9). Use touch to convey respect and sensitivity. Do not use it

in a condescending way such as patting an older adult on the head. When you reach out to an older adult, do not be surprised if he or she reciprocates.

Reality Orientation. Reality orientation is a communication technique that makes an older adult more aware of person, place, and time. The purposes of reality orientation include restoring a sense of reality; improving the level of awareness; promoting socialization; elevating independent functioning; and minimizing confusion, disorientation, and physical regression. Although you use reality orientation techniques in any health care setting, they are especially useful in the acute care setting. The older adult experiencing a change in environment, surgery, illness, or emotional stress is at risk for becoming disoriented (Chiu et al., 2018). Environmental changes such as bright lights, unfamiliar noises, and lack of windows in specialized units of a hospital often lead to disorientation and confusion. Absence of familiar caregivers is also disorienting. The use of anesthesia, sedatives, tranquilizers, analgesics, and physical restraints in older patients increases disorientation. Anticipate and monitor for disorientation and confusion as possible consequences of hospitalization, relocation, surgery, loss, or illness, and incorporate interventions on the basis of reality orientation into the plan of care.

The principles of reality orientation offer useful guidelines for communicating with individuals who are acutely confused. The key elements of reality orientation include frequent reminders of person, place, and time; the use of familiar environmental aids such as clocks, calendars, and personal belongings; and stability of the environment, routine, and staff (Chiu et al., 2018).

Validation Therapy. Validation therapy is an alternative approach to communication with an older adult who is confused. Whereas reality orientation insists that the confused older adult agree with statements of time, place, and person, validation therapy accepts the description of time and place as stated by the older adult. You do not challenge or argue with statements and behaviors of the older adult. Instead the focus is the emotional aspect of the conversation, which represents an inner need or feeling (Scales, 2018). For example, a patient insists that the day is actually a different day because of high anxiety. Caregivers should acknowledge the distress the individual is experiencing. Validation does not involve reinforcing the older adult's misperceptions; it reflects sensitivity to hidden meanings in statements and behaviors. By listening with sensitivity and validating what the patient is expressing, you convey respect, reassurance, and understanding. Validating or respecting older adults' feelings in the time and place that is real to them is more important than insisting on the literally correct time and place.

Reminiscence. Reminiscence is recalling the past. Many older adults enjoy sharing past experiences. As a therapy, reminiscence uses the recollection of the past to bring meaning and understanding to the present and resolve current conflicts. Looking back to positive resolutions of problems reminds an older adult of coping strategies used successfully in the past. Reminiscing is also a way to express personal identity. Reflection on past achievements supports self-esteem (Scales, 2018). For some older adults the process of looking back on past events uncovers new meanings for those events.

During the assessment process use reminiscence to assess self-esteem, cognitive function, emotional stability, unresolved conflicts, coping ability, and expectations for the future. For example, have a patient talk about a previous loss to assess coping. You can also reminisce during direct care activities. Taking time to ask questions about past experiences and listening attentively conveys to an older adult your attitudes of respect and concern.

Although many use reminiscence in a one-on-one situation, it is also used as a group therapy for older adults who are cognitively impaired or depressed (Siverova and Buzgova, 2018). You begin by organizing the group and selecting strategies to start a conversation. For example, you ask the group to discuss family activities or childhood memories, adapting questions to the group's size, structure, process, goals, and activities to meet its members' needs.

Body Image Interventions. The way older adults present themselves influences body image and feelings of isolation (see Chapter 33). Some physical characteristics of older adulthood such as distinguished-looking gray hair are socially desirable. Other features, such as a lined face that displays character or wrinkled hands that show a lifetime of hard work, are also impressive.

Consequences of illness and aging that threaten an older adult's body image include invasive diagnostic procedures, pain, surgery, loss of sensation in a body part, skin changes, and incontinence. The use of devices such as dentures, hearing aids, artificial limbs, indwelling catheters, ostomy devices, and enteral feeding tubes also affects body image.

You need to consider the importance to an older adult of presenting a socially acceptable image. When older adults have acute or chronic illnesses, the related physical dependence makes it difficult for them to maintain body image. Help them with grooming and hygiene. It takes little effort to help an older adult comb hair, clean dentures, shave, or change clothing. He or she does not choose to have an objectionable appearance. Be sensitive to odors in the environment. Odors created by urine and some illnesses are often present. By controlling odors you may prevent visitors from shortening their stay or not coming at all.

OLDER ADULTS AND THE ACUTE CARE SETTING

Older adults in the acute care setting need special attention to help them adjust to the acute care environment and meet their basic needs. The acute care setting poses increased risk for adverse events such as delirium, dehydration, malnutrition, health care–associated infections (HAIs), urinary incontinence, and falls. The risk for delirium increases when hospitalized older adults experience immobilization, sleep deprivation, infection, dehydration, pain, sensory impairment, drug interactions, anesthesia, and hypoxia. Nonmedical causes of delirium include unfamiliar surroundings, unfamiliar staff, bed rest, separation from support systems, and stress. Refer to the discussion of delirium, dementia, and depression earlier in the chapter on distinguishing between these three conditions. Impaired vision or hearing contributes to confusion and interferes with attempts to reorient an older adult.

When the prevention of delirium fails, nursing management begins with identifying and treating the cause. Supportive interventions include encouraging family visits, providing memory cues (clocks, calendars, and name tags), and compensating for sensory deficits. Reality orientation techniques are often useful.

Older adults are at greater risk for dehydration and malnutrition during hospitalization because of standard procedures such as limiting food and fluids in preparation for diagnostic tests and medications that decrease appetite. The risk for dehydration and malnutrition increases when older adults are unable to reach beverages or feed themselves while in bed or connected to medical equipment. Interventions include getting the patient out of bed, providing beverages and snacks frequently, and including favorite foods and beverages in the diet plan.

The increased risk for HAIs in older adults is associated with the decreased immune system response related to advancing age in addition to other chronic conditions that make older adults more susceptible, along with invasive procedures and devices. The most common HAI are central line-associated bloodstream infections (CLABSIs), catheter-associated UTIs (CAUTIs), surgical site infection, and ventilator-associated pneumonia (VAP) (CDC, 2018). The leading preventive measure is hand hygiene combined with proper isolation policy and procedures to prevent and control the transmission of infection (see Chapter 28).

Older hospitalized adults are at risk for becoming incontinent of urine (transient incontinence). Causes of incontinence include delirium, untreated UTIs, medications, restricted mobility, or need for assistance to get to the bathroom. Individualized interventions to decrease incontinence include voiding opportunities and modification of the environment to improve access to the toilet. It is important to avoid indwelling urinary catheterization (see Chapter 46).

The increased risk for skin breakdown and the development of pressure injuries is related to changes in aging skin and to situations that occur in the acute care setting such as immobility, incontinence, and malnutrition. The key points in the prevention of skin breakdown are using a mattress appropriate for the risk of skin breakdown with proper positioning, reducing shear and friction, providing meticulous skin care and moisture management, and providing nutritional support (see Chapter 48).

Older adults in the acute care setting are also at greater risk for falling and sustaining injuries. The cause of a fall is typically multifactorial and composed of intrinsic or extrinsic factors (see Box 14.7). Sedative and hypnotic medications increase unsteadiness. Lower extremity weakness and general fatigue and deconditioning can make it difficult for a patient to get out of bed. Once the patient does get out of bed, often he or she is very unsteady and prone to falling. Medications causing orthostatic hypotension also increases the risk for falls because the blood pressure drops when an older adult gets out of a bed or chair. The increase in urine output from diuretics increases the risk for falling by increasing the number of attempts to get out of bed to void. Equipment such as wires from monitors, intravenous tubing, urinary catheters, and other medical devices become obstacles to safe ambulation. Impaired vision prevents an older adult from seeing tripping hazards such as trash cans.

Physical restraints are used only as an intervention of last resort and require a health care provider's order. Many hospitals use bed and chair alarms. Making hourly rounds focusing on toileting needs, pain management, and personal needs of the patient often reduces falls (Christiansen, et al., 2018).

OLDER ADULTS AND RESTORATIVE CARE

Restorative care refers to two types of ongoing care: the continuation of the recovery from acute illness or surgery that began in the acute care setting and support of chronic conditions that affect day-to-day functioning. Both types of restorative care take place in private homes and long-term care settings.

Interventions during convalescence from acute illness or surgery aim at regaining or improving patients' prior level of independence in ADLs. Continue interventions that began in the acute care setting and later modify them as convalescence progresses. To achieve this continuation, ensure that discharge information provided by the acute care setting includes information on required ongoing interventions (e.g., exercise routines, wound care routines, medication schedules, and blood glucose monitoring). Interventions also need to address the restoration of interpersonal relationships and activities at either their previous level or the level desired by the older adult. When restorative care addresses chronic conditions, the goals of care include stabilizing the chronic condition and maximizing independence in ADLs.

Interventions to promote independence in ADLs address a person's physical and cognitive ability and safety. The physical ability to perform ADLs requires strength, flexibility, and balance. You need to make accommodations for impairments of vision, hearing, and touch. The cognitive ability to perform ADLs requires the ability to recognize, judge, and remember. Cognitive impairments such as dementia interfere with safe performance of ADLs, although an older adult is still physically capable of the activities. Adapt interventions to promote independence in ADLs to meet the needs and lifestyle of the older adult. Although safety is paramount, an older adult needs to be able to perform ADLs with a level of risk that is acceptable to him or her. Collaborate with an occupational therapist, who is trained in selecting the correct type of assistive devices for patients.

You need to support an older adult's ability to perform IADLs such as using a telephone, doing laundry, cleaning the home or apartment, handling money, paying bills, and driving an automobile. To live independently at home or in an apartment, older adults need to be able to perform IADLs, purchase services by outside workers, or have a supportive network of family and friends who help with these tasks. Occupational therapists are an important resource for helping people adapt when IADLs are difficult to perform. Also, it might be appropriate to have a family caregiver assume more responsibility by completing IADLs for patients.

Restorative care measures focus on activities that allow older adults to remain functional and safe within their living environments. Collaborate with an older adult to establish priorities of care and patient goals, determine expected outcomes, and select appropriate interventions. Patient collaboration promotes a patient's understanding about care and minimizes conflicts. Consideration of an older adult's lifetime experiences, values, and sociocultural patterns serves as the basis for planning individual care. When an older adult's cognitive status prevents participation in health care decisions, you need to include the family caregivers. Family and friends are rich sources of data because they knew the older adult before the impairment. Frequently they provide explanations for the older adult's behaviors and suggest methods of management. Thoughtful assessment and planning lead to goals of care that consider the influence of normal aging changes, facilitate an optimal level of comfort and coping, and promote independence in self-care activities.

■ KEY POINTS

- Nurses must be aware of and avoid any preconceived biases against older adults. Instead they must promote a positive perception of older adults.
- Nurses collaborate with older adults in assisting them to achieve their developmental tasks in a healthy manner.
- It is important to differentiate normal changes in aging with disease manifestations.
- Delirium, dementia, and depression share some common symptoms, but an accurate diagnosis is essential for appropriate management.
- Nurses can assist older adults to adapt to psychosocial issues commonly seen in aging.
- There are different types of elder mistreatment; nurses must be alert to cues of mistreatment and report appropriately.
- Nurses should be alert to atypical presentation of illness in older adults.
- Nursing interventions should focus on maintaining maximal functioning and independence.

■ REFLECTIVE LEARNING

Consider an older patient you have recently encountered and consider the following:
- What safety concerns might you have for this person? If the older adult were to return to his or her previous living arrangement, what safety concerns will exist there?
- Describe any concerns you have about how they are adapting to the aging process.
- How have you adapted your communication strategies for this person? Was it effective?

■ REVIEW QUESTIONS

1. A patient's family member is considering having her mother placed in a nursing center. The nurse has talked with the family before and knows that this is a difficult decision. Which of the following criteria does the nurse recommend in choosing a nursing center? (Select all that apply.)
   1. The center needs to be clean, and rooms should look like a hospital room.
   2. Adequate staffing is available on all shifts.
   3. Social activities are available for all residents.
   4. The center provides three meals daily with a set menu and serving schedule.
   5. Staff encourage family involvement in care planning and assisting with physical care.
2. A nurse conducted an assessment of a new patient who came to the medical clinic. The patient is 82 years old and has had osteoarthritis for 10 years and diabetes mellitus for 20 years. He is alert but becomes easily distracted during the assessment. He recently moved to a new apartment, and his pet beagle died just 2 months ago. He is most likely experiencing:
   1. Dementia.
   2. Depression.
   3. Delirium.
   4. Anxiety.
3. A nurse is completing a health history with the daughter of a newly admitted patient who is confused and agitated. The daughter reports that her mother was diagnosed with Alzheimer's disease 1

year ago but became extremely confused last evening and was hallucinating. She was unable to calm her, and her mother thought she was a stranger. On the basis of this history, the nurse suspects that the patient is experiencing:

1. Normal aging.
2. Delirium.
3. Depression.
4. Worsening dementia.

4. Older adults frequently experience a change in sexual activity. Which best explains this change?
    1. The need to touch and be touched is decreased.
    2. The sexual preferences of older adults are not as diverse.
    3. Medication side effects often impact sexual functioning.
    4. Frequency and opportunities for sexual activity may decline.

5. A nurse sees a 76-year-old woman in the outpatient clinic. She states that she recently started to notice a glare in the lights at home. Her vision is blurred, and she is unable to play cards with her friends, read, or do her needlework. Which of the following nursing interventions are appropriate? (Select all that apply.)
    1. Refer her to an ophthalmologist.
    2. Suggest large-print books and playing cards.
    3. Reassure her that this is part of normal aging.
    4. Suggest lower-wattage light bulbs to decrease glare.
    5. Assess her home environment for safety.

6. A 63-year-old patient is retiring from his job at an accounting firm where he was in a management role for the past 20 years. He has been with the same company for 42 years and was a dedicated employee. His wife is a homemaker. She raised their five children, babysits for her grandchildren as needed, and belongs to numerous church committees. What are the major concerns for this patient? (Select all that apply.)
    1. The loss of his work role
    2. The risk of social isolation
    3. A determination on whether the wife will need to start working
    4. How the wife expects household tasks to be divided in the home in retirement
    5. The age the patient chose to retire

7. A nurse is assessing an older adult brought to the emergency department following a fall and wrist fracture. The patient is very thin and unkempt, has a stage 3 pressure injury on her coccyx, and has old bruising to the extremities in addition to her new bruises from the fall. She defers all of the questions to her caregiver son, who accompanied her to the hospital. What is the nurse's next step?
    1. Call social services to begin nursing home placement.
    2. Ask the son to step out of the room so that she can complete her assessment.

3. Call adult protective services because you suspect elder mistreatment.
4. Assess the patient's cognitive status.

8. A nurse is participating in a health and wellness event at the local community center. A woman approaches and relates that she is worried that her widowed father is becoming more functionally impaired and may need to move in with her. The nurse asks about his ability to complete activities of daily living (ADLs). ADLs include independence with: (Select all that apply.)
    1. Driving.
    2. Toileting.
    3. Bathing.
    4. Daily exercise.
    5. Eating.

9. During a home health visit a nurse talks with a patient and his family caregiver about the patient's medications. The patient has hypertension and renal disease. Which of the following findings place him at risk for an adverse drug event? (Select all that apply.)
    1. Taking two medications for hypertension
    2. Taking a total of eight different medications during the day
    3. Having one physician who reviews all medications
    4. Patient's health history of renal disease
    5. Involvement of the caregiver in helping with medication administration

10. A 71-year-old patient enters the emergency department after falling down stairs at church. The nurse is conducting a fall history with the patient and his wife. They live in a one-level ranch home. He has had diabetes for over 15 years and experiences some numbness in his feet. He wears bifocal glasses. His blood pressure is stable at 130/70. The patient does not exercise regularly and states that he experiences weakness in his legs when climbing stairs. He is alert, oriented, and able to answer questions clearly. What are the fall risk factors for this patient? (Select all that apply.)
    1. Impaired vision
    2. Residence design
    3. Blood pressure
    4. Leg weakness
    5. Exercise history

Answers: 1. 2, 3, 5; 2. 2, 3; 3. 2, 4; 4. 5; 5. 1, 2, 5; 6. 1, 4; 7. 2; 8. 2, 3, 5; 9. 2, 4; 10. 1, 4, 5.

Rationales for Review Questions can be found on the Evolve website.

REFERENCES

Administration on Aging (AOA): *A profile of older Americans*, 2017. https://www.acl.gov/sites/default/files/Aging%20and%20Disability%20in%20America/2017OlderAmericansProfile.pdf. Accessed June 15, 2019.

Alderman J: Pain. In Meiner S, Yeager JJ, editors: *Gerontologic nursing*, ed 6, Mosby, 2019.

Alzheimer's Association: *Types of Dementia*, 2018. https://www.alz.org/alzheimers-dementia/what-is-dementia/types-of-dementia. Accessed June 15, 2019.

American Cancer Society (ACS): *Key Statistics for prostate cancer*, 2018. https://www.cancer.org/cancer/prostate-cancer/about/key-statistics.html. Accessed June 15, 2019.

American Foundation for Suicide Prevention: *Suicide statistics*, 2018. https://afsp.org/about-suicide/suicide-statistics/. Accessed June 15, 2019.

American Heart Association: *Understand YOUR risks to prevent a heart attack*, 2016. https://www.heart.org/en/health-topics/heart-attack/understand-your-risks-to-prevent-a-heart-attack. Accessed June 15, 2019.

American Heart Association: *Understanding stroke risk*, 2018. http://www.strokeassociation.org/STROKEORG/AboutStroke/UnderstandingRisk/Understanding-Stroke-Risk_UCM_308539_SubHomePage.jsp. Accessed June 15, 2019.

American Lung Association: How serious is COPD? 2018a. http://www.lung.org/lung-disease/copd/resources/facts-figures/COPD-Fact-Sheet.html. Accessed June 15, 2019.

American Lung Association: *Physical activity and COPD*, 2018b. http://www.lung.org/lung-health-and-diseases/lung-disease-lookup/copd/living-with-copd/physical-activity.html. Accessed June 15, 2019.

Brook S: Nutritional consideration in older adults, *Br J Community Nursing* 23(9):449, 2018.

Bub L: Loss and end-of-life issues. In Meiner S, Yeager JJ, editors: *Gerontologic nursing* ed 6, Mosby, 2019.

Centers for Disease Control and Prevention (CDC): *Compendium of effective fall interventions: what works for community-dwelling older adults*, ed 3, 2015. https://www.cdc.gov/homeandrecreationalsafety/falls/compendium.html. Accessed June 15, 2019.

Centers for Disease Control and Prevention (CDC): *Important facts about falls*, 2017. http://www.cdc.gov/homeandrecreationalsafety/Falls/adultfalls.html. Accessed June 15, 2019.

Centers for Disease Control and Prevention (CDC): Healthcare-associated infections, 2018. https://www.cdc.gov/hai/. Accessed June 15, 2019.

Centers for Disease Control and Prevention (CDC): *National center for injury prevention and control: understanding elder abuse*, 2016. https://www.cdc.gov/violenceprevention/pdf/em-factsheet-a.pdf. Accessed June 15, 2019.

Centers for Medicare and Medicaid Services (CMS): Drug coverage—Part D, (n.d.). http://www.medicare.gov/-/part-d/index.html. Accessed June 15, 2019.

Centers for Medicare & Medicaid Services (CMS): *Your guide to choosing a nursing home or other long-term care*, Baltimore, MD, 2018, CMS. https://www.medicare.gov-/Pubs/pdf/02174-Nursing-Home-Other-Long-Term-Services.pdf. Accessed June 15, 2019.

Davis A: Health promotion and illness/disability prevention. In Meiner S, Yeager JJ, editors: *Gerontologic nursing*, ed 6, Mosby, 2019.

Federal Interagency Forum on Aging-Related Statistics: *Older Americans 2016: key indicators of well-being*, 2016. https://agingstats.gov/docs/LatestReport/Older-Americans-2016-Key-Indicators-of-WellBeing.pdf. Accessed June 15, 2019.

Fulmer T: *Fulmer SPICES: an overall assessment tool for older adults*, 2019. https://consultgeri.org/try-this/general-assessment/issue-1.pdf. Accessed June 15, 2019.

Health in Aging: *home safety tips for older adults*, 2019. http://www.healthinaging.org/resources/resource:home-safety-tips-for-older-adults/. Accessed June 15, 2019.

Jett K: Assessment and documentation for optimal care. In Touhy T, Jett K, editors: *Ebersole and Hess' gerontological nursing and healthy aging*, ed 5, St Louis, 2018a, Mosby.

Jett K: Biological theories of aging and age-related physiological changes. In Touhy T, Jett K, editors: *Ebersole and Hess' gerontological nursing and healthy aging*, ed 5, St Louis, 2018b, Elsevier.

National Cancer Institute (NCI): US National Cancer Institute fact sheet: harms of smoking and health benefits of quitting, 2017. http://www.cancer.gov-/cancertopics/factsheet/Tobacco/cessation. Accessed June 15, 2019.

National Center on Elder Abuse: Adult protective services, n.d. https://ncea.acl.gov/What-We-Do/Practice/Intervention-Partners/APS.aspx. Accessed June 15, 2019.

National Council on Aging: Falls free initiative, n.d. https://www.ncoa.org/healthy-aging/falls-prevention/falls-free-initiative/. Accessed June 15, 2019.

National Institute of Health (NIH): *National Institute on aging: elder abuse*, 2016. https://www.nia.nih.gov-/health/elder-abuse. Accessed June 15, 2019.

National Institute of Health (NIH): *National Institute on aging: aging in place: growing old at home*, 2017. https://www.nia.nih.gov/health/aging-place-growing-old-home. Accessed June 15, 2019.

National Osteoporosis Foundation: *Bone health basics: get the facts*, 2018. https://www.nof.org/preventing-fractures/general-facts/. Accessed June 15, 2019.

National Prevention: *Health promotion, and public health Council: healthy aging in action*, 2016. https://www.surgeongeneral.gov/priorities/prevention/about/healthy-aging-in-action-final.pdf. Accessed June 15, 2019.

Office of Disease Prevention and Health Promotion: *Healthy People 2020, older adults*, 2019. https://www.healthypeople.gov/2020/topics-objectives/topic/older-adults. Accessed June 15, 2019.

Population Reference Bureau: Fact sheet: *Aging in the United States*, 2018. https://www.prb.org/aging-united-states-fact-sheet/. Accessed June 15, 2019.

Touhy T: Psychosocial, spiritual, and cognitive aspects of aging. In Touhy T, Jett K, editors: *Ebersole and Hess' gerontological nursing and healthy aging*, ed 5, St Louis, 2018a, Mosby.

Touhy T: Relationships, roles, and transitions. In Touhy T, Jett K, editors: *Ebersole and Hess' gerontological nursing and healthy aging*, ed 5, St Louis, 2018b, Mosby.

Touhy T: Caregiving. In Touhy T, Jett K, editors: *Ebersole and Hess' gerontological nursing and healthy aging*, ed 5, St Louis, 2018c, Mosby.

Touhy T: Care of individuals with neurocognitive disorders. In Touhy T, Jett K, editors: *Ebersole and Hess' gerontological nursing and healthy aging*, ed 5, St. Louis, 2018d, Mosby.

Touhy T: Hydration and oral care. In Touhy T, Jett K, editors: *Ebersole and Hess' gerontological nursing and healthy aging*, ed 5, St. Louis, 2018e, Mosby.

US Census Bureau: *Income and poverty in the United States: 2016*, 2017. https://www.census.gov/library/publications/2017/demo/p60-259.html. Accessed June 15, 2019.

World Health Organization: *Health promotion: health literacy: the Mandate for health literacy*, 2018. http://www.who.int/healthpromotion/conferences/9gchp/health-literacy/en/. Accessed June 15, 2019.

Xu J, et al: Deaths: Final data for 2016. National Vital Statistics Reports: 67(5). https://www.cdc.gov/nchs/data/nvsr/nvsr67/nvsr67_05.pdf. Accessed June 15, 2019.

Yeager JJ: Sexuality and aging. In Meiner S, Yeager JJ, editors: *Gerontologic nursing*, ed 6, 2019a, Mosby.

Yeager JJ: Drugs and aging. In Meiner S, Yeager JJ, editors: *Gerontologic nursing*, ed 6, 2019b, Mosby.

Yeager JJ: Assessment of the older adult. In Meiner S, Yeager JJ, editors: *Gerontologic nursing*, ed 6, 2019c, Mosby.

RESEARCH REFERENCES

Acierno R, et al.: The national elder mistreatment study: an 8-year longitudinal study of outcomes, *J Elder Abuse Negl* 29(4):254, 2018.

American Geriatrics Society: American geriatrics society 2015 updated Beers criteria for potentially inappropriate medication use in older adults, *J Am Geriatr Soc* 63(11):2227, 2015.

Andrew MK, et al.: Polypharmacy and use of potentially inappropriate medications in long-term care facilities: does coordinated primary care make a difference, *Int J Pharm Pract* 26:318, 2018.

Campbell J, et al.: Assessing statewide need for older adult health promotion services: the Oklahoma experience, *J Soc Serv Res* 44(2), 2018.

Chiu HY, et al.: Reality orientation therapy benefits cognition in older people with dementia: a meta-analysis, *Int J Nurs Stud* 86:20, 2018.

Christiansen A, et al.: Intentional rounding in acute adult healthcare settings: a systematic mixed-method review, *J Clin Nurs* 27:1759–1792, 2018.

Cutilli C, et al.: Health literacy, health disparities, and sources of health information in U.S. older adults, *Orthop Nurs* 37(1):54–64, 2018.

Emiliussen J, et al.: Identifying risk factors for late-onset (50+) alcohol use disorder and heavy drinking: a systematic review, *Subst Use Misuse* 52(12):1575, 2017.

Gibson KM, et al.: Understanding old problem drinkers: the role of drinking to cope, *Addict Behav* 64:101, 2017.

Kaushal N, et al.: The effects of multi-component exercise training on cognitive functioning and health-related quality of life in older adults, *Int J Behav Med* 25(6):617, 2018.

Kendrick D, et al.: Keeping active: maintenance of physical activity after exercise programmes for older adults, *Publish Health* 164:118, 2018.

Kovacevic SV, et al.: Elderly polypharmacy patients' needs and concerns regarding medication assessed using the structured patient-pharmacist consultation model, *Patient Educ Couns* 100:1714, 2017.

Lenander C, et al.: Effects of medication reviews on use of potentially inappropriate medications in elderly patients; a cross-sectional study in Swedish primary care, *BMC Health Serv Res* 18:616, 2018.

Lewis B, et al.: Drinking patterns and adherence to "low-risk" guidelines among community -residing older adults, *Drug Alcohol Depend* 187(1):285, 2018.

O'Mahony D, et al.: STOPP/START criteria for potentially inappropriate prescribing in older people: Version 2, *Age and Aging* 44(2):213, 2015.

Roller M, et al.: Pilates reformer exercises for fall risk reduction in older adults: a randomized controlled trial, *J Bodyw Mov Ther* 22:983, 2018.

Rosen T, et al.: Improving quality of care in hospitals for victims of elder mistreatment: development of the vulnerable elder protection team, *Joint Comm J Qual Patient Saf* 44(3):164, 2018.

Scales K, et al.: Evidence-based nonpharmacological practices to address behavioral and psychological symptoms of dementia, *Gerontol* 58(S1):S88–S102, 2018.

Siverova J, Buzgova R: The effect of reminiscence therapy on quality of life, attitudes to ageing, and depressive symptoms in institutionalized elderly with cognitive impairment: a quasi-experimental study, *Int J Ment Health Nurs* 27(5):1430, 2018.

Tyndall A, et al.: Protective effects of exercise on cognition and brain health in older adults, *Exerc Sport Sci Rev* 46(4):215, 2018.

Van der Linden L, et al.: Medication review versus usual care to improve drug therapies in older inpatients not admitted to geriatric wards: a quasi-experimental study (RASP-IGCT), *BMC Geriatr* 18 (155), 2018.

15

Critical Thinking in Nursing Practice

OBJECTIVES

- Describe the nature of clinical judgments in nursing practice.
- Explain how questioning promotes critical thinking.
- Discuss how reflection improves a nurse's capacity for making future clinical decisions.
- Compare and contrast the three levels of critical thinking.
- Explain the importance of problem solving in nursing practice.
- Describe processes of inductive and deductive reasoning in decision making.
- Describe the components of a critical thinking model for clinical decision making.
- Describe approaches for developing critical thinking skills.

KEY TERMS

Clinical decision making, p. 197
Clinical judgment, p. 197
Concept map, p. 207
Critical thinking, p. 197
Decision making, p. 201

Deductive reasoning, p. 202
Diagnostic reasoning, p. 201
Evidence-based knowledge, p. 197
Inductive reasoning, p. 202
Inference, p. 202

Knowing the patient, p. 202
Nursing process, p. 202
Problem solving, p. 200
Reflection, p. 198
Scientific method, p. 200

MEDIA RESOURCES

http://evolve.elsevier.com/Potter/fundamentals/
- Review Questions
- Case Study with Questions

- Audio Glossary
- Content Updates
- Answers to QSEN Activity and Review Questions

Being a nurse is very challenging. Nurses frequently begin their clinical experiences in hospital settings. In the acute care hospital environment there is a great emphasis on patient-centered care, recognizing a patient or family member as the source of control and full partner in providing compassionate and coordinated care based on a patient's preferences, values, and needs (QSEN, 2018). In addition, hospitals expect evidence-based practice (see Chapter 5) to be routinely applied to ensure better patient outcomes. Amid these expectations is the need to also address patients' satisfaction in care while dealing with ongoing and demanding staffing issues (Chan, 2013). Outpatient clinics, home care agencies, and community health programs also have many of the same expectations as hospitals but with different types of demands. To be competent within any complex health care environment, critical thinking is an essential skill (Chan, 2013).

Every day you think critically without realizing it. If your computer flashes an error warning or your cell phone does not take you to the application you wish, you think about the actions you took before the error, consider possible causes of the problem, and correct a key stroke or reboot the device. If you decide to walk your dogs, go to the door, and notice that it is raining, you decide to change into your raincoat. These simple examples show how you use basic critical thinking skills each day.

As a professional nurse, critical thinking is a bit more complicated. You care for patients with unique, complex health care problems that can change within minutes. Critical thinking becomes embedded in your everyday practice, as it involves knowing as much as possible about each patient and sorting out the information into patterns to clarify problems, recognize changes, and make appropriate care decisions under pressure. Critical thinking is an essential process for safe, efficient, and skillful nursing intervention (Papathanasiou, 2014). Sound critical thinking enables you to face each new experience and problem involving a patient's care with open-mindedness, confidence, and continual inquiry. Critical thinkers do not passively accept information from others or look at information in a cursory way. Instead, thinkers question, seek, and look for answers and deeper meanings (Chan, 2013).

Critical thinking improves patients' outcomes because it helps nurses perform evidence-based practices rather than guessing the facts (Profetto-McGrath, 2005; Chan, 2013). Critical thinking is not a simple step-by-step, linear process that you learn overnight. It is a process gained only through experience, commitment, and an active curiosity toward learning.

CLINICAL JUDGMENT IN NURSING PRACTICE

Registered nurses (RNs) are responsible for making accurate and appropriate clinical decisions or judgments that ensure patients receive appropriate, timely, and effective nursing interventions. A clinical judgment is a conclusion about a patient's needs or health problems and/or the decisions to take or avoid action, use or modify standard approaches, or create new approaches based on the patient's response (Tanner, 2006). Clinical decision making separates professional nurses from assistive personnel (AP). For example, an RN observes for changes in patient's conditions, collects data about the changes, recognizes and identifies new and potential problems, plans nursing strategies, and takes immediate action when a patient's clinical condition worsens. Nurses direct AP to perform basic aspects of care based on patient need; AP do not have the knowledge or critical thinking skills to analyze why or when patients' clinical conditions change and what strategies are required. Good clinical decision making requires you to investigate and analyze all aspects of a clinical problem and then apply scientific and nursing knowledge to choose the best course of action.

In 2006, Dr. Christine Tanner described a research-based model of clinical judgment in nursing. It included the following conclusions:

- Clinical judgments are influenced more by a nurse's experience and knowledge than by the objective data about the situation at hand. Experience is crucial is knowing how to interpret the data.
- Sound clinical judgment partly relies on knowing the patient and his or her typical pattern of responses, as well as engaging with the patient about his or her concerns.
- Clinical judgments are influenced by the context of clinical situations and the culture of patient care settings.
- Nurses use a variety of reasoning approaches in combination, such as problem solving and reflection to understand patient problems and create an individualized plan of care.

Most patients have health care problems for which there are no clear textbook solutions. Each patient's health problems are unique, a product of the patient's physical health, lifestyle, culture, relationship with family and friends, living environment, and experiences. Thus, as a nurse you do not always have a clear picture of a patient's needs and the appropriate actions to take when first meeting a patient. Instead you must learn to question, wonder, and explore different perspectives and interpretations to find a solution that benefits the patient. With experience you learn to creatively seek new knowledge, act quickly when events change, and make quality decisions for patients' well-being.

CRITICAL THINKING DEFINED

Mr. Lawson is a 68-year-old patient who had abdominal surgery for a colon resection and removal of a tumor yesterday. His nurse, Tonya, finds the patient lying supine in bed with his arms held tightly over his abdomen. His facial expression is tense. When Tonya checks the patient's surgical wound, she notes that he winces when she gently places her hands to palpate around the surgical incision. She asks Mr. Lawson when he last turned onto his side, and he responds, "Not since last night." Tonya asks Mr. Lawson if he is having pain around his incision, and he nods yes, saying, "It hurts too much to move." Tonya assesses Mr. Lawson with a pain-rating scale. He rates his pain at a 7 on a scale of 0 to 10. Tonya considers the information she observed and learned from the patient to determine that he is in pain and has reduced mobility because of it. She decides to take action by administering an ordered analgesic. In this case example Tonya observes the patient's clinical situation. She asks questions and reflects on her previous experiences caring for patients who had abdominal surgery. She considers what she knows and has learned about managing postoperative pain and about preventing complications

related to immobility. Tonya makes a clinical decision by applying critical thinking, the ability to think in a systematic and logical manner with openness to question and reflect on the reasoning process.

Critical thinking involves open-mindedness, continual inquiry, and perseverance, combined with a willingness to look at each unique patient situation and determine which identified assumptions are true and relevant. A nurse learns to recognize that a patient problem exists, analyzes information about the problem (e.g., clinical data, observation of patient behavior), interprets the information (reviewing assumptions and evidence, recognizing patterns), and makes conclusions so that he or she can act appropriately. A critical thinker considers what is important in each clinical situation, imagines and explores alternatives, considers ethical principles, and makes informed decisions about the care of patients. The aim of critical thinking is the ability to focus on the important issues at hand in any clinical situation and make decisions that produce desired outcomes (Raterink, 2011).

Critical thinkers question, seek, and examine information for answers and deeper meanings in order to understand their patients (Chan, 2013). *Tonya first learned about the importance of early mobility after surgery when she read the nursing and scientific literature on the concept of mobility and deconditioning. She also learned that pain reduces mobility when she cared for previous patients.* Critical thinking is a way of thinking about clinical situations by asking questions such as:

- "Why does the patient have this condition?"
- "Are the signs and symptoms shown by the patient what I would expect for the condition or situation?"
- "What do I really know about this patient's situation?"
- "What other ways can I collect data to help me understand the problem?"
- "What care options do I have?"

Evidence-based knowledge, or knowledge based on research or clinical expertise, makes nurses better informed critical thinkers (see Chapter 5). Thinking critically and learning about the scientific concepts of deconditioning, comfort, and mobility prepare Tonya to better anticipate Mr. Lawson's needs, identify problems more quickly, and provide appropriate care.

Tonya's review of her observations and the patient's report of pain confirmed her knowledge that pain was likely a problem. Her decision is to give Mr. Lawson an ordered analgesic and wait until it takes effect so that she is able to reposition and make him more comfortable. Once he has less acute pain, Tonya plans to teach Mr. Lawson some relaxation exercises to maintain his comfort. As the patient gains relief, Tonya will consider when to begin the mobility protocol to increase Mr. Lawson's activity level.

You learn to think critically early in your practice. For example, as you learn about giving baths and providing other hygiene measures, take time to read your textbook, online resources, and the scientific literature about the concept of comfort. What are the criteria for comfort? How does a patient's culture affect perceptions of comfort? What are the many factors that promote comfort? When you apply core critical thinking skills to your nursing care, you are using the complex process of clinical decision making (Table 15.1). Being able to apply all of these skills takes practice. You also need to have a sound knowledge base and thoughtfully consider what you learn when caring for patients.

Nurses who apply critical thinking in their work are able to see the big picture from all possible perspectives. They focus clearly on options for solving problems and making decisions rather than quickly and carelessly forming quick solutions (Kataoka-Yahiro and Saylor, 1994). Learning to think critically helps you care for patients as their advocate, or supporter, and make better-informed choices about their care. Facione and Facione (1996) identified concepts for thinking critically (Table 15.2). Critical thinking is more than just problem solving. It is

TABLE 15.1   Critical Thinking and Clinical Judgment Skills

Skill	Nursing Practice Applications
Interpretation	Be orderly in collecting data about patients. Apply reasoning while looking for patterns to emerge. Categorize the data (e.g., nursing diagnoses [see Chapter 17]). Gather additional data and clarify any data about which you are uncertain.
Analysis	Be open-minded as you look at information about a patient. Do not make careless assumptions. Does the data reveal a problem or trend that you believe is true, or are there other options?
Inference	Look at the meaning and significance of findings. Are there relationships among findings? Do data about the patient help you see that a problem exists?
Evaluation	Look at all situations objectively. Use criteria (e.g., expected outcomes, pain characteristics, learning objectives) to determine results of nursing actions. Reflect on your own behavior.
Explanation	Support your findings and conclusions. Use knowledge and experience to choose strategies to use in the care of patients.
Self-regulation	Reflect on your experiences. Be responsible for connecting your actions with outcomes. Identify the ways you can improve your own performance. What will make you believe that you have been successful?

Modified from Facione P: Critical thinking: a statement of expert consensus for purposes of educational assessment and instruction. *The Delphi report: research findings and recommendations prepared for the American Philosophical Association,* ERIC Doc No. ED 315, Washington, DC, 1990, ERIC.; and Tanner CA: Thinking like a nurse: a research-based model of clinical judgment in nursing, *J Nurs Educ* 45(6):204, 2006.

a continuous attempt to improve how you apply your knowledge and experience when faced with problems in patient care (Erickson, 2017).

REFLECT NOW

Consider a patient you have been assigned to recently. Based on that individual patient's needs and health problems, what evidence-based information might you seek to provide evidence-based nursing care?

Reflection

As you care for patients, you will often review your practice experiences to describe, analyze, and evaluate results (Barksby et al., 2015). Such a review is **reflection,** a part of critical thinking that involves purposefully reviewing a situation to discover its purpose or meaning. After caring for a patient, you might ask yourself:

- How did I act?
- Why did I choose such an action?
- What could I have done differently?
- Were the results what I expected?
- What should I do in a similar situation in the future?

As a nurse you will reflect on the purpose and meaning of each patient's situation, as well as the purpose and meaning of your actions in that situation. *For example, before Tonya makes a conclusion about Mr. Lawson's problems, she thinks about previous surgical patients for whom she cared and how they responded to incisional pain. She recalls a patient who had a serious pulmonary embolus (clot in the lung) after surgery and how that pain differed from incisional pain. Reflecting on previous clinical situations prepares Tonya to act knowledgeably and quickly in caring for Mr. Lawson.* Research has shown that when nurses reflect on past experiences, they perceive that their knowledge increases, and their critical thinking moves to a higher level (Kaddoura, 2013).

Reflection is like instant replay. It is not intuitive. It involves purposefully visualizing a past situation and taking the time to honestly review everything you remember about it. This reflection allows you to gain new knowledge and raise questions about your practice, which can lead to a search for better approaches using evidence for practice (Barksby et al., 2015) Research shows that reflective reasoning improves the accuracy of making diagnostic conclusions (see Chapter 17) (Mamede et al., 2012). This means that gathering information about a patient, reflecting on the meaning of your findings, and exploring the possible meaning of those findings improve your ability

TABLE 15.2   Concepts for a Critical Thinker

Concept	Critical Thinking Behavior
Truth seeking	Seek the true meaning of a situation. Be courageous, honest, and objective about asking questions.
Open-mindedness	Be tolerant of different views; be sensitive to the possibility of your own prejudices; respect the right of others to have different opinions.
Analyticity	Analyze potentially problematic situations; anticipate possible results or consequences; value reason; use evidence-based knowledge.
Systematicity	Be organized, focused; work hard in any inquiry.
Self-confidence	Trust in your own reasoning processes.
Inquisitiveness	Be eager to acquire knowledge and learn explanations even when applications of the knowledge are not immediately clear. Value learning for learning's sake.
Maturity	Multiple solutions are acceptable. Reflect on your own judgments; have cognitive maturity.

Modified from Facione N, Facione P: Externalizing the critical thinking in knowledge development and clinical judgment, *Nurs Outlook* 44(3):129, 1996.

to problem solve. Reflection lessens the guesswork in decision making. By reviewing your previous actions, you see successes and opportunities for improvement. Always be cautious in using reflection. Reliance on it can block thinking and not allow you to look at newer evidence or subtle aspects of situations that you have not encountered. Box 15.1 lists steps of a model for using reflection in your practice.

QSEN Building Competency in Patient-Centered Care Think about a patient you recently cared for. Describe how you would use each of the elements of the REFLECT model to incorporate principles of patient-centered care.

Answers to QSEN Activities can be found on the Evolve website.

LEVELS OF CRITICAL THINKING IN NURSING

Your ability to think critically grows as you gain new knowledge and experience in nursing practice. Kataoka-Yahiro and Saylor (1994)

BOX 15.1   Model for Reflection

REFLECT: This model can be used individually or as a process shared with others.

R **Recall** the events. Review the facts about a situation and describe what happened.

E **Examine your responses.** Think about or discuss your thoughts and actions at the time of the situation.

F Acknowledge **Feelings:** Identify any feelings you had during the situation.

L **Learn** from the experience: Review and highlight what you learned from the situation—for example, your patient's responses and your actions.

E **Explore options:** Think about or discuss your options for similar situations in the future.

C **Create** a plan of action: Create a plan for how to act in future similar situations.

T Set a **Time:** Set a time by which your plan of action will be completed.

Adapted from Barksby J, et al: A new model of reflection for clinical practice, *Nurs Times* 111(34/35):21-23, 2015.

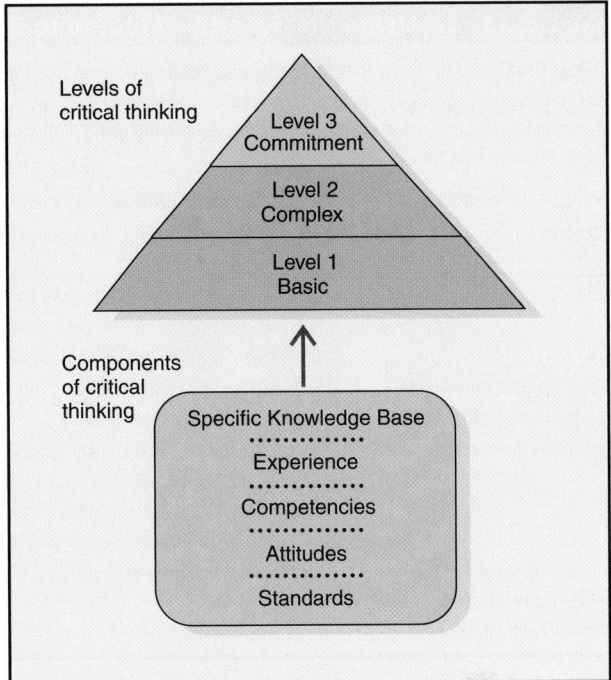

FIG. 15.1 Critical thinking model for nursing judgment. (Redrawn from Kataoka-Yahiro M, Saylor C: A critical thinking model for nursing judgment, *J Nurs Educ* 33(8):351, 1994. Modified from Glaser E: *An experiment in the development of critical thinking,* New York, 1941, Bureau of Publications, Teachers College, Columbia University; Miller M, Malcolm N: Critical thinking in the nursing curriculum, *Nurs Health Care* 11:67, 1990; Paul RW: The art of redesigning instruction. In Willsen J, Blinker AJA, editors: *Critical thinking: how to prepare students for a rapidly changing world,* Santa Rosa, CA, 1993, Foundation for Critical Thinking; and Perry W: *Forms of intellectual and ethical development in the college years: a scheme,* New York, 1979, Holt, Rinehart, & Winston.)

developed a critical thinking model (Fig. 15.1) that includes three levels: basic, complex, and commitment.

Basic Critical Thinking

Beginning nursing students are task oriented as they focus on performing skills and organizing nursing care activities. At the basic level of critical thinking a learner trusts that experts have the right answers for every problem. Thinking is concrete and based on a set of rules or principles. For example, as a nursing student you use a hospital procedure manual to confirm how to change an intravenous (IV) dressing. You are likely to follow the procedure step by step without adjusting it to meet a patient's unique needs (e.g., positioning to minimize the patient's pain or mobility restrictions). You do not have enough experience to anticipate how to individualize the procedure when problems arise. At this level answers to complex problems are perceived as either right or wrong (e.g., when the IV is not infusing correctly, the rate must be regulated correctly), and a single solution usually resolves each problem (e.g., adjusting the rate instead of trying to position the patient's arm to prevent catheter kinking). Basic critical thinking is an early step in developing reasoning (Kataoka-Yahiro and Saylor, 1994). A basic critical thinker learns to accept the diverse opinions and values of experts (e.g., instructors and staff nurse preceptors). However, inexperience, weak competencies, and inflexible attitudes restrict a person's ability to move to the next level of critical thinking (Erickson, 2017).

Complex Critical Thinking

Complex critical thinkers begin to rely less on experts and trust their own decisions more. For example, while teaching a patient how to use an inhaler, you recognize that your patient cannot deliver a dose correctly. Rather than refer to a procedure manual and repeat the same approach, you adapt by offering an inhaler the patient can activate and instruct the patient on how to better coordinate inhaling with delivery of a medication dose. You analyze the clinical situation (e.g., weakness in patient's hands) and examine choices more independently. Critical thinking combined with creativity allows nurses to become more flexible and find original solutions to specific problems when traditional interventions are not effective (Papathanasiou et al., 2014). Creativity also allows nurses to generate many ideas quickly, be able to change viewpoints, and create original problem solutions. A person's thinking abilities and initiative to look beyond expert opinion begin to change. As a nurse you learn that alternative and perhaps conflicting solutions exist.

Consider Mr. Lawson's case. His pain was partially relieved after receiving an analgesic (rating of 4 on scale of 0 to 10), and Tonya has helped him out of bed and into a chair. However, the patient becomes restless, cannot get comfortable, and begins to feel short of breath. Tonya wonders if something other than the incision is causing Mr. Lawson's discomfort. She sits down next to him and asks, "Is the pain you're feeling now different from before I gave you your medication?" The patient tells her that the pain feels sharper, in his chest. Tonya quickly takes a set of vital signs. His heart rate, which was 88 and regular 1 hour ago, is now 102 and irregular. Tonya calls the physician and notifies her of the changes in Mr. Lawson's condition. Tonya thought outside the box. Rather than assume that Mr. Lawson's continued pain was from his incision, she gathered more data and recognized that the patient possibly was experiencing a life-threatening condition, a pulmonary embolus.

In complex critical thinking each solution has benefits and risks that you weigh before making a final decision. There are options. Thinking becomes more innovative. A complex critical thinker considers different options from routine procedures. You gather additional information and take a variety of different approaches for the same therapy.

Commitment

The third level of critical thinking is commitment (Kataoka-Yahiro and Saylor, 1994). At this level you anticipate when to make choices without assistance from others and accept accountability for decisions made. As a nurse you do more than just consider the complex alternatives that a problem poses. At the commitment level you choose an

TABLE 15.3	Using the Scientific Method to Solve Nursing Practice Questions
Clinical Problem: The incidence of a health care–associated infection, *Clostridium difficile* infection, has increased on a hospital general medicine unit. The nursing staff on the unit practice committee, an infection control specialist, and a clinical nurse specialist in medicine meet to discuss factors that may be contributing to the problem. They note that visitors are inconsistent in the use of antiseptic hand rubs. A staff member questions whether the use of hand rubs is the best approach for this type of infection.	
Identify the problem.	The incidence of *C. difficile* has increased among patients on a general medicine unit.
Collect data.	Staff members review the literature about the nature of *C. difficile* infection and the hand antiseptic techniques recommended to prevent the infection.
	Staff members search the literature for studies that have investigated hand-hygiene practices of visitors of hospitalized patients.
	Staff members review performance improvement reports to monitor the occurrence of *C. difficile* on the unit.
	The infection control specialist is asked to discuss the trends within the hospital in the incidence of *C. difficile*.
Form a research question to study the problem.	Does visitor use of antiseptic hand rub with chlorhexidine vs. handwashing with soap and water reduce incidence of *C. difficile* infection in medical patients?
Answer the question.	The nurse specialist and a small team of staff members create a 4-month study approved by the hospital research board.
	Patients' visitors are asked to use a chlorhexidine rub on their hands before entering and leaving patient rooms.
	Visitors switch to handwashing with soap and water for the next 2 months.
	The infection control specialist tracks the incidence of *C. difficile* infection over the 4 months.
Evaluate the results of the study. Does the study answer the research question?	Compare the incidence of *C. difficile* infection for the 2-month period when each hand-hygiene method was used.

action or belief that is based on the available alternatives and support it. Sometimes an action is your decision to not act or to delay an action until a later time based on your experience and knowledge. Because you take accountability for the decision, you consider the results of the decision and determine whether it was appropriate.

CRITICAL THINKING COMPETENCIES

Critical thinking competencies are the cognitive processes a nurse uses to make judgments about the clinical care of patients (Kataoka-Yahiro and Saylor, 1994). These include general critical thinking, specific critical thinking in clinical situations, and specific critical thinking in nursing. General critical thinking processes are not unique to nursing. They include the scientific method, problem solving, and decision making. Specific critical thinking competencies include diagnostic reasoning, clinical inference, and clinical decision making. The specific critical thinking competency in nursing is the nursing process, which involves each of the specific critical thinking competencies.

General Critical Thinking

Scientific Method. The scientific method is a methodical way to solve problems using reasoning. It is a systematic, ordered approach to gather data and solve problems. This approach looks for the truth or verifies that a set of facts agrees with reality. Health care researchers, including nurse scientists, use the scientific method when testing research questions (see Chapter 5). The scientific method has five steps:
1. Identify the problem.
2. Collect data.
3. Formulate a question or hypothesis.
4. Test the question or hypothesis.
5. Evaluate results of the test or study.

Table 15.3 offers an example of a nursing practice issue solved by applying the scientific method in a research study.

Problem Solving. Patients routinely present problems in nursing practice. For example, a home care nurse learns that a patient has difficulty taking her medications regularly. The patient is unable to describe which medications she has taken for the past 3 days. The medication

bottles are labeled and filled. The nurse has to solve the problem of why the patient is not adhering to or following her medication schedule. The nurse knows that when the patient was discharged from the hospital, she had five medications ordered. The patient tells the nurse that she also takes two over-the-counter medications regularly. When the nurse asks her to show the medications that she takes in the morning, the nurse notices that the patient has difficulty seeing the medication labels. The patient is able to describe the medications that she is to take but is uncertain about the times of administration. The nurse recommends having the patient's pharmacy relabel the medications in larger lettering. In addition, the nurse shows the patient examples of pill organizers that will help her sort her medications by time of day for a period of 7 days.

A problem is an unsettled or unsteady state. Effective **problem solving** requires one to obtain information that clarifies the nature of a problem, suggest possible solutions, and try the solution over time to make sure that it is effective. In the case of patient care, a solution to a problem should be consistently effective, allowing a patient to return to a stable condition or situation. It becomes necessary to try different options if a problem recurs. From the previous example, during a follow-up visit the nurse finds that the patient has organized her medications correctly and is able to read the labels without difficulty. The nurse obtained information that correctly clarified the cause of the patient's problem and tested a solution that proved successful. Having solved a problem in one situation adds to a nurse's experience in practice, which allows the nurse to apply that knowledge in future patient situations (Papathanasiou et al, 2014).

Decision Making. When you face a problem and choose a course of action from several options, you are making a decision. Decision making goes hand in hand with problem solving and problem resolution. Following a set of criteria helps you make a thorough and thoughtful decision. The criteria may be personal, based on an organizational policy or standard, or in the case of nursing, based on a professional standard.

For example, a person makes a decision when he or she chooses a health care provider. The individual must first recognize and define the problem (the need for a health care provider) and assess all options (e.g., consider a recommended health care provider or choose one whose office is close to home). The person weighs each option against a set of personal criteria (experience, friendliness, reputation, location), tests possible options (talks directly with the different health care providers), considers the consequences of the decision (examines pros and cons of selecting one provider over another), and makes a final decision. Although the set of criteria follows a sequence of steps, decision making involves moving back and forth when considering all criteria. This process leads to informed conclusions that are supported by evidence and reason. A similar process occurs in clinical nursing.

Specific Critical Thinking

Diagnostic Reasoning. Once you gather information about a patient, as Tonya did in collecting information about Mr. Lawson's discomfort, **diagnostic reasoning** begins. It is a form of decision making. Diagnostic reasoning involves being able to understand and think through clinical problems, look for clues, understand the meaning of evidence, and know when there is enough information to make an accurate diagnosis, consider different causes of the problem, and then select interventions that best meet the needs of a patient (Resnick, 2016; Croskerry and Nimmo, 2011). Accurate recognition of a patient's problems (e.g., nursing diagnoses, collaborative problems) is necessary before choosing solutions and implementing action (Erickson, 2017). The Institute of Medicine (2015) reports that the right diagnosis is a key aspect of health care because it explains a patient's health problem(s) and informs subsequent health care decisions. It requires you to assign meaning to the behaviors and physical signs and symptoms presented by a patient. *For example, what does Mr. Lawson's restlessness, shortness of breath, and developing chest pain indicate? Diagnostic reasoning begins when you interact with a patient or make physical or behavioral observations. An expert nurse sees the context of a patient situation (e.g., Mr. Lawson just had major surgery; has been inactive; and is at risk for blood pooling in the lower extremities, which can cause clots to form in the circulation), observes patterns and themes (e.g., symptoms that include shortness of breath, sharp chest pain, and irregular heart rate), and makes decisions quickly (e.g., a clot may have dislodged and traveled to the patient's lung, requiring a quick medical response).* The information that a nurse collects and analyzes leads to a diagnosis of a patient's condition. Nurses do not make medical diagnoses, but they do assess and monitor each patient closely and compare a patient's signs and symptoms with those that are common to a medical diagnosis (e.g., in the case of Mr. Lawson, a pulmonary embolus). Nurses make nursing diagnoses (see Chapter 17). Through diagnostic reasoning nurses understand the nature of a problem more quickly and select proper therapies.

Part of diagnostic reasoning is the decision-making skill of clinical inference. When making an inference, you form patterns of information from data before making a diagnosis. *In the initial scenario Tonya noted that Mr. Lawson was lying in a position to splint movement of his incision, had a tense facial expression, and experienced tenderness when his wound was palpated. Tonya infers that Mr. Lawson has a level of discomfort.* She demonstrates diagnostic reasoning by identifying the nursing diagnosis *Acute Pain* (see Chapter 17).

Through diagnostic reasoning Tonya gathered and analyzed patient data logically, considered evidence as to the typical problems to expect in a patient after surgery, and recognized a problem. As a student, confirm any judgments you make about nursing diagnoses or a medical problem you believe is developing with experienced nurses. At times you may be wrong, but consulting with nurse experts gives you feedback to build on future clinical situations. Communication is essential with peers due to the complex nature of many clinical problems nurses face.

Often you cannot make a precise diagnosis during your first meeting with a patient. Sometimes you sense that a problem exists but do not have enough data to make a specific diagnosis. Some patients' physical conditions limit their ability to tell you about symptoms. Others choose to not share sensitive and important information during your initial assessment. Some patients' behaviors and physical responses become observable only under conditions not present during your initial assessment. When uncertain of a diagnosis, continue to collect data. Critically analyze changing clinical situations until you are able to determine a patient's unique situation (Croskerry and Nimmo, 2011). Any diagnostic conclusions that you make will help health care providers identify the nature of a problem more quickly and select appropriate medical therapies.

Clinical Decision Making. When you face a clinical problem or situation with a patient and need to choose a course of action from several options, you are making a clinical decision. **Decision making** is a product of critical thinking that focuses on resolving a patient's problem such as a nursing diagnosis (see Chapter 17). When you approach a clinical problem, such as a patient who is less mobile and develops an area of redness over the hip, you make a decision that identifies the problem (impaired skin integrity in the form of a pressure injury) and choose the best nursing interventions (skin care, special bed surface, and a turning schedule). Nurses make clinical decisions all the time to improve a patient's health or maintain wellness by reducing the severity of the problem or resolving the problem completely.

Effective clinical decision making requires inductive and deductive reasoning and making valid inferences. A nurse faces a problem or situation by critically analyzing data to determine important information and ideas and then discards unnecessary data until a later time (Papathanasiou et al., 2014). Following a set of questions or criteria about the data helps a nurse make thorough and thoughtful decisions (Box 15.2). Socratic questioning is a technique for looking beneath the surface, recognizing and examining assumptions, searching for inconsistencies, examining multiple points of view, and differentiating what one knows from what one merely believes (Papathanasiou et al., 2014). These types of questions are common when a nurse completes an end of shift or reviews a patient's history and progress.

After you answer decision-making questions, you begin to form inferences and make conclusions. A set of assessment facts (e.g.,

---

BOX 15.2 Decision-Making Questions

Questions About a Problem
- Is the problem clear and understandable?
- Is the problem important or a priority in the patient's care?

Questions About Your Perspective
- You are looking at the problem from the view of _____. Why?
- How might someone with an opposite view see the problem?
- How does your view compare with that of the patient?

Questions About Assumptions
- You are assuming _____. How does that affect your analysis of the problem?
- What might you assume instead? Is there another option?

Questions About Evidence
- What evidence supports your assumption?
- Is there a reason to doubt the evidence? Does it apply to this specific situation?
- What further evidence is needed?

objective clinical findings, diagnostic test results) and observations about a patient leads a nurse to begin making generalizations and to then perform inductive reasoning. When viewed together, the facts and observations suggest a particular interpretation. Inductive reasoning moves from reviewing specific data elements to making an inference by forming a conclusion about the related pieces of evidence. Previous experience with the evidence is also considered. For example, a nurse who observes a patient who has weakness of lower extremities, an unsteady gait, and a previous history of a fall, considers previous patients cared for and concludes this specific patient is at risk for falling. In contrast, deductive reasoning moves from the general to the specific. A nurse will start analysis of the facts and observations from a conceptual viewpoint, such as prioritization of needs by Maslow or Nola Pender's health promotion model. Then the nurse forms an inference and eventually interprets the patient's condition with respect to the conceptual view (Papathanasiou et al., 2014).

Skilled clinical decision making occurs through knowing the patient (Zolnierek, 2014). Knowing the patient is an in-depth knowledge of a patient's patterns of responses within a clinical situation and knowing the patient as a person (Tanner et al., 1993). While nurses use prior clinical experiences and interactions with patients as key sources of knowledge, these sources are limited for nurses with less experience and in care situations in which the patient's ability to interact may be affected by developmental age (e.g., an infant) or medical state (e.g., intubated) (Kelley et al., 2013). Nonetheless, you need to know your patients to develop your clinical expertise. Knowing a patient has two components: a nurse's understanding of a specific patient and his or her subsequent selection of interventions. It relates to a nurse's experience with caring for patients, time spent in a specific clinical area, and having a sense of closeness with patients. For example, an expert nurse who has worked on a general surgery unit for many years has cared for a patient the past 2 days. The nurse is familiar with how the patient is progressing physically and mentally. When the patient begins to experience a change (e.g., a slight fall in blood pressure, becoming less responsive), the nurse knows that something is wrong, suspects the patient may be bleeding internally, and takes action. Because of the nurse's clinical experience and knowing the patient, the expert nurse can make a clinical decision and act more quickly than a new nurse can be expected to act.

Knowing the patient is central to individualizing nursing care so that a patient feels cared for and cared about (Zolnierek, 2014). Knowing offers a nurse "the big picture" and "knowing the whole person" so that he or she can make suitable decisions to protect patients from harm. Henneman et al. (2010) found that knowing the patient enabled nurses to identify problems and potential errors and thus rescue their patients from potential adverse events. A critical aspect to knowing patients and thus being able to make timely and appropriate decisions is spending time establishing relationships with them (Zolnierek, 2014). Forming relationships builds your ability to make clinical decisions and enhances your ability to know your patients. Follow these tips:

- Spend enough time during initial and follow-up patient assessments to observe patient behavior and measure physical and psychosocial findings as a way to improve knowledge of your patients. Determine what is important to them, and make a positive emotional connection. Patients perceive meaningful time as that involving personal rather than task-oriented conversation.
- Know trends and normative patterns in a patient's clinical condition over time so that you can identify when patients require a change in their treatment plan (Kelley et al., 2013).
- Know a patient's typical behaviors, schedules, and preferences at home to help guide you with their stay in a hospital or extended-care

setting (Kelley et al., 2013). This allows you to adjust and provide individualized patient-centered care.

- When talking with patients, listen to their accounts of their experiences with illness, watch them, and come to understand how they typically respond (Tanner, 2006).
- Consistently check on patients to assess and monitor problems to help you identify how clinical changes develop over time.
- Ask to have the same patient assigned to you over consecutive days. Researchers have noted that a nurse-patient relationship develops from getting to know a patient and building a foundation for connecting on the first day of care, to deepening understanding of the patient and sustaining a connection by the second day, to being comfortable with the patient by the third day (Lotzkar and Bottorff, 2010).
- Engaging patients in conversations and being able to care for them over time (e.g., days or visits) develops knowing and nurse-patient relationships (Zolnierek, 2014).

Always keep a patient as your center of focus when solving clinical problems. Making accurate patient-centered clinical decisions allows you to prioritize the interventions to implement first (see Chapter 18). Do not assume that certain health situations produce automatic priorities. For example, a patient who has surgery is anticipated to experience a certain level of postoperative pain, which often becomes a priority for care. However, if a patient is having severe anxiety that increases pain perception, you need to focus on ways to relieve the anxiety before pain-relief measures will be effective.

Critical thinking and clinical decision making are complicated because nurses care for multiple patients in fast-paced and unpredictable environments. When you provide patient care, use decision criteria that include the clinical condition of the patient, Maslow's hierarchy of needs (see Chapter 6), the risks involved in treatment delays, environmental factors (staff resources available), and patients' expectations of care to determine which patients have the greatest priorities. For example, a patient who is having a sudden drop in blood pressure along with a change in consciousness requires your immediate attention as opposed to a patient who needs you to collect a urine specimen or one who needs your help to walk down the hallway. Critical thinking in decision making allows you to attend to a patient whose condition is changing quickly and delegate the specimen collection and ambulation to assistive personnel. For you to manage the wide variety of problems associated with groups of patients, skillful, prioritized clinical decision making is critical (Box 15.3).

REFLECT NOW

Ask a nurse who works in one of the health care agencies where you have clinicals to spend a moment talking to you about knowing patients. Ask the nurse what he or she does to know patients. Also discuss the barriers that make knowing patients difficult.

NURSING PROCESS COMPETENCY

Nurses apply the nursing process as a competency when delivering patient care (Kataoka-Yahiro and Saylor, 1994). The American Nurses Association (ANA) (2010) standards provide the framework necessary for critical thinking in the application of the five-step nursing process: assessment, diagnosis, planning, implementation, and evaluation. The purpose of the nursing process is to diagnose and treat human responses (e.g., patient symptoms, need for knowledge) to actual or potential health problems (ANA, 2010). Use of the process allows nurses to help patients meet agreed-on outcomes for better health (Fig. 15.2). The nursing process requires a nurse to use the general and specific critical thinking competencies described earlier to focus on a patient's unique needs. The format for the nursing process is unique to the discipline of nursing and provides a common language and process for nurses to "think through" patients' clinical problems (Kataoka-Yahiro and Saylor, 1994).

A CRITICAL THINKING MODEL FOR CLINICAL DECISION MAKING

Because critical thinking is complex, a model helps explain the steps in making clinical decisions and judgments about your patients. Kataoka-Yahiro and Saylor (1994) developed a model of critical thinking for nursing judgment based in part on previous works by Paul (1993) and Miller and Malcolm (1990) (see Fig. 15.1). This model is still relevant today. It defines the outcome of critical thinking: nursing judgment that is relevant to nursing problems in a variety of health care settings. The model includes five elements of critical thinking in nursing judgment: competence (e.g., problem solving and clinical decision-making ability), knowledge, experience, attitudes, and standards (intellectual and professional). The five elements combined guide nurses in making clinical decisions that lead to safe, effective nursing care (Box 15.4). Throughout this text the model helps you to apply critical thinking as part of the nursing process. Graphic illustration of the model in the clinical chapters shows you how to apply critical thinking in assessing patients, planning and delivering interventions, and evaluating the results. Applying elements of the model will help you become a more confident and effective professional.

Competence

The first element of critical thinking is competence—in this case, competence in the use of the nursing process. Competence also involves the ability to perform nursing skills (e.g., hands-on procedures, physical examination techniques) proficiently. Until your nursing skills become like second nature, they create a distraction, making it difficult for you as a new nurse to focus on important critical thinking competencies such as gathering data, problem solving, and clinical decision making. You will develop competence as you continue to practice and perform nursing skills.

Specific Knowledge Base

A nurse's specific knowledge base varies according to educational experience that includes basic nursing education, continuing education courses, and additional college degrees. A nurse also builds knowledge by reading the nursing literature (especially research-based literature) to maintain current knowledge of nursing science and theory. Knowledge prepares a nurse to better anticipate and identify patient problems by understanding their origin and nature.

A nurse's knowledge base includes information and theory from the basic sciences, humanities, behavioral sciences, and nursing science. Nurses use this knowledge base in a different way than other health care disciplines because they think holistically about patient problems. For example, a nurse's broad knowledge base offers a physical, psychological, social, moral, ethical, and cultural view of patients and their health care needs. The depth and extent of knowledge influence your ability to think critically about nursing problems.

BOX 15.3 Clinical Decision Making for Groups of Patients

- Identify the nursing diagnoses and collaborative problems of each patient (see Chapter 17).
- Analyze the diagnoses/problems and decide which are most urgent on the basis of basic needs, the patients' changing or unstable status, and problem complexity (see Chapter 18).
- Consider the time it will take to care for patients whose problems are of high priority (e.g., do you have the time to restart a critical intravenous [IV] line when medication is due for a different patient?).
- Consider the resources you have to manage each problem, assistive personnel assigned with you, other health care providers, and patients' family members.
- Involve patients and/or their family as decision makers and participants in care.
- Decide how to combine activities to resolve more than one patient problem at a time.
- Decide which, if any, nursing care procedures to delegate to assistive personnel so that you are able to spend your time on activities requiring professional nursing knowledge.
- Discuss complex cases with other members of the health care team. This ensures a smooth transition in care throughout a patient's health care experience.

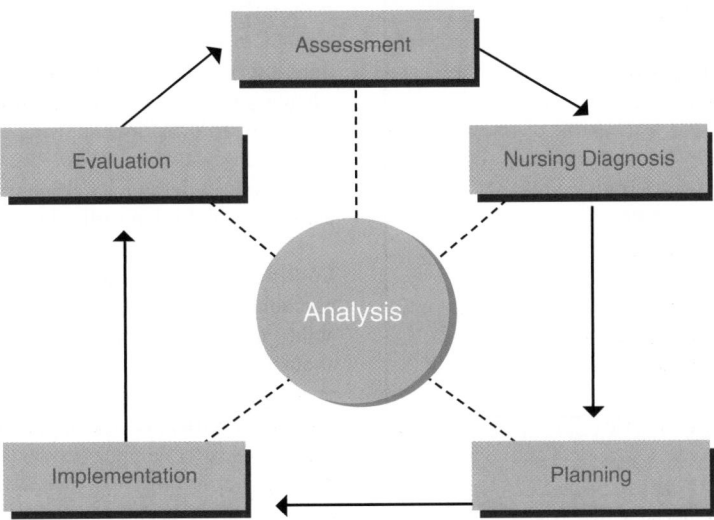

FIG. 15.2 Five-step nursing process model.

Tonya previously earned a bachelor's degree in education and taught high school for 1 year. She is now in her second year as an RN. She is taking additional classes to further her education, including courses in health ethics and population health. Her experience as a staff nurse has allowed her to develop knowledge about a variety of surgical procedures, the effects of different medications, and responses patients typically show to their treatment. Although she is still new to nursing, her experiences as a teacher and her preparation and knowledge base in nursing help her know how to interact and form relationships with patients that help her make clinical decisions about patients' health promotion practices.

Experience

Nursing is a practice discipline. Clinical learning experiences are necessary to acquire clinical decision-making skills. Knowledge combined with clinical expertise from experience defines critical thinking. In clinical situations you learn from observing, sensing, talking with patients and families, and reflecting actively on all experiences. Clinical experience is the laboratory for developing and testing approaches that you safely adapt or revise to fit the setting, a patient's unique qualities, and

---

BOX 15.4 Components of Critical Thinking in Nursing

I. Specific knowledge base in nursing
II. Experience
III. Critical thinking competencies
   A. General critical thinking
   B. Specific critical thinking
   C. Specific critical thinking in nursing: nursing process
IV. Attitudes for critical thinking
   Confidence, independence, fairness, responsibility, risk taking, discipline, perseverance, creativity, curiosity, intellectual integrity, humility
V. Standards for critical thinking
   A. Intellectual standards
     Clear—Plain and understandable (e.g., clarity in how one communicates).
     Precise—Exact and specific (e.g., focusing on one problem and possible solution).
     Specific—To mention, describe, or define in detail
     Accurate—True and free from error; getting to the facts (objective and subjective)
     Relevant—Essential and crucial to a situation (e.g., a patient's changing clinical status)
     Plausible—Reasonable or probable
     Consistent—Expressing consistent beliefs or values
     Logical—Engaging in correct reasoning from what one believes in a given instance to the conclusions that follow
     Deep—Containing complexities and multiple relationships
     Broad—Covering multiple viewpoints (e.g., patient and family)
     Complete—Thoroughly thinking and evaluating
     Significant—Focusing on what is important and not trivial
     Adequate (for purpose)—Satisfactory in quality or amount
     Fair—Being open-minded and impartial
   B. Professional standards
     1. Ethical criteria for nursing judgment
     2. Criteria for evaluation
     3. Professional responsibility

Modified from Kataoka-Yahiro M, Saylor C: A critical thinking model for nursing judgment, *J Nurs Educ* 33(8):351, 1994. Data from Paul RW: The art of redesigning instruction. In Willsen J, Blinker AJA, editors: *Critical thinking: how to prepare students for a rapidly changing world*, Santa Rosa, CA, 1993, Foundation for Critical Thinking.

---

the experiences you have from caring for previous patients. Research has shown that a clinical environment that is safe and encourages free discussion and expression of thought promotes critical thinking (Chan, 2013). With experience you begin to understand clinical situations, anticipate and recognize cues of patients' health patterns, and interpret the cues as relevant or irrelevant. Learn to value all patient experiences, which become stepping-stones for building new knowledge and inspiring innovative thinking.

When Tonya was finishing her last year in nursing school, she worked as a nurse assistant in a nursing home. Through this experience she spent time interacting with older-adult patients and giving basic nursing care. Each patient provided her with valuable learning experiences, which she applied in her work with other patients. Specifically, she developed good interviewing skills, gained an understanding of the importance of the family in an individual's health, and learned to become a patient advocate. She also learned that older adults need more time to perform activities such as eating, bathing, and grooming; therefore, she has adapted these skill techniques.

The Nursing Process Competency

The nursing process competency is the third component of the critical thinking model. In your practice you will apply critical thinking components during each step of the nursing process. Chapters 16 through 20 describe each step of the nursing process.

Attitudes for Critical Thinking

The fourth component of the critical thinking model is attitudes. Paul (1993) defined 11 attitudes that define the central features of a critical thinker and how a successful critical thinker approaches a problem (see Box 15.4). In a consensus statement on critical thinking in nursing, an international panel of nurse experts defined additional attitudes that included contextual perspective, flexibility, and open-mindedness (Scheffer and Rubenfeld, 2000). Papathanasiou and colleagues (2014) also describe spiritual courage as a critical thinking attitude.

An example of applying critical thinking attitudes involves a patient who complains of anxiety before a diagnostic procedure. A curious nurse seeks an explanation and information by asking several questions to learn what the patient does not know and the nature of the patient's concerns (Kaddoura, 2013). The nurse shows discipline in forming questions and collecting a thorough assessment to find the source of the patient's anxiety. Attitudes of inquiry involve an ability to recognize that problems exist, to consider the context of those problems, and to recognize that there is a need for evidence to support what you think is true. Critical thinking attitudes are guidelines for how to approach a problem or decision-making situation. Important parts of critical thinking are interpreting, evaluating, and making judgments about the adequacy of various arguments and available data. Knowing when you need more information, knowing when information is misleading, and recognizing your own knowledge limits are examples of how critical thinking attitudes guide decision making. Table 15.4 summarizes the use of critical thinking attitudes in nursing practice.

Confidence. Confidence is the belief in oneself, one's judgment and psychomotor skills, and one's possession of the knowledge and the ability to think critically. When you are confident, you feel certain about accomplishing a task or goal such as performing a procedure or making a diagnosis. Confidence grows with experience in recognizing your strengths and limitations. You shift your focus from your own needs (e.g., remembering what assessment data mean or how to perform a procedure) to a patient's needs. When you are not confident in knowing whether a patient is clinically changing or in performing a nursing skill, you become anxious about not knowing what to do.

TABLE 15.4 Critical Thinking Attitudes and Applications in Nursing Practice

Critical Thinking Attitude	Application in Practice
Confidence	The nurse, gaining more experience in reasoning and decision making, does not hesitate to disagree and be troubled, thereby acting as a role model to colleagues (Papathanasiou et al., 2014). Speak with conviction to a patient when you begin an intervention. Do not lead a patient to think that you are unable to perform care safely. Always be well prepared before performing a nursing activity. Encourage a patient to ask questions.
Thinking independently	As you acquire new knowledge and experiences, examine your beliefs under new evidence (Papathanasiou et al., 2014). Be open-minded about different interventions. Read the scientific literature, especially when there are different views on the same subject. Talk with other nurses and share ideas about nursing interventions.
Fairness	Listen to both sides of a discussion. If a patient or family member complains about a co-worker, listen to the story and speak with the co-worker as well. If a staff member labels a patient uncooperative, assume the care of that patient with openness and a desire to meet the patient's needs.
Responsibility and authority	Ask for help if you are uncertain about how to perform a nursing skill. Refer to a policy and procedure manual to review steps of a skill. Report any problems immediately. Follow standards of practice in your care.
Risk taking	If your knowledge causes you to question a health care provider's order, do so. Be willing to recommend alternative approaches to nursing care when colleagues are having little success with patients, especially if your ideas are supported with scientific evidence.
Discipline	Be thorough in whatever you do. Use known scientific and practice-based criteria for activities such as assessment and evaluation. Take time to be thorough and manage your time effectively.
Perseverance	Be cautious of an easy answer that avoids uncomfortable situations. If co-workers give you information about a patient and some fact seems to be missing, clarify the information or talk to the patient directly. If problems of the same type continue to occur on a nursing division, bring co-workers together, look for a pattern, and find a solution.
Creativity	Look for different approaches if interventions are not working for a patient. For example, a patient in pain may need a different positioning or distraction technique. When appropriate, involve the patient's family in adapting your approaches to care methods used at home.
Curiosity	Always ask why. Be willing to challenge tradition. A clinical sign or symptom often indicates a variety of problems. Explore and learn more about a patient so as to make appropriate clinical judgments.
Integrity	Recognize when your opinions conflict with those of a patient; review your position and decide how best to proceed to reach outcomes that will satisfy everyone. Do not compromise nursing standards or honesty in delivering nursing care.
Humility	Recognize when you need more information to make a decision. When you are new to a clinical division, ask for an orientation to the area. Ask registered nurses (RNs) regularly assigned to the area for assistance with approaches to care.

This prevents you from attending to the patient. Always be aware of the extent and limits of your knowledge. If you question the meaning of a clinical situation and you don't know whether the information you have is important, discuss it with your nursing instructor first. Never perform a procedure unless you have the knowledge base and feel confident. Patient safety is of the utmost importance. When you show confidence, your patients recognize it by how you communicate and the way you perform nursing care. Confidence builds trust between you and your patients.

Thinking Independently. As you gain new knowledge, you learn to consider a wide range of ideas and concepts before forming an opinion or making a judgment. You are not limited by what you learn in school but become open-minded to new concepts and interventions (Papathanasiou et al., 2014). This does not mean that you ignore other people's ideas. Instead you learn to consider all sides of a situation. A critical thinker does not accept another person's ideas without question. When thinking independently, you challenge the ways that others think and look for rational and logical answers to problems. You raise important questions about your practice. For example, why is one type of surgical dressing ordered over another, or why do patients on your nursing unit fall? When nurses ask questions and look for the evidence behind clinical problems, they are thinking independently; this is an important step in evidence-based practice (see Chapter 5). Independent thinking and reasoning are essential to the improvement and expansion of nursing practice.

Fairness. A critical thinker deals with situations justly. This means that you do not let bias or prejudice affect your decisions. For example, regardless of how you feel about obesity, you do not allow personal attitudes to influence the way you care for a patient who is overweight. Look at a situation objectively and consider all viewpoints to understand the situation completely before making a decision. Having a sense of imagination helps you develop an attitude of fairness. Imagining what it is like to be in your patient's situation helps you see it with new eyes and appreciate its complexity.

Responsibility and Accountability. Responsibility is the knowledge that you are accountable for your decisions, actions, and critical thinking. When caring for patients, you are responsible for correctly performing nursing care activities on the basis of standards of practice. Standards of practice are the minimum level of performance accepted to ensure high-quality care. For example, you do not take shortcuts or work-arounds when you give a patient a medication (e.g., skipping a step—failing to identify a patient, preparing medication doses for multiple patients at the same time). Professional nurses are responsible for competently performing nursing therapies and making clinical decisions about patients. As a nurse you are answerable or accountable for your decisions, the outcomes of your actions, and knowing the limits and scope of your practice.

Risk Taking. People often associate taking risks with danger. Driving 30 miles an hour over the speed limit is a risk that sometimes results in injury to a driver and an unlucky pedestrian. But risk taking does not always have negative outcomes. Risk taking is desirable, particularly when the result is a positive outcome. A critical thinker will take risks when trying different ways to solve problems. The willingness to take risks comes from experience with similar problems. Risk taking often leads to advances in patient care. In the past nurses have taken risks when trying different approaches to skin and wound care and pain management, to name a few. When taking a risk, follow safety guidelines, analyze any potential dangers to a patient, and act in a well-reasoned, logical, and thoughtful manner. Risk taking does not eliminate the need to incorporate evidence into practice approaches.

Discipline. A disciplined thinker misses few details and is orderly or systematic when collecting information, making decisions, or taking action. For example, you have a patient who is in pain. Instead of only asking the patient, "How severe is your pain on a scale of 0 to 10?" you also ask more specific questions about the character of pain (e.g., "What makes the pain worse? Where does it hurt? How long have you noticed it?"). Being disciplined helps you identify problems more accurately and select the most appropriate interventions.

Perseverance. A critical thinker is determined to find effective solutions to patient care problems. This is especially important when problems remain unresolved or recur. Learn as much as possible about a problem and try various approaches to care. Persevering means to keep looking for more resources until you find a successful approach. It often requires creativity. For example, a patient who is unable to speak following throat surgery poses challenges for the nurse to communicate effectively. Perseverance leads the nurse to try different communication approaches (e.g., message boards or alarm bells) until he or she finds a method that is effective. A critical thinker who perseveres is not satisfied with minimal effort but works to achieve the highest level of quality care.

Creativity. Creativity involves original thinking. This means that you find solutions outside the standard routines of care while still following standards of practice. Creativity motivates you to think of options and unique approaches. A patient's clinical problems, social support systems, and living environment are just a few examples of factors that make the simplest nursing procedure more complicated. For example, a home care nurse has to find a way to help an older patient with arthritis have greater mobility in the home. The patient has difficulty lowering and raising herself in a chair because of pain and limited range of motion in her knees. The nurse uses wooden blocks to elevate the chair legs so that the patient is able to sit and stand with little discomfort while making sure that the chair is safe to use.

Curiosity. A critical thinker's favorite question is "Why?" In any clinical situation you learn a great deal of information about a patient. As you analyze patient information, data patterns appear that are not always clear. Having a sense of curiosity (asking yourself, "What if?") motivates you to inquire further (e.g., question family or physician, review the scientific literature) and investigate a clinical situation so that you get all the information you need to make a decision.

Integrity. Critical thinkers question and test their own knowledge and beliefs. Your personal integrity as a nurse builds trust from your co-workers. Nurses face many dilemmas or problems in everyday clinical practice, and everyone makes mistakes at times. A person of integrity is honest and willing to admit to mistakes or inconsistencies in his or her own behavior, ideas, and beliefs. A professional nurse always tries to follow the highest standards of practice.

Humility. It is important for you to admit to any limitations in your knowledge and skill. Critical thinkers admit what they do not know and try to find the knowledge needed to make proper decisions. It is common for a nurse to be an expert in one area of clinical practice but a novice in another because the knowledge in all areas of nursing is unlimited. A patient's safety and welfare are at risk if you do not admit your inability to deal with a practice problem. You have to rethink a situation; learn more; and use the new information to form opinions, draw conclusions, and take action.

Mr. Lawson continues to have chest pain and shortness of breath. As Tonya waits for the medical team to arrive, she knows that she is responsible for his welfare until treatment can be initiated. Tonya acts independently by keeping Mr. Lawson comfortable in the chair, not moving him (to avoid worsening of his condition) and gathering additional assessment data. She displays discipline in further assessing Mr. Lawson's condition: rechecking vital signs, observing his abdominal wound and incision, and talking with him to notice if there is a change in consciousness. Tonya knows that she cannot diagnose medically. When the health care provider arrives, she objectively reports what happened with Mr. Lawson once he sat up in the chair, the symptoms he displayed, and how those symptoms have changed.

Standards for Critical Thinking

The fifth component of the critical thinking model includes intellectual and professional standards (Kataoka-Yahiro and Saylor, 1994).

Intellectual Standards. Paul (1993) identified 14 intellectual standards (see Box 15.4) universal for critical thinking. An intellectual standard is a guideline or principle for rational thought. You apply these standards during all steps of the nursing process. For example, when you consider a patient problem, apply the intellectual standards of preciseness, accuracy, and consistency in measurement to make sure that you have all the data you need to make sound clinical decisions. During planning, apply standards such as being logical and significant so that the plan of care is meaningful and relevant to a patient's needs. A thorough use of intellectual standards in clinical practice prevents you from performing critical thinking haphazardly.

The health care provider orders a lung scan and chest x-ray and places Mr. Lawson on bed rest. Blood tests are also ordered in anticipation of placing the patient on anticoagulation (to prevent further clot formation). Tonya asks the physician whether there are risks to be considered regarding Mr. Lawson's wound should the patient receive an anticoagulant (relevant question). She also asks if she can give additional pain medication at this time to manage the patient's surgical incision pain during the x-ray procedures (logical decision). By applying intellectual standards, Tonya is a competent partner in managing the patient's care, showing her ability to anticipate possible clinical problems.

Professional Standards. Professional standards for critical thinking refer to ethical criteria for nursing judgments, evidence-based criteria used for evaluation, and criteria for professional responsibility (Paul, 1993). Application of professional standards requires you to use critical thinking for the good of individuals or groups (Kataoka-Yahiro and Saylor, 1994). Professional practice standards improve patient outcomes and maintain a high level of quality nursing care.

Excellent nursing practice is a reflection of ethical standards (see Chapter 22). Being able to focus on a patient's values and beliefs helps you make clinical decisions that are just, respectful of a patient's choices, and beneficial to a patient's well-being. Critical thinkers maintain a sense of self-awareness through conscious awareness of their own beliefs, values, and feelings and the multiple perspectives that patients, family members, and peers present in clinical situations.

Critical thinking also requires the use of evidence-based criteria for making clinical judgments. These criteria are sometimes scientifically based on research findings (see Chapter 5) or practice based on standards developed by clinical experts and performance improvement initiatives of an institution. Examples are the clinical practice guidelines developed by individual clinical agencies and national organizations such as the American Association of Critical Care Nurses (AACN) or Oncology Nursing Society (ONS). A clinical practice guideline includes standards for the treatment of select clinical conditions such as stroke, deep vein thrombosis, and pressure injuries. Another example is clinical criteria used to categorize clinical conditions such as the criteria for staging pressure injuries (see Chapter 48) and rating phlebitis (see Chapter 42). Evidence-based evaluation criteria set the minimum requirements necessary to ensure appropriate and high-quality care.

The standards of professional responsibility that a nurse tries to achieve are the standards cited in Nurse Practice Acts, institutional practice guidelines, and professional organizations' standards of practice (e.g., The ANA Standards of Professional Performance (see Chapter 1). These standards "raise the bar" for the responsibilities and accountabilities that a nurse assumes in guaranteeing quality health care to the public.

DEVELOPING CRITICAL THINKING SKILLS

Although you will need time to develop critical thinking skills, start now by actively engaging patients who are in your care. Apply the principles of the critical thinking model that have been presented in this chapter. Many factors in health care settings pose barriers to critical thinking. Rising patient acuity, decreasing length of stay, and conflicts in professional relationships are a few of the factors that challenge even experienced nurses who are adept at critical thinking.

Reflective Journaling

Reflective journaling is a tool for developing critical thought and reflection by clarifying concepts (Raterink, 2016). It involves keeping a written record of your clinical experiences in your own words in a personal journal. Remember to keep your journal entries confidential so that if someone else reads your journal, patient identity is protected. Returning to the journal after each clinical experience gives you the chance to record the perceptions you had during patient care and better develop the ability to apply theory in practice. Oftentimes reflections are on things that go wrong; however, reflecting on things that went well can be just as rewarding and useful to build confidence in your practice (Kiron et al., 2017). Journaling also improves your observational and descriptive skills. Writing skills improve as you learn to clearly describe concepts applied in practice (e.g., suffering, hope, powerlessness). A journal increases your experiential learning during clinical experiences (Silvia, 2013). Here are examples of questions to pose in a journal:

- What did I learn from the experience?
- Did I respond appropriately in this situation? If not, how should I have responded?
- What were the consequences of my actions? Whom did they affect and in what way?
- How might I act differently in the future?
- Was I working from tradition or evidence-based practices?

Meeting with Colleagues

A way to develop critical thinking skills is to regularly meet with colleagues such as fellow students or nurses, faculty members, or preceptors to discuss and examine work experiences and validate decisions.

Connecting with others helps you learn that you do not need to know everything because support is available from other colleagues. When nurses have a formal means to discuss their experiences, such as a staff meeting or unit practice council, the dialogue allows for questions, differing viewpoints, and sharing of experiences. When they are able to discuss their practices, the process validates good practice and also offers challenges and constructive criticism. A discussion of critical incidents that occur in the live clinical setting is invaluable for developing critical thinking (LaMartina and Ward-Smith, 2014). Much can be learned by drawing from others' experiences and perspectives to promote reflective critical thinking.

Concept Mapping

As a nurse you will care for patients who have multiple nursing diagnoses and/or collaborative problems. A concept map is a visual representation of patient problems and interventions that shows their relationships to one another. It is a nonlinear picture of a patient to be used for comprehensive care planning. Research shows that when compared with traditional educational methods, concept mapping can improve students' critical thinking ability as measured by various critical thinking skills tests and scales (Yue et al., 2017). However, more high-quality studies are needed to support these findings.

Concept maps help you better synthesize relevant data about a patient, including assessment data, nursing diagnoses, health needs, nursing interventions, and evaluation measures. Through drawing a concept map, you learn to organize or connect information in a unique way, so the diverse information that you have about a patient begins to form meaningful patterns and concepts. You begin to see a more holistic view of a patient. When you see the relationship between the various patient diagnoses and the data that support them, you better understand a patient's clinical situation. Sample concept maps can be found in the clinical chapters of this text (see Units V and VI).

MANAGING STRESS

The connection between stress in a health care setting and its effects on a nurse's mental and physiological state is receiving more attention. Autonomic control of decision making, error detection, speech, memory, and emotions during stressful situations are disrupted because of continued sympathetic nervous system stimulation. Research has shown that the stress of working 12-hour shifts, for example, can impair nursing judgment, in part because of the way stress affects attention (McClelland et al., 2013). The work of professional nursing is difficult as you see patients endure suffering from disease and painful therapies and as you try to manage care responsibilities in busy, fast-paced work settings (Box 15.5). Stress over a prolonged period or when extreme can lead to poor work productivity, impaired decision making and communication, and reduced ability to cope with clinical situations. Chapter 37 offers perspectives on ways to better manage stress so that you can make clear, thoughtful decisions and communicate effectively with health care colleagues.

CRITICAL THINKING SYNTHESIS

Critical thinking is a reasoning process by which you reflect on and analyze your thoughts, action, and knowledge. As a beginning nurse, it is important to learn the steps of the nursing process and incorporate the elements of critical thinking (Fig. 15.3). The two processes go hand in hand in making quality decisions about patient care. This text provides a model to show you how important critical thinking is in the practice of the nursing process.

BOX 15.5   EVIDENCE-BASED PRACTICE

Stress Management

PICOT Question: For staff nurses who experience stress in clinical settings, does stress management compared with no intervention reduce stress?

Evidence Summary

In a qualitative study by van Graan and colleagues (2016), practicing nurses recognized clinical practice as a stressful experience, more so for a novice nurse. A positive relationship between the nursing staff on a unit and nursing students is a crucial factor in creating a positive learning environment. The study participants proposed that the first clinical experience of novice nursing students should be positive and an example of what nursing entails (van Graan et al., 2016). A high level of anxiety can lead to decreased learning as students focus on their anxiety and being accepted rather than on learning. Concern regarding the stress nurses face has resulted in the American Nurses Association (ANA) creating the goal of improving the work life of health care providers, along with an original aim of improving the care experience (Cipriano, 2016). Improving work life means ensuring an ethical practice environment and one that supports emotional caregiving; that is free of the toxic effects of workplace incivility, violence, and bullying; and that promotes safe staffing and safe patient handling. A randomized controlled trial of a web-based program designed to reduce nurses' perceived stress was successful in building staff resiliency (Hersch et al., 2016).

Application to Nursing Practice:

Hersch and colleagues (2016) recommend the following:

- Nurses should take advantage of educational and self-help programs for stress management. Programs such as *BREATHE* focus on areas of nursing stress that nurses could address either by changing the way they view stressors, changing how they respond to stress, or, when possible, changing the stressful situation.
- Exercises on grieving and coping with the demands of caring for dying patients can minimize stress and improve overall care of patients who are terminally or critically ill.
- Nurses should learn assertive communication, conflict resolution, and problem solving strategies to reduce the stress associated with different interactions with other nurses or health care providers.

KEY POINTS

- Clinical judgments are influenced by a nurse's experience and knowledge and a reliance on knowing the patient and his or her typical pattern of responses, as well as engaging with the patient and his or her concerns.
- The ability to ask questions and to seek and examine information for answers and deeper meanings is essential in critical thinking.
- Purposefully reflecting on a past situation and taking the time to honestly review everything you remember about it allows you to gain new knowledge and raise questions about your practice.
- A basic critical thinker learns to accept the diverse opinions and values of experts, while complex critical thinkers begin to rely less on experts.
- Effective problem solving involves obtaining information that clarifies the nature of a problem, suggesting possible solutions, and trying the solution over time to ensure it is effective, thus adding to nurses' knowledge in future patient situations.
- In inductive reasoning one reviews a specific set of facts and observations about a patient, forms generalizations, and then interprets the data and makes a conclusion about the related pieces of evidence.
- In deductive reasoning one analyzes facts and observations from a conceptual viewpoint, then forms an inference and interprets the patient's condition with respect to the conceptual view.
- The critical thinking model for decision making includes five elements of critical thinking in nursing judgment: competence, knowledge, experience, attitudes, and standards (intellectual and professional).
- Competence involves the ability to perform nursing skills proficiently, while knowledge prepares a nurse to better anticipate and identify patient problems by understanding their origin and nature.
- Intellectual standards provide guidelines for rational thought and decision making that you apply during all steps of the nursing process.
- Reflective journaling involves keeping a written record of clinical experiences to develop critical thought and reflection so that you can improve practices and apply theory in practice in the future.

REFLECTIVE LEARNING

- Consider a patient you recently cared for during a clinical experience. Identify three critical thinking attitudes you applied as you implemented the nursing process.
- Have a conversation with a staff nurse on the clinical unit to which you are assigned. Ask the nurse the type of stressors in the workplace that affect his or her ability to think and make clinical decisions correctly.
- Make a journal entry of your most recent clinical experience. Remember to respect your patients' confidentiality. Review it and compare the elements you included with elements of the REFLECT model.

REVIEW QUESTIONS

1. A nurse enters a patient's room at the beginning of a shift to conduct an assessment of his condition following a blood transfusion. The nurse cared for the patient on the previous day as well. The patient has a number of issues he wishes to share with the nurse, who takes time to explore each issue. The nurse also assesses the patient and finds no signs or symptoms of a reaction to the blood product. The

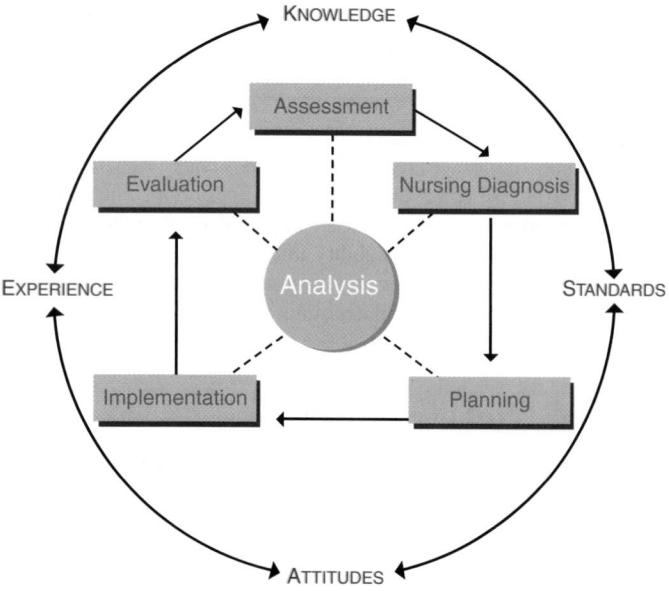

FIG. 15.3 Synthesis of critical thinking with the nursing process competency.

nurse observed the patient the prior day and sees a change in his behavior, a reluctance to get out of bed and ambulate. Which of the following actions improve the nurse's ability to make clinical decisions about this patient? (Select all that apply.)
1. Working the same shift each day
2. Spending time during the patient assessment
3. Knowing the early mobility protocol guidelines
4. Caring for the patient on consecutive days.
5. Knowing the pattern of patient behavior about ambulation

2. Match the concepts for a critical thinker on the right with the application of the term on the left.

Term Application	Concepts for Critical Thinkers
a. Anticipate how a patient might respond to a treatment.	___ 1. Truth seeking
b. Organize assessment on the basis of patient priorities.	___ 2. Open-mindedness
c. Be objective in asking questions of a patient.	___ 3. Analyticity
d. Be tolerant of the patient's views and beliefs.	___ 4. Systematicity

3. A nurse has seen many cancer patients struggle with pain management because they are afraid of becoming addicted to the medicine. Pain control is a priority for cancer care. By helping patients focus on their values and beliefs about pain control, a nurse can best make clinical decisions. This is an example of:
1. Creativity.
2. Fairness.
3. Clinical reasoning.
4. Applying ethical criteria.

4. The REFLECT model can improve learning after providing patient care. Place the steps of this model in the correct order:
1. Think about your thoughts and actions at the time of a situation.
2. Review the knowledge you gained from the experience.
3. Review the facts of the situation.
4. Set a schedule for completing your plan of action.
5. Consider options for handling a similar situation in the future.
6. Recall any feelings you had at the time of the situation.
7. Create a plan for future situations.

5. One element of clinical decision making is knowing the patient. Which of the following activities affect a nurse's ability to know patients better? (Select all that apply.)
1. Caring for similar groups of patients over time
2. Reading the evidence-based practices appropriate to patients
3. Learning how patients typically respond to their clinical situations
4. Observing patients
5. Engaging with patients experiencing illness

6. A nurse is preparing medications for a patient. The nurse checks the name of the medication on the label with the name of the medication on the doctor's order. At the bedside the nurse checks the patient's name against the medication order as well. The nurse is following which critical thinking attitude?
1. Responsibility
2. Humility
3. Accurate
4. Fairness

7. A nurse has been caring for a patient with a chronic wound that has not been healing. The nurse talks with a nurse specialist in wound care to find alternative approaches from what the health care provider ordered for dressing the wound. The two decide that because of the patient's allergy to tape a nonallergenic dressing will be used. The nurse obtains an order from the health care provider for the new dressing. After two days there is improvement in the wound. This is an example of which critical thinking standards? (Select all that apply.)
1. Clear
2. Broad
3. Relevant
4. Risk taking
5. Creativity

8. A nurse is assigned to care for a woman who is expecting her first child. The nurse organizes herself and plans to gather data about the patient by applying Pender's health promotion model, including the patient's characteristics and experiences and situational influences. She plans to observe patient behavior and consider the patient's psychosocial issues. Such data will offer a clear understanding to help the nurse identify the patient's needs. This is an example of which of the following concepts? (Select all that apply.)
1. Diagnostic reasoning
2. Deductive reasoning
3. Inductive reasoning
4. Assessment
5. Problem solving

9. A nurse is caring for a patient who has poor pain control. The patient has a history of opioid abuse. During the day the patient made frequent requests for a pain medication. In order to make an effective clinical decision about this patient, the nurse needs to ask questions about the data available on the patient to make a thorough and thoughtful decision. The nurse asks herself, "How does my view about the patient's pain tolerance compare with the patient's, and does that pose a problem?" This is an example of:
1. A question about assumptions.
2. A question about evidence.
3. A question about procedure.
4. A question about perspective.

10. Which of the following describes a nurse's application of a specific knowledge base during critical thinking? (Select all that apply.)
1. Initiative in reading current evidence from the literature
2. Application of nursing theory
3. Reviewing a policy and procedure manual
4. Considering a colleague's view of a patient's needs
5. Previous time caring for a specific group of patients

Answers: 1. 2, 4, 5; **2.** 1c, 2d, 3a, 4b; **3.** 4; **4.** 3, 1, 6, 2, 5, 7, 4; **5.** 1, 3, 4, 5; **6.** 1; **7.** 3, 4, 5; **8.** 2, 4, 5; **9.** 4; **10.** 1, 2.

Rationales for Review Questions can be found on the Evolve website.

REFERENCES

American Nurses Association (ANA): *Nursing's social policy statement: the essence of the profession*, Washington, DC, 2010, The Association.

Barksby J, et al.: A new model of reflection for clinical practice, *Nurs Times* 111(34/35):21, 2015.

Cipriano P: *Safe nurses safe patients*, 2016. http://www.theamericannurse.org/2016/12/14/safe-nurses-safe-patients/. Accessed June 2019.

Croskerry P, Nimmo GR: Better clinical decision making and reducing diagnostic error, *J R Coll Physicians Edinb* 41(2):155, 2011.

Erickson K: *The importance of critical thinking skills in nursing*, 2017. http://www.rasmussen.edu/degrees/nursing/blog/understanding-why-nurses-need-critical-thinking-skills/. Accessed November 2018.

Facione N, Facione P: Externalizing the critical thinking in knowledge development and clinical judgment, *Nurs Outlook* 44:129, 1996.

Institute of Medicine (IOM): *Improving diagnosis in health care*, 2015. Institute of Medicine. http://www.nationalacademies.org/hmd/Reports/2015/Improving-Diagnosis-in-Healthcare.aspx. Accessed November 2018.

Kataoka-Yahiro M, Saylor C: A critical thinking model for nursing judgment, *J Nurs Educ* 33(8):351, 1994.

Kiron K, et al.: Reflective practice in health care and how to reflect effectively, *Int J Surg Oncol* 2(6):e20, 2017.

Miller M, Malcolm N: Critical thinking in the nursing curriculum, *Nurs Health Care* 11:67, 1990.

Paul RW: The art of redesigning instruction. In Willsen J, Blinker AJA, editors: *Critical thinking: how to prepare students for a rapidly changing world*, Santa Rosa, CA, 1993, Foundation for Critical Thinking.

Papathanasiou IV, et al.: Critical thinking: the development of an essential skill for nursing students, *Acta Informatica Med* 22(4):283, 2014.

Profetto-McGrath J: Critical thinking and evidence-based practice, *J Prof Nurs* 21(6):364, 2005.

QSEN Institute: *QSEN competencies*, 2018. http://qsen.org/competencies/pre-licensure-ksas/. Accessed November 2018.

Raterink G: Reflective journaling for critical thinking development in advanced practice registered nurse students, *J Nurs Educ* 55(2):101, 2016.

Resnick B: Improving care through diagnostic reasoning, *Geriatric Nurs* 37(2):91, 2016.

RESEARCH REFERENCES

Chan ZC: A systematic review of critical thinking in nursing education, *Nurse Educ Today* 33(2013):236, 2013.

Henneman EA, et al.: Strategies used by critical care nurses to identify, interrupt, and correct medical errors, *Am J Crit Care* 19:500, 2010.

Hersch RK, et al.: Reducing nurses' stress: a randomized controlled trial of a web-based stress management program for nurses, *Appl Nurs Res* 32:18, 2016.

Kaddoura M: New graduate nurses' perceived definition of critical thinking during their first nursing experience, *Educ Res Q* 36(3):3, 2013.

Kelley T, et al.: Information needed to support knowing the patient, *ANS Adv Nurs Sci* 36(4):351, 2013.

LaMartina K, Ward-Smith P: Developing critical thinking skills in undergraduate nursing students: the potential for strategic management simulations, *J Nurs Educ Pract* 4(9):155, 2014.

Lotzkar M, Bottorff JL: An observational study of the development of a nurse-patient relationship, *Clin Nurs Res* 10:275, 2010.

Mamede S, et al.: Exploring the role of salient distracting clinical features in the emergence of diagnostic errors and the mechanisms through which reflection counteracts mistakes, *BMJ Qual Saf* 21(4):295, 2012.

McClelland LE, et al.: Changes in nurses' decision making during a 12-h day shift, *Occup Med* 63(1):60, 2013.

Raterink G: Critical thinking: reported enhancers and barriers by nurses in long-term care: implications for staff development, *J Nurses Staff Dev* 27(3):136, 2011.

Scheffer B, Rubenfeld M: A consensus statement on critical thinking in nursing, *J Nurs Educ* 39:352, 2000.

Silvia B, et al.: The reflective journal: a tool for enhancing experience-based learning in nursing students in clinical practice, *J Nurs Educ Pract* 3(3), 2013.

Tanner CA: Thinking like a nurse: a research-based model of clinical judgment in nursing, *J Nurs Educ* 45(6):204, 2006.

Tanner CA, et al.: The phenomenology of knowing the patient, *J Nurs Scholarsh* 25:273, 1993.

Van Graan AC, et al.: Professional nurses' understanding of clinical judgement: a contextual inquiry, *Health SA Gesondheid* 21:280, 2016.

Yue M, et al.: The effectiveness of concept mapping on development of critical thinking in nursing education: a systematic review and meta-analysis, *Nurs Edu Today* 52:87, 2017.

Zolnierek CD: An integrative review of knowing the patient, *J Nurs Scholarsh* 46(1):3, 2014.

16

Nursing Assessment

OBJECTIVES

- Explain the two steps involved in nursing assessment.
- Describe the three types of nursing assessments.
- Explain principles to follow in the use of data sources during assessment.
- Explain the importance of building a nurse-patient relationship before a formal nursing assessment.
- Describe skills to apply when conducting a patient interview during a nursing history.

- Explain communication approaches to use during the working phase of a patient-centered interview.
- Explain how to maintain professionalism during history taking.
- Identify components of a nursing health history.
- Describe elements of the assessment process.

KEY TERMS

Assessment, p. 212
Back channeling, p. 218
Closed-ended questions, p. 218
Cue, p. 222

Inference, p. 222
Nursing health history, p. 219
Nursing process, p. 211
Objective data, p. 214

Open-ended questions, p. 218
Review of systems (ROS), p. 221
Subjective data, p. 214
Validation, p. 223

MEDIA RESOURCES

http://evolve.elsevier.com/Potter/fundamentals/
- Review Questions
- Concept Map Creator
- Case Study with Questions

- Audio Glossary
- Content Updates
- Answers to QSEN Activity and Review Questions

The **nursing process** is a critical thinking five-step process that professional nurses use to apply the best available evidence to deliver nursing care. The steps of the nursing process (assessment, diagnosis, planning and outcome identification, implementation, and evaluation [Fig. 16.1]) are the essential core of nursing practice developed by the American Nurses Association (ANA) that all registered nurses, regardless of role, population, or specialty, are expected to competently perform (ANA, n.d.). The nursing process enables nurses to deliver holistic, patient-centered care (ANA, n.d.). The Quality and Safety Education for Nurses (QSEN) Institute defines patient-centered care as recognizing a patient or a person selected by the patient as a full partner in providing compassionate and coordinated care based on respect for a patient's preferences, values, and needs (QSEN, 2018). Thus, you use the essential first step of the nursing process, assessment, to learn as much as you can about each patient's health condition and health problems by partnering with the patient and family caregivers in a therapeutic relationship. Consider the following case study that was also described in Chapter 15.

Mr. Lawson is a 62-year-old patient who had abdominal surgery for a colon resection and removal of a tumor 1 day ago. His nurse, Tonya, completed an initial assessment when she first cared for Mr. Lawson yesterday. She noted from the previous shift's nurses

notes that the patient had been having fairly good control of his postoperative pain. She implemented pain control strategies to help him become more mobile so that recovery could proceed. His recovery plan involves early ambulation, and up until now he has had a pain rating at a level of 4 on a scale of 0 to 10. Mr. Lawson continues to guard his incision by placing his hand over the wound when he gets out of bed.

Mr. Lawson weighs 109 kg (240 lb) and is 5 feet, 11 inches tall. He has tried to cough more during his postoperative deep-breathing exercises. Tonya is caring for him for the second day in a row and begins the evening shift by inspecting his surgical wound. The wound is approximately 15 cm (6 inches) in length and closed with steel sutures. Tonya notices separation of the wound between two sutures at the bottom of the incision. There is a small amount of serous drainage. The area is inflamed, and Tonya asks the patient if the incision is tender when she gently palpates it. Mr. Lawson states, "Ow, that feels sore there. I think I pulled it when I coughed last night." He also rates pain at this time as being at a level of 5. Tonya checks the patient's vital signs and notes that his temperature is 37.5°C (99.6°F), slightly above his average temperature of 37.2°C (99.0°F). Tonya also inspects the intravenous (IV) access site in the patient's left forearm. It is intact, and there are no signs of phlebitis.

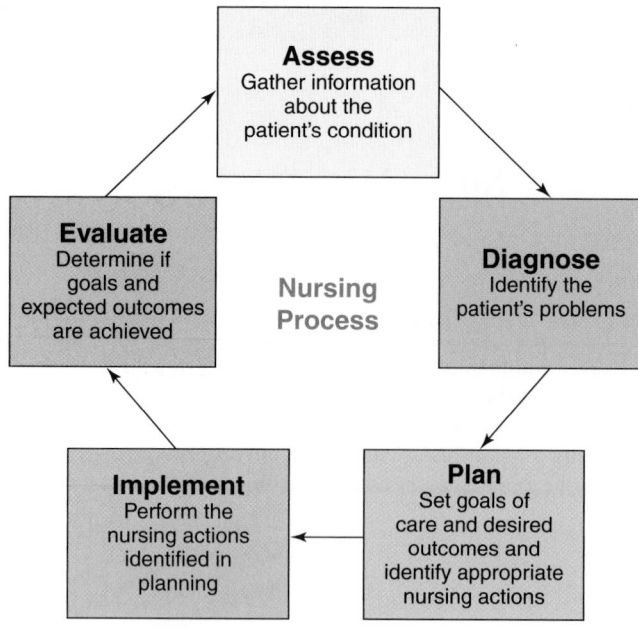

FIG. 16.1 Five-step nursing process.

The nursing process is a type of scientific reasoning. Practicing the five steps of the nursing process ensures a rigorous, systematic, and dynamic way to approach your practice. During the first step of assessment, you collect a comprehensive set of data about a patient and recognize and identify patterns that begin to reflect the meaning of a patient's response to health problems. In the case study involving Tonya and Mr. Lawson, Tonya gathers information to fully understand Mr. Lawson's condition, using observational and interview techniques. Having an accurate and complete database about a patient allows you to make a clinical judgment in the form of a nursing diagnosis and then plan and implement relevant and appropriate nursing interventions. Your assessment also provides the standards for later evaluating the outcomes of care. Each time you interact with a patient you apply the nursing process, as you will see Tonya do throughout the case study.

CRITICAL THINKING IN ASSESSMENT

Think about what you do when you study or consider a problem. For example, why is my child or spouse acting this way? You collect data about the problem. In the case of a family member behaving differently, you consider his or her previous behavior, specifically how he or she is behaving now (voice tone, mannerisms, what he or she says to you) and perhaps how the behavior is affecting others in the family. You assess the situation. You gather as much information as possible in an effort to understand the true nature of the problem (e.g., my family member does not feel well, is angry, or just received bad news at work). The collection, review, and analysis of data make up the process of assessment.

A nursing assessment is the deliberate and systematic collection of data about a patient. Assessment includes not only physiological data but also psychosocial, cultural, spiritual, and lifestyle factors (ANA, n.d.). The data you gather during an assessment reveal your patient's current and past health status, functional status, and present and past coping patterns (Carpenito, 2017). Nursing assessment involves two steps:

- Collection of information from a primary source (a patient) and secondary sources (e.g., family caregiver, family members or friends, health professionals, medical record).

- The interpretation and validation of data to determine whether more data are needed or the database is complete.

In the case study Tonya collects information from Mr. Lawson through observation and asking questions. She saw the inflammation in the incisional area and validated its presence by asking the patient whether it was tender. She begins to interpret the meaning of her findings. An open area of an incision (skin breakdown), draining fluid, and tenderness around the site indicate a pattern of localized and altered wound healing. She also measured Mr. Lawson's body temperature to determine whether an early sign of a systemic infection is present.

If you practice in a hospital setting, you will usually care for more than one patient, and any of your patients' conditions can change quickly. In the home and community setting, your patients' conditions will also change. Sometimes their changes will be acute, but most often the change they experience is subtle and develops over time. An assessment database changes as a patient's condition changes. Thus assessment is an ongoing process.

Mr. Lawson presents with signs of altered wound healing. Tonya reports these findings to the patient's surgeon, who orders antibiotics intravenously (IV) for 24 hours but also plans for the patient's discharge tomorrow. Mr. Lawson's priorities are to transition from immediate recovery from surgery to planning for discharge home. Tonya also needs to assess the patient's response to the IV therapy. She continues to manage Mr. Lawson's pain but also has to further assess the patient's knowledge, observe his behaviors, ask questions about his ability to care for his wound when he goes home, observe the nonverbal cues he provides, and determine whether there are problems that will affect discharge planning.

Critical thinking is a vital part of assessment (see Chapter 15). While gathering data about a patient, you synthesize relevant knowledge, recall prior clinical experiences, apply critical thinking standards and attitudes, and use professional standards of practice to direct your assessment in a meaningful and purposeful way (Fig. 16.2). You apply knowledge from the physical, biological, and social sciences to ask relevant questions and collect a complete history and physical. Clinical decision making is complex, requiring a broad knowledge base and access to reliable sources of information, as well as working in a supportive environment (Bjørk and Hamilton, 2011). Your ultimate goal in assessment is to gather all of the information necessary to reveal a patient's health care needs.

Tonya knows that Mr. Lawson had a colectomy to remove the part of his colon that had a cancerous tumor. She reviewed her medical-surgical nursing textbook and learned how a colectomy alters gastrointestinal function and poses risks for blood clots in the legs (venous thrombosis) after surgery. This knowledge leads her to assess Mr. Lawson's bowel sounds, ask him if he is passing flatus, and assess the circulation in his legs. Tonya has learned from previous experiences in caring for patients with abdominal surgery that they have activity restrictions after surgery to reduce strain on the incision. Mr. Lawson's incision has a small separation; thus Tonya knows that she needs to assess what he has learned so far about activity restrictions in the home. Using good communication skills through interviewing and applying critical thinking intellectual standards, such as relevance (which activities the patient performs at home) and a broad review (including patient's wife in assessment), will enable Tonya to collect a complete, accurate, and relevant database.

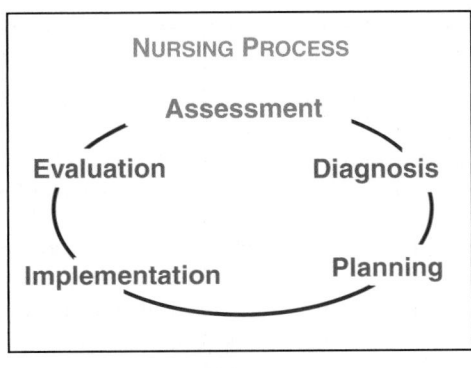

KNOWLEDGE
Underlying disease process
Normal growth and development
Normal physiology and psychology
Normal assessment findings
Health promotion
Assessment skills
Communication skills

EXPERIENCE
Previous patient care experience
Validation of assessment findings
Observation of assessment techniques

NURSING PROCESS

Assessment

Evaluation   Diagnosis

Implementation   Planning

STANDARDS
ANA Scope and Standards of Nursing Practice
Specialty standards of practice
Intellectual standards of
measurement

ATTITUDES
Perseverance
Fairness
Integrity
Confidence
Creativity

FIG. 16.2 Critical thinking and the assessment process.

The decisions nurses make while assessing their patients influence their effectiveness in clinical practice and make an impact on patients' lives and experiences with health care in any setting in which they practice (Bjørk and Hamilton, 2011).

Types of Assessments

Assessment requires accurate and thorough data collection. There are different types of assessments:

- Patient-centered interview (conducted during a nursing history)
- Periodic assessments (conducted during ongoing contact with patients)
- Physical examination (conducted during a nursing history and at any time a patient presents a symptom)

Each type of assessment is either comprehensive or problem focused. Use a patient-centered interview when you conduct a comprehensive nursing history (i.e., a detailed assessment of a patient's physical, psychosocial, cultural, spiritual, and lifestyle needs). Usually you include categories of information in the patient's history that follow a structured database format based on an accepted framework or practice standard. Marjory Gordon's "Functional Health Patterns" (1994), Nola Pender's "Health Promotion Model" (2015), and the Long Term Care Minimum Data Set (Centers for Medicare and Medicaid Services, 2010) for residents in certified Medicare long-term care agencies are a few examples. A theory or practice standard provides the categories of information for you to assess. Pender's model is outlined in Chapter 6. Gordon's 11 functional health patterns include health perception and management, nutritional-metabolic, elimination, activity-exercise, sleep-rest, cognitive-perceptual, self-concept, role-relationship, sexuality-reproduction, coping-stress tolerance, and value-beliefs. A health care agency often relies on the nursing history model included in the electronic health record (EHR) as the organizing framework for an assessment. Often EHR frameworks are medically driven. Frameworks developed from nursing theories are holistic and provide for a comprehensive patient review. *Tonya plans to further assess Mr. Lawson's cognitive-perceptual pattern using the questions included in her agency's EHR assessment form. She wants to learn more about what the patient knows about recovery from surgery, restrictions recommended by his surgeon, and how Mr. Lawson prefers to learn and make decisions about his care.*

Periodic problem-focused assessments collected during rounding or while you administer patient care include quick screenings to rule out or follow up on patient problems. For example, an emergency department nurse uses the Airway, Breathing, Circulation, Disability, Exposure (ABCDE) approach in all clinical emergencies for immediate assessment and treatment of patients who are injured or critically ill (Thim et al., 2012). This quick screening approach allows nurses to assess critical physiologic functions and make quick treatment decisions. Another example is a medical-surgical nurse who performs a quick screening of a patient who is demonstrating incisional pain. The quick screening focuses on the patient's incisional pain, which is a priority problem.

Another type of problem-focused approach begins with a patient's presenting situation and specific problematic areas (expected as well as unexpected), such as incisional pain or limited understanding of postoperative recovery. You ask the patient follow-up questions to clarify and expand your assessment so that you better understand the full nature of the problem. Then you perform a physical examination focusing on the same problem areas to confirm your observations. *For example, Tonya chooses to focus on Mr. Lawson's symptoms the first 48 hours after surgery, the expected healing response, and signs of potential complications. She inspects the condition of the patient's surgical wound,*

TABLE 16.1	Example of Problem-Focused Patient Assessment: Pain	
Problem and Associated Factors	**Questions for Assessment**	**Physical Examination**
Nature of pain	Describe your pain. Tell me how the pain is affecting your daily life.	Observe for nonverbal cues (e.g., facial grimacing, crying).
Precipitating factors causing pain	What causes your pain to worsen during the day? Is your pain associated with movement? Anything else?	Observe if patient demonstrates nonverbal signs of pain during movement (e.g., positioning, swallowing, walking).
Severity of pain	Rate your pain on a scale of 0 to 10.	Inspect area of discomfort. Palpate area for tenderness.

looking for signs of healing and observes his progress in ambulating. She later expands her assessment to determine how Mr. Lawson is adjusting emotionally to surgery and his cancer diagnosis and whether he is prepared for discharge. Table 16.1 offers an example of a problem-focused assessment.

A physical examination is a comprehensive review of all major body systems (see Chapter 30), providing objective data about a patient's clinical status. Portions of a physical exam are typically included in a nursing history (e.g., height and weight, inspection of the skin, lung sounds). You also use physical examination techniques to validate your observations with data, as in the case of Tonya when she palpated Mr. Lawson's tender incision line. Patient symptoms such as pain, shortness of breath, or nausea will direct you to examine various bodily functions (shortness of breath: long sounds and chest excursion; nausea: bowel sounds, abdominal distention).

Types of Data

There are two primary types of data: subjective and objective. Subjective data are your patients' verbal descriptions of their health problems. Subjective data include patient feelings, perceptions, and self-reported symptoms. For example, Mr. Lawson's self-report of pain at the area where his incision slightly separated is an example of subjective data. Only patients provide subjective data relevant to their health condition. The data often reflect physiological or psychological changes. You explore physiological changes through objective physical examination of body systems.

Objective data are the findings resulting from direct observation or measurement, including what you see, hear, and touch (Ball et al., 2019). Inspecting the condition of a wound, observing a patient walk down the floor, measuring blood pressure, and describing specifically an observed behavior (patient seizure) are examples of objective data. Objective data are measured on the basis of an accepted standard such as the Fahrenheit or Celsius measure on a thermometer, inches or centimeters on a measuring tape, or a pain rating scale. When you collect objective data, apply critical thinking intellectual standards (e.g., clear, precise, and consistent) so that you can correctly interpret your findings.

Assessment Data Sources

A variety of sources provide information about a patient's current and past level of wellness and functional status, anticipated prognosis, risk factors for health problems, health and lifestyle practices, goals, cultural background, responses to previous treatment, and patterns of health and illness.

Patient. A patient is your best source of information. Patients who are conscious, alert, and able to answer questions appropriately provide the most accurate information. Those with cognitive changes—such as patients who are inattentive or easily distracted, those who are diagnosed with dementia, or who have psychological symptoms such as

anxiety or fear—can be less reliable sources. When a patient is not a reliable source, you may refer to the family. Always consider the setting for your assessment and your patient's condition. A patient experiencing acute symptoms in an emergency department will not offer as much information as one who comes to an outpatient clinic for a routine checkup. Also, know your patient's health literacy level. A patient with limited health literacy has difficulty obtaining, processing, and understanding basic health information (AHRQ, 2016). This means that patients do not always understand some of the questions you use during assessment, especially if you use more clinically focused words or terms or do not speak their language. You will not gather accurate information if a patient does not understand assessment questions. The Agency for Healthcare Research and Quality (2016) offers tools for assessment of health literacy, including Short Assessment of Health Literacy (Spanish and English), Rapid Estimate of Adult Literacy in Medicine (short form), and Short Assessment of Health Literacy for Spanish Adults (Box 16.1).

An older adult often requires more time for assessment than a younger patient if his or her hearing or cognitive function is impaired. However, physiological age and chronological age may not match. It is important to recognize that not all adults experience the same changes and that changes occur at different rates (Ball et al., 2019). Some older adults have sensory alterations (visual and hearing) that make it more difficult to communicate. Use short (but not leading) questions, keep your language uncomplicated, and listen to a patient carefully (Ball et al., 2019) (Box 16.2). Consult family members, when appropriate, to fill in any gaps in information. Always be attentive, be engaged, and show a caring presence with patients (see Chapter 7). Patients are more likely to fully reveal the nature of health care problems when you show interest, avoid distractions by activities around them, and focus on their concerns.

Family Caregivers and Significant Others. Family caregivers, other family members, and significant others are primary sources of information for infants or children, critically ill adults, and patients who have intellectual disabilities or cognitive impairments. In cases of severe illness or emergency situations, family members are often your only source of information. The family and significant others are also important secondary sources of information for alert and responsive patients. They confirm findings or identify important health patterns (e.g., whether a patient takes medications regularly, is able to sleep well, and the type of diet the patient regularly eats). Include the family in an assessment when appropriate. Patients do not always want you to question or involve their families. In some cultures, including the family is inappropriate. Some health care agencies require a patient's oral or written permission to collect data from family members. A spouse or close friend who sits in during an assessment can provide his or her view of a patient's health problems or needs. Not only do they supply information about a patient's current health status, but they are also able to tell when changes in the patient's condition have occurred. Family

BOX 16.1 EVIDENCE-BASED PRACTICE

Assessment of Health Literacy

PICOT Question: In adults does the use of formal literacy screening tools versus asking basic screening questions identify patients with inadequate health literacy?

Evidence Summary

Numerous instruments are available to assess health literacy. However, most were developed for use in research. Although they capture health literacy comprehensively and measure many factors associated with health literacy, they are not always useful in clinical practice, especially when time is limited (Altin et al., 2014). Commonly used instruments include the Rapid Estimate of Adult Literacy in Medicine (REALM), the Short Test of Functional Health Literacy in Adults (S-TOFHLA), and the Newest Vital Sign (NVS) (Weiss et al., 2005). However, the Single Item Literacy Screener (SILS) asks respondents only one question: How often do you need to have someone help you when you read instructions, pamphlets, or other written material from your doctor or pharmacy? This question allows health care providers to do an initial quick screen and then target additional assessment of health literacy skills (Morris et al., 2006). Routinely screening patients for health literacy has not been shown to improve outcomes. Instead, using universal health literacy precautions to provide understandable and accessible information to all patients is recommended, regardless of their literacy or education levels (Hersh et al., 2015).

Application to Nursing Practice

- Use the literacy screening tools made available at your health care institution with all patients.
- Follow universal health literacy precautions (Hersh et al., 2015):
- Avoid use of medical jargon.
- Break down information or instructions into small concrete steps.
- Limit the focus of a visit (such as a patient assessment) to three key points.
- Assess a patient's understanding of any instruction.
- Ensure printed information is written at or below a fifth- to sixth-grade reading level.

BOX 16.2 FOCUS ON OLDER ADULTS

Approaches for Assessing Older Adults

- Listen patiently; older adults are a rich source of wisdom and experience.
- Allow for pauses and give patients time to tell their story.
- Recognize normal changes associated with aging (see Chapter 14). Older adults' symptoms are often muted or less obvious, vague, or nonspecific compared with younger adults.
- Some patients may not report symptoms because they attribute them to old age or they think nothing can be done for them (Ball et al., 2019).
- If a patient has limited hearing or visual deficits, use nonverbal communication when conducting your interview (see Chapter 49):
  - **Patient-directed eye gaze:** Maintain eye contact with the patient. This allows you or a patient who is speaking to check whether information is understood. It is a signal for readiness to initiate interaction with a patient. Eye contact shows interest in what the other person is saying.
  - **Affirmative head nodding:** This has an important social function. It regulates an interaction (especially when alternate people speak), supports spoken language, and allows for comments on the interaction.
  - **Smiling:** A positive sign that indicates good humor, warmth, and immediacy. Smiles help when first establishing the nurse-patient relationship.
  - **Forward leaning:** This shows awareness, attention, and immediacy. During an interaction it also suggests interest in the person.

BOX 16.3 Hand-Off Communication

- Patient safety is at risk when the receiver of a hand-off report gets information that is inaccurate, incomplete, not timely, misinterpreted, or unneeded.
- A hand-off is an opportunity for care providers to share information: the patient's condition, care, treatment, medications, services, and any recent or anticipated changes.
- Hand-offs need to be structured and focused to ensure continuity of care. Many agencies use forms or structured processes for hand-offs, such as the program I-PASS (Illness severity, Patient summary, Action list, Situation awareness and contingency plans, and Synthesis by receiver).
- Avoid barriers to effective hand-offs when possible, such as delays in reporting, inattention, or lack of knowledge about the patient being transferred from receivers.
- Provide hand-offs through face-to-face communication; do not make hand-offs using solely electronic or paper communications.

Adapted from The Joint Commission: *The Joint Commission Center for Transforming Healthcare. Improving transitions of care: hand-off communications.* Oakbrook Terrace, IL: The Joint Commission, 2014.

members are often well informed because of their experiences living with a patient and observing how his or her health affects daily living activities. They can make important observations about patients' needs that will influence the way you deliver care (e.g., how a patient eats a meal, makes choices, or performs hygiene). A strong nurse-family relationship is important for you to gather the information you need.

Health Care Team. You will frequently communicate with other health care team members when gathering information about patients. In acute care settings the change-of-shift report or patient hand-off is the way for nurses to communicate the most recent information about patients to nurses or other health care providers on oncoming shifts (see Chapter 26). A hand-off report is defined by The Joint Commission (TJC) as a transfer and acceptance of patient care responsibility achieved through effective communication. It is a real-time process of passing patient-specific information from one caregiver to another or from one team of health care providers to another for the purpose of ensuring the continuity and safety of the patient's care (TJC, 2014). Hand-offs also occur when patients are transferred from one unit or area of care to another. Effective communication through hand-offs can improve health care providers' perceptions of accuracy, completeness, and types of interventions provided to patients during a previous shift or level of care. Typically when nurses and other health care providers consult on a patient's condition, each contributes

information about the patient. There can be problems with hand-off communication unless each member of the team assumes responsibility for either giving or receiving a complete and accurate report (TJC, 2017) (Box 16.3). Potential for patient harm is introduced when the receiver gets information that is inaccurate, incomplete, not timely, misinterpreted, or otherwise not what is needed to provide care (TJC, 2017). Hand-off information is vital for you to be able to assess and understand a patient's most current health care needs.

Medical Records. The medical record is a valuable resource for your patient assessment. It contains a patient's medical history, laboratory and diagnostic test results, current physical findings, and a health care provider's treatment plan. In some cases medical records also contain consultation notes. There are health care agencies that hold medical records for all of a patient's visits within the agency system, including inpatient and outpatient. Data in the records offer baseline and ongoing information about a patient's response to illness and progress to date. The Health Insurance Portability and Accountability Act (HIPAA) of 1996 has a privacy rule that came into effect in 2003 to set standards for the protection of health information (USDHHS, 2003). Information in a patient's medical record is confidential. A nurse can review a patient's medical record for assessment data but needs to know the agency policies governing how to share the information with other staff. The record is a valuable tool to check the consistency and similarities of your own observations and measurements.

Other Records and the Scientific Literature. Educational, military, and employment records often contain significant data about a patient (e.g., immunizations, prior illnesses). If a patient received services at a community clinic or a different hospital, you need written permission from the patient or guardian to access the record. The HIPAA regulations protect access. The privacy rule allows health care providers to share protected information as long as they use reasonable safeguards. Consult agency policies and participate in annual HIPAA training as required.

Reviewing recent nursing, medical, and pharmacological literature abut a patient's illness or treatments provides up-to-date information that helps you to anticipate patient needs and to implement evidence-based interventions (see Chapter 18). This review increases your knowledge about expected signs and symptoms, treatment options, and established standards of therapeutic practice. Always be sure to review the most current literature available (see Chapter 5).

Nurse's Experience. Your experience in caring for patients is a source of data. Through clinical experience you observe other patients' behaviors and physical signs and symptoms; track trends and recognize clinical changes; and learn the types of questions to ask, choosing the questions that will give the most useful information. This experience builds your ability to know patients, knowing the pattern of responses shown by similar patients. As a new nurse, you will use a systematic and analytical method to make decisions when you analyze data and ultimately make a nursing diagnosis (Muntean, 2012) (see Chapter 17). The tendency for a new nurse is to just focus on data and not consider the whole context of a patient's situation. New nurses have not had that kind of experience. However, as you gain more practice, you will eventually make fluid intuitive decisions that account for all of the patient's data and the mental connections to data gained from previous experiences. That intuition is a feeling of knowing something without conscious use of reason, but is a critical part of clinical decision making (Muntean, 2012). Practical experience and the opportunity to make clinical decisions strengthen your critical thinking.

REFLECT NOW

The next time you assess a patient, consider the data you collect and identify what information is subjective versus objective. Is the information you collect complete, and if not, how might you gather additional information?

THE NURSE-PATIENT RELATIONSHIP IN ASSESSMENT

Effective communication is the foundation for creating nurse-patient relationships that enable patients to tell their stories and nurses to understand patients and the experiences they express (Kourkouta and Papathanasiou, 2014). It requires skills and simultaneously the sincere intention of a nurse to understand what concerns a patient. Only to understand a patient is insufficient; the nurse must also convey the message that the patient is understandable and acceptable (Kourkouta and Papathanasiou, 2014). Trust is central to an effective nurse-patient relationship and necessary to ensure that you are able to learn the information needed to care for a patient.

Typically there is much information to consider about a patient. Where should you begin? Start by taking quality time to be present with a patient, even if it is for a few minutes. This can be difficult when you are faced with interruptions, the care of other patients, other home visits, or the restricted time given to you in a health care provider's office. Having quality time should occur during admission of a patient to a hospital unit, during rounds when you begin a shift of care, during a follow-up home or clinic visit, or in any encounter with a patient. Connecting with a patient by showing interest in his or her problems and concerns helps you collect a relevant database. Research shows that hearing accounts of patients' health and illness experiences, watching them, and coming to understand how they typically respond develops a type of knowing that fosters good clinical judgments (Tanner, 2006). Visiting a hospitalized patient at set intervals (called rounding) allows you to address essential care needs and patient experiences and helps organize your workload. Rounding is a vital opportunity to build trust with patients, increasing the likelihood that you will gain more information that will help you identify and communicate their health-related problems. Chapter 24 reviews how to establish a nurse-patient relationship and the skills of effective communication.

THE PATIENT-CENTERED INTERVIEW

When conducting an assessment of a patient you will use interview and observational skills. A patient-centered interview is relationship based and is an organized conversation focused on learning about a patient's concerns and needs. If you are to prevent misinterpretation of information and misperceptions, you must make every effort to sense the world of an individual patient as he or she senses it (Ball et al., 2019). An empathic, patient-centered interview strengthens a patient's sense of self-esteem and lessens the feelings of helplessness that often accompany an episode of illness. Research has shown that interview skills contribute significantly to problem detection, diagnostic accuracy, patient satisfaction, patient adjustment to stress and illness, patient recall of information, patient adherence to therapy, and patient health outcomes (Keifenheim et al., 2015). The most extensive patient-centered interview is the one used during collection of a nursing history. Primary objectives while taking an initial nursing history are to discover details about a patient's concerns, explore expectations for the health care visit, and display genuine interest and partnership.

One type of patient-centered interview is motivational interviewing. It is a technique used often in counseling and patient education that allows you to become a helper in the change process. Motivational interviewing addresses a patient's ambivalence or uncertainty about following medically indicated behavioral changes and supports patients in making health care decisions in cases in which there is more than one reasonable option (Elwyn et al., 2014).

Interview Preparation

Before you begin an interview, especially for a nursing history, be prepared. Review a patient's medical record when information is available. If your interview is performed at patient admission, there may be little information in the record except for an admitting diagnosis and the patient's chief complaint. In other cases review the previous medical entries or nurses' notes. Were problems identified that remain a part of the patient's treatment plan? Do any of those problems require clarification or follow-up? Does a patient's admitting diagnosis or do other diagnoses suggest lines of questioning? For example, in the case of a patient with a history of chronic lung disease, you would include questions about the patient's respiratory status, effects of disease symptoms on lifestyle, and the patient's acceptance and understanding of a chronic disease. The information you obtain during a hand-off report at the beginning of a shift will help you frame clinical questions to address the problems you decide to explore.

Communication Skills. Effective communication with patients during an assessment interview requires the following skills (Ball et al., 2019):

- **Courtesy**
  - Greet patients by the name by which they prefer to be addressed. Ask, "Would you prefer I call you by Mrs. Silver or by your first name?" It is all right to shake hands.
  - Introduce yourself and explain your role the first time you meet. For example, "My name is Julia, and I will be your nursing student today. I would like to ask you questions about how you are feeling right now. Is that okay with you?"
  - Ensure confidentiality of the information the patient chooses to share.
  - Meet and acknowledge visitors in the patient's room and learn their names and roles.
  - Sit down next to the patient and do not make an effort to exit the room too soon.
  - Remember to ask the patient's permission to conduct an interview in a visitor's presence.
  - Try to take notes sparingly; remember key words.
- **Comfort**
  - Ensure that your patient is comfortable. If a patient is in pain or has nausea or fatigue, it is difficult to gather a thorough and accurate history. Provide necessary comfort measures before beginning the interview. When patients have symptoms, keep questions short and focused.
  - Maintain privacy. Close room curtains or doors and provide a comfortable room temperature.
  - Select a location for the interview that is quiet and free of interruptions. Do not answer your pager during the interview unless there is an emergency. If possible, set aside a 10- to 15-minute period when no other activities are planned.
  - Avoid overtiring the patient. You do not need to complete the interview in one session.
- **Connection**
  - It is important to make a good first impression. Avoid staring at a computer screen while filling in required data fields or talking on a cell phone; patients will perceive you are uncaring or uninterested in what they have to say.
  - Stiff formality may inhibit a patient, but being too casual may not instill confidence. Do not be careless with your choice of words; what you think is a harmless or innocent phrase may seem very important to a patient who is anxious to understand you.
  - Begin with open-ended questions that encourage patients to tell their stories (e.g., "How have you been feeling?" "What questions would you like to discuss?" "Tell me how you want us to help you").
  - Allow patients to fully describe their symptoms without interrupting them (Muhrer, 2014).
  - Do not dominate a discussion or assume that you know the nature of a patient's problems. Listen and be attentive.
  - Use your observational skills. Note the patient's tone of voice, posture, and level of energy when talking.

- Respect silence and be flexible. Let the patient's needs, concerns, or questions guide your follow-up questions. Health problems can have multiple causes; do not leap to one cause too quickly.
- **Confirmation**
  - At the end of an interview, ask the patient to summarize the discussion so that there are no uncertainties. Be open to further clarification or discussion. Ask the patient, "Is there something else you want to talk about?" (Muhrer, 2014).
  - If there are questions you cannot answer, say so and promise that you will return with follow-up if possible.

Phases of the Interview

When you begin a formal patient-centered interview for the purpose of collecting a nursing history, you will go through the traditional three interview phases: (1) orientation or setting an agenda, (2) working phase—collecting assessment data, and (3) termination of the interview (see Chapter 24).

Orientation and Setting an Agenda. Begin by introducing yourself, and explain why you are collecting data. Assure patients that information will be kept confidential. Your aim is to set an agenda for the interview, including how you will gather information about a patient's chief concerns or problems (e.g., asking questions and performing a physical exam). Focus on a patient's goals, preferences, and concerns, not your personal agenda. This is a time that allows a patient to feel comfortable speaking with you and becoming an active partner in decisions about care. The professionalism and competence that you show when interviewing strengthens the nurse-patient relationship.

Tonya is doing a follow-up interview to learn more about Mr. Lawson's home situation. She explains, "Mr. Lawson, it looks as if your doctor wants to send you home tomorrow. It's important for us to know more about how you care for yourself at home. Are you comfortable, and can I take a few minutes to talk about your discharge now?" Mr. Lawson replies, "I feel a bit better, and, yes, I've been thinking about some questions I want to ask." Tonya replies, "Good. We'll start there."

Working Phase—Collecting Data. Whether you are conducting a complete nursing history or gathering ongoing assessment information, the working phase of a relationship involves gathering accurate, relevant, and complete information about a patient's condition. Beginning an interview with open-ended questions allows patients to describe their concerns and problems clearly. For example, begin by having patients explain their symptoms or physical or psychological concerns. Ask them to describe what they know about their health problems or to describe their health care expectations. Use attentive listening and summarize key issues to validate your understanding with the patient, and encourage him or her to tell a full story (see Chapter 24). Do not rush to an opinion about what the patient tells you. When a patient describes a symptom, such as dizziness, queasy stomach, or weakness, clarify what the patient means. For example, say, "Describe how you feel when you are dizzy." Be willing to wait for the patient to respond no matter how long it takes (Muhrer, 2014). If you ask direct questions (e.g., "Does the room spin?" or "Do you feel faint?" in the case of dizziness), most patients will say yes to most of your questions (Muhrer, 2014). However, this may not reveal the true problem. This is important because symptoms often reflect multiple disorders. Dizziness can indicate the patient has an ear disorder, cardiovascular disease, an anxiety disorder, or a neurological problem. Unless you listen and get a full description of the patient's symptoms and how they affect him or her, you will not identify the true problem.

The verbal cues that a patient expresses will help you stay focused so that you can direct an assessment appropriately. Do not rush a patient. An initial interview is more extensive. Gather information about a patient's concerns and then complete all relevant sections of the nursing history. Ongoing interviews, which occur each time you interact with your patient, do not need to be as extensive. Organize your time with a patient and focus on priority areas to assess. An ongoing interview also allows you to update a patient's status and concerns, focus on changes previously identified, and review new problems.

> Tonya: "Mr. Lawson, you said you had some questions. Can you tell me what they are?"
>
> Mr. Lawson: "Well, the doctor told me that I would not be able to lift anything heavy for a while, and I'm not sure if I understand. The way my incision looks, will I need to do something to it?"
>
> Tonya: "Let's start with your question about lifting. Tell me what you think that means."
>
> Mr. Lawson: "Well, I suppose it is anything big, but I do not plan to move furniture or do any work around the house until I feel better."
>
> Tonya: "Tell me the types of things you lift regularly at home and approximately how much they weigh."
>
> Mr. Lawson: "Well, when our grandchildren visit, they like to be picked up. We have a pet schnauzer, but he just jumps up on the chair with me. My wife does grocery shopping, but I come out to unload the car."
>
> Tonya: "Anything else?"
>
> Mr. Lawson: "Hmmm, occasionally I lift the laundry basket and take it downstairs."
>
> Tonya: "Okay, and about your incision, yes, you will need to care for it. Can you tell me the signs of infection?"
>
> Mr. Lawson: "Not sure I can, but I guess it would hurt more. Is infection common?"
>
> Tonya: "No, but you and your wife need to know the signs, so if something happens once you return home, you can know to call your doctor quickly. Has your doctor or the nurse practitioner talked to you about incision care?"
>
> Mr. Lawson: "No, they have not mentioned anything about that yet."
>
> Tonya: "Okay, I'll explain everything you need to know and take the time to be sure you understand. Do you think you learn best by reading information or listening to explanations?"
>
> Mr. Lawson: "I think I do okay with both."
>
> Tonya's assessment focuses on the patient's questions and how they pertain to the information he will need to learn to go home and assume self-care.

Interview Techniques. How you conduct the interview is just as important as the questions you ask. During an interview you direct the flow of the discussion so that patients have the opportunity to freely describe their health problems to enable you to get a detailed picture of their needs. Remember, some interviews are focused, while others are more comprehensive. Because a patient's report will contain subjective information, validate subjective data later with objective information. For example, if a patient reports difficulty breathing, you will further assess the patient's respiratory rate and lungs sounds during the physical examination.

Observation. Observation is powerful. Observe a patient's verbal and nonverbal behaviors, such as the use of eye contact, body language and positioning, or tone of voice. While observing nonverbal behavior, appearance, and the patient's interaction with the environment, determine whether the data you obtained are consistent with what the patient states verbally. Your observations will lead you to pursue further

objective information to form thorough and accurate conclusions. Patients are also observant during interviews. If you establish trust, the patient feels comfortable asking you questions about the health care environment, planned treatments, diagnostic testing, and available resources. A patient needs this information to partner in making decisions and planning the goals of care.

An important aspect of observation includes a patient's level of function: the physical, developmental, psychological, and social aspects of everyday living. Observation of level of function involves watching what a patient does when eating, performing hygiene, or making a decision about preparing a medication. It is not what the patient tells you that he or she can do. Observation of function often occurs in the home or in a health care setting during a return demonstration.

Open-Ended Questions. During a patient-centered interview you try to learn, in the patient's own words, his or her concerns or problems, possible causes, and any health care goals. Open-ended questions elicit the patient's unique story. An open-ended question gives a patient discretion about the extent of his or her answer (Ball et al., 2019). For example, "So, tell me more about ...." or "What are your concerns about this?" or "Tell me how you have been feeling." This approach does not presuppose a specific answer. You are exploring with the patient. The use of open-ended questions prompts patients to describe a situation in more than just one or two words, allowing patients to actively describe their health status. This interaction strengthens your relationship together. The open-ended question shows that you want to hear a patient's thoughts and feelings. Listen carefully and do not interrupt the patient. When you interrupt, you will not gather complete information and you also may end up disagreeing with the patient about his or her views of the illness or purpose of the health visit (Muhrer, 2014).

Direct Closed-Ended Questions. As you obtain information from a patient you will sometimes ask direct closed-ended questions to seek specific information about a problem or situation. Direct questions are not ideal when you wish a patient to be thorough in describing a health problem. However, this problem-seeking technique reveals details to identify a patient's specific problems accurately and more fully. For example, a patient reports having indigestion over the course of several days and acknowledges having some diarrhea and loss of appetite. The patient's explanation for the cause relates to a recent series of trips that changed his eating habits. The nurse focuses on the symptoms the patient identifies and the general indigestion problem by asking closed-ended questions that limit answers to one or two words such as "yes" or "no" or a number or frequency of a symptom. For example, the nurse asks, "How often does the diarrhea occur?" and "Do you have pain or cramping?" This technique requires short answers and clarifies previous information to provide a more comprehensive database. The questions do not encourage patients to volunteer more information than you request.

Leading Questions. These types of interview questions are risky because they can limit the information a patient will provide to what a patient thinks you want to know (Ball et al., 2019). Two examples of leading questions are (1) "It seems to me this is bothering you quite a bit. Is that true?" and (2) "That wasn't very hard to do, was it?" When asking how often a symptom or problem occurs, allow a patient to define "often." Do not ask, "It didn't happen too often, did it?" A patient may not understand what you are asking and may say so (Ball et al., 2019).

Back Channeling. Reinforce your interest in what a patient has to say through the use of good eye contact and listening. Also use back channeling, which includes active listening prompts such as "all right," "go on," or "uh-huh." This technique shows that you have heard what a patient says, are interested in hearing the full story, and are encouraging the patient to give more details.

Probing. As a patient tells his or her story, encourage a full description without trying to control the story's direction. This requires you to probe with more open-ended questions, such as "Is there anything else you can tell me?" or "What else is bothering you?" Each time a patient offers more detail, probe again until the patient has nothing else to say and has told the full description. Always be observant. If a patient becomes fatigued or uncomfortable, know that it is time to postpone the interview until later.

Interpret. Ultimately it is important to come to the correct conclusion and decision about a patient's problems based on your assessment. By interpreting, you repeat what you have heard to confirm the patient's meaning (Ball et al., 2019). Clarity is critical before you analyze your data to make a diagnostic conclusion (see Chapter 17).

QSEN **Building Competency in Patient-Centered Care**
Describe how you would conduct a patient-centered interview with Mr. Lawson about his expectations for going home after surgery during the working phase of the interview.

Answers to QSEN Activities can be found on the Evolve website.

Termination Phase. You summarize your discussion with a patient and check for accuracy of the information you collected during the termination phase of an interview. Let your patient know when the interview is coming to an end. For example, say, "I have just two more questions. We'll be finished in a few more minutes." This helps a patient maintain direct attention without being distracted by wondering when the interview will end. This approach also gives the patient an opportunity to ask additional questions. End the interview in a friendly manner, telling the patient when you will return to provide care.

Tonya: *"You've given me a good idea of which topics we need to cover and the plans we need to make to get you ready to go home. And we'll include your wife in these decisions if that is okay?"*
Mr. Lawson: *"Yes, for sure. She always helps me when I need it."*
Tonya: *"I'll come back after I check on two other patients, okay?"*
Mr. Lawson: *"Yes, you have already been very helpful."*

REFLECT NOW

Before your next clinical assignment, consider how to plan a patient-centered interview. What ways can you connect early with a patient? What questions might be appropriate based on the patient's health situation?

NURSING HEALTH HISTORY

The nursing health history typically contains similar information regardless of the health care setting and EHR software or form used to gather and document patient information. Data gleaned from the health history are used to inform a patient's nursing care. You will gather a nursing health history during an initial or early contact with a patient. The history is a key component of your comprehensive assessment. Most health history forms (electronic and manual) are structured. However, on the basis of information you gain as you conduct the patient-centered interview, you learn which components of the history to explore fully and which require less detail. As you gain more experience, you will learn to refine and broaden questions as needed to correctly identify a patient's unique needs. Your patient's priorities and needs and the amount of time you have available determine how complete a history will be. A comprehensive history covers all health dimensions (Fig. 16.3).

Cultural Considerations

Obtaining a nursing health history requires cultural competence (see Chapter 9). This involves self-awareness, reflective practice, and knowledge of a patient's core cultural background. It is critical for you to adapt each assessment to the uniqueness of each patient. Cultural humility requires you to recognize your own knowledge limitations and cultural perspective and thus be open to new perspectives (Ball et al., 2019). Without humility you are at risk for being biased and misinterpreting assessment findings.

Show your patients respect and understand their individual needs and differences; do not impose your own attitudes, biases, and beliefs. Having a genuine curiosity about a patient's beliefs and values lays a foundation for a trusting and strong nurse-patient relationship (Ball et al., 2019). Consider a patient's cultural background when you begin history taking. For clarity, explain the intent of any questions you have. Avoid making stereotypes; the assumptions tied to stereotypes (e.g., obese patients do not exercise regularly) can lead to the collection of inaccurate information. Draw on knowledge gained from your assessment and ask questions in a constructive and probing way to allow you to truly know who a patient is (Box 16.4).

Professionalism in History Taking

Most health care institutions use computerized software programs to enter data into the Electronic Health History (EHR). In many cases computers are at each patient's bedside. To display professionalism and a caring approach during an interview, look at the patient and not the computer screen. Use the computer if you must, but position it in a way that does not distract from your focus on the patient (Ball et al., 2019). In an observational study involving physicians and patients during routine clinic visits, fewer than half (48%) of the patients who had physicians with heavy computer use and focus during clinical encounters rated the care they received as excellent on patient experience surveys. In contrast the majority (83%) of patients whose physicians were less engaged (more patient focused) with their computers during the clinic visit felt the care they received was excellent (Ratanawongsa et al., 2016). The same study showed that high computer use by physicians was associated with observable communication differences—less patient engagement and more negative rapport. Do not let a computer program guide your assessment. Ask patients to explain why they have come for health care, listen actively, proceed at a reasonable pace, and ask open-ended questions (Ball et al., 2019).

Components of the Nursing Health History

Biographical Information. Biographical information is factual demographic data that include a patient's age, gender, address, insurance information, occupation, working status, marital status, and referral source. The staff who work in the admitting office usually collect this information.

Chief Concern or Reason for Seeking Health Care. The chief concern is a brief statement about why a patient (in his or her own words) is seeking health care (Ball et al., 2019). This information offers a focus to explore a patient's concerns and issues. Once you learn a patient's chief concerns, you will compare those findings with what you learn during your assessment. Often you will learn much more. Ask a patient why he or she is seeking health care (e.g., "Tell me, Ms. Richard, what brought you to the clinic today?"). Once you learn a chief concern, you then gather more comprehensive data and probe for a full description of the patient's health status. You record a patient's response in quotations to indicate a subjective statement. As you explore a patient's

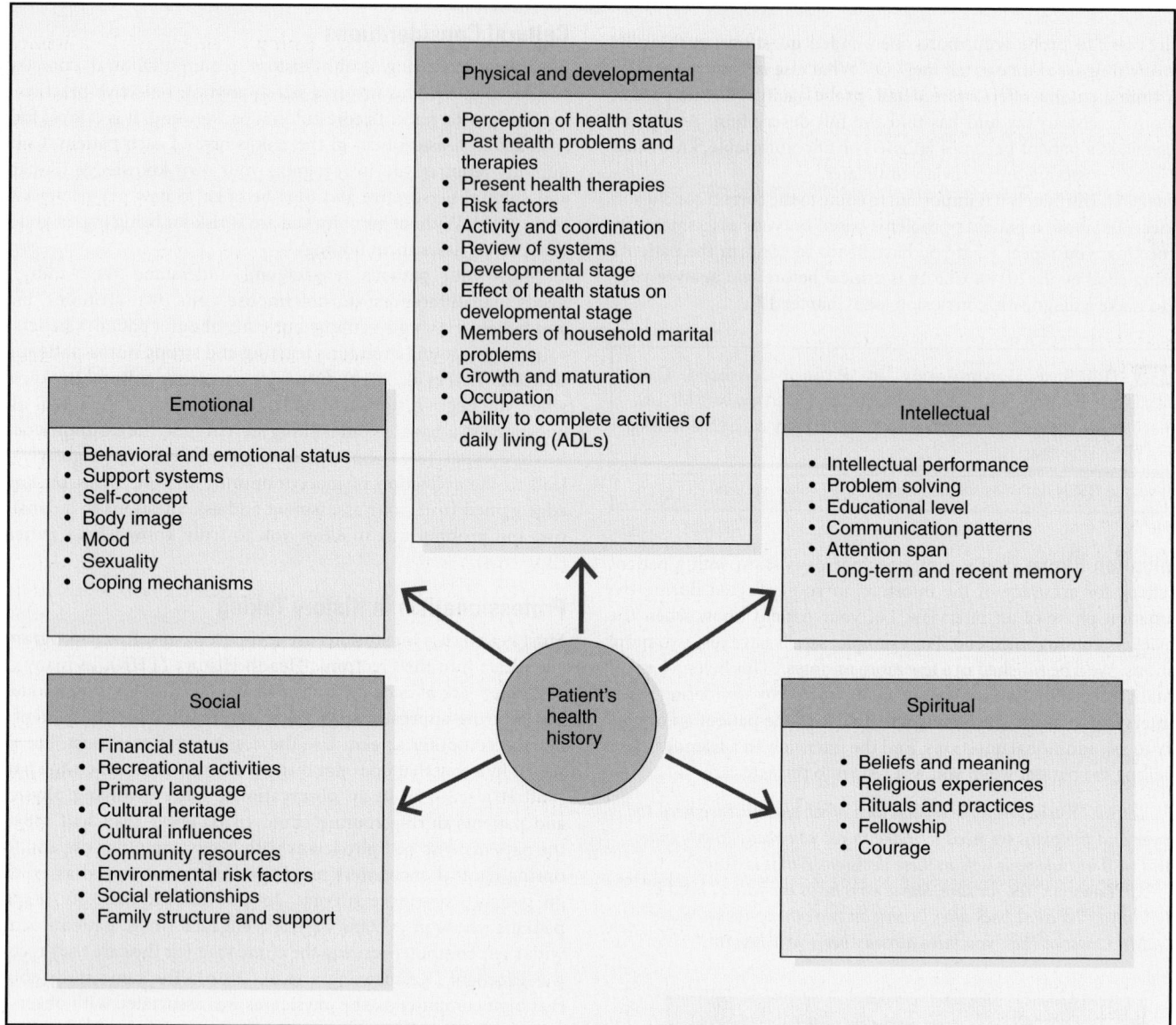

FIG. 16.3 Dimensions for gathering data for a health history.

reason for seeking health care, you will learn the chronological and sequential history of his or her health problems.

Patient Expectations. It is important to assess a patient's expectations of health care providers (e.g., being diagnosed correctly, obtaining pain relief, or being treated for a disease). Patient satisfaction, a standard measure of quality for all hospitals throughout the country, can be perceived by patients as poor if their expectations are unmet (see Chapter 2). Patients typically expect to receive information about their treatments, prognosis, and a plan of care for their return home (whether they are inpatients or outpatients). In addition, they expect relief of pain and other symptoms and to have caring expressed by health care providers. During the initial interview have a patient express expectations when entering the health care setting. Later, as the patient interacts with health care providers, assess whether these expectations changed or were met.

Present Illness or Health Concerns. If a patient presents with an illness, collect essential and relevant data about its course and symptoms. Go slowly as you try to give context to the present illness or problem,

giving it a chronological and sequential framework (Ball et al., 2019). Apply critical thinking intellectual standards (see Chapter 15), and use the acronym (PQRST) to guide your assessment:

P—Provokes (precipitating and relieving factors): How did it come about? What might be the causes for the symptom? What makes it better or worse? Are there activities (e.g., exercise, sleep) that affect it?

Q—Quality What does the symptom feel like? (Have the patient explain in his or her own words.) If the patient has difficulty in describing symptoms, offer probes (e.g., "Is the pain sharp? Dull?" or "Do you feel light-headed, dizzy, off balance?"). What does the illness or symptom mean to the patient?

R—Radiate: Where is the symptom located? Is it in one place? Does it go anywhere else? Have the patient be as precise as possible.

S—Severity: Ask a patient to rate the severity of a symptom on a scale of 0 to 10 (with no symptom at 0 and the worst intensity at 10). This gives you a baseline with which to compare in follow-up assessments.

T—Time: Assess the onset and duration of symptoms. When did a symptom start? Does it come and go? If so, how often and for how long? What time of day or on what day of the week does it occur?

BOX 16.4 CULTURAL ASPECTS OF CARE

Developing a Patient-Centered Approach

To successfully explore a patient's illness or health care problems, use a patient-centered approach. Elicit patient values, preferences, and expressed needs as part of your clinical interview (QSEN, 2018). Ensure the interview is inclusive. When patients desire involvement of family members, remove any barriers to having families present (QSEN, 2018). Use a professional interpreter if there is a language difference.

Implications for Patient-Centered Care
- When talking about a patient's illness, try to understand it "through the patient's eyes."
  - What do you think is wrong with you?
  - What worries you most about your illness?
  - How do you define health and illness? How do you feel about pain, your illness, or death?
- When talking about treatments, value a patient's expertise with own health and symptoms.
  - What should we do to control or eliminate your problem?
  - Which types of treatment do you use at home?
  - What benefits do you expect from the planned treatment?
- Learn about a patient's sources of support (Ball et al., 2019).
  - Who makes decisions in the family?
  - What is the family composition? How many generations are considered part of the family?
  - Are there individuals in the patient's social network that can influence perception of health and illness?
  - Is there a particular cultural group with which the patient identifies?

Also assess whether the patient is experiencing other symptoms along with the primary symptom. For example, does nausea accompany pain? Does the patient have pain along with shortness of breath?

Past Health History. A health history provides a holistic view of a patient's health care experiences and current health habits (see Fig. 16.3). Assess whether a patient has ever been hospitalized or injured or has had surgery. Has any illness or injury limited the patient's ability to function? Include a complete medication history (including past, current, and recent medications). Review the use of any prescription medications, herbal supplements, and over-the-counter (OTC) drugs. Also essential are descriptions of allergies, including allergic reactions to food, latex, drugs, or contact agents (e.g., soap). Asking patients whether they have had problems with medications or food clarifies the type and amount of agent, the specific reaction, and whether a patient has required treatment. If the patient has an allergy, note the specific reaction and treatment on the assessment form and the special armband provided. When considering allergies, also ask if the patient has ever had a blood product transfusion and whether any reactions occurred.

The history also includes a description of a patient's habits, emotional status, and lifestyle patterns. Assessing for the use of alcohol, tobacco, caffeine, or recreational drugs (e.g., methamphetamine or cocaine) determines a patient's risk for diseases involving the liver, lungs, heart, or nervous system. It is essential to gather information about the type of habit and the frequency and duration of use. Assessing patterns of coping (see Chapter 37), sleep (see Chapter 43), exercise (see Chapter 38), and nutrition (see Chapter 45) are also important when planning nursing care. Your aim is to match a patient's lifestyle patterns with interventions in the plan of care as much as possible.

Family History. The family history includes data about immediate and blood relatives. Your objective is to determine whether a patient is at risk for illnesses of a genetic or familial nature and to identify areas of health promotion and illness prevention (see Chapter 6). A complete and accurate family history guides your risk assessment and recommendations for risk-guided prevention strategies (Orlando et al., 2013). There are clinical treatment guidelines for patients and family members based on risk factors for conditions such as breast and ovarian cancer, colon cancer, thrombosis, cardiovascular disease, cerebrovascular disease, inherited cardiomyopathies and arrhythmias, and inherited neurological conditions. For example, a patient with a strong family history of breast cancer will be recommended to pursue mammography more often, and female children may be recommended for genetic counseling.

A patient's family history also reveals information about family structure, interaction, support, and function that is useful in planning care, such as when a family caregiver is needed (see Chapter 10). *In the case study Tonya assesses the level of support that Mrs. Lawson is willing to provide. Mrs. Lawson tells Tonya that the two have been married 32 years and states, "I feel I can do whatever is needed for him." Tonya's assessment shows a pattern that Mrs. Lawson is supportive and able to help her husband adjust to activity limitations when he returns home. Tonya's assessment ultimately allows her to include Mrs. Lawson when she provides patient education.* If a patient's family is not supportive, do not involve the family in care. Stressful family relationships are sometimes a significant barrier when you try to help patients with problems involving loss, self-concept, spiritual health, and personal relationships.

Psychosocial History. A psychosocial history provides information about a patient's support system, which often includes a spouse or partner, children, other family members, and close friends. The history also includes information about ways in which a patient and family typically cope with stress (see Chapter 37). Behaviors that patients use at home to cope with stress such as walking, reading, or talking with a friend can also be used as nursing interventions if the patient experiences stress while receiving health care. In addition, you need to learn whether the patient has experienced any recent losses that create a sense of grief (see Chapter 36).

Spiritual Health. Life experiences and events shape a person's spirituality. The spiritual dimension represents the totality of one's being and is difficult to assess quickly (see Chapter 35). Review with patients their beliefs about life, their source for guidance in acting on beliefs, and the relationship they have with family in exercising their faith. Also assess rituals and religious practices that patients use to express their spirituality. Patients may request availability of these practices while in a health care setting.

Review of Systems. The review of systems (ROS) is a systematic approach for collecting subjective information from patients about the presence or absence of health-related issues in each body system (Ball et al., 2019). During the ROS ask the patient about the normal functioning of each body system and any noted changes. You are more likely to conduct a comprehensive review of all systems during a nonemergent admission to a clinic or an initial home visit. A problem-focused review is common in emergent situations within acute care. Use a series of questions to assess each system as needed. For example, the review of the skin, hair, and nails includes assessment of whether a patient has noticed any rash or skin lesions or has itching or abnormal nail or hair growth. When using a structured admission form, you probably will not cover all of the questions for each body system every time you collect a history. When a patient mentions any unexpected signs or symptoms, explore the affected system(s) more in depth. The systems you assess thoroughly depend on a patient's condition and the urgency in starting care.

Along with the ROS, you conduct a physical examination (see Chapter 30) to further explore and confirm patient information. The physical examination involves use of the techniques of inspection, palpation, percussion, auscultation, and smell. An accurate history helps focus the physical examination, making it more productive and time efficient. As you gain experience, you will learn to look for more data, challenge any interpretations that you made solely based on the history, and persevere to gather accurate and complete assessment data.

Observation of Patient Behavior. Throughout a patient-centered interview and physical examination it is important to closely observe a patient's verbal and nonverbal behaviors. This information adds depth to your objective database. You determine whether data obtained by observation matches what a patient communicates verbally. For example, a patient expresses no concern about an upcoming diagnostic test but shows poor eye contact, shakiness, and restlessness, all suggesting anxiety and verbal and nonverbal data conflict. Observations direct you to gather additional objective information to form accurate conclusions about the patient's condition.

An important aspect of observation includes a patient's level of function: the physical, developmental, psychological, and social aspects of everyday living. Observation of level of function differs from observations you make during an interview. You assess level of function by watching what a patient does when eating or making a decision about preparing a medication rather than what the patient tells you that he or she can do. Observation of function often occurs in the home or in a health care setting during a return demonstration.

Diagnostic and Laboratory Data. The results of diagnostic and laboratory tests provide further explanation of alterations or problems identified during the health history and physical examination. For example, during the history a patient reports having a bad cold for 6 days and currently has a productive cough with brown sputum and mild shortness of breath. On physical examination you notice an elevated temperature, increased respirations, and decreased breath sounds in the right lower lobe. You review the results of a complete blood count and note that the white blood cell count is elevated (indicating an infection). You report your results to the patient's health care provider, who orders a chest x-ray film. When the results of the x-ray film show the presence of a right lower lobe infiltrate, the health care provider makes the medical diagnosis of pneumonia. Your assessment leads to the associated nursing diagnosis of *Impaired Gas Exchange*.

Some patients collect and monitor laboratory data in the home. For example, patients with diabetes mellitus often measure blood glucose daily and those with asthma measure forced expiratory volumes. Ask patients about their routine results to determine their response to illness and information about the effects of treatment measures. Compare laboratory data with the established norms for a particular test, age-group, and gender.

Data Documentation

Record the results of the nursing health history and physical examination in a clear, concise manner using appropriate terminology. This information becomes the baseline to identify a patient's nursing diagnoses and health problems, to plan and implement care, and to evaluate a patient's response to interventions. Standardized forms, especially electronic forms, make it easy to enter assessment data as a patient responds to questions. A timely clear, concise record is necessary for use by other health care professionals (see Chapter 26). If you

do not record an assessment finding or a suspected problem, it is lost and unavailable to anyone else caring for the patient. If information is not specific, the reader is left with only general impressions. Observing and recording patient status are legal and professional responsibilities for all nurses. The Nurse Practice Acts in all states and the American Nurses Association Nursing's Social Policy Statement (ANA, 2010) require accurate data collection and recording as independent functions essential to the role of the professional nurse.

A basic rule in documentation of an assessment is to record all observations succinctly. When recording data, pay attention to facts, and be as descriptive as possible. You need to report anything you hear, see, feel, or smell precisely. Record objective information in accurate terminology (e.g., weighs 77.2 kg [170 lb], abdomen is soft and nontender to palpation). Record any subjective information by using quotation marks. Do not generalize or form judgments through written communication when entering data. Conclusions about such data become nursing diagnoses and thus must be factual and accurate. As you gain experience and learn clusters and patterns of signs and symptoms, you will correctly conclude the existence of a health problem. Review Chapter 26 for details on documentation.

THE ASSESSMENT PROCESS

When you conduct an assessment, think critically about what to assess for a patient's specific situation. As you form your relationship with a patient during the working phase of your interview, the quality of your connection with your patient will affect what the patient chooses to share with you. Determine which questions or measurements are appropriate on the basis of what you initially learn from a patient about his or her health concerns and history, your clinical knowledge, and your experience with other patients.

Data Collection. Use information about a patient's needs to adapt your data collection. Whether you conduct a comprehensive or problem-focused assessment, be sure your data are as thorough as possible. Support subjective findings with objective information. Use all sources for data gathering.

Interpretation. As you gather data, you begin to differentiate important data from all the data you collect. Critically interpret assessment data to determine whether abnormal findings are present. Your clinical reasoning allows you to recognize that further observations are needed to clarify information and begin to identify a patient's health problems. A cue is information you obtain through the use of senses. The cues you gather are the signs and symptoms that you obtain through observation and measurement. You begin to cluster cues that relate together, make inferences, and identify emerging patterns. Clinical inference is part of the clinical decision-making process that occurs before you determine what your patient's problems are. It is the interpretation of the cues (Fig. 16.4). For example, a patient crying is a cue that possibly infers fear, pain, or sadness. You ask the patient about any concerns and make known any nonverbal expressions that you notice in an effort to direct the patient to share his or her feelings. As you see patterns in a patient's signs and systems, you may confirm a pattern by adding more data or refute a pattern based on a different assessment finding. Eventually you will identify potential problems and nursing diagnoses from the patient's data (see Chapter 17).

To assess a patient well you critically anticipate, which means that you continuously think about what the data tell you and decide whether more data are needed. Remember to always have supporting signs and symptoms before you make an inference. Your inferences direct you to further questions. Once you ask a patient a question or

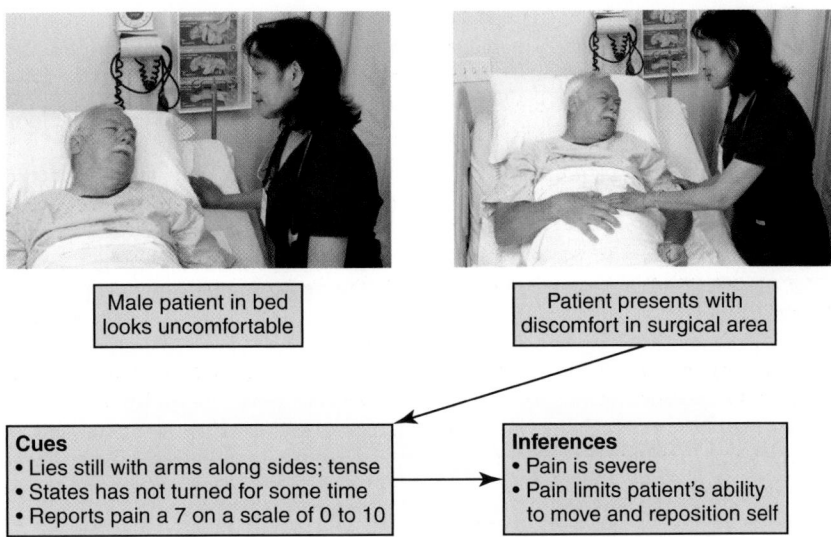

FIG. 16.4 Use of cues to form inferences.

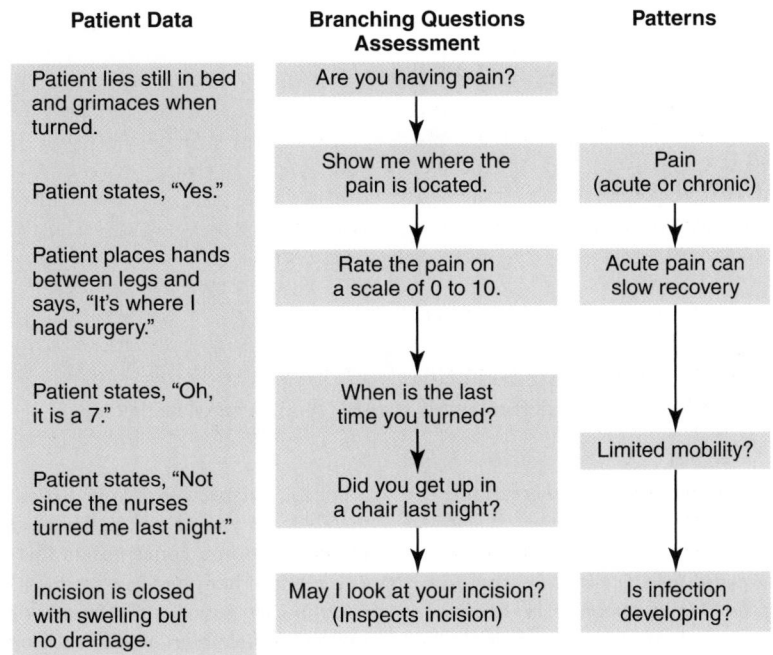

FIG. 16.5 Example of branching logic for selecting additional assessment questions.

make an observation, patterns form, and the information branches to an additional series of questions or observations (Fig. 16.5). Knowing how to probe and frame questions is an assessment skill that grows with experience. You learn to decide which questions are relevant to a situation and attend to accurate data interpretation on the basis of inferences and experience.

Validation. Before you complete data interpretation, validate the information you have collected to avoid making incorrect inferences. Validation of assessment data is the comparison of data with another source to determine data accuracy. For example, you observe a patient crying and logically infer that it is related to hospitalization or a medical diagnosis. Making such an initial inference is not wrong, but problems result if you do not validate the inference with the patient. Instead ask, "I notice that you have been crying. Can you tell me about it?" By validating you discover the real reason for the patient's crying behavior.

Ask patients to validate unclear information obtained during an interview and history. Validate findings from the physical examination and observation of patient behavior by comparing data in the medical record and consulting with other nurses or health care team members. Often family or friends validate your assessment information.

Validation opens the door for gathering more assessment data because it involves clarifying vague or unclear data. Occasionally you need to reassess previously covered areas of the nursing history or gather further physical examination data. Continually analyze to make concise, accurate, and meaningful interpretations. Critical thinking applied to assessment enables you to fully understand a patient's problems, judge the extent of the problems carefully, and discover possible relationships among the problems.

Tonya has gathered assessment data to better understand Mr. Lawson's health care needs. The focus of her assessment switched from

CONCEPT MAP

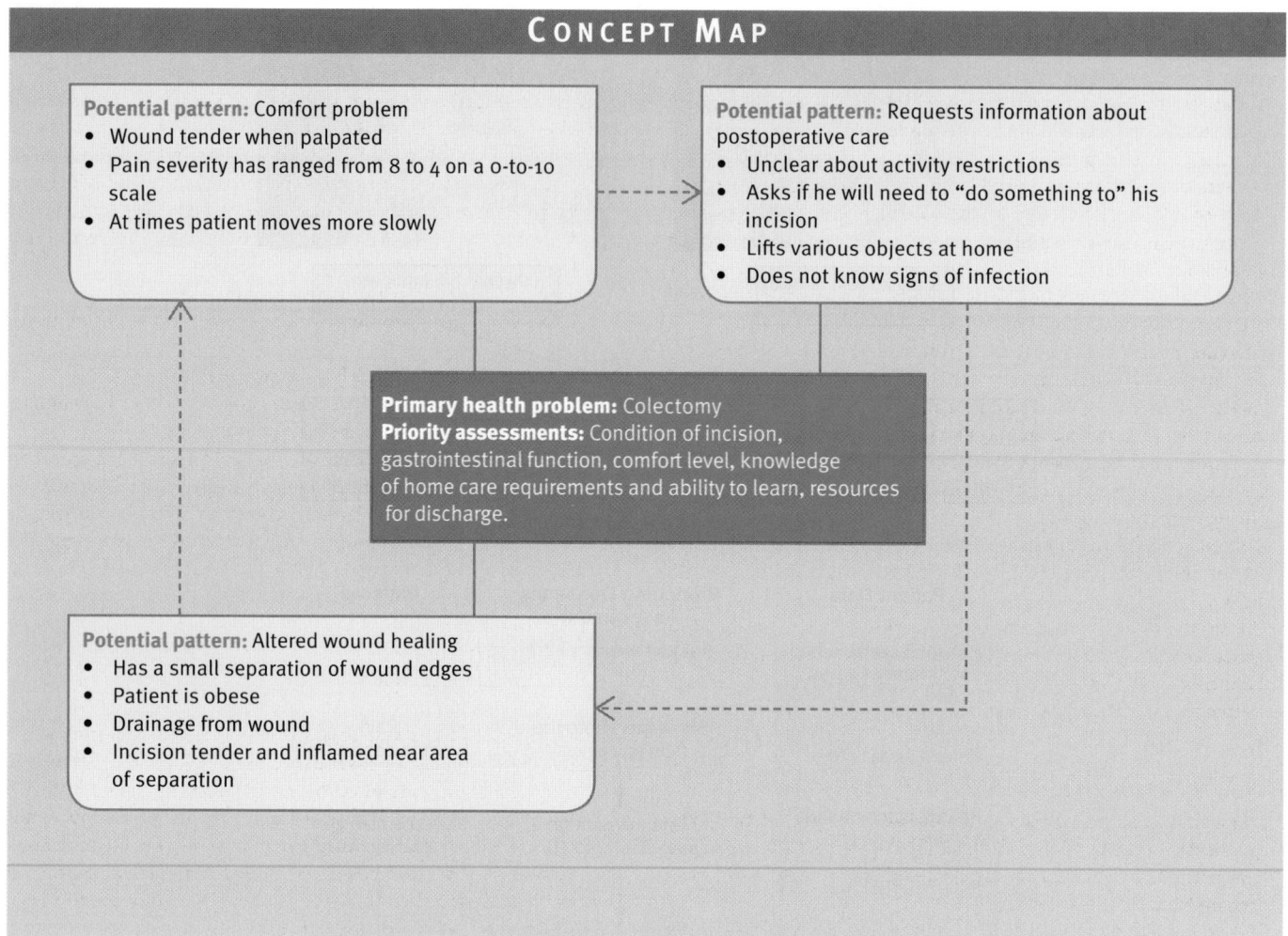

FIG. 16.6 Concept map for Mr. Lawson: Assessment data patterns.

pain to that of physical characteristics of the surgical incision because the patient's condition changed. Her findings suggest that the patient is at risk for infection. She also assessed the patient's knowledge and learning needs so that she can adequately formulate a plan of care to prepare him for discharge. She applied critical thinking in her assessment as she considered the need to include Mr. Lawson's wife in the assessment. In addition, she reflected on her knowledge base concerning the care of patients following a colectomy and anticipated what she needed to assess to plan Mr. Lawson's discharge teaching. When Tonya saw the need for more information, she directed her assessment to learn more about Mr. Lawson's concerns about the success of his surgery and what to expect during recovery.

Concept Mapping

Most patients will present with more than one health problem. A concept map is a visual representation that allows you to graphically show the connections among a patient's many health problems. The concept map is a strategy that develops critical thinking skills by helping a learner understand the relationships that exist among patient problems (Bittencourt et al., 2013). Concept maps foster reflection and help students evaluate critical thinking patterns and see the reasons for nursing care. Your first step in concept mapping is to organize the assessment data you collect. Placing all of the cues together into the clusters that form patterns leads you to the next step of the nursing process, nursing diagnosis (see Chapter 17). Through concept mapping you obtain

a holistic perspective of your patient's health care needs, which ultimately leads you to making better clinical decisions. Fig. 16.6 shows the first step in a concept map that Tonya develops for Mr. Lawson as a result of her nursing assessment. *Tonya begins to identify patterns reflecting Mr. Lawson's problems. As a result of the assessment, she has continuing discomfort over the incision, the risk for development of infection, and the need for instruction about surgical postoperative care. The next step (see Chapter 17) is to identify specific nursing diagnoses so you can plan appropriate nursing interventions.*

■ KEY POINTS

- Nursing assessment includes the collection of information from primary and all secondary sources and the interpretation and validation of the data collected.
- A patient-centered interview is utilized when you conduct a comprehensive nursing history about a patient.
- Periodic assessments collected during rounding or while you administer patient care include quick screenings to rule out or follow up on patient problems.
- A physical examination, conducted during a nursing history and at any time a patient presents a symptom, provides objective data about a patient's clinical status.
- A patient is the primary source of assessment information. Be sure to consider the setting for your assessment and your patient's condition.

- Family members, when appropriate, are useful data sources for confirming assessment findings or identifying important health patterns of the patient.
- A therapeutic nurse-patient relationship enables patients to tell their stories and enables nurses to understand patients and the experiences they express.
- Demonstrate courtesy by introducing yourself, ensuring confidentiality of information shared by the patient, and sitting down next to the patient. Avoid exiting the room too soon. Take time to be present during patient interactions.
- When making a connection with patients, begin with open-ended questions that encourage patients to tell their stories, and do not interrupt patients to allow them to fully describe their symptoms.
- During the working phase of a patient interview use open-ended questions, attentively listen to the patient's response, and summarize key issues to validate your understanding of the patient's story.
- To display professionalism during an interview, look at the patient, not the computer screen, and do not let the computer distract you during history taking.
- A nursing health history includes a patient's chief concern, expectations, and a thorough review of present illness and past health history.
- During the assessment process you determine which questions or measurements are appropriate based on what you initially learn from a patient. You identify cues and form patterns as you make inferences and interpret the clinical meaning of the data.

REFLECTIVE LEARNING

- Think about a patient you recently were assigned to care for during a clinical experience. How did you apply critical thinking when you engaged your patient in a patient-centered interview? How did you prepare in advance for the interview?
- Did you conduct the interview to understand the patient's health concerns "through the patient's eyes"? If yes, explain how you accomplished this. If no, explain why you had difficulty with this aspect of patient assessment. How would you approach this patient differently in the future to better understand the patient's concerns?
- What information did you gather from your patient's family and psychosocial history? How did this information guide your care?

REVIEW QUESTIONS

1. A nurse completes the following steps during her shift of care. Which are the steps of nursing assessment? (Select all that apply.)
   1. The review of patient data in the medical record
   2. Confirming a patient's self-report of abdominal pain by inspecting the abdomen
   3. Reporting results of an ongoing assessment to a nurse working the next scheduled shift
   4. Analyzing a set of signs revealing lower leg weakness and unsteady gait with a pattern of mobility alteration
   5. Conducting an interview of a family caregiver
2. Match the assessment activity on the left with the type of assessment on the right.
   1. Assessment conducted at beginning of a nurse's shift   A. Problem focused
   2. Review of a patient's chief complaint   B. Comprehensive
   3. Completion of admitting history at time of patient admission to a hospital
   4. Completion of the Long Term Care Minimum Data Set during an elderly patient admission to a nursing home

3. A nurse initiates a brief interview with a patient who has come to the medical clinic because of self-reported hoarseness, sore throat, and chest congestion. The nurse observes that the patient has a slumped posture and is using intercostal muscles to breathe. The nurse auscultates the patient's lungs and hears crackles in the left lower lobe. The patient's respiratory rate is 20 per minute compared with an average of 16 per minute during previous clinic visits. The patient tells the nurse, "It is hard for me to get a breath." Which of the following data sets are examples of subjective data? (Select all that apply.)
   1. Heart rate of 20 per minute and chest congestion
   2. Lung sounds revealing crackles and use of intercostal muscles to breathe
   3. Patient statement, "It's hard for me to get a breath"
   4. Slumped posture and previous respiratory rate of 16 per minute
   5. Patient report of sore throat and hoarseness
4. The nurse asks a patient the following series of questions: "Describe for me how much you exercise each day." "How do you tolerate the exercise?" "Is the amount of exercise you get each day the same, less, or more than what you did a year ago?" This series of questions would likely occur during which phase of a patient-centered interview?
   1. Orientation
   2. Working phase
   3. Data interpretation
   4. Termination
5. A young male patient enters the emergency department with fever and signs of a possible sexually transmitted infection. The nurse enters the patient's cubicle and begins to enter a history on the computer screen. Before beginning the nurse introduces himself and tells the patient all information will be held confidentially. The nurse starts data collection by establishing eye contact with the patient and then looks at the computer prompts to select a series of questions. As the nurse fills out questions on the computer, the patient asks a question about his treatment. The nurse states, "Let me get through these questions first." Which action interferes with the nurse's ability to use connection as a communication skill.
   1. Introducing self to patient
   2. Using the computer as a prompt for questions
   3. Making the nurse's questions a priority
   4. Assuring the patient all information is confidential
6. A nurse observes a patient walking down the hall with a shuffling gait. When the patient returns to bed, the nurse checks the strength in both of the patient's legs. The nurse applies the information gained to suspect that the patient has a mobility problem. This conclusion is an example of:
   1. Reflection.
   2. Clinical inference.
   3. Cue.
   4. Validation.
7. Place the following steps of the assessment process in the correct order.
   1. Compare data with another source to determine data accuracy.
   2. As a pattern forms, probe and frame further questions.
   3. Interview a patient, observe behavior, and gather physical assessment findings.
   4. Cluster cues that relate together, make inferences, and identify emerging patterns.
   5. Differentiate important data from the total data you collect.
8. In preparing to collect a nursing history for a patient admitted for elective surgery, which of the following data are part of the review of present illness in the nursing health history?

1. Current medications
2. Patient expectations of planned surgery
3. Review of patient's family support system
4. History of allergies
5. Patient's explanation for what might be the cause of symptoms that require surgery

9. A nurse is conducting a patient-centered interview. Place the statements from the interview in the correct order, beginning with the first statement a nurse would ask.
    1. "You say you've lost weight. Tell me how much weight you've lost in the past month."
    2. "My name is Terry. I'll be the nurse taking care of you today."
    3. "I have no further questions. Is there anything else you wish to ask me?"
    4. "Tell me what brought you to the hospital."
    5. "So, to summarize, you've lost about 6 pounds in the past month, and your appetite has been poor—correct?"

10. Which of the following approaches are recommended when gathering assessment data from an 82-year-old male patient entering a primary care clinic for the first time? (Select all that apply.)
    1. Recognize normal changes associated with aging.
    2. Avoid direct eye contact.
    3. Lean forward and smile as you pose questions.
    4. Allow for pauses as patient tells his story.
    5. Use the list of questions from the clinic assessment form to complete all data.

Answers: 1. 1, 2, 4, 5; **2.** 1A, 2A, 3B, 4B; **3.** 3, 5; **4.** 2, 5; **6.** 2; **7.** 3, 5, 4, 2, 1; **8.** 5, 9, 2, 4, 1, 5, 3; **10.** 1, 3, 4.

Rationales for Review Questions can be found on the Evolve website.

REFERENCES

Agency for Healthcare Research and Quality (AHRQ): *Health literacy measurement tools (revised)*, Rockville, MD, February 2016, Agency for Healthcare Research and QualityFebruary 2016. http://www.ahrq.gov/professionals/quality-patient-safety/quality-resources/tools/literacy/index.html. Accessed April 24, 2018.

American Nurses Association (ANA): *Nursing's social policy statement: the essence of the profession*, ed 3, Washington, DC, 2010, The Association.

American Nurses Association (ANA): *The nursing process*, n.d. , https://www.nursingworld.org/practice-policy/workforce/what-is-nursing/the-nursing-process/. Accessed April 24, 2018.

Ball JW, et al.: *Seidel's guide to physical examination: an interprofessional approach*, ed 9, St Louis, 2019, Elsevier.

Bjørk IT, Hamilton GA: Clinical decision making of nurses working in hospital settings, Nursing Research and Practice, 2011. Available at: https://www.hindawi.com/journals/nrp/2011/524918/. Accessed April 24, 2018.

Carpenito LJ: *Nursing diagnosis: application to clinical practice*, ed 15, Philadelphia, 2017, Lippincott, Williams & Wilkins.

Centers for Medicare and Medicaid Services: *Long term care Minimum data set (MDS) 3.0*, 2010. https://www.resdac.org/cms-data/files/mds-3.0. Accessed August 1, 2019.

Elwyn G, et al.: Shared decision making and motivational interviewing: achieving patient-centered care across the spectrum of health care problems, *Ann Fam Med* 12(3):270, 2014.

Gordon M: *Nursing diagnosis: process and application*, ed 3, St. Louis, 1994, Mosby.

Hersh L, et al.: Health literacy in primary care practice, *Am Fam Physician* 92(2):118, 2015.

Kourkouta L, Papathanasiou IV: Communication in nursing practice, *Mater Sociomed* 26(1):65, 2014.

Muhrer JC: History and physical diagnosis, *Nurse Pract* 39(4):30, 2014.

Pender NJ, et al.: *Health promotion in nursing practice*, ed 7, Upper Saddle River, NJ, 2015, Pearson.

Quality and Safety Education for Nurses Institute (QSEN): *QSEN Competencies*, 2018. http://qsen.org/competencies/pre-licensure-ksas/#patient-centered_care. Accessed April 24, 2018.

The Joint Commission (TJC): *The Joint Commission Center for Transforming Healthcare. Improving transitions of care: hand-off communications*, Oakbrook Terrace, IL, 2014, The Joint Commission.

The Joint Commission (TJC): Sentinel Event Alert: Inadequate hand-off communication, Issue 58, September 12, 2017, https://www.jointcommission.org/assets/1/18/SEA_58_Hand_off_Comms_9_6_17_FINAL_(1).pdf. Accessed November 8, 2018.

Thim T, et al.: Initial assessment and treatment with the Airway, breathing, circulation, disability, Exposure (ABCDE) approach, *Int J Gen Med* 5:117, 2012.

US Department of Health and Human Services (USDHHS): *Standards for privacy of individually identifiable health information*, 2003. https://biotech.law.lsu.edu/cases/medrec/hipaa_combinedrules-08-03.pdf. Accessed April 25, 2018.

RESEARCH REFERENCES

Altin SV, et al.: The evolution of health literacy assessment tools: a systematic review, *BMC Public Health* 14:1207, 2014.

Bittencourt GK, et al.: Concept maps of the graduate programme in nursing: experience report, *Rev Gaucha Enferm* 34(2):172, 2013.

Keifenheim KE, et al.: Teaching history taking to medical students: a systematic review, *BMC Med Educ* 15:159, 2015.

Morris NS, et al.: The Single Item Literacy Screener: evaluation of a brief instrument to identify limited reading ability, *BMC Fam Pract* 7:21, 2006.

Muntean WJ: Nursing clinical-decision making, a literature review, *National Council of State Boards of Nursing*, 2012, Available at: https://www.ncsbn.org/Clinical_Judgment_Lit_Review_Executive_Summary.pdf. Accessed April 25, 2018.

Orlando LA, et al.: Development and validation of a primary care-based family health history and decision support program (MeTree), *N C Med J* 74(4):287, 2013.

Ratanawongsa N, et al.: Association between clinician computer use and communication with patients in safety-net clinics, *JAMA Internal Med* 176(1):125, 2016.

Tanner CA: Thinking like a nurse: a research-based model of clinical judgment in nursing, *J Nurs Educ* 45(6):204, 2006.

Weiss BD, et al.: Quick assessment of literacy in primary care: the newest vital sign, *Ann Fam Med* 3:514, 2005.

Nursing Diagnosis

Nurses continuously collect assessment data. Data collection begins when a nurse cares for a patient the first time, and it continues every time the nurse cares for that patient. Other health care providers also collect data when caring for the patient. All members of the health care team need to share and review the data they collect to provide safe and effective patient care. The nurse constantly observes, interacts, and applies physical examination techniques (Chapter 30) to gather information about a patient's condition to identify accurate and relevant health problems. The American Nurses Association defines nursing as "the protection, promotion, and optimization of health and abilities, prevention of illness and injury, alleviation of suffering through the diagnosis and treatment of human response, and advocacy in the care of individuals, families, communities, and populations" (ANA, 2015). A key word in this definition is *diagnosis*. A nursing diagnosis is made when a nurse identifies a health-related problem or the potential to develop a problem based on patient data. Unless a nurse correctly identifies or diagnoses the nature of a patient's illness or health condition, a patient's real problems will remain unidentified and untreated. While gathering information about a patient, a nurse is constantly sorting data to determine what the data mean. What are the patterns of data that ultimately point to a clear problem or phenomenon? Nursing diagnosis is the second step of the nursing process. Nurses deliberately use critical thinking to make nursing diagnoses that accurately identify a patient's responses to illness.

TYPES OF DIAGNOSES

When making a diagnosis, a clear label or term that is familiar to all those involved in a patient's care is necessary to understand a patient's needs. For example, the terms *anger* or *impaired breathing* are terms that will prompt nurses to consider similar problem areas: emotional and behavioral versus respiratory or ventilatory. Using standardized terminology is essential for diagnostic clarity and effective team communication. Standard nursing terminology allows nurses to formulate nursing diagnoses with associated interventions and to assess the outcomes of nursing care (Mynaříková and Žiaková, 2014). Using nursing diagnosis in practice is supported by health care technologies. For example, it is critical that electronic health records contain standard terminologies that nurses, health care providers, and others can use to communicate a patient's condition and the impact of his or her care to the entire interprofessional team. Within nursing practice there are three types of diagnoses or problem statements.

Medical Diagnoses

The use of medical diagnosis began in ancient China, Egypt, and Greece. Practitioners used diagnoses to describe the symptoms for many illnesses thousands of years ago. When physicians or certified advanced practice nurses identify and confirm common medical diagnoses such as rheumatoid arthritis or diabetes mellitus today, they know the meaning of the diagnoses, the implications, and the standard approaches for treatment. A medical diagnosis is the identification of a disease condition based on a specific evaluation of physical signs and symptoms, a patient's medical history, and the results of diagnostic tests and procedures (Table 17.1). Physicians and advanced practice nurses, such as nurse practitioners and midwives, are licensed to treat diseases and conditions described in medical diagnostic statements. For example, in the case of diabetes, health care practitioners will order various medications and tests such as a hemoglobin A1c (HbA1c) to manage a patient's blood glucose. Medical diagnosis is the language medical practitioners use to communicate a patient's health problem and associated treatments and response.

TABLE 17.1   Example of a Diagnosis With Diagnostic and Assessment Findings

Medical Diagnosis	Diagnostic Findings	Nursing Diagnostic Label	Assessment Findings
Pneumonia	Abnormal lung sounds: crackles, rales Chest x-ray Chest pain with productive cough Confusion Shortness of breath Positive blood culture for pneumococcus	Impaired Respiratory System—impaired gas exchange (ICNP, 2017)	Irregular respirations Tachycardia Orthopnea Hypercapnia Diaphoresis Productive cough Restlessness Confusion Dyspnea

Nursing Diagnosis

A **nursing diagnosis** is a clinical judgment made by a nurse to describe a patient's response or vulnerability to health conditions or life events that a nurse is licensed and competent to treat (NANDA-I, 2018b). It is a diagnostic label that classifies an individual's, family's, or community's response to illness so that all nurses understand a specific patient's health care needs. Nursing prescribes for and treats client and group *responses* to situations that include five categories (Carpenito, 2017): pathophysiological (e.g., myocardial infarction, borderline personality), treatment-related (e.g., anticoagulant therapy, dialysis), personal (e.g., dying, divorce), environmental (e.g., overcrowded school, safety barriers in home), and maturational (e.g., peer pressure, parenthood). Just as health care providers make a medical diagnosis, a nurse identifies a nursing diagnosis by recognizing patterns of assessment data associated with a specific problem (see Table 17.1). Nurses cannot treat medical diagnoses; they cannot order an HgA1c or insulin. Nurses instead treat patients' responses to health conditions. A patient with rheumatoid arthritis will have pain and mobility alterations. Nurses provide interventions to minimize and control pain (e.g., application of heat or cold to an injured area) and improve mobility (e.g., implement early mobility protocols). Nursing diagnoses such as *Acute Pain* or *Activity Intolerance* provide clear direction as to the type of nursing interventions (see Chapter 19) nurses are licensed to provide independently.

Collaborative Problems

A **collaborative problem** is a problem that requires both medicine and nursing interventions to treat (Carpenito, 2017). Nurses practice with other health care professions to manage certain types of collaborative problems using physician-prescribed and nursing-prescribed interventions to minimize complications of the events (Carpenito, 2017). For example, in the case of a patient who enters a clinic with an infected leg wound, the patient's health care provider prescribes antibiotics, the nurse monitors for fever and provides wound care, a dietitian recommends an appropriate therapeutic diet high in protein, and the patient collaborates in learning good hand hygiene and wound care practices. In the case of a patient who is paralyzed from a spinal cord injury, a nurse uses proper positioning and transfer techniques for patient safety while a physical therapist recommends exercises for the patient's extremities.

All physiological complications are not collaborative problems. If a nurse can prevent the onset of a complication or provide the primary treatment for it, then the diagnosis is a nursing diagnosis (Carpenito, 2017). For example:

Nurses Can Prevent	Nursing Diagnosis (ICNP, 2017)
Pressure injuries	*Risk for Pressure Ulcer*
Thrombophlebitis	*Impaired Circulatory System Function*
Aspiration	*Risk for Aspiration*

Nurses Can Treat	Nursing Diagnosis
Stage I or II pressure injuries	*Impaired Tissue Integrity*
Swallowing problems	*Impaired Swallowing*

Nurses Cannot Prevent	Collaborative Problems
Seizures	Seizures
Bleeding	Bleeding

Interprofessional collaboration in managing patient problems is based on the assumption that when health care providers from various disciplines and patients communicate and consider one another's unique perspectives, they will better manage the multiple factors that influence the health of individuals, families, and communities (Sullivan et al., 2015).

REFLECT NOW

Review the electronic health record of a patient to whom you are assigned to care for. Look at the list of all health problems identified. Sort those problem out by nursing diagnoses, medical diagnoses, and collaborative problems.

TERMINOLOGIES FOR NURSING DIAGNOSES

Nurses work in a variety of settings, even within a single health care institution such as a hospital. Therefore, in order for you to be able to communicate knowledge in a meaningful way that can be shared across all disciplines and care settings, common terminologies are necessary. Using standard terms when communicating nursing diagnoses and the associated interventions and patient outcomes resulting from nursing care contributes to effective communication. Health care communicated in unspecific, unclear wording leads to inconsistencies due to differences in naming patients' care needs (nursing diagnoses), nursing interventions, and treatment goals among providers, teams, or facilities (Rabelo-Silva et al., 2016). Standard terminology is a key component of electronic health record systems (EHRs) (see Chapter 26). Common terminologies in EHRs used in the United States include the NANDA International (NANDA-I) (formerly known as the North American Nursing Diagnosis Association), Nursing Intervention Classification (NIC), Nursing Outcome Classification (NOC), Omaha System, and the SNOMED CT for clinical terminology (Lundberg et al., 2008). A standard terminology system used across the world is the International Classification for Nursing Practice (ICNP®), which was developed by The International Council of Nurses (ICN, 2017). The ICN is a federation of more than 130 national nurses associations (NNAs), representing more than 20 million nurses worldwide (ICN, 2017).

It is common for a health care institution to work with vendors of EHRs to create a standard language or set of terminologies unique to the institution. At times these terminologies are based on medical diagnoses only and the opinions or expertise of the institution's health care staff. Nursing diagnosis terminology may or may not be integrated. When it is not integrated, it is up to an individual nurse to specifically identify a patient's relevant nursing diagnoses as they pertain to the patient's health condition.

The nursing diagnosis classification and taxonomy system of NANDA-I was developed in 1982, when nurse educators recognized that assessment data needed to be analyzed and clustered into patterns and interpreted before nurses could make accurate nursing diagnoses (NANDA-I, 2018a). Soon diagnosis became part of the five-step nursing process. The NANDA-I diagnostic classification system has grown to currently include 244 diagnoses (NANDA-I, 2018b). You cannot plan and intervene correctly for patients if you do not know the health problems or conditions you are dealing with. The NANDA-I terminology is one system that provides standard, formal diagnostic statements (including definitions, defining characteristics, and related or risk factors). The NANDA-I system aims to achieve the following outcomes (NANDA-I, 2018b):

- Provide a precise definition of a patient's human responses to health problems and life processes.
- Develop, refine, and disseminate evidence-based terminology representing clinical judgments by professional nurses.
- Allow nurses to communicate (e.g., verbally and in writing) what to do among themselves and with other health care professionals and the public.
- Foster the development of nursing knowledge through research.
- Contribute to the development of informatics and information standards.
- Document care for reimbursement of nursing services.

Many of these same outcomes describe the purposes of the ICNP® system. The ICN developed the International Classification for Nursing Practice (ICNP®) as a unified nursing language system to support standardized nursing documentation at the patient's bedside or point of care (ICN, 2017). It is a wide-ranging, understandable reference terminology that can adapt to multiple purposes (e.g., documentation, research categories, practice guidelines) in different countries and that serves as a primary resource to describe nursing practices (Rabelo-Silva et al., 2016). The ICNP is a classification of nursing phenomena (diagnoses), nursing actions or interventions, and nursing outcomes that describes nursing practice. The ICNP® system currently uses a model that has 7 axes (Box 17.1). With multi-axial terminology, terms from different axes are combined to create a concept. For example, the term "pain" (from the ICNP® Focus of Nursing Practice Axis) can be combined with "chronic" (from the ICNP® Duration Axis) to create the diagnosis "chronic pain." Nurses and other hospital staff can use the data-based information from ICNP® for planning and managing nursing care, financial forecasting, analysis of patient outcomes, and health policy development (ICN, 2017).

BOX 17.1 ICNP 7 Axes With Definitions

- **Focus:** The area of attention that is relevant to nursing (e.g., pain, homelessness, elimination, life expectancy, knowledge).
- **Judgment:** Clinical opinion or determination related to the focus of nursing practice (e.g., decreasing level, risk, enhanced, interrupted, abnormal).
- **Client:** Subject to whom a diagnosis refers and who is the recipient of an intervention (e.g., newborn, caregiver, family, community).
- **Action:** An intentional process applied to or performed by a client (e.g., educating, changing, administering, monitoring).
- **Means:** A manner or method of accomplishing an intervention (e.g., bandage, bladder-training technique)
- **Location:** Anatomical and spatial orientation of a diagnosis or intervention (e.g., posterior, abdomen, school, community health center).
- **Time:** The point, period, instance, interval, or duration of an occurrence (e.g., admission, childbirth, chronic).

Adapted from Garcia TR, Nobrega MML: The International Classification for Nursing Practice: participation of Brazilian nurses in the project of the International Council of Nurses, *Acta Paul Enferm* 22(Especial - 70 Anos):875-9, 2009.

In addition to improving communication among health care providers, using standard nursing terminology creates a scientific knowledge base for nursing. Advances in the discipline of nursing involve the development of interconnections among three elements: theory, research, and nursing practice. The use of a clear, well-established terminology system such as nursing diagnoses forms the basis of classification systems in nursing care. Such classification systems help nurses recognize phenomena, make correct decisions, and perform research activities in clinical settings that build new knowledge within the profession of nursing (Mynaříková and Žiaková, 2014).

There are similarities in the language of NANDA-I and the ICNP. The ICNP taxonomy or model refers to nursing diagnoses, while NANDA-I officially refers to diagnostic labels. The two classification systems have many of the same labels for certain diagnoses, while there is also much variation in labels describing similar responses to health conditions.

QSEN **Building Competency in Teamwork and Collaboration** A nurse is caring for a 73-year-old patient who fell while in the hospital. The patient has cardiac and respiratory health problems that affect her ability to tolerate exercise. The nurse is attending a discharge planning conference with the physical therapist and social worker. Describe how this nurse can enhance interprofessional collaboration with the other health care providers in the use of nursing diagnosis.

Answers to QSEN Activities can be found on the Evolve website.

Types of Nursing Diagnostic Statements

NANDA-I categorizes nursing diagnoses into three types: problem-focused, risk diagnosis, and health promotion (NANDA-I, 2018b). The ICNP® categorizes diagnoses as positive or negative nursing diagnoses with associated outcomes. The focus of diagnoses from both classifications is similar. Problem-focused nursing diagnoses or negative diagnoses identify an undesirable human response to existing problems or concerns of a patient. Examples include *Acute Pain* or *Urinary Retention* (NANDA-I, 2018b) or *Acute Pain* and *Impaired Urination* (ICN, 2017). Risk nursing diagnoses are diagnoses that apply when there is an increased potential or vulnerability for a patient to develop a problem or complication (NANDA-I, 2018b). Examples include *Risk for Fall* (ICN, 2017) and *Risk for Unstable Blood Pressure* (NANDA-I,

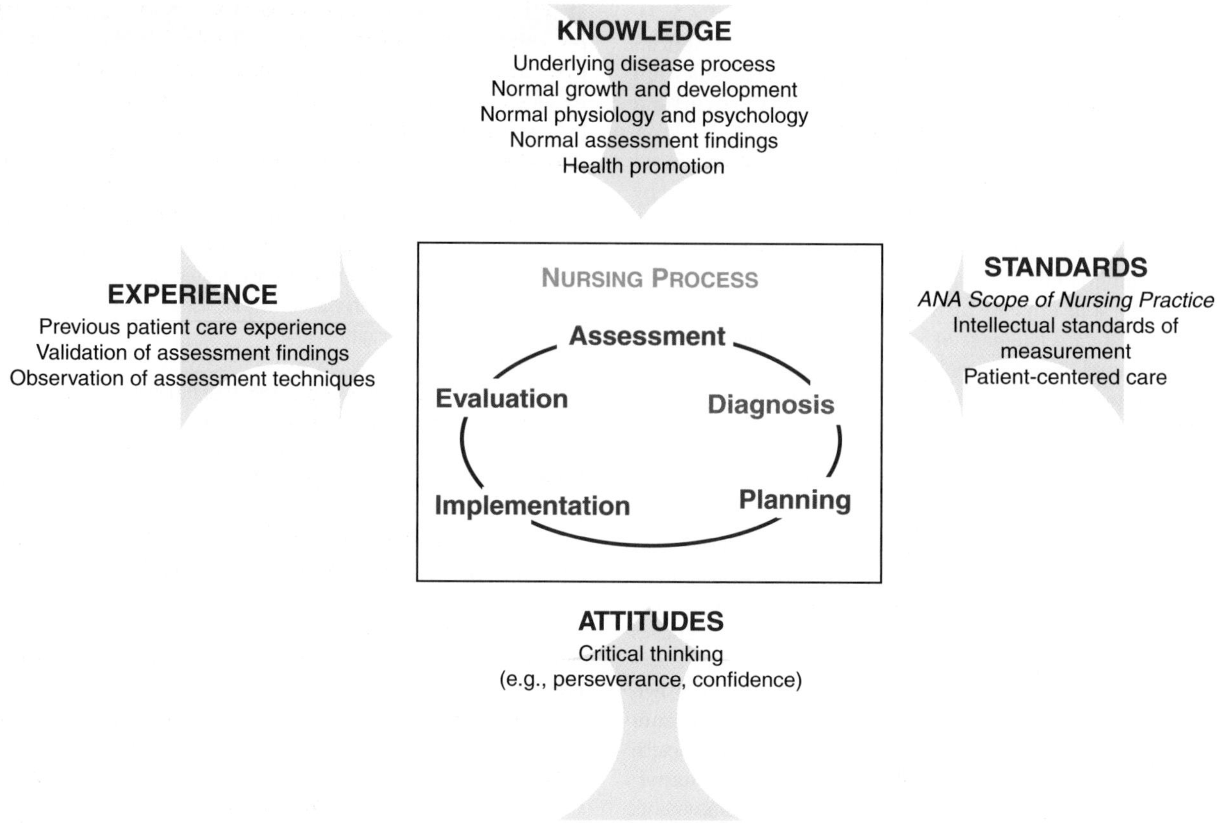

KNOWLEDGE
Underlying disease process
Normal growth and development
Normal physiology and psychology
Normal assessment findings
Health promotion

EXPERIENCE
Previous patient care experience
Validation of assessment findings
Observation of assessment techniques

NURSING PROCESS

Assessment

Evaluation   **Diagnosis**

Implementation   **Planning**

STANDARDS
ANA Scope of Nursing Practice
Intellectual standards of
measurement
Patient-centered care

ATTITUDES
Critical thinking
(e.g., perseverance, confidence)

FIG. 17.1 Critical thinking and the nursing diagnostic process.

2018b). Health promotion nursing diagnoses and positive diagnoses identify the desire or motivation to improve health status through a positive behavioral change. Examples include *Readiness for Enhanced Relationship* and *Readiness for Enhanced Power* (NANDA-I, 2018b) and *Positive Family Support* and *Hope* (ICN, 2017). Although many nursing diagnoses are used to identify problems being experienced by individual patients, you will apply some nursing diagnoses to families, groups of individuals, and communities.

CRITICAL THINKING AND THE NURSING DIAGNOSTIC PROCESS

Use the nursing diagnostic process to accurately identify a patient's nursing diagnoses. Critical thinking (see Chapter 15), with the application of knowledge, experience, critical thinking attitudes, and intellectual standards during the collection of a comprehensive assessment database about a patient, will improve diagnostic accuracy (Fig. 17.1). When practicing nursing, it is important for you to know the nursing diagnosis classification system used within your school and clinical practice sites. You will also need to become familiar with the definitions, related or causative factors, and the defining characteristics or assessment findings that apply to each diagnosis. It is impossible to memorize the information needed for every type of nursing diagnosis, no matter what system you use. However, you need to know how to access this information easily within the agency in which you work. Sources of information about nursing diagnoses include faculty, advanced practice nurses, clinical staff, documentation systems, and practice guidelines.

Use patient assessment data during the diagnostic reasoning process to logically explain a clinical judgment, in this case a nursing diagnosis. You gather a comprehensive set of data, validate your information, and add additional data if you find information is lacking. You

then interpret the data by identifying clusters or patterns that lead to identification of nursing diagnoses and other problems. The diagnostic process flows from the assessment process and includes decision-making steps (Fig. 17.2).

Data Clustering and Finding Patterns

Your review and analysis of assessment data involve critically organizing all data elements about a patient into meaningful patterns, also called **data clusters** or sets of assessment findings/defining characteristics. A set of assessment findings is a group of data elements, the signs or symptoms gathered during assessment. Each data element is an objective or subjective sign, symptom, or risk factor that leads you into making a diagnostic conclusion (see Chapter 16). As you analyze data, you begin to see data elements that offer cues to a type of health problem. For example, shortness of breath, walking only 100 feet before becoming breathless, and an increased respiratory rate suggest a breathing problem pattern. A patient who reports having no immediate family, does not initiate conversation, and who just lost his vision shows a coping problem pattern. It is these patterns or data clusters that begin to shape a more formal label or description.

While looking for a pattern, compare a patient's data with information that is consistent with normal, healthy patterns. Use accepted norms as the basis for comparison and judgment, norms such as laboratory test values, professional standards, and normal physiological limits. Also determine whether the grouped signs and symptoms are expected for a patient (e.g., consider current condition and history) and whether they are within the range of healthy responses. Separate out data that are not within healthy norms to allow you to identify a pattern correctly.

During assessment you collect individual data points either intentionally or unintentionally. An intentional assessment includes the deliberate collection of data through physical examination or

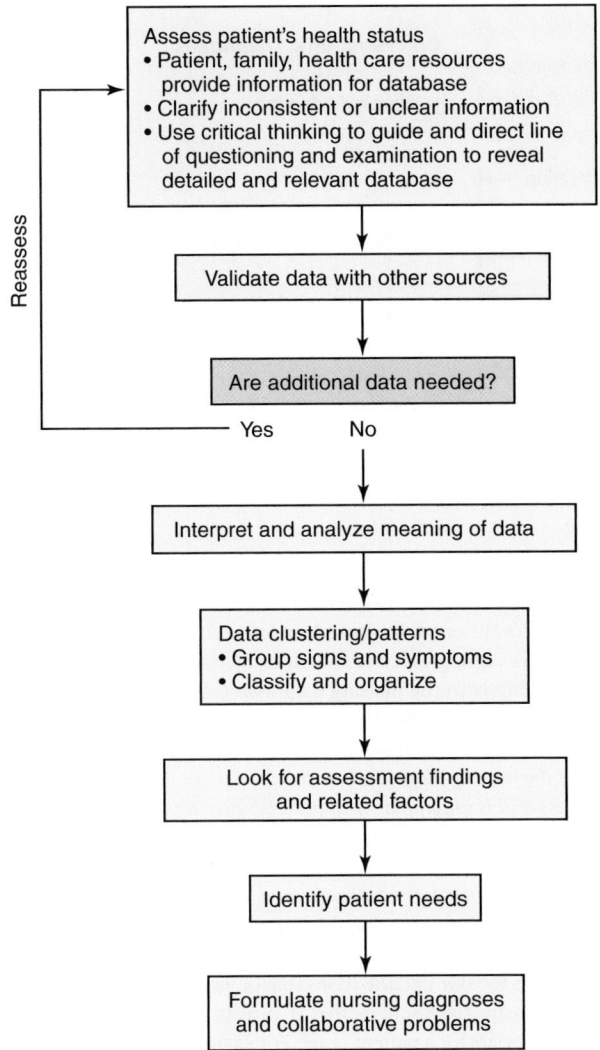

FIG. 17.2 Nursing diagnostic process.

When assessment data reveal risk factors (i.e., the factors that increase a patient's vulnerability to an unhealthy event), you will recognize patterns, compare the patterns with expected data for a risk diagnosis, and then select the correct risk nursing diagnosis.

During her assessment in Chapter 16 Tonya gathered information suggesting that Mr. Lawson possibly has several health problems. The data about Mr. Lawson are cues that form patterns in three areas: comfort, requesting information about postoperative care for impending discharge, and the potential for infection at his wound site. Selecting specific diagnoses for these problem areas will allow Tonya to develop a relevant and appropriate plan of care.

Data Interpretation

Data interpretation involves placing a label on your data pattern or cluster to clearly identify a patient's response to health problems. Selecting a diagnosis cannot be casual or simply intuitive. Critical thinking is necessary. Your interpretation of data clusters or patterns leads to the selection of various nursing diagnoses that apply to your patient. It is important to compare the data in a cluster with the data standards for a diagnosis to come to a reasoned conclusion about a patient's response to a health problem.

In the case of the NANDA-I classification, the standards are the defining characteristics or risk factors (NANDA-I, 2018b) used to form a diagnosis. When ICNP® is used as the diagnosis system, the institution where you work will have set standards for the assessment findings and risk factors that form a pattern for a nursing diagnosis (Fig. 17.3). Nurses who use ICNP® in their care settings have contributed to the development of clinically relevant sets of diagnosis, outcome, and intervention statements for a variety of health priorities and delivery settings (Coenen et al., 2012). Users of ICNP have created catalogs of nursing data subsets for specified health phenomena (nursing diagnoses such as pain), diseases (e.g., HIV/AIDS, depression), care specialties (e.g., palliative care), and care settings (e.g., neonatal nursery). These catalogs are then used to build health information systems (Rabelo-Silva et al., 2016).

Regardless of the diagnostic system you use, you compare your data with the assessment findings standard for select nursing diagnoses to select the specific diagnosis that fits your patient. The recognition of data in a logical cluster or pattern reveals the nursing diagnoses, how a patient is responding to a health condition or life process.

*Tonya clusters the data she has learned from Mr. Lawson, analyzes the data, and recognizes patterns of a knowledge problem. As Tonya considers Mr. Lawson's request for information, there are different nursing diagnoses for problems related to knowledge, including **Lack of Knowledge, Readiness for Enhanced Knowledge, and Adequate Knowledge.** Knowing the differences among these diagnoses and identifying which one applies comes from thoughtful interpretation of data. Lack of Knowledge suggests the patient has insufficient knowledge about a topic or area of interest. Readiness for Enhanced Knowledge or Adequate Knowledge infers that the individual has knowledge about a topic but needs further information to strengthen understanding. Tonya learns that this was Mr. Lawson's first experience with major surgery. His earlier questions about lifting and incision care suggest he has limited knowledge of postoperative care.*

interviewing during a health history. Unintentional assessment is noticing data points that are important without planning to collect them (NANDA-I, 2018b). For example, an unintentional data point is seeing a patient grimace and hold a body part while you turn and reposition the patient in bed.

Finding a data cluster helps you think less about individual data points and instead focus on pattern recognition. Your ability to recognize a pattern or cluster comes with clinical experience and intentional practice. At first you will not notice some of the subtleties you find when observing or examining patients. For example, the first time you look at a patient's surgical wound you will notice the length of an incision and general color of the surrounding skin, but you might not notice an individual suture that has loosened or minor swelling at the end of the incision.

While clustering data you will find that some data are descriptive (e.g., patient's age) and do not necessarily fit a pattern with other data. You also will find data that relate to the cause or nature of a patient's problem (e.g., history of stroke, poor adherence to therapy). A specific assessment finding may apply to one or more patterns of data (e.g., moving a limb slowly can reveal a mobility problem, as well as a problem with comfort). As you recognize data elements, you will cluster or group them together in patterns in a logical way that during interpretation will reveal the nursing diagnoses that describe how a patient is responding to a health condition or life process.

Working with similar patients over a period of time helps you recognize patterns of assessment findings, but remember that each patient is unique and requires an individualized diagnostic approach. It can be a challenge to select a diagnosis when assessment findings for two different diagnoses are similar. For example, having insufficient knowledge to set up a medication schedule and being unable to identify the purpose of a medication might be considered assessment

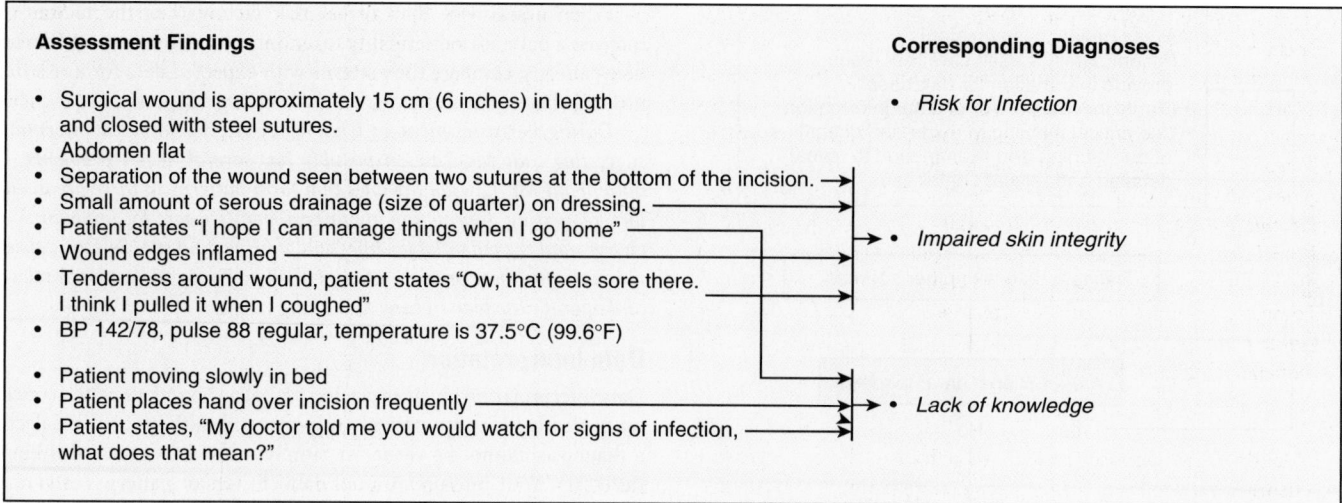

Assessment Findings

- Surgical wound is approximately 15 cm (6 inches) in length and closed with steel sutures.
- Abdomen flat
- Separation of the wound seen between two sutures at the bottom of the incision. →
- Small amount of serous drainage (size of quarter) on dressing. ——
- Patient states "I hope I can manage things when I go home" ——
- Wound edges inflamed ——
- Tenderness around wound, patient states "Ow, that feels sore there. I think I pulled it when I coughed"
- BP 142/78, pulse 88 regular, temperature is 37.5°C (99.6°F)

- Patient moving slowly in bed
- Patient places hand over incision frequently ——
- Patient states, "My doctor told me you would watch for signs of infection, —— what does that mean?"

Corresponding Diagnoses

- *Risk for Infection*

- *Impaired skin integrity*

- *Lack of knowledge*

FIG. 17.3 Comparing assessment data with standards.

findings for the diagnoses of *Lack of Knowledge* (ICNP, 2017) or *Impaired Ability To Manage Medication Regime* (ICNP, 2017). Further exploration is needed to determine if the patient's problem is a knowledge issue only or if the patient has physical limitations that prevent him or her from following a medication schedule. Remember, as you gather data and see clusters or patterns, confirm your data with your source of standards for the diagnostic system you use. It is critical to select the correct diagnosis for each of a patient's health problem responses.

Formulating the Diagnostic Statement

The way you phrase or word a nursing diagnostic statement affects how you communicate a patient's problems to other health care staff, which nursing interventions you choose, and how you evaluate patient outcomes. Clarity and precision are essential. When forming a diagnosis, each type of diagnosis has a different format. You write problem-focused nursing diagnostic statements with three parts: a diagnosis label, related factors, and major defining characteristics (NANDA-I, 2018b, p. 113). Risk nursing diagnoses have two segments: a diagnosis and the associated risk factors preceded by the phrase *as evidenced by* (NANDA-I, 2018b, p. 114). Health promotion nursing diagnoses also are written with only two sections: the diagnosis label and defining characteristics or assessment findings. Unless you use the correct format for a nursing diagnosis, the label for the diagnosis is meaningless and can easily be misunderstood (NANDA-I, 2018b).

The same formats can be used for ICNP® diagnoses as well. However, establishing a nursing diagnosis in the ICNP system requires that a clinical nurse select at least one term from two axes, namely, the axes "focus" and "judgment" (Rabelo-Silva et al., 2016). The focus is the area of relevance to nursing practice, e.g., physiological status or knowledge, whereas judgment is the clinical opinion related to the selected focus, e.g., decreasing level, risk, or enhanced. If you use ICNP® diagnoses, choose among the assessment findings that have formed a pattern for a specific diagnosis; then you can also include a related factor from the data gathered.

Components

Diagnostic Label or Diagnosis—A diagnostic label or diagnosis is the name of a nursing diagnosis approved by NANDA-I, ICNP®, or any other system used by your institution. The NANDA-I system offers definitions for each diagnosis to describe the characteristics of the human response identified.

Related Factors—A patient's response to a health problem is related to a set of conditions that caused or influenced the response. Related factors are etiologies, circumstances, facts, or influences that have a relationship with the nursing diagnosis (NANDA-I, 2018b).

*Tonya uses a critical thinking approach to identify the correct diagnosis that applies to Mr. Lawson's situation. She selects **Lack of Knowledge** as the nursing diagnosis because the patient has not undergone surgery and is unfamiliar with postoperative routines. She further clarifies the statement as **Lack of Knowledge regarding postoperative care**. She then selects the related factor as the patient's inexperience. She words the formal diagnosis as **Lack of Knowledge regarding postoperative care related to inexperience with surgery**.*

A review of your assessment data will identify the related factor that applies to your patient. The value of having a related factor in the diagnostic statement is that it directs the type of interventions appropriate for a patient's care. For example, the nursing diagnosis *Body Weight Problem* from the ICNP® system is a clearer statement when written as *Body Weight Problem related to nausea and inadequate nutrient intake*. Appropriate interventions for this diagnosis include adjusting the type of diet (e.g., switching from solid foods to liquids), controlling the patient's mealtime environment by eliminating noxious odors, and administering prescribed antiemetics (collaborative intervention). In contrast, for the diagnosis *Body Weight Problem related to excess calorie intake and limited knowledge about healthy food choices*, the choice of interventions is very different (e.g., patient education regarding healthy diet, patient creating a weekly menu, adding an exercise plan).

Related factors for NANDA-I diagnoses have been categorized into four groups: pathophysiological (biological or psychological), treatment-related, situational (environmental or personal), and maturational (Carpenito, 2017). The ICNP® system has not defined sets of possible related factors for nursing diagnoses. A related factor is not intended as a cause-and-effect statement. It instead indicates that the etiology contributes to or is associated with the patient's diagnosis (Fig. 17.4). Risk diagnoses do not have related factors because you are identifying a vulnerability in a patient for a potential problem; a problem does not yet exist (NANDA-I, 2018b).

Major Assessment Findings—Further clarity is added to a diagnostic statement if you list major assessment findings or defining characteristics that were used to select a diagnosis. Highlighting a patient's major assessment findings offers guidelines for how you will evaluate the efficacy of nursing care. For example, in the diagnosis *Body*

Weight Problem: Underweight related to nausea and inadequate nutrient intake, adding the phrase "*as evidenced by 10-lb weight loss in 1 month and oral pain*" offers more information to plan nursing care. Outcomes for a patient with this problem will include a specific targeted monthly weight gain and the patient's report of reduced or absent oral pain (see Chapter 20).

In the case of Mr. Lawson, Tonya offers further clarity to the patient's diagnosis, entering the final diagnostic statement in his plan of care, "Lack of Knowledge regarding postoperative care related to inexperience with surgery as evidenced by frequent queries about postoperative routines."

A complete, accurate diagnostic statement is necessary to deliver appropriate patient-centered care. Table 17.2 shows further examples of the benefits of diagnostic clarity.

Diagnostic Validity

Before identifying a diagnosis, refer to the official ICNP® or NANDA-I list to ensure accuracy of the diagnostic statement. This is essential for

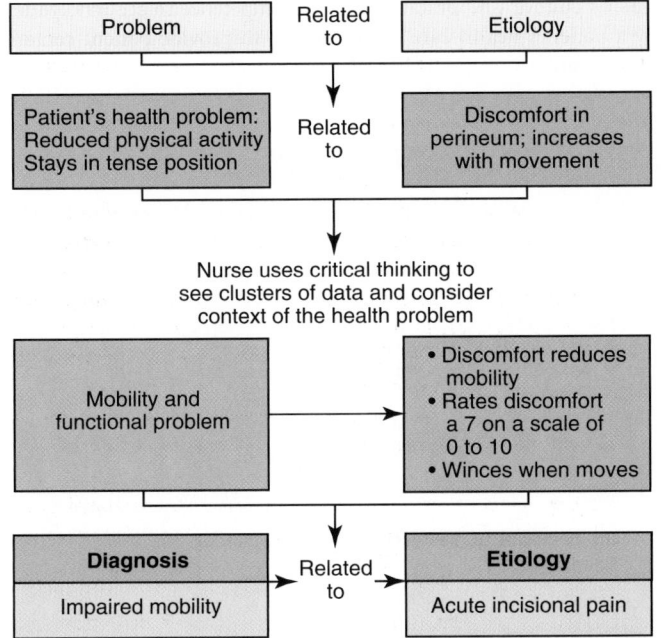

FIG. 17.4 Relationship between a diagnosis and related factor or etiology.

clear communication with all health care team members. Standard diagnostic terminology must be used in any electronic health record using nursing diagnosis. Accurate nursing diagnoses are foundational to the development of an effective, personalized plan of care (Yoost and Crawford, 2020).

> **REFLECT NOW**
>
> Share a case summary of assessment findings from a patient you cared for with a student colleague. Compare the nursing diagnoses you make with those your colleague makes. Discuss the similarities and differences.

USE OF NURSING DIAGNOSIS IN PRACTICE

Patients usually present with a variety of health problems, and these problems can cause numerous types of human responses. For example, a medical diagnosis of cerebrovascular accident or stroke often results in altered human responses, including changes in mobility, speech, thought processes, behavioral coping, and family support. Therefore, a single nursing diagnosis such as altered mobility is insufficient to truly design a comprehensive patient-centered approach to care. The assessment findings you obtain will often apply to one or more nursing diagnoses. For example, the subjective finding of "Patient hesitant to perform range-of-motion exercises" may apply to the diagnoses of *Impaired Exercise Behaviour* and *Lack of Knowledge*. The patient's hesitancy to perform the exercise may be due to the patient's unwillingness to accept his health problem, or it may also be due to the patient's insufficient knowledge to perform the exercise correctly. Thoroughly interpreting assessment findings leads to a broader picture of a patient's various health responses. One way to communicate the relationship between a patient's multiple nursing diagnoses is through Concept Mapping.

Concept Mapping

In Chapter 16 you learned how concept mapping offers a graphic look at the connections among patients' multiple health responses to problems. It is challenging to prioritize and focus on all of a patient's nursing diagnoses. The challenge is compounded when you care for multiple patients in clinical practice. A concept map helps you critically think about a patient's diagnoses and how they relate to one another. Many

TABLE 17.2	Comparison of Interventions for Nursing Diagnoses With Different Related Factors		
Nursing Diagnoses	**Related Factor**	**Assessment Findings**	**Interventions**
Patient A			
Anxiety	Uncertainty over surgery	Patient asks, "What type of pain will I have?" Restless and unable to sleep	Provide detailed instruction about surgery, recovery process, expected postoperative care. Plan formal time for patient to ask questions.
Impaired Mobility	Acute pain	Pain rated a 7 on scale of 1 to 10 Limits movement of right leg	Administer analgesic 30 minutes before planned exercise. Instruct patient on how to splint painful site during activity.
Patient B			
Anxiety	Loss of Job	Fired from position 1 month ago Primary source of family income	Consult with social worker to arrange for job counseling. Encourage health promotion activities (e.g., exercise, routine social activities).
Impaired Mobility	Musculoskeletal injury	Weakness in right leg Reduced extension in right leg	Perform active range-of-motion exercises to right leg every 2 hours. Instruct patient on use of 3-point crutch gait.

educators use concept mapping to help students develop critical thinking (Aein and Aliakbari, 2017). Concept mapping organizes and links data about a patient's multiple diagnoses in a logical way. It graphically represents the connections among concepts (e.g., nursing diagnoses, assessment findings, and interventions) that relate to a central subject (the patient's primary health problems). In Fig. 17.5 the dotted lines between nursing diagnoses show that one diagnosis is directly related to another. Concept mapping develops skills that provide nurses with expertise in flexible, individualized, situation-specific problem solving for each patient (Aein and Aliakbari, 2017).

*In Fig. 17.5, the concept map for Mr. Lawson, three nursing diagnoses have been developed and linked together to communicate Mr. Lawson's health care needs. The diagnosis of **Acute Pain** has a direct impact on the patient's **Lack of Knowledge,** which will require Tonya and the other nurses to consider teaching approaches that take Mr. Lawson's comfort level into consideration (see Chapter 18). Pain reduces a patient's attentiveness. The patient's **Lack of Knowledge** affects his **Risk for Infection** because Mr. Lawson must understand wound care before he goes home. As Tonya reviews the concept map, she sees the interrelationships of his nursing diagnoses and ultimately the interventions that she includes in his plan of care.*

An advantage of a concept map is its central focus on a patient rather than on a disease or health alteration, even though the patient's health problems are central. This holistic focus encourages nurses to concentrate on patients' specific health problems and nursing diagnoses rather than using one approach for all patients with similar problems.

Cultural Relevance in Diagnostics

When you select nursing diagnoses, consider your patients' cultural diversity, including ethnicity, values, beliefs, language, and health practices (see Chapter 9). This includes knowing the cultural differences that affect how your patients define health and illness and their preferences or choices for treatment. For example, Lai et al. (2013) explored how nursing diagnoses affected the quality of professional nursing from the perspective of Taiwanese nurses. Their work found that certain diagnoses were difficult for nurses to apply considering the cultural beliefs of the traditional Chinese health care setting, which emphasizes holistic harmony and balance. It is important to know yourself, consider your patient's culture, and practice cultural competence to accurately identify a patient's health care problems and to provide patient-centered nursing care.

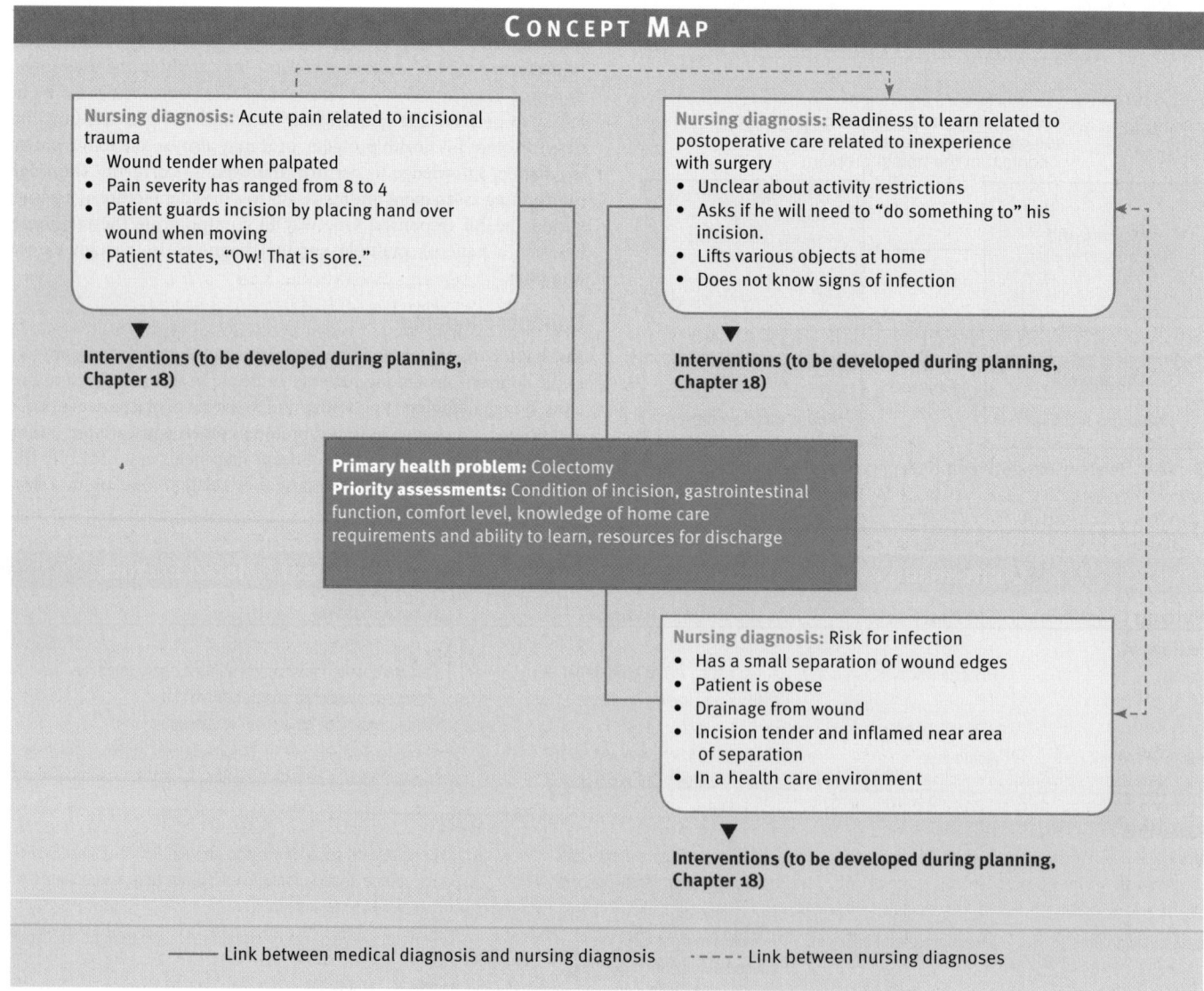

FIG. 17.5 Concept map for Mr. Lawson: Nursing diagnoses identified.

Consider the example of the ICNP* nursing diagnosis *Conflicting Caregiver Attitude,* where differences of opinion are found to exist between family caregivers of a patient near the end of life. It would be easy to apply your own cultural bias in selecting this diagnosis, depending on your beliefs, past experiences, and comfort in counseling caregivers about death. It would also be easy to apply the diagnosis inappropriately without considering the patient's and family members' values and beliefs. Attitudes and behaviors of families and care providers toward patients and their relationships with patients can affect patients' dignity significantly (Guo and Jacelon, 2014). The inappropriate selection of a nursing diagnosis based on your values or beliefs potentially results in the implementation of interventions that a patient or family caregiver is unlikely to accept. Consider asking these questions to make culturally competent nursing diagnoses:

- How has this health problem affected you and your family?
- What do you believe will help or fix the problem?
- What worries you the most about this problem?
- Which cultural practices do you observe to keep yourself and your family well?

When you ask questions such as these, you use a patient-centered approach that allows you to see a patient's health situation through his or her eyes. This is necessary to identify relevant assessment data pertaining to a patient's health problems.

SOURCES OF DIAGNOSTIC ERROR

Errors occur in the nursing diagnostic process during data collection, analysis of data clusters or patterns, and interpretation in choosing a nursing diagnostic statement (Mynaříková and Žiaková, 2014). Accuracy is a critical thinking element for selection of a nursing diagnosis. Do not skip any of the steps in the nursing diagnostic process, and be sure you complete every step.

Errors in Data Collection

During assessment (see Chapter 16) be knowledgeable, thorough, and skillful. Avoid inaccurate or missing data. Be willing to confirm a finding with another nurse. If you do not think you have complete data, consider what other questions you might ask the patient or family. Was your physical examination thorough and relevant to the symptoms a patient reported? Be thorough as you collect data applicable to the patient's health problems. Validate that your measurable, objective physical findings support subjective data. For example, when a patient reports "difficulty breathing," you also listen to lung sounds, assess respiratory rate, and measure a patient's chest excursion (see Chapter 30). Current evidence shows that insufficient identification of defining characteristics/assessment findings or related factors is common when making diagnoses (Mynaříková and Žiaková, 2014).

Errors in Data Clustering

Errors occur if you cluster data prematurely, incorrectly, or not at all. Premature clustering occurs when you make a nursing diagnosis before grouping all patient data. For example, a patient reports having occasional incontinence and urinary frequency. You cluster the available data and begin to identify an alteration in urination. Incorrect clustering occurs when you try to make a diagnosis fit a limited set of signs and symptoms that you gather. In this example, further assessment reveals that the patient has incontinence in small volumes with coughing or exercise. The patient does not leak urine at nighttime. The complete data cluster helps you to focus more specifically on an incontinence problem. Before analyzing your assessment data to identify clusters or patterns, validate the accuracy and completeness of your data one more

time. You can do this by reassessing for a particular symptom, confirming data from the health record, or consulting with another nurse. When you are unable to validate data, this is a warning that there may be an inaccurate match between clinical data elements and the nursing diagnosis you want to select.

Errors in Analysis and Interpretation of Data

During analysis and interpretation, be careful to consider any conflicting data elements and determine whether there are sufficient data to form a diagnosis. Remember, a single symptom is insufficient for selecting a nursing diagnosis. For example, a patient wincing may be responding to pain, nausea, or even fear, all valid nursing diagnoses.

In the example of the patient displaying incontinence symptoms of urinary frequency and occasional incontinence in small volumes following exercise and coughing, a review of assessment findings for associated urinary alteration diagnoses is necessary. The assessment findings identified for this patient best fit criteria for *Stress Incontinence of Urine.* The patient does not leak urine during nighttime or report a constant urge to void, so a nursing diagnosis of *Urge Incontinence of Urine* is probably inappropriate. You learn to sort out the data you have collected and match them with assessment findings standard to a diagnosis to select an appropriate nursing diagnosis. Interpretation is accurate only when you carefully review nursing diagnoses with similar assessment findings to choose the one that best fits your patient's condition.

Errors in a Diagnostic Statement

Clinical reasoning leads to an accurate nursing diagnosis, which eventually leads to individualized, specific, and effective nursing interventions. Successful selection of nursing interventions depends on having the correct related or etiologic factors or risk factors for a nursing diagnosis. An accurate diagnostic statement with relevant assessment findings guides you and the patient in the selection of appropriate patient outcomes. Unfortunately, research shows that nurses are not always methodical in the way they form nursing diagnoses (Box 17.2). You can reduce errors in diagnostic statements by selecting appropriate, concise, and precise language. Be sure that the etiology or related factor is within the scope of nursing practice to diagnose and treat. The following guidelines will assist you in reducing diagnostic errors.

- Identify a patient's response to a health problem, not a medical diagnosis (Carpenito, 2017). A medical diagnosis requires medical interventions; thus, it is inappropriate to include your patient's medical diagnosis in a nursing diagnostic statement. For example, instead of the diagnosis of hypertension, select the nursing diagnosis *Altered Blood Pressure* (ICN, 2017).
- Identify a diagnostic statement rather than a symptom. Identify nursing diagnoses from a cluster of assessment findings and not just a single symptom. One assessment finding is insufficient for diagnosis identification. For example, dyspnea alone does not lead you to a diagnosis. A pattern of dyspnea, reduced chest excursion, and tachypnea are assessment findings for the diagnosis of *Impaired Breathing.*
- Identify a related factor or risk factor treatable through nursing intervention. A diagnostic test or a chronic condition is not an etiology that a nursing intervention is able to treat. A patient with fractured ribs probably has pain when inhaling, impaired chest excursion, and slower, shallow respirations. An x-ray may show collapse of alveoli in the affected area. The nursing diagnosis of *"Impaired Breathing* related to shallow respirations" is incorrect. There are no interventions that directly make respirations less

Sources of Error and Frequency of Nursing Diagnoses Used in Clinical Practice

PICOT Question: Among practicing nurses what is the level of accuracy in the making of nursing diagnostic statements?

Evidence Summary

A review of 39 studies conducted internationally examined the most frequently occurring mistakes in nursing diagnostics and the frequency of nursing diagnoses used in clinical practice (Mynaříková and Žiaková, 2014). The literature review included formal studies as well as expert reviews and educational texts. The review found deficiencies in the formation of nursing diagnostic conclusions, including identification of diagnostic elements (e.g., defining characteristics or related factors). In addition, the researchers found that nursing diagnoses are very often determined based on irrelevant or invalid data (Mynaříková and Žiaková, 2014). Studies that examined documentation of nursing diagnoses in a wide variety of settings found that diagnoses pertaining to dysfunctional body functions were more commonly identified, whereas diagnoses from the psychosocial area are identified much less often. Because nurses commonly use the same nursing diagnoses for individual medical diagnoses or conditions, they may be less comfortable identifying mental, social, and spiritual diagnoses. For example, any time a patient has a hip replacement, nurses will identify acute pain and impaired mobility regardless of what other data may indicate.

Application to Nursing Practice

- Because accuracy in selecting nursing diagnoses involves critical thinking, take the time to analyze data carefully before forming a statement.
- Avoid identifying irreversible related factors, which cannot be changed with nursing interventions.
- Do not predefine a nursing diagnosis based on a patient's medical diagnosis. Base your diagnosis selection on complete patient-specific data.

shallow. The diagnosis of "*Impaired Breathing* related to chest pain from rib fracture evidenced by reduced excursion and dyspnea" is correct. Nursing interventions directed toward pain relief will lead to improved breathing.

- Identify a problem caused by the treatment or diagnostic study rather than the treatment or study itself. Patients experience many responses to diagnostic tests and medical treatments. These responses are the focus of nursing care. The patient who has chest pain and is scheduled for a cardiac catheterization possibly has a nursing diagnosis of "*Anxiety* related to lack of knowledge about cardiac testing, evidenced by inability to describe cardiac catheterization after repeated questioning." An incorrect diagnosis is "*Anxiety* related to cardiac catheterization."
- Identify a patient response to the equipment rather than the equipment itself. Patients are often unfamiliar with medical technology and its use. The diagnosis of "*Lack of Knowledge* regarding the need for cardiac monitoring related to inexperience" is accurate compared with the statement "*Lack of Knowledge* related to cardiac monitoring."
- Identify a patient's problems rather than your problems with nursing care. Nursing diagnoses are patient-centered and form the basis for goal-directed care. Consider a patient with a peripheral intravenous (IV) infusion. "*Potential Intravenous Complications* related to poor vascular access" indicates a nursing problem in maintaining the infusion. The diagnosis "*Risk for Infection* evidenced by swollen IV site, pain at site, and slowed infusion" properly centers attention on the patient's potential needs.

- Identify a patient problem rather than a nursing intervention. You plan nursing interventions after identifying a nursing diagnosis. The intervention "Offer bedpan frequently because of incontinence" is not a diagnostic statement. Instead, with the proper assessment data, the correct diagnostic statement would be "*Diarrhea* related to food intolerance evidenced by 3 stools daily and soft formed stools." A correct diagnosis will more likely result in the selection of appropriate interventions to solve the patient's problem.
- Identify a patient need rather than the goal of care. You establish goals during the planning step of the nursing process (Chapter 18). Goals based on accurate identification of a patient's problems serve as a basis to determine problem resolution. Change the goal-phrased statement of "Patient needs high-protein diet related to potential alteration in nutrition" to "*Impaired Nutritional Intake* related to difficulty swallowing evidenced by inability to eat solid foods and painful mouth."
- Make professional rather than prejudgmental statements. Base nursing diagnoses on subjective and objective patient data and do not include your personal beliefs and values. Remove your judgment from "*Impaired Skin Integrity* related to poor hygiene habits" by changing the diagnostic statement to read "*Impaired Skin Integrity* related to inadequate knowledge about perineal care evidenced by inability to cleanse perineum and inability to explain cleansing techniques."
- Avoid legally inadvisable statements in a diagnostic statement (Carpenito, 2017). Statements that imply blame, negligence, or malpractice (see Chapter 23) have the potential to result in a lawsuit. The statement "*Acute Pain* related to insufficient medication" implies an inadequate prescription by a health care provider. Correct problem identification is *Acute Pain* related to insufficient knowledge of analgesic schedule evidenced by self-report of pain intensity and inability to describe dosage plan.
- Identify the problem and etiology to avoid a circular statement. Circular statements are vague and give no direction to nursing care. Change the statement "*Impaired Breathing* related to shallow breathing" to identify the real patient problem and cause, *Impaired Breathing* related to incision pain evidenced by splinting and increased respiratory rate.
- Identify only one patient problem in the diagnostic statement. Every problem has different expected outcomes (see Chapter 18). Confusion during the planning of care occurs when you include multiple problems in a nursing diagnosis. It also can result in choosing an insufficient number of nursing interventions or inappropriate interventions. For example, *Pain* and *Anxiety* related to difficulty in ambulating are two diagnoses combined in this example of one nursing diagnosis statement. Two separate diagnoses for *Pain* and *Anxiety* are more accurate. It is permissible to include multiple etiologies contributing to one patient problem, as in *Dysfunctional Grief* related to diagnosis of a terminal illness and change in family role.

DOCUMENTATION AND INFORMATICS

Accuracy and consistency in the way information is shared among health care providers are essential. Standardized formats used in electronic health records (EHRs) enable nurses and other care providers to share information about the care they provide to sustain life, enable recovery, and promote health (Lundberg et al., 2008). The use of standard, familiar terminology in an EHR can provide nurses greater ease in their selection of nursing diagnoses and interventions in planning patient care (Estrada and Dunn, 2012). Many state-of-the-art EHRs contain nursing diagnoses with NANDA-I diagnoses, related factors, defining characteristics, and Nursing Intervention Classifications (NIC) and Nursing Outcome Classifications (NOC) (NANDA-I,

2018b). The ICNP develops catalogs (nursing data subsets) for specified health situations that are used in building health information systems for a variety of settings (Tastan et al., 2014; Rabelo-Silva, 2016). The use of standard language in an EHR is also valuable for making it easier to capture and analyze nursing practice information for research (Rabelo-Silva, 2016).

Once you identify a patient's nursing diagnoses, enter them in the EHR of the agency. The agency information system will dictate how the diagnosis is disseminated throughout the record, such as in a formal care plan, a daily task sheet, or nurses' notes. In advanced systems a nurse enters assessment data into the EHR, and the computer software program organizes the data into patterns that enhance the ability to select accurate nursing diagnoses. Once diagnoses are selected, the computer system directs the nurse to outcome and intervention options to select for the specific patient, allowing for individualized care. The value of the NANDA-I system is that many of the nursing diagnoses are evidence based. Select diagnoses developed since 2002 are based on the research and work of professional nurses around the world (NANDA-I, 2018b).

List nursing diagnoses chronologically as you identify them. When initiating an original care plan, place the highest-priority nursing diagnosis first. This will depend on a patient's condition and the nature of the nursing diagnosis (see Chapter 18). Thereafter add nursing diagnoses to the list. Date a nursing diagnosis at the time of initiation. When caring for a patient, review the list and first identify nursing diagnoses with the greatest priority, regardless of chronological order.

NURSING DIAGNOSES APPLICATION TO CARE PLANNING

Nursing diagnosis provides a universal and standardized way for professional nurses to communicate among themselves and across other health care disciplines. It enhances interprofessional collaboration (see Chapter 18). Diagnoses direct the planning process and the selection of nursing interventions to achieve desired outcomes for patients. Just as a medical diagnosis of diabetes leads a health care provider to prescribe a low-carbohydrate diet and medication for blood glucose control, the nursing diagnosis of *Impaired Health Maintenance* will lead a nurse to design appropriate educational and social support interventions. In Chapter 18 you will learn how combining nursing diagnostic statements with the Nursing Interventions Classification (NIC) and Nursing Outcomes Classification (NOC) systems facilitates the process of patient-centered care planning. The care plan (see Chapter 18) is a road map for delivering nursing care and demonstrates your accountability for patient care. By making accurate nursing diagnoses, your subsequent care plan communicates a patient's health care responses to problems to all health care professionals and ensures high-quality care.

▌ KEY POINTS

- When making a diagnosis, a clear label or term that is familiar to all those involved in a patient's care is necessary to understand a patient's needs.
- Nursing diagnoses provide clear direction as to the types of nursing interventions nurses are licensed to provide independently.
- Nurses cannot treat medical diagnoses; instead, they treat patients' responses to the medical health conditions.
- Nurses intervene in collaboration with personnel from other health care professions to manage collaborative problems.
- Using standardized terminology leads to diagnostic clarity and effective communication and enables nurses to formulate nursing diagnoses, associated interventions, and to assess the outcomes of nursing care.

- The nursing diagnostic reasoning process involves using the assessment data gathered about a patient to logically explain a clinical judgment in the form of a nursing diagnosis.
- Your review and analysis of assessment data involve critically organizing all data elements about a patient into meaningful patterns, also called data clusters or sets of assessment findings/defining characteristics.
- As you recognize data elements from an assessment, you will cluster or group them together in meaningful patterns in a logical way that during interpretation will reveal the nursing diagnoses.
- Data interpretation involves placing a label on a data pattern or cluster to clearly identify a patient's responses to health problems.
- Errors occur in the nursing diagnostic process during data collection; analysis of data, clusters, or patterns; and interpretation in choosing a nursing diagnostic statement.
- Identify nursing diagnoses from a cluster of assessment findings and not just a single symptom.
- Identify a patient need rather than the goal of care when forming a diagnostic statement.

▌ REFLECTIVE LEARNING

After you complete an assessment of a patient in a clinical area or in a simulation laboratory, review your data and apply critical thinking.

- What patterns of data appear logically together as you analyze all the information?
- As you look at the data in each pattern, are there cases in which an individual data element falls into more than one pattern? What does that suggest?
- Take a data pattern that you have identified and form a nursing diagnostic statement.

▌ REVIEW QUESTIONS

1. A nursing student is working with a faculty member to identify a nursing diagnosis for an assigned patient. The student has assessed that the patient is undergoing radiation treatment, has liquid stool, and the skin is clean and intact. The student selects the nursing diagnosis *Impaired Skin Integrity*. The faculty member explains that the student has made a diagnostic error for which of the following reasons?
   1. Incorrect clustering of data
   2. Wrong diagnosis
   3. Condition is a collaborative problem
   4. Premature ending assessment
2. A nurse conducts an assessment of a 42-year-old woman at a health clinic. The woman is married and lives in a condo with her husband. She reports having frequent voiding and pain when she passes urine. The nurse asks whether she has to go to the bathroom at night, and the patient responds, "Yes, usually twice or more." The patient had an episode of diarrhea 1 week ago. She weighs 300 lb and reports having difficulty cleansing herself after voiding or passing stool. Which of the following demonstrate assessment findings that cluster to indicate the nursing diagnosis *Impaired Urination*. (Select all that apply.)
   1. Age 42
   2. Dysuria
   3. Difficulty performing perineal hygiene
   4. Nocturia
   5. Episode of diarrhea
3. Review the following nursing diagnoses and identify the diagnoses that are stated correctly. (Select all that apply.)
   1. Offer frequent skin care because of *Impaired Skin Integrity*
   2. *Risk of Infection*

3. *Chronic Pain* related to osteoarthritis
4. *Activity Intolerance* related to physical deconditioning
5. *Lack of Knowledge* related to laser surgery

4. Which of the following best describe a collaborative health problem? (Select all that apply.)
   1. An actual or potential physiological complication that nurses monitor to detect the onset of changes in a patient's health status
   2. The language medical practitioners use to communicate a patient's health problem and associated treatments and response
   3. A diagnostic label that classifies a patient's response to illness so that all nurses can be familiar with a specific patient's health care needs
   4. A language used by health care providers to communicate and consider each other's unique perspective, so they can better manage the multiple factors that influence the health of individuals
   5. A diagnosis that provides clear direction as to the type of nursing interventions nurses are licensed to provide independently

5. Which of the following is a diagnostic error involving identification of a goal of care rather than a patient need?
   1. Patient obtains social support care related to caregiver stress
   2. *Fear* related to open-heart surgery
   3. *Acute Pain* related to splinting of incision
   4. *Impaired Family Coping* related to insufficient caregiver support

6. A nurse is assigned to a new patient admitted to the medical unit. The nurse collects a nursing history and interviews the patient. Place the following steps for making a nursing diagnosis in the correct order.
   1. Consider the context of patient's health problem and select a related factor.
   2. Review assessment data, noting objective and subjective clinical information.
   3. Cluster clinical data elements that form a pattern.
   4. Identify appropriate assessment findings for diagnosis.
   5. Identify a nursing diagnosis.

7. A nurse interviews and conducts a physical examination of a patient that includes the following findings: reduced movement of lower leg, reduced range of motion in left knee, and difficulty turning in bed without assistance. This data set is an example of:
   1. Collaborative data set.
   2. Diagnostic label.
   3. Related factors.
   4. Data cluster.

8. A nurse reviews data gathered regarding a patient's response to a diagnosis of cancer. The nurse notes that the patient is restless, avoids eye contact, has increased blood pressure, and expresses a sense of helplessness. The nurse compares the pattern of assessment findings for *Anxiety* with those of *Fear* and selects *Anxiety* as the correct diagnosis. This is an example of the nurse avoiding an error in? (Select all that apply.)
   1. Data collection
   2. Data clustering
   3. Data interpretation
   4. Making a diagnostic statement
   5. Goal setting

9. A nursing assessment reveals a patient in the home setting who has reduced mobility following recovery from a stroke. The patient has weakness in the left leg and arm. The patient has a walker, which he has never used before, and his wife tells the nurse that he is unsteady in using the walker. The patient fell while in the hospital. The physical therapist came to the home, but the wife tells the nurse, "We are not sure how to get my husband upstairs. The therapist explained how to use the walker, but we have questions." The nurse developed the following concept map. Place the links between the nursing diagnoses in the correct direction.

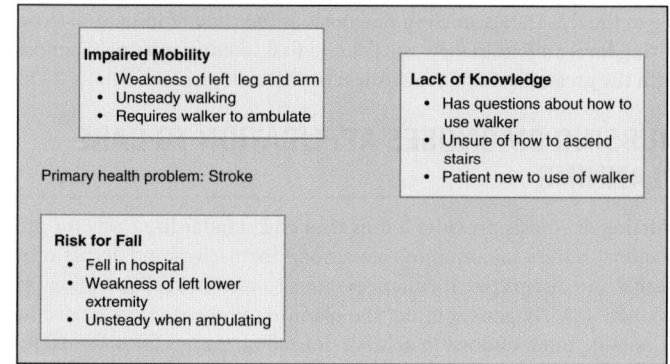

10. Fill in the Blank:

    A(n) _____ diagnosis is one that applies when there is an increased potential or vulnerability for a patient to develop a problem.

Rationales for Review Questions can be found on the Evolve website.

REFERENCES

American Nursing Association (ANA): *Nursing scope and standards of practice*, ed 3, Washington DC, 2015, American Nurses Association.

Carpenito LJ: *Nursing diagnosis: application to clinical practice*, ed 15, Wolters Kluwer, 2017.

Lundberg CB, et al.: Selecting a standardized terminology for the electronic health record that reveals the impact of nursing on patient care, *On-Line J Nurs Inf* 12(2), 2008, Available at https://ojni.org/12_2/lundberg.pdf. Accessed June 22, 2019.

Mynaříková E, Žiaková K: The use of nursing diagnoses in clinical practice, *Cent Eur J Nurs Midw* 5(3):117–126, 2014.

North American Nursing Diagnosis International (NANDA-I): *NANDA international history*, 2018a, http://kb.nanda.org/category/43/0/10/English-/About-NANDA-International/NANDA-International-History/. Accessed June 22, 2019.

North American Nursing Diagnosis International (NANDA-I): In Herdman TH, Kamitsuru S, editors: *Nursing Diagnoses: definitions and classification 2018-2020*, ed 11, New York, 2018b, Thieme.

International Council of Nurses (ICN): *Nursing diagnosis and outcome statements – international classification for nursing practice Catalogue*, Geneva, 2017, Switzerland.

Yoost B, Crawford L: *Fundamentals of nursing: active learning for collaborative practice*, ed 2, St Louis, 2020, Elsevier.

RESEARCH REFERENCES

Aein F, Aliakbari F: Effectiveness of concept mapping and traditional linear nursing care plans on critical thinking skills in clinical pediatric nursing course, *J Educ Health Promot* 6:13, 2017.

Coenen A, et al.: ICNP Catalogues for supporting nursing content in electronic health records, *Stud Health Technol Inform* 180:1075–1078, 2012.

Estrada NA, Dunn CR: Standardized nursing diagnoses in an electronic health record: nursing survey results, *Int J Nurs Knowl* 23(2):86–95, 2012.

Guo Q, Jacelon CS: An integrative review of dignity in end-of-life care, *Palliat Med* 28(7):931–940, 2014.

Lai W, et al.: Does one size fit all? Exploring the cultural applicability of NANDA-I nursing diagnoses to Chinese nursing practice, *J Transcult Nurs* 24(1):43, 2013.

Rabelo-Silva ER, et al.: Advanced nursing process quality: comparing the international classification for nursing practice (ICNP) with the NANDA international (NANDA-I) and nursing interventions classification (NIC), *J Clin Nurs* 26(3–4):379–387, 2016.

Sullivan M, et al.: Interprofessional collaboration and education, *AJN* 115(3):47–54, 2015.

Tastan S, et al.: Evidence for the existing American Nurses Association-recognized standardized nursing terminologies: a systematic review, *Int J Nurs Stud* 1:1160–1170, 2014.

18

Planning Nursing Care

OBJECTIVES

- Explain the relationship of planning to nursing diagnosis.
- Discuss criteria used in priority setting.
- Discuss the difference between a goal and an expected outcome.
- Use the SMART model for writing goal and outcome statements.
- Discuss the differences between independent and dependent nursing interventions.
- Discuss benefits of nursing care plans.
- Describe the consultation process.
- Explain the process of interprofessional collaboration.

KEY TERMS

Consultation, p. 253
Dependent nursing interventions, p. 246
Expected outcome, p. 244
Goal, p. 242
Independent nursing interventions, p. 246
Interprofessional care plans, p.249
Interprofessional collaboration, p. 244

Long-term goal, p. 243
Nursing care plan, p. 249
Nursing Interventions Classification (NIC), p. 247
Nursing Outcomes Classification (NOC), p. 245
Nursing-sensitive patient outcome, p. 245

Other provider interventions, p. 246
Patient-centered goal, p. 240
Planning, p. 240
Priority setting, p. 241
Scientific rationale, p. 246
Short-term goal, p. 243

MEDIA RESOURCES

- Review Questions
- Concept Map Creator
- Case Study with Questions

- Audio Glossary
- Content Updates
- Answers to QSEN Activity and Review Questions

---

*Tonya conducted a thorough assessment of Mr. Lawson's health status and identified three nursing diagnoses: **Acute Pain** related to trauma of surgical incision, **Lack of Knowledge** regarding postoperative care related to inexperience with surgery, and **Risk for Infection**. Tonya is responsible for the initial planning of Mr. Lawson's nursing care after identifying relevant nursing diagnoses. The care that she plans will continue to be implemented and updated during Mr. Lawson's hospital stay by the other nurses involved in Mr. Lawson's' care. If Tonya plans well, the individualized interventions that she selects will prepare the patient for a smooth transition home. Collaboration with the patient and his wife will be critical for a plan of care to be successful. Using input from Mr. Lawson, Tonya identifies the goals and expected outcomes for each of his nursing diagnoses. The goals and outcomes direct Tonya in selecting appropriate therapeutic nursing interventions. Tonya knows that Mrs. Lawson must be involved in her husband's care because of the ongoing support that she provides and because she will be a key care provider once Mr. Lawson returns home. Consultation and collaboration with other health care providers such as home health ensures that the right resources will be used in planning care. In addition, Tonya poses a PICOT question about Mr. Lawson: Does the use of visual aids compared with standard discharge literature affect adult patients' ability to learn infection control principles? Tonya will use results of her literature search to build interventions for Mr. Lawson's care. Careful planning involves seeing the*

relationships among a patient's problems, recognizing that certain problems take precedence over others, identifying the most appropriate interventions, and proceeding with planning a safe and efficient approach to care.

How well do you plan? After reviewing the food products in your kitchen pantry, do you make a list and plan meals over the course of a week? As a mother or father do you collaborate with a spouse after considering a week's activities and plan for what to do over a weekend? Planning is the process of identifying a problem (missing food products in the pantry) and making or carrying out a plan of action that is often goal oriented. You select foods you need for the kitchen pantry, plan the trip to the grocery store, and then select and prepare the types of meals that best use the products you purchased.

Planning nursing care is much more complicated, but it involves basic elements of reviewing a patient's problems or needs, determining the best course of action to meet those problems, setting goals and outcomes to guide the plan of care, and developing a plan of interventions to be used in patient care.

After identifying a patient's nursing diagnoses and collaborative problems, you begin the planning step of the nursing process. Planning involves setting priorities based on patient diagnoses and collaborative problems, identifying patient-centered goals and expected outcomes, and prescribing nursing interventions appropriate for each diagnosis. The most important principle in planning is the individualization of a patient-centered plan of care for each patient's unique needs. The patient's nursing diagnoses direct your mutual selection of nursing interventions and the goals and outcomes you hope your patient achieves (Flagg, 2015). Planning requires critical thinking applied through deliberate decision making and problem solving. It also requires communicating closely with patients, their families, and the health care team and ongoing collaboration with team members. Know that any plan of care is dynamic and changes as a patient's needs change.

ESTABLISHING PRIORITIES

A single patient often has multiple nursing diagnoses and collaborative problems. When you enter nursing practice, you will care for multiple patients. You must collaborate with patients and family caregivers (as applicable) and health care team members to determine the urgency of an identified problem for each patient and to prioritize patient diagnoses (Ackley et al., 2017). Priority setting is the ordering of nursing diagnoses or patient problems to establish a preferential order for nursing interventions. Generally, problem-focused diagnoses and problems take priority over wellness, possible risk, and health promotion problems. Short-term acute patient care needs and problems typically take priority over longer-term chronic needs (NCLEX, n.d.). Priority setting is not the ordering of a list of care tasks but an organization of the desired outcomes for a patient.

Use your nursing and scientific knowledge base to recognize patterns of symptoms from your patient assessment and certain knowledge triggers to help you understand which diagnoses require intervention and when you need to intervene to plan effective nursing care (Ackley et al., 2017). This requires you to identify symptoms that patients have related to their illness, understand which symptom patterns require action, and identify the associated time frame for effective intervention. Some knowledge triggers include pathophysiology and pharmacology, your experiences with other patients who have had similar problems, and what you know about your select patient you are caring for now. For example, a nurse is caring for a patient who suddenly spikes a fever following surgery. The nurse connects this symptom with other symptoms of purulent drainage and tenderness over a surgical wound and an inflamed incision. The pattern of symptoms tells the nurse that the patient most likely has developed an infection, which requires immediate action.

As you care for a patient or multiple patients, you must deal with certain aspects of care before others. By ranking a patient's nursing diagnoses in order of importance and always monitoring changing signs and symptoms of patient problems, you attend to each patient's most important needs and better organize ongoing care activities. Priorities help you anticipate and sequence nursing interventions when a patient has multiple nursing diagnoses and collaborative problems. You also set priorities by selecting mutually agreed-on priorities with a patient based on the urgency of the problems, the patient's safety and desires, the nature of the treatment indicated, and the relationship among the diagnoses. Priority setting is not a matter of numbering the nursing diagnoses based on severity or physiological importance. Such a numbering system does not always reflect actual clinical changes in patients. Instead, you establish priorities in relation to their ongoing clinical importance.

Methods for Prioritizing

Classify patients' priorities as high, intermediate, or low importance. Nursing diagnoses that, if untreated, result in harm to a patient or others (e.g., those related to airway status, circulation, safety, and pain) have the highest priorities. Prioritize nursing diagnoses first by considering patients' immediate needs based on ABC (airway, breathing, and circulation) (Ackley et al., 2017). The highest priority can also be determined by using Maslow's hierarchy of needs (see Chapter 6).

For example, *Risk for Violence, Impaired Gas Exchange,* and *Impaired Cardiac Function* are examples of high-priority nursing diagnoses that drive the priorities of safety, adequate oxygenation, and adequate circulation. However, it is always important to consider each patient's unique situation. Avoid classifying only physiological nursing diagnoses as high priority. *Consider Mr. Lawson's case. Among his nursing diagnoses,* **Acute Pain** *was an initial priority because Tonya knew that she needed to relieve Mr. Lawson's acute pain for him to be ready for discharge education. Now that his pain is controlled reasonably well,* **Lack of Knowledge** *became the priority because of the patient's expressed concern for how to care for himself and the urgent need to prepare him adequately for his upcoming discharge.*

Intermediate-priority nursing diagnoses are nonemergent and not life threatening. In Mr. Lawson's case, *Risk for Infection* is an intermediate diagnosis. The nursing staff will continue to monitor his wound healing, and it is important for Mr. and Mrs. Lawson to learn the signs of infection and understand what to observe once the patient returns home. In this case focused and individualized instruction from all members of the health care team about infection prevention is necessary throughout the patient's hospitalization.

Low-priority nursing diagnoses are not always directly related to a specific illness or prognosis but affect a patient's future well-being. Many low-priority diagnoses focus on a patient's long-term health care needs. *You learned in Chapter 17 that Mr. Lawson shares a concern with Tonya, "I'm worried about being able to return to work on time." When instructing the patient, Tonya noticed that he was having trouble attending to what she had to say. Tonya has not yet identified a nursing diagnosis related to Mr. Lawson's concern about returning to work. She will need to assess him more fully, but a nursing diagnosis such as* **Anxiety** *may be of low priority compared with others. However, if the patient's anxiety is left unaddressed, it could become a higher priority if it interferes with his ability to learn discharge information.*

Patients' priorities change as their conditions and needs change, sometimes within a matter of minutes. Each time you begin to care for a patient, such as at the beginning of a hospital shift or during a clinic visit, review patient priorities. *For example, when Tonya first met Mr. Lawson, he rated his pain at a 7, and it was apparent that administering an analgesic and repositioning the patient were greater priorities than trying to prepare him for instruction. Later, after receiving the analgesic, Mr. Lawson's pain lessened to a level of 4, and Tonya was able to gather more assessment information and begin to focus on his problem of* **Lack of Knowledge**. *Ongoing patient assessment is critical to determine the status of a patient's nursing diagnoses. The appropriate ordering of priorities ensures that you meet a patient's needs in a safe, timely, and effective way.*

Priority setting includes determining which nursing interventions you plan to use with a patient and the order in which you need to implement them. *For example, as Tonya considers the high-priority diagnosis of* **Acute Pain** *for Mr. Lawson, she includes in her plan of care these options: timely administration of an analgesic, repositioning, and teaching relaxation exercises. With each clinical encounter, Tonya applies critical thinking to prioritize which intervention to use first. Tonya knows that a certain degree of pain relief is necessary before a patient can participate in relaxation exercises. When she is in the patient's room, she might decide to turn and reposition Mr. Lawson first and then prepare the analgesic. However, if Mr. Lawson expresses that pain is a high level and he is too uncomfortable to turn, Tonya chooses obtaining and administering the analgesic as her first priority. Later, with Mr. Lawson's pain more under control, she considers whether relaxation is appropriate.*

Involve patients in priority setting whenever possible. Patient-centered care requires you to know a patient's preferences, values, and expressed needs. Sometimes a patient assigns priorities differently from those you select. Resolve these differences through open communication. Consulting with and knowing a patient's concerns do not relieve you of the responsibility to act in a patient's best interests. Always assign priorities based on good nursing judgment.

Ethical care is a part of priority setting (see Chapter 22). When ethical issues cloud priorities, you must maintain an open dialogue with the patient, family members, and other health care providers. For example, when caring for patients with cancer, discuss the situation with them and understand their expectations, understand your professional responsibility in protecting the patients from harm, know their health care provider's therapeutic or palliative goals, and then form appropriate plans of care.

Priorities in Practice

Many factors within the health care environment affect your ability to set priorities (Fig. 18.1). For example, in a hospital setting the model for delivering care (see Chapter 21), the workflow routine of a nursing unit, staffing levels, availability of material resources, and interruptions from other care providers affect the minute-by-minute determination of patient care priorities. In the home health setting the number of visits scheduled for a day and the availability of family caregivers and resources within a patient's home affect a patient's priorities. Nurses should have a plan of action to effectively manage their time, avoid unnecessary interruptions, and avoid helping others when this could potentially jeopardize their patients' priorities of care (NCLEX, n.d.). Remember, however, a colleague might ask for assistance when his or her patient has a priority needing immediate attention.

Successful priority setting involves collaborating with the health care team. When you work with assistive personnel (AP), discuss the purpose of each patient's hospitalization, the picture of how the patient should look at the end of the shift, the plan for achieving desired outcomes, and the part you and the AP will play. You agree on priorities at the beginning of a shift, but you will most likely need to change them several times before the next shift due to changes in your patients' needs and changes in your patient assignment due to discharges, transfers, and admissions.

The same factors that influence your ability to prioritize nursing actions minute by minute affect your ability to prioritize nursing diagnoses and plan care for groups of patients. The nature of nursing work challenges you to attend to a given patient's priorities when you care for more than one patient. The nursing care process is nonlinear. Often you complete an assessment and identify nursing diagnoses for one patient,

leave the room to perform an intervention for a second patient, and move on to evaluate the care of a third patient. Nurses exercise "cognitive shifts" (i.e., shifts in attention from one patient to another during the conduct of the nursing process). This shifting of attention occurs in response to changing patient needs, new procedures being ordered, or environmental processes interacting (e.g., call lights, alarms). Because of these cognitive shifts, it becomes important to stay organized and know your patients' priorities. Work from your plan of care and use patients' priorities to organize the order for delivering interventions and organizing documentation of care.

CRITICAL THINKING IN SETTING GOALS AND EXPECTED OUTCOMES

The planning process involves application of your knowledge, knowledge about a specific patient, clinical experiences, standards, and critical thinking attitudes (Fig. 18.2). It is a dynamic process, changing as a patient's needs change. Apply critical thinking after you identify a patient's nursing diagnoses or collaborative problems and ask yourself these questions:

- What is the best approach to address and resolve the problem?
- What does my patient need to achieve (physically, psychologically, socially, and spiritually)? What are the goals and outcomes related to these needs?
- How will I know when my patient has achieved the goals and outcomes?

Goals and expected outcomes are specific statements of patient behavior or physiological responses that you select to resolve a nursing diagnosis or collaborative problem. They serve two purposes: to set a clear direction for the selection and use of nursing interventions and to set specific measures for evaluating the effectiveness of meeting goals and outcomes. In the case of Mr. Lawson, Tonya sets the goal of the patient being "infection free." The expected outcomes for achieving that goal include the patient remaining afebrile, without wound drainage, and with wound edges healing. Expected outcomes are time limited, measurable ways of determining whether a goal is met (Table 18.1).

Goals

A **goal** is a broad statement that describes a desired change in a patient's condition, perceptions, or behavior. Mr. Lawson has the diagnosis of *Lack of Knowledge*. A goal of care for this diagnosis includes, "Patient

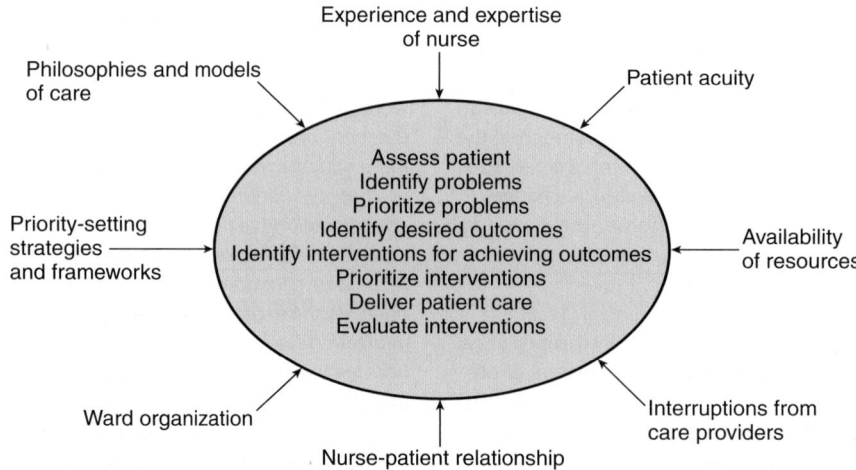

FIG. 18.1 A model for priority setting. (Modified from Hendry C, Walker A: Priority setting in clinical nursing practice, *J Adv Nurs* 47(4):427, 2004.)

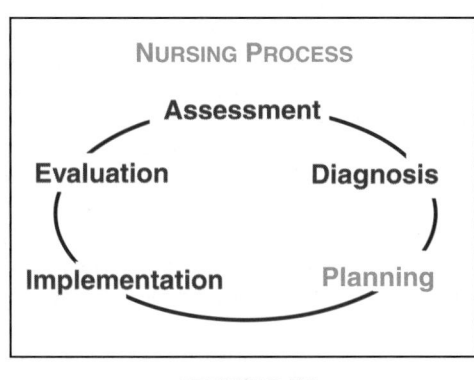

KNOWLEDGE
Patient's database and selected nursing diagnoses
Anatomy and physiology
Psychology
Pathophysiology
Normal growth and development
Evidence-based nursing interventions
Role of other health care disciplines
Community resources
Family dynamics
Teaching/learning process
Delegation principles
Priority-setting principles

EXPERIENCE
Previous patient care experience
Personal experience in
organizing activities

NURSING PROCESS

Assessment

Evaluation   Diagnosis

Implementation   Planning

STANDARDS
ANA Scope of Nursing Practice
Specialty standards of practice
Patient-centered goals and outcomes
Intellectual standards
Agency's policies and procedures

ATTITUDES
Creativity
Responsibility
Perseverance
Discipline

FIG. 18.2 Critical thinking and the process of planning care.

TABLE 18.1 Examples of Goal Setting with Expected Outcomes for Mr. Lawson

Nursing Diagnoses	Goals	Expected Outcomes
Acute Pain related to trauma of surgical incision	Mr. Lawson will achieve pain relief by day of discharge.	Mr. Lawson reports pain at a level of 3 or below by discharge. Mr. Lawson walks to chair with no increase in pain in 24 hours. Mr. Lawson's incisional area shows signs of wound healing by discharge.
Lack of Knowledge regarding postoperative care related to inexperience with surgery	Mr. Lawson will express understanding of how to minimize postoperative risks by discharge.	Mr. Lawson describes activity restrictions to follow by discharge in 48 hours. Mr. Lawson demonstrates how to cleanse surgical wound by discharge day. Mr. Lawson describes three risks for infection in 24 hours.
Risk for Infection	Mr. Lawson will remain infection free by discharge.	Mr. Lawson remains afebrile by discharge. Mr. Lawson's wound shows no purulent drainage by discharge. Mr. Lawson's wound closes at site of incision separation by discharge

will express understanding of how to minimize postoperative risks within 24 hours." A goal is realistic and based on patient needs, preferences, and resources. It predicts resolution of a problem, evidence of progress toward problem resolution, progress toward improved health status, or continued maintenance of good health or function (Carpenito, 2017).

Each goal is time limited, so the health care team has a common timeline for problem resolution. The time frame depends on the nature of the problem, etiology, overall condition of the patient, and treatment setting. A short-term goal is an objective behavior or response that you expect the patient to achieve in a short time, usually less than a week. In an acute care setting short-term goals may be set for just a few hours. A long-term goal is an objective behavior or response that you expect the patient to achieve, usually over several days, weeks, or months.

Goals are often based on standards of care or clinical guidelines established for minimal safe practice. For example, the Infusion Nurses Society (INS) has standards of care to prevent IV complications of

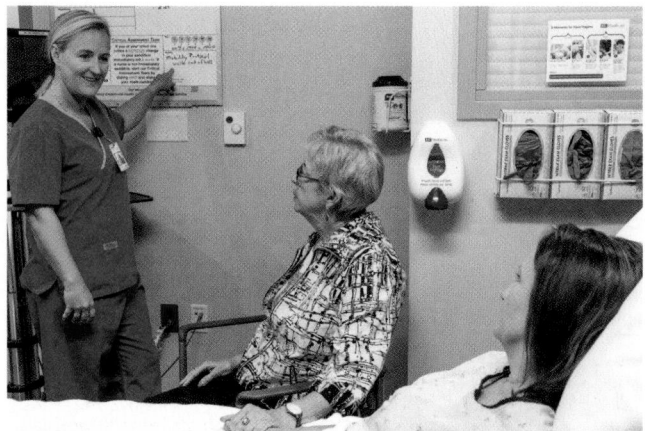
FIG. 18.3 Collaborative goal setting with patient and family member.

phlebitis, and the Association of Operating Room Nurses (AORN) has standards of care for patient recovery after surgery.

Role of Patients in Goal Setting. Patient-centered care includes the involvement of patient, family, and friends (as appropriate) (QSEN, 2018). Always collaborate with your patients during goal setting. Mutual goal setting helps you prioritize the goals of care and develop a realistic and relevant plan of care for a patient (Fig. 18.3). Unless goals are mutually set and include a clear plan of action, patients or family caregivers may not fully participate. Patients need to understand and see the value of nursing therapies even though they are often totally dependent on you as the nurse.

Role of Health Care Team in Goal Setting. Interprofessional collaboration is a complex process that is formed between two or more people from various professional fields to achieve common goals for a patient (Mahdizadeh et al., 2015). The need for interprofessional team collaboration is increasing as a result of an aging population with more complex needs associated with chronic diseases, increasing complexity of skills required to deliver care, knowledge required to provide comprehensive care to patients, and increasing specialization within health professions (Nancarrow et al., 2013). The elements that must be in place before interprofessional collaboration can be successful are interprofessional education, role awareness as a member of the team, interpersonal relationship skills, deliberate intervention, and support of the interprofessional team (Petri, 2010). Nancarrow and colleagues (2013) add that positive leadership and management attributes, communication structures, personal rewards, appropriate resources and procedures, appropriate skill mix, and clarity of vision are also necessary. Interprofessional team-based care involves care delivered by intentionally created, usually small work groups in health care who are recognized by others as well as by themselves as having a collective identity and shared responsibility for a group of patients (e.g., rapid response team, palliative care team) (Interprofessional Education Collaborative, 2016).

Nurses play a key role in interprofessional collaboration, especially in communicating patient needs to all members of the health care team, clarifying priorities, and ensuring a continuum of care. When interprofessional collaboration functions well, the outcomes are improvements in patient care, improvements in health care providers' and nurses' satisfaction, control of costs, reduction in clinical errors, and improvements in patient safety (Mahdizadeh et al., 2015).

Expected Outcomes

The goal for Mr. Lawson to understand the risks associated with his type of surgery gives Tonya a clear focus on the topics to include in her instruction (e.g., wound care, activity restriction). For Tonya to know whether Mr. Lawson understands his postoperative risks, the patient must meet expected outcomes. An expected outcome is the measurable change (patient behavior, physical state, or perception) that must be achieved to reach a goal. *In Mr. Lawson's case, after Tonya provides an educational intervention, the expected outcome would be "Patient identifies signs and symptoms of wound infection before discharge." Tonya will perform teach-back after instruction to determine whether outcomes are met. In this case she wishes to have Mr. Lawson learn three different signs of wound infection— wound drainage, fever, and increased tenderness around the wound.* Sometimes an outcome includes several measures that must be met for a single outcome. In all cases the goal and expected outcomes should align with the patient's nursing diagnoses or collaborative problems.

In health care, the terms *goals* and *outcomes* are sometimes interchanged and thus cause confusion. Outcome measurement is a priority within health care institutions; however, the way in which electronic health records (EHRs) label goal/outcome categories that nurses use to complete care plans can be unclear. Think of a *goal* as an ultimate outcome and *expected outcomes* as the measurable changes that a patient achieves to reach a goal.

Planning nursing care requires you to critically assess your patient's nursing diagnoses, the urgency or priority of the problems, and the resources of the patient and the health care delivery system. Apply knowledge from the medical, sociobehavioral, and nursing sciences to plan patient care. When Tonya selected her PICOT question about approaches for teaching infection control, she applied the knowledge she gained in selecting a specific teaching approach. The selection of goals, expected outcomes, and interventions requires consideration of your previous experience with patients who had similar problems and any established standards for clinical problem management. The goals and outcomes need to meet established intellectual standards by being relevant to patient needs, specific, singular, observable, measurable, and time limited. You also use critical thinking attitudes in selecting interventions with the greatest likelihood of success.

*Tonya has a discussion with Mr. Lawson and his wife about setting the plan for the diagnosis of **Lack of Knowledge**. Tonya explains the topics that they need to discuss so that the couple understands Mr. Lawson's postoperative risks. In addition, she talks about a program available on hospital TV about infection control that the couple can watch in their room. Tonya applied knowledge learned from her PICOT question literature search and chose the visual aid strategy. They plan for the couple to view the TV program when Mrs. Lawson visits. Mr. Lawson asks Tonya to also provide specific instruction about the activities he can and cannot do once he returns home. Tonya agrees and consults with the surgeon to be sure that her information is accurate and realistic.*

Selecting Goals and Expected Outcomes

A patient-centered goal reflects a patient's highest possible level of wellness and independence in function. It is realistic and based on patient needs, abilities, and resources. A patient-centered goal and associated outcome reflect a patient's specific behavior, not your own goals or nursing interventions. Typically all health care providers contribute to achievement of patient outcomes. However, nurses monitor and manage patient conditions and diagnose problems that can be treated with nursing interventions. The clinical reasoning and decision making of nurses are key parts of quality health care (Moorhead et al., 2018). Thus it becomes important to measure patient outcomes that are influenced by nursing care. A nursing-sensitive patient outcome is a measurable patient, family, or community behavior or perception that is measured along a continuum in response to nursing interventions (Moorhead et al., p viii, 2018). Examples of nursing-sensitive outcomes include reduction in pain frequency and severity and incidence of pressure injuries and falls. In comparison, medical outcomes are largely influenced by medical interventions. Examples include patient mortality, surgical wound infection, and hospital readmissions. For the nursing profession to become a full participant in clinical evaluation research, policy development, and interprofessional collaboration, nurses need to identify and measure patient outcomes influenced by nursing interventions.

Nursing Outcomes Classification. A valuable resource in selecting patient goals and outcomes is the Nursing Outcomes Classification (NOC), which links outcomes to NANDA International (NANDA-I) nursing diagnoses (Moorhead et al., 2018). This resource is an option that you can use in selecting goals and outcomes for your patients. For each nursing diagnosis there are multiple evidence-based outcomes (goals). The outcomes have labels for describing the focus of nursing care and include indicators (expected outcomes) to use in evaluating the success with nursing interventions. The indicators for each NOC outcome allow for measurement at any point on a five-point Likert scale from most negative to most positive (Moorhead et al., 2018). The rating system adds objectivity to judging a patient's progress. The use of NOC facilitates the evaluation of the effects of nursing interventions over time and across a variety of health care settings. Using a common language for outcomes allows nurses to plan effective patient care and provides a standardized way to measure whether nursing interventions are successful.

What NOC describes as an outcome, such as anxiety level, appetite, or physical comfort, is a very abstract term, which in real clinical practice comes closer to a goal statement. For example, in NOC terminology the outcome for the nursing diagnosis of *Acute Pain* is described as "pain control" or pain relief, the goal set for Mr. Lawson. The NOC outcome indicators are the same for what most clinicians set as expected outcomes. In the example of pain control, the expected outcomes include symptom severity measured on a pain scale or mobility level. Table 18.2 offers more examples of how to use NOC terminology for describing the focus or goals of nursing care and outcome indicators as they relate to nursing diagnoses.

Writing Goals and Expected Outcomes

Goals and expected outcomes direct your nursing care. After you set a patient-centered goal for a nursing diagnosis, the expected outcomes set the desired physiological, psychological, social, developmental, or spiritual responses that indicate resolution of the patient's health problems. Use the *SMART* acronym (*S*pecific, *M*easurable, *A*ttainable, *R*ealistic, *T*imed) to write goals and outcome statements (Ackley et al., 2017).

1. **Specific**—Outcomes and goals reflect a specific patient behavior or response. A correct goal statement is: "Patient will ambulate independently in 3 days." A correct outcome statement is: "Patient ambulates in the hall 3 times a day by 4/22." A common error is to write an intervention: "Ambulate patient in the hall."

   A specific outcome addresses only one behavior or response. For example, an incorrect outcome reads, "Patient's lungs are clear to auscultation, and respiratory rate is 24 breaths/minute by 8/22." How would you evaluate the outcome when you determine that

TABLE 18.2 Examples of Nursing Diagnoses and Suggested NOC Linkages

Nursing Diagnosis	Examples of NOC Outcomes (Consider as Goal Statements)	Outcome Indicators (Examples)
Impaired Oral Mucous Membrane	Oral Health	Knowledge of infection management Self-care oral hygiene
	Tissue Integrity	Hydration Infection severity
Activity Intolerance	Activity Tolerance	Oxygen saturation with activity Pulse rate with activity Respiratory rate with activity
	Self-Care Status	Bathes self Dresses self Prepares food and fluid for eating

NOC, Nursing Outcomes Classification.
Adapted from Moorhead S, et al: *Nursing Outcomes Classification (NOC),* ed 6, St Louis, 2018, Elsevier.

the lungs are clear but the respiratory rate is 28 breaths/min? You would be unable to do so. It is preferable that each outcome be separate. A focus on a single outcome enables you to decide whether you need to modify a plan of care.

2. **Measurable**—You must be able to measure or observe whether a change takes place in a patient's status. Changes occur in physiological findings and in a patient's knowledge, perceptions, and behavior. Examples such as "Body temperature will remain below 98.6°F (37°C)" and "Apical pulse will remain between 60 and 100 beats/min" allow you to objectively measure physical changes in a patient's status. The outcome statement "Patient's pain is less than 4 on a scale of 0 to 10 in 48 hours" allows you to objectively measure patient perception using a pain-rating scale. Do not use vague qualifiers such as "normal," "acceptable," or "stable" in an expected outcome statement. Vague terms result in guesswork in determining a patient's response to care. Terms describing quality, quantity, frequency, length, or weight allow you to evaluate outcomes precisely.

3. **Attainable**—A goal and an outcome are more attainable or achievable when you mutually set them with a patient. This ensures that you and your patient agree on the direction and time limits of care. Mutual goal setting (e.g., distance to walk, topics to learn about, medications) increases a patient's motivation and cooperation. As a patient advocate, apply standards of practice, evidence-based knowledge, safety principles, and basic human needs when helping patients set goals. Use your knowledge about and experience with patients' typical responses to clinical interventions to help your patients select goals and outcomes. Always consider patients' desires to recover and their physical and psychological condition to set goals and outcomes.

4. **Realistic**—Set goals and expected outcomes that are realistic or relevant for patients. Consider the patient's preferences and needs and the resources of the health care agency, family, and patient. Be aware of a patient's physiological, emotional, cognitive, and sociocultural potential and the economic cost and resources available to reach expected outcomes in a timely manner. For example, are the patient's cultural beliefs reflected in the goals you set? Does the patient have a family caregiver to assist with an intervention to be performed in the home? You set realistic goals and outcomes within the patient's limitations and abilities. For example, an initial goal is

"Patient will wash hands and face in 72 hours." Your assessment and collaboration with occupational therapy will determine whether the goal is realistic for the level of the patient's weakness. Setting realistic goals and outcomes often requires you to communicate these goals and outcomes to caregivers in other settings who will assume responsibility for patient care (e.g., home health, rehabilitation).

5. **Timed**—Set a time for each goal and outcome to be met. This helps the health care team collaborate to resolve patient problems. For example, the goal of "patient will achieve pain relief" for Mr. Lawson is complete by adding the time frame "by day of discharge." With this goal in place, all members of the nursing team will aim to manage and reduce the patient's pain while he is hospitalized. At the time of discharge, evaluation of expected outcomes (e.g., pain-rating score, signs of grimacing, level of movement) show whether the goal was met. Always collaborate with patients to set realistic and reasonable time frames. Time frames also help you and a patient determine whether the patient is making progress at a reasonable rate. If not, you must revise the plan of care. Time frames also promote accountability in delivering and managing nursing care.

CRITICAL THINKING IN PLANNING NURSING CARE

During planning you make clinical decisions by choosing the nursing interventions most appropriate for a patient's nursing diagnosis and collaborative problems. The actual implementation of these interventions occurs during implementation, the fourth step of the nursing process (see Chapter 19). Choosing suitable nursing interventions involves critical thinking and applying the best evidence for a patient's health problems. Nursing interventions are any treatments or actions based on clinical judgment and knowledge that nurses perform to enhance patient outcomes (Butcher et al., 2018). During planning you select interventions designed to help patients move from their present level of health to the level described in the goal and measured by the expected outcomes.

Tonya identified a PICOT question to help her select instructional interventions for enhancing Mr. and Mrs. Lawson's knowledge about infection control. She also chooses interventions based on what she has learned about the related factors behind his learning needs. Mr. Lawson has not experienced postoperative care, he is facing restrictions with which he is unfamiliar, and the condition of his incision requires wound care at home. Tonya will plan instructional topics to address postoperative risks in a way that will be relevant to Mr. Lawson and his usual routines. She learned the patient enjoys walking his dog, household maintenance, and gardening. Some of these activities will be limited or not allowed until the patient recovers. The instruction will include Mrs. Lawson since she is the patient's family caregiver.

Types of Interventions

Nursing interventions include direct and indirect care measures aimed at individual patients, families, and/or the community (Butcher et al., 2018). In addition, nursing interventions are classified as nurse-initiated, health care provider–initiated, and other provider–initiated (e.g., pharmacist, respiratory therapist) interventions (Butcher et al., 2018). Some patients require all three classifications, whereas others need only nurse- and health care provider–initiated interventions. Direct care measures are those treatments or procedures performed through interaction with a patient involving the laying on of hands. Examples include bathing, wound care, and inserting an IV catheter. Indirect care measures are those treatments or procedures performed away from a patient but on behalf of a patient (Butcher et al., 2018). Examples include managing the patient care environment and consultation.

Nurse-initiated interventions are the independent nursing interventions that a nurse initiates in response to a nursing diagnosis without supervision, direction, or orders from others. Examples include positioning patients to prevent pressure injury formation, initiating early mobility protocols, offering counseling for coping, or instructing patients in side effects of medications. Nurse-initiated interventions are autonomous actions based on scientific rationale. Such interventions benefit a patient in a predicted way related to nursing diagnoses and patient goals (Butcher et al., 2018). Each state within the United States has a Nurse Practice Act that defines the legal scope of nursing practice (see Chapter 23). According to the Nurse Practice Acts in a majority of states, independent nursing interventions pertain to activities of daily living, health education and promotion, and counseling. *For Mr. Lawson, Tonya selects the following nursing interventions to resolve his acute pain: positioning, relaxation therapy, and exercise promotion.*

Health care provider–initiated interventions are dependent nursing interventions that require an order from a health care provider. The interventions are based on a physician's or nurse practitioner's choices for treating or managing a medical diagnosis. Advanced practice nurses who work under collaborative agreements with physicians or who are licensed independently by state practice acts are able to write dependent interventions. As a nurse you intervene by carrying out the health care provider's written and/or verbal orders. Administering a medication, implementing an invasive procedure (e.g., inserting a Foley catheter, starting an IV infusion), and preparing a patient for diagnostic tests are examples of health care provider–initiated interventions.

Each health care provider–initiated intervention requires specific nursing responsibilities and technical nursing knowledge. You are often the one performing the intervention, and you must know the types of observations and precautions to take for the intervention to be delivered safely and correctly. For example, when administering a medication, you are responsible for not only giving the medicine correctly but also knowing the classification of the drug; its physiological action, normal dosage, and side effects; and the nursing interventions related to its action or side effects (see Chapter 31). You are responsible for knowing when an invasive procedure is necessary, the clinical skills necessary to complete it, and its expected outcome and possible side effects. You are also responsible for adequate preparation of a patient and proper communication of the results. You perform dependent nursing interventions, like all nursing actions, with appropriate knowledge, clinical reasoning, and good clinical judgment.

Other provider interventions, or interdependent interventions, are therapies that require the combined knowledge, skill, and expertise of multiple health care providers. Typically when you plan care for a patient, you review the necessary interventions and determine whether the collaboration of other health care disciplines (e.g., social work, rehabilitation, pharmacy) is necessary. A patient care conference with an interprofessional health care team results in selection of interdependent interventions.

In the case study involving Mr. Lawson, Tonya plans independent interventions to continue managing Mr. Lawson's pain and to begin teaching him about postoperative care activities. Among the dependent interventions Tonya plans to implement are the administration of an ordered analgesic and wound care. Tonya's other-initiated intervention involves collaborating with the unit discharge coordinator, who will help Mr. and Mrs. Lawson plan for their return home, and the home health department to ensure that the Lawsons have home health visits.

When preparing for health care provider–initiated or other provider–initiated interventions, do not automatically implement the therapies but determine whether they are appropriate for each patient.

Every nurse faces an inappropriate or incorrect order at some time. The nurse with a strong knowledge base and clinical experience recognizes an error and seeks to correct it. The ability to recognize incorrect therapies is particularly important when administering medications or procedures. Errors occur in writing orders or transcribing them to a documentation form or computer screen. Clarifying an order is competent nursing practice, and it protects a patient and members of the health care team. When you carry out an incorrect or inappropriate intervention, it is as much your error as the person who wrote or transcribed the original order. You are legally responsible for any complications resulting from an error (see Chapter 23).

> ### REFLECT NOW
>
> Consider that Tonya has independent, dependent, and other provider-initiated interventions to perform for Mr. Lawson. How does this affect her prioritization of nursing care for the patient?

Selection of Interventions

During planning do not select interventions randomly. For example, patients with the diagnosis of *Anxiety* do not always need care involving the same interventions. You treat *Anxiety related to the uncertainty of surgical recovery* very differently from *Anxiety related to a threat to loss of job*. When choosing interventions, consider six important factors: (1) desired patient outcomes, (2) characteristics of the nursing diagnosis, (3) research base knowledge for the intervention, (4) feasibility for doing the intervention, (5) acceptability to the patient, and (6) your own competency (Butcher et al., 2018) (Box 18.1).

When developing a plan of care, review resources such as the scientific literature, standard protocols or guidelines, the Nursing Outcomes Classification (NOC) and Nursing Interventions Classification (NIC), policy or procedure manuals, other health professionals, or textbooks. As you select interventions, review your patient's needs, priorities, and previous experiences to select the interventions that have the best potential for achieving the expected outcomes.

Nursing Interventions Classification. Just as with the standardized NOC, the Iowa Intervention Project developed a set of nursing interventions that provides a level of standardization to enhance communication of nursing care across all health care settings and compare outcomes (Butcher et al., 2018). The NIC model includes three levels: domains, classes, and the interventions for ease of use. The seven domains are the highest level (level 1) of the model, using broad terms (e.g., safety and basic physiological) to organize the more specific classes and interventions (Table 18.3). The second level of the model includes 30 classes or groups of related interventions, which offer useful clinical categories to reference when selecting interventions. An example of a class is *Physical Comfort Promotion*. The third level of the model includes the 565 interventions, defined as any treatment based on clinical judgment and knowledge that a nurse performs to enhance patient outcomes (Butcher et al., 2018) (Box 18.2). The interventions can be used with various diagnostic

---

BOX 18.1 Choosing Nursing Interventions

Desired Patient Outcomes
- Outcomes serve as the criteria against which to judge efficacy of interventions.
- Nursing Outcomes Classification (NOC) outcomes are linked to NANDA Nursing Diagnoses and ICNP diagnoses with the same label.
- NOC outcomes are also linked to Nursing Interventions Classification (NIC) interventions (Moorhead et al., 2018). Use these resources to develop care plans.

Characteristics of the Nursing Diagnosis
- Choose interventions to alter the etiological (related to) factor or causes of the diagnosis. **Example:** *Acute Pain* related to trauma of surgical incision—choose interventions for Mr. Lawson that relieve swelling and strain on the incision site (positioning and turning measures) and that lower pain reception (analgesic).
- When an etiological factor cannot change, direct the interventions toward treating the signs and symptoms (e.g., assessment findings for a diagnosis). **Example:** *Lack of Knowledge* regarding postoperative care related to inexperience with surgery and impending discharge with self-care needs—choose interventions that provide information that answers Mr. and Mrs. Lawson's questions about recovery procedures and wound care, and that prepares them to monitor Mr. Lawson's progress at home.
- For risk diagnoses, direct interventions at altering or eliminating the risk factors for the diagnosis. **Example:** *Risk for Infection* requires interventions for keeping Mr. Lawson's incisional area clean and free from further trauma, and for maintaining good nutrition.

Research Base
- Be familiar with the research evidence for an intervention, and use it for the appropriate patient group and/or setting (see Chapter 5).

- Research evidence in support of a nursing intervention will indicate the effectiveness of using the intervention with certain types of patients.
- When research is unavailable, use scientific principles (e.g., infection control, learning) or consult a clinical expert about your patient.

Feasibility
- A specific intervention has the potential to interact with other interventions provided by the nurse and other health professionals.
- Know and be involved in a patient's total plan of care.
- Consider cost of an intervention and the amount of time required for implementation (in consideration of patient's condition). **Example:** If you plan to get a patient up into a chair three times a day, will there be staff to assist with the transfer? Is the patient becoming weaker?

Acceptability to the Patient
- When possible, offer a patient a choice of interventions to assist in reaching outcomes.
- Promote informed choice; give patients information about each intervention and how they are expected to participate.
- Consider a patient's values, beliefs, and culture for a patient-centered approach to selecting interventions.

Capability of the Nurse
- Have knowledge of the scientific rationale for the intervention.
- Have the necessary psychosocial and psychomotor skills to complete the intervention.
- Be able to function within the specific setting to effectively use health care resources.

Modified from Butcher GM, et al: *Nursing interventions classification (NIC)*, ed 7, St Louis, 2018, Elsevier.

TABLE 18.3   Examples of Nursing Interventions Classification (NIC) Taxonomy—Domains 1-4 and Accompanying Classes of Interventions

Domain 1	Domain 2	Domain 3	Domain 4
Level 1 Domains			
1. **Physiological: Basic**	2. **Physiological: Complex**	3. **Behavioral**	4. **Safety**
Care that supports physical functioning	Care that supports homeostatic regulation	Care that supports psychosocial functioning and facilitates lifestyle changes	Care that supports protection against harm
Level 2 Classes			
A *Activity and Exercise Management:* Interventions to organize or assist with physical activity and energy conservation and expenditure	G *Electrolyte and Acid-Base Management:* Interventions to regulate electrolyte/acid-base balance and prevent complications	O *Behavior Therapy:* Interventions to reinforce or promote desirable behaviors or alter undesirable behaviors	U *Crisis Management:* Interventions to provide immediate short-term help in both psychological and physiological crises
B *Elimination Management:* Interventions to establish and maintain regular bowel and urinary elimination patterns and manage complications caused by altered patterns	H *Drug Management:* Interventions to facilitate desired effects of pharmacological agents	P *Cognitive Therapy:* Interventions to reinforce or promote desirable cognitive functioning or alter undesirable cognitive functioning	V *Risk Management:* Interventions to initiate risk-reduction activities and continue monitoring risks over time
C *Immobility Management:* Interventions to manage restricted body movement and the sequelae	I *Neurologic Management:* Interventions to optimize neurological function	Q *Communication Enhancement:* Interventions to facilitate delivering and receiving verbal and nonverbal messages	
D *Nutrition Support:* Interventions to modify or maintain nutritional status	J *Perioperative Care:* Interventions to provide care before, during, and immediately after surgery	R *Coping Assistance:* Interventions to assist another to build on own strengths, adapt to a change in function, or achieve a higher level of function	
E *Physical Comfort Promotion:* Interventions to promote comfort using physical techniques	K *Respiratory Management:* Interventions to promote airway patency and gas exchange	S *Patient Education:* Interventions to facilitate learning	
F *Self-Care Facilitation:* Interventions to provide or assist with routine activities of daily living	L *Skin/Wound Management:* Interventions to maintain or restore tissue integrity	T *Psychological Comfort Promotion:* Interventions to promote comfort using psychological techniques	
	M *Thermoregulation:* Interventions to maintain body temperature within a normal range		
	N *Tissue Perfusion Management:* Interventions to optimize circulation of blood and fluids to the tissue		

From Butcher GM, et al: *Nursing interventions classification (NIC)*, ed 7, St Louis, 2018, Mosby.

BOX 18.2   Example of Interventions for Physical Comfort Promotion

Class: Physical Comfort Promotion (Level 2)
Interventions to promote comfort using physical techniques

Interventions (Examples)
Aromatherapy
Cutaneous Stimulation
Environmental Management
Heat/Cold Application
Nausea Management
Pain Management
Progressive Muscle Relaxation

Examples of Linked Nursing Diagnoses
Acute Pain
Chronic Pain

From Butcher GM, et al: *Nursing interventions classification (NIC)*, ed 7, St Louis, 2018, Mosby.

BOX 18.3   Example of an Intervention and Associated Nursing Activities

Intervention—Environmental Management: Comfort
Examples of Activities

- Create a calm and supportive environment.
- Provide a single room if it is the patient's preference to offer quiet and rest.
- Adjust room temperature to that most comfortable for the individual.
- Provide a safe and clean environment.
- Determine sources of discomfort: damp dressing, positioning on tubing, wrinkled linen.
- Position patient to facilitate comfort.
- Provide prompt attention to call lights, which should always be within reach.

From Butcher GM, et al: *Nursing interventions classification (NIC)*, ed 7, St Louis, 2018, Mosby.

---

classifications, including NANDA, ICNP, and others (Butcher et al., 2018). Each intervention then includes a variety of nursing activities from which to choose (Box 18.3) and which a nurse commonly uses in a plan of care. For example, if a patient has a nursing diagnosis of *Acute Pain,* the class of interventions that would apply to the patient is *Physical Comfort Promotion.* That class includes 18 interventions,

such as aromatherapy, cutaneous stimulation, and pain management: acute. Each class has a variety of activities. The intervention for *Pain Management: Acute* has 20 recommended nursing activities, such as ensuring that the patient receives prompt analgesic care or using combination analgesics. NIC is a valuable resource for selecting appropriate interventions and activities for your patient. It is evolving and practice oriented. The classification is comprehensive, including independent and collaborative interventions. It remains your decision to determine which interventions and activities best suit your patient's individualized needs and situation.

SYSTEMS FOR PLANNING NURSING CARE

Systems exist for developing and communicating a nurse's plan of care to other nurses and collaborating health care providers. Good planning ensures the safety and quality of care (QSEN, 2018). Each of the systems that exist within health care agencies promotes continuity and use of best practices in patient care.

Health Care Agency Care Plans

In any health care setting nurses are responsible for providing a nursing plan of care for each patient. The plan of care can take several forms (e.g., individual electronic care plan or standardized care plans). With the growth of EHRs within health care institutions, documentation systems typically include software programs for creating individualized and standard nursing care plans. These programs use standardized nursing language, including nursing diagnostic language (e.g., NANDA or ICNP), and NOC and NIC taxonomies, enabling nurses to clearly identify a plan of care using appropriate nursing diagnoses, outcomes, and interventions. This enables nurses and other health care providers to quickly identify a patient's needs and situation. Although EHR plans often follow a standard format, a nurse customizes each plan to the unique needs of each patient. Standardized care plans have typically been developed by a health care agency's clinical experts based on clinical experience and scientific evidence. The standardized plans are usually based on common medical or surgical conditions. They outline the nursing care to be provided for patients with such conditions. A standardized care plan is more difficult to individualize since it is based on agreed standards of care, but such plans are believed to improve the quality of care and are easy to understand (Jansson et al., 2010).

A **nursing care plan** includes nursing diagnoses, goals and/or expected outcomes, individualized nursing interventions, and a section for evaluation findings (see Chapter 20). The plan promotes continuity of care and better communication because it informs all health care providers about a patient's needs and interventions and reduces the risk for incomplete, incorrect, or inappropriate care measures. Nurses revise a plan when a patient's status changes. Preprinted standardized care plans and EHR care plans follow a standardized format, but you can individualize each plan to a patient's unique needs. The plan gives all nurses a central document that outlines a patient's diagnoses/problems, the plan of care for each diagnosis/problem, and the outcomes for monitoring and evaluating patient progress. The plan of care communicates nursing care priorities to nurses and other health care providers. It also identifies and coordinates resources for delivering nursing care. For example, in a care plan you list specific supplies necessary to use in a dressing change or names of clinical nurse specialists who are caring for a patient.

In hospitals and community-based settings, patients receive care from more than one nurse, health care provider, or allied health professional. Thus more institutions are developing **interprofessional care plans**, which include contributions from all disciplines involved in patient care. The interprofessional plan focuses on patient priorities and improves the coordination of all patient therapies and communication among all disciplines.

The Nursing Care Plan provided below is an example of a care plan for Mr. Lawson, using the standard format found throughout this text.

◎ NURSING CARE PLAN

Anxiety

ASSESSMENT

Mr. Lawson continues to recover, but Tonya observes behaviors that suggest he is worried about recovery. She waits about an hour after administering a pain medication and enters his room. She wants to have a discussion about how the patient is emotionally coping with surgery.

Assessment Activities	Assessment Findings[a]
Ask patient to clarify concerns he has about his recovery from surgery.	Patient **reports concern** about his wound not healing and keeping him from being able to return to work in 6 weeks. Has difficulty explaining what to expect during recovery.
Assess patient's cognitive function.	Patient **does not attend** to Tonya's explanation of risk factors for infection and shows **poor eye contact** when discussing condition.
Observe patient's behaviors during discussion.	Patient is observed to be **irritable** and **displays facial tension** when discussing surgical recovery process.

[a]**Assessment Findings** are shown in bold type.

NURSING DIAGNOSIS: Anxiety related to uncertainty over ability to return to work

PLANNING

Goals	Expected Outcomes (NOC)[b]
	Anxiety Level
Mr. Lawson will experience reduced anxiety during instruction.	Patient shows less facial tension during discussions about recovery from surgery in 24 hours.
	Patient maintains attention during instruction about wound care within 24 hours.
	Coping
Mr. Lawson will obtain a clear understanding of what to expect following surgery.	Patient will be able to describe expected progression of his wound healing by discharge.
	Patient will express confidence in being able to recover successfully.
Mr. Lawson will accept ability to recover as planned.	

[b]Outcomes classification labels from Moorhead S, et al: *Nursing outcomes classification (NOC)*, ed 6, St Louis, 2018, Mosby.

Continued

⊚ NURSING CARE PLAN—CONT'D

INTERVENTIONS (NIC)[c]	RATIONALE
Anxiety Reduction	
Use a calm, reassuring approach while explaining expectations for recovery; listen attentively to patient's questions.	For patients to be able to express concerns and ask questions, they must see nurses as being nonthreatening, reliable, and willing to have a human connection (Varcarolis, 2017).
Encourage patient to express concerns.	
Collaborate with health care provider to provide information about wound care, normal progress of wound healing, and signs of poor wound healing as these factors affect expectations for patient's ability to return to work.	Providing information about the processes of surgical recovery helps patients handle symptoms of anxiety (Johnson, 2017).
Teach patient relaxation exercise using deep breathing and reading relaxing sentences while sitting in chair.	Systematic relaxation technique involving reading relaxing sentences significantly reduced anxiety in older patients undergoing abdominal surgery (Rejeh et al., 2013).

[c]Intervention classification labels from Butcher HK, et al: *Nursing interventions classification (NIC)*, ed 7, St Louis, 2018, Mosby.

EVALUATION

Evaluation Activity	Patient Response/Finding	Outcome Status
Observe Mr. Lawson's verbal and nonverbal behavior during instructional session.	Mr. Lawson is able to attend to discussion about his recovery and shows good eye contact. Asks relevant questions and able to perform relaxation during a discussion with nurse.	Patient maintains attention during discussion; shows less facial tension.
Ask Mr. Lawson to describe how his wound is expected to heal during the next 2 weeks.	Patient able to describe normal inflammation, how wound should look and feel as it heals, and signs of infection.	Patient able to describe expected progression of wound healing and signs of infection.
Ask patient how he feels about managing his wound.	Patient states, "I do feel better about it. I now know what to watch out for, and I know my wife will help."	Patient expresses confidence in managing wound care.

A care plan includes a patient's short- and long-term goals and outcomes, making it an important part of discharge planning. Thus you need to involve the family in planning care if the patient is agreeable. The family is often a resource to help a patient meet health care goals. In addition, meeting some of the family's needs can improve a patient's level of wellness. Discharge planning is especially important for a patient with a disability or injury that was not present before hospitalization. As a result, the patient must undergo long-term rehabilitation in the community and often will require home health care. Same-day surgeries and earlier discharges from hospitals require you to begin planning discharge from the moment the patient enters the health care agency. The complete care plan is the blueprint for nursing action.

Student Care Plans

Student care plans help you learn problem solving, the nursing process, skills of written communication, and organizational skills for nursing care. Most important, a student care plan helps you apply knowledge gained from the scientific literature and the classroom to a practice situation. Students typically write a care plan for each nursing diagnosis, using a table format with columns for assessment findings, goals, expected outcomes, nursing interventions with supporting rationales, and criteria to evaluate outcomes. Similar to health care agency care plans, the student care plan focuses on substantiating interventions with rationales so that students can learn the scientific basis for their practice. Each school uses a different format for student care plans. Often the format used is similar to the one used by the health care agency that provides clinical experiences for the students. The following questions will help you complete a student care plan:

- *What* is the intervention? Is it evidence based and connected to an outcome?
- *When* should each intervention be implemented?
- *How* should the intervention be performed for the specific patient?
- *Who* should be involved in each aspect of intervention? Is interprofessional collaboration necessary?

Each scientific rationale that you use to support a nursing intervention needs to include a reference, whenever possible, to document the source from the scientific literature. This reinforces the importance of evidence-based nursing practice. It is also important that each intervention be specific and unique to a patient's situation. The planning of nonspecific nursing interventions results in incomplete or inaccurate nursing care, lack of continuity among caregivers, and poor use of resources. Common omissions that nurses make in writing nursing interventions include action, frequency, quantity, method, or person to perform them (see Chapter 19). These errors occur when nurses are unfamiliar with the planning process. The fifth column of the care plan includes a section for you to evaluate the plan of care: Was each goal/outcome fully or only partially met? Use the evaluation column to document whether the plan requires revision or when outcomes are met, thus indicating when a nursing diagnosis is no longer relevant to a patient's plan of care (see Chapter 20).

Care Plans for Community-Based Settings

Planning care for patients who are in community-based settings (e.g., clinics or patients' homes) applies the same principles of nursing practice as those for patients who are hospitalized. However, in community-based settings you complete a more comprehensive community, home, and family assessment. Ultimately a patient/family unit must be able to provide the majority of health care independently. You design a plan to (1) educate the patient and designated family caregiver about the necessary care techniques and precautions, (2) teach a patient and family caregiver how to integrate care within family activities, and (3) guide the patient and family caregiver on how to assume a greater percentage of care over time. Finally, the plan includes nurses' and the patient's/family caregiver's evaluation of expected outcomes.

Hand-Off Reporting

Part of planning is transferring essential information (along with responsibility and authority) from one nurse to the next during

BOX 18.4 EVIDENCE-BASED PRACTICE

Nursing Hand-Off Reports

PICOT Question: Does the use of bedside hand-off communication compared with standard end-of shift report between nurses in acute care settings improve patient outcomes?

Evidence Summary

A nursing hand-off during change of shift involves a nurse-to-nurse verbal exchange of information about patients. This contrasts with nurses gaining report from taped summaries or written reviews of electronic records. Hand-off reporting became a provision of care standard by The Joint Commission (TJC) in 2010, which states that a health care "organization's process for hand-off communication provides for the opportunity for discussion between the giver and receiver of patient information" (TJC, 2017). A systematic review of scientific articles discussing nursing hand-offs identified strategies for and barriers to effective hand-offs (Riesenberg et al., 2010). A recent qualitative study found that off-going nurses' ability to grasp a patient's story intra-shift was essential to convey the full picture during a hand-off (Birmingham et al., 2015). This emphasizes the importance of knowing patients (see Chapter 16) and being able to understand the full context of a patient's clinical situation. Hand-offs have multiple purposes, including information transfer, shared decision making, review of treatment options, and shared planning (Riesenberg, 2012; Birmingham et al., 2015). Carefully consider the following strategies and decide whether they are useful and fit your institutional setting and resources.

Application to Nursing Practice
Strategies for Effective Nursing Hand-Offs

- Do prework; manage your time so that you are prepared to give report and be concise.
- Provide information on how to reduce risks to patients so that the receiving nurse is better prepared to coordinate patient care, prevent errors, and detect

and intervene if a patient's status deteriorates. Patient-specific details such as abnormal vital signs or a risk for falls enable the receiving nurse to cue-in more effectively to signs and symptoms of deterioration (Birmingham et al., 2015).
- Keep report patient centered; ask questions and clarify. Use prompts to gather details.
- Standardize the process using tools, forms, and checklists, and be sure that essential information is consistently included. Written notes based on a nurse's own structured method help him or her remember large amounts of information, stay organized, and prepare for the next end-of-shift handoff (Birmingham et al., 2015).
- During walking rounds include patient and family in discussion of goals.
- Limit interruptions, distraction, and noise.
- Acknowledge information received and transfer of responsibility (Riesenberg, 2012).

Barriers to Effective Nursing Hand-Offs

- Delaying hand-off reports is a barrier caused when nurses arrive late to work and/or off-going nurses are detained in patient care responsibilities (Birmingham et al., 2015). This results in a rushed and incomplete report.
- Communication barriers result when the receiver gets information that is inaccurate, incomplete, untimely, misinterpreted, or otherwise not what is needed (TJC, 2017).
- Social problems, including a culture of blame on the patient care unit that inhibits questioning, may result. Research has shown that off-going nurses may feel the need to defend themselves and that important information may not be communicated when nurses feel flustered, doubted, or unable to think.

---

transitions in care (e.g., end of shift, during a patient transfer to a new care unit, discharge to another setting). Hand-off reporting is a real-time process that offers a health care provider accepting the care of a patient the opportunity to ask questions to clarify and confirm important details about a patient's plan of care, patient progress, and continuing needs during the transfer of information. Quality hand-off information enables nurses to quickly recognize changes in patient status and to anticipate risks, thereby promoting safe patient care (Birmingham et al., 2015). A correctly formulated nursing care plan facilitates a hand-off report as one nurse communicates to another. You learn to focus your reports on the nursing care, treatments, patient goals, and expected outcomes documented in your care plans. During a hand-off report always provide accurate, up-to-date, and pertinent information to the next nurse assuming patient care. The hand-off is a critical time to ensure continuity of care for a patient and prevent errors or delays in providing nursing interventions. Recent research identifies approaches to use for effective hand-offs and barriers to their effectiveness (Box 18.4).

Concept Maps

Because nurses care for patients who have multiple health problems and related nursing diagnoses, it is often not realistic to have a written care plan developed for each nursing diagnosis. In addition, care plans usually do not allow you to show the associations among different nursing diagnoses and different nursing interventions. A concept map is a visual representation of all of a patient's nursing diagnoses (including supportive assessment findings) that allows you to diagram interventions for each. A concept map makes a patient's diagnoses more meaningful because it shows the cognitive connections you make

between diagnoses and interventions. Using a concept map has been shown to improve self-reflection and critical thinking (Daley et al., 2016). A map shows you the relationships within the nursing process (i.e., how nursing interventions often apply to more than one nursing diagnosis). Concept maps group and categorize nursing concepts to give you a holistic view of your patient's health care needs.

In Chapter 17 you learned how to add nursing diagnostic labels to a concept map. When planning care for each nursing diagnosis, analyze the relationships among the diagnoses. Draw dotted lines between nursing diagnoses to indicate their relationships to one another (Fig. 18.4). It is important for you to make meaningful associations between one concept and another. The links need to be accurate, meaningful, and complete so that you can explain why nursing diagnoses are related. Mr. Lawson's concept map has a new, fourth nursing diagnosis, *Anxiety*. Mr. Lawson's *Anxiety* and *Acute Pain* are interrelated; in addition, *Acute Pain* has an influence on his *Lack of Knowledge*.

Finally, on a separate sheet of paper or on the map itself, list nursing interventions to attain the measurable outcomes for each nursing diagnosis. This step corresponds to the planning phase of the nursing process. While caring for a patient, use the map to write his or her responses to each nursing activity. Also write your clinical impressions regarding the patient's progress toward expected outcomes and the effectiveness of interventions. Keep the concept map with you throughout the clinical day. As you revise the plan, take notes and add or delete nursing interventions. Use the information recorded on the map to document patient care. Critical thinkers learn by organizing and relating cognitive concepts. Concept maps help you learn the interrelationships among nursing diagnoses to create a unique meaning and organization of information collected.

CONCEPT MAP

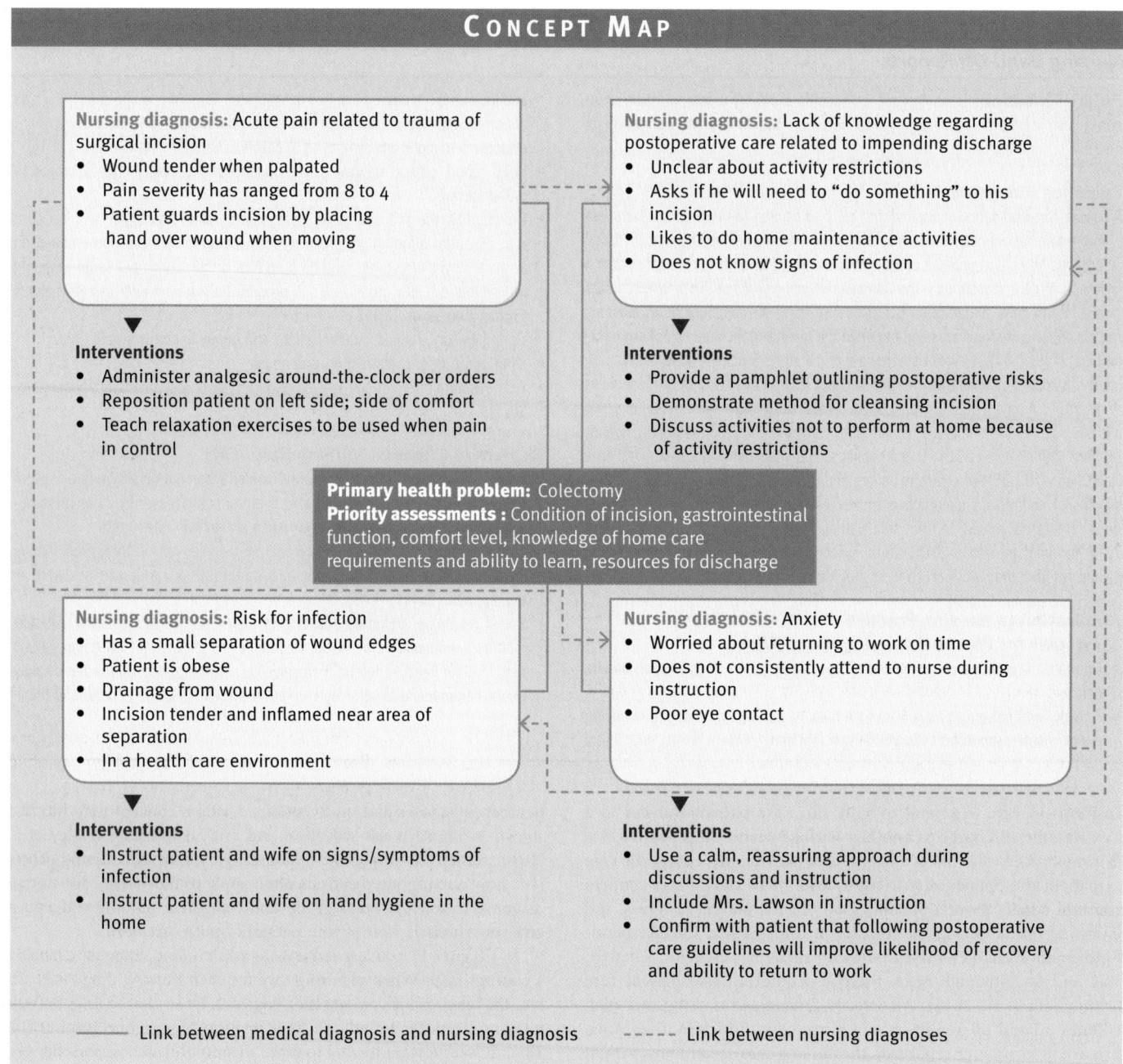

Nursing diagnosis: Acute pain related to trauma of surgical incision
- Wound tender when palpated
- Pain severity has ranged from 8 to 4
- Patient guards incision by placing hand over wound when moving

Interventions
- Administer analgesic around-the-clock per orders
- Reposition patient on left side; side of comfort
- Teach relaxation exercises to be used when pain in control

Nursing diagnosis: Lack of knowledge regarding postoperative care related to impending discharge
- Unclear about activity restrictions
- Asks if he will need to "do something" to his incision
- Likes to do home maintenance activities
- Does not know signs of infection

Interventions
- Provide a pamphlet outlining postoperative risks
- Demonstrate method for cleansing incision
- Discuss activities not to perform at home because of activity restrictions

Primary health problem: Colectomy
Priority assessments : Condition of incision, gastrointestinal function, comfort level, knowledge of home care requirements and ability to learn, resources for discharge

Nursing diagnosis: Risk for infection
- Has a small separation of wound edges
- Patient is obese
- Drainage from wound
- Incision tender and inflamed near area of separation
- In a health care environment

Interventions
- Instruct patient and wife on signs/symptoms of infection
- Instruct patient and wife on hand hygiene in the home

Nursing diagnosis: Anxiety
- Worried about returning to work on time
- Does not consistently attend to nurse during instruction
- Poor eye contact

Interventions
- Use a calm, reassuring approach during discussions and instruction
- Include Mrs. Lawson in instruction
- Confirm with patient that following postoperative care guidelines will improve likelihood of recovery and ability to return to work

——— Link between medical diagnosis and nursing diagnosis   - - - - - Link between nursing diagnoses

FIG. 18.4 Concept map for Mr. Lawson: Planning.

Critical Pathways

Many hospitals are using critical pathways and enhanced recovery after surgery (ERAS) protocols to reduce variations in clinical practice, standardize evidence-based care, reduce patient length of stay, and improve patient outcomes. An ERAS incorporates evidence-based practices and includes a comprehensive projected plan for a patient's journey through the surgical process from preoperative screening through postoperative care (Woolfrey et al., 2018). For example, an ERAS will set time frames for when patients are to progress with mobility, advance diets, receive specific types of medications, and have therapies (such as IV infusion, Foley catheterization) discontinued. A pathway is a clinical management tool that provides a road map for best practices based on clinicians' expertise and clinical guidelines shaped by interprofessional teams (Hipp et al., 2016). Traditionally, critical pathways and ERAS have been developed for medical

and surgical conditions that are high volume and shown to be consistent and relatively predictable (e.g., total hip replacement, low back pain, palliative care). Although pathways and recovery protocols offer an approach to a consistent workflow, it is still imperative to individualize patient care. There is a risk that clinical pathways can contribute to fragmentation of care if clinicians focus on the disease rather than on the person as a whole (Beaulieu, 2013).

REFLECT NOW

Consider three ways that the use of a critical pathway might enhance the quality of a hand-off report.

CONSULTING WITH HEALTH CARE PROFESSIONALS

You consult with members of the health care team when you face problems in providing nursing or collaborative care or in delivering dependent interventions. A consultation is vital if you need to seek procedural assistance or clinical expertise for a specific problem to ensure a patient receives needed clinical interventions or insights (Stevens et al., 2015).

Consultation can occur at any time, but you usually consult most often during planning and implementation. During these times you are more likely to identify a problem requiring additional knowledge, skills, or resources. One way to initially consult is by using the ISBAR approach, a mechanism for framing conversations, especially critical ones, requiring a clinician's immediate attention and action. ISBAR is an acronym for *Identify, Situation, Background, Assessment,* and *Recommendation* (IHI, 2018).

Consultation requires you to be aware of your strengths and limitations as a team member. During a consultation you seek the expertise of a specialist such as your nursing instructor, a health care provider, or a clinical nurse specialist to identify ways to handle specific problems in patient management or the planning and implementation of therapies. A nurse in practice will consult with dietitians, therapists, or pharmacists, for example. The consultation process offers new insight and specific recommendations for a patient's plan of care. It differs from interprofessional collaboration in that it is often a onetime event. However, consultation can lead to the health care professionals involved collaborating as part of the interprofessional team.

An experienced nurse is a valuable consultant when you face an unfamiliar patient care situation, such as a new procedure or a patient presenting a set of symptoms that you cannot identify. In clinical nursing consultation helps to solve problems in the delivery of nursing care. For example, a nursing student consults a clinical specialist for wound care techniques, a home care nurse on how to help a patient adapt to restrictions in the home, or an educator for useful teaching resources. Nurses are consulted for their clinical expertise, patient education skills, or staff education skills. Be prepared before you make a consultation. Consultation is based on the problem-solving approach, and the consultant is the stimulus for change.

QSEN **Building Competency in Teamwork and Collaboration** Tonya consults with the unit discharge coordinator, who will help Mr. and Mrs. Lawson plan for their return home. What does Tonya know about Mr. Lawson's situation that should be communicated to the coordinator? Identify three ways in which the coordinator might be most helpful to the Lawson family.

Answers to QSEN Activities can be found on the Evolve website.

When to Consult

Consultation occurs when you identify a problem that you or the interprofessional team are unable to solve. However, the process requires good interprofessional collaboration. Consultation with other care providers increases your knowledge about a patient's problems and helps you learn skills and use additional resources. A good time to consult with another health care provider is when the exact problem remains unclear. An objective consultant enters a clinical situation and more clearly assesses and identifies the nature of a problem, whether it is patient, personnel, or equipment oriented. Most often you consult with health care providers who are working in your clinical area. However, sometimes you consult over the telephone (Box 18.5).

BOX 18.5   Tips for Making Phone Consultations

- Have the information you need (e.g., medical record notes, medication sheets, recent nurse summary) available BEFORE you make a call.
- Assess the patient yourself before making the call. For example, when you consult with health care providers, they rely heavily on your assessment so that they can give appropriate advice.
- Address both the clinical history and patient's perspective, including social and cultural context.
- Give a diagnosis or interpretation of the patient's problem with an explanation or a summary. Use of the ISBAR approach in reporting is helpful.
- Understand why you are calling for consultation and think through some possible solutions. Your experience in caring for the patient allows you to make useful suggestions.

Data from Maison D: Effective communications are more important than ever: a health care provider's perspective, *J Home Care Hospice Professional* 24(3):178, 2006; Males T: In the dark: risks of telephone consultations, *Sessional GP* 4(2):2012, http://www.medicalprotection.org/docs/default-source/pdfs/uk-sessional-gp/oct-2012.pdf. Accessed June 29, 2019.

How to Consult

Begin with your own understanding of a patient's clinical problems. The following list contains important steps to follow in the consultation process.

- Identify the general problem area.
- Choose the appropriate professional, such as another nurse or social worker, to help resolve the problem.
- Provide a consultant with relevant information and resources about the problem area. Provide a summary of the problem, methods used to resolve the problem so far, and outcomes of these methods. Share information from the patient's medical record and conversations with other nurses and the patient's family.
- Do not prejudice or influence consultants. Biasing or showing prejudice blocks problem resolution. Avoid bias by not overloading consultants with subjective and emotional conclusions about the patient and the problem.
- Be available to discuss a consultant's findings and recommendations. Provide a private, comfortable atmosphere for the consultant and patient to meet. However, this does not mean that you leave the environment. A common mistake is turning the whole problem over to the consultant. The consultant is not there to take over the problem but to help you resolve it. Request the consultation for a time when both you and the consultant are able to discuss the patient's situation with minimal interruptions or distractions.
- Incorporate the consultant's recommendations into the care plan. Always give the consultant feedback regarding the outcome of the recommendations.

Successful Planning Equals Patient Participation

The process of planning is comprehensive, evidence-based, and patient outcome oriented. But critical to success is patient participation, involving patients in the decisions that affect their health care. Research has shown factors that influence patient participation include relationships with health care professionals, allocation of sufficient time for participation in planning care, and the recognition of the patient's own knowledge, physical and cognitive ability, and emotional connections, beliefs, values, and experiences in relation to health services (Shaghayegh et al., 2014). Applying the principles of planning discussed in this chapter will address these factors and ensure your patients quality care.

KEY POINTS

- After identifying a patient's nursing diagnoses and collaborative problems, you begin planning, which involves setting priorities based on patient diagnoses and problems, identifying patient-centered goals and expected outcomes, and prescribing nursing interventions for each diagnosis.

- Symptom pattern recognition from patient assessment and certain knowledge triggers (e.g., pathophysiology or knowing patients) help you understand which diagnoses require intervention and the associated time frame during which you need to intervene.

- By ranking a patient's nursing diagnoses in order of importance and always monitoring changing signs and symptoms of patient problems, you attend to each patient's most important needs and better organize ongoing care activities.

- A goal is a broad statement that describes a desired change in a patient's condition, perceptions, or behavior, while an outcome is the measurable change needed to reach a goal.

- Goals and outcomes must be measurable so that you can measure or observe whether a change takes place in a patient's physiological status or in a patient's knowledge, perceptions, and behavior.

- Mutual goal setting increases a patient's motivation and cooperation to achieve a goal.

- Nurse-initiated interventions are autonomous actions based on scientific rationale.

- Dependent nursing interventions require an order from a health care provider to perform.

- Care plans identify a plan of care based on a patient's appropriate nursing diagnoses, outcomes, and interventions individualized to the patient's unique needs.

- You initiate a consult when your patient is experiencing a problem you cannot solve independently as a professional nurse or when you need the advice of another health care professional to provide quality patient care.

- Interprofessional collaboration is a process that is formed between two or more people from various professional fields to achieve common goals for a patient.

REFLECTIVE LEARNING

Ask to spend some time shadowing an RN who is caring for a group of patients on a hospital unit. If possible, ask the RN to give a brief summary of the patients' needs. After observing the RN performing care, consider these questions:

- What was the priority nursing diagnosis or health care problem for each patient the RN cared for?
- Did any of those priorities change as you observed the RN; if so, why?
- In what way did the RN communicate or collaborate with other care providers for the benefit of his/her patients?

REVIEW QUESTIONS

1. Setting priorities for a patient's nursing diagnoses or health problems is an important step in planning patient care. Which of the following statements describe elements to consider in planning care? (Select all that apply.)
   1. Priority setting establishes a preferential order for nursing interventions.
   2. In most cases wellness problems take priority over problem-focused problems.
   3. Recognition of symptom patterns helps in understanding when to plan interventions.
   4. Longer-term chronic needs require priority over short-term problems.
   5. Priority setting involves creating a list of care tasks.

2. Match the elements for correct identification of outcome statements with the SMART acronym terms below.
   1. Specific
   2. Measurable
   3. Attainable
   4. Realistic
   5. Timed

   a. Mutually set an outcome that a patient agrees to meet.
   b. Set an outcome that a patient can meet based upon his or her physiological, emotional, economic, and sociocultural resources.
   c. Be sure an outcome addresses only one patient behavior or response.
   d. Include when an outcome is to be met.
   e. Use a term in an outcome statement that allows for observation as to whether a change takes place in a patient's status.

3. A nursing student is providing a hand-off report to the RN assuming her patient's care. She explains, "I ambulated him twice during the shift; he tolerated walking to end of hall each time and back with no shortness of breath. Heart rate was 88 and regular after exercise. The patient said he slept better last night after I closed his door and gave him a chance to have some uninterrupted sleep. I changed the dressing over his intravenous (IV) site and started a new bag of D₅½NS. Which intervention is a dependent intervention?
   1. Providing hand-off report at change of shift
   2. Enhancing the patient's sleep hygiene
   3. Administering IV fluids
   4. Taking vital signs

4. A nurse is assigned to care for six patients at the beginning of the night shift. The nurse learns that the floor will be short by one registered nurse (RN) as a result of a call-in. A patient care technician from another area is coming to the nursing unit to assist. Because the unit requires hourly rounds on all patients, the nurse begins to make rounds on a patient who recently asked for a pain medication. The nurse is interrupted by another registered nurse who asks about another patient. Which factors in this nurse's unit environment will affect the ability to set priorities? (Select all that apply.)
   1. Policy for conducting hourly rounds
   2. Staffing level
   3. Interruption by staff nurse colleague
   4. Type of hospital unit
   5. Competency of patient care technician

5. A nursing student is providing a hand-off report to a registered nurse (RN) who is assuming her patient's care at the end of the clinical day. The student states, "The patient had a good day. His intravenous (IV) fluid is infusing at 124 mL/hr with D₅½NS infusing in left forearm. The IV site is intact, and no complaints of tenderness. I ambulated him twice during the shift; he tolerated walking to the visitors lounge and back with no shortness of breath, respirations 14, heart rate 88 after exercise. He uses his walker without difficulty, gait normal. The patient ate ¾ of his dinner with no gastrointestinal complaints. For the goal of improving the patient's activity tolerance, which expected outcomes were shared in the hand-off? (Select all that apply.)
   1. IV site not tender
   2. Uses walker to walk
   3. Walked to visitors lounge
   4. No shortness of breath
   5. Tolerated dinner meal

6. Which of the following factors should be considered when choosing an intervention for a patient's plan of care? (Select all that apply.)
   1. The specific patient outcome against which to judge effectiveness of interventions
   2. The timing of care activities routinely conducted on the care unit
   3. The scientific evidence available in support of an intervention
   4. The amount of time required for implementation in consideration of patient's condition
   5. The patient's values and beliefs regarding the intervention

7. A nurse on a hospital unit is preparing to hand off care of a patient being discharged to a home health nurse. Match the activities on the left with the hand-off report categories on the right.

Activities
1. Use a standard checklist for the report.
2. Encourage questions and clarification.
3. Offer specific information on how to reduce patient's risks.
4. Give report at time when shift has ended and other nurses are requesting information.
5. Explain how patient's discharge was delayed by insufficient numbers of staff.
6. Organize time by preparing in advance what to report.

Categories
A. Strategy for Effective Hand-off
B. Strategy for Ineffective Hand-off

8. A patient diagnosed with colon cancer has been receiving chemotherapy for 6 weeks. The patient visits the outpatient infusion center twice a week for infusions. The nurse assigned to the patient is having difficulty accessing the patient's intravenous (IV) port used to administer the chemotherapy. Despite attempts to flush the port, it is obstructed. This also occurred 2 weeks earlier. What steps should the nurse follow to make a consultation with a member of the IV infusion team? (Select all that apply.)
   1. Ask the IV nurse to come to the infusion center at a time when the nurse starts care for a second patient.
   2. Specifically identify the problem of port obstruction, and attempt to flush the port to resolve the problem.
   3. Explain to the IV nurse the frequency in which this port has obstructed in the past.
   4. Tell the IV nurse the problem is probably related to the physician who inserted the port.
   5. Describe to the IV nurse the type and condition of the port currently in use.

9. A nurse assesses a 78-year-old patient who weighs 108.9 kg (240 lb) and is partially immobilized because of a stroke. The nurse turns the patient and finds that the skin over the sacrum is very red and the patient does not feel sensation in the area. The patient has had fecal incontinence on and off for the past 2 days. The nurse identifies the nursing diagnosis of *Risk for Impaired Skin Integrity*. Which of the following outcomes is appropriate for the patient?
   1. Patient will be turned every 2 hours within 24 hours.
   2. Patient will have normal formed stool within 48 hours.
   3. Patient's ability to turn self in bed improves.
   4. Erythema of skin will be mild to none within 48 hours.

10. An 82-year-old patient who resides in a nursing home has the following three nursing diagnoses: *Risk for Fall, Impaired Physical Mobility related to pain,* and *Imbalanced Nutrition: Less Than Body Requirements related to reduced ability to feed self.* The nursing staff identified several goals of care. Match the goals on the left with the appropriate outcome statements on the right.

Goals
1. _____ Patient will ambulate independently in 3 days.
2. _____ Patient will be injury free for 1 month.
3. _____ Patient will achieve 5-pound weight gain in 1 month.
4. _____ Patient will achieve pain relief by discharge.

Outcomes
a. Patient expresses fewer nonverbal signs of discomfort within 24 hours.
b. Patient increases caloric intake to 2500 calories daily.
c. Patient walks 20 feet using a walker in 24 hours.
d. Patient identifies barriers to remove in the home within 1 week.

Answers: 1. 3; **2.** 1c, 2e, 3a, 4b, 5d; **3.** 3, 4, 2, 3, 5; **4.** 3; **5.** 3, 4; **6.** 1, 3, 4, 5; **7.** 1A, 2A, 3A, 4B, 5B, 6A; **8.** 2, 3, 5; **9.** 4; **10.** 1c, 2d, 3b, 4a.

Rationales for Review Questions can be found on the Evolve website.

REFERENCES

Ackley BJ, et al.: *Nursing diagnosis handbook,* ed 11, St Louis, 2017, Mosby.
Beaulieu M: Clinical pathways: unique contribution of family medicine, *Can Fam Physician* 59(6):705, 2013.
Butcher GM, et al.: *Nursing interventions classification (NIC),* ed 7, St Louis, 2018, Elsevier.
Carpenito LJ: *Nursing diagnoses: application to clinical practice,* ed 15, Philadelphia, 2017, Lippincott, Williams & Wilkins.
Daley BJ, et al.: Concept maps in nursing education: a historical literature review and research directions, *J Nurs Educ* 55(11):631–639, 2016.
Flagg AJ: The role of patient-centered care in nursing, *Nurs Clin North Am* 50(1):75, 2015.
Hipp R, et al.: A primer on clinical pathways, *Hosp Pharm* 51(5):416–421, 2016.
Institute for Healthcare Improvement (IHI): ISBAR trip tick, 2018, http://www.ihi.org/resources/Pages/Tools/ISBARTripTick.aspx. Accessed June 29, 2019.

Interprofessional Education Collaborative: Core competencies for interprofessional collaborative practice: 2016 update, Washington D.C., 2016, https://nebula.wsimg.com/2f68a39520b03336b41038c370497473?AccessKeyId=DC06780E69ED19E2B3A5&disposition=0&allow-origin=1. Accessed June 29, 2019.
Johnson J: *Depression after surgery: what you need to know,* Medical News Today, 2017, https://www.medicalnewstoday.com/articles/317616.php. Accessed June 29, 2019.
Moorhead S, et al.: *Nursing outcomes classification,* ed 6, St Louis, 2018, Mosby.
Nancarrow SA, et al.: Ten principles of good interprofessional team work, *Hum Resour Health* 11:19, 2013.
NCLEX: Establishing priorities: NCLEX-RN, Registered Nursing.org, n.d, https://www.registerednursing.org/nclex/establishing-priorities/. Accessed June 29, 2019.

Petri L: Concept analysis of interprofessional collaboration, *Nurs Forum* 45(2):73–82, 2010.
QSEN Institute: *QSEN competencies: patient-centered care,* 2018, http://qsen.org/competencies/pre-licensure-ksas/. Accessed June 29, 2019.
Stevens JP, et al.: Variation in inpatient consultation among older adults in the United States, *J Gen Intern Med* 30(7):992–999, 2015.
The Joint Commission (TJC): Sentinel Event Alert: Inadequate hand-off communication, issue 58, 2017, https://www.jointcommission.org/assets/1/18/SEA_58_Hand_off_Comms_9_6_17_FINAL_(1).pdf. Accessed June 29, 2019.
Varcarolis EM: *Essentials of psychiatric mental health nursing: a communication approach to evidence-based care,* ed 3, St Louis, 2017, Elsevier.

RESEARCH REFERENCES

Birmingham P, et al.: Handoffs and patient safety: grasping the story and painting a full picture, *West J Nurs Res* 37(11):1458–1478, 2015.

Jansson I, et al.: Factors and conditions that influence the implementation of standardized nursing care plans, *Open Nurs J* 4:25–34, 2010.

Mahdizadeh M, et al.: Clinical interprofessional collaboration models and frameworks from similarities to differences: a systematic review, *Glob J Health Sci* 7(6):170–180, 2015.

Rejeh N, et al.: Effect of systematic relaxation techniques on anxiety and pain in older patients undergoing abdominal surgery, *Int J Nurs Pract* 19(5):462–470, 2013.

Riesenberg LA: Shift-to-shift handoff research: where do we go from here? *J Grad Med Educ* 4(1):4, 2012.

Riesenberg LA, et al.: Nursing handoffs: a systematic review of the literature, *Am J Nurs* 110(4):24, 2010.

Shaghayegh V, et al.: Patient involvement in health care decision making: a review, *Iran Red Crescent Med J* 16(1):e12454, 2014.

Woolfrey MR, et al: Optimisation of enhanced rapid recovery after surgery (ERAS) for total joint arthroplasty: a Canadian community hospital perspective, Orthopedic Proceedings, Vol 98B, No. Supp 20, published online Feb 2018, https://online.boneandjoint.org.uk/doi/abs/10.1302/1358-992X.98BSUPP_20.COA2016-060. Accessed June 29, 2019.

19

Implementing Nursing Care

OBJECTIVES

- Explain the relationship between nursing interventions and nursing's scope of practice.
- Explain the benefits of standard nursing interventions.
- Describe implications for use of standard care bundles.
- Describe the association between critical thinking and selecting nursing interventions.
- Explain a nurse's role in the implementation process.
- Explain how a nurse balances organizational and patient priorities in time management.
- Describe how nurses anticipate and prevent complications.
- Define the three implementation skills as they relate to direct and indirect nursing interventions.
- Describe common forms of direct and indirect nursing interventions.

KEY TERMS

MEDIA RESOURCES

*You first met Tonya and Mr. Lawson in Chapter 15. Mr. Lawson is a 68-year-old patient who had abdominal surgery for a colon resection and is preparing to be discharged soon from the hospital. His nurse Tonya developed a plan of care to address four different nursing diagnoses: **Acute Pain, Anxiety, Lack of Knowledge,** and **Risk for Infection.** Mr. Lawson is interested in learning about his postoperative activity restrictions and in being able to care for his incision, which had a small separation. However, he also shared with Tonya that he is worried about his wound healing and being able to return to work after surgery. Tonya and the other nursing staff have consistently applied the nursing process. Tonya identified the diagnosis of **Anxiety** while planning for Mr. and Mrs. Lawson's education. During implementation Tonya, along with her health care colleagues, will provide planned interventions to achieve the goals and expected outcomes identified in Mr. Lawson's plan of care. Critical thinking, which includes good clinical decision making, is important for the successful implementation of nursing interventions.*

Implementation, the fourth step of the nursing process, begins after you develop a patient's plan of care. It involves the performance of nursing and collaborative interventions necessary to achieve the goals and expected outcomes needed to support or improve a patient's health status. A nursing intervention is any treatment based on clinical judgment and knowledge that a nurse performs to enhance patient outcomes (Butcher et al., 2018). Nursing interventions include direct and indirect care measures, which are either nurse-initiated, physician (health care provider)-initiated, or other provider–initiated (see Chapter 18). Ideally a nurse chooses nursing interventions that are evidence based (see Chapter 5), providing the most current, scientifically supported, up-to-date approaches for delivering patient-centered care.

Direct care interventions are treatments nurses provide through interactions with patients or a group of patients (Butcher et al., 2018). For example, a patient receives direct intervention in the form of medication administration, insertion of a urinary catheter, discharge instruction, or counseling during a time of grief. Indirect care interventions are treatments performed away from a patient but on behalf of the patient or group of patients (e.g., managing a patient's environment [e.g., safety and infection control]), documentation, and interprofessional collaboration (Butcher et al., 2018) (Fig. 19.1).

Within the scope of nursing practice, the American Nurses Association (ANA, n.d.) describes what a nurse is licensed to perform: "Nursing is the protection, promotion, and optimization of health and abilities; prevention of illness and injury; facilitation of healing; alleviation of suffering through the diagnosis and treatment of human response; and advocacy in the care of individuals, families, groups, communities, and populations."

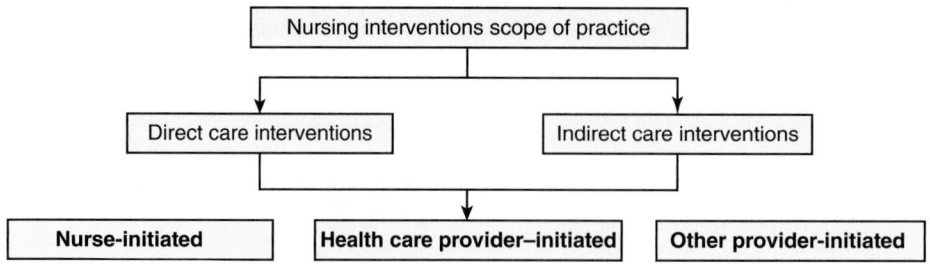

Examples of Interventions by Initiation

DOMAINS			
Helping	Conducting family care plan conference		Discharge planning conference
Teaching-Coaching	1:1 instruction, interpersonal skills	1:1 instruction	Exercise, ADL training
Diagnostic/Patient Monitoring	VS monitoring during clinical change	Blood glucose testing	Diet calorie count
Managing Rapidly Changing Situations	Measuring oxygen saturation	Oxygen therapy	Comforting family during patient emergency
Administering/Monitoring Treatments	Pressure ulcer prevention measures	Wound irrigation	Review of wound culture reports
Monitoring/Ensuring Quality Health Care Practices	Following fall prevention protocol	Monitoring surgical infection rates	Gathering data on fall occurrence
Organizational/Work-Role Competence	Hand-off reporting/Delegation	Physician credentialing	Interdisciplinary rounding

FIG. 19.1 Nursing interventions scope of practice.

BOX 19.1 Domains of Nursing Practice

- The Helping Role
- The Teaching-Coaching Function
- The Diagnostic and Patient-Monitoring Function
- Effective Management of Rapidly Changing Situations
- Administering and Monitoring Therapeutic Interventions and Regimens
- Monitoring and Ensuring the Quality of Health Care Practices
- Organizational and Work-Role Competencies

From Benner P: *From novice to expert,* Menlo Park, CA, 1984, Addison Wesley.

The professional scope of practice identifies the nature and intent of the ways nurses intervene for patients, described by Benner (1984) as the domains of practice (Box 19.1). How do the scope of practice, nursing domains, and nursing interventions relate? Here is an example: for a nurse to promote a patient's health status (scope of practice), he or she provides a teaching-coaching function (domain of practice) by delivering 1:1 patient education sessions (direct care).

The challenges and complexities within health care organizations can make it difficult for nurses to fully fulfill the scope and domains of practice (see Chapter 2). Nurses are required to have effective organizational skills and to maintain competencies in advanced nursing care. In addition, nurses must manage conflict and effectively advocate for patients in challenging interprofessional relationships. Thus it is important for implementation to be patient-centered. Nursing is an art and a science. It is not simply a task-based profession. You must learn to intervene for a patient within the context of his or her unique situation. Consider these factors during implementation: Who is the patient? How do a patient's attitudes, values, and cultural background affect how you provide care? What does an illness mean to a patient and his or her family? Which clinical situation requires you to intervene? How does a patient perceive the interventions that you will deliver? In what way do you best support or show caring as you intervene? The answers to these questions enable you to deliver care compassionately and effectively with the best outcomes for your patients.

STANDARD NURSING INTERVENTIONS

Health care settings offer opportunities for nurses to create and individualize patients' care plans. Although it is critical for each patient to have his or her unique set of interventions, many health care systems have mechanisms for developing standard interventions for more common health care problems. Standard interventions allow nurses to intervene more quickly and appropriately. When clinical expertise and scientific evidence are used to form standard interventions, nurses are able to deliver the most clinically effective care to improve patient outcomes (see Chapter 5). The creation of standard interventions is supported in health information documentation systems. Using standard interventions helps capture patient care information that can be shared across disciplines and care settings, making it easier to measure the quality of care delivered and supporting ongoing research and analysis (MBL Technologies, 2017).

As a nurse, you are accountable for individualizing standardized interventions based on your patients' needs and preferences. Nurse- and health care provider–initiated standard interventions include clinical practice guidelines and protocols, care bundles, standing orders, Nursing Interventions Classification (NIC) interventions, and standards of practice. The ANA defines standards of professional nursing practice, while the Quality and Safety Education for Nurses (QSEN) defines skills competencies (QSEN, 2019). These standards are authoritative statements of the duties that all registered nurses (RNs) are expected to perform competently, regardless of role, patient population they serve, or specialty (ANA, 2010) (see Chapter 1).

Clinical Practice Guidelines and Protocols

A clinical practice guideline or protocol is a systematically developed set of statements about appropriate health care for specific health care problems or clinical situations (e.g., pressure injury prevention, DVT prevention, fall prevention). Evidence-based research provides the basis for sound clinical practice guidelines and associated recommendations that often improve quality of care. A nurse individualizes nursing interventions for each patient.

Clinicians within a health care agency formally review the scientific literature and their own standard of practice to develop guidelines and

BOX 19.2 EVIDENCE-BASED PRACTICE

Use of Care Bundles

PICOT Question: Does the use of care bundles compared with standard practice improve hospitalized patients' recovery outcomes?

Evidence Summary

Care bundles are a set of evidence-based interventions performed collectively and reliably to improve the quality of patient care (Lavallée et al., 2017). Common care bundles include those for deep vein thrombosis, ventilator-associated pneumonia, and surgical site infection (SSI) prevention. A review of studies designed to reduce SSI involved use of core interventions such as antibiotic administration, appropriate hair removal, glycemic (blood glucose) control, and temperature management. The SSI rate in the bundle groups was 7.0% compared with 15.1% in a standard care group. The research showed that surgical care bundles help reduce the risk of SSI compared with standard care (Tanner et al., 2015). In a review of studies designed to better manage chronic obstructive pulmonary disease it was found that the use of discharge bundles reduced hospital readmissions, but there was insufficient evidence that care bundles influenced long-term mortality (Ospina et al., 2017). Care bundles are becoming more common in acute care hospitals and show promising benefits. However, clinical staff do not always perform all interventions within a bundle (Juknevicius et al., 2012). General benefits of care bundles include simplification of clinical decisions, reduced omissions of interventions, and reduced errors in medical decision making.

Application to Nursing Practice

The following are recommendations when implementing care bundles (Camporota and Brett, 2011).

- Perform the full set of interventions in a care bundle.
- Use clinical judgment when practicing within guidelines of a care bundle.
- If the interventions in a bundle are scientifically sound, perform the interventions, but if the evidence is conflicting, use a critical common-sense approach.
- Consistent use of care bundles for routine and common practices is probably beneficial and unlikely to cause significant harm to patients.
- The optimal balance between care bundle interventions versus individualized care will vary among institutions, depending on staffing and the availability of new research.

BOX 19.3 Purposes of Nursing Interventions Classification (NIC)

1. Standardize the language nurses use to describe sets of actions in delivering patient care.
2. Expand nursing knowledge about connections among nursing diagnoses, treatments, and outcomes.
3. Develop a nursing language for software of health care information systems.
4. Provide a standard set of interventions for effectiveness research, productivity measurement, and competency evaluation.
5. Link with the classification systems of other health care providers.

From Butcher HK, et al: *Nursing interventions classification (NIC)*, ed 7, St Louis, 2018, Elsevier.

agreement with a physician identifies protocols for the medical conditions that APRNs are permitted to treat, such as controlled hypertension, and the types of treatment that they are permitted to administer, such as antihypertensive medications. These protocols vary by physician and APRN. APRNs are also able to act independently, developing and applying clinical protocols that outline independent nursing interventions. Databases such as Up-to-Date and the Cochrane library provide valuable treatment guidelines supported by rigorous systematic reviews to provide evidence-based treatment guidelines.

Standing Orders

A standing order is a preprinted document containing medical orders for routine therapies, monitoring guidelines, and/or diagnostic procedures for specific patients with identified clinical problems. A standing order directs patient care in a specific clinical setting. Licensed prescribing health care providers in charge of care at the time of implementation approve and sign standing orders. These orders reflect health care provider treatment preferences and are common in critical care settings and other specialized acute care settings where patients' needs change rapidly and require immediate attention. An example of such a standing order is one specifying certain medications such as diltiazem (Cardizem) and amiodarone (Cordarone) for an irregular heart rhythm. After assessing a patient and identifying the irregular rhythm, the critical care nurse gives the specified medication without first notifying the health care provider because his or her standing order covers the nurse's action. After completing a standing order, the nurse notifies the health care provider. Standing orders are also common in community health settings, where nurses face situations that do not permit immediate contact with a health care provider. Standing orders give nurses legal protection to intervene appropriately in the best interests of patients with rapidly changing needs.

REFLECT NOW

What do you see as a limitation of standard orders when compared with clinical practice guidelines?

Nursing Interventions Classification (NIC) Interventions

The NIC system developed by the University of Iowa differentiates nursing practice from that of other health care disciplines (Box 19.3) by offering a language that nurses can use to identify treatments nurses perform, organize this information into an understandable structure, and provide a language to communicate with patients, families, communities, and all health care providers (Butcher et al., 2018). The NIC interventions offer a level of standardization to enhance

protocols to improve the standard of care at their agency. For example, a hospital develops a rapid-assessment medical protocol to improve the identification and early treatment of patients suspected of having a stroke or sepsis. Some guidelines are already developed by professional health care organizations. In the case of nursing clinical guidelines, the Association of Critical Care Nurses, the Oncology Nursing Society, and the University of Iowa Hartford Center developed evidence-based practice (EBP) guidelines for their specialties.

Ongoing review of the scientific literature and best practices within a health care organization may result in the development of care bundles, a type of clinical guideline. A care bundle is a group of interventions related to a disease process or condition. The interventions, when implemented together, result in better patient outcomes than when the interventions are implemented individually (Box 19.2). Care bundles improve quality of care while preventing the most common complications associated with their conditions or diagnoses (Goldstone et al., 2015). You will implement care bundle interventions during your clinical experiences.

Advanced practice registered nurses (APRNs), who provide primary care for patients in a variety of settings, frequently follow diagnostic and treatment protocols for their interventions. A collaborative

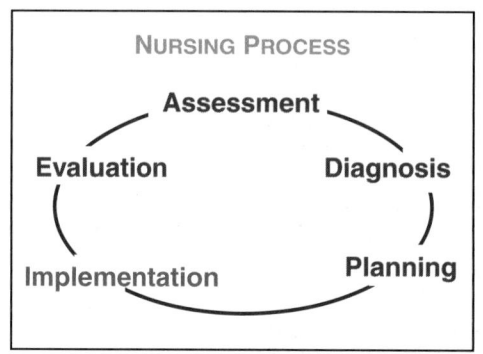

KNOWLEDGE
Expected effects of interventions
Techniques used in performing interventions
Nursing Interventions Classification
Role of other health care disciplines
Health care resources (e.g., equipment, personnel)
Anticipated patient responses to care
Interpersonal skills
Counseling theory
Teaching/learning principles
Delegation and supervision principles

EXPERIENCE
Previous patient care experience
Knowledge of
successful interventions

NURSING PROCESS

Assessment

Evaluation   **Diagnosis**

Implementation   **Planning**

STANDARDS
Standards of practice (e.g., ANA,
subspecialty) and evidence-
based practice guidelines
(e.g., AHRQ, APS)
Agency's policies/procedures
for guidelines of nursing
practice and delegation
Intellectual standards
Patient's expected outcomes

ATTITUDES
Independent thinking
Responsibility
Authority
Creativity
Discipline

FIG. 19.2 Critical thinking and the process of implementing care. *AHRQ*, Agency for Healthcare Research Quality; *ANA*, American Nurses Association; *APS*, American Pain Society.

communication of nursing care across settings and to compare outcomes. Many health care information systems incorporate the NIC system. By using NIC you will learn the common interventions recommended for various nursing diagnoses. Chapter 18 describes the NIC system in more detail.

Standards of Practice

Nurses use the ANA Standards of Professional Nursing Practice (ANA, 2010) as evidence of the standard of care provided to patients (see Chapter 1). The standards are formally reviewed on a regular basis. The newest standards include competencies for establishing professional and caring relationships, using evidence-based interventions and technologies, providing ethical holistic care across the life span to diverse groups, and using community resources and systems. The standards emphasize implementing a timely plan following patient safety goals (ANA, 2010).

Quality and Safety Education for Nurses (QSEN)

The QSEN Institute established standard competencies in knowledge, skills, and attitudes (KSAs) for the preparation of future nurses (QSEN, 2019). The goal of QSEN is to prepare nurses so that they can continuously improve the quality and safety of the health care systems within which they work. Examples of QSEN skills include providing patient-centered care with sensitivity and respect for the diversity of the human experience, initiating effective treatments to relieve pain and suffering, and participating in building consensus or resolving conflict in the context of patient care (QSEN, 2019).

CRITICAL THINKING IN IMPLEMENTATION

Selecting nursing interventions for your patient is part of clinical decision making. Strong clinical reasoning and decision-making skills help you accurately identify appropriate nursing interventions for a patient's specific nursing diagnoses. The critical thinking model discussed in Chapter 15 is a framework for how to make decisions when implementing nursing care. You learn how to implement nursing care by applying appropriate knowledge, experience, attitudes, and standards of care (Fig. 19.2). Delivering nursing interventions is complex. It is based on the knowledge you have about a patient and the social context of the health care setting where you work. Interprofessional relationships between nurses and health care providers contribute to nursing judgments for understanding a patient's problems and intervening effectively. The context in which you deliver care to each patient and the many interventions required result in decision-making approaches for each clinical situation. Critical thinking allows you to consider the complexity of interventions, changing priorities, alternative approaches, and the amount of time available to act. Always prepare well before providing any intervention.

*Tonya identified four relevant nursing diagnoses for Mr. Lawson: **Acute Pain** related to trauma of surgical incision, **Lack of Knowledge** regarding postoperative care related to inexperience with surgery, **Risk for Infection**, and **Anxiety** related to uncertainty over ability to return to work. The diagnoses are interrelated, and* *sometimes a planned intervention (e.g., promoting relaxation exercises) treats or modifies more than one of the patient's health problems (anxiety and acute pain). Tonya applies critical thinking and uses her time with Mr. Lawson wisely by anticipating his priorities, applying the knowledge she has about his problems and the interventions planned, and implementing care strategies skillfully.*

Apply what you have learned during previous clinical experiences in performing specific interventions. Consider which interventions have worked before and which have not worked in previous clinical situations. With experience you become more proficient in anticipating what to expect in a given clinical situation and how to modify your approach. Be aware of professional and agency standards of practice, which offer guidelines for selection of interventions, their frequency and timing, and whether interventions can be delegated. Also be aware of a patient's changing condition and what you would expect after caring for patients with similar conditions. Then adjust the interventions based on ongoing evaluation (see Chapter 20). Maintain organization and time management skills to provide safe and effective patient care (see Chapter 21).

Exercise critical judgment and decision making while delivering each intervention: think before you act. Consider the resources you have and the scheduling of activities in a health care setting, which often influence when and how to complete an intervention. You are responsible for having the necessary knowledge and clinical competency to safely and effectively perform interventions for your patients. Follow these tips for making decisions during implementation:

- Review the set of all possible nursing interventions for a patient's problem (e.g., for Mr. Lawson's pain Tonya considered analgesic administration, positioning and splinting, progressive relaxation, and other nonpharmacological approaches).
- Review all possible consequences associated with each possible nursing action (e.g., Tonya considers that the analgesic will relieve pain; have little or insufficient effect; or cause an adverse reaction, including sedating the patient and increasing the risk of falling).
- Determine the probability of all possible consequences (e.g., if Mr. Lawson's pain continues to decrease with analgesia and positioning and there have been no side effects, it is unlikely that adverse reactions will occur, and the intervention will be successful; however, if the patient continues to remain highly anxious, his pain may not stay relieved, and Tonya needs to consider an alternative).
- Judge the value of the consequence to the patient (e.g., if the administration of an analgesic is effective, Mr. Lawson will probably become less anxious and more responsive to postoperative instruction and counseling about his anxiety).

QSEN Building Competency in Evidence-Based Practice

Explore the scientific literature for current evidence on what Tonya might provide to best manage Mr. Lawson's anxiety. What evidence-based strategies can you identify that reduce anxiety with the outcome of improving attention and learning?

Answers to QSEN Activities can be found on the Evolve website.

As you perform a nursing intervention, apply intellectual standards, which are the guidelines for rational thought and responsible action (see Chapter 15). *For example, before Tonya begins to teach Mr. Lawson, she considers how to make her instructions relevant, clear, logical, and complete to promote patient learning.* A critical thinker applies critical thinking attitudes when intervening. For example, show confidence in performing an intervention. When you are unsure of how to perform a procedure, be responsible. Seek assistance from others. Confidence in performing interventions builds trust with patients. Creativity and self-discipline

are attitudes that guide you in reviewing, modifying, and implementing interventions. As a beginning nursing student, seek out supervision from instructors or experienced nurses or review agency policy and procedures to guide you in the decision-making process for implementation.

IMPLEMENTATION PROCESS

Preparation for implementation ensures more efficient, safe, and effective nursing care. Perform these five preparatory activities: (1) reassess the patient, (2) review and revise the existing nursing care plan, (3) organize resources and care delivery, (4) anticipate and prevent complications, and (5) implement nursing interventions.

Tonya returns to Mr. Lawson's room to begin instruction. His wife is present, and Mr. Lawson reports that his incisional pain is currently a level of 3. Tonya helps the patient sit up in a chair. She sets up the teaching program on the hospital educational TV system and the evidence-based booklets she wants to use to prepare the patient and his wife for infection control, wound care, and activity restrictions in the home. Because Mr. Lawson still has concerns about returning to work, Tonya wants to incorporate discussion about wound care with expected postoperative recovery. Tonya sees the opportunity of using Mr. Lawson's desire to return to work to increase the likelihood of his adherence to postoperative restrictions. If Mrs. Lawson understands how she can help Mr. Lawson in recovery, positive outcomes should be achieved.

Reassessing a Patient

Assessment is a continuous process that occurs each time you interact with a patient. It involves the collection of new data. Reassessment is not the same as evaluating care or determining a patient's response to an intervention (see Chapter 20). Instead, it is the gathering of additional information to ensure that the plan of care is still complete, current, and appropriate. When you collect new data about a patient, you sometimes identify a new nursing diagnosis or determine that additional interventions might be necessary for not only the new diagnosis but also existing diagnoses. Creating a concept map helps you better understand the relationship between different nursing diagnoses and interventions appropriate to a patient's care (Fig. 19.3). During the initial phase of implementation reassess the patient to confirm that you have selected appropriate interventions. The reassessment helps you decide if the proposed nursing actions are still appropriate for a patient's level of wellness. *For example, Tonya begins to talk with Mr. and Mrs. Lawson about wound care and the patient's activity restrictions. Mrs. Lawson shares that Mr. Lawson's employer called to ask how he was doing. Tonya notices that Mr. Lawson begins to show more anxiety; as Tonya explains restrictions on lifting, the patient is not able to teach back what he can and cannot do. Tonya decides to redirect the discussion. She says to Mr. Lawson, "Let's talk about going back to work. Tell me more about when they expect you to return and what your work actually involves." Tonya realizes that to be effective with instruction she needs an attentive learner. Gaining more detail about the patient's work will help him express his concerns while at the same time allow Tonya to explain how activity restrictions fit into daily routines.*

Reviewing and Revising the Existing Nursing Care Plan

After you reassess a patient and determine there is a need to add to or modify the plan of care, you revise the care plan. An out-of-date, incomplete, or incorrect care plan compromises the quality of nursing care. When you gather evaluation data (see Chapter 20) to determine if previously selected interventions were successful and whether outcomes were met, similar types of revisions can be made. Review and

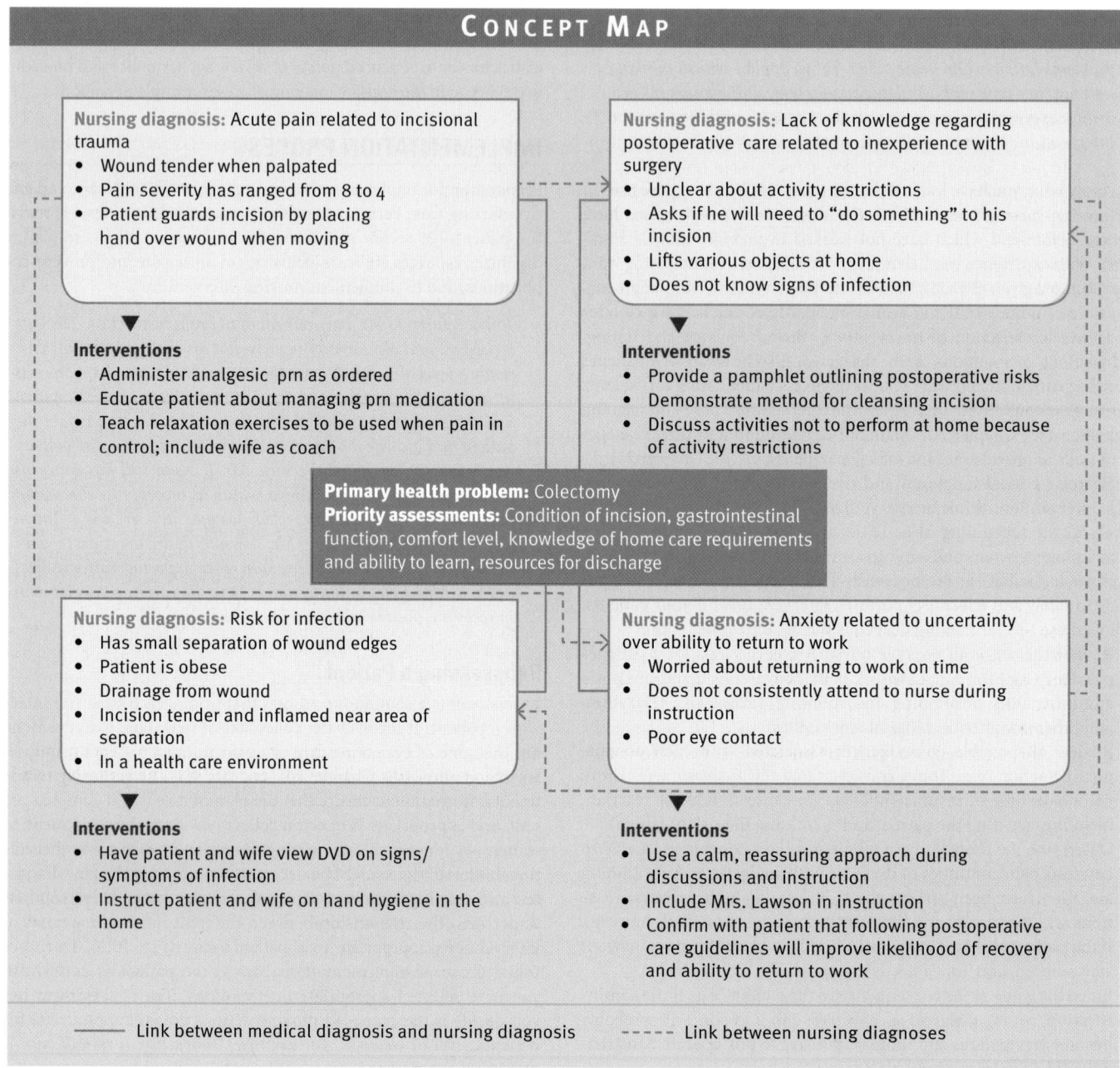

CONCEPT MAP

Nursing diagnosis: Acute pain related to incisional trauma
- Wound tender when palpated
- Pain severity has ranged from 8 to 4
- Patient guards incision by placing hand over wound when moving

Interventions
- Administer analgesic prn as ordered
- Educate patient about managing prn medication
- Teach relaxation exercises to be used when pain in control; include wife as coach

Nursing diagnosis: Lack of knowledge regarding postoperative care related to inexperience with surgery
- Unclear about activity restrictions
- Asks if he will need to "do something" to his incision
- Lifts various objects at home
- Does not know signs of infection

Interventions
- Provide a pamphlet outlining postoperative risks
- Demonstrate method for cleansing incision
- Discuss activities not to perform at home because of activity restrictions

Primary health problem: Colectomy
Priority assessments: Condition of incision, gastrointestinal function, comfort level, knowledge of home care requirements and ability to learn, resources for discharge

Nursing diagnosis: Risk for infection
- Has small separation of wound edges
- Patient is obese
- Drainage from wound
- Incision tender and inflamed near area of separation
- In a health care environment

Interventions
- Have patient and wife view DVD on signs/symptoms of infection
- Instruct patient and wife on hand hygiene in the home

Nursing diagnosis: Anxiety related to uncertainty over ability to return to work
- Worried about returning to work on time
- Does not consistently attend to nurse during instruction
- Poor eye contact

Interventions
- Use a calm, reassuring approach during discussions and instruction
- Include Mrs. Lawson in instruction
- Confirm with patient that following postoperative care guidelines will improve likelihood of recovery and ability to return to work

——— Link between medical diagnosis and nursing diagnosis   - - - - - Link between nursing diagnoses

FIG. 19.3 Concept map for Mr. Lawson: Implementation.

revision of a plan enable you to provide more appropriate and timely nursing interventions to best meet a patient's needs. Modification of an existing written care plan includes four steps:

1. Revise data in the assessment column to reflect the patient's current status. Date any new data to inform other members of the health care team of the time that the change occurred.
2. Revise the nursing diagnoses, goals and outcomes. Add any new nursing diagnoses that have been identified and select appropriate goals and outcomes. For existing nursing diagnoses, revise related factors and the patient's goals, outcomes, and priorities as necessary. Date any revisions.
3. Select or revise specific interventions that correspond to the new nursing diagnoses or that are necessary for existing diagnoses. Be sure that revisions reflect the patient's present status.
4. Choose the methods of evaluation that will be used to determine whether the patient achieves his or her outcomes.

As Tonya continues to prepare Mr. Lawson for discharge, she evaluates his pain status. His pain has been controlled well on around-the-clock analgesics and use of relaxation. Tonya reassesses whether Mr. Lawson has ever taken analgesics at home and what works best. In consultation with the physician and in preparation for discharge, the physician decides to discontinue the around-the-clock analgesic and orders an analgesic prn instead. Tonya plans to explain to Mr. and Mrs. Lawson how best to take a prn medication (see Chapter 25). Tonya also decides to include Mrs. Lawson as a coach to facilitate relaxation exercises for Mr. Lawson.

Preparing for Implementation

The organization of time and resources is an important part of implementation of nursing care. Always be sure that a patient is physically and psychologically ready for any interventions or procedures.

Time Management. Providing patient-centered care is the focus of your nursing practice. You will practice within work environments that are part of the sociocultural context of a health care organization (see Chapter 21). These are busy environments, and you will assume dual roles: a patient care provider and an organizational employee. In this dual role you need to be aware of the organization's goals of efficiency and cost control. However, you need to competently provide timely, thoughtful, safe, and efficient care. The ability to manage care in a timely way conveys caring and concern to your patients. Poor patient care results when you are hurried, experience interruptions, or are disorganized. Time devoted to nursing care has three components: physical (the physical amount of time consumed in the completion of nursing activities), psychological (what nursing care patients experience and how they experience it), and sociological (the sequential ordering of events within the daily routines of a practice setting) (Jones, 2010). All components of time occur within the context of an organization and the resources available. As a new nurse, understand that the decisions you make about how your time is allocated, prioritized, and sequenced are always interpreted by the patients you serve (Jones, 2010). Be aware of factors affecting time with patients and apply time-management principles (see Chapter 21).

Equipment. Most nursing procedures require some equipment or supplies. Before performing an intervention, decide which supplies you need and determine their availability. Is the equipment in working order to ensure safe use, and do you know how to use it? Place supplies in a convenient location to provide easy access during a procedure. Keep extra supplies available in case of errors or mishaps, but do not open them unless you need them. This controls health care costs, allowing you to be a fiscally responsible member of the health care team. After a procedure return any unopened supplies to storage areas.

REFLECT NOW

Think about a procedure you recently performed in the lab or with an assigned patient. Did you manage your time well in preparing for the skill? What might you have done differently?

Personnel. Nursing care practice models determine how nursing personnel are organized to deliver patient care, including staff RNs, auxiliary staff such as assistive personnel (APs), and RNs in special roles (e.g., nurse specialists). A practice model reflects nursing values that exemplify the culture of a health care organization (Chamberlain et al., 2013). Common values shared among models include nursing autonomy; empowerment; and cost-effective, quality care. A practice model designates a nurse's role and accountability to patients and other members of the nursing team. Traditional models include team and primary nursing. More recently patient- and family-centered care models and case management have been adopted by nursing departments. Chapter 21 offers details on the various models of care.

Regardless of the practice model, as a nurse you are responsible for deciding whether to perform an intervention, delegate it to an unlicensed member of the nursing team, or have an RN colleague assist you. Your ongoing assessment of each patient, the priorities of care (see Chapter 18), the activities occurring in the workplace, and not an intervention alone direct your decision about delegation. You have a legal duty to follow delegation guidelines and only delegate interventions within the delegate's training and ability according to the state Nurse Practice Act.

BOX 19.4   Physical Environmental Factors That Promote Patient Healing

- Standardization of patient rooms and equipment for making routine tasks simpler, thus decreasing errors.
- Improving light illumination in areas where medications are dispensed.
- Features of a patient room and bath that reduce falls: no slippery floors, appropriate door openings, correct placement of rails and accessories, correct toilet and furniture height, single-bed rooms, easy-to-clean surfaces, automated sinks, and smooth edges in rooms (for easier cleaning).
- Self-supporting systems, such as control over the position of the bed, control over the temperature, control over the lights (including dimmers), control over the sound (music and television), and control over the natural light.
- Privacy and single-patient rooms

Adapted from Huisman ERCM, et al: Healing environment: a review of the impact of physical environmental factors on users, *Building and Environment* 58:70, 2012.

Patient care staff work together as patients' needs demand it. If a patient makes a request such as use of a bedpan or assistance in feeding, help the patient if you have time rather than trying to find an AP who is in a different room. Nursing staff respect colleagues who show initiative, collaborate, and communicate with one another on an ongoing reciprocal basis as patients' needs change. When interventions are complex or physically difficult, you will need assistance from colleagues. For example, a nurse will be more effective in changing a dressing for a large gaping wound when an AP can assist with patient positioning and handing off supplies.

Environment. A patient's care environment, especially in hospitals, rehabilitation units, and skilled care facilities, needs to be safe and conducive to implementing therapies. Patient safety is your first concern. You can make the environment safer by removing clutter and unnecessary furniture or equipment, creating clear paths for patients to ambulate, and making sure patients' personal items are easily accessible when they lie in bed. If a patient has sensory deficits, physical disabilities, or an alteration in level of consciousness, it is especially important to arrange the environment to prevent injury. For example, provide a patient's assistive devices (e.g., walker or eyeglasses), rearrange furniture and equipment when ambulating a patient, or make sure that the water temperature is not too warm before a bath. Patients benefit most from nursing interventions when surroundings are compatible with care activities. When you need to expose a patient's body parts, do so privately by closing room doors or curtains because the patient will then be more relaxed. Ask visitors to leave as you complete care. Reduce distractions during teaching to enhance a patient's learning opportunities.

The environment influences the ability of a patient to heal and recover. Hospitals and other health care settings are using evidence-based design to create healing environments (Huisman et al., 2012). This concept is being applied with the building and renovation of hospitals and other care settings. How a nursing unit is designed impacts both patients and care providers. For example, a well-designed hospital unit can contribute to patient outcomes through no errors, safety and security, control, privacy, and comfort (Huisman et al., 2012) (Box 19.4).

Patient. Make sure that your patients are physically and psychologically comfortable before you implement care. Physical symptoms such as nausea, dizziness, fatigue, or pain often interfere with a patient's full concentration and ability to cooperate. Offer comfort measures before initiating interventions to help patients participate more fully. If you need a patient to be alert, administer a dose of pain medication strong enough to relieve discomfort but not to impair mental faculties (e.g., ability to follow instruction and communication). If a patient is fatigued, delay ambulation or transfer to a chair until after he or she has had a chance to rest. Also consider a patient's level of endurance, and plan only the amount of activity that he or she is able to tolerate comfortably.

Awareness of a patient's psychosocial needs helps you create a favorable emotional climate. *Do not rush your care.* Some patients feel reassured by having a significant other present to lend encouragement and moral support. Other strategies include planning sufficient time or multiple opportunities for a patient to work through and ventilate feelings and anxieties. Adequate preparation allows a patient to obtain maximal benefit from each intervention.

Anticipating and Preventing Complications

Risks to patients come from both illness and treatment. Observe for and recognize these risks, adapt your choice of interventions to each situation, assess the relative benefit of the intervention versus the risk, and take risk-prevention measures. Many conditions place patients at risk for complications. For example, a patient with preexisting left-sided paralysis following a stroke is at risk for developing a pressure injury following orthopedic surgery that requires traction and bed rest. A patient with obesity and diabetes mellitus who has major abdominal surgery is at risk for poor wound healing. Nurses are often the first ones to detect and document changes in patients' conditions. Expert nurses learn to anticipate changes in patient conditions even before confirming that diagnostic signs of complications develop.

Your knowledge of pathophysiology and experience with previous patients help you identify complications that can occur. A thorough assessment reveals the level of a patient's current risk. The evidence or scientific rationale for how interventions (e.g., pressure-relief devices, repositioning, or wound care) prevent or minimize complications help you select the most appropriate preventive measures. For example, if a patient who is obese has uncontrolled postoperative pain, the risk for pressure injury development increases because the patient is unwilling or unable to change position frequently. The nurse anticipates when a patient's pain will increase, administers ordered analgesics, and then positions the patient to remove pressure on the skin and underlying tissues. If a patient continues to have difficulty turning or repositioning, the nurse selects a pressure-relief device to place on the patient's bed.

Some nursing procedures pose risks. Be aware of potential complications and take precautions. For example, the patient with a urinary catheter is at risk for infection. In this case implementing catheter-associated urinary tract infection (CAUTI) care guidelines for UTI prevention reduces infection risk (Chapter 46).

Identifying Areas of Assistance.

Certain patient care situations require you to obtain assistance by seeking additional personnel, knowledge, and/or nursing skills. Before beginning care, review the plan to determine the need for assistance and the type required. Sometimes you need assistance in performing a procedure, providing comfort measures, or preparing a patient for a diagnostic test. Do not take shortcuts if assistance is not immediately available to avoid injury to you and the patient. For example, when you care for a patient who is overweight and immobilized, you require additional personnel and transfer equipment to turn and position the patient safely. Be sure to determine in advance the number of additional personnel needed. Discuss your need for assistance with other nurses or the APs.

You will require additional knowledge and skills in situations in which you are less familiar or experienced. For example, seek additional knowledge when you give a new medication or perform a new procedure. Because of the continual growth in health care technology, you may lack the motor skills to manipulate new equipment for a procedure. When you are faced with administering an unfamiliar therapy or operating a new piece of equipment, follow these steps.

1. Seek the information you need to be informed about a procedure. Check the scientific literature for evidence-based information, review resource manuals (e.g. hospital formulary or procedure manuals), or consult with experts (e.g., pharmacists, clinical nurse specialists).
2. Collect all equipment necessary for the procedure in order to be organized.
3. Consider the consequences of performing the procedure on each specific patient.
4. Have another nurse (e.g., staff nurse, faculty member, clinical nurse specialist) who has completed the procedure correctly and safely provide assistance and guidance. Requesting assistance occurs frequently in all types of nursing practice. It is a learning process that continues throughout educational experiences and into professional development. One tip is to verbalize with an instructor or staff nurse the steps you will take before performing the procedure to improve your confidence and ensure accuracy.

Implementation Skills

Nursing practice requires cognitive, interpersonal, and psychomotor skills to implement direct and indirect nursing interventions. You are responsible for knowing when one type of implementation skill is preferred over another and for having the necessary knowledge and skill to perform each. For example, interpersonal skills of silence and listening are effective as indirect nurse-initiated interventions within the domains of helping and coaching to better facilitate patient adherence (see Fig. 19.1).

Cognitive Skills. Cognitive skills include the critical thinking and decision-making skills such as problem solving and clinical decision making described in Chapter 15. Always use good judgment and sound clinical decision making when performing any intervention. This ensures that no nursing action is automatic but instead is thoughtful and patient-centered. Grasp each clinical situation at hand, interpret the information you observe, and anticipate a patient's response so that you individualize patient care appropriately. A cognitive skill involves knowing the rationale for therapeutic interventions and understanding normal and abnormal physiological and psychological responses. Also know the evidence in nursing science to ensure that you deliver current and relevant nursing interventions.

> *Tonya knows the pathophysiology of colon cancer, the anatomy of the abdomen and surrounding structures, and the normal mechanisms for pain. She considers each of these as she observes Mr. Lawson, noting how the patient's movement and position either aggravate or lessen his incisional pain. Tonya focused initially on relieving Mr. Lawson's acute pain with an analgesic, but now that pain has become well managed, she considers additional nonpharmacological approaches to keep him comfortable and help lessen any anxiety.*

Interpersonal Skills. Interpersonal skills are essential for effective nursing intervention. Apply interpersonal communication skills by developing a trusting relationship, expressing caring, and communicating clearly with patients and their families (see Chapter 24). Good interpersonal communication keeps patients informed and engaged in decision making, provides individualized instruction, and supports patients who have challenging emotional needs.

Proper use of interpersonal skills enables you to be perceptive of your patients' verbal and nonverbal communication, understand their needs and desires, and improve your ability to correctly select relevant interventions. As a member of the health care team, communicate patient problems and needs clearly, intelligently, and in a timely way.

Psychomotor Skills. Psychomotor skills require the integration of cognitive and motor activities. For example, when giving an injection, you need to understand anatomy and pharmacology (cognitive) and use good coordination and precision to administer the injection correctly (motor). With time and practice you learn to perform skills correctly, smoothly, and confidently. This is critical in establishing patient trust. You are responsible for acquiring necessary psychomotor skills through your experience in the nursing laboratory, the use of interactive instructional technology, or actual hands-on care of patients. When performing a new skill, assess your level of competency, and obtain the necessary resources to ensure that your patients receive safe treatment.

DIRECT CARE

Nurses provide a wide variety of direct care measures, treatments, or procedures performed through interaction with a patient(s) involving the laying-on of hands. How a nurse applies implementation skills affects the success of any direct care activity. Remain sensitive to a patient's clinical condition, previous experiences, expectations, and cultural views as you deliver interventions. All direct care measures require competent safe practice. Show a caring approach each time you provide direct care.

Activities of Daily Living

Activities of daily living (ADLs) are direct care measures usually performed during a normal day; they include ambulation, toileting, eating, dressing, bathing, personal device care, functional mobility (getting into/out of a bed or bathtub), and grooming (Lyon, 2018). A patient's need for assistance with ADLs is temporary, permanent, or rehabilitative. For example, a patient with impaired physical mobility because of bilateral arm casts temporarily needs assistance with eating and bathing. A patient with dementia may initially require coaching to complete tasks, but later require direct assistance (Box 19.5). A patient with an irreversible cervical spinal cord injury is paralyzed and has a permanent need for full assistance. When patients have difficulty performing ADLs or need to learn new ways to perform self-care activities, occupational and physical therapists play key roles in rehabilitation to restore ADL function.

When a patient is experiencing fatigue, a limitation in mobility, confusion, and/or pain, assistance with ADLs is probably needed. For example, a patient who experiences shortness of breath avoids eating because of associated fatigue. Help the patient by setting up meals, offering to cut up food, and planning for smaller, more frequent meals to maintain his or her nutrition. Assistance with ADLs ranges from partial assistance to complete care. Remember to always respect a patient's wishes and determine his or her preferences. Patients from some cultures prefer to receive assistance with ADLs from family members. If a patient is stable and alert, it is appropriate to allow family to help with care. Most patients want to remain independent in meeting their basic needs. Allow a patient to participate to the level that he or she is able. Involving patients in planning the timing and types of interventions boosts their self-esteem and willingness to become more independent.

BOX 19.5 Assisting Patients With Dementia in Performing Activities of Daily Living

- Patients with early dementia may need reminding to have a bath or complete other grooming.
- Be present in case patients have problems. For example, be sure the person is soaping and rinsing adequately or eating a complete meal; if not, you may prompt them to do so.
- As dementia progresses, a patient may need to be reminded of specific tasks in a bath (such as soap yourself, rinse yourself) in the right sequence. The objects needed for the bath may need to be prepared for them (basin with water at the right temperature, shaving mug is accessible, towel and clean gown/clothes are on the towel bar).
- Patients may need help for some actions, such as applying soap on the back, washing the toes, or shampooing the hair. Help may be given by guiding the person's wrist or holding the elbow to guide the arm. They often are able to do the task if you help them start the task.
- After dementia continues to progress, patients will need help with trickier tasks, such as tying shoelaces or putting in hearing aids.
- After some days, you may find the person looking at the bath basin in a puzzled way. The amount of assistance needed increases.
- The person may also lose interest in doing anything.

Adapted from *Dementia care notes: helping with activities of daily living,* 2018, https://dementiacarenotes.in/caregivers/toolkit/adl/. Accessed July 19, 2018.

Instrumental Activities of Daily Living

Illness or disability sometimes alters a patient's ability to be independent in society. Instrumental activities of daily living (IADLs) refer to activities that support daily life and are oriented toward interacting with the environment, e.g., shopping, caring for pets, home maintenance, preparing meals, housecleaning, writing checks, and taking medications (Lyon, 2018). IADLs are typically more complex than ADLs and generally are managed by occupational therapists. However, nurses within home care and community health settings frequently help patients adapt ways to perform IADLs (such as providing appropriate assistive devices or creating medication organization systems). Often family and friends are excellent resources for helping patients. In acute care it is important to anticipate how patients' illnesses will affect their ability to perform IADLs so that you can make appropriate referrals to be sure they have the resources they need at home.

Physical Care Techniques

Physical care techniques involve the safe and competent administration of nursing procedures (e.g., turning and positioning, inserting a feeding tube, administering medications, inserting an intravenous catheter, and providing comfort measures). The specific knowledge and skills needed to perform these procedures are in subsequent clinical chapters of this text. All physical care techniques require you to protect yourself and patients from injury, use safe patient-handling techniques during preparation, use proper infection control practices, stay organized, and follow applicable practice guidelines.

You are responsible to be knowledgeable about the procedure itself, the standard frequency, the associated risks, and the necessary assessments/evaluations before, during, and after performing a skill. Always remain thoughtful of a patient's condition and how the patient has responded to the procedure in the past. Know how the procedure is going to affect the patient and which expected outcomes you and the patient desire. For example, if you are going to ambulate a patient, discuss how far you wish the patient to walk and whether there will be opportunity to sit or stop to rest. Ask the patient to tell you if he or she becomes short of breath.

In a hospital you perform many procedures each day, often for the first time. Before performing a new procedure, assess the situation and your personal competencies to determine whether you need assistance, new knowledge, or new skills. Performing any procedure correctly requires critical thinking and thoughtful decision making.

Lifesaving Measures

A lifesaving measure is a physical care technique that you use when a patient's physiological or psychological state is threatened (see Chapter 41). The purpose of lifesaving measures is to restore physiological or psychological homeostasis. Such measures include administering emergency medications, instituting cardiopulmonary resuscitation, intervening to protect a patient who is confused or violent, and obtaining immediate counseling from a crisis center for a patient who is severely anxious. If a nurse faces a situation requiring emergency measures, the proper nursing actions are to stay with the patient, maintain support, and have another staff member obtain an experienced professional.

Counseling

Counseling is a direct care method that helps patients use problem-solving processes to recognize and manage stress and facilitate interpersonal relationships. As a nurse you counsel patients to accept actual or impending changes resulting from stress (see Chapter 37). Examples include patients who are facing terminal or chronic illness. Counseling involves emotional, intellectual, spiritual, and psychological support. A patient and family who need nurse counseling have normal adjustment difficulties and are upset or frustrated, but they are not necessarily psychologically disabled. An example is the stress that a young woman faces when caring for her aging mother. Family caregivers need assistance in adjusting to the physical and emotional demands of caregiving. Sometimes they need respite (i.e., a break from providing care). The recipient of care also needs assistance in adjusting to his or her disability. Patients with psychiatric diagnoses require therapy from nurses specializing in psychiatric nursing or social workers, psychiatrists, or psychologists.

Many counseling techniques foster cognitive, behavioral, developmental, experiential, and emotional growth in patients. Counseling encourages individuals to examine available alternatives and decide which choices are useful and appropriate. When patients are able to examine alternatives, they develop a sense of control and are able to better manage stress.

Teaching

Patient education is key to patient-centered care. A teaching plan is essential for every patient, especially when patients need to manage health problems they are facing for the first time. Counseling and teaching closely align. Both involve using good interpersonal skills to create a change in a patient's knowledge and behavior. Counseling results in changes in the development of new attitudes, behaviors, and feelings, whereas teaching focuses on intellectual growth or the acquisition of psychomotor skills.

When you educate patients, respect their expertise with their own health and symptoms, their daily routines, the diversity of their human experiences, their values and preferences as to how they learn, and the importance of shared decision making. As an educator you present health care principles, procedures, and techniques to inform patients about their health status in such a way that patients can adapt what they learn to their daily routines at

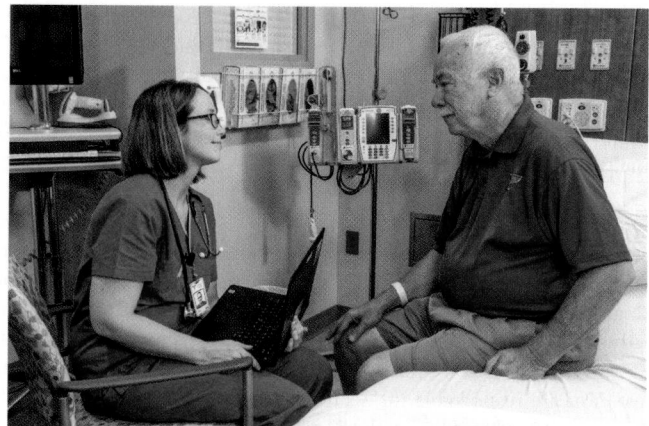

FIG. 19.4 Nurse providing discharge instructions.

home to achieve self-care. Emphasis has been placed on patient education in acute care since 2006, when the Hospital Consumer Assessment of Healthcare Providers and Systems (HCAHPS) standardized survey began to be used across the country by hospitals to measure patients' perspectives on hospital care (HCAHPS, 2018). The survey results currently are a standard for measuring and comparing quality of hospitals. Hospitals stress the importance of nurses addressing the topics covered by the survey, including patient education for discharge preparation.

The HCAHPS initiative stresses the importance of patient education. But remember, teaching is an ongoing process of keeping patients informed. Patients want to know why you do what you do. When performing a procedure, engage your patient and explain the procedure, why it is being done, the expected outcomes, and any problems to look for afterward. Encourage patients to ask questions. Here is an example of incorporating teaching in your daily work. When starting an intravenous (IV) infusion, explain what the IV fluid bag contains, how long the bag should last, sensations the patient will feel if the IV site becomes inflamed, the fact that a small flexible catheter is in the arm, and any potential side effects of medications in the bag.

Teaching takes place in all health care settings (Fig. 19.4). As a nurse you are accountable for the quality of education you deliver. Chapter 25 provides a thorough overview of patient education principles and practices. Follow these basic patient education tips (Nurse Journal, 2018):

- Delegate more responsibilities to support staff and be more focused on patient education.
- Begin educating patients with every encounter from admission.
- Based on what a patient already knows, correct any misinformation.
- Provide information in layman's terms. Use visual activities as often as possible. People remember what they see far more than what they hear or read.
- Question their understanding of the care, and plan for the next lesson. It is all part of the nursing process.
- Use return demonstration when administering care. Involve the patient from the very first treatment.
- Ask patients to tell you how they would explain (step by step) their disease or treatment to their spouse, partner, or friend.
- Repeat as needed and build upon the teaching with every opportunity throughout a hospitalization or stay.

- Provide patients with information about signs and symptoms to report to their physicians and ensure that they know to do this promptly, without waiting for another crisis to act.

Know your patient; be aware of the cultural and social factors that influence a patient's willingness and ability to learn. It is also important to know your patient's health literacy level (see Chapter 25). Do not assume that patients understand their illness or disease. If they seem uneasy or refuse a treatment, simply ask what concerns them. This gives you the chance to provide further teaching and correct knowledge deficiencies.

Controlling for Adverse Reactions

An adverse reaction is a harmful or unintended effect of a medication, diagnostic test, or therapeutic intervention. Adverse reactions can result from any nursing intervention; thus learn to anticipate and know which adverse reactions to expect. Nursing actions that control for adverse reactions reduce or counteract a reaction. For example, when applying a moist heat compress, you know that burning the patient's skin is a possible adverse reaction unless you protect the skin. First assess the condition of the area where you plan to place the compress. Following application of the compress, inspect the area every 5 minutes for any adverse reaction such as excessive reddening of the skin from the heat or skin maceration from the moisture (see Chapter 48). Taking the right precautions can prevent adverse reactions.

When completing a health care provider–directed intervention such as medication administration, always know the potential side effects of the drug. After you administer a medication, evaluate the patient for adverse effects. Also be aware of drugs that counteract the side effects. For example, a patient has an unknown hypersensitivity to penicillin and develops hives after three doses. You record the reaction, stop further administration of the drug, and consult with the physician. You then administer an ordered dose of diphenhydramine, an antihistamine and antipruritic medication, to reduce the allergic response and relieve the itching.

When caring for patients who undergo diagnostic tests, you need to understand the test and any potential adverse effects. Although adverse effects are not common, they do occur. It is important that you recognize the signs and symptoms of an adverse reaction and intervene in a timely manner.

Preventive Interventions

Preventive nursing interventions promote health and prevent illness to avoid the need for acute or rehabilitative health care (see Chapter 2). Changes in the health care system are leading to greater emphasis on health promotion and illness prevention. Primary prevention aimed at health promotion includes health education programs, immunizations, and physical and nutritional fitness activities. Secondary prevention focuses on people who are experiencing health problems or illnesses and who are at risk for developing complications or worsening conditions. It includes screening techniques and treating early stages of disease. Tertiary prevention involves minimizing the effects of long-term illness or disability, including rehabilitation measures.

INDIRECT CARE

Indirect care measures are nursing treatments or procedures performed away from a patient(s) but on behalf of a patient(s) (Butcher et al., 2018). Examples include interventions that manage the patient care environment and interprofessional collaborative actions that support the effectiveness of direct care interventions (Butcher et al., 2018) (Box 19.6). Nurses spend much time in indirect unit management activities. Communicating information about patients (e.g., hand-off report, hourly rounding, and consultation) is critical, ensuring that direct care

---

BOX 19.6 Examples of Indirect Care Activities

- Documentation (electronic or written)
- Delegation of care activities to assistive personnel
- Medical order transcription
- Infection control (e.g., proper handling and storage of supplies, use of protective isolation)
- Environmental safety management (e.g., making patient rooms safe)
- Telephone consultations with health care providers
- Hand-off reports to other health care team members
- Collecting, labeling, and transporting specimens
- Transporting patients to procedural areas and other nursing units

From Butcher HK, et al: *Nursing interventions classification (NIC)*, ed 7, St Louis, 2018, Elsevier.

---

activities are planned, coordinated, and performed with the proper resources. Delegation of care to APs is another indirect care activity (see Chapter 21). When performed correctly, delegation ensures that the right care provider performs the right tasks so that the nurse and APs work together most efficiently for a patient's benefit.

Communicating Nursing Interventions

Any intervention that you provide for a patient is communicated in an electronic, written, or oral format (see Chapter 26). Electronic health records (EHRs) or written charts have sections for individualized interventions that are part of the nursing care plan (see Chapter 18) and a patient's permanent medical record. The record entry usually includes a brief description of pertinent assessment findings, the specific intervention(s), and the patient's response. An EHR or written record validates that you performed a procedure and provides valuable information to subsequent caregivers about the approaches needed to provide successful care. Some institutions have interprofessional care plans (i.e., plans representing the contributions of all disciplines caring for a patient). You enter nursing interventions into the plan, documenting the treatment and patient's response.

Effective communication and good teamwork reduce medical errors and prevent adverse patient outcomes (ECRI Institute, 2019). Miscommunication is often the root cause for most reported adverse or sentinel events that occur in health care organizations. Communication with other health care professionals needs to be timely, accurate, and relevant to a patient's clinical situation. Ineffective or incomplete communication often results in caregivers being uninformed, interventions duplicated needlessly, procedures delayed, or tasks left undone. Chapter 26 explains the approach for effective hand-off communication. Always be clear, concise, and to the point when you communicate nursing interventions.

Delegating, Supervising, and Evaluating the Work of Other Staff Members

A nurse who develops a patient's care plan frequently does not personally perform all of the nursing interventions. Some activities you coordinate and delegate to other members of the health care team, including other RNs, LPNs, or assistive personnel. Remember that RNs delegate care tasks but not the nursing process (ANA and National Council of State Boards of Nursing [NCBSN], 2012). You can assign noninvasive and repetitive interventions to certified nurse assistants and other APs. Such activities include skin care, transfer and mobility skills, hygiene, and vital signs for patients who are stable. Evidence shows that the better the communication and collaborative relationship between a nurse and the delegatee, the better the outcome of the delegation process (National Council State Boards of Nursing, 2016). Delegation requires clinical judgment and accountability for patient care. The frequency and way nursing care activities are delegated often depends on a nursing unit delivery of care model.

Delegation allows you to use your time more wisely and to have other care providers assist. When you delegate tasks to an AP, you are responsible for ensuring that you assign each task appropriately and that the AP completes each task according to the standard of care. This requires ongoing supervision to be sure the AP has performed the task on time without difficulty. You must be sure that any delegated action was completed correctly, documented, and evaluated. You only delegate direct care interventions to personnel who are competent. Chapter 21 describes the principles to follow in delegation.

ACHIEVING PATIENT GOALS

You implement interventions to achieve patient goals and expected outcomes (see Chapter 18). In most clinical situations multiple interventions are needed to achieve select outcomes. In addition, patients' conditions often change minute by minute. Therefore it is important to apply principles of care coordination such as good time management, organizational skills, and appropriate use of resources to ensure that you deliver interventions effectively and meet desired outcomes (see Chapter 21). Priority setting is critical in successful implementation. Priorities help you to anticipate and sequence nursing interventions when a patient has multiple nursing diagnoses and collaborative problems.

Another way to help patients achieve their goals is to help them adhere to their treatment plan. Patient adherence means that patients and families invest time in carrying out required health care treatments. Przemyslaw and colleagues (2013) explain that adherence is complicated because, in the case of medication adherence, it includes willingness of a patient to implement a regimen (daily drug-taking) and persistence (continuity of treatment) in taking the medication. Whether a patient chooses to adhere to a treatment relates in part to the values and perceptions placed on the treatment. When a treatment is seen as beneficial and making a difference in a patient's quality of life, adherence is more likely. Similarly, when there is a risk of negative consequences if a treatment is not followed, adherence is more likely. The majority of research on patient adherence has focused on medication management and chronic disease management. Studies on medication management suggest that presence of family and social support, as well as the use of simple treatment regimens, favorably impacts adherence. In contrast, economic factors such as unemployment, poverty, and a lack of or inadequate medical/prescription coverage, as well as a high out-of-pocket cost of drugs, contribute to nonadherence (Przemyslaw et al., 2013). Interventions that improve adherence have been shown to be technical (e.g., simplification of drug regimen and packaging, pill organizers), behavioral (e.g., memory aids and reminders), educational (e.g., motivational techniques), and multicomponent (Przemyslaw et al., 2013; van Dulmen et al., 2007).

To ensure that patients have a smooth transition across different health care settings (e.g., hospital to home and clinic, hospital to rehabilitation agency, or hospital to assisted living), it is important to introduce interventions that patients are willing and able to follow. Adequate and timely discharge planning with collaborative patient and family education are the first steps in promoting a smooth transition from one health care setting to another or to the home. Individualize your care and take into consideration the various factors that influence a patient's health beliefs (see Chapter 6). *For example, for Tonya to effectively help Mr. Lawson follow the activity limitations required after surgery, she needs to know whether Mr. Lawson understands the risks to wound healing if limitations are not followed. His anxiety about being able to return to work on time will probably improve his motivation to adhere.* You are responsible for delivering interventions in a way that reflects your understanding of a patient's health beliefs, culture, lifestyle pattern, and

patterns of wellness. In addition, reinforcing successes with the treatment plan encourages a patient to follow his or her care plan.

KEY POINTS

- A nursing intervention is any treatment based on clinical judgment and knowledge that a nurse is licensed to perform within the professional scope of practice.
- Standard interventions, based on scientific evidence and clinical expertise, are developed for patients with common health problems to assist nurses to intervene more efficiently and appropriately.
- Use of care bundles shows promising benefits but requires implementation of the full set of interventions and use of clinical judgment when practicing within guidelines of a care bundle.
- Nurses use critical thinking in implementation when considering the complexity of interventions, changing priorities, alternative approaches, and the amount of time available to act.
- As a nurse you are responsible for deciding whether to perform an intervention, delegate it to an unlicensed member of the nursing team, or have an RN colleague assist you.
- Time management allows you to competently provide timely, thoughtful, safe, and efficient care.
- The decisions a nurse makes about how time is allocated, prioritized, and sequenced are always interpreted by the patients you serve within the sociocultural context of a health care institution.
- Expert nurses learn to anticipate changes in patients' conditions even before confirming that diagnostic signs of complications develop.
- Knowledge of pathophysiology and experience with previous patients helps nurses identify the risk of complications.
- Nursing practice requires cognitive, interpersonal, and psychomotor skills to implement direct and indirect nursing interventions.
- Direct care interventions include providing ADLs, assisting with IADLs, performing physical care, lifesaving measures, counseling, teaching, preventive interventions, and controlling for adverse reactions.
- Communication of information about patients (e.g., hand-off report, hourly rounding, and consultation) is critical, ensuring that direct care activities are planned, coordinated, and performed with the proper resources.

REFLECTIVE LEARNING

After your next clinical experience review the interventions you provided for your patient(s).
- Which of the interventions were direct nurse-initiated versus indirect nurse-initiated?
- In what way did you communicate the interventions you provided your patient to members of the health care team?
- What nursing skills did you apply in your implementation of patient care?

REVIEW QUESTIONS

1. A nurse is assigned to five patients, including one who was recently admitted and one returning from a diagnostic procedure. It is currently mealtime. The other three patients are stable, but one has just requested a pain medication. The nurse is working with an assistive personnel. Which of the following are appropriate delegation actions on the part of the nurse? (Select all that apply.)
   1. The nurse directs the assistive personnel to obtain a set of vital signs on the patient returning from the diagnostic procedure.

2. The nurse directs the patient care technician to go to the patient in pain and to reposition and offer comfort measures until the nurse can bring an ordered analgesic to the patient.
3. The nurse directs the patient care technician to set up meal trays for patients.
4. The nurse directs the patient care technician to gather a history from the newly admitted patient about his medications.
5. The nurse directs the patient care technician to assist one of the stable patients up in a chair for his meal.

2. A nurse working the evening shift has five patients and is teamed up with an assistive personnel. One of the assigned patients has just returned from surgery, three others are stable and resting, and one has requested a pain medication. The patient in pain has two analgesics ordered prn for pain and has been using cold applications on his surgical site for pain relief. The last time an analgesic was given was 4 hours ago. The patient is scheduled for a physical therapy visit in 2 hours. Which of the following demonstrate good clinical decision making during intervention? (Select all that apply.)
   1. The nurse reviews the options for pain relief for the patient.
   2. The nurse assesses whether the prn medication, ordered every 4 to 6 hours and last given 4 hours ago, is effective and whether a new type of medication is needed.
   3. The nurse reviews the policy and procedure for the cold application.
   4. The nurse considers how the patient might react if the pain medication is held until an hour before physical therapy.
   5. The nurse delegates vital sign assessment of the patient returning from surgery to the assistive personnel.

3. A nurse working the evening shift has five patients and is teamed up with an assistive personnel. One of the assigned patients has just returned from surgery, one is newly admitted, and one has requested a pain medication. The patient who has returned from surgery just minutes ago has a large abdominal dressing, is still on oxygen by nasal cannula, and has an intravenous line. One of the other patients has just called out for assistance in setting up a meal tray. Another patient is stable and resting comfortably. Which patient is the nurse's current greatest priority?
   1. Patient in pain
   2. Patient newly admitted
   3. Patient who returned from surgery
   4. Patient requesting assistance with meal tray

4. The nurse administers a tube feeding via a patient's nasogastric tube. This is an example of which of the following?
   1. Physical care technique
   2. Activity of daily living
   3. Indirect care measure
   4. Lifesaving measure

5. Which principle is most important for a nurse to follow when using a clinical practice guideline for an assigned patient?
   1. Knowing the source of the guideline
   2. Reviewing the evidence used to develop the guideline
   3. Individualizing how to apply the clinical guideline for a patient
   4. Explaining to a patient the purpose of the guideline

6. A nurse is visiting a patient who lives alone at home. The nurse is assessing the patient's adherence to medications. While talking with the family caregiver, the nurse learns that the patient has been missing doses. The nurse wants to perform interventions to improve the patient's adherence. Which of the following will affect how this nurse will make clinical decisions about how to implement care for this patient? (Select all that apply.)
   1. Reviewing the family caregiver's availability during medication administration times
   2. Determining the value the patient places on taking medications
   3. Reviewing the number of medications and time each is to be taken
   4. Determining all consequences associated with the patient missing specific medicines
   5. Reviewing the therapeutic actions of the medications

7. The nurse enters a patient's room and finds that the patient was incontinent of liquid stool. Because the patient has recurrent redness in the perineal area, the nurse worries about the risk of the patient developing a pressure injury. The nurse cleanses the patient, inspects the skin, and applies a skin barrier ointment to the perineal area. The nurse consults the ostomy and wound care nurse specialist for recommended skin care measures. Which of the following correctly describe the nurse's actions? (Select all that apply.)
   1. The application of the skin barrier is a dependent care measure.
   2. The call to the ostomy and wound care specialist is an indirect care measure.
   3. The cleansing of the skin is a direct care measure.
   4. The application of the skin barrier is an instrumental activity of daily living.
   5. Inspecting the skin is a direct care activity.

8. Match the category of direct care on the left with the specific direct care activity on the right.
   1. Counseling ____
   2. Lifesaving measure ____
   3. Physical care technique ____
   4. Activity of daily living ____

   a. Assisting patient with oral care
   b. Discussing a patient's options in choosing palliative care
   c. Protecting a violent patient from injury
   d. Using safe patient handling during positioning of a patient

9. Which measures does a nurse follow when being asked to perform an unfamiliar procedure? (Select all that apply.)
   1. Checks scientific literature or policy and procedure
   2. Determines whether additional assistance is needed
   3. Collects all necessary equipment
   4. Delegates the procedure to a more experienced nurse
   5. Considers all possible consequences of the procedure

10. A nurse is conferring with another nurse about the care of a patient with a stage II pressure injury. The two decide to review the clinical practice guideline of the hospital for pressure injury care. The use of a clinical practice guideline achieves which of the following? (Select all that apply.)
   1. Allows nurses to act more quickly and appropriately
   2. Sets a level of clinical excellence for practice
   3. Eliminates need to create an individualized care plan for the patient
   4. Incorporates evidence-based interventions for stage II pressure injury
   5. Provides for access to patient care information within the electronic health record

Answers: 1. 2, 3, 5; **2.** 1, 2, 4; **3.** 3, 4; **4.** 1; **5.** 3; **6.** 2, 4; **7.** 2, 3; **8.** 1 b, 2 c, 3 d, 4 a; **9.** 1, 2, 3; **10.** 1, 2, 4.

Rationales for Review Questions can be found on the Evolve website.

REFERENCES

American Nurses Association (ANA): *Scope and standards of practice: nursing*, ed 2, Silver Spring, MD, 2010, American Nurses Association.

American Nurses Association (ANA): Scope of practice, n.d., https://www.nursingworld.org/practice-policy/scope-of-practice/. Accessed July 14, 2018.

American Nurses Association (ANA) and National Council of state Boards of nursing (NCSBN): Joint statement on delegation, 2012, https://www.ncsbn.org/Delegation_joint_statement_NCSBN-ANA.pdf. Accessed July 21, 2018.

Butcher HK, et al.: *Nursing interventions classification (NIC)*, ed 7, St Louis, 2018, Elsevier.

Chamberlain B, et al.: Practice models: a concept analysis, *Nurs Manage* 44(10):16, 2013. http://www.njha.com/media/278946/NursingMgmt1013.pdf. Accessed July 17, 2018.

ECRI Institute: Top 10 patient safety concerns for 2019, 2019, ECRI Institute: Top 10 patient safety concerns. Accessed July 21, 2019.

Goldstone L, et al.: Bundle up: introducing care bundles to increase knowledge and confidence of senior nursing students, *Teach Learn Nurs* 10(3):143, 2015.

Hospital Consumer Assessment of Healthcare Providers and Systems (HCAHPS): HCAHPS, 2018, https://www.surveyvitals.com/start/hcahps?gclid=EAIaIQobChMI5deBqMCw3AIVBrbACh34_w6VEAAYASAAEgIh-7vD_BwE. Accessed July 21, 2018.

Jones TL: A holistic framework for nursing time: implications for theory, practice and research, *Nurs Forum* 45(3):185, 2010.

Lyon S: Occupational therapy: what to know about ADLs and IADLS, VeryWell Health, 2018. https://www.verywellhealth.com/what-are-adls-and-iadls-2510011. Accessed July 21, 2018.

MBL Technologies: Standard nursing terminologies: a landscape analysis, 2017, https://www.healthit.gov/sites/default/files/snt_final_05302017.pdf. Accessed January 20, 2019.

National Council of State Boards of Nursing: *National Guidelines for Nursing Delegation* 7(1):5, 2016. https://www.journalofnursingregulation.com/article/S2155-8256(16)31035-3/pdf. Accessed August 1, 2019.

Nurse Journal: Tips to improve patient education, 2018, https://nursejournal.org/community/tips-to-improve-patient-education/. Accessed July 21, 2018.

Przemyslaw K, et al.: Determinants of patient adherence: a review of systematic reviews, *Front Pharmacol*, 2013. https://doi.org/10.3389/fphar.2013.00091. Accessed July 21, 2018.

Quality Safety Education for Nurses (QSEN): 2019, update, http://qsen.org/competencies/pre-licensure-ksas/. Accessed July 21, 2019.

RESEARCH REFERENCES

Benner P: *From novice to expert*, Menlo Park, CA, 1984, Addison-Wesley.

Camporota L, Brett S: Care bundles: implementing evidence or common sense? *Crit Care* 15(3):159, 2011.

Huisman ERCM, et al.: Healing environment: a review of the impact of physical environmental factors on users, *Build Environ* 58:70, 2012.

Juknevicius G, et al.: Implementation of evidence-based care bundles in the ICU, *Crit Care* 16(Suppl 1):524, 2012.

Lavallée JF: The effects of care bundles on patient outcomes: a systematic review and meta-analysis, *Implement Sci* 12:142, 2017.

Ospina MB, et al.: A systematic review of the effectiveness of discharge care bundles for patients with COPD, *Thorax* 72:31, 2017.

Tanner J, et al.: Do surgical care bundles reduce the risk of surgical site infections in patients undergoing colorectal surgery? A systematic review and cohort meta-analysis of 8,515 patients, *Surgery* 158(1):66, 2015.

van Dulmen S, et al.: Patient adherence to medical treatment: a review of reviews, *BMC Health Serv Res* 7:55, 2007.

20

Evaluation

OBJECTIVES

- Discuss the relationship between critical thinking and evaluation.
- Explain the difference between evaluative measures and assessment.
- Explain the importance of using the right evaluative measures.
- Explain the relationship among goals of care, expected outcomes, and evaluative measures when evaluating nursing care.
- Explain how evaluation reveals errors or omissions in care.
- Discuss the process of determining the need to revise a plan of care.

KEY TERMS

MEDIA RESOURCES

Evaluation is the crucial fifth step of the nursing process that determines whether a patient's condition or well-being improved after nursing interventions were delivered. It is imperative for nurses to monitor on an ongoing basis a patient's clinical progress. Critical thinking in nursing practice strengthens your clinical performance and reflects your ability to resolve patients' health-related problems (Shu-Yuan et al., 2013). Evaluation monitors the progress of each of your patients and gives you valuable information about the efficacy of your interventions. The outcomes of nursing practice are the measurable conditions of patient, family, or community status; behavior; or perception. These outcomes are the criteria for judging the success in delivering nursing care.

Nurses are responsible for evaluating the effect of nursing practice on patient outcomes in the areas of health promotion, injury and illness prevention, and alleviation of suffering (Jones, 2016). Outcome evaluation is a part of every health care organization's quality assessment to determine what clinical practices and nursing care standards are effective. Nurses who provide direct care to patients are the best source of information about nursing practice and patient outcomes on an organizational level (Jones, 2016).

Evaluation is critical to knowing a patient's health status. A patient is diagnosed with pneumonia based on clinical signs such as productive cough, fever, and a chest x-ray showing lung consolidation. After the patient completes a course of antibiotics, the health care provider repeats the chest x-ray and looks for an improvement in cough and lowering of body temperature to determine whether the pneumonia has resolved. When a nurse provides wound care, including application of a warm compress, several steps are involved. He or she assesses the appearance of the wound, determines its severity, applies the appropriate form of compress, and returns later to inspect the wound to determine whether the condition has improved. These scenarios depict what ultimately occurs during the process of evaluation: comparing assessment measures at two different time points to determine a patient's condition and whether the desired outcome of treatment has been achieved. *The nurse performs evaluative measures (e.g., reinspection of wound) to determine whether a patient met expected outcomes (e.g., wound heals within 2 weeks), not whether nursing interventions were completed.* The expected outcomes established during planning (see Chapter 18) are the standards against which a nurse judges whether goals (e.g., wound healing) have been met and care is successful.

In the continuing case study Mr. Lawson is going home in a couple of hours. Tonya organizes her care so that she can take the time needed to evaluate the outcomes of her plan of care. Mr. Lawson took two doses of the prn analgesic ordered for his pain over the past 8 hours. Thirty minutes after the last dose he rated his pain a 3 on a scale of 0 to 10. He states, "I only really notice now when I move too quickly." Mrs. Lawson is in the room, so Tonya takes time to inspect and evaluate Mr. Lawson's wound, describes what she sees, and asks the Lawsons to explain the signs of infection and how to care for the wound at home. Tonya gives the Lawsons the discharge instruction sheet that is part of the standard of care of her nursing unit. She asks Mr. Lawson to explain the types of activity he needs to avoid for the first 2 weeks that he is home.

STANDARDS FOR EVALUATION

Nursing care helps patients resolve actual health problems, prevent the occurrence of potential problems, and maintain a healthy state. Evaluation is an integral step to that end. The American Nurses Association (ANA) defines standards of professional nursing practice (see Chapter 1), which include standards for the evaluation step of the nursing process. The standards are authoritative statements of the duties that all registered nurses, regardless of role, patient population

271

they serve, or specialty, are expected to perform competently (ANA, 2010). The competencies for evaluation include being systematic and using criterion-based evaluation, collaborating with patients and health care professionals, using ongoing assessment data to revise a plan, and communicating results to patients and families. Always deliver interventions responsibly and appropriately to minimize unwarranted or unwanted treatment (ANA, 2010).

CRITICAL THINKING IN EVALUATION

Critical thinking is key to evaluation (Fig. 20.1). In Chapter 15 you learned that clinical decision making is complex, requiring flexibility and the ability to know and recognize subtle changes or aspects of a patient's condition. A literature review of studies examining critical thinking indicators identified four actions that show a nurse is competent to perform evaluation (Shu-Yuan et al., 2013):

- Examine the results of care according to clinical data collected.
- Compare achieved effects or outcomes with goals and expected outcomes.
- Recognize errors or omissions.
- Understand a patient situation, reflect on the situation, and correct errors.

The evaluation process is comprehensive and complex. It requires more than making a quick check of a patient to be sure that he or she is stable or without further problems. It is a methodical approach for determining whether nursing implementation effectively influenced a patient's progress or condition favorably.

Examine Results

Nurses are accountable for and obligated to evaluate interventions and outcomes in the areas of health promotion, prevention of illness and injury, and alleviation of suffering (Jones, 2016).

Evaluation occurs whenever you have contact with a patient. It is an ongoing process that includes a before-and-after comparison or an after comparison with an established standard. For example, after assessing a patient's behaviors reflecting anxiety, you offer counseling and instructional support, then compare the behaviors with those shown after interventions are completed. After a patient undergoes tracheal suctioning, comparing the patient's actual oxygen saturation with the presuctioning level and the saturation level you anticipate (standard of >90%) informs you about the efficacy of suctioning and the patient's response.

Once you deliver an intervention, you continuously examine results by gathering subjective and objective data from a patient, family, and health care team members (as appropriate). At the same time you reflect on your knowledge regarding a patient's current condition, the treatment, and the resources available for recovery. By also reflecting on previous experiences caring for similar patients, you are in a better position to know how to evaluate your patient. You can anticipate what to evaluate.

You need to have an open mind, keen observation skills, and a neutral perspective to effectively evaluate patient outcomes (Shu-Yuan et al., 2013). Do not form a judgment about a patient's progress or response without gathering data pertinent to the health care problem. *For example, because Mr. Lawson is being discharged and there have been no delays, Tonya might assume that his pain is under control. However, until Tonya reassesses the patient's pain character and severity, evaluation is not complete.* Be thorough in gathering all clinical information needed to adequately evaluate a patient's condition.

Evaluative Measures. Although you may measure or observe patient data in the same way during assessment and evaluation, an assessment identifies what, if any, problems exist while an evaluation determines whether the problems you identified during assessment have remained the same, improved, or otherwise changed. Evaluative measures are similar to and often the same assessment skills and techniques (e.g., observations, physiological measurements, use of measurement scales, patient interview) you perform during a patient assessment (Fig. 20.2). However, evaluative and assessment measures differ based on when you perform them. Evaluative measures are made following nursing interventions, when you make decisions about a patient's status and progress (Table 20.1).

In many clinical situations it is important to collect evaluative measures over a period of time. You look for trends to determine whether a pattern of improvement or change exists. A one-time observation of a pressure injury is insufficient to determine that the ulcer is healing. It is important to note a consistency in change. For example, over a period of 3 days is the pressure injury gradually decreasing in size, is the amount of drainage declining, and is the redness of inflammation resolving? Recognizing a pattern of improvement or deterioration allows you to reason and decide whether a patient's problems (expressed as nursing diagnoses or collaborative problems) are resolved. This is very important in the home care or nursing home setting. It may take weeks or even months to determine whether interventions led to a pattern of improvement. For example, when evaluating a patient's risk for falls over time, has the patient, family, or health care team successfully reduced fall risks in the home, such as eliminating barriers in the home, removing factors impairing the person's vision, or providing direction for proper use of assistive devices?

It is important to use the right evaluative measure. For example, pain scales are valid and reliable for assessing pain severity (see Chapter 44) and change over time. The European Pressure Ulcer Advisory Panel (EPUAP) and National Pressure injury Advisory Panel (NPIAP) and Pan Pacific Pressure Injury Alliance (2019a, b) has specific criteria for the accurate staging of pressure injuries (see Chapter 48) that allow you to identify whether a treated pressure injury has changed. By using the right measure you are more likely to accurately identify a change, if any, in a patient's condition.

Being able to evaluate behavioral change is more difficult. The information about behavior (e.g., taking medications correctly, following a diet, perceiving less grief) often relies on a patient's self-report. An example of a behavioral measure is any survey or interview that evaluates a patient's ability to perform self-care and achieve self-management. Self-report is a measure of a patient's own perceptions or beliefs and may not truly reflect whether change has occurred. Your willingness to use self-report as an outcome measure of behavior or patient perception reflects trust in the patient. When using self-report, it is very important that the patient understands questions posed and why his or her response is important to gauge behavioral change.

Much emphasis in health care today is on patients and their family caregivers to achieve self-management to improve the quality of their lives. The aim of self-management is to minimize the impact of chronic disease or sudden acute illness on physical health status and functioning and to enable people to cope with the psychological effects of an illness. *In Mr. Lawson's case, Tonya planned and implemented educational interventions designed to improve his ability to adopt the behaviors needed for self-care, specifically to follow activity restrictions and perform correct wound care. Tonya evaluates the patient's ability by measuring what he is able to either explain or demonstrate.* There are relevant, objective, and appropriate evaluative indicators of self-management, including knowledge (information relevant to a patient's situation), independence (independence over areas of health and well-being and other areas that patients feel confident to manage, *and* being independent from others), skills (i.e., ability to manage stress and make decisions), bio-psychosocial markers of health (i.e., quality of life), and positive social networks (Boger et al., 2015) (Table 20.2).

KNOWLEDGE
Characteristics of improved physiological, psychological, spiritual, and sociocultural status
Expected outcomes of pharmacological, medical, nutritional, and other therapies
Unexpected outcomes of pharmacological, medical, nutritional, and other therapies
Characteristics of improved family and group dynamics
Community resources

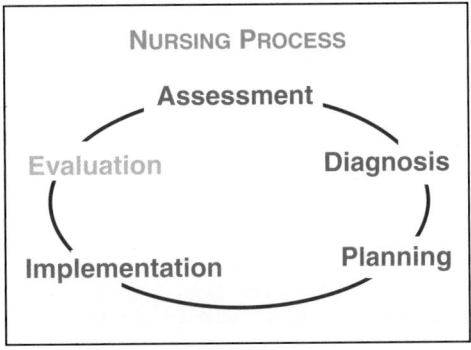

EXPERIENCE
Previous patient care experience

NURSING PROCESS
Assessment
Evaluation   Diagnosis
Implementation   Planning

STANDARDS
Expected outcomes of care
Specialty standards of practice (e.g., American Pain Society; University of Iowa Evidence-Based Protocols, Intravenous Nursing Society)
Intellectual standards

ATTITUDES
Creativity
Responsibility
Perseverance
Humility

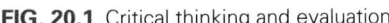

FIG. 20.1 Critical thinking and evaluation.

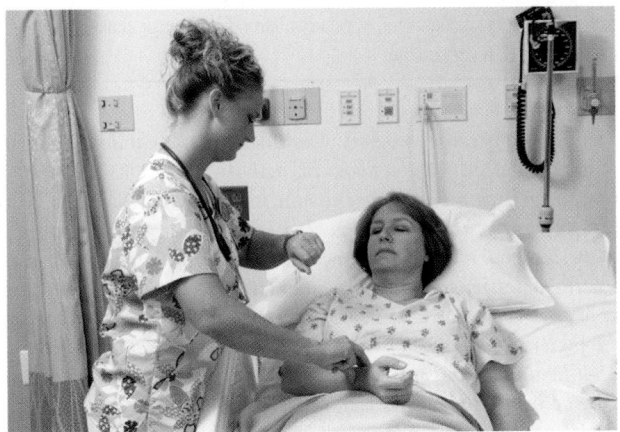

FIG. 20.2 Evaluative measures. Nurse evaluates patient's vital signs.

During planning a valuable resource for selecting outcomes is the Nursing Outcomes Classification (NOC) (see Chapter 18). The classification offers a standard nursing language (SNL) for the outcomes used in the evaluation step of the nursing process (Box 20.1). The benefits of NOC include (Moorhead et al., 2018):

- Providing a means for nurses and other health care providers to evaluate the status of patients, family, or community
- Providing an outcome measurement system using SNL for all health care settings, specialties, and patients across the life span
- Offering a means to quantify the change in patient status after nursing interventions and to monitor patient progress

The NOC system includes 540 outcomes, with each outcome having a set of evaluation indicators that describe specific states, perceptions, or behaviors related to the outcome, and Likert-type measurement scales (Moorhead et al., 2018) (Table 20.3). The outcomes are very broadly defined, while the indicators are defined in terms like those used to write patient goal statements. For example, the outcome "Comfort Status: Physical" is a broad category, but indicators such as "symptom control," "physical well-being," and "fluid intake" could be used as specific patient goal statements. The five-point Likert-type scales are used with all indicators to demonstrate variability in the state, behavior, or perception patients describe when measuring outcomes. For example, the outcome *Gait* is measured on a scale of "severely compromised to not compromised," while the outcome *Knowledge: Fall Prevention* is measured on a scale of "no knowledge to extensive knowledge." The NOC system was designed to be used with the NANDA-I nursing diagnoses (see Chapter 17) and the Nursing Interventions Classification (NIC) (see Chapter 19). However, the outcome indicators are totally appropriate for use with the International Classification for Nursing Practice (ICNP) diagnoses.

> **QSEN Building Competency in Informatics** Explain how use of the NOC classification in an electronic health record could improve patient safety. How would such a system help you monitor patient outcomes over time?
>
> Answers to QSEN Activities can be found on the Evolve website.

TABLE 20.1   Evaluative Measures To Determine the Success of Goals and Expected Outcomes

Goals	Evaluative Measures	Expected Outcomes
Patient's pressure injury will heal within 7 days.	Inspect color, condition, and location of pressure injury. Measure diameter of ulcer daily. Note odor and color of drainage from ulcer.	Erythema is reduced in 2 days. Diameter of ulcer decreases in 5 days. Ulcer has no drainage in 2 days. Skin overlying ulcer is closed in 7 days.
Patient will tolerate ambulation to end of hall with a safe maximal heart rate by 11/20.	Measure patient's radial pulse after patient ambulates and compare with baseline and the safe maximal heart rate (age-predicted HR max equation equals $208 - [0.7 \times Age]$). Assess respiratory rate during exercise. Observe patient for dyspnea or breathlessness during exercise.	Pulse remains below age-predicted HR during exercise. Pulse rate returns to resting baseline within 10 minutes after exercise. Respiratory rate remains within two breaths of patient's baseline rate. Patient denies feeling of breathlessness.
Patient adheres to medication regimen in 1 week.	Ask patient to fill a pill organizer for 7 days. Have patient identify the schedule for daily medications. Have patient explain purpose and benefits of each ordered medication.	Patient fills a pill organizer correctly for 7 days. Patient identifies daily medication schedule in 2 days. Patient discusses purpose and benefits of ordered medications in 1 day.

TABLE 20.2   Self-Management Evaluation

Evaluation Indicator	Examples of Measures
Self-Efficacy	General self-efficacy (GSE) scale; disease-specific self-efficacy scales (e.g., arthritis, diabetes, cardiac); medication-adherence self-efficacy scale
Health Behavior	Adherence to medication administration (e.g., pill count; number of injections); demonstrated psychomotor skill (e.g., dressing change, self-injection); adherence to medical follow-up visits
Physical Health Status	Clinical indicators (e.g., exercise tolerance, blood pressure control, blood glucose control [HgA1C])
Health Service Utilization	Readmission to hospital in 30 days; admission to emergency department
Quality of Life	Quality-of-life scales (e.g., for chronic illness, cancer, chronic pain)
Psychological Indicators	Perceived-stress scale, self-control, or other validated surveys or scales (e.g., Impulsivity Teen Conflict survey)

Compare Achieved Effect with Goals and Outcomes. A nursing plan of care includes mutually established goals and nurse-sensitive outcomes relevant to a patient's health status. In Chapter 18 you learned that a nurse-sensitive outcome is a state, behavior, or perception that is measured along a continuum in response to a nursing intervention (Moorhead et al., 2018). During evaluation you perform evaluative measures that allow you to compare clinical assessment data, patient behavioral measures, and patient self-report measures collected before implementation with measures gathered after administering nursing care. Next you decide whether the results of care match the expected outcomes and goals set for a patient. If outcomes are met, the overall goals for the patient also are met. Critical thinking directs you to analyze the findings from evaluation (Fig. 20.3). Has the patient's condition improved? Is the patient able to progress, or are there physical factors preventing recovery? Does this patient's motivation or willingness to pursue healthier behaviors influence responses to therapies?

Outcomes are statements of progressive, step-by-step physical, emotional, or behavioral responses that a patient needs to accomplish to achieve the goals of care. When your patients achieve outcomes, the related factors for a problem-focused nursing diagnosis or the risk factors for an at-risk nursing diagnosis usually no longer exist or are better managed. *In Mr. Lawson's case the nursing diagnosis of* **Anxiety related to uncertainty over ability to return to work** *has the goal of* "Mr. Lawson will be able to assume activity restrictions at home." *Tonya has planned and implemented nursing care to prepare Mr. Lawson for*

a smooth postoperative recovery. She intervenes to minimize his anxiety and provides instruction about his activity restrictions so that he will adhere to his treatment plan. The aim is to achieve adherence so that return to work is a reasonable goal. Two of the expected outcomes for Mr. Lawson's goal include that the patient will maintain attention during instructional sessions and that the patient will explain how activity restrictions aid recovery. Tonya uses evaluative measures, including observation of the patient's behavior during instruction and then patient self-report of what he understands about his activity restrictions. If Tonya's plan of care is successful, the related factor of "uncertainty over ability to return to work" was managed. Tonya will know that, because Mr. Lawson was able to attend during instruction and explain how adherence to activity restrictions will hasten his recovery, one source of anxiety has lessened.

REFLECT NOW

What evaluative measures and outcomes might you anticipate for a patient who has the nursing diagnosis *Risk for Fall?*

Interpreting and Summarizing Findings. A patient's clinical condition often changes during an acute illness. In contrast, chronic illness results in slow, subtle changes, although acute exacerbations can occur. When you compare achieved effects of interventions with goals and outcomes, you interpret or learn to recognize relevant evidence

BOX 20.1 EVIDENCE-BASED PRACTICE

Improved Care Plans Using Standardized Nursing Language

PICOT Question: Does the use of standard nursing language (SNL) compared with no SNL improve the accuracy of nursing care plans for adult patients?

Evidence Summary

One of the essential characteristics of a quality nursing care plan is accuracy. Nursing care plan content must be comprehensive, which is defined as "documentation according to the different phases of the nursing process," and accurate, which pertains to how precisely the data describe a patient's situation (Thoroddsen et al., 2013). For example, describing a patient's pain as moderate is less accurate than noting the patient's pain severity rating. Also a nursing care plan must contain accurate nursing diagnoses based on the assessment data gathered from a patient.

An international study involving a systematic review of research examined the impact SNL has on nursing documentation and care plans (Johnson et al., 2018). Nurses use SNL in electronic health care records (EHRs) to label the clinical judgments they make during a nursing assessment. The review of articles concluded that critical thinking improved the accurateness of nursing diagnoses when the nurses used SNL (Johnson et al., 2018).

Application to Nursing Practice

- The consistent use of SNL ensures quality data collection that enables care providers and health care organizations to evaluate nursing care practices.
- Accuracy of nursing care plans depends on accuracy, content, and degree to which plans are based on data (Johnson et al., 2018).
- In certain EHRs it is increasingly difficult to describe the nursing care that is taking place without SNL (Johnson et al., 2018).
- Using SNL makes documenting nursing care more efficient and facilitates communication of nursing care across health care disciplines and health care environments (Johnson et al., 2018).

TABLE 20.3 Examples of Nursing Outcome Classification Outcomes and Indicators

NOC Outcomes	Indicators (Examples)
Anxiety level	Level of restlessness Decreased productivity Level of verbalized anxiety
Knowledge: treatment procedures	Description of treatment procedures Follows restrictions related to procedure Correct use of equipment
Risk control: aspiration	Cleans dentures daily Selects foods based on swallowing ability
Sleep	Hours of sleep Sleep pattern

Adapted from Moorhead S, et al: *Nursing outcomes classification (NOC)*, ed 6, St Louis, 2018, Elsevier.

about a patient's condition, even evidence that sometimes does not match clinical expectations. By applying your clinical knowledge and experience, you learn to recognize complications or adverse responses to illness and treatment in addition to expected outcomes.

Careful monitoring and early detection of problems are a nurse's first line of defense. Always make clinical judgments based on your observations of what is occurring with a specific patient and not merely on what happens to patients in general. Gather detailed,

patient-specific evaluation measures because change in a patient's status frequently is not obvious. Make your evaluation based on your understanding of each patient's behavior, physical status, and reaction to caregivers. Perceptive clinical judgment involves interpreting and summarizing evaluation measures to determine whether a patient's status is improving. Comparing expected and actual findings allows you to interpret and judge a patient's condition and whether predicted changes occurred (Table 20.4). Perform the following steps to objectively evaluate the level of your patient's success in achieving outcomes of care:

1. Examine the outcome criteria to identify the exact desired patient behavior or response.
2. Evaluate a patient's actual behavior or response.
3. Compare the established outcome criteria with the actual behavior or response.
4. Judge the degree of agreement between outcome criteria and the actual behavior or response.
5. If there is no agreement (or only partial agreement) between the outcome criteria and the actual behavior or response, what is the reason? Why did they not agree? What is your next action?

Evaluation is easier to perform after you care for a patient over a long period. You are then able to make subtle comparisons of patient responses and behaviors. When you have not cared for a patient over an extended time, evaluation improves by referring to previous experiences or asking colleagues who are familiar with the patient to confirm evaluation findings. The accuracy of any evaluation improves when you are familiar with a patient's behavior and physiological status or have cared for more than one patient with a similar problem.

Recognize Errors or Unmet Outcomes

During evaluation the recognition of errors or unmet outcomes requires you to have an open mind, to actively pursue truth, to be patient and confident, and to engage in self-reflection (Shu-Yuan et al., 2013). You cannot assume that your treatment approaches will be successful. You must apply observational skills, critical thinking intellectual standards (see Chapter 15), knowledge, and reflection to recognize the actual results of your care. Reflection is a conscious effort to think about your interventions and outcomes, consider what was positive or challenging, and consider how the plan of care might be enhanced, improved, or done differently in the future (Royal College of Nursing, 2015). It usually occurs in the presence of a trigger event, which involves a breakdown or perceived breakdown in practice. For example, a nurse observes how a patient reacts to a treatment (e.g., exercise, positioning, or teaching) and realizes that the approach is ineffective. Or a nurse reviewing a patient's progress identifies that planned interventions were not done or not completed, described in the literature as "missed care" (Ball and Griffiths, 2018). Reflection involves a nurse's ability to recognize how a patient is responding and then adjust interventions as a result. A nurse will change the frequency of an intervention, change how the intervention is delivered, or select a new intervention based on a patient's response.

Often evaluation reveals patients who have unmet needs. Patients with the same health care problem are not treated the same way. As a result you sometimes make errors in judgment. The systematic use of evaluation provides a way for you to catch these errors. By consistently incorporating evaluation into practice, you minimize errors and ensure that a patient's plan of care is appropriate and relevant and changes according to met and unmet needs.

Correction of Errors

Reflection and subsequent clinical learning are also parts of evaluation. What a nurse gains from caring for patients and carefully evaluating the

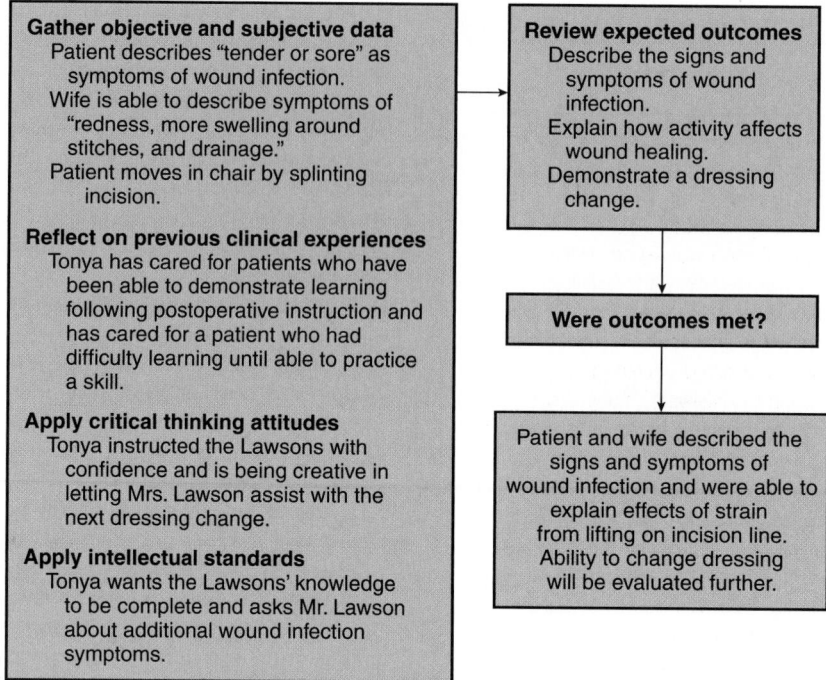

FIG. 20.3 Critical thinking and the evaluation process.

TABLE 20.4   Examples of Objective Evaluation of Goal Achievement

Goals	Outcomes	Patient Response	Evaluation Findings
Patient will change surgical dressing correctly by 12/18.	Patient demonstrates correct hand hygiene by 12/16. Patient describes material to use in dressing change by 12/17. Patient demonstrates dressing change by 12/18.	Patient used antiseptic hand rub correctly to wash hands. Patient applied clean gauze correctly and taped securely in place over incision.	Patient shows progression toward outcomes and achieved desired behavior.
Patient's lungs will be free of secretions by 11/30.	Coughing is nonproductive by 11/29. Lungs are clear to auscultation by 11/30. Respirations are 20/min by 11/30.	Patient coughed frequently and productively on 11/29 following nebulization. Lungs were clear to auscultation on 11/30. Respirations were 18/min on 11/29.	Patient will require continued nebulizer therapy. Condition is improving.

outcomes of care later contributes to ongoing clinical knowledge development and capacity for making clinical judgments about future patients (Tanner, 2006). This process helps correct and prevent errors. Reflective reasoning improves the accuracy of clinical decisions and making diagnostic conclusions. This means that, when you gather evaluative measures about a patient, reflection on the findings and exploration about what the findings mean improve your ability to problem solve. Reflection lessens the likelihood that reasoning is based on assumptions or guesswork and increases the likelihood that it is based on objective critical thinking.

REFLECT NOW

Think about an experience in a simulation lab or a recent encounter with a patient. What was your approach and how successful were you? Were there errors made? What might you have done differently to achieve a desired outcome?

Revising the Care Plan

The result of an evaluation helps you decide whether to continue, discontinue, or revise the plan of care. The patient and sometimes family members can tell you how interventions helped or did not help (Ackley et al., 2017). This information adds to the evaluative measures you collect. If your patient meets a goal successfully, either maintain treatment as planned or discontinue that part of the care plan if intervention is no longer required. For example, in the case of a patient achieving a desired level of exercise, you will still continue an exercise regimen. In the case of a patient who is able to demonstrate knowledge of a topic after instruction, further instruction is not needed. When there are unmet or partially met goals, or if you determine that perhaps a new problem has developed, reassessment is necessary. A complete reassessment of patient factors relating to an existing nursing diagnosis and etiology is necessary when modifying a plan. If outcomes have not been met, it is helpful to consider the SMART acronym discussed in Chapter 18 (Ackley et al., 2017). For example, were the outcomes **S**pecific? Were the outcomes **M**easurable? You will often modify or add nursing diagnoses or collaborative problems with appropriate goals and expected outcomes. You then select interventions and redefine priorities of care. Reassessment ensures that the database is accurate and current. It also reveals any missing links (i.e., a critical piece of new information that was overlooked and thus interfered with goal achievement). You sort, validate, and cluster all new data to analyze and interpret differences from the original database (see Chapter 16). An important step in critical thinking in evaluation is knowing how a patient is progressing and how problems resolve or worsen.

Tonya evaluates through teach-back Mr. Lawson's understanding of how activity restrictions aid recovery. Tonya states, "I want to know how well you understand your activity restrictions. Describe for me the restrictions your doctor explained." The patient states, "My doctor doesn't want me to do any heavy lifting. It could affect how my wound heals." As Tonya listens to Mr. and Mrs. Lawson further discuss going home, Mrs. Lawson comments, "It will be great for my husband to see the grandkids soon. He's really close to them. He loves playing with the 3-year-old." Tonya uses the evaluative measure of patient self-report to determine what Mr. Lawson understands about his activity restrictions. She recognizes that playing with grandkids could involve picking up the children. Tonya decides to modify her plan of care by reassessing the types of activities Mr. Lawson does at home (e.g., type of lifting, exercise, manual work) and adapting her instructions to be more comprehensive.

Discontinuing a Care Plan. After you determine that your patient met expected outcomes and goals, confirm your evaluation with the patient when possible. If you and the patient agree, you discontinue that part of the care plan. Documentation of a discontinued plan ensures that other nurses will not unnecessarily continue interventions for that part of the plan. Continuity of care assumes that care provided to patients is relevant and timely. You waste time and energy when you do not communicate achieved goals with other nurses.

Modifying a Care Plan. When patients do not meet goals and outcomes, you perform a reassessment and identify the factors that interfere with their achievement. Usually a change in a patient's condition, needs, or abilities makes alteration of the care plan necessary. This will require you to continue interventions either as planned or less/more often, or you will choose to add interventions focused on the factors affecting goal achievement. For example, when teaching self-administration of insulin, a nurse discovers that a patient has developed a new problem, a tremor associated with a side effect of a medication. The patient is unable to draw medication from a syringe or inject the needle safely. As a result, the original outcomes of "Patient correctly prepares insulin in a syringe" and "Patient administers insulin injection independently" are no longer appropriate because they cannot be met. The nurse introduces new interventions (instructing a family member in insulin preparation and administration) and revises outcomes—"Family caregiver correctly prepares insulin in syringe" and "Family caregiver administers insulin injection correctly"—to meet the goal of care.

At times a lack of goal achievement results from an error in nursing judgment or failure to follow each step of the nursing process. Patients often have multiple and complex problems. Always remember the possibility of overlooking or misjudging something. When a goal is not met, no matter what the reason, repeat the nursing process sequence for that nursing diagnosis. Reassess the patient; determine accuracy of the nursing diagnosis; and establish a plan with new goals, expected outcomes, and appropriate priority interventions.

Redefining Diagnoses. After reassessment determine which nursing diagnoses are accurate for the situation. Ask yourself whether you selected the correct diagnosis and if the related factor or risk factor is accurate and current. Then revise the problem list to reflect the patient's changed status. Sometimes you form a new diagnosis or change the prioritization of diagnoses. You base your nursing care on an accurate list of nursing diagnoses. Accuracy is more important than the number of diagnoses selected. As a patient's condition changes, the diagnoses also change.

Revising Goals and Expected Outcomes. When revising a care plan, review the goals and expected outcomes for necessary changes. For example, does the time frame for outcomes need to be revised? Does your reassessment reveal a goal that is unrealistic? Is a more specific measure needed to determine outcome achievement? Examine the appropriateness of goals for any unchanged nursing diagnoses and remember that a change in one health care problem sometimes affects the goals for others. *In Mr. Lawson's case, if his anxiety were to worsen again, Tonya probably would have to not only revise the plan for managing the anxiety but also consider whether her selection of teaching strategies needs to be changed.* Determining that each goal and expected outcome is realistic for the problem, etiology, and time frame is important. Unrealistic expected outcomes and time frames make goal achievement difficult.

Revising Interventions. The evaluation of interventions examines two factors: the appropriateness of the intervention selected and the correct application of the intervention. Appropriateness is based on the nursing standards of care for a patient's health problem (see Chapter 19). Standards of care (i.e., standard interventions, clinical guidelines, care bundles) are the minimum level of care accepted to ensure high-quality patient care. Standards of care define the types of therapies typically administered to patients with defined problems or needs. For example, if a patient who is receiving chemotherapy for leukemia has the nursing diagnosis *Acute Pain related to oral mucosa inflammation from mucositis,* the standard of care established by the nursing department for this problem includes pain-control measures, mouth care guidelines, and diet therapy. Professional organizations such as the Oncology Nursing Society often have clinical guidelines as standards of care for select health problems. The nurse reviews the standard of care and decides which interventions have been chosen and whether additional ones are required to achieve expected outcomes.

Increasing or decreasing the frequency of an intervention is another approach to ensure appropriateness of the intervention. You adjust interventions based on a patient's actual response to therapy and your previous experience with similar patients. For example, if a patient continues to have congested lung sounds, you increase the frequency of coughing and deep-breathing exercises to remove secretions and add positioning to ensure airway clearance.

During evaluation you find that some planned interventions are designed for an inappropriate level of nursing care. If you need to change the level of care, substitute a different action verb such as *assist* in place of *provide* or *demonstrate* in place of *instruct*. For example, helping a patient walk requires you to assist the patient during ambulation, whereas providing an assistive device (e.g., a cane or walker) suggests that the patient is more independent. In addition, demonstration requires you to show a patient how a skill is performed rather than simply telling the patient how to perform it. Sometimes the level of care is appropriate, but the interventions are unsuitable because of a change in the expected outcome. In this example discontinue the interventions and plan new ones.

Make any changes in the plan of care based on the nature of a patient's unfavorable response. Consulting with other health care team members often suggests ways to improve the care delivery approach.

Experienced nurses are often excellent resources and can provide valuable insight. Simply changing a care plan is not enough. Implement the new plan and reevaluate the patient's response to the nursing actions. *Evaluation is continuous, occurring through each step of the nursing process.*

COLLABORATE AND EVALUATE EFFECTIVENESS OF INTERVENTIONS

An important aspect of evaluation is collaboration. Patient-centered care is achieved only when a patient and family are actively involved in the evaluation process. This requires you to consider what is important to your patients, including their values, preferences, and expressed needs. When you develop patient care goals and expected outcomes with patients, they are an important resource for being able to tell you whether outcomes are being met. They are able to share their perspective of whether an intervention is successful. For example, a patient knows best if pain has lessened or if breathing is easier. The same holds true for the family, who often can recognize changes in patient behavior sooner than you can because of their familiarity with the patient.

It is essential for nurses to collaborate closely with all members of the health care team during evaluation. Successful collaboration involves interactions in which professionals work together cooperatively with shared responsibility and interdependence toward achieving patient outcomes. Members of the health care team who contribute to the patient's care also gather evaluative findings. Communicating openly and on a regular basis with the health care team improves the likelihood of staying informed about a patient's responses to care.

Proper evaluation determines the effectiveness of nursing interventions. This includes evaluating whether each patient reaches a level of wellness or recovery that the health care team and patient established in the goals of the care plan. In addition, it is important to evaluate whether you have met a patient's expectations of care. Begin by asking patients about their perceptions of care with questions such as "Are you receiving the type of pain relief you expect?" "Do you have enough information to change your dressing when you return home?" "What is your most important need before going home?" Evaluating patient expectations determines a patient's satisfaction with care and strengthens partnering between you and the patient.

DOCUMENT OUTCOMES

Documentation and reporting are important parts of evaluation because it is crucial to share information about a patient's progress and current status. Accurate information needs to be present in a patient's medical record and shared during hand-off communication so that nurses and other health care team members know whether a patient is progressing and can make ongoing clinical decisions. For example, clearly documented goals and expected outcomes for new or revised nursing diagnoses are necessary so that all team members are aware of a revised care plan. In settings in which the same nurse will not be providing care throughout a patient's stay, it becomes very important to have consistent, thorough documentation of a patient's progress toward expected outcomes. The use of nursing diagnostic language and the NIC and NOC is becoming more common in electronic medical records, improving the quality, consistency, and accuracy of what is documented. In addition, electronic systems provide linkages to make it easier to interpret cues regarding whether interventions led to expected patient outcomes. When documenting a patient's response to your interventions, describe the interventions, the evaluative measures used, the outcomes achieved, and the continued plan of care. *Here is an example of Tonya's documentation of evaluation of care:*

> 1430: Instructed patient on importance of handwashing and need to observe surgical wound daily for signs of redness or drainage from incision. Discussed ways to reduce strain on suture line by avoiding lifting any object over 20 lb, including his grandchildren. Asked patient to describe when it is necessary to call doctor about wound. Patient and wife were able to identify signs of infection and occurrence of pain as reasons to notify doctor. Wife was able to demonstrate proper handwashing technique. Patient was able to verbalize several examples of objects not to lift (grandchild, groceries, trash). Provided patient additional instruction in form of pamphlet with outline of wound care steps. Will recommend to home health the need to observe patient and wife perform wound care at home.

Your documentation should present a clear argument from the evaluative data as to whether a patient is progressing. One of the ANA standards for evaluation is to share results of care with patients and their families according to federal and state regulations (ANA, 2010). Keep patients and families informed about the patients' progress. Be aware of guidelines of your agency for the type of clinical information (e.g., diagnostic findings, results of treatment) that you can communicate.

EVALUATION OF HEALTH CARE

The Centers for Medicaid and Medicare (CMS) do not reimburse health care agencies for the costs associated with treating preventable adverse outcomes such as air embolism, blood incompatibility, or stages III and IV pressure injuries. The occurrence of such outcomes can be potentially fatal to patients. There are 11 preventable adverse outcomes; four of those (severe pressure injuries, falls and trauma, catheter-associated urinary tract infections [CAUTI], and vascular catheter-associated infections) are nursing-sensitive quality outcomes that can potentially be decreased with greater and better nursing care (Burston, et al., 2014; Sung-Heui, 2016). These nursing-sensitive quality outcomes are significant health care problems because they increase patient pain and suffering, prolong hospital stays, and increase health care costs (Burston et al., 2014). As a practicing nurse you will become involved in implementing clinical guidelines, care bundles, and other evidence-based interventions to prevent these outcomes. Health care organizations gather monthly data on the rates of nursing-sensitive preventable outcomes. All patient care units regularly evaluate their progress in reducing these preventable outcomes and implement ongoing quality improvement efforts (see Chapter 5).

A nurse can be most effective in impacting these organization-wide preventable outcomes by delivering patient-centered care and conducting ongoing evaluation of the efficacy of interventions. Learning what is effective for individual patients builds your knowledge of both evidence-based and practical approaches for improving quality of care.

KEY POINTS

- Critical thinking is integral to evaluation as evidenced by the following nursing actions: (1) examining the results of care according to clinical data collected; (2) comparing achieved effects with goals and expected outcomes; (3) recognizing errors or omissions; and (4) understanding a patient situation, participating in self-reflection, and correcting errors.

- Although you may measure or observe assessment and evaluation data in the same way, your assessment identifies what, if any, problems exist while your evaluation determines whether the problems you identified during assessment have remained the same, improved, worsened, or otherwise changed.
- By using the right evaluative measure you are more likely to accurately identify whether there has been a change in a patient's condition.
- During the evaluation phase of the nursing process you perform evaluative measures to compare clinical assessment data, patient behavior, and patient self-reported data collected before implementation with data gathered after administering nursing care to determine whether the results of care match the expected outcomes and goals set for a patient.
- The evaluation process involves the use of observational skills, critical thinking intellectual standards, knowledge, and reflection to recognize errors or omissions so that adjustments to interventions can be made in care plan revision.
- Conducting evaluation involves reviewing evaluative measures to determine whether goals and outcomes are met successfully so that decisions can be made to either continue, discontinue, or revise a plan of care.
- When patients do not meet goals and outcomes, you perform a reassessment and identify the factors that interfere with their achievement, which usually involves a change in a patient's condition, needs, or abilities.

■ REFLECTIVE LEARNING

Tonya organizes herself so that she can take the time needed to evaluate the outcomes of her plan of care. Mr. Lawson has the nursing diagnosis of *Acute Pain related to trauma of surgical incision.* The patient has taken two doses of the prn analgesic ordered for his pain over the past 8 hours. Thirty minutes after the last dose Mr. Lawson rated his pain a 3 on a scale of 0 to 10; he states, "I only really notice the pain now when I move too quickly." An outcome for the patient's goal of achieving pain relief is for pain scores to be at 4 or less. Mrs. Lawson is in the room, so Tonya takes time to give the Lawsons the discharge instruction sheet that is part of the standard of care of her nursing unit. She asks Mr. Lawson to explain the types of activity he must avoid for the first 2 weeks he is at home.

- Describe the type of evaluation measure Tonya uses when asking Mr. Lawson to explain the types of activities he should avoid. What limitations are there in using this type of evaluation measure?
- Explain how Tonya can determine whether the patient's nursing diagnosis of *Acute Pain* has been resolved. Describe how this affects her other priorities.
- Explain how Tonya's evaluation of the patient's ability to learn about activity restrictions can be patient centered.

■ REVIEW QUESTIONS

1. A nurse admits a 32-year-old patient for treatment of acute asthma. The patient has labored breathing, a respiratory rate of 28 per minute, and lung sounds with bilateral wheezing. The nurse makes the patient comfortable and starts an ordered intravenous infusion to administer medication that will relax the patient's airways. The patient tells the nurse after the first medication infusion, "I feel as if I can breathe better." The nurse auscultates the patient's lungs and notes decreased wheezing with a respiratory rate of 22 per minute. Which of the following is an evaluative measure? (Select all that apply.)

   1. Asking patient to breathe deeply during auscultation
   2. Counting respirations per minute
   3. Asking the patient to describe how his breathing feels
   4. Starting the intravenous infusion
   5. Auscultating lung sounds

2. A patient has labored breathing, a respiratory rate of 28 per minute, and lung sounds that reveal wheezing bilaterally. The nurse starts an ordered intravenous infusion to administer medication that will relax the patient's airways. When the nurse asks how the patient feels, he responds by saying, "I feel as if I can breathe better." The nurse auscultates the patient's lungs and notes decreased wheezing with a respiratory rate of 22 per minute. Which of the following evaluative measures may not reflect change in a patient's condition?

   1. Counting respirations per minute
   2. Asking the patient to describe how his breathing feels
   3. Observing breathing pattern
   4. Auscultating lung sounds

3. Which of the following statements correctly describes the evaluation process? (Select all that apply.)

   1. Evaluation involves reflection on the approach to care.
   2. Evaluation involves determination of the completion of a nursing intervention.
   3. Evaluation involves making clinical decisions.
   4. Evaluation requires the use of assessment skills.
   5. Evaluation is performed only when a patient's condition changes.

4. A nurse in a community health clinic has been caring for a young female teenager with diabetes for several months. The nurse's goal of care for this patient is to achieve self-management of insulin medication. Identify appropriate evaluative measures for self-management for this patient. (Select all that apply.)

   1. Quality of life
   2. Patient satisfaction
   3. Clinic follow-up visits
   4. Adherence to self-administration of insulin
   5. Description of side effects of medications

5. From the following list of indicators, determine which indicators are goals (**G**) and which indicators are outcomes (**O**).

   1. _____ Will achieve pain relief
   2. _____ Ambulates 10 feet down hallway
   3. _____ Will remain free of infection
   4. _____ Will be afebrile
   5. _____ Reports pain severity reduced from 6 to a 4 on scale of 0 to 10
   6. _____ Will gain improved mobility

6. A nurse has been caring for a patient over 2 consecutive days. During that time the patient had an intravenous (IV) catheter in the right forearm. At the end of shift on the second day the nurse inspects the catheter site, observes for redness, and asks whether the patient feels tenderness when the site is palpated. The nurse reviews the medical record from 24 hours ago and finds the catheter site was without redness or tenderness. Which of the activities below reflect the nurse's ability to perform patient evaluation? (Select all that apply.)

   1. Comparing patient response with previous response
   2. Examining results of clinical data
   3. Recognizing error
   4. Self-reflection
   5. Checking medical record for when IV was inserted.

7. A nurse asks how a patient's condition from a serious infection changed since yesterday while receiving a hand-off report. The

nurse leaving the shift reports the patient has two priority nursing diagnoses—fluid imbalance and fever. The receiving nurse begins to provide care by measuring the patient's body temperature, inspecting the condition of the skin, reviewing the intake and output record, and checking the summary notes describing the patient's progress since the day before. The nurse asks a technician to measure intake and output during the shift. What critical thinking indicators reflect the nurse's ability to perform evaluation? (Select all that apply.)

1. Checking the summary notes
2. Asking the leaving RN about the patient's condition.
3. Assigning the technician to measure intake and output
4. Comparing current outcomes with those set for the patient's goals
5. Reflecting on patient's progress

8. A nurse in the recovery room is monitoring a patient who had a left knee replacement. The patient arrived in recovery 15 minutes ago. The nurse observes the patient to be restless, turning frequently, and groaning; the patient's heart rate is 92 compared with 76 preoperatively. Blood pressure is stable since admission to the recovery room. The nurse reviews the medical orders for analgesic therapy. The nurse notes that the postop dose of an ordered analgesic has not yet been given. What is most likely to cause the nurse to reflect on the patient's situation?
1. The patient is recovering normally.
2. The symptoms reflecting restlessness
3. The patient's blood pressure trend
4. The delay in administration of the analgesic

9. A nurse enters a patient's room and begins a conversation. During this time the nurse evaluates how a patient is tolerating a new diet plan. The nurse decides to also evaluate the patient's expectations of care. Which of the following is appropriate for evaluating a patient's expectations of care?
1. On a scale of 0 to 10 rate your level of nausea.
2. The nurse weighs the patient.
3. The nurse asks, "Did you believe that you received the information you needed to follow your diet?"
4. The nurse states, "Tell me four different foods included in your diet."

10. Which of the following statements correctly describe the evaluation process? (Select all that apply.)
1. Evaluation is an ongoing process.
2. Evaluation involves the gathering of data for recognizing errors or omissions in care.
3. Evaluation involves making clinical decisions.
4. Evaluation requires the use of assessment skills.
5. Evaluation is done only when a patient's condition changes.

Answers: 1. 2, 3, 5; **2.** 3; **3.** 1, 3, 4; **4.** 1, 3, 4, 5; 1G, 2O, 3G, 4G, 5O, 6G; **6.** 1, 2, 7; **7.** 1, 2, 4, 5; **8.** 4; **9.** 3; **10.** 1, 2, 3, 4.

Rationales for Review Questions can be found on the Evolve website.

REFERENCES

Ackley BJ, et al.: *Nursing diagnosis handbook*, ed 11, St Louis, 2017, Elsevier.

American Nurses Association (ANA): *Scope and standards of practice: nursing*, ed 2, Silver Spring, MD, 2010, American Nurses Association.

Ball J, Griffiths P: *Missed nursing care: a key measure for patient safety*, Agency for Healthcare Research and Quality Patient Safety Network, 2018. https://psnet.ahrq.gov/perspectives/perspective/245/missed-nursing-care-a-key-measure-for-patient-safety. Accessed July 27, 2018.

Burston S, et al.: Nurse-sensitive indicators suitable to reflect nursing care quality: a review and discussion of issues, *J Clin Nurs* 23(13/14):1785, 2014.

European Pressure Ulcer Advisory Panel (EPUAP) and National Pressure Injury Advisory Panel (NPIAP), and Pan Pacific Pressure Injury Alliance: *Treatment of pressure ulcers/injuries: Clinical Practice Guideline. The International Guideline*, Emily Haesler (ED). EPUAP/NPIAP/PPPIA, 2019a.

European Pressure Ulcer Advisory Panel (EPUAP) and National Pressure Injury Advisory Panel (NPIAP), and Pan Pacific Pressure Injury Alliance: *Treatment of pressure*

ulcers/injuries: Quick Reference Guide*, Emily Haesler (ED). EPUAP/NPIAP/PPPIA, 2019b.

Jones T: Outcome measurement in nursing: imperatives, ideals, history, and challenges, *Online J Issues Nurs* 21(2):1, 2016.

Moorhead S, et al.: *Nursing outcomes classification (NOC)*, ed 6, St Louis, 2018, Elsevier.

Royal College of Nursing: *Reflection in action*, 2015. http://rcnhca.org.uk/personal-and-people-development/reflection/reflection-in-action/. Accessed July 27, 2018.

RESEARCH REFERENCES

Boger E, et al.: Self-management and self-management support outcomes: a systematic review and mixed research synthesis of stakeholder views, *PLoS One* 10(7):e0130990, 2015.

Johnson L, et al.: A systematic literature review of accuracy in nursing care plans and using standardised nursing language, *Collegian* 25(3):355, 2018.

National Pressure Ulcer Advisory Panel (NPUAP): *NPUAP pressure injury stages*, 2016. http://www.npuap.org/re-

sources/educational-and-clinical-resources/npuap-pressure-injury-stages/. Accessed July 25, 2018.

Shu-Yuan C, et al.: Identifying critical thinking indicators and critical thinker attributes in nursing practice, *J Nurs Res* 21(3):204, 2013.

Sung-Heui B: The Centers for Medicare & Medicaid services reimbursement policy and nursing-sensitive adverse patient outcomes, *Nurs Econ* 34(4):161, 2016.

Tanner CA: Thinking like a nurse: a research-based model of clinical judgment in nursing, *J Nurs Educ* 45(6):204, 2006.

Thoroddsen A, et al.: Accuracy, completeness and comprehensiveness of information on pressure ulcers recorded in the patient record, *Scand J Caring Sci* 27:84, 2013.

21

Managing Patient Care

OBJECTIVES

- Describe the characteristics and traits of a transformational leader.
- Differentiate among the types of nursing care delivery models.
- Identify the elements of patient- and family-centered care.
- Discuss the ways in which a nurse manager supports staff involvement in a decentralized decision-making model.
- Differentiate among the different elements of the decision-making process

- Create a plan to develop your own leadership.
- Discuss ways to prioritize patient care effectively.
- Discuss evidence-based methods to ensure accurate communication for building teams.
- Discuss principles to follow in the appropriate delegation of patient care activities.

KEY TERMS

Accountability, p. 284
Authority, p. 284
Autonomy, p. 284
Case management, p. 283

Delegation, p. 289
Patient- and family-centered care, p. 283
Responsibility, p. 284
Shared governance, p. 284

Transformational leadership, p. 281

MEDIA RESOURCES

http://evolve.elsevier.com/Potter/fundamentals/
- Review Questions
- Case Study with Questions

- Audio Glossary
- Content Updates
- Answers to QSEN Activity and Review Questions

It is important for you to acquire the necessary knowledge and competencies that ultimately allow you to practice as a nurse. The National Council of State Boards of Nursing (NCSBN, 2018) develops licensure examinations for registered nurses (RNs) and licensed practical nurses (LPNs) to ensure entry-level nurses can safely practice nursing. Although nurse practice acts and professional nursing standards vary, you will be expected to possess certain knowledge, skills, and attitudes when you enter the nursing profession (Box 21.1). Wherever you practice nursing, you use critical thinking to implement professional standards of care, use health care resources appropriately, use time productively, set priorities, collaborate with the health care team, and apply leadership skills. Delivering nursing care within a health care system is a challenge because of the changes that influence health professionals, patients, and health care organizations (see Chapter 2). However, change offers opportunities. As you develop the knowledge and skills to become a nurse, you learn what it takes to effectively manage the patients for whom you care and to take the initiative in becoming a leader among your professional colleagues.

BUILDING A NURSING TEAM

Nurses who work in health care institutions and on units that have cultures that promote autonomy, quality, and collaboration are more satisfied and experience lower levels of moral distress (Hiler et al., 2018; Shimp, 2017). Professional nurses are self-directed and, with proper leadership and motivation, work together to solve complex problems. Your education and commitment to practice nursing within established standards and guidelines help you become part of a cohesive and strong nursing team that values mentoring, integrity, and teamwork. A strong nursing team works together to achieve the best outcomes for patients. Effective team development requires team building and training, trust, communication, and a workplace that facilitates collaboration (Huber, 2018). Patient care units where teamwork is stronger are associated with improved patient safety and nurse well-being (Welp and Manser, 2016). Stronger levels of teamwork among nurses often contribute to higher levels of job satisfaction among nurses (Kaiser and Westers, 2018).

An empowering work environment brings out the best in nurses. It concentrates on effective patient care systems, supports risk taking and innovation, focuses on results and rewards, and offers professional opportunities for growth and advancement. Building an empowered nursing team begins with the nurse executive, who is often a chief nursing officer. The executive's position within an organization is critical in uniting the strategic direction of an organization with the philosophical values and goals of nursing. The nurse executive is a clinical and business leader who is concerned with maximizing quality of care and cost-effectiveness while maintaining relationships and professional satisfaction of the staff. Perhaps the most important responsibility of the nurse executive is to establish a philosophy for nursing that enables managers and staff to provide quality nursing care.

Effective nurse managers play a critical role in developing successful teams that work together (Huber, 2018; James, 2018; Kivland, 2018) (Box 21.2). The nurse manager who uses transformational leadership is focused on change and innovation through team development,

---

BOX 21.1 Entry-Level Nurse Knowledge, Skills, and Attitudes

- Value placing the patient at the center of care.
- Respect patients' rights, beliefs, culture, spirituality, preferences, values, and needs.
- Understand the health care system and processes to promote safety, reduce harm, and enhance efficiency and effectiveness.
- Manage patient care.
- Think critically and make clinical decisions using the nursing process.
- Use data to monitor outcomes, assess problems, identify and implement solutions, evaluate care, and follow up appropriately.
- Communicate effectively with patients and health care team members, and document events and activities surrounding patient care appropriately in written and/or electronic records.
- Use evidence-based interventions when providing patient care.
- Promote change in patient behavior when needed using appropriate teaching and learning strategies.
- Demonstrate nursing knowledge and display confidence in knowledge base.
- Work effectively in nursing and interprofessional teams, recognizing the contributions of all team members, encouraging open communication, and fostering shared decision making.
- Recognize own limitations and seek help as needed.

Modified from NCSBN: NCLEX-RN® examination test plan for the National Council Licensure Examination for Registered Nurses, 2018, https://www.ncsbn.org/2019_RN_TestPlan-English.pdf; QSEN Institute: QSEN Competencies, 2018, http://qsen.org/competencies/pre-licensure-ksas/. Accessed September 2018.

BOX 21.2 Characteristics of Effective Leaders

- Develop interpersonal trust and ensure effective communication with individuals and teams.
- Have awareness of personal strengths and weaknesses, allowing vulnerabilities to show.
- Take initiative and sustain motivation, especially during times of uncertainty.
- Seek multiple perspectives and opinions to generate options and solutions when problem solving.
- Rebound from setbacks with positivity.
- Understand what they can and cannot change.
- Schedule time and space to regularly reflect, recharge, and reframe.
- Take responsibility for decisions.
- Display caring, understanding, and empathy for others.
- Motivate and empower others.
- Identify need to change and support change effectively.
- Use different leadership styles (e.g., transformational, authentic, value-based) appropriately.

Modified from James AH: Action learning can support leadership development for undergraduate and postgraduate nurses, *Br J Nurs* 27(15):876, 2018; Kivland C: Successfully managing emotions and behavior: emotional intelligence matters more than ever to your leadership career, *Healthc Exec* 33(1):68, 2018; Huber DL: *Leadership & nursing care management*, ed 6, St Louis, 2018, Elsevier.

---

serves as a mentor for staff, and develops and supports the moral agency of nurses (Grace, 2018; Huber, 2018). Transformational leaders spend time on the unit with the staff sharing ideas, empowering the staff, supporting opportunities to enhance the team, showing appreciation and recognizing team members for a job well done, and holding team members accountable.

Together a manager and the nursing staff share a philosophy of care for their work unit. A philosophy of care includes the professional nursing staff's values and concerns for the way they view and care for patients. For example, a philosophy addresses the purpose of the nursing unit, how staff members work with patients and families, and the standards of care for the work unit. Selection of a nursing care delivery model and a management structure that supports professional nursing practice are essential to the philosophy of care.

A nurse manager's leadership style affects the work environment and patient outcomes. Contemporary nurse leaders have a shared vision that leads the team to a common goal. Because nurses have specialized knowledge, they need leaders who value and foster the attainment of new knowledge (Huber, 2018). Nurse managers who use interactional and relationship-based leadership styles create a positive work environment by fostering interaction and generating stability to create the energy a team needs to adapt to and grow with a constantly changing health care environment (Huber, 2018).

One contemporary relationship-based leadership style is servant leadership. Servant leaders choose to serve others before they decide to become leaders. Their priority is putting the needs of others first and promoting personal growth and autonomy by ensuring their individual employee's highest priority needs are met (Huber, 2018; Savel and Munro, 2017). Servant nurse leaders work closely with their team to understand individual member's strengths and weaknesses. A servant leader creates teams based on this understanding and ensures that the nurses on

a unit are working in the positions that best use their strengths (Savel and Munro, 2017). Servant nurse leaders also practice humility. They understand that although they possess a great deal of knowledge, they do not know all the answers. They remain modest and calm, and they give credit to their staff for successes (Savel and Munro, 2017). Effective nurse leaders use a variety of evidence-based strategies to create healthy work environments and lead their teams through change (Box 21.3).

Magnet Recognition Program®

One way of creating an empowering work environment is through the Magnet Recognition Program (see Chapter 2). The Magnet Recognition Program is based on five model components—transformational leadership; structural empowerment; exemplary professional practice, new knowledge, innovation, and improvements; and empirical quality results (American Nurses Credentialing Center [ANCC], n.d.). A hospital that is Magnet® certified has a transformed culture with a practice environment that is dynamic, autonomous, collaborative, and positive for nurses. The culture focuses on concern for patients. Typically, a Magnet hospital has clinical promotion systems and research- and evidence-based practice programs. The nurses have professional autonomy over their practice and control over the practice environment (Stimpfel et al., 2016). A Magnet hospital empowers a nursing team to make changes and be innovative (Nelson-Brantley et al., 2018). Professional nurse councils at the organizational and unit level help to create an empowerment model. This culture and empowerment combine to produce a strong collaborative relationship among team members and improve patient quality outcomes (ANCC, n.d.; Stimpfel et al., 2016).

Nursing Care Delivery Models

A nursing care delivery model allows you to help your patients achieve desirable outcomes. Nursing care delivery models contain the common components of nurse-patient relationship, clinical decision making, methods for patient assignments and work allocation, interprofessional communication, and management of the environment of care (Huber, 2018).

BOX 21.3 EVIDENCE-BASED PRACTICE

Nurses Work Engagement

PICOT Question: Do nurse leaders who use transformational or relationship-based leadership strategies create healthier work environments and improve patient outcomes?

Evidence Summary

Creating healthy work environments and improving patient outcomes requires effective nursing leadership at all levels in an organization, from the nurse executive to the nurse manager to the staff nurses. Effective nurse leaders often use transformational or relationship-based leadership to create workplaces that promote better outcomes for patients and nurses (Alilyyani et al., 2018; Boamah et al., 2018).

Nurses who attend professional leadership development programs have improved collaboration and communication skills, which ultimately leads to a healthy work environment and better patient outcomes (Lacey et al., 2017). Focusing on transformational or relationship-based leadership is supported by current evidence. For example, authentic leadership, a type of relationship-based leadership, has been shown to improve the work environment (e.g., job satisfaction, employee health and well-being) and patient outcomes (Alilyyani et al., 2018). Authentic leaders choose a leadership style consistent with their personalities. They are dedicated to their own growth and build strong relationships with others. Regardless of the leadership strategy used, strong clinical leaders who encourage collaboration and regular interaction among nurse experts within the same health care organization or across different organizations create environments that have a positive impact on patient outcomes, quality of care, and the culture of the workplace (Brown et al., 2016).

Application to Nursing Practice

- Build positive relationships with colleagues on your nursing unit (Nelson-Bratley, 2018; Alilyyani et al., 2018) as well as with colleagues who work in other health care organizations (Brown et al., 2016).
- Attend professional conferences to stimulate your personal and professional growth and develop your leadership and communication skills (Lacey et al., 2017; Boamah et al., 2018).
- Be engaged with initiatives in your organization that focus on reducing hospital-acquired conditions (e.g., falls, pressure injuries, catheter-associated urinary tract infections) (Lacey et al., 2017).
- Respect the contributions of all members of the health care team and make a conscious commitment to make a positive impact in your workplace every day (Alilyyani et al., 2018; Boamah et al., 2018).

Two classic nursing models used in some health care institutions are team nursing and primary nursing. In team nursing, care is provided by a group of people led by an RN. The team often includes other RNs, practical nurses, and assistive personnel (APs). To be successful, this model requires effective team leadership, collaboration, and communication (Huber, 2018).

In primary nursing, one RN assumes the responsibility for a caseload of patients from admission to discharge. The same nurse provides care for the same patients throughout their hospitalization. When the nurse is not scheduled to work on the unit, directions are left (in plan of care or other communication mode) for other RNs to follow the plan of care. The model became more popular in the 1970s and early 1980s as hospitals began to employ more RNs. It is typically not practiced today because of the high cost of an all-RN staffing model (Huber, 2018). Total patient care is similar to primary nursing. In this model an RN is responsible for all aspects of care for one or more patients during a shift of care, working directly with patients, families, and health team members.

More common models used today are patient- and family-centered care and case management. **Patient- and family-centered care** promotes mutual partnerships among the patient, family, and health care team to plan, implement, and evaluate nursing and health. At the center of patient-centered care is the patient or family member as the source of control and full partner in providing care (QSEN Institute, 2018). An RN is the health care leader that assesses patient needs, recognizes clinical changes, and directs care. The Institute for Patient-and Family-Centered Care identified four core concepts for patient-centered care (IPFCC, n.d.):

1. *Dignity and respect,* ensuring that the care provided is given on the basis of a patient's and family's knowledge, values, beliefs, and cultural backgrounds
2. *Information sharing,* meaning that health care providers communicate and share information so that patients and families receive timely, complete, and accurate information to effectively participate in care and decision making
3. *Participation,* whereby patients and families are encouraged and supported in participating in care and decision making
4. *Collaboration,* demonstrated by the health care leaders collaborating with patients and families in policy and program development, implementation, and evaluation and patients who are fully engaged in their health care

Nurses support and promote patient engagement and empowerment when using patient- and family-centered communication, bedside shift report, and patient- and family-centered interprofessional rounds (IPFCC, n.d.; Bigani and Correia, 2018).

Case management coordinates and links health care services across all levels of care for patients and their families while streamlining costs and maintaining quality (see Chapter 2). The case-management system is focused on achieving patient outcomes within effective time frames and with available resources (Huber, 2018). Case managers work with patients to identify issues and overcome barriers to help patients become healthier (CMSA, 2015). Current evidence shows case managers link and coordinate health care services to patients and their families while achieving quality cost-effective outcomes (Brown et al., 2017). Case managers, either individually or as part of a team, oversee the management of patients with complex nursing and medical problems (e.g., patients with diabetes or traumatic brain injury) across all levels of care. Case managers are often advanced practice nurses who, through specific interventions, help to improve patient outcomes, optimize patient safety by facilitating care transitions, decrease length of stay, and lower health care costs. They are accountable for cost management and quality.

For example, a case manager coordinates a patient's acute care in the hospital and follows up with the patient after discharge, either to home, rehabilitation, or a long-term care setting. Case managers do not provide direct care. Instead, they collaborate with direct-care providers and actively coordinate patient discharge planning. Ongoing communication with team members facilitates a patient's transition to home. Case managers help patients identify health needs, determine the services and resources that are available, and make cost-efficient choices.

Decision Making

Decision making is a critical skill for an effective leader and manager (Huber, 2018). A nurse executive supports nurse managers by advocating a nursing governance structure that incorporates policies and procedures for decision making needed to achieve organizational goals. A nurse manager directs and supports a group of staff in applying an organization's nursing philosophy. Thus, it takes a committed nurse executive, excellent nurse managers, and an empowered nursing staff to create an enriching work environment. Box 21.4 highlights the diverse responsibilities of nursing managers.

BOX 21.4 Responsibilities of a Nurse Manager

- Collaborate with staff to establish annual goals for the unit and the systems needed to accomplish goals (e.g., assignment methods, quality improvement activities, patient education methods).
- Monitor professional nursing standards of practice on the unit.
- Develop an ongoing staff development plan, including one for new employees.
- Recruit new employees (interview and hire).
- Conduct routine staff evaluations.
- Role model positive customer service (customers include patients, families, and other health care team members).
- Submit staffing schedules for the unit.
- Advocate for the nursing staff to the administration of the organization.
- Conduct regular patient rounds and problem solve patient or family complaints.
- Establish, monitor, and implement a quality improvement (QI) plan for the unit.
- Review and recommend new equipment for the unit.
- Conduct regular staff meetings.
- Make rounds with health care providers.
- Establish and support staff and interprofessional committees.

Decentralization is a component of the hierarchical level of decision making found in health care institutions. This management approach allows decisions to be made at the staff level. Shared governance is the typical decentralized structure used within health care organizations today (Huber, 2018). This structure creates an environment in which managers and staff become more actively involved in making decisions to shape the identity and determine the success of a health care organization. Working in a decentralized structure has the potential for greater collaborative effort, increased competency of staff, increased staff motivation, and ultimately a greater sense of professional accomplishment and satisfaction (Huber, 2018; Sulit Oriza et al., 2016).

Progressive organizations achieve more when employees at all levels are empowered and actively involved in decision making. As a result, the role of a nurse manager is critical in the management of effective nursing units or groups. To make shared governance work, managers move decision making down to the lowest level possible. On a nursing unit it is important for all nursing staff members (RNs, LPNs, and LVNs), nursing assistants, and unit secretaries to become engaged and provide input on practice issues and unit operations. They need to be kept well informed of unit and organizational initiatives. Giving staff the opportunity to participate in problem-solving activities related to direct patient care and unit activities promotes a high level of employee engagement—a key factor in promoting teamwork and collaboration and a healthy work environment (Sulit Oriza et al., 2016). Important elements of the decision-making process are responsibility, autonomy, authority, and accountability.

Responsibility refers to the duties and activities that you are employed to perform. A position description outlines your responsibilities as a professional nurse and your expected level of participation as a member of a nursing unit.

Responsibility reflects ownership and obligation. An individual who manages employees distributes responsibility, and the employees accept it. Managers need to ensure that staff clearly understand their responsibilities, particularly in the face of change. For example, when hospitals participate in work redesign, patient care delivery models change significantly. A manager is responsible for clearly defining an RN's role within a new care delivery model. If decentralized decision making is in place, the professional nursing staff needs to be engaged to define the new RN role. Each RN on the team is responsible for knowing his or her role and how to perform that role on the busy nursing unit. For example, nurses are responsible for completing a nursing assessment of all assigned patients and developing a plan of care that addresses each of the patient's nursing diagnoses (Huber, 2018) (see Chapters 16 to 20). As the staff implements the plan of care, the nurse evaluates whether the plan is successful. This responsibility becomes a work ethic for the nurse in delivering excellent patient care.

Autonomy is freedom of choice and responsibility for the choices. Autonomy consistent with the scope of professional nursing practice maximizes a nurse's effectiveness (Huber, 2018). With clinical autonomy you make independent decisions about patient care, plan patient care within the scope of professional nursing practice, and implement independent nursing interventions (see Chapter 19). Another type of autonomy for nurses is work autonomy. In work autonomy a nurse makes independent decisions about the work of the unit such as scheduling or unit governance. Autonomy is not an absolute; it occurs in degrees. For example, you have the autonomy to develop and implement a discharge teaching plan based on specific patient needs for your patients and their family caregivers. However, if your unit does not use self-scheduling, you do not have the autonomy to create your own schedule.

Authority refers to the legal ability to perform a task (Huber, 2018). It provides the power for a nurse to make final decisions and give instructions related to the decisions. You use authority to determine whether collaboration was successful. For example, while managing the care of a patient, you discover that one of the members of the health care team, the registered dietitian, did not follow through on a discharge teaching plan. You have the authority to consult with the dietitian to learn why the recommendations on the plan of care were not implemented and to review the established plan to ensure recommended patient teaching is completed.

Accountability refers to individuals being answerable for their actions. It involves follow-up and a reflective analysis of decisions and an evaluation of their effectiveness. It means that as a nurse you take responsibility to provide excellent patient care by following standards of practice and institutional policies and procedures. You assume responsibility for the outcomes of the actions, judgments, and omissions in providing that care. You are not accountable for the overall outcomes of patient care, but you are accountable for what you do (i.e., performing the nursing process, performing nursing procedures correctly, communicating effectively with health care team colleagues, and staying current on nursing practice issues). You will sometimes delegate responsibility, but you remain accountable for the care you delegated. For example, you delegate taking your patient's vital signs to an AP. You are responsible for knowing what your patient's vital signs are normally and for providing appropriate care if the vital signs are not in the expected range (e.g., verifying the temperature and giving acetaminophen as ordered when your patient's temperature is elevated).

Members of a successful nursing unit support the four elements of decision making: responsibility, autonomy, authority, and accountability. An effective nurse manager sets expectations for the staff in how decisions are made. Staff members need to feel comfortable in expressing differences of opinion and challenging ways in which the team functions. Ultimately shared governance helps the staff on a nursing unit to implement its philosophy and vision of professional nursing care.

Staff Involvement. When transformational or relationship-based leadership and decentralized decision making exist on a nursing unit, all staff members actively participate in unit activities (Fig. 21.1).

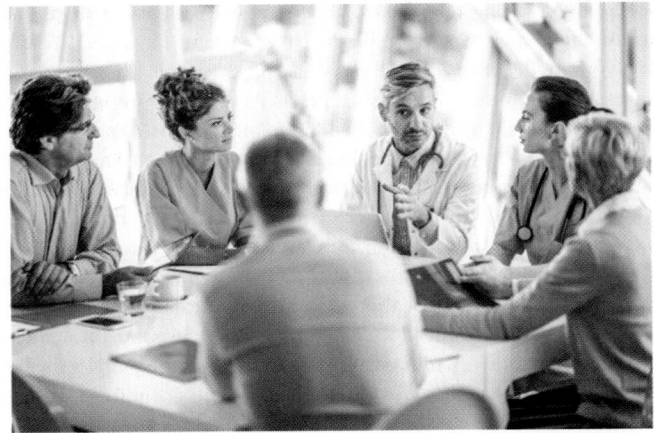

FIG. 21.1 Staff collaborating on practice issues. (Copyright © iStock/skynesher.)

Because the work environment promotes participation, all staff members benefit from the knowledge and skills of the entire work group. If the staff learns to value the pursuit of knowledge and the contributions of co-workers, better patient care results. Recognizing nurses' exceptional work with patients helps reinforce these behaviors, creates a healthy work environment, and reduces nurse burnout (Kelly and Lefton, 2017). Healthy work environments have nurses who are skilled in communication, promote true collaboration among health care team members, encourage effective decision making, have appropriate levels of staffing to meet patient needs, recognize nurses in a meaningful way, and have an authentic nurse leader (AACN, n.d.). Authentic leadership results in greater nurse empowerment, improved culture and climate, increased implementation of evidence-based practice, better teamwork between nurses and physicians, greater role clarity, and reduced conflict and ambiguity. The nursing manager supports staff involvement through a variety of approaches:

1. **Establishing nursing practice through problem-solving committees or professional shared governance councils.** Staff committees establish and maintain care standards for nursing practice on their unit. Shared governance is a dynamic process that promotes decision making, accountability, and empowerment in staff nurses and enables them to make meaningful and sustainable changes in patient care (Huber, 2018; Gordon, 2016). The committees review ongoing clinical care issues, identify problems, apply evidence-based practice in establishing standards of care, develop policy and procedures, implement new practice approaches, resolve patient satisfaction issues, or develop new documentation tools. It is important for the committees to balance their focus between patient outcomes and work issues to ensure quality care on the unit. Quality of care is improved when nurses control their own practice. The committee establishes methods to ensure that all staff have input on practice issues. Managers do not always sit on a committee, but they receive regular reports of committee progress. The nature of work on the nursing unit determines committee membership. At times members of other disciplines (e.g., pharmacy, respiratory therapy, or clinical nutrition) participate in practice committees or shared governance councils.

2. **Interprofessional collaboration among nurses and health care providers.** Interprofessional collaboration among nurses and health care providers (e.g., medical doctors, physical therapists, respiratory therapists) is critical to the delivery of quality, safe patient care and the creation of a positive work culture for practitioners (McBeth et al., 2017; Interprofessional Education Collaborative Expert Panel [IECEP], 2016). Interprofessional collaboration involves bringing various disciplines together to work with patients and families to deliver quality care (IECEP, 2016). Interprofessional collaboration involves all professions bringing different points of view to the table to identify, clarify, and solve complex patient problems together, providing integrated and cohesive patient care (Goldsberry, 2018). The nurse plays a unique role within the team and is often viewed as the team leader because it is the nurse who takes on the responsibilities of coordination of communication and patient care (QSEN Institute, 2018). Open communication, cooperation, trust, mutual respect, and understanding of team member roles and responsibilities are critical for successful interprofessional collaboration (QSEN Institute, 2018; IECEP, 2016). The IECEP (2016) identified four competencies that health care practitioners need to be effective team members in interprofessional collaboration. The development of these competencies comes through interprofessional education (Homeyer et al., 2018). Competencies needed for effective interpersonal collaboration include:

   - *Values/ethics for interprofessional practice:* Work with individuals of other professions to maintain a climate of mutual respect and shared values.
   - *Roles/responsibilities:* Use the knowledge of one's own role and those of other professions to appropriately assess and address the health care needs of patients and to promote and advance the health of populations.
   - *Interprofessional communication:* Communicate with patients, families, communities, and professionals in health and other fields in a responsive and responsible manner that supports a team approach to promote and maintain health and prevent and treat disease.
   - *Teams and teamwork:* Apply relationship-building values and the principles of team dynamics to perform effectively in different team roles to plan, deliver, and evaluate patient- or population-centered care and population health programs and policies that are safe, timely, efficient, effective, and equitable.

3. **Interprofessional rounding.** Many institutions that focus on patient- and family-centered care conduct interprofessional rounding to encourage patient and family involvement in planning care, improve patient care coordination, and enhance communication among the health care team (Bigani and Correia, 2018). During rounding members of the team meet and share patient information, answer questions asked by other team members, discuss a patient's clinical progress and plans for discharge, and focus all team members on the same patient goals (Prystajecky et al., 2017; McBeth, 2017). Interprofessional rounding improves decision making, nurses' job satisfaction, and quality of care (Perry et al., 2016). For interprofessional rounding to be successful, health care team members need to be flexible and open to ideas, questions, and suggestions offered by others.

4. **Staff communication.** A manager's greatest challenge, especially if a work group is large, is communication with staff. It is difficult to make sure that all staff members receive consistent, clear, accurate, and timely information. Lack of communication about planned changes often leads to mistrust among staff members. However, a manager cannot assume total responsibility for all communication. An effective manager uses a variety of approaches to communicate quickly and accurately to all staff. For example, many managers distribute biweekly or monthly newsletters of ongoing unit or agency activities. Minutes of committee meetings are usually in an accessible location for all staff to read or are sent to individuals via e-mail. When the team needs to discuss important issues regarding the operations of the unit, the manager conducts staff meetings. When the unit has practice- or quality-improvement committees, each committee member has the responsibility to communicate directly to a select number of staff members. Thus, all staff members are contacted and given the opportunity for input.

5. **Staff education.** A professional nursing staff needs to always grow in knowledge. It is impossible to remain knowledgeable about current medical and nursing practice trends without ongoing education. A nurse manager is responsible for making learning opportunities available, so staff members remain competent in their practice and empowered in their decision making. This involves planning in-service programs, sending staff to continuing education classes and professional conferences, and having staff present case studies or evidence-based practice issues during staff meetings. Staff members are responsible for pursuing educational opportunities for relicensure/recertification and changing information regarding their patient population.

LEADERSHIP SKILLS FOR NURSING STUDENTS

It is important to prepare yourself for leadership roles from the time you decide to become a nurse. Begin by being a dependable, respectful, and competent team member. As a nursing student you are responsible and accountable for the care you give to your patients. Learn to become a leader by consulting with instructors and nursing staff to obtain feedback in making good clinical decisions, learning from mistakes and seeking guidance, working closely with professional nurses, and trying to improve your performance during each patient interaction. These skills require you to think critically and solve problems in the clinical setting (see Chapter 15). Thinking critically allows you to provide high-quality care, meet the needs of your patients while considering their preferences, consider alternatives to problems, understand the rationale for performing nursing interventions, and evaluate the effectiveness of care. Clinical experiences develop these critical thinking skills (Benner et al., 2010). Important leadership skills to learn include clinical care coordination, team communication, delegation, and knowledge building.

> ### REFLECT NOW
>
> Think about what you have learned about leadership development so far. Create a personal plan you can use to help you develop your own leadership skills.

Clinical Care Coordination

You acquire necessary knowledge and skills so you can deliver patient care competently and effectively. In the beginning you will probably care for only one patient, but eventually you will be able to care for groups of patients. To coordinate the clinical care of patients, you need to learn how to make clinical decisions, set priorities, delegate safely, gain organizational skills, use resources, manage time, and evaluate your patient's outcomes. Clinical care coordination requires you to use critical reflection and reasoning and clinical judgment (Benner et al., 2010). These are important first steps in developing a caring relationship with a patient. Use a critical thinking approach, applying previous knowledge and experience to the decision-making process (see Chapter 15).

Clinical Decisions. You will make clinical decisions by applying the nursing process (see Chapters 16 to 20). You begin caring for a patient by conducting a focused but complete assessment so that you know your patient and can make accurate clinical judgments (see Chapter 16). Knowing the patient involves more than gathering formal assessment data. It requires learning a patient's typical patterns of responses and his or her current situation and knowing the patient as an individual. Your initial contact with a patient is an important first step in developing a caring relationship. Encouraging patients to share their stories about their health problems is very useful (e.g., say, "Tell me how you are dealing with …" or "Can you share what has been your biggest problem since becoming ill?"). After obtaining a thorough assessment and identifying a patient's nursing diagnoses and problems, you develop a plan of care, implement nursing interventions, and evaluate patient outcomes. The process requires clinical decision making using a critical thinking approach (see Chapter 15).

Accurate clinical decision making ensures therapeutic nursing care, especially when a patient's condition changes. An important lesson in organizational skills is to be thorough. Learn to attend and listen to the patient, look for any cues (obvious or subtle) that point to a pattern of findings, and direct your assessment to explore the pattern further. Never hesitate to ask for assistance when a patient's condition changes.

Priority Setting. After forming a picture of a patient's total needs, you set priorities by deciding which patient needs or problems need attention first (see Chapter 18). Priority setting is not the ordering of a list of care tasks but rather a way to organize your care. Symptom pattern recognition from your assessment database and your knowledge help you understand which diagnoses require intervention and the associated time frame to intervene effectively (Ackley and Ladwig, 2017). It is important to set priorities whenever you provide patient care because it allows you to see the most important issues as well as the relationships among patient problems and avoid delays in taking action that can lead to serious complications for a patient. If a patient is experiencing serious physiological or psychological problems, the priority becomes clear. You need to act immediately to stabilize his or her condition.

Nurses prioritize care in different ways. If you use Maslow's hierarchy of needs, you meet a patient's physiological needs such as oxygen, food, water, sleep, and elimination first. Once physiological needs are met, you help patients meet their higher-level needs, such as safety, security, belonging, esteem, and self-actualization. To prioritize your care, evaluate and weigh each competing task by reflecting on the following three questions:

- Is this a life-threatening situation? Will this patient or another patient be endangered if this task is not done immediately or is left for later?
- Is this task essential to patient or staff safety?
- Is this task essential to the patient's plan of care?

When prioritizing care, you need to understand the "big picture" of your patient's problems and goals. Once you know all your patient's problems, determine the relationships among the problems. Remember that setting priorities is a dynamic process; it changes frequently (Alfaro-Lefevre, 2017). Always give high priority to patient and caregiver safety (e.g., fall prevention, safe medication administration, and patient education needs). Use the following steps to classify problems into one of three priority levels, and use this information to help you set priorities (Alfaro-Lefevre, 2017):

1. Assign high priority to first-level problems using *ABC+VL* (**a**irway, **b**reathing, **c**ardiac and circulation problems, **v**ital signs concerns, and **l**ife-threatening laboratory values) and attend to these immediately.
2. Next address second-level problems, which immediately follow the first level and include concerns such as changes in mental status, untreated medical issues, acute pain, acute elimination problems, abnormal laboratory results, and risks.
3. Then tend to third-level problems, which are health problems other than those at the first two levels, such as long-term issues in health management, rest, and family coping.

Many patients have all three levels of problems, requiring you to make careful judgments in choosing a course of action. High-priority needs demand immediate attention. When a patient has diverse priority needs, it helps to focus on his or her basic needs. For example, a patient who just ambulated down the hall is short of breath. The dietary assistant arrives in the room to deliver a meal tray. Instead of immediately helping the patient with the meal, you position him comfortably in bed, offer basic hygiene measures, and then evaluate his breathlessness. The patient is likely to become more interested in eating after he is more comfortable. He also is more receptive to any instruction you need to provide.

Eventually you will be required to meet the priority needs of a group of patients. This means that you need to know the priorities of each patient within the group, assessing each patient's needs as soon as possible while addressing high priorities first. Use information from the change-of-shift or hand-off report, the patient acuity classification system, and information from the medical record to determine which patient to assess first. Over time you learn to spontaneously rank patients' needs by priority or urgency. Priorities do not remain stable but change as a patient's condition changes. It is important to think about the resources available, be flexible in recognizing that priority needs often change, and consider how to use time wisely.

You also set priorities based on your patient's expectations. Sometimes you establish an excellent plan of care; however, if a patient resists certain therapies or disagrees with your approach, your care will not be effective or safe. Be caring and work closely with a patient and family caregiver when setting priorities to establish trust and cooperation.

> ### REFLECT NOW
>
> Think about a patient you cared for recently. How did you prioritize the care you provided your patient? Did you provide care that was effective and efficient? What could you have done differently to improve your prioritization?

Organizational Skills. Implementing a plan of care requires you to be effective and efficient. Effective use of time means doing the right things, whereas efficient use of time means doing things right. Learn to become efficient by combining various nursing activities (i.e., doing more than one thing at a time). For example, during medication administration or while obtaining a specimen, combine therapeutic communication, teaching interventions, and assessment and evaluation. Always establish and strengthen relationships with patients and use any patient contact as an opportunity to convey important information. Patient interaction gives you the chance to show caring and interest. Always attend to a patient's behaviors and responses to therapies to assess whether new problems are developing and to evaluate responses to interventions.

It is easier to provide patient care if you are organized. A well-organized nurse approaches any procedure by having all the necessary equipment available and making sure that the patient is prepared. If the patient is comfortable and well informed, the procedure will probably go smoothly. Sometimes you need help from colleagues to perform or complete a procedure. Keep the work area organized and complete preliminary steps before asking co-workers for assistance.

Although you plan and deliver care based on established priorities, events sometimes occur that interfere with your plans. For example, just as you begin to bathe a patient, an x-ray technician enters to take a chest x-ray film. Once the technician takes the x-ray, a phlebotomist arrives to draw a blood sample. In this case your priorities conflict with the priorities of other health care personnel. It is important to always keep a patient's needs at the center of attention. If the patient experienced symptoms earlier that required a chest x-ray film and laboratory work, it is important to be sure that the diagnostic tests are completed. In another example a patient is waiting to visit family, and a chest x-ray film is a routine order. The patient's condition is stable, and the x-ray technician is willing to return later to shoot the film. In this case attending to the patient's hygiene and comfort so that family members can visit is the higher priority.

Use of Resources. Appropriate use of resources is an important aspect of clinical care coordination. Resources include members of the health care team. In any setting providing patient care occurs more smoothly when staff members work together. Never hesitate to have staff help you, especially when there is an opportunity to make a procedure or activity more comfortable and safer for patients. For example, assistance in turning, positioning, and ambulating patients is frequently necessary when patients have mobility limitations. Having a staff member such as an AP assist with handling equipment and supplies during complicated procedures such as catheter insertion or dressing changes makes procedures more efficient. In addition, you need to recognize personal limitations and use professional resources for assistance. For example, you assess a patient and find relevant clinical signs and symptoms but are unfamiliar with the physical condition. Consulting with an experienced RN confirms findings and ensures that you take the proper course of action for the patient. Leaders know their limitations and seek professional colleagues for guidance and support.

Time Management. Shorter hospital stays, early discharges, same-day surgeries, and increasing complexity in patient's needs create stress for nurses as they work to meet patient needs in hospital settings (Huber, 2018). One way to manage this stress is to use time-management skills. These skills involve learning how, where, and when to use your time. Because you have a limited amount of time with patients, it is essential to remain goal oriented and use time wisely. Managing yourself better leads to better time management and reduces the risk of developing burnout (Moss and Good, 2016). Effective time management includes being prepared, being organized, and managing priorities.

Make efficient and effective use of your time by remaining focused on your patient's goals. However, also learn how to establish personal goals and realistic time frames. For example, you are caring for two patients on a busy surgical nursing unit. One had surgery the day before, and the other will be discharged the next day. The first patient's goals center on restoring physiological function that is impaired because of surgery. The second patient's goals center on adequate preparation to assume self-care at home. In reviewing the therapies required for both patients, you learn how to organize your time so that you complete your nursing care and your patients achieve their goals. Anticipate when care will be interrupted for medication administration and diagnostic testing, and determine the best time for planned therapies such as dressing changes, patient education, and patient ambulation. Delegating tasks is another way to help improve time management.

One useful time-management skill involves making a to-do list. When you begin to work with patients, it helps to make a list that sequences the nursing activities you need to perform. The hand-off report at the change of shift helps you prioritize activities based on what you learn about a patient's condition and the care provided before you arrived on the unit.

Consider activities that have specific time limits in terms of addressing patient needs such as administering a pain medication before a scheduled procedure or instructing patients before their discharge home. You also analyze the items on the list that are scheduled by agency policies or routines (e.g., medications or intravenous [IV] tubing changes). Note which activities need to be done on time and which

---

BOX 21.5 Principles of Time Management

Goal setting: Review a patient's goals of care for the day and any goals you have for activities such as completing documentation, attending a patient care conference, giving a hand-off report, or preparing medications for administration.

Time analysis: Reflect on how you use your time. While working on a clinical area, keep track of how you use your time in different activities. This helps you become more aware of how well organized you really are and areas you may need to improve upon.

Priority setting: Set the priorities that you have established for patients within set time frames. For example, determine when is the best time to have teaching sessions, plan ambulation, and provide rest periods based on what you know about a patient's condition. For example, if a patient is nauseated or in pain, it is not a good time for a teaching session.

Interruption control: Everyone needs time to socialize or discuss issues with colleagues. However, do not let this interrupt important patient care activities such as medication administration (see Chapter 31), ordered treatments, or teaching sessions. Use time during report, mealtime, or team meetings to your advantage. In addition, plan time to help fellow colleagues so that it complements your patient care schedule.

Evaluation: At the end of each day take time to think and reflect about how effectively you used your time. If you are having difficulties, discuss them with an instructor or a more experienced staff member.

BOX 21.6 Key TeamSTEPPS® Principles

Team Structure: Identify the complex parts of the health care system that have to work together effectively to promote patient safety.

Communication: Use structured processes to clearly and accurately exchange information among members of the health care team.

Leadership: Ensure that all members of the health care team understand the team's actions, receive information about changes, and have resources needed to perform their jobs.

Situation Monitoring: Actively assess any situation to gather information, improve your understanding, or maintain awareness to support the functioning of the team.

Mutual Support: Understand the responsibilities and workload of all team members so that you can anticipate and support their needs.

Modified from Agency for Healthcare Research and Quality (AHRQ): Pocket guide: TeamSTEPPS®, 2014, https://www.ahrq.gov/team-stepps/instructor/essentials/pocketguide.html#frame. Accessed September 2018.

activities you can do at your discretion. You need to administer medication within a specific schedule, but you are also able to perform other activities while in the patient's room. Finally, estimate the amount of time needed to complete the various activities. Activities requiring the assistance of other staff members usually take longer because you have to plan around their schedules.

Good time management also involves setting goals to help you complete one task before starting another. You will always deliver care to a group of patients, moving back and forth between patients as needs and priorities change. If possible, complete an activity started with one patient before moving on to the next. Care is less fragmented, and you are better able to focus on what you are doing for each patient. As a result, you will be less likely to make errors. Time management requires you to anticipate the activities of the day and combine activities when possible. When you practice good time management, you focus on organization and setting priorities. Other strategies include keeping your work area clean and clutter free and trying to decrease interruptions as you are completing tasks. Box 21.5 summarizes principles of time management.

Evaluation. Evaluation is one of the most important aspects of clinical care coordination (see Chapter 20). You constantly evaluate a patient's condition and progress toward an expected patient outcome. Evaluation is an ongoing process. It does not occur only at the end of an activity. Once you assess a patient's needs and implement interventions for a patient's problem, immediately evaluate whether the interventions were effective and the patient's response. The process of evaluation compares actual patient outcomes with expected outcomes. For example, a clinic nurse assesses a foot ulcer of a patient who has diabetes to determine whether healing has progressed since the last clinic visit. When expected outcomes are not met, evaluation reveals the need to continue current therapies for a longer period, revise approaches to care, or introduce new therapies. As you care for a patient throughout the day, anticipate when to return to the bedside to evaluate care (e.g., 30 minutes after an oral medication was administered, 15 minutes after an IV fluid has begun infusing, or 60 minutes after discussing discharge instructions with the patient and family).

Focusing on evaluation of a patient's progress lessens the chance of becoming distracted by the tasks of care. It is common to assume that staying focused on planned activities ensures that you will perform care appropriately. However, task orientation does not ensure positive patient outcomes. Learn that at the heart of good organizational skills is the constant inquiry into a patient's condition and progress toward an improved level of health.

Team Communication

Effective communication is critical to all teams (QSEN Institute, 2018). As a part of a health care team, you are responsible for using open, professional communication. Regardless of the setting, an enriching professional environment is one in which staff members respect one another's ideas, share information, and keep one another informed (Kaiser and Westers, 2018).

Some health care organizations use evidence-based teamwork principles to improve communication, teamwork, and patient safety. The TeamSTEPPS® system provides training for all health care staff to guide communication, increase team awareness, and eliminate barriers to patient safety (AHRQ, 2017). Use TeamSTEPPS® principles to promote professional communication and teamwork in your practice setting (Box 21.6).

Strategies to improve your communication with health care providers include addressing the colleague by name, having the patient and medical record available when discussing patient issues, focusing on the patient problem, and being professional and assertive but not aggressive or confrontational. One way of fostering good team communication is to understand the roles and responsibilities of everyone on the health care team (AHRQ, 2014). A professional nurse treats colleagues with respect, listens to the ideas of other staff members without interruption, explores the way other staff members think, and is honest and direct while communicating. Part of good communication is clarifying what others are saying and building on the merits of co-workers' ideas. An effective team knows that it is able to count on all members when needs arise.

Sharing expectations of what, when, and how to communicate is a step toward establishing a strong work team (AHRQ, 2014). Examples of effective team communication strategies include briefings or short discussions among team members, group rounds on patients, callouts to share critical information such as vital signs with all team members at the same time, and check-backs to restate what a person has said to verify understanding of information. The two-challenge rule allows

---

BOX 21.7 SBAR As a Communication Tool

Case Study: A nurse caring for patients on an orthopedic surgery unit administered 1 tablet of oxycodone HCl 5 mg/ibuprofen 400 mg PO to a patient 30 minutes ago for postsurgical pain. The nurse returns to the patient's room to evaluate the effectiveness of the medication. The patient rates his pain as an 8 on a scale of 0–10. The nurse uses SBAR to contact the patient's health care provider.

Situation: The patient is rating his pain as an 8 on a scale of 0–10. He had his pain medication 30 minutes ago.

Background: The patient had a knee replacement and returned from the postanesthesia care unit 6 hours ago. He has 1 tablet of oxycodone HCl 5 mg/ibuprofen 400 mg PO ordered every 6 hours. This is the first pain medication he has taken since being admitted to the unit.

Assessment: His current medication order is not sufficiently managing the patient's pain. He does not want to sit up or move because of the pain he is experiencing.

Recommendation: Request a change of the pain medication order for the patient.

---

concerns about safety to be voiced twice. Some patient care settings use different tools to communicate a change in a patient's condition. For example, some use the CUS Tool, which means I am Concerned, I am Uncomfortable, and this is a Safety issue (AHRQ, 2014). Another tool often used by health care organizations to share information is Situation-Background-Assessment-Recommendation (SBAR) (Box 21.7; see Chapter 27) (AHRQ, 2014). When using electronic communication, it is important to communicate the appropriate information to the correct person, always maintaining patient privacy and confidentiality.

QSEN **Building Competency in Teamwork and Collaboration** You are caring for Mrs. Saucer, who had a stroke 3 days ago. Upon your initial assessment, she was oriented, smiling, and joking with her visitors. You enter her room 2 hours later and find that Mrs. Saucer remains oriented, but she is tearful, and her emotional status has changed. She states, "I'm not sure what is wrong with me. I feel so much different than I did earlier today." Your intuition tells you that although Mrs. Saucer's physical status and orientation have not changed, there is something that is not quite right. You know that even the slightest neurological change in a patient who has had a stroke could be a sign of worsening neurological status. Using the CUS tool, how would you communicate this change in status to Mrs. Saucer's health care provider?

Answers to QSEN Activities can be found on the Evolve website.

Delegation

The art of effective delegation is a skill that you need to observe and practice to improve your own management skills. **Delegation** is the process of assigning part of your responsibility to another qualified person in a specific situation (NCSBN and ANA, 2019). Your state's Nurse Practice Act, along with principles of authority, accountability, and responsibility, provides the basis for effective delegation. Effective delegation results in the achievement of quality, safe patient care; improved efficiency; increased productivity; empowered staff; and skill development (Yoder-Wise, 2015). For example, asking a staff member to obtain an ordered specimen while you administer a patient's pain medication effectively prevents a delay in the patient gaining pain relief. Delegation also provides job enrichment. You show trust in colleagues by delegating tasks to them and showing staff members that they are important players in the delivery of care (Riisgaard et al.,

---

BOX 21.8 The Five Rights of Delegation

Right Task
The right tasks to delegate are ones that are included in the delegatee's job description or are included in the health care agency's policies and procedures. Policies and procedures need to describe expectations, limits, and required competency training for the activity.

Right Circumstance
Consider the patient's status. The patient needs to be stable in order to delegate tasks. The delegatee must report changes in patient condition to the licensed nurse. The licensed nurse must reassess and evaluate the situation and appropriateness of delegation when a patient's condition changes.

Right Person
The licensed nurse, employer, and delegatee are all responsible for ensuring the delegatee has the knowledge and skills required to perform the activity.

Right Directions and Communication
Give a clear, concise description of a task, including its objective, limits, and expectations. Communication needs to be ongoing between the licensed nurse and delegatee. The delegatee is responsible to ask questions to clarify information.

Right Supervision and Evaluation
Provide appropriate monitoring, evaluation, intervention as needed, and feedback. The licensed nurse must follow up with the delegatee at the end of the activity to evaluate patient outcomes, be available and ready to intervene when appropriate, and ensure appropriate documentation.

Modified from National Council of States Boards of Nursing and American Nurses Association (NCSBN & ANA): *National guidelines for nursing delegation,* 2019, https://www.ncsbn.org/NGND-PosPaper_06.pdf. Accessed July 28, 2019.

2017). Successful delegation is important to the quality of the relationship you have with all team members, including LPNs and APs (Lyman et al., 2017). Delegating a task that you dislike doing or would not do yourself creates negative feelings and poor working relationships. For example, if a patient asks to be placed on a bedpan and there are no urgent care issues, you assist the patient rather than leave the room to find the LPN or AP. Remember that even though the delegation of a task transfers the responsibility and authority to another person, you are accountable for the delegated task.

As a nurse you are responsible and accountable for providing care to patients and delegating care activities to others (Huber, 2018). Use the five rights of delegation to ensure you stay within an RN's legal scope of practice (Box 21.8). Never delegate clinical reasoning, nursing judgment (e.g., the steps of the nursing process of assessment, diagnosis, planning, intervention, and evaluation or patient teaching), and critical decision making to APs (NCSBN and ANA, 2019). Remember that when you delegate to another member of the health care team, you delegate tasks, not patients. Although LPNs can manage the majority of patient care on their own, do not give APs sole responsibility for the care of patients. One way to accomplish safe delegation is to conduct rounds with LPNs and APs who are assigned to work with you. APs attend to basic patient needs (e.g., hygiene, meal assistance, ambulation) while LPNs can provide basic direct nursing care (e.g., observe and report clinical changes, perform wound care, and ADLs). You delegate care based on assessment findings and priority setting.

As a leader of the health care team, you give clear instructions, effectively prioritize patient needs and therapies, and give staff timely and meaningful feedback. Do not automatically delegate a task because it is a task. Rather delegate it because it is appropriate for LPNs or APs to perform it. For example, as a nurse, you are always responsible for the assessment of a patient's ongoing status; but if a patient is stable, you delegate administration of medications (exception: IV medications in most states) to the LPN and the taking of vital signs to the AP.

Effective delegation begins with knowing which skills you are able to delegate. Thus you need to be familiar with the Nurse Practice Act of your state, institutional policies and procedures, and institutional job descriptions for LPNs and APs. These standards define the necessary level of education and competency of all staff and contain specific guidelines regarding which tasks or activities you can delegate. A job description identifies any required education and the types of tasks LPNs and APs can perform, either independently or with direct supervision. Institutional policies define the training required for APs. Procedures detail who is qualified to perform a given nursing procedure, whether supervision is necessary, and the type of reporting required.

As a professional nurse you cannot delegate without considering the implications. Assess the patient and determine a plan of care before identifying which tasks someone else is able to perform. Determine how much supervision is necessary. For example, you are working with an AP who was recently hired. When deciding which tasks to delegate to the AP, determine whether the patient has a complicating factor that makes your assistance necessary. Ask the AP, "Is this the first time you have performed this task?" "Have you cared for patients with similar needs?" "Have you had the chance to do this skill during orientation?" If you decide you can delegate the skill, you need to evaluate whether the AP performed the task properly and whether the desired outcomes were met.

Efficient delegation requires ongoing communication (i.e., sending clear messages and listening so that all participants understand expectations regarding patient care) (Huber, 2018). Provide clear instructions and desired outcomes when delegating tasks. Focus your instructions on the procedure itself, what will be accomplished, when it should be completed, and the unique needs of the patient. You also communicate when and which information to report such as expected observations and specific patient concerns (NCSBN and ANA, 2019). Communication is a two-way process in delegation; thus create a trusting relationship so that the staff you work with (e.g., LPNs, APs) feel comfortable and are able to ask questions and clarify your expectations (NCSBN and ANA, 2019). Effective communication, shared decision making, and sharing of knowledge promote safe patient care (O'Leary, 2016). As you become more familiar with a staff member's competency, trust builds, and the staff member needs fewer instructions. Always clarify patients' specific needs.

When delegating patient care, you evaluate a staff member's performance, achievement of the patient's outcomes, the communication process used, and any problems or concerns that occurred (NCSBN and ANA, 2019). For example, when a newly hired AP performs a task correctly and does a good job, it is essential to provide praise and recognition. If a staff member's performance is not satisfactory, give constructive and appropriate feedback. Always give specific feedback regarding any mistakes that staff members make, explaining how to avoid the mistake or a better way to handle the situation. Giving feedback in private is professional and preserves the staff member's dignity. When giving feedback, focus on what can be changed, choose only one issue at a time, and give specific details. Frequently when a staff member's performance does not meet expectations, it is the result of inadequate training or assignment of too many tasks. In this case, review the procedure and offer demonstration or even recommend additional training with the education department. If too many tasks are being delegated, this might be a nursing practice issue. All staff need to discuss the appropriateness of delegation on their unit. Sometimes staff need help to learn how to prioritize. In some cases, you discover that you are over delegating. It is your responsibility to complete documentation of the delegated task. Here are a few tips on appropriate delegation to assistive personnel (Yoder-Wise, 2015; NCSBN and ANA, 2019):

- *Assess the knowledge and skills of the person to whom you are delegating:* Assess the person's knowledge and skills by asking open-ended questions that elicit conversation and details about what he or she knows (e.g., "How do you usually apply the cuff when you measure a blood pressure?" or "Tell me how you prepare the tubing before you give an enema.")

- *Match tasks to the person's skills:* Know which tasks and skills the training program includes for APs in your organization. Determine whether APs have learned critical thinking skills such as knowing when a patient is in harm or the difference between normal clinical findings and changes to report.

- *Communicate clearly:* Always provide clear directions by describing a task, the desired outcome, and the time period within which the AP needs to complete the task. Never give instructions through another staff member. Make APs feel as though they are part of the team. Begin requests for help with *please* and end with *thank you.* For example, "I'd like you to please help me by getting Mr. Floyd up to ambulate before lunch. Be sure to check his blood pressure before he stands and record it in his chart. Thank you for your help." Ask the AP to report back to you after completing the task.

- *Listen attentively:* Listen to an AP's response after you provide directions. Does the AP feel comfortable in asking questions or requesting clarification? Does the AP understand your request? Ask the AP for suggestions in patient care and listen to his or her response. Be especially attentive if the AP is helping another nurse. Help sort out priorities.

- *Provide feedback:* Always give the AP feedback regarding performance, regardless of outcome. Let them know of a job well done. A "thank you" increases the likelihood of the AP helping in the future. If an outcome is undesirable, find a private place to discuss what occurred, any miscommunication, and how to achieve a better outcome in the future.

Knowledge Building

As a professional and accountable nurse, you are responsible for lifelong learning and maintaining your competency (Zittel et al., 2016). Lifelong learning allows you to continuously provide safe, effective, quality care. A leader recognizes that there is always something new to learn. Opportunities for learning occur with each patient interaction, each encounter with a professional colleague, and each meeting or class session in which health care professionals meet to discuss clinical care issues. People always have different experiences and knowledge to share. Listen to the contributions of others and value the information they share. In-service programs, workshops, professional conferences, professional reading, and taking classes to further your education offer innovative and current information on the rapidly changing world of health care. To be a safe and competent nurse you need to actively pursue learning opportunities, both formal and informal, and to respectfully interact with the professional colleagues you encounter.

▌ KEY POINTS

- A transformational leader develops effective teams on the nursing unit, empowers staff members, communicates effectively with the nursing team, and guides and supports the nursing team in shared decision making.

- Nursing care delivery models vary according to the responsibility and autonomy of the nurse in coordinating care delivery and the roles other staff members play in assisting with care.
- Patient- and family-centered care is composed of the core concepts of respect and dignity, information sharing, participation of family members, and collaboration.
- Shared governance, a type of decentralized decision-making model, empowers nursing staff to make decisions about how they practice and deliver patient care.
- Important elements of professional nursing and the decision-making process include responsibility (activities you perform), autonomy (freedom of choice), authority (your legal ability to perform a task), and accountability (being answerable for your actions).
- Nursing students and nurses develop their own leadership skills by being responsible and accountable, thinking critically, reflecting upon and learning from mistakes, and being an engaged member of the health care team.
- Nurses prioritize patient care in different ways. For example, to prioritize patient care, evaluate and weigh each competing task by reflecting on whether the patient is in a life-threatening situation, whether the task is essential to patient or staff safety, and whether the task is essential to the patient's plan of care.
- Nurses use evidence-based communication strategies such as SBAR and CUS to accurately communicate patient problems to other members of the health care team.
- Effective delegation requires effective communication skills and improves productivity and job enrichment. Using the five rights of delegation helps you delegate care appropriately.

REFLECTIVE LEARNING

- Reflect on a recent clinical experience. Which nursing care delivery model was used in this setting? What contributed to the effectiveness of this model? What challenges do you think the team may experience with this model?
- Describe how you prioritized care for a recent patient or group of patients during a recent clinical or simulation experience. Evaluate the effectiveness of your care and the decisions you made. Reflecting on this experience, is there anything you would have done differently? Explain your answer.
- Reflect on a clinical experience. What are some examples of teamwork and collaboration you witnessed? Did you observe any situations in which the health care team did not work well together? If so, what do you think caused this situation and what could be done to improve the work environment to reduce conflict and improve patient care? What effect did the lack of teamwork have on your patient?

REVIEW QUESTIONS

1. At 1200 the registered nurse (RN) says to the assistive personnel (AP), "You did a good job walking Mrs. Taylor by 0930. I saw that you recorded her pulse before and after the walk. I saw that Mrs. Taylor walked in the hallway barefoot. For safety, the next time you walk a patient, you need to make sure that the patient wears slippers or shoes. Please walk Mrs. Taylor again by 1500." Which characteristics of positive feedback did the RN use when talking to the AP? (Select all that apply.)
   1. Feedback is given immediately.
   2. Feedback focuses on one issue.
   3. Feedback offers concrete details.
   4. Feedback identifies ways to improve.
   5. Feedback focuses on changeable things.
   6. Feedback is specific about what is done incorrectly only.
2. A nurse received change-of-shift report on these four patients and starts rounding. Which patient does the nurse need to focus on as a priority?
   1. The patient who had abdominal surgery 2 days ago who is requesting pain medication
   2. A patient admitted yesterday with atrial fibrillation who now has a decreased level of consciousness
   3. A patient with a wound drain who needs teaching before discharge in the early afternoon
   4. A patient going to surgery for a mastectomy in 3 hours who has a question about the surgery
3. A nurse asks an AP to help the patient in Room 418 walk to the bathroom right now. The nurse tells the AP that the patient needs the assistance of one person and the use of a walker. The nurse also tells the AP that the patient's oxygen can be removed while he goes to the bathroom but to make sure that when it is put back on the flowmeter is still at 2 L. The nurse also instructs the AP to make sure the side rails are up and the bed alarm is reset after the patient gets back in bed. Which of the following components of the "Five Rights of Delegation" were used by the nurse? (Select all that apply.)
   1. Right task
   2. Right circumstance
   3. Right person
   4. Right directions and communication
   5. Right supervision and evaluation
4. While administering medications, a nurse realizes that a prescribed dose of a medication was not given. The nurse acts by completing an incident report and notifying the patient's health care provider. Which of the following is the nurse exercising?
   1. Authority
   2. Responsibility
   3. Accountability
   4. Decision making
5. Which task is appropriate for a registered nurse (RN) to delegate to an AP?
   1. Explaining to the patient the preoperative preparation before the surgery in the morning
   2. Administering the ordered antibiotic to the patient before surgery
   3. Obtaining the patient's signature on the surgical informed consent
   4. Helping the patient to the bathroom before leaving for the operating room
6. A nurse performs the following four steps in delegating a task to an AP. Place the steps in the order of appropriate delegation.
   1. Do you have any questions about walking Mr. Malone?
   2. Before you take him for his walk to the end of the hallway and back, please take and record his pulse rate.
   3. In the next 30 minutes please assist Mr. Malone in Room 418 with his afternoon walk.
   4. I will make sure that I check with you in about 40 minutes to see how the patient did.
7. Which example demonstrates a nurse performing the skill of evaluation?
   1. The nurse explains the side effects of the new blood pressure medication ordered for the patient.
   2. The nurse asks a patient to rate pain on a scale of 0 to 10 before administering a pain medication.
   3. After completing a teaching session, the nurse observes a patient drawing up and administering an insulin injection.
   4. The nurse changes a patient's leg ulcer dressing using aseptic technique.

8. The nurse manager from the surgical unit was awarded the nursing leadership award for practice of transformational leadership. Which of the following are characteristics or traits of transformational leadership displayed by the award winner? (Select all that apply.)
   1. The nurse manager regularly rounds on staff to gather input on unit decisions.
   2. The nurse manager sends thank-you notes to staff in recognition of a job well done.
   3. The nurse manager sends memos to staff about decisions that the manager has made regarding unit policies.
   4. The nurse manager has an "innovation idea box" to which staff are encouraged to submit ideas for unit improvements.
   5. The nurse manager develops a philosophy of care for the staff.

9. A new nurse graduate is in orientation on a surgical unit and is being mentored by an experienced nurse. Which action completed by the new nurse graduate requires intervention by the experienced nurse? (Select all that apply.)
   1. The new nurse stops documenting about a dressing change to take a patient some water.
   2. The new nurse gathered the medications for two different patients at the same time.
   3. The new nurse asked an AP to help transfer a patient from the bed to a wheelchair before discharge.
   4. The new nurse educates a patient about pain management when administering a pain medication to a patient.
   5. The new nurse gathers all equipment necessary to start a new IV site before entering a patient's room.

10. A nurse is calling a patient's health care provider about a problem the patient is having following surgery. The health care organization uses the SBAR system in reporting patient problems. Put the statements in order according to the SBAR system.
    1. Would it be possible to give the patient an antiemetic to help with the patient's nausea and comfort?
    2. The patient is experiencing nausea right now. The nausea has worsened over the past hour. He states he feels as though he is going to get sick.
    3. The patient had surgery earlier today to remove a tumor in the colon. He was admitted to the surgical unit 4 hours ago. He has a nasogastric (NG) tube in place. There is no postoperative order for an antiemetic.
    4. The patient denies pain and vital signs are stable. B/P 114/68; pulse 76; respiratory rate 20; temperature 98.6° F. The surgical dressing is dry and intact. The NG tube is intact and draining light brown fluid. It flushes well, and placement was confirmed using pH testing of gastric contents. The patient does not want to roll onto his side because of the nausea.

Answers: 1. 1, 2, 3, 4, 5; **2.** 2, 3; **3.** 1, 2, 3, 4; **4.** 3, 5; **5.** 4, 6; **6.** 3, 2, 4, 1; **7.** 3; **8.** 1, 2, 4, 9; **9.** 1, 2; **10.** 2, 3, 4, 1

Rationales to Review Questions can be found on the Evolve website.

REFERENCES

Ackley BJ, Ladwig G: *Nursing diagnosis handbook*, ed 11, St Louis, 2017, Mosby.

Agency for Healthcare Research and Quality (AHRQ): *Pocket guide*, TeamSTEPPS®, 2014, https://www.ahrq.gov/teamstepps/instructor/essentials/pocketguide.html#frame. Accessed September 2018 .

Agency for Healthcare Research and Quality (AHRQ): *About TeamSTEPPS* ®, 2017, https://www.ahrq.gov/teamstepps/about-teamstepps/index.html. Accessed September 2018.

Alfaro-Lefevre R: *Critical thinking, clinical reasoning, and clinical judgment: a practical approach*, ed 6, St Louis, 2017, Saunders.

American Association of Critical Care Nurses (AACN): Is your work environment healthy? n.d., https://www.aacn.org/nursing-excellence/healthy-work-environments. Accessed September 2018.

American Nurses Credentialing Center (ANCC): Magnet Recognition Program®, n.d., https://www.nursingworld.org/organizational-programs/magnet/. Accessed September 2018.

Benner P, et al.: *Educating nurses: a call for radical transformation*, San Francisco, CA, 2010, Josey-Bass.

Case Management Society of America (CMSA): *What is case management?* 2015, http://solutions.cmsa.org/acton/fs/blocks/showLandingPage/a/10442/p/p-0003/t/page/fm/0/r/l-0264:3/s/l-0264?sid=VBd1pHNyI.

Goldsberry JW: Advanced practice nurses leading the way: interprofessional collaboration, *Nurse Educ Today* 65(1), 2018.

Gordon JN: Empowering oncology nurses to lead change through a shared governance project, *Oncol Nurs Forum* 43(6):688, 2016.

Grace P: Enhancing nurse moral agency: the leadership promise of doctor of nursing practice preparation, *Online J Issues Nurs* 23(1):1, 2018.

Huber DL: *Leadership and nursing care management*, ed 6, St Louis, 2018, Saunders.

Institute for Patient and Family Centered Care (IPFCC): Patient- and family-centered care, http://www.ipfcc.org/about/pfcc.html. Accessed September 2018.

Interprofessional Education Collaborative Expert Panel (IECEP): *Core competencies for interprofessional collaborative practice: 2016 update*, 2016, https://www.ipecollaborative.org/resources.html. Accessed September 2018.

James AH: Action learning can support leadership development for undergraduate and postgraduate nurses, *Br J Nurs* 27(15):876, 2018.

Kivland C: Successfully managing emotions and behavior: emotional intelligence matters more than ever to your leadership career, *Healthc Exec* 33(1):68, 2018.

Moss M, Good VS: An official Critical Care Societies Collaborative statement: burnout syndrome in critical care health care professionals: a call to action, *Am J Crit Care* 25(4):368, 2016.

National Council of State Boards of Nursing (NCSBN): *History*, 2018, https://www.ncsbn.org/history.htm. Accessed September 2018.

National Council of States Boards of Nursing and American Nurses Association (NCSBN & ANA): *National guidelines for nursing delegation*, 2019, https://www.ncsbn.org/NGND-PosPaper_06.pdf. Accessed July 28 2019.

QSEN Institute: *QSEN competencies*, 2018. http://qsen.org/competencies/pre-licensure-ksas/.

Savel RH, Munro CL: Servant leadership: the primacy of service, *Am J Crit Care* 26(2):97, 2017.

Yoder-Wise PS: *Leading and managing in nursing*, ed 6, St Louis, 2015, Mosby.

Zittel B, et al.: Registered nurses as professionals: accountability for education and practice, *Online J Issues Nurs* 21(3):8, 2016.

RESEARCH REFERENCES

Alilyyani B, et al.: Antecedents, mediators, and outcomes of authentic leadership in healthcare: a systematic review, *Int J Nurs Stud* 83:34, 2018.

Bigani DK, Correia AM: On the same page: nurse, patient, and family perceptions of change-of-shift bedside report, *J Pediatr Nurs* 41:84, 2018.

Boamah SA, et al.: Effect of transformational leadership on job satisfaction and patient safety outcomes, *Nurs Outlook* 66(2):180, 2018.

Brown BB, et al.: The effectiveness of clinical networks in improving quality of care and patient outcomes: a systematic review of quantitative and qualitative studies, *BMC Health Serv Res* 16:360, 2016.

Brown K, et al.: Grandparents raising grandchildren with disabilities: assessing health status, home environment and impact of a family support case management model, *Int Public Health* 9(2):181, 2017.

Hiler CA, et al.: Predictors of moral distress in a US sample of critical care nurses, *Am J Crit Care* 27(1):59, 2018.

Homeyer S, et al.: Effects of interprofessional education for medical and nursing students: enablers, barriers and expectations for optimizing future interprofessional collaboration—a qualitative study, *BMC Nurs* 17(1), 2018.

Kaiser JA, Westers JB: Nursing teamwork in a health system: a multisite study, *J Nurs Manage* 26(5):555, 2018.

Kelly LA, Lefton C: Effect of meaningful recognition on critical care nurses' compassion fatigue, *Am J Crit Care* 26(6):438, 2017.

Lacey SR, et al.: Driving organizational change from the bedside: the AACN clinical Scene Investigator Academy, *Crit Care Nurse* 37(4):e12, 2017.

Lyman B, et al.: Organizational learning in a cardiac intensive care unit, *DCCN* 36(2):78, 2017.

McBeth CL, et al.: Interprofessional huddle: one children's hospital's approach to improving patient flow, *Pediatr Nurs* 43(2):71, 2017.

Nelson-Brantley HV, et al.: Nurse executives leading change to improve critical access hospital outcomes: a literature review with research-informed recommendations, *Online J Rural Nurs Health Care* 18(1):148, 2018.

O'Leary DF: Exploring the importance of team psychological safety in the development of two interprofessional teams, *J Interprof Care* 30(1):29, 2016.

Perry V, et al.: CNE series. A daily goals tool to facilitate indirect nurse-physician communication during morning rounds on a medical-surgical unit, *Medsurg Nurs* 25(2):83, 2016.

Prystajecky M, et al.: A case study of healthcare providers' goals during interprofessional rounds, *J Interprof Care* 31(4):463, 2017.

Riisgaard H, et al.: Associations between degrees of task delegation and job satisfaction of general practitioners and their staff: a cross-sectional study, *BMC Health Serv Res* 17:44, 2017.

Shimp KM: Systematic review of turnover/retention and staff perception of staffing and resource adequacy related to staffing, *Nurs Econ* 35(5):239, 2017.

Stimpfel AW, et al.: Hospitals known for nursing excellence associated with better hospital experience for patients, *Health Serv Res* 51(3):1120, 2016.

Sulit Oriza N, et al.: Shared governance for a healthy work environment in a pediatric cardiothoracic intensive care unit, *AACN Adv Crit Care* 27(2):152, 2016.

Welp A, Manser T: Integrating teamwork, clinician occupational well-being and patient safety – development of a conceptual framework based on a systematic review, *BMC Health Serv Res* 16:1, 2016.

22

Ethics and Values

OBJECTIVES

- Discuss the role of ethics in professional nursing.
- Use values clarification when you apply ethics in practice.
- Define the principles and approaches commonly used in health care ethics discussions.
- Describe the difference between an ethical dilemma and moral distress.
- Apply a stepwise approach to ethical problems.
- Discuss contemporary ethical issues that nurses face.

KEY TERMS

Accountability, p. 296
Advocacy, p. 296
Autonomy, p. 295
Beneficence, p. 295
Bioethics, p. 294
Casuistry, p. 297
Code of ethics, p. 296

Confidentiality, p. 296
Deontology, p. 297
Ethics, p. 294
Ethics of care, p. 298
Feminist ethics, p. 298
Fidelity, p. 295
Justice, p. 295

Morals, p. 294
Nonmaleficence, p. 295
Utilitarianism, p. 297
Value, p. 294

MEDIA RESOURCES

http://evolve.elsevier.com/Potter/fundamentals/

- Review Questions
- Case Study with Questions

- Audio Glossary
- Content Updates
- Answers to QSEN Activity and Review Questions

Ethics is the study of what is right and wrong in our conduct. It concerns our obligations to individuals, groups and society. Acts that are ethical reflect a commitment to standards that individuals, professions, and societies strive to meet. When decisions must be made about health care, understandable disagreement can occur among health care professionals, families, patients, friends, and people in the community. The right thing to do can be hard to determine, particularly when individual values, beliefs, and perceptions conflict. This chapter describes concepts that will help you embrace the role of ethics in your professional life and promote resolution when ethical problems develop.

BASIC TERMS IN HEALTH ETHICS

Ethical issues differ from legal issues. Legal issues are resolved by reference to laws that are usually concrete and publicly determined. Breaking a law results in a public consequence such as a ticket for speeding or jail time for stealing. However, ethics has a broader base of interest than the law, referring more to issues of behavior and character. The terms *ethics* and *morals* sometimes are used interchangeably. Morals usually refer to judgment about behavior, based on specific beliefs, and ethics refers to the study of the ideals of right and wrong behavior.

Values play an important role in understanding ethics. A value is a deeply held personal belief about the worth a person holds for an idea, a custom, or an object. The values that a person holds reflect cultural and social influences. For example, a person who makes a living in a rural place may value the environment differently than someone who visits rural areas for recreation. Ethical codes grow from shared values, negotiated and discussed over time through religious groups, ethnic groups, or work groups. As you enter the nursing profession, you undergo a similar process of learning shared values. Clarity about your values and your own point of view will guide you in making effective ethical decisions.

The study of bioethics represents a branch of ethics within the field of health care. The study of bioethics has grown over the last 50 years, beginning with the emergence of technologies related to organ transplant. When researchers perfected kidney transplant procedures in the early 1970s, only a limited number of kidneys were available for transplant compared with the number of patients in need. This lack of resources became an immediate ethical concern. The health care community in the United States began to address this issue by means of ethical discussion in local and national groups.

Changing medical technologies continue to require societies to face difficult ethical questions. Why should we do genetic testing for diseases we cannot cure? How shall we define quality of life? Who should decide? In the study of bioethics, health care professionals agree to negotiate these difficult and important questions by referring to a common set of ethical principles.

An understanding of the concepts common in ethical discourse will help you participate thoughtfully in discussions with others and may help you shape your own thoughts about ethical issues. The application of the concepts is fundamental to developing skills in ethical decision making. During the ethical decision-making process, you will apply the concepts of autonomy, beneficence, nonmaleficence, justice, and fidelity.

Autonomy

Autonomy refers to freedom from external control. In health care the concept applies to respect for the autonomy of patients. It can also apply to institutional respect for the autonomy of health care professionals. A commitment to respect the autonomy of others is a fundamental principle of ethical practice.

Respect for patient autonomy refers to the commitment to include patients in decisions about all aspects of care (Klugman, 2017). It is a key feature of patient-centered care. In respecting patient autonomy, you acknowledge and protect a patient's independence. Respect for autonomy reflects a movement away from paternalistic patient care in which health care providers made all decisions. Involving patients in decisions about their care is now standard practice. We often demonstrate respect for patient autonomy through the informed consent process. Rather than the health care team making choices about the patient's care, the team's role is to inform patients about risks and benefits of treatment options and then, with the patient, determine a plan of care that matches their goals and values. In many cases (e.g., surgery and diagnostic procedures), the consent of a patient is documented by the patient's signature.

Another way nurses show respect for patient autonomy is by explaining nursing procedures such as obtaining a blood pressure or administering medications. Nurses also demonstrate respect for patient autonomy by supporting patients who raise questions about procedures and by ensuring that they get the information they request. In addition, your conversations with patients and families can help them to articulate their preferences, values, and goals. Clarifying what is important to them is a key step in making autonomous health care decisions.

Respect for professional autonomy refers to the relationship between members of the health care team and the institutions in which they work. What happens when a health care professional is asked to perform duties that conflict with a religious or personal belief? Institutions have developed policies that accommodate respect for health care professionals by finding a way to reassign duties when this conflict occurs. However, the reassignment is conducted so that the patient is protected from abandonment and patient care is not compromised. What happens when an individual employee takes issue with policies or practices of an institution and is concerned that a practice is unsafe? Employees may be concerned about reporting information because of potential retaliation. Some organizations have an anonymous reporting system for this reason. Institutional whistle blower protections prohibit retaliation against an employee who makes a legitimate report about clinical safety issues. These protections represent expressions of respect for professional autonomy.

REFLECT NOW

Consider decisions that you make about the activities you engage in or the people you are friends with. Do these decisions reflect autonomous choices or do factors outside your own preference influence them?

Beneficence

Beneficence refers to taking positive actions to help others (Klugman, 2017). The concept of beneficence is fundamental to the practice of nursing and medicine. The agreement to act with beneficence implies that the best interests of the patient remain more important than self-interest. It implies that nurses practice primarily as a service to others, even in the details of daily work.

Nonmaleficence

Maleficence refers to harm or hurt. Nonmaleficence refers to the avoidance of harm or hurt. In health care, ethical practice involves not only the will to do good but the equal commitment to do no harm (Klugman, 2017). A health care professional tries to balance the risks and benefits of care while striving at the same time to do the least harm possible. A bone marrow transplant procedure may offer a chance at cure; but the process involves periods of suffering, and it may not be possible to guarantee a positive outcome. Decisions about the best course of action can be difficult and uncertain precisely because nurses agree to avoid harm at the same time as they commit to promoting benefit.

Justice

Justice refers to fairness and the distribution of resources (Klugman, 2017). The term is most often used in discussions about access to health care, including the just distribution of scarce services and resources. Discussions about health insurance, hospital locations and services, and organ transplants generally are among the issues that cite the concept of justice. The term itself is open to interpretation, as people interpret fairness differently. Does the concept of justice mean that health care resources should be available to those who have earned them? Or is it fairer to distribute them equally? Should those with a greater need for resources receive more than others? Especially as health care costs continue to rise, the issue of justice remains a critical part of the discussion about health care reform and access to care.

The term *just culture* refers to the promotion of open discussion without fear of recrimination whenever mistakes, especially those involving adverse events, occur or nearly occur. Blame is withheld at least at first so that system issues and other elements can be investigated for their contributions to the error. By fostering open discussion about errors, members of the health care team become more richly informed participants, able to design new systems that prevent harm.

Fidelity

Fidelity refers to faithfulness or the agreement to keep promises (Doherty and Purtilo, 2016). As a nurse you have a duty to be faithful to the patients you care for, to the institution you work for, and to yourself. If you assess a patient for pain and offer a plan to manage the pain, the standard of fidelity encourages you to initiate the interventions in the plan as soon as possible and to monitor the patient's response to the plan. Fidelity is honored when we strive to provide excellent care to all patients, including those whose values are different from our own. We recognize a professional duty to apply the same skills and knowledge to the care of patients and families, regardless of their background, lifestyle, or past or present choices. When our need to exercise our own autonomy leads us to remove ourselves for a particular treatment or situation, fidelity demands that we not abandon the patient but instead find an equally qualified professional to provide the care we are unable to give.

Our duty to be faithful to the institution employing us means that we follow the policies and procedures set forth, or in the event that the policy or procedure is not appropriate, we seek to correct it and improve the standard of care provided by the institution. Finally, fidelity to oneself is honored when we attend to our own needs for emotional support, mentoring, or continuing education. Honoring our commitment to ourselves is essential to the delivery of safe and effective care to patients.

PROFESSIONAL NURSING CODE OF ETHICS

A code of ethics is a set of guiding principles that all members of a profession accept. It is a collective statement about the group's expectations and standards of behavior. The American Nurses Association (ANA) established its first Code of Ethics for Nursing in 1950, and the organization has continued to review and revise it periodically. The provisions of the Code of Ethics describe the nurse's obligation to the patient, the role of the nurse as a member of the health care team, and the duties of the nurse to the profession and to society (ANA, 2015). A few of the key principles in the code include advocacy, responsibility, accountability, and confidentiality.

Advocacy

Advocacy refers to the application of one's skills and knowledge for the benefit of another person. Lawyers are sometimes called "advocates" because they use their expertise to advance their clients' best interests. As a nurse you advocate for the health, safety, and rights of patients, including their right to privacy and their right to refuse treatment (Giuliante, 2017). Your special relationship with patients provides you with knowledge that is specific to your role as a registered nurse and as such with the opportunity to make a unique contribution to understanding a patient's point of view.

Responsibility

The word *responsibility* refers to a willingness to respect one's professional obligations and to follow through. As a nurse you are responsible for your actions, the care you provide, and the tasks that you delegate to others. This responsibility also means maintaining your competence to provide care and seeking guidance when you are uncertain of your skills and knowledge. You also demonstrate responsibility by applying your workplace's policies and procedures to the care you provide.

Accountability

Accountability refers to answering for your own actions. You ensure that your professional actions are explainable to your patients and your employer. Health care institutions also exercise accountability by monitoring individual and institutional compliance with national standards established by agencies such as The Joint Commission (TJC). TJC establishes national patient safety guidelines to ensure patient and workplace safety through consistent, effective nursing practices (TJC, 2019). The ANA Code of Ethics promotes ethical decision making by setting standards for collaborative interprofessional communication (ANA, 2015).

Confidentiality

Patients have the right to keep their personal health information private. Confidentiality refers to the health care team's obligation to respect patient privacy. Confidentiality is a fundamental part of the trusting relationship between a nurse and a patient (Doherty and Purtilo, 2016). Federal legislation known as the Health Insurance Portability and Accountability Act of 1996 (HIPAA) mandates confidentiality and protection of patients' personal health information. The legislation defines the rights and privileges of patients for protection of privacy. It establishes fines for violations (USDHHS, 2017). In practice, you cannot share information about a patient's medical condition or personal information with anyone who is not involved in the care of the patient. HIPAA calls this the "right to know." HIPAA also regulates communication of patient information contained in medical records (see Chapter 26).

VALUES

Nursing is a work of intimacy. Nursing practice requires you to be in contact with patients physically, emotionally, psychologically, and spiritually. In most other intimate relationships, you choose to enter the relationship anticipating that at least some of your values will align with those of the other person. But as a nurse you agree to provide care to your patients solely on the basis of their need for your services. The ethical concepts of beneficence and fidelity shape the practice of health care and distinguish it from other common human relationships such as friendship, marriage, and employer-employee. By its very nature, relationships in health care sometimes occur in the presence of conflicting values.

A value is a deeply held belief about the worth of an idea, attitude, custom, or object that affects choices and behaviors. While values reflect cultural and social influences, they can change over time as individuals become part of different groups. For example, you have personal values from your family, education, and other experiences, and then, as a nurse, you develop professional values as a member of the nursing profession and the health care team. Recognizing your own values is like seeing the bubble you live in; most of the time, we look at the world through the lens of our values without acknowledging them. Values are intrinsic to our view of the world. Learning to appreciate your values as your own individual perspective is the first step to working effectively with other health care professionals, patients, and families whose values are different.

Values Clarification

Ethical dilemmas almost always occur in the presence of conflicting values. To resolve ethical conflicts, one needs to distinguish among value, fact, and opinion. Facts are supported by objective data, and opinions are views or ideas that are not necessarily based on facts. Sometimes people have such strong values that they consider them to be facts. However, when people express a strong emotional reaction, this is often a sign that their values are threatened. Sometimes people are so passionate about their values that they become judgmental in a way that intensifies conflict. Clarifying values—your own, your patients', your co-workers'—is an important and effective part of ethical discourse.

Examine the cultural values exercise in Box 22.1. The values in the exercise are in neutral terms so that you can appreciate how differing values need not indicate "right" or "wrong." For example, for some people it is important to remain silent and stoic in the presence of great pain, and for others it is important to talk about it to understand and control it. Identifying values as something separate from facts can help you understand others even when there are differences that set you apart.

APPROACHES TO ETHICS

Historically, health care ethics constituted a search for fixed standards that would determine correct actions. Over time ethics has grown into a field of study that is more flexible and is filled with differences of opinion and deeply meaningful efforts to understand human interaction. The following review introduces you to some of the philosophical approaches to ethics that you may encounter during ethical discussions in health care settings. These approaches can be intentionally adopted to help you interpret and address ethical problems in practice. *To illustrate how these approaches work, consider a situation in which a nurse is caring for an older adult, Stella, who has dementia and whose son, David, does not adhere to the unit's visitation policy, namely, that he leave her bedside for half an hour during change of shift.*

Deontology

Deontology proposes a system of ethics that is perhaps most familiar to health care practitioners. Deontology defines actions as right or wrong based on their adherence to rules and principles such as fidelity to promises, truthfulness, and justice (Klugman, 2017). Instead of looking at consequences of actions to determine whether they are right or wrong, deontology examines a situation for the existence of essential right or wrong. *In the situation of Stella and David, the nurse applying a deontology approach may see the right action as seeking help in enforcing the visitation policy. Her fidelity to the institution supports a duty to enforce its regulations. Making an exception for David when other family members are following the rules is an injustice.*

Deontology requires a mutual understanding of justice, autonomy, and goodness. But it still leaves room for confusion to surface. The principle of respect for autonomy can be complicated when dealing with children and patients, like Stella, who may be unable to voice their preferences. *If Stella stated clearly that she desired David's presence at all times, a respect for her autonomy could be the guiding principle. In this case, the nurse should advocate for an exception to the visitation policy.* A commitment to respect the "rightness" of autonomy is a guiding principle in deontology, but adherence to the principle alone does not always provide clear answers for complicated situations.

Utilitarianism

A utilitarian system of ethics proposes that the value of something is determined by its usefulness. This philosophy is sometimes called consequentialism because its main emphasis is on the outcome or consequence of action. The greatest good for the greatest number of people is the guiding principle for determining right action in a utilitarian system (Klugman, 2017). As with deontology, utilitarianism relies on the application of a certain principle (i.e., measures of "good" and "greatest"). The difference between utilitarianism and deontology is the focus on outcomes. Utilitarianism measures the effect that an act will have; deontology looks at the act itself and judges its "rightness" by the rules or principles it upholds.

> *In the case of Stella and David, a nurse applying a utilitarian approach may determine that resolving the issue about David's visit should be done in a manner that creates the least risk of disturbing the rest of the patients and the other staff members on the unit. The nurse interprets the greatest good for the greatest number as the absence of conflict and thus negotiates an exception to the visitation policy. While violating the policy is unacceptable in a deontological approach because that action itself is not good, in utilitarianism, if the outcome, a peaceful interaction with the son, is good, then the action itself is correct.*

As with deontology, the utilitarian approach has some flaws, mainly that it can be taken too far. Do the ends always justify the means? A classic example in health care is the idea of removing organs from a perfectly healthy person to save the lives of seven other people who are awaiting transplantation. Seven people are more than one, so the outcome is good, but does that make the action, killing that one person, right? In addition, people have conflicting definitions of "greatest good." As with deontology, utilitarianism provides guidance, but it does not guarantee agreement.

Casuistry

Casuistry, or case-based reasoning, turns away from conventional principles of ethics as a way to determine best actions and focuses instead on the details of a situation. People who take this approach to ethics find similar precedent cases and determine a course of action on the basis of what was done to manage that prior situation (Strong, 2013). *A nurse applying this approach to the case of Stella and David would consider past instances in which families were permitted to stay at the bedside, even during change of shift, or other instances in which families made a similar request but were asked to follow the policy as it stands. A key step in applying this approach is comparing the details of Stella and David's situation, such as her prognosis and his ability to contribute to her care, to determine which prior situation is the closest match.* A weakness of the casuistry approach is that finding a similar precedent case may be challenging, particularly in complex situations with unique features.

Feminist Ethics

Noting the limitations of deontology and utilitarianism, scholars who focused on differences between genders, especially women's points of view, developed a critique of conventional ethical philosophies. Called feminist ethics, it looks to the nature of relationships to guide participants in making difficult decisions, especially relationships in which power is unequal or in which a point of view has become ignored or invisible (Green, 2012). Writers with a feminist perspective tend to concentrate more on practical solutions than on theory and to ask questions about the people involved and their relationships rather than looking to underlying principles.

For Stella and David, a nurse taking the feminist approach might look for a power imbalance and seek to take action that addresses it. Is David's presence at the bedside intimidating for Stella? Are staff members seeking to enforce the policy assuming a position of unjustified power over David? These questions, which may not surface in a traditional approach, will help determine the action that is right from a feminist ethics perspective.

Critics of feminist ethics worry about the lack of appeal to traditional ethical principles. Without guidance from concepts such as autonomy and beneficence, they argue, solutions to ethical questions will depend too much on subjective judgment.

Ethics of Care

The ethics of care offers an alternative view to utilitarianism and deontology. Similar to feminist ethics, care-based ethics focuses on understanding relationships, personal narratives and the context in which ethical problems arise. Unlike feminism, ethics of care emphasizes the role of the decision maker in the situation. With deontology and utilitarianism, the decision maker is detached and objective, gathering facts, identifying principles, or predicting outcomes. In the ethics of care, the decision maker lies in the context of the situation, relating to the people involved (Lachman, 2012). This philosophy often resonates with nurses who, in their intimate experiences with patients, are often making ethical decisions while engaged in caring relationships.

A nurse taking the ethics of care approach with Stella and David first learns more about the relationships involved in the current situation and then identifies the course of action that best supports them. Stella and David have a relationship to each other, and the nurses caring for Stella also have a relationship with each of them. What action, allowing David to stay or asking that he leave, will have the best impact on those relationships? Are there additional actions, such as listening to David's reasons for wanting to stay, that might have a positive impact on these relationships?

NURSING POINT OF VIEW

All patients in health care systems interact with nurses at some point, and they interact in ways that are unique to nursing. Nurses generally engage with patients over longer periods of time than other disciplines. They are involved in intimate physical acts such as bathing, feeding, and special procedures. As a result, patients and families may feel more comfortable in revealing information or asking questions they have not shared with other health care providers. Details about family life, information about coping styles, personal preferences, and details about fears and insecurities are likely to come out during the course

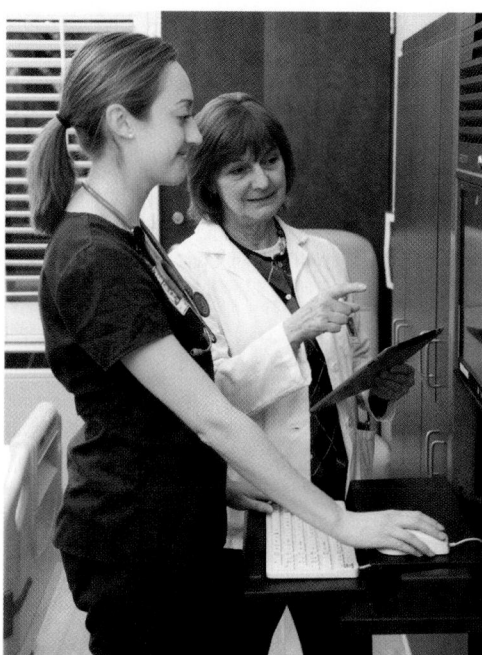

FIG. 22.1 Nurses collaborate with other professionals in making ethical decisions.

of nursing interventions. Your ability to shape your care based on this special knowledge provides an indispensable contribution to the overall care of your patient.

The care of any patient involves the collaboration of many disciplines. Therapists, physicians, surgeons, social workers, and pharmacists are some of the interprofessional team members who will provide care to patients with you and bring their own points of view. In addition, managers and administrators from many different professional backgrounds contribute to ethical discourse with their knowledge of systems, distribution of resources, financial possibilities, and limitations (Fig. 22.1).

REFLECT NOW

Consider a time in which you disagreed with a family member or a friend about the correct action to take in a situation. What factors helped you or prevented you from honestly expressing your own point of view? What did it feel like to listen to the other person's perspective?

Types of Ethical Problems

Two common ethical problems that nurses encounter are ethical dilemmas and moral distress (Robichaux, 2017). As an example, take a situation in which a nursing student working with an older adult finds that the patient refuses to take her morning pills. "I won't take a single one until you give me my hormone medicine." The patient has several medical problems, but none of her morning pills fit the description of "hormone medicine." In relating the issue to another member of the health care team, she is advised, "Why don't you go in there with one of the pills she needs and tell her it is her hormone pill? Then she'll cooperate with you."

Ethical Dilemma

The nursing student immediately feels conflicted by this advice. If the student follows the suggestion, the student can accomplish the task of delivering the medications, a task that is in the patient's interest and so could be justified by the principle of beneficence. At the same time, the student feels uncomfortable lying to the patient. Lying to her is a violation of the patient's autonomy, a betrayal of her trust. This interpretation of the situation is a classic example of an ethical dilemma. The student cannot do both options—take the advice to lie so that the patient gets the benefit of the medications *and* be truthful in identifying the pills to the patient. An ethical problem is called a dilemma when two opposing courses of action can both be justified by ethical principles (Robichaux, 2017).

Moral Distress

Now imagine the same situation with a change in details. The person the nursing student consults for help is the patient's attending physician, and the advice to lie about the pills feels to the student like a specific direction—not so much a suggestion but more of an order. At the same time, envision that at this moment during the clinical day, there is no one else the student can turn to for help. The student was told by her clinical instructor about the need to be more efficient in completing tasks and the medications were due to be given 30 minutes ago. Given the pressure of time and the source of the advice, the student might feel compelled to lie to the patient. But what if, based on her values, the student feels that action is morally wrong? Now the student is at risk for moral distress, a different ethical problem. In moral distress, instead of competing options for action, the nurse feels the need to take a specific action while believing that action to be wrong (Robichaux, 2017).

Distinguishing between ethical dilemmas and moral distress is important to achieving resolution. When the problem is a dilemma, with two opposing but justifiable options, often the application of the nursing process will include identifying more options. For example, the student might be able to succeed in giving the patient her medications without lying if the student builds trust with the patient by spending time with her. With moral distress, as this example shows, the environment often contributes to the problem. Discuss situations that generate moral distress with another person when they are identified. Additional resources, such as nursing colleagues, managers, and other health care professionals, can work together to address the factors that contribute to moral distress (Box 22.2).

Processing an Ethical Problem

Resolving an ethical problem is similar to the nursing process in its methodical approach to a clinical issue. However, it differs from the nursing process in that it requires negotiation of differences of opinion and clarity about situations where there may not be a single right answer. Finding clarity and consensus can occur when the following elements remain essential to the process: the presumption of goodwill on the part of all participants, strict adherence to confidentiality, patient-centered decision making, and the welcome participation of families and primary caregivers.

Because they involve values and obligations, ethical problems can raise troubling emotions. Processing an ethical problem begins with recognizing that an ethical problem exists (Doherty and Purtilo, 2016). Sometimes communication problems look like ethical problems, and taking the time to speak openly and listen to others achieves resolution. You then gather pertinent information about the case, including recent clinical evaluations, the views of colleagues, and the values and perspectives of the patient and family involved. Examining your personal values at this point can help to differentiate between fact and opinion, an important part of the process. Once information is gathered and ethical elements identified, developing a statement of the problem will facilitate discussion. The next step, listing all possible courses of action, requires some creativity and is best done in a conversation with

---

BOX 22.2   EVIDENCE-BASED PRACTICE

Moral Distress

PICOT Question: Do strategies that build moral resilience reduce moral distress among acute care nurses?

Evidence Summary

Moral distress describes the anguish experienced when a person feels unable to act according to closely held core values. Evidence indicates that causes of moral distress among acute care nurses include inadequate staffing, poor communication between members of the health care team, and situations that involve end-of-life care (Rodney, 2017). Nurses need to be aware of moral distress and recognize the need for moral reasoning (Rushton, 2017). While multiple studies document the existence of moral distress and its association with aspects of the work environment, interventions to address moral distress are an area of evolving research (Rushton, 2017). Strategies to address moral distress consider not only the individual experiencing the problem but also the work environment. Institutions often offer services such as an ethics resource or a moral distress service to specifically address the needs of nurses. Hamric and Epstein (2017) described a Moral Distress Consult Service that is accessible to all units in the hospital and helps address pervasive or persistent issues that are causing moral distress. On the unit level, proactive interventions may be applied to prevent moral distress. For instance, an assessment tool to identify patient care situations with a high likelihood of generating ethical problems allows early allocation of resources, such as multidisciplinary discussion, to reduce the risk (Pavlish et al., 2015). An additional unit-level strategy is to find and correct problems in the work environment (Sofer, 2017). The American Association of Critical-Care Nurses (AACN) created the Standards for Establishing and Sustaining Healthy Work Environments and an Assessment Tool that health care teams can use to identify and address gaps (AACN, 2016). Moral resilience is the ability to grow and even gain confidence from adverse and complex ethical problems (Rushton, 2017). While further study is needed, deliberate attention to building moral resilience among nurses may reduce their susceptibility to moral distress.

Application to Nursing Practice

- Develop and practice skilled communication. Learning to talk with colleagues, patients, and families in a professional manner that conveys a desire to share your own views and an openness to theirs can help prevent conflicts and reduce moral distress.
- Be aware of the resources available to help you reduce moral distress. Find out whether your hospital has an ethics committee or other resource for support and how that resource is consulted (Hamric and Epstein, 2017).
- Find a mentor or leader on your unit with a particular skill in examining ethical problems to help you process ethical situations.
- After you've had some experience on a unit, you may notice a pattern in which certain clinical situations repeatedly lead to moral distress. When caring for a patient in that kind of situation, seek support before conflict arises. Early action may help reduce your distress (Pavlish et al., 2015).

---

others. Deciding on an action and implementing it sometimes requires courage. The final step is an evaluation of the outcome (Doherty and Purtilo, 2016) (Box 22.3).

If the process involves a family conference or changes in the treatment plan, you document all relevant information in the medical record. Some institutions use a special ethics consultation form to structure documentation. However, if the ethical concern does not directly affect patient care, you may document the discussion in meeting minutes or in an e-mail to those involved in the discussion.

To review the process of ethical decision making, consider the following situation:

You are caring for Miguel, an 18-year-old with diabetes. Another nurse tells you that his parents are supportive, involved, and knowledgeable about his condition, but Miguel is mostly angry and uninterested in diabetes education. You walk into the room and find that a friend from Miguel's high school is visiting and has brought in candy and other snacks that contradict Miguel's prescribed diet. What is the best action to take?

Step 1. Ask: Is this an ethical problem?

While feeling uncertain about how to respond can be an indication of an ethical problem, not all uncertainty involves values and obligations. Some uncertainty can resolve with asking for advice or gathering more information. When strong emotions are triggered and when you are in a situation in which the action you take will demonstrate your personal or professional values, then you may have an ethical problem. If the problem is an ethical dilemma, you will likely feel conflicted between opposing courses of action, which each seem right in some ways and wrong in others. Moral distress often manifests as anger or frustration (Rushton et al., 2017).

In this case, more clinical information alone will not resolve the problem; you know that Miguel's health could be harmed if he ate all the candy and snacks his friends brought him. You may feel angry that Miguel is threatening his own health, which, as a member of the health care team, you feel obligated to protect. At the same time, you may also value Miguel's autonomy; he is technically an adult and has a right to select his diet, as long as he is informed of the risks and benefits. If you feel compelled to allow him to enjoy the snacks his friend brought while also feeling that it is wrong to do so, the situation may become morally distressing. There could be an ethical dilemma because two opposing actions—to try to stop Miguel from eating the snacks or to leave him alone—can both be justified. The situation is an ethical problem.

Step 2. Gather information that is relevant to the case.

Resolution of ethical problems can come from unlikely sources. Helpful information may include clinical information about the patient's current state of health, literature about his disease process, and information about his religious, cultural, and family background. A key strategy in gathering information is asking open-ended questions and taking time to listen. Because our interpretation of a situation is based on our own values, we need focused interaction to hear the perspectives of others.

A review of Miguel's chart shows that his diabetes is poorly controlled. There is a note from the hospital's diabetes education program indicating that Miguel and his parents were given information about a diabetic diet and appeared to understand the information. There is also a note by the social worker concerned that Miguel is having trouble accepting this diagnosis.

Step 3. Identify the ethical elements in the problem and examine your values.

Part of the goal is to accurately identify your own perspective, and an equally critical goal is to form respect for the perspectives of others. Consider whether the principles discussed earlier support a particular course of action. Take a moment to examine whether there are relationships involved that need to be supported or that could be adversely affected by actions to resolve the problem.

Reflect on your values. You want to ensure that Miguel manages his diabetes because you value his health. At the same time, you recognize that as a teenager, he wants the freedom to make his own choices, unrestrained by his disease process. You value him as a person and recognize that in addition to his physical health problems, he has developmental needs. Beneficence, the obligation to do good, supports you in seeking the action that is best for Miguel. The concept of autonomy supports actions that respect his right to make his own choices, while fidelity to the health care team supports actions that adhere to the current treatment plan.

Step 4. Name the problem.

This step is harder than it sounds and often goes better if you involve others—either a friend, another nurse, or the health care team. While it is possible to develop a statement that specifically describes the problem on your own, speaking aloud encourages you to use the right language and allows you to get feedback from others. As you will find in Step 5, you may need to collaborate in later steps too, and so identifying someone to talk to at this step may facilitate a faster resolution.

After reviewing Miguel's medical record, you find a colleague who has a few minutes to hear your story. As you talk to her, you say, "On the one hand, I want to go in there and take away that food because he really shouldn't have it, and I know he knows that. On the other hand, I can see where he may be trying to show his independence from his parents and do things that other teenagers do." You arrive at the conclusion that you have an ethical dilemma between acting with beneficence to protect Miguel's health and respecting his autonomy.

Step 5. Consider possible courses of action.

In a dilemma, there are two courses of action that can be justified, but they are opposing, so it is often helpful to think of other options. At this stage, it is important to know your resources. Ask yourself what the options are and also ask who is available to help. Like most aspects of health care, ethics is best managed as a team and not in isolation. Knowing the resources available to help you with ethical problems is similar to knowing the resources for clinical issues. Box 22.4 lists some of the resources to consider.

As you talk to your colleague, you identify the option of taking a tough stance with Miguel and removing the food and the option of avoiding his room and pretending to be unaware of his behavior. Your colleague points out that another option is to ask him about his behavior but in a kind way, not punitive or threatening. You also consider calling in Miguel's doctor to talk to him, calling his parents and asking that they intervene, or pulling Miguel's friend out of the room and explaining to him that he needs to leave and take the food with him because he is disrupting Miguel's care.

Step 6. Create an action plan and carry it out.

Often through the process of articulating the problem and listing the options, the course of action that is the best fit becomes clear. Rather than determining a single action to take, it may be helpful to select what to do first and then what to do later if that first step is ineffective in achieving resolution. For instance, if in identifying options for action you decide to call on a particular resource, such as a manager, for help, you may also decide that if the manager validates the issue, you will go on to consult the hospital ethics committee.

This step requires courage. Because ethics deals with values and obligations, unpleasant emotions such as fear and anger can occur. As much as possible, focus on your desired outcome, which is resolution of the ethical issue, to help you enact the plan.

You decide to take your colleague's advice and go to the room to speak to Miguel. If that is ineffective, then you will call on other members of the health care team. Your colleague helps you to plan the words you will use. Despite your nervousness, you enter the room and tell Miguel, "I don't want to stop you from enjoying your friend's visit, but I'm concerned about the snacks he brought. I know you've had education about your diet. Can we can talk about that?"

Miguel shrugs and says, "I don't really care." You then ask, "Well, what do you care about?" Miguel looks surprised. His friend smiles and says the name of a computer game Miguel likes. "That's what Miguel cares about," the friend says. A conversation ensues among you, Miguel, and his friend, and for the first time Miguel seems content rather than sullen and angry. After the conversation, you ask Miguel if his friend can take the snacks with him when he leaves, telling him, "It sounds as if you have things to do that are better than being in the hospital, and these snacks won't help you get out of here." Miguel nods and helps you pack the food back into the friend's grocery bag.

Step 7. Evaluate the action plan.

This is the step where you decide whether further action is needed or resolution has been achieved. If the evaluation shows that the issue has resolved, be sure to consider what aspects of your actions and the

actions of others made that happen. These are lessons to apply in the future. If the situation is not resolved, then further action is required.

In evaluating the outcome with Miguel, you realize that spending a few minutes to learn more about him made it easier to negotiate the removal of the snacks. He came to trust you because of the interest you showed in him as a person; this is often more effective than education that tells the patient what he or she can and cannot do. This is a strategy you can apply in the future.

Ethics Committees

Most hospitals have an ethics committee devoted to the teaching and processing of ethical issues and dilemmas. An ethics committee involves individuals from different disciplines and backgrounds who support health care institutions with three major functions: providing clinical ethics consultation, developing and/or revising policies pertaining to clinical ethics and hospital policy (e.g., advance directives, withholding and withdrawing life-sustaining treatments, informed consent, organ procurement), and facilitating education about topical issues in clinical ethics (University of Washington, 2018). In most institutions, any person seeking ethical advice, including nurses, physicians, health care providers, patients, and family members, can request access to an ethics committee.

Ethics committees often conduct their work by calling a meeting with the members of the team and the patient and family involved in the situation. When you attend an ethics meeting, be sure to articulate a personal point of view and at the same time to show respect for the points of view of others. A successful meeting is one in which every perspective is heard. Sometimes these meetings result in consensus around a specific course of action; other times the meeting ends without a clear plan but with an improved understanding of one another's perspectives.

You may also process ethical issues in settings other than a committee. Nurses provide insight about ethical problems at family conferences, staff meetings, or even in one-on-one meetings. As a member of a health care community, regardless of your work setting, you can reduce the risk for moral distress by promoting discourse even when disagreements or confusion are profound. You will find it helpful when engaged in these conversations to assume that all the participants want to do good, even if they may have different ideas about what that means.

> **QSEN** **Building Competency in Patient-Centered Care** You are assigned to care for a 75-year-old patient who is readmitted to the hospital after having knee surgery a week ago. He was brought to the hospital by ambulance because his family could not wake him up. In the emergency department, he responds well to treatment for opioid overdose, becoming more awake and alert. When you enter the room to do an initial assessment, the daughter expresses anger at her father's situation, namely that he was discharged after surgery with "too much medication." She states her belief that the care on the last hospital stay was "really inappropriate, especially since the news tells us we are in an opioid crisis." How will a focus on patient-centered care help you address this patient's needs and the daughter's concern?
>
> Answers to QSEN Activities can be found on the Evolve website.

ISSUES IN HEALTH CARE ETHICS

Ethical issues change as society and technologies change, but common denominators remain: the basic process used to address the issues and your responsibility to deal with them. The following section describes a few of the many current sources of ethical concerns.

Social Media

The access to Internet-based social networks, such as Facebook, Twitter, Snapchat, and Instagram, may present ethical challenges for nurses. On one hand, social media can be a supportive source of information about patient care or professional nursing activities and can provide you with emotional support when you encounter hardships at work. Social media can also be a source of support to your patients, to connect with friends and loved ones who cannot be physically present. On the other hand, the risk to patient privacy with social media is great (NCSBN, 2018). Posting information or pictures about patients, even without specific identifiers, is a violation of confidentiality.

Interactions between health care professionals and patients on social media is also problematic. Online "friendship" with a patient risks clouding your ability to remain objective in your clinical perceptions. This crosses the professional boundary between the patient and professional, and the relationship becomes more personal. The public nature of online interactions poses the additional risk that other users will recognize the nature of your relationship with the patient and learn more than they should about that person's health (NCSBN, 2018). Workplace policies may help to answer questions you have about when and where it is appropriate to engage in social media. In addition, the ANA (n.d.) has created a webpage with principles to guide nurses' use of social media (see https://www.nursingworld.org/social/).

Quality of Life

Quality of life is deeply personal. Health care researchers use quality-of-life measures to scientifically define the value and benefits of medical interventions. Any intervention creates a burden for the patient and family, and this must be offset by the benefit that they will receive from that care. Injections of flu vaccine, for instance, cause pain, but the short-term nature of this burden is offset by the large benefit of potentially avoiding infection with the flu or spreading of the flu, which are low-quality experiences. A more complex intervention, such as a 6-month course of chemotherapy, creates a greater burden and so impacts the quality of the patient's life to a greater degree. That impact is acceptable if the treatment outcome is a return to quality of life, based on the patient's definition. In the event that the treatment is unlikely to result in a quality of life that the patient finds acceptable, a different plan of care is considered.

Objective measures of quality of life can include the age of a patient, the patient's ability to live independently, or the ability to contribute to society in a gainful way. Subjective measures involve asking patients to identify their priorities, what they enjoy, and what matters most to them. Increasingly, scientists incorporate not just observed measurement but also patient self-reports about quality of life and other outcomes, referred to as Patient-Reported Outcomes (Basch et al., 2017). As a nurse, you can facilitate conversations about treatment choices by encouraging patients to articulate their definition of quality of life.

> ### REFLECT NOW
> What matters most to you and so should be included in your own personal definition of quality of life? What roles, relationships, or activities are you engaged in that are most meaningful to you?

Care At the End of Life

Providing care to patients at the end of life and to those with serious illness who may be nearing end of life is a frequent source of ethical problems. While everyone can agree that a "good death" is desirable, there are a variety of opinions about what a "good death" looks like.

In addition, patients and families may have goals for end of life, such as adequate pain control or being with family, but expect that this will happen much later and not now. Predictions about health outcomes are not always accurate, and thus health care providers may have difficulty conveying to patients with serious illness that end of life is at hand. Because views about death and dying are part of deeply held spiritual and cultural beliefs, conflicts about end-of-life care are common in health care. These conflicts can occur between members of the health care team and between patients, families, and team members (Giuliante, 2017).

The term *futile* refers to something that is hopeless or serves no useful purpose. In health care discussions, the term *futile* refers to interventions unlikely to produce benefit for a patient (Giuliante, 2017). The concept is slippery when applied to clinical situations. If a patient is dying of a condition with little or no hope of recovery, almost any intervention beyond symptom management and comfort measures is seen as futile. In this situation an agreement to label an intervention as futile can help the health care team members, families, and patients turn to palliative care measures as a more constructive approach to the situation (see Chapter 36).

Access to Health Care

Access to health care is an ethical issue of justice (Kub, 2017). The questions of "Is health care a right that everyone can claim?" and "How can we best divide the health care resources we have?" involve fairness and justice. In the United States, the cost of care is such that few can afford services unless they are enrolled in an insurance plan. In some cases, health insurance is provided as a benefit of employment. Those who do not have employer-based health insurance may qualify for state-based Medicaid programs on the basis of need or for Medicare, a federal insurance program available to all individuals over the age of 65. Because of conflicting views about what is fair and because of its effect on everyone, access to health care is a controversial issue.

While the nature of insurance coverage varies, most plans allow an individual to access some basic preventive care and more expensive urgent services when unexpected changes in health occur. In the latter part of the 20th century, as health care costs increased at a dramatic rate, the number of people with insurance declined. In 2010, the Affordable Care Act (ACA) was passed to create regulations that control costs and improve the availability of insurance. This legislation has facilitated access to care for millions of formerly uninsured individuals in the United States. According to a 2017 report by the National Health Center for Health Statistics, part of the US Department of Health and Human Services, the number of uninsured people in the United States declined by 20 million between 2010 and 2016 (Cohen et al., 2017). The ACA also offered changes in payment for services to reward practices that reduce harm and promote quality outcomes. The aim of this part of the legislation was to expand access to less expensive preventive health services and so reduce the incidence of expensive, burdensome chronic illness. How people access health care in the United States will continue to evolve. Staying knowledgeable about affordable care in your community as a way to ensure healthy outcomes is an important part of your role as advocate for your patients and will reflect your ethical commitment to justice (Box 22.5).

The courage and intelligence to act as both an advocate for patients and a professional member of the health care community come from a committed effort to learn and understand ethical principles. As a professional nurse, you provide a unique point of view regarding patients, the systems that support patients, and the institutions that make up the health care system. You have an obligation and a privilege to articulate that point of view. Learning how to identify and discuss ethical issues are some of the skills necessary to exercise this privilege. Review and consideration of various ethical principles help you form personal points of view, a necessary skill in the negotiation of difficult ethical situations.

🌐 BOX 22.5 CULTURAL ASPECTS OF CARE

Access to Affordable Health Care

Since the implementation of the Affordable Care Act, more residents in the United States have access to care than ever before. But according to the National Healthcare Disparities Report (NHDR), people of color, ethnic minorities, and low-income residents are "disproportionately represented among those with access problems." Reports from the National Healthcare Quality Report and NHDR reveal that lack of health insurance is the most significant contributing factor to poor quality of care (AHRQ, 2016).

Implications for Patient-Centered Care

- Issues of justice and the just distribution of resources help to inform the discussion about access to care and its effect on health care outcomes.
- Health outcomes often correlate directly to health care access.
- Know and respect patients' cultural practices regarding health promotion and health care needs (see Chapter 9).
- Identify culturally appropriate resources for patients and families in their communities.

KEY POINTS

- Learning and applying the language of ethics is an essential element of nursing practice.
- Understanding our own values and encouraging patients, families, and colleagues to clarify their values promote productive discussion of ethical problems.
- You apply fundamental concepts such as autonomy, justice, fidelity, and beneficence to ethical decision making.
- Approaches to ethics include deontology, utilitarianism, and a relationship-based perspective.
- In an ethical dilemma, a nurse faces two equally justifiable courses of action, whereas in moral distress the nurse feels unable to take the action that is correct.
- Using a systematic approach similar to the nursing process promotes resolution of ethical issues. While the specific ethical issues nurses face evolve and change over time, the values and obligations remain constant.

REFLECTIVE LEARNING

- Do you think there are situations in which maintaining confidentiality and withholding private information are not the right actions? Discuss why.
- Think about your first impression of a patient early in the day, when you first met. How did this impression change over the course of spending a shift involved in their care? How do you think this change in your perspective relates to your ethical obligations as a nurse?
- What questions might you ask a patient if you wanted to better understand the patient's view of quality of life?

REVIEW QUESTIONS

1. The nurse is caring for a patient who needs a liver transplant to survive. This patient has been out of work for several months, does not have health insurance, and cannot afford the procedure. Which of the following statements speaks to the ethical elements of this case?
   1. The health care team should select a plan that considers the principle of justice as it pertains to the distribution of health care resources.
   2. The patient should enroll in a clinical trial of a new technology that can do the work of the liver, similar to the way dialysis treats kidney disease.
   3. The social worker should look into enrolling the patient in Medicaid, since many states offer expanded coverage.
   4. A family meeting should take place in which the details of the patient's poor prognosis are made clear to his family so that they can adopt a palliative approach.
2. When designing a plan for pain management for a patient following surgery, the nurse assesses that the patient's priority is to be as free of pain as possible. The nurse and patient work together to identify a plan to manage the pain. The nurse continually reviews the plan with the patient to ensure that the patient's priority is met. If the nurse's actions are driven by respect for autonomy, what aspect of this scenario best demonstrates that?
   1. Assessing the patient's pain on a numeric scale every 2 hours
   2. Asking the patient to establish the goal for pain control
   3. Using alternative measures such as distraction or repositioning to relieve the pain
   4. Monitoring the patient for oversedation as a side effect of his pain medication
3. The application of deontology does not always resolve an ethical problem. Which of the following statements best explains one of the limitations of deontology?
   1. The emphasis on relationships feels uncomfortable to decision makers who want more structure in deciding the best action.
   2. The single focus on power imbalances does not apply to all situations in which ethical problems occur.
   3. In a diverse community it can be difficult to find agreement on which principles or rules are most important.
   4. The focus on consequences rather than on the "goodness" of an action makes decision makers uncomfortable.
4. The *ethics of care* suggests that ethical dilemmas can best be solved by attention to relationships. How does this differ from other approaches to ethical problems? (Select all that apply.)
   1. Ethics of care pays attention to the context in which caring occurs.
   2. Ethics of care is used only by nurses because it is part of the Nursing Code of Ethics.
   3. Ethics of care requires understanding the relationships between involved parties.
   4. Ethics of care considers the decision maker's relationships with other involved parties.
   5. Ethics of care is an approach that suggests a greater commitment to patient care.
   6. Ethic of care considers the decision maker to be in a detached position outside the ethical problem.
5. The following are steps in the process to help resolve an ethical problem. What is the best order of these steps to achieve resolution?
   1. List all the possible actions that could be taken to resolve the problem.
   2. Articulate a statement of the problem or dilemma that you are trying to resolve.
   3. Develop and implement a plan to address the problem.
   4. Gather all relevant information regarding the clinical, social, and spiritual aspects of the problem.
   5. Take time to clarify values and identify the ethical elements, such as principles and key relationships involved.
   6. Recognize that the problem requires ethics.

6. What is the best response for the nurse to give if a patient asks the nurse to send a photo of an x-ray to him via a messaging tool in a social media site?
   1. Yes, if you remove all patient identifiers before sending
   2. No, because the patient's x-ray results should be discussed with a provider
   3. Yes, because respect for autonomy means honoring this patient's request
   4. No, because health information of any kind should not be shared on social media

7. Resolution of an ethical problem involves discussion with the patient, the patient's family, and participants from appropriate health care disciplines. Which statement best describes the role of the nurse in the resolution of ethical problems?
   1. To articulate the nurse's unique point of view, including knowledge based on clinical and psychosocial observations
   2. To study the literature on current research about the possible clinical interventions available for the patient in question
   3. To hold a point of view but realize that respect for the authority of administrators and physicians takes precedence over personal views
   4. To allow the patient and the physician private time to resolve the dilemma on the basis of ethical principles

8. Which statements reflect the difficulty that can occur for agreement on a common definition of the word *quality* when it comes to quality of life? (Select all that apply.)
   1. Community values influence definitions of quality, and they are subject to change over time.
   2. Individual experiences influence perceptions of quality in different ways, making consensus difficult.
   3. The value of elements such as cognitive skills, ability to perform meaningful work, and relationship to family is difficult to quantify using objective measures.
   4. Statistical analysis is difficult to apply when the outcome cannot be quantified.
   5. Whether a person has a job is an objective measure, but it does not play a role in understanding quality of life.

9. Which statements properly apply an ethical principle to justify access to health care? (Select all that apply.)
   1. Access to health care reflects the commitment of society to principles of beneficence and justice.
   2. If low income compromises access to care, respect for autonomy is compromised.
   3. Access to health care is a privilege in the United States, not a right.
   4. Poor access to affordable health care causes harm that is ethically troubling because nonmaleficence is a basic principle of health care ethics.
   5. If a new drug is discovered that cures a disease but at great cost per patient, the principle of justice suggests that the drug should be made available to those who can afford it.

10. Match the following actions (1 through 4) with the terms (a through d) listed below:

    a. Advocacy
    b. Responsibility
    c. Accountability
    d. Confidentiality

    1. You see an open medical record on the computer and close it so that no one else can read the record without proper access.
    2. You administer a once-a-day cardiac medication at the wrong time, but nobody sees it. However, you contact the provider and your head nurse and follow agency procedure.
    3. A patient at the end of life wants to go home to die, but the family wants every care possible. The nurse contacts the primary care provider about the patient's request.
    4. You tell your patient that you will return in 30 minutes to give him his next pain medication.

Answers: 1. 1; 2. 3; 3. 4; 1; 3; 4; 5; 6. 4; 5; 2; 1; 3; 6. 4; 7. 1; 8. 1, 2, 4; 9. 1, 2, 4; 10. 1d, 2c, 3a, 4b.

Rationales for Review Questions can be found on the Evolve website.

REFERENCES

Agency for Healthcare Research and Quality (AHRQ): *National Healthcare Disparities report*, 2016. https://www.ahrq.gov/research/findings/nhqrdr/nhqdr16/index.html. Accessed July 28, 2019.

American Nurses Association (ANA): Code of ethics, revised 2015, http://www.nursingworld.org/MainMenu-Categories/EthicsStandards/CodeofEthicsforNurses/Code-of-Ethics-For-Nurses.html. Accessed July 28, 2019.

American Nurses Association (ANA): Social networking principles, n.d. https://www.nursingworld.org/social/. Accessed July 28, 2019.

Basch E, et al.: Overall survival results of a trial assessing patient-Reported outcomes for symptom monitoring during Routine Cancer treatment, *J Am Med Assoc* 318(2):197–198, 2017.

Cohen RA, et al.: Health insurance coverage: early release of estimates from the National Health Interview Survey 2016. 2017. https://www.cdc.gov/nchs/data/nhis/earlyrelease/insur201705.pdf. Accessed July 28, 2019.

Doherty RF, Purtilo RB: A six-step process of ethical decision making. In *Ethical Dimensions in the health professions*, ed 6, St Louis, 2016, Elsevier.

Green B: Applying feminist ethics of care to nursing practice, *Nurs Care* 1:3, 2012, https://doi.org/10.4172/2167-1168.1000111.

Giuliante MM: Exploring ethical issues encountered with the older adult. In Robichaux C, editor: *Ethical competence in nursing practice: competencies, skills and decision making*, New York, 2017, Springer Publishing Company.

Klugman CM: Recognizing ethical terms, theories and principles. In Robichaux C, editor: *Ethical competence in nursing practice: competencies, skills and decision making*, New York, 2017, Springer Publishing Company.

Kub J: Public health ethics and social justice in the community. In Robichaux C, editor: *Ethical competence in nursing practice: competencies, skills and decision making*, New York, 2017, Springer Publishing Company.

Lachman V: Applying the ethics of care to your nursing practice, *Medsurg Nurs* 21(2):112–116, 2012.

National Council of State Boards of Nursing (NCSBN): *A nurse's guide to the use of social media*, 2018, https://www.ncsbn.org/NCSBN_SocialMedia.pdf. Accessed July 28, 2019.

Robichaux C: Recognizing and addressing moral distress in nursing practice: personal, professional and organizational factors. In Robichaux C, editor: *Ethical competence in*

nursing practice: competencies, skills and decision making, New York, 2017, Springer Publishing Company.

Rushton C, et al.: A collaborative state of the science initiative: transforming moral distress into moral resilience in nursing, 2017, American Journal of Nursing "State of the Science: Transforming Moral Distress into Moral Resilience in Nursing" February 2017 VOL 117 Supplement 1. S2-S6, https://journals.lww.com/ajnonline/toc/2017/02001. Accessed July 28, 2019.

Strong C: *Casuistry. The international encyclopedia of ethics*, 2013, https://doi.org/10.1002/9781444367072.wbiee344. Accessed July 28, 2019.

The Joint Commission (TJC): *Facts about the national patient safety goals*, 2019, https://www.jointcommission.org/assets/1/6/NPSG_Chapter_HAP_Jan2019.pdf. Accessed July 28, 2019.

University of Washington: Ethics committees, programs and consultations, Ethics in Medicine. 2018, Available at https://depts.washington.edu/bhdept/ethics-medicine. Accessed July 28, 2019.

US Department of Health and Human Services (USDHHS): *HIPAA for professionals*, 2017, https://www.hhs.gov/hipaa/for-professionals/index.html. Accessed July 28, 2019.

RESEARCH REFERENCES

American Association of Critical-Care Nurses: *AACN standards for establishing and sustaining healthy work environments*, ed 2, 2016, https://www.aacn.org/~/media/aacn-website/nursing-excellence/standards/hwestandards.pdf. Accessed July 28, 2019.

Hamric AB and Epstein EG: A health system-wide moral distress consultation service: development and evaluation, *HEC Forum* 29(2): 127-143, 2017, https://doi.org/10.1007/s10730-016-9315-y.

Pavlish C, et al.: Screening situations for risk of ethical conflicts: a pilot study, 2015, *Am J Crit Care* 24(3):248–256, 2015.

Rodney P: What we know about moral distress, 2017, *Am J Nurs* 117(2):S7–S10, 2017, https://doi.org/10.1097/01.NAJ.0000512204.85973.04.

Rushton C: Cultivating moral resilience, 2017, *Am J Nurs* 117(2):S11–S15, 2017, https://doi.org/10.1097/01.NAJ.0000512205.93596.00.

Sofer D: Panel discussion 2: promising system and environmental strategies for addressing moral distress and building moral resilience. 2017, *Am J Nurs* 117(2):S18–S20, 2017, https://doi.org/10.1097/01.NAJ.0000512207.39339.01.

23

Legal Implications in Nursing Practice

OBJECTIVES

- Compare constitutional, civil, and criminal law.
- Describe statutory law as it affects nursing practice.
- Define the scope of nursing practice and the standards of nursing care.
- Define the standard of proof required to establish a nurse's negligence.
- Discuss examples of federal statutes that affect nursing practice.
- Analyze under what circumstances a patient can be chemically or physically restrained.

- Explain what a nurse's witnessing of a patient's informed consent indicates.
- List the elements needed to establish negligence and malpractice.
- Determine nursing actions most often associated in a breach of nursing practice.
- Identify proactive measures nurses can take to help reduce their legal risks.

KEY TERMS

Administrative law, p. 307
Battery, p. 314
Case law, p. 307
Civil law, p. 306
Common law, p. 307
Constitutional law, p. 306
Criminal law, p. 306
Defamation of character, p. 314
Durable power of attorney for health care (DPAHC), p. 310

Informed consent, p. 313
Intentional tort, p. 314
Libel, p. 315
Malpractice, p. 315
Neglect, p. 314
Negligence, p. 315
Nurse Practice Acts, p. 306
Occurrence report, p. 318
Professional licensure defense, p. 312
Risk management, p. 317

Scope of nursing practice, p. 307
Slander, p. 314
Standard of proof, p. 307
Standards of nursing care, p. 307
Statutory law, p. 306
Torts, p. 314
Unintentional torts, p. 315

MEDIA RESOURCES

http://evolve.elsevier.com/Potter/fundamentals/
- Review Questions
- Case Study with Questions

- Audio Glossary
- Content Updates
- Answers to QSEN Activity and Review Questions

Safe evidence-based and competent nursing practice requires nurses to know laws, policies, and other valid, reliable, and applicable sources that define their practice. Laws, standards, and policies help to frame the health care system in which nurses practice. They include state Nurse Practice Acts, the scope and standards of nursing care, and the code of ethics for nursing practice. Understanding where you fit in the health care system demands clinical judgment skills. Society expects safe health care delivery, especially from nurses, who typically are perceived as being part of the most ethical and trusted profession. As patient care becomes more complex and practice innovations and new health care technologies emerge, the principles of negligence and malpractice liability are being applied to challenging new situations. Thus, you need to know laws governing nursing practice to provide evidence-based care that keeps the patient at the center of decision making.

LEGAL LIMITS OF NURSING

Sources of Law

Many types of law govern nursing practice, including constitutional law, statutory law, common law, administrative law, and case law. Knowing these sources of law informs your practice and identifies why it is important to provide current evidence-based care when working with your clients.

Constitutional law is derived from federal and state constitutions. For example, in the United States, a constitutional right afforded to every citizen is the right to refuse treatment (Furrow et al., 2018). As a nurse, you must know the parameters of the right of your patients to refuse treatment even when you may not agree with their decisions.

Statutory law is derived from statutes passed by the US Congress and state legislatures. These laws are either civil or criminal. **Civil laws** protect the rights of individuals and provide for fair and equitable treatment when civil wrongs or violations occur (Furrow et al., 2018; Pozgar, 2016). **Nurse Practice Acts** are civil state laws that define nursing and the standards you must meet within individual states. As a nursing student, you will find your scope of practice, the educational requirements you must have, and information you may need in the future when you want to take the NCLEX exam in your state's Nurse Practice Act (Oyeleye, 2019; Pozgar, 2016). Nurse Practice Acts also distinguish nursing from other health professions (e.g., medicine, therapists, and alternative medicine providers).

Criminal laws protect society and provide punishment for crimes, which are defined by municipal, state, and federal legislation (Furrow et al., 2018). Typically, actions that violate criminal laws are defined as either misdemeanors or felonies. Criminal mistreatment of vulnerable adults is an example of criminal statutory law. Criminal mistreatment is classified as either a misdemeanor or felony offense depending on the severity of harm done to a vulnerable patient.

Administrative law, or regulatory law, more clearly defines expectations of civil and criminal laws. For example, a Nurse Practice Act, as a civil statutory law, states that you have a duty to care for your patients. Regulations typically state that duty means you will observe, assess, diagnose, plan, intervene, and evaluate patient care. Providing current, evidence-based care is essential to meeting nursing statutory duty and regulations. Regulatory law also describes the process to report incompetent or unethical nursing conduct to the State Board of Nursing or Nursing Commission. A nurse who does not report unethical or incompetent conduct violates regulatory law. Nurses can appeal violations to the State Board of Nursing or the Nursing Commission. In comparison, criminal mistreatment statutes have regulations to determine the intent of the person who commits the crime. The degree of offense often distinguishes whether the person intentionally committed the mistreatment, knew or should have known harm would result, or didn't consider that harm would result. Nurses who are accused of violating a regulatory law typically knew or should have known their actions could result in patient harm.

Common law originates from decisions that were made in the absence of law. For example, the right to privacy is implied in the US Constitution. Thus, patient confidentiality originated as common law. Prior to the passage of multiple related laws, a patient's right to confidentiality, which prevents nurses and health care providers from sharing patient information with others who are not caring for the patient, was implied through common law (Furrow et al., 2018; Busch, 2019; McGuire et al., 2019).

Case law describes decisions made in legal cases that were resolved in courts. After a case is presented to a judge or jury, there is a report of the issue, facts, findings, and subsequent decision that was made to resolve the issue. For example, In Re: Estate of Turner v. M. Medical Center (2018), the guardian of the estate of Ms. Turner alleged that her health care providers did not meet the standard of practice when caring for a tracheostomy required to assist her to breathe. Subsequently, she died. At trial, the jury concurred and awarded the estate $22 million. After an appeal and a lengthy analysis, the court awarded in favor of the estate for $7 million in light of past damages, but it denied the request for future damages in the amount of $15 million.

Scope and Standards of Nursing

The scope of nursing practice defines nursing and reflects the values of the nursing profession. Standards of nursing care reflect the knowledge and skill ordinarily possessed and used by nurses (Furrow et al., 2018; Black, 2020) (see Chapter 1). Standards of nursing care are derived from health care laws, best practice guidelines, professional organization white papers, evidence-based nursing knowledge, and citizen advocacy groups.

The American Nurses Association (ANA) (2015a) and specialty nursing organizations develop standards for nursing practice, the code of ethics for nurses, and policy statements. For example, the scope of nursing and 17 standards of practice that describe what nurses do are published by the ANA (2015a). Nursing is defined, and the responsibilities and expectations of a registered nurse (RN) are clearly explained. They define the scope, function, and role of the nurse in practice and guide your practice. Sometimes they are used when legal actions are taken against nurses.

Nursing policies and procedures within health care agencies are based on the scope and standards of nursing practice. They must reflect current best practice and the evidence that supports the processes that they describe. The Joint Commission (TJC) (2019) requires written nursing policies and procedures that are accessible on all nursing units. Agency policies and procedures must conform to state and federal laws and community standards (TJC, 2019; Furrow et al., 2018).

For example, bedside report is a best practice for health care settings because it places patients at the center of decision making and emphasizes the importance of clear communication with patients and their families. When a hospital establishes a policy and procedure to implement bedside hand-off reporting, the nurse who is transferring care of a patient to another nurse, the nurse accepting the care of the patient, and the patient should be involved in the reporting process. If the nurses decide not to follow the policy and procedure and conduct the report without including the patient, the nurses are not following the policy and procedure. Thus, the nurses may be at risk for litigation, especially if harm occurs to the patient because of not following the hospital's policy. Thus, it is important to know the scope and standards of nursing practice as well as the health care agency's policies and procedures intended to implement them.

Standard of Proof

The standard of proof is typically what a reasonably prudent nurse would do under similar circumstances in the geographic area in which the alleged breach occurred. Malpractice is the result of nursing care falling below a standard of care. In a malpractice lawsuit, it is typically required that the nurse had a duty of care (i.e., Nurse Practice Act), that the duty was breached (i.e., nursing regulations), that physical harm occurred (i.e., testimony and records), and that in that state damages or monetary compensation are allowed. The standard of proof in this case is the degree to which the evidence must show that a duty of care was violated, resulting in harm to the patient.

During a malpractice suit, a nurse's actual conduct is compared with nursing standards of care (i.e., Scope and Standards of Nursing Care [ANA, 2015a, b]) to determine whether the nurse acted as any reasonably prudent nurse would act under the same or similar circumstances (Furrow et al., 2018; Philo et al., 2015). For example, if a patient is burned from a warm compress application, negligence is determined by reviewing whether the nurse followed the correct procedure for applying the compress. If a procedure is not followed, the policy is reviewed. It there is no policy, this could reflect a systemic problem because the nurses are not provided information regarding current evidence-based knowledge to guide them on how to appropriately apply warm compresses. There is a greater possibility that other patients are at risk for, or have already had, burns due to erroneous application of warm compresses. The scope and standards of nursing practice are also being violated; subsequently, litigation would encompass more than failure to simply follow a procedure. The policies and procedures that guide your practice need to be updated regularly and reflect current best practice evidence. When you follow your agency's policies and procedures, you ensure that your care is similar to what other reasonable, prudent nursing colleagues would provide under the same or similar circumstances.

FEDERAL STATUTES IMPACTING NURSING PRACTICE

Federal statutes and regulations affect nursing practice in many ways. Typically, they are linked to certification contracts for Medicare and Medicaid reimbursement. They are often expanded when states pass laws that increase application of the federal statute to others in that state. For example, the Omnibus Reconciliation Act of 1987 mandated that skilled nursing facility residents are given rights, including but not limited to being able to vote, receiving visitors privately, receiving a

30-day notice of discharge before moving from the facility, and being able to participate in meetings to develop their plan of care. Many states subsequently passed laws where these same rights were given to patients in retirement homes, assisted-living facilities, and adult family homes. Thus, it is important to consider federal statutes in context with how they are implemented in each state.

Patient Protection and Affordable Care Act

The Patient Protection and Affordable Care Act (PPACA) was passed in 2010. Its name was later changed to the Affordable Care Act (ACA). The ACA is characterized by four themes embedded in nursing practice: (1) consumer rights and protections, (2) affordable health care coverage, (3) increased access to care, and (4) quality of care that meets the needs of patients. The ACA has been challenged in court many times since its enactment. Examples of issues discussed in court around the ACA include mandatory enrollment in health care insurance and eligibility for insurance for patients with a pre-existing condition.

A new Patient's Bill of Rights, created by the ACA, prohibits patients from being denied health care coverage because of prior existing conditions, limits on the amount of care for those conditions, and/or an accidental mistake in paperwork when a patient got sick (PPACA, 2010). More than 17.6 million children with preexisting conditions became eligible for health care and more than 105 million Americans no longer have lifetime limits to receive care when they are ill because of the ACA.

The ACA intended to reduce overall medical costs by (1) providing tax credits, (2) increasing insurance company accountability for premiums and rate increases, and (3) increasing the number of choices available to patients to select insurers that best meet their needs. In addition, the ACA increased access to health care. Patients now receive recommended preventive services such as screenings for cancer, blood pressure, and diabetes without having to pay copays or deductibles. The ACA improved Medicare coverage for vulnerable populations by improving access to care and prescriptions, decreasing costs of medications, extending the life of the Medicare Trust Fund until 2024, and addressing fraud and abuse in billing practices (USDHHS, 2015).

The ACA reduced the number of uninsured Americans from over 44 million people in 2013, right before the act's health care coverage provisions began, to just below 27 million people in 2016. In 2017, however, the number of uninsured people went up by almost 700,000 people (KFF, 2018). The high cost of medical insurance and not having access to medical coverage through an employer are the main reasons people remain uninsured. Other adults are ineligible for financial assistance for health care coverage, especially those who live in states that did not expand Medicaid coverage. Those who remain uninsured typically are in families who have at least one family member who works, who are in families that have a low income, and who are adults under 65 years of age. The largest increases in the number of people who are uninsured occurred in non-Hispanic blacks and people living above poverty (KFF, 2018).

Like all statutes, the ACA has and will continue to change. For example, the Centers for Medicare & Medicaid Services (CMS, 2019) proposed changes in the act to increase the affordability of coverage, to allow people the choice to join Qualified Health Plans (QHPs) that do not cover termination of pregnancy services, and to provide greater flexibility in how people shop for QHPs. It is especially important that nurses have current factual knowledge about these changes and provide accurate information to patients when they seek guidance about their health care. Nurses are often at the center of those decisions with their patients. It is critical that when helping patients make decisions about their care, the decisions are clinically sound and based on the patient's preferences, values, and beliefs.

Emergency Medical Treatment and Active Labor Act

The Emergency Medical Treatment and Active Labor Act (EMTALA) (1986) prohibits the transfer of patients from private to public hospitals without appropriate screening and stabilization. It is intended to prevent what is referred to as patient dumping. This act ensures that when patients come to the emergency department or the hospital, an appropriate medical screening occurs. Staff must assess all patients who enter the hospital and cannot discharge or transfer them until their conditions stabilize. Exceptions to this provision include if a patient requests transfer or discharge in writing after receiving information about the benefits and risks of the transfer or if a physician or nurse practitioner certifies that the benefits of transfer outweigh the risks.

Health Insurance Portability and Accountability Act

The Health Insurance Portability and Accountability Act (HIPAA, 1996) provides rights to patients and protects employees. It includes standards regarding accountability in the health care setting. Notably, it establishes patient rights regarding privacy of their health care information and records.

HIPAA established a patient's right to consent to the use and disclosure of protected health information, to inspect and copy one's medical record, and to amend mistaken or incomplete information (Privacy Rights Clearinghouse, 2014). It limits who can access a patient's record. It establishes the basis for privacy and confidentiality concerns, viewed as two basic rights within the US health care system. Privacy is the right of patients to keep personal information from being disclosed. Confidentiality protects private patient information once it is disclosed in health care settings. Nurses help health care agencies protect patients' rights to privacy and confidentiality. Although HIPAA does not require extreme measures such as soundproof rooms in hospitals, it does mean that nurses and health care providers need to avoid discussing patients in public hallways and provide reasonable levels of privacy when communicating with and about patients in any manner. For example, message boards used in hospital rooms to post daily patient care information can no longer contain information revealing a patient's medical condition. Thus, nurses must be especially vigilant to assure that patients are afforded the privacy they are entitled to and that is mandated in law.

Health care information privacy is also protected by standards set by the Centers for Medicare and Medicaid Services (CMS) for hospitals and health care providers who participate in Medicare and Medicaid (CMS, 2018; Furrow et al., 2018). These standards require that hospitals and health care providers give notice to patients of their rights to decisions about their care, grievances regarding their care management, personal freedom and safety, confidentiality, access to their own medical records, and freedom from physical or chemical restraints that are not clinically necessary (see Chapter 14). In addition, many state laws allow patients to access their medical records. Exceptions apply to psychotherapy notes or when a health care provider has determined that access would result in harm to the patient or another party (Privacy Rights Clearinghouse, 2018).

Health Information Technology Act

The Health Information Technology for Economic and Clinical Health Act (HITECH Act, 2009) was passed with HIPAA in response to new technology and social media. HITECH expands the principles extended under HIPAA, especially when a security breach of personal health information (PHI) occurs. Under the HITECH Act, nurses must

BOX 23.1 EVIDENCE-BASED PRACTICE

Social Media and Legal Liability

PICOT Question: Do nurses who use social media as a part of their professional practice put themselves at greater risk for legal liability compared with nurses who do not use social media?

Evidence Summary

Social media is used today to reach millions of patients, colleagues, and peers. It is a useful tool for promoting collaboration, disseminating and sharing information, and providing education. Nurses are ultimately responsible and accountable for understanding the use, implications, and guidelines associated with the use of social media (NCSBN, 2018; Scruth et al., 2015). The NCSBN (2018) and the International Nurse Regulators Collaborative (INRC) identified nurses' behaviors for appropriate use of social media. Nurses who follow current professional guidelines and laws can use social media to enhance their practice and do not place themselves at greater risk for liability (NCSBN, 2018; Scruth et al., 2015).

Application to Nursing Practice

- Understand the risks and benefits of using social media (NCSBN, 2018).
- Maintain professional boundaries (NCSBN, 2018).
- Present a professional image in all social media interactions (Scruth et al., 2015).
- Maintain privacy and confidentiality (NCSBN, 2018).
- Understand the implications of identifying yourself as a nurse (NCSBN, 2018).
- Know state laws governing use of social media (NCSBN, 2018).

ensure that patient PHI is not inadvertently conveyed on social media and that protected data are not disclosed other than as permitted by patients (Box 23.1). Best practice, regardless of patient consent, is to never enter patient information on social media. Electronic data are accessible, regardless of assurances to the contrary. Civil and criminal sanctions may be brought against both a nurse and an organization if either or both violate HIPAA or the HITECH Act. Report violations of patient confidentiality to your supervisor.

Americans With Disabilities Act

The Americans With Disabilities Act (ADA) of 1990 and amended in 2008 is a civil rights statute that protects the rights of people with physical or mental disabilities (ADANN, 2018; Dupler et al., 2012). The ADA prohibits discrimination and ensures equal opportunities for people with disabilities in employment, state and local government services, public accommodations, commercial facilities, and transportation. As defined by the statute and the US Supreme Court, a disability is a mental or physical condition that substantially limits a major life activity, including seeing, hearing, speaking, walking, breathing, performing manual tasks, learning, caring for oneself, and/or working. Employers must provide reasonable accommodations to employees or applicants who are qualified to hold a job. Reasonable accommodations enable a person to perform the essential functions of a job (ADA, 2019). For example, as expanded under the ADA, an employer must consider the needs of a person with diabetes mellitus as a potential disability and reasonably accommodate that person's needs. A person with a disability makes the choice whether to tell others of his or her disability. By exception, several cases have held that a health care provider must disclose if he or she has human immunodeficiency virus (HIV). Despite these rulings and as enforced by the Office of Equal Employment Opportunity, the ADA protects health care workers in the workplace with disabilities such as HIV infection. Likewise, health care workers cannot discriminate against patients who are HIV-positive (Furrow et al., 2018).

Mental Health Parity and Addiction Equity Act

The Mental Health Parity and Addiction Equity Act of 2008 (MHPAEA) (as amended by the Health Care and Education Reconciliation Act of 2010 and collectively part of the ACA) requires health insurance companies to provide coverage for mental health and substance use disorder (SUD) treatment, just as they do for medical coverage. The ACA extended these requirements to small group and individual health insurance plans (US Department of Treasury, 2013). The ACA requires parity (the state or condition of being equal) in the provision of 10 specific services, including mental health, behavioral health, and SUD services. Insurers may not discriminate or deny coverage to patients with mental illness or SUD because of preexisting conditions. However, the ACA does not clearly define mental illness or SUD. Thus, many believe that insurers will provide services; however, the cost of the insurance may be so high that the services will not be affordable to those who need them.

The Mental Health and Substance Use Disorder Parity Task Force first met in March 2016. It facilitates coordination of services among federal agencies and assures that consumers receive the care and treatment they require. The task force improved awareness of the benefits that parity for mental health and substance use disorders provides. For example, to increase transparency, the task force has helped stakeholders (e.g., insurers, regulators, and consumers) understand what equality means in relation to treatment of mental health illnesses and substance use disorders. The task force also provides resources to ensure that coverage is consistent with the intent of the MHPAEA (https://www.hhs.gov/programs/topic-sites/mental-health-parity/index.html).

Admission of a patient to a mental health or SUD unit occurs involuntarily or on a voluntary basis. Involuntary admission to a mental health center usually occurs when patients are a danger to themselves (e.g., patients who are suicidal) or others. Typically, this determination is made by a mental health professional (MHP) in the emergency room. In some states, patients with a SUD can also be placed in a treatment center by a SUD professional if they are a danger to themselves or others. In either case, the professional who assessed the patient, a court-appointed guardian ad litem, a family member, or another interested party can ask the court to determine whether a longer stay is required to protect the patient from continuing to harm self or others. A judge may order the patient to be hospitalized for 21 more days for treatment. From a legal perspective this is viewed as taking away a patient's constitutional rights. Nurses must clearly and accurately document the patient's behaviors. The court will review this evidence when making its decisions (Furrow et al., 2018; Barr et al., 2019). Under constitutional law, having the right to move from place to place is at the very basis of being a US citizen. When removing that constitutionally protected right, the case must be made that not doing so would result in significant or deadly harm.

When patients attempt suicide within health care settings, it is typically alleged that nurses failed to provide appropriate individualized care, supervise the patient adequately, and adhere to existing policies and procedures to keep the patient safe. When providing care to patients with mental illnesses and SUDs, consider the scope and standards of nursing care as well as the specific statutes and regulations associated with their care. You also need to know your employer's policies and procedures when caring for patients at risk of harm. Integrate this knowledge to provide evidence-based nursing and to ensure that your documentation reflects the care you provided.

Patient Self-Determination Act

The Patient Self-Determination Act (PSDA) enacted in 1991 requires health care institutions to provide written information to patients concerning their rights to make decisions about their care, including the right to refuse treatment and to formulate an advance directive. A patient's record must indicate whether a patient has signed an advance directive and include a copy of the directive if it is available. Patients must also be offered information about advance directives.

An advance directive is a document developed by the patient that instructs others to do tasks before, during, and after his or her death. At a minimum, an advance directive includes a statement of the patient's wishes if a respiratory or cardiac arrest occurs and a copy of the patient's durable power of attorney for health care (DPAHC). Instructions regarding care before or during cardiac or respiratory arrest should be signed by either a physician or nurse practitioner. Unless otherwise specified by state law, the document should be treated as an order; it may direct whether to provide lifesaving measures such as cardiopulmonary resuscitation (CPR) or to provide comfort care only.

Most DPAHCs begin with a statement that says the designated person can make decisions when the patient becomes incapacitated. This means that patients cannot be bypassed—they retain the ability and the right to make their own decisions whenever they can. This is true whether they are at home, in the emergency room, or in an inpatient setting. Decisional capacity is the patient's ability to make choices about his or her care. The health care provider, working in conjunction with information from nurses and family members, can make the determination of decisional capacity. The power of attorney for health care may not be asked and cannot make health care decisions until a provider makes an assessment that the patient no longer has the capacity to make decisions. The assessment that triggers the beginning of the DPAHC should be reflected in the record.

When the physician or nurse practitioner is unable to determine capacity or there is disagreement regarding the patient's capacity, a competency hearing is conducted in court on the patient's behalf. As in involuntary commitment hearings, the court is asked to deny a US citizen the constitutional right to make decisions, which essentially takes away all rights and privileges provided as a US citizen. When a patient is determined to be incompetent, a guardian is appointed to make decisions regarding care the patient will or will not receive. No other person, including family members or providers, has the power to override the guardian's decisions. To do so, that person must return to court and explain why the guardian's decision should not be honored. Thus, under the Patient Self-Determination Act and state specific statutes, advance directives that include a DPAHC and orders whether to provide or not provide resuscitation must be clear and in compliance with law. Nursing care is individualized based on the patient's instructions and on the state in which the patient resides at the time a directive is implemented. The DPAHC's ability to make decisions for the patient ends at the time of death. Thus, it is important that patients and their families arrange their after-life care in advance when possible.

Living wills also include information about a patient's preferences regarding end-of-life care (Furrow et al., 2018; Touhy & Jett, 2018). Some include physician orders about sustaining life, such as use of enteral feedings. Others contain information on whether to initiate CPR on cessation of breathing. It is important to thoroughly read documents titled "living will." They are based on values of informed consent, patient autonomy over end-of-life decisions, truth telling, and control over the dying process. A patient must be capable to make decisions regarding his or her own health care treatment when creating a living will. Many resources are available to help create a living will. For example, Five Wishes is an organization that helps patients write their directives when responding to five questions (https://fivewishes.org/). The questions help patients identify a DPAHC, the kind of medical treatment wanted or not wanted, comfort measures they wish to receive, how they want to be treated by those around them, and what they want those who love them to know. Providing this information and assisting patients in recording their wishes is rewarding for the patient, empowering to their loved ones, and humbling to the nurses who help them.

Patients make difficult decisions when writing a living will. Sometimes family and friends have difficulty in understanding and adhering to those decisions. The ethical doctrine of autonomy, which has been upheld in court, ensures the patient right to refuse medical treatment. For example, courts upheld a patient's right to refuse medical treatment in the *Bouvia v Superior Court* case (1986). Courts have also upheld the right of a legally competent patient to refuse medical treatment for religious reasons. The US Supreme Court stated in the *Cruzan v Director of Missouri Department of Health* case (1990) that "we assume that the US Constitution would grant a constitutionally protected competent person the right to refuse lifesaving hydration and nutrition." In the Terri Schiavo case, (*Schindler & Schindler v Schiavo*, 2003) Schiavo's husband, who was her legal guardian, argued that his wife would not want to have her life artificially prolonged. Her parents disagreed and wanted her to continue to receive artificial nutrition and hydration. The court noted that it understood "why a parent who had raised and nurtured a child from conception would hold out hope that some level of cognitive function remained." However, after more than 10 years, the court upheld the guardianship court's initial decision to allow Ms. Schiavo's husband, as her guardian, to make medical decisions on her behalf in the absence of her wishes being known before her death.

In cases involving a patient's right to refuse or withdraw medical treatment, the courts balance the patient's interest with the interest of the state in protecting life, preserving medical ethics, preventing suicide, and protecting innocent third parties. Children are generally innocent third parties. Although the courts will not force adults to undergo treatment refused for religious reasons, they will grant an order allowing hospitals and health care providers to treat children of parents or groups who have denied consent for treatment of their minor children for religious reasons. This is based on the legal doctrine of *parens patriae* in which the state or government makes decisions on behalf of those who are unable to make decisions for themselves.

In addition to patient refusals of treatment, nurses frequently encounter "do not resuscitate" (DNR) or "no code" DNR orders. The state of New York was the first to develop legislation based on the recommendations of the New York State Task Force on Life and the Law in 1986. These recommendations, which went into effect in 1988, allow competent adults to authorize a DNR order (Golden, 1988). Documentation that the health care provider has consulted with the patient and/or family is required before writing a DNR order in the patient's medical record (Furrow et al., 2018; Touhy & Jett, 2018). Patient conditions change, and patients have the right to change their minds. The health care provider needs to review DNR orders with the patient periodically to assure that the order reflects current wishes.

When patients have living wills or advance directives remember that the "do not resuscitate" designation does not mean "do not care." Although the patient has made the choice to refuse CPR and other acts (stated on DNR order) in the event of a cardiopulmonary arrest, you must provide patient care and meet the patient's needs. Health care providers are required to make every effort to revive patients who arrest and do not have a DNR order. Some states offer DNR Comfort Care and DNR Comfort Care Arrest protocols. Protocols in these instances list specific actions that health care providers will take when providing CPR.

CPR is an emergency treatment provided without patient consent (see Chapter 41). Health care providers perform CPR when needed unless there is a DNR order in the patient's chart. The statutes assume that all patients want to be resuscitated unless there is a written DNR order in the medical record. Legally, capable adult patients consent to a DNR order verbally or in writing after receiving the appropriate information by the health care provider. Be familiar with the DNR protocols of your state.

REFLECT NOW

You are caring for a patient who is terminally ill and has a "do not resuscitate" order, but the medical record does not have an entry regarding the physician's discussion with the patient prior to writing the order. How would you respond if the patient has a cardiac arrest? How would your response differ if the patient were 8 versus 80 years old?

Uniform Anatomical Gift Act

The Uniform Anatomical Gift Act (UAGA) (1987) was developed more than 50 years ago by the National Conference of Commissioners on Uniform Laws and was approved by the American Bar Association (Sadler & Sadler, 2018). The UAGA provides the foundation for the national organ donation system. Patient autonomy, individual autonomy, and public trust remain the ethical principles on which organ donation occurs. An individual who is at least 18 years of age can make an organ donation (defined as a "donation of all or part of a human body to take effect upon or after death"). Donors make the gift in writing. In many states adults sign the back of their driver's license, indicating consent to organ donation.

In most states Required Request laws mandate that, at the time of admission to a hospital, a qualified health care provider must ask each patient over age 18 whether he or she is an organ or tissue donor. If the answer is affirmative, the health care provider obtains a copy of the document. If the answer is negative, the health care provider discusses the option to make or refuse an organ donation and places such documentation in the patient's medical record. In most states there is a law requiring that at the time of death a qualified health care provider asks a patient's family members to consider organ or tissue donation (National Organ Transplant Act, 1984). Individuals are approached in the following order: (1) spouse, (2) adult son or daughter, (3) parent, (4) adult brother or sister, (5) grandparent, and (6) guardian. The health care provider who certifies death is not involved in the removal or transplantation of organs (see Chapter 36).

The National Organ Transplant Act (1984) prohibits the purchase or sale of organs (Korobkin, 2017). The act provides civil and criminal immunity to the hospital and health care provider who perform in accordance with the act. It also protects the donor's estate from liability for injury or damage that results from the use of the gift. Organ transplantation is extremely expensive. Patients in end-stage renal disease are eligible for Medicare coverage for a kidney transplant. Sometimes private insurance pays for other transplants. The United Network for Organ Sharing (UNOS) has a contract with the federal government and sets policies and guidelines for the procurement of organs. Recently UNOS changed policy regarding transplant eligibility. The patient with the most urgent need for a transplant will have first claim on any organ from a compatible donor within a 150-mile radius, then a 250-mile radius, and on up to a 500-mile radius (Luthi, 2018). This process will continue with the priority given to the sickest people. Older laws based on geographic proximity arguably reduced access to many critically ill people. Geography is still a factor, but patient need is now the priority (Luthi, 2018). Be familiar with the policies and procedures of your agency regarding organ donation.

The Omnibus Budget Reconciliation Act (1987)

The Omnibus Reconciliation Act (OBRA) of 1987 significantly altered the way in which health care is provided to older adults. It focused on patient rights, quality of life, quality of care, and the physical environment in which patients lived. One change focused on the use of restraints intended to change older adult behavior.

OBRA 1987 addressed the use of both physical and chemical restraint use (see Chapter 14). The legal definition of a restraint is any manual method, physical or mechanical device, or material or equipment that immobilizes or reduces the ability of a patient to move freely, with a chemical restraint including the use of medication to alter the behavior of a patient (CMS, 2008). The use of restraints has been associated with serious complications and even death. The Centers for Medicare and Medicaid Services (CMS) (2008), ANA (2012), and TJC (2018) set standards to reduce the use of all types of restraints in health care settings. All patients have a US constitutional right to be free from seclusion and physical or chemical restraints, except on rare occasions, to ensure the safety of patients, staff, and others in emergency situations.

Application of a physical restraint or administration of a chemical restraint must be the intervention of last resort and not the first intervention of choice when a patient is nonadherent, aggressive, or combative. Chapter 14 describes interventions for a restraint-free environment and the conditions that ultimately allow restraints to be ordered. You must know current evidence-based and legal procedures related to both the use of restraints and their discontinuation. It is critical to know who can legally order the use of restraints, the assessments required, and the length of time restraints can be used. You are required to continuously monitor patients who are restrained or secluded to assure they are safe. A physician, nurse practitioner, physician assistant, or RN who has been trained in CMS restraint and seclusion requirements is required to assess the patient face to face within 1 hour or less of applying the restraints (CMS, 2018).

Restraints can be used (1) only to ensure the physical safety of the patient or other patients, (2) when less restrictive interventions are unsuccessful, and (3) only on the written order of a health care provider (CMS, 2018). The regulations also describe documentation of restraint use and follow-up assessments. Litigation from improper restraint use may include allegations of unlawful imprisonment and/or harm associated with injury due to restraint use (Pozgar, 2016). Knowing when and how to use restraints correctly is key (see Chapter 27).

STATE STATUTES IMPACTING NURSING PRACTICE

State law directs how health care will be delivered and regulates and licenses health care agencies and health care professionals providing care to citizens. Thus, when harm occurs to patients, malpractice suits are filed primarily under state law, actions are taken against facilities to no longer operate, and charges are made against a nurse's license when it is determined that the nurse contributed to the harm. In *Gibbons v Ogden* (1824) the US Supreme Court established that regulation and licensure of local matters belong to the states under powers afforded to them under the US Constitution. Nursing licenses are issued and enforced by states.

Nurse Practice Act

Nurse Practice Acts are state laws intended to protect citizens, make nurses accountable, and ensure that care is consistent with best practice within the scope and standards of nursing. Creation of a state board of nursing, sometimes called the nursing commission, is part of a state

Nurse Practice Act. Members of the boards and the boards' responsibilities are written in the statute and in the regulations that more clearly delineate their duties. State boards of nursing educate the public and nurses as the profession changes. For example, white papers to clarify administration of conscious sedation by a nurse have been shared with stakeholders when practice acts are revised or challenged. State boards regulate and disseminate information related to nursing practice.

A State Board of Nursing or Nursing Commission licenses all RNs in the state in which they practice. The requirements for licensure vary among states. States use the National Council Licensure Examinations (NCLEX®) for nursing examinations. Legally, a license to practice nursing is considered a privilege and not a right. Licensure permits people to offer special skills to the public, and it also provides legal guidelines for protection of the public.

The enhanced nurse licensure compact (eNLC) enables a nurse to practice in multiple states under one license; an individual license from each participating state is not required (NCSBN, n.d.). Having an eNLC license allows nurses to provide telehealth care when working in one state and the patient is in another state. It also facilitates care when nurses cross state lines to provide care during emergencies. As practice acts change, more states are participating in the eNLC process (NCSBN, n.d.).

The State Board of Nursing investigates, suspends, and/or revokes a license if a nurse's conduct violates the Nurse Practice Act. For example, a nurse who wrongfully administers a medication that results in permanent harm to a patient may have a restriction placed on his or her license. If this occurs and the nurse has an eNLC license, other states may also investigate and take action in their jurisdictions, even though the act occurred in another state. Actions taken in other states may be less, worse, or the same as that taken in the originating state where the violation occurred. In part, this demonstrates the importance of having professional liability insurance.

While a license may be considered a privilege, it is also a means by which a person is employed. As such, when penalties are taken against a nurse's license, right to employment statutes may be triggered to protect the person's ability to work. Thus, actions taken to restrict, suspend, and/or revoke a nursing license may become daunting to the nurse who wishes to remain in practice.

The State Board of Nursing must provide notice and follow due process before revoking or suspending a license. Notice means that affirmative actions are taken to inform the nurse that a charge has been made and will be investigated by the Board. It also means that reasonable efforts will be made to inform the nurse of the date, time, and place where an action may be taken to restrict, suspend, or revoke the nurse's license. Due process means that the state is required to inform the nurse of the allegations and the investigation process, including who is being asked to provide information about the allegations. The name of the complainant is disclosed only under court order when anonymity is requested. Nurses should attend and respond to allegations during hearings regarding any allegations. They may and should request an attorney to represent and defend them in a hearing. Hearings for suspension or revocation of a license do not occur in court. Usually a panel of professionals conducts the hearing. Most states provide administrative and judicial review of these cases after nurses have exhausted all other forms of appeal. Actions and decisions by State Boards of Nursing are published and accessible by health care agencies and the public. When administrative appeals have been exhausted, nurses can bring their cases forward to the court for review of the actions taken by the Board in their respective states.

Professional licensure defense is expensive when nurses do not have insurance that covers the costs of keeping their licenses to practice nursing. On average, $12,000 or more is required to respond to a complaint and effectively defend a claim. Nurses often presume that either their personal or their employer's malpractice insurance will include costs of defending and retaining their nursing license. In most instances this is not true. Professional licensure defense insurance is a contract between a nurse and an insurance company. When a complaint is made to the State Board of Nursing, an action is initiated that could result in a restriction, suspension, or revocation of the nurse's license to practice. When a nurse specifically has professional licensure defense insurance, the nurse notifies the company. In response, the company will refer the nurse to an attorney, usually a nurse attorney, who will then represent the nurse when interacting with the state board. The insurance company will cover costs of representing the nurse when responding to allegations the state board is investigating.

Malpractice insurance is a contract between an insurance company and a nurse or employer. It is intended to cover costs incurred when a patient sues the employer and/or the nurse. Malpractice insurance provides for a defense of the nurse and the employer in a lawsuit. The insurance company pays for costs, attorney's fees, settlement, and other related fees generated in the representation of the nurse. It covers the costs to the patient; it does not cover the costs when a complaint is filed with the state licensing board. These are two different actions, and different laws apply. Therefore, it is suggested that nurses carry both professional licensure defense and malpractice insurance or one policy that specifically includes both actions. It is also often recommended that nurses have their own personal insurance policy. Relying on the employer's malpractice insurance is often inadequate.

Health care agencies have insurance intended to provide financial assistance when it is alleged that a patient was permanently harmed in one of their facilities. As an employee or agent of the agency, the actions of the nurse when caring for the patient are examined. It is important to remember in these cases that the lawyer is representing the employer and not the nurse. The insurance provided by the employing agency covers nurses only while they are working within the scope of their employment.

REFLECT NOW

Consider your role as a nursing student as it is defined in your state's Nurse Practice Act. What are you required to do when working in a hospital? In your state, is it different if you are working in a skilled nursing facility or nursing home? What about if you are in a retirement center? What can you do in one place that you cannot do in another?

Informed Consent and Health Care Acts

Health care acts within each state describe and define the minimum standards of care that will be provided within their geographic region. These acts and the regulations associated with them are interrelated with other laws governing the practice of nursing. For example, these acts include expectations regarding consent.

A patient's signed consent form is necessary for admission to a health care agency, invasive procedures such as intravenous central line insertion, surgery, some treatment programs such as chemotherapy, and participation in research studies (Furrow et al., 2018). State laws designate individuals who are legally able to give consent to medical treatment (Medical Patient Rights Act, 1994). Nurses need to know the law in their states and be familiar with the policies and procedures of their employing agency regarding consent (Box 23.2). Special consideration is used when a patient is deaf, illiterate, or speaks a foreign language. A professional interpreter must be present in person or remotely to explain the terms of consent. A family member or acquaintance who

BOX 23.2   Statutory Guidelines for Legal Consent for Medical Treatment

Those who may consent to treatment are governed by state law but generally include the following:

I. Adults
   A. Any competent individual 18 years of age or older for himself or herself
   B. Any parent for his or her unemancipated minor
   C. Any guardian for his or her ward
   D. Any adult for the treatment of his or her minor brother or sister (if an emergency and parents are not present)
   E. Any grandparent for a minor grandchild (in an emergency and if parents are not present)

II. Minors
   A. Ordinarily minors may not consent to medical treatment without a parent. However, emancipated minors may consent to medical treatment without a parent. Emancipated minors include:
      1. Minors who are designated emancipated by a court order
      2. Minors who are married, divorced, or widowed
      3. Minors who are in active military service
   B. Unemancipated minors may consent to medical treatment if they have specific medical conditions
      1. Pregnancy and pregnancy-related conditions (Various states differ in characterizing a pregnant minor as either emancipated or unemancipated. Know your state rules in this matter.)
      2. A minor parent for his or her custodial child
      3. Sexually transmitted infection (STI) information and treatment
      4. Substance abuse treatment
      5. Outpatient and/or temporary sheltered mental health treatment
   C. The issue of emancipated or unemancipated minors does not relieve the health care provider's duty to attempt to obtain meaningful informed consent.

speaks a patient's language should not interpret health information. Make every effort to help the patient make an informed choice.

In addition, health care acts have been amended to include more specific direction to assure that patients receive information that the typical person would reasonably want to know when providing consent to medical care. **Informed consent** is a patient's agreement to have a medical procedure after receiving full disclosure of risks, benefits, alternatives, and consequences of refusal (Furrow et al., 2018; Pozgar, 2016). Informed consent requires a health care provider to disclose information in terms a patient can understand to make an informed choice (Cruzan, 1990; Furrow et al., 2018). Failure to obtain consent in situations other than emergencies can result in a claim of battery.

Informed consent is part of the health care provider–patient relationship. It must be obtained and witnessed when the patient is not under the influence of medication such as opioids. In most situations obtaining patients' informed consent does not fall within the nurse's responsibility. The person responsible for performing the procedure is responsible for obtaining the informed consent.

Key elements of informed consent include the following (Furrow et al., 2018):

1. The patient receives an explanation of the procedure or treatment.
2. The patient receives the names and qualifications of people performing and assisting in the procedure.
3. The patient receives a description of the serious harm, including death, that may occur as a result of the procedure and anticipated pain and/or discomfort.
4. The patient receives an explanation of alternative therapies to the proposed procedure/treatment and the risks of doing nothing.

5. The patient knows that he or she has the right to refuse the procedure/treatment without discontinuing other supportive care.
6. The patient knows that he or she may refuse the procedure/treatment even after the procedure has begun.

Nurses witness consent; they do not obtain consent for procedures performed by others (Furrow et al., 2018). The nurse's signature as a witness to the consent means that the patient appeared to voluntarily give consent, he or she appeared capable to give consent, and that the patient signed the consent in the nurse's presence. If you suspect that the patient does not understand or did not voluntarily and/or knowingly give consent, notify the health care provider and nursing supervisor. If necessary to assure valid consent, contact the medical director. If a patient refuses the treatment, ensure that documentation of the rejection is written, signed, and witnessed. Nursing students cannot and should not be responsible for or asked to witness consent forms because of the legal nature of the document.

Parents are usually the legal guardians of pediatric patients; they typically are the people who sign consent forms for treatment. Occasionally a parent or guardian refuses treatment for a child. For example, you are caring for a child whose parents do not want their child to receive the measles, mumps, rubella (MMR) vaccine. The court may intervene on the child's behalf. Courts generally consider the child's ultimate safety and well-being as the most important factors. Under these circumstances, the court may also order the child to be vaccinated under the doctrine of *parens patriae*, in the best interests of the child and those who may be exposed to the disease if the unvaccinated child is exposed to and develops measles.

In some instances, obtaining informed consent is difficult. For example, if a patient is unconscious, you must obtain consent from a person legally authorized to give it on the patient's behalf. Sometimes a patient has legally designated surrogate decision makers through special power of attorney documents or court guardianship procedures. In emergencies, if it is impossible to obtain consent from the patient or an authorized person, a health care provider may perform a procedure required to benefit the patient or save a life without liability for failure to obtain consent. In such cases the law assumes that the patient would wish to be treated.

Patients with mental illnesses or substance use disorders must also give consent. They have the right to refuse treatment until a court has determined legally that they are incompetent to decide for themselves. Informed consent is one aspect of health care statutes. Implications related to informed consent are influenced by many related statutes.

Good Samaritan Laws

Good Samaritan laws encourage health care professionals to assist in emergencies (Furrow et al., 2018). These laws limit liability and offer legal immunity if a nurse helps at the scene of an accident. For example, if you stop at the scene of an automobile accident and give appropriate emergency care such as applying pressure to stop hemorrhage, you are acting within accepted standards, even though proper equipment is unavailable. If the patient subsequently develops complications due your actions, you are immune from liability if you acted without gross negligence (Furrow et al., 2018; Good Samaritan Act, 1997). Although Good Samaritan laws provide immunity to a nurse who does what is reasonable to save a person's life, if you perform a procedure exceeding your scope of practice and for which you have no training, you are liable for injury that may result from that act. You should only provide care that is consistent with your level of knowledge and experience. In addition, once you have committed to providing emergency care to a patient, you must stay with that patient until you can safely transfer his or her care to someone who can provide needed care, such as emergency medical technicians (EMTs) or emergency department staff. If you leave the patient without properly transferring or handing him or her off to a capable person, you may be liable for patient abandonment and responsible for any injury suffered after you leave him or her (Furrow et al., 2018; Pozgar, 2016).

Public Health Laws

Public health laws affect individuals, populations, and communities. They may be either federal or state statutes that are intended to improve the health of people. State legislatures enact statutes under health codes, which describe the requirements for reporting communicable diseases, school immunizations, and other conditions intended to promote health and reduce health risks in communities. The Centers for Disease Control and Prevention (CDC) (http://www.CDC.gov) and the Occupational Health and Safety Act (OHSA) (http://www.osha.gov) provide guidelines on a national level for safe and healthy communities and work environments. Public health laws protect populations, advocate for the rights of people, regulate health care and health care financing, and ensure professional accountability for care provided.

Nurses have the legal duty to provide care to protect public health (see Chapter 3). These laws include reporting suspected abuse and neglect of a child, older adult, or victim of domestic violence; reporting communicable diseases; ensuring that patients in the community have received required immunizations; and reporting other health-related issues to protect public health. In most states, all nurses are mandatory reporters of abuse or neglect of patients when they have reasonable suspicion to believe an individual is at risk of harm. In most states, neglect means a pattern of conduct by a person with a duty of care to provide services that maintain the physical and/or mental health of a child or vulnerable adult (Adigun & Hatcher, 2019). It may also be a one-time act that is a clear and present danger to another's health, welfare, or safety. Neglect does not usually require that a nurse intentionally acts to harm a patient; rather, the nurse knew or should have known that neglect would occur under the circumstances. Abuse means the willful act or inaction that inflicts injury, confinement, intimidation, or punishment on a child or an adult. Of note in situations of neglect or abuse, the standard of proof to report is that a nurse has a reasonable suspicion that the person may be at risk of harm. Nurses must place the health and safety of the patient above that of the caregiver when making the decision to report. Health care professionals who do not report instances when they have suspicion of abuse or neglect may be liable for civil or criminal legal action. Some State Boards of Nursing now require mandatory continuing education on abuse and neglect for license renewal or before obtaining a new nursing license.

The Uniform Determination of Death Act

Many legal issues surround the event of death, including a basic definition of the actual point at which a person is legally dead. The definitions vary by state law. There are two standards for the determination of death. The cardiopulmonary standard requires irreversible cessation of circulatory and respiratory functions. The whole-brain standard requires irreversible cessation of all functions of the entire brain, including the brainstem. Most states have statutes like the proposed language in the Uniform Determination of Death Act (1980). It states that health care providers can use either the cardiopulmonary or the whole-brain definition to determine death. Be aware of legal definitions of death in your state because you need to document relevant information when the patient is in your care. Nurses have a specific legal obligation to treat the deceased person's remains with dignity (see Chapter 36). Wrongful handling of a deceased person's remains causes emotional harm to the surviving family.

LEGAL IMPLICATIONS AND ISSUES ASSOCIATED WITH NURSING PRACTICE

Some patients or their families, especially those who experience poor health outcomes, believe that care provided by nurses failed to fall within the scope of nursing practice or failed to meet the standards of nursing practice. Sometimes in these cases, patients or their families file torts or lawsuits in the courts, alleging that the nurses knew, or should have known, that their behavior was less than what a reasonably prudent nurse would do under similar circumstances.

Torts

Torts are civil wrongful acts or omissions made against a person or property. They are classified as intentional, quasi-intentional, or unintentional.

Intentional torts are deliberate acts against a person or his or her property that may result in both civil and criminal actions. Assault is an intentional threat toward another person that places the person in reasonable fear of harmful, imminent, or unwelcome contact (Furrow et al., 2018). No actual contact is required for an assault to occur. For example, if a nurse threatens to give a patient an injection or to restrain a patient for an x-ray film procedure when the patient has refused consent, the nurse's action is considered an assault. Likewise, assault occurs when a patient threatens a nurse. **Battery** is any intentional offensive touching without consent or lawful justification (Furrow et al., 2018; Nuse, 2017). The contact can be harmful to the patient and cause an injury, or it merely can be offensive to the patient's personal dignity. In the example of a nurse threatening to give a patient an injection without the patient's consent, if the nurse gives the injection, it is battery. Battery also results if the health care provider performs a procedure that goes beyond the scope of a patient's consent. For example, if a patient gives consent for an appendectomy and the surgeon performs a tonsillectomy, battery has occurred. The key component is the patient's consent. False imprisonment occurs when a patient is restrained without a legal reason. False imprisonment happens when nurses restrain a patient in a confined area, preventing the ability to move freely in a bed, chair, room, or other area in which the patient wishes to be (Furrow et al., 2018; Yeung et al., 2019).

Quasi-Intentional Torts. **Quasi-intentional torts** are acts in which a person may not intend to cause harm to another but does. Typically, the person invades another's privacy or in some way defames his or her character. Quasi-intentional torts are alleged when a person should have known that harm to another person could occur.

Invasion of privacy is usually the release of a patient's health care information to an unauthorized person, such as a member of the press, the patient's employer, the patient's family, or online. HIPAA and the HITECH Act privacy standards have raised awareness of the need for health care professionals to provide confidentiality and privacy. The information that is in a patient's medical record is a confidential communication that may be shared only with health care providers to provide treatment. This includes electronic communication by e-mail, text, or other devices. All communications become part of the health care record and must be considered confidential. They may not be released without permission of the patient. Individuals who insist on receiving information without patient consent must immediately be referred to a supervisor. It is not within the nurse's scope of practice to determine when information should or should not be disclosed.

Defamation of character is the publication of false statements that result in damage to a person's reputation. **Slander** occurs when one speaks falsely about another. For example, if a nurse tells people erroneously that a patient has gonorrhea and the disclosure affects the patient's business, the nurse is liable for slander. Libel is the written defamation of character (e.g., charting false defamatory entries in a medical record) (Furrow et al., 2018; Philo et al., 2015).

Unintentional Torts. Unintentional torts arise when a person is harmed and the person inflicting the harm knew, or should have known, that his or her actions were less than the accepted scope and standard of practice.

Negligence is conduct that falls below the generally accepted standard of care of a reasonably prudent person (Furrow et al., 2018). Anyone, including people not in the medical field, can be liable for negligence. A nurse is negligent when he or she had a duty of care that is breached and a patient is physically harmed. A reasonably prudent nurse under similar circumstances would have provided care differently. The law establishes the standard of care to protect others against an unreasonably great risk of harm (Furrow et al., 2018). Negligent acts, such as hanging the wrong intravenous solution for a patient, often result in disciplinary action by the State Board of Nursing and a lawsuit for negligence against the nurse and his or her employer. Most lawsuits allege negligence.

Malpractice is a type of negligence. A person being held liable for malpractice must be a professional. Certain criteria are necessary to establish nursing malpractice: (1) the nurse (defendant) owed a duty of care to the patient (plaintiff), (2) the nurse did not carry out or breached that duty, (3) the patient was injured due to the breach in duty, and (4) damages or remedies are allowed under state law to "make the person whole" in the eyes of the court. Even though nurses do not intend to injure patients, some patients file claims of malpractice if nurses give care that does not meet the appropriate standards. Most malpractice and professional licensure claims occur in hospital settings. Common causes of malpractice against nurses include failure to follow the standard of care (e.g., not implementing a pressure injury or fall prevention protocol), failure to communicate important information to another health care provider, failure to document appropriately, failure to assess and monitor a patient, and inappropriate delegation of nursing tasks.

More health care agencies are using medication administration technology, such as bar coding, to try to reduce medication administration errors. However, the capacity to override or work around intended safeguards has contributed to significant harm to patients. It is essential that you always follow the policies and procedures at your agency and never override safeguards intended to promote safe patient care. In Tennessee (2018), a nurse and medical center were found in violation of federal and state law after a "help-all" nurse erroneously retrieved and administered the wrong medication to a patient in radiology. The patient was left unsupervised, went into cardiac arrest, and later died. Subsequently, civil and criminal indictments have been filed.

Malpractice sometimes involves failing to check a patient's identification correctly before administering blood and then giving the blood to the wrong patient. It also involves administering a medication to a patient even though the medical record contains documentation that the patient has an allergy to that medication. In general, courts define nursing malpractice as the failure to use a degree of skill or learning ordinarily used under the same or similar circumstances by members of the nursing profession (Furrow et al., 2018).

Another area of potential risk is associated with the use of electronic monitoring devices. No monitor is always reliable. Therefore, do not depend on them completely. Continual assessment of a patient is necessary to help determine the accuracy of electronic monitoring. There are also electrical hazards to the nurse and the patient. Biomedical engineers check equipment to ensure that it is in proper working order

and that a patient will not receive an electrical shock. Document when calibration of equipment occurs.

The best way for nurses to avoid malpractice is to follow evidence-based standards of care, deliver care competently, and communicate with other health care providers. You also avoid malpractice by developing a caring rapport with patients and thoroughly documenting assessments, interventions, and evaluation of care. Generate and act on your spirit of inquiry to provide the best care in conjunction with your patients' preferences and values. Know and follow the policies and procedures of the agency where you work. Be sensitive to your patients' risks and the common sources of patient injury such as pressure injuries, falls, and medication errors. Finally, communicate with your patients; explain all tests, medications, and treatments; document patient education you provide; and listen to your patients' concerns about treatments. You are accountable to report any significant changes in your patient's condition in a timely manner to the health care provider and to document these changes in the patient's electronic health record (see Chapter 26). Timely and truthful documentation is important to provide communication necessary among health care team members. Documentation must be accurate (Furrow et al., 2018). In the electronic health record (EHR), assure that assessments are complete and consistent with those completed previously. Ensure that you conduct your own assessment rather than copying the previous assessment in the patient's medical record to ensure accuracy of information. Investigate and do not override safeguards built into each program to alert you to concerns such as black box warnings when administering medications. Notify other team members in a timely manner when changes in condition are triggered within the record. If you are named in a malpractice suit, you need to know your rights and understand the legal process (Box 23.3). Work with your health care agency's legal team, and be sure to advocate for yourself.

If a health care provider negligently alters or loses medical records relevant to a malpractice claim, the health care provider must explain why these events occurred. An agency must maintain nursing records according to specific statutes and accreditation regulations. Nursing notes contain substantial evidence needed to understand the care received by a patient. If records are lost, incomplete, or altered, there is a presumption that the care was negligent and therefore the cause of the patient's injuries. In addition, incomplete or illegible records make a health care provider less credible or believable. Determine changes in patient conditions documented by prior nursing staff, and document timely responses to those changes. In addition, it is essential to provide and document patient decision making; the patient is the primary decision maker, regardless of setting, when care is provided. EHRs can be retrieved in their existent form on any day. Thus, it is apparent when you have viewed or altered records documentation. In addition, EHRs can be retrieved and compared as they existed in real time from one moment to another. When making a late entry into an electronic record, it is essential that the amended note be entered as such; never delete and then reenter different language representative of the same date and time as had been previously erased. Regardless of intent, the record subsequently may be considered altered to protect the agency and hide information from the court regarding care received or not received by the patient.

Beginning- and End-of-Life Nursing Issues

Termination of Pregnancy. In 1973 in the case of *Roe v Wade*, the US Supreme Court ruled that there is a fundamental right to privacy, which includes a woman's decision to terminate a pregnancy. The court ruled that during the first trimester a woman could end her pregnancy without state regulation because the risk of natural

---

BOX 23.3 Anatomy of a Lawsuit

Pleadings Phase

Petition: Elements of the claim. The plaintiff outlines what the defendant nurse did wrong and, because of that alleged negligence, how the plaintiff was injured.

Answer: The nurse admits or denies each allegation in the petition. The plaintiff must establish anything that the nurse does not admit.

Discovery: The process of discovering all the facts of the case involves using interrogatories, full access to the medical records in question, and the depositions. The patient and the health care staff are asked questions by counsel for the defense. They answer under oath, and their testimony is recorded and kept for reference.

Interrogatories: Written questions requiring answers under oath. Typically opposing counsel requests a list of possible witnesses, insurance experts, and which health care providers the plaintiff saw before and after the event.

Requests for productions: Opposing parties request relevant documents, pictures, or related materials such as medical records for treatment before and after the event.

Depositions: Questions are posed to opposing parties, witnesses, and experts under oath to obtain all relevant, nonprivileged information about the case. Experts establish the elements of the case and the applicable standard of care.

Medical records: The defendant obtains all the plaintiff's relevant medical records for treatment before and after the event. Everything written by the nurses and the health care provider in the medical record is open to examination by both the plaintiff and the defendants. This includes all e-mails, texts, and other social media communications.

Witnesses' deposition: Questions are posed to the witnesses under oath to obtain all relevant, nonprivileged information about the case.

Parties' depositions: The plaintiff and defendants (health care provider, nurse, and hospital personnel) are almost always deposed.

Other witnesses: Factual witnesses, both neutral and biased, are deposed to obtain information about their version of the case. They may include family members on the plaintiff's side and other medical personnel (e.g., nurses) on the defendant's side.

Experts: The plaintiff selects experts to establish the essential legal elements of the case against the defendant. The defendant selects experts to establish the appropriateness of the nursing care. Nursing experts are asked to testify to the reasonableness or inappropriate actions of the health care staff once the patient's condition began to change. The expert is asked to compare the actions of the nursing staff to the standard of care.

Trial: The trial usually occurs 3 years after the filing of the petition. Most are settled before trial.

---

mortality from abortion is less than with normal childbirth. During the second trimester the state has an interest in protecting maternal health, and it enforces regulations regarding the person terminating the pregnancy and the agency where it is done. By the third trimester, when the fetus becomes viable, the interest of the state is to protect the fetus; therefore, it prohibits termination except when necessary to save the mother.

In *Webster v Reproductive Health Services* (1989), the court substantially narrowed Roe v Wade. Some states require viability tests before conducting abortions. Other states require a minor's parental consent or a judicial decision that the minor is mature and can self-consent, while other states do not require parental consent. Recently, some states have passed "heartbeat" laws, which state a pregnancy may not be terminated after a heartbeat is heard. Thus it is critical to know the law in your state related to termination of pregnancy before working in this area of practice.

Death With Dignity or Physician-Assisted Suicide. Providing end-of-life care in today's world is challenging for health care professionals because people are living longer (see Chapter 36). The Oregon Death with Dignity Act (1994) was the first statute that legislatively defined "death with dignity," sometimes called *physician-assisted suicide.* The statute stated that a competent individual with a terminal disease could make an oral and written request for medication to end his or her life in a humane and dignified manner. A terminal disease is defined as an "incurable and irreversible disease that has been medically confirmed and will, within reasonable medical judgment, produce death within 6 months."

The ANA (2019a) believes that nurses' participation in assisted suicide violates the code of ethics for nurses. The American Association of Colleges of Nursing (AACN) has historically supported the International Council of Nurses' mandate to ensure an individual's peaceful end of life. The positions of these two national organizations are not considered contradictory and require nurses to approach a patient's end of life with openness to listening to a patient's expressions of fear and to attempt to control a patient's pain during his or her last months of life. You need to know your state's laws and ensure that your practice falls within the laws' requirements.

Nursing Workforce Issues

Nursing Students. Nursing students are liable if their actions exceed their scope of practice and cause harm to patients. Regardless of intent, students are expected to know what they can and cannot do when providing care to patients. If a student harms a patient as a direct result of a lack of action, the student, instructor, hospital or health care agency, and university or educational institution generally share the liability for the incorrect action. Nursing students should never be assigned to perform tasks for which they are unprepared, and instructors should supervise them carefully as they learn new skills. Although nursing students are not employees of the hospital, the agency has a responsibility to monitor their acts. They are expected to perform as professional nurses would in providing safe patient care. Faculty members are usually responsible for instructing and observing students, but in some situations staff nurses serving as preceptors share these responsibilities. Every nursing school should provide clear definitions of preceptor and faculty responsibility. It is equally important that nursing preceptors be aware of state laws applicable to nursing students, faculty, and the educational institution when supervising students.

Nursing students should perform only tasks that have been delegated to them and that are included in their titled job description when they are employed in health care settings (e.g., as nursing assistants, medication technicians). For example, if a student who also works as a medication technician has learned to administer intramuscular (IM) medications in a nursing class, the student cannot administer IM injections when working as a medication technician unless this is allowed under the state's Nurse Practice Act and the student's job description. If a staff nurse assigns a nursing student work without regard for the student's ability to safely conduct the task defined in the job description, the staff nurse is also liable. A student employed in the agency as a nurse's aide must refuse to perform tasks that he or she is not prepared to complete safely. The student employee must tell the supervisor so that the task can be assigned to an appropriate health care professional. Patient safety is essential. Nursing students must assure that their actions meet the scope of nursing required of them. Their actions must meet the standards of practice required for safe care of a patient whether they are at school, in the community, or employed at health care agency. While you may have learned about a nursing task, it does not mean that you can safely perform the task on a patient. Err on the side of caution. Do not exceed your scope of practice whether you are a nurse's aide, nursing assistant, medication assistant, nursing student medication technician, or any other title.

Staffing and Nurse-to-Patient Ratios.

Adequate staffing is required to assure patient safety and satisfaction with care. Nurse-to-patient ratios are determined in different ways. Legal issues occur when there are not enough nurses to provide competent care or when nurses work excessive overtime. In the case of *Spires v Hospital Corporation of America* (2006), poor patient care due to insufficient RN staffing resulting in the death of a patient was alleged. This suit emphasized the potential seriousness of short staffing and the importance of nurses' asserting employee rights.

Many states require that safe staffing nursing committees in acute care settings determine safe staffing based on the needs of patients admitted to their facilities. While staffing committees have worked to determine appropriate staffing needs, employers have inappropriately asked some committees to make budgetary recommendations to pay for the staffing. In California, fixed nurse-patient ratios in acute care settings are mandated by law. The safe staffing ratio debate is occurring throughout the country and demands close attention by all nurses (ANA, 2019b).

The ANA and other professional nursing organizations have supported federal legislation titled the Safe Staffing for Nurse and Patient Safety Act of 2018 (ANA, 2019b). Ideally, hospitals receiving Medicare reimbursement will be required to have staffing committees, 55% of which will be direct-care nurses. Committees will develop and implement staffing plans for each unit. Patients will receive better care, and it is anticipated that a decrease will occur in adverse events, nurse turnover, and hospital readmissions. Under this act, nurses become an integral part of ensuring that patients receive care from nurses qualified to meet their needs in a safe environment.

Nursing Assignments.

Nurses are sometimes required to work on a unit where they do not typically care for patients. In this practice, often called "floating," nurses temporarily work in another area because there are not enough nurses to care for the number of patients and the acuity of the patients' needs on that unit at that time. If you are asked to float, you must inform the supervisor if you do not have the required education or experience to care for the patients assigned to you. You should request and receive an orientation to the unit. Supervisors are responsible if they give a staff nurse an assignment that he or she cannot handle safely. Before accepting employment, learn the policies of the agency regarding floating and understand what is expected (ANA, 2018).

Patient Abandonment.

Patient abandonment occurs when a nurse refuses to provide care for a patient after having established a patient-nurse relationship. Before having established that relationship, a nurse may refuse an assignment when (1) the nurse lacks the knowledge or skill to provide competent care; (2) care exceeding the Nurse Practice Act is expected; (3) health of the nurse or the nurse's unborn child is directly threatened by the type of assignment; (4) orientation to the unit has not been completed and safety is at risk; (5) the nurse clearly states and documents a conscientious objection on the basis of moral, ethical, or religious grounds; or (6) the nurse's clinical judgment is impaired as a result of fatigue, resulting in a safety risk for the patient (ANA, 2015a; NSO, 2017).

When refusing an assignment, it is important to give your immediate supervisor specific reasons for the refusal and to determine whether other alternatives, such as reassignment, are available. Document in your personal notes the specifics of the incident, to whom you reported it, and actions you took to ensure that patients were safe and that you did not abandon your patients.

Nurse Delegation.

Nurse delegation is defined in Nurse Practice Acts; regulations vary from state to state. Generally, **nurse delegation** means that an RN educates, observes, and verifies that a non-nurse can do a specific task that is usually completed by a nurse (see Chapter 21). Several requirements assure patient safety when delegating care. The RN retains responsibility to supervise care received by the patient and to periodically reassess whether nurse delegation continues to be appropriate. RNs usually delegate to nursing assistants who work in specified settings. Delegated tasks may include administration of prescription medications or blood glucose monitoring. It is important to know delegation requirements, including patient consent, caregiver education and experience, and the role and responsibilities of the RN. Some State Boards of Nursing or commissions define responsibilities of the RN specifically and develop position statements and guidelines to help licensed nurses delegate safely to assistive personnel (NCSBN, 2016; NCSBN & ANA, 2019).

Risk Management and Performance/Quality Improvement

Risk-management and performance improvement (PI) and quality improvement (QI) programs help to reduce a nurse's legal risk for malpractice and negligence because they help to identify potential hazards and eliminate them before harm occurs. The two processes are similar, but PI places more emphasis on human performance, whereas QI focuses on work processes. These programs also promote a "just culture" environment that encourages honest disclosure and systemwide resolution to prevent occurrence or reoccurrence of circumstances surrounding a concern. Risk management involves several components, including identifying possible risks, analyzing them, acting to reduce the risks, and evaluating the steps taken to reduce them (TJC, 2019). QI, PI, and risk-management procedures are essential; they require documentation of information to facilitate resolution of questions regarding care.

Nurses are risk managers. For example, surgeons rely on operating room nurses to compare the consent form with the indicated and prepped surgical site for accuracy. TJC's Universal Protocol helps prevent errors due to patients undergoing the wrong surgery or having surgery performed on the wrong site (TJC, 2020). The protocol requires mandatory time-outs before beginning any surgery. Nurses are responsible to implement this protocol whenever an invasive surgical procedure is to be performed, regardless of the location (hospital, ambulatory surgical center [ASC], or health care provider office). The three principles of the protocol are (1) preoperative verification that relevant documents and studies are available before the start of the procedure and that these documents are consistent with the patient's expectations; (2) marking the operative site with indelible ink to mark left and right distinction, multiple structures (e.g., fingers), and levels of the spine; and (3) a *time-out* just before starting the procedure for final verification of the correct patient, procedure, site, and any implants (see Chapter 50).

Patient safety and improved care are the goals of QI, PI, and risk management (TJC, 2019). Professional groups such as the Institute of Medicine focus on patient safety as major goals. *Never events* are preventable errors, which include falls, urinary tract infections from improper use of catheters, and pressure injuries (AHRQ, 2018). The federal government and health care insurance companies have developed policies to withhold reimbursement for never events (AHRQ, 2018) (see Chapter 27). All inpatient health care settings conduct routine monthly monitoring of the incidence of never events, and health care staff are expected to maintain standards for prevention of these events. When trending shows an increase in never events, QI and PI activities are quickly implemented. Know your agency's policies and procedures to help develop a system and culture of patient safety.

One tool used in risk management is the occurrence report or incident report. Occurrence reporting provides a database to determine deviations from standards of care, to identify corrective measures needed to prevent recurrence, and to alert risk management to a potential claim (see Chapter 23). Examples of an occurrence include patient or visitor falls or injury; failure to follow health care provider orders; a significant complaint by patient, family, health care provider, or other hospital department; an error in technique or procedure; and a malfunctioning device or product. Agencies generally have specific guidelines to direct health care providers in how to complete occurrence reports. A report is confidential and separate from the health care record. However, it is discoverable by court order during a legal proceeding. Risk managers work with nurses to provide safe care and to determine how to prevent reoccurrence of circumstances when a patient is potentially or actually harmed.

Nurse Experts

A nursing expert testifies about the standards of nursing care as applied to the facts of a case (Box 23.4). An expert has education and experience related to the alleged complaint of the patient and accurately and concisely describes the pertinent scope and standards of practice required of a nurse under similar circumstances. For example, when a patient sustains an injury from a fall, a nurse with experience in risk management and fall prevention will be asked to consult as an expert on the case. The expert nurse must determine that no conflict of interest exists before accepting a case. For example, the expert nurse could not work for either party's employer. The expert will review all evidence before giving an opinion, including relevant laws and regulations, policies and procedures, patient records, other expert reports, and depositions. Depositions are interviews in which lawyers can ask questions of others who are under oath to provide honest and complete answers. These interviews are transcribed by a court reporter who is present during the sessions. For example, opposing counsel will depose the expert nurse. During the deposition, the nurse will respond to the questions that are asked. The court reporter will record the session in writing, on audiotape, and sometimes on videotape. Within a couple of weeks, the deposition document will be given to all parties to make corrections. Once completed, the document is finalized and will be entered into the case record (Furrow et al., 2018). Nurse experts base their opinions on existing standards of practice established by Nurse Practice Acts, federal and state licensing laws, TJC standards, professional organizations, institutional policies and procedures, job descriptions, and current evidence-based literature. Nurses must meet the same standards as other nurses practicing in similar settings and under similar circumstances. Specialized nurses such as critical care nurses, wound care specialists, or surgical nurses have specially defined standards of care and skills. Ignorance of the law or of standards of care is not a defense against malpractice (Furrow et al., 2018). Nurses are required to know valid, reliable, and credible evidence that is applicable to their practice and the settings in which they work, including current standards of care and the policies and procedures of their employing agency (ANA, 2015a; TJC, 2019). Expert nurses offer opinions on whether others have met the standard of practice; they do not make legal decisions.

One of the first and most important cases to discuss a nurse's liability was *Darling v Charleston Community Memorial Hospital* (1965). It involved an 18-year-old man with a fractured leg. The emergency department physician applied a cast with insufficient padding. The man's toes became swollen and discolored, and he developed decreased sensation. He reported the decreased sensation to nursing staff many times. Although the nurses recognized the symptoms as signs of impaired circulation, they failed to tell their supervisor that the physician did not respond to their calls or the patient's needs. Gangrene

---

BOX 23.4   Proof of Negligence

- The nurse owed a duty of care to the patient.
- The nurse did not carry out the duty or breached it (failed to use that degree of skill and learning ordinarily used under the same or similar circumstances by members of the profession).
- The patient was physically injured or harmed because the nurse breached the duty.
- The patient's injury resulted in compensable damages that can be qualified as medical bills, lost wages, and pain and suffering.

Common Sources of Negligence

Be aware of the common negligent acts that have resulted in lawsuits against hospitals and nurses.

- Failure to assess and/or monitor, including making a nursing diagnosis
- Failure to observe, assess, correctly diagnose, or treat in a timely manner
- Failure to use, calibrate, or replace equipment required to safely care for the patient
- Failure to document care and evaluation of care provided to the patient in a timely manner
- Failure to notify the health care provider of significant changes in a patient's status
- Failure to respond to or correctly implement new and existing orders
- Failure to follow the seven rights of medication administration
- Failure to convey discharge instructions to the patient, his or her family, or providers who are assuming responsibility for the patient
- Failure to ensure patient safety, especially patients who have a history of falling, are sedated or confused, are frail, are mentally impaired, get up in the night, or are uncooperative
- Failure to follow policies and procedures
- Failure to properly delegate and supervise

---

developed, and the man's leg was amputated. Although the physician was held liable for incorrectly applying the cast, the nursing staff were also held liable for failing to adhere to the standards of care for monitoring and reporting the patient's symptoms. Even though the nurses attempted to contact the physician, the jury and subsequent judges held that when the physician failed to respond, the nurses should have acted on behalf of the patient's safety and obtained assistance from the charge nurse, nursing supervisor, and the chief medical officer to make sure that the patient received appropriate care. Almost every state uses this 1965 Illinois Supreme Court case as a legal precedent.

QSEN **Building Competency in Quality Improvement** You are a member of your unit's task force focusing on quality improvement and reduction in sentinel events. The chairperson explains to the task force that quality improvement relates to data collection, evaluation, and improvement in patient outcomes. One of the nurses asks, "How can we reduce the number of occurrence reports being filed on the unit related to patient falls?" How would you respond?

Answers to QSEN Activities can be found on the Evolve website.

Professional Involvement

As a professional nurse, it is important to remain aware of current issues in health care. Become involved in professional organizations and committees that define the standards of care for nursing practice. If current laws, rules and regulations, or policies under which nurses practice are not evidence based, advocate to ensure that the scope of nursing practice is defined accurately. Be willing to represent nursing and the patient's perspective in the community as well. The voice of nursing is powerful and effective when the organizing focus is the protection and welfare of the public entrusted to nurses' care.

KEY POINTS

- Constitutional law refers to rights granted to citizens in the US Constitution and state constitutions. Civil laws are passed by Congress and state legislatures to protect the rights of individuals. Criminal laws are passed by Congress and state legislatures to protect society and provide punishment for crimes.
- Statutory law is civil or criminal. Civil laws protect the rights of individuals as in the case of a Nurse Practice Act, which defines the scope of nursing practice and the standards you must meet within individual states to ensure safe evidence-based and competent nursing practice.
- The scope of nursing practice defines nursing and reflects the values of the nursing profession. Standards of nursing care reflect the knowledge and skill ordinarily possessed and used by nurses.
- A nurse has a duty of care. When a nurse's performance is questioned, the standard of proof in nursing is typically what a reasonably prudent nurse would do under similar circumstances in the geographic area in which the alleged breach occurred.
- The Health Insurance Portability and Accountability Act, Health Information Technology Act, and Americans with Disabilities Act are examples of federal statutes that affect nursing practice.
- The Patient Self-Determination Act is a federal statute that requires health care institutions to provide information to patients regarding their rights to make informed decisions about their care, including the right to create an advanced directive. When a patient has an advanced directive that includes a "do not resuscitate" (DNR) order, you need to ensure that the patient and provider have discussed end-of-life choices and that the discussion is documented in the patient's medical record.
- Physical or chemical restraints are used only as a last resort to ensure the physical safety of the patient or other patients when less restrictive interventions are unsuccessful and require a written order from a health care provider.
- A nurse's witness to a patient's informed consent indicates that the patient appeared to voluntarily give consent, that he or she appeared capable to give consent, and that the patient signed the consent in the nurse's presence.
- Negligence occurs when a nurse had a duty of care that is breached, a patient is physically harmed, and damages are provided to "make the person whole"; a reasonably prudent nurse under similar circumstances would have done care differently.
- Worsening pressure injuries, failure to contact the provider as conditions change, and medication errors often trigger complaints of negligence or malpractice against nurses.
- It is important to know your Nurse Practice Act, to implement and follow agency policies and procedures, to delegate care appropriately, and to participate in risk-management and quality improvement activities to reduce your legal risk when practicing nursing.

REFLECTIVE LEARNING

You are working in an outpatient clinic where you meet a 34-year-old married mother of two small children who is seeing the doctor for numbness and tingling in her right leg. Over the next 6 months, she has critically high glucose levels, she doesn't take her medication, and the provider is significantly concerned. She continues to have numbness and tingling that migrate from her left hip, leg, and foot. The physician orders scans of her leg and lower spine. Each scan is negative. She continues to have pain and numbness and tingling in her neck, back, and legs. During her most recent visit, the provider orders a scan of her thoracic spine and right knee. One week later, the patient e-mails the provider that while the knee scan was completed, no one has contacted her about the other scan. The nurse checks the record and responds, "My bad…. I missed it…. I'll order it now." The next day the patient unexpectedly appears at the clinic, where you observe her staggering at the desk and slurring her speech, asking to see you. You and the receptionist place her immediately into a wheelchair. After being assessed, she is admitted to the hospital, where she is diagnosed with a slow bleed into the spinal column. The patient has irreparable damage to the spine and will be quadriplegic the remainder of her life.

- What standards of practice apply in this scenario?
- Does this situation establish negligence? Specifically, what is the duty, the breach in duty, the permanent harm, and damages in this case?
- What is the standard of proof that would be applied to this situation to determine whether the nurse is liable for the harm incurred by this patient? Make a case for either side.

REVIEW QUESTIONS

1. A nurse is planning care for a patient going to surgery. Who is responsible for informing the patient about the surgery along with possible risks, complications, and benefits?
   1. Family member
   2. Surgeon
   3. Nurse
   4. Nurse manager
2. A woman has severe life-threatening injuries, is unresponsive, and is hemorrhaging following a car accident. The health care provider ordered two units of packed red blood cells to treat the woman's anemia. The woman's husband refuses to allow the nurse to give his wife the blood for religious reasons. What is the nurse's responsibility?
   1. Obtain a court order to give the blood.
   2. Convince the husband to allow the nurse to give the blood.
   3. Call security and have the husband removed from the hospital.
   4. Gather more information about the wife's preferences and determine whether the husband is her power of attorney for health care.
3. A nurse sends a text message to the oncoming nurse to report that a patient refuses to take medication as ordered. What should the oncoming nurse do? (Select all that apply).
   1. Add this information to the board hanging at the patient's bedside.
   2. Tell the nurse who sent the text that the text is a HIPAA violation.
   3. Inform the nursing supervisor.
   4. Forward the text to the charge nurse.
   5. Thank the nurse for sending the information.
4. Which of the following actions, if performed by a registered nurse, could result in both criminal and administrative law sanctions against the nurse? (Select all that apply.)
   1. Reviewing the electronic health record of a family member who is a patient in the same hospital on a different unit
   2. Refusing to provide health care information to a patient's child
   3. Reporting suspected abuse and neglect of children
   4. Applying physical restraints without a written order
   5. Completing an occurrence report on the unit
5. A nurse received bedside report at the change of shift with the night-shift nurse and the patient. The nursing student assigned to

the patient asks to review the patient's medical record. The nurse lists patients' medical diagnoses on the message boards in the patients' rooms. Later in the day the nurse discusses the plan of care for a patient who is dying with the patient's family. Which of these actions describes a violation of the Health Insurance Portability and Accountability Act (HIPAA)?

1. Discussing patient conditions at the bedside at the change of shift
2. Allowing the nursing student to review the assigned patient's chart before providing care during the clinical experience
3. Posting medical information about the patient on a message board in the patient's room
4. Releasing patient information regarding terminal illness to family when the patient has given permission for information to be shared

6. A patient is in skeletal traction and has a plaster cast due to a fractured femur. The patient experiences decreased sensation and a cold feeling in the toes of the affected leg. The nurse observes that the patient's toes have become pale and cold but forgets to document this because one of the nurse's other patients experienced cardiac arrest at the same time. Two days later the patient in skeletal traction has an elevated temperature, and he is prepared for surgery to amputate the leg below the knee. Which of the following statements regarding a breach of duty apply to this situation? (Select all that apply.)

1. Failure to document a change in assessment data
2. Failure to provide discharge instructions
3. Failure to provide patient education about cast care.
4. Failure to use proper medical equipment ordered for patient monitoring
5. Failure to notify a health care provider about a change in the patient's condition

7. A man who is homeless enters the emergency department seeking health care. The health care provider indicates that the patient needs to be transferred to the city hospital for care before assessing the patient. This action is most likely a violation of which of the following laws?

1. Health Insurance Portability and Accountability Act (HIPAA)
2. Americans with Disabilities Act (ADA)
3. Patient Self-Determination Act (PSDA)
4. Emergency Medical Treatment and Active Labor Act (EMTALA)

8. A home health nurse notices significant bruising on a 2-year-old patient's head, arms, abdomen, and legs. The patient's mother describes the patient's frequent falls. What is the best nursing action for the home health nurse to take?

1. Document her findings and treat the patient.
2. Instruct the mother on safe handling of a 2-year-old child.
3. Contact a child abuse hotline.
4. Discuss this story with a colleague.

9. Which of the following statements indicate that the new nursing graduate understands ways to remain involved professionally? (Select all that apply.)

1. "I am thinking about joining the health committee at my church."
2. "I need to read newspapers, watch news broadcasts, and search the Internet for information related to health."
3. "I will join nursing committees at the hospital after I have completed orientation and better understand the issues affecting nursing."
4. "Nurses do not have very much voice in legislation in Washington, DC, because of the nursing shortage."
5. "I will go back to school as soon as I finish orientation."

10. You are floated to work on a nursing unit where you are given an assignment that is beyond your capability. Which is the best nursing action to take first?

1. Call the nursing supervisor to discuss the situation.
2. Discuss the problem with a colleague.
3. Leave the nursing unit and go home.
4. Say nothing and begin your work.

Answers: 1. 2; **2.** 4; **3.** 2; **4.** 1; **5.** 3; **6.** 1,4; **7.** 4; **8.** 3; **9.** 1,2,3; **10.** 1.

Rationales for Review Questions can be found on the Evolve website.

REFERENCES

Adigun OO, Hatcher JD: *Abuse and neglect*, 2019. https://www.ncbi.nlm.nih.gov/books/NBK436015/. Accessed 8 August 2019.

Agency for Healthcare Research and Quality (AHRQ): *Never events*, US Department of Health and Human Services, 2018. https://psnet.ahrq.gov/primers/primer/3/Never-Events. Accessed October 2018.

American Disabilities Act National Network (ADANN): What is the American with disabilities act? https://adata.org/learn-about-ada, 2019. Accessed August 4, 2019.

American Nurses Association (ANA): *Position statement: reduction of patient restraint and seclusion in health care settings*, Silver Spring, MD, 2012, Author. https://www.nursingworld.org/practice-policy/nursing-excellence/official-position-statements/id/reduction-of-patient-restraint-and-seclusion-in-health-care-settings/. Accessed August 4, 2019.

American Nurses Association (ANA): *Nursing: scope and standards of practice*, ed 3, Silver Spring, MD, 2015a, The Association.

American Nurses Association (ANA): *Position statement: risk and responsibility in providing nursing care*, Silver Spring, MD, 2015b, Author. https://www.nursingworld.org/~4af23e/globalassets/docs/ana/ethics/riskandresponsibilitypositionstatement2015.pdf. Accessed August 4, 2019.

American Nurses Association (ANA): *Position statement: questions to ask about safe staffing before accepting employment*, 2018, Silver Spring, MD https://www.nursingworld.org/practice-policy/workforce/questions-to-ask-about-safe-staffing-before-accepting-employment/. Accessed October 2018.

American Nurses Association (ANA): *Nurse staffing*, 2019a. https://www.nursingworld.org/practice-policy/advocacy/state/nurse-staffing/. Accessed August 4, 2019.

American Nurses Association (ANA): *Position statement: nurse's role when a patient requests medical aid in dying*, 2019b. https://www.nursingworld.org/~49e869/globalassets/practiceandpolicy/nursing-excellence/ana-position-statements/social-causes-and-health-care/the-nurses-role-when-a-patient-requests-medical-aid-in-dying-web-format.pdfthe. Accessed August 5, 2019.

Barr L, et al.: Promoting positive and safe care in forensic mental health inpatient settings: evaluating critical factors that assist nurses to reduce the use of restrictive practices, *Int J Mental Health Nurs* 28(4):888, 2019.

Busch C: Implementing Personalized law: personalized disclosures in consumer law and data privacy law, *Univ Chicago Law Rev* 86(2):309, 2019. https://www.jstor.org/stable/26590557. Accessed 8 August 2019.

Centers for Medicare and Medicaid Services (CMS): *Revisions to Medicare conditions of participation*, 482. Bethesda, Md, 2008, US Department of Health and Human Services, p 13.

Centers for Medicare and Medicaid Services (CMS): *State operations manual appendix a—survey protocol, regulations and interpretive guidelines for hospitals*, 2018. https://www.cms.gov/Regulations-and-Guidance/Guidance/Manuals/downloads/som107ap_a_hospitals.pdf. Accessed July 16, 2019.

Centers for Medicare and Medicaid Services (CMS): *Patient protection and affordable care act; HHS notice of benefit and Payment parameters for 2020*, 2019. https://www.federalregister.gov/documents/2019/01/24/2019-00077/patient-protection-and-affordable-care-act-hhs-notice-of-benefit-and-payment-parameters-for-2020. Accessed August 4, 2019.

Dupler A, et al.: Leveling the playing field for nursing students with disabilities: implications of the amendments to the American with Disabilities Act, *J Nurs Educ* 51:144, 2012.

Furrow BR, et al.: *Health law: cases, materials and problems*, ed 8, St. Paul, MN, 2018, West Academic Publishing.

Golden S: Do not resuscitate orders: a matter of life and death in New York, *J Contemp Health Law Policy* 4(1):449, 1988.

KFF Henry J Kaiser Family Foundation (KFF): Key facts about the uninsured population, 2018, https://www.kff.org/uninsured/fact-sheet/key-facts-about-the-uninsured-population/. Accessed August 4, 2019.

Korobkin R: Property rights and the control of human biospecimens. In Lynch HF, et al.: *Specimen science: ethics and policy implications*, Cambridge, MA, 2017, The MIT Press, p 47. https://books.google.com/books?hl=en&lr=&id=8rM5DwAAQBAJ&oi=fnd&pg=PA47&dq=selling+huan+organs&ots=9gp4Z_gMj-&sig=psikkPlRGj2bduT_4gjXbpfzvlw#v=onepage&q=selling%20human%20organs&f=false. Accessed October 2018.

Luthi S: U. S. Organ transplant rules get an overhaul, Modern Healthcare, December 7, 2018. https://www.modernhealthcare.com/article/20181207/NEWS/181209931/u-s-organ-transplant-rules-get-an-overhaul. Accessed July 18, 2019.

McGuire AL, et al.: Who owns the data in a medical information commons? *J Law Med Ethics* 47(1):62, 2019. https://doi.org/10.1177%2F1073110519840485. Accessed 8 August 2019.

National Council of State Boards of Nursing (NCSBN): *White paper: national guidelines for nursing delegation*, 2016. https://www.ncsbn.org/NCSBN_Delegation_Guidelines.pdf. Accessed August 5, 2019.

National Council of State Boards of Nursing (NCSBN): *eNLC Fast Facts*, n.d.,2019. https://www.ncsbn.org/NLC_Fast_Facts.pdf. Accessed August 4, 2019.

National Council of State Boards of Nursing (NCSBN): *White paper: a nurse's guide to the use of social media*, 2018. https://www.ncsbn.org/NCSBN_SocialMedia.pdf. Accessed October 2018.

National Council of State Boards of Nursing (NCSBN) & American Nurses Association (ANA): *National guidelines for nursing delegation*, 2019. https://www.ncsbn.org/NGND-PosPaper_06.pdf. Accessed August 5, 2019.

Nurses' Service Organization: *When to refuse an assignment*, 2017, Affinity Insurance Services. https://www.nso.com/Learning/Artifacts/Articles/when-to-refuse-an-assignment. Accessed July 20, 2019.

Oyeleye OA: The nursing licensure compact and its disciplinary provisions: what nurses should know, *Online J Issues Nurs* 24(2), 2019. https://doi.org/10.3912/OJIN.Vol24No02PPT09.

Philo H, et al.: *Lawyers desk reference*, ed 9, Eagan, MN, 2015, Thomson West Publishing.

Pozgar GD: *Legal and ethical issues for health professionals*, Burlington, MA, 2016, Jones & Bartlett Publishing, p 2016.

Privacy Rights Clearinghouse: *The HIPAA privacy rule: patients' rights*, 2014. https://www.privacyrights.org/consumer-guides/hipaa-privacy-rule-patients-rights. , Accessed October 2018.

Sadler BL, Sadler Jr AM: Organ transplantation and the Uniform Anatomical gift act: a fifty–year perspective, *Hastings Cent Rep* 48(2):14–18, 2018.

Scruth E, et al.: Electronic and social media: the legal and ethical issues for healthcare, *Clin Nurse Spec* 29(1):10, 2015.

The Joint Commission (TJC): *Restraint and seclusion—enclosure beds, side rails and mitts. Is an enclosure bed, side rails or hand mitts a restraint?* 2018. https://www.jointcommission.org/standards_information/jcfaqdetails.aspx?StandardsFaqId=1566&ProgramId=46. Accessed October 2018.

The Joint Commission (TJC): *Comprehensive accreditation manual for hospitals: the official handbook*, Oak Brook Terrace, IL, 2019, The Joint Commission.

The Joint Commission (TJC): *2020 National patient safety goals*, Oakbrook Terrace, IL, 2020, The Commission. https://www.jointcommission.org/en/standards/national-patient-safety-goals/. Accessed January 2, 2020.

Touhy TA, Jett F: *Ebersole and Hess' gerontological nursing & healthy aging*, ed 5, St Louis, 2018, Elsevier, p 2018.

US Department of Health and Human Services (USDHHS): Key features of the affordable care act by year, 2015, HHS.gov/HealthCare (website), http://www.hhs.gov/healthcare/facts/timeline/timeline-text.html. Accessed October 2018.

US Department of the Treasury: Final rules under the Paul Wellstone and Pete Domenici Mental Health Parity and Addiction Equity Act of 2008; technical amendment to external review for multi-state plan program; final rule, *Federal Register* Document number 2013-27086 , 2013, https://www.federalregister.gov/documents/2013/11/13/2013-27086/final-rules-under-the-paul-wellstone-and-pete-domenici-mental-health-parity-and-addiction-equity-act. Accessed July 16, 2019.

Yeung AS, et al.: Capacity assessment and involuntary commitment in psychiatric and medical settings: clinical, legal and cultural considerations. https://www.ncbi.nlm.nih.gov/pubmed/31265769. Accessed August 8, 2019.

STATUTES

Americans with Disabilities Act (ADA), 42 USC §§121.010-12213 (1990)

Emergency Medical Treatment and Active Labor Act (EMTALA), 42 USC §1395 (dd) (1986)

Good Samaritan Act, IL Compiled Statutes, 745 ILCS 49/ (1997)

Health Insurance Portability and Accountability Act of 1996 (HIPAA), Public Law No. 104 (1996)

Health Information Technology for Economic and Clinical Health Act (HITECH Act) 45 C.F.R. § 164.304.n8

Health Information Technology for Economic and Clinical Health Act (HITECH Act), Pub. L. No. 111-5, 123 Stat. 115 (Feb. 17, 2009), § 13401(a) (codified at 42 U.S.C. § 17931(a); 45 C.F.R. § 160.103).

Medical Patient Rights Act, IL Compiled Statutes, 410 ILCS 50 (1994)

Mental Health Parity Act of 1996, 29 USC §1885 (1996)

National Organ Transplant Act: Public Law 98–507, 1984.

Omnibus Budget Reconciliation Act of 1987 (Federal Nursing Home Reform Act). Retrieved from https://www.govtrack.us/congress/bills/99/hr5300.

Oregon Death With Dignity Act, Ore Rev Stat §§127.800-127.897 (1994)

Patient Protection and Affordable Care Act, 42 USC 18001 (2010)

Patient Self-Determination Act, 42 CFR 417 (1991)

Uniform Anatomical Gift Act (1987)

Uniform Determination of Death Act (1980)

CASES

Bouvia v Superior Court, 225 Cal Rptr 297 (1986)

Cruzan v Director of Missouri Department of Health, 497 U.S. 261 (1990)

Darling v Charleston Community Memorial Hospital, 33 Ill 2d 326 (Ill 1965)

Gibbons v. Ogden, 22 US 1, 6 L. Ed. 23, 1824 US LEXUS 370 – Supreme Court, 1824

In Re: *Estate of Jeanette Turner v Mercy Hospital and Medical Center*, 2018 IL App (1st) https://scholar.google.com/scholar_case?case=5606201838084968189&q=nursing-+care &hl=en&as_sdt=2006&as_ylo=2018

Roe v Wade, 410 U.S. 113 (1973)

Schindler R, Schindler M, *Appellants v: Michael Schiavo, as guardian of the person of Theresa Marie Schiavo, appellee*. https://scholar.google.com/scholar_case?case=14050841824849133847&q=Terri+Schiavo&hl=en&as_sdt=4,10,60&as_ylo=2000&as_yhi=2019. Accessed August 2019.

Spires v Hospital Corporation of America, 28 U.S.C. §1391(b) Kansas (2006), W. L. 1642701 (2006).

State v. Nurse Appellant's Brief Dckt. 44574, 2017. https://digitalcommons.law.uidaho.edu/cgi/viewcontent.cgi?article=7695&context=idaho_supreme_court_record_briefs.

Webster v Reproductive Health Services, 492 U.S. 490 (1989)

24

Communication

OBJECTIVES

- Identify ways to apply critical thinking to the communication process.
- Use the five levels of communication with patients.
- Describe features of the circular transactional communication process.
- Describe features of the verbal communication process
- Identify key aspects of nonverbal communication process.
- Incorporate features of a helping relationship when interacting with patients.
- Identify a nurse's communication approaches within the four phases of a nurse-patient helping relationship.

- Identify desired outcomes of nurse–health care team member relationships.
- Demonstrate professional communication while interacting with patients.
- Identify opportunities to improve communication with patients while giving care.
- Engage in effective communication techniques for older patients.
- Offer alternative communication devices when appropriate to promote communication with patients who have impaired communication.
- Implement nursing care measures for patients with special communication needs.

KEYTERMS

Active listening, p. 333
Assertiveness, p. 330
Autonomy, p. 330
Channel, p. 325
Circular transactional communication process, p. 325
Circular transactional model, p. 325
Communication, p. 322

Complementary, p. 325
Empathy, p. 334
Environment, p. 326
Feedback, p. 325
Interpersonal variables, p. 325
Lateral violence, p. 329
Message, p. 325
Motivational interviewing, p. 328

Perceptual biases, p. 323
Receiver, p. 325
Referent, p. 325
Sender, p. 325
Stereotypes, p. 323
Symmetrical, p. 325
Therapeutic communication, p. 333

MEDIA RESOURCES

http://evolve.elsevier.com/Potter/fundamentals/
- Review Questions
- Case Study with Questions

- Audio Glossary
- Content Updates
- Answers to QSEN Activity and Review Questions

COMMUNICATION AND NURSING PRACTICE

Communication is a lifelong learning process. Nurses make intimate journeys with patients and their families from the miracle of birth to the mystery of death. As a nurse you communicate with patients and families to develop meaningful relationships. Within those relationships you collect relevant assessment data, provide education and counseling and interact during nursing interventions. The use of therapeutic communication promotes personal growth and helps patients reach their health-related goals. Despite the complexity of technology and the multiple demands on nurses' time, it is the intimate moment of connection that makes all the difference in the quality of care and meaning for a patient and a nurse. Communication is essential when establishing nurse-patient relationships and delivering patient-centered care.

Patient safety also requires effective communication among members of the health care team as patients move from one caregiver to another or from one care setting to another. Good communication

skills help to reduce the risk of errors. These skills promote improved patient outcomes and increased patient satisfaction (Sethi and Rani, 2017). Effective team communication and collaboration skills are essential to ensure patient safety and optimum patient care (Lazure et al., 2014). Competent communication maintains effective relationships within the entire sphere of professional practice and meets legal, ethical, and clinical standards of care. The qualities and behaviors of therapeutic communication described in this chapter characterize professionalism in caring relationships.

Communication and Interpersonal Relationships

Caring relationships formed by a nurse and those affected by the nurse's practice are at the core of nursing (see Chapter 7). All behavior communicates, and all communication influences behavior. Nurses demonstrate caring by being with, doing for, and enabling patient well-being (Lillykutty and Samson, 2018). The following nursing actions reflect caring:

- Becoming sensitive and supportive to self and others
- Being present and encouraging the expression of positive and negative feelings
- Developing healing relationships
- Instilling faith and hope
- Promoting interpersonal teaching and learning
- Providing for nursing care needs in a supportive way
- Respecting and allowing for spiritual expression

A nurse's ability to relate to others is important for interpersonal communication. This includes the ability to take initiative in establishing and maintaining communication, to be authentic (one's self), and to respond appropriately to the other person. Effective interpersonal communication also requires a sense of mutuality (i.e., a belief that the nurse-patient relationship is a partnership and that both are equal participants). Nurses honor the fact that people are very complex and ambiguous. Often more is communicated than first meets the eye, and patient responses are not always what you expect. Each patient is a unique individual, with specific communication needs. Nurses need to embrace a nonjudgmental, holistic view of people and understand the need for effective, supportive communication and human interaction. When patients and nurses work together, much can be accomplished. Patient- and family-centered communication, such as involving the patient in conversations about transitions in care, contributes to a culture of safety (Johnson, 2015). When these conversations occur at the bedside, providing for privacy is essential.

Therapeutic communication occurs within a healing relationship between a nurse and patient (Arnold and Boggs, 2016). Like any powerful therapeutic agent, a nurse's communication can result in both harm and good. Every nuance of posture, every small expression and gesture, every word chosen, every attitude held—all have the potential to hurt or heal, affecting others through the transmission of human energy. Knowing that intention and behavior directly influence health gives nurses the ethical responsibility to do no harm to those entrusted to their care. Respect the potential power of communication and do not misuse communication carelessly to hurt, manipulate, or coerce others. Skilled communication empowers others to express what they believe and make their own choices; these are essential aspects of the individualized healing process. Nurses have wonderful opportunities to bring about good things for themselves, their patients, and their colleagues through therapeutic communication.

Developing Communication Skills

Gaining expertise in communication requires both an understanding of the communication process and reflection about one's communication experiences as a nurse. Nurses who develop critical thinking skills make the best communicators. They form therapeutic relationships to gather relevant and comprehensive information about their patients. Then they draw on theoretical knowledge about communication and integrate this knowledge with knowledge previously learned through personal clinical experience. They interpret messages received from others to obtain new information, correct misinformation, promote patient understanding, and plan patient-centered care (Arnold and Boggs, 2016).

Critical thinking attitudes and ethical standards of care promote effective communication. When you consider a patient's problems, it is important to apply critical thinking and critical reasoning skills to improve communication in assessment and care of the patient (Arnold and Boggs, 2016). For example, curiosity motivates a nurse to communicate and learn more about a person. Patients are more likely to communicate with nurses who express an interest in them.

Perseverance and creativity are also attitudes that motivate a nurse to communicate and identify innovative solutions. A self-confident attitude is important because a nurse who conveys confidence and comfort while communicating more readily establishes an interpersonal caring relationship. In addition, an independent attitude encourages a nurse to communicate with colleagues and share ideas about nursing interventions. Integrity allows nurses to recognize when their opinions conflict with others (e.g., patients, co-workers), review positions of those involved, and decide how to communicate to reach mutually beneficial decisions. It is also very important for a nurse to communicate responsibly and ask for help if uncertain or uncomfortable about an aspect of patient care. An attitude of humility is necessary to recognize when you need to better communicate and intervene with patients, especially related to their cultural needs (Isaacson, 2014).

It is challenging to understand human communication within interpersonal relationships. Each individual bases his or her perceptions about information received through the five senses of sight, hearing, taste, touch, and smell (Arnold and Boggs, 2016). An individual's culture and education also influence perception. Critical thinking helps nurses overcome perceptual biases or stereotypes that interfere with accurately perceiving and interpreting messages from others. People often incorrectly assume that they understand an individual's culture. They tend to distort or ignore information that goes against their expectations, preconceptions, or stereotypes (Isaacson, 2014). By thinking critically about personal communication habits, you learn to control these tendencies and become more effective in interpersonal relationships.

You become more competent in the nursing process as your communication skills develop. You learn to integrate communication skills throughout the nursing process as you collaborate with patients and health care team members to achieve goals (Box 24.1). Use communication skills to gather, analyze, and transmit information and accomplish the work of each step of the process. Each step of the nursing process depends on effective communication among nurse, patient, family, and others on the health care team. Although the nursing process is a reliable framework for patient care, it does not work well unless you master the art of effective interpersonal communication.

Patients often experience high levels of anxiety when they are ill or receiving treatment. Nurses use self-awareness, motivation, empathy, and social skills to build therapeutic relationships with patients (Marquis and Huston, 2017). Patients' emotions can negatively influence their self-care behaviors. When you understand a patient's perceptions and motivations, you can help the patient make healthy behavior changes.

The nature of the communication process requires you to constantly decide what, when, where, why, and how to convey a message. A nurse's decision making is always contextual (i.e., the unique features of any situation influence the nature of the decisions made). For example, the explanation of the importance of following a prescribed diet to a patient with a newly diagnosed medical condition differs from the explanation to a patient who has repeatedly chosen not to follow diet restrictions. Effective communication techniques are easy to learn, but their application is difficult. Deciding which techniques best fit each unique nursing situation is challenging. Communicating with patients and families about illness such as cancer or advance care planning can be stressful. Nurses may experience grief and fatigue related to emotional exhaustion when discussing these topics, especially when they have developed a bond with patients or families. However, discussion of these important and sensitive topics is linked to an increased quality of life for patients and family members (Zajac et al., 2017).

BOX 24.1 Communication Throughout the Nursing Process

Assessment
- Verbal interviewing and history taking
- Visual and intuitive observation of nonverbal behavior
- Visual, tactile, and auditory data gathering during physical examination
- Written medical records, diagnostic tests, and literature review

Nursing Diagnosis
- Intrapersonal analysis of assessment findings
- Validation of health care needs and priorities via verbal discussion with patient
- Documentation of nursing diagnosis

Planning
- Interpersonal or small-group health care team planning sessions
- Interpersonal collaboration with patient and family to determine implementation methods
- Written documentation of expected outcomes
- Written or verbal referral to health care team members

Implementation
- Delegation and verbal discussion with health care team
- Verbal, visual, auditory, and tactile health teaching activities
- Provision of support via therapeutic communication techniques
- Contact with other health resources
- Written documentation of patient's progress in medical record

Evaluation
- Acquisition of verbal and nonverbal feedback
- Comparison of actual and expected outcomes
- Identification of factors affecting outcomes
- Modification and update of care plan
- Verbal and/or written explanation of care plan revisions to patient

---

BOX 24.2 Challenging Communication Situations

- People who are silent, withdrawn, and have difficulty expressing feelings or needs
- People who are sad and depressed
- People who require assistance with visual or speech disabilities (special needs)
- People who are angry or confrontational and cannot listen to explanations
- People who are uncooperative and resent being asked to help others
- People who are talkative or lonely and want someone to be with them all the time
- People who are demanding and expect others to meet their requests
- People who are frightened, anxious, and having difficulty coping
- People who are confused and disoriented
- People who speak and/or understand little English
- People who are flirtatious or sexually inappropriate

Throughout this chapter, brief clinical examples will guide you in learning how to use effective communication techniques. Situations that challenge your decision-making skills and call for careful use of therapeutic techniques involve a variety of human behaviors, described in Box 24.2. Because the best way to acquire skill is through practice, it is useful for you to discuss and role-play these scenarios before experiencing them in the clinical setting. Effective communication and collaboration are imperative for success.

Levels of Communication

Nurses use different levels of communication in their professional role. A competent nurse uses a variety of techniques in each level.

Intrapersonal communication is a powerful form of communication that you use as a professional nurse. This level of communication is also called *self-talk*. People's thoughts and inner communications strongly influence perceptions, feelings, behavior, and self-esteem. Always be aware of the nature and content of your own thinking. Positive self-talk provides a mental rehearsal for difficult tasks or situations so that you can deal with them more effectively and with increased confidence (Arnold and Boggs, 2016). You use intrapersonal communication to develop self-awareness and a positive self-esteem to enhance appropriate self-expression. Positive self-talk can diminish cognitive distortions that lead to a decrease in self-esteem and impact your ability to work with patients. Transforming statements from "I'm scared to work with this type of patient" into "This is my opportunity to learn about this patient, and I can ask for help when it's needed" is an example of positive self-talk.

Interpersonal communication is one-on-one interaction between a nurse and another person that most often occurs face-to-face. It is the level most frequently used in nursing situations and lies at the heart of nursing practice. It takes place within a social context and includes all the symbols and cues used to give and receive meaning. Because meaning resides in people and not in words, messages received are sometimes different from intended messages. Nurses work with people who have different opinions, experiences, values, and belief systems; thus it is important to validate meaning or mutually negotiate it between participants. For example, use interaction to assess understanding and clarify misinterpretations when teaching a patient about a health concern. Meaningful interpersonal communication results in an exchange of ideas, problem solving, expression of feelings, decision making, goal accomplishment, team building, and personal growth.

Small-group communication is the interaction that occurs when a small number of people meet. This type of communication is usually goal directed and requires an understanding of group dynamics. When nurses work on committees with nurses or other disciplines and participate in patient care conferences, they use a small-group communication process. Communication in these situations should be organized, concise, and complete. All participating disciplines are encouraged to contribute and provide feedback. Good communication skills help each participant better meet a patient's needs and promote a safer care environment.

Public communication is interaction with an audience. Nurses often speak with groups of consumers about health-related topics, present scholarly work to colleagues at conferences, or lead classroom discussions with peers or students. Public communication requires special adaptations in eye contact, gestures, voice inflection, and the use of media materials to communicate messages effectively. Effective public communication increases audience knowledge about health-related topics, health issues, and other issues important to the nursing profession.

Electronic communication is the use of technology to create ongoing relationships with patients and their health care team. Secure messaging provides an opportunity for frequent and timely communication with a patient's physician or nurse via a patient portal. An electronic portal enables patients to stay engaged and informed, though the empathetic nature of the therapeutic relationship with the health care team may be more challenging (Brandt et al., 2018).

ELEMENTS OF THE COMMUNICATION PROCESS

Communication is an ongoing and continuously changing process. You are changing, the people with whom you are communicating are

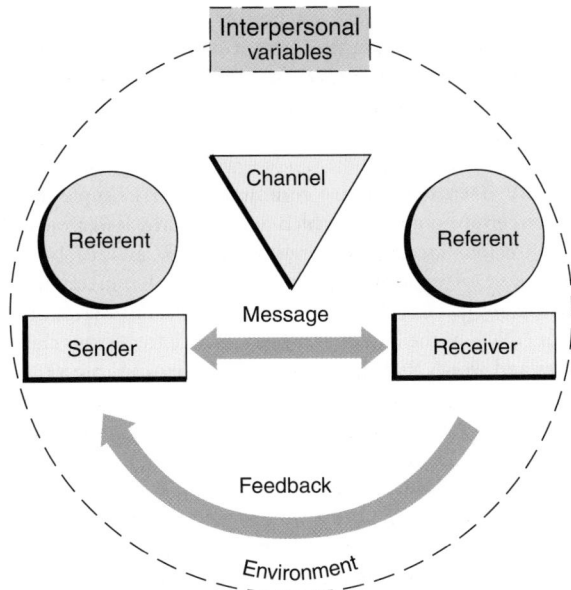

FIG. 24.1 Circular transactional model of communication.

changing, and your environment is also continually changing. Fig. 24.1 shows an example of a **circular transactional communication process** model. The model shows the situational contextual inputs, channels of communication, interpersonal contextual concepts, and factors affecting the sender and receiver. Nursing situations have many unique aspects that influence the nature of communication and interpersonal relationships. As a professional you will use critical thinking to focus on each aspect of communication so that your interactions are purposeful and effective.

Circular Transactional Model

The **circular transactional model** includes several elements: the referent, sender and receiver, message, channels, context or environment in which the communication process occurs, feedback, and interpersonal variables (see Fig. 24.1). In this model each person in the communication interaction is both a speaker and a listener and can be simultaneously sending and receiving messages. Both parties view the perceptions, attitudes, and potential reactions to a sent message. Communication becomes a continuous and interactive activity. Feedback from the receiver or environment enables the communicators to correct or validate the communication. This model also describes the role relationship of the communicators as **complementary** and **symmetrical**. Complementary role relationships function with one person holding an elevated position over the other person. Symmetrical relationships are more equal. A complementary role occurs when a nurse provides education to a patient about a new medication. A group of patients discussing their plans after discharge is an example of a symmetrical role relationship (Arnold and Boggs, 2016).

Referent. The **referent** motivates one person to communicate with another. In a health care setting sights, sounds, sensations, perceptions, and ideas are examples of cues that initiate the communication process. Knowing a stimulus or referent that initiates communication allows you to develop and organize messages more efficiently. For example, a patient request for help prompted by his difficulty in breathing causes a different response than a patient request resulting from hunger.

Sender and Receiver. The **sender** is the person who encodes and delivers a message, and the **receiver** is the person who receives and decodes the message. The sender puts the message into verbal and nonverbal symbols that the receiver can understand (Arnold and Boggs, 2016). The sender's message acts as a referent for the receiver. Transactional communication involves the role of sender and receiver switching back and forth between nurse and patient. A decoding process includes the receiver interpreting the meaning of the word symbols. Active listening is important to accurately decode and understand a message. The more the sender and receiver have in common and the closer the relationship, the more likely they will accurately perceive one another's meaning and respond accordingly (Arnold and Boggs, 2016). Establishing rapport with a patient ensures more effective communication.

Message. The **message** is the content of the communication. It contains verbal and nonverbal expressions of thoughts and feelings. Effective messages are clear, direct, and in understandable language. Individuals with communication barriers may need assistance via clarification devices such as hearing aids, interpreters, or pictures to ensure that messages sent and received are understandable. Personal perceptions may also distort the receiver's interpretation of a message. As a nurse you send effective messages by expressing clearly, directly, and in a manner familiar to a patient. You determine the need for clarification by watching the patient listen for nonverbal cues that suggest confusion or misunderstanding. Communication is difficult when participants have different levels of education literacy and experience. For example, statements such as "Your incision is well approximated without purulent drainage" means the same as "Your wound edges are close together, and there are no signs of infection," but the latter is easier to understand. You can also send messages in writing, but make sure that patients are able to read.

Channels. Individuals use communication **channels** to send and receive messages through visual, auditory, and tactile senses. Facial expressions send visual messages; spoken words travel through auditory channels. Touch uses tactile channels. Individuals usually understand a message more clearly when the sender uses more channels to send it.

Feedback. **Feedback** is the message a sender receives from the receiver. It indicates whether the receiver understood the meaning of the sender's message. Feedback occurs continuously between a sender and receiver. A sender seeks verbal and nonverbal feedback to evaluate the receiver's response and effectiveness of a communicated message. The type of feedback a sender or receiver gives depends on factors such as their background, prior experiences, attitudes, cultural beliefs, and self-esteem. A sender and receiver need to be sensitive and open to one another's messages, to clarify the messages, and to modify behavior accordingly for successful communication.

Interpersonal Variables. **Interpersonal variables** are factors within both the sender and receiver that influence communication. Perception provides a uniquely personal view of reality formed by an individual's culture, expectations, and experiences. Each person senses, interprets, and understands events differently. A nurse says, "You haven't been talking very much since your family left. Is there something on your mind?" One patient may perceive the nurse's question as caring and concerned; another perceives the nurse as invading privacy and is less willing to talk. Cultural sensitivity enables you to explore the interpersonal variables such as educational and developmental level, sociocultural background, values and beliefs, emotions, gender, physical health status, and roles and relationships that affect how a patient communicates. Interpersonal variables associated with illness such as pain, anxiety, and medication effects also affect nurse-patient communication.

Environment. The environment is the setting for sender-receiver interaction. An effective communication setting provides participants with physical and emotional comfort and safety. Noise, temperature extremes, distractions, and lack of privacy or space create confusion, tension, and discomfort. Environmental distractions are common in health care settings and interfere with messages sent between people. You control the environment as much as possible to create favorable conditions for effective communication.

FORMS OF COMMUNICATION

Messages are conveyed verbally and nonverbally, concretely and symbolically. As people communicate, they express themselves through words, movements, voice inflection, facial expressions, and use of space. These elements work in harmony to enhance a message or conflict with one another to contradict and confuse it.

Verbal Communication

Verbal communication uses spoken or written words. Verbal language is a code that conveys specific meaning through a combination of words. The most important aspects of verbal communication are presented in the following paragraphs.

Vocabulary. Communication is unsuccessful if senders and receivers cannot translate one another's words and phrases. When you care for a patient who speaks another language, a professional interpreter is necessary. Even those who speak the same language use subcultural variations of certain words (e.g., *dinner* means a noon meal to one person and the last meal of the day to another). Medical jargon (technical terminology used by health care providers) sounds like a foreign language to patients unfamiliar with the health care setting. Limiting use of medical jargon to conversations with other health care team members improves communication. Children have a more limited vocabulary than adults and often use special words to describe bodily functions or a favorite blanket or toy. Teenagers often use words in unique ways that are unfamiliar to adults.

Denotative and Connotative Meaning. Some words have several meanings. Individuals who use a common language share the denotative meaning: *baseball* has the same meaning for everyone who speaks English, but *code* denotes cardiac arrest primarily to health care providers. The connotative meaning is the shade or interpretation of the meaning of a word influenced by the thoughts, feelings, or ideas that people have about the word. For example, health care providers tell a family that a loved one is in serious condition and they believe that death is near; but to nurses *serious* simply describes the nature of the illness. You need to select words carefully, avoiding easily misinterpreted words, especially when explaining a patient's medical condition or therapy. Even a much-used phrase such as "I'm going to take your vital signs" may be unfamiliar to an adult or frightening to a child. "I'm going to check your blood pressure, heart rate, and temperature" may be more appropriate.

Pacing. Conversation is more successful at an appropriate speed or pace. Speak moderately slowly and enunciate clearly. Talking rapidly, using awkward pauses, or speaking excessively slowly and deliberately conveys an unintended message. Long pauses and rapid shifts to another subject give the impression that you are hiding the truth. Think before speaking and develop an awareness of the rhythm of your speech to improve pacing.

Intonation. Tone of voice dramatically affects the meaning of a message. Depending on intonation, even a simple question or statement expresses enthusiasm, anger, concern, or indifference. Be aware of voice tone to avoid sending unintended messages. If a patient interprets your patronizing tone of voice as condescending, this will inhibit further communication. A patient's tone of voice provides information about his or her emotional state or energy level.

Clarity and Brevity. Effective communication is simple, brief, and direct. For certain populations such as the elderly, fewer words result in less confusion. Speak slowly, enunciate clearly, and use brief examples to make explanations easier to understand. Repeating important parts of a message also clarifies communication. Phrases such as "you know" or "OK?" at the end of every sentence detract from clarity. Use sentences and words that express an idea simply and directly. "Where is your pain?" is much better than "I would like you to describe for me the location of your discomfort."

Timing and Relevance. Timing is critical in communication. Even though a message is clear, poor timing prevents it from being effective. For example, you do not begin routine teaching when a patient is in severe pain or emotional distress. Often the best time for interaction is when a patient expresses an interest in communicating. If messages are relevant or important to the situation at hand, they are more effective. When a patient is facing emergency surgery, discussing the risks of smoking is less relevant than explaining presurgical procedures. Face-to-face time while performing assessments, administering medications, or performing procedures offers an excellent opportunity to talk with patients and provide support or education. Patients report improved satisfaction, understanding, and perception of safety with registered nurses (RNs) who provide a bedside hand-off and communicate information about the plan of care (Ford et al., 2014).

Nonverbal Communication

Nonverbal communication includes the five senses and everything that does not involve the spoken or written word. Nonverbal aspects of communication such as voice tone, eye contact, and body positioning are often as important as verbal messages (Lorié, 2017). Thus nonverbal communication is unconsciously motivated and more accurately indicates a person's intended meaning than spoken words (Varcarolis, 2017). When there is incongruity between verbal and nonverbal communication, the receiver usually "hears" the nonverbal message as the true message.

All nonverbal communication is important, but interpreting it is often problematic. Sociocultural background is a major influence on the meaning of nonverbal behavior. In the United States, with its diverse cultural communities, nonverbal messages between people of different cultures are easily misinterpreted. Assessing and responding to nonverbal messages are important aspects of nursing care (Sethi and Rani, 2017).

Personal Appearance. Personal appearance includes physical characteristics, facial expression, and manner of dress and grooming. These factors are a powerful means of nonverbal communications to patients and the health care team. In the health care setting research shows patients prefer that nurses employed in an agency all wear a single uniform and that the "RN" or "LPN" tag be displayed prominently (West et al., 2016). Many health care agencies restrict how much jewelry you can wear and whether certain types of tattoos need to be covered. For hygienic reasons nurses should have long hair pulled back and off the shoulders and short clean fingernails. Remember, first impressions are largely based on appearance. Nurses learn to develop a general impression of patient health and emotional status through appearance, and patients develop a general impression of the nurse's professionalism and caring in the same way.

Posture and Gait. Posture and gait (manner or pattern of walking) can be forms of self-expression. The way people sit, stand, and move reflects attitudes, emotions, self-concept, and health status. For example, an erect posture and a quick, purposeful gait communicate a sense of well-being and confidence. Leaning forward conveys attention. A slumped posture and slow, shuffling gait indicate depression, illness, or fatigue.

Facial Expression. The face is the most expressive part of the body. Facial expressions convey emotions such as surprise, fear, anger, happiness, and sadness. Some people have an expressionless face, or flat affect, which reveals little about what they are thinking or feeling. An inappropriate affect is a facial expression that does not match the content of a verbal message (e.g., smiling when describing a sad situation). People are sometimes unaware of the messages their expressions convey. For example, a nurse frowns in concentration while doing a procedure, and the patient interprets this as anger or disapproval. Patients closely observe nurses. Consider the impact your facial expression could have on a person who asks, "Am I going to die?" The slightest change in the eyes, lips, or facial muscles reveals your feelings. Although it is hard to control all facial expressions, try to avoid showing shock, disgust, dismay, or other distressing reactions in a patient's presence.

Eye Contact. People signal readiness to communicate through eye contact. Maintaining eye contact during conversation shows respect and willingness to listen. Eye contact also allows people to closely observe one another. Lack of eye contact sometimes indicates anxiety, defensiveness, discomfort, or lack of confidence in communicating. However, people from some cultures consider eye contact intrusive, threatening, or harmful and minimize or avoid its use (see Chapter 9). Always consider a person's culture when interpreting the meaning of eye contact. Eye movements communicate feelings and emotions. Looking down on a person establishes authority, whereas interacting at the same eye level indicates equality in the relationship. Rising to the same eye level as an angry person helps establish autonomy.

Gestures. Gestures emphasize, punctuate, and clarify the spoken word. Gestures alone carry specific meanings, or they create messages with other communication cues. A finger pointed toward a person communicates several meanings, but when accompanied by a frown and stern voice, the gesture becomes an accusation or a threat. Pointing to an area of pain is sometimes more accurate than describing its location.

Sounds. Sounds such as sighs, moans, groans, or sobs also communicate feelings and thoughts. Combined with other nonverbal communication, sounds help to send clear messages. They have several interpretations. For example, moaning can convey pleasure or suffering, and crying can communicate happiness, sadness, or anger. Validate nonverbal messages with patients to interpret them accurately. For example, "I notice you frowning as you move, are you having pain?"

Territoriality and Personal Space. Territoriality is the need to gain, maintain, and defend one's right to space. Territory is important because it provides people with a sense of privacy, identity, security, and control. It is sometimes separated and made visible to others, as with a fence around a yard or a curtain around a bed in a hospital room. Personal space is invisible and individual and travels with a person. During interpersonal interaction people maintain varying distances between one another, depending on their culture, the nature of their relationship, and the situation. When personal space becomes threatened, people respond defensively and communicate less effectively. Situations dictate whether the interpersonal distance between nurse and patient is appropriate. Box 24.3

BOX 24.3   Zones of Personal Space

Zones Of Personal Space
Intimate Distance (0–18 inches)
- Holding a crying infant
- Performing physical assessment
- Bathing, grooming, dressing, feeding, and toileting a patient
- Changing a patient's surgical dressing

Personal Distance (18 inches–40 inches)
- Sitting at a patient's bedside
- Taking a patient's nursing history
- Teaching an individual patient

Social Distance (4–12 feet)
- Giving directions to visitors in the hallway
- Asking whether families need assistance from the patient doorway
- Giving verbal report to a group of nurses

Public Distance (12 feet and more)
- Speaking at a community forum
- Lecturing to a class of students
- Testifying at a legislative hearing

Special Zones of Touch
Social Zone (Permission Not Needed)
Hands, arms, shoulders, back

Consent Zone (Permission Needed)
Mouth, wrists, feet

Vulnerable Zone (Special Care Needed)
Face, neck, front of body

Intimate Zone (Permission and Great Sensitivity Needed)
Genitalia, rectum

---

provides examples of nursing actions within communication zones (Varcarolis, 2017). Nurses frequently move into patients' territory and personal space because of the nature of caregiving. You need to convey confidence, gentleness, and respect for privacy, especially when your actions require intimate contact or involve a patient's vulnerable zone.

Metacommunication

Metacommunication is a broad term that refers to all factors that influence communication. Awareness of influencing factors helps people better understand what is communicated (Arnold and Boggs, 2016). For example, a nurse observes a young patient holding his body rigidly, and his voice is sharp as he says, "Going to surgery is no big deal." The nurse replies, "You say having surgery doesn't bother you, but you look and sound tense. I'd like to hear more about how you're feeling." Awareness of the tone of the verbal response and the nonverbal behavior results in further exploration of the patient's feelings and concerns.

PROFESSIONAL NURSING RELATIONSHIPS

Your application of knowledge, understanding of human behavior and communication, and commitment to ethical behavior create professional relationships. Having a philosophy based on caring and respect for others helps you be more successful in establishing relationships of this nature.

Nurse-Patient Caring Relationships

Caring relationships are the foundation of clinical nursing practice. In such relationships you assume the role of a professional who cares about each patient and his or her unique health needs, human responses, and patterns of living. Therapeutic relationships promote a psychological climate that promotes positive change and growth, such as your patients ability to attain health-related goals (Arnold and Boggs, 2016). The goals of a therapeutic relationship focus on a patient achieving optimal personal growth related to personal identity, ability to form relationships, and ability to satisfy needs and achieve personal goals (Varcarolis, 2017). There is an explicit time frame, a goal-directed approach, and a high expectation that what you discuss together is kept confidential among only members of the health care team involved in the patient's care. You establish, direct, and take responsibility for the interaction, and a patient's needs take priority over your needs. Your nonjudgmental acceptance of a patient is an important characteristic of the relationship. Acceptance conveys a willingness to hear a message or acknowledge feelings. It does not mean that you always agree with the other person or approve of the patient's decisions or actions. A caring relationship between you and a patient does not just happen; you create it with skill and trust.

There is a natural progression of four goal-directed phases that characterize the nurse-patient relationship (Box 24.4). The relationship often begins before you meet a patient and continues until the caregiving relationship ends. Even a brief interaction uses an abbreviated version of preinteraction, orientation, working, and termination (Varcarolis, 2017). For example, a nursing student gathers patient information to prepare in advance for caregiving, meets the patient and establishes trust, accomplishes health-related goals through use of the nursing process, and says goodbye at the end of the day.

Socializing is an important initial component of interpersonal communication. It helps people get to know one another and relax. It is easy, superficial, and not deeply personal, whereas therapeutic interactions are often more intense, difficult, and uncomfortable. A nurse often uses social conversation to lay a foundation for a closer relationship: "Hi, Mr. Simpson, I hear it's your birthday today. How old are you?" A friendly, informal, and warm communication style establishes trust, but you need to move beyond social conversation to talk about issues or concerns affecting the patient's health. During social conversation, some patients ask personal questions such as those about your family or place of residence. Students often wonder whether it is appropriate to reveal such information. The skillful nurse uses judgment about what to share and provides minimal information or deflects such questions with gentle humor and refocuses conversation back to the patient.

In a therapeutic relationship, it may be helpful to encourage patients to share personal stories. Sharing stories is called *narrative interaction*. Through listening to stories, you begin to understand the context of others' lives and learn what is meaningful for them from their perspective. For example, a nurse listens to a patient's perception of what it means to refuse medication treatment for breast cancer and is then better able to articulate the patient's wishes Taking adequate time to listen to patients' stories positively impacts the patient care experience (Sethi and Rani, 2017). This information is not usually revealed with a standard history form that elicits short answers.

As a nurse, you can also tell stories to enhance communication. Telling good stories frames important messages you wish to send and makes messages memorable for your patients. Purposeful storytelling brings across factual information along with a human interest perspective that draws on an individual's emotions, such as a patient's desire to get well or feel a sense of hope. Be mindful not to divulge confidential information while using a story to illustrate a point. Emotions play a significant role in helping adults learn the ability to grasp new ideas.

BOX 24.4 Phases of the Helping Relationship

Preinteraction Phase

Before meeting a patient:
- Review available data, including the medical and nursing history.
- Talk to other caregivers who have information about the patient.
- Anticipate health concerns or issues that arise.
- Identify a location and setting that fosters comfortable, private interaction.
- Plan enough time for the initial interaction.

Orientation Phase

When you and a and patient meet and get to know one another:
- Set the tone for the relationship by adopting a warm, empathetic, caring manner.
- Recognize that the initial relationship is often superficial, uncertain, and tentative.
- Expect the patient to test your competence and commitment.
- Closely observe the patient and expect to be closely observed by the patient.
- Begin to make inferences and form judgments about patient messages and behaviors.
- Assess the patient's health status.
- Prioritize the patient's problems and identify his or her goals.
- Clarify the patient's and your roles.
- Form contracts with the patient that specify who will do what.
- Let the patient know when to expect the relationship to be terminated.

Working Phase

When you and a patient work together to solve problems and accomplish goals:
- Encourage and help the patient express feelings about his or her health.
- Encourage and help the patient with self-exploration.
- Provide information needed to understand and change behavior.
- Encourage and help the patient set goals.
- Take action to meet the goals set with the patient.
- Use therapeutic communication skills to facilitate successful interactions.
- Use appropriate self-disclosure and confrontation.

Termination Phase

During the ending of the relationship:
- Remind the patient that termination is near.
- Evaluate goal achievement with the patient.
- Reminisce about the relationship with the patient.
- Separate from the patient by relinquishing responsibility for his or her care.
- Achieve a smooth transition for the patient to other caregivers as needed.

Motivational Interviewing

Motivational interviewing (MI) is a technique that encourages patients to share their thoughts, beliefs, fears, and concerns with the aim of changing their behavior. MI provides a way of working with patients who may not seem ready to make behavioral changes that are considered necessary by their health practitioners. You can use it to evoke change talk, which links to improved patient outcomes (Copeland et al., 2015). For example, an interviewer uses information about a patient's personal goals and values to promote the patient's adherence to a new medication or exercise plan. The interviewing is delivered in a nonjudgmental, guided communication approach. When using MI, a nurse tries to understand a patient's motivations and values using an empathic and active listening approach. The nurse identifies differences between a patient's current health goals and behaviors and his or her current health status. The patient is supported even though a phase of resistance and ambivalence often occurs. Communication then focuses on recognizing the patient's strengths and supporting those strengths to make positive changes. This can result in dramatic improvements in health outcomes and patient satisfaction (Stawnychy et al., 2014).

Nurse-Family Relationships

Many nursing situations, especially those in community and home care settings, require you to form caring relationships with entire families. The same principles that guide one-on-one helping relationships also apply when the patient is a family unit, although communication within families requires additional understanding of the complexities of family dynamics, needs, and relationships (see Chapter 10).

Nurse–Health Care Team Relationships

Your communication with other members of the health care team affects patient safety and the work environment. According to Hannawa (2018), patient health outcomes are optimized when health care team members communicate well. Problems occur when communication is ineffective. The acronym SACCIA is one way to assist nurses in communicating effectively. The acronym stands for *Sufficiency, Accuracy, Clarity, Contextualization,* and *Interpersonal Adaptation.*

When patients move from one nursing unit to another or from one provider to another, there is a risk for miscommunication. To address this risk, health care providers provide detailed hand-off reports at the end of shifts or when patients transfer off care units to ensure that patients have a safe and smooth transition in care (Bucknall, 2016). Standardized discharge or transfer procedures and forms reduce the risk of errors during patient transitions. Timely follow-up after discharge or transfer is also appropriate.

Use of a common language such as the SBAR technique for communicating critical information improves the perception of communication and information about patients among health care providers (IHI, 2018; Stewart, 2017). This technique is a popular communication tool that standardizes communication. SBAR is the acronym for *Situation, Background, Assessment,* and *Recommendation* (IHI, 2018). Some organizations have added an Identify step (ISBAR) into the SBAR process. The Identify step is used when health care providers do not actively know one another. They start with an introduction, a description of their location, and their role in caring for the patient (IHI, 2018). The use of these easy-to-remember, orderly techniques relays relevant information in a structured and timely manner (Marquis and Huston, 2017). Evidence identifies nursing actions that increase the effectiveness of nurse-to-nurse interaction and interprofessional communication (Box 24.5).

QSEN Building Competency in Patient-Centered Care You are assigned to work with Mr. Rodriguez, a patient with a recent fracture of the femur, who is having surgery later today. Mr. Rodriguez fractured his femur on the job as a landscaper. He is a legal immigrant whose family is from Mexico. Mr. Rodriguez speaks English but has limited literacy. The registered nurse (RN) providing a handover report to you gives the relevant objective data about the patient. As an aside, the RN complains about how demanding and difficult the patient has been and how she does not believe people like him belong here, and she berates his insistence on the inclusion of a family member in all conversations. You recognize that providing patient-centered care, including integration of many dimensions of care, as well as respect for diverse cultural, ethnic, and social backgrounds, may contribute to positive patient care outcomes. What possible values, preferences, and needs may the patient be experiencing? Describe communication strategies and approaches that you would use to facilitate effective patient-centered care. How should every nurse recognize and address personally held beliefs and attitudes about patients from diverse backgrounds?

Answers to QSEN Activities can be found on the Evolve website.

BOX 24.5 EVIDENCE-BASED PRACTICE
Bedside Nurse to Nurse Handover Report

PICOT Question: In the hospital setting, do nurses who use bedside nursing handover report improve patient satisfaction and patient care outcomes compared with nurses who do not use bedside nursing handover report?

Evidence Summary

It has been widely argued that many of the adverse events occurring during hospitalization may have been prevented with a complete and effective nurse-to-nurse handover report conducted by nurses with effective training (Slade et al., 2018). Nurse-to-nurse bedside handover report has been used as a tool to improve patient-centered care, enhance patient understanding of the care plan, and enhance the completeness of report, among other benefits (Bains et al., 2018). In a systematic review of the literature on bedside handover, Gregory et al. (2014) identified six potential areas of positive impact: enhanced team collaboration, effective dyadic relationships, individual patient benefit, satisfaction, accountability, and cost containment. In a more recent systematic review of bedside shift-to-shift handovers, Mardis et al. (2016) found that the nurse-to-nurse bedside handover methodology enhanced patient and nurse satisfaction, improved communication, and helped patients understand their condition. However, the evidence of improved safety outcomes was weak and was identified as an area for future controlled study.

Application to Nursing Practice

- Failure to completely and accurately communicate during nurse-to-nurse handovers is a course of miscommunication that can lead to patient care errors.
- Bedside nurse-to-nurse shift reporting is an important tool that may enhance patient-centered care, patient and nurse satisfaction, and patient understanding (Bains et al., 2018).
- Nurses who complete education on a standardized approach to bedside reporting are well prepared to use this important intervention (Slade et al., 2018).
- More study is needed to establish a clear link between bedside nurse-to-nurse shift reporting and patient care outcomes in many areas (Mardis et al., 2016).

Lateral Violence. Professional nursing care requires nurses to interact with members of the nursing team and interprofessional health care providers. Communication focuses on team building, facilitating group processes, collaborating, consulting, delegating, supervising, leading, and managing (see Chapter 21). Social, informational, and therapeutic interactions help team members build morale, accomplish goals, and strengthen working relationships. Lateral violence or workplace bullying between colleagues sometimes occurs and includes behaviors such as withholding information, backbiting, making snide remarks or put-downs, and nonverbal expressions of disapproval such as raising eyebrows or making faces. Lateral violence adversely affects the work environment, leading to job dissatisfaction, a decreased sense of value, poor teamwork, poor retention of qualified nurses, and nurses leaving the profession. New nurses are especially prone to bullying behavior (Frederick, 2014). Lateral violence can be a precursor to compassion fatigue, when health care workers perceive a threat during interactions with colleagues and react emotionally rather than communicating intentionally in a professional manner.

Lateral violence interferes with effective health care team communication and jeopardizes patient safety (Marquis and Huston, 2017). Intimidation decreases the likelihood that a nurse will report a near-miss event, question an order, or act to improve the quality of patient care. There must be zero tolerance of lateral violence. Develop skills in conflict management and assertive communication to stop the spread of lateral violence in the workplace. Requesting a mentor can help a new nurse learn skills to address the perpetrators of bullying. The mentor can also be a personal support for the nurse and serve as a role model for the department (Frederick, 2014). The nurse experiencing lateral violence can also use additional techniques such as the following:

- Address the behavior when it occurs in a calm manner.
- Describe how the behavior affects your functioning.
- Ask for the abuse to stop.
- Notify the manager to get support for the situation.
- Plan for taking action in the future.
- Document the incidents in detail in your personal notes, not patient records.

Nurse-Community Relationships

Many nurses form relationships with community groups by participating in local organizations, volunteering for community service, or becoming politically active. As a nurse, learn to establish relationships with your community to be an effective change agent. Providing clear and accurate information to members of the public is the best way to prevent errors, reduce resistance, and promote change. Communication within the community occurs through channels such as neighborhood newsletters, health fairs, public bulletin boards, newspapers, radio, television, and electronic information sites. Use these forms of communication to share information and discuss issues important to community health (see Chapter 3).

ELEMENTS OF PROFESSIONAL COMMUNICATION

Professional appearance, demeanor, and behavior are important in establishing trustworthiness and competence. A professional is expected to be clean, neat, well groomed, conservatively dressed, and odor free. Visible tattoos and piercings may not be considered acceptable in some professional settings. Professional behavior reflects warmth, friendliness, confidence, and competence. Professionals speak in a clear, well-modulated voice; use good grammar; listen to others; help and support colleagues; and communicate effectively. Being on time, organized, well prepared, and equipped for the responsibilities of the nursing role also communicate professionalism.

Courtesy

Common courtesy is part of professional communication. To practice courtesy, say hello and goodbye to patients and knock on doors before entering. State your purpose, address people by name, and say "please" and "thank you" to team members. Introduce yourself and state your title. When a nurse is discourteous, others perceive him or her as rude or insensitive. It sets up barriers to forming helping relationships between nurse and patient and causes friction among team members.

Use of Names

Always introduce yourself. Failure to give your name and status (e.g., nursing student, RN, or licensed practical nurse) or to acknowledge a patient creates uncertainty about an interaction and conveys an impersonal lack of commitment or caring. Making eye contact and smiling are ways to recognize others. Addressing people by name conveys respect for human dignity and uniqueness. Because using last names is respectful in most cultures, nurses usually use a patient's last name in an initial interaction and then use the first name if the patient requests it. Ask how your patients and co-workers prefer to be addressed and honor their personal preferences. Using first names is appropriate for infants, young children, patients who are confused or unconscious, and close team members. Avoid terms of endearment such as "honey,"

"dear," "grandma," or "sweetheart." Even the closest nurse-patient relationships rarely progress to identities beyond first names. Avoid referring to patients by diagnosis, room number, or another attribute, which is demeaning and sends the message that you do not care enough to know the person as an individual.

Trustworthiness

Trust is relying on someone without doubt or question. Being trustworthy means helping others without hesitation. To foster trust, communicate warmth and demonstrate consistency, reliability, honesty, competence, and respect. Sometimes it isn't easy for a patient to ask for help. Trusting another person involves risk and vulnerability, but it also fosters open, therapeutic communication and enhances the expression of feelings, thoughts, and needs. Without trust a nurse-patient relationship rarely progresses beyond social interaction and superficial care. Avoid dishonesty at all costs. Withholding key information, lying, or distorting the truth violates both legal and ethical standards of practice. Sharing personal information or gossiping about others sends the message that you cannot be trusted and damages interpersonal relationships.

Autonomy and Responsibility

Autonomy is being self-directed and independent in accomplishing goals and advocating for others. Professional nurses make choices and accept responsibility for the outcomes of their actions (Varcarolis, 2017). They take initiative in problem solving and communicate in a way that reflects the importance and purpose of a therapeutic conversation (Arnold and Boggs, 2016). Professional nurses also recognize their patients' autonomy.

Assertiveness

Assertiveness allows you to express feelings and ideas without judging or hurting others. Assertive behavior includes intermittent eye contact; nonverbal communication that reflects interest, honesty, and active listening; spontaneous verbal responses with a confident voice; and culturally sensitive use of touch and space. An assertive nurse communicates self-assurance; communicates feelings; takes responsibility for choices; and is respectful of others' feelings, ideas, and choices (Gultekin et al., 2018). Assertive behavior increases self-esteem and self-confidence, increases the ability to develop satisfying interpersonal relationships, and increases goal attainment. Assertive individuals make decisions and control their lives more effectively than nonassertive individuals. They deal with criticism and manipulation by others and learn to say no, set limits, and resist intentionally imposed guilt. Assertive responses contain "I" messages such as "I want," "I need," "I think," or "I feel" (Arnold and Boggs, 2016). Nurses may experience ethical issues that make it difficult to use their assertiveness skills for fear of retaliation (e.g., identifying an error made by another health care provider). In such a situation the individual needs to take steps to resolve this ethical dilemma (see Chapter 22).

AIDET® is a technique developed by the Studer Group to enable health care workers to provide accurate and timely communication to patients and families while focusing on excellent patient service. It is a technique commonly used in hospitals today. The acronym stands for *Acknowledge, Introduce, Duration, Explain,* and *Thank* you. When using AIDET, you first acknowledge the person standing in front of you with a positive attitude and make the person feel comfortable. Introduce yourself and let the person know what his or her role is in the department and in the person's care. It is important to always wear a name badge when working in a health care setting. When possible, give a patient or family an idea of how long a procedure may take. This keeps the patient informed of any delays that may occur. It is also helpful to let a patient know how long it will take to get results if they are related to testing. When explaining procedures, describe what the patient will experience with the treatment, procedure, or test. Inform him or her of any safety precautions. When using AIDET, thank a patient for coming to your organization for care and let the patient know how much you enjoyed working with him or her (Rubin, 2014).

❖ NURSING PROCESS

Apply the nursing process and use a critical thinking approach in your care of patients. The nursing process provides a clinical decision-making approach for you to develop and implement an individualized plan of care. It guides care for patients who need special assistance with communication. Use therapeutic communication techniques as an intervention in any interpersonal nursing situations.

◆ Assessment

During the assessment process thoroughly assess each patient and critically analyze findings to ensure that you make patient-centered clinical decisions required for safe nursing care.

Through the Patient's Eyes. Patient-centered care requires careful assessment of a patient's values; preferences; and cultural, ethnic, and social backgrounds (Harvey and Ahmann, 2014). During assessment a nurse also explores any personal biases and experiences that might affect his or her ability to form a therapeutic relationship. If the nurse cannot resolve his or her bias related to a patient, care should be transferred to another individual. Internal and external factors also affect a patient's ability to communicate (Box 24.6). Assessing these factors keeps your focus on a patient and helps you make patient-centered decisions during the communication process. Seek to understand the patient's viewpoint as you provide patient-centered care.

Physical and Emotional Factors. It is especially important to assess the psychophysiological factors that influence communication. Many altered health states and human responses limit communication. People with hearing or visual impairments often have difficulty receiving messages (see Chapter 49). Facial trauma, laryngeal cancer, or endotracheal intubation often prevents movement of air past vocal cords or mobility of the tongue, resulting in inability to articulate words. An extremely breathless person needs to use oxygen to breathe rather than speak. People with aphasia after a stroke or in late-stage Alzheimer's disease cannot understand or form words. Some mental illnesses such as psychoses or depression cause patients to jump from one topic to another, constantly verbalizing the same words or phrases or exhibiting a slowed speech pattern. People with high anxiety are sometimes unable to perceive environmental stimuli or hear explanations. Finally patients who are unresponsive or heavily sedated cannot send or respond to verbal messages.

Review of a patient's medical record provides relevant information about his or her ability to communicate. The medical history and physical examination document physical barriers to speech, neurological deficits, and pathophysiology affecting hearing or vision. Reviewing a patient's medication record is also important. For example, opiates, antidepressants, neuroleptics, hypnotics, or sedatives may cause a patient to slur words or use incomplete sentences. The nursing progress notes in the electronic health record (EHR) sometimes reveal other factors that contribute to communication difficulties, such as the absence of family members to provide more information about a patient who is confused.

Communicate directly with patients during assessment to determine their ability to attend to, interpret, and respond to stimuli. If

---

BOX 24.6 Assessment: Factors Influencing Communication

Psychophysiological Context (Internal Factors Affecting Communication)
- Physiological status (e.g., pain, hunger, nausea, weakness, dyspnea)
- Emotional status (e.g., anxiety, anger, hopelessness, euphoria)
- Growth and development status (e.g., age, developmental tasks)
- Unmet needs (e.g., safety/security, love/belonging)
- Attitudes, values, and beliefs (e.g., meaning of illness experience)
- Perceptions and personality (e.g., optimist/pessimist, introvert/extrovert)
- Self-concept and self-esteem (e.g., positive or negative)

Relational Context (Nature of the Relationship Among Participants)
- Social, helping, or working relationship
- Level of trust among participants
- Level of caring expressed
- Level of self-disclosure among participants
- Shared history of participants
- Balance of power and control

Situational Context (Reason for Communication)
- Information exchange
- Goal achievement
- Problem resolution
- Expression of feelings

Environmental Context (Physical Surroundings in Which Communication Occurs)
- Privacy level
- Noise level
- Comfort and safety level
- Distraction level

Cultural Context (Sociocultural Elements That Affect an Interaction)
- Educational level of participants
- Language and self-expression patterns
- Customs and expectations

---

patients have difficulty communicating, assess the effect of the problem. Patients who are unable to speak are at risk for injury unless nurses identify an alternate communication method. If barriers exist that make it difficult to communicate directly with patients, family or friends become important sources concerning the patients' communication patterns and abilities.

Developmental Factors. Aspects of a patient's growth and development also influence nurse-patient interaction. For example, an infant's self-expression is limited to crying, body movement, and facial expression, whereas older children express their needs more directly. Adapt communication techniques to the special needs of infants and children and their parents. Depending on a child's age, include the parents, child, or both as sources of information about the child's health. Giving a young child toys or other distractions allows parents to give you their full attention. Children are especially responsive to nonverbal messages. Sudden movements, loud noises, or threatening gestures are frightening. Children often prefer to make the first move in interpersonal contacts and do not like adults who stare or look down at them. A child who has received little environmental stimulation possibly is behind in language development, thus making communication more challenging.

BOX 24.7 FOCUS ON OLDER ADULTS

Tips for Improved Communication With Older Adults Who Have Hearing Loss

- Make sure the patient knows that you are talking.
- Face the patient, be sure that your face/mouth is visible to him or her, and do not chew gum or talk while chewing.
- Speak clearly but do not exaggerate lip movement or shout.
- Speak a little more slowly but not excessively slow.
- Check whether patient uses hearing aids, glasses, or other adaptive equipment.
- Choose a quiet, well-lit environment with minimal distractions.
- Allow time for the patient to respond. Do not assume that patient is being uncooperative if he or she does not reply or takes a long time to reply.
- Give the patient a chance to ask questions.
- Keep communication short and to the point. Ask one question at a time.

Data from Arnold E, Boggs KU: *Interpersonal relationships: professional communication skills for nurses,* ed 7, St Louis, 2016, Saunders; and Blevins S: Nurses as educators: teaching patients with hearing loss, *Medsurg Nurs* 24(2):128-129, 2015.

Age alone does not determine an adult's capacity for communication. Hearing loss and visual impairments are changes that may occur during aging that contribute to communication barriers (Dowd, 2015). Communicate with older adults on an adult level and avoid patronizing or speaking in a condescending manner. Simple measures facilitate communication with older individuals who have hearing loss (Box 24.7).

Sociocultural Factors. Culture influences thinking, feeling, behaving, and communicating. Be aware of the typical patterns of interaction that characterize various ethnic groups, but do not allow this information to bias your response. Know each patient individually (e.g., does he or she feel comfortable with eye contact or in sharing information with others?). You will approach a patient very differently if he or she is open and willing to discuss private family matters versus others who are reluctant to reveal personal or family information to strangers.

People from other countries do not always speak or understand English. Those who speak English as a second language often have trouble with self-expression or language comprehension. To practice cultural sensitivity in communication, understand that people of different ethnic origins use different degrees of eye contact, personal space, gestures, loud voice, pace of speech, touch, silence, and meaning of language. Make a conscious effort not to interpret messages through your cultural perspective, but consider the communication within the context of the other individual's background. Avoid stereotyping, patronizing, and making fun of other cultures. Language and cultural barriers are not only frustrating but also dangerous, causing delay in care (Box 24.8).

Gender. Gender influences how we think, act, feel, and communicate. Men tend to use less verbal communication but are more likely to initiate communication and address issues more directly. They are also more likely to talk about issues. Women tend to disclose more personal information and use more active listening, answering with responses that encourage the other person to continue the conversation. It is important for you to recognize a patient's gender communication pattern. Being insensitive blocks therapeutic nurse-patient relationships. Assess communication patterns of each individual and do not make assumptions based simply on gender, race, sexuality, or cultural differences.

REFLECT NOW

As you think back on a recent experience interacting with a patient or family member, describe the unique personal factors that you observed. How should you tailor your own communication to create an effective interaction?

BOX 24.8 CULTURAL ASPECTS OF CARE

Cultural Diversity and Communication

- Differences in language comprehension may impede understanding and negatively impact the quality and safety of nursing care.
- Even among native speakers, variability in word usage, vocabulary, and literacy may skew patient and nurse understanding.
- Differences in nonverbal communication styles may create misunderstanding or discomfort, including practices regarding personal space, privacy, eye contact, and touch.
- Among people of different cultures decision-making authority for patient care decisions may vary.
- Variability in religious and spiritual beliefs affects how individuals perceive the health care experience.
- Incorporating the patient's beliefs and practices into the health care situation contributes to a patient-centered care experience.

Implications for Patient-Centered Care
- Understand your own cultural values and biases.
- Assess the patient's primary language and level of fluency in English.
- Speak directly to the patient even if an interpreter is present.
- Nodding or statements such as "OK" do not necessarily mean that the patient understands.
- Provide written information in English and primary language.
- Learn about other cultures, especially those commonly encountered in your work area.
- Incorporate the patient's communication methods or need into plan of care.

Communication with Non–English-Speaking Patients
Patients who speak little or no English present challenges for nurse-patient communication. Federal and state laws require that hospitals that receive federal funding, including Medicare, Medicaid, and SCHIP, are required to provide language access services for their patients. For hospitals unable to provide on-site interpreters, telephone interpretation services must be available (Marcus, 2014). Use of family members, friends, or bilingual staff members to interpret for patients is strongly discouraged. Sometimes communication with patients is needed in sudden crucial interactions. Use family members or friends cautiously when there is a delay in acquiring interpretive services. Use of family members, children, or auxiliary personnel poses legal liabilities. Language is not the only barrier. Cultural differences also lead to misunderstanding and have been identified as an important factor impacting patient satisfaction (Sethi and Rani, 2017).

◆ Nursing Diagnosis

Most individuals experience difficulty with some aspect of communication. Patients sometimes lack skills in attending, listening, responding, and self-expression as a result of illness, treatment effects, or cultural or language barriers. The primary nursing diagnostic label used to describe a patient with limited or no ability to communicate verbally is *Impaired Verbal Communication.* This occurs when an individual experiences difficulty receiving, processing, transmitting, and using symbols for a variety of reasons. Use this diagnosis if your patient is unable to articulate words or experiences inappropriate verbalization, difficulty in forming words, and difficulty in comprehending (ICNP, 2017). This diagnosis is useful for a wide variety of patients with special problems and needs related to communication, such as impaired perception, reception, and articulation. Although a patient's primary problem is *Impaired Verbal Communication,* the associated difficulty in self-expression or altered communication patterns may also contribute to other nursing diagnoses such as:

- *Communication Barrier*
- *Difficulty Coping*
- *Powerlessness*
- *Impaired Socialization*

Assessment findings in a patient with *Impaired Verbal Communication* focus on the causes of a communication disorder, which often include physiological, mechanical, anatomical, psychological, cultural, or developmental factors. Accuracy in identifying assessment findings is necessary so that you select interventions that effectively resolve the diagnostic problem. For example, you manage the diagnosis of *Impaired Verbal Communication related to cultural difference (Hispanic heritage)* very differently from the diagnosis of *Impaired Verbal Communication related to hearing loss.*

◆ Planning

Once you have identified the nature of a patient's communication issues, consider several factors when designing the care plan. Motivation is a factor in improving communication, and patients often require encouragement to try different approaches that involve significant change. It is especially important to involve the patient and family in decisions about the plan of care to determine whether suggested methods are acceptable. Consider ways to meet basic comfort and safety needs before introducing new communication methods and techniques. Allow adequate time for practice. Participants need to be patient with themselves and one another to achieve effective communication. When the focus is on practicing communication, arrange for a quiet, private place that is free of distractions such as television or visitors.

Goals and Outcomes. Once you identify a diagnosis, select a goal that is relevant and achievable for the patient, such as being able to express needs or achieving understanding of physical condition. Next select expected outcomes that are very specific and measurable. Outcomes identify ways to determine whether a broader goal is met. For example, outcomes for a patient possibly include the following:

- Patient initiates conversation about diagnosis or health care problem.
- Patient is able to attend to appropriate stimuli.
- Patient conveys clear and understandable messages with health care team.
- Patient expresses increased satisfaction with the communication process.

At times you care for patients whose difficulty in sending, receiving, and interpreting messages interferes with healthy interpersonal relationships. In this case impaired communication is a contributing factor to other nursing diagnoses such as *Impaired Socialization* or *Difficulty Coping.* Plan interventions to help these patients improve their communication skills. Expected outcomes for a patient in this situation possibly include demonstrating the ability to appropriately express needs, feelings, and concerns; communicating thoughts and feelings more clearly; engaging in appropriate social conversation with peers and staff; and increasing feelings of autonomy and assertiveness.

Setting Priorities. It is essential to always maintain an open line of communication so that a patient can express emergent needs or problems. This sometimes involves an intervention as simple as keeping the nurse call system in reach for a patient restricted to bed or providing communication augmentative devices (e.g., message board or Braille computer). When you plan to have lengthy interactions with a patient, it is important to address physical care priorities first so that the discussion is not interrupted. Make the patient comfortable by ensuring that any symptoms are under control and elimination needs have been met.

Teamwork and Collaboration. To ensure an effective plan of care, you sometimes need to collaborate with other health care team members who have expertise in communication strategies. Speech language pathologists help patients with aphasia, professional interpreters are necessary for patients who speak a foreign language, and mental health nurse specialists help angry or highly anxious patients to communicate more effectively.

◆ Implementation

In carrying out any plan of care, use communication techniques that are appropriate for a patient's individual needs. Before learning how to adapt communication methods to help patients with serious communication impairments, it is necessary to learn the communication techniques that serve as the foundation for professional communication. It is also important to understand communication techniques that create barriers to effective interaction.

Therapeutic Communication Techniques. Therapeutic communication techniques are specific responses that encourage the expression of feelings and ideas and convey acceptance and respect. These techniques apply in a variety of different situations. Although some of the techniques seem artificial at first, skill and comfort increase with practice. Tremendous satisfaction results from developing therapeutic relationships that achieve desired patient outcomes.

Active Listening. Active listening means being attentive to what a patient is saying both verbally and nonverbally. It facilitates patient communication. Inexperienced nurses sometimes feel the need to talk to prove that they know what they are doing or to decrease anxiety (Varcarolis, 2017). It is often difficult at first to be quiet and really listen. Active listening enhances trust because you communicate acceptance and respect for a patient. The SURETY Model is one model you can use to facilitate attentive listening and therapeutic communication with your patients (Stickley, 2011).

- **S**—Sit at an angle facing the patient. Sitting at a slight angle to the patient creates a nonconfrontational seating arrangement that is conducive to communication. This posture conveys the message that you are there to listen and are interested in what the patient is saying.
- **U**—Uncross legs and arms. This position suggests that you are "open" to what the patient says. A "closed" position such as crossing arms conveys a defensive attitude, possibly provoking a similar response in the patient.
- **R**—Relax. It is important to communicate a sense of being relaxed and comfortable with the patient. Restlessness communicates a lack of interest and a feeling of discomfort to the patient.
- **E**—Eye contact—Establish and maintain intermittent eye contact to convey your involvement in and willingness to listen to what the patient is saying (Fig. 24.2). Absence of eye contact or shifting the eyes gives the message that you are not interested in what the patient is saying.

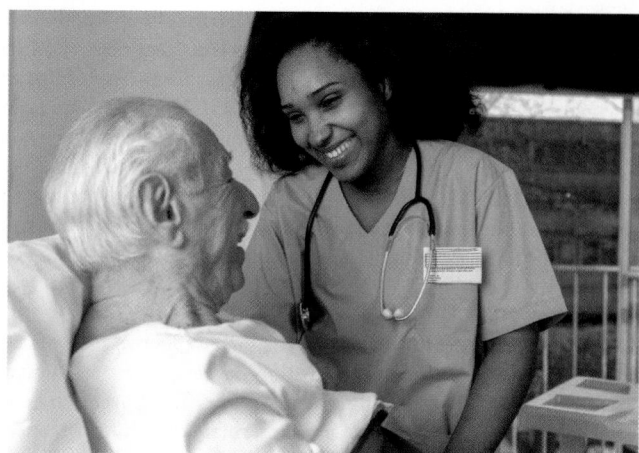

FIG. 24.2 Maintain eye contact when communicating with patients. (Copyright © iStock).

- **T**—*Touch.* Use touch that is respectful to communicate empathy and understanding to the patient. Ensure that your use of touch is therapeutic and acceptable to the patient.
- **Y**—*Your intuition.* Trust your intuition as you grow in confidence to individualize, adapt, and apply communication techniques in your interpersonal encounters with your patients.

Sharing Observations. Nurses make observations by commenting on how the other person looks, sounds, or acts. Stating observations often helps a patient communicate without the need for extensive questioning, focusing, or clarification. This technique can help start a conversation with a patient who is quiet or withdrawn. Do not state observations that will embarrass or anger a patient, such as telling someone, "You look a mess!" Even if you make such an observation with humor, the patient can become resentful.

Sharing observations differs from making assumptions, which means drawing unnecessary conclusions about the other person without validating them. Making assumptions puts a patient in the position of having to contradict you. Examples include interpreting a patient's fatigue as depression or assuming that untouched food indicates lack of interest in meeting nutritional goals. Making observations is a gentler and safer technique: "You look tired …," "You seem different today …," or "I see you haven't eaten anything."

Sharing Empathy. Empathy is the ability to understand and accept another person's reality, accurately perceive feelings, and communicate this understanding to the other. This is a therapeutic communication technique that enables you to understand a patient's situation, feelings, and concerns (Lorié, 2017). To express empathy, you reflect that you understand and feel the importance of the other person's communication. Empathetic understanding requires you to be sensitive and imaginative, especially if you have not had similar experiences. Strive to be empathetic in every situation because it is a key to unlocking concern and communicating support for others. Statements reflecting empathy are highly effective because they tell a person that you heard both the emotional and the factual content of the communication. Empathetic statements are neutral and nonjudgmental and help establish trust in difficult situations. For example, a nurse says to an angry patient who has low mobility after a stroke, "It must be very frustrating to not be able to do what you want."

Sharing Hope. Nurses recognize that hope is essential for healing and learn to communicate a "sense of possibility" to others. Appropriate encouragement and positive feedback are important in fostering hope and self-confidence and for helping people achieve their potential and reach their goals. You give hope by commenting on the positive aspects of the other person's behavior, performance, or response. Sharing a vision of the future and reminding others of their resources and strengths also strengthen hope. Reassure patients that there are many kinds of hope and that meaning and personal growth can come from illness experiences. For example, a nurse says to a patient discouraged about a poor prognosis, "I believe that you'll find a way to face your situation because I've seen your courage and creativity."

Sharing Humor. Humor is an important but often underused resource in nursing interactions. It is a coping strategy that can reduce anxiety and promote positive feelings (Haydon et al., 2015). It is a perception and attitude in which a person can experience joy even when facing difficult times. It provides emotional support to patients and professional colleagues and humanizes the illness experience. It enhances teamwork and relieves tension. Bonds develop between people who laugh together (Mills et al., 2019). Patients use humor to release tension, cope with fear related to pain and suffering, communicate a fear or need, or cope with an uncomfortable or embarrassing situation. The goals of using humor as a health care provider are to bring hope and joy to a situation and enhance a patient's well-being and the therapeutic relationship. It makes you seem warmer and more approachable (Haydon et al., 2015). Use humor during the orientation phase to establish a therapeutic relationship and during the working phase as you help a patient cope with a situation.

You will care for patients from different cultural backgrounds. Humor often has a cultural context. When you interact with patients, be sensitive and realize that they may misunderstand or misinterpret jokes and statements meant to be humorous. It is never appropriate, with any patient, to joke about sexual orientation, race, economic status, disability, or any cultural attribute.

Health care professionals sometimes use a kind of dark, negative humor after difficult or traumatic situations to deal with unbearable tension and stress. This coping humor has a high potential for misinterpretation as uncaring by people not involved in the situation. For example, nursing students are sometimes offended and wonder how staff are able to laugh and joke after unsuccessful resuscitation efforts. When nurses use coping humor within earshot of patients or their loved ones, great emotional distress results.

Sharing Feelings. Emotions are subjective feelings that result from one's thoughts and perceptions. Feelings are not right, wrong, good, or bad, although they are pleasant or unpleasant. If individuals do not express feelings, stress and illness may worsen. Help patients express emotions by making observations, acknowledging feelings, encouraging communication, giving permission to express "negative" feelings, and modeling healthy emotional self-expression. At times patients will direct their anger or frustration prompted by their illness toward you. Do not take such expressions personally. Acknowledging patients' feelings communicates that you listened to and understood the emotional aspects of their illness situation.

When you care for patients, be aware of your own emotions because feelings are difficult to hide. Students sometimes wonder whether it is helpful to share feelings with patients. Sharing emotion makes nurses seem more human and brings people closer. It is appropriate to share feelings of caring or even to cry with others if you are in control of the expression of these feelings and express them in a way that does not burden the patient or break confidentiality. Patients are perceptive and sense your emotions. It is usually inappropriate to discuss negative personal emotions such as anger or sadness with patients. A social support system of colleagues is helpful. Employee assistance programs, peer group meetings, and the use of interprofessional teams, such as social work and pastoral care, provide other means for nurses to safely express feelings away from patients.

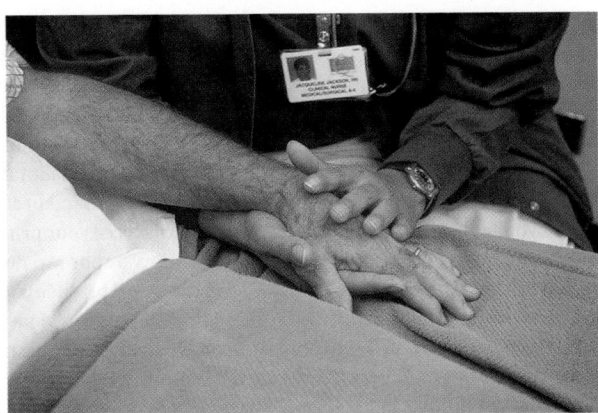

FIG. 24.3 The nurse uses touch to communicate.

Using Touch. Because of modern fast-paced technical environments in health care, nurses face major challenges in bringing the sense of caring and human connection to their patients (see Chapter 7). Touch is one of the most potent and personal forms of communication. It expresses concern or caring to establish a feeling of connection and promote healing (Varcarolis, 2017). Touch conveys many messages, such as affection, emotional support, encouragement, tenderness, and personal attention. Comfort touch such as holding a hand is especially important for vulnerable patients who are experiencing severe illness with its accompanying physical and emotional losses (Fig. 24.3).

Some students initially find giving intimate care to be stressful, especially when caring for patients of the opposite gender. They learn to cope with intimate contact by changing their perception of the situation. Since much of what nurses do involves touching, you need to learn to be sensitive to others' reactions to touch and use it wisely. It should be as gentle or as firm as needed and delivered in a comforting, non-threatening manner. Sometimes you withhold touch for highly suspicious or angry persons who respond negatively or even violently to you.

Nurses need to be aware of patients' nonverbal cues and ask permission before touching them to ensure that touch is an acceptable way to provide comfort. Some individuals may be sensitive to physical closeness and uncomfortable with touch. When this occurs, share the information with other nurses who will care for the patient. Nurses should be aware of a patient's concern and act accordingly. A nod, gesture, body position, or eye contact can also convey interest and acceptance of touch, which promotes a bonding moment with a patient (Varcarolis, 2017).

Using Silence. It takes time and experience to become comfortable with silence. Most people have a natural tendency to fill empty spaces with words, but sometimes these spaces really allow time for a nurse and patient to observe one another, sort out feelings, think about how to say things, and consider what has been communicated. Silence prompts some people to talk. It allows a patient to think and gain insight (Varcarolis, 2017). In general, allow a patient to break the silence, particularly when he or she has initiated it.

Silence is particularly useful when people are confronted with decisions that require much thought. For example, it helps a patient gain the necessary confidence to share the decision to refuse medical treatment. It also allows the nurse to pay attention to nonverbal messages, such as worried expressions or loss of eye contact. Remaining silent demonstrates patience and a willingness to wait for a response when the other person is unable to reply quickly. Silence is especially therapeutic during times of profound sadness or grief.

Providing Information. Providing relevant information tells other people what they need or want to know so that they are able to make decisions, experience less anxiety, and feel safe and secure. It is also an integral aspect of health teaching (see Chapter 25). It usually is not helpful to hide information from patients, particularly when they seek it. If a health care provider withholds information, the nurse clarifies the reason with him or her. Patients have a right to know about their health status and what is happening in their environment. Information of a distressing nature needs to be communicated with sensitivity, at a pace appropriate to a patient's ability to absorb it, and in general terms at first: "John, your heart sounds have changed from earlier today, and so has your blood pressure. I'll let your doctor know." A nurse provides information that enables others to understand what is happening and what to expect: "Mrs. Evans, John is getting an echocardiogram right now. This test uses painless sound waves to create a moving picture of his heart structures and valves and should tell us what's causing his murmur."

Clarifying. To check whether you understand a message accurately, restate an unclear or ambiguous message to clarify the sender's meaning. In addition, ask the other person to rephrase it, explain further, or give an example of what the person means. Without clarification you may make invalid assumptions and miss valuable information. Despite efforts at paraphrasing, you still may not understand a patient's message. Let the patient know if this is the case: "I'm not sure I understand what you mean by 'sicker than usual.' What is different now?"

Focusing. Focusing involves centering a conversation on key elements or concepts of a message. If conversation is vague or rambling or patients begin to repeat themselves, focusing is a useful technique. Do not use focusing if it interrupts patients while they are discussing important issues. Rather use it to guide the direction of conversation to important areas: "We've talked a lot about your medications; now let's look more closely at the trouble you're having in taking them on time."

Paraphrasing. Paraphrasing is restating another's message more briefly using one's own words. Through paraphrasing you send feedback that lets a patient know that he or she is actively involved in the search for understanding. Accurate paraphrasing requires practice. If the meaning of a message is changed or distorted through paraphrasing, communication becomes ineffective. For example, a patient says, "I've been overweight all my life and never had any problems. I can't understand why I need to be on a diet." Paraphrasing this statement by saying "You don't care if you're overweight" is incorrect. It is more accurate to say, "You're not convinced that you need to make different food choices because you've stayed healthy."

Validation. This is a technique that nurses use to recognize and acknowledge a patient's thoughts, feelings, and needs. Patients and families know they are being heard and taken seriously when the caregiver addresses their issues (Harvey and Ahmann, 2014). For example, a nurse validates a patient's comments by asking, "Tell me if I understand your concerns regarding your surgery. You're worried that you will not be able to do some of the things you can do before your surgery." This type of statement enables a nurse to convey empathy and interest in the patient's thoughts, feelings, and perceptions.

Asking Relevant Questions. Ask relevant questions to seek information needed for decision making. Ask only one question at a time, and fully explore one topic before moving to another area. During patient assessment you ask questions that follow a logical sequence and usually proceed from general to more specific. Open-ended questions allow patients to take the conversational lead and introduce pertinent information about a topic. For example, "What's your biggest problem at the moment?" Use focused questions when more specific information is needed in an area: "How has your pain affected your life at home?" Allow patients to respond fully to open-ended questions before asking more focused questions. Closed-ended questions elicit a yes, no, or one-word response: "How many times a day are you taking pain medication?" Although they are helpful during assessment, they are generally less useful during therapeutic exchanges.

Sometimes asking too many questions is dehumanizing. Seeking factual information does not allow a nurse or patient to establish a meaningful relationship or deal with important emotional issues. It is a way for a nurse to ignore uncomfortable areas in favor of more comfortable, neutral topics. A useful exercise is to try to converse without asking the other person a single question. By using techniques such as giving general leads ("Tell me about it …"), making observations, paraphrasing, focusing, and providing information, you discover important information that would have remained hidden if you had limited the communication process to questions alone.

Summarizing. Summarizing is a concise review of key aspects of an interaction. It brings a sense of satisfaction and closure to an individual conversation and is especially helpful during the termination phase of a nurse-patient relationship. By reviewing a conversation, participants focus on key issues and add relevant information as needed. Beginning a new interaction by summarizing a previous one helps patients recall topics discussed and shows that you analyzed their communication. Summarizing also clarifies expectations, as in this example of a nurse manager who has been working with an unsatisfied employee: "You've told me a lot of things about why you don't like this job and how unhappy you've been. We've also come up with some possible ways to make things better, and you've agreed to try some of them and let me know if any help."

Self-Disclosure. Self-disclosures are subjectively true personal experiences about the self that are intentionally revealed to another person. This is not therapy for a nurse; rather it shows a patient that the nurse understands his experiences and that they are not unique. You choose to share experiences or feelings that are like those of the patient and emphasize both the similarities and differences. This kind of self-disclosure is indicative of the closeness of the nurse-patient relationship and indicates respect for the patient. You offer self-disclosure as an expression of sincerity and honesty; it is an aspect of empathy (Lorié, 2017). Self-disclosures need to be relevant and appropriate and made to benefit the patient rather than yourself. Use them sparingly so that the patient is the focus of the interaction.

Confrontation. When you confront someone in a therapeutic way, you help the other person become more aware of inconsistencies in his or her feelings, attitudes, beliefs, and behaviors (Varcarolis, 2017). This technique improves patient self-awareness and helps him or her recognize growth and deal with important issues. Use confrontation only after you have established trust, and do it gently with sensitivity: "You say you've already decided what to do; yet you're still talking a lot about your options."

Nontherapeutic Communication Techniques.
Certain communication techniques hinder or damage professional relationships. These specific techniques are referred to as *nontherapeutic* or *blocking* and often cause others to activate defenses to avoid being hurt or negatively affected. Nontherapeutic techniques discourage further expression of feelings and ideas and engender negative responses or behaviors in others.

Asking Personal Questions. "Why don't you and John get married?" Asking personal questions that are not relevant to a situation simply to satisfy your curiosity is inappropriate professional communication. Such questions are nosy, invasive, and unnecessary. If patients wish to share private information, they will. To learn more about a patient's interpersonal roles and relationships, ask questions such as: "How would you describe your relationship with John?"

Giving Personal Opinions. "If I were you, I'd put your mother in a nursing home." When a nurse gives a personal opinion, it takes decision making away from the other person. It inhibits spontaneity, stalls problem solving, and creates doubt. Personal opinions differ from professional

advice. At times people need suggestions and help to make choices. Suggestions that you present are options; the other person makes the final decision. Remember that the problem and its solution belong to the other person and not to you. A much better response is: "Let's talk about which options are available for your mother's care." The nurse also should not make promises to a patient about situations that require collaboration. For example, "I can't recommend that you stop taking the medications because of your side effects, but I would be happy to inform your primary care provider and ask whether a change in medication is appropriate."

Changing the Subject. "Let's not talk about your problems with the insurance company. It's time for your walk." Changing the subject when another person is trying to communicate his or her story is rude and shows a lack of empathy. It blocks further communication, and the sender then withholds important messages or fails to openly express feelings. In some instances, changing the subject serves as a face-saving maneuver. If this happens, reassure the patient that you will return to his or her concerns: "After your walk let's talk some more about what's going on with your insurance company."

Automatic Responses. "Older adults are always confused." "Administration doesn't care about the staff." Stereotypes are generalized beliefs held about people. Making stereotyped remarks about others reflects poor nursing judgment and threatens nurse-patient or team relationships. A cliché is a stereotyped comment such as "You can't win them all" that tends to belittle the other person's feelings and minimize the importance of his or her message. These automatic phrases communicate that you are not taking concerns seriously or responding thoughtfully. Another kind of automatic response is parroting (i.e., repeating what the other person has said word for word). Parroting is easily overused and is not as effective as paraphrasing. A simple "oh?" gives you time to think if the other person says something that takes you by surprise.

A nurse who is task oriented automatically makes the task or procedure the entire focus of interaction with patients, missing opportunities to communicate with them as individuals and meet their needs. Task-oriented nurses are often perceived as cold, uncaring, and unapproachable. When students first perform technical skills, it is difficult to integrate therapeutic communication because of the need to focus on the procedure. In time you learn to integrate communication with high-visibility tasks and accomplish several goals simultaneously.

False Reassurance. "Don't worry; everything will be all right." When a patient is seriously ill or distressed, you may be tempted to offer hope to him or her with statements such as "You'll be fine" or "There's nothing to worry about." When a patient is reaching for understanding, false reassurance discourages open communication. Offering reassurance not supported by facts does more harm than good. Although you are trying to be kind, it has the secondary effect of helping you avoid the other person's distress, and it tends to block conversation and discourage further expression of feelings. To use a more facilitative response you can say, "It must be difficult not to know what the surgeon will find. What can I do to help?"

Sympathy. "I'm so sorry about your mastectomy; you probably feel devastated." Sympathy is concern, sorrow, or pity felt for another person. A nurse often takes on a patient's problems as if they were his or her own. Sympathy is a subjective look at another person's world that prevents a clear perspective of the issues confronting that person. If a nurse overidentifies with a patient, objectivity is lost, and the nurse is unable to help the patient work through the situation (Varcarolis, 2017). Although sympathy is a compassionate response to another's situation, it is not as therapeutic as empathy. A nurse's own emotional issues sometimes prevent effective problem solving and impair good judgment. A more empathetic approach is: "The loss of a breast is a major change. Do you feel comfortable talking about how it will affect your life?"

Asking for Explanations. "Why are you so anxious?" Some nurses are tempted to ask patients why they believe, feel, or act in a certain way. Patients frequently interpret "why" questions as accusations or think nurses know the reasons and are simply testing them. Regardless of a patient's perception of your motivation, asking "why" questions causes resentment, insecurity, and mistrust. If you need additional information, it is best to phrase a question to avoid using the word "why." For example, "You seem upset. What's on your mind?" is more likely to help an anxious patient communicate.

Approval or Disapproval. "You shouldn't even think about assisted suicide; it's not right." Do not impose your own attitudes, values, beliefs, and moral standards on others while in the professional helping role. Other people have the right to be themselves and make their own decisions. Judgmental responses often contain terms such as *should, ought, good, bad, right,* or *wrong.* Agreeing or disagreeing sends the subtle message that you have the right to make value judgments about patient decisions. Approving implies that the behavior being praised is the only acceptable one. Often a patient shares a decision with you not to seek approval but to provide a means to discuss feelings. Disapproval implies that the patient needs to meet your expectations or standards. Instead help patients explore their own beliefs and decisions. For example, the response of "I'm surprised you're considering assisted suicide; tell me more about it" gives the patient a chance to express ideas or feelings without fear of being judged.

Defensive Responses. "No one here would intentionally lie to you." Becoming defensive in the face of criticism implies that the other person has no right to an opinion. The sender's concerns are ignored when the nurse focuses on the need for self-defense, defense of the health care team, or defense of others. When patients express criticism, listen to what they have to say. Listening does not imply agreement. Listen nonjudgmentally to discover reasons for a patient's anger or dissatisfaction. By avoiding a defensive attitude, you are able to defuse anger and uncover deeper concerns. A better response would be: "You believe that people are dishonest with you. It must be hard to trust anyone."

Passive or Aggressive Responses. "Things are bad, and there's nothing I can do about it." "Things are falling apart, and it's all your fault." Passive responses serve to avoid conflict or sidestep issues. They reflect feelings of sadness, depression, anxiety, powerlessness, and hopelessness. Aggressive responses provoke confrontation at the other person's expense. They reflect feelings of anger, frustration, resentment, and stress. Nurses who lack assertive skills also use triangulation (i.e., complaining to a third party rather than confronting the problem or expressing concerns directly to the source). This lowers team morale and draws others into the conflict situation. Assertive communication is a far more professional approach for a nurse to take.

Arguing. "How can you say you didn't sleep a wink when I heard you snoring all night long?" Challenging or arguing against perceptions denies that they are real and valid. A skillful nurse gives information or presents reality in a way that avoids argument, with a statement such as "You feel as if you didn't get any rest at all last night, even though I thought you slept well since I heard you snoring."

REFLECT NOW

Learning to avoid nontherapeutic communication techniques is difficult, as they are often a part of everyday conversation. As you reflect on a recent conversation with a patient, which nontherapeutic communication techniques did you catch yourself using? What therapeutic response could you have used?

Adapting Communication Techniques for the Patient with Special Needs. As the population ages, more patients have difficulty in communicating. Hearing loss increases with age. Approximately 16% of the US population has hearing loss (CDC, 2018). Vision loss affects communication and presents a challenge for many individuals, particularly over the age of 65. Vision loss is among the top 10 disabilities in the United States and impacts activities of daily living, sometimes leading to depression and isolation (Kirtland et al., 2015).

Interacting with people who have conditions that impair communication requires special thought and sensitivity. For example, patients who have had a stroke or laryngectomy may require communication aids such as a writing or picture board or a special call system. Such patients benefit greatly when you adapt communication techniques to their unique circumstances, developmental level, or cognitive and sensory deficits. A nurse caring for a patient with *Impaired Verbal Communication related to cognitive impairment* can use several techniques such as pictures or demonstration to enable the patient to understand the caregiver. The nurse interacts with the patient and family caregiver, aiming to facilitate as much clarity of understanding as possible without causing undue frustration related to conveying a message that is too complex (Dooley et al., 2015).

A nurse directs actions toward meeting the goals and expected outcomes identified in the plan of care, addressing both the communication impairment and its contributing factors. Box 24.9 lists methods available to encourage, enhance, restore, or substitute for verbal communication. Be sure that a patient is physically able to use the chosen method and that it does not cause frustration by being too complicated or difficult. Patients and families who do not speak English need assistance with communication. You use interpretation services to facilitate communication, which improves patient safety and patient outcomes (Weldon et al., 2014).

Because nursing care of the older adult ideally is delivered through an interprofessional model, the primary goal is to establish a reliable communication system that all health care team members can understand easily. Effective communication involves adapting to special needs resulting from sensory, motor, or cognitive impairments. Encouraging older adults to share life stories and reminisce about the past has a therapeutic effect and increases their sense of well-being. Avoid sudden shifts from subject to subject. It is helpful to include a patient's family and friends and to become familiar with a patient's favorite topics for conversation.

◆ Evaluation

Evaluate the effectiveness of your own communication by videotaping practice sessions with peers or by making process recordings—written records of your verbal and nonverbal interactions with patients. Process recording analysis reveals how to improve personal communication techniques to make them more effective. Box 24.10 contains a sample communication analysis of such a record. Analysis of a process recording enables you to evaluate the following:

- Determine whether you encouraged openness and allowed the patient to "tell his story," expressing both thoughts and feelings.
- Identify any missed verbal or nonverbal cues or conversational themes.
- Examine whether nursing responses facilitated or blocked the patient's efforts to communicate.
- Determine whether nursing responses were positive and supportive or superficial and judgmental.
- Examine the type and number of questions asked.
- Determine the type and number of therapeutic communication techniques used.
- Discover any missed opportunities to use humor, silence, or touch.

BOX 24.9 Communicating With Patients Who Have Special Needs

Patients Who Cannot Speak Clearly (Aphasia, Dysarthria, Muteness)

- Listen attentively, be patient, and do not interrupt.
- Ask simple questions that require "yes" or "no" answers.
- Allow time for understanding and response.
- Use visual cues (e.g., words, pictures, and objects) when possible.
- Allow only one person to speak at a time.
- Encourage patient to converse.
- Let patient know if you have not understood him or her.
- Collaborate with speech therapist as needed.
- Use communication aids: letter boards, flash cards, computer-generated speech program).

Patients Who Have a Cognitive Impairment

- Use simple sentences and avoid long explanations.
- Ask one question at a time.
- Allow time for patient to respond.
- Be an attentive listener.
- Include family and friends in conversations, especially in subjects known to patient.
- Use picture or gestures that mimic the action desired.

Patients Who Have a Hearing Impairment

- Check for hearing aids and glasses.
- Reduce environmental noise.
- Get patient's attention before speaking.
- Face patient with mouth visible.
- Do not chew gum.
- Speak at normal volume—do not shout.

- Rephrase rather than repeat if misunderstood.
- Provide a sign-language interpreter if indicated.

Patients Who Are Visually Impaired

- Check for use of glasses or contact lenses.
- Identify yourself when you enter the room, and notify the patient when you leave the room.
- Speak in a normal tone of voice.
- Do not rely on gestures or nonverbal communication.
- Use indirect lighting, avoiding glare.
- Use at least 14-point print.

Patients Who Are Unresponsive

- Call patient by name during interactions.
- Communicate both verbally and by touch.
- Speak to patient as though he or she can hear.
- Explain all procedures and sensations.
- Provide orientation to person, place, and time.
- Avoid talking about patient to others in his or her presence.

Patients Who Do Not Speak English

- Speak to patient in normal tone of voice.
- Establish method for patient to ask for assistance (call light or bell).
- Provide a professional interpreter as needed.
- Avoid using family members, especially children, as interpreters.
- Use communication board, pictures, or cards.
- Translate words from native language into English list for patient to make basic requests.
- Have dictionary (e.g., English/Spanish) available if patient can read.

BOX 24.10 Sample Communication Analysis

Nurse: Good morning, Mr. Simpson."
(Smiles, approaches bed holding clipboard)
Acknowledged by name, social greeting to begin conversation

Patient: "What's good about it?"
(Arms crossed over chest, frowning, direct stare)
Nonverbal signs of anger

Nurse: "You sound unhappy."
(Pulls up chair and sits at bedside)
Sharing observation, nonverbal communication of availability

Patient: "You'd be unhappy, too, if nobody would answer your questions. That girl wouldn't tell me my blood sugar."
(Angry voice tone, challenging expression)
Further expression of feelings facilitated by nurse making accurate observation

Nurse: "This hospital has a fine staff, Mr. Simpson. I'm sure no one would intentionally keep information from you."
Feeling threatened and being defensive, a nontherapeutic technique

Nurse: "I'm going to test your glucose in a minute, and I'll tell you the results." (Does test) "Your blood sugar was 350."

Providing information, demonstrating trustworthiness

Patient: "I'm so afraid complications will set in since my blood sugar is high."
(Stares out window)
Feels free to express deeper concerns, but they are hard to face

Nurse: "What kinds of things are you worried about?"
Open-ended question to seek information

Patient: "I could lose a leg, like my mother did, or go blind or have to live hooked up to a kidney machine for the rest of my life.

Nurse: "You've been thinking about all kinds of things that could go wrong, and it adds to your worry not to be told what your blood sugar is."
Summarizing to let patient "hear" what he has communicated

Patient: "I always think the worst."
(Shakes head in exasperation)
Expressing insight into his "inner dialogue"

Nurse: "I'll pass along to the technician that it's OK to tell you your glucose levels. And later this afternoon I'd like us to talk more about some things you can do to help avoid these complications and set some goals for controlling your glucose."
Providing information, encouraging collaboration, and goal setting

Through the Patient's Eyes. You and your patient determine the success of the plan of care by evaluating patient communication outcomes together. You determine which strategies or interventions were effective and which patient changes (behaviors or perceptions) resulted because of the interventions. Ask the patient whether you and other members of the interprofessional health care team met his or her expectations. For example, does the patient believe that nurses responded in a timely way when the call light was turned on? Does the patient feel able to express his needs clearly? Is the patient satisfied with the information that has been provided about his condition or hospitalization? Successful nursing care related to patients' communication needs results in clear and effective communication between patients and all members of the health care team and can favorably impact patient satisfaction and the delivery of safe care.

Patient Outcomes. If expected outcomes for the patient's plan of care are not met or if progress is unsatisfactory, you determine which factors influenced the outcomes and modify the plan of care. If your evaluation data indicate that a patient perceives difficulty in communicating, you explore contributing factors so that they can be addressed. For example, if using a pen and paper is frustrating for a patient who is nonverbal and whose handwriting is shaky, you revise the care plan to include the use of a picture board instead. Possible questions you ask when a patient does not meet expected outcomes include:

- You seem to be having difficulty communicating right now. What do you think is contributing to this?
- You're telling me that you don't feel anxious right now, but your face appears tense. Help me better understand how you're feeling right now.
- You seem frustrated with the use of pencil and paper to communicate. Would you like to try a letter board or a picture board to see whether either of these is easier for you to use?

Evaluation of the communication process helps nurses gain confidence and competence in interpersonal skills. Becoming an effective communicator greatly increases your professional satisfaction and success. There is no skill more basic, no tool more powerful.

KEY POINTS

- Effective use of critical thinking promotes good communication.
- Nurses use the five levels of communication in their interactions: intrapersonal, interpersonal, small group, public, and electronic.
- The circular transactional communication process demonstrates the ever-changing nature of communication, and includes the sender, the receiver, and referents.
- Verbal communication involves spoken or written words, and the vocabulary, pacing, tone, clarity, and brevity of the message.
- Nonverbal communication occurs through the five senses and includes everything except the written or spoken word.
- Nurse-patient caring relationships are the foundation of the nursing process.
- The four phases of a nurse-patient helping relationship are: preinteraction, orientation, working, and termination.
- Effective nurse–health care team relationships promote safe and effective care and contribute to satisfying professional working relationships.
- Use of both professional and therapeutic communication techniques contributes to achievement of patient outcomes. Practicing these techniques is essential in your development as a nurse.
- Nontherapeutic communication techniques damage professional and caring relationships; therefore pay attention to your own communication to remove these blocking techniques from your responses.
- Adapting your communication with older adults to meet their unique needs ensures an effective nurse-patient relationship.
- Patients with impaired communication benefit from the use of devices that overcome barriers to understanding and communicating.
- Patients with special communication needs such as an inability to speak, cognitive impairment, and hearing or vision loss require the nurse to employ specific techniques to facilitate mutual understanding.

REFLECTIVE LEARNING

- Compare and contrast the similarities and differences in factors that affect communication among two patients that you have cared for recently and describe how you altered your own communication style to create an effective nurse-patient communication.
- Describe a recent nurse-to-nurse handover that you observed or participated in. What were the elements of effective communication you observed? How might this interaction have been improved?
- Describe a recent patient care experience in which the patient demonstrated *Impaired Verbal Communication*. What were the impairments that you observed and how was nursing care adjusted to provide for mutual understanding and respect?

REVIEW QUESTIONS

1. When working with an older adult who is hearing-impaired, the use of which techniques would improve communication? (Select all that apply.)
   1. Check for needed adaptive equipment.
   2. Exaggerate lip movements to help the patient lip-read.
   3. Give the patient time to respond to questions.
   4. Keep communication short and to the point.
   5. Communicate only through written information.
2. Nurses must communicate effectively with the health care team for which of the following reasons? (Select all that apply.)
   1. To improve the nurse's status with the health team members
   2. To reduce the risk of errors to the patient
   3. To provide an optimum level of patient care
   4. To improve patient outcomes
   5. To prevent issues that need to be reported to outside agencies
3. Motivational interviewing (MI) is a technique that applies understanding a patient's values and goals in helping the patient make behavioral changes. When using motivational interviewing, what outcomes does the nurse expect? (Select all that apply.)
   1. Gaining an understanding of the patient's motivations
   2. Directing the patient to avoid poor health choices
   3. Recognizing the patient's strengths and supporting his or her efforts
   4. Providing assessment data that can be shared with families to promote change
   5. Identifying differences in patient's health goals and current behaviors
4. The nurse therapeutically responds to an adult patient who is anxious by: (Select all that apply.)
   1. Matching the rate of speech to be the same as that of the patient
   2. Providing good eye contact
   3. Demonstrating a calm presence
   4. Spending time attentively with the patient
   5. Assuring the patient that all will be well
5. A nurse prepares to contact a patient's physician about a change in the patient's condition. Put the following statements in the correct order using SBAR (Situation, Background, Assessment, and Recommendation) communication.
   1. "She is a 53-year-old female who was admitted 2 days ago with pneumonia and was started on levofloxacin at 5 PM yesterday. She states she has a poor appetite; her weight has remained stable over the past 2 days."
   2. "The patient reported feeling very nauseated after her dose of levofloxacin an hour ago."

3. "Is it possible to make a change in antibiotics, or could we give her a nutritional supplement before her medication?"

4. "The patient started to complain of nausea yesterday evening and has vomited several times during the night."

6. The patient states, "I don't have confidence in my doctor. She looks so young." The nurse therapeutically responds: (Select all that apply.)
   1. Tell me more about your concern.
   2. You have nothing to worry about. Your doctor is perfectly competent.
   3. You are worried about your care?
   4. You can go online and see how others have rated your doctor. I do that.
   5. You should ask your doctor to tell you her background.

7. The nurse applying effective communication skills throughout the nursing process should: (Place the following interventions in the correct order.)
   1. Validate health care needs through verbal discussion with the patient.
   2. Compare actual and expected patient care outcomes with the patient.
   3. Provide support through therapeutic communication techniques.
   4. Complete a nursing history using verbal communication techniques.

8. A nurse works with a patient using therapeutic communication and the phases of the therapeutic relationship. Place the nurse's statements in order according to these phases.
   1. The nurse states, "Let's work on learning injection techniques."
   2. The nurse is mindful of his/her own biases and knowledge in working with the patient with B$_{12}$ deficiency.

3. The nurse summarizes progress made during the nursing relationship.

4. After providing introductions, the nurse defines the scope and purpose of the nurse-patient relationship.

9. Which strategies should a nurse use to facilitate a safe transition of care during a patient's transfer from the hospital to a skilled nursing facility? (Select all that apply.)
   1. Collaboration between staff members from sending and receiving departments
   2. Requiring that the patient visit the facility before a transfer is arranged
   3. Using a standardized transfer policy and transfer tool
   4. Arranging all patient transfers during the same time each day
   5. Relying on family members to share information with the new facility

10. The nurse uses silence as a therapeutic communication technique. What are the purposes of the nurse's silence? (Select all that apply.)
    1. Allows the nurse time to focus and avoid saying the wrong thing
    2. Prompts the patient to talk when he or she is ready
    3. Allows the patient time to think and gain insight
    4. Allows time for the patient to drift off to sleep
    5. Determines whether the patient would prefer to talk with another staff member

Answers: 1. 1, 3, 4; **2.** 2, 3, 4; **3.** 1, 3, 5; **4.** 2, 3, 4; **5.** 4S; 1B, 2A, 3R; **6.** 1, 3; **7.** 4, 1, 3, 2; **8.** 2, 4, 1, 3; **9.** 1, 3; **10.** 2, 3.

Rationales to Review Questions can be found on the Evolve website.

REFERENCES

Arnold E, Boggs KU: *Interpersonal relationships: professional communication skills for nurses*, ed 7, St Louis, 2016, Saunders.

Brandt C, et al.: Determinants of successful eHealth coaching for consumer lifestyle changes: qualitative interview study among health care professionals, *JMIR* 20(7):76–85, 2018.

Bucknall TK, et al.: Engaging patients and families in communication across transitions of care: an integrative review protocol, *J Adv Nurs* 72(7):1689–1700, 2016.

Centers for Disease Control (CDC): CDC estimates U.S. hearing loss prevalence at 16 percent, *ASHA Leader* 23(2):14, 2018.

Copeland L, et al.: Mechanisms of change within motivational interviewing in relation to health behavior outcomes: a systematic review, *Patient Educ Couns* 98(4):401, 2015.

Dooley J, et al.: Communication in healthcare interactions in dementia: a systematic review of observational studies, *Int Psychogeriatr* 27(8):1277–1300, 2015.

Dowd K: When hearing loss goes unnoticed, *ASHA Leader* 20(6):44–49, 2015.

Ford Y, et al.: Patients' perceptions of bedside handoff: the need for a culture of always, *J Nurs Care Qual* 29(4):1, 2014.

Frederick D: Bullying, mentoring and patient care, *AORN J* 99(5):587, 2014.

Gultekin A, et al.: The effect of assertiveness education on communication skills given to nursing students, *Int J Caring Sci* 11(1):395–401, 2018.

Hannawa AF: "SACCIA Safe Communication": five core competencies for safe and high-quality care, *J Patient Saf Risk Manag* 23(3):99–107, 2018.

Harvey P, Ahmann E: Validation: a family-centered communication skill, *Pediatr Nurs* 40(3):143, 2014.

Haydon G, et al.: A narrative inquiry: humour and gender differences in the therapeutic relationship between nurses and their patients, *Contemp Nurse* 50(2/3):214–226, 2015.

Institute for Healthcare Improvement (IHI): *ISBAR trip tick*, 2018, http://www.ihi.org/resources/Pages/Tools/IS-BARTripTick.aspx. Accessed June 29, 2019.

International Council of Nurses (ICNP*): *Nursing diagnosis and outcome statements*, 2017, https://www.icn.ch/sites/default/files/inline-files/icnp2017-dc.pdf. Accessed July 14, 2019.

Isaacson M: Clarifying concepts: cultural humility or competency, *J Prof Nurs* 30(3):251, 2014.

Johnson E: Clinical communication: is patient involvement warranted? *J Nurs Care Qual* 30(2):104–105, 2015.

Kirtland KA, et al.: Geographic disparity of severe vision loss - United States, 2009-2013, *MMWR* 64(19):513–517, 2015.

Lazure P, et al.: Communication – the foundation for collaborative relationships amongst providers, and between providers and patients: a case in breast and colorectal cancer, *J Commun Healthc* 7(1):41, 2014.

Lillykutty MJ, Samson R: Insights from Kristen M Swanson's Theory of Caring, *AJNER* 8(1):173–177, 2018.

Lorié A: Culture and nonverbal expressions of empathy in clinical settings: a systematic review, *Patient Educ Couns* 100(3):411–424, 2017.

Marcus V: Are hospitals required to provide language access services? *NWI Global*, August 2014, http://www.nwiglobal.com/blog/hospitals-required-provide-language-access-services/. Accessed July 14, 2019.

Marquis BL, Huston CJ: *Leadership roles and management functions in nursing: theory and application*, ed 9, Philadelphia, 2017, Lippincott Williams & Wilkins.

Mills CB, et al.: No laughing matter: workplace bullying, humor orientation, and leadership styles, *Workplace Health & Safety* 67(4):159–167, 2019.

Rubin R: *AIDET* in the medical practice: more important than ever*, 2014, https://www.studergroup.com/resources/news-media/healthcare-publications-resources/insights/november-2014/aidet-in-the-medical-practice-more-important-than. Accessed July 14, 2019.

Sethi D, Rani MK: Communication barrier in health care setting as perceived by nurses and patient, *Int J Nurs Educ* 9(4):30–35, 2017, https://doi.org/10.5958/0974-9357.2017.00092.7.

Stickley T: From SOLER to SURETY for effective nonverbal communication, *Nurse Education in Practice* 11:395, 2011.

Stawnychy M, et al.: Using brief motivational interviewing to address the complex needs of a challenging patient with heart failure, *J Cardiovasc Nurs* 29(5):E1, 2014, Lippincott Williams & Williams, 2014.

Stewart KR: SBAR, communication, and patient safety: an integrated literature review, *Medsurg Nurs* 26(5):297–305, 2017.

Varcarolis E: *Essentials of psychiatric mental health nursing*, ed 3, St Louis, 2017, Elsevier.

Weldon JM, et al.: Special needs populations: overcoming language barriers for pediatric surgical patients and their family members, *AORN J* 99(5):616, 2014.

West MM, et al.: Contributing to a quality patient experience: applying evidence based practice to support changes in nursing dress code policies, *Online J Issues Nurs* 21(1), 3–3, 2016.

Zajac LM, et al.: Confronting compassion fatigue: assessment and intervention in inpatient oncology, *Clin J Oncol Nurs* 21(4):446–453, 2017.

RESEARCH REFERENCES

Bains VK, et al.: Bedside shift report: benefits, barriers, and strategies for adopting a patient centered approach to nurse handover, *Can J Crit Care Nurs* 29(2):20–21, 2018.

Gregory S, et al.: Bedside shift reports, *JONA* 44(10):541–545, 2014.

Mardis T, et al.: Bedside shift-to-shift handoffs: a systematic review of the literature, *J Nurs Care Qual* 31(1):54–60, 2016.

Slade D, et al.: Benefits of health care communication training for nurses conducting bedside handovers: an Australian hospital case study, *J Contin Educ Nurs* 49(7):329–336, 2018.

Patient Education

Patient education is one of the most important nursing interventions in any health care setting. Shorter hospital stays, increased demands on nurses' time, an increased number of chronically ill patients, and the need to give acutely ill patients meaningful information quickly emphasize the importance of quality patient education. As nurses try to find the best way to educate patients, the public has become more assertive in seeking knowledge, understanding health, and finding resources available within the health care system. Through education, nurses empower their patients to prevent acute and chronic disease, decrease disability, and improve wellness (Miller & Stoeckel, 2019). Patient education is a key component in terms of enhancing a patient's quality of life, improving self-care, reducing hospital admissions, and improving medication adherence (Flanders, 2018).

Patients have the right to know and be informed about their health risks, diagnoses, prognoses, and available treatments to help them make intelligent, informed decisions about their health and lifestyle. Part of patient-centered care is to integrate educational approaches that acknowledge patients' understanding of their own health. The goals of a well-designed, comprehensive teaching plan include providing a good fit with each patient's unique learning needs, reducing health care costs, improving quality of care, and ultimately changing behaviors to improve patient outcomes. In due course this helps patients make informed decisions about their care and become healthier and more independent (Flanders, 2018).

STANDARDS FOR PATIENT EDUCATION

Patient education has long been a standard for professional nursing practice. All state Nurse Practice Acts recognize that patient teaching falls within the scope of nursing practice (Bastable, 2017). In addition, various accrediting agencies set guidelines for providing patient education in health care institutions. For example, The Joint Commission (TJC, 2018a) sets standards for patient and family education. These standards require nurses and all health care providers to assess patients' learning needs and provide education on a variety of topics, including medications, nutrition, use of medical equipment, pain management, and the patient's plan of care. Implementing the standards successfully requires collaboration among health care professionals and enhances patient safety. Ensure that your educational efforts are patient centered by taking into consideration your patients' literacy level and own education and experience on the topic to be discussed. Do not assume that because your patient is educated that he or she has knowledge regarding this topic. For example, a nurse with 20 years' experience in obstetrics and gynecology may not be up-to-date regarding the latest treatment recommendations for colon cancer. Also consider patients' desire to actively participate in the educational process, as well as their psychosocial, spiritual, and cultural values. It is important to document patient education interventions and a patient's response to teaching in the medical record. These standards help to direct patient education and ensure the best outcomes.

PURPOSES OF PATIENT EDUCATION

The primary goal of patient education is to help individuals, families, or communities achieve optimal levels of health (Miller & Stoeckel, 2019). Patient education through active patient participation and decision making is an essential component of providing safe, patient-centered care (QSEN, 2019). In addition, providing education about preventive health care helps reduce health care costs for individuals. Because most patients now know more about their health, they want to be actively involved in their health maintenance. Comprehensive patient education includes three important purposes, each involving a separate phase of health care: health promotion and illness prevention, health restoration, and coping.

Maintenance and Promotion of Health and Illness Prevention

As a nurse you are a visible, competent resource for patients who want to improve their physical and psychological well-being. In the school, home, clinic, or workplace you provide information and skills to help *patients* adopt healthier behaviors. For example, in childbearing classes you teach expectant parents about physical and psychological changes in a woman. After learning about normal childbearing, the mother who applies new knowledge is more likely to eat healthy foods, engage in physical exercise, and avoid substances that can harm the fetus. Success in patient education is not the ability of a patient to simply recall information that is provided to him or her but is the ability of the patient to incorporate knowledge into everyday life activities in a way that promotes health. Not only can nurses provide knowledge in terms of health maintenance or disease management, but nurses can also help patients come up with a plan to incorporate that knowledge into their own lives.

Restoration of Health

Patients recovering from and adapting to changes resulting from illness or injury often seek information about their conditions and need information and skills to help them regain or maintain their levels of health. However, some patients find it difficult to adapt to illness and become disinterested in learning. As the nurse you learn to identify patients' willingness to learn and motivate interest in learning (Bastable, 2017). The family often is a vital part of a patient's return to health if a patient chooses to involve them. Family caregivers usually require as much education as the patient, including information on how to perform skills within the home. If you exclude a family from a teaching plan, conflicts can occur. However, do not assume that a family should be involved; assess the patient-family relationship before providing education for family caregivers.

Coping With Impaired Functions

Not all patients fully recover from illness or injury. In addition, patients with preexisting mental illness or those who have lower literacy skills have difficulty understanding patient education (Bastable, 2017). Many patients with impaired function have to learn to cope with permanent health alterations. New knowledge and skills are often necessary for patients to continue activities of daily living. For example, a patient loses the ability to speak after larynx surgery and has to learn new ways of communicating. Changes in function are physical and/or psychosocial. In the case of serious disability such as following a stroke or a spinal cord injury, the patient's family (as defined by the patient) needs to understand and accept many changes in his or her physical capabilities. The family's ability to provide support results in part from education, which begins as soon as you identify the patient's needs and the family displays a willingness to help. Teach family members to help the patient with health care management (e.g., giving medications through gastric tubes and doing passive range-of-motion exercises). Families

of patients with alterations such as alcohol use disorder, intellectual disability, or substance abuse disorder learn to adapt to the emotional effects of these chronic conditions and provide psychosocial support to facilitate the patient's health. Comparing a realistic desired level of health with the actual state of health enables you to identify deficits and needs and then plan effective teaching programs.

TEACHING AND LEARNING

It is impossible to separate teaching from learning. Teaching is the concept of imparting knowledge through a series of directed activities. It consists of a conscious, deliberate set of actions that help individuals gain new knowledge, change attitudes, adopt new behaviors, or perform new skills (Billings and Halstead, 2016). An educator needs to be knowledgeable about the subject matter and patient teaching principles in order to provide individuals with guidance, appropriately set the learning pace, and creatively introduce concepts to successfully achieve the objectives of new knowledge, behaviors, or changed attitudes.

Learning is defined as a "conscious or unconscious permanent change in behavior as a result of a lifelong, dynamic process by which individuals acquire new knowledge, skills, and/or attitudes that can be measured and can occur at any time or in any place through exposure to environmental stimuli" (Bastable, 2017). It is a process of both understanding and applying newly acquired concepts. For example, an adult exhibits learning when he demonstrates how to set up his weekly pillbox correctly. He shows transfer of learning when he demonstrates how to set up his wife's pillbox. Teaching and learning begin when a person identifies a need for knowing or acquiring an ability to do something. Teaching is most effective when it responds to a learner's needs. An educator assesses these needs by asking questions and determining a learner's interests. Interpersonal communication is essential for successful teaching (see Chapter 24).

Role of the Nurse in Teaching and Learning

Nurses are legally responsible for providing education to all patients, regardless of gender, culture, age, literacy level, religion, or any other defining characteristics (Bastable, 2017). In The Patient Care Partnership, the American Hospital Association (2018) indicates that patients have the right to make informed decisions about their care. The information required to make informed decisions must be accurate, complete, and relevant to patients' needs, language, and literacy. Medicare (medicare.gov, n.d.) also has standards for residents' rights in nursing homes, including the right to be informed about one's medical condition, medications, and to see one's own doctor.

The Joint Commission's Speak Up program helps patients understand their rights when receiving medical care (TJC, 2018b). The assumption is that patients who ask questions and are aware of their rights have a greater chance of getting the care they need when they need it. The program offers the following Speak Up tips to help patients become more involved in their treatment:

- **S**peak up if you have questions or concerns. If you still do not understand, ask again. It is your body, and you have a right to know.
- **P**ay attention to the care you get. Always make sure that you are getting the right treatments and medicines by the right health care professionals. Do not assume anything.
- **E**ducate yourself about your illness. Learn about the medical tests that are prescribed and your treatment plan.
- **A**sk a trusted family member or friend to be your advocate (adviser or supporter).
- **K**now which medicines you take and why you take them. Medication errors are the most common health care mistakes.

- *U*se a hospital, clinic, surgery center, or other type of health care organization that you have researched or checked carefully.
- *P*articipate in all decisions about your treatment. You are the center of the health care team.

In addition, patients are advised that they have a right to be informed about the care they will receive, obtain information about care in their preferred language, know the names of their caregivers, receive treatment for pain, receive an up-to-date list of current medications, and expect that they will be heard and treated with respect.

Teach information that patients and their families need. You frequently clarify information provided by health care providers, such as how a patient can limit lifting heavy objects upon returning home or how to restrict activities as prescribed by the health care provider. You are the primary source of information to help patients adjust to health problems (Bastable, 2017). It is also important to understand patients' preferences for what they wish to learn. For example, a patient requests information about a new medication, or family members question the reason for their mother's pain. Identifying the need for teaching is easy when patients request information. However, a patient's need for teaching (such as how to avoid complications from an illness) is often less obvious to the patient. To be an effective educator, the nurse has to do more than just pass on facts. Carefully determine what patients need to know, their preferences, and existing knowledge and then find the time to educate them when they are ready to learn. When you value and provide education, patients are better prepared to assume health care responsibilities. Nursing research about patient education supports the positive impact of patient education on patient outcomes (Box 25.1).

Teaching as Communication

The teaching process closely parallels the communication process (see Chapter 24). Effective teaching depends in part on effective interpersonal communication. An educator applies each element of the communication process while providing information to learners. Thus the educator and learner become involved together in a teaching process that increases the learner's knowledge and skills.

The steps of the teaching process are similar to those of the communication process. You use patient requests for information or perceive a need for information because of a patient's health restrictions or the recent diagnosis of an illness. Then you identify specific **learning objectives** to describe the behaviors the learner will exhibit as a result of successful instruction (Bastable, 2017).

The nurse is the sender who conveys a message to the patient. Many intrapersonal variables influence your style and approach. Attitudes, values, emotions, cultural perspective, and knowledge influence the way information is delivered. Past experiences with teaching are also helpful for choosing the best way to present necessary content.

The receiver in the teaching-learning process is the learner. A number of intrapersonal variables affect the motivation and ability to learn. Patients are ready to learn when they express a desire to do so and are more likely to receive your message when they understand the content. Attitudes, anxiety, physical symptoms, literacy level, and values influence the ability to understand a message. The ability to learn depends on factors such as emotional and physical health, education, cultural perspective, patients' values about their health, the stage of development, and previous knowledge.

Effective communication involves feedback. An effective educator provides a mechanism for evaluating the success of a teaching plan and then provides positive reinforcement (Bastable, 2017). This type of response reinforces health behavior and promotes continued self-management. You need to provide feedback both during and at the completion of each instructional encounter. Feedback needs to affirm the level of success of the learner in achieving objectives (i.e., the learner

---

BOX 25.1 EVIDENCE-BASED PRACTICE

The Effectiveness of the Teach-Back Method to Reduce Hospital Readmissions

PICOT Question: In adult patients who are discharged from the hospital, does utilizing the teach-back method compared with standard review of teaching content result in fewer hospital readmissions?

Evidence Summary

As of 2016, there were approximately 39 million inpatient hospital discharges in the United States each year, and almost 1 in 5 patients covered by Medicare are readmitted within 30 days, which has been an increasing trend (Axon et al., 2016). There is a nationwide focus on how to improve care transitions from the hospital to home or treatment center, such as a nursing home or rehabilitation center. The Centers for Medicare and Medicaid (CMS) has sponsored more than 100 projects to explore the best practice in terms of care transitions. Research has shown that effective education that includes ensuring the patient understands the discharge plan may decrease the likelihood of readmission by 30% (Almkuist, 2017). The teach-back method has been linked to a more effective discharge process, which helps ensure safer transitions from the hospital (Peter et al., 2015). The importance of understanding discharge instructions is imperative as patients need to know how to take medications and when to make follow-up appointments once leaving the hospital. When patients understand discharge information, current evidence supports that patient readmissions or visits the emergency department after discharge are reduced. Some research has focused on specific patient diagnoses, such as heart failure, while other studies have looked at generalized patient populations. For example, heart failure affects 5.7 million people and 1 in 4 patients discharged with heart failure are readmitted within 30 days (Almkuist, 2017). Almkuist (2017) conducted a systematic review of patients with heart failure and found that using the teach-back method during discharge can reduce readmission rates and also improve self-care abilities and increase the patient and family's knowledge about a specific disease. Peter et al. (2015) found that when a nurse used the teach-back method for patients with heart failure, it improved the patients' understanding of their disease, improved adherence to patient education, and caused a decline in readmission rates. While examining the impact of the teach-back method in general patient populations in terms of reducing readmission, Axon (2016) found decreases in readmission rates for several patient populations, including acute myocardial infarction, heart failure, and chronic obstructive pulmonary disease.

Application to Nursing Practice

- Implement the teach-back method when teaching about complex chronic illnesses, such as heart failure (Almkuist, 2017).
- The use of teach-back is an effective tool to use during hospitalization to help prepare patients for self-care after discharge (Almkuist, 2017).
- The teach-back method increases patients' and caregivers' understanding of and adherence to postdischarge instructions, which helps decrease readmissions (Peter et al., 2015).
- Not utilizing the teach-back method can lead to gaps in understanding between health care providers, patients, and family caregivers.

---

successfully verbalizes information or provides a return demonstration of skills learned). Feedback you receive from the learner is also important because it indicates the effectiveness of instruction and whether you need to modify your approach.

DOMAINS OF LEARNING

Learning occurs in three domains: cognitive (understanding), affective (attitudes), and psychomotor (motor skills) (Bastable, 2017). The most effective learning takes place when all three of these domains are utilized (Miller & Stoeckel, 2019). You often work with patients who need to learn in each domain. For example, patients who have undergone surgery for colon cancer and who have an ostomy to manage need to learn how the ostomy is affected by diet, medications, and activity (cognitive domain). In addition, a patient begins to learn coping skills to accept the change in body image created by the ostomy (affective domain). The patient with an ostomy needs to learn how to change an ostomy pouch and provide skin care (psychomotor domain). The characteristics of learning within each domain influence your teaching and evaluation methods. Understanding each learning domain prepares you to select proper teaching techniques and apply the basic principles of learning (Box 25.2).

Cognitive Learning

Cognitive learning occurs when an individual gains information to further develop his or her intellectual abilities, mental capacities, understanding, and thinking processes (Bastable, 2017). Bloom's revised taxonomy of six cognitive behaviors is a hierarchy, which increases in complexity (Anderson and Krathwohl, 2001; Krathwohl, 2002) (Fig. 25.1). Each simpler category was originally a prerequisite to mastery of the next more complex one. For example, knowledge or remembering has to be mastered before someone can master the higher level of understanding or comprehension. Each of the cognitive behaviors is divided into subcategories. For example, remembering (formerly *Knowledge*) includes factual, conceptual, procedural, and metacognitive knowledge (Krathwohl, 2002). The revised taxonomy includes these domains:

- Remember (formerly *Knowledge*): Recognizing or recalling knowledge from memory
- Understand (formerly *Comprehension*): Constructing meaning from different types of messages or activities, such as interpreting, exemplifying, classifying, summarizing, inferring, comparing, or explaining
- Apply: Carrying out or using a procedure through executing or implementing
- Analyze: Breaking materials or concepts into parts, then determining how the parts relate to one another or how they interrelate, or how the parts relate to an overall structure or purpose
- Evaluate: Making judgments based on criteria and standards through checking and critiquing
- Create (formerly *Synthesis*): Putting elements together to form a coherent or functional whole; reorganizing elements into a new pattern or structure through generating, planning, or producing

Affective Learning

Affective learning deals with the expression of feelings and emotions and the development of values, attitudes, and beliefs (Billings and Halstead, 2016). Values clarification (see Chapter 22) is an example of affective learning. The affective domains of learning were developed by Krathwohl and Bloom (Krathwohl et al., 1956) The simplest behavior in affective learning is receiving, and the most complex is characterizing. Affective learning includes the following (Wilson, 2019):

- Receiving: Learner is passive but is aware of stimuli and willing to receive information.
- Responding: Requires active participation. This refers to a learner's active attention to stimuli, verbal and nonverbal responses, and motivation to learn.
- Valuing: Attaching worth and value to the acquired knowledge as demonstrated by the learner's behavior through acceptance, preference, or commitment.

BOX 25.2 Appropriate Teaching Methods Based on Domains of Learning

Cognitive
- Discussion (one-on-one or group)
  - Involves nurse and one patient or a nurse with several patients
  - Promotes active participation and focuses on topics of interest to patient
  - Allows peer support
  - Enhances application and analysis of new information
- Lecture
  - Is more formal method of instruction because it is educator controlled
  - Helps learner acquire new knowledge and gain comprehension
- Question-and-answer session
  - Addresses patient's specific concerns
  - Helps patient apply knowledge
- Role play, discovery
  - Allows patient to actively apply knowledge in controlled situation
  - Promotes synthesis of information and problem solving
- Independent project (computer-assisted instruction), field experience
  - Allows patient to assume responsibility for completing learning activities at own pace
  - Promotes analysis, synthesis, and evaluation of new information and skills

Affective
- Role play
  - Allows expression of values, feelings, and attitudes
- Discussion (group)
  - Allows patient to receive support from others in group
  - Helps patient learn from others' experiences
  - Promotes responding, valuing, and organization
- Discussion (one-on-one)
  - Allows discussion of personal, sensitive topics of interest or concern

Psychomotor
- Demonstration
  - Provides presentation of procedures or skills by nurse
  - Permits patient to incorporate modeling of nurse's behavior
  - Allows nurse to control questioning during demonstration
- Practice
  - Gives patient opportunity to perform skills using equipment in a controlled setting
  - Provides repetition
- Return demonstration
  - Permits patient to perform skill as nurse observes
  - Provides excellent source of feedback and reinforcement
  - Assists in determining patient's ability to correctly perform a skill or technique
- Independent projects, games
  - Requires teaching method that promotes adaptation and origination of psychomotor learning
  - Permits learner to use new skills

- Organizing: Developing a value system. Learner internalizes values and beliefs involving (1) the conceptualization of values and (2) the organization of a value system.
- Characterizing: Highest level of internalization. Acting and responding with a consistent value system; requires introspection and self-examination of one's own values in relation to an ethical issue or particular experience

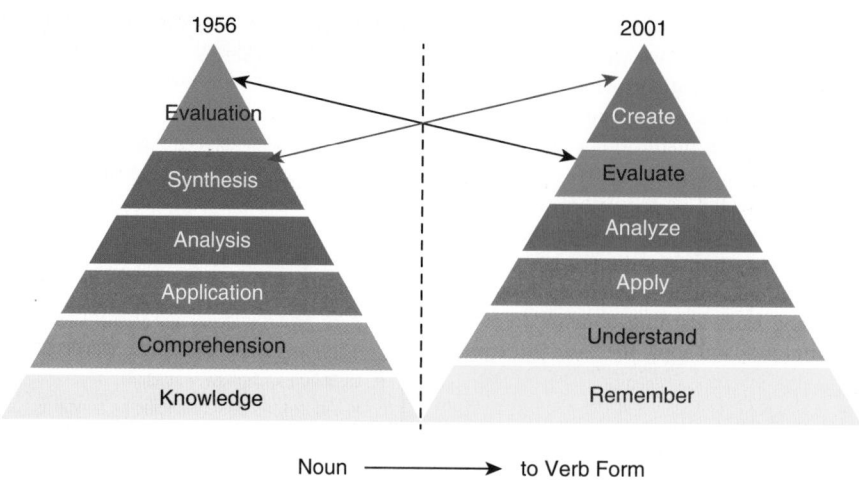

FIG. 25.1 Bloom's taxonomy: Bloom vs. Anderson/Krathwohl. (From Wilson LO: Anderson and Krathwohl — Bloom's taxonomy revised, The Second Principle, available at: https://thesecondprinciple.com/teaching-essentials/beyond-bloom-cognitive-taxonomy-revised/.)

Psychomotor Learning

Psychomotor learning involves the development of manual or physical skills, such as learning how to walk or how to type on a computer (Billings and Halstead, 2016; Wilson, 2019). The simplest behavior in the hierarchy is fundamental (depending on the hierarchical model), whereas the most complex is origination. Psychomotor learning includes the following:

- Fundamental: Skills, movements, or behaviors related to walking, running, jumping, pushing, pulling, and manipulating. They are often components for more complex actions.
- Perception: Skills related to kinesthetic (bodily movements), visual, auditory, tactile (touch), or coordination abilities as they are related to the ability to take in information from the environment and react
- Guided response: Early stages of learning a particular skill under the guidance of an instructor that involves imitation and practice of a demonstrated act
- Mechanism: Higher level of behavior in which a person gains confidence and proficiency in performing a skill that is more complex or involves several more steps than a guided response
- Complex overt response: Smoothly and accurately performing a motor skill that requires complex movement patterns
- Adaptation: Motor skills are well developed and movements can be modified when unexpected problems occur
- Origination: Using existing psychomotor skills to create new movement patterns and perform them as needed in response to a particular situation or problem

BASIC LEARNING PRINCIPLES

To teach effectively and efficiently you must first be aware of the principles that influence how a person learns (Bastable, 2017). Achievement of the desired learning outcomes (objectives) depends on a number of principles, including an individual's motivation, readiness and ability to learn, and the environment where learning will take place. The ability to learn depends on physical and cognitive attributes, developmental level, physical wellness, and intellectual thought processes. All of these principles influence your teaching approach.

A person's learning style may affect his or her preferences for learning. People process information in a number of ways: through seeing, touch and hearing, reflecting and acting, reasoning logically and intuitively, and analyzing and visualizing. Effective teaching plans incorporate a combination of activities that target a variety of learning styles (Savage et al., 2017; Miller and Stoeckel, 2019). When you tailor your teaching approach to meet your patient's needs and learning style, you will optimize the learning experience at the individual level.

Motivation to Learn

Motivation is an internal state (e.g., an idea, emotion, or a physical need) that helps arouse, direct, and sustain human behavior (Miller and Stoeckel, 2019). A patient's motivation to learn is influenced by his or her belief of the need to know something. Patients who need knowledge for survival have a stronger motivation to learn than patients who need it for promoting health (Bastable, 2017). Unfortunately not all people are interested in maintaining health. Many do not adopt new health behaviors or change unhealthy behaviors unless they perceive a disease as a threat, overcome barriers to changing health practices, and see the benefits of adopting a healthy behavior. For example, some patients with lung disease continue to smoke. No therapy has an effect unless a person believes that health is important and that the therapy will improve health.

Motivational interviewing is a counseling and educational technique that is focused on patient goals and is goal directed and patient centered (Stewart and Fox, 2011). It is based on the principle that the motivation for change must come from the patient rather than the health care provider. As health care providers we may think we know what a patient "needs to learn." However, if the information we choose to deliver does not meet a patient's own personal goals or values, teaching efforts may be ineffective. Motivational interviewing (MI) is often particularly successful with patients who are not motivated to change (Miller and Rollnick, 2002). Solid evidence exists for the efficacy of MI to address lifestyle behaviors such as diet, exercise, and smoking cessation, as well as the psychosocial needs of patients living with cancer (Spencer and Wheeler, 2016). MI has also been shown to be effective in primary care settings with improvement in patient management of body weight, alcohol and tobacco use, sedentary behavior, and self-monitoring (Lundahl et al., 2013). The objective of MI is not to solve a patient's problem or even to develop a plan; the goal is to help patients resolve their ambivalence about adopting new self-care behaviors, develop some momentum, and believe that behavioral change is possible (Stewart and Fox, 2011). MI interview questions are also useful in the assessment process for determining patients' learning needs.

TABLE 25.1 Learning Theories

Learning Theory	Definition	Application
Cognitive Dissonance	Individuals desire consistency and will make necessary changes and adaptations to gain that consistency (Festinger, 1957; Gruber, 2003). Cognitive dissonance is experienced in situations in which a patient is challenged by an inconsistency requiring a life change.	A patient with a recent myocardial infarction (MI) faces stressors associated with potential and actual health risks and changes needed as result of diagnosis. There are lifelong implications. The patient needs to change beliefs, attitudes, and values to regain consistency in life during recovery.
Health Belief Model	A patient will perceive a certain susceptibility and severity of their disease. Modifying factors include knowledge, as well as demographics and social and psychological variables. Likelihood of action is based on the perceived barriers and benefits of the situation (Hochbaum, 1958).	How a patient who has an MI copes with illness will depend on all modifying factors. If the patient does not feel threatened, believes that he or she will not benefit from interventions, or is not confident that he or she will be effective in the management of the condition, the patient may not be as receptive to teaching.
Transtheoretical Model of Change	Model is used to define how individuals initiate change in their lives, progress through those changes, and process and maintain behaviors. There are five stages in the model: precontemplation, contemplation, preparation, action, and maintenance (Prochaska, et al., 1998).	If the patient has experienced serious damage to the heart and requires cardiac rehabilitation, there are lifestyle changes to consider, such as diet, exercise, and medication management. With each stage of the model the patient makes decisions weighing the pros and cons and probable outcomes. Positive outcomes must outweigh negative aspects of change.
Self-Efficacy	Model focuses on the patient's belief in his or her own abilities to make and maintain changes and positive outcomes in the patient's life (Bandura, 1977). Self-efficacy is based on self-confidence and is a good indicator for motivation to make behavioral changes.	If a patient who has an MI is discharged home, he or she must provide some level of self-care. Break down any skill into manageable steps with encouragement and support from others. The patient moves from self-doubt and anxiety to comfort and confidence in his or her abilities.
Health Promotion	Model is based on the premise that characteristics and experiences of an individual affect actions specific to behaviors and in turn affect outcomes specific to behavior (Pender, 1975). The model applies general information from social learning theory to build on the nursing perspective of the holistic patient.	The behaviors of a patient who has an MI are driven by prior health promotion behaviors, as well as personal factors (biological, psychological, and sociocultural). Patients must be active participants in initiating and maintaining health promotion.

Adapted from Syx RL: The practice of patient education: the theoretical perspective, *Orthop Nurs* 27(1):50-54, 2008.

Use of Theory to Enhance Motivation and Learning.

Health education often involves changing attitudes and values that are not easy to change simply through transfer of information. Therefore it is important for you to use theory-based interventions when developing patient education plans. Learning theories focus on how individuals learn. Such theories are typically based on learning research. The use of theory facilitates the teaching-learning process by creating the desired climate for learning and guiding the selection of instructional strategies. Because patient education is complex, there are different theories and models available to guide patient education (Table 25.1). Using a theory that matches a patient's needs and personal learning preferences allows the patient to become an active participant, leading to effective instruction.

Among the various theories, social learning theory is one of the most useful approaches to patient education. It considers the personal characteristics of the learner, behavioral patterns, and the environment and guides the educator in developing effective teaching interventions that motivate and enhance learning (Bastable, 2017). According to social learning theory, a person's state of mind and intrinsic motivational factors (i.e., sense of accomplishment, pride, or confidence) reinforce behaviors and influence learning (Miller and Stoeckel, 2019). This type of internal reward system allows a person to attain desired outcomes and avoid undesired outcomes, resulting in improved motivation. Self-efficacy, a concept included in social learning theory, refers to a person's perceived ability to successfully complete a task. When people believe that they can achieve a particular behavior, they are more likely to perform the behavior consistently and correctly. Motivational interviewing techniques incorporate self-efficacy principles.

Self-efficacy beliefs come from four sources: verbal persuasion, vicarious experience, enactive mastery experience, and psychological and affective states (Bandura, 1997; Miller and Stoeckel, 2019). For example, a nurse who is teaching a child recently diagnosed with asthma how to correctly use an inhaler expresses personal belief in the child's ability to use the inhaler (verbal persuasion). Then the nurse demonstrates how to use the inhaler (vicarious experience). Once the demonstration is complete, the child uses the inhaler (enactive mastery experience). As the child's wheezing and anxiety decrease after the correct use of the inhaler, he or she experiences positive feedback, further enhancing his or her confidence to use it (physiological and affective states). Interventions such as these enhance perceived self-efficacy, which in turn improves the achievement of desired outcomes.

Self-efficacy is a concept included in many health promotion theories because it often is a strong predictor of healthy behaviors and because many interventions improve self-efficacy, resulting in improved lifestyle choices (Bandura, 1997). For example, Kate Lorig (2015), as the director of the Stanford Patient Education Research Center, developed a Chronic Disease Self-Management Program based on self-efficacy theory. The program uses skill mastery, modeling, reinterpretation, and social persuasion to enhance a person's self-efficacy. Dr. Lorig's programs have been especially effective for patients with diabetes, chronic lung problems and those in cardiac rehabilitation (see Chapter 8). When nurses implement interventions to enhance self-efficacy, their patients frequently experience positive outcomes. For example, researchers associated increased self-efficacy scores and increased achievement of health goals when patients had follow-up education through telephone encounters over a period of 6 months (Zhou et al., 2018). In another study, researchers found that a self-care education program was effective at reducing all unplanned readmission for patients with heart failure (Boyde et al., 2018).

TABLE 25.2   Relationship Between Psychosocial Adaptation to Illness, Grief, and Learning

Stage	Patient's Behavior	Learning Implications for Nurse and Family Caregiver	Rationale
Denial or disbelief	Patient avoids discussion of illness ("I'm fine; nothing is wrong with me"), withdraws from others, and disregards physical restrictions. Patient suppresses and distorts information that has not been presented clearly.	Provide support, empathy, and careful explanations of all procedures while they are being done. Remain available and accessible for discussion. Explain situation to family or significant other if appropriate. Teach in present tense (e.g., explain current therapy).	Patient is not prepared to deal with problem. Any attempt to convince or tell patient about illness results in further anger or withdrawal. Provide only information patient pursues or absolutely requires.
Anger	Patient blames and directs anger toward nurse or others.	Do not argue with patient. Listen to concerns. Use good eye contact. Teach in present tense. Reassure family and significant others that patient's anger is normal.	Patient needs opportunity to express feelings and anger; he or she is still not prepared to face the future.
Bargaining	Patient offers to live better life in exchange for promise of better health. ("If God lets me live, I promise to quit smoking.")	Continue to introduce only reality. Teach only in present tense.	Patient is still unwilling to accept limitations.
Resolution	Patient begins to express emotions openly, realizes that illness has created changes, and begins to ask questions.	Encourage expression of feelings. Find out what patient wants to learn. Begin to share information needed for future and set aside formal times for discussion.	Patient begins to perceive need for assistance and is ready to be responsible for learning.
Acceptance	Patient recognizes reality of condition, actively pursues information, and strives for independence.	Focus teaching on future skills and knowledge required. Continue to teach about present occurrences. Involve family/significant other in teaching information for discharge.	Patient is more easily motivated to learn. Acceptance of illness reflects willingness to deal with its implications.

Cultural Factors. Knowing your patients' cultural preferences (see Chapter 9) and health beliefs (Chapter 6) helps you develop patient-centered interventions that will motivate your patients to learn. Carefully assess a patient's cultural needs and preferences for instructional methods to enhance learning and adherence. Using a model such as ACCESS helps you to focus on cultural factors that influence patient education outcomes. The six ACCESS model components are (Purnell, 2014):

1. **Assessment** of a patient's lifestyle, health beliefs, cultural traditions, and health practices.
2. **Communication** with an awareness of the many variations in verbal and nonverbal responses.
3. **Cultural** negotiation and compromise that encourages awareness of characteristics of a patient's culture and one's own biases.
4. **Establishment** of respect for a patient's cultural beliefs and values; creating a caring rapport.
5. **Sensitivity** to how patients from diverse backgrounds perceive their care needs and the patterns of communication they use.
6. **Safety** that enables patients to feel culturally secure and avoids disempowerment of their cultural identity.

Active Participation. Learning occurs when a patient is motivated to be actively involved in an educational session (Edelman and Kudzma, 2017). A patient's involvement in learning implies an eagerness to acquire knowledge or skills. It also improves the opportunity for the patient to make decisions during teaching sessions. For example, when teaching car-seat safety during a parenting class, hold a teaching session in the parking lot where the participants park their cars. Encourage active participation by providing the learners with several different car seats for them to place in their cars. At the completion of this session, the parents are able to determine which type of car seat fits best in their cars and which is the easiest to use. This provides participants with the information needed to purchase the appropriate car seat.

Readiness to Learn

Readiness to learn is based on a patient's willingness to engage in learning (Miller and Stoeckel, 2019). Many factors affect readiness to learn. A loss of health is usually very difficult for patients to accept. Grief is a complex process that patients experience during illness (see Chapter 36). The process of grieving gives individuals time to adapt psychologically to the emotional and physical implications of their illnesses. Readiness to learn is affected by each stage of grieving (Table 25.2). Patients cannot learn when they are unwilling or unable to accept their illness. However, properly timed teaching during the grieving process facilitates adjustment to illness or disability.

A patient's health status also affects readiness to learn. Patients move along a continuum of health. As a patient moves along this continuum, the readiness to learn changes as well (Miller and Stoeckel, 2019). For example, a patient who is acutely ill is concerned with survival and will likely be most interested in a treatment plan before learning about long-term implications of illness. A patient who has had a stroke will be most ready to learn about self-care skills when receiving rehabilitation care.

An **attentional set** is the mental state that allows a learner to focus on and comprehend a learning activity. Before learning anything, patients must be able to pay attention to or concentrate on the information to be learned. Physical discomfort, anxiety, confusion, and environmental distractions influence the ability to concentrate. Therefore determine a patient's level of comfort before beginning a teaching plan, and ensure that the patient is able to focus on the information. As anxiety increases, a patient's ability to pay attention often decreases. A mild level of anxiety can be conducive to learning. However, a high level of anxiety prevents learning from occurring. At times when a patient is unable to attend, a family caregiver often becomes the recipient of education. Simple facts, rather than detailed teaching strategies, are most important during these times. For example, a patient in pain is reception to learning about how to use a patient-controlled analgesia pump but not how to use crutches.

Ability to Learn

A patient's developmental level and cognitive and physical capabilities influence the ability to learn. In addition the learning environment is a significant factor affecting learning ability.

Developmental Capability. Cognitive development influences a patient's ability to learn. You can be a competent educator, but if you do not consider a patient's intellectual abilities, teaching is unsuccessful. Learning, like developmental growth, is an evolving process. Assess a patient's level of knowledge and intellectual skills (e.g., simple problem solving, decision making, applying a concept such as infection control in the home) before beginning a teaching plan. Learning occurs more readily when new information complements existing knowledge. For example, measuring liquid or solid food portions requires the ability to perform mathematical calculations. When caring for a patient in the home setting, first determine whether the patient understands what a portion consists of and then observe the patient prepare the liquid or solid food. Reading a medication label or discharge instructions requires reading and comprehension skills. Assessing a patient's health literacy level will help determine the patient's existing ability.

Learning in Children. The capability for learning and the type of behaviors that children are able to learn depend on the child's maturation (Chapter 12). Without proper physiological, motor, language, and social development, many types of learning cannot take place. In addition, every child learns in different ways. However, learning occurs in children of all ages. Intellectual growth moves from the concrete to the abstract as the child matures. Therefore information presented to children needs to be understandable, and the expected outcomes must be realistic based on the child's developmental stage (Box 25.3). Remember that a child's developmental stage may not correspond to the child's chronological age. Use teaching methods that are evidence-based. Some evidence-based teaching strategies include creating clear lesson goals, using questions to check understanding, summarizing learning in a graphic way (with charts or concept maps), providing feedback, and being flexible in terms of how long it takes to learn (Killian, 2013). Use teaching aids that are developmentally appropriate (Fig. 25.2). Learning occurs when behavior changes as a result of experience or growth (Miller and Stoeckel, 2019).

Adult Learning. Teaching adults differs from teaching children. Adults are able to reflect on their current situation critically but sometimes need help to see their problems and change their perspectives. Because adults become independent and self-directed as they mature, they are often able to identify their own learning needs (Billings and Halstead, 2016). Learning needs come from problems or tasks that result from real-life situations. Although adults tend to be self-directed learners, they often become dependent in new learning situations. The amount of information you provide and the amount of time you spend with an adult patient vary depending on the patient's personal situation and readiness to learn. An adult's readiness to learn is often associated with his or her developmental stage and other events that are occurring in his or her life. Help patients resolve any needs they perceive as important so that learning can occur.

Adults have a wide variety of personal life experiences. Adult learners do best when asked to both use their previous experiences

and apply new knowledge to solve a real-life problem (Billings and Halstead, 2016). Adult learners are more successful when they view the information as personally relevant and important to their daily lives (Billings and Halstead, 2016). For example, if you instruct a patient to limit certain activities after surgery, learn what activities a person normally performs that may conflict with the restrictions. Find ways that will help the patient adhere to the restrictions. Assessing what an adult patient currently knows or does, teaching what the patient wants to know, and setting mutual goals improve the outcomes of patient education (Bastable, 2017).

Health Literacy and Learning Disabilities. Research shows that not only is health literacy a strong predictor of a person's health status but that it is a stronger predictor compared with several other factors,

---

BOX 25.3 Teaching Methods Based on Patient's Developmental Capacity

Infant
- Keep routines (e.g., feeding, bathing) consistent.
- Hold infant firmly while smiling and speaking softly to convey sense of trust.
- Have infant touch different textures (e.g., soft fabric, hard plastic).

Toddler
- Use play to teach procedure or activity (e.g., handling examination equipment, applying bandage to doll).
- Offer picture books that describe story of children in hospital or clinic.
- Use simple words such as "cut" instead of "laceration" to promote understanding.

Preschooler
- Use role play, imitation, and play to make learning fun.
- Encourage questions and offer explanations. Use simple explanations and demonstrations.
- Encourage children to learn together through pictures and short stories about how to perform hygiene.

School-Age Child
- Teach psychomotor skills needed to maintain health. (Complicated skills such as learning to use a syringe take considerable practice.)
- Offer opportunities to discuss health problems and answer questions.

Adolescent
- Help adolescent learn about feelings and need for self-expression.
- Use teaching as collaborative activity.
- Allow adolescent to make decisions about health and health promotion (safety, sex education, substance abuse).
- Use problem solving to help adolescent make choices.

Young or Middle Adult
- Encourage participation in teaching plan by setting mutual goals.
- Encourage independent learning.
- Offer information so adult understands effects of health problem.

Older Adult
- Teach when patient is alert and rested.
- Involve adult in discussion or activity.
- Focus on wellness and person's strength.
- Use approaches that enhance patient's reception of stimuli when he or she has a sensory impairment (see Chapter 49).
- Keep teaching sessions short.

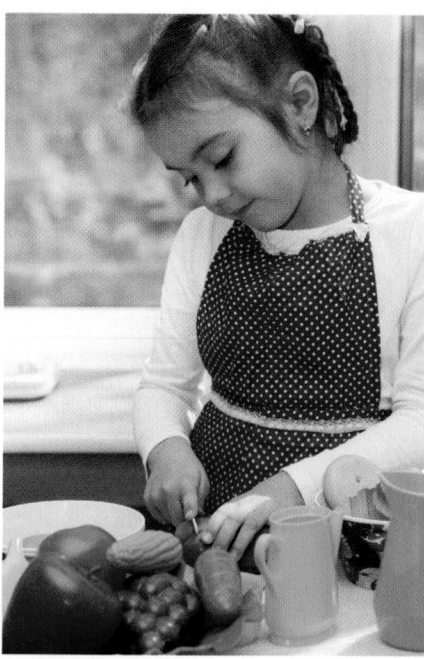

FIG. 25.2 Young child learning about healthy foods with plastic food models. (Copyright © iStock/alkir.)

including age, income, employment status, educational level, and race (Parnell, 2015). The World Health Organization (WHO, 2018) defines health literacy as the cognitive and social skills that determine the ability of individuals to gain access to, understand, and use information in ways that promote and maintain good health. Health literacy pertains not only to a patient's ability to read and comprehend health-related information but also to having the skills to problem solve, articulate, and make appropriate health care decisions (Parnell, 2015). People most likely to be at risk for low health literacy include older adults, minority populations, immigrant populations, people of low income, people without a high school education, and people with chronic mental and/or physical health conditions (US Department of Education, 2015). According to the Centers for Disease Control and Prevention (2016) 9 of 10 adults struggle to understand and use health information if it is unfamiliar, complex, or uses jargon.

The US Department of Health and Human Services (USDHHS, n.d.b) reports that only 12 percent of adults have proficient health literacy, meaning nearly 9 of 10 adults may lack the skills needed to manage their health and prevent disease. To compound the problem, research has shown that health materials are often written at complex levels that exceed not only the general public's reading level but also the reading level of average high school graduates (Parnell, 2015). This discrepancy results in unsafe health care. Health literacy is one of the most important predictors of health outcomes. Low health literacy can lead to more emergency department visits, along with more hospital admissions and readmissions (Miller and Stoeckel, 2019). To ensure patient safety, all health care providers need to ensure that information is presented clearly and in a culturally sensitive manner (TJC, 2018a). Many people need printed health information at a fifth-grade level or lower and people often read at a level or two lower than their highest level of education (Miller and Stoeckel, 2019).

Physical Capability. Readiness to learn often depends on a patient's level of physical development and overall physical health. Many factors impair the ability to learn, including preexisting physical or mental illness, fatigue, body temperature, electrolyte imbalance, oxygenation status, and blood glucose level. To learn psychomotor skills a patient

must possess a certain level of strength, coordination, and sensory acuity. For example, it is useless to teach a patient to transfer from a bed to a wheelchair if he or she has insufficient upper body strength. An older patient with poor eyesight or the inability to grasp objects tightly cannot learn to apply an elastic bandage. Therefore do not overestimate the patient's physical development or status. The following physical characteristics are necessary to learn psychomotor skills:

- Size (patient's height and weight should match the task to be performed or the equipment being used)
- Strength (ability of the patient to follow a strenuous exercise program)
- Coordination (dexterity needed for complicated motor skills such as using utensils or changing a bandage)
- Sensory acuity (visual, auditory, tactile, gustatory, and olfactory; sensory resources needed to receive and respond to messages taught)

Determining a patient's ability to perform psychomotor skills is best assessed by a physical therapist or occupational therapist. Also, consider how a patient adapts any physical limitations to performing skills at home.

Any condition or symptom (e.g., pain, nausea, or fatigue) that depletes a patient's energy also impairs the ability to learn. For example, a patient who spends a morning having rigorous diagnostic studies is unlikely to be able to learn later in the day because of fatigue. Postpone teaching when an illness becomes aggravated by complications such as a high fever or respiratory difficulty. As you work with a patient, assess energy level by noting the patient's willingness to communicate, the amount of activity initiated, and responses to questions. Temporarily stop teaching if the patient needs rest. You achieve better outcomes when patients are physically able to actively participate in learning.

Learning Environment

Factors in the physical environment where teaching takes place make learning either a pleasant or a difficult experience (Bastable, 2017). The ideal setting helps a patient focus on the learning task. The number of people included in the teaching session; the need for privacy; the room temperature; and the lighting, noise, ventilation, and furniture in the room are important factors when choosing a setting. The ideal environment for learning is well lit and has good ventilation, appropriate furniture, and a comfortable temperature. A darkened room interferes with a patient's ability to watch your actions, especially when demonstrating a skill or using visual aids such as posters or pamphlets. A room that is cold, hot, or stuffy makes a patient too uncomfortable to focus on the information being presented.

It is also important to choose a quiet setting. A quiet setting offers privacy; infrequent interruptions are best. Provide privacy even in a busy hospital by closing cubicle curtains or taking the patient to a quiet spot. Family caregivers often need to share in discussions in the home setting. However, patients who are reluctant to discuss the nature of the illness when others are in the room benefit from receiving education in a room separate from household activities, such as a bedroom.

Teaching a group of patients requires a room that allows everyone to be seated comfortably and within hearing distance of the educator. Make sure that the size of the room does not overwhelm the group. Arranging the group to allow participants to observe one another further enhances learning. More effective communication occurs as learners observe others' verbal and nonverbal interactions.

❖ NURSING PROCESS

Apply the nursing process and use a critical thinking approach in your care of patients. The nursing process provides a clinical decision-making approach for you to develop and implement an individualized plan of care. There are distinct similarities between the nursing process and the teaching process. During the assessment phase of the nursing process, you determine a patient's health care needs (see Unit 3). Like the nursing process, the teaching process requires assessment—in this case analyzing a patient's learning needs, motivation, and ability to learn. Your findings regarding the type of information, skill, or behavioral change that a patient needs to learn will lead to a nursing diagnostic statement. An example is *Lack of Knowledge* regarding a newly diagnosed condition related to insufficient information. A diagnosis such as *Anxiety* will often identify factors interfering with learning. Instead of outcomes, you develop specific learning objectives for a teaching plan. The nursing and teaching processes differ in that the nursing process requires assessment of all sources of data to determine a patient's total health care needs. The teaching process focuses on a patient's learning needs and willingness and capability to learn.

Implementation involves the use of appropriate patient-centered and evidence-based teaching strategies. Incorporate learning principles to ensure that your patient acquires the necessary knowledge and skills. Finally, the teaching process requires an evaluation of learning, including patient feedback based on learning objectives. Table 25.3 compares the teaching and nursing processes.

◆ Assessment

Through the Patient's Eyes. When providing patient education, it is important to partner with the patient to ensure safe, compassionate, and coordinated care (QSEN, 2019). This means that during the assessment you determine a patient's expectations for any teaching encounter. What does the patient expect to learn? What type of information does the patient perceive will be needed to maintain self-care at home or in a transitional care setting? During the assessment process thoroughly assess a patient and critically analyze your findings to ensure that you make patient-centered clinical decisions required for appropriate patient education. Assess the patient's preferences, values, and expressed needs in order to see the health care situation through his or her eyes (QSEN, 2019). In this way you gain a better appreciation of your patient's knowledge, expectations, and preferences for learning. Teaching will be more effective.

Learning Needs. Learning needs are defined as "gaps in knowledge that exist between a desired level of performance and the actual level of performance" (Miller & Stoeckel, 2019). Box 25.4 summarizes examples of specific assessment questions to use in determining a patient's unique learning needs.

Sometimes nurses use formal educational assessment tools to determine their patients' perceived learning needs. Other times they identify their patients' expectations during routine assessments. Patients often identify their own learning needs on the basis of the implications of living with their illness. To meet these learning needs, assess what patients view as important information to know. When a patient has a need to know something, he or she is likely to be receptive to information presented. For example, new parents need to know how to care for their baby. Therefore they are often very receptive to information about infant care (e.g., how to feed the infant and make sure that he or she gets enough sleep).

Determine information that is critical for patients to learn. Learning needs change, depending on a patient's current health status. Because health status is dynamic, assessment is an ongoing activity. Assess the following:

- Information or skills needed by a patient to perform self-care and to understand the implications of a health problem: Health care team members anticipate learning needs related to specific health problems. For example, you teach a young man who has just entered high school how to prevent sexually transmitted infections (STIs).
- Patient experiences (e.g., new or recurring problem, past hospitalization) that influence the willingness and need to learn.
- Information that family caregivers require to support the patient's needs: The amount of information needed depends on the extent of a family member's role in helping the patient.

Motivation to Learn. Ask questions to identify and define a patient's motivation. These questions determine whether a patient is prepared and willing to learn. Assess the following factors:

- Behavior (e.g., attention span, tendency to ask questions, memory, and ability to concentrate during the teaching session)
- Health beliefs and sociocultural background: Norms, values, experiences, and traditions all influence a patient's beliefs and values about health and various therapies, communication patterns, and perceptions of time (see Chapter 9).
- Perception of the severity and susceptibility of a health problem and the benefits and barriers to treatment
- Identification of patient goals for learning, which must originate from the patient and not be imposed from outside by health care providers (Stewart and Fox, 2011)
- Perceived ability to perform needed health behaviors
- Desire to learn

TABLE 25.3	Comparison of the Nursing and Teaching Processes	
Basic Steps	**Nursing Process**	**Teaching Process**
Assessment	Collect data about patient's physical, psychological, social, cultural, developmental, and spiritual needs from patient, family, diagnostic tests, medical record, nursing history, and literature.	Gather data about patient's learning needs, motivation, ability to learn, health literacy, and teaching resources from patient, family, learning environment, medical record, nursing history, and literature.
Nursing diagnosis	Identify appropriate nursing diagnoses on basis of assessment findings.	Identify patient's learning needs on basis of three domains of learning. Nursing diagnoses may identify learning need or conditions that interfere with learning.
Planning	Develop an individualized care plan. Set diagnosis priorities on basis of patient's immediate needs, expected outcomes, and patient-centered goals. Collaborate with patient on care plan.	Establish learning objectives stated in behavioral terms. Identify priorities regarding learning needs. Collaborate with patient about teaching plan. Identify type of teaching method(s) to use.
Implementation	Perform nursing care therapies. Include patient as active participant in care. Involve family/significant other in care as appropriate.	Implement teaching methods. Actively involve patient in learning activities. Include family caregiver as appropriate.
Evaluation	Identify success in meeting desired outcomes and goals of nursing care. Alter interventions as indicated when goals are not met.	Determine outcomes of teaching-learning process. Measure patient's achievement of learning objectives. Reinforce information as needed.

BOX 25.4 Nursing Assessment Questions

Motivation to Learn

- If you had one habit that you wanted to change to improve your health, what would that be?
- What goal for your health would you like to set that you are willing to achieve?
- Listen reflectively—let patients express their thoughts and then, instead of telling them what they need to learn, capture the essence of what they have said, with the purpose of eliciting conversation and helping them arrive at an idea for change.

Previous Learning and Identification of Learning Needs and Preferences

- What do you want to know about _____?
- What do you know about your illness and your treatment plan?
- Which experiences have you had in the past that are similar to those you are experiencing now?
- Together we can choose the best way for you to learn about your disease. How can I best help you?
- When you learn new information, do you prefer to have it given to you in pictures or written down in words?
- When you give someone directions to your house, do you tell the person how to get there, write out the instructions, or draw a map?

Self-Management

- How does (or will) your illness affect your current lifestyle?
- Which barriers currently exist that prevent you from managing your illness the way you would like to manage it?
- What role do you believe your health care providers should take in helping you manage your illness or maintain health?
- How involved do you want a family member to be in the management of your illness? Who is that family member?

Cultural and Spiritual Influences

- Which cultural or spiritual beliefs do you have about your illness and its treatment?

For Family Caregivers

- When are you available to help, and how do you plan to help your loved one?
- Your spouse needs some help. How do you feel about learning how to assist him or her?
- Tell me how you feel about performing the care activities that your family member requires.

- Attitudes about health care providers (e.g., role of patient and nurse in making decisions)
- Learning style preference: As the nurse, any educational effort will be more effective if the chosen method of instruction aligns with your patient's preferred learning style (Billings and Halstead, 2016). Education may require more than one instructor as each instructor may excel at different types of teaching (verbal versus role-playing). Patients who are visual-spatial learners enjoy learning through pictures, visual charts, or any exercise that allows them to visualize concepts. The verbal/linguistic learner demonstrates strength in the language arts and therefore prefers learning by listening or reading information. Kinesthetic learners process knowledge by moving and participating in hands-on activities. Role-play and return demonstrations are popular activities for the kinesthetic learner. Patients who learn through logical-mathematical reasoning think in terms of cause and effect and respond best when required to

predict logical outcomes. If a patient is unable to identify a preferred learning style, delivering a combination of strategies will be more effective than just focusing on one type of learning style.

Readiness and Ability to Learn. Determine a patient's physical and cognitive ability to learn. Health care providers often underestimate patients' cognitive and physical deficits. Assess the following factors:

- Physical strength, endurance, movement, dexterity, and coordination: Determine the extent to which a patient can perform skills by having him or her practice with equipment that will be used in self-care at home (Chapter 30).
- Sensory deficits (see Chapter 49) that affect a patient's ability to understand or follow instruction
- Patient's reading level: This is often difficult to assess because patients who are functionally illiterate are often able to conceal it by using distractors such as not having the time to read or not being able to see the print. Two ways to assess a patient's reading level and level of understanding are to ask the patient to read instructions from an educational handout and then explain their meaning or to complete a health literacy screening tool (see the discussion of health literacy below).
- Patient's developmental level, which influences the selection of teaching approaches (see Box 25.3). Consider age-appropriate abilities.
- Patient's cognitive function, including memory, knowledge, association, and judgment
- Pain, fatigue, depression, anxiety, or other physical or psychological symptoms that interfere with the ability to maintain attention and participate: In acute care and rehab settings a patient's physical condition can easily prevent a patient from learning.

Teaching Environment. The environment for a teaching session needs to be conducive to learning. Assess the following environmental factors:

- Distractions or persistent noise: A quiet area is essential for focusing on the topic and effective learning.
- Comfort of the room, including ventilation, temperature, lighting, furniture, and size
- Room facilities and available equipment

Resources for Learning. A patient often requires the support of family members or significant others. Determine who is the patient's primary family caregiver. If this support is necessary, assess the readiness and ability of family caregivers to learn the information necessary for the care of the patient. Also review resources within the home environment. Assess the following:

- Patient's willingness to have family caregivers involved in the teaching plan and provide health care: Information about a patient's health care is confidential unless the patient chooses to share it. Sometimes it is difficult for a patient to accept the help of family caregivers, especially when bodily functions are involved.
- Family caregiver's perceptions and understanding of a patient's illness and its implications: Conflict occurs in a teaching plan if the family caregiver's perceptions do not match those of the patient.
- Family caregiver's willingness and ability to participate in care: If a patient chooses to share information about his or her health status with family members, they need to be responsible, willing, and physically and cognitively able to assist in care activities such as bathing or administering medications. Not all family members meet these requirements.
- Resources, including financial or material, such as having the ability to obtain health care equipment

- Teaching tools, including brochures, audiovisual materials, or posters: Materials should be current, written clearly and logically, and match the patient's reading level.

Health Literacy. Because health literacy influences how you deliver teaching strategies, it is critical for you to assess a patient's health literacy before providing instruction. Assessing health literacy is challenging, especially in busy clinical settings where often there is little time to conduct a thorough health literacy assessment. However, all health care providers need to identify problems and provide appropriate education to people who have special health literacy needs (TJC, 2018a).

To assess health literacy, ask patients to perform simple literacy skills. For example, can a patient read a medication label back to you correctly? After you give a simple 1-minute explanation of a diet or exercise program, can the patient explain it back to you? Can a patient correctly describe in his or her own words the information in a written handout? A variety of screening tools are available to test literacy. The Wide Range Achievement Test (WRAT 3) is a word-recognition screening test that evaluates reading, spelling, and arithmetic skills for patients from 5 to 74 years of age. The Rapid Estimate of Adult Literacy in Medicine (REALM) uses pronunciation of health care terms to determine a patient's ability to read medical vocabulary. The Cloze test, used to assess comprehension of health education materials, asks patients to fill in the blanks that are in a written paragraph.

In addition to literacy level, assess patients for learning disabilities. For example, many self-care behaviors require an understanding of mathematics, including computation and fractions. If a learning disability impairs a patient's ability to effectively use mathematics skills, teaching is challenging, especially when trying to teach him or her about complex medication dosages and frequencies. Although not considered a learning disability, attention-deficit hyperactivity disorder (ADHD) also affects a patient's ability to learn. Patients with ADHD frequently experience inattention, hyperactivity, and impulsivity, which makes it difficult for them to stay focused during educational sessions, making learning challenging (Learning Disabilities Association of America, 2018).

Patients who have low health literacy or learning disabilities may be ashamed of not being able to understand you and often try to mask their inability to comprehend information. Therefore make sure that you are sensitive and maintain a therapeutic relationship with your patients while assessing their ability to learn. Appreciating the unique qualities of your patients helps to ensure safe and effective patient care (QSEN, 2019).

REFLECT NOW

You are creating a teaching plan for your local community regarding road safety. The plan will be presented at a weekly community safety class for older adults and for a group of sixth graders at a local school. How do you differentiate your teaching plan for adults versus children?

◆ Nursing Diagnosis

After assessing information related to the patient's motivation, readiness, and ability to learn, interpret data and cluster assessment findings to form diagnoses that reflect his or her specific learning needs or factors affecting the ability to learn (Box 25.5). This ensures that teaching will be goal directed and individualized. If a patient has several learning needs, the nursing diagnoses guide priority setting. When the nursing diagnosis is *Lack of Knowledge,* the diagnostic statement describes the specific type of learning need and its cause (e.g., *Lack of Knowledge* regarding a surgical procedure). Providing a related factor (e.g., related to lack of recall and exposure to information) for a problem-oriented

---

BOX 25.5 Nursing Diagnostic Process

Lack of Knowledge (Psychomotor) Regarding Use of Crutches Related to Lack of Experience

Assessment activities	Assessment findings
Have patient describe how to walk with crutches.	Patient states that he or she has not received information about use of crutches.
	Patient asks questions about how to use crutches.
Have patient demonstrate three-point crutch walking on level surfaces and up stairs.	Patient uses crutches inappropriately.
	Patient cannot go up or down stairs on crutches.

---

or negative diagnosis offers further specificity in how to design teaching strategies. Patients often require education to support resolution of their various health problems. Examples of nursing diagnoses that indicate a need for education include the following:

- *Decisional Conflict*
- *Lack of Knowledge (Affective, Cognitive, Psychomotor)*
- *Impaired Health Maintenance*
- *Impaired Ability to Manage Dietary/Exercise Regime*
- *Self Care Deficit*

When you can manage or eliminate health care problems through education, the related factor of a diagnostic statement is *Lack of Knowledge.* For example, an older adult woman is having difficulty managing a medication regimen that involves a number of newly prescribed medications that she has to take at different times of the day. The nursing diagnosis is *Impaired Health Maintenance regarding scheduling of medications related to lack of knowledge.* In this case educating the patient about her medications and the correct dosage schedules improves her ability to schedule and take them as directed. When you identify conditions that cause barriers to effective learning (e.g., nursing diagnosis of *Acute Pain* or *Activity Intolerance),* teaching is inappropriate. In these cases delay teaching until the nursing diagnosis is resolved or the health problem is controlled.

◆ Planning

After determining the nursing diagnoses that identify a patient's learning needs, develop a teaching plan, determine goals and expected outcomes, and involve the patient in selecting learning experiences (see the Nursing Care Plan). Expected outcomes of an education plan are learning objectives. They guide the choice of teaching strategies and approaches with a patient. Patient participation ensures a more relevant, meaningful plan.

Goals and Outcomes. Goals of patient education identify what a patient needs to achieve to gain a better understanding of a health care topic and to better manage his or her illness (e.g., "achieves ostomy self-care"). Outcomes describe the specific behaviors that a patient must achieve to meet each goal, such as "empties colostomy bag" and "describes diet options to reduce diarrhea." When developing outcomes, conditions or time frames need to be realistic and meet the patient's needs (e.g., "will identify the side effects of aspirin by discharge"). Consider conditions under which the patient or family will typically perform the behavior (e.g., "will walk from bedroom to bathroom using crutches"). Include the patient when establishing learning goals and outcomes, and serve as a resource in setting the minimum criteria for success.

In some health care settings nurses develop teaching plans in the electronic health record. The teaching plan includes standard topics for

◎ NURSING CARE PLAN

Anxiety Related to Lack of Knowledge About Impending Surgery

ASSESSMENT

Connie, a nurse who practices in a surgeon's office, is preparing Mr. Holland for a colon resection that is scheduled in 1 week. Mr. Holland is 75 years old, alert and oriented. He is married and lives with his wife of 45 years. He was recently diagnosed with colorectal cancer and has not had surgery in the past. He displays a number of behaviors that Connie wishes to further assess to determine their impact on his ability to learn.

Assessment Activities	*Assessment Findings[a]*
Ask Mr. Holland to describe his planned surgery.	Mr. Holland responds, "**I can't remember** what the doctor told me when I saw him last week, but I know it is for my cancer."
Observe the patient's verbal and nonverbal behavior.	Patient has **poor eye contact**, **restless** in chair. States, "**I am a bit worried about all of this.**"
Ask the patient if his wife can be included in discussion. Ask Mrs. Holland, "Tell me if you feel your husband is ready for surgery?"	Patient consents to wife's participation. Wife explains, "He has **not been sleeping well** since knowing he had to have surgery. He has looked at a booklet the doctor gave him, but he **has already forgotten what to do before he comes to the hospital. I am not sure he know how serious this is.**"
Assess Mr. Holland's previous coping strategies.	Mr. Holland states, "The last time I felt stressed was when a good friend died. I found it helped to talk about it."

[a]**Assessment Findings** are shown in bold type.

NURSING DIAGNOSIS: Anxiety related to lack of knowledge about impending surgery

PLANNING

Goals	*Expected Outcomes (NOC)[b]*
	Anxiety Self-Control
Patient will attend to teaching session.	Patient will ask relevant questions specific to surgery.
	Patient will perform relaxation exercises during instructional session.

[b]Outcome classification labels from Moorhead S et al: *Nursing outcomes classification (NOC)*, ed 6, St Louis, 2018, Elsevier.

INTERVENTIONS (NIC)[c]	RATIONALE
Learning Readiness Enhancement	
Provide planned time for patient and wife to ask questions and clarify what is expected. Show your interest, and ask patient to describe his feelings and fear about surgery.	Establishes a trusting relationship. Aids in gaining understanding of patient's perspective of stressful situation so that clarification can be provided (Butcher et al., 2018)
Use a calm, reassuring approach to explain purpose of surgery. Be factual and clarify any patient misconceptions. Use plain language and follow EDUCATE model (see Table 25.4).	EDUCATE model is an evidence-based model to improve outcomes from verbal instruction (Marcus, 2014).
Learning Facilitation	
Use visual charts of colectomy and website that explains preoperative and postoperative activities, including exercises and ambulation while teaching patient and wife.	Preoperative educational interventions can help reduce preoperative anxiety, particularly when information is given by a nurse expert (Alanazi, 2014).
Instruct patient on relaxation exercise using controlled breathing during times of perceived stress.	Offers coping mechanism to reduce sympathetic stimulation accompanying stress.

[c]Intervention classification labels from Butcher HK, et al: *Nursing interventions classification (NIC)*, ed 7, St Louis, 2018, Elsevier.

EVALUATION

Evaluation Activity	*Patient Response/Finding*	*Outcome Status*
Observe patient's behaviors during teaching sessions.	Patient asks relevant questions about activity restriction after surgery. States, "I'm still really worried about my surgery though. I just don't know if I'm going to need a colostomy or not."	Patient asks relevant questions specific to surgery. Still has concerns about outcome of surgery.
Observe patient performing deep breathing and relaxation.	Patient describes and demonstrates deep breathing technique.	Patient demonstrates deep breathing.

instruction, resources (e.g., equipment, teaching booklets, and referrals to special educational programs), recommendations for involving family, and objectives of the teaching plan. Some plans are very detailed, whereas others are in outline form. Use the plan to provide continuity of instruction. The more specific the plan, the easier it is to follow.

The setting influences the complexity of any teaching plan. In an acute care setting plans are concise and focused on the primary learning needs of the patient because there is limited time for teaching. Home care and outpatient clinic teaching plans are usually more comprehensive in scope because you often have more time to instruct patients and patients are often less anxious in outpatient settings.

Setting Priorities. Include the patient when determining priorities for patient education. Base priorities on a patient's nursing diagnoses or collaborative problems and the goals and outcomes established for him or her. Priorities also depend on what a patient perceives to be most important, his or her anxiety or physical comfort level, and the amount of time available to teach. You set a patient's learning needs in order of priority. For example, a patient recently diagnosed with coronary artery disease has *Lack of Knowledge regarding newly diagnosed illness*. The patient benefits most by first learning about the correct way to take nitroglycerin and how long to wait before calling for help when chest pain occurs. Once you assist in meeting patient needs related to basic survival, you can discuss other topics such as exercise and nutritional changes.

Timing. When is the right time to teach? Before a patient enters a hospital? When a patient first enters a clinic? At discharge? At home? Each is appropriate because patients continue to have learning needs for as long as they stay in a health care system. Plan teaching activities for a time when a patient is most attentive, receptive, and alert and organize the patient's activities to provide time for rest and teaching-learning interactions.

In acute care, timing instruction is sometimes difficult because the emphasis is on a patient's timely discharge from a hospital. For example, it takes several hours after surgery for a patient to be alert and comfortable enough to learn. By the time a patient feels ready to learn, discharge is already scheduled. Limited time is available for short teaching sessions and opportunity for patient feedback. Therefore, to improve patient outcomes, anticipate patients' educational needs before they enter the hospital, and involve family if possible.

Although prolonged teaching sessions reduce concentration and learner attentiveness, make sure that teaching sessions are not too brief. A patient needs time to comprehend the information and give feedback. It is easier for patients to tolerate and retain interest in the material during frequent sessions lasting 10 to 15 minutes. However, factors such as shorter hospital stays and lack of insurance reimbursement for outpatient education sessions often necessitate longer teaching sessions. Follow-up care in the form of referrals to home health or rehab can help provide continuity of instruction after a patient goes home.

The frequency of teaching sessions depends on a learner's abilities and the complexity of the material. For example, a child newly diagnosed with diabetes requires more visits to an outpatient center than the older adult who has had diabetes for 15 years and lives at home. Make sure that intervals between teaching sessions are not so long that the patient forgets information. Home care nurses frequently reinforce learning during home visits after patients are discharged from the hospital.

Organizing Teaching Material. An effective educator carefully considers the order of information to present. When a nurse has an ongoing relationship with a patient, as in the case of home health or case management, an outline of content helps organize information into a logical sequence. Material needs to progress from simple to complex because a person must learn the simple facts and concepts before learning how to make associations or complex interpretations of ideas. Staff nurses in acute care settings often focus on the simpler, more essential concepts, whereas home health nurses can better address complex issues. For

example, a nurse plans to teach a wife how to feed her husband, who has a gastric tube. The nurse will first teach the wife how to measure the tube feeding and manipulate the equipment. Once the wife has accomplished this, instruction on how to administer the feeding will occur.

Begin instruction with essential content because patients are more likely to remember information that you teach early in a teaching session. For example, immediately after surgical removal of a malignant breast tumor, a patient has many learning needs. To ensure that all essential material is covered, start with content considered to be high priority, such as how to monitor an incision site for signs of infection. Deal with the emotional aspects of a cancer diagnosis and complete the teaching session with informative but less critical content, such as how often follow-up appointments will occur. Repetition reinforces learning. A concise summary of key content helps the learner remember the most important information (Bastable, 2017). Using instructional materials that contain the same summaries is very helpful.

Teamwork and Collaboration. During planning choose appropriate teaching methods that match the topics to be presented. Encourage the patient to offer suggestions about timing and methods and make referrals to other health care professionals (e.g., dietitians and physical, speech, or occupational therapists) when appropriate. As a nurse you are the member of the health care team primarily responsible for ensuring that all patient educational needs are met. However, sometimes patient needs are highly complex. In these cases identify appropriate health system educational resources available in the patient's community during planning. Examples of resources for patient education include diabetes education clinics, cardiac rehabilitation programs, prenatal classes, and support groups. When patients receive education and support from these types of resources, the nurse obtains a referral order (if necessary), encourages patients to attend educational sessions, and reinforces information taught. Resources that specialize in a particular health need (e.g., wound care or ostomy specialists) are integral to successful patient education.

REFLECT NOW

Your patient is a 44-year-old single man who was recently hospitalized due to an embolic stroke with residual left-sided weakness. He is left-handed and does not currently have any fine motor skills on the left side. He was found to have untreated hypertension and high cholesterol, so he was started on clopidogrel for secondary stroke prevention along with lisinopril for hypertension and atorvastatin for high cholesterol. What disciplines would you include when providing his discharge education?

◆ Implementation

The implementation of patient education depends on the accuracy of the nursing diagnoses identified for the patient's learning needs. On the basis of the nursing diagnoses, you develop a teaching plan (see Nursing Care Plan). Carefully evaluate the learning objectives and determine which teaching and learning principles most effectively and efficiently help the patient meet expected goals and outcomes. Implementation involves believing that each interaction with a patient is an opportunity to teach. Use evidence-based interventions to create an effective learning environment.

Maintaining Learning Attention and Participation. Active participation is key to learning. People learn better when more than one of the senses is stimulated. Audiovisual aids, group discussion, and role-playing are good teaching strategies. By actively experiencing a learning event, a person is more likely to retain knowledge. An educator's actions also increase learner attention and interest. When conducting a discussion with a learner, an educator stays active by changing the tone and intensity of his or her voice, making eye contact, and using gestures that accentuate key points of discussion. An effective educator engages learners, includes active learning strategies, and talks and moves among a group rather than remaining stationary behind a lectern or table. A learner remains interested in an educator who is actively enthusiastic about the subject under discussion.

If a patient is anxious or inattentive, implement strategies such as relaxation and deep breathing to decrease the patient's anxiety (see Chapter 37). Have the patient practice these skills before instruction to improve his or her comprehension and understanding of the information given (Bastable, 2017). Also remember to manage any symptoms, such as pain or nausea, before beginning a teaching session so that a patient can better relax during instruction.

Building on Existing Knowledge.

A patient learns best on the basis of preexisting cognitive abilities and knowledge. Thus an educator is more effective when he or she presents information that builds on a learner's existing knowledge. For example, a patient who has lived with multiple sclerosis for several years is beginning a new medication that is given subcutaneously. Before teaching the patient how to prepare the medication and give the injection, the nurse asks about the patient's previous experience with injections. On assessment the nurse learns that the patient's father had diabetes and that the patient administered the insulin injections. The nurse thus individualizes the teaching plan by building on the patient's previous knowledge and experience with insulin injections and focuses on the unique approach the patient will use for self-injection.

Teaching Approaches.

A nurse's teaching approach is different from teaching methods. Some situations require an educator to be directive. Others require a nondirective approach. An effective educator concentrates on the task and uses teaching approaches appropriate to the learner's needs. A learner's needs and motives frequently change over time. Thus the effective educator is always aware of the need to modify teaching approaches.

Telling. Use the telling approach when there is limited time for teaching information (e.g., preparing a patient for an emergent diagnostic procedure). If a patient is highly anxious but it is vital for information to be given, telling is effective. When using telling, the nurse outlines the task that a patient will perform and gives simple, explicit instructions. There is no opportunity for feedback with this method.

Participating. In the participating approach a nurse and patient set objectives and become involved in the learning process together. The patient helps decide content, and the nurse guides and counsels the patient with pertinent information. In this method there is opportunity for discussion, feedback, mutual goal setting, and revision of the teaching plan. For example, a parent caring for a child with leukemia must learn how to care for the child at home and recognize problems that need to be reported immediately. The parent and nurse collaborate on developing an appropriate teaching plan for how to recognize and manage complications, maintain a healthy diet for the child, and maximize the child's ability to remain active. After each teaching session is completed, the parent and nurse review the objectives together, determine whether the objectives were met, and plan what will be covered in the next session.

Entrusting. The entrusting approach provides a patient the opportunity to manage self-care. The aim of the instructional approach is to provide the knowledge and skills that enable a patient to accept responsibilities and perform tasks correctly and consistently. The nurse observes the patient's progress and remains available to assist without introducing more new information. For example, a patient has been managing type 2 diabetes well for 10 years with oral medications, diet, and exercise. However, 1 year ago his diabetes changed, and it was difficult to control his hemoglobin A1c level (which reflects glucose control). As a result, the oral medications were discontinued, and insulin was added to his self-management plan. After initial instruction on dose management and injections, the nurse now monitors the patient's A1c level, offers reinforcement, and asks the patient if any new learning needs have developed. The nurse trusts the patient has become self-sufficient with managing insulin doses and injections.

Reinforcing. Reinforcement requires the use of a stimulus to increase the probability of a desired response. A learner who receives reinforcement before or after a desired learning behavior is more likely to repeat that behavior. Reinforcers are positive or negative. Positive reinforcement such as a smile or verbal praise promotes desired behaviors. Although negative reinforcement such as frowning or criticizing can decrease an undesired response, it may also discourage participation and cause the learner to withdraw (Bastable, 2017). The effects of negative reinforcement are less predictable and often undesirable.

Reinforcers can come in the form of social acknowledgments (e.g., nods, smiles, words of encouragement), pleasurable activities (e.g., walks or play time), and tangible rewards (e.g., toys or food). Choosing an appropriate reinforcer to alter behavior requires careful observation of an individual's response to specific stimuli. When a nurse works with a patient, most reinforcers are social; however, material reinforcers may work well with young children. In adults reinforcement is more effective when the nurse has established a therapeutic relationship with the patient. Whatever the form, it is important that reinforcement closely follows the desired behavior. Timing is essential so that a clear correlation between the desired behavior and reward is established (Bastable, 2017).

Incorporating Teaching With Nursing Care.

Many nurses find that they are able to teach more effectively while delivering nursing care. This becomes easier as you gain confidence in your clinical skills. For example, while hanging blood, you explain to the patient why the blood is necessary and the symptoms of a transfusion reaction that need to be reported immediately. Another example is to explain the side effects of a medication while administering it. An informal, unstructured style relies on the positive therapeutic relationship between nurse and patient, which fosters spontaneity in the teaching-learning process. Teaching during routine care is efficient and cost-effective (Fig. 25.3).

Instructional Methods.

Choose instructional methods that match a patient's learning needs, the time available for teaching, the setting, the resources available, and your comfort level with teaching. Skilled educators are flexible in altering teaching methods according to a learner's responses. An experienced educator uses a variety of techniques and teaching aids. Specific teaching strategies should include open-ended questioning and problem-solving exercises. Do not expect to be an expert educator when first entering nursing practice. Learning to become an effective educator takes time and practice.

When first starting to teach patients, it helps to remember that patients perceive you as an expert. However, this does not mean that they expect you to have all of the answers. It simply means that they expect that you will keep them appropriately informed. Effective nurses keep the teaching plan simple and focused on patients' needs.

Verbal One-on-One Discussion. The most common method of instruction is a one-on-one verbal discussion. This approach involves sharing information directly with a patient. Verbal education of patients and family members requires an interdisciplinary approach that takes into account learning styles, literacy, and culture to apply clear communication and instructional methods (Marcus, 2014). This approach typically is done in an informal manner, allowing a patient to ask questions and share concerns. Speaking with an "expert" nurse or health care provider is a preferred educational modality for many

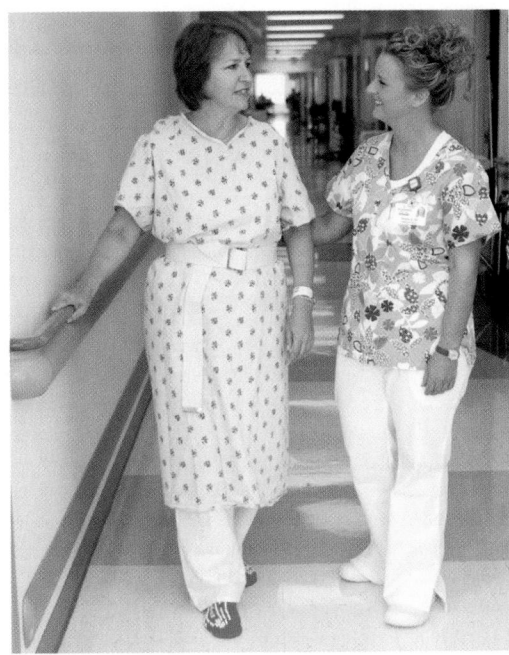

FIG. 25.3 Teaching postoperative care while walking with the patient uses time efficiently.

patients (Kit Delgado et al., 2010). However, education is ineffective if verbal instruction is not done well. Instructional information must be accurate, timely, complete, and unambiguous when presented. Research has shown that verbal communication is often partly understood, misunderstood, or misinterpreted (Marcus, 2014). Also, nurses today often do not have the time to fully listen to patients and engage in quality verbal instruction. The Brigham and Women's Faulkner Hospital (BWFH) Patient/Family Education Committee reviewed research on verbal instruction and developed the EDUCATE Model (Table 25.4) (Marcus, 2014). It is a process-based model that leads a nurse educator through five stages of verbal education to reach teaching and education goals. The EDUCATE model is simple but enables all health care providers to better guide verbal education and ensure that education is more patient- and family-centered.

Group Instruction. You may choose to teach patients in groups because of the advantages associated with group teaching. Groups are an economical way to teach a number of patients at one time. Patients are able to interact with one another and learn from the experiences of others. Learning in a group of six or less is most effective and avoids distracting behaviors (Bastable, 2017). Group-based instruction benefits include deeper understanding, longer retention, increased social support, and more active participation (Bastable, 2017). Group instruction often involves both lecture and discussion. Lectures are highly structured and efficient in helping groups of patients learn standard content about a subject. A lecture does not ensure that learners are actively thinking about the material presented; thus discussion and practice sessions are essential. After a lecture, learners need the opportunity to share ideas and seek clarification. Group discussions allow patients and families to learn from one another as they review common experiences. A productive group discussion helps participants solve problems and arrive at solutions toward improving each member's health. To be an effective group leader, you guide participation. Acknowledging a look of interest, asking questions, and summarizing key points foster group involvement. However, not all patients benefit from group discussions; sometimes the physical or emotional level of wellness makes participation difficult or impossible.

Preparatory Instruction. Patients frequently face unfamiliar tests or procedures that create significant anxiety about the procedure and outcome. Providing information about procedures often decreases anxiety because this gives patients a better idea of what to expect during their procedures, enhancing their sense of control. The known is less threatening than the unknown. Follow these guidelines for giving preparatory explanations:

- Describe physical sensations during a procedure. For example, when drawing a blood specimen, explain that the patient will feel a sticking sensation as the needle punctures the skin.
- Describe the cause of the sensation, preventing misinterpretation of the experience. For example, explain that a needlestick burns because the alcohol used to clean the skin enters the puncture site.
- Prepare patients only for aspects of the experience that others have commonly noticed. For example, explain that it is normal for a tight tourniquet to cause a person's hand to tingle and feel numb.
- Be sure the patients know when the results will be available and who will give them the results of their tests and/or procedures.

A cognitive regulation technique called "reappraisal" can be effective in reducing anticipatory anxiety. This cognitive change strategy involves changing the meaning of a stimulus in a way that alters its emotional impact (Sheppes and Gross, 2011). For example, rather than saying to a patient during the insertion of an intravenous catheter, "You are going to feel a stick," say instead, "The catheter I am about to place in your arm will be our way of giving you the fluids and medications you need." Reappraisal typically includes reconsideration or reframing of an emotional event in less emotional terms (Yoshimura et al., 2014).

Demonstrations. Use demonstrations when teaching psychomotor skills such as preparing a syringe, bathing an infant, crutch walking, or taking a pulse. Demonstrations are most effective when learners first observe the educator and during a return demonstration have the chance to practice the skill. Combine a demonstration with discussion to clarify concepts and feelings. An effective demonstration requires advanced planning:

1. Be sure that the learner can see each step of the demonstration easily. Position the learner to provide a clear view of the skill being performed.
2. Assemble and organize the equipment. Make sure that all equipment works.
3. Perform each step slowly and accurately in sequence while analyzing the knowledge and skills involved, and allow the patient to handle the equipment.
4. Review the rationale and steps of the procedure.
5. Encourage the patient to ask questions so that he or she understands each step.
6. Judge proper speed and timing of the demonstration on the basis of the patient's cognitive abilities and anxiety level.
7. To demonstrate mastery of the skill, have the patient perform a return demonstration under the same conditions that will be experienced at home or in the place where the skill is to be performed. For example, when a patient needs to learn to walk with crutches, simulate the home environment. If the patient's home has stairs, the patient would practice going up and down a staircase in the hospital.

Analogies. Learning occurs when an educator translates complex language or ideas into words or concepts that a patient understands. Analogies supplement verbal instruction with familiar images that make complex information more real and understandable. For example, when explaining arterial blood pressure, use an analogy of the flow of water through a hose. Follow these general principles when using analogies:

- Be familiar with the concept.

TABLE 25.4	**EDUCATE Model**					
E	**D**	**U**	**C**	**A**		**T E**
Enhance Comprehension and Retention	**Deliver Patient-Centered Education**	**Understand the Learner**	**Communicate Clearly and Effectively**	**Address Health Literacy and Cultural Competence**		**Teaching and Education Goals**
Use a question list so that patients can ask questions and providers can answer them (Posma et al., 2009).	Talk to—NOT AT—people (Behar-Horenstein et al., 2005).	Find out what the patient already knows before providing information; ask, "What do you already know about high blood pressure?" (Kripalani and Weiss, 2006).	New communication skills require practice to use them effectively, and structured skill development exercises may be helpful for providers (Kripalani and Weiss, 2006).	Ask patients, "Do you need help understanding health information?" (TJC, 2010).		Adequate preparation for teaching and learning
Repeat the most important information (Margolis, 2004; Ronco et al., 2012; Takemura et al., 2011).	Practice empathetic skills, especially when the view of the patient is different from that of the provider (Cant and Aroni, 2008; Posma et al., 2009; Skorpen and Malterud, 1997).	Be aware of nonverbal messages when delivering verbal communication, including gestures, body language, and dress (Cant and Aroni, 2008).	Present the most important information first (Margolis, 2004). Emphasize one to three key points (Kripalani & Weiss, 2006). Focus on one issue at a time (Avitzur, 2011). Present the information in logical blocks (Remshardt, 2011). Use concrete instructions (Margolis, 2004).	Supplement and reinforce verbal education with simple written and visual materials (Behar-Horenstein et al., 2005; Margolis, 2004); however, the materials should be used for reinforcement and not to replace verbal instruction or direct interaction.		Effective teaching methods
Ask patients to repeat information in their own words (Engel et al., 2009).	Ask patients about their life experiences and build upon them when teaching (Montin et al., 2010). Use metaphors comparing the patient's care to his or her life situation (Behar-Horenstein et al., 2005).	Determine the patient's barriers to health literacy (Paasche-Orlow, 2011). Use interviews and observation to assess a patient's ability to learn (Behar-Horenstein et al., 2005).	Use easy-to-understand language (Kripalani and Weiss, 2006; Margolis, 2004; Posma et al., 2009).	Use an interpreter if a patient requires one due to language or disability (Dreger, 2001; Lieu et al., 2007). Avoid using technical terminology or medical jargon (The Joint Commission, 2010).		Overcoming barriers to learning
Provide information in several different ways to make sure the patient understands (Skorpen & Malterud, 1997). Digital recordings of patient consultations can be effective for patient recall of verbal education (Friedman, et al., 2011).	Pay attention to the patient's worries and fears and try to dispel them (Posma et al., 2009).	Include family members in your education when appropriate. On many occasions (e.g., for pain management) family members also need to be educated (Behar-Horenstein et al., 2005).	Patients must be given an opportunity to ask questions before discharge. Give them time to speak (Behar-Horenstein et al., 2005).	Consider using a scripted tool to make patient education clearer and more understandable (Piazza et al., 2012).		Teaching as an interactive process
Use the teach-back method (Anonymous, 2008; Kripalani and Weiss, 2006; The Joint Commission, 2010).	Ask patients to state their goals of medical care to begin a discussion (Paasche-Orlow, 2011).	Realize that patients may not be aware that they do not understand what is being communicated to them (Engel et al., 2009).	Consider using audio recordings of patient consultations to improve patient recall of important information (Friedman et al., 2011).	Do not just ask the patient, "Do you understand?" Regardless of their ability to understand, many patients may still answer, "Yes" (The Joint Commission, 2010).		Assessment of learning

Note: The last column of the EDUCATE model stands for T and E, Teaching and Education goals; it outlines principles of the model as they relate to the model's individual components.

From Marcus C: Strategies for improving the quality of verbal patient and family education: a review of the literature and creation of the EDUCATE model, *Health Psychol Behav Med.* 2(1): 482–495, 2014.

- Know the patient's background, experience, and culture so that you can make an analogy relevant.
- Keep the analogy simple and clear.

Role-Playing. In role-playing people are asked to play themselves or someone else. Patients learn required skills and feel more confident in being able to perform them independently. The technique involves rehearsing a desired behavior. For example, a nurse who is teaching a parent how to respond to a child's behavior pretends to be a child who is having a temper tantrum. The parent responds to the nurse who is pretending to be the child. Afterward the nurse evaluates the parent's response and determines whether an alternative approach would have been more appropriate.

Simulation. Simulation is a useful technique for teaching problem solving, application, and independent thinking. During individual or group discussion you pose a pertinent problem or situation for patients to solve. For example, patients with heart disease plan a meal that is low in cholesterol and fat. The patients in the group decide which foods are appropriate. You ask the group members to present their diet, providing an opportunity to identify mistakes and reinforce correct information.

Illiteracy and Other Disabilities. Patients with low health literacy, illiteracy, and learning disabilities have an impaired ability to analyze instructions or synthesize information. Many of these patients have not acquired or are unable to acquire the problem-solving skills of drawing conclusions and inferences from experience, and they do not ask questions to obtain or clarify information that has been presented. Using strategies to promote health literacy creates a more patient-centered approach to health education and can have a significant impact on patient outcomes (Edelman and Kudzma, 2017) (Box 25.6). You can promote health literacy by creating a safe, shame-free environment, using clear and purposeful communication techniques, using visual aids to reinforce spoken material, and by taking special care to evaluate patient understanding of the content. Follow the EDUCATE model (see Table 25.4).

Sometimes patients have sensory deficits that affect how you present information (see Chapter 49). For example, patients who are deaf may require a sign language interpreter. Not all people who are deaf read lips. Therefore it is very important to provide clear written materials that match the patients' reading level. Visual impairments also affect the teaching strategy you use. Many people who are blind have acute listening skills. Avoid shouting, and announce your presence to patients with visual impairments before approaching them. If the patient has partial vision, use colors and a print font size (14-point font or greater) that the patient is able to see. Be sure to use proper lighting. Other helpful interventions include audio recording teaching sessions and providing structured, well-organized instructions (Bastable, 2017).

BOX 25.6 PATIENT TEACHING

Teaching a Patient With Literacy or Learning Disability Problems

Objective
- Patient will perform desired behaviors accurately.

Teaching Strategies
- Establish trust with patient before beginning the teaching-learning session.
- Face patient when speaking. Sit at his or her level to maintain eye contact.
- Speak slowly and encourage questions.
- Use simple terminology. If necessary, explain medical terms using basic one- or two-syllable words.
- Keep teaching sessions short and to the point and minimize distractions. Include the most important information at the beginning of the session.
- Teach in increments and organize information into sections.
- Provide teaching materials written in plain language that reflect the reading level of the patient, with attention given to short words and sentences, large type, and simple format (generally, information written on a fifth-grade reading level is recommended for adult learners).
- Relate practical information to personal experiences or real-life situations.
- Use visual aids when appropriate and simple analogies or stories to personalize messages.
- Model appropriate behavior and use role-playing to help patient learn how to ask questions and ask for help effectively.
- Frequently ask patient for feedback to determine whether he or she comprehends information.
- Ask for return demonstrations, use the teach-back method, and clarify instructions when needed.
- Keep motivation high and recognize progress with positive reinforcement.
- Reinforce the most important information at the end of the session.
- Schedule teaching sessions at frequent intervals.

Evaluation

Use the principles of teach back to evaluate patient/family caregiver learning:
- I want to make sure I explained this information clearly. Please tell me why it is important for you to manage your illness.
- We discussed how it will be important for you to prepare a diet at home with the right type of foods. Let me see you prepare a sample menu for a breakfast, lunch, and dinner.

Data from Bastable S: *Nurse as educator: principles of teaching and learning for nursing practice,* ed 5, Burlington, VT, 2017, Jones & Bartlett.

🌐 BOX 25.7   CULTURAL ASPECTS OF CARE

Patient Education

Patient-centered education needs to be culturally sensitive for learning to occur. Sociocultural norms, values, and traditions often determine the importance of different health education topics and the preference of one learning approach over another. Educational efforts are especially challenging when patients and educators do not speak the same language or when written materials are not culturally sensitive and are written above patients' reading abilities.

Implications for Patient-Centered Care

- Develop a cultural awareness to establish and maintain respectful relationships with culturally diverse patients to encourage trust and communication (Bastable, 2017) (see Chapter 9).
- Implement the National CLAS Standards (https://www.thinkculturalhealth.hhs.gov/clas), a set of 15 action steps intended to advance health equity, improve quality, and help eliminate health care disparities (USDHHS, n.d.a).
- When you and the patient do not speak the same language, use trained and certified health care interpreters to provide health care information.
- Sociocultural factors influence a patient's perception of health and illness and how patients seek health care information (Bastable, 2017).
- Nurses need to have access to a variety of culturally diverse health care resources and should select teaching strategies that are relevant to the individual patient.

QSEN **Building Competency in Patient-Centered Care** You are assessing a 62-year-old patient named Betty at an outpatient neurology clinic; Betty was recently discharged from the hospital following an ischemic stroke. Betty was recently started on several new medications for secondary stroke prevention, including medications for high cholesterol and high blood pressure and thrombolytic therapy. While reviewing her medications, you find that she has difficulty understanding print ed teaching sheets. Betty discloses to you, "I had to drop out of school when I was 13 years old to take care of my younger siblings. I really haven't been to the doctor since my old doctor retired and I didn't like his replacement, and that was over 10 years ago." When asked where she keeps her medication, Betty shows you a grocery bag that has prescription bottles inside, and it includes both current and expired prescriptions. Which assessment questions and teaching strategies, approaches, and tools do you need to enhance Betty's learning and ability to take her medications as prescribed?

Answers to QSEN Activities can be found on the Evolve website.

Cultural Diversity. Accept a patient's cultural background and belief system and be prepared to offer culturally sensitive approaches in a patient's native language (see Chapter 9 and Box 25.7). Be careful not to generalize or stereotype patients solely on the basis of their culture. Collaborate with other nurses and educators to develop appropriate teaching approaches, and ask people from their cultural group to help by sharing their values and beliefs. Ethnic nurses are excellent resources who are able to provide input through their experiences to improve the care provided to members of their own community.

In addition, be aware of intergenerational conflicts of values. This occurs when immigrant parents uphold their traditional values and their children, who are exposed to American values in social encounters, develop beliefs similar to those of their American peers. Consider this conflict in values when providing information

to families or groups who have members from different generations. To enhance patient education in culturally diverse populations, know when and how to provide education while respecting cultural values. Modify teaching to accommodate for cultural differences. Research has shown that health outcomes are improved when education is given in the context of each person's specific cultural beliefs and practices (Bastable, 2017).

Using Teaching Tools. Many teaching tools are available for patient education. Selection of the right tool depends on the instructional method, a patient's learning needs, and the ability to learn (Table 25.5). For example, a printed pamphlet is not the best tool to use for a patient with poor reading comprehension, but an audio recording is a good choice for a patient with visual impairment. Health care agencies often provide clinicians with access to a variety of teaching resources. Be knowledgeable about what is available in your agency to better serve your patients. Also, if patients show interest in seeking information about their health from the Internet, inform them of the most reliable sources. For example, the American Cancer Society, American Lung Association, American Heart Association, and Centers for Disease Control and Prevention offer excellent information for laypeople.

Special Needs of Children and Older Adults. Children, adults, and older adults learn differently. You adapt teaching strategies to each learner. Children pass through several developmental stages (see Unit 2). In each developmental stage children acquire new cognitive and psychomotor abilities that respond to different types of teaching methods. Incorporate parental input in planning health education for children.

Older adults experience numerous physical and psychological changes as they age (see Chapter 14). These changes not only increase their educational needs but also create barriers to learning unless adjustments are made in nursing interventions. Sensory changes such as visual and hearing changes require adaptation of teaching methods to enhance functioning. Older adults learn and remember effectively if you pace the learning properly and if the material is relevant to the learner's needs and abilities. Although many older adults have slower cognitive function and reduced short-term memory, you facilitate learning in several ways to support behaviors that maximize the individual's capacity for self-care (Box 25.8).

Establish short-term goals when teaching older patients. Include family members who assume care for the patient. However, be sensitive to a patient's desire for assistance because offering unwanted support often results in negative outcomes and perceptions of nagging and interference. Not all relationships between older adults and other family members are therapeutic.

◆ Evaluation

Through the Patient's Eyes. An important part of evaluation is to determine whether the patient's expectations, identified during assessment, were met. You engage patients to determine if they perceive having learned what they expected. Be sure their expectations have been fully met. Does the patient have the sense that he or she can maintain self-care based on the information received? It is important to evaluate through the patient's eyes, considering the types of situations and environments that patients return to after receiving care. Evaluation helps the educator determine adequacy of teaching. If expectations have not been met, you revise the plan of care and offer additional instruction or reinforcement.

Patient Outcomes. Evaluation of any instructional approach involves measuring whether learning objectives were met. You gather data to

TABLE 25.5 Teaching Tools for Instruction

Description	Learning Implications
Written Materials	
Printed and Online Materials	
Written teaching tools available as pamphlets, booklets, brochures	Material needs to be easy to read. Information needs to be accurate and current. Method is ideal for understanding complex concepts and relationships.
Programmed Instruction	
Written sequential presentation of learning steps requiring that learners answer questions and educators tell them whether they are right or wrong	Instruction is primarily verbal, but the educator sometimes uses pictures or diagrams. Method requires active learning, giving immediate feedback, correcting wrong answers, and reinforcing right answers. Learner works at own pace.
Computer Instruction	
Use of programmed instruction format in which computers store response patterns for learners and select further lessons on basis of these patterns (programs can be individualized)	Method requires reading comprehension, psychomotor skills, and familiarity with computer.
Nonprint Materials	
Diagrams	
Illustrations show interrelationships by means of lines and symbols	Method demonstrates key ideas, summarizes, and clarifies key concept.
Graphs (Bar, Circle, or Line)	
Visual presentations of numerical data	Graphs help learner grasp information quickly about single concept.
Charts	
Highly condensed visual summary of ideas and facts that highlights series of ideas, steps, or events	Charts demonstrate relationship of several ideas or concepts. Method helps learners know what to do.
Pictures	
Photographs or drawings used to teach concepts in which the third dimension of shape and space is not important	Photographs are more desirable than diagrams because they more accurately portray the details of the real item.
Physical Objects	
Use of actual equipment, objects, or models to teach concepts or skills	Models are useful when real objects are too small, large, or complicated or are unavailable. Allows learners to manipulate objects that they will use later in skill.
Other Audiovisual Materials	
Slides, audiotapes, television, and videotapes used with printed material or discussion	Materials are useful for patients with reading comprehension problems and visual deficits.

measure whether the patient has the new knowledge, behaviors, or skills that education aimed to provide. You observe a patient's performance of any expected behavior or skill. You also ask evaluative questions, phrased carefully, then guide the patient to identity or describe information so that you can determine whether the established goals and learning objectives were met. For example, you might say, "Tell me specifically the times of day you are to take this new medication" or "We discussed the safety risks in your home; tell me what you plan to do to remove them." Consider these questions as you evaluate a patient's education plan.

- Were the patient's goals or outcomes realistic and observable?
- Is the patient able to perform the behavior or skill in the natural setting (e.g., home)?
- How well is the patient able to answer questions about the topic?
- Does the patient continue to have problems understanding the information or performing a skill? If so, how can you change the interventions to enhance knowledge or skill performance?

Evaluate a patient's learning in a timely manner so that you can make adjustments or changes as needed.

The nurse is legally responsible for providing accurate, timely patient information that promotes continuity of care; therefore, it is essential to document the outcomes of teaching. Documentation of patient teaching also supports quality improvement efforts, meets TJC standards, and promotes third-party reimbursement. Teaching flow sheets and written plans of care (e.g., CareMaps) are excellent records that document the plan, implementation, and evaluation of learning.

Teach-Back. It is imperative to assess whether a patient understands information during an educational session. One way to evaluate patient understanding is with the teach-back method. Teach-back is a closed-loop communication technique that assesses patient retention of the information given during a teaching session. To perform teach-back, ask the patient to explain material that was discussed, such as the role of diet and exercise in managing blood glucose levels, or to demonstrate a skill, such as self-monitoring blood glucose. The response allows you to determine the degree to which the patient remembers and understands what was taught or demonstrated. Use nonjudgmental language so that patients do not feel tested (Flanders, 2018). For example, say, "I want to

BOX 25.8 FOCUS ON OLDER ADULTS

Providing Patient Education

Facilitate learning by using the following teaching strategies when providing patient education to older adults:

- Promote concentration and learner readiness by scheduling teaching sessions when the patient is comfortable and well rested. Provide medication for pain relief when necessary. Ensure that the patient is not drowsy from medication during the education session.
- Create a casual and relaxed learning environment.
- Establish personalized, realistic short-term learning goals.
- Provide sufficient lighting with low glare.
- If using visual aids or written materials to supplement instruction, assess the patient's reading ability and make sure that information is printed in a large-size font and in a color that contrasts with the background (e.g., black 14-point print on matte white paper). Avoid blues and greens because these colors can become more difficult to distinguish with age.
- To accommodate for hearing loss, present information slowly and in a clear, low tone of voice. Eliminate any extraneous noises and directly face the learner when speaking. Do not place your hand near your mouth while a

hearing-impaired patient is trying to hear (or lip-read) instructions. Mustaches can make lipreading difficult for a hearing-impaired patient.

- Encourage the use of prosthesis (i.e., glasses, hearing aid), and ensure proper fit and working condition.
- Allow sufficient time to process and comprehend new information.
- Build on existing knowledge and present content in a way that relates to relevant past life experiences.
- Make information meaningful by using concrete examples that apply to current situations.
- Present only the most significant information to avoid overwhelming the learner. Use repetition to reinforce content.
- When giving instructions or teaching a new skill, give concise, step-by-step directions. Assess understanding of each step before moving ahead.
- Provide regular positive reinforcement.
- Keep teaching sessions short and allow for frequent breaks. Schedule follow-up sessions as needed to ensure learning.
- Conclude with a brief summary and allow sufficient time for questions and feedback.

Data from Touhy TA, Jett KF: *Ebersole and Hess' toward healthy aging*, ed 9, St Louis, 2015, Mosby; Edelman C, Kudzma EC: *Health promotion throughout the life span*, ed 9, St Louis, 2017, Mosby.

be certain that I taught this well. Can you please describe some symptoms of a stroke?" Examples of teach-back prompts and questions include:

1. "Tell me in your own words how you will take this medication at home."
2. "Please demonstrate how to use this blood glucose monitor."
3. "What are some of the side effects that you should watch for?"
4. "When will you call the office regarding your blood pressure?"
5. "Please show me how to request a refill of this medication online."

If the patient has difficulty recalling the material or demonstrating a skill, modify and repeat the content and reassess his or her retention. Also, take ownership of the teaching experience by responding, "I must not have explained stroke symptoms very well. Let me try again." Patient understanding is confirmed when the patient can accurately restate the information in his or her own words (Bastable, 2017).

KEY POINTS

- The three purposes of patient education are health promotion and illness prevention, health restoration, and coping.
- Teaching and learning generally begin when a person identifies a need for knowing or acquiring an ability to do something.
- Nurses have a legal responsibility to provide education to all patients.
- The Joint Commission's Speak Up initiatives help patients understand their rights when receiving medical care.
- An effective educator provides a mechanism for evaluating the success of a teaching plan and then provides positive reinforcement.
- The three domains of learning including cognitive, affective, and psychomotor.
- The ability to learn depends on physical and cognitive attributes, developmental level, physical wellness, and intellectual thought processes. A person's learning style affects his or her preferences for learning.
- Self-efficacy is a concept included in many health promotion theories because it often is a strong predictor of healthy behaviors.
- An adult's readiness to learn is often associated with his or her developmental stage and other events occurring in his or her life.
- Both the nursing and teaching processes require assessment and evaluation. The nursing and teaching processes differ in that the

nursing process requires assessment of all sources of data to determine a patient's total health care needs.

- A nurse bases educational priorities on a patient's immediate needs, nursing diagnoses, and the goals and outcomes established for the patient. Priorities also depend on what a patient perceives to be most important.
- The ideal environment for learning is well lit and has good ventilation, appropriate furniture, and a comfortable temperature.
- At the end of the session, the nurse uses the teach-back technique to evaluate learning by asking the patient to explain the material that was discussed.

REFLECTIVE LEARNING

- Reflect on a patient you cared for recently. How did you determine if the patient understood the care you provided during that experience?
- Consider that you have a young adult patient who has to take an antibiotic three times a day. How would your teaching approach be different if the patient were an older adult and had difficulty seeing and hearing?
- Go to a website that provides patient information about an illness (e.g., heart disease, diabetes). Is the information easy to understand? How could the information be presented in a way that would enhance its readability?

REVIEW QUESTIONS

1. A patient asks a nurse to provide instruction on how to perform a breast self-exam. Which domains are required to learn this skill? (Select all that apply.)
   1. Affective domain
   2. Sensory domain
   3. Cognitive domain
   4. Attentional domain
   5. Psychomotor domain

2. A patient suddenly experiences a severe headache with numbness and decreased movement in the left arm. The emergency room physician suspects a stroke and is going to have the patient undergo an emergent angiogram to remove the clot. Which teaching approach is most appropriate?
   1. Selling approach
   2. Telling approach
   3. Entrusting approach
   4. Participating approach

3. A nurse is caring for a young patient who has been told he has multiple sclerosis. The nurse has planned time to conduct a teaching session that will focus on the disease and principles of management. The nurse chooses to use the EDUCATE model to proceed with instruction. Which of the following are components of the model? (Select all that apply.)
   1. State goals of the session for the patient.
   2. Repeat the most important information.
   3. Practice empathetic skills.
   4. Be aware of nonverbal messages.
   5. Use a standard question list for the chosen topic.

4. A nurse is teaching an older adult patient about ways to detect a melanoma. Which of the following are age-appropriate teaching techniques for this patient? (Select all that apply.)
   1. Speak in a low tone.
   2. Begin and end the session with the most important information regarding melanoma.
   3. Provide a pamphlet about melanoma with large font in blues and greens.
   4. Provide specific information in frequent, small amounts for older adult patients.
   5. Speak quickly so that you do not take up much of the patient's time.

5. A 55-year-old adult male has been in the hospital over a week following surgical complications. The patient has had limited activity but is now finally ordered to begin a mobility program. The patient just returned from several diagnostic tests and tells the nurse he is feeling quite fatigued. The nurse prepares to instruct the patient on the mobility program protocol. Which of the following learning principles will likely be affected by this patient's condition?
   1. Motivation to learn
   2. Developmental stage
   3. Stage of grief
   4. Readiness to learn

6. A patient recovering from open heart surgery is taught how to cough and deep breathe using a pillow to support or splint the chest incision. Following the teaching session, which of the following is the best way for the nurse to evaluate whether learning has taken place?
   1. Verbalization of steps to use in splinting
   2. Selecting from a series of flash cards the images showing the correct technique
   3. Return demonstration
   4. Cloze test

7. A patient's cultural background affects the motivation for learning. Using the ACCESS model, match the nursing approach with the correct model component.

ACCESS model component	Nursing approach
1. Assessment	A. Help patients feel culturally secure and able to maintain their cultural identity.
2. Communication	B. Remain aware of verbal and nonverbal responses.
3. Cultural	C. Be aware of how patients from diverse backgrounds perceive their care needs.
4. Establishment	D. Become aware of your patient's culture and your own cultural biases.
5. Sensitivity	E. Learn about the patient's health beliefs and practices.
6. Safety	F. Show respect by creating a caring rapport.

8. A 63-year-old woman is a family caregiver for her 88-year-old mother who has dementia. The caregiver asked the home health nurse how to manage her mother when she becomes confused and violent. The best instructional method a nurse can use for this situation is:
   1. Demonstration
   2. Preparatory instruction
   3. Role-playing
   4. Group instruction with other family caregivers

9. A nurse is preparing to teach a patient who has sleep apnea how to use a CPAP machine at night. Which action is most appropriate for the nurse to perform first?
   1. Allow patient to manipulate machine and look at parts.
   2. Provide a teach-back session.
   3. Set mutual goals for the education session.
   4. Discuss the purpose of the machine and how it works.

10. Which of the following scenarios demonstrate that learning has taken place? (Select all that apply.)
   1. A patient listens to a nurse's review of the warning signs of a stroke.
   2. A patient describes how to set up a pill organizer for newly ordered medicines.
   3. A patient attends a spinal cord injury support group.
   4. A patient demonstrates how to take his blood pressure at home.
   5. A patient reviews written information about resources for cancer survivors.

Answers: 1. 3, 5; 2. 3; 3. 2, 3, 4; 4. 1, 2, 4; 5. 4; 6. 3; 7. 1E, 2B, 3D, 4F, 5C, 6A; 8. 3; 9. 3; 10. 2, 4.

Rationales for Review Questions can be found on the Evolve website.

REFERENCES

American Hospital Association: *The patient care partnership: understanding expectations, rights, and responsibilities*, 2018, http://www.aha.org/aha/issues/Communicating-With-Patients/pt-care-partnership.html. Accessed January 2, 2019.

Bastable SB: *Nurse as educator: principles of teaching and learning for nursing practice*, ed 5, Burlington, VT, 2017, Jones & Bartlett.

Billings DM, Halstead JA: *Teaching in nursing: a guide for faculty*, ed 5, St Louis, 2016, Elsevier.

Centers for Disease Control and Prevention: *Health literacy*, 2016, https://www.cdc.gov/healthliteracy/shareinteract/TellOthers.html. Accessed August 26, 2019.

Edelman C, Kudzma EC: *Health promotion throughout the life span*, ed 9, St Louis, 2017, Mosby.

Flanders SA: Effective patient education: evidence and common sense, *Medsurg Nurs* 27(1):55–58, 2018.

The Joint Commission: *Advancing effective communication, cultural competence, and patient- and family-centered care: A roadmap for hospitals*, Oakbrook Terrace, IL, 2010, The Commission, http://www.jointcommission.org/assets/1/6/aroadmapforhospitalsfinalversion727.pdf. Accessed August 26, 2019.

Killian S: *Top 10 evidence-based teaching strategies*, 2013, http://www.evidencebasedteaching.org.au/evidence-based-teaching-strategies/. Accessed December 6, 2019.

Krathwohl DR, et al.: *Taxonomy of educational objectives: the classification of educational goals. Handbook II: affective domain*, New York, 1956, David McKay Co., Inc.

Krathwohl DR: A revision of Bloom's taxonomy: an overview, *Theory into Practice* 41(4), Autumn 2002, College of Education, The Ohio State University, https://www.depauw.edu/files/resources/krathwohl.pdf. Accessed January 3, 2019.

Learning Disabilities Association of America: *ADHD*, 2018, http://ldaamerica.org/types-of-learning-disabilities/adhd/. Accessed July 10, 2018.

Lorig K: Chronic disease self-management program: insights from the eye of the storm, *Front Public Health* 2:253, 2015.

Medicare: *Resident rights*, n.d., https://www.medicare.gov/nursinghomecompare/resources/resident-rights.html. Accessed August 18, 2019.

Miller M, Stoeckel P: *Client education: theory and practice*, ed 3, Sudbury, MA, 2019, Jones & Bartlett.

Miller WR, Rollnick S: *Motivational interviewing: preparing people for change*, ed 2, New York, 2002, Guilford Press.

Parnell TA: *Health literacy in nursing: providing person-centered care*, New York, NY, 2015, Springer Publishing.

Purnell LD: *Guide to culturally competent health care*, Philadelphia, 2014, F.A. Davis.

Quality and Safety Education for Nurses (QSEN): *Competency KSAs (pre-licensure)*, 2019, http://qsen.org/competencies/pre-licensure-ksas/#patient-centered_care. Accessed January 4, 2019.

Stewart FE, Fox C: Encouraging patients to change unhealthy behaviors with motivational interviewing, *Fam Pract Manag* 18(3):21–25, 2011.

The Joint Commission (TJC): *Comprehensive accreditation manual for hospitals: the official handbook (E-dition)*, The Joint Commission, 2018a.

The Joint Commission (TJC): *Speak up initiatives*, 2018b, http://www.jointcommission.org/speakup.aspx. Accessed June 12, 2018.

US Department of Education: *Adult education and literacy*, 2015, http://www2.ed.gov/about/offices/list/ovae/pi/AdultEd/index.html. Accessed June 25, 2015.

US Department of Health: Human Services, office of minority health (USDHHS): National CLAS standards, n.d.a., https://www.thinkculturalhealth.hhs.gov/clas. Accessed January 8, 2019.

Wilson LO: *Three domains of learning : Cognitive, affective, psychomotor*, The Second Principle, 2019, https://thesecondprinciple.com/instructional-design/threedomainsoflearning/. Accessed January 3, 2019.

World Health Organization (WHO): *Health promotion. Track 2: health literacy and health behavior*, 2018, http://www.who.int/healthpromotion/conferences/7gchp/track2/en/. Accessed January 5, 2019.

RESEARCH REFERENCES

Alanazi AA: Reducing anxiety in preoperative patients: a systematic review, *Br J Nurs* 23(7):387–393, 2014.

Almkuist KD: Using teach-back method to prevent 30-day readmissions in patients with heart failure: a systematic review, *Medsurg Nurs* 26(5):309–314, 2017.

Anderson LW, Krathwohl DR, editors: *A taxonomy for learning, teaching, and assessing: a revision of Bloom's taxonomy of educational objectives*, Boston, MA, 2001, Allyn & Bacon.

Anonymous: Create a standard for communication despite patient's level of health literacy, *Patient Educ Manage* 15(4):37, 2008.

Avitzur O: How to make your doctor listen, *Consum Rep* 76(7):13, 2011.

Axon RN, et al.: Evolution and initial experience of a statewide care transitions quality improvement collaborative: preventing avoidable readmissions together, *Popul Health Manag* 19(1):4–10, 2016.

Bandura A: *Self-efficacy: the exercise of control*, New York, 1997, WH Freeman.

Behar-Horenstein LS, et al.: Improving patient care through patient–family education programs, *Hosp Top* 83(1):21–27, 2005.

Boyde M, et al.: Self-care educational intervention to reduce hospitalizations in heart failure: a randomized controlled trial, *Eur J Cardiovasc Nurs* 17(2):178–185, 2018.

Cant RP, Aroni RA: Exploring dietitians' verbal and nonverbal communication skills for effective dietitian–patient communication, *J Hum Nutr Diet* 21(5):502–511, 2008.

Dreger V: Communication: an important assessment and teaching tool, *Insight* 26(2):57–60, 2001.

Engel KG, et al.: Patient comprehension of emergency department care and instructions: are patients aware of when they do not understand? *Ann Emerg Med* 53(4):454–461, 2009.

Festinger L: *A theory of cognitive dissonance*, Palo Alto, CA, 1957, Stanford University Press.

Friedman AJ, et al.: Effective teaching strategies and methods of delivery for patient education: a systematic review and practice guideline recommendations, *J Cancer Educ* 26(1):12–21, 2011.

Gruber, M.: Cognitive dissonance theory and motivation for change: A case study, *Gastroenterol Nurs*, 26(6), 242, 2003.

Hochbaum GM: *Public participation in medical screening programs: a sociopsychological study, PHS Publication No. 572*, Washington, DC, 1958, US Government Printing Office.

Kit Delgado M, et al.: Multicenter study of preferences for health education in the emergency department population, *Acad Emerg Med* 17(6):652–658, 2010.

Kripalani S, Weiss BD: Teaching about health literacy and clear communication, *J Gen Intern Med* 21(8):888–890, 2006, http://www.ncbi.nlm.nih.gov/pmc/articles/PMC1831575/.

Lieu CC, et al.: Communication strategies for nurses interacting with deaf patients, *Medsurg Nurs* 16(4):239–245, 2007.

Lundahl B, et al.: Motivational interviewing in medical care settings: a systematic review and meta-analysis of randomized controlled trials, *Patient Educ Couns* 93(2):157–168, 2013.

Marcus C: Strategies for improving the quality of verbal patient and family education: a review of the literature and creation of the EDUCATE model, *Health Psychol Behav Med* 2(1):482–495, 2014.

Margolis RH: Boosting memory with information counseling: helping patients understand the nature of disorders and how to manage them, *The ASHA Leader* 9(14):10–13, 2004, https://leader.pubs.asha.org/doi/10.1044/leader.FTR5.09142004.10. Accessed August 18, 2019.

Montin L, et al.: Total joint arthroplasty patient perception of received knowledge of care, *Orthop Nurs* 29(4):246–253, 2010.

Paasche-Orlow M: Caring for patients with limited health literacy: a 76-year-old man with multiple medical problems, *JAMA* 306(10):1122–1129, 2011.

Pender NJ: A conceptual model for preventive health behavior, *Nurs Outlook* 23(6):385–390, 1975.

Peter D, et al.: Reducing readmissions using teach-back: enhancing patient and family education, *J Nurs Adm* 45(1):35–42, 2015.

Piazza G, et al.: Patient education program for venous thromboembolism prevention in hospitalized patients, *Am J Med* 125(3):258–264, 2012.

Posma ER, et al.: Older cancer patients' information and support needs surrounding treatment: an evaluation through the eyes of patients, relatives and professionals, *BMC Nurs* 8(1), 2009.

Prochaska JO, et al.: The transtheoretical model of behavior change. In Shumaker SS, Schron EB, editors: *The hand-book of health behavior change*, ed 2, New York, 1998, Springer Publishing Company, pp 59–84.

Remshardt MA: The impact of patient literacy on healthcare practices, *Nurs Manage* 42(11):24–29, 2011.

Ronco M, et al.: Patient education outcomes in surgery: a systematic review from 2004 to 2010, *Int J Evid Based Healthc* 10(4):309–323, 2012.

Savage K, et al.: Preferences in learning styles and modes of information delivery in patients receiving first-day education for radiation therapy, *J Med Imaging Radiat Sci* 48(2):193–198, 2017.

Sheppes G, Gross JJ: Is timing everything? Temporal considerations in emotional regulation, *Pers Soc Psychol Rev* 15:319–331, 2011.

Skorpen JB, Malterud K: What did the doctor say – what did the patient hear? Operational knowledge in clinical communication, *Fam Pract* 14(5):382–386, 1997.

Spencer JC, Wheeler SB: A systematic review of motivational interviewing interventions in cancer patients and survivors, *Patient Educ Couns* 99(7):1099–1105, 2016.

Takemura M, et al.: Relationships between repeated instruction on inhalation therapy, medication adherence, and health status in chronic obstructive pulmonary disease, *Int J Chronic Obstr Pulm Dis* 6:97–104, 2011. http://www.ncbi.nlm.nih.gov/pmc/articles/PMC3048085/.

The Joint Commission: *Advancing effective communication, cultural competence, and patient- and family-centered care: a roadmap for hospitals*, Oakbrook Terrace, IL, 2010, Author. http://www.jointcommission.org/assets/1/6/aroadmapforhospitalsfinalversion727.pdf. Accessed January 8, 2019.

US Department of Health and Human Services (USDHHS): Quick guide to health literacy, n.d.b., https://health.gov/communication/literacy/quickguide/factsbasic.htm. Accessed January 5, 2019.

Yoshimura S, et al.: Neural basis of anticipatory anxiety reappraisals, *PLoS One* 9(7), 2014.

Zhou Y, et al.: Effects of a nurse-led phone follow-up education program based on the self-efficacy among patients with cardiovascular disease, *J Cardiovasc Nurs* 33(1):E15–E23, 2018.

26

Informatics and Documentation

OBJECTIVES

- Identify the purposes of a health care record.
- Discuss the relationship between documentation and financial reimbursement for health care.
- Discuss legal guidelines for documentation.
- Identify ways to maintain confidentiality of health care record data.
- Describe guidelines for quality documentation.
- Identify appropriate and inappropriate use of abbreviation(s) in health care documentation.

- Describe different methods used in record keeping.
- Identify elements to include when documenting a patient's discharge plan.
- Describe elements to include in documentation of telephone conversations with providers.
- Discuss the relationship between informatics and quality health care.
- Discuss the specific competencies in informatics for new graduate nurses entering the workforce.

KEY TERMS

Accreditation, p. 370
Acuity rating system, p. 376
Case management, p. 377
Charting by exception (CBE), p. 374
Clinical decision support system (CDSS), p. 379
Clinical information system (CIS), p. 378
Clinical practice guidelines (CPG), p. 375
Computerized provider order entry (CPOE), p. 378
Critical pathways, p. 377
Diagnosis-related group (DRG), p. 366

Documentation, p. 365
Electronic health record (EHR), p. 368
Electronic health record system (EHRS), p. 368
Electronic medical record (EMR), p. 368
Firewall, p. 369
Flow sheets, p. 372
Health care informatics, p. 379
Health care information system (HIS), p. 378
Health information technology (HIT), p. 377

Health record, p. 365
Incident (occurrence) report, p. 376
Meaningful use, p. 368
Narrative documentation, p. 372
Nursing clinical information system (NCIS), p. 378
Nursing informatics, p. 379
Password, p. 369
Protected health information (PHI), p. 369
Standardized care plans, p. 375
Variances, p. 377

MEDIA RESOURCES

http://evolve.elsevier.com/Potter/fundamentals/
- Review Questions
- Case Study with Questions

- Audio Glossary
- Content Updates
- Answers to QSEN Activity and Review Questions

Documentation is a key communication strategy that produces a written account of pertinent patient data, clinical decisions and interventions, and patient responses in a health record. Documentation in a patient's health record is a vital aspect of nursing practice. Health care documentation consists of all information entered into a health record, which may be electronic, paper, or a combination of both formats. Nursing documentation systems should reflect current standards of nursing practice and minimize the risk of errors. Documentation systems need to be flexible enough to allow members of the health care team to efficiently document and retrieve clinical data, track patient outcomes, and facilitate continuity of care. Information in a patient's record provides a detailed account of the level of quality of care delivered. The quality of care, the standards of regulatory agencies and nursing practice, the reimbursement structure in the health care system, and legal guidelines make documentation and reporting an extremely important nursing responsibility.

The information you enter into a patient's individual medical record communicates within the patient's integrated health record the type and frequency of patient care delivered and provides accountability for the care you implemented. This information is then available for all members of the health care team in all settings to review.

It is necessary to document all the nursing care you provide for each patient, including assessment data, nursing problems or diagnoses, interventions, and evaluation of patient responses, in the health record. Your data enable providers and outside reviewers of the medical record to track a patient's clinical course. In 2008, the Centers for Medicare and Medicaid (CMS) implemented a policy under which hospitals are no longer reimbursed for the treatment of 11 specific hospital-acquired conditions (HAC) or preventable adverse events, commonly known as "never events" (Cantrell, 2017). Four of these preventable adverse events are considered "nurse-sensitive": stage III and IV pressure injuries, falls with injury, catheter-associated urinary tract infections (CAUTIs), and central line–catheter-associated bloodstream infections (CLABSIs) (Bae & Yoder, 2015). Identifying the progress of a patient and how events develop is crucial to clinical care and ultimately hospital reimbursement. It is also crucial that your documentation accurately reflects the status of the patient and responses to interventions, especially upon admission, transfer, or discharge.

PURPOSES OF THE HEALTH CARE RECORD

The health care record is a valuable source of data for all members of the health care team. Data entered into the health care record serve many purposes, including facilitating interprofessional communication among health care providers, providing a legal record of care provided, justification for financial billing and reimbursement of care. Data are also used to audit, monitor, and evaluate care provided to support the process needed for quality and performance improvement (Wager, et al., 2017). In addition the health care record is a resource for education and research. There are privacy and ethical considerations to address when accessing health care information and when health records serve as resources for nursing and health care education and for research data (Hwang, 2017).

INTERPROFESSIONAL COMMUNICATION WITHIN THE HEALTH RECORD

The health care record provides a way for members of the interprofessional health care team to communicate about multiple aspects of patient care, including patient needs and response to care and therapies; clinical decision making; and the content and outcomes of consultations, patient education, and discharge planning. Information communicated in the health care record allows health care providers to know a patient thoroughly, facilitating safe, effective, timely, and patient-centered clinical decision making. The health care record is the most current and accurate, continuous source of information about a patient's health care status, allowing the plan of care to be clear to anyone who accesses the record. To enhance communication and promote safe patient care, you document assessment findings and patient information as soon as possible after you provide care (e.g., immediately after providing a nursing intervention or completing a patient assessment). The quality of patient care depends on your ability to communicate with other members of the health care team (see Chapter 24). When a plan is not communicated to all members of the health care team, care becomes fragmented, tasks are repeated, and delays or omissions in care often occur. The health record is an important means of communication because it is a confidential, permanent, legal documentation of information relevant to a patient's health care. The record is an ongoing current and accurate account of a patient's health care status and is available to all members of the health care team.

The record is one resource that prepares the health care provider to know a patient thoroughly so that timely and appropriate care decisions can be made. All health records contain the following information:
- Patient identification and demographic data
- Existence of "living will" or "durable power of attorney for health care" documents
- Informed consent for treatment and procedures
- Admission data
- Nursing diagnoses or problems and the nursing or interprofessional care plan
- Record of nursing care treatment and evaluation
- Medical history
- Medical diagnoses
- Therapeutic orders, including code status (i.e., provider order for "do not resuscitate")

- Medical and interprofessional progress notes (including treatments administered)
- Physical assessment findings
- Diagnostic study results
- Patient education
- Summary of operative procedures
- Discharge summary and plan

Legal Documentation

Accurate documentation is one of the best defenses for legal claims associated with nursing care. Documentation is an important professional responsibility. To limit liability, your documentation needs to follow organizational standards, which include a clear description of individualized and goal-directed nursing care you provide based on your nursing assessment. Always document patient care in a timely manner following agency standards. Documenting all aspects of the nursing process is a critical nursing responsibility that limits nursing liability by providing evidence that you maintained or exceeded practice standards while taking care of patients (Lewis et al., 2017; Wager et al., 2017).

Mistakes in documentation that can result in malpractice include the following examples: (1) failing to record pertinent health or drug information, (2) failing to record nursing actions, (3) failing to record medication administration, (4) failing to record drug reactions or changes in patients' conditions, (5) incomplete or illegible records, and (6) failing to document discontinued medications. Table 26.1 provides guidelines for avoiding these mistakes and gives some examples of basic criteria for legally sound documentation in a health record.

Reimbursement

Documentation of patient care by all members of the health care team allows one to determine the severity of a patient's illness, the intensity of services received, and the quality of care provided during an episode of care. Insurance companies use this information to determine payment or reimbursement for health care services. Diagnosis-related groups (DRGs) are classifications based on a hospitalized patient's primary and secondary medical diagnoses that are used as the basis for establishing Medicare reimbursement for patient care. Hospitals are reimbursed a predetermined dollar amount by Medicare for each DRG. Private insurance carriers and auditors from federal agencies review records to determine the reimbursement that a patient or a health care agency receives (Bauder et al., 2017). Accurate documentation of nursing services provided, as well as the supplies and equipment used in a patient's care, clarifies the type of treatment a patient received and supports accurate and timely reimbursement to a health care agency and/or patient.

Auditing and Monitoring

Quality patient care depends on the ability of all members of the interprofessional team to communicate effectively and in a timely manner. As a member of that team, you are held accountable for the accuracy of the documentation you enter into the patient's record. Regulations from agencies such as The Joint Commission (TJC) and the Centers for Medicare and Medicaid Services (CMS) require health care institutions to monitor and evaluate the quality and appropriateness of patient care (TJC, 2018; US Centers for Medicare & Medicaid Services, 2019). Audits of health records offer information on recurrent health care problems, specific patient incidents, and whether health care providers follow standards of care. Health care record audits help to identify areas for improvement and staff development. For example, a quality improvement (QI) nurse may monitor a unit's records to determine whether nurses consistently and accurately documented

TABLE 26.1 Legal Guidelines for Documentation

Guidelines for Electronic and Written Documentation	Rationale	Correct Action
Do not document retaliatory or critical comments about a patient or care provided by another health care professional. Do not enter personal opinions.	Statements can be used as evidence for nonprofessional behavior or poor quality of care.	Enter only objective and factual observations of a patient's behavior or the actions of another health care professional. Quote all patient statements.
Correct all errors promptly.	Errors in recording can lead to errors in treatment or may imply an attempt to mislead or hide evidence.	Avoid rushing to complete documentation; be sure that information is accurate and complete.
Record all facts.	Record must be accurate, factual, and objective.	Be certain that each entry is thorough. A person reading your documentation needs to be able to determine that a patient received adequate care.
Document discussions with providers that you initiate to seek clarification regarding an order that is questioned.	If you carry out an order that is written incorrectly, you are just as liable for prosecution as the health care provider.	Do not record "physician made error." Instead document that "Dr. Smith was called to clarify order for analgesic." Include the date and time of the phone call, with whom you spoke, and the outcome.
Document only for yourself.	You are accountable for information that you enter into a patient's record.	Never enter documentation for someone else (exception: if caregiver has left unit for the day and calls with information that needs to be documented; include date and time of entry and reference specific date and time to which you are referring and name of source of information in entry; include that information was provided via telephone).
Avoid using generalized, empty phrases such as "status unchanged" or "had good day."	This type of documentation is subjective and does not reflect patient assessment.	Use complete, concise descriptions of assessments and care provided so that documentation is objective and factual.
Begin each entry with date and time and end with your signature and credentials.	Ensures that the correct sequence of events is recorded; signature documents who is accountable for care delivered.	Do not wait until the end of shift to record important changes that occurred several hours earlier; sign each entry according to agency policy (e.g., M. Marcus, RN).
Protect the security of your password for computer documentation.	Maintains security and confidentiality of patient health records.	Once logged into a computer, do not leave computer screen unattended. Log out when you leave the computer. Make sure that a computer screen is not accessible for public viewing.

Guidelines Specific to Written Documentation	Rationale	Correct Action
Do not erase or scratch out errors made while recording.	Charting becomes illegible: it appears as if you were attempting to hide information or deface a written record.	Draw single line through error, write word "error" above it, and sign your name or initials and date it. Then record note correctly.
Do not leave blank spaces or lines in a written nurses' progress note.	Allows another person to add incorrect information in open space.	Chart consecutively, line by line; if space is left, draw a line horizontally through it and place your signature and credentials at the end.
Record all written entries legibly using black ink. Do not use pencils, felt-tip pens, or erasable ink.	Illegible entries are easily misinterpreted, causing errors and lawsuits; ink from felt-tip pen can smudge or run when wet and may destroy documentation; erasures are not permitted in clinical documentation; black ink is more legible when records are photocopied or scanned.	Write clearly and include appropriate abbreviations using black ink.

implementation of fall precautions or evaluation of pain management interventions. Any deficiencies identified are shared with all members of the nursing staff so that changes in policy or practice can occur.

Education

Health care records are a rich source of information about a patient's health care. Reading the record of a patient for whom you are assigned to care is an effective way to learn the nature of a patient's condition and response to treatment. Over time, as you care for patients with similar diagnoses or problems, the information gained from those patients' records allows you to identify patterns and trends and to build your clinical knowledge. As you identify patterns associated with specific diseases and conditions, you are able to anticipate the type of care your patients require and how patients respond to treatment (Fig. 26.1).

Research

De-identification is a process used to prevent a person's identity from being connected with information. For example, when a data form is used to collect information from a health record a patient's name or Social Security number is not entered; instead a random number is used for labeling and categorizing the form. De-identified data obtained from health records can be used for statistical analysis (e.g., frequency of clinical disorders, complications, use of specific medical and nursing therapies, clinical outcomes

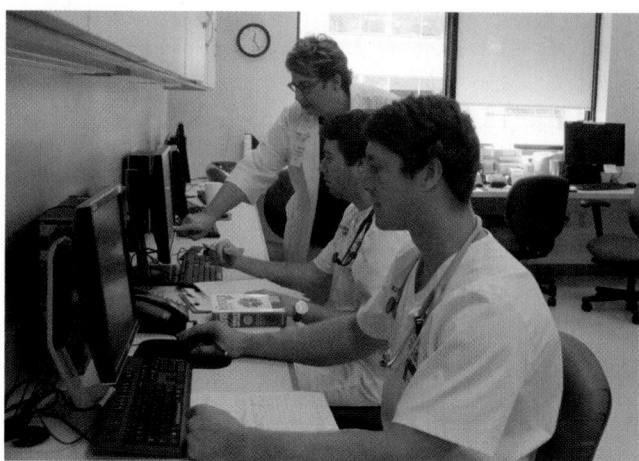

FIG. 26.1 Nursing students and nursing faculty at computer screens.

achieved during care for specific illnesses, and patient mortality). Analysis of the data contributes to evidence-based nursing practice and quality health care (Polit & Beck, 2018). After obtaining appropriate approval from an Institutional Review Board (IRB) of a health care agency or hospital, a nurse researcher reviews patients' records in a research study to collect information on a particular health problem. For example, if a nurse researcher suspects that early ambulation decreases the complication rate in postoperative patients, the researcher could review the records of select surgical patients to compare the rates of postoperative complications following early versus late ambulation.

The Shift To Electronic Documentation

Historically, health care professionals documented on paper health care records. Paper records were episode oriented, with a separate record created for each patient visit to a health care agency. Because a health care provider could not easily review a previous record, key information such as patient allergies, current medications, and complications from treatment were lost from one episode of care (e.g., hospitalization or clinic visit) to the next, jeopardizing a patient's safety (Hebda et al., 2019).

To facilitate communication among health care providers and improve patient safety, the American Recovery and Reinvestment Act (ARRA) of 2009 set a goal that all health care records would be kept electronically as of 2014 (Hebda et al., 2019). Since 2011, the Health Information Technology for Economic and Clinical Health Act (HITECH), enacted under Title XIII of ARRA, has been a major driver in the adoption and use of electronic health records (EHRs) across the United States. HITECH established provisions to promote the meaningful use of health information technology (HIT) to improve the quality and value of health care (Compliancy Group: HIPAA Done Right, 2019). Meaningful use requires that use of an electronic health record system (EHRS) results in improved quality, safety, and efficiency of health care; increases health care consumers' active involvement in their care; increases coordination of health care delivery; advances public health; and safeguards the privacy and security of personal health records (Stimson & Bodruff, 2017). The goal of the ARRA was to have all health care records maintained electronically by 2014. Although the goal has not been fully met, the Office of the National Coordinator for Health Information Technology (2018) reports the following as of 2017:

- Ninety-six percent of all nonfederal acute care hospitals possessed certified health IT.
- Small rural and critical access hospitals had the lowest rates at 93%.

- Ninety-nine percent of large hospitals (more than 300 beds) had certified health IT, while 97 percent of medium-sized hospitals (more than 100 beds) had certified health IT.

Although the terms *EHR* and *EMR* have been used interchangeably in practice, there are differences between them. The term electronic health record (EHR) has become the favored term for an individual's lifetime computerized record; it means both the displayed or printed record. The addition of an "S" at the end of the acronym (EHRS) indicates the supporting software system. The term electronic medical record (EMR) refers to a patient's record within an integrated health care information system for an individual visit to a health care provider's office or for an individual admission to an acute care setting that allows for seamless documentation of the progression of care. To meet agreed-on standards, EHRs are expected to have the following attributes or components (Hebda et al., 2019):

- Provide a longitudinal or lifetime patient record by linking all patient data from previous health care encounters.
- Contain a problem list that indicates current clinical problems for each health care encounter, the number of occurrences associated with all past and current problems, and the current status of each problem.
- Use accepted standardized measures to evaluate and record health status and functional levels.
- Provide a method for documenting the clinical reasoning or rationale for diagnoses and conclusions that allows clinical decision making to be tracked by all providers who access the record.
- Support confidentiality, privacy, and audit trails.
- Provide continuous access to authorized users at any time, and allow multiple health care providers access to customized views of patient data at the same time.
- Support links to local or remote information resources such as databases using the Internet or intranet resources based within an organization.
- Support the use of decision analysis tools.
- Support direct entry of patient data by providers.
- Include mechanisms for measuring the cost and quality of care.
- Support existing and evolving clinical needs by being flexible and expandable.

A unique feature of an EHR is its ability to integrate all patient information into one record, regardless of the number of times a patient enters a health care system. An EHR also includes results of diagnostic studies that may include diagnostic images (e.g., x-ray or ultrasound images) and decision support software programs. Because an unlimited number of patient records potentially can be stored within an EHR system, health care providers can access clinical data to identify quality issues, link interventions with positive outcomes, and make evidence-based decisions (Rajkovića et al., 2018) The key advantages of an EHR for nursing include a means for nurses to compare current clinical data about a patient with data from previous health care encounters, maintain ongoing symptom management, and provide an ongoing record of health education provided to a patient and the patient's response to that information (Ostrovsky, et al., 2016; Ozkaynak, et al., 2017).

Maintaining Privacy, Confidentiality, and Security of the Health Care Record

Nurses are legally and ethically obligated to keep information about patients confidential. Only members of the health care team who are directly involved in a patient's care have legitimate access to a patient's health record. You discuss a patient's diagnosis, treatment, assessment, and any personal conversations only with members of the health care team who are specifically involved in the patient's care. Do not share information with other patients or with health care team members who are not caring for the patient. Patients have the right to request copies of their medical record and read the information. Each institution has policies that describe how medical records are shared with patients or other people who request them. In most situations, patients are required to give written permission for release of their medical information.

The Health Insurance Portability and Accountability Act (HIPAA) of 1996 was the first federal legislation to provide protection for patient records; it governs all areas of patient information and management of that information. To eliminate barriers that potentially delay access to care, HIPAA requires providers to notify patients of privacy policies and to obtain written acknowledgment from patients indicating they received this information. Under HIPAA, the Privacy Rule requires that disclosure or requests regarding health information are limited to the specific information required for a particular purpose (Hebda et al., 2019). For example, if you need a patient's home telephone number to reschedule an appointment, access to the health record is limited solely to telephone information. Of equal importance under HIPAA is the Security Rule, which specifies administrative, physical, and technical safeguards for 18 specific elements of protected health information (PHI) in electronic form (HIPAA Journal, 2019).

Nurses are permitted to use health records for data gathering, research, or continuing education as long as records are used as specified and permission is granted from an Institutional Review Board (for research) or appropriate administrative department. When you are a student learning in a clinical setting, maintaining patient confidentiality and adherence to HIPAA are required as part of professional practice. You can review patient health records only for information needed to provide safe and effective patient care. For example, when you are assigned to care for a patient, you need to review the patient's health record and the interprofessional plan of care. You *do not* share this information with classmates (except for clinical conferences) and *do not* access the health records of other patients on the unit. Access to an EHR is traceable through user log-in information. It is unethical to view health records of other patients, and breaches of confidentiality will lead to disciplinary action by employers and potentially dismissal from work or nursing school. To protect patient confidentiality, you must ensure that any electronic or written materials you use in your student clinical practice *do not* include patient identifiers (e.g., name, room number, date of birth, demographic information). *Never* print material from an EHR for personal use; any information printed must be for professional use only and should not include identifiable information.

Privacy, Confidentiality, and Security Mechanisms

There are legal implications associated with the use of electronic documentation. It is possible for anyone to access a computer within a health care agency and gain information about almost any patient. Under HIPAA, ensuring appropriate access to and confidentiality of personal health information (PHI) is the responsibility of all persons working in health care. Personal health information is individually identifiable information relating to an individual's past, present, or future health status that is created, collected, transmitted, or maintained by a HIPAA-covered entity in relation to the provision of health care, payment for health care services, or use in health care operations (HIPAA Journal, 2019). Protection of information and computer systems is one of your top priorities.

Most computer information system security mechanisms use a combination of logical and physical restrictions to protect information. For example, an automatic sign-off is a safety mechanism that logs a user off a computer system after a specified period of inactivity

(Hebda et al., 2019). Other security measures include firewalls and the installation of antivirus and spyware-detection software. A firewall is a combination of hardware and software that protects private network resources (e.g., the information system of the hospital) from outside hackers, network damage, and theft or misuse of information.

Physical security measures include placing computers or file servers in restricted areas or using privacy filters for computer screens that are visible to visitors or other people who should not have access to the information displayed. This form of security has limited benefit, especially if an organization uses mobile wireless devices such as notebooks, tablets, personal computers (PCs), and smartphones. These devices are easily misplaced or lost, and at risk for falling into the wrong hands.

Access or log-in codes along with passwords are frequently used for authenticating authorized access to electronic records. A password is a collection of alphanumeric characters and symbols that a user types into a computer sign-on screen before accessing a program after the entry and acceptance of an access code or user name. Strong passwords use combinations of letters, numbers, and symbols that are difficult to guess. When using a health care agency computer system, it is essential that you do not share your computer password with anyone under any circumstances. A good system requires frequent changes in personal passwords to prevent unauthorized persons from tampering with records. A password does not appear on the computer screen when it is typed, and it should not be known to anyone but the user and information system administrators (Hebda et al., 2019). Most health care personnel are given access only to patients in their work area. Some staff (e.g., administrators or risk managers) have authority to access all patient records. To protect patient privacy, health care agencies track who accesses patient records and when they access them. Failure to adhere to HIPAA can result in civil and criminal penalties for health care agencies and providers. Depending on the nature of a violation, civil penalties can result in minimal fines of $100 per violation and maximum fines of $50,000 per violation with an annual maximum of $1.5 million (American Medical Association, 2017). Thus employers have policies for disciplinary action.

Handling and Disposing of Information

Maintaining the confidentiality of health records is a fundamental responsibility of all members of the health care team. It is essential to safeguard any information that is printed from the record or extracted for report purposes. For example, you print a copy of a nursing activities work list to use in planning your shift while providing patient care. You refer to information on the list and write notes to record into the computer and share later during hand-off report. Information on the list is PHI; you must not leave it out for view by unauthorized persons. Destroy (e.g., shred or place in a locked receptacle designated for collection of material that is to be shredded) anything that is printed when the information is no longer needed. Nursing students should not print information from the health record to take away from the clinical agency to complete written assignments for clinical. Instead, patient information needed for clinical assignments should be transcribed to academic forms or notebooks directly from viewing the health record on the computer screen or the physical chart. All patient data must be de-identified when transcribed onto forms or used for academic papers for clinical courses in nursing school. Any information that is transcribed and must be removed from the clinical setting and any documents that must be printed out must be kept secure and destroyed through shredding or disposal in a locked receptacle as soon as possible.

Historically, information printed from a patient record and/or faxed to other health care providers has been the primary source for accidental, unauthorized disclosure of PHI. All papers containing PHI must be destroyed after use or after being faxed. Nurses also work in settings where they may be responsible for erasing files from a computer hard drive that contains calendars, schedules for surgery or diagnostic procedures, or other daily records that contain PHI (Hebda et al., 2019). You are responsible to know and follow disposal policies for these types of records in the agency where you work.

Health care facilities and departments should have policies for the use of fax machines that specify the kinds of information that can be faxed, who can receive faxed information, where information can be sent, and the process used to verify that information was sent to and received by the appropriate person or persons. Information sent by fax should not exceed what was requested or required for immediate clinical needs. Following are some steps that can be taken to enhance fax security (Touchstone Compliance, 2017):

- Always use a cover letter.
- To prevent numbers from being misdialed, use saved speed-dial numbers for frequently used fax recipients. Check those numbers regularly.
- For any new recipient, verify the number with a test fax before sending PHI.
- Follow policies for what to do if a fax is sent to the wrong number.
- Set up fax machines to never save copies of faxes sent or received.
- Make sure that faxes containing PHI are promptly delivered to the intended recipient.
- Follow agency policies for storing, copying, and disposing of faxes containing PHI.
- Use a fax machine designated exclusively for PHI, and keep it separate from other fax machines.

STANDARDS AND GUIDELINES FOR QUALITY NURSING DOCUMENTATION

Whether the transfer of patient information occurs through verbal reports or electronic or written documents, you need to follow basic guidelines and standards for nursing documentation. Every health care organization has standards that govern the type of information nurses document and for which they are held accountable. Agency standards or policies often dictate the frequency of documentation, such as how often you record a nursing assessment or a patient's level of pain. You are responsible for knowing the standards of care for every nursing procedure and the standards for providing complete and accurate documentation. Information in patient health records can be used as evidence in a court of law to demonstrate whether nursing standards of practice were, or were not, met.

In addition, your documentation needs to conform to the standards of the National Committee for Quality Assurance (NCQA) and accrediting bodies such as TJC to maintain institutional accreditation and to minimize liability. Health care organizations usually incorporate accreditation standards into policies and revise documentation systems and forms to suit these standards. Current documentation standards require that all patients admitted to a health care agency be assessed for physical, psychosocial, environmental, self-care, spiritual, cultural, knowledge level, and discharge planning needs. Your documentation needs to demonstrate application of the nursing process, describe clinical decision making, and include evidence of patient and family teaching and discharge planning (TJC, 2018). In addition to HIPAA standards, health care documentation is affected by standards from state and federal regulatory agencies, the Department of Justice, and CMS.

Guidelines for Quality Documentation

Quality nursing documentation enhances efficient, individualized patient care and has five important characteristics: factual, accurate, current, organized, and complete. It is easier to maintain these characteristics in your documentation if you continually seek to express ideas clearly and succinctly by doing the following:

- Stick to the facts.
- Write in short sentences.
- Use simple, short words.
- Avoid the use of jargon or abbreviations.

Factual

A factual record contains clear descriptive, objective information about what a nurse observes, hears, palpates, and smells. Avoid vague terms such as *appears, seems,* or *apparently.* These words suggest you are stating an opinion; they do not accurately communicate facts and do not inform other caregivers about the details regarding the behaviors exhibited by a patient. Objective data are obtained through direct observation and measurement and include description of a patient's behaviors, for example, *"BP 90/50, heart rate 115 and regular, patient diaphoretic and holding both hands over abdominal dressing."* The only subjective data included in the record are statements made by a patient. When recording subjective data, document a patient's exact words within quotation marks whenever possible. Include objective data to support subjective data so that your documentation is as descriptive as possible. For example, instead of documenting *"the patient seems anxious,"* provide objective signs of anxiety and document the patient's statement about the feelings experienced: *"patient's heart rate 110 beats/min, respiratory rate is slightly labored at 22 breaths/min, and patient states, 'I feel very nervous.'"*

Accurate

Using exact measurements establishes accuracy and helps you determine whether a patient's condition has changed in a positive or negative way. For example, a description such as *"Intake, 360 mL of water"* is more accurate than *"Patient drank an adequate amount of fluid."* Documenting that an abdominal incision is *"Approximated, 5 cm in length without redness, drainage, or edema"* is more descriptive than *"Large abdominal incision healing well."* Documentation of concise data is clear and easy to understand. Avoid using unnecessary words and irrelevant detail. For example, the fact that the patient is watching television is necessary only when this activity is significant to the patient's status and plan of care. Examples of criteria for documentation or reporting specific situations can be found in Table 26.2.

Appropriate Use of Abbreviations in Health Care Documentation

Use abbreviations carefully to avoid misinterpretation and promote patient safety. TJC (2018) developed a list of "do not use" abbreviations in 2004 that is still used by all health care providers today to promote patient safety (Table 26.3). In addition, TJC requires that health care institutions develop a list of standard abbreviations, symbols, and

TABLE 26.2   Examples of Criteria for Documentation and Reporting

Topic	Criteria To Report or Record
Subjective assessment data	Patient's description of episode in quotation marks (e.g., *"I feel like an elephant is sitting on my chest, and I can't catch my breath."*) Describe in patient's own words the onset, location, description of condition (severity, duration, frequency, precipitating, aggravating, and relieving factors) (e.g., *"The pain in my left knee started last week after I knelt on the ground. Every time I bend my knee, I have a shooting pain on the inside of the knee."*).
Objective assessment data (e.g., rash, tenderness, breath sounds, or descriptions of patient behavior [e.g., anxiety, confusion, hostility])	Onset, location, description of condition (e.g., 11:00: 2-cm raised pale, red area noted on back of left hand). Precipitating factors, behaviors exhibited (e.g., Physician informed patient of diagnosis, patient pacing in room, avoiding eye contact with nurse), patient statements (e.g., repeatedly stating, *"I have to go home now."*)
Nursing interventions, treatments, and evaluation (e.g., enema, bath, dressing change)	Time administered, equipment used, patient's response (subjective and objective response) compared with previous treatment (e.g., denied incisional pain during abdominal dressing change, ambulated 300 feet in hallway without assistance)
Medication administration	At time of administration when using a computerized bar-code medication administration program (or immediately after administration), document: time medication given, medication name, dose, route, preliminary assessment (e.g., pain level, vital signs), patient response, or effect of medication (e.g., 1500: Reports *"throbbing headache all over my head."* Rates pain at 6 (scale 0 to 10). Tylenol 650 mg given PO. 1530: Patient reports pain level 2 (scale 0 to 10) and states, *"the throbbing has stopped."*
Patient and/or family teaching	Information presented; method of instruction (e.g., discussion, demonstration, videotape, booklet); and patient response, including questions and evidence of understanding such as teach-back, return demonstration, or change in behavior
Discharge planning	Measurable patient goals or expected outcomes, progress toward goals, need for referrals.

TABLE 26.3   The Joint Commission's Official "Do Not Use" List of Abbreviations

Do Not Use	Potential Problem	Use Instead
U, u (unit)	Mistaken for "0" (zero), the number "4" (four) or "cc"	Write "unit."
IU (International Unit)	Mistaken for "IV" (intravenous) or the number "10" (ten)	Write "International Unit."
Q.D., QD, q.d., qd (daily)	Mistaken for each other	Write "daily."
Q.O.D., QOD, q.o.d., qod (every other day)	Period after the Q mistaken for "I" and the "O" mistaken for "I"	Write "every other day."
Trailing zero (X.0 mg)[a]	Decimal point is missed	Write X mg.
Lack of leading zero (.X mg)		Write 0.X mg.
MS	Can mean morphine sulfate or magnesium sulfate	Write "morphine sulfate."
MSO_4 and $MgSO_4$	Confused for one another	Write "magnesium sulfate."

[a]Exception: A "trailing zero" may be used only where required to demonstrate the level of precision of the value being reported, such as for laboratory results, imaging studies that report size of lesions, or catheter/tube sizes. It may not be used in medication orders or other medication-related documentation.

From https://www.jointcommission.org/facts_about_do_not_use_list/. Accessed June 10, 2019.

acronyms to be used by all members of the health care team when documenting or communicating patient care and treatment. To minimize errors, spell out abbreviations in their entirety when they become confusing.

Correct spelling demonstrates a level of competency and attention to detail. Many terms are easily misinterpreted (e.g., *dysphagia* or *dysphasia*). Some spelling errors can result in serious treatment errors (e.g., the names of medications such as lamotrigine and lamivudine or hydromorphone and hydrocodone are similar). Transcribe medication information carefully to ensure a patient receives the correct medication.

All health care record entries should be dated and timed, and the author of each entry must be clearly identified (TJC, 2018). Each entry in a patient's record must end with the caregiver's full name or initials and credentials/title/role such as "Jane Cook, RN." If initials are used in a signature, the full name and credentials/title/role of the individual needs to be documented at least once in the health care record to allow others to readily identify that individual. As a nursing student, enter your full name and nursing student abbreviation, such as "David Jones, NS" or "David Jones, SN." The abbreviation for *nursing student* varies between *NS* for *nursing student* or *SN* for *student nurse*. Include information about your educational institution at the end of your signature when required by agency policy.

Current

Timely entries are essential in a patient's ongoing care, as delays in documentation can lead to unsafe patient care. Many health care agencies keep records or computers near a patient's bedside to facilitate immediate documentation of information. Document the following activities or findings at the time of occurrence:

- Vital signs
- Pain assessment
- Administration of medications and treatments

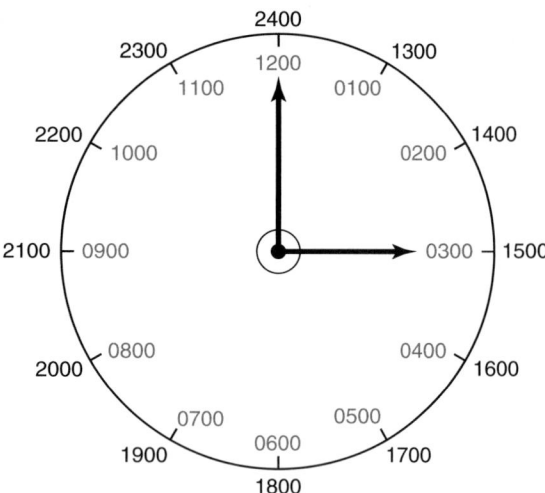

FIG. 26.2 Comparison of 24 hours of military time with the hourly positions for civilian time on the clockface.

- Preparation for diagnostic tests or surgery, including preoperative checklist
- Change in patient's status, treatment provided, and who was notified (e.g., health care provider, manager, patient's family)
- Admission, transfer, discharge, or death of a patient
- Patient's response to treatment or intervention

Most health care agencies use military time, a 24-hour system that avoids misinterpretation of AM and PM times (Fig. 26.2). Instead of two 12-hour cycles in standard time, the military clock is one 24-hour time cycle. The military clock ends with midnight at 2400 and begins at 1 minute after midnight as 0001. For example, 10:22 AM is 1022 military time, and 10:22 PM is 2222 military time.

Organized

Documentation is more effective when notes are concise, clear and to the point, and presented in a logical order. To document notes about complex situations in an organized fashion, first think about the situation, and then make decisions about what information and words you need to include before beginning to enter data in the health care record. Application of your critical thinking skills and the nursing process will help you document clearly and comprehensively in a logical order. For example, an organized entry would describe a patient's pain, your assessment and interventions, and the patient's response to treatment.

Complete

Be sure the information within a recorded entry or a report is complete, containing appropriate and essential information. Follow established criteria and standards for thorough communication within the health care record or when reporting certain health problems or nursing activities.

METHODS OF DOCUMENTATION

There are several documentation methods for recording patient assessment data and progress notes. Regardless of whether documentation is entered electronically or on paper, each health care agency selects a documentation system that reflects the philosophy of nursing at that agency. The same system is used throughout a specific agency and sometimes is used throughout a health care system as well.

Documentation of Patient Assessment Data

Within the EHR, nurses routinely document patient physiologic data and routine care using **flow sheets** (graphic records) that are organized by body system and navigated through use of the computer mouse with a series of tabs or rows (Fig. 26.3). These forms allow you to quickly and easily enter assessment data about a patient, such as vital signs, admission and daily weights, and percentage of meals eaten. They also facilitate the documentation of routine, repetitive care, such as hygiene measures, ambulation, and safety and restraint checks. These documents provide current patient information accessible to all members of the health care team and help team members quickly see patient trends over time.

Describe any routine data in greater detail when a change in a patient's functional ability or status occurs. For example, if your patient's blood pressure, pulse, and respirations are elevated above expected values after a walk down the hall, you would first complete and record a focused assessment in the flow sheet, and then document additional, detailed information about the patient's status and response to the walk in the appropriate place in the health care record using narrative free text within the flow sheet, or in a narrative progress note.

Progress Notes. Health care team members monitor and record the progress made toward resolving a patient's problems in progress notes. Health care providers write narrative progress notes in one of several formats or structured notes within the EHR. Notes may take the form of traditional narrative documentation or make use of precise formats such as (1) focus charting, incorporating data, action, and response (DAR); (2) SOAP notes, identifying interprofessional problems; or (3) notes with a specific nursing focus, identifying nursing problems or diagnoses (PIE). See Box 26.1 for examples of nursing documentation using these formats. Narrative documentation is the format traditionally used by nurses and health care providers to record patient assessment, clinical decisions, and care provided; it consists of a storylike format to document information. In an electronic nursing information system, this is accomplished through the use of free text entry or menu selections (Hebda et al., 2019). An example of a comprehensive narrative note written by a nurse looks like this:

> 1915: Adhering to bed rest as ordered. Left lower extremity is swollen; calf circumference is 30 inches. Areas of redness that are warm and tender to touch are noted over anterior (3 cm by 4 cm) and medial areas (3 cm by 3 cm) of left leg. Left lower leg elevated on one pillow. Heparin infusing at 3600 units/hour via 20-gauge peripheral IV in left lower forearm. Site without redness, swelling, or drainage. Verbalizes sharp throbbing leg pain rated at 8 on a 0-to-10 scale. Pedal pulses 3+ bilaterally. Capillary refill in toes of both feet is less than 3 seconds. Oxycodone/acetaminophen 2 tablets (PO) given for pain as ordered. Chris Banks, RN.
> 2000: States, "The pain medication really helped." Rates pain in left lower leg at 4 on a 0-to-10 scale. Comfort level goal is 4/10. Chris Banks, RN.

While the nursing patient assessment flow sheet section of the EHR allows users to enter descriptive details through the use of short, narrative comments, these sections of the EHR are primarily designed to allow the use of multiple checkboxes or drop-down lists. Research has shown that some nurses believe flow sheet data may not adequately convey the details of significant events that result in a change in patient condition (Brown, 2016; Topaz et al., 2016). When entering a narrative progress note in the EHR, be clear and accurate when describing subjective and objective patient assessment findings, as well as any interventions taken to resolve patient problems and maintain patient safety. Health care providers review nursing documentation for details about changes in a patient's condition, and use of narrative documentation within the EHR may provide more detail than charting by exception when trying to document complex situations. EHRs that enable all health care providers to easily retrieve important patient information

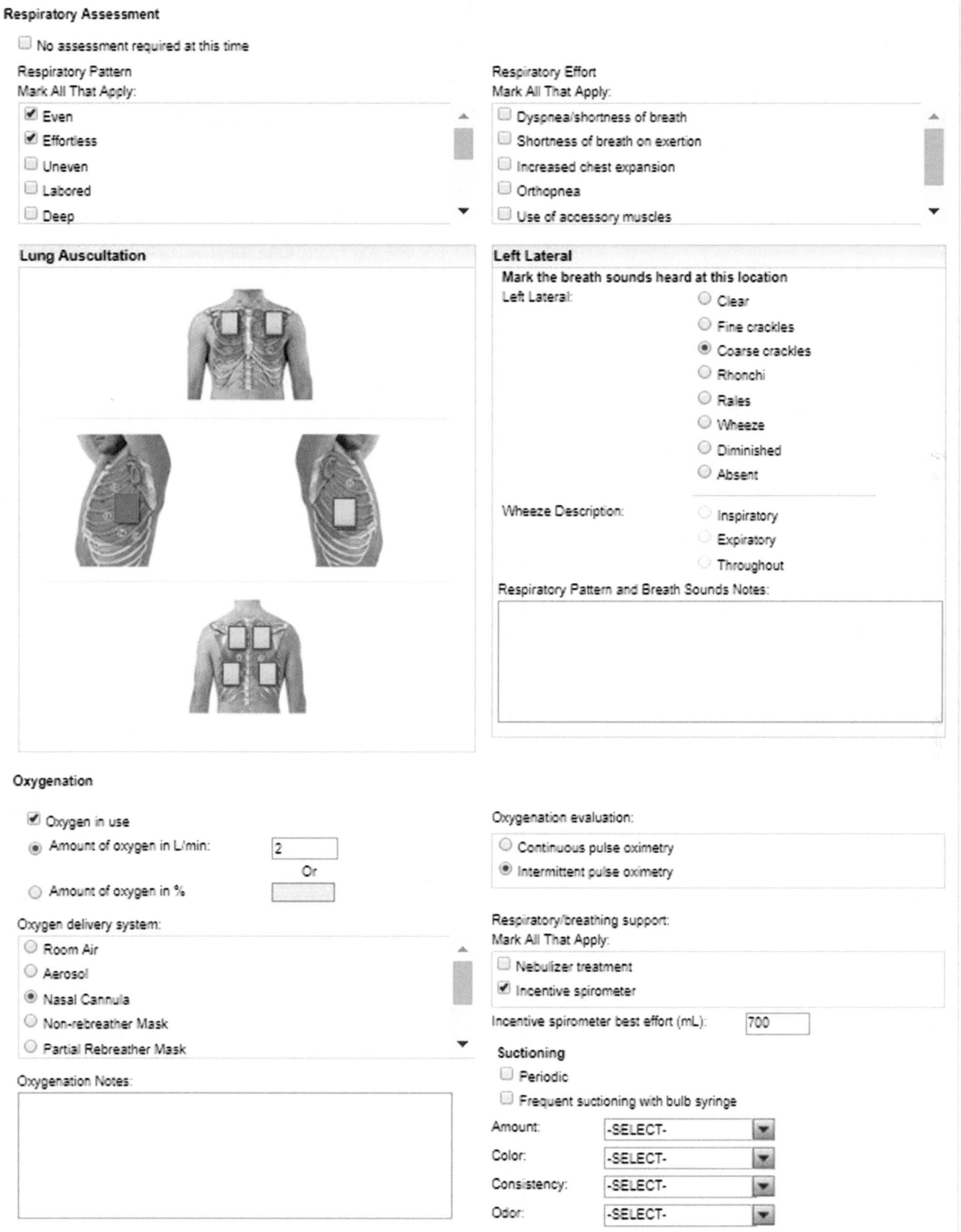

Respiratory Assessment

☐ No assessment required at this time

Respiratory Pattern
Mark All That Apply:

☑ Even
☑ Effortless
☐ Uneven
☐ Labored
☐ Deep

Respiratory Effort
Mark All That Apply:

☐ Dyspnea/shortness of breath
☐ Shortness of breath on exertion
☐ Increased chest expansion
☐ Orthopnea
☐ Use of accessory muscles

Lung Auscultation

Left Lateral

Mark the breath sounds heard at this location

Left Lateral:
○ Clear
○ Fine crackles
◉ Coarse crackles
○ Rhonchi
○ Rales
○ Wheeze
○ Diminished
○ Absent

Wheeze Description:
○ Inspiratory
○ Expiratory
○ Throughout

Respiratory Pattern and Breath Sounds Notes:

Oxygenation

☑ Oxygen in use
◉ Amount of oxygen in L/min: [2]
                            Or
○ Amount of oxygen in % [   ]

Oxygen delivery system:
○ Room Air
○ Aerosol
◉ Nasal Cannula
○ Non-rebreather Mask
○ Partial Rebreather Mask

Oxygenation Notes:

Oxygenation evaluation:
○ Continuous pulse oximetry
◉ Intermittent pulse oximetry

Respiratory/breathing support:
Mark All That Apply:
☐ Nebulizer treatment
☑ Incentive spirometer

Incentive spirometer best effort (mL): [700]

Suctioning
☐ Periodic
☐ Frequent suctioning with bulb syringe

Amount: [-SELECT- ▼]
Color: [-SELECT- ▼]
Consistency: [-SELECT- ▼]
Odor: [-SELECT- ▼]

FIG. 26.3 Example of documentation of nursing assessment of respiratory system within the electronic health record (EHR). (Copyright © Elsevier 2019. SimChart® www.evolve.elsevier.com.)

BOX 26.1 Examples of Nursing Documentation in Different Formats

Narrative Note

- Patient states, "My leg is so swollen. I'm worried about this blood clot." Is asking question about medications and how DVT will be treated. Alert and oriented; responds appropriately to instruction. Discussed importance of bed rest and the reason for treatment with heparin infusion. Explained need for daily blood tests to check anticoagulation levels. Provided brochure on anticoagulation therapy for DVT. Used teach-back method to validate patient understanding; he is able to describe that the heparin infusion will be stopped when his PT/INR is therapeutic on warfarin and he can expect to take warfarin for about 6 months after discharge until clot is resolved.

PIE

- A PIE note has a specific nursing focus.
- **P: Nursing problem or diagnosis**—*Lack of Knowledge* related to inexperience with disease condition
- **I: Interventions that will be used to address the problem**—Provided brochure on anticoagulation therapy for DVT. Explained rationale for bed rest and daily blood tests to check anticoagulation levels. Explained that heparin infusion will be stopped when PT/INR is at therapeutic level and that he can expect to take warfarin for about 6 months until clot resolves.
- **E: Nursing evaluation**: Patient states, "I'm worried about the blood clot, but I understand how it is being treated." Able to teach back and verbalize that the heparin infusion will be stopped when PT/INR tests are "normal." Also states that he expects to take warfarin for about 6 months until clot in leg dissolves.

Focus Charting

- Uses a DAR format to report problems. DAR notes address patient concerns such as a sign or symptom, condition, nursing diagnosis, behavior, significant event or change in condition.
- **D: Data** (subjective and objective)—Patient states, "My leg is so swollen. I'm worried about this blood clot. Do you know how they are going to treat it?"
- **A: Action or nursing intervention**—Provided brochure on anticoagulation therapy for DVT. Explained rationale for bed rest and daily blood tests to check anticoagulation levels. Explained that heparin infusion will be stopped when PT/INR is at therapeutic level.
- **R: Response of the patient**—Able to teach back and verbalized that heparin infusion will be stopped when PT/INR reaches "normal level" and that he can expect to take warfarin for 6 months after discharge until clot is fully resolved.

SOAP Note—Used By All Health Care Disciplines

- **S: Subjective**—Patient states, "My leg is so swollen. I'm worried about this blood clot. Do you know how they are going to treat it?"
- **O: Objective**—Patient asking question about medications and how DVT will be treated. Alert and oriented; responds appropriately to instruction.
- **A: Assessment**—Patient lacks knowledge regarding anticoagulation therapy, seeking information about therapy.
- **P: Plan**: Discussed importance of bed rest and the reason for treatment with heparin infusion. Provided brochure on anticoagulation therapy for DVT. Explained rationale for bed rest and daily blood tests to check anticoagulation levels. Explained that heparin infusion will be stopped when PT/INR is at therapeutic level and that he can expect to take warfarin for about 6 months until clot resolves.

---

from narrative notes, as well as flow sheet data, may augment clinician communication and interprofessional understanding for patient care (Bardach et al., 2017).

REFLECT NOW

What patient situations have you observed in the clinical setting that might be more appropriately documented through use of a narrative note versus use of flow sheet documentation within the EHR? Think of a recent patient situation you observed that you believe should be documented in narrative fashion. Practice writing a narrative note about that situation, and ask your clinical faculty to review and comment on your work.

Charting By Exception

The philosophy behind charting by exception (CBE) is that all standards for normal assessment findings or for routine care activities are met unless otherwise documented. Exception-based documentation systems incorporate standards of care and use clearly, predefined statements for the nursing documentation of "normal" body system findings. These normal findings called "within defined limits" (WDL) or "within normal limits" (WNL) consist of written criteria for a "normal" assessment for each body system. Documentation within a computerized system allows nurses to select a WDL statement or to choose other statements from a drop-down menu that allow description of any unexpected assessment findings or assessment findings that deviate from the WDL definition (Elliott et al., 2018). Well-designed flow sheets are a key part of a good exception-based documentation system within the EHR. But this form of documentation also calls for use of narrative notes concerning any significant indicator of the patient's condition or change in status, any subsequent interventions, and the patient's response (Nurses Service Organization, 2018). When

an exception occurs, if a nurse's note offers few explanations, little description of key findings, or no mention of periodic patient checks, a patient's lawyer could claim negligence on the part of the nurse (Nurses Service Organization, 2018).

The SBAR or ISBAR format is a commonly used framework for a narrative note when exceptions occur. Both are also popular formats for verbal reporting (see Chapter 24). When changes in a patient's condition develop, a narrative progress note must include a thorough and precise description of the effects of the changes on the patient and the actions taken to address those changes.

COMMON RECORD-KEEPING FORMS WITHIN THE ELECTRONIC HEALTH RECORD

Nurses use a variety of electronic or paper forms for the type of information routinely documented within the EHR. The categories or data fields within a form are usually derived from institutional standards of practice or guidelines established by accrediting agencies.

Admission Nursing History Form

A nurse completes a nursing history form when a patient is admitted to a nursing unit. The fields in the form guide you through a comprehensive assessment to identify relevant nursing diagnoses or problems (see Chapters 16 and 30). Completion of this form provides baseline data that you use for comparison when a patient's condition changes.

Patient Care Summary

Many computerized documentation systems generate a patient care summary document that you review (and sometimes print) for each patient at the beginning and/or end of each shift to use as a worksheet for organizing care and in giving hand-off report (Fig. 26.4). The document automatically updates and provides the most current information

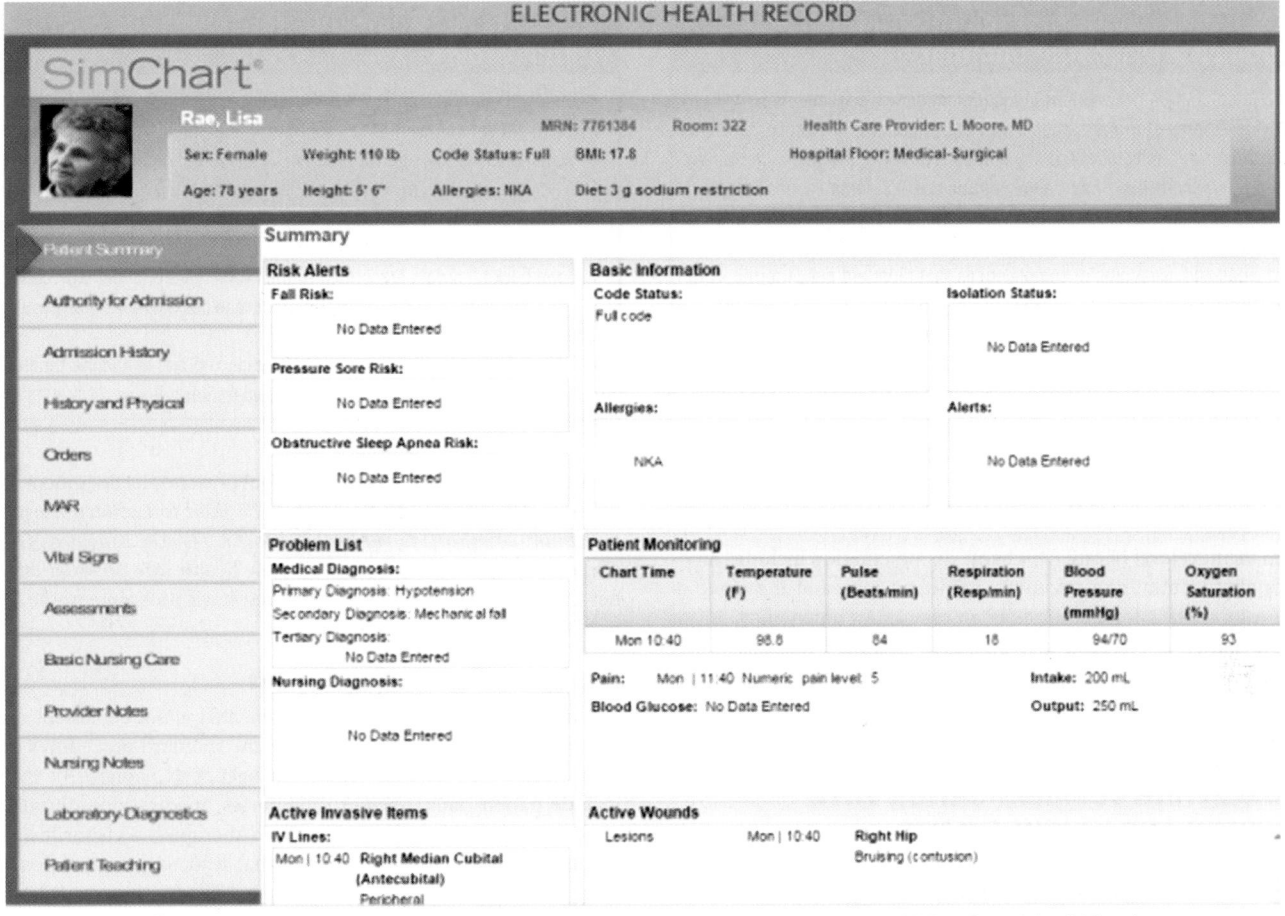

FIG. 26.4 Example of sections/information available in an electronic health record (EHR). (Copyright © Elsevier 2019. SimChart® www.evolve.elsevier.com.)

that was entered into the EHR and usually includes the following information:

- Basic demographic data (e.g., age, religion)
- Health care provider's name
- Primary medical diagnosis
- Medical and surgical history
- Current orders from the health care provider (e.g., dressing changes, ambulation, glucose monitoring)
- Nursing care plan
- Nursing orders (e.g., education needed, symptom relief measures, counseling)
- Scheduled tests and procedures
- Safety precautions used in a patient's care
- Factors that affect patient independence with activities of daily living
- Nearest relative/guardian or person designated as a patient's health care power of attorney to contact in an emergency
- Emergency code status (e.g., indication of do-not-resuscitate order)
- Allergies

Care Plans

Many computerized documentation systems include standardized care plans or clinical practice guidelines (CPGs) to facilitate the creation and documentation of a nursing and or interprofessional plan of care (see Chapter 18). Each standardized plan facilitates safe and consistent care for an identified problem by describing or listing institutional standards and evidence-based guidelines that are easily accessed and included within a patient's EHR (Khokhar et al., 2017). After completing a nursing assessment, you identify and select the standardized

plans that are appropriate for the patient and are to be included in the individualized plan of care. Most computer documentation systems allow these care plans to be modified by creating individualized interventions, goals, and outcomes for each patient.

Standardized care plans are useful when conducting QI audits. They also improve continuity of care among professional nurses. When they are used, the nurse still remains responsible for providing individualized care to each patient. Standardized care plans cannot replace a nurse's professional judgment and decision making. You update care plans on a regular basis to ensure that the documents are appropriate and evidence-based.

Discharge Summary Forms

Nurses help ensure cost-effective care and appropriate reimbursement by preparing patients for a safe, effective, and timely discharge from a health care institution. Developing a comprehensive plan for a safe discharge relies on interprofessional discharge planning. This process includes identification of key clinical outcomes and appropriate timelines for reaching them, the appropriate level of care for discharge, and all necessary resources.

Ideally discharge planning begins at admission, which requires partnering with the patient and family to identify goals for recovery and identifying potential discharge needs. Nursing and other health care professionals then begin to plan with the patient for discharge to the appropriate level of care. Consideration is given to the support services (i.e., home care, physical therapy) required and whether any health care equipment is needed in the home setting. Involvement of the patient and family in the discharge planning process ensures that they have the necessary information and resources to return home or

---

BOX 26.2   Guidelines for Information to Include on a Discharge Summary

- Use clear, concise descriptions in the patient's own language.
- Provide step-by-step instructions for how to perform any procedure that the patient or family will be doing independently (e.g., emptying a urinary catheter drainage bag or self-administration of an injectable medication).
- Identify precautions to follow when performing self-care or administering medications.
- List signs and symptoms of complications that a patient needs to report to a health care provider.
- List names and phone numbers of health care providers and community resources that the patient can contact.
- Identify any unresolved problems, including plans for follow-up and continuous treatment.
- List actual time of discharge, mode of transportation, and who accompanied the patient.

---

move to the next level of care. Discharge documentation includes medications, diet, community resources, follow-up care, and the name of a person to contact for questions or in case of an emergency. All of this information is included in a discharge summary document that is printed out and given to the patient on discharge. The information remains in the EHR as a record of the discharge teaching that was provided (Box 26.2).

DOCUMENTING COMMUNICATION WITH PROVIDERS AND UNIQUE EVENTS

Telephone Calls Made to a Provider

Document every phone call you make to a health care provider. Your documentation needs to include when the call was made, the number called, who made the call, who was called, to whom information was given, what information was given, and what information was received. For example: *"08/25/2018 (2130): Called Dr. Banks' office at 123-456-7890. Spoke with L. Matthews, RN, who will inform Dr. Banks that Mr. Andrews' potassium level drawn at 2000 was 5.9 mEq/dL. Informed that Dr. Banks will call back after he is finished seeing his current patient. R. Jenner, RN."*

Telephone and Verbal Orders

Telephone orders (TOs) occur when a health care provider gives therapeutic orders over the phone to an RN. Verbal orders (VOs) occur when a health care provider gives therapeutic orders to an RN face-to-face while they are standing in proximity to each other. The potential for verbal orders to be misunderstood, misheard, or transcribed incorrectly makes them error prone, particularly given different care provider accents, dialects, and drug name pronunciations (Institute for Safe Medication Practices [ISMP], 2017) Use of VOs is discouraged except in urgent or emergent situations. TOs and VOs should be used only when absolutely necessary and not for the sake of convenience for the health care provider. In some situations, it is wise to have a second person listen on the telephone line as a TO is given by a health care provider; some agency policies require this. Check your agency's policy. Box 26.3 provides guidelines that promote accurate documentation of TOs or VOs.

A nurse receiving a TO or VO enters the complete order into the computer using the computer provider order entry (CPOE) software or writes it out on a physician's order sheet for entry into the computer as soon as possible. The Joint Commission requires the receiver of a VO or TO record it and read (not repeat) it back to the prescriber. This helps assure that one has not only heard an order correctly but also

---

BOX 26.3   Guidelines for Telephone and Verbal Orders

- Clearly identify the patient's name, room number, and diagnosis.
- Use clarification questions to avoid misunderstandings.
- Document "TO" (telephone order) or "VO" (verbal order), including date and time, name of patient, the complete order; the name and credentials of the health care provider giving the order(s); and your name and credentials as the nurse taking the order.
- Read back all orders prescribed to the health care provider who gave them and document "TORB" (telephone order read back) when signing your name and credentials.
- Follow agency policies; some institutions require telephone (and verbal) orders to be reviewed and signed by two nurses.

---

transcribed it accurately (ISMP, 2017). For example, document a TO as follows: *"09/30/2016 (1015), Change IV fluid to Lactated Ringers with potassium 20 mEq/L to run at 125 mL/hr. TO: Dr. Knight/K. Day, RN, telephone order read back (TORB)."* The health care provider later verifies the TO or VO legally by co-signing it within a time frame (e.g., 24 hours) set by agency policy.

Incident or Occurrence Reports

An incident or occurrence is any event that is not consistent with the routine, expected care of a patient or the standard procedures in place on a health care unit or within an agency (Chapter 23). Examples include patient falls, needlestick injuries, medication administration errors, accidental omission of ordered therapies, a visitor losing consciousness, and any circumstances that lead to injury or pose a risk for patient injury such as a "near miss." There are several definitions for "near miss"; however, there is consensus that this term should be used to indicate incidents in which a patient is exposed to a hazardous situation with the potential to cause harm but in which, for a variety of reasons (luck or early detection), no harm did occur (Agency for Healthcare Research and Quality, 2019).

An **incident report (occurrence report)** is completed whenever an incident occurs. Analysis of incident reports helps to identify system and/or individual human issues in which educational or in-service programs or changes in policies and procedures are needed to reduce the risk of future occurrences. Incident reports are an important part of the QI program of a unit or agency; however, they are not part of the health care record. Incident reports contain confidential information; distribution of the report is limited to the individuals responsible for reviewing the forms.

Follow agency policy when completing an incident report, and file the report with your agency's risk-management department. When an incident occurs, document an objective description of what happened, what you observed, and the follow-up actions taken, including notification of the patient's health care provider in the patient's health care record. Remember to evaluate and document the patient's response to the incident in the health care record as well. Do not label this as an "incident," "near miss," or "sentinel event" in the health care record, and do not make any reference to these types of documents. A notation about an incident, near miss, or sentinel event report in a patient's health care record makes it easier for a lawyer to argue that the reference makes the incident report part of the health care record and therefore admissible for attorney review.

ACUITY RATING SYSTEMS

Nurses use **acuity rating systems** to determine the hours of care and number of staff required for a given group of patients every shift or every 24 hours. A patient's acuity level, usually determined by the assessment data an RN enters into a computer program, is based on the type and number of nursing interventions (e.g., IV therapy, wound care, or ambulation assistance) required by that patient over a 24-hour period. Although acuity ratings are not part of a patient's health care record, nursing documentation within the health care record provides evidence that supports the assessment of an acuity rating for an individual patient.

The acuity level is a classification that compares one or more patients with another group of patients. An acuity system classifies patients from 1 (independent in all but one or two aspects of care; almost ready for discharge) to 5 (totally dependent in all aspects of care; requiring intensive care). Using this system, a patient returning from surgery requiring frequent monitoring and extensive care has an acuity level of 3, compared with another patient awaiting discharge after a successful recovery from surgery who has an acuity level of 1. Accurate acuity ratings justify the number and qualifications of staff needed to safely care for patients. The patient-to-staff ratios established for a unit depend on a composite gathering of 24-hour acuity data for all patients receiving care (Sir et al., 2015).

DOCUMENTATION IN THE LONG-TERM HEALTH CARE SETTING

Long-term health care settings include skilled nursing facilities (SNFs), in which patients receive 24-hour-a-day care, including housing, meals, specialized (skilled) nursing care, treatment services, and long-term care facilities, in which patients with chronic conditions receive 24-hour-a-day care, including housing, meals, personal care, and basic nursing care. Requirements for documentation in these facilities are governed by individual state regulations, TJC, and CMS. CMS mandates use of the Resident Assessment Instrument (RAI), which includes the Minimum Data Set (MDS) and the Care Area Assessment (CAA) to document data in long-term care facilities. MDS assessment forms are completed on admission and then periodically within specific guidelines and time frames for all residents in certified nursing homes (Ahn et al., 2015). MDS data also determine the reimbursement level under the prospective payment system for Medicare Part A residents in an SNF (Chapter 2).

Communication among nurses; social workers; dietitians; and recreational, speech, physical, and occupational therapists is essential. Documentation in the long-term care setting supports an interprofessional approach to the assessment and planning process for all patients. Adherence to state and federal requirements as well as reimbursement for care provided in a long-term care facility is dependent on accurate completion of the required documentation to justify the care provided (Hebda et al., 2019).

DOCUMENTATION IN THE HOME HEALTH CARE SETTING

Documentation in the home care setting is different from other areas of nursing. The use of laptop and tablet computers makes it possible for home health care records to be available in multiple locations (i.e., the patient's home and the home care agency). This system improves accessibility to information and facilitates interprofessional collaboration. Medicare has specific guidelines to establish eligibility for home care reimbursement. Information used for reimbursement is gathered from documentation of care provided in the home care setting. Documentation is the quality control and the justification for reimbursement from Medicare, Medicaid, or private insurance companies. Information in the home care health care record includes patient assessment, referral and intake forms, the interprofessional plan of care, a list

of medications, and reports to third-party payers. Nurses document all their services for payment (e.g., direct skilled care, patient teaching, skilled observation, and evaluation visits) (TJC, 2018).

Nurses use two different data sets to document clinical assessments and care provided in the home care setting. Assessment using the Outcome and Assessment Information Set (OASIS) is required for all patients age 18 years and older (with the exception of patients receiving prenatal or postnatal care) who are receiving skilled care through a home health agency that is reimbursed by Medicare or Medicaid (Shang et al., 2015). OASIS includes a comprehensive admission assessment and allows for the calculation of clinical, functional, and service scores that provide justification for reimbursement of services (Research Data Assistance Center, 2016). The Omaha System is a research-based, comprehensive, standardized taxonomy or classification designed to enhance practice, documentation, and information management. It consists of three components (Problem Classification Scheme, Intervention Scheme, and Problem Rating Scale for Outcomes) and provides a useful model for comprehensive evaluation of the quality of nursing care provided in the home care setting (Hebda et al., 2019; Martin & Monsen, 2018).

CASE MANAGEMENT AND USE OF CRITICAL PATHWAYS

The case management model incorporates an interprofessional approach to delivery and documentation of patient care (see Chapter 2). Critical pathways (also known as clinical pathways, practice guidelines, or CareMap tools) are interprofessional care plans that identify patient problems, key interventions, and expected outcomes within an established time frame (AHC Media, 2015). Critical pathway documents facilitate integration of care because all members of the health care team use the same document to monitor a patient's progress during each shift or, in the case of home care, every visit. Evidence-based critical pathways can improve patient outcomes. For example, use of critical pathways has been shown to improve adherence to evidence-based guidelines for administration of antibiotics for community-acquired pneumonia (Almatar et al., 2016).

Unexpected outcomes, unmet goals, and interventions not specified within a critical pathway are called variances. A variance occurs when the activities on the critical pathway are not completed as predicted or a patient does not meet the expected outcomes. Variances sometimes result from a change in a patient's health or because of other health complications not associated with the primary reason for which a patient requires care. Once you identify a variance, you modify the patient's care to meet the needs associated with the variance. A positive variance occurs when a patient makes progress faster than expected (e.g., an indwelling urethral catheter is discontinued a day earlier than anticipated according to the critical pathway). An example of a negative variance is when a patient develops pulmonary complications after surgery, requiring oxygen therapy and monitoring with pulse oximetry. Variances to expected outcomes are documented with a progress note (Box 26.4). Documentation allows trends to be identified and analyzed, which can provide data to develop an effective action plan for responding to identified patient problems. Over time health care teams sometimes revise critical pathways if similar variances reoccur.

INFORMATICS AND INFORMATION MANAGEMENT IN HEALTH CARE

Health information technology (HIT) is the use of information systems and other information technology to record, monitor, and deliver patient care, and to perform managerial and organizational functions

---

BOX 26.4   Example of Variance Documentation

An RN working in the case management role is using a critical pathway for "Routine Postoperative Care" for a 56-year-old man who had abdominal surgery yesterday. One of the expected outcomes for postoperative day 1 on the critical pathway document is "Afebrile with lungs clear bilaterally." This patient has an elevated temperature, his breath sounds are decreased bilaterally in the bases of both lobes of the lungs, and he is slightly confused.

The following is an example of how the RN case manager documents this variance on the pathway:

"Breath sounds diminished bilaterally at the bases. T-100.4; P-92; R-28/min; pulse oximetry 84% on room air. Daughter states he is "confused" and did not recognize her when she arrived a few minutes ago. Oxygen 2 L nasal cannula started per standing orders. Oxygen saturation improved to 92% after 5 minutes. Dr. Lopez notified of change in status. Daughter remains at bedside."

---

in health care (Hebda et al., 2019). The focus of HIT is the patient and the process of care, and the goal of using HIT is to enhance the quality and efficiency of care provided.

Health Care Information System

A **health care information system (HIS)** consists of "computer hardware and software dedicated to the collection, storage, processing, retrieval, and communication of patient care information in a healthcare organization" (Hebda et al., 2019). An HIS consists of two major types of information systems: a clinical information system and an administrative information system. Together the two systems operate to make the entry and communication of data and information more efficient. Individual health care agencies sometimes use one or several clinical information systems and administrative information systems. Administrative information systems include databases such as payroll, financial, and quality improvement systems (Hebda et al., 2019).

Clinical Information System

A **clinical information system (CIS)** (also known as a patient care information system) is a large, computerized database management system that is used to access patient data needed to plan, implement, and evaluate care (Hebda et al., 2019). A CIS can include monitoring systems; order entry systems; and laboratory, radiology, and pharmacy systems. A monitoring system can include devices that automatically monitor and record biometric measurements (e.g., vital signs and oxygen saturation) in acute care, critical care, and specialty care areas. Some of these devices can be programmed to electronically send measurements directly to a nursing documentation system, decreasing nursing workload.

One example of an order-entry system is a computer program that allows nurses to order supplies and services from another department, such as sterile supplies from the central supply department. This eliminates the use of written order forms and expedites the delivery of needed supplies to a nursing unit. Another example is a **computerized provider order entry (CPOE)** system that allows health care providers to directly enter standardized, legible, and complete orders for patient care into a medical record from any computer in the HIS. Advanced CPOE systems have built-in clinical decision support tools and alerts to help a health care provider select the most appropriate medication or diagnostic test and automatically check for drug interactions, medication allergies, and other potential problems (HealthIT.gov, 2018). The direct entry of orders by providers eliminates safety issues related to illegible handwriting and transcription errors. In addition, a CPOE

system potentially speeds the implementation of ordered diagnostic tests and treatments, which contributes to quality care and better patient outcomes. A CPOE system improves reimbursements since some orders require preapprovals from insurance plans. CPOE, when integrated with an electronic practice management system, can flag orders that require preapproval, helping a health care institution reduce denied insurance claims (HealthIT.gov, 2018). Use of a CPOE system has been shown to improve productivity and cost-effectiveness in the communication and implementation of health care provider orders. More important, most CPOE systems have significant potential to reduce medication errors associated with illegibility and inappropriate drug use and dosing (Hebda et al., 2019).

Nursing Clinical Information Systems

A well-designed **nursing clinical information system (NCIS)** incorporates the principles of nursing informatics to support the work that nurses do by facilitating documentation of nursing process activities and offering resources for managing nursing care delivery (Box 26.5). It is important for nurses to be able to access computer programs easily, review patients' medical histories and health care provider orders, and then go to the patients' bedsides to conduct comprehensive assessments. Once you complete an assessment, you enter data into the computer terminal at the patient's bedside and develop a plan of care from the information gathered. This allows you to quickly share the plan of care with your patient and other health care providers. You will periodically return to the computer to check on laboratory test results and document the care you deliver. The computer screens and optional pop-up windows make it easy to locate information, enter and compare data, and make changes.

NCISs have two designs. The nursing process design is the most traditional. It organizes documentation within well-established formats such as admission and postoperative assessment problem lists, care plans, intervention lists or notes, and discharge planning instructions. The nursing process design facilitates the following:

- Generation of a nursing work list that outlines routine scheduled care activities for a patient
- Documentation of routine aspects of patient care such as hygiene, positioning, fluid intake and output, wound care measures, and blood glucose measurements
- Progress note entries: narrative notes, charting by exception, and/or flow sheets
- Documentation of medication administration (see Chapter 31)

More advanced systems incorporate standardized nursing languages such as the International Classification of Nursing Practice (ICNP), the North American Nursing Diagnosis Association–International (NANDA-I) nursing diagnoses, the Nursing Interventions Classification (NIC), and the Nursing Outcomes Classification (NOC) into the software (Hebda et al., 2019).

The other model for an NCIS is the protocol or critical pathway design (Hebda et al., 2019). This design facilitates interprofessional management of information because all health care providers use evidenced-based protocols or critical pathways to document the care they provide. The information system allows a user to select one or more appropriate protocols for a patient. An advanced system merges multiple protocols, using a master protocol or path to direct patient care activities. Standard health care provider order sets are included in the protocols and automatically processed. The system also integrates appropriate information into the medication delivery process to enhance patient safety. In addition, the system identifies variances of the anticipated outcomes on the protocols as documentation is entered. This provides all caregivers the ability to analyze variances and offer an accurate clinical picture of a patient's progress.

BOX 26.5 EVIDENCE-BASED PRACTICE
Effect of EHR Documentation on Nursing Practice

PICOT Question: For nurses working in acute care settings, what is the effect of using the electronic health record for documentation on time spent at the bedside providing patient care?

Evidence Summary

Nurses have long perceived that the time needed to complete documentation of patient care has negatively impacted the quality and time available for provision of direct patient care (Michel et al., 2017). However, technologies such as electronic health record systems have increasingly become integrated in the support of nursing practice, including direct patient care, health care administration, and health care education and research. There are few current studies demonstrating effective ways to integrate use of today's health information technology with the concept of caring. In a study by Schenk and colleagues (2016) clinical RNs were surveyed about ease of use, usefulness, and attitude before and after implementation of an EHR. While participants commented on both their frustration and optimism about EHRs, on average, one year after adoption, nurses believed that the EHR did not improve patient care, that the learning curve was steep, and they had lower confidence in using the EHR than anticipated. However, a second study surveyed nurses from eight medical-surgical units working 12-hour shifts, across four hospitals in two states, 6 months after implementation of an EHR (Gomes et al, 2016). Data demonstrated that after implementation nurses spent more time in patient rooms engaged in purposeful interaction with patients and that time required for nursing documentation decreased by 4%, which may have been related to increased skill in using the EHR for documentation.

In a systematic review conducted by Baumann and colleagues (2018), the proportion of staff time spent on documentation was higher in the presence of an EHR system compared with settings without EHR implementation for physicians, nurses, and interns, and this difference was statistically significant for nurses. Study results indicated that pre-EHR, interns had the largest proportion of total workload spent on documentation tasks, followed by physicians, and that nurses had the lowest workload time spent completing documentation. After implementation of an EHR, physicians had the largest proportion of total workload spent on documentation tasks, followed by interns and then nurses. However, there is some evidence that over a longer period of time with full implementation of an EHR, documentation time may ultimately decrease, accompanied by improved work and information flow, significant decreases in multitasking, and improved patient safety (Baumann et al., 2018).

Application to Nursing Practice
- More studies are needed to clearly demonstrate the percentage of time needed for nurses to satisfactorily document the care they provide. Institutions should monitor clinical nurses' perceptions of EHR functions.
- Using technology, including electronic documentation systems for patient intake and assessment, can help enhance quality and safety in nursing. However, establishing a therapeutic nurse-patient relationship is essential to quality care.

Advantages of a Nursing Clinical Information System. Anecdotal reports and descriptive studies suggest that NCISs offer important advantages to nurses in practice. According to Hebda et al. (2019), some specific advantages include:
- Better access to information.
- Enhanced quality of documentation through prompts.
- Reduced errors of omission.
- Reduced hospital costs.
- Increased nurse job satisfaction.
- Adherence to requirements of accrediting agencies (e.g., TJC).
- Development of a common clinical database.
- Enhanced ability to track records.

Many NCISs include content-importing technologies that allow the use of templates, macros, automated data points, and the ability to copy forward either parts of or entire nursing shift assessments that enable nurses to quickly document their assessment or the care they provided. These features have benefits and risks associated with their use. When allergy and current medication lists are automatically imported into nursing admission documentation from a previous hospital encounter, you need to meticulously review this information for accuracy and update it as needed to avoid documentation errors and patient safety concerns. When nursing shift assessment data is copied forward from a previous shift or day, it must be updated so that it accurately reflects a patient's current clinical status (National Institute of Standards and Technology - US Department of Commerce, 2017).

Clinical Decision Support Systems

A **clinical decision support system (CDSS)** is a computerized program that aids and supports clinical decision making. The knowledge base within a CDSS contains rules and logic statements that link information required for clinical decisions to generate tailored recommendations for individual patients; the recommendations are presented to health care providers as alerts, warnings, or other information for consideration (Hebda et al., 2019). For example, an effective CDSS notifies health care providers of patient allergies before entering a medication order using CPOE to increase patient safety during the medication-ordering process.

CDSSs also improve nursing care. When patient assessment data are combined with patient care guidelines, nurses are better able to implement evidence-based nursing care. These programs are called a *nursing CDSS (NCDSS)* when used to support nursing decisions.

An example of an NCDSS is a program that requires entry of data regarding a patient's risk factors for falls and provides evidence-based alternatives for fall prevention interventions. The interventions are displayed through the decision support system based on a patient's fall risk score and are selected for the plan of care, thus supporting clinical decision making (Ahamed et al., 2016). Use of nursing-specific CDSSs has not been implemented as often as CDSSs in other disciplines. However, CDSSs are in development for acute care nursing settings (Ahamed et al., 2016; Rudolph et al., 2016).

Nursing Informatics

You need to be knowledgeable in the science and application of nursing informatics. **Nursing informatics** is the specialty that integrates nursing science, computer science, and information science to manage and communicate data, information, knowledge, and wisdom in nursing and informatics practice (American Nursing Informatics Association, 2019). Nursing informatics is recognized as a specialty area of nursing practice at the graduate level. Nurses who specialize in informatics have advanced knowledge in information management and demonstrate proficiency with informatics to support all areas of nursing practice, including QI, research, project management, and system design (American Nursing Informatics Association, 2019). Through the application of nursing informatics, technology is put to practical use to enhance bedside care and education. It offers an efficient and effective nursing information system that facilitates the integration of data, information, and knowledge to support patients, nurses, and other providers in patient care decision making.

Informatics Competencies for Nursing Graduates Entering the Workforce

Nursing competence in **health care informatics** is a priority as health care providers and agencies across the United States shift

BOX 26.6   QSEN Competencies for Informatics

QSEN Competency in Informatics: Use information and technology to communicate, manage knowledge, mitigate error, and support decision making.

Knowledge:
Explain why information and technology skills are essential for safe patient care.

Skills:
Seek education about how information is managed in care settings before providing care.
Apply technology and information management tools to support safe processes of care.

Attitudes:
Appreciate the necessity for all health professionals to seek lifelong, continuous learning of information technology skills.

Knowledge:
Identify essential information that must be available in a common database to support patient care.
Contrast benefits and limitations of different communication technologies and their impact on safety and quality.

Skills:
Navigate the electronic health record.
Document and plan patient care in an electronic health record.
Employ communication technologies to coordinate care for patients.

Attitudes:
Value technologies that support clinical decision making, error prevention, and care coordination.
Protect confidentiality of protected health information in electronic health records.

Knowledge:
Describe examples of how technology and information management are related to the quality and safety of patient care.
Recognize the time, effort, and skill required for computers, databases, and other technologies to become reliable and effective tools for patient care.

Skills:
Respond appropriately to clinical decision-making supports and alerts.
Use information management tools to monitor outcomes of care processes.
Use high-quality electronic sources of health care information.

Attitudes:
Value nurses' involvement in design, selection, implementation, and evaluation of information technologies to support patient care.

From QSEN Institute: *QSEN competencies.* http://qsen.org/competencies/pre-licensure-ksas/#informatics. Accessed June 10, 2019.

to the use of electronic documentation. You need informatics competencies to deliver safe and efficient care and to facilitate the implementation of evidence-based practice. Professional organizations such as the American Association of Colleges of Nursing, the National League for Nursing, and the Quality and Safety Education for Nurses (QSEN) Institute recommend that all nurses acquire a minimal level of awareness and competence in informatics and the use of information technology (Hebda et al., 2019). The American Association of Colleges of Nursing (2008) established a framework

that outlines curricular goals and informatics competencies for baccalaureate, master's, and doctoral programs of nursing that remains current today.

QSEN defined the scope of RN competencies for informatics as "the use of information and technology to communicate, manage knowledge, mitigate error, and support decision making" and outlined specific knowledge, skills, and attitudes that nursing students need to learn to use informatics technology to provide patient care in an effective and safe manner (QSEN Institute, 2018). Competence in informatics is not the same as computer competency. To become competent in informatics, you must use evolving methods of discovering, retrieving, and using information in practice (Hebda et al., 2019). Patients' records contain multiple types of data, and you need to know how to record, interpret, and report data and use critical thinking to apply your knowledge when providing patient care. You must also recognize when information is needed and have the skills to find, evaluate, and use that information effectively. QSEN competencies in informatics for prelicensure nursing students are outlined in Box 26.6.

As a nurse you need to know how to use clinical databases within your institution and apply the information so that you can deliver high-quality, appropriate patient care. You will collect data, including numbers, characters, or facts, according to a perceived need for analysis and possible action. You gain knowledge from gathering and using information from several sources. For example, you review several consecutive assessments of a wound documented within the EHR. Reviewing changes in the descriptions of the wound's edges, color of drainage, and measurements over several days allows you to evaluate and identify a pattern that indicates that the wound is not healing. Based on evidence available in the scientific literature, you apply knowledge of wound care principles and intervene to develop new nursing interventions to manage the patient's wound and promote healing.

QSEN **Building Competency in Informatics** A patient diagnosed with a deep vein thrombosis in the left lower leg was admitted 3 days ago and has been receiving a continuous heparin infusion of 1300 units/hr via the peripheral IV located in the left lower forearm. You are the RN caring for this patient from 1500 to 2300 today, and you learn during hand-off report that the patient's most recent partial thromboplastin time (PTT) is 70 seconds, indicating that the current dose of heparin infusing at 1300 units/hr is therapeutic (Pagana et al., 2019). The goal for this patient is to establish therapeutic anticoagulation levels using warfarin (an oral anticoagulant) so that the heparin infusion can be discontinued. The patient will be discharged with a prescription for warfarin, which will be taken daily for 6 months until the DVT has resolved. The patient received the first dose of warfarin 10 mg PO yesterday evening.

The patient's next dose of warfarin 10 mg PO is due at 1800. You log on to the computer located in the patient's room at that time and open the medication administration record in the patient's EHR. As you scan the package of warfarin using the bar code medication administration function, a warning statement, "Review most recent PT/INR results before administration," pops up on the computer screen. You switch screens in the EHR to review the patient's laboratory results and note that the patient's most recent prothrombin time (PT) is 21 seconds, and the international normalized ration (INR) is 2.3, indicating that the dose of warfarin that the patient received yesterday was too high and that the patient has a critically increased risk for bleeding (Pagana et al., 2019). The abnormal results are displayed in red font in the EHR, and a notation reading "Critical Value" is displayed next to each of the results displayed in red. What does the warning statement that popped up on the computer screen represent? What is the most appropriate action for you to take in this situation?

Answers to QSEN Activities can be found on the Evolve website.

KEY POINTS

- The health care record provides a legal and financial record of care, aids in clinical education and research, and guides professional and organizational performance improvement.
- Nursing documentation supports reimbursement to health care agencies through accurate accounting of the use of services and equipment and medications administered.
- Effective nursing documentation limits liability through objective description of what happened to a patient and clearly indicates that individualized, goal-directed nursing care was provided based on nursing assessment.
- Nurses must understand and be able to implement administrative, physical, and technical safeguards for protected health information (PHI) found in all forms of the health care record.
- Quality documentation is accurate, detailed, timely, and incorporates precise measurements, correct spelling, and proper use of abbreviations.
- Patient safety is enhanced when health care professionals eliminate the use of dangerous abbreviations, acronyms, symbols, and dose designations from their documentation.
- Documentation in the electronic health record requires nurses to be skilled in the use of flow sheets and narrative formats for recording patient information.
- Documentation of a safe plan for discharge includes information given on medications, diet, community resources, follow-up care, and contact information for whom to call with questions or in case of an emergency.
- When information relevant to care is communicated by telephone, verification of information through use of a read-back process should be documented in the health care record.
- Health care informatics facilitates the integration of data, information, knowledge, and wisdom to support patients, nurses, and other providers in decision making in all roles and settings.
- Nursing students must develop the knowledge, skills, and attitudes that will enable them to facilitate safe patient care and maintain patient confidentiality when using electronic documentation systems.

REFLECTIVE LEARNING

- Describe the actions you will take to protect the privacy of patient information if you need to print information from an EHR during clinical to complete your clinical paperwork after returning to campus.
- Using a recent clinical experience, describe how a clinical decision support system could support evidence-based practice allowing you to make decisions that would result in safe and effective nursing actions.
- Imagine there is an increased incidence of pressure injuries among the patients on the unit where you have clinical. Describe what data you could collect from the agency's nursing information system to determine why these patients are at greater risk for skin breakdown and what factors related to the nursing care provided on the unit are influencing the prevalence of hospital-acquired pressure injuries. Discuss why this information is important to collect.

REVIEW QUESTIONS

1. The nurse contacts a provider about a change in a patient's condition and receives several new orders for the patient over the phone. When documenting telephone orders in the electronic health record, most hospitals require a nurse to do which of the following?
   1. Print out a copy of all telephone orders entered into the electronic health record in order to keep them in personal records for legal purposes.
   2. "Read back" all telephone orders to the provider over the phone to verify all orders were heard, understood, and transcribed correctly before entering the orders in the electronic health record.
   3. Record telephone orders in the electronic health record, but wait to implement the order(s) until they are electronically signed by the health care provider who gave them.
   4. Implement telephone order(s) immediately, but insist that the health care provider come to the patient care unit to personally enter the order(s) into the electronic health record within the next 24 hours.

2. The nurse is working in an agency that has recently implemented an electronic health record. Which of the following are acceptable practices for maintaining the security and confidentiality of electronic health record information? (Select all that apply.)
   1. Using a strong password and changing your password frequently according to agency policy
   2. Allowing a temporary staff member to use your computer user name and password to access the electronic record
   3. Ensuring that work lists (and any other data that must be printed from the electronic health record) are protected throughout the shift and disposed of in a locked receptacle designated for documents that are to be shredded when no longer needed
   4. Ensuring that the patient information that is displayed on the computer monitor that you are using is not visible to visitors and other health care providers who are not involved in that patient's care
   5. Remaining logged in to a computer to save time if you only need to step away to administer a medication

3. When documenting an assessment of a patient's cardiac system in an electronic health record, the nurse uses the computer mouse to select the "WNL" statement to document the following findings: *"Heart sounds S1 & S2 auscultated. Heart rate between 80–100 beats per minute, and regular. Denies chest pain."* This is an example of using which of the following documentation formats?
   1. Focus charting incorporating "Data, Action & Response" (DAR)
   2. Problem-intervention-evaluation (PIE)
   3. Charting-by-exception (CBE)
   4. Narrative documentation

4. The nurse works at an agency where military time is used for documentation, and needs to document that a patient was transported to the operating room for an emergency procedure at 8 in the evening. Point to the area on the clockface below that indicates 8 in the evening in military time:

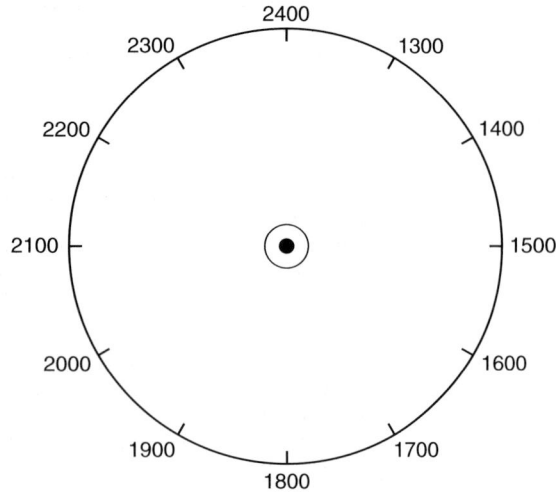

5. The nurse who works at the local hospital is transferring a patient to an acute rehabilitation center in another town. To complete the transfer, information from the patient's electronic health record must be printed and faxed to the acute rehabilitation center. Which of the following actions is most appropriate for the nurse to take to maintain privacy and confidentiality of the patient's information when faxing this information? (Select all that apply.)
   1. Confirm that the fax number for the acute rehabilitation center is correct before sending the fax.
   2. Use the encryption feature on the fax machine to encode the information and make it impossible for staff at the acute rehabilitation center to read the information unless they have the encryption key.
   3. Fax the patient's information without a cover sheet so that the person receiving the information at the acute rehabilitation center can identify it more quickly.
   4. After sending the fax, place the information that was printed out in a standard trash can after ripping it into several pieces.
   5. After sending the fax, place the information that was printed out in a secure canister marked for shredding.
6. The nurse is administering a dose of metoprolol to a patient, and is completing the steps of bar code medication administration within the EHR. As the bar code information on the medication is scanned, an alert that states "Do not administer dose if apical heart rate (HR) is <60 beats/minute or systolic blood pressure (SBP) is <90 mm Hg" appears on the computer screen. The alert that appeared on the computer screen is an example of what type of system?
   1. Electronic health record (EHR)
   2. Charting by exception
   3. Clinical decision support system (CDSS)
   4. Computerized physician order entry (CPOE)
7. The nurse is writing a narrative progress note. Identify each of the following statements as subjective data (S) or objective data (O):
   1. April 24, 2019 (0900)
   2. Repositioned patient on left side.

3. Medicated with hydrocodone-acetaminophen 5/325 mg, 2 tablets PO.
4. "The pain in my incision increases every time I try to turn on my right side."
5. S. Eastman, RN
6. Surgical incision right lower quadrant, 3 inches in length, well approximated, sutures intact, no drainage
7. Rates pain 7/10 at location of surgical incision.
8. The nurse is discussing the advantages of using computerized provider order entry (CPOE) with a nursing colleague. Which statement best describes the major advantage of a CPOE system within an electronic health record?
   1. CPOE reduces the time necessary for health care providers to write orders.
   2. CPOE reduces the time needed for nurses to communicate with health care providers.
   3. Nurses do not need to acknowledge orders entered by CPOE in an electronic health record.
   4. CPOE improves patient safety by reducing transcription errors.
9. The nurse is reviewing health care provider orders that were handwritten on paper when all computers were down during a system upgrade. Which of the following orders contain an inappropriate abbreviation included on The Joint Commission's "Do Not Use" list and should be clarified with the health care provider?
   1. Change open midline abdominal incision daily using wet-to-moist normal saline and gauze.
   2. Lorazepam 0.5 mg PO every 4 hours prn anxiety
   3. Morphine sulfate 1 mg IVP every 2 hours prn severe pain
   4. Insulin aspart 8u SQ every morning before breakfast
10. The nurse is changing the dressing over the midline incision of a patient who had surgery. Assessment of the incision reveals changes from what was documented by the previous nurse. After documenting the current wound assessment, the nurse contacts the surgeon (Dr. Oakman) by telephone to discuss changes in the incision that are of concern. Which of the following illustrates the most appropriate way for the nurse to document this conversation?
    1. Health care provider notified about change in assessment of abdominal incision. T. Wright, RN
    2. 09-3-18: Notified Dr. Oakman by phone that there is a new area of redness around the patient's incision. T. Wright, RN
    3. 1015: Contacted Dr. Oakman and notified about changes in abdominal incision. T. Wright, RN
    4. 09-3-18 (1015): Dr. Oakman contacted by phone. Notified about new area of bright red erythema extending approximately 1 inch around circumference of midline abdominal incision and oral temperature of 101.5 F. No orders received. T. Wright, RN

Answers: 1. 2; **2.** 1, 3, 4; **3.** 3; **4.** 2000; **5.** 1, 2, 5; **6.** 3; **7.** O: 1, 2, 3, 5, 6, 7; S: 4; **8.** 4; **9.** 4; **10.** 4.

Rationales for Review Questions can be found on the Evolve website.

REFERENCES

Agency for Healthcare Research and Quality: *Patient Safety Network: Adverse events, near misses, and errors*, 2019. https://psnet.ahrq.gov/primers/primer/34/Adverse-Events-Near-Misses-and-Errors. Accessed July 20, 2019.

Ahamed T, et al.: Towards a methodology for nursing-specific clinical decision support systems, *Journal of Decision Systems* 25:23–34, 2016.

AHC Media: They're back! Clinical pathways are in favor again, *Hosp Case Manag* 23(2):13–15, 2015.

American Association of Colleges of Nursing: *The essentials of baccalaureate education for professional nursing practice*, Washington, DC, 2008, American Association of Colleges of Nursing.

American Medical Association: *HIPAA violations & enforcement*, 2017. https://www.ama-assn.org/practice-management/hipaa-violations-enforcement. Accessed July 20, 2019.

American Nursing Informatics Association: *Mission statement of the American Nursing Informatics Association*, 2019. https://www.ania.org/sites/default/files/assets/documents/factSheet.pdf. Accessed July 20, 2019.

Bae SH, Yoder LH: Implementation of the Centers for Medicare & Medicaid Services' nonpayment policy for preventable hospital-acquired conditions in rural and nonrural US hospitals, *J Nurs Care Qual* 30(4):313–322, 2015.

Brown G: Averting malpractice issues in today's nursing practice, *ABNF J* 27(2):25–27, 2016.

Cantrell S: Cultivating a culture of safety: communication and technology working together to reduce Never Events, *Healthcare Purchasing News* 41(6):38–44, 2017.

Compliancy Group: *HIPAA Done Right: What is the HITECH Act?* 2019. https://compliancy-group.com/what-is-the-hitech-act/. Accessed July 20, 2019.

Elliott L, et al.: Standardizing documentation: a place for everything, *Medsurg Nurs* 27(1):32–37, 2018.

gov HealthIT: What is computerized provider order entry? https://www.healthit.gov/faq/what-computerized-provider-order-entry, 2018. Accessed July 20, 2019.

Hebda T, et al.: *Handbook of informatics for nurses and health care professionals*, ed 6, New York, 2019, Pearson.

HIPAA Journal: *What is considered protected health information under HIPAA?* https://www.hipaajournal.com/what-is-considered-protected-health-information-under-hipaa/, 2019. Accessed July 20, 2019.

Hwang K: *Sources of big data in medicine*, 2017. https://www.verywellhealth.com/sources-of-big-data-in-health-care-1739184. Accessed July 20, 2019.

Institute for Safe Medication Practices (ISMP): *Despite technology, verbal orders persist, read back is not widespread, and errors continue*, 2017. https://www.ismp.org/resources/despite-technology-verbal-orders-persist-read-back-not-widespread-and-errors-continue. Accessed July 20, 2019.

Khokhar A, et al.: Framework for mining and analysis of standardized nursing care plan data, *West J Nurs Res* 39(1):20–41, 2017.

Lewis SL, et al.: *Medical-surgical nursing: assessment and management of clinical problems*, ed 10, St Louis, 2017, Elsevier-Mosby2017.

Martin KS, Monsen KA: *The Omaha System: solving the clinical data-information puzzle*, 2018. http://www.omahasystem.org/overview.html. Accessed July 20, 2019.

National Institute of Standards and Technology - US Department of Commerce: Examining the 'copy and paste' function in the use of electronic health records, *NISTIR* 8166:1–57, 2017.

Office of the National Coordinator for Health Information Technology: Health IT Dashboard: percent of hospitals, by type, that possess certified health IT, dashboard.healthit.gov/quickstats/pages/certified-electronic-health-record-technology-in-hospitals.php, 2018. Accessed July 20, 2019.

Ostrovsky Y, et al.: Technology and dynamic pathways: how to improve nursing care, documentation, and efficiency, *IPROC* 2(1), 2016.

Pagana K, et al.: *Mosby's diagnostic and laboratory test reference*, ed 13, St Louis, 2019, Mosby.

Polit DF, Beck CT: *Essentials of nursing research: appraising evidence for nursing practice*, ed 9, Philadelphia, 2018, Wolters Kluwer: Lippincott Williams & Wilkins.

QSEN Institute: *QSEN competencies: informatics*, 2018. http://qsen.org/competencies/pre-licensure-ksas/#informatics. Accessed July 20, 2019.

Rajković P, et al.: Checking the potential shift to perceived usefulness -the analysis of users' response to the updated electronic health record core features, *Int J Med Inform* 115:80–91, 2018.

Nurses Service Organization: *Charting by exception: the legal risks*, 2018. https://www.nso.com/Learning/Artifacts/Articles/Charting-by-exception-the-legal-risks. Accessed July 20, 2019.

Research Data Assistance Center: *Home Health Outcome and Assessment Information Set*, 2016. https://www.resdac.org/cms-data/files/oasis. Accessed July 20, 2019.

Sir MY, et al.: Nurse–patient assignment models considering patient acuity metrics and nurses' perceived workload, *J Biomed Inform* 55:237–248, 2015.

Stimson CE, Bodruff AL: Daily electronic health record reports meet meaningful use requirements, improve care efficiency, and provide a layer of safety for trauma patients, *J Trauma Nurs* 24(1):53–56, 2017.

The Joint Commission (TJC): Comprehensive accreditation manual for hospitals: the official handbook. (E-dition), The Joint Commission 2018.

Touchstone Compliance: *9 safeguards for a HIPAA compliant fax*, 2017. https://www.touchstonecompliance.com/9-safeguards-for-a-hipaa-compliant-fax/. Accessed July 20, 2019.

US Centers for Medicare and Medicaid Services: Clinical quality measures basics, https://www.cms.gov/regulations-and-Guidance/Legislation/EHRIncentivePrograms/ClinicalQualityMeasures.html, 2019. Accessed July 20, 2019.

Wager KA, et al.: *Health care information systems: a practical approach for health care management*, ed 4, San Francisco, CA, 2017, Jossey-Bass.

RESEARCH REFERENCES

Ahn H, et al.: Bodily pain intensity in nursing home residents with pressure ulcers: analysis of national Minimum Data Set 3.0, *Res Nurs Health* 38(3):207–212, 2015.

Almatar M, et al.: Clinical pathway and monthly feedback improve adherence to antibiotic guideline recommendations for community-acquired pnuemonia, *PloS One* 11(7):e0159467, 2016.

Bardach SH, et al.: Perspectives of health care practitioners: an exploration of interprofessional communication using electronic medical records, *J Interprof Care* 31(3):300–306, 2017.

Bauder R, et al.: A survey on the state of health care upcoding fraud analysis and detection, *Health Serv Outcomes Res Methodol* 17(1):31–55, 2017.

Baumann LA, et al.: The impact of electronic health record systems on clinical documentation times: a systematic review, *Health Policy* 122(8):827–836, 2018.

Gomes M, et al.: Connecting professional practice and technology at the bedside: nurses' beliefs about using an electronic health record and their ability to incorporate professional and patient-centered nursing activities in patient care, *Comput Inform Nurs* 34(12):578–586, 2016.

Michel L, et al.: The content and meaning of administrative work: a qualitative study of nursing practices, *J Adv Nurs* 73(9):2179–2190, 2017.

Ozkaynak M, et al.: Use of electronic health records by nurses for symptom management in inpatient settings: a systematic review, *Comp Inform Nurs* 35(9):465–472, 2017.

Rudolph JL, et al.: Validation of a delirium risk assessment using electronic medical record information, *J Am Med Dir Assoc* 17(3):244–248, 2016.

Schenk EC, et al.: RN perceptions of a newly adopted electronic health record, *J Nurs Admin* 46(3):139–145, 2016.

Shang J, et al.: Infection in home health care: results from national Outcome and Assessment Information Set data, *Am J Infect Control* 43:454–459, 2015.

Topaz M, et al.: Nurse informaticians report low satisfaction and multi-level concerns with electronic health records: results from an international survey, *AMIA Annu Symp Proc* 2016–2025, 2016, 2016.

27

Patient Safety and Quality

OBJECTIVES

- Discuss the key factors in patient-centered care that can improve patient safety.
- Discuss the vulnerable populations most at risk for threats to safety.
- Discuss common physical hazards and methods for preventing them.
- Discuss how an individual's developmental age creates safety risks.
- Explain the mobility alterations that pose risks for falling.
- Describe ways to prevent procedure-related accidents.

- Describe assessment activities that identify the physical, psychosocial, and cognitive status of a patient as it pertains to his or her safety.
- Discuss how to select environmental interventions for fall prevention for the home environment.
- Identify evidence-based alternatives to restraints for patients who are alert, oriented, and low risk.
- Identify factors to assess before placing patients in physical restraints.
- Identify the factors to assess when a patient is in restraints.

KEY TERMS

Aura, p. 407
Immunization, p. 388
Pathogen, p. 388
Poison, p. 386

Restraint, p. 405
Root cause analysis, p. 392
Seizure, p. 407
Seizure precautions, p. 407

Status epilepticus, p. 407
Workplace violence, p. 393

MEDIA RESOURCES

http://evolve.elsevier.com/Potter/fundamentals/
- Review Questions
- Video Clips
- Concept Map Creator
- Case Study with Questions

- Skills Performance Checklists
- Audio Glossary
- Content Updates
- Answers to QSEN Activity and Review Questions

Safety, often defined as freedom from psychological and physical injury, is a basic human need. Health care provided in a safe manner and in a safe community environment is essential for a patient's survival and well-being. A safe environment reduces the risk for illness and injury and helps to contain the cost of health care by preventing extended lengths of treatment and/or hospitalization, improving or maintaining a patient's functional status, and increasing a patient's sense of well-being. Nurses are responsible for incorporating critical thinking skills to promote patient safety. This involves using the nursing process—assessing patients' risks for injury in their home or health care environment, assessing for hazards that threaten safety, accurately diagnosing problems, and then planning and intervening appropriately to maintain a safe environment.

As members of the health care team, nurses are professionally responsible for engaging in activities that support a patient-centered safety culture. Patient-centered care promotes safety and requires you to recognize your patients or their designee as the source of control and full partner in providing compassionate and coordinated care based on respect for patient preferences, values, and needs (QSEN, 2018). Partnership is the key factor. The National Academy of Medicine's scientific panel defined patient and family engaged care (PFEC) as care planned, delivered, managed, and continuously improved in active partnership with patients and their families to ensure integration of their health and health care goals, preferences, and values (Frampton et al., 2017). It is difficult to achieve positive patient outcomes without nurses actively involving patients and families in safety promotion.

Health care organizations use a variety of processes and approaches to improve the quality of care delivered to patients. Much of the force behind the focus on safety comes from regulatory and accrediting agencies such as the Centers for Medicare and Medicaid Services (CMS) and The Joint Commission (TJC). The Joint Commission's 2020 National Patient Safety Goals (Box 27.1) are standards for all health care institutions and are specifically directed at reducing the risk of medical errors (TJC, 2020).

A culture of safety within a health care institution is important for minimizing adverse events even as nurses perform complex and

BOX 27.1 The Joint Commission 2020 Hospital National Patient Safety Goals

- Identify patients correctly.
- Improve staff communication.
- Use medicines safely.
- Use alarms safely.
- Prevent infection.
- Identify patient safety risks.
- Prevent mistakes in surgery.

hazardous work. The Agency for Healthcare Research and Quality (AHRQ, 2018a) describes key features of a "culture of safety":

- Acknowledgment of the high-risk nature of an organization's activities and the determination to achieve consistently safe operations
- A blame-free environment where individuals are able to report errors or near misses without fear of reprimand or punishment
- Encouragement of collaboration across levels of employees and disciplines to seek solutions to patient safety problems
- Organizational commitment of resources to address safety concerns

Recently the Joint Commission issued a safety alert, emphasizing the importance of identifying and reporting unsafe conditions before they cause harm, trusting that other health care staff and leadership will act on the report, and taking personal responsibility for one's actions to create a safety culture within a health care organization (TJC, 2018d). Organizations that support a culture of safety continually focus on performance improvement efforts, empowering employees to actively participate in the safety activities of the organization, risk-management findings, and safety reports to design safer work environments (see Chapter 23) (Boysen, 2013).

SCIENTIFIC KNOWLEDGE BASE

Environmental Safety

A patient's environment includes physical and psychosocial factors that influence or affect the life and survival of that patient. This broad definition of environment crosses the continuum of care for settings in which the nurse and patient interact, such as the hospital, long-term care facility, clinic, community center, school, and home. A safe environment protects the staff as well, allowing them to function optimally. Vulnerable populations are especially at risk for alterations in safety because of reduced access to health care, fewer resources, and increased morbidity. Those vulnerable groups most affected include infants, children, older adults, individuals with a chronic disease or a physical or mental disability, individuals who have difficulty communicating, and individuals who have a low-income or are homeless (Joszt, 2018; CDC, 2018a). A safe environment meets basic needs, reduces physical hazards as well as the transmission of pathogens, and controls pollution.

Basic Human Needs. Physiological needs, including the need for sufficient oxygen, nutrition, and optimum temperature, influence a person's safety. According to Maslow's hierarchy of needs, these basic needs must be met before physical and psychological safety and security can be addressed (see Chapter 6).

Oxygen. Supplemental oxygen is sometimes needed to meet a person's oxygenation needs. Patients who require supplemental oxygen in health care settings are at risk because oxygen is highly flammable. Fire can occur when a patient on oxygen therapy chooses to smoke or is exposed to a heat source. Strict codes regulate the use and storage

of medical oxygen in health care agencies. This is not the case in home environments. Be sure to administer oxygen safely and provide patients and family caregivers the information needed to manage oxygen correctly in the home (see Chapter 41). Oxygen can build up in a home and on a patient's clothing and hair. If a person smokes in an environment that has supplemental oxygen, such as a house, even a small spark can cause a fire that will spread very quickly, resulting in extensive burns and even death. Thus it is essential that no one smokes in a home equipped with supplemental oxygen.

Know factors in a patient's environment that decrease the amount of available oxygen. An improperly functioning heating system is a hazard in the home. A furnace, fireplace, or stove that is not properly vented introduces carbon monoxide (CO) into the environment. Carbon monoxide affects oxygenation by binding strongly with hemoglobin, preventing the formation of oxyhemoglobin and reducing the supply of oxygen delivered to tissues. Low concentrations of oxygen cause nausea, dizziness, headache and fatigue. Unintentional, non–fire-related (UNFR) carbon monoxide poisoning is one of the most common causes of poisoning in the United States. The (CDC 2018b) reports that every year approximately 50,000 people in the United States visit the emergency department due to accidental CO poisoning.

Nutrition. Meeting nutritional needs of patients requires knowledge about healthy food and food safety. Chapter 45 details the principles of balanced nutrition. Health care agencies are required to meet State Board of Health regulations for the storage, preparation, and provision of food to patients. In the home some patients do not know how to properly refrigerate, store, and prepare food. The (CDC 2018c) estimates that 48 million people get sick from a foodborne illness, 128,000 are hospitalized, and 3000 die each year. When you care for patients returning home or if you work in home health, educate them about food safety principles. Also, patients require an adequate, clean water supply for drinking and to wash fresh produce and dishes. If a patient does not prepare or store foods properly, it increases the risk for infections and food poisoning from norovirus or bacteria such as *Escherichia coli, Salmonella,* or *Listeria.*

Temperature. Temperature extremes that frequently occur during the winter and summer pose safety risks for vulnerable populations. Exposure to severe cold for prolonged periods causes frostbite and accidental hypothermia. Older adults, the young, patients with cardiovascular conditions, patients who have ingested drugs or alcohol in excess, and people who are homeless are at high risk for hypothermia. In contrast, exposure to extreme heat changes the electrolyte balance of the body and raises the core body temperature, potentially resulting in heatstroke or heat exhaustion. Chronically ill patients, older adults, and infants are at greatest risk for injury from extreme heat.

Physical Hazards. Physical hazards in the home and work environment threaten a person's safety and often result in physical or psychological injury or death. In 2016 unintentional injuries became the third leading cause of death (Kochanek et al., 2017). Motor vehicle accidents, poisonings, and falls were the leading causes of unintentional injuries. Additional environmental hazards include fire and disasters. In the work setting, repetitive motion injuries, vehicle accidents, falling objects and falls are common causes of injuries. A nurse's role is to educate patients about the common safety hazards in the home and at work, teaching them how to prevent injury and emphasizing the hazards to which patients are the most vulnerable.

Motor Vehicle Accidents. Vehicle design and equipment such as seat belts, airbags, laminated windshields, and accident prevention systems have improved vehicular safety. State laws relating to licensing of young drivers, safety belt use, child restraint use, and motorcycle helmets exist for driver protection. It is important that children ride in

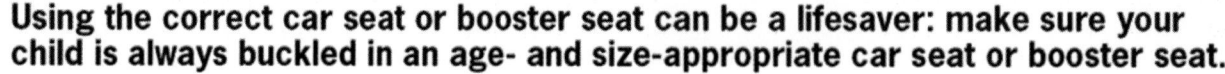
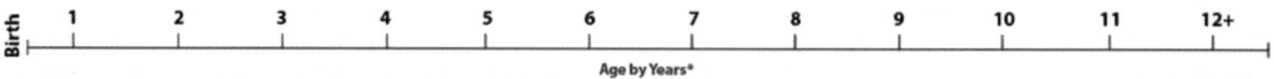

Using the correct car seat or booster seat can be a lifesaver: make sure your child is always buckled in an age- and size-appropriate car seat or booster seat.

Birth   1   2   3   4   5   6   7   8   9   10   11   12+

Age by Years*

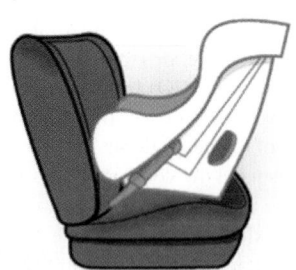
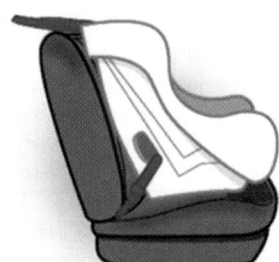
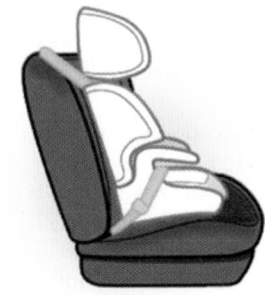
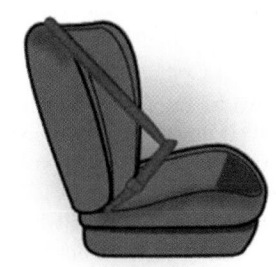

REAR-FACING CAR SEAT

FORWARD-FACING CAR SEAT

BOOSTER SEAT

SEAT BELT

Birth up to Age 2*
Buckle children in a rear-facing seat until age 2 or when they reach the upper weight or height limit of that seat.

Age 2 up to at least age 5*
When children outgrow their rear-facing seat, they should be buckled in a forward-facing car seat until at least age 5 or when they reach the upper weight or height limit of that seat.

Age 5 up until seat belts fit properly*
Once children outgrow their forward-facing seat, they should be buckled in a booster seat until seat belts fit properly. The recommended height for proper seat belt fit is 57 inches tall.

Once seat belts fit properly without a booster seat
Children no longer need to use a booster seat once seat belts fit them properly. Seat belts fit properly when the lap belt lays across the upper thighs (not the stomach) and the shoulder belt lays across the chest (not the neck).

Keep children ages 12 and under in the back seat. Never place a rear-facing car seat in front of an active air bag.

*Recommended age ranges for each seat type vary to account for differences in child growth and height/weight limits of car seats and booster seats. Use the car seat or booster seat owner's manual to check installation and the seat height/weight limits, and proper seat use.

Child safety seat recommendations: American Academy of Pediatrics.
Graphic design: adapted from National Highway Traffic Safety Administration.

FIG. 27.1 Car seat and booster seat guidelines. (From https://www.cdc.gov/injury/features/child-passenger-safety/. Accessed January 9, 2020.)

child safety seats and booster seats appropriate for their age and weight and type of car. The American Academy of Pediatrics (AAP, 2018a) recommends the following:

- Infants and toddlers should ride in a rear-facing car safety seat (Fig. 27.1) as long as possible, until they reach the highest weight or height allowed by their seat (see manufacturer's directions). Most convertible seats have limits that will allow children to ride rear-facing for 2 years or more.
- Once they are facing forward, children should use a forward-facing car safety seat with a harness for as long as possible, until they reach the height and weight limits for their seats. Many seats can accommodate children up to 65 lb or more.
- When children exceed these limits, they should use a belt-positioning booster seat until the vehicle's lap and shoulder seat belt fits properly. This is often when they have reached at least 4 feet, 9 inches in height and are 9 to 12 years of age.
- When children are old enough and large enough to use the vehicle seat belt alone, they should always use lap and shoulder seat belts for optimal protection.
- All children 12 years of age and younger should be restrained in the rear seats of vehicles for optimal protection.

According to the (CDC 2018d), the risk of motor vehicle accidents is higher among 16- to 19-year-old drivers than any other age-group,

with motor vehicle crashes being the leading cause of death for this age-group. Teens often underestimate dangerous situations or are unable to recognize hazardous situations (e.g., texting or talking on a phone while driving). In addition, they tend to speed and allow shorter headways, ride with intoxicated drivers, drive at night, and drive after using alcohol or drugs. Teens also have the lowest rate of seat belt use.

Elderly drivers are keeping their licenses longer and driving more miles than in the past. Driving is an important way in which older adults remain independent. But there are often risks, the longer an older adult drives. Age-related decline in vision and cognitive functioning (ability to reason and remember) and physical changes affect driving abilities of some older adults (CDC, 2017a). Ways to promote safety among older adult drivers include:

- Exercising regularly to increase strength and flexibility.
- Asking the doctor or pharmacist to review medications—both prescription and over-the-counter—to reduce side effects and interactions.
- Having eyes checked by an eye doctor at least once a year and wearing glasses and corrective lenses as required.
- Driving during daylight and in good weather.
- Finding the safest route, with well-lit streets, intersections with left-turn arrows, and easy parking.

Poison. A **poison** is any substance that impairs health or results in death when ingested, inhaled, injected, or absorbed into the body. Poisons often impair the function of every major organ system. Almost any substance is poisonous if too much is taken. Sources of poison in a person's home may include medicines, solid or liquid cleaning substances, gases, and vapors. Toddlers, preschoolers, and young school-age children are at greatest risk because of their curiosity, often ingesting household cleaning solutions, medications, or personal hygiene products in the home. Medications are commonly packaged in containers that hold multiple doses. As a result a child who is able to open a medicine container has access to multiple tablets or capsules. Emergency treatment is necessary when a person ingests a poisonous substance or comes into contact with a chemical that is absorbed through the skin. Every day, over 300 children in the United States ages 0 to 19 are treated in an emergency department as a result of being poisoned (CDC, 2016a). A poison control center is the best resource for patients and parents needing information about the treatment of an accidental poisoning. The nationwide poison control hotline center phone number is 1-800-222-1222.

Although lead has not been used in house paint or plumbing materials since the US Consumer Product Safety Commission banned it in 1978, some older homes still contain high lead levels. Soil and water systems are sometimes contaminated. Lead is emitted into the environment from industrial sources and contaminated sites, such as former lead smelters (EPA, 2018). Poisoning occurs from swallowing or inhaling lead. Fetuses, infants, and children are more vulnerable to lead poisoning than adults because their bodies absorb lead more easily, and small children are more sensitive to the damaging effects of lead. Exposure to excessive levels of lead affects a child's growth or causes learning and behavioral problems and brain and kidney damage.

Falls. A fall is an event that results in a person coming to rest inadvertently on the ground or floor or other lower level (WHO, 2018). Falls have been a major health problem, ranking as the second leading cause of accidental or unintentional injury deaths worldwide (WHO, 2018). Falls contribute to disability, lost work time, and in the case of many older adults, long-term care and institutionalization. Fall prevention has been a major quality health care initiative for community-dwelling older adults, as well as those in health care settings.

Falls are multifactorial; numerous factors increase the risk of falls. Older adults have the highest risk of death or serious injury following a fall (WHO, 2018). Other risk factors include (WHO, 2018; National Institute on Aging 2017):

- Occupations at elevated heights or other hazardous working conditions.
- Alcohol or substance use.
- Socioeconomic factors, including poverty, overcrowded housing, sole parenthood, or young maternal age.
- Underlying medical conditions, such as neurological, cardiac (orthostatic hypotension), or other disabling conditions.
- Polypharmacy and side effects of medications.
- Physical inactivity and loss of balance, particularly among older adults.
- Poor mobility (impaired balance, gait, coordination), cognition, and vision, particularly among those living in an institution, such as a nursing home or chronic care facility.
- Unsafe environments (e.g., broken stairs, icy sidewalks, inadequate lighting, throw rugs, exposed electrical cords, barriers along walking paths, and improper equipment for ambulation).
- Foot problems that cause pain and unsafe footwear, such as backless shoes or high heels.

Hospitals throughout the country carefully monitor the incidence of falls and fall-related injuries as part of their ongoing performance improvement work. Some of the agencies that provide education, monitoring guidelines, and fall prevention resources include:

- The Joint Commission—https://www.jointcommission.org/.
- The Institute for Healthcare Improvement—www.ihi.org.
- The US Department of Veterans Affairs Center for Patient Safety— https://www.patientsafety.va.gov/index.asp?_ga=2.255699786.35041262.1543845065-460341664.1543845065.
- US Department of Health and Human Services—www.HHS.gov.

Falls often lead to serious injuries such as fractures or internal bleeding. Patients most at risk for injury are those with osteoporosis or with bleeding tendencies resulting from disease or medical treatments. Fear of falling is a concern of community-dwelling older adults, and many avoid activities because of their fear.

Fire. A total of 358,500 structure fires were reported in the United States in 2011 to 2015, resulting in 2510 deaths, 12,300 injuries, and $6.7 billion in direct damage (NFPA, 2017a). The leading cause of fire-related death is careless smoking, especially when people smoke in bed at home. Cooking equipment was the leading cause of home structure fires and home fire injuries and the second leading cause of home fire deaths. Heating equipment (e.g., space heaters) was the second most common cause of home fires and fire injuries and the third leading cause of fire deaths (NFPA, 2017a). The improper use of cooking equipment and appliances, particularly stoves, is a major cause of in-home fires and fire injuries. Nurses play a role in educating the public about fire prevention measures.

Fires occur in health care facilities each year, with most occurring in nursing homes, followed by mental health facilities, hospitals, and hospices. Because patients in health care facilities are sick, disabled, or elderly, health care staff must know how to protect patients and respond to fires appropriately. Health care agencies have routine fire drills to measure staff responsiveness and understanding of fire safety protocols (NFPA, 2017b).

Disasters. Natural disasters such as floods, tsunamis, hurricanes, tornadoes, and wildfires are a major cause of death and injury. These types of disasters may result in death and can leave many people homeless. Every year millions of Americans are affected by natural disasters and their terrifying consequences. Bioterrorism is another cause of disaster and refers to biological agents (microbes or toxins) used as weapons to further personal or political agendas. A bioterrorist attack could be caused by virtually any pathogenic microorganism. The agents of greatest concern are anthrax (a bacterium) and smallpox (a virus). Both can be lethal. Anthrax is not communicable from direct contact but is transmitted in spores that become aerosolized. Smallpox is readily transmitted from person-to-person contact. Symptoms caused by these pathogens vary depending upon how the person was exposed but generally occur within 7 days of the exposure. Hospitals that are accredited by The Joint Commission must demonstrate they have proper plans and response mechanisms in place if a disaster occurs. The hospitals conduct annual disaster-preparedness exercises and must monitor the following six critical factors (Response Systems, n.d.):

- Communications—internal and external to community care partners, state/federal agencies
- Supplies—adequate levels and appropriateness to hazard vulnerabilities
- Security—enabling normal hospital operations and protection of staff and property
- Staff—roles and responsibilities within a standard hospital incident command structure
- Utilities—enabling self-sufficiency for as long as possible, with a goal of 96 hours

- Clinical activity—maintaining care, supporting vulnerable populations, and alternate standards of care

Transmission of Pathogens. Pathogens and parasites pose an ongoing threat to an individual's safety (see Chapter 28). Both patients and health care providers are at risk for exposure to pathogens. A pathogen is any microorganism capable of producing an illness. The most common means of transmission of pathogens is by the hands. For example, if an individual infected with hepatitis A does not wash his or her hands thoroughly after having a bowel movement, the risk for transmitting the disease to others during food preparation is increased. Nurses must educate patients about their unique risks for developing infection, such as immunosuppression from medications, chronic disease, or older age.

When a patient acquires an infection in a health care setting, it is called a nosocomial infection or health care–acquired infection (HAI). An HAI is one not present in the patient at the time of admission to the health care agency but that develops during the course of the stay. Health care facilities have standards for infection prevention in a variety of clinical situations, such as prevention of surgical site infections or catheter-associated urinary tract infections. One of the most effective methods for limiting the transmission of pathogens in health care is the medically aseptic practice of hand hygiene (see Chapter 28). It is important that nurses adhere to the practice of hand hygiene, follow standard and transmission-based isolation precautions, and educate patients, families, and caregivers about the importance of incorporating hand hygiene in all aspects of their lives.

Immunizations. Childhood vaccination has proven to be one of the most effective public health strategies to control and prevent disease (Ventola, 2016). Immunization reduces, and in some cases prevents, the transmission of disease from person to person. Recently, however, parents have shown concerns about immunizing their children. For example, some parents have had concerns that autism might be linked to the vaccines children receive, but studies have shown that there is no link between receiving vaccines and developing autism (CDC, 2016b). Another parental concern has been whether the timing of the 2-month and 4-month vaccinations is associated with sudden infant death syndrome, which commonly occurs in that same time frame. Studies have found that vaccines do not cause and are not linked to SIDS (CDC, 2016b). Currently, early childhood vaccination rates continue to improve among commercially insured children in the United States, with 77% of children born in 2013 completing their CDC-recommended seven-vaccine series by 2016, up from 69% for children born in 2010 (Blue Cross Blue Shield, 2018). Adherence to childhood vaccinations is a problem for vulnerable populations. In 2014, black children were less likely to be fully vaccinated than white or Hispanic children, and children in families with incomes below the poverty level were less likely than those in families with incomes at or above the poverty level to receive the combined-series vaccination (Child Trends Data Bank, 2015). Missed well-child visits are a primary driver of undervaccinated children (Blue Cross Blue Shield, 2018). Nurses play a role in informing parents about the importance of adhering to vaccination schedules for their children.

Adults require regular vaccinations depending on their age, job, lifestyle, travel, or health conditions (CDC, 2018e). For example, older adults are at risk for infectious disease if not regularly immunized for the flu and pneumonia. People in this age-group should also consult with their health care providers about receiving the vaccine for shingles as it is recommended for healthy adults 50 years and older (CDC, 2018e), Health care workers who are at risk for being exposed to blood or other body fluids should receive the three-dose series of vaccinations for hepatitis B.

NURSING KNOWLEDGE BASE

Factors Influencing Patient Safety

In addition to being knowledgeable about the home and health care environment and the inherent safety risks, nurses need to know a patient's developmental level; mobility, sensory, and cognitive status; lifestyle choices; and knowledge of common safety precautions. Nurses apply scientific evidence in managing developmental risks and the unique safety risks that are found in health care settings.

Developmental Stages and Risks. A patient's developmental stage can create threats to safety because of lifestyle, cognitive and mobility status, sensory impairments, and safety awareness. With this information safety-prevention programs are tailored to address the needs, preferences, and life circumstances of particular age-groups. Unfortunately, all age-groups are subject to physical and mental abuse. Child abuse, domestic violence, and elder abuse are serious threats to safety (see Chapters 11 to 14).

Infant, Toddler, and Preschooler. Injuries are the leading cause of death in children over age 1. The nature of the injury sustained is closely related to normal growth and development. For example, because of improved motor skills, coordination, and balance, preschoolers are less prone to falls than toddlers (Hockenberry et al., 2019). Infants and toddlers explore the environment and, because of their increased level of oral activity, put objects in their mouths. This increases their risk for poisoning or aspiration and choking on foreign material such as small toys. Parents do not always recognize the danger in seemingly harmless items, such as remote control devices and keyless remote door openers for vehicles. Button batteries if swallowed can cause serious injury or death (National Safety Council, 2019).

A safe sleep environment for an infant involves the placement of the infant on his back on a firm mattress in a safety-approved crib that is free of pillows, toys, and blankets, as these are suffocation hazards. Instruct patents about the hazards of sleeping with an infant in bed, on the sofa, or on the floor (National Institutes of Health, 2014).

Fortunately, preschoolers are generally less reckless and are aware of potential dangers such as hot objects or sharp instruments (Hockenberry et al., 2019). Limited physical coordination in preschoolers contributes to falls from riding bicycles and using playground equipment. Other injuries include burns and drowning. Most drowning or near-drowning incidents happen when a child falls into a pool or is left alone in the bathtub (National Safety Council, 2019). Accidents involving children are largely preventable. But accident prevention requires health education for parents and the removal of dangers whenever possible.

School-Age Child. School-age children enter a period of less intense emotions, secure in their dependency on parents and family and with self-confidence tempered by a more realistic perspective. They have energy to explore the environment beyond the home and to gradually increase the scope of interpersonal interaction (Hockenberry et al., 2019). When a child enters school, the environment expands to include the school, transportation to and from school, school friends, and after-school activities. School-age children are learning how to perform more complicated motor activities and often are uncoordinated. They are also expanding their cognitive and psychosocial skills. A child at this age needs to learn to cope with the rules and expectations of schools and peers. School-age children involved in team and contact sports may not consistently follow the rules for playing safely and may fail to use protective safety equipment, such as helmets and other protective gear. School-agers are exposed to more environments in which they need protection, they have less supervision, and they take more responsibility as they participate in a more adult world (Hockenberry et al., 2019).

The incidence of school violence, including fighting/assaults (with or without weapons by two or more individuals); bullying; physical, sexual, and psychological abuse; and violence against one-self (intentional nonsuicidal self-injury) has increased. The CDC's Youth Risk Behavior Survey found that nearly 24% of students had been in a physical fight on school property one or more times during the 12 months before the survey (CDC, 2018f). Violence in any form disrupts a child's ability to learn and may have a negative effect on health throughout life (National Association of School Nurses, 2018). School nurses are able to recognize the multiple factors that may increase or decrease a youth's risk of becoming a perpetrator or victim of school violence and may be able to identify students at risk (Box 27.2).

Adolescent. As children enter adolescence, they develop greater independence and a sense of identity. Adolescents begin to separate emotionally from their families, and peer groups begin to have a stronger influence. Adolescents typically have wide variations that swing from childlike to mature behavior. They test their boundaries by trying risky behaviors. Experimentation with the use of tobacco, alcohol, and other substances is common. By the 12th grade, approximately 63% of students have used alcohol, 45% have used electronic vapor cigarettes, 32% have smoked tobacco, 39% have tried cannabis, and 6% have tried illicit drugs (Kann et al., 2016). Trends such as the current opioid epidemic have alerted school communities to the dangers of prescription painkillers, as overdoses among young adults in the United States have quadrupled in the past decade (National Institute on Drug Abuse [NIDA], 2016). Without appropriate health literacy skills, misinformed parents and students can overlook or downplay the risks of substance use (NIDA, 2016). Environmental clues of substance abuse include the presence of drug-oriented magazines, beer and liquor bottles, or drug paraphernalia and the wearing of long-sleeved shirts in hot weather. Psychosocial clues include failing grades, change in dress, absenteeism from school, isolation, and changes in interpersonal relationships. Substance abuse increases the risks for accidents such as drowning and motor vehicle accidents. The Insurance Institute for Highway Safety ([IIHS], 2016) reports that males ages 20 to 24 and adults ages 85 and older had the highest rates of crash deaths.

Adolescents are also at risk for suicide because of feelings of decreased self-worth and hopelessness. Risk factors include (Kaslow, 2018):

- A recent or serious loss, such as the death of a family member, a friend, or a pet.
- A psychiatric disorder, particularly a mood disorder, such as depression, or a trauma- and stress-related disorder.
- Prior suicide attempts.
- Alcohol and other substance abuse disorders, as well as getting into a lot of trouble, having disciplinary problems, or engaging in high-risk behaviors
- Struggling with sexual orientation in an environment that is not respectful of or accepting of that orientation.

BOX 27.2 Risk Factors for Violence

- History of victimization
- Disabilities
- Emotional problems
- Substance abuse
- Low IQ
- Authoritarian parenting
- Low family involvement and low income
- Gang involvement
- School failure
- Transient lifestyle
- Diminished economic opportunities

Adapted from Centers for Disease Control and Prevention, Youth Violence: Risk and Protective Factors, 2017, https://www.cdc.gov/ViolencePrevention/youthviolence/riskprotectivefactors.html. Accessed December 16, 2019.

- A family history of suicide, as well as a history of domestic violence, child abuse, or neglect.
- Lack of social support. A child who doesn't feel support from significant adults in her life, as well as her friends, can become isolated.
- Bullying. It is known that being a victim of bullying is a risk factor, but there's also some evidence that kids who are bullies may be at increased risk for suicidal behavior.
- Access to lethal means, such as firearms and pills.

Adult. The threats to an adult's safety are frequently related to lifestyle habits. For example, a person who uses alcohol excessively is at greater risk for motor vehicle accidents or sustaining an injury at home. People who smoke long-term have a greater risk of cardiovascular or pulmonary disease because of the inhalation of smoke and the effect of nicotine on the circulatory system. Likewise, the adult experiencing a high level of stress is more likely to have an accident or illness such as headaches, gastrointestinal (GI) disorders, and infections.

Older Adult. The physiological changes associated with aging, the effects of multiple medications, psychological and cognitive factors, and the effects of acute or chronic disease increase an older adult's risk for falls and other types of accidents (e.g., burn injuries, vehicular crashes). More than one out of four adults 65 years of age and older falls each year, but fewer than half tell their health care providers (CDC, 2017b). Falls are the major cause of injury leading to disability and death among adults 65 years of age and older. Once a patient falls, the risk of falling a second time is increased (CDC, 2017b).

There are multiple reasons for cognitive changes in older adults. Some cognitive changes are part of the natural aspect of aging. For example, an older adult may walk into a room and forget the purpose of going to the room or begin to leave the home and find the car keys are misplaced. However, there are also reasons for abnormal cognitive changes that need to be assessed in the older adult. For example, the changes may be associated with treatment for a disease process (such as chemotherapy for cancer). Lange et al. (2018) studied patients who were 65 years or older with newly diagnosed early-stage breast cancer (EBC). The researchers noted five significant patterns of cognitive decline and impairment after the patients had completed their treatments.

Dementia is a clinical syndrome caused by neurodegeneration and characterized by progressive deterioration in cognitive ability and capacity for independent living. A systematic review of the literature estimated that 35.6 million people lived with dementia worldwide in 2010, with numbers expected to almost double every 20 years, to 65.7 million in 2030 and 115.4 million in 2050 (Prince et al., 2013). Dementia limits the ability to process information cognitively that normally allows people to perform tasks and prevent injury. Older adults who develop dementia often suffer from wandering. Wandering is the meandering, aimless, or repetitive locomotion that exposes a person to harm and is often in conflict with boundaries (such as doors), limits, or obstacles (Herdman and Kamitsuru, 2018). Wandering is dangerous. Individuals can walk away from home or off care units or enter restricted or closed areas without the knowledge of caregivers. Interrupting a wandering patient can increase his or her distress. Family caregivers, as well as professional caregivers, must apply safety principles to reduce patients' tendencies to wander and to provide safe living environments.

Mind-wandering is common among all older adults. It involves engaging in task-irrelevant thoughts that can have negative functional consequences, such as falls, and impaired task performance. In a study by Nagamatsu and colleagues (2013), falls were associated with an increased frequency of mind-wandering, involving an inability to actively control attention to align with current behavioral goals while simultaneously inhibiting task-unrelated thoughts. The tendency to mind-wander poses an obstacle for individuals to safely navigate their environments. Research is needed to explore whether mind-wandering is related to changes in gait.

Individual Risk Factors.
Other risk factors posing threats to safety include lifestyle, impaired mobility, sensory or communication impairment, limited economic resources, and the lack of safety awareness. Know patients' risks when you plan nursing care.

Lifestyle. Some lifestyle choices increase safety risks. People who drive or operate machinery while under the influence of chemical substances (drugs or alcohol), who work at dangerous jobs, or are risk takers are at greater risk of injury. In addition, people experiencing stress, anxiety, fatigue, or alcohol or drug withdrawal or those taking prescribed medications are sometimes more accident prone. Because of these factors, some people are too preoccupied to notice the source of potential accidents, such as cluttered stairs or a stop sign.

Impaired Mobility. A patient with impaired mobility has many kinds of safety risks. Muscle weakness, paralysis, abnormal gait, and poor coordination or balance are major factors in placing patients at risk for falls. Immobilization predisposes patients to physical deconditioning and emotional hazards, which in turn further restrict mobility and independence. People who are physically challenged are at greater risk for injury when entering motor vehicles and buildings that are not handicap accessible.

Sensory or Communication Impairment. Cognitive impairments associated with delirium, dementia, and depression alter concentration and attention span and cause impaired memory and orientation changes. Patients with these alterations become easily confused about their surroundings and are more likely to have falls and burns. This is a common problem when such patients temporarily or permanently move to a health care setting. Patients with visual, hearing, tactile, or communication impairment, such as aphasia or a language barrier, are not always able to perceive a potential danger or express their need for assistance (see Chapter 49). Patients with reduced health literacy are unable to understand the information needed to make the decisions required for providing safe home environments.

Economic Resources. People with lower incomes (including the homeless) are more likely to have behavioral health issues, such as depression or substance use problems, that place them at risk for injury. They also do not have access to the health care resources (such as medications and treatments) that those with higher incomes have (see Chapter 9). Those who are homeless are less likely to report having a regular source of health care and are more likely to have forgone needed care (McInnes et al., 2013). Those who are homeless may also not have a safe place to stay. When a patient who has a lower income enters a health care agency, ensure you assess all the patient's safety risks.

Lack of Safety Awareness. Some patients are unaware of or inexperienced in following safety precautions in the home, such as keeping medicine or poisons away from children or reading the expiration dates on food products. You cannot assume a patient's knowledge about a safety topic. A nursing assessment that includes a home inspection will help to identify a patient's level of knowledge about home safety. Use this information to guide patient education and when creating an individualized nursing care plan.

Risks in Health Care Agencies.
The prevention of medical errors continues to be one of the most pressing health care challenges in the nation. Medical errors occur when planned actions are not completed as intended or wrong plans of care are used. They occur in all health care settings. Be aware of the organizational and regulatory patient safety measures that have been established in the health care setting where you work. The AHRQ lists 20 tips for patients to become partners and help prevent medical errors (AHRQ, 2018b). The patient fact sheet can be viewed at the AHRQ website, https://www.ahrq.gov/patients-consumers/care-planning/errors/20tips/index.html.

TJC and the Centers for Medicare and Medicaid Services (CMS) emphasize error prevention and patient safety. Their "Speak Up" campaign encourages patients to take a role in preventing health care errors by becoming active, involved, and informed participants on the health care team (TJC, 2018a). For example, patients are encouraged to ask health care workers whether they have washed their hands before providing care. The National Patient Safety Goals of The Joint Commission (2019) highlight specific improvements in patient safety and ongoing problematic areas in health care. These evidence-based recommendations require health care agencies to focus their attention on a series of specific actions.

Another national organization, the National Quality Forum (NQF), leads the national collaboration among health care agencies and the public to improve health and health care quality through measurement (NQF, 2018a).The NQF brings key public- and private-sector leaders together to establish national priorities and goals to achieve health care that is safe, effective, patient-centered, timely, efficient, and equitable. In addition the organization creates NQF-endorsed standards used to measure and report on the quality and efficiency of health care in the United States. Many of the NQF measurement standards for patient safety (e.g., patient falls with injury, incidence of pressure injuries, and central line bloodstream infection [CLBSI]) are standards for judging the quality of care of health care organizations. Among the safety measures, the NQF endorsed a select list of serious reportable events (SREs) that include a range of clinical settings where patients receive care, including office-based practices, ambulatory surgery centers, and skilled nursing facilities (Box 27.3) (NQF, 2018b). The 29 events are a major focus of health care providers for patient safety initiatives.

The CMS selects some SREs as their *Never Events* (Box 27.4). Many of the hospital-acquired conditions (e.g., fall or stage III pressure injury) are nurse-sensitive indicators, meaning that a nurse directly affects their development. These indicators are the focus of performance improvement efforts by nursing departments across the country. The NQF released 34 Safe Practices for Better Healthcare (last updated in 2010) are effective in reducing the occurrence of adverse health care events across a variety of environments (NQF, 2018c). Scientific evidence supports the effectiveness of these practices in reducing the occurrence of adverse health care events.

Health care agencies often conduct a failure mode and effect analysis (FMEA) to identify problems with health care processes and products before they occur. When an actual or potential adverse event occurs, the nurse or health care provider involved completes an incident or occurrence report. An incident report is a confidential document that

BOX 27.3 National Quality Forum Serious Reportable Events in Health Care

1. Surgical or Invasive Procedure Events

A. Surgery or other invasive procedure performed on the wrong site (updated)

B. Surgery or other invasive procedure performed on the wrong patient

C. Wrong surgical or other invasive procedure performed on a patient (updated)

D. Unintended retention of a foreign object in a patient after surgery or other invasive procedure (updated)

E. Intraoperative or immediately postoperative/postprocedure death in an ASA Class 1 patient (updated)

2. Product or Device Events

A. Patient death or serious injury associated with the use of contaminated drugs, devices, or biologics provided by the health care setting (updated)

B. Patient death or serious injury associated with the use or function of a device in patient care, in which the device is used or functions other as intended (updated)

C. Patient death or serious injury associated with intravascular air embolism that occurs while being cared for in a health care setting (updated)

3. Patient Protection Events

A. Discharge or release of a patient/resident of any age who is unable to make decisions to other than an authorized person (updated)

B. Patient death or serious injury associated with patient elopement (disappearance) (updated)

C. Patient suicide, attempted suicide, or self-harm that results in serious injury, while being cared for in a health care setting (updated)

4. Care Management Events

A. Patient death or serious injury associated with a medication error (e.g., errors involving the wrong drug, wrong dose, wrong patient, wrong time, wrong rate, wrong preparation, or wrong route of administration) (updated)

B. Patient death or serious injury associated with unsafe administration of blood products (updated)

C. Maternal death or serious injury associated with labor or delivery in a low-risk pregnancy while being cared for in a health care setting (updated)

D. Death or serious injury of a neonate associated with labor or delivery in a low-risk pregnancy (new)

E. Patient death or serious injury associated with a fall while being cared for in a health care setting (updated)

F. Any Stage 3, Stage 4, and unstageable pressure ulcers acquired after admission/presentation to a health care setting (updated)

G. Artificial insemination with the wrong donor sperm or wrong egg (updated)

H. Patient death or serious injury resulting from the irretrievable loss of an irreplaceable biological specimen (new)

I. Patient death or serious injury resulting from failure to follow up or communicate laboratory, pathology, or radiology test results (new)

5. Environmental Events

A. Patient or staff death or serious injury associated with an electric shock in the course of a patient care process in a health care setting (updated)

B. Any incident in which systems designated for oxygen or other gas to be delivered to a patient contain no gas, the wrong gas, or are contaminated by toxic substances (updated)

C. Patient or staff death or serious injury associated with a burn incurred from any source in the course of a patient care process in a health care setting (updated)

D. Patient death or serious injury associated with the use of physical restraints or bedrails while being cared for in a health care setting (updated)

6. Radiologic Events

A. Death or serious injury of a patient or staff associated with the introduction of a metallic object into the MRI area (new)

7. Potential Criminal Events

A. Any instance of care ordered by or provided by someone impersonating a physician, nurse, pharmacist, or other licensed health care provider (updated)

B. Abduction of a patient/resident of any age (updated)

C. Sexual abuse/assault on a patient or staff member within or on the grounds of a health care setting (updated)

D. Death or serious injury of a patient or staff member resulting from a physical assault (i.e., battery) that occurs within or on the grounds of a health care setting (updated)

BOX 27.4 The 2014 Centers for Medicare and Medicaid Services Hospital-Acquired Conditions (Present-on-Admission Indicator)

For discharges occurring on or after October 1, 2008, hospitals will not receive additional payment for cases in which one of the selected conditions was not present on admission:

- Foreign object retained after surgery
- Air embolism
- Blood incompatibility
- Pressure injury Stages 3 or 4
- Falls and trauma (fracture, dislocation, intracranial injury, crushing injury, burn, electric shock)
- Catheter-associated urinary tract infections
- Vascular catheter-associated infections

- Manifestations of poor glycemic control (diabetic ketoacidosis, nonketotic hyperosmolar coma, hypoglycemic coma, secondary diabetes with ketoacidosis, secondary diabetes with hyperosmolarity)
- Surgical site infections following:
  - Mediastinitis following coronary artery bypass graft
  - Certain orthopedic procedures (spine, neck, shoulder, elbow)
  - Bariatric surgery for obesity (laparoscopic gastric bypass, gastroenterostomy, laparoscopic gastric restrictive surgery)
  - Cardiac implantable medical device
  - Deep-vein thrombosis (DVT)/pulmonary embolism (PE) following certain orthopedic procedures (total knee replacement, hip replacement)
  - Iatrogenic pneumothorax with venous catheterization

From Centers for Medicare and Medicaid Services (CMS): *Hospital-acquired conditions (present on admission indicator)*, 2018, http://www.cms.gov/HospitalAcqCond/06_Hospital-Acquired_Conditions.asp. Accessed December 2018.

completely describes any patient accident occurring on the premises of a health care agency (see Chapter 23). Reporting allows an organization to identify trends or patterns throughout the agency and areas to improve. Focusing on the root cause of an event instead of the individual involved promotes a culture of safety that helps in specifically identifying what contributed to an error. The evidence shows that the use of evidence-based practices can have a favorable impact on patient safety. The strongest evidence exists for interventions that are effective in preventing delirium, adverse drug events, infections, and falls (Zegers et al., 2016).

Chemical Exposure. Both patients and health care workers face serious environmental health risks within health care agencies. An example of a risk to health care workers is exposure to various forms of chemicals. Chemicals found in some medications (e.g., chemotherapy), anesthetic gases, cleaning solutions, and disinfectants are potentially toxic if ingested, absorbed into the skin, or inhaled. A health care provider or family caregiver who becomes exposed to a chemotherapeutic agent, especially one in liquid form, has an increased risk for leukemia, other cancers, and adverse reproductive outcomes and chromosomal damage (CDC, 2018g). When exposure to a chemical occurs, material safety data sheets (MSDSs) provide detailed information about the chemical, the precautions for safe handling and use, health hazards related to exposure, first aid guidelines, and steps for containment and removal in case of release or spillage. MSDSs are required resources available in any health care agency (OSHA, n.d.a). Nurses need to know the location of the MSDSs and how to follow safety guidelines within their agencies.

Falls. Falls result in minor-to-severe injuries such as bruises, hip fractures, or head trauma that result in reduced mobility and independence and increase the risk for premature death. Falls often occur in health care settings. As is the case in home and community environments, falls are multifactorial in health care settings. Approximately 30% to 35% of patients who fall sustain injuries ([The Joint Commission Center for Transforming Healthcare TJCCTH, 2018]). Common factors within the hospital environment that contribute to falls include sleep deprivation, a new environment, a change in medications, or deterioration in physical strength brought on by change in a disease process. A fall contributes to a patient's functional decline and increased health care use. A fall can cause lasting pain and suffering and may limit physical, psychological, and social function, placing burdens on patients, families, and society. Each injury resulting from a fall, on average, adds 6.3 days to a hospital stay and costs about $14,056 (TJCCTH, 2018). When a patient death or serious injury is associated with a fall while the patient is being cared for in a health care setting, it is called a *Never Event*. The Centers for Medicare and Medicaid will not pay for additional costs associated with *Never Events*. When a fall occurs within a health care setting, The Joint Commission (TJC) mandates the organization perform a thorough root cause analysis after the event in an effort to find approaches to prevent similar events in the future (AHRQ, 2018c). Health care agencies have initiatives in place to reduce falls, including use of special fall risk assessment tools, evidence-based fall prevention protocols, fall alert room signs, and special identification bands (Box 27.5).

Patient-Inherent Accidents. Patient-inherent accidents are accidents (other than falls) in which a patient is the primary reason for the accident. Examples include self-inflicted cuts, injuries, and burns; ingestion or injection of foreign substances; self-mutilation or setting fires; and pinching fingers in drawers or doors. A diagnosis of a seizure disorder places a patient at risk for a patient-inherent accident. Place patients with seizure disorders on seizure precautions to reduce risk of injury.

Procedure-Related Accidents. Procedure-related accidents are caused by health care providers and include medication and fluid administration errors, improper application of external devices,

---

BOX 27.5 EVIDENCE-BASED PRACTICE

Fall Prevention

PICOT Question: Does a multifactorial fall-intervention program compared with single interventions reduce the incidence of falls among hospitalized adult patients?

Evidence Summary

Research shows that fall prevention is successful with an interprofessional approach; however, using only one intervention is not successful (TJC, 2016). A systematic review revealed that using multiple interventions along with exercise is most successful at preventing falls (Zegers, 2016). Hospitals use multiple evidence-based fall prevention interventions aimed at each patient's fall risk factors to reduce falls and falls with injuries. Interventions include fall risk assessments, purposeful interprofessional hourly rounding, bed exit alarms and sensor technology, environmental and equipment modifications (e.g., bedside commode, low beds), improved medication management (evaluating polypharmacy), assistance with transfer and activities of daily living (e.g., showering and toileting), and post-fall evaluations (Hempel et al., 2013; Potter et al., 2017; Stanford Health Care, 2017; CDC, 2017b). The TJCCTH targeted solutions online tool allows organizations to use a systematic approach to fall prevention. The use of the tool has reduced the rate of patient falls by 35% and the rate of patients injured in a fall by 62% (TJCCTH, 2018). Use of the tool involves selection of multiple interventions.

Application to Nursing Practice

- All clinical and nonclinical staff within a health care agency need to attend a mandatory in-service program describing the purpose and goals of the fall management program (ECRI, 2017).
- Implement a fall prevention bundle that includes multiple interventions (fall risk armband, skidproof socks, gait belt use) (TJCCTH, 2018).
- Purposeful rounding as part of a staff-led quality improvement intervention can decrease fall rates by up to 50% with hospitalized patients (Morgan et al., 2017). Purposeful or hourly rounding is a work process that structures time with patients by using an actual standard or mental checklist of procedures meant to promote optimal outcomes in a clean, comfortable, safe environment (McLeod and Tetzlaff, 2015).
- Interventions shown to be effective in preventing falls in the acute care setting include fall risk cards, short-term administration of vitamin D supplementation, one-on-one patient-centered education focusing on the individual patient's risk factors and preventive strategies, and targeted risk factor reduction intervention that includes screening for fall risk factors (Avanacean et al., 2017).

---

and accidents related to improper performance of procedures such as dressing changes or urinary catheter insertion. Always follow the policies and procedures of a health care agency and the standards of nursing practice to prevent these accidents. For example, proper preparation and administration of medications, use of patient and medication bar coding, and "smart" intravenous (IV) pumps reduce medication errors (see Chapters 31 and 42). All staff need to be aware that distractions and interruptions contribute to procedure-related accidents and need to be limited, especially during high-risk procedures such as medication administration. Another common procedure that places patients at risk for injury is transferring to a bed or chair. Correct use of safe patient handling techniques and equipment reduces the risk of injuries when moving and lifting patients (see Chapter 38).

Equipment-Related Accidents. Equipment-related accidents result from an electrical hazard or malfunction, disrepair, or misuse of equipment. To avoid rapid infusion of IV fluids, all general-use and patient-controlled analgesic pumps need to have free-flow protection devices. To avoid accidents, do not operate medical equipment without adequate instruction. If you discover a faulty piece of equipment, replace it with properly working equipment, place a tag on the faulty one, take it out of service, and promptly report any malfunctions. Assess potential electrical hazards to reduce the risk of electrical fires, electrocution, or injury from faulty equipment. Clinical engineering staff in health care settings regularly make safety checks of equipment. Agencies must report all suspected medical device–related deaths to the US Food and Drug Administration (FDA, 2018a) and the product manufacturer.

Workplace Safety. Violence is a familiar occurrence in health care settings. The sources of violence include patients, visitors, intruders, and co-workers. The National Institute for Occupational Safety and Health (NIOSH, 2018) defines workplace violence as the act or threat of violence, ranging from verbal abuse to physical assault, directed toward persons at work or on duty. The impact of workplace violence ranges from psychological issues (e.g., posttraumatic stress disorder [PTSD], compassion fatigue) to physical injury or death. When subjected to workplace violence, health care staff experience anger, frustration, fear, stress and irritability.

From 2002 to 2013, incidents of serious workplace violence (incidents requiring victims to take days off to recuperate) were four times more common in health care than in private industry (OSHA, n.d.b). However, workplace violence occurs on a continuum. Bullying, verbal threats, and name calling are common. In health care settings patients are most commonly the source of violence resulting from hitting, kicking, beating, and shoving (OSHA, n.d.b). Risk factors for workplace violence caused by patients include working with patients who have a history of violence, overcrowded waiting areas, poor lighting in hallways, working in isolation from co-workers, inadequate security staff, work setting located in high-crime neighborhood, having a mobile workplace, transporting or lifting patients, and presence of firearms (OSHA, n.d.b). Many incidents of violence are not reported, but violence can be prevented with proper safety policies and environmental adaptations.

QSEN Building Competency in Safety A nurse is caring for a patient who is receiving chemotherapy. The patient becomes confused and pulls out her IV line, and the chemotherapy drug leaks into the bed linens and all over the floor. What risks are posed for this patient? What risks are posed for the nurse? How should the nurse manage the situation?

Answers to QSEN Activities can be found on the Evolve website.

CRITICAL THINKING

Successful critical thinking requires a synthesis of knowledge, experience, critical thinking attitudes, reflective reasoning, and adherence to professional standards. Clinical judgments that are based on critical thinking require nurses to anticipate necessary information, analyze the data, and make decisions regarding patient care. During an assessment (Fig. 27.2) all critical thinking elements and information about a specific patient should be considered to make appropriate nursing diagnoses.

In the case of safety, nurses integrate knowledge from nursing and other scientific disciplines, previous experiences in caring for patients who were at risk for or had an injury, critical thinking attitudes such as responsibility and discipline, and any standards of practice that are applicable. The American Nurses Association (ANA) standards for nursing practice address the nurse's responsibility in maintaining patient safety. (TJC 2018b) also provides standards for safety. Critical thinking allows nurses to anticipate the needs of their patients and make conclusions about available data. For example, while assessing a patient's home environment,

Knowledge
- Basic human needs
- Potential risks to patient safety from physical hazards, lifestyle, risks associated with health care environment, environmental risks, and biohazards
- Influence of developmental stage on safety needs
- Influence of illness/medications on patient safety

Experience
- Caring for patients whose medical conditions or mobility, cognitive, or sensory impairments increase threats to safety
- Personal experience in caring for younger siblings or children

ASSESSMENT
- Identify patient's perceptions of safety needs and risks
- Identify actual and potential threats to the patient's safety
- Determine impact of the underlying illness on the patient's safety
- Identify the presence of risks for the patient's developmental stage and patient's environment
- Determine medication history and side effects posing safety risks

Standards
- Apply intellectual standards such as accuracy, significance, and completeness when assessing for threats to the patient's safety
- Apply ANA standards for nursing practice
- Apply agency practice standards (e.g., fall prevention or restraint protocols)
- Review and apply the most current TJC patient safety goals

Attitudes
- Demonstrate perseverance when necessary to identify all safety threats
- Be responsible for collecting unbiased, accurate data regarding threats to the patient's safety
- Show discipline in conducting a thorough review of the patient's home environment

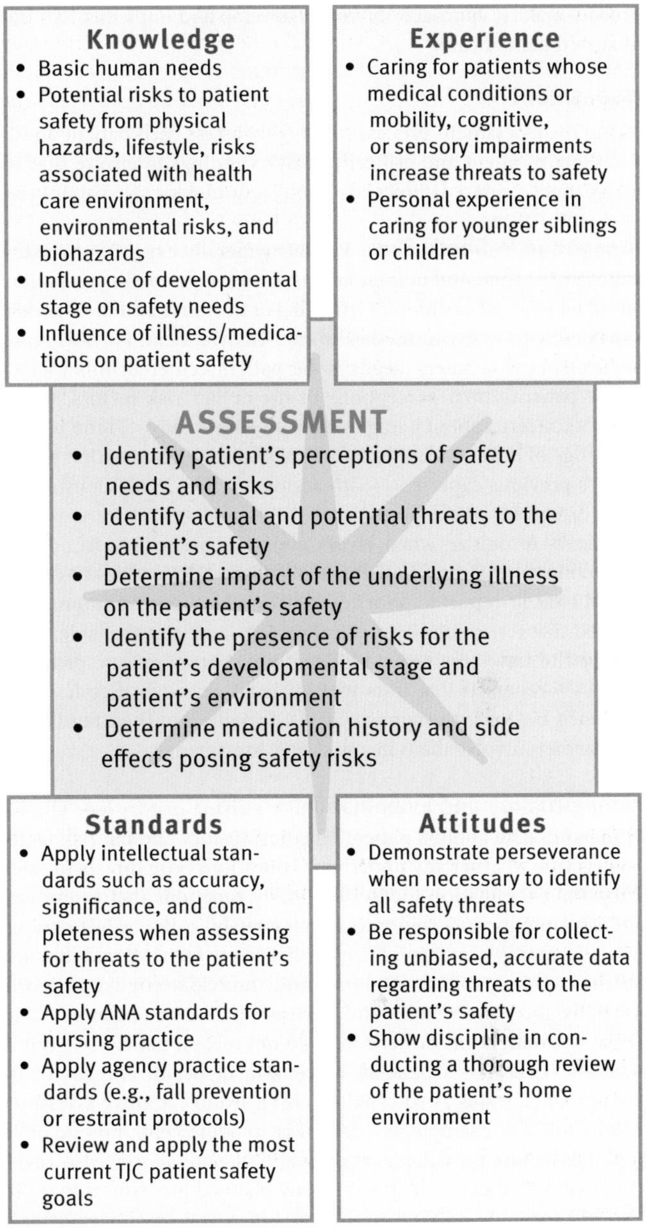

FIG. 27.2 Critical thinking model for safety assessment. *ANA,* American Nurses Association; *TJC,* The Joint Commission.

you consider typical locations within the home where dangers commonly exist. If a patient has a visual impairment, you apply previous experiences in caring for patients with visual changes to anticipate how to thoroughly assess his or her needs.

REFLECT NOW

Reflect on your last clinical experience. What risks to patient safety did you observe? Describe interventions taken to reduce risks to patient safety.

❖ NURSING PROCESS

Apply the nursing process and use a critical thinking approach in your care of patients. The nursing process provides a clinical decision-making approach for you to develop and implement an individualized plan of care.

◆ Assessment

During the assessment process thoroughly assess each patient and his or her environment and critically analyze findings to ensure that you make patient-centered clinical decisions required for safe patient care.

Through the Patient's Eyes. Patients generally expect to be safe in health care settings and in their homes. However, sometimes a patient's view of what is safe is different from that of the nurse and the standards associated with safety in the health care environment. For this reason your nursing assessment needs to be patient centered; this includes (1) the patient's own perceptions of his or her risk factors, (2) the patient's concerns about being in a health care setting, (3) the patient's knowledge of how to adapt to safety risks, and (4) information about a patient's previous experience with accidents (Box 27.6). Consult with family caregivers when appropriate.

Patients recognize when errors occur or when they feel at risk. Research involving over 19,000 patients from 11 countries has shown that patient self-report of poor coordination of care is common: 10.9% reported that test results or medical records were not available, 19.6% perceived to have received conflicting information by care providers, and 10.5% reported that tests were ordered although they had been performed before (Schwappach, 2014). Patients and their families are your partner; involve them in any safety assessment.

Nursing History and Examination. A nursing history (see Chapter 30) includes data about a patient's medical history and fall risk factors to determine whether any underlying conditions pose threats to safety. A physical examination focuses on bodily functions that can affect a patient's mobility and ability to interact safely in his or her environment. For example, an assessment with a safety focus should include a patient's cognitive status, gait, lower-body muscle strength and coordination, balance, and visual status. Measure balance and gait by having the patient walk in his or her room; do not rely on patient self-report. Include a review of a patient's perception of health and his or her developmental status as you analyze physical and cognitive assessment information. For example, if a patient is an adolescent, does he or she show risk factors for suicide or drug and alcohol abuse? Also review the patient's medication history and any planned procedures that pose risks. For example, the use of diuretics increases frequency of voiding and results in the patient having to use toilet facilities more often. Frequent toileting is a risk factor for falls, especially when patients get out of bed quickly without assistance.

Health Care Environment. When caring for patients within a health care setting, determine whether any hazards exist in the immediate care environment:

- Does the placement of equipment (e.g., drainage bags, IV pumps) or furniture pose barriers when the patient tries to ambulate?
- Does positioning of the patient's bed allow him or her to reach items on a bedside table or stand easily? Does the patient need help with ambulation?
- Is there a gait belt or an assist device available for when the patient ambulates?
- Are health care workers and family visitors following hand hygiene guidelines?
- Are there multiple tubes or IV lines?
- Is the nurse call system within reach?

Contact the clinical engineering staff if there are questions as to whether equipment is functioning properly and in good condition.

Risk for Falls. Assessing a patient's risk factors for falling is essential to determine specific needs and develop targeted interventions to prevent falls. Many fall risk–assessment instruments are available; use the tool chosen by your health care agency. Most tools include risk categories on age, fall history, elimination habits, high-risk medications, mobility, and cognition. At a minimum the assessment needs to be completed on admission, following a change in a patient's condition, after a fall, and when transferred. If it is determined that a patient is at risk for falling, ongoing assessments are required. When a patient has a previous history of falling, ask about the nature of the fall and what the patient thinks precipitated it. Focus the assessment on that information to determine whether a condition or risk persists. In many cases family members are important resources in assessing a patient's fall risk. Families often can report on the patient's level of confusion and ability to ambulate or safely toilet. Based on the results of a fall risk assessment, you will implement multiple evidence-based interventions for fall prevention. It is very important that you inform the patient and family members about the fall risks that you identify from the assessment. Often younger patients are not aware of how

---

BOX 27.6 Nursing Assessment Questions

Activity and Exercise
- Do you use any assistive devices, such as a wheelchair, walker, or cane, to help you move or get around? Did someone show you how to use them safely? (Have patient demonstrate use.)
- Describe for me any difficulties you have with bathing, dressing, or toileting.
- Describe for me the type of exercise or physical activity you do regularly. How often do you exercise?
- Explain how you prepare meals at home (e.g., use stove and appliances safely).
- Do you do your own laundry? How do you do this, and where are these appliances located?
- Do you drive a car or motorcycle? When do you normally drive? How far?
- How often do you wear a seat belt when in the car or a helmet when on your bike?

Medication History
- Which medications (prescription, over-the-counter, herbal) do you take?
- Has your doctor or pharmacist reviewed your medicines with you in the last year?
- Describe for me any side effects that you have after taking your medications.

History of Falls
- Have you ever fallen or tripped over anything in your home? Have you had any near misses?
- Tell me what you think caused you to fall. Which activity were you performing before the fall?
- Have you ever suffered an injury from a fall? What was it and how did it happen?
- Did you have any symptoms right before you fell? What were they?

Home Maintenance and Safety
- Who does your simple home maintenance or minor home repairs?
- Who shovels your snow? Mows your lawn?
- Do you feel safe in your home? Describe anything in your environment that makes you feel unsafe.
- If you have an emergency at home, whom can you call for help?
- How do you feel about modifying your home to make it safer? Do you need help finding resources to help you do this?

medications and treatments cause dizziness, orthostatic hypotension, or changes in balance. When patients are unaware of their risks, they are less likely to ask for assistance. If family members are informed, they will often call for help (when they are visiting patients) to be sure that patients have appropriate assistance.

Risk for Medical Errors. Be alert to factors within your own work environment that create conditions in which medical errors are more likely to occur. Distractions during medication preparation or nursing procedures in the form of phone calls, alarms, or staff needing assistance are common. Studies show that overwork and fatigue, particularly when working consecutive 12 hour-shifts, cause a significant decrease in alertness and concentration, leading to errors (Geiger-Brown et al., 2012). It is important for you to be aware of risk factors in the workplace and to include checks and balances when working under stress. For example, to reduce the chance for a medical error, it is essential that a patient's identification be checked by using two identifiers (e.g., name and birthday or name and medical record number) according to agency policy before beginning any procedure or administering a medication (see Chapter 31).

Disasters. Hospitals must be prepared to respond to and care for a sudden influx of patients at the time of a community disaster. Although the occurrence of bioterrorism attacks has been limited to the anthrax deaths following September 11, 2001, the threat is very real. Be prepared to make accurate and timely assessments in any type of setting. Initially, a bioterrorist attack is likely to resemble a natural outbreak. Acutely ill patients representing the earliest cases after a covert attack seek care in emergency departments. Patients less ill at the onset of an illness possibly seek care in primary care settings. Rapid detection of a bioterrorism attack occurs through syndrome surveillance and reporting of suspected cases. The early signs of a bioterrorism-related illness often include nonspecific symptoms (e.g., nausea, vomiting, diarrhea, skin rash, fever, confusion) that may persist for several days before the onset of more severe disease. Patients with prodromal illnesses seek outpatient care and are assigned nonspecific diagnoses such as "viral syndrome." Data on patients fitting various syndromic criteria are then transferred to a health department and tested.

Patient's Home Environment. When caring for a patient in the home, a home hazard assessment is necessary. A thorough hazard assessment includes all the rooms in a home and the outdoor entrance areas. Each room assessment covers topics such as adequacy of lighting (inside and outdoors), condition of flooring and walking surfaces, presence of safety devices (e.g., alarms, side rails on steps, safety bars in bath tubs), and placement of furniture or other items that can create barriers. Know where medications and cleaning supplies are located. Walking through the home with the patient and discussing how he or she normally conducts daily activities and whether the environment poses problems is important. Additional assessment includes the presence of locks on doors and windows. Getting a sense of a patient's routines helps you recognize less obvious hazards. It is also important to learn the patient's willingness to make changes in his or her environment. Decisions on changing the environment require the patient's full participation.

Assessment for risk of food-borne illness includes assessing a patient's knowledge of food preparation and storage practices. For example, does a patient know to check expiration dates of prepared food and milk products? Does he or she keep foods in the refrigerator that are fresh and not spoiled? Does the patient clean fresh fruits and vegetables correctly before eating them? Assess for clinical signs of infection by conducting an examination of GI and central nervous system function, observing for a fever, and analyzing the results of cultures of feces and emesis. Further assessment includes inspecting the food and water sources and assessing the patient's and family members' handwashing practices.

Assessment of the environmental comfort of a patient's home includes a review of when the patient normally has heating and cooling systems serviced. Does the patient have a functional furnace or space heater? Does the home have air conditioning or fans? Inform patients who use space heaters of the risk for fires. Are smoke detectors and carbon monoxide detectors up-to-date and functional, and are fire extinguishers present and placed strategically throughout the home and checked routinely?

When patients live in older homes, encourage them to have inspections for lead in paint, dust, or soil. Because lead also comes from the solder or plumbing fixtures in a home, patients need to have water from each faucet tested. Local health offices will help homeowners locate a trained lead inspector who takes samples from various locations and has them analyzed at a laboratory for lead content.

It is important that your nursing assessment and interventions help individuals focus on avoiding losses and reducing their risk for injury associated with disasters. The Federal Emergency Management Agency (http://www.fema.gov/) and the American Red Cross (http://www.red-cross.org/) provide nationwide education to help community members prepare for disasters of all types.

REFLECT NOW

Go to the CDC website (https://www.cdc.gov/HomeandRecreational Safety/pubs/English/booklet_Eng_desktopa.pdf) and conduct a home risk assessment on your own home or the home of someone you know who is 65 years of age or older. Once completed, think about how to minimize safety risks.

◆ Nursing Diagnosis

Gather data from your nursing assessment and analyze clusters of assessment findings, including risk factors, to identify relevant nursing diagnoses (Box 27.7). In addition to the accurate clustering of assessment data, an important part of formulating nursing diagnoses is identifying the relevant causative or related factor (when a diagnosis is *negative* or problem focused) or risk factors (when a diagnosis is a risk diagnosis). You choose interventions that treat or modify the related factor *or risk* for the diagnosis to be resolved. For example, the nursing diagnosis of *Risk for Fall* might be associated with altered mobility or a visual alteration as risk factors. Altered mobility will lead you to select such nursing interventions

---

BOX 27.7 Nursing Diagnostic Process

Risk for Fall

Assessment Activities	Assessment Findings
Observe patient's posture, range of motion, gait, strength, balance, and body alignment.	Decrease in left lower-extremity strength; demonstrates unsteady gait, impaired balance when standing
Assess patient's visual acuity— ability to read, identify distant objects.	Reports difficulty seeing at night
	Vision blurred, unable to identify near objects without glasses
Complete a home hazard appraisal.	Poorly lighted home
	Excessive amount of furniture in living room
	Rugs not secure throughout home
	No grab bars in bath

as range-of-motion (ROM) exercises; more frequent supervised ambulation; or teaching the proper use of safety devices such as side rails, canes, or crutches. Also consult with a patient's health care provider about a physical therapy referral. If visual impairment is the risk factor, select different interventions, such as keeping the living area well lit; orienting the patient to the surroundings; or keeping eye glasses clean, handy, and well protected. When you do not identify the correct risk factors for the diagnosis *Risk for Fall,* the use of inappropriate interventions or omission of proper interventions may increase a patient's risk for falling. Examples of additional nursing diagnoses for patients with safety risk include the following:

- *Risk for Injury*
- *Impaired Cognition: Confusion*
- *Lack of Knowledge*
- *Risk for Poisoning*
- *Risk for Trauma*

◆ Planning

Patients with actual or potential risks to safety require a nursing care plan with interventions that prevent and minimize threats to their safety. Design your interventions to help a patient feel safe to move about and interact freely within the environment. The plan of care addresses all aspects of patient needs and uses resources of the health care team and the community when appropriate. Critically synthesize information from multiple sources (Fig. 27.3). Critical thinking ensures that a patient's plan of care integrates all that you learned about the patient and the key critical thinking elements. For example, you reflect on knowledge regarding the services that other health professions (e.g., occupational therapy, case management) provide to help patients return to their home environments safely. Also reflect on previous experiences when patients benefited from safety interventions. Such experience helps you adapt approaches with each new patient. Applying critical thinking attitudes such as creativity helps you to collaborate with a patient in planning interventions that are relevant and most useful, particularly when making changes in the home environment.

Goals and Outcomes. You collaborate with a patient, family, and other members of the health care team when setting goals and expected outcomes during the planning process (see the Nursing Care Plan). The patient who actively participates in reducing threats to safety becomes more alert to potential hazards and is more likely to adhere to the plan. Make sure that goals and outcomes for each nursing diagnosis are measurable and realistic, with consideration of the resources available to the patient. For example, in the case of the nursing diagnosis of *Impaired Walking related to left-sided paralysis,* the goal is the patient "will remain free of injury throughout hospitalization." Examples of expected outcomes include:

- Patient uses tripod cane correctly within 24 hours.
- Patient describes approach to rise up from bed correctly with assistance by end of the teaching session today.

Setting Priorities. Prioritize a patient's nursing diagnoses and interventions to provide safe and efficient care. For example, the concept map (Fig. 27.4) has several nursing diagnoses that apply to promoting a patient's safety. The patient's mobility problem is an obvious priority because of its influence on risk for fall. Plan individualized interventions based on the severity of risk factors and the patient's developmental stage, level of health, lifestyle, and cultural needs (Box 27.8). Planning involves an understanding of the patient's need to maintain independence within physical and cognitive capabilities. Build a consensus with the patient and family (when appropriate) as to the type of interventions to deliver (QSEN, 2018). Collaborate to establish ways

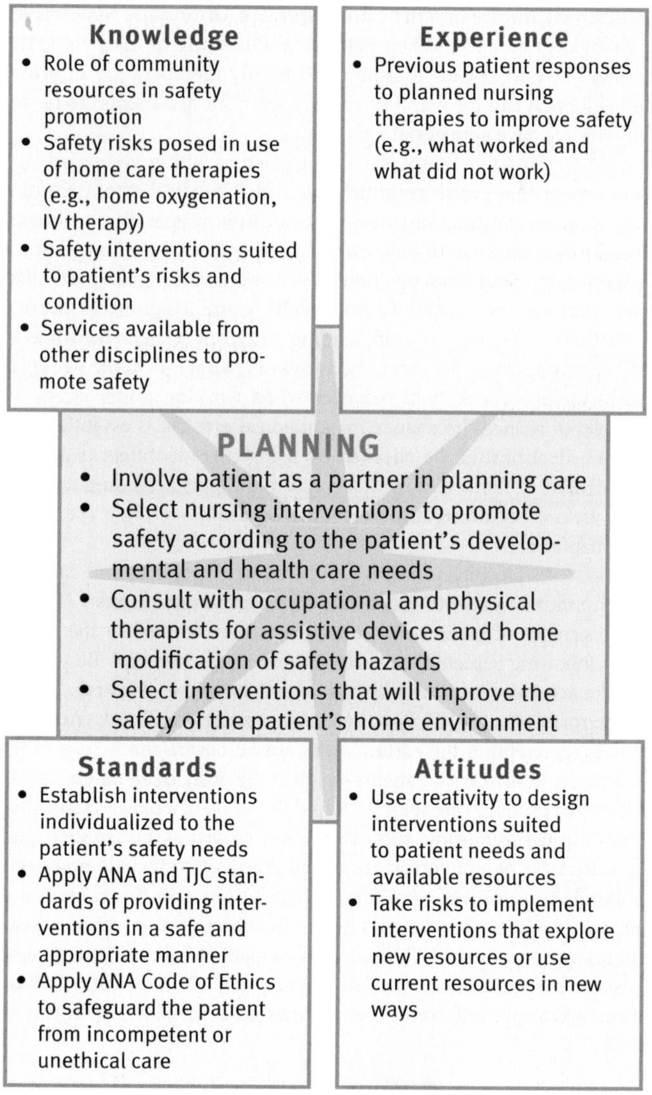

Knowledge
- Role of community resources in safety promotion
- Safety risks posed in use of home care therapies (e.g., home oxygenation, IV therapy)
- Safety interventions suited to patient's risks and condition
- Services available from other disciplines to promote safety

Experience
- Previous patient responses to planned nursing therapies to improve safety (e.g., what worked and what did not work)

PLANNING
- Involve patient as a partner in planning care
- Select nursing interventions to promote safety according to the patient's developmental and health care needs
- Consult with occupational and physical therapists for assistive devices and home modification of safety hazards
- Select interventions that will improve the safety of the patient's home environment

Standards
- Establish interventions individualized to the patient's safety needs
- Apply ANA and TJC standards of providing interventions in a safe and appropriate manner
- Apply ANA Code of Ethics to safeguard the patient from incompetent or unethical care

Attitudes
- Use creativity to design interventions suited to patient needs and available resources
- Take risks to implement interventions that explore new resources or use current resources in new ways

FIG. 27.3 Critical thinking model for safety planning. (*ANA,* American Nurses Association; *IV,* intravenous; *TJC,* The Joint Commission.)

of maintaining the patient's active involvement within the home and health care environment. Education of the patient and family is also an important intervention to plan for reducing safety risks over the long term.

REFLECT NOW

Consider a patient you cared for recently. How did you prioritize meeting the patient's safety needs?

Teamwork and Collaboration. Collaboration with the patient, family, and other health care professions, such as social work and occupational and physical therapy, becomes an important part of a patient's plan of care. For example, a patient in a hospital needs to go to a rehabilitation center to gain strength and endurance before being discharged home. An occupational therapist is helpful in the home setting for making recommendations for installation of stairway railings, slip-resistant surfacing in the bathroom, and provision of lighting (Stark et al., 2017). Communication with all participants in the plan of care is essential. You

⊚ NURSING CARE PLAN

Risk for Fall

ASSESSMENT

Mr. Key, a home health nurse, is visiting Ms. Cohen, an 85-year-old woman living at home. The patient is recovering from a stroke affecting her left side. Ms. Cohen lives alone but receives regular help from her daughter and son, who both live within 10 miles of the patient.

Assessment Activities	*Assessment Findings[a]*
Ask how the stroke has affected her mobility.	She responds, "**I bump into things,** and **I'm afraid I'm going to fall.**"
Conduct a home hazard assessment.	Kitchen table is cluttered with unopened mail, plastic bags, and papers. Cabinets in kitchen are **cluttered** and full of breakable items that could fall out. **Throw rugs are on floors;** bathroom **lighting is poor** (40-watt bulbs); bathtub **lacks safety strips** or grab bars; **home is cluttered** with furniture and small objects.
Observe gait and posture.	She has **kyphosis** and a **hesitant, uncoordinated gait;** frequently holds walls for support.
Ask patient her age.	Patient is 85 years old.
Assess visual acuity with corrective lenses.	She has **trouble reading and seeing familiar objects at a distance** while wearing current glasses. The patient confirms that her vision has been getting worse over the last year; things are not "clear and crisp," almost like there is a layer of "cotton candy" blurring her vision.

[a]**Assessment Findings** are shown in bold type.

NURSING DIAGNOSIS: Risk for fall

PLANNING

Goals	*Expected Outcomes (NOC)[b]* *Knowledge: Personal Safety*
Patient and family will understand patient's fall risks and develop a plan to reduce risks within 1 month.	Patient and daughter will identify personal and environmental risks for falls in 1 week. Patient and daughter will select prevention methods to avoid falls in home at conclusion of teaching session next week.
	Fall Prevention Behavior
Patient will be free of injury at 1 month.	Patient will safely ambulate throughout the home within 1 week.

[b]Outcome classification labels from Moorhead S et al: *Nursing outcomes classification (NOC)*, ed 6, St Louis, 2018, Elsevier.

INTERVENTIONS (NIC)[c] *Fall Prevention*	*RATIONALE*
Review findings from home hazard assessment with patient and her daughter, and collaborate with an occupational therapist on proposed changes.	Home hazard assessment highlights extrinsic factors that lead to falls and that can be changed. Home modifications, when delivered by occupational therapists, can reduce falls among high-risk community-dwelling older adults (Stark et al., 2017)
Establish a list of patient's priorities to modify the home.	Implementing home modifications based on home assessment decreases falls. Successful home modifications, such as bathroom safety devices, are tailored to the participant's needs and expressed wishes (Stark et al., 2017).
Discuss with patient and daughter the normal changes of aging, effects of recent stroke, associated risks for injury, and how to reduce risks.	Education regarding hazards reduces fear of falling (Olsen and Bergland, 2014).
Encourage daughter to schedule vision testing for new prescription within 2 to 4 weeks.	Studies have found correlations between the aging of visual functions and falls in elderly people (Saftari and Kwon, 2018).
Refer to physical therapist to assess need for strengthening and endurance training and use of assistive devices for kyphosis, left-sided weakness, and gait.	A multicomponent exercise intervention composed of strength, endurance, and balance training has been shown to be the best strategy to improve rate of falls, gait ability, balance, and strength performance in physically frail older adults (Cadore et al., 2013).

[c]Intervention classification labels from Butcher HK, et al: *Nursing interventions classification (NIC)*, ed 7, St Louis, 2018, Elsevier.

EVALUATION

Evaluation Activity	*Patient Response/Finding*	*Outcome Status*
Ask patient and daughter to identify fall risks and the plan for changes in home.	Patient identified the piles of magazines and mail cluttered in family room and throw rugs on floors as safety hazards. Daughter identified bathroom hazards, including bathroom lighting and lack of grab bars. Have plan to install grab bars in bathroom.	Patient and family have gained knowledge of modifiable hazards in the home. Need to reinforce value of installing safety strips in bath tub.
Reassess if patient has experienced a fall in the last month.	Patient has not experienced a fall	Fall prevention achieved.

CONCEPT MAP

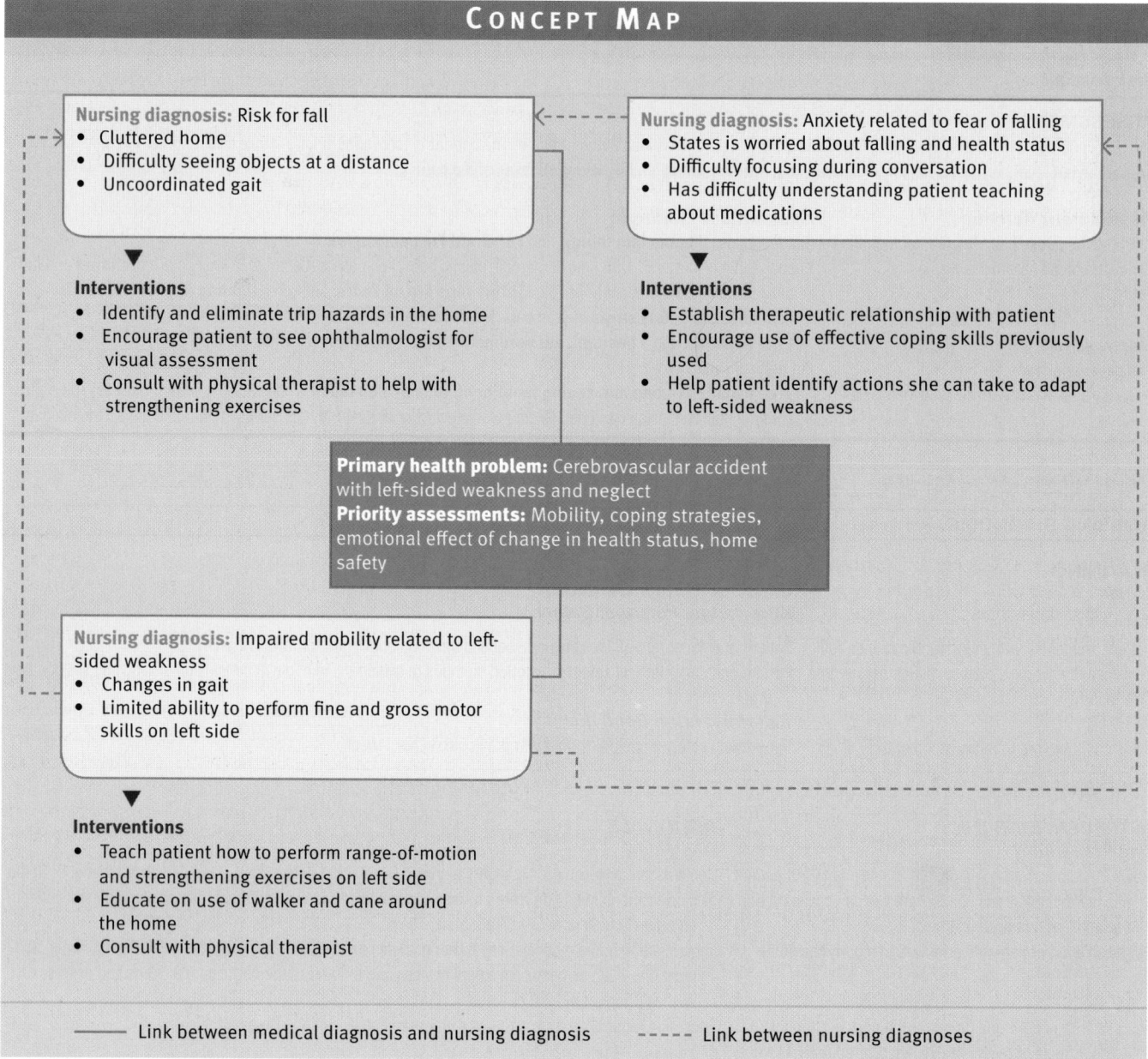

FIG. 27.4 Concept map for Ms. Cohen. *ADLs,* Activities of daily living; *CVA,* cerebrovascular accident.

BOX 27.8   CULTURAL ASPECTS OF CARE

A Patient-Centered Care Approach

Hospitalization places patients at risk for injury in an unfamiliar and confusing environment. The experience is usually at least minimally frightening. Normal life cues such as a bed without side rails and the direction one usually takes to the bathroom are absent. Thought processes and coping mechanisms are affected by illness and its accompanying emotions. Thus patients are more vulnerable to injury. This vulnerability is often intensified for patients of diverse backgrounds. It is a nurse's responsibility to diligently protect all patients, regardless of their socioeconomic status and cultural background. Most untoward events are related to failures of communication. Patients who have low health literacy create challenges for nurses during assessments and efforts at implementing safe care measures. Screen all patients for health literacy. Ensure that you use an approach that recognizes a patient's cultural background so that you ask appropriate questions to reveal health behaviors and risks. Be aware of cultural beliefs about physical restraints when caring for patients who need them. A physical restraint is a way of purposely limiting or obstructing the freedom of a person's bodily movement and can be seen as a significant threat by anyone who comes from a culture of violence. Patient safety is enhanced when you consider the whole person and value seeing each care situation through "the patient's eyes" and not just through your own perspective. Some specific patient-centered safety guidelines about the use of restraints follow.

Implications for Patient-Centered Care

- When restraints are needed, assess their meaning to the patient and the family. Some cultures may find restraints to be disrespectful. Similarly, some survivors of war or persecution or those suffering from posttraumatic stress disorder may view restraints as imprisonment or punishment.
- Collaborate with family members in accommodating a patient's cultural perspectives about restraints. Removing the restraints when family members are present shows respect and caring for the patient.
- Define the protocol of the nursing unit on the use of restraints. Identify potential areas for negotiation with the patient's/family's preferences for using restraints, including having family members stay with the patient.

communicate risk factors and the plan of care with the patient, family, and other health care providers, including other disciplines and nurses on other shifts. Permanent dry-erase boards in the patient's room with patient information such as activity and level of assistance communicate information to all health care providers. A standard approach to communication such as ISBAR or SBAR ([*Introduction*], *Situation*, *Background*, *Assessment*, *Recommendation*, *Request*, or *Readback*) helps you obtain and organize information about patients when problems develop (see Chapter 24).

QSEN **Building Competency in Patient-Centered Care.** A 78-year-old patient comes to the outpatient medicine clinic for a follow-up visit after being hospitalized for pneumonia. The patient's 45-year-old daughter accompanies him. The patient asks to have the daughter in the examination room. The patient answers questions readily, is oriented, and shows appropriate nonverbal expressions during conversation. What assessment factors does the clinic nurse include in determining whether the patient is at risk for fall in the home?

Answers to QSEN Activities can be found on the Evolve website.

Patients need to be able to identify, select, and know how to use resources within their communities (e.g., neighborhood block homes, local police departments, and neighbors willing to check on their well-being) that enhance safety. Make sure that the patient and family understand the need for these resources and how to contact these resources, and determine whether they are willing to make changes that promote their safety.

◆ Implementation

QSEN (2018) outlines recommended skills to ensure nurse competency in patient safety. Among these skills are those involving safe nursing practice during direct care:

- Demonstrate effective use of technology and standardized practices that support safety and quality.
- Demonstrate effective use of strategies to reduce risk of harm to self or others.
- Use appropriate strategies (e.g., forcing functions, checklists) to reduce reliance on memory.
- Communicate observations or concerns related to hazards and errors to patients, families, and the health care team.

Direct your nursing interventions toward maintaining a patient's safety in all types of settings. You implement health promotion and illness prevention measures in the community setting, whereas prevention is a priority in the acute care setting.

Health Promotion. Health promotion requires a person to be in a safe environment and practice a lifestyle that minimizes risk of injury. There are both passive and active strategies aimed at health promotion. Passive strategies include public health measures (e.g., public education about neighborhood safety, closing schools during inclement weather, issuing travel restrictions and screening travelers) and governmental legislative interventions (e.g., sanitation and clean water laws) (see Chapter 3). Active strategies are those in which an individual is actively involved through changes in lifestyle (e.g., engaging in better nutritional health or exercise programs, wearing seat belts) and participation in wellness programs.

Nurses promote individual and community health by supporting legislation, acting as positive role models, and working in community-based settings. Because environmental and community values have the greatest influence on health promotion, community and home health nurses can assess and recommend safety measures in the home, school, neighborhood, and workplace.

Developmental Interventions

Infant, Toddler, and Preschooler. Growing, curious children need adults to protect them from injury. Educate parents or guardians about reducing risks of disease and injuries to children, and teach ways to promote safety in the home (Table 27.1). One area that is crucial is the encouragement of parents to follow immunization guidelines for their children. The (American Academy of Pediatrics 2018b) recommends these steps for vaccine-hesitant parents:

- Listen to parents' concerns and acknowledge them in a nonconfrontational manner. This will increase their willingness to listen to a pediatrician's views.
- Promote partnerships with parents in decision making. Make sure the parent understands the information about vaccines. Clarify and reaffirm parents' correct beliefs about immunization and modify misconceptions.
- Discuss the benefits of vaccines and the possibility of adverse events. Be open about what is known about immunizations and what is not known.
- Stress the number of lives saved by immunization, as a positive approach.

Nurses working in prenatal and postpartum settings routinely incorporate safety into the care plans of childbearing families. Community health nurses assess the home and show parents how to promote safety.

School-Age Child. School-age children increasingly explore their environment (see Chapter 12). They have friends outside their immediate neighborhood, and they become more active in school, church, and community activities. The school-age child needs specific teaching regarding safety in school and at play. See Table 27.1 for nursing interventions to help guide parents in providing for the safety of school-age children.

Adolescent. Risks to the safety of adolescents involve many factors outside the home because much of their time is spent away from home and with their peer group (see Chapter 12). Adults who serve as positive role models for adolescents provide examples of how to behave, set expectations, and provide education to minimize risks to the adolescent's safety. Because of peer pressure this age group is at risk for alcohol and drug use. In addition, this age-group has a high incidence of suicide. Be aware of the risks posed at this time and be prepared to teach adolescents and their parents the measures needed to prevent accidents and injury. You can also help parents be aware of ways to minimize risk of adolescent suicide, including the promotion of good problem-solving abilities (e.g., conflict with peers); support for strong connections to their families, friends, and people in the community; restricted access to highly lethal means of suicide; and demonstration of cultural and religious beliefs that discourage suicide and that support self-preservation (Kaslow, 2018).

Adult. Risks to young and middle-age adults frequently result from lifestyle factors such as childrearing, high stress levels, inadequate nutrition, use of firearms, excessive alcohol intake, and substance abuse (see Chapter 13). In this fast-paced society there also appears to be more expression of anger, which can quickly precipitate accidents related to "road rage." Help adults understand their safety risks and guide them in making lifestyle modifications by referring them to resources such as classes to help quit smoking or for stress management, including employee-assistance programs. Also encourage adults to exercise regularly, maintain a healthy diet, practice relaxation techniques, and get adequate sleep (see Chapter 43).

Older Adult. Nursing interventions for older adults reduce patients' risk for falls and other accidents and compensate for the physiological changes of aging (Box 27.9). The American Geriatric Society (2015) developed an algorithm for fall prevention (Fig. 27.5).

TABLE 27.1 Interventions to Promote Safety for Children and Adolescents

Intervention	Rationale
Infants and Toddlers	
Keep soft objects, toys, crib bumpers, and loose bedding out of a baby's sleep area to reduce the risk of sudden infant death syndrome (SIDS). Make sure nothing covers the baby's head.	Possibility exists for these items to cause risk of suffocation, strangulation, or entrapment.
Use a firm sleep surface, such as a mattress in a safety-approved crib covered by a fitted sheet.	Reduces suffocation.
Prepare a baby's sleep area next to where parents sleep. A baby should not sleep in an adult bed, on a couch, or on a chair alone or with a parent or anyone else.	
Infants should be immunized and have regular health checkups.	Evidence suggests that immunization reduces the risk of SIDS and other preventable diseases. Access the American Academy of Pediatrics current immunization schedule at https://www.aap.org/en-us/advocacy-and-policy/aap-health-initiatives/immunizations/Pages/Immunization-Schedule.aspx.
Do not attach pacifiers to string or ribbon and place around a child's neck.	String or ribbon around the neck increases risk for choking.
Follow all instructions for preparing and storing formula.	Proper formula preparation and storage prevent contamination. Following product directions ensures proper concentration of formula. Undiluted formula causes fluid and electrolyte disturbances; much-diluted formula does not provide sufficient nutrients.
Use large, soft toys without small parts such as buttons.	Small parts become dislodged, and choking and aspiration can occur.
Do not leave the mesh sides of playpens lowered; spaces between crib slats need to be less than 2⅜ inches (6 cm) apart.	Possibility exists for a child's head to become wedged in the lowered mesh side or between crib slats, and asphyxiation may occur.
Never leave crib sides down or babies unattended on changing tables or in infant seats, swings, strollers, or high chairs.	Infants and toddlers roll or move and fall from changing tables or out of accessories such as infant seats or swings.
Discontinue using accessories such as infant seats and swings when the child becomes too active or physically too big and/or according to the manufacturer's directions.	When physically active or too big, the child can fall out of or tip over these accessories and suffer an injury.
Never leave a child alone in the bathroom, tub, or near any water source (e.g., pool).	Supervision reduces risk for accidental drowning.
Baby-proof the home; remove small or sharp objects and toxic or poisonous substances, including plants; install safety locks on floor-level cabinets.	Babies explore their world with their hands and mouth. Choking and poisoning can occur.
Remove plastic bags from the cleaners or grocery store from the home.	Removal reduces risk for suffocation from plastic bags.
Cover electrical outlets.	Covers reduce opportunity for crawling babies to insert objects into outlets and experience an electrical shock.
Install keyless locks (e.g., deadbolts) on doors above a child's reach, even when they are standing on a chair.	Deadbolts prevent a toddler from leaving the house and wandering off. Keyless locks allow for rapid exit in case of fire.
Follow the American Academy of Pediatrics guidelines for rear-facing car safety seats.	Protects infants and toddlers from injury during motor vehicle accidents.
Caregivers need to learn cardiopulmonary resuscitation (CPR) and the Heimlich maneuver.	Caregivers need to be prepared to intervene in acute emergencies such as choking.
Preschoolers	
Teach children to swim at an early age, but always provide supervision near water.	Learning to swim is a useful skill that can someday save a child's life. However, all children need constant supervision.
Teach children how to cross streets and walk in parking lots. Instruct them to never run out after a ball or toy.	Pedestrian accidents involving young children are common.
Teach children not to talk to, go with, or accept any item from a stranger.	Avoiding strangers reduces the risk of injury and stranger abduction.
Teach children basic physical safety rules such as proper use of safety scissors, never running with an object in their mouth or hand, and never attempting to use the stove or oven unassisted.	Risk of injury is lower if children know basic safety procedures.
Teach children not to eat items found in the street or grass.	Avoiding these items reduces risk for possible poisoning.
Remove doors from unused refrigerators and freezers. Instruct children not to play or hide in a car trunk or unused appliances.	If a child cannot freely exit from appliances and car trunks, asphyxiation can occur.
School-Age Children	
Teach children proper bicycle and skate board safety, including use of helmet and rules of the road.	Reduces injuries from falling off a bike or skateboard or being hit by a car.

TABLE 27.1   Interventions to Promote Safety for Children and Adolescents—cont'd

Intervention	Rationale
Teach children proper techniques for specific sports and the need to wear proper safety gear (e.g., helmets, eyewear, mouth guards).	Using proper techniques, correct equipment, and protective gear prevents injuries.
Teach children not to operate electrical equipment while unsupervised.	If an electrical mishap were to occur, no one would be available to help.
Do not allow children access to firearms or other weapons. Keep all firearms in locked cabinets.	Children are often fascinated by firearms and often try to play with them.
Adolescents	
Encourage enrollment in driver education classes.	Many injuries in this age-group are related to motor vehicle accidents.
Provide information about the effects of smoking and using alcohol and drugs.	Adolescents are highly prone to risk-taking behaviors and are subject to peer pressures.
Refer adolescents to community- and school-sponsored activities.	The adolescent needs to socialize with peers, yet needs some supervision.
Encourage mentoring relationships between adults and adolescents.	Adolescents are in need of role models after whom they can pattern their behavior.
Teach them safe use of the Internet.	Avoids overuse and possible exposure to inappropriate websites.

Modified from Hockenberry M, Wilson D: *Wong's nursing care of infants and children*, ed 11, St Louis, 2019, Elsevier.

BOX 27.9   FOCUS ON OLDER ADULTS

Physiological Changes of Aging and Their Effect on Patient Safety

As people age, physiological changes occur. They experience visual and hearing alterations, slowed reaction time, and decreased range of motion, flexibility, and strength. In addition, reflexes are slowed, and the ability to respond to multiple stimuli is reduced. Memory can become impaired, and nocturia and incontinence are more frequent in older adults. The family plays a significant role in the care of older adults. There are nearly 44 million family caregivers in the United States, nearly 20% of the US adult population (National Alliance for Caregiving, 2019). Educate family members on how to best support the older adult.

The high prevalence of chronic conditions in older adults results in the use of a high number of prescription and over-the-counter medications. Coupled with age-related changes in pharmacokinetics, there is a greater risk of serious adverse effects. Medications typically prescribed for older adults include anticholinergics, diuretics, anxiolytic and hypnotic agents, antidepressants, antihypertensives, vasodilators, analgesics, and laxatives, all of which pose risks or interact to increase the risk for falls.

Implications for Practice

- Encourage family caregivers to allow older adult to remain as independent as possible.
- Offer family caregivers resources from the CDC on the STEADI fall prevention program (CDC, 2017c). Available at https://www.cdc.gov/steadi/patient.html.

- Encourage annual vision and hearing examinations and frequent cleaning of glasses and hearing aids as a means of preventing falls and burns.
- Teach patients safety tips for avoiding automobile accidents. Sometimes driving needs to be restricted to daylight hours or temporarily or permanently suspended.
- Encourage supervised strengthening and balance exercise classes for older adults.
- Install safety features in the home such as grab bars and smoke alarms.
- Be sure that adults know how to use assistive devices (e.g., walkers and canes) correctly. Consult with a physical therapy staff member.
- Consult with an occupational therapist to help patients make adaptations needed to feed, bathe, eat, and toilet independently.
- Institute a regular toileting schedule for the patient. A recommended frequency is every 2 or 3 hours. Give diuretics in the morning. Provide assistance, along with adequate lighting, to patients who need to go to the bathroom at night.
- Encourage patients to use medication organizers, which can be purchased at any drugstore at a very reasonable cost. Fill these dispensers once a week with the proper medications to be taken at a specific time during the day.
- Review the patient's drug profile to ensure that these drugs are used cautiously, and assess the patient regularly for any adverse effects that increase fall risk.

Use this resource to reduce risks in the home. Provide information about neighborhood resources to help an older adult maintain an independent lifestyle. Older adults frequently relocate to new neighborhoods and need to become acquainted with new resources, such as modes of transportation, church schedules, and food resources (e.g., Meals on Wheels).

Educate older adults about safe driving tips (e.g., driving shorter distances, using side and rearview mirrors carefully, and looking behind them toward their "blind spot" before changing lanes). If hearing is a problem, encourage the patient to keep a window rolled down while driving or to reduce the volume of the radio. Counseling is often necessary to help older patients decide when to stop driving. At that time help locate resources in the community that provide transportation.

Burns and scalds are also more apt to occur with older people because they sometimes forget and leave hot water running or become confused when turning the dials on a stove or other heating appliance. Nursing measures for preventing burns minimize the risk from impaired vision. Hot-water faucets and dials are color coded to make it easier for an adult to know which is hot and which is cold. Reducing the temperature of the hot water heater is also very beneficial.

Many older adults love to walk. Reduce pedestrian accidents for older adults and all other age-groups by persuading people to wear reflectors on garments when walking at night; to stand on the sidewalk and not in the street when waiting to cross a street; to always cross at corners and not in the middle of the block (particularly if the street is a major one); to cross with the traffic light and not against it; and to

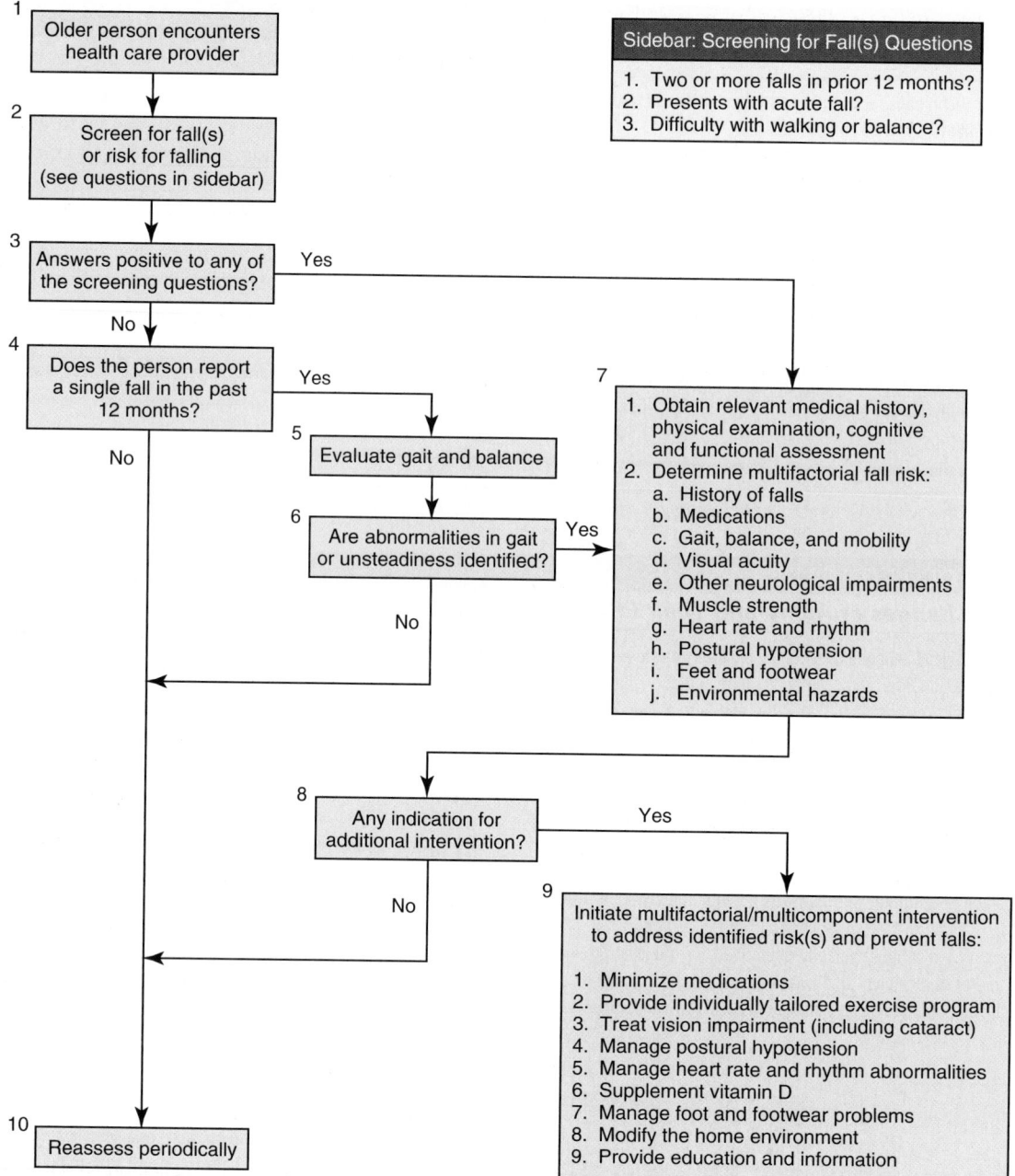

FIG. 27.5 American Geriatrics Society Clinical Practice Guideline Fall Prevention Algorithm 2010. (From American Geriatrics Society/British Geriatrics Society. (2010). *AGS/BGS Clinical Practice Guideline: Prevention of falls in older persons algorithm.* New York: American Geriatrics Society.)

look left, right, and left again before entering the street or crosswalk. Also encourage people to assess their walking route for hazards such as unequal or damaged walkways, unrestrained dogs, and excessive toys; all of these increase the risk for falls.

Environmental Interventions. Nursing interventions directed at eliminating environmental threats include those associated with a person's basic needs and general preventive measures.

Basic Needs. When administering oxygen, take appropriate precautions to prevent fire. In home settings, post "No Smoking" and "Oxygen in Use" signs. Do not use oxygen around electrical equipment or flammable products. Store oxygen tanks upright in carts or stands to prevent tipping or falling over. Chapter 41 outlines guidelines for proper oxygen administration. In the home setting a home medical

provider and home health nurse educate patients who require oxygen in the home about safe oxygen use.

Fire safety in the home requires education of patients and families about the importance of purchasing modern space heaters that include safety features, placing smoke detectors and carbon monoxide detectors strategically throughout the home, and keeping multipurpose fire extinguishers in close proximity to the kitchen and workshop areas. Recommend that patients have annual inspections of heating systems, chimneys, and fuel-burning appliances in the home. Carbon monoxide detectors are not expensive but are not a replacement for proper use and maintenance of fuel-burning appliances. Space heaters are a fire risk. Instruct patients on proper use in the home (Electrical Safety Foundation International, 2015):

- Be sure a space heater has a label showing that it is listed by a recognized testing laboratory.
- Before using any space heater, read the manufacturer's instructions carefully.
- Inspect heaters for cracked or broken plugs or loose connections before each use. If frayed, worn, or damaged, do not use the heater.
- Never leave a space heater unattended. Turn it off when you're leaving a room or going to sleep, and don't let pets or children play too close to a space heater.
- Space heaters are only meant to provide supplemental heat and should never be used to warm bedding, cook food, dry clothing or thaw pipes.
- Install smoke alarms on every floor of your home and outside all sleeping areas.
- Proper placement of space heaters is critical. Heaters must be kept at least 3 feet away from anything that can burn, including papers, clothing, and rugs.
- Plug space heaters directly into a wall outlet. Do not use an extension cord or power strip, which could overheat and result in a fire.

Food safety requires a patient and family to understand the principles of food preparation and storage. Patients should follow four basic safety tips (CDC, 2018c).

- First, wash hands and food preparation and cooking surfaces often. This includes cooking utensils and cutting boards thoroughly.
- Second, do not cross contaminate food while preparing or while stored in a refrigerator. Keep raw meat, poultry, seafood, and their juices away from other foods. Use separate cutting boards. Rinse fruits and vegetables thoroughly.
- Third, always cook food to the proper temperature. Refrigerate leftovers promptly.
- Fourth, be sure a patient living at home has a functioning refrigerator with a freezer compartment to keep perishable foods fresh. Keep a refrigerator below 40° F, and know when to throw leftovers or opened containers of food away.

Fall Safety in the Home. Modifications in the home environment easily reduce the risk of falls. Collaborate with patient and family caregiver to make changes based on their home fall risk assessment and the patient's risk factors. For example, remove all obstacles (e.g., furniture, piles of magazines or boxes) from halls and other heavily traveled areas. Be sure that end tables are secure and have stable, straight legs. Place nonessential items in drawers to eliminate clutter. Patients who have problems stumbling or tripping should never have small area rugs in the home. If small area rugs are used, secure them with a nonslip pad or skid-resistant adhesive strips. Make sure that carpeting on the stairs is secured with carpet tacks. If patients have a history of falling and live alone, recommend that they wear an electronic safety alert device. When activated by the wearer, this device alerts a monitoring site to call emergency services for assistance.

Observe patients using assistive devices (e.g., canes, walkers) in the home to ensure the devices are held and used correctly. Inform patients about how to keep these devices in safe working order.

General Preventive Measures. Neighborhood safety is important. Often patients are not aware of basic safety tips. Proper lighting and locks on windows and doors help reduce the risk of injury from crime. The local police department and community organizations often have safety classes available for residents to learn how to take precautions to minimize the chance of becoming involved in a crime. For example, some useful tips include always parking the car near a bright light or busy public area, carrying a whistle attached to the car keys, keeping car doors locked while driving, and always paying attention while driving to notice if anyone starts to follow the car.

Accidental home fires typically result from smoking in bed, placing cigarettes in trash cans, grease fires, improper use of candles or space

---

BOX 27.10 PATIENT TEACHING
Prevention of Electrical Hazards

Objective
- Patient will recognize and eliminate electrical hazards in the home.

Teaching Strategies
- Discuss importance of checking for grounding of electrical appliances and other equipment.
- Provide examples of common hazards: frayed cords, damaged equipment, and overloaded outlets.
- Discuss guidelines to prevent electrical shocks:
  - Use extension cords only when necessary and use electrical tape to secure the cord to the floor, preferably against baseboards.
  - Do not run wires under carpeting.
  - Grasp the plug, not the cord, when unplugging items.
  - Keep electrical items away from water.
  - Do not operate unfamiliar equipment.
  - Disconnect items before cleaning.

Evaluation
Use the principles of teach-back to evaluate patient/family caregiver learning:
- I want to be sure I explained fire hazards clearly. What electrical hazards exist in your home right now, and what steps can you take to eliminate them?
- What can you do to prevent getting an electrical shock?

---

heaters, or electrical fires resulting from faulty wiring or appliances. Teach patients and families how to reduce the risk of electrical injury in the home (Box 27.10) and how to use a home fire extinguisher (Box 27.11). To reduce the risk of fires in the home, counsel patients to quit smoking or to smoke outside the home. Have them inspect the condition of cooking equipment and appliances, particularly irons and stoves. Have patients with visual deficits install dials with large numbers or symbols on temperature controls. Make sure that smoke detectors are in strategic positions throughout the home so that the alarm will alert the occupants in a home in case of fire. All patients, even young children, need to know the phrase "stop, drop, and roll," which describes what to do when a person's clothing or skin is burning.

Help parents reduce the risk of accidental poisoning by teaching them to keep hazardous substances such as medications, cleaning fluids, and batteries out of the reach of children. Drug and other substance poisonings in adolescents and adults are commonly related to suicide attempts or drug experimentation. Teach parents that calling a poison control center for information before attempting home remedies will save their child's life. Guidelines for accepted interventions for accidental poisonings are available to teach a parent or guardian (Box 27.12). Older adults are also at risk for poisoning because diminished eyesight may cause an accidental ingestion of a toxic substance. In addition, the impaired memory of some older adults results in an accidental overdose of prescription medications. In health care settings it is important for you to know how to respond when exposure to a poisonous substance occurs. In addition, adhere to guidelines for intervening in accidental poisoning.

Be sure that a patient's home medications are kept in their original containers and labeled in large print. Recommend the use of medication organizers that are filled once a week by the patient and/or family caregiver. Have patients keep poisonous substances out of the bathroom and discard old or unused medications appropriately.

To prevent the transmission of pathogens, nurses teach aseptic practices. Medical asepsis, which includes hand hygiene and environmental cleanliness, reduces the transfer of organisms (see Chapter 28).

BOX 27.11 PATIENT TEACHING

Correct Use of a Fire Extinguisher in the Home

Objective
- Patient will use a fire extinguisher in the home correctly.

Teaching Strategies
- Discuss how to choose a correct location for an extinguisher: Place on each level of the home, near an exit, in clear view, away from stoves and heating appliances, and above the reach of small children.
- Keep a fire extinguisher in the kitchen, near the furnace, and in the garage.
- Make sure that patients read instructions after purchasing the extinguisher and that they know how often to review the instructions.
- Describe considerations to make before using a fire extinguisher. Attempt to fight the fire only when all occupants have left the home, the fire department has been called, the fire is confined to a small area, there is an exit route readily available, the extinguisher is the right type for the fire, and the patient knows how to use it.
- Instruct the patient to memorize the mnemonic *PASS*:
  - *P*ull the pin to unlock handle,
  - *A*im low at the base of the fire,
  - *S*queeze the handles,
  - *S*weep the unit from side to side (see Fig. 27.9).

Evaluation
Use the principles of teach-back to evaluate patient/family caregiver learning:
- When would it be appropriate to use a fire extinguisher at home?
- Explain for me what the mnemonic *PASS* means.

BOX 27.12 Intervening in Accidental Poisoning

1. If the person is conscious and alert, go online at https://www.poison.org/ or call the national toll-free poison control center number (**1-800-222-1222**) before trying any intervention. **Post this number in a visible area in the home.** Poison control centers have information needed to treat poisoned patients or offer referral to treat. *The administration of ipecac syrup or induction of vomiting is no longer recommended for routine home treatment of poisoning.*
2. Assess for signs or symptoms of ingestion of harmful substance, such as nausea, vomiting, foaming at the mouth, drooling, difficulty breathing, sweating, and lethargy.
3. Stop exposure to the poison. Have the person empty his or her mouth of pills, plant parts, or other material.
4. If poisoning is caused by skin or eye contact, irrigate the skin or eye with copious amounts of cool tap water for 15 to 20 minutes. In the case of an inhalation exposure, safely remove the victim from the potentially dangerous environment.
5. Identify the type and amount of substance ingested to help determine the correct type and amount of antidote needed.
6. If the victim has collapsed or stopped breathing, call 911. Initiate CPR if indicated until emergency personnel arrive. Ambulance personnel can provide emergency measures if needed. In addition, a parent or guardian is sometimes too upset to drive safely.
7. Position the victim with head turned to the side to reduce risk for aspiration.
8. Never induce vomiting if the victim has ingested the following poisonous substances: lye, household cleaners, hair care products, grease or petroleum products, furniture polish, paint thinner, or kerosene.

CPR, Cardiopulmonary resuscitation.
Modified from Hockenberry MJ, Wilson D: *Wong's essentials of pediatric nursing,* ed 11, St Louis, 2019, Elsevier; American Academy of Pediatrics, Committee on Injury, Violence and Poison Prevention: Gastrointestinal decontamination of the poisoned patient, *Pediatr Emerg Care* 24(3):176, 2008.

Patients and family members need to learn how to perform thorough hand hygiene (handwashing or use of a hand rub) and when to use it (i.e., before and after caring for a family member, before food preparation, before preparing a medication for a family member, after using the bathroom, and after contacting any bodily fluids). Patients also need to know how to dispose of infectious material such as wound dressings and used needles in the home setting. Heavy plastic containers such as hard, colored plastic liquid detergent bottles are excellent for needle disposal. The US Food and Drug Administration (2018b) recommends a two-step process:
- Place all needles and other sharps (e.g., lancets) in a sharps container immediately after use.
- Dispose of used sharps disposal containers according to community guidelines, including drop box or supervised collection sites, household hazardous waste collection sites, mail-back programs, or residential special waste pickup services.

Acute and Restorative Care. Within hospital and long-term care settings nurses take various measures to maintain patient safety, including fall prevention strategies, prevention of injuries from use of restraints and side rails, and precautions to prevent fires and exposure to poisoning and electrical hazards. Special precautions are also necessary to prevent injury in patients susceptible to having seizures. Radiation injuries are also a specific safety concern in hospitals.

Nurses are responsible for making a patient's bedside safe. Explain and demonstrate to patients how to use the call light or nurse call system device, and always place the device close to the patient. Respond quickly to call lights and bed/chair alarms. Keep the environment free from clutter around the bedside.

Fall Prevention. Patient falls continue to be a top adverse event in hospitals, often resulting in injury and even death (Joint Commission International, 2017b). Falls are also a serious concern in skilled nursing and long-term care settings. Fall reduction programs are a routine part of any hospital and long-term care setting. Implementing such a program begins with the nurse and patient partnering in recognizing the patient's fall risks. A fall reduction program includes a fall risk assessment of every patient, conducted routinely (see hospital policy) until a patient's discharge. Many hospitals have implemented hourly/purposeful rounding to reduce falls (see Box 27.5). In addition, most organizations apply yellow color-coded wristbands to patients' wrists to communicate to all health care providers that a patient is a fall risk. The American Hospital Association recommended that hospitals standardize wristband colors: red for patient allergies, yellow for fall risk, and purple for do-not-resuscitate preferences (AHA, 2008). Most hospitals have adopted this practice. However, wristbands can be difficult to discern at a distance, in low light, or when obscured, and can go unnoticed during a crisis (Wood and Bagian, 2011); therefore, additional measures are needed.

Patient-centered care is an important component of any fall reduction plan, with nurses making patients and families their partners in taking preventive action. A fall reduction plan should include individualized nursing interventions (see Skill 27.1). For example, if a patient has postural hypotension, the nurse will place the bed in the low position and have the patient dangle his or her feet on the side of bed for 3 to 5 minutes before ambulation. A patient with a history of urinary urgency or incontinence should be provided a bedside commode instead of being expected to walk to the bathroom unassisted.

Gait belts and additional safety equipment should be used as needed when moving, transferring, and ambulating patients (see Chapter 38).

When patients use assistive aids such as canes, crutches, or walkers, it is important to routinely check the condition of rubber tips and the integrity of the aid. Additionally, it is important to ensure that patients use their devices correctly. Remove excess furniture and equipment and instruct patients to wear rubber-soled shoes or slippers for walking or transferring. Safety bars near toilets (Fig. 27.6), locks on beds and wheelchairs (Fig. 27.7), and a nurse call system are additional safety features found in health care settings.

Another area of fall risk includes wheelchair-related falls involving older adults or patients with disabilities. Patients are at risk for falls during transfer tasks and reaching while seated in a wheelchair. An example of a wheelchair characteristic that increases risk for falls is having smaller and harder front wheels that cause a chair to tip when striking uneven terrain (such as an uneven floor surface moving into an elevator). Tripping over the front foot or leg rest and leaning over the back of a wheelchair to engage or disengage the wheel lock are common causes of injury.

Restraints. Patients who are confused or agitated or who repeatedly try to remove medical devices (e.g., IV lines, urinary catheters, or wound dressings) may temporarily require physical restraints to keep them safe. In the nursing home environment, research shows restraints being used when there are increases in the degree of care dependency as well as mobility limitations (Hofmann et al., 2015). A physical restraint is any manual method, physical or mechanical device, material, or equipment that immobilizes or reduces the ability of a patient to move arms, legs, body, or head freely. A restraint does not include devices such as orthopedically prescribed devices, protective helmets, or methods that involve physically holding a patient to conduct an examination or test, protecting a patient from falling out of bed or permitting a patient to participate in activities without risk of physical harm (TJC, 2018b). Chemical restraints are medications such as anxiolytics and sedatives used to manage a patient's behavior and are not a standard treatment for a patient's condition. Restraints are not a solution to a patient problem, rather a temporary means to provide safety. You must use all alternatives before placing patients in restraints. Federal and state laws prohibit Medicare- and Medicaid-certified nursing homes from using restraints unless they are medically needed. Only in emergencies can restraints be applied without a resident's or family member's informed consent.

Patients who are confused or disoriented, who repeatedly wander or fall, or who try to remove medical devices may require the temporary use of restraints to keep them safe. *However, the use of alternatives to restraints is preferred, and if a restraint is required, use the least restrictive type (e.g., soft mitt versus a limb restraint).* Individualize your choice of a restraint alternative based on each patient's situation (Box 27.13). An interprofessional approach that includes individualized assessments and development of structured treatment plans reduces restraint use. The optimal goal for all patients is a restraint-free environment.

The use of restraints is associated with serious complications resulting from immobilization, such as pressure injuries, pneumonia, constipation, and incontinence. Loss of self-esteem, humiliation, and agitation are also serious problems. In some cases, death has resulted because of restricted breathing and circulation. A study from Australia revealed that neck compression and entrapment by a restraint was the mechanism of harm in all reported cases, resulting in patient asphyxia (Bellenger et al., 2017). Because of these risks, legislation and regulatory standards have reduced the use of restraints. The Joint Commission and Centers for Medicare and Medicaid enforce standards for safe use of restraint devices. Many health care agencies have eliminated the use of the once-common jacket (vest) restraint (Ealey and Cameron, 2016). One standard involves staff training. All direct care staff must receive training in a health care

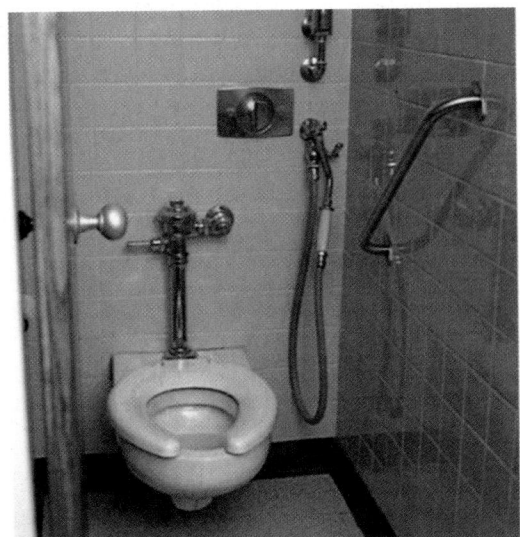

FIG. 27.6 Safety bars around toilets and showers.

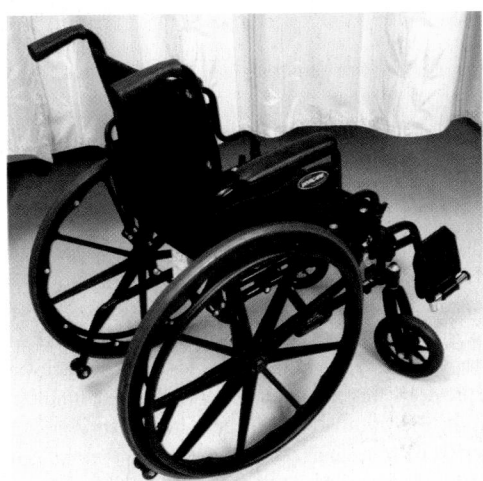

FIG. 27.7 Wheelchair with safety locks and anti-tip bars.

setting's restraint and seclusion policies and procedures, and all staff who may be involved in the use of restraints must be trained in safe use of mechanical restraint devices (CMS, 2007).

For patients who continue to try to ambulate without assistance, use low beds and electronic bed/chair alarms (see Skill 27.1). An alarm device warns nursing staff that a patient is attempting to leave a bed or chair unassisted. There are a variety of devices, including one with a knee band that sounds an alarm when the patient reaches a near-vertical position. An infrared type of alarm is affixed to a headboard or bedframe, allowing a patient to move freely with a bed. If a patient tries to leave the bed, the infrared beam detects motion and sends out an alarm. Alarm devices help avoid physical restraints and, when responded to promptly, can prevent patient falls and subsequent injuries.

When restraints are required to protect a patient (or nursing staff from being assaulted), involve the patient and family in the decision to use them. Help them adapt to this change by explaining the purpose of the restraint, expected care while the patient is in restraints, and that the restraint is temporary and protective. For legal purposes know agency-specific policy and procedures for appropriate use and monitoring of restraints. The use of a restraint must be clinically justified and part of a patient's prescribed medical treatment and plan of care. A health care

BOX 27.13 Alternatives to Restraints

- Orient patients and family members to the environment; explain all procedures.
- Provide companionship and supervision; use trained sitters; adjust staffing and involve family.
- Offer diversional activities: music, puzzles, activity aprons, folding towels. Use ideas of the patient and/or family.
- Assign confused or disoriented patients to rooms near nurses' stations, and observe frequently.
- Use de-escalation, time-out, and other verbal intervention techniques when managing aggressive behaviors.
- Provide visual and auditory stimuli (e.g., family pictures, a clock, music).
- Remove cues that promote leaving the room (e.g., close doors to block view of stairs; do not allow inpatient to wear street clothes).
- Promote relaxation techniques and normal sleep patterns.
- Institute exercise and ambulation schedules as allowed by patient's condition.
- Attend frequently to patient's needs for toileting, food and liquid, and pain management.
- Camouflage intravenous lines with clothing, stockinette, or Kling gauze dressing.
- Evaluate all medication effects and ensure timely and effective pain management.
- Discontinue bothersome treatments (e.g., nasogastric tubes or Foley catheters) as soon as possible.
- Use protective devices such as hip pads, helmet, skidproof slippers, and nonskid strips near bed.

provider's order based on a face-to-face assessment of a patient is required (TJC, 2018b). The order must be current (within 24 hours), stating the type and location of the restraint, and specify the duration and circumstances (e.g., preventing removal of medical device) under which it will be used. For restraints applied for violent or self-destructive behavior, a health care provider must assess the patient within 60 minutes. The orders need to be renewed within a specific time frame according to agency policy. In hospitals each original restraint order and renewal is limited to 4 hours for adults (18 years of age and older), 2 hours for children 9 through 17 years of age, and 1 hour for children younger than 9 years of age (CMS, 2016; TJC, 2018b). Orders may be renewed to the time limits for a maximum of 24 consecutive hours. Restraints are not to be ordered prn.

Nurses are responsible for making ongoing assessments of patients who are restrained. After a restraint is applied, monitor a patient closely (i.e., every 15 minutes for a violent patient and every 2 hours for a nonviolent patient). Monitoring should include vital signs, skin integrity underneath the restraint, nutrition, hydration, circulation to an extremity, range of motion, hygiene, elimination needs, cognitive functioning, psychological status, and need for restraint. Remove restraints periodically per agency policy. Assess patients who are violent continuously via audio or video monitors.

Skill 27.2 includes guidelines for the proper use and application of restraints. Their use must meet one of the following objectives:
- Reduce the risk of patient injury from falls.
- Prevent interruption of therapy such as traction, IV infusions, nasogastric (NG) tube feeding, or Foley catheterization.
- Prevent patients who are confused or combative from removing life-support equipment.
- Reduce the risk of injury to others by the patient.

Collaborate with other members of the health care team to design fall prevention approaches and a restraint-free environment for patients. The goal is to discontinue the use of restraints as soon as possible.

Side Rails. When used correctly, side rails help to increase a patient's mobility and/or stability when repositioning or moving in bed or moving from bed to chair. Although side rails are the most commonly used physical restraint, they increase the risk of falls when patients attempt to get out of bed or crawl over a rail. Side rails also can lead to patients becoming caught, trapped, entangled, or strangled, especially in the frail, elderly, or confused (FDA, 2017). Therefore an assessment of a patient's mobility and responsiveness to instructions helps determine whether using a side rail is safe. The same bedrail may have the effect of restraining one individual but not another, depending on the patient's condition.

A patient needs to have a route to exit a bed safely and to maneuver freely within the bed; in this case side rails are not considered a restraint. For example, raising only the two side rails at the top of a bed so that the lower part of the bed is open gives a patient room to exit the bed safely. Side rails used to prevent a patient such as one who is sedated from falling out of bed are not considered a restraint. Always know agency policy about the use of side rails. Be sure a bed is in the lowest position possible when side rails are raised. Check the condition or rails; bars between the bedrails need to be closely spaced to prevent entrapment. A potential exists for trapping a person's head and body in gaps and openings between the bedframe and mattress.

The use of side rails alone for a patient who is disoriented usually causes more confusion and further injury. Frequently a patient who is confused or determined to get out of bed because of pain or toileting needs tries to climb over a side rail or out at the foot of the bed. Either attempt often results in a fall. To reduce a patient's confusion, focus your interventions first on the cause, such as a response to a new medication, dehydration, or pain. Frequently nurses mistake a patient's attempt to explore his or her environment or to self-toilet as confusion. Additional safety measures include the use of a low bed with a nonskid mat placed alongside the bed on the floor. A low bed reduces the distance between the bed and floor, facilitating a roll rather than a fall from the bed.

Fires. Although smoking is not allowed in hospital and long-term care settings, smoking-related fires continue to pose a significant risk because of unauthorized smoking in beds or bathrooms. Institutional fires also may result from an electrical or anesthetic-related fire. The best intervention is to prevent fires. Nursing measures include complying with the smoking policies of an agency and keeping combustible material away from heat sources. Box 27.14 highlights fire intervention guidelines in health care agencies. Health care agencies are required to have practice fire drills annually.

If a fire occurs in a health care agency, protect patients from immediate injury, report the exact location of the fire, contain it, and extinguish it if possible. Fig. 27.8 demonstrates the process of using an extinguisher. Some agencies have fire doors that are held open by magnets and close automatically when a fire alarm sounds. It is important to keep equipment from blocking these doors. All personnel evacuate patients when appropriate. Patients who are close to a fire, regardless of its size, are at risk of injury and need to be moved to another area. If a patient is on life support, maintain his or her respiratory status manually with a bag-valve-mask device (e.g., Ambu-bag) (see Chapter 41) until he or she is moved away from the fire. Direct all ambulatory patients to walk by themselves to a safe area. In some cases, they can help move patients in wheelchairs. Move patients who cannot get out of bed from the scene of a fire by a stretcher, their bed, or a wheelchair. Try to avoid carrying patients. If you overextend your physical limits for lifting, injuring yourself results in further injury to the patient. If fire department personnel are on the scene, they help evacuate the patients.

BOX 27.14   Fire Intervention Guidelines

- Always keep the phone number for reporting fires visible on the telephone.
- Know the fire drill and evacuation plan of the agency.
- Know the locations of all fire alarms, exits, extinguishers, and oxygen shut-offs in your work area.
- Use the mnemonic *RACE* to set priorities in case of fire:

  R—Rescue and remove all patients in immediate danger.

  A—Activate the alarm. Always do this before attempting to extinguish even a minor fire.

  C—Confine the fire by closing doors and windows and turning off oxygen and electrical equipment.

  E—Extinguish the fire with an appropriate extinguisher.

Electrical Hazards. Much of the equipment used in health care settings is electrical and must be well maintained. The clinical engineering departments of hospitals inspect biomedical equipment such as hospital beds, infusion pumps, or ventilators regularly. You know that a piece of equipment is safe to use when you see a safety inspection sticker with an expiration date. Decrease the risk for electrical injury and fire by using properly grounded and functional electrical equipment. The ground prong of an electrical outlet carries any stray electrical current back to the ground. Remove equipment that is not in proper working order or that sparks when plugged in for service, and notify the appropriate hospital staff.

Seizures. Patients who have experienced some form of neurological injury or metabolic disturbance are at risk for a seizure. A **seizure** is hyperexcitation and disorderly discharge of neurons in the brain, leading to a sudden, violent, involuntary series of muscle contractions that is episodic, causing loss of consciousness, falling, tonicity (rigidity of muscles), and clonicity (jerking of muscles). At the time of a seizure patients are at risk for musculoskeletal or head injury as a result of a fall or striking a body part against a hard object. Patients with a history of seizures should be placed on seizure precautions so that if a seizure occurs, the risk of injury can be minimized.

Know the signs and symptoms of seizures. A generalized tonic-clonic, or grand mal, seizure lasts approximately 2 minutes (no longer than 5) and is characterized by a cry and loss of consciousness with falling, tonicity, clonicity, and incontinence. Before a convulsive episode a few patients report an aura, which serves as a warning or sense that a seizure is about to occur. An **aura** is often a bright light or a smell or taste. During a seizure the patient often experiences shallow breathing, cyanosis, and loss of bladder and bowel control. A postictal phase follows the seizure, during which the patient has amnesia or confusion and falls into a deep sleep. A person in the community needs immediate medical attention if he or she has repeated seizures, if a seizure lasts 5 minutes or longer, if one seizure occurs right after another without the person regaining consciousness between seizures, if seizures occur closer together than usual for that person, if breathing is difficult or the person appears to be choking, if the seizure occurs in water, or if an injury is suspected (Epilepsy Foundation, 2018). Instruct family members in the steps to take when a patient experiences a seizure. Assess a patient's home for environmental hazards considering a seizure condition.

Prolonged or repeated seizures indicate **status epilepticus**, a medical emergency that requires intensive monitoring and treatment. It is important that you observe the patient carefully before, during, and after the seizure so that you can document the episode accurately. **Seizure precautions** encompass nursing interventions to protect a

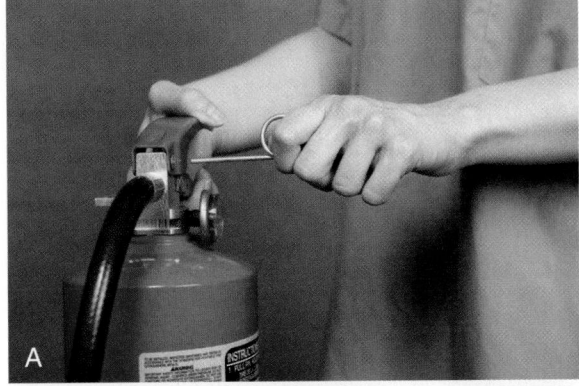
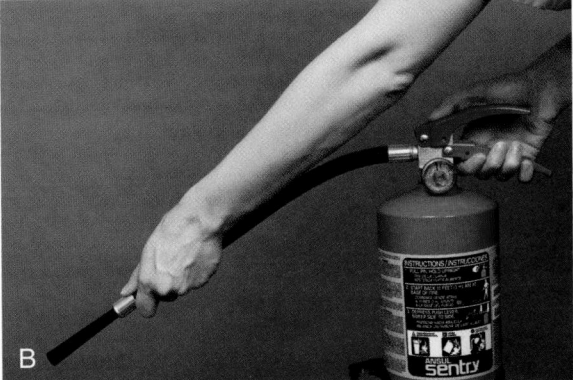
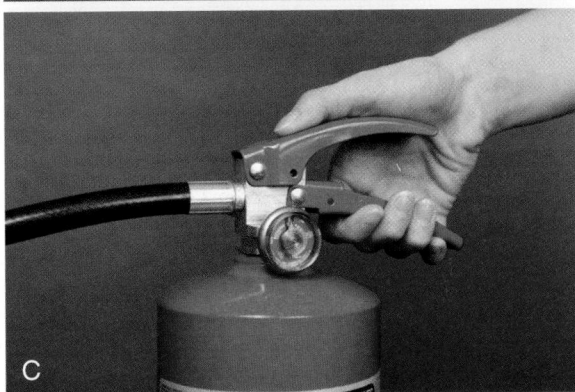

FIG. 27.8 Correct use of a fire extinguisher. A, *P*ull pin. B, *A*im at base of fire. C, *S*queeze handles and *S*weep from side to side to coat area evenly.

patient from traumatic injury, to position for adequate ventilation and drainage of oral secretions, and to provide privacy and support following a seizure (Box 27.15).

Disasters. As a nurse be prepared to respond and care for a sudden influx of patients during a disaster. The Joint Commission (2018b) requires hospitals to have an emergency-management plan that addresses the identification of possible emergency situations and their probable impact, maintenance of an adequate amount of supplies, and a formal response plan that includes actions to be taken by staff and steps to restore essential services and resume normal operations following the emergency. Infection control practices are critical in the event of a biological attack. You must manage all patients with suspected or confirmed bioterrorism-related illnesses with standard precautions (see Chapter 28). Additional precautions including airborne or contact isolation are needed for diseases such as smallpox and pneumonic plague. Most infections associated with biological agents are not transmissible from patient to patient. However, limit the transport and movement of patients only to movement that is essential for treatment. An important

---

BOX 27.15 Tips for Protecting Patients During a Seizure

1. When a seizure begins, note the time, stay with the patient, and call for help. Track duration of seizure. Notify health care provider immediately.
2. Position patient safely. If standing or sitting, ease the patient safely to the floor and protect head by cradling in your lap or placing a pad under head.
3. Do not lift patient from floor to bed while seizure is in progress. Clear surrounding area of furniture and anything else that is hard or sharp.
4. If patient is in bed, remove pillows and raise side rails.
5. If possible, turn patient onto one side, head tilted slightly forward.
6. Do not restrain patient; hold limbs loosely if they are flailing. Loosen clothing. Remove eyeglasses.
7. Never force apart a patient's clenched teeth. Do not place any objects into patient's mouth such as fingers, medicine, tongue depressor, or airway when teeth are clenched. **Insert a bite-block or oral airway in advance only if you recognize the possibility of a tonic-clonic seizure.**
8. Stay with patient, observing sequence and timing of seizure activity.
9. As patient regains consciousness, reorient and reassure. Assist patient to position of comfort in bed with side rails up (one rail down for easy exit) and bed in lowest position.
10. Conduct a head-to-toe evaluation, including an inspection of oral cavity for breaks in mucous membranes from bites or broken teeth; look for bruising of skin or injury to bones and joints.

---

aspect of care for patients who have a bioterrorism-related illness is postexposure management.

Preventing Workplace Violence. Being able to work in a safe environment is central to job satisfaction. As a nurse, be aware of your risks of being exposed to violence in the setting where you work. Nurses do not always know what acts constitute violence. A study involving nurses in emergency departments found that nurses often underreport violence, and as a direct result resources are not recognized or provided (Stene et al., 2015). It is important to recognize the patients who are most likely to enact violence. Jackson and colleagues (2014) reported from an observational study, conducted in an acute care setting, six key behaviors that predict patient violence: (1) increased volume of speech, (2) irritability, (3) prolonged or intense glaring, (4) mumbling, (5) abusive language toward caregivers (e.g., name calling/swearing), and (6) pacing around waiting area or bed. In a study that reviewed hospital incident reports involving patient violence, health care staff reported these causal factors for violence (Arnetz et al., 2015):

- Patient behavior—cognitive impairment and demanding to leave.
- Patient care issues—use of needles, pain/discomfort, and physical transfers.
- Situational events—restraints (holding or use of physical/chemical restraint), transitions in care, intervening (attempts to stop a patient from acting), and redirecting (helping a patient back into bed/back to hospital room).

Assessment tools are available for nurses to predict patients who are likely to act violently (see agency procedure). If you face a violent situation, use the following tips for reducing violence (CPI, n.d.):

1. Be nonjudgmental and empathic of the patient's feelings.
   - Whatever the patient's problem is, it can be highly important to him or her.

2. Respect personal space.
   - Stand 1.5 to 3 feet away from a patient who is escalating. This helps reduce a patient's anxiety and can help you prevent acting-out behavior.
   - If you must enter personal space to provide care, first explain what you are doing and why.
3. Use nonthreatening nonverbal communication.
   - As a patient loses control, he or she does not listen to what you have to say. Instead the patient reacts to your nonverbal communication (see Chapter 24).
   - Keep your voice tone, facial expressions, and movements neutral.
4. Do not overreact.
   - Stay calm, rational, and professional. Use positive thoughts, such as "I can manage this."
5. Focus on feelings.
   - Some people cannot identify how they really feel in a situation. Watch and listen carefully for the patient's real message.
6. Redirect or refocus any challenging questions, such as "Why does it always take so long for the doctor to see me?" or "Who's going to make me go to that test?"
   - Restate your request or directive; do not ignore the patient.
   - Bring the discussion back to how you can work together.
7. Set limits.
   - If patients become belligerent, defensive, or disruptive, give them *clear, simple, enforceable limits.*
   - Speak clearly, and offer a positive choice first.
8. Choose wisely what you insist on.
   - Be thoughtful in deciding *which rules are negotiable and which are not.* For example, if a patient is unwilling to walk at a given time, can you let the patient choose a better time?
   - When patients have options and flexibility, you may avoid an altercation.
9. Allow silence for reflection.
   - Silence gives a person a chance to think about what is happening and how to proceed.
10. Allow time for the patient to make a decision.
    - Give patients a few moments *to think through what you have said.* A person's stress increases when they feel rushed.

If you find that you work in a setting where violence is common, be sure to take care of yourself. Dealing with patients who are potentially violent is stressful and sometimes dangerous. Find positive ways to care for yourself away from work using stress-management approaches (see Chapter 37).

REFLECT NOW

Consider the following situation. You are caring for a 10-year-old child who has recently been diagnosed with acute lymphocytic leukemia. The child has started receiving treatment and is experiencing many side effects. The child's father is extremely angry about his child's diagnosis and perceives that family and friends are not providing appropriate support. You walk into the patient's room to administer a medication and the father begins to yell at you because he believes you are not providing appropriate care to his son. How would you respond to the father at this time? Role play your response with a peer.

◆ **Evaluation**

Through the Patient's Eyes. Patient-centered care involves a thorough evaluation of a patient's perspective related to safety and whether his or her expectations have been met. Ask the patient questions, such as "Are you satisfied with the changes you have chosen to make for your home? Do

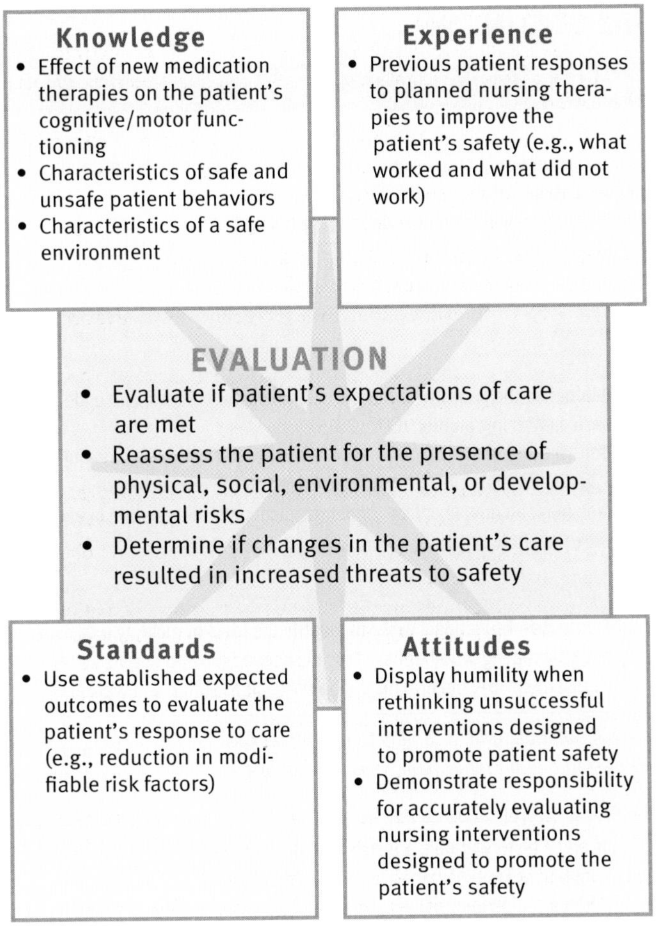

Knowledge
- Effect of new medication therapies on the patient's cognitive/motor functioning
- Characteristics of safe and unsafe patient behaviors
- Characteristics of a safe environment

Experience
- Previous patient responses to planned nursing therapies to improve the patient's safety (e.g., what worked and what did not work)

EVALUATION
- Evaluate if patient's expectations of care are met
- Reassess the patient for the presence of physical, social, environmental, or developmental risks
- Determine if changes in the patient's care resulted in increased threats to safety

Standards
- Use established expected outcomes to evaluate the patient's response to care (e.g., reduction in modifiable risk factors)

Attitudes
- Display humility when rethinking unsuccessful interventions designed to promote patient safety
- Demonstrate responsibility for accurately evaluating nursing interventions designed to promote the patient's safety

FIG. 27.9 Critical thinking model for safety evaluation.

you feel safer because of the changes? Are you still afraid of falling? In what way could we make you feel safer?" Involve the family in your evaluation, especially if they live with the patient and provide assistance in the home.

Patient Outcomes. Evaluation involves monitoring the actual care delivered by the health care team based on the expected outcomes (Fig. 27.9). For each nursing diagnosis measure whether the outcomes of care have been met. If your patient meets the goals, the diagnosis is resolved, and your nursing interventions were effective and appropriate. If not, determine whether new safety risks to the patient have developed or whether previous risks remain. For example, if the patient has a recurrent fall, reassess the conditions surrounding that fall and determine whether contributing factors can be removed or managed. The patient and family need to participate to find permanent ways to reduce risks to safety. When patient outcomes are not met, ask the following questions:
- What factors led to your fall/injury?
- Help me understand what makes you feel unsafe in your environment.
- What questions do you have about your safety?
- Do you need help locating community resources to help make your home safer?
- What changes have you recently experienced that you believe contribute to your risk for falling or lack of safety?

Continually reassess a patient's and family's need for additional support services, such as home care, physical therapy, counseling, and further teaching. A safe environment is essential to promoting, maintaining, and restoring health. Overall your expected outcomes include a safe physical environment and a patient whose expectations have been met, who is knowledgeable about safety factors and precautions, and who is free of injury.

SAFETY GUIDELINES FOR NURSING SKILLS

Ensuring patient safety is an essential role of the professional nurse. To ensure patient safety, communicate clearly with members of the health care team, assess and incorporate the patient's priorities of care and preferences, and use the best evidence when making decisions about the interventions to use in patient care delivery. When performing the skills in this chapter, remember the following points to ensure safe, individualized patient care:
- Anticipate a patient's fall risks based on your assessment and knowledge of physiological and behavioral factors when choosing fall prevention strategies.
- Involve patients and families in the selection of fall prevention strategies to improve adherence.
- Always try restraint alternatives before using a restraint. Involve family in your approach.
- Implement fall prevention protocols and provide patient and family education about fall prevention.

SKILL 27.1   FALL PREVENTION IN HEALTH CARE SETTINGS

Delegation and Collaboration
The skill of assessing and communicating a patient's risks for falling cannot be delegated to assistive personnel (AP). Skills used to prevent falls can be delegated. The nurse directs the AP by:
- Explaining a patient's specific fall risks and associated prevention measures needed to minimize risks.
- Explaining environmental safety precautions to use.
- Explaining specific patient behaviors (e.g., disorientation, wandering) that are precursors to falls and that should be reported to the RN immediately.

Equipment
- Standardized and valid fall risk assessment tool (TJC, 2018b)
- Hospital bed with side rails; *option*—low bed
- Wedge cushion
- Nurse call system
- Gait belt for assisting with ambulation
- Wheelchair and seat belt (as needed)
- Optional safety devices: bed alarm pad, nonslip floor mat, head protective gear, hip protector

SKILL 27.1   FALL PREVENTION IN HEALTH CARE SETTINGS—cont'd

STEP	RATIONALE

ASSESSMENT

1. Identify patient using at least two identifiers (e.g., name and birthday or name and medical record number) according to agency policy.

2. Review medical record and determine whether patient has a recent history of a fall or risks for injury (ABCs) (IHI, n.d.):

   *A*ge over 85

   *B*one disorders (e.g., metastasis, osteoporosis)

   *C*oagulation disorders (e.g., leukemia, thrombocytopenia, anticoagulant use)

   *S*urgery (specifically, thoracic or abdominal surgery or lower limb amputation)

3. Assess patient and family health literacy.

4. Perform hand hygiene. Assess for fall risks using a validated fall risk assessment tool. Compute fall risk score. Conduct a comprehensive individualized patient assessment and consider patient's unique fall risks (TJC, 2018b) Perform a fall risk assessment in general acute care settings on admission, on transfer from one unit to another or with a significant change in a patient's condition, or after a fall (AHRQ, 2013).

5. Perform the Banner Mobility Assessment Tool (BMAT) (Boynton et al., 2014) or the "timed get up and go (TUG)" test (CDC, n.d.) if patient is able to ambulate. At a minimum, observe patient walk in room (with or without help).

Rationale column:

Ensures correct patient. Complies with The Joint Commission standards and improves patient safety (TJC, 2020).

Conditions increase likelihood of serious injury from a fall such as fracture or internal hemorrhage.

Ensures patient has the capacity to obtain, communicate, process, and understand basic health information (CDC, 2019).

Reduces transmission of microorganisms. A variety of intrinsic physiological factors predispose patients to falls. Tools based on the risk factors of a population (e.g., elderly, oncology, or neurological patient) are more likely to be sensitive to predicting falls.

The BMAT assesses 4 functional tasks to identify the level of mobility a patient can achieve, revealing whether assistance is needed (Boynton et al., 2014). The TUG test measures the progress of balance, sit to stand, and walking.

CLINICAL DECISION: *Do not ask patient to provide a self-report of balance, gait, or ability to ambulate. Ask patient to walk a short distance using Timed Get Up and Go (Podsiadlo and Richardson, 1991), or complete the BMAT (Boynton, 2014) assessment, and observe each factor.*

---

6. Assess patient's pain severity (use rating scale ranging 0 to 10).

7. Ask patient or family caregiver whether patient has a history of recent falls or other injuries within the home. Assess previous falls using the acronym SPLATT (Touhy and Jett, 2018).

   *S*ymptoms at time of fall

   *P*revious fall

   *L*ocation of fall

   *A*ctivity at time of fall

   *T*ime of fall

   *T*rauma after fall

8. Review patient's medications (including over-the-counter [OTC] medications and herbal products) for drugs that create risk for falls. Also assess for polypharmacy (unnecessary use of multiple [five or more] and/or redundant medications in management of the same condition and drugs inappropriate for condition).

9. Assess patient's fear of falling: consider if patient is female, older age, lower level of education, chronic illness (more than three chronic illnesses), poor subjective health, functional impairment, a history of falling, and depression.

10. Assess condition of equipment (e.g., legs on bedside commode, end tips on a walker).

11. Use patient-centered approach to determine what patient already knows about risks for falling. Show patient and family caregiver results of fall risk assessment and explain significance of risk factors. Explain how a plan for fall prevention will be developed.

Rationale column:

Fear of falls and a history of falls are substantially more common among older adults with bothersome pain than in those without pain (Patel et al., 2014).

Symptoms are helpful in identifying cause for fall. Onset, location, and activity offer details on how to prevent future falls.

Effects of certain medications, such as those that depress the central nervous system (e.g., benzodiazepines, antipsychotics, antidepressants, opioids and barbiturates, antihistamines, and anticonvulsants), antihypertensives, diuretics, and laxatives, increase risk for falls (Severo et al., 2014). Over a 2-year period polypharmacy was significantly associated with a 21% increased rate of falls in a study involving adults over 60 years (Dhalwani et al., 2017).

Factors found to be associated with a severe fear of falling (Park et al., 2017)

Equipment in poor repair increases risk for fall.

Knowledge of fall risks influences one's ability to take necessary precautions in reducing falling. Matching interventions with factors that patient perceives as relevant may increase success in preventing falls.

STEP	**RATIONALE**
12. If patient is a fall risk, apply color-coded wristband (see illustration). Some agencies institute fall risk signs on doors, while others may use color-coded socks or gowns.	Color-coded yellow bands, socks, and gowns are easily recognizable.
13. If patient is in a wheelchair, assess his or her level of comfort, fatigue, boredom, mental status, or level of engagement with others.	These factors can cause patient to make an attempt to exit wheelchair without help.

PLANNING

1. Prepare equipment, being sure all is functional.	A well-equipped room with functioning equipment promotes safety.
2. Provide patient privacy and drape as appropriate for comfort.	Maintaining privacy promotes patient dignity and respect.
3. Position the patient in a comfortable position, depending on mobility restrictions.	Appropriate positioning allows for increased participation in care activities.
4. Explain safety measures taken as they pertain to patient's specific fall risks.	Clear, concise information with explanations for purpose, benefits, and expectations results in increased patient participation.

IMPLEMENTATION

1. Conduct hourly purposeful rounds on all patients to determine status of pain, need to toilet, comfort of position, and need to relocate personal items for easy reach; provide pain relief intervention.	Effective purposeful rounding can promote patient safety, encourage team communication, and improve staff ability to provide efficient patient care (McLeod and Tetzlaff, 2015).
2. Implement early mobility protocols within health care agency (see Chapter 38). Follow protocols to ensure that patient increases level of mobility progressively. Consider use of accelerometers, small devices that can be worn by a patient and that quantify biomechanical body movement and number of steps per shift (Growdon et al., 2017).	A patient's functional decline (loss of the ability to perform self-care activities or activities of daily living) may result from deconditioning, which is associated with inactivity (Gorman et al., 2014). Deconditioning is a risk for hospitalized patients who spend most of their time in bed, even when they are able to walk.
3. Adjust bed to low position with wheels locked (AHRQ, 2013). *Option:* Place nonslip padded floor mats at exit side of bed.	Height of bed allows ambulatory patient to get in and out of bed easily and safely. Mats provide nonslippery surface for preventing falls and injuries.
4. Encourage use of properly fitted skidproof footwear (AHRQ, 2013).	Prevents falls from slipping on floor.
5. Orient patient to surroundings, nurse call system, and routines to expect in plan of care (AHRQ, 2013).	Orientation to room and plan of care provides familiarity with environment and activities to anticipate.
a. Provide patient's hearing aid and glasses. Be sure that each is functioning/clean (AHRQ, 2013). If patient states he or she is having visual or hearing problems, refer to appropriate health care provider.	Enables patient to remain alert to conditions in environment.
b. Place nurse call system in an accessible location within patient's reach (see illustration). Explain and demonstrate how to use system at bedside and in bathroom. Have patient perform return demonstration.	Knowledge of location and use of nurse call system is essential for patient to be able to call for help quickly. Reaching for an object when in bed can lead to an accidental fall.
c. Explain to patient/family member when and why to use nurse call system (e.g., report pain, assistance needed to get out of bed or go to bathroom). Provide clear instructions regarding mobility restrictions.	Increases likelihood that patient/family caregiver will call for help and allows nurse to respond to patient's needs in a timely way.
6. Safe use of side rails:	
a. Explain to patient and family caregiver reason for patient to use side rails: moving and turning self in bed.	Promotes a feeling of comfort and security. Aids in turning and repositioning and provides easy access to bed controls (FDA, 2017).
b. Check agency policy regarding use of side rails.	
(1) Dependent, less mobile patients: In two–side rail bed, keep both rails up. (**Note:** Rails on newer hospital beds allow for room at foot of bed for patient to safely exit bed.) In four–side rail bed, leave two upper rails up.	Side rails are restraint devices if they restrict a patient's freedom of movement and therefore do not promote the individual's independent functioning (TJC, 2017a).

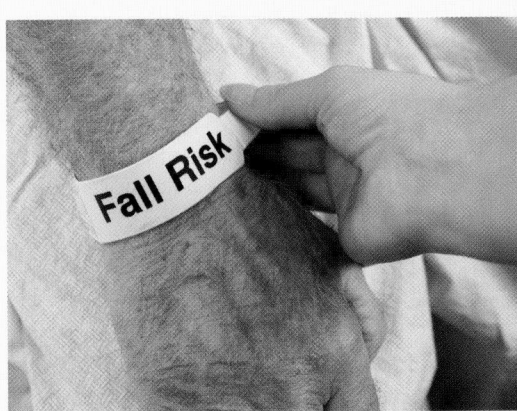

STEP 12 A "fall risk" armband alerts health care staff to patient's risk of falling.

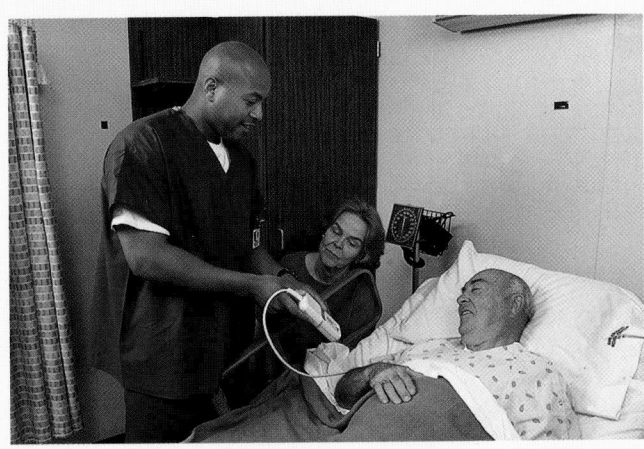

STEP 5b Nurse demonstrates use of nurse call system to patient.

Continued

SKILL 27.1	FALL PREVENTION IN HEALTH CARE SETTINGS—cont'd

STEP	RATIONALE
(2) Patient able to get out of bed independently: In four–side rail bed, leave two upper side rails up. In two–side rail bed, keep only one rail up.	Allows for safe exit from bed.
c. Use a proper-size mattress or mattress with raised foam edges (FDA, 2017).	Prevent patients from being trapped between the mattress and rail.
d. Reduce the gaps between the mattress and side rails (FDA, 2017)	Prevent patient entrapment.
7. Make patient's environment safe:	
a. Remove excess equipment, supplies, and furniture from rooms and halls.	Reduces likelihood of falling or tripping over objects.
b. Keep floors free of clutter and obstacles (e.g., intravenous [IV] pole, electrical cords), particularly path to bathroom (AHRQ, 2013).	Reduces likelihood of falling or tripping over objects.
c. Coil and secure excess electrical, telephone, and any other cords or tubing.	Reduces risk of entanglement.
d. Clean all spills on floors promptly (AHRQ, 2013). Post sign indicating wet floor. Remove sign when floor is dry (usually done by housekeeping).	Reduces risk of falling on slippery, wet surfaces.
e. Ensure adequate glare-free lighting; use a night-light at night.	Glare may be a problem for older adults because of vision changes.
f. Have assistive devices (e.g., cane, walker, bedside commode) on exit side of bed. Have chair back of a bedside commode placed against wall of room if possible.	Provides added support when transferring out of bed. Stabilizes commode.
g. Arrange personal items (e.g., water pitcher, telephone, reading materials, dentures) within patient's easy reach and in logical way (AHRQ, 2013).	Facilitates independence and self-care; prevents falls related to reaching for hard-to-reach items.
h. Secure locks on beds, stretchers, and wheelchairs (AHRQ, 2013).	Prevents accidental movement of devices during patient transfer.
8. Provide nonpharmacological comfort measures (Chapter 44); offer ordered analgesics for patients experiencing pain, preferably around-the-clock.	Pain can cause patients to exit bed and increases risk for falls (Patel et al., 2014). Be cautious as opioids further increase fall risk.
9. **Interventions for patients at moderate-to-high risk for falling** (based on fall risk assessment):	
a. Prioritize nurse call system responses to patients at high risk; use a team approach with all staff knowing responsibility to respond.	Ensures rapid response by care provider when patient calls for help; decreases chance of patient trying to get out of bed on own.
b. Establish elimination schedule; use bedside commode when appropriate.	Proactive toileting keeps patients from being unattended with sudden urge to use toilet.

CLINICAL DECISION: *Toileting is a common event leading to a patient's fall (Berry and Kiel, 2016).*

STEP	RATIONALE
c. Stay with patient during toileting (standing outside bathroom door). Increase availability and use of raised toilet seats (VA Healthcare, 2015).	Patients often try to get up to stand and walk back to their beds from the bathroom without help. Raised seats make it easier to sit on or stand up from toilet.
d. Place patient in a geri-chair or wheelchair with wedge cushion. Use wheelchair only for transport, not for sitting an extended time.	Maintains alignment and comfort and makes it difficult to exit chair.
e. Consider use of a low bed that has lower height than standard hospital bed. *Option:* Apply nonskid floor mats (VA Healthcare, 2015).	Low beds may reduce fall-related injuries by making it difficult for patients with lower extremity weakness or pain in lower joints to exert effort needed to stand. Mats prevent slipping when walking and standing.
f. Activate a bed alarm or camera monitoring system for patient (VA Healthcare, 2015).	Alarm activates when patient rises off sensor. Alarm sounds alert to staff. Camera can detect falls.

CLINICAL DECISION: *Use judgment in choosing use of a bed alarm. Bed alarms alert nursing staff so that if a patient exits a bed, a quick response may prevent a fall. If a patient exits a bed quickly and falls, the alarm alerts staff to respond so that further injury does not occur while patient lies on floor. However, bed and chair alarms can restrict patient activity. Reports have shown that patients perceive an alarm as restraining (Growdon et al., 2017). Determine whether use of bed or chair alarm is limiting frequency of patient getting up and remaining active.*

STEP	RATIONALE
g. Confer with physical therapy about gait training, strength and balance training, and regular weight-bearing activities.	Exercise can reduce falls, fall-related fractures, and several risk factors for falls in individuals with low bone density and older adults. Strength and balance training reduces the rate of falls with injuries in older adults (Uusi-Rasi et al., 2015).
h. Use sitters or restraints only when alternatives are exhausted.	A sitter is a nonprofessional staff member or volunteer who stays in a patient room to closely observe patients who are at risk for falling. Restraints should be used only as a final option (see Skill 27.2).

STEP	RATIONALE

(1) Consider having patient wear head protective gear (e.g., patient with cancer or patients at risk for bleeding) or hip protectors (patients at risk for fracture) (VA Healthcare, 2015).

Contains impact-resistant material within the hat that surrounds the head and protects against head injury. Hip protectors have padding to reduce fall impact.

10. When ambulating patient, have patient wear a gait belt or walking sling, and walk along his or her side (see Chapter 38).

Safe patient-handling techniques allow for safe patient ambulation and prevention of injury to you and patient.

11. Safe use of wheelchair:

   a. Be sure that wheelchair is correct fit for patient: patient thighs are level while sitting, feet flat on floor; back of chair comes up to midshoulder, elbows rest on armrests without leaning over or tucking arms in, and two fingerwidths of space between patient and side of chair.

Correctly fitted chair promotes comfort, making it less likely for patient to try to exit it.

   b. Transfer patient to wheelchair using safe handling techniques (see Chapter 38). Use a wedge cushion in chair (see illustration).

Cushion prevents patient from slipping out of chair.

   c. Back wheelchair into and out of elevator or door, leading with large rear wheels first (see illustration).

Prevents smaller front wheels from catching in crack between elevator and floor, causing chair to tip.

   d. Manage patient's pain and do not allow him or her to sit in wheelchair an extended amount of time; provide alternative sitting option.

Reduces restlessness and discomfort that can lead to wheelchair exit.

12. Schedule oral medication administration for at least 2 hours before "bedtime" (TJC, 2016).

Reduces risk created by medications that can cause patients to have to use bathroom during night.

13. Remove unnecessary supplies at bedside from patient room. Perform hand hygiene.

Reduces clutter. Reduces transmission of microorganisms.

EVALUATION

1. Ask patient/family caregiver to identify patient's fall risks.

Demonstrates learning.

2. Ask patient/family caregiver to describe fall prevention interventions to implement.

Demonstrates learning.

3. Evaluate patient's ability to use assistive devices such as walker or bedside commode at different times during the day.

Adjustments in devices may become necessary. Evaluating at different times can help identify strengths and weaknesses.

4. Evaluate for changes in motor, sensory, and cognitive status, and review if any falls or injuries have occurred.

May require different interventions to be added. Fall outcomes determine success of plan.

5. Evaluate patient's level of pain using a pain rating scale.

Determines whether patient's pain is under adequate control.

6. Continue hourly purposeful rounding.

Reduces patient anxiety, lessens need for patient to exit bed independently

7. Use Teach-Back: "I want to be sure I explained clearly to you why you are at risk to fall. Tell me some of those reasons." Revise your instruction now or develop plan for revised patient/family caregiver teaching if patient/family caregiver is not able to teach back correctly.

Determines patient's/family caregiver's level of understanding of instructional topic.

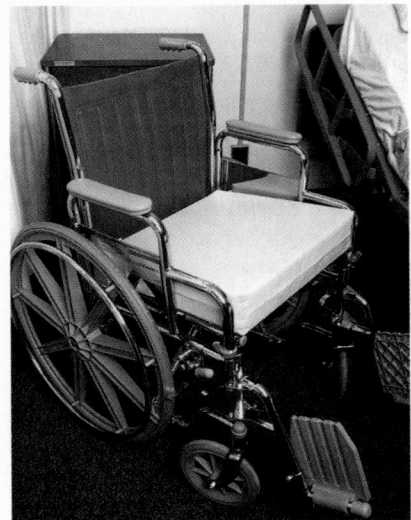

STEP 11b Wheelchair with footplates raised and wedge cushion in place.

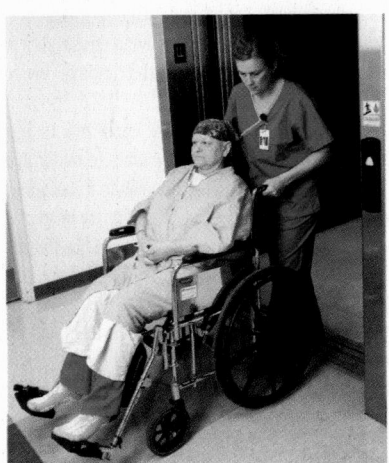

STEP 11c Nurse backing wheelchair into elevator.

Continued

SKILL 27.1 FALL PREVENTION IN HEALTH CARE SETTINGS—cont'd

UNEXPECTED OUTCOMES AND RELATED INTERVENTIONS

1. Patient/family caregiver unable to identify fall risks or fall prevention strategies.
   - Reinforce identified risks, and review safety measures with patient and family caregiver.
   - Consider using other instructional options.
2. Patient found after falling.
   - Call for assistance.
   - Assess patient for injury, and stay with him or her until help arrives.
   - Notify primary health care provider and family caregiver.
   - Complete an agency occurrence or incident event report (see agency policy).
   - Conduct a huddle/debrief as soon as possible after the fall. Involve staff at all levels and the patient if possible. Discuss whether appropriate interventions were in place, considerations as to why fall occurred, staffing at time of fall, which environment of care factors were in place, and how care plan will change (VA Healthcare, 2015; TJC, 2016).

RECORDING AND REPORTING

- Record in the plan of care specific fall prevention interventions. Use white boards in patient rooms to communicate patient fall risks to all staff (TJC, 2016).
- Document what patient is able to explain or not explain about fall risks and interventions taken.
- Complete a facility safety event or incident report noting objective details of a fall (time, location, patient's condition, treatment, treatment response). Do not place the report in patient's medical record.
- Use a hand-off communication tool that includes specific patient risks for falls and falls with injury between caregivers. Discuss patient specific interventions taken. (VA Healthcare, 2015; TJC, 2016).
- Report immediately to the health care provider if patient sustains a fall or an injury.

SKILL 27.2 APPLYING PHYSICAL RESTRAINTS

Delegation and Collaboration

The skill of assessing a patient's behavior, orientation to the environment, need for restraints, and appropriate use of restraints cannot be delegated. The application and routine checking of a restraint can be delegated to assistive personnel (AP). CMS (2016) requires training of all direct care staff who apply restraints. The nurse instructs the AP about:

- Appropriate restraint to use and correct placement of restraint.

- When and how to change patient's position and provide range-of-motion exercises, hydration, toileting, skin care, and time for socialization.
- When to report signs and symptoms of patient not tolerating restraint and what to do.

Equipment
- Proper-sized restraint
- Padding (if needed)

STEP	RATIONALE

ASSESSMENT

1. Identify patient using at least two identifiers (e.g., name and birthday or name and medical record number) according to agency policy.

   Ensures correct patient. Complies with The Joint Commission standards and improves patient safety (TJC, 2020).

2. Review medical record to assess for underlying cause(s) of agitation and cognitive impairment leading to patient-initiated medical device removal (Bradas et al., 2012).

   a. Assess for life-threatening physiological impairments, e.g., respiratory, neurological, fever and sepsis, hypoglycemia or hyperglycemia, alcohol or substance withdrawal, or fluid and electrolyte imbalance.

   Physiological alterations might lead to accidental patient-initiated medical device removal (Bradas et al., 2012). Identification of conditions might lead to more appropriate medical or pharmacological treatment, eliminating need for restraints.

   b. If there is abrupt change in perception, attention, or level of consciousness, perform hand hygiene and assess for these same life-threatening conditions.

   Reduces transmission of microorganisms. Factors that affect patient cognition can develop quickly.

   c. Notify health care provider of change in mental status and compromised physiological status.

3. Assess patient's or family caregiver's health literacy level and then determine knowledge about use of restraints and experience.

   Ensures patient has the capacity to obtain, communicate, process, and understand basic health information (CDC, 2019).

4. Obtain baseline or premorbid cognitive function from family caregivers.

   Excellent sources of information for patient's behavioral patterns and history.

5. Establish whether patient has history of dementia or depression (Bradas et al., 2012).

   Patients who are cognitively impaired are at risk for exiting bed without asking for assistance.

6. Review medications that can cause risk for falling (e.g., antiemetics, opioid analgesics, anticholinergic agents acting on the bladder, and benzodiazepines/hypnotics) (Bradas et al., 2012; Browne et al., 2014).

   Medications can alter cognition, cause postural hypotension, and create other risks.

7. Review current laboratory values (e.g., electrolytes, blood glucose, blood culture, urinalysis).

   May reveal a fluid and electrolyte imbalance or other problems, such as a blood glucose imbalance or an infection, all of which can cause sudden confusion in the elderly (National Health Service [NHS, 2015]).

STEP	RATIONALE
8. Assess patient's current behavior (e.g. confusion, disorientation, agitation, restlessness, combativeness, inability to follow directions, or repeated removal of therapeutic devices). Does patient create a risk to other patients?	If patient's behavior continues despite treatment or restraint alternatives, use of least restrictive restraint might be indicated.

CLINICAL DECISION: *In the case of alcohol withdrawal, the use of restraints can increase agitation and worsen neuropsychiatric disturbances (Rainier, 2014).*

9. If restraint alternatives failed earlier, confer with health care provider. Review agency policies and state laws regarding restraints. **Obtain current health care provider's order for restraint,** including purpose, type, location, and time or duration of restraint. Determine whether signed consent for use of restraint is necessary (long-term care). For patients who are nonviolent/non–self-destructive, orders are renewed per hospital policy.	A restraint order that is being used for violent or self-destructive behavior has a definite time limit (e.g., every 4 hours for adults, every 2 hours for children); these orders may be renewed according to the prescribed time limits for a maximum of 24 consecutive hours (TJC, 2017b). A health care provider's order for least restrictive type of restraint is required. (TJC, 2018b).

CLINICAL DECISION: *A licensed independent health care provider responsible for the care of the patient evaluates the patient in person within 1 hour of the initiation of restraint used for the management of **violent or self-destructive behavior** that jeopardizes the physical safety of the patient, staff, or others. A registered nurse or a physician assistant may conduct the in-person evaluation if he or she is trained in accordance with the requirements and consults with the above health care provider after the evaluation as determined by hospital policy (**TJC, 2018b**).*

10. Review manufacturer instructions for restraint application. Determine most appropriate size restraint. Be familiar with all devices.	Incorrect sizing and application of restraint device can result in patient injury or death.

PLANNING

1. Prepare restraint, being sure it is intact.	Ensures restraint is in condition for correct use.
2. Provide patient privacy, and drape as appropriate for comfort.	Promotes patient comfort.
3. Explain purpose of restraint, how it will be applied, length of time to be used, and procedure for ongoing assessment.	Promotes patient cooperation and helps to minimize any anxiety.

IMPLEMENTATION

1. Perform hand hygiene. Adjust bed to proper height and lower side rail on side of patient contact. Be sure that patient is comfortable and in proper body alignment.	Reduces transmission of microorganisms. Allows you to reposition patient during restraint application without injuring self or patient. Proper alignment prevents contracture formation when restraints are in place.
2. Inspect area where restraint is to be placed. Note whether there is any nearby tubing or device. Assess condition of skin, sensation, adequacy of circulation, and range of joint motion.	Restraints sometimes compress and interfere with functioning of devices or tubes. Assessment provides baseline to monitor patient's response to restraint.
3. Pad skin and bony prominences (as necessary) that will be under restraint.	Reduces friction and pressure from restraint to skin and underlying tissue.
4. Apply proper-sized restraint. **NOTE:** Refer to manufacturer directions.	
a. *Mitten restraint:* Thumbless mitten device restrains patient's hands. Place hand in mitten, being sure that Velcro strap is around wrist and not forearm (see illustration).	Prevents patient from dislodging or removing medical device, removing dressings, or scratching but allows greater movement than wrist restraint. It is considered a restraint alternative if untethered and patient is physically and cognitively able to remove it.
b. *Elbow restraint (freedom splint):* Restraint consists of rigidly padded fabric that wraps around arm and is closed with Velcro. The upper end has a clamp that hooks to sleeve of patient's gown or shirt (see illustration). Insert arm so that elbow joint rests against padded area, keeping joint extended.	The restraint makes it difficult to remove or disrupt a medical device near the face or neck. It does not impede removing abdominal or urinary medical devices.

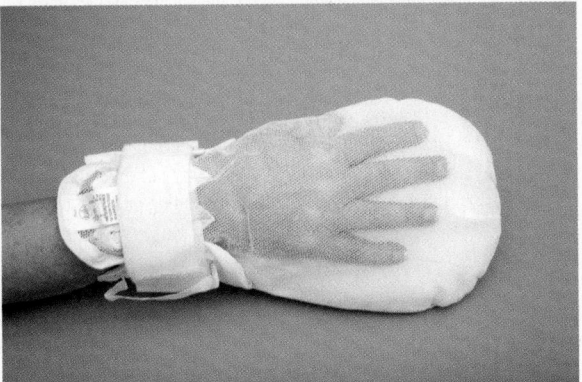

STEP 4a Mitten restraint. (From Sorrentino SA, Remmert LN: *Mosby's textbook for nursing assistants*, ed 10, St Louis, 2021, Elsevier.)

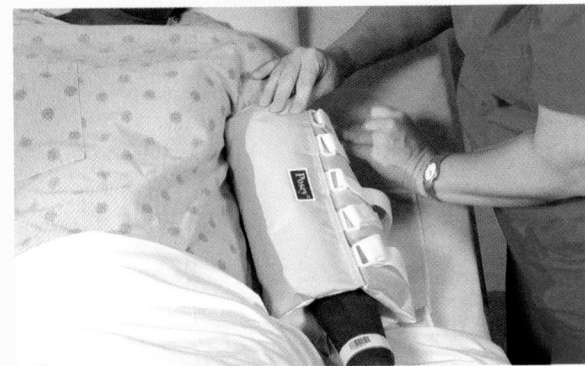

STEP 4b Freedom elbow restraint. (Copyright © Mosby's Clinical Skills: Essentials Collection.)

Continued

SKILL 27.2   APPLYING PHYSICAL RESTRAINTS—cont'd

STEP	RATIONALE

c. *Belt or body restraint:* Have patient in sitting position in bed. Apply belt over clothes, gown, or pajamas. Be sure to place restraint at waist, not chest or abdomen. Slot in belt may be positioned in front for limited movement or rear for increased movement. Remove wrinkles or creases in clothing. Bring ties through slots in belt. Help patient lie down in bed. Have patient roll to side and avoid applying belt too tightly. Ensure that straps secured to bedframe are snug so that belt does not slide to sides of bed. *Option:* Apply restraint net if intent is to limit patient turning.

Restrains center of gravity and prevents patient from rolling off stretcher, sitting up while on stretcher, or from falling out of bed. Tight application interferes with ventilation if belt moves up over abdomen or chest.

d. *Soft extremity (ankle or wrist) restraint:* Restraint made of soft quilted material or sheepskin with foam padding. Wrap limb restraint around wrist or ankle with soft part toward skin and secure snugly (not tightly) in place by Velcro strap. Insert two fingers under secured restraint (see illustration).

Restraint designed to immobilize one or all extremities. Maintain immobilization of extremity to protect patient from fall or accidental removal of therapeutic device (e.g., IV tube, Foley catheter). Tight application interferes with circulation and potentially causes neurovascular injury.

CLINICAL DECISION: *Patient with wrist and ankle restraints is at risk for aspiration if positioned supine. Place patient in lateral position or with head of bed elevated rather than supine.*

---

5. Attach restraint straps to part of bedframe that moves when raising or lowering head of bed. Be sure that straps are secure. *Do not attach to side rails.* Attach restraint to chair frame for patient in chair or wheelchair, being sure that buckle is out of patient's reach.

Properly positioned strap does not tighten and restrict circulation when bed is raised or lowered.

6. Secure restraints on bedframe with quick-release buckle (see illustration). *Do not tie strap in a knot.* Be sure that buckle is out of patient's reach.

Allows for quick release in emergency.

7. Double-check and insert two fingers under secured restraint one more time. Assess proper placement of restraint, including skin integrity, pulses, skin temperature and color, and sensation of restrained body part. Place bed in lowest position after restraint(s) applied.

Provides baseline to later evaluate if injury develops from restraint. Provides safest environment in which to leave a patient who is restrained.

8. Perform hand hygiene. Remove restraint at least every 2 hours (TJC, 2018b) or more frequently as determined by agency policy. Reposition patient, provide comfort and toileting measures, and evaluate patient condition each time. If patient is agitated, violent or noncompliant, remove one restraint at a time and/or have staff assistance while removing restraints.

Provides opportunity to attend to patient's basic needs and determine need for continuation of restraints.

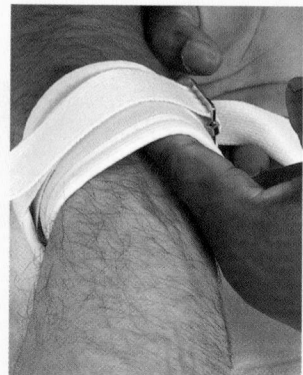

STEP 4d Soft extremity restraint. Check restraint for constriction by inserting two fingers under restraint.

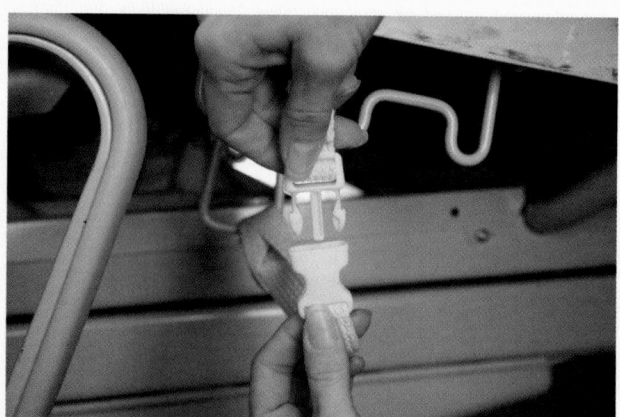

STEP 6 Quick-release buckle makes it easier to disconnect and evacuate patients in an emergency.

STEP	RATIONALE

CLINICAL DECISION: *Do not leave a patient who is violent or aggressive unattended while restraints are off. Monitoring of violent/self-destructive patients placed in restraints is continuous (by way of video or audio) versus every 2 hours for nonviolent patients.*

9. Be sure nurse call system is within patient's reach.	Allows patient, family, or caregiver to get help quickly.
10. Leave bed or chair with wheels locked. Keep bed in lowest position.	Prevents bed or chair from moving if patient tries to get out. If patient falls with bed in lowest position, this reduces chance of injury.
11. Remove and dispose of any supplies. Perform hand hygiene.	Reduces transmission of microorganisms.

EVALUATION

1. After restraint application, evaluate patient's response to restraints:
   a. For patients who are nonviolent, conduct evaluation for signs of injury (e.g., circulation, ROM, vital signs, skin condition), behavior and psychological status, and readiness for discontinuation (frequency based on agency policy) (TJC, 2018b).
   b. For patients who are violent/self-destructive, conduct same evaluation every 15 minutes. Perform visual checks if patient is too agitated to approach (TJC, 2018b).
	Frequent evaluation prevents injury to patient and ensures removal of restraint at earliest possible time. Frequency of monitoring guides staff in determining appropriate intervals for evaluation based on patient's needs and condition, type of restraint used, risk associated with use of chosen intervention, and other relevant factors.

2. Evaluate patient's need for toileting, nutrition and fluids, hygiene, and elimination, and release restraint at least every 2 hours.	Prevents injury to patient and attends to basic needs.
3. Evaluate patient for any complications of immobility.	Early detection of skin irritation, restricted breathing, or reduction in mobility prevents serious adverse events.

4. Renewal of restraints:
   a. Patients who are not violent may have renewal of restraints based on hospital policy. However, the restraint must be discontinued at the earliest possible time, regardless of the scheduled expiration of the order.
   b. Patients who are violent/self-destructive may have restraints renewed within the following limits:
     • 4 hours for adults 18 years of age or older
     • 2 hours for children and adolescents 9 to 17 years of age
     • 1 hour for children under 9 years of age
   These orders may be renewed according to the time limits for a maximum of 24 consecutive hours.
	Ensures that restraint application continues to be medically appropriate.

5. Observe IV catheters, urinary catheters, and drainage tubes to determine that they are positioned correctly and that therapy remains uninterrupted.	Reinsertion is uncomfortable and increases risk for infection or interrupts therapy.
6. **Use Teach-Back:** "We've talked about the reason we're using restraints on your father. Tell me that reason. I want to be sure you understand." Revise your instruction now or develop a plan for revised family caregiver teaching if family caregiver is not able to teach back correctly.	Determines family caregiver's level of understanding of instructional topic.

UNEXPECTED OUTCOMES AND RELATED INTERVENTIONS

1. Patient experiences impaired skin integrity.
   • Evaluate need for continued use of restraint and whether alternatives can be used.
   • If restraint is still needed, be sure that it is applied correctly, and provide adequate padding.
   • Check skin under restraint for abrasions, and remove restraints more often. Provide appropriate skin care and change wet or soiled restraints.
2. Patient becomes more confused or agitated.
   • Try to determine cause of behavior and eliminate if possible; consult with health care provider.
   • Determine need for more or less sensory stimulation and make stimulation meaningful.
   • Reorient as needed and try restraint-free options.
3. Patient has neurovascular injury (e.g., cyanosis, pallor, and coldness of skin or complaints of tingling, pain, or numbness).
   • Remove restraint immediately, stay with patient, and have health care provider notified.
   • Protect extremity from further injury.

Continued

SKILL 27.2 APPLYING PHYSICAL RESTRAINTS—cont'd

RECORDING AND REPORTING

- Record restraint alternatives tried, patient's behavior, level of orientation, and patient or family member's statement of understanding of the purpose of restraint and consent for application (if required by the agency).
- Record placement and purpose for restraint, type and location of restraint, time applied, time restraint ended, and all routine assessments made in nurses' notes and flow sheet.
- Record patient's behavior after restraint application. Record times patient was assessed, attempts to use alternatives to restraint and patient's response, times restraint was released (temporarily and permanently), and patient's response when restraint was removed.
- Document evaluation of patient learning.
- Report any injury resulting from a restraint to RN in charge and health care provider immediately.
- During handoff, report location of restraint, last time assessment was conducted, and findings.

HOME CARE CONSIDERATIONS

- A physical restraint is a device that requires a health care provider's order. Do not send a patient home with intent of restraining unless device is necessary to protect patient from injury. If patient's family wishes to use restraint at home, a health care provider's order is required, and you need to give clear instructions regarding proper application, care needed while in restraints, and complications for which to look. Carefully assess the family for competency and understanding of intent for using restraint.

KEY POINTS

- Patient-centered care involves a patient as a full partner in providing coordinated care based on respect for a patient's preferences, values, and needs, with partnership as the essential factor.
- Patient-centered care is planned, delivered, managed, and continuously improved in active partnership with patients and their families to promote safety.
- Vulnerable populations such as infants, children, older adults, individuals with chronic disease or a physical or mental disability, individuals who have difficulty communicating, and individuals with a low income or who are homeless are at risk for threats in safety because of reduced access to health care, fewer resources, and increased morbidity.
- Motor vehicle accidents, poisonings, and falls are the leading causes of unintentional injuries and can be prevented by following recommended precautions such as child safety seat use, safe driving practices for older adults, and reducing exposure to poisonous substances in the home.
- School-age children are expanding their cognitive and psychosocial skills and need to learn to cope with the rules and expectations of schools and peers, such as rules for playing safely and using protective safety equipment.
- Adolescents begin to separate emotionally from their families, and the peer group begins to have a stronger influence, increasing the risk for experimentation with alcohol, tobacco, and drugs.
- Muscle weakness, paralysis, abnormal gait, and poor coordination or balance are major factors in placing patients at risk for falls.
- Distractions and interruptions contribute to accidents and need to be limited, especially during high-risk procedures such as medication administration.
- Correct use of safe patient-handling techniques and equipment reduces the risk of injuries when moving and lifting patients.
- The assessment of a patient's medical history, current physical condition (e.g., alertness, gait, lower-body muscle strength, and vision), medication history, developmental status, and safety risk factors determines whether any underlying conditions exist that pose threats to a patient's safety.

- When caring for a patient in the home, a home hazard assessment and a review of a patient's home routines help you recognize less obvious hazards and the type of environmental changes needed.
- It is important to learn the patient's willingness to make changes in his or her environment since decisions on ways to change the environment require the patient's full participation.
- Restraint alternatives for patients at low risk include adjusting beds to low position with wheels locked, providing properly fitted skidproof footwear, providing clear walking paths, and orienting patients to surroundings with easy access to assistive devices and the nurse call system.
- Before applying restraints, review the medical record for underlying cause(s) of agitation and cognitive impairment, assess whether the patient has a history of dementia or depression, and review medications and current laboratory values.
- When a patient is in a physical restraint, assess the placement of the restraint, and note skin integrity, pulses, skin temperature and color, and sensation of the restrained body part.

REFLECTIVE LEARNING

- Consider the patients you interacted with today and describe their age-specific safety risks.
- Thinking back over your past week of interacting with patients, identify factors that created a culture of safety as well as opportunities you saw for creating or improving a culture of safety.
- Consider the patients you interacted with today and their safety risks. What types of interventions would you include in your nursing care plan to help prevent and minimize the intrinsic and extrinsic threats to their safety?

REVIEW QUESTIONS

1. Which of the following are safe practices to follow in the safe preparation and storage of food? (Select all that apply.)
   1. Always use a single cutting board to prepare foods for cooking.
   2. Refrigerate leftovers as soon as possible.
   3. Always buy vegetables in packages marked "prewashed."
   4. Cook meats to the proper temperature.
   5. Wash hands thoroughly before food preparation.

2. A nurse enters the hospital room of a patient who had a total knee replacement the day before. Which of the following pose potential safety risks? (Select all that apply.)
    1. A current safety inspection sticker is on the IV fluids pump.
    2. A walker is positioned near the patient's bedside.
    3. The hospital bed is in the high position.
    4. There is no gait belt at the bedside.
    5. The overbed table with the patient's glasses is positioned against the wall opposite the end of the bed.

3. A nurse working on a medicine unit in the hospital hears the fire alarm go off. As the nurse walks down the hallway, there is smoke coming from the family waiting area. Which of the following steps should the nurse take? (Select all that apply.)
    1. Immediately phone in to the hospital alert system the exact location of the fire.
    2. Direct the nurse technician to place empty stretchers behind the fire doors.
    3. Go to each patient room, and direct ambulatory patients to walk themselves to a safe area.
    4. Work with the nurse technician to help move patients requiring wheelchairs from their rooms.
    5. Close the room doors of patients who cannot get out of bed, and keep them in their rooms.

4. Match the threats to safety on the right to the category of risk factors on the left.

    A. Individual Risks
    B. Developmental Risks

    1. An older adult has limited finances.
    2. A young toddler likes to explore objects by placing them in his mouth.
    3. A 55-year-old patient has a residual gait change due to a stroke.
    4. A school-age child chooses to play ice hockey.
    5. A patient newly diagnosed with diabetes has low health literacy.

5. A nurse working on a surgery floor is assigned four patients. The nurse assesses each patient, noting behaviors and physical signs and symptoms. Which of the following patients is more likely to be violent toward the nurse?
    1. The first patient maintains eye contact with the nurse, is calm during the nurse's assessment, and asks questions frequently.
    2. The second patient is very drowsy, loses attention span when the nurse asks questions, and mumbles when speaking.
    3. The third patient moves nervously in bed, swears and grimaces when trying to cough, and speaks in a low volume.
    4. The fourth patient speaks in a loud voice and becomes irritable when the nurse arrives to help walk the patient.

6. A nurse working the night shift is assigned a patient who has a history of having fallen in the hospital during a previous admission. The nurse wants to review the admission assessment completed by the nurse on the day shift. Which of the following sections in the assessment are most likely to provide information about the patient's current fall risks? (Select all that apply.)
    1. Allergy history
    2. Medication history
    3. Patient age
    4. Patient's occupation
    5. Physical exam of neuromuscular function

7. Match the intervention for promoting child safety on the left with the correct developmental stage on the right.

    1. Teach children proper bicycle and skate board safety.
    2. Teach children how to cross streets and walk in parking lot.
    3. Teach children proper techniques for specific sports.
    4. Teach children not to operate electric toothbrushes while unsupervised.
    5. Teach children not to talk to or go with a stranger.
    6. Teach children not to eat items found in the grass.

    A. School-age child
    B. Preschooler

8. The nurse finds a 68-year-old woman wandering in the hallway and exhibiting confusion. The patients says she is looking for the bathroom. Which interventions are appropriate for this patient? (Select all that apply.)
    1. Ask the health care provider to order a restraint.
    2. Recommend insertion of a urinary catheter.
    3. Provide scheduled toileting rounds every 2 to 3 hours.
    4. Institute a routine exercise program for the patient.
    5. Keep the bed in high position with side rails down.
    6. Keep the pathway from the bed to the bathroom clear.

9. Place the following steps for applying a wrist restraint in the correct order:
    1. Pad the skin overlying the wrist.
    2. Insert two fingers under the secured restraint to be sure that it is not too tight.
    3. Be sure that the patient is comfortable and in correct anatomical alignment.
    4. Secure restraint straps to bedframe with quick-release buckle.
    5. Wrap limb restraint around wrist or ankle with soft part toward skin and secure snugly.

10. Match the fall prevention intervention on the left with the scientific rationale on the right.

    1. Prioritize nurse call system responses to patients at high risk.
    2. Place patient in a wheelchair with wedge cushion.
    3. Establish elimination schedule with bedside commode.
    4. Use a low bed for patient.
    5. Provide a hip protector.
    6. Place nonskid floor mat on floor next to bed.

    A. Maintains comfort and makes exit difficult
    B. Makes it difficult for patients with lower extremity weakness to stand
    C. Reduces slipping when walking
    D. Reduces fall impact
    E. Ensures rapid response for help
    F. Reduces chance of patient trying to get out of bed on own

Answers: 1. 2, 4, 5; 2. 3, 4, 5; 3. 1, 3, 4; 4. 1A, 2B, 3A, 4B, 5A; 5. 4.; 6. 2, 3, 5; 7. A: 1, 2, 3 B: 4, 5, 6; 8. 3, 4, 6; 9. 3, 4, 1, 5, 2; 4; 10. 1E, 2A, 3F, 4B, 5D, 6C.

Rationales for Review Questions can be found on the Evolve website.

REFERENCES

Agency for Healthcare Research and Quality (AHRQ): *Culture of safety,* 2018a, https://psnet.ahrq.gov/primers/primer/5/Culture-of-Safety. Accessed November 29, 2018.

Agency for Healthcare Research and Quality (AHRQ): *20 tips to help prevent medical errors: a patient fact sheet,* 2018b, https://www.ahrq.gov/patients-consumers/care-planning/errors/20tips/index.html. Accessed December 3, 2018.

Agency for Healthcare Research and Quality (AHRQ): *Patient safety Network: never events,* 2018c, https://psnet.ahrq.gov/primers/primer/3/never-events. Accessed November 29, 2018.

Agency for Healthcare Research and Quality (AHRQ): *Preventing falls in hospitals: a toolkit for improving quality of care,* AHRQ Publication No. 13-0015-EF, 2013, available https://www.ahrq.gov/sites/default/files/publications/files/fallpxtoolkit.pdf. Accessed December 17, 2018.

American Academy of Pediatrics (AAP): *AAP updates recommendations on car seats for children,* 2018a, https://www.aap.org/en-us/about-the-aap/aap-press-room/Pages/AAP-Updates-Recommendations-on-Car-Seats-for-Children.aspx. Accessed November 29, 2018.

American Academy of Pediatrics (AAP): *Immunizations: vaccine hesitant parents,* 2018b, https://www.aap.org/en-us/advocacy-and-policy/aap-health-initiatives/immunizations/Pages/vaccine-hesitant-parents.aspx. Accessed December 10, 2018.

American Geriatric Society: *Clinical practice guideline fall prevention in older persons,* 2015, http://www.americangeriatrics.org/health_care_professionals/clinical_practice/clinical_guidelines_recommendations/prevention_of_falls_summary_of_recommendations. Accessed September 2015.

American Hospital Association: *Quality advisory: implementing standardized colors for patient alert wristbands,* 2008, https://www.scha.org/files/documents/patient_wristband_alert_advisory_aha.pdf. Accessed December 11, 2018.

Blue Cross Blue Shield: *Early childhood vaccination trends in America,* 2018. https://www.bcbs.com/the-health-of-america/reports/early-childhood-vaccination-trends-america. Accessed December 11, 2018.

Boysen P: Just culture: a foundation for balanced accountability and patient safety, *Ochsner J* 13(3):400, 2013, https://www.ncbi.nlm.nih.gov/pmc/articles/PMC3776518/. Accessed November 28, 2018.

Bradas CM, et al.: Physical restraints and side rails in acute and critical care settings. In Boltz M, et al.: *Evidence-based geriatric nursing protocols for best practice,* ed 4, New York, 2012, Springer Publishing Company, pp 229–245.

Centers for Disease Control and Prevention (CDC): *Poisoning prevention,* 2016a, https://www.cdc.gov/safechild/poisoning/index.html. Accessed November 29, 2018.

Centers for Disease Control and Prevention (CDC): *Common vaccine safety concerns,* 2016b, https://www.cdc.gov/vaccinesafety/concerns/index.html. Accessed December 1, 2018.

Centers for Disease Control and Prevention (CDC): *Older adult drivers,* 2017a, https://www.cdc.gov/motorvehiclesafety/older_adult_drivers/index.html. Accessed November 29, 2018.

Centers for Disease Control and Prevention (CDC): *Important facts about falls,* 2017b, https://www.cdc.gov/homeandrecreationalsafety/falls/adultfalls.html. Accessed December 1, 2018.

Centers for Disease Control and Prevention (CDC): *STEADI materials for your older adult patients,* 2017c, Available at https://www.cdc.gov/steadi/patient.html. Accessed December 18, 2018.

Centers for Disease Control and Prevention (CDC): *Center for preparedness and response: emergency preparedness & vulnerable populations: planning for those most at risk,* 2018a, https://www.cdc.gov/cpr/whatwedo/vulnerable.htm. Accessed November 29, 2018.

Centers for Disease Control and Prevention (CDC): *Carbon monoxide (CO) Poisoning Prevention,* 2018b, https://www.cdc.gov/features/copoisoning/index.html. Accessed November 29, 2018.

Centers for Disease Control and Prevention (CDC): *Food safety: foodborne illnesses and Germs,* 2018c, https://www.cdc.gov/foodsafety/foodborne-germs.html. Accessed November 29, 2018.

Centers for Disease Control and Prevention (CDC): *Teen drivers: get the facts,* 2018d, https://www.cdc.gov/motor-vehiclesafety/teen_drivers/teendrivers_factsheet.html. Accessed November 29, 2018.

Centers for Disease Control and Prevention (CDC): *What vaccines are recommended for you,* 2018e, https://www.cdc.gov/vaccines/adults/rec-vac/index.html. Accessed January 12, 2018.

Centers for Disease Control and Prevention (CDC): *About school violence,* 2018f, https://www.cdc.gov/violenceprevention/youthviolence/schoolviolence/index.html. Accessed December 1, 2018.

Centers for Disease Control and Prevention (CDC): *Antineoplastic drug administration – effects of organizational safety practices and perceived safety climate on Use of exposure controls and adverse events,* 2018g, https://www.cdc.gov/niosh/topics/healthcarehsps/antidrugeffects.html. Accessed December 7, 2018.

Centers for Disease Control and Prevention (CDC): *What is health literacy,* 2019, https://www.cdc.gov/healthliteracy/learn/index.html. Accessed December 23, 2019.

Centers for Disease Control and Prevention (CDC): *The timed get up and go test (TUG),* n.d. https://www.cdc.gov/steadi/pdf/STEADI-Assessment-TUG-508.pdf. Accessed December 17, 2017.

Centers for Medicare and Medicaid Services (CMS): *Revisions to Medicare conditions of participation,* 482.13, Bethesda, MD, 2007, US, Department of Health and Human Services.

Centers for Medicare and Medicaid Services (CMS): *The CMS restraint training Requirements Handbook,* HCPro, Inc, a division of BLR, 2016, https://hcmarketplace.com/aitdownloadablefiles/download/aitfile/aitfile_id/1880.pdf. Accessed December 18, 2018.

Child Trends Databank: *Immunization,* 2015. https://www.childtrends.org/?indicators=immunization. Accessed November 30, 2018.

Crisis Prevention Institute (CPI): *CPI's top 10- de-escalation tips,* n.d., https://www.crisisprevention.com/Blog/October-2017/CPI-s-Top-10-De-Escalation-Tips-Revisited. Accessed January 4, 2019.

Ealey R, Cameron E: *Restraints: patient safety and regulatory compliance – extended version,* SSRN, 2016, https://doi.org/10.2139/ssrn.2712831. Accessed December 14, 2018.

ECRI: *Fall prevention training program achieves results in reducing falls and related injuries,* 2017. https://www.ecri.org/components/HRCAlerts/Pages/HRCAlerts100417_Fall.aspx. Accessed December 7, 2018.

Environmental Protection Agency (EPA): *Learn about lead,* 2018, https://www.epa.gov/lead/learn-about-lead. Accessed November 29, 2018.

Epilepsy Foundation: *Seizure first aid,* 2018, https://www.epilepsy.com/learn/seizure-first-aid-and-safety/adapting-first-aid-plans/seizure-first-aid. Accessed December 17, 2018.

Electrical Safety Foundation International: *Space heater safety tips,* 2015. https://www.esfi.org/resource/space-heater-safety-tips-146. Accessed December 10, 2018.

Frampton SB, et al.: *Harnessing evidence and experience to change culture: a guiding Framework for patient and family engaged care,* Washington, DC, 2017, Discussion Paper, National Academy of Medicine. https://nam.edu/wp-content/uploads/2017/01/Harnessing-Evidence-and-Experience-to-Change-Culture-A-Guiding-Framework-for-Patient-and-Family-Engaged-Care.pdf. Accessed September 6, 2019.

Gorman G, et al.: Physical activity, exercise and aging, *Wellbeing* 4(7):1, 2014.

Growdon ME, et al.: Viewpoint: the tension between promoting mobility and preventing falls in the hospital, *JAMA Internal Medicine* 177(6):759, 2017.

Herdman TH, Kamitsuru S, editors: *NANDA International nursing diagnoses: definitions and classification,* ed 11, New York, 2018, Thieme, pp 2018–2020.

Hockenberry MJ, et al.: *Wong's nursing care of infants and children,* ed 11, St Louis, 2019, Elsevier.

Institute for Healthcare Improvement (IHI): The ABCs of Reducing Harm from Falls, n.d., http://www.ihi.org/resources/Pages/ImprovementStories/ABCsofReducingHarmfromFalls.aspx.

Insurance Institute for Highway Safety (IIHS): *General Statistics-Fatality facts 2016,* 2016, Arlington, vol. A https://www.iihs.org/iihs/topics/t/general-statistics/fatalityfacts/overview-of-fatality-facts. Accessed December 1, 2018.

Joszt L: *5 vulnerable populations in healthcare,* AJMC, 2018, https://www.ajmc.com/newsroom/5-vulnerable-populations-in-healthcare. Accessed November 29, 2018.

Kann L, et al.: Youth risk behavior surveillance-United States, 2015. *Morbid Mortal Wkly Rep Surveill Summ* 65:1, 2016.

Kaslow N: Teen Suicides: What Are the Risk Factors? 2018, https://childmind.org/article/teen-suicides-risk-factors/. Accessed December 20, 2018.

Kochanek KD, et al.: *Mortality in the United States, 2016,* Centers for Disease Control and Prevention: National Center for Health Statistics, 2017. https://www.cdc.gov/nchs/products/databriefs/db293.htm. Accessed November 29, 2018.

McLeod J, Tetzlaff S: The value of purposeful rounding, *Am Nurse Today* 10(11), 2015, https://www.americannursetoday.com/value-purposeful-rounding/. Accessed December 20, 2018.

National Alliance for caregiving: research, 2019, http://www.caregiving.org/research/. Accessed September 2, 2019.

National Association of School Nurses: *School violence - the role of the school nurse: position Statement,* 2018, https://www.nasn.org/advocacy/professional-practice-documents/position-statements/ps-violence. Accessed December 1, 2018.

National Fire Protection Association [NFPA]: *Fact sheet – research; US home structure fires,* 2017a, Retrieved from https://www.nfpa.org/News-and-Research/Fire-statistics-and-reports/Fire-statistics/Fires-by-property-type/Residential/Home-Structure-Fires. Accessed November 30, 2018.

National Fire Protection Association [NFPA]: *Fires in healthcare facilities,* 2017b, https://www.nfpa.org/News-and-Research/Data-research-and-tools/Building-and-Life-Safety/Fires-in-Health-Care-Facilities. Accessed November 30, 2018.

National Health Service (NHS): *Sudden confusion: delirium,* 2015. https://www.nhs.uk/conditions/confusion/. Accessed December 18, 2018.

National Institute on Aging: *Prevent falls and fractures,* 2017, https://www.nia.nih.gov/health/prevent-falls-and-fractures. Accessed December 3, 2018.

National Institute on Drug Abuse: *Abuse of prescription drugs affect young adults most,* 2016, https://www.drugabuse.gov/related-topics/trends-statistics/infographics/abuse-prescription-rx-drugs-affects-young-adults-most. Accessed December 18, 2018.

National Institute for Occupational Safety and Health (NIOSH): *Workplace violence prevention for nurses,* 2018, https://www.cdc.gov/niosh/topics/violence/training_nurses.html. Accessed January 3, 2019.

National Institutes of Health: *Safe sleep for your Baby,* NIH Pub. No. 12-5759, August 2014. https://www.nichd.nih.gov/sites/default/files/publications/pubs/Documents/Safe_Sleep_Environment_English.pdf.

National Safety Council: *Safety at home,* 2019. https://www.nsc.org/home-safety/safety-topics/child-safety. Accessed January 3, 2019.

National Quality Forum (NQF): *NQF's Mission and vision,* 2018a, Washington DC, https://www.qualityforum.org/about_nqf/mission_and_vision/. Accessed December 3, 2018.

National Quality Forum (NQF): *List of SRE's,* 2018b, Washington DC, https://www.qualityforum.org/Topics/SREs/List_of_SREs.aspx. Accessed December 3, 2018.

National Quality Forum (NQF): *Patient safety: safe practices - 2010,* 2018c, Washington DC, http://www.qualityforum.org/Projects/Safe_Practices_2010.aspx. Accessed December 3, 2018.

Occupational Safety and Health Administration (OSHA): Hazard communication, n.d. a, United States Department of Labor, https://www.osha.gov/dsg/hazcom/. Accessed December 2, 2018.

Occupational Safety and Health Administration (OSHA): Workplace violence in healthcare - Understanding the challenge, n.d.b, https://www.osha.gov/Publications/OSHA3826.pdf. Accessed December 8, 2018.

Podsiadlo D, Richardson S: The timed "Up & Go": a test of basic functional mobility for frail elderly persons, *J Am Geriatr Soc* 39(2):142, 1991.

Quality and Safety Education for Nurses (QSEN): *QSEN competencies: patient-centered care,* NC, 2018, University of North Carolina at Chapel Hill, Chapel Hill. http://qsen.org/competencies/pre-licensure-ksas/#patient-centered_care. Accessed November 28, 2018.

Response Systems: JCAHO Compliance, n.d. http://www.disasterpreparation.net/resources.html. Accessed November 30, 2018.

Saftari LN, Kwon O: Ageing vision and falls: a review, *J Physiol Anthropol* 37:11, 2018.

Stanford Health Care: *Nursing: patient centered care and education,* 2017, https://stanfordhealthcare.org/health-care-professionals/nursing/patient-care/fall-prevention.html. Accessed January 4, 2019.

Stene J, et al.: Workplace violence in the emergency department: giving staff the tools and support to report, *The Permanente J* 19(2):e113, 2015.

The Joint Commission (TJC): *Preventing patient falls: a systematic approach from The Joint Commission center for Transforming healthcare Project,* October 2016, http://www.hpoe.org/Reports-HPOE/2016/preventing-patient-falls.pdf. Accessed December 10, 2018.

The Joint Commission (TJC): *Standards FAQ details: restraint and seclusion -side rails,* 2017a, https://www.jointcommission.org/standards_information/jcfaqdetails.aspx?StandardsFaqId=1362&ProgramId=46. Accessed December 18, 2018.

The Joint Commission (TJC): Joint Commission Resources Quality & Safety Network (JCRQSN) *Resource Guide*: Be Prepared: Maximizing Behavioral Healthcare-Related Tracer Activities, April 27, 2017b.

The Joint Commission (TJC): *Speak up initiatives,* 2018a, https://www.jointcommission.org/speakup.aspx. Accessed November 28, 2018.

The Joint Commission (TJC): *Comprehensive accreditation manual for hospitals,* Oakbrook Terrace, IL, 2018b, TJC.

The Joint Commission: Sentinel Event Alert - Developing a reporting culture: learning from close calls and hazardous conditions, issue 60, 2018d, https://www.jointcommission.org/assets/1/18/SEA_60_Reporting_culture_FINAL.pdf. Accessed December 17, 2018.

The Joint Commission (TJC): *2020 National Patient Safety Goals,* Oakbrook Terrace, IL, 2020, The Commission.

https://www.jointcommission.org/en/standards/national-patient-safety-goals/Accessed January 2, 2020.

The Joint Commission Center for Transforming Healthcare (TJCCTH): *Targeted solutions tool for preventing falls,* 2018, https://www.centerfortransforminghealthcare.org/tst_pfi.aspx. Accessed December 3, 2018.

Touhy T, Jett K: *Ebersole and Hess' gerontological nursing and health care,* ed 5, St Louis, 2018, Elsevier.

US Food and Drug Administration (FDA): *A guide to bed safety bed rails in hospitals, nursing homes and home health care: the facts,* 2017, Revised, https://www.fda.gov/medicaldevices/productsandmedicalprocedures/generalhospitaldevicesandsupplies/hospitalbeds/ucm123676.htm. Accessed December 15, 2018.

US Food and Drug Administration (FDA): *Report a problem to the FDA,* 2018a, https://www.fda.gov/safety/reportaproblem/default.htm. Accessed December 7, 2018.

US Food and Drug Administration (FDA): *Best way to get Rid of used needles and other sharps,* 2018b, https://www.fda.gov/medicaldevices/productsandmedicalprocedures/homehealthandconsumer/consumerproducts/sharps/ucm263240.htm. Accessed December 11, 2018.

Ventola CL: Immunization in the United States: recommendations, barriers, and measures to improve compliance, Part 1: childhood vaccinations, *Pharm Therapeut* 41(7):426, 2016.

Veterans Administration (VA): *Healthcare: Implementation guide for fall injury reduction,* 2015, https://www.patientsafety.va.gov/docs/fallstoolkit14/falls_implementation_%20guide%20_02_2015.pdf. Accessed December 18, 2018.

World Health Organization (WHO): *Falls,* 2018, http://www.who.int/news-room/fact-sheets/detail/falls. Accessed November 29, 2018.

RESEARCH REFERENCES

Arnetz JE, et al.: Understanding patient-to-worker violence in hospitals: a qualitative analysis of documented incident reports, *J Adv Nurs* 71(2):338–348, 2015.

Avanacean D, et al.: Effectiveness of patient-centered interventions on falls in the acute care setting: a quantitative systematic review protocol, *JBI Database System Rev Implement Rep* 15(1):55, 2017.

Bellenger E, et al.: Physical restraint deaths in a 13-year national cohort of nursing home residents, *Age Ageing* 46(4):688, 2017.

Berry S, Kiel D: *Falls: prevention in nursing care facilities and the hospital setting,* UpToDate, 2016, http://www.uptodate.com/contents/falls-prevention-in-nursing-care-facilities-and-the-hospital-setting. Accessed December 18, 2018.

Boynton T, et al.: Implementing a mobility assessment tool for nurses: a nurse-driven assessment tool reveals the patient's mobility level and guides SPHM technology choices, *Am Nurse Today* 13, 2014, https://americannursetoday.com/wp-content/uploads/2014/09/ant9-Patient-Handling-Supplement-821a_Implementing.pdf. Accessed December 17, 2018.

Browne C, et al.: Falls prevention focused medication review by a pharmacist in an acute hospital: implications for future practice, *Int J Clin Pharm* 36(5):969, 2014.

Cadore EL, et al.: Effects of different exercise interventions on risk of falls, gait ability, and balance in physically frail older adults: a systematic review, *Rejuvenation Res* 16(2):105, 2013.

Dhalwani NN, et al.: Association between polypharmacy and falls in older adults: a longitudinal study from England, *BMJ Open* 7:e016358, 2017, https://bmjopen.bmj.com/content/7/10/e016358. Accessed December 18, 2018.

Geiger-Brown J, et al.: Sleep, sleepiness, fatigue, and performance of 12-hour shift nurses, *Chronobiol Int* 29(2):211, 2012.

Hempel S, et al.: Hospital fall prevention: a systematic review of implementation, components, adherence, and effectiveness, *J Am Geriatr Soc* 61(4):483, 2013.

Hofmann H, et al.: Use of physical restraints in nursing homes: a multicentre cross-sectional study, *BMC Geriatr* 15:129, 2015.

Jackson D, et al.: Cues that predict violence in the hospital setting: findings from an observational study, *Collegian* 21:65, 2014.

Lange M, et al.: Cognitive changes after adjuvant treatment in older adults with early-stage breast cancer, *The Oncologist* 23(9), 2018, epub ahead of print.

McInnes DK, et al.: Opportunities for engaging low-income, vulnerable populations in health care: a systematic review of homeless persons' access to and use of information technologies, *Am J Public Health* 103(Suppl 2):e11, 2013.

Morgan L, et al.: Intentional rounding: a staff-led quality improvement intervention in the prevention of patient falls, *J Clin Nurs* 26(1–2):115, 2017.

Nagamatsu LS, et al.: Mind-wandering and falls risk in older adults, *Psychol Aging* 28(3):685, 2013.

Olsen CF, Bergland A: The effect of exercise and education on fear of falling in elderly women with osteoporosis and a history of vertebral fracture: results of a randomized controlled trial, *Osteoporos Int* 25(8):2017, 2014.

Park J, et al.: Risk factors associated with the fear of falling in community-living elderly people in Korea: role of psychological factors, *Psychiatry Investig* 14(6):894, 2017.

Patel KV, et al.: High prevalence of falls, fear of falling, and impaired balance among older adults with pain in the

United States: findings from the 2011 National Health and Aging Trends Study, *J Am Geriatr Soc* 62(10):1844–1852, 2014.

Potter P, et al.: Evaluation of sensor technology to detect fall risk and prevent falls in acute care, *Jt Comm J Qual Patient Saf* 43(8):414, 2017.

Prince M, et al.: The global prevalence of dementia: a systematic review and metaanalysis, *Alzheimer's Dementia* 9:63, 2013, https://www.alzheimersanddementia.com/article/S1552-5260(12)02531-9/pdf. Accessed December 3, 2018.

Rainier NC: Reducing physical restraint use in alcohol withdrawal patients: a literature review, *Dim Crit Care Nurs* 33(4):201, 2014.

Schwappach DLB: Risk factors for patient–reported medical errors in eleven countries, *Health Expect* 17(3):321, 2014.

Severo IM, et al.: Risk factors for falls in hospitalized adult patients: an integrative review, *Rev Esc Enferm USP* 48(3):537, 2014.

Stark S, et al.: Protocol for the home hazards removal program (HARP) study: a pragmatic, randomized clinical trial and implementation study, *BMC Geriatr,* 2017, https://bmcgeriatr.biomedcentral.com/articles/10.1186/s12877-017-0478-4. Accessed December 8, 2018.

Uusi-Rasi K, et al.: Exercise and vitamin D in fall prevention among older women: a randomized clinical trial, *JAMA Intern Med* 175(5):703, 2015.

Wood SD, Bagian JP: A cognitive analysis of color-coded wristband use in health care, *Proc Hum Factors Ergon Soc Annu Meet* 55(1):281, 2011.

Zegers M, et al.: Evidence-based interventions to reduce adverse events in hospitals: a systematic review of systematic reviews, *BMJ Open* 6(9):e012555, 2016.

28

Infection Prevention and Control

OBJECTIVES

- Explain the relationship between the infection chain and transmission of infection.
- Give an example of preventing infection for each element of the infection chain.
- Describe the signs/symptoms of a localized infection and those of a systemic infection.
- Identify the normal defenses of the body against infection.
- Discuss the events in the inflammatory response.
- Explain conditions that promote the transmission of health care–associated infection.
- Identify patients most at risk for infection.
- Explain the difference between medical and surgical asepsis.
- Explain the rationale for Standard Precautions.
- Perform proper procedures for hand hygiene.
- Explain procedures for each isolation category.
- Explain how infection control measures differ in the home versus the hospital.
- Properly apply a disposable mask and sterile gloves.
- Understand the definition of occupational exposure.
- Explain the postexposure process.

KEY TERMS

Aerobic, p. 424
Anaerobic, p. 424
Asepsis, p. 435
Bactericidal, p. 424
Bacteriostasis, p. 424
Broad-spectrum antibiotics, p. 426
Colonization, p. 423
Communicable disease, p. 423
Cough etiquette, p. 437
Disinfection, p. 436
Endogenous infection, p. 428
Exogenous infection, p. 428

Hand hygiene, p. 439
Handwashing, p. 439
Health care–associated infections (HAIs), p. 427
Iatrogenic infections, p. 428
Immunocompromised, p. 424
Infection, p. 423
Infectious, p. 423
Invasive, p. 423
Localized, p. 425
Medical asepsis, p. 435
Multidrug-resistant organism, p. 427

Pathogens, p. 423
Reservoir, p. 424
Standard Precautions, p. 440
Sterile field, p. 448
Sterilization, p. 436
Suprainfection, p. 426
Surgical asepsis, p. 446
Susceptibility, p. 425
Systemic, p. 425
Vector, p. 425
Virulence, p. 423

MEDIA RESOURCES

http://evolve.elsevier.com/Potter/fundamentals/
- Review Questions
- Video Clips
- Concept Map Creator
- Concept Care Map

- Case Study with Questions
- Skills Performance Checklists
- Audio Glossary
- Content Updates
- Answers to QSEN Activity and Review Questions

The incidence of infectious diseases such as AIDS, influenza, pneumonia, measles, and sexually transmitted infections are a significant public health problem in the United States and around the world (Centers for Disease Control and Prevention [CDC], 2017d). In 2016 there were 15.5 million visits to physician offices, with infectious and parasitic diseases as the primary diagnosis (CDC, 2017d). Multiple factors affect the spread of infectious diseases, such as humans' susceptibility, drug resistance, human tendency to avoid vaccination, and drug immunosuppression. The effects of infectious disease are constantly evolving; an infection that is considered a national or global threat one year could be eliminated the next (Contagion Live, 2019). For example, the opioid crisis has increased the number of people diagnosed with infective endocarditis as a result of IV injections, subsequently requiring cardiac valve replacements

(CDC, 2017d). As a nurse it is critical to understand how infections develop, your patients' risk for infection, and how to institute preventive measures.

The incidence of patients who develop infections as the direct result of contact with health care personnel is an increasing health problem. Based on a large sample of US acute care hospitals, a CDC survey found that, on any given day, about 1 in 25 patients who are hospitalized has at least one health care–associated infection (HAI) (CDC, 2018a). Current trends, public awareness, and rising costs of health care have increased the importance of infection prevention and control. The Joint Commission (TJC) (2020) views HAIs as a patient safety issue. Nurses are essential to infection prevention and control when creating a safe health care environment for patients, families, and health care staff. Patients in all health care settings are at risk for acquiring infections because of lower resistance to pathogens; increased exposure to pathogens, some of which may be resistant to most antibiotics; and invasive procedures. Health care workers are at risk for exposure to pathogens as a result of contact with patient blood, body fluids, and contaminated equipment and surfaces. By practicing basic infection prevention and control techniques, you avoid spreading pathogens to patients and sustaining an exposure when providing direct care.

Patients and their families need to be able to recognize sources of infection and understand measures used to protect themselves. Patient teaching must include basic information about infection, the various modes of transmission, and appropriate methods of prevention such as hand hygiene and covering the mouth during a cough.

Health care workers protect themselves from contact with infectious material, sharps injury, and/or exposure to communicable diseases by applying knowledge of the infectious process and using appropriate personal protective equipment (PPE). Increases in multidrug-resistant organisms (MDROs), health care–acquired infections (HAIs), and concern about diseases such as hepatitis B virus (HBV) and hepatitis C virus (HCV), human immunodeficiency virus (HIV) infection, and tuberculosis (TB) require a greater emphasis on infection prevention and control techniques (CDC, 2007, 2013a, 2017).

SCIENTIFIC KNOWLEDGE BASE

Nature of Infection

It is important to know the difference between an infection and a colonization. An infection results when a pathogen invades tissues and begins growing within a host. Colonization is the presence and growth of microorganisms within a host but without tissue invasion or damage (Tweeten, 2018). Disease or infection results only if the pathogens multiply and alter normal tissue function. Some infectious diseases such as viral meningitis and pneumonia have a low risk or no risk for transmission. Although these illnesses can be serious for patients, they do not pose a risk to others, including caregivers.

If an infectious disease can be transmitted directly from one person to another, it is termed a communicable disease (Tweeten, 2018). If the pathogens multiply and cause clinical signs and symptoms, the infection is symptomatic. If clinical signs and symptoms are not present, the illness is termed asymptomatic. HCV is an example of a communicable disease that can be asymptomatic. It is most efficiently transmitted through the direct passage of blood into the skin from a percutaneous exposure, even if the source patient is asymptomatic (CDC, 2018b).

Chain of Infection

The presence of a pathogen does not mean that an infection will occur. Infection occurs in a cycle that depends on the presence of all of the following elements:

- An infectious agent or pathogen
- A reservoir or source for pathogen growth
- A port of exit from the reservoir
- A mode of transmission
- A port of entry to a host
- A susceptible host

Infection can develop if this chain remains uninterrupted (Fig. 28.1). Preventing infections involves breaking the chain of infection.

Infectious Agent. Microorganisms include bacteria, viruses, fungi, and protozoa (Table 28.1). Microorganisms on the skin are either resident or transient flora. Resident organisms (normal flora) are permanent residents of the skin and within the body, where they survive and multiply without causing illness (CDC, 2008; World Health

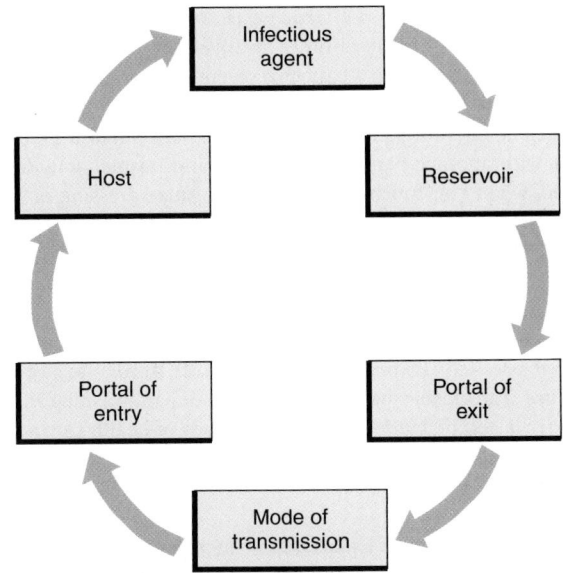

FIG. 28.1 Chain of infection.

TABLE 28.1 Infections and Common Causative Organisms

Infection Site	Common Organisms
Bronchitis	*S. pneumoniae, H. influenzae*, respiratory viruses
Device-related	Coagulase-negative staphylococci, *Corynebacterium* sp.
Empyema	*S. aureus*, streptococci, anaerobes
Endocarditis	*S. viridans, S. aureus*, enterococci
Gastroenteritis	*Salmonella* sp., *Shigella* sp., *Campylobacter* sp.,
Meningitis	*E. coli* O157:H7, viruses
Pelvic inflammatory disease	*H. influenzae, N. meningitides, S. pneumoniae*
Peritonitis	*C. trachomatis, N. gonorrhoeae, Bacteroides* sp., Enterobacteriaceae
Pneumonia (community)	*S. pyogenes*, respiratory viruses
Pneumonia (health care–associated)	*S. pneumoniae, H. influenzae, M. pneumoniae, C. pneumoniae, M. tuberculosis*
Osteomyelitis	*Pseudomonas* sp., *S. aureus*, Enterobacteriaceae
Septic arthritis	*S. aureus*
Septicemia	*S. aureus, N. gonorrhoeae*
Skin	*S. pneumoniae, H. influenzae, S. pyogenes, S. aureus*
Urinary tract	*S. aureus, S. pyogenes, Candida* sp., dermatophytes

Modified from Brown M: Microbiology basics. In Grota P, editor: *APIC text of infection control and epidemiology*, Washington, DC, 2018, Association for Professionals in Infection Control and Epidemiology.

Organization [WHO], 2009). The potential for microorganisms or parasites to cause disease depends on the number of microorganisms present; their virulence, or ability to produce disease; their ability to enter and survive in a host; and the susceptibility of the host. Resident skin microorganisms are not virulent. However, they can cause serious infection when surgery or other invasive procedures allow them to enter deep tissues or when a patient is severely immunocompromised (has an impaired immune system).

Transient microorganisms attach to the skin when a person has contact with another person or object during normal activities. For example, when you touch a contaminated gauze dressing or cleanse a patient following a diarrheal episode, transient bacteria adhere to your skin. These organisms may be readily transmitted unless removed using hand hygiene (Ellingson et al., 2014). If hands are visibly soiled with proteinaceous material or care is being provided to a patient with *Clostridium difficile (C. difficile)*, washing with soap and water is the preferred practice (Dubberke et al., 2014). If hands are not visibly soiled, use of an alcohol-based hand product or handwashing with soap and water is acceptable for disinfecting hands of health care workers. Hand hygiene is the most effective way to break the chain of infection (CDC, 2008; WHO, 2009).

Reservoir.
A reservoir is a place where microorganisms survive, multiply, and await transfer to a susceptible host. Common reservoirs are humans and animals (hosts), insects, food, water, and organic matter on inanimate surfaces (fomites). Frequent reservoirs for HAIs include health care workers, especially their hands; patients; equipment; and the environment. Human reservoirs are divided into two types: those with acute or symptomatic disease and those who show no signs of disease but are carriers of it. Humans can transmit microorganisms in either case. Animals, food, water, insects, and inanimate objects can also be reservoirs for infectious organisms. To thrive organisms require a proper environment, including appropriate food, oxygen, water, temperature, pH, and light.

Food. Microorganisms require nourishment. Some such as *Clostridium perfringens,* the microbe that causes gas gangrene, thrive on organic matter. Others such as *Escherichia coli* consume undigested foodstuff in the bowel. Carbon dioxide and inorganic material such as soil provide nourishment for other organisms.

Oxygen. Aerobic bacteria require oxygen for survival and for multiplication sufficient to cause disease. Aerobic organisms cause more infections in humans than anaerobic organisms. An example of an aerobic organism is *Staphylococcus aureus.* Anaerobic bacteria thrive where little or no free oxygen is available. Anaerobes typically cause infections deep within the pleural cavity, in a joint, or in a deep sinus tract. An example of an anaerobic organism is *Bacteroides fragilis,* an organism that is part of the normal flora of the human colon but that can cause infection if displaced into the bloodstream or surrounding tissue following surgery or injury.

Water. Most organisms require water or moisture for survival. For example, a frequent place for microorganisms is the moist drainage from a surgical wound. Some bacteria assume a form, called a *spore,* that is resistant to drying and can live on inanimate surfaces for long periods. A common spore-forming bacterium is *C. difficile,* an organism that causes antibiotic-induced diarrhea.

Temperature. Microorganisms can live only in certain temperature ranges. Each species of bacteria has a specific temperature at which it grows best. The ideal temperature for most human pathogens is 20° to 43° C (68° to 109° F). For example, *Legionella pneumophila* grows best in water at 25° to 42° C (77° to 108° F). Cold temperatures tend to prevent growth and reproduction of bacteria (bacteriostasis). A temperature or chemical that destroys bacteria is bactericidal.

pH. The acidity of an environment determines the viability of microorganisms. Most microorganisms prefer an environment within a pH range of 5.0 to 7.0. Bacteria thrive in urine with an alkaline pH.

Light. Microorganisms thrive in dark environments such as those under dressings and within body cavities.

Portal of Exit.
After microorganisms find a site to grow and multiply, they need to find a portal of exit if they are to enter another host and cause disease. Portals of exit include sites such as blood, skin and mucous membranes, respiratory tract, genitourinary (GU) tract, gastrointestinal (GI) tract, and transplacental (mother to fetus). Some viruses such as Ebola virus are transmitted through direct contact with the blood or body fluids of a person who is sick with Ebola. However, droplets (e.g., splashes or sprays) of respiratory or other secretions from a person who is sick with Ebola could also be infectious. Therefore, certain precautions (called Standard, Contact, and Droplet Precautions) are recommended for use in health care settings to prevent the transmission of the virus from patients who are sick with Ebola to health care personnel and other patients or family members (CDC, 2015a).

Skin and Mucous Membranes. The skin is considered a portal of exit because any break in the integrity of the skin and mucous membranes allows pathogens to exit the body. This may be exhibited by the presence of purulent drainage.

Respiratory Tract. Pathogens that infect the respiratory tract, such as the influenza virus, are released from the body when an infected person sneezes or coughs.

Urinary Tract. Normally urine is sterile. However, when a patient has a urinary tract infection (UTI), microorganisms exit during urination.

Gastrointestinal Tract. The mouth is one of the most bacterially contaminated sites of the human body, but most of the organisms are normal floras. A common flora in the stomach is *Helicobacter pylori, the organism that can cause peptic ulcers.* The *Lactobacillus* and *Enterococcus* are bacteria found in the duodenum. Organisms that are normal floras in one person can be pathogens in another. For example, organisms exit when a person expectorates saliva. In addition, gastrointestinal portals of exit include emesis, bowel elimination, drainage of bile via surgical wounds, or drainage tubes.

Reproductive Tract. The female reproductive tract contains normal microbial flora that are developmentally and age related. *Lactobacilli* are typically the dominant organism in adult females, but other organisms present in the vagina include staphylococci, *Coryneform* bacteria, *Candida,* and *Streptococcus.* Organisms such as *Neisseria gonorrhea* and HIV exit through a man's urethral meatus or a woman's vaginal canal during sexual contact.

Blood. The blood is normally a sterile body fluid; however, in the case of communicable diseases such as HBV, HCV, or HIV, it becomes a reservoir for pathogens. Organisms exit from wounds, venipuncture sites, hematemesis, and bloody stool.

Modes of Transmission.
Each disease has a specific mode of transmission. Often, you are able to do little about the infectious agent or the susceptible host, but by practicing infection prevention and control techniques such as hand hygiene, you interrupt the mode of transmission (Box 28.1). The same microorganism is sometimes transmitted by more than one route. For example, varicella zoster (chickenpox) is spread by the airborne route in droplet nuclei or by direct contact.

The major route of transmission for pathogens identified in the health care setting is the unwashed hands of the health care worker (Ellingson et al., 2014; WHO, 2009). Equipment used within the environment (e.g., a stethoscope, blood pressure cuff, or bedside commode) often becomes a source for the transmission of pathogens.

Portal of Entry.
Organisms enter the body through the same routes they use for exiting. For example, during venipuncture when a needle

pierces a patient's skin, organisms enter the body if proper skin preparation is not performed first. Factors such as a depressed immune system that reduce body defenses enhance the chances of pathogens entering the body.

Susceptible Host. Susceptibility to an infectious agent depends on an individual's degree of resistance to pathogens. Although everyone is constantly in contact with large numbers of microorganisms, an infection does not develop until an individual becomes susceptible to the strength and numbers of the microorganisms. A person's natural defenses against infection and certain risk factors (e.g., age, nutritional

status, presence of chronic disease, trauma, and smoking) affect susceptibility (resistance) (Tweeten, 2018). Organisms such as *S. aureus* with resistance to key antibiotics are becoming more common in all health care settings but especially acute care. The increased resistance is associated with the frequent and sometimes inappropriate use of antibiotics over the years in all settings (i.e., acute care, ambulatory care, clinics, and long-term care) (Arnold, 2018).

The Infectious Process

By understanding the chain of infection, you have knowledge that is vital in preventing infections. When a patient acquires an infection, observe for signs and symptoms of infection and take appropriate action to prevent its spread. Infections follow a progressive course (Box 28.2).

If an infection is localized (e.g., a wound infection), a patient usually experiences localized symptoms such as pain, tenderness, warmth, and redness at the wound site. An infection that affects the entire body instead of just a single organ or part is systemic and can become fatal if undetected and untreated.

The course of an infection influences the level of nursing care provided. The nurse is responsible for implementing infection control practices, properly administering antibiotics, monitoring the response to drug therapy (see Chapter 31), using proper hand hygiene, following Standard Precautions, and using Isolation Precautions when necessary. Supportive therapy includes providing adequate nutrition and rest to bolster defenses of the body against the infectious process. The course of care for the patient often has additional effects on body systems affected by the infection.

Defenses Against Infection. The body has natural defenses that protect against infection. Normal floras, body system defenses, and inflammation are all nonspecific defenses that protect against microorganisms regardless of prior exposure. If any of these body defenses fail, an infection usually occurs and leads to a serious health problem.

Normal Floras. The body normally contains microorganisms that reside on the surface and deep layers of skin, in the saliva and oral

---

BOX 28.1 Modes of Transmission

Contact

Direct
- Person-to-person (fecal, oral) physical contact between source and susceptible host.
- A health care provider's hands become contaminated by touching germs present on a patient, medical equipment, or high-touch surfaces, and the health care worker then carries the germs on his or her hands and spreads to a susceptible person.

Indirect
- Personal contact of susceptible host with contaminated inanimate object (e.g., needles or sharp objects, soiled linen, dressings, environment)

Droplet
- An infected person coughs or sneezes, creating droplets that carry germs short distances (within approximately 6 feet). These germs can land on a susceptible person's eyes, nose, or mouth and can cause infection (e.g., pertussis or meningitis).

Airborne
- Organisms are carried in droplet nuclei or residue or evaporated droplets suspended in air during coughing or sneezing. Germs are aerosolized by medical equipment or by dust from a construction zone (e.g., nontuberculous mycobacteria or Aspergillus).

Vehicles
- Contaminated items. For example, sharps injuries can lead to infections (e.g., HIV, HBV, HCV) when bloodborne pathogens enter a person through a skin puncture by a used needle or sharp instrument.
- Water
- Drugs, solutions
- Blood
- Food (improperly handled, stored, or cooked; fresh or thawed meats)

Vector
- External mechanical transfer (flies)
- Internal transmission such as parasitic conditions between vector and host such as:
  - Mosquito
  - Louse
  - Flea
  - Tick

Modified from Tweeten S: General principles of epidemiology. In Grota P, editor: *APIC text of infection control and epidemiology,* Washington, DC, 2018, Association for Professionals in Infection Control and Epidemiology; Centers for Disease Control and Prevention (CDC): How infections spread, 2016, https://www.cdc.gov/infectioncontrol/spread/index.html.

BOX 28.2 Course of Infection by Stage

Incubation Period
Interval between entrance of pathogen into body and appearance of first symptoms (e.g., chickenpox, 14 to 16 days after exposure; common cold, 1 to 2 days; influenza, 1 to 4 days; measles, 10 to 12 days; mumps, 16 to 18 days; Ebola 2 to 21 days (CDC, 2015a).

Prodromal Stage
Interval from onset of nonspecific signs and symptoms (malaise, low-grade fever, fatigue) to more specific symptoms. (During this time microorganisms grow and multiply, and patient may be capable of spreading disease to others.) For example, herpes simplex begins with itching and tingling at the site before the lesion appears.

Illness Stage
Interval when patient manifests signs and symptoms specific to type of infection. For example, strep throat is manifested by sore throat, pain, and swelling; mumps is manifested by high fever and parotid gland swelling.

Convalescence
Interval when acute symptoms of infection disappear. (Length of recovery depends on severity of infection and patient's host resistance; recovery may take several days to months.)

mucosa, and in the GI and GU tracts. A person normally excretes trillions of microbes daily through the intestines. Normal floras do not usually cause disease when residing in their usual area of the body but instead participate in maintaining health.

Normal floras of the large intestine exist in large numbers without causing illness. They also secrete antibacterial substances within the walls of the intestine. The normal floras of the skin exert a protective, bactericidal action that kills organisms landing on the skin. The mouth and pharynx are also protected by floras that impair growth of invading microbes. Normal floras maintain a sensitive balance with other microorganisms to prevent infection. Any factor that disrupts this balance places a person at increased risk for acquiring a disease. For example, the use of broad-spectrum antibiotics for the treatment of infection can lead to suprainfection. A suprainfection develops when broad-spectrum antibiotics eliminate a wide range of normal flora organisms, not just those causing infection. When normal bacterial floras are eliminated, body defenses are reduced, which allows disease-producing microorganisms to multiply, causing illness (Arnold, 2018).

Body System Defenses. A number of body organ systems have unique defenses against infection (Table 28.2). The skin, respiratory tract, and GI tract are easily accessible to microorganisms. Pathogenic organisms can adhere to the surface skin, be inhaled into the lungs, or be ingested with food. Each organ system has defense mechanisms physiologically suited to its specific structure and function. For example, the lungs cannot completely control the entrance of microorganisms. However, the airways are lined with moist mucous membranes and cilia, or hairlike projections, that rhythmically beat to move mucus or cellular debris up to the pharynx to be expelled through swallowing.

Inflammation. The cellular response of the body to injury, infection, or irritation is termed *inflammation*. Inflammation is a protective vascular reaction that delivers fluid, blood products, and nutrients to an area of injury. The process neutralizes and eliminates pathogens or dead (necrotic) tissues and establishes a means of repairing body cells and tissues. Signs of localized inflammation include swelling, redness, heat, pain or tenderness, and loss of function in the affected body part. When inflammation becomes systemic, other signs and symptoms

TABLE 28.2 Natural Defense Mechanisms Against Infection

Defense Mechanisms	Action	Factors That May Alter Defense Mechanisms
Skin		
Intact multilayered surface (first line of defense against infection)	Provides barrier to microorganisms and antibacterial activity	Cuts, abrasions, puncture wounds, areas of maceration
Shedding of outer layer of skin cells	Removes organisms that adhere to outer layers of skin	Failure to bathe regularly, improper handwashing technique
Sebum	Contains fatty acid that kills some bacteria	Excessive bathing
Mouth		
Intact multilayered mucosa	Provides mechanical barrier to microorganisms	Lacerations, trauma, extracted teeth
Saliva	Washes away particles containing microorganisms Contains microbial inhibitors (e.g., lysozyme)	Poor oral hygiene, dehydration
Eye		
Tearing and blinking	Provides mechanisms to reduce entry (blinking) or help wash away (tearing) particles containing pathogens, thus reducing dose of organisms	Injury, exposure—splash/splatter of blood or other potentially infectious material into eye
Respiratory Tract		
Cilia lining upper airway, coated by mucus	Traps inhaled microbes and sweeps them outward in mucus to be expectorated or swallowed	Smoking, high concentration of oxygen and carbon dioxide, decreased humidity, cold air
Macrophages	Engulf and destroy microorganisms that reach alveoli of lung	Smoking
Urinary Tract		
Flushing action of urine flow	Washes away microorganisms on lining of bladder and urethra	Obstruction to normal flow by urinary catheter placement, obstruction from growth or tumor, delayed micturition
Intact multilayered epithelium	Provides barrier to microorganisms	Introduction of urinary catheter, continual movement of catheter in urethra can facilitate migration of organisms to bladder
Gastrointestinal Tract		
Acidity of gastric secretions	A gastric fluid pH of 1 to 2 is deleterious to many microbial pathogens	Administration of antacids Inhibition of acid secretion by various drugs
Rapid peristalsis in small intestine	Prevents retention of bacterial contents	Delayed motility resulting from impaction of fecal contents in large bowel or mechanical obstruction by masses
Vagina		
At puberty normal flora causing vaginal secretions to achieve low pH	Inhibit growth of many microorganisms	Antibiotics and oral contraceptives disrupting normal flora

develop, including fever, increased white blood cells (WBCs), malaise, anorexia, nausea, vomiting, lymph node enlargement, or organ failure.

Physical agents, chemical agents, or microorganisms trigger the inflammatory response. Mechanical trauma, temperature extremes, and radiation are examples of physical agents. Chemical agents include external and internal irritants such as harsh poisons or gastric acid. Sometimes microorganisms also trigger this response.

After tissues are injured, a series of well-coordinated events occurs. The inflammatory response includes vascular and cellular responses, formation of inflammatory exudates (fluid and cells that are discharged from cells or blood vessels [e.g., pus or serum]), and tissue repair.

Vascular and Cellular Responses. Acute inflammation is an immediate response to cellular injury. Rapid vasodilation occurs, allowing more blood to be delivered near the location of the injury. The increase in local blood flow causes the redness and localized warmth at the site of inflammation.

Injury causes tissue damage and possibly necrosis. As a result, the body releases chemical mediators that increase the permeability of small blood vessels, and fluid, protein, and cells enter interstitial spaces. The accumulation of fluid appears as localized swelling (edema). Another sign of inflammation is pain, which is caused by the swelling of inflamed tissues that increases pressure on nerve endings. As a result of the physiological inflammatory response, the involved body part may have a temporary loss of function. For example, a localized infection of the hand causes the fingers to become swollen, painful, and discolored. Joints become stiff because of swelling, but function of the fingers returns when inflammation subsides.

During the cellular response of inflammation, WBCs arrive at the site. WBCs pass through blood vessels and into the tissues. Phagocytosis is a process that involves the destruction and absorption of bacteria. Through the process of phagocytosis, specialized WBCs, called neutrophils and monocytes, ingest and destroy microorganisms or other small particles. If inflammation becomes systemic, other signs and symptoms develop. Leukocytosis, or an increase in the number of circulating WBCs, is the response of the body to WBCs leaving blood vessels. In the adult a serum WBC count is normally 5,000 to 10,000/mm^3 but typically rises to 15,000 to 20,000/mm^3 and higher during inflammation. Fever is caused by phagocytic release of pyrogens from bacterial cells, which causes a rise in the hypothalamic set point (see Chapter 29).

Inflammatory Exudate. Accumulation of fluid, dead tissue cells, and WBCs forms an exudate at the site of inflammation. Exudate may be serous (clear, like plasma), sanguineous (containing red blood cells), or purulent (containing WBCs and bacteria). Usually the exudate is cleared away through lymphatic drainage. Platelets and plasma proteins such as fibrinogen form a meshlike matrix at the site of inflammation to prevent its spread.

Tissue Repair. When there is injury to tissue cells, healing involves the defensive, reconstructive, and maturative stages (see Chapter 48). Damaged cells eventually are replaced with healthy new cells. The new cells undergo a gradual maturation until they take on the same structural characteristics and appearance as the previous cells. If inflammation is chronic, tissue defects sometimes fill with fragile granulation tissue that eventually takes the form of a scar at the completion of the healing process. The scar and surrounding tissues are not as strong as normal tissue and may be more susceptible to injury from pressure, shear, or friction, which increase the risk for pressure injury development (see Chapter 48).

Health Care–Associated Infections

Patients in health care settings, especially hospitals and long-term care facilities, have an increased risk of acquiring infections.

Health care–associated infections (HAIs) result from the delivery of health services in a health care agency. They occur as the result of invasive procedures, antibiotic administration, the presence of multidrug-resistant organisms (MDROs), and breaks in infection prevention and control activities. The number of health care employees having direct contact with a patient, the type and number of invasive procedures, the therapy received, and the length of hospitalization further influence the risk of infection. Major sites for HAIs include surgical or traumatic wounds, urinary and respiratory tracts, and the bloodstream (Box 28.3).

HAIs significantly increase the cost of health care. This is especially true in older adults, who have increased susceptibility to these infections because of their affinity to chronic disease and the aging process (Box 28.4). Extended stays in health care institutions, increased disability, increased costs of antibiotics, and prolonged recovery times add to the expenses both of the patient and the health care institution and funding bodies (e.g., Medicare). Costs for HAIs are often not

---

BOX 28.3 Examples of Sites for and Causes of Health Care–Associated Infections

Improperly performing hand hygiene increases patient risk for all types of health care–associated infections.

Urinary Tract
- Unsterile insertion of urinary catheter
- Improper positioning of the drainage tubing
- Open drainage system
- Catheter and tube becoming disconnected
- Drainage bag port touching contaminated surface
- Improper specimen collection technique
- Obstructing or interfering with urinary drainage
- Urine in catheter or drainage tube being allowed to reenter bladder (reflux)
- Repeated catheter irrigations
- Improper perineal hygiene

Surgical or Traumatic Wounds
- Improper skin preparation before surgery (e.g., shaving versus clipping hair; not performing a preoperative bath or shower)
- Failure to clean skin surface properly
- Failure to use aseptic technique during operative procedures and dressing changes
- Use of contaminated antiseptic solutions

Respiratory Tract
- Contaminated respiratory therapy equipment
- Failure to use aseptic technique while suctioning airway
- Improper disposal of secretions

Bloodstream
- Contamination of intravenous (IV) fluids by tubing
- Insertion of drug additives to IV fluid
- Addition of connecting tube or stopcocks to IV system
- Improper care of needle insertion site
- Contaminated needles or catheters
- Failure to change IV access at first sign of infection or at recommended intervals
- Improper technique during administration of multiple blood products
- Improper care of peritoneal or hemodialysis shunts
- Improperly accessing an IV port

BOX 28.4   FOCUS ON OLDER ADULTS

Risks for Infection

- An age-related functional deterioration in immune system function, termed immune senescence, increases the susceptibility of the body to infection and slows overall immune response (Meiner and Yeager, 2019; Pawelec, 2018).
- Older adults are less capable of producing lymphocytes to combat challenges to the immune system. When antibodies are produced, the duration of their response is shorter, and fewer cells are produced (Roach, 2018).
- Risks associated with the development of infections or health care–associated infections in older patients include poor nutrition, unintentional weight loss, lack of exercise, poor social support, and low serum albumin levels (Meiner and Yeager, 2019).
- Flu and pneumonia vaccinations are recommended for the older adult population to reduce their risk for infectious diseases.
- Teach older adults and their families how to reduce the risk for infections by using proper hand hygiene practices.

reimbursed; as a result, prevention has a beneficial financial impact and is an important part of patient care. TJC lists several national safety goals focusing on the care of older adults (e.g., ensuring that older adults receive influenza and pneumonia vaccines, preventing infection after surgery) (TJC, 2020).

Patients who develop HAIs often have multiple illnesses, are older adults, or are poorly nourished and may have a compromised immune system; thus, they are more susceptible to infections. In addition, many patients have a lowered resistance to infection because of underlying medical conditions (e.g., diabetes mellitus or cancer) that impair or damage the immune response of the body. Invasive treatment devices such as IV catheters or indwelling urinary catheters impair or bypass the natural defenses of the body against microorganisms. Critical illness increases patients' susceptibility to infections, especially multidrug-resistant bacteria. Meticulous hand hygiene practices, the use of chlorhexidine washes for bathing and personal hygiene care, advances in intensive care unit (ICU) infection prevention, and the creation of evidence-based bundles help to prevent these infections (Donskey and Deshpande, 2016; Mehta et al., 2014).

HAI infections are either exogenous or endogenous. An exogenous infection comes from microorganisms found outside the individual, such as *Salmonella*, *Clostridium tetani*, and *Aspergillus*. These microorganisms do not exist as normal floras. An endogenous infection occurs when part of the patient's flora becomes altered and an overgrowth occurs (e.g., staphylococci, enterococci, yeasts, and streptococci). This often happens when a patient receives broad-spectrum antibiotics that alter the normal floras. When sufficient numbers of microorganisms normally found in one body site move to another site, an endogenous infection develops. The number of microorganisms needed to cause an HAI depends on the virulence of the organism, the susceptibility of the host, and the body site affected.

Iatrogenic infections are a type of HAI caused by an invasive diagnostic or therapeutic procedure. For example, procedures such as a bronchoscopy and treatment with broad-spectrum antibiotics increase the risk for certain infections (Arnold, 2018; Day, 2018). Use critical thinking when practicing aseptic techniques during the performance of procedures. Follow basic infection prevention and control policies and procedures to reduce the risk of HAIs. Always consider the patient's risks for infection and anticipate how the approach to care increases or decreases the risk.

REFLECT NOW

What are the nursing strategies you can use to break the chain of infection when you care for a patient at risk for a urinary tract infection?

NURSING KNOWLEDGE BASE

Body substances such as feces, urine, and wound drainage contain potentially infectious microorganisms. Health care workers are at risk for exposure to microorganisms in the hospital and/or home setting (Fiutem, 2018). The meticulous use of specific infection prevention practices reduces the risk of cross-contamination and transmission of infection to noninfected patients when caring for a patient with a known or suspected infection.

Serious infections are ongoing challenges to clinicians, and they create feelings of anxiety, frustration, loneliness, and anger in patients and/or their families (Nesher et al., 2014). These feelings worsen when patients are isolated to prevent transmission of a microorganism to other patients or health care staff. Isolation disrupts normal social relationships with visitors and caregivers. Patient safety is usually an additional risk for a patient on isolation precautions (Monsees, 2018). For example, an older patient with a chronic illness is more at risk for an HAI. When family members fear the possibility of developing the infection, they may avoid contact with the patient. Some patients perceive the simple procedures of proper hand hygiene and gown and glove use as evidence of rejection. Help patients and families reduce some of these feelings by discussing the disease process; explaining isolation procedures; and maintaining a friendly, understanding manner.

When establishing a plan of care, it is important to know how a patient reacts to an infection or infectious disease. The challenge is to identify and support behaviors that maintain human health or prevent infection.

Factors Influencing Infection Prevention and Control

Multiple factors influence a patient's susceptibility to infection. It is important to understand how each of these factors alone or in combination increases this risk. When more than one factor is present, a patient's susceptibility often increases, which affects length of stay, recovery time, and/or overall level of health following an illness. Understanding these factors helps you to assess and care for a patient who has an infection or is at risk for one.

Age. Throughout life a person's susceptibility to infection changes. For example, an infant has immature defenses against infection. Born with only the antibodies provided by the mother, an infant's immune system is incapable of producing the necessary immunoglobulins and WBCs to adequately fight some infections. However, breastfed infants often have greater immunity than bottle-fed infants because they receive their mother's antibodies through the breast milk. As the child grows, the immune system matures but the child is still susceptible to organisms that cause the common cold, intestinal infections, and infectious diseases such as mumps, measles, and chickenpox (if not vaccinated). Since 2000, there has been a major effort to vaccinate all children against all infectious diseases for which vaccines are available. Vaccine-preventable disease levels are at or near record lows (CDC, 2018c).

The young or middle-age adult has refined defenses against infection. Viruses are the most common cause of communicable illness in young or middle-age adults. Young women are most likely to develop urinary tract infections (UTIs), vaginal yeast infections, and human papillomavirus (HPV). Although UTIs are relatively uncommon in men, prostatitis (infection of the prostate gland) affects men of all ages but tends to be more common in men 50 or younger (Mayo Clinic, 2018).

Defenses against infection change with aging (Roach, 2018). The immune response, particularly cell-mediated immunity, declines. Older adults also undergo alterations in the structure and function of the skin, urinary tract, and lungs. For example, the skin loses its turgor, and the epithelium thins. As a result, it is easier to tear or abrade the skin, which increases the potential for invasion by pathogens. In addition, older adults who are hospitalized or reside in an assisted-living or residential care facility are at risk for airborne infections. Ensuring that health care workers are vaccinated against influenza reduces the transmission of this illness in older adults (Thomas et al., 2013).

Sex. Women and men differ in their immune responses to infections. This applies to infections with viruses, bacteria, and parasites, including the pathogens such as malaria, TB, AIDS, hepatitis, and influenza (Lunzen and Altfeld, 2014). Only recently have the biological pathways responsible for these sex-based differences in the manifestations of infectious diseases been researched. Besides genetic factors, these differences can be explained through the greatly divergent and changing levels of sex steroid hormones and their interplay with the immune system. Estrogens promote (but androgens suppress) immune responses during infections and after vaccination. They also increase the risk for autoimmune diseases (Giefing-Kröll, et al., 2015). In vaccinated adults, sex-related differences have been observed in immunogenicity (ability of an antigen to provoke an immune response in the body of a human) and clinical effectiveness of influenza, pneumococcal polysaccharide, hepatitis A and B, tetanus, diphtheria, measles, rabies, and smallpox vaccines (Giefing-Kröll, et al., 2015).

Nutritional Status. A patient's nutritional health directly influences susceptibility to infection. A reduction in the intake of protein and other nutrients such as carbohydrates and fats reduces body defenses against infection and impairs wound healing (see Chapter 48). Patients with illnesses or problems that increase protein requirements, such as extensive burns and febrile conditions, are at further risk. For example, patients who have undergone surgery require increased protein. A thorough diet history is necessary. Determine a patient's normal daily nutrient intake and whether preexisting problems such as nausea, impaired swallowing, or oral pain alter food intake. Confer with a registered dietitian to assist in calculating the calorie count of foods ingested.

Stress. The body responds to emotional or physical stress by the general adaptation syndrome (see Chapter 37). During the alarm stage the basal metabolic rate increases as the body uses energy stores. Adrenocorticotropic hormone increases serum glucose levels and decreases unnecessary antiinflammatory responses through the release of cortisone. If stress continues or becomes intense, elevated cortisone levels result in decreased resistance to infection. Continued stress leads to exhaustion, which causes depletion in energy stores, and the body has no resistance to invading organisms. The same conditions that increase nutritional requirements, such as surgery or trauma, also increase physiological stress.

Disease Process. Patients with diseases of the immune system are at particular risk for infection. Leukemia, AIDS, lymphoma, and aplastic anemia are conditions that compromise a host by weakening defenses against infectious organisms. For example, patients with leukemia are unable to produce enough WBCs to fight off infection. Patients with HIV are often unable to ward off simple infections and are prone to opportunistic infections.

Patients with chronic diseases such as diabetes mellitus and multiple sclerosis are also more susceptible to infection because of general debilitation and nutritional impairment. Diseases that impair body system defenses such as emphysema and bronchitis (which impair ciliary action and thicken mucus), cancer (which alters the immune response), and peripheral vascular disease (which reduces blood flow to injured tissues) increase susceptibility to infection. Patients with burns have a high susceptibility to infection because of the damage to skin surfaces. The greater the depth and extent of the burns, the higher is the risk for infection.

> **REFLECT NOW**
>
> Consider the care of an older adult patient who is receiving chemotherapy for a recent cancer diagnosis. What risk factors for infection would you need to address when planning care for this patient?

❖ NURSING PROCESS

Apply the nursing process and use a critical thinking approach in your care of patients. The nursing process provides a clinical decision-making approach for you to develop and implement an individualized plan of care.

◆ Assessment

Perform a thorough assessment of each patient and critically analyze findings to ensure that you make patient-centered clinical decisions required for safe nursing care. You will assess a patient's current condition as well as review any history of previous health problems involving infection. As you conduct your assessment, apply knowledge of the infectious process and the patient's diagnosed medical problem(s) to focus on your physical examination.

Through the Patient's Eyes. Determine how the patient feels about his or her illness or risk for infection. Has the patient had experiences in the past that will affect expectations for care? For example, a patient undergoing a second surgical procedure might have different expectations than a first-time surgery patient regarding the prevention of wound infection. Assess a patient's knowledge of his or her risk factors that increase the susceptibility for developing an infection (Table 28.3) to help you plan appropriate patient education.

Some patients with infection have a variety of problems, including physical, psychological, social, or economic needs. Patients with chronic or serious infection, especially communicable infections such as TB or AIDS, experience psychological and social problems from self-imposed isolation or rejection by friends and family. Ask the patient how an infection affects the ability to maintain relationships and perform activities of daily living. Determine whether chronic infection has drained the patient's financial resources. Ask about his or her expectations of care (e.g., how a procedure should be performed) and determine how much he or she wants to be involved in planning care. Some patients and their families wish to know more about the disease process, whereas others only want to know the interventions necessary to treat the infection. Encourage patients to verbalize their expectations so that you are able to establish interventions to meet patients' priorities.

Risk Factors. A review of a patient's clinical condition can begin with the identification of risk factors. Ask specific questions to determine the patient's and family's awareness of any risks for infection (Box 28.5). Assess the patient's age, nutritional status, presence of chronic illnesses or stress, and presence of disease processes to identify factors that influence susceptibility to infection. Gather information about each factor through your interview and the patient's medical history.

TABLE 28.3 Host Characteristics Influencing Susceptibility To and Severity of Disease

Characteristic	Examples
Age	"Childhood diseases" (e.g., measles, chickenpox) are seen more frequently in children, whereas chronic diseases, such as heart disease or chronic obstructive pulmonary disease, occur more frequently in older patients.
Sex	Reproductive diseases are sex-specific. Sex influences immune response and susceptibility to certain infections.
Ethnicity	Tay-Sachs disease occurs in Jews of European descent.
Socioeconomic status	Socioeconomic status influences the ability to purchase food, pay for immunizations, and obtain health care services
Marital status	Some studies of stress-related diseases have shown marital status to be a factor influencing susceptibility.
Lifestyle	Homelessness increases susceptibility due to poor nutrition and exposure to pathogens.
Heredity	Sickle cell anemia influences susceptibility.
Nutritional status	Inadequate nutrition reduces immune function.
Occupation	Coal miners are at risk for black lung. Prison guards or social workers involved with immigrants or asylum seekers originating from areas with a high tuberculosis (TB) prevalence are at risk for contacting TB.
Immunization status	Those who have not been vaccinated for measles are at risk for the disease.
Diagnostic/therapeutic procedures	Transplant patients have an increased risk of infection.
Medications	Steroid use increases the risk of infection.
Pregnancy	Tuberculosis-positive women who are pregnant are more likely to reactivate.
Trauma	Injury may provide a portal of entry for organisms and triggers an inflammatory response that may increase the risk of infection.

Modified from Tweeten SM: General principles of epidemiology. In Grota P, editor: *APIC text of infection control and epidemiology*, Washington, DC, 2018, Association for Professionals in Infection Control and Epidemiology.

BOX 28.5 Nursing Assessment Questions

Risk Factors
- Do you have any recent cuts or lacerations? Show me the location.
- Describe for me any illnesses or diseases that you have and those for which you receive treatment.
- Tell me about any recent diagnostic testing you have undergone, such as colonoscopy or cystoscopy?

Possible Existing Infections
- Do you have or feel as if you have a fever?
- Do you have any cuts or wounds with drainage?
- Do you have any pain/burning during urination?
- Do you have a cough? Is there any sputum?

Recent Travel History
- Have you traveled outside the United States in the past 6 months?
- Are you a resident of or have you traveled within the past 21 days to a country where an Ebola outbreak is occurring (CDC, 2015b)?
- Were any of the people you visited or traveled with ill?

Medication History
- List for me the medications you are currently taking.
- Describe for me the doses of each medication you are supposed to take daily.
- Describe any over-the-counter medications or herbals that you are currently taking.

Stressors
- Tell me about any major lifestyle change occurring, such as the loss of employment or place of residence, divorce, or disability.

Clinical Appearance. Perform a physical assessment (see Chapter 30) of a patient, examining areas involved in an infection as well as areas where risk of infection exists. The signs and symptoms of infection may be local or systemic. Localized infections are most common in areas of skin or mucous membrane breakdown, such as surgical and traumatic wounds, pressure injuries, oral lesions, and abscesses.

To assess an area for localized infection, first inspect it for redness, warmth, and swelling caused by inflammation. Because there may be drainage from open lesions or wounds, wear clean gloves. Infected drainage may be yellow, green, or brown depending on the pathogen. For example, green nasal secretions often indicate a sinus infection. Ask the patient about pain or tenderness around the site. Some patients complain of tightness and pain caused by edema. If the infected area is large enough, movement is restricted. Gentle palpation of an infected area usually results in some degree of tenderness. Wear protective eyewear and a surgical mask when there is a risk for splash or spray with blood or body fluids.

Systemic infections cause more generalized symptoms than local infection. These symptoms often include fever, fatigue, nausea/vomiting, and malaise. Lymph nodes that drain the area of infection often become enlarged, swollen, and tender during palpation. For example, an abscess in the peritoneal cavity causes enlargement of lymph nodes in the groin. An infection of the upper respiratory tract causes cervical lymph node enlargement. If an infection is serious and widespread, all major lymph nodes may enlarge.

Systemic infections sometimes develop after treatment for localized infection has failed. Be alert for changes in a patient's level of activity and responsiveness. As systemic infections develop, an elevation in body temperature can lead to episodes of increased heart and respiratory rates and low blood pressure. Involvement of major body systems produces specific symptoms. For example, a pulmonary infection results in a productive cough with purulent sputum. A UTI results in cloudy, foul-smelling urine.

An infection does not always present with typical signs and symptoms in all patients. For example, in some older adults an infection may be advanced before it is identified. Because of the aging process, there is a reduced inflammatory and immune response. Older adults have increased fatigue and diminished pain sensitivity. A reduced or absent fever response often occurs from chronic use of aspirin or nonsteroidal antiinflammatory drugs. Atypical symptoms such as confusion, incontinence, or agitation may be the only symptoms of an infectious illness (Roach, 2018). For example, as many as 20% of older adults with pneumonia do not have the typical signs and symptoms of fever, shaking, chills, and colored productive sputum. Often the only symptoms are an unexplained increase in heart rate, confusion, or generalized fatigue. A pneumonia vaccine is available and recommended for all people with chronic respiratory problems and those over 65 years of age.

Status of Defense Mechanisms. As you conduct your physical assessment, determine the status of normal defense mechanisms against infection. For example, any break in the skin such as an ulcer on the foot of a patient who has diabetes is a potential site for infection. Any reduction in the primary or secondary defenses of the body against infection such as a weakened ability to cough places a patient at increased risk.

Medical Therapy. Some drugs and medical therapies compromise immunity, increasing the risk for infection. Assess your patient's medication history to determine whether he or she takes any medications that increase infection susceptibility (see Box 28.5). This includes any over-the-counter medications and herbal supplements. A review of therapies received within the health care setting further reveals risks. For example, adrenal corticosteroids, prescribed for several conditions, are antiinflammatory drugs that cause protein breakdown and impair the inflammatory response against bacteria and other pathogens. Corticosteroids and TNF (tumor necrosis factor) inhibitors are two medications that increase the chance of getting a fungal infection (CDC, 2017e). Cytotoxic and antineoplastic drugs attack cancer cells but also cause the side effects of bone marrow depression and normal cell toxicity, which affects the response of the body against pathogens.

Travel History. Conduct a review of a patient's recent travel history to determine possible exposure to communicable diseases. Also assess if any immediate family members have traveled and presented risks to the patient (see Box 28.5). A person's exposure depends on the presence of infectious agents in the area visited. The risk of becoming infected will vary according to the purpose of the trip and the itinerary within the area; the standards of accommodation, hygiene, and sanitation; and the behavior of the traveler (WHO, 2019a).

Laboratory Data. Review laboratory data as soon as the results are available. Laboratory values such as increased WBCs and/or a positive blood culture often indicate infection (Table 28.4). However, laboratory values are not enough to detect infection. It is possible that a contaminated specimen was collected because of poor technique (e.g., a blood sample is mixed with IV fluid because it is improperly collected from an indwelling line; a urine specimen is contaminated because of poor perineal cleansing). You need to assess other clinical signs of infection. A culture result may show growth of an organism in the absence of infection. For example, in the older adult bacterial growth in urine without clinical symptoms does not always indicate the presence of a UTI (Roach, 2018). Also know that laboratory values often vary from laboratory to laboratory. Be sure to know the standard range of laboratory values for the laboratory in your facility.

REFLECT NOW

What questions would you ask a patient who just returned from a mission trip from another country when assessing for a possible infection?

◆ **Nursing Diagnosis**

During assessment gather objective data such as inspection of an open incision or a reduced caloric intake record and subjective data such as a patient's complaint of tenderness over a surgical wound site. Review the data carefully, looking for clusters of assessment findings or risk factors that create a pattern. This pattern suggests a specific nursing diagnosis (Box 28.6). The following are examples of nursing diagnoses that often apply to patients with infection:

- *Risk for Infection*
- *Impaired Nutritional Status: Deficient Food Intake*
- *Impaired Oral Mucous Membrane*
- *Social Isolation*
- *Impaired Tissue Integrity*

TABLE 28.4 Laboratory Tests To Screen for Infection

Laboratory Value	Normal (Adult) Values	Indication of Infection
White blood cell (WBC) count	5000-10,000/mm³	Increased in acute infection, decreased in certain viral or overwhelming infections
Erythrocyte sedimentation rate	Up to 15 mm/hr for men and 20 mm/hr for women	Elevated in presence of inflammatory process
Iron level	80-180 mcg/mL for men 60-160 mcg/mL for women	Decreased in chronic infection
Cultures of urine and blood	Normally sterile, without microorganism growth	Presence of infectious microorganism growth
Cultures and Gram stain of wound, sputum, and throat	No WBCs on Gram stain, possible normal flora	Presence of infectious microorganism growth and WBCs on Gram stain
Differential Count (Percentage of Each Type of White Blood Cell)		
Neutrophils	55%-70%	Increased in acute suppurative (pus-forming) infection, decreased in overwhelming bacterial infection (older adult)
Lymphocytes	20%-40%	Increased in chronic bacterial and viral infection, decreased in sepsis
Monocytes	2%-8%	Increased in protozoan, rickettsial, and tuberculosis infections
Eosinophils	1%-4%	Increased in parasitic infection
Basophils	0.5%-1.5%	Normal during infection

Adapted from Pagana KD, et al: *Mosby's diagnostic and laboratory test reference*, ed 13, St Louis, 2017, Elsevier.

BOX 28.6 Nursing Diagnostic Process

Risk for Infection

Assessment Activities	Assessment Findings
Check results of laboratory tests.	WBC count 5000/mm^3
Review current medications.	Patient receiving antibiotics and oral antidiabetic medications
Identify potential sites of infection.	IV catheter in right forearm, in place for 3 days
	Foley catheter draining cloudy amber-colored urine

IV, Intravenous; *WBC,* white blood cell.

It is necessary to validate data such as inspecting the integrity of a wound more carefully and to review laboratory findings to confirm a diagnosis. Success in planning appropriate nursing interventions depends on the accuracy of the diagnostic statement and the ability to meet the patient's needs. A patient will have assessment findings for a problem-focused or a negative diagnosis. You individualize the diagnosis with the addition of an accurate *related* factor in the diagnostic statement. For example, minimizing the risk for infection in a patient with a diagnosis of *Impaired Oral Mucous Membrane related to mouth breathing* requires frequent and proper oral hygiene measures. Minimizing the risk for infection in a patient with a nursing diagnosis of *Impaired Nutritional Status: Deficient Food Intake related to inability to absorb nutrients* requires good nutritional support and fluid balance. At-risk diagnoses such as *Risk for Infection* require careful identification of relevant risk factors.

◆ Planning

Goals and Outcomes. The patient's care plan is based on each nursing diagnosis and any related or risk factors (see the Nursing Care Plan). Develop a plan that sets realistic outcomes, so interventions are purposeful, direct, and measurable. For example, when you care for a patient with broken skin and obesity, the nursing diagnosis of *Risk for Infection* requires you to implement skin and wound care measures to promote healing. The expected outcome of "absence of drainage" sets an expected outcome for measuring the patient's improvement. A goal for this situation would be "Patient remains free of infection at discharge." Additional goals of care applicable to patients with infection often include the following:

- Preventing further exposure to infectious organisms
- Controlling or reducing the extent of infection
- Maintaining resistance to infection
- Verbalizing understanding of infection prevention and control techniques (e.g., hand hygiene)

REFLECT NOW

How would you begin setting goals with a patient in the hospital who is experiencing an infection?

Patients often have multiple nursing diagnoses that are interrelated, and one diagnosis often affects other diagnoses. A concept map for the patient, Mrs. Andrews, helps to show the relationships among multiple nursing diagnoses (Fig. 28.2).

Setting Priorities. Establish priorities for each diagnosis and related goals of care. For example, you are caring for a patient with cancer who develops an open wound and is unable to tolerate solid foods.

The priority of administering therapies to promote wound healing such as improved nutritional intake overrides the goal of educating the patient to assume self-care therapies at home. When the patient's condition improves, the priorities change, and patient education will then become an essential intervention. Patient priorities change quickly, especially in the acute care environment. In the home setting, priorities may remain appropriate for weeks at a time.

Teamwork and Collaboration. The development of a care plan includes prevention and infection control practices provided by multiple disciplines. Select interventions in collaboration with the patient, the family caregiver, and health care providers such as the registered dietitian or respiratory therapist. Know the patient's sociocultural preferences to help you identify the most appropriate types of interventions (Box 28.7). In addition, consult with an expert in infection control in planning the patient's care. Before discharge, consult with case management to complete a home assessment and identify home health needs. Case managers work with the patient, family, and home care services to ensure that the transition from the hospital goes smoothly and that a safe discharge plan is in place.

When care continues into the patient's home, the home health nurse plans to ensure that the home environment supports good infection prevention and control practices. For example, if a patient does not have running water yet requires wound care, even simple hand hygiene with soap and water is difficult to achieve. Home health nurses instruct patients to perform hand hygiene with either bottled water and soap or alcohol-based hand products. In addition, in the home it is common to use clean instead of sterile asepsis. Consult with the patient's health care provider if you have questions about proper aseptic technique.

◆ Implementation

By identifying relevant nursing diagnoses and implementing a plan of care with appropriate evidence-based measures, you can effectively reduce the risk of infection.

Health Promotion. Use your critical thinking skills to prevent an infection from developing or spreading. In the home and community settings, review with and teach patients and their family caregivers about ways to strengthen a potential host's defenses against infection. Nutritional support, rest, personal hygiene, maintenance of physiological protective mechanisms, and recommended immunizations protect patients. Explain how to perform infection prevention and control principles such as hand hygiene and methods for proper disposal of medical waste. Based on your assessment of a patient's cultural practices, integrate infection prevention and control measures into the patient's daily lifestyle practices.

Nutrition. Nutritional requirements for your patients will vary depending on their age and condition. A proper diet helps the immune system function and consists of a variety of foods from all food groups (see Chapter 45). Collaborate with registered dietitians, the patient, and the family to select the correct foods. Recommend ways to prepare foods that the patient will enjoy. Teach patients the importance of a proper diet in maintaining immunity and preventing infection.

Hygiene. Personal hygiene measures (see Chapter 40) reduce microorganisms on the skin and maintain the integrity of mucous membranes such as the mouth and vagina. Patients and family caregivers need to understand techniques for cleansing the skin and how to avoid the spread of microorganisms in body secretions or excretions. For example, teach female patients how to wash their perineum from clean to dirty, from the urethra down toward the rectum, using a clean washcloth with each wipe. Another example is to teach patients the proper technique to cleanse around a wound (see Chapter 48).

◎ NURSING CARE PLAN

Risk for Infection

ASSESSMENT

Mrs. Andrews has diabetes mellitus, urinary incontinence, and degenerative disk disease. She had surgery on her lower spine yesterday and is now experiencing pain along her incision and difficulty walking. Mrs. Andrews needs to wear a brace when she is out of bed and needs an incisional dressing change because of contamination from urinary incontinence. The health care provider removes the dressing, leaving the incision open to air. The physical therapist plans to help Mrs. Andrews transfer to a chair after breakfast.

Assessment Activities	*Assessment Findings[a]*
Review Mrs. Andrews' chart for laboratory data that reflects infection (e.g., white blood cell [WBC] count).	The WBC count is 9500/mm^3.
Inspect incision area.	**Incision** edges are slightly pink; edges approximated but edematous; no drainage noted.
Review risk factors for infection.	Has had **diabetes mellitus** for past 16 years; states blood sugars have been "poorly controlled" for the past year. Dietary assessment reflects malnutrition before surgery. Is **taking a glucocorticosteroid,** which reduces inflammation and suppresses the immune system.

[a]**Assessment Findings** are shown in bold type.

NURSING DIAGNOSIS: Risk for infection

PLANNING

Goals	*Expected Outcomes (NOC)[b]*
	Immune Status
Mrs. Andrews will remain free from symptoms of infection.	Mrs. Andrews has no signs or symptoms of infection (e.g., remains afebrile; incision intact; edges approximated; no redness, swelling, or drainage).
	Knowledge: Infection Management
Mrs. Andrews will describe ways to prevent infection before discharge.	Mrs. Andrews demonstrates appropriate hand hygiene before discharge.
	Mrs. Andrews identifies who will help assess incisional site when she goes home.

[b]Outcome classification labels from Moorhead S, et al.: *Nursing outcomes classification (NOC),* ed 6, St Louis, 2018, Elsevier.

Interventions (NIC)[c]	*Rationale*
Infection Protection	
Teach Mrs. Andrews how to perform hand hygiene correctly.	Meticulous hand hygiene reduces bacterial counts on the hands (Hass, 2018). Patient can easily come in contact with organisms in the health care environment that can cause infection.
Monitor Mrs. Andrews frequently to prevent urine contamination of the incision site.	Offer bedpan/restroom hourly to decrease risk for incontinence.
Provide Mrs. Andrews with incontinence panties that she wears at home.	Absorbent padding will wick away urine from Mrs. Andrew's incision.
Help Mrs. Andrews identify a family member to check the incision until it is healed and teach Mrs. Andrews and the family member signs and symptoms of infection.	Mrs. Andrews will be unable to visualize incision since it is on her back; she will need a family member to help monitor healing of the surgical site.

[c]Intervention classification labels from Butcher HK, et al.: *Nursing interventions classification (NIC),* ed 7, St Louis, 2018, Elsevier.

EVALUATION

Evaluation Activity	*Patient Response/Finding*	*Outcome Status*
Compare Mrs. Andrews' body temperature with baseline.	Mrs. Andrews has an oral temperature of 38°C (100.4°F).	Mrs. Andrews is suspected to have infection at this time.
Ask Mrs. Andrews to describe signs and symptoms to report to health care provider.	Mrs. Andrews is unable to identify temperature range to report; unable to identify signs of wound infection.	Mrs. Andrews has minimal understanding of signs and symptoms to report. Will require additional instruction and include an information sheet on signs and symptoms of infection. Family member caring for Mrs. Andrews incision will also need instruction on signs and symptoms to report.
Observe for signs of infection at incisional site (e.g., redness, warmth, and wound discharge).	Incision shows signs of infection: redness, warmth, and a small amount of tan drainage.	Incision is showing signs of infection at this time.

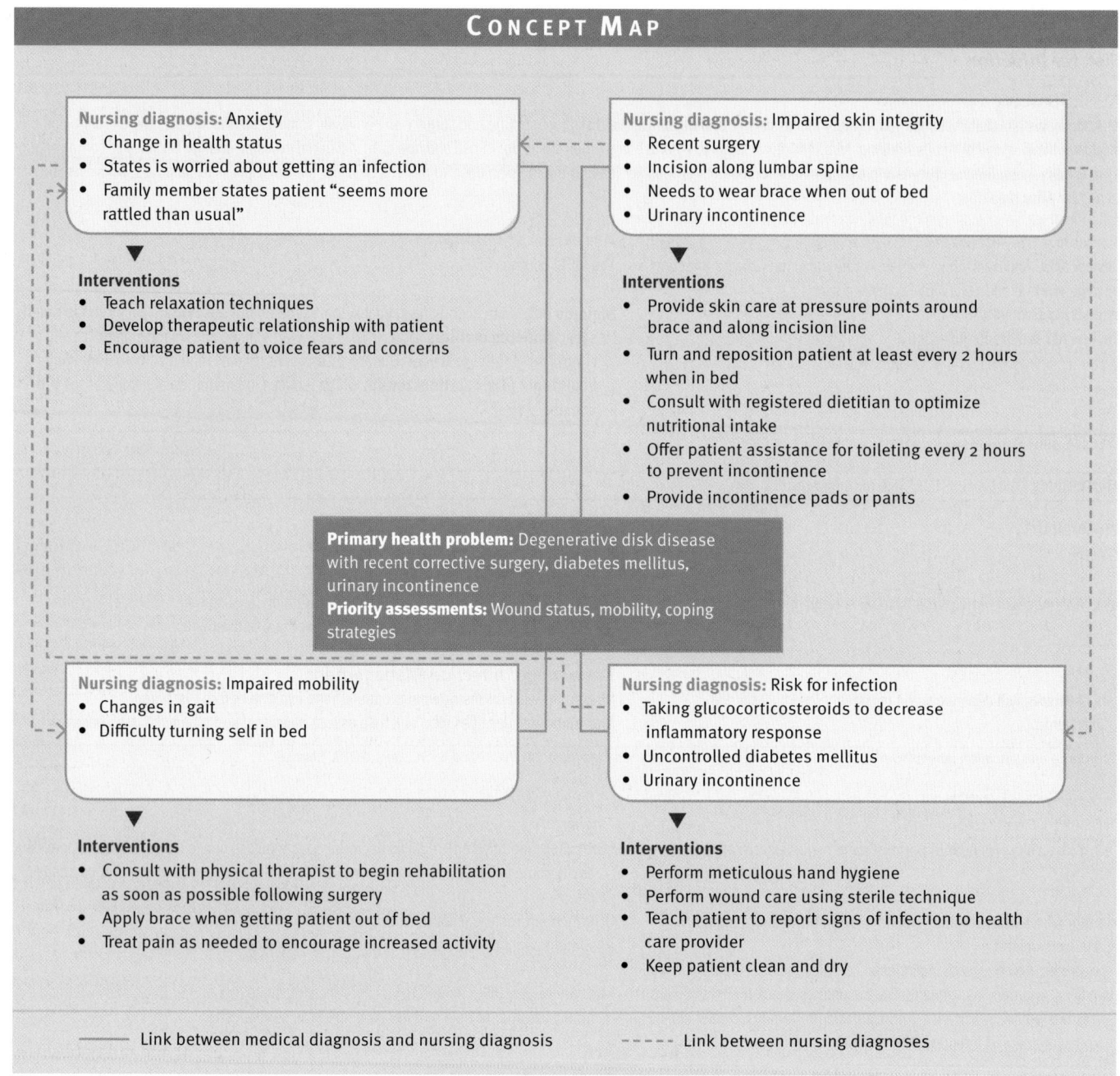

CONCEPT MAP

Nursing diagnosis: Anxiety
- Change in health status
- States is worried about getting an infection
- Family member states patient "seems more rattled than usual"

Interventions
- Teach relaxation techniques
- Develop therapeutic relationship with patient
- Encourage patient to voice fears and concerns

Nursing diagnosis: Impaired skin integrity
- Recent surgery
- Incision along lumbar spine
- Needs to wear brace when out of bed
- Urinary incontinence

Interventions
- Provide skin care at pressure points around brace and along incision line
- Turn and reposition patient at least every 2 hours when in bed
- Consult with registered dietitian to optimize nutritional intake
- Offer patient assistance for toileting every 2 hours to prevent incontinence
- Provide incontinence pads or pants

Primary health problem: Degenerative disk disease with recent corrective surgery, diabetes mellitus, urinary incontinence
Priority assessments: Wound status, mobility, coping strategies

Nursing diagnosis: Impaired mobility
- Changes in gait
- Difficulty turning self in bed

Interventions
- Consult with physical therapist to begin rehabilitation as soon as possible following surgery
- Apply brace when getting patient out of bed
- Treat pain as needed to encourage increased activity

Nursing diagnosis: Risk for infection
- Taking glucocorticosteroids to decrease inflammatory response
- Uncontrolled diabetes mellitus
- Urinary incontinence

Interventions
- Perform meticulous hand hygiene
- Perform wound care using sterile technique
- Teach patient to report signs of infection to health care provider
- Keep patient clean and dry

——— Link between medical diagnosis and nursing diagnosis   - - - - - Link between nursing diagnoses

FIG. 28.2 Concept map for Mrs. Andrews.

Immunization. The CDC's Advisory Committee on Immunization Practices recommends routine vaccination by age 24 months against 14 potentially serious illnesses (CDC, 2018). Immunization programs for infants and children have historically decreased the occurrence of childhood diphtheria, whooping cough, and measles. In 2017, coverage with most recommended vaccines among children 19 to 35 months of age remained stable and high, but coverage was lower in more rural areas and among children who were uninsured or on Medicaid (CDC, 2018). A small but increasing proportion of children received no vaccines by age 24 months (CDC, 2018d).

More recently developed vaccines for meningococcal pneumonia and rotavirus provide immunity to adults and children. Another important vaccine for adults is the shingles vaccine. Recombinant zoster vaccine (RZV, Shingrix) has been in use since 2017 and is recommended by the CDC's Advisory Committee on Immunization Practices (ACIP) as the preferred shingles vaccine (CDC, 2018f). Inform patients

that their risk of shingles and postherpetic neuralgia (PHN) increases as they get older and that just because they may have had shingles does not mean they cannot acquire the virus a second time. Advise parents about the advantages of immunizations but also make them aware of the contraindications for certain vaccines, especially in pregnant and lactating women. You can access the most current immunization schedules at http://www.cdc.gov/vaccines/schedules/hcp/index.html.

Adequate Rest and Regular Exercise. Adequate rest and regular exercise help prevent infection. Physical exercise increases lung capacity, circulation, energy, and endurance. It also decreases stress and improves appetite, sleeping, and elimination. Help patients with a schedule that balances regular exercise with the need for rest and sleep.

Acute Care. Treatment of an infectious process includes eliminating the infectious organisms and supporting a patient's defenses. To identify the causative organisms, you will collect specimens of body fluids such

BOX 28.7 CULTURAL ASPECTS OF CARE

Implications for Infection Control and Isolation Procedures

Various cultural practices and beliefs present challenges to health care providers when infection control and isolation procedures are needed. Patients' health care practices and beliefs influence their decisions to seek treatment for an infection or to use methods to prevent infections. In the United States cities and rural areas have immigrant populations that hold on to the health care practices of their countries of origin. Some members of the immigrant population may come from war-torn countries where health care was limited and infections were rampant. In addition, some of these patients may fear isolation equipment, which for some may indicate that they have a deadly disease or that harm will come to them or their families. It is important to meet the cultural needs of the patients but also to integrate best practices related to infection control and, when needed, isolation procedures. Although gender-congruent caregivers are important for many cultures, the cultural aspects of care for infection control must expand beyond that premise (San Patten and Associates, 2016).

Implications for Patient-Centered Care

- Assess a patient's literacy level and identify the best method for communication and patient teaching for the patient and family. This may include a community elder, an interpreter, or a family member.
- Determine initially whether the patient has any signs of fear, anxiety, or confusion about his condition and treatment plan.
- Reinforce that infection control and isolation procedures are designed for patient safety. Use simple language to explain.
- Explain each item used for infection control and isolation procedures, and obtain feedback from the patient to determine his or her level of understanding.
- Be aware that in some cultures touch from a person who is not a family member is not appropriate. Prepare the patient by explaining why you need to touch; when possible, ask permission. For example, say, "I need to check your arm that has an IV line. May I do that now?"
- If the patient seems fearful of the isolation equipment, continually reinforce why you are wearing the equipment.
- Culturally sensitive care is necessary to identify unique approaches to help patients who are on isolation precautions to understand why the precautions are necessary, answer any questions, and allay patient's and/or family's fear.

IV, Intravenous.

as sputum or drainage from infected body sites for lab cultures. When the disease process or causative organism is identified, the health care provider prescribes the most effective treatment (e.g., antimicrobials).

Systemic infections require measures to prevent complications of fever (see Chapter 29). Maintaining intake of fluids prevents dehydration resulting from diaphoresis. The patient's increased metabolic rate requires an adequate nutritional intake, which may be provided through IV parenteral nutrition. Rest preserves energy for the healing process.

Localized infections often require measures to assist removal of debris to promote healing. You apply principles of wound care to remove infected drainage from wound sites and support the integrity of healing wounds (see Chapter 48). When changing a dressing, wear a mask and goggles or a mask with a face shield if splashing or spraying with blood or body fluids is anticipated. Apply gloves to reduce the transmission of microorganisms into the wound. Apply special dressings to facilitate removal of drainage and promote healing of wound margins. Sometimes a surgeon will insert drainage tubes to remove infected drainage from body cavities (see Chapter 48). Use medical and surgical aseptic techniques appropriately to manage wounds and ensure correct handling of all drainage or body fluids.

During the course of infection, support the patient's body defense mechanisms. For example, if a patient has diarrhea, maintain skin integrity by frequent cleansing of the skin, application of a skin-barrier cream, and frequent repositioning to prevent breakdown and the entrance of additional microorganisms. Other routine hygiene measures such as cleaning the oral cavity and bathing protect the skin and mucous membranes from invasion and overgrowth of organisms.

Medical Asepsis. Asepsis is the absence of pathogenic (disease-producing) microorganisms. Aseptic technique refers to the practices/procedures that help reduce the risk for infection. The two types of aseptic technique are medical and surgical asepsis. Basic medical aseptic techniques break the chain of infection. Use these techniques for all patients, even when no infection is diagnosed. Aggressive preventive measures are highly effective in reducing HAIs. Hand hygiene, barrier techniques, and routine environmental cleaning are examples of medical asepsis. Principles of medical asepsis are also commonly followed in the home; examples are performing hand hygiene with soap and water before preparing food, after using the bathroom, or after touching what are interpreted as dirty objects. It is important to include cultural or social beliefs of the patient and family.

Control or Elimination of Infectious Agents. With the increased use of disposable equipment, nurses are often less aware of disinfection and sterilization procedures. The proper cleaning, disinfection, and sterilization of contaminated objects significantly reduce and/or eliminate microorganisms (Chetan, 2018). In health care agencies a sterile processing department is responsible for the disinfection and sterilization of reusable supplies and equipment. However, nurses sometimes need to perform these functions in the home care setting. Many principles of cleaning and disinfection also apply to the home, so it is important to educate patients and family caregivers on these techniques.

Cleaning. Cleaning is the removal of organic material (e.g., blood) or inorganic material (e.g., soil) from objects and surfaces (Chetan, 2018). In general, cleaning involves the use of water, a detergent/disinfectant, and proper mechanical scrubbing. Cleaning occurs before disinfection and sterilization procedures.

When an object comes in contact with an infectious or potentially infectious material, it is contaminated. If the object is disposable, it is discarded. Reusable objects need to be cleaned thoroughly before reuse and then either disinfected or sterilized according to manufacturer recommendations. Failure to follow manufacturer recommendations transfers liability from the manufacturer to the health care agency if an infection results from improper processing.

Apply protective eyewear (or a face shield) and utility (dishwashing style) gloves when cleaning equipment that is soiled by organic material such as blood, fecal matter, mucus, or pus. Protective barriers provide protection from potentially infectious organisms. A brush and detergent or soap are necessary for cleaning. The following steps ensure that an object is clean:

1. Rinse the contaminated object or article with cold running water to remove organic material. Hot water causes the protein in organic material to coagulate and stick to objects, making removal difficult.
2. After rinsing, wash the object with soap and warm water. Soap or detergent reduces the surface tension of water and emulsifies dirt or remaining material. Rinse the object thoroughly.
3. Use a brush to remove dirt or material in grooves or seams. Friction dislodges contaminated material for easy removal. Open hinged items for cleaning.
4. Rinse the object in warm water.
5. Dry the object and prepare it for disinfection or sterilization if indicated by classification of the item (i.e., critical, semicritical, or noncritical).
6. The brush, gloves, and sink used to clean the equipment are considered contaminated and are cleaned and dried according to policy.

Disinfection and Sterilization. Disinfection and sterilization use both physical and chemical processes that disrupt the internal functioning of microorganisms by destroying cell proteins. **Disinfection** describes a process that eliminates many or all microorganisms, with the exception of bacterial spores, from inanimate objects (Chetan, 2018).

There are two types of disinfection: (1) the disinfection of surfaces, and (2) high-level disinfection, which is required for some patient care items such as endoscopes and bronchoscopes. **Sterilization** eliminates or destroys all forms of microbial life, including spores (Chetan, 2018). Sterilization methods include processing items using steam, dry heat, hydrogen peroxide plasma, or ethylene oxide (ETO). The decision to clean, clean and disinfect, or sterilize depends on the intended use of a contaminated item (Box 28.8). Be familiar with the policies and procedures of your health care agency for cleaning, handling, and delivering care items for eventual disinfection and sterilization. Workers in the central processing area who are specially trained in disinfection and sterilization perform most of the procedures. The following factors influence the efficacy of the disinfecting or sterilizing method:

- *Concentration of solution and duration of contact.* A weakened concentration or shortened exposure time lessens its effectiveness.
- *Type and number of pathogens.* The greater the number of pathogens on an object, the longer the required disinfecting time.
- *Surface areas to treat.* All dirty surfaces and areas need to be fully exposed to disinfecting and sterilizing agents. The type of surface is an important factor. Is the surface porous or nonporous?
- *Temperature of the environment.* Disinfectants tend to work best at room temperature.
- *Presence of soap.* Soap causes certain disinfectants to be ineffective. Thorough rinsing of an object is necessary before disinfecting.
- *Presence of organic material.* Disinfectants become inactivated unless blood, saliva, pus, or body excretions are washed off.

Table 28.5 lists processes for disinfection and sterilization and their characteristics. Some delicate instruments requiring sterilization cannot tolerate steam and must be processed with gas or plasma.

Protection of the Susceptible Host. A patient's resistance to infection improves as you protect normal body defenses against infection. Intervene to maintain the normal reparative processes of the body (Box 28.9). Nurses also protect themselves and others through the use of isolation precautions.

Control or Elimination of Reservoirs of Infection. To control or eliminate the numbers and types of organisms in reservoir sites, eliminate sources of body fluids, drainage, or solutions that possibly harbor microorganisms. Eliminating reservoirs of infection (e.g., emptying urinary drainage bags), controlling portals of exit and entry (e.g., using antiseptic wipes on IV tubing ports), and avoiding actions that transmit microorganisms prevent bacteria from finding a new

---

BOX 28.8 Categories for Sterilization, Disinfection, and Cleaning

Critical Items

Items that enter sterile tissue or the vascular system present a high risk of infection if they are contaminated with microorganisms, especially bacterial spores. *Critical items* must be *sterile*. These items include:
- Surgical instruments
- Cardiac or intravascular catheters
- Urinary catheters
- Implants

Semicritical Items

Items that come in contact with mucous membranes or nonintact skin also present a risk. These objects must be free of all microorganisms (except bacterial spores). *Semicritical items* must be *high-level disinfected (HLD)* or *sterilized*. These items include:
- Respiratory and anesthesia equipment
- Endoscopes
- Endotracheal tubes
- GI endoscopes
- Diaphragm fitting rings

After rinsing, dry items and store in a manner to protect from damage and contamination.

Noncritical Items

Items that come in contact with intact skin, but not mucous membranes must be clean. *Noncritical items* must be *disinfected*. These items include:
- Bedpans
- Blood pressure cuffs
- Bedrails
- Linens
- Stethoscopes
- Bedside trays and patient furniture
- Food utensils

TABLE 28.5 Examples of Disinfection and Sterilization Processes

Characteristics	Examples of Use
Moist Heat	
Steam is moist heat under pressure. When exposed to high pressure, water vapor reaches a temperature above boiling point to kill pathogens and spores.	Autoclave sterilizes heat-tolerant surgical instruments and semicritical patient care items.
Chemical Sterilants—High-Level Disinfection (HLD)	
A number of chemical disinfectants are used in health care. These include alcohols, chlorines, formaldehyde, glutaraldehyde, hydrogen peroxide, iodophors, phenolics, and quaternary ammonium compounds. Each product performs in a unique manner and is used for a specific purpose.	Chemicals disinfect heat-sensitive instruments and equipment such as endoscopes and respiratory therapy equipment.
Ethylene Oxide (ETO) Gas	
This gas destroys spores and microorganisms by altering the metabolic processes of cells. Fumes are released within an autoclave-like chamber. ETO gas is toxic to humans, and aeration time varies with products.	This gas sterilizes most medical materials.
Boiling Water	
Boiling is least expensive for use in the home. Bacterial spores and some viruses resist boiling. It is not used in health care facilities.	Boiling is commonly used in the home for items such as urinary catheters, suction tubes, and drainage collection devices.

BOX 28.9 Infection Prevention and Control: Protecting the Susceptible Host

Protecting Natural Defense Mechanisms

- Regular bathing removes transient microorganisms from the surface of the skin. Lubrication helps keep the skin hydrated and intact. In many intensive care settings, a chlorhexidine (CHG) bath is recommended if there is a risk for methicillin-resistant Staphylococcus aureus (MRSA) or other resistant bacteria (CDC, 2013b; Popovich, 2017)).
- Perform regular oral hygiene. Saliva contains enzymes that promote digestion and has a bactericidal action to maintain control of bacteria. Flossing removes tartar and plaque that cause germ infection.
- Maintenance of adequate fluid intake promotes normal urine formation and a resultant outflow of urine to flush the bladder and urethral lining of microorganisms.
- For patients who are physically dependent or immobilized, encourage routine coughing and deep breathing to keep lower airways clear of mucus.
- Encourage proper immunization of children or adult patients who are exposed to certain infectious microorganisms. Children are vaccinated for measles, mumps, rubella, chickenpox, diphtheria, and other vaccine-preventable diseases. Adults receive one booster of tetanus-diphtheria-acellular pertussis (Tdap), annual flu vaccine, and others as recommended by the Centers for Disease Control and Prevention (CDC) (2010). Older adults should receive a pneumococcal vaccine, shingles vaccine, and an annual influenza vaccine.

Maintaining Healing Processes

- Promote intake of adequate fluids and a well-balanced diet containing essential proteins, vitamins, carbohydrates, and fats. Use measures to increase the patient's appetite.
- Promote a patient's comfort and sleep so that energy stores are replaced daily.
- Help the patient learn techniques to reduce stress.

BOX 28.10 Infection Prevention and Control to Reduce Reservoirs of Infection

Bathing

- Use soap and water to remove drainage, dried secretions, or excess perspiration.

Dressing Changes

- Change dressings that become wet and/or soiled (see Chapter 48).

Contaminated Articles

- Place tissues, soiled dressings, or soiled linen in fluid-resistant bags for proper disposal.

Contaminated Sharps

- Place all needles, safety needles, and needleless systems into puncture-proof containers, which should be located at the site of use. Federal law requires the use of needle-safe technology. Blood tube holders are single use only (OSHA, 2012a).

Bedside Unit

- Keep table surfaces clean and dry.

Bottled Solutions

- Do not leave bottled solutions open.
- Keep solutions tightly capped.
- Date bottles when opened and discard in 24 hours.

Surgical Wounds

- Keep drainage tubes and collection bags patent to prevent accumulation of serous fluid under the skin surface.

Drainage Bottles and Bags

- Wear gloves and protective eyewear if splashing or spraying with contaminated blood or body fluids is anticipated.
- Empty and dispose of drainage suction bottles according to agency policy.
- Empty all drainage systems on each shift unless otherwise ordered by a health care provider.
- Never raise a drainage system (e.g., urinary drainage bag) above the level of the site being drained unless it is clamped off.

site in which to grow (Box 28.10). Be aware of the state regulations for the handling and disposal of medical (infectious) waste. Occupational Safety and Health Administration (OSHA) regulations address the handling and disposal of blood and body fluids that potentially pose a risk for the transmission of bloodborne pathogens. These regulations defer to state laws and regulations (OSHA, 2012a).

Control of Portals of Exit/Entry. To control organisms exiting via the respiratory tract, cover your mouth or nose when coughing or sneezing. Teach patients, health care staff, patient's families, and visitors about respiratory hygiene or cough etiquette. The use of posters and written material explaining cough etiquette to learners is beneficial. Cough etiquette has become more important because of concern for transmission of respiratory infections such as *Mycobacterium tuberculosis*, severe acute respiratory syndrome (SARS), and H1N1 influenza (CDC, 2007). The elements of respiratory hygiene and cough etiquette are summarized in Table 28.6 (CDC, 2007).

Another way of controlling the exit of microorganisms is by using Standard Precautions (see Table 28.6) when handling body fluids such as urine, feces, and wound drainage. Wear clean gloves if there is any chance of contact with any blood or body fluids, and perform hand hygiene after providing care. Be sure to bag contaminated items (e.g., linen placed in fluid-resistant linen bags) appropriately.

Many measures that control the exit of microorganisms also control their entrance. Maintaining the integrity of skin and mucous membranes reduces the chances of microorganisms reaching a host. Keep a patient's skin well lubricated by using lotion as appropriate. Patients who are

immobilized and debilitated are particularly susceptible to skin breakdown. Do not position patients on tubes or objects that cause breaks in the skin. It is important to turn and position patients before their skin becomes reddened. Frequent oral hygiene prevents the drying of mucous membranes. A water-soluble ointment keeps a patient's lips well lubricated.

After elimination instruct women to clean the rectum and perineum by wiping from the urinary meatus toward the rectum. Cleaning in a direction from the least to the most contaminated area helps reduce GU infections. Meticulous and frequent perineal care is especially important in older-adult women who wear disposable incontinence pads.

Another cause for entrance of microorganisms into a host is improper handling and management of urinary catheters and drainage sets (see Chapter 46) (Box 28.11). Keep the point of connection between a catheter and drainage tube closed and intact. If such systems are closed, their contents are considered sterile. Outflow spigots on drainage bags should also remain closed to prevent entrance of bacteria. Minimize movement of the catheter at the urethra by stabilizing it with tape or a securing device to reduce the chance of microorganisms ascending the urethra into the bladder. Do not share urine-measuring containers among patients. Sometimes you care for patients with closed

TABLE 28.6 Centers for Disease Control and Prevention Isolation Guidelines

Standard Precautions (Tier One) for Use With All Patients

- Standard Precautions apply to blood, blood products, all body fluids, secretions, excretions (except sweat), nonintact skin, and mucous membranes.
- Perform hand hygiene before direct contact with patients; between patient contacts; after contact with blood, body fluids, secretions, and excretions and with equipment or articles contaminated by them; and immediately after gloves are removed.
- When hands are visibly soiled or contaminated with blood or body fluids, wash them with either a nonantimicrobial soap or antimicrobial soap and water.
- When hands are not visibly soiled or contaminated with blood or body fluids, use an alcohol-based hand rub to perform hand hygiene.
- Wash hands with nonantimicrobial or antimicrobial soap and water if contact with spores (e.g., *Clostridium difficile*) is likely to have occurred.
- Do not wear artificial fingernails or extenders if duties include direct contact with patients at high risk for infection and associated adverse outcomes.
- Wear gloves when touching blood, body fluids, secretions, excretions, nonintact skin, mucous membranes, or contaminated items or surfaces. Remove and dispose of gloves and perform hand hygiene between patient care encounters and when going from a contaminated to a clean body site.
- Wear PPE when your anticipated patient interaction is likely to involve contact with blood or body fluids.
- A private room is unnecessary. Check with the infection prevention and control professional of your agency.
- Discard all contaminated sharp instruments and needles in a puncture-resistant container. Health care facilities must make needleless devices available. Activate the mechanical safety device, if present. If needle recapping is necessary, use the one-handed scoop method and dispose of the capped needle as soon as possible.
- Respiratory hygiene and cough etiquette: Have patients cover the nose or mouth when sneezing or coughing; use tissues to contain respiratory secretions and dispose in nearest waste container; perform hand hygiene after contact with respiratory secretions and contaminated objects or materials; contain respiratory secretions with procedure or surgical mask; sit at least 3 feet away from others if coughing.

Transmission-Based Precautions (Tier Two) for Use With Specific Types of Patients

Category	Disease	Barrier Protection
Airborne Precautions (Droplets <5 μm)	Measles, chickenpox (varicella), disseminated herpes zoster, *Mycobacterium tuberculosis*, rubeola	Private room; negative-pressure airflow of at least 6-12 exchanges per hour via HEPA filtration; mask or respiratory protection device, N95 respirator
Droplet Precautions (Droplets >5 μm; being within 3 feet of the patient)	Influenza, adenovirus, group A streptococcus, *Neisseria meningitides*, pertussis, rhinovirus, mycoplasma pneumoniae, pertussis, diphtheria, pneumonic plague, rubella, mumps, respiratory syncytial virus	Private room or cohort patients; mask or respirator (refer to agency policy)
Contact Precautions (Direct patient or environmental contact)	Colonization or infection with multidrug-resistant organisms, such as VRE and MRSA, *Clostridium difficile*, shigella and other enteric pathogens, major wound infections, herpes simplex, scabies, varicella zoster (disseminated), respiratory syncytial virus	Private room or cohort patients (see agency policy); gloves, gowns
Protective environment	Allogeneic hematopoietic stem cell transplants	Private room; positive airflow with ≥12 air exchanges per hour; HEPA filtration for incoming air; mask, gloves, gowns

HEPA, High-efficiency particulate air; *MRSA,* methicillin-resistant *Staphylococcus aureus*; *PPE,* personal protective equipment; *VRE,* vancomycin-resistant enterococcus.

Modified from Centers for Disease Control and Prevention (CDC) Hospital Infection Control Practice Advisory Committee: *Guidelines for isolation precautions in hospitals,* 2017; Association of periOperative Registered Nurses (AORN): *AORN guidelines for perioperative practice,* Denver, 2019; US Food and Drug Administration (FDA): *What to do if you can't find a sharps disposal container,* 2016, https://www.fda.gov/medicaldevices/productsandmedicalprocedures/homehealthandconsumer/consumerproducts/sharps/default.htm.

drainage systems that collect wound drainage, bile, or other body fluids. Make sure that the site from which a drainage tube exits remains clear of excess moisture or accumulated drainage. Keep all tubing connected throughout use and open drainage receptacles only when it is necessary to discard or measure the volume of drainage (see Chapter 46).

Control of Transmission. Effective prevention and control of infection requires you to remain aware of the modes of transmission of microorganisms and ways to control them. The use of Standard Precautions (Table 28.6) for all patients is a step toward preventing transmission of infection. In any health care setting a patient usually has a personal set of care items. Sharing bedpans, urinals, bath basins, and eating utensils among patients easily leads to cross-infection by indirect contact. When using a stethoscope, always wipe off the bell, diaphragm, and ear tips with a disinfectant such as an alcohol wipe before proceeding to the next patient. Diaphragms and ear tips are a

common location for staphylococcal organisms (Adesanya et al., 2017). In facilities where HAI diarrhea occurs, electronic thermometers are not recommended for rectal temperatures. You usually use oral or tympanic thermometers to assess temperature. Do not use electronic thermometers for patients on contact isolation.

Always be careful when handling exudate such as urine, feces, emesis, and blood. Contaminated fluids easily splash while being discarded in toilets or hoppers. Urinals and bedpans need to be emptied at water level to reduce the risk of splash or splatter, and gloves and protective eyewear are worn. Appropriately dispose of disposable soiled items in trash bags. Dispose of items contaminated with large amounts of blood in biohazard bags. Know the location of biohazard bags; it will differ among facilities. Handle laboratory specimens from all patients as if they were infectious and place them in designated biohazard containers or bags for transport or disposal. Because certain microorganisms

BOX 28.11 EVIDENCE-BASED PRACTICE

Daily Unit Rounds to Reduce CAUTI

PICOT Question: Does the implementation of routine root cause analysis compared with routine daily rounds reduce the incidence of catheter-associated urinary tract infections?

Evidence Summary

Among urinary tract infections (UTI) acquired in the hospital, approximately 75% are associated with a urinary catheter, and between 15% and 25% of hospitalized patients receive urinary catheters during their hospital stay (CDC, 2017b). The most important risk factor for developing a catheter-associated urinary tract infection (CAUTI) is prolonged use of the urinary catheter. CAUTIs are a common infection in hospitals across the United States, with many hospitals demonstrating high CAUTI rates and high urinary catheter utilization rate for several years. CAUTIs are usually preventable, so numerous studies have examined strategies for decreasing CAUTI rates. Strategies have included the development of CDC guidelines for the prevention of CAUTIs (CDC, 2009), the use of a CAUTI guide with questions regarding proper indwelling catheter use (Fletcher et al., 2016), and a quality improvement collaboration of health care centers throughout the United States (Fakih et al., 2014). One successful strategy implemented by Graziano-Husser and colleagues (2018) involved implementing daily huddle rounds for urinary catheter justification. The project team started to implement mini root cause analyses (RCAs) to review CAUTI cases, identify issues that contributed to the CAUTI, and educate nurses and nursing assistants to generate awareness of why and how CAUTIs occur and strategies to prevent them. After a CAUTI was found, the chart was reviewed by unit staff for key factors, including necessity of catheter, appropriate culturing, and appropriate care and maintenance. Findings were then discussed among the unit staff on challenges and concerns related to the urinary catheter and maintenance and opportunities for improvement. Through the intervention, the unit's CAUTI rate was decreased by 38.5%.

Application to Nursing Practice

- Insert catheters only for appropriate indications, such as acute urinary retention or strict output monitoring (Graziano-Husser et al, 2018).
- Leave catheters in place only as long as needed and remove within 24 hours unless there are appropriate indications for continued use (Fakih et al, 2014).
- Ensure that only properly trained persons insert and maintain urinary catheters (Fakih et al, 2014).
- Insert urinary catheters using aseptic technique and sterile equipment (CDC, 2009).
- Following aseptic insertion, maintain a closed drainage system (CDC, 2009).
- Use hand hygiene and Standard (or appropriate isolation) Precautions.

---

travel easily through the air, do not shake linens or bedclothes. Dust with a treated or dampened cloth to prevent dust particles from entering the air.

To prevent transmission of microorganisms through indirect contact, do not allow soiled items and equipment to touch your clothing. A common error is to carry dirty linen in the arms against your uniform. Use fluid-resistant linen bags or carry soiled linen with hands held out from the body. Cover laundry hampers and empty them before they become overloaded. **Never put clean or soiled linens on the floor.**

Hand Hygiene. The most effective basic technique in preventing and controlling the transmission of infection is hand hygiene (see Skill 28.1) (Hass, 2018; WHO, 2017). Hand hygiene is a general term that applies to four techniques: handwashing, antiseptic hand wash,

antiseptic hand rub, or surgical hand antisepsis. Handwashing is defined by the CDC (2008) as the vigorous, brief rubbing together of all surfaces of lathered hands followed by rinsing under a stream of warm water for 15 seconds. The fundamental principle behind handwashing is removing microorganisms mechanically from the hands and rinsing with water. Handwashing does not kill microorganisms.

An antiseptic hand wash means washing hands with warm water and soap or other detergents containing an antiseptic agent; some antiseptics kill bacteria and some viruses. An antiseptic hand rub means applying an antiseptic hand-rub product to all surfaces of the hands to reduce the number of microorganisms present. Ethanol-based hand antiseptics containing 60% to 90% alcohol appear to be the most effective against common pathogens found on the hands (CDC, 2008). Alcohol-based products are more effective for standard handwashing or hand antisepsis (nonsoiled hands) by health care workers than regular soap or antimicrobial soaps (CDC, 2008). Surgical hand antisepsis is an antiseptic hand-wash or hand-rub technique that surgical personnel perform before surgery to eliminate transient and reduce resident hand flora. Antiseptic detergent preparations have persistent antimicrobial activity (CDC, 2008; WHO, 2009).

According to the WHO (2009), hand cleansing practices are likely to be established in the first 10 years of a person's life. This imprinting affects an individual's attitudes about hand cleansing throughout life. This is called inherent hand hygiene (WHO, 2009). Attitudes toward handwashing in situations such as the delivery of health care are called elective handwashing practices (WHO, 2009). In many patient populations, inherent and elective handwashing is influenced by cultural factors. Thus, hand hygiene is often performed for hygienic reasons, rituals, and symbolic reasons. It is important to learn the significance hand hygiene holds for an individual.

The use of alcohol-based hand rubs is recommended by the CDC (2008) to improve hand hygiene practices, protect health care workers' hands, and reduce the transmission of pathogens to patients and personnel in health care settings. Alcohols have excellent germicidal activity and are as effective as soap and water. However, alcohol-based hand antiseptics are not effective on hands that are visibly dirty or are contaminated with organic material (CDC, 2013a). WHO (2017) recommends the following hand hygiene guidelines:

1. When hands are visibly dirty, when hands are soiled with blood or other body fluids, before eating, and after using the toilet, wash hands with water and either a nonantimicrobial or antimicrobial soap.
2. Wash hands if exposed to spore-forming organisms such as *C. difficile*, *Bacillus anthracis*, or *Norovirus* (CDC, 2014).
3. If hands are not visibly soiled (WHO, 2017), use an alcohol-based, waterless antiseptic agent for routinely decontaminating hands in the following clinical situations:
   - Before, after, and between direct patient contact (e.g., taking a pulse, lifting a patient)
   - Before putting on sterile gloves and before inserting invasive devices such as a peripheral vascular catheter or urinary catheter
   - After contact with body fluids or excretions, mucous membranes, nonintact skin, and wound dressings (even if gloves are worn)
   - When moving from a contaminated to a clean body site during care
   - After contact with surfaces or objects in the patient's room (e.g., overbed table, IV pump)
   - After removing gloves (CDC, 2008)

Remember, contaminated hands of health care workers are a primary source of infection transmission in health care settings. It is recommended that health care workers have well-manicured nails and refrain from wearing artificial nails to reduce microorganism transmission.

Infection can easily be transmitted by visitors of patients in health care settings. A study by Birnbach and colleagues (2015) included hand hygiene observations of visitors and collection of cultures as visitors entered patient rooms. Thirty-five of 55 visitors did not perform hand hygiene before entering the patient room, and all 55 visitors agreed to providing hand cultures. All of the cultures from visitors not doing hand hygiene grew a significantly higher number of bacteria than the cultures from visitors doing hand hygiene. The study demonstrates the need for education of visitors on the importance of hand hygiene and evaluation of corresponding changes in hand hygiene behavior. Instruct patients and visitors about proper hand hygiene technique, the reason for it, and the times for performing it. If health care is to continue at home, teach patients and family caregivers to wash their hands before eating or handling food; after handling contaminated equipment, linen, or organic material; and after elimination. In health care settings, encourage visitors to wash their hands before eating or handling food; after coming in contact with infected patients; and after handling contaminated equipment, patient furniture, or organic material (Gould et al., 2011).

You are responsible for providing the patient and family with a safe environment. The CDC (2015d) launched a Clean Hands Save Lives Campaign that highlights for consumers the five simple and effective steps (Wet, Lather, Scrub, Rinse, Dry) to take to reduce the spread of diarrheal and respiratory illnesses and thus to stay healthy. Many hospitals encourage patients to follow the recommendations of TJC's "Speak Up" campaign. TJC together with the Centers for Medicare and Medicaid Services urges patients to take a role in preventing health care errors by becoming active, involved, and informed participants on the health care team. The program features brochures, posters, and buttons on a variety of patient safety topics. One recommendation is to have patients speak up to be sure the health care provider has cleaned his or her hands or wears gloves when providing care.

The effectiveness of infection prevention practices such as hand hygiene depends on the conscientiousness and consistency in using proper technique by all health care providers. It is human nature to forget key procedural steps or, when hurried, to take shortcuts that break aseptic procedures. However, failure to adhere to basic procedures places patients at risk for infections that can seriously impair recovery or lead to death.

Isolation and Isolation Precautions. In 2007 the Hospital Infection Control Practices Advisory Committee (HICPAC) of the CDC published revised guidelines for isolation precautions. HICPAC recommended that facilities modify the guidelines according to need and as dictated by federal, state, or local regulations. The guidelines contain recommendations for respiratory hygiene/cough etiquette as part of Standard Precautions. The CDC recommendations contain two tiers of precautions (see Table 28.6). The first and most important tier is called *Standard Precautions,* which are designed to be used for the care of all patients, in all settings, regardless of risk or presumed infection status. Standard Precautions are the primary strategies (including barrier precautions) for prevention of infection transmission and apply to contact with blood, body fluids, nonintact skin, mucous membranes, and equipment or surfaces contaminated with potentially infectious materials. In the acute care setting, nurses follow Standard Precautions in all aspects of care. This includes barrier precautions and the appropriate use of PPE such as gowns, gloves, masks, eyewear, and other protective devices or clothing. The choice of barriers depends on the task being performed and the patient's disease. Standard Precautions apply to all patients because every patient has the potential to transmit infection

via blood and body fluids, and the risk for infection transmission is unknown. Respiratory hygiene/cough etiquette applies to any person with signs of respiratory infection, including cough, congestion, rhinorrhea, or increased production of respiratory secretions, when entering a health care site. Educating health care staff, patients, and visitors to follow respiratory hygiene/cough etiquette protects both patients and health care workers.

The second tier of precautions (see Table 28.6) includes precautions designed for the care of patients who are known or suspected to be infected or colonized with microorganisms transmitted by droplet, airborne, or contact routes (Berends and Walesa, 2018; CDC, 2007). There are four types of transmission-based precautions, which are based on the mode of transmission of a disease: **Airborne, Droplet, Contact,** and **Protective Environment Precautions.** These precautions are for patients with highly transmissible pathogens. The protective environment category is designed for patients who have undergone transplants and gene therapy, making them highly vulnerable to infection(CDC, 2007).

- *Contact Precautions:* Used for direct and indirect contact with patients and their environment. Direct contact refers to the care and handling of contaminated body fluids. Contact Precautions require a gown and gloves. An example includes blood or other body fluids from an infected patient that enter the health care worker's body through direct contact with compromised skin or mucous membranes. Indirect contact involves the transfer of an infectious agent through a contaminated intermediate object such as contaminated instruments or hands of health care workers. The health care worker may transmit microorganisms from one patient site to another if hand hygiene is not performed between patients (CDC, 2007).
- *Droplet Precautions:* Focus on diseases that are transmitted by large droplets (greater than 5 microns) expelled into the air and by being within 3 feet of a patient. Droplet Precautions require the wearing of a surgical mask when within 3 feet of the patient, proper hand hygiene, and some dedicated-care equipment. An example is a patient with influenza.
- *Airborne Precautions:* Focus on diseases that are transmitted by smaller droplets, which remain in the air for longer periods of time. Airborne Precautions require a specially equipped room with a negative airflow referred to as an *airborne infection isolation room.* Air is not returned to the inside ventilation system but is filtered through a high-efficiency particulate air (HEPA) filter and exhausted directly to the outside. For example, all health care personnel wear an N95 respirator every time they enter the room of a patient with TB.
- *Protective environment:* Focuses on a very limited patient population, all of whom are highly susceptible to infection. This form of isolation requires a specialized room with positive airflow. The airflow rate is set at greater than 12 air exchanges per hour, and all air is filtered through a HEPA filter. One example of a patient requiring a protective environment is a patient who received a kidney transplant. The patient wears a mask when out of his or her room during transportation to x-ray.

Health care facilities are required to have the capability of isolating patients. However, not all communicable diseases require placing a patient in a special private room. You can conduct many isolation practices in standard rooms using barrier precautions.

Because of the resurgence of TB, the CDC (2007) developed guidelines to prevent its transmission to health care workers and stresses the importance of isolation for the patient with known or suspected TB in a special negative-pressure room. Close the doors to the patient's room to control the direction of airflow. You must wear a special high-filtration particulate respirator on entering a respiratory isolation room. A respirator must be fitted to your facial size and characteristics. When worn correctly, particulate respirators and masks have a tighter face seal and filter at a higher level than routine surgical masks.

MDROs such as methicillin-resistant *Staphylococcus aureus* (MRSA), vancomycin-resistant enterococcus (VRE) and *C. difficile* are more common as a cause of colonization and HAIs. MDROs have developed a resistance to one or more broad-spectrum antibiotics, making the organisms hard to treat effectively. Major efforts have been in place for a number of years to reduce the incidence of HAIs caused by these dangerous organisms. For example, evidence shows that the percentage of central line bloodstream infections (see Chapter 42) caused by MRSA, VRE, and gram-negative bacteria has declined (CDC, 2011). Unlike MRSA and VRE, *C. difficile* (which is transmitted by the fecal-oral route) is harder to eliminate from the environment. It is a spore-forming microorganism, meaning it can remain on surfaces (e.g., bedside table, stethoscope) in a dormant state for long periods. To reduce the risk of cross-contamination among patients, use Contact Precautions in addition to Standard Precautions when caring for patients with MDROs.

Regardless of the type of isolation or barrier protection you use, follow these basic principles when caring for patients:

- Understand how certain diseases are transmitted and which protective barriers to use.
- Use thorough hand hygiene before entering and leaving the room of a patient in isolation.
- Dispose of contaminated supplies and equipment in a manner that prevents spread of microorganisms to other people as indicated by the mode of transmission of the organism.
- Protect all people who might be exposed during transport of a patient outside the isolation room.

Psychological Implications of Isolation. Consider the psychological effects of being in an isolation room. Many patients find positive aspects of being in a single room; however, the overall experience of isolation is commonly viewed negatively (Mehrotra et al., 2013). Isolation imposes barriers to the expression of a patient's identity and normal interpersonal relationships and affects the delivery of quality care. When a patient requires isolation in a private room, a sense of loneliness sometimes develops because normal social relationships become disrupted. This situation can be psychologically harmful, especially for children. A study noted that patients in isolation experienced more depression and anxiety and were less satisfied with their care (Sprague et al., 2016). Patients' body images become altered as a result of the infectious process. Some feel unclean, rejected, lonely, or guilty. Infection prevention and control practices further intensify these beliefs of difference or undesirability. Isolation disrupts normal social relationships with visitors and caregivers. Take the opportunity to listen to a patient's concerns or interests. If you rush care or show a lack of interest in a patient's needs, he or she feels rejected and even more isolated.

Before you institute isolation measures, the patient and family need to understand the nature of the disease or condition, the purposes of isolation, and steps for following specific precautions. If they are able to participate in maintaining infection prevention and control practices, the chances of reducing the spread of infection increase. Teach the patient and family to perform hand hygiene and use barrier protection if appropriate. Demonstrate each procedure; be sure to give the patient and family an opportunity for practice. It is also important to explain how infectious organisms are transmitted so that the patient and family understand the difference between contaminated and clean objects. Explaining and demonstrating these procedures, especially hand hygiene, help the family to consistently practice correct hand hygiene and prescribed isolation measures (Gould et al., 2011).

Take measures to improve a patient's sensory stimulation during isolation. Make sure that the room environment is clean and pleasant. Open drapes or shades and remove excess supplies and equipment. Listen to the patient's concerns or interests. Mealtime is a particularly good opportunity for conversation. Providing comfort measures such as repositioning, a back massage, or a warm sponge bath increases physical stimulation. Depending on the patient's condition, encourage him or her to walk around the room or sit up in a chair. Recreational activities such as board games, reading, and playing cards are options for keeping a patient mentally stimulated.

Explain to the family the patient's risk for depression or loneliness. Encourage visiting family members to avoid expressions or actions that convey revulsion or disgust related to infection prevention and control practices. Discuss ways to provide meaningful stimulation.

The Isolation Environment. Private rooms used for isolation sometimes provide negative-pressure airflow to prevent infectious particles from flowing out of a room to other rooms and the air handling system. Special rooms with positive-pressure airflow are also used for patients who are immunocompromised, such as recipients of transplanted organs. On the door or wall outside the room a nurse posts a card listing precautions for the isolation category in use according to health care agency policy. The card is a handy reference for health care personnel and visitors and alerts anyone who enters the room that special precautions must be followed.

An area immediately outside an isolation room or an adjoining anteroom needs to contain hand hygiene and PPE supplies. Soap and antiseptic (antimicrobial) solutions also should be available. Personnel and visitors perform hand hygiene before entering a patient's room and again before leaving the room. If toilet facilities are unavailable, there are special procedures for handling portable commodes, bedpans, or urinals.

All patient care rooms, including those used for isolation, should contain an impervious bag for soiled or contaminated linen and a trash container with plastic liners. Impervious receptacles prevent transmission of microorganisms by preventing leaking and soiling of the outside surface. A disposable rigid container needs to be available in the room to discard used sharps such as safety needles and syringes.

Remain aware of infection prevention and control techniques while working with patients in protected environments. You need to feel comfortable performing all procedures and yet remain conscious of infection prevention and control principles. Depending on the microorganism and mode of transmission, evaluate which articles or equipment to take into an isolation room. For example, the CDC (2017c) recommends the dedicated use of articles such as stethoscopes, sphygmomanometers, and thermometers in the isolation room of a patient infected or colonized with VRE. Do not use these devices on other patients unless they are first adequately cleaned and disinfected.

Personal Protective Equipment. The PPE, specialized clothing or equipment (e.g., gowns, masks or respirators, protective eyewear, and gloves) that you wear for protection against exposure to infectious materials, should be readily available in a patient care area (CDC, 2017c). You choose the equipment to use depending on the task to be performed.

Gowns. The primary reason for gowning is to prevent soiling clothes during contact with a patient. Gowns or cover-ups protect health care personnel and visitors from coming in contact with infected material and blood or body fluids. Gowns are often required, depending on the expected amount of exposure to infectious material. Gowns used for barrier protection are made of a fluid-resistant material. Change gowns immediately if damaged or heavily contaminated.

Isolation gowns usually open at the back and have ties or snaps at the neck and waist to keep the gown closed and secure. Gowns need to be long enough to cover all outer garments. Long sleeves with tight-fitting cuffs provide added protection. No special technique is required for applying clean gowns if they are fastened securely. However, carefully remove gowns to minimize contamination of the hands and uniform and discard them after removal.

Masks. Masks provide respiratory protection. Wear full-face protection (with eyes, nose, and mouth covered) when you anticipate splashing or spraying of blood or body fluid into the face. Also wear masks when working with a patient placed on Airborne or Droplet Precautions. If a patient is on Airborne Precautions for TB, apply an OSHA-approved respirator-style mask. The mask protects you from inhaling microorganisms and small-particle droplet nuclei that remain suspended in the air from a patient's respiratory tract. The surgical mask protects a wearer from inhaling large-particle aerosols that travel short distances (3 feet). When caring for patients on Droplet or Airborne Precautions, apply a mask (surgical or respirator) when entering the isolation room.

At times, a patient who is susceptible to infection wears a mask to prevent inhalation of pathogens. Patients on Droplet or Airborne Precautions who are transported outside their rooms need to wear a surgical mask to protect other patients and personnel. Masks prevent transmission of infection by direct contact with mucous membranes (CDC, 2005a). A mask discourages the wearer from touching the eyes, nose, or mouth (Box 28.12).

If a person wears glasses, the top edge of the mask fits below the glasses so that they do not cloud over as the person exhales. Keep talking to a minimum while wearing a mask to reduce respiratory airflow. A mask that becomes moist does not provide a barrier to microorganisms and is ineffective. You need to discard it. Never reuse a disposable mask. Warn patients and family members that a mask can cause a sensation of smothering. If family members become uncomfortable, they should leave the room and discard the mask.

Specially fitted respiratory protective devices (N95 respirator masks) are required when caring for patients on Airborne Precautions such as patients with known or suspected TB (Fig. 28.3) (CDC, 2005a). The mask must have a higher filtration rating than regular surgical masks and be fitted snugly to prevent leakage around the sides. Be aware of health care agency policy regarding the type of respiratory protective device required. Special fit testing is required to establish the size and ability of the nurse to wear this type of mask (CDC, 2005a).

Eye Protection. Use either special glasses or goggles when performing procedures that generate splash or splatter. Examples of such procedures include irrigation of a large abdominal wound or insertion of an arterial catheter when the nurse assists a health care provider. A nurse who wears prescription glasses uses removable, reusable, or disposable side shields over them (OSHA, 2011). Eyewear is available in the form of plastic glasses or goggles. The eyewear needs to fit snugly around the face so that fluids cannot enter between the face and the glasses.

BOX 28.12   PROCEDURAL GUIDELINES

Applying a Disposable Mask

Delegation and Collaboration

The skill of applying a surgical mask can be delegated when assistive personnel (AP) are trained in required sterile procedure. The nurse informs AP to:

- Put on the mask following the appropriate steps.
- Change the mask if it becomes moist or contaminated.
- Remove the mask when leaving the patient's room.

Equipment

Disposable mask

Steps

1. Find top edge of mask (some have a thin metal strip along edge). Pliable metal fits snugly against bridge of nose. Others offer an occlusive fit that does not require an adjustment.
2. Hold mask by top two strings or loops. Secure two top ties at top of back of head (see illustration), with ties above ears. (*Alternative:* Slip loops over each ear.)

3. Tie two lower ties snugly around neck with mask well under chin (see illustration).
4. Gently pinch upper metal band around bridge of nose.
   NOTE: Change mask when it becomes wet, moist, or contaminated.
5. Remove mask by untying *bottom* mask strings and then top strings; pull mask away from face and drop into trash receptacle. (Do not touch outer surface of mask.)

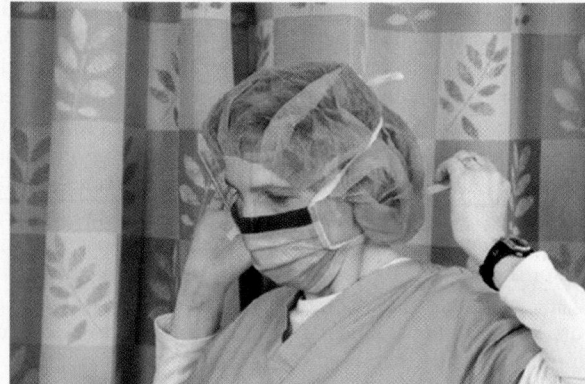

STEP 3 Securing lower ties of a tie-on mask.

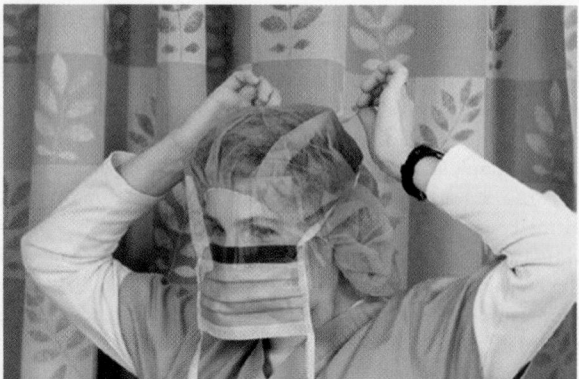

STEP 2 Securing top two ties of a tie-on mask.

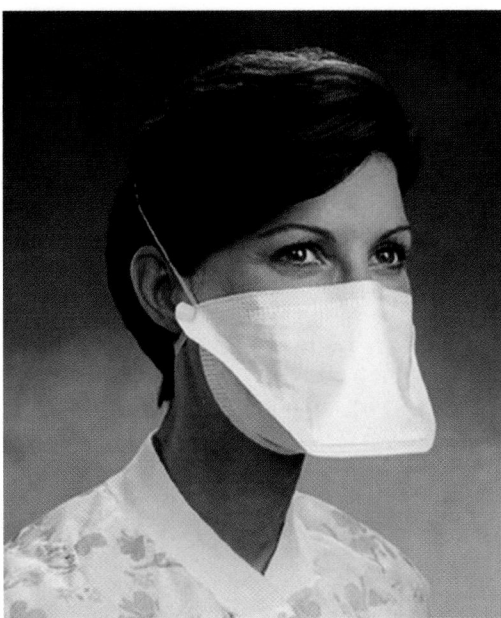

FIG. 28.3 N95 respirator mask. (Courtesy of Halyard Health, Inc., Alpharetta, GA.)

Gloves. Gloves help to prevent the transmission of pathogens by direct and indirect contact. The CDC (2007) notes that you need to wear clean gloves when touching blood, body fluid, secretions, excretions (except sweat), moist mucous membranes, nonintact skin, and contaminated items or surfaces. Follow these guidelines:

- Change and dispose of gloves and perform hand hygiene between tasks and procedures on the same patient after contact with material that contains a high concentration of microorganisms.
- Remove and dispose of gloves promptly after use, before touching noncontaminated items and environmental surfaces, and before going to another patient.
- Perform hand hygiene immediately after removing gloves to avoid transfer of microorganisms to other patients or environments.

To reduce the incidence of health care providers developing a sensitivity or allergy to the latex in gloves, health care agencies provide nonlatex gloves to employees. Most health care agencies are working to become latex free to protect health care providers and patients.

Box 28.13 describes the steps to follow for applying full PPE. During a procedure, be sure PPE remains in place. If you notice a break or tear in a glove while providing care, change gloves. If you do not plan to have additional contact with a patient after a care activity, reapplying gloves is unnecessary. Perform hand hygiene when gloves are removed.

Instruct family members visiting patients on isolation precautions on how to apply gloves properly. Demonstrate the application of gloves to family members, and explain the reason for the use of gloves. Emphasize the importance of performing hand hygiene after removing gloves.

Specimen Collection. Many laboratory studies are often necessary when a patient is suspected of having an infectious or communicable disease (Box 28.14). You collect body fluids and secretions suspected of containing infectious organisms for culture and sensitivity tests. After a specimen is sent to a laboratory, the laboratory technologist identifies the microorganisms growing in the culture. Additional test results indicate the antibiotics to which the organisms are resistant or sensitive. Sensitivity reports determine which antibiotics used in treatment are effective and need to be ordered for treatment.

Obtain all culture specimens using clean gloves and sterile equipment. Blood cultures are taken from two separate venipuncture sites and before initiation of antimicrobials. Collecting fresh material such as wound drainage from the site of infection ensures that neighboring microbes do not contaminate a specimen. Seal all specimen containers tightly to prevent spillage and contamination of the outside of the container.

Bagging Trash or Linen. Bagging contaminated items prevents accidental exposure of personnel and contamination of the surrounding environment. Double bagging is not recommended (CDC, 2007). The use of a single intact, standard-size linen bag that is not overfilled and that is tied securely is adequate to prevent infection transmission. Check the color code of bag that your agency uses for bagging these items.

Transporting Patients. Before transferring patients to wheelchairs or stretchers, give them clean gowns to serve as robes. Patients infected with organisms transmitted by the airborne route normally leave their rooms only for essential purposes such as diagnostic procedures or surgery. When a patient has an airborne infection, he or she must wear a mask when leaving the room. Notify personnel in diagnostic or procedural areas or the operating room of the type of isolation precautions the patient requires. Some patients being transported drain body fluids onto a stretcher or wheelchair. Use an extra layer of sheets to cover the stretcher or seat of the wheelchair. Be sure to clean the equipment with an approved germicide after patient use and before another patient uses the shared equipment.

QSEN **Building Competency in Evidence-Based Practice** You are asked to participate on a unit-based team to help your fellow health care workers be more adherent to hand hygiene before and after patient care. Your unit's current rate of adherence to hand hygiene is 74%, and the unit manager has been directed by administration to improve the rate by the next quarter. Your team meets, and many team members offer opinions on how best to improve the unit hand hygiene adherence rates, but no one is sure where to start. You know that implementing an evidence-based plan will be more successful than a trial and error approach. How can you guide the team in a way that will provide an evidence-based approach to the problem?

Answers to QSEN Activities can be found on the Evolve website.

Role of the Infection Control Professional. An infection control professional is a valuable resource for helping nurses control HAIs. These professionals are specially trained in infection prevention and control. They are responsible for advising health care personnel regarding infection prevention and control practices and monitoring infections within the hospital. An infection control professional's responsibilities often include (Friedman, 2018):

- Collection and analysis of infection data
- Evaluation of products and procedures
- Development and review of policies and procedures
- Consultation on infection risk assessment, prevention, and control strategies (includes activities related to occupational health, construction, and emergency management)
- Educational efforts directed at interventions to reduce infection risks
- Education of patients and families
- Implementation of changes mandated by regulatory, accrediting, and licensing agencies (includes reporting communicable diseases to health departments)
- Application of epidemiological principles, including activities directed at improving patient outcomes using implementation science
- Antimicrobial management
- Participation in research projects
- Monitoring antibiotic-resistant organisms in the institution

Delegation and Collaboration

The skill of caring for a patient on isolation precautions can be delegated to assistive personnel (AP). However, it is the nurse who assesses the patient's status and isolation indications. Instruct AP about:

- Reason patient is on isolation precautions
- Use of the correct personal protective equipment (PPE) for the specific isolation type
- Precautions about bringing equipment into the patient's room
- Reporting abnormal findings and any high-risk behaviors (e.g., patient does not adhere to secretion control when coughing)
- Special precautions regarding individual patient needs such as transportation to diagnostic tests.

Equipment

PPE—gloves, gowns, masks, protective eyewear, or face shield—is determined by the type of isolation that is needed. Other patient care equipment depends on procedures performed in room (e.g., hygiene items; disposable blood pressure (BP) cuff, thermometer, and stethoscope; sharps container; soiled linen bag; and trash receptacle).

Steps

1. Assess patient's health history for isolation indications (e.g., tuberculosis [TB], diarrhea, major draining wound or purulent cough).
2. Review laboratory test results (e.g., wound culture; acid-fast bacillus [AFB] smears) to identify the type of microorganism for which the patient is isolated and whether the patient is immunocompromised.
3. Review agency policies and precautions necessary for the specific isolation system, and consider care measures you will perform and necessary equipment to use while in the patient's room.
4. Review nurses' notes or speak with colleagues regarding patient's emotional state and adjustment to isolation.
5. Determine whether patient has latex allergy to avoid sensitivity or allergic reaction. If allergy exists, refer to agency policy to provide full latex-free care.
6. Perform hand hygiene and prepare all equipment that you need to take into patient's room. In some cases, equipment remains in the room (stethoscope or BP cuff).
7. Prepare for entrance into isolation room. Ideally, before applying PPE, step into patient's room and stay by door. Introduce yourself and explain the care that you are providing. If this is not possible, apply PPE outside of room.
   a. Apply cover gown, being sure that it covers all outer garments. Pull sleeves down to wrist. Tie securely at neck and waist (see illustration).

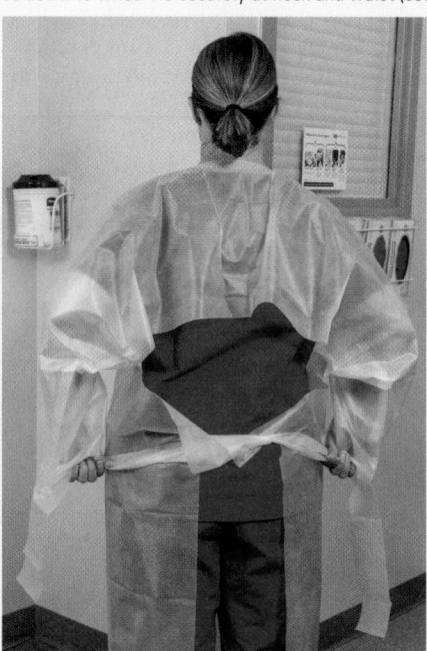

STEP 7a Tie gown at waist.

b. Apply either surgical mask or fitted respirator around mouth and nose. (Type depends on type of precautions and agency policy.) You must have a medical evaluation and be fit tested before using a respirator (OSHA, 2011).

c. If needed, apply eyewear, goggles, or face shield securely around face and eyes. If prescription glasses are worn, side shield may be used.

d. Apply clean gloves. (NOTE: Wear unpowdered latex-free gloves if you, patient, or another health care worker has a history of latex allergy.) Secure glove cuffs over edge of gown sleeves (see illustration).

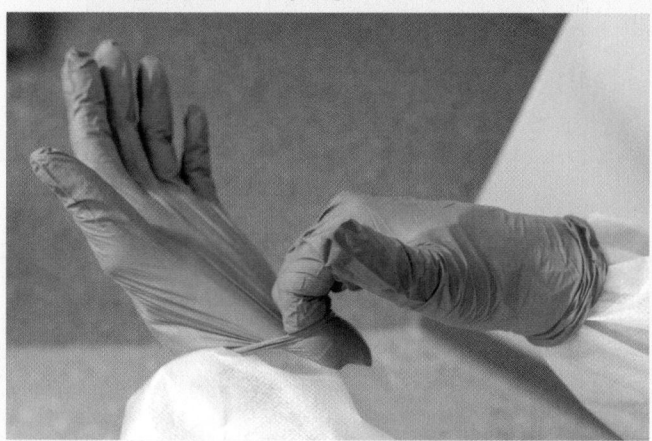

STEP 7d Apply gloves over gown sleeves.

8. Enter patient's room. Arrange supplies and equipment. (If equipment will be removed from room for reuse, place on clean paper towel.)
9. Identify patient using at least two identifiers (e.g., name and birthday, or name and medical record number) according to agency policy.
10. Assess patient's or family caregiver's knowledge, experience, and health literacy level.
11. Explain purpose of isolation and necessary precautions for patient and family to take. Offer opportunity to ask questions. Discuss types of activities patient may wish to do to try to stay occupied. Assess for evidence of emotional problems that can occur from isolation. If TB precautions are in use, instruct patient to cover mouth with tissue when coughing and to wear disposable surgical mask when leaving room.
12. Assess vital signs (see Chapter 29).
    a. If patient is infected or colonized with a resistant organism (e.g., vancomycin-resistant enterococci, methicillin-resistant *Staphylococcus aureus* or *Clostridium difficile*), use disposable equipment that remains in room. This includes thermometer, stethoscope, and BP cuff.
    b. If stethoscope is to be reused, clean diaphragm or bell with alcohol. Set aside on clean surface.
    c. Use individual electronic or disposable thermometer.

CLINICAL DECISION: If disposable thermometer indicates a fever, assess for other signs/symptoms. Confirm fever using an alternative thermometer. Do not use electronic thermometer if patient is suspected or confirmed to have *C. difficile* (Amitra et al., 2018).

13. Administer medications (see Chapter 31).
    a. Give oral medication in wrapper or cup.
    b. Dispose of wrapper or cup in plastic-lined receptacle.
    c. Wear gloves when administering an injection.
    d. Discard safety needle and syringe or uncapped needle into sharps container.
    e. Place reusable syringe (e.g., Carpujet) on a clean towel for eventual removal and disinfection.
    f. If you are not wearing gloves and hands come into contact with contaminated article or body fluids, perform hand hygiene as soon as possible.
14. Administer hygiene, encouraging patient to discuss questions or concerns about isolation. Provide informal teaching at this time.

BOX 28.13 **PROCEDURAL GUIDELINES—cont'd**

Caring for a Patient on Isolation Precautions

    a. Avoid allowing isolation gown to become wet. Carry wash basin out away from gown; avoid leaning against any wet surface.

    b. Help patient remove own gown; discard in leakproof linen bag.

    c. Remove linen from bed; avoid contact with isolation gown. Place in linen bag according to agency policy.

    d. Provide clean bed linen and a set of towels.

    e. Remove and dispose of gloves, perform hand hygiene, and reglove if further care is necessary.

15. Collect specimens.

    a. Place specimen containers on clean paper towel in patient's bathroom. Follow procedure for collecting specimen of body fluids.

    b. Transfer specimen to container without soiling outside of container. Label specimen in front of patient. All specimen containers must be placed in a double-sided, self-sealing polythene bag with one compartment containing the laboratory request form and the other the specimen (Nukifora, 2015).

    c. Perform hand hygiene and reglove if additional procedures are needed.

    d. Check label on specimen for accuracy. Send to laboratory. Be sure containers are labeled with a biohazard label (see illustration).

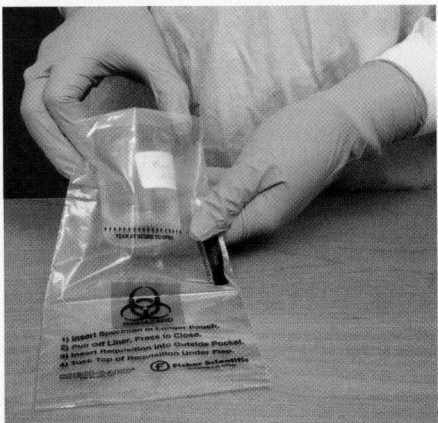

STEP 15d Specimen container placed in biohazard bag.

16. Assist patient to comfortable position. Place nurse call system in an accessible location within patient's reach. Instruct patient in its use.

17. Raise side rails (as appropriate) and lower bed to lowest position.

18. Dispose of linen, trash, and disposable items.

    a. Empty trash bag as it becomes full.

    b. Use sturdy, moisture-resistant single bags to contain soiled articles. Use double bag if outside of bag is contaminated.

    c. Tie bags securely at top in knot (see illustration).

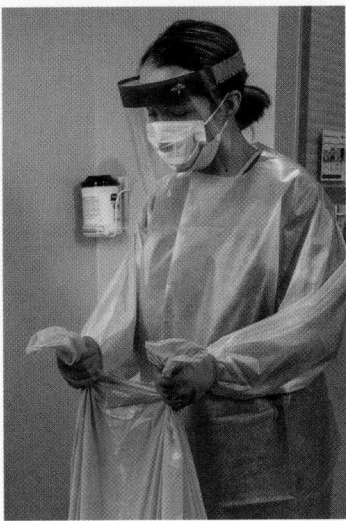

STEP 18c Tie trash bag securely.

19. Retrieve and clean nondedicated reusable equipment. Clean any contaminated surfaces (see health care agency policy).

20. Resupply room as needed. Have a staff member outside the isolation room hand you new supplies.

21. Explain to patient when you plan to return to room. Ask whether patient requires any personal care items, books, or magazines.

22. Leave isolation room. The order for removing PPE depends on what was needed for the type of isolation. The sequence listed is based on full PPE being required.

    a. Remove and dispose of gloves. Remove one glove by grasping cuff and pulling glove inside out over hand. With ungloved hand tuck finger inside cuff of remaining glove and pull it off, inside out (see illustration).

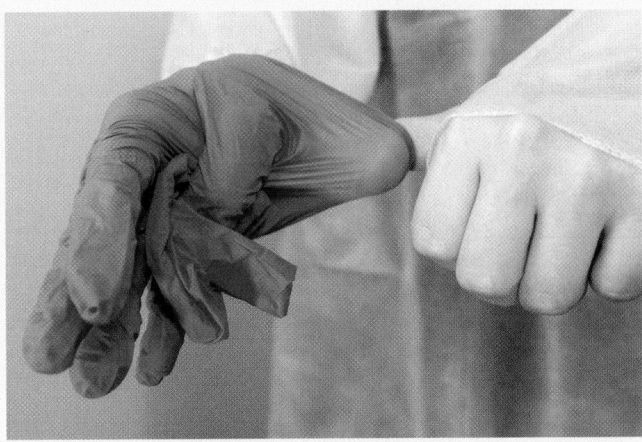

STEP 22a Remove glove.

    b. Remove eyewear/face shield or goggles.

    c. Untie waist and neck strings of gown. Allow gown to fall from shoulders. Remove hands from sleeves without touching outside of gown. Hold gown inside at shoulder seams and fold inside out. Discard in laundry bag if fabric or in trash can if gown is disposable.

    d. Remove mask: If mask loops over your ears, remove from ears and pull away from face. For a tie-on mask, untie *top* mask strings; hold strings; untie bottom strings, pull mask away from face, and drop it into trash receptacle. Do not touch outer surface of mask (see illustrations).

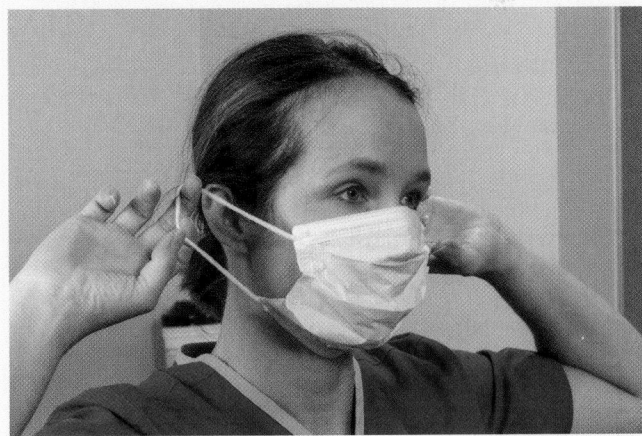

STEP 22d Remove mask.

    e. Perform hand hygiene.

    f. Leave room and close door if necessary. (Make sure that door is closed if patient is on airborne precautions.)

    g. Dispose of all contaminated supplies and equipment in a manner that prevents spread of microorganisms to other people (see health care agency policy).

BOX 28.14 Specimen Collection Techniques[a]

Ensure that all specimen containers used have the biohazard symbol on the outside (Pagana et al., 2018). Also follow agency policy in confirming proper labeling of all specimen containers (i.e., labeling in front of patient (TJC, 2020).

Wound Specimen

Perform hand hygiene and apply clean gloves. Clean site with sterile water or saline before wound specimen collection with a clean swab. Wipe from edges outward to remove old exudate (see Chapter 48). Remove and dispose of gloves, perform hand hygiene, and apply gloves and use sterile cotton-tipped swab or syringe to collect as much drainage as possible. Have clean test tube or culture tube on clean paper towel. After swabbing center of wound site, grasp collection tube with a paper towel. Carefully insert swab without touching outside of tube. After securing top of tube, label specimen container with patient name and identifying information, then transfer tube into labeled biohazard bag for transport and perform hand hygiene.

Blood Specimen

(This procedure is often performed by a laboratory technician.)

Wearing gloves, clean venipuncture site with antiseptic swab; move the first swab back and forth on horizontal plane, another swab on the vertical plane, and the last swab in a circular motion from site outward for 5 cm (2 inches), lasting a total of 30 seconds. Allow area to dry. Clean tops of culture bottles for 15 seconds with agency-approved cleansing solution. Use a 20-mL needle-safe syringe and collect up to 10 to 15 mL of blood per culture bottle (check health care agency policy). Perform venipuncture at two different sites to decrease likelihood of both specimens being contaminated with skin flora. Place blood culture bottles on a clean paper towel on bedside table or other surface; swab off bottle tops with alcohol. Inject an appropriate amount of blood into each bottle. If collecting aerobic and anaerobic specimens, inject blood into the aerobic bottle first and the anaerobic bottle second. Transfer labeled specimen into clean, labeled biohazard bag for transport. Remove and dispose of gloves and perform hand hygiene.

Stool Specimen

Wearing gloves, use clean cup with seal top (need not be sterile) and a tongue blade to collect a small amount, approximately 2 to 3 cm (1 inch) of stool. Place cup on clean paper towel in patient's bathroom. Using tongue blade, collect needed amount of feces from patient's bedpan. Transfer feces to cup without touching outside surface of cup. Dispose of tongue blade and place seal on cup. Transfer labeled specimen into clean labeled biohazard bag for transport. Remove and dispose of gloves and perform hand hygiene.

Urine Specimen

Apply gloves, cleanse needleless port on urinary catheter and, using a needleless safety syringe, collect 1 to 5 mL of urine. Fill sterile specimen tube and place on clean towel in patient's bathroom. Instruct patient to follow procedure to obtain a clean voided specimen (see Chapter 46) if not catheterized. Secure top of transfer container, label container in front of patient, and place in a biohazard bag with label attached. Remove and dispose of gloves and perform hand hygiene.

[a]Health care agency policies may differ on types of containers and amounts of specimen material required.

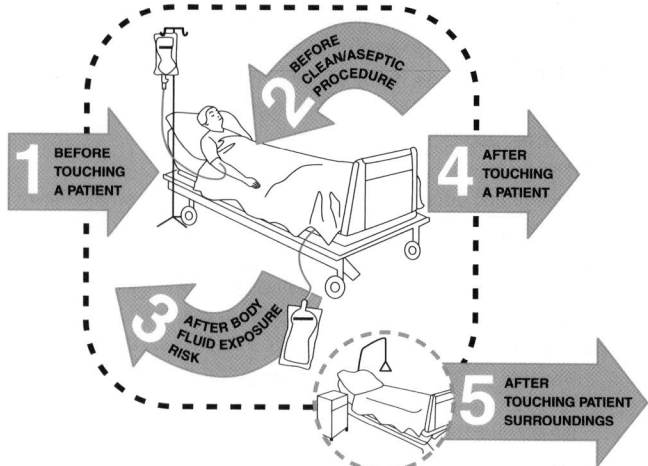

FIG. 28.4 Five Moments for Hand Hygiene. (From World Health Organization: *About SAVE Lives: Clean Your Hands: 5 moments for hand hygiene,* 2017, http://www.who.int/gpsc/5may/background/5moments/en/.)

WHO recently released a new initiative for improving adherence of health care workers to hand hygiene. The WHO's Five Moments for Hand Hygiene has emerged from the WHO Guidelines on Hand Hygiene in Health Care to add value to any hand hygiene improvement strategy (WHO, 2019b). The Five Moments defines the key moments for hand hygiene, overcoming misleading language and complicated descriptions (Fig. 28.4).

Patient Education. Often patients need to learn to use infection prevention and control practices at home (Box 28.15). Preventive technique becomes almost second nature to the nurse who practices it daily. However, patients are less aware of factors that promote the spread of infection or ways to prevent its transmission. The home environment may not always lend itself to infection prevention and control. Often you help a patient adapt according to the resources available to maintain hygienic techniques. Generally, patients in a home care setting have a decreased risk of infection because of decreased exposure to resistant organisms such as those found in a health care setting and fewer invasive procedures. However, it is important to educate patients and their family caregivers about infection prevention and control techniques.

Surgical Asepsis. Surgical asepsis or sterile technique prevents contamination of an open wound, serves to isolate an operative or procedural area from an unsterile environment, and maintains a sterile field for surgery or procedural intervention. Surgical asepsis includes procedures used to eliminate all microorganisms, including pathogens and spores, from an object or area (Chetan, 2018). In surgical asepsis an area or object is considered contaminated if touched by any object that is not sterile. It demands the highest level of aseptic technique and requires that all areas be kept free of infectious microorganisms.

Use surgical asepsis in the following situations:

- During procedures that require intentional perforation of the patient's skin, such as insertion of peripheral IV catheters or a central IV line
- When the integrity of the skin is broken as a result of trauma, surgical incision, or burns
- During invasive procedures, such as the insertion of a urinary catheter or the insertion of surgical instruments into sterile body cavities (e.g., placement of a wound drain)

Infection Prevention and Control for Hospital Personnel.

Health care workers are continually at risk for exposure to infectious microorganisms. Numerous efforts have been made by health care agencies to improve health care provider adherence to hand hygiene, including increased access to automatic alcohol-based hand sanitizers, posted reminders, and sensor monitoring of sanitizer use. The

BOX 28.15 Patient Teaching

Infection Prevention and Control

Objective

- Patient and/or caregiver will use proper infection prevention and control practices when performing a clean dressing change.

Teaching Strategies

- Demonstrate proper hand hygiene, explaining that patient and/or caregiver needs to perform it before and after all treatments and when infected body fluids are contacted.
- Instruct patient and/or caregiver about the signs and symptoms of wound infection and when to notify the health care provider.
- Instruct patient and/or caregiver to place contaminated dressings and other disposable items containing infectious body fluids in impervious plastic or brown paper bags. Place needles in metal or hard plastic containers, such as coffee cans or laundry detergent bottles, and tape the openings shut. *Some states have specific requirements for sharps disposal. Check local regulations.*
- Instruct patient and/or caregiver to separate linen soiled with wound drainage from other laundry. Wash in warm water with detergent. There are no special recommendations for setting a dryer temperature (CDC, 2007).

Evaluation

Use the principles of teach-back to evaluate patient/family caregiver learning:

- Tell me how what you will do to decrease the transmission of infection at home. Show me how you do hand hygiene before the dressing change.
- Show me how you would change your dressing.
- Tell me three signs or symptoms of wound infection that you will watch for. Tell me the signs and symptoms that you might develop that would require you to call your health care provider.

Although surgical asepsis is common in the operating room, labor and delivery area, and major diagnostic/procedural areas, you also use surgical aseptic techniques at the patient's bedside (e.g., when inserting IV or urinary catheters, suctioning the tracheobronchial airway, and sterile dressing changes). A nurse in an operating room follows a series of steps to maintain sterile technique, including applying a mask, protective eyewear, and a cap; performing a surgical hand scrub; and applying a sterile gown and gloves. In contrast, a nurse performing a dressing change at a patient's bedside only performs hand hygiene and applies sterile gloves. For certain procedures (e.g., changing a central line dressing) the nurse also uses a mask and gown (see agency policy). Regardless of the procedures followed or the setting, the nurse always recognizes the importance of strict adherence to aseptic principles (Iwamoto and Post, 2018).

Patient Preparation for a Sterile Procedure. Because surgical asepsis requires exact techniques, you need to have the patient's full cooperation. Therefore, assess a patient's understanding of the sterile procedure, and explain the reasons for not moving or interfering with the procedure. Certain patients fear moving or touching objects during a sterile procedure, whereas others try to help. Explain how you will perform a procedure and what the patient can do to avoid contaminating sterile items, including the following:

- Avoid sudden movements of body parts covered by sterile drapes.
- Refrain from touching sterile supplies, drapes, or the nurse's gloves and gown.
- Avoid coughing, sneezing, or talking over a sterile area.

Certain sterile procedures last an extended time. Assess a patient's needs and anticipate factors that may disrupt a procedure. If a patient

is in pain, administer ordered analgesics about a half an hour before a sterile procedure begins. Ask a patient whether he or she needs to use the bathroom or a bedpan. Often patients have to assume relatively uncomfortable positions during sterile procedures. Help a patient assume the most comfortable position possible. Finally, a patient's condition sometimes results in actions or events that contaminate a sterile field. For example, a patient with a respiratory infection transmits organisms by coughing or talking. Anticipate such a problem and place a surgical mask on him or her before the procedure begins.

Principles of Surgical Asepsis. Performing sterile aseptic procedures requires a work area in which objects can be handled with minimal risk of contamination. A sterile field provides a sterile surface for placement of sterile equipment. It is an area considered free of microorganisms and consists of a sterile kit or tray, a work surface draped with a sterile towel or wrapper, or a table covered with a large sterile drape (Murphy, 2018). When beginning a surgically aseptic procedure, nurses follow certain principles to ensure maintenance of asepsis. Failure to follow these principles places patients at risk for infection. The following principles are important:

1. *A sterile object remains sterile only when touched by another sterile object.* This principle guides a nurse in placement of sterile objects and how to handle them.
    a. Sterile touching sterile remains sterile (e.g., use sterile gloves or sterile forceps to handle objects on a sterile field).
    b. Sterile touching clean becomes contaminated (e.g., if the tip of a syringe or other sterile object touches the surface of a clean disposable glove, the object is contaminated).
    c. Sterile touching contaminated becomes contaminated (e.g., when a nurse touches a sterile object with an ungloved hand, the object is contaminated).
    d. Sterile state is questionable (e.g., when you find a tear or break in the covering of a sterile object). Discard it regardless of whether the object itself appears untouched.
2. *Only sterile objects may be placed on a sterile field.* All items are properly sterilized before use. Sterile objects are kept in clean, dry storage areas. The package or container holding a sterile object must be intact and dry. A package that is torn, punctured, wet, or open is considered unsterile.
3. *A sterile object or field out of the range of vision or an object held below a person's waist is contaminated.* Nurses never turn their back on a sterile field or tray or leave it unattended. Contamination can occur accidentally by a dangling piece of clothing or an unknowing patient touching a sterile object. Any object held below waist level is considered contaminated because it cannot always be viewed. Keep sterile objects in front with the hands as close together as possible.
4. *A sterile object or field becomes contaminated by prolonged exposure to air.* Avoid activities that create air currents such as excessive movements or rearranging linen after a sterile object or field becomes exposed. When you open sterile packages, it is important to minimize the number of people walking into an area. Microorganisms also travel by droplet through the air. Do not talk, laugh, sneeze, or cough over a sterile field or when gathering and using sterile equipment. When opening sterile packages, hold the item or piece of equipment as close as possible to the sterile field without touching the sterile surface.
5. When a sterile surface comes in contact with a wet, contaminated surface, the sterile object or field becomes contaminated by capillary action. If moisture leaks through the protective covering of a sterile package, microorganisms travel to the sterile object. When stored sterile packages become wet, discard the objects immediately or send the equipment for resterilization. When working with a sterile field or tray, you may have to pour sterile solutions. Any spill is a

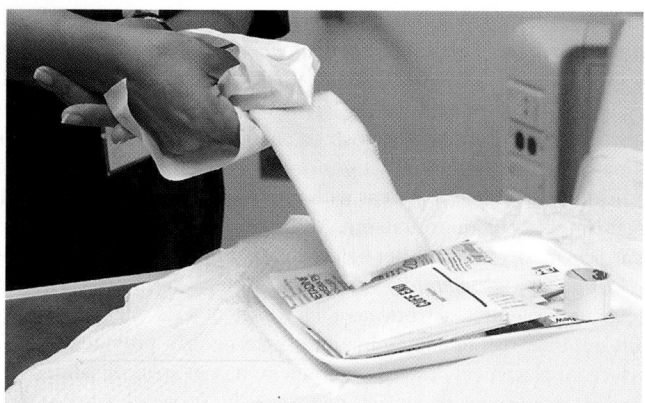

FIG. 28.5 Placing sterile item on sterile field.

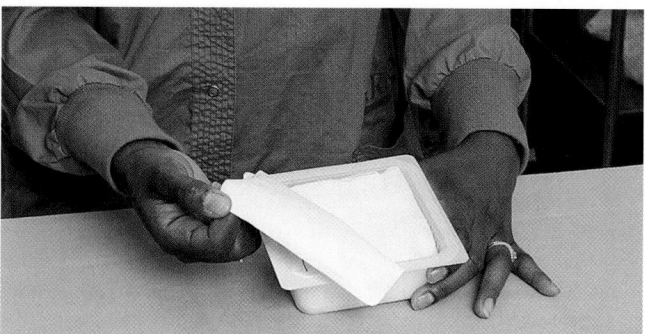

FIG. 28.6 Nurse opens sterile package on work area above waist level.

source of contamination unless on a sterile surface that moisture cannot penetrate. Urinary catheterization trays contain sterile supplies that rest in a sterile, plastic container. In contrast, if you place a piece of sterile gauze in its wrapper on a patient's bedside table and the table surface is wet, the gauze is considered contaminated.

6. *Fluid flows in the direction of gravity.* A sterile object becomes contaminated if gravity causes a contaminated liquid to flow over the surface of the object. To avoid contamination during a surgical hand scrub, hold your hands above your elbows. This allows water to flow downward without contaminating your hands and fingers. The principle of water flow by gravity is also the reason for drying from fingers to elbows, with hands held up, after the scrub.

7. *The edges of a sterile field or container are considered to be contaminated.* Frequently you place sterile objects on a sterile towel, drape, or tray (Fig. 28.5). Because the edge of the drape touches an unsterile surface such as a table or bed linen, a 2.5-cm (1-inch) border around the drape is considered contaminated. Objects placed on the sterile field need to be *inside* this border. The edges of sterile containers become exposed to air after they are open and thus are contaminated. After you remove a sterile needle from its protective cap or forceps from a container, the objects must not touch the edge of the container.

Performing Sterile Procedures. Assemble all the equipment that will be needed before a procedure. Have a few extra supplies available in case objects accidentally become contaminated. Do not leave a sterile area, because you will not know if the area was contaminated during your absence. Before a sterile procedure, explain each step so that the patient can cooperate fully. If an object becomes contaminated during the procedure, do not hesitate to discard it immediately.

Donning and Removing Caps, Masks, and Eyewear. Wear a surgical mask and eyewear without a cap for any sterile procedures on a general nursing unit. Eyewear is worn as a part of Standard Precautions if there is a risk of fluid or blood splashing into your eyes. For sterile surgical procedures, you first apply a clean cap that covers all your hair and then the surgical mask and eyewear. A mask must fit snugly around the face and nose. After wearing a mask for several hours, the area over the mouth and nose often becomes moist. Because moisture promotes the growth of microorganisms, change the mask if it becomes moist.

Protective glasses or goggles fit snugly around the forehead and face to fully protect the eyes. Wear eyewear only for procedures that create the risk of body fluids splashing into the eyes. Remove PPE in the following order: gloves, face shield or goggles, gown, and mask or respirator (CDC, 2005b). After removing all PPE, perform hand hygiene.

Opening Sterile Packages. Sterile items such as syringes, gauze dressings, or catheters are packaged in paper or plastic containers and are impervious to microorganisms as long as they are dry and intact.

These items have expiration labels on the packages. Do not use an item after the expiration date. Some institutions wrap reusable supplies (e.g., operating room instruments) in a double thickness of paper, linen, or muslin. These packages are permeable to steam and thus allow for steam autoclaving. Sterile items are kept in clean, enclosed storage cabinets and separated from dirty equipment.

Sterile supplies that have been autoclaved have chemical tapes indicating that a sterilization process has taken place. The tapes change color during the process. Failure of the tapes to change color means that the item is not sterile. Health care agencies follow the principles of event-related sterility, a concept that items are considered sterile if the packaging is uncompromised (Jefferson and Young, 2018). Never use a sterile item if the packaging is open or soiled, shows evidence that the package has been wet, or has dropped to the floor. Before opening a sterile item, perform hand hygiene. Inspect the supplies for package integrity and sterility and assemble the supplies in the work area such as the bedside table or treatment room before opening packages. A bedside table or countertop provides a large, clean working area for opening items. Keep the work area above waist level. Do not open sterile supplies in a confined space where contamination might occur.

Opening a Sterile Item on a Flat Surface. You must open sterile packages without contaminating the contents. Commercially packaged items are usually designed so that you only have to tear away or separate the paper or plastic cover. Hold the item in one hand while pulling the wrapper away with the other (Fig. 28.6). Take care to keep the inner contents sterile before use. You may use a sterile wrapper from a commercial kit or a sterile paper or linen wrapper from an institutional pack to create a sterile field on which to work. Use the inner surface of the package (except for the 2.5-cm [1-inch] border around the edges) as a sterile field to add sterile items. You can grasp the 2.5-cm (1-inch) border to maneuver the field on a table surface (see Skill 28.2).

Opening a Sterile Item While Holding It. To open a small sterile item, hold the package in your nondominant hand while opening the top flap and pulling it away from you. Using the dominant hand, carefully open the sides and innermost flap away from the enclosed sterile item in the same order as opening a sterile item on a flat surface (see Skill 28.2). You open the item in a hand so that you can pass it to a person wearing sterile gloves or transfer it to a sterile field.

Preparing a Sterile Field. When performing sterile procedures, you need a sterile work area that provides room for handling and placing sterile items. A sterile field is an area free of microorganisms and prepared to receive sterile items. You prepare the field by using the inner surface of a sterile wrapper as the work surface or by using a sterile drape or dressing tray. After creating the surface for the sterile field, add sterile items by placing them directly on the field or transferring them with sterile forceps (see Skill 28.2). Discard an object that comes in contact with the 2.5-cm (1-inch) border.

BOX 28.16 Hepatitis B Vaccination and Postexposure Follow-Up After Hepatitis C and Human Immunodeficiency Virus Exposure

- Health care employers shall make available the hepatitis B vaccine and vaccination series to all employees who may have occupational exposures. If an employee declines the vaccine, he or she must sign a declination form. Evaluation and follow-up care is available to all employees who have been exposed.
- Hepatitis B vaccinations are made available to employees within 10 working days of assignment—this means before starting to provide patient care and after receiving education and training on the vaccine.
- A blood test (titer) is offered in some facilities 1 to 2 months after completing the three-dose vaccine series (check the health care agency policy).
- Vaccine is offered at no cost to employees. At present the vaccine does not require any boosters.
- After exposure no treatment is needed if there is a positive blood titer on file. If no positive titer is on file, follow CDC guidelines.

Exposure to Hepatitis C Virus
- If the source patient is positive for hepatitis C virus (HCV), the employee receives a baseline test.
- At 4 weeks after exposure the employee should be offered an HCV-RNA test to determine whether he or she contracted HCV.
- If positive, the employee starts treatment.
- There is no prophylactic treatment for HCV after exposure.
- Early treatment for infection can prevent chronic infection.

Exposure to Human Immunodeficiency Virus
- If the patient is positive for human immunodeficiency virus (HIV) infection, a viral load study should be performed to determine the amount of virus present in the blood.
- If the exposure meets the CDC criteria for HIV PEP, it should be started as soon as possible, preferably within 24 hours after the exposure (CDC, 2013c).

  All medical evaluations and procedures, including the vaccine and vaccination series and evaluation after exposure (prophylaxis), are made available at no cost to at-risk employees.

  A confidential written medical evaluation will be available to employees with exposure incidents.

CDC, Centers for Disease Control and Prevention; *RNA,* ribonucleic acid; *PEP,* postexposure prophylaxis.
From Occupational Safety and Health Administration: Occupational Safety and Health Act of 2001, 2001, 2005, http://www.cdc.gov.

Sometimes you will wear sterile gloves while preparing items on a sterile field. If you do this, you can touch the entire drape, but sterile items must be handed over by an assistant. The gloves cannot touch the wrappers of sterile items.

Pouring Sterile Solutions. Often you need to pour sterile solutions into sterile containers. A bottle containing a sterile solution is sterile on the inside and contaminated on the outside; the neck of the bottle is also contaminated, but the inside of the bottle cap is considered sterile. After you remove the cap or lid, hold it in your hand or place its sterile side (inside) up on a *clean* surface. This means that you can see the inside of the lid as it rests on the table surface. Never rest a bottle cap or lid on a sterile surface. The outer edge of the cap is unsterile and contaminates the surface. Placing a sterile cap down on an unsterile surface increases the chances of the inside of the cap becoming contaminated.

Hold the bottle with its label in the palm of the hand to prevent the possibility of the solution wetting and fading the label. Keep the edge of the bottle away from the edge or inside of the receiving container. Pour the solution slowly to avoid splashing the underlying drape or field. Never hold the bottle so high above the container that even slow pouring causes splashing. Hold the bottle outside the edge of the sterile field. Any remaining fluids should be discarded. The edge of a container is considered contaminated after the contents have been poured. Reuse of open containers may contaminate solutions due to drops contacting unsterile areas and then running back over container openings (AORN, 2019).

Surgical Scrub. Patients undergoing operative procedures are at an increased risk for infection. Nurses working in operating rooms perform surgical hand antisepsis (see Skill 28.3) to decrease and suppress the growth of skin microorganisms under gloved hands in case of glove tears. A surgical hand scrub must eliminate the transient flora and reduce the resident flora on the hands. For maximum elimination of bacteria, remove all jewelry and keep the nails clean and short. Do not wear chipped nail polish, artificial nails, or extenders because they often hold a greater number of bacteria (AORN, 2019; WHO, 2009). Nurses who have active skin infections, open lesions or cuts, or respiratory infections should be excluded from the surgical or procedure team.

During surgical hand antisepsis the nurse scrubs from fingertips to elbows with an antiseptic soap before each surgical procedure. Research studies vary on the optimum duration of a surgical hand scrub (WHO, 2009). Chlorhexidine gluconate has been found to be more effective than povidone-iodine as a cleansing agent, although both can be found in health care agencies. Thus, the type of product used for cleansing will influence the time required for hand antisepsis (CDC, 2008; WHO 2009). The traditional scrub time in the United States for both the initial and the subsequent scrub is 5 minutes, but research has shown effectiveness can be gained when scrubs are performed for 2, 3, and 6 minutes (WHO, 2009). Follow the manufacturer recommendation for scrub solutions. For many years preoperative handwashing protocols required nurses to scrub with a brush. However, this practice damages the skin. Scrubbing with a disposable sponge or combination sponge-brush reduces bacterial counts on the hands as effectively as scrubbing with a brush. However, several studies suggest that neither a brush nor a sponge is necessary to reduce bacterial counts on the hands, especially when using an alcohol-based product (CDC, 2008).

Applying Sterile Gloves. Sterile gloves are an additional barrier to bacterial transfer. There are two gloving methods: open and closed. Nurses who work on general nursing units use open gloving before procedures such as dressing changes or urinary catheter insertions. The glove cuffs are placed over a gown sleeve (when worn). The closed-gloving method, which you perform after applying a sterile gown, is practiced in operating rooms and special procedure areas (see Skills 28.4 and 28.5). In this case, the glove cuffs remain under the surgical gown cuffs. Make sure to select the proper glove size; the glove should not stretch so tightly that it can tear easily, yet it must be tight enough that you can pick up objects easily.

Donning a Sterile Gown. Nurses wear sterile gowns when assisting at the sterile field in the operating room, delivery room, and special procedure areas. It allows the nurse to handle sterile objects and also be comfortable with less risk of contamination. The sterile gown acts as a barrier to decrease shedding of microorganisms from skin surfaces into the air and thus prevents wound contamination. Nurses caring for patients with large open wounds or assisting health care providers during major invasive procedures (e.g., inserting an arterial catheter) also wear sterile gowns. The circulating nurse generally does not wear one.

The nurse does not apply a sterile gown until after applying a mask and surgical cap and completing surgical handwashing. He or she picks up the gown from a sterile pack, or an assistant hands the gown to the nurse. Only a certain portion of the gown (i.e., the area from the anterior waist to, but not including, the collar and the anterior surface of the sleeves) is considered sterile. The back of the gown, the area under the arms, the collar, the area below the waist, and the underside of the sleeves are not sterile because the nurse cannot keep these areas in constant view and ensure their sterility (see Skill 28.4).

Exposure Issues. Patients and health care personnel, including housekeepers and maintenance personnel, are at risk for acquiring infections from accidental needlesticks. In the past, a stray needle lying in bed linen or carelessly thrown into a wastebasket served as a prime source for exposure to bloodborne pathogens. With the passage of the Needlestick Safety and Prevention Act in 2000 (OSHA, 2012b) and the implementation of safety needle devices, the incidence rate of sharps injuries has decreased. All sharps must now be either needle safe or needleless. After administering an injection or inserting an IV catheter, place the used needle safety device in a puncture-resistant box (see Chapter 31). Sharps boxes must be at the site of use; this is an OSHA requirement (OSHA, 2012b).

HBV and HCV are the infections most commonly transmitted by contaminated needles (Box 28.16). Report any contaminated needlestick immediately. Additional criteria for exposure reporting include blood or other potentially infectious materials (OPIMs) that come into direct contact with an open area of the skin, blood or OPIM that is splashed into a health care worker's eye or mouth or up the nose, and cuts with a sharp object that is covered with blood or OPIM.

Follow-up for risk of acquiring infection begins with source patient testing. Access to testing the source patient is stated in the testing law for each state. Some states have deemed consent, which means that the state has granted the patient's consent to be tested. Other states require that the patient consent to testing for the presence of bloodborne pathogens. Know the testing policies in the agency and state in which you practice. Health care agencies and workers' compensation require exposed employees to complete an injury report and seek appropriate treatment if needed. The need for treatment is linked to the results of a risk assessment and the testing of the patient. Test the patient for HIV, HBV, and HCV. If positive for HIV or HCV, testing for syphilis may be indicated because of the incidence of coinfection (CDC, 2015e). It is required that an exposed employee be given the patient's testing results. This is *not* a violation of the Health Insurance Portability and Accountability Act (HIPAA) of 1996. Both the CDC and OSHA state that this information must be given to the exposed health care worker contingent on the health care worker's willingness to be tested.

Testing the exposed employee at the time of the exposure is not needed immediately unless required by the state testing law. If the patient tests positive for a bloodborne pathogen or if the source patient is unknown, prophylactic treatment is recommended for the employee.

Exposures also occur involving nonbloodborne pathogens. Airborne and droplet diseases pose a risk to the nonimmune nurse. The CDC (2016) has published a list of recommended immunizations and vaccinations for health care workers, including hepatitis B vaccine; TB testing; annual influenza vaccine; measles, mumps, and rubella (MMR); chickenpox vaccine; and tetanus, diphtheria, and pertussis. Employee health should review your health history and offer appropriate prevention. Declination forms are needed if these are declined (OSHA, 2011)

◆ Evaluation

Measure the success of infection prevention and control techniques by determining whether you achieved the goals for reducing or preventing infection. Document the patient's response to therapies for infection prevention and control. A clear description of any signs and symptoms of systemic or local infection is necessary to give all nurses a baseline for comparative evaluation.

Through the Patient's Eyes. Patients generally expect to be safe and protected when receiving health care. Ask patients about whether their expectations for care have been met. A patient at risk for infection needs to understand the measures needed to reduce or prevent microorganism growth and spread. Providing patients and/or family caregivers the opportunity to discuss infection prevention and control measures or to demonstrate procedures such as hand hygiene reveals their ability to adhere to therapy. Be sure that you understand the patient's perceptions of how infection spreads, his or her expectations for self-care, and how it can affect him or her as you evaluate the results of your instruction. Sometimes patients require new information, or previously instructed information needs reinforcement.

Patient Outcomes. A comparison of a patient's response before and after an infection control measure, such as the absence of fever or wound infection, is an example of an expected outcome for measuring the success of nursing interventions. Observe wounds during dressing changes to determine the degree of wound healing. Monitor patients, especially those at risk, for signs and symptoms of infection. For example, a patient who has undergone a surgical procedure is at risk for infection at the surgical site and other invasive sites such as the venipuncture site or central line sites. In addition, the patient is at risk for a respiratory tract infection as a result of decreased mobility and for a UTI if an indwelling catheter is present. Observe all invasive and surgical sites for swelling, erythema (redness), or purulent drainage. Monitor breath sounds for changes and observe sputum character for change in color or consistency. Review laboratory test results for leukocytes. For example, leukocytosis in the urine often indicates a UTI. The absence of signs or symptoms of infection is the expected outcome of infection prevention and control.

SAFETY GUIDELINES FOR NURSING SKILLS

Ensuring patient safety is an essential role of the professional nurse. To ensure patient safety, communicate clearly with members of the health care team, assess and incorporate the patient's priorities of care and preferences, and use the best evidence when making decisions about your patient's care. When performing the skills in this chapter, remember the following points to ensure safe, individualized patient care.

- Apply Standard Precautions when performing all nursing care activities.
- Use clean gloves when you anticipate contact with body fluids and nonintact skin or mucous membranes when there is a risk of drainage.

- Use gown, mask, and eye protection when there is a risk for splash.
- Keep bedside table surfaces clutter-free, clean, and dry when performing aseptic procedures.
- Clean all equipment that is shared between patients.
- Ensure that patients cover mouth and nose when coughing or sneezing, use tissues to contain respiratory secretions, and dispose of tissues in waste receptacle.

SKILL 28.1   HAND HYGIENE

Delegation and Collaboration

The skill of hand hygiene is performed by all caregivers. Hand hygiene is not optional.

Equipment

- Antiseptic hand rub
  - Alcohol-based waterless antiseptic
- Handwashing
  - Easy-to-reach sink with warm running water
  - Antimicrobial or regular soap
  - Paper towels
  - Disposable nail cleaner *(optional)*

STEP	RATIONALE
ASSESSMENT	
1. Inspect surface of hands for breaks or cuts in skin or cuticles. Cover any skin lesions with a dressing before providing care. If lesions are too large to cover, you may be restricted from direct patient care.	Open cuts or wounds can harbor high concentrations of microorganisms. Agency policy may prevent nurses from caring for high-risk patients if open lesions are present on hands (WHO, 2017).
2. Inspect hands for visible soiling.	Visible soiling requires handwashing with soap and water (CDC, 2017a).
3. Inspect condition of nails. Natural tips should be no longer than 0.625 cm (¼ inch) long. Be sure that fingernails are short, filed, and smooth.	Microorganisms can live under artificial nails after handwashing and using an alcohol-based sanitizer and should not be worn by health care providers having direct contact with patients (CDC, 2017b).
PLANNING	
1. Ensure that a filled hand sanitizer dispenser is available and/or a sink with running water and soap.	Having needed hand hygiene supplies readily available and visible increases hand hygiene adherence.
IMPLEMENTATION	
1. Push wristwatch and long uniform sleeves above wrists. Avoid wearing rings. If worn, remove during hand hygiene.	Provides complete access to fingers, hands, and wrists. The skin underneath jewelry may carry a higher bacterial count (AORN, 2019).
2. Antiseptic hand rub	
a. Following manufacturer directions, dispense ample amount of product into palm of one hand (see illustration).	Use enough product to cover hands thoroughly.
b. Rub hands together covering all surfaces of hands and fingers with antiseptic (see illustration).	Ensures even bacteriostatic action.
c. Rub hands together (approximately 20 seconds) until alcohol is dry. Allow hands to dry completely before applying gloves.	Provides enough time for product to work (CDC, 2017a).
3. Handwashing using regular or antimicrobial soap:	
a. Stand in front of sink, keeping hands and uniform away from sink surface. (If hands touch sink during handwashing, repeat sequence.)	Inside of sink is a contaminated area. Reaching over sink increases risk of touching edge, which is contaminated.
b. Turn on water. Turn on faucet (see illustration). It is best if sinks have knee, foot, or electronic sensor controls.	Knee pads within operating room and treatment areas are preferred to prevent hand contact with faucet. Faucet handles are likely to be contaminated with organic debris and microorganisms (AORN, 2019).
c. Avoid splashing water against uniform.	Microorganisms travel and grow in moisture.
d. Regulate flow of water so that temperature is warm.	Warm water removes less of protective oils on hands than hot water.
e. Wet hands and wrists thoroughly under running water. Keep hands and forearms lower than elbows during washing.	Hands are most contaminated parts to wash. Water flows from least to most contaminated area, rinsing microorganisms into sink.
f. Apply the amount of antiseptic soap recommended by the manufacturer and rub hands together (see illustration).	Ensure that all surfaces of hands and fingers are cleaned.

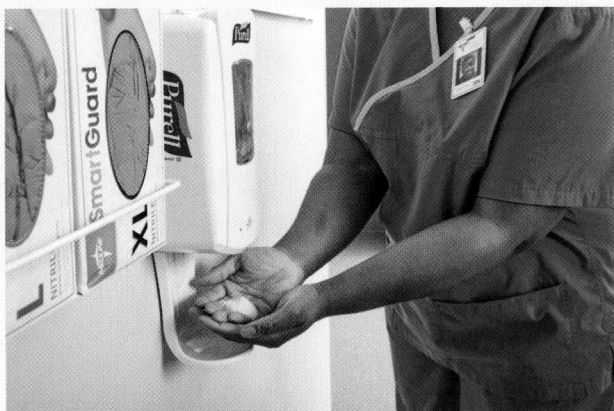

STEP 2a Apply waterless antiseptic to hands.

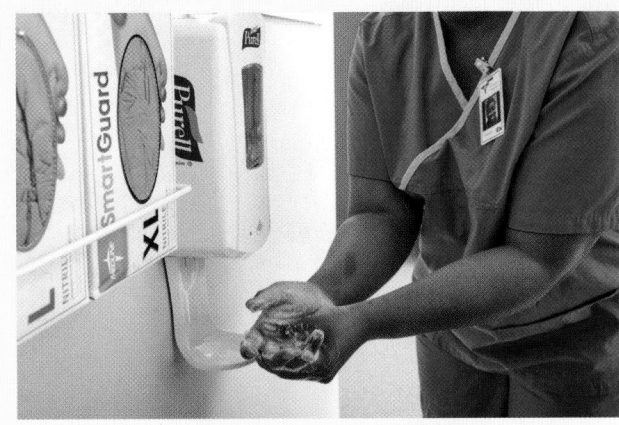

STEP 2b Rub hands thoroughly.

Continued

SKILL 28.1   HAND HYGIENE—cont'd

STEP	RATIONALE

CLINICAL DECISION: *The decision whether to use an antiseptic soap or an alcohol-based hand rub depends on whether the hands are visibly soiled, the type of infectious microorganism, the procedure you will perform, and the patient's immune status.*

g. Perform hand hygiene using plenty of lather and friction for at least 15 seconds. Interlace fingers and rub palms and back of hands with circular motion at least five times each. Keep fingertips down to facilitate removal of microorganisms.

Soap cleans by emulsifying fat and oil and lowering surface tension. Friction and rubbing mechanically loosen and remove dirt and transient bacteria. Interlacing fingers and thumbs ensures that all surfaces are cleaned. Adequate time is needed to expose skin surfaces to antimicrobial agent.

h. Areas underlying fingernails are often soiled. Clean them with fingernails of other hand and additional soap or with disposable nail cleaner.

Area under nails can be highly contaminated, which increases risk for transmission of infection from nurse to patient.

i. Rinse hands and wrists thoroughly, keeping hands down and elbows up (see illustration).

Rinsing mechanically washes away dirt and microorganisms.

j. Dry hands thoroughly from fingers to wrists with paper towel or single-use cloth.

Drying from cleanest (fingertips) to least clean (wrist) avoids contamination. Drying hands prevents chapping and roughened skin. Do not tear or cut skin under or around nail.

k. If paper towel is used, discard in proper receptacle.

Prevents transfer of microorganisms.

l. To turn off hand faucet, use clean, dry paper towel; avoid touching handles with hands (see illustration). Turn off water with foot or knee pedals (if applicable).

Wet towel and hands allow transfer of pathogens from faucet by capillary action.

m. If hands are dry or chapped, use small amount of lotion or barrier cream.

Helps to minimize skin dryness. Only use lotions or creams approved by your health care agency as they have been selected to not interact with hand sanitizing products (CDC, 2017a).

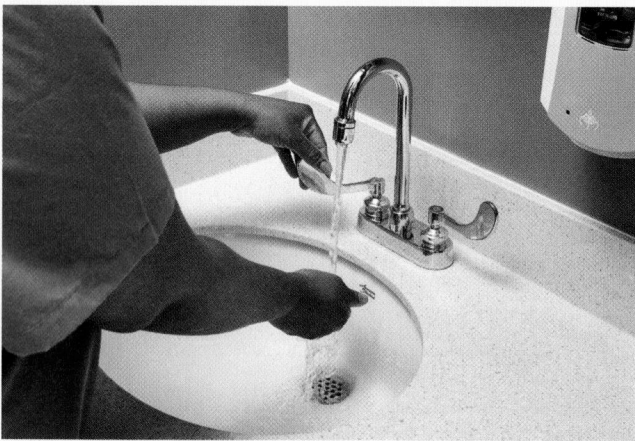

STEP 3b Turn on water.

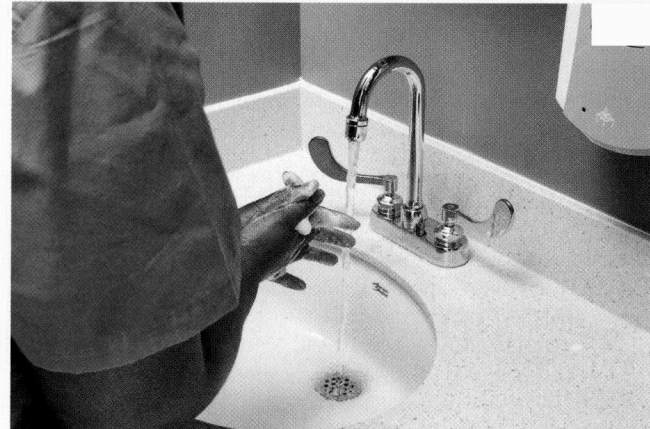

STEP 3f Lather hands thoroughly.

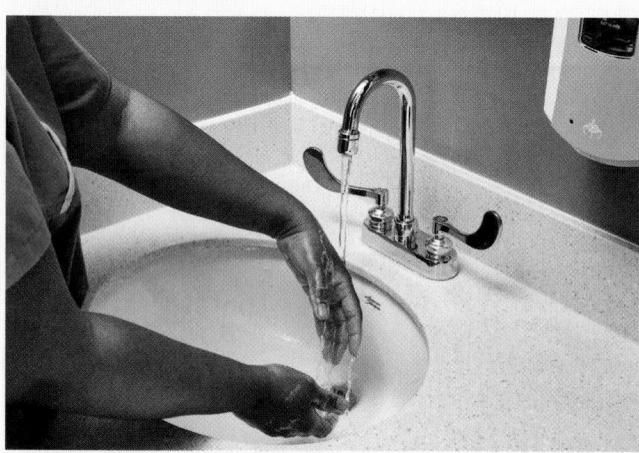

STEP 3i Rinse hands.

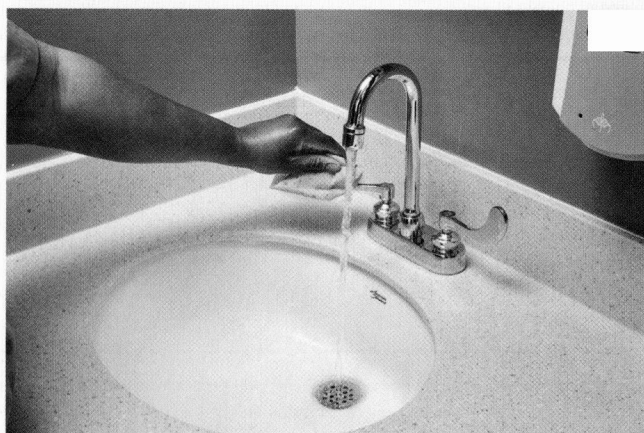

STEP 3l Turn off faucet.

STEP	**RATIONALE**

EVALUATION

1. Inspect surface of hands for obvious signs of dirt or other contaminants.
2. Inspect hands for dermatitis or cracked skin.

Determines if hand hygiene is adequate.
Breaks in skin integrity increase risk for transmission of microorganisms.

UNEXPECTED OUTCOMES AND RELATED INTERVENTIONS

1. Hands or areas under fingernails remain soiled.
   - Repeat handwashing with soap and water.
2. Repeated use of soaps or antiseptics causes dermatitis or cracked skin.
   - Rinse and dry hands thoroughly after using soap and water; avoid excessive amounts of soap or antiseptic; try various products.
   - Use approved hand lotions or barrier creams that will not interfere with hand sanitizing products (CDC, 2017a).

RECORDING AND REPORTING

- It is unnecessary to document handwashing.
- Report dermatitis, psoriasis, and/or cuts to your agency's employee health or infection control department.

HOME CARE CONSIDERATIONS

- Evaluate the handwashing facilities in a patient's home, including the availability of warm running water and soap, to determine the potential for contamination, how close the facilities are to the patient, and available supplies in the area.
- Anticipate the need for alternative handwashing products such as alcohol-based hand rubs and/or detergent-containing towels.
- Instruct the patient and primary caregiver in proper techniques and situations for handwashing. Use teach-back to confirm learning.

SKILL 28.2	**PREPARATION OF STERILE FIELD**	◗

Delegation and Collaboration

Nurses prepare sterile fields for some sterile procedures, such as urinary catheter insertion and performing tracheostomy care and suctioning, while other health care providers usually prepare sterile fields in the operating room (see agency's policy). The skill of preparing a sterile field cannot be delegated to assistive personnel (AP). The nurse can direct the AP to:

- Help with patient positioning and obtain any necessary supplies.

Equipment

- Sterile pack (commercial or facility wrapped)
- Sterile drape or kit that will be used as a sterile field
- Sterile gloves (if not included in kit)
- Sterile solution and equipment specific to procedure
- Waist-high table/countertop surface
- Appropriate personal protective equipment (PPE): gown, mask, cap, protective eyewear (see agency policy)

STEP	**RATIONALE**

ASSESSMENT

1. Identify patient using at least two identifiers (e.g., name and birthday or name and medical record number) according to agency policy.
2. Assess type of aseptic technique needed for procedure.
3. Assess patient's comfort, positioning, oxygen requirements, and elimination needs before preparing for procedure.

4. Assess patient for latex allergies.

5. Check sterile package integrity for punctures, tears, discoloration, moisture, or any other signs of contamination. Check the expiration date. Check sterile package for sterilization indicator (marker that changes color when exposed to heat or steam).
6. Anticipate supplies needed for procedure.

7. Assess patient's or family caregiver's knowledge, experience, and health literacy level.
8. Instruct patient (and family caregiver, if present) not to touch work surface or equipment during procedure.

Ensures correct patient. Complies with The Joint Commission standards and improves patient safety (TJC, 2020).
Some procedures require medical, whereas others require surgical aseptic technique.
Certain procedures requiring a sterile field may last a long time. Anticipates patient's needs so that patient can relax and avoid any unnecessary movement that might disrupt procedure.
A review of the patient's health history may reveal a latex allergy. Determine the need to use latex-free supplies.
Inspection of packaging ensures that sterile field is not contaminated (AORN, 2019).

Not all sterile kits contain sufficient amounts or types of supplies needed for all procedures. Failure to have the proper supplies may cause you to leave sterile field, increasing risk for contamination and potential need to set up another sterile field.
Ensures patient has the capacity to obtain, communicate, process, and understand basic health information (CDC, 2019).
Prevents contamination of sterile field. Promotes patient understanding and cooperation.

Continued

SKILL 28.2	PREPARATION OF STERILE FIELD—cont'd	

STEP	RATIONALE

PLANNING

1. Complete all other nursing interventions (e.g., medication administration, hygiene) before beginning procedure.

2. Suggest that visitors step out of room briefly during procedure. Discourage movement of staff assisting with procedure.

3. Provide privacy. Arrange equipment/supplies at bedside or in a location convenient to the procedure.

4. Position patient comfortably for specific procedure to be performed. If a body part is to be examined or treated, position patient so area is accessible. Have AP help with positioning as needed.

5. Provide an explanation of procedure.

Prepare sterile field as close as possible to time of use to reduce potential for contamination (AORN, 2019).

Traffic or movement can increase potential for contamination through spread of microorganisms by air currents.

Surgical preparation often includes full or partial skin exposure before draping. Ensures availability of equipment before procedure and prevents break in sterile technique. (**NOTE:** Povidone-iodine and chlorhexidine are not considered sterile solutions and require separate work surfaces for preparation).

Patient should be able to lie still in one position comfortably during procedure. Movement can disrupt the sterile field.

Preparing patient for procedure improves adherence and decreases patient stress.

IMPLEMENTATION

1. Perform hand hygiene (see Skill 28.1.)

2. Apply PPE as needed (check agency policy).

3. Select a clean, flat, dry work surface above waist level.

4. Prepare sterile work surface.
   a. Use sterile commercial kit or package containing sterile items.

   (1) Place sterile kit or package on the prepared work surface.

   (2) Open outside cover (see illustration) and remove package from dust cover. Place on work surface.

   (3) Grasp outer surface of tip of outermost flap.

   (4) Open outermost flap away from body, keeping arm outstretched and away from sterile field (see illustration).

   (5) Grasp outside surface of edge of first side flap.

   (6) Open side flap, pulling to side, allowing it to lie flat on table surface. Keep arm to side and not over sterile surface (see illustration).

   (7) Repeat Step (6) for second side flap (see illustration).

Hand hygiene reduces number of microorganisms on hands, thus reducing transmission to patient. Do not allow rinse water to run down arms onto clean hands (i.e., arms are considered dirty).

PPE controls microorganism transmission.

A dry surface is needed for a sterile field. A sterile object placed below a person's waist is considered contaminated.

Outside of kit is not sterile. Inner kit remains sterile.

Outer surface of package is considered unsterile. There is a 2.5-cm (1-inch) border around any sterile drape or wrap that is considered contaminated and can be touched with clean fingers.

Reaching over sterile field contaminates it.

Outer border is considered unsterile.

Drape or wrapper should lie flat, so it does not accidentally rise up and contaminate inner surface or sterile contents.

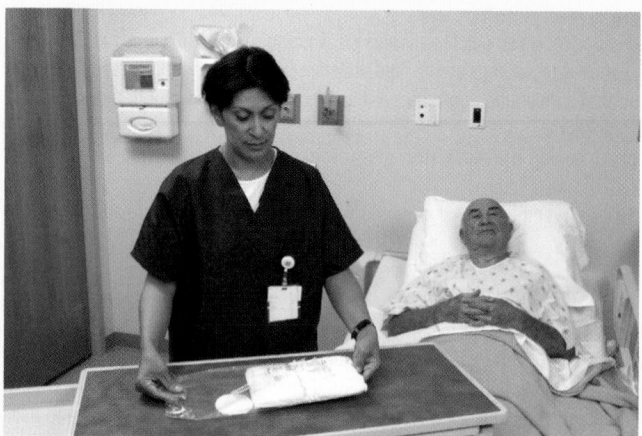

STEP 4a(2) Open outside cover of sterile kit.

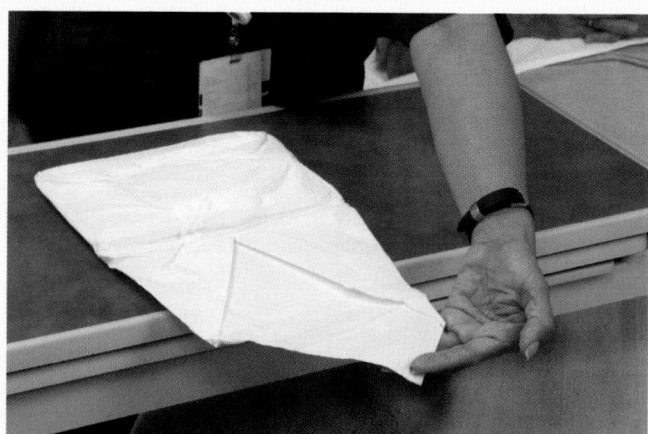

STEP 4a(4) Open outermost flap of sterile kit away from body.

STEP	RATIONALE

(8) Grasp outside border of last and innermost flap (see illustration). Stand away from sterile package and pull flap back, allowing it to fall flat on table. Kit is ready to be used.

Outer border is considered unsterile.
Never reach over a sterile field.

b. Open sterile linen-wrapped package.
   (1) Place package on clean, dry, flat work surface above waist level.
   (2) Remove sterilization tape seal and unwrap both layers following same steps (see Steps 4a [2] through 4a [8]) as for sterile kit (see illustration).
   (3) Use opened package wrapper as sterile field.

Sterile items placed below waist level are considered contaminated.
Linen-wrapped items have two layers. The first is a dust cover. The second layer must be opened to view sterilization indicator.

Inside of package wrapper is considered sterile.

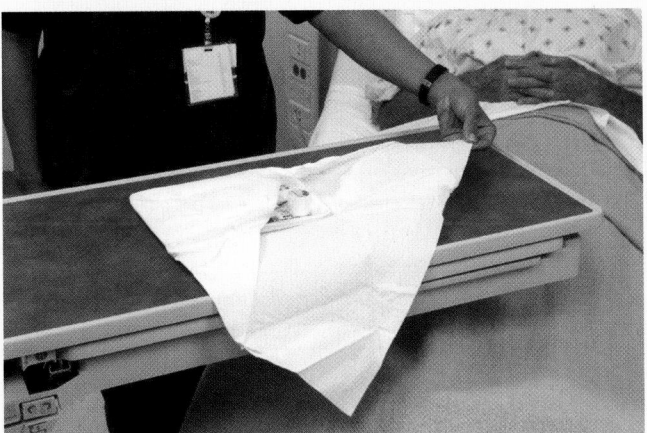

STEP 4a(6) Open first side flap, pulling to side.

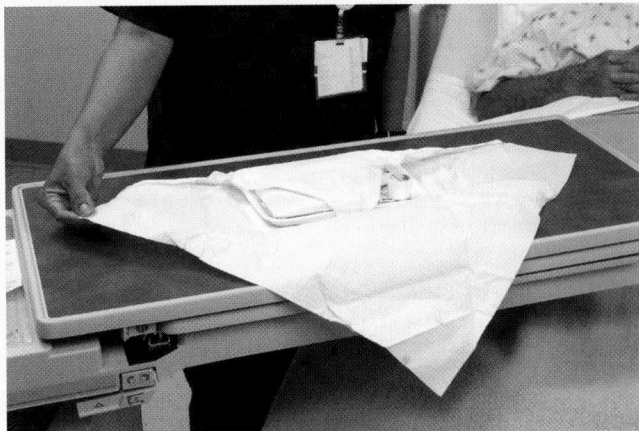

STEP 4a(7) Open second side flap, pulling to side.

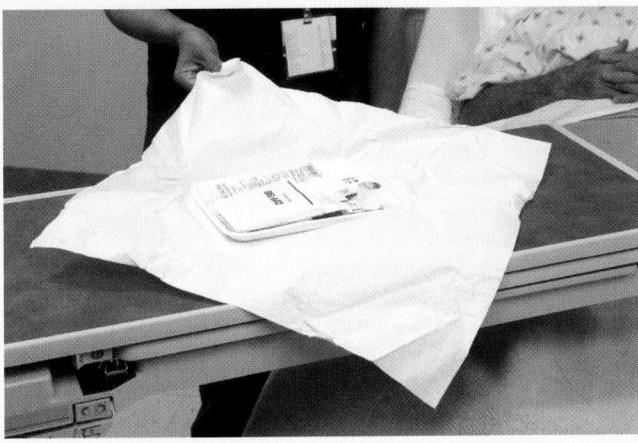

STEP 4a(8) Open Last and innermost flap.

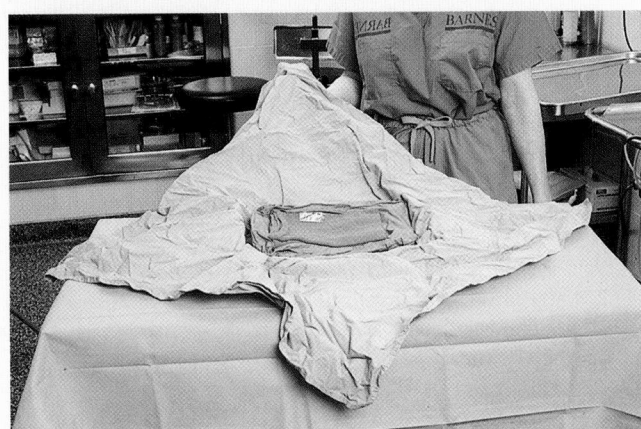

STEP 4b(2) Open sterile linen-wrapped package.

Continued

SKILL 28.2	PREPARATION OF STERILE FIELD—cont'd	◗

STEP	RATIONALE

   c. Prepare sterile drape.

      (1) Place pack containing sterile drape on flat, dry surface and open as described (see Steps 4a [2] through 4a[8]) for sterile package.

Packaged drape remains sterile.

      (2) Apply sterile gloves (*optional,* see agency policy). The outer 2.5-cm (1-inch) border of drape may be touched without wearing gloves.

Sterile object remains sterile only when touched by another sterile object. Gloves are not necessary as long as fingers grasp the 2.5-cm (1-inch) unsterile border of the drape.

      (3) Using fingertips of one hand, pick up folded top edge of drape along 2.5-cm (1-inch) border. Gently lift drape up from its wrapper without touching any object. Discard wrapper with other hand.

If sterile object touches any nonsterile object, it becomes contaminated.

      (4) With other hand, grasp an adjacent corner of drape and hold it straight up and away from body. Allow drape to unfold, keeping it above waist and work surface and away from body (see illustration).

An object held below a person's waist or above chest is contaminated. Drape can now be placed properly with two hands.

      (5) Holding drape, position bottom half over top half of intended work surface (see illustration).

Proper positioning prevents nurse from reaching over sterile field.

      (6) Allow top half of drape to be placed over bottom half of work surface (see illustration). Sterile field is ready to use.

Proper positioning creates flat, sterile work surface for placement of sterile supplies.

CLINICAL DECISION: *Use slow movements when setting up sterile drapes. Fast movements can stir up dust, lint, and infectious microorganisms, which can contaminate the sterile field.*

---

5. Add sterile items to sterile field.

   a. Open sterile item (following package directions) while holding outside wrapper in nondominant hand.

Use of nondominant hand frees dominant hand for unwrapping outer wrapper.

   b. Carefully peel wrapper over nondominant hand.

Item remains sterile. Inner surface of wrapper covers hand, making it sterile.

   c. Be sure that the wrapper does not fall onto the sterile field. Place the item onto the field at an angle (see illustration). **Do not hold arms over sterile field.**

Secured wrapper edges prevent flipping wrapper and contaminating contents of sterile field (AORN, 2019).
Skin is a source of bacteria and shedding.

   d. Dispose of outer wrapper.

Disposal prevents accidental contamination of sterile field.

6. Pour sterile solutions.

   a. Verify contents and expiration date of solution.

Verification ensures proper solution and sterility of contents.

   b. Place receptacle for solution near table/work surface edge. Sterile kits have cups or plastic molded sections into which fluids can be poured.

Proper placement prevents reaching over sterile field during pouring of solution.

   c. Remove sterile seal and cap from bottle in upward motion.

Upward movement prevents contamination of bottle lip.

   d. With solution bottle held away from field and bottle lip 2.5 to 5 cm (1 to 2 inches) above inside of sterile receiving container, slowly pour needed amount of solution into container. Hold bottle with label facing palm of hand (see illustration).

Edge and outside of bottle are considered contaminated. Slow pouring prevents splashing. Sterility of contents cannot be ensured if cap is replaced.
Prevents label from becoming wet and illegible.

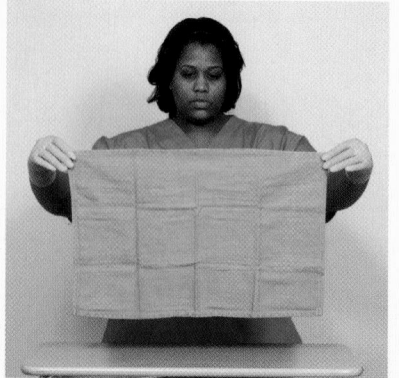

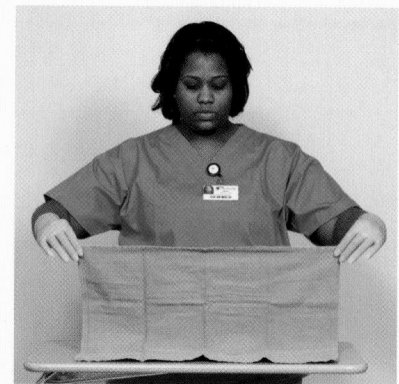

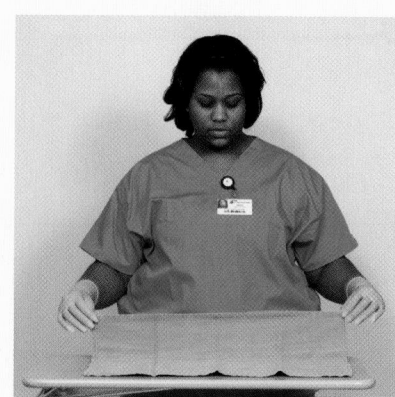

STEP 4c(4) Grasp corners of sterile drape, then hold up and away from body.

STEP 4c(5) Position bottom half of sterile drape over top half of work space.

STEP 4c(6) Allow top half of drape to be placed over bottom half of work surface.

CLINICAL DECISION: *When liquids permeate sterile field or barrier, it is called a strikethrough, resulting in contamination of the sterile field.*

7. Remove and dispose of gloves and perform hand hygiene.	Reduces transmission of infection.

EVALUATION

1. Observe for breaks in sterile technique throughout the procedure.	A break in sterile technique requires you to repeat the procedure.
2. **Use Teach-Back:** "I want to be sure I explained the procedure that I just performed and steps I took to prevent any infection. Please tell me in what way the procedure will help you." Revise your instruction now or develop a plan for revised patient/family caregiver teaching if patient/family caregiver is not able to teach back correctly.	Determines patient's/family caregiver's level of understanding of instructional topic.

UNEXPECTED OUTCOMES AND RELATED INTERVENTIONS

1. Sterile field comes in contact with contaminated object or liquid splatters onto drape, causing strikethrough.
   - Discontinue field preparation and start over with new equipment.
2. Sterile item falls off sterile field.
   - Open another package containing new sterile item and add to field. Apply a new pair of sterile gloves. If field becomes contaminated, a new sterile field needs to be established. Apply a new pair of sterile gloves.

RECORDING AND REPORTING

- Record the procedure performed and that sterile technique was used.
- Discuss with nurses and other pertinent health care providers the sterile procedure performed, outcome, patient's response, and any necessary follow-up. This assures quality continuation of care and provides for optimal patient outcomes.

SKILL 28.3	**SURGICAL HAND ASEPSIS**

Delegation and Collaboration

The skill of surgical hand asepsis can be delegated to properly trained surgical technicians (know the state Nurse Practice Act).

Equipment
- Deep sink with foot or knee controls for dispensing water and soap (faucets should be high enough for hands and forearms to fit comfortably)
- Antimicrobial agent approved by the health care agency
- Surgical scrub sponge with plastic nail pick *(optional)*
- Paper face mask, cap or hood, surgical shoe covers
- Sterile towel
- Sterile pack containing sterile gown
- Protective eyewear (glasses or goggles)

STEP	RATIONALE
1. Consult manufacturer policy regarding required length of time and antiseptic to use for hand antisepsis. Chlorhexidine has been found to be more effective than povidone iodine (WHO, 2009).	Guidelines vary regarding ideal time needed and antiseptic to use for surgical scrub. Most facilities in the United States follow 5 minutes for hand scrub (WHO, 2015).
2. Remove bracelets, rings, and watches.	Jewelry may harbor or protect microorganisms from removal. Allergic skin reactions may occur as a result of scrub agent or glove powder accumulating under jewelry (Association of Surgical Technologists [AST], 2017).
3. Be sure that fingernails are short, clean, and healthy. Artificial nails should be removed. Natural nails should be less than ¼ inch long from fingertip.	Long nails and chipped or old polish increase number of bacteria residing on nails. Long fingernails can puncture gloves, causing contamination. Artificial nails are known to harbor gram-negative microorganisms and fungus (AORN, 2019; CDC, 2008).

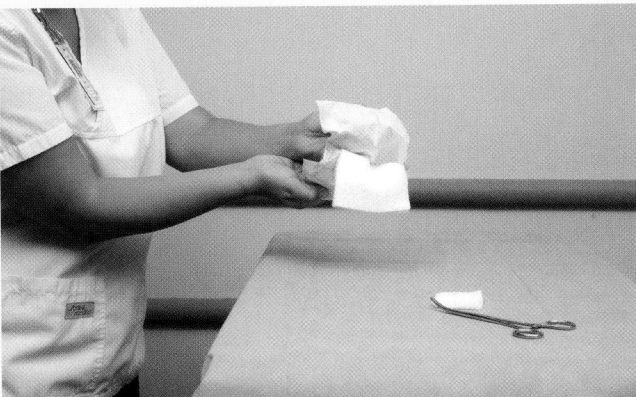

STEP 5c Add items to sterile field.

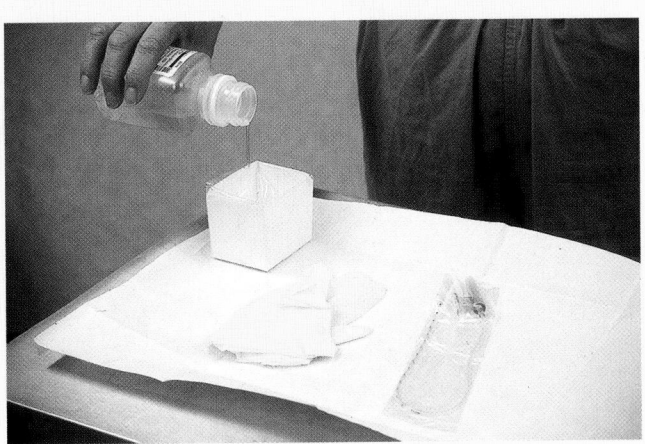

STEP 6d Pour solution into receiving container on sterile field.

Continued

SKILL 28.3	SURGICAL HAND ASEPSIS—cont'd
STEP	**RATIONALE**

CLINICAL DECISION: *Remove nail polish if chipped or worn longer than 4 days because it is likely to harbor microorganisms (AORN, 2019).*

STEP	RATIONALE
4. Inspect condition of cuticles, hands, and forearms for abrasions, cuts, or open lesions.	These conditions increase likelihood of more microorganisms residing on skin surfaces. Broken skin permits microorganisms to enter layers of the skin, providing deeper microbial breeding grounds (AORN, 2019).
5. Apply surgical shoe covers, cap or hood, face mask, and protective eyewear (depends on procedure; see agency policy).	Mask prevents escape into air of microorganisms that can contaminate hands. Other protective wear prevents exposure to blood and body fluid splashes during the procedure.
6. Turn on water using knee or foot controls and adjust to comfortable temperature.	Knee or foot controls prevent contamination of hands after scrub.
7. Prescrub wash/rinse: Wet hands and arms under running lukewarm water and lather with detergent to 5 cm (2 inches) above elbows. (Hands need to be above elbows at all times.)	Water runs by gravity from fingertips to elbows. Hands become cleanest part of upper extremity. Keeping hands elevated allows water to flow from least to most contaminated areas. Washing a wide area reduces risk of contaminating overlying gown that the nurse later applies.
8. Rinse hands and arms thoroughly under running water. Remember to keep hands above elbows.	Rinsing removes transient bacteria from fingers, hands, and forearms.
9. Under running water clean under nails of both hands with nail pick. Discard after use (see illustration).	Removes dirt and organic material that harbor large numbers of microorganisms.
10. Surgical hand scrub (with sponge)	
a. Wet clean sponge and apply antimicrobial agent. Visualize each finger, hand, and arm as having four sides. Wash all four sides effectively. Scrub the nails of one hand with 15 strokes. Scrub the palm, each side of thumb and fingers, and posterior side of hand with 10 strokes each.	Friction loosens resident bacteria that adhere to skin surfaces. Ensures coverage of all surfaces. Scrubbing is performed from cleanest area (hands) to marginal area (upper arms).
c. Discard sponge. Flex arms and rinse from fingertips to elbows in one continuous motion, allowing water to run off at elbow (see illustration).	Hands remain the cleanest part of upper extremities.
d. Turn off water with foot or knee control, with hands elevated in front of and away from body. Enter operating room suite by backing into room.	Keeps hands free of microorganisms.
b. Divide the arm mentally into thirds: scrub each third 10 times (AORN, 2019) (see illustration). Some health care agency policies require scrub by total time (e.g., 5 minutes) rather than number of strokes. Rinse sponge and repeat sequence for the other arm. A two-sponge method may be substituted (check health care agency policy).	Eliminates transient microorganisms and reduces resident hand flora.
e. Approach sterile setup; grasp sterile towel, taking care not to drip water onto sterile setup.	Water contaminates sterile setup.

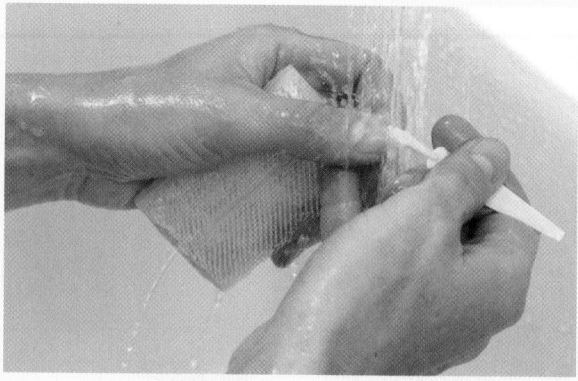

STEP 9 Clean under fingernails.

STEP	**RATIONALE**
f. Bending slightly at waist, keeping hands and arms above waist and outstretched, grasp one end of sterile towel and dry one hand, moving from fingers to elbow in a rotating motion (see illustrations).	Avoids sterile towel from contacting unsterile scrub attire and transferring contamination to hands. Dry skin from cleanest (hands) to least clean (elbows).
g. Repeat drying method for other hand by carefully reversing towel or using a new sterile towel.	Prevents accidental contamination.
h. Drop towel into linen hamper or circulating nurse's hand.	Prevents accidental contamination.
11. *Optional:* Brushless antiseptic hand rub	
a. After prescrub wash (see Step 7), dry hands and forearms thoroughly with paper towel.	Promotes reduction in microorganisms on all surfaces of hands and arms.
b. Dispense 2 mL of antimicrobial agent hand preparation into palm of one hand. Dip fingertips of opposite hand into hand preparation and work it under nails. Spread remaining hand preparation over hand and up to just above elbow, covering all surfaces (see illustrations).	
c. Using another 2 mL of hand preparation, repeat with other hand.	
d. Dispense another 2 mL of hand preparation into either hand and reapply to all aspects of both hands up to wrist. Allow to dry thoroughly before donning gloves.	Ensures complete antiseptic coverage of all hand surfaces.
12. Proceed with sterile gowning (see agency policy).	

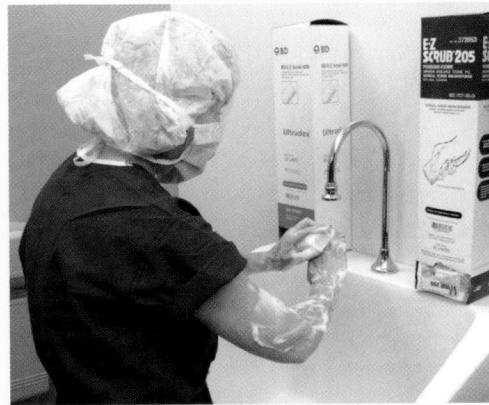

STEP 10b Scrub forearms.

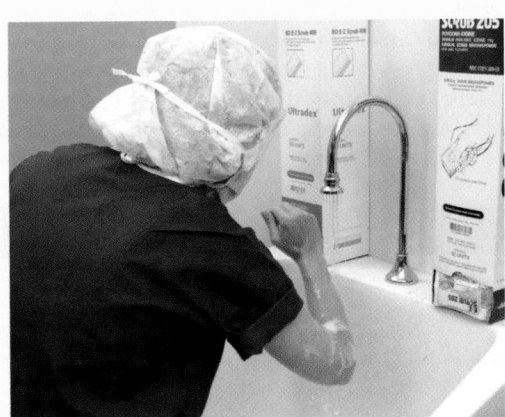

STEP 10c Rinse arms.

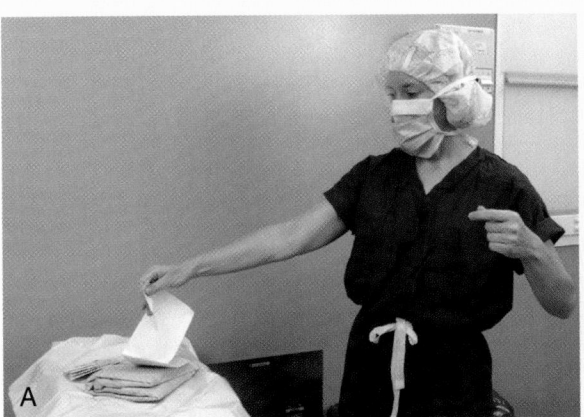

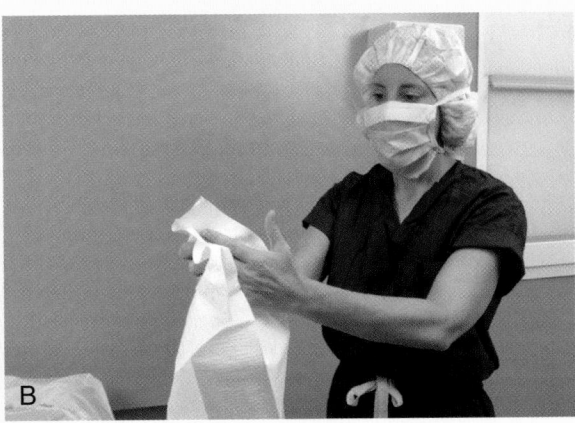

STEP 10f A, Grasp sterile towel. **B,** Drying sequence.

Continued

| SKILL 28.3 | SURGICAL HAND ASEPSIS—cont'd | |

| **STEP** | **RATIONALE** |

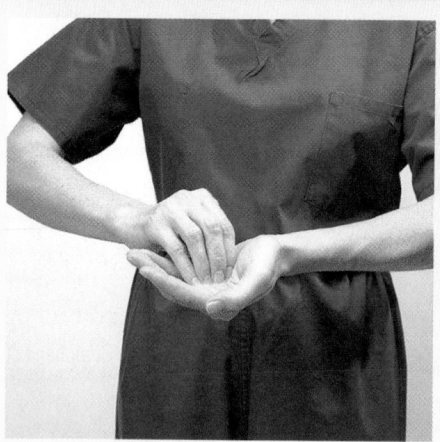
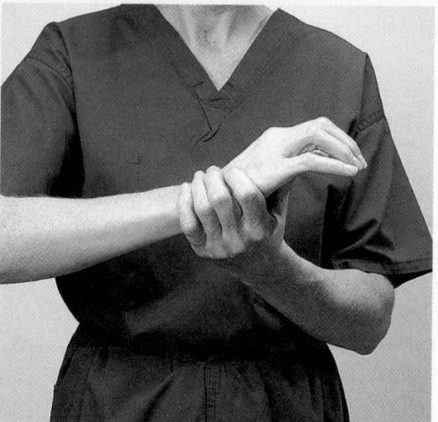

STEP 11b Application of antimicrobial agent for brushless hand scrub. Nurse using 3M Avagard. (Photos courtesy 3M Health Care.)

RECORDING AND REPORTING

- It is not necessary to record or report this procedure.
- Report any skin dermatitis to employee health or infection control per agency policy.

| SKILL 28.4 | OPEN GLOVING | |

Delegation and Collaboration

Assisting with skills that include the application and removal of sterile gloves may be delegated to assistive personnel (AP). However, most procedures that require the use of sterile gloves cannot be delegated to AP. The nurse instructs the AP about:

- The reason sterile gloves are being used for a specific procedure.

Equipment

- Package of proper-size sterile gloves, latex or synthetic nonlatex. If patient has a latex allergy, ensure that gloves are latex free and powder free.

| **STEP** | **RATIONALE** |

ASSESSMENT

1. Consider the type of procedure to be performed and consult agency policy on use of sterile gloves. In some facilities, double gloving is recommended for the operating room and if exposure to blood, body fluids, or infectious microorganisms is anticipated (AORN, 2019).

   Ensures proper use of sterile gloves. Evidence supports the use of double gloving and double gloving with an indicator glove system to decrease the risk of percutaneous injury and therefore be an effective barrier to bloodborne pathogen exposure (AORN, 2019).

2. Consider patient's risk for infection (e.g., preexisting condition, immunosuppressed, type of procedure).

   Knowledge of risk directs you to follow necessary precautions (e.g., use of additional protective barriers) if necessary.

3. Select correct size and type of gloves and examine glove package to determine if it is dry and intact with no visible stains.

   Torn or wet package is considered contaminated. Visible stains on package indicate previous contamination by water or other liquid.

4. Use nonpowdered gloves.

   The FDA passed a ruling that powdered gloves may no longer be used due to increased risks of hypersensitivity and allergic reactions (FDA, 2016).

5. Inspect condition of hands for cuts, hangnails, open lesions, or abrasions. In some settings, you can cover any open lesion with a sterile, impervious transparent dressing (check agency policy). In some cases, presence of such lesions may prevent you from participating in a procedure.

   Cuts, abrasions, and hangnails tend to ooze serum, which possibly contains pathogens. Breaks in skin integrity permit microorganisms to enter and increase the risk for infection for both patient and nurse (AORN, 2019).

6. Assess patient for the following risk factors before applying latex gloves:

   Risk factors determine level of patient's risk for latex allergy.

   a. Previous reaction to the following items within hours of exposure: adhesive tape, dental or face mask, golf club grip, ostomy bag, rubber band, balloon, bandage, elastic underwear, intravenous (IV) tubing, rubber gloves, condom.

   Items are known to lead to latex allergy.

   b. Personal history of asthma, contact dermatitis, eczema, urticaria, rhinitis.

   Patients with a history of these conditions are at higher risk of having a reaction.

   c. History of food allergies, especially avocado, banana, peach, chestnut, raw potato, kiwi, tomato, papaya.

   Patients with a history of food allergies are at higher risk of developing a reaction.

   d. Previous history of adverse reactions during surgery or dental procedure.

   Previous history suggests allergic response.

   e. Previous reaction to latex product.

   Previous reaction suggests allergic response.

7. Assess patient's or family caregiver's knowledge, experience and health literacy level.

   Ensures patient has the capacity to obtain, communicate, process, and understand basic health information (CDC, 2019).

STEP	RATIONALE

PLANNING

1. Provide privacy.

2. Set up equipment.

3. Explain procedure.

Assures patient is comfortable answering assessment questions.
Having needed supplies readily available decreases time patient needs to be exposed.
Preparing patient for procedure improves adherence and decreases patient stress.

IMPLEMENTATION

1. Apply sterile gloves.

   a. Remove outer glove package wrapper by carefully separating and peeling apart sides (see illustration).

   b. Grasp inner package and place on clean, dry, flat surface at waist level. Open package, keeping gloves on inside surface of wrapper (see illustration).

   c. Identify right and left glove. Each glove has a cuff approximately 5 cm (2 inches) wide. Glove dominant hand first.

   d. With thumb and first two fingers of nondominant hand, grasp glove for dominant hand by touching only inside surface of cuff.

   e. Carefully pull glove over dominant hand, leaving a cuff and being sure that cuff does not roll up wrist. Be sure that thumb and fingers are in proper spaces (see illustration).

   f. With gloved dominant hand, slip fingers underneath cuff of second glove (see illustration).

   g. Carefully pull second glove over fingers of nondominant hand (see illustration).

   h. After second glove is on, interlock hands together and hold away from body above waist level until beginning procedure (see illustration).

Proper removal prevents inner glove package from accidentally opening and touching contaminated objects.

Sterile object held below waist is contaminated. Inner surface of glove package is sterile.

Proper identification of gloves prevents contamination by improper fit. Gloving of dominant hand first improves dexterity.

Inner edge of cuff will lie against skin and thus is not sterile.

If outer surface of glove touches hand or wrist, it is contaminated.

Cuff protects gloved fingers. Sterile touching sterile prevents glove contamination.

Contact of gloved hand with exposed hand results in contamination.

Ensures smooth fit over fingers and prevents contamination.

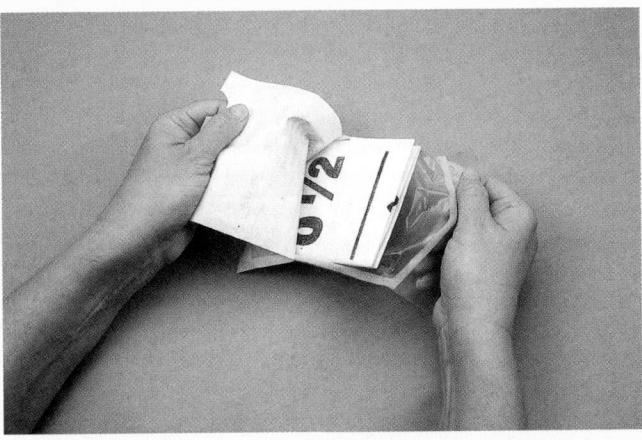

STEP 1a Open outer glove package wrapper.

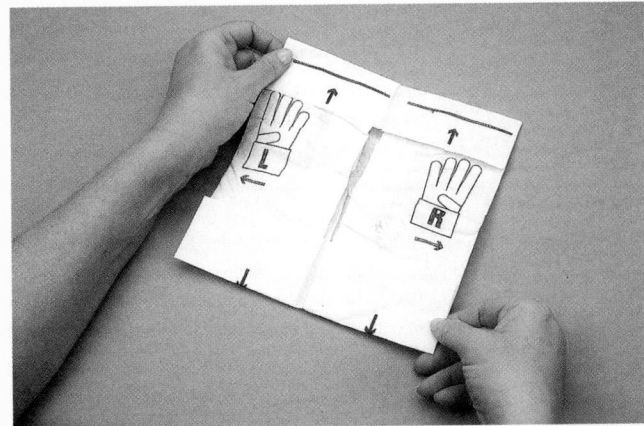

STEP 1b Open inner glove package on work surface.

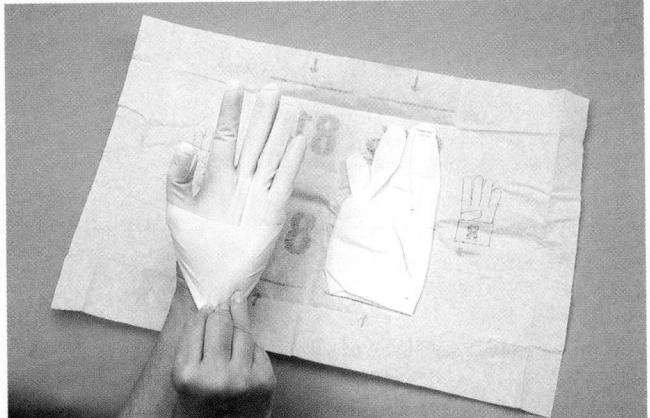

STEP 1e Pick up glove at cuff of dominant hand and insert fingers. Pull glove completely over dominant hand (example is for left-handed person).

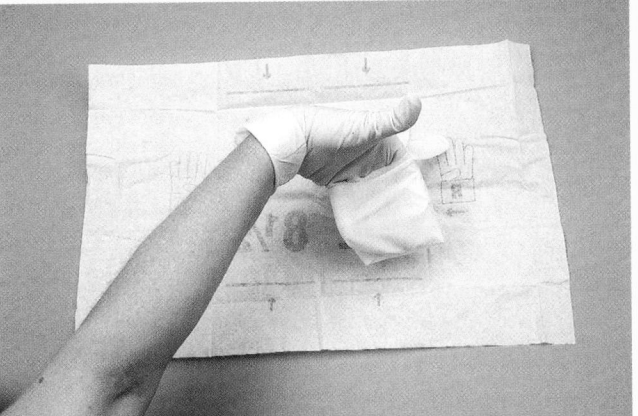

STEP 1f Pick up glove for nondominant hand.

Continued

SKILL 28.3	SURGICAL HAND ASEPSIS—cont'd
STEP	**RATIONALE**

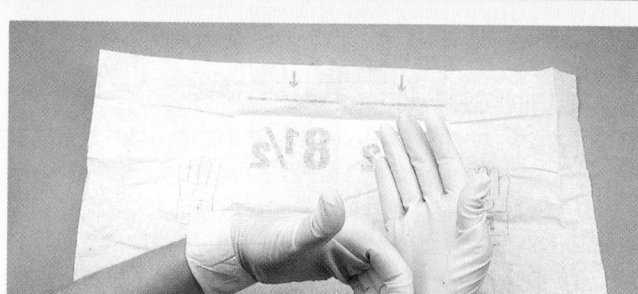

STEP 1g Pull second glove over nondominant hand.

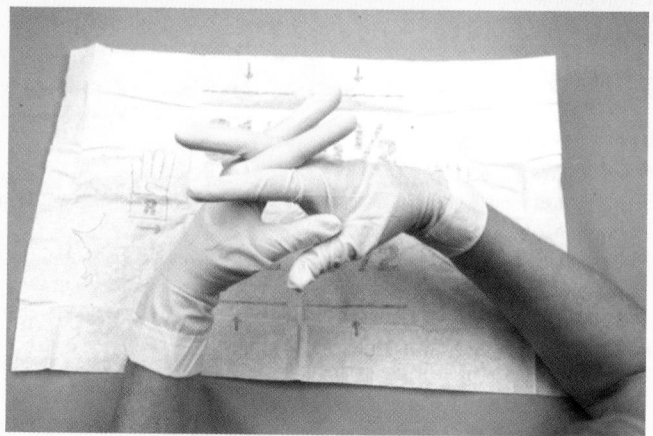

STEP 1h Interlock gloved hands.

CLINICAL DECISION: *Do not allow fingers and thumb of gloved dominant hand to touch any part of exposed nondominant hand. Keep thumb of dominant hand abducted back.*

2. Perform procedure.
3. Remove and dispose of gloves.
   a. Grasp outside of one cuff with other gloved hand; avoid touching wrist.   Procedure minimizes contamination of underlying skin.
   b. Pull glove off, turning it inside out, and place it in gloved hand.   Outside of glove does not touch skin surface.
   c. Take fingers of bare hand and tuck inside remaining glove cuff (see illustration). Peel glove off inside out and over previously removed glove. Discard both gloves in trash receptacle.   Fingers do not touch contaminated glove surface.

   d. Perform thorough hand hygiene.   Hand hygiene protects health care provider from contamination resulting from any unseen tears or pinholes in gloves.

EVALUATION

1. Assess patient for signs/symptoms of infection, focusing on area treated.   Improper sterile technique contributes to development of an infection.
2. Assess patient for signs/symptoms of latex allergy.   Assessment establishes baseline for patient's reaction to latex.
3. **Use Teach-Back:** "I want to be sure I explained why I used sterile gloves for this procedure. Please explain to me why I needed to use sterile gloves." Revise your instruction now or develop a plan for revised patient/family caregiver teaching if patient/family caregiver is not able to teach back correctly.   Determines patient's/family caregiver's level of understanding of instructional topic.

UNEXPECTED OUTCOMES AND RELATED INTERVENTIONS

1. Patient develops localized signs of infection (e.g., urine becomes cloudy or odorous; wound becomes painful, edematous, or reddened).
   • Contact health care provider and implement appropriate interventions as prescribed.
2. Patient develops systemic signs of infection (e.g., fever, malaise, increased white blood cell count).
   • Contact health care provider and implement appropriate interventions as prescribed.
3. Patient develops allergic reaction to latex.
   • Immediately remove source of latex, if known.
   • Bring emergency equipment to bedside. Have epinephrine injection ready for administration and be prepared to initiate IV fluids and oxygen.
   • Alert the health care team following agency protocol.

RECORDING AND REPORTING

• No recording or reporting is required for sterile gloving.
• Record the procedure performed and patient's response.
• Discuss with nurses and other pertinent health care providers the sterile procedure performed, patient's response, outcome, and any necessary follow-up.

STEP	RATIONALE

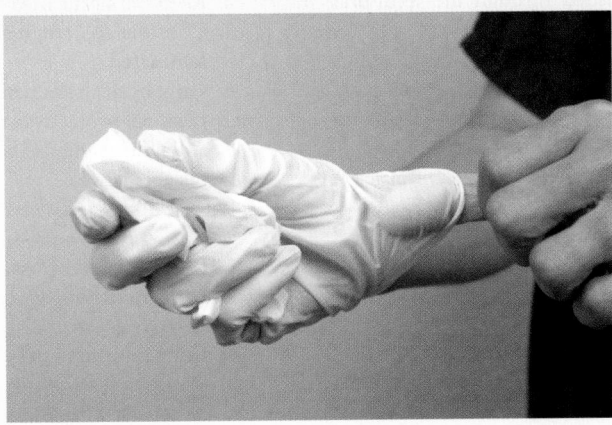

STEP 3c Remove second glove by turning it inside out.

KEY POINTS

- Transmission of infection can occur if the six elements of the infection chain are present and uninterrupted.
- Prevention of infection involves breaking an element of the chain of transmission.
- The severity of an infection determines the level and type of nursing care provided.
- Normal body flora and body system defenses help the body resist infection by reducing the number of pathogenic organisms.
- The inflammatory response neutralizes and eliminates pathogens and promotes healing to the damaged cells and tissue.
- Health care–associated infections can lead to adverse patient events and higher health care costs.
- Advanced age, poor nutrition, stress, inherited conditions, chronic disease, and treatments that compromise the immune response increase susceptibility to infection.
- Surgical asepsis requires more stringent techniques than medical asepsis.
- Standard Precautions are applied in all patient care activities to prevent patients and health care workers from transmitting infection.
- Hand hygiene is the most effective basic technique in preventing and controlling infection transmission.
- Transmission-based precautions are used in addition to Standard Precautions for patients with highly transmissible pathogens.

- Educating patients and caregivers on infection prevention in the home should include adaptations made for the home environment.
- Proper application of protective personal equipment protects the patient and health care worker from transmission of pathogens.
- Understanding and practicing infection prevention and control decreases the risk of the health care worker to infectious organisms.
- Understanding the postexposure process allows health care workers to access early intervention and decrease risk of transmission.

REFLECTIVE LEARNING

- Per best practice guidelines, hand hygiene is required before donning both clean and sterile gloves. How would you explain the rationale to a co-worker who states that hand hygiene is not necessary when wearing gloves?
- What would you include in an assessment of a patient with a large, stapled abdominal wound that is open to air?
- What are some infection-related factors to consider when providing care to older adults?

REVIEW QUESTIONS

1. A patient who has been placed on Contact Precautions for *Clostridium difficile* (*C. difficile*) asks you to explain what he should

know about this organism. What is the most appropriate information to include in patient teaching? (Select all that apply.)
1. The organism is usually transmitted through the fecal-oral route.
2. Hands should always be cleaned with soap and water versus alcohol-based hand sanitizer.
3. Everyone coming into the room must be wearing a gown and gloves.
4. While the patient is in Contact Precautions, he cannot leave the room.
5. *C. difficile* dies quickly once outside the body.

2. A patient is diagnosed with meningitis. Which type of isolation precaution is *most* appropriate for this patient?
1. Reverse isolation
2. Droplet Precautions
3. Standard Precautions
4. Contact Precautions

3. A patient is placed on Airborne Precautions for pulmonary tuberculosis. The nurse notes that the patient seems to be angry, but he knows that this is a normal response to isolation. Which is the best intervention?
1. Provide a dark, quiet room to calm the patient.
2. Reduce the level of precautions to keep the patient from becoming angry.
3. Explain the reasons for isolation procedures and provide meaningful stimulation.
4. Limit family and other caregiver visits to reduce the risk of spreading the infection.

4. Which type of personal protective equipment should the nurse wear when caring for a pediatric patient who is placed on Airborne Precautions for confirmed chickenpox/herpes zoster? (Select all that apply.)
1. Disposable gown
2. N95 respirator mask
3. Face shield or goggles
4. Disposable mask
5. Gloves

5. The infection control nurse has asked the staff to work on reducing the number of iatrogenic infections on the unit. Which of the following actions on your part would contribute to reducing health care–acquired infections? (Select all that apply.)
1. Teaching correct handwashing to assigned patients
2. Using correct procedures in starting and caring for an intravenous infusion
3. Providing perineal care to a patient with an indwelling urinary catheter
4. Isolating a patient on antibiotics who has been having loose stool for 24 hours
5. Decreasing a patient's environmental stimuli to decrease nausea

6. Which of the following actions by the nurse demonstrate the practice of core principles of surgical asepsis? (Select all that apply.)
1. The front and sides of the sterile gown are considered sterile from the waist up.
2. Keep the sterile field in view at all times.
3. Consider the outer 2.5 cm (1 inch) of the sterile field as contaminated.
4. Only health care personnel within the sterile field must wear personal protective equipment.
5. After cleansing the hands with antiseptic rub, apply clean disposable gloves.

7. Put the following steps for removal of protective barriers after leaving an isolation room in order.
1. Remove and dispose of gloves.
2. Perform hand hygiene.
3. Remove eyewear or goggles.
4. Untie top and then bottom mask strings and remove from face.
5. Untie waist and neck strings of gown. Remove gown, rolling it onto itself without touching the contaminated side.

8. A patient is diagnosed with a multidrug-resistant organism (MDRO) in his surgical wound and asks the nurse what this means. What is the nurse's best response? (Select all that apply.)
1. There is more than one organism in the wound that is causing the infection.
2. The antibiotics the patient has received are not strong enough to kill the organism.
3. The patient will need more than one type of antibiotic to kill the organism.
4. The organism has developed a resistance to one or more broad-spectrum antibiotics, indicating that the organism will be hard to treat effectively.
5. There are no longer any antibiotic options available to treat the patient's infection.

9. Which of these statements are true regarding disinfection and cleaning? (Select all that apply.)
1. Proper cleaning requires mechanical removal of all soil from an object or area.
2. General environmental cleaning is an example of medical asepsis.
3. When cleaning a wound, wipe around the wound edge first and then clean inward toward the center of the wound.
4. Cleaning in a direction from the least to the most contaminated area helps reduce infections.
5. Disinfecting and sterilizing medical devices and equipment involve the same procedures.

10. Patient-to-patient transmission of infection cannot occur if gloves are routinely used.
1. True
2. False

Answers: 1. 1, 2, 3; **2.** 2, 3; **3.** 4; **4.** 1, 2, 5; **5.** 1, 2, 3; **6.** 2, 3; **7.** 1, 3, 5, 4, 2; **8.** 2, 4; **9.** 1, 2, 4; **10.** 2.

Rationales for Review Questions can be found on the Evolve website.

REFERENCES

Arnold F: Antimicrobials and resistance. In Grota P, editor: *APIC text of infection control and epidemiology*, Washington, DC, 2018, Association for Professionals in Infection Control and Epidemiology.

Association of periOperative Registered Nurses (AORN): *Guidelines for perioperative practice*, Denver, 2019, AORN2019.

Association of Surgical Technologists (AST): *AST guidelines for best practices for wearing jewelry*, 2017. http://www.ast.org/uploadedFiles/Main_Site/Content/About_Us/Standard%20Wearing%20Jewelry.pdf. Accessed June 10, 2018.

Berends C, Walesa B: Isolation precautions (transmission precautions). In Grota P, editor: *APIC text of infection control and epidemiology*, Washington, DC, 2018, Association for Professionals in Infection Control and Epidemiology.

Centers for Disease Control and Prevention (CDC): *Guideline for preventing the transmission of mycobacterium tuberculosis in health-care facilities*, Washington, DC, 2005a, CDC.

Centers for Disease Control and Prevention (CDC): *Updated US Public Health Service guidelines for the management of occupational exposures to HIV and recommendations for post exposure prophylaxis*, Washington, DC, 2005b, CDC.

Centers for Disease Control and Prevention (CDC): *Guideline for isolation precautions: preventing transmission of infectious agents in healthcare settings—recommendations to the Healthcare Infection Control Practices Advisory Committee (HICPAC)*, Washington, DC, 2007, CDC. http://www.cdc.gov/hicpac/2007IP/2007isolationPrecautions.html. Accessed June 10, 2018.

Centers for Disease Control and Prevention (CDC): *Hospital infection control practice advisory committee and the HICPAC/SHEA/APIC/IDSA: hand hygiene task force guidelines for hand hygiene in health care settings*, Atlanta, 2008, Centers for Disease Control and Prevention.

Centers for Disease Control and Prevention (CDC): *Guidelines for the prevention of catheter-associated urinary tract infections*, CDC, 2009. https://www.cdc.gov/infectioncontrol/guidelines/cauti/index.html. Accessed August 27, 2019.

Centers for Disease Control and Prevention (CDC): *Recommended vaccines for healthcare workers*, CDC, 2016. https://www.cdc.gov/vaccines/adults/rec-vac/hcw.html. Accessed August 27, 2019.

Centers for Disease Control and Prevention (CDC): *CDC vital signs: making health care safer*, 2011. http://www.cdc.gov/vitalsigns/pdf/2011-03-vitalsigns.pdf. Accessed June 10, 2018.

Centers for Disease Control and Prevention (CDC): *Wash your hands*, 2013a. http://www.cdc.gov/features/handwashing, 2013a. Accessed June 10, 2018.

Centers for Disease Control and Prevention (CDC): *Precautions to prevent the spread of MRSA in healthcare settings*, 2013b. http://www.cdc.gov/mrsa/index.html. Accessed June 10, 2018.

Centers for Disease Control and Prevention (CDC): *Updated US Public Health Service guidelines for the management of occupational exposures to HIV and recommendations for postexposure prophylaxis*, Washington, DC, 2013c, CDC.

Centers for Disease Control and Prevention (CDC): *Show me the science—when to use hand sanitizers*. 2014, http://www.cdc.gov/handwashing/show-me-the-science-hand-sanitizer.html. Accessed June 10, 2018.

Centers for Disease Control and Prevention (CDC): *Ebola virus disease*, August 2015a. http://www.cdc.gov/vhf/ebola/index.html. Accessed June 10, 2018.

Centers for Disease Control and Prevention (CDC): *Fact sheet: screening and monitoring travelers to prevent the spread of Ebola*, September 2015b. http://www.cdc.gov/vhf/ebola/travelers/ebola-screening-factsheet.html. Accessed June 10, 2018.

Centers for Disease Control and Prevention (CDC): *Long-term effectiveness of whooping cough vaccines*, June 2015c. http://www.cdc.gov/pertussis/pregnant/mom/vacc-effectiveness.html. Accessed June 7, 2018.

Centers for Disease Control and Prevention (CDC): *Handwashing: clean hands save lives*, 2015d. http://www.cdc.gov/handwashing/. Accessed June 10, 2018.

Centers for Disease Control and Prevention (CDC): *2015 Sexually transmitted disease treatment guidelines*, 2015e. https://www.cdc.gov/std/tg2015/default.htm. Accessed June 10, 2018.

Centers for Disease Control and Prevention (CDC): *What is health literacy*, 2019, https://www.cdc.gov/healthliteracy/learn/index.html. Accessed December 23, 2019.

Centers for Disease Control and Prevention (CDC): *Clean hands count for healthcare providers*, 2017a. https://www.cdc.gov/handhygiene/providers/index.html. Accessed June 10, 2018.

Centers for Disease Control and Prevention (CDC): *HAI data and statistics*, 2017b. https://www.cdc.gov/hai/surveillance/index.html. Accessed June 10, 2018.

Center for Disease Control and Prevention (CDC): *Transmission-based precaustions*, 2017c. https://www.cdc.gov/infectioncontrol/basics/transmission-based-precautions.html. Accessed 10 June 2018.

Centers for Disease Control and Prevention (CDC): *National center for health statistics: infectious diseases*, 2017d. https://www.cdc.gov/nchs/fastats/infectious-disease.htm. Accessed July 27, 2019.

Centers for Disease Control and Prevention (CDC): *Medications that weaken your immune system and fungal infections*, 2017e. https://www.cdc.gov/fungal/infections/immune-system.html. Accessed July 27, 2019.

Centers for Disease Control and Prevention (CDC): *Healthcare-associated infections, HAI data*, 2018a. https://www.cdc.gov/hai/data/index.html. Accessed July 27, 2019.

Centers for Disease Control and Prevention (CDC): *Hepatitis overview and statistics*, 2018b. https://www.cdc.gov/hepatitis/hcv/hcvfaq.htm#section2. Accessed June 7, 2018.

Centers for Disease Control and Prevention (CDC): *Vaccination laws*, CDC, 2018c. Accessed https://www.cdc.gov/phlp/publications/topic/vaccinationlaws.html. Accessed June 7, 2018.

Centers for Disease Control and Prevention (CDC): *Vaccination coverage among children aged 19-35 months: United States 2017*, 2018d. https://www.cdc.gov/mmwr/volumes/67/wr/mm6740a4.htm. Accessed July 27, 2019.

Centers for Disease Control and Prevention (CDC): *What everyone should know about shingles vaccine*, 2018e. https://www.cdc.gov/vaccines/vpd/shingles/public/index.html. Accessed July 27, 2019.

Chetan J: Cleaning, disinfection and sterilization. In Grota P, editor: *APIC text of infection control and epidemiology*, Washington, DC, 2018, Association for Professionals in Infection Control and Epidemiology.

Live C: *Top 5 infectious disease concerns to watch in 2019*, January 1, 2019. https://www.contagionlive.com/news/top-5-infectious-disease-concerns-to-watch-in-2019. Accessed 27 July 2019.

Day M: Endoscopy. In Grota P, editor: *APIC text of infection control and epidemiology*, Washington, DC, 2018, Association for Professionals in Infection Control and Epidemiology.

Ellingson K, et al.: Strategies to prevent healthcare-associated infections through hand hygiene, *Infect Control Hosp Epidemiol* 35(8):937, 2014.

Fiutem C: Risk factors facilitating transmission of infectious agents. In Grota P, editor: *APIC text of infection control and epidemiology*, Washington, DC, 2018, Association for Professionals in Infection Control and Epidemiology.

Food and Drug Administration (FDA): *Banned devices; ban powdered surgeon's gloves, powdered patient examination gloves, and absorbable powder for lubricating a surgeon's glove*, 2016, Docket No. FDA-2015-N-5017 https://www.fda.gov/downloads/aboutfda/reportsmanualsforms/reports/economicanalyses/ucm532959.pdf. Accessed June 10, 2018.

Friedman C: Infection prevention and control programs. In Grota P, editor: *APIC text of infection control and epidemiology*, Washington, DC, 2018, Association for Professionals in Infection Control and Epidemiology.

Hass J: Hand hygiene. In Grota P, editor: *APIC text of infection control and epidemiology*, Washington, DC, 2018, Association for Professionals in Infection Control and Epidemiology.

Iwamoto P, Post M: Aseptic technique. In Grota P, editor: *APIC text of infection control and epidemiology*, Washington, DC, 2018, Association for Professionals in Infection Control and Epidemiology.

Giefing-Kröll C, et al.: How sex and age affect immune responses, susceptibility to infections, and response to vaccination, *Aging Cell* 14:309–321, 2015.

Jefferson J, Young M: Sterile processing. In Grota P, editor: *APIC text of infection control and epidemiology*, Washington, DC, 2018, Association for Professionals in Infection Control and Epidemiology.

The Joint Commission (TJC): *2020 National patient safety goals*, Oakbrook Terrace, IL, 2020, The Commission. https://www.jointcommission.org/en/standards/national-patient-safety-goals/. Accessed January 2, 2020.

Lunzen J, Altfeld M: Sex differences in infectious diseases: common but neglected, *J Infect Dis* 209(Suppl 3):S79–S80, 2014.

Mayo Clinic: *Prostatitis*, 2018. https://www.mayoclinic.org/diseases-conditions/prostatitis/symptoms-causes/syc-20355766. Accessed July 27, 2019.

Mehta Y, et al.: Guidelines for prevention of hospital acquired infections, *Indian J Crit Care Med* 18(3):149, 2014.

Meiner S, Yeager JJ: *Gerontologic nursing*, ed 6, St Louis, 2019, Elsevier.

Monsees E: Patient safety. In Grota P, editor: *APIC text of infection control and epidemiology*, Washington, DC, 2018, Association for Professionals in Infection Control and Epidemiology.

Murphy R: Surgical services. In Grota P, editor: *APIC text of infection control and epidemiology*, Washington, DC, 2018, Association for Professionals in Infection Control and Epidemiology.

Nesher L, et al.: The current spectrum of infection in cancer patients with chemotherapy-related neutropenia, *Infection* 42(5), 2014.

Nukifora K: *The importance of proper specimen collection and handling*, 2015. http://www.labtestingmatters.org/the-importance-of-proper-specimen-collection-and-handling/. Accessed June 11, 2018.

Occupational Safety and Health Administration (OSHA): *Respiratory protective devices: final rules and notice*, *Fed Regist* 33606, 2011.

Occupational Safety and Health Administration (OSHA): *Enforcement procedures for the occupational exposure to bloodborne injury final rule*, *Fed Regist* 33606, 2012a.

Occupational Safety and Health Administration (OSHA): *Needlestick safety and prevention Act*, *Fed Regist* 19934, 2012b.

Pagana KD, Pagana TJ: *Manual of diagnostic and laboratory tests*, ed 6, St Louis, 2018, Mosby.

Pawelec G: Age and immunity: what is "immunosenescence"? *Exp Gerontol* 105:4–9, 2018. https://www.sciencedirect.com/science/article/pii/S0531556517306599.

Popovich KJ: Another look at CHG bathing in a surgical intensive care unit, *Ann Transl Med* 5(1):13, 2017.

Roach R: Geriatrics. In Grota P, editor: *APIC text of infection control and epidemiology*, Washington, DC, 2018, Association for Professionals in Infection Control and Epidemiology.

San Patten and Associates: *International literature review for newcomer, migrant and refugee health*, 2016, The Interagency Coalition on AIDs and Development. http://www.icad-cisd.com/pdf/NMRH/NMRH-International-Lit-Review-FINAL.pdf. Accessed June 18, 2018.

Tweeten SM: General principles of epidemiology. In Grota P, editor: *APIC text of infection control and epidemiology*, Washington, DC, 2018, Association for Professionals in Infection Control and Epidemiology.

World Health Organization (WHO): *WHO guidelines on hand hygiene in healthcare*, Geneva, Switzerland, 2009, WHO Press2009.

World Health Organization (WHO): *Clean care is safer care: about SAVE LIVES: clean your hands*, 2017. http://www.who.int/gpsc/5may/background/5moments/en/. Accessed August 27, 2019.

World Health Organization (WHO): *International travel and health*, 2019a. https://www.who.int/ith/other_health_risks/infectious_diseases/en/. Accessed July 27, 2019.

World Health Organization (WHO): *My 5 moments for hand hygiene*, 2019b. https://www.who.int/infection-prevention/campaigns/clean-hands/5moments/en/. Accessed July 27, 2019.

RESEARCH REFERENCES

Adesanya OA, et al.: Bacterial contamination of stethoscopes at a tertiary care hospital in southwestern Nigeria, *Afr J Clin Exp Microbiol* 8(2):59, 2017.

Amitra J, et al.: Evaluation of the potential for electronic thermometers to contribute to spread of healthcare-associated pathogens, *Am J Infect Control* 46(6):708, 2018.

Birnbach DJ, et al.: An evaluation of hand hygiene in an intensive care unit: are visitors a potential vector for pathogens? *J Infect Public Health* 8(6):570, 2015.

Donskey E, Deshpande A: Effect of chlorhexidine bathing in preventing infections and reducing skin burden and environmental contamination: a review of the literature, *Am J Infect Control* 44(Suppl 5):17, 2016.

Dubberke E, et al.: Strategies to prevent Clostridium difficile infections in acute care hospitals: 2014 update, *Infect Control Hosp Epidemiol* 35(S2):S48, 2014.

Fakih M, et al.: Engaging health care workers to prevent catheter-associated urinary tract infection and avert patient harm, *Am J Infect Control* 42(Suppl 10):S223, 2014.

Fletcher K, et al.: Qualitative validation of the CAUTI Guide to patient safety assessment tool, *Am J Infect Control* 44(10):1102, 2016.

Gould D, et al: Interventions to improve hand hygiene compliance in patient care, *Cochrane Database Syst Rev* volume 8, *The Cochrane Library*, 2011, The Cochrane Collaboration.

Graziano-Husser J, et al.: Does including front line staff in root cause analyses reduce the incidence of catheter associated urinary tract infections? *Am J Infect Control* 46(Suppl 6):S77, 2018.

Mehrotra P, et al.: Effects of contact precautions on patient perception of care and satisfaction: a prospective cohort study, *Infect Control Hosp Epidemiol* 34(10):1087, 2013.

Sprague E, et al.: Patient isolation precautions: are they worth it? *Can Respir J* 5352625, 2016.

Thomas R, et al: Influenza vaccination for healthcare workers who care for people aged 60 or older living in long-term care institutions, The Cochrane Library, Issue 7, 2013, The Cochrane Collaboration. http://onlinelibrary.wiley.com/doi/10.1002/14651858.CD005187.pub4/pdf. Accessed June 10, 2018.

29

Vital Signs

OBJECTIVES

- Explain the principles and mechanisms of thermoregulation.
- Describe nursing measures that promote heat loss and heat conservation.
- Discuss physiological changes associated with fever.
- Describe factors that cause variations in body temperature, pulse, oxygen saturation, respirations, capnography, and blood pressure measurement.
- Describe an ethnic variation with blood pressure assessment.
- Identify ranges of acceptable vital sign values for an infant, a child, and an adult.

- Explain variations in technique used to assess an infant's, a child's, and an adult's vital signs.
- Describe the benefits and precautions involving self-measurement of blood pressure.
- Identify when to measure vital signs.
- Accurately record and report vital sign measurements.
- Appropriately delegate measurement of vital signs to assistive personnel.

KEY TERMS

Afebrile, p. 471
Antipyretics, p. 477
Auscultatory gap, p. 488
Blood pressure, p. 483
Bradycardia, p. 479
Capnography, p. 483
Conduction, p. 469
Convection, p. 470
Core temperature, p. 468
Diaphoresis, p. 470
Diastolic pressure, p. 484
Dysrhythmia, p. 479
Eupnea, p. 481
Evaporation, p. 470
Febrile, p. 471

Fever, p. 471
Fever of unknown origin (FUO), p. 472
Frostbite, p. 472
Heat exhaustion, p. 472
Heatstroke, p. 472
Hematocrit, p. 484
Hypertension, p. 485
Hyperthermia, p. 472
Hypotension, p. 486
Hypothermia, p. 472
Hypoxemia, p. 481
Malignant hyperthermia, p. 472
Nonshivering thermogenesis, p. 469
Orthostatic hypotension, p. 486
Oxygen saturation, p. 482

Postural hypotension, p. 486
Pulse deficit, p. 479
Pulse pressure, p. 484
Pyrexia, p. 471
Pyrogens, p. 471
Radiation, p. 469
Shivering, p. 469
Sphygmomanometer, p. 486
Systolic pressure, p. 484
Tachycardia, p. 479
Thermogenesis, p. 469
Thermoregulation, p. 469
Ventilation, p. 480
Vital signs, p. 467

MEDIA RESOURCES

http://evolve.elsevier.com/Potter/fundamentals/
- Review Questions
- Video Clips
- Case Study with Questions

- Skills Performance Checklists
- Audio Glossary
- Content Updates
- Answers to QSEN Activity and Review Questions

The most frequent and routine measurements obtained by health care providers are those of temperature, pulse, blood pressure (BP), respiratory rate, and oxygen saturation. As indicators of health status, these measures indicate the effectiveness of circulatory, respiratory, neural, and endocrine body functions. Because of their importance, they are referred to as vital signs (VS). Pain, a subjective symptom, is often called another vital sign and is frequently measured with the others (see Chapter 44).

Measurement of vital signs provides data to determine a patient's usual state of health (baseline data). Many factors such as the temperature of the environment, the patient's physical exertion, and the effects of illness cause vital signs to change, sometimes outside an acceptable range. An alteration in vital signs signals a change in physiological function. Assessment of vital signs provides data to identify nursing diagnoses, implement planned interventions, and evaluate outcomes of care.

Vital signs are a quick and efficient way of monitoring a patient's condition or identifying problems and evaluating his or her response to intervention. When you learn the physiological variables influencing vital signs and recognize the relationship of their changes to one another and to other physical assessment findings, you can make precise determinations about a patient's health status and the need for medical or nursing interventions. Vital signs and other physiological measurements are the basis for clinical decision making and problem solving. Many agencies adopt Early Warning Scores (EWS) determined by vital signs data entered into the electronic medical record (EMR) to alert nurses to potential changes in a patient's condition. An EWS system responds to multiple vital sign parameters at the same time and identifies at-risk patients at the first sign of a subtle change in vital signs (IHI, 2018).

GUIDELINES FOR MEASURING VITAL SIGNS

Vital signs are a part of the assessment database. You include them in a complete physical assessment (see Chapter 30), routinely per a health care provider's order, or obtain them individually to assess a patient's condition. Establishing a database of vital signs during a routine physical examination serves as a baseline for future assessments. A patient's condition determines when, where, how, and by whom vital signs are measured. You need to measure them correctly, and at times you appropriately delegate their measurement. You also need to know expected values (Box 29.1), interpret your patient's values, communicate findings appropriately, and begin interventions as needed. Use the following guidelines to incorporate measurements of vital signs into nursing practice:

- Measuring vital signs is your responsibility. You may delegate these measurements in selected situations (e.g., in stable patients). However, it is your responsibility to review vital sign data, interpret their significance, and critically think through decisions about interventions.
- Assess equipment to ensure that it is working correctly to provide accurate findings.
- Select equipment on the basis of the patient's condition and characteristics (e.g., do not use an adult-size BP cuff for a child).
- Know the patient's usual range of vital signs. These values can differ from the acceptable range for a patient's age or health status. The patient's usual values serve as a baseline for comparison with later findings. Thus you are able to detect a change in condition over time.
- Know your patient's health history, therapies, and prescribed and over-the-counter medications. Some illnesses or treatments cause predictable changes in vital signs. Some medications affect one or more vital signs.
- Control or minimize environmental factors that affect vital signs. For example, assessing a patient's temperature in a warm, humid room may yield a value that is not a true indicator of his or her condition.

- Use an organized, systematic approach. Each vital sign procedure requires a step-by-step approach to ensure accuracy.
- On the basis of a patient's condition, collaborate with health care providers to decide the frequency of vital sign assessment. In the hospital health care providers order a minimum frequency of vital sign measurements for each patient. As a patient's physical condition worsens, it is often necessary to monitor more frequently, such as every 5 to 10 minutes. The nurse is responsible for judging whether more frequent assessments are necessary (Box 29.2).
- Use vital sign measurements to determine indications for medication administration. For example, give certain cardiac drugs only within a range of pulse or BP values. Administer antipyretics when temperature is elevated outside the acceptable range for the patient. Know the acceptable vital sign ranges for your patients before administering medications.
- Analyze the results of vital sign measurements on the basis of patient's condition and past health history.
- Verify and communicate significant changes in vital signs. Baseline measurements provide a starting point for identifying and accurately interpreting possible changes. When VS appear abnormal, have another nurse or health care provider repeat the measurement to verify readings. Inform the charge nurse or health care provider immediately, document findings in your patient's record, and report changes to nurses during hand-off communication (TJC, 2020).
- Educate the patient or family caregiver in vital sign assessment and the significance of findings.

BODY TEMPERATURE

Physiology

Body temperature is the difference between the amount of heat produced by body processes and the amount lost to the external environment.

$$\text{Heat Produced} - \text{Heat Lost} = \text{Body Temperature}$$

Despite extremes in environmental conditions and physical activity, temperature-control mechanisms of humans keep body **core temperature** (temperature of the deep tissues) relatively constant (Fig. 29.1). However, surface temperature varies, depending on blood flow to the skin and the amount of heat lost to the external environment. Body

---

BOX 29.1　Vital Signs

Acceptable Ranges for Adults

Temperature Range
Average temperature range: 36° to 38° C (96.8° to 100.4° F)
Average oral/tympanic: 37° C (98.6° F)
Average rectal: 37.5° C (99.5° F)
Axillary: 36.5° C (97.7° F)

Pulse
60 to 100 beats/min, strong and regular

Pulse Oximetry (SpO₂)
Normal: SpO_2 ≥95%

Respirations
12 to 20 breaths/min, deep and regular

Blood Pressure
Systolic <120 mm Hg
Diastolic <80 mm Hg
Pulse pressure: 30 to 50 mm Hg

Capnography (EtCO₂)
Normal: 35-45 mm Hg

BOX 29.2　When to Measure Vital Signs

- On admission to a health care facility
- When assessing a patient during home care visits
- In a clinic setting before a health care provider examines the patient and after any invasive procedures
- In a hospital on a routine schedule according to the health care provider's order or hospital standards of practice
- Before, during, and after a surgical procedure or invasive diagnostic/treatment procedure
- Before, during, and after a transfusion of any type of blood product
- Before, during, and after the administration of medication or therapies that affect cardiovascular, respiratory, or temperature-control functions
- When a patient's general physical condition changes (e.g., loss of consciousness or increased intensity of pain)
- Before, during, and after nursing interventions influencing a vital sign (e.g., before a patient previously on bed rest ambulates or before a patient performs range-of-motion exercises)
- When a patient reports nonspecific symptoms of physical distress (e.g., feeling "funny" or "different")

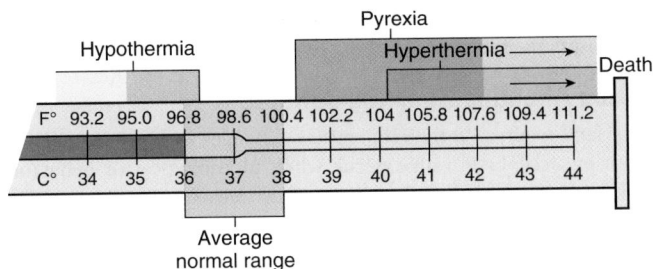

FIG. 29.1 Ranges of normal temperature values and abnormal body temperature alterations.

tissues and cells function efficiently within a narrow range, from 36° to 38° C (96.8° to 100.4° F), but no single temperature is normal for all people.

The site of temperature measurement (oral, rectal, tympanic membrane, temporal artery, esophageal, pulmonary artery, axillary, or even urinary bladder) is one factor that determines a patient's temperature. For healthy young adults the average oral temperature is 37° C (98.6° F). In the elderly population the average core temperature ranges from 35° to 36.1° C (95° to 97° F) as a result of changes in temperature regulation. The time of day also affects body temperature, with the lowest temperature at 6:00 AM and the highest temperature at 4:00 PM in healthy people. Invasive measurements obtained with a pulmonary artery or esophageal catheter are considered core temperatures, whereas axillary temperatures are reflective of the surface temperature of the body. It is important to remember that a consistent body temperature measurement from a single site allows you to monitor patterns of your patient's body temperature. As you assess and document these temperature trends, you collaborate with the health care team to determine whether a specific body temperature measurement site is more appropriate.

Body Temperature Regulation. Physiological and behavioral mechanisms regulate the balance between heat lost and heat produced, or **thermoregulation**. For the body temperature to stay constant and within an acceptable range, various mechanisms maintain the relationship between heat production and heat loss. Apply knowledge of temperature-control mechanisms to promote temperature regulation.

Neural and Vascular Control. The hypothalamus, located between the cerebral hemispheres, controls body temperature the same way a thermostat works in the home. A comfortable temperature is the "set point" at which a heating system operates. In the home a drop in environmental temperature activates the furnace, whereas a rise in temperature shuts the system down.

The hypothalamus senses minor changes in body temperature. The anterior hypothalamus controls heat loss, and the posterior hypothalamus controls heat production. When nerve cells in the anterior hypothalamus become heated beyond the set point, impulses are sent out to reduce body temperature. Mechanisms of heat loss include sweating, vasodilation (widening) of blood vessels, and inhibition of heat production. The body redistributes blood to surface vessels to promote heat loss.

If the posterior hypothalamus senses that body temperature is lower than the set point, the body initiates heat-conservation mechanisms. Vasoconstriction (narrowing) of blood vessels reduces blood flow to the skin and extremities to reduce heat loss. Compensatory heat production is stimulated through voluntary muscle contraction and muscle shivering. When vasoconstriction is ineffective in preventing additional heat loss, shivering begins. Disease or trauma to the hypothalamus or the spinal cord, which carries hypothalamic messages, causes serious alterations in temperature control.

Heat Production. Temperature regulation depends on normal heat production processes. Heat produced by the body is a by-product of metabolism, which is the chemical reaction in all body cells. Activities requiring additional chemical reactions increase the metabolic rate. As metabolism increases, additional heat is produced. When metabolism decreases, less heat is produced. Heat production occurs during rest, voluntary movements, involuntary shivering, and nonshivering **thermogenesis**.

- Basal metabolism accounts for the heat produced by the body at absolute rest. The average basal metabolic rate (BMR) depends on the body surface area. Thyroid hormones also affect the BMR. By promoting the breakdown of body glucose and fat, thyroid hormones increase the rate of chemical reactions in almost all cells of the body. When large amounts of thyroid hormones are secreted, the BMR can increase 100% above normal. The absence of thyroid hormones reduces the BMR by half, causing a decrease in heat production. The male sex hormone testosterone increases BMR. Men have a higher BMR than women.
- Voluntary movements such as muscular activity during exercise require additional energy. The metabolic rate increases during activity, sometimes causing heat production to increase up to 50 times normal.
- Shivering is an involuntary body response to temperature differences in the body. The skeletal muscle movement during shivering requires significant energy. Shivering sometimes increases heat production 4 to 5 times greater than normal. The heat that is produced helps equalize the body temperature, and the shivering ceases. In vulnerable patients shivering seriously drains energy sources, resulting in further physiological deterioration.
- Nonshivering thermogenesis occurs primarily in neonates because they cannot shiver (Hockenberry et al, 2019). A limited amount of vascular brown tissue, present at birth, is metabolized for heat production.

Heat Loss. Heat loss and heat production occur simultaneously. The structure of the skin and exposure to the environment result in constant, normal heat loss through radiation, conduction, convection, and evaporation.

Radiation is the transfer of heat from the surface of one object to the surface of another without direct contact between the two. As much as 85% of the surface area of the human body radiates heat to the environment. Peripheral vasodilation increases blood flow from the internal organs to the skin to increase radiant heat loss. Peripheral vasoconstriction minimizes radiant heat loss. Radiation increases as the temperature difference between the objects increases. Radiation heat loss can be considerable during surgery when the patient's skin is exposed to a cool environment. However, if the environment is warmer than the skin, the body absorbs heat through radiation.

The patient's position enhances radiation heat loss (e.g., standing exposes a greater radiating surface area, and lying in a fetal position minimizes heat radiation). Help promote heat loss through radiation by removing clothing or blankets. Covering the body with dark, closely woven clothing decreases the amount of heat lost from radiation.

Conduction is the transfer of heat from one object to another with direct contact. Solids, liquids, and gases conduct heat through contact. When the warm skin touches a cooler object, heat is lost. Conduction normally accounts for a small amount of heat loss. Applying an ice pack or bathing a patient with a cool cloth increases conductive heat loss. Applying several layers of clothing reduces conductive loss. The body loses heat by conduction when it makes contact with materials cooler than skin temperature (e.g., application of an ice pack).

Convection is the transfer of heat away by air movement. A fan promotes heat loss through convection. The rate of heat loss increases when moistened skin comes into contact with slightly moving air.

Evaporation is the transfer of heat energy when a liquid is changed to a gas. The body continuously loses heat by evaporation. Approximately 600 to 900 mL a day evaporates from the skin and lungs, resulting in water and heat loss. By regulating perspiration or sweating, the body promotes additional evaporative heat loss. When body temperature rises, the anterior hypothalamus signals the sweat glands to release sweat through tiny ducts on the surface of the skin. During physical exercise over 80% of the heat produced is lost by sweat evaporation.

Diaphoresis is visible perspiration primarily occurring on the forehead and upper thorax, although it occurs in other places on the body. For each hour of exercise in hot conditions up to 2 L of body fluid can be lost in sweat. Excessive evaporation causes skin scaling and itching and drying of the nares and pharynx. A lowered body temperature inhibits sweat gland secretion. People who have a congenital absence of sweat glands or a serious skin disease that impairs sweating are unable to tolerate warm temperatures because they cannot cool themselves adequately.

Skin in Temperature Regulation. The skin regulates temperature through insulation of the body, vasoconstriction (which affects the amount of blood flow and heat loss to the skin), and temperature sensation. The skin, subcutaneous tissue, and fat keep heat inside the body. People with more body fat have more natural insulation than do slim and muscular people.

The way the skin controls body temperature is similar to the way an automobile radiator controls engine temperature. An automobile engine generates a great deal of heat. Water is pumped through the engine to collect the heat and carry it to the radiator, where a fan transfers the heat from the water to the outside air. In the human body the internal organs produce heat; during exercise or increased sympathetic stimulation (such as in the stress response) the amount of heat produced is greater than the usual core temperature. Blood flows from the internal organs, carrying heat to the body surface. The skin has many blood vessels, especially the areas of the hands, feet, and ears. Blood flow through these vascular areas of the skin varies from minimal flow to as much as 30% of the blood ejected from the heart. Heat transfers from the blood, through vessel walls, and to the surface of the skin and is lost to the environment through heat-loss mechanisms. The core temperature of the body remains within safe limits.

The degree of vasoconstriction determines the amount of blood flow and heat loss to the skin. If the core temperature is too high, the hypothalamus inhibits vasoconstriction, thus blood vessels dilate, and more blood reaches the surface of the skin. On a hot, humid day the blood vessels in the hands are dilated and easily visible. In contrast, if the core temperature becomes too low, the hypothalamus initiates vasoconstriction, and blood flow to the skin lessens to conserve heat.

Behavioral Control. Healthy individuals maintain a comfortable body temperature when exposed to temperature extremes. The ability of a person to control body temperature depends on (1) the degree of temperature extreme, (2) the person's ability to sense feeling comfortable or uncomfortable, (3) thought processes or emotions, and (4) the person's mobility or ability to remove or add clothes. Individuals are less able to control body temperature if any of these abilities are lost. For example, infants are able to sense uncomfortable warm conditions but need help to change their environment. Older adults sometimes need help to detect cold environments and minimize heat loss. Illnesses, a decreased level of consciousness, or impaired thought processes result in an inability to recognize the need to change behavior for temperature control. When temperatures become extremely hot or cold, health-promoting behaviors such as removing or adding clothing have a limited effect on controlling temperature.

Factors Affecting Body Temperature

Many factors affect body temperature. Changes in body temperature within an acceptable range occur when physiological or behavioral mechanisms alter the relationship between heat production and heat loss. Be aware of these factors when assessing temperature variations and evaluating deviations from normal.

Age. At birth the newborn leaves a warm, relatively constant environment and enters one in which temperatures fluctuate widely. Temperature-control mechanisms are immature. An infant's temperature responds drastically to changes in the environment. Take extra care to protect newborns from environmental temperatures. A newborn loses up to 30% of body heat through the head and therefore needs to wear a cap to prevent heat loss (Hockenberry et al., 2019). When protected from environmental extremes, the newborn's body temperature is usually within 35.5° to 37.5°C (95.9° to 99.5°F).

Temperature regulation is unstable until children reach puberty. The usual temperature range gradually drops as individuals approach older adulthood. The older adult has a narrower range of body temperatures than the younger adult. Oral temperatures of 35°C (95°F) are sometimes found in older adults in cold weather. However, the average body temperature of older adults is approximately 35° to 36.1°C (95° to 97°F). Older adults are particularly sensitive to temperature extremes because of deterioration in control mechanisms, particularly poor vasomotor control (control of vasoconstriction and vasodilation), reduced amounts of subcutaneous tissue, reduced sweat gland activity, and reduced metabolism.

Exercise. Muscle activity requires an increased blood supply and carbohydrate and fat breakdown. Any form of exercise increases metabolism and heat production and thus body temperature. Prolonged strenuous exercise such as long-distance running temporarily raises body temperature.

Hormone Level. Women generally experience greater fluctuations in body temperature than men. Hormonal variations during the menstrual cycle cause body temperature fluctuations. Progesterone levels rise and fall cyclically during the menstrual cycle. When progesterone levels are low, the body temperature is a few tenths of a degree below the baseline level. The lower temperature persists until ovulation occurs. During ovulation greater amounts of progesterone enter the circulatory system and raise the body temperature to previous baseline levels or higher. These temperature variations help to predict a woman's most fertile time to achieve pregnancy.

Body temperature changes also occur in women during menopause (cessation of menstruation). Women who have stopped menstruating often experience periods of intense body heat and sweating lasting from 30 seconds to 5 minutes. During these periods skin temperature can increase as much as 4°C (7.2°F), referred to as hot flashes. This is caused by the instability of the vasomotor controls for vasodilation and vasoconstriction.

Circadian Rhythm. Body temperature normally changes 0.5° to 1°C (0.9° to 1.8°F) during a 24-hour period. However, temperature is one of the most stable rhythms in humans. The temperature is usually lowest between 1:00 and 4:00 AM (Fig. 29.2). During the day body temperature rises steadily to a maximum temperature value at about 4:00 PM and then declines to early-morning levels. Temperature patterns are not automatically reversed in people who work at night and sleep during the day. It takes 1 to 3 weeks for the cycle to reverse. In general the circadian temperature rhythm does not change with age.

Stress. Physical and emotional stress increase body temperature through hormonal and neural stimulation (see Chapter 37). These physiological changes increase metabolism, which increases heat production. A patient who is anxious about entering a hospital or a health care provider's office often has a higher normal temperature.

Environment. Environment influences body temperature. When placed in a warm room a patient may be unable to regulate body temperature by heat-loss mechanisms, and the body temperature may elevate. If the patient is outside in the cold without warm clothing, body temperature may be low as a result of extensive radiant and conductive heat loss. Environmental temperatures affect infants and older adults more often because their temperature-regulating mechanisms are less efficient.

Temperature Alterations. Changes in body temperature outside the usual range are related to excessive heat production, excessive heat loss, minimal heat production, minimal heat loss, or any combination of these alterations.

Fever. Fever, or *pyrexia*, occurs because heat-loss mechanisms are unable to keep pace with excessive heat production, resulting in an abnormal rise in body temperature. In general, a fever is a temperature above 100.4° F (38° C) for an adult or child, depending on the type of thermometer used (Ward, 2019; Mayo Clinic, 2017). The height of a child's fever is not always the best indicator of whether the child needs to be treated. Instead, it is important to note how a child behaves and appears because fever is usually accompanied by other symptoms

(Ward, 2019). These are the cutoffs for fever in children using different types of thermometers (Seattle Children's Hospital, 2019):

- Rectal (bottom), ear, or forehead temperature: 100.4° F (38.0° C) or higher
  - Caution: Ear temperatures are not accurate before 6 months of age.
- Oral (mouth) temperature: 100° F (37.8° C) or higher
- Under the arm (armpit) temperature: 99° F (37.2° C) or higher

A single temperature reading does not always indicate a fever (Bijur et al., 2016). In addition to physical signs and symptoms of infection, fever determination is also based on several temperature readings at different times of the day compared with the usual value for that person at that time.

A true fever results from an alteration in the hypothalamic set point. **Pyrogens** such as bacteria and viruses elevate body temperature by acting as antigens to trigger the immune system. The hypothalamus reacts to raise the set point, and the body responds by producing and conserving heat. Several hours pass before the body temperature reaches the new set point. During this period a person experiences the physical signs and symptoms of chills, shivers, and feeling cold, even though the body temperature is rising (Fig. 29.3). The chill phase resolves when the new set point, a higher temperature, is achieved. During the next phase, the plateau, the chills subside, and the person feels warm and dry. If the new set point is "overshot" or the pyrogens are removed (e.g., destruction of bacteria by antibiotics), the third phase of a **febrile** episode occurs. The hypothalamus set point drops, initiating heat-loss responses. The skin becomes warm and flushed because of vasodilation. Diaphoresis assists in evaporative heat loss. When the fever "breaks," the patient becomes **afebrile.**

Fever is an important defense mechanism. Mild temperature elevations as high as 39° C (102.2° F) enhance the immune system of the body. However, during a fever cellular metabolism increases; for every 1° C rise in body temperature, the body's chemical reactions increase 10% (Mordiffi et al., 2016). During a febrile episode white blood cell production is stimulated. Increased temperature reduces the concentration of iron in the blood plasma, suppressing the growth of bacteria. Fever also fights viral infections by stimulating interferon, the natural virus-fighting substance of the body.

The body responds to the increase in metabolic needs during a fever by increasing heart and respiratory rates. The increased metabolism uses energy to produce additional heat. If a patient has a cardiac or respiratory problem, the stress of a fever is great. A prolonged fever weakens a patient by exhausting energy stores. Increased metabolism

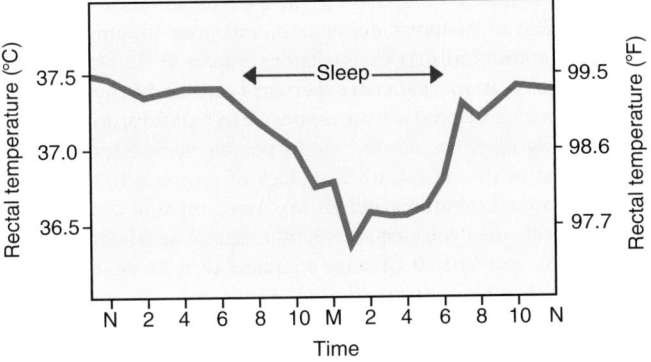

FIG. 29.2 Temperature cycle for 24 hours.

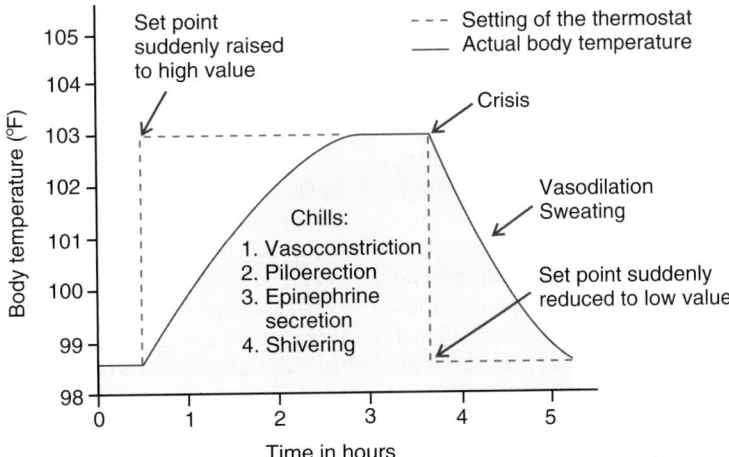

FIG. 29.3 Effect of changing set point of hypothalamic temperature control during a fever. (Modified from Guyton AC, Hall JE: *Textbook of medical physiology,* ed 13, Philadelphia, 2016, Saunders.)

BOX 29.3 Patterns of Fever

Sustained: A constant body temperature continuously above 38° C (100.4° F) that has little fluctuation

Intermittent: Fever spikes interspersed with usual temperature levels (Temperature returns to acceptable value at least once in 24 hours.)

Remittent: Fever spikes and falls without a return to acceptable temperature levels.

Relapsing: Periods of febrile episodes and periods with acceptable temperature values (Febrile episodes and periods of normothermia are often longer than 24 hours.)

TABLE 29.1 Classification of Hypothermia by Core Temperature

	Celsius	Fahrenheit
Mild	32°-35°	90.0°-95°
Moderate	28°-32°	82°-90°
Severe	<28°	<82°

From Zafren K, Mechem CC: *Accidental hypothermia in adults*, UpToDate, 2018, https://www.uptodate.com/contents/accidental-hypothermia-in-adults.

---

requires additional oxygen. If the body cannot meet the additional oxygen demand, cellular hypoxia (inadequate oxygen) occurs. Myocardial hypoxia produces angina (chest pain). Cerebral hypoxia produces confusion. When water loss through increased respiration and diaphoresis is excessive, the patient is at risk for fluid volume deficit. Dehydration is a serious problem for older adults and children with low body weight. Maintaining optimum fluid volume status is an important nursing action (see Chapter 42).

Fevers and fever patterns serve a diagnostic purpose. Fever patterns differ, depending on the causative pyrogen (Box 29.3). The increase or decrease in pyrogen activity results in fever spikes and declines at different times of the day. The duration and degree of fever depend on the strength of the pyrogen and the ability of the individual to respond. The term fever of unknown origin (FUO) refers to a fever with an undetermined cause.

Hyperthermia. An elevated body temperature related to the inability of the body to promote heat loss or reduce heat production is hyperthermia. Whereas fever is an upward shift in the set point, hyperthermia results from an overload of the thermoregulatory mechanisms. Any disease or trauma to the hypothalamus impairs heat-loss mechanisms. Malignant hyperthermia is a hereditary condition of uncontrolled heat production that occurs when susceptible people receive certain anesthetic drugs (see Chapter 50).

Heatstroke. Heat depresses hypothalamic function. Prolonged exposure to the sun or a high environmental temperature overwhelms the heat-loss mechanisms of the body. These conditions cause heatstroke, defined as a body temperature of 40° C (104° F) or more accompanied by hot, dry skin and central nervous system abnormalities, such as delirium, convulsions, or coma (Hifumi et al., 2018). Heatstroke is a dangerous heat emergency with a high mortality rate. There are two groups of heatstroke. Exertional heatstroke develops in able-bodied individuals, such as athletes, soldiers, or laborers who are performing rigorous physical activities. In contrast, nonexertional heatstroke can develop during low-level physical activities among elderly, ambulatory individuals with comorbidities (e.g., diabetes or cardiovascular disease) (Gaudio and Grissom, 2016). Also at risk are those who take medications that decrease the ability of the body to lose heat (e.g., phenothiazines, anticholinergics, diuretics, amphetamines, and beta-adrenergic receptor antagonists).

Signs and symptoms of heatstroke include giddiness, confusion, delirium, excessive thirst, nausea, muscle cramps, visual disturbances, and even incontinence. Vital signs reveal a body temperature sometimes as high as 45° C (113° F), with an increase in heart rate (HR) and lowering of BP. The most important sign of heatstroke is hot, dry skin. Victims of heatstroke do not sweat because of severe electrolyte loss and hypothalamic malfunction. If the condition progresses, a patient with heatstroke becomes unconscious, with fixed, nonreactive pupils. Permanent neurological damage occurs unless cooling measures are rapidly started.

Heat Exhaustion. Heat exhaustion occurs when profuse diaphoresis results in excess water and electrolyte loss. Caused by environmental heat exposure, a patient exhibits signs and symptoms of deficient fluid volume (see Chapter 42).

Hypothermia. Heat loss during prolonged exposure to cold overwhelms the ability of the body to produce heat, causing hypothermia. Hypothermia is classified by core temperature measurements (Table 29.1). Hypothermia contributes to poor patient outcomes such as increased infection complications, clotting disorders, and prolonged length of hospitalization (Salota et al., 2016). Preventing hypothermia increases patient comfort and prevents complications.

Hypothermia can be unintentional, such as falling through the ice of a frozen lake, or intentionally induced during surgical or emergency procedures to decrease metabolism and the body's need for oxygen. Accidental hypothermia usually develops gradually and goes unnoticed for several hours. Older adults are more susceptible to accidental hypothermia (Salota et al., 2016). When skin temperature drops below 34° C (93.2° F), the patient suffers uncontrolled shivering, loss of memory, depression, and poor judgment. As the body temperature falls, HR, respiratory rate, and BP also fall. The skin becomes cyanotic. Patients experience cardiac dysrhythmias and loss of consciousness and are unresponsive to painful stimuli if hypothermia progresses. In severe cases a person demonstrates clinical signs similar to those of death (e.g., lack of response to stimuli and extremely slow respirations and pulse). Assessment of core temperature is critical when you suspect hypothermia. A special low-reading thermometer is required because standard devices do not register below 35° C (95° F).

Frostbite occurs when the body is exposed to subnormal temperatures. Ice crystals form inside the cells, and permanent circulatory and tissue damage occurs. Areas particularly susceptible to frostbite are the earlobes, tip of the nose, and fingers and toes. The injured area becomes white, waxy, and firm to the touch. The patient loses sensation in the affected area. Interventions include gradual warming measures, analgesia, and protection of the injured tissue.

❖ NURSING PROCESS

Apply the nursing process and use a critical thinking approach in your care of patients. The nursing process provides a clinical decision-making approach for you to develop and implement an individualized plan of care.

Knowledge of the physiology of body temperature regulation is essential to assess and evaluate a patient's response to temperature alterations and to intervene safely. Implement independent nursing measures to increase or minimize heat loss, promote heat conservation, and increase comfort. These measures complement the effects of medically ordered therapies during illness. You also provide education to family members, parents of children, or other caregivers.

◆ Assessment

During the assessment process thoroughly assess each patient and critically analyze findings to ensure that you make patient-centered clinical decisions required for safe nursing care.

Through the Patient's Eyes. Identify your patient's values, beliefs, current treatments, and expectations regarding fever management. When possible, select the temperature site preferred by the patient. Include the patient's preferences when selecting nonpharmacological interventions for hyperthermia (e.g., cooling blankets, tepid baths, fans).

Temperature Measurement Sites. Core and surface body temperature can be measured at several sites. Intensive care units use the core temperatures of the pulmonary artery, esophagus, and urinary bladder. These measurements require the use of continuous invasive devices placed in body cavities or organs and continually display readings on an electronic monitor.

Use a thermometer for the mouth, rectum, tympanic membrane, or temporal artery to obtain intermittent temperature measurements.

Axillary temperature measurements, obtained by placing a thermometer under the axillae, require longer measurement time and are only reliable for stable infants (Charafeddine et al., 2014). You can apply noninvasive chemically prepared thermometer patches to the skin to screen for temperature alterations.

Oral, rectal, and skin temperature sites rely on effective blood circulation at the measurement site. The heat of the blood is conducted to the thermometer probe. Tympanic temperature relies on the radiation of body heat to an infrared sensor. Because the tympanic membrane shares the same arterial blood supply as the hypothalamus, it is a core temperature. Temporal artery measurements detect the temperature of cutaneous blood flow.

To ensure accurate temperature readings, measure each site correctly (see Skill 29.1). The temperature obtained varies, depending on the site used, but it is usually between 36° C (96.8° F) and 38° C (100.4° F). Rectal temperatures are usually 0.5° C (0.9° F) higher than oral temperatures. Each of the common temperature measurement sites has advantages and disadvantages (Table 29.2). Choose the safest and most accurate site for each patient. When possible, use the same site when repeated measurements are necessary.

TABLE 29.2   Advantages and Disadvantages of Select Temperature Measurement Sites

Site Advantages	Site Limitations
Oral Easily accessible—requires no position change Comfortable for patient Provides accurate surface temperature reading Reflects rapid change in core temperature Reliable route to measure temperature in patients who are intubated	Causes delay in measurement if patient recently ingested hot/cold fluids or foods, smoked, or is receiving oxygen by mask/cannula Not for patients who had oral surgery, trauma, history of epilepsy, or shaking chills Not for infants, small children, or patients who are confused, unconscious, or uncooperative Risk of body fluid exposure
Tympanic Membrane Easily accessible site Found to be most accurate method in critically ill patients when compared with oral, axillary, and rectal (Asadian et al., 2016). Minimal patient repositioning required Obtained without disturbing, waking, or repositioning patients Used for patients with tachypnea without affecting breathing Sensitive to core temperature changes Very rapid measurement (2 to 5 seconds) Unaffected by oral intake of food or fluids or smoking Not influenced by environmental temperatures	More variability of measurement than with other core temperature devices Requires removal of hearing aids before measurement Requires disposable sensor cover with only one size available Otitis media and cerumen impaction distorts readings Not used in patients who have had surgery of the ear or tympanic membrane Does not accurately measure core temperature changes during and after exercise Does not obtain continuous measurement Affected by ambient temperature devices such as incubators, radiant warmers, and facial fans Use in infants older than 6 months (Seattle Children's Hospital, 2019) and children under 3 years of age; use care to position device correctly because anatomy of ear canal makes it difficult to position. Inaccuracies reported caused by incorrect positioning of handheld unit
Rectal Argued to be more reliable when oral temperature is difficult or impossible to obtain	Lags behind core temperature during rapid temperature changes Not for patients with diarrhea, rectal disorders, or bleeding tendencies or those who had rectal surgery Requires positioning and is often source of patient embarrassment and anxiety Risk of body fluid exposure and injury to rectal lining Requires lubrication Not for routine vital signs in newborns Readings influenced by impacted stool
Skin Inexpensive Provides continuous reading Safe and noninvasive Used for neonates	Measurement lags behind other sites during temperature changes, especially during hyperthermia Adhesion impaired by diaphoresis or sweat Reading affected by environmental temperature Cannot be used for patients with allergy to adhesives

Continued

TABLE 29.2	Advantages and Disadvantages of Select Temperature Measurement Sites—cont'd
Site Advantages	**Site Limitations**
Temporal Artery	
Easy to access without position change	Inaccurate with head covering or hair on forehead
Very rapid measurement	Affected by skin moisture such as diaphoresis or sweating
Comfortable with no risk of injury to patient or nurse	
Eliminates need to disrobe or be unbundled	
Comfortable for patient	
Used in premature infants, newborns, and children (Reynolds et al., 2014)	
Reflects rapid change in core temperature	
Sensor cover not required	
Axillary	
Safe and inexpensive	Long measurement time
Reliable in stable term and preterm infants (Charafeddine et al., 2014)	Requires continuous positioning
	Measurement lags behind core temperature during rapid temperature changes
	Not recommended for detecting fever
	Requires exposure of thorax that can result in temperature loss, especially in newborns
	Affected by exposure to environment, including time to place the thermometer
	Underestimates core temperature

Thermometers. Two types of thermometers are available for measuring body temperature: electronic and disposable. The mercury-in-glass thermometer, once the standard device, has been eliminated from health care facilities because of the environmental hazards of mercury. However, some patients still use mercury-in-glass thermometers at home. When you find a mercury-in-glass thermometer in the home, teach the patient about safer temperature devices and encourage the disposal of mercury products at appropriate neighborhood hazardous disposal locations. Disposable digital thermometers are readily available for use in the home setting. Home disposable thermometers are useful for temperature screening but are not as accurate as nondisposable electronic thermometers.

Each device measures temperature using the Celsius or Fahrenheit scale. Electronic thermometers convert the temperature scales by activating a switch. When it is necessary to convert temperature readings, use the following formulas:

1. To convert Fahrenheit to Celsius, subtract 32 from the Fahrenheit reading and multiply the result by 5/9.

$$C = (F - 32) \times \frac{5}{9}$$

$$\text{Example} : 40° \, C = \left(104° \, F - 32\right) \times \frac{5}{9}$$

2. To convert Celsius to Fahrenheit, multiply the Celsius reading by 9/5 and add 32 to the product.

$$F = \left(\frac{9}{5} \times °C\right) + 32$$

$$\text{Example} : 104° \, F = \left(\frac{9}{5} \times 40°C\right) + 32°$$

Electronic Thermometer. The electronic thermometer consists of a rechargeable battery-powered display unit, a thin wire cord, and a temperature-processing probe covered by a disposable probe cover (Fig. 29.4A). Separate unbreakable reusable probes with single-use disposable covers are available for oral and rectal use. Electronic thermometers provide two modes of operation: a 4-second predictive temperature and a 3-minute standard temperature. Nurses use the 4-second predictive mode, which improves measurement accuracy. A sound signals, and a reading appears on the display unit when the peak temperature reading has been measured.

Another form of electronic thermometer is used exclusively for tympanic temperature. An otoscope-like speculum with an infrared sensor tip detects heat radiated from the tympanic membrane (Fig. 29.4B). The tip is covered by a single patient-use cover. Within seconds of placement in the auditory canal, a sound signals, and a reading appears on the display unit when the peak temperature reading has been measured.

There is an electronic thermometer that measures the temperature of the superficial temporal artery. A handheld scanner with an infrared sensor tip detects the temperature of cutaneous blood flow by sweeping the sensor across the forehead and just behind the ear (Fig. 29.4C). After scanning is complete, a reading appears on the display unit. Temporal artery temperature is a reliable noninvasive measure of core temperature.

The greatest advantages of electronic thermometers are that their readings appear within seconds and they are easy to read. The plastic sheath is unbreakable and ideal for children. Their expense is a major disadvantage. Maintaining cleanliness of the probes is an important consideration. For example, if not properly cleaned between patients, gastrointestinal contamination of a rectal probe causes disease transmission. Wipe the thermometer device daily with alcohol and the thermometer probe with an alcohol swab after each patient, paying particular attention to the ridges where the probe cover is secured to the probe.

Chemical Dot Thermometers. Single-use or reusable chemical dot thermometers (Fig. 29.4D) are thin strips of plastic with a temperature sensor at one end. The sensor consists of a matrix of chemically impregnated dots that change color at different temperatures. In the Celsius version there are 50 dots, each representing a temperature increment of 0.1° C, over a range of 35.5° C to 40.4° C. The Fahrenheit version has 45 dots with increments of 0.2° F and a range of 96° F to 104.8° F. Chemical dots on the thermometer change color to reflect temperature reading, usually within 60 seconds. Most are for single use. In one reusable brand for a single patient, the chemical dots return

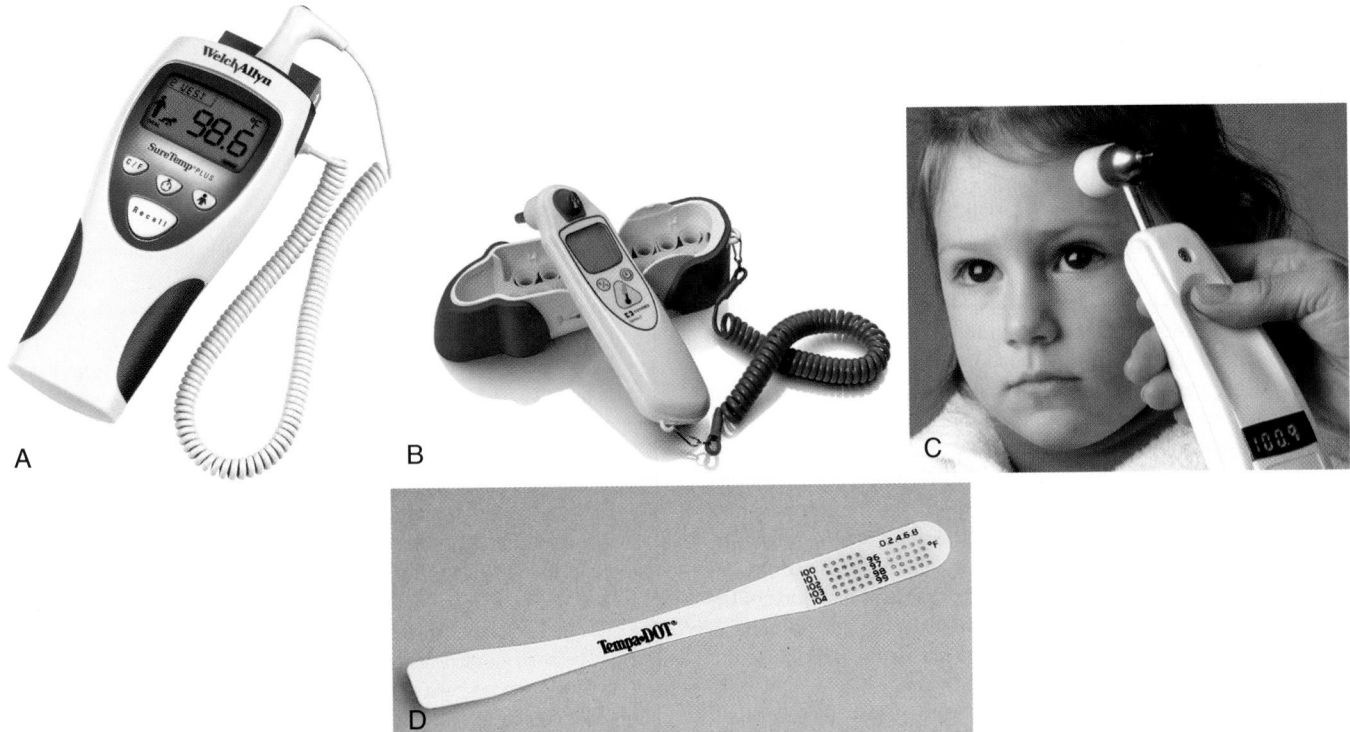

FIG. 29.4 A, Electronic thermometer with disposable probe. **B,** Genius 3 Tympanic Thermometer. **C,** Temporal artery thermometer. **D,** Chemical dot disposable single-use thermometer. (**A,** Courtesy Hillrom; **B,** Copyright © 2018 Courtesy of Cardinal Health UK Ltd.; **C,** photo courtesy Exergen.)

to the original color within a few seconds. Chemical dot thermometers are for oral use and are useful for screening temperatures, especially in infants, young children, and patients who are intubated. Chemical dot thermometers often underestimate oral temperature by 0.4° C (0.7° F) or more. Use an electronic thermometer to confirm measurements made with a chemical dot thermometer when treatment decisions are involved. Chemical dot thermometers are useful when caring for patients who have sores in the mouth or who are on protective isolation to avoid the need to take electronic instruments into patient rooms (see Chapter 28).

Another disposable thermometer useful for screening temperature is a temperature-sensitive patch or tape. Applied to the forehead or abdomen, chemical-sensitive areas of the patch change color at different temperatures. This type of thermometer can also be affected by environmental temperature.

REFLECT NOW

You are planning interventions for a patient with hyperthermia who has entered the emergency department. How will the patient's characteristics influence your care plan?

◆ Nursing Diagnosis

After concluding your assessment, cluster assessment findings to form a nursing diagnosis (Box 29.4). For example, a decrease in body temperature, shivering, skin cool to touch, tachycardia and lowered SpO₂ indicate the nursing diagnosis of *Hypothermia*. State a nursing diagnosis as either an at-risk or problem-focused (negative) temperature alteration. Implement actions to minimize or eliminate risk factors if

---

BOX 29.4 Nursing Diagnostic Process

Impaired Thermoregulation Related to Aging and Inability to Adapt to Environmental Temperature

Assessment Activities	Assessment Findings
Obtain vital signs, including temperature, pulse (see Skill 29.2), respirations (see Skill 29.3), SpO₂ (see Skill 29.4).	Increased body temperature above usual range
	Tachycardia
	Tachypnea
Palpate skin.	Warm, dry skin
Observe patient's appearance and behavior while talking and resting.	Confusion
	Mild shivering
	Flushed skin
Review health history.	Found in unventilated apartment during heat wave; 85 years old with history of dementia

---

the patient has an at-risk diagnosis. Examples of nursing diagnoses for patients with body temperature alterations include the following:

- *Risk for Impaired Thermoregulation*
- *Hyperthermia*
- *Hypothermia*
- *Impaired Thermoregulation*
- *Fever*

Once you determine a diagnosis, accurately select the related factor for problem-focused (negative) diagnoses. The related factor allows you to develop/set appropriate patient goals and select appropriate nursing interventions. In the example of hyperthermia, a related factor of *vigorous activity* results in interventions that are much different from those used with a related factor of *decreased ability to perspire*.

◆ Planning

During planning integrate the knowledge gathered from assessment and the patient history to develop an individualized plan of care. Match the patient's needs with interventions that are supported and recommended in the clinical research literature.

Goals and Outcomes. The plan of care for a patient with alteration in temperature includes realistic and individualized goals along with relevant outcomes. This requires collaboration with the patient and family in setting patient-centered goals and outcomes while selecting nursing interventions. Establish expected outcomes to gauge progress toward returning the body temperature to an acceptable range. In cases in which the temperature alteration requires helping patients modify their environment, goals may be long term (e.g., obtaining appropriate clothing to wear in cold weather). Short-term goals such as regaining normal range of body temperature improve patient health. In the example of a patient who has an elevated fever and excessive diaphoresis, the goal of care is attaining fluid and electrolyte balance. The outcome is that the patient's intake and output are balanced for the next 24 hours.

Setting Priorities. Set priorities of care with regard to the extent that the temperature alteration affects a patient. The severity of a temperature alteration and its effects, together with the patient's general health status, influence your priorities in his or her care. Safety is a top priority. Often other medical problems complicate the care plan. For instance, body temperature imbalance affects body requirements for fluids. Patients with heart problems often have difficulty tolerating required fluid replacement therapy.

Teamwork and Collaboration. Patients at risk for imbalanced body temperature require an individualized care plan directed at maintaining normothermia and reducing risk factors. For example, it is important to establish the outcome that a patient who is homeless can explain appropriate actions to take (e.g., fluid intake, type of clothing) and available community resources to use (e.g., cooling stations) during a heat wave. In contrast, an older adult living at home may need encouragement and reminders from family to use fans or window air conditioner units and to drink appropriate amounts of fluids. Teach the patient and caregiver the importance of thermoregulation and actions to take during excessive environmental heat. Education is particularly important for parents, who need to know how to take action at home and whom to call (e.g., health care provider's office, home care nurse) when an infant or child develops a temperature imbalance.

◆ Implementation

Health Promotion. By maintaining balance between heat production and heat loss you promote the health of patients at risk for imbalanced body temperature. Consider patient activity, temperature of the environment, and appropriate clothing. Teach patients to avoid strenuous exercise in hot, humid weather; to drink fluids such as water or clear fruity juices before, during, and after exercise; and to wear lightweight, loose-fitting, light-colored clothes. Also teach patients to avoid exercising in areas with poor ventilation, to wear a protective covering over the head when outdoors, and to expose themselves to hot climates gradually.

Prevention is key for patients at risk for hypothermia. It involves educating patients, family members, and friends. Patients at risk include the very young; the very old; and people debilitated by trauma,

---

BOX 29.5 Nursing Interventions for Patients With a Fever

Interventions (Unless Contraindicated by Medical Condition)

- Obtain cultures of body fluids such as urine, sputum, or blood (before beginning antibiotics) if ordered. Obtain blood specimens to coincide with temperature spikes, when the antigen-producing organism is most prevalent.
- Minimize heat production: reduce frequency of activities that increase oxygen demand such as excessive turning and ambulation; allow rest periods; limit physical activity.
- Maximize heat loss: reduce external covering on patient's body without causing shivering; keep patient, clothing, and bed linen dry.
- Satisfy requirements for increased metabolic rate: provide supplemental oxygen therapy as ordered to improve oxygen delivery to body cells; provide measures to stimulate appetite and offer well-balanced meals; provide fluids (at least 8 to 10 [8-oz] glasses for patients with normal cardiac and renal function) to replace fluids lost through insensible water loss and sweating.
- Promote patient comfort: encourage oral hygiene because oral mucous membranes dry easily from dehydration; control temperature of the environment without inducing shivering; apply damp cloth to patient's forehead.
- Identify onset and duration of febrile episode phases: examine previous temperature measurements for trends.
- Initiate health teaching as indicated.
- Control environmental temperature to 21° to 27° C (70° to 80° F).

---

stroke, diabetes, drug or alcohol intoxication, and sepsis. Patients who are mentally ill or handicapped sometimes fall victim to hypothermia because they are unaware of the dangers of cold conditions. People with inadequate home heating, shelter, diet, or clothing are also at risk. Fatigue, dark skin color, malnutrition, and hypoxemia contribute to the risk of frostbite.

Prevention is also the focus for individuals at risk for heatstroke, with prevention strategies such as using air conditioners; limiting outdoor activities during the daytime; consuming ample fluids; wearing loose-fitting and light-colored clothing; being aware of medication side effects that may cause fluid losses, decrease sweating, or decrease heart rate; and never leaving impaired adults or children in a car unattended (Peiris et al., 2017).

Acute Care

Fever. When an elevated body temperature develops, initiate interventions to treat fever. The objective of therapy is to increase heat loss, reduce heat production, and prevent complications. The choice of interventions depends on the cause; adverse effects; and the strength, intensity, and duration of the temperature elevation. The health care provider attempts to determine the cause of the elevated temperature by isolating the causative pyrogen. Sometimes it is necessary to obtain culture specimens for laboratory analysis such as urine, blood, sputum, and wound sites (see Chapter 28). Some antibiotic medications are ordered to be given after the cultures have been obtained. Administering antibiotics destroys pyrogenic bacteria and eliminates body stimulus for the elevated temperature. Nurses are essential in assessing and implementing temperature-reducing strategies (Box 29.5).

Most fevers in children are of a viral origin, last only briefly, and have limited effects. However, children still have immature temperature-control mechanisms, and temperatures can rise rapidly. Dehydration and febrile seizures occur during rising temperatures of children between 6 months and 3 years of age. Febrile seizures are unusual in children over 5 years old. The extent of the temperature, often exceeding 38.8° C (101.8° F), seems to be a more important factor in regard to seizures than the rapidity of the temperature increase. Children are at particular risk for fluid volume deficit because they can quickly lose large amounts of fluids in proportion to their body weight. It is important to maintain accurate intake and output records, weigh the patient daily, encourage fluids, and provide regular mouth/oral care.

Sometimes a fever is a hypersensitivity response to a drug. Drug fevers are often accompanied by other allergy symptoms such as rash or pruritus (itching). Treatment involves withdrawing the medication, treating any skin integrity impairment, and educating the patient and family about the allergy.

Antipyretics are medications that reduce fever. Acetaminophen and nonsteroidal antiinflammatory drugs such as ibuprofen, salicylates, and indomethacin reduce fever by increasing heat loss. Although not used to treat fever, corticosteroids reduce heat production by interfering with the hypothalamic response. It is important to remember that steroids mask signs and symptoms of infection (Frenkel et al., 2018). Therefore patients who are prescribed steroids need to be monitored closely, especially if they are at risk for infection.

Nonpharmacological therapies for fever increase heat loss by evaporation, conduction, convection, or radiation. Make sure that nursing measures to enhance body cooling do not stimulate shivering. Shivering is counterproductive and increases energy expenditure up to 400%. Tepid sponge baths, bathing with alcohol-water solutions, applying ice packs to axillae and groin areas, and cooling fans were previously used to reduce fever; however, *avoid these therapies because they lead to shivering*. There is no advantage of these methods over antipyretic medications.

Blankets cooled by circulating water delivered by motorized units increase conductive heat loss. Follow manufacturer instructions for applying these hypothermia blankets because of the risk for skin breakdown and "freeze burns." Placing a bath blanket between the patient and the hypothermia blanket and wrapping distal extremities (fingers, toes, and genitalia) reduces the risk of injury to the skin and tissue from hypothermia therapy. Wrapping the patient's extremities reduces the incidence and intensity of shivering. Medications such as meperidine or butorphanol reduce shivering.

Heatstroke. Heatstroke is an emergency situation, First aid treatment includes moving the patient to a cooler environment; removing excess body clothing; placing cool, wet towels over the skin; and using oscillating fans to increase convective heat loss. Emergency medical treatment also includes administering intravenous (IV) fluids, irrigating the stomach and lower bowel with cool solutions, and applying hypothermia blankets.

Hypothermia. The priority treatment for hypothermia is to prevent a further decrease in body temperature. Removing wet clothes, replacing them with dry ones, and wrapping patients in blankets are key nursing interventions. In emergencies away from a health care setting, have the patient lie under blankets next to a warm person. A conscious patient benefits from drinking hot liquids such as soup and by avoiding alcohol and caffeinated fluids. It is also helpful to keep the head covered, place the patient near a fire or in a warm room, or place heating pads next to areas of the body (head and neck) that lose heat the quickest.

REFLECT NOW

You implement an order for acetaminophen for an elderly patient with a fever of 100.6°F. What additional measures can you implement to improve comfort care? What vital sign changes do you expect if your interventions are successful?

Restorative and Continuing Care. Educate the patient with a fever about the importance of taking and continuing any antibiotics as directed until the course of treatment is completed. Children and older adults are at risk for deficient fluid volume because they can quickly lose large amounts of fluids in proportion to their body weight. Provide education on signs of dehydration such as dry mouth, sunken eyes, and decreased urine output. Identifying preferred fluids and encouraging oral fluid intake are important ongoing nursing interventions.

◆ Evaluation

Through the Patient's Eyes. Evaluate your patient's perspectives about the care provided. Is he or she satisfied with the outcomes of care or does the care plan need to be modified? Including the patient in the evaluation demonstrates that you value his or her perspective and contributes to patient safety.

Patient Outcomes. Evaluate all nursing interventions by comparing the patient's actual response to the expected outcomes of the care plan. Determine whether goals of care were met and make revisions to the care plan when necessary. After an intervention, measure the patient's temperature to evaluate for change. In addition, use other evaluative measures such as palpating the skin and assessing pulse and respirations. If therapies are effective, body temperature returns to an acceptable range, other vital signs stabilize, and the patient reports a sense of comfort.

PULSE

The pulse is the palpable bounding of blood flow in a peripheral artery. Blood flows through the body in a continuous circuit. The pulse is an indirect indicator of circulatory status.

Physiology and Regulation

Electrical impulses originating from the sinoatrial (SA) node travel through heart muscle to stimulate cardiac contraction. Approximately 60 to 70 mL of blood enters the aorta with each ventricular contraction (stroke volume [SV]). With each SV ejection, the walls of the aorta distend, creating a pulse wave that travels rapidly toward the distal ends of the arteries. The pulse wave moves 15 times faster through the aorta and 100 times faster through the small arteries than the ejected volume of blood. When a pulse wave reaches a peripheral artery, you can feel it by palpating the artery lightly against underlying bone or muscle. The number of pulsing sensations occurring in 1 minute is the pulse rate.

The volume of blood pumped by the heart during 1 minute is the cardiac output, the product of HR and the ventricular SV. In an adult the heart normally pumps 5000 mL of blood per minute. A change in HR or SV does not always change the output of the heart or the amount of blood in the arteries. For example, if a person's HR is 70 beats/min and the SV is 70 mL, the cardiac output is 4900 mL/min (70 beats/min × 70 mL/beat). If the HR drops to 60 beats/min and the SV rises to 85 mL/beat, the cardiac output increases to 5100 mL or 5.1 L/min (60 beats/min × 85 mL/beat).

Mechanical, neural, and chemical factors regulate the strength of ventricular contraction and the SV. SV depends on the time available to fill the ventricle with blood. When the contraction strength or SV cannot be altered, a change in HR causes a change in cardiac output. As HR increases, there is less time for the ventricular chambers of the heart to fill. When SV cannot change when the HR increases, the BP will decrease. As HR slows, filling time is increased, and BP increases.

An abnormally slow, rapid, or irregular pulse alters cardiac output. Assess the ability of the heart to meet the demands of body tissue for nutrients by palpating a peripheral pulse or using a stethoscope to listen to heart sounds (apical pulse) (see Skill 29.2).

TABLE 29.3   Pulse Sites

Site	Location	Assessment Criteria
Temporal	Over temporal bone of head, above and lateral to eye	Easily accessible site used to assess pulse in children
Carotid	Along medial edge of sternocleidomastoid muscle in neck	Easily accessible site used during physiological shock or cardiac arrest when other sites are not palpable
Apical	Fourth to fifth intercostal space at left midclavicular line	Site used to auscultate for apical pulse
Brachial	Groove between biceps and triceps muscles at antecubital fossa	Site used to assess status of circulation to lower arm and to auscultate blood pressure
Radial	Radial or thumb side of forearm at wrist	Common site used to assess character of pulse peripherally and status of circulation to hand
Ulnar	Ulnar or little finger side of forearm at wrist	Site used to assess status of circulation to hand; also used to perform an Allen's test
Femoral	Below inguinal ligament, midway between symphysis pubis and anterior superior iliac spine	Site used to assess character of pulse during physiological shock or cardiac arrest when other pulses are not palpable; used to assess status of circulation to leg
Popliteal	Behind knee in popliteal fossa	Site used to assess status of circulation to lower leg
Posterior tibial	Inner side of ankle, below medial malleolus	Site used to assess status of circulation to foot
Dorsalis pedis	Along top of foot, between extension tendons of great and first toe	Site used to assess status of circulation to foot

❖ NURSING PROCESS

◆ Assessment of Pulse

You can assess any artery for pulse rate, but you typically use the radial artery because it is easy to palpate. When a patient's condition suddenly worsens, the carotid artery site is recommended for quickly finding and assessing the pulse. The heart continues to deliver blood through the carotid artery to the brain as long as possible. When cardiac output declines significantly, peripheral pulses weaken and are difficult to palpate.

The radial and apical locations are the most common sites for pulse rate assessment. Use the radial pulse to teach patients how to monitor their own HRs (e.g., athletes, people taking heart medications, and patients starting a prescribed exercise regimen). If the radial pulse is abnormal or intermittent resulting from dysrhythmias or if it is inaccessible because of a dressing or cast, assess the apical pulse. When a patient takes medication that affects the HR, the apical pulse provides a more accurate assessment of heart function. The brachial or apical pulse is the best site for assessing an infant's or a young child's pulse because other peripheral pulses are deep and difficult to palpate accurately.

Assessment of other peripheral pulse sites such as the brachial or femoral artery is unnecessary when routinely obtaining vital signs. You assess other peripheral pulses when conducting a complete physical, when surgery or treatment has impaired blood flow to a body part, or when there are clinical indications of impaired peripheral blood flow (see Chapter 30). Table 29.3 summarizes pulse sites and criteria for measurement.

Use of a Stethoscope. Assessing the apical rate requires a stethoscope. The five major parts of the stethoscope are the earpieces, binaurals, tubing, bell chest piece, and diaphragm chest piece (Fig. 29.5). The plastic or rubber earpieces should fit snugly and comfortably in your ears. The binaurals should be angled and strong enough that the earpieces stay firmly in the ears without causing discomfort. To ensure the best reception of sound, the earpieces follow the contour of the ear canal, pointing toward the face when the stethoscope is in place.

The polyvinyl tubing is flexible and 30 to 40 cm (12 to 18 inches) in length. Longer tubing decreases the transmission of sound waves.

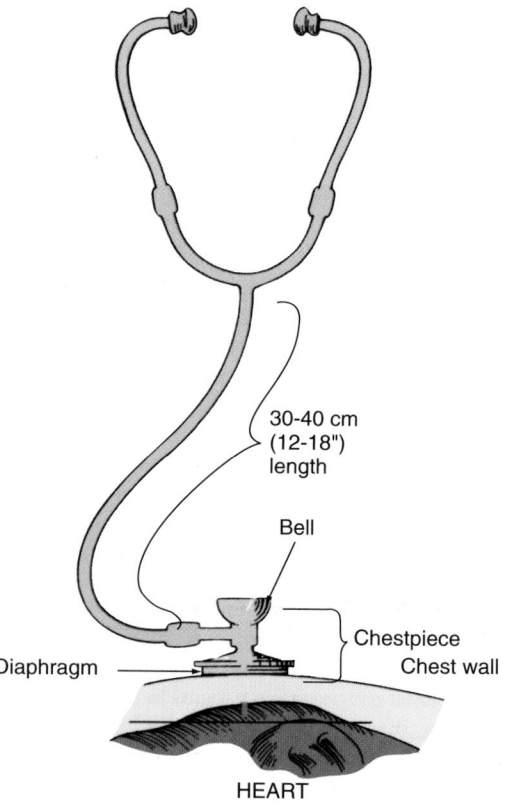

FIG. 29.5 Parts of stethoscope.

Thick-walled and moderately rigid tubing eliminates the transmission of environmental noise and prevents the tubing from kinking, which distorts sound-wave transmission. Stethoscopes have single or dual tubes.

The chest piece consists of a bell and a diaphragm that you rotate into position. The diaphragm or bell needs to be in proper position during use to hear sounds through the stethoscope. With the earpieces in your ears, tap lightly on the diaphragm to determine which side of the chest piece is functioning. The diaphragm is the circular, flat portion of the chest piece covered with a thin plastic disk. It transmits

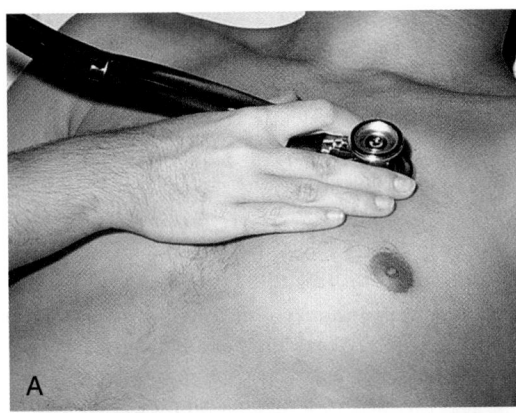

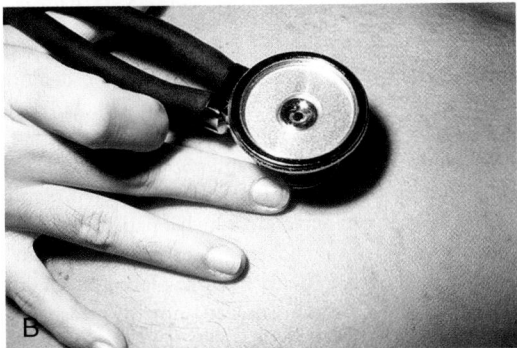

FIG. 29.6 A, Place the diaphragm firmly and securely when auscultating high-pitched lung and bowel sounds. **B,** The bell must be placed lightly on the skin to hear low-pitched vascular and heart sounds.

TABLE 29.4	Acceptable Ranges of Heart Rate
Age	**Heart Rate (beats/min)**
Infant	120-160
Toddler	90-140
Preschooler	80-110
School-age child	75-100
Adolescent	60-90
Adult	60-100

high-pitched sounds created by the high-velocity movement of air and blood. Auscultate bowel, lung, and heart sounds with the diaphragm. Place the stethoscope directly on the skin because clothing obscures the sound. Position the diaphragm to make a tight seal and press firmly against the patient's skin (Fig. 29.6A). Do not use your thumb to hold the diaphragm in place because you may hear the pulse being transmitted through it.

The bell is the bowl-shaped chest piece usually surrounded by a rubber ring. The ring avoids chilling patients with cold metal when placed on the skin. The bell transmits low-pitched sounds created by the low-velocity movement of blood. Auscultate heart and vascular sounds with the bell. Apply the bell lightly, resting the chest piece on the skin (Fig. 29.6B).

Compressing the bell against the skin reduces low-pitched sound amplification and creates a "diaphragm of skin." Some stethoscopes have one chest piece that combines features of the bell and diaphragm. When you use light pressure, the chest piece is a bell; exerting more pressure converts the bell into a diaphragm.

The stethoscope is a delicate instrument and requires proper care for optimal function. Remove the earpieces regularly and clean them of cerumen (earwax). Clean the bell and diaphragm between patients thoroughly with an antiseptic swab to remove microorganisms. Clean the tubing regularly with mild soap and water. A study examined the cross-contamination of physicians' hands with MRSA microorganisms following a physical examination of patients. The study showed that the contamination level of the stethoscope was substantial after a single physical examination and comparable to the contamination of parts of the physician's dominant hand (Longtin et al., 2014)

Character of the Pulse. Assessment of the radial pulse includes measuring the rate, rhythm, strength, and equality. When auscultating an apical pulse, assess rate and rhythm only.

Rate. Before measuring a pulse, review the patient's baseline rate for comparison (Table 29.4). Some practitioners prefer to make baseline measurements of the pulse rate as a patient assumes a sitting, standing, and lying position. Postural changes affect the pulse rate because of alterations in blood volume and sympathetic activity. The HR temporarily increases when a person changes from a lying to a sitting or standing position.

When assessing the pulse, consider the variety of factors influencing the heart rate (Table 29.5). A single factor or a combination of these factors often causes significant changes. If you detect an abnormal rate while palpating a peripheral pulse, the next step is to assess the apical rate. The apical rate requires auscultation of heart sounds, which provides a more accurate assessment of cardiac contraction.

Assess the apical rate by listening to heart sounds (see Chapter 30). Identify the first and second heart sounds (S_1 and S_2). At normal slow rates S_1 is low pitched and dull, sounding like a "lub." S_2 is higher pitched and shorter, creating the sound "dub." Count each set of "lub-dub" as one heartbeat. Using the diaphragm or bell of the stethoscope, count the number of lub-dubs occurring in 1 minute.

Peripheral and apical pulse rate assessment often reveals variations in HR. Two common abnormalities in pulse rate are tachycardia and bradycardia. Tachycardia is an abnormally elevated HR, above 100 beats/min in adults. Bradycardia is a slow rate, below 60 beats/min in adults.

An inefficient contraction of the heart that fails to transmit a pulse wave to the peripheral pulse site creates a pulse deficit. To assess a pulse deficit you and a colleague assess radial and apical rates simultaneously and then compare rates (see Skill 29.2). The difference between the apical and radial pulse rates is the pulse deficit. For example, an apical rate of 92 with a radial rate of 78 leaves a pulse deficit of 14 beats. Pulse deficits are often associated with abnormal rhythms.

Rhythm. Normally a regular interval occurs between each pulse or heartbeat. An interval interrupted by an early or late beat or a missed beat indicates an abnormal rhythm, or dysrhythmia. A dysrhythmia threatens the ability of the heart to provide adequate cardiac output, particularly if it occurs repetitively. You identify a dysrhythmia by palpating an interruption in successive pulse waves or auscultating an interruption between heart sounds. If a dysrhythmia is present, assess the regularity of its occurrence and auscultate the apical rate (see Chapter 30). Dysrhythmias are described as regularly irregular or irregularly irregular.

To document a dysrhythmia, the health care provider often orders an electrocardiogram (ECG), Holter monitor, or telemetry monitor. An ECG records the electrical activity of the heart for a 12-second interval. This test requires placement of electrodes across a patient's chest followed by recording of the heart rhythm. A patient wears the Holter monitor, which records and stores 24 hours of electrical activity. Access to the information recorded is not available until after the 24 hours have passed and the data are reviewed. Cardiac telemetry provides continuous monitoring of the electrical activity of the heart

TABLE 29.5   Factors Influencing Heart Rate

Factor	Increases Pulse Rate	Decreases Pulse Rate
Exercise	Short-term exercise	Heart conditioned by long-term exercise, resulting in lower resting pulse and quicker return to resting level after exercise (AHA, 2015)
Temperature	Fever and heat	Hypothermia
Acute pain	Increased sympathetic activity increases heart rate, stroke volume, and peripheral resistance, all of which increase myocardial work and oxygen demand.	Effect of chronic pain on heart rate varies; parasympathetic stimulation increased by unrelieved severe pain lowers heart rate
Emotions	Sympathetic stimulation increased by anxiety affects heart rate.	
Medications	Positive chronotropic drugs such as epinephrine	Negative chronotropic drugs such as digitalis; beta-adrenergic and calcium channel blockers
Hemorrhage	Sympathetic stimulation increased by loss of blood	
Postural changes	Standing or sitting	Lying down
Pulmonary conditions	Diseases causing poor oxygenation such as asthma, chronic obstructive pulmonary disease (COPD)	

transmitted to a stationary monitor. Telemetry permits continuous observation of heart rhythm during all of a patient's daily activities and thus allows for immediate treatment if the rhythm becomes erratic or unstable.

Children often have a sinus dysrhythmia, which is an irregular heartbeat that speeds up with inspiration and slows with expiration. This is a normal finding that you can verify by having the child hold his or her breath; the HR usually becomes regular.

Strength. The strength or amplitude of a pulse reflects the volume of blood ejected against the arterial wall with each heart contraction and the condition of the arterial vascular system leading to the pulse site. Normally the pulse strength remains the same with each heartbeat. Document the pulse strength as bounding (4); full or strong (3); normal and expected (2); diminished or barely palpable (1); or absent (0). Include assessment of pulse strength in the assessment of the vascular system (see Chapter 30).

Equality. Assess radial pulses on both sides of the peripheral vascular system, comparing the characteristics of each. A pulse in one extremity is sometimes unequal in strength or absent in many disease states (e.g., thrombus [clot] formation). Assess all symmetrical pulses simultaneously except for the carotid pulse. Never measure the carotid pulses simultaneously because excessive pressure occludes blood supply to the brain.

◆ Nursing Diagnosis

Pulse assessment determines the general state of cardiovascular health and the response of the body to other system imbalances. Tachycardia,

bradycardia, and dysrhythmias are assessment findings found for many nursing diagnoses, including the following:

- *Activity Intolerance*
- *Dehydration*
- *Hypervolaemia*
- *Impaired Cardiac Function*
- *Impaired Peripheral Tissue Perfusion*

◆ Planning and Implementation

The nursing care plan includes independent nursing interventions based on the nursing diagnosis identified and the risk factors or related factors. For example, the assessment findings of an abnormal HR in response to activity, exertional dyspnea, and a patient's verbal report of fatigue lead to a diagnosis of *Activity Intolerance*. When the related factor is *inactivity following a prolonged illness*, interventions focus on increasing the patient's daily exercise routine. If the diagnosis has a related factor of *sedentary lifestyle*, interventions include an exercise routine with adaptions during activities of daily living that increase the patient's overall activity level. Chapter 38 details standards for promoting early activity and exercise. A patient-centered plan of care is key to developing an exercise plan to which a patient will adhere. Also educate patients about the benefits of exercise and how to measure heart rate during exercise. Patients who are placed on medications to improve heart function should also learn how to measure their own pulse.

A patient's nursing diagnoses (e.g., *Activity Intolerance*) will often develop as a result of medical conditions, such as heart failure, chronic lung diseases, or myocardial infarction. Therefore the plan of care includes dependent interventions that focus on the timely administration of medications (e.g., cardiotonics, beta-adrenergic blocking agents, and oxygen) and careful management of fluid balance.

◆ Evaluation

Patient Outcomes. Once a plan of care is implemented, evaluate the patient's outcomes, which will involve evaluation of the character of the pulse in response to interventions. For example, if a patient is beginning to ambulate after prolonged immobility, measure the pulse as the patient ambulates and when ambulation is completed to identify any change. Basically the patient's goal is to stay within 10 to 20 beats above normal resting rate (AHA, 2015). Exercise intensity is a subjective measure of how hard physical activity feels to a person while he or she is exercising (Mayo Clinic, 2019). It is important to always ask patients how they feel, especially when exercising the first time after a prolonged illness or surgery. For example, during low to moderate exercise a patient may perceive that breathing quickens, but he or she is not out of breath. The patient may develop a light sweat after about 10 minutes of activity (Mayo Clinic, 2019). A more objective measure of activity tolerance is measuring a patient's actual heart rate compared with his or her target heart rate. The target heart rate is useful for evaluating a patient's exercise intensity and tolerance (see Chapter 50).

RESPIRATION

Human survival depends on the ability of oxygen (O_2) to reach body cells and carbon dioxide (CO_2) to be removed from the cells. Respiration is the mechanism the body uses to exchange gases between the atmosphere and the blood and the blood and the cells. Respiration involves **ventilation** (the movement of gases in and out

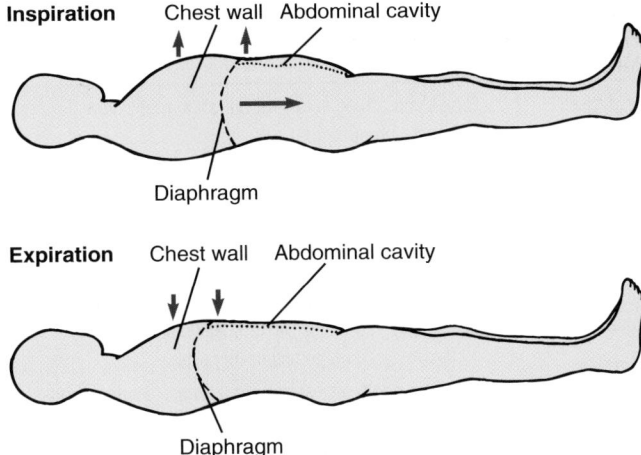

FIG. 29.7 Illustration of diaphragmatic and chest wall movement during inspiration and expiration.

of the lungs), diffusion (the movement of oxygen and carbon dioxide between the alveoli and the red blood cells), and perfusion (the distribution of red blood cells to and from the pulmonary capillaries). Analyzing respiratory efficiency requires integrating assessment data from all three processes. Assess ventilation by determining respiratory rate, depth, rhythm, and end-tidal carbon dioxide ($EtCO_2$) value. Assess diffusion and perfusion by determining oxygen saturation (SpO_2).

Physiological Control

Breathing generally is a passive process. Normally a person thinks little about it. The respiratory center in the brainstem regulates the involuntary control of respirations. Adults normally breathe in a smooth, uninterrupted pattern 12 to 20 times a minute.

The body regulates ventilation using levels of CO_2, O_2, and hydrogen ion concentration (pH) in the arterial blood. The most important factor in the control of ventilation is the level of CO_2 in the arterial blood. An elevation in the CO_2 level causes the respiratory control system in the brain to increase the rate and depth of breathing. The increased ventilatory effort removes excess CO_2 (hypercarbia) by increasing exhalation. However, patients with chronic lung disease have ongoing hypercarbia. For these patients chemoreceptors in the carotid artery and aorta become sensitive to hypoxemia, or low levels of arterial O_2. When arterial oxygen levels fall, these receptors signal the brain to increase the rate and depth of ventilation. Hypoxemia thus helps to control ventilation in patients with chronic lung disease. However, when arterial oxygen levels fall below 88%, supplemental low dose oxygen may be required. Continuous long-term oxygen administration improves survival of patients with COPD (Koczulla et al., 2018)

Mechanics of Breathing

Although breathing is normally passive, muscular work is involved in moving the lungs and chest wall. Inspiration is an active process. During inspiration the respiratory center sends impulses along the phrenic nerve, causing the diaphragm to contract. Abdominal organs move downward and forward, increasing the length of the chest cavity to move air into the lungs. The diaphragm moves approximately 1 cm (4/10 inch), and the ribs retract upward from the midline of the body approximately 1.2 to 2.5 cm (1/2 to 1 inch). During a normal, relaxed breath, a person inhales 500 mL of air. This amount is referred to as the tidal volume. During expiration the diaphragm relaxes, and the abdominal organs return to their original positions. The lung and chest wall return to a relaxed position (Fig. 29.7). Expiration is a passive

process. Sighing interrupts the normal rate and depth of ventilation, eupnea. The sigh, a prolonged deeper breath, is a protective physiological mechanism for expanding small airways and alveoli not ventilated during a normal breath.

The accurate assessment of respirations depends on the recognition of normal thoracic and abdominal movements. During quiet breathing the chest wall gently rises and falls. Contraction of the intercostal muscles between the ribs or contraction of the muscles in the neck and shoulders (the accessory muscles of breathing) is not visible. During normal quiet breathing diaphragmatic movement causes the abdominal cavity to rise and fall slowly.

❖ NURSING PROCESS

◆ Assessment of Ventilation

Respirations are the easiest of all vital signs to assess, but they are often the most haphazardly measured. Do not estimate respirations. Accurate measurement requires observation and palpation of chest wall movement.

A sudden change in the character of respirations is important. Because respiration is tied to the function of numerous body systems, consider all variables when changes occur (Box 29.6). For example, a decrease in respirations occurring in a patient after head trauma often signifies injury to the brainstem.

Do not let a patient know that you are assessing respirations. Quietly observe the patient's breathing and when appropriate begin to count the rate A patient aware of the assessment can alter the rate and depth of breathing (Hill et al., 2018). Assess respirations immediately after measuring pulse rate, with your hand still on the patient's wrist as it rests over the chest or abdomen. In children, measure respirations first, before other vital signs. When assessing a patient's respirations, keep in mind the patient's usual ventilatory rate and pattern, the influence any disease or illness has on respiratory function, the relationship between respiratory and cardiovascular function, and the influence of therapies on respirations. The objective measurements of respiratory status include the rate and depth of breathing and the rhythm of ventilatory movements (see Skill 29.3).

Respiratory Rate. Observe a full inspiration and expiration when counting ventilation or respiration rate. The usual respiratory rate varies with age (Table 29.6). The usual range of respiratory rate declines throughout life. A patient's respiratory rate can be used to help predict a risk for cardiac arrest. For example a respiratory rate greater than 27 breaths/min in an adult is a better predictor of cardiac arrest within 72 hours than heart rate or blood pressure (Kelly, 2018).

The apnea monitor is a device that aids respiratory rate assessment. This device uses leads attached to a patient's chest wall; the leads sense movement. The absence of chest wall movement triggers the apnea alarm. Apnea monitoring is used often with infants in the hospital and at home to observe the risk for prolonged apneic events.

Ventilatory Depth. Assess the depth of respirations by observing the degree of excursion or movement of the chest. Describe ventilatory movements as deep or shallow, normal or labored. A deep respiration involves a full expansion of the lungs with full exhalation. Respirations are shallow and difficult to observe when only a small quantity of air passes through the lungs. Use more objective techniques if you observe that chest excursion is unusually shallow (see Chapter 30). Table 29.7 summarizes types of breathing patterns.

Ventilatory Rhythm. Determine breathing pattern by observing the chest or the abdomen. Diaphragmatic breathing results from the

BOX 29.6 Factors Influencing Character of Respirations

Exercise
- Exercise increases rate and depth to meet the need of the body for additional oxygen and to rid the body of CO_2.

Acute Pain
- Pain alters rate and rhythm of respirations; breathing becomes shallow.
- Patient inhibits or splints chest wall movement when pain is in area of chest or abdomen.

Anxiety
- Anxiety increases respiration rate and depth as a result of sympathetic stimulation.

Smoking
- Chronic smoking changes pulmonary airways, resulting in increased rate of respirations at rest when not smoking.

Body Position
- A straight, erect posture promotes full chest expansion.
- A stooped or slumped position impairs ventilatory movement.
- Lying flat prevents full chest expansion.

Medications
- Opioid analgesics, general anesthetics, and sedative hypnotics depress rate and depth.
- Amphetamines and cocaine sometimes increase rate and depth.
- Bronchodilators slow rate by causing airway dilation.

Neurological Injury
- Injury to brainstem impairs respiratory center and inhibits respiratory rate and rhythm.

Hemoglobin Function
- Decreased hemoglobin levels (anemia) reduce oxygen-carrying capacity of the blood, which increases respiratory rate.
- Increased altitude lowers amount of saturated hemoglobin, which increases respiratory rate and depth.
- Abnormal blood cell function (e.g., sickle cell disease) reduces ability of hemoglobin to carry oxygen, which increases respiratory rate and depth.

TABLE 29.7 Alterations in Breathing Pattern

Alteration	Description
Bradypnea	Rate of breathing is regular but abnormally slow (less than 12 breaths/min).
Tachypnea	Rate of breathing is regular but abnormally rapid (greater than 20 breaths/min).
Hyperpnea	Respirations are labored, increased in depth, and increased in rate (greater than 20 breaths/min) (occurs normally during exercise).
Apnea	Respirations cease for several seconds. Persistent cessation results in respiratory arrest.
Hyperventilation	Rate and depth of respirations increase. Hypocarbia sometimes occurs.
Hypoventilation	Respiratory rate is abnormally low, and depth of ventilation is depressed. Hypercarbia sometimes occurs.
Cheyne-Stokes respiration	Respiratory rate and depth are irregular, characterized by alternating periods of apnea and hyperventilation. Respiratory cycle begins with slow, shallow breaths that gradually increase to abnormal rate and depth. The pattern reverses; breathing slows and becomes shallow, concluding as apnea before respiration resumes.
Kussmaul's respiration	Respirations are abnormally deep, regular, and increased in rate.
Biot's respiration	Respirations are abnormally shallow for two to three breaths, followed by irregular period of apnea.

TABLE 29.6 Acceptable Ranges of Respiratory Rate

Age	Rate (breaths/min)
Newborn	30-60
Infant (6 months)	30-50
Toddler (2 years)	25-32
Child	20-30
Adolescent	16-20
Adult	12-20

contraction and relaxation of the diaphragm, and you observe it best by watching abdominal movements. Healthy men and children usually demonstrate diaphragmatic breathing. Women tend to use thoracic muscles to breathe, assessed by observing movements in the upper chest. Labored respirations usually involve the accessory muscles of respiration visible in the neck. When something such as a foreign body interferes with the movement of air in and out of the lungs, the intercostal spaces retract during inspiration. A longer expiration phase is evident when the outward flow of air is obstructed (e.g., asthma, chronic obstructive pulmonary disease (COPD).

With normal breathing a regular time interval occurs after each respiratory cycle. Infants tend to breathe less regularly. A young child often breathes slowly for a few seconds and then suddenly breathes more rapidly. Respiration is regular or irregular in rhythm.

◆ Assessment of Diffusion and Perfusion

Assess the respiratory processes of diffusion and perfusion by measuring the oxygen saturation of the blood. Blood flow through the pulmonary capillaries delivers red blood cells for oxygen attachment. After oxygen diffuses from the alveoli into the pulmonary blood, most of the oxygen attaches to hemoglobin molecules in red blood cells. Red blood cells carry the oxygenated hemoglobin molecules through the left side of the heart and out to the peripheral capillaries, where the oxygen detaches, depending on the needs of the tissues.

The percent of hemoglobin that is bound with oxygen in the arteries is the percent of saturation of hemoglobin (or SaO_2). It is usually between 95% and 100%. It is affected by factors that interfere with ventilation, perfusion, or diffusion (see Chapter 41). The saturation of venous blood (SvO_2) is lower because the tissues have removed some of the oxygen from the hemoglobin molecules. Factors that interfere with or increase tissue oxygen demand affect the usual value for SvO_2, which is 70%.

Measurement of Arterial Oxygen Saturation. A pulse oximeter permits the indirect measurement of oxygen saturation (see Skill 29.4) by measuring the hemoglobin saturation in peripheral blood. The pulse oximeter is a probe with a light-emitting diode (LED)

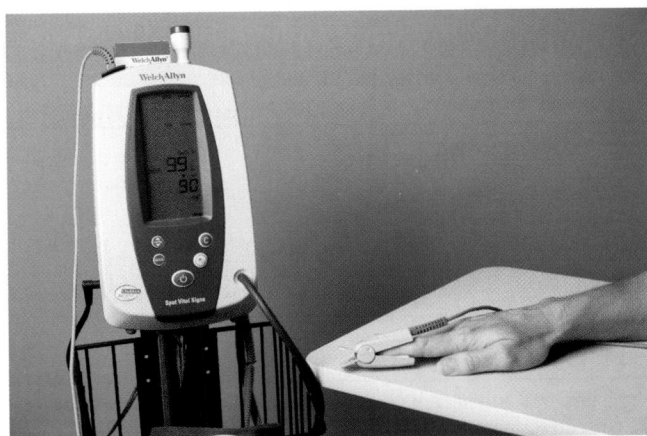

FIG. 29.8 Portable pulse oximeter with digit probe.

BOX 29.7 **Factors Affecting Determination of Pulse Oxygen Saturation (SpO$_2$)**

Interference with Light Transmission

- Outside light sources interfere with ability of oximeter to process reflected light.
- Carbon monoxide (caused by smoke inhalation or poisoning) artificially elevates SpO$_2$ by absorbing light similar to oxygen.
- Patient motion interferes with ability of oximeter to process reflected light.
- Jaundice interferes with ability of oximeter to process reflected light.
- Intravascular dyes (methylene blue) absorb light similar to deoxyhemoglobin and artificially lower saturation.
- Black or brown nail polish or metal studs in nails and thickened nails (e.g., artificial) can interfere with light absorption and the ability of the oximeter to process reflected light.
- Dark skin pigment sometimes results in signal loss or overestimation of saturation.

Interference with Arterial Pulsations

- Peripheral vascular disease (atherosclerosis) reduces pulse volume.
- Hypothermia at assessment site decreases peripheral blood flow.
- Pharmacological vasoconstrictors (e.g., epinephrine) decrease peripheral pulse volume.
- Low cardiac output and hypotension decrease blood flow to peripheral arteries.
- Peripheral edema obscures arterial pulsation.
- Tight probe records venous pulsations in finger that compete with arterial pulsations.

connected by a cable to an oximeter (Fig. 29.8). The LED emits light wavelengths that the oxygenated and deoxygenated hemoglobin molecules absorb differently. A photodetector in the probe detects the amount of oxygen bound to hemoglobin molecules, and the oximeter calculates the peripheral saturation (SpO$_2$). SpO$_2$ is a reliable estimate of SaO$_2$ when the SaO$_2$ is over 70%. A saturation greater than 93% is acceptable while a saturation of less than 90% is a clinical emergency (WHO, 2011). Values obtained with pulse oximetry are less accurate at saturations less than 70%.

Selecting the appropriate pulse oximeter probe is important to reduce measurement error. Digit probes are spring-loaded and conform to various sizes. Earlobe probes have greater accuracy at lower saturations and are least affected by peripheral vasoconstriction. You can apply disposable sensor pads to a variety of sites, including the forehead, the bridge of an adult's nose, or the sole of an infant's foot. These pads are less likely than the spring-loaded probes to cause pressure injuries. Oxygen saturation measurement using a forehead probe is quicker than finger probes and more accurate in conditions that decrease blood flow. Factors that affect light transmission or peripheral arterial pulsations affect the ability of the photodetector to measure SpO$_2$ correctly (Box 29.7). An awareness of these factors allows accurate interpretation of abnormal SpO$_2$ measurements.

Capnography

Capnography is the measurement of exhaled carbon dioxide throughout exhalation. At the end of exhalation, the EtCO$_2$ measurement approximates the PaCO$_2$ in a healthy patient, normally 35 to 45 mm Hg. In nonintubated patients EtCO$_2$ can be obtained from a special nasal cannula (see Chapter 41) connected to a monitor that detects the percentage of carbon dioxide exhaled at the end of each respiratory cycle. The EtCO$_2$ can be used to assess respiratory and cardiac status, whereas interpretation of a continuous recording, or capnogram, can detect changes in ventilation.

◆ Nursing Diagnosis

Measurement of respiratory rate, pattern, and depth, along with SpO$_2$, assesses ventilation, diffusion, and perfusion. You also conduct other assessments to measure respiratory status (see Chapter 30). Use assessment data to determine the nature of a patient's problem. Respiratory assessment data are assessment findings for many nursing diagnoses, including the following:

- *Activity Intolerance*
- *Impaired Airway Clearance*
- *Impaired Breathing*
- *Impaired Gas Exchange*

◆ Planning and Implementation

The nursing care plan includes interventions based on the nursing diagnosis identified and the related factors. For example, the assessment findings of tachycardia, dyspnea, restlessness, and an increase in CO$_2$ level lead to a diagnosis of *Impaired Gas Exchange*. Related factors could include *alveolar capillary membrane changes from infection or a ventilator-perfusion imbalance*.

You select interventions (e.g., coughing, positioning, and fluid management) on the basis of the related factor. As in the case of pulse alterations, medical diagnoses associated with respiratory changes require dependent nursing interventions. Chapter 41 details oxygen therapies.

◆ Evaluation

Patient Outcomes. After providing interventions designed to improve a patient's activity tolerance, breathing pattern, and/or gas exchange, evaluate patient outcomes by evaluating the respiratory rate, ventilatory depth, rhythm, and SpO$_2$. Consider the physiological changes expected from nursing interventions as you evaluate patient outcomes. For example, after suctioning secretions from a patient's airway, the respiratory rate should decrease and the respiratory depth should increase. The administration of bronchodilators, which relax constricted airways, can reduce respiratory rate and improve respiratory depth.

BLOOD PRESSURE

Blood pressure is the force exerted on the walls of an artery by the pulsing blood under pressure from the heart. Systemic or arterial BP, the BP in the system of arteries in the body, is a good indicator of cardiovascular health. Blood flows throughout the circulatory system because of pressure changes. It moves from an area of high pressure to one of low pressure.

The contraction of the heart forces the blood under high pressure into the aorta. The peak of maximum pressure when ejection occurs is the **systolic pressure**. When the ventricles relax, the heart fills, and the pressure of blood in the arteries is the **diastolic pressure**. Diastolic pressure is the minimal pressure exerted against the arterial walls at all times.

The standard unit for measuring BP is millimeters of mercury (mm Hg). The measurement indicates the height to which the BP raises a column of mercury. Record BP with the systolic reading before the diastolic reading (e.g., 120/80). The difference between systolic and diastolic pressure is the **pulse pressure**. For example, for a BP of 120/80, the pulse pressure is 40.

Physiology of Arterial Blood Pressure

Blood pressure reflects the interrelationships of cardiac output, peripheral vascular resistance, blood volume, blood viscosity, and artery elasticity. Your knowledge of these hemodynamic variables helps in the assessment of BP alterations.

Cardiac Output. The BP depends on the cardiac output. When volume increases in an enclosed space such as a blood vessel, the pressure in that space rises. Thus as cardiac output increases, more blood is pumped against arterial walls, causing the BP to rise. Cardiac output increases as a result of an increase in HR, greater heart muscle contractility, or an increase in blood volume. Changes in HR occur faster than changes in heart muscle contractility or blood volume. A rapid or significant increase in HR decreases the filling time of the heart, which decreases the volume in the left ventricle, and BP decreases.

Peripheral Resistance. The BP depends on peripheral vascular resistance. Blood circulates through a network of arteries, arterioles, capillaries, venules, and veins. Arteries and arterioles are surrounded by smooth muscle that contracts or relaxes to change the size of the lumen. The size of arteries and arterioles changes to adjust blood flow to the needs of local tissues. For example, when a major organ needs more blood, the peripheral arteries constrict, decreasing their supply of blood. More blood becomes available to the major organ because of the resistance change in the periphery. Normally arteries and arterioles remain partially constricted to maintain a constant flow of blood. Peripheral vascular resistance is the resistance to blood flow determined by the tone of vascular musculature and diameter of blood vessels. The smaller the lumen of a vessel, the greater is the peripheral vascular resistance to blood flow. As resistance rises, arterial BP rises. When vessels dilate and resistance falls, arterial BP falls.

Blood Volume. Blood pressure depends on the volume of circulating blood. Most adults have a circulating blood volume of 5000 mL. Normally the blood volume remains constant. However, an increase in blood volume exerts more pressure against arterial walls. For example, the rapid, uncontrolled infusion of IV fluids elevates BP. When a person's circulating blood volume falls, as in the case of hemorrhage or dehydration, the BP also falls.

Viscosity. The thickness or viscosity of blood affects the ease with which blood flows through small vessels. The **hematocrit**, or percentage of red blood cells in the blood, determines blood viscosity. When the hematocrit rises and blood flow slows, arterial BP increases. The heart contracts more forcefully to move the viscous blood through the circulatory system.

Elasticity. Normally the walls of an artery are elastic and easily distensible. As pressure within the arteries increases, the diameter of vessel walls increases to accommodate the pressure change. The ability of arteries to dilate prevents wide fluctuations in BP. However, in certain

TABLE 29.8	Average Optimal Blood Pressure for Age
Age	**Blood Pressure (mm Hg)**
Newborn (3000 g [6.6 lb])	40 (mean)
1 month	85/54
1 year	95/65
6 years[a]	105/65
10-13 years[a]	110/65
14-17 years[a]	119/75
18 years and older	<120/<80

[a]In children and adolescents, hypertension is defined as blood pressure that on repeated measurement is at the 95th percentile or greater adjusted for age, height, and gender.
From James PA et al: Evidence-based guideline for the management of high blood pressure in adults: report by the panel appointed to the Eighth Joint National Committee (JNC 8), *JAMA* 31:507, 2014.

diseases such as arteriosclerosis, the vessel walls lose their elasticity and are replaced by fibrous tissue that cannot stretch well. Reduced elasticity results in greater resistance to blood flow. As a result, when the left ventricle ejects its SV, the vessels no longer yield to pressure. Instead a given volume of blood is forced through the rigid arterial walls, and the systemic pressure rises. Systolic pressure is more significantly elevated than diastolic pressure as a result of reduced arterial elasticity.

Each hemodynamic factor significantly affects the others. For example, as arterial elasticity declines, peripheral vascular resistance increases. The complex control of the cardiovascular system normally prevents any single factor from permanently changing the BP. For example, if the blood volume falls, the body compensates with an increased vascular resistance.

Factors Influencing Blood Pressure

Blood pressure is not constant. With many influencing factors one BP measurement cannot adequately reflect a patient's health status. Even under the best conditions, BP changes from heartbeat to heartbeat. BP trends, not individual measurements, guide nursing interventions. Understanding these factors ensures a more accurate interpretation of BP readings.

Age. Normal BP levels vary throughout life (Table 29.8). BP increases during childhood. You assess the level of a child's or adolescent's BP with respect to their percentile of height and their age (Hockenberry et al., 2019). Larger children (heavier and/or taller) have higher BPs than smaller children of the same age. During adolescence BP continues to vary according to body size. An adult's BP tends to rise with advancing age. The optimal BP for a healthy, middle-age adult is less than 120/80 mm Hg. A systolic value of 120 to 129 and a diastolic greater than 80 is considered to be an elevated blood pressure.

Stress. Emotional stress (e.g., anxiety and fear) and acute pain result in sympathetic stimulation, which increases HR, cardiac output, and vascular resistance. The effect of sympathetic stimulation increases BP.

Ethnicity and Genetics. Ethnic and genetic characteristics influence blood pressure. The prevalence of hypertension (high blood pressure) in African Americans in the United States is among the highest in the world. In addition, more than 40% of non-Hispanic African-American men and women have high blood pressure

TABLE 29.9   Antihypertensive Medications

Medication Type	Example	Action
Diuretics	Furosemide, spironolactone, metolazone, polythiazide, hydrochlorothiazide	Lower blood pressure by reducing resorption of sodium and water by the kidneys, thus lowering circulating fluid volume
Beta-adrenergic blockers	Atenolol, nadolol, timolol maleate, metoprolol	Combines with beta-adrenergic receptors in the heart, arteries, and arterioles to block response to sympathetic nerve impulses; reduces heart rate and thus cardiac output
Vasodilators	Hydralazine hydrochloride, minoxidil	Acts on arteriolar smooth muscle to cause relaxation and reduce peripheral vascular resistance
Calcium channel blockers	Diltiazem, verapamil hydrochloride, nifedipine, nicardipine	Reduces peripheral vascular resistance by systemic vasodilation
Angiotensin-converting enzyme (ACE) inhibitors	Captopril, enalapril, lisinopril, benazepril	Lowers blood pressure by blocking the conversion of angiotensin I to angiotensin II, preventing vasoconstriction; reduces aldosterone production and fluid retention, lowering circulating fluid volume
Angiotensin-II receptor blockers (ARBs)	Losartan, olmesartan	Lowers blood pressure by blocking the binding of angiotensin II, which prevents vasoconstriction

(AHA, 2016). However, other ethnic groups are at risk as well. A study by Carson and colleagues (2011) has shown that among adults 45 to 84 years of age there is a higher incidence of hypertension among Hispanics compared with whites; however, hypertension incidence did not differ for Chinese and white participants. In a study involving prevalence of hypertension among Asian and Hispanics adults in New York City, two major racial/ethnic minority groups had higher odds of hypertension than non-Hispanic whites: non-Hispanic black and Asian individuals (Fei et al., 2017). There is the need for specifically targeted interventions for hypertension, because of ethnic differences (Fei et al., 2017). Genetic factors also contribute to a patient's blood pressure. Assess the patient's family history for early hypertension and any complications related to hypertension. Individuals with a family history of high blood pressure may share common environments and other potential factors that increase their risk of hypertension (CDC, 2014).

Gender. There is no clinically significant difference in BP levels between boys and girls. After puberty males tend to have higher BP readings. After menopause women tend to have higher BP levels than men of similar age There are no specific guidelines for treating hypertension in men and women. However, numerous human studies have shown differences in the mechanisms responsible for blood pressure control between the sexes (Reckelhoff, 2018). Both men and women require education on the risk for hypertension and hypertension-related complications.

Daily Variation. Blood pressure varies throughout the day, with lower BP during sleep between midnight and 3:00 AM. Between 3:00 AM and 6:00 AM there is a slow and steady rise in BP. When a patient awakens, there is an early-morning surge. It is highest during the day between 10:00 AM and 6 PM. No two people have the same pattern or degree of variation.

Medications. Some medications directly or indirectly affect BP. Before BP assessment ask whether the patient is receiving antihypertensive, diuretic, or other cardiac medications, which lower BP (Table 29.9). Another class of medications that lower BP is opioid analgesics. Vasoconstrictors and an excess volume of IV fluids increase BP.

Activity and Weight. A period of exercise can reduce BP for several hours afterward. An increase in oxygen demand by the body

TABLE 29.10   Categories of BP in Adults[a]

BP Category	SBP		DBP
Normal	<120 mm Hg	and	<80 mm Hg
Elevated	120-129 mm Hg	and	<80 mm Hg
Hypertension			
Stage 1	130-139 mm Hg	or	80-89 mm Hg
Stage 2	≥140 mm Hg	or	≥90 mm Hg

[a]Individuals with SBP and DBP in 2 categories should be designated to the higher BP category.
BP indicates blood pressure (based on an average of ≥2 careful readings obtained on ≥2 occasions, as detailed in diastolic blood pressure (DBP) and systolic blood pressure (SBP).
Data from Whelton et al: Guideline for the prevention, detection, evaluation, and management of high blood pressure in adults, *J Am Coll Cardiol* 71(19):2199-2269, 2018.

during activity increases BP. Inadequate exercise frequently contributes to weight gain, and obesity is a factor in the development of hypertension.

Smoking. Smoking results in vasoconstriction, a narrowing of blood vessels. BP rises when a person smokes and returns to baseline about 15 minutes after stopping smoking.

Hypertension

The most common alteration in BP is hypertension. Hypertension is often asymptomatic. An elevated blood pressure or hypertension is diagnosed in adults when an average of two or more readings on at least two subsequent health care visits is above 120/80 mm Hg. One elevated BP measurement does not qualify as a diagnosis of hypertension. A systolic blood pressure between 120 and 129 with a diastolic blood pressure less than 80 is considered elevated. Hypertension is classified as Stage 1 or Stage 2, depending on systolic and diastolic values (Table 29.10). Hypertension increases the risk of hypertension-related illness, including stroke, heart attack, and damage to kidneys, retinas, and the peripheral nervous system. The categories of hypertension determine nonpharmacological and pharmacological intervention. Table 29.11 summarizes recommended follow-up for patients diagnosed with BP alterations.

TABLE 29.11   Recommendations for Blood Pressure Follow-Up

Initial Blood Pressure	Follow-Up Recommended[a]
Normal	Recheck in 1 year.
Elevated	Recheck in 3-6 months.[b]
Stage 1 hypertension	Evaluate therapy within 3-6 months.[b]
Stage 2 hypertension	Evaluate therapy within 1 month.[b] For those with higher pressure (e.g., >180/110 mm Hg), evaluate and treat immediately or within 1 week, depending on clinical situation and complications.

[a]Modify the scheduling of follow-up according to reliable information about past blood pressure measurements, other cardiovascular risk factors, or target organ damage.
[b]Provide advice about lifestyle modifications.
Data from Whelton et al: Guideline for the prevention, detection, evaluation, and management of high blood pressure in adults-executive summary, *J Am Coll Cardiol* 71:(19): 2199, 2018.

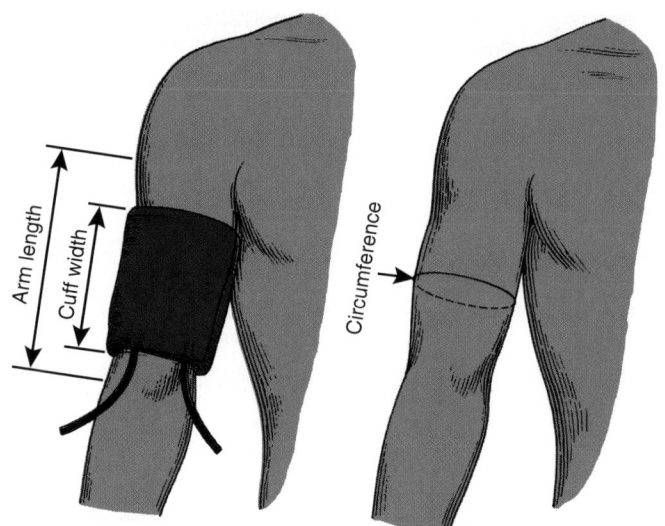

FIG. 29.9 Guidelines for proper blood pressure cuff size. Cuff width 20% more than upper-arm diameter or 40% of circumference and two-thirds of arm length.

Hypertension is associated with thickening and loss of elasticity in the arterial walls. Peripheral vascular resistance increases within thick and inelastic vessels. The heart continually pumps against greater resistance. As a result blood flow to vital organs such as the heart, brain, and kidney decreases with untreated or chronic hypertension.

Multiple risk factors are associated with hypertension. Modifiable risk factors include obesity, cigarette smoking, heavy alcohol consumption, and high sodium (salt) intake. Sedentary lifestyle and continued exposure to stress are also linked to hypertension. The incidence of hypertension is greater in patients with diabetes and in older adults. Hypertension contributes to deaths from strokes and myocardial infarctions (heart attacks).

Hypotension

Hypotension is present when the systolic BP falls to 90 mm Hg or below. Although some adults have a low BP normally, for most people low BP is an abnormal finding associated with illness.

Hypotension occurs because of the dilation of the arteries in the vascular bed, the loss of a substantial amount of blood volume (e.g., hemorrhage), or the failure of the heart muscle to pump adequately (e.g., myocardial infarction). Hypotension associated with pallor, skin mottling, clamminess, confusion, increased HR, or decreased urine output is life threatening and is reported to a health care provider immediately.

When a healthy individual changes from a lying–to sitting–to standing position, the peripheral blood vessels in the legs constrict. When standing, the lower-extremity vessels constrict, preventing the pooling of blood in the legs caused by gravity. Thus an individual normally does not feel any symptoms when standing. Orthostatic hypotension, also referred to as postural hypotension, occurs when a normotensive person develops symptoms and a drop in systolic pressure by at least 20 mm Hg or a drop in diastolic pressure by at least 10 mm Hg within 3 minutes of rising to an upright position (Shibao et al., 2013). Orthostatic hypotension occurs when patients are unable to constrict their lower extremity blood vessels to maintain their BP. Patients who are dehydrated, anemic, or have experienced prolonged bed rest or recent blood loss are at risk for orthostatic hypotension, particularly in the morning (Shibao et al., 2013). Some medications cause orthostatic hypotension, especially in older adults or young patients.

❖ NURSING PROCESS

◆ Assessment of Blood Pressure

Arterial BP measurements are obtained either directly (invasively) or indirectly (noninvasively). The direct method requires the insertion of a thin catheter into an artery. Tubing connects the catheter with electronic hemodynamic monitoring equipment. The monitor displays a constant arterial pressure waveform and reading. Because of the risk of sudden blood loss from an artery, invasive BP monitoring is used only in intensive care settings. The common indirect methods require either a sphygmomanometer and stethoscope with auscultation or an automated oscillometric device without auscultation. The use of a sphygmomanometer and stethoscope has been considered the gold standard for BP measurement when properly used and maintained (Stergiou, 2012). The technique for measuring BP by auscultation is described in Skill 29.5.

Blood Pressure Equipment for Auscultation. Before assessing BP, make sure that you are comfortable using the equipment. For more than half a century health care settings relied on a sphygmomanometer and stethoscope to measure BP by auscultation. A sphygmomanometer includes a pressure manometer, an occlusive cuff that encloses an inflatable rubber bladder, and a pressure bulb with a release valve that inflates the bladder manually. The aneroid manometer has a glass-enclosed circular gauge containing a needle that registers millimeter calibrations. Before using the aneroid model, make sure that the needle points to zero and that the manometer is correctly calibrated. Aneroid sphygmomanometers require biomedical calibration every 6 months to verify their accuracy.

An occlusive cuff comes in different sizes. The size selected is proportional to the circumference of the limb being assessed (Fig. 29.9). Ideally the width of the cuff is 40% of the circumference (or 20% wider than the diameter) of the midpoint of the limb on which the cuff is used to measure BP. The inflatable bladder, contained in the occlusive cuff, encircles at least 80% of the upper arm of an adult and the entire arm of a child.

Measure a blood pressure in the arm by placing the lower edge of the cuff above the antecubital fossa, allowing room for positioning the stethoscope bell or diaphragm over the brachial artery. Many adults require a large adult cuff. Using the forearm when a larger cuff is not readily available is not recommended and can result in an overestimate

TABLE 29.12 Common Errors in Blood Pressure Assessment

Error	Effect
Bladder or cuff too wide	False-low reading
Bladder or cuff too narrow or too short	False-high reading
Cuff wrapped too loosely or unevenly	False-high reading
Deflating cuff too slowly	False-high diastolic reading
Deflating cuff too quickly	False-low systolic and false-high diastolic reading
Arm below heart level	False-high reading
Arm above heart level	False-low reading
Arm not supported	False-high reading
Stethoscope that fits poorly or impairment of examiner's hearing, causing sounds to be muffled	False-low systolic and false-high diastolic reading
Stethoscope applied too firmly against antecubital fossa	False-low diastolic reading
Inflating too slowly	False-high diastolic reading
Repeating assessments too quickly	False-high systolic reading
Inadequate inflation level	False-low systolic reading
Multiple examiners using different sounds for diastolic readings	False-high systolic and false-low diastolic reading

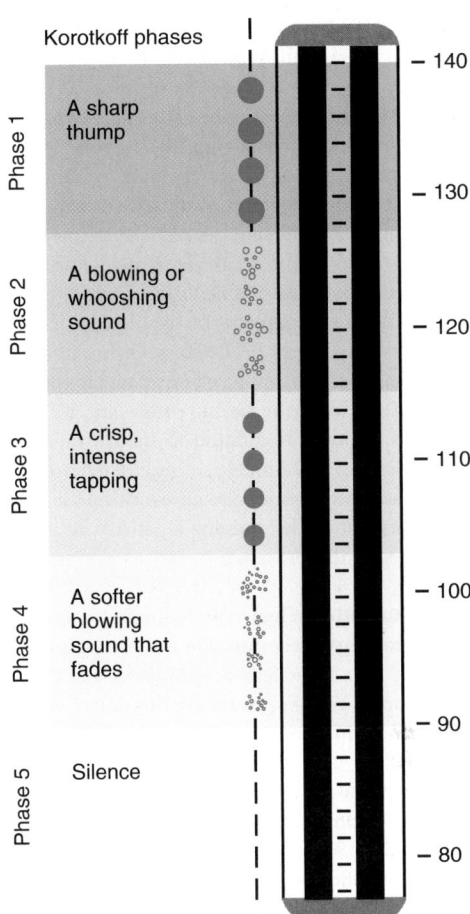

FIG. 29.10 The sounds auscultated during blood pressure measurement can be differentiated into five phases. In this example blood pressure is 140/90 mm Hg.

of systolic blood pressure up to 20 mm Hg (Schimanski et al., 2014). An improperly fitting cuff causes inaccurate BP measurements (Table 29.12). The release valve of the sphygmomanometer needs to be clean and freely movable in either direction. A closed valve holds the pressure constant. A sticky valve makes pressure cuff deflation hard to regulate.

Auscultation. The best environment for BP measurement by auscultation is a quiet room at a comfortable temperature. Although the patient may lie or stand, sitting is the preferred position. In most cases BP readings obtained with the patient in the supine, sitting, and standing positions are similar.

The patient's position during routine BP determination needs to be the same during each measurement to permit a meaningful comparison of values. Before obtaining the patient's BP, attempt to control factors responsible for artificially high readings such as pain, anxiety, or exertion. The patient's perception that the physical or interpersonal environment is stressful affects the BP measurement. BP measurements taken at the patient's place of employment or in a health care provider's office are often higher than those taken at the patient's home.

During the initial assessment obtain and record the BP in both arms. Normally there is a difference of 5 to 10 mm Hg between the arms. In subsequent assessments, measure the BP in the arm with the higher pressure. Pressure differences greater than 10 mm Hg indicate vascular problems and are reported to the health care provider or nurse in charge.

Ask the patient to state his or her usual BP. If the patient does not know, inform him or her after measuring and recording it. This is a good opportunity to educate a patient about optimal values of BP, risk factors for developing hypertension, and dangers of hypertension.

Indirect measurement of arterial BP works on a basic principle of pressure. Blood flows freely through an artery until an inflated cuff applies pressure to tissues and causes the artery to collapse. After release of the cuff pressure, the point at which blood flow returns and sound appears through auscultation is the systolic pressure.

In 1905 Korotkoff, a Russian surgeon, first described the sounds heard over an artery distal to the BP cuff when the cuff was deflated. The first sound is a clear rhythmical tapping corresponding to the pulse rate that gradually increases in intensity. *Onset of the sound corresponds to the systolic pressure.* A blowing or swishing sound occurs as the cuff continues to deflate, resulting in the second sound. As the artery distends there is turbulence in blood flow. The third sound is a crisper and more intense tapping. The fourth sound becomes muffled and low pitched as the cuff is further deflated. At this point the cuff pressure has fallen below the pressure within the vessel walls; *this sound is the diastolic pressure in infants and children.* The fifth sound marks the disappearance of sound. *In adolescents and adults the fifth sound corresponds with the diastolic pressure* (Fig. 29.10). In some patients the sounds are clear and distinct. In others only the beginning and ending sounds are clear.

The manual auscultatory method for BP measurement is prone to observer bias and requires clinical skill (MHRA, 2013). Obtaining an accurate measurement is essential because BP assessment results in many medical decisions and nursing interventions. There are several sources for error (see Table 29.12). When you are unsure of a reading, have a colleague reassess the BP.

The American Heart Association recommends recording two numbers for a BP measurement: the point on the manometer when you hear the first sound for systolic and the point on the manometer when you hear the fifth sound for diastolic. Some institutions recommend recording the point when you hear the fourth sound as well, especially for patients with hypertension. Divide the numbers by slashed lines (e.g., 120/70 or 120/100/70). Note the arm used to measure the BP (e.g., right arm [RA] 130/70) and the patient's position (e.g., sitting).

Orthostatic Hypotension. Assess for orthostatic hypotension during measurements of vital signs by obtaining BP and pulse in sequence with the patient supine, sitting, and standing. Obtain BP readings within 3 minutes after the patient changes position. In most cases orthostatic hypotension is detected within a minute of standing. If it occurs, help the patient to a lying position and notify the health care provider or nurse in charge. While obtaining orthostatic measurements, monitor for changes in pulse rate and observe for other symptoms of hypotension such as fainting, weakness, blurred vision, or light-headedness. Orthostatic hypotension is a risk factor for falls, especially among elderly patients with hypertension (Angelousi et al., 2014). When recording orthostatic BP measurements, record the patient's position in addition to the BP measurement (e.g., 140/80 mm Hg supine, 132/72 mm Hg sitting, 108/60 mm Hg standing). The skill of orthostatic measurements requires critical thinking and ongoing nursing judgment when determining a patient's response to repositioning. Do not delegate this procedure.

Ultrasonic Stethoscope. When you are unable to auscultate sounds because of a weakened arterial pulse, you can use an ultrasonic stethoscope (see Chapter 30). This stethoscope allows you to hear low-frequency systolic sounds. You frequently use this device when measuring the BP of infants and children or low BP in adults.

Palpation. Indirect measurement of BP by palpation is useful for patients whose arterial pulsations are too weak to create sounds that are audible by auscultation. Severe blood loss and decreased heart contractility are examples of conditions that result in BPs too low to auscultate accurately. In these cases you can assess the systolic BP by palpation (see Skill 29.5, Step 10). The diastolic BP is difficult to determine by palpation. When using the palpation technique, record the systolic value and how you measured it (e.g., RA 90/-, palpated, supine).

In some patients with hypertension the sounds usually heard over the brachial artery when the cuff pressure is high disappear as pressure is reduced and then reappear at a lower level. This temporary disappearance of sound is the auscultatory gap. It typically occurs between the first and second sounds. The gap in sound covers a range of 40 mm Hg and thus causes an underestimation of systolic pressure or overestimation of diastolic pressure. The examiner needs to be certain to inflate the cuff high enough to hear the true systolic pressure before the auscultatory gap. Palpation of the radial artery helps to determine how high to inflate the cuff. The examiner inflates the cuff 30 mm Hg above the pressure at which the radial pulse was palpated. Record the range of pressures in which the auscultatory gap occurs (e.g., BP RA 180/94 mm Hg with an auscultatory gap from 180 to 160 mm Hg, sitting).

Equipment for Oscillometric Measurement. More common today is the use of automated electronic oscillometric devices that do not require use of a stethoscope for auscultation. The devices include an electronic monitor with a pressure sensor, a digital display, and an upper arm cuff (Fig. 29.11). An electrically driven pump raises the pressure in the cuff (MHRA, 2013). There are also devices that fit around a patient's wrist. Devices usually have an adjustable set inflation pressure or they will automatically inflate to the appropriate level, usually about 30 mm Hg above an estimated systolic reading (MHRA, 2013). When started, the device automatically inflates, then deflates the cuff and displays the systolic and diastolic values. These devices rely on oscillometric principle to measure mean blood pressure and apply a manufacturer- and device-specific algorithm to estimate systolic and diastolic blood pressure (Stergiou, 2012).

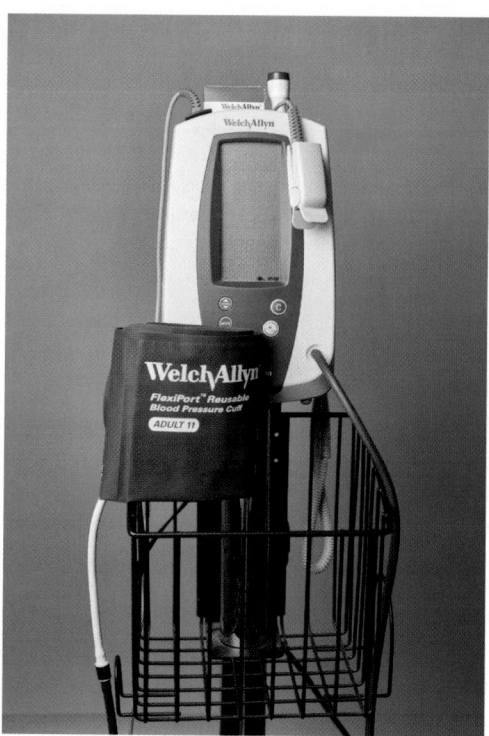

FIG. 29.11 Automatic blood pressure monitor.

Blood Pressure Measurement Using Oscillometric Device. Many different styles of electronic oscillometric devices are available to determine BP automatically. The arm cuff is placed around the upper arm, just above the brachial artery. A push of a button activates the inflation of the cuff. The electronic pressure sensor detects the vibrations caused by the rush of blood through an artery (Box 29.8). Once a BP is sensed, a reading will be shown on the electronic display. Oscillometric devices are mercury-free, lightweight, compact, portable, easy to use, and offer no observer bias (MHRA, 2013). More of these devices can be found in physician offices and clinics and even on hospital inpatient units. The devices are particularly useful when frequent BP assessment is necessary, such as in patients who are critically ill or unstable, during or after invasive procedures, or when therapies require frequent monitoring (e.g., IV heart and BP medications). Box 29.9 lists conditions that are not appropriate for automatic BP devices. If a BP result is questionable based on a patient's condition, ensure accurate BP measurement by obtaining manual measurements using auscultation with a sphygmomanometer

Blood Pressure Assessment in Children. Blood pressure measurement in the ambulatory setting begins at 3 years of age during every wellness visit. For otherwise healthy children, BP need only be measured annually rather than during every health care encounter (Flynn et al., 2017). If a child has obesity, diabetes, renal disease, or vascular problems, obtain readings during every health encounter (Flynn et al., 2017). BP in children changes with growth and development. The prevalence of BP elevations and hypertension in children, especially among children who are overweight, has increased (Flynn et al., 2017). Help parents understand the importance of routine BP screening to detect children who are at risk for hypertension. The measurement of BP in infants and children is difficult for several reasons:

- Different arm size requires careful and appropriate cuff size selection. Do not choose a cuff on the basis of the name of the cuff. An "infant" cuff can be too small for some infants.

BOX 29.8   PROCEDURAL GUIDELINES

Electronic Blood Pressure Measurement

Delegation and Collaboration

The skill of blood pressure measurement using an electronic blood pressure machine can be delegated to assistive personnel (AP) unless the patient is considered unstable (i.e., hypotensive). The nurse instructs the AP by:

- Explaining the frequency and the extremity to use for measurement.
- Reviewing how to select appropriate-size blood pressure cuff for designated extremity and appropriate cuff for the machine.
- Reviewing patient's usual blood pressure and directing AP to report significant changes or abnormalities to the nurse.

Equipment

Electronic oscillometric blood pressure device; blood pressure cuff of appropriate size as recommended by machine manufacturer; pen and vital sign flow sheet in chart or electronic health record (EHR)

Steps

1. Identify patient using at least two identifiers (e.g., name and birthday or name and medical record number), according to agency policy (TJC, 2020).
2. Assess need to measure blood pressure (see Skill 29.5 Assessment Steps 2, 3, and 5), and determine patient's baseline blood pressure.
3. Determine appropriateness of using electronic blood pressure measurement. Patients with irregular heart rate, known hypertension, peripheral vascular disease, seizures, tremors, and shivering are not candidates for the device (Wang et al., 2016).
4. Collect and bring appropriate equipment to patient's bedside. Select appropriate cuff size for patient extremity. Electronic blood pressure cuff and device must be matched by manufacturer and are not interchangeable.
5. Perform hand hygiene and determine best site for cuff placement; inspect condition of extremities.
6. Assist patient to comfortable position, either lying or sitting. Plug device into electrical outlet and place it near patient, ensuring that connector hose between cuff and machine reaches.
7. Locate on/off switch and turn on machine to enable device to self-test computer systems.
8. Remove constricting clothing to ensure proper cuff application.
9. Prepare blood pressure cuff by manually squeezing all the air out of the cuff and connecting it to connector hose.
10. Wrap flattened cuff snugly around extremity, verifying that only one finger can fit between cuff and patient's skin. Make sure that "artery" arrow marked on outside of cuff is placed correctly (see illustration).

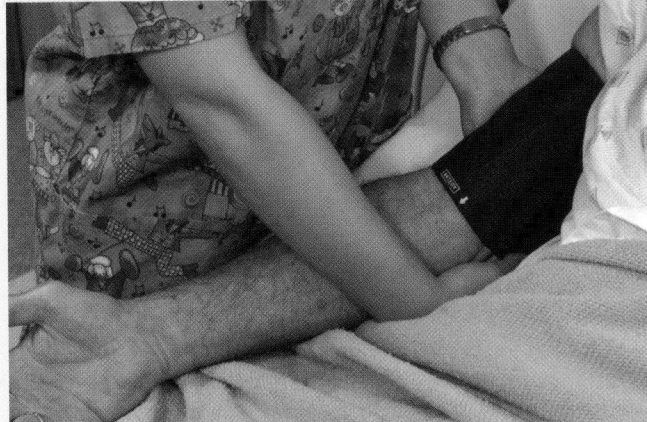

STEP 10 Aligning blood pressure cuff arrow with brachial artery.

11. Verify that connector hose between cuff and machine is not kinked. Kinking prevents proper inflation and deflation of cuff.

12. Following manufacturer directions, set frequency control for automatic or manual and press the start button. The first blood pressure measurement pumps cuff to a peak pressure of approximately 180 mm Hg. After this pressure is reached, the machine begins a deflation sequence that determines the blood pressure. The first reading determines peak pressure inflation for additional measurements.
13. When deflation is complete, digital display provides most recent values and flashes time in minutes that have elapsed since the measurement occurred (see illustration).

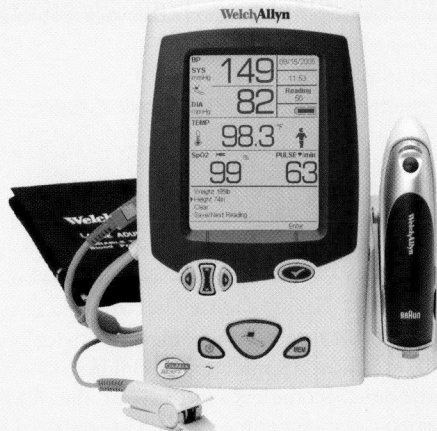

STEP 13 Digital electronic blood pressure display. (Image courtesy of Hillrom.)

> **CLINICAL DECISION:** If unable to obtain blood pressure with electronic device, verify machine connections (e.g., plugged into working electrical outlet, hose-cuff connections tight, machine on, correct cuff). Repeat electronic blood pressure; if unable to obtain, use auscultatory technique (see Skill 29.5).

14. Set frequency of measurements and upper and lower alarm limits for systolic, diastolic, and mean blood pressure readings. Intervals between measurements can be set from 1 to 90 minutes. A nurse determines frequency and alarm limits on the basis of patient's acceptable range of blood pressure, nursing judgment, and health care provider order.
15. Obtain additional readings at any time by pressing the start button. Pressing the cancel button immediately deflates the cuff.
16. If frequent measurements are required, the cuff may be left in place. Remove it at least every 2 hours to assess underlying skin integrity and, if possible, alternate measurement sites.

> **CLINICAL DECISION:** Frequent measurement by electronic blood pressure machines increases the risk of extremity pressure injuries, especially in vulnerable elders. Patients with abnormal bleeding tendencies are at risk for microvascular rupture from repeated inflations. Inspect the skin under the blood pressure cuff at regular intervals, depending on the frequency of use.

17. When patient no longer requires frequent blood pressure monitoring:
    a. Assist patient in return to comfortable position and cover upper arm or leg if previously clothed to restore comfort and provide sense of well-being.
    b. Place nurse call system within reach and instruct patient in its use to promote safety and prevent falls.
    c. Raise side rails (as appropriate) and lower bed to lowest position to promote safety and prevent falls.
    d. Wipe cuff with agency-approved disinfectant to reduce transmission of infection. Clean and store electronic blood pressure machine.

Continued

BOX 29.8   PROCEDURAL GUIDELINES—cont'd

Electronic Blood Pressure Measurement

18. Perform hand hygiene.
19. Compare electronic blood pressure readings with auscultatory measurements to verify accuracy of electronic device. Electronic measurements can underestimate measurements (Drawz, 2017).
20. **Use Teach-Back:** "I want to be sure I explained why you need to keep your arm straight while the machine is taking your blood pressure. Tell me why it is important to remain still." Revise your instruction now or develop a plan for revised patient/family caregiver teaching if patient/family caregiver is not able to teach back correctly.
21. Record blood pressure, site assessed, and use of electronic device; record any signs or symptoms of blood pressure alterations.
22. Notify nurse in charge or health care provider of abnormal findings.

BOX 29.9   Patient Conditions Not Appropriate for Electronic Blood Pressure Measurement

- Irregular heart rate
- Known hypertension
- Peripheral vascular obstruction (e.g., clots, narrowed vessels)
- Shivering
- Seizures
- Excessive tremors
- Inability to cooperate
- Blood pressure less than 90 mm Hg systolic

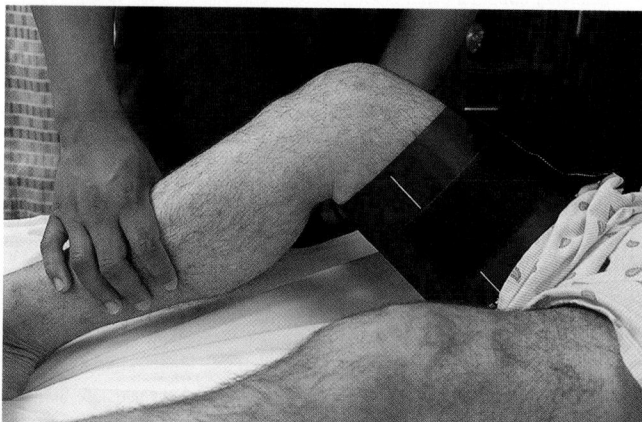

FIG. 29.12 Lower-extremity blood pressure cuff positioned above popliteal artery at midthigh with knee flexed.

- Readings are difficult to obtain in restless or anxious infants and children. Allow at least 15 minutes for children to recover from recent activities and become less apprehensive. The child's cooperation is increased when you or the parent have prepared him or her for the unusual sensation of the BP cuff. Most children understand the analogy of a "tight hug on your arm."
- Placing the stethoscope too firmly on the antecubital fossa causes errors in auscultation. Sounds are difficult to hear in children because of low frequency and amplitude. A pediatric stethoscope bell is often helpful.

Lower-Extremity Blood Pressure. Dressings, casts, IV catheters, or arteriovenous fistulas or shunts make the upper extremities inaccessible for BP measurement. You then need to obtain the BP in a lower extremity. Comparing upper-extremity BP with that in the legs is also necessary for patients with certain cardiac and BP abnormalities. The popliteal artery, palpable behind the knee in the popliteal space, is the site for auscultation or oscillometric measurement. The cuff needs to be wide and long enough to allow for the larger girth of the thigh. Placing the patient in a prone position is best. If such a position is impossible, ask the patient to flex the knee slightly for easier access to the artery. Position the cuff 2.5 cm (1 inch) above the popliteal artery, with the bladder over the posterior aspect of the midthigh (Fig. 29.12). The procedure is identical to brachial artery measurement. Systolic pressure in the legs is usually higher by 10 to 40 mm Hg than in the brachial artery, but the diastolic pressure is the same.

Self-Measurement of Blood Pressure. Electronic monitoring devices allow individuals to measure their own BPs in their home with the push of a button. The devices are mercury-free, lightweight, compact, portable, easy to use, and have no observer bias (MHRA, 2013). The most common portable home devices are electronic digital readout devices that do not require use of a stethoscope. The electronic devices are easy to manipulate but require frequent recalibration, more than once a year.

Stationary automatic BP devices are often found in public places such as grocery stores, fitness clubs, airports, or work sites. Users simply rest their arms within the inflatable cuff of the machine, which contains a pressure sensor. A visual display tells users their BP within 60 to 90 seconds. The reliability of the stationary machines is limited. BP values can vary by 5 to 10 mm Hg or more (for both systolic and diastolic values) compared with pressures taken with a manual sphygmomanometer.

Self-measurement of BP has several benefits. Sometimes elevated BP is detected in people previously unaware of a problem. People with prehypertension provide information about the pattern of BP values to their health care provider. Patients with hypertension benefit from participating actively in their treatment through self-monitoring, which helps adherence with treatment. The disadvantages of self-measurement include improper use of the device and risk of inaccurate readings. Some patients are needlessly alarmed with one elevated reading. Some patients with hypertension become overly conscious of their BP and inappropriately self-adjust medications.

◆ Nursing Diagnosis

The assessment of BP along with pulse assessment evaluates the general state of cardiovascular health and responses to other system imbalances. Hypotension, hypertension, orthostatic hypotension, and narrow or wide pulse pressures are assessment findings of certain nursing diagnoses, including the following:
- *Activity Intolerance*
- *Anxiety*
- *Impaired Cardiac Output*
- *Fluid Imbalance*
- *Acute Pain*

◆ Planning and Implementation

The nursing care plan includes interventions based on the nursing diagnosis identified and the related factors. For example, the assessment findings of hypotension, bradycardia or tachycardia, edema, fatigue, or weight gain lead to a diagnosis of *Impaired Cardiac Output*. Related factors might include deconditioning or altered fluid intake. The related factor guides the choice of nursing interventions.

BOX 29.10 PATIENT TEACHING

Health Promotion

Objective
- Patient identifies measures to promote cardiovascular health.

Teaching Strategies
- Instruct patient about the importance of diet, exercise, and remaining tobacco free.
- Demonstrate self-assessment of heart rate using the carotid pulse. Patients taking certain prescribed cardiac medications need to learn to assess their own pulse rate to detect side effects of medications. Patients undergoing cardiac rehabilitation need to learn to assess their own pulse rate to determine their response to exercise.
- Instruct patient about normal blood pressure values, risk factors for hypertension, and usual lack of hypertension symptoms.
- Demonstrate how to obtain blood pressure to the patient/patient's family caregiver using an appropriate-size blood pressure cuff for home use:
  - Do not take a measurement over clothing (AHA, 2017).
  - Sit correctly with your back straight and supported (on a dining chair, rather than a sofa). The feet should be flat on the floor and the legs should not be crossed (AHA, 2017).
  - Measure at the same time each day, after patient has had a brief rest, and in the same position and arm each time pressure is taken.
  - Take two or three readings 1 minute apart, and record the results at each measurement (AHA, 2017).

Evaluation
Use the principles of teach-back to evaluate patient/family caregiver learning:
- Tell me three activities you will do to promote cardiovascular health.
- Observe patient obtaining carotid pulse rate.
- Observe patient or family caregiver's measurement of blood pressure.

Health Promotion. The emphasis on health promotion and maintenance and early discharge from hospital settings has resulted in an increase in the need for patients and their families to monitor vital signs in the home and to know how to take medications correctly for management of cardiovascular problems. Teaching considerations affect all vital sign measurements. Incorporate them within the patient's plan of care (Box 29.10).

When patients are diagnosed with an elevated blood pressure or hypertension, educate them about BP values, long-term follow-up care and therapy, the usual lack of symptoms (the fact that it may not be "felt"), the ability of therapy to control but not cure high BP, and a consistently followed treatment plan that ensures a relatively normal lifestyle (James et al., 2014).

Consumers can learn to use self-measurement devices if they have the information needed to perform the procedure correctly and if they know when to seek a health care provider. Advise patients of possible inaccuracies in the BP devices, help them understand the meaning and implications of readings, and teach them proper measurement techniques. Encourage them to record the date of their BP readings to assess BP over time and share findings with their health care provider.

When considering how to teach patients and their families about vital sign measurements and their importance and significance, a patient's age is an important factor. With an increase in the older-adult population there is a greater need for family caregivers to be aware of changes that are unique to older adults. Box 29.11 identifies some of these variations.

◆ Evaluation

Patient Outcomes. Know a patient's baseline trend when evaluating blood pressure values in response to therapies. Know the expected effects of an intervention for blood pressure alterations. For example, if a patient is receiving an antihypertensive medication or an increased infusion of IV fluids, has the BP responded appropriately? The antihypertensive medication should lower BP while an increase in fluids can raise the BP. Evaluate outcomes of teaching interventions by having

BOX 29.11 FOCUS ON OLDER ADULTS

Factors Affecting Vital Signs of Older Adults

Temperature
- The temperature of older adults is at the lower end of the normal temperature range, 36° to 36.8° C (96.8° to 98.3° F) orally and 36.6° to 37.2° C (98° to 99° F) rectally. Therefore temperatures considered within normal range sometimes reflect a fever in an older adult. In an older adult fever is present when a single oral temperature is over 37.8° C (100° F); repeated oral temperatures are over 37.2° C (99° F); rectal temperatures are over 37.5° C (99.5° F); or temperature has increased more than 1° C (2° F) over baseline.
- Older adults are very sensitive to slight changes in environmental temperature because their thermoregulatory systems are not as efficient.
- A decrease in sweat gland reactivity in the older adult results in a higher threshold for sweating at high temperatures, which leads to hyperthermia and heatstroke.
- Be especially attentive to subtle temperature changes and other manifestations of fever in this population such as tachypnea, anorexia, falls, delirium, and overall functional decline.
- Older adults without teeth or with poor muscle control may be unable to close their mouths tightly to obtain accurate oral temperature readings.

Pulse Rate
- If it is difficult to palpate the pulse of an obese older adult, a Doppler device provides a more accurate reading.
- Pedal pulses are often difficult to palpate in older adults.

- The older adult has a decreased heart rate at rest.
- It takes longer for the heart rate to rise in the older adult to meet sudden increased demands that result from stress, illness, or excitement. Once elevated, the pulse rate takes longer to return to normal resting rate.
- Heart sounds are sometimes muffled or difficult to hear in older adults because of an increase in air space in the lungs.

Blood Pressure
- Older adults who have lost upper arm mass, especially the frail elderly, require special attention to selection of a smaller-size blood pressure cuff.
- Older adults sometimes have an increase in systolic pressure related to decreased vessel elasticity, whereas the diastolic pressure remains the same, resulting in a wider pulse pressure.
- Instruct older adults to change position slowly and wait after each change to avoid postural hypotension and prevent injuries.
- Skin of older adults is more fragile and susceptible to cuff pressure during frequent measurements. More frequent assessment of skin under the cuff or rotating blood pressure sites is recommended.

Respirations
- Aging causes ossification of costal cartilage and downward slant of ribs, resulting in a more rigid rib cage, which reduces chest wall expansion. Kyphosis and scoliosis that occur in older adults also restrict chest expansion and decrease tidal volume.

BOX 29.11 FOCUS ON OLDER ADULTS—cont'd

Factors Affecting Vital Signs of Older Adults

- Older adults depend more on accessory abdominal muscles during respiration than on weaker thoracic muscles.
- The respiratory system matures by the time a person reaches 20 years of age and begins to decline in healthy people after the age of 25. Despite this decline older adults are able to breathe effortlessly as long as they are healthy.

However, sudden events that require an increased demand for oxygen (e.g., exercise, stress, illness) create shortness of breath in the older adult.
- Identifying an acceptable pulse oximeter probe site is difficult with older adults because of the likelihood of peripheral vascular disease, decreased cardiac output, cold-induced vasoconstriction, and anemia.

---

patients or family caregivers explain the importance of BP measurement and BP medications. Request a demonstration of the blood pressure measurement device.

Recording Vital Signs. Special electronic and paper graphic flow sheets exist for recording vital signs (see Chapter 26). Identify institution procedure for documenting on a graphic. In addition to the actual vital sign values, record in the nurses' notes any accompanying or precipitating symptoms such as chest pain and dizziness with changes in pulse rate, abnormal BP, shortness of breath with abnormal respirations, or flushing and diaphoresis with elevated temperature. Document any interventions initiated as a result of vital sign measurement such as administration of oxygen therapy, cooling blankets, or an antihypertensive medication.

Patients being managed on critical paths often have vital sign values listed as outcomes. If a vital sign value is above or below the anticipated outcome, write a variance note to explain the nature of the variance and the nursing course of action. For example, a path for a patient who has undergone lung surgery often has an outcome during the postoperative period of "afebrile." If the patient has a fever, the nurse's variance note addresses possible sources of fever (e.g., retained pulmonary secretions) and nursing interventions (e.g., increased suctioning, postural drainage, or hydration).

QSEN Building Competency in Informatics The team leader notifies you that your patient has achieved a critical Early Warning Score, a computer-generated value that reflects a patient's condition on the basis of the vital signs entered by the assistive personnel within the past 15 minutes. After completing a focused assessment of the patient, you review the vital signs and compare the most recent with baseline readings. Which vital signs that are included in the Early Warning Score indicate a potential change in the patient's condition? Which actions should you take next?

Baseline Vital Signs	Vital Signs During the Past 15 Minutes
Heart rate 86 and regular	Heart rate 92 and regular
Blood pressure 120/84 in right arm via electronic blood pressure machine	Blood pressure 92/76 in right arm via electronic blood pressure machine
Oxygen saturation 95% on 2 L nasal cannula	Oxygen saturation 89% on 2 L nasal cannula
Respiratory rate 16, regular and deep	Respiratory rate 22, regular and deep
Temperature 37.2° C via temporal artery	Temperature 37.6° C via temporal artery

Answers to QSEN Activities can be found on the Evolve website.

SAFETY GUIDELINES FOR NURSING SKILLS

Ensuring patient safety is an essential role of the professional nurse. To ensure patient safety, communicate clearly with the members of the health care team, assess and incorporate the patient's priorities of care and preferences, and use the best evidence when making decisions about your patient's care. When performing the skills in this chapter, remember the following points to ensure safe, individualized patient-centered care.

- Devices for measuring vital signs are often shared among patients. Cleaning each device carefully between patients decreases patients' risk of infection.

- Blood pressure cuffs and pulse oximetry sensors can apply excessive pressure on fragile skin. Rotating sites during repeated measurements decreases risk for skin breakdown.
- Analyze trends for measuring vital signs, and report abnormal findings to the health care provider.
- Determine frequency of measuring vital signs on the basis of the patient's condition.
- Determine a patient's status before delegating a vital sign skill.

SKILL 29.1 MEASURING BODY TEMPERATURE

Delegation and Collaboration

The skill of temperature measurement can be delegated to assistive personnel (AP). The nurse instructs the AP by:

- Communicating the appropriate route, device, and frequency of temperature measurement.
- Explaining any precautions needed in positioning the patient (e.g., for rectal temperature measurement).
- Reviewing the patient's usual temperature values and significant changes to report to the nurse.

Equipment

- Thermometer (selected on the basis of site used)
- Soft tissue or wipe
- Alcohol swab
- Water-soluble lubricant (for rectal measurements only)
- Pen and vital sign flow sheet, record form, or electronic health record (EHR)
- Clean gloves (optional), plastic thermometer sleeve, disposable probe or sensor cover
- Towel

STEP	RATIONALE
ASSESSMENT	
1. Identify patient using at least two identifiers (e.g., name and birthday or name and medical record number) according to agency policy.	Ensures correct patient. Complies with The Joint Commission standards and improves patient safety (TJC, 2020).
2. Obtain data from patient's electronic health record (EHR) to determine need to measure patient's body temperature:	

STEP	RATIONALE
a. Note patient's risks for temperature alterations: • Expected or diagnosed infection • Open wounds or burns • White blood cell count below 5000/mm³ or above 12,000/mm³ • Immunosuppressive drug therapy • Injury to hypothalamus • Exposure to temperature extremes • Blood product infusion • Hypothermia or hyperthermia therapy	Certain conditions place patients at risk for temperature alterations and require more frequent temperature measurement and nursing assessment.
b. Perform hand hygiene. Assess for signs and symptoms that indicate a temperature alteration: • *Hyperthermia:* Decreased skin turgor, dry mucous membranes; tachycardia; hypotension; decreased venous filling; concentrated urine • *Heatstroke:* Body temperature of 40° C (104° F) or more (Hifumi et al., 2018); hot, dry skin; tachycardia; hypotension; excessive thirst; muscle cramps; visual disturbances; confusion or delirium • *Hypothermia:* Pale skin; skin cool or cold to touch; bradycardia and dysrhythmias; uncontrollable shivering; reduced level of consciousness; shallow respirations	Reduces transmission of microorganisms. Physical signs and symptoms alert you to alterations in body temperature.
c. Assess for factors that normally influence temperature: • Age	Allows you to accurately assess for presence and significance of temperature alteration. Older adults have narrower range of temperature than younger adults.

CLINICAL DECISION: *No single temperature is normal for all people. A temperature within an acceptable range in an adult may reflect a fever in an older adult. Undeveloped temperature-control mechanisms in infants and children cause temperature to rise and fall rapidly.*

STEP	RATIONALE
• Exercise	Muscle activity increases metabolism, which increases heat production and raises temperature.
• Hormones	Women have wider temperature fluctuations than men because of menstrual cycle hormonal changes, because body temperature varies during menopause, and because women have thicker layer of subcutaneous fat.
• Stress	Stress elevates temperature.
• Environmental temperature	Infants and older adults are more sensitive to environmental temperature changes.
• Medications	Some drugs impair or promote sweating, vasoconstriction, or vasodilation or interfere with ability of hypothalamus to regulate temperature.
• Daily fluctuations	Body temperature normally changes 0.5° to 1° C (0.9° to 1.8° F) during 24-hour period. Temperature is lowest during early morning. Most patients have maximum temperature elevation between 4 PM and 7 PM; temperature falls gradually during night.
3. Determine appropriate measurement site and device for patient (Table 29.2). Use disposable thermometer for patient on isolation precautions.	Determines whether patient's status contraindicates selection of a specific method or site.
4. Determine previous baseline temperature and measurement site (if available) from patient's electronic health record.	Allows you to assess for change in condition. Provides comparison with future temperature measurements.
5. Assess patient's or family caregiver's knowledge, experience, and health literacy level.	Ensures patient has the capacity to obtain, communicate, process, and understand basic health information (CDC, 2019).

PLANNING

STEP	RATIONALE
1. Provide privacy: draw curtain around bed and/or close room door. Prepare bedside environment for patient safety.	Maintains patient comfort and removes barriers that may interfere with procedure.
2. Collect and bring appropriate supplies to the patient's bedside.	Ensures an organized approach for body temperature measurement.
3. If measuring oral temperature, verify that patient has not had anything to eat or drink and has not chewed gum or smoked within the past 20 minutes.	Oral food and fluids, smoking, and gum can alter oral temperature measurement.
4. Explain to patient the way you will measure temperature and the importance of maintaining proper position until reading is complete.	Promotes patient cooperation.

IMPLEMENTATION

STEP	RATIONALE
1. Perform hand hygiene.	Reduces transmission of infection.
2. Help patient to a comfortable position that provides easy access to temperature measurement site. **a.** Sitting or lying supine (oral, tympanic, temporal, axillary) **b.** Side lying with upper leg flexed (rectal)	Ensures patient's comfort and accuracy of temperature reading.

Continued

SKILL 29.1	MEASURING BODY TEMPERATURE—cont'd
STEP	**RATIONALE**

3. Obtain temperature reading.

   a. Oral temperature (electronic):

      (1) *Optional:* Apply clean gloves when there is risk for exposure to respiratory secretions or facial or mouth wound drainage.

      (2) Remove thermometer pack from charging unit. Attach oral thermometer probe stem (blue tip) to thermometer unit. Grasp top of probe stem, being careful not to apply pressure on ejection button.

      (3) Slide disposable plastic probe cover over thermometer probe stem until cover locks in place (see illustrations).

      (4) Ask patient to open mouth; gently place thermometer probe under tongue in posterior sublingual pocket lateral to center of lower jaw (see illustration).

      (5) Ask patient to hold thermometer probe with lips closed.

      (6) Leave thermometer probe in place until audible signal indicates completion and patient's temperature appears on digital display; remove thermometer probe from under patient's tongue.

      (7) Push ejection button on thermometer probe stem to discard plastic probe cover into appropriate receptacle.

An oral probe cover is removable without physical contact; thus does not require gloves.

Charging provides battery power. Ejection button releases plastic cover from probe stem.

Soft plastic cover will not break in patient's mouth and prevents transmission of infection between patients.

Heat from superficial blood vessels in sublingual pocket results in temperature reading. With electronic thermometer, temperatures in right and left posterior sublingual pocket are significantly higher than in area under front of tongue.

Maintains proper position of thermometer during recording.

Probe must stay in place until signal occurs to ensure accurate reading.

Reduces transmission of infection.

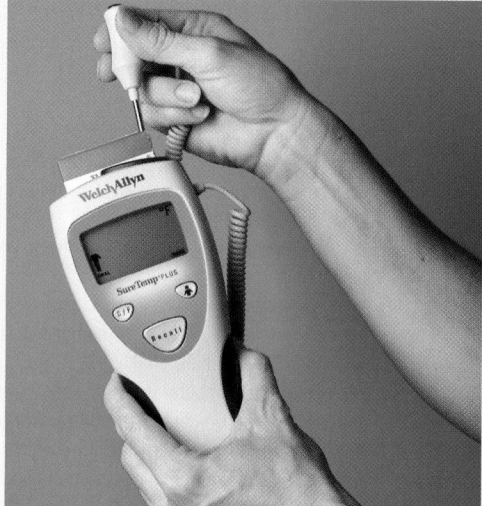 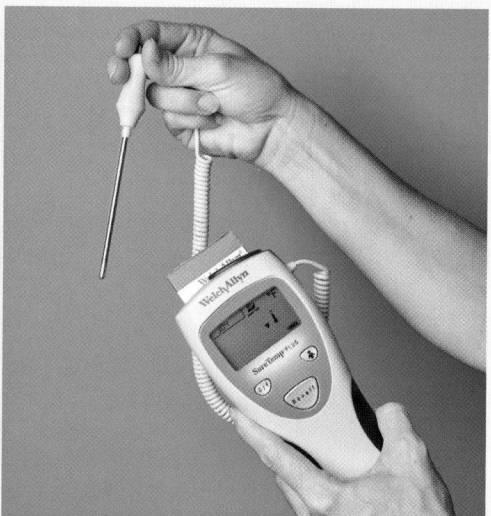

STEP 3a(3) Disposable plastic cover is placed over probe.

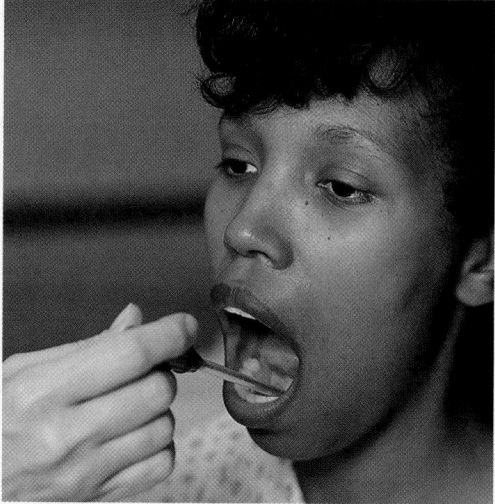

STEP 3a(4) Probe placed under tongue in posterior sublingual pocket.

STEP	RATIONALE

(8) If wearing gloves, remove, dispose in appropriate receptacle, and perform hand hygiene.

Reduces transmission of infection.

(9) Return thermometer probe stem to storage position of thermometer unit.

Protects probe stem from damage. Returning thermometer probe stem automatically causes digital reading to disappear.

b. **Rectal temperature (electronic):**

(1) Move aside bed linen to only expose anal area. Keep patient's upper body and lower extremities covered with sheet or blanket.

Maintains patient's privacy, minimizes embarrassment, and promotes comfort.

(2) Apply clean gloves. Cleanse anal region when feces and/or secretions are present. Remove soiled gloves, perform hand hygiene, and reapply clean gloves.

Maintains Standard Precautions when exposed to items soiled with body fluids (e.g., feces).

(3) Remove thermometer pack from charging unit. Attach rectal thermometer probe stem (red tip) to thermometer unit. Grasp top of probe stem, being careful not to apply pressure on ejection button.

Ejection button releases plastic cover from probe stem.

(4) Slide disposable plastic probe cover over thermometer probe stem until cover locks in place.

Soft plastic probe cover prevents transmission of infection between patients.

(5) Using a single-use package, squeeze a liberal amount of lubricant on tissue. Dip probe cover of thermometer, blunt end, into lubricant, covering 2.5 to 3.5 cm (1 to 1½ inches) for adult.

Lubrication minimizes trauma to rectal mucosa during insertion. Using a tissue allows adequate lubrication of probe.

(6) With nondominant hand separate patient's buttocks to expose anus. Ask patient to breathe slowly and relax.

Fully exposes anus for thermometer insertion. Relaxes anal sphincter for easier thermometer insertion.

(7) Gently insert thermometer into anus in direction of umbilicus 3.5 cm (1½ inches) for adult. Do not force thermometer.

Ensures adequate exposure against blood vessels in rectal wall.

(8) If you feel resistance during insertion, withdraw immediately. Never force thermometer.

Prevents trauma to mucosa.

CLINICAL DECISION: *If you cannot adequately insert thermometer into rectum or resistance is felt during insertion, remove thermometer and consider alternative method for obtaining temperature.*

---

(9) Once positioned, hold thermometer probe in place until audible signal indicates completion and patient's temperature appears on digital display; remove thermometer probe from anus (see illustration).

Probe must stay in place until signal occurs to ensure accurate reading.

(10) Push ejection button on thermometer stem to discard plastic probe cover into appropriate receptacle. Wipe probe stem with alcohol swab, paying particular attention to ridges where probe stem connects to probe.

Reduces transmission of infection.

(11) Return thermometer stem to storage position of recording unit.

Protects probe stem from damage. Returning thermometer stem automatically causes digital reading to disappear.

(12) Wipe patient's anal area with soft tissue to remove lubricant or feces and discard tissue. Perform perineal hygiene as needed.

Provides for comfort and hygiene.

(13) Remove and dispose of gloves in appropriate receptacle. Perform hand hygiene.

Reduces transmission of infection.

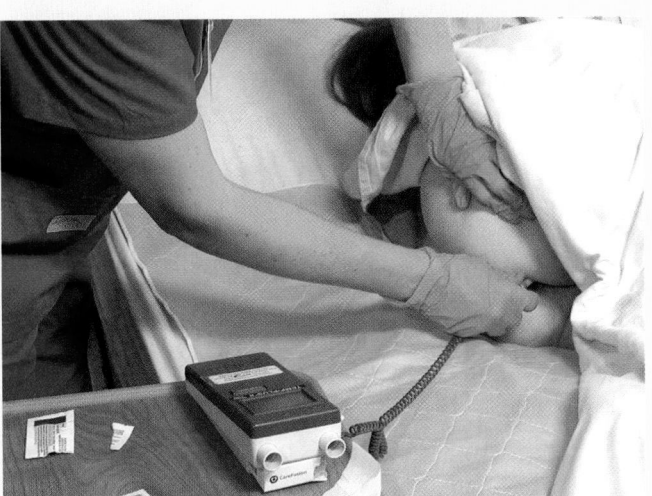

STEP 3b(9) Probe inserted into anus. (Copyright © Mosby's Clinical Skills: Essentials Collection.)

Continued

SKILL 29.1 **MEASURING BODY TEMPERATURE—cont'd**

STEP	RATIONALE

c. **Axillary temperature (electronic):**

(1) Move clothing or gown away from shoulder and arm.

Exposes axilla for correct thermometer probe placement.

(2) Remove thermometer pack from charging unit. Attach oral thermometer probe stem (blue tip) to thermometer unit. Grasp top of thermometer probe stem, being careful not to apply pressure on ejection button.

Charging provides battery power. Ejection button releases plastic cover from probe stem.

(3) Slide disposable plastic probe cover over thermometer stem until cover locks in place.

Soft plastic probe cover prevents transmission of infection between patients.

(4) Raise patient's arm away from torso. Inspect for skin lesions and excessive perspiration; if needed, dry axilla or select alternative site. Place thermometer probe into center of axilla (see illustration), lower arm over probe, and place arm across patient's chest.

Maintains proper position of thermometer against blood vessels in axilla.

CLINICAL DECISION: *Do not use axilla if skin lesions are present because local temperature can be altered, and area may be painful to touch.*

(5) Once thermometer probe is positioned, hold it in place until audible signal indicates completion and patient's temperature appears on digital display; remove thermometer probe from axilla.

Thermometer probe must stay in place until signal occurs to ensure accurate reading.

(6) Push ejection button on thermometer stem to discard plastic probe cover into appropriate receptacle.

Reduces transmission of microorganisms.

(7) Return thermometer stem to storage position of recording unit.

Returning thermometer stem to storage position automatically causes digital reading to disappear. Protects stem from damage.

(8) Replace linen or gown.

Restores comfort and sense of well-being.

(9) Perform hand hygiene.

Reduces transmission of infection.

d. **Tympanic membrane temperature:**

(1) Instruct patient to turn head toward side, away from you. If patient has been lying on one side, use upper ear. Note if there is an obvious presence of cerumen (earwax) in patient's ear canal.

Ensures comfort and facilitates exposure of auditory canal for accurate temperature measurement.

Heat trapped in ear facing down causes false-high temperature reading.

Cerumen impedes lens cover of speculum. Switch to other ear or select alternative measurement site.

(2) Obtain temperature from patient's right ear if you are right-handed. Obtain temperature from patient's left ear if you are left-handed.

The less acute the angle of approach, the better the probe seal.

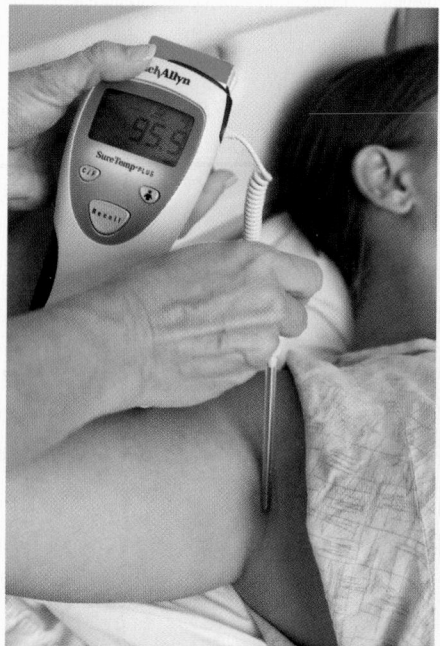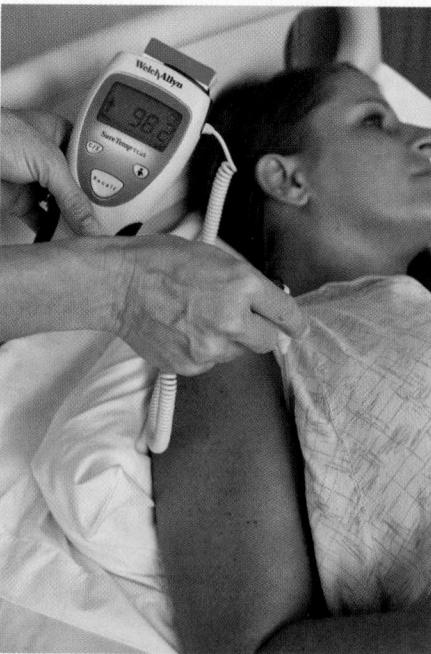

STEP 3c(4) Insert thermometer probe into center of axilla.

STEP	RATIONALE

(3) Remove thermometer handheld unit from charging base, being careful not to apply pressure to ejection button.

Charging base provides battery power. Removal of handheld unit from base prepares it to measure temperature. Ejection button releases plastic probe cover from thermometer tip.

(4) Slide disposable speculum cover over otoscope-like lens tip until it locks in place. Be careful not to touch lens cover.

Soft plastic probe cover prevents transmission of infection between patients. Lens cover should not have dust, fingerprints, or cerumen obstructing optical pathway.

(5) Insert speculum into ear canal following manufacturer instructions for tympanic probe positioning (see illustration):

Correct positioning of probe with respect to ear canal allows maximal exposure of tympanic membrane.

(a) Pull ear pinna backward, up, and out for an adult. For children less than 3 years of age, pull pinna down and back; point covered probe toward mid-point between eyebrow and sideburns. For children older than 3 years, pull pinna up and back (Hockenberry et al., 2019).

Ear tug straightens external auditory canal, allowing maximum exposure of tympanic membrane and therefore correctly positioning speculum (Hockenberry et al., 2019).

(b) Fit speculum tip snug in canal, pointing toward nose.

Gentle pressure seals ear canal from ambient air temperature, which alters readings as much as 2.8° C (5° F).

Optional: Move thermometer in figure-eight pattern.

Some manufacturers recommend movement of speculum tip in figure-eight pattern that allows sensor to detect maximum tympanic membrane heat radiation.

(6) Once positioned, press scan button on handheld unit. Leave speculum in place until audible signal indicates completion and patient's temperature appears on digital display.

Pressing scan button causes detection of infrared energy. Speculum probe tip must stay in place until device has detected infrared energy noted by audible signal.

(7) Carefully remove speculum from auditory meatus. Note temperature. Push ejection button on handheld unit to discard speculum cover into appropriate receptacle.

Reduces transmission of infection. Automatically causes digital reading to disappear.

(8) If temperature is abnormal or second reading is necessary, replace probe cover and wait 2 minutes before repeating in same ear or repeat measurement in other ear. Consider an alternative temperature site or instrument.

Lens cover must be free of cerumen to maintain optical path. Time allows ear canal to regain usual temperature.

(9) Return handheld unit to thermometer base.

Protects sensor tip from damage.

(10) Perform hand hygiene and assist patient to a comfortable position.

Reduces transmission of infection.

e. Temporal artery temperature:

(1) Ensure that forehead is dry; dry with towel if needed.

Moisture interferes with thermometer sensor.

(2) Place sensor firmly on patient's forehead.

Firm contact avoids measurement of ambient temperature.

(3) Press red scan button with your thumb. Slowly slide thermometer straight across forehead while keeping sensor flat and firmly on skin (see illustration). Keeping scan button depressed, lift sensor after sweeping forehead and touch sensor on neck just behind earlobe. Read temperature when clicking sound during scanning stops. Release scan button.

Thermometer continuously scans for highest temperature when scan button is depressed. Area behind earlobe is less affected by diaphoresis and verifies temperature.

(4) Gently clean sensor with alcohol swab, return to storage unit, and perform hand hygiene.

Prevents transmission of infection.

(5) Return thermometer to charger.

Maintains battery charge of thermometer unit.

4. Assist patient to comfortable position.

Ensures comfort and well-being.

5. Inform patient of temperature reading and record per agency policy.

Promotes participation in care and understanding of health status

6. Place nurse call system within reach; instruct patient in use.

Promotes safety and prevents falls.

7. Raise side rails (as appropriate) and place bed in lowest position.

Promotes safety and prevents falls.

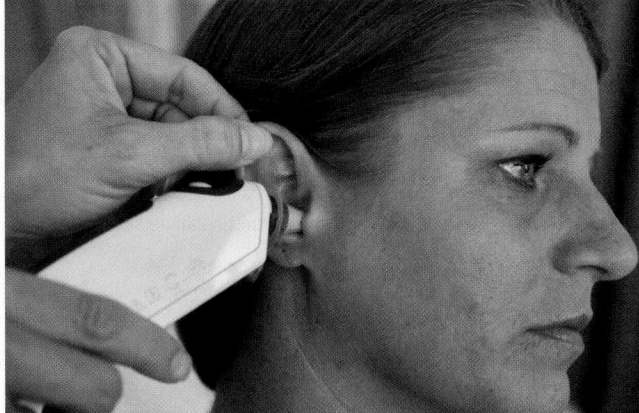

STEP 3d(5) Tympanic thermometer with probe cover inserted into auditory canal.

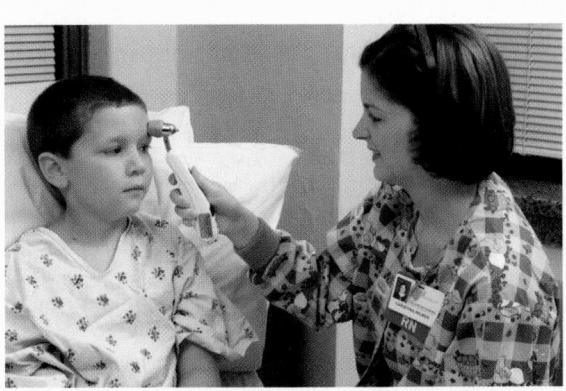

STEP 3e(3) Scanning the forehead with a temporal artery thermometer.

Continued

SKILL 29.1   MEASURING BODY TEMPERATURE—cont'd

STEP	RATIONALE

EVALUATION

1. If you are assessing temperature for the first time, establish it as baseline if it is within acceptable range.

Used to compare future temperature measurements.

2. Compare temperature reading with patient's previous baseline and acceptable temperature range for patient's age-group.

Body temperature fluctuates within narrow range; comparison reveals presence of abnormality. Improper placement or movement of thermometer can cause inaccuracies. Second measurement confirms initial findings of abnormal body temperature.

3. If patient has fever, take temperature approximately 30 minutes after administering antipyretics and every 4 hours until temperature stabilizes.

Determines whether temperature begins to fall in response to therapy.

4. **Use Teach-Back.** "I want to be sure I explained how to check your child's temperature at home. Show me how to swipe his forehead using the temporal thermometer." Revise your instruction now or develop a plan for revised patient/family caregiver teaching if patient/family caregiver is unable to teach back correctly.

Determines patient's/family caregiver's level of understanding of instructional topic.

UNEXPECTED OUTCOMES AND RELATED INTERVENTIONS

1. Patient has temperature 1° C (1.8° F) or more above usual range.
   Initiate measures to lower body temperature:
   - Cool room envixronment.
   - Reduce external covering on patient's body to promote heat loss, but do not induce shivering.
   - Keep clothing and bed linen dry.
   - Apply hypothermia blanket as ordered.
   - Limit physical activity and sources of emotional stress.
   - Administer antipyretics as ordered.
   - Increase fluid intake to at least 3 L daily (unless contraindicated).
2. Patient has temperature 1° C (1.8° F) or more below usual range.
   Initiate measures to raise body temperature:
   - Apply warm blankets and, unless contraindicated, offer warm liquids.
   - Apply hyperthermia blankets if ordered.
   - Remove wet clothing or linen.
3. Unable to obtain temperature.
   - Reassess correct placement of temperature probe or sensor.
   - Choose alternative temperature measurement site.
   - Obtain alternative temperature measurement device.

RECORDING AND REPORTING

- Record temperature and route and any signs or symptoms of temperature alteration in the EHR.
- Record temperature after administration of specific therapies, such as blood or blood product transfusions.
- Document your evaluation of patient learning.
- Report type of temperature, abnormal findings and any measures used to reduce or increase temperature to health care provider.

HOME CARE CONSIDERATIONS

- Assess temperature and ventilation of patient's environment to determine existence of any environmental condition that influences patient's temperature.

SKILL 29.2   ASSESSING APICAL AND RADIAL PULSE

Delegation and Collaboration

The skill of apical pulse measurement cannot be delegated to assistive personnel (AP). This measurement is often taken when you suspect an irregularity in the radial pulse or when a patient's condition requires more accurate pulse assessment.

The skill of radial pulse measurement can be delegated to assistive personnel (AP) if a patient's condition is stable. The skill cannot be delegated when a patient's condition is unstable because the patient is at high risk for acute or serious cardiac problems or when the nurse is evaluating a patient's response to a treatment or medication. The nurse instructs the AP by:

- Indicating the appropriate site for measuring pulse rate; frequency of measurement; and factors related to the patient history such as risk for abnormally slow, rapid, or irregular pulse.
- Reviewing patient's usual pulse rate and specific changes or abnormalities to report to the nurse.

Equipment

- Stethoscope
- Wristwatch with second hand or digital seconds display
- Pen and vital sign flow sheet in chart or electronic health record (EHR)
- Alcohol swab

STEP	RATIONALE

ASSESSMENT

Apical pulse or radial pulse:

1. Identify patient using at least two identifiers (e.g., name and birthday or name and medical record number) according to agency policy.

Ensures correct patient. Complies with The Joint Commission standards and improves patient safety (TJC, 2020).

2. Obtain data from patient's EHR to determine need to assess pulse:

   a. Assess for history of the following: heart or peripheral vascular disease, onset of sudden chest pain or acute pain from any site, invasive cardiovascular diagnostic tests, surgery, sudden infusion of large volume of intravenous (IV) fluid, internal or external hemorrhage, administration of medications that alter heart function.

   Certain conditions are risk factors for pulse alterations. A history of peripheral vascular disease often alters pulse rate and quality.

   b. Perform hand hygiene. Assess for signs and symptoms of altered cardiac function such as dyspnea, fatigue, chest pain, orthopnea, syncope, palpitations, edema of dependent body parts.

   Reduces transmission of infection. Physical signs and symptoms indicate alteration in conduction of cardiac electrical impulses, cardiac output, or stroke volume, all of which can affect radial pulse and rhythm.

   c. Assess for factors that normally influence pulse rate and rhythm:

   Allows you to anticipate factors that alter pulse, ensuring an accurate interpretation.

   * Age

   Newborn's heart rate (HR) ranges from 120-140 beats/min at rest; by age 2 pulse rate slows to 70 to 120 beats/min; by adolescence rate varies between 60 and 90 beats/min and remains so throughout adulthood (Hockenberry et al., 2019).

   * Exercise

   Physical activity increases HR; a well-conditioned patient may have a slower-than-usual resting HR that returns more quickly to resting rate after exercise.

   * Position changes

   HR increases temporarily when changing from lying to sitting or standing position.

   * Medications

   Antidysrhythmics, sympathomimetics, and cardiotonics affect rate and rhythm of pulse; large doses of opioid analgesics can slow HR; general anesthetics slow HR; central nervous system stimulants such as caffeine can increase HR.

   * Temperature

   Fever or exposure to warm environments increases HR; HR declines with hypothermia.

   * Sympathetic stimulation

   Emotional stress, anxiety, or fear stimulates sympathetic nervous system, which increases HR.

   d. Determine previous baseline pulse rate (if available).

   Allows you to assess for change in condition.

3. If obtaining apical pulse, determine any report of latex allergy. If patient has latex allergy, ensure that stethoscope is latex free.

Reduces risk of allergic reaction to stethoscope.

4. Assess patient's or family caregiver's knowledge, experience, and health literacy level.

Ensures patient has the capacity to obtain, communicate, process, and understand basic health information (CDC, 2019).

PLANNING

1. Provide privacy for patient; if necessary, draw curtain around bed and/or close door.

Maintains privacy and minimizes embarrassment, helping patient relax.

2. Collect appropriate equipment and bring to patient's bedside.

Ensures an organized approach for assessing pulse.

3. Explain to patient that you will assess radial pulse rate or apical pulse rate. Encourage patient to relax as much as possible. If patient has been active, wait 5 to 10 minutes before assessing pulse rate. If patient has been smoking or ingesting caffeine, wait 15 minutes before assessing pulse rate.

Anxiety, activity, smoking and caffeine elevate heart rate.

IMPLEMENTATION

1. **Apical pulse**

   a. Perform hand hygiene.

   Reduces transmission of infection.

   b. Have patient assume a sitting or supine position. Locate anatomical landmarks to identify point of maximal impulse (PMI), also called apical *impulse* (see Chapter 30). The heart is located behind and to left of sternum with base at top and apex at bottom. Find angle of Louis just below suprasternal notch between sternal body and manubrium; it feels like a bony prominence (see illustration A). Slip fingers down each side of angle to find second intercostal space (ICS) (see illustration B). Carefully move fingers down left side of sternum to fifth ICS and laterally to left midclavicular line (MCL) (see illustration C). A light tap felt within area 1 to 2.5 cm (½ to 1 inch) of PMI is reflected from apex of heart (see illustration D).

   Provides easy access to pulse sites. Use of anatomical landmarks allows correct placement of stethoscope over apex of heart. This position enhances ability to hear heart sounds clearly. If unable to palpate PMI, reposition patient on left side. In presence of serious heart disease, you may locate PMI to left of MCL or at sixth ICS. PMI may not be palpated in obese adults or patients with severe pulmonary disease that has changed shape of thorax.

   c. Place diaphragm of stethoscope in palm of hand for 5 to 10 seconds.

   Warming of metal or plastic diaphragm prevents patient from being startled and promotes comfort.

   d. Place diaphragm of stethoscope over PMI at fifth ICS, at left MCL, and auscultate for normal S_1 and S_2 heart sounds (heard as "lub-dub") (see illustrations).

   Allow stethoscope tubing to extend straight without kinks that would distort sound transmission. Normal sounds S_1 and S_2 are high pitched and best heard with diaphragm.

Continued

SKILL 29.2   **ASSESSING APICAL AND RADIAL PULSE—cont'd**

STEP	RATIONALE
e. When you hear S_1 and S_2 with regularity, use second hand of watch and begin to count rate; when sweep hand hits number on dial, start counting with zero, then one, two, and so on.	Apical rate is determined accurately only after you are able to auscultate sounds clearly. Timing begins with zero. Count of one is first sound auscultated after timing begins.
f. If apical rate is regular, count for 30 seconds and multiply by 2.	You can assess regular apical rate within 30 seconds.

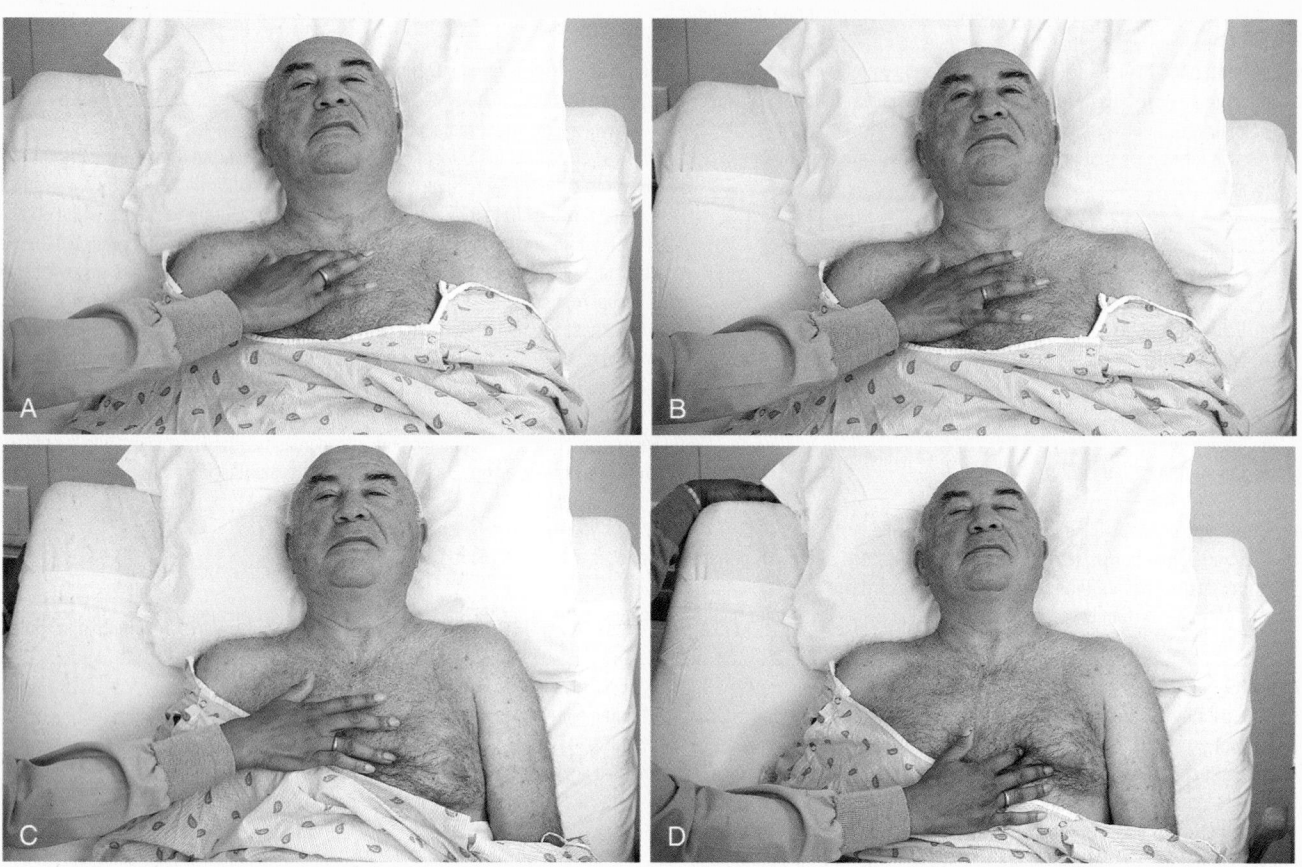

STEP 1b A, Nurse locates sternal notch. **B,** Nurse locates second intercostal space. **C,** Nurse locates fifth intercostal space. **D,** Nurse locates point of maximal impulse at fifth intercostal space at left midclavicular line.

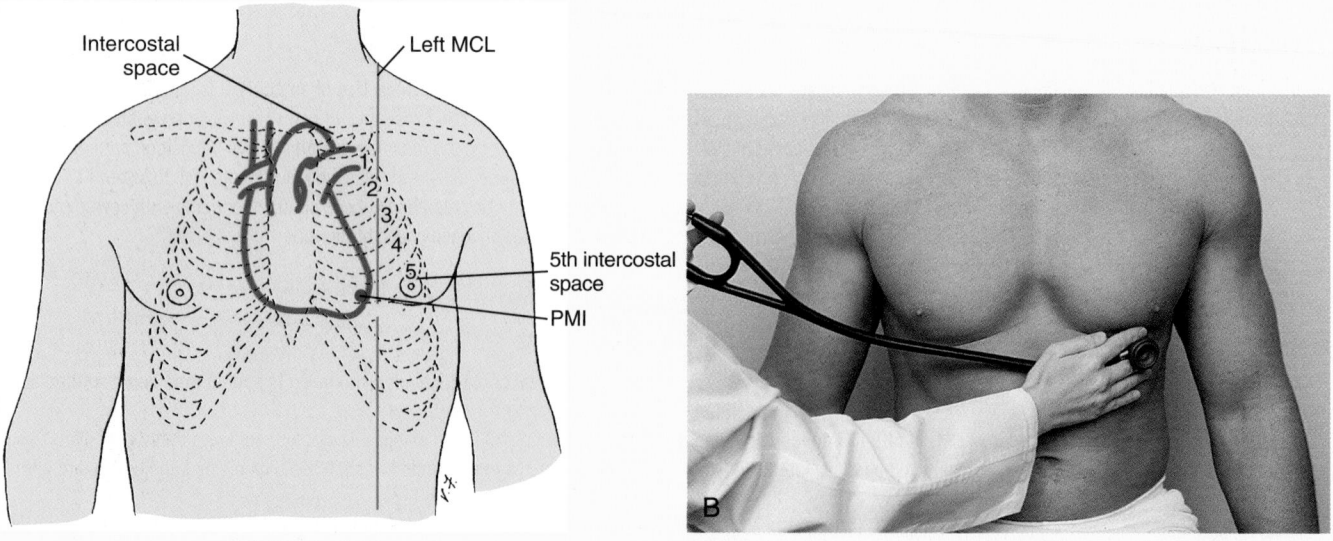

STEP 1d A, Location of point of maximal impulse (PMI) in adult. **B,** listening to PMI in adult.

STEP	RATIONALE
g. If HR is irregular or patient is receiving cardiovascular medication, count for a full 60 seconds.	Irregular rate is more accurately assessed when measured over longer interval.
h. Note regularity of any dysrhythmia (S_1 and S_2 occurring early or late after previous sequence of sounds) (e.g., every third or every fourth beat is skipped).	Regular occurrence of dysrhythmia within 1 minute indicates inefficient contraction of heart and potential alteration in cardiac output.

CLINICAL DECISION: *If apical rate is abnormal or irregular, repeat measurement or have another nurse conduct measurement. Original measurement may be incorrect. Second measurement confirms initial findings of an abnormal HR.*

i. Replace patient's gown and bed linen.	Restores comfort and promotes sense of well-being.
2. Radial pulse	
a. Perform hand hygiene.	Reduces transmission of infection.
b. Help patient to assume a supine or sitting position.	Provides easy access to pulse sites.
c. If patient is supine, place his or her forearm straight alongside or across lower chest or upper abdomen (see illustration A). If sitting, bend patient's elbow 90 degrees and support lower arm on chair or on your arm. Place tips of first two or middle three fingers of hand over groove along radial or thumb side of patient's inner wrist (see illustration B). Slightly extend or flex wrist with palm down until you note strongest pulse.	Fingertips are most sensitive parts of hand to palpate arterial pulsation. Your thumb has pulsation that interferes with accuracy.
d. Lightly compress pulse against radius, losing pulse initially; relax pressure so that pulse becomes easily palpable.	Pulse assessment is more accurate when using moderate pressure. Too much pressure occludes pulse and impairs blood flow.
e. Determine strength of pulse. Note whether thrust of vessel against fingertips is bounding (4+); full, strong (3+); expected (2+); barely palpable, diminished (1+); or absent, not palpable (0).	Strength reflects volume of blood ejected against arterial wall with each heart contraction. Accurate description of strength improves communication among nurses and other health care providers.
f. After palpating a regular pulse, look at watch second hand and begin to count rate. Count the first beat after the second hand hits the number on the dial; count as one, then two, and so on.	Rate is determined accurately only after pulse has been palpated. Timing begins with zero. Count of one is first beat palpated after timing begins.
(1) If pulse is regular, count rate for 30 seconds and multiply total by 2.	A 30-second count is accurate for rapid, slow, or regular pulse rates.
(2) If pulse is irregular, count rate for a full 60 seconds. Assess frequency and pattern of irregularity.	Inefficient contraction of heart fails to transmit pulse wave, resulting in irregular pulse. Longer time ensures accurate count.
(3) When pulse is irregular, compare radial pulses bilaterally and compare with apical pulse.	A marked difference between pulses indicates that arterial flow is compromised to one extremity; as a nurse you need to take action.
3. Assist patient to comfortable position.	Promotes comfort and sense of well-being.
4. Discuss findings with patient	Promotes participation in care and understanding of health status.
5. Place nurse call system within reach; instruct patient in use.	Promotes safety and prevents falls.
6. Raise side rails (as appropriate) and lower bed to lowest position.	Promotes safety and prevent falls.
7. Store reusable equipment. Perform hand hygiene.	Reduces transmission of infection.

EVALUATION

1. If assessing pulse for first time, establish apical or radial rate as baseline if it is within an acceptable range.	Used to compare future pulse assessments.
2. Compare apical or radial rate and character with patient's previous baseline and acceptable range of HR for patient's age.	Allows you to assess for change in patient's condition and for presence of cardiac alteration.

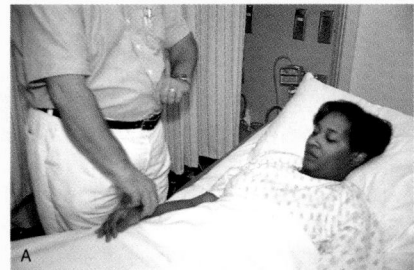
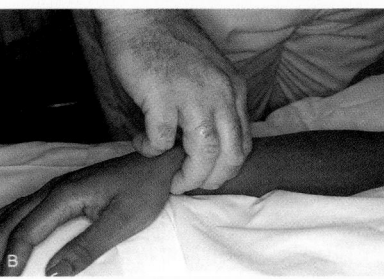

STEP 2c A, Pulse check with patient's forearm at side with wrist extended. **B,** Hand placement for pulse check.

Continued

SKILL 29.2   ASSESSING APICAL AND RADIAL PULSE—cont'd

STEP	RATIONALE
3. **Use Teach-Back:** "I want to be sure I explained why it is important to check your heart rate at home. Tell me which medication you are taking that would decrease your heart rate." Revise your instruction now or develop a plan for revised patient/family caregiver teaching if patient/family caregiver is not able to teach back correctly.	Determines patient's/family caregiver's level of understanding of instructional topic.

UNEXPECTED OUTCOMES AND RELATED INTERVENTIONS

1. Adult patient's apical or radial pulse is greater than 100 beats/min (tachycardia).
   - Identify related data, including fever, pain, fear or anxiety, recent exercise, low blood pressure, blood loss, or inadequate oxygenation.
   - Observe for signs and symptoms associated with abnormal cardiac function, including dyspnea, fatigue, chest pain, orthopnea, syncope, palpitations, edema of body parts.
2. Patient's apical or radial pulse is less than 60 beats/min (bradycardia).
   - Assess for factors that decrease HR such as beta blockers and antiarrhythmic drugs.
   - Observe for signs and symptoms associated with abnormal cardiac function, including dyspnea, fatigue, chest pain, orthopnea, syncope, palpitations, edema of body parts, or dizziness.
   - Have another nurse assess apical pulse.
   - Report findings to nurse in charge and/or health care provider. It may be necessary to withhold prescribed medications that alter HR until health care provider can evaluate need to adjust dosage.
3. Patient's apical pulse is irregular.
   - Assess for signs and symptoms of decreased cardiac output.
   - Report findings to nurse in charge and/or health care provider, who may order an electrocardiogram to detect cardiac conduction alteration.
4. Patient's radial pulse is irregular.
   Assess for Pulse Deficit.
   - One nurse auscultates apical pulse while a second provider palpates radial pulse; one nurse begins 60-second pulse count by calling out loud when both should begin to count pulses. The two pulse rates are compared.
   - If pulse count differs by more than 2, a deficit exists. Assess for other signs and symptoms of decreased cardiac output (see Chapter 30).

RECORDING AND REPORTING

- Record pulse rate and character routinely and after administration of specific therapies in the EHR.
- Record any signs and symptoms of alteration in cardiac function.
- Document your evaluation of patient learning.
- Report bradycardia, tachycardia, or irregular pulse to nurse in charge or health care provider immediately.

HOME CARE CONSIDERATIONS

- Assess home environment to determine room that affords quiet environment for auscultating apical rate.

SKILL 29.3   ASSESSING RESPIRATIONS

Delegation and Collaboration

The skill of counting respirations can be delegated to assistive personnel (AP) unless the patient is considered unstable (i.e., complaints of dyspnea). The nurse instructs the AP by:
- Communicating the frequency of measurement and factors related to patient history or risk for increased or decreased respiratory rate or irregular respirations.
- Reviewing any unusual respiratory values and significant changes to report to the nurse.

Equipment
- Wristwatch with second hand or digital seconds display
- Pen and vital sign flow sheet in chart or electronic health record (EHR)

STEP	RATIONALE
ASSESSMENT	
1. Identify patient using at least two identifiers (e.g., name and birthday or name and medical record number) according to agency policy.	Ensures correct patient. Complies with The Joint Commission standards and improves patient safety (TJC, 2020).
2. Obtain data from patient's electronic health record (EHR) to assess for factors that influence character of patient's respirations:	Allows you to anticipate factors that influence respirations, ensuring a more accurate interpretation.

STEP	RATIONALE
• Fever	Elevated body temperature increases oxygen demand and increases respiration rate and depth.
• Exercise	Respirations increase in rate and depth to meet need for additional oxygen and rid body of carbon dioxide.
• Anxiety	Increases oxygen demand, respiratory rate and depth because of sympathetic nervous system stimulation.
• Diseases/trauma of chest wall or muscles	Certain conditions (e.g., fractured ribs, thoracic surgery, asthma, chronic lung disease) affect inspiration and/or expiration.
• Constrictive chest or abdominal dressings	Dressings can restrict ease with which a patient is able to breathe deeply.
• Acute pain	Pain increases oxygen demand and alters rate and rhythm of respirations; breathing becomes shallow. Patient inhibits or splints chest wall movement when pain is in area of chest or abdomen.
• Smoking	Chronic smoking changes pulmonary airways, resulting in increased respiratory rate at rest when not smoking.
• Medications	Opioid analgesics, general anesthetics, and sedative hypnotics depress rate and depth; amphetamines and cocaine increase rate and depth; bronchodilators cause dilation of airways, which ultimately slows respiratory rate.
• Body position	Standing or sitting erect promotes full ventilatory movement and lung expansion; stooped or slumped posture impairs ventilatory movement; lying flat prevents full chest expansion.
• Neurological injury	Damage to brainstem impairs respiratory center and inhibits rate and rhythm.
• Anemia, decreased hemoglobin	Decreased hemoglobin levels lower amount of oxygen carried in blood, which results in increased respiratory rate to increase oxygen delivery.
• Increased altitude	An increase in altitude lowers the amount of saturated hemoglobin, which increases respiratory rate and depth.

3. Perform hand hygiene. Assess for signs and symptoms of respiratory alterations such as:
  • Bluish or cyanotic appearance of nail beds, lips, mucous membranes, and skin
  • Restlessness, irritability, confusion, reduced level of consciousness
  • Pain during inspiration
  • Labored or difficult breathing
  • Orthopnea
  • Use of accessory muscles
  • Adventitious breath sounds (see Chapter 30)
  • Inability to breathe spontaneously
  • Thick, frothy, blood-tinged, or copious sputum production
	Reduces transmission of infection. Physical signs and symptoms indicate alterations in respiratory status (see Chapter 30).

4. Review EHR and assess pertinent laboratory/clinical values:
  a. *Arterial blood gases (ABGs):* Normal ranges (values vary slightly among agencies) (Pagana et al., 2019):
    • pH, 7.35–7.45
    • $PaCO_2$, 35–45 mm Hg
    • HCO_3, 21–28 mEq/L
    • PaO_2, 80–100 mm Hg
    • SaO_2, 95%–100%
	ABG values measure arterial blood pH, partial pressure of oxygen and carbon dioxide, and arterial oxygen saturation, which reflect patient's ventilation and oxygenation status (see Chapter 41).

b. *Pulse oximetry (SpO_2):* Normal SpO_2 ≥95%–100%; less than 90% is a clinical emergency (see Skill 29.4).	SpO_2 less than 90% is often accompanied by changes in respiratory rate, depth, and rhythm.

c. *Complete blood count (CBC):* Normal ranges for adults (values vary among agencies)(Pagana et al., 2019):
    • Hemoglobin: 14–18 g/100 mL, males; 12–16 g/100 mL, females
    • Hematocrit: 42%–52%, males; 37%–47%, females
    • Red blood cell count: 4.7–6.1 million/mm^3, males; 4.2–5.4 million/mm^3, females
	CBC measures red blood cell count; volume of red blood cells; and concentration of hemoglobin, which reflects patient's capacity to carry oxygen.

5. Determine previous baseline respiratory rate (if available in the EHR).	Assesses for change in condition. Provides comparison with future respiratory measurements.

Continued

SKILL 29.3   ASSESSING RESPIRATIONS—cont'd

STEP	RATIONALE
6. Assess patient's or family caregiver's knowledge, experience, and health literacy level.	Ensures patient has the capacity to obtain, communicate, process, and understand basic health information (CDC, 2019).

PLANNING

1. Provide privacy; close curtains or room door.	Promotes relaxation and provides privacy.
2. If patient has been active, wait 5 to 10 minutes before assessing respirations.	Exercise increases respiratory rate and depth. Assessing respirations while patient is at rest allows for objective comparison of values.
3. In an adult, assess respirations after pulse rate; in children assess respirations first.	Inconspicuous assessment after pulse assessment prevents patients from consciously or unintentionally altering rate and depth of breathing. Assess respirations before invasive procedures in children, which may cause anxiety.
4. Position patient in a comfortable position, preferably sitting or lying with the head of the bed elevated 45 to 60 degrees.	Sitting erect promotes full ventilator movement. A position of discomfort causes patient to breath more rapidly.

CLINICAL DECISION: *Assess patients with difficulty breathing, dyspnea, heart failure, or abdominal ascites and patients in the late stages of pregnancy in the position of greatest comfort. Repositioning may increase the work of breathing, which increases respiratory rate.*

IMPLEMENTATION

1. Perform hand hygiene.	Prevents transmission of infection.
2. Be sure that patient's chest is visible. If necessary, move bed linen or gown.	Ensures clear view of chest wall and abdominal movements.
3. Place patient's arm in relaxed position across abdomen or lower chest or place your hand directly over patient's upper abdomen.	A similar position used during pulse assessment allows respiratory rate assessment to be inconspicuous. Patient awareness of monitoring reduces respiratory rate by 2 breaths per minute (Hill et al., 2018). The patient's or your hand rises and falls during respiratory cycle.
4. Observe complete respiratory cycle (one inspiration and one expiration).	Rate is accurately determined only after viewing a complete respiratory cycle.
5. After observing a cycle, look at second hand of watch and begin to count rate: when sweep hand hits number on dial, begin time frame, counting one with first full respiratory cycle.	Timing begins with count of one. Respirations occur more slowly than pulse; thus timing does not begin with zero.
6. If rhythm is regular, count number of respirations in 30 seconds and multiply by 2. If rhythm is irregular, less than 12, or greater than 20, count for **1 full minute** (Box 29.12).	Respiratory rate is equivalent to number of respirations per minute. Suspected irregularities require assessment for at least 1 minute (Table 29.7).

BOX 29.12   EVIDENCE-BASED PRACTICE

Reliability in Assessing Respiratory Rate

PICOT Question: Do nurses who count respirations for 15 or 30 seconds accurately assess the respiratory rate compared with nurses who count respirations for 60 seconds?

Evidence Summary

Respiratory rate is a strong predictor of adverse events and strongly correlated with in-hospital mortality. Some experts believe that respiratory rate is a stronger predictor of mortality than blood pressure or pulse. Many Early Warning Scores include respiratory rate measurements. Therefore it is important that respiratory rate be measured accurately and reliably. Brabrand and colleagues (2018) presented experienced nurses with five 60-second patient videos and asked them to measure respiratory rate. In each case measurements had a wide range of more than 10 breaths per minute. Daw et al (2017) conducted a similar study using 169 emergency room pediatric patients. Three health care professionals, a nurse, physician, and respiratory therapist, measured respiratory rate. Measurements varied from 11 breaths below to 18 breaths above the known respiratory rate. Higher respiratory rates resulted in less agreement. Nurses who count for 15 seconds and multiply by 4 or count for 30 seconds and multiply by 2 round down or round up, which contributes to the measurement error. Convenient electronic devices exist for pulse, blood pressure, oxygen saturation, and temperature for prompt and accurate measurement. Respiratory rate remains a subjective assessment full of human error.

Application to Nursing Practice

- 15-second assessments of respiratory rates are not reliable.
- High respiratory rates require a 60-second assessment of respiratory rate.
- Abnormal respiratory rates should be reassessed before initiating therapies.

STEP	RATIONALE
7. Note depth of respirations by observing degree of chest wall movement while counting rate. In addition, assess depth by palpating chest wall excursion or auscultating posterior thorax after you have counted rate (see Chapter 30). Describe depth as shallow, normal, or deep.	Character of ventilatory movement reveals specific disease states restricting volume of air from moving into and out of lungs.
8. Note rhythm of ventilatory cycle. Normal breathing is regular and uninterrupted. Do not confuse sighing with abnormal rhythm.	Character of ventilations reveals specific types of alterations. Periodically people unconsciously take single deep breaths or sighs to expand small airways prone to collapse.

CLINICAL DECISION: *Any irregular respiratory pattern or periods of apnea (cessation of respiration over 5 seconds) are symptoms of underlying disease in an adult; report this to the health care provider or nurse in charge. Further assessment and immediate intervention are often necessary.*

9. Replace bed linen and patient's gown.	Restores comfort and promotes sense of well-being.
10. Assist patient to comfortable position.	Promotes comfort and sense of well-being.
11. Place nurse call system within reach and instruct patient in use.	Promotes safety and prevents falls.
12. Raise side rails (as appropriate) and lower bed to lowest position.	Promotes safety and prevents falls.
13. Perform hand hygiene.	Reduces transmission of infection.
14. Discuss results with patient.	Promotes participation in care and understanding of health.

EVALUATION

1. If assessing respirations for the first time, establish rate, rhythm, and depth as baseline if within acceptable range.	Used to compare future respiratory assessments.
2. Compare respirations with patient's previous baseline and usual rate, rhythm, and depth.	Allows you to assess for changes in patient's condition and presence of respiratory alterations.
3. Correlate respiratory rate, depth, and rhythm with data obtained from pulse oximetry and ABG measurements if available.	Evaluation of ventilation, perfusion, and diffusion is interrelated.
4. **Use Teach-Back**: "I want to be sure I explained why you need to take deep breaths after your surgery. Tell me why deep breathing is important." Revise your instruction now or develop a plan for revised patient/family caregiver teaching if patient/family caregiver is not able to teach back correctly.	Determines patient's/family caregiver's level of understanding of instructional topic.

UNEXPECTED OUTCOMES AND RELATED INTERVENTIONS

1. Adult patient's respiratory rate is below 12 breaths/min (bradypnea) or above 20 breaths/min (tachypnea). Breathing pattern is irregular (see Table 29.7). Depth of respirations is increased or decreased. Patient complains of dyspnea.
   - Assess for related factors, including obstructed airway, abnormal breath sounds, productive cough, restlessness, anxiety, and confusion (see Chapter 30).
   - Help patient to supported sitting position (semi- or high-Fowler's) unless contraindicated.
   - Provide oxygen as ordered (see Chapter 41).
   - Assess for environmental factors that influence patient's respiratory rate such as secondhand smoke, poor ventilation, or gas fumes.
   - Notify health care provider or nurse in charge if alteration continues.

2. Patient demonstrates Kussmaul's, Cheyne-Stokes, or Biot's respirations (see Table 29.7).
   - Notify health care provider for additional evaluation and possible medical intervention.

RECORDING AND REPORTING

- Record respiratory rate and character, noting any abnormalities.
- Record respiratory rate after administration of specific therapies.
- Record type and amount of oxygen therapy if used by patient during assessment.
- Document your evaluation of patient learning.
- Report bradypnea, tachypnea, abnormal depth or rhythm to nurse in charge or health care provider immediately.

HOME CARE CONSIDERATIONS

- Assess for environmental factors in the home that influence respiratory rate such as secondhand smoke, poor ventilation, gas or fireplace fumes, dust, and pets.

SKILL 29.4	MEASURING OXYGEN SATURATION (PULSE OXIMETRY)	▶

Delegation and Collaboration

The skill of SpO_2 measurement can be delegated to assistive personnel (AP). The nurse instructs the AP by:
- Communicating specific factors related to the patient that can falsely lower SpO_2.
- Informing AP about appropriate sensor site and probe and about reporting any skin irritation from probe placement to nurse.
- Notifying about frequency of SpO_2 measurements for a specific patient.
- Informing AP to notify the nurse immediately of any reading lower than SpO_2 of 95% or value for specific patient.

- Instructing to refrain from using pulse oximetry to obtain heart rate because oximeter will not detect an irregular pulse.

Equipment
- Oximeter
- Oximeter probe appropriate for patient and recommended by oximeter manufacturer
- Acetone or nail-polish remover if needed
- Pen and vital sign flow sheet in chart or the EHR

Continued

STEP	RATIONALE
ASSESSMENT	
1. Identify patient using at least two identifiers (e.g., name and birthday or name and medical record number) according to agency policy.	Ensures correct patient. Complies with The Joint Commission standards and improves patient safety (TJC, 2020).
2. Determine previous baseline SpO$_2$ (if available) from patient's medical record.	Provides basis for comparison and assists in the assessment of current status and evaluation of interventions.
3. Determine need to assess patient's oxygen saturation:	Certain conditions place patients at risk for decreased oxygen saturation.
a. Review the EHR to identify conditions that can cause decreased oxygen saturation, including acute or chronic compromised respiratory function, recovery from general anesthesia or conscious sedation, traumatic injury to chest wall, collapse of lung tissue, ventilator dependence, or a change in oxygen therapy.	
b. Perform hand hygiene. Assess for signs and symptoms of alteration in oxygen saturation such as altered respiratory rate, depth or rhythm; abnormal breath sounds (see Chapter 30); cyanotic appearance of nail beds, lips, mucous membranes; restlessness, irritability, confusion; reduced level of consciousness; and labored or difficult breathing.	Reduces transmission of infection. Physical signs and symptoms often indicate low oxygen saturation.
4. Assess for factors that influence measurement of SpO$_2$ (e.g., oxygen therapy, respiratory therapy such as postural drainage and percussion, hemoglobin level, hypotension, temperature, nail polish, and medications such as bronchodilators).	Allows you to accurately assess oxygen saturation variations.
5. Determine if patient has a latex allergy.	Disposable adhesive sensors may contain latex.
6. Determine most appropriate patient-specific probe site (e.g., finger, toe, earlobe, forehead, nose) for sensor placement by evaluating capillary refill (see Chapter 30). If capillary refill is greater than 2 seconds, select alternative site.	Sensor requires pulsating vascular bed to identify light-absorbing hemoglobin molecules. Patients requiring vasopressors or who are critically ill may have increased peripheral capillary refill; forehead sensors are preferred. Moisture and black or brown nail polish alter readings. Motion artifact is the most common cause of inaccurate measurements. Clip-on probe may be too small for obese patient.
7. Assess patient's or family caregiver's knowledge, experience, and health literacy level.	Ensures patient has the capacity to obtain, communicate, process, and understand basic health information (CDC, 2019).
PLANNING	
1. Provide privacy and prepare bedside environment for patient safety.	Maintains patient comfort and removes barriers that may interfere with procedure.
2. Collect and bring appropriate supplies to the patient's bedside.	Ensures an organized approach for oxygen saturation measurement.
3. Explain to patient the way you will measure oxygen saturation and the importance of breathing normally until reading is complete.	Promotes patient cooperation and increases adherence. Prevents large fluctuations in minute ventilation and possible error in SpO$_2$ readings
IMPLEMENTATION	
1. Perform hand hygiene.	Prevents transmission of infection.
2. Position patient in a comfortable position, preferably sitting or lying with the head of the bed elevated 45 to 60 degrees.	Sitting erect promotes full ventilation. A position of discomfort causes patient to breath more rapidly.
3. Attach sensor to monitoring site (see illustrations). If using finger, remove fingernail polish from digit with acetone or polish remover. Instruct patient that clip-on probe will feel like a clothes pin on the finger but will not hurt.	Nail polish falsely alters saturation.

CLINICAL DECISION: *Do not attach probe to finger, ear, or bridge of nose if area is edematous or skin integrity is compromised. Do not use earlobe and bridge of nose sensors for infants and toddlers because of skin fragility. Do not attach sensor to fingers that are hypothermic. Select ear or bridge of nose if adult patient has a history of peripheral vascular disease. Do not use disposable adhesive sensors if patient has a latex allergy. Do not place sensor on same extremity as electronic blood pressure cuff because blood flow to finger will be interrupted temporarily when cuff inflates and cause inaccurate reading that can trigger alarms.*

4. Once sensor is in place, turn on oximeter by activating power. Observe pulse waveform/intensity display and audible beep. Correlate oximeter pulse rate with patient's radial pulse.	Pulse waveform and audible beep enables detection of valid pulse. Pitch of audible beep is proportional to SpO$_2$ value. Correlating pulse rates ensures oximeter accuracy; difference requires reassessment of sensor placement site.
5. Leave sensor in place 10 to 30 seconds or until oximeter readout reaches constant value and pulse display reaches full strength during each cardiac cycle. Inform patient that oximeter alarm will sound if sensor falls off or patient moves it. Read SpO$_2$ on digital display.	Sensor alarm may frighten patient or visitors.

STEP	**RATIONALE**
6. For continuous SpO$_2$ monitoring:	Sensor tension and sensitivity to disposable sensor adhesive cause skin irritation and lead to disruption of skin integrity.
• Verify SpO$_2$ alarm limits preset by manufacturer at a low of 85% and a high of 100%.	
• Determine limits for SpO$_2$ and pulse rate as indicated by patient's condition.	
• Verify that alarms are on.	
• Assess skin integrity under sensor probe every 2 hours; relocate sensor at least every 4 hours and more frequently if skin integrity is altered or tissue perfusion compromised.	
7. If you plan intermittent checking or spot-checking of SpO$_2$, remove probe and turn oximeter power off. Clean sensor and store sensor in appropriate location.	Prevents transmission of infection. Sensor probes are vulnerable to damage.
8. Assist patient to comfortable position.	Restores comfort and promotes a sense of well-being.
9. Place nurse call system within patient's reach and instruct patient in use.	Promotes safety and prevents falls.
10. Raise side rails (as appropriate) and lower bed to lowest position.	Promotes safety and prevents falls.
11. Perform hand hygiene.	Prevents transmission of infection.
12. Discuss results with patient.	Promotes participation in care and understanding of health.

EVALUATION

1. If assessing oxygen saturation for the first time, establish it as baseline if within acceptable range.	Used to compare future SpO$_2$ measurements.
2. Compare SpO$_2$ reading with patient's previous baseline and acceptable values. Note use of oxygen therapy, which can affect SpO$_2$.	Allows you to assess for changes in patient's condition and presence of respiratory alterations.
3. Correlate SpO$_2$ with SaO$_2$, obtained from ABG measurements if available.	Documents reliability of noninvasive assessment.
4. Correlate reading with data obtained from respiratory rate, depth and rhythm assessment (see Skill 29.3).	Measurements assessing ventilation, perfusion, and diffusion are interrelated.
5. **Use Teach Back:** "I want to be sure I explained the reasons for a low oxygen saturation. Can you tell me two actions that could improve the oxygen level in your blood?" Revise your instruction now or develop a plan for revised patient/family caregiver teaching if patient/family caregiver is unable to teach back correctly.	Determines patient's/family caregiver's level of understanding of instructional topic.

UNEXPECTED OUTCOMES AND RELATED INTERVENTIONS

1. SpO$_2$ is less than 90%.
   - Verify that oximeter sensor is intact and properly applied.
   - Observe for signs and symptoms of decreased oxygenation such as anxiety, restlessness, tachycardia.
   - Verify that supplemental oxygen is delivered as ordered and that system is functioning properly.
   - Assist patient to a position that maximizes ventilator effort (e.g., position an obese patient in a high-Fowler position).
   - Report SpO$_2$ to nurse in charge or health care provider to initiate appropriate evaluation and treatment.

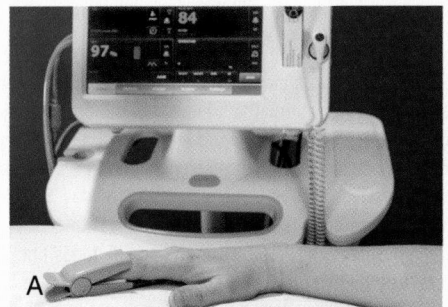 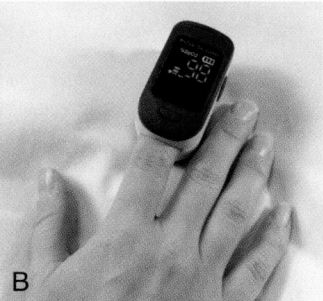

STEP 3 A, Pulse oximetry machine. B, Clip-on pulse oximetry sensor.

Continued

SKILL 29.4	MEASURING OXYGEN SATURATION (PULSE OXIMETRY)—cont'd

STEP	RATIONALE

2. Sensor device results in pressure injury.
   - Rotate oximetry probe sites more frequently.
   - Change type or location of sensor device.
   - Increase frequency of skin assessment under sensor.

RECORDING AND REPORTING

- Record type and amount of oxygen therapy used by patient during assessment, SpO_2 readings, and any signs or symptoms of alterations in oxygenation in EHR.
- Document your evaluation of patient learning.
- Report alterations in SpO_2 to health care provider.

SKILL 29.5	MEASURING BLOOD PRESSURE BY AUSCULTATION

Delegation and Collaboration

The skill of BP measurement can be delegated to assistive personnel (AP) unless the patient is considered unstable (i.e., hypotensive). The nurse instructs the AP by:

- Explaining the appropriate limb for measurement, BP cuff size, and equipment (manual or electronic) to be used.
- Communicating the frequency of measurement and factors related to the patient's history such as risk for orthostatic hypotension.
- Reviewing the patient's usual BP values and significant changes or abnormalities to report to the nurse.

Equipment

- Aneroid sphygmomanometer
- Cloth or disposable vinyl pressure cuff of appropriate size for patient's extremity (see Planning Step 2)
- Stethoscope
- Alcohol swab
- Pen and vital sign flow sheet in chart or electronic health record (EHR)

STEP	RATIONALE

ASSESSMENT

1. Identify patient using at least two identifiers (e.g., name and birthday or name and medical record number) according to agency policy.

Ensures correct patient. Complies with The Joint Commission standards and improves patient safety (TJC, 2020).

2. Obtain data from the patient's electronic record (EHR) to:

Certain conditions place patients at risk for BP alteration.

   a. Assess for presence of
      - History of cardiovascular disease
      - Renal disease
      - Diabetes mellitus
      - Circulatory shock (hypovolemic, septic, cardiogenic, or neurogenic)
      - Acute or chronic pain
      - Rapid intravenous (IV) infusion of fluids or blood products
      - Increased intracranial pressure
      - Postoperative status
      - Toxemia of pregnancy

   b. Assess for factors that influence BP:

   Allows you to anticipate factors that influence BP, ensuring a more accurate interpretation.

      - Age

      Acceptable values for BP vary throughout life. Older patients experience greater "white coat" effect as BP increases when in the presence of a provider (Kallioinen et al., 2017).

      - Gender

      During and after menopause women often have higher BPs than men of same age.

      - Daily (diurnal) variation

      BP varies throughout day; pressure is highest during the day between 10:00 AM and 6:00 PM and lowest in early morning.

      - Position

      BP falls as person moves from lying to sitting or standing position; acceptable postural variations are less than 10 mm Hg (Hale et al., 2017).

      - Exercise

      Increases in oxygen demand by body during activity increases BP. BP can be increased if patient does not rest at least 15 minutes before measurement (Kallioinen et al., 2017).

      - Weight

      Obesity is an independent predictor of hypertension.

      - Sympathetic stimulation

      Pain, anxiety, or fear stimulates sympathetic nervous system, causing BP to rise. A full bladder increases systolic and diastolic BP (Kallioinen et al., 2017).

      - Medications

      Antihypertensives, diuretics, beta-adrenergic blockers, vasodilators, calcium channel blockers, angiotensin-converting enzyme (ACE) inhibitors, angiotensin receptor blockers (ARBs), and antidysrhythmics lower BP; opioids and general anesthetics also cause a drop in BP (Soyal et al., 2016).

STEP	RATIONALE

- Smoking

Smoking results in vasoconstriction, a narrowing of blood vessels. SBP and DBP rises acutely and returns to baseline approximately 20-30 minutes after stopping smoking, 30 minutes after snuff chewing, and 40-60 minutes after a nicotine tablet (Kallioinen et al., 2017).

- Ethnicity

Incidence of hypertension is higher in African-Americans and Hispanics than in European Americans. African-Americans tend to develop more severe hypertension at an earlier age and have twice the risk for the complications of hypertension (i.e., stroke and heart attack). Hypertension-related deaths are also higher among African-Americans (Moughrabi, 2017).

- Temperature

Cold exposure increases systolic BP (Kallioinen et al., 2017).

3. Perform hand hygiene. Assess for signs and symptoms of BP alterations (especially patients at high risk for hypertension): headache (usually occipital), flushing of face, nosebleed, and fatigue in older adults. Hypotension is associated with dizziness; mental confusion; restlessness; pale, dusky, or cyanotic skin and mucous membranes; and cool, mottled skin over extremities.

Reduces transmission of infection. Physical signs and symptoms indicate alterations in BP. Hypertension is often asymptomatic until pressure is very high.

4. Determine best site for BP assessment. Avoid applying cuff to extremity when IV fluids are infusing, an arteriovenous shunt or fistula is present, or breast or axillary surgery has been performed on that side. In addition, avoid applying cuff to traumatized or diseased extremity or one that has a cast or bulky bandage. Use lower extremities when brachial arteries are inaccessible.

Inappropriate site selection may result in poor amplification of sounds, causing inaccurate readings. Application of pressure from inflated cuff bladder temporarily impairs blood flow and can further compromise circulation in extremity that already has impaired blood flow.

5. Determine previous baseline BP and site (if available). Determine any report of latex allergy.

Assesses for change in condition. Provides comparison with future BP measurements. If patient has latex allergy, verify that stethoscope and BP cuff are latex free.

6. Assess patient's or family caregiver's knowledge, experience, and health literacy level.

Ensures patient has the capacity to obtain, communicate, process, and understand basic health information (CDC, 2019).

PLANNING

1. Provide privacy and prepare bedside environment for patient safety.

Maintains patient comfort and removes barriers that may interfere with procedure.

2. Select appropriate cuff size (see Fig. 29.9) and insure that sphygmomanometer is in patient's room.

Use of improper cuff can cause measurement errors (see Table 29.12).

3. Ensure that patient has not exercised, ingested caffeine, or smoked for 30 minutes before assessing BP.

Exercise causes false elevation in BP. Smoking increases BP immediately and up to 15 minutes. Caffeine increase BP for up to 3 hours (James et al., 2014).

4. Explain to patient that you will be measuring blood pressure. Have patient rest at least 5 minutes before measuring lying or sitting BP and one minute before measuring standing BP. Ask patient to uncross legs and not to speak when BP being measured.

Promotes patient cooperation and increases adherence. Crossed legs or talking during assessment increases BP (AACN Practice Alert, 2016).

IMPLEMENTATION

1. Perform hand hygiene. Clean stethoscope earpieces and diaphragm with alcohol swab.

Reduces transmission of infection.

2. Position Patient

a. *Upper extremity:* With patient sitting or lying, position his or her forearm at heart level with palm turned up (see illustration). Support arm on a table or under your arm. If sitting, support back and instruct patient to keep feet flat on floor without legs crossed. If supine, patient should not have legs crossed.

If arm is extended and not supported, patient will perform isometric exercise that can increase diastolic pressure. Placement of arm above level of heart causes false-low reading; arm below the level of the heart creates a false-high reading (Kallioinen et al., 2017). Not supporting the arm can falsely elevate systolic BP (Gunes and Efteli, 2016). BP readings measured with the back unsupported are higher than those with the back supported (Ringrose et al., 2017). Legs crossed at the knees can significantly increase BP (Kallioinen et al., 2017).

b. *Lower extremity:* With patient prone, position patient so that knee is slightly flexed. If the patient cannot be placed in prone position, position him or her supine with knee slightly bent.

3. Expose extremity (arm or leg) fully by removing constricting clothing. Cuff may be placed over a sleeve as long as stethoscope rests on skin (Kallioinen et al., 2017).

Ensures proper cuff application.

4. Palpate brachial artery in arm (see illustration A) or popliteal artery in leg. With cuff fully deflated, apply bladder of cuff above artery by centering arrows marked on cuff over artery (see illustration B). If cuff does not have any center arrows, estimate center of bladder and place this center over artery. Position cuff 2.5 cm (1 inch) above site of pulsation (antecubital or popliteal space). With cuff fully deflated, wrap it evenly and snugly around upper arm (see illustration C) or leg (see illustration D).

Brachial artery is along groove between biceps and triceps muscles above elbow at antecubital fossa. Popliteal artery is just below patient's thigh, behind knee.

Placing bladder directly over artery ensures that you apply proper pressure during inflation. Loose-fitting cuff causes false-high readings.

Continued

SKILL 29.5   MEASURING BLOOD PRESSURE BY AUSCULTATION—cont'd

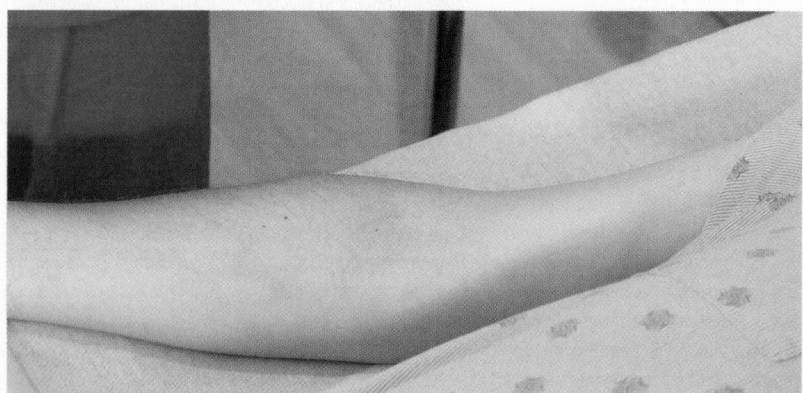

STEP 2a Patient's forearm supported on bed. (*Copyright © Mosby's Clinical Skills: Essentials Collection.*)

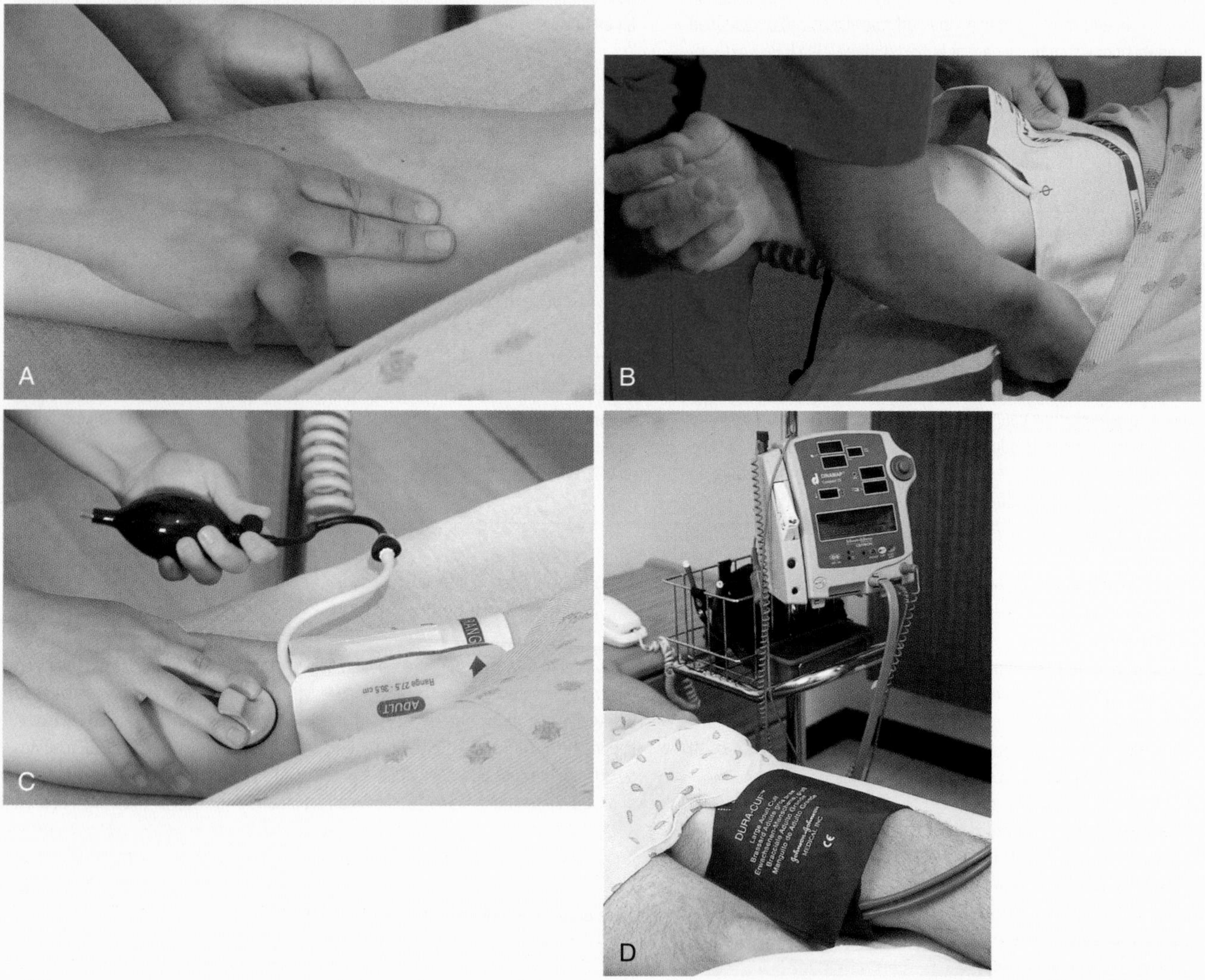

STEP 4 A, Palpating brachial artery. **B,** Aligning blood pressure cuff arrow with brachial artery. **C,** Blood pressure cuff wrapped around upper arm. **D,** Blood pressure cuff applied around thigh. (*A-C Copyright © Mosby's Clinical Skills: Essentials Collection.*)

STEP	RATIONALE
5. Position manometer gauge vertically at eye level. You should be no farther than 1 meter (approximately 1 yard) away.	Looking up or down at scale can result in distorted readings.
6. **Measure BP.**	
a. **Two-step method:**	
(1) Relocate brachial or popliteal pulse. Palpate artery distal to cuff with fingertips of nondominant hand while inflating cuff rapidly to pressure 30 mm Hg above point at which pulse disappears. Slowly deflate cuff and note point when pulse reappears. Deflate cuff fully and wait 30 seconds.	Estimating prevents false-low readings. Determine maximal inflation point for accurate reading by palpation. If unable to palpate artery because of weakened pulse, use ultrasonic stethoscope (see Chapter 30). Deflating the cuff completely prevents venous congestion and false-high readings.
(2) Place stethoscope earpieces in ears and be sure that sounds are clear, not muffled.	Ensure that each earpiece follows angle of ear canal to facilitate hearing.
(3) Relocate artery and place bell or diaphragm chest piece of stethoscope over it. Do not allow chest piece to touch cuff or clothing.	Proper stethoscope placement ensures best sound reception. Stethoscope improperly positioned causes muffled sounds that often result in false-low systolic and false-high diastolic readings. The bell provides better sound reproduction, whereas the diaphragm is easier to secure with fingers and covers a larger area. Placing the stethoscope under the cuff increases the systolic and decreases the diastolic BP measurement (Kallioinen et al., 2017).
(4) Close valve of pressure bulb clockwise until tight. Quickly inflate cuff to 30 mm Hg above patient's estimated systolic pressure.	Tightening valve prevents air leak during inflation. Rapid inflation ensures accurate measurement of systolic pressure.
(5) Slowly release pressure bulb valve and allow manometer needle to fall at rate of 2 to 3 mm Hg/second.	Too-rapid a decline decreases systolic BP and increases diastolic BP measurement (Kallioinen et al., 2017).
(6) Note point on manometer when you hear first clear sound. Sound will slowly increase in intensity.	First sound reflects systolic BP.
(7) Continue to deflate cuff gradually, noting point at which sound disappears in adults. Note pressure to nearest 2 mm Hg. Listen for 20 to 30 mm Hg after last sound and allow remaining air to escape quickly.	Beginning of last or fifth sound is indication of diastolic pressure in adults (Thomas and Pohl, 2017). In children distinct muffling of sounds indicates diastolic pressure (Thomas and Pohl, 2017).
b. **One-step method:**	
(1) Place stethoscope earpieces in ears and be sure that sounds are clear, not muffled.	Earpieces should follow angle of ear canal to facilitate hearing.
(2) Relocate brachial or popliteal artery and place bell or diaphragm chest piece of stethoscope over it. Do not allow chest piece to touch cuff or clothing.	Proper stethoscope placement ensures optimal sound reception. Stethoscope improperly positioned causes muffled sounds that often result in false readings. Bell provides better sound reproduction, whereas diaphragm is easier to secure with fingers and covers a larger area. Placing the stethoscope under the cuff increases the systolic and decreases the diastolic BP measurement (Kallioinen et al., 2017).
(3) Close valve of pressure bulb clockwise until tight. Quickly inflate cuff to 30 mm Hg above patient's usual systolic pressure.	Tightening valve prevents air leak during inflation. Inflation above systolic level ensures accurate measurement of systolic pressure.
(4) Slowly release pressure bulb valve and allow manometer needle to fall at rate of 2 to 3 mm Hg/second. Note point on manometer when you hear first clear sound. Sound will slowly increase in intensity.	A too-rapid decline decreases systolic BP and increases diastolic BP measurement (Kallioinen et al., 2017). First sound reflects systolic pressure.
(5) Continue to deflate cuff gradually, noting point at which sound disappears in adults. Note pressure to nearest 2 mm Hg. Listen for 10 to 20 mm Hg after last sound, and allow remaining air to escape quickly.	Beginning of fifth sound is indication of diastolic pressure in adults (Thomas and Pohl, 2017). In children distinct muffling of sounds indicates diastolic pressure (Thomas and Pohl, 2017).
7. The American Heart Association recommends average of two sets of BP measurement, 2 minutes apart. Use second set of BP measurements as baseline. If readings are different by more than 5 mm Hg, additional readings are necessary.	Two sets of BP measurements help to prevent false-positive readings based on patient's sympathetic response (alert reaction). Averaging minimizes effect of anxiety, which often causes first reading to be higher than subsequent measures (Kallioinen et al., 2017).
8. Remove cuff from patient's arm or leg unless patient condition requires repeated measurements.	Continuous cuff inflation causes arterial occlusion, resulting in numbness and tingling of patient's arm/leg.
9. If this is first assessment of patient, repeat procedure on other arm or leg.	Comparison of BP in both arms and legs detects circulatory problems. (Normal difference of 5 to 10 mm Hg exists between arms.) Use arm with higher pressure for repeated measurements (AACN Practice Alert, 2016).
10. **Assess systolic BP by palpation:**	
a. Follow Steps 2-5.	
b. Locate and then continually palpate brachial, radial, or popliteal artery with fingertips of one hand. Inflate cuff to pressure 30 mm Hg above point at which you can no longer palpate pulse.	Ensures accurate detection of true systolic pressure once pressure valve is released.

Continued

STEP	RATIONALE

CLINICAL DECISION: *If unable to palpate artery because of weakened pulse, use a Doppler ultrasonic stethoscope (see Chapter 30).*

c. Slowly release valve and deflate cuff, allowing manometer needle to fall at rate of 2 mm Hg/second. Note point on manometer when pulse is again palpable, which indicates systolic pressure.	A too-rapid decline decreases systolic BP and increases diastolic BP measurement (Kallioinen et al., 2017). Palpation helps identify systolic pressure only.
d. Deflate cuff rapidly and completely. Remove cuff from patient's extremity unless patient condition requires repeated measurements.	Continuous cuff inflation causes arterial occlusion, resulting in numbness and tingling of extremity.
11. Assist patient return to comfortable position and cover upper arm or leg if previously clothed.	Restores comfort and provides sense of well-being.
12. Discuss results with patient.	Promotes participation in care and understanding of health.
13. Place nurse call system within reach and instruct patient in use.	Promotes safety and prevents falls.
14. Raise side rails (as appropriate) and lower bed to lowest position.	Promotes safety and prevents falls.
15. Wipe cuff with agency-approved disinfectant if used between patients.	Reduces transmission of infection.
16. Clean earpieces and diaphragm of stethoscope with alcohol swab.	Reduces transmission of infection when nurses share stethoscope.
17. Perform hand hygiene.	Reduces transmission of infection.

EVALUATION

1. If assessing BP for first time, establish baseline BP if it is within acceptable range.	Used to compare future BP measurements.
2. Compare BP reading with patient's previous baseline and usual BP for patient's age.	Allows you to assess for change in condition. Provides comparison with future BP measurements.
3. **Use Teach-Back** "I want to be sure I explained why it is important to stand up slowly since you are taking blood pressure medications. Tell me which of your medications might make you dizzy if you stand up too fast." Revise your instruction now or develop a plan for revised patient/family caregiver teaching if patient/family caregiver is not able to teach back correctly.	Determines patient's/family caregiver's level of understanding of instructional topic.

UNEXPECTED OUTCOMES AND RELATED INTERVENTIONS

1. Patient's BP is above acceptable range.
   - Repeat measurement in other extremity and compare findings. When a clinically significant difference greater than 10 mm Hg exists, use the arm with the higher pressure (AACN Practice Alert, 2016).
   - Verify correct size and placement of BP cuff.
   - Have another nurse repeat measurement in 1 to 2 minutes.
   - Observe for related symptoms that are not apparent unless BP is extremely high, including headache, facial flushing, nosebleed, and fatigue in an older patient.
   - Report BP to nurse in charge or health care provider to initiate appropriate evaluation and treatment.
   - Administer antihypertensive medications as ordered.
2. Patient's BP is below acceptable range.
   - Compare BP value with baseline.
   - Position patient in supine position to enhance circulation and restrict activity that decreases BP further.
   - Assess for signs and symptoms associated with hypotension, including tachycardia; weak, thready pulse; weakness; dizziness; confusion; and cool, pale, dusky, or cyanotic skin.
   - Assess for factors that contribute to low BP, including hemorrhage, dilation of blood vessels resulting from hyperthermia, anesthesia, or medication side effects.
   - Report BP to nurse in charge or health care provider to initiate appropriate interventions.
   - Increase rate of IV infusion or administer vasoconstriction drugs if ordered.
   - If patient stabilizes, assess for postural hypotension.
3. Unable to obtain BP reading.
   - Determine that no immediate crisis is present by obtaining pulse and respiratory rate.
   - Assess for signs and symptoms of decreased cardiac output; if present, notify nurse in charge or health care provider immediately.
   - Use alternative sites or procedures to obtain BP: use Doppler ultrasonic instrument (see Chapter 30); palpate systolic BP.

STEP	RATIONALE

RECORDING AND REPORTING

- Record BP, extremity assessed, method of assessment, and any signs and symptoms of BP alterations in EHR.
- Record measurement of BP after administration of specific therapies.
- Document assessment of patient learning.
- Report elevated or low blood pressure, a difference of more than 20 mm Hg between extremities or more than 20 mm Hg drop in systolic blood pressure or a 10 mm Hg drop in diastolic blood pressure when rising from a supine to a sitting or standing position.

HOME CARE CONSIDERATIONS

- Assess home noise level to determine room that provides most quiet environment for assessing BP.
- Consider use of an electronic BP cuff for home if patient has hearing difficulties, sufficient financial resources, and adequate dexterity.
- Blood pressure taken in the home may differ from the measurements assessed in a health care facility because the equipment and environment are different.
- Home blood pressure readings predict cardiovascular events and are particularly useful for monitoring the effects of treatment.

◼ KEY POINTS

- For the body temperature to stay constant and within an acceptable range, various mechanisms maintain the relationship between heat production and heat loss.
- Body temperature will decrease using measures that increase radiation, evaporation, convection, and conduction of heat.
- Fever serves as an important mechanism to enhance the immune system's ability to fight infection.
- Fever increases metabolism, which requires additional energy and oxygen.
- Vital sign assessment requires an organized approach.
- Patient age, gender, activity, medications, and health status influence vital signs.
- Measurement location and time of day influence vital signs.
- Hypertension occurs more frequently among African Americans.
- Acceptable vital signs fall within a normal range, with infant and children values higher for pulse and respirations and lower in blood pressure, compared with adults.
- Changes related to aging influence the vital sign values of older adults.
- Assessment of a child's vital signs requires you to consider that the brachial or apical pulse is the best site for assessing an infant's or a young child's pulse, and when measuring respirations, infants tend to breathe less regularly.
- Self-measurement of blood pressure helps patients adhere to treatment regimens, but findings should not be used for treatment decisions.
- Report route and site when measuring temperature, blood pressure, pulse, and oxygen saturation.
- When vital signs are above or below expected values, enter a note in the patient's record regarding the finding, any intervention, and the patient's response.
- Vital signs can be delegated to assistive personnel when the patient's condition is stable; however, the skill of apical pulse measurement cannot be delegated.

◼ REFLECTIVE LEARNING

- Consider your experience with vital sign delegation and how you met the rights of delegation.
- Consider the vital sign measurement equipment you used and describe how you prevented the spread of infection.
- Consider a patient you cared for today and provide your rationale for the frequency and order of the vital sign measurements you completed.

◼ REVIEW QUESTIONS

1. A 52-year-old woman is admitted with pneumonia, dyspnea, and discomfort in her left chest when taking deep breaths. She has smoked for 35 years and recently lost over 10 lb. She is started on intravenous antibiotics, high-protein shakes, and 2 L O_2 via nasal cannula. Her most recent vital signs are HR 112, BP 138/82, RR 22, tympanic temperature 37.9° C (100.2° F), and oxygen saturation 94%. Which vital signs reflect a positive outcome of the treatment interventions? (Select all that apply.)
   1. Temperature: 37° C (98.6° F)
   2. Radial pulse: 98
   3. Respiratory rate: 18
   4. Oxygen saturation: 96%
   5. Blood pressure: 134/78

2. The licensed practical nurse (LPN) provides you with the change-of-shift vital signs on four of your patients. Which patient does the nurse need to assess first?
   1. 84-year-old man recently admitted with pneumonia, RR 28, SpO_2 89%
   2. 54-year-old woman admitted after surgery for repair of a fractured arm, BP 160/86 mm Hg, HR 72
   3. 63-year-old man with venous ulcers from diabetes, temperature 37.3° C (99.1° F), HR 84
   4. 77-year-old woman with left mastectomy 2 days ago, RR 22, BP 148/62

3. A patient has been hospitalized for the past 48 hours with a fever of unknown origin. His medical record indicates tympanic temperatures of 38.7° C (101.6° F) at 0400, 36.6° C (97.9° F) at 0800, 36.9° C (98.4° F) at 1200, 37.6° C (99.6° F) at 1600, and 38.3° C (100.9° F) at 2000. How would the nurse describe this pattern of temperature measurements?
   1. Usual range of circadian rhythm measurements
   2. Sustained fever pattern
   3. Intermittent fever pattern
   4. Resolving fever pattern

4. A patient presents in the clinic with dizziness and fatigue. The assistive personnel (AP) reports a slow but regular radial pulse of 44. Place the following care activities in priority order.
   1. Direct the AP to obtain a blood pressure.
   2. Request that the patient lie on the clinical stretcher.
   3. Assess the patient's apical pulse for a full minute.
   4. Prepare to administer cardiac-stimulating medications.

5. Which of the following patients are at most risk for tachypnea? (Select all that apply.)
   1. Patient just admitted with four rib fractures
   2. Woman who is 9 months' pregnant
   3. A patient admitted with hypothermia
   4. Postoperative patient waking from general anesthesia
   5. Three-pack–per-day smoker with pneumonia

6. Which number marks the location where the nurse would auscultate the point of maximal impulse (PMI)?

   1. 1
   2. 2
   3. 3
   4. 4
   5. 5
   6. 6

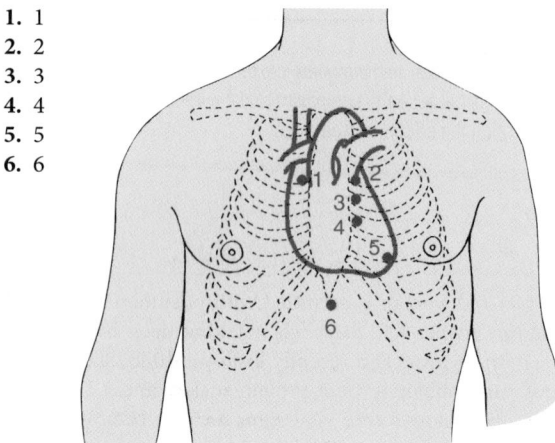

7. During admission of an obese patient with heart failure the assistive personnel (AP) reports to the nurse that the blood pressure (BP) is 140/76 on the left arm and 128/72 on the right arm. What actions do you take on the basis of this information? (Select all that apply.)
   1. Notify the health care provider immediately.
   2. Repeat the measurements on both arms using a stethoscope.
   3. Ask the patient if she has taken her blood pressure medications recently.
   4. Obtain blood pressure measurements on lower extremities.
   5. Verify that the correct cuff size was used during the measurements.
   6. Review the patient's record for her baseline vital signs.
   7. Compare right and left radial pulses for strength.

8. The assistive personnel (AP) informs the nurse that the electronic blood pressure machine on the patient who has recently returned from surgery after removal of her gallbladder is flashing a blood pressure of 65/46 and alarming. Place the care activities in priority order.
   1. Press the start button of the electronic blood pressure machine to obtain a new reading.
   2. Obtain a manual blood pressure with a stethoscope.
   3. Check the patient's pulse distal to the blood pressure cuff.
   4. Assess the patient's mental status.
   5. Remind the patient not to bend her arm with the blood pressure cuff.

9. A healthy adult patient tells the nurse that he obtained his blood pressure in "one of those quick machines in the mall" and was alarmed that it was 152/72 when his normal value ranges from 114/72 to 118/78. The nurse obtains a blood pressure of 116/76. What would account for the blood pressure of 152/92? (Select all that apply.)
   1. Cuff too small
   2. Arm positioned above heart level
   3. Slow inflation of the cuff by the machine
   4. Patient did not remove his long-sleeved shirt
   5. Insufficient time between measurements

10. A patient is admitted for dehydration caused by pneumonia and shortness of breath. He has a history of heart disease and cardiac dysrhythmias. The assistive personnel reports his admitting vital signs to the nurse. Which measurements should the nurse reassess? (Select all that apply.)
    1. Right arm BP: 118/72
    2. Radial pulse rate: 72 and irregular
    3. Temporal temperature: 37.4° C (99.3° F)
    4. Respiratory rate: 28
    5. Oxygen saturation: 99%

Answers: 1. 1,2,3,4,2. 1:3 3,4. 2,1,3,5,4,5 1,2,5,6. 5,7, 2, 6:8. 4,1,3,2,5,9. 1,5,10. 2,4,5.

Rationales for Review Questions can be found on the Evolve website.

REFERENCES

AACN Practice Alert: Obtaining accurate noninvasive blood pressure measurements in adults, *Crit Care Nurse* 36(3):e12, 2016.

American Heart Association (AHA): Know your target heart rates for exercise, losing weight and health, 2015, http://www.heart.org/en/healthy-living/fitness/fitness-basics/target-heart-rates. Accessed March 20, 2019.

American Heart Association (AHA): High blood pressure and African Americans, 2016, https://www.heart.org/en/health-topics/high-blood-pressure/why-high-blood-pressure-is-a-silent-killer/high-blood-pressure-and-african-americans. Accessed March 20, 2019.

American Heart Association (AHA): Monitoring your blood pressure at home, 2017, https://www.heart.org/en/health-topics/high-blood-pressure/understanding-blood-pressure-readings/monitoring-your-blood-pressure-at-home. Accessed March 21, 2019.

Centers for Disease Control and Prevention (CDC): *What is health literacy*, 2019, https://www.cdc.gov/healthliteracy/learn/index.html. Accessed December 23, 2019.

Centers for Disease Control and Prevention (CDC): Family history and other characteristics that increase risk for high blood pressure, 2014, https://www.cdc.gov/bloodpressure/family_history.htm. Accessed March 16, 2019.

Drawz P: Clinical implications of different blood pressure measurement techniques, *Curr Hypertens Rep* 19:54, 2017.

Gaudio FG, Grissom CK: Cooling methods in heat stroke, *J Emerg Med* 50:607, 2016.

Gunes UY, Efteli EU: Does errors made during indirect blood pressure measurement affect the results? *Int J Caring Sciences* 9(2):520, 2016.

Hale G, et al.: Treatment of primary orthostatic hypotension, *Ann Pharmacother* 51(5):417, 2017.

Hifumi T, et al.: Heat stroke, *J Intensive Care* 6:30, 2018. https://www.ncbi.nlm.nih.gov/pmc/articles/PMC5964884/. Accessed March 16, 2019.

Hockenberry MJ, et al.: *Wong's nursing care of infants and children*, ed 11, St Louis, 2019, Elsevier.

Institute for Healthcare Improvement (IHI): Early Warning Systems: scorecards that save lives, 2018. http://www.ihi.org/resources/Pages/ImprovementStories/EarlyWarningSystemsScorecardsThatSaveLives.aspx. Accessed December 31, 2018.

James P, et al.: Evidence-based guideline for the management of high blood pressure in adults: report from the panel members appointed to the Eighth Joint National Committee (JNC8), *JAMA* 311:507, 2014.

Kelly C: Respiratory rate 1: why accurate measurement and recording are crucial, *Nursing Times* 114(4):23, 2018.

Mayo Clinic: Exercise intensity: how to measure it, 2019, Mayo Foundation for Medical Education and Research, https://www.mayoclinic.org/healthy-lifestyle/fitness/in-depth/exercise-intensity/art-20046887. Accessed August 6, 2019.

Medicines and Healthcare Products Regulatory Agency (MHRA): Blood pressure measurement devices, 2013, https://assets.publishing.service.gov.uk/government/uploads/system/uploads/attachment_data/file/403448/Blood_pressure_measurement_devices.pdf. Accessed March 21, 2019.

Mordiffi Z, et al.: The use of non-invasive thermometers in healthcare facilities: a scoping review protocol, *JBI Database System Rev Implement Rep* 14(11):106, 2016.

Moughrabi S: Nonadherence to hypertension medications in African-American adolescents, *Pediatr Nurs* 43:223, 2017.

Pagana DK, et al.: *Mosby's diagnostic & laboratory test reference*, ed 14, St. Louis, 2019, Elsevier.

Peiris AN, et al.: Heat stroke, *JAMA* 318(24):2503, 2017.

Reckelhoff JF: Gender differences in hypertension, *Curr Opin Nephrol Hypertens* 27(3):176, 2018.

Seattle Children's Hospital: Fever-How to take the temperature, 2019, https://www.seattlechildrens.org/conditions/a-z/fever-how-to-take-the-temperature/. Accessed August 6, 2019.

Shibao C, et al.: Evaluation and treatment of orthostatic hypotension, *J Am Soc Hypertens* 7:317, 2013.

Soyal P, et al.: When should orthostatic blood pressure changes be evaluated in elderly: 1st, 3rd or 5th minute? *Arch Gerontol and Geriatr* 65:199, 2016.

Stergiou GS, et al.: Requirements for professional office blood pressure monitors, *J Hypertens* 30:537–542, 2012.

The Joint Commission (TJC): *2020 National Patient Safety Goals*, Oakbrook Terrace, IL, 2020, The Commission. http://www.jointcommission.org/en/standards/national-patient-safety-goals/. Accessed January 2, 2020.

Thomas G, Pohl MA: Blood pressure measurement in the diagnosis and management of hypertension in adults, 2017, UpToDate (website). https://www.uptodate.com/contents/blood-pressure-measurement-in-the-diagnosis-and-management-of-hypertension-in-adults. Accessed December 31, 2018.

Wang X, et al.: How to evaluate BP measurements using the oscillometric method in atrial fibrillation: the value of pulse rate variation, *Hypertens Res* 39:588, 2016.

Ward MA: Patient education: fever in children (beyond the basics), UpToDate (website), 2019, https://www.uptodate.com/contents/fever-in-children-beyond-the-basics. Accessed March 16, 2019.

World Health Organization (WHO): WHO pulse oximetry training manual, 2011, http://www.who.int/patientsafety/safesurgery/pulse_oximetry/who_ps_pulse_oximetry_training_manual_en.pdf. Accessed December 26, 2018.

RESEARCH REFERENCES

Angelousi A, et al.: Association between orthostatic hypotension and cardiovascular risk, cerebrovascular risk, cognitive decline and falls, as well as overall mortality: a systematic review and meta-analysis, *J Hypertens* 32:1562, 2014.

Asadian S, et al.: Accuracy and precision of four common peripheral temperature measurement methods in intensive care patients, *Med Devices (Auckl)* 9:301, 2016.

Bijur P, et al.: Temperature measurement in the adult emergency department: oral, tympanic membrane and temporal artery temperatures versus rectal temperature, *Emerg Med J* 33:843, 2016.

Brabrand M, et al.: Measurement of respiratory rate by multiple raters in a clinical setting is unreliable: a cross-sectional simulation study, *J Crit Care* 44:404, 2018.

Carson A, et al.: Ethnic differences in hypertension incidence among middle-aged and older U. S. adults: the multi-ethnic study of atherosclerosis, *Hypertension* 57(6):1101, 2011.

Charafeddine L, et al.: Axillary and rectal thermometry in the newborn: do they agree? *BMC Res Notes* 31(7):584, 2014.

Daw W, et al.: Poor inter-observer agreement in the measurement of respiratory rate in children: a prospective observational study, *BMJ Paediatr Open* 1:e000173, 2017.

Fei K, et al.: Racial and ethnic subgroup disparities in hypertension prevalence, New York City Health and Nutrition Examination Survey, 2013–2014, *Prev Chronic Dis* 14:160478, 2017. https://www.cdc.gov/pcd/issues/2017/16_0478.htm. Accessed March 20, 2019.

Flynn JT, et al.: Clinical practice guideline for screening and management of high blood pressure in children and adolescents, *Pediatrics* 140(3), 2017, http://pediatrics.aappublications.org/content/140/3/e20171904. Accessed December 31, 2018.

Frenkel A, et al.: Estimations of a degree of steroid induced leukocytosis in patients with acute infections, *Am J Emerg Med* 36(5):749, 2018.

Hill A, et al.: The effects of awareness and count duration on adult respiratory rate measurements: an experimental study,, *J Clin Nurs* 27:546, 2018.

Kallioinen N, et al.: Sources of inaccuracy in the measurement of adult patients' resting blood pressure in clinical settings: a systematic review, *J Hypertens* 35:421, 2017.

Koczulla A, et al.: Long-term oxygen therapy, *Dtsch Arztebl Int* 115(51-52):871, 2018.

Longtin Y, et al.: Contamination of stethoscopes and physicians' hands after a physical examination, *Mayo Clin Proc* 89(3):291, 2014.

Mayo Clinic: Fever: first aid. 2017, https://www.mayoclinic.org/first-aid/first-aid-fever/basics/art-20056685. Accessed March 16, 2019.

Reynolds M, et al.: Are temporal artery temperatures accurate enough to replace rectal temperature measurement in pediatric ED patients? *J Emerg Nurs* 40:46, 2014.

Ringrose J, et al.: The effect of back and feet support on oscillometric blood pressure measurements,, *Blood Pres Monit* 22(4):213, 2017.

Salota V, et al.: Is postoperative tympanic membrane temperature measurement effective? *Br J Nurs* 25:490, 2016.

Schimanski K, et al.: Comparison study of upper arm and forearm non-invasive blood pressures in adult emergency department patients, *Int J Nurs Stud* 51(12):1575, 2014.

30

Health Assessment and Physical Examination

OBJECTIVES

- Discuss the purpose of a physical assessment.
- Discuss how cultural diversity influences a nurse's approach to and findings from a health assessment.
- List techniques for preparing a patient physically and psychologically before and during an examination.
- Describe interview techniques used to enhance communication during history taking.
- Make environmental preparations before an examination.
- Identify data to collect from the nursing history before an examination.
- Demonstrate the techniques used with each physical assessment skill.

- Discuss normal physical findings in a young, middle-age, and older adult.
- Discuss ways to incorporate health promotion and health teaching into an examination.
- Identify ways to use physical assessment skills during routine nursing care.
- Describe physical measurements made in assessing each body system.
- Identify self-screening examinations commonly performed by patients.
- Identify preventive screenings and the appropriate age(s) for each screening to occur.

KEY TERMS

Adventitious sounds, p. 552
Alopecia, p. 532
Aphasia, p. 582
Apical impulse or point of maximal impulse (PMI), p. 554
Arcus senilis, p. 537
Atrophied, p. 580
Auscultation, p. 523
Borborygmi, p. 569
Bruit, p. 558
Cerumen, p. 539
Clubbing, p. 561
Conjunctivitis, p. 537
Distention, p. 568
Dysrhythmia, p. 556
Ectropion, p. 537
Edema, p. 530

Entropion, p. 537
Erythema, p. 528
Excoriation, p. 542
Goniometer, p. 577
Hypertonicity, p. 578
Hypotonicity, p. 578
Indurated, p. 529
Inspection, p. 522
Jaundice, p. 528
Kyphosis, p. 576
Lordosis, p. 576
Malignancy, p. 547
Murmurs, p. 557
Nystagmus, p. 536
Olfaction, p. 522
Orthopnea, p. 551
Osteoporosis, p. 576

Ototoxicity, p. 541
Palpation, p. 522
Percussion, p. 523
Peristalsis, p. 569
PERRLA, p. 538
Petechiae, p. 530
Polyps, p. 542
Ptosis, p. 537
Scoliosis, p. 576
Stenosis, p. 558
Striae, p. 568
Syncope, p. 558
Thrill, p. 557
Turgor, p. 530
Ventricular gallop, p. 556
Vocal or tactile fremitus, p. 552

MEDIA RESOURCES

http://evolve.elsevier.com/Potter/fundamentals/
- Review Questions
- Video Clips
- Case Study with Questions

- Audio Glossary
- Content Updates
- Answers to QSEN Activity and Review Questions

Completing a health assessment and physical examination is an important step toward providing safe and competent nursing care. The nurse is in a unique position to determine each patient's current health status, distinguish variations from the norm, and recognize improvements or deterioration in the patient's condition. Nurses must be able to recognize and interpret each patient's behavioral and physical presentation. You perform health assessments and physical examinations to identify health patterns and evaluate each patient's response to treatments and therapies.

You gather assessment data about patients' past and current health conditions in a variety of ways, using a comprehensive or focused approach, depending on the patient situation. Nurses perform assessments at health fairs, at screening clinics, in a health provider's office, in acute care agencies, or in patients' homes. Depending on the outcome of an assessment, a nurse considers evidence-based recommendations for care based on a patient's values, the health provider's clinical expertise, or personal experience.

A complete health assessment involves a nursing history (see Chapter 16) and behavioral and physical examination. Through the health history interview you gather subjective data about a patient's condition. Objective data is obtained while observing a patient's behavior and overall presentation. Gather additional objective data through a head-to-toe body system review during the physical examination. You make clinical judgments based on all of the gathered data to create a plan of care for each situation. With accurate data you create a patient-centered care plan, identifying the nursing diagnoses, desired patient outcomes, and nursing interventions.

PURPOSES OF THE PHYSICAL EXAMINATION

Nurses conduct physical examinations for many reasons, such as an initial evaluation in triage for emergency care; for routine screening to promote wellness behaviors and preventive health care measures; to determine eligibility for health insurance, military service, or a new job; or to admit a patient to a hospital or long-term care facility. After considering a patient's current condition, a nurse selects a focused physical examination on a specific system or area. For example, when a patient is having a severe asthma episode, the nurse first focuses on the pulmonary and cardiovascular systems so that treatments can begin immediately. When the patient is no longer at risk for a poor outcome or injury, the nurse performs a more comprehensive examination of the other body systems.

For patients who are hospitalized, a nurse integrates the collection of physical assessment data during routine patient care, validating findings with what is known about the patient's health history. For example, on entering a patient's room a nurse may notice behavioral patient cues that indicate sadness or may observe swallowing difficulties while administering medications. Use physical examination to do the following:

- Gather baseline data about a patient's health status.
- Supplement, confirm, or refute subjective data obtained.
- Identify and confirm nursing diagnoses.
- Make clinical decisions about a patient's changing health status and management.
- Evaluate the outcomes of care.

Cultural Sensitivity

Respect the cultural differences among patients from a variety of backgrounds when completing an examination. It is important to remember that cultural differences influence patient behaviors. Consider the patient's health beliefs, use of alternative therapies, nutritional habits, relationships with family, and comfort with physical closeness during the examination and history. These factors will affect both your approach and the type of findings you might expect.

Be culturally aware and avoid stereotyping based on gender, race, education, or other cultural factors. There is a difference between cultural and physical characteristics. Learn to recognize common characteristics and disorders among members of ethnic populations within the community. It is equally important to recognize variations in physical characteristics such as in the skin and musculoskeletal system. Recognize the impact of cultural difference in racial and ethnic aspects. Be aware of cultural humility and recognize your own knowledge deficits related to different cultures. Consider how the illness may impact the patient, adaptations that may be needed for the physical assessment, mode of communication, health beliefs and practices, familial relationships and nutritional practices. (Ball et al., 2019). By addressing cultural diversity, you show respect for each patient's uniqueness, leading to higher-quality care and improved clinical outcomes (see Chapter 9).

PREPARATION FOR EXAMINATION

Physical examination is a routine and integral part of a nurse's patient assessment. In many care settings a head-to-toe physical assessment is required daily. You perform a reassessment when a patient's condition changes, as it improves or worsens. In some health care settings, such as during a home health visit, a focused physical examination is preferred. A proper physical examination will take into consideration cultural aspects, infection control, preparation of the environment, patient position, age of the patient, equipment, and explanation of assessment procedures. This will provide a smooth physical examination with few interruptions. A disorganized approach could cause errors and incomplete findings. Safety for patients who are confused should be a priority; never leave a patient who is confused or combative alone during an examination.

Infection Control

Some patients present with open skin lesions, infected wounds, or other communicable diseases. Use Standard Precautions throughout an examination (see Chapter 28). When an open sore or microorganism is present, wear gloves to reduce contact with contaminants. If a patient has excessive drainage or there is a risk of splattering from a wound, use additional personal protective equipment, such as an isolation gown or eye shield. Follow the agency's hand hygiene policies before initiating and after completing a physical assessment.

Although most health care agencies make nonlatex gloves available, it is your responsibility to identify latex allergies in patients and use equipment items that are latex free. By recognizing risk factors for latex allergies, patients remain free of a natural rubber latex (NRL) allergy. Three types of allergic responses appear with NRL. The most immediate is an immunological reaction. This is a type 1 response, for which the body develops antibodies known as *immunoglobulin E* that can lead to an anaphylactic response. The second is type IV (delayed-type) hypersensitivity, which is T cell–mediated and appears 48 to 96 hours after exposure (AAFA, 2015). Irritant contact dermatitis is a nonallergic reaction and presents with dry, irritated, or fissured skin. The severity of the response varies among individuals. Table 30.1 provides a short list of products that contain latex and suggests available alternatives.

Environment

A respectful, considerate physical examination requires privacy. In the acute setting nurses perform assessments in a patient's room while examination rooms are used in clinics or offices. In the home the examination is performed in a space where privacy can be established such as the patient's bedroom.

Examination spaces need to be well equipped for any procedures. Adequate lighting is necessary to properly illuminate body parts. The hospital room can be secured for privacy so that patients are comfortable discussing their condition. Eliminate extra noise and take precautions to prevent interruptions from others. The room must be warm enough to maintain comfort.

Depending on the body part being assessed, it may be difficult to perform a selected assessment skill when a patient is in bed or on a stretcher. Special examination tables make positioning easier and body areas more easily accessible. By helping patients on and off examination tables, injury can be avoided. Examination tables can be uncomfortable; elevate the head of the table about 30 degrees. A small pillow helps with head and neck comfort. If the examination is completed in the patient room, raise the height of the patient's bed to be able to reach the patient more comfortably.

Equipment

Perform hand hygiene thoroughly before handling equipment and starting an examination. Arrange any necessary equipment so that it is

TABLE 30.1 Products Containing Latex and Nonlatex Substitutes[a]

Products Containing Latex	Nonlatex Substitutes
Medical Equipment	
Disposable gloves	Vinyl, nitrile, or neoprene gloves
Blood pressure cuffs	Covered cuffs
Stethoscope tubing	Covered tubing
Intravenous injection ports	Needleless system, stopcocks, covered latex ports
Tourniquets	Latex-free or cloth-covered tourniquets
Syringes	Glass syringes
Adhesive tape	Nonlatex tapes
Oral and nasal airways	Nonlatex tubes
Endotracheal tubes	Hard plastic tubes
Catheters	Silicone catheters
Eye goggles	Silicone eye goggles
Anesthesia masks	Silicone masks
Respirators	Nonlatex respirators
Rubber aprons	Cloth-covered aprons
Wound drains	Silicone drains
Medication vial stoppers	Stoppers removed
Household Items	
Rubber bands	String; latex-free bands
Erasers	Silicone erasers
Motorcycle and bicycle handgrips	Handgrips removed or covered
Carpeting	Other types of flooring
Swimming goggles	Silicone construction
Shoe soles	Leather shoes
Expandable fabric (e.g., waistbands)	Fabric removed or covered
Dishwashing gloves	Vinyl gloves
Condoms	Nonlatex condoms
Diaphragms	Synthetic rubber diaphragms
Balloons	Mylar balloons
Pacifiers and baby bottle nipples	Silicone, plastic, or nonlatex pacifiers and nipples

[a]This list is intended to provide examples of products and alternatives. It is not complete.
Modified from Ball JW, et al: *Mosby's guide to physical examination*, ed 9, St Louis, 2019, Elsevier; and U.S. National Library of Medicine Medline Plus: *Latex allergies: for hospital patients*, 2019. https://medlineplus.gov/ency/patientinstructions/000499.htm. Accessed October 7, 2019.

BOX 30.1 Equipment and Supplies for Physical Assessment

- Cervical brush or broom devices (if needed)
- Cotton applicators
- Disposable pad/paper towels
- Drapes/cover
- Eye chart (e.g., Snellen chart)
- Flashlight and spotlight
- Forms (e.g., physical, laboratory)
- Nonlatex gloves (clean)
- Gown for patient
- Ophthalmoscope
- Otoscope
- Papanicolaou (Pap) liquid preparation (if needed)
- Percussion (reflex) hammer
- Pulse oximeter
- Ruler
- Scale with height measurement rod
- Specimen containers, slides, wooden or plastic spatula, and cytological fixative (if needed)
- Sphygmomanometer and cuff
- Sterile swabs
- Stethoscope
- Tape measure
- Thermometer
- Tissues
- Tongue depressors
- Tuning fork
- Vaginal speculum (if needed)
- Water-soluble lubricant
- Watch with second hand or digital display

Physical preparation involves making certain that patient privacy is maintained with proper dress and draping. The patient in the hospital is probably wearing a hospital gown. In the clinic or health care provider's office the patient needs to undress and usually is provided a disposable paper cover or gown. If the examination is limited to certain body systems, it is not always necessary for the patient to undress completely. Provide the patient privacy and plenty of time to undress to lessen the patient's anxiety. After changing, the patient sits or lies down on the examination table with a light drape over the lap or lower trunk. Make sure that drafts are eliminated, temperature is controlled, and blankets are provided. Routinely ask whether he or she is comfortable.

Positioning. During the examination ask the patient to assume proper positions so that body parts are accessible and he or she stays comfortable. Table 30.2 lists the preferred positions for each part of the examination and contains figures illustrating the positions. Patients' abilities to assume positions depend on their physical strength, mobility, ease of breathing, age, and degree of wellness. After explaining a position, help the patient to assume it correctly. Take care to maintain respect and show consideration by adjusting the drapes so that only the area examined is accessible. During the examination a patient may need to assume more than one position. To decrease the number of position changes, organize the examination so that all techniques requiring a sitting position are completed first, followed by those that require a supine position next, and so forth. Use extra care when positioning older adults with disabilities and limitations.

Psychological Preparation of a Patient

Many patients find an examination stressful or tiring, or they experience anxiety about possible findings. A thorough explanation of the purpose and steps of each assessment lets a patient know what to expect and how to cooperate. Adapt your explanations to the patient's level of understanding, and encourage him or her to ask questions and comment on any discomfort. Convey an open, professional approach while remaining relaxed. A quiet, formal demeanor inhibits a patient's ability to communicate, but a style that is too casual may cause him or her to doubt an examiner's competence (Ball et al., 2019).

Consider cultural or social norms when performing an examination on a person of the opposite gender. When this situation occurs,

readily available and easy to use. Prepare equipment as appropriate (e.g., warm the diaphragm of the stethoscope between the hands before applying it to the skin). Be sure that equipment functions properly before using it (e.g., ensure that the ophthalmoscope and otoscope have good batteries and light bulbs). Box 30.1 lists typical equipment used during a physical examination.

Physical Preparation of the Patient

Show respect for a patient by ensuring that physical comfort needs, such as using the restroom, are met before starting the exam. An empty bladder and bowel facilitate a more comfortable examination of the abdomen, genitalia, and rectum. Collect urine or fecal specimens at this time if needed.

TABLE 30.2   Positions for Examination

Position	Areas Assessed	Rationale	Limitations
Sitting	Head and neck, back, posterior thorax and lungs, anterior thorax and lungs, breasts, axillae, heart, vital signs, and upper extremities	Sitting upright provides full expansion of lungs and better visualization of symmetry of upper body parts.	Physically weakened patient sometimes is unable to sit. Use supine position with head of bed elevated instead.
Supine	Head and neck, anterior thorax and lungs, breasts, axillae, heart, abdomen, extremities, pulses	This is normally a relaxed position. It provides easy access to pulse sites.	If patient becomes short of breath easily, raise head of bed.
Dorsal recumbent	Head and neck, anterior thorax and lungs, breasts, axillae, heart, abdomen	Position is for abdominal assessment because it promotes relaxation of abdominal muscles.	Patients with painful disorders are more comfortable with knees flexed.
Lithotomy[a]	Female genitalia and genital tract	Position provides maximal exposure of female genitalia and facilitates insertion of vaginal speculum.	Lithotomy position is embarrassing and uncomfortable; thus examiner minimizes time that patient spends in it. Keep patient well draped.
Sims'	Rectum and vagina	Flexion of hip and knee improves exposure of rectal area.	Joint deformities hinder patient's ability to bend hip and knee.
Prone	Musculoskeletal system	Position is only for assessing extension of hip joint, skin, and buttocks.	Patients with respiratory difficulties do not tolerate this position well.
Lateral recumbent	Heart	Position aids in detecting murmurs.	Patients with respiratory difficulties do not tolerate this position well.
Knee-chest[a]	Rectum	Position provides maximal exposure of rectal area.	This position is embarrassing and uncomfortable.

[a]Some patients with arthritis or other joint deformities are unable to assume this position.

another person of the patient's gender or a culturally approved family member needs to be in the room. By taking this step you demonstrate cultural awareness for a patient's individual needs. As a side benefit, the second person acts as a witness to the conduct of the examiner and the patient should any question arise.

During the examination watch the patient's emotional responses by observing whether his or her facial expressions show fear or concern or whether body movements indicate anxiety. When you remain calm, the patient is more likely to relax. Especially if the patient is weak or elderly, it is necessary to pace the examination, pausing at intervals to ask how he or she is tolerating the assessment. If the patient feels all right, the examination can proceed. However, do not force the patient to cooperate based on your schedule. Postpone the examination when needed; your findings may be more accurate when the patient can cooperate and relax.

Assessment of Age-Groups

Use different interview styles and approaches to physical examination for patients of different age-groups. When assessing children, show sensitivity and anticipate a child's perception of the examination as a strange and unfamiliar experience. Routine pediatric examinations focus on health promotion and illness prevention, particularly for well children who receive competent parenting and have no serious health problems (Hockenberry and Wilson, 2019). This examination focuses on growth and development, sensory screening, dental examination, and behavioral assessment. When examining children, the following tips help in data collection:

- Gather all or part of the history on infants and children from parents or guardians. Use open-ended questions to allow parents to share more information and describe more of the children's situation. This will allow observation of parent-child interactions. Older children can be interviewed and provide details about their health history and severity of symptoms.
- Gain a child's trust before doing any type of an examination. Perform the examination in a nonthreatening area. Talk and play with the child first. Do the visual parts of the examination before touching the child. Start the examination from the periphery and then move to the center (e.g., start with the extremities before moving to the chest).
- Because parents sometimes think the examiner is testing them, offer support during the examination and do not pass judgment.
- Call children by their first names and address the parents as "Mr., Mrs., or Ms." rather than by their first names unless instructed differently.
- Treat adolescents as adults and individuals because they tend to respond best when treated as such. Remember that adolescents have the right to confidentiality. After talking with parents about historical information, speak alone with adolescents.

A comprehensive health assessment and examination of older adults includes physical data; family relationships; religious and occupational pursuits; and a review of the patient's cognitive, affective, and social level. An important aspect is to assess the patient's ability to perform basic activities of daily living (e.g., bathing, grooming) and complex instrumental activities of daily living (e.g., making a phone call).

Throughout an examination, recognize that older adults often present with subtle or atypical signs and symptoms (Touhy and Jett, 2017). Principles to follow during examination of an older adult include the following:

- Do not stereotype about aging patients' level of cognition. Most older adults are reliable historians and are able to adapt to change and learn about their health.
- Recognize that some older adults have sensory or physical limitations that affect how quickly they can be interviewed and examinations can be conducted. It might be necessary to plan for more than one examination session. Sometimes it helps to give patients an initial health questionnaire before they come to a clinic or office.
- Perform the examination with adequate space; this is especially important for patients with mobility aids such as a cane or walker.
- During the examination use patience, allow for pauses, and observe for details. Recognize normal physiological and behavioral changes that are characteristic of later life.
- Giving certain types of health information is stressful for older patients. Some view illness as a threat to independence and a step toward institutionalization.
- Be aware of the location of the closest bathroom in case the patient has an urgent need to eliminate.
- Be alert to signs of increasing fatigue such as sighing, grimacing, irritability, leaning against objects for support, and drooping head and shoulders.

> ### REFLECT NOW
>
> As the nurse preparing to begin the physical examination, verbalize your opening statement to your older adult patient. Reflect on your knowledge of culture, aging, and developing a safe environment of trust. What nursing strategies should you use during the physical examination?

ORGANIZATION OF THE EXAMINATION

Assess each body system during a physical examination. Use judgment to ensure that an examination is relevant and includes the correct assessments. Patients with focused symptoms or needs require only parts of an examination; thus, when a patient comes to a clinic with symptoms of a severe chest cold, a neurological assessment is not usually required. When a patient is admitted to the hospital, you perform a complete examination at the time of admission and at least once each day to maintain and monitor the patient's baseline. Agency guidelines may define the components of a complete examination (see agency policy). A patient in the community seeks screening for specific conditions, often dependent on his or her age or health risks listed in Table 30.3.

Follow a systematic routine when you perform a physical examination to avoid missing important findings. A head-to-toe approach includes all body systems, and the examiner recalls and performs each step in a predetermined order. For an adult the examination begins with an assessment of the head and neck and progresses methodically down the body to incorporate all body systems. The following tips help keep an examination well organized:

- Compare both sides of the body for symmetry. A degree of asymmetry is occasionally normal (e.g., the biceps muscles in the dominant arm are sometimes more developed than the same muscles in the nondominant arm).
- If the patient is seriously ill, first assess the systems of the body most at risk for being abnormal. For example, complete a cardiovascular assessment first when caring for a patient with chest pain.
- If the patient becomes fatigued, offer rest periods between assessments.
- Perform painful procedures near the end of an examination.
- Record assessments in specific terms in the electronic or paper record. A standard form allows for recording information in the same sequence that it is gathered.
- Use common and accepted medical terms and abbreviations to keep notes accurate, brief, and concise.
- Record quick notes during the examination to avoid delays. Complete any larger documentation notes at the end of the examination.

TABLE 30.3   Recommended Preventive Screenings

Disease/Condition	Age-Group	Screening Measures
Breast cancer [a] (Women at average risk)	Ages 40-44	Should have the choice to start annual breast cancer screening with mammograms if they wish to do so. The risks of screening as well as the potential benefits should be considered.
		Monthly BSE dependent on health care provider recommendations (not recommended by ACS)
	Ages 45-54	Monthly BSE dependent upon health care provider recommendations (not recommended by ACS)
		Should get mammogram every year
	Ages 55 and older	Should switch to mammograms every 2 years or have the choice to continue yearly screening.
	Women with a personal history of breast cancer, a family history of breast cancer, a genetic mutation known to increase the risk of breast cancer (such as *BRCA*), and women who have had radiation therapy to the chest before the age of 30 are at a higher risk for breast cancer, not average risk. These women require earlier and more extensive screening.	
Colon/rectal cancer [b]	Ages 45 and older	Men and women need to have one of the following sensitive tests that look for signs of cancer: fecal occult blood test (FOBT) or flexible sigmoidoscopy (FSIG) or colonoscopy. Earlier screening is necessary if risk factors exist.
Ear disorders	All ages	Periodic hearing checks as needed
	Over age 65	Regular hearing checks
Eye disorders	Age 40 and under	Complete eye examination every 3 to 5 years (more if positive history for eye disease [e.g., diabetes])
	Ages 40 to 64	Complete eye examination every 2 years to screen for conditions that may go unnoticed (e.g., glaucoma)
		Annual eye examinations if patient has diabetes
	Age 65 and older	Complete eye examination every year
Heart/vascular disorders	Men age 45 to 65	Regular measurement of total blood cholesterol levels, lipids, and triglycerides; blood pressure screenings (If patient has risk factors for coronary artery disease [CAD], blood pressure screening needs to begin at age 20-35 for men, 20-45 for women.)
	Women age 45 to 65	
Obesity	All ages	Periodic height and weight measurements
Oral cavity/pharyngeal disorders/cancer	All ages (children, adults, older adults)	Regular dental examinations every 6 months
Ovarian cancer [c]	Age 18 and up or on becoming sexually active	Annual pelvic examinations by health care provider (This screening rarely detects ovarian cancer unless it is in its advanced stage. Those at high risk need to have a thorough pelvic examination, a transvaginal ultrasound, and a blood test [tumor marker CA 125]) (ACS, 2018d).
Prostate cancer [b]	Ages 50 and up	Men who have at least a 10-year life expectancy need to have a digital rectal examination (DRE) and prostate-specific antigen (PSA) blood test annually. Men at high risk require earlier screening.
Skin cancer [b]	Ages 20 to 40	See specialist every 3 years
	Over 40	Annual skin checkups with biopsy of suspicious lesions
Testicular cancer [b]	Age 15 and up	Monthly testicular self-examination (TSE)
Uterine cancer [b]	Screening begins 3 years after having vaginal intercourse but not later than age 21	[d]Annual pelvic examination by health care provider plus annual Papanicolaou (Pap) test
Cervical cancer	An **annual** Pap test is no longer recommended by the American Cancer Society (ACS, 2016).	
	Ages 21-29	Pelvic examination by health care provider plus Pap test with cytology every 3 years; human papillomavirus (HPV) needed only if Pap test is abnormal (ACS, 2016)
	Ages 30-65	Preferred screening is with a Pap test combined with an HPV test every 5 years. This is called co-testing (ACS, 2016).
	Over 65	No testing needed if previous regular testing was competed and normal. If a high risk for cervical cancer or previous perchance then screening should be continued (ACS, 2016).
Endometrial cancer	Same as for cervical cancer	Endometrial biopsy at age 35 for high-risk patients (those with or at risk for hereditary nonpolyposis colon cancer [HNPCC]) (At menopause women at average and high risk need to be informed about signs and symptoms to report.)

[a]Data from American Cancer Society (ACS): *Breast cancer early detection and diagnosis,* 2018. https://www.cancer.org/cancer/breast-cancer/screening-tests-and-early-detection.html. Accessed October 30, 2018.
[b]American Cancer Society (ACS): *Cancer A-Z,* n.d. https://www.cancer.org/cancer.html. Accessed September 17, 2019.
[c]Data from American Cancer Society (ACS): *Can ovarian cancer be found early?* 2018. https://www.cancer.org/cancer/ovarian-cancer/detection-diagnosis-staging/detection.html?_ga=2.29301694.34924562.1540912089-41350218.1539106062. Accessed October 30, 2018.
[d]Data from American Cancer Society (ACS): *Uterine sarcoma early detection, diagnosis, and staging.* https://www.cancer.org/cancer/uterine-sarcoma/detection-diagnosis-staging/detection.html. Accessed December 13, 2019.

TABLE 30.4 Assessment of Characteristic Odors

Odor	Site or Source	Potential Causes
Alcohol	Oral cavity	Ingestion of alcohol, diabetes
Ammonia	Urine	Urinary tract infection, renal failure
Body odor	Skin, particularly in areas where body parts rub together (e.g., underarms and under breasts)	Poor hygiene, excess perspiration (hyperhidrosis), foul-smelling perspiration (bromhidrosis)
	Wound site	Wound abscess
	Vomitus	Abdominal irritation, contaminated food
Feces	Vomitus/oral cavity (fecal odor)	Bowel obstruction
	Rectal area	Fecal incontinence
Foul-smelling stools in infant	Stool	Malabsorption syndrome
Halitosis	Oral cavity	Poor dental and oral hygiene, gum disease
Sweet, fruity ketones	Oral cavity	Diabetic acidosis
Stale urine	Skin	Uremic acidosis
Sweet, heavy, thick odor	Draining wound	*Pseudomonas* (bacterial) infection
Musty odor	Casted body part	Infection inside cast
Fetid, sweet odor	Tracheostomy or mucus secretions	Infection of bronchial tree (*Pseudomonas* bacteria)

TECHNIQUES OF PHYSICAL ASSESSMENT

The four techniques used in a physical examination are inspection, palpation, percussion, and auscultation.

Inspection

To inspect, carefully look, listen, and smell to distinguish normal from abnormal findings. To do so, you must be aware of any personal visual, hearing, or olfactory deficits. It is important to deliberately practice this skill and learn to recognize all the possible pieces of data that can be gathered through inspection alone. Inspection occurs when interacting with a patient, watching for nonverbal expressions of emotional and mental status and assessing physical movements and structural components. Most important, be deliberate and pay attention to detail. Follow these guidelines to achieve the best results during inspection:

- Make sure that adequate lighting is available, either direct or indirect.
- Use a direct lighting source (e.g., a penlight or lamp) to inspect body cavities.
- Inspect each area for size, shape, color, symmetry, position, and abnormality.
- Position and expose body parts as needed so that all surfaces can be viewed but privacy can be maintained.
- When possible, check for side-to-side symmetry by comparing each area with its match on the opposite side of the body.
- Validate findings with the patient.

While assessing a patient, recognize the nature and source of body odors (Table 30.4). An unusual odor often indicates an underlying pathology. Olfaction helps to detect abnormalities. For example, when a patient's breath has a sweet, fruity odor, assess for signs of diabetes. Continue to inspect various parts of the body during the entire physical examination. Palpation may be used concurrently with inspection, or it may follow in a more deliberate fashion.

Palpation

Palpation involves using the sense of touch to gather information. Through touch you make judgments about expected and unexpected findings of the skin or underlying tissue, muscle, and bones. For example, you palpate the skin for temperature, moisture, texture, turgor, tenderness, and thickness and the abdomen for tenderness, distention, or masses. Use different parts of the hand to detect different characteristics (Table 30.5). The palmar surface of the hand and finger pads is more sensitive than the fingertips and is used to determine position, texture, size, consistency, masses, fluid, and crepitus (Fig. 30.1A). Assess body temperature by using the dorsal surface or back of the hand (Fig. 30.1B). Vibration is best felt on the palmar surface of the hand and fingers (Fig. 30.1C).

Touching a patient is a personal experience for both you and the patient. Display respect and concern throughout an examination. Before palpating consider the patient's condition and ability to tolerate the assessment techniques, paying close attention to areas that are painful or tender. In addition, always be conscious of the environment and any threats to the patient's safety.

Prepare for palpation by warming hands, keeping fingernails short, and using a gentle approach. Palpation proceeds slowly, gently, and deliberately. Encourage the patient to relax, and help the patient feel comfortable since tense muscles make assessment more difficult. To promote relaxation, have him or her take slow, deep breaths and place both arms along the sides of the body. Ask the patient to point to more sensitive areas, watching for nonverbal signs of discomfort. *Palpate tender areas last.*

Two types of palpation, light and deep, are used for physical examination. Perform light palpation by placing the hand on the body part being examined; it also involves pressing inward about 1 cm (½inch). Light, superficial palpation of structures such as the abdomen gives the patient the chance to identify areas of tenderness (Fig. 30.2A). Inquire about areas of tenderness and assess them further for potentially serious pathologies. Use deep palpation to examine the condition of organs such as those in the abdomen (Fig. 30.2B). Depress the area under examination approximately 4 cm (2 inches) (Ball et al., 2019), using one or both hands (bimanually). When using bimanual palpation, relax one hand (sensing hand) and place it lightly over the patient's skin. The other hand (active hand) helps apply pressure to the sensing hand. The lower hand does not exert pressure directly and thus remains sensitive to detect organ characteristics. For safety deep palpation should be used with caution in a patient with discomfort in the area to be palpated.

TABLE 30.5 Examples of Characteristics Measured By Palpation

Area Examined	Criteria Measured	Portion of Hand To Use
Skin	Temperature	Dorsum of hand/fingers
	Moisture	Palmar surface
	Texture	Palmar surface
	Turgor and elasticity	Grasping with fingertips
	Tenderness	Finger pads/palmar surface of fingers
	Thickness	Palmar surface
Organs (e.g., liver and intestine)	Size	Entire palmar surface of hand or palmar surface of fingers
	Shape	
	Tenderness	
	Absence of masses	
Glands (e.g., thyroid and lymph)	Swelling	Pads of fingertips
	Symmetry and mobility	
Blood vessels (e.g., carotid or femoral artery)	Pulse amplitude	Palmar surface/pads of fingertips
	Elasticity	
	Rate	
	Rhythm	
Thorax	Excursion	Palmar surface
	Tenderness	Finger pads/palmar surface of fingers
	Fremitus	Palmar or ulnar surface of entire hand

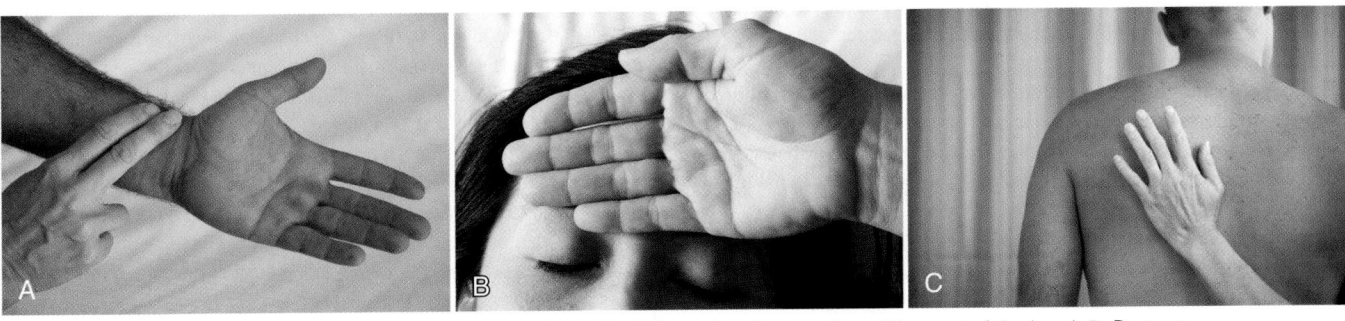

FIG. 30.1 **A,** Radial pulse is detected with pads of fingertips, the most sensitive part of the hand. **B,** Dorsum of hand detects temperature variations in skin. **C,** Bony part of palm at base of fingers detects vibrations.

Percussion

Percussion involves tapping the skin with the fingertips to vibrate underlying tissues and organs. The vibration travels through body tissues, and the character of the resulting sound reflects the density of the underlying tissue. The denser the tissue, the quieter is the sound. By knowing how various densities influence sound, it is possible to locate organs or masses, map their edges, and determine their size. An abnormal sound from what is expected in that area suggests a mass or substance such as air or fluid within an organ or body cavity. The skill of percussion is used more often by advanced practice nurses than by nurses in daily practice at the bedside.

Auscultation

Auscultation involves listening to sounds the body makes to detect variations from normal. Some sounds such as speech and coughing can be heard without additional equipment, but a stethoscope is necessary to hear internal body sounds.

Internal body sounds are created by blood, air, or gastric contents as they move against the body structures. For example, normal heart sounds are created when the heart valves close, moving blood to the next part of the cardiovascular system. Normal sounds for each body system are discussed later in this chapter. Learn to recognize abnormal sounds after learning normal variations. Becoming more proficient in auscultation occurs by knowing the types of sounds each body structure makes and the location in which the sounds are heard best.

To auscultate internal sounds, you need to hear well, have a good stethoscope, and know how to use it properly. Nurses with hearing disorders can obtain stethoscopes with extra sound amplification. There are two aspects to the stethoscope. The bell is best for hearing low-pitched sounds such as vascular and certain heart sounds, and the diaphragm is best for listening to high-pitched sounds such as bowel and lung sounds.

By practicing with the stethoscope, you become proficient at using it and realize when sounds are clear and when there are extraneous sounds. Extraneous sounds created by rubbing against the tubing or chest piece interfere with auscultation of body organ sounds. By deliberately producing these sounds, you learn to recognize and disregard them during the actual examination. Box 30.2 contains ways to practice using the stethoscope and techniques for caring for the

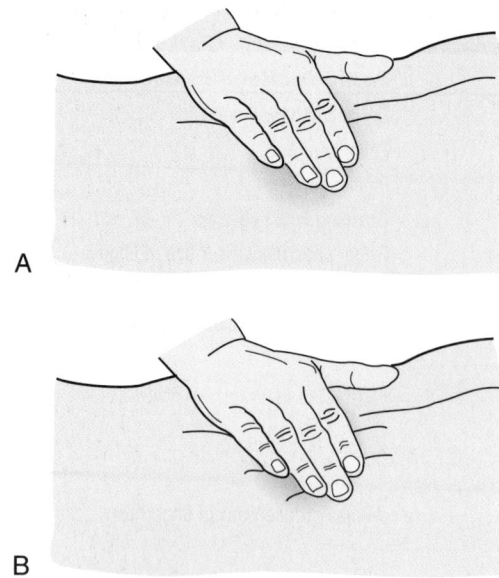

FIG. 30.2 A, During light palpation gentle pressure against underlying skin and tissues can detect areas of irregularity and tenderness. B, During deep palpation depress tissue to assess condition of underlying organs.

stethoscope. Describe any sound you hear using the following characteristics:

- Frequency indicates the number of sound wave cycles generated per second by a vibrating object. The higher the frequency, the higher the pitch of a sound and vice versa.
- Loudness refers to the amplitude of a sound wave. Auscultated sounds range from soft to loud.
- Quality refers to sounds of similar frequency and loudness from different sources. Terms such as *blowing* or *gurgling* describe the quality of sound.
- Duration means the length of time that sound vibrations last. The duration of sound is short, medium, or long. Layers of soft tissue dampen the duration of sounds from deep internal organs.

Auscultation requires concentration and practice. While listening, know which sounds are expected in certain parts of the body and what causes the sounds. Expected sounds are discussed in each body system section of this chapter. After understanding the cause and character of normal auscultated sounds, it becomes easier to recognize abnormal sounds and their origins.

GENERAL SURVEY

When a patient first enters an examination room, observe his or her walk and general appearance and be attentive to his or her behavior and dress. A general survey, or appraisal, of the patient's presentation and behavior provides information about characteristics of an illness, the patient's ability to function independently, body image, emotional state, recent changes in weight, and developmental status. If there are abnormalities or problems, assess the affected body system more closely during the full examination.

General Appearance and Behavior

Assess appearance and behavior while preparing the patient for the examination. For this review include:

- *Gender and race:* A person's gender affects the type of examination performed and the order of the assessments. Different physical features are related to gender and race. Certain illnesses are more likely

BOX 30.2 Use and Care of the Stethoscope

- Ensure that the earpiece follows the contour of the ear canals. Learn which fit is best for you by comparing amplification of sounds with the earpieces in both directions.
- Place the earpieces in your ears with the tips turned toward the face. *Lightly* blow into the diaphragm. Again, place the earpieces in your ears, this time with the ends turned toward the back of the head. *Lightly* blow into the diaphragm. You will find that you hear clearer sounds with the earpiece turned toward the face. After you have learned the right fit for the loudest amplification, wear the stethoscope the same way each time.
- Put on the stethoscope and *lightly* blow into the diaphragm. If the sound is barely audible, *lightly* blow into the bell. Sound is carried through only one part of the chest piece at a time. If the sound is greatly amplified through the diaphragm, the diaphragm is in position for use. If the sound is barely audible through the diaphragm, the bell is in position for use. Rotation of the diaphragm and bell places the chest piece in the desired position. Leave the diaphragm in position for the next exercise.
- Place the diaphragm over the anterior part of your chest. Ask a friend to speak in a normal conversational tone. Environmental noise seriously detracts from hearing the noise created by body organs. When using a stethoscope, the patient and the examiner need to remain quiet.
- Put on the stethoscope and gently tap the tubing. It is often difficult to avoid stretching or moving the stethoscope tubing. The examiner is in a position so that the tubing hangs free. Moving or touching the tubing creates extraneous sounds.
- *Care of the stethoscope:* Remove earpieces regularly and clean; remove cerumen (earwax). Keep the bell and diaphragm free of dust, lint, and body oils. Keep the tubing away from any body oils. Avoid draping the stethoscope around the neck next to the skin. Clean daily or after soiling by wiping the entire stethoscope (e.g., diaphragm, tubing) with alcohol. Be sure to dry all parts thoroughly. Follow manufacturer recommendations.
- *Infection control:* Harmful bacteria such as gram-positive bacilli, methicillin-resistant *Staphylococcus aureus* (MRSA), nonaureus *Staphylococcus, Enterobacter cloacae,* and methicillin-sensitive *S. aureus* can be transferred from patient to patient when using portable equipment such as stethoscopes. Clean the stethoscope (diaphragm/bell) *before* reuse on another patient. Using a disinfectant such as isopropyl alcohol (with or without chlorhexidine), benzalkonium, or sodium hypochlorite is effective in reducing the number of bacterial colonies. Hand foam serves this purpose well. Earpieces of stethoscopes are sources of transferable bacteria. When you inadvertently touch your ears and care for the patient, potential pathogens could contaminate the earpieces. Using hand hygiene before and after patient contact decreases the risk of transmitting microorganisms from your ear to your patient. Follow the institution's infection control guidelines, especially Contact Precautions, to decrease this risk.

to affect a specific gender or race (e.g., the incidence of skin cancer is more common in whites than in blacks, prostate cancer is higher in black men than in white men, and cancer of the bladder is higher in men than in women) (ACS, 2018b).

- *Age:* Age influences normal physical characteristics and a person's ability to participate in some parts of the examination.
- *Signs of distress:* Sometimes obvious signs or symptoms indicate pain (grimacing, splinting painful area), difficulty breathing (shortness of breath, sternal retractions), or anxiety. Set priorities and examine the related physical areas first.
- *Body type:* Observe whether the patient appears trim and muscular, obese, or excessively thin. Body type reflects the level of health, age, and lifestyle.

- *Posture:* Normal standing posture shows an upright stance with parallel alignment of the hips and shoulders. Normal sitting posture involves some degree of rounding of the shoulders. Observe whether the patient has a slumped, erect, or bent posture, which reflects mood or pain. Changes in older adult physiology often result in a stooped, forward-bent posture, with the hips and knees somewhat flexed and the arms bent at the elbows.
- *Gait:* Observe as the patient walks into the room or stands at the bedside (if the patient is ambulatory). Note whether movements are coordinated or uncoordinated. A person normally walks smoothly, with the arms swinging freely at the sides and the head and face leading the body.
- *Body movements:* Observe whether movements are purposeful, noting any tremors involving the extremities. Determine whether any body parts are immobile.
- *Hygiene and grooming:* Note the patient's level of cleanliness by observing the appearance of the hair, skin, and fingernails. Determine whether his or her clothes are clean. Grooming depends on the patient's cognitive and emotional function, daily or social activities, and occupation. Observe for excessive use of cosmetics or colognes that could indicate a change in self-perception.
- *Dress:* Culture, lifestyle, socioeconomic level, and personal preference affect the selection and wearing of clothing. However, you assess whether the clothing is appropriate for the temperature, weather conditions, or setting. People who are depressed or mentally ill may not be able to select proper clothing, and an older adult might tend to wear extra clothing because of sensitivity to cold.
- *Body odor:* An unpleasant body odor can result from physical exercise, poor hygiene, or certain disease states. Validate any odors that might indicate a health problem.
- *Affect and mood:* Affect is how a person appears to others. Patients express mood or emotional state verbally and nonverbally. Determine whether verbal expressions match nonverbal behavior and whether the mood is appropriate for the situation. By maintaining eye contact you can observe facial expressions while asking questions.
- *Speech:* Normal speech is understandable and moderately paced and shows an association with the person's thoughts. However, emotions or neurological impairment sometimes causes rapid or slowed speech. Observe whether the patient speaks in a normal tone with clear inflection of words.
- *Signs of patient abuse:* During the examination observe whether the patient fears his or her spouse or partner, a caregiver, a parent, or an adult child. Abuse of children, women, and older adults is a growing health problem. Consider any obvious physical injury or neglect as signs of possible abuse (e.g., evidence of malnutrition or presence of bruising on the extremities or trunk) (WHO, 2018). Abuse occurs in many forms: physical, mental or emotional, sexual, social, and financial or economic. Observe the behavior of the individual for any signs of frustration, explanations that do not fit his or her physical presentation, or signs of injury. Most states mandate a report to a social service center when abuse or neglect is suspected (Box 30.3). It is difficult to detect abuse because victims often do not report that they are in abusive situations. If you suspect abuse, find a way to interview the patient in private; patients are more likely to reveal any problems when the suspected abuser is absent from the room. It is imperative that you, the health care team, and the proper authorities help the patient find safe housing or seek protection from the abuser since the risk for further abuse is high once the victim has reported it or tries to leave the abusive situation.
- *Substance abuse:* Unusual or inconsistent behavior may be an indicator of substance abuse, which can affect all socioeconomic groups. Although a single patient visit to a clinic does not always reveal the problem, investigate unusual behaviors further with a well-focused history and physical examination. Always approach the patient in a caring and nonjudgmental way; substance abuse involves both emotional and lifestyle issues. Box 30.4 lists characteristics of patients who should be further assessed for potential substance abuse. A tool such as the online Tobacco, Alcohol, Prescription medication, and other Substance use (TAPS) tool can be used to assess a patient's risk for substance abuse (NIDA, 2018). If you suspect that alcohol abuse is a major problem, the CAGE questionnaire provides a useful set of questions to guide assessment. CAGE is an acronym for the following:

- Have you ever felt the need to **Cut down** on your drinking or drug use?
- Have people **Annoyed** you by criticizing your drinking or drug use?
- Have you ever felt bad or **Guilty** about your drinking or drug use?
- Have you ever used or had a drink first thing in the morning as an **Eye-opener** to steady your nerves or feel normal?

Among older adults, risk factors for development of alcohol-related problems include chronic medical disorders, sleep disorders, social isolation, loneliness, bereavement, and acute or chronic pain. When assessing adolescents there are brief online tools to screen substance use, such as the Brief Screener for Tobacco, Alcohol, and other Drugs (BSTAD) and Screening to Brief Intervention (S2BI) (NIDA, 2017).

Vital Signs

After completing the general survey, measure the patient's vital signs. Measurement of vital signs is more accurate if completed before beginning positional changes or movements. If there is a chance that the vital signs are inaccurate when you first take them, recheck them later during the rest of the examination. Assess for pain, the fifth vital sign, whenever you take a patient's vital signs.

Height and Weight

The relationship of height and weight reflects a person's general health status. Assess every patient to identify whether he or she is at a healthy weight, underweight, overweight, or obese. Weight is routinely measured during health screenings, visits to physicians' offices or clinics, and on admission to the hospital. Infants and children are measured for both height and weight at each health care visit to assess for healthy growth and development. If older adults are underweight, difficulty with feeding and other functional activities is a possibility. Measuring height and weight of older adults, along with obtaining a dietary history (Box 30.5), shows risk factors for chronic diseases.

Evaluate a patient's weight and height, and assess for trends in weight changes. Assessments screen for abnormal weight changes. A patient's weight normally varies daily because of fluid loss or retention. Use the nursing history to identify possible causes for a change in weight (Table 30.6). For example, a downward trend in an older adult who is frail indicates a serious reduction in nutritional reserves. Ask the patient to report current height and weight, along with a history of any substantial weight gain or loss. A weight gain of 2 to 3 lb (0.9-1.4 kg) in 1 day indicates fluid-retention problems. A weight loss is considered significant if the patient has lost more than 5% of body weight in a month or 10% in 6 months.

When a patient is hospitalized, daily weight is measured at the same time of day and on the same scale (Ball et al., 2019). This allows an objective comparison of subsequent weights. Accuracy of weight measurement is important because health care providers base medical and nursing decisions (e.g., drug dosage, medications) on changes.

Several different scales are available for use. Patients capable of bearing their own weight use a standing scale. You calibrate a standard

BOX 30.3   Clinical Indicators of Abuse

Physical Findings	Behavioral Findings
Child Abuse	
Vaginal or penile discharge	Problem sleeping or eating, anxiety, depression
Blood on underclothing	Fear of certain people or places
Pain, itching, or unusual odor in genital area	Play activities recreate the abuse situation
Genital injuries	Regressed behavior
Difficulty sitting or walking	Sexual acting out Knowledge of explicit sexual matters
Pain while urinating; recurrent urinary tract infections	Preoccupation with others' or own genitals
Foreign bodies in rectum, urethra, or vagina	Profound and rapid personality changes
Sexually transmitted infections	Rapidly declining school performance
Pregnancy in young adolescent	Poor relationship with peers
Intimate Partner Violence	
Injuries and trauma inconsistent with reported cause	Overuse of health services
Multiple injuries involving head, face, neck, breasts, abdomen, and genitalia (black eyes, orbital fractures, broken nose, fractured skull, lip lacerations, broken teeth, vaginal tears)	Thoughts of or attempted suicide
X-ray films showing old and new fractures in different stages of healing	Eating or sleeping disorders
Abrasions, lacerations, bruises/welts	Anxiety and panic attacks
Burns from cigarettes or other	Pattern of substance abuse (follows physical abuse)
Human bites	Low self-esteem
Unexplained injuries (e.g., bruises, fractures, and welts)	Depression, problems with eating or sleeping
Strangulation marks on neck from rope burns or bruises; throat pain, voice changes, trouble swallowing; damage to hyoid bone	Sense of helplessness
Stress-related disorders such as irritable bowel syndrome, exacerbation of asthma, or chronic pain	Guilt
	Smoking
	Stress-related complaints (headache, anxiety)
	Financial dependence on abuser
	Isolation from others
	Unsafe sexual behaviors
Older-Adult Abuse	
Injuries and trauma inconsistent with reported cause (scratch, bruise, or bite)	Dependent on caregiver
Hematomas, bruises at various stages of resolution	Physically and/or cognitively impaired
Unexplained bruises or welts, pattern bruises	Combative, verbally aggressive
Burns	Wandering
Bruises, chafing, excoriation on wrist or legs (restraints)	Minimal social support
Fractures inconsistent with cause described	Prolonged interval between injury and medical treatment
Dried blood	Life circumstances do not match size of patient's estate
Overmedication or undermedication	Uncommunicative or isolated
Exposure to severe weather, cold or hot	
Torn, bloody underwear or vaginal and anal bruises	
Sunken eyes or loss of weight	
Extreme thirst	
Bed sores	

Data from Cooper C, et al: The prevalence of elder abuse and neglect: a systematic review, *Age Aging* 37(2):151, 2008; Hockenberry MJ, Wilson P: *Wong's nursing care of infants and children*, ed 10, St Louis, 2019, Mosby; World Health Organization (WHO): *Intimate partner violence*, 2012, http://www.who.int/reproductivehealth/publications/violence/rhr12_36/en/index.html. Accessed October 27, 2018.

platform scale by moving the large and small weights to zero. By adjusting the calibrating knob, the balance beam is leveled and steadied. The patient stands on the scale platform and remains still as the nurse adjusts the largest solid weight to the 50-lb or 22.5-kg increment under the patient's weight. Next the smaller weight is moved to balance the scale at the nearest ¼ lb or 0.1 kg (Ball et al., 2019). Electronic scales are calibrated automatically each time they are used and automatically display the weight within seconds.

Bed and chair scales are available for patients who are unable to bear weight. Newer electronic hospital beds have built-in electronic scales for weighing patients who are not able to get out of bed.

You can use a basket or platform scale to weigh infants. Keep the room warm to prevent chills. Before weighing the infant, clean the infant scale and place a light cloth or paper cover on the surface to prevent cross-infection from urine or feces. Place a dry diaper on the scale and zero the scale so that the weight of the items on the scale will not be represented in the infant's weight. Once the scale is at zero, the naked infant can be placed on the scale and the diaper secured. When placing an infant in a basket or on a platform, hold a hand lightly above him or her to detect movements and prevent accidental falls. Measure an infant's weight in both ounces and grams.

In patients who can stand, measure height by having them remove their shoes. The standing surface should be clean. Use a measuring rod attached vertically to a weight scale, or use a tape ruler on the wall. As the patient stands erect, place a flat surface on his or her head that is even with the vertical measure. Then read the number on the scale or ruler that indicates his or her height in centimeters or inches.

BOX 30.4 Behaviors That Are Suspicious for Substance Abuse

Among adolescents and adults: Agitation; inappropriate behavior; problems thinking clearly, remembering, and paying attention; poor coordination; seizure; respiratory depression; coma; asphyxiation; aspiration; pulmonary edema; cardiac arrhythmias; immune system impairment; self-inflicted trauma; and suicidal ideation

Red flags:
- The risk of suicide, seizures, and violent behavior is high among substance abusers.
- Intoxicated patients, particularly those with phencyclidine (PCP) or methamphetamine intoxication, are at significant risk for becoming agitated and violent, placing themselves and others at risk for injury.

Observe for combinations or repetition of these behaviors:
- Frequently misses appointments
- Frequently requests written excuses for absence from school or work
- Drops out of school
- Chief complaints of insomnia, "bad nerves," or pain that do not fit a particular pattern
- Reports lost prescriptions (e.g., tranquilizers or pain medications) or asks for frequent refills
- Frequent emergency department visits
- History of changing health care providers or brings in medication bottles prescribed by several different providers
- History of gastrointestinal bleeds, peptic ulcers, pancreatitis, cellulitis, or frequent pulmonary infections
- Frequent sexually transmitted infections (STIs), complicated pregnancies, multiple abortions, or sexual dysfunction
- Complaints of chest pains or palpitations or has a history of admissions to rule out heart attacks
- History of activities that place the patient at risk for human immunodeficiency virus (HIV) infection (multiple partners, multiple rapes)
- Family history of addiction; history of childhood sexual, physical, or emotional abuse; or social and financial or marital problems
- Intimate partner violence

Data from American Psychiatric Association: *Diagnostic and statistical manual of mental disorders*, ed 5, text revision, Washington, DC, 2013, The Association; American Society of Addiction Medicine and Widlitz M, Marin D: Substance abuse in older adults: an overview, *Geriatrics* 57(12):29, 2002; and Walsh K, et al: Examining the interface between substance misuse and intimate partner violence, *Substance Abuse Res Treatment* 3:25, 2009; and National Institute on Drug Abuse: *Drugs, brains and behavior: the science of addiction*, 2018, https://www.drugabuse.gov/publications/drugs-brains-behavior-science-addiction/introduction. Accessed January 22, 2019.

BOX 30.5 Dietary History for Older Adults

- Does the older adult need or have help shopping for or preparing meals?
- Is income adequate for food purchasing? Food stamps or public assistance required?
- Does the patient ever skip meals?
- Are the five primary food groups from MyPlate (fruits, grains, protein, vegetables, dairy) represented in the daily diet (see Chapter 45) (USDA, 2018)?
- Does the older adult take nutritional supplements such as multivitamins?
- Does the older adult take any medication affecting appetite or absorption of nutrients?
- Does the older adult have any religious or cultural beliefs and practices that influence diet?
- Does the older adult have a special diet, food intolerances, or allergies? Does the patient's diet contain an unusual amount of alcohol, sweets, or fried food?
- Does the older adult have problems with chewing, swallowing, or salivation?
- Does the older adult have gastrointestinal problems that interfere with food intake?

Data from Meiner SE, Yeager JJ: *Gerontologic nursing*, ed 6 , St Louis, 2019, Elsevier; and US Department of Agriculture and US Department of Health and Human Services: *2015-2020 Dietary guidelines for Americans*, ed 8, Washington, DC, 2015, https://health.gov/dietaryguidelines/2015/resources/2015-2020_Dietary_Guidelines.pdf. Accessed September 22, 2019.

Skin

Begin an assessment of the skin by focusing on the health history questions found in Table 30.7. Then inspect all visible skin surfaces; assess less visible surfaces when you examine other body systems. Use the senses of sight, smell, and touch while inspecting and palpating the skin.

Assessment of the skin reveals the patient's health status related to oxygenation, circulation, nutrition, local tissue damage, and hydration. Check the condition of the patient's skin to determine the need for nursing care. If there is an alteration in integumentary status, then adequate nutrition and hydration may become priority goals of therapy (see Chapter 45).

Every patient has a risk for skin impairment in a hospital setting. This risk increases in certain situations, such as pressure against the skin when the patient is immobile, reactions to various medications used in treatment, and moisture if the patient is incontinent or has wound drainage. Patients at high risk are those who have neurological impairments, chronic illnesses, decreased mental status, poor tissue oxygenation, low cardiac output, or inadequate nutrition or those who have had orthopedic or vascular injuries. Patients who are homebound, in nursing homes, or in extended-care facilities are often at risk for pressure injuries, depending on their level of mobility and the presence of chronic illness. Routinely assess the skin of all patients, especially those at risk, to look for primary or initial lesions that develop. Without identification and appropriate care, primary lesions can quickly deteriorate to become secondary lesions that require more extensive nursing care. For example, the development of a pressure injury lengthens a hospital stay unless it is prevented or discovered and treated early (see Chapter 48).

Adequate lighting is required when assessing the skin. Daylight is the best choice for identifying variations in skin color, especially for detecting skin changes in patients with dark skin. When sunlight is unavailable, fluorescent lighting is the next best choice. Room temperature also affects skin assessment. A room that is too warm causes superficial vasodilation, resulting in increased redness of the skin. A

Remove the shoes of a patient who cannot bear weight, and position the patient (such as an infant) supine on a firm surface. When measuring an infant, hold his or her head and make sure that his or her legs are straight at the knees. After positioning the infant, use a tape measure to measure length from the head to the bottom of the feet (Fig. 30.3). Record the infant's length to the nearest 0.5 cm (¼ inch).

SKIN, HAIR, AND NAILS

The integumentary system refers to the skin, hair, scalp, and nails. To assess, you first gather a health history to guide your examination and use the techniques of inspection and palpation.

TABLE 30.6   Nursing History for Weight Assessment

Assessment	Rationale
Ask about total weight lost or gained; compare with usual weight; note time period for loss and whether it was planned (e.g., gradual, sudden, desired, or undesired).	Assessment determines severity of problem and reveals whether weight change is related to disease process, change in eating pattern, or pregnancy.
If weight loss desired, ask about eating habits, diet plan followed, food preparation, calorie intake, appetite, exercise pattern, support group participation, weight goal.	Assessment helps to determine appropriateness of diet plan followed.
If weight loss undesired, ask about anorexia; vomiting; diarrhea; thirst; frequent urination; and change in lifestyle, activity, and stress levels.	Assessment focuses on problems that cause weight loss (e.g., gastrointestinal problems).
Assess whether patient has noted changes in social aspects of eating: more meals in restaurants, rushing to eat meals, stress at work, or skipping meals.	Lifestyle changes sometimes contribute to weight changes.
Assess whether patient takes chemotherapy, diuretics, insulin, fluoxetine, prescription and nonprescription appetite suppressants, laxatives, oral hypoglycemics, or herbal supplements (weight loss); steroids, oral contraceptives, antidepressants, insulin (weight gain).	Weight gain or loss is a side effect of these medications.
Assess for preoccupation with body weight or body shape such as fasting, never feeling thin enough, unusually strict caloric intake or restrictions, laxative abuse, induced vomiting, amenorrhea, excessive exercise, alcohol intake.	Excesses indicate an eating disorder.

cool environment causes a sensitive patient to develop cyanosis around the lips and nail beds (Ball et al., 2019).

Although you inspect the skin over each part of the body during an examination, it is helpful to make a brief but careful overall visual sweep of the entire body. This approach provides a good idea of the distribution and extent of any lesions and the overall symmetry of skin color. Inspect all skin surfaces, making a point to do so when examining other body systems. Often overlooked, inspection of the feet is absolutely essential for patients with poor circulation or diabetes. If any abnormalities are found during an examination, palpate the involved areas. Use disposable gloves for palpation if open, moist, or draining lesions are present.

Throughout the examination remain alert for skin odors. Black and white adolescents and adults ordinarily have body odor because they have a greater number of functioning apocrine glands. In contrast, Asians and Native Americans/American Indians often do not (Ball et al., 2019). Fig. 30.4 illustrates a normal cross-section of the skin.

Color. Skin color varies from body part to body part and from person to person. Despite individual variations, it is usually uniform over the body. Table 30.8 lists common variations. Normal skin pigmentation ranges in tone from ivory or light pink to ruddy pink in light skin and from light to deep brown or olive in dark skin. In older adults, pigmentation increases unevenly, causing discolored skin. While inspecting the skin, be aware that cosmetics or tanning agents sometimes mask normal skin color.

The assessment of color first involves areas of the skin not exposed to the sun such as the palms of the hands. Note whether the skin is unusually pale or dark. Areas exposed to the sun such as the face and arms are darker. It is more difficult to note changes such as pallor or cyanosis in patients with dark skin. Usually color hues are most evident in the palms, soles of the feet, lips, tongue, and nail beds. Areas of increased (hyperpigmentation) and decreased (hypopigmentation) color are common. Skin creases and folds are darker than the rest of the body in patients with dark skin.

Inspect sites where abnormalities are more easily identified. For example, pallor is more evident in the face, buccal (mouth) mucosa, conjunctiva, and nail beds. Observe for cyanosis (bluish discoloration) in the lips, nail beds, palpebral conjunctivae, and palms. In recognizing pallor in a patient with dark skin, observe that normal brown skin

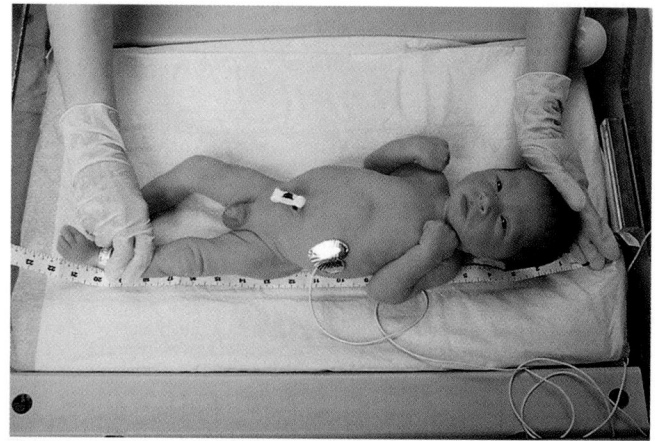

FIG. 30.3 Measurement of infant length. (From Murray SS, McKinney ES: *Foundations of maternal-newborn and women's health nursing,* ed 7, St Louis, 2019, Elsevier.)

appears to be yellow-brown and normal black skin appears to be ashen gray. Also assess the lips, nail beds, and mucous membranes for generalized pallor; if pallor is present, the mucous membranes are ashen gray. Assess for cyanosis in a patient with dark skin in areas where pigmentation occurs the least (conjunctiva, sclera, buccal mucosa, tongue, lips, nail beds, and palms and soles). In addition, verify these findings with clinical manifestations (Ball et al., 2019).

Discoloration of the skin occurs on different areas of the body for varying reasons. A patient's sclera is the best site to inspect for *jaundice* (yellow-orange discoloration). Normal reactive hyperemia, or redness, is most often seen in regions exposed to pressure such as the sacrum, heels, and greater trochanter. Inspect for any patches or areas of skin color variation. Localized skin changes such as pallor or *erythema* (red discoloration) indicate circulatory changes. It is difficult to observe erythema in a patient with dark skin; thus palpate the area for heat and warmth to note the presence of skin inflammation. For example, you notice an area of erythema in a patient with dark skin that is caused by localized vasodilation resulting from a sunburn, inflammation, or fever. Compare the area with a different part of the skin to detect a

TABLE 30.7 Nursing History for Skin Assessment

Assessment	Rationale
Ask patient about history of changes in skin: dryness, pruritus, sores, rashes, lumps, color, texture, odor, and lesion that does not heal.	Patient is best source to recognize change. Usually skin cancer is first noticed as a localized change in skin color.
Consider whether patient has the following history: fair, freckled, ruddy complexion; light-colored hair or eyes; tendency to burn easily.	Characteristics are risk factors for skin cancer.
Determine whether patient works or spends excessive time outside. If so, ask whether patient wears sunscreen and the level of protection.	Exposed areas such as face and arms are more pigmented than rest of body. The American Cancer Society (2018b) recommends sun safety and use of sunscreen and lip balm with broad-spectrum protection and a sun protection factor (SPF) of 30 or higher and not sunbathing or indoor tanning.
Determine whether patient has noted lesions, rashes, or bruises.	Most skin changes do not develop suddenly. Change in character of lesion can indicate cancer. Bruising indicates trauma or bleeding disorder.
Question patient about frequency of bathing and type of soap used.	Excessive bathing and use of harsh soaps cause dry skin.
Ask whether patient has had recent trauma to skin.	Some injuries cause bruising and changes in skin texture.
Determine whether patient has history of allergies.	Skin rashes commonly occur from allergies.
Ask whether patient uses topical medications or home remedies on skin.	Incorrect use of topical agents causes inflammation or irritation.
Ask whether patient goes to tanning parlors, uses sunlamps, or takes tanning pills.	Overexposure of skin to these irritants can cause skin cancer.
Ask whether patient has family history of serious skin disorders such as skin cancer or psoriasis.	Family history can reveal information about patient's condition.
Determine whether patient works with creosote, coal, tar, petroleum products, arsenic compounds, or radium.	Exposure to these agents creates risk for skin cancer.

difference in temperature. An area of an extremity that appears unusually pale results from arterial occlusion or edema. Be sure to ask whether the patient has noticed any changes in skin coloring.

There is also a pattern of findings associated with patients who are chemically dependent or abuse intravenous (IV) drugs (Table 30.9). It is sometimes difficult to recognize signs and symptoms through an isolated examination. A patient who takes repeated IV injections has edematous, reddened, and warm areas along the arms and legs. This pattern suggests recent injections. Areas of old injection sites appear as hyperpigmented and shiny or scarred.

Moisture. The hydration of skin and mucous membranes helps to reveal body fluid imbalances, changes in the environment of the skin, and regulation of body temperature. Moisture refers to wetness and oiliness. The skin is normally smooth and dry. Skinfolds such as the axillae are normally moist. Minimal perspiration or oiliness is often present (Ball et al., 2019). Increased perspiration can be associated with activity, exposure to warm environments, obesity, anxiety, or excitement. Use ungloved fingertips to palpate skin surfaces. Observe for dullness, dryness, crusting, and flaking that resembles dandruff when the skin surface is lightly rubbed. Excessively dry skin is common in older adults because their sebaceous and sweat gland activity decreases, reducing perspiration (Ball et al., 2019). Other factors causing dry skin include lack of humidity, exposure to sun, smoking, stress, excessive perspiration, and dehydration. Excessive dryness worsens existing skin conditions such as eczema and dermatitis. Patients with large abdominal skinfolds are at high risk for moisture within the skinfolds. Excessive moisture may cause maceration of the skin or softening of the tissues, resulting in an increased risk for breakdown (see Chapter 48).

Temperature. The temperature of the skin depends on the amount of blood circulating through the dermis. Increased or decreased skin temperature indicates an increase or decrease in blood flow. An increase in skin temperature often accompanies localized erythema or redness of the skin. A reduction in skin temperature often accompanies pallor

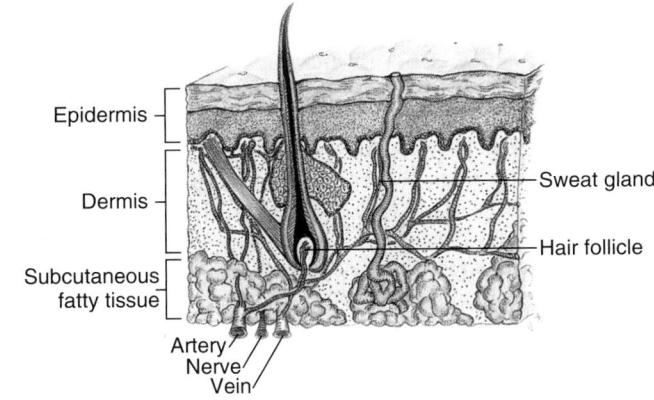

FIG. 30.4 Cross-section of skin reveals three layers: epidermis, dermis, and subcutaneous fatty tissues.

and reflects a decrease in blood flow. Remember that a cold or excessively warm examination room can cause changes in the patient's skin temperature and color.

Accurately assess temperature by palpating the skin with the dorsum or back of the hand and compare symmetrical body parts. Normally the skin temperature is warm. Sometimes it is the same throughout the body, and other times it varies in one area. Always assess skin temperature for patients at risk of having impaired circulation such as after a cast application or vascular surgery. A stage I pressure injury can be identified early by noting warmth over an area of erythema on the skin (see Chapter 48).

Texture. Texture refers to the appearance of the surface of the skin and how the deeper layers feel. By palpating lightly with the fingertips, you determine whether the patient's skin is smooth or rough, thin or thick, tight or supple, and indurated (hardened) or soft. The texture of the skin is normally smooth, soft, even, and flexible in children and adults. However, the texture is usually not uniform throughout, with thicker

TABLE 30.8   Skin Color Variations

Color	Condition	Causes	Assessment Locations
Bluish (cyanosis)	Increased amount of deoxygenated hemoglobin (associated with hypoxia)	Heart or lung disease, cold environment	Nail beds, lips, mouth, skin (severe cases)
Pallor (decrease in color)	Reduced amount of oxyhemoglobin	Anemia	Face, conjunctivae, nail beds, palms of hands
	Reduced visibility of oxyhemoglobin resulting from decreased blood flow	Shock	Skin, nail beds, conjunctivae, lips
Loss of pigmentation	Vitiligo	Congenital or autoimmune condition causing lack of pigment	Patchy areas on skin over face, hands, arms
Yellow-orange (jaundice)	Increased deposit of bilirubin in tissues	Liver disease, destruction of red blood cells	Sclera, mucous membranes, skin
Red (erythema)	Increased visibility of oxyhemoglobin caused by dilation or increased blood flow	Fever, direct trauma, blushing, alcohol intake	Face, area of trauma, sacrum, shoulders, other common sites for pressure injuries
Tan-brown	Increased amount of melanin	Suntan, pregnancy	Areas exposed to sun: face, arms, areolas, nipples

texture over the palms of the hand and soles of the feet. In older adults the skin becomes wrinkled and leathery because of a decrease in collagen, subcutaneous fat, and sweat glands.

Localized skin changes result from trauma, surgical wounds, or lesions. When there are irregularities in texture such as scars or indurations, ask the patient about recent injury to the skin. Deeper palpation sometimes reveals irregularities such as tenderness or localized areas of induration, which can be caused by an injury or repeated injections.

Turgor. Turgor refers to the elasticity of the skin. To assess skin turgor, grasp a fold of skin on the back of the forearm or sternal area with the fingertips and release (Fig. 30.5). Normally the skin loses its elasticity with age, but fluid balance can also affect skin turgor. Edema or dehydration diminishes turgor and makes the skin tauter. Since the skin on the back of the hand is normally loose and thin, turgor is not assessed reliably at that site (Ball et al., 2019). Normally the skin lifts easily and falls immediately back to its resting position. When turgor is poor, it stays pinched and shows tenting. Evaluate the ease with which the skin moves and the speed at which it returns to its resting state. Failure of the skin to reassume its normal contour or shape indicates dehydration. A patient with poor skin turgor does not have resilience to the normal wear and tear on the skin, and a decrease in turgor predisposes him or her to skin breakdown.

Vascularity. The circulation of the skin affects color in localized areas and leads to the appearance of superficial blood vessels. Vascularity occurs in localized pressure areas when patients remain in one position. Vascularity appears reddened, pink, or pale (see Chapter 48). With aging, capillaries become fragile and more easily injured. Petechiae are nonblanching, pinpoint-size, red or purple spots on the skin caused by small hemorrhages in the skin layers. Many petechiae have no known cause; but some may indicate serious blood-clotting disorders, drug reactions, or liver disease.

Edema. Edema is present when areas of the skin become swollen or edematous from a buildup of fluid in the tissues. Direct trauma and impairment of venous return are two common causes of edema. Inspect edematous areas for location, color, and shape. The formation of edema separates the surface of the skin from the pigmented and

TABLE 30.9   Physical Findings of the Skin Indicative of Substance Abuse

Skin Finding	Commonly Associated Drug
Diaphoresis	Sedative hypnotic (including alcohol)
Spider angiomas	Alcohol, stimulants
Burns (especially fingers)	Alcohol
Needle marks	Opioids
Contusion, abrasions, cuts, scars	Alcohol, other sedative hypnotics, intravenous (IV) opioids
"Homemade" tattoos	Cocaine, IV opioids (prevents detection of injection sites)
Vasculitis	Cocaine
Red, dry skin	Phencyclidine (PCP)

Modified from Burchum J, Rosenthal L, *Lehne's pharmacology for nursing care*, ed 10, St Louis, 2019, Saunders; Ries R, Wilford B: *Principles of addiction medicine*, ed 5, Chevy Chase, MD, 2014, Lippincott Williams & Wilkins.

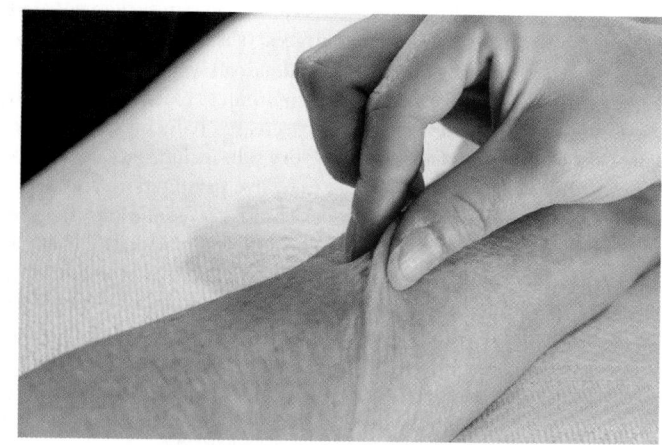

FIG. 30.5 Assessment for skin turgor.

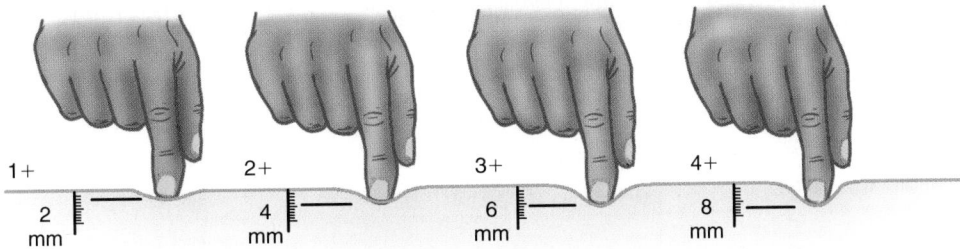

FIG. 30.6 Assessing for pitting edema. (From Ball JW, et al: *Seidel's guide to physical examination*, ed 9, St Louis, 2019, Elsevier.)

vascular layers, masking skin color. Edematous skin also appears stretched and shiny. Palpate edematous areas to determine mobility, consistency, and tenderness. When pressure from the examiner's fingers leaves an indentation in the edematous area, it is called pitting edema. To assess the degree of pitting edema, press the edematous area firmly with the thumb for several seconds and release. The depth of pitting, recorded in millimeters, determines the degree of edema (Ball et al., 2019). For example, 1+ edema equals a 2-mm depth, 2+ edema equals a 4-mm depth, 3+ equals 6 mm, and 4+ equals 8 mm (Fig. 30.6).

Lesions. The term *lesion* refers broadly to any unusual finding of the skin surface. Normally the skin is free of lesions, except for common freckles or age-related changes such as skin tags, senile keratosis (thickening of skin), cherry angiomas (ruby red papules), and atrophic warts. Lesions that are primary occur as an initial spontaneous sign of a pathological process such as with an insect bite. Secondary lesions result from later formation or trauma to a primary lesion such as a pressure injury. When you find a lesion, collect standard information about its color, location, texture, size, shape, type, grouping (clustered or linear), and distribution (localized or generalized). Next observe for any exudate, odor, amount, and consistency. Measure the size of the lesion in centimeters by using a small, clear, flexible ruler. Measure each lesion for height, width, and depth.

Palpation helps determine the mobility, contour (flat, raised, or depressed), and consistency (soft or indurated) of a lesion. Certain types of lesions present characteristic patterns. For example, a tumor is usually an elevated, solid lesion larger than 2 cm (1 inch). Primary lesions such as macules and nodules come from some stimulus to the skin (Box 30.6). Secondary lesions such as ulcers occur as alterations in primary lesions. After you identify a lesion, closely inspect it in good lighting. Palpate gently, covering the entire area of the lesion. If it is moist or draining fluid, wear gloves during palpation and pay attention to whether the patient identifies any areas of tenderness.

Skin (cutaneous) malignancies are the most common neoplasms. For this reason you need to complete a thorough skin assessment on all patients. Cancerous lesions have distinct features and over time undergo changes in color and size (Box 30.7). Basal cell carcinoma is most common in areas exposed to the sun and frequently occurs with a history of sun damage; it almost never spreads to other parts of the body. Squamous cell carcinoma is more serious than basal cell and develops on the outer layers of sun-exposed skin; these cells may travel to lymph nodes and throughout the body. Malignant melanoma, a skin cancer that develops from melanocytes, begins as a mole or other area that has changed in appearance and is usually located on normal skin. (**NOTE:** Melanoma also can originate in noncutaneous primary sites, including mucosal epithelium [GI tract], retinas, and leptomeninges.) In African Americans (more than in other races) it can also appear under fingernails or on the palms of the hands and soles of the feet. Use

the *ABCD* mnemonic to assess the skin for any type of carcinoma (ACS, 2018b):

- *Asymmetry*—Look for an uneven shape. One half of mole does not match the other half.
- *Border irregularity*—Look for edges that are blurred, notched, or ragged.
- *Color*—Look for pigmentation that is not uniform; variegated areas of blue, black, and brown and areas of pink, white, gray, blue, or red are abnormal.
- *Diameter*—Look for areas greater than 6 mm (about the size of a typical pencil eraser).

Report abnormal lesions to the health care provider for further examination. Since ultraviolet light of the sun or tanning beds increases the risk for development of skin cancers, teach patients about the risks that exist. In addition, using individualized teaching materials, teach patients how to perform a skin self-examination.

Hair and Scalp

Assess a patient's hair during all parts of the examination. Two types of hair cover the body: soft, fine, vellus hair, which covers the body; and coarse, long, thick terminal hair, which is easily visible on the scalp, axillae, and pubic areas and in the facial beard on men. First obtain health history information listed in Table 30.10. Prepare to inspect the condition and distribution of hair and the integrity of the scalp by first obtaining a good light source.

Inspection. During inspection explain that it is necessary to separate parts of the hair to detect abnormalities. Wear a pair of clean gloves if open lesions or lice are noted.

First inspect the color, distribution, quantity, thickness, texture, and lubrication of body hair. Scalp hair is coarse or fine and curly or straight; it should be shiny, smooth, and pliant. While separating sections of scalp hair, observe characteristics of color and coarseness. Color varies from very light blond to black to gray and is sometimes altered by rinses or dyes. In older adults the hair sometimes becomes dull gray, white, or yellow.

Be aware of the normal distribution of hair growth in a man and a woman. At puberty an increase in the amount and distribution of hair occurs for both genders. During the aging process the hair may thin over the scalp, axillae, and pubic areas. Facial hair of older men decreases. A woman with hirsutism has hair growth on the upper lip, chin, and cheeks, with vellus hair becoming coarser over the body; this may be related to an endocrine disorder. For some a change in hair growth negatively affects body image and emotional well-being. The amount of hair covering the extremities is sometimes reduced as a result of aging, or it could result from arterial insufficiency that could reduce hair growth over the lower extremities. In the United States and some other cultures, women commonly shave their legs and axilla,

BOX 30.6   Types of Primary Skin Lesions

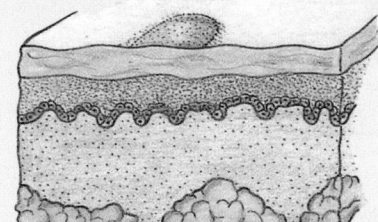

Macule: Flat, nonpalpable change in skin color; smaller than 1 cm (e.g., freckle, petechiae)

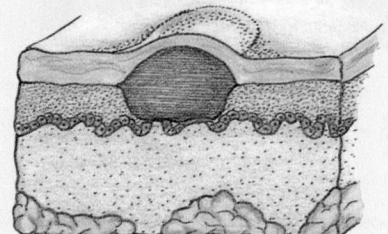

Papule: Palpable, circumscribed, solid elevation in skin; smaller than 1 cm (e.g., elevated nevus)

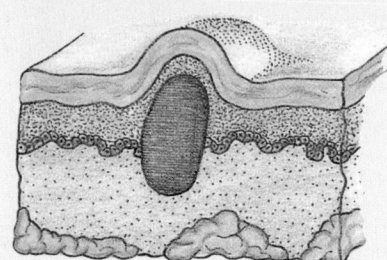

Nodule: Elevated solid mass, deeper and firmer than papule; 1-2 cm (e.g., wart)

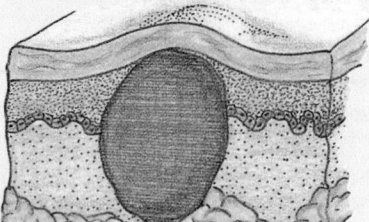

Tumor: Solid mass that extends deep through subcutaneous tissue; larger than 1-2 cm (e.g., epithelioma)

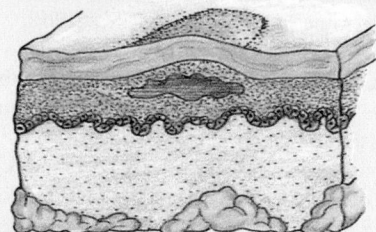

Wheal: Irregularly shaped, elevated area or superficial localized edema; varies in size (e.g., hive, mosquito bite)

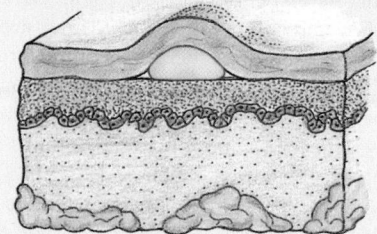

Vesicle: Circumscribed elevation of skin filled with serous fluid, smaller than 1 cm (e.g., herpes simplex, chickenpox)

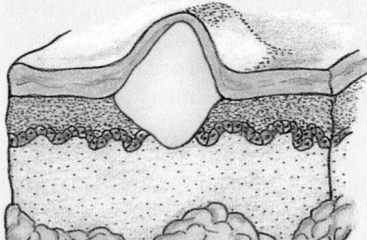

Pustule: Circumscribed elevation of skin similar to vesicle but filled with pus; varies in size (e.g., acne, staphylococcal infection)

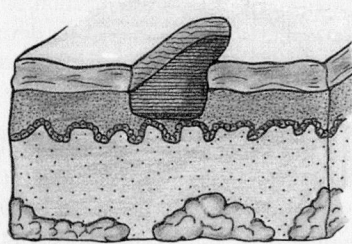

Ulcer: Deep loss of skin surface that extends to dermis and frequently bleeds and scars; varies in size (e.g., venous stasis ulcer)

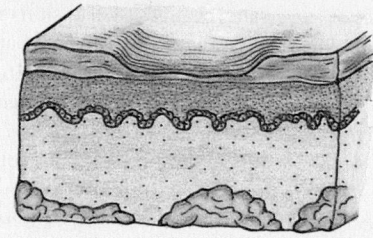

Atrophy: Thinning of skin with loss of normal skin furrow, with skin appearing shiny and translucent; varies in size (e.g., arterial insufficiency)

although shaving remains a matter of personal preference among women from all cultures.

Assess for causes of changes in the thickness, texture, and lubrication of scalp hair. At times these are a result of febrile illnesses or scalp diseases that result in hair loss. Conditions such as thyroid disease alter the condition of the hair, making it fine and brittle. Hair loss (alopecia) or thinning of the hair is usually related to genetic tendencies, endocrine disorders such as diabetes, thyroiditis, and menopause. Poor nutrition causes stringy, dull, dry, and thin hair. The oil of sebaceous glands lubricates the hair, but excessively oily hair is associated with androgen hormone stimulation. Dry, brittle hair occurs with aging and excessive use of chemical agents.

Normally the scalp is smooth and inelastic with even coloration. Carefully separate strands of hair and thoroughly inspect the scalp for lesions, which are not easy to notice in thick hair. Note the characteristics of any scalp lesion. For lumps or bruises, ask whether the patient has experienced recent head trauma. Moles on the scalp are common, but they can bleed as a result of vigorous combing or brushing. Dandruff or psoriasis frequently causes scaliness or dryness of the scalp.

Careful inspection of hair follicles on the scalp and pubic areas can reveal lice or other parasites. The three types of lice are *Pediculus humanus capitis* (head lice), *Pediculus humanus corporis* (body lice), and *Pediculus pubis* (crab lice). The presence of lice does not mean that a person practices poor hygiene. Lice spread easily, especially among children who play closely together. Head and crab lice attach their eggs to hair. The tiny eggs look like oval particles of dandruff, although the lice themselves are difficult to see (Fig. 30.7). Head and body lice are very small with grayish-white bodies, whereas crab lice have red legs. To better identify infestations, observe for small, red, pustular eruptions in the hair follicles and areas where skin surfaces meet, such as behind the ears and in the groin. A person often has intense itching of the scalp, especially on the back of the head or neck. Combing with a fine-tooth comb reveals the small oval-shaped lice; discovery of lice requires immediate treatment. Teach the patient to perform hair and scalp hygiene practices (Box 30.8).

Nails

The condition of the nails reflects a person's general health, state of nutrition, occupation, and habits of self-care. Before assessing the nails, gather a brief history (Table 30.11). The most visible part of the nail is the nail plate, the transparent layer of epithelial cells covering the nail bed (Fig. 30.8). The vascularity of the nail bed creates the underlying color of the nail. The semilunar whitish area at the base of the nail bed is called the *lunula*, from which the nail plate grows.

BOX 30.7 Skin Malignancies

Basal Cell Carcinoma
- 0.5- to 1-cm crusted lesion that is flat or raised and has a rolled, somewhat scaly border
- Frequent appearance of underlying, widely dilated blood vessels within the lesion

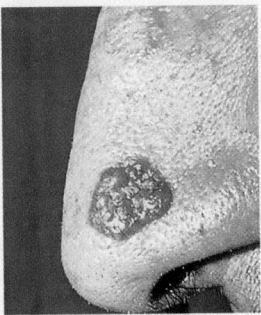

Squamous Cell Carcinoma
- Occurs more often on mucosal surfaces and nonexposed areas of skin than basal cell
- 0.5- to 1.5-cm scaly lesion sometimes ulcerated or crusted; appears frequently and grows more rapidly than basal cell

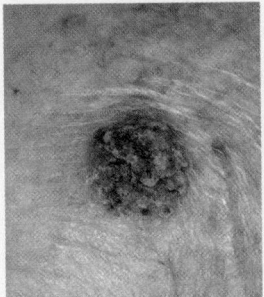

Melanoma
- 0.5- to 1-cm brown, flat lesion; appears on sun-exposed or nonexposed skin; variegated pigmentation, irregular borders, and indistinct margins
- Ulceration, recent growth, or recent changes in long-standing mole are ominous signs

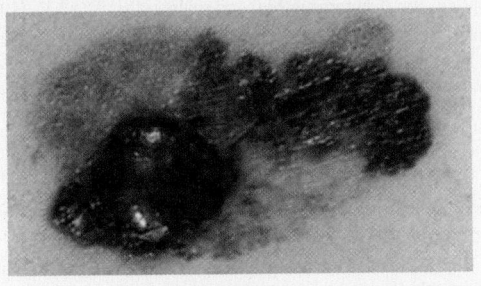

Illustrations from Belcher AE: *Cancer nursing,* St Louis, 1992, Mosby; Habif TP: *Clinical dermatology: a color guide to diagnosis and therapy,* ed 3, St Louis, 1996, Mosby; and Zitelli BJ, et al: *Zitelli and Davis' atlas of pediatric physical diagnosis,* ed 7, St Louis, 2018, Saunders.

TABLE 30.10 Nursing History for Hair and Scalp Assessment

Assessment	Rationale
Ask patient whether he or she is wearing a wig or hairpiece; if so, ask him or her to remove it.	Wigs or hairpieces interfere with inspection of hair and scalp. (Patient sometimes requests to omit this part of examination.)
Determine whether patient has noted change in growth, loss of hair, or change in texture or color.	Change often occurs slowly over time.
Identify type of hair-care products used for grooming.	Excessive use of chemical agents and burning of hair causes drying and brittleness.
Determine whether patient has had chemotherapy (drugs that cause hair loss) recently or taken a vasodilator (minoxidil) for hair growth.	Chemotherapeutic agents kill cells that rapidly multiply such as tumor and normal hair cells. Minoxidil causes excessive hair growth.
Has patient noted changes in diet or appetite?	Nutrition influences condition of hair.

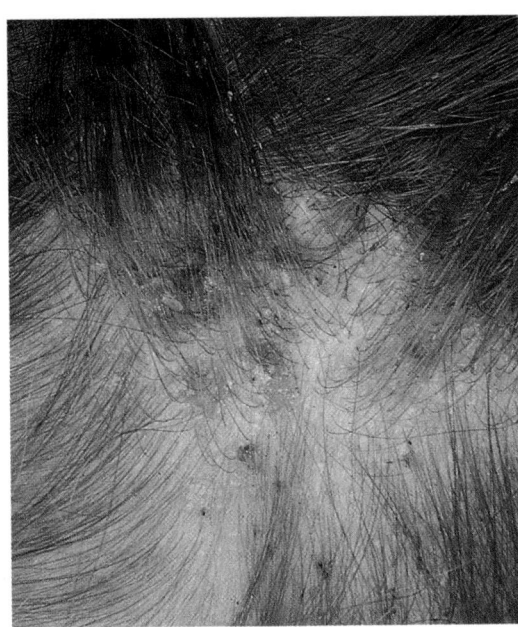

FIG. 30.7 Head lice infestation. (From Habif TP: *Clinical dermatology: a color guide to diagnosis and therapy,* ed 4, Philadelphia, 2004, Mosby.)

Inspection and Palpation. Inspect the nail bed for color, length, symmetry, cleanliness, and configuration. The shape and condition of the nails can give clues to pathophysiological problems. Assess the thickness and shape of the nail, its texture, the angle between the nail and the nail bed, and the condition of the lateral and proximal nail folds around the nail. When inspecting the nails, you gather a sense of a patient's hygiene practices. The nails are normally transparent, smooth, well rounded, and convex, with a nail bed angle of about 160 degrees (Box 30.9). A larger angle and softening of the nail bed indicate chronic oxygenation problems. The surrounding cuticles are smooth, intact, and without inflammation. When you assess for basic care of the nails, you recognize that nail biting, stains, and jagged edges either represent poor nail care or are caused by habits or occupational exposure to grease or dirt. Jagged, bitten, or broken nail edges or cuticles predispose a patient to localized infection.

When palpating, expect to find a firm nail base, and check for any abnormalities such as erythema or swelling. For patients with impaired circulation, especially observe for early signs of infection or open lesions. To palpate, gently grasp the patient's finger and observe the color of the nail bed. The nail bed and nails appear pink with white nail tips in white patients. In patients with darker skin, the nail beds are darkly pigmented with a blue or reddish hue. A brown or black pigmentation is normal with longitudinal streaks (Fig. 30.9). Trauma, cirrhosis, diabetes mellitus, and hypertension cause splinter hemorrhages while vitamin, protein, and electrolyte changes cause various lines or bands to form on the nail beds.

Nails normally grow at a constant rate, but direct injury or generalized disease changes growth patterns. With aging the nails of the fingers and toes become harder and thicker, longitudinal striations develop, and the rate of nail growth slows. In older adults with insufficient calcium nails become more brittle, dull, turn opaque-yellow and the cuticle becomes thick and wide.

Calluses and corns commonly are found on the toes or fingers. A callus is flat and painless, resulting from a thickening of the epidermis. Friction and pressure from shoes cause corns, usually over bony prominences. During the examination instruct the patient in proper nail care (Box 30.10).

HEAD AND NECK

An examination of the head and neck includes assessment of the head, eyes, ears, nose, mouth, pharynx, and neck (lymph nodes, carotid arteries, thyroid gland, and trachea). Assessment of the head and neck uses inspection, palpation, and auscultation. Many times, you will inspect and palpate the head and neck at the same time.

Head

Inspection and Palpation. The nursing history screens for intracranial injury and local or congenital deformities (Table 30.12). Inspect the patient's head, noting the position, size, shape, and contour. The head is normally held upright and midline to the trunk. A patient who tilts the head to one side may have unilateral hearing or visual loss or muscle weakness in the neck. A horizontal jerking or bobbing may indicate a tremor.

Note the patient's facial features, looking at the eyelids, eyebrows, nasolabial folds, and mouth for shape and symmetry. It is normal for slight asymmetry to exist. If there is facial asymmetry, note whether all features on one side of the face are affected or if only a part of the face is involved. Various neurological disorders (e.g., facial nerve paralysis) affect different nerves that innervate muscles of the face.

Examine the size, shape, and contour of the skull. The skull is generally round with prominences in the frontal area anteriorly and the occipital area posteriorly. Trauma typically causes local skull deformities. In infants a large head results from congenital anomaly or the buildup of cerebrospinal fluid in the ventricles (hydrocephalus). Some adults have enlarged jaws and facial bones resulting from acromegaly, a disorder caused by excessive secretion of growth hormone. Palpate the skull for nodules or masses. Gently rotate the fingertips down the midline of the scalp and along the sides of the head to identify abnormalities. Palpate the temporomandibular joint (TMJ) space bilaterally. Place the fingertips just anterior to the tragus of each ear. The fingertips should slip into the joint space as the patient's mouth opens to gently palpate the joint spaces. Normally the movements should be smooth, although it is not unusual to hear or feel a clicking, grating, or snapping in the TMJ, indicating degenerative joint disease (Ball et al., 2019).

BOX 30.8 PATIENT TEACHING
Hair and Scalp Assessment

Objective
- Patient will perform proper hygiene practices for care of hair and scalp.

Teaching Strategies
- Instruct patient about basic hygiene practices for hair and scalp care.
- Instruct patients who have head lice to shampoo thoroughly with pediculicide (shampoo available at drugstores) in cold water at a basin or sink. Do not use a tub or shower, where the medication can reach other body parts. Comb thoroughly with a fine-tooth comb (following product directions) and discard comb. *Caution: Do not use products containing Lindane, a toxic ingredient known to cause adverse reactions.* Repeat shampoo treatment 12 to 24 hours later.
- After shampooing, remove any detectable nits or nit cases with tweezers or a metal nit comb. A dilute solution of vinegar and water helps loosen nits.
- Instruct patients and parents about ways to reduce transmission of lice:
  - Do not share hairbrushes, combs, hairpieces, hats, bedding, towels, or clothing with someone who has head lice.
  - Vacuum all rugs, car seats, pillows, furniture, and flooring thoroughly and discard vacuum bag.
  - Seal nonwashable items in plastic bags for 14 days if unable to dry-clean or vacuum.
  - Use thorough hand hygiene practices.
  - Launder all clothing, linen, and bedding in hot water and detergent; then dry in a hot dryer for at least 31 minutes. Dry clean nonwashable items.
  - Do not use insecticide.
- Instruct patient to notify his or her partner if lice were sexually transmitted.
- Avoid physical contact with infested individuals and their belongings, especially clothing and bedding.
- Soak any comb or brush used to remove lice for 15 minutes in very hot ammonia water (1 tsp ammonia to 2 cups hot water) or boiling water for 10 minutes.

Evaluation
Use the principles of teach-back to evaluate patient/family caregiver learning:
- Tell me how you care for your hair and scalp.
- Explain to me the steps you will take to reduce lice transmission in your home.

Eyes

Examination of the eyes includes assessment of visual acuity, visual fields, extraocular movements, and external and internal eye structures. Fig. 30.10 shows a cross-section of the eye. The eye assessment detects visual alterations and determines the general level of assistance that patients require when ambulating or performing self-care activities. Some patients with visual problems also need special aids for reading educational materials or instructions (e.g., medication labels). Table 30.13 reviews the nursing history for an eye examination. Box 30.11 describes common types of visual problems.

Visual Acuity. Assessing visual acuity (i.e., the ability to see small details) tests central vision. The easiest way to assess near vision is to ask patients to read printed material under adequate lighting. If patients wear glasses, make sure that they wear them during the assessment.

TABLE 30.11 Nursing History for Nail Assessment

Assessment	Rationale
Ask whether patient has experienced recent trauma or changes in nails (splitting, breaking, discoloration, thickening).	Trauma changes shape and growth of nail. Systemic conditions cause changes in color, growth, and shape.
Has patient had other symptoms of pain, swelling, presence of systemic disease with fever, or psychological or physical stress?	Alterations sometimes occur slowly over time.
Question patient's nail care practices. Determine whether patient has acrylic nails or silk wraps.	Change in nails can be caused by local or systemic problem. Acrylic nails and silk wraps are areas for fungal growth.
Determine whether patient has risks for nail or foot problems (e.g., diabetes, peripheral vascular disease, older adulthood, obesity).	Chemical agents cause drying of nails. Improper care damages nails and cuticles. Vascular changes associated with diabetes and peripheral vascular disease reduce blood flow to peripheral tissues; foot lesions and thickened nails are common. Some older adults have trouble performing foot and nail care because of poor vision, lack of coordination, or inability to bend over. Patients who are obese often have difficulty bending.

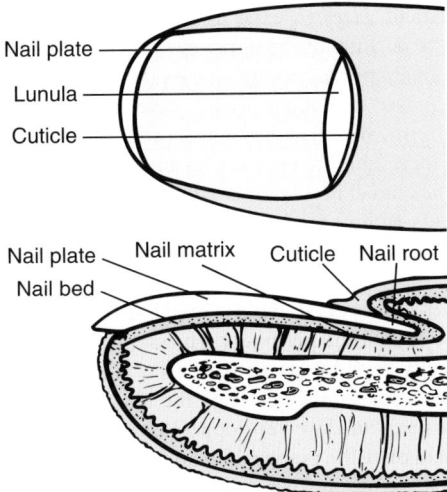

FIG. 30.8 Components of nail unit. (From Lewis SL, et al: *Medical-surgical nursing*, ed 9, St Louis, 2014, Mosby.)

Asking patients to read aloud helps to determine literacy. If the patient has difficulty reading, move to the next step.

Assessment of distant vision requires using a Snellen chart (paper chart or projection screen). The chart should be well lit. Test vision without corrective lenses first. Have the patient sit or stand 6.1 m (20 feet) away from the chart and try to read all of the letters beginning at any line with both eyes open. Then have the patient read the line with each eye separately (patient covers the opposite eye with an index card or eye cover to avoid applying pressure to the eye). Note the smallest line for which the patient can read all of the letters correctly and record the visual acuity for that line. Repeat the test with the patient wearing corrective lenses. Complete the test rapidly enough so that the patient does not memorize the chart (Ball et al., 2019). If a patient is unable to read, use an E chart or one with pictures of familiar objects. Instead of reading letters, patients tell which direction each E is pointing or the name of the object.

The Snellen chart has standardized numbers at the end of each line of the chart. The numerator is the number 20, or the distance the patient stands from the chart. The denominator is the distance from which the normal eye is able to read the chart. Normal visual acuity is 20/20. The larger the denominator, the poorer the patient's visual acuity. For example, a value of 20/40 means that the patient, standing 20 feet away, can read a line that a person with normal vision can read from 40 feet away. Record visual acuity for each eye and both eyes and

BOX 30.9 Abnormalities of the Nail Bed

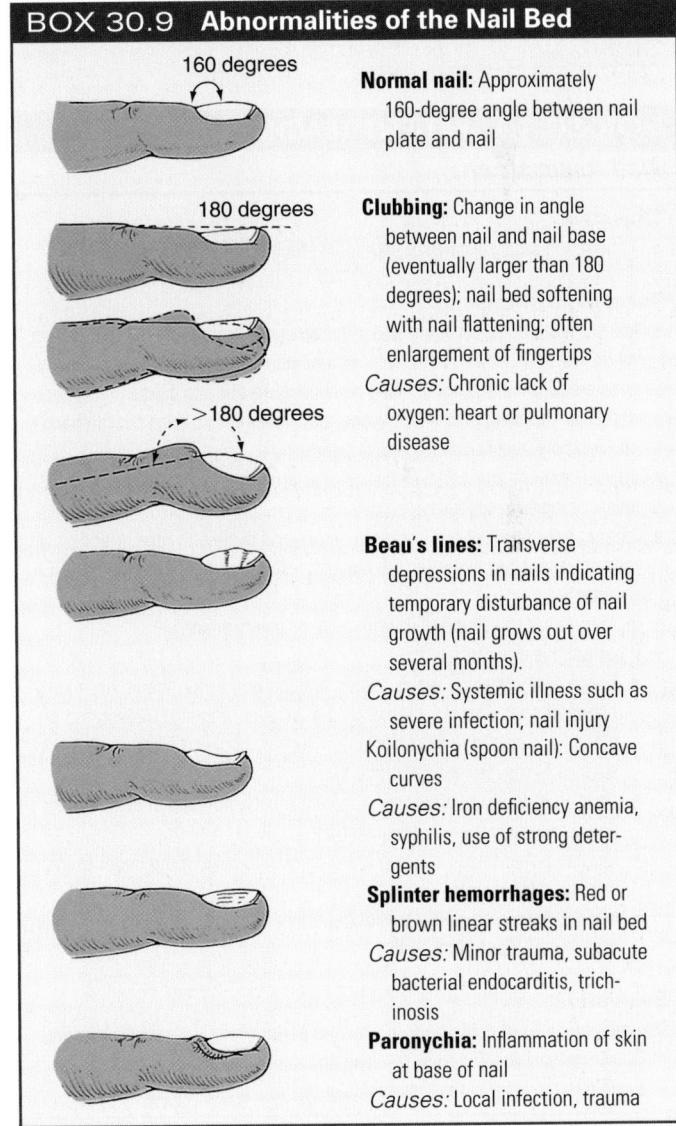

Normal nail: Approximately 160-degree angle between nail plate and nail

Clubbing: Change in angle between nail and nail base (eventually larger than 180 degrees); nail bed softening with nail flattening; often enlargement of fingertips
Causes: Chronic lack of oxygen: heart or pulmonary disease

Beau's lines: Transverse depressions in nails indicating temporary disturbance of nail growth (nail grows out over several months).
Causes: Systemic illness such as severe infection; nail injury
Koilonychia (spoon nail): Concave curves
Causes: Iron deficiency anemia, syphilis, use of strong detergents
Splinter hemorrhages: Red or brown linear streaks in nail bed
Causes: Minor trauma, subacute bacterial endocarditis, trichinosis
Paronychia: Inflammation of skin at base of nail
Causes: Local infection, trauma

record whether the test was performed with or without correction (including glasses or contact lenses).

If patients cannot read even the largest letters or figures of a Snellen chart, test their ability to count upraised fingers or to distinguish light.

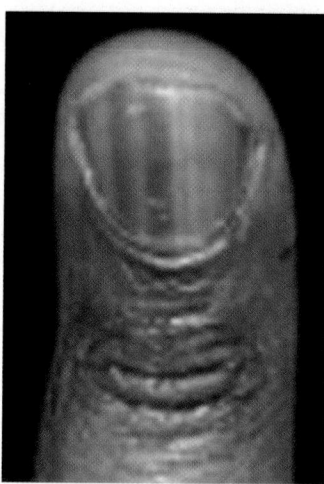

FIG. 30.9 Pigmented bands in nail of patient with dark skin. (From Habif TP: *Clinical dermatology: a color guide to diagnosis and therapy,* ed 5, St Louis, 2010, Mosby.)

BOX 30.10 PATIENT TEACHING

Nail Assessment

Objective
- Patient will properly care for fingernails, feet, and toenails.

Teaching Strategies
- Instruct patient to cut nails only after soaking them about 10 minutes in warm water. (*Exception:* Patients with diabetes or peripheral vascular disease are warned against soaking nails because this can cause maceration of the skin, leading to infection. Long-term soaking also dries out the hands and feet; dry, cracked skin leads to infection.)
- Caution patient against over-the-counter preparations to treat corns, calluses, or ingrown toenails.
- Instruct patient to cut nails straight across and even with tops of fingers or toes. If patient has diabetes, tell him or her to file rather than cut nails (see Chapter 40).
- Instruct patient to shape nails with a file or emery board.
- If patient has diabetes:
  - Wash feet daily in warm water and carefully dry them, especially between toes. Inspect feet each day in good lighting, looking for dry places and cracks in skin. Soften dry feet by applying a cream or lotion such as Nivea, Eucerin, or Alpha Keri.
  - Do not put lotion between toes; moisture between toes allows microorganisms to grow, leading to infections.
  - Caution patient against using sharp objects to poke or dig under toenail or around the cuticle.
  - Have patient see a podiatrist for treatment of ingrown toenails and nails that are thick or tend to split.

Evaluation
Use the principles of teach-back to evaluate patient/family caregiver learning:
- Show me how you are going to clean and moisturize your hands and feet.
- Explain the measures that you will take to avoid injury to your feet.

Hold a hand 31 cm (1 foot) from the patient's face and have him or her count the upraised fingers. To check light perception, shine a penlight into the eye and turn off the light. If the patient notes when the light is turned on or off, light perception is intact.

Assess near vision by asking the patient to read a handheld card containing a vision screening chart. The patient holds the card a comfortable distance (31.7 to 35.5 cm [about 12½ to 14 inches]) from the eyes and reads the smallest line possible. This part of the examination is a good time to discuss the need for routine eye examinations (Box 30.12).

Extraocular Movements. Six small muscles guide the movement of each eye. Both eyes move parallel to one another in each of the six directions of gaze (Fig. 30.11). To assess extraocular movements, a patient sits or stands, and the nurse faces the patient from 60 cm (2 feet) away. The nurse holds a finger at a comfortable distance (15 to 31 cm [6 to 12 inches]) from the patient's eyes. While the patient maintains his or her head in a fixed position facing forward, the nurse directs him or her to follow with the eyes only as the nurse's finger moves to the right, left, and diagonally up and down to the left and right. The nurse moves the finger smoothly and slowly within the normal field of vision.

As the patient gazes in each direction, observe for parallel eye movement, the position of the upper eyelid in relation to the iris, and the presence of abnormal movements. As the eyes move through each direction of gaze, the upper eyelid covers the iris only slightly. Nystagmus, an involuntary, rhythmical oscillation of the eyes, occurs as a result of local injury to eye muscles and supporting structures or a disorder of the cranial nerves innervating the muscles. Initiate nystagmus in patients with normal eye movements by having them gaze to the far left or right.

Visual Fields. As a person looks straight ahead, he or she normally can see all objects in the periphery. To assess visual fields, direct the patient to stand or sit 60 cm (2 feet) away at eye level. The patient gently closes or covers one eye (e.g., the left) and looks at your eye directly opposite. You close your opposite eye (in this case the right) so that the field of vision is superimposed on that of the patient. Next move a finger equidistant between you and the patient outside the field of vision and slowly bring it back into the visual field. The patient reports when he or she can see the finger. If you see the finger before the patient does, a part of the patient's visual field is reduced. To test temporal field vision, hold an object or your finger slightly behind the patient. Repeat the procedure for each field of vision for the other eye. Patients with visual field problems are at risk for injury because they cannot see all of the objects in front of them. Older adults commonly have loss of peripheral vision caused by changes in the lens.

External Eye Structures. To inspect external eye structures, stand directly in front of the patient at eye level and ask him or her to look at your face.

Position and Alignment. Assess the position of the eyes in relation to one another. Normally they are parallel to one another. Bulging eyes (exophthalmos) usually indicate hyperthyroidism. Crossed eyes (strabismus) result from neuromuscular injury or inherited abnormalities. Tumors or inflammation of the orbit often cause abnormal eye protrusion.

For the remainder of the eye examination have the patient remove contact lenses.

Eyebrows. Inspect the eyebrows for size, extension, texture of hair, alignment, and movement. Normally the eyebrows are symmetrical. Coarseness of hair and failure to extend beyond the temporal canthus possibly reveals hypothyroidism. Thin brows may be a result of waxing or plucking. Aging causes loss of the lateral third of the eyebrows. To assess movement, ask the patient to raise and lower the eyebrows. The

TABLE 30.12 Nursing History for Head Assessment

Assessment	Rationale
Determine whether patient experienced recent head trauma. If so, assess state of consciousness after injury (immediately on return and 5 minutes later), duration of unconsciousness, and predisposing factors (e.g., seizure, poor vision, blackout).	Trauma is major cause for lumps, bumps, cuts, bruises, or deformities of scalp or skull. Loss of consciousness following head injury indicates possible brain injury.
Ask whether patient has history of headache; note onset, duration, character, pattern, and associated symptoms.	Character of headache helps to reveal causative factors such as sinus infection, migraine, or neurological disorders.
Determine length of time patient has experienced neurological symptoms.	Duration of signs or symptoms reveals severity of problem.
Review patient's occupational history for use of safety helmets.	Nature of some occupations creates a risk for head injury.
Ask whether patient participates in contact sports, cycling, rollerblading, or skateboarding.	These activities require use of safety helmets.

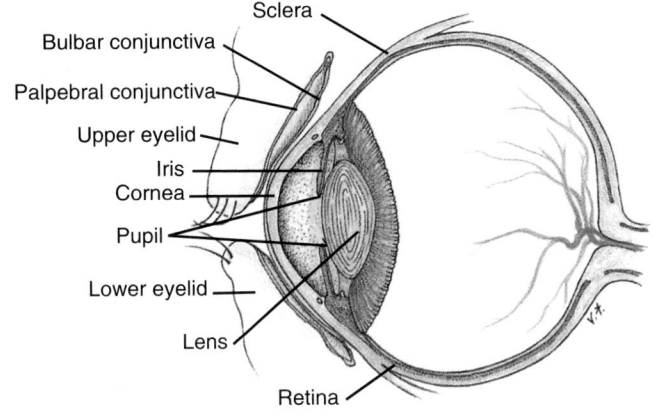

FIG. 30.10 Cross-section of eye.

Labels: Sclera, Bulbar conjunctiva, Palpebral conjunctiva, Upper eyelid, Iris, Cornea, Pupil, Lower eyelid, Lens, Retina

brows normally raise and lower symmetrically. An inability to move them indicates a facial nerve paralysis (cranial nerve VII).

Eyelids. Inspect the eyelids for position; color; condition of the surface; condition and direction of the eyelashes; and the patient's ability to open, close, and blink. When the eyes are open in a normal position, the lids cover the sclera above the iris but not the pupil. The lids are also close to the eyeball. An abnormal drooping of the lid over the pupil is called ptosis (pronounced "toe-sis") and is caused by edema or impairment of the third cranial nerve. In the older adult ptosis results from a loss of elasticity that accompanies aging. An older adult frequently has lid margins that turn out (ectropion) or in (entropion). Entropion sometimes leads to the lashes of the lid irritating the conjunctiva and cornea, increasing the risk of infection. Normally the eyelashes are distributed evenly and curved outward away from the eye. An erythematous or yellow lump (hordeolum or sty) on the follicle of an eyelash indicates an acute suppurative inflammation.

To inspect the surface of the upper lids, ask the patient to close his or her eyes while observing for lid tremors. Normally the lids are smooth and the same color as the surrounding skin. Redness indicates inflammation or infection. Lid edema is sometimes caused by allergies or heart or kidney failure. Edema of the eyelids prevents them from closing. Inspect any lesions for typical characteristics and discomfort or drainage. Wear clean gloves if drainage is present.

The lids normally close symmetrically. Their failure to close exposes the cornea to drying. This condition is common in unconscious patients or those with facial nerve paralysis. To inspect the lower lids, ask the patient to open the eyes again while you look for the same characteristics noted for the upper lids. Normally a patient blinks involuntarily and

bilaterally up to 20 times a minute. The blink reflex lubricates the cornea. Report absent, infrequent, rapid, or monocular (one-eyed) blinking.

Lacrimal Apparatus. The lacrimal gland (Fig. 30.12), located in the upper outer wall of the anterior part of the orbit, is responsible for tear production. Tears flow from the gland across the surface of the eye to the lacrimal duct, which is in the nasal corner or inner canthus of the eye. The lacrimal gland is sometimes the site of tumors or infections and should be inspected for edema and redness. Palpate the gland gently to detect tenderness; normally tenderness cannot be felt.

The nasolacrimal duct sometimes becomes obstructed, blocking the flow of tears. Observe for evidence of edema in the inner canthus. Gentle palpation of the duct at the lower eyelid just inside the lower orbital rim causes a regurgitation of tears.

Conjunctivae and Sclerae. The bulbar conjunctiva covers the exposed surface of the eyeball up to the outer edge of the cornea. Observe the sclera under the bulbar conjunctiva; normally it has the color of white porcelain in patients with light skin and is light yellow in patients with dark skin. Sclerae become pigmented and appear either yellow or green if liver disease is present.

Take care when inspecting the conjunctivae. For adequate exposure of the bulbar conjunctiva, retract the eyelids without placing pressure directly on the eyeball. Gently retract both lids, with the thumb and index finger pressed against the lower and upper bony orbits. Ask the patient to look up, down, and from side to side. Many patients begin to blink, making the examination difficult. Inspect for color, texture, and the presence of edema or lesions. Normally the conjunctivae are free of erythema. The presence of redness indicates an allergic or infectious conjunctivitis. Bright red blood in a localized area surrounded by normal-appearing conjunctiva usually indicates subconjunctival hemorrhage. Conjunctivitis is a highly contagious infection. It is easy to spread the crusty drainage that collects on eyelid margins from one eye to the other. When drainage is present wear clean gloves during the examination and perform proper hand hygiene before and after the eye examination.

Corneas. The cornea is the transparent, colorless part of the eye covering the pupil and iris. From a side view it looks like the crystal of a wristwatch. While the patient looks straight ahead, inspect the cornea for clarity and texture while shining a penlight obliquely across its entire surface. The cornea is normally shiny, transparent, and smooth. In older adults it loses its luster. Any irregularity in the surface indicates an abrasion or tear that requires further examination by a health care provider. Both conditions are very painful. Note the color and details of the underlying iris. In an older adult the iris becomes faded. A thin white ring along the margin of the iris, called an arcus senilis, is common with aging but is abnormal in anyone under age 40. To test for the corneal blink reflex, see the cranial nerve test section of this chapter.

TABLE 30.13   Nursing History for Eye Assessment

Assessment	Rationale
Determine whether patient has history of eye disease (e.g., glaucoma, retinopathy, cataracts), eye trauma, diabetes, hypertension, or eye surgery.	Some diseases or trauma cause risk for partial or complete visual loss. Patient may have had surgery for a visual disorder.
Determine problems that prompted patient to seek health care. Ask patient about eye pain, photophobia (sensitivity to light), burning or itching, excess tearing or crusting, diplopia (double vision) or blurred vision, awareness of a "film" or "curtain" over field of vision, floaters (small black spots that seem to float across field of vision), flashing lights, or halos around lights.	Common symptoms of eye disease indicate need for health care provider.
Determine whether there is family history of eye disorders or diseases.	Certain eye problems such as glaucoma or retinitis pigmentosa are inherited.
Review patient's occupational history and recreational hobbies. Are safety glasses worn?	Performance of close, intricate work causes eye fatigue. Working with computers causes eye strain. Certain occupational tasks (e.g., working with chemicals) and recreational activities (e.g., fencing, motorcycle riding) place people at risk for eye injury unless they take precautions.
Ask patient whether he or she wears glasses or contacts and, if so, how often.	Patients need to wear glasses or contacts during certain parts of examination for accurate assessment.
Determine when patient last visited ophthalmologist or optometrist.	Date of last eye examination reveals level of preventive care patient takes.
Assess medications patient is taking, including eyedrops or ointment.	Determines need to assess patient's knowledge of medications. Certain medications cause visual symptoms.

Pupils and Irises. Observe the pupils for size, shape, equality, accommodation, and reaction to light. They are normally black, round, regular, and equal in size (3 to 7 mm in diameter) (Fig. 30.13). The iris should be clearly visible.

Cloudy pupils indicate cataracts. Dilated pupils result from glaucoma, trauma, neurological disorders, eye medications (e.g., atropine), or withdrawal from opioids. Inflammation of the iris or use of drugs (e.g., pilocarpine, morphine, or cocaine) causes constricted pupils. Pinpoint pupils are a common sign of opioid intoxication. Shining a beam of light through the pupil and onto the retina stimulates the third cranial nerve, causing the muscles of the iris to constrict. Any abnormality along the nerve pathways from the retina to the iris alters the ability of the pupils to react to light. Changes in intracranial pressure, lesions along the nerve pathways, locally applied ophthalmic medications, and direct trauma to the eye alter pupillary reaction.

Test pupillary reflexes (to light and accommodation) in a dimly lit room. Instruct the patient to avoid looking directly at the light. While the patient looks straight ahead, bring a penlight from the side of his or her face, directing the light onto the pupil (Fig. 30.14). A directly illuminated pupil constricts, and the opposite pupil constricts consensually. Observe the quickness and equality of the reflex. Repeat the examination for the opposite eye.

To test for accommodation, ask the patient to gaze at a distant object (the far wall) and then at a test object (finger or pencil) held approximately 10 cm (4 inches) from the bridge of his or her nose. The pupils normally converge and accommodate by constricting when looking at close objects. The pupillary responses are equal. Testing for accommodation is important only if the patient has a defect in the pupillary response to light (Ball et al., 2019). If assessment of pupillary reaction is normal in all tests, record the abbreviation PERRLA (pupils equal, round, reactive to light, and accommodation).

Internal Eye Structures. The examination of the internal eye structures through the use of an ophthalmoscope is beyond the scope of new graduate nurses' practice. Advanced nurse practitioners use the ophthalmoscope to inspect the fundus (Fig. 30.15), which includes the retina, choroid, optic nerve disc, macula, fovea centralis, and retinal vessels. Patients in greatest need of an examination are those with diabetes, hypertension, and intracranial disorders.

Ears

The ear assessment determines the integrity of ear structures and hearing acuity. The three parts of the ear are the external, middle, and inner ear (Fig. 30.16). Inspect and palpate external ear structures, which consist of the auricle, outer ear canal, and tympanic membrane (eardrum). The ear canal is normally curved and approximately 2.5 cm (1 inch) long in an adult. It is lined with skin containing fine hairs, nerve endings, and glands secreting cerumen. The middle ear is inspected with an otoscope. It is an air-filled cavity containing the three bony ossicles (malleus, incus, and stapes). The eustachian tube connects the middle ear to the nasopharynx. Pressure between the outer atmosphere and the middle ear is stabilized through this tube. Finally, the inner ear is tested by measuring a patient's hearing acuity. The inner ear contains the cochlea, vestibule, and semicircular canals. Assessing the ears determines the integrity of ear structures and the condition of hearing. Use nursing history data to identify patients' risks for hearing disorders (Table 30.14).

Understanding the mechanisms for sound transmission helps identify the nature of hearing disorders. Sound travels through the ear by air and bone conduction. Nerve impulses from the cochlea travel to the auditory nerve (eighth cranial nerve) and the cerebral cortex. Disorders of the ear result from several types of problems, including mechanical dysfunction (blockage by cerumen or foreign body), trauma (foreign bodies or noise exposure), neurological disorders (auditory nerve damage), acute illnesses (viral infection), and toxic effects of medications.

Auricles. With the patient sitting comfortably, inspect the size, shape, symmetry, landmarks, position, and color of the auricle (Fig. 30.17). The auricles are normally of equal size and level with each other. The upper point of attachment is in a straight line with the lateral canthus, or corner of the eye. The position of the auricle is almost vertical. Ears that are low set or at an unusual angle are a sign of chromosomal abnormality such as Down syndrome. Ear color is usually the same as that of the face, without moles, cysts, deformities, or nodules. Redness is a sign of inflammation or fever. Extreme pallor indicates frostbite.

BOX 30.11 Common Eye and Vision Problems

Hyperopia
Hyperopia is farsightedness, a refractive error in which rays of light enter the eye and focus behind the retina. People are able to clearly see distant objects but not close objects.

Myopia
Myopia is nearsightedness, a refractive error in which rays of light enter the eye and focus in front of the retina. People are able to clearly see close objects but not distant objects.

Presbyopia
Presbyopia is impaired near vision in middle-age and older adults caused by loss of elasticity of the lens and associated with the aging process.

Retinopathy
Retinopathy is a noninflammatory eye disorder resulting from changes in retinal blood vessels. It is a leading cause of blindness.

Strabismus
Strabismus is a (congenital) condition in which both eyes do not focus on an object simultaneously; these eyes appear crossed. Impairment of the extraocular muscles or their nerve supply causes strabismus.

Cataracts
A cataract is an increased opacity of the lens, which blocks light rays from entering the eye. Cataracts sometimes develop slowly and progressively after age 35 or suddenly after trauma. They are one of the most common eye disorders. Most older adults (65 years old and older) have some evidence of visual impairment from cataracts.

Glaucoma
Glaucoma is intraocular structural damage resulting from elevated intraocular pressure. Obstruction of the outflow of aqueous humor causes this. Without treatment the disorder leads to blindness.

Macular Degeneration
Macular degeneration is associated with aging and results in severe loss of a patient's central vision. It is the leading cause of blindness and low vision in the United States in those 65 years of age and older (CDC, 2018b). There is no cure, but there are injections and laser treatments that may slow the progression.

BOX 30.12 PATIENT TEACHING

Eye Assessment

Objective
- Patient will follow recommendations for regular eye examinations and prevention of injury.

Teaching Strategies
- Explain recommended frequency for eye testing with a Snellen chart and examination (see Table 30.3).
- Describe the typical symptoms of eye disease.
- Instruct older adult to take the following precautions because of normal vision changes: avoid or use caution while driving at night, increase lighting in the home to reduce risk of falls, and paint the first and last steps of a staircase and the edge of each of the other steps a bright color to aid depth perception.
- Remind patient that wearing protective eyewear prevents injury from debris and splashes.

Evaluation
Use the principles of teach-back to evaluate patient/family caregiver learning:
- Tell me how often you should schedule an eye examination.
- Describe for me the symptoms you should watch for and when you should call the health care provider.
- Tell me what changes you are making in your home that will improve your safety.

Modified from Ball JW, et al: *Seidel's guide to physical examination*, ed 9, St Louis, 2019, Elsevier.

Make sure that the patient avoids moving the head during the examination to avoid damage to the canal and tympanic membrane. Infants and young children might need to be held securely to prevent movement. Lay infants supine with head turned to one side and arms held securely at the sides. Have young children sit on their parents' laps with their legs held between the parents' knees.

Turn on the otoscope by rotating the dial at the top of the handle. To insert the speculum properly, ask the patient to tip the head slightly toward the opposite shoulder. Hold the handle of the otoscope in the space between the thumb and index finger, supported on the middle finger. This leaves the ulnar side of the hand to rest against the patient's head, stabilizing the otoscope as you insert it into the canal (Ball et al., 2019). There are two ways to grip the otoscope: (1) hold the handle along the patient's face with the fingers against the face or neck, and (2) lightly brace the inverted otoscope against the side of the patient's head or cheek. This latter grip, used with children, prevents accidental movement of the otoscope deeper into the ear canal. Insert the scope while pulling the auricle upward and backward in the adult and older child (Fig. 30.18). This maneuver straightens the ear canal. For infants the auricle should be pulled down and back.

Insert the speculum slightly down and forward 1 to 1.5 cm (½ inch) into the ear canal. Take care not to scrape the sensitive lining, which is painful. The ear canal normally has little cerumen and is uniformly pink with tiny hairs in the outer third of the canal. Observe for color, discharge, scaling, lesions, foreign bodies, and cerumen. Normally cerumen is dry (light brown to gray and flaky) or moist (dark yellow or brown) and sticky. Dry cerumen is common in Asians and Native Americans (Ball et al., 2019). A reddened canal with discharge is a sign of inflammation or infection. In other adults accumulated cerumen is a common problem; buildup creates a mild hearing loss. During the examination ask the patient about methods he or she uses to clean the ear canal (Box 30.13).

Palpate the auricles for texture, tenderness, and skin lesions. Auricles are normally smooth and without lesions. If a patient has pain, gently pull the auricle, press on the tragus, and palpate behind the ear over the mastoid process. If palpating the external ear increases the pain, an external ear infection is likely. If palpating the auricle and tragus does not influence the pain, the patient may have a middle ear infection. Tenderness in the mastoid area indicates mastoiditis.

Inspect the opening of the ear canal for size and presence of discharge. If discharge is present, wear clean gloves. A swollen or occluded meatus is not normal. A yellow, waxy substance called cerumen is common. Yellow or green, foul-smelling discharge indicates infection or a foreign body.

Ear Canals and Eardrums. Observe the deeper structures of the external and middle ear with the use of an otoscope. A special ear speculum attaches to the handle of the ophthalmoscope. For best visualization select the largest speculum that fits comfortably in the patient's ear. Before inserting the speculum, check for foreign bodies in the opening of the auditory canal.

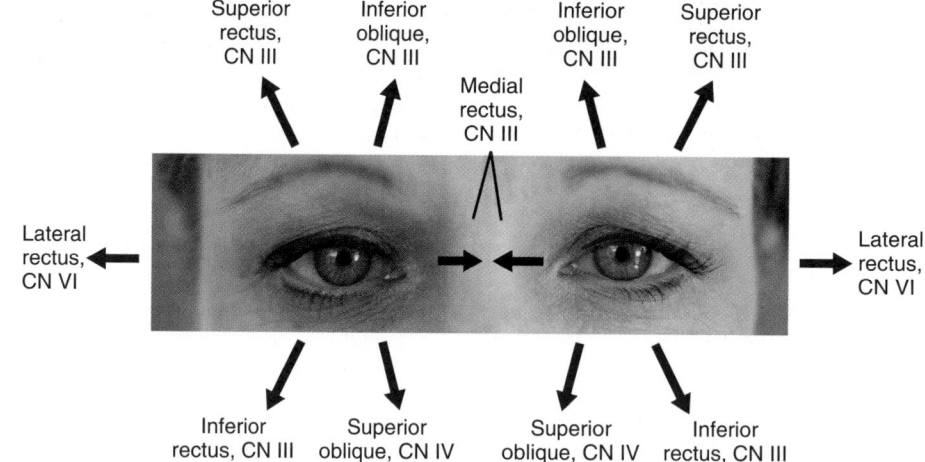

FIG. 30.11 Six directions of gaze. Direct patient to follow finger movement through each gaze. *CN,* Cranial nerve.

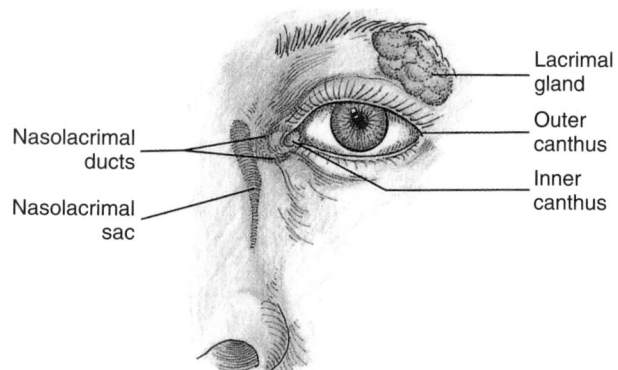

FIG. 30.12 The lacrimal apparatus secretes and drains tears, which moisten and lubricate eye structures.

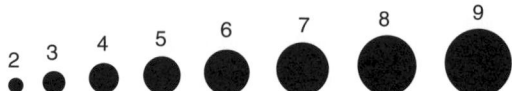

FIG. 30.13 Chart depicting pupillary size in millimeters.

The light from the otoscope allows visualization of the tympanic membrane. Know the common anatomical landmarks and their appearances (Fig. 30.19). Gently move the otoscope so that the entire tympanic membrane and its periphery are visible. Because the tympanic membrane is angled away from the ear canal, the light from the otoscope appears as a cone shape rather than a circle. A ring of fibrous cartilage surrounds the oval membrane. The umbo is near the center of the membrane, behind which is the attachment of the malleus. The underlying short process of the malleus creates a knoblike structure at the top of the drum. Check carefully to make sure that there are no tears or breaks in the membrane. The normal tympanic membrane is translucent, shiny, and pearly gray. It is free from tears or breaks. A pink or red bulging membrane indicates inflammation. A white color reveals pus behind it. The membrane is taut, except for the small triangular pars flaccida near the top. If cerumen is blocking the tympanic membrane, warm water irrigation safely removes the wax.

Hearing Acuity. A patient with a hearing loss often fails to respond to conversation. The three types of hearing loss are conduction,

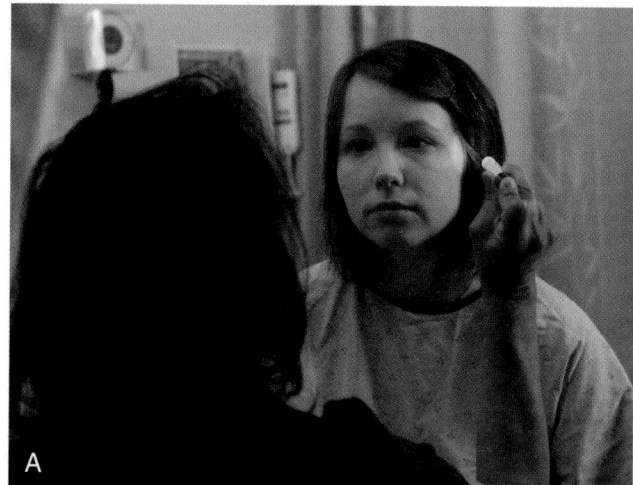

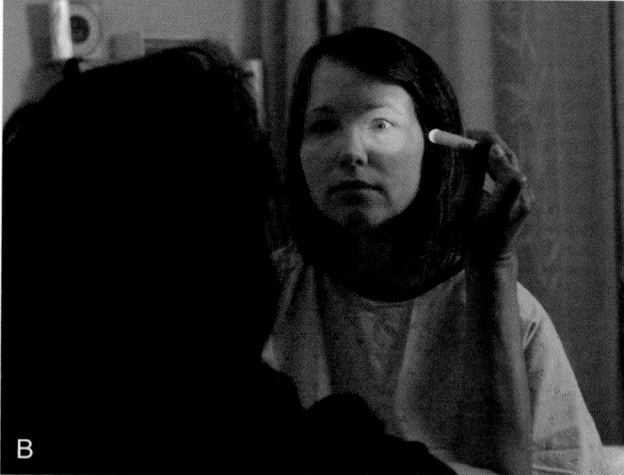

FIG. 30.14 **A,** To check pupillary reflexes the nurse first holds penlight to side of patient's face. **B,** Illumination of pupil causes pupillary constriction.

sensorineural, and mixed. A conduction loss interrupts sound waves as they travel from the outer ear to the cochlea of the inner ear because the sound waves are not transmitted through the outer and middle ear structures. Causes of a conduction loss include swelling of the auditory canal and tears in the tympanic membrane. A sensorineural loss involves the inner ear, auditory nerve, or hearing center of the brain. Sound is conducted through the outer and middle ear structures, but the continued transmission of sound becomes interrupted at some point beyond the bony ossicles. A mixed loss involves a combination of conduction and sensorineural loss. Patients working or living around loud noises and those who listen to loud music are at risk for hearing loss.

Older adults experience an inability to hear high-frequency sounds and consonants (e.g., *S, Z, T,* and *G*). Deterioration of the cochlea and thickening of the tympanic membrane cause older adults to gradually lose hearing acuity. They are especially at risk for hearing loss caused by **ototoxicity** (injury to auditory nerve) resulting from high maintenance doses of antibiotics (e.g., aminoglycosides).

To conduct a hearing assessment, have the patient remove any hearing aid if worn. Note his or her response to questions. Normally he or she responds without excessive requests to have the questions repeated. If a hearing loss is suspected, check the patient's response to the whispered voice. Test one ear at a time while the patient occludes the other ear with a finger. Ask him or her to gently move the finger up and down during the test in response to the whispered sound. While standing 31 to 60 cm (1 to 2 feet) from the testing ear, speak while covering the mouth so that the patient is unable to read lips. After exhaling fully, whisper softly toward the unoccluded ear, reciting random numbers with equally accented syllables, such as *nine-four-ten*. If necessary, gradually increase voice intensity until the patient correctly repeats the numbers. Then test the other ear for comparison. Ball et al. (2019) report that patients normally hear numbers clearly when whispered, responding correctly at least 50% of the time.

If a hearing loss is present, test the hearing using a tuning fork. A tuning fork of 256 to 512 hertz (Hz) is most commonly used. The

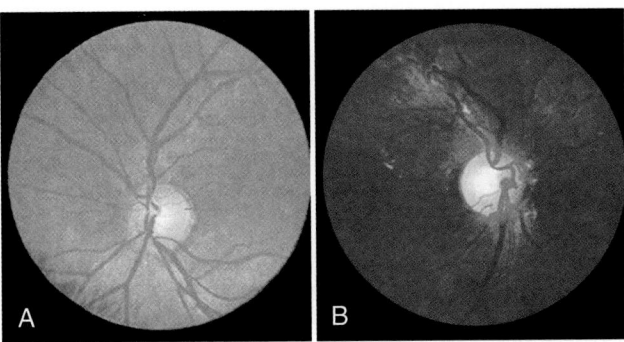

FIG. 30.15 Fundus of white patient (**A**) and black patient (**B**). (Courtesy of MEDCOM, Cypress, CA.)

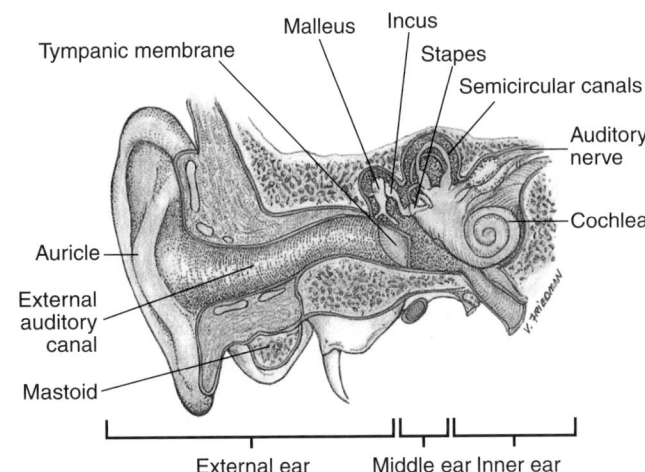

FIG. 30.16 Structures of external, middle, and inner ear.

TABLE 30.14 Nursing History for Ear Assessment	
Assessment	**Rationale**
Ask whether patient has experienced ear pain, itching, discharge, vertigo, tinnitus (ringing in ears), or change in hearing.	These signs and symptoms indicate infection or hearing loss.
Assess risks for hearing problem. *Infants/children:* Hypoxia at birth, meningitis, birth weight less than 1500 g, family history of hearing loss, congenital anomalies of skull or face, nonbacterial intrauterine infections (rubella, herpes), maternal drug use, excessively high bilirubin, head trauma *Adolescents:* Frequent exposure to loud music from concerts, car radios, and cell phone or iPods while wearing headphone, earbuds, or other devices *Adults:* Exposure to industrial or recreational noise, genetic disease (Ménière's disease), neurodegenerative disorder	Risk factors predispose patient to permanent hearing loss. It is difficult to assess infant's hearing status with examination only.
Determine patient's exposure to loud noises at work and availability of protective devices.	Prolonged noise exposure causes temporary or permanent hearing loss.
Note behaviors indicative of hearing loss such as failure to respond when spoken to, requests to repeat comments, leaning forward to hear, and child's inattentiveness or use of a monotonous voice tone.	People with hearing loss cope with sensory deficit through a variety of behavioral cues.
Assess whether patient takes large doses of aspirin or other ototoxic drugs (e.g., aminoglycosides, furosemide, streptomycin, cisplatin, ethacrynic acid).	Medications have side effects of hearing loss.
Determine whether patient uses hearing aid.	Determination allows you to assess patient's ability to care for device and adjust voice tone to communicate.
If patient had recent hearing problem, note onset, contributing factors, affected ear, and effect on activities of daily living.	Helps determine nature and severity of hearing problem.
Determine whether patient has repeated history of cerumen buildup in ear.	Cerumen impaction is common cause for conduction deafness.

tuning fork allows for comparison of hearing by bone conduction with that of air conduction. Hold the base of the tuning fork with one hand without touching the tines. Tap the fork lightly against the palm of the other hand to set it in vibration (Table 30.15).

Nose and Sinuses

Use inspection and palpation to assess the integrity of the nose and sinuses. The patient sits during the examination. A penlight allows for gross examination of each naris. A more detailed examination requires use of a nasal speculum to inspect the deeper nasal turbinates. Do not use a speculum unless a qualified practitioner such as a nurse educator or an advanced practice nurse is present. Table 30.16 lists components of the nursing history.

Nose. When inspecting the external nose, observe for shape, size, skin color, and the presence of deformity or inflammation. The nose is normally smooth and symmetrical with the same skin color as the face. Recent trauma sometimes causes edema and discoloration. If swelling or deformities exist, gently palpate the ridge and soft tissue of the nose by placing one finger on each side of the nasal arch and gently moving the fingers from the nasal bridge to the tip. Note any tenderness, masses, or underlying deviations. Nasal structures are usually firm and stable.

Air normally passes freely through the nose when a person breathes. To assess patency of the nares, place a finger on the side of the patient's nose and occlude one naris. Ask the patient to breathe with the mouth closed. Repeat the procedure for the other naris.

While illuminating the anterior nares, inspect the mucosa for color, lesions, discharge, swelling, and evidence of bleeding. If discharge is present, apply gloves. Normal mucosa is pink and moist without lesions. Pale mucosa with clear discharge indicates allergy. A mucoid discharge indicates rhinitis. An infection (viral or bacterial) results in yellowish or greenish discharge. Habitual use of intranasal cocaine and opioids causes puffiness and increased vascularity of the nasal mucosa. For the patient with a nasogastric tube, routinely check for local skin breakdown (excoriation) of the naris, characterized by redness and skin sloughing.

To view the septum and turbinates, have the patient tip the head back slightly to provide a clear view. Illuminate the septum and observe for alignment, perforation, or bleeding. Normally the septum is close to the midline and thicker anteriorly than posteriorly. The turbinates are covered with mucous membranes that warm and moisten inspired air. Normal mucosa is pink and moist, without lesions. A deviated septum obstructs breathing and interferes with passage of a nasogastric tube. Perforation of the septum often occurs after repeated use of intranasal cocaine. Note any polyps (tumorlike growths) or purulent drainage.

Sinuses. Examination of the sinuses involves palpation. In cases of allergies or infection, the interior of the sinuses becomes inflamed and swollen. The most effective way to assess for tenderness is by externally palpating the frontal and maxillary facial areas (Fig. 30.20). Palpate the frontal sinus by exerting pressure with the thumb up and under the

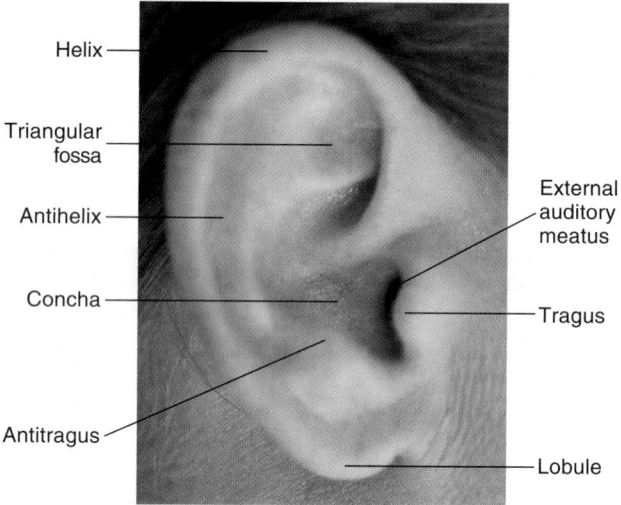

FIG. 30.17 Anatomical structures of auricle.

Helix — Triangular fossa — Antihelix — Concha — Antitragus — External auditory meatus — Tragus — Lobule

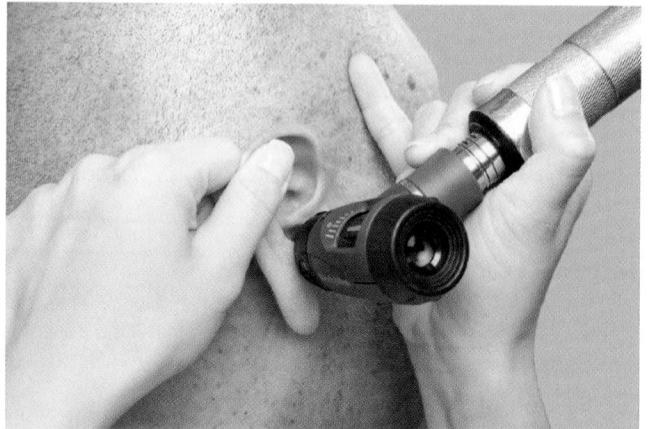

FIG. 30.18 Otoscopic examination. (From Wilson S, Giddens J: *Health assessment for nursing practice*, ed 6, St Louis, 2016, Elsevier.)

BOX 30.13 PATIENT TEACHING
Ear Assessment

Objective
- Patient will follow preventive guidelines for screening of hearing loss and proper cleaning technique for the ears.

Teaching Strategies
- Explain that noise-induced hearing loss can lead to communication difficulties, learning difficulties, pain or ringing in the ears (tinnitus), distorted or muffled hearing, and an inability to hear some environmental sounds and warning signals.
- Encourage patients to adopt behaviors to protect their hearing (CDC, 2017):
  - Avoid or limit exposure to excessively loud sounds.
  - Turn down the volume of music systems.
  - Move away from the source of loud sounds when possible.
  - Use hearing protection devices when it is not feasible to avoid exposure to loud sounds or to reduce them to a safe level.
- Instruct patient in the proper way to clean the outer ear (see Chapter 40), avoiding use of cotton-tipped applicators and sharp objects such as hairpins, which cause impaction of cerumen deep in the ear canal or trauma.
- Tell patient to avoid inserting pointed objects into the ear canal.
- Encourage patients over age 65 to have regular hearing checks. Explain that a reduction in hearing is a normal part of aging (see Chapter 49).
- Instruct family members of patients with hearing loss to avoid shouting; to speak in slower, low tones; and to be sure that the patient is able to see the speaker's face.

Evaluation
Use the principles of teach-back to evaluate patient/family caregiver learning:
- Describe two ways to protect hearing while you are home.
- Show me how you will safely clean your ears.
- Tell me how often you will get your hearing checked.

patient's eyebrow. Gentle, upward pressure elicits tenderness easily if sinus irritation is present. Do not apply pressure to the eyes. If sinus tenderness is present, the sinuses may be transilluminated. However, this procedure requires advanced experience. Box 30.14 describes teaching guidelines during nose and sinus assessment.

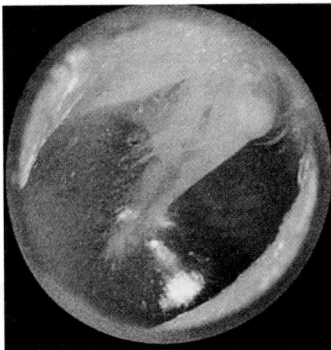

FIG. 30.19 Normal right tympanic membrane. (Courtesy Dr. Richard A. Buckingham, Abraham Lincoln School of Medicine, University of Illinois, Chicago.)

Mouth and Pharynx

Assess the mouth and pharynx to detect signs of overall health. Determine a patient's oral hygiene needs and therapies needed if he or she has dehydration, restricted intake, oral trauma, or oral airway obstruction. To assess the oral cavity, use a penlight and tongue depressor or gauze square. Wear clean gloves during the examination. Have the patient sit or lie down. Assess the oral cavity also while administering oral hygiene (see Chapter 40). Table 30.17 describes the nursing history for assessment of the mouth and pharynx.

Lips. Inspect the lips for color, texture, hydration, contour, and lesions. With the patient's mouth closed, view the lips from end to end. Normally they are pink, moist, symmetrical, and smooth (Fig. 30.21). Lip color in a patient with dark skin varies from pink to plum. Have female patients remove their lipstick before the examination. Anemia causes pallor of the lips, with cyanosis caused by respiratory or cardiovascular problems. Cherry-colored lips indicate carbon monoxide poisoning. When you inspect any lesion, consider the potential of it being an infection, irritation, or skin cancer.

TABLE 30.15 Tuning Fork Tests

Tests and Steps	Rationale
Weber's Test (Lateralization of Sound) Hold fork at its base and tap it lightly against heel of palm. Place base of vibrating fork on midline vertex of patient's head or middle of forehead (see illustration *A*). Ask patient whether he or she hears the sound equally in both ears or better in one ear (lateralization).	Patient with normal hearing hears sound equally in both ears. In conduction deafness sound is heard best in impaired ear. In sensorineural hearing loss, sound is heard better in normal ear.
Rinne Test (Comparison of Air and Bone Conduction) Place stem of vibrating tuning fork against patient's mastoid process (see illustration *B*). Begin counting the interval with your watch. Ask patient to tell you when he or she no longer hears the sound; note number of seconds. Quickly place still-vibrating tines 1 to 2 cm (½ to 1 inch) from ear canal and ask patient to tell you when he or she no longer hears the sound (see illustration *C*). Continue counting time the sound is heard by air conduction. Compare number of seconds the sound is heard by bone conduction versus air conduction.	Patient should hear air-conducted sound twice as long as bone-conducted sound (2:1 ratio). For example, if patient hears bone-conducted sound for 10 seconds, he or she should hear air-conducted sound for an additional 10 seconds. In conduction deafness patient hears bone conduction longer than air conduction in affected ear. In sensorineural loss patient hears air conduction longer than bone conduction in affected ear, but at less than a 2:1 ratio (Ball et al., 2019).

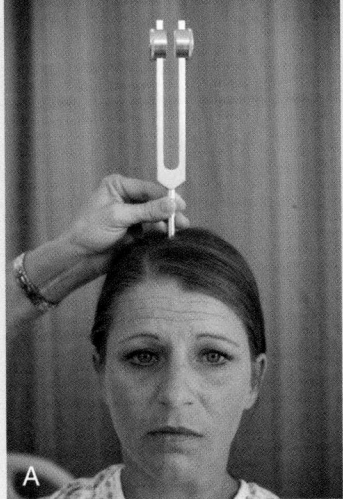

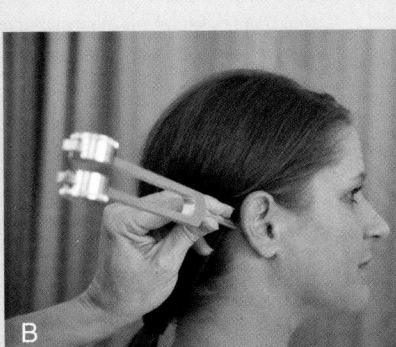

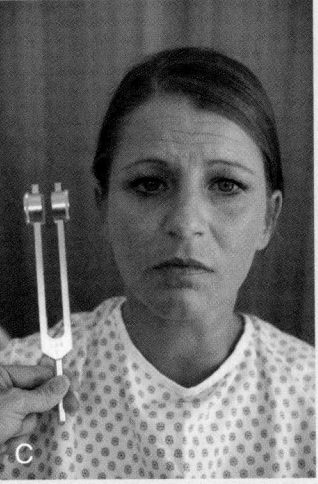

Buccal Mucosa, Gums, and Teeth. Ask the patient to clench the teeth and smile to observe teeth occlusion. The upper molars normally rest directly on the lower molars, and the upper incisors slightly override the lower incisors. A symmetrical smile reveals normal facial nerve function.

Inspect the teeth to determine the quality of dental hygiene (Box 30.15). Note the position and alignment of the teeth. To examine the posterior surface of the teeth, have the patient open the mouth with the lips relaxed. Use a tongue depressor to retract the lips and cheeks, especially when viewing the molars. Note the color of teeth and presence of dental caries (cavities), tartar, and extraction sites. Normal, healthy teeth are smooth, white, and shiny. A chalky white discoloration of the enamel is an early indication of caries formation. Brown or black discolorations indicate the formation of caries. A stained yellow color is from tobacco use; coffee, tea, and colas cause a brown stain. In the older adult loose or missing teeth are common because bone resorption increases. An older adult's teeth often feel rough when tooth enamel calcifies. Yellow or darkened teeth are also common in the older adult because of the general wear and tear that exposes the darker underlying dentin.

To view the mucosa and gums, ask the patient to first remove any dental appliance. View the inner oral mucosa by having the patient open and relax the mouth slightly and then gently retract his or her

lower lip away from the teeth (Fig. 30.22). Repeat this process for the upper lip. Inspect the mucosa for color; hydration; texture; and lesions such as ulcers, abrasions, or cysts. Normally the mucosa is glistening, pink, smooth, and moist. Some common small, yellow-white raised lesions on the buccal mucosa and lips are Fordyce spots, or ectopic sebaceous glands (Ball et al., 2019). If lesions are present, palpate them gently with a gloved hand for tenderness, size, and consistency.

To inspect the buccal mucosa, ask the patient to open the mouth and then gently retract the cheeks with a tongue depressor (Fig. 30.23). View the surface of the mucosa from right to left and top to bottom. A penlight illuminates the most posterior part of the mucosa. Normal mucosa is glistening, pink, soft, moist, and smooth. Varying shades of hyperpigmentation are normal in 10% of whites after age 50 and as many as 90% of blacks by the same age. For patients with

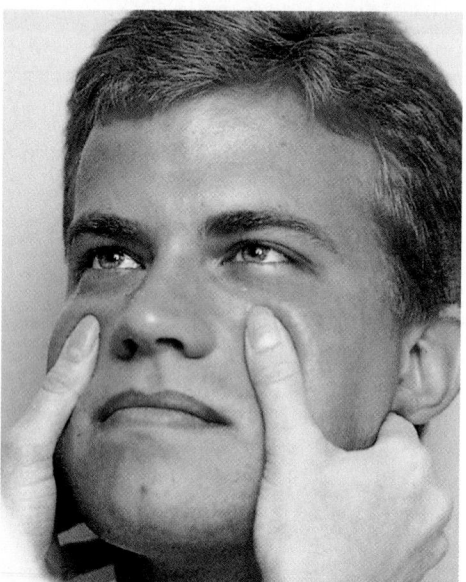

FIG. 30.20 Palpation of maxillary sinuses.

BOX 30.14 **Patient Teaching**

Nose and Sinus Assessment

Objective
- Patient will explain self-care measures to address and minimize loss of olfaction.

Teaching Strategies
- Caution patient against overuse of over-the-counter nasal sprays, which leads to "rebound" effect, causing excess nasal congestion.
- Instruct parents in care of a child with nosebleeds: have child sit up and lean forward to avoid aspiration of blood, apply pressure to the anterior nose with the thumb and forefinger as the child breathes through the mouth, and apply ice or a cold cloth to the bridge of the nose if pressure fails to stop bleeding.
- Instruct older adults with loss of olfaction to follow safety precautions:
  - Install smoke detectors on each floor of their home.
  - Ask others to advise them when food smells pungent.
- Instruct older adults to always check dated labels on food to ensure against spoilage.

Evaluation
Use the principles of teach-back to evaluate patient/family caregiver learning:
- Show me how you will instill the nasal spray you purchased at the pharmacy.
- Show me the techniques that you will use to stop a nosebleed.
- Show me the smoke detector locations in your home and how you check to make sure they are working properly.

TABLE 30.16	Nursing History for Nose and Sinus Assessment
Assessment	**Rationale**
Ask whether patient has had trauma to nose.	Trauma causes septal deviation and asymmetry of external nose.
Ask whether patient has history of allergies, nasal discharge, epistaxis (nosebleeds), or postnasal drip.	History is useful in determining source or nature of nasal and sinus drainage.
If there is history of nasal discharge, assess color, amount, odor, duration, and associated symptoms (e.g., sneezing, nasal congestion, obstruction, or mouth breathing).	Aids in ruling out presence of infection, allergy, or drug use.
Assess for history of nosebleed, including site, frequency, amount of bleeding, treatment, and difficulty stopping bleeding.	Characteristics sometimes reveal trauma, medication use, or excessive dryness as causative factors.
Ask whether patient uses nasal spray or drops, including amount, frequency, and duration of use.	Overuse of over-the-counter nasal preparations causes physical change in mucosa.
Ask whether patient snores at night or has difficulty breathing.	Difficulty breathing or snoring indicates septal deviation or obstruction.

TABLE 30.17 Nursing History for Mouth and Pharyngeal Assessment

Assessment	Rationale
Determine whether patient wears dentures or retainers and whether they are comfortable.	Patient needs to remove dentures to visualize and palpate gums. Ill-fitting dentures chronically irritate mucosa and gums.
Determine whether patient has had recent change in appetite or weight.	Symptoms result from painful mouth conditions or poor hygiene.
Determine whether patient uses tobacco products: • Smoking cigarettes, cigars, or pipe; smokeless tobacco; chewing tobacco and snuff • E-cigarettes or vapor cigarettes	Tobacco use in any form (smoked and smokeless) increases the risk for oral-pharyngeal cancer (ACS, 2018b). Long-term smokeless tobacco users have an increased risk for cancer of the gums and cheeks (ACS, 2018b). Electronic nicotine delivery systems (e-cigarettes) are on the rise in adolescence and may contribute to the use of combustible tobacco products because the flavorings desensitize the lungs' negative response to nicotine inhalation (ACS, 2018b; Cancer.Net, 2018).
Review history for alcohol consumption.	Oral and pharyngeal cancers are more common in people who use alcohol. Those who both smoke and drink have a 15 times greater risk of developing oral cancer than others (ACS, 2018b; Oral Cancer Foundation, 2018).
Assess dental hygiene practices, including use of fluoride toothpaste, frequency of brushing and flossing, and frequency of dental visits.	Assessment reveals patient's need for education and/or financial support. Periodontal disease has a higher prevalence in older adults who have history of high plaque buildup, use tobacco, and visit the dentist infrequently.
Ask whether patient has pain from chewing or eating. If so, ask whether mouth lesions are present, including duration and associated symptoms.	Pain is often associated with broken tooth, teeth grinding, or temporomandibular joint problems. Extra care is needed during oral hygiene administration.
Review a patient's medical history for a previous diagnosis of the human papilloma virus (HPV).	HPV, particularly HPV16, has been definitively implicated as a risk for oral cancers, particularly those that occur in the back of the mouth (oropharynx, base of tongue, tonsillar pillars and crypt, and the tonsils themselves) (Oral Cancer Foundation, 2018; ACS, 2018b).

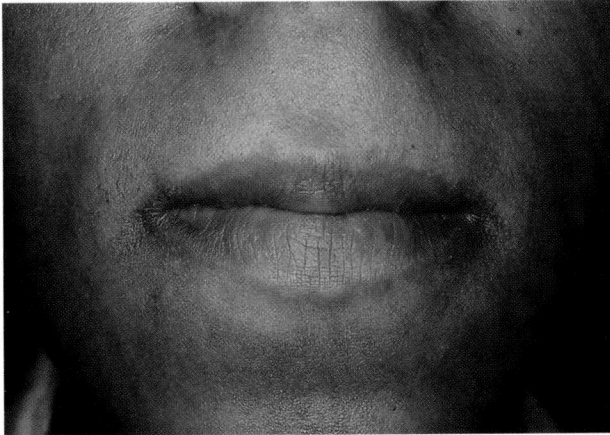

FIG. 30.21 Lips are normally pink, symmetrical, smooth, and moist.

normal pigmentation, the buccal mucosa is a good site to inspect for jaundice and pallor. In older adults the mucosa is normally dry because of reduced salivation. Thick white patches (leukoplakia) are often a precancerous lesion seen in heavy smokers and alcoholics. Palpate for any buccal lesions by placing the index finger within the buccal cavity and the thumb on the outer surface of the cheek. Patients who smoke cigarettes, cigars, or pipes and those who use smokeless tobacco have an increased risk of oral, pharyngeal, laryngeal, and esophageal cancer. These individuals may have leukoplakia or other lesions anywhere in their oral cavity (e.g., lips, gums, or tongue) at an early age. These usually appear as cream-white patches throughout the inner mouth area.

Inspect the gums (gingivae) for color, edema, retraction, bleeding, and lesions while retracting the cheeks. Healthy gums are pink, smooth, and moist and fit tightly around each tooth. Patients with dark skin often have patchy pigmentation. In older adults the gums are usually pale. Using clean gloves, palpate the gums to assess for lesions,

BOX 30.15 PATIENT TEACHING

Mouth and Pharyngeal Assessment

Objective
- Patient will practice proper oral hygiene/dental care measures and identify symptoms of oral cancer.

Teaching Strategies
- Discuss proper techniques for oral hygiene, including brushing and flossing (see Chapter 40).
- Explain the early warning signs of oral cavity and pharynx cancer that should be checked by a health care professional, including a mouth sore that bleeds easily and does not heal, a lump or thickening in the cheek, a white or red patch on the mucosa that persists, a sore throat or a feeling that something is caught in the throat, numbness of the tongue or other area of the mouth, or a swelling of the jaw that causes dentures to not fit (Oral Cancer Foundation, 2018).
- Late symptoms of oral cancer are difficulty in chewing, swallowing, or moving the tongue or jaw (ACS, 2018b).
- Encourage regular dental examination every 6 months for children, adults, and older adults.

Evaluation
Use the principles of teach-back to evaluate patient/family caregiver learning:
- Show me the technique you use to brush your teeth.
- Explain to me how often you should have regular dental checkups.
- Tell me the warning signs of mouth cancer and when you should call the health care provider.

thickening, or masses. Normally there is no tenderness. Spongy gums that bleed easily indicate periodontal disease and vitamin C deficiency. If a patient has loose or mobile teeth, swollen gums, or pockets containing debris at the tooth margins, a dental referral is necessary to check for periodontal disease or gingivitis.

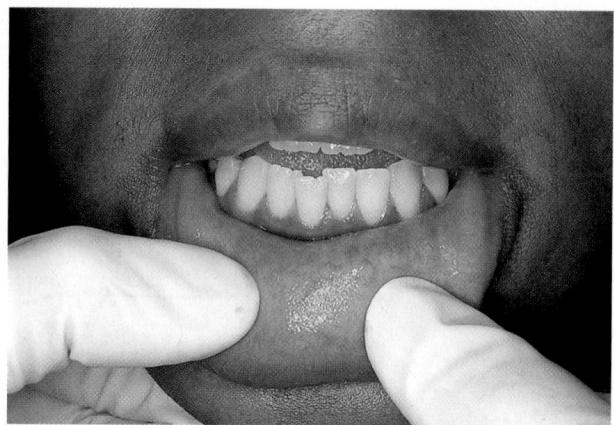

FIG. 30.22 Inspection of inner oral mucosa of lower lip.

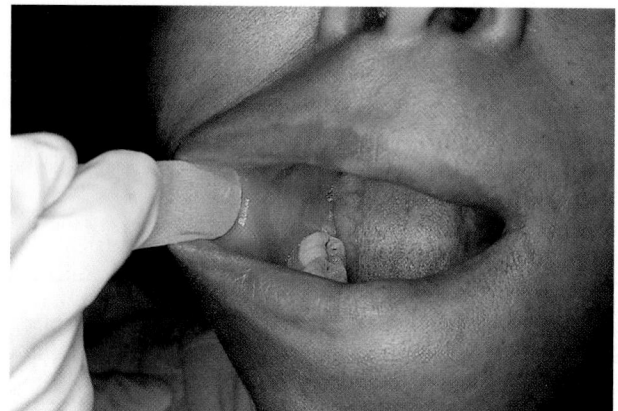

FIG. 30.23 Retraction of buccal mucosa allows for clear visualization.

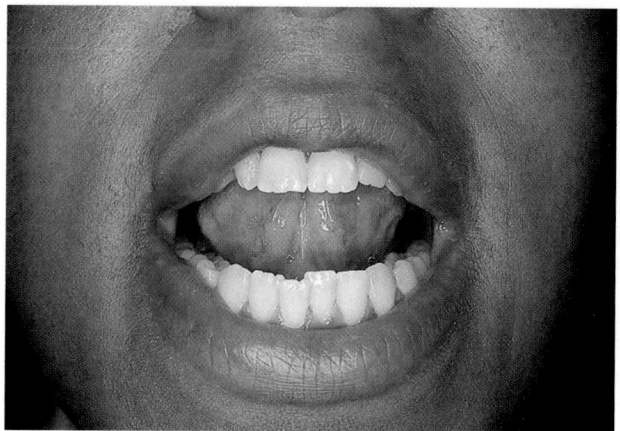

FIG. 30.24 Undersurface of tongue is highly vascular.

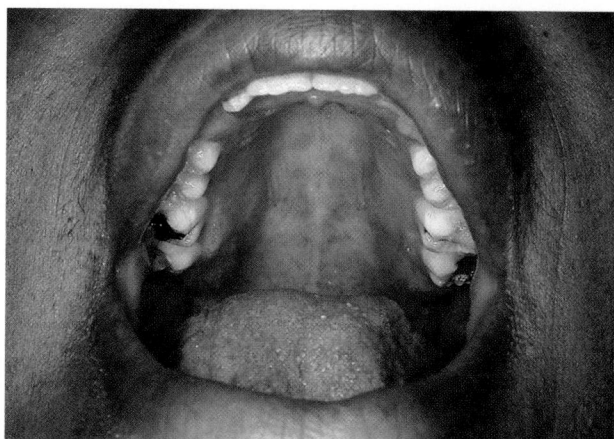

FIG. 30.25 Hard palate is located anteriorly in roof of mouth.

Tongue and Floor of Mouth. Carefully inspect the tongue on all sides and the floor of the mouth. Have the patient relax the mouth and stick the tongue out halfway. Note any deviation, tremor, or limitation in movement. This tests hypoglossal nerve function. If a patient protrudes the tongue too far, it elicits the gag reflex. When the tongue protrudes, it lays midline. To test for tongue mobility, ask the patient to raise it up and move it from side to side. It should move freely.

Using a penlight for illumination, examine the tongue for color, size, position, texture, and coatings or lesions. A normal tongue is medium or dull red in color, moist, slightly rough on the top surface, and smooth along the lateral margins. The undersurface of the tongue and the floor of the mouth are highly vascular (Fig. 30.24). Take extra care to inspect this area, a common site for oral cancer lesions. The patient lifts the tongue by placing its tip on the palate behind the upper incisors. Inspect for color, swelling, and lesions such as nodules or cysts. The ventral surface of the tongue is pink and smooth, with large veins between the frenulum folds. To palpate the tongue, explain the procedure and ask the patient to protrude it. Grasp the tip with a gauze square and gently pull it to one side. With a gloved hand palpate the full length of the tongue and the base for any areas of hardening or ulceration. Varicosities (swollen, tortuous veins) are common in the older adult and rarely cause problems.

Palate. Have the patient extend the head backward, holding the mouth open to inspect the hard and soft palates. The hard palate, or roof of the mouth, is located anteriorly. The whitish hard palate is dome shaped. The soft palate extends posteriorly toward the pharynx. It is normally light pink and smooth. Observe the palates for color, shape, texture,

and extra bony prominences or defects (Fig. 30.25). A bony growth, or exostosis, between the two palates is common.

Pharynx. Perform an examination of pharyngeal structures to rule out infection, inflammation, or lesions. Have the patient tip the head back slightly, open the mouth wide, and say "ah" while you place the tip of a tongue depressor on the middle third of the tongue. Take care not to press the lower lip against the teeth. By placing the tongue depressor too far anteriorly, the posterior part of the tongue mounds up, obstructing the view. Placing the tongue depressor on the posterior tongue elicits the gag reflex.

With a penlight first inspect the uvula and soft palate (Fig. 30.26). Both structures, which are innervated by the tenth cranial (vagus) nerve, should rise centrally as the patient says "ah." Examine the anterior and posterior pillars, soft palate, and uvula. View the tonsils in the cavities between the anterior and posterior pillars and note the presence or absence of tissue. The posterior pharynx is behind the pillars. Normally pharyngeal tissues are pink and smooth and well hydrated. Small irregular spots of lymphatic tissue and small blood vessels are normal. Note edema, petechiae (small hemorrhages), lesions, or exudate. Patients with chronic sinus problems frequently exhibit a clear exudate that drains along the wall of the posterior pharynx. Yellow or green exudate indicates infection. A patient with a typical sore throat has a red and edematous uvula and tonsillar pillars with possible presence of yellow exudate.

Neck

Assessment of the neck includes assessing the neck muscles, lymph nodes of the head and neck, carotid arteries, jugular veins, thyroid gland, and

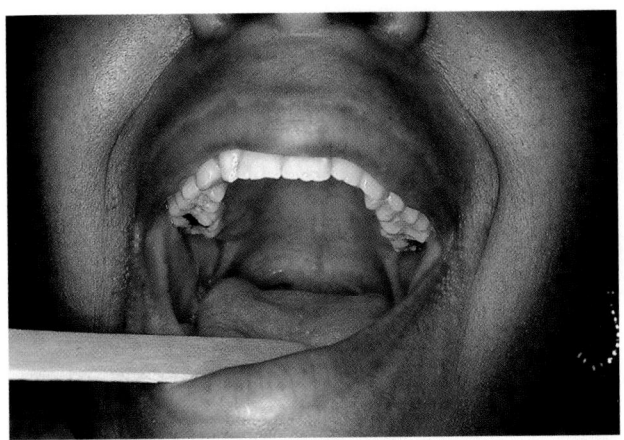

FIG. 30.26 Penlight and tongue depressor allow visualization of uvula and posterior soft palate.

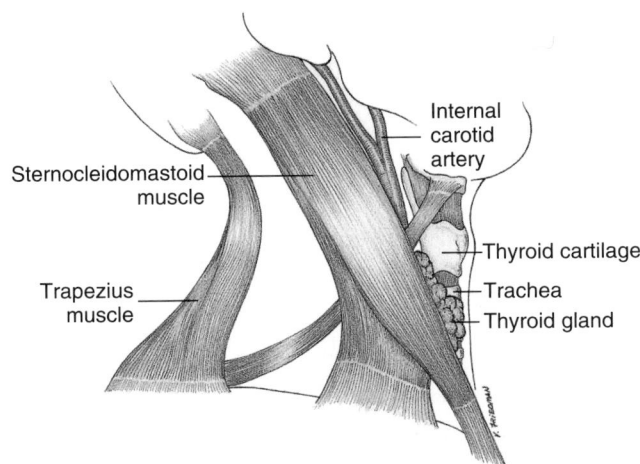

FIG. 30.27 Anatomical position of major neck structures. Note triangles formed by sternocleidomastoid muscle, lower jaw, and anterior neck anteriorly and sternocleidomastoid muscle, trapezius muscle, and lower neck posteriorly.

trachea (Fig. 30.27). You may postpone the examination of the jugular veins and carotid arteries until the vascular system assessment. Inspect and palpate the neck to determine the integrity of its structures and examine the lymphatic system. An abnormality of superficial lymph nodes sometimes reveals the presence of an infection or malignancy. Examine the lymphatic system region by region during the assessment of other body systems (head and neck, breast, genitalia, and extremities). Examination of the thyroid gland and trachea also aids in ruling out malignancies. Perform this examination with the patient sitting. The sternocleidomastoid and trapezius muscles outline the areas of the neck, dividing each side of the neck into two triangles. The anterior triangle contains the trachea, thyroid gland, carotid artery, and anterior cervical lymph nodes. The posterior triangle contains the posterior lymph nodes. Table 30.18 reviews the nursing history for the head and neck examination.

Neck Muscles. First inspect the neck in the usual anatomical position, with slight hyperextension. Observe for symmetry of the neck muscles. Ask the patient to flex the neck with the chin to the chest, hyperextend the neck backward, and move the head laterally to each side and then sideways with the ear moving toward the shoulder. This tests the sternocleidomastoid and trapezius muscles. The neck normally moves without discomfort. Perform other tests for muscle strength and function during assessment of the musculoskeletal system.

Lymph Nodes. An extensive system of lymph nodes collects lymph from the head, ears, nose, cheeks, and lips (Fig. 30.28). The immune system protects the body from foreign antigens, removes damaged cells from the circulation, and provides a partial barrier to growth of malignant cells within the body. Assessing the lymph nodes requires competence when caring for patients with a compromised immune system, which is often linked to allergies, human immunodeficiency virus (HIV) infection, autoimmune disease (e.g., lupus erythematosus), or serious infection.

With the patient's chin raised and head tilted slightly, first inspect the area where lymph nodes are distributed and compare both sides. This position stretches the skin slightly over any possible enlarged nodes. Inspect visible nodes for edema, erythema, or red streaks. Nodes normally are not visible.

Use a methodical approach to palpate the lymph nodes to avoid overlooking any single node or chain. The patient relaxes with the neck flexed slightly forward. Inspect and palpate both sides of the neck for

TABLE 30.18 Nursing History for Neck Assessment

Assessment	Rationale
Assess for history of recent cold, infection, or enlarged lymph nodes or exposure to radiation or toxic chemicals.	Colds or infections cause temporary or permanent lymph node enlargement. Lymph nodes are also enlarged in various diseases such as cancer.
If there is an enlarged lymph node, consider reviewing history of intravenous drug use, hemophilia, sexual contact with people infected with human immunodeficiency virus (HIV), history of blood transfusion, multiple and indiscriminate sexual contacts, or male with homosexual or bisexual activities.	These are risk factors for HIV infection.
Ask whether patient has had history of neck pain with restriction in movement.	This indicates muscle strain, head injury, local nerve injury, or enlarged or swollen lymph node.
Ask whether patient has had change in temperature preference (more or less clothing); swelling in neck; change in texture of hair, skin, or nails; or change in emotional stability.	Symptoms indicate thyroid disease.
Ask whether patient has history of hypothyroidism or hyperthyroidism, takes thyroid medication, or has a family history of thyroid disease.	Disease or medications influence tissue growth of gland.
Review medical history of pneumothorax (collapsed lung) or bronchial tumor.	Conditions place patient at risk for tracheal displacement or lateral deviation.

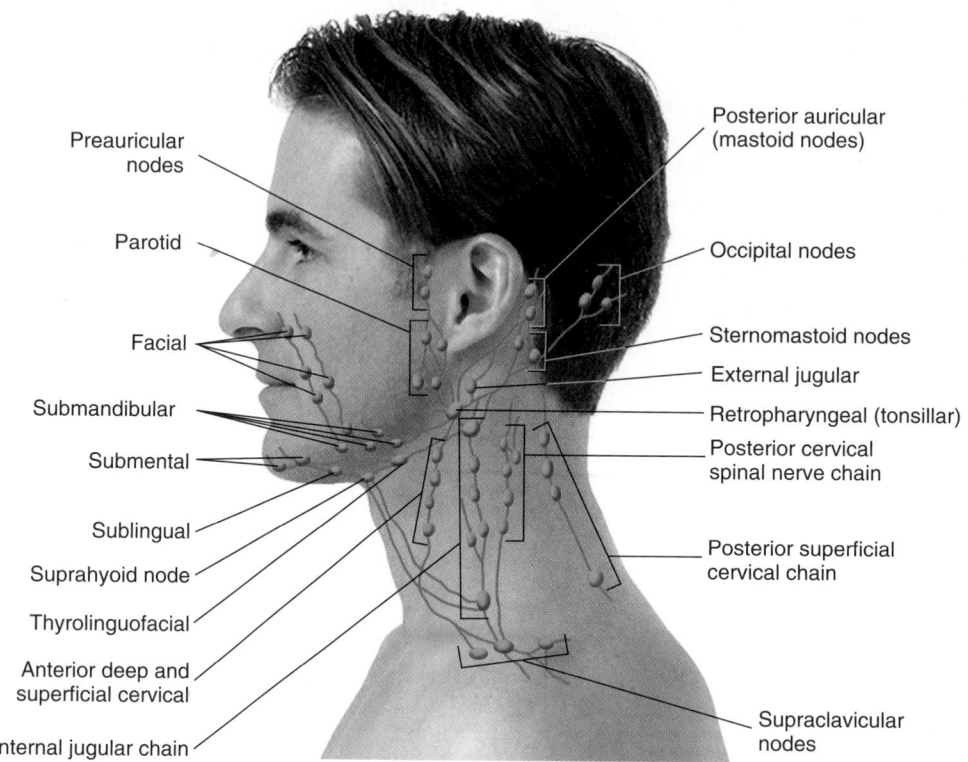

FIG. 30.28 Palpable lymph nodes in head and neck. (From Ball JW, et al: *Seidel's guide to physical examination*, ed 9, St Louis, 2019, Mosby.)

comparison. During palpation either face or stand to the side of the patient for easy access to all nodes. Use the pads of the middle three fingers of each hand to gently palpate in a circular motion over the nodes (Fig. 30.29). Check each node methodically in the following sequence: occipital nodes at the base of the skull, postauricular nodes over the mastoid, preauricular nodes just in front of the ear, retropharyngeal nodes at the angle of the mandible, submandibular nodes, and submental nodes in the midline behind the mandibular tip. Try to detect enlargement and note the location, size, shape, surface characteristics, consistency, mobility, tenderness, and warmth of the nodes. If the skin is mobile, move it over the area of the nodes. It is important to press underlying tissue in each area and not simply move the fingers over the skin. However, if you apply excessive pressure, you miss small nodes and destroy palpable nodes.

To palpate supraclavicular nodes, ask the patient to bend the head forward and relax the shoulders. Palpate these nodes by hooking the index and third finger over the clavicle lateral to the sternocleidomastoid muscle. Palpate the deep cervical nodes only with the fingers hooked around the sternocleidomastoid muscle.

Normally lymph nodes are not easily palpable. However, small, mobile, nontender nodes are common. Lymph nodes that are large, fixed, inflamed, or tender indicate a problem such as local infection, systemic disease, or neoplasm (Ball et al., 2016) (Box 30.16). When you find enlarged nodes, explore the adjacent areas and regions that they drain. Tenderness almost always indicates inflammation. A problem involving a lymph node of the head and neck means an abnormality in the mouth, throat, abdomen, breasts, thorax, or arms. These are the areas drained by the head and neck nodes.

Thyroid Gland. The thyroid gland lies in the anterior lower neck, in front of and to both sides of the trachea. The gland is fixed to the trachea, with the isthmus overlying the trachea and connecting the two

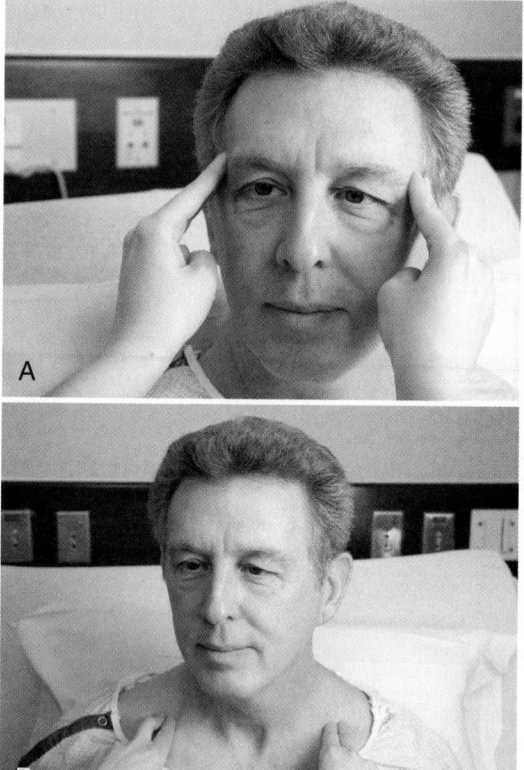

FIG. 30.29 A, Palpation of preauricular lymph nodes. B, Palpation of supraclavicular lymph nodes.

BOX 30.16 PATIENT TEACHING
Neck Assessment

Objective
- Patient will take proper preventive action if he or she notices a mass in the neck.

Teaching Strategies
- Stress the importance of regular adherence with the medication schedule to patients with thyroid disease.
- Instruct patient about the lymph nodes and how infection commonly causes node tenderness and mild enlargement.
- Instruct patient to call a health care provider when he or she notices a fixed, enlarged lump or mass in the neck.
- Teach patient the risk factors for HIV infection and other sexually transmitted diseases.

Evaluation
Use the principles of teach-back to evaluate patient/family caregiver learning:
- Tell me what signs and symptoms in the neck area would require you to contact your health care provider.

HIV, Human immunodeficiency virus.

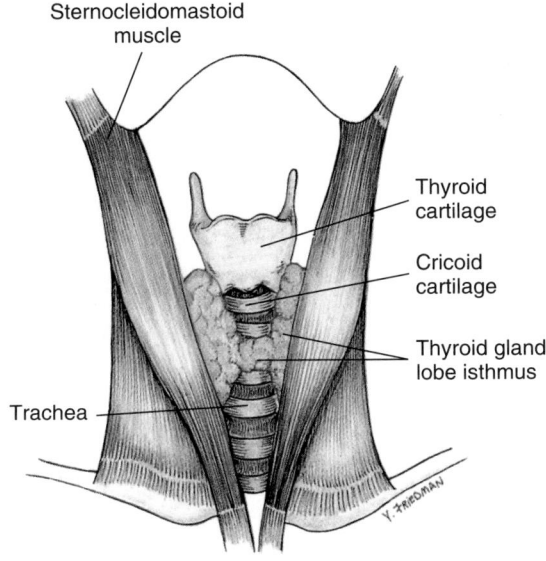

FIG. 30.30 Anatomical position of thyroid gland.

Labels: Sternocleidomastoid muscle; Thyroid cartilage; Cricoid cartilage; Thyroid gland lobe isthmus; Trachea

BOX 30.17 PATIENT TEACHING
Lung Assessment

Objective
- The patient will practice preventive care measures for lung health.

Teaching Strategies
- Explain risk factors for chronic lung disease and lung cancer, including cigarette smoking; history of smoking for over 20 years; exposure to environmental pollution; and radiation exposure from occupational, medical, and environmental sources. Exposure to radon and asbestos also increases risk. Other risk factors include exposure to certain metals (e.g., arsenic, cadmium, chromium), some organic chemicals, and tuberculosis. Exposure to secondhand cigarette smoke increases risk for nonsmokers (ACS, 2018b).
- Share brochures on lung cancer, asthma, and COPD from American Cancer Society with patient and family.
- Instruct patient with asthma to identify and tell family members and friends which triggers cause asthma episodes.
- Discuss warning signs of lung cancer such as a persistent cough, sputum streaked with blood, chest pains, and recurrent attacks of pneumonia or bronchitis.
- Counsel older adult about benefits of receiving influenza and pneumonia vaccinations because of a greater susceptibility to respiratory infection.
- Instruct patient with COPD how to perform coughing and pursed-lip breathing exercises.
- Refer people at risk for tuberculosis to visit clinics or health care centers for skin testing.

Evaluation
Use the principles of teach-back to evaluate patient/family caregiver learning:
- Tell me three risk factors for lung disease and lung cancer.
- Describe for me the warning signs of lung cancer.
- Explain to me the importance of receiving a pneumonia and annual influenza vaccine.
- Show me how you perform your deep breathing and coughing exercises.

COPD, Chronic obstructive pulmonary disease.

irregular, cone-shaped lobes (Fig. 30.30). Inspect the lower neck overlying the thyroid gland for obvious masses, symmetry, and any subtle fullness at the base of the neck. Ask the patient to hyperextend the neck, which helps tighten the skin for better visualization. Offer the patient a glass of water, and, while observing the neck, have him or her swallow. This maneuver helps to visualize an abnormally enlarged thyroid. Normally the thyroid cannot be visualized. Advanced practice nurses examine the thyroid by palpating for more subtle masses.

Carotid Artery and Jugular Vein. This part of the examination is described under examination of the vascular system (see later section).

Trachea. The trachea is a part of the upper respiratory system that you directly palpate. It is normally located in the midline above the suprasternal notch. Masses in the neck or mediastinum and pulmonary abnormalities cause displacement laterally. Have the patient sit or lie down during palpation. Determine the position of the trachea by palpating at the suprasternal notch, slipping the thumb and index fingers to each side. Note if the finger and thumb shift laterally. Do not apply forceful pressure because this elicits coughing.

THORAX AND LUNGS

Accurate physical assessment of the thorax and lungs requires review of the ventilatory and respiratory functions of the lungs. Diseases of the lungs affect other body systems. For example, the brain is very sensitive to oxygen levels. When a patient has reduced oxygenation, changes in level of consciousness and mental alertness result. Use data from all body systems to determine the nature of pulmonary alterations. You use inspection, palpation, and auscultation to examine the thorax and lungs. Diagnostic equipment such as x-ray films, magnetic resonance imaging (MRI), and computed tomography (CT) scans create little need for the use of percussion as an assessment measure. Risk factors for lung disease are reviewed at the time of respiratory assessment (Box 30.17).

First identify the landmarks of the chest to assess the thorax and lungs correctly (Fig. 30.31A-C). A patient's nipples, angle of Louis, suprasternal notch, costal angle, clavicles, and vertebrae are key landmarks that provide a series of imaginary lines for sign identification. Keep a mental image of the location of the lobes of the lung and the position of each rib (Fig. 30.32A-C). Your understanding of the

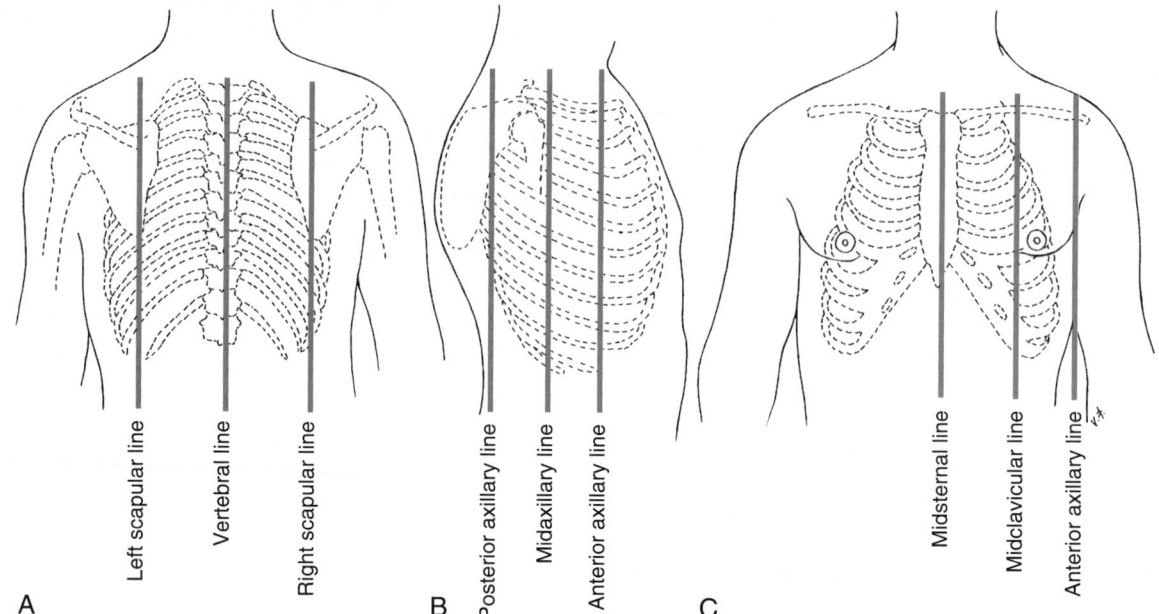

FIG. 30.31 Anatomical chest wall landmarks. **A,** Posterior chest landmarks. **B,** Lateral chest landmarks. **C,** Anterior chest landmarks.

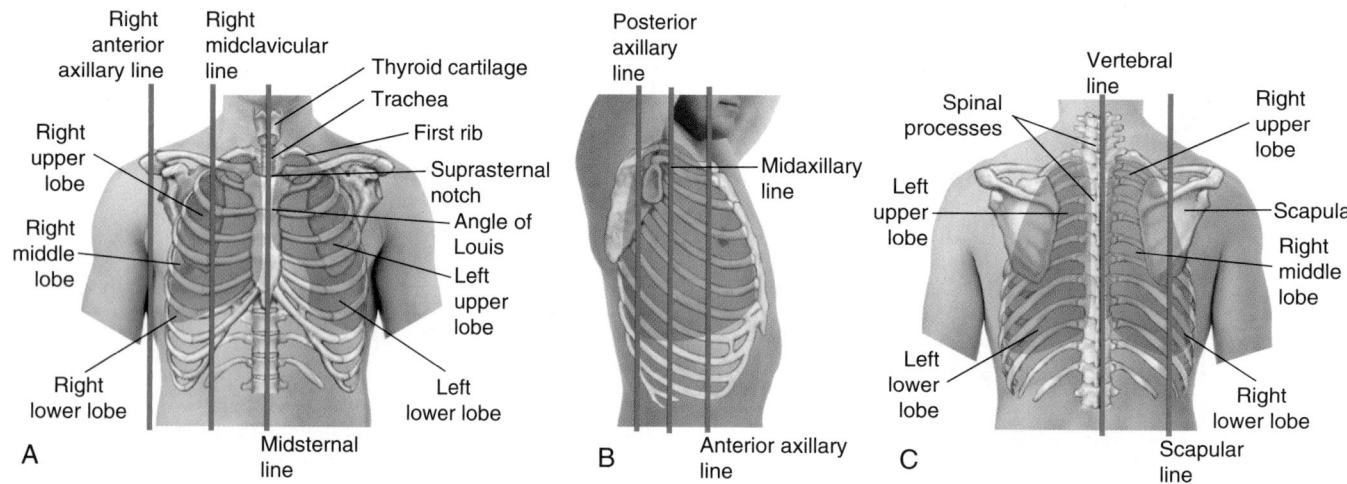

FIG. 30.32 Position of lung lobes in relation to anatomical landmarks. **A,** Anterior position. **B,** Lateral position. **C,** Posterior position. (From Ball JW, et al: *Seidel's guide to physical examination*, ed 9, St Louis, 2019, Elsevier.)

anatomical structures ensures a thorough assessment of the anterior, lateral, and posterior thorax.

Locate the position of each rib to visualize the lobe of the lung being assessed. To begin, find the angle of Louis at the manubriosternal junction. The angle is a visible and palpable angulation of the sternum and is the point at which the second rib articulates with the sternum. Count the ribs and intercostal spaces (between the ribs) from this point. The number of each intercostal space corresponds with that of the rib just above it. The spinous process of the third thoracic vertebra and the fourth, fifth, and sixth ribs help to locate the lobes of the lung laterally. The lower lobes project laterally and anteriorly (see Fig. 30.32B). Posteriorly the tip or inferior margin of the scapula lies approximately at the level of the seventh rib (see Fig. 30.32C). After identifying the seventh rib, count upward to locate the third thoracic vertebra and align it with the inner borders of the scapula to locate the posterior lobes.

Ensure the patient is undressed to the waist, and ensure the room has good lighting when performing your assessment. Begin with the patient sitting to assess the posterior and lateral chest if possible. Have him or her sit or lie down for assessment of the anterior chest. Table 30.19 reviews the nursing history for lung examination.

Posterior Thorax

Begin examination of the posterior thorax by observing for any signs or symptoms in other body systems that indicate pulmonary problems. Reduced mental alertness, nasal flaring, somnolence, and cyanosis are examples of assessed signs that indicate oxygenation problems. Inspect the posterior thorax by observing the shape and symmetry of the chest from the patient's back and front. Note the anteroposterior diameter. Body shape or posture significantly impairs ventilatory movement. Normally the chest contour is symmetrical, with the anteroposterior diameter one-third to one-half of the transverse, or side-to-side, diameter. A barrel-shaped chest (anteroposterior diameter equals transverse diameter) characterizes aging and chronic lung disease. Infants have an almost round shape. Congenital and postural alterations cause abnormal contours in which a patient may

TABLE 30.19   Nursing History for Lung Assessment

Assessment	Rationale
Assess history of tobacco or marijuana use, including type of tobacco, duration, and amount (Pack-years = Number of years smoking × Number of packs per day), age started, efforts to quit, and length of time since smoking stopped.	Smoking is a risk factor for lung cancer, heart disease, cerebrovascular disease, emphysema, or chronic bronchitis. It accounts for a significant percentage of all cancer deaths. It increases the risk for 12 types of cancer (ACS, 2018b).
Ask whether patient has had a *persistent cough* (productive or nonproductive), *sputum streaked with blood, voice change, chest pain,* shortness of breath, orthopnea, dyspnea during exertion or at rest, poor activity tolerance, or *recurrent attacks of pneumonia or bronchiti*s.	Symptoms of cardiopulmonary alterations help localize objective physical findings. (Warning signals for lung cancer are in italic type.) The diaphragm of the lungs expands more easily when the individual is sitting upright, as for patients who must be in an upright position to breathe.
Determine whether patient works in environment containing pollutants (e.g., asbestos, arsenic, coal dust) or requiring exposure to radiation. Does patient have exposure to secondhand smoke?	These risk factors increase chance for various lung diseases.
Review history for known or suspected human immunodeficiency virus (HIV) infection; substance abuse; low income; or being homeless, a resident or employee of a nursing home or shelter, a recent prison inmate, a family member of a tuberculosis (TB) patient, or an immigrant to the United States from a country where TB is prevalent.	These are risk factors for TB.
Ask whether patient has history of persistent cough, hemoptysis, unexplained weight loss, fatigue, night sweats, or fever.	These are risk factors for both TB and HIV infection.
Does patient have history of chronic hoarseness?	Hoarseness indicates laryngeal disorder or abuse of cocaine or opioids (sniffing).
Assess history of allergies to pollens, dust, or other airborne irritants and to foods, drugs, or chemical substances.	Symptoms such as choking feeling, bronchospasm with respiratory stridor, wheezes on auscultation, and dyspnea are often caused by allergic response.
Review family history for cancer, TB, allergies, or chronic obstructive pulmonary disease.	Conditions place patient at risk for lung disease.
Ask whether patient has had a pneumonia or influenza vaccine and a TB test; if not, educate him or her on need to do so.	The very young, the very old, and those with chronic respiratory problems or immunosuppressive diseases are at increased risk for respiratory disease.

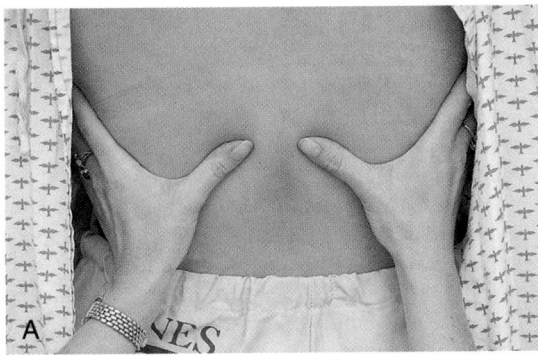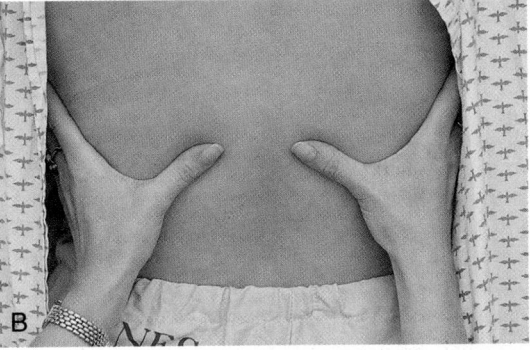

FIG. 30.33 A, Hand position for palpation of posterior thorax excursion. B, As patient inhales, movement of chest excursion separates thumbs.

lean over a table or splint the side of the chest because of a breathing problem. Pain sometimes causes a patient to splint or hold the chest wall and bend toward the affected side, resulting in impaired ventilatory movement.

Standing at a midline position behind the patient, look for deformities, position of the spine, slope of the ribs, retraction of the intercostal spaces during inspiration, and bulging of the intercostal spaces during expiration. The scapulae are normally symmetrical and closely attached to the thoracic wall. The normal spine is straight without lateral deviation. Posteriorly the ribs tend to slope across and down. The ribs and intercostal spaces are easier to see in a thin person. Normally no bulging or active movement occurs within the intercostal spaces during breathing. Bulging indicates that a patient is using great effort to breathe.

Also assess the rate and rhythm of breathing. Observe the thorax as a whole. It normally expands and relaxes regularly with equal movement bilaterally. In healthy adults the normal respiratory rates vary from 12 to 20 respirations per minute.

Palpation of the posterior thorax provides further information about a patient's health status. Palpate the thoracic muscles and skeleton for lumps, masses, pulsations, and unusual movement. If the patient voices pain or tenderness, avoid deep palpation. Fractured rib fragments could be displaced against vital organs. Normally the chest wall is not tender. If there is a suspicious mass or swollen area, lightly palpate it for size, shape, and the typical qualities of a lesion.

To measure chest excursion or depth of breathing, stand behind the patient and place the thumbs along the spinal processes at the 10th rib, with the palms lightly contacting the posterolateral surfaces. Place thumbs 5 cm (2 inches) apart, pointing toward the spine with fingers pointing laterally (Fig. 30.33A). Press the hands toward the spine so that a small skinfold appears between the thumbs. Do not slide the hands over the skin. Instruct the patient to exhale and then take a deep breath. Note movement of the thumbs during inhalation (see Fig. 30.33B). Chest excursion is symmetrical, separating the thumbs 3 to 5 cm (1¼ to 2 inches). Reduced chest excursion may be caused by pain, postural

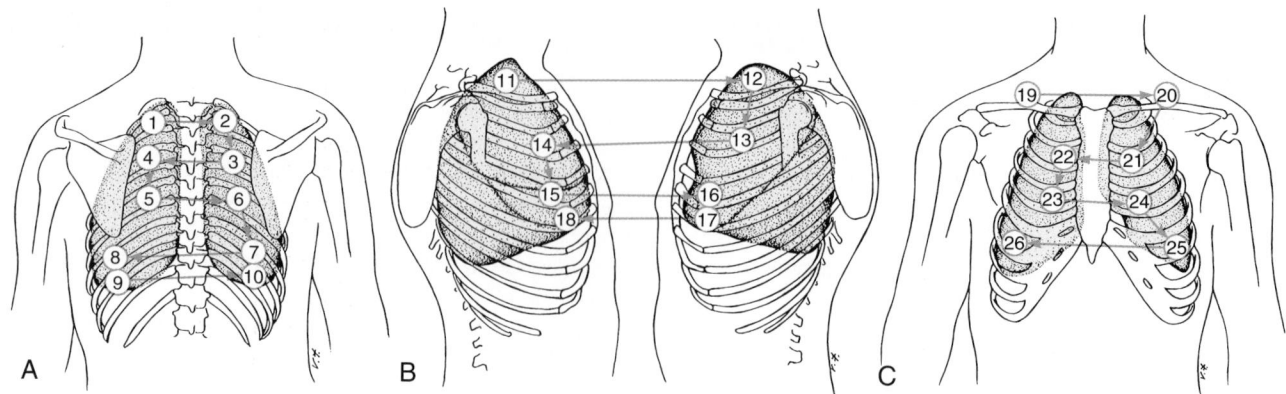

FIG. 30.34 A to C, Systematic pattern (posterior-lateral-anterior) is followed when palpating and auscultating thorax.

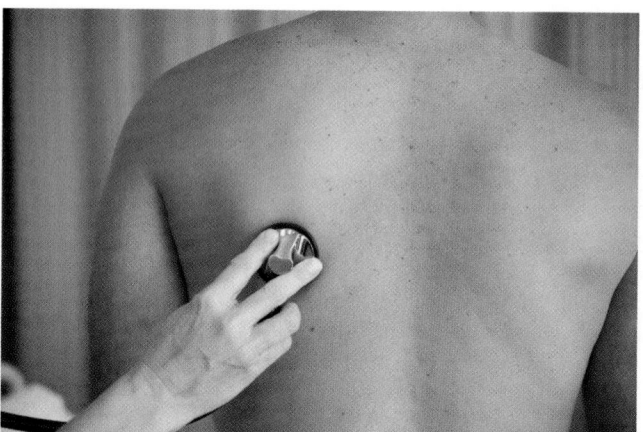

FIG. 30.35 Use diaphragm of stethoscope to auscultate breath sounds.

deformity, or fatigue. In older adults chest movement normally declines because of costal cartilage calcification and respiratory muscle atrophy.

During speech the sound created by the vocal cords is transmitted through the lungs to the chest wall. The sound waves create vibrations that you palpate externally. These vibrations are called vocal or tactile fremitus. The accumulation of mucus, the collapse of lung tissue, or the presence of one or more lung lesions blocks the vibrations from reaching the chest wall.

To palpate for tactile fremitus, use a firm, light touch and place the palmar surfaces of the fingers or the ulnar part of the hand over symmetrical intercostal spaces, beginning at the lung apex (Fig. 30.34A). Ask the patient to say "ninety-nine" or "one-one-one." Palpate both sides simultaneously and symmetrically (from top to bottom) for comparison or use one hand, quickly alternating between the two sides (Ball et al., 2019). Normally a faint vibration is present as a patient speaks. If fremitus is faint, ask the patient to speak in a louder or lower tone of voice. Normally fremitus is symmetrical. Vibrations are strongest at the top, near the level of the tracheal bifurcation. Strong vibrations through the chest wall occur in crying infants.

Use auscultation to assess the movement of air through the tracheobronchial tree and detect mucus or obstructed airways. Normally air flows through the airways in an unobstructed pattern. Recognizing the sounds created by normal airflow allows you to detect sounds caused by airway obstruction. Follow the same systematic approach you used for palpation when auscultating the lungs (see Fig. 30.34A).

Place the diaphragm of the stethoscope firmly on the skin, over the posterior chest wall between the ribs (Fig. 30.35). Have the patient fold the arms in front of the chest and keep the head bent forward while taking slow, deep breaths with the mouth slightly open. Listen to an entire inspiration and expiration at each position of the stethoscope. If sounds are faint, as in a patient who is obese, ask the patient to breathe harder and faster temporarily. Breath sounds are much louder in children because of their thin chest walls. The bell works best in children because of a child's small chest. Auscultate for normal breath sounds and abnormal or adventitious sounds (Fig. 30.36). Normal breath sounds differ in character, depending on the area you are auscultating and the age of the patient. Bronchovesicular and vesicular sounds are normally heard over the posterior thorax (Table 30.20).

Abnormal sounds result from air passing through moisture, mucus, or narrowed airways. They also result from alveoli suddenly reinflating or an inflammation between the pleural linings of the lung. Adventitious sounds often occur superimposed over normal sounds. The four types of adventitious sounds are crackles, rhonchi, wheezes, and pleural friction rub (see Fig. 30.36). Each sound has a specific cause and typical auditory features (Table 30.21). During auscultation note the location and characteristics of the sounds and listen for the absence of breath sounds (found in patients with collapsed or surgically removed lobes).

If there are abnormalities in tactile fremitus or auscultation, perform the vocal resonance tests (spoken and whispered voice sounds). Place the stethoscope over the same locations used to assess breath sounds and have the patient say "ninety-nine" in a normal voice tone. Normally the sound is muffled. If fluid is compressing the lung, the vibrations from the patient's voice are transmitted to the chest wall, and the sound becomes clear (bronchophony). Then ask the patient to whisper "ninety-nine." The whispered voice is usually faint and indistinct. Certain lung abnormalities cause the whispered voice to become clear and distinct (whispered pectoriloquy).

Lateral Thorax

After assessing the posterior thorax, move to the lateral sides of the chest. The patient sits during examination of the lateral chest whenever possible. Have the patient raise the arms to improve access to lateral thoracic structures. Use inspection, palpation, and auscultation skills to examine the lateral thorax (see Fig. 30.34B). Do not assess excursion laterally. Normally the breath sounds you hear are vesicular.

Anterior Thorax

Inspect the anterior thorax for the same features as the posterior thorax. The patient sits or lies down with the head elevated. Observe the accessory muscles of breathing: sternocleidomastoid, trapezius, and abdominal muscles. The accessory muscles move little with normal passive breathing. However, patients who use a great deal of effort to breathe as a result of strenuous exercise or

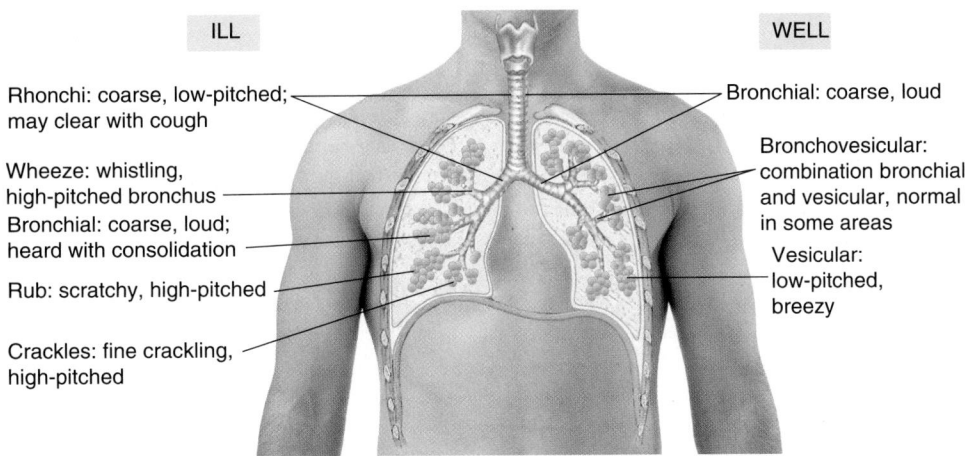

FIG. 30.36 Schema of breath sounds in the ill and well patient. (From Ball JW, et al: *Seidel's guide to physical examination*, ed 9, St Louis, 2019, Elsevier.)

TABLE 30.20 Normal Breath Sounds

Description	Location	Origin
Vesicular Vesicular sounds are soft, breezy, and low pitched. Inspiratory phase is 3 times longer than expiratory phase.	Best heard over periphery of lung (except over scapula)	Created by air moving through smaller airways
Bronchovesicular Bronchovesicular sounds are blowing sounds that are medium pitched and of medium intensity. Inspiratory phase is equal to expiratory phase.	Best heard posteriorly between scapulae and anteriorly over bronchioles lateral to sternum at first and second intercostal spaces	Created by air moving through large airways
Bronchial Bronchial sounds are loud and high pitched with hollow quality. Expiration lasts longer than inspiration (3:2 ratio).	Heard only over trachea	Created by air moving through trachea close to chest wall

TABLE 30.21 Adventitious Breath Sounds

Sound	Site Auscultated	Cause	Character
Crackles	Most common in dependent lobes: right and left lung bases	Random, sudden reinflation of groups of alveoli; disruptive passage of air through small airways	Fine crackles are high-pitched fine, short, interrupted crackling sounds heard during end of inspiration; usually not cleared with coughing. Medium crackles are lower, moister sounds heard during middle of inspiration; not cleared with coughing. Coarse crackles are loud, bubbly sounds heard during inspiration; not cleared with coughing.
Rhonchi (sonorous wheeze)	Primarily heard over trachea and bronchi; if loud enough, able to be heard over most lung fields	Muscular spasm, fluid, or mucus in larger airways; new growth or external pressure causing turbulence	Loud, low-pitched, rumbling, coarse sounds are heard either during inspiration or expiration; sometimes cleared by coughing.
Wheezes (sibilant wheeze)	Heard over all lung fields	High-velocity airflow through severely narrowed or obstructed airway	High-pitched, continuous musical sounds are like a squeak heard continuously during inspiration or expiration; usually louder on expiration.
Pleural friction rub	Heard over anterior lateral lung field (if patient is sitting upright)	Inflamed pleura; parietal pleura rubbing against visceral pleura	Dry, rubbing, or grating quality is heard during inspiration or expiration; does not clear with coughing; heard loudest over lower lateral anterior surface.

Data from Ball JW, et al: *Seidel's guide to physical examination*, ed 9, St Louis, 2019, Elsevier.

TABLE 30.22   Nursing History for Heart Assessment

Assessment	Rationale
Determine history of smoking, alcohol intake, caffeine intake, use of prescriptive and recreational drugs, exercise habits, and dietary patterns and intake (including fat and sodium intake).	Smoking; alcohol ingestion; cocaine use; lack of regular exercise; intake of foods high in carbohydrates, fats, and cholesterol are risk factors for cardiovascular disease. Caffeine can cause heart dysrhythmias.
Determine whether patient is taking medications for cardiovascular function (e.g., antidysrhythmics, antihypertensives) and whether he or she knows their purpose, dosage, and side effects.	Knowledge allows nurse to assess adherence with drug therapies. Medications sometimes affect vital sign values.
Assess for chest pain or discomfort, palpitations, excess fatigue, cough, dyspnea, leg pain or cramps, edema of feet, cyanosis, fainting, and orthopnea. Ask whether symptoms occur at rest or during exercise.	These are key symptoms of heart disease. Cardiovascular function is sometimes adequate during rest but not during exercise. Positions affect how well lungs can expand.
If patient reports chest pain, determine whether it is cardiac in nature. Anginal pain is usually a deep pressure or ache that is substernal and diffuse, radiating to one or both arms, neck, or jaw.	Assessment determines nature of pain and need to initiate care immediately.
Determine whether patient has stressful lifestyle. Which physical demands and/or emotional stress exist?	Repeated exposure to stress increases risk for heart disease.
Assess family history for heart disease, diabetes, high cholesterol levels, hypertension, stroke, or rheumatic heart disease.	Factors increase risk for heart disease.
Ask patient about history of heart trouble (e.g., heart failure, congenital heart disease, coronary artery disease, dysrhythmias, murmurs).	Knowledge reveals patient's level of understanding of condition. Preexisting condition influences examination techniques used and findings to expect.
Determine whether patient has preexisting diabetes, lung disease, obesity, or hypertension.	These disorders alter heart function.

pulmonary disease (e.g., chronic obstructive pulmonary disease) rely on the accessory and abdominal muscles to contract to inhale and exhale. Some patients who require great effort produce a grunting sound.

Observe the width of the costal angle. It is usually larger than 90 degrees between the two costal margins. Observe a patient's breathing pattern. Normal breathing is quiet and barely audible near the open mouth. You most often assess respiratory rate and rhythm anteriorly. The male patient's respirations are usually diaphragmatic, whereas a female's are more costal. Accurate assessment occurs as the patient breathes passively.

Palpate the anterior thoracic muscles and skeleton for lumps, masses, tenderness, or unusual movement. The sternum and xiphoid are relatively inflexible. Place the thumbs parallel approximately along the costal margin 6 cm (2½ inches) apart with the palms touching the anterolateral chest. Push the thumbs toward the midline to create a skinfold. As the patient inhales deeply, the thumbs normally separate approximately 3 to 5 cm (1¼ to 2 inches), with each side expanding equally.

Assess tactile fremitus over the anterior chest wall. Anterior findings differ from posterior findings because of the heart and female breast tissue. Fremitus is felt next to the sternum at the second intercostal space, at the level of the bronchial bifurcation. It decreases over the heart, lower thorax, and breast tissue.

Auscultation of the anterior thorax follows a systematic pattern (see Fig. 30.34C) comparing right and left sides. This allows you to compare lung sounds in one region on one side of the body with sounds in the same region on the opposite side of the body.

If possible, have the patient sit to maximize chest expansion. Give special attention to the lower lobes, where mucus secretions commonly gather. Listen for bronchovesicular and vesicular sounds above and below the clavicles and along the lung periphery. In addition, auscultate for bronchial sounds, which are loud, high pitched, and hollow sounding, with expiration lasting longer than inspiration (3:2 ratio). This sound is normally heard over the trachea.

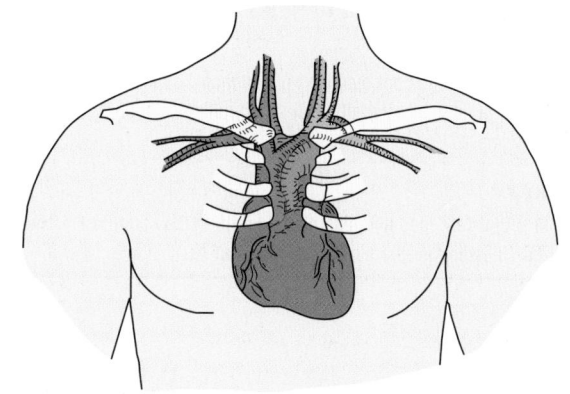

FIG. 30.37 Anatomical position of heart.

HEART

Compare your assessment of a patient's heart with findings from the vascular assessment (see later section). Alterations in either system sometimes manifest as changes in the other. Some patients with signs or symptoms of heart (cardiac) problems have a life-threatening condition requiring immediate attention. In this case act quickly and conduct only the parts of the examination that are necessary. Conduct a more thorough assessment when the patient is more stable. The nursing history (Table 30.22) provides data to help interpret physical findings.

Assess cardiac system through the anterior thorax. Form a mental image of the exact location of the heart (Fig. 30.37). In the adult it is located in the center of the chest (precordium), behind and to the left of the sternum, with a small section of the right atrium extending to the right of the sternum. The base of the heart is the upper part, and the apex is the bottom tip. The surface of the right ventricle composes most of the anterior surface of the heart. A section of the left ventricle shapes the left anterior side of the apex. The apex touches the anterior chest wall at approximately the fourth to fifth intercostal space just medial to the left midclavicular line. This is the apical impulse or point of maximal impulse (PMI).

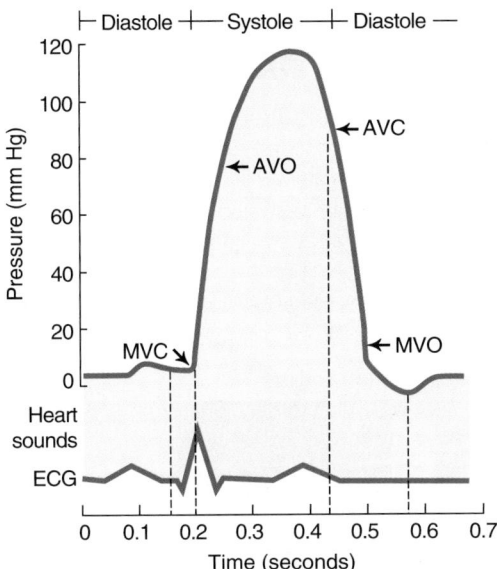

FIG. 30.38 Cardiac cycle. *AVC,* Aortic valve closes; *AVO,* aortic valve opens; *ECG,* electrocardiogram; *MVC,* mitral valve closes; *MVO,* mitral valve opens.

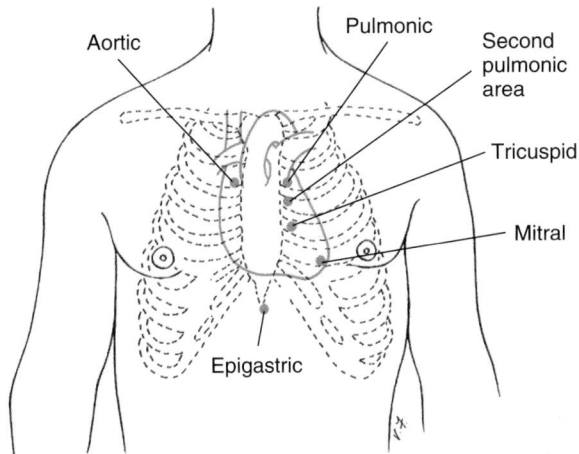

FIG. 30.39 Anatomical sites for assessment of cardiac function.

An infant's heart is positioned more horizontally. The apex of the heart is at the third or fourth intercostal space, just to the left of the midclavicular line. By the age of 7 a child's PMI is in the same location as the adult's. In tall, slender people the heart lies more vertically and centrally. In shorter or stockier individuals, the heart tends to lie more to the left and horizontally (Ball et al., 2019).

To assess the heart, you need a clear understanding of the cardiac cycle and associated physiological events (Fig. 30.38). The heart normally pumps blood through its four chambers in a methodical, even sequence. Events on the left side occur just before those on the right. As blood flows through each chamber, the valves open and close, the pressures within chambers rise and fall, and the chambers contract. Each event creates a physiological sign. Both sides of the heart function in a coordinated fashion.

There are two phases to the cardiac cycle: systole and diastole. During systole the ventricles contract and eject blood from the left ventricle into the aorta and from the right ventricle into the pulmonary artery. During diastole the ventricles relax, and the atria contract to move blood into the ventricles and fill the coronary arteries.

Heart sounds occur in relation to physiological events in the cardiac cycle. As systole begins, ventricular pressure rises and closes the mitral and tricuspid valves. Valve closure causes the first heart sound (S_1), often described as "lub." The ventricles then contract, and blood flows through the aortic and pulmonary valves into circulation. After the ventricles empty, ventricular pressure falls below that in the aorta and pulmonary artery. This allows the aortic and pulmonic valves to close, causing the second heart sound (S_2), described as "dub." As ventricular pressure continues to fall, it drops below that of the atria. The mitral and tricuspid valves reopen to allow ventricular filling. When the heart attempts to fill an already distended ventricle, a third heart sound (S_3) can be heard, as with heart failure. An S_3 is considered abnormal in adults over 31 years of age but can often be heard normally in children and young adults. It can also be present among women in the late stages of pregnancy. A fourth heart sound (S_4) occurs when the atria contract to enhance ventricular filling. An S_4 is often heard in healthy older adults, children, and athletes, but it is not normal in adults. Because S_4 also indicates an abnormal condition, report it to a health care provider.

Inspection and Palpation

Provide a relaxed and comfortable environment for the examination. Explain the assessment procedure to help decrease a patient's anxiety. An anxious or uncomfortable patient can have mild tachycardia, which leads to inaccurate findings.

Use the skills of inspection and palpation simultaneously. Begin the examination with the patient in the supine position or with the upper body elevated 45 degrees. Patients with heart disease frequently experience shortness of breath while lying flat. Stand at the patient's right side. Do not let the patient talk, especially when auscultating heart sounds. Good lighting in the room is essential.

Direct your attention to the anatomical sites best suited for assessment of the cardiac area. During inspection and palpation look for visible pulsations and exaggerated lifts and palpate for the apical impulse and any source of vibrations (thrills). Follow an orderly sequence, beginning with assessment of the base of the heart (top) and moving toward the apex (bottom). First inspect the angle of Louis, which lies between the sternal body and manubrium, and feel the ridge in the sternum approximately 5 cm (2 inches) below the sternal notch. Slip the fingers along the angle on each side of the sternum to feel adjacent ribs. The intercostal spaces are just below each rib. The second intercostal space allows identification of each of the six anatomical landmarks (Fig. 30.39). The second intercostal space on the right is the *aortic area,* and the left second intercostal space is the *pulmonic area.* You need to use deeper palpation to feel the spaces in obese or heavily muscled patients. After locating the pulmonic area, move the fingers down the patient's left sternal border to the third intercostal space, called the *second pulmonic area.* The *tricuspid area* is located at the fourth or fifth intercostal space along the sternum. To find the *apical* or *mitral area,* locate the fifth intercostal space just to the left of the sternum and move the fingers laterally to the left midclavicular line. Locate the apical area with the palm of the hand or the fingertips. Normally you feel the apical impulse as a light tap in an area 1 to 2 cm (½ to 1 inch) in diameter at the apex (Fig. 30.40). Another landmark is the epigastric area at the tip of the sternum. Palpate there if you suspect aortic abnormalities.

Locate the six anatomical landmarks of the heart and inspect and palpate each area. Look for the appearance of pulsations, viewing each area over the chest at an angle to the side. Normally you do not see pulsations except perhaps at the PMI in thin patients or at the epigastric area as a result of abdominal aorta pulsation. Use the proximal halves of the four fingers together and alternate this with the ball of the hand to palpate for pulsations. Touch the areas gently to allow movements to lift the hand. Normally no pulsations or vibrations are felt in the second, third, or fourth intercostal spaces. Loud murmurs cause a vibration.

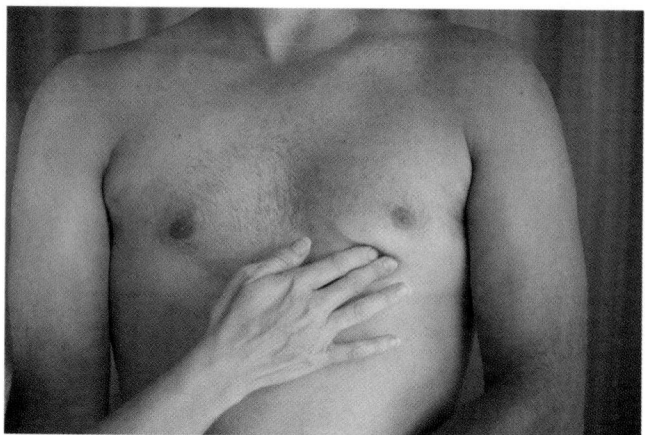

FIG. 30.40 Palpation of apical pulse.

Just medial to the left midclavicular line, at the fourth or fifth intercostal space, is the PMI. If you cannot locate it with the patient in a supine position, have him or her roll onto the left side, moving the heart closer to the chest wall. Estimate the size of the heart by noting the diameter of the PMI and its position relative to the midclavicular line. In cases of serious heart disease, the cardiac muscle enlarges, with the PMI found more to the left of the midclavicular line. The PMI is sometimes difficult to find in the older adult because the chest deepens in its anteroposterior diameters. It is also difficult to find in muscular or overweight patients. An infant's PMI is located near the third or fourth intercostal space. It is easy to palpate because of the child's thin chest wall.

Auscultation

You may hear normal heart sounds, extra heart sounds, and/or murmurs during auscultation of the heart. Concentrate on detecting the normal low-intensity sounds created by valve closures. Before auscultating the heart, eliminate all sources of room noise and explain the procedure to reduce the patient's anxiety. Follow a systematic pattern, beginning at the aortic area and inching the stethoscope across each of the anatomical sites. Listen for the complete cycle ("lub-dub") of heart sounds clearly at each location. Repeat the sequence with the bell of the stethoscope. Sometimes you will have a patient assume three different positions during the examination to hear sounds clearly (Fig. 30.41A-C): sitting up and leaning forward (good for all areas and to hear high-pitched murmurs), supine (good for all areas), and left lateral recumbent (good for all areas; best position to hear low-pitched sounds in diastole).

Learn to identify the first (S_1) and second (S_2) heart sounds. At normal rates S_1 occurs after the long diastolic pause and before the short systolic pause. S_1 is high pitched, dull in quality, and heard best at the apex. If it is difficult to hear S_1, time it in relation to the carotid pulsation. S_2 follows the short systolic pause and precedes the long diastolic pause; it is best heard at the aortic area.

Auscultate for rate and rhythm after hearing both sounds clearly. Each combination of S_1 and S_2 or "lub-dub" counts as one heartbeat. Count the rate for 1 minute and listen for the interval between S_1 and S_2 and then the time between S_2 and the next S_1. A regular rhythm involves regular intervals of time between each sequence of beats. There is a distinct silent pause between S_1 and S_2. Failure of the heart to beat at regular successive intervals is a dysrhythmia. Some dysrhythmias are life threatening.

When assessing an irregular heart rhythm, compare apical and radial pulse rates simultaneously to determine whether a pulse deficit exists. Auscultate the apical pulse first and then immediately palpate

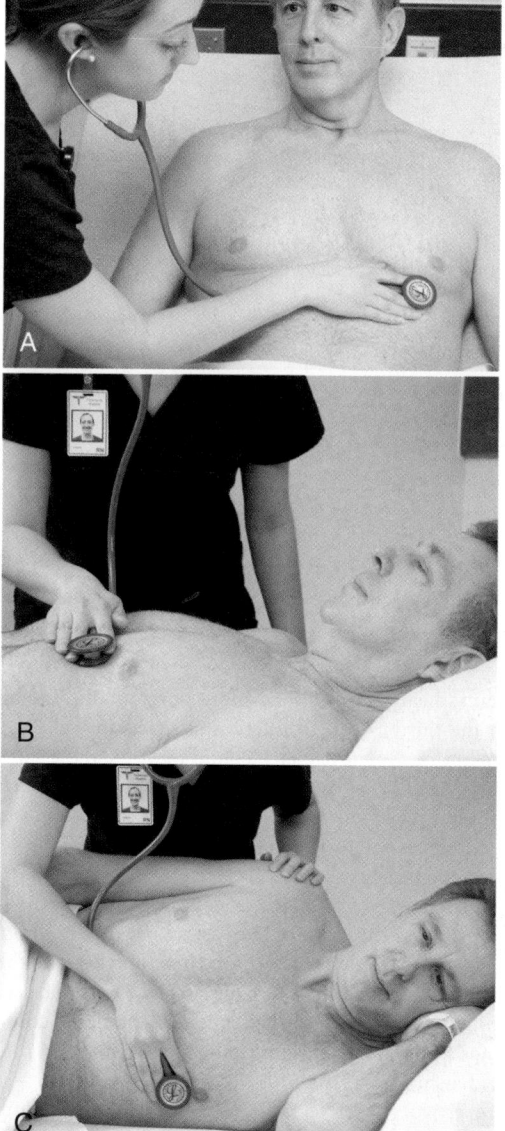

FIG. 30.41 Sequence of patient positions for heart auscultation. **A,** Sitting. **B,** Supine. **C,** Left lateral recumbent.

the radial pulse (one examiner present). When two examiners are present, assess the apical and radial rates at the same time. When a patient has a pulse deficit, the radial pulse is slower than the apical pulse because ineffective contractions fail to send pulse waves to the periphery. Report a difference in pulse rates to the health care provider immediately.

Assess for extra heart sounds at each auscultatory site. Use the bell of the stethoscope and listen for low-pitched extra heart sounds such as S_3 and S_4 gallops, clicks, and rubs. Auscultate over all anatomical areas. S_3, or a **ventricular gallop**, occurs after S_2. It is caused by a premature rush of blood into a ventricle that is stiff or dilated as a result of heart failure and hypertension. The combination of S_1, S_2, and S_3 sounds like "Ken-TUCK-y."

S_4, or an atrial gallop, occurs just before S_1 or ventricular systole. The sound of an S_4 is similar to that of "TEN-nes-see." Physiologically it is caused by an atrial contraction pushing against a ventricle that is not accepting blood because of heart failure or other alterations. You can hear extra heart sounds more easily with the patient lying on the left side and the stethoscope at the apical site.

BOX 30.18 PATIENT TEACHING

Heart Assessment

Objective
- Patient will describe risk factors for heart disease and take appropriate steps to eliminate risks from lifestyle.

Teaching Strategies
- Explain risk factors for heart disease, including high dietary intake of saturated fat or cholesterol, lack of regular aerobic exercise, smoking, excess weight, stressful lifestyle, hypertension, and family history of heart disease.
- Refer patient (if appropriate) to resources available for controlling or reducing risks (e.g., nutritional counseling, exercise class, stress-reduction programs).
- Teach patient to eat a well-rounded healthy diet. Explain that a healthy pattern emphasizes variety, including fruits and vegetables, whole grains, low-fat dairy products, skinless poultry and fish, nuts and legumes, and nontropical vegetable oils. Limit saturated and trans fats, sodium, red meats, sweets, and sugar-sweetened beverages (AHA, 2015).
- Encourage patient who is over 20 years old to have his or her cholesterol checked every 4 to 6 years. A complete cholesterol test, also called a lipid profile, will give the results of HDL (good), LDL (bad), triglycerides, and total blood cholesterol. The health care provider will look at these numbers in relation to your other risk factors to assess overall cardiovascular risk (AHA, 2017).
- Encourage patient to discuss with health care provider the need for periodic C-reactive protein (CRP) testing. CRP levels assess a patient's risk for cardiovascular disease.
- Advise patient to avoid cigarette smoke because nicotine causes vasoconstriction.
- Advise patient to quit smoking to lower the risk for coronary heart disease and coronary vascular disease.
- Patients who are at risk benefit from taking a daily low dose of aspirin. Consult health care provider before starting therapy.

Evaluation
Use the principles of teach-back to evaluate patient/family caregiver learning:
- List for me the risk factors for heart disease.
- Show me the meal plan you developed that helps you follow a diet low in cholesterol and saturated fat.
- Describe for me how you have reduced risk factors for heart disease in your life.

TABLE 30.23 Nursing History for Vascular Assessment

Assessment	Rationale
Determine whether patient experiences leg cramps; numbness or tingling in extremities; sensation of cold hands or feet; pain in legs; or swelling or cyanosis of feet, ankles, or hand.	These signs and symptoms indicate vascular disease.
If patient experiences leg pain or cramping in lower extremities, ask whether walking or standing for long periods or sleeping aggravates or relieves it.	Relationship of symptoms to exercise clarifies whether problem is vascular or musculoskeletal. Pain caused by vascular condition tends to increase with activity. Musculoskeletal pain usually is not relieved when exercise ends.
Ask patients whether they wear tight-fitting garters, socks, or hosiery and sit or lie in bed with legs crossed.	Tight hosiery around lower extremities and crossing legs can impair venous return.
Reconsider previous heart risk factors (e.g., smoking, exercise, nutritional problems).	These predispose patient to vascular disease.
Assess medical history for heart disease, hypertension, phlebitis, diabetes, or varicose veins.	Circulatory and vascular disorders influence findings gathered during examination.

- To assess for radiation, listen over other areas in addition to where it is heard best. Murmurs can also be heard over the neck or back.
- Intensity or loudness is related to the rate of blood flow through the heart or the amount of blood regurgitated. Feel for a thrust or intermittent palpable sensation at the auscultation site in serious murmurs. A **thrill** is a continuous palpable sensation that resembles the purring of a cat. Intensity is recorded using the following grades (Ball et al., 2019):
  - *Grade 1:* Barely audible in a quiet room
  - *Grade 2:* Quiet but clearly audible
  - *Grade 3:* Moderately loud
  - *Grade 4:* Loud, with associated thrill
  - *Grade 5:* Very loud; thrill easily palpable
  - *Grade 6:* Very loud; audible with stethoscope not in contact with chest; thrill palpable and visible
- A murmur is low, medium, or high in pitch, depending on the velocity of blood flow through the valves. A low-pitched murmur is best heard with the bell of the stethoscope. If the murmur is best heard with the diaphragm, it is high pitched.

The quality of a murmur refers to its characteristic pattern and sound. A crescendo murmur starts softly and builds in loudness. A decrescendo murmur starts loudly and becomes less intense.

The final part of the auscultation examination includes assessment for heart murmurs. **Murmurs** are sustained swishing or blowing sounds heard at the beginning, middle, or end of the systolic or diastolic phase. They are caused by increased blood flow through a normal valve, forward flow through a stenotic valve or into a dilated vessel or heart chamber, or backward flow through a valve that fails to close. A murmur is asymptomatic or a sign of heart disease (Box 30.18). It is common in children. Keep the following factors in mind when auscultating to detect murmurs:
- When a murmur is detected, auscultate the mitral, tricuspid, aortic, and pulmonic valve areas for placement in the cardiac cycle (timing); the place it is heard best (location); radiation; loudness; pitch; and quality.
- If a murmur occurs between S_1 and S_2, it is a systolic murmur.
- If it occurs between S_2 and the next S_1, it is a diastolic murmur.
- The location of a murmur is not necessarily directly over the valves. Experience with hearing murmurs helps with better understanding of where each type of murmur is best heard. For example, mitral murmurs are best heard at the apex of the heart.

VASCULAR SYSTEM

Examination of the vascular system includes measuring the blood pressure and assessing the integrity of the peripheral vascular system. Table 30.23 reviews the nursing history data collected before the examination. Use the skills of inspection, palpation, and auscultation. Perform parts of the vascular examination during other body system assessments. For example, check the carotid pulse after palpating the cervical lymph nodes. Assess the skin, as part of the vascular system, for signs and symptoms of arterial and venous insufficiency.

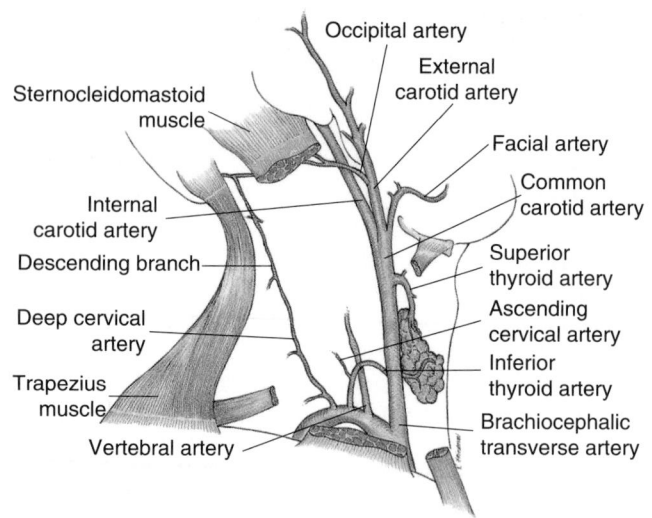

FIG. 30.42 Anatomical position of carotid artery.

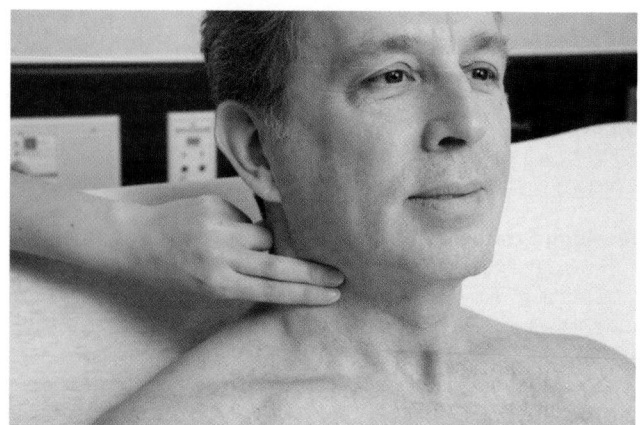

FIG. 30.43 Palpation of internal carotid artery along margin of sterno-cleidomastoid muscle.

Blood Pressure

When auscultating blood pressure, know that readings between the arms vary by as much as 10 mm Hg and tend to be higher in the right arm (Ball et al., 2019). Always record the higher reading. Repeated systolic readings that differ by 15 mm Hg or more suggest atherosclerosis or disease of the aorta.

Carotid Arteries

When the left ventricle pumps blood into the aorta, the arterial system transmits pressure waves. The carotid arteries reflect heart function better than peripheral arteries because their pressure correlates with that of the aorta. The carotid artery supplies oxygenated blood to the head and neck (Fig. 30.42). The overlying sternocleidomastoid muscle protects it.

To examine the carotid arteries, have the patient sit or lie supine with the head of the bed elevated 30 degrees. Examine one carotid artery at a time. If both arteries are occluded simultaneously during palpation, the patient loses consciousness as a result of inadequate circulation to the brain. *Do not palpate or massage the carotid arteries vigorously* because the carotid sinus is located at the bifurcation of the common carotid arteries in the upper third of the neck. This sinus sends impulses along the vagus nerve. Stimulating it causes a reflex drop in heart rate and blood pressure, which causes syncope or circulatory arrest. This is a particular problem for older adults.

Begin inspection of the neck for obvious pulsation of the artery. Have the patient turn the head slightly away from the artery being examined. Sometimes the wave of the pulse is visible. The carotid is the only site for assessing the quality of a pulse wave. An absent pulse wave indicates arterial occlusion (blockage) or stenosis (narrowing).

To palpate the pulse, ask the patient to look straight ahead or turn the head slightly toward the side you are examining. Turning relaxes the sternocleidomastoid muscle. Slide the tips of the index and middle fingers around the medial edge of the sternocleidomastoid muscle. Gently palpate to avoid occlusion of circulation (Fig. 30.43).

The normal carotid pulse is localized and strong rather than diffuse. It has a thrusting quality. As a patient breathes, no change occurs. Rotating the neck or going from a sitting to a supine position does not change the quality of the carotid impulse. Both carotid arteries are normally equal in pulse rate, rhythm, and strength and are equally elastic. Diminished or unequal carotid pulsations indicate atherosclerosis or other forms of arterial disease.

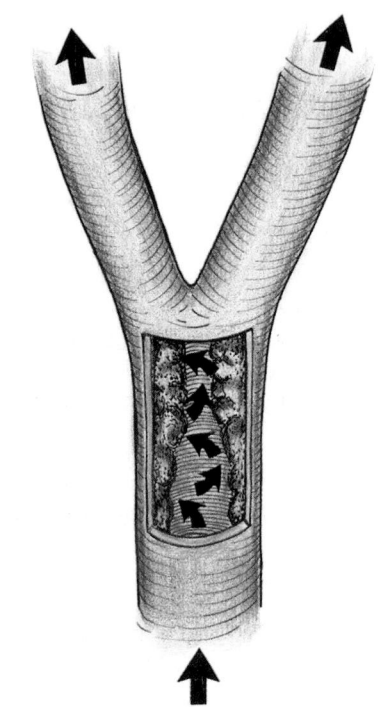

FIG. 30.44 Occlusion or narrowing of the carotid artery disrupts normal blood flow. The resultant turbulence creates a sound (bruit) that is auscultated.

The carotid is the most commonly auscultated pulse. Auscultation is especially important for middle-age or older adults or patients suspected of having cerebrovascular disease. When the lumen of a blood vessel is narrowed, it disturbs blood flow. As blood passes through the narrowed section, it creates turbulence, causing a blowing or swishing sound. The blowing sound is called a bruit (pronounced "brew-ee") (Fig. 30.44).

Place the bell of the stethoscope over the carotid artery at the lateral end of the clavicle and the posterior margin of the sternocleidomastoid muscle. Have the patient turn his or her head slightly away from the side being examined (Fig. 30.45). Ask him or her to hold the breath for a moment so that breath sounds do not obscure a bruit. Normally you do not hear any sounds during carotid auscultation. Palpate the artery lightly for a thrill (palpable bruit) if you hear a bruit.

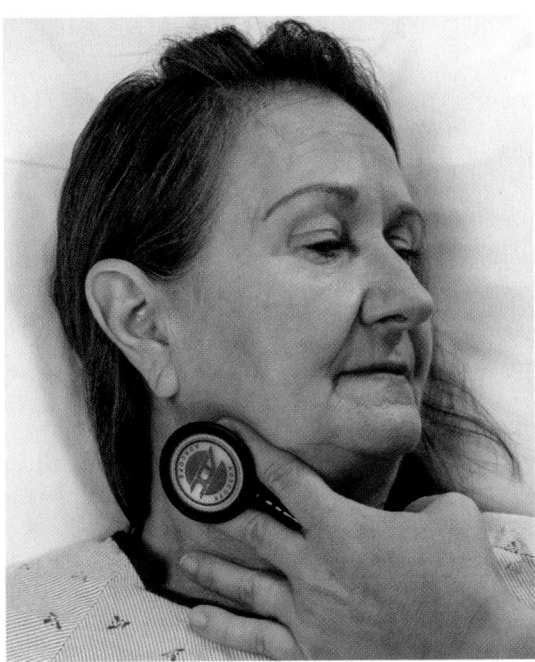

FIG. 30.45 Auscultation for carotid artery bruit.

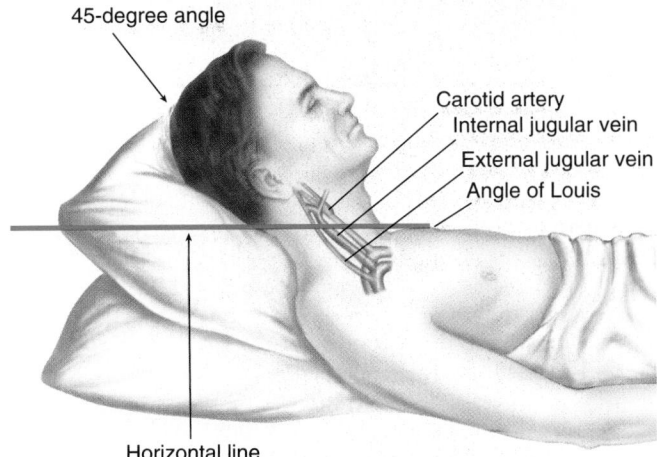

FIG. 30.46 Position of patient to assess jugular vein distention. (From Thompson JM, et al: *Mosby's manual of clinical nursing*, ed 5, St Louis, 2001, Mosby.)

Jugular Veins

The most accessible veins for examination are the internal and external jugular veins in the neck. Both veins drain bilaterally from the head and neck into the superior vena cava. The external jugular vein lies superficially and is just above the clavicle. The internal jugular vein lies deeper, along the carotid artery.

It is best to examine the right internal jugular vein because it follows a more direct anatomical path to the right atrium of the heart. The column of blood inside the internal jugular vein serves as a manometer, reflecting pressure in the right atrium. The higher the column, the greater is the venous pressure. Raised venous pressure reflects right-sided heart failure.

Normally, when a patient lies in the supine position, the external jugular vein distends and becomes easily visible. In contrast, the jugular veins normally flatten when the patient changes to a sitting or standing position. However, for some patients with heart disease the jugular veins remain distended when sitting.

Venous pressure is influenced by blood volume (i.e., the capacity of the right atrium to receive blood and send it to the right ventricle and the ability of the right ventricle to contract and force blood into the pulmonary artery). Any factor resulting in greater blood volume within the venous system results in elevated jugular venous pressure. You can observe for elevation in jugular venous pressure by using the following steps:

1. Have the patient lie flat in the supine position. Expose the neck and upper thorax. Use a pillow to align the head. Avoid neck hyperextension or flexion to ensure that the vein is not stretched or kinked (Fig. 30.46). Observe for engorgement of the jugular veins.
2. Gradually raise the head of the bed until the jugular venous pulsations become evident between the angle of the jaw and the clavicle. **NOTE:** Palpating a carotid pulse helps to distinguish venous pulsations from carotid palpations. The jugular pulse can only be visualized, not palpated.
3. Inspect the jugular veins. Usually pulsations are not evident with the patient sitting up. As he or she slowly leans back into a supine position, the level of venous pulsations begins to rise above the level of the manubrium as much as 1 or 2 cm (½ to 1 inch) as the patient reaches a 45-degree angle.

TABLE 30.24	Indicators for Assessing Local Blood Flow	
Indicator	**Rationale**
Systemic diseases (e.g., arteriosclerosis, atherosclerosis, diabetes)	Diseases result in changes in integrity of walls of arteries and smaller blood vessels.
Coagulation disorders (e.g., thrombosis, embolus)	Blood clot causes mechanical obstruction to blood flow.
Local trauma or surgery (e.g., contusion, fracture, vascular surgery)	Direct manipulation of vessels or localized edema impairs blood flow.
Application of constricting devices (e.g., casts, dressings, elastic bandages, restraints)	Constriction causes tourniquet effect, impairing blood flow to areas below site of constriction.

Peripheral Arteries and Veins

To examine the peripheral vascular system, first assess the adequacy of blood flow to the extremities by measuring arterial pulses and inspecting the condition of the skin and nails. Next assess the integrity of the venous system. Assess the arterial pulses in the extremities to determine sufficiency of the entire arterial circulation.

Factors such as coagulation disorders, local trauma or surgery, constricting casts or bandages, and systemic diseases impair circulation to the extremities (Table 30.24). Discuss risk factors and ways to monitor for circulatory problems with the patient (Box 30.19).

Peripheral Arteries. Examine each peripheral artery using the distal pads of your second and third fingers. The thumb helps anchor the brachial and femoral artery. Apply firm pressure but avoid occluding a pulse. When a pulse is difficult to find, it helps to vary pressure and feel all around the pulse site. Be sure not to palpate your own pulse.

Routine vital signs usually include assessment of the rate and rhythm of the radial artery because it is easily accessible. Count the pulse for either 30 seconds or a full minute, depending on the character of the pulse. Always count an irregular pulse for 60 seconds. With palpation, the pulse waves are normally felt at regular intervals. When an interval is interrupted by an early, a late, or a missed beat, the pulse rhythm is irregular. During cardiac emergencies health care providers usually assess the carotid artery because it is accessible and most

BOX 30.19 PATIENT TEACHING

Vascular Assessment

Objective

- Patient with vascular insufficiency will avoid activities that worsen circulatory status.

Teaching Strategies

- Instruct patient with risk or evidence of vascular insufficiency in the lower extremities to avoid tight clothing over the lower body or legs, to avoid sitting or standing for long periods, to avoid sitting with legs crossed, to walk regularly, and to elevate feet when sitting.
- Advise patient to avoid or stop the smoking of cigarettes, cigars, or pipes or the use of nicotine products (e.g., chewing tobacco, nicotine patches or gum) because nicotine causes vasoconstriction. Offer a referral to a reliable stop-smoking program.
- Instruct patient with hypertension about the benefits of regular monitoring of blood pressure (daily, weekly, or monthly). Teach patient how to use home monitoring kits.

Evaluation

Use the principles of teach-back to evaluate patient/family caregiver learning:

- Explain to me what precautions you are taking to avoid further decrease in your peripheral circulation.
- Explain to me what your normal limits for blood pressure are. Tell me when you would contact your health care provider.
- Show me how you take your blood pressure at home.

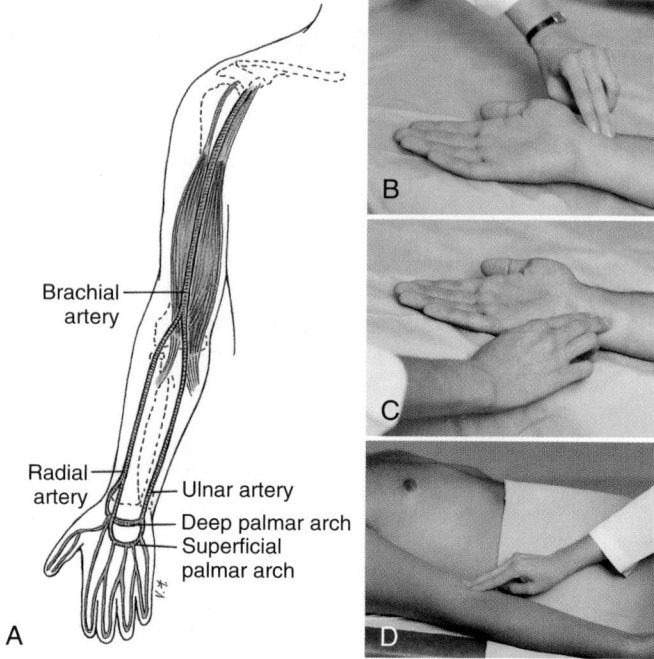

FIG. 30.47 **A,** Anatomical positions of brachial, radial, and ulnar arteries. **B,** Palpation of radial pulse. **C,** Palpation of ulnar pulse. **D,** Palpation of brachial pulse.

useful in evaluating heart activity. To check local circulatory status of tissues (e.g., when a leg cast is in place or following vascular surgery), palpate the peripheral arteries long enough to note that a pulse is present.

Assess each peripheral artery for elasticity of the vessel wall, strength, and equality. The arterial wall normally is elastic, making it easily palpable. After depressing the artery, it springs back to shape when the pressure is released. An abnormal artery is hard, inelastic, or calcified.

The strength of a pulse is a measurement of the force at which blood is ejected against the arterial wall. Some examiners use a scale rating from 0 to 4 for the strength of a pulse (Ball et al., 2019):

0: Absent, not palpable
1: Pulse diminished, barely palpable
2: Expected
3: Full, increased
4: Bounding, aneurysmal

Measure all peripheral pulses for equality and symmetry. Compare the left radial pulse with that of the right and so on. Lack of symmetry indicates impaired circulation such as a localized obstruction or an abnormally positioned artery.

In the upper extremities the brachial artery channels blood to the radial and ulnar arteries of the forearm and hand. If circulation in this artery becomes blocked, the hands do not receive adequate blood flow. If circulation in the radial or ulnar arteries becomes impaired, the hand still receives adequate perfusion. An interconnection between the radial and ulnar arteries guards against arterial occlusion (Fig. 30.47A).

To locate pulses in the arm, have the patient sit or lie down. Find the radial pulse along the radial side of the forearm at the wrist. Thin individuals have a groove lateral to the flexor tendon of the wrist. Feel the radial pulse with light palpation in the groove (see Fig. 30.47B). The ulnar pulse is on the opposite side of the wrist and feels less prominent (see Fig. 30.47C). Palpate the ulnar pulse when evaluating arterial insufficiency to the hand.

To palpate the brachial pulse, find the groove between the biceps and triceps muscle above the elbow at the antecubital fossa (see Fig. 30.47D). The artery runs along the medial side of the extended arm. Palpate it with the fingertips of the first three fingers in the muscle groove.

The femoral artery is the primary artery in the leg, delivering blood to the popliteal, posterior tibial, and dorsalis pedis arteries (Fig. 30.48A). An interconnection between the posterior tibial and dorsalis pedis arteries guards against local arterial occlusion.

Find the femoral pulse with the patient lying down with the inguinal area exposed (see Fig. 30.48B). The femoral artery runs below the inguinal ligament, midway between the symphysis pubis and the anterosuperior iliac spine. Sometimes deep palpation is necessary to feel the pulse. Bimanual palpation is effective in patients who are obese. Place the fingertips of both hands on opposite sides of the pulse site. Feel a pulsatile sensation when the arterial pulsation pushes the fingertips apart.

The popliteal pulse runs behind the knee. Have the patient slightly flex the knee with the foot resting on the examination table or assume a prone position with the knee slightly flexed (see Fig. 30.48C) and leg muscles relaxed. Palpate with the fingers of both hands deeply into the popliteal fossa, just lateral to the midline. The popliteal pulse is difficult to locate.

With the patient's foot relaxed, locate the dorsalis pedis pulse. The artery runs along the top of the foot in line with the groove between the extensor tendons of the great toe and first toe (see Fig. 30.48D). To find the pulse, place the fingertips between the first and second toes and slowly move up the dorsum of the foot. This pulse is sometimes congenitally absent.

Find the posterior tibial pulse on the inner side of each ankle (Fig. 30.48E). Place the fingers behind and below the medial malleolus (ankle bone). With the foot relaxed and slightly extended, palpate the artery.

Ultrasound Stethoscopes. If a pulse is difficult to palpate, an ultrasound (Doppler) stethoscope is a useful tool that amplifies the sounds of a pulse wave. Factors that weaken a pulse or make palpation difficult include obesity, reduction in the stroke volume of the heart, diminished blood volume, or

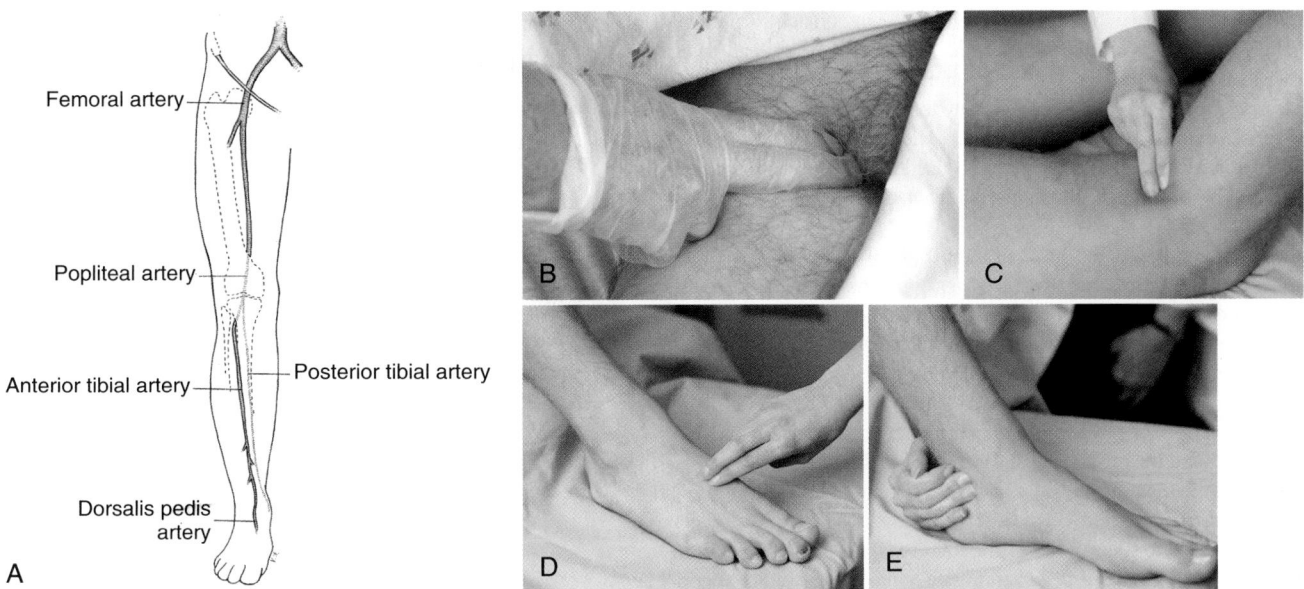

FIG. 30.48 A, Anatomical position of femoral, popliteal, dorsalis pedis, and anterior and posterior tibial arteries. B, Palpation of femoral pulse. C, Palpation of popliteal pulse. D, Palpation of dorsalis pedis pulse. E, Palpation of posterior tibial pulse.

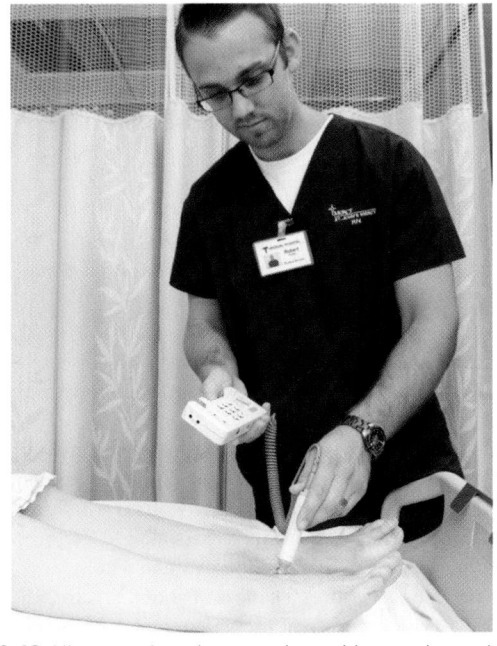

FIG. 30.49 Ultrasound stethoscope in position on the pedal pulse.

arterial obstruction. Apply a thin layer of transmission gel to the patient's skin at the pulse site or directly onto the transducer tip of the probe. Turn on the volume control and place the tip of the transducer at a 45- to 90-degree angle on the skin (Fig. 30.49). Move the transducer until you hear a pulsating "whooshing" sound that indicates that arterial blood flow is present.

REFLECT NOW

How would you respond if while completing an assessment you found a severe abnormality in a body system? Think through your body language, facial expression, and the conversation you would have with the patient through this situation. What further assessments might you need to complete?

TABLE 30.25   Signs of Venous and Arterial Insufficiency

Assessment Criterion	Venous	Arterial
Color	Normal or cyanotic	Pale; worsened by elevation of extremity; dusky red when extremity is lowered
Temperature	Normal	Cool (blood flow blocked to extremity)
Pulse	Normal	Decreased or absent
Edema	Often marked	Absent or mild
Skin changes	Brown pigmentation around ankles	Thin, shiny skin; decreased hair growth; thickened nails

Tissue Perfusion. The condition of the skin, mucosa, and nail beds offers useful data about the status of circulatory blood flow. Examine the face and extremities, looking at the color of the skin, lips, mucosa, and nail beds. Bluish color of lips or nail beds or decrease in pallor sometimes indicate cyanosis. When cyanosis is present, obtain a patient's oxygen saturation to determine the severity of the problem. Health care providers sometimes order additional blood tests to further evaluate oxygenation status. Examination of the nails involves inspection for **clubbing**, a bulging of the tissues at the nail base, which causes an abnormal curvature of the nail. Clubbing suggests a chronic problem such as emphysema and congenital heart disease.

Inspect the lower extremities for changes in color, temperature, and condition of the skin, indicating either arterial or venous alterations (Table 30.25). Ask if the patient has pain in the legs. If an arterial occlusion is present, the patient will experience pain distal to the occlusion. The five *P*s—pain, pallor, pulselessness, paresthesias, and paralysis—characterize an occlusion. Venous congestion causes tissue changes that indicate an inadequate circulatory flow back to the heart.

While examining the lower extremities, also inspect skin and nail texture; hair distribution on the lower legs, feet, and toes; the venous pattern; and scars, pigmentation, or ulcers. Absence of hair on the legs may indicate circulatory insufficiency; remember to consider whether the patient has shaved legs or wears tight socks, which can lead to a decrease in hair on the legs. Chronic recurring ulcers of the feet or lower legs are a serious sign of circulatory insufficiency and require a health care provider's intervention. Palpate the legs and feet for color, temperature, and edema. Capillary refill is used to determine adequacy of peripheral blood flow to the digits (Ball et al., 2019).

Peripheral Veins. Assess the status of the peripheral veins by asking the patient to assume sitting and standing positions. Assessment includes inspection and palpation for varicosities, peripheral edema, and phlebitis. Varicosities are superficial veins that become dilated, especially when the legs are in a dependent position. They are common in older adults because the veins normally fibrose, dilate, and stretch. They are also common in people who stand for prolonged periods. Varicosities in the anterior or medial part of the thigh and the posterolateral part of the calf are abnormal.

Dependent edema around the area of the feet and ankles is a sign of venous insufficiency or right-sided heart failure. It is common in older adults and people who spend a lot of time standing (e.g., waitresses, security guards, and nurses). To assess for pitting edema, use the index finger to press firmly for several seconds and release over the medial malleolus or the shins. A depression left in the skin indicates edema. Grading 1+ through 4+ characterizes the severity of the edema (see Fig. 30.6).

Phlebitis is an inflammation of a vein that occurs commonly after trauma to the vessel wall, infection, immobilization, and prolonged insertion of IV catheters. To assess for phlebitis in the leg, inspect the calves for localized redness, tenderness, and swelling over vein sites. Gentle palpation of calf muscles reveals warmth, tenderness, and firmness of the muscle. Unilateral edema of the affected leg is one of the most reliable findings of phlebitis. The Homan sign is not a reliable indicator of phlebitis or deep vein thrombosis (DVT) and is present in other conditions (Ambesh, 2017). To confirm DVT, other diagnostic tests are used whether or not the Homan sign is positive (Ambesh, 2017).

Lymphatic System

Assess the lymphatic drainage of the lower extremities during examination of the vascular system or during the female or male genital examination. Superficial and deep nodes drain the legs, but only two groups of superficial nodes are palpable. With the patient supine, palpate the area of the superficial inguinal nodes in the groin area (Fig. 30.50A). Then move the fingertips toward the inner thigh, feeling for any inferior nodes. Use a firm but gentle pressure when palpating over each lymphatic chain. Multiple nodes normally are not palpable, although a few soft nontender nodes are not unusual. Enlarged, hardened, tender nodes reveal potential sites of infection or metastatic disease.

In the upper extremities, lymph is carried by the collecting ducts from the upper extremities to the subclavian lymphatic trunk. To assess this lymph system, gently palpate the epitrochlear nodes, located on the medial aspect of the arms near the antecubital fossa (see Fig. 30.50B). The proximal part of the upper-extremity lymph system is located in the axilla and is usually assessed during examination of the breasts.

BREASTS

It is important to examine the breasts of both female and male patients. Men have a small amount of glandular tissue in the breast, which is a potential site for the growth of cancer cells. In contrast, the majority of the female breast is glandular tissue.

Female Breasts

New cases of invasive breast cancer were predicted to affect an estimated 231,840 women in the United States during 2015; about 2,350

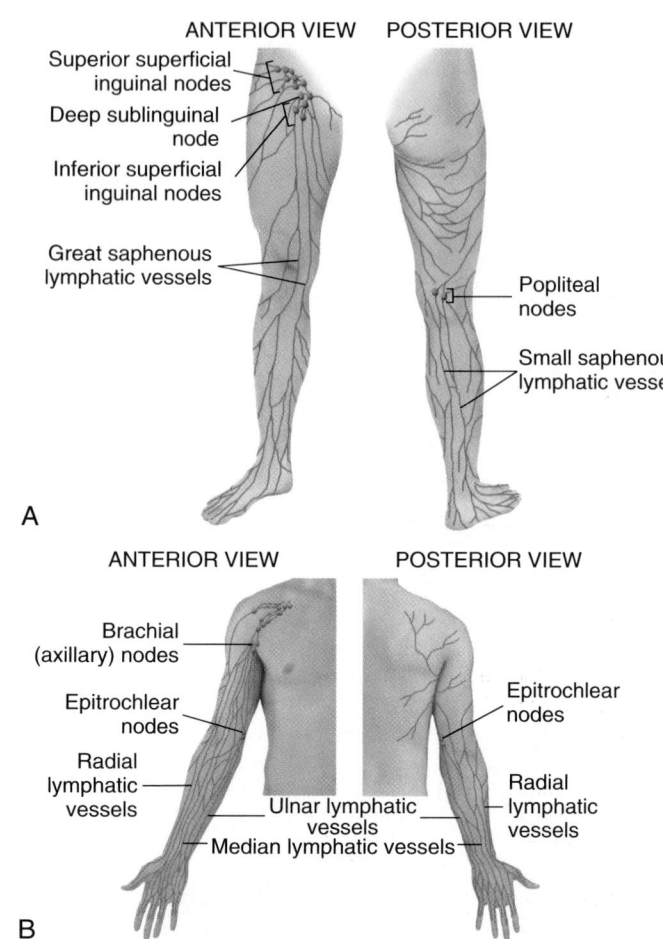

FIG. 30.50 **A,** Lymphatic drainage for lower extremities. **B,** Lymphatic drainage for upper extremities. (From Ball JW, et al: *Seidel's guide to physical examination*, ed 9, St Louis, 2019, Mosby.)

new cases were expected in men (ACS, 2018b). The disease is second to lung cancer as the leading cause of death in women with cancer. Early detection is the key to cure.

Table 30.3 outlines the American Cancer Society (ACS, 2018a) guidelines for the early detection of breast cancer in women at average risk. The ACS (2018b) recommends that women who are at high risk for breast cancer based on certain factors should get an MRI and a mammogram every year. This includes women who:

- Have a lifetime risk of breast cancer of about 20% to 25% or greater, according to risk assessment tools that are based mainly on family history
- Have a known *BRCA1* or *BRCA2* gene mutation
- Have a first-degree relative (parent, brother, sister, or child) with a *BRCA1* or *BRCA2* gene mutation and have not had genetic testing themselves
- Had radiation therapy to the chest when they were between 10 and 30 years of age

Monthly breast self-examination (BSE) is no longer recommended by the ACS (2018a) for women at any age because there is limited evidence to benefits in locating cancerous tumors, but other health organizations encourage BSE as an important option for women (National Breast Cancer Foundation, 2016). Encourage women to ask their personal physician what he or she recommends. If a female patient chooses to perform BSE, assess the method she uses and when she does the examination in relation to her menstrual cycle (Box 30.20). The best time for a BSE is the fourth through seventh day of the menstrual cycle

BOX 30.20 Breast Self-Examination

Procedure

- Help patient identify the appropriate time of the month to perform breast self-examination (BSE).
- Describe normal findings and what findings require notification of health care provider.
- Teach patient the steps to perform BSE:
  1. Examine your right breast. Lie on your back and place your right arm behind your head. The examination is best completed lying down, not standing up, because when you lie down the breast tissue spreads evenly over the chest wall and is as thin as possible, making it much easier to feel all of it.
  2. Use finger pads of the three middle fingers on your left hand to feel for lumps in the right breast. Use overlapping dime-size circular motions of the finger pads to feel the breast tissue. Use three different levels of pressure to feel all the breast tissue. Light pressure is needed to feel the tissue closest to the skin, medium pressure to feel a little deeper, and firm pressure to feel the tissue closest to the chest and ribs. It is normal to feel a firm ridge in the lower curve of each breast, but you should tell your health care provider if you feel anything else out of the ordinary. If you are not sure how hard to press, discuss this with your health care provider. Use each pressure level to feel the breast tissue before moving on to the next spot.
  3. Move around the breast in an up-and-down pattern starting at an imaginary line drawn straight down your side from the underarm and moving across the breast to the middle of the chest bone (sternum or breastbone).

Be sure to check the entire breast area, going down until you feel only ribs and up to the neck or collarbone (clavicle). Evidence shows that the up-and-down pattern is the most effective pattern for covering the entire breast.
  4. Repeat self-examination in the left breast, putting your left arm behind your head and examining the left breast as noted in Steps 1 to 3.
  5. While standing in front of a mirror with your hands pressing firmly down on your hips, look at your breasts, observing for any changes in size, shape, contour, dimpling, redness, or scaliness of the nipple or breast tissue. Pressing down on your hips contracts the chest wall muscles and enhances any breast changes.
  6. Examine each underarm while sitting or standing and with your arm only slightly raised so that you can feel any lumps or changes in this area easily. Raising your arm straight tightens the tissue in this area, making it harder to examine.
      - **NOTE:** If implants are present, help the patient determine the edges of each implant and how to evaluate each breast.
  7. Instruct patient to call the health care provider if she finds a lump or other abnormality.
  8. **Use Teach Back:** "I want to be sure I explained to you how to conduct a breast self-examination. Can you show me how to conduct an examination on both of your breasts?" Document your evaluation of patient learning. Revise your instruction or develop a plan for revised patient teaching to be implemented at an appropriate time if patient is not able to teach back correctly.

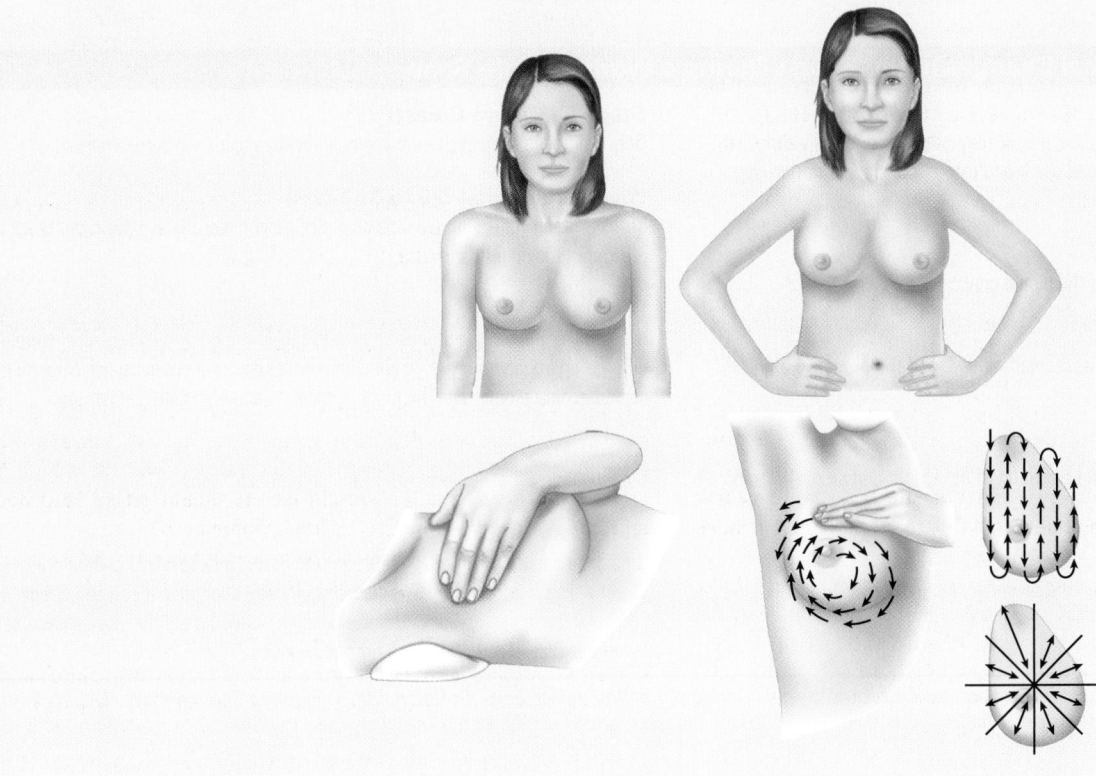

Images from Silvestri LA, Silvestri AE: *Saunders comprehensive review for the NCLEX-PN ® Examination*, ed 7, St Louis, 2019, Elsevier.

or right after the menstrual cycle ends, when the breasts are no longer swollen or tender from hormone elevations. If the woman does not menstruate (e.g., due to pregnancy or menopause), advise her to check her breasts on the same day each month.

Older women require special attention when reviewing the need for regular BSE. Unfortunately, many older women ignore changes in their breasts, assuming that they are a part of aging. In addition,

physiological factors affect the ease with which older women perform a BSE. Musculoskeletal limitations, diminished peripheral sensation, reduced eyesight, and changes in joint range of motion (ROM) limit palpation and inspection abilities.

The patient's history (Table 30.26) reveals normal developmental changes and signs of breast disease. Because of its glandular structure, the breast undergoes changes during a woman's life. Knowing these

TABLE 30.26 Nursing History for Breast Assessment

Assessment	Rationale
Determine whether woman is over age 40; has a personal or family history of breast cancer, especially with the *BRCA1* or *BRCA2* inherited gene mutations; early-onset menarche (before age 12) or late-age menopause (after age 55); has never had children or gave birth to first child after age 31; or has recently used oral contraceptives.	These are risk factors for breast cancer (ACS, 2018a; ACS, 2018b).
Ask whether patient (both sexes) has noticed lump, thickening, pain, or tenderness of breast; discharge, distortion, retraction, or scaling of the nipple; or change in size of breast.	Potential signs and symptoms of breast cancer allow nurse to focus on specific areas of breast during assessment.
Determine patient's use of medications (oral contraceptives, digitalis, diuretics, steroids, or estrogen). Determine his or her caffeine intake.	Some medications cause nipple discharge. Hormones and caffeine cause fibrocystic changes in breast.
Determine patient's level of activity, alcoholic intake, and weight.	Breast cancer incidence rates correlate with being overweight or obese (postmenopausal), physical inactivity, and consumption of alcoholic beverages (ACS, 2018b).
Ask whether patient performs monthly breast self-examination (BSE). If so, determine time of month she performs examination in relation to menstrual cycle. Have her describe or demonstrate method used.	Nurse's role is to educate patient about breast cancer and correct techniques for BSE.
If patient reports a breast mass, ask about length of time since she first noticed the lump. Does lump come and go, or is it always present? Have there been changes in the lump (e.g., size, relationship to menses), and are there associated symptoms?	Assessment helps to determine nature of mass (e.g., breast cancer versus fibrocystic disease).

BOX 30.21 Normal Changes in the Breast During a Woman's Life Span

Puberty (8 to 20 Years)
Breasts mature in five stages. One breast may grow more rapidly than the other. The ages at which changes occur and rate of developmental progression vary.

Stage 1 (Preadolescent)
This stage involves elevation of the nipple only.

Stage 2
The breast and nipple elevate as a small mound, and the areolar diameters enlarge.

Stage 3
There is further enlargement and elevation of the breast and areola, with no separation of contour.

Stage 4
The areola and nipple project into the secondary mound above the level of the breast (does not occur in all girls).

Stage 5 (Mature Breast)
Only the nipple projects, and the areola recedes (varies in some women).

Young Adulthood (20 to 31 Years)
Breasts reach full (nonpregnant) size. Shape is generally symmetrical. Breasts are sometimes unequal in size.

Pregnancy
Breast size gradually enlarges to two to three times the previous size. Nipples enlarge and become erect. Areolas darken, and diameters increase. Superficial veins become prominent. The nipples expel a yellowish fluid (colostrum).

Menopause
Breasts shrink. Tissue becomes softer, sometimes flabby.

Older Adulthood
Breasts become elongated, pendulous, and flaccid as a result of glandular tissue atrophy. The skin of the breasts tends to wrinkle, appearing loose and flabby.
Nipples become smaller and flatter and lose erectile ability. They sometimes invert because of shrinkage and fibrotic changes.

Data from Touhy TA, Jett KF: *Ebersole and Hess' gerontological nursing & healthy aging*, ed 5, St Louis, 2019, Elsevier; Hockenberry MJ, Wilson D: *Wong's nursing care of infants and children*, ed 10, St Louis, 2017, Elsevier; and Ball JW, et al: *Seidel's guide to physical examination*, ed 9, St Louis, 2019, Elsevier.

changes (Box 30.21) allows complete and accurate assessment. Encourage both men and women to observe their breasts for changes and to report any changes to their health care provider.

Inspection. Have the patient remove the top gown or drape to allow simultaneous visualization of both breasts. Have her stand or sit with her arms hanging loosely at her sides. If the patient chooses to perform BSE, place a mirror in front of her if possible during inspection so that she sees what to look for when performing a BSE. Describe observations or findings in relation to imaginary lines that divide the breast into four quadrants and a tail. The lines cross at the center of the nipple. Each tail extends outward from the upper outer quadrant (Fig. 30.51).

Inspect the breasts for size and symmetry. Normally they extend from the third to the sixth ribs, with the nipple at the level of the fourth intercostal space. It is common for one breast to be smaller. However, inflammation or a mass causes a difference in size. As a woman ages, the ligaments supporting the breast tissue weaken, causing the breasts to sag and the nipples to lower.

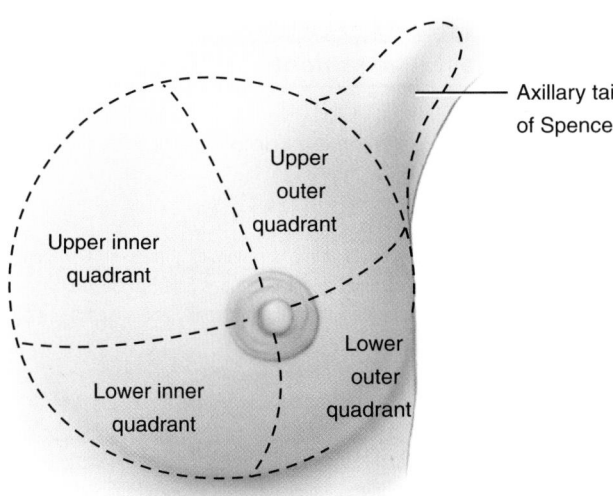

FIG. 30.51 Quadrants of left breast and axillary tail of Spence. (From Shiland BJ: *Medical terminology and anatomy for coding*, ed 3, St Louis, 2017, Mosby.)

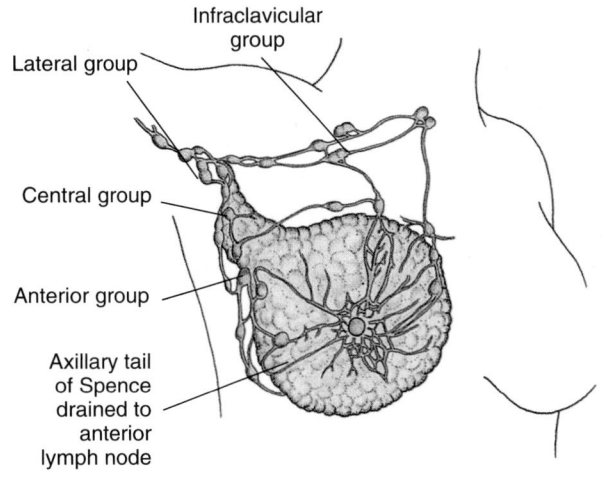

FIG. 30.52 Anatomical position of axillary and clavicular lymph nodes.

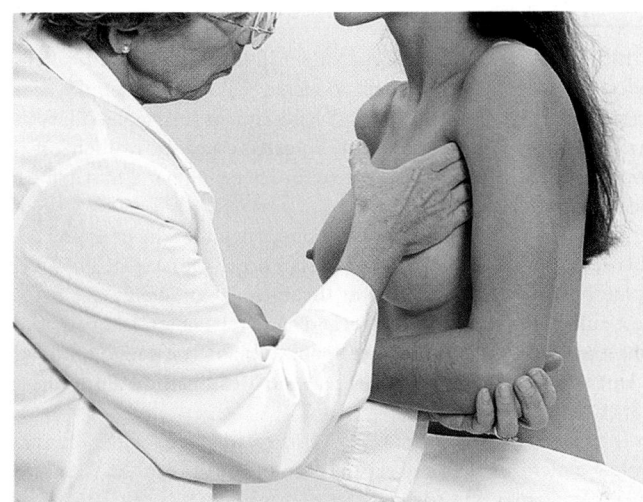

FIG. 30.53 Support patient's arm and palpate axillary lymph nodes. (From Wilson S, Giddens J: *Health assessment for nursing practice*, ed 6, St Louis, 2016, Elsevier.)

Observe the contour or shape of the breasts and note masses, flattening, retraction, or dimpling. Breasts vary in shape from convex to pendulous or conical. Retraction or dimpling can result from invasion of underlying ligaments by tumors. The ligaments fibrose and pull the overlying skin inward toward the tumor. Edema also changes the contour of the breasts. To bring out retraction or changes in the shape of breasts, ask the patient to assume three positions: raise arms above the head, press hands against the hips, and extend arms straight ahead while sitting and leaning forward. Each maneuver causes a contraction of the pectoral muscles, which accentuates the presence of any retraction.

Carefully inspect the skin for color; venous pattern; and the presence of lesions, edema, or inflammation. Lift each breast when necessary to observe lower and lateral aspects for color and texture changes. The breasts are the color of neighboring skin, and venous patterns are the same bilaterally. Venous patterns are easily visible in thin or pregnant women. Women with large breasts often have redness and excoriation of the undersurfaces caused by rubbing of skin surfaces.

Inspect the nipple and areola for size, color, shape, discharge, and the direction in which the nipples point. The normal areolas are round or oval and nearly equal bilaterally. Color ranges from pink to brown. In light-skinned women the areola turns brown during pregnancy and remains dark. In dark-skinned women the areola is brown before pregnancy (Ball et al., 2019). Normally the nipples point in symmetrical directions, are everted, and have no drainage. If the nipples are inverted, ask whether this has been a lifetime history. A recent inversion or inward turning of the nipple indicates an underlying growth. Rashes or ulcerations are not normal on the breast or nipples. Note any bleeding or discharge from the nipple. Clear yellow discharge 2 days after childbirth is common. While inspecting the breasts, explain the characteristics you see. Teach patients the significance of abnormal signs or symptoms.

Palpation. Use palpation to assess the condition of underlying breast tissue and lymph nodes. Breast tissue consists of glandular tissue, fibrous supportive ligaments, and fat. Glandular tissue is organized into lobes that end in ducts that open onto the surface of the nipple. The largest part of glandular tissue is in the upper outer quadrant and tail of each breast. Suspensory ligaments connect to skin and fascia underlying the breast to support the breast and maintain its upright position. Fatty tissue is located superficially and to the sides of the breast.

A part of the lymph system of the breasts drains into axillary lymph nodes. If cancerous lesions metastasize (spread), the nodes commonly become involved. Study the location of supraclavicular, infraclavicular, and axillary nodes (Fig. 30.52). The axillary nodes drain lymph from the chest wall, breasts, arms, and hands. A tumor of one breast sometimes involves nodes on the same and opposite sides.

To palpate the lymph nodes, have the patient sit with her arms at her sides and muscles relaxed. While facing the patient and standing on the side you are examining, support her arm in a flexed position and abduct it from the chest wall. Place the free hand against the patient's chest wall and high in the axillary hollow. With the fingertips press gently down over the surface of the ribs and muscles. Palpate the four areas of the axilla and the axillary nodes with the fingertips, gently rolling soft tissue (Fig. 30.53).

Normally lymph nodes are not palpable. Carefully assess each area and note their number, consistency, mobility, and size. One or two small, soft, nontender palpable nodes are normal. An abnormal palpable node feels like a small mass that is hard, tender, and immobile. Continue to palpate along the upper and lower clavicular ridges. Reverse the procedure for the patient's other side.

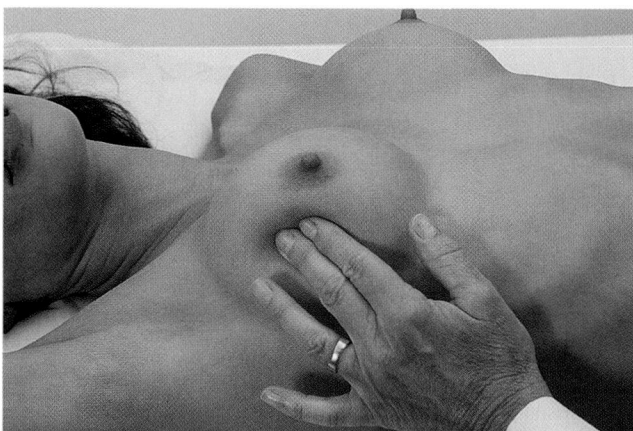

FIG. 30.54 Patient lies flat with arm abducted and hand under head to help flatten breast tissue evenly over chest wall. Each breast is palpated in a systematic fashion. (From Wilson S, Giddens J: *Health assessment for nursing practice*, ed 6, St Louis, 2016, Elsevier.)

It is sometimes difficult for a patient to learn to palpate for lymph nodes. Lying down with the arm abducted makes the area more accessible. Instruct the patient to use her left hand for the right axillary and clavicular areas. Take the patient's fingertips and move them in the proper fashion. Then have the patient use her right hand to palpate for nodes on the left side.

With the patient lying supine and one arm under the head and neck (alternating with each breast), palpate her breast tissue (Fig. 30.54). The supine position allows the breast tissue to flatten evenly against the chest wall. The position of the arm and hand further stretches and positions breast tissue evenly. Place a small pillow or towel under the patient's shoulder blade to further position breast tissue. Palpate the tail of Spence.

The consistency of normal breast tissue varies widely. The breasts of a young patient are firm and elastic. In an older patient the tissue sometimes feels stringy and nodular. A patient's familiarity with the texture of her own breasts is very important. Teach patients about strategies to promote breast health (Box 30.22).

If you or the patient palpate a mass, examine the opposite breast to ensure an objective comparison of normal and abnormal tissue. Use the pads of the first three fingers to compress breast tissue gently against the chest wall, noting tissue consistency. Perform palpation systematically in one of three ways: (1) using a vertical technique with the fingers moving up and down each quadrant; (2) clockwise or counterclockwise, forming small concentric circles with the fingers along each quadrant and the tail; or (3) palpating from the center of the breast in a radial fashion, returning to the areola to begin each spoke (Fig. 30.55A-C). Whichever approach you use, be sure to cover the entire breast and tail, directing attention to any areas of tenderness. Use a bimanual technique when palpating large, pendulous breasts. Support the inferior part of the breast in one hand while using the other hand to palpate breast tissue against the supporting hand.

During palpation note the consistency of breast tissue. It normally feels dense, firm, and elastic. With menopause breast tissue shrinks and becomes softer. The lobular feel of glandular tissue is normal. The lower edge of each breast sometimes feels firm and hard. This is the normal inframammary ridge and not a tumor. It helps to move the patient's hand so that she can feel normal tissue variations. Palpate abnormal masses to determine location in relation to quadrants, diameter in centimeters, shape (e.g., round or discoid), consistency (soft, firm, or hard), tenderness, mobility, and discreteness (clear or unclear boundaries).

BOX 30.22 **PATIENT TEACHING**

Female Breast Assessment

Objective
- Patient will follow prevention and detection practices to ensure breast health.

Teaching Strategies
- Have patient perform return demonstration of breast self-examination (BSE) and offer the opportunity to ask questions (see Box 30.20).
- Explain recommended frequency of mammography and assessment by the patient's health care provider.
- Discuss signs and symptoms of breast cancer.
- Discuss signs and symptoms of benign (fibrocystic) breast disease.
- Inform a woman who is obese or has a family history of breast cancer that she is at higher risk for the disease (ACS, 2018b). Encourage dietary changes, including limiting meat consumption to well-trimmed, lean beef, pork, or lamb; removing skin from cooked chicken before eating it; selecting tuna and salmon packed in water and not oil; and using low-fat dairy products.
- Encourage patient to reduce intake of caffeine and theophyllines. Although this approach is controversial, it can reduce symptoms of benign (fibrocystic) breast disease.

Evaluation
Use the principles of teach-back to evaluate patient/family caregiver learning:
- Tell me when was your last mammogram? Explain to me how often you should get a mammogram.
- Describe for me the signs and symptoms of breast cancer and when you should contact your health care provider.

Cancerous lesions are hard, fixed, nontender, irregular in shape, and usually unilateral. A common benign condition of the breast is benign (fibrocystic) breast disease. Bilateral lumpy, painful breasts and sometimes nipple discharge characterize this condition. Symptoms are more apparent during the menstrual period. When palpated, the cysts (lumps) are soft, well differentiated, and movable. Deep cysts feel hard.

Give special attention to palpating the nipple and areola. Palpate the entire surface gently. Use the thumb and index finger to compress the nipple and note any discharge. During the examination of the nipple and areola, the nipple sometimes becomes erect with wrinkling of the areola. These changes are normal. Continue by positioning the patient and examining the other breast.

Male Breasts

Inspect the nipple and areola for nodules, edema, and ulceration. An enlarged male breast results from obesity or glandular enlargement. Breast enlargement in young males results from steroid use. Fatty tissue feels soft, whereas glandular tissue is firm. Use the same techniques to palpate for masses used in examination of the female breast. Because breast cancer in men is relatively rare, routine self-examinations are unnecessary. However, men who have a first-degree relative (e.g., mother or sister) with breast cancer are at risk for breast cancer and may be scheduled by their health care provider for routine mammograms.

ABDOMEN

The abdominal examination is complex because of the number of organs located within and near the abdominal cavity. A thorough nursing history (Table 30.27) helps interpret physical signs. The

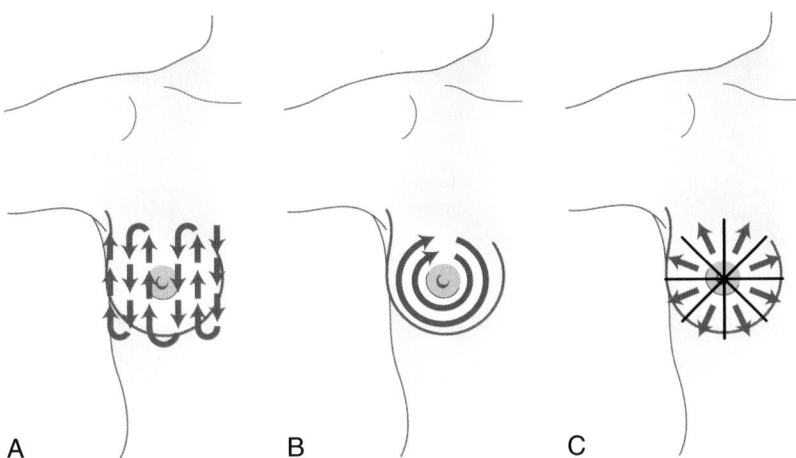

FIG. 30.55 Various methods for palpation of breast. **A,** Palpate from top to bottom in vertical strips. **B,** Palpate in concentric circles. **C,** Palpate out from center in wedge sections.

TABLE 30.27 Nursing History for Abdominal Assessment

Assessment	Rationale
If patient has abdominal or low back pain, assess character of pain in detail (location, onset, frequency, precipitating factors, aggravating factors, type of pain, severity, course).	Pattern of characteristics of pain helps determine its source.
Carefully observe patient's movement and position, including lying still with knees drawn up, moving restlessly to find comfortable position, and lying on one side or sitting with knees drawn to chest.	Positions assumed by patient reveal nature and source of pain, including peritonitis, renal stone, and pancreatitis.
Assess normal bowel habits and stool character; ask whether patient uses laxatives.	Data compared with physical findings help identify cause and nature of elimination problems.
Determine whether patient has had abdominal surgery, trauma, or diagnostic tests of gastrointestinal (GI) tract.	Surgical or traumatic alterations of abdominal organs cause changes in expected findings (e.g., position of underlying organs). Diagnostic tests change character of stool.
Assess whether patient has had recent weight changes or intolerance to diet (e.g., nausea, vomiting, cramping, especially in last 24 hours).	Data can indicate alterations in upper GI tract (stomach or gallbladder) or lower colon.
Assess for difficulty in swallowing, belching, flatulence (gas), bloody emesis (hematemesis), black or tarry stools (melena), heartburn, diarrhea, or constipation.	These characteristic signs and symptoms indicate GI alterations.
Ask whether patient takes antiinflammatory medication (e.g., aspirin, ibuprofen, steroids) or antibiotics.	Pharmacological agents cause GI upset or bleeding.
Ask patient to locate tender areas before examination begins.	Assess painful areas last to minimize discomfort and anxiety.
Inquire about family history of cancer, kidney disease, alcoholism, hypertension, or heart disease.	Data can reveal risk for alterations identifiable during examination.
Determine whether female patient is pregnant; note last menstrual period.	Pregnancy causes changes in abdominal shape and contour.
Assess patient's usual intake of alcohol.	Chronic alcohol ingestion causes GI and liver problems, including liver, colon, and pancreatic cancer (ACS, 2018b).
Review patient's history for the following: health care occupation, hemodialysis, intravenous drug user, household or sexual contact with hepatitis B virus (HBV) carrier, heterosexual person with more than one sex partner in previous 6 months, sexually active homosexual or bisexual male, international traveler in area of high HBV infection rate.	Risk factors for HBV exposure.

examination includes an assessment of structures of the lower gastrointestinal (GI) tract in addition to the liver, stomach, uterus, ovaries, kidneys, and bladder. Abdominal pain is one of the most common symptoms that patients report when seeking medical care. An accurate assessment requires matching patient history data with a careful assessment of the location of physical symptoms.

Assess the organs anteriorly and posteriorly. A system of landmarks helps map out the abdominal region. The xiphoid process (tip of the sternum) is the upper boundary of the anterior abdominal region. The symphysis pubis marks the lower boundary. Divide the abdomen into four imaginary quadrants (Fig. 30.56A); refer to assessment findings

and record them in relation to each quadrant. Posteriorly the lower ribs and heavy back muscles protect the kidneys, which are located from the T12 to L3 vertebrae (see Fig. 30.56B). The costovertebral angle formed by the last rib and vertebral column is a landmark used during kidney palpation.

During the abdominal examination the patient needs to relax. A tightening of abdominal muscles hinders palpation. Ask the patient to void before beginning. Be sure that the room is warm and drape upper chest and legs. The patient lies supine or in a dorsal recumbent position with the arms at the sides and knees slightly bent. Place small pillows beneath the knees. If the patient places the arms under the head, the

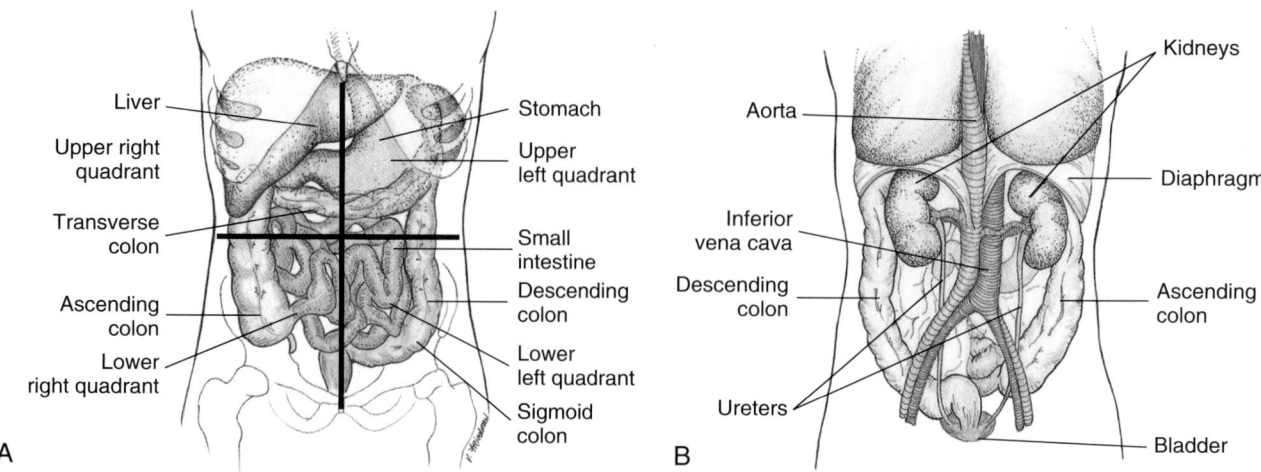

FIG. 30.56 **A,** Anterior view of abdomen divided by quadrants. **B,** Posterior view of abdominal section.

abdominal muscles tighten. Proceed calmly and slowly, being sure that there is adequate lighting. Expose the abdomen from just above the xiphoid process down to the symphysis pubis. Warm hands and stethoscope further promote relaxation. Ask the patient to report pain and point out tender areas. Assess tender areas last.

The order of an abdominal examination differs slightly from previous assessments. Begin with inspection and follow with auscultation. By completing palpation last there is less chance of altering the frequency and character of bowel sounds. Be sure to have a tape measure and marking pen available during the examination.

Inspection

Make it a habit to observe the patient during routine care activities. Note his or her posture and look for evidence of abdominal splinting: lying with the knees drawn up or moving restlessly in bed. A patient free from abdominal pain does not guard or splint the abdomen. To inspect the abdomen for abnormal movement or shadows, stand on the patient's right side and inspect from above the abdomen. After sitting or stooping down to look across the abdomen, assess abdominal contour. Direct the examination light over the abdomen.

Skin. Inspect the skin over the abdomen for color, scars, venous patterns, lesions, and striae (stretch marks). The skin is subject to the same color variations as the rest of the body. Venous patterns are normally faint, except in thin patients. Striae result from stretching of tissue by obesity or pregnancy. Artificial openings indicate drainage sites resulting from surgery (see Chapter 50) or an ostomy (see Chapters 46 and 47). Scars reveal evidence of past trauma or surgery that has created permanent changes in underlying organ anatomy. Bruising indicates accidental injury, physical abuse, or a type of bleeding disorder. If needle marks or bruises are present, ask whether the patient self-administers injections (e.g., low-molecular-weight heparin or insulin). Unexpected findings include generalized color changes such as jaundice or cyanosis. Shiny abdominal skin with a taut (tight) appearance can indicate ascites.

Umbilicus. Note the position; shape; color; and signs of inflammation, discharge, or protruding masses. A normal umbilicus is flat or concave, with the color the same as that of the surrounding skin. Underlying masses cause displacement of the umbilicus. An everted (pouched-out) umbilicus usually indicates distention. Hernias (protrusion of abdominal organs through the muscle wall) cause upward protrusion of the umbilicus. Normally the umbilical area does not emit discharge.

Contour and Symmetry. Inspect for contour, symmetry, and surface motion of the abdomen, noting any masses, bulging, or distention. A flat abdomen forms a horizontal plane from the xiphoid process to the symphysis pubis. A round abdomen protrudes in a convex sphere from the horizontal plane. A concave abdomen appears to sink into the muscular wall. Each of these findings is normal for the individual patient if the shape of the abdomen is symmetrical. In older adults there is often an overall increased distribution of adipose tissue. The presence of masses on only one side, or asymmetry, can indicate an underlying pathological condition.

Intestinal gas, a tumor, or fluid in the abdominal cavity causes distention (swelling). When distention is generalized, the entire abdomen protrudes. The skin often appears taut, as if it were stretched over the abdomen. When gas causes distention, the flanks (side muscles) do not bulge. However, if fluid is the source of the problem, the flanks bulge. Ask the patient to roll onto one side. A protuberance forms on the dependent side if fluid is the cause of the distention. Ask the patient whether the abdomen feels unusually tight. Be careful not to confuse distention with obesity. In obesity the abdomen is large, rolls of adipose tissue are often present along the flanks, and the patient does not complain of tightness in the abdomen. If distention is expected, measure the abdomen by placing a tape measure around it at the level of the umbilicus (this may require the patient to roll side-to-side as you position the tape measure). Consecutive measurements show any increase or decrease in distention. Use a marking pen to indicate the location of the tape measure.

Enlarged Organs or Masses. Observe the contour of the abdomen while asking the patient to take a deep breath and hold it. Normally the contour remains smooth and symmetrical. This maneuver forces the diaphragm downward and reduces the size of the abdominal cavity. Any enlarged organs in the upper abdominal cavity (e.g., liver or spleen) descend below the rib cage to cause a bulge. Perform a closer examination with palpation. To evaluate the abdominal musculature have the patient raise the head. This position causes superficial abdominal wall masses, hernias, and muscle separations to become more apparent.

Movement or Pulsations. Inspect for movement. Normally men breathe abdominally, and women breathe more costally. A patient with severe pain has diminished respiratory movement and tightens the abdominal muscles to guard against the pain. Closely inspect for peristaltic movement and aortic pulsation by looking across the abdomen from the side. These movements are visible in thin patients; otherwise no movement is present.

BOX 30.23 EVIDENCE-BASED PRACTICE

Detection of Gastrointestinal Complications

PICOT Question: Are patients with general medical problems more at risk for gastrointestinal (GI) complications compared with patients who are critically ill?

Evidence Summary

A well-performed, complete GI assessment can identify changes that lead to complications and guide care of the patient. The subjective component of the GI assessment requires questions to determine history, normal routine, food consumption, elimination patterns, and discomfort. It is recommended to use multiple objective assessment techniques such as auscultation, inspection, and palpation as well as more detailed tests such as computed tomography (CT), ultrasound, endoscopy and real-time bowel sound analysis using acoustic sensors (Goto et al., 2015). Using only one component of the exam, such as auscultation of bowel sounds is not a good indicator of complications (Felder et al., 2014). Bowel sounds can vary greatly depending on the patient situation. An increase in the frequency of bowel sounds can present because the patient is chewing gum (Frazer et al., 2018), or an increase in blood sugar can slow motility and decrease the frequency of bowel sounds (Ladopoulos et al., 2018). Over the years the physical GI exam has been scaled down while imaging techniques have increased (Zuin et al., 2017). Scales such as the sequential failure assessment (SOFA) and GI failure (GIF) can be used in combination with a physical exam to help identify complications (Moonen et al., 2018).

GI complications contribute to a high risk of mortality, increased length of stay, and medical costs (Frazer et al., 2018). Patients in intensive care units are more likely to have more GI devices, such as nasogastric (NG) tubes to suction, a tube for feedings, and parenteral feeding, and require additional monitoring (Jacob, 2017).

These aspects of care contribute to a patient in the intensive care area having an increased risk for complications when compared to a general medicine patient. Current and preexisting conditions, such as obesity, advancing age, chronic alcohol use, altered fluid and electrolytes, or kidney issues, make the patient more likely to experience GI complications (Bond and Hallmark, 2018). Patients with a decreased level of consciousness have an increased risk of GI complications; therefore, different assessment techniques may be needed (Li et al., 2014). Goto and colleagues (2015) discuss the use of a real-time bowel sound analysis system for continuous monitoring of bowel sounds through recording equipment and acoustic sensors. This monitoring allows for the initial change in bowel sound to be addressed as soon as possible to assist with the identification of complications.

Application to Nursing Practice

- GI complications are common in patients admitted to the hospital (Jacob, 2017).
- A complete GI assessment needs to be completed, including subjective and objective information because an assessment finding as minor as hiccups can be an indication of a complication (Bond and Hallmark, 2018).
- Auscultation of bowel sounds should be completed but should not be the sole indicator of a complication (Zuin et al., 2017).
- Education should be completed on standard practice for auscultation of bowel sounds and evaluation conducted to make sure standards are being followed (Li et al., 2014).
- Movement can help decrease GI complications in patients (Morisawa et al., 2017).

Auscultation

Auscultate before palpation during the abdominal assessment because manipulation of the abdomen alters the frequency and intensity of bowel sounds. Ask patients not to talk. Patients with GI tubes connected to suction need them temporarily turned off before beginning an examination.

Bowel Motility. Peristalsis, or the movement of contents through the intestines, is a normal function of the small and large intestine. Bowel sounds are the audible passage of air and fluid that peristalsis creates. Place the warmed diaphragm of the stethoscope lightly over each of the four quadrants. Normally air and fluid move through the intestines, creating soft gurgling or clicking sounds that occur irregularly 5 to 35 times per minute (Ball et al., 2019). It normally takes 5 to 20 seconds to hear a bowel sound. However, it takes 5 minutes of continuous listening before determining that bowel sounds are absent (Ball et al., 2019). Auscultate all four quadrants to be sure that you do not miss any sounds. The best time to auscultate is between meals. Sounds are generally described as normal, audible, absent, hyperactive, or hypoactive. Absent sounds indicate a lack of peristalsis, possibly the result of late-stage bowel obstruction; paralytic ileus; or peritonitis. Absent or hypoactive bowel sounds may be normal after surgery following general anesthesia. Hyperactive sounds are loud, "growling" sounds called borborygmi, which indicate increased GI motility and can be caused by inflammation of the bowel, anxiety, diarrhea, bleeding, excessive ingestion of laxatives, and reaction of the intestines to certain foods. Assessment findings vary based on patient situation and level of care (Box 30.23). Teach patients practices that promote normal elimination patterns (Box 30.24).

Vascular Sounds. Bruits indicate narrowing of the major blood vessels and disruption of blood flow. The presence of bruits in the

BOX 30.24 PATIENT TEACHING

Abdominal Assessment

Objective

- Patient will maintain normal bowel elimination.

Teaching Strategies

- Explain factors that promote normal bowel elimination such as diet (fruits, vegetables, fiber), regular exercise, limited use of over-the-counter drugs causing constipation, establishment of regular elimination schedule, and a good fluid intake (see Chapter 47). Stress importance for older adults.
- Caution patients about the dangers of excessive use of laxatives or enemas.
- Instruct patient to have acute abdominal pain evaluated by a health care provider.

Evaluation

Use the principles of teach-back to evaluate patient/family caregiver learning:
- Describe for me your bowel elimination pattern and what the stool looks like.
- Describe for me the high-fiber foods that you have added to your diet.

abdominal area can reveal aneurysms or stenotic vessels. Use the bell of the stethoscope to auscultate in the epigastric region and each of the four quadrants. Normally there are no vascular sounds over the aorta (midline through the abdomen) or femoral arteries (lower quadrants). You can hear renal artery bruits by placing the stethoscope over each upper quadrant anteriorly or over the costovertebral angle posteriorly. Report a bruit immediately to a health care provider.

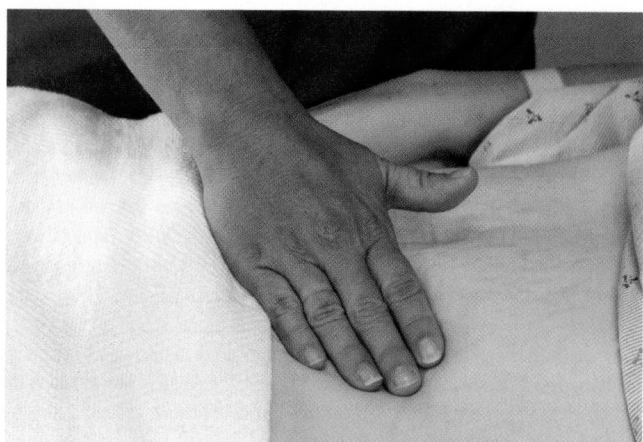

FIG. 30.57 Light palpation of abdomen.

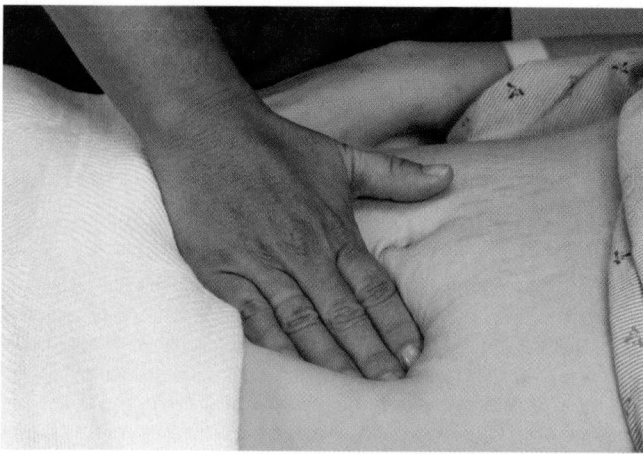

FIG. 30.58 Deep palpation of abdomen.

Kidney Tenderness. With the patient sitting or standing erect, use direct or indirect percussion to assess for kidney inflammation. With the ulnar surface of the partially closed fist, percuss posteriorly the costovertebral angle at the scapular line. If the kidneys are inflamed, the patient feels tenderness during percussion.

Palpation

Palpation primarily detects areas of abdominal tenderness, distention, or masses. As your skill base increases, learn to palpate for specific organs by using light and deep palpation.

Use light palpation over each abdominal quadrant to detect areas of tenderness. Initially avoid areas previously identified as problem spots. Lay the palm of the hand with fingers extended and approximated lightly on the abdomen. Explain the maneuver to the patient and, with the palmar surface of the fingers, depress approximately 1.3 cm (½ inch) in a gentle dipping motion (Fig. 30.57). Avoid quick jabs and use smooth, coordinated movements. If the patient is ticklish, first place his or her hand on the abdomen with your hand on the patient's; continue this until the patient tolerates palpation.

Use a systematic palpation approach for each quadrant and assess for muscular resistance, distention, tenderness, and superficial organs or masses. Observe the patient's face for signs of discomfort. The abdomen is normally smooth with consistent softness and nontender without masses. In contrast to firm muscles found among young adults, an older adult often lacks abdominal tone. Guarding or muscle tenseness sometimes occurs while palpating a sensitive area. If tightening remains after the patient relaxes, peritonitis, acute cholecystitis, or appendicitis is sometimes the cause. It is easy to detect a distended bladder with light palpation because the bladder lies below the umbilicus and above the symphysis pubis. Routinely check for a distended bladder if the patient has been unable to void (e.g., because of anesthesia or sedation, has been incontinent, or if an indwelling urinary catheter is not draining well).

With practice and experience perform deep palpation to delineate abdominal organs and detect less obvious masses. You need short fingernails. It is important for the patient to be relaxed while the hands depress approximately 2.5 to 7.5 cm (1 to 3 inches) into the abdomen (Fig. 30.58). Never use deep palpation over a surgical incision, over tender organs, or on abnormal masses. Deep pressure causes tenderness in a healthy patient over the cecum, sigmoid colon, aorta, and the midline near the xiphoid process (Ball et al., 2019).

Survey each quadrant systematically. Palpate masses for size, location, shape, consistency, tenderness, pulsation, and mobility. Test for rebound tenderness by pressing a hand slowly and deeply into the involved area and letting go quickly; if discomfort is present, then the test is positive. Be careful with this examination technique if pain is present. Rebound tenderness occurs in patients with peritoneal irritation such as occurs in appendicitis; pancreatitis; or any peritoneal injury causing bile, blood, or enzymes to enter the peritoneal cavity.

Aortic Pulsation. Palpate with the thumb and forefinger of one hand deeply into the upper abdomen just left of the midline to assess aortic pulsation. Normally a pulsation is transmitted forward. If the aorta is enlarged because of an aneurysm (localized dilation of a vessel wall), the pulsation expands laterally. Do not palpate a pulsating abdominal mass. When enlargement from an aneurysm is present, palpate this area only lightly, referring the finding to the health care provider. In patients who are obese, it is often necessary to palpate with both hands, one on each side of the aorta.

FEMALE GENITALIA AND REPRODUCTIVE TRACT

Examination of the female genitalia can be embarrassing to a patient unless you use a calm, relaxed approach. The gynecological examination is one of the most difficult experiences for adolescents. A person's cultural background further adds to apprehension. For example, female Mexican Americans have a strong social value that women do not expose their bodies to men or even to other women. Similarly, Chinese Americans believe that the examination of genitalia is offensive. Muslim women value respect for female modesty. Provide a thorough explanation of the reason for the procedures used in an examination. The lithotomy position assumed during the examination is an added source of embarrassment and can increase anxiety. A patient is more comfortable when you use correct positioning and draping. Be sure to explain each part of the examination in advance so that patients anticipate necessary actions. Adolescents sometimes choose to have parents present in the examination room.

Sometimes a patient requires a complete examination of the female reproductive organs, including assessing the external genitalia and performing a vaginal examination. You can examine external genitalia while performing routine hygiene measures or when preparing to insert a urinary catheter. An internal examination is part of each woman's preventive health care because ovarian cancer causes more deaths than any other cancer of the female reproductive system (ACS, 2018b).

Adolescents and young adults are examined because of the growing incidence of sexually transmitted infections (STIs). The average age of menarche among young girls has declined, and the majority of male and female teenagers are sexually active by age 19 (Hockenberry and Wilson, 2019). It is important to assess a patient's level of anxiety when obtaining the nursing history (Table 30.28). Combine rectal and anal assessments with the pelvic examination since the patient is situated in a lithotomy or dorsal recumbent position.

TABLE 30.28 Nursing History for Female Genitalia and Reproductive Tract Assessment

Assessment	Rationale
Determine whether patient has had previous illness or surgery involving reproductive organs, including STIs.	Illness or surgery influences appearance and position of organs being examined.
Determine whether patient has received HPV vaccine.	HPV increases patient's risk for development of cervical cancer.
Review menstrual history, including age at menarche, frequency and duration of menstrual cycle, character of flow (e.g., amount, presence of clots), presence of dysmenorrhea (painful menstruation), pelvic pain, dates of last two menstrual periods, and premenstrual symptoms.	This information helps to reveal level of reproductive health, including normalcy of menstrual cycle.
Ask patient to describe obstetrical history, including each pregnancy and history of abortions or miscarriages.	Observed physical findings vary, depending on woman's history of pregnancy.
Determine whether patient uses safe sex practices; have patient describe current and past contraceptive practices and problems encountered. Discuss risk of STIs and HIV infection.	Use of certain types of contraceptives influences reproductive health (e.g., sensitivity reaction to spermicidal jelly). Sexual history reveals risk for and understanding of STIs.
Assess whether patient has signs and symptoms of vaginal discharge, painful or swollen perianal tissues, or genital lesions.	These signs and symptoms may indicate STI or other pathological condition.
Determine whether patient has symptoms or history of genitourinary problems, including burning during urination, frequency, urgency, nocturia, hematuria, incontinence, or stress incontinence (see Chapter 46).	Urinary problems are associated with gynecological disorders, including STIs.
Ask whether patient has had signs of bleeding outside of normal menstrual period or after menopause or has had unusual vaginal discharge.	These are warning signs for cervical and endometrial cancer or vaginal infection.
Determine whether patient has history of HPV (condyloma acuminatum, herpes simplex, or cervical dysplasia), has multiple sex partners, smokes cigarettes, has had multiple pregnancies, or was young at first intercourse.	These are risk factors for cervical cancer (ACS, 2018b).
Ask if patient has a strong personal or family history of breast or ovarian cancer; women who have had breast cancer or who have tested positive for inherited mutations in BRCA1 or BRCA2 genes are at increased risk. Other medical conditions associated with increased risk include pelvic inflammatory disease and Lynch syndrome. The use of estrogen alone as menopausal hormone therapy has been shown to increase risk. Tobacco smoking increases the risk of mucinous ovarian cancer. Heavier body weight may be associated with increased risk of ovarian cancer.	These are risk factors for ovarian cancer (ACS, 2018b).
Determine whether patient is postmenopausal, is obese, has abdominal fat, or is infertile. Assess whether patient received menopausal estrogen therapy, had late menopause, never had children, and had a history of polycystic ovary syndrome. Tamoxifen, a drug used to reduce breast cancer risk, increases the risk slightly because it has estrogen-like effects on the uterus. Medical conditions that increase the risk include Lynch syndrome and diabetes.	These are risk factors for endometrial cancer (ACS, 2018b).

HIV, Human immunodeficiency virus; *HPV*, human papillomavirus (HPV) vaccine; *STI*, sexually transmitted infection.

Preparation of the Patient

As a new nurse, you are responsible for assisting a patient's health care provider with a pelvic examination. For a complete examination the following equipment is needed: examination table with stirrups, vaginal speculum of correct size, adjustable light source, sink, clean disposable gloves, sterile cotton swabs, glass slides, plastic or wooden spatula, cervical brush or broom device, cytological fixative, and culture plates or media (Ball et al., 2019).

Make sure that the equipment is ready before the examination begins. Ask the patient to empty her bladder so that the uterus and ovaries are readily palpable. Often it is necessary to collect a urine specimen. Help the patient to the lithotomy position in bed or on an examination table for the external genitalia assessment. Assist her into stirrups for a speculum examination. Have a woman stabilize each foot in a stirrup and slide the buttocks down to the edge of the examining table. Place a hand at the edge of the table and instruct the patient to move until touching the hand. The patient's arms should be at her sides or folded across the chest to prevent tightening of abdominal muscles.

Sometimes women who have pain or a deformity of the joints are unable to assume a lithotomy position. In this situation have the patient abduct only one leg or have another person assist in separating the patient's thighs. In addition, use the side-lying position with the patient on the left side with the right thigh and knee drawn up to her chest.

Give the patient a square drape or sheet. She holds one corner over her sternum, the adjacent corners fall over each knee, and the fourth corner covers the perineum. After the examination begins, lift the drape over the perineum. A male examiner always needs to have a female attendant present during the examination, whereas a female examiner may choose to work alone. An additional woman should be present if the patient requests it.

External Genitalia

You can perform this examination independently of a health care provider. Make sure that the perineal area is well illuminated. Follow standard precautions and wear clean gloves to prevent contact with infectious organisms. The perineum is sensitive and tender; do not touch the area suddenly without warning a patient. It is best to touch the inner thigh first before touching the perineum.

While sitting at the end of the examination table or bed, inspect the quantity and distribution of hair growth. Preadolescents have no pubic hair. During adolescence hair grows along the labia, becoming darker, coarser, and curlier. In an adult hair grows in a triangle over the female

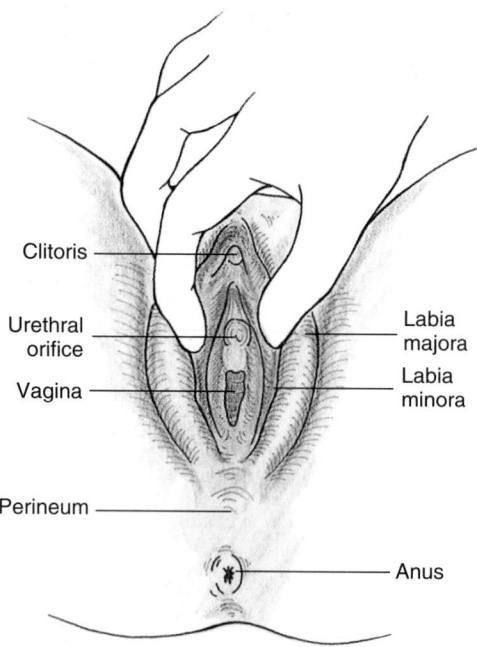

FIG. 30.59 Female external genitalia.

perineum and along the medial surfaces of the thighs. The underlying skin is free of inflammation, irritation, or lesions.

Inspect surface characteristics of the labia majora. The skin of the perineum is smooth, clean, and slightly darker than other skin. The mucous membranes appear dark pink and moist. The labia majora can be gaping or closed, appear dry or moist, and are usually symmetrical. After childbirth the labia majora separate, causing the labia minora to become more prominent. When a woman reaches menopause, the labia majora become thinned; they become atrophied in older age. The labia majora are normally without inflammation, edema, lesions, or lacerations.

To inspect the remaining external structures, use your nondominant hand and gently place the thumb and index finger inside the labia minora and retract the tissues outwardly (Fig. 30.59). Be sure to have a firm hold to avoid repeated retraction against the sensitive tissues. Use the other hand to palpate the labia minora between the thumb and second finger. On inspection the labia minora are normally thinner than the labia majora, and one side is sometimes larger. The tissue feels soft on palpation and without tenderness. The size of the clitoris varies, but it normally does not exceed 2 cm (1 inch) in length and 0.5 cm (¼ inch) in width. Look for atrophy, inflammation, or adhesions. If inflamed, the clitoris is a bright cherry red. In young women it is a common site for an abnormal finding such as syphilitic lesions, or chancres, which appear as small open ulcers that drain serous material.

Inspect the urethral orifice carefully for color and position. It is normally intact without inflammation. The urethral meatus is anterior to the vaginal orifice and is pink. It appears as a small slit or pinhole opening just above the vaginal canal. Note any discharge, polyps, or fistulas.

Inspect the vaginal orifice for inflammation, edema, discoloration, discharge, and lesions. Normally the opening is a thin, vertical slit, and the tissue is moist. While inspecting the vaginal orifice, note the condition of the hymen, which is just inside the opening. In the virgin female the hymen restricts the opening of the vagina, but the tissue retracts or disappears after sexual intercourse or with normal growth in adolescence (Ball et al., 2019).

BOX 30.25 PATIENT TEACHING

Female Genitalia and Reproductive Tract Assessment

Objective
- Patient will use measures to maintain sexual health and prevent acquisition and transmission of sexually transmitted infections (STIs).

Teaching Strategies
- Instruct patient about purpose and recommended frequency of Papanicolaou (Pap) smears and gynecological examinations. Explain that a pelvic examination is needed yearly for women who are sexually active or over the age of 21. Patients are screened more often if certain risk factors exist such as a weak immune system, multiple sex partners, smoking, and a history of infections (e.g., human papillomavirus [HPV]).
- Counsel patient with an STI about the implications of diagnosis and treatment.
- Counsel young males and females and their parents about genital HPV infection and the need to receive the HPV vaccine before becoming sexually active. The vaccine is recommended for preteen boys and girls at age 11 or 12 (CDC, 2018a). Adolescent boys and girls who did not start or finish the HPV vaccine series when they were younger should get it now. Young women can get an HPV vaccine through age 26, and young men can get vaccinated through age 21 (CDC, 2018b).
- Instruct in genital self-examination (GSE). Using a mirror, position self to examine the area covered by the pubic hair. Spread the hair apart, looking for bumps, sores, or blisters. Also look for any warts, which appear as small, bumpy spots and enlarge to fleshy, cauliflower-like lesions. Next spread the outer vaginal lips apart and look at the clitoris for bumps, blisters, sores, or warts. Look at both sides of the inner vaginal lips. Inspect the area around the urinary and vaginal opening for bumps, blisters, sores, or warts.
- Explain warning signs of STIs: pain or burning on urination, pain during sex, pain in pelvic area, bleeding between menstruation, itchy rash around vagina, and abnormal vaginal discharge.
- Teach measures to prevent STIs: male partner's use of condoms, restricting number of sexual partners, avoiding sex with people who have several other partners, and perineal hygiene measures.
- Tell patients with an STI to inform sexual partners of the need for an examination.
- Reinforce the importance of performing perineal hygiene (as appropriate).

Evaluation
Use the principles of teach-back to evaluate patient/family caregiver learning:
- Explain to me the rationale for obtaining the HPV vaccination for your child.
- Explain to me why a routine gynecological examination and Pap test are important.
- Describe measures you can take to prevent transmission of an STI.
- Since you were diagnosed with an STI, describe for me the safe sexual practices that you are using to prevent further infections.

Inspect the anus, looking for lesions and hemorrhoids (see rectal examination). After completion of the external examination, dispose of examination gloves and offer the patient soft disposable cloths for perineal hygiene.

Patients who are at risk for contracting an STI need to learn to perform a genital self-examination (Box 30.25). The purpose of the examination is to detect any signs or symptoms of an STI. Many people do not know that they have an STI (e.g., chlamydia), and some STIs (e.g., syphilis) remain undetected for years.

Speculum Examination of Internal Genitalia

An examination of the internal genitalia requires much skill and practice. Advanced nurse practitioners and primary care providers

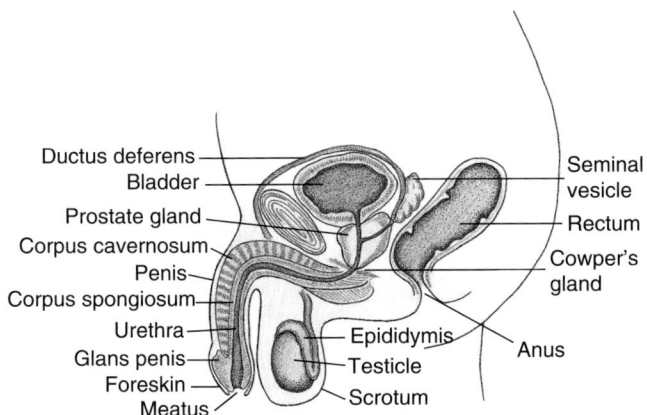

FIG. 30.60 External and internal male sex organs.

Labels: Ductus deferens, Bladder, Prostate gland, Corpus cavernosum, Penis, Corpus spongiosum, Urethra, Glans penis, Foreskin, Meatus, Seminal vesicle, Rectum, Cowper's gland, Epididymis, Testicle, Scrotum, Anus

perform this examination. As a nursing student you observe the procedure or assist the examiner by helping the patient with positioning, handing off specimen supplies, and providing emotional support for the patient.

The examination involves use of a plastic or metal speculum consisting of two blades and an adjustment device. The examiner inserts the speculum into the vagina to assess the internal genitalia for cancerous lesions and other abnormalities. During the examination the examiner collects a specimen for a Papanicolaou (Pap) test for cervical and vaginal cancer. The cervix is inspected for color, position, size, surface characteristics, and discharge (Ball et al., 2019).

MALE GENITALIA

An examination of the male genitalia assesses the integrity of the external genitalia (Fig. 30.60), inguinal ring, and canal. Because the incidence of STIs in adolescents and young adults is high, an assessment of the genitalia needs to be a routine part of any health maintenance examination for this age-group (Box 30.26). The examination begins by having the patient void. Make sure the examination room is warm. During the examination have the patient stand or lie supine with the chest, abdomen, and lower legs draped. Apply clean gloves.

Use a calm, gentle approach to lessen the patient's anxiety. The position and exposure of the body during the examination is embarrassing for some men. To minimize his anxiety, it often helps to offer explanation of the steps of examination so that he anticipates all actions. Manipulate the genitalia gently to avoid causing erection or discomfort. Obtain a thorough history (Table 30.29) before the examination, ensuring that the assessment is complete.

Sexual Maturity

First note the sexual maturity of the patient by observing the size and shape of the penis and testes; the size, color, and texture of the scrotal skin; and the character and distribution of pubic hair. The testes first increase in size in preadolescence and there is no pubic hair. By the end of puberty, the testes and penis enlarge to adult size and shape, and scrotal skin darkens and becomes wrinkled. Hair becomes coarser and more abundant in the pubic area. The penis has no hair, and the scrotum has very little hair (Fig. 30.61A-B). Also inspect the skin covering the genitalia for lice, rashes, excoriations, or lesions. Normally it is clear, without lesions.

Penis

To inspect penile surfaces, manipulate the genitalia or have the patient assist. Inspect the shaft, corona, prepuce (foreskin), glans, and urethral

---

BOX 30.26 PATIENT TEACHING

Male Genitalia Assessment

Objective
- Patient will use measures to maintain sexual health and prevent acquisition and transmission of sexually transmitted infections (STIs).

Teaching Strategies
- Teach patient how to perform genital self-examination (see Box 30.27).
- Counsel patient who has an STI about diagnosis implications and treatment.
- Explain warning signs of STIs: pain on urination and during sex, abnormal penile discharge (different from usual), swollen lymph nodes, or rash or ulcer on skin or genitalia.
- Teach measures to prevent STIs: HPV immunization, use of condoms, avoiding sex with infected partner, restricting number of sexual partners, avoiding sex with people who have multiple partners, and using regular perineal hygiene.
- Recommend HPV vaccine for preteen boys age 11 or 12; young men can get vaccinated through age 21 (CDC, 2018c).
- Tell patients with an STI to inform their sexual partners of the need to have an examination.
- Instruct patient to seek treatment as soon as possible if partner becomes infected with an STI.

Evaluation
Use the principles of teach-back to evaluate patient/family caregiver learning:
- Describe measures you can take to prevent transmission of an STI.
- Since you were diagnosed with an STI, describe for me the safe sexual practices that you are using to prevent further infections.

---

meatus. The dorsal vein is apparent on inspection. In uncircumcised males retract the foreskin to reveal the glans and urethral meatus. The foreskin usually retracts easily. A small amount of white, thick smegma sometimes collects under this foreskin. Obtain a culture if abnormal discharge is present. The urethral meatus is slitlike in appearance and positioned on the ventral surface just millimeters from the tip of the glans. In some congenital conditions the meatus is displaced along the penile shaft. The area between the foreskin and glans is a common site for venereal lesions. Gently compress the glans between the thumb and index finger; this opens the urethral meatus for inspection of lesions, edema, and inflammation. Normally the opening is glistening and pink without discharge. Palpate any lesion gently to note tenderness, size, consistency, and shape. When inspection and palpation of the glans is complete, pull the foreskin down to its original position.

Continue by inspecting the entire shaft of the penis, including the undersurface, looking for lesions, scars, or edema. Palpate the shaft between the thumb and first two fingers to detect localized areas of hardness or tenderness. A patient who has lain in bed for a prolonged time sometimes develops dependent edema in the penis shaft.

It is important for any male patient to learn to perform a genital self-examination to detect signs or symptoms of STIs, especially men who have had more than one sexual partner or whose partner has had other partners. It is common for men to have an STI but not be aware of it; self-examination is a routine part of self-care (Box 30.27).

Scrotum

Be particularly cautious while inspecting and palpating the scrotum because the structures lying within the scrotal sac are very sensitive. The scrotum is divided internally into two halves. Each half contains a testicle, epididymis, and the vas deferens, which travels upward into

TABLE 30.29 Nursing History for Male Genitalia Assessment

Assessment	Rationale
Review normal urinary elimination pattern, including frequency of voiding; history of nocturia; character and volume of urine; daily fluid intake; symptoms of burning, urgency, and frequency; difficulty starting stream; and hematuria (see Chapter 46).	Urinary problems are directly associated with genitourinary problems because of anatomical structure of men's reproductive and urinary systems.
Assess patient's sexual history and use of safe sex habits (multiple partners, infection in partners, failure to use condom).	Sexual history reveals risk for and understanding of sexually transmitted diseases (STIs) and human immunodeficiency virus (HIV).
Determine whether patient has received the human papillomavirus (HPV) vaccine.	HPV is associated with genital warts in males and can lead to cervical cancer in females (CDC, 2018a).
Determine whether patient has had previous surgery or illness involving urinary or reproductive organs, including STI.	Alterations resulting from disease or surgery are sometimes responsible for symptoms or changes in organ structure or function.
Ask whether patient has noted penile pain or swelling, genital lesions, or urethral discharge.	These signs and symptoms may indicate STI.
Determine whether patient has noticed heaviness or painless enlargement of testis or irregular lumps.	These signs and symptoms are early warning signs for testicular cancer.
If patient reports an enlargement in inguinal area, assess whether it is intermittent or constant, associated with straining or lifting, and painful; and whether pain is affected by coughing, lifting, or straining at stool.	Signs and symptoms reflect potential inguinal hernia.
Ask whether patient has difficulty achieving erection or ejaculation; also review whether patient is taking diuretics, sedatives, antihypertensives, or tranquilizers.	These medications influence sexual performance.

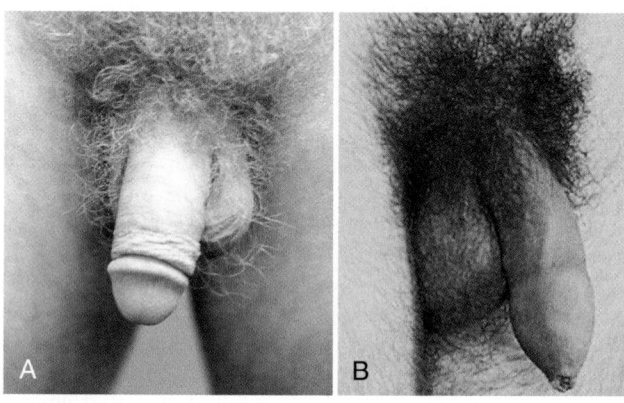

FIG. 30.61 Appearance of male genitalia. **A,** Circumcised. **B,** Uncircumcised. (From Ball JW et al: *Seidel's guide to physical examination,* ed 9, St Louis, 2019, Mosby.)

the inguinal ring. Normally the left testicle is lower than the right. Inspect the size, shape, and symmetry of the scrotum while observing for lesions or edema. Gently lift the scrotum to view the posterior surface. The scrotal skin is usually loose, and the surface is coarse. The scrotal skin is more deeply pigmented than body skin. Tightening of the skin or loss of wrinkling reveals edema. The size of the scrotum normally changes with temperature variations because the dartos muscle contracts in cold and relaxes in warm temperatures. Lumps in the scrotal skin are commonly sebaceous cysts.

Testicular cancer is a solid tumor common in young men ages 18 to 34 years. Early detection is critical. Explain testicular self-examination (see Box 30.27) while examining the patient. The testes are normally sensitive but not tender. The underlying testicles are normally ovoid and approximately 2 to 4 cm (1 to 1½ inch) in size. Gently palpate the testicles and epididymis between the thumb and first two fingers. The testes feel smooth, rubbery, and free of nodules. The epididymis is resilient. Note the size, shape, and consistency of the organs. The most common symptoms of testicular cancer are a painless enlargement of one testis and the appearance of a small, hard palpable lump, about the size of a pea, on the front or side of the testicle. In the older adult the

testicles decrease in size and are less firm during palpation. Continue to palpate the vas deferens separately as it forms the spermatic cord toward the inguinal ring, noting nodules or swelling. It normally feels smooth and discrete.

Inguinal Ring and Canal

The external inguinal ring provides the opening for the spermatic cord to pass into the inguinal canal. The canal forms a passage through the abdominal wall, a potential site for hernia formation. A hernia is a protrusion of a part of intestine through the inguinal wall or canal. Sometimes an intestinal loop enters the scrotum. Have the patient stand during this part of the examination.

During inspection ask the patient to strain or bear down. The maneuver helps to make a hernia more visible. Look for obvious bulging in the inguinal area. Complete the examination by palpating for inguinal lymph nodes. Normally small, nontender, mobile horizontal nodes are palpable. Any abnormality indicates local or systemic infection or malignant disease.

RECTUM AND ANUS

A good time to perform the rectal examination is after the genital examination. Usually this examination is not performed for young children or adolescents. It detects colorectal cancer in its early stages. The rectal examination also detects prostatic tumors in men. Collect a health history (Table 30.30) to detect the patient's risk for bowel or rectal disease (men and women) or prostate disease (men). Teach the patient about the purpose of the examination (Box 30.28).

The rectal examination is uncomfortable; thus explaining all steps helps a patient relax. Use a calm, slow-paced, gentle approach during the examination. Female patients remain in the dorsal recumbent position following genitalia examination or they assume a side-lying (Sims') position. The best way to examine men is to have the patient stand and bend over forward with hips flexed and upper body resting across an examination table. Examine a patient who cannot stand in the Sims' position. Use nonlatex clean gloves.

BOX 30.27 Male Genital Self-Examination

All men 15 years and older need to perform this examination monthly using the following steps.

Genital Examination

- Perform the examination after a warm bath or shower when the scrotal skin is less thick.
- Stand naked in front of a mirror, hold the penis in your hand, and examine the head. Pull back the foreskin if uncircumcised to expose the glans.
- Inspect and palpate the entire head of the penis in a clockwise motion, looking carefully for any bumps, sores, or blisters (bumps and blisters may be light colored or red, resemble pimples).
- Look also for any genital warts.
- Look at the opening (urethral meatus) at the end of the penis for discharge (see illustration).
- Look along the entire shaft of the penis for the same signs.
- Be sure to separate pubic hair at the base of the penis and carefully examine the skin underneath.

Testicular Self-Examination

- Look for swelling or lumps in the skin of the scrotum while looking in the mirror.
- Use both hands, placing the index and middle fingers under the testicles and the thumb on top (see illustration).
- Gently roll the testicle, feeling for lumps, swelling, soreness, or a harder consistency.
- Find the epididymis (a cordlike structure on the top and back of the testicle; it is not a lump).
- Feel for small, pea-size lumps on the front and side of the testicle. Abnormal lumps are usually painless.
- Call your health care provider for abnormal findings.

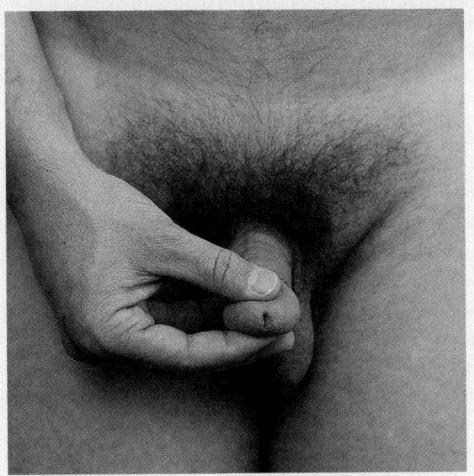

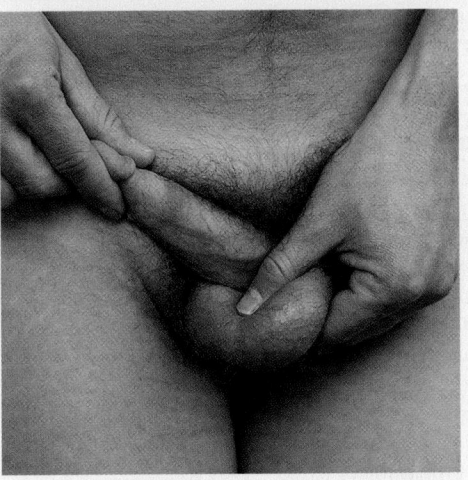

Illustrations from Ball JW, et al: *Seidel's guide to physical examination*, ed 9, St Louis, 2019, Elsevier.

TABLE 30.30 Nursing History for Rectal and Anal Assessment

Assessment	Rationale
Determine whether patient has experienced bleeding from rectum, black or tarry stools (melena), rectal pain, or change in bowel habits (constipation or diarrhea).	These are warning signs of colorectal cancer or other gastrointestinal alterations.
Determine whether patient has personal or strong family history of colorectal cancer, polyps, or chronic inflammatory bowel disease. Ask whether patient is over age 40.	These are risk factors for colorectal cancer (ACS, 2018c).
Assess dietary habits, including high fat intake, diet high in processed or red meats, or deficient fiber content (inadequate fruits and vegetables).	Bowel cancer is often linked to dietary intake of fat or insufficient fiber intake (ACS, 2018b).
Determine whether patient is obese, is physically inactive, smokes, or consumes alcohol.	These are risk factors for colorectal cancer (ACS, 2018c).
Determine whether patient has undergone screening for colorectal cancer (digital examination, fecal occult blood test, flexible sigmoidoscopy, and colonoscopy).	Undergoing this screening reflects understanding and adherence with preventive health care measures.
Assess medication history for use of laxatives or cathartic medications.	Repeated use causes diarrhea and eventual loss of intestinal muscle tone.
Assess for use of codeine or iron preparations.	Codeine causes constipation. Iron turns the color of feces black and tarry.
Ask male patient whether he has experienced weak or interrupted urine flow, inability to urinate, difficulty starting or stopping urine flow, polyuria, nocturia, hematuria, or dysuria. Does patient have continuing pain in lower back, pelvis, or upper thighs?	These are warning signs of prostate cancer (ACS, 2018b). Symptoms also suggest infection or prostate enlargement.

BOX 30.28 PATIENT TEACHING
Rectal and Anal Assessment

Objective
- Patient will be able to identify symptoms of colorectal and prostatic cancer.

Teaching Strategies
- Discuss the guidelines of the American Cancer Society (ACS, 2018b) for early detection of colorectal cancer. **Beginning at age 45,** both men and women of average risk should use one of these screening tests (ACS, 2018c):
  - Fecal occult blood test (FOBT) or fecal immunochemical test (FIT) annually
  - Stool DNA test performed every 3 years
  - Flexible sigmoidoscopy (FSIG): Visual inspection of the rectum and lower colon with a hollow, lighted tube performed by a health care provider every 5 years OR
  - Double-contrast barium enema every 5 years if recommended by health care provider
  - Colonoscopy every 10 years if recommended
  - Computed tomography (CT) colonoscopy every 5 years if recommended
- Individuals at increased risk should discuss options with their health care provider.

- Discuss warning signs of colorectal cancer (see Table 30.30).
- Discuss with male patient the ACS guidelines (2018b) for early detection of prostate cancer:
  - For men ages 50+, digital rectal examination (DRE) and prostate-specific antigen test (PSA). The ACS recommends that men who have at least a 10-year life expectancy should have an opportunity to make an informed decision with their health care provider about whether to be screened for prostate cancer after receiving information about the potential benefits, risks, and uncertainties of testing.
- Discuss warning signs of prostate cancer.

Evaluation
Use the principles of teach-back to evaluate patient/family caregiver learning:
- Tell me what screening tests for colorectal cancer that you have had done and when they were completed.
- Describe for me the warning signs of colorectal and prostate cancer and when you should contact your health care provider.

Inspection

Using the nondominant hand, gently retract the buttocks to view the perianal and sacrococcygeal areas. Perianal skin is smooth, more pigmented, and coarser than skin over the buttocks. Inspect anal tissue for skin characteristics, lesions, external hemorrhoids (dilated veins that appear as reddened protrusions), ulcers, fissures and fistulas, inflammation, rashes, or excoriation. Anal tissues are moist and hairless, and the voluntary external muscle sphincter holds the anus closed. Next ask a patient to bear down as though having a bowel movement. Any internal hemorrhoids or fissures appear at this time. Use clock reference (e.g., 3 o'clock or 8 o'clock) to describe location of findings. Normally there is no protrusion of tissue.

Digital Palpation

Examine the anal canal and sphincters with digital palpation, and in male patients palpate the prostate gland to rule out enlargement. Usually advanced practitioners perform this part of the examination. This technique is not discussed here.

MUSCULOSKELETAL SYSTEM

The musculoskeletal assessment can be performed as a separate examination or integrated with other parts of the total physical examination. In addition, you can assess the patient's movements while performing other nursing care measures such as bathing or positioning. The assessment of musculoskeletal function focuses on determining range of joint motion, muscle strength and tone, and joint and muscle condition. Assessing musculoskeletal integrity is especially important when a patient reports pain or loss of function in a joint or muscle. Because muscular disorders are often the result of neurological disease, you may choose to perform a simultaneous neurological assessment.

While examining a patient's musculoskeletal function, visualize the anatomy of bone and muscle placement and joint structure (see Chapter 38). Joints vary in degree of mobility, depending on the type of joint.

For a complete examination expose the muscles and joints, so they are free to move. Have the patient assume a sitting, supine, prone, or standing position while assessing specific muscle groups. Table 30.31 lists the information gathered in the nursing history.

General Inspection

Observe a patient's gait when he or she enters the examination room. When the patient is unaware of the nature of your observation, gait is more natural. Later have the patient walk in a straight line away from and returning to the point of origin. Note how the patient walks, sits, and rises from a sitting position. Normally patients walk with the arms swinging freely at the sides and the head leading the body. Older adults often walk with smaller steps and a wider base of support. Note foot dragging, limping, shuffling, and the position of the trunk in relation to the legs.

Observe the patient from the side and while facing him or her in a standing position. The normal standing posture is upright with parallel alignment of the hips and shoulders (Fig. 30.62 A-C). There is an even contour of the shoulders, level scapulae and iliac crests, alignment of the head over the gluteal folds, and symmetry of extremities. While observing from the side of the patient, note the normal cervical, thoracic, and lumbar curves. Holding the head erect is normal. As the patient sits, some degree of rounding of the shoulders is normal. Older adults tend to assume a stooped, forward-bent posture with the hips and knees somewhat flexed and arms bent at the elbows, raising the level of the arms.

Common postural abnormalities include kyphosis, lordosis, and scoliosis (Fig. 30.63A-C). Kyphosis, or hunchback, is an exaggeration of the posterior curvature of the thoracic spine. This postural abnormality is common in older adults. Lordosis, or swayback, is an increased lumbar curvature. A lateral spinal curvature is called scoliosis. Loss of height is frequently the first clinical sign of osteoporosis, in which height loss occurs in the trunk as a result of vertebral fracture and collapse. Osteoporosis is a systemic skeletal condition that is noted to have both decreased bone mass and deterioration of bone tissue, making bones fragile and at risk for fracture (Ball et al., 2019). Osteopenia, characterized by low bone mass of the hip, puts people at risk for osteoporosis, fractures, and potential complications later in life. Approximately 80% of people with osteoporosis are women. It can affect any age-group, including children. Teach patients ways to reduce the chance of developing this disease (Box 30.29).

TABLE 30.31 Nursing History for Musculoskeletal Assessment

Assessment	Rationale
Determine whether patient is involved in competitive sports (particularly involving collision and contact), fails to warm up adequately, is in poor physical condition, or has had a rapid growth spurt (adolescents).	These are risk factors for sports injury.
Assess for risk factors of osteoporosis. Uncontrollable risk factors: • Over age 50 • Female • Nulliparous • Menopause before age 45 • Family history of osteoporosis • Low body weight/being small and thin/constant dieting • Broken bones or height loss Controllable risk factors: • Not getting enough calcium (less than 500 mg) and vitamin D • Not eating enough fruits and vegetables • Getting too much protein, sodium, and caffeine • Having an inactive lifestyle • Smoking • Drinking too much alcohol • Losing weight Long-term use of certain medications: aluminum-containing antacids; antiseizure medicines such as phenytoin or phenobarbital; aromatase inhibitors such as anastrozole, exemestane and letrozole; cancer chemotherapeutic drugs; and heparin.	These are risk factors for osteoporosis (USPSTF, 2018).
Ask patient to describe history of problems in bone, muscle, or joint function (e.g., recent fall, trauma, lifting of heavy objects, history of bone or joint disease with sudden or gradual onset, location of alteration).	History helps to assess nature of musculoskeletal problem.
Assess nature and extent of pain, including location, duration, severity, predisposing and aggravating factors, relieving factors, and type.	Pain frequently accompanies alterations in bone, joints, or muscle. This has implications not only for comfort, but also for ability to perform activities of daily living.
Assess patient's normal activity pattern, including type of exercise routinely performed.	Provides baseline in assessment. Sedentary lifestyle and lack of appropriate exercise increase bone loss and risk of fractures.
Determine how alteration influences ability to perform activities of daily living (e.g., bathing, feeding, dressing, toileting, ambulating) and social functions (e.g., household chores, work, recreation, sexual activities).	The extent to which patient is able to perform self-care determines the level of nursing care. Type and degree of restriction in continuing social activities influence topics for patient education and ability of nurse to identify alternative ways to maintain function.
Assess height loss of woman over age 50 by subtracting current height from recall of maximum adult height. Refer to physician for bone density exam (women 65 years and older).	Measurement is useful screening tool to predict osteoporosis. Bone measurement testing recommended by USPSTF (2018).

During general inspection look at the extremities for overall size, gross deformity, bony enlargement, alignment, and symmetry. Normally there is bilateral symmetry in length, circumference, alignment, and position and in the number of skinfolds (Ball et al., 2019). A general review can identify areas requiring a more specialized assessment.

Palpation

Apply gentle palpation to all bones, joints, and surrounding muscles during a complete examination. For a focused assessment examine only the involved area. Note any heat, tenderness, edema, or resistance to pressure. The patient should not feel any discomfort when you palpate. Muscles should be firm.

Range of Joint Motion

The examination includes comparison of both active and passive ROM. Ask the patient to put each major joint through active and passive full

ROM (see Chapter 38). Learn the correct terminology for the movements that the joints can make (Table 30.32) and teach the patient how to move through each ROM. Demonstrate ROM to the patient when possible. To assess ROM passively, ask the patient to relax and then passively move the extremities through their ROM. Compare the same body parts for equality in movement. Fig. 30.64A-F, shows an example of ROM positions for the hand and wrist. Do not force a joint into a painful position. Know the normal range of each joint and the extent to which you can move the patient's joints. ROM is equal between contralateral joints. Ideally assess the patient's normal range to determine a baseline for assessing later change.

Joints are typically free from stiffness, instability, swelling, or inflammation. There should be no discomfort when applying pressure to bones and joints. In older adults, joints often become swollen and stiff, with reduced ROM resulting from cartilage erosion and fibrosis of synovial membranes (see Chapter 38). If a joint appears swollen and inflamed, palpate it for warmth. A goniometer is an

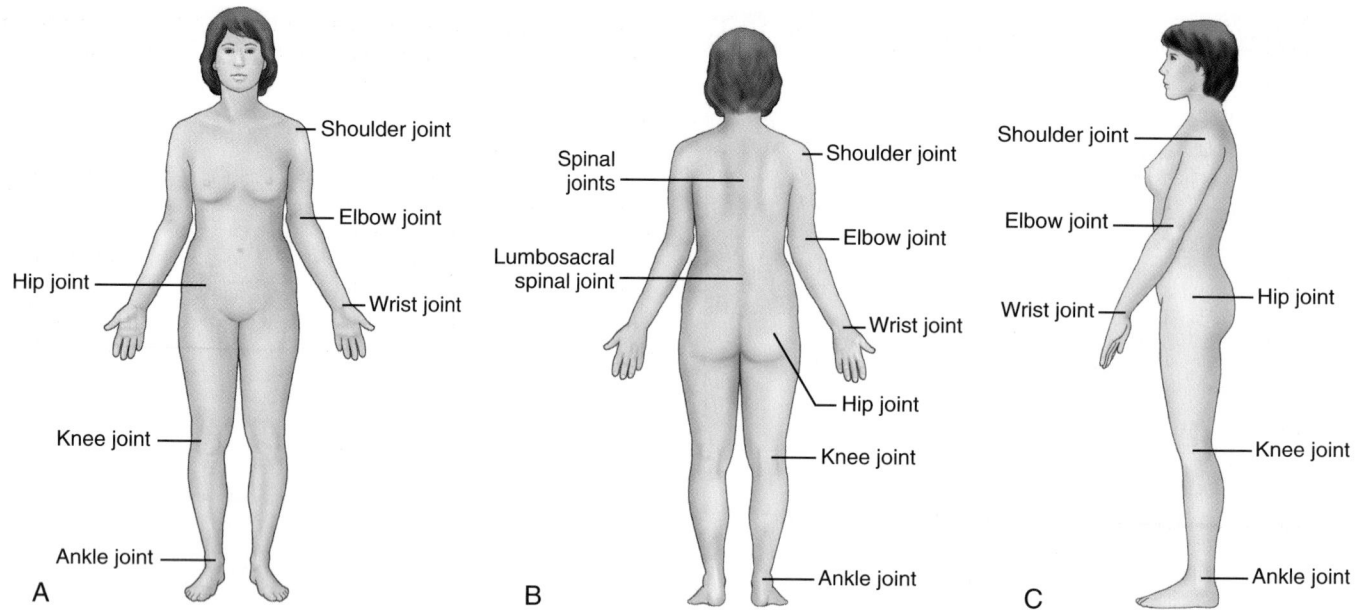

FIG. 30.62 Inspection of overall body posture. **A**, Anterior view. **B**, Posterior view. **C**, Lateral view. (From Muscolino: JE: *Kinesiology: the skeletal system and muscle function*, ed 2, St Louis, 2011, Elsevier.)

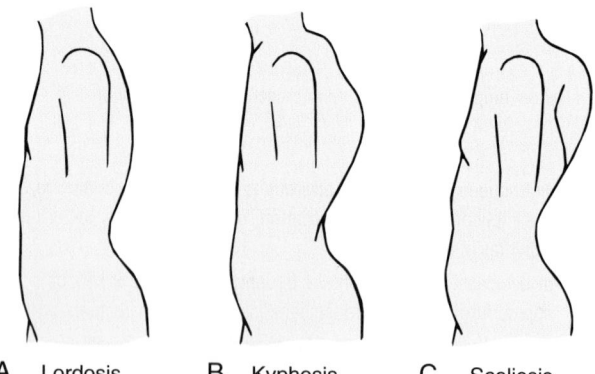

A   Lordosis   **B**   Kyphosis   **C**   Scoliosis

FIG. 30.63 Common postural abnormalities. **A**, Lordosis. **B**, Kyphosis. **C**, Scoliosis.

instrument with two flexible arms and a 180-degree protractor in the center. It is frequently used by physical and occupational therapists to measure the precise degree of motion in a joint and is mainly for patients who have a suspected reduction in joint movement.

Muscle Tone and Strength

Assess muscle strength and tone during ROM measurement. Integrate these findings with those from the neurological assessment. Note muscle tone, the slight muscular resistance felt as you move the relaxed extremity passively through its ROM.

Ask the patient to allow an extremity to relax or hang limp. This is often difficult, particularly if the patient feels pain in it. Support the extremity and grasp each limb, moving it through the normal ROM (Fig. 30.65). Normal tone causes a mild, even resistance to movement through the entire range.

If a muscle has increased tone, or **hypertonicity,** there is considerable resistance with any sudden passive movement of a joint. Continued movement eventually causes the muscle to relax. A muscle that has little tone (**hypotonicity**) feels flabby. The involved extremity hangs loosely in a position determined by gravity.

BOX 30.29   PATIENT TEACHING

Health Promotion to Prevent Osteoporosis in Women

Objective
- Patient will follow measures to prevent or minimize osteoporosis.

Teaching Strategies
- Recommend women age 65 and older for routine screening for osteoporosis (USPSTF, 2018). Recommend men for screening as well; they are at risk for development of osteoporosis equally as they age.
- To reduce bone demineralization, instruct older adults in a proper exercise program (e.g., weight-bearing, muscle-strengthening, and balance-training exercises) to be followed 3 or more times a week.
- Encourage intake of calcium to meet the recommended daily allowance. Increased vitamin D aids calcium absorption.
- Recommendation for calcium supplements for adults over age 25 is 1000 to 1500 mg/day. Instruct patient to take no more than 500 mg of calcium at one time.
- Instruct older adults and those with osteoporosis in proper body mechanics and range-of-motion and moderate weight-bearing exercises (e.g., swimming and walking) to minimize trauma and subsequent fracture of bones.
- Instruct older patients to pace activities to compensate for loss in muscle strength.

Evaluation
Use the principles of teach-back to evaluate patient/family caregiver learning:
- Show me how you maintain correct posture when you are sitting, standing, and walking.
- Describe for me what therapies you use for preventing osteoporosis.
- Show me how you do your range-of-motion exercises.

For assessment of muscle strength, have the patient assume a stable position. He or she performs maneuvers demonstrating strength of major muscle groups (Table 30.33). Use a grading scale of 0 to 5 to compare symmetrical muscle pairs for strength (Table 30.34). The

TABLE 30.32 Terminology for Normal Range-Of-Motion Positions

Term	Range of Motion	Examples of Joints
Flexion	Movement decreasing angle between two adjoining bones; bending of limb	Elbow, fingers, knee
Extension	Movement increasing angle between two adjoining bones	Elbow, knee, fingers
Hyperextension	Movement of body part beyond its normal resting extended position	Head
Pronation	Movement of body part so that front or ventral surface faces downward	Hand, forearm
Supination	Movement of body part so that front or ventral surface faces upward	Hand, forearm
Abduction	Movement of extremity away from midline of body	Leg, arm, fingers
Adduction	Movement of extremity toward midline of body	Leg, arm, fingers
Internal rotation	Rotation of joint inward	Knee, hip
External rotation	Rotation of joint outward	Knee, hip
Eversion	Turning of body part away from midline	Foot
Inversion	Turning of body part toward midline	Foot
Dorsiflexion	Flexion of toes and foot upward	Foot
Plantar flexion	Bending of toes and foot downward	Foot

arm on the dominant side normally is stronger than the arm on the nondominant side. In older adults a loss of muscle mass causes bilateral weakness, but muscle strength remains greater in the dominant arm or leg.

Examine each muscle group. Ask the patient to first flex the muscle you are examining and then to resist when you apply an opposing force against that flexion. It is important to not allow the patient to move the joint. Gradually increase pressure to a muscle group (e.g., elbow extension). Have the patient resist the pressure you apply by attempting to move against resistance (e.g., elbow flexion) until instructed to stop. Vary the amount of pressure applied and observe the joint move. If you identify a weakness, compare the size of the muscle with its opposite

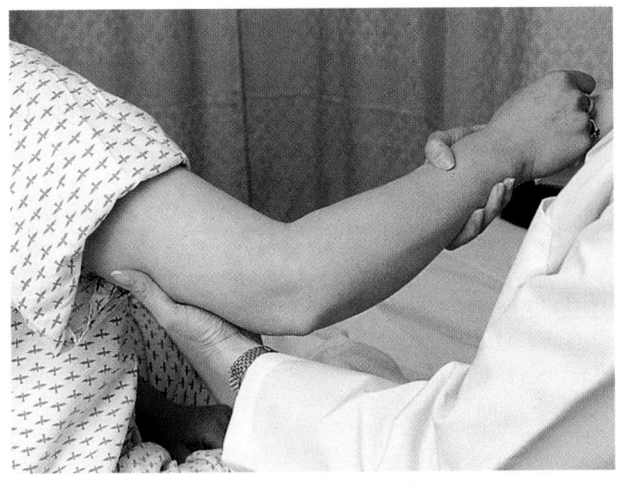

FIG. 30.65 Assessing muscle tone.

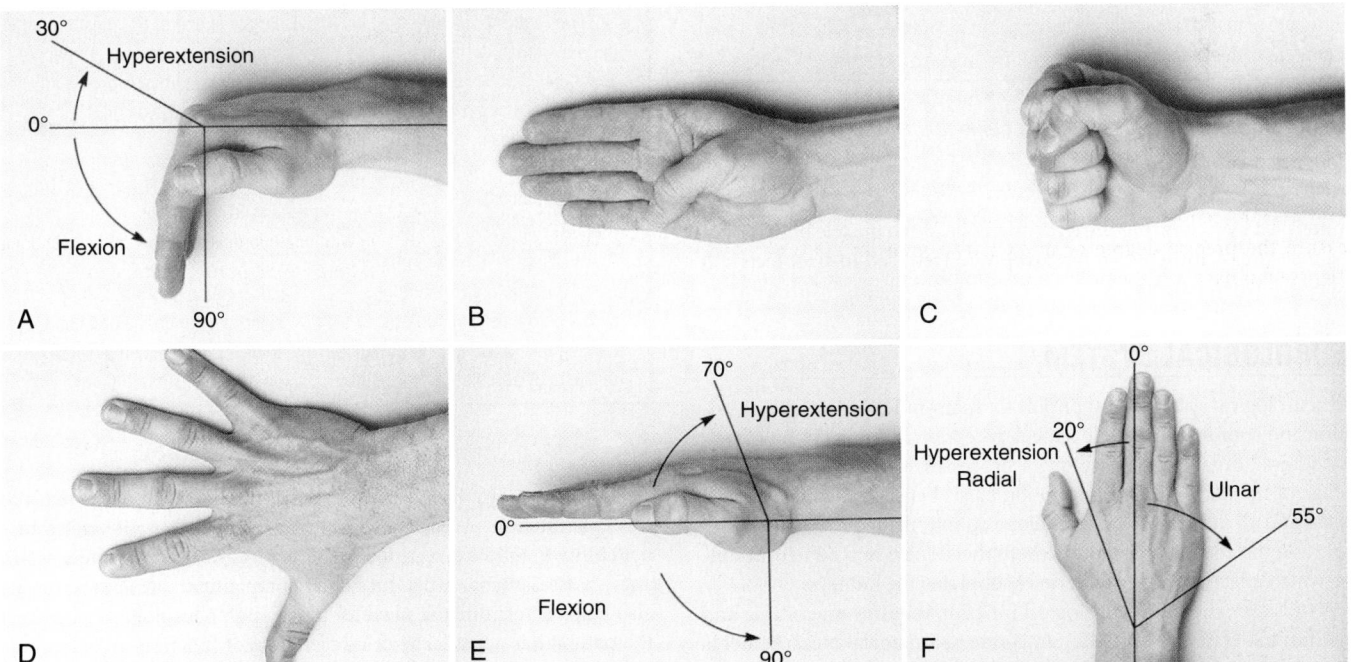

FIG. 30.64 Range of motion of hand and wrist. **A,** Metacarpophalangeal flexion and hyperextension. **B,** Finger flexion: thumb to each fingertip and to base of little finger. **C,** Finger flexion, fist formation. **D,** Finger abduction. **E,** Wrist flexion and hyperextension. **F,** Wrist radial and ulnar movement. (From Ball JW et al: *Seidel's guide to physical examination,* ed 9, St Louis, 2019, Mosby.)

TABLE 30.33 Maneuvers to Assess Muscle Strength

Muscle Group	Maneuver
Neck (sternocleidomastoid)	Place hand firmly against patient's upper jaw. Ask patient to turn head laterally against resistance.
Shoulder (trapezius)	Place hand over midline of patient's shoulder, exerting firm pressure. Have patient raise shoulders against resistance.
Elbow	
Biceps	Pull down on forearm as patient attempts to flex arm.
Triceps	As you flex patient's arm, apply pressure against forearm. Ask patient to straighten arm.
Hip	
Quadriceps	When patient is sitting, apply downward pressure to thigh. Ask patient to raise leg up from table.
Gastrocnemius	Patient sits while examiner holds shin of flexed leg. Ask patient to straighten leg against resistance.

TABLE 30.34 Muscle Strength

Muscle Function Level	SCALES		
	Grade	% Normal	Lovett Scale
No evidence of contractility	0	0	0 (zero)
Slight contractility, no movement	1	10	T (trace)
Full range of motion, gravity eliminated[a]	2	25	P (poor)
Full range of motion with gravity	3	50	F (fair)
Full range of motion against gravity, some resistance	4	75	G (good)
Full range of motion against gravity, full resistance	5	100	N (normal)

[a]Passive movement.
Modified from Ball JW, et al: *Seidel's guide to physical examination*, ed 9, St Louis, 2019, Elsevier.

counterpart by measuring the circumference of the muscle body with a tape measure. A muscle that has **atrophied** (reduced in size) feels soft and boggy when palpated.

NEUROLOGICAL SYSTEM

The neurological system is responsible for many functions, including initiation and coordination of movement, reception and perception of sensory stimuli, organization of thought processes, control of speech, and storage of memory. A close integration exists between the neurological system and all other body systems. For example, urine production relies in part on the adequacy of blood flow to the kidneys and on neural control, which affects the size of arterioles supplying the kidneys.

A full assessment of neurological function requires much time and attention to detail. For efficiency, integrate neurological measurements with other parts of the physical examination. For example, test cranial nerve function while assessing the head and neck. Observe mental and emotional status during the initial interview.

TABLE 30.35 Nursing History for Neurological Assessment

Assessment	Rationale
Determine whether patient uses analgesics, alcohol, sedatives, hypnotics, antipsychotics, antidepressants, nervous system stimulants, or recreational drugs.	These medications alter level of consciousness or cause behavioral changes. Abuse sometimes causes tremors, ataxia, and changes in peripheral nerve function.
Determine whether patient has recent history of seizures/convulsions: clarify sequence of events (aura, fall to ground, motor activity, loss of consciousness); character of any symptoms; and relationship of seizure to time of day, fatigue, or emotional stress.	Seizure activity often originates from central nervous system alteration. Characteristics of seizure help determine its origin.
Screen patient for symptoms of headache, tremors, dizziness, vertigo, numbness or tingling of body part, visual changes, weakness, pain, or changes in speech. Presence of any symptom requires more detailed review (onset, severity, precipitating factors or sequence of events).	These symptoms frequently originate from alterations in central or peripheral nervous system function. Identification of specific patterns aids in diagnosis of pathological condition.
Discuss with patient's family any recent changes in patient's behavior (e.g., increased irritability, mood swings, memory loss, change in energy level).	Behavioral changes sometimes result from intracranial pathological states.
Assess patient for history of change in vision, hearing, smell, taste, or touch.	Major sensory nerves originate from brainstem. These symptoms help to localize nature of problem.
If an older patient displays sudden acute confusion (delirium), review history for drug toxicity (anticholinergics, diuretics, digoxin, cimetidine, sedatives, antihypertensives, antiarrhythmics), serious infections, metabolic disturbances, heart failure, and severe anemia.	Delirium is one of the most common mental disorders in older people. Condition is always potentially reversible (see Box 30.31).
Review past history for head or spinal cord injury, meningitis, congenital anomalies, neurological disease, or psychiatric counseling.	Factors cause neurological symptoms or behavioral changes to develop, focusing assessment on possible cause.

Consider many variables when deciding the extent of the neurological examination. A patient's level of consciousness influences his or her ability to follow directions. General physical status influences tolerance to assessment. A patient's chief complaint or presenting problem also helps determine the need for a thorough neurological assessment. If a patient has a headache or a recent loss of function in an extremity, he or she needs a complete neurological review. Table 30.35 lists the data collected in the nursing history. You will need the following items for a complete examination:

- Reading material
- Vials containing aromatic substances (e.g., vanilla extract and coffee)
- Opposite tip of cotton swab or tongue blade broken in half
- Snellen eye chart
- Penlight
- Vials containing sugar, salt, lemon with applicators
- Tongue blade
- Two test tubes, one filled with hot water and the other with cold water
- Cotton balls or cotton-tipped applicators
- Tuning fork
- Reflex hammer

Mental and Emotional Status

You learn a great deal about mental capacities and emotional state simply by interacting with a patient. Ask questions during an examination to gather data and observe the appropriateness of emotions and thoughts. Special assessment tools are designed to assess a patient's mental status. The Mini-Mental State Examination (MMSE) is an instrument developed by Folstein et al. (1975) that measures orientation and cognitive function. The questions in Box 30.30 offer examples of questions found on the MMSE. The maximum score on the MMSE is 31. Patients with scores of 21 or less generally reveal cognitive impairment requiring further evaluation.

To ensure an objective assessment, consider a patient's cultural and educational background, values, beliefs, and previous experiences. Such factors influence response to questions. An alteration in mental or emotional status reflects a disturbance in cerebral functioning. The cerebral cortex controls and integrates intellectual and emotional functioning. Primary brain disorders, medication, and metabolic changes are examples of factors that change cerebral function.

Delirium is an acute mental disorder that occurs among patients who are hospitalized. Obtain a thorough history of a patient's behavior before delirium develops to recognize the condition early. Family members are usually a good resource. It is characterized by confusion, disorientation, and restlessness. It is often a sign of an impending or underlying physical illness in older adults; it may be related to serious injury, impaired senses, poor pain management, medications, or restraint use (Ball et al., 2019). The acute condition differs from dementia, a more progressive, organic mental disorder such as Alzheimer's disease. You need to recognize the difference so that you can try to learn the underlying cause of delirium. Fortunately, the condition often reverses when it is correctly assessed and the underlying cause is treated (i.e., central nervous system [CNS], metabolic, or cardiopulmonary disorders; systemic illnesses; or sensory deprivation or overload). To avoid misdiagnosis, you need to adequately assess mental status. Frequently patients who develop delirium are labeled with "sundown syndrome" because the delirium frequently worsens at night. Many practitioners mistake this as being common with old age. Children can also be vulnerable to delirium due to illness, medications, trauma, or surgeries (Hockenberry and Wilson, 2019). Box 30.31 summarizes clinical criteria for delirium.

Level of Consciousness. A person's level of consciousness exists along a continuum from full awakening, alertness, and cooperation to unresponsiveness. Talk with the patient, asking questions about events involving his or her concerns about any health problems. A fully conscious patient responds to questions quickly and expresses ideas logically. With a lowering of a patient's consciousness, use the Glasgow Coma Scale (GCS) for an objective measurement of consciousness on a numerical scale (Table 30.36). The patient needs to be

---

BOX 30.30 Mini-Mental State Examination Sample Questions

- Orientation to time
  "What is the date?"
- Registration
  "Listen carefully. I am going to say three words. Say them back after I stop. Ready? Here they are . . .
  HOUSE (pause), CAR (pause), LAKE (pause). Now repeat these words back to me."
  (Repeat up to 5 times but score only the first trial.)
- Naming
  "What is this?" (Point to a pencil or pen.)
- Reading
  "Please read this and do what it says." (Show examinee the words on the stimulus form.)
  CLOSE YOUR EYES

Reproduced by special permission of the publisher, Psychological Assessment Resources, Inc., 16204 North Florida Avenue, Lutz, FL 33549, from *Mini-Mental State Examination,* by Marshal Folstein and Susan Folstein, Copyright 1975, 1998, 2001 by Mini Mental, LLC, Inc. Published 2001 by Psychological Assessment Resources, Inc. Further reproduction is prohibited without permission of PAR, Inc. The MMSE can be purchased from PAR, Inc. by calling (800) 331-8378 or (813) 968-3103.

BOX 30.31 Clinical Criteria for Delirium

Definition: An acute disturbance of consciousness that is accompanied by a change in cognition. It is not caused by a preexisting or evolving dementia. Delirium develops over a short period of time, usually hours to days, and tends to fluctuate during the course of the day. It is usually a direct physiological consequence of a general medical condition. It is most common in older adults but occasionally occurs in younger patients.

- There is reduced clarity of awareness of the environment.
- Ability to focus, sustain, or shift attention is impaired (questions must be repeated).
- Irrelevant stimuli easily distract the person.
- There is an accompanying change in cognition (memory impairment, disorientation, or language disturbance).
- Recent memory commonly is affected.
- Disorientation usually occurs, with patient disoriented to time, place, or person.
- Language disturbance involves impaired ability to name objects or ability to write; speech is sometimes rambling.
- Perceptual disturbances include misinterpretations, delusions, or visual and auditory hallucinations. Neurological signs include tremor, unsteady gait, asterixis, or myoclonus.

Reprinted with permission from the *Diagnostic and statistical manual of mental disorders,* ed 5, text revision, Copyright © 2013, American Psychiatric Association.

---

as alert as possible before testing. Take care when using the scale if the patient has sensory losses (e.g., vision or hearing). The GCS allows evaluation of a patient's neurological status over time. The higher the score, the better the patient's neurological function. Ask short, simple questions such as "What is your name?" "Where are you?" and "What day is this?" Also ask the patient to follow simple commands such as "Move your toes."

If the patient is not conscious enough to follow commands, try to elicit the pain response. Apply firm pressure with the thumb over the root of the patient's fingernail. The normal response to the painful

TABLE 30.36 Glasgow Coma Scale

(The total score is the sum of the scores in the three categories.)

Action	Response	Score
Eyes open	Spontaneously	4
	To speech	3
	To pain	2
	None	1
Best verbal response	Oriented	5
	Confused	4
	Inappropriate words	3
	Incomprehensible sounds	2
	None	1
Best motor response	Obeys commands	6
	Localized pain	5
	Flexion withdrawal	4
	Abnormal flexion	3
	Abnormal extension	2
	Flaccid	1
	TOTAL SCORE	**3 to 15**

stimuli is withdrawal of the body part from the stimulus. A patient with serious neurological impairment exhibits abnormal posturing in response to pain. A flaccid response indicates the absence of muscle tone in the extremities and severe injury to brain tissue.

Behavior and Appearance. Behavior, moods, hygiene, grooming, and choice of dress reveal pertinent information about mental status. Remain perceptive of a patient's mannerisms and actions during the entire physical assessment. Note nonverbal and verbal behaviors. Does the patient respond appropriately to directions? Does his or her mood vary with no apparent cause? Does he or she show concern about appearance? Is his or her hair clean and neatly groomed, and are the nails trim and clean? The patient should behave in a manner expressing concern and interest in the examination. He or she should make eye contact with you and express appropriate feelings that correspond to the situation. Normally the patient shows some degree of personal hygiene.

Choice and fit of clothing reflect socioeconomic background or personal taste rather than deficiency in self-concept or self-care. Avoid being judgmental and focus assessment on the appropriateness of clothing for the weather. Older adults sometimes neglect their appearance because of finances, reduced vision, or a lack of energy.

Language. Normal cerebral function allows a person to understand spoken or written words and express the self through written words or gestures. Assess the patient's voice inflection, tone, and manner of speech. Normally a patient's voice has inflections, is clear and strong, and increases in volume appropriately. Speech is fluent. When communication is clearly ineffective (e.g., omission or addition of letters and words, misuse of words, or hesitations), assess for aphasia. Injury to the cerebral cortex results in aphasia.

The two types of aphasia are sensory (or receptive) and motor (or expressive). With receptive aphasia a person cannot understand written or verbal speech. With expressive aphasia a person understands written and verbal speech but cannot write or speak appropriately when attempting to communicate. A patient sometimes suffers a combination of receptive and expressive aphasia. Assess language

capabilities when a patient is communicating ineffectively. Some simple assessment techniques include the following:

- Point to a familiar object and ask the patient to name it.
- Ask the patient to respond to simple verbal and written commands such as "Stand up" or "Sit down."
- Ask the patient to read simple sentences out loud.

Normally a patient names objects correctly, follows commands, and reads sentences correctly.

Intellectual Function

Intellectual function includes memory (recent, immediate, and past), knowledge, abstract thinking, association, and judgment. Testing each aspect of function involves a specific technique. However, because cultural and educational background influences the ability to respond to test questions, do not ask questions related to concepts or ideas with which a patient is unfamiliar.

Memory. Assess immediate recall and recent and remote memory. Patients demonstrate immediate recall by repeating a series of numbers (e.g., 7, 4, 1) in the order they are presented or in reverse order. Patients normally recall a series of five to eight digits forward and four to six digits backward.

First ask to test the patient's memory. Then state clearly and slowly the names of three unrelated objects. After mentioning all three, ask the patient to repeat each. Later in the assessment ask the patient to repeat the three words again. He or she should be able to identify them. Another test for recent memory involves asking the patient to recall events occurring during the same day (e.g., what was eaten for breakfast). Validate information with a family member.

To assess past memory, ask the patient to recall his or her mother's maiden name, a birthday, or a special date in history. It is best to ask open-ended rather than simple yes-or-no questions. A patient usually has immediate recall of such information. With older adults do not interpret hearing loss as confusion. Good communication techniques are essential throughout the examination to ensure that a patient clearly understands all directions and testing.

Knowledge. Assess knowledge by asking how much the patient knows about his or her illness or the reason for seeking health care. A knowledge assessment allows you to determine a patient's ability to learn or understand. If there is an opportunity to teach, test a patient's mental status by asking for feedback during a follow-up visit.

Abstract Thinking. Interpreting abstract ideas or concepts reflects the capacity for abstract thinking. For an individual to explain common phrases such as "A stitch in time saves nine" or "Don't count your chickens before they're hatched" requires a higher level of intellectual function. Note whether a patient's explanations are relevant and concrete. A patient with altered mental status probably interprets the phrase literally or merely rephrases the words.

Association. Another higher level of intellectual functioning involves finding similarities or associations between concepts: a dog is to a beagle as a cat is to a Siamese. Name related concepts and ask the patient to identify their associations. Ask questions that are appropriate to the patient's level of intelligence, using simple concepts.

Judgment. Judgment requires a comparison and evaluation of facts and ideas to understand their relationships and form appropriate conclusions. Attempt to measure the patient's ability to make logical decisions with questions such as "Why did you seek health care?" or "What

TABLE 30.37 Cranial Nerve Function and Assessment

Number	Name	Type	Function	Method
I	Olfactory	Sensory	Sense of smell	Ask patient to identify different nonirritating aromas such as coffee and vanilla.
II	Optic	Sensory	Visual acuity	Use Snellen chart or ask patient to read printed material while wearing glasses.
III	Oculomotor	Motor	Extraocular eye movements: inward, up and inward, up and outward, down and outward	Assess six directions of gaze.
			Pupil constriction and dilation	Measure pupillary reaction to light reflex and accommodation.
			Opening the eye	
IV	Trochlear	Motor	Downward, inward eye movements	Assess six directions of gaze.
V	Trigeminal	Sensory and motor	Sensory nerve to skin of face	Lightly touch cornea with wisp of cotton. Assess corneal reflex. Measure sensation of light pain and touch across skin of face.
			Motor nerve to muscles of jaw	Palpate temples as patient clenches teeth.
VI	Abducens	Motor	Lateral movement of eyeballs	Assess six directions of gaze.
VII	Facial	Sensory and motor	Facial expression	As patient smiles, frowns, puffs out cheeks, and raises and lowers eyebrows, look for asymmetry.
			Taste	Have patient identify salty or sweet taste on front of tongue.
VIII	Auditory	Sensory	Hearing	Assess ability to hear spoken word.
IX	Glossopharyngeal	Sensory and motor	Taste	Ask patient to identify sour or sweet taste on back of tongue.
			Ability to swallow	Use tongue blade to elicit gag reflex.
X	Vagus	Sensory and motor	Sensation of pharynx	Ask patient to say "ah." Observe movement of palate and pharynx.
			Movement of vocal cords	Assess speech for hoarseness.
			Parasympathetic innervation to glands of mucous membranes of the pharynx, larynx, organs in the neck, thorax (heart and lungs), and abdomen	Assess heart rate, presence of peristalsis.
XI	Spinal accessory	Motor	Movement of head and shoulders	Ask patient to shrug shoulders and turn head against passive resistance.
XII	Hypoglossal	Motor	Position of tongue	Ask patient to stick out tongue to midline and move it from side to side.

would you do if you became ill at home?" Normally a patient makes logical decisions.

Cranial Nerve Function

To assess cranial nerve function, you may test all 12 cranial nerves, a single nerve, or a related group of nerves. A dysfunction in one nerve reflects an alteration at some point along the distribution of the cranial nerve. Measurements used to assess the integrity of organs within the head and neck also assess cranial nerve function. A complete assessment involves testing the 12 cranial nerves in their numerical order. To remember the order of the nerves, use this simple phrase: "On old Olympus' towering tops, a Finn and German viewed some hops." The first letter of each word in the phrase is the same as the first letter of the names of the cranial nerves listed in order (Table 30.37).

Sensory Function

The sensory pathways of the CNS conduct sensations of pain, temperature, position, vibration, and crude and finely localized touch. Different nerve pathways relay the sensations. Most patients require only a quick screening of sensory function unless there are symptoms of reduced sensation, motor impairment, or paralysis. The risk of skin breakdown is greater in a patient with impaired sensation. When assessing decreased sensation, complete a skin assessment of the area affected by

the sensory loss. In addition, teach the patient to avoid pressure, thermal, and/or chemical trauma to the area.

Normally a patient has sensory responses to all stimuli that are tested. He or she feels sensations equally on both sides of the body in all areas. Assess the major sensory nerves by knowing the sensory dermatome zones (Fig. 30.66A-B). Some areas of the skin are innervated by specific dorsal root cutaneous nerves. For example, if assessment reveals reduced sensation when checking for light touch along an area of the skin (e.g., the lower neck), this determines in general where a neurological lesion exists (e.g., fourth cervical spinal cord segment).

Perform all sensory testing with the patient's eyes closed so that he or she is unable to see when or where a stimulus touches the skin (Table 30.38). Then touch the patient's skin in a random, unpredictable order to maintain his or her attention and prevent detection of a predictable pattern. Ask the patient to describe when, what, and where he or she feels each stimulus. Compare symmetrical areas of the body while applying stimuli to the patient's arms, trunk, and legs.

Motor Function

An examination of motor function includes assessments made during the musculoskeletal examination. In addition, you assess the patient's cerebellar function. The cerebellum coordinates muscular activity, maintains balance and equilibrium, and controls posture.

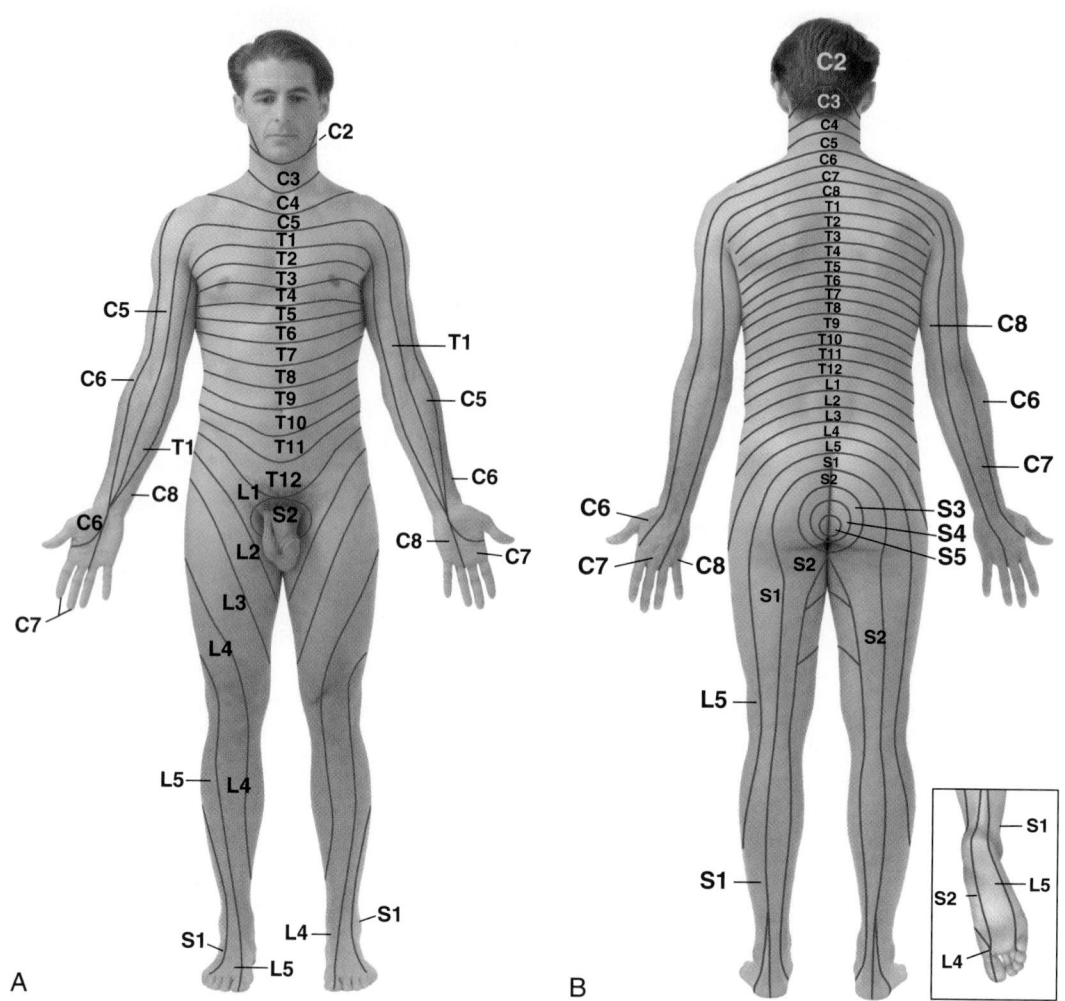

FIG. 30.66 Dermatomes of body (body surface areas innervated by particular spinal nerves); C1 usually has no cutaneous distribution. **A,** Anterior view. **B,** Posterior view. It appears that there is a distinct separation of surface area controlled by each dermatome, but there is almost always overlap between spinal nerves. (From Ball JW, et al: *Seidel's guide to physical examination,* ed 9, St Louis, 2019, Mosby.)

Coordination. To avoid confusion, demonstrate each maneuver and have the patient repeat it, observing for smoothness and balance in his or her movements (Box 30.32). In older adults, normally slow reaction time causes movements to be less rhythmical.

To assess fine-motor function, have the patient extend the arms out to the sides and touch each forefinger alternately to the nose (first with eyes open, then with eyes closed). Normally a patient alternately touches the nose smoothly. Performing rapid, rhythmical, alternating movements demonstrates coordination in the upper extremities. While sitting, the patient begins by patting the knees with both hands. Then he or she alternately turns up the palm and back of the hands while continuously patting the knees. Normally patients perform the maneuver smoothly and regularly with increasing speed.

An additional maneuver for upper-extremity coordination involves touching each finger with the thumb of the same hand in rapid sequence. A patient moves from the index finger to the little finger and back, with one hand tested at a time. The dominant hand is slightly less awkward when performing this movement. Movement is smooth and in succession.

Test lower-extremity coordination with the patient lying supine, legs extended. Place a hand at the ball of the patient's foot. The patient taps the hand with the foot as quickly as possible. Test each foot for speed and smoothness. The feet do not move as rapidly or evenly as the hands.

Balance. Use one or two of the following tests to assess balance and gross-motor function. When examining the older adult for balance and equilibrium, be aware of the risk for falls. Some older adults need help with this part of the examination.

Have the patient perform a Romberg's test by standing with feet together, arms at the sides, both with eyes open and eyes closed. Protect the patient's safety by standing at the side; observe for swaying. Expect slight swaying of the body in the Romberg's test. A loss of balance (positive Romberg) causes a patient to fall to the side. Normally he or she does not break the stance.

Have the patient close his or her eyes, with arms held straight at the sides, and stand on one foot and then the other. Normally patients are able to maintain balance for 5 seconds with slight swaying. Another test involves asking the patient to walk a straight line by placing the heel of one foot directly in front of the toes of the other foot.

Reflexes

Eliciting reflex reactions provides data about the integrity of sensory and motor pathways of the reflex arc and specific spinal cord segments. Assessment of reflexes does not determine higher neural center functioning but helps to assess peripheral-spinal nerve function. Fig. 30.67 traces the pathway of the reflex arc. Each muscle contains a small

TABLE 30.38 Assessment of Sensory Nerve Function

Function	Equipment	Method	Precautions
Pain	End of paper clip or wooden end of cotton applicator	Ask patients to voice when they feel dull or sharp sensation. Alternately apply sharp and blunt ends of the paper clip or broken cotton applicator to surface of skin. Note areas of numbness or increased sensitivity.	Remember that areas where skin is thick such as heel or sole of foot are less sensitive to pain.
Temperature	Two test tubes, one filled with hot water and another with cold	Touch skin with tube. Ask patient to identify hot or cold sensation.	Omit test if pain sensation is normal.
Light touch	Cotton ball or cotton-tip applicator	Apply light wisp of cotton to different points along surface of skin. Ask patients to voice when they feel a sensation.	Apply at areas where skin is thin or more sensitive (e.g., face, neck, inner aspect of arms, top of feet and hands).
Vibration	Tuning fork	Apply stem of vibrating fork to distal interphalangeal joint of fingers and interphalangeal joint of great toe, elbow, and wrist. Have patients voice when and where they feel vibration.	Be sure that patient feels vibration and not merely pressure.
Position		Grasp finger or toe, holding it by its sides with thumb and index finger. Alternate moving finger or toe up and down. Ask patient to state when finger is up or down. Repeat with toes.	Avoid rubbing adjacent appendages as you move finger or toe. Do not move joint laterally; return to neutral position before moving again.
Two-point discrimination	Two ends of paper clips	Lightly apply one or both ends of paper clips simultaneously to the surface of the skin. Ask patients whether they feel one or two pricks. Find the distance at which patient can no longer distinguish two points.	Apply blade tips to same anatomical site (e.g., fingertips, palm of hand, or upper arms). Minimum distance at which patient discriminates two points varies (2 to 8 mm on fingertips).

BOX 30.32 PATIENT TEACHING

Neurological Assessment

Objective
- Patient and family or significant others will understand relationship of patient's behavioral and mental changes to physical status.

Teaching Strategies
- Explain to family caregiver the implications of any behavioral or mental impairment shown by patient.
- If patient has sensory or motor impairments, explain measures to ensure safety (e.g., wearing glasses or hearing aids, use of ambulation aids or safety bars in bathrooms or stairways) (see Chapter 49).
- Teach older adult to plan enough time to complete tasks because reaction time is slow.
- Teach older adult to observe skin surfaces for areas of trauma since pain perception is reduced.

Evaluation
Use the principles of teach-back to evaluate patient/family caregiver learning:
- Describe for me behaviors that can indicate a neurological impairment.
- Describe for me the safety measures you are using to avoid injury because of your sensory and motor limitations.
- Explain to me why it is important as an older adult that you inspect your skin surface regularly.

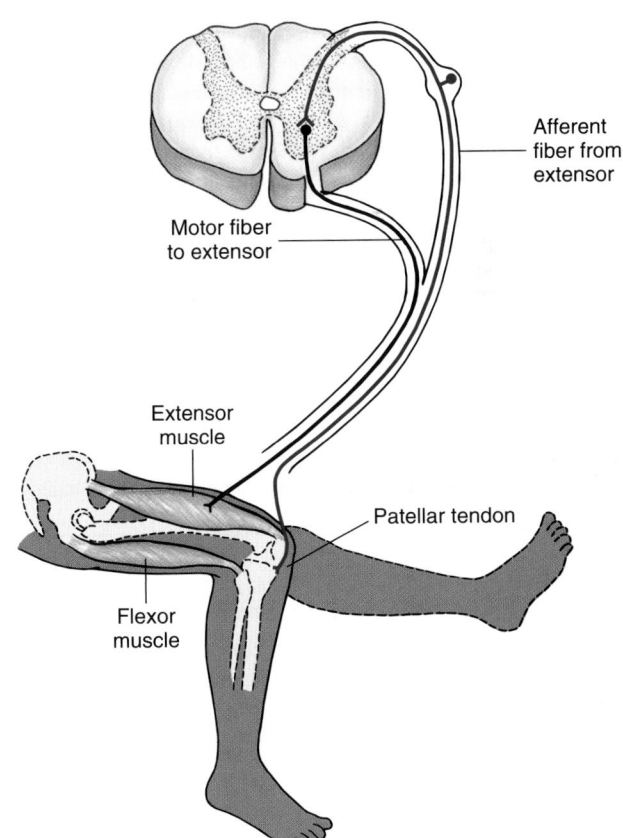

FIG. 30.67 Pathway of reflex arc.

sensory unit called a *muscle spindle*, which controls muscle tone and detects changes in the length of muscle fibers. Tapping a tendon with a reflex hammer stretches the muscle and tendon, lengthening the spindle. The spindle sends nerve impulses along afferent nerve pathways to the dorsal horn of the spinal cord segment. Within milliseconds the impulses reach the spinal cord and synapse to travel to the efferent motor neuron in the spinal cord. A motor nerve sends the impulses back to the muscle, causing the reflex response.

The two categories of normal reflexes are deep tendon reflexes, elicited by mildly stretching a muscle and tapping a tendon, and cutaneous reflexes, elicited by stimulating the skin superficially. Grade reflexes as follows (Ball et al., 2019):

0: No response
1+: Sluggish or diminished
2+: Active or expected response
3+: More brisk than expected, slightly hyperactive
4+: Brisk and hyperactive with intermittent or transient clonus

When assessing reflexes, have the patient relax as much as possible to avoid voluntary movement or tensing of muscles. Position the limbs to slightly stretch the muscle being tested. Hold the reflex hammer loosely between the thumb and fingers so it can swing freely and tap the tendon briskly (Fig. 30.68). Compare the responses on corresponding sides. Normally the older adult presents with diminished reflexes. Reflexes are hyperactive in patients with alcohol, cocaine, or opioid intoxication. Table 30.39 summarizes common deep tendon and cutaneous reflexes.

AFTER THE EXAMINATION

Record findings from the physical assessment either during the examination or after it has been completed. Special forms are available to record data both electronically and on printed forms. Review all findings before helping patients dress in case it is necessary to recheck any information or gather additional data. Integrate physical assessment findings into the plan of care.

After completing an assessment, give the patient time to dress. A patient in a hospital sometimes needs help with hygiene and returning to bed. When the patient is comfortable, it helps to share a summary of the assessment findings. If the findings have revealed serious abnormalities such as a mass or highly irregular heart rate, consult the patient's health care provider before revealing them. It is the health care provider's responsibility to make definitive medical diagnoses. Explain the type of abnormality found and the need for the health care provider to conduct an additional examination.

Delegate the cleanup of the examination area to support staff if needed. Use infection control practice to remove materials or instruments soiled with potentially infectious wastes. If the patient's bedside was the examination site, clear away soiled items from the bedside table and make sure that the bed linen is dry and clean. A patient appreciates

a clean gown and the opportunity to wash the face and hands. Afterward be sure to perform hand hygiene.

Be sure to record a complete assessment. Review the documents for accuracy and thoroughness. Communicate significant findings to appropriate personnel, either verbally or in the patient's written care plan.

> **QSEN** **Building Competency in Safety** A 38-year-old female patient presents to the examination room via a wheelchair. You notice that she is frail, her feet are curled up into the chair, and both of her arms are across her stomach and pressing into her stomach in a firm manner. The patient is sitting in the fetal position within the wheelchair. When you ask her whether she needs help getting on the table in the exam room, she answers in Spanish and you see tears in her eyes. She is accompanied by a younger woman who explains that the patient said, "My stomach hurts, and I don't think I can get to the table." Which aspects of the QSEN competency of safety would be used to best care for this patient throughout the entire physical examination related to culture and physical assessment of the abdomen? How does the competency of patient-centered care play a role in the patient's safety?
>
> Answers to QSEN Activities can be found on the Evolve website.

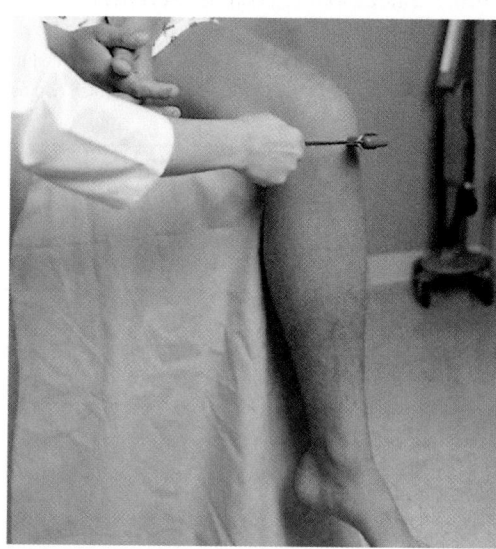

FIG. 30.68 Position for eliciting patellar tendon reflex. Lower leg normally extends.

TABLE 30.39 Assessment of Common Reflexes

Type	Procedure	Normal Reflex
Deep Tendon Reflexes		
Biceps	Flex patient's arm up to 45 degrees at elbow with palms down. Place your thumb in antecubital fossa at base of biceps tendon and your fingers over biceps muscle. Strike biceps tendon with reflex hammer.	Flexion of arm at elbow
Triceps	Flex patient's arm at elbow, holding arm across chest, or hold upper arm horizontally and allow lower arm to go limp. Strike triceps tendon just above elbow.	Extension at elbow
Patellar	Have patient sit with legs hanging freely over side of table or chair or have him or her lie supine and support knee in a flexed 90-degree position. Briskly tap patellar tendon just below patella.	Extension of lower leg
Achilles	Have patient assume same position as for patellar reflex. Slightly dorsiflex patient's ankle by grasping toes in palm of your hand. Strike Achilles tendon just above heel at ankle malleolus.	Plantar flexion of foot
Cutaneous Reflexes		
Plantar	Have patient lie supine with legs straight and feet relaxed. Take handle end of reflex hammer and stroke lateral aspect of sole from heel to ball of foot, curving across ball of foot toward big toe.	Plantar flexion of all toes
Abdominal	Have patient stand or lie supine. Stroke abdominal skin with base of cotton applicator over lateral borders of rectus abdominis muscle toward midline. Repeat test in each abdominal quadrant.	Contraction of rectus abdominis muscle with pulling of umbilicus toward stimulated side

KEY POINTS

- Knowing the purpose of the overall assessment is important so that you can focus and organize the history and physical.
- Your patient's cultural background will impact how you conduct your health assessment and physical examination, ensuring that you show cultural respect.
- Having an organized approach plan for the entire assessment helps ensure the mental and physical comfort of the patient.
- Using open-ended, focused questions helps you gather current information and history to complete a full assessment.
- Before the exam, set up the room and make sure it is a comfortable temperature for the patient.
- Review the nursing history to assist in the knowledge you will need to best complete the physical exam.
- Each assessment area has different techniques and normal and abnormal findings that you will use to interpret data.
- Recognize that the normal aging process impacts physical and assessment findings in older adults.
- During each part of the examination converse with the patient. Teaching health promotion activities related to the area being assessed is a good way to build a relationship of trust and to help the patient.
- Physical assessment can be incorporated into routine care. For example, skin assessment can be completed while helping the patient transfer or prepare for bathing.
- Physical measurements (i.e., height, weight, vital signs, evaluation scales) are used to assess the overall patient condition and within specific areas.

REFLECTIVE LEARNING

- Describe the order in which you completed the assessment on a patient that you cared for during your last clinical rotation. Explain the rationale for completing the assessment in this manner.
- Describe any abnormal assessment findings you obtained when assessing your patient during your clinical experience. What might these findings indicate? Describe the steps you took after obtaining the abnormal findings.
- Consider a patient that you cared for on the clinical unit. Describe how this patient's assessment findings varied based on his or her age.

REVIEW QUESTIONS

1. The nurse prepares to conduct a general survey on an adult patient. Which assessment is performed first while the nurse initiates the nurse-patient relationship?
   1. Appearance and behavior
   2. Measurement of vital signs
   3. Observing specific body systems
   4. Conducting a detailed health history
2. Which number corresponds to the area of the chest where you would auscultate for the tricuspid valve?

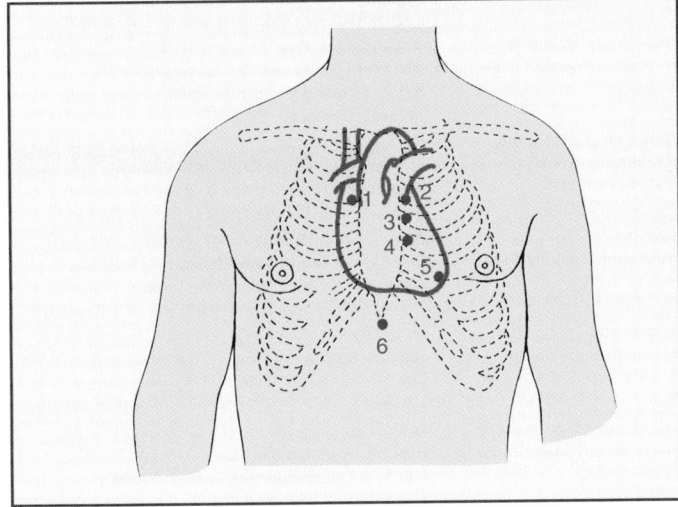

3. The nurse is assessing a patient who returned 1 hour ago from surgery for an abdominal hysterectomy. Which assessment finding would require immediate follow-up?
   1. Auscultation of an apical heart rate of 76
   2. Absence of bowel sounds on abdominal assessment
   3. Respiratory rate of 8 breaths/min
   4. Palpation of dorsalis pedis pulses with strength of +2
4. Which statement made by a patient who is at average risk for colorectal cancer indicates an understanding about teaching related to early detection of colorectal cancer?
   1. "I'll make sure to schedule my colonoscopy annually after the age of 60."
   2. "I'll make sure to have a colonoscopy every 2 years."
   3. "I'll make sure to have a flexible sigmoidoscopy every year once I turn 55."
   4. "I'll make sure to have a fecal occult blood test annually once I turn 45.
5. The nurse is teaching a patient to prevent heart disease. Which information should the nurse include? (Select all that apply.)
   1. Add salt to every meal.
   2. Talk with your health care provider about taking a daily low dose of aspirin.
   3. Work with your health care provider to develop a regular exercise program.
   4. Limit daily intake of fats to less than 25% to 35% of total calories.
   5. Review strategies to encourage the patient to quit smoking.
6. The nurse is assessing the cranial nerves. Match the cranial nerve with its related function.

Cranial Nerves	Cranial Nerve Function
1. XII Hypoglossal	a. Motor innervation to the muscles of the jaw
2. V Trigeminal	b. Lateral movement of the eyeballs
3. VI Adducens	c. Sensation of the pharynx
4. IV Trochlear	d. Downward, inward eye movements
5. X Vagus	e. Position of the tongue

7. The nurse is teaching a patient how to perform a testicular self-examination. Which statement made by the patient indicates a need for further teaching?
   1. "I'll recognize abnormal lumps because they are very painful."
   2. "I'll start performing testicular self-examination monthly after I turn 15."
   3. "I'll perform the self-examination in front of a mirror."
   4. "I'll gently roll the testicle between my fingers."

8. The nurse is observing as the student nurse performs a respiratory assessment on a patient. Which action by the student nurse requires the nurse to intervene?
   1. The student stands at a midline position behind the patient, observing for position of the spine and scapula.
   2. The student palpates the thoracic muscles for masses, pulsations, or abnormal movements.
   3. The student places the bell of the stethoscope on the anterior chest wall to auscultate breath sounds.
   4. The student places the palm of the hand over the intercostal spaces and asks the patient to say "ninety-nine."

9. A patient has undergone surgery for a femoral artery bypass. The surgeon's orders include assessment of dorsalis pedis pulses. The nurse will use which of the following techniques to assess the pulses? (Select all that apply.)

1. Place the fingers behind and below the medial malleolus.
2. Have the patient slightly flex the knee with the foot resting on the bed.
3. Have the patient relax the foot while lying supine.
4. Palpate the groove lateral to the flexor tendon of the wrist.
5. Palpate along the top of the foot in a line with the groove between the extensor tendons of the great and first toes.

10. The faith community nurse is teaching the community center women's group about breast cancer risk factors. Which factors does the nurse include? (Select all that apply.)
    1. First child at the age of 26 years
    2. Menopause onset at the age of 49 years
    3. Family history with *BRCA1* inherited gene mutation
    4. Age over 40 years
    5. Onset of menses before the age of 12
    6. Recent use of oral contraceptives

Answers: 1. 1; **2.** 4; **3.** 3; **4.** 2; **5.** 2; **6.** 1e, 2a, 3b, 4d, 5c; **7.** 1; **8.** 3; **9.** 3, 5; **10.** 3, 4, 5, 6.

Rationales for Review Questions can be found on the Evolve website.

REFERENCES

Ambesh P: Homan's sign for deep vein thrombosis: a grain of salt? *Indian Heart J* 69(3):418, 2017.

American Cancer Society (ACS): *The American Cancer Society Guidelines for the Prevention and Early Detection of Cervical Cancer*, 2016. https://www.cancer.org/cancer/cervical-cancer/prevention-and-early-detection/cervical-cancer-screening-guidelines.html. Accessed October 30, 2018.

American Cancer Society (ACS): *American Cancer Society recommendations for early breast cancer detection in women without breast symptoms*, 2018a. http://www.cancer.org/cancer/breastcancer/more-information/breastcancerearlydetection/breast-cancer-early-detection-acs-recs. Accessed October 9, 2018.

American Cancer Society (ACS): *Cancer facts and figures*, 2018b. https://www.cancer.org/content/dam/cancer-org/research/cancer-facts-and-statistics/annual-cancer-facts-and-figures/2018/cancer-facts-and-figures-2018.pdf. Accessed October 9, 2018.

American Cancer Society (ACS): *Colorectal cancer: what are the risk factors for colorectal cancer?* 2018c. http://www.cancer.org/cancer/colonandrectumcancer/detailedguide/colorectal-cancer-risk-factors. Accessed October 9, 2018.

American Cancer Society (ACS): *Ovarian cancer*, 2018d. http://www.cancer.org/cancer/ovariancancer/detailedguide/ovarian-cancer-key-statistics. Accessed October 9, 2018.

American Heart Association (AHA): *The American Heart Association's diet and lifestyle recommendations*, 2015. https://www.heart.org/en/healthy-living/healthy-eating/eat-smart/nutrition-basics/aha-diet-and-lifestyle-recommendations. Accessed October 30, 2018.

American Heart Association (AHA): *What your cholesterol levels mean*, 2017. https://www.heart.org/en/health-topics/cholesterol/about-cholesterol/what-your-cholesterol-levels-mean. Accessed October 30, 2018.

Asthma and Allergy Foundation of America (AAFA): *Latex allergy*, 2015. https://www.aafa.org/latex-allergy/. Accessed October 7, 2019.

Ball JW, et al.: *Seidel's guide to physical examination*, ed 9, St Louis, 2019, Mosby.

Cancer.Net: *Health risks of e-cigarettes, smokeless tobacco, and waterpipes*, Alexandria, VA, 2018, American Society of Clinical Oncology, The Association. http://www.cancer.net/navigating-cancer-care/prevention-and-healthy-living/tobacco-use/health-risks-e-cigarettes-smokeless-tobacco-and-waterpipes. Accessed October 9, 2018.

Centers for Disease Control and Prevention (CDC): *Loud noise can cause hearing loss*, 2017. https://www.cdc.gov/nceh/hearing_loss/. Accessed October 30, 2018.

Centers for Disease Control and Prevention (CDC): *HPV vaccines: vaccinating your preteen or teen*, 2018a. http://www.cdc.gov/hpv/parents/vaccine.html. Accessed October 9, 2018.

Centers for Disease Control and Prevention (CDC): *Learn about age-related macular degeneration*, 2018b. https://www.cdc.gov/features/healthyvisionmonth/index.html. Accessed October 30, 2018.

Centers for Disease Control and Prevention (CDC): *Vaccines and immunizations: HPV vaccine questions and answers*, 2018c. http://www.cdc.gov/vaccines/vpd-vac/hpv/vac-faqs.htm. Accessed October 30, 2018.

Hockenberry MJ, Wilson P: *Wong's nursing care of infants and children*, ed 10, St Louis, 2019, Mosby.

National Breast Cancer Foundation: *Breast self-exam*, 2016. http://www.nationalbreastcancer.org/breast-self-exam. Accessed October 30, 2018.

National Institute on Drug Abuse (NIDA): *Screening tools for adolescent substance use*, 2017. https://www.drugabuse.gov/nidamed-medical-health-professionals/screening-tools-for-adolescent-substance-use. Accessed October 30, 2018.

National Institute on Drug Abuse (NIDA): *New clinical screening tool available for substance use*, 2018. https://www.drugabuse.gov/news-events/news-releases/2018/06/new-clinician-screening-tool-available-substance-use. Accessed October 30, 2018.

Oral Cancer Foundation: *Oral cancer facts*, 2018. http://oralcancerfoundation.org/facts/index.htm. Accessed October 9, 2018.

Touhy T, Jett K: *Ebersole and Hess' gerontological nursing & healthy aging*, ed 5, St Louis, 2017, Mosby.

US Department of Agriculture (USDA): *Let's eat for the health of it, Pub No: Home & Garden Bulletin No. 232-CP*, 2018. http://www.choosemyplate.gov/food-groups/downloads/MyPlate/DG2010Brochure.pdf. Accessed October 30, 2018.

US Preventive Services Task Force (USPSTF): Screening for osteoporosis to prevent fractures, US Preventive Services Task Force recommendation statement, *JAMA* 319(24):2521–2531, 2018.

World Health Organization: *Understanding and addressing violence against women*, 2018. http://apps.who.int/iris/bitstream/handle/10665/77432/WHO_RHR_12.36_eng.pdf;jsessionid=9C1C7A48DE-6DAFA56FEEAE0846EA9E97?sequence=1. Accessed October 30, 2018.

RESEARCH REFERENCES

Bond L, Hallmark B: Educating nurses in the intensive care unit about gastrointestinal complications, *Crit Care Nurs Clin North Am* 30(1):75–85, 2018.

Felder S, et al.: Usefulness of bowel sounds auscultation: a prospective evaluation, *J Surg Educ* 71(5):768–773, 2014.

Folstein MF, et al.: "Mini-mental state": a practical method for grading the cognitive state of patients for the clinician, *J Psychiatr Res* 12(3):189, 1975.

Frazer C, et al.: Gastrointestinal motility problems in critically ill patients, *Crit Care Nurs Clin North Am* 30(1):109–121, 2018.

Goto J, et al.: Usefulness of real-time bowel sound analysis system in patients with severe sepsis (pilot study), *J Artif Organs* 18(1):86–91, 2015.

Jacob L: Auscultation of bowel sounds in critical care: the role of the nurse, Br J Nurs 26(17):962-963.

Ladopoulos T, et al.: Gastrointestinal dysmotility in critically ill patients, *Ann Gastroenterol* 3(31):273–281, 2018.

Li B, et al.: Analysis of bowel sounds application status for gastrointestinal function monitoring in the intensive care unit, *Crit Care Nurs Q* 37(2):199–206, 2014.

Moonen P, et al.: The black box revelation: monitoring gastrointestinal function, *Anaesthesiol Intensive Ther* 50(1):72–81, 2018.

Morisawa T, et al.: Passive exercise of the lower limbs and trunk alleviates decreased intestinal motility in patients in the intensive care unit after cardiovascular surgery, *J Phys Ther Sci* 29:312–316, 2017.

Zuin M, et al.: Is abdominal auscultation a still relevant part of the physical examination? *Eur J Intern Med* 43:e24–e25, 2017.

31

Medication Administration

OBJECTIVES

- Discuss nursing roles and responsibilities in medication administration.
- Discuss legal responsibilities in medication administration.
- Describe the physiological mechanisms of medication action.
- Differentiate among different types of medication actions.
- Discuss developmental factors that influence pharmacokinetics.
- Identify the characteristics of adverse medication events.
- Discuss factors that influence medication actions.
- Discuss methods used to educate patients about prescribed medications.

- Compare and contrast the roles of the health care provider, pharmacist, and nurse in medication administration.
- Implement nursing actions to prevent medication errors.
- Describe factors to consider when choosing routes of medication administration.
- Calculate prescribed medication doses correctly.
- Discuss factors to include in assessing a patient's needs for and response to medication therapy.
- Identify the seven rights of medication administration and apply them in clinical settings.
- Correctly and safely prepare and administer medications.

KEY TERMS

Absorption, p. 592
Adverse effects, p. 594
Anaphylactic reactions, p. 594
Biological half-life, p. 595
Biotransformation, p. 593
Buccal, p. 596
Detoxify, p. 593
Idiosyncratic reaction, p. 594
Infusions, p. 595
Injection, p. 592
Instillation, p. 598
Intraarticular, p. 596
Intracardiac, p. 596
Intradermal (ID), p. 596
Intramuscular (IM), p. 596
Intraocular, p. 598

Intravenous (IV), p. 596
Irrigations, p. 599
Medication allergy, p. 594
Medication error, p. 605
Medication interaction, p. 594
Medication reconciliation, p. 606
Medication tolerance, p. 594
Minimum effective concentration (MEC), p. 595
Ophthalmic, p. 620
Parenteral administration, p. 596
Peak, p. 595
Pharmacokinetics, p. 592
Polypharmacy, p. 615
Prescriptions, p. 604

Pressurized metered-dose inhalers (pMDIs), p. 620
Side effect, p. 594
Solution, p. 599
Subcutaneous, p. 596
Sublingual, p. 596
Synergistic effect, p. 594
Therapeutic effect, p. 593
Therapeutic range, p. 595
Toxic effects, p. 594
Transdermal disk, p. 597
Trough, p. 595
Verbal order, p. 602
Z-track method, p. 633

MEDIA RESOURCES

http://evolve.elsevier.com/Potter/fundamentals/
- Review Questions
- Video Clips
- Case Study with Questions

- Skills Performance Checklists
- Audio Glossary
- Content Updates
- Answers to QSEN Activity and Review Questions

Patients with health problems use a variety of strategies to restore or maintain their health. One strategy they often use is medication, a substance used in the diagnosis, treatment, cure, relief, or prevention of health problems. No matter where patients receive health care (i.e., hospitals, clinics, or home), nurses play an essential role in preparing, administering, and evaluating the effects of medications. Family caregivers, friends, or home care personnel often administer medications when patients cannot administer them themselves at home. In all settings nurses are responsible for evaluating the effects of medications on the patient's ongoing health status, providing education about

medications and side effects, encouraging adherence to the medication regimen, and evaluating the patient's and family caregiver's ability to administer medications.

SCIENTIFIC KNOWLEDGE BASE

Because medication administration and evaluation are a critical part of nursing practice, nurses need to understand the actions and effects of all medications taken by their patients. Administering medications safely requires an understanding of legal aspects of health care, pharmacology, pharmacokinetics (the movement of drugs in the human body), the life sciences, pathophysiology, human anatomy, and mathematics.

Medication Legislation and Standards

Federal Regulations. The US government protects the health of the people by ensuring that medications are safe and effective. The first American law to regulate medications was the Pure Food and Drug Act. This law simply requires all medications to be free of impure products. Subsequent legislation created standards related to safety, potency, and efficacy. Currently the Food and Drug Administration (FDA) enforces medication laws that ensure that all medications on the market undergo vigorous testing before they are sold to the public. Federal medication laws also control medication sales and distribution; testing, naming, and labeling; and the use of controlled substances. Official publications such as the *United States Pharmacopeia* (USP) and the *National Formulary* set standards for medication strength, quality, purity, packaging, safety, labeling, and dose form. In 1993 the FDA instituted the MedWatch program. This voluntary program encourages nurses and other health care professionals to report when a medication, product, or medical event causes serious harm to a patient by completing the MedWatch form. The form is available on the MedWatch website (USFDA, 2018a).

State and Local Regulation of Medication. State and local medication laws must conform to federal legislation. States often have additional controls, including control of substances not regulated by the federal government. Local governmental bodies regulate the use of alcohol and tobacco.

Health Care Institutions and Medication Laws. Health care agencies establish individual policies to meet federal, state, and local regulations. The size of the agency, the services it provides, and the professional personnel it employs influence these policies. Agency policies are often more restrictive than governmental controls. For example, a common agency policy is the automatic discontinuation of narcotics after a set number of days. Although a health care provider can reorder the narcotic, this policy helps to control unnecessarily prolonged medication therapy because it requires the health care provider to regularly review the need for the medication.

Medication Regulations and Nursing Practice. State Nurse Practice Acts (NPAs) define the scope of nurses' professional functions and responsibilities. Most NPAs are purposefully broad so that nurses' professional responsibilities are not limited. Health care agencies can interpret specific actions allowed under NPAs, but they cannot modify, expand, or restrict the intent of the act. The primary intent of NPAs is to protect the public from unskilled, undereducated, and unlicensed personnel.

A nurse is responsible for following legal provisions when administering controlled substances such as opioids, which are carefully controlled through federal and state guidelines. Violations of the Controlled Substances Act are punishable by fines, imprisonment, and loss of nurse licensure. Hospitals and other health care agencies have policies for the proper storage and distribution of narcotics (Box 31.1).

Pharmacological Concepts

Medication Names. Some medications have as many as three different names. The chemical name of a medication provides an exact description of its composition and molecular structure. Nurses rarely use chemical names in clinical practice. An example of a chemical name is N-acetyl-para-aminophenol, which is commonly known as Tylenol. The manufacturer who first develops the medication gives the generic

---

BOX 31.1 Guidelines for Safe Opioid (Narcotic) Administration and Control

- Store all narcotics in a locked, secure cabinet or container (e.g., computerized, locked cabinets are preferred).
- Maintain a running count of opioids by counting them whenever dispensing them. If you find a discrepancy, correct and report it immediately.
- Use a special inventory record each time an opioid is dispensed. Records are often kept electronically and provide an accurate ongoing count of narcotics used, wasted, and remaining.
- Use the record to document the patient's name, date, time of medication administration, name of medication, and dosage. If the agency keeps a paper record, the nurse dispensing the medication signs the record. If the agency uses a computerized system, the computer records the nurse's name.
- If a nurse gives only part of a dose of a controlled substance, a second nurse witnesses the disposal of the unused part. Computerized systems record the nurses' names electronically. If paper records are kept, both nurses sign their names on the form.
- Follow agency policy for appropriate waste of opioids. Do not place wasted parts of medications in sharps containers.

---

or nonproprietary name, with United States Adopted Names (USAN) Council approval (AMA, 2018). Acetaminophen is an example of the generic name for Tylenol. The generic name becomes the official name listed in official publications such as the United States Pharmacopeia (USP). The trade name, brand name, or proprietary name is the name under which a manufacturer markets a medication. The trade name has the symbol (™) at the upper right of the name, indicating that the manufacturer has trademarked the name of the medication (e.g., Panadol™ and Tempra™).

Manufacturers choose trade names that are easy to pronounce, spell, and remember. Many companies produce the same medication, and similarities in trade names are often confusing. Therefore, be careful to obtain the exact name and spelling for each medication you administer to your patients. Because similarities in medication names are a common cause of medical errors, the Institute for Safe Medication Practices (ISMP) (2015a; 2018a) publishes a list of medications that are frequently confused with one another. The ISMP recommends the use of Food and Drug Administration (FDA)-approved tall-man or mixed-case letters when possible (e.g., aMILoride versus amLODIPine) to help health care providers easily recognize the difference between these commonly confused medications.

Classification. Medication classification indicates the effect of a medication on a body system, the symptoms a medication relieves, or its desired effect. Usually each class contains more than one medication that is used for the same type of health problem. For example, patients who have asthma often take a variety of medications, such as beta$_2$-adrenergic agonists, to control their illness. The *beta$_2$-adrenergic* classification contains more than 15 different medications (Burchum and Rosenthal, 2019). Some medications are in more than one class. For example, aspirin is an analgesic, an antipyretic, and an antiinflammatory medication.

Medication Forms. Medications are available in a variety of forms, or preparations. The form of the medication determines its route of administration. The composition of a medication enhances its absorption and metabolism. Many medications come in several forms, such as tablets, capsules, elixirs, and suppositories. When administering a medication, be certain to use the proper form (Table 31.1).

TABLE 31.1 Forms of Medication

Form	Description
Medication Forms Commonly Prepared for Administration by Oral Route	
Solid Forms	
Caplet	Shaped like capsule and coated for ease of swallowing
Capsule	Medication encased in gelatin shell
Tablet	Powdered medication compressed into hard disk or cylinder; in addition to primary medication, contains binders (adhesive to allow powder to stick together), disintegrators (to promote tablet dissolution), lubricants (for ease of manufacturing), and fillers (for convenient tablet size)
Enteric-coated tablet	Coated tablet that does not dissolve in stomach; coatings dissolve in intestine, where medication is absorbed
Liquid Forms	
Elixir	Clear fluid containing water and/or alcohol; often sweetened
Extract	Syrup or dried form of pharmacologically active medication, usually made by evaporating solution
Aqueous solution	Substance dissolved in water and syrups
Aqueous suspension	Finely dissolved medication particles dispersed in liquid medium; when suspension is left standing, particles settle to bottom of container
Syrup	Medication dissolved in a concentrated sugar solution
Tincture	Alcohol extract from plant or vegetable
Other Oral Forms and Terms Associated with Oral Preparations	
Troche (lozenge)	Flat, round tablets that dissolve in mouth to release medication; not meant for ingestion
Aerosol	Aqueous medication sprayed and absorbed in mouth and upper airway; not meant for ingestion
Sustained release	Tablet or capsule that contains small particles of a medication coated with material that requires a varying amount of time to dissolve
Medication Forms Commonly Prepared for Administration by Topical Route	
Ointment (salve or cream)	Semisolid, externally applied preparation, usually containing one or more medications
Liniment	Usually contains alcohol, oil, or soapy emollient applied to skin
Lotion	Semiliquid suspension that usually protects, cools, or cleanses skin
Paste	Medication preparation that is thicker than ointment; absorbed through skin more slowly than ointment; often used for skin protection
Transdermal disk or patch	Medicated disk or patch absorbed through skin slowly over long period of time (e.g., 24 hours)
Medication Forms Commonly Prepared for Administration by Parenteral Route	
Solution	Sterile preparation that contains water with one or more dissolved compounds
Powder	Sterile particles of medication that are dissolved in a sterile liquid (e.g., water, normal saline) before administration
Medication Forms Commonly Prepared for Instillation Into Body Cavities	
Intraocular disk	Small, flexible oval (similar to contact lens) consisting of two soft, outer layers and a middle layer containing medication; slowly releases medication when moistened by ocular fluid
Suppository	Solid dosage form mixed with gelatin and shaped in form of pellet for insertion into body cavity (rectum or vagina); melts when it reaches body temperature, releasing medication for absorption

Pharmacokinetics as the Basis of Medication Actions

For a medication to be useful therapeutically, it must be taken into a patient's body; be absorbed and distributed to cells, tissues, or a specific organ; and alter physiological functions. Pharmacokinetics is the study of how medications enter the body, reach their site of action, metabolize, and exit the body. You use knowledge of pharmacokinetics when timing medication administration, selecting the route of administration, and evaluating a patient's response.

Absorption. Absorption occurs when medication molecules pass into the blood from the site of medication administration. Factors that influence absorption are the route of administration, ability of the medication to dissolve, blood flow to the site of administration, body surface area (BSA), and lipid solubility of medication.

Route of Administration. Each route of medication administration has a different rate of absorption. When applying medications on the skin, absorption is slow because of the physical makeup of the skin. Because orally administered medications pass through the gastrointestinal (GI) tract, the overall rate of absorption is usually slow. Medications placed on the mucous membranes and respiratory airways are absorbed quickly because these tissues contain many blood vessels. Intramuscular (IM) and subcutaneous medications absorb more quickly than oral medications, with IM injections entering the bloodstream more quickly than medications in subcutaneous injections. Intravenous (IV) injection produces the most rapid absorption because medications are available immediately when they enter the systemic circulation.

Ability of a Medication To Dissolve. The ability of an oral medication to dissolve depends largely on its form or preparation. The body absorbs solutions and suspensions already in a liquid state more readily than tablets or capsules. Acidic medications pass through the gastric mucosa rapidly. Medications that are basic are not absorbed before reaching the small intestine.

Blood Flow to the Site of Administration. The blood supply to the site of administration will determine how quickly the body can absorb a medication. Medications are absorbed as blood comes in contact with the site of administration. The richer the blood supply to the site of administration, the faster a medication is absorbed.

Body Surface Area. When a medication comes in contact with a large surface area, it is absorbed at a faster rate. This helps explain why most of medications are absorbed in the small intestine rather than the stomach (Burchum and Rosenthal, 2019).

Lipid Solubility. Because the cell membrane has a lipid layer, highly lipid-soluble medications cross cell membranes easily and are absorbed quickly. Another factor that often affects medication absorption is whether food is in the stomach. Some oral medications are absorbed more easily when administered between meals because food changes the structure of a medication and sometimes impairs its absorption. When some medications are administered together, they interfere with one another, impairing the absorption of both medications.

Safe medication administration requires knowledge of factors that alter or impair absorption of prescribed medications. You need to understand medication pharmacokinetics, a patient's health history, physical examination data, and knowledge gained through daily patient interactions. Use your knowledge and agency policy to plan medication administration times that will promote optimal absorption. For example, plan medication administration times around meals (e.g., before or after meals) when medications interact with food. When they interact with one another, make sure that you do not give them at the same time. Consult and collaborate with your patient's health care provider or a pharmacist when setting medication times to ensure that the patient achieves the therapeutic effect of all medications. Before administering any medication, check pharmacology books, medication references, or package inserts or consult with pharmacists to identify medication-medication or medication-food interactions.

Distribution. After a medication is absorbed, it is distributed within the body to tissues and organs and ultimately to its specific site of action. The rate and extent of distribution depend on the physical and chemical properties of the medication and the physiology of the person taking it.

Circulation. Once a medication enters the bloodstream, it is carried throughout the tissues and organs. How fast it reaches a site depends on the vascularity of the various tissues and organs. Conditions that limit blood flow or blood perfusion inhibit the distribution of a medication. For example, patients with heart failure have impaired circulation, which slows medication delivery to the intended site of action. Therefore, the effectiveness of medications in these patients is often delayed or altered.

Membrane Permeability. Membrane permeability refers to the ability of a medication to pass through tissues and membranes to enter target cells. To be distributed to an organ, a medication must pass through all of the tissues and biological membranes of the organ. Some membranes serve as barriers to the passage of medications. For example, the blood-brain barrier allows only fat-soluble medications to pass into the brain and cerebral spinal fluid. Therefore, central nervous system infections often require treatment with antibiotics injected directly into the subarachnoid space in the spinal cord. Some older adults experience adverse effects (e.g., confusion) because of the change in the permeability of the blood-brain barrier, with easier passage of fat-soluble medications.

Protein Binding. The degree to which medications bind to serum proteins such as albumin affects their distribution. Most medications partially bind to albumin, reducing the ability of a drug to exert pharmacological activity. The unbound or "free" medication is its active form. Older adults and patients with liver disease or malnutrition have decreased albumin in the bloodstream. Because more medication is unbound in these patients, they are at risk for an increase in medication activity, toxicity, or both.

Metabolism. After a medication reaches its site of action, it becomes metabolized into a less active or an inactive form that is easier to excrete. Biotransformation occurs under the influence of enzymes that detoxify, break down, and remove biologically active chemicals. Most biotransformation occurs within the liver, although the lungs, kidneys, blood, and intestines also metabolize medications. The liver is especially important because its specialized structure oxidizes and transforms many toxic substances. The liver degrades many harmful chemicals before they become distributed to the tissues. If a decrease in liver function occurs such as with aging or liver disease, a medication is usually eliminated more slowly, resulting in its accumulation. Patients are at risk for medication toxicity if organs that metabolize medications are not functioning correctly. For example, a small sedative dose of a barbiturate sometimes causes a patient with liver disease to lapse into a coma.

Excretion. After medications are metabolized, they exit the body through the kidneys, liver, bowel, lungs, and exocrine glands. The chemical makeup of a medication determines the organ of excretion. Gaseous and volatile compounds such as nitrous oxide and alcohol exit through the lungs. Deep breathing and coughing (see Chapter 41) help patients eliminate anesthetic gases more rapidly after surgery. The exocrine glands excrete lipid-soluble medications. When medications exit through sweat glands, the skin often becomes irritated, requiring you to teach patients good hygiene practices (see Chapter 40). If a medication is excreted through the mammary glands, there is a risk that a nursing infant will ingest the chemicals. Check the safety of any medication used in breastfeeding women.

The GI tract is another route for medication excretion. Medications that enter the hepatic circulation are broken down by the liver and excreted into the bile. After chemicals enter the intestines through the biliary tract, the intestines resorb them. Factors that increase peristalsis (e.g., laxatives and enemas) accelerate medication excretion through the feces, whereas factors that slow peristalsis (e.g., inactivity and improper diet) often prolong the effects of a medication.

The kidneys are the main organs for medication excretion. Some medications escape extensive metabolism and exit unchanged in the urine. Others undergo biotransformation in the liver before the kidneys excrete them. Maintenance of an adequate fluid intake (50 mL/kg/hr) promotes proper elimination of medications for the average adult. If a patient's renal function declines, the kidneys cannot adequately excrete medications. Thus, the risk for medication toxicity increases. Health care providers usually reduce medication doses when this happens.

Types of Medication Action

Medications vary considerably in the way they act and their types of action. Patients do not always respond in the same way to each successive dose of a medication. Sometimes the same medication causes very different responses in different patients. Therefore, you need to understand all the effects that medications you administer have on patients.

Therapeutic Effects. The therapeutic effect is the expected or predicted physiological response caused by a medication. For example, nitroglycerin reduces cardiac workload and increases myocardial oxygen supply. Some medications have more than one therapeutic effect. For example, prednisone, a steroid, decreases swelling, inhibits inflammation, reduces allergic responses, and prevents rejection of transplanted organs. Knowing the desired therapeutic effect for each medication allows you to provide patient education and accurately evaluate the desired effect of a medication.

Adverse Effects. Every medication can harm a patient. Undesired, unintended, and often unpredictable responses to medication are referred to as adverse effects. Adverse medication effects range from mild to severe. Some happen immediately, whereas others develop over time. Be alert and assess for unusual individual responses to medications, especially with newly prescribed medications. Patients most at risk for adverse medication reactions include the very young and older adults, pregnant women, patients taking multiple medications, patients who are extremely underweight or overweight, and patients with renal or liver disease. If adverse effects are mild and tolerable, patients often remain on the medications. However, if they are not tolerated and are potentially harmful, stop giving the medication immediately. When adverse responses to medications occur, the health care provider discontinues the medication immediately. Health care providers report adverse effects to the FDA using the MedWatch program (USFDA, 2018a).

Side Effects. A side effect is a predictable and often unavoidable adverse effect produced at a usual therapeutic dose. For example, some antihypertensive medications cause impotence in men. Side effects range from being harmless to causing serious symptoms or injury. If the side effects are serious enough to negate the beneficial effects of the therapeutic action of the medication, the health care provider discontinues the medication. Patients often stop taking medications because of side effects, the most common of which are anorexia, nausea, vomiting, constipation, drowsiness, and diarrhea.

Toxic Effects. Toxic effects often develop after prolonged intake of a medication or when a medication accumulates in the blood because of impaired metabolism or excretion. Excess amounts of a medication within the body sometimes have lethal effects, depending on its action. For example, toxic levels of morphine, an opioid, cause severe respiratory depression and death. Antidotes are available to treat specific types of medication toxicity. For example, naloxone, an opioid antagonist, reverses the effects of opioid toxicity.

Idiosyncratic Reactions. Medications sometimes cause unpredictable effects such as an idiosyncratic reaction, in which a patient overreacts or underreacts to a medication or has a reaction different from normal. For example, a child who receives diphenhydramine, an antihistamine, becomes extremely agitated or excited instead of drowsy. At present, it is not possible to predict whether a patient will have an idiosyncratic response to a medication.

Allergic Reactions. Allergic reactions are unpredictable responses to a medication. Some patients become immunologically sensitized to the initial dose of a medication. With repeated administration the patient develops an allergic response to it, its chemical preservatives, or a metabolite. The medication or chemical acts as an antigen, triggering the release of the antibodies in the body. A patient's medication allergy symptoms vary, depending on the individual and the medication (Table 31.2). Among the different classes of medications, antibiotics cause a high incidence of allergic reactions. Severe or anaphylactic reactions, which are life threatening, are characterized by sudden constriction of bronchiolar muscles, edema of the pharynx and larynx, and severe wheezing and shortness of breath. Immediate medical attention is required to treat anaphylactic reactions. A patient with a known history of an allergy to a medication needs to avoid taking that medication in the future and wear an identification bracelet or medal (Fig. 31.1), which alerts nurses and other health care providers to the allergy if a patient is unable to communicate when receiving medical care.

TABLE 31.2   Mild Allergic Reactions

Symptom	Description
Urticaria (hives)	Raised, irregularly shaped skin eruptions with varying sizes and shapes; eruptions have reddened margins and pale centers
Rash	Small, raised vesicles that are usually reddened; often distributed over entire body
Pruritus	Itching of skin; accompanies most rashes
Rhinitis	Inflammation of mucous membranes lining nose; causes swelling and clear, watery discharge

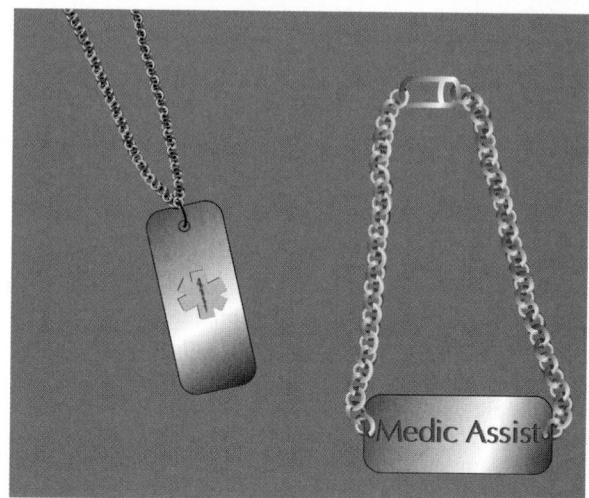

FIG. 31.1 Allergy identification bracelet and medal.

Medication Interactions. When one medication modifies the action of another, a medication interaction occurs. Medication interactions are common when individuals take several medications. Some medications increase or diminish the action of others or alter the way another medication is absorbed, metabolized, or eliminated from the body. When two medications have a synergistic effect, their combined effect is greater than the effect of the medications when given separately. For example, alcohol is a central nervous system depressant that has a synergistic effect on antihistamines, antidepressants, barbiturates, and narcotic analgesics. Sometimes a medication interaction is desired. Health care providers often combine medications to create an interaction that has a beneficial effect. For example, a patient with high blood pressure takes several medications such as diuretics and vasodilators that act together to control blood pressure when one medication is not effective on its own.

Medication Tolerance and Dependence. Medication tolerance occurs over time. It is usually noted clinically when patients receive more and more medication (higher doses) to achieve the same therapeutic effect. Medications that produce tolerance include opium alkaloids (e.g., morphine), nitrates, and ethyl alcohol. Patients hospitalized for acute illnesses usually do not develop medication tolerance. It may take a month or longer for tolerance to occur.

Medication tolerance is not the same as medication dependence. Two types of medication dependence (addiction) exist: physical and psychological. In psychological dependence a patient desires the medication for benefit other than the intended effect. Physical dependence is a physiological adaptation to a medication that manifests by intense physical disturbance when the medication is withdrawn. If a patient is

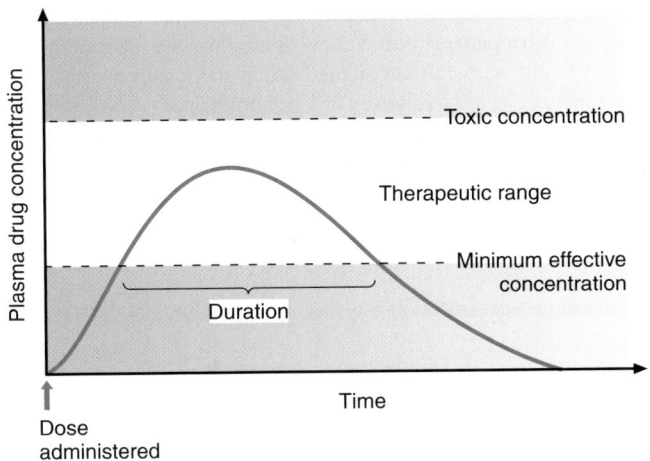

FIG. 31.2 The therapeutic range of a medication occurs between the minimum effective concentration and the toxic concentration. (From Burchum JR, Rosenthal LD: *Pharmacology for nursing care*, ed 10, St Louis, 2019, Elsevier.)

TABLE 31.3 Common Dosage Administration Schedules

Dosage Schedule (Meaning)	Abbreviation
Before meals	AC, ac
As desired	ad lib
Twice each day	BID, bid
After meals	PC, pc
Whenever there is a need	prn
Every morning, every AM	q am
Every hour	qh
Every day	Daily
Every 4 hours	q4h
4 times per day	QID, qid
Give immediately	STAT, stat
3 times per day	TID, tid

dependent on alcohol, a higher-than-usual medication dose is necessary for the desired effect of the medication.

Nurses and other health care professionals play an important role in the care of patients with drug addiction. Patients need to be approached with positive attitudes, so the patient may be more open to learning about treatment options. Using the newest evidence-based treatment options can help patients with addictions receive the care and treatment they need.

Timing of Medication Dose Responses

Medications administered intravenously enter the bloodstream and act immediately, whereas those given in other routes take time to enter the bloodstream and have an effect. The quantity and distribution of a medication in different body compartments change constantly. Medications are ordered at various times, depending on when their response begins, becomes most intense, and ceases.

The minimum effective concentration (MEC) is the plasma level of a medication below which the effect of the medication does not occur. The toxic concentration is the level at which toxic effects occur. When a medication is prescribed, the goal is to achieve a constant blood level within a safe therapeutic range, which falls between the MEC and the toxic concentration (Fig. 31.2). When a medication is administered repeatedly, its serum level fluctuates between doses. The highest level is called the peak concentration, and the lowest level is called the trough concentration. After reaching its peak, the serum concentration of the medication falls progressively. With IV infusions the peak concentration occurs quickly, but the serum level also begins to fall immediately. Some medication doses (e.g., vancomycin) are based on peak and trough serum levels. The trough level is generally drawn 30 minutes before administering the medication, and the peak level is drawn whenever the medication is expected to reach its peak concentration. The time it takes for a medication to reach its peak concentration varies, depending on the pharmacokinetics of the medication.

All medications have a biological half-life, which is the time it takes for excretion processes to lower the serum medication concentration by half. To maintain a therapeutic plateau, a patient needs to receive regular fixed doses. For example, pain medications are most effective for some cancer patients when they are given around-the-clock (ATC) rather than when a patient intermittently complains of pain because the body maintains an almost constant level of pain medication (Burchum and Rosenthal, 2019). After an initial medication dose, the patient receives each successive dose when the previous dose reaches its half-life. The patient and nurse need to follow regular dosage schedules and administer prescribed doses at correct intervals. Know the following time intervals of medication action to anticipate the effect of a medication:

1. *Onset of medication action*: Period of time it takes after you administer a medication for it to produce a therapeutic effect
2. *Peak action*: Time it takes for a medication to reach its highest effective peak concentration
3. *Trough*: Minimum blood serum concentration of medication reached just before the next scheduled dose
4. *Duration of action*: Length of time during which a medication is present in a concentration great enough to produce a therapeutic effect
5. *Plateau*: Blood serum concentration reached and maintained after repeated, fixed doses

You and your patient follow prescribed doses and dosage intervals (Table 31.3). Health care agencies usually set schedules for medication administration. However, you can change this schedule based on your knowledge about a medication. For example, you work at an agency where medications ordered once a day are given at 0800. Your patient has a medication ordered once a day that works better when given before bedtime; therefore, you adjust the time to give the medication accordingly, based on agency policy. Acute care agencies also follow guidelines from the ISMP to determine safe, effective, and timely administration of medications (CMS, 2014; ISMP, 2011a). According to the guidelines, hospitals determine whether medications are time critical. Medications that are time critical most likely cause harm or have subtherapeutic effects if they are not administered on time (usually 30 minutes before or after the scheduled dose). Non–time-critical medications most likely do not cause harm if they are given within 1 to 2 hours before or after the scheduled time. Thus, you need to administer time-critical medications at a precise time, within 30 minutes before or after their scheduled time. You administer non–time-critical medications within 1 to 2 hours of their scheduled time. Ensure that you follow your agency medication policies about the timing of medications to ensure that your patients receive their medications at the right time (CMS 2014; ISMP, 2011a).

When you teach patients about dosage schedules, use familiar language. For example, when teaching a patient about twice-daily medication dosing, instruct him or her to take the medication in the morning

TABLE 31.4 Terms Associated with Medication Actions

Term	Meaning
Onset	Time it takes after a medication is administered for it to produce a response
Peak	Time it takes for a medication to reach its highest effective concentration
Trough	Minimum blood serum concentration of medication reached just before the next scheduled dose
Duration	Time during which medication is present in concentration great enough to produce a response
Plateau	Blood serum concentration of medication reached and maintained after repeated fixed doses

and again in the evening. Knowledge of the time intervals of medication action help you anticipate the effect of the medication (Table 31.4). With this knowledge, instruct the patient when to expect a response.

Routes of Administration

The route prescribed for administering a medication depends on the properties and desired effect of the medication and the patient's physical and mental condition (Table 31.5). Work with the health care provider to determine the best route for a patient's medication.

QSEN Building Competency in Evidence-Based Practice

A nursing student is caring for a patient being treated for multiple fractures after a recent fall. The health care provider writes a new medication order for morphine sulfate liquid suspension 20 mg orally STAT and then q4h as needed for pain. The patient is having difficulty swallowing pills as a result of the trauma; thus, the medications are ordered in liquid suspension.

1. What does the student need to know about morphine sulfate before administering it?
2. Four unit-dose containers of liquid morphine sulfate arrive on the patient care unit. The labels on the medication say: "40 mg morphine sulfate/5 mL." You will need to waste some of the liquid morphine before administering it to the patient. What are the procedures for wasting a narcotic?
3. You collect the appropriate equipment to administer the medication, perform hand hygiene, prepare the medication, take it to the patient at the correct time, and use two unique patient identifiers to ensure that this is the right patient. Which step do you need to take next in administering the medication?

Answers to QSEN Activities can be found on the Evolve website.

Oral Routes. The oral route is the easiest and the most commonly used route of medication administration. Medications are given by mouth and swallowed with fluid. Oral medications have a slower onset of action and a more prolonged effect than parenteral medications. Patients generally prefer the oral route.

Sublingual Administration. Some medications (e.g., nitroglycerin) are readily absorbed after being placed under the tongue to dissolve (Fig. 31.3). Instruct patients not to swallow a medication given by the sublingual route or drink anything until the medication is completely dissolved to ensure that the medication will have the desired effect.

Buccal Administration. Administration of a medication by the buccal route involves placing the solid medication in the mouth against the mucous membranes of the cheek until it dissolves (Fig. 31.4). Teach patients to alternate cheeks with each subsequent dose to avoid mucosal irritation. Warn patients not to chew or swallow the medication or to take any liquids with it. A buccal medication acts locally on the mucosa or systemically as it is swallowed in a person's saliva.

Parenteral Routes. Parenteral administration involves injecting a medication into body tissues. The following are the four major sites of injection:

1. Intradermal (ID): Injection into the dermis just under the epidermis
2. Subcutaneous: Injection into tissues just below the dermis of the skin
3. Intramuscular (IM): Injection into a muscle
4. Intravenous (IV): Injection into a vein

Some medications are administered into body cavities through other routes, including epidural, intrathecal, intraosseous, intraperitoneal, intrapleural, and intraarterial. Nurses usually are not responsible for the administration of medications through these advanced techniques. Whether or not you actually administer a medication, you remain responsible for monitoring the integrity of the medication delivery system, understanding the therapeutic value of the medication, and evaluating a patient's response to the therapy.

Epidural. Epidural medications are administered in the epidural space via a catheter, which is placed by a nurse anesthetist or an anesthesiologist. This route is used for the administration of regional analgesia for surgical procedures (see Chapters 44 and 50). Nurses who have advanced education in the epidural route can administer medications by continuous infusion or a bolus dose.

Intrathecal. Physicians and specially educated nurses administer intrathecal medications through a catheter surgically placed in the subarachnoid space or one of the ventricles of the brain. Intrathecal medication administration often is a long-term treatment.

Intraosseous. This method of medication administration involves the infusion of medication directly into the bone marrow. It is used most commonly in infants and toddlers who have poor access to their intravascular space or when an emergency arises, and IV access is impossible.

Intraperitoneal. Medications administered into the peritoneal cavity are absorbed into the circulation. Chemotherapeutic agents, insulin, and antibiotics are administered in this fashion.

Intrapleural. A syringe and needle or a chest tube is used to administer intrapleural medications directly into the pleural space. Chemotherapeutic agents are the most common medications administered via this method. Physicians also instill medications that help resolve persistent pleural effusion to promote adhesion between the visceral and parietal pleura. This is called *pleurodesis*.

Intraarterial. Intraarterial medications are administered directly into the arteries. Intraarterial infusions are common in patients who have arterial clots and receive clot-dissolving agents. A nurse manages a continuous infusion of the clot-dissolving agent and carefully monitors the integrity of the infusion to prevent inadvertent disconnection of the system and subsequent bleeding.

Other methods of medication administration that are usually limited to physician administration are intracardiac, an injection of a medication directly into cardiac tissue, and intraarticular, an injection of a medication into a joint.

Topical Administration. Medications applied to the skin and mucous membranes generally have local effects. You apply topical medications to the skin by painting or spreading the medication over an area, applying moist dressings, soaking body parts in a solution, or giving

TABLE 31.5 Factors Influencing Choice of Administration Routes

Advantages By Route	Disadvantages/Contraindications
Oral, Buccal, Sublingual Routes Convenient and comfortable Economical Easy to administer Often produce local or systemic effects Rarely cause anxiety for patient	Oral route is avoided when patient has alterations in gastrointestinal (GI) function (e.g., nausea, vomiting), reduced GI motility (after general anesthesia or bowel inflammation), and surgical resection of the GI tract. Oral administration is contraindicated in patients unable to swallow (e.g., patients with neuromuscular disorders, esophageal strictures, mouth lesions). Oral administration is contraindicated in patients who are unconscious, confused, or unable or unwilling to swallow or hold medication under tongue. Oral medications cannot be administered when patients have gastric suction; are contraindicated before some tests or surgery. Oral medications sometimes irritate lining of GI tract, discolor teeth, or have unpleasant taste. Gastric secretions destroy some medications.
Parenteral Routes (Subcutaneous, Intramuscular, Intravenous, Intradermal) Can be used when oral medications are contraindicated More rapid absorption than with topical or oral routes Intravenous (IV) infusion provides medication delivery when patient is critically ill or long-term therapy is necessary; if peripheral perfusion is poor, IV route preferred over injections	There is risk of introducing infection. Some medications are expensive. Some patients experience pain from repeated needlesticks. Subcutaneous, intramuscular (IM), and intradermal (ID) routes are avoided in patients with bleeding tendencies. There is risk of tissue damage. IM and IV routes have higher absorption rates, thus placing patient at higher risk for reactions. They often cause considerable anxiety in many patients, especially children.
Topical Routes ***Skin*** Primarily provides local effect Painless Limited side effects	Patients with skin abrasions are at risk for rapid medication absorption and systemic effects. Medications are absorbed through skin slowly.
Transdermal Prolonged systemic effects with limited side effects	Medication leaves oily or pasty substance on skin and sometimes soils clothing.
***Mucous Membranes*[a]** Therapeutic effects provided by local application to involved sites Aqueous solutions readily absorbed and capable of causing systemic effects Potential route of administration when oral medications are contraindicated	Mucous membranes are highly sensitive to some medication concentrations. Patients with ruptured eardrum cannot receive ear irrigations. Insertion of rectal and vaginal medication often causes embarrassment. Rectal suppositories contraindicated if patient has had rectal surgery or if active rectal bleeding is present.
Other Routes ***Inhalation*** Provides rapid relief for local respiratory problems Used for introduction of general anesthetic gases	Some local agents cause serious systemic effects.
Intraocular Disk Route advantageous because it does not require frequent administration as eyedrops do	Local reactions possible; expensive Patients must be taught to insert and remove disk Contraindicated in eye infections

[a]Includes eyes, ears, nose, vagina, rectum, and ostomy.

medicated baths. Systemic effects often occur if a patient's skin is thin or broken down, the medication concentration is high, or contact with the skin is prolonged. A **transdermal disk** or patch (e.g., nitroglycerin, scopolamine, and estrogens) has systemic effects. The disk secures the medicated ointment to the skin. These topical applications are left in place for as little as 12 hours or up to 7 days.

You apply topical medications to mucous membranes in the following ways:
1. Direct application of a liquid or ointment (e.g., eyedrops, gargling, or swabbing the throat)
2. Insertion of a medication into a body cavity (e.g., placing a suppository in rectum or vagina or inserting medicated packing into vagina)

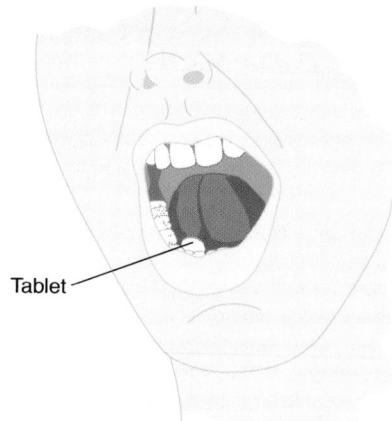

FIG. 31.3 Sublingual administration of a tablet.

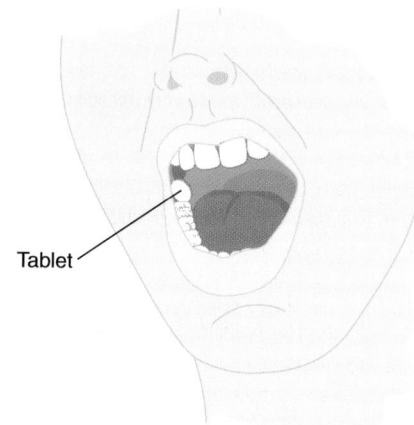

FIG. 31.4 Buccal administration of a tablet.

3. Instillation of fluid into a body cavity (e.g., eardrops, nose drops, or bladder and rectal instillation [fluid is retained])
4. Irrigation of a body cavity (e.g., flushing eye, ear, vagina, bladder, or rectum with medicated fluid [fluid is not retained])
5. Spraying a medication into a body cavity (e.g., instillation into nose and throat)

Inhalation Route. The deeper passages of the respiratory tract provide a large surface area for medication absorption. Nurses administer inhaled medications through the nasal and oral passages or endotracheal or tracheostomy tubes. Endotracheal tubes enter the patient's mouth and end in the trachea, whereas tracheostomy tubes enter the trachea directly through an incision made in the neck. Inhaled medications are readily absorbed and work rapidly because of the rich vascular alveolar capillary network present in the pulmonary tissue. Many inhaled medications have local or systemic effects.

Intraocular Route. Intraocular medication delivery involves inserting a medication similar to a contact lens into a patient's eye. The eye medication disk has two soft outer layers that have medication enclosed in them. The nurse inserts the disk into the patient's eye, much like a contact lens. The medication remains in the eye for up to 1 week.

Systems of Medication Measurement

Safely administering medications requires the ability to compute medication doses accurately and measure medications correctly. A careless mistake in placing a decimal point or adding a zero to a dose can lead to a fatal error. Check every dose carefully before giving a medication.

The health care industry in the United States uses primarily the metric system of measurement for medication therapy. Globally most nations use the metric system as their standard of measurement. However, the household system may still be used in medication orders when health care providers write prescriptions, or orders for medications, that are to be administered at home by patients in household measures. The ISMP (2011b) recommends that a household measure can be listed in parentheses in an order immediately following the metric measure, such as 5 mL (1 teaspoonful). Health care providers rarely use the apothecary system, a measurement system that includes ounces, pounds, and pints.

Metric System. As a decimal system, the metric system is the most logically organized. You convert and compute metric units using simple multiplication and division. Each basic unit of measurement is organized into units of 10. Multiplying or dividing by 10 forms secondary units. In multiplication the decimal point moves to the right; in division the decimal moves to the left. For example:

$$10 \, \text{mg} \times 10 = 100 \, \text{mg}$$

$$10 \, \text{mg} \div 10 = 1 \, \text{mg}$$

The basic units of measurement in the metric system are the meter (length), the liter (volume), and the gram (weight). For medication calculations only use the volume and weight units. The metric system uses lowercase or capital letters or a combination of lowercase and capital letters to designate basic units:

Gram = g or GM
Liter = l or L
Milligram = mg
Milliliter = mL

A system of Latin prefixes designates subdivision of the basic units: *deci-* (1/10 or 0.1), *centi-* (1/100 or 0.01), and *milli-* (1/1000 or 0.001). Greek prefixes designate multiples of the basic units: *deka-* (10), *hecto-* (100), and *kilo-* (1000). When writing medication doses in metric units, health care providers and nurses use fractions or multiples of a unit. Convert fractions to decimals.

$$500 \, \text{mg or } 0.5 \, \text{g}, \textit{not } \tfrac{1}{2} \, \text{g}$$

$$10 \, \text{mL or } 0.01 \, \text{L}, \textit{not } 1/100 \, \text{L}$$

Many actual and potential medication errors happen with the use of fractions and decimal points. Follow practice standards when medications are ordered in fractions to prevent these errors. For example, to make the decimal point more visible, a leading zero is *always* placed in front of a decimal (e.g., use 0.25, *not* .25). *Never* use a trailing zero (i.e., a zero after a decimal point) because if a health care worker does not see the decimal point, the patient may receive 10 times more medication than that prescribed (e.g., use 5, *not* 5.0) (ISMP, 2017a).

Household Measurements. Most people are familiar with household measures, which include liquid measures such as drops, teaspoons, tablespoons, cups, pints, and quarts. Even though household measurements are convenient and familiar, they are inaccurate. Dose errors have occurred when household measures are used (ISMP, 2018a, Consumer Med Safety, 2018a). As a result, the ISMP recommends a best practice for all oral liquids that are not commercially available as unit-dose products. The liquids should be dispensed by the pharmacy in an oral syringe using metric measurement (ISMP, 2018a). The ISMP also recommends that patients or family caregivers purchase oral liquid dosing devices (oral syringes/cups/droppers) that display only the metric scale. Encourage patients to never use household measuring

TABLE 31.6 Equivalents of Measurement

Metric	Household
1 mL	15 drops (gtt)
5 mL	1 teaspoon (tsp)
15 mL	1 tablespoon (tbsp)
30 mL	2 tablespoons (tbsp)
240 mL	1 cup (c)
480 mL (approximately 500 mL)	1 pint (pt)
960 mL (approximately 1 L)	1 quart (qt)
3785 mL (approximately 4 L)	1 gallon (gal)

devices with liquid medications (Table 31.6). Today's over-the-counter (OTC) liquid medications almost always have their own measuring devices (Consumer Med Safety, 2018a).

Solutions. Nurses use solutions of various concentrations for injections, *irrigations*, and infusions. A *solution* is a given mass of solid substance dissolved in a known volume of fluid or a given volume of liquid dissolved in a known volume of another fluid. When a solid is dissolved in a fluid, the concentration is in units of mass per units of volume (e.g., g/L, mg/mL). You can also express a concentration of a solution as a percentage. For example, a 10% solution is 10 g of solid dissolved in 100 mL of solution. A proportion also expresses concentrations. A $^1/_{1000}$ solution represents a solution containing 1 g of solid in 1000 mL of liquid or 1 mL of liquid mixed with 1000 mL of another liquid.

REFLECT NOW

You are teaching a family caregiver of a 5-year-old about administering an oral antibiotic after discharge. What are some important concepts to teach the family caregiver about administering oral medications to children in the home?

NURSING KNOWLEDGE BASE

In 1999 the Institute of Medicine (IOM) published the book *To Err Is Human: Building a Safer Health System*. This book created national awareness about the effect of medical errors within the health care system. Recently, researchers from Johns Hopkins estimated that more than 250,000 Americans die each year from medical errors (Makary and Daniel, 2016). According to the CDC (2016) more people die from medical errors (e.g., surgical complications, health care–acquired infections, and medication errors) than from chronic lower respiratory diseases, accidents, stroke, Alzheimer's disease, and diabetes mellitus.

Nurses play an important role in patient safety, especially in the area of medication administration. The safe administration of medications is also an important topic for current nursing researchers (Box 31.2). As a nurse you need to know how to calculate medication doses accurately and understand the different roles that members of the health care team play in prescribing and administering medications. Apply your knowledge and think critically to ensure safe medication administration.

Clinical Calculations

To administer medications safely, you need to understand basic mathematics skills to calculate medication doses, mix solutions,

BOX 31.2 EVIDENCE-BASED PRACTICE
Reducing Errors During Medication Administration

PICOT Question: In health care agencies does the use of computerized prescription order entry (CPOE), automated medication dispensers (AMDs), and bar-code medication administration (BCMA) during medication administration decrease the incidence of medication errors made by nurses when compared with nurses who do not use these health technologies?

Evidence Summary

Adverse medication effects account for about 19% of adverse effects patients experience in health care agencies. They can occur before admission, during the stay, or after discharge. A multisystem approach, including the provider, nurse, and health care system, should be used to prevent medication errors (Zhu and Weingart, 2018).

Application to Nursing Practice

- Everyone administering medications should review the medication list at each patient encounter.
- Be vigilant when handling and administering high-risk medications.
- Consider medications as the cause of any new symptoms.
- Use computerized physician order entry (CPOE) when possible to
  - Standardize practice.
  - Improve legibility of orders.
  - Alert and update health care providers on side effects, drug-drug interactions, and new orders (Rochon, 2019; Zhu and Weingart, 2018).
- Use an electronic medical record when possible and interface this with CPOE if available to improve communication and alert all providers to administration times (Rochon, 2019; Zhu and Weingart, 2018).
- Bar-coding medications linked to patient identification bracelets improves safety and provides one last opportunity to identify a medication error (Fanning et al, 2016; Zhu and Weingart, 2018).
- Use smart pumps to administer intravenous medications.
- Medication reconciliation identifies medication discrepancies and prevents errors.
- Patient, family caregiver, and provider education can be used to prevent medication errors.

and perform a variety of other activities. This is important because medications are not always dispensed in the unit of measure in which they are ordered. Medication companies package and bottle medications in standard dosages. For example, a patient's health care provider orders 20 mg of a medication that is available only in 40-mg vials. Nurses frequently convert available units of volume and weight to desired doses. You use equivalents when performing other nursing actions such as when calculating patients' intake and output and IV flow rates. You are responsible for converting available units of volume and weight to the desired doses. Know the approximate equivalents in all major measurement systems.

Conversions Within One System. Converting measurements within one system is relatively easy; simply divide or multiply in the metric system. To change milligrams to grams, divide by 1000, moving the decimal 3 points to the left.

$$1000\ mg = 1\ g$$

$$350\ mg = 0.35\ g$$

To convert liters to milliliters, multiply by 1000 or move the decimal 3 points to the right.

$$1 \text{ L} = 1000 \text{ mL}$$

$$0.25 \text{ L} = 250 \text{ mL}$$

To convert units of measurement within the household system, consult an equivalence table. For example, when converting fluid ounces to quarts, you first need to know that 32 ounces is the equivalent of 1 quart. To convert 8 ounces to a quart measurement, divide 8 by 32 to get the equivalent, ¼ or 0.25 quart.

Conversion Between Systems. The conversion between systems is becoming less common because of the ISMP (2018a) recommendations for use of the metric system for liquid medication dosing. Even though health care providers are encouraged to order using the metric system, you may encounter a situation when you calculate the correct dose of a medication by converting weights or volumes from one system of measurement to another. For example, metric units are sometimes converted to equivalent household measures for medication administration at home. To convert from one measurement system to another, always use equivalent measurements. Tables of equivalent measurements are available in all health care agencies. The pharmacist is also a good resource.

The liquids should be dispensed by the pharmacy in an oral syringe using metric measurement (ISMP, 2018a). The ISMP (2018a) also recommends that patients or family caregivers purchase oral liquid dosing devices (oral syringes/cups/droppers) that display only the metric scale. Encourage patients to never use household measuring devices with liquid medications (Table 31.6). Today's over-the-counter (OTC) liquid medications almost always have their own measuring devices (Consumer Med Safety, 2018a).

Dose Calculations. Dosage calculation methods include the ratio and proportion method, the formula method, and dimensional analysis. Use the method that is the most logical and comfortable for you. Use this same method consistently. Before you begin any calculation, make a mental estimate of the approximate and reasonable dosage. If your estimate does not closely match the answer you calculate, you need to recheck your math before preparing and administering the medication. Many nursing students feel uncomfortable or anxious when they have to do medication calculations. To enhance accuracy and decrease your anxiety, think critically about the steps you go through in calculating medications, and practice doing calculations to feel more confident about your math skills.

Most health care agencies require a nurse to double-check calculations with another nurse before giving medications, especially when the risk for giving the wrong medication dose is high (e.g., heparin or insulin). Always have another nurse or health care professional double-check your work if the answer to a medication calculation seems unreasonable or inappropriate.

The Ratio and Proportion Method. A ratio indicates the relationship between two numbers separated by a colon (:). The colon in the ratio indicates the need to use division. Think of a ratio as a fraction; the number to the left is the numerator, and the number to the right is the denominator. For example, the ratio 1:2 is the same as 1/2. A proportion is an equation that has two ratios of equal value. Write a proportion in one of three ways:

Example 1 1:2 = 4:8
Example 2 1:2::4:8
Example 3 1/2 = 4/8

In a proportion the first and last numbers are called the *extremes,* and the second and third numbers are called the *means.* When multiplying the extremes, the answer is the same as when multiplying the means. For example, in the previous proportions, multiplying the extremes ($1 \times 8 = 8$) yields the same result as multiplying the means ($2 \times 4 = 8$). Because of this relationship, if you know three of the numbers in the proportion, calculating the unknown fourth number is easy. The numbers need to all be in the same unit and system of measurement. To solve a calculation using the ratio and proportion method, first estimate the answer in your mind. Then set up the proportion, labeling all the terms. Put the terms of the ratio in the same sequence (e.g., mg : mL = mg : mL). Cross-multiply the means and the extremes and divide both sides by the number before the *x* to obtain the dosage. *Always* label the answer; if the answer is not close to the estimate, recheck the calculation.

Example: The health care provider orders 500 mg of amoxicillin to be administered in a gastric tube every 8 hours. The bottle of amoxicillin is labeled 400 mg/5 mL. Use the following steps to calculate how much amoxicillin to give:

1. **Estimate the answer:** The amount to be given is a little more than the labeled dose per 5 mL (unit dose) that is provided in the solution; therefore, the answer is a little more than 5 mL.
2. **Set up the proportion:**

$$\frac{400 \text{ mg}}{5 \text{ mL}} = \frac{500 \text{ mg}}{x \text{ mL}}$$

3. **Cross-multiply the means and the extremes:**

$$400x = 500 \times 5$$
$$400x = 2500$$

4. **Divide both sides by the number before x:**

$$\frac{400x}{400} = \frac{2500}{400}$$
$$x = \frac{2500}{400}$$
$$x = 6.25 \text{ mL}$$

5. **Compare the estimate in Step 1 with the answer in Step 4:** The answer (6.25 mL) is close to the estimated amount (a little more than 5 mL). Therefore, the answer is correct; prepare and administer 6.25 mL in the patient's gastric tube.

The Formula Method. Using this method requires you to first memorize the formula. Estimate the answer and then place all the information from the medication order into the formula. Label all the parts of the formula and ensure that all measures in the formula are in the same units and system of measurement before calculating the dosage. If the measures are not in the same measurement system, convert the numbers to the same system before calculating the dose. Calculate and label the answer and compare the answer with the estimated answer. If the estimate is not similar to the answer, recheck the calculation. Use the following basic formula when using the formula method:

$$\frac{\text{Dose ordered}}{\text{Dose on hand}} \times \text{Amount on hand} = \text{Amount to administer}$$

The dose ordered is the amount of medication prescribed. The dose on hand is the dose (e.g., mg, units) of medication supplied by the pharmacy. The amount on hand is the basic unit or quantity of the medication that contains the dose on hand. For solid medications the amount on hand is often one capsule; the amount of liquid on hand is sometimes 1 mL or 1 L, depending on the container. For example, a liquid medication comes in the strength of 125 mg per 5 mL. In this case 125 mg is the dose on hand, and 5 mL is the amount on hand. The amount to administer is the actual amount of medication the nurse administers. Always express the amount to administer in the same unit as the amount on hand.

Example: The health care provider orders morphine sulfate 2 mg IV. The medication is available in a vial containing 10 mg/mL. The formula is applied as follows:

1. **Estimate the answer:** The medication is a liquid; thus, the answer will be in milliliters (mL). The amount to be given is less than ½ of the dose; thus, the answer will be less than ½ mL.

2. **Set up the formula:**

$$\frac{\text{Dose ordered}}{\text{Dose on hand}} \times \text{Amount on hand} = \text{Amount to administer}$$

$$\frac{2\text{ mg}}{10\text{ mg}} \times 1\text{ mL} = \text{Amount to administer}$$

3. **Calculate the answer:**

$$\frac{2\text{ mg}}{10\text{ mg}} \times 1\text{ mL} = 0.2\text{ mL}$$

4. **Compare the estimate in Step 1 with the answer in Step 3:** The answer is less than ½ mL; thus, it is close to the estimated answer. Prepare 0.2 mL of the medication in a syringe and administer it to the patient.

Dimensional Analysis. Dimensional analysis is the factor-label or the unit-factor method. There is no need to memorize a formula since only one equation is needed and the same steps are used in solving every medication calculation. Nursing students who use dimensional analysis to calculate medication dosages often find it easier to calculate medications than when they use the formula method. Use the following steps to calculate medication doses by dimensional analysis:

1. Identify the unit of measure that you need to administer. For example, if you are giving a pill, you usually give a tablet or a capsule; for parenteral or liquid oral medications, the unit is milliliters.

2. Estimate the answer.

3. Place the name or appropriate abbreviation for x on the left side of the equation (e.g., x tab, x mL).

4. Place available information from the problem in a fraction format on the right side of the equation. Place the abbreviation or unit that matches what you are going to administer (determined in Step 1) in the numerator.

5. Look at the medication order and add other factors into the problem. Set up the numerator so it matches the unit in the previous denominator.

6. Cancel out like units of measurement on the right side of the equation. You should end up with only one unit left in the equation, and it should match the unit on the left side of the equation.

7. Reduce to the lowest terms if possible and solve the problem or solve for x. Label your answer.

8. Compare your estimate from Step 1 with your answer in Step 2.

Example: The health care provider orders 0.45 g penicillin V potassium through a gastric tube. The vial label reads: penicillin V potassium 125 mg/5 mL.

1. **Identify the unit of measure that you need to administer.** This medication is given in a gastric tube, which is a liquid medication; therefore, the answer will be in milliliters (mL).

2. **Estimate the answer.** The medication order is more than 3 times but less than 4 times the unit dose in the vial; thus, the answer is more than 15 mL but less than 20 mL.

3. **Place the name or appropriate abbreviation for x on the left side of the equation.**

$$x\text{ mL} =$$

4. **Place available information from the problem in a fraction format on the right side of the equation.** Since the medication will be administered in milliliters, place mL in the numerator.

$$x\text{ mL} = \frac{5\text{ mL}}{125\text{ mg}}$$

5. **Look at the medication order and add other factors into the problem.** Set up the numerator so it matches the unit in the previous denominator. The order is for 0.45 g, and the medication is available in 125-mg bottles. Knowing that 1 g = 1000 mg, add this conversion to the calculation.

$$x\text{ mL} = \frac{5\text{ mL}}{125\text{ mg}} \times \frac{1000\text{ mg}}{1\text{ g}} \times \frac{0.45\text{ g}}{1}$$

6. **Cancel out like units of measurement on the right side of the equation.**

$$x\text{ mL} = \frac{5\text{ mL}}{125\text{ \sout{mg}}} \times \frac{1000\text{ \sout{mg}}}{1\text{ \sout{g}}} \times \frac{0.45\text{ \sout{g}}}{1}$$

7. **Reduce to the lowest terms if possible and solve the problem or solve for x.** Label your answer.

$$x\text{ mL} = \frac{5 \times 1000 \times 0.45}{125}$$
$$x = \frac{2250}{125}$$
$$x = 18\text{ mL}$$

8. **Compare the estimate from Step 2 with the answer in Step 7.** The calculated answer is 18 mL, which is between 15 mL and 20 mL. This matches the estimate made in Step 2. Prepare and administer 18 mL of medication as ordered.

Pediatric Doses. Current evidence shows that children are at a much higher risk for experiencing a medication error than adults, and medication errors in children have a much greater chance of causing serious and even fatal consequences. To prevent medication errors in children (Beal, 2017):

- Use only the metric system on prescriptions, medication labels, and dosing instruments.
- Never administer medications using household spoons.
- Round all dosing instructions to the nearest 0.1, 0.5, or 1 mL.
- Provide education using hands-on demonstration and return demonstration.
- Consider using picture-based education if low health literacy is a possibility.

Calculating children's medication doses requires caution (Hockenberry et al., 2019). Even small errors or discrepancies in medication amounts can affect a child's health negatively. A child's age, weight, and maturity of body systems affect the ability to metabolize and excrete medications. Nurses sometimes have difficulty in evaluating a child's response to a medication, especially when he or she cannot communicate verbally. For example, a side effect of vancomycin is ototoxicity. If a child cannot talk yet, it is challenging to assess for ototoxicity. Use the following guidelines when calculating pediatric doses:

1. Most pediatric medications are ordered in milligrams per kilogram (mg/kg). Therefore, weigh the patient in kilograms before administering medications. Avoid converting the patient's weight from pounds to kilograms to prevent errors.

2. Pediatric doses are usually a lot smaller than adult doses for the same medication. You frequently use micrograms and small syringes (e.g., tuberculin or 1 mL).

3. IM doses are very small and usually do not exceed 1 mL in small children or 0.5 mL in infants.

4. Subcutaneous dosages are also very small and do not usually exceed 0.5 mL.

5. Most medications are not rounded off to the nearest tenth. Instead they are rounded to the nearest thousandth.

6. Measure dosages that are less than 1 mL in syringes that are marked in tenths of a milliliter if the dosage calculation comes out even and does not need to be rounded. Use a tuberculin syringe for medication preparation when the medication needs to be rounded to the nearest thousandth.

7. Estimate the patient's dose before beginning the calculation; label and compare the answer with the estimate before preparing the medication.

8. To determine if a dose is safe before giving the medication, compare and evaluate the amount of medication ordered over 24 hours with the recommended dosage.

Different formulas and methods are used to calculate medication dosages in children. The two most common methods of calculating pediatric dosages are based on a child's weight or BSA. BSA is used in rare situations (e.g., determining chemotherapy doses). Refer to a pediatric or pharmacology resource and consult with the patient's health care provider or the pharmacist if you must calculate a medication based on BSA.

Most of the time you calculate medications based on a child's weight. You can use the ratio and proportion method, the formula method, or dimensional analysis to calculate a pediatric dose using body weight. Refer to the previous sections on ratio and proportion, formula method, and dimensional analysis to select the method easiest for you to use.

Health Care Provider's Role

A physician, nurse practitioner, or physician's assistant prescribes medications by writing an order on a form in a patient's medical record, in an order book, or on a legal prescription pad. Some health care providers use a desktop, laptop, or handheld electronic device to enter medication orders. Many health care agencies implement computerized physician order entry (CPOE) to handle medication orders to decrease medication errors (Zhu and Weingart, 2018). In these systems the health care provider completes all computerized fields before the order for the medication is filled, thus avoiding incomplete or illegible orders.

Sometimes a health care provider orders a medication by telephone or by talking to a nurse in person. An order for a medication or medical treatment made over the telephone is called a *telephone order*. If the order is given verbally to the nurse, it is called a verbal order. When a verbal or telephone order is received, the nurse who took the order writes the complete order or enters it into a computer, reads it back, and receives confirmation from the health care provider to confirm accuracy. The nurse indicates the time and the name of the health care provider who gave the order, signs it, and follows agency policy to indicate that it was read back. The health care provider countersigns the order later, usually within 24 hours after giving it. Follow guidelines for taking telephone or verbal orders for medications safely (Box 31.3). Agency policies vary regarding personnel who can take telephone or verbal orders. Nursing students cannot take medication orders of any kind. They give newly ordered medications only after a registered nurse has written and verified the order.

Common abbreviations are often used when writing orders. Abbreviations indicate dosage frequencies or times, routes of administration, and special information for giving the medication (see Table 31.3). Medication errors frequently involve the use of abbreviations. Table 31.7 lists abbreviations that are associated with a high incidence of medication errors. Do *not* use these abbreviations when documenting medication orders or other information about medications (ISMP,

2017a; TJC, 2017). Sometimes abbreviations used by different agencies vary. Check agency policy to determine which abbreviations are acceptable to use and their meaning.

BOX 31.3 **Guidelines for Telephone and Verbal Orders**

- Only authorized staff receive and record telephone or verbal orders. The health care agency identifies in writing the staff who are authorized.
- Clearly identify patient's name, room number, and diagnosis.
- Read back all orders to health care provider (TJC, 2020).
- Use clarification questions to avoid misunderstandings.
- Write "TO" (telephone order) or "VO" (verbal order), including date and time, name of patient, and complete order; sign the name of the health care provider and nurse.
- Follow agency policies; some agencies require documentation of the "read-back" or require two nurses to review and sign telephone or verbal orders.
- The health care provider co-signs the order within the time frame required by the agency (usually 24 hours; verify agency policy).

QSEN **Building Competency in Safety** The health care provider has written the following orders for a 4-year-old patient with otitis media of the right ear. Which orders do you need to clarify before administering the medication? Provide a rationale for your answers, and rewrite the order so that it follows the ISMP current medication order safety guidelines.

Floxin otic solution AS twice a day
Amoxicillin 25 mg/kg/day in divided doses
Acetaminophen 1 teaspoon for fever greater than 38.3° C (101° F)

Answers to QSEN Activities can be found on the Evolve website.

Types of Orders in Acute Care Agencies

A medication cannot be given to a patient without a health care provider order. The frequency and urgency of medication administration forms the basis for medication orders. Some conditions change the status of a patient's medication orders. For example, in some agencies a patient's preoperative medications are discontinued automatically, and the health care provider writes new medication orders after surgery (see Chapter 50). Agency policies that surround medication orders vary. Nurses need to be aware of and follow these policies.

Standing Orders or Routine Medication Orders. A standing order is carried out until the health care provider cancels it by another order or a prescribed number of days elapse. Some standing orders indicate a final date or number of treatments or doses. Know your agency policies surrounding the discontinuation of standing orders. The following are examples of standing orders:

Tetracycline 500 mg PO q6h
Decadron 10 mg daily × 5 days

prn Orders. Sometimes the health care provider orders a medication to be given only when a patient requires it. This is a prn order. Use objective and subjective assessment (e.g., severity of pain, body temperature) and discretion in determining whether the patient needs the medication. An example of a prn order is:

Morphine sulfate 2 mg IV q2h prn for incisional pain

This order indicates that the patient needs to wait at least 2 hours between doses and can take the medication if experiencing pain at the incision. When administering prn medications, document assessment findings to show why the patient needs the medication and the time

TABLE 31.7 Prohibited and Error-Prone Abbreviations[a]

The abbreviations, symbols, and dose designations found in this table have been reported to ISMP through the USP-ISMP Medication Error Reporting Program as being frequently misinterpreted and involved in harmful medication errors. They should NEVER be used when communicating medical information. This includes internal communications, telephone/verbal prescriptions, computer-generated labels, labels for medication storage bins, medication administration records, and pharmacy and prescriber computer order entry screens. The Joint Commission (TJC) has established a National Patient Safety Goal that specifies that certain abbreviations must appear on the do-not-use list of the accredited organization; they are highlighted with a superscript "b" ([b]). However, we hope that you will consider others beyond the minimum TJC requirements. By using and promoting safe practices and educating one another about hazards, we can better protect our patients.

Abbreviations	Intended Meaning	Misinterpretation	Correction
µg	Microgram	Mistaken as "mg"	Use "mcg"
AD, AS, AU	Right ear, left ear, each ear	Mistaken as OD, OS, OU (right eye, left eye, each eye)	Use "right ear," "left ear," or "each ear"
OD, OS, OU	Right eye, left eye, each eye	Mistaken as AD, AS, AU (right ear, left ear, each ear)	Use "right eye," "left eye," or "each eye"
BT	Bedtime	Mistaken as "BID" (twice daily)	Use "bedtime"
HS	Half-strength	Mistaken as bedtime	Use "half-strength" or "bedtime"
hs	At bedtime, hours of sleep	Mistaken as half-strength	Use "bedtime" or "half-strength"
IU[b]	International unit	Mistaken as IV (intravenous) or 10 (ten)	Use "units"
o.d. or OD	Once daily	Mistaken as "right eye" (OD—oculus dexter), leading to oral liquid medications administered in the eye	Use "daily"
Per os	By mouth, orally	The "os" can be mistaken as "left eye" (OS—oculus sinister)	Use "PO," "by mouth," or "orally"
q.d. or QD[b]	Every day	Mistaken as q.i.d., especially if the period after the "q" or the tail of the "q" is misunderstood as an "I"	Use "daily"
qhs	Nightly at bedtime	Mistaken as "qhr" or every hour	Use "nightly"
SC, SQ, sub q	Subcutaneous	SC mistaken as SL (sublingual); SQ mistaken as "5 every"; the "q" in "sub q" has been mistaken as "every" (e.g., a heparin dose ordered "sub q 2 hours before surgery" misunderstood as every 2 hours before surgery)	Use "subcut" or "subcutaneously"
TIW or tiw	3 times a week	Mistaken as "3 times a day" or "twice in a week"	Use "3 times weekly"
U or u[b]	Unit	Mistaken as the number 0 or 4, causing a 10-fold overdose or greater (e.g., 4 U seen as "40" or 4 u seen as "44"); mistaken as "cc" so dose given in volume instead of units (e.g., 4 u seen as 4 cc)	Use "unit"

Dose Designations and Other Information	Intended Meaning	Misinterpretation	Correction
Trailing zero after decimal point (e.g., 1.0 mg)[c]	1 mg	Mistaken as 10 mg if the decimal point is not seen	Do not use trailing zeros for doses expressed in whole numbers
"Naked" decimal point (e.g., .5 mg)[b]	0.5 mg	Mistaken as 5 mg if the decimal point is not seen	Use zero before a decimal point when the dose is less than a whole unit
Abbreviations such as mg. or mL. with a period following the abbreviation	mg mL	The period is unnecessary and could be mistaken as the number 1 if written poorly	Use mg, mL, etc. without a terminal period

Drug Name Abbreviations	Intended Meaning	Misinterpretation	Correction
HCl	hydrochloric acid or hydrochloride	Mistaken as potassium chloride (The "H" is misinterpreted as "K")	Use complete drug name unless expressed as a salt of a drug
HCT	hydrocortisone	Mistaken as hydrochlorothiazide	Use complete drug name
HCTZ	hydrochlorothiazide	Mistaken as hydrocortisone (seen as HCT250 mg)	Use complete drug name
MgSO4[b]	magnesium sulfate	Mistaken as morphine sulphate	Use complete drug name
MS, MSO4[b]	morphine sulfate	Mistaken as magnesium sulphate	Use complete drug name
PCA	procainamide	Mistaken as patient-controlled analgesia	Use complete drug name

Stemmed Drug Names	Intended Meaning	Misinterpretation	Correction
"Nitro" drip	nitroglycerin infusion	Mistaken as sodium nitroprusside infusion	Use complete drug name

Continued

TABLE 31.7   Prohibited and Error-Prone Abbreviations[a]—cont'd

Symbols	Intended Meaning	Misinterpretation	Correction
ʒ	Dram	Symbol for dram mistaken as "3"	Use metric system
×3d	For three days	Mistaken as "3 doses"	Use "for three days"
> and <	Greater than and less than	Mistaken as opposite of intended; mistakenly use incorrect symbol; "<10" mistaken as "40"	Use "greater than" or "less than"
@	At	Mistaken as "2"	Use "at"
&	And	Mistaken as "2"	Use "and"
+	Plus or and	Mistaken as "4"	Use "and"
°	Hour	Mistaken as a zero (e.g., q2° seen as q20)	Use "hr," "h," or "hour"

[a]Applies to all orders and medication-related documentation that is handwritten (including free-text computer entry or on preprinted forms).
[b]These abbreviations are included on The Joint Commission "minimum list" of dangerous abbreviations, acronyms, and symbols that must be included on the "Do Not Use" list of an organization.
[c]Exception: A "trailing zero" may be used only where required to show precision of a reported value (e.g., laboratory test results), in studies that report the size of lesions, or for catheter and tube sizes. A "trailing zero" cannot be used in medication orders or medication-related documentation (ISMP, 2017a).
From The Joint Commission (TJC): *Facts about the Official "Do Not Use" List of Abbreviations*, 2017, https://www.jointcommission.org/facts_about_do_not_use_list/. Accessed May 6, 2018. Reprinted with permission.

of administration. Frequently evaluate the effectiveness of the medication and record evaluation data appropriately. Unclear orders for prn medications that include a range (e.g., morphine sulfate IM 5-10 mg every 4-6 hours) are a source of medication errors. If a range order is written, ensure that the order follows agency policy for these types of orders. An example of a safer range order is to increase morphine dosage 50% to 100% if pain is moderate to severe based on use of the agency pain scale.

When multiple prn medications with the same action are ordered, the orders need to identify when to use each medication and how to use the medications in relationship to each other. The order below provides an example of a safe prn order for two medications used for treatment of constipation:

Docusate 100 mg PO TID prn constipation for two days and if no results then administer magnesium hydroxide 30 mL PO prn constipation

Single (One-Time) Orders. Sometimes a health care provider orders a medication to be given once at a specified time. This is common for preoperative medications or medications given before diagnostic examinations. The following is an example of a single order:

Ativan 1 mg IV on call to MRI

STAT Orders. A STAT order signifies that a single dose of a medication is to be given immediately and only once. STAT orders are often written for emergencies when a patient's condition changes suddenly. For example:

Apresoline 10 mg IV STAT

Now Orders. A now order is more specific than a 1-time order and is used when a patient needs a medication quickly but not right away, as in a STAT order. When receiving a now order, the nurse has up to 90 minutes to administer the medication. Only administer now medications 1 time. For example:

Vancomycin 1 g IV piggyback now

Prescriptions. The health care provider writes prescriptions for patients who are to take medications outside the hospital. The prescription includes more detailed information than a medication order because the patient needs to understand how to take the medication and when to refill the prescription if necessary. Some agencies require health care providers to write prescriptions for controlled substances on a special prescription pad that is different (e.g., a different color) than the prescription pad used for other medications. Fig. 31.5 illustrates the parts of a prescription.

Pharmacist's Role

The pharmacist prepares and distributes prescribed medications. Pharmacists work with nurses, physicians, and other health care providers to evaluate the effectiveness of patients' medications. They are responsible for filling prescriptions accurately and being sure that prescriptions are valid. Pharmacists in health care agencies rarely mix compounds or solutions, except in the case of IV solutions. Most medication companies deliver medications in a form ready for use. Dispensing the correct medication, in the proper dosage and amount, with an accurate label is the pharmacist's main task. Pharmacists also provide information about medication side effects, toxicity, interactions, and incompatibilities.

Distribution Systems

Systems for storing and distributing medications vary. Health care agencies have a special area for stocking and dispensing medications. Examples of storage areas include special medication rooms, portable locked carts, computerized medication cabinets, and individual storage units next to patients' rooms. Medication storage areas need to be locked when unattended.

Unit Dose. A unit-dose system is a storage system that varies by health care agency. Pharmacists provide the medications in single-unit packages that contain the ordered dose of medication that a patient receives at one time. Nurses distribute the medications to patients. Each tablet or capsule is wrapped separately. Usually no more than a 24-hour supply of medication is available at any given time. Some unit-dose systems use carts containing a drawer with a 24-hour supply of medications for each patient. Each drawer is labeled with the name of the patient in his or her designated room. At a designated time, each day the pharmacist or a pharmacy technician refills the drawers in the cart with a fresh medication supply. The cart also contains limited amounts of prn and

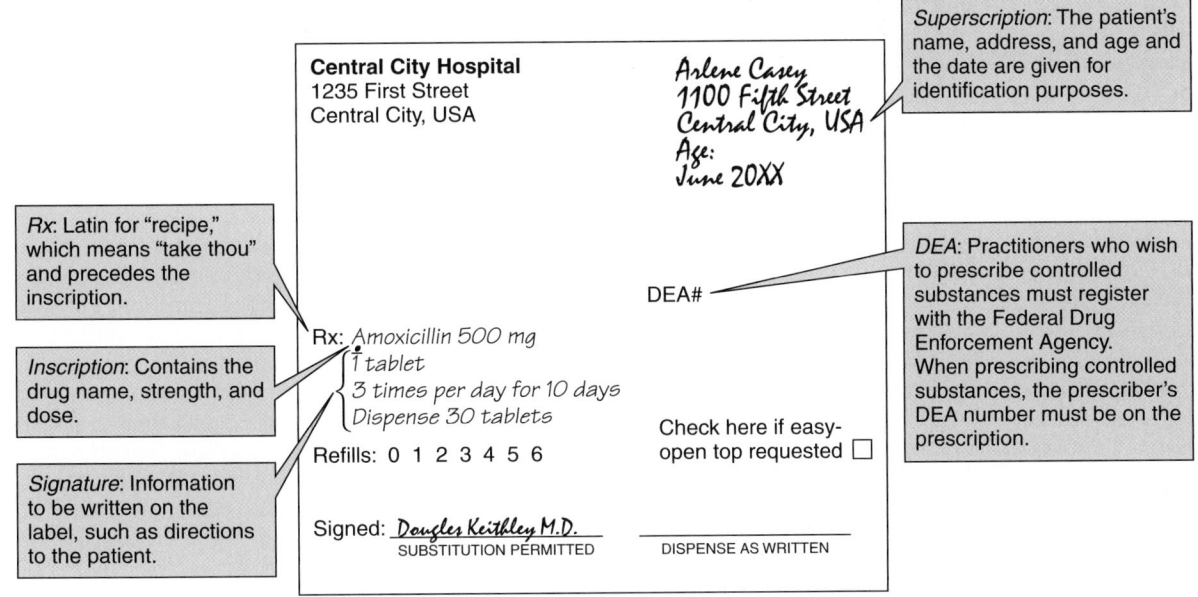

Superscription: The patient's name, address, and age and the date are given for identification purposes.

Central City Hospital
1235 First Street
Central City, USA

Arlene Casey
1100 Fifth Street
Central City, USA
Age:
June 20XX

Rx: Latin for "recipe," which means "take thou" and precedes the inscription.

Inscription: Contains the drug name, strength, and dose.

Signature: Information to be written on the label, such as directions to the patient.

Rx: *Amoxicillin 500 mg*
1 tablet
3 times per day for 10 days
Dispense 30 tablets

Refills: 0 1 2 3 4 5 6

Signed: *Douglas Keithley M.D.*
SUBSTITUTION PERMITTED

DEA#

Check here if easy-open top requested ☐

DISPENSE AS WRITTEN

DEA: Practitioners who wish to prescribe controlled substances must register with the Federal Drug Enforcement Agency. When prescribing controlled substances, the prescriber's DEA number must be on the prescription.

FIG. 31.5 Example of a medication prescription.

stock medications for special situations. Controlled substances are not kept in an individual patient drawer. Instead they are kept in a larger locked drawer to keep them secure. The unit-dose system reduces medication errors, decreases the amount of medication that is stocked in patient care areas, and saves time for nurses and pharmacists.

Automated Medication Dispensing Systems. Automated medication dispensing systems (AMDSs) are used throughout the country (Fig. 31.6). The systems within an agency are networked with one another and with other agency computer systems (e.g., computerized medical record). AMDSs control the dispensing of all medications, including narcotics. Each nurse accesses the system by entering a security code. Some systems require bio-identification as well. In these systems you place your finger on a screen to access the computer. You select the patient's name and his or her medication profile before the AMDS dispenses a medication. In these systems you can select the desired medication, dosage, and route from a list displayed on the computer screen. The system causes the drawer containing medication to open, records it, and charges it to the patient. Systems that are connected to the patient's computerized medical record then record information about the medication (e.g., medication name, dose, time) and the nurse's name in the patient's medical record. The bar-code medication administration (BCMA) system is often used with AMDSs. BCMA requires nurses to scan bar codes to identify the patient, the medication, and an identification tag of the nurse administering the medication before recording this information in the patient's computerized medical record. Agencies that implement AMDS with BCMA often reduce the incidence of medication errors (see Box 31.2).

Nurse's Role

Administering medications requires unique nursing knowledge and skills. You first determine that the medication ordered is the correct medication. As a nurse you need to assess the patient's ability to self-administer medications, determine whether a patient should receive a medication at a given time, administer medications correctly, and then closely monitor their effects. Do not delegate any part of the medication administration process to assistive personnel (AP), and use the nursing process to integrate medication therapy into care.

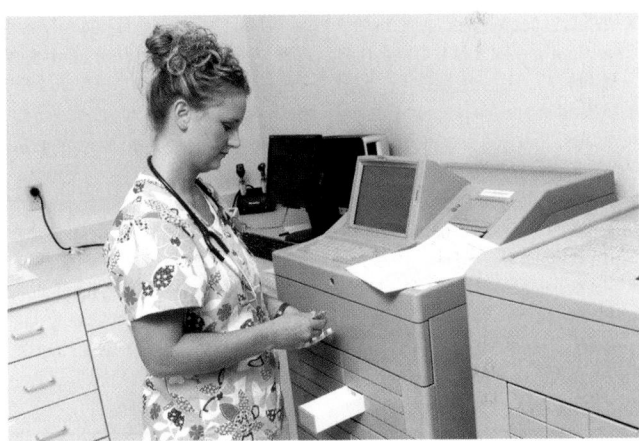

FIG. 31.6 Automated medication dispensing system (AMDS).

Patient and family caregiver education about proper medication administration and monitoring is an integral part of your role. Begin instruction about medications that the patient will be taking home as soon as possible. This often does not occur until the day of discharge, but if you can obtain this information sooner, the patient will benefit.

Medication Errors

The National Coordinating Council for Medication Error Reporting and Prevention (2018) defines a **medication error** as any preventable event that may cause inappropriate medication use or jeopardize patient safety. Medication errors include inaccurate prescribing, administering the wrong medication, giving the medication using the wrong route or time interval, administering extra doses, and/or failing to administer a medication. Preventing medication errors is essential. The process of administering medications has many steps and involves many members of the health care team. Because nurses play an essential role in preparing and administering medications, they need to be vigilant in preventing errors (Box 31.4). Advances in health care informatics have helped to decrease the occurrence of medication errors (Box 31.5).

Medication errors can be caused by many factors, such as technology work-arounds, the design of medication labels, and medication

BOX 31.4 Steps to Take to Prevent Medication Errors

- Follow the seven rights of medication administration.
- Prepare medications for only one patient at a time.
- Be sure to read labels at least 3 times (comparing MAR with label): (1) when removing medication from storage, (2) before taking to patient's room, and (3) before giving medication.
- Use at least two patient identifiers every time you administer medications (e.g., patient name, birthday, hospital number) whenever administering a medication (TJC, 2020).
- Do not allow any other activity to interrupt administration of medication to a patient (e.g., phone call, pager, discussion with other staff).
- Double check all calculations and other high-risk medication administration processes (e.g., patient-controlled analgesia) and verify with another nurse.
- Do not interpret illegible handwriting; clarify with the health care provider.
- Question unusually large or small doses.
- Document all medications as soon as they are given.
- When you have made or discovered an error, reflect on what went wrong and ask how you could have prevented it. Complete an occurrence report per agency policy.
- Evaluate the context or situation in which a medication error occurred. This helps to determine whether nurses have the necessary resources for safe medication administration.
- When repeated medication errors occur within a work area, identify and analyze the factors that may have caused the errors and take corrective action.
- Attend in-service programs on the medications you commonly administer.
- Ensure that you are well rested when caring for patients. Nurses make more errors when they are tired.
- Involve and educate patients when administering medications. Address patients' concerns about medications before administering them (e.g., concerns about their appearance or side effects).
- Follow established agency policies and procedures when using technology to administer medications (e.g., automated medication dispensing system [AMDS] and bar-code scanning). Medication errors occur when nurses "work around" the technology (e.g., override alerts without thinking about them) (Zhu and Weingart, 2018).

AMDS, Automated medication dispensing system; *MAR,* medication administration record.

BOX 31.5 Informatics and Medication Safety

Many medication errors occur when a nurse incorrectly administers medications at the patient's bedside. The following innovations and advances in technology have helped reduce the number of medication errors in nursing practice.

- Networked computers allow all the patient's health care providers to see a current list of ordered and discontinued medications.
- Internet and intranet access allows nurses and other health care providers to access current information about medications (e.g., indications, desired effects, adverse effects) and specific agency policies that address medication administration (e.g., how fast to administer an intravenous [IV] push medication, how to administer medications through a nasogastric tube).
- In some agencies health care providers use computerized prescription order entry (CPOE), allowing them to enter medication orders directly into a networked computer system or a personal handheld computer (Zhu and Weingart, 2018).
- Automated medication dispensers (AMDs) and electronic medication administration records (eMARs) help with medication reconciliation, administration, and documentation (Fanning et al, 2016; Zhu and Weingart, 2018).
- Bar-coding technology requires nurses to scan the medication, the patient's identification bracelet, and the nurse's identification badge before administering the medication, which helps ensure the seven rights of medication administration.

Application to Nursing Practice
- Actively participate in selecting and evaluating advanced technologies and creating nursing policies and protocols used for medication administration.
- Always follow agency policies when administering medications.
- Implement agency policies when the technology cannot be used (e.g., during down time or power outages).
- Follow manufacturer guidelines for care of electronic equipment, and report problems with technology immediately.

distribution systems. When an error occurs, the patient's safety and well-being are the top priorities. You first assess and examine the patient's condition and notify the health care provider of the incident as soon as possible. Once the patient is stable, report the incident to the appropriate person in the agency (e.g., manager or supervisor). You are responsible for preparing and filing an occurrence or incident report as soon as possible after the error occurs. The report includes patient identification information; the location and time of the incident; an accurate, factual description of what occurred and the actions taken; and your signature. The occurrence report is not a permanent part of the medical record and is not referred to anywhere in a patient's medical record to legally protect the nurse and health care agency (see Chapters 23 and 26). Occurrence reports track incident patterns and indicate the need to implement quality improvement actions.

Report all medication errors that reach the patient, including those that do not cause harm. You also need to report near misses. For example, you are caring for a patient who has a urinary tract infection and is allergic to sulfa medications. The patient's health care provider orders trimethoprim/sulfamethoxazole (TMP/SMZ). You know TMP/SMZ contains sulfa. You contact the health care provider before you administer the medication to obtain an order for a different medication. This type of medication error is a near miss because it did not actually reach the patient. All health care workers, including nurses, need to feel comfortable in reporting an error and not fear repercussions from managers or administrators. Even when a patient suffers no harm from a medication error, the agency can still learn why the mistake occurred and what can be done to avoid similar errors in the future.

Some medication errors happen when patients experience a transition in care such as when a patient is admitted or discharged from a hospital, is transferred from an intensive care unit to a general patient care unit, or sees a new health care provider. During these times the risk of unintended changes in medication orders increases. Thus, reconciling medication information is a key Hospital National Patient Safety Goal (TJC, 2020). During medication reconciliation nurses, pharmacists, and other health care providers compare the medication that a patient is taking currently with what the patient should be taking and any newly ordered medications (Box 31.6). Throughout this process you identify and resolve orders that are duplicated and omitted. You also evaluate the risk for unintended medication interactions. Creating and maintaining an accurate list of all patient medications helps to ensure safe and effective patient care. For example, when you admit a patient who is having a hip replacement to an orthopedic unit, you compare the medications that the patient took at home with those ordered in the hospital. When the patient is discharged to a rehabilitation unit, you communicate the patient's current medications with the nurse who is accepting the patient. The nurse on the rehabilitation unit reconciles the patient's medications when the patient is discharged with

BOX 31.6 Process for Medication Reconciliation

1. **Obtain, Verify, Document:** Obtain a comprehensive and current list of a patient's medications whenever he or she experiences a change in health care setting (e.g., during admission, transfer, discharge). Include all current prescriptions, over-the-counter (OTC) medications, and homeopathic products.

2. **Consider and Compare:** Review what the patient was taking at home or preadmission, and make sure that the list of medications, dosages, and frequencies is accurate. Compare this list to the current ordered medications and treatment plan to ensure accuracy. Include family caregiver in this discussion when appropriate.

3. **Reconcile:** Compare new medication orders with the current list; investigate any discrepancies with the patient's health care provider. Document any changes.

4. **Communicate:** Ensure that all the patient's health care providers have the most updated list of medications. Communicate and verify changes in medications as with the patient.

Data from Zhu J, Weingart S: Prevention of adverse drug events in hospitals, *UpToDate*, 2018, https://www.uptodate.com/contents/prevention-of-adverse-drug-events-in-hospitals. Accessed May 13, 2018.

the home health nurse. Many agencies have computerized or written forms to facilitate the process of medication reconciliation. The process is challenging and takes a lot of time and concentration. Eliminate distractions and go slowly when reconciling patients' medications. Always clarify information when needed and question for accuracy. Accurate medication reconciliation requires consulting with the patient, family caregivers, other clinicians, pharmacists, and other members of the health care team.

CRITICAL THINKING

Knowledge

You use knowledge from many disciplines when administering medications. Your knowledge helps you understand why a medication is prescribed for a patient and how it will alter the patient's physiology to have a therapeutic effect. For example, in physiology you learn that potassium is a major intracellular ion. When patients do not have enough potassium in their body (hypokalemia), they experience signs and symptoms such as muscle fatigue or weakness. In some cases, severe hypokalemia is fatal because of associated cardiac dysrhythmias. Prescribed medications help to restore the patient's potassium level to normal, which relieves the signs and symptoms of hypokalemia. In another example knowledge about child development indicates that children often associate medication administration with a negative experience. Use principles from child development to ensure that the child cooperates with the medication experience.

Patients take a variety of medications, and new medications are constantly approved. As a result, you will not always understand all the medications ordered for a patient. Critical thinkers admit what they do not know and acquire the knowledge needed to safely administer unfamiliar medications. This means that, when you do not know all the medications you need to administer, you will consult a reliable source (e.g., a more expert nurse, pharmacist, the health care provider, or a reference book) *before* administering the medication.

Experience

Nursing students have limited experience with medication administration as it applies to professional practice. Clinical experiences give you opportunities to use the nursing process as it applies to medication administration. As you gain experience, your psychomotor skills ("the how-to") become more refined. However, psychomotor skills represent a small part of medication administration. Patient attitudes, knowledge, physical and mental status, and responses make medication administration a complex responsibility.

Attitudes

Use your critical thinking skills to administer medications safely. Be disciplined and take adequate time to prepare and administer medications. Take the time to read your patient's medical record before administering medications, and carefully review the patient's history, physical examination, and orders. Look up medications that you do not know in a medication reference, and determine why each patient is taking each of the prescribed medications. Every step of safe medication administration requires a disciplined attitude and a comprehensive, systematic approach. Following the same procedure each time medications are administered ensures safe administration.

Responsibility and accountability are other critical thinking attitudes essential to safe medication administration. Accept full accountability and responsibility for all actions surrounding the administration of medications. Do not assume that a medication that is ordered for a patient is the correct medication or the correct dose. Be responsible for knowing that the medications and doses ordered are correct and appropriate. You are accountable if you give an ordered medication that is not appropriate for a patient. Therefore, be familiar with each medication, including its therapeutic effect, usual dosage, anticipated changes in laboratory data, and side effects. You are also responsible for ensuring that patients or caregivers who administer medications have been properly informed about all aspects of self-administration (TJC, 2020). If you determine that a patient cannot self-administer medications safely, design interventions such as involving family caregivers to ensure safe administration.

Standards

Standards are actions that ensure safe nursing practice. Standards for medication administration are set by health care agencies and the nursing profession. Agency policy sets limits on a nurse's ability to administer medications in certain units of the acute care setting. Sometimes nurses are limited by certain medication routes or dosages. Most agencies have nursing procedure manuals and formularies that contain policies that define the types of medications nurses can and cannot administer. The types and dosages of some medications that nurses deliver vary from unit to unit within the same agency. For example, phenytoin, a medication for treating seizures, may be administered by mouth or IV push. In large dosages phenytoin affects heart rhythm. Therefore, some agencies place limits on how much nurses can administer to a patient on a nursing unit that does not have the ability to monitor a patient's heart rate and rhythm. Not all health care providers are aware of the limitations and sometimes prescribe medications that nurses cannot give in a particular health care setting. Recognize these limitations and inform the health care provider accordingly. Take appropriate actions to ensure that patients receive medications as prescribed and within the time prescribed in the appropriate environment.

Professional standards such as *Nursing: Scope and Standards of Practice* (ANA, 2015) (see Chapters 1 and 23) apply to the activity of medication administration. To prevent medication errors, follow the seven rights of medication administration consistently every time you administer medications. Many medication errors can be linked in some way to an inconsistency in adhering to these seven rights:

1. The right medication
2. The right dose
3. The right patient
4. The right route

5. The right time
6. The right documentation
7. The right indication

Right Medication. A medication order is required for every medication that you administer to a patient. Sometimes health care providers write orders by hand in the patient's medical record. Alternatively, some agencies use CPOE. CPOE allows a health care provider to order medications electronically, eliminating the need for written orders and enhancing medication safety (Zhu and Weingart, 2018). Regardless of how a nurse receives a medication order, he or she compares the health care provider's written orders with the medication administration record (MAR) or electronic MAR (eMAR) when it is ordered initially. Nurses verify medication information whenever new MARs are created or distributed or when patients transfer from one nursing unit or health care setting to another.

Once you determine that information on a patient's MAR is accurate, use it to prepare and administer medications. When preparing medications from bottles or containers, compare the label of the medication container with the MAR 3 times: (1) before removing the container from the drawer or shelf, (2) as the amount of medication ordered is removed from the container, and (3) at the patient's bedside before administering the medication to the patient. Never prepare medications from unmarked containers or containers with illegible labels (TJC, 2020). With unit-dose prepackaged medications, check the label with the MAR when taking medications out of the medication dispensing system. Finally verify all medications at the patient's bedside with the patient's MAR and use at least two identifiers before giving the patient any medications (TJC, 2020).

Patients who self-administer medications need to keep them in their original labeled containers, separate from other medications, to avoid confusion. Many health care agencies require that nurses administer all medications rather than letting patients self-administer to enhance accuracy and patient safety. Because the nurse who administers the medication is responsible for any errors related to it, nurses administer only the medications they prepare. You cannot delegate preparation of medication to another person and then administer the medication to the patient. If a patient questions the medication, do not ignore these concerns. A patient or a family caregiver familiar with a patient's medications often knows whether a medication is different from those received before. In most cases a patient's medication order has changed; however, sometimes patient questions reveal an error. When this occurs, withhold the medication and recheck it against the health care provider's orders. If a patient refuses a medication, discard it rather than returning it to the original container. Unit-dose medications can be saved if they are not opened. If a patient refuses opioids or any controlled substance, follow proper agency procedure by having someone else witness the "wasted" medication.

Right Dose. The unit-dose system is designed to minimize errors. When preparing a medication from a larger volume or strength than needed or when the health care provider orders a system of measurement different from that which the pharmacy supplies, the chance of error increases. You need to have another qualified nurse check the calculated doses when performing medication calculations or conversions. Prepare medications using standard measurement devices such as graduated cups, syringes, and scaled droppers to measure medications accurately. Educate patients to use similar measurement devices at home, such as measuring spoons with metric calibrations rather than household teaspoons and tablespoons, which are inaccurate.

Medication errors occur when pills need to be split. Studies show that the accuracy of split tablets is questionable, even if a tablet is scored (ISMP, 2017c). In addition, in the home setting patients may assume that tablets in containers have already been split when they have not or split them again when they have been split already (ISMP, 2017c). The US FDA (USFDA, 2018b) developed suggestions to help patients split pills. They include ensuring that the tablet is designed to be split, using a tablet splitter and not splitting the entire prescription at one time, and determining whether the patient has the motor dexterity or visual acuity to split tablets. If possible, health care providers need to avoid ordering medications that require splitting.

Tablets are sometimes crushed and mixed with food. Be sure to completely clean a crushing device before crushing the tablet. Remnants of previously crushed medications increase the concentration of a medication or result in the patient receiving part of a medication that was not prescribed. Mix crushed medications with very small amounts of food or liquid (e.g., a single tablespoon). Do not use a patient's favorite foods or liquids because medications alter their taste and decrease the patient's desire for them. This is especially a concern for pediatric patients.

Not all medications are suitable for crushing. Some medications (e.g., extended-release capsules) have special coatings to prevent them from being absorbed too quickly. These medications should not be crushed. Refer to the "Do Not Crush List" (ISMP, 2016a) to ensure that a medication is safe to crush.

Right Patient. Medication errors often occur because a patient gets a medication intended for another patient. Therefore, an important step in safe medication administration is being sure that you give the right medication to the right patient. It is difficult to remember every patient's name and face. Before administering a medication, use at least two patient identifiers (TJC, 2020). Acceptable patient identifiers include the patient's name, his or her medical record number assigned by a health care agency, or a telephone number. Do not use the patient's room number or physical complaint as an identifier. To identify a patient correctly, you usually compare the patient identifiers on the MAR with the patient's identification bracelet while at the patient's bedside. If an identification bracelet becomes smudged or illegible or is missing, obtain a new one. All agencies in all health care settings need to use a system that verifies the patient's identification with at least two identifiers before administering medications and other treatments.

Patients do not need to state their names and other identifiers when you administer medications. Collect patient identifiers reliably when he or she is admitted to a health care setting. Once the identifiers are assigned to the patient (e.g., putting identifiers on an armband and placing the armband on the patient), you use the identifiers to match the patient with the MAR, which lists the correct medications. Asking patients to state their full names and identification information provides a third way to verify that the nurse is giving medications to the right patient.

In addition to using two identifiers, some agencies use BCMA to help identify the right patient (Fig. 31.7). This system requires nurses to scan a personal bar code that is commonly placed on their name tag first. Then the nurse scans a bar code on the single-dose medication package. Finally, the nurse scans the patient's armband. All this information is then stored in a computer for documentation purposes. This system helps eliminate medication errors because it provides another step to ensure that the right patient receives the right medication (Hutton et al, 2017).

Right Route. Always consult the health care provider if an order does not include a route of administration. Likewise alert the health care provider immediately if the specified route is not the recommended route. Recent evidence shows that medication errors involving the wrong route are common. For example, when nurses need to prepare an oral medication in a syringe, the risk to administer the medication via the wrong route (e.g., intravenously) is very high and often results in fatal consequences. Thus, the ISMP (2018a) recommends that pharmacists, *not nurses*, prepare all oral

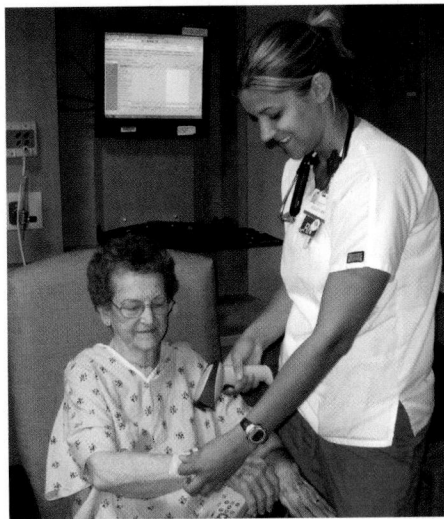

FIG. 31.7 Nurse using bar-code scanner to identify patient during medication administration.

medications that are not prepared commercially as a unit product to enhance patient safety.

The accidental IV injection of a liquid designed for oral use produces local complications, such as sterile skin abscess, or systemic effects, such as a fatality. If you work in a setting that requires you to prepare oral medications, use only enteral syringes (e.g., ENFit) when you prepare oral medications (ISMP, 2015c). Enteral syringes often use a color different from the parenteral syringes and are clearly labeled for oral or enteral use. The syringe tips of enteral syringes will not connect with parenteral medication administration systems. Needles do not attach to enteral syringes, and the syringes cannot be inserted into any type of IV line. Label the syringe after preparing the medication and be sure to remove any caps from the tip of an oral syringe before administering the medication.

Right Time. To administer medications safely, you need to know why a medication is ordered for certain times of the day and whether you can alter the time schedule. For example, two medications are ordered, one q8h (every 8 hours) and the other 3 times a day. Both medications are scheduled for 3 times within a 24-hour period. You need to give the q8h medication every 8 hours ATC to maintain therapeutic blood levels of the medication. In contrast, you need to give the 3-times-a-day medication at 3 different times while the patient is awake. Each agency has a recommended time schedule for medications ordered at frequent intervals. You can alter these recommended times if necessary or appropriate.

The health care provider often gives specific instructions about when to administer a medication. A preoperative medication to be given "on call" means that you give the medication when the operating room staff members notify you that they are coming to get a patient for surgery. Give a medication ordered PC (after meals) within half an hour after a meal, when a patient has a full stomach. Give a STAT medication immediately.

Give priority to time-critical medications that must act and therefore be given at certain times. Hospitals designate which medications are time critical and which are non–time critical (CMS, 2014; ISMP, 2011a). You administer time-critical medications within 30 minutes before or after their scheduled time. For example, give insulin (a time-critical medication) at a precise interval before a meal. Give antibiotics 30 minutes before or after they are scheduled ATC to maintain therapeutic blood levels. Give all routinely ordered non–time-critical medications within 1 to 2 hours before or after the scheduled time or per agency policy (CMS, 2014; ISMP, 2011a).

Some medications require a nurse's clinical judgment in deciding the proper time for administration. Administer a prn sleeping medication when a patient is prepared for bed. In addition, use judgment when administering prn analgesics. For example, you may need to obtain a STAT order from the health care provider if a patient requires a medication before the prn interval has elapsed. Always document when you call a patient's health care provider to obtain a change in a medication order.

Before discharge from the hospital setting, evaluate a patient's need for home care, especially if he or she was admitted to the hospital because of a problem with medication self-administration. Patients often leave the hospital with a basic knowledge of their medications but are unable to remember or implement this knowledge once back home. Before patients are discharged from the hospital, evaluate whether the medications are adequate or prescribed at therapeutic levels for them.

At home some patients take several medications throughout the day. Help to plan schedules based on preferred medication intervals, the pharmacokinetics of the medications, and the patient's daily schedule. For patients who have difficulty remembering when to take medications, make a chart that lists the times to take each one, or prepare a special container to hold each timed dose.

Right Documentation. Nurses and other health care providers use documentation to communicate with one another. Many medication errors result from inaccurate documentation. Therefore, always document medications accurately at the time of administration and identify any inaccurate documentation before you give medications.

Before you administer a medication, ensure that the MAR clearly shows:

- *The patient's full name*
- *The full name of the ordered medication (without abbreviations of medication names)*
- *The time the medication is to be administered*
- *The dosage, route, and frequency of administration*

Common problems with medication orders include incomplete information; inaccurate dosage form or strength; illegible order or signature; incorrect placement of decimals, leading to the wrong dosage; and nonstandard terminology. If there is any question about a medication order because it is incomplete, illegible, vague, or not understood, contact the health care provider before administering the medication. The health care provider is responsible to provide accurate, complete, and understandable medication orders. If he or she is unable to do this, nurses implement agency policy (usually a "chain of command" policy) to determine whom to contact until they resolve issues related to patients' medications. You are responsible to begin this chain of command to ensure that patients receive the correct medication. You are also responsible for documenting any preassessment data required of certain medications such as a blood pressure measurement for antihypertensive medications or laboratory values, as in the case of warfarin, before giving the medication.

After administering a medication, immediately document which medication was given on a patient's MAR per agency policy to verify that it was given as ordered. Inaccurate documentation, such as failing to document giving a medication or documenting an incorrect dose, leads to errors in subsequent decisions about patient care. For example, errors in documentation about insulin often result in negative patient outcomes. Consider the following situation: a patient receives insulin before breakfast, but the nurse who gave the insulin forgot to document it. The nurse caring for the patient goes home, and you are the patient's new nurse for the day. You notice that the insulin is not documented, you assume that the previous nurse did not give the insulin, and you give the patient another dose of insulin. Approximately 2 hours later, the patient experiences a low blood glucose level, which results in seizure activity. Accurate documentation and following up with the nurse from the previous shift to verify that the insulin was given as ordered would have prevented this situation from happening.

Never document that you have given a medication until you have actually given it. Document the name of the medication, the dose, the time of administration, and the route on the MAR. Also document the site of any injections and the patient's responses to medications, either positive or negative. Notify a patient's health care provider of any negative responses to medications, and document the time, date, and name of the health care provider who was notified in the patient's medical record. The efforts you make to ensure proper documentation help provide safe care.

Maintaining Patients' Rights. In accordance with *The Patient Care Partnership* (American Hospital Association, n.d.) and because of the potential risks related to medication administration, a patient has the following rights:

- To be informed of the name, purpose, and action of a medication and its potential for undesired effects
- To refuse a medication regardless of the consequences
- To have qualified nurses or physicians assess a medication history, including allergies and use of herbals
- To be properly advised of the experimental nature of medication therapy and give written consent for its use
- To receive labeled medications safely and without discomfort in accordance with the seven rights of medication administration
- To receive appropriate supportive therapy in relation to medication therapy
- To receive no unnecessary medications
- To be informed if medications are a part of a research study

Know these rights and handle all patient and family caregiver questions courteously and professionally. Do not become defensive if a patient refuses medication therapy, recognizing that every person of consenting age has a right to refusal.

Right Indication. ISMP (2016b) is considering a seventh right of medication administration that would enhance the safety of every medication order, the *right indication*. Indication-based prescribing would narrow medication choices, dosage forms, and dosing regimens, which reduces the risk of a wrong medication being chosen (Schiff et al., 2016). In addition, indication-based prescribing would empower and educate patients, which can improve medication adherence. Communication would be improved between the interprofessional team and the patients and family caregivers. Medication reconciliation would improve as indication-based prescribing would aid in preventing represcribing.

REFLECT NOW

You have three patients in need of 0800 medication administration. One needs a STAT medication on call for the operating room, the second needs routine 0800 medications, and the third needs pain medication, complaining of pain of a 4 on a scale of 0 to 10. Considering the seven rights of medication administration, how do you decide in what order to administer these medications?

❖ NURSING PROCESS

Apply the nursing process and use a critical thinking approach in your care of patients. The nursing process provides a clinical decision-making approach for you to develop and implement an individualized plan of care.

◆ Assessment

Thoroughly assess each patient and critically analyze findings to ensure that you make patient-centered clinical decisions required for safe nursing care.

Through the Patient's Eyes. Use professional knowledge, skills, and attitudes to provide compassionate and coordinated care. Consider patients' preferences and values while determining their need for and possible responses to medication therapy. Assess their experiences and encourage them to express their beliefs, feelings, and concerns about their medications. For example, ask them how their religious or family backgrounds influence their beliefs about taking medications. Putting patients in the center of their care helps you to see the situation through their eyes and contributes to safe medication administration. Begin your assessment by asking a variety of questions to help you better understand your patients' current medication management routine, their ability to afford medications, and their beliefs and expectations about medications.

History. Before you administer medications, review a patient's medical history to help you understand the indications or contraindications for medication therapy. Some illnesses place patients at risk for adverse medication effects. For example, if a patient has a gastric ulcer, medications containing aspirin increase the likelihood of bleeding. Long-term health problems (e.g., diabetes or arthritis) require specific medications. This knowledge helps you anticipate the type of medications that a patient requires. A patient's surgical history also sometimes indicates the need for medications. For example, after a thyroidectomy a patient requires thyroid hormone replacement.

Allergies. Inform the other members of the health care team if a patient has a history of allergies to medications and foods. Many medications have ingredients also found in food sources. For example, propofol, which is used for anesthesia and sedation, includes egg lecithin and soybean oil as inactive ingredients. Therefore, patients who have an egg or soy allergy should not receive propofol (Skidmore-Roth, 2018). In most health care settings patients wear identification bands listing medication and food allergies. Ensure that all your patient's allergies and their allergic reactions are documented appropriately in the patient's medical record (e.g., history and physical, MAR) to facilitate communication of this essential information to members of the health care team.

Medications. Ask your patients questions to find out about each medication they take (Box 31.7). Possible questions include: How long have you been taking these medications? What is the current dosage of each medication? Do you experience side effects or adverse effects from your medications? In addition, review the action, purpose, normal dosage, routes, side effects, and nursing implications for administering and monitoring each medication. You often need to consult several resources such as pharmacology textbooks; medication manuals available on a computer, electronic tablet, or AMDS; nursing journals; the *Physicians' Desk Reference* (PDR); medication package inserts; and pharmacists to gather necessary information. As a nurse you are responsible for knowing as much as possible about each medication your patients take.

BOX 31.7 Nursing Assessment Questions

- Which prescription and nonprescription medications and herbal and nutritional supplements do you take? When do you take them? How do you take them? Do you have a list of medications from your pharmacy or health care provider's office?
- Why do you take these medications?
- Which side effects do you experience? Which of the side effects bother you or affect you negatively?
- What have you been told to do if a side effect develops?
- Have you ever stopped taking your medications? If so, why?
- What do you do to help remember to take your medications?
- Do you have any allergies to medications or foods? If so, which ones? Describe what happens when you take the medication or eat the food.
- Describe your normal eating patterns. Which foods and at what times do you normally eat?
- How do you pay for your medications? Do you sometimes have to stretch your budget to afford them or space them out to save money?
- What questions do you have about your medications?

BOX 31.8 CULTURAL ASPECTS OF CARE

Influences in Medication Administration

Health beliefs vary by culture and often influence how patients manage and respond to medication therapy. Significant differences in attitudes, regional differences, and socioeconomic status affect a patient's adherence to or preference for medication therapy (Ball et al., 2019). Some cultures attach different symbolic meanings to medications and medication therapy. Herbal remedies and alternative therapies are common in various cultures and ethnic groups and sometimes interfere with prescribed medications (Saper, 2018). Some people stop taking medications when their symptoms are resolved, even if the medications are still needed for management of a chronic illness. In addition, health beliefs often differ markedly between health providers and patients, further affecting a patient's adherence to medical therapy (Ball et al., 2019). In addition to the psychosocial aspect of medication therapy, pharmacological research has shown that differences in medication response, metabolism, and side effects may be affected by patients' ethnicity, genetics, gender, and age (Ball et al., 2019).

Implications for Patient-Centered Care

- Assess cultural beliefs, attitudes, and values when administering medications and teaching patients about self-administration.
- Establish trust with patients and resolve conflicts between medications and cultural beliefs to achieve optimal patient outcomes (Ball et al., 2019).
- Investigate whether the patient practices any alternative therapies or is taking any herbal preparations (Saper, 2018).
- Consider cultural influences on medication response, metabolism, and side effects if a patient is not responding to medication therapy as expected. Confer with health care provider because a change in the patient's medication is sometimes necessary.
- Assess food preferences that may interfere with patients' medication therapy (Betancourt et al., 2018; Saper, 2018).

Diet History. A diet history reveals a patient's normal eating patterns and food preferences. Use your patient's diet history to plan an effective and individualized medication dosage schedule. Teach your patient to avoid foods that interact with medications. In addition, provide education when your patients take medications that need to be taken before, with, or after meals.

Patient's Perceptual or Coordination Problems. Patients with perceptual, fine-motor, or coordination limitations often have difficulty self-administering medications. For example, a patient who takes insulin to manage blood glucose and has arthritis has difficulty manipulating a syringe. Assess the patient's ability to prepare doses and take medications correctly. If a patient is unable to self-administer medications, assess whether a family caregiver or friends are available to help, or make a home care referral.

Patient's Current Condition.

The ongoing physical or mental status of a patient affects whether a medication is given and how it is administered. *Assess a patient carefully before giving any medication.* For example, check a patient's blood pressure before giving an antihypertensive. A patient who is vomiting is unable to take medications by mouth. Notify the patient's health care provider when this happens. Assessment findings serve as a baseline in evaluating the effects of medication therapy.

Patient's Attitude About Medication Use.

A patient's attitudes about medications (e.g., benefit, risk, likelihood to cure) sometimes reveal a level of medication dependence or medication avoidance. Some patients do not express their feelings about taking a medication, particularly if dependence is a problem. Listen carefully when a patient describes how he or she uses medications to identify evidence of dependence or avoidance. Also, be aware that cultural beliefs about Western medicine sometimes interfere with medication adherence (Box 31.8; see Chapter 9).

Factors Affecting Adherence To Medication Therapy.

Many complex factors affect a patient's ability to adhere to prescribed medication therapy. For example, a patient's knowledge and understanding of medication therapy influence the willingness or ability to follow a medication regimen. If a patient has a history of poor adherence (e.g., frequently missed doses or failure to fill prescriptions), investigate whether he or she can afford prescribed medications, and review resources available for the purchase of medications if indicated. Also determine whether the patient understands the purpose of the medication, the importance of regular dosage schedules, proper administration methods, and the possible side effects. Without adequate funding, knowledge, and motivation, adherence to medication schedules is unlikely (Ball et al., 2019).

Patient's Learning Needs.

Health-related information is difficult to understand because of the use of technical terminology. Serious errors can occur when patients do not understand information about their medications. Assess patients' health literacy regarding medication administration to determine their need for instruction (Betancourt et al., 2018) (see Chapter 25). Have the patient explain the medication schedule of a typical day. Have him or her read a medication label and explain what it includes. Health literacy also includes numeracy. Have a patient show how to give a medication dose if it is necessary to split a pill or give more than one in a container. Consider patient responses to your medication assessment questions such as those listed in Box 31.7. When a patient is unable to answer questions about medications appropriately, assess his or her health literacy.

◆ Nursing Diagnosis

Assessment provides data about the patient's condition, ability to self-administer medications, and medication adherence. Use these data to determine a patient's actual or potential problems with medication therapy. Certain data are assessment findings that, when clustered together, reveal actual nursing diagnoses. For example, *Complex Medication Regimen related to complexity of medication schedule* is indicated when patients have a complex medication schedule and admit to having difficulty integrating their medications into their daily routine. This list of nursing diagnoses may apply during medication administration in a variety of settings:

- *Impaired Health Maintenance*
- *Lack of Knowledge (Medication)*
- *Nonadherence (Medication Regimen)*
- *Adverse Medication Interaction*
- *Complex Medication Regimen (Polypharmacy)*

After selecting the diagnosis, identify the related factor (if applicable) that drives the selection of nursing interventions. In the example of *Nonadherence*, the related factors of *financial barriers* versus *lack of knowledge about the regimen* require different interventions. If a patient's nursing diagnosis is related to inadequate finances, you collaborate with family caregivers, social workers, case managers, or community agencies to connect the patient with necessary financial resources and develop a medication regimen the patient can afford. If the related factor is *lack of knowledge*, you implement a teaching plan with appropriate follow-up.

◆ Planning

Always organize your care activities to ensure the safe administration of medications. Rushing to give patients medications leads to errors (Westbrook et al., 2017). It is important to minimize distractions or interruptions when preparing and administering medications (Bravo and Cochran, 2016; Yoder et al., 2015). No-interruption zones (NIZs) have been recommended to reduce distractions and interruptions during medication administration (Yoder et al., 2015). NIZs are created by placing signs, red tape, or some type of border on the floor around medication carts or areas. Nurses standing in these areas are not to be interrupted.

Goals and Outcomes. Setting goals and related outcomes contributes to patient safety and allows for effective use of time during medication administration. For example, a nurse establishes the following goal and related outcomes for a patient with newly diagnosed type 2 diabetes who has the diagnosis of *Lack of Knowledge related to insufficient medication information*:

Goal: The patient will safely self-administer all ordered medications before discharge.

Outcomes:

- The patient verbalizes understanding of desired and adverse effects of medications.
- The patient states signs, symptoms, and treatment of hypoglycemia.

- The patient can monitor blood glucose levels to determine whether it is safe to take medication or an alteration in dose is needed.
- The patient prepares a dose of ordered medication.
- The patient describes a daily routine that will integrate timing of medication with daily activities.

Setting Priorities. Prioritize care when administering medications. Use patient assessment data to determine which medications to give first, whether it is time to evaluate a patient's response to a medication, or whether it is appropriate to administer prn medications. For example, if a patient is in pain, it is important to provide pain medication as soon as possible. If the patient's blood pressure is elevated, administer the blood pressure medication before other medications. Nurses also prioritize when providing patient education about medications. Provide the most important information about the medications first. For example, hypoglycemia is a serious side effect of insulin. A patient taking insulin needs to be able to identify and treat hypoglycemia immediately; thus, first teach how to recognize and treat hypoglycemia before teaching how to administer an injection.

Teamwork and Collaboration. Collaboration during medication administration is essential. You need to collaborate with a patient's family caregivers whenever possible. Family caregivers and significant others often reinforce the importance of medication schedules when a patient is at home. Nurses often collaborate with patients' health care providers, pharmacists, and case managers to ensure that patients can afford their medications. On discharge ensure that patients know where and how to obtain medications. Be sure that patients can read medication labels and medication teaching information. Some patients also need to understand how to calculate dosages and prepare complex medication regimens. Collaborate with community resources (e.g., agency on aging, public health department, medical interpreters) when patients have significant literacy issues or difficulty in understanding medication instructions (see Chapter 25).

◆ Implementation

Health Promotion. In promoting or maintaining a patient's health, nurses identify factors that improve or diminish well-being. Health beliefs, personal motivation, socioeconomic factors, and habits influence a patient's adherence with medications. Several nursing interventions promote adherence to the medication regimen and foster independence. Teach a patient and family caregiver about the benefit of a medication and the knowledge needed to take it correctly. Integrate a patient's health beliefs and cultural practices into the treatment plan. Help a patient and family caregiver establish a medication routine that fits into the patient's normal schedule. Make referrals to community resources if a patient is unable to afford or cannot arrange transportation to obtain necessary medications.

Patient and Family Caregiver Teaching. Some patients take medications incorrectly or not at all because they do not understand their medications. When this happens, you need to provide patient education using language your patient understands (see Chapter 25). Include information about the purpose, actions, timing, dosages, and side effects of medications. Many health care agencies offer easy-to-read teaching sheets written at the sixth-grade level about specific types of medications. Patients need to know how to take medications properly and the risks associated when they fail to do so. For example, after receiving a prescription for an antibiotic, a patient needs to understand the importance of taking the full prescription. Failure to do this can lead to a worsening of the condition and the development of bacteria resistant to the medication. Current recommendations suggest the use of teach-back as a method to confirm patient learning and improve health care provider education (Betancourt et al., 2018). Have the patient explain the topic about which you instructed him or her, so you can confirm understanding.

Nurses teach patients how to administer their medications correctly. For example, teach a patient how to measure a liquid medication accurately. Provide special education to patients who depend on daily injections (Box 31.9). The patient learns to prepare and administer an injection correctly using aseptic technique. Teach family caregivers how to give injections in case the patient becomes ill or physically unable to handle a syringe. Provide specially designed equipment such as syringes with enlarged calibrated scales or medications with labels in braille when patients have visual alterations.

Patients need to know the symptoms of medication side effects or toxicity. For example, patients taking anticoagulants learn to notify their health care providers immediately when signs of bleeding or bruising develop. Inform family caregivers or friends of medication side effects such as changes in behavior because they are often the first to recognize these effects. Patients cope better with problems caused by medications if they understand how and when to act. All patients need to learn the basic guidelines for medication safety, which ensure the proper use and storage of medications in the home.

Acute Care. Patients are often hospitalized to receive expert nursing assessment and documentation of responses to medications. When a nurse receives a medication order, several nursing interventions are essential for safe and effective medication administration.

Receiving, Transcribing, and Communicating Medication Orders. A medication order is required to administer any medication to a patient. In the absence of CPOE, health care providers handwrite orders onto order sheets in a patient's chart. If orders are handwritten, be sure that medication names, dosages, and symbols are legible. Clarify and then rewrite any unclear or illegible transcribed orders.

The process of verifying medical orders varies among health care agencies. Nurses follow agency policy and current national patient safety standards when receiving, transcribing, and communicating medication orders. *Nursing students are prohibited from transcribing or receiving verbal and telephone orders.*

Medication orders need to contain all the elements in Box 31.10. If a medication order is incomplete, inform the health care provider and ensure completeness before carrying it out. Nurses read back verbal or telephone orders to health care providers to ensure that the correct order is obtained. The registered nurse follows agency policy regarding receiving, recording, and transcribing verbal and telephone orders. Generally, the health care provider must sign them within 24 hours.

Nurses and pharmacists check all medication orders for accuracy and thoroughness several times during the transcription process. They also take patients' current problems, treatments, laboratory values, and other prescribed medications into consideration. Once the nurse and pharmacist determine that a medication order is safe and appropriate, it is placed on the appropriate medication form, usually called the *MAR*. The MAR is either printed on paper or available electronically. An electronic version of the MAR is called an *eMAR*. Whether it is handwritten, printed from a computer, or in an electronic version, it includes the patient's name, room, and bed number; medical record number; medical and food allergies; other patient identifiers (e.g., birthday); and

---

BOX 31.9 PATIENT TEACHING
Safe Insulin Administration

Objective
- Patient will correctly self-administer subcutaneous insulin.

Teaching Strategies
- Teach patient how to determine whether insulin is expired.
- Instruct patient to keep medication in its original labeled container and refrigerated if needed.
- Demonstrate how to prepare insulin in a syringe, assessing visual acuity to ensure that patient can draw up the correct amount of insulin.
- Coach patient through the steps of administering subcutaneous insulin injection.
- Demonstrate how to rotate insulin injection sites.
- Help patient determine the amount of insulin required based on the results of home capillary glucose monitoring as ordered by the health care provider.
- Show patient how to keep a daily log for insulin injections, including results of home capillary glucose monitoring, type and amount of insulin given, expiration date on insulin vial, time of insulin injection, and injection site used.

Evaluation
Use the principles of teach-back to evaluate patient/family caregiver learning:
- Describe for me the procedure you use at home for determining the correct dose of insulin you need and how you select your injection site.
- Please show me how you draw up your insulin based on the results of your capillary glucose monitoring result. Show me how you select your injection site and administer your insulin.
- Review your log with me so I can evaluate it for completeness.

BOX 31.10 Components of Medication Orders

A medication order needs to have all the following parts:

Patient's full name: A patient's full name distinguishes the patient from other people with the same last name. In the acute care setting patients are sometimes assigned special identification numbers (e.g., medical record number) to help distinguish patients with the same names. This number is often included on the order form.

Date and time that the order is written: The day, month, year, and time need to be included. Designating the time that an order is written clarifies when certain orders are to start and stop. If an incident occurs involving a medication error, it is easier to document what happened when this information is available.

Medication name: A health care provider orders a medication by its generic or trade name. Correct spelling is essential to prevent confusion with medications with similar spelling.

Dosage: The amount or strength of the medication is included.

Route of administration: A health care provider uses only accepted abbreviations for medication routes. Accuracy is important to ensure that patients receive medications by the intended route.

Time and frequency of administration: A nurse needs to know what time and how frequently to administer medications. Orders for multiple doses establish a routine schedule for medication administration.

Signature of health care provider: The signature makes an order a legal request.

medication name, dose, frequency, and route and time of administration. Each time a medication dose is prepared, the nurse refers to the MAR.

It is essential to verify the accuracy of every medication you give to your patients with the patients' orders. If the medication order is incomplete, incorrect, or inappropriate or if there is a discrepancy between the original order and the information on the MAR, consult with the health care provider. Do not give a medication until you are certain that you can follow the seven rights of medication administration. When you give the wrong medication or an incorrect dose, *you* are legally responsible for the error.

Accurate Dose Calculation and Measurement. You calculate each dose when preparing medications. To avoid calculation errors, pay close attention to the process of calculation and avoid interruptions from other people or nursing activities. Ask another nurse to double-check your calculations against the health care provider's order if you are in doubt about the accuracy of your calculation or if you are calculating a new or unusual dose.

Avoidance of Distractions.
Research reveals that nurses are frequently distracted during three phases of medication administration—the acquisition of the medication, transportation to the bedside, and during actual administration (Bravo and Cochran, 2016). Distraction comes from a variety of sources such as a page, a phone call, or a request from a colleague that draws away, disturbs, or diverts attention from a current desired task or forces attention on a new task at least temporarily. Follow these tips:

- Reduce distractions (e.g., turn off pager) and interruptions around automated medication dispensing machines (Bravo and Cochran, 2016).
- In areas where medications are being prepared, use a brightly colored sign or tape to alert staff to avoid interruptions (e.g., discussions) (Connor et al., 2016).
- Establish a no-interruption zone (NIZ).
- Provide staff education about the risks of interruptions.
- Create checklists for critical procedures requiring medication administration
- Turn off or manage mobile devices.
- Gather supplies before prescribing, preparing, or administering medication.

REFLECT NOW

Observe two RNs administering medications on the clinical unit to which you are assigned. What types of distractions occurred while the RNs were setting up morning medications? What can you take away from this experience to help you safety set up and administer medications in the future?

Correct Administration. For safe administration follow the seven rights of medication administration. Verify the patient's identity by using at least two patient identifiers (TJC, 2020). In the acute care setting identifiers are usually on a patient's armband. Carefully compare patient identifiers with the MAR to ensure that you are giving the medication to the right patient. Use aseptic technique and proper procedures when handling and giving medications, and perform necessary assessments (e.g., heart rate for antidysrhythmic medications) before administering a medication to a patient. Carefully monitor a patient's response to a medication, especially when the first dose of a new medication is administered.

Recording Medication Administration. Follow all agency policies when documenting medication administration. After administering a medication, appropriately document the name of the medication, dose, route, and exact time of administration immediately. Include the site of any injections per agency policy.

If a patient refuses a medication or is undergoing tests or procedures that result in a missed dose, explain the reason that a medication was not given in the nurses' notes. Some agencies require the nurse to circle the prescribed administration time on the medication record or to notify the health care provider when a patient misses a dose. Be aware of the effects that missing doses may have on a patient (e.g., with hypertension or diabetes). Coordinating care with health care providers and other services when testing or diagnostic procedures are being completed helps ensure patient safety and therapeutic control of the disease.

Restorative Care. Because of the numerous types of restorative care settings, medication administration activities vary. Patients with functional limitations often require a nurse to fully administer all medications. In the home care setting patients usually administer their own medications or receive assistance from family caregivers. Regardless of the type of medication activity, the nurse is responsible for instructing patients and family caregivers in medication action, administration, and side effects. He or she is also responsible for monitoring adherence with medication and determining the effectiveness of medications that have been prescribed.

Special Considerations for Administering Medications To Specific Age-Groups. A patient's developmental level is a factor to consider when administering medications. Knowledge of developmental needs helps you anticipate responses to medication therapy.

Infants and Children. In many pediatric settings the standard of practice is to have another nurse verify all pediatric dose calculations before administration. All children require special psychological preparation before receiving medications. A child's parents are often valuable resources for determining the best way to give a child medication. Sometimes it is less traumatic for a child if a parent gives the medication and the nurse supervises. Supportive care is necessary if a child is expected to cooperate. Explain the procedure to a child, using words appropriate to his or her level of comprehension. Long explanations increase a child's anxiety, especially for painful procedures such as an injection. Providing a child with choices when possible can result in greater success. For example, saying "It's time to take your pill now. Do you want it with water or juice?" allows a child to make a choice. Do not give the child the option of not taking a medication. After the medication has been administered, praise the child and offer a simple reward such as a star or token. Tips for administering medication to children are in Box 31.11.

Older Adults. Adverse medication events occur in 22% or more of older adult patients presenting to health care agencies (Rochon, 2019). The most common serious manifestations include falls, orthostatic hypotension, heart failure, and delirium. Older adults require special nursing considerations during medication administration (Box 31.12). Be vigilant when administering medications and know the physiological changes of aging (Fig. 31.8) so that you can anticipate adverse reactions. Nurses can collaborate with health care providers to minimize adverse medication events in older adults by discontinuing medications, prescribing new medications sparingly, reducing the number of prescribers, and frequently reconciling medications (Rochon, 2019).

BOX 31.11 Tips for Administering Medications to Children

Oral Medications

- Liquids are safer to swallow than pills to avoid aspiration.
- Use calibrated droppers for administering liquids to infants; the use of straws often helps older children or patients who have difficulty swallowing pills.
- Offer juice, a soft drink, or frozen juice bar, if allowed, after the child swallows a medication.
- When mixing medications in other foods or liquids, use only a small amount. The child may refuse to take all of a larger mixture.
- Avoid mixing a medication in a child's favorite foods or liquids because the child may later refuse them.
- A plastic disposable oral syringe is the most accurate device for preparing liquid doses, especially those less than 10 mL. (Cups, teaspoons, and droppers are inaccurate.)

Injections

- Use caution when selecting intramuscular (IM) injection sites. Infants and small children have underdeveloped muscles. Follow agency policy.
- Children are sometimes unpredictable and uncooperative. Make sure that someone (preferably another nurse) is available to restrain a child if needed. Have the parent act as a comforter, not restrainer, if restraint is necessary.
- Always awaken a sleeping child before giving an injection.
- Distracting a child with conversation, bubbles, or a toy reduces pain perception.
- If time allows, apply a lidocaine ointment (e.g., EMLA cream) to an injection site before the injection to reduce pain perception during the injection.

BOX 31.12 FOCUS ON OLDER ADULTS

Safety in Medication Administration

- Frequently review a patient's medication history, including use of over-the-counter medications, and consult with health care provider to simplify the medication therapy plan whenever possible (Rochon et al., 2018).
- Keep instructions clear and simple, provide memory aids (e.g., calendar, medication schedule), and ensure that written information about medications is in print large enough for a patient to see (Rochon, 2019; Touhy and Jett, 2017).
- Assess functional status (including vision, hand grasp, fine-motor skills) to determine whether patient will require assistance in taking medications (Touhy and Jett, 2017).
- Some older adults have a greater sensitivity to medications, especially those that act on the central nervous system. Therefore, carefully monitor patients' responses to medications and anticipate dosage adjustments as needed (Touhy and Jett, 2017).
- If patient has difficulty swallowing a capsule or tablet, ask the health care provider to substitute a liquid medication or instruct patient to place medication on the front of the tongue and then swallow fluid to help wash it to the back of the throat. If the patient continues to have problems, have him or her try taking medication with a very small amount of semisolid food (e.g., applesauce) (Touhy and Jett, 2017).
- Teach alternatives to medications such as a proper diet instead of vitamins and exercise instead of laxatives (Rochon, 2019; Touhy and Jett, 2017).

Polypharmacy. Polypharmacy is the use of multiple medications, the use of potentially inappropriate or unnecessary medications, or the use of a medication that does not match a diagnosis (Touhy and Jett, 2017). For example, polypharmacy exists when a patient takes two medications from the same chemical class to treat the same illness. Suspect polypharmacy if your patient uses two or more medications with the same or similar actions to treat several illnesses simultaneously and mixes nutritional supplements or herbal products with medications. Older adults also often experience polypharmacy when they seek relief from a variety of symptoms (e.g., pain, constipation, insomnia, and indigestion) by using OTC preparations. Sometimes polypharmacy is unavoidable. For example, some patients need to take more than one medication to control their high blood pressure. When a patient experiences polypharmacy, the risk of adverse reactions and medication interactions with other medications and food is increased.

Because many older adults suffer chronic health problems, polypharmacy is common. However, it is also becoming more common in children and patients with mental illnesses. Taking OTC medications frequently, lack of knowledge about medications, incorrect beliefs about medications, and visiting several health care providers to treat different illnesses increase the risk for polypharmacy. To minimize risks associated with polypharmacy, frequent communication among health care providers is essential to make sure that the patients' medication regimen is as simple as possible (Rochon, 2019).

◆ Evaluation

Evaluation of medication administration is an essential role of professional nursing that requires assessment skills; critical thinking; analysis; and knowledge of medications, physiology, and pathophysiology. You need to thoroughly and accurately gather data to complete a holistic evaluation. The goal of safe and effective medication administration is met when a patient responds appropriately to medication therapy and assumes responsibility for self-care. When patients do not experience expected outcomes of medication therapy, investigate possible reasons and determine appropriate revisions to the plan of care.

Through the Patient's Eyes. Evaluation is more effective when you value your patients' participation. Therefore, partner with your patients and include them in the evaluation process. Ensure that they understand and can safely administer their medications. For example, if you are caring for a child who needs an inhaler, be sure to watch the patient use the inhaler. To determine whether patients understand their medication schedules, ask them to explain when they take their medications and whether they can take them as prescribed. When patients struggle with their medication schedule, determine barriers to adherence (e.g., cost, lack of knowledge) and remove these barriers if possible. Also remember that patients have different values and define health differently. These values and beliefs influence their perception of the effectiveness of their medications. Therefore, ask patients to describe this effectiveness. Ask whether they are satisfied with their medications and how they make them feel. Use patients' statements and responses to questions (e.g., "I feel less anxious now") when determining the effectiveness of medications. Including patients in the evaluation process empowers them and helps them become more actively involved in their care.

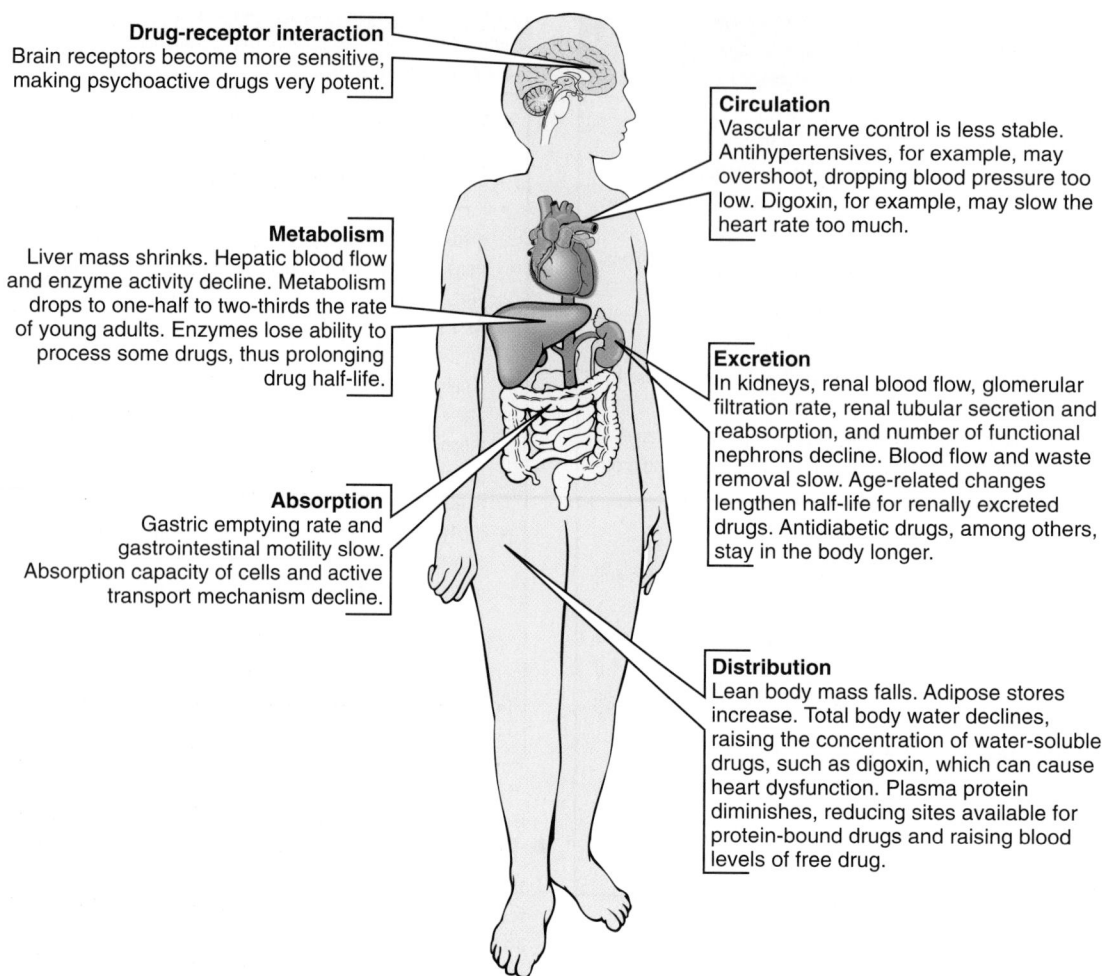

Drug-receptor interaction
Brain receptors become more sensitive, making psychoactive drugs very potent.

Circulation
Vascular nerve control is less stable. Antihypertensives, for example, may overshoot, dropping blood pressure too low. Digoxin, for example, may slow the heart rate too much.

Metabolism
Liver mass shrinks. Hepatic blood flow and enzyme activity decline. Metabolism drops to one-half to two-thirds the rate of young adults. Enzymes lose ability to process some drugs, thus prolonging drug half-life.

Excretion
In kidneys, renal blood flow, glomerular filtration rate, renal tubular secretion and reabsorption, and number of functional nephrons decline. Blood flow and waste removal slow. Age-related changes lengthen half-life for renally excreted drugs. Antidiabetic drugs, among others, stay in the body longer.

Absorption
Gastric emptying rate and gastrointestinal motility slow. Absorption capacity of cells and active transport mechanism decline.

Distribution
Lean body mass falls. Adipose stores increase. Total body water declines, raising the concentration of water-soluble drugs, such as digoxin, which can cause heart dysfunction. Plasma protein diminishes, reducing sites available for protein-bound drugs and raising blood levels of free drug.

FIG. 31.8 Effects of aging on medication metabolism. (From Lewis SM, et al: *Medical-surgical nursing,* ed 9, St Louis, 2014, Mosby.)

Patient Outcomes. A patient's clinical condition can change minute by minute. Use knowledge of the desired effect and common side effects of each medication to compare expected outcomes with actual findings. A change in a patient's condition is often physiologically related to changes in health status or results from medications or both. Be alert for reactions in a patient taking several medications. To evaluate patient responses to medications nurses use a variety of measures, such as direct observation of physiological measures (e.g., blood pressure or laboratory values), behavioral responses (e.g., agitation), and rating scales (e.g., rating on a pain or nausea scale). The type of measurement used varies with the medication action being evaluated, the reading skill and knowledge level of the patient, and the patient's cognitive and psychomotor ability. The most common type of measurement is physiological. Examples of physiological measures are blood pressure, heart rate, and visual acuity. Nurses also use patient statements as evaluative measures. Table 31.8 contains examples of goals, expected outcomes, and corresponding evaluative measures.

MEDICATION ADMINISTRATION

A sound knowledge base is required for medications to be administered safely. Nurses need to be prepared to administer medications using a variety of routes.

Oral Administration

The easiest and most desirable route for administering medications is by mouth (see Skill 31.1). Patients usually can self-administer oral medications. Food sometimes affects the absorption, so give oral medications on an empty stomach if absorption is decreased. Likewise, give medications with meals if absorption is enhanced by food (Burchum and Rosenthal, 2019). Most tablets and capsules need to be swallowed and administered with approximately 60 to 240 mL of fluid (as allowed).

Oral medication administration is contraindicated in some situations (see Table 31.5). Many medications interact with nutritional and herbal supplements. You need to be knowledgeable about these interactions to determine the best time to give oral medications.

An important precaution to take when administering any oral preparation is to protect patients from aspiration. Aspiration occurs when food, fluid, or medication intended for GI administration inadvertently enters the respiratory tract. Protect a patient from aspiration by assessing his or her ability to swallow. Box 31.13 provides techniques that protect patients from aspiration. Proper positioning is essential. Position a patient in a seated position at a 90-degree angle when administering oral medications if not contraindicated by his or her condition. Usually having the patient slightly flex the head in a chin-down position reduces aspiration. Use a multidisciplinary approach (e.g., speech therapist, registered dietitian, and occupational therapist) to determine the best techniques for patients who have difficulty swallowing.

TABLE 31.8 Example Evaluation for Patient Goals

Goal	Expected Outcomes	Evaluative Measure with Example
Patient and family caregiver will understand medication therapy.	Patient and family caregiver describe information about medication, dosage, schedule, purpose, and adverse effects.	Written measurement: Have patient write out medication schedule for a 24-hour period. Oral questioning: Use teach-back and ask patient to describe purpose, dosage, and adverse effects of each prescribed medication.
	Patient and family caregiver identify situations that require medical intervention.	Oral questioning: Use teach-back and have family caregiver describe what to do when a patient has adverse effects from a medication.
	Patient and family caregiver demonstrate appropriate administration technique.	Direct observation: Have patient complete return demonstration by filling insulin syringe and administering injection.
Patient will safely self-administer medications.	Patient follows prescribed treatment regimen.	Anecdotal notes: Have family caregiver keep log of patient's adherence to therapy for 1 week.
	Patient performs administration techniques correctly.	Direct observation: Observe patient instill eyedrops.
	Patient identifies available resources for obtaining necessary medication.	Oral questioning: Use teach-back and ask family caregiver to identify how to contact local pharmacy or community clinic for necessary medications.

BOX 31.13 Protecting a Patient From Aspiration

- Allow patient to self-administer medications if possible.
- Know signs of dysphagia (difficulty swallowing): cough, change in voice tone or quality after swallowing, delayed swallowing, incomplete oral clearance or pocketing of food, regurgitation.
- Assess patient's ability to swallow and cough by checking for presence of gag reflex and then offering 50 mL of water in 5-mL allotments. Stop if patient begins to cough.
- Prepare oral medication in form that is easiest to swallow.
- Position the patient in an upright seated position at a 90-degree angle with feet on the floor, hips and knees at 90 degrees, head midline, and back erect if possible and if not contraindicated by his or her condition.
- Suggest that the patient slightly flex the head in a chin-down position before swallowing.
- Prepare oral medications in the form that is easiest to swallow.
- If patient has unilateral (one-sided) weakness, place medication in stronger side of mouth.
- Administer pills one at a time, ensuring that each medication is properly swallowed before next one is introduced.
- Thicken regular liquids or offer fruit nectars if patient cannot tolerate thin liquids.
- Some medications can be crushed and mixed with pureed foods if necessary. Refer to a medication reference to identify medications that are safe to crush.
- Avoid straws because they decrease the control the patient has over volume intake, which increases risk of aspiration.
- Have patient hold and drink from a cup if possible.
- Time medications, if possible, to coincide with mealtimes or when patient is well rested and awake.
- Administer medications using another route if risk of aspiration is severe (see agency policy).

Special consideration is needed when administering medications to patients with enteral or small-bore feeding tubes (Box 31.14). Failing to follow current evidence-based recommendations from the American Society for Parenteral and Enteral Nutrition (ASPEN) can result in tube obstruction, reduced medication effectiveness, and increased risk of medication toxicity (Boullata et al., 2017). Tubing misconnections continue to cause patient injury because tubes with different functions can be connected with Luer connectors (TJC, 2014). In response to this issue the International Organization for Standardization (ISO) (ISMP, 2015c) has developed tubing connector standards in which the enteral connector will no longer be Luer compatible. A new enteral-only connector (ENFit) is available, and health care agencies have changed enteral nutrition practices, policies, procedures, and processes per the new guidelines (TJC, 2014). Before giving a medication by this route, verify that the location of the tube (e.g., stomach or jejunum) is compatible with medication absorption. For example, iron dissolves in the stomach and is mostly absorbed in the duodenum. If it is administered through a jejunal tube, it has poor bioavailability.

Use liquid medications when possible. When liquid medications are unavailable, crush simple tablets or open capsules and dilute them in water. Pierce a gel cap with a sterile needle and empty the contents into 30 mL of warm water or other solution as designated by the manufacturer of the medication. You can dissolve gel caps in warm water, but this often takes 15 to 20 minutes. Only use oral syringes when preparing medications for this route to prevent accidental parenteral administration. Flush tubes with at least 30 mL of water before and after giving medications. When administering more than one medication at a time, give each separately and flush between medications with 15 to 30 mL of water. Determine whether medications need to be given on an empty stomach or if they are compatible with the patient's enteral feeding. If a medication needs to be given on an empty stomach or is incompatible with the feeding (e.g., phenytoin, carbamazepine, warfarin, fluoroquinolones, proton pump inhibitors), hold the feeding for at least 30 minutes before or 30 minutes after medication administration. Verify the time with a medication reference or consult with a pharmacist. Monitor the patient closely for adverse reactions. The risk for drug-drug interactions is high when two or more medications are given in this route because they can interact together as soon as they are administered.

Topical Medication Applications

Topical medications are medications that are applied locally, most often to intact skin. They come in many forms (see Table 31.1). They are also applied to mucous membranes.

BOX 31.14 PROCEDURAL GUIDELINES

Administering Medications Through an Enteral Tube (Nasogastric Tube, G-Tube, J-Tube, or Small-Bore Feeding Tube)

Delegation and Collaboration

The skill of administering medications by enteral feeding tubes cannot be delegated to assistive personnel (AP). The nurse instructs the AP to:

- Keep the head of the bed elevated a minimum of 30 degrees (preferably 45 degrees) for 1 hour after medication administration; follow agency policy.
- Report immediately to the nurse coughing, choking, gagging, or drooling of liquid or dissolved pills.
- Report to the nurse any occurrence of possible medication side effects (specific to medication).

Equipment

Medication administration record (MAR) (electronic or printed), appropriate medication syringe or 60-mL Asepto syringe for large-bore tubes only, enteral-only connector (ENFit) designed to fit the specific enteral tube (TJC, 2014) (see illustration), gastric pH test strip (scale of 0 to 11.0), graduated container, medication to be administered, pill crusher if medication in tablet form, water or sterile water for immunocompromised patients, tongue blade or straw to stir dissolved medication, clean gloves, and pulse oximeter (for evaluation).

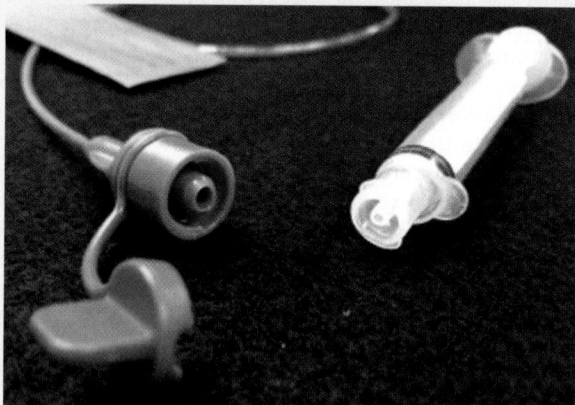

Enteral-only connector (ENFit).

Steps

1. Check accuracy and completeness of each MAR or computer printout with health care provider's written medication order. Check patient's name, medication name and dosage, route of administration, and time for administration. Clarify incomplete or unclear orders with health care provider before administration.
2. Review pertinent information related to medication, including action, purpose, normal dose and route, side effects, time of onset and peak action, indication and nursing implications.
3. Assess for any contraindications to receiving enteral medications, including presence of bowel inflammation, reduced peristalsis, recent gastrointestinal (GI) surgery, and gastric suction that cannot be turned off.
4. Avoid complicated medication schedules that often interrupt enteral feedings. Use alternative routes of medication administration if possible (e.g., transdermal, rectal, IV).
   a. Determine where medication is absorbed and ensure that point of absorption is not bypassed by feeding tube. For example, some medications such as antacids are absorbed in stomach, not jejunum.
   b. Determine whether medication interacts with enteral feeding. If so, hold the feeding for at least 30 minutes before giving the medication (see agency policy or consult pharmacist).

5. Assess patient's medical, medication, and diet history and history of allergies. List patient's food and medication allergies on each page of the MAR, and prominently display it on the patient's medical record per agency policy. When patient has allergy, provide allergy bracelet. If you identify contraindications, withhold medication and inform health care provider.
6. For a postoperative patient, review the postoperative orders for type of enteral tube care.
7. Perform hand hygiene. Gather and review physical assessment data (e.g., bowel sounds, abdominal distention) and laboratory data (e.g., renal and liver function) that may influence medication administration.
8. Check with pharmacy for availability of liquid preparation for patient's medications. The health care provider may need to change dosage form.
9. Before administration of enteral medications, verify placement of feeding tube according to agency policy and determine that tube is placed in the stomach or small intestine correctly.
10. Assess patient's or family caregiver's knowledge, experience, and health literacy.
11. Perform hand hygiene. Collect equipment and MAR.
12. Prepare medications for instillation into feeding tube. Attend to procedure and avoid distractions. Check medication label against MAR two times—when removing medication from unit dose or automated medication dispensing system (AMDS) and before leaving medication preparation area. *These are the first and second checks for accuracy.* Fill graduated container with 50 to 100 mL of tepid water. Use sterile water for immunocompromised or critically ill patients (Boullata et al., 2017).

    CLINICAL DECISION: Whenever possible, use liquid medications instead of crushed tablets. If you must crush tablets, flush the tubing before and after the medication administration to prevent the medication from adhering to the inside of the tube. In addition, make sure that concentrated medications are thoroughly diluted. Never add crushed medications directly to a tube feeding (Boullata et al., 2017).

    a. *Tablets:* Crush each tablet into a fine powder, using pill-crushing device or two medication cups. Dissolve each tablet in separate cup of 30 mL of warm water.
    b. *Capsules:* Apply clean gloves. Ensure that contents of capsule (granules or gelatin) can be expressed from covering (consult with pharmacist). Open capsule or pierce gel cap with sterile needle and empty contents into 30 mL of warm water (or solution designated by drug company). Gel caps dissolve in warm water, but this may take 15 to 20 minutes. Remove and dispose of gloves.
    c. Prepare liquid medication (prepared by pharmacy in appropriate syringe).
    d. Perform hand hygiene.
13. Take medication(s) to patient at correct time (see agency policy). Consider if medication is time critical. During administration apply seven rights of medication administration.
14. Identify patient using at least two identifiers (e.g., name and birthday or name and medical record number) according to agency policy. Compare identifiers with information on patient's MAR or medical record.
15. At patient's bedside again compare MAR or computer printout with names of medications on medication labels and patient name. Ask patient whether he or she has allergies. *This is the third check for accuracy.*
16. Explain procedure to patient and discuss purpose of each medication, action, and possible adverse effects. Allow patient to ask any questions about medications.

BOX 31.14 PROCEDURAL GUIDELINES

Administering Medications Through an Enteral Tube (Nasogastric Tube, G-Tube, J-Tube, or Small-Bore Feeding Tube)—cont'd

17. Assist patient to sitting position. Elevate head of bed to minimum of 30 degrees and preferably 45 degrees (unless contraindicated) or sit patient up in a chair (Boullata et al., 2017).
18. If continuous enteral tube feeding is infusing, adjust infusion pump setting to hold tube feeding.
19. Perform hand hygiene. Apply clean gloves. Check placement of feeding tube by observing gastric contents and checking pH of aspirate contents. *Gastric pH less than 5.0 is a good indicator that tip of tube is correctly placed in stomach* (Boullata et al., 2017; Clifford et al., 2015).
20. Check for gastric residual volume (GRV). Draw up 10 to 30 mL of air into a 60-mL syringe and connect syringe to feeding tube. Flush tube with air and pull back slowly to aspirate gastric contents. Determine GRV using either scale on syringe or a graduated container. If GRV exceeds 500 mL, hold feeding for 2 hours and recheck (Boullata et al., 2017) (check agency policy). When GRV is excessive, hold medication and contact health care provider.
21. Irrigate the tubing.
    a. Pinch or clamp enteral tube and remove syringe. Draw up 30 mL of water into syringe. Reinsert tip of syringe into tube, release clamp, and flush tubing. Clamp tube again and remove syringe.
    b. Using the appropriate enteral connector, attach to enteral tube.
22. Remove bulb or plunger of syringe and reinsert syringe into tip of feeding tube.
23. Administer dose of first liquid or dissolved medication by pouring into syringe. Allow to flow by gravity.

CLINICAL DECISION: Verify that the connector meets the ISO tubing connector standards (Boullata et al., 2017; TJC, 2014). Do not attach the enteral tubing to a standardized Luer syringe or needleless device (Guenther, 2015; TJC, 2014).

CLINICAL DECISION: Sometimes it is necessary to transfer oral medications into a medication cup for enteral administration. If medication does not flow freely, raise the height of the syringe to increase the rate of flow or try having the patient change position slightly because the end of the feeding tube may be against the gastric mucosa. If these measures do not improve the flow, a gentle push with bulb of Asepto syringe or plunger of the syringe may facilitate flow of fluid.

a. If giving only one dose of medication, flush tubing with 30 to 60 mL of water after administration.
b. To administer more than one medication, give each separately and flush between medications with 15 to 30 mL of water.
c. Follow last dose of medication with 30 to 60 mL of water.
24. Clamp proximal end of feeding tube if tube feeding is not being administered, and cap end of tube.
25. When continuous tube feeding is being administered by infusion pump, follow medication administration policy for turning off feedings prior to administering medications. If medications are not compatible with feeding solution, hold feeding for additional 30 to 60 minutes (Boullata et al., 2017).
26. Help patient to comfortable position and keep head of bed elevated, if not contraindicated, for 1 hour (see agency policy).
27. Be sure nurse call system is in an accessible location within patient's reach.
28. Raise side rails (as appropriate) and lower bed to lowest position.
29. Dispose of soiled supplies, rinse graduated container and syringe with tap water, remove and dispose of gloves, and perform hand hygiene.
30. Document name of medication, dose, route, and time administered on MAR. Document patient's response in nurses' notes of MAR in the electronic health record (EHR) or chart.
31. Record patient teaching and validation of patient's understanding on flow sheet or nurses' notes in electronic health record (EHR) or chart.
32. Observe patient for signs of aspiration such as choking, gurgling, gurgling speech, breath sounds, and difficulty breathing.
33. Return within 30 minutes to evaluate patient's response to medications.
34. **Use Teach-Back:** "I want to be sure I explained clearly why your father must take his medications through his feeding tube. Tell me why he is receiving his medications through his feeding tube." Revise your instruction now or develop a plan for revised patient/family caregiver teaching if patient/family caregiver is not able to teach back correctly. Determines patient's/family caregiver's level of understanding of instructional topic.

Skin Applications. Because many locally applied medications such as lotions, pastes, and ointments create systemic and local effects, apply these medications with gloves and applicators. Use sterile technique if a patient has an open wound. Skin encrustation and dead tissues harbor microorganisms and block contact of medications with the tissues to be treated. Before applying medications, clean the skin thoroughly by washing the area gently with soap and water, soaking an involved site, or locally debriding tissue.

Apply each type of medication according to directions to ensure proper penetration and absorption. When applying ointments or pastes, spread the medication evenly over the involved surface and cover the area well without applying an overly thick layer. Health care providers sometimes order a gauze dressing to be applied over the medication to prevent soiling clothes and wiping away the medication. Lightly spread lotions and creams onto the surface of the skin; rubbing often causes irritation. Apply a liniment by rubbing it gently but firmly into the skin. Dust a powder lightly to cover the affected area with a thin layer.

Some topical medications are applied in the form of a transdermal patch that remains in place for an extended amount of time (e.g., 12 hours or 7 days). Before applying a new patch, don disposable gloves and remove the old one. Medication remains on the patch even after its recommended duration of use. Nurses and patients have inadvertently left old transdermal patches in place, resulting in the patient receiving an overdose of the medication. For example, patients who use fentanyl transdermal patches for pain management can experience respiratory depression, coma, and death when the patches are not removed. In addition, some people, especially children, have experienced life-threatening harm from accidental exposure to fentanyl patches that were not disposed of properly. Many patches are clear, which makes them difficult to see. Therefore, carefully assess the patient's skin and be sure to remove the existing patch before applying a new one. Follow these guidelines to ensure safe administration of transdermal or topical medications:

- When taking a medication history or reconciling medications, specifically ask patients if they take any medications in the forms of patches, topical creams, or any route other than the oral route.
- When applying a transdermal patch, ask the patient whether he or she has an existing patch.
- Wear disposable clean gloves when removing and applying transdermal patches.

- If the dressing or patch is difficult to see (e.g., clear), apply a noticeable label to the patch.
- Document on the MAR the location on the patient's body where the medication was placed.
- Document removal of the patch or medication on the MAR. Fold sticky sides of the patch together and dispose of the patch in a child-proof container. There are exceptions; a fentanyl patch, an adhesive patch that delivers a potent pain medication through the skin, comes with instructions to flush used or leftover patches (USFDA, 2018a). Always read package directions.

Nasal Instillation. Patients with nasal sinus alterations sometimes receive medications by spray, drops, or tampons (Box 31.15). The most common form of nasal instillation is via decongestant spray or drops, used to relieve symptoms of sinus congestion and colds. Caution patients to avoid abuse of medications because overuse leads to a rebound effect in which the nasal congestion worsens. When excess decongestant solution is swallowed, serious systemic effects also develop, especially in children. Saline drops are safer than nasal preparations that contain sympathomimetics (e.g., oxymetazoline or phenylephrine) as a decongestant for children.

It is easier to have patients self-administer sprays because they can control the spray and inhale as the medication enters the nasal passages. For patients who use nasal sprays repeatedly, check the nares for irritation. When used to treat a sinus infection, position patients to permit the nasal medication to reach the affected sinus. Severe nosebleeds are usually treated with packing or nasal tampons, which are treated with epinephrine, to reduce blood flow. Usually a health care provider places nasal tampons.

Eye Instillation. Some patients use OTC eyedrops and ointments such as artificial tears and vasoconstrictors (e.g., Visine and Murine). Other patients, especially older adults, receive prescribed ophthalmic medications for eye conditions such as glaucoma or after cataract extraction. Age-related problems, including poor vision, hand tremors, and difficulty grasping or manipulating containers, affect an older adult's ability to self-administer eye medications. Educate your patients and family caregivers about the proper techniques for administering them (see Skill 31.2). Evaluate a patient's and family caregiver's ability to self-administer through a return demonstration of the procedure. Show patients each step for instilling eyedrops to help them understand the procedure. Follow these principles when administering eye medications:

- Avoid instilling any form of eye medications directly onto the cornea. The cornea of the eye has many pain fibers and thus is very sensitive to anything applied to it.
- Avoid touching the eyelids or other eye structures with eyedroppers or ointment tubes. The risk of transmitting infection from one eye to the other is high.
- Use eye medication only for the patient's affected eye.
- Never allow a patient to use another patient's eye medications.

Intraocular Administration. One less common way to administer eye medications is by the intraocular route (see Skill 31.2). These medications resemble a contact lens. You place the medication into the conjunctival sac, where it remains for up to 1 week. You need to teach patients how to insert and remove the disk and to monitor for adverse medication reactions.

Ear Instillation. Because internal ear structures are very sensitive to temperature extremes, you need to instill eardrops at room temperature to prevent vertigo, dizziness, or nausea. Although the structures of the outer ear are not sterile, sterile solutions are used in case the eardrum is ruptured. The entrance of nonsterile solutions into middle ear structures often results in infection.

If a patient has ear drainage, check with the health care provider to be sure that the patient does not have a ruptured eardrum before instilling the drops. Never occlude or block the ear canal with the dropper or irrigating syringe. Forcing medication into an occluded ear canal creates pressure that injures the eardrum. Box 31.16 provides guidelines for administering eardrops.

Ear irrigations are performed when the external ear canal becomes occluded with cerumen that cannot be removed by more conservative measures such as wax softeners. Typically, an irrigation is performed only when the patient has a hearing deficit, ear discomfort, or if it is necessary to visualize the tympanic membrane. You should not perform an ear irrigation if there is a history of middle ear infection in the last 6 weeks, if the patient has undergone *any* form of ear surgery, if the patient has a perforation, or if there is a history of a mucous discharge in the last year.

Vaginal Instillation. Vaginal medications are available as suppositories, foam, jellies, or creams. Solid, oval-shaped suppositories (Fig. 31.9) are packaged individually in foil wrappers and are sometimes stored in the refrigerator to prevent them from melting. After a suppository is inserted into the vaginal cavity, body temperature causes it to melt and be distributed and absorbed. Foam, jellies, and creams are administered with an applicator inserter (Box 31.17)

Insert the suppository with a gloved hand in accordance with Standard Precautions (see Chapter 28). Patients often prefer administering their own vaginal medications and need privacy. Because vaginal medications are often given to treat infection, discharge is usually foul smelling. Follow aseptic technique and offer the patient frequent opportunities to maintain perineal hygiene (see Chapter 40).

Rectal Instillation. Rectal suppositories are thinner and more bullet-shaped than vaginal suppositories. The rounded end prevents anal trauma during insertion. Rectal suppositories contain medications that exert local effects such as promoting defecation or systemic effects such as reducing nausea. They are stored in a refrigerator until administered. Sometimes it is necessary to clear the rectum with a small cleansing enema before inserting a suppository (Box 31.18).

Administering Medications By Inhalation

Medications administered with handheld inhalers are dispersed through an aerosol spray, mist, or powder that penetrates lung airways. The alveolar-capillary network absorbs medications rapidly.

Pressurized metered-dose inhalers (pMDIs), breath-actuated metered-dose inhalers (BAIs), and dry powder inhalers (DPIs) deliver medications that produce local effects such as bronchodilation. Some medications create serious systemic side effects. pMDIs use a chemical propellant to push the medication out of the inhaler and require the patient to apply approximately 5 to 10 pounds of pressure to the top of the canister to administer the medication. Children or older adults with chronic respiratory diseases often use pMDIs. These two populations have diminished hand strength; therefore, it is essential to assess whether they have enough strength to use the pMDI.

Sometimes patients use a spacer with the pMDI. A spacer is a tube that is 10.16 to 20.32 cm (4 to 8 inches) in length that attaches to the pMDI and allows the particles of medication to slow down and break into smaller pieces. This helps the medication get deeper into the lungs and enhances absorption. Spacers are helpful when a patient has difficulty coordinating the steps involved in self-administering medications.

BOX 31.15 PROCEDURAL GUIDELINES

Administering Nasal Medications

Delegation and Collaboration

The skill of administering nasal medications cannot be delegated to assistive personnel (AP). The nurse instructs the AP about:

- Potential side effects of medications and to report their occurrence to the nurse.
- Reporting any bloody nasal drainage to the nurse.

Equipment

Medication administration record (MAR) (electronic or printed), prepared medication with clean dropper or spray container, facial tissue, small pillow *(optional)*, washcloth *(optional)*, clean gloves

Steps

1. Check accuracy and completeness of each MAR with health care provider's medication order. Check patient's name and medication name, dosage, route (which sinus), and time of administration. Clarify incomplete or unclear orders with health care provider before administration.
2. Review pertinent information related to medication, including action, purpose, normal dose and route, side effects, time of onset and peak action, and nursing implications.
3. Assess patient's medical history (e.g., hypertension, heart disease, diabetes, and hyperthyroidism), medication history, and history of allergies. List medication allergies on each page of the MAR and prominently display any allergies on the patient's medical record per agency policy. When patient has allergy, provide allergy bracelet.
4. Perform hand hygiene. Using a penlight, inspect condition of nose and sinuses. Palpate sinuses for pain or tenderness (see Chapter 30). Note type of drainage if present.
5. Assess patient's knowledge regarding use of nasal instillation, technique for instillation, and willingness to learn self-administration.
6. Perform hand hygiene. Collect appropriate equipment and MAR.
7. Prepare medications for instillation. Attend to procedure to avoid distractions. Check label of medication against MAR two times (see Skill 31.1). Preparation usually involves checking label when removing nasal drops or sprays out of storage and before leaving preparation area. Check expiration date on container. *These are the first and second checks for accuracy.* Perform hand hygiene.
8. Take medication(s) to patient at correct time (see agency policy). Consider whether medication is time critical. During administration, apply seven rights of medication administration.
9. Identify patient using two identifiers (e.g., name and birthday or name and medical record number) according to agency policy. Compare identifiers with information on patient's MAR or medical record.

10. At patient's bedside again compare MAR or computer printout with names of medications on medication labels and patient name. Ask patient whether he or she has allergies. *This is the third accuracy check.*
11. Explain procedure to patient and sensations to expect. Discuss purpose of each medication, action, and possible adverse effects. Allow patient to ask any questions about medications. Patients who self-instill medications may be allowed to give drops under nurse's supervision (check agency policy). Tell patients receiving nasal instillation that they may experience burning or stinging of mucosa or choking sensation as medication trickles into throat.
12. Arrange supplies and medications at bedside. Perform hand hygiene and apply clean gloves (if nasal drainage is present).
13. Gently roll or shake container. Instruct patient to clear or blow nose gently unless contraindicated (e.g., risk of increased intracranial pressure or nosebleeds).
14. *Administer nasal drops:*
    a. Help patient to supine position and position head properly.
       (1) For access to posterior pharynx, tilt patient's head backward.
       (2) For access to ethmoid or sphenoid sinus, tilt head back over edge of bed or place small pillow under patient's shoulder and tilt head back (see illustration).
       (3) For access to frontal and maxillary sinus, tilt head back over edge of bed or pillow with head turned toward side to be treated (see illustration).
    b. Support patient's head with nondominant hand.
    c. Instruct patient to breathe through mouth.
    d. Hold dropper 1 cm (½ inch) above nares and instill prescribed number of drops toward midline of ethmoid bone.
    e. Have patient remain in supine position 5 minutes.
    f. Offer facial tissue to blot runny nose, but caution patient against blowing nose for several minutes.
15. *Administer nasal spray:*
    a. Help patient into upright position with head tilted slightly forward.
    b. Instruct or assist patient to insert tip of nasal spray into appropriate nares and occlude other nostril with finger. Point spray tip toward side and away from center of nose.
    c. Have patient spray medication into nose while inhaling. Help patient remove nozzle from nose and instruct to breathe out through the mouth.
    d. Offer facial tissue to blot runny nose, but caution patient against blowing nose for several minutes.

CLINICAL DECISION: Some medications are designed for one spray per dose. Examples include calcitonin, desmopressin, and sumatriptan. It is essential to ensure that the patient understands the correct number of sprays to use per dose to prevent overdosing.

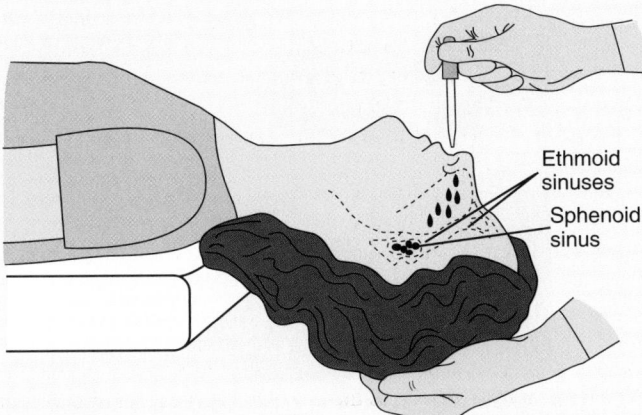

STEP 14a(2) Position for instilling nose drops into ethmoid or sphenoid sinus.

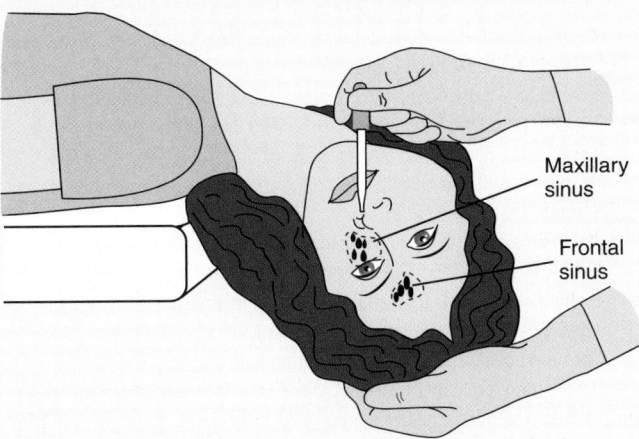

STEP 14a(3) Position for instilling nose drops into frontal and maxillary sinus.

Continued

BOX 31.15   PROCEDURAL GUIDELINES

Administering Nasal Medications—cont'd

16. Help patient to a comfortable position after medication is absorbed.
17. Dispose of soiled supplies, remove and dispose of gloves, and perform hand hygiene.
18. Document name of medication, dose, route, and time of administration on MAR.
19. Observe patient for onset of side effects 15 to 30 minutes after administration.
20. Ask whether patient can breathe through nose after decongestant administration. It may be necessary to have patient occlude one nostril at a time and breathe deeply.
21. Reinspect condition of nasal passages between instillations.
22. Ask patient to describe risks of overuse of decongestants and methods for administration.
23. Feedback ensures that patient can self-administer medications properly.
24. Have patient demonstrate self-administration of nasal medication.

25. Record patient response to medication, patient teaching, and validation of patient understanding and self-administration on flow sheet or nurses' notes in electronic health record (EHR) or chart.
26. **Use Teach-Back:** "I want to be sure I explained your nasal spray correctly. Can you tell me the best time for you to use this spray? What side effects may you get from using the spray?" If patient self-administers medications at home, state, "Show me how you're going to take this medication at home." Revise your instruction now or develop plan for revised teaching if patient/family caregiver is not able to teach back correctly. Determines patient's/family caregiver's level of understanding of instructional topic.

BOX 31.16   PROCEDURAL GUIDELINES

Administering Ear Medications

Delegation and Collaboration

The skill of administering ear medications cannot be delegated to assistive personnel (AP). The nurse instructs the AP about:
- Potential side effects of medications and to report their occurrence.
- The potential for dizziness or irritation after administration of ear medications.

Equipment

Medication administration record (MAR) (electronic or printed)
Drops: Medication bottle with dropper, cotton-tipped applicator, cotton balls, clean gloves if drainage is present
Irrigation: Irrigating solution and syringe, kidney basin, towel

Steps

1. Check accuracy and completeness of each MAR with health care provider's medication order. Check patient's name, medication name and dosage, route, and time for administration. Clarify incomplete or unclear orders with health care provider before administration.
2. Review pertinent information related to medication, including action, purpose, normal dose and route (one or both ears), side effects, time of onset and peak action, and nursing implications.
3. Assess patient's medical history, medication history, and history of allergies (including latex). List medication allergies on each page of the MAR and prominently display any allergies on the patient's medical record per agency policy. When patient has allergy, provide allergy bracelet.
4. Perform hand hygiene. Assess condition of external ear structures (see Chapter 30). This may be done just before medication instillation (apply clean gloves if drainage is present).
5. Determine whether patient has any symptoms of ear discomfort or hearing impairment.
6. Assess patient's level of consciousness (LOC) and ability to follow directions.
7. Assess patient's knowledge regarding medication therapy and desire to self-administer medication.
8. Assess patient's ability to manipulate and hold ear dropper.
9. Perform hand hygiene. Collect appropriate equipment and MAR.
10. Prepare medications for instillation. Attend to procedure and avoid distractions. Check label of medication against MAR two times (see Skill 31.1). Take eardrops out of refrigerator and rewarm to room temperature before administering to patient. Preparation usually involves checking label when removing eardrops out of storage and before leaving preparation area. Check expiration date on container. *These are the first and second checks for accuracy.* Perform hand hygiene.

11. Take medication(s) to patient at correct time (see agency policy). Consider whether medication is time critical. During administration apply seven rights of medication administration.
12. Arrange supplies at bedside.
13. Identify patient using at least two identifiers (e.g., name and birthday or name and medical record number) according to agency policy. Compare identifiers with information on patient's MAR or medical record.
14. At patient's bedside again compare MAR or computer printout with names of medications on medication labels and patient name. Ask patient whether he or she has allergies.
    This is the third check for accuracy
15. Explain procedure to patient and sensations to expect. Discuss purpose of each medication, action, and possible adverse effects. Allow patient to ask any questions about the medications. Patients who self-instill medications may be allowed to give drops under nurse's supervision (check agency policy).
16. Perform hand hygiene.
17. **Administer eardrops**
    a. Position patient on side (if not contraindicated) with ear to be treated facing up, or patient may sit in chair or at bedside. *Option:* Apply clean gloves if ear drainage is present.
    b. If cerumen or drainage occludes outermost part of ear canal, wipe out gently with cotton-tipped applicator (see illustration) or washcloth. Take care not to force cerumen into canal.

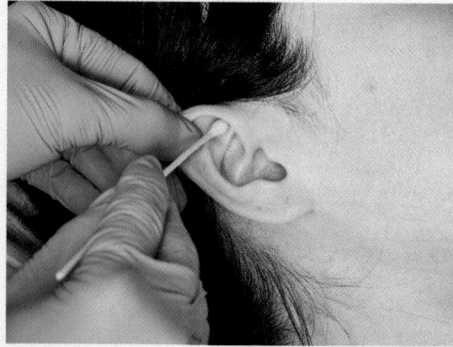

STEP 17b Always clean only outer canal. Do not push cerumen or secretions into ear.

BOX 31.16 PROCEDURAL GUIDELINES

Administering Ear Medications—cont'd

c. Hold the container in the palm of your hands for a few minutes to warm the contents to body temperature. Then, if the eardrops are in a cloudy suspension, shake bottle for about 10 seconds.

d. Straighten ear canal by pulling pinna up and back to 10 o'clock position (adult or child older than age 3) or down and back to 6 to 9 o'clock position (child under age 3).

e. Instill prescribed drops holding dropper 1 cm (½ inch) above ear canal. Avoid contact of dropper tip against external ear canal (see illustration).

f. Ask patient to remain in side-lying position for a few minutes. Apply gentle massage or pressure to tragus of ear with finger (see illustration).

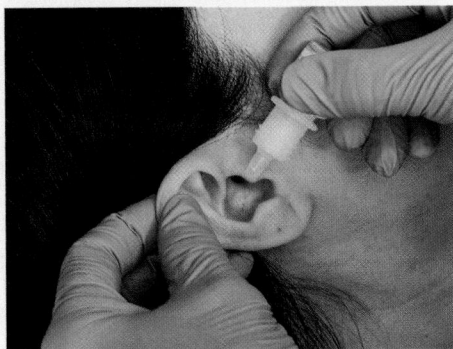

STEP 17e Pull pinna up and back for adults and children older than 3 years.

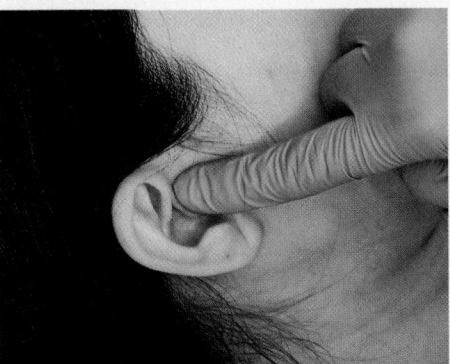

STEP 17f Nurse applies gentle pressure to tragus of ear after instilling drops.

g. If ordered, gently insert part of cotton ball into outermost part of canal. Do not press cotton into canal.

h. Remove cotton after 15 minutes. Help patient to comfortable position after drops are absorbed.

18. **Administer Ear Irrigations**

a. Assess the tympanic membrane or review medication record for history of eardrum perforation, which contraindicates ear irrigation.

b. Help patient into sitting position or lying position with head tilted or turned toward affected ear. Place towel under patient's head and shoulder and have patient hold basin under affected ear.

c. Fill irrigating syringe with solution (approximately 50 mL) at room temperature.

d. Gently grasp auricle and straighten ear by pulling pinna down and back for children younger than 3 years or upward and outward for patients 3 years of age and older.

e. Slowly instill irrigating solution by holding tip of syringe 1 cm (½ inch) above opening of ear canal. Allow fluid to drain out during instillation. Continue until you use all solution.

19. Clean area and put supplies away.

20. Remove and dispose of gloves and perform hand hygiene.

21. Record medication, concentration, dose or strength, number of drops, site of application (left, right, or both ears), and time of administration on MAR immediately after administration.

22. Observe response to medication by assessing hearing changes, asking whether symptoms are relieved, and noting any side effects or discomfort felt.

23. Ask patient to discuss purpose of medication, action, side effects, and technique of administration.

24. Record patient response to medication, patient teaching, and validation of patient understanding and self-administration on flow sheet or nurses' notes in electronic health record (EHR) or chart.

25. **Use Teach-Back:** "I want to be sure I clearly showed you how to administer eardrops. Let's take this time we have for you to show me how to place eardrops in your right ear." Revise your instruction now or develop a plan for revised patient/family caregiver teaching if patient/family caregiver is not able to teach back correctly. Determines patient's/family caregiver's level of understanding of instructional topic.

However, patients who do not use their spacers correctly do not receive the full effect of the medication. BAIs and DPIs do not use spacers.

BAIs release medication when a patient raises a lever and inhales. Release of the medication depends on the strength of the patient's breath on inspiration, and a BAI is a good choice for patients who have difficulty in using pMDIs because it eliminates the need for hand-breath coordination (Ari, 2015).

DPIs hold dry powder medication and create an aerosol when the patient inhales through a reservoir that contains a dose of the medication. The reservoir holds a dose of the medication. Compared with MDIs, DPIs deliver more medication to the lungs (Burchum and Rosenthal, 2019). Some DPIs are unit dosed. These inhalers require patients to load a single dose of medication into the inhaler with each

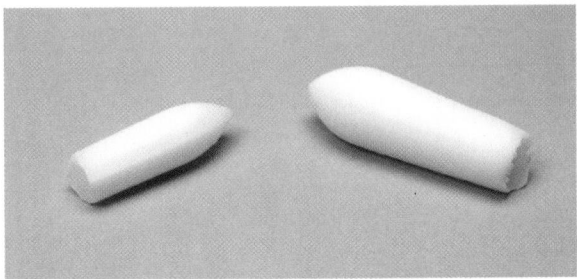

FIG. 31.9 Vaginal suppositories (right) are larger and more oval than rectal suppositories (left). (From Lilley LL, et al: *Pharmacology and the nursing process*, ed 9, St Louis, 2020, Elsevier.)

use. Other DPIs hold enough medication for 1 month. DPIs require less manual dexterity. Because the device is activated with the patient's breath, there is no need to coordinate puffs with inhalation. However, the medication inside the DPI can clump if the patient is in a humid climate, and some patients cannot inspire fast enough to administer the entire dose of the medication.

Patients who receive medications by inhalation frequently suffer from chronic respiratory disease such as chronic asthma, emphysema, or bronchitis. Different respiratory problems require different inhaled medication. For example, patients with asthma usually receive antiin-flammatory medications because asthma is primarily an inflammatory disease, whereas patients with chronic obstructive pulmonary disease

---

BOX 31.17   PROCEDURAL GUIDELINES

Administering Vaginal Medications

Delegation and Collaboration

The skill of administering vaginal medications cannot be delegated to assistive personnel (AP). The nurse instructs the AP about:

- Potential side effects of medications and to report their occurrence to the nurse.
- Reporting any change in comfort level or new or increased vaginal discharge or bleeding to the nurse.

Equipment

Medication administration record (MAR) (electronic or printed); vaginal cream, foam, jelly, tablet, suppository, or irrigating solution; applicators (Fig. 31.10) (if needed); clean gloves; tissues; towels and/or washcloths; perineal pad; drape or sheet; water-soluble lubricants; bedpan; irrigation or douche container (if needed); gooseneck lamp *(optional)*

Steps

1. Check accuracy and completeness of each MAR with health care provider's medication order. Check patient's name, medication name and dosage, route, and time for administration. Clarify incomplete or unclear orders with health care provider before administration.
2. Review pertinent information related to medication, including action, indication, purpose, normal dose and route, side effects, time of onset and peak action, and nursing implications.
3. Assess patient's medical and medication history and history of allergies. List medication allergies on each page of the MAR and prominently display any allergies on the patient's medical record per agency policy. When patient has allergy, provide allergy bracelet.
4. Perform hand hygiene and apply clean gloves. During perineal care inspect condition of vaginal tissues; note if drainage is present. Remove and dispose of gloves and perform hand hygiene.
5. Ask whether patient is experiencing any symptoms of pruritus, burning, or discomfort.
6. Review patient's knowledge of medication and readiness to learn (e.g., asks questions about medication, requests education in use of suppository).
7. Assess patient's ability to manipulate applicator, suppository, or irrigation equipment and to properly position self to insert medication (may be done just before insertion).
8. Perform hand hygiene. Collect appropriate equipment and MAR.

9. Prepare suppository for administration. Attend to the procedure and avoid distraction. Preparation usually involves checking the label when removing suppository from refrigerator and before leaving preparation area. Check expiration date on container. *These are the first and second checks for accuracy.* Perform hand hygiene.
10. Take medication(s) to patient at correct time (see agency policy). Consider whether medication is time critical. During administration apply seven rights of medication administration.
11. Identify patient using at least two identifiers (e.g., name and birthday or name and medical record number) according to agency policy. Compare identifiers with information on patient's MAR or medical record.
12. At patient's bedside again compare MAR or computer printout with names of medications on medication labels and patient name. Ask patient whether he or she has allergies. *This is the third check for accuracy.*
13. Explain procedure to patient. Be specific if patient plans to self-administer medication. Discuss purpose of each medication, action, and possible adverse effects. Allow patient to ask any questions about medication.
14. Close door or pull curtain. Perform hand hygiene and apply clean gloves. Have patient void (using bathroom agencies or bedpan). Help her lie in dorsal recumbent position. Patients with restricted mobility in knees or hips may lie supine with legs abducted.
15. Keep abdomen and lower extremities draped.
16. Be sure that vaginal orifice is well illuminated by room light. Otherwise position portable gooseneck lamp.
17. Insert vaginal suppository.
    a. Remove suppository from wrapper and apply liberal amount of water-soluble lubricant to smooth or rounded end (see illustration). Be sure that suppository is at room temperature. Lubricate gloved index finger of dominant hand.
    b. With nondominant gloved hand gently separate labial folds in front-to-back direction.

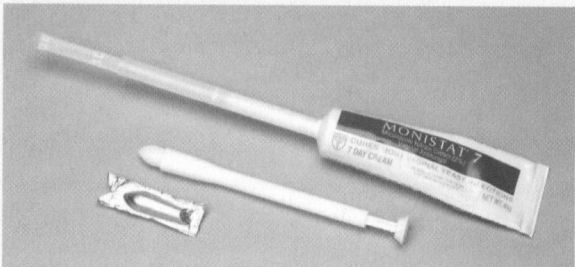

FIG. 31.10 From top: Vaginal cream with applicator, applicator, and vaginal suppository. (From Lilley LL, et al: *Pharmacology and the nursing process*, ed 9, St Louis, 2020, Elsevier.)

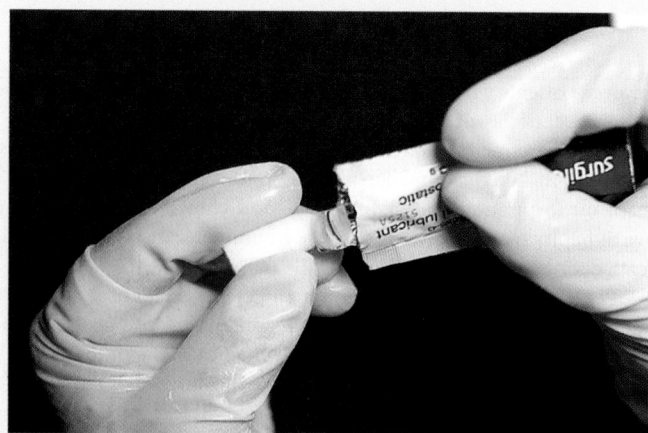

STEP 17a Lubricate tip of suppository.

BOX 31.17 PROCEDURAL GUIDELINES

Administering Vaginal Medications—cont'd

c. With dominant gloved hand insert rounded end of suppository along posterior wall of vaginal canal the entire length of finger (7.5 to 10 cm [3 to 4 inches]) (see illustration).

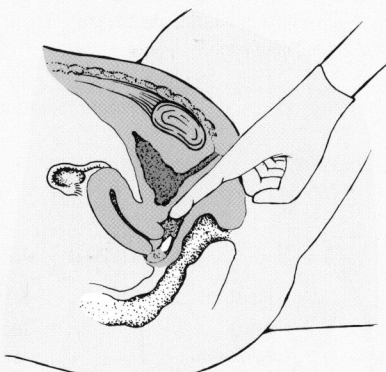

STEP 17c Angle of vaginal suppository insertion.

d. Withdraw finger and wipe away remaining lubricant from around orifice and labia with tissue or cloth.
e. Remove and dispose of gloves and perform hand hygiene

18. Apply cream or foam.
    a. Perform hand hygiene and apply clean gloves. Fill cream or foam applicator following package directions.
    b. With nondominant gloved hand gently separate labial folds.
    c. With dominant gloved hand gently insert applicator approximately 5 to 7.5 cm (2 to 3 inches). Push applicator plunger to deposit medication into vagina (see illustration).

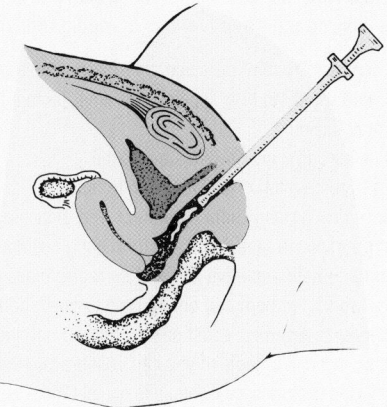

STEP 18c Applicator inserted into vaginal canal. Plunger pushed to instill medication.

d. Withdraw applicator and place on paper towel. Wipe off residual cream from labia or vaginal orifice with tissue or cloth.
e. Remove and dispose of gloves and perform hand hygiene.

19. Administer irrigation or douche.
    a. Place patient on bedpan with absorbent pad underneath.
    b. Be sure that irrigation or douche fluid is at body temperature. Run fluid through container nozzle (priming the tubing).
    c. Perform hand hygiene and apply gloves
    d. Gently separate labial folds and direct nozzle toward sacrum, following floor of vagina.
    e. Raise container approximately 30 to 50 cm (12 to 20 inches) above level of vagina. Insert nozzle 7 to 10 cm (3 to 4 inches). Allow solution to flow while rotating nozzle. Administer all irrigating solution.
    f. Withdraw nozzle and help patient to comfortable sitting position.
    g. Allow patient to remain on bedpan for a few minutes. Clean perineum with soap and water.
    h. Help patient off bedpan. Dry perineal area.
    i. Remove and dispose of gloves and perform hand hygiene

20. Instruct patient who received suppository, cream, or tablet to remain on her back for at least 10 minutes.
21. If using an applicator, wash with soap and warm water, rinse, air dry, and then store for future use.
22. Offer perineal pad when patient resumes ambulation.
23. Dispose of supplies, remove and dispose of gloves, perform hand hygiene. Help patient to comfortable position.
24. Record the medication, dosage, route, and actual time and date of administration on MAR immediately after administration, not before. Include initials or signature
25. Thirty minutes after administration perform hand hygiene and apply clean gloves. Then inspect condition of vaginal canal and external genitalia. Assess vaginal discharge if present. Remove and dispose of gloves and perform hand hygiene.
26. Question patient regarding continued pruritus, burning, discomfort, or discharge.
27. Ask patient to discuss purpose, action, and side effects of medication.
28. Record patient response to medication, patient teaching and validation of patient understanding and self-administration of suppository on flow sheet or nurses' notes in electronic health record (EHR) or chart.
29. **Use Teach-Back:** "I want to be sure I explained how to use the vaginal cream applicator. Tell me how you will draw the correct amount of cream into the applicator." Revise your instruction now or develop a plan for revised patient/family caregiver teaching if patient/family caregiver is not able to teach back correctly. Determines patient's/family caregiver's level of understanding of instructional topic.

(COPD) receive bronchodilators because they usually have problems with bronchoconstriction. Inhaled medications are also often described as "rescue" or "maintenance" medications. Rescue medications are short acting and taken for immediate relief of acute respiratory distress. Maintenance medications are used on a daily schedule to prevent acute respiratory distress. The effects of maintenance medications start within hours of administration and last for a longer period of time than rescue medications. Some inhalers contain combinations of rescue and maintenance medications. Because patients depend on

inhaled medications for disease control and current evidence shows that many patients do not use their inhalers correctly, nurses need to teach and reteach their patients about their safe and effective use (Ari, 2015) (see Skill 31.3).

One important aspect of patient teaching is to help the patient determine when the MDI, BAI, or DPI is empty and needs to be replaced. Floating an MDI in water to determine how much medication is left is not recommended because extra propellant causes the container to float even if no medication remains in the inhaler. Devices that count

BOX 31.18 PROCEDURAL GUIDELINES

Administering Rectal Suppositories

Delegation and Collaboration

The skill of rectal medication administration cannot be delegated to assistive personnel (AP). The nurse instructs the AP to:

- Report expected fecal discharge or bowel movement to the nurse.
- Report the occurrence of any potential side effects of medications to the nurse.
- Inform the nurse of any rectal pain or bleeding.

Equipment

Medication administration record (MAR) (electronic or printed); rectal suppository; water-soluble lubricating jelly; clean gloves; tissue; drape

Steps

1. Check accuracy and completeness of each MAR or computer printout with health care provider's written medication order. Check patient's name, medication name and dosage, route of administration, and time of administration. Clarify incomplete or unclear orders with health care provider before administration.

2. Review pertinent information related to medication, including action, purpose, normal dose and route, side effects, time of onset and peak action, indication, and nursing implications.

3. Review patient's medical history (e.g., history of rectal surgery or bleeding, cardiac problems), medication history, and history of allergies. List medication allergies on each page of the MAR and prominently display the list of allergies on the patient's medical record per agency policy. When patient has allergy, provide allergy bracelet.

4. Review any presenting signs and symptoms of GI alterations (e.g., constipation or diarrhea).

5. Assess patient's ability to hold suppository and position self to insert medication.

6. Review patient's knowledge of purpose of medication therapy and interest in self-administering suppository.

7. Perform hand hygiene. Collect appropriate equipment and MAR.

8. Prepare suppository for administration. Attend to procedure and avoid distraction. Check label of medication against MAR two times (see Skill 31.1). Preparation usually involves checking label when taking suppository out of refrigerator and before leaving preparation area. Check expiration date on container. *These are the first and second checks for accuracy.*

9. Take medication(s) to patient at correct time (see agency policy). Consider whether medication is time critical. During administration apply seven rights of medication administration.

10. Identify patient using at least two identifiers (e.g., name and birthday or name and medical record number) according to agency policy. Compare identifiers with information on patient's MAR or medical record.

11. At patient's bedside again compare MAR or computer printout with names of medications on medication labels and patient name. Ask patient whether he or she has allergies. *This is the third check for accuracy.*

12. Explain procedure to patient. Be specific if patient wishes to self-administer medication. Discuss purpose of each medication, action, and possible adverse effects. Allow patient to ask any questions about the medications. Explain procedure if patient plans to self-administer medication.

13. Perform hand hygiene. Arrange supplies at bedside and apply clean gloves. Close door or pull curtain.

14. Help patient assume left side-lying Sims' position with upper leg flexed upward.

15. If patient has mobility impairment, help into lateral position. Obtain help to turn patient and use pillows under upper arm and leg.

16. Keep patient draped with only anal area exposed.

17. Examine condition of anus externally. *Option:* Palpate rectal walls as needed (e.g., if impaction is suspected) (see Chapter 30). If you palpate rectal walls, dispose of gloves by turning them inside out and placing them in proper receptacle if they become soiled. Otherwise keep gloves on your hands and proceed to Step 19.

18. Perform hand hygiene and apply new pair of clean gloves (if previous gloves were soiled and discarded).

CLINICAL DECISION: Do not palpate patient's rectum if there is a recent history of rectal surgery. A suppository is contraindicated in the presence of active bleeding and diarrhea (Burchum and Rosenthal, 2019).

19. Remove suppository from foil wrapper and lubricate rounded end with water-soluble lubricant. Lubricate gloved index finger of dominant hand. If patient has hemorrhoids, use liberal amount of lubricant and touch area gently.

20. Ask patient to take slow, deep breaths through mouth and relax anal sphincter.

21. Retract patient's buttocks with nondominant hand. With gloved index finger of dominant hand, insert suppository gently through anus, past internal sphincter, and against rectal wall, 10 cm (4 inches) in adults (see illustration) or 5 cm (2 inches) in infants and children. You should feel rectal sphincter close around your finger.

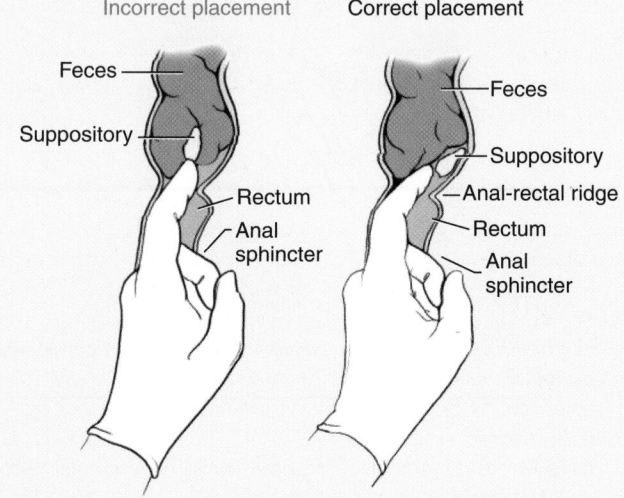

STEP 21 Inserting rectal suppository past sphincter and against rectal wall. (From DeWit S, O'Neill P: *Fundamental concepts and skills for nursing*, ed 4, Philadelphia, 2014, Saunders.)

CLINICAL DECISION: Do not insert suppository into a mass of fecal material; this will reduce effectiveness of medication.

22. *Option:* A suppository may be given through a colostomy (not ileostomy) if ordered. Patient should lie supine. Use small amount of water-soluble lubricant for insertion.

23. Withdraw finger and wipe patient's anal area.

24. Ask patient to remain flat or on side for 5 minutes.

25. Discard gloves by turning them inside out and dispose of them and used supplies in appropriate receptacle. Perform hand hygiene.

26. If suppository contains laxative or fecal softener, place nurse call system within reach so that patient can obtain help to reach bedpan or toilet.

27. If suppository was given for constipation, remind patient *not* to flush commode after bowel movement, so you can observe characteristics of stool.

28. Record the medication, dosage, route, and actual time and date of administration on MAR immediately after administration, not before. Include initials or signature.

29. Return to bedside within 5 minutes to determine whether suppository was expelled.

30. Ask whether patient experienced localized anal or rectal discomfort during insertion.

31. Evaluate patient at time of peak medication effect for relief of symptoms for which medication was prescribed.

32. Record patient response to medication, patient teaching, and validation of patient understanding of self-administration of suppository on flow sheet or nurses' notes in electronic health record (EHR) or chart.

33. **Use Teach-Back:** "I want to be sure I explained clearly to you how to insert a rectal suppository. Describe the steps you will follow to insert the suppository." Revise your instruction now or develop a plan for revised patient/family caregiver teaching if patient/family caregiver is not able to teach back correctly. Determines patient's/family caregiver's level of understanding of instructional topic.

down the number of remaining doses are available for MDIs. Some DPIs have mechanisms that indicate how many doses are left. However, these mechanisms are not always accurate. Therefore, to calculate how long medication in an inhaler will last, divide the number of doses in the container by the number of doses the patient takes per day. For example, a patient is to take albuterol 2 puffs 4 times a day. The canister has a total of 200 puffs. Complete the following calculation to determine how long the MDI will last:

$$2 \text{ puffs} \times 4 \text{ times a day} = 8 \text{ puffs per day}$$
$$200 \text{ puffs} \div 8 \text{ puffs per day} = 25 \text{ days}$$

The canister in this example will last 25 days. To ensure that the patient does not run out of medication, teach him or her to refill it at least 7 to 10 days before it runs out.

Administering Medications By Irrigations

Some medications irrigate or wash out a body cavity and are delivered through a stream of solution. Irrigations most commonly use sterile water, saline, or antiseptic solutions on the eye, ear, throat, vagina, or urinary tract. Use aseptic technique if there is a break in the skin or mucosa. Use clean technique when the cavity to be irrigated is not sterile, as in the case of the ear canal or vagina. Irrigations cleanse an area, instill a medication, or apply hot or cold to injured tissue (see Chapter 48).

Parenteral Administration of Medications

Parenteral administration of medications is the administration of medications by injection into body tissues. This is an invasive procedure that is performed using aseptic techniques (Box 31.19). A risk of infection occurs after a needle pierces the skin. This is an invasive procedure that is performed with the following aseptic techniques:

- Draw up medication quickly to avoid contaminating solutions. Do not allow ampules to stand open.
- Avoid letting a needle touch contaminated surfaces (e.g., outer edges of ampule or vial, outer surface of needle cap).
- Avoid touching length of plunger or inner part of barrel. Keep tip of syringe covered with cap or needle.
- Prepare skin by washing with soap and water if soiled. Use friction and a circular motion when cleaning with an antiseptic swab. Swab from center of site and move outward in a 5-cm (2-inch) radius.

Each type of injection requires certain skills to ensure that the medication reaches the proper location. The effects of a parenteral medication develop rapidly, depending on the rate of medication absorption. You must closely observe a patient's response to parenteral medications.

Equipment. You will administer parenteral medications by using a needle and a syringe, available in a variety of sizes. Each is designed to deliver a certain volume of a medication to a specific type of tissue. Determine the appropriate size of syringe, length and gauge of needle, volume of solution, and medication route based on the quantity and type of medication prescribed and the body size of a patient. Most syringes come with needleless systems or safety needles that help prevent needlestick injuries.

Syringes. Syringes consist of a cylindrical barrel with a tip designed to fit the hub of a hypodermic needle and a close-fitting plunger. Syringes are single use, disposable, and classified as being Luer-Lok or non–Luer-Lok. This terminology is based on the design of the tip of the syringe. Luer-Lok syringes have needles that are twisted onto the tip and lock themselves in place (Fig. 31.11, A and B). This design prevents the inadvertent removal of the needle. Non–Luer-Lok syringes (Fig. 31.11, C and D) have needles that slip onto the tip. Syringes come with or without a sterile needle and with a needleless sharp with engineered sharps injury protection (SESIP) device.

Syringes come in a variety of sizes, from 0.5 to 60 mL. It is unusual to use a syringe larger than 5 mL for an injection. A 1- to 3-mL syringe is usually adequate for a subcutaneous or IM injection. A larger volume creates discomfort. Use larger syringes to administer certain IV medications and to irrigate wounds or drainage tubes. Syringes often come prepackaged with a needle attached. However, you sometimes change a needle based on the route of administration and size of a patient.

The tuberculin syringe (see Fig. 31.11, C) is calibrated in sixteenths of a minim and hundredths of a milliliter and has a capacity of 1 mL. Use a tuberculin syringe to prepare small amounts of medications (e.g., ID or subcutaneous injections). A tuberculin syringe is also useful when preparing small, precise doses for infants or young children.

Insulin syringes (see Fig. 31.11, *D*) hold 0.3 mL to 1 mL, and low-dose insulin syringes (30 units per 0.3 mL or 50 units per 0.5 mL) hold 0.3 mL to 1 mL. Both come with preattached needles and are calibrated in units. Most insulin syringes are U-100s, designed for use with U-100–strength insulin. Each milliliter of solution contains 100 units of insulin.

Fill a syringe by pulling the plunger outward while the needle tip remains immersed in the prepared solution. Touch only the outside of the syringe barrel and the handle of the plunger to maintain sterility. Avoid letting any unsterile object touch the tip or inside of the barrel, the hub, the shaft of the plunger, or the needle (Fig. 31.12).

Needles. Some needles come packaged in individual sheaths to allow flexibility in choosing the right needle for a patient, whereas others are preattached to standard-size syringes. Most needles are made of stainless steel, and all are disposable. A needle has three parts: the hub, which fits onto the tip of a syringe; the shaft, which connects to the hub; and the bevel, or slanted tip (Fig. 31.13). The tip of a needle, or the

---

BOX 31.19 Preventing Infection During an Injection

- To prevent contaminating the solution, draw up medication quickly. Do not allow ampules to stand open.
- To prevent needle contamination, avoid letting a needle touch contaminated surfaces (e.g., outer edges of ampule or vial, outer surface of needle cap, nurse's hands, countertop, table surface).
- To prevent syringe contamination, avoid touching length of plunger or inner part of barrel. Keep tip of syringe covered with cap or needle.
- To prepare skin, wash with soap and water if soiled with dirt, drainage, or feces, and dry. Use friction and a circular motion while cleaning with an antiseptic swab. Swab from center of site and move outward in a 5-cm (2-inch) radius.

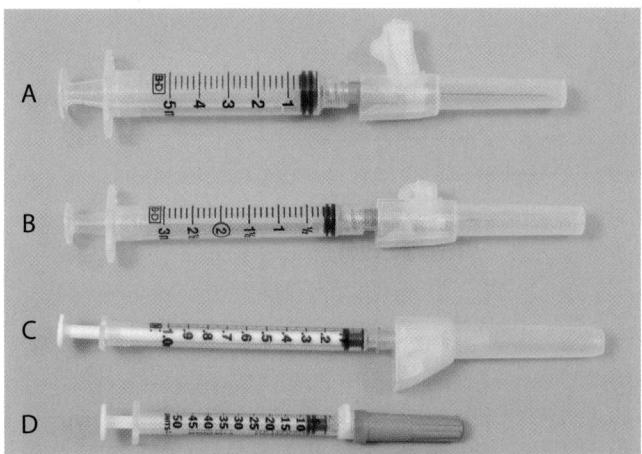

FIG. 31.11 Types of syringes. **A**, 5-mL syringe. **B**, 3-mL syringe. **C**, Tuberculin syringe marked in 0.01 (hundredths) for doses less than 1 mL. **D**, Insulin syringe marked in units (50).

bevel, is always slanted. The bevel creates a narrow slit when injected into tissue that quickly closes when the needle is removed to prevent leakage of medication, blood, or serum. Long, beveled tips are sharper and narrower, minimizing discomfort when entering tissue used for subcutaneous or IM injections.

Most needles vary in length from ¼ to 3 inches (Fig. 31.14). Choose the needle length according to a patient's size and weight and the type of tissue into which the medication is to be injected. Current evidence suggests that needle length should be based on a patient's weight (Holliday et al., 2019). There should be a 5-mm depth of muscle penetration for an IM injection (Hibbard et al., 2017). A child or slender adult generally requires a shorter needle. Use longer needles (1 to 1½ inches) for IM injections and a shorter needle (⅜ to ⅝ inch) for subcutaneous injections. As the needle gauge becomes smaller, the diameter becomes larger. The selection of a gauge depends on the viscosity of fluid to be injected or infused.

Disposable Injection Units. Single-dose, prefilled, disposable syringes are available for some medications. You do not need to prepare medication doses except perhaps to expel unneeded portions of medication or air. However, it is important to check the medication and concentration carefully because prefilled syringes appear very similar. Prefilled unit-dose systems such as Tubex and Carpuject include reusable plastic syringe holders and disposable, prefilled, sterile, glass cartridge units (Fig. 31.15). To assemble a prefilled system, place the cartridge barrel first into the plastic syringe holder. Following manufacturer's instructions, turn the plunger rod to the left (counterclockwise) and the lock to the right (clockwise) until it "clicks." Finally, remove the needle guard and advance the plunger to expel air and excess medication, as with a regular syringe. The cartridge may be used with SESIP needles. After administering a medication, dispose of the glass cartridge safely in a puncture-proof and leak-proof container. This design reduces the risk for needlestick injury.

Preparing an Injection From an Ampule. Ampules contain single doses of medication in a liquid. They are available in several sizes, from 1 mL to 10 mL or more (Fig. 31.16, *A*). An ampule is made of glass with a constricted neck that must be snapped off to allow access to the medication. A colored ring around the neck indicates where the ampule is prescored so that you can break it easily. Carefully aspirate the medication into a syringe (see Skill 31.4) with a filter needle. Filter needles

must be used when preparing medication from a glass ampule to prevent glass particles from being drawn into the syringe (Joo et al., 2016). *Do not* use a filter needle to administer a medication. Place an appropriate-size needle on the syringe after withdrawing the medication.

Preparing an Injection From a Vial. A vial is a single-dose or multi-dose container with a rubber seal at the top (see Fig. 31.16, *B*). A metal cap protects the seal until it is ready for use. Vials contain liquid or dry forms of medications. Medications that are unstable in solution are packaged dry. The vial label specifies the solvent or diluent used to dissolve the medication and the amount of diluent needed to prepare a desired medication concentration. Normal saline and sterile distilled water are commonly used to dissolve medications.

Unlike the ampule, the vial is a closed system, and air needs to be injected into it to permit easy withdrawal of the solution. Failure to inject air when withdrawing creates a vacuum within the vial that makes withdrawal difficult. If concerned about drawing up parts of the rubber stopper or other particles into the syringe, use a filter needle when preparing medications from vials (ISMP, 2015d). Some vials contain powder, which is mixed with a diluent during preparation and before injection (see Skill 31.4). After mixing multidose vials, make a label that includes the date and time of mixing and the concentration of medication per milliliter. Some multidose vials require refrigeration after the contents are reconstituted.

Mixing Medications. If two medications are compatible, it is possible to mix them in one injection if the total dose is within accepted limits. This prevents a patient from having to receive more than one injection at a time. Most nursing units have charts that list common compatible medications. If there is any uncertainty about medication compatibilities, consult a pharmacist or a medication reference.

Mixing Medications From a Vial and an Ampule. When mixing medication from both a vial and ampule, prepare medication from the vial first. Using the same syringe and filter needle, next withdraw medication from the ampule. Nurses prepare the combination in this

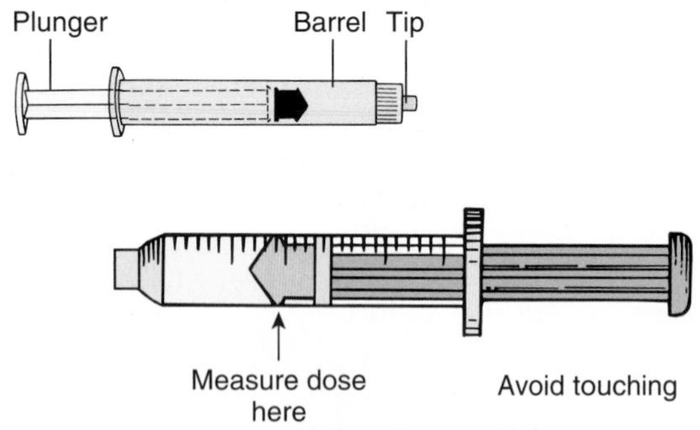

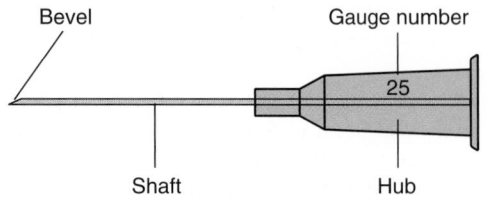

Plunger   Barrel Tip

Measure dose here   Avoid touching

FIG. 31.12 Parts of a syringe.

Bevel   Gauge number

25

Shaft   Hub

FIG. 31.13 Parts of the needle.

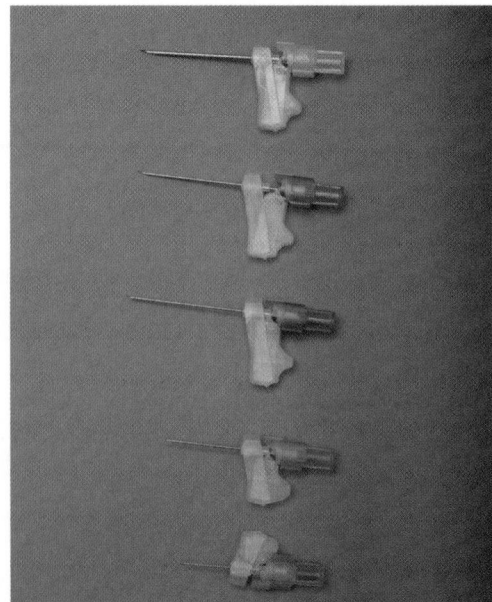

FIG. 31.14 Hypodermic needles *(top to bottom)*: 18 gauge, 1½-inch length; 21 gauge, 1½-inch length; 22 gauge, 1½-inch length; 23 gauge, 1-inch length; and 25 gauge, 5/8-inch length.

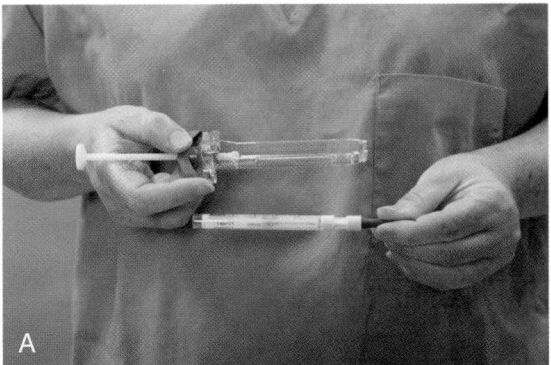

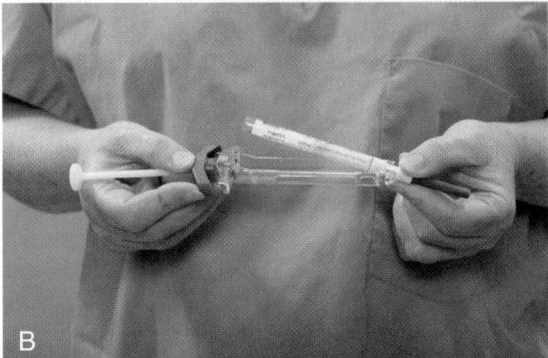

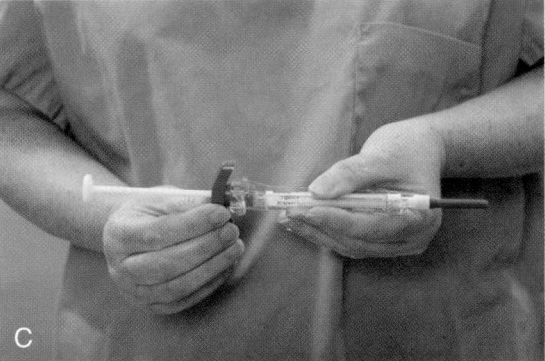

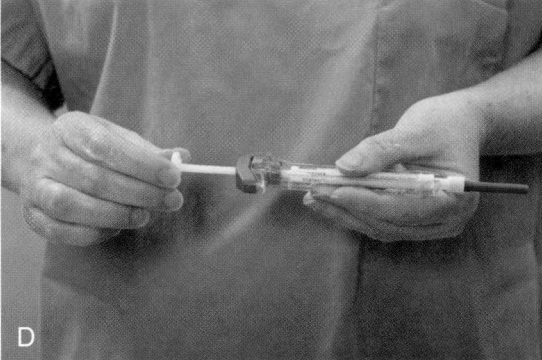

FIG. 31.15 **A,** Carpuject syringe and prefilled sterile cartridge with needle. **B,** Assembling the Carpuject. **C,** Cartridge slides into syringe barrel. Turn and lock syringe into cartridge. **D,** Screw plunger into end of cartridge. Expel excess medication to obtain accurate dose (not pictured).

order because it is not necessary to add air to withdraw medication from an ampule.

Mixing Medications From Two Vials. Apply these principles when mixing medications from two vials:

1. Do not contaminate one medication with another.
2. Ensure that the final dose is accurate.
3. Maintain aseptic technique.

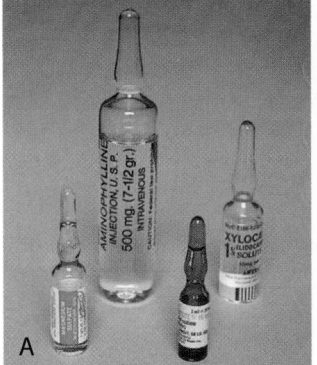
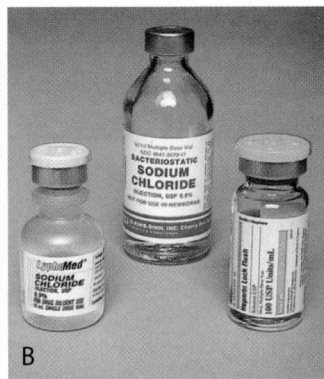

FIG. 31.16 **A,** Medication in ampules. **B,** Medication in vials.

Use only one syringe with a needle or needleless access device attached to mix medications from two vials (Fig. 31.17). Aspirate the volume of air equivalent to the dose of the first medication (vial A) (see Fig. 31.17, *A*). Inject the air into vial A, making sure that the needle does not touch the solution. Withdraw the needle and aspirate air equivalent to the dose of the second medication (vial B). Inject the volume of air into vial B (see Fig. 31.17, *B*). Immediately withdraw the medication from vial B into the syringe and insert the needle back into vial A, being careful not to push the plunger and expel the medication within the syringe into the vial. Withdraw the desired amount of medication from vial A into the syringe (see Fig. 31.17, *C*). After withdrawing the necessary amount, withdraw the needle and apply a new safety needle or needleless access device suitable for injection.

Insulin Preparation. Insulin is the hormone used to treat diabetes mellitus. It is administered by injection because the GI tract breaks down and destroys an oral form of insulin. Most patients with diabetes mellitus who take insulin injections learn to administer their own injections. In the United States and Canada, health care providers usually prescribe insulin in concentrations of 100 units per milliliter of solution. This is called *U-100 insulin*. Insulin is also commercially available in concentrations of 500 units per milliliter of solution; it is called *U-500 insulin*. U-500 insulin is 5 times as strong as U-100 insulin and is used only in rare cases when patients are very resistant to insulin. Insulin injection guidelines have been developed and modified over the past several years in response to increasing evidence and research about best practices for patient assessment and site selection (McCulloch et al., 2018). Based on this evidence:

- Use the same technique for both insulin syringes and insulin pens.
- Use a body area where 2.5 cm (1 inch) of subcutaneous fat can be pinched.
- Use a 27-gauge needle, perpendicular to the pinched skin.
- Do not aspirate the injection and hold needle in place for several seconds. This is especially important with insulin pens to prevent leakage of medication.
- Insulin is absorbed rapidly through the abdominal wall, so the abdomen should be the first choice for sites when using rapid-acting insulin.

Use the correct syringe when preparing insulin. Use a 100-unit insulin syringe or an insulin pen to prepare U-100 insulin. Until recently there was no syringe designed to prepare U-500 insulin, and many medication errors resulted with this kind of insulin. To prevent errors, ensure that the health care provider order for U-500 specifies units and that the patient is taught the difference between

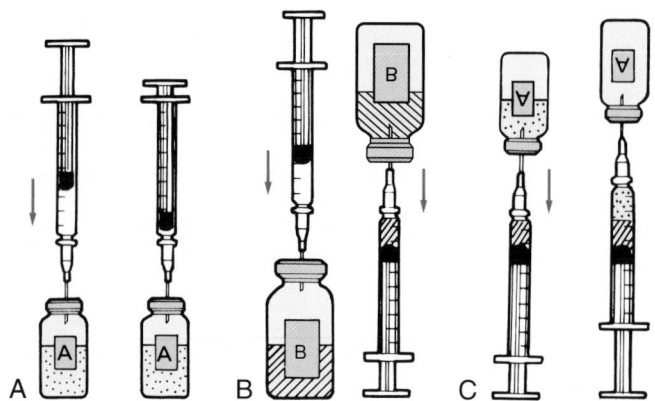

FIG. 31.17 **A,** Injecting air into vial A. **B,** Injecting air into vial B and withdrawing dose. **C,** Withdrawing medication from vial A; medications are now mixed.

U-500 and U-100 syringes (Consumer Med Safety, 2018b; ISMP, 2017b). Verify every injection you prepare with another nurse before administering it. Additional safety measures common with U-500 insulin include listing the insulin as being concentrated in computerized medication dispensing systems, making health care providers and pharmacists verify that a patient is to receive U-500 insulin when it is ordered, and stocking U-500 insulin on patient care units only when it is ordered for a specific patient (ISMP, 2017b; ISMP, 2018c).

Insulin is classified by rate of action, including rapid-acting, short-acting, intermediate-acting, and long-acting. To provide safe and effective care, you need to know the onset, peak, and duration for each of your patients' ordered insulin doses. Refer to a medication reference or consult with a pharmacist if you are unsure of this information. Regular insulin is the only type of insulin that can be given intravenously.

A patient with diabetes mellitus sometimes requires more than one type of insulin. For example, by receiving a short-acting (regular) and intermediate-acting (NPH) insulin, a patient receives more sustained control of blood glucose levels over 24 hours. The timing of insulin injections attempts to imitate the normal pattern of insulin release from the pancreas. Some insulins come in a stable premixed solution (e.g., 70/30 insulin is 70% NPH [intermediate] and 30% regular), eliminating the need to mix the insulins in a syringe. Other patients use an insulin pen. The insulin pen provides multiple doses and allows a patient to dial in the dose, avoiding the need to use a syringe for insulin preparation. Research shows that different types of a patient's blood cells can enter into the insulin pen after an injection. Several US health care agencies recently reported that the same insulin pen was inadvertently used on multiple patients, exposing the patients to bloodborne illnesses (e.g., human immunodeficiency virus [HIV], hepatitis B, and hepatitis C). Thus, the ISMP (2017b) recommends that insulin pens be used only at home and that inpatient settings provide an insulin pen for a single patient use.

Insulin is ordered by a specific dose at select times. Correction or correctional insulin, also known as sliding-scale insulin, provides a dose of insulin based on the patient's blood glucose level (Box 31.20). The term *correctional insulin* is preferred because it indicates that small doses of rapid- or short-acting insulin are needed to correct a patient's elevated blood sugar. Reliance on correctional insulin is unlikely to achieve long-term glucose control; therefore, it should be ordered only on a temporary basis (ISMP, 2017b).

Before drawing up insulin doses, gently roll all cloudy insulin preparations between the palms of the hands to resuspend the insulin.

Do not shake insulin vials; shaking causes bubbles to form. Bubbles take up space in the syringe and alter the dose.

If more than one type of insulin is required to manage the patient's diabetes, you mix two different types of insulin into one syringe *if* they are compatible (Box 31.21). If regular and intermediate-acting insulins are ordered, prepare the regular insulin first to prevent it from becoming contaminated with the intermediate-acting insulin (ISMP, 2017b). Use the following principles when mixing insulins (ISMP, 2017b; McCulloch et al., 2018):

- Patients whose blood glucose levels are well controlled on a mixed-insulin dose need to maintain their individual routine when preparing and administering their insulin.
- Do not mix insulin with any other medications or diluents unless approved by the health care provider.
- Never mix insulin glargine or insulin detemir with other types of insulin.
- Inject rapid-acting insulins mixed with NPH insulin within 15 minutes before a meal.
- Verify insulin doses with another nurse while you are preparing the injection.

Administering Injections

Each injection route differs based on the type of tissues the medication enters. The characteristics of the tissues influence the rate of medication absorption, affecting the onset of medication action. Before injecting a medication, know the volume of the medication to administer, the characteristics and viscosity of the medication, and the location of anatomical structures underlying injection sites (see Skill 31.5).

If you do not administer injections correctly, negative patient outcomes result. Failure to select an injection site in relation to anatomical landmarks results in nerve or bone damage during needle insertion. Inability to maintain stability of the needle and syringe unit can result in pain and tissue damage. If you fail to aspirate the syringe before injecting an IM medication, the medication may be injected accidentally directly into an artery or vein. Injecting too large a volume of medication for the site selected causes extreme pain and results in local tissue damage.

Many patients, particularly children, fear injections. Patients with serious or chronic illness often are given several injections daily. Minimize discomfort in the following ways:

- Use a sharp-beveled needle in the smallest suitable length and gauge.
- Position a patient as comfortably as possible to reduce muscular tension.
- Select the proper injection site, using anatomical landmarks.
- Apply a vapocoolant spray (e.g., Fluori-Methane spray or ethyl chloride) or topical anesthetic (e.g., EMLA cream) to the injection

BOX 31.21   PROCEDURAL GUIDELINES

Mixing Two Types of Insulin in One Syringe

Delegation and Collaboration

The skill of mixing two types of insulin in one syringe cannot be delegated to assistive personnel (AP). The nurse directs the AP about:

- Potential side effects of medications and the need to immediately report their occurrence to the nurse.

Equipment

Medication administration record (MAR) (printed or electronic); insulin vials, insulin syringe, antiseptic swab

Steps

1. Check accuracy and completeness of MAR or computer printout with health care provider's written medication order. Check patient's name, medication name and dosage, route of administration, and time of administration. Clarify incomplete or unclear orders with health care provider before administration.
2. Review medication and medical history (e.g., type of diabetes, reason for elevated blood sugar) and allergies to medications, food, and latex.
3. Verify insulin labels carefully against MAR before preparing the dose to ensure that you give the correct type of insulin. *This is the first check for accuracy.*
4. Perform hand hygiene.
5. If patient takes insulin that is cloudy, roll the bottle of insulin between the hands to resuspend the insulin preparation.
6. Wipe off tops of both insulin vials with alcohol swabs and allow to dry.
7. Verify insulin dosages against MAR a second time. *This is the second accuracy check.*
8. If mixing rapid- or short-acting insulin with intermediate-acting insulin, take insulin syringe and aspirate volume of air equivalent to dose to be withdrawn from intermediate-acting insulin first. If two intermediate-acting insulins are mixed, it makes no difference which vial you prepare first.
9. Insert needle and inject air into vial of intermediate-acting insulin. Do not let the tip of the needle touch the insulin.
10. Remove the syringe from the vial of intermediate-acting insulin without aspirating medication.
11. With the same syringe, inject air equal to the dose of rapid- or short-acting insulin into the vial and withdraw the correct dose into the syringe.
12. Remove the syringe from the rapid- or short-acting insulin and get rid of air bubbles to ensure accurate dosing.
13. After verifying insulin dosages with MAR a third time, show insulin prepared in syringe to another nurse to verify that you prepared correct dosage of insulin. *This is the third accuracy check.* Determine which point on syringe scale combined units of insulin measure by adding the number of units of both insulins together (e.g., 5 units regular + 10 units NPH = 15 units total).
14. Place the needle of the syringe back into the vial of intermediate-acting insulin. Be careful not to push plunger and inject insulin in syringe into the vial.
15. Invert the vial and carefully withdraw the desired amount of insulin into syringe.
16. Withdraw needle and check fluid level in syringe. Keep needle of prepared syringe sheathed or capped until ready to administer medication. Show another nurse the syringe to verify that you prepared the correct dose.
17. Dispose of soiled supplies in proper receptacle. Place empty vials in puncture-proof and leak-proof container and perform hand hygiene.
18. Because rapid- or short-acting insulin binds with intermediate-acting insulin, which reduces the action of the faster-acting insulin, administer mixture within 5 minutes of preparing it.

Modified from McCulloch D, et al: *General principles of insulin therapy in diabetes mellitus,* UpToDate, 2018. http://www.uptodate.com/contents/general-principles-of-insulin-therapy-in-diabetes-mellitus. Accessed May 16, 2018.

site before giving the medication when possible (see agency policy).

- Divert the patient's attention from the injection through conversation using open-ended questioning.
- Insert the needle quickly and smoothly to minimize tissue pulling.
- Hold the syringe steady while the needle remains in tissues.
- Inject the medication slowly and steadily.

Subcutaneous Injections. Subcutaneous injections involve placing medications into the loose connective tissue under the dermis (see Skill 31.5). Because subcutaneous tissue is not as richly supplied with blood as the muscles, medication absorption is somewhat slower than with IM injections. Physical exercise or application of hot or cold compresses influences the rate of drug absorption by altering local blood flow to tissues. Any condition that impairs blood flow is a contraindication for subcutaneous injections. Because subcutaneous tissue contains pain receptors, a patient often experiences slight discomfort.

The best subcutaneous injection sites include the outer posterior aspect of the upper arms, the abdomen from below the costal margins to the iliac crests, and the anterior aspects of the thighs (Fig. 31.18). The site most frequently recommended for heparin injections is the abdomen (Fig. 31.19). Alternative subcutaneous sites for other medications include the scapular areas of the upper back and the upper ventral or dorsal gluteal areas. The injection site you choose needs to be free of skin lesions, bony prominences, and large underlying muscles or nerves.

The administration of low-molecular-weight heparin (LMWH) (e.g., enoxaparin) requires special considerations. When injecting the medication, use the right or left side of the abdomen at least 5 cm (2 inches) from the umbilicus (the patient's "love handles") and pinch the injection site as you insert the needle. Administer LMWH in its prefilled syringe with the attached needle, and do not expel the air bubble in the syringe before giving the medication.

Use U-100 insulin syringes with preattached 31- to 25-gauge needles when giving U-100 insulin and U-500 insulin syringes when giving U-500 insulin. ISMP (2017b; 2018c) recommends the use of individual patient insulin pens for all insulin administration. Recommended sites for insulin injections include the upper arm and the anterior and lateral parts of the thigh, buttocks, and abdomen. Rotating injections within the same body part (intrasite rotation) provides more consistency in the absorption of the insulin. For example, if a patient receives morning insulin in the right arm, give the next injection in a different place in the same arm. The injections are to be given at least 2.5 cm (1 inch) away from the previous site. Injection sites should not be used again for at least 1 month (McCulloch et al., 2018). The rate of insulin absorption varies based on the site; the abdomen has the quickest absorption, followed by the arms, thighs, and buttocks (McCulloch et al., 2018).

Subcutaneous tissue is sensitive to irritating solutions and large volumes of medications. Thus, you administer only small volumes (0.5 to 1.5 mL) of water-soluble medications subcutaneously to adults. You give smaller volumes up to 0.5 mL to children (Hockenberry et al.,

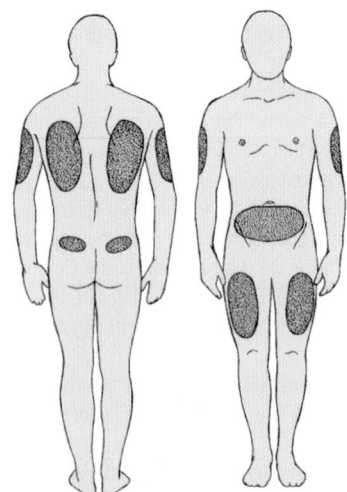

FIG. 31.18 Sites recommended for subcutaneous injections.

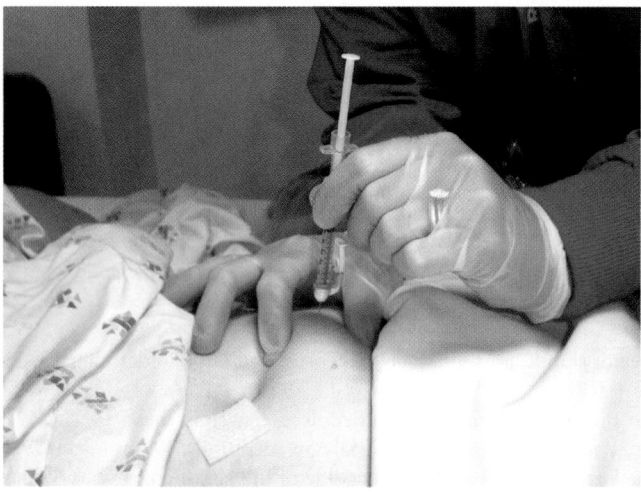

FIG. 31.19 Giving subcutaneous heparin in abdomen.

2019). Hardened, painful lumps called *sterile abscesses* occur under the skin if medication collects within the tissues.

A patient's body weight indicates the depth of the subcutaneous layer. Therefore, choose the needle length and angle of insertion based on a patient's weight and an estimation of the amount of subcutaneous tissue (Larkin et al., 2018). Nurses typically use a 25-gauge, ⅝-inch (16-mm) needle inserted at a 45-degree angle (Fig. 31.20) or a ½-inch (12-mm) needle inserted at a 90-degree angle to administer subcutaneous medications to a normal-size adult patient. Some children require only a ½-inch needle. If the patient is obese, pinch the tissue and use a needle long enough to insert through fatty tissue at the base of the skinfold. Thin patients often do not have sufficient tissue for subcutaneous injections; the upper abdomen is usually the best site in this case. To ensure that a subcutaneous medication reaches the subcutaneous tissue, follow this rule: If you can grasp 2 inches (5 cm) of tissue, insert the needle at a 90-degree angle; if you can grasp 2.5 cm (1 inch) of tissue, insert the needle at a 45-degree angle.

Newer research in insulin administration shows that insulin needles that are ⁵⁄₁₆ (8 mm) or longer often enter the muscles of men and people with a body mass index (BMI) of 25 or less. Shorter (³⁄₁₆-inch or 4- to 5-mm) needles were associated with less pain, adequate control of blood sugars, and minimal leakage of medication (ISMP, 2017b). Thus, when administering insulin, you should use needles of ³⁄₁₆ inch (4 to 5 mm) administered at a 90-degree angle to reduce pain and achieve adequate control of blood sugars with minimal adverse effects for people of all BMIs, including children (Levitsky et al., 2017).

Several new technologies are available for administration of subcutaneous injections. *Injection pens* are a technology that patients can use to self-administer medications (e.g., epinephrine, insulin, or interferon) subcutaneously (Fig. 31.21). They offer a convenient delivery method using prefilled, disposable cartridges. The patient pinches the skin, inserts the needle, and injects a predetermined medication dose. Teaching is essential to ensure that patients use the correct injection technique and deliver the correct dose of medication. Patients need to be taught the importance of purging the pen before a dose is given. The disadvantages to this technology include increased risk for needlestick injury and user's lack of knowledge and skill in administration technique (ISMP, 2017b). One new technology is a *needleless jet injection system* that administers subcutaneous medications without the use of needles. Needle-free injections use high pressure to penetrate the skin with the medication into the subcutaneous tissue (Fig. 31.22). Another new advance in subcutaneous injection is the *subcutaneous injection device* (e.g.,

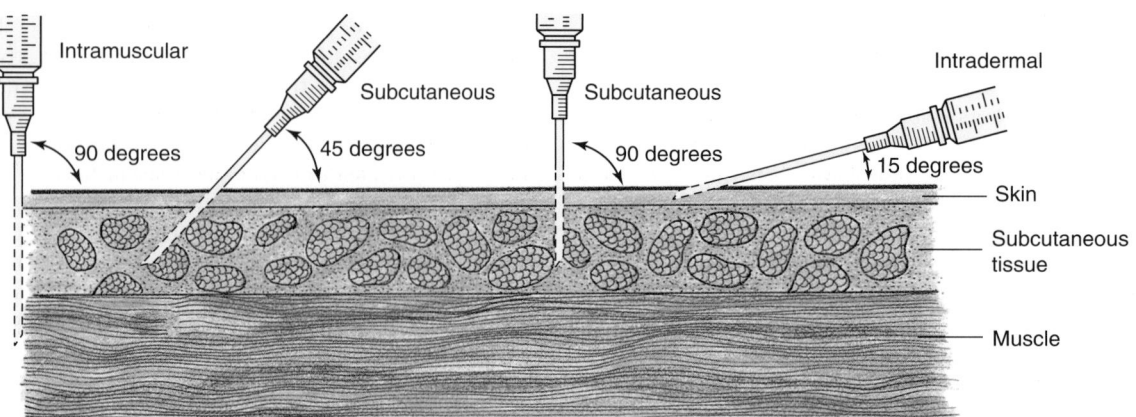

FIG. 31.20 Comparison of angles of insertion for intramuscular (90 degrees), subcutaneous (45 to 90 degrees), and intradermal (15 degrees) injections.

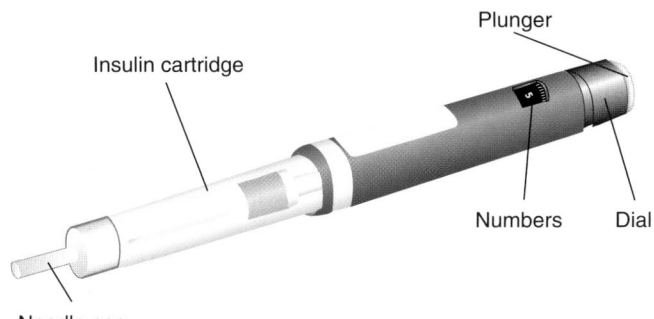

FIG. 31.21 Insulin injection pen. (From Lewis SM, et al: *Medical-surgical nursing,* ed 10, St Louis, 2017, Elsevier.)

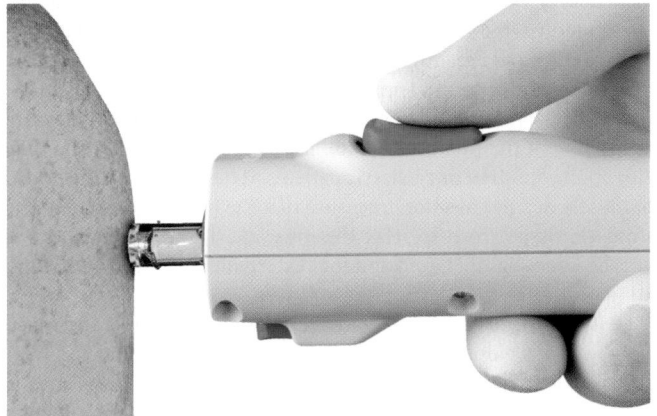

FIG. 31.22 Jet injection system is held perpendicular to skin. (Image courtesy Pharmajet. All rights reserved.)

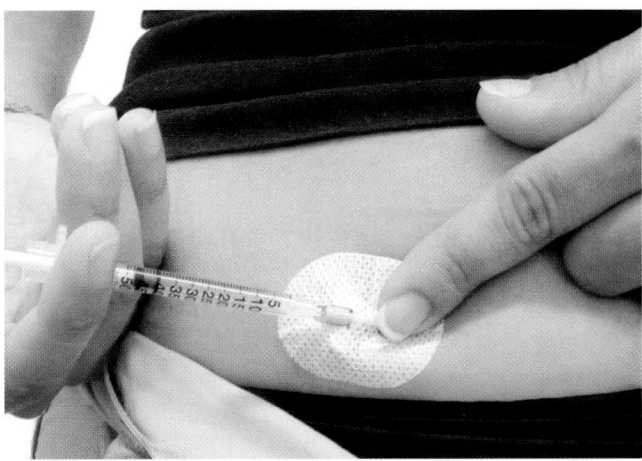

FIG. 31.23 Subcutaneous device. (Image courtesy IntraPump Infusion Systems. All rights reserved.)

insuflon) (Fig. 31.23), which is inserted into the subcutaneous tissue; the needle is then removed, leaving the cannula in the tissue to provide an avenue for administering medications for up to 3 days without having to puncture the skin with each injection.

Intramuscular Injections. The intramuscular (IM) injection route deposits medication into deep muscle tissue, which has a rich blood supply, allowing medication to absorb faster than by the subcutaneous route. However, there is a risk for injecting medications directly into blood vessels. Any factor that interferes with local tissue blood flow affects the rate and extent of medication absorption. In addition, if a medication is not injected correctly into a muscle, complications can arise such as abscess, hematoma, ecchymosis, pain, and vascular and nerve injury (Kaya et al., 2015).

The viscosity of the medication, injection site, patient's weight, and amount of adipose tissue influence needle size selection. Determine needle gauge by the medication to be administered. Therefore, whenever administering a medication by the IM route, first verify that the injection is justified (CDC, 2017; WHO, 2016). Some medications, such as hepatitis B and tetanus, diphtheria, and pertussis (Tdap) immunizations, are given only intramuscularly.

Use a longer and heavier-gauge needle to pass through subcutaneous tissue and penetrate deep muscle tissue (see Skill 31.5). A patient's BMI and the amount of adipose tissue influence needle size selection. The choice of needle length and site of injection must be made based on the size of the muscle, the thickness of adipose tissue at the injection site, the volume to be administered, injection technique, and the depth below the muscle surface to be injected (CDC, 2017). Investigate other medication routes, especially when IM injections are ordered for obese

patients (Larkin et al., 2018). Note that the most common intramuscular injections are immunizations.

The angle of insertion for an IM injection is 90 degrees (see Fig. 31.20). Muscle is less sensitive to irritating and viscous medications. A normal, well-developed adult patient tolerates 2 to 5 mL of medication into a larger muscle without severe muscle discomfort (Hopkins and Arias, 2013). However, larger volumes of medication (4 to 5 mL) are unlikely to be absorbed properly. Children, older adults, and thin patients tolerate only 2 mL of an IM injection. Do not give more than 1 mL to small children and older infants, and do not give more than 0.5 mL to smaller infants (Hockenberry et al., 2019).

Assess a muscle before giving an injection. Properly identify the site for the IM injection by palpating bony landmarks, and be aware of the potential complications associated with each site. The site needs to be free of tenderness because repeated injections in the same muscle cause severe discomfort. With the patient relaxed, palpate the muscle to rule out any hardened lesions. Minimize discomfort during an injection by helping a patient assume a position that helps to reduce muscle strain. Other interventions such as distraction and applying pressure to an IM site decrease pain during an injection.

Rotate IM injection sites to decrease the risk for tissue hypertrophy. Emaciated or atrophied muscles absorb medication poorly; thus, avoid their use when possible. The Z-track method, a technique for pulling the skin during an injection, is recommended for IM injections (Ogston-Tuck, 2014b; Yilmaz, et al., 2016). It prevents leakage of medication into subcutaneous tissues, seals medication in the muscle, and minimizes irritation. To use the Z-track method, apply the appropriate-size needle to the syringe and select an IM site, preferably in a large, deep muscle such as the ventrogluteal. Pull the overlying skin and subcutaneous tissues approximately 2.5 to 3.5 cm (1 to 1 ½ inches) laterally to the side with the ulnar side of the nondominant hand. Hold the skin in this position until you have administered the injection (Fig. 31.24A). After cleaning a site, inject the needle deeply into the muscle. To reduce injection site discomfort, there is no longer any need to aspirate after the needle is injected when *administering vaccines* (CDC, 2017). It is the nurse's responsibility to follow agency policy for aspirating vaccines after injecting the needle. Keep the needle inserted for 10 seconds to allow the medication to disperse evenly. Release the skin after withdrawing the needle. This leaves a zigzag path that seals the needle track wherever tissue planes slide across one another see (Fig. 31.24B). The medication is sealed in the muscle tissue.

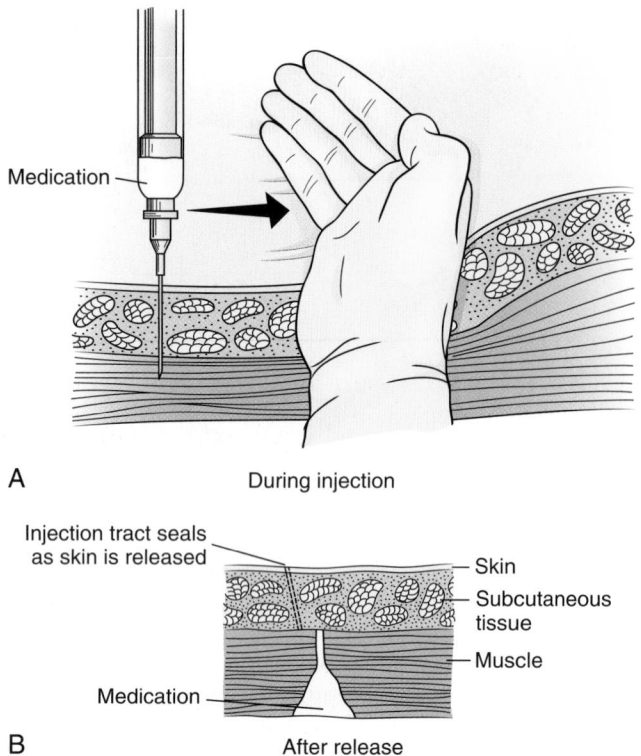

A   During injection

B   After release

FIG. 31.24 A, Pulling on overlying skin during intramuscular injection moves tissue to prevent later tracking. **B,** Z-track method of injection prevents deposit of medication into sensitive tissue.

Sites. When selecting an IM site, consider the following: Is the area free of infection or necrosis? Are there local areas of bruising or abrasions? What is the location of underlying bones, nerves, and major blood vessels? What volume of medication is to be administered? Each site has different advantages and disadvantages.

Ventrogluteal. The ventrogluteal muscle is the preferred and safest injection site for all adults, children, and infants, especially for large-volume, viscous, and irritating medications (CDC, 2017; Hockenberry et al., 2019; Hopkins and Arias, 2013; Kara et al., 2015). The site involves the gluteus medius where the thickness of subcutaneous tissue is less than other injection sites and there are relatively fewer nerves and blood vessels (Kara et al., 2015). Furthermore, in this site, the muscles are large, well established, and the muscle limit points are easy to find (Kara et al., 2015). Locate the ventrogluteal muscle by positioning the patient in a supine or lateral position. One way to locate the ventrogluteal muscle site to use is by the "V" method (Kara et al., 2015). You position a patient in a supine or lateral position with the knee and hip flexed to relax the muscle. Use your right hand for the left hip and your left hand for the right hip. For example, if you are administering the injection into the patient's left hip, place the palm of your right hand over the greater trochanter of the patient's hip with your wrist perpendicular to the femur. Then move your thumb toward the patient's groin and your index finger toward the anterior superior iliac spine. Extend or open your middle finger back along the iliac crest toward the patient's buttock. The index finger, middle finger and the iliac crest form a V-shaped triangle, with the injection site in the center of the triangle (Fig. 31.25A-C) (Kara et al., 2015; Larkin et al., 2018).

There has been some evidence to suggest that the "V" technique is not always reliable because of differences in nurses' hand structure and patients' body structure, especially when a patient is obese (Kara et al., 2015; Larkin et al., 2017). Thus, the "G" method, or geometric

method, is another option for identifying the correct ventrogluteal site (Fig. 31.26). With a patient in the sidelying position you reference three bone prominences and draw imaginary lines between the ends of the bones (Kara et al., 2015). You imagine lines drawn from the patient's greater trochanter to the iliac crest, and then to the anterosuperior iliac spine, and from the greater trochanter to the anterosuperior iliac spine. Thus, a triangle is created by the imaginary lines. After that, draw median lines from every single corner of triangle to the opposite side. The convergence point of the three median lines is the center for the triangle, the needle entry point for intramuscular injections (Kaya et al., 2015).

Vastus Lateralis. The vastus lateralis muscle is another injection site used in adults and is the preferred site for administration of biologicals (e.g., immunizations) to infants, toddlers, and children (CDC, 2017; Hockenberry et al., 2019). The muscle is thick and well developed; it is located on the anterolateral aspect of the thigh. It extends in an adult from a hand breadth above the knee to a hand breadth below the greater trochanter of the femur (Fig. 31.27). Use the middle third of the muscle for injection. The width of the muscle usually extends from the midline of the thigh to the midline of the outer side of the thigh. With young children or cachectic patients, it helps to grasp the body of the muscle during injection to ensure that the medication is deposited in muscle tissue. To help relax the muscle, ask the patient to lie flat with the knee slightly flexed and foot externally rotated or to assume a sitting position.

Deltoid. Although the deltoid site is easily accessible, the muscle is not well developed in many adults. There is potential for injury because the axillary, radial, brachial, and ulnar nerves and the brachial artery lie within the upper arm under the triceps and along the humerus (Fig. 31.28). *Carefully assess the condition of the deltoid muscle, consult medication references for suitability of medication, and carefully locate the injection site using anatomical landmarks.* Use this site for small medication volumes (less than 2 mL); administration of routine immunizations in toddlers, older children, and adults; or when other sites are inaccessible because of dressings or casts (CDC, 2017; Hopkins and Arias, 2013).

Locate the deltoid muscle by fully exposing the patient's upper arm and shoulder and asking him or her to relax the arm at the side or by supporting the patient's arm and flexing the elbow. Do not roll up any tight-fitting sleeve. Allow the patient to sit or lie down. Palpate the lower edge of the acromion process, which forms the base of a triangle in line with the midpoint of the lateral aspect of the upper arm. The injection site is in the center of the triangle, about 3 to 5 cm (1 to 2 inches) below the acromion process (see Fig. 31.28B). You locate the apex of the triangle by placing four fingers across the deltoid muscle, with the top finger along the acromion process. The injection site is three finger widths below the acromion process.

Intradermal Injections. ID injections typically are used for skin testing (e.g., tuberculin screening and allergy tests). Because these medications are potent, they are injected into the dermis, where blood supply is reduced and medication absorption occurs slowly. Some patients have a severe anaphylactic reaction if medications enter the circulation too rapidly. You need to choose skin-testing sites that allow you to easily assess for changes in color and tissue integrity. Thus, ID sites need to be lightly pigmented, free of lesions, and relatively hairless. The inner forearm and upper back are ideal locations.

Use a tuberculin or small hypodermic syringe for skin testing. The angle of insertion for an ID injection is 5 to 15 degrees (see Fig. 31.20), and the bevel of the needle is pointed up. As you inject the medication, a small bleb resembling a mosquito bite appears on the surface of the skin. If a bleb does not appear or if the site bleeds after needle

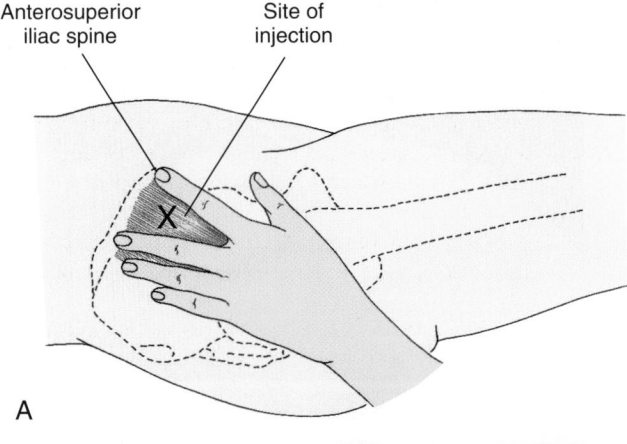

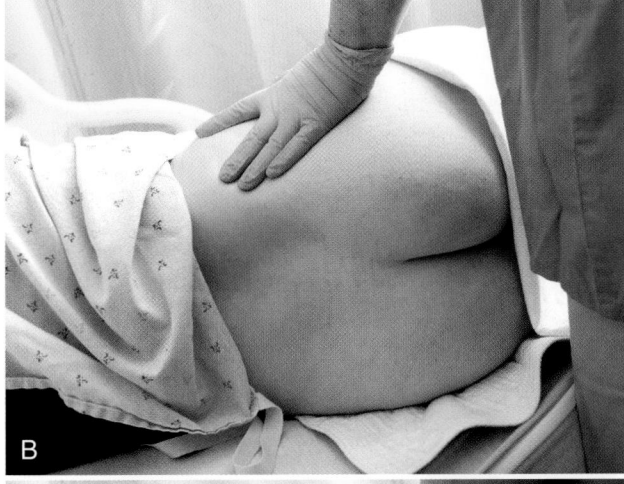

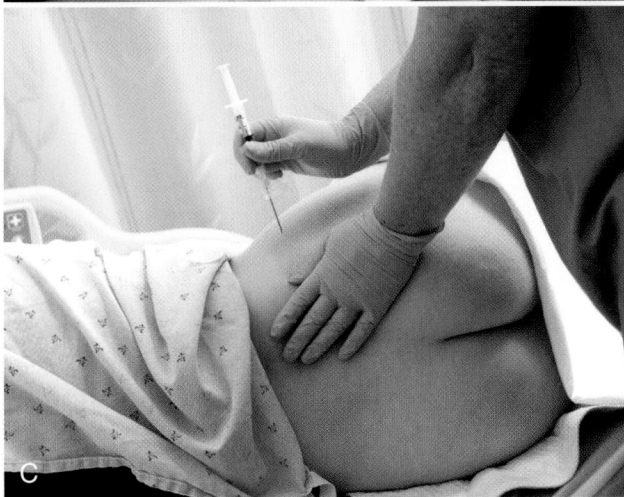

FIG. 31.25 A, Landmarks for ventrogluteal site. B, Locating ventrogluteal site in patient. C, Giving intramuscular injection in ventrogluteal muscle using Z-track method.

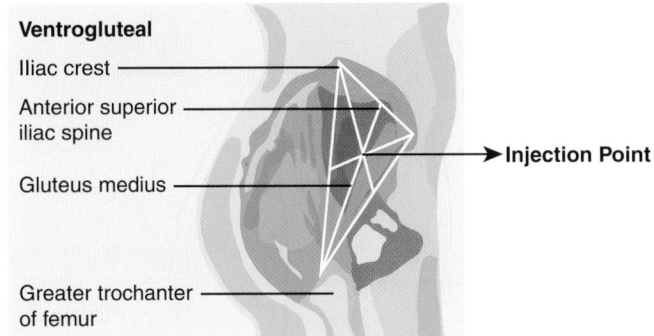

FIG. 31.26 Determination of intramuscular injection site using the G method. (From Kaya N, et al: The reliability of site determination methods in ventrogluteal area injection: a cross-sectional study, *Int J Nurs Stud* 52:355, 2015.)

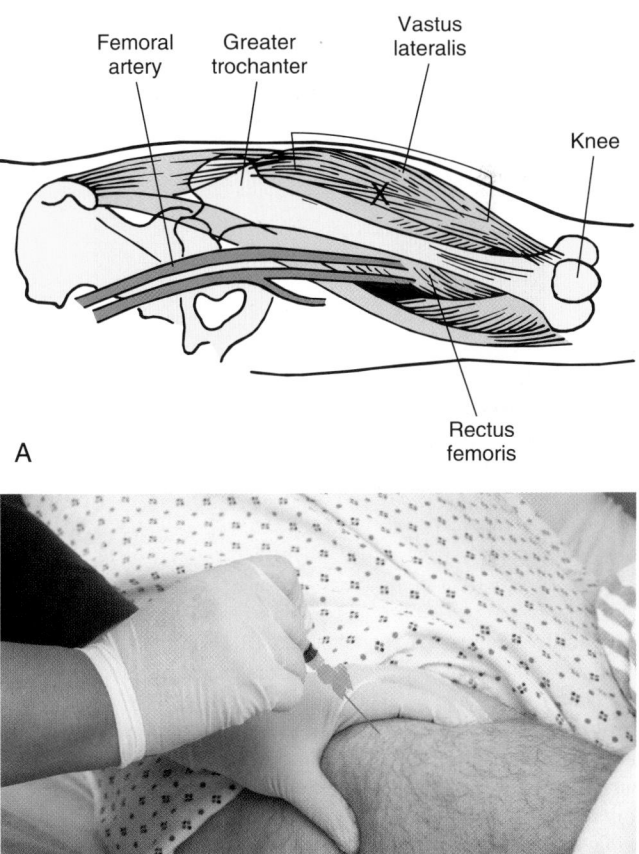

FIG. 31.27 A, Landmarks for vastus lateralis site. B, Giving intramuscular injection in vastus lateralis muscle.

withdrawal, there is a good chance that the medication entered subcutaneous tissues. In this case test results will not be valid.

Safety in Administering Medications by Injection

Needleless Devices. Approximately 5.6 million health care workers in the United States are at risk of occupational exposure to bloodborne pathogens such as HIV and the hepatitis B virus (Occupational Safety and Health Administration [OSHA], n.d.). Occupational exposure often occurs through accidental needlesticks and sharps injuries. Needlestick injuries commonly occur when health care workers recap

needles, mishandle IV lines and needles, or leave needles at a patient's bedside. Exposure to bloodborne pathogens is one of the deadliest hazards to which nurses are exposed daily. Most needlestick injuries are preventable with the implementation of safe needle devices. The Needlestick Safety and Prevention Act mandates the use of special needle safety devices to reduce the frequency of needlestick injuries.

Safety syringes have a sheath or guard that covers a needle immediately after it is withdrawn from the skin (Fig. 31.29A-B). This eliminates the chance for a needlestick injury. The syringe and sheath are disposed of together in a receptacle. Use needleless devices whenever

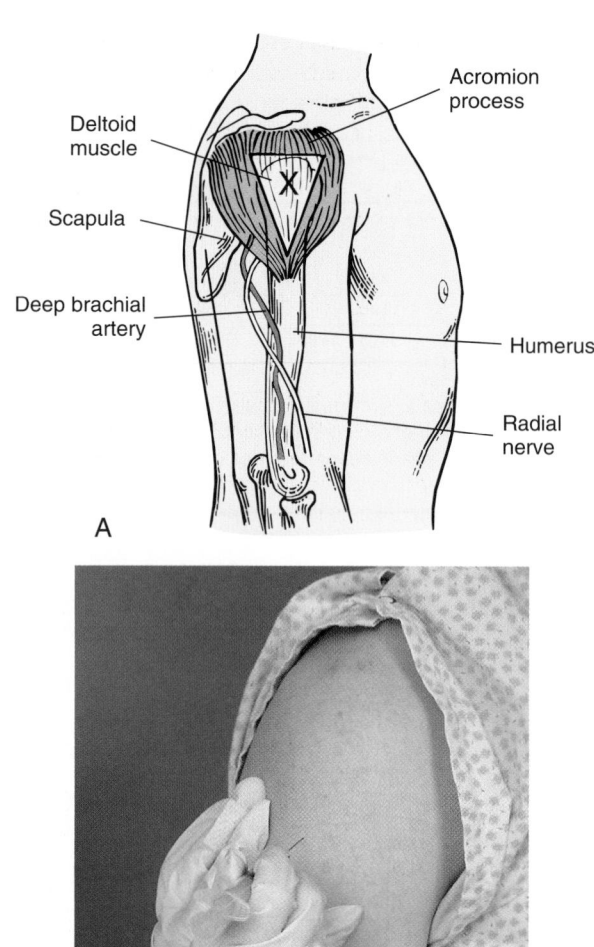

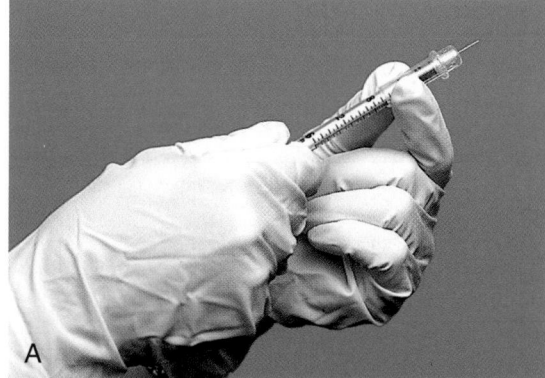

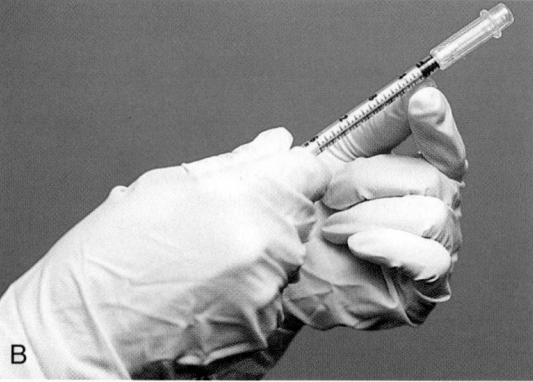

FIG. 31.29 Needle with plastic guard to prevent needlesticks. **A,** Position of guard before injection. **B,** After injection guard locks in place, covering needle.

FIG. 31.28 A, Landmarks for deltoid site. **B,** Giving intramuscular injection in deltoid muscle.

possible to reduce the risk of needlestick and sharps injuries (OSHA, n.d.). Always dispose of needles and other instruments considered sharps into clearly marked, appropriate containers (Fig. 31.30). Containers need to be puncture proof and leak proof. Never force a needle into a full needle disposal receptacle. Never place used needles and syringes in a wastebasket, in your pocket, on a patient's meal tray, or at the patient's bedside. Box 31.22 summarizes the recommendations for the prevention of needlestick injuries.

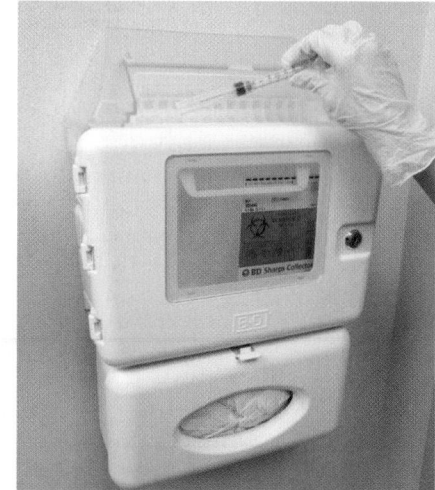

FIG. 31.30 Sharps disposal using only one hand.

Intravenous Administration. Nurses administer medications intravenously by the following methods:

1. Infusion of large volumes of IV fluid containers that contain medications mixed, labeled, and dispensed by pharmacy
2. Injection of a bolus or small volume of medication through an existing IV infusion line or intermittent venous access (heparin or saline lock)
3. "Piggyback" infusion of a solution containing the prescribed medication and a small volume of IV fluid through an existing IV line

In all three methods a patient has either an existing IV infusion running continuously or an IV access site for intermittent infusions.

Most policies and procedures list who can administer IV medications and in which patient care units they can be given. These policies are made based on the medication, capability, and availability of staff and the type of monitoring equipment available.

Chapter 42 describes the technique for performing venipuncture and establishing continuous IV fluid infusions. Medication administration is only one reason for supplying IV fluids. IV fluid therapy is used primarily for fluid replacement in patients unable to take oral fluids and as a means of supplying electrolytes and nutrients.

When using any method of IV medication administration, observe patients closely for symptoms of adverse reactions. After a medication

BOX 31.22 Recommendations for Prevention of Needlestick Injuries

- Avoid using needles when effective needleless systems or SESIP devices are available.
- Do not recap needles after medication administration.
- Plan safe handling and disposal of needles before beginning a procedure that requires the use of a needle.
- Immediately dispose of used needles, needleless systems, and SESIP into puncture- and leak-proof sharps disposal containers.
- Maintain a sharps injury log that reports the following: type and brand of device involved in the incident; location of the incident (e.g., department or work area); description of the incident; privacy of the employees who have had sharps injuries (see agency policy).
- Attend educational offerings regarding bloodborne pathogens, and follow recommendations for infection prevention, including receiving the hepatitis B vaccine.
- Report all needlestick and sharps-related injuries immediately, according to agency policies.
- Participate in the selection and evaluation of SESIP devices with safety features within your agency whenever possible.

Data from Occupational Safety and Health Administration (OSHA): Bloodborne pathogens and needlestick injuries, *Fed Regist 77(64):19934,* 2012. https://www.osha.gov/FedReg_osha_pdf/FED-20120403.pdf. Accessed May 17, 2018.

enters the bloodstream, it begins to act immediately, and there is no way to stop its action. Thus, take special care to avoid errors in dose calculation and preparation. Carefully follow the seven rights of safe medication administration, double-check medication calculations with another nurse, and know the desired action and side effects of every medication you give. If the medication has an antidote, make sure that it is available during administration. When administering potent medications, assess vital signs before, during, and after infusion. There are situations where it is recommended to do an independent double check of a medication dosage, especially high-risk medications given IV. The ISMP (2018a) describes how to do an independent double check:

- A double check must be conducted independently by a second person. A single person preparing and checking a medication is likely to see what he or she expects to see, even if an error has occurred.
- Two people must *separately* check each component of the work process. For example, a pharmacist calculates a dose, prepares a syringe of medication, and compares the product to the order; then a nurse *independently* checks the order, calculates the dose, and compares the results with the dispensed product for verification.
- Two people are unlikely to make the same mistake if they work independently. Holding up a syringe and a vial while saying "This is 5 units of insulin; can you check it?" is ineffective. The person asking for the double check must not influence the individual checking the product in any way.
- Use a double check only for very selective high-risk tasks or high-alert medications (not all) that most warrant their use (see agency policy).
- Fewer double checks performed strategically at the most vulnerable points of the medication use process are more effective than too many.

Administering medications by the IV route has advantages. Nurses often use this route in emergencies when a fast-acting medication needs to be delivered quickly. The IV route is also best when it is necessary to give medications to establish constant therapeutic blood levels.

Some medications are highly alkaline and irritating to muscle and subcutaneous tissue. These medications cause less discomfort when given intravenously. Because IV medications are immediately available to the bloodstream once they are administered, verify the rate of administration with a medication reference or a pharmacist before giving them to ensure that you give them safely over the appropriate amount of time. Patients experience severe adverse reactions if IV medications are administered too quickly.

Large-Volume Infusions. In the past nurses often, mixed medications into large volumes of intravenous (IV) fluids (500 to 1000 mL). However, today's safety standards and scientific evidence no longer support this practice (Infusion Nurses Society [INS], 2016; TJC, 2020). Many patient safety risks such as incorrect calculation, poor aseptic technique, incorrect labeling, pump programming errors, lack of medication knowledge, and mix-up with another medication occur when nurses must prepare medications in IV containers on patient care units. Box 31.23 summarizes current best practices for preparation and administration of IV medication.

Pharmacies prepare medications in large volumes (500 or 1000 mL) of compatible IV fluids such as normal saline or lactated Ringer's solution. Vitamins and potassium chloride are two types of medications often added to IV fluids. Continuous infusion carries a risk: if the IV fluid is infused too rapidly, the patient is at risk for medication overdose and circulatory fluid overload.

Nurses mix medications into IV fluids only in emergency situations. The nurse *never* prepares high-alert medications (e.g., heparin, dopamine, dobutamine, nitroglycerin, potassium, antibiotics, or magnesium) on a patient care unit. Check with a pharmacist before mixing a medication in an IV container. If a pharmacist confirms that you need to prepare the medication, ask another nurse to verify your medication calculations and have that nurse watch you during the entire procedure to ensure that you prepare the medication safely. First ensure that the IV fluid and medication are compatible. Then prepare the medication in a syringe (see Skill 31.4) using strict aseptic technique. *Do not* add medications to IV bags that are already hanging because there is no way to tell the exact concentration of the medication. Add medications *only* to new IV bags.

When administering medications in large IV infusions, regulate the IV rate according to the health care provider's order. Monitor patients closely for adverse reactions to the medication and fluid volume overload. Also check the site frequently for infiltration and phlebitis (see Chapter 42).

Intravenous Bolus. An IV bolus involves introducing a concentrated dose of a medication directly into the systemic circulation (see Skill 31.6). Because a bolus requires only a small amount of fluid to deliver the medication, it is an advantage when the amount of fluid that the patient can take is restricted. The IV bolus, or "push," is the most dangerous method for administering medications because there is no time to correct errors. In addition, a bolus may cause direct irritation to the lining of blood vessels. Before administering a bolus confirm placement of the IV line. Never give a medication intravenously if the insertion site appears swollen or edematous or the IV fluid cannot flow at the proper rate. Accidental injection of a medication into the tissue around a vein causes pain, sloughing of tissue, and abscesses, depending on the composition of the medication. Medications that carry a risk of adverse effects if administered too quickly should be diluted and administered as a piggyback or via an infusion pump.

Determine the rate of administration of an IV bolus medication by the amount of medication that can be given each minute. For example, if a patient is to receive 4 mL of a medication over 2 minutes, give 2 mL of the IV bolus medication every minute. Look up each medication to

BOX 31.23 Best Practices for Administration of Intravenous Solutions and Medications

- Review medication orders for standardized concentrations and dosages of medication.
- Use standardized procedures for ordering, preparing, and administering intravenous (IV) medications.
- Administer solutions and medications prepared and dispensed from the pharmacy or as commercially prepared when possible.
- Never prepare high-alert medications (e.g., heparin, dopamine, dobutamine, nitroglycerin, potassium, antibiotics, or magnesium) on a patient care unit.
- Review medication order for use of standardized infusion concentrations of "high-alert" medications.
- Standardize the storage of IV medications.
- Use the mnemonic CATS PRRR to help remember safety checks for administering IV medications: *C,* compatibilities; *A,* allergies; *T,* tubing correct; *S,* site checked; *P,* pump safety checked; *R,* right rate; *R,* release clamps; *R,* return and reassess the patient.
- Use standardized label practices. Bold patient name, generic medication name, and patient-specific dose.
- Correctly use technology such as intelligent-infusion devices, bar code–assisted medication administration, and electronic medication administration record.

Adapted from Infusion Nurses Society: Infusion nursing standards of practice, *J Intraven Nurs* 39(1S), 2016; Gorski L: *Phillips's manual of I.V. therapeutics: evidence-based practice for infusion therapy,* ed 7, Philadelphia, 2019, FA Davis; and The Joint Commission (TJC): *2020 National Patient Safety Goals,* Oakbrook Terrace, IL, 2020, The Joint Commission. http://www.jointcommission.org/standards_information/npsgs.aspx.

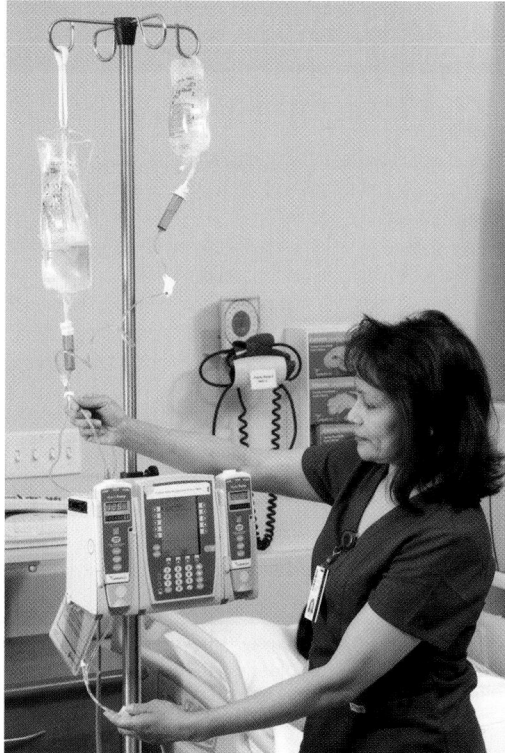

FIG. 31.31 Piggyback setup.

determine the recommended concentration and rate of administration. The ISMP (2015d) recommends avoiding the use of terms such as "IV push," "IVP," or "bolus" in orders with medications that require administration over 1 minute or longer. Use more descriptive terms such as "IV over 5 minutes." Remember, consider the purpose for which an IV medication is prescribed and any potential adverse effects related to the rate or route of administration.

Volume-Controlled Infusions. Another way of administering IV medications is through small amounts (50 to 100 mL) of compatible IV fluids. The fluid is within a secondary fluid container separate from the primary fluid bag. The container connects directly to the primary IV line or to separate tubing that inserts into the primary line (see Skill 31.7). Three types of containers are volume-control administration sets (e.g., Volutrol or Pediatrol), piggyback sets, and syringe pumps. Using volume-controlled infusions has several advantages:

- It reduces risk of rapid-dose infusion by IV push. Medications are diluted and infused over longer time intervals (e.g., 30 to 60 minutes).
- It allows for administration of medications (e.g., antibiotics) that are stable for a limited time in solution.
- It allows for control of IV fluid intake.

Piggyback. A piggyback is a small (25 to 250 mL) IV bag or bottle connected to a short tubing line that connects to the *upper* Y-port of a primary infusion line or to an intermittent venous access (Fig. 31.31). The label on the medication follows the ISMP IV piggyback medication label format (ISMP, 2018d) (Fig. 31.32). The piggyback tubing is a microdrip or macrodrip system (see Chapter 42). The set is called a

piggyback because the small bag or bottle is higher than the primary infusion bag or bottle. In the piggyback setup the main line does not infuse when the piggybacked medication is infusing. The port of the primary IV line contains a back-check valve that automatically stops flow of the primary infusion once the piggyback infusion flows. After the piggyback solution infuses and the solution within the tubing falls below the level of the primary infusion drip chamber, the back-check valve opens, and the primary infusion again flows.

Volume-Control Administration. Volume-control administration (e.g., Buretrol) sets are small (150-mL) containers that attach just below the primary infusion bag or bottle. The set is attached and filled in a manner similar to that used with a regular IV infusion. Follow package directions for priming sets (see Chapter 42).

Syringe Pump. The syringe pump is battery operated and allows medications to be given in very small amounts of fluid (5 to 60 mL) within controlled infusion times using standard syringes.

Intermittent Venous Access. An intermittent venous access (commonly called a *saline lock*) is an IV catheter capped off on the end with a small chamber covered by a rubber diaphragm or a specially designed cap. Special rubber-seal injection caps usually accept needle safety devices (see Chapter 42). Advantages to intermittent venous access include the following:

- Cost savings resulting from the omission of continuous IV therapy
- Effectiveness of nurse's time enhanced by eliminating constant monitoring of flow rates
- Increased mobility, safety, and comfort for the patient

Before administering an IV bolus or piggyback medication, assess the patency and placement of the IV site. After the medication has been administered through an intermittent venous access, the access must

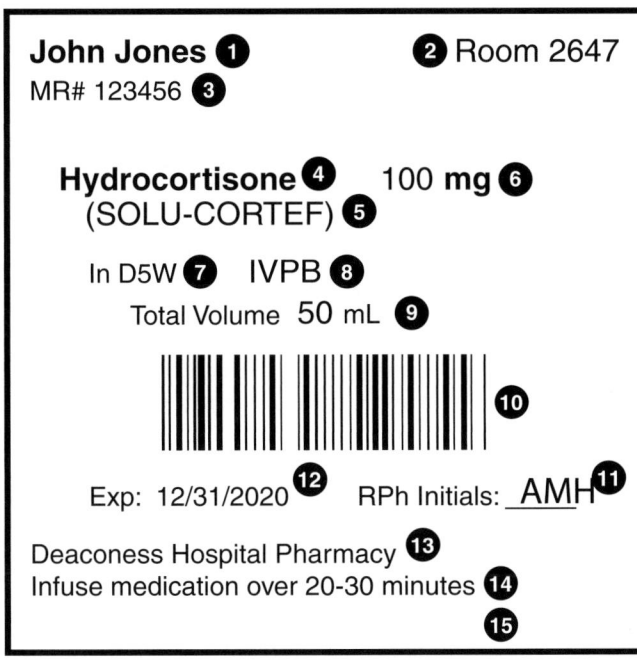

FIG. 31.32 IV piggyback medication with label following ISMP safe-labeling guidelines.

be flushed with a solution to keep it patent. Generally normal saline is an effective flush solution for peripheral catheters. Some agencies require the use of heparin. Nurses need to verify and follow agency policies regarding the care and maintenance of the IV site.

Administration of Intravenous Therapy in the Home. Sometimes patients need IV therapy at home. Common infusions that patients receive include antimicrobials, chemotherapy, total parenteral nutrition, biological therapy, and other medications (Gorski, 2019). Most patients typically receive their home IV therapy through a long-term central venous catheter (CVC) (see Chapter 42). Home health nurses assess patients' responses to the medication, monitor the CVC site, and teach patients and their family caregivers how to administer infusions and maintain the CVC.

Carefully assess patients and their family caregivers to determine their ability to manage IV therapy at home. Begin instruction on IV care management as soon as you know that a patient will have IV therapy at home. Your instruction often begins while a patient is hospitalized. Patients and family caregivers need to learn how to check their catheter for signs of complications and to flush, lock, and ensure the patency of the IV catheter (Gorski, 2019). If the patient has a tunneled catheter (see Chapter 42), site care including dressing changes may be taught as well. Patients also need to know when to notify the home care nurse or health care provider. Plan to teach patients and their family caregivers how to maintain IV administration equipment, including the infusion pump.

SAFETY GUIDELINES FOR NURSING SKILLS

Ensuring patient safety is an essential role of a professional nurse. To ensure patient safety, communicate clearly with members of the interprofessional team, assess and incorporate the patient's priorities of care and preferences, and use the best evidence when making decisions about your patient's care. When performing the skills in this chapter, remember the following points to ensure safe, individualized patient care.

Follow these guidelines to ensure safe medication administration:

- Be vigilant during medication administration. Avoid distractions while preparing all medications. No-interruption zones (NIZs) have been recommended to reduce distractions during medication preparation and administration (Bravo and Cochran, 2016; Yoder et al., 2015). NIZs are created by placing signs, red tape, or tile borders on the floor around medication carts or areas. Nurses standing in these zones are not to be interrupted.
- Be sure that your patients receive the appropriate medications.

- Know why your patient is receiving each medication; know what you need to do before, during, and after medication administration; and evaluate the effectiveness of medications and any adverse effects.
- Verify that medications have not expired by checking labels.
- Use at least two identifiers before administering medications, and check against the medication administration record (MAR). Follow agency policy for patient identification.
- Before administering medication, it is critical to ensure that all information is correct. You should check for accuracy three times:
  1. The first check is when the medications are pulled or retrieved from the automated dispensing machine, the medication drawer, or whatever system is in place at the agency.
  2. The second check is when preparation of the medications for administration takes place.
  3. The final check occurs at the patient's bedside just before medications are given.

- Clarify unclear medication orders and ask for help whenever you are uncertain about an order or calculation. Consult with your peers, pharmacists, and other health care providers, and be sure that you have resolved all concerns related to medication administration before preparing and giving medications.
- Use the technology (e.g., bar scanning, electronic MARs) available in your agency when preparing and giving medications. Follow all policies related to use of the technology, and do not use "work-arounds." A *work-around* bypasses a procedure, policy, or problem in a system. Nurses who use "work-arounds" fail to follow agency protocols, policies, or procedures during medication administration in an attempt to get medications administered to patients in a timelier fashion.
- Use strict aseptic technique during parenteral medication preparation and administration.
- Educate patients about each medication they take while you are administering medications. It is important for a patient to know each medication with respect

to purpose, daily dose and when to take the medications, most common side effects, and the problems to report to the health care provider. Make sure that you answer all their questions before administering medications. Educate family caregivers if appropriate.
- Most of the time you cannot delegate medication administration. Ensure that you follow standards set by the Nurse Practice Act in your state and guidelines established by your health care agency. Licensed practical nurses or licensed vocational nurses usually can administer medications via the oral (po), subcutaneous, IM, and ID routes. Sometimes they can give medications intravenously if they have had special training and if the medications are not high-alert medications. Some states also allow certified medical assistants to administer some types of medications (e.g., oral medications) in long-term care agencies.
- Follow safety guidelines to prevent needlestick injuries. Use engineered devices and dispose of all sharps in safety containers.

SKILL 31.1   ADMINISTERING ORAL MEDICATIONS

Delegation and Collaboration

The skill of administering oral medications cannot be delegated to assistive personnel (AP). The nurse instructs the AP about:

- Potential side effects of medications and to report their occurrence.
- Informing nurse if patient condition changes or worsens (e.g., pain, itching, or rash) after medication administration.

Equipment

- Automated, computer-controlled medication dispensing system or medication cart
- Disposable medication cups (mL only cup)
- Glass of water, juice, or preferred liquid and drinking straw
- Pill-crushing device *(optional)*
- Paper towels
- Medication administration record (MAR) (electronic or printed)
- Clean gloves (if handling an oral medication)

STEP	RATIONALE

ASSESSMENT

1. Check accuracy and completeness of each MAR or computer printout with health care provider's written medication order. Check patient's name, medication name and dosage, route of administration, and time of administration. Clarify incomplete or unclear orders with health care provider before administration.

2. Review pertinent information related to medication, including action, purpose, normal dose and route, side effects, time of onset and peak action, indications, and nursing implications.

3. Assess for any contraindications to patient receiving oral medication, including being on NPO status, inability to swallow, nausea/vomiting, bowel inflammation, reduced peristalsis, recent gastrointestinal (GI) surgery, gastric suction, and decreased level of consciousness (LOC). Notify health care provider if any contraindications are present.

4. Assess patient's medical, medication, and diet history, and history of allergies. List any medication allergies on each page of MAR and prominently display on patient's medical record. When allergies are present, patient should wear an allergy bracelet.

5. Perform hand hygiene. Gather and review physical assessment findings, including patient's weight (in metric units), vital signs, and laboratory data that influence medication administration such as results of renal and liver function studies.

6. Assess risk for aspiration using a dysphagia screening tool if available (see Chapter 45). Protect patient from aspiration by assessing swallowing ability.

7. Assess patient's symptoms before initiating medication therapy.

8. Assess patient's preference for fluids and determine whether medications can be given with these fluids. Maintain fluid restrictions as prescribed.

9. Assess patient's and family caregiver's knowledge regarding health and medication use, medication schedule, and ability to prepare medications.

The order sheet is the most reliable source and only legal record of medications that patient is to receive. Ensures that patient receives the correct medications (Westbrook et al., 2017). Transcription errors are a source of medication errors (Truitt et al., 2016).

Allows you to anticipate effects of medication and observe patient's response.

Alterations in GI function can interfere with medication absorption, distribution, and excretion. Patients with GI suction do not receive actions of oral medications because the medications are suctioned from the GI tract before they are absorbed.

These factors influence how certain medications act. Information reveals previous problems with medication administration. Allergy alert helps prevent adverse events.

Many medication doses are based on patient's weight. Physical examination findings or laboratory data may contraindicate medication administration. Renal and liver function status affects metabolism and excretion of medications (Burchum and Rosenthal, 2019).

Aspiration occurs when food, fluid, or medication intended for GI administration is inadvertently administered into the respiratory tract. Patients with altered ability to swallow are at higher risk for aspiration (Forough et al.,2018).

Provides information to evaluate desired effect of medication.

Some fluids interfere with medication absorption (e.g., dairy products affect tetracycline). Offering fluids during medication administration is an excellent way to increase patient's fluid intake. Fluids ease swallowing and facilitate absorption from the GI tract. However, if fluid restriction exists, skillful planning of fluid intake must coordinate with medication times and types of medications.

Determines patient's and family caregiver's need for medication education and guidance to achieve medication adherence.

STEP	RATIONALE

PLANNING

1. Perform hand hygiene. Collect appropriate equipment and MAR.

   Promotes time management and efficiency when preparing medications for all patients.

2. Plan preparation to avoid interruptions. Create a quiet environment. Do not take phone calls or talk with others. Follow agency "No-interruption zone" (NIZ) policy.

   Interruptions contribute to medication errors (Westbrook et al., 2017; Yoder et al., 2015) (see Box 31.4).

IMPLEMENTATION

1. Prepare medications.

   a. Perform hand hygiene. Arrange medication tray and cups in medication preparation area or move medication cart to position outside patient's room.

      Reduces transfer of microorganisms. Organization of equipment saves time and reduces error.

   b. Log on to automated medication dispensing system (AMDS) or unlock medicine drawer or cart.

      Medications are safeguarded when locked in cabinet, cart, or AMDS.

   c. Perform hand hygiene and prepare medications for *one patient at a time* using aseptic technique. Follow the seven rights of medication administration. Keep all pages of MARs or computer printouts for one patient together or look at only one patient's electronic MAR screen.

      Ensures that medications remain sterile. Prevents preparation errors.

   d. Select correct medication from AMDS, unit-dose drawer, or stock supply. Compare name of medication on label with MAR or computer printout (see illustration). Exit AMDS after removing medication.

      Reading label and comparing it against transcribed order reduces errors. Exiting AMDS ensures no one else can remove medications using your identify. *This is the first check for accuracy.*

   e. Check or calculate medication dose as necessary. Double-check any calculation. Check expiration date on all medications and return outdated medication to pharmacy.

      Double-checking pharmacy calculations reduces risk for error. Agency policy may require you to check calculations of certain medications such as insulin with another nurse. Expired medications may be inactive or harmful to patient.

   f. If preparing a controlled substance, check record for previous medication count and compare current count with available supply. Controlled medications may be stored in computerized locked cart.

      Controlled substance laws require nurses to carefully monitor and count dispensed controlled medications (e.g., opioids).

   g. Prepare solid forms of oral medications.

      (1) To prepare unit-dose tablets or capsules, place packaged tablet or capsule directly into medication cup without removing wrapper. Administer medications only from containers with labels that are clearly marked.

         Wrappers maintain cleanliness and identify medication name and dose, which can facilitate teaching.

      (2) When using a blister pack, "pop" medications through foil or paper backing into a medication cup (see illustration).

         Packs provide a 1-month supply, with each "blister" usually containing a single dose.

      (3) If it is necessary to give half the dose of medication, pharmacy should split, label, package, and send medication to unit. If you must split medication, use clean, gloved hand to cut with clean pill-cutting device. Only cut tablets that are prescored by the manufacturer (line traverses the center of the tablet).

         Reduces contamination of the tablet. In health care agencies, only pharmacy should split tablets to ensure patient safety (USDHHS, 2015). If a tablet is FDA-approved to be split, this information will be printed in the "HOW SUPPLIED" section of the manufacturer's label insert.

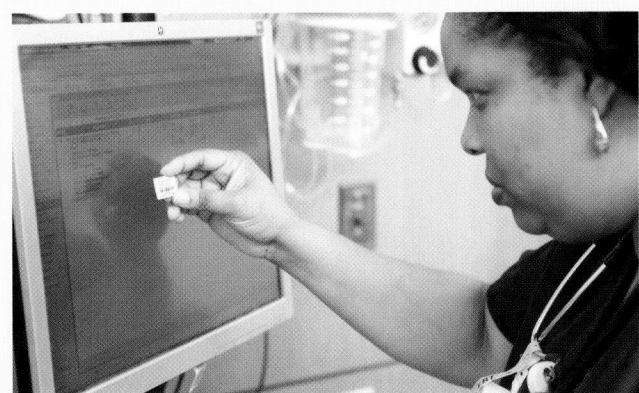

STEP 1d Nurse compares label of medication with transcribed medication order on computerized MAR.

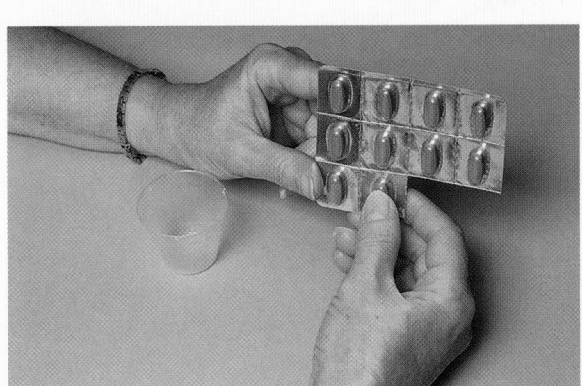

STEP 1g(2) Place tablet from blister pack into medicine cup without removing wrapper.

Continued

SKILL 31.1   ADMINISTERING ORAL MEDICATIONS—cont'd

STEP	RATIONALE
(4) Place all tablets or capsules that patient will receive in one medicine cup, except for those requiring pre-administration assessments (e.g., pulse rate or blood pressure). Place those medications in separate additional cup with wrapper intact.	Keeping medications that require pre-administration assessments separate from others serves as a reminder and makes it easier to withhold medications as necessary.
(5) If patient has difficulty swallowing and liquid medications are not an option, use a pill-crushing device (see illustration A). Clean device before using. If device is unavailable, place medication between two cups, and grind and crush (see illustration B). Mix ground tablet in small amount (teaspoon) of soft food (custard or applesauce).	Large tablets are often difficult to swallow. A ground tablet mixed with palatable soft food is usually easier to swallow.

CLINICAL DECISION: *Not all medications can be crushed safely. Consult with a pharmacist or the ISMP Do Not Crush List (ISMP, 2018a).*

---

h. Prepare liquids.	
(1) Use unit-dose container with correct amount of medication. Gently shake container. Administer medication packaged in a single-dose cup directly from the single-dose cup. Do not pour medicine into another cup.	Using unit-dose container with correct dosage of medication provides most accurate dose of medication (ISMP, 2018a). Shaking container ensures that medication is mixed before administration.
(2) Unit-dose oral syringe (see illustration): Be sure to use only oral syringes marked "Oral Use Only" dispensed by pharmacy.	Ensures that all oral medications that are not commercially available as unit-dose products are dispensed by the pharmacy in an oral syringe (ISMP, 2018a).

CLINICAL DECISION: *Based on current best practice (ISMP, 2018a), liquid medications that are not available or are not in correct dose in a unit-dose container should be dispensed by the pharmacy in special oral syringes marked "Oral Use Only." These syringes do not connect to any type of parenteral (e.g., intravenous [IV]) tubing. Additionally, current evidence shows that liquid measuring devices on patient care units result in inaccurate dosing. Having oral medications prepared in the pharmacy ensures that you give the most accurate dose of a medication possible and prevents parenteral administration of oral medications. Ensure that the small plastic ring on the syringe (especially 1-mL syringes) has been removed (ISMP, 2018b).*

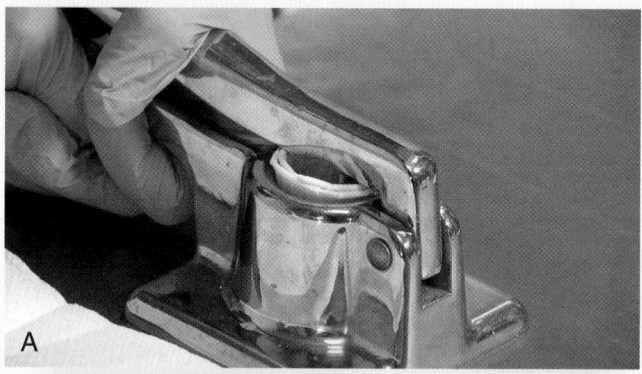

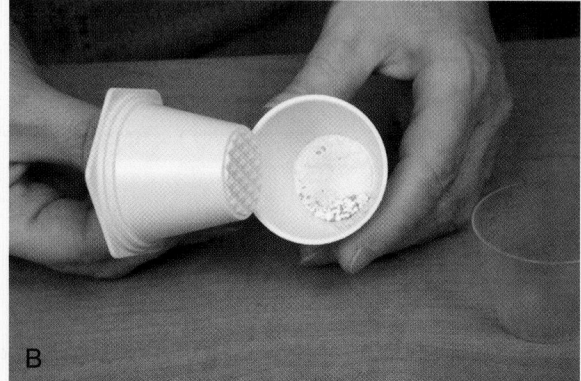

STEP 1g(5) A, Pill crushing device. **B,** Crushing tablet with pill-crushing device.

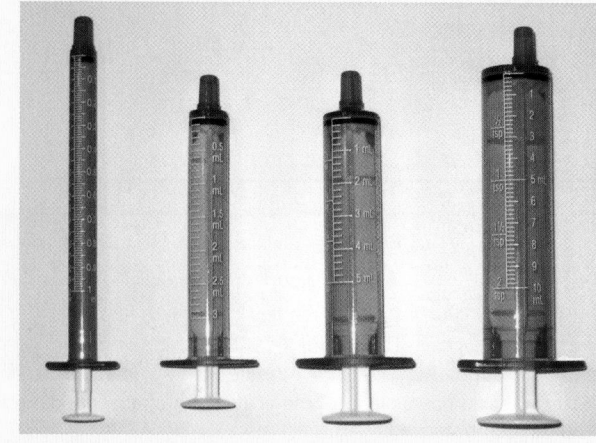

STEP 1h(2) Use special oral medication syringes to prepare small amounts of liquid medications.

STEP	RATIONALE
i. Return stock containers or unused unit-dose medications to shelf or drawer. Label medication cups and poured medications with patient's name before leaving medication preparation area. Do not leave medications unattended.	Ensures that correct medications are prepared for correct patient.
j. Before going to patient's room, compare patient's name and name of medication on label of prepared medications with MAR.	Comparing labels a second time reduces errors. *This is the second check for accuracy.*
2. Administer medications.	
a. Take medication to patient at correct time (see agency policy). Medications that require exact timing include STAT doses, first-time or loading doses, and one-time doses. Give time-critical scheduled medications (e.g., antibiotics, anticoagulants, insulin, anticonvulsants, or immunosuppressive agents) at exact time ordered (no more than 30 minutes before or after scheduled dose). Give non–time-critical scheduled medications within a range of 1 or 2 hours of scheduled dose (ISMP, 2011a). During administration apply seven rights of medication administration.	Hospitals must adopt medication administration policy and procedure for timing of medication administration that considers nature of the prescribed medication, specific clinical application, and patient needs (DHHS, 2011; ISMP, 2011a). Time-critical scheduled medications are those for which early or delayed administration of maintenance doses of greater than 30 minutes before or after the scheduled dose may cause harm or result in substantial suboptimal therapy or pharmacological effect. Non–time-critical medications are those for which early or delayed administration within a specified range of either 1 or 2 hours should not cause harm or result in substantial suboptimal therapy or pharmacological effect (DHHS, 2011; ISMP, 2011a).
b. Identify patient using at least two identifiers (e.g., name and birthday or name and medical record number) according to agency policy. Compare identifiers with information on patient's MAR or medical record.	Ensures correct patient. Complies with The Joint Commission standards and improves patient safety (TJC, 2020).
c. At patient's bedside, again compare MAR or computer printout with name of medication on medication labels and patient name. Ask patient whether he or she has allergies.	*This is the third check for accuracy* and ensures that patient receives correct medication. Confirms patient's allergy history.
d. Explain the purpose of each medication, action, and most common adverse effects. Allow sufficient time for patient to ask questions. Include family caregiver if appropriate.	Patient has the right to be informed, and patient and family caregiver understanding of each medication improves adherence with medication therapy.
e. Perform hand hygiene. Perform necessary pre-administration assessment (e.g., blood pressure, pulse) for specific medications. Ask patient again whether he or she has allergies.	Reduces transmission of microorganisms. Determines whether specific medications should be withheld at that time. Confirms patient's allergy history.

CLINICAL DECISION: *If patient expresses concern regarding accuracy of a medication, do not give the medication. Explore patient's concern and verify health care provider's order before administering. Listening to patient's concerns may prevent a medication error.*

STEP	RATIONALE
f. Help patient to sitting or Fowler's position. Use side-lying position if he or she is unable to sit. Have patient stay in this position for 30 minutes after administration.	Decreases risk for aspiration during swallowing.
g. *For tablets:* Patient may wish to hold solid medications in hand or cup before placing in mouth. Offer water or preferred liquid to help patient swallow medications.	Patient can become familiar with medications by seeing each medication. Choice of fluid can improve fluid intake.
h. *For orally disintegrating formulations (tablets or strips):* Remove medication from packet just before use. Do not push tablet through foil. Place medication on top of patient's tongue. Caution against chewing it.	Orally disintegrating formulations begin to dissolve when placed on tongue. Water is not needed. Careful removal from packaging is necessary because tablets and strips are thin and fragile.
i. *For sublingually administered medications:* Have patient place medication under tongue and allow it to dissolve completely (see Fig. 31.3). Caution patient against swallowing tablet.	Medication is absorbed through blood vessels of undersurface of tongue. If swallowed, it is destroyed by gastric juices or rapidly detoxified by liver, preventing therapeutic blood level.
j. *For buccal administered medications:* Have patient place medication in mouth against mucous membranes of cheek and gums until it dissolves (see Fig. 31.4).	Buccal medications act locally or systemically as they are swallowed in saliva.

CLINICAL DECISION: *Avoid administering anything by mouth, including other oral medications, until orally disintegrating buccal or sublingual medication is completely dissolved.*

Continued

SKILL 31.1 **ADMINISTERING ORAL MEDICATIONS—cont'd**

STEP	RATIONALE
k. *For powdered medications:* Mix with liquids at bedside and give to patient to drink.	When prepared in advance, powdered medications thicken; some even harden, making swallowing difficult.
l. *For crushed medications mixed with food:* Give each medication separately in teaspoon of food.	Ensures that patient swallows all of medicine. *Never mix medication in a meal serving of food.*
m. *For lozenge:* Caution patient against chewing or swallowing lozenges.	Lozenges act through slow absorption through oral mucosa, not gastric mucosa.
n. *For effervescent medication:* Add tablet or powder to glass of water. Administer immediately after dissolving.	Effervescence improves unpleasant taste and often relieves GI problems.
o. If patient is unable to hold medications, place medication cup or oral syringe to lips and gently introduce each medication into mouth one at a time. Administer each tablet or capsule one at a time. Inject liquid from oral syringe slowly. A spoon can also be used to place pill in patient's mouth. Do not rush or force medications.	Administering a single-dose tablet, capsule, or oral syringe dose eases swallowing and decreases risk for aspiration.
p. Stay until patient swallows each medication completely or takes it by the prescribed route. Ask patient to open mouth if uncertain whether medication has been swallowed.	Ensures that patient receives ordered dose. If left unattended, patient may not take dose or may save medications, causing health risks.
q. For highly acidic medications (e.g., aspirin), offer patient a nonfat snack (e.g., crackers) if not contraindicated by his or her condition.	Reduces gastric irritation. Fat content of foods may delay medication absorption.
r. Help patient return to position of comfort.	Maintains patient's comfort.
s. Stay with patient for several minutes and observe for any allergic reactions.	Dyspnea, wheezing, and circulatory collapse are signs of severe anaphylactic reaction.
3. Dispose of soiled supplies and perform hand hygiene. Return cart to medication room and clean work area.	Reduces transmission of microorganisms.

EVALUATION

1. Return within an appropriate time to evaluate patient's response to medications, including therapeutic effects, side effects or allergic reactions, and adverse effects.	Evaluates therapeutic benefit of medication and helps to detect onset of side effects or allergic reactions. Sublingual medications act in 15 minutes; most oral medications act in 30 to 60 minutes.
2. Ask patient or family caregiver to identify medication name and explain purpose, indication, action, dose schedule, and potential side effects.	Determines level of knowledge gained by patient and family caregiver.
3. **Use Teach-Back:** "I want to be sure I showed you how to use your sublingual nitroglycerin. Show me where you will place the tablet in your mouth." Revise your instruction now or develop a plan for revised patient/family caregiver teaching if patient/family caregiver is not able to teach back correctly.	Determines patient's/family caregiver's level of understanding of instructional topic.

UNEXPECTED OUTCOMES AND RELATED INTERVENTIONS

1. Patient exhibits adverse effects (e.g., side effect, toxic effect, allergic reaction).
   - Notify health care provider and pharmacy.
   - Withhold further doses.
   - Assess vital signs.
   - Symptoms such as urticaria, rash, pruritus, rhinitis, and wheezing may indicate an allergic reaction and need for emergency medications.
   - Add allergy information to patient's medical record.
2. Patient refuses medication.
   - Assess reason for patient refusing medication.
   - Provide further instruction
   - Do not force patient to take medications.
   - Document and notify health care provider.
3. Patient or family caregiver is unable to explain medication information.
   - Further assess patient's or family caregiver's knowledge of medications and guidelines for medication safety.
   - Further instruction or different approach to instruction is necessary.

RECORDING AND REPORTING

- Record medication, dose, route, and time administered on patient's MAR immediately *after* administration, not before. Include initials or signature.
- If you do not administer the medication, record reason on flow sheet or nurses' notes in electronic health record (EHR) or chart, and follow agency policy for noting withheld medication.
- Record patient response to medication, instructions (including teach-back), and validation of understanding on flow sheet or nurses' notes in electronic health record (EHR) or chart.
- Report adverse effects and patient response and/or withheld medications to nurse in charge or health care provider.

SKILL 31.2   ADMINISTERING EYE (OPHTHALMIC) MEDICATIONS

Delegation and Collaboration

The skill of administering eye medications cannot be delegated to assistive personnel (AP). The nurse instructs the AP about:

- The specific potential side effects of medications and to report their occurrence.
- The potential for temporary burning or blurring of vision after administration of eye medications.

Equipment

- Appropriate medication (eyedrops with sterile dropper, ointment tube, or medicated intraocular disk)
- Clean gloves (for eyedrops)
- Medication administration record (MAR) (electronic or printed)
- Eyedrops or Ointment
- Cotton balls or facial tissue
- Warm water and washcloth
- Eye patch and tape *(optional)*

STEP	RATIONALE

ASSESSMENT

1. Check accuracy and completeness of each MAR or computer printout with health care provider's written medication order. Check patient's name, medication name and dosage, route of administration, and time of administration. Clarify incomplete or unclear orders with health care provider before administration.

The order sheet is the most reliable source and only legal record of medications that patient is to receive. Ensures that patient receives the correct medications (Westbrook et al., 2017). Transcription errors are a source of medication errors (Truitt et al., 2016).

2. Review pertinent information related to medication, including action, purpose, normal dose and route, side effects, time of onset and peak action, indication, and nursing implications.

Allows you to anticipate effects of medication and observe patient's response.

3. Assess patient's medical and medication history and history of allergies. List any medication allergies on each page of the MAR and prominently display it on the patient's medical record per agency policy. When allergies are present, patient should wear allergy bracelet.

Factors influence how certain medications act. Reveals patient's need for medication. Allergy alert prevents adverse effects.

4. Perform hand hygiene. Assess condition of external eye and structures (see Chapter 30). This may be done just before medication instillation (if drainage is present, apply clean gloves).

Provides baseline to determine whether local response to medications occurs. Also indicates need to clean eye before medication application.

5. Determine whether patient has any symptoms of eye discomfort or visual impairment.

Certain eye medications act to either lessen or increase these symptoms.

6. Assess patient's level of consciousness (LOC) and ability to follow directions.

If patient becomes restless or combative during procedure, greater risk for accidental eye injury exists.

7. Assess patient's and family caregiver's knowledge regarding medication therapy and patient's desire to self-administer medication.

Indicates need for health teaching. Motivation influences teaching approach.

8. Assess patient's ability to manipulate and hold dropper or ocular disk.

Reflects patient's ability to learn to self-administer medication.

PLANNING

1. Perform hand hygiene. Collect appropriate equipment and MAR.

Promotes time management and efficiency when preparing medications for all patients.

2. Plan preparation to avoid interruptions. Create a quiet environment. Do not take phone calls or talk with others. Follow agency "No-interruption zone" policy.

Interruptions contribute to medication errors (Westbrook et al., 2017; Yoder et al., 2015) (see Box 31.4).

IMPLEMENTATION

1. Prepare medications for *one patient at a time*. Attend to procedure and avoid distraction. Check label of medication against MAR two times, when removing medication from unit dose or AMDS and before leaving preparation area (see Skill 31.1). Prepare eyedrops by taking container out of refrigerator and rewarming to room temperature before administering to patient. Check expiration date on container. Perform hand hygiene.

Warming eyedrops reduces eye irritation. *These are the first and second checks for accuracy.* Process ensures that right patient receives right medication.

2. Take medication(s) to patient at correct time (see agency policy). Medications that require exact timing include STAT doses, first-time or loading doses, and one-time doses. Give time-critical scheduled medications (e.g., antibiotics, anticoagulants, insulin, anticonvulsants, or immunosuppressive agents) at exact time ordered (no more than 30 minutes before or after scheduled dose). Give non–time-critical scheduled medications within a range of 1 or 2 hours of scheduled dose (ISMP, 2011a). During administration apply seven rights of medication administration.

Hospitals must adopt medication administration policy and procedure for timing of medication administration that considers nature of the prescribed medication, specific clinical application, and patient needs (DHHS, 2011; ISMP, 2011a). Time-critical scheduled medications are those for which early or delayed administration of maintenance doses of greater than 30 minutes before or after the scheduled dose may cause harm or result in substantial suboptimal therapy or pharmacological effect. Non–time-critical medications are those for which early or delayed administration within a specified range of either 1 or 2 hours should not cause harm or result in substantial suboptimal therapy or pharmacological effect (DHHS, 2011; ISMP, 2011a).

Continued

SKILL 31.2   **ADMINISTERING EYE (OPHTHALMIC) MEDICATIONS—cont'd**

STEP	RATIONALE
3. Identify patient using at least two identifiers (e.g., name and birthday or name and medical record number) according to agency policy. Compare identifiers with information on patient's MAR or medical record.	Ensures correct patient. Complies with The Joint Commission standards and improves patient safety (TJC, 2020).
4. At patient's bedside again compare MAR or computer printout with names of medications on medication labels and patient name. Ask patient whether he or she has allergies.	*This is the third check for accuracy* and ensures that patient receives correct medication. Confirms patient's allergy history.
5. Discuss purpose of each medication, action, and possible adverse effects. Allow patient to ask any questions about the medications. Patients who self-instill medications may be allowed to give drops under nurse's supervision (check agency policy).	Patient has right to be informed, and patient's understanding of each medication improves adherence to medication therapy.
6. Tell patients receiving eyedrops (e.g., mydriatics) that vision will be blurred temporarily and that sensitivity to light may occur.	May relieve patient's anxiety.

CLINICAL DECISION: *Instruct and reinforce that patient should not drive or operate machinery or perform any activity that requires clear vision until vision and sensitivity to light return to normal.*

---

7. Instill eye medications.	
a. Apply clean gloves. Ask patient to lie supine or sit back in chair with head slightly hyperextended, looking up.	Position provides easy access to eye for medication instillation and minimizes drainage of medication into tear duct.

CLINICAL DECISION: *Do not hyperextend the neck of a patient with cervical spine injury.*

---

b. If drainage or crusting is present along eyelid margins or inner canthus, gently wash away. Soak any dried crusts with warm, damp washcloth or cotton ball over eye for several minutes. Always wipe clean from inner to outer canthus (see illustration). Remove and dispose of gloves and perform hand hygiene.	Soaking allows easy removal of crusts without applying pressure to eye. Cleaning from inner to outer canthus avoids entrance of microorganisms into lacrimal duct (Burchum and Rosenthal, 2019).
c. Explain that there might be temporary burning sensation from drops.	Corneas are highly sensitive.
d. Instill eyedrops.	
(1) Hold clean cotton ball or tissue in nondominant hand on patient's cheekbone just below lower eyelid.	Cotton or tissue absorbs medication that escapes eye.
(2) With tissue or cotton ball resting below lower lid, gently press downward with thumb or forefinger against bony orbit, exposing conjunctival sac. Never press directly against patient's eyeball.	Prevents pressure and trauma to eyeball and prevents fingers from touching eye.
(3) Ask patient to look at ceiling. Rest dominant hand on patient's forehead; hold filled medication eyedropper approximately 1 to 2 cm (0.5 to 1.0 inch) above conjunctival sac.	Action moves cornea up and away from conjunctival sac and reduces blink reflex. Prevents accidental contact of eyedropper with eye and reduces risk of injury and transfer of microorganisms to dropper (ophthalmic medications are sterile).
(4) Drop prescribed number of drops into conjunctival sac (see illustration).	Conjunctival sac normally holds 1 or 2 drops. Provides even distribution of medication across eye.

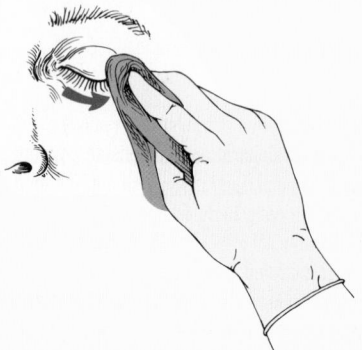

STEP 7b Clean eye, washing from inner to outer canthus before administering drops or ointment.

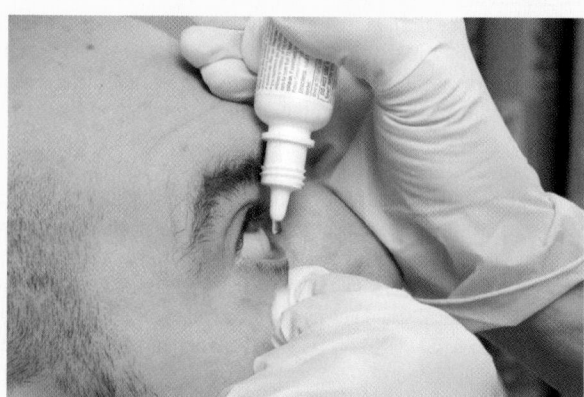

STEP 7d(4) Hold eyedropper over lower conjunctival sac.

STEP	RATIONALE

(5) If patient blinks or closes eye, causing drops to land on outer lid margins, repeat procedure.

Drops must enter conjunctival sac to achieve therapeutic effect.

(6) When administering drops that have systemic effects, apply gentle pressure to patient's nasolacrimal duct with clean tissue for 30 to 60 seconds over each eye, one at a time (see illustration). Avoid pressure directly against patient's eyeball.

Prevents overflow of medication into nasal and pharyngeal passages. Prevents absorption into systemic circulation (Lilley et al., 2020).

(7) After instilling drops, ask patient to close eyes gently.

Helps distribute medication. Squinting or squeezing eyelids forces medication from conjunctival sac (Lilley et al., 2020).

e. Instill ophthalmic ointment.

(1) Holding applicator above lower lid margin, apply thin ribbon of ointment evenly along inner edge of lower eyelid on conjunctiva (see illustration) from inner to outer canthus.

Reduces transmission of infection. Distributes medication evenly across eye and lid margin.

(2) Have patient close eye and rub lid lightly in circular motion with cotton ball if not contraindicated. Avoid placing pressure directly against patient's eyeball.

Further distributes medication without traumatizing eye.

(3) If excess medication is on eyelid, gently wipe it from inner to outer canthus.

Promotes comfort and prevents trauma to eye.

(4) If patient needs an eye patch, apply clean one by placing it over affected eye so that entire eye is covered. Tape securely without applying pressure to eye.

Clean eye patch reduces risk of infection.

f. Insert intraocular disk.

(1) Open package containing disk. Gently press your fingertip against disk so that it adheres to your finger. It may be necessary to moisten gloved finger with sterile saline. Position convex side of disk on your fingertip.

Allows you to inspect disk for damage or deformity.

(2) With your other hand gently pull patient's lower eyelid away from eye. Ask patient to look up.

Prepares conjunctival sac for receiving medicated disk and moves sensitive cornea away.

(3) Place disk in conjunctival sac so that it floats on sclera between iris and lower eyelid (see illustration).

Ensures delivery of medication.

(4) Pull patient's lower eyelid out and over disk (see illustration). You should not be able to see disk at this time. Repeat if you can see disk.

Ensures accurate medication delivery.

8. Remove intraocular disk.

a. Perform hand hygiene and apply clean gloves. Gently pull downward on lower eyelid using your nondominant hand.

Exposes disk.

b. Using forefinger and thumb of your dominant hand, pinch disk and lift it out of patient's eye (see illustration).

9. After administering eye medications, remove and dispose of gloves and soiled supplies; perform hand hygiene.

Reduces transmission of microorganisms.

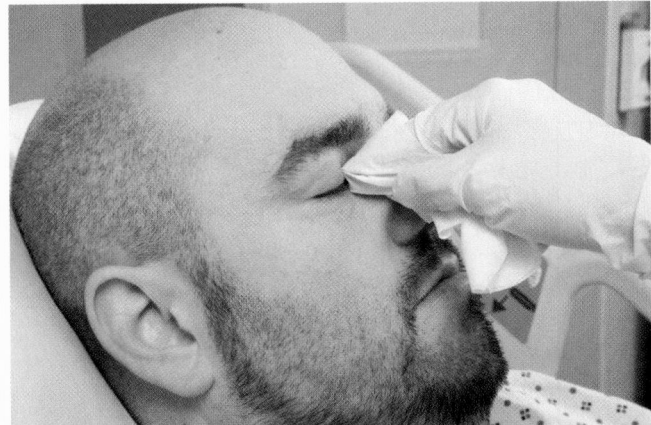

STEP 7d(6) Apply gentle pressure against nasolacrimal duct after giving eye medications.

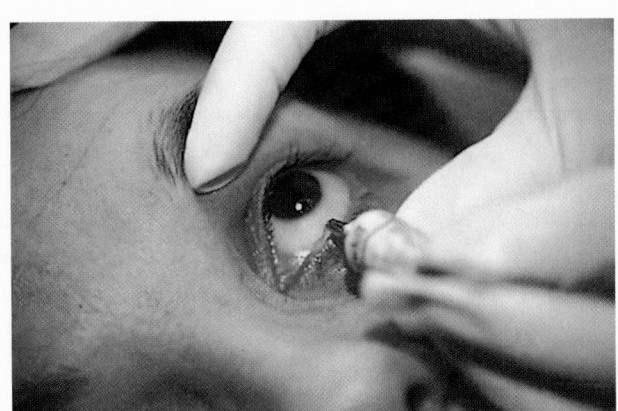

STEP 7e(1) Nurse applies ointment along inner edge of lower eyelid from inner to outer canthus.

Continued

SKILL 31.2	ADMINISTERING EYE (OPHTHALMIC) MEDICATIONS—cont'd

STEP	RATIONALE

EVALUATION

1. Observe response to medication by assessing visual changes, asking whether symptoms are relieved, and noting any side effects or discomfort felt.

Evaluates effects of medication.

2. Ask patient to discuss purpose of medication, indication, action, side effects, and technique of administration.

Determines patient's level of understanding.

3. **Use Teach-Back:** "I want to be sure I showed you how to insert the intraocular disk. Show me how to insert it into your left eye." Revise your instruction now or develop a plan for revised patient/family caregiver teaching if patient/family caregiver is not able to teach back correctly.

Determines patient's/family caregiver's level of understanding of instructional topic.

UNEXPECTED OUTCOMES AND RELATED INTERVENTIONS

1. Patient complains of burning or pain or experiences local side effects (e.g., headache, bloodshot eyes, local eye irritation). Medication concentration and patient's sensitivity both influence chances of side effects developing.
   - Eyedrops may have been instilled onto cornea, or dropper touched surface of eye.
   - Notify health care provider for possible adjustment in medication type and dosage.
2. Patient experiences systemic effects from drops (e.g., increased heart rate and blood pressure from epinephrine, decreased heart rate and blood pressure from timolol).
   - Notify health care provider immediately.
   - Remain with patient. Assess vital signs.
   - Withhold further doses.
3. Patient or family caregiver is unable to explain medication information or steps for administering eyedrops or has trouble manipulating dropper.
   - Repeat instructions as appropriate. Include return demonstration.

RECORDING AND REPORTING

- Record medication, concentration, dose or strength, number of drops, site of application (e.g., right eye, left eye, or both eyes), and time administered on MAR immediately after administration, not before. Include initials or signature.
- Record patient teaching (including teach-back) and validation of understanding on flow sheet or nurses' notes in electronic health record (EHR) or chart.
- Record objective data related to tissues involved (e.g., redness, drainage, irritation), any subjecStive data (e.g., pain, itching, altered vision), and patient's response to medications. Note evidence of any side effects experienced on flow sheet or nurses' notes in electronic health record (EHR) or chart.
- Report adverse effects and patient response and/or withheld medications to nurse in charge or health care provider.

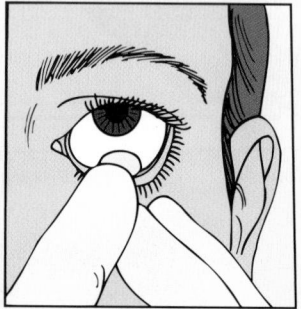

STEP 7f(3) Place intraocular disk in conjunctival sac between iris and lower eyelid.

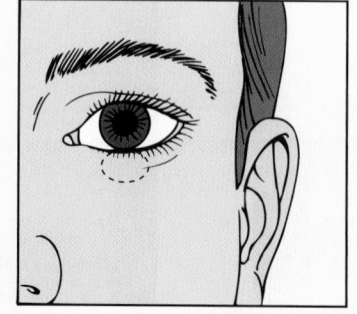

STEP 7f(4) Gently pull patient's lower eyelid over disk.

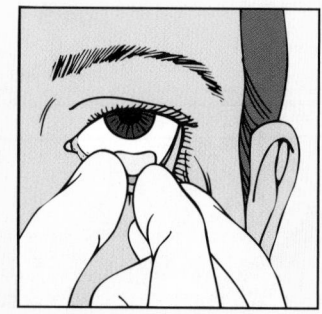

STEP 8b Carefully pinch disk to remove it from patient's eye.

SKILL 31.3   USING METERED-DOSE OR DRY POWDER INHALERS

Delegation and Collaboration

The skill of administering inhaled medications cannot be delegated to assistive personnel (AP). The nurse instructs the AP about:

- Potential side effects of medications and to report their occurrence to the nurse.
- Reporting breathing difficulty (e.g., paroxysmal or sustained coughing, audible wheezing) to the nurse.

Equipment

- Inhaler device with medication canister (metered-dose inhaler [MDI], breath-actuated inhaler [BAI], or dry powder inhaler [DPI]) (Fig. 31.33)
- Spacer device such as AeroChamber or InspirEase (optional for MDI)
- Facial tissues *(optional)*
- Medication administration record (MAR) (electronic or printed)
- Stethoscope
- Pulse oximeter *(optional)*

STEP	RATIONALE

ASSESSMENT

1. Check accuracy and completeness of each MAR or computer printout with health care provider's written medication order. Check patient's name, medication name and dosage, route of administration, and time of administration. Clarify incomplete or unclear orders with health care provider before administration.

2. Review pertinent information related to medication, including action, purpose, normal dose and route, side effects, time of onset and peak action, indication, and nursing implications.

3. Assess patient's medical and medication history and history of allergies. List medication allergies on each page of the MAR and prominently display it on the patient's medical record. When allergies are present, patient should wear an allergy bracelet.

4. Perform hand hygiene. Assess respiratory status and auscultate breath sounds (see Chapter 30). Also assess exercise tolerance; does patient develop shortness of breath easily?

5. Measure the patient's peak expiratory flow rate using a peak flow meter. Have patient measure if done so at home. Use patient's peak flow meter if available (see Chapter 41).

6. Assess patient's symptoms before initiating medication therapy.

7. Assess patient's ability to hold, manipulate, and depress canister and inhaler.

8. If patient was previously instructed in self-administration, have patient demonstrate how to use the device.

The order sheet is the most reliable source and only legal record of medications that patient is to receive. Ensures that patient receives the correct medications (Westbrook et al., 2017). Transcription errors are a source of medication errors (Truitt et al., 2016).

Allows you to anticipate effects of medication while observing patient's response.

Factors influence how certain medications act. Reveals patient's need for medication.

Allergy alert helps prevent adverse effects.

Reduces transmission of microorganisms. Establishes baseline of airway status for comparison during and after treatment.

A peak flow meter is used to measure air flow or peak expiratory flow rate and aids in monitoring airway status of patients with chronic asthma (AAAAI, 2016).

Provides information to evaluate desired effect of medication.

Any impairment of grasp or presence of hand tremors interferes with patient's ability to depress canister within inhaler. Spacer device is often necessary with an MDI.

Patients who have adequate understanding of how to use an inhaler may forget the procedure. Ongoing assessment of inhaler technique identifies areas for further education and reinforcement (Ari, 2015).

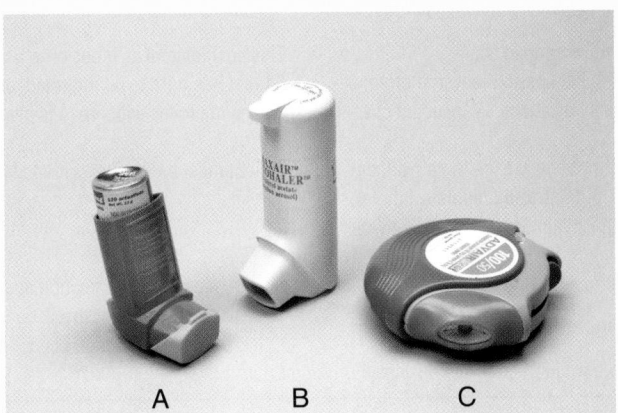

FIG. 31.33 Types of inhalers. **A,** Metered-dose inhaler (MDI). **B,** Breath-actuated inhaler (BAI). **C,** Dry powder inhaler (DPI).

Continued

SKILL 31.3   USING METERED-DOSE OR DRY POWDER INHALERS—cont'd

STEP	RATIONALE
9. Assess patient's readiness and ability to learn and use inhaler. Determine type of device patient may prefer, considering portability, access to obtain, and cost. Ask questions about medication and its availability. Determine whether patient is alert, able to participate in own care, and is not fatigued, in pain, or in respiratory distress.	When selecting an aerosol delivery device, consider several factors, such as medication availability and administration time, patient age and ability to use the device correctly, portability of device, convenience in both outpatient and inpatient settings, and costs, as well as health care provider and patient preference (Barrons et al., 2015; Bonini and Usmani, 2015). In some situations, mental or physical limitations affect patient's ability to learn and methods used for instruction.
10. Assess patient's knowledge and understanding of disease and purpose and action of prescribed medications.	Knowledge of disease is essential for patient to realistically understand when to use inhaler.

PLANNING

1. Perform hand hygiene. Collect appropriate equipment and MAR.	Promotes time management and efficiency when preparing medications for all patients.
2. Plan preparation to avoid interruptions. Create a quiet environment. Do not take phone calls or talk with others. Follow agency "No-interruption zone" policy.	Interruptions contribute to medication errors (Westbrook et al., 2017; Yoder et al., 2015) (see Box 31.4).

IMPLEMENTATION

1. Prepare medications for inhalation. Attend to procedure and avoid distraction. Check label of medication against MAR two times, when removing inhaler from unit dose or AMDS and before leaving medication preparation area (see Skill 31.1). Preparation usually involves taking inhaler device out of storage and into patient room. Check expiration date on container. Perform hand hygiene.	*These are the first and second checks for accuracy.* Process ensures that right patient receives right medication.
2. Take medication to patient at correct time (see agency policy). Medications that require exact timing include STAT dose, first-time or loading doses, and one-time doses. Give time-critical scheduled medications (e.g., antibiotics, anticoagulants, insulin, anticonvulsants, or immunosuppressive agents) at exact time ordered (no more than 30 minutes before or after scheduled dose). Give non–time-critical scheduled medications within a range of 1 or 2 hours of scheduled dose (ISMP, 2011a). During administration apply seven rights of medication administration.	Hospitals must adopt medication administration policy and procedure for timing of medication administration that considers nature of the prescribed medication, specific clinical application, and patient needs (DHHS, 2011; ISMP, 2011a). Time-critical scheduled medications are those for which early or delayed administration of maintenance doses of greater than 30 minutes before or after the scheduled dose may cause harm or result in substantial suboptimal therapy or pharmacological effect. Non–time-critical medications are those for which early or delayed administration within a specified range of either 1 or 2 hours should not cause harm or result in substantial suboptimal therapy or pharmacological effect (DHHS, 2011; ISMP, 2011a).
3. Identify patient using at least two identifiers (e.g., name and birthday or name and medical record number) according to agency policy. Compare identifiers with information on patient's MAR or medical record.	Ensures correct patient. Complies with The Joint Commission standards and improves patient safety (TJC, 2020).
4. At patient's bedside again compare MAR or computer printout with names of medications on medication labels and patient name. Ask patient whether he or she has allergies.	*This is the third check for accuracy* and ensures that patient receives correct medication. Confirms patient's allergy history.
5. Help patient to sit up into high-Fowler's position or up in chair.	This position makes it easier to use inhaler.
6. Discuss purpose of each medication, action, and possible adverse effects. Allow patient to ask any questions about the medications. Warn about overuse of inhaler and side effects.	Patient has right to be informed, and patient's understanding of each medication improves adherence to medication therapy.
7. Explain procedure to patient. Be specific if patient wishes to self-administer medication. Allow adequate time for patient to manipulate inhaler, canister, and/or spacer device (if provided). Explain where and how to set up at home.	Patient must be familiar with how to use equipment.
8. Explain and demonstrate steps for administering MDI without spacer.	Simple one-on-one instruction and demonstration of step-by-step administration allow patient to ask questions at any point during procedure and increase patient adherence to inhaler use (Ari, 2015).
a. Insert MDI canister into holder. Then remove mouthpiece cover from inhaler.	

CLINICAL DECISION: *If using an MDI that is new or has not been used for several days, push a "test spray" into the air to prime the device before using. This ensures that the MDI is patent and that the metal canister is positioned properly.*

b. Shake inhaler well for 2 to 5 seconds (five or six shakes).	Aerosolizes fine particles of medication.
c. Have patient hold inhaler in dominant hand.	Easier position to activate device.

STEP	**RATIONALE**

   d. Instruct patient to position inhaler in one of two ways:

     (1) Have patient place close mouth around mouthpiece with opening toward back of throat, closing lips tightly around it (see illustration). Do not block the mouthpiece with the teeth or tongue

Proper positioning of inhaler is essential to administering medication correctly.

     (2) Position mouthpiece 2 to 4 cm (1 to 2 inches) in front of widely opened mouth (see illustration), with opening of inhaler toward back of throat. Lips should not touch inhaler.

Directs aerosol spray toward airway. This is best way to deliver medication without a spacer.

   e. While holding the mouthpiece away from the mouth, have patient take deep breath and exhale completely.

Empties lung volume and prepares airway to receive medication.

   f. With inhaler positioned correctly, be sure patient holds inhaler with thumb at mouthpiece and index and middle fingers at top. *This is a three-point or lateral hand position.*

MDIs are easier to activate when patients use a three-point or lateral hand position to activate canister (Burchum and Rosenthal, 2019).

   g. Instruct patient to tilt head back slightly and inhale slowly and deeply through mouth for 3 to 5 seconds while depressing canister fully.

Medication is distributed to airways during inhalation.

   h. Have patient hold breath for as long as comfortable, up to 10 seconds.

Allows aerosol spray droplets to reach deeper branches of airways.
Keeps small airways open during exhalation.

   i. Have patient remove MDI from mouth before exhaling and exhale slowly through nose or pursed lips.

9. Explain and demonstrate steps to administer MDI using spacer device.

Simple one-on-one instruction and demonstration of step-by-step administration allows patient to ask questions at any point during procedure and increases patient adherence to inhaler use (Ari, 2015).

   a. Remove mouthpiece cover from MDI and mouthpiece of spacer device.

Inhaler fits into end of spacer device.

   b. Shake inhaler well for 2 to 5 seconds (five or six shakes).

Aerosolizes fine particles of medication.

   c. Insert MDI into end of spacer device.

Spacer device traps medication released from MDI; patient then inhales medication from device. These devices resolve hand-breath coordination difficulty to improve delivery of correct dose of inhaled medication (Barrons et al., 2015).

   d. Instruct patient to place spacer device mouthpiece in mouth and close lips. Do not insert beyond raised lip on mouthpiece. Avoid covering small exhalation slots with lips.

Medication should not escape through mouth.

   e. Have patient take a deep breath, exhale, and then breathe normally through spacer device mouthpiece (see illustration).

Allows patient to empty lungs and relax before delivering medication.

   f. Instruct patient to depress medication canister 1 time, spraying one puff into spacer device.

Spacer contains fine spray and allows patient to inhale more medication. The spacer increases medication delivery and deposition of the medication on the oropharyngeal mucosa (Burchum and Rosenthal, 2019).

   g. Have patient breathe slowly and fully through mouth for 5 seconds.

Ensures that particles of medication are distributed to deeper airways.

   h. Instruct patient to hold full breath for 10 seconds.

Ensures full medication distribution through airways.

   i. Have patient remove MDI and spacer and then exhale.

10. Explain steps to administer a DPI or breath-actuated (BAI) inhaler

   a. If DPI has an external counter, note number indicated.

Determines doses remaining.

   b. Remove mouthpiece cover. *Do not shake* inhaler

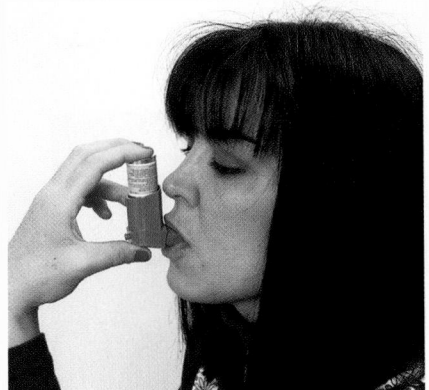

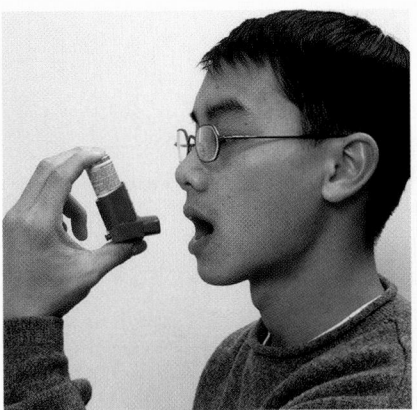

STEP 8d(1) Patient opens lips and places inhaler mouthpiece in mouth with opening toward back of throat.

STEP 8d(2) Patient positions inhaler mouthpiece 2 to 4 cm (1 to 2 inches) from widely open mouth. This is considered the best way to deliver medication without a spacer.

Continued

SKILL 31.3	USING METERED-DOSE OR DRY POWDER INHALERS—cont'd
STEP	RATIONALE

   c. Prepare medication. Some DPIs require loading medication before administration; some require rotation of a lever to load medication or insertion of a capsule; and some require insertion of a disk into inhaler device. Follow manufacturer specific instructions.

Primes inhaler, ensuring that medication is delivered to patient effectively.

   d. Have patient take a breath and exhale away from the inhaler.

Prevents loss of powder.

   e. Have patient position mouthpiece of DPI between lips and inhale quickly and deeply through mouth (see illustration).

Keeps medication from escaping through mouth. Forceful inhalation creates an aerosol.

   f. Have patient hold breath for 5 to 10 seconds.

Distributes medication.

11. Instruct patient to wait 20 to 30 seconds between inhalations (if same medication) or 2 to 5 minutes between inhalations (if different medications). Be sure patient inhales correct number of prescribed puffs.

Medications must be inhaled sequentially. Always administer bronchodilators before steroids so that dilators can open airway passages (Burchum and Rosenthal, 2019).

12. Instruct patient to not repeat inhalations before next scheduled dose.

Medications are prescribed at intervals during day to provide constant medication levels and minimize side effects. Beta-adrenergic MDIs are used either on an "as needed" basis or regularly every 4 to 6 hours.

13. Warn patients that they may feel gagging sensation in throat caused by droplets of medication on pharynx or tongue.

This occurs when medication is sprayed and inhaled incorrectly.

14. About 2 minutes after last dose, instruct patient to rinse mouth with warm water and spit water out.

Steroids may alter normal flora of oral mucosa and lead to development of fungal infection. Rinsing out patient's mouth reduces risk of fungal infection (Ari, 2015).

15. Instruct patient how to clean the inhaler.

Removes residual medication and reduces transmission of microorganisms.

   a. Once a day remove MDI canister and cap from the mouthpiece. Do not wash the canister or immerse it in water. Run warm tap water through the top and bottom of the plastic mouthpiece for 30 to 60 seconds. Make sure that inhaler is completely dry before reusing. Do not get valve mechanism of canister wet.

Water damages valve mechanism of canister. Accumulation of medication around mouthpiece interferes with proper medication distribution during use.

   b. Instruct patient to clean mouthpiece of MDI and spacer twice a week with a mild dishwashing soap, rinse thoroughly, and dry completely before storage.

Provides better antimicrobial removal. Pressurized metered-dose inhalers are potential reservoirs for bacteria.

16. Help patient to comfortable position and perform hand hygiene.

Reduces transmission of microorganisms and promotes patient comfort.

EVALUATION

1. Auscultate patient lungs, listen for abnormal breath sounds, and obtain peak flow measures if ordered.

Determines patient response to medication.

2. Have patient explain and demonstrate steps in use and cleaning of inhaler.

Return demonstration provides feedback for measuring patient's learning.

3. Ask patient to explain medication schedule and dose of medication.

Improves likelihood of adherence to therapy.

4. Ask patient to describe side effects of medication and criteria for calling health care provider.

Allows patient to recognize signs of overuse and need to seek medical support when medications are ineffective.

5. **Use Teach-Back:** "I want to be sure I clearly showed you how to use your inhaler. Let's take this time; show me how you will use the inhaler to take your medicine." Revise your instruction now or develop a plan for revised patient/family caregiver teaching if patient/family caregiver is not able to teach back correctly.

Determines patient's/family caregiver's level of understanding of instructional topic.

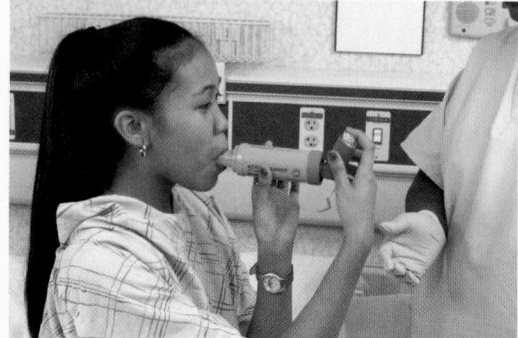

STEP 9e Using spacer device with an MDI.

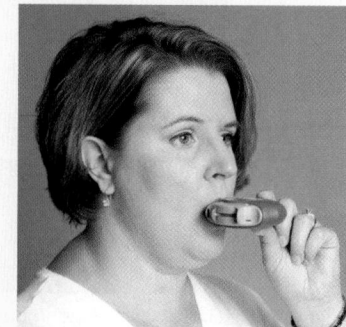

STEP 10e Have patient place mouthpiece of dry powder inhaler (DPI) between lips.

UNEXPECTED OUTCOMES AND RELATED INTERVENTIONS

1. Patient's respirations are rapid and shallow; breath sounds indicate wheezing.
   - Evaluate vital signs and respiratory status.
   - Notify health care provider.
   - Reassess type of medication and/or delivery method.
2. Patient needs bronchodilator more than every 4 hours (may indicate respiratory problem).
   - Reassess type of medication and delivery methods needed.
   - Notify health care provider.
3. Patient experiences cardiac dysrhythmias (e.g., light-headedness, syncope), especially if receiving beta-adrenergic medications.
   - Withhold all further doses of medication.
   - Evaluate cardiac and pulmonary status (see Chapter 30).
   - Notify health care provider for reassessment of type of medication and delivery method.

RECORDING AND REPORTING

- Record medication administered, dose or strength, number of inhalations, and actual time administered immediately after administration, not before. Include initials or signature.
- Record patient and family caregiver teaching (use of teach-back) and validation of understanding on flow sheet or nurses' notes in electronic health record (EHR) or chart.
- Record on flow sheet or nurses' notes in electronic health record (EHR) or chart the patient's response to inhaled medication (e.g., respiratory rate and pattern, breath sounds), evidence of side effects (e.g., arrhythmia, patient's feelings of anxiety), and patient's ability to use inhaler.
- Report adverse effects and patient response and/or withheld medications to nurse in charge or health care provider.

SKILL 31.4	PREPARING INJECTIONS FROM VIALS AND AMPULES

Delegation and Collaboration

The skill of preparing injections from ampules and vials cannot be delegated to assistive personnel (AP).

Equipment
Medication in an Ampule
- Syringe, needle, and filter needle
- Small sterile gauze pad or alcohol swab

Medication in a Vial
- Syringe and two needles
- Needles:
  - Needleless blunt-tip vial-access cannula or needle (with safety sheath) for drawing up medication (if needed)
  - Filter needle if indicated
- Small sterile gauze pad or alcohol swab
- Diluent (e.g., 0.9% sodium chloride or sterile water if indicated)

Both
- Sharps with engineered sharps injury protection (SESIP) safety needle for injection
- Medication administration record (MAR) or computer printout
- Medication in vial or ampule
- Puncture-proof container for disposal of syringes, needles, and glass

STEP	RATIONALE

ASSESSMENT

1. Check accuracy and completeness of each MAR or computer printout with health care provider's written medication order. Check patient's name, medication name and dosage, route of administration, and time of administration. Clarify incomplete or unclear orders with health care provider before administration.

   The order sheet is the most reliable source and only legal record of medications that patient is to receive. Ensures that patient receives the correct medications (Westbrook et al., 2017). Transcription errors are a source of medication errors (Truitt et al., 2016).

2. Review pertinent information related to medication, including action, purpose, normal dose and route, side effects, time of onset and peak action, indication and nursing implications.

   Allows you to anticipate effects of medication while observing patient's response.

3. Assess patient's medical and medication history and history of allergies. List medication allergies on each page of the MAR and prominently display it on the patient's medical record. When allergies are present, patient should wear an allergy bracelet.

   Factors influence how certain medications act. Reveals patient's need for medication.
   Allergy alert helps prevent adverse effects.

4. Review medication reference information for action, purpose, side effects, and nursing implications.

   Allows you to administer medication properly and monitor patient's response.

5. Assess patient's body build, muscle size, weight, and viscosity of medication if giving subcutaneous or intramuscular (IM) medication.

   Determines type and size of syringe and needle for injection.

PLANNING

1. Perform hand hygiene. Collect appropriate equipment and MAR.

   Promotes time management and efficiency when preparing medications for all patients.

2. Plan preparation to avoid interruptions. Create a quiet environment. Do not take phone calls or talk with others. Follow agency "No-interruption zone" policy. Keep all pages of MARs or computer printouts for one patient together or look at only one patient's electronic MAR at a time.

   Interruptions contribute to medication errors (Westbrook et al., 2017; Yoder et al., 2015) (see Box 31.4).

Continued

SKILL 31.4	**PREPARING INJECTIONS FROM VIALS AND AMPULES—cont'd**

STEP	**RATIONALE**

IMPLEMENTATION

1. Perform hand hygiene and prepare medications.
   a. If using a medication cart, move it outside patient's room.
   b. Unlock medication drawer or cart or log onto AMDS.
   c. Select correct medication from stock supply or unit-dose drawer. Compare label of medication with MAR computer printout or computer screen.
   d. Check expiration date on each medication, one at a time.

   e. Calculate medication dose as necessary. Double-check your calculation. In the case of high-risk medications ask another nurse to perform an independent double check of dosage (see agency policy).
   f. If preparing a controlled substance, check record for previous medication count and compare with supply available.
   g. Do not leave medications unattended.
2. Prepare ampule.
   a. Tap top of ampule lightly and quickly with finger until fluid moves from its neck (see illustration).
   b. Place small gauze pad around neck of ampule (see illustration).

   c. Snap neck of ampule quickly and firmly away from hands (see illustration).
   d. Draw up medication quickly, using filter needle long enough to reach bottom of ampule to access medication.
   e. Hold ampule upside down or set it on flat surface. Insert filter needle into center of ampule opening. Do not allow needle tip or shaft to touch rim of ampule.
   f. Aspirate medication into syringe by gently pulling back on plunger (see illustrations).

Organization of equipment saves time and reduces error.
Medications are safeguarded when locked in cabinet, cart, or AMDS.
Reading label and comparing it with transcribed order reduce errors. *This is the first check for accuracy.*
Medications used past their expiration date are sometimes inactive, less effective, or harmful to patients.
Double-checking may help reduce error. Independent double checks should be used only for very selective high-alert medications (not all) that most warrant their use (ISMP, 2018a).
Controlled substance laws require careful monitoring of dispensed narcotics.

Nurse is responsible for safekeeping of medications.

Dislodges any fluid that collects above neck of ampule. All solution moves into lower chamber.
Protects fingers from trauma as glass tip is broken off. Do not use opened alcohol swab to wrap around top of ampule because alcohol may leak into ampule.
Protects your fingers and face from shattering glass.
System is open to airborne contaminants. Filter needles filter out any fragments of glass (Joo et al., 2016).
Broken rim of ampule is considered contaminated. When ampule is inverted, solution dribbles out if needle tip or shaft touches rim of ampule.
Withdrawal of plunger creates negative pressure within syringe barrel, which pulls fluid into syringe.

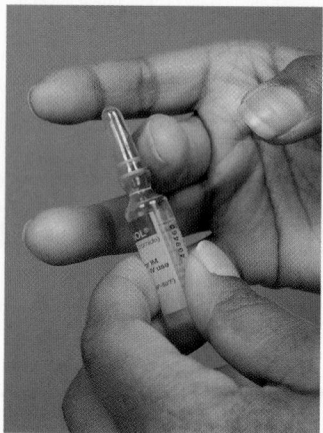

STEP 2a Tapping ampule moves fluid down neck.

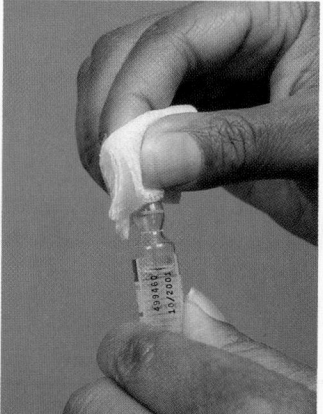

STEP 2b Gauze pad placed around neck of ampule.

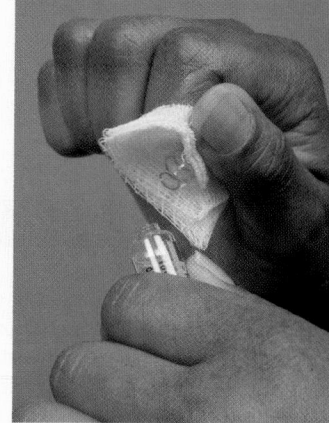

STEP 2c Neck snapped away from hands.

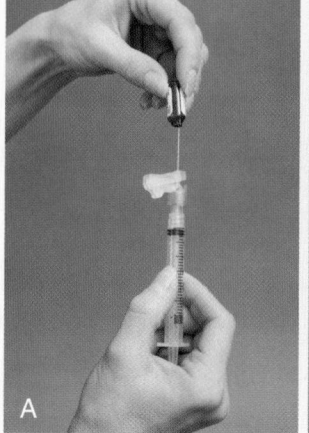
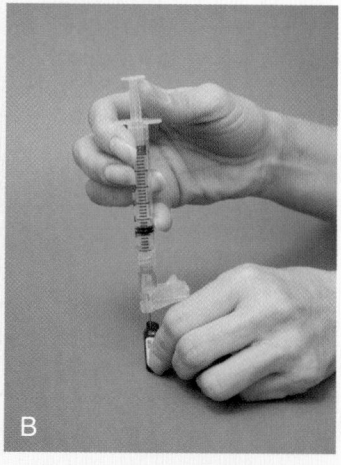

STEP 2f A, Medication aspirated with ampule inverted. **B,** Medication aspirated with ampule on flat surface

STEP	**RATIONALE**

g. Keep needle tip under surface of liquid. Tip ampule to bring all fluid within reach of needle.

Prevents aspiration of air bubbles.

h. If you aspirate air bubbles, do not expel air into ampule.

Air pressure forces fluid out of ampule, and medication will be lost.

i. To expel excess air bubbles, remove needle from ampule. Hold syringe vertically with needle pointing up. Tap side of syringe to cause bubbles to rise toward needle. Draw back slightly on plunger and push plunger upward to eject air. Do not eject fluid.

Withdrawing plunger too far removes it from barrel. Holding syringe vertically allows fluid to settle in bottom of barrel. Pulling back on plunger allows fluid within needle to enter barrel so that fluid is not expelled. Then expel air at top of barrel and within needle.

j. If syringe contains excess fluid, use sink for disposal. Hold syringe vertically with needle tip up and slanted slightly toward sink. Slowly eject excess fluid into sink. Recheck fluid level in syringe by holding it vertically.

Safely disperses excess medication into sink. Position of needle allows you to expel medication without having it flow down needle shaft. Rechecking fluid level ensures proper dose.

k. Cover needle with its safety sheath or cap. Replace filter needle with regular SESIP needle.

Minimizes needlesticks. Filter needles cannot be used for injection.

3. Prepare vial containing a solution.

a. Remove cap covering top of unused vial to expose sterile rubber seal. If a multi-dose vial has been used before, cap is already removed. Firmly and briskly wipe surface of rubber seal with alcohol swab and allow it to dry.

Vial comes packaged with cap that cannot be replaced after seal removal. Not all medication manufacturers guarantee that rubber seals of unused vials are sterile. Swabbing with alcohol reduces transmission of microorganisms. Allowing alcohol to dry prevents alcohol from coating needle and mixing with medication.

b. Pick up syringe and remove needle cap or cap covering needleless access device (see illustration). Pull back on plunger to draw amount of air into syringe equivalent to volume of medication to be aspirated from vial.

Injecting air into vial prevents buildup of negative pressure in vial when aspirating medication.

c. With vial on flat surface, insert tip of needle or needleless device through center of rubber seal (see illustration). Apply pressure to tip of needle during insertion.

Center of seal is thinner and easier to penetrate. Using firm pressure prevents dislodging rubber particles that could enter vial or needle.

d. Inject air into air space of vial, holding on to plunger. Hold plunger firmly; plunger is sometimes forced backward by air pressure within vial.

Injection of air creates vacuum needed to get medication to flow into syringe. Injecting into air space of vial prevents formation of bubbles and an inaccurate dose.

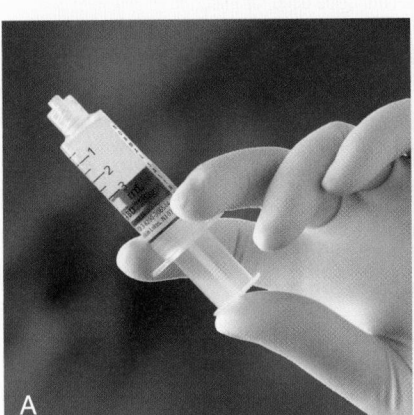
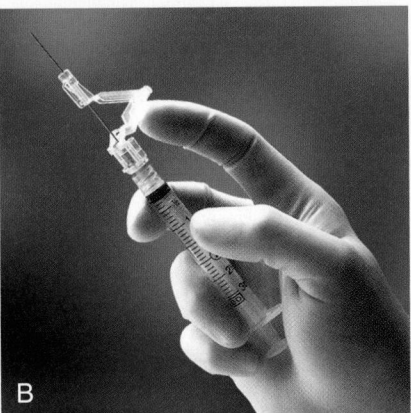
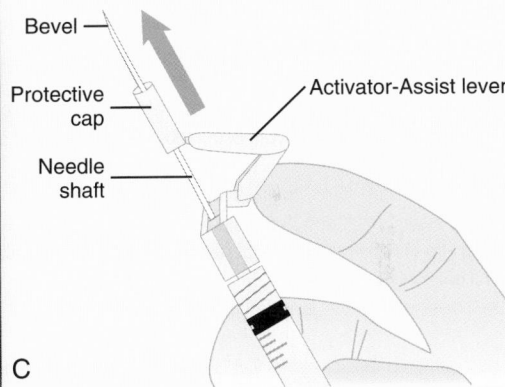

STEP 3b A, Needleless system. **B,** Safety needle system. **C,** Detail of safety needle system. (**A** and **B** Courtesy and © Becton, Dickinson and Company.)

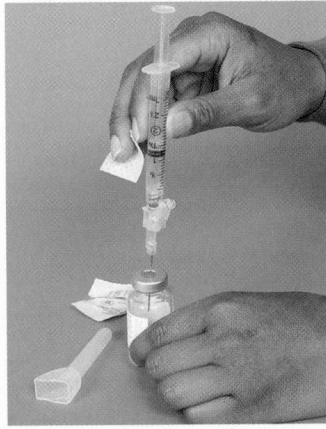
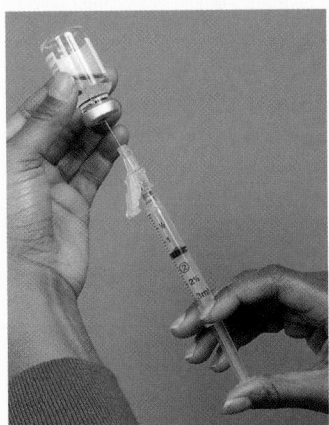
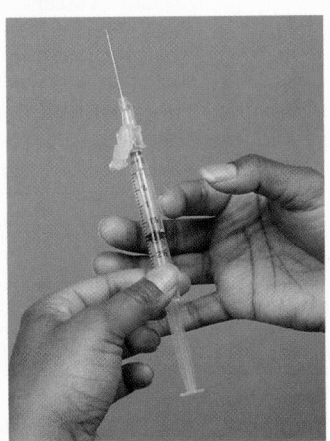

STEP 3c Insert safety needle through center of vial diaphragm (with vial flat on table).

STEP 3e Withdraw fluid with vial inverted.

STEP 3h Hold syringe upright; tap barrel to dislodge air bubbles.

Continued

SKILL 31.4   PREPARING INJECTIONS FROM VIALS AND AMPULES—cont'd

STEP	RATIONALE
e. Invert vial while keeping firm hold on syringe and plunger. Hold vial between thumb and middle fingers of nondominant hand (see illustration). Grasp end of syringe barrel and plunger with thumb and forefinger of dominant hand to counteract pressure in vial.	Inverting vial allows fluid to settle in lower half of container. Position of hands prevents forceful movement of plunger and permits easy manipulation of syringe.
f. Keep tip of needle or needleless device below fluid level.	Prevents aspiration of air.
g. Allow air pressure from vial to fill syringe gradually with medication. If necessary, pull back slightly on plunger to obtain correct amount of medication.	Positive pressure within vial forces fluid into syringe.
h. When you obtain desired volume, position needle or needleless device into air space of vial; tap side of syringe barrel gently to dislodge any air bubbles (see illustration). Eject any air remaining at top of syringe into vial.	Forcefully striking barrel while needle is inserted in vial may bend needle. Accumulation of air displaces medication and causes dose errors.
i. Remove needle or needleless access device from vial by pulling back on barrel of syringe.	Pulling plunger rather than barrel causes plunger to separate from barrel, resulting in loss of medication.
j. Hold syringe at eye level at 90-degree angle to ensure correct volume and absence of air bubbles. Remove any remaining air by tapping barrel to dislodge any air bubbles. Draw back slightly on plunger; then push it upward to eject air. Do not eject fluid. Recheck volume of medication.	Holding syringe vertically allows fluid to settle in bottom of barrel. Tapping dislodges air to top of barrel. Pulling back on plunger allows fluid within needle to enter barrel so that you do not expel fluid. You then expel air at top of barrel and within needle.

CLINICAL DECISION: *When preparing medication from single-dose vial, do not assume that volume listed on label is total volume in vial. Some manufacturers provide small amount of extra liquid, expecting loss during preparation. Be sure to draw up only desired volume.*

k. Before you inject medication into patient's tissue, change needle with regular SESIP to appropriate gauge and length according to route of medication administration.	Inserting needle through rubber stopper dulls beveled tip. New needle is sharper and, because no fluid is along shaft, does not track medication through tissues. Filter needles cannot be used for injection.
l. Cover needle with its safety sheath or cap.	Minimizes needlesticks.
m. For multi-dose vial, make label that includes date of opening, concentration of medication per milliliter, and your initials.	Ensures that nurses will prepare future doses correctly. You discard some medications within a certain time frame after mixing.
4. Prepare vial containing powder (reconstituting medications).	
a. Remove cap covering vial of powdered medication and cap covering vial of proper diluent. Firmly swab both rubber seals with alcohol swab and allow alcohol to dry.	Allowing alcohol to dry prevents it from coating needle and mixing with medication.
b. Draw up manufacturer suggestion for volume and type of diluent into syringe following Steps 3b through 3j.	Prepares diluent for injection into vial containing powdered medication.
c. Insert tip of needle or needleless device through center of rubber seal of vial of powdered medication. Inject diluent into vial. Remove needle.	Diluent begins to dissolve and reconstitute medication.
d. Mix medication thoroughly. Roll in palms. Do not shake.	Ensures proper dispersal of medication throughout solution and prevents formation of air bubbles.
e. Reconstituted medication in vial is ready to be drawn into new syringe. Read label carefully to determine dose after reconstitution.	Once you add diluent, concentration of medication (mg/mL) determines dose you give. Reading medication label carefully decreases medication errors.
f. Draw up reconstituted medication into syringe. Insert needleless device/needle into vial. Do not add air. Then follow Steps 3e through 3l.	Prepares medication for administration.

CLINICAL DECISION: *Some agencies require that doses of certain medications (e.g., insulin and heparin) be checked using an independent double check by another nurse (ISMP, 2018a). Check policies and procedures before administering medication.*

5. Compare label of medication with MAR, computer screen, or computer printout.	*This is the second check for accuracy.*
6. Dispose of soiled supplies. Place broken ampule and/or used vials and used needle or needleless device in puncture- and leak-proof container. Clean work area and perform hand hygiene.	Proper disposal of glass and needle prevents accidental injury to staff. Controls transmission of infection.

EVALUATION

1. Just before administering medication to patient, compare MAR with label of prepared medication and compare dose in syringe with desired dose.	Ensures that dose is accurate. *This is the third check for accuracy.*

UNEXPECTED OUTCOMES AND RELATED INTERVENTIONS

1. Air bubbles remain in syringe.
   - Expel air from syringe and add medication to it until you prepare correct dose.
2. Incorrect dose of medication is prepared.
   - Discard prepared dose.
   - Prepare correct new dose.

SKILL 31.5   ADMINISTERING INJECTIONS

Delegation and Collaboration

The skill of administering injections cannot be delegated to assistive personnel (AP). The nurse instructs the AP about:

- Potential medication side effects and allergic responses and the need to report their occurrence along with any changes in patient's vital signs or level of consciousness (e.g., sedation).

Equipment

- Proper size syringe and (SESIP) needle:
  - *Subcutaneous:* syringe (1- to 3-mL) and needle (25- to 27-gauge, ⅜- to ⅝-inch)
  - *Immunizations:* 5/8-inch, 23- to 25-gauge needle (CDC, 2017)

- *Subcutaneous U-100 insulin:* insulin syringe (1 mL) with preattached needle (28- to 31-gauge, ⅜- to ⅝-inch)
- *Subcutaneous U-500 insulin:* insulin syringe (1 mL) with preattached needle (28- to 31-gauge, ⅜- to ⅝-inch) (Consumer Med Safety, 2018b).
- *Intramuscular (IM):* Syringe 2 to 3 mL for adult, 0.5 to 1 mL for infants and small children
- Needle length typically corresponds to site of injection, age, gender, and size of patient. Refer to following guidelines for vaccine administration; length needed may vary outside of these guidelines for patients who are smaller or larger than average.

NEEDLE LENGTH FOR IMMUNIZATIONS*

Site	Child	Adult
Ventrogluteal	Not recommended	1½ inches
Vastus lateralis	⅝-1.25 inch	⅝-1 inch
Deltoid	⅝-1 inch	1-1½ inches

Gender-Male	Gender-Female	Needle Length
Less than 130 pounds	Less than 130 pounds	⅝-1 inch
130-152 pounds	130-152 pounds	1 inch
153-260 pounds	153-200 pounds	1-1½ inches
260+ pounds	200+ pounds	1½ inches

Age-Group	Needle Length	Site
Neonates[a]	⅝ inch (16 mm)[b]	Vastus lateralis
Infants, 1-12 months	1 inch (25 mm)	Vastus lateralis
Toddlers, 1-2 years	1-1.25 inch (25-32 mm)	Vastus lateralis [c]
	⅝ [b]-1 inch (16-25 mm)	Deltoid muscle of arm
Children, 3-10 years	⅝ [b]-1 inch (16-25 mm)	Deltoid muscle of arm[c]
	1-1.25 inches (25-32 mm)	Vastus lateralis
Children, 11-18 years	⅝ [b]-1 inch (16-25 mm)	Deltoid muscle of arm[c]
	1-1.5 inches (25-38 mm)	Vastus lateralis
Men and women, <60 kg (130 lb)	1 inch (25 mm)	Deltoid muscle of arm
Men and women, 60-70 kg (130-152 lb)	1 inch (25 mm)	Deltoid muscle of arm
Men, 70-118 kg (152-260 lb)	1-1.5 inches (25-38 mm)	Deltoid muscle of arm
Women, 70-90 kg (152-200 lb)	1-1.5 inches (25-38 mm)	Deltoid muscle of arm
Men, >118 kg (260 lb)	1.5 inches (38 mm)	Deltoid muscle of arm
Women, >90 kg (200 lb)	1.5 inches (38 mm)	Deltoid muscle of arm

*Centers for Disease Control and Prevention (CDC): *Vaccine administration,* 2017, https://www.cdc.gov/vaccines/hcp/acip-recs/general-recs/administration.html.
[a]First 28 days of life.
[b]If skin is stretched tightly and subcutaneous tissues are not bunched.
[c]Preferred site.

Based on CDC, 2017 Guidelines

- Needle gauge often depends on length of needle; administer biologic and medication in aqueous solution with a 20- to 25-gauge needle. Use 18- to 21-gauge needles for medications in oil-based solutions
- *Intradermal (ID):* 1-mL tuberculin syringe with needle (25- to 27-gauge, ½- to ⅝-inch)

All Injections

- Small gauze pad
- Alcohol swab
- Vial or ampule of medication or skin test solution
- Clean gloves
- Medication administration record (MAR) (electronic or printed)
- Puncture-proof container for sharps

Continued

SKILL 31.5   ADMINISTERING INJECTIONS—cont'd

STEP	RATIONALE

ASSESSMENT

1. Check accuracy and completeness of each MAR with health care provider's medication order. Check patient's name, medication name and dosage, and route and time of administration. Clarify incomplete or unclear orders with health care provider before administration.

   The order sheet is the most reliable source and only legal record of medications that patient is to receive. Ensures that patient receives the correct medications (Westbrook et al., 2017). Transcription errors are a source of medication errors (Truitt et al., 2016).

2. Assess patient's medical and medication history and history of allergies. List medication allergies on each page of the MAR and prominently display any allergies on the patient's medical record. When allergies are present, patient should wear an allergy bracelet.

   Factors influence how certain medications act. Reveals patient's need for medication.

   Allergy alert helps prevent adverse effects.

3. Review medication reference information for medication action, purpose, normal dose, side effects, time and peak of onset, and nursing implications. In the case of an intradermal injection, review expected reaction and/or anticipated effects when testing skin with specific allergen and appropriate time to read site.

   Allows you to administer medication safely and monitor patient's response to therapy. Type of reaction to an immunization depends on patient's ability to mount a cell-mediated immune response. Knowledge of expected and adverse reactions to skin testing helps you determine for which symptoms to monitor, how frequently, and when to reassess patient.

4. Assess for contraindications to injections.
   a. For ID injections
      (1) Reduced local tissue perfusion. Assess for history of severe adverse reactions that occurred after previous ID injection.

   Decreased tissue perfusion reduces absorption of ID medications. Prior history of severe reactions increases the risk for future severe reactions.

   b. For subcutaneous injections
      (1) Assess for factors such as circulatory shock or reduced local tissue perfusion. Assess adequacy of patient's adipose tissue.

   Reduced tissue perfusion interferes with medication absorption and distribution. Physiological changes of aging or patient illness often influence amount of subcutaneous tissue that patient possesses.

   c. For IM injections
      (1) Assess for factors such as muscle atrophy, reduced blood flow, or circulatory shock.

   Atrophied muscle absorbs medication poorly. Factors interfering with blood flow to muscles impair medication absorption.

5. Assess patient's knowledge of purpose and expected response to medication or skin testing.

   Patients need to know when to return for follow-up reading of skin test and when and how to report any reaction. Poses implications for patient education.

6. Assess patient's symptoms before initiating medication therapy.

   Provides information to evaluate desired effect of medication.

7. Assess patient's knowledge about medication.

   Determines whether there is a need for patient education.

8. For subcutaneous insulin or heparin, assess relevant laboratory results (e.g., blood glucose, partial thromboplastin).

   Provides baseline for measuring medication response.

9. Observe patient's previous verbal and nonverbal responses toward injection.

   Anticipating patient's anxiety allows you to use distraction to reduce pain awareness.

10. Check expiration date on medication.

    Dose potency increases or decreases when expired.

PLANNING

1. Perform hand hygiene. Collect appropriate equipment and MAR

   Promotes time management and efficiency when preparing medications for all patients.

2. Plan preparation to avoid interruptions. Create a quiet environment. Do not take phone calls or talk with others. Follow agency "No-interruption zone" policy. Keep all pages of MARs or computer printouts for one patient together or look at only one patient's electronic MAR at a time.

   Interruptions contribute to medication errors (Westbrook et al., 2017; Yoder et al., 2015) (see Box 31.4).

IMPLEMENTATION

1. Prepare medications for injection. Attend to procedure and avoid distraction. Check label of medication against MAR two times, when removing medication from unit dose or AMDS and before leaving medication preparation area (see Skill 31.1). Perform hand hygiene.

   Ensures that medication is sterile. Preventing distractions reduces medication preparation errors. *These are the first and second checks for accuracy* and ensure that correct medication is administered. Reduces transmission of microorganisms. Hand hygiene decreases transfer of microorganisms.

2. Take medications to patient at correct time (see agency policy). Medications that require exact timing include STAT doses, first-time, loading, and one-time doses. Give time-critical scheduled medications (e.g., antibiotics, anticoagulants, insulin, anticonvulsants, or immunosuppressive agents) at exact time ordered (within 30 minutes before or after scheduled dose). Give non–time-critical scheduled medications within a range of either 1 or 2 hours of scheduled doses (ISMP, 2011a). Apply the seven rights of medication administration throughout medication administration.

   Ensures intended therapeutic effect and complies with professional standards. Hospitals need to adopt a medication administration policy and procedure for the timing of medication administration that considers patient needs, prescribed medication, and specific clinical indications (CMS, 2014; ISMP, 2011a). Time-critical scheduled medications are medications in which early or delayed administration of maintenance doses of more than 30 minutes before or after the scheduled dose may cause harm or result in suboptimal therapy or pharmacological effect. Non–time-critical medications are medications in which early or delayed administration of 1 to 2 hours should not cause harm or result in suboptimal therapy or pharmacological effects (CMS, 2014; ISMP, 2011a).

STEP	RATIONALE
3. Close room curtain or door.	Provides privacy.
4. Identify patient using at least two identifiers (e.g., name and birthday or name and medical record number) according to agency policy. Compare identifiers with information on patient's MAR or medical record.	Ensures correct patient. Complies with The Joint Commission standards and improves patient safety (TJC, 2020).
5. At patient's bedside, compare MAR or computer printout with names of medications on medication labels and patient name. Ask patient whether he or she has allergies.	*This is the third accuracy check* and ensures that patient receives correct medication. Confirms patient's allergy history.
6. Discuss purpose of each medication and/or skin test, action, and possible adverse effects. Allow patient to ask any questions. Tell patient that injection will cause slight burning or sting. An intradermal injection will create a small bleb on the skin.	Patient has right to be informed, and patient's understanding of each medication improves adherence to medication therapy. Helps minimize patient's anxiety.
7. Perform hand hygiene and apply clean gloves. Keep sheet or gown draped over body parts not requiring exposure.	Reduces transmission of microorganisms. Draping the patient provides privacy.
8. Select appropriate injection site. Inspect skin surface over sites for bruises, inflammation, or edema.	Injection sites need to be free of abnormalities that interfere with medication absorption. Sites used repeatedly become hardened from lipohypertrophy (increased growth in fatty tissue). Do not use an area that is bruised or has signs associated with infection.
a. Intradermal (ID): (1) Note lesions or discolorations of skin. If possible, select site three to four finger widths below antecubital space and a hand width above wrist. If you cannot use forearm, inspect upper back. If necessary, use sites for subcutaneous injections.	An ID site needs to be clear, so you can see results of skin test and interpret them correctly (WHO, 2016).
b. Subcutaneous: (1) Do not use an area that is bruised or has signs associated with infection. Palpate sites and avoid those with masses or tenderness. Be sure that needle is correct size by grasping skinfold at site with thumb and forefinger. Measure fold from top to bottom. Make sure that needle is one-half length of fold.	You can mistakenly give subcutaneous injections in muscle, especially in abdomen and thigh sites. Appropriate size of needle ensures that you inject medication into subcutaneous tissue (Ogston-Tuck, 2014a).
(2) When administering insulin or heparin, use abdominal injection sites first, followed by thigh injection site. Choose site on right or left side of abdomen at least 5 cm (2 inches) away from umbilicus.	Injecting LMWH on side of abdomen helps decrease pain and bruising at injection site (RCN, 2016).
c. IM: (1) Note integrity and size of muscle and palpate for tenderness or hardness. Avoid these areas. If injections are given frequently, rotate sites. Use ventrogluteal site if possible.	Ventrogluteal is the preferred injection site for adults (CDC, 2017). The anterolateral thigh can be used for children of all ages but the ventrogluteal site is the preferred choice as it causes fewer reactions (Hockenberry et al, 2019; Ogston-Tuck, 2014b).
9. Help patient to comfortable position:	
a. ID: Have patient extend elbow and support it and forearm on flat surface.	Stabilizes injection site for easiest accessibility.
b. Subcutaneous: Have patient relax arm, leg, or abdomen, depending on site selection.	Relaxation of site minimizes discomfort.
c. IM: Position patient depending on site chosen (e.g., sit or lie flat, on side, or prone).	Reduces strain on muscle and minimizes discomfort of injections.

CLINICAL DECISION: *Ensure that medical condition (e.g., circulatory shock, orthopedic surgery) does not contraindicate patient's position for injection.*

STEP	RATIONALE
10. Relocate site using anatomical landmarks. For subcutaneous insulin, rotate site within anatomical area (e.g., abdomen) and systematically rotate sites within area.	Injection into correct anatomical site prevents injury to nerves, bones, and blood vessels.
11. Clean site with an antiseptic swab. Apply swab at center of site and rotate outward in circular direction for approximately 5 cm (2 inches) (see illustration). *Option for IM injection*: Apply eutectic mixture of local anesthetic (EMLA) cream on injection site at least 1 hour before IM injection or use vapocoolant spray (e.g., ethyl chloride) just before injection (see agency policy).	Mechanical action of swab removes secretions containing microorganisms. Decreases pain at injection site.
12. Hold swab or gauze between third and fourth fingers of nondominant hand.	Gauze or swab remains readily accessible when withdrawing needle after injection.
13. Remove needle cap or sheath from needle by pulling it straight off.	Preventing needle from touching sides of cap prevents contamination.
14. Hold syringe between thumb and forefinger of dominant hand:	
a. ID: Hold syringe with bevel of needle pointing up.	With bevel up, medication is less likely to be deposited into tissues below dermis.
b. Subcutaneous and IM: Hold as dart, palm up (see illustration).	Quick, smooth injection requires proper manipulation of syringe parts.

Continued

SKILL 31.5	ADMINISTERING INJECTIONS—cont'd

STEP	RATIONALE

15. Administer injection:
   a. Intradermal
      (1) With nondominant hand stretch skin over site with forefinger or thumb.

Needle pierces tight skin more easily.

      (2) With needle almost against patient's skin, insert it slowly with bevel up at 5- to 15-degree angle until resistance is felt. Advance needle through epidermis to approximately 3 mm (⅛ inch) below skin surface. You will see needle tip through skin.

Ensures that needle tip is in dermis. You obtain inaccurate results if you do not inject needle at correct angle and depth (WHO, 2016).

      (3) Inject medication slowly. Normally you feel resistance. If not, needle is too deep; remove and begin again.

Slow injection minimizes discomfort at site. Dermal layer is tight and does not expand easily when solution is injected.

      (4) While injecting medication, notice that small bleb approximately 6 mm (¼ inch) in diameter (resembling mosquito bite) appears on surface of skin (see illustration). Instruct patient that this is normal finding.

Bleb indicates that medication is deposited in dermis.

   b. Subcutaneous
      (1) For average-size patient, pinch skin with nondominant hand.

Needle penetrates taut skin more easily than loose skin. Pinching skin elevates subcutaneous tissue and desensitizes area.

      (2) Inject needle quickly and firmly at 45- to 90-degree angle (see Fig. 31.19). Release skin. *Option:* If using injection pen or administering heparin, continue to pinch skin while injecting medication.

Quick, firm insertion minimizes discomfort. (Injecting medication into compressed tissue irritates nerve fibers.) Correct angle prevents accidental injection into muscle.

      (3) For obese patient pinch skin at site and inject needle at 90-degree angle below tissue fold.

Obese patients have fatty layer of tissue above subcutaneous layer.

      (4) After needle enters site, grasp lower end of syringe barrel with nondominant hand to stabilize it. Move dominant hand to end of plunger and slowly inject medication over several seconds (see illustration). When giving heparin, inject over 30 seconds (Mohammady et al., 2017; RCN, 2016). Avoid moving syringe.

Movement of syringe may displace needle and cause discomfort. Slow injection of medication minimizes discomfort.

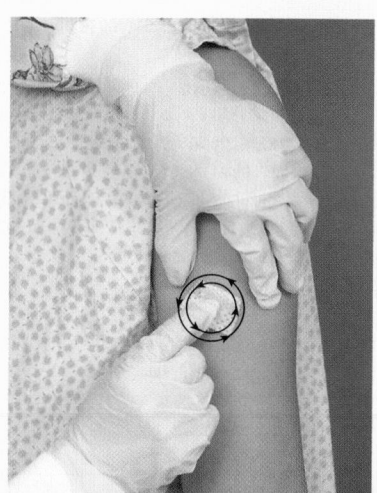

STEP 11 Clean site with circular motion.

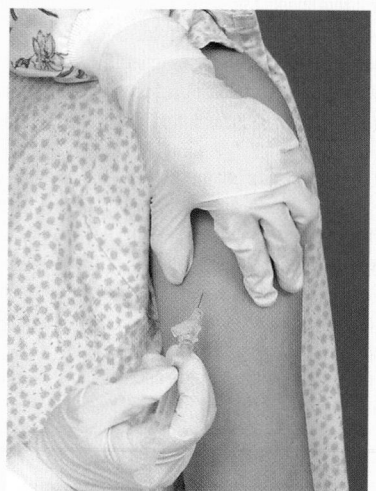

STEP 14b Hold syringe as if grasping a dart.

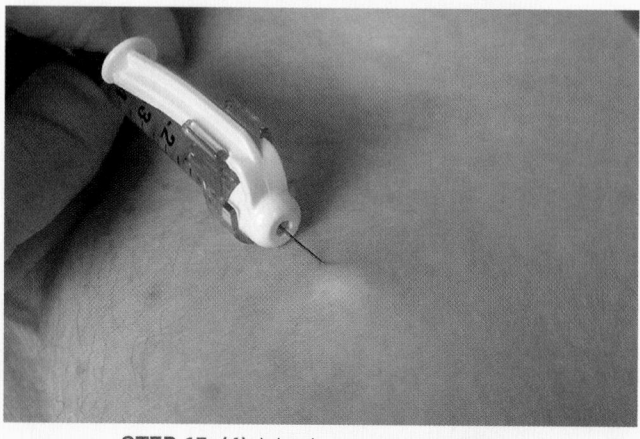

STEP 15a(4) Injection creates small bleb.

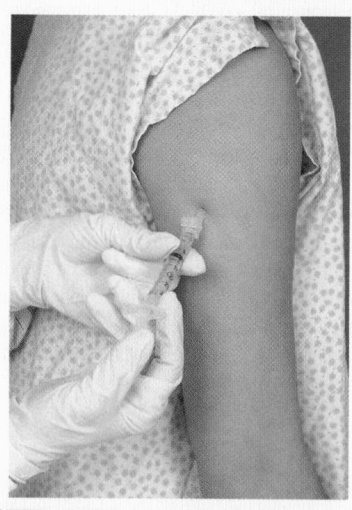

STEP 15b(4) Inject medication slowly.

STEP	RATIONALE

CLINICAL DECISION: *Aspiration after injecting a subcutaneous medication is not necessary. Piercing a blood vessel in a subcutaneous injection is very rare. Aspiration after injecting heparin and insulin is not recommended (CDC, 2017; Sepah, 2017).*

c. Intramuscular

(1) Position ulnar aspect of your nondominant hand just below site and pull skin approximately 2.5 to 3.5 cm (1 to 1.5 inches) down or laterally to administer in a Z-track. Hold position until medication is injected (see Fig. 31.24). With dominant hand inject needle quickly at 90-degree angle into muscle (see Fig. 31.20).

Z-track creates zigzag path through tissues that seals needle track to avoid tracking of medication. Use Z-track for all IM injections (Ogston-Tuck, 2014b; Yilmaz et al., 2016). A quick, dartlike injection reduces discomfort.

(2) *Option:* If patient's muscle mass is small, grasp body of muscle between thumb and fingers.

Ensures that medication reaches muscle mass (CDC, 2017; Hockenberry et al., 2019).

CLINICAL DECISION: *When giving immunizations to adults, to avoid injection into subcutaneous tissue, spread the skin of the selected vaccine administration site taut between the thumb and forefinger, isolating the muscle (CDC, 2017).*

(3) After needle pierces skin, still pulling on skin with nondominant hand, grasp lower end of syringe barrel with fingers of nondominant hand to stabilize it. Move dominant hand to end of plunger. Avoid moving syringe.

Smooth manipulation of syringe reduces discomfort from needle movement. Skin remains pulled until after medication is injected to ensure Z-track administration.

(4) Pull back on plunger 5 to 10 seconds. If no blood appears, inject medicine slowly, at rate of 1 mL/10 seconds. **NOTE:** Do not aspirate if administering immunizations (CDC, 2017).

Aspiration of blood into syringe indicates possible placement of needle into a vein. Slow injection rate reduces pain and tissue trauma and reduces chance of leakage of medication back through needle track (Hockenberry et al., 2019). The CDC (2017) no longer recommends aspiration when administering an immunization.

CLINICAL DECISION: *If blood appears in syringe, remove needle and dispose of medication and syringe properly. Prepare another dose of medication for injection.*

(5) Once medication is injected, wait 10 seconds; then smoothly and steadily withdraw needle, release skin, and apply gauze gently over site.

Allows time for medication to absorb into muscle before removing syringe. Dry gauze minimizes discomfort associated with alcohol on nonintact skin.

16. Apply gentle pressure to site. Do not massage site. Apply bandage if needed.

Massage causes underlying tissue damage. Massaging ID site disperses medication into underlying tissue layers and alters test results.

17. Help patient to comfortable position.

Gives patient sense of well-being.

18. Discard uncapped needle or needle enclosed in safety shield and attached syringe into puncture-proof, leak-proof receptacle.

Prevents injury to patient and health care personnel. Recapping needles increases risk of needlestick injury (OSHA, n.d.).

19. Remove and dispose of gloves and perform hand hygiene.

Reduces transmission of microorganisms.

20. Stay with patient and observe for any allergic reactions.

Dyspnea, wheezing, and circulatory collapse are signs of severe anaphylactic reaction, which is life-threatening emergency.

EVALUATION

1. Return to room in 15 to 30 minutes and ask whether patient feels any acute pain, burning, numbness, or tingling at injection site.

After an ID injection, continued discomfort could indicate injury to underlying tissue. After a subcutaneous or IM injection continued discomfort may indicate injury to underlying bones or nerves.

2. After an ID injection ask patient to discuss implications of skin testing and signs of hypersensitivity.

Patient's ability to recognize signs of skin testing helps to ensure timely reporting of results.

Continued

SKILL 31.5 ADMINISTERING INJECTIONS—cont'd

STEP	RATIONALE
3. Inspect ID bleb. *Option:* Use skin pencil and draw circle around perimeter of injection site. Read TB test site at 48 to 72 hours; look for induration (hard, dense, raised area) of skin around injection site of: • 15 mm or more in patients with no known risk factors for tuberculosis. • 10 mm or more in patients who are recent immigrants; injection medication users; residents and employees of high-risk settings; patients with certain chronic illnesses; children younger than 4 years of age; and infants, children, and adolescents exposed to high-risk adults. • 10 mm or more in patients who are recent immigrants; injection medication users; residents and employees of high-risk settings; patients with certain chronic illnesses; children younger than 4 years of age; and infants, children, and adolescents exposed to high-risk adults. • 5 mm or more in patients who are human immunodeficiency virus (HIV) positive, have fibrotic changes on chest x-ray film consistent with previous tuberculosis infection, have had organ transplants, or are immunosuppressed.	Determines whether reaction to antigen occurs; indication positive for tuberculosis or tested allergens. Site must be read at various intervals to determine test results. Pencil marks make site easy to find. You determine results of skin testing at various times, based on type of medication used or type of skin testing completed. Manufacturer directions determine when to read test results. Degree of reaction varies based on patient condition.
4. Inspect subcutaneous or IM site, noting any bruising or induration. Document bruising or induration if present. Notify health care provider and provide warm compress to site.	Bruising or induration indicates complication associated with injection. Document findings and notify health care provider.
5. Observe patient's response to medication at times that correlate with onset, peak, and duration of medication. Review laboratory results as appropriate (e.g., blood glucose, partial thromboplastin).	Adverse effects of parenteral medications develop rapidly. Evaluate effect of medication on basis of onset, peak, and duration of action.
6. **Use Teach-Back:** "I want to be sure I explained about your injection. Can you explain why you need this injection and the side effects to watch for and report to me if they occur?" Revise your instruction now or develop plan for revised patient/family caregiver teaching if patient/family caregiver is not able to teach back correctly.	Determines patient's/family caregiver's level of understanding of instructional topic.

UNEXPECTED OUTCOMES AND RELATED INTERVENTIONS

1. Raised, reddened, or hard zone (induration) forms around an ID test site.
   • Notify patient's health care provider.
   • Document sensitivity to injected allergen or positive test if tuberculin skin testing was completed.
2. Patient has adverse reaction with signs of urticaria, pruritus, wheezing, and dyspnea.
   • Notify patient's health care provider immediately.
   • Follow agency policy for appropriate response to medication reactions (e.g., administration of antihistamine such as diphenhydramine or epinephrine).
   • Add allergy information to patient's record.
3. Patient complains of localized pain, numbness, tingling, or burning at injection site, indicating possible injury to nerve or tissues.
   • Assess injection site.
   • Document findings.
   • Notify patient's health care provider.

RECORDING AND REPORTING

• Record medication, dose, route, site, time, and date on MAR in the electronic health record (EHR) or chart immediately after administration, not before. Correctly sign MAR according to agency policy.
• Record patient teaching, validation of understanding, and patient's response to medication in the electronic health record (EHR) or chart.
• Record area of ID injection and appearance of skin in the electronic health record (EHR) or chart.
• Report any undesirable effects from injection to patient's health care provider and document adverse effects in record.
• Document immunizations in patient's permanent record, including date of administration, vaccine manufacturer and lot number, expiration date, name and title of the person who administered the vaccine and the address of the agency where the permanent record will reside, vaccine information statement (VIS) and date printed on the VIS, and date VIS given to patient or parent/guardian (CDC, 2018).

SKILL 31.6 ADMINISTERING MEDICATIONS BY INTRAVENOUS BOLUS

Delegation and Collaboration

The skill of administering medications by IV bolus cannot be delegated to assistive personnel (AP). The nurse directs the AP about:

- Potential medication actions and side effects and to immediately report their occurrence to the nurse.
- Reporting any patient complaints of moisture or discomfort around IV insertion site.
- Obtaining any required vital signs and reporting them to the nurse.

Equipment

- Watch with second hand
- Clean gloves
- Antiseptic gloves
- Medication in vial or ampule
- Proper-size syringes for medication and saline flush with needleless device or SESIP needle (21- to 25- gauge)
- Intravenous lock: Vial of normal saline flush solution (saline recommended [Gorski, 2019]); if agency continues to use heparin flush, the most common concentration is 10 units/mL; check agency policy.
- Medication administration record (MAR) or computer printout
- Puncture-proof container

STEP	RATIONALE

ASSESSMENT

1. Check accuracy and completeness of each MAR or computer printout with health care provider's written medication order. Check patient's name, medication name and dosage, route of administration, and time of administration. Clarify incomplete or unclear orders with health care provider before administration.

The order sheet is the most reliable source and only legal record of medications that patient is to receive. Ensures that patient receives the correct medications (Westbrook et al., 2017). Transcription errors are a source of medication errors (Truitt et al., 2016).

CLINICAL DECISION: *Some IV medications can be pushed safely only when a patient is monitored continuously for dysrhythmias, blood pressure changes, or other adverse effects. Therefore, some medications can be pushed only in specific patient care units. Confirm agency guidelines.*

2. Assess patient's medical and medication history and history of allergies. List medication allergies on each page of the MAR and prominently display any allergies on the patient's medical record. When allergies are present, patient should wear an allergy bracelet.

Determines need for medication or possible contraindications for medication administration. IV bolus delivers medication rapidly. Allergic response is immediate.

3. Review medication reference information for medication action, purpose, side effects, normal dose, time of peak onset, how slowly to give medication, and nursing implications such as need to dilute medication or administer it through a filter.

Knowledge of medication allows you to give it safely and monitor patient's response to therapy.

4. If you give medication through an existing IV line, determine compatibility of medication with IV fluids and any additives within IV solution.

IV medication is not always compatible with IV solution and/or additives, and a new site may need to be initiated.

5. Assess patient's symptoms before initiating medication therapy.

Provides information to evaluate desired effects of medication.

6. Perform hand hygiene. (Apply clean gloves if risk of contact with body fluids). Assess condition of IV needle insertion site for signs of infiltration or phlebitis.

Reduces transmission of microorganisms. Do not administer medication if site is edematous or inflamed.

7. Assess patency of patient's existing IV infusion line or saline lock (see Chapter 42).

For medication to reach venous circulation effectively, IV line must be patent, and fluids must infuse easily.

8. Assess patient's understanding of purpose of medication therapy.

Poses implication for education.

PLANNING

1. Perform hand hygiene. Collect appropriate equipment and MAR.

Reduces transmission of microorganisms. Ensures organized procedure.

2. Follow agency's "No-interruption zone" policy. Prepare medications for one patient at a time. Keep all pages of MARs or computer printouts for one patient together, or look at only one patient's electronic MAR at a time.

Interruptions contribute to medication errors (Westbrook et al, 2017; Yoder et al., 2015) (see Box 31.4).

IMPLEMENTATION

1. Prepare medications for intravenous bolus administration. Attend to procedure and avoid distraction. Check label of medication against MAR two times, when removing medication from unit dose or AMDS and before leaving medication preparation area. Perform hand hygiene.

Ensures that medication is sterile. *These are the first and second checks for accuracy* and ensure that correct medication is administered. Reduces transmission of microorganisms.

CLINICAL DECISION: *Some IV medications require dilution before administration. Verify with agency policy or pharmacy if dilution is permitted. If a small amount of medication is given (e.g., less than 1 mL), dilute medication in small amount (e.g., 5 mL) of normal saline or sterile water so that it does not collect in the "dead spaces" (e.g., Y-site injection port, IV cap) of the IV delivery system.*

Continued

SKILL 31.6   ADMINISTERING MEDICATIONS BY INTRAVENOUS BOLUS—cont'd

STEP	RATIONALE
2. Take medication(s) to patient at correct time (see agency policy). Medications that require exact timing include STAT doses, first-time or loading doses, and one-time doses. Give time-critical scheduled medications (e.g., antibiotics, anticoagulants, insulin, anticonvulsants, or immunosuppressive agents) at exact time ordered (no more than 30 minutes before or after scheduled dose). Give non–time-critical scheduled medications within a range of 1 or 2 hours of scheduled dose (ISMP, 2011a). During administration apply seven rights of medication administration.	Hospitals must adopt medication administration policy and procedure for timing of medication administration that considers nature of the prescribed medication, specific clinical application, and patient needs (DHHS, 2011; ISMP, 2011a). Time-critical scheduled medications are those for which early or delayed administration of maintenance doses of greater than 30 minutes before or after the scheduled dose may cause harm or result in substantial suboptimal therapy or pharmacological effect. Non–time-critical medications are those for which early or delayed administration within a specified range of either 1 or 2 hours should not cause harm or result in substantial suboptimal therapy or pharmacological effect (DHHS, 2011; ISMP, 2011a).
3. Close room curtain or door.	Provides privacy.
4. Identify patient using at least two identifiers (e.g., name and birthday or name and medical record number) according to agency policy. Compare identifiers with information on patient's MAR or medical record.	Ensures correct patient. Complies with The Joint Commission standards and improves patient safety (TJC, 2020).
5. At patient's bedside again compare MAR or computer printout with names of medications on medication labels and patient name. Ask patient whether he or she has allergies.	*This is the third check for accuracy* and ensures that patient receives correct medication. Confirms patient's allergy history.
6. Discuss purpose of each medication, action, and possible adverse effects. Allow patient to ask questions. Explain that you will give medication through existing IV line. Encourage patient to report symptoms of discomfort at IV site.	Keep patient informed of planned therapies, minimizing anxiety. Patients who verbalize pain at IV site help detect IV infiltrations early, lessening damage to surrounding tissue.
7. Perform hand hygiene and apply clean gloves.	Reduces transmission of microorganisms.
8. IV push (existing IV line):	
a. Select injection port of IV tubing closest to patient. Use needleless injection port.	Follows provisions of Needle Safety and Prevention Act of 2001 (OSHA, n.d.).

CLINICAL DECISION: *Never administer IV medications through tubing that is infusing blood, blood products, or parenteral nutrition solutions.*

STEP	RATIONALE
b. Clean injection port with antiseptic swab. Allow to dry.	Prevents transfer of microorganisms during blunt cannula insertion.
c. Connect syringe to IV line: Insert needleless tip of syringe containing medication through center of port (see illustration).	Prevents introduction of microorganisms. Prevents damage to port diaphragm and possible leakage from site.
d. Occlude IV line by pinching tubing just above injection port (see illustration). Pull back gently on plunger of syringe to aspirate for blood return.	Final check ensures that medication is being delivered into bloodstream.

CLINICAL DECISION: *In the case of smaller-gauge IV needles, blood return sometimes is not aspirated even if IV line is patent. If IV site does not show signs of infiltration and IV fluid is infusing without difficulty, give IV push.*

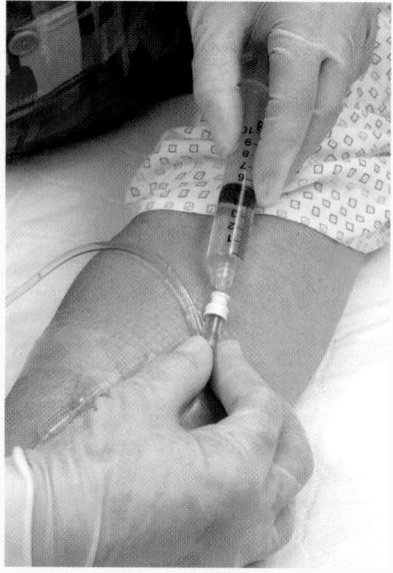

STEP 8c Connect syringe to IV line with needleless blunt cannula tip.

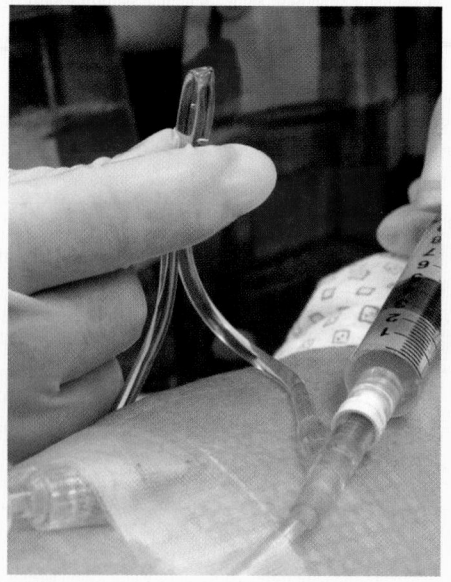

STEP 8d Occlude IV tubing above injection port.

STEP	RATIONALE

e. Release tubing and inject medication within amount of time recommended by agency policy, pharmacist, or medication reference manual. Use watch to time administrations (see illustration). You can pinch IV line while pushing medication and release it when not pushing medication. Allow IV fluids to infuse when not pushing medication.

Ensures safe medication infusion. Rapid injection of IV medication can be fatal. Allowing IV fluids to infuse while pushing IV medication enables medication to be delivered to patient at prescribed rate.

f. After injecting medication, withdraw syringe and recheck IV fluid infusion rate.

Injection of bolus may alter rate of fluid infusion. Rapid fluid infusion can cause circulatory fluid overload.

g. If IV medication is incompatible with IV fluids, stop IV fluids, clamp IV line, and flush with 10 mL of normal saline or sterile water (see agency policy). Then give IV bolus over appropriate amount of time and flush with another 10 mL of normal saline or sterile water at *same rate* as medication was administered.

Allows IV bolus to be administered without risks associated with IV incompatibilities. Ensure that agency guidelines permit flushing lines with incompatible medications. A new site may need to be initiated.

h. If IV line that currently is hanging is a medication, disconnect it and administer IV push medication as outlined in Step 9. Verify agency policy for stopping IV fluids or continuous IV medications. If unable to stop IV infusion, start new IV site (see Chapter 42) and administer medication using IV push (IV lock) method.

Avoids giving patient sudden bolus of medication in existing IV line.

9. IV push (IV lock):

  a. Prepare flush solutions according to agency policy.

    (1) *Saline flush method (preferred method):* Prepare two syringes filled with 2 to 3 mL of normal saline (0.9%). Many agencies do not provide prefilled normal saline syringes for flushing IV lines.

Normal saline is effective in keeping IV locks patent and is compatible with wide range of medications (Gorski, 2019).

    (2) Heparin flush method (prepare heparin flush and saline syringe according to agency policy).

  b. Administer medication:

    (1) Clean injection port with antiseptic swab.

    (2) Insert needleless tip of syringe with normal saline 0.9% through center of injection port of IV lock (see illustrations).

Prevents transfer of microorganisms during needle insertion.

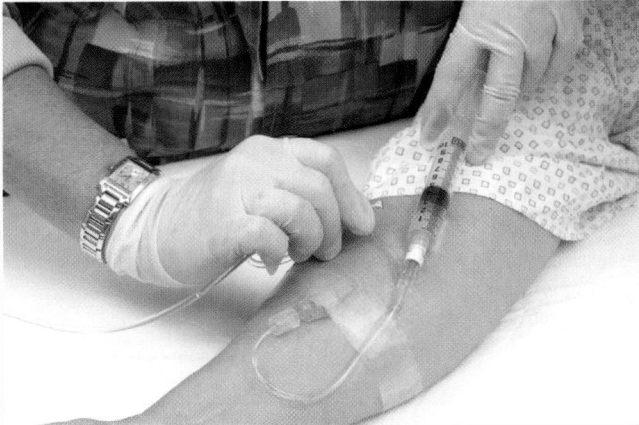

STEP 8e Use watch to time IV push medication.

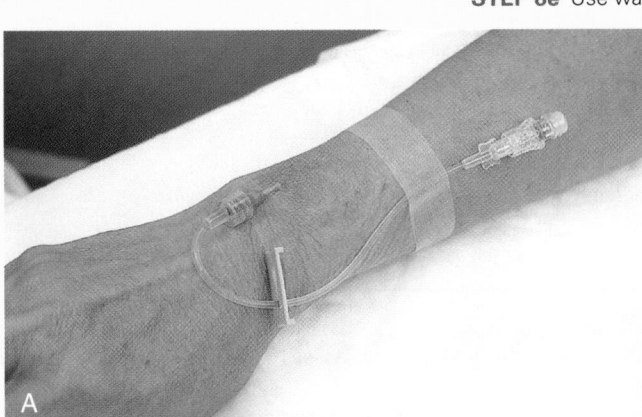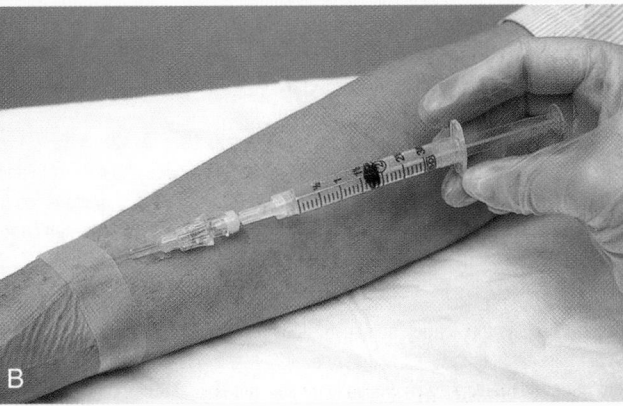

STEP 9b(2) A, IV catheter with saline lock adapter. **B,** Syringe inserted into injection port.

Continued

SKILL 31.6	ADMINISTERING MEDICATIONS BY INTRAVENOUS BOLUS—cont'd

STEP	RATIONALE
(3) Pull back gently on syringe plunger and check for blood return.	Indicates if needle or catheter is in vein.
(4) Flush IV site with normal saline by pushing slowly on plunger.	Clears needle and reservoir of blood. Flushing without difficulty indicates patent IV line.

CLINICAL DECISION: *Carefully observe the area of skin above the IV catheter. Note any puffiness or swelling as the IV site is flushed, which could indicate infiltration into the vein, requiring removal of catheter.*

STEP	RATIONALE
(5) Remove saline-filled syringe.	
(6) Clean injection port with antiseptic swab.	Prevents transmission of microorganisms.
(7) Insert needleless tip of syringe containing prepared medication through injection port of IV lock.	Allows administration of medication.
(8) Inject medication within amount of time recommended by agency policy, pharmacist, or medication reference manual. Use watch to time administration.	Many medication errors are associated with IV pushes being administered too quickly. Following guidelines for IV push rates promotes patient safety.
(9) After administering bolus, withdraw syringe.	
(10) Clean injection port with antiseptic swab.	Prevents transmission of microorganisms.
(11) Flush injection port.	
(a) Attach syringe with normal saline and inject flush at same rate that medication was delivered.	Flushing IV line with saline prevents occlusion of IV access device and ensures that all medication is delivered. Flushing IV site at same rate as medication ensures that any medication remaining within IV needle is delivered at the correct rate.
10. Help patient to comfortable position.	Gives patient sense of well-being.
11. Discard uncapped needle or needle enclosed in safety shield and attached syringe into puncture- and leak-proof receptacle.	Prevents injury to patients and health care personnel. Recapping needles increases risk for needlestick injury (OSHA, n.d.).
12. Remove and dispose of gloves and perform hand hygiene.	Reduces transmission of microorganisms.
13. Stay with patient for several minutes and observe for any allergic reactions.	Dyspnea, wheezing, and circulatory collapse are signs of severe anaphylactic reaction.

EVALUATION

1. Observe patient closely for adverse reactions during administration and for several minutes thereafter.	IV medications act rapidly.
2. Observe IV site during injection for sudden swelling and for 48 hours after IV push.	Swelling indicates infiltration into tissue surrounding vein. Signs of infiltration may not occur for 48 hours.
3. Assess patient's status after giving medication to evaluate effectiveness of the medication.	Some IV bolus medications can cause rapid changes in patient's physiological status, thus requiring careful monitoring and assessment and possibly future laboratory testing (e.g., vasopressors and antiarrhythmics require blood pressure and heart rate monitoring, and heparin requires laboratory studies after administration to determine therapeutic levels).
4. **Use Teach-Back:** "I want to be sure I explained to you why you are receiving this IV medication. Can you explain to me what the medication is for and when to call the nurse?" Revise your instruction now or develop a plan for revised patient/family caregiver teaching if patient/family caregiver is not able to teach back correctly.	Determines patient's/family caregiver's level of understanding of instructional topic.

UNEXPECTED OUTCOMES AND RELATED INTERVENTIONS

1. Patient develops adverse reaction to medication.
   - Stop delivering medication immediately and follow agency policy or guidelines for appropriate response to allergic reaction (e.g., administration of antihistamine such as diphenhydramine or epinephrine) and reporting of adverse medication reactions.
   - Notify patient's health care provider of adverse effects immediately.
   - Add allergy information to patient's record.
2. IV site shows symptoms of infiltration or phlebitis (see Chapter 42).
   - Stop IV infusion immediately or discontinue access device and restart in another site.
   - Determine how much damage IV medication can produce in subcutaneous tissue.
   - Provide IV extravasation care as indicated by agency policy; use a medication reference and consult pharmacist to determine appropriate follow-up care.

RECORDING AND REPORTING

- Immediately record medication administration, including medication, dose, route, time instilled, and date and time administered on MAR in the electronic health record (EHR) or chart. Include initials or signature.
- Record patient's medication response in nurses' notes.
- Record patient teaching and validation of understanding on the flow sheet or nurses' notes in the electronic health record (EHR) or chart.
- Report any adverse reactions to patient's health care provider. Patient's response sometimes indicates need for additional medical therapy.

SKILL 31.7	ADMINISTERING INTRAVENOUS MEDICATIONS BY PIGGYBACK, INTERMITTENT INTRAVENOUS INFUSION SETS, AND MINI-INFUSION (SYRINGE) PUMPS

Delegation and Collaboration

The skill of administering IV medications by piggyback, intermittent infusion sets, and mini-infusion (syringe) pumps cannot be delegated to assistive personnel (AP). The nurse directs the AP about:

- Potential medication actions and side effects and to immediately report their occurrence to the nurse.
- Reporting any patient complaints of moisture or discomfort around IV insertion site.
- Reporting any change in patient's condition or vital signs to the nurse.

Equipment

- Adhesive tape *(optional)*
- Antiseptic swab
- Clean gloves
- IV pole
- MAR or computer printout
- Puncture-proof container

Piggyback or Mini-Infusion (Syringe) Pump.

- Medication prepared in 5- to 250-mL labeled infusion bag or syringe
- Prefilled syringe containing normal saline flush solution (for saline lock only)
- Short microdrip, macrodrip, or syringe IV tubing set, with blunt-end needleless cannula attachment
- Needleless device
- Syringe pump if indicated

Volume-Control Administration Set.

- Volutrol or Buretrol
- Infusion tubing with needleless system attachment
- Syringe (1 to 20 mL)
- Vial or ampule of ordered medication

STEP	RATIONALE

ASSESSMENT

1. Check accuracy and completeness of each MAR or computer printout with health care provider's written medication order. Check patient's name, medication name and dosage, route of administration, and time of administration. Clarify incomplete or unclear orders with health care provider before administration.

The order sheet is the most reliable source and only legal record of medications that patient is to receive. Ensures that patient receives the correct medications (Westbrook et al., 2017). Transcription errors are a source of medication errors (Truitt et al., 2016).

2. Assess patient's medical and medication history and history of allergies. List medication allergies on each page of the MAR and prominently display any allergies on the patient's medical record. When allergies are present, patient should wear an allergy bracelet.

Determines need for medication or possible contraindications for medication administration. IV bolus delivers medication rapidly. Allergic response is immediate.

3. Review medication reference information for medication action, purpose, side effects, normal dose, time of peak onset, how slowly to give medication, and nursing implications such as need to dilute medication or administer it through a filter.

Allows you to administer medication safely and monitor patient's response to therapy.

4. If you give medication through existing IV line, determine compatibility of medication with IV fluids and any additional additives within IV solution.

IV medication is sometimes not compatible with IV solution and/or additives.

CLINICAL DECISION: *Never administer IV medications through tubing that is infusing blood, blood products, or parenteral nutrition solutions.*

5. Perform hand hygiene. Assess patency and placement of patient's existing IV infusion line or saline lock (see Chapter 42).

Do not administer medication if site is edematous or inflamed. For medication to reach circulation effectively, IV line must be patent, and fluids must infuse easily.

CLINICAL DECISION: *If patient's IV site is saline locked, clean the port with alcohol and assess the patency of the IV line by flushing it with 2 to 3 mL of sterile sodium chloride.*

6. Assess patient's symptoms before initiating medication therapy.

Provides information to evaluate desired effects of medication.

7. Assess patient's knowledge of medication.

Poses implications for education.

PLANNING

1. Perform hand hygiene. Collect appropriate equipment and MAR.

Reduces transmission of microorganisms. Ensures organized procedure.

2. Follow agency's "No-interruption zone" policy. Prepare medications for one patient at a time. Keep all pages of MARs or computer printouts for one patient together or look at only one patient's electronic MAR at a time.

Interruptions contribute to medication errors (Westbrook et al., 2017; Yoder et al., 2015) (see Box 31.4).

IMPLEMENTATION

1. Prepare medications for intravenous administration. Attend to procedure and avoid distraction. Check label of medication against MAR two times, when removing medication from unit dose or AMDS and before leaving medication preparation area. Pharmacy prepares piggyback and prefilled syringes. You will prepare medication for a volume administration set. Perform hand hygiene.

Ensures that medication is sterile.
These are the first and second checks for accuracy and ensure that correct medication is administered. Reduces transmission of microorganisms.

Continued

SKILL 31.7　ADMINISTERING INTRAVENOUS MEDICATIONS BY PIGGYBACK, INTERMITTENT INTRAVENOUS INFUSION SETS, AND MINI-INFUSION (SYRINGE) PUMPS —cont'd

STEP	RATIONALE
2. Take medication(s) to patient at correct time (see agency policy). Medications that require exact timing include STAT doses, first-time or loading doses, and one-time doses. Give time-critical scheduled medications (e.g., antibiotics, anticoagulants, insulin, anticonvulsants, or immunosuppressive agents) at exact time ordered (no more than 30 minutes before or after scheduled dose). Give non–time-critical scheduled medications within a range of 1 or 2 hours of scheduled dose (ISMP, 2011a). During administration apply seven rights of medication administration.	Hospitals must adopt medication administration policy and procedure for timing of medication administration that considers nature of the prescribed medication, specific clinical application, and patient needs (DHHS, 2011; ISMP, 2011a). Time-critical scheduled medications are those for which early or delayed administration of maintenance doses of greater than 30 minutes before or after the scheduled dose may cause harm or result in substantial suboptimal therapy or pharmacological effect. Non–time-critical medications are those for which early or delayed administration within a specified range of either 1 or 2 hours should not cause harm or result in substantial suboptimal therapy or pharmacological effect (DHHS, 2011; ISMP, 2011a).
3. Close room curtain or door.	Provides privacy.
4. Identify patient using at least two identifiers (e.g., name and birthday or name and medical record number) according to agency policy. Compare identifiers with information on patient's MAR or medical record.	Ensures correct patient. Complies with The Joint Commission standards and improves patient safety (TJC, 2020).
5. At patient's bedside again compare MAR or computer printout with names of medications on medication labels and patient name. Ask patient whether he or she has allergies.	*This is the third check for accuracy* and ensures that patient receives correct medication. Confirms patient's allergy history.
6. Discuss purpose of each medication, action, and possible adverse effects. Allow patient to ask any questions. Explain that you will give medication through existing IV line. Encourage patient to report symptoms of discomfort at site.	Keep patient informed of planned therapies, minimizing anxiety. Patients who verbalize pain at IV site help detect IV infiltrations early, lessening damage to surrounding tissues.
7. Perform hand hygiene and apply clean gloves. Administer infusion:	Reduces transmission of microorganisms.
a. Piggyback infusion:	
(1) Connect infusion tubing to medication bag (see Chapter 42). Fill tubing by opening regulator flow clamp. Once tubing is full, close clamp and cap end of tubing.	Filling infusion tubing with solution and freeing air bubbles prevent air embolus. Capping reduces transmission of microorganisms.
(2) Hang piggyback (see illustration) medication bag above level of primary fluid bag. (Use hook to lower main bag.) Primary line continues to infuse.	Height of fluid bag affects rate of flow to patient.

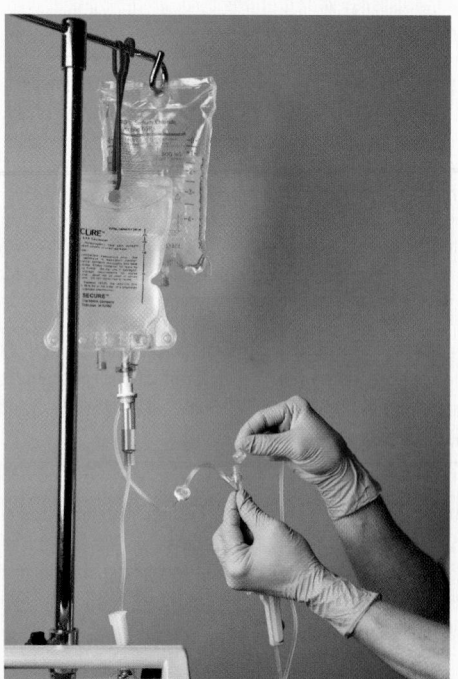

STEP 7a(2) Small-volume minibag for piggyback infusion.

STEP	RATIONALE
(3) Connect tubing of piggyback infusion to appropriate connector on upper Y-port of primary infusion line:	Connection allows IV medication to enter main IV line.
(a) *Needleless system:* Wipe off needleless port of main IV line with alcohol swab, allow to dry, and insert cannula tip of piggyback infusion tubing.	Use needleless connections to prevent accidental needlestick injuries (INS, 2016; OSHA, n.d.).
(b) *Normal saline lock:* Follow steps to flush and prepare lock (see Skill 31.6). Wipe off port with alcohol swab, let dry, and insert tip of piggyback infusion tubing via needleless access (see illustrations).	Flushing of lock ensures patency.
(4) Regulate flow rate of medication solution by adjusting regulator clamp or IV pump infusion rate. Infusion times vary. Refer to medication reference or agency policy for safe flow rate.	Provides slow, safe, intermittent infusion of medication and maintains therapeutic blood levels.
(5) Once medication has infused:	
(a) Continuous infusion: Check flow rate of primary infusion. Primary infusion automatically begins after piggyback solution is empty.	Back-check valve on piggyback prevents flow of primary infusion until medication infuses. Checking flow rate ensures proper administration of IV fluids.
(b) Normal saline lock: Disconnect tubing, clean port with alcohol, and flush IV line with 2 to 3 mL of sterile 0.9% sodium chloride. Maintain sterility of IV tubing between intermittent infusions.	
(6) Regulate continuous main infusion line to ordered rate.	Infusion of piggyback sometimes interferes with main line infusion rate.
(7) Leave IV piggyback and tubing in place for future medication administration (see agency policy) or discard it and the uncapped needle/ needle enclosed safety shield of flushing syringe in puncture- and leak-proof container.	Establishing secondary line produces route for microorganisms to enter main line. Repeated changes in tubing increase risk for infection transmission.

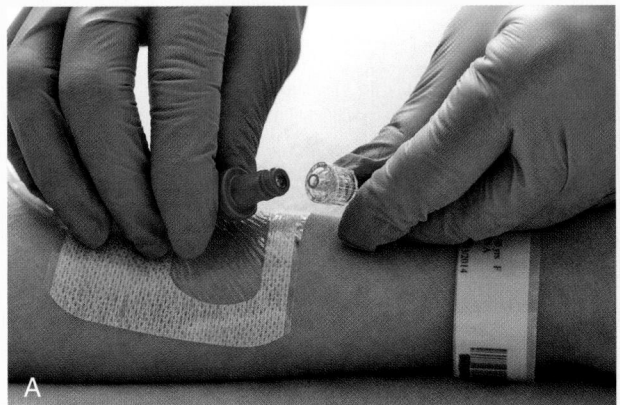 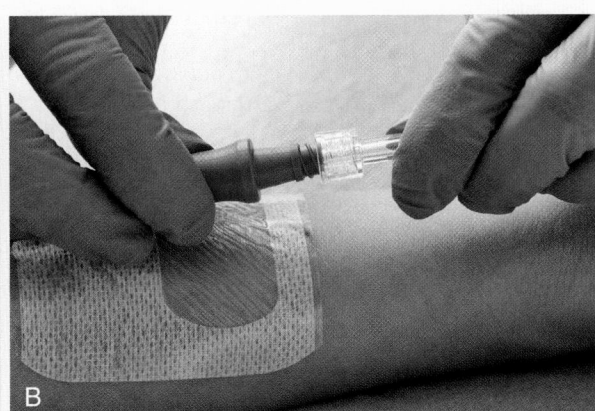

STEP 7a(3)(b)   **A,** Needleless lock cannula system. **B,** Blunt-ended cannula inserts into port and locks.

Continued

SKILL 31.7   **ADMINISTERING INTRAVENOUS MEDICATIONS BY PIGGYBACK, INTERMITTENT INTRAVENOUS INFUSION SETS, AND MINI-INFUSION (SYRINGE) PUMPS —cont'd**

STEP	RATIONALE
b. Volume-control administration set (e.g., Volutrol):	
(1) Fill Volutrol with desired amount of IV fluid (50 to 100 mL) by opening clamp between Volutrol and main IV bag (see illustration).	Small volume of fluid dilutes IV medication and reduces risk of fluid infusing too rapidly.
(2) Close clamp and check to be sure that clamp on air vent Volutrol chamber is open.	Prevents additional leakage of fluid into Volutrol. Air vent allows fluid in Volutrol to exit at regulated rate.
(3) Clean injection port on top of Volutrol with antiseptic swab.	Prevents introduction of microorganisms during needle insertion.
(4) Remove needle cap or sheath and insert needleless syringe or syringe needle through port and inject medication (see illustration). Gently rotate Volutrol between hands.	Rotating mixes medication with solution to ensure equal distribution in Volutrol.
(5) Regulate IV infusion rate to allow medication to infuse in time recommended by agency policy, pharmacist, or medication reference manual.	For optimal therapeutic effect, medication should infuse in prescribed time interval.
(6) Label Volutrol with name of medication; dosage; total volume, including diluent; and time of administration following ISMP (2018d) safe-medication label format.	Alerts nurses to medication being infused. Prevents other medications from being added to Volutrol.
(7) If patient is receiving continuous IV infusion, check infusion rate after Volutrol infusion is complete.	Ensures appropriate rate of administration.
(8) Dispose of uncapped needle or needle enclosed in safety shield and syringe in puncture- and leak-proof container. Discard supplies in appropriate container. Perform hand hygiene.	Prevents accidental needlesticks (OSHA, n.d.). Reduces transmission of microorganisms.
c. Mini-infusion administration:	
(1) Connect prefilled syringe to mini-infusion tubing; remove end cap of tubing.	Special tubing designed to fit syringe delivers medication to main IV line.
(2) Carefully apply pressure to syringe plunger, allowing tubing to fill with medication.	Ensures that tubing is free of air bubbles to prevent air embolus.
(3) Place syringe into mini-infusion pump (follow product directions) and hang on IV pole. Be sure that syringe is secured.	Secure placement is needed for proper infusion.

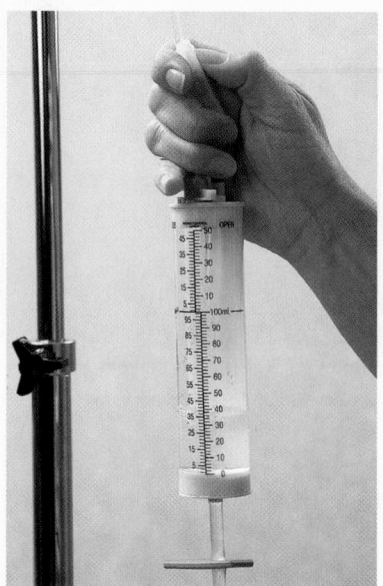

STEP 7b(1) Fill volume-control administration device.

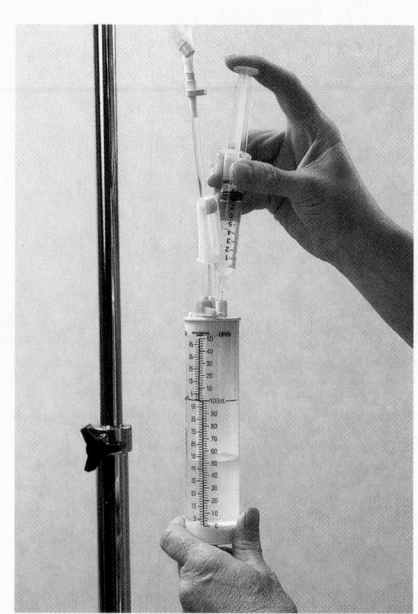

STEP 7b(4) Medication injected into device.

STEP	RATIONALE
(4) Connect end of mini-infusion tubing to main IV line or saline lock:	Establishes route for IV medication to enter main IV line.
(a) *Existing IV line:* Wipe off needleless port on main IV line with alcohol swab, allow to dry, and insert tip of mini-infusion tubing through center of port.	Needleless connections reduce risk for accidental needlestick injuries (OSHA, n.d.).
(b) *Normal saline lock:* Follow steps to flush and prepare lock (see Skill 31.6). Wipe off port with alcohol swab, allow to dry, and insert tip of mini-infusion tubing.	Flushing of lock ensures patency.
(5) Set pump to deliver medication within time recommended by agency policy, pharmacist, or medication reference manual. Press button on pump to begin infusion.	Pump automatically delivers medication at safe, constant rate based on volume in syringe.
(6) Once medication has infused:	
(a) *Main IV infusion:* Check flow rate. Infusion automatically begins to flow once pump stops. Regulate infusion to desired rate as needed.	Maintains patent primary IV fluids.
(b) *Normal saline lock:* Disconnect tubing, clean port with alcohol, and flush IV line with 2 to 3 mL of sterile 0.9% sodium chloride. Maintain sterility of IV tubing between intermittent infusions.	
(c) Dispose of uncapped needle or needle enclosed in safety shield of flushing syringe in puncture- and leak-proof container. Discard supplies in appropriate container. Perform hand hygiene.	
8. Help patient to comfortable position.	Gives patient sense of well-being.
9. Stay with patient for several minutes and observe for any allergic reactions.	Dyspnea, wheezing, and circulatory collapse are signs of severe anaphylactic reaction.

EVALUATION

1. Observe patient for signs or symptoms of adverse reaction.	IV medications act rapidly.
2. During infusion periodically check infusion rate and condition of IV site.	IV must remain patent for proper medication administration. Infiltration of IV site requires discontinuing infusion.
3. Ask patient to explain purpose and side effects of medication.	Evaluates patient's understanding of instruction.
4. **Use Teach-Back:** "I want to be sure I explained to you the reason for this IV medication. Can you explain to me why you are receiving the medication and what to report to the nurse?" Revise your instruction now or develop a plan for revised patient/family caregiver teaching if patient/family caregiver is not able to teach back correctly.	Determines patient's/family caregiver's level of understanding of instructional topic.

UNEXPECTED OUTCOMES AND RELATED INTERVENTIONS

1. Patient develops adverse or allergic reaction to medication.
   - Stop medication infusion immediately.
   - Follow agency policy or guidelines for appropriate response to allergic reaction (e.g., administration of antihistamine such as diphenhydramine or epinephrine) and reporting of adverse medication reactions.
   - Notify patient's health care provider of adverse effects immediately.
   - Add allergy information to patient record per agency policy.
2. Medication does not infuse over established time frame.
   - Determine reason (e.g., improper calculation of flow rate, poor positioning of IV needle at insertion site, infiltration).
   - Take corrective action as indicated by agency policy or health care provider.
3. IV site shows signs of infiltration or phlebitis (see Chapter 42).
   - Stop IV infusion and discontinue access device.
   - Treat IV site as indicated by agency policy.
   - Insert new IV catheter if therapy continues.
   - For infiltration determine how harmful IV medication is to subcutaneous tissue. Provide IV extravasation care (e.g., injecting phentolamine around IV infiltration site) as indicated by agency policy, or consult pharmacist to determine appropriate follow-up care.

RECORDING AND REPORTING

- Immediately record medication administration, including medication, dose, route, time instilled, and date and time administered on MAR in the electronic health record (EHR) or chart. Include initials or signature.
- Record volume of fluid in medication bag or syringe pump as fluid intake.
- Record patient teaching and validation of understanding on the flow sheet or nurses' notes in the electronic health record (EHR) or chart
- Report any adverse reactions to patient's health care provider. Patient's response sometimes indicates need for additional medical therapy.

KEY POINTS

- Apply knowledge of the four major pharmacokinetic processes—medication absorption, distribution, metabolism, and excretion—to time medication administration, select the route of administration, and evaluate a patient's response.
- Prompt recognition and reporting of adverse medication events prevents serious patient injury.
- In health care agencies, patients with known medication allergies have their allergy information recorded in a clearly identifiable place.
- A health care provider prescribes a patient's medications while the pharmacist prepares and distributes prescribed medications. Nurses, physicians, and other health care providers work together to evaluate the effectiveness of medication therapy.
- When a medication is prescribed, the goal is a constant blood level within a safe therapeutic range.
- Medications that are time critical most likely cause harm or have subtherapeutic effects if they are not administered on time (usually 30 minutes before or after the scheduled dose).
- The route prescribed for administering a medication depends on the medication's properties and desired effect and on a patient's physical and mental condition.
- Metric units are easy to convert and calculate using simple multiplication and division, with each basic unit of measurement organized into units of 10.
- Responsibilities of medication administration include knowing medication therapeutics, assessing a patient before administration, calculating doses, administering medications using the seven rights, monitoring and evaluating medication effects, and assessing a patient's ability to self-administer medications.
- The seven rights of medication administration include the right medication, right dose, right patient, right route, right time, right documentation, and right indication.
- Before administering medications, perform a physical assessment, which will reveal physical findings for any indications or contraindications for medication therapy.
- Factors contributing to medication nonadherence in older adults include depression, problems with cognitive or functional abilities, dislike for medication side effects, a busy and active lifestyle, and inability to afford medications.
- Distractions may cause a medication error. Distractions include a page, phone call, or request from a colleague or patient that draws away, disturbs, or diverts attention from a current desired task, or forces attention on a new task at least temporarily.
- Collaboration with patients and their family caregivers is essential, particularly if patients will require assistance with self- administration and if medication regimens are complicated.
- For patient safety it is essential that you refer to the MAR each time you prepare a medication and have it available at the patient's bedside when administering medications.
- Rotate IM injection sites to decrease the risk for tissue hypertrophy, and use the Z-track method for administration.

REFLECTIVE LEARNING

- You are a new nurse and have started a staff nurse position on a busy medical-surgical unit. You must administer many medications to four different patients throughout the shift and feel overwhelmed. How would you organize safe medication administration for these patients?

- Consider all the nonparenteral routes of medication your patients may be receiving during their admission to a health care agency. Consider the need for different approaches to administering these medications. When might it be acceptable to allow a patient to administer some of these routes of medications themselves?
- Consider a time when you were caring for patients who required a variety of routes for administering IV medication. How might you ensure you are correctly assessing for medication compatibility, rate of infusion, and route of administration?

REVIEW QUESTIONS

1. It is important to take precautions to prevent medication errors. A nurse is administering an oral tablet to a patient. Which of the following steps is the second check for accuracy in determining the patient is receiving the right medication?
   1. Logging on to automated dispensing system (ADS) or unlocking medicine drawer or cart.
   2. Before going to patient's room, comparing patient's name and name of medication on label of prepared drugs with MAR.
   3. Selecting correct medication from ADS, unit-dose drawer, or stock supply and comparing name of medication on label with MAR or computer printout.
   4. Comparing MAR or computer printout with names of medications on medication labels and patient name at patient's bedside.
2. The health care provider has written the following orders. Which orders does the nurse need to clarify before administering the medication? Provide rationale for your answers, and rewrite the order so that it follows the ISMP current medication order safety guidelines.
   Timoptic .25% solution 1 drop OD BID
   Metoprolol 12.50 mg QD
   Insulin Glargine 6 u SC twice a day
   Enalapril 2.5 mg. PO three times a day, hold for systolic blood pressure <100
3. An older adult states that she cannot see her medication bottles clearly to determine when to take her prescription. What should the nurse do? (Select all that apply.)
   1. Provide a dispensing system for each day of the week.
   2. Provide larger, easier-to-read labels.
   3. Tell the patient what is in each container.
   4. Have a family caregiver administer the medication.
   5. Use teach-back to ensure that the patient knows what medication to take and when.
4. The nurse must take a verbal order during an emergency on the unit. Which of the following guidelines can be used for taking verbal or telephone orders? (Select all that apply).
   1. Only authorized staff may receive and record verbal or telephone orders. The health care agency identifies in writing the staff who are authorized.
   2. Clearly identify patient's name, room number, and diagnosis.
   3. Read back all orders to health care provider.
   4. Use clarification questions to avoid misunderstandings.
   5. Write "VO" (verbal order) or "TO" (telephone order), including date and time, name of patient, and complete order; sign the name of the health care provider and nurse.
5. A nurse is administering ophthalmic ointment to a patient. Place the following steps in correct order for the administration of the ointment.
   1. Clean eye, washing from inner to outer canthus.

2. Assess patient's level of consciousness and ability to follow instructions.

3. Apply thin ribbon of ointment evenly along inner edge of lower eyelid on conjunctiva.

4. Have patient close eye and rub lightly in a circular motion with a cotton ball.

5. Ask patient to look at ceiling, and explain the steps to patient.

6. The nurse is administering an IV push medication to a patient who has a compatible IV fluid running through intravenous tubing. Place the following steps in the appropriate order.

   1. Release tubing and inject medication within amount of time recommended by agency policy, pharmacist, or medication reference manual. Use watch to time administration.

   2. Select injection port of IV tubing closest to patient. Whenever possible, injection port should accept a needleless syringe. Use IV filter if required by medication reference or agency policy.

   3. After injecting medication, release tubing, withdraw syringe, and recheck fluid infusion rate.

   4. Connect syringe to port of IV line. Insert needleless tip or small-gauge needle of syringe containing prepared drug through center of injection port

   5. Clean injection port with antiseptic swab. Allow to dry.

   6. Occlude IV line by pinching tubing just above injection port. Pull back gently on syringe plunger to aspirate blood return.

7. A nurse is administering a metered-dose inhaler (MDI) with a spacer to a patient with chronic obstructive pulmonary disease. Place the steps of the procedure in the correct order.

   1. Insert MDI into end of spacer.

   2. Perform a respiratory assessment.

   3. Remove mouthpiece from MDI and spacer device.

   4. Place the spacer mouthpiece into patient's mouth, and instruct patient to close lips around the mouthpiece.

   5. Depress medication canister, spraying 1 puff into spacer device.

   6. Shake inhaler for 2-5 seconds.

   7. Instruct patient to hold breath for 10 seconds.

   8. Instruct patient to breathe in slowly through mouth for 3 to 5 seconds.

8. A patient is to receive medications through a small-bore nasogastric feeding. Which nursing actions are appropriate? (Select all that apply.)

   1. Verifying tube placement after medications are given

   2. Mixing all medications together to give all at once

   3. Using an enteral tube syringe to administer medications

   4. Flushing tube with 30 to 60 mL of water after the last dose of medication

   5. Checking for gastric residual before giving the medications

   6. Keeping the head of the bed elevated 30 to 60 minutes after the medications are given

9. Place the steps of administering an intradermal injection in the correct order.

   1. Inject medication slowly.

   2. Note the presence of a bleb.

   3. Advance needle through epidermis to 3 mm.

   4. Using nondominant hand, stretch skin over site with forefinger.

   5. Insert needle at a 5- to 15-degree angle into the skin until resistance is felt.

   6. Cleanse site with antiseptic swab.

10. After receiving an intramuscular (IM) injection in the deltoid, a patient states, "My arm really hurts. It's burning and tingling where I got my injection." What should the nurse do next? (Select all that apply.)

   1. Assess the injection site.

   2. Administer an oral medication for pain.

   3. Notify the patient's health care provider of assessment findings.

   4. Document assessment findings and related interventions in the patient's medical record.

   5. This is a normal finding, so nothing needs to be done.

   6. Apply ice to the site for relief of burning pain.

Answers: 1. 2; **2.** See Evolve; **3.** 1, 2, 5; **4.** 1, 2, 3, 4; **5.** 5, 2, 1, 5, 3, 4; **6.** 2, 5, 4, 6, 1, 3; **7.** 2, 3, 6, 1, 4, 5, 8, 7; **8.** 3, 4, 5, 6; **9.** 6, 4, 5, 3, 1, 2; **10.** 1, 3, 4.

Rationales for Review Questions can be found on the Evolve website.

REFERENCES

American Academy of Allergy, Asthma and Immunology (AAAAI): *Peak flow meter*, 2016. https://www.aaaai.org/conditions-and-treatments/library/asthma-library/peak-flow-meter. Accessed May 18, 2018.

American Hospital Association: *The patient care partnership*, n.d. http://www.aha.org/advocacy-issues/communicatingpts/pt-care-partnership.shtml. Accessed May 13, 2018.

American Medical Association (AMA): *Generic naming*, 2018. https://www.ama-assn.org/procedure-us-an-name-selection. Accessed May 6, 2018.

American Nurses Association (ANA): *Nursing: scope and standards of practice*, ed 3, Silver Spring, MD, 2015, The Association.

Ari A: Patient education and adherence to aerosol therapy, *Respir Care* 60(6):941, 2015.

Ball J, et al.: *Seidel's guide to physical examination: an interprofessional approach*, ed 9, St Louis, 2019, Elsevier.

Barrons R, et al.: Opportunities for inhaler device selection in elderly patients with asthma or COPD, *Patient Intell* 7:53–65, 2015.

Beal J: Pediatric medication errors, *Am J Matern Child Nurs* 42(2):116, 2017.

Bonini M, Usmani OS: The importance of inhaler devices in the treatment of COPD, *COPD Res Pract* 1(9), 2015.

Burchum J, Rosenthal L: *Lehne's pharmacology for nursing care*, ed 10, St Louis, 2019, Elsevier.

Centers for Disease Control and Prevention (CDC): *Deaths and mortality: number of deaths for leading causes of death*, 2016. http://www.cdc.gov/nchs/fastats/deaths.htm. Accessed May 20, 2018.

Centers for Disease Control and Prevention (CDC): *Vaccine recommendations and guidelines of the ACIP: Vaccine administration*, 2017. https://www.cdc.gov/vaccines/hcp/acip-recs/general-recs/administration.html. Accessed May 19, 2018.

Centers for Disease Control and Prevention (CDC): *Epidemiology and prevention of vaccine-preventable diseases: Vaccine administration*, 2018. https://www.cdc.gov/vaccines/pubs/pinkbook/vac-admin.html. Accessed August 20, 2019.

Centers for Medicare and Medicaid Services (CMS): *CMS manual system*, 2014. https://www.cms.gov/Regulations-and-Guidance/Guidance/Transmittals/downloads/R3011CP.pdf. Accessed September 2019.

Consumer Med Safety: *Tips for measuring liquid medicines safely*, Institute for Safe Medicine Practices, 2018a. http://www.consumermedsafety.org/tools-and-resources/medication-safety-tools-and-resources/taking-your-medicine-safely/measure-liquid-medications. Accessed May 12, 2018.

Consumer Med Safety: *U-500 insulin errors*, Institute for Safe Medicine Practices, 2018b. http://consumermedsafety.org/tools-and-resources/insulin-safety-center/u-500-insulin-errors. Accessed December 7, 2018.

Department of Health and Human Services, Centers for Medicare & Medicaid (DHHS): *Updated guidance on medication administration, Hospital Appendix A of State Operations Manual*, Baltimore, 2011, Department of Health and Human Services.

Gorski L: *Phillips's manual of I.V. therapeutics: evidence-based practice for infusion therapy*, ed 7, Philadelphia, PA, 2019, FA Davis.

Guenther, P: New enteral connectors: raising awareness, *Nutr Clin Pract* 29:612, 2015.

Hockenberry MJ, et al.: *Wong's nursing care of infants and children*, ed 11, St Louis, 2019, Elsevier.

Hutton K, et al.: The effects of bar-coding technology on medication errors: a systematic literature review, *J Patient Saf* 24, 2017.

Infusion Nurses Society (INS): Infusion therapy standards of practice, *J Infus Nurs* 39(Suppl 1):S1, 2016.

Institute for Safe Medication Practices (ISMP): *ISMP acute care guidelines for timely administration of scheduled medications*, 2011a. http://www.ismp.org/Tools/guidelines/acutecare/tasm.pdf. Accessed May 20, 2018.

Institute for Safe Medication Practices (ISMP): *ISMP statement on use of metric measurements to prevent errors with oral liquids*, 2011b. https://www.ismp.org/news/ismp-statement-use-metric-measurements-prevent-errors-oral-liquids. Accessed December 2018.

Institute for Safe Medication Practices (ISMP): *List of confused drug names*, 2015a. https://www.ismp.org/recommendations/confused-drug-names-list. Accessed December 2018.

Institute for Safe Medication Practices (ISMP): *ENFit enteral devices are on their way: important safety considerations for hospitals*, MSA, 2015c. https://www.ismp.org/resources/enfit-enteral-devices-are-their-wayimportant-safety-considerations-hospitals. Accessed May 14, 2018.

Institute for Safe Medication Practices (ISMP): *Guidelines for safe practice of adult IV push medication*, 2015d. https://www.ismp.org/guidelines/iv-push. Accessed May 20, 2018.

Institute for Safe Medication Practices (ISMP): *Oral dosage forms that should not be crushed*, 2016a. http://www.ismp.org/tools/donotcrush.pdf. Accessed May 13, 2018.

Institute of Safe Medication Practices (ISMP): *Is an indication-based prescribing system in our future?*

2016b. https://www.ismp.org/Newsletters/acutecare/showarticle.aspx?id=1153. Accessed May 13, 2018.

Institute for Safe Medication Practices (ISMP): *ISMP's list of error-prone abbreviations, symbols, and dose designations*, 2017a. https://www.ismp.org/recommendations/error-prone-abbreviations-list. Accessed May 6, 2018.

Institute for Safe Medication Practices (ISMP): *ISMP guidelines for optimizing safe subcutaneous insulin use in adults*, Horsham, PA, 2017b, The Institute for Safe Medication Practices.

Institute for Safe Medication Practices (ISMP): Crushing or splitting the wrong tablet can be a deadly errors, *ISMP Long-term care Advice ERR* 5(4):2, 2017c.

Institute for Safe Medication Practices (ISMP): *2018-2019 targeted medication safety best practices for hospitals*, 2018a. https://www.ismp.org/guidelines/best-practices-hospitals. Accessed May 12, 2018.

Institute for Safe Medication Practices (ISMP): ISMP medication safety alert: caution advised with tamper-evident caps, *ISMP* 23(8), 2018b, AA1.

Institute for Safe Medication Practices (ISMP): Hardwiring safety into the computer, *ISMP* 21(9):2, 2018c.

Institute for Safe Medication Practices (ISMP): *Part II: Survey results suggest action is needed to improve safety with adult IV push medications*, 2018d. https://www.ismp.org/resources/part-ii-survey-results-suggest-action-needed-improve-safety-adult-iv-push-medications. Accessed September 27, 2019.

Lilley LL, et al.: *Pharmacology and the nursing process*, ed 9, St Louis, 2020, Elsevier.

Makary MA, Daniel M: Medical error—the third leading cause of death in the US, *BMJ* 353, 2016, https://doi.org/10.1136/bmj.i2139. Accessed May 2018.

McCulloch D, et al.: General principles of insulin therapy in diabetes mellitus, *UpToDate*, 2018. http://www.uptodate.com/contents/general-principles-of-insulin-therapy-in-diabetes-mellitus. Accessed May 16, 2018.

National Coordinating Council for Medication Error Reporting and Prevention (NCCMERP): *What is a medication error?* 2018. http://www.nccmerp.org/about-medication-errors. Accessed May 13, 2018.

Occupational Safety and Health Administration (OSHA): *Bloodborne pathogens and needlestick prevention*, n.d.

https://www.osha.gov/SLTC/bloodbornepathogens/index.html. Accessed May 20, 2018.

Rochon P: Drug prescribing for older adults, *UpToDate*, 2019. https://www.uptodate.com/contents/drug-prescribing-for-older-adults. Accessed September 27, 2019.

Schiff G, et al.: Incorporating indications into medication ordering—time to enter the age of reason, *N Engl J Med* 375(4):306, 2016.

Skidmore-Roth L: *Mosby's 2019 nursing drug reference*, ed 32, St Louis, 2018, Elsevier.

The Joint Commission (TJC): *Sentinel alert event: managing risk during transition to new ISO connector standards*, 2014. http://www.jointcommission.org/assets/1/6/SEA_53_Connectors_8_19_14_final.pdf. Accessed May 20, 2018.

The Joint Commission (TJC): *Facts about the official "Do Not Use" list of abbreviations*, 2017. https://www.jointcommission.org/facts_about_do_not_use_list/. Accessed May 6, 2018.

The Joint Commission (TJC): *2020 National Patient Safety Goals*, Oakbrook Terrace, IL, 2020, The Commission. https://www.jointcommission.org/en/standards/national-patient-safety-goals/.

Touhy TA, Jett KF: *Ebersole and Hess' gerontological nursing & healthy aging*, ed 5, St Louis, 2017, Elsevier.

US Department of Health and Human Services (USDHHS): *Tablet splitting a risky practice*, 2015. https://www.fda.gov/ForConsumers/ConsumerUpdates/ucm171492.htm. Accessed May 18, 2018.

US Food and Drug Administration (USFDA): *MedWatch: the FDA safety information and adverse event reporting program*, 2018a. https://www.fda.gov/safety/medwatch/default.htm. Accessed May 6, 2018.

US Food and Drug Administration (USFDA): *Safe use initiative - current projects*, 2018b. https://www.fda.gov/drugs/drugsafety/safeuseinitiative/ucm188762.htm#adherence. Accessed May 6, 2018.

World Health Organization (WHO): *WHO guideline on the use of safety-engineered syringes for intramuscular, intradermal, and subcutaneous injection in health care settings*, World Health Organization, 2016.

RESEARCH REFERENCES

Betancourt J: *Cross-cultural care and communication*, *UpToDate*, 2018. https://www.uptodate.com/contents/cross-cultural-care-and-communication#!. Accessed May 2018.

Boullata J, et al.: ASPEN safe practices for enteral nutrition therapy, *J Parenter Enteral Nutr* 41(1):15, 2017.

Bravo K, Cochran G: Nursing strategies to increase medication safety in inpatient settings, *J Nurs Care Qual* 31(4):335, 2016.

Clifford P, et al.: Following the evidence: enteral tube placement and verification in neonates and young children, *J Perinat Neonatal Nurs* 29(2):149, 2015.

Connor J, et al.: Implementing a distraction-free practice with the red zone medication safety initiative, *Dimens Crit Care Nurs* 35(3):116, 2016.

Fanning L, et al.: Impact of automated dispensing cabinets on medication selection and preparation error rates in an emergency department: a prospective and direct observational before-and-after study, *J Eval Clin Pract* 22(2):156, 2016.

Forough A, et al.: Nurses' experiences of medication administration to people with swallowing difficulties

in aged care agencies: a systematic review protocol, *JBI Database System Rev Implement Rep* 15(4):932, 2018.

Hibbard P, et al.: Approach to immunizations in healthy adults, *UpToDate*, 2017. https://www.uptodate.com/contents/approach-to-immunizations-in-healthy-adults. Accessed May 16, 2018.

Holliday R, et al.: Body mass index: a reliable predictor of subcutaneous fat thickness and needle length for ventral gluteal intramuscular injections, *Am J Ther* 26(1):e72, 2019.

Hopkins U, Arias C: Large-volume IM injections: a review of best practices, *Oncol Nurse Advis* 32, 2013. http://www.oncologynurseadvisor.com/chemotherapy/large-volume-im-injections-a-review-of-best-practices/article/281208/. Accessed May 17, 2018.

Joo G, et al.: The effect of different methods of intravenous injection on glass particle contamination from ampules, *SpringerPlus* 5:15, 2016.

Kara D, et al.: Using ventrogluteal site in intramuscular injections is a priority or an alternative? *Int J Caring Sciences* 8(2):507–513, 2015.

Kaya N, et al.: The reliability of site determination methods in ventrogluteal area injection: a cross-sectional study, *Int J Nurs Stud* 52(1):355–360, 2015.

Larkin T, et al.: Comparison of the V and G methods for ventrogluteal site identification: muscle and subcutaneous fat thickness and considerations for successful intramuscular injection, *Int J Ment Health Nurs*, 27(2):631, 2017.

Larkin T, et al.: Influence of gender, BMI, and body shape on theoretical injection outcome at the ventrogluteal and dorsogluteal sites, *J Clin Nurs* 27(1/2):e242, 2018.

Levitsky L, et al.: Management of type 1 diabetes mellitus in children and adolescents, *UpToDate*, 2017. https://www.uptodate.com/contents/management-of-type-1-diabetes-mellitus-in-children-and-adolescents. Accessed May 2018.

Mohammady M, et al.: Slow versus fast subcutaneous heparin injections for prevention of bruising and site-pain intensity, *Cochrane Database Syst Rev* 10:CD008077, 2017.

Ogston-Tuck S: Subcutaneous injection technique: an evidence-based approach, *Nurs Stand* 29(3):53–58, 2014a.

Ogston-Tuck S: Intramuscular injection technique: an evidence-based approach, *Nurs Stand* 29(4):55, 2014b.

Royal College of Nursing (RCN): *Infusion therapy standards: rapid evidence review*, London, 2016, Royal College of Nursing.

Saper R: Overview of herbal medicine and dietary supplements, *UpToDate*, 2018. https://www.uptodate.com/contents/overview-of-herbal-medicine-and-dietary-supplements. Accessed May 2018.

Sepah Y, et al.: Aspiration in injections: should we continue or abandon the practice? *F1000Research* 3(157), 2017, https://doi.org/10.12688/f1000research.1113.3. Accessed May 2018.

Truitt E, et al.: Effect of the implementation of barcode technology and an electronic medication administration record on adverse drug events, *Hosp Pharm* 51(6):474–483, 2016.

Westbrook J, et al.: Effectiveness of a 'Do not interrupt' bundled intervention to reduce interruptions during medication administration: a cluster randomized controlled feasibility study, *BMJ Qual Saf* 26(9):734, 2017.

Yilmaz D, et al.: The effect of the Z-track technique on pain and drug leakage in intramuscular injections, *Clin Nurse Spec* 30(6):e7, 2016.

Yoder M, et al.: The effect of a safe zone on nurse interruptions, distractions, and medication administration errors, *J Infus Nurs* 38(2):140, 2015.

Zhu J, Weingart S: Prevention of adverse drug events in hospitals, *UpToDate*, 2018. https://www.uptodate.com/contents/prevention-of-adverse-drug-events-in-hospitals. Accessed August 20, 2019.

32

Complementary Therapies and Integrative Health

OBJECTIVES

- Differentiate between the use of therapies as complementary versus alternative treatments.
- Describe integrative health as applied to nursing practice.
- Describe the clinical applications of relaxation therapies.
- Discuss the relaxation response and its effect on somatic ailments.
- Identify the principles and effectiveness of imagery, meditation, and breathwork.

- Describe the purpose and principles of biofeedback.
- Describe the methods of and the psychophysiological responses to therapeutic touch.
- Discuss the principles and applications of acupuncture.
- Describe safe and unsafe herbal therapies.

KEY TERMS

Acupoints, p. 683
Acupuncture, p. 683
Allopathic or biomedicine, p. 676
Alternative therapies, p. 677
Biofeedback, p. 682
Chiropractic therapy, p. 684
Complementary therapies, p. 676
Creative visualization, p. 681
Cupping, p. 683

Imagery, p. 681
Integrative health care, p. 677
Integrative nursing, p. 677
Integrative therapies, p. 677
Meditation, p. 680
Moxibustion, p. 683
Passive relaxation, p. 680
Progressive relaxation, p. 679
Qi gong, p. 683

Relaxation response, p. 679
Stress response, p. 677
Tai chi, p. 683
Therapeutic touch (TT), p. 683
Traditional Chinese medicine (TCM), p. 682
Vital energy (*qi*), p. 683
Whole medical systems, p. 677
Yin and yang, p. 682

MEDIA RESOURCES

With few exceptions, the general health of North American people has steadily improved over the course of the past century, as evidenced by lower mortality rates and increased life expectancies. Changes in knowledge, technology, science, and health care have altered the course of many illnesses. Although allopathic or biomedicine (conventional Western medicine) is quite effective in treating numerous physical ailments (e.g., bacterial infections, structural abnormalities, and acute emergencies), it is generally less effective in decreasing stress-induced illnesses, managing symptoms of chronic disease, caring for the emotional and spiritual needs of individuals, and improving quality of life and general well-being. As a result, patients continue to seek complementary (non-biomedical) treatments in increasing numbers, integrating these therapies with biomedicine.

The most recent comprehensive national survey estimates that between 33.2% and 50.6% of the US population integrate complementary and biomedical treatments to reduce symptom burden and improve overall well-being (Clarke et al., 2015). In part, this use corresponds to (1) a desire for less invasive, less toxic, "more natural" treatments; (2) lack of satisfaction with biomedical treatments; (3) an increasing desire by patients to take a more active role in their treatment process; (4) beliefs that a combination of treatments (biomedical and complementary) result in better overall results; (5) the increased

number of research articles in journals such as *Journal of Alternative and Complementary Medicine* and the *Journal of Holistic Nursing;* and (6) beliefs and values that are consistent with an approach to health that incorporates the mind, body, and spirit or a holistic approach (Koithan, 2018).

COMPLEMENTARY AND INTEGRATIVE APPROACHES TO HEALTH

The National Institutes of Health/National Center for Complementary and Integrative Health (NIH/NCCIH, 2018) identifies complementary and integrative approaches as an array of health care approaches with a history of use or origins outside of mainstream or conventional medicine. Complementary therapies are therapies used together with conventional treatment recommended by a person's health care provider. As the name implies, complementary therapies complement conventional treatments. Many of them, such as therapeutic touch, contain diagnostic and therapeutic methods that require special training. Others, such as guided imagery and breathwork, are easily learned and applied. Complementary therapies also include relaxation; exercise; massage; reflexology; prayer; biofeedback; hypnotherapy; creative therapies, including art, music, or dance therapy; meditation; chiropractic therapy; and herbs/supplements (Lindquist et al., 2018). Another term that is used to describe interventions used in this fashion, particularly by licensed health care providers, is integrative therapies (Kreitzer and Koithan, 2019).

When nonpharmacologic therapies such as exercise, chiropractic, and herb supplements are used in place of conventional pharmacologic or other medical procedures, they are considered alternative therapies (NCCIH, 2018). These therapies then become primary treatments, replacing biomedical care. For example, most of the time a person with chronic pain uses yoga to encourage flexibility and relaxation at the same time in which nonsteroidal antiinflammatory or opioid medications are prescribed. Both sets of interventions are based on conventional pathophysiology and anatomy while acknowledging the mind-body connection that contributes to the physiological pain response. In this case, yoga is used as a complementary intervention. However, when that same patient decides to use a meditative practice that includes yoga and other lifestyle changes rather than medication, yoga now becomes an alternative therapy and is perceived as more helpful than an allopathic approach for chronic pain. Some patients, particularly those from different cultural backgrounds, may choose to use whole medical systems such as traditional Chinese medicine (TCM), Ayurveda, or naturopathy as alternative systems of care to biomedicine. When used in this fashion, these approaches are always considered alternative because they are based on completely different philosophies and life systems than those used by allopathic medicine. Table 32.1 presents types of complementary therapies.

Because of the increased interest in complementary therapies, many institutions, including medical and nursing schools, have integrated conventional "biomedical" education with programs that incorporate complementary therapy content. These integrative health care programs graduate practitioners who recommend a full spectrum of possible treatments, both biomedical and complementary. In an integrative health care system consumers are treated by a team of providers consisting of both biomedical and complementary practitioners. More fully defined, integrative health care emphasizes the importance of the relationship between practitioner and patient; focuses on the whole person; is informed by evidence; and makes use of appropriate therapeutic approaches, health care professionals, and disciplines to achieve optimal health (Rakel, 2018).

Nurses have historically practiced in an integrative fashion; a review of nursing theory (see Chapter 4) reveals the values of holism, relational care, and evidence-informed practice. Until recently, nursing identified its practice as holistic rather than integrated. Holistic nursing treats the mind-body-spirit of the patient, using interventions such as relaxation therapy, music therapy, touch therapies, and guided imagery (Dossey and Keegan, 2016). The American Holistic Nurses Association maintains Standards of Holistic Nursing Practice, which defines and establishes the scope of holistic practice and describes the level of care expected from a holistic nurse (AHNA/ANA, 2013).

Kreitzer and Koithan (2019) challenge the profession to embrace its long-standing roots of integrative care, standing alongside colleagues to help transform the current health care system and operationalize our collective wisdom to offer whole person care that is patient-centered, relationship-based, and supported by evidence that incorporates the best of all possible interventions. Grounded in six principles, integrative nursing is defined as "a way of being-knowing-doing that advances the health and well-being of persons, families, and communities through caring-healing relationships. Integrative nurses use evidence to inform traditional and emerging interventions that support whole person/whole systems healing" (Kreitzer and Koithan, 2019).

Increasing interest in integrative health care is evident in the increased number of publications in respected health care journals and the continued support of research. The mission of the National Institutes of Health/National Center for Complementary and Integrative Health (NIH/NCCIH) supports the investigation of the benefits and safety of complementary interventions. Although the body of evidence about complementary therapies is growing, limited data make it difficult to establish the benefits of specific therapies. Reasons are varied but reflect the growing and developing nature of the science. More research is needed. Therefore nurses need to weigh the risk and benefits of each intervention and consider the following when recommending complementary therapies: (1) the history of each therapy (many have been used by cultures for thousands of years to support health and ameliorate suffering); (2) nursing's history and experience with a particular therapy; (3) other forms of evidence reporting outcomes and safety data, including case study and qualitative research; and (4) the cultural influences and context for certain patient populations.

This chapter discusses several types of complementary therapies, including a description, the clinical applications, and the limitations of each therapy. The therapies are organized into two categories. The first are nursing-accessible therapies that you can begin to learn and apply in patient care. The second category includes training-specific therapies such as chiropractic therapy or acupressure that a nurse cannot perform without additional training and/or certification.

> **REFLECT NOW**
>
> Reflect on your own life experiences. Do you personally use a variety of therapeutic strategies (e.g., massage for a sore back or neck), and do your own practices influence your acceptance of this approach to care?

NURSING-ACCESSIBLE THERAPIES

Some complementary therapies and techniques are general in nature and use natural processes (e.g., breathing, thinking and concentration, presence, movement) to help people feel better and cope with both acute and chronic conditions (Box 32.1). You can learn about these techniques and integrate them into your independent nursing practice with patients. Ongoing assessment and evaluation of response to these interventions will determine both the appropriateness and usefulness of these complementary therapies. Sometimes changes to physician-prescribed therapies, such as medication doses, are needed when complementary therapies alter physiological responses and lead to therapeutic responses (Ringdahl, et al., 2018).

Complementary therapies teach individuals ways to change their behavior to help alter physical responses to stress and improve symptoms such as muscle tension, gastrointestinal discomfort, pain, or sleep disturbances. Active involvement is a primary principle for these therapies; individuals achieve better responses if they commit to practice the techniques or exercises daily. Therefore, to achieve effective outcomes, therapeutic strategies need to be matched with an individual's lifestyle, his or her beliefs and values, and the context within which the care is to be delivered (acute or community-based).

Relaxation Therapy

People face situations in everyday life that evoke the stress response (see Chapter 37). The mind modifies the biochemical functions of the major organ systems in response to feedback. Thoughts and feelings influence the production of chemicals (i.e., neurotransmitters, neurohormones, and peptides) that circulate throughout the body and convey messages via cells to various systems within the body. The stress response is a good example of the way in which systems cooperate to protect an individual from harm. Physiologically, the cascade of changes associated with the

TABLE 32.1   Complementary Therapies

Types	Definitions
Biologically Based Therapies *(Natural products)*	
Dietary supplements	Defined by the Dietary Supplement Health and Education Act of 1994 and used to supplement dietary/nutritional intake by mouth; contain one or more dietary ingredients, including vitamins, minerals, herbs, or other botanical products
Herbal medicines	Plant-based therapies used in whole systems of medicine or as individual preparations by allopathic providers and consumers for specific symptoms or issues
Macrobiotic diet	Predominantly a vegan diet (no animal products except fish); initially used in the management of a variety of cancers; emphasis placed on whole cereal grains, vegetables, and unprocessed foods
Mycotherapies	Fungi-based (mushroom) products
Orthomolecular medicine (megavitamin)	Increased intake of nutrients such as vitamin C and beta-carotene; treats cancer, schizophrenia, autism, and certain chronic diseases such as hypercholesterolemia and coronary artery disease
Probiotics	Live microorganisms (in most cases, bacteria) that are similar to beneficial microorganisms found in the human gastrointestinal system; also called *good bacteria*
The "Zone"	Dietary program that requires eating protein, carbohydrate, and fat in a 30:40:30 ratio—30% of calories from protein, 40% from carbohydrate, and 30% from fat; used to balance insulin and other hormones for optimal health
Energy Therapies *(Use or manipulation of energy fields)*	
Acupuncture	Traditional Chinese method of producing analgesia or altering the function of a body system by inserting thin needles along a series of lines or channels, called meridians; direct needle manipulation of energetic meridians influences deeper internal organs by redirecting *qi*
Healing touch	Biofield therapy; uses gentle touch directly on or close to body to influence and support the human energy system and bring balance to the whole body (physical, spiritual, emotional, and mental); a formal educational and certification system provides credentials for practitioners
Reiki therapy	Biofield therapy derived from ancient Buddhist rituals; practitioner places hands on or above a body area and transfers "universal life energy," providing strength, harmony, and balance to treat a patient's health disturbances
Therapeutic touch	Biofield therapy involving direction of a practitioner's balanced energies in an intentional manner toward those of a patient; practitioner's hands lay on or close to a patient's body
Magnet therapy	Bioelectromagnetic therapy; devices (magnets) applied to the body surface, producing a measurable magnetic field; used primarily to alleviate pain associated with musculoskeletal injuries or disorders
Manipulative and Body-Based Methods *(Involve movement of body with focus on body structures and systems)*	
Acupressure	Applying digital pressure in a specified way on designated points on the body to relieve pain, produce analgesia, or regulate a body function
Chiropractic medicine	Manipulating the spinal column; includes physiotherapy and diet therapy
Craniosacral therapy	Assessing the craniosacral motion for rate, amplitude, symmetry, and quality and attuning/aligning the spinal column, cerebrospinal fluid, and rhythmic processes, releasing restrictions or abnormal barriers to motion
Massage therapy	Manipulating soft tissue through stroking, rubbing, or kneading to increase circulation, improve muscle tone, and provide relaxation
Simple touch	Touching the patient in appropriate and gentle ways to make connection, display acceptance, and give appreciation
Mind-Body Interventions *(Honor connections between thoughts and physiological functioning using emotion to influence health and well-being)*	
Art therapy	Use of art to reconcile emotional conflicts, foster self-awareness, and express patients' unspoken and frequently unconscious concerns about their disease
Biofeedback	Process providing a person with visual or auditory information about autonomic physiological functions of the body such as muscle tension, skin temperature, and brain wave activity through the use of instruments
Breathwork	Using a variety of breathing patterns to relax, invigorate, or open emotional channels
Guided imagery	Concentrating on an image or series of images to treat pathological conditions
Meditation	Self-directed practice for relaxing the body and calming the mind using focused rhythmic breathing
Music therapy	Using music to address physical, psychological, cognitive, and social needs of individuals with disabilities and illnesses; improves physical movement and/or communication, develops emotional expression, evokes memories, and distracts people who are in pain

Continued

TABLE 32.1 Complementary Therapies—cont'd

Types	Definitions
Tai chi	Incorporating breath, movement, and meditation to cleanse, strengthen, and circulate vital life energy and blood; stimulate the immune system; and maintain external and internal balance
Yoga	Focuses on body musculature, posture, breathing mechanisms, and consciousness; goal is attainment of physical and mental well-being through mastery of body achieved through exercise, holding of postures, proper breathing, and meditation

Movement Therapies
(Eastern or Western approaches to promote well-being)

Dance therapy	Intimate and powerful medium because it is a direct expression of the mind and body; treats persons with social, emotional, cognitive, or physical problems
Feldenkrais method	A complementary therapy based on establishment of good self-image through awareness and correction of body movements; integrates the understanding of the physics of body movement patterns with an awareness of the way people learn to move, behave, and interact
Pilates	Method of body movement used to strengthen, lengthen, and improve the voluntary control of muscles and muscle groups, especially those used for posture and core strengthening; awareness of breathing and precise movements are integral components

Whole Medical Systems
(Complete systems of theory and practice that have evolved independently from or parallel to conventional biomedicine)

Ayurvedic medicine	One of the oldest systems of medicine, practiced in India since the first century AD. There are eight branches of Ayurvedic medicine, including internal medicine; surgery; treatment of head and neck disease; gynecology, obstetrics, and pediatrics; toxicology; psychiatry; elder care and rejuvenation; and sexual vitality. Treatments balance the doshas using a combination of dietary and lifestyle changes, herbal remedies and purgatives, massage, meditation, and exercise.
Homeopathic medicine	Developed in Germany and practiced in the United States since the mid-1800s. It is a system of medical treatments based on the theory that certain diseases can be cured by giving small, highly diluted doses of substances that in a healthy person would produce symptoms like those of the disease. Prescribed substances called *remedies* are made from naturally occurring plant, animal, or mineral substances and are used to stimulate the vital force of the body so that it can heal itself.
Latin American traditional healing	*Curanderismo* is a Latin American traditional healing system that includes a humoral model for classifying food, activity, drugs, and illnesses and a series of folk illnesses. The goal is to create a balance between the patient and his or her environment, thereby sustaining health.
Native American traditional healing	Tribal traditions are individualistic, but similarities across traditions include the use of sweating and purging, herbal remedies, and ceremonies in which a shaman (a spiritual healer) makes contact with spirits to ask their direction in bringing healing to people to promote wholeness and healing.
Naturopathic medicine	A system of therapeutics focused on treating the whole person and promoting health and well-being rather than an individual disease. Therapeutics include herbal medicine, nutritional supplementation, physical medicine, homeopathy, lifestyle counseling, and mind-body therapies with an orientation toward assisting the person's internal capacity for self-healing (vitalism).
Traditional Chinese medicine (TCM)	An ancient healing tradition identified in the first century AD focused on balancing yin/yang energies. It is a set of systematic techniques and methods, including acupuncture, herbal medicines, massage, acupressure, moxibustion (use of heat from burning herbs), qi gong (balancing energy flow through body movement), cupping, and massage. Fundamental concepts are from Taoism, Confucianism, and Buddhism.

stress response causes increased heart and respiratory rates; tightened muscles; increased metabolic rate; and a general sense of foreboding, fear, nervousness, irritability, and negative mood. Other physiological responses include elevated blood pressure; dilated pupils; stronger cardiac contractions; and increased levels of blood glucose, serum cholesterol, circulating free fatty acids, and triglycerides. Although these responses prepare a person for short-term stress, the effects on the body of long-term stress may include structural damage and chronic illness such as angina, tension headaches, cardiac arrhythmias, pain, ulcers, and atrophy of the immune system organs (Voss and Kreitzer, 2018).

The **relaxation response** reduces generalized cognitive, physiological, and/or behavioral arousal. The process of relaxation elongates the muscle fibers, reduces the neural impulses sent to the brain, and thus decreases the activity of the brain and other body systems. Decreased heart and respiratory rates, blood pressure, and oxygen consumption and increased alpha brain activity and peripheral skin temperature characterize the relaxation response. The relaxation response occurs through a variety of techniques that incorporate a repetitive mental focus and the adoption of a calm, peaceful attitude (Bee et al., 2018).

Relaxation helps individuals develop cognitive skills to reduce the negative ways in which they respond to situations within their environment. Cognitive skills include the following:

- Focusing (the ability to identify, differentiate, maintain attention on, and return attention to simple stimuli for an extended period)
- Passivity (the ability to stop unnecessary goal-directed and analytic activity)
- Receptivity (the ability to tolerate and accept experiences that are uncertain, unfamiliar, or paradoxical)

The long-term goal of relaxation therapy is for people to continually monitor themselves for indicators of tension and consciously let go and release the tension contained in various body parts.

Progressive relaxation training teaches the individual how to effectively rest and reduces tension in the body. The person learns to detect subtle localized muscle tension sequentially, one muscle group at a time (e.g., the upper arm muscles, the forearm muscles). In doing so the individual learns to differentiate between high-intensity tension (strong fist clenching), very subtle tension, and relaxation (Bee et al., 2018). A person practices this activity using different muscle groups. One active

BOX 32.1   EVIDENCE-BASED PRACTICE

Pain in Hospitalized Children

PICOT Question: Do complementary therapies versus biomedical therapies safely and effectively reduce pain and discomfort in hospitalized children?

Evidence Summary

Pain is a complex phenomenon for children, involving psychological, biological, and sociological factors. Hospitalization and pain are often linked in the minds of children. Despite advances in pediatric pain management, recent studies demonstrate that many children continue to have uncontrolled moderate-to-severe pain when they are in the hospital. Several systematic analyses focusing on the use of complementary therapies to control pain show that many complementary and nonpharmacological therapies, such as relaxation, repositioning, distraction, focused breathing, art therapy, and humor, are effective in reducing discomfort in children who are hospitalized (Buratti et al., 2015; Kahsay, 2017; Thrane et al., 2016). Barriers to the use of complementary therapies included nurses' heavy workloads and the need for further education about how to use these techniques.

Application to Nursing Practice

- Children who are hospitalized often respond positively to complementary therapies, experience reduced pain, and need fewer medications to control their pain.
- Instructing parents on specific complementary therapies used for their child's pain control (e.g., breathing techniques, art therapy) allows the parents to use these techniques.
- Nurses need to learn about and use complementary therapies such as breathing techniques and distraction to alleviate the pain associated with painful and stressful procedures, especially among children.

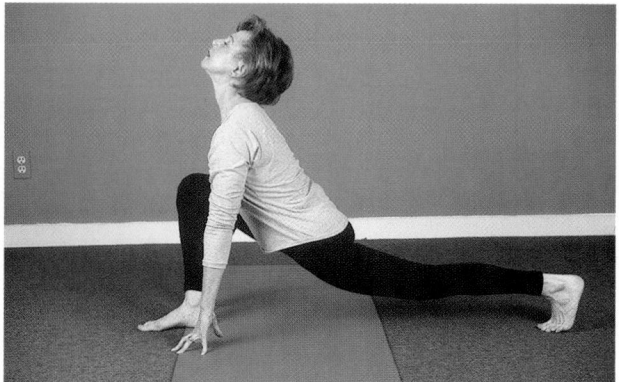

FIG. 32.1 Yoga is a discipline that focuses on muscles, posture, breathing, and consciousness.

progressive relaxation technique involves the use of slow, deep abdominal breathing while tightening and relaxing an ordered succession of muscle groups, focusing on the associated bodily sensations while letting go of extraneous thoughts. When guiding a patient, you may decide to begin with the muscles in the face, followed by those in the arms, hands, abdomen, legs, and feet. Conversely you may also guide a patient to tense and relax muscles, beginning with the feet and working up the body.

The goal of *passive relaxation* is to still the mind and body intentionally without the need to tighten and relax any particular body part. One effective passive relaxation technique incorporates slow abdominal breathing exercises while imagining warmth and relaxation flowing through specific body parts such as the lungs or hands. Passive relaxation is useful for persons for whom the effort and energy expenditure of active muscle contracting leads to discomfort or exhaustion.

Clinical Applications of Relaxation Therapy. Research shows relaxation techniques effectively lower blood pressure (Nagele et al., 2014) and heart rate, decrease muscle tension, improve well-being, and reduce symptom distress in persons experiencing a variety of situations (e.g., complications from medical treatments, chronic illness, or loss of a significant other) (Golding, et al., 2016; Meyer et al, 2016). Research also indicates that relaxation, alone or in combination with imagery, yoga (Fig. 32.1), and music, reduces pain and anxiety while improving well-being (Charalambous et al., 2016). Other benefits of relaxation include the reduction of depression (Pospos et al., 2018) and breathlessness in persons with chronic respiratory illnesses (Brighton et al., 2018).

Relaxation enables individuals to exert control over their lives. Some experience a decreased feeling of helplessness and a more positive psychological state overall. For example, relaxation also reduces

workplace stress experienced by nurses working on nursing units. Deep-breathing exercises, centering, and focusing attention often lead to improved staff satisfaction, staff relationships and communication, and workload perceptions (Clarke et al., 2009). Nursing units that incorporate relaxation activities into daily routines experience reduced turnover and improved patient satisfaction scores (Kreitzer and Zbrowsky, 2018).

Limitations of Relaxation Therapy. During relaxation training individuals learn to differentiate between low and high levels of muscle tension. During the first months of training sessions, when the person is learning how to focus on body sensations and tensions, there are reports of increased sensitivity in detecting muscle tension. Usually these feelings are minor and resolve as the person continues with the training. However, be aware that on occasion some relaxation techniques result in continued intensification of symptoms or the development of altogether new symptoms (Dossey and Keegan, 2016).

An important consideration when choosing any type of relaxation technique is the physiological and psychological status of the individual. Some patients with advanced disease such as cancer or acquired immunodeficiency syndrome (AIDS) seek relaxation training to reduce their stress response. However, techniques such as active progressive relaxation training require a moderate expenditure of energy, which often increases fatigue and limits an individual's ability to complete relaxation sessions and practice. Therefore, active progressive relaxation is not appropriate for patients with advanced disease or those who have decreased energy reserves. Passive relaxation or guided imagery is more appropriate for these individuals.

REFLECT NOW

Reflect on a time when you were experiencing a substantial stress response. What physical and mental/cognitive sensations did you feel? What strategies (passive or progressive) did you use to relax or reduce this stress response?

Meditation and Breathing

Meditation is any activity that limits stimulus input by directing attention to a single unchanging or repetitive stimulus so that the person is able to become more aware of self (Gross et al., 2018). It is a general term for a wide range of practices that involve relaxing the body and stilling the mind. Although meditation has its roots in Eastern religious practices (Hinduism, Buddhism, and Taoism), conventional health care practitioners began to recognize its healing potential in the early 1970s (Gross et al., 2018). According to Benson (1975), the four components of meditation are (1) a quiet space, (2) a comfortable position, (3) a receptive attitude, and (4) a focus of attention. He described meditation as a process that anyone can use to calm down; cope with stress; and, for those with spiritual inclinations, feel one with God or the universe.

Meditation is different from relaxation; the purpose of meditation is to become "mindful," increasing our ability to live freely and escape destructive patterns of negativity. Meditation is self-directed; it does not necessarily require a teacher and can be learned from books or audiotapes (Kabat-Zinn, 2018). Most meditation techniques involve slow, relaxed, deep abdominal breathing that evokes a restful state, lowers oxygen consumption, reduces respiratory and heart rates, and reduces anxiety (Hilton et al., 2017).

Clinical Applications of Meditation. Several studies support the clinical benefits of meditation. For example, meditation reduces overall systolic and diastolic blood pressures and significantly reduces hypertensive risk (Park and Han, 2017). It also successfully reduces relapses in alcohol treatment programs (Wilson et al., 2017). Patients with cancer who use mindfulness-based cognitive therapies often experience less depression, anxiety, and distress and report an improved quality of life (Carlson, 2017). Patients who have posttraumatic stress disorders and chronic pain also benefit from mindfulness meditation (Cushing and Braun, 2018). In addition, meditation increases productivity, improves mood, increases sense of identity, and lowers irritability (Bee et al., 2018).

Considerations for the appropriateness of meditation include the person's degree of self-discipline; it requires ongoing practice to achieve lasting results. Most meditation activities are easy to learn and do not require memorization or particular procedures. Patients typically find mindfulness and meditation self-reinforcing. The peaceful, positive mental state is usually pleasurable and provides an incentive for individuals to continue to meditate.

Limitations of Meditation. Although meditation contributes to improvement in a variety of physiological and psychological ailments, it is contraindicated for some people. For example, a person who has a strong fear of losing control will possibly perceive it as a form of mind control and thus will be resistant to learning the technique. Some individuals also become hypertensive during meditation and require a much shorter session than the average session of 15 to 20 minutes.

Meditation may also increase the effects of certain drugs. Therefore monitor individuals learning meditation closely for physiological changes with respect to their medications. Prolonged practice of meditation techniques sometimes reduces the need for antihypertensive, thyroid-regulating, and psychotropic medications (e.g., antidepressants and anti-anxiety agents). In these cases, adjustment of the medication is necessary (Gross et al., 2018).

Imagery

Imagery or visualization is a mind-body therapy that uses the conscious mind to create mental images to stimulate physical changes in the body, improve perceived well-being, and/or enhance self-awareness. Frequently imagery, combined with some form of relaxation training, facilitates the effect of the relaxation technique. Imagery is self-directed, in which individuals create their mental images, or guided, during which a practitioner leads an individual through a particular scenario (Fitzgerald and Langevin, 2016. When guiding an imagery exercise, direct the patient to begin slow abdominal breathing while focusing on the rhythm of breathing (see Chapter 44). Then direct the patient to visualize a specific image such as ocean waves coming to shore with each inspiration and receding with each exhalation. Next instruct the patient to take notice of the smells, sounds, and temperatures that he or she is experiencing. As the imagery session progresses, instruct the patient to visualize warmth entering the body during inspiration and tension leaving the body during exhalation. Individualize imagery scenarios for each patient to ensure that the image does not evoke negative memories or feelings.

Imagery often evokes psychophysiological responses such as alterations in gastric secretions, body chemistry, internal and superficial blood flow, wound healing, and heart rate/heart rate variability (Pincus and Sheikh, 2009). Although most imagery techniques involve visual images, they also include the auditory, proprioceptive, gustatory, and olfactory senses. An example of this involves visualizing a lemon being sliced in half and squeezing the lemon juice on the tongue. This visualization produces increased salivation as effectively as the actual event. People typically respond to their environment according to the way they perceive it and by their own visualizations and expectancies. Therefore you need to help patients individualize imagery based on their preferences and expectations (Fitzgerald and Langevin, 2016).

Creative visualization is one form of self-directed imagery that is based on the principle of mind-body connectivity (i.e., every mental image leads to physical or emotional changes) (Gawain, 2016). Box 32.2 lists patient teaching strategies for creative visualization.

Clinical Applications of Imagery. Imagery has applications in a number of pediatric and adult patient populations. For example, it helps control or relieve pain, decrease nightmares, and improve sleep (Pincus and Sheikh, 2009). It also aids in the treatment of chronic conditions such as asthma, cancer, sickle cell anemia, migraines, autoimmune disorders, atrial fibrillation, functional urinary disorders, menstrual and premenstrual syndromes, gastrointestinal disorders such as irritable bowel syndrome and ulcerative colitis, and rheumatoid arthritis (Fitzgerald and Langevin, 2018).

BOX 32.2 PATIENT TEACHING

Creative Visualization

Objective
- The patient will demonstrate skills in creative visualization.

Teaching Strategies
- Set mutual goals the patient can meet. Success leads to confidence and increased self-esteem.
- Create a clear image. Although it is sometimes difficult to develop a visual image, if the patient views the goals of the imagery with clear thoughts and in the present tense, the patient will be more successful in creating an effective image.
- Have the patient frequently visualize the image. Have him or her perform this visualization during relaxing states and throughout the day but particularly before bedtime or on wakening, when his or her mind usually is more relaxed.
- Have the patient repeat encouraging statements while focusing on the image. This alleviates any doubts about his or her ability to achieve established goals.

Evaluation
Use the principles of teach-back to evaluate patient/family caregiver learning:
- Describe when you plan to use visualization.
- I want to be sure I described this therapy well. Please explain to me the steps you are going to take to practice visualization.

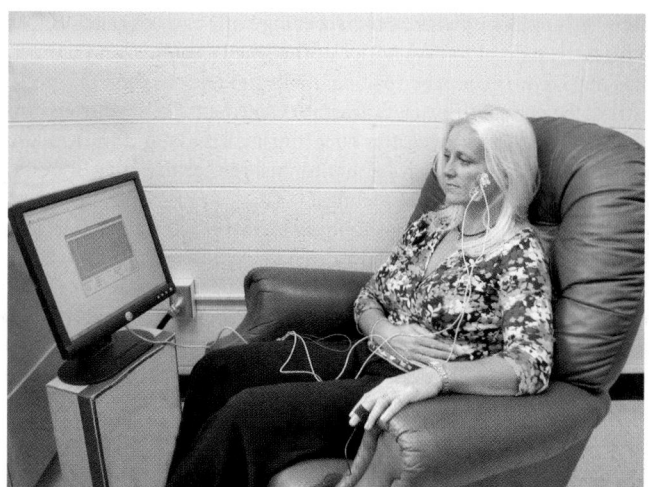

FIG. 32.2 A patient using biofeedback can visually see how relaxation affects physiological functions. (From Okeson JP: *Management of temporomandibular disorders and occlusion,* ed 8, St Louis, 2020, Elsevier.)

Limitations of Imagery. Imagery is a behavioral intervention that has relatively few side effects (Fitzgerald and Langevin, 2018). Yet increased anxiety and fear sometimes occur when imagery is used to treat posttraumatic stress disorders and social anxiety disorders (Bisson et al, 2013). Some patients with chronic obstructive pulmonary disease (COPD) and asthma experience increased airway constriction when using guided imagery (Volpato et al., 2015). Thus you need to closely monitor patients when using this therapy.

TRAINING-SPECIFIC THERAPIES

Training-specific therapies are complementary treatments that nurses administer only after completing a specific course of study and training. These therapies require postgraduate certificates or degrees indicating completion of additional education and training, national certification, or additional licensure beyond the registered nurse (RN) to practice and administer them. Several training-specific therapies (e.g., biofeedback and acupuncture) are very effective and often recommended by conventional health care practitioners (NIH/NCCIH, 2018; Qaseem et al., 2017). However, others (e.g., homeopathy and naturopathy) have not been adequately studied, and their effectiveness in many conditions has been questioned (National Health and Medical Research Council, 2015; NIH/NCCIH, 2018). Although many of these complementary therapies elicit positive effects, all therapies carry some risk, particularly when used in conjunction with conventional medical therapies. Therefore, you need advanced knowledge to effectively talk about them with patients and provide education about their safe use.

Biofeedback

Biofeedback is a mind-body technique that uses instruments to teach self-regulation and voluntary self-control over specific physiological responses. Electronic or electromechanical instruments measure, process, and provide information to patients about their muscle tension, cardiac activity, respiratory rates, brain-wave patterns, and autonomic nervous system activity. This information, or feedback, is given in physical, physiological, auditory, and/or visual feedback signals that increase a person's awareness of internal processes that are linked to illness and distress. Biofeedback therapies are used to change thinking, emotions, and behaviors, which in turn support beneficial physiological changes, resulting in improved health and well-being. For example, patients connected to a biofeedback device sometimes hear a sound if their pulse rate or blood pressure increases out of their therapeutic

zone. Practitioners then help patients interpret these sounds and use a variety of breathing, relaxation, and imaging exercises to gain voluntary control over their racing heart or their increasing systolic blood pressure (Good and Zauszmiewski, 2016).

Biofeedback is an effective addition to more traditional relaxation programs because it immediately demonstrates to patients their ability to control some physiological responses and the relationship among thoughts, feelings, and physiological responses (Fig 32.2). It helps individuals focus on and monitor specific body parts. Biofeedback helps patients control the physiological functions that are most difficult to control by providing immediate feedback about which stress relaxation behaviors work most effectively. Eventually patients notice positive physiological changes without the need for instrument feedback.

Clinical Applications of Biofeedback. Biofeedback in a variety of forms has application in numerous situations, with evidence supporting its effectiveness dating back to the 1980s. Initial studies suggest that it may be helpful in stroke recovery, smoking cessation, attention-deficit/hyperactivity disorder (ADHD), epilepsy, headache disorders, and a variety of gastrointestinal and urinary tract disorders (Secic et al., 2016; Stanton et al, 2011, 2017). One of the most critical components of any behavioral program is adherence to the treatment regimen. Patients who adhere to the treatment regimen have more positive results.

Limitations of Biofeedback. Although biofeedback produces effective outcomes in many patients, there are several precautions, particularly in those with psychological or neurological conditions. During biofeedback sessions the repressed emotions or feelings for which coping is difficult sometimes surface. For this reason, practitioners who offer biofeedback need to be trained in more traditional psychological methods or have qualified professionals available for referral. In addition, long-term use of biofeedback sometimes lowers blood pressure, heart rates, and other physiological parameters. As with other biobehavioral interventions, monitor patients closely to determine the need for medication adjustments.

Traditional Chinese Medicine

Traditional Chinese medicine (TCM) is a whole system of medicine that began as an ethnic healing system approximately 3600 years ago. Chinese medicine views health as "life in balance," which manifests as lustrous hair, a radiant complexion, engaged interactions, a body that functions without limitations, and emotional balance. Health promotion encourages a healthy diet, moderate regular exercise, regular meditation/introspection, healthy family and social relationships, and avoidance of environmental toxins such as cigarette smoke.

Several concepts and principles guide the TCM system of assessment, diagnosis, and intervention. The most important of these is the concept of yin and yang, which represent opposing yet complementary phenomena that exist in a state of dynamic equilibrium. Examples are night/day, hot/cold, and shady/sunny. Yin represents shade, cold, and inhibition, whereas yang represents fire, light, and excitement. Yin also represents the inner part of the body, specifically the viscera, liver, heart, spleen, lung, and kidney, whereas yang represents the outer part, specifically the bowels, stomach, and bladder. Harmony and balance in every aspect of life are the keys to health, including yin/yang balance. Practitioners believe that disease occurs when there is an imbalance in these two paired opposites (Holland, 1999). Imbalance occurs as excess or deficiencies in three areas: external (six "evils" linked to weather and climate, including wind, cold, fire, damp, summer heat, and dryness), internal (originate in emotions and affect different organs, such as anger [liver], joy [heart], or fear [kidney]), or neither internal nor external (congenital weak constitutions, such as birth defects, trauma, overexertion, excessive sexual activity, poor-quality diet, and poisons). Imbalance ultimately leads to disruption of vital energy, *qi*, which then compromises the body-mind-spirit of the person, causing "disease." Disruptions in *qi* along the meridians can be systematically evaluated and treated by TCM practitioners.

TCM is an individualized treatment system based on a very specific assessment process. Practitioners use four methods to evaluate a patient's condition: observing, hearing/smelling, asking/interviewing, and touching/palpating. In TCM, outward manifestations reflect the internal environment. For example, the color, shape, and coating of the tongue reflect the general condition of the internal organs. The pulses provide information about the condition and balance of *qi*, blood, yin and yang, and internal organs. Therapeutic modalities include acupuncture, Chinese herbs, tui na massage, moxibustion (burning moxa, a cone or stick of dried herbs that have healing properties on or near the skin), cupping (placing a heated cup on the skin to create a slight suction), tai chi (originally a martial art that is now viewed as a moving meditation in which patients move their bodies slowly, gently, and with awareness while breathing deeply), *qi gong* (originally a martial art, now viewed as a series of carefully choreographed movements or gestures that are designed to promote and manipulate the flow of qi within the body), lifestyle modifications, and dietary changes.

Clinical Applications of Traditional Chinese Medicine.
In spite of widespread use of TCM in Asia, evidence about its effectiveness as a whole system of care is limited. Most research in this field focuses on the study of individual treatment components of TCM such as acupuncture and herbal therapies. However, some evidence shows that TCM is helpful in treating fibromyalgia (Deare et al., 2013) and in addressing symptoms associated with menopause (Taylor-Swanson et al., 2015).

Limitations of Traditional Chinese Medicine.
TCM is not currently regulated in most states, although acupuncture is. The federal government recognizes the Accreditation Commission for Acupuncture and Oriental Medicine (ACAOM) as responsible for accrediting schools that teach acupuncture and TCM, and approximately one-third of the states that license acupuncture require graduation from an ACAOM-accredited school. The National Certification Commission for Acupuncture and Oriental Medicine (NCCAOM) offers a certification examination for acupuncture and Chinese herbal and manipulative therapies. Refer patients requesting TCM to a qualified practitioner found at http://www.nccaom.org/find-a-practitioner-directory/.

There is some concern about the safety of Chinese herbal treatments that are used in teas, remedies, and supplements. The US Food and Drug Administration (FDA) does not regulate, inspect, or ensure that the ingredients of these herbs are safe and without toxins. Recent reports about these products suggest that many Chinese herbs are contaminated with drugs, toxins, or heavy metals or that their ingredients may not be clearly listed or labeled. Further, these herbs can be very powerful, interacting with drugs and causing serious complications. When assessing a person using TCM, you always need to ask about the full complement of therapies, including the types of herbs that the patient is using. Some patients consider these as teas or dietary additives, powders, or supplements and not as over-the-counter medications.

Acupuncture

As a key component of TCM, acupuncture is an ancient practice shared by other Asian systems of care. When applied outside the system practice of TCM, acupuncture is viewed as a mind-body therapy and is referred to as medical acupuncture. In the United States, medical acupuncture is often provided as an individual treatment by conventionally trained physicians, nurses, chiropractors, dentists, and acupuncturists for many chronic conditions. Many states now have regulations and licensure requirements to practice as an acupuncturist.

Acupuncture regulates or realigns the vital energy (*qi*), which flows like a river through the body in channels that form ta system of pathways called meridians. Twelve primary and eight secondary meridians are used by medical acupuncturists. An obstruction in these channels blocks energy flow in other parts of the body. Acupuncturists insert needles in specific areas along the channels called acupoints, through which the *qi* can be influenced and flow reestablished. Application of heat or weak electrical currents enhances the effects of the needles.

Clinical Applications of Acupuncture.
Current evidence shows that acupuncture modifies the body's response to pain and how pain is processed by central neural pathways and cerebral function (NIH/NCCIH, 2018). Acupuncture is effective for low back pain, myofascial pain (e.g., temporomandibular joint disorder and trigeminal neuralgia), hot flashes, simple and migraine headaches, osteoarthritis, plantar heel pain, and chronic shoulder pain (Frisk et al., 2014; Reinstein et al., 2017). It is also used to treat sinusitis, gastrointestinal disorders, chronic pruritus, perimenstrual symptoms, menopausal symptoms, clinical depression, smoking, and other addictions with varying effectiveness (NIH/NCCIH, 2018).

Limitations of Acupuncture.
Acupuncture is a safe therapy when the practitioner has the appropriate training and uses sterilized needles. Although needle complications occur, they are rare if the practitioner takes appropriate steps to ensure the safety of the equipment and the patient. Reported complications include infections resulting from inadequately sterilized needles or those that are left in place for an extended length of time, broken needles, puncture of an internal organ, bleeding, fainting, seizures, and posttreatment drowsiness.

Caution is necessary when using acupuncture with pregnant patients and those who have a history of seizures, are carriers of hepatitis, or are infected with human immunodeficiency virus (HIV). Treatment is contraindicated in persons who have bleeding disorders and skin infections. Further, semipermanent needles should not be used with patients who have valvular heart disease because of the increased risk of infection. Electroacupuncture is not recommended for persons with a pacemaker and those who have cardiac arrhythmias or epilepsy or are pregnant (Fontaine, 2018).

Therapeutic Touch

Therapeutic touch (TT), developed in the 1970s by Delores Krieger and Dora Kunz, is one of the "touch therapies" identified by NCCIH. It affects the energy fields that surround and penetrate the human body with the conscious intent to help or heal (Dossey and Keegan, 2016). Other touch therapies include acupressure, healing touch (HT), and reiki. Blending ancient Eastern traditions with modern nursing theory, TT uses the energy of the provider to positively influence the patient's energy field.

TT consists of placing the practitioner's open palms either on or close to the body of a person (Fig. 32.3). It occurs in five phases: centering, assessing, unruffling, treating, and evaluating. To begin, the practitioner centers physically and psychologically, becoming fully present in the moment and quieting outside distractions. Then the practitioner scans the body of the patient with the palms (roughly 2 to 6 inches [5 to 15 cm] from the body) from head to toe. While assessing the energetic biofield of the patient, the practitioner focuses on the quality of the *qi*, identifying areas of accumulated energetic tensions, uneasiness, sluggishness, or congestion that manifest as sensations of congestion, pressure, warmth, coolness, blockage, pulling or drawing, or static or tingling. The practitioner then redirects these energetic patterns to harmonize distressed areas or to stimulate movement of *qi* in areas that are stuck and congested. Using long downward strokes over the energy fields of the body, the practitioner touches the body or maintains the hands in a position a few inches away from the body. The final phase

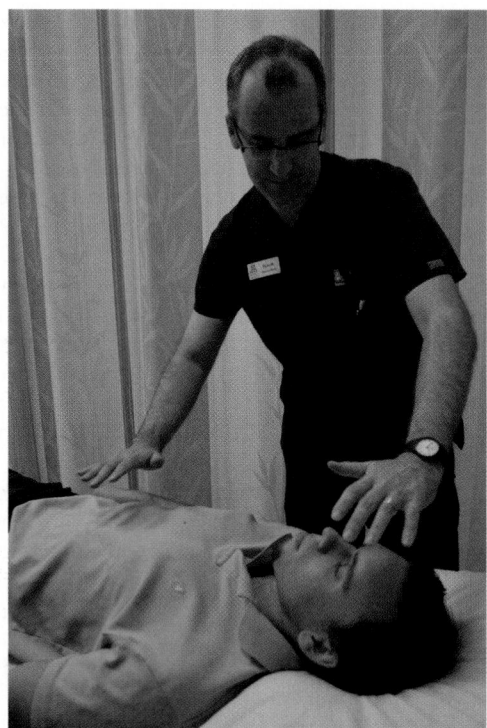

FIG. 32.3 During a therapeutic touch session, the practitioner intentionally directs energy to facilitate the patient's healing process.

consists of evaluating the patient, reassessing the energy field to ensure that energy is flowing freely, and determining additional outcomes and responses to the treatment (Krieger, 1975, 1979).

Clinical Applications of Touch Therapies. The evidence supporting the effectiveness of touch therapies, including therapeutic and healing touch, is inconclusive, although it may be effective in treating pain in adults and children, dementia, trauma, and anxiety during acute and chronic illnesses (Baldwin and Trent, 2017). Box 32.3 summarizes the importance of touch in older adults.

Limitations of Touch Therapies. Although touch therapies cause very few complications or side effects, they may be contraindicated in certain patient populations. For example, people who are sensitive to human interaction and touch (e.g., those who have been physically abused or have psychiatric disorders) often misinterpret the intent of the treatment and feel threatened and anxious by it. Determining if your patient has experienced trauma is important before using touch therapies (see https://www.samhsa.gov/trauma-violence for additional information). Other patients, including pregnant women, neonates, patients with cardiovascular and neurological instabilities, or patients who are dying, sometimes are sensitive to energy repatterning. Sessions with these populations need to be time limited and particularly gentle (Umbreit and Johnson, 2018).

Chiropractic Therapy

Chiropractic therapy, a manipulative or body-based therapy, was developed in 1895 in Iowa. Chiropractors graduate from well-established postbaccalaureate educational programs similar to medical schools. The central belief of the chiropractic profession is that body structure (primarily that of the spine and spinal cord) and the ability of the body to function normally are closely related. Thus when the spine is misaligned, energy flow is impeded, and the innate healing abilities of the body are impaired. Chiropractic therapy aims to normalize the relationship between structure and function by a series of

manipulations. Practitioners use their hands or a device to provide manipulation, which is the application of a controlled, sudden forceful movement to a joint, moving it beyond its passive range of motion. Often manipulations are combined with additional therapeutic modalities, including ice and heat, electrical stimulation, deep tissue massage, joint immobilization, lifestyle counseling, and medications.

Chiropractic care is a popular form of complementary therapy in the United States; 8.4% of the adult and 3.3% of the pediatric population visit chiropractors each year, representing almost 20 million health care visits (Clarke et al., 2015). Compared with other forms of complementary therapies, chiropractic care is often covered by insurance plans, including Medicare, Medicaid, state workers' compensation plans, health maintenance organizations (HMOs), and private insurance plans. Licensure is regulated by individual state governments, and scopes of practice and prescriptive authority vary from state to state.

Clinical Applications of Chiropractic Therapy. The basic goals of chiropractic therapy focus on restoring structural and functional imbalances. Chiropractors believe that structure and function coexist with one another and that alterations or distortions in structure ultimately lead to abnormalities in function. A major structural problem that chiropractors treat is vertebral (neck/back) subluxation with its accompanying symptom of pain.

Chiropractic therapy improves acute pain and disability in some patients. This therapy is also sometimes effective over longer periods to reduce acute and subacute low back pain and joint pain caused by osteoarthritis (Globe et al., 2016). Chiropractic care may also enhance the effects of conventional treatments in pediatric asthma (Gleberzon et al., 2012). Chiropractic interventions are also used to treat headaches, dysmenorrhea, vertigo, tinnitus, and visual disorders (Bryans et al., 2014).

Limitations of Chiropractic Therapy. Although chiropractic therapies are safe for a variety of conditions, chiropractors do not treat several diseases or conditions with manipulation. Bone and joint infections require pharmaceutical or surgical intervention because the structural integrity of the bone is compromised if excessive force is used. Other contraindications include acute myelopathy, fractures, dislocations, rheumatoid arthritis, and osteoporosis.

Some risks are associated with chiropractic therapy. A variety of injuries, ranging in severity from mild adverse responses (e.g., mild transient headache, increased pain and stiffness) to more serious injuries (e.g., vertebral artery dissection), have been reported (Shekelle et al., 2017). Degree and risk of injury depend on the type of manipulation performed, location of the manipulation (cervical spine is more susceptible to serious injury), overall health of the patient, and expertise of the provider. When educating patients about chiropractic care, you need to include educational and licensure credentials of qualified chiropractors, typical treatments, and possible complications.

Natural Products and Herbal Therapies

It is estimated that approximately 25,000 plant species are used medicinally throughout the world. It is the oldest form of medicine known to man, and archeological evidence suggests that herbal remedies have been used for over 60,000 years. Herbal medicines are a prominent part of health care among indigenous populations worldwide. Interest in natural products also continues to increase in countries where biomedicine is dominant (Clarke, et al., 2015).

Nonvitamin, nonmineral natural products are used by 18% of the US population to prevent disease and illness and to promote health and well-being (Clarke et al., 2015). A natural product is a chemical compound or substance produced by a living organism and includes herbal medicines (also known as botanicals), dietary supplements, vitamins, minerals, mycotherapies (fungi-based products), essential oils (aromatherapy), and probiotics. Many are sold over the counter as dietary supplements. The most frequently used products are fish oil/omega-3 fatty acids, glucosamine, probiotics/prebiotics, melatonin, coenzyme Q10, echinacea, cranberry, garlic, ginseng, and ginkgo biloba (Clarke et al., 2015).

Herbal medicines are not approved for use as drugs and are not regulated by the FDA. For this reason, many are sold as foods or food supplements. The Dietary Supplement Health and Education Act (1994) allows companies to sell herbs as dietary supplements as long as there are no health claims written on their labels. Natural products in the United States are prepared primarily from plant materials. They are provided as tinctures or extracts, elixirs, syrups, capsules, pills, tablets, lozenges, powders, ointments or creams, drops, and suppositories.

Clinical Applications of Herbal Therapy. A number of herbs are safe and effective for a variety of conditions (Table 32.2). Cranberry juice has been sometimes used to treat urinary tract infections for decades. The effectiveness evidence supporting cranberry supplements to prevent urinary tract infections is mixed although clinicians continue to cite case studies that suggest its effectiveness, particularly in postmenopausal women with incontinence because cranberry molecules bind with the iron that bacteria need to grow and reproduce and substances in cranberry block adherence of bacteria to the walls of the bladder (Wang, et al., 2012). Curcumin is a yellow plant substance associated with turmeric as well as ginger. A polyphenol, curcumin appears to have a potent antiinflammatory effect, with suggested use in cancer prevention and progression as well as other chronic conditions. Clinical trials have recently found that curcuminoids are effective in lowering fasting blood sugars in persons with dysglycemia, including prediabetes and other metabolic syndromes (Melo et al., 2018).

Limitations of Herbal Therapy. Simply because a product is "natural" does not make it "safe." Although herbal medicines provide beneficial effects for a variety of conditions, a number of problems exist. Because they are not regulated, concentrations of the active ingredients vary considerably. Contamination with other herbs or chemicals, including pesticides and heavy metals, is also problematic. Not all companies follow strict quality control and manufacturing guidelines that set standards for acceptable levels of pesticides, residual solvents, bacterial levels, and heavy metals. For this reason, teach patients to purchase herbal medicines only from reputable manufacturers. This means that labels on herbal products need to contain the scientific name of the botanical, the name and address of the actual manufacturer, a batch or lot number, the date of manufacture, and the expiration date. Using natural products that have been verified by the US Pharmacopeia (USP) is another way to ensure product safety, quality, and purity. Look for the USP Verified Dietary Supplement mark on product labels when buying or recommending natural products.

Some herbs also contain toxic products that have been linked to cancer. Table 32.3 lists several unsafe herbs. Some herbal substances contain powerful chemicals. As with any other medication, examine herbs for interaction and compatibility with other prescribed or over-the-counter substances that are being used simultaneously.

THE INTEGRATIVE NURSING ROLE

The interest in complementary therapies and an integrative approach to care continues to increase, fueled in part by the explosion in opioid addictions, the increase in chronic disease, and the need to consider nonpharmacological treatment options (National Academies of Sciences, Engineering, and Medicine, 2017). In North America and Europe, professional groups increasingly support the use of complementary therapies and monitor research in this area. The American College of Physicians issued new clinical practice guidelines for the management of acute, subacute, and chronic low back pain in 2017, recommending the use of nonpharmacological interventions that include tai chi, yoga, and other mind/body techniques (Qaseem et al., 2017). In January 2018, The Joint Commission (TJC, 2019a) implemented new pain assessment and management standards, requiring accredited hospitals to offer nonpharmacological (complementary) therapy to effectively manage patients' pain. All providers, including nurses, need to encourage open, honest dialogue with patients about the use of complementary therapies. Providers also need to actively engage patients to accept integrative care to prevent disease, manage illness, and improve whole person well-being by employing the full spectrum of possible therapeutics rather than relying solely on surgery or drugs.

The integrative approach to health care is consistent with nursing's patient-centered, relationship-based legacy, which is focused on whole person well-being and health. Nurses have the potential for becoming essential participants in this type of health care delivery system. Many nurses already practice the use of touch, relaxation techniques, imagery, and breathwork and practice using the principles of integrative nursing (Kreitzer and Koithan, 2019). Familiarize yourself with the evidence in each modality that you incorporate into your practice. Know which patient is most likely to benefit from each therapy, when to use the various therapies, which complications might occur, and which precautions are needed when using these therapies.

In addition, you need enough knowledge to discuss the full range of biomedical and complementary therapeutic options so that you can help patients make informed health care decisions. Always ask patients directly about their use of complementary therapies, including self-care activities such as yoga, meditation, or dietary supplements. Be knowledgeable about the evidence for different complementary therapies so that you can make appropriate recommendations about which therapies are possibly useful for patients. Know about the different credentialing processes and how to refer patients to competent providers. Understand thoroughly the potential benefits and risks so that information is clearly and fully disclosed. Be knowledgeable, so you can give advice to patients about when to seek conventional care and when it is safe to consider complementary care services. For example, if a patient has right lower abdominal pain, nausea, and vomiting, be suspicious of conditions such as appendicitis or colitis and recommend consultation with a health care provider. However, if the patient has a chronic gastrointestinal disorder and has a diagnosis of irritable bowel

TABLE 32.2	Safe or Effective Herbs Determined By Non–United States Regulatory Authorities	
Common Name and Uses	**Effects**	**Potential Drug Interactions**
Aloe		
Skin disorders, including burns, inflammation and acute injuries (used topically)	Acceleration of wound healing	Furosemide (Lasix) and loop diuretics
GI ulcerations, including Crohn's disease and ulcerative colitis (taken orally)	Unknown mechanism, although there is a known laxative effect	May enhance the effects of laxatives when taken orally
Chamomile		
Inflammatory diseases of GI and upper respiratory tracts	Antiinflammatory	Drugs that cause drowsiness (alcohol, barbiturates, benzodiazepines, narcotics, antidepressants)
Generalized anxiety disorder	Calming agent	
Echinacea		
Upper respiratory tract infections	Stimulant of immune system	Anti-rejection and other drugs that weaken immune system May interact with antiretrovirals and other drugs used in the treatment of HIV/AIDS
Feverfew		
Wound healing	Antiinflammatory	Warfarin and other anticoagulants
Arthritis	Inhibition of serotonin and prostaglandins	Aspirin and ibuprofen
Garlic		
Elevated cholesterol levels	Inhibition of platelet aggregation	Warfarin and blood thinners
Hypertension		Saquinavir and other anti-HIV drugs
Ginger		
Nausea and vomiting	Antiemetic	Warfarin and anticoagulants Aspirin and NSAIDs
Ginkgo biloba		
Alzheimer's disease and dementia	Memory improvement, although these effects are now in question given results in two recent clinical trials	Warfarin and anticoagulants Aspirin and NSAIDs
Ginseng		
Age-related diseases	Increased physical endurance, improved immune function	Warfarin and anticoagulants Aspirin and NSAIDs MAO inhibitors
Licorice		
GI disorders, including gastric ulcers and hepatitis C	Unknown	Corticosteroids and other immunosuppressive drugs Digoxin Antihypertensive drugs
Saw palmetto		
Benign prostatic hyperplasia	Prevention of conversion of testosterone to dihydrotestosterone (needed for prostate cell multiplication)	Finasteride and antiandrogen drugs
Chronic pelvic pain	Unknown mechanism	None known
Valerian		
Sleep disorders, mild anxiety and restlessness	Central nervous system depression	Barbiturates and other sleep medications Alcohol Antihistamines

AIDS, Acquired immunodeficiency disease; *GI,* gastrointestinal; *HIV,* human immunodeficiency virus; *MAO,* monoamine oxidase; *NSAIDs,* nonsteroidal antiinflammatory drugs.
Data from National Institutes of Health/National Center for Complementary and Integrative Health: *Herbs at a glance,* 2018. https://nccih.nih.gov/health/herbsataglance.htm. Accessed August 19, 2018.

TABLE 32.3 Unsafe Herbs

Common Name	Effects	Comments
Calamus (Indian type most toxic)	Fever Digestive aid	Contains varying amounts of carcinogenic *cis*-isoasarone Documented cases of kidney damage and seizures with oral preparations
Chaparral	Anticancer Used for bronchitis in traditional healing systems (Native American and Hispanic folk medicine) Found in "natural" weight-loss products	No proven efficacy Induces severe liver toxicity in some cases Severe uterine contractions
Coltsfoot	Antitussive	Contains carcinogenic pyrrolizidine alkaloids Hepatotoxic
Comfrey	Wound healing and acute injuries Used for antiinflammatory effects in osteoarthritis and rheumatoid arthritis	Contains carcinogenic pyrrolizidine alkaloids May induce venoocclusive disease Hepatotoxic
Ephedra (ma huang)	Central nervous system stimulant Bronchodilator Cardiac stimulation Weight loss	Unsafe for people with hypertension, diabetes, or thyroid disease Avoid consumption with caffeine
Life root	Menstrual flow stimulant	Hepatotoxic
Pokeweed	Antirheumatic Anticancer	Do not use with children, but many websites state that it is safe with observation and monitoring and proper dosing; often used with folk remedies and in Native American healing

Data from National Institutes of Health/National Center for Complementary and Integrative Health: *Herbs at a glance,* 2018. http://nccam.nih.gov/health/herbsataglance.htm; Accessed August 19, 2018; Natural Standard, 2018, accessed November 18, 2018, from https://naturalmedicines.therapeuticresearch.com/databases/food,-herbs-supplements.aspx; US Pharmacopeia, 2018. from http://www.usp.org/. November August 18, 2018.

syndrome, the patient may benefit from relaxation and herbal therapy. Be aware of the safety precautions for each complementary therapy, and incorporate these in your teaching plans. Finally, understand your state Nurse Practice Act with regard to complementary therapies and practice only within the scope of these laws.

Nurses work very closely with their patients and are in the unique position of becoming familiar with the patient's spiritual and cultural viewpoints. They are often able to determine which complementary therapies are more appropriately aligned with these beliefs and offer recommendations accordingly. Being knowledgeable about complementary therapies will help you provide accurate information to patients and other health care professionals.

QSEN Building Competency in Patient-Centered Care You are caring for a 48-year-old woman, Carmen, with stage 3 breast cancer who has returned to the hospital after being discharged after a mastectomy. She developed an infection in her suture line and around her drain site. Just before changing her dressings, you notice that she is more withdrawn and unwilling to speak more than one or two words and only to answer direct questions. When you question her further, she states that she can't stop thinking about her future and fears that "this will be how it's going to be … one hospital visit after another." She also says that she's concerned about the amount of pain medication that she's taking and that she's "tired of feeling drowsy and out-of-it" when her family comes to visit but doesn't know how else to manage her fear and pain. Which techniques could you offer Carmen to alleviate her suffering? Are there strategies that would help address her fears of the future and begin to view it in a more positive light?

Answers to QSEN Activities can be found on the Evolve website.

KEY POINTS

- Integrative health care programs use the full complement of treatment approaches (biomedical and complementary) to provide patient-centered care to patients.
- The stress response is an adaptive response that allows individuals to respond to stressful situations.
- A chronic stress response is often maladaptive, leading to chronic muscle tension, mood changes, and immune changes.
- Complementary therapies require commitment and regular involvement by the patient to be most effective and have prolonged beneficial outcomes.
- Choose complementary therapies appropriately according to a patient's overall health status, presenting symptom severity and distress, beliefs and cultural values, access to health care options, and insurance coverage/ability to pay.
- Continuously evaluate a patient's response to complementary therapies, as medication doses may need to change based on physiological responses.
- Complementary therapies accessible to nursing include relaxation, meditation and mindfulness techniques, and imagery. Evidence supports their use to decrease the effects of stress and improve overall patient well-being.
- Many complementary therapies require additional education and certification, including biofeedback, touch therapies (therapeutic touch, reiki, and healing touch), and acupuncture.
- Although there is increasing evidence to support the use of complementary therapies, additional research of sufficient quality and rigor is needed.

REFLECTIVE LEARNING

- You are completing an admission assessment for a surgical patient. What types of assessment questions would you ask to determine whether your patient is using any natural products or complementary therapies?
- Reflect on a recent clinical experience. Were there situations when the integrative approach to care would be helpful or perhaps inappropriate? For example, think about whether an integrative approach would be just as useful in the emergency department as it is in hospice care?
- Reflect on a couple of relaxation techniques discussed in this chapter. How could you use these techniques to help you prepare for your current courses and clinical experiences?

REVIEW QUESTIONS

1. When planning patient education, it is important to remember that patients with which of the following illnesses often find relief in complementary therapies?
   1. Lupus and diabetes
   2. Ulcers and hepatitis
   3. Heart disease and pancreatitis
   4. Chronic back pain and arthritis
2. Which complementary therapies are most easily learned and applied by a nurse? (Select all that apply.)
   1. Therapeutic massage therapy
   2. Traditional Chinese medicine
   3. Progressive relaxation
   4. Breathwork and guided imagery
   5. Therapeutic touch
3. While planning care for a patient, a nurse understands that providing integrative care includes treating which of the following?
   1. Disease, spirit, and family interactions
   2. Desires and emotions of the patient
   3. Mind-body-spirit of patients and their families
   4. Muscles, nerves, and spine disorders
4. In addition to a thorough patient assessment, when a nurse uses one of the nursing-accessible complementary therapies, he or she must ensure that which of the following has occurred?
   1. The family has provided permission.
   2. The patient has provided permission and consent.
   3. The health care provider has given approval or provided orders for the therapy.
   4. The nurse has received specialized training in the therapeutic technique.
5. A nurse is caring for a patient with chronic arthritis pain. The patient wants to add some complementary therapies to help with pain management. Which therapies might be most effective for controlling pain (Select all that apply):
   1. Biofeedback
   2. Acupuncture
   3. Therapeutic touch
   4. Chiropractic therapy
   5. Herbal medicines
6. A nurse is caring for a patient experiencing a stress response. The nurse plans care with the knowledge that systems respond to stress in what manner? (Select all that apply.)
   1. Always fail and cause illness and disease
   2. Cause negative responses over time
   3. React the same way for all individuals
   4. Protect an individual from harm in the short term
   5. Tolerate the stress response indefinitely
7. Meditation may intensify the effects of which of these medications? (Select all that apply.)
   1. Steroid medications
   2. Insulin
   3. Thyroid-regulating medications
   4. Cough syrups
   5. Antihypertensive medications
8. Which of the following statements best explains therapeutic touch (TT)?
   1. Intentionally mobilizes energy to balance, harmonize, and repattern the recipient's biofield
   2. Intentionally heals tissue damage or corrects certain disease symptoms
   3. Is overwhelmingly effective in many conditions
   4. Is completely safe and does not warrant any special precautions
9. Traditional Chinese medicine (TCM) is used by many patients. Which statement most accurately describes intervention(s) offered by TCM providers?
   1. Uses acupuncture as its primary intervention modality
   2. Uses many modalities based on the individual's needs
   3. Uses primarily herbal remedies and exercise
   4. Is the equivalent of medical acupuncture
10. The nurse manager of a community clinic arranges for staff in-services about various complementary therapies available in the community. What is the purpose of this training? (Select all that apply.)
    1. Nurses play an essential role in the safe use of complementary therapies.
    2. Nurses are often asked for recommendations and strategies that promote well-being and quality of life.
    3. Nurses learn how to provide all of the complementary modalities during their basic education.
    4. Nurses play an essential role in patient education to provide information about the safe use of these healing strategies.
    5. Nurses appreciate the cultural aspects of care and recognize that many of these complementary strategies are part of a patient's life.

Answers: 1. 4; **2.** 1, 3, 4; **3.** 3; **4.** 3; **5.** 1, 2, 3; **6.** 2, 4; **7.** 2, 3, 5; **8.** 1; **9.** 2; **10.** 1, 2, 4, 5.

Rationales for Review Questions can be found on the Evolve website.

REFERENCES

American Holistic Nursing Association/American Nurses Association (AHNA/ANA): *Holistic nursing: scope and standards of practice*, ed 2, Silver Spring, MD, 2013, American Nurses Publishing.

Benson H: *The relaxation response*, New York, 1975, Avon.

Dossey B, Keegan L: *Holistic nursing: a handbook for practice*, ed 7, Boston, MA, 2016, Jones & Bartlett.

Fitzgerald M, Langevin M: Imagery. In Dossey B, Keegan L, editors: *Holistic nursing: a handbook for practice*, ed 7, Boston, MA, 2016, Jones & Bartlett.

Fontaine K: *Complementary and integrative therapies for nursing practice*, ed 5, Upper Saddle River, NJ, 2018, Prentice Hall.

Gawain S: *Creative visualization: use the power of your imagination to create what you want in your life*, Novato, CA, 2016, New World Library.

Good M, Zauszmiewski J: Biofeedback. In Dossey B, Keegan L, editors: *Holistic nursing: a handbook for practice*, ed 7, Boston, MA, 2016, Jones & Bartlett.

Gross C, et al.: Meditation. In Lindquist R, et al.: *Complementary and alternative therapies in nursing*, ed 8, New York, 2018, Springer.

Holland A: *Voices of qi: an introductory guide to Traditional Chinese Medicine*, Berkeley, 1999, North Atlantic Books1999.

Kabat-Zinn J: *Falling awake: how to practice mindfulness in everyday life*, New York, NY, 2018, Hachette Books.

Koithan M: Concepts and principles of integrative nursing. In Kreitzer MJ, Koithan M, editors: *Integrative Nursing*, ed 2, New York, 2018, Oxford Press.

Kreiger D: Therapeutic touch: the imprimatur of nursing, *Am J Nurs* 25:784, 1975.

Kreiger D: Searching for evidence of physiological change, *Am J Nurs* 79:660, 1979.

Kreitzer MJ, Koithan M: *Integrative nursing*, ed 2, New York, 2019, Oxford Press.

Lindquist R, et al.: *Complementary and alternative therapies in nursing*, ed 8, New York, 2018, Springer.

National Academies of Sciences: Engineering, and Medicine: *Pain management and the opioid epidemic: balancing societal and individual benefits and risks of prescription opioid use*, Washington, DC, 2017, The National Academies Press.

National Health and Medical Research Council: *NHMRC information paper: evidence on the effectiveness of homeopathy for treating health conditions*, Canberra, 2015, National Health and Medical Research Council.

National Institutes of Health/National Center for Complementary and Integrative Health (NIH/NCCIH) 2018. https://nccih.nih.gov/. Accessed August 20, 2018.

Pincus D, Sheikh AA: *Imagery for pain relief: a scientifically grounded guidebook for clinicians*, New York, 2009, Routledge, Taylor & Francis Group.

Qaseem A, et al.: Noninvasive treatments for acute, subacute, and chronic low back pain: a clinical practice guideline from the American College of Physicians, *Ann Intern Med* 166(7):514–530, 2017.

Rakel D: *Integrative medicine*, ed 4, Philadelphia, PA, 2018, Elsevier Saunders.

Ringdahl D, et al.: Integrative nursing practice. In Kreitzer MJ, Koithan M, editors: *Integrative Nursing*, ed 2, New York, 2018, Oxford Press.

Voss M, Kreitzer MJ: Stress, resilience and wellbeing. In Kreitzer MJ, Koithan M, editors: *Integrative Nursing*, ed 2, New York, 2018, Oxford Press.

RESEARCH REFERENCES

Baldwin AL, Trent NL: An integrative review of scientific evidence for reconnective healing, *J Altern Complement Med* 23(8):590–598, 2017.

Bee SM, et al.: Relaxation therapies. In Lindquist R, et al.: *Complementary and alternative therapies in nursing*, ed 8, New York, 2018, Springer.

Bisson JI, et al.: Psychological therapies for chronic post-traumatic stress disorder (PTSD) in adults, *Cochrane Database Syst Rev* 12:CD003388, 2013.

Brighton LJ, et al.: Holistic services for people with advanced disease and chronic breathlessness: a systematic review and meta-analysis, *BMJ*, 2018. https://doi.org/10.1136/thoraxjnl-2018-211589, Thorax, thoraxjnl-2018-211589.

Bryans R, et al.: Evidence-based guidelines for the chiropractic treatment of adults with neck pain, *J Manipulative Physiol Ther* 37(1):42–63, 2014.

Buratti V, et al.: Distraction as a technique to control pain in pediatric patients during venipuncture. A narrative review of literature, *Prof Inferm* 68(1):52–62, 2015.

Carlson LE: Distress management through mind-body therapies in oncology, *J Natl Cancer Inst Monogr* 2017(52):37–41, 2017.

Charalambous A, et al.: Guided imagery and progressive muscle relaxation as a cluster of symptoms management intervention in patients receiving chemotherapy: a randomized trial, *PLoS One* 11(6), 2016:e0156911.

Clarke T, et al.: Trends in the use of complementary health approaches among adults: United States, 2002–2012, *Natl Health Stat Report* 79:1–16, 2015.

Cushing RM, Braun KL: Mind-body therapy for military veterans with post-traumatic stress disorder: a systematic review, *J Altern Complement Med* 24(2):106–114, 2018.

Deare JC, et al.: Acupuncture for treating fibromyalgia, *Cochrane Database Syst Rev* 5(CD007070), 2013.

Frisk JW, et al.: How long do the effects of acupuncture on hot flashes persist in cancer patients? *Support Care Cancer* 22(5):1409–1415, 2014.

Gleberzon BJ, et al.: The use of spinal manipulative therapy for pediatric health conditions: a systematic review of the literature, *J Can Chiropr Assoc* 56(2):128–141, 2012.

Globe G, et al.: Clinical practice guidelines: chiropractic care for low back pain, *J Manipulative Physiol Ther* 39(1):1–22, 2016.

Golding K, et al.: Self-help relaxation for post-stroke anxiety: a randomized, controlled pilot study, *Clin Rehabil* 30(2):372–378, 2016.

Hilton L, et al.: Mindfulness meditation for chronic pain: systematic review and meta-analysis, *Ann Behav Med* 51(2):199–213, 2017.

Kahsay H: Assessment and treatment of pain in pediatric patients, *Curr Pediatric Res* 21(1):148–157, 2017.

Kreitzer MJ, Zbrowsky T: Creating optimal healing environments. In Lindquist R, et al.: *Complementary and alternative therapies in nursing*, ed 8, New York, 2018, Springer.

Melo I, et al.: Curcumin or combined curcuminoids are effective in lowering the fasting blood glucose concentrations of individuals with dysglycemia: systematic review and meta-analysis of randomized controlled trials, *Pharmacol Res* 128:137–144, 2018.

Meyer B, et al.: Progressive muscle relaxation reduces migraine frequency and normalizes amplitudes of continuous negative variation, *J Headache Pain* 17(7):1–9, 2016.

Nagele E, et al.: Clinical effectiveness of stress-reduction techniques in patients with hypertension: systematic review and meta-analysis, *J Hypertens* 32(10):1936–1944, 2014.

National Center for Complementary and Integrative Health: Complementary, alternative, or integrative health: what's in a name?, 2018. https://nccih.nih.gov/health/integrative-health. Accessed August 6, 2019.

Park SH, Han KS: Blood pressure response to meditation and yoga: a systematic review and meta-analysis, *J Altern Complement Med* 23(9):685–695, 2017.

Pospos S, et al.: Web-based tools and mobile applications to mitigate burnout, depression, and suicidality among healthcare students and professionals: a systematic review, *Acad Psychiatry* 42(1):109–120, 2018.

Reinstein AS, et al.: Acceptability, adaptation, and clinical outcomes of acupuncture provided in the emergency department: a retrospective pilot study, *Pain Med* 18(1):169–178, 2017.

Secic A, et al.: Biofeedback training and tension type headache, *Acta Clin Croat* 55(1):156–160, 2016.

Shekelle PG, et al: The effectiveness and harms of chiropractic care for the treatment of acute neck and lower back pain: a systematic review, *VA ESP Project #05-226*, 2017.

Stanton R, et al.: Biofeedback improves activities of lower limb after stroke: a systematic review, *J Physiother* 57(3):145–155, 2011.

Stanton R, et al.: Biofeedback improves performance in lower limb activities more than usual therapy in people following stroke: a systematic review, *J Physiother* 63(1):11–16, 2017.

Taylor-Swanson L, et al.: Effects of traditional Chinese medicine on symptom clusters during the menopausal transition, *Climacteric* 18(2):142–156, 2015.

The Joint Commission (TJC): *Pain management standards for accredited organizations*, 2019a. https://www.jointcommission.org/topics/pain_management_standards_hospital.aspx. Accessed July 27, 2019.

Thrane SE, et al.: The assessment and non-pharmacologic treatment of procedural pain from infancy to school age through a developmental lens: a synthesis of evidence with recommendations, *J Pediatr Nurs* 31(1):e23–32, 2016.

Umbreit A, Johnson L: Healing touch. In Lindquist R, et al.: *Complementary and alternative therapies in nursing*, ed 8, New York, 2018, Springer.

Volpato E, et al.: Relaxation techniques for people with chronic obstructive pulmonary disease: a systematic review and a meta-analysis, *Evid Based Complement Alternat Med* 628365, 2015.

Wang CH, et al.: Cranberry-containing products for prevention of urinary tract infections in susceptible populations: a systematic review and meta-analysis of randomized controlled trials, *Arch Intern Med* 172(13):988–996, 2012.

Wilson AD, et al.: Mindfulness-based interventions for addictive behaviors: implementation issues on the road ahead, *Psychol Addict Behav* 31(8):888–896, 2017.

33

Self-Concept

OBJECTIVES

- Discuss factors that influence the components of self-concept and self-esteem.
- Identify stressors that affect self-concept and self-esteem.
- List the components of self-concept as related to psychosocial and cognitive developmental stages.
- Explore ways in which a nurse's self-concept and nursing actions affect a patient's self-concept and self-esteem.
- Discuss evidence-based care for patients with identity confusion, disturbed body image, altered self-concept, low self-esteem, and role conflict.
- Examine cultural considerations that affect self-concept and self-esteem.
- Apply the nursing process to promote a patient's self-concept.

KEY TERMS

Body image, p. 692
Identity, p. 692
Identity confusion, p. 694
Role ambiguity, p. 695

Role conflict, p. 695
Role overload, p. 695
Role performance, p. 693
Role strain, p. 695

Self-concept, p. 690
Self-esteem, p. 693
Sick role, p. 695

MEDIA RESOURCES

http://evolve.elsevier.com/Potter/fundamentals/
- Review Questions
- Concept Map Creator
- Case Study with Questions

- Audio Glossary
- Content Updates
- Answers to QSEN Activity and Review Questions

Self-concept is an individual's view of self. It is subjective and involves a complex mixture of unconscious and conscious thoughts, attitudes, and perceptions. Self-concept, or how a person *thinks* about oneself, directly affects self-esteem, or how one *feels* about oneself. Although these two terms often are used interchangeably, nurses need to differentiate the two so that they correctly and completely assess a patient and develop an individualized plan of care based on a patient's needs.

Patients face a variety of health problems that threaten their self-concept and self-esteem. A loss of bodily function, decline in activity tolerance, and difficulty in managing a chronic illness are examples of situations that change a patient's self-concept. You will help patients adjust to alterations in self-concept and strengthen components of self-concept to promote successful coping and positive health outcomes.

SCIENTIFIC KNOWLEDGE BASE

The development and maintenance of self-concept and self-esteem begin at a young age and continue across the life span. Parents and other primary caregivers not only influence the development of a child's self-concept and self-esteem, but research suggests that self-concept

clarity is transmitted from parents to children (Crocetti et al., 2016). In addition, individuals learn and internalize cultural influences on self-concept and self-esteem in childhood and adolescence. There is a significant emphasis on fostering a school-age child's self-concept. In general young children tend to rate themselves higher than they rate other children, suggesting that their view of themselves is positively inflated (Thomaes et al., 2017). Adolescence is a particularly critical developmental period when many variables, including school, family, and friends, affect self-concept and self-esteem (Rosenberg, 1965). The adolescent experience can adversely affect self-esteem, often more strongly for girls than for boys (Bleidorn et al., 2016). Boys often have better overall self-concepts than girls, particularly in physical and social domains (Agrahari and Kinra, 2017). Some adolescent girls are more sensitive about their appearance and how others view them (Vartanian et al., 2018). It is during adolescence that the search for an enduring sense of self turns into a core developmental task impacted by biological changes (e.g., puberty) and psychosocial changes (e.g., new interactions with peers and modifications in parent-adolescent relationships) (Erikson, 1963). During adolescence, individuals may rethink their previous sense of self and experiment with new roles and life plans. Thus, it is important to assess changes in identity formation

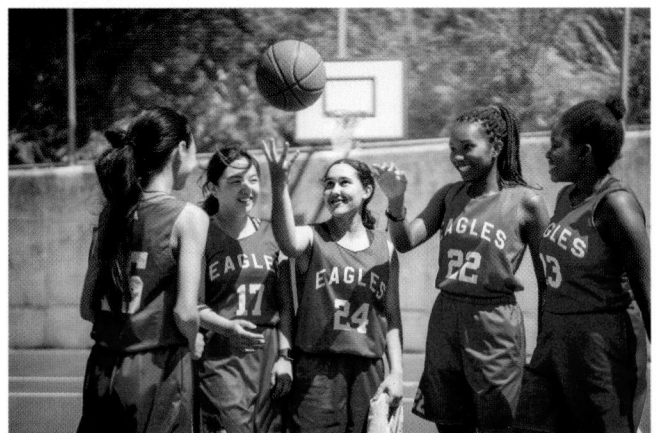

FIG. 33.1 Adolescents' participation in group activities can foster self-esteem. (iStock.com/hraun.)

and self-esteem among early, middle, and late adolescence because changes in self-concept occur over time (Fig. 33.1).

Most individuals cope with the transition from childhood through adolescence to adulthood successfully and become healthy and productive adults (Kann et al., 2018). Job satisfaction and overall performance in adulthood are also linked to self-esteem. Self-enhancing opportunities such as exploring new ideas, solving problems in creative ways, and learning new skills predict job satisfaction and commitment and promote self-concept clarity and self-esteem (Touhy and Jett, 2016). Sometimes when individuals lose a job, their sense of self diminishes, they lose motivation to be socially active, and they even become depressed. They lose their job identity, altering their self-perceptions and self-care practices. Establishing a stable sense of self that transcends relationships and situations is a developmental goal of adulthood.

Cultural variations in self-concept and self-esteem across the life span can impact health behaviors. In adolescent girls, culture, class, and self-esteem serve as protective factors against risk-taking behaviors, including unhealthy sexual behaviors (Kerpelman et al., 2016; Wilkins and Miller, 2017). Similarly, cultural identity of older adults is one of the major elements of self-concept and a key aspect of self-esteem (Touhy and Jett, 2016). Be aware of the cultural perspectives of aging when providing patient care. Sensitivity to factors that affect self-concept and self-esteem in diverse cultures is essential to ensure an individualized approach to health care.

There is a close relationship between how individuals view themselves and their perception of their health. Lower self-esteem is a risk factor that leaves one vulnerable to health problems, whereas higher self-esteem and strong social relationships support good health (Halter, 2018). A patient's belief in personal health often enhances his or her self-concept. Statements such as "I can get through anything" or "I've never been sick a day in my life" indicate that a person's thoughts about personal health are positive. Illness, hospitalization, and surgery affect self-concept. Chronic illness often affects the ability to provide financial support and maintain relationships, which then affects an individual's self-esteem and perceived identity and roles. Negative perceptions regarding health status are reflected in such statements as "It's not worth it anymore" or "I'm a burden to my family." Chronic illness affects identity and body image as reflected by verbalizations such as "I'll never get any better" or "I can't stand to look at myself anymore."

What individuals think and how they feel about themselves affect the way in which they approach self-care physically and emotionally and how they care for others. A person's behaviors are generally consistent with both self-concept and self-esteem. Individuals who have

a poor self-concept often do not feel in control of situations and worthy of care, which influences decisions regarding health care. Patients often have difficulty making even simple decisions, such as what to eat. Knowledge of variables that affect self-concept and self-esteem is critical to provide effective treatment.

> **REFLECT NOW**
>
> Reflect on a statement a patient made recently about identity, body image, role performance, or self-esteem for which you felt unprepared to respond.

NURSING KNOWLEDGE BASE

When providing evidence-based patient care, incorporate professional nursing knowledge developed from the humanities, sciences, nursing research, and clinical practice. A broad knowledge base allows nurses to have a holistic view of patients, thus promoting quality patient care that best meets the self-concept needs of each patient and family. Understanding a patient's self-concept is a necessary part of all nursing care (Halter, 2018).

Factors Influencing the Development of Self-Concept

The development of self-concept is a complex lifelong process that involves many factors. Erikson's psychosocial theory of development (1963) remains beneficial in understanding key tasks that individuals face at various stages of development. Each stage builds on the tasks of the previous stage. Successful mastery of each stage leads to a solid sense of self (Box 33.1).

Learn to recognize an individual's failure to achieve an age-appropriate developmental stage or his or her regression to an earlier stage in a period of crisis. This understanding allows you to individualize care and determine appropriate nursing interventions. Self-concept is always changing and is based on the following:

- Sense of competency
- Perceived reactions of others to one's body
- Ongoing perceptions and interpretations of the thoughts and feelings of others
- Personal and professional relationships
- Academic and employment-related identity
- Personality characteristics that affect self-expectations
- Perceptions of events that have an impact on self
- Mastery of prior and new experiences
- Cultural identity

Self-esteem usually increases in early and middle childhood, fluctuates or remains constant in adolescence, increases strongly in young adulthood, continues to increase in middle adulthood, and peaks between ages 60 and 70 years. Depending on self-concept clarity, self-esteem diminishes or stays constant in old age with a sharp drop in very old age (Orth et al., 2018). Although this pattern varies, in general it holds true across gender, socioeconomic status, and culture. Children often report high self-esteem because their sense of self is inflated by a variety of extremely positive sources, and periodic declines may be associated with shifts to more realistic information about the self. Adolescence is a time of marked maturational changes and shifting levels of self-esteem that set the stage for rises in self-concept from adolescence to young adulthood (Bleidorn et al., 2016).

Erikson's (1963) emphasis on the generativity stage explains the rise in self-esteem and self-concept in adulthood (see Chapter 11). The individual focuses on being increasingly productive and creative at work while at the same time promoting and guiding the

BOX 33.1 Self-Concept: Developmental Tasks

Trust versus Mistrust (Birth to 18 Months)
- Develops trust following consistency in caregiving and nurturing interactions
- Distinguishes self from environment

Autonomy versus Shame and Doubt (18-24 Months to 3 Years)
- Begins to communicate likes and dislikes
- Increasingly independent in thoughts and actions
- Appreciates body appearance and function (e.g., dressing, feeding, talking, and walking)

Initiative versus Guilt (3 to 5 Years)
- Identifies with a gender
- Enhances self-awareness
- Increases language skills, including identification of feelings

Industry versus Inferiority (6 to 11 Years)
- Incorporates feedback from peers and teachers
- Increases self-esteem with new skill mastery (e.g., reading, mathematics, sports, music)
- Aware of strengths and limitations

Identity versus Role Confusion (12 to 18 Years)
- Accepts body changes/maturation
- Examines attitudes, values, and beliefs; establishes goals for the future
- Feels positive about expanded sense of self

Intimacy versus Isolation (Late Teens to Mid-40s)
- Has stable, positive feelings about self
- Experiences successful role transitions and increased responsibilities

Generativity versus Self-Absorption (Mid-40s to Mid-60s)
- Able to accept changes in appearance and physical endurance
- Reassesses life goals
- Shows contentment with aging

Ego Integrity versus Despair (Mid-Late 60s to Death)
- Feels positive about life and its meaning
- Interested in providing a legacy for the next generation

next generation. On the basis of Erikson's stages of development, a decline in self-concept in later adulthood reflects a diminished need for self-promotion and a shift in self-concept to a more modest and balanced view of self. Many report a decline in self-esteem in later adulthood caused in part by physical and emotional changes associated with aging, but older adults with self-concept clarity demonstrate psychological well-being (Touhy and Jett, 2018). When aging is associated with deterioration of health, nursing interventions must focus on health behavior changes to promote self-care and self-concept (Touhy and Jett, 2016). Identifying specific nursing interventions to address the unique needs of patients at various life stages is essential.

Components and Interrelated Terms of Self-Concept

A positive self-concept gives a sense of meaning, wholeness, and consistency to a person. A healthy self-concept provides a high degree of stability, which generates positive feelings toward self. The components of self-concept are identity, body image, and role performance.

Identity. Identity involves the internal sense of individuality, wholeness, and consistency of a person over time and in different situations. It implies being distinct and separate from others. Being "oneself" or living an authentic life is the basis of true identity. Children learn culturally accepted values, behaviors, and roles through identification and modeling. They often gain an identity from self-observations and from what individuals tell them. An individual first identifies with parenting figures and later with other role models such as teachers or peers (Hockenberry et al., 2019). Relationships with parents, teachers, and peers have unique and combined effects on young children's general, academic, and social self-concept. To form an identity, a child must be able to bring together learned behaviors and expectations into a coherent, consistent, and unique whole (Erikson, 1963).

The achievement of identity is necessary for intimate relationships because individuals express identity in relationships with others (Halter, 2018). Sexuality is a part of identity, and its focus differs across the life span. For example, as an adult ages, the focus shifts from procreation to companionship, physical and emotional intimacy, and pleasure seeking (Touhy and Jett, 2018). Gender identity is a person's private view of maleness or femaleness; gender role is the masculine or feminine behavior exhibited. This image and its meaning depend on culturally determined values (see Chapters 9 and 34).

Cultural differences in identity exist (Box 33.2). Cultural identity develops from identification and socialization within an established group and through the experience of integrating the response of individuals outside the group into one's self-concept. Differences in cultural identity exist through identification with traditions, customs, and rituals within one's cultural group. When cultural identity is central to self-concept and is positive, cultural pride and self-esteem tend to be strong. In contrast, internalization of prejudice and devaluation of one's racial minority group can result in social isolation, which can negatively influence self-concept (Benninger and Savahl, 2017). An individual who experiences discrimination, prejudice, or environmental stressors such as low-income or high-crime neighborhoods can conceptualize himself or herself differently than an individual who experiences privilege. One's perception of social class also affects self-esteem (Wilkins and Miller, 2017).

Body Image. Body image involves attitudes related to the body, including physical appearance, structure, or function. Feelings about body image include those related to sexuality, femininity and masculinity, youthfulness, health, and strength. These mental images are not always consistent with a person's actual physical structure or appearance. Some body image distortions have deep psychological origins, such as the eating disorder anorexia nervosa. Other alterations occur as a result of situational events, such as the loss or change in a body part. Be aware that most men and women experience some degree of dissatisfaction with their bodies, which affects body image and overall self-concept. Individuals often exaggerate disturbances in body image when a change in health status occurs. The way others view a person's body and the feedback offered are also influential. For example, a controlling, violent husband tells his wife that she is ugly and that no one else would want her. Over the years of marriage she incorporates this devaluation into her self-concept.

Cognitive growth and physical development also affect body image. Normal developmental changes such as puberty and aging have a more apparent effect on body image than on other aspects of self-concept. Hormonal changes during adolescence influence body image. The development of secondary sex characteristics and the changes in body fat distribution have a tremendous impact on an adolescent's self-concept. For both male and female adolescents, appearance comparisons can result in a negative body image that impacts health behaviors,

BOX 33.2 CULTURAL ASPECTS OF CARE

Promoting Self-Concept and Self-Esteem in Culturally Diverse Patients

Cultural identity is an essential component of a person's self-concept and self-esteem. Early in growth and development an individual develops this identity within the context of family (Crocetti et al., 2016). As an individual matures, the cultural aspects of his or her self-concept are reinforced through social, family, or cultural experiences. In addition, a person's self-concept is strengthened or questioned through political, social, or cultural influences experienced in the home, school, and workplace environments. Positive or negative cultural role modeling, identity, and past experiences influence self-care, self-concept, and self-esteem. Social media also has a significant impact on the development of self-concept and identity (Eleuteri et al., 2017). Bullying, including cyberbullying, is one type of youth violence that threatens young people's self-concept and well-being. Nationwide, electronic bullying is rising, particularly among youth of color, including through e-mail, chat rooms, instant messaging, websites, or texting (Kann et al., 2018).

Implications for Patient-Centered Care

- Develop an open, nonrestrictive attitude for assessing and encouraging cultural practices to improve patients' self-concept.
- Understand that the relationship among self-esteem, stress, and social support can facilitate the development of nursing strategies to promote effective coping in culturally diverse adolescents (Bleidorn et al., 2016).
- Ask patients what they think is important to help them feel better or gain a stronger sense of self.
- Encourage cultural identity and pride by individualizing self-care practices and offering treatment choices to meet patients' self-concept needs.
- Facilitate culturally sensitive health promotion activities that address at-risk behaviors identified through evidence-based practice (e.g., smoking, vaping, drinking, eating disorder risks, premature sexual experiences, excessive and violent video gaming) (Eleuteri et al., 2017).
- When completing a social history, a priority nursing action is the assessment of child and adolescent coping strategies, conflict resolution, and stress management as it relates to the use of social media and texting (Kann et al., 2018).

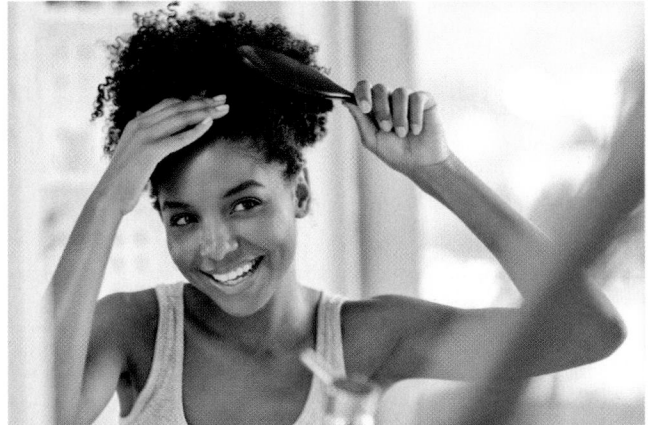

FIG. 33.2 An individual's appearance influences self-concept. (iStock.com/katleho Seisa.)

including disordered eating and exercise (Vartanian et al., 2018). For example, an adolescent girl may have a distorted body image and view herself as fat, which signals an eating disorder. Your assessment may reveal that an adolescent engages in self-harmful behaviors such as cutting; self-mutilation can indicate self-concept and self-esteem issues that warrant nursing intervention (Halter, 2018). A threat to body image and overall self-concept can affect adherence to recommended health regimens, including diet, exercise, health screening practices, and taking medications as prescribed. Changes associated with aging (e.g., menopause; wrinkles; graying hair; and decrease in visual acuity, hearing, and mobility) also affect body image in an older adult (Touhy and Jett, 2018).

Cultural and societal attitudes and values influence body image. Culture and society dictate the accepted norms of body image and influence one's attitudes (Fig. 33.2). Cultural background plays an integral role in body satisfaction in adolescent girls and is reflected in differences in body satisfaction among groups. Body image is more favorable in cultures in which girls describe more reasonable views about physical appearance, report less social pressure for thinness, and have less tendency to base self-esteem on body image. Low self-concept clarity increases vulnerability to body image issues as a result of the internalization of the thin ideal and appearance-related social comparisons (Vartanian et al., 2018). Values such as ideal body weight and shape and

attitudes toward piercing and tattoos are culturally based. American society emphasizes youth, beauty, and wholeness. Western cultures have been socialized to dread the normal aging process, whereas Eastern cultures view aging positively and respect older adults. Body image issues are often associated with impaired self-concept and self-esteem.

Role Performance. Role performance is the way in which individuals perceive their ability to carry out significant roles (e.g., parent, supervisor, partner, or close friend). Normal changes associated with maturation result in changes in role performance. For example, when a man has a child, he becomes a father. The new role of father requires many changes in behavior if the man is going to be successful. Roles that individuals follow in given situations involve socialization, expectations, or standards of behavior. The patterns are stable and change only minimally during adulthood.

Ideal societal role behaviors are often hard to achieve in real life. Individuals have multiple roles and personal needs that sometimes conflict. Successful adults learn to distinguish between ideal role expectations and realistic possibilities. To function effectively in multiple roles, a person must know the expected behavior and values, desire to conform to them, and be able to meet the role requirements. Fulfillment of role expectations leads to an enhanced sense of self. Difficulty or failure to meet role expectations leads to deficits and often contributes to decreased self-esteem or altered self-concept.

Self-Esteem. Because how one thinks about oneself (self-concept) affects how one feels about oneself (self-esteem), you need to understand both concepts. Self-esteem is an individual's overall feeling of self-worth or the emotional appraisal of self-concept. It is the most fundamental self-evaluation because it represents the overall judgment of personal worth or value. Self-esteem is positive when one feels capable, worthwhile, and competent. A person's self-esteem is related to his or her evaluation of his or her effectiveness at school, within the family, and in social settings. The evaluation of others also is likely to have a profound influence on a person's self-esteem.

Considering the relationship between a person's actual self-concept and his or her ideal self enhances understanding of that person's self-esteem. The ideal self consists of the aspirations, goals, values, and standards of behavior that a person considers ideal and strives to attain. In general, a person whose self-concept comes close to matching the ideal self has high self-esteem, whereas a person whose self-concept varies widely from the ideal self suffers from low self-esteem (Halter, 2018). Once established, basic feelings about the self tend to be constant, even though a situational crisis can temporarily affect self-esteem.

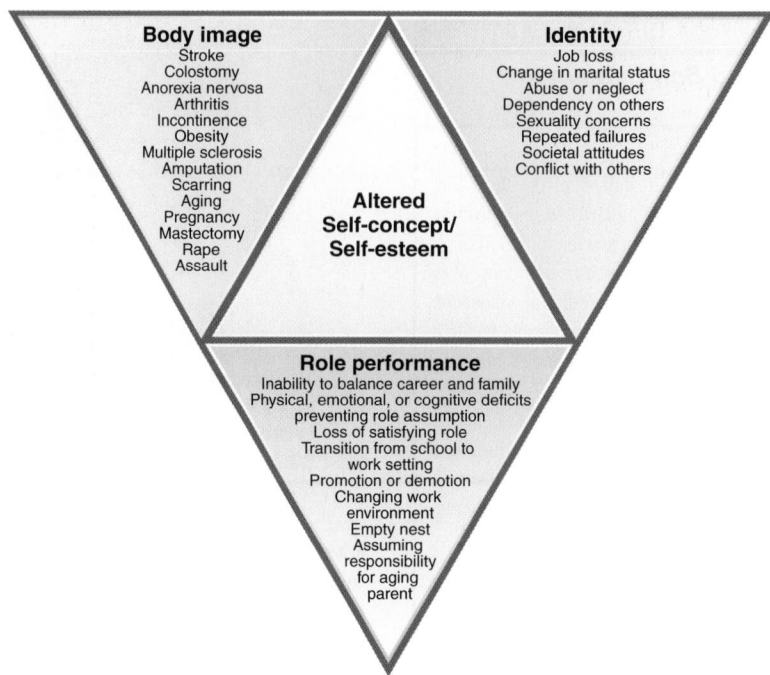

FIG. 33.3 Common stressors that influence self-concept.

Factors Influencing Self-Concept

A self-concept stressor is any real or perceived change that threatens identity, body image, or role performance (Fig. 33.3). An individual's perception of the stressor is the most important factor in determining his or her response. The ability to reestablish balance following a stressor is related to numerous factors, including the number of stressors, duration of the stressor, and health status (see Chapter 37). Stressors challenge a person's adaptive capacities. Changes that occur in physical, spiritual, emotional, sexual, familial, and sociocultural health affect self-concept. Being able to successfully adapt to stressors is likely to lead to a positive sense of self, whereas failure to adapt often leads to a negative self-concept.

Any change in health is a stressor that potentially affects self-concept. A physical change in the body sometimes leads to an altered body image, affecting identity and self-esteem (White and Taliaferro, 2016). Chronic illness often alters role performance, which changes an individual's identity and self-esteem. An essential process in the adjustment to loss is the development of a new self-concept. A loss of a partner can lead to a loss of identity and a lower self-esteem. Unlike the loss in self-esteem shown in vulnerable older adults, the resiliency demonstrated in some older adults may reflect more sophisticated cognitive strategies to manage losses (Touhy and Jett, 2018).

The stressors created as a result of a crisis also affect a person's health. If the resulting identity confusion, disturbed body image, low self-esteem, or role conflict is not relieved, illness can result. For example, the diagnosis of cancer places additional demands on a person's established living pattern. It changes his or her appraisal of and satisfaction with the current level of physical, emotional, and social functioning (see Chapter 37). Assess self-esteem, effectiveness of coping strategies, and social support in all patients. During self-concept crises, supportive and educational resources are valuable in helping a person learn new ways of coping with and responding to the stressful event or situation to maintain or enhance self-concept.

Identity Stressors. Stressors affect an individual's identity throughout life, but individuals are particularly vulnerable during adolescence. Adolescents need to adjust to the physical, emotional, and mental changes of increasing maturity, which results in insecurity and anxiety. Adolescents also develop academic and psychosocial competence at this time. The use of social media affects identity development as adolescents attempt to navigate relationships and express themselves in a way others will accept and like (Eleuteri et al., 2017).

Compared with an adolescent, an adult generally has a more stable identity and thus a more firmly developed self-concept (Orth et al., 2018). Cultural and social stressors rather than personal stressors have more impact on an adult's identity. For example, an adult has to balance career and family or make choices regarding honoring religious traditions from one's family of origin. Identity confusion results when people do not maintain a clear, consistent, and continuous consciousness of personal identity. Inability to adapt to identity stressors can result in identity confusion regardless of stage of life.

Body Image Stressors. A change in the appearance, structure, or function of a body part requires an adjustment in body image. An individual's perception of the change and the relative importance placed on body image affects the significance of a loss of function or change in appearance. For example, if a woman's body image incorporates reproductive organs as the ideal, a hysterectomy needed because of a diagnosis of uterine cancer is a significant alteration and can result in a perceived loss of femininity or wholeness. Changes in the appearance of the body such as an amputation, facial disfigurement, or scars from burns are obvious stressors affecting body image. Mastectomy and colostomy are surgical procedures that alter the appearance and function of the body, yet the changes typically are not apparent to others when the individual is dressed. Although potentially undetected by others, these changes significantly impact the individual. Even some elective changes such as breast augmentation or reduction affect body image. Chronic illnesses such as heart and renal disease affect body image because the body no longer functions at an optimal level. The patient has to adjust to a decrease in activity tolerance that impacts his or her ability to perform normal activities of daily living. In addition, pregnancy, significant weight gain or loss, pharmacological management of illness, or radiation therapy changes body image. Negative body image often leads to adverse health outcomes.

The response of society to physical changes in an individual often depends on the conditions surrounding the alteration. Some social changes have allowed the public to respond more favorably to illness and altered body image. For example, the media frequently present positive stories about people adjusting in a healthy manner to serious injuries, debilitating illness, or chronic disease (e.g., surfer Bethany Hamilton with her loss of a limb, actor Michael J. Fox with Parkinson's disease, and singer and actress Selena Gomez with lupus). These stories change public awareness and the perception of what constitutes a disability, and provide positive role models for individuals undergoing self-concept stressors and their families, friends, and society as a whole. In view of the growing epidemic of obesity in Western cultures, parents and health care providers need to address weight-management issues without causing further injury to body image. Providing a social environment that focuses on health and fitness rather than a drive for thinness for girls or muscularity for boys can potentially increase adolescent satisfaction with their bodies.

Role Performance Stressors.
Throughout life a person undergoes numerous role changes. Situational transitions occur when parents, spouses, children, or close friends die or people move, marry, divorce, or change jobs. It is important to recognize that a shift along the continuum from illness to wellness is as stressful as a shift from wellness to illness. Any of these transitions may lead to role conflict, role ambiguity, role strain, or role overload.

Role conflict results when a person has to simultaneously assume two or more roles that are inconsistent, contradictory, or mutually exclusive. For example, when a middle-age woman with teenage children assumes responsibility for the care of her older parents, conflicts occur in relation to being both a parent to her children and the child of her parents. Negotiating a balance of time and energy between her children and parents creates role conflicts (see Chapter 13). The perceived importance of each conflicting role influences the degree of conflict experienced. The sick role involves the expectations of others and society regarding how an individual behaves when sick. Role conflict occurs when general societal expectations (take care of yourself, and you will get better) and the expectations of co-workers (need to get the job done regardless of illness) collide. The conflict of taking care of oneself while getting everything done is often a major challenge.

Role ambiguity involves unclear role expectations, which makes people unsure about what to do or how to do it, creating stress and confusion. Role ambiguity is common in the adolescent years. Parents, peers, and the media pressure adolescents to assume adultlike roles; yet many lack the resources to move beyond the role of a dependent child. Role ambiguity is also common in employment situations. In complex, rapidly changing, or highly specialized organizations, employees often become unsure about job expectations.

Role strain combines role conflict and role ambiguity. Some express role strain as a feeling of frustration when a person feels inadequate or unsuited to a role such as providing care for a disabled child or a family member with dementia or terminal cancer (see Chapter 14).

Role overload involves having more roles or responsibilities within a role than are manageable. This is common in an individual who unsuccessfully attempts to meet the demands of work and family while carving out some personal time. Often during periods of illness or change, those involved either as the one who is ill or as a significant other find themselves in role overload.

Self-Esteem Stressors.
Individuals with high self-esteem generally are more resilient and better able to cope with demands and stressors than those with low self-esteem. Low self-worth contributes to feeling unfulfilled and disconnected from others. Decreased self-worth potentially can result in depression and unremitting uneasiness or anxiety. Illness, surgery, or accidents that change life patterns also influence feelings of self-worth. Chronic illnesses such as diabetes, arthritis, and cardiac disease require changes in accepted and long-assumed behavioral patterns. Female children and adolescents with chronic illness are particularly vulnerable to low self-esteem. The more the chronic illness interferes with the person's ability to engage in activities contributing to feelings of worth or success, the more it affects self-esteem.

Self-esteem stressors vary with developmental stages. Perceived inability to meet parental expectations, harsh criticism, inconsistent discipline, and unresolved sibling rivalry reduce the level of self-worth of children. A developmental milestone such as pregnancy introduces unique self-esteem stressors and has significant health care implications. Self-esteem and health behaviors are intertwined (Tonsing and Ow, 2018). Self-concept guides health behaviors and organizes health-related actions. Stressors affecting the self-esteem of an adult include failure in work and unsuccessful relationships. Self-esteem stressors in older adults include health problems, declining socioeconomic status, spousal loss or bereavement, loss of social support, and decline in achievement experiences following retirement (Box 33.3).

Family Effect on Self-Concept Development

The family plays a key role in creating and maintaining the self-concepts of its members. Children develop a basic sense of who they are from their family caregivers. A child also gains accepted norms for thinking, feeling, and behaving from family members (Hockenberry et al., 2019). Sometimes well-meaning parents cultivate negative self-concepts in children. Some literature (e.g., Crocetti et al., 2016) suggests that parents are the most important influences on a child's development, yet variations in parenting approach depend on the culture. Specifically a child's positive self-esteem and school achievement are fostered by parents who respond in a firm, consistent, and warm manner. High parental support and parental monitoring are related to greater self-esteem and lower risk behaviors. Parents who are harsh, inconsistent, or have low self-esteem themselves often behave in ways that foster negative self-concepts in their children. Positive communication and social support foster self-esteem and well-being in adolescence. To reverse a patient's negative self-concept, first assess the family's style of relating (see Chapter 10). Family and cultural factors sometimes influence negative health practices such as excessive drinking (Box 33.4). Change in self-concept demands an evidence-based practice approach supported by the entire health care team.

Nurse's Effect on Patient's Self-Concept

Your acceptance of a patient with an altered self-concept can promote positive change. Often this simply involves sitting with a patient and forming a therapeutic relationship. When a patient's physical appearance has changed, it is likely that both the patient and the family look to nurses and observe their verbal and nonverbal responses and reactions to the changed appearance. You need to remain aware of your own feelings, ideas, values, expectations, and judgments. Self-awareness is critical in understanding and accepting others. Nurses derive their self-concepts and professional identity from their public image; work environment; education; and their professional, social, and cultural values. Positive self-esteem and interprofessional collaboration appear to protect nurses from burnout and emotional exhaustion, which in

---

BOX 33.3   FOCUS ON OLDER ADULTS
Enhancing Self-Esteem in Older Adults

In some older adults, self-esteem can be negatively affected due to a number of life changes. However, in other individuals aging promotes improved coping strategies that protect against the declining feelings of low self-esteem, despite the physical and emotional changes associated with aging (Touhy and Jett, 2018). High levels of self-esteem and sexual quality of life are associated with successful aging in postmenopausal women (White and Taliaferro, 2016). Nursing interventions aimed at enhancing self-concept and self-esteem in older adults are essential, particularly during illness, injury, or disability. Encouraging physical exercise can enhance the global well-being needed for successful aging and health-related quality of life (Hsu and Lu, 2018). Changing negative attitudes toward the elderly on the part of health care providers is essential to assure positive patient outcomes (Haesler et al., 2016).

Implications for Practice

- Clarify what the life changes mean and the effect on self-esteem. Discuss perceptions of health problems, declining socioeconomic status, spousal loss or bereavement, and loss of social support following retirement (Haesler et al., 2016).
- Conduct supportive conversations to understand challenges to the patient's perceptions of body image adjustments as part of aging and changes associated with illness, injury, or disability (Hsu and Lu, 2018).

- Assess for preoccupation with physical complaints. Thoroughly assess patient's complaints and, if no physical explanation exists, encourage him or her to verbalize needs (e.g., fear, insecurity, loneliness) in a nonphysical way.
- Identify positive and negative coping mechanisms. Support effective strategies (Halter, 2018).
- Provide resources to help patient learn new positive coping mechanisms, including self-care practices of nutrition, sleep, and exercise (Leão et al., 2017).
- Encourage the use of storytelling and review of old photographs.
- Modify nursing interventions with patients experiencing dementia to support self-concept; recognize that self-concept in early dementia is largely intact (Touhy and Jett, 2018).
- Communicate that the older adult is worthwhile by actively listening to and accepting the person's feelings, being respectful, and praising healthy behaviors.
- Allow additional time to complete tasks. Reinforce the older adult's efforts at independence.

BOX 33.4   EVIDENCE-BASED PRACTICE
Self-Concept and the Impact on Adolescent Drinking Behaviors and Drug Use

PICOT Question: How does self-concept influence drinking behaviors and drug use in at-risk adolescents?

Evidence Summary

Adolescents experience changes in their physical appearance, social interactions, confidence, and independence. All of these influence self-concept. A low self-concept may precede or perhaps increase the risk for adolescent drinking (Bartsch et al., 2017). Because many teens engage in behaviors that increase the potential for morbidity and mortality, helping youth develop a healthy self-concept may prevent health risk behaviors, including teen drinking and drug use (Kann et al., 2018). In 2017, the CDC reported that 29.8% of high school students endorsed current alcohol use, and 19.8% reported current marijuana use. In addition, 14.0% of students had taken prescription pain medicine without a health care provider's prescription or differently than how the prescriber told them to use it. Nationwide, 8.8% of high school students had smoked cigarettes and 13.2% had used an electronic vapor product on at least 1 day during the 30 days before the survey (Kann et al., 2018). Identifying risk and protective factors is important when creating drinking, cigarette and electronic vapor products, and drug prevention programs, as well as harm reduction programs (Eleuteri et al 2017). Enhancing opportunities

to learn skills to increase self-compassion, self-awareness, resiliency, and self-worth, as well as to improve relationships with peers and families, may reduce the risk behaviors in adolescents (Bartsch et al, 2017).

Application to Nursing Practice

- Drinking prevention efforts should include stress management and improvement in self-esteem (Bartsch et al., 2017).
- A priority nursing action is the assessment of child and adolescent coping strategies. Appropriate techniques include effective communication, conflict resolution, and stress management (Leão et al., 2017).
- Families, peers, teachers, and health care providers should instill students' cultural pride, which promotes self-concept and the use of protective factors against risk behaviors such as drinking and drug use (Benninger and Savahl, 2017).
- Family, social, and behavioral factors are important issues to address during preadolescence and adolescence (Benninger and Savahl, 2017; Halter, 2018).
- Identifying risk factors for early drug and alcohol use, including genetic predisposition, family environment, and cultural identity, needs to be a priority for health care providers.

---

turn allows nurses to deliver quality patient care (Manomenidis et al., 2017). You need to assess and clarify the following self-concept issues about yourself before caring for patients:

- Thoughts and feelings about lifestyle, health, and illness
- Awareness of how your nonverbal communication affects patients and families
- Personal values and expectations and how these affect patients
- Ability to convey a nonjudgmental attitude toward patients and families
- Preconceived attitudes toward cultural differences in self-concept and self-esteem

Some patients with a change in body appearance or function are extremely sensitive to the verbal and nonverbal responses of the health care team. A positive, matter-of-fact approach to care provides a model for the patient and family to follow. For example, when you observe a positive change in a patient's behavior, note it and allow the patient to establish its meaning. Nurses have a significant effect on patients by conveying genuine interest and acceptance. Including self-concept issues in the planning and delivery of care can influence patient outcomes positively. Building a trusting nurse-patient relationship that incorporates both the patient and family in the decision-making process enhances self-concept and self-esteem. You can individualize your approach by highlighting a patient's unique needs and incorporating alternative health care practices or methods of spiritual expression into the plan of care. It is important that health care providers understand the degree to which self-esteem and sexuality affect patient outcomes.

Your nursing care significantly affects a patient's body image. For example, the body image of a woman following a mastectomy is positively influenced by showing acceptance of the mastectomy scar. On the other hand, a nurse who has a shocked or disgusted facial expression contributes to the woman developing a negative body image. Patients closely watch the reactions of others to their wounds and scars, and it is very important to be aware of your responses toward the patient. Statements such as "This wound is healing nicely" or "This tissue looks healthy" are affirmations for the body image of the patient. Nonverbal behaviors convey the level of caring that exists for a patient and affect self-esteem. Anticipate personal reactions, acknowledge them, and focus on the patient instead of the unpleasant task or situation. Nurses who put themselves in the patient's situation incorporate measures to ease embarrassment, frustration, anger, and denial.

Preventive measures against self-concept stressors, early identification of existing stressors, and appropriate treatment minimize the intensity of self-concept stressors and the potential effects for a patient's self-esteem. Learn to design specific self-concept interventions to fit a patient's profile of risk factors. It is essential to assess a patient's perception of a problem and work collaboratively to resolve self-concept issues. Interventions designed to promote active living and healthy eating may be beneficial for preventing childhood obesity, improving self-esteem, preventing chronic diseases, and improving health outcomes in adulthood.

CRITICAL THINKING

Successful critical thinking requires a synthesis of knowledge, experience, information gathered from patients and families, critical thinking attitudes, and intellectual and professional standards. Clinical judgments require you to anticipate information, analyze the data, and make decisions regarding your patient's care. During assessment consider all elements that build toward making an appropriate nursing diagnosis.

In the case of self-concept, it is essential to integrate knowledge from nursing and other disciplines, including self-concept theory, communication principles, and a consideration of cultural and developmental factors. Previous experience in caring for patients with self-concept alterations helps to individualize care. Self-concept profoundly influences a person's response to illness. A critical thinking approach to care is essential.

REFLECT NOW

Describe a situation you encountered recently in which your own self-concept or self-esteem negatively influenced the care you provided.

❖ NURSING PROCESS

Apply the nursing process and use a critical thinking approach in your care of patients. The nursing process provides a clinical decision-making approach for you to develop and implement an individualized plan of care.

◆ Assessment

During the assessment process thoroughly assess each patient and critically analyze findings to ensure that you make patient-centered

---

BOX 33.5 Behaviors Suggestive of Altered Self-Concept

- Avoidance of eye contact
- Slumped posture
- Unkempt appearance
- Overly apologetic
- Hesitant speech
- Overly critical or angry
- Frequent or inappropriate crying
- Negative self-evaluation
- Excessively dependent
- Hesitant to express views or opinions
- Lack of interest in what is happening
- Passive attitude
- Difficulty in making decisions
- Self-harm behaviors

---

clinical decisions required for safe nursing care. In assessing self-concept and self-esteem, first focus on each component of self-concept (identity, body image, and role performance). Then determine the patient's perceptions of these factors to reveal his or her level of self-esteem. Assessment also includes identifying the patient's self-concept stressors (Fig. 33.3), the number and intensity of stressors, observing the range of behaviors suggesting an altered self-concept (Box 33.5), and identifying coping resources and patterns. Gathering comprehensive assessment data requires the critical synthesis of information from multiple sources (Fig. 33.4). In addition to direct questioning (Box 33.6), gather much of the data regarding self-concept through observation of the patient's nonverbal behavior and by paying attention to the content of the patient's conversations. Take note of the manner in which patients talk about the people in their lives because this provides clues to both stressful and supportive relationships and key roles the patient assumes. Use knowledge of developmental stages to determine which areas are likely to be important to the patient, and inquire about these aspects of the person's life. For example, ask a 70-year-old patient about his life and what has been important to him. The individual's conversation likely provides data relating to role performance, identity, self-esteem, stressors, and coping patterns.

Through the Patient's Eyes. An important factor in assessing self-concept is the person's viewpoint of his or her health condition and its influence on self-concept. Give patients the opportunity to tell their stories of how they perceive their illness or condition affecting their identity, their image of themselves, and their ability to lead a normal lifestyle. Assess their expectations of health care by asking them how interventions will make a difference. This is also an opportunity to discuss the patient's goals. For example, a nurse teaching relaxation exercises to a patient who is experiencing anxiety related to an upcoming diagnostic study asks the patient about his expectations of the relaxation exercise that they have been practicing together. The patient's response gives the nurse valuable information about his beliefs and attitudes regarding the efficacy of the interventions and the potential need to modify the nursing approach.

QSEN Building Competency in Patient-Centered Care You are caring for a patient who is recovering from a stroke. As you prepare to assess his self-esteem and self-concept, which questions might you ask him and his family to identify the factors that currently are influencing his self-esteem and self-concept?

Answers to QSEN Activities can be found on the Evolve website.

Coping Behaviors. Assessment of a patient's coping behaviors includes a review of his or her internal and external resources. Knowledge of how a patient has dealt with stressors in the past provides

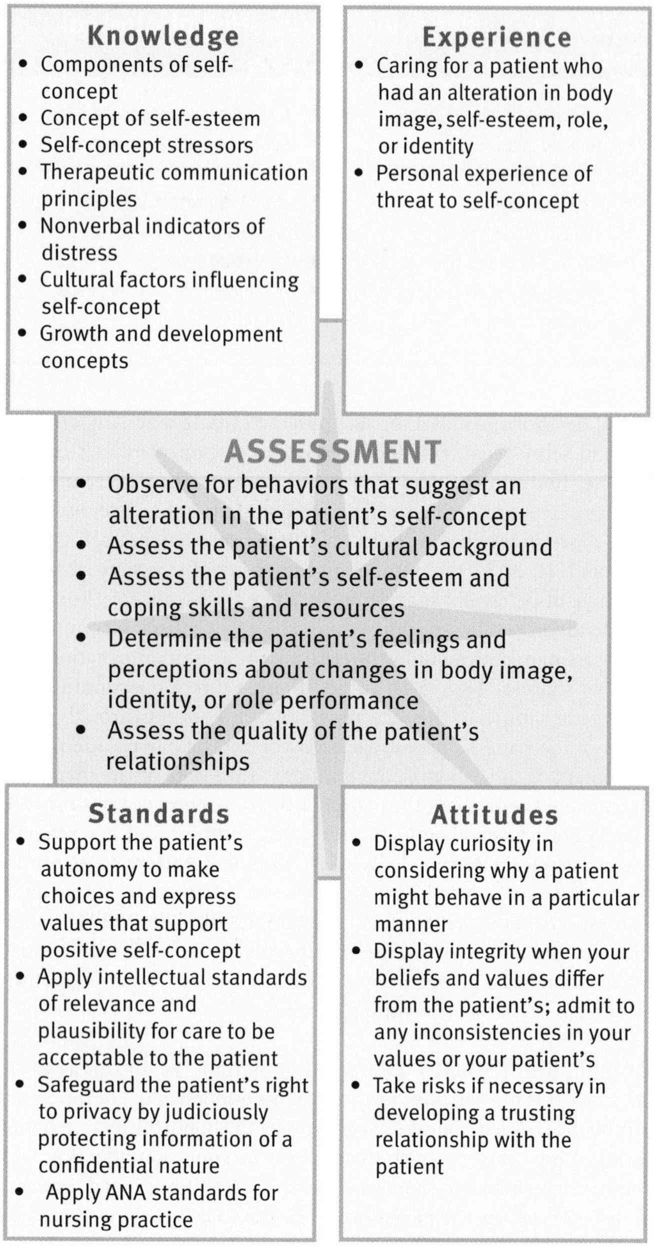

Knowledge
- Components of self-concept
- Concept of self-esteem
- Self-concept stressors
- Therapeutic communication principles
- Nonverbal indicators of distress
- Cultural factors influencing self-concept
- Growth and development concepts

Experience
- Caring for a patient who had an alteration in body image, self-esteem, role, or identity
- Personal experience of threat to self-concept

ASSESSMENT
- Observe for behaviors that suggest an alteration in the patient's self-concept
- Assess the patient's cultural background
- Assess the patient's self-esteem and coping skills and resources
- Determine the patient's feelings and perceptions about changes in body image, identity, or role performance
- Assess the quality of the patient's relationships

Standards
- Support the patient's autonomy to make choices and express values that support positive self-concept
- Apply intellectual standards of relevance and plausibility for care to be acceptable to the patient
- Safeguard the patient's right to privacy by judiciously protecting information of a confidential nature
- Apply ANA standards for nursing practice

Attitudes
- Display curiosity in considering why a patient might behave in a particular manner
- Display integrity when your beliefs and values differ from the patient's; admit to any inconsistencies in your values or your patient's
- Take risks if necessary in developing a trusting relationship with the patient

FIG. 33.4 Critical thinking model for self-concept assessment.

BOX 33.6 Nursing Assessment Questions

Nature of the Problem
- How would you describe yourself?
- Which aspects of your appearance do you like?
- Tell me about the things you do that make you feel good about yourself.
- Tell me about your primary roles. How effective are you at carrying out each of these roles?

Onset and Duration
- When did you start to think or feel differently about yourself?
- How long have you struggled with _____ (specify identity, body image, role performance, or self-esteem)?
- Can you remember a time when you felt good about yourself?

Effect on Patient
- Tell me how your (e.g., loss of a breast, loss of hand function) affects your ability to take care of yourself.
- What impact does your self-esteem have on relationships?
- How does your self-esteem affect other areas of your life, such as decision making, socializing with friends?
- Have you considered hurting yourself (specify self-mutilation, suicidal gestures)?

REFLECT NOW

Reflect on how you could have improved your self-concept assessment of a patient who was either under 18 or over 50.

◆ Nursing Diagnosis

Carefully consider the assessment data to identify a patient's actual or potential problem areas. Rely on knowledge and experience, apply appropriate professional standards, and look for clusters of assessment findings that indicate a nursing diagnosis. The following list provides examples of self-concept–related nursing diagnoses:
- *Disturbed Body Image*
- *Disturbed Personal Identity*
- *Impaired Role Performance*
- *Situational Low Self-Esteem*

Making nursing diagnoses about self-concept is complex. Often isolated data are assessment findings for more than one nursing diagnosis (Box 33.7). For example, a patient expresses feelings of uncertainty and inadequacy. These assessment data may be found in both *Anxiety* and *Situational Low Self-Esteem*. Realizing that the patient is demonstrating assessment findings of more than one nursing diagnosis guides you to gather specific data to validate and differentiate the underlying problem. To further assess the possibility of *Anxiety* as a nursing diagnosis, consider whether the person has any of the following assessment findings: Is the person experiencing increased muscle tension, shakiness, a sense of being "rattled," or restlessness? These symptoms suggest *Anxiety* as the more appropriate diagnosis. On the other hand, if he or she expresses a predominantly negative self-appraisal, including inability to handle situations or events and difficulty in making decisions, these findings suggest that *Situational Low Self-Esteem* is more appropriate. To further aid in differentiating between the two provisional diagnoses, information regarding recent events in the person's life and how he or she has viewed himself or herself in the past provide insight into the most appropriate nursing diagnosis. As you gather additional data, usually the priority nursing diagnosis becomes evident.

---

insight into his or her style of coping. Patients do not address all issues in the same way, but they often use a familiar coping pattern for newly encountered stressors. Identify previous coping strategies to determine whether these patterns have contributed to healthy functioning or created more problems. For example, the use of drugs or alcohol during times of stress often creates additional stressors (see Chapter 37).

Significant Others. Exploring resources and strengths such as availability of significant others or prior use of community resources is important in formulating a realistic and effective plan of care. Valuable information comes from conversations with family and significant others. Significant others sometimes have insights into the person's way of dealing with stressors. They also have knowledge about what is important to the person's self-concept. The way in which a significant other talks about the patient and the significant other's nonverbal behaviors provide information about which kind of support is available for the patient.

BOX 33.7 Nursing Diagnostic Process

Situational Low Self-Esteem

Assessment Activities	Assessment Findings
Ask patient to explain thoughts and feelings about self.	Patient is tearful and reports negative thoughts about self. She reports not wanting to have any visitors.
Observe patient's behavior and ask family whether she is experiencing emotional or behavioral changes.	Spouse describes withdrawal and avoidance of intimacy. He describes wife as unable to make decisions.
Determine whether patient has had issues with self-esteem in the past and her plans to improve her self-esteem.	Patient denies experiencing self-esteem issues during adulthood. She is receptive to counseling to discuss ways to return to high self-esteem.

Validate the nursing diagnosis by sharing observations with the patient and allowing him or her to verify perceptions. This approach often results in the patient providing additional data, which further clarifies the situation. For example, "I noticed that you jumped when I touched your arm. Are you feeling uneasy today?" allows the patient to verify whether he or she is in fact anxious and to describe his or her concerns.

◆ Planning

During planning synthesize knowledge, experience, critical thinking attitudes, and standards (Fig. 33.5). Critical thinking ensures that a patient's plan of care integrates information known about the individual and key critical thinking elements (see the Nursing Care Plan). Professional nursing scope and standards of practice (e.g., ANA, 2015) establish ethical and evidence-based practice guidelines for selecting effective nursing interventions.

Another method to help plan care is a concept map. An example of an illustrative concept map (Fig. 33.6) shows the relationship of a primary health problem (postoperative bilateral radical mastectomy) and four nursing diagnoses and several interventions. The concept map shows how the nursing diagnoses are interrelated. It also helps to show the interrelationships among nursing interventions. A single nursing intervention can be effective for more than one diagnosis.

Goals and Outcomes. Develop an individualized plan of care for each nursing diagnosis. Work collaboratively with the patient to set realistic expectations for care. Make sure that goals are individualized and realistic with measurable outcomes. In establishing goals consult with the patient about whether they are achievable. Consultation with significant others, mental health clinicians, and community resources results in a more comprehensive and workable plan. When you set goals, consider the data necessary to demonstrate that the patient's problem would change if the nursing diagnosis were managed. The outcome criteria should reflect these changes. For example, a patient is diagnosed with *Situational Low Self-Esteem related to a recent job layoff.* Establish a goal: "Patient's self-esteem will improve in 1 week." Examples of expected outcomes directed toward that goal include the following:

- The patient discusses a minimum of three areas of her life in which she is functioning well.
- The patient is able to voice the recognition that losing her job is not reflective of her worth as a person.
- The patient reports the ability to discuss her feelings in a support group.

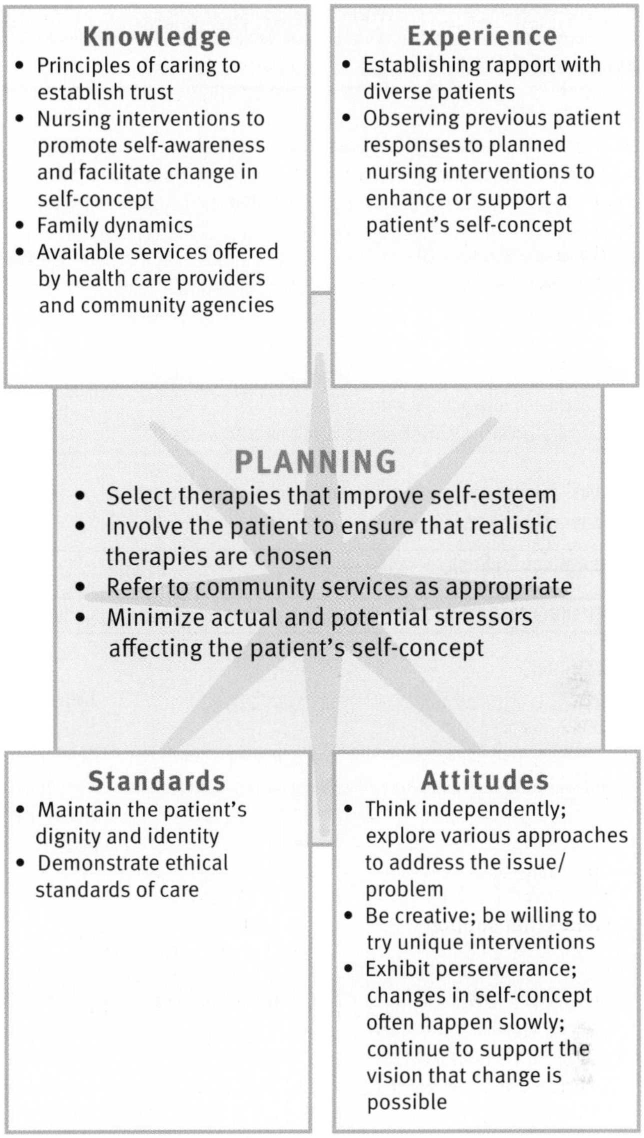

Knowledge
- Principles of caring to establish trust
- Nursing interventions to promote self-awareness and facilitate change in self-concept
- Family dynamics
- Available services offered by health care providers and community agencies

Experience
- Establishing rapport with diverse patients
- Observing previous patient responses to planned nursing interventions to enhance or support a patient's self-concept

PLANNING
- Select therapies that improve self-esteem
- Involve the patient to ensure that realistic therapies are chosen
- Refer to community services as appropriate
- Minimize actual and potential stressors affecting the patient's self-concept

Standards
- Maintain the patient's dignity and identity
- Demonstrate ethical standards of care

Attitudes
- Think independently; explore various approaches to address the issue/problem
- Be creative; be willing to try unique interventions
- Exhibit perserverance; changes in self-concept often happen slowly; continue to support the vision that change is possible

FIG. 33.5 Critical thinking model for self-concept planning.

Setting Priorities. A care plan presents the goals, expected outcomes, and interventions for a patient with an alteration in self-concept. Interventions help a patient adapt to the stressors that led to the self-concept disturbance and support and reinforce the development of coping methods. Often a patient perceives a situation as overwhelming and feels hopeless about returning to the level of previous functioning. He or she often needs time to adapt to physical changes but can work toward progressive improvement in self-concept and self-esteem.

Establishing priorities includes using therapeutic communication to address self-concept issues, which ensures that the patient's ability to address physical needs is maximized. Look for strengths in both the individual and the family, and provide resources and education to turn limitations into strengths. Patient teaching creates understanding of the normalcy of certain situations (e.g., nature of a chronic disease; change in relationships; effect of a loss). Often, once patients understand their situations, their sense of hopelessness and helplessness is lessened.

REFLECT NOW

Reflect about some self-concept priorities for an adolescent with facial trauma following a motor vehicle accident.

NURSING CARE PLAN

Disturbed Body Image

ASSESSMENT

Mrs. Johnson is recovering from a left radical mastectomy. She is in her room requesting that the curtains remain drawn at the window and lights off. She doesn't initiate any interaction with hospital staff when they enter her room. She received pain medication about 30 minutes ago, and the nurse sits with Mrs. Johnson to discuss how the impact of the mastectomy is affecting her body image and self-esteem.

Assessment Activities	*Assessment Findings[a]*
Assess identity and body image concerns (e.g., sexual role, femininity). Ask how the loss of her breast has affected her sense of self.	Mrs. Johnson **looks away, shakes her head**, and states, "**I feel like less of a woman**. My husband says I'm still attractive, but I don't believe him. I really **don't want to talk** with him."
Observe Mrs. Johnson's mood and affect and her nonverbal communication and interactions with others.	Mrs. Johnson demonstrates intermittent eye contact, frequent **crying when alone,** pulling hospital gown tightly across chest, and superficial conversations with family members.
Assess Mrs. Johnson's involvement in self-care activities.	Mrs. Johnson is unable to decide when to bathe, comb her hair, or apply typical makeup. **She avoids looking in a mirror.**
Ask Mrs. Johnson if she would like opportunities to participate in treatment activities.	**Mrs. Johnson avoids** looking at or touching her chest and **does not ask questions** about her condition. "I don't know if I want to do anything right now."

[a]**Assessment findings** are shown in bold type.

NURSING DIAGNOSIS: Disturbed body image related to negative view of self after mastectomy

PLANNING

Goals	*Expected Outcomes (NOC)[b]*
	Self-Esteem
Mrs. Johnson will demonstrate self-care practices within 2 days and will verbalize improved self-esteem within 4 days.	Mrs. Johnson meets basic grooming and hygiene needs within 2 days.
	Mrs. Johnson verbalizes improved feelings of self-acceptance and self-worth within 4 days.
	Body Image
	Mrs. Johnson demonstrates positive adjustments to changes in body appearance within 1 week.

[b]Outcome classification labels from Moorhead S, et al: *Nursing Outcomes Classification (NOC): measurement of health outcomes,* ed 6, St Louis, 2018, Elsevier.

INTERVENTIONS (NIC)[c]	**RATIONALE**
Self-Esteem Enhancement	
Use communication techniques to facilitate an environment that will increase self-esteem.	A therapeutic nurse-patient relationship promotes positive patient outcome, including the patient assuming responsibility for her own care (Halter, 2018).
Engage patient in discussion about her changed physical appearance and how she can select attractive clothing.	Self-esteem and body image are strong predictors of depression. The nurse must assess thoughts and feelings, including depression and risk for suicide, to ensure the patient's safety and make appropriate referrals (Smith, 2018).
Encourage increased responsibility for self, and help patient assume self-care practices.	Promoting self-care practices, including improved sleep, exercise, and nutrition, enhances self-esteem and overall health (Leão et al., 2017).
Body Image Enhancement	
Provide patient-centered care to support self-care practices and acceptance of alterations in physical appearance.	A threat to body image and overall self-concept often influences self-care practices and acceptance of changes in physical appearance (Halter, 2018).

[c]Intervention classification labels from Butcher HK, et al: *Nursing Interventions Classification (NIC),* ed 7, St Louis, 2018, Elsevier.

EVALUATION

Evaluation Activity	*Patient Response/Finding*	*Outcome Status*
Ask Mrs. Johnson how effective she feels in her ability to identify and express feelings verbally and nonverbally.	Mrs. Johnson reports, "I've been able to talk with my husband, even about my concerns that he won't find me attractive anymore."	Mrs. Johnson demonstrates a positive adjustment to changes in body appearance within 1 week.
Monitor changes in Mrs. Johnson's statements about herself.	Mrs. Johnson is making fewer negative comments and evaluating body image more realistically but remains dissatisfied with appearance.	Mrs. Johnson demonstrates a positive adjustment to changes in body appearance within 1 week.
Observe Mrs. Johnson's participation in self-care related to mastectomy.	Mrs. Johnson is more assertive in completing basic hygiene; uses a mirror to examine mastectomy scar.	Mrs. Johnson meets basic grooming and hygiene needs within 2 days and verbalizes improved feelings of self-acceptance and self-worth within 4 days.

CONCEPT MAP

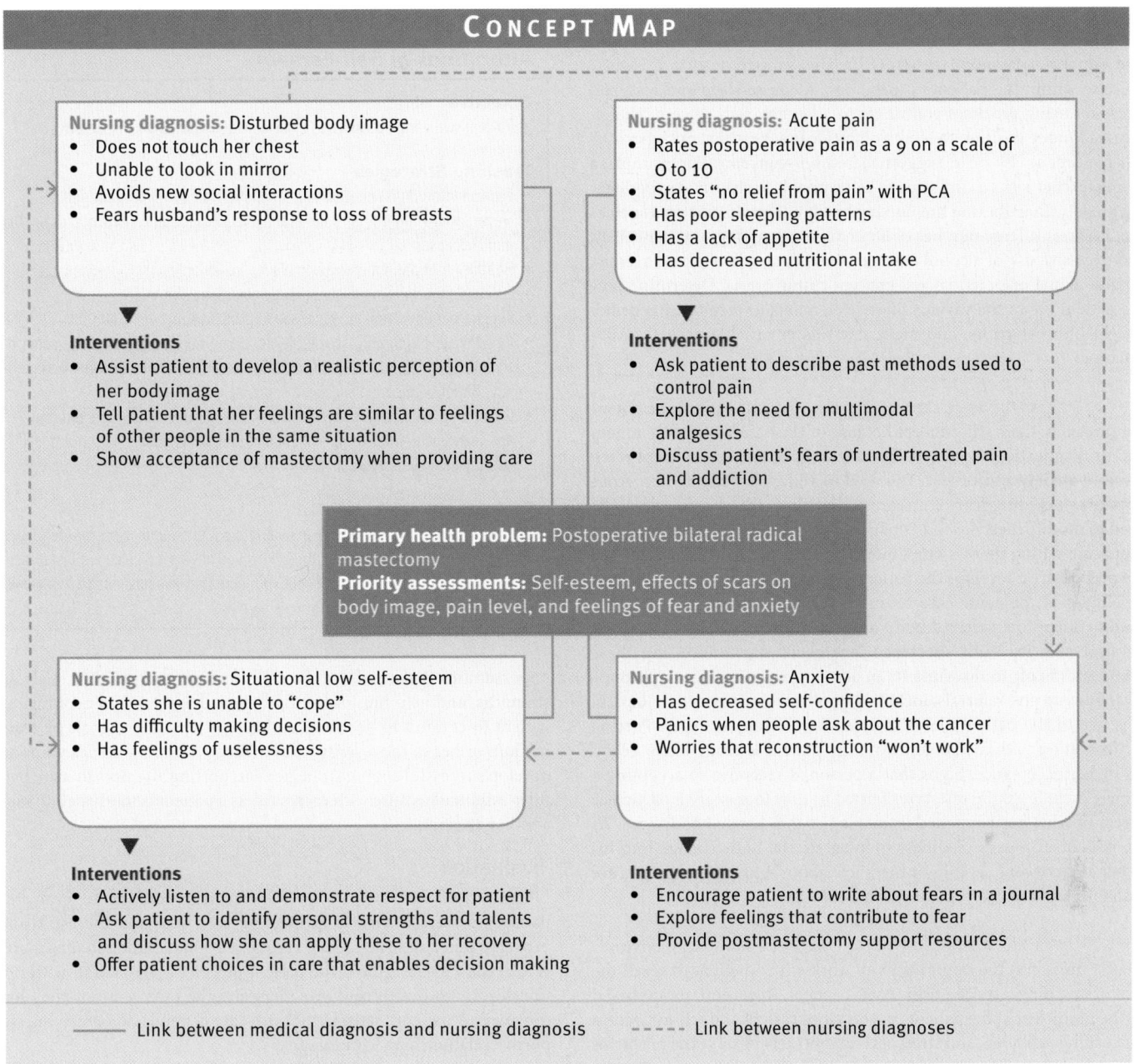

Nursing diagnosis: Disturbed body image
- Does not touch her chest
- Unable to look in mirror
- Avoids new social interactions
- Fears husband's response to loss of breasts

Interventions
- Assist patient to develop a realistic perception of her body image
- Tell patient that her feelings are similar to feelings of other people in the same situation
- Show acceptance of mastectomy when providing care

Nursing diagnosis: Acute pain
- Rates postoperative pain as a 9 on a scale of 0 to 10
- States "no relief from pain" with PCA
- Has poor sleeping patterns
- Has a lack of appetite
- Has decreased nutritional intake

Interventions
- Ask patient to describe past methods used to control pain
- Explore the need for multimodal analgesics
- Discuss patient's fears of undertreated pain and addiction

Primary health problem: Postoperative bilateral radical mastectomy
Priority assessments: Self-esteem, effects of scars on body image, pain level, and feelings of fear and anxiety

Nursing diagnosis: Situational low self-esteem
- States she is unable to "cope"
- Has difficulty making decisions
- Has feelings of uselessness

Interventions
- Actively listen to and demonstrate respect for patient
- Ask patient to identify personal strengths and talents and discuss how she can apply these to her recovery
- Offer patient choices in care that enables decision making

Nursing diagnosis: Anxiety
- Has decreased self-confidence
- Panics when people ask about the cancer
- Worries that reconstruction "won't work"

Interventions
- Encourage patient to write about fears in a journal
- Explore feelings that contribute to fear
- Provide postmastectomy support resources

———— Link between medical diagnosis and nursing diagnosis   - - - - - Link between nursing diagnoses

FIG. 33.6 Concept map for Mrs. Johnson. *PCA*, Patient-controlled analgesia.

Teamwork and Collaboration. A patient's perceptions of significant others are important to incorporate into the plan of care. Individuals who have experienced deficits in self-concept before the current episode of treatment have often established a system of support that includes mental health clinicians, clergy, and other community resources. Before including family members, consider the patient's desires for their involvement and cultural norms regarding who most frequently makes decisions in the family. Patients who are experiencing threats to or alterations in self-concept often benefit from collaboration with mental health and community resources to promote increased awareness. Additional resources include physical therapy, occupational therapy, behavioral health, social services, and pastoral care. Knowledge of available resources allows appropriate referrals. Improving your own self-esteem and professional identity through effective interprofessional teamwork can promote resilience and prevent burnout, which in turn can promote better patient outcomes (Manomenidis et al., 2017).

◆ Implementation

As with all the steps of the nursing process, a therapeutic nurse-patient relationship is central to the implementation phase. Collaboratively you develop the goals and outcome criteria and then consider nursing interventions for promoting a healthy self-concept and helping a patient move toward his or her goals. To identify effective nursing interventions, consider each nursing diagnosis and individualize interventions that address the diagnosis. Collaborating with members of the health care team maximizes the comprehensiveness of the approach to self-concept issues. Regardless of the health care setting, it is important to work with patients and their families or significant others to promote a healthy self-concept. For example, select nursing interventions that help patients regain or restore the elements that contribute to a strong and secure sense of self. The approaches chosen vary according to the level of care required.

Health Promotion. Work with patients to help them develop healthy lifestyle behaviors that contribute to a positive self-concept. Measures that support adaptation to stress such as proper nutrition, regular exercise within the patient's capabilities, adequate sleep and rest, and stress-reducing practices contribute to a healthy self-concept. Nurses are in a unique position to identify lifestyle practices that put a person's self-concept at risk or to suggest altered self-concepts. For example, a young teacher visits a clinic due to being unable to sleep and experiencing anxiety. In gathering the nursing history, lifestyle practices such as too little rest, a large number of life changes occurring simultaneously, and excessive use of alcohol emerge. These data, when taken together, suggest actual or potential self-concept disturbances. Determine how the patient views the various lifestyle elements to facilitate his or her insight into behaviors, and make referrals or provide needed health teaching.

Acute Care. In the acute care setting some patients experience potential threats to their self-concept because of the nature of the treatment and/or diagnostic procedures. Threats to a person's self-concept often result in anxiety and/or fear. You need to address a patient's numerous stressors, including fear of unknown diagnoses (diagnostic tests), the need to modify lifestyle, and anticipated changes in functioning. In the acute care setting there is often more than one stressor, thus increasing the overall stress level for the patient and family.

Nurses in the acute care setting encounter patients who face the need to adapt to an altered body image as a result of surgery or other physical change. With shortened lengths of stay, addressing these needs is difficult to do while in an acute care setting; thus appropriate follow-up and referrals, including home care, are essential. Remain sensitive to the patient's level of acceptance of any changes. Forcing confrontation with a change before the patient is ready likely delays his or her acceptance. Signs that a person is receptive to accepting a change include asking questions related to how to manage a particular aspect of what has happened or looking at the changed body area. As the patient expresses readiness to integrate the body change into his or her self-concept, let him or her know about support groups that are available, and offer to make the initial contact.

Restorative and Continuing Care. Often in a home care environment a nurse has the opportunity to work with a patient to reach the goal of attaining a more positive self-concept. Interventions are based on the premise that the patient first develops insight and self-awareness concerning problems and stressors and then acts to solve the problems and cope with the stressors. One way to achieve this is by reframing the patient's thoughts and feelings in a more positive way. Incorporate this approach into patient teaching for alterations in self-concept, including situational low self-esteem, that sometimes are present in the home care setting (Box 33.8).

Increase a patient's self-awareness by allowing him or her to openly explore thoughts and feelings. A priority nursing intervention is the expert use of therapeutic communication skills to clarify the expectations of a patient and family. Open exploration makes the situation less threatening for a patient and encourages behaviors that expand self-awareness. Use a nonjudgmental approach when accepting a patient's thoughts and feelings, help the patient clarify interactions with others, and be empathic.

Help the patient define problems clearly and apply those coping mechanisms most suitable for the problem. Work closely with him or her to analyze adaptive and maladaptive responses, contrast alternatives, devise a plan, and discuss outcomes. Collaborate with the patient to identify alternative solutions and develop realistic goals to facilitate real change and encourage further goal-setting behaviors. Design

---

BOX 33.8 PATIENT TEACHING
Alterations in Self-Esteem

Objective
- Patient will verbalize ways to improve situational low self-esteem.

Teaching Strategies
- Provide information needed to allow patient to better care for self.
- Have patient identify strengths and weaknesses and reinforce strengths and successes.
- Reaffirm that patient is responsible for behavior.
- Discuss situations in which patient's stress may intensify.
- Explore patient's coping responses to problems.
- Incorporate psychiatric co-morbidities (e.g., depression, anxiety, somatoform disorders) and alterations to self-esteem and body image when planning patient education sessions.
- Collaboratively identify alternative solutions and encourage alternatives not previously tried (e.g., communication skills, decision-making skills, healthy coping strategies).

Evaluation
Use the principles of teach-back to evaluate patient/family caregiver learning.
- Describe the new communication skills you have tried since we last met.
- Tell me about the decisions about your care that you have made this week.
- Which coping strategies are you using now?

---

opportunities that result in success, reinforce the patient's skills and strengths, and help him or her find needed assistance. Encourage the patient to commit to decisions and actions to achieve goals by teaching him or her to move away from ineffective coping mechanisms and develop successful coping strategies. Supporting attempts that are helpful is essential because with each success a patient is motivated to make another attempt.

◆ Evaluation

Through the Patient's Eyes. Use critical thinking to evaluate a patient's perceived success in meeting each goal and the established expected outcomes (Fig. 33.7). Frequent evaluation of patient progress is necessary. Determine if the patient perceives satisfaction with relationships with health care providers and the interventions they have provided. A patient's satisfaction with care depends on perceiving supportive relationships with caregivers.

Patient Outcomes. Expected outcomes for a patient with a self-concept disturbance include displaying behaviors indicating a positive self-concept, verbalizing statements of self-acceptance, and validating acceptance of change in appearance or function. Key indicators of a patient's self-concept are nonverbal behaviors. For example, a patient who has difficulty in making eye contact demonstrates a more positive self-concept by making more frequent eye contact during conversation. Social interaction, adequate self-care, acceptance of the use of prosthetic devices, and statements indicating understanding of teaching all indicate progress. Investing in satisfying activities, exerting choices in daily life, understanding their own needs during transitions, and adapting to life circumstances are evidence of self-esteem and self-efficacy in older adults (Touhy and Jett, 2016). A positive attitude toward rehabilitation and increased movement toward independence facilitate a return to preexisting roles at work or at home. Patterns of interacting also reflect changes in self-concept. For example, a patient who has been hesitant to express personal views more readily offers opinions and ideas as self-esteem increases.

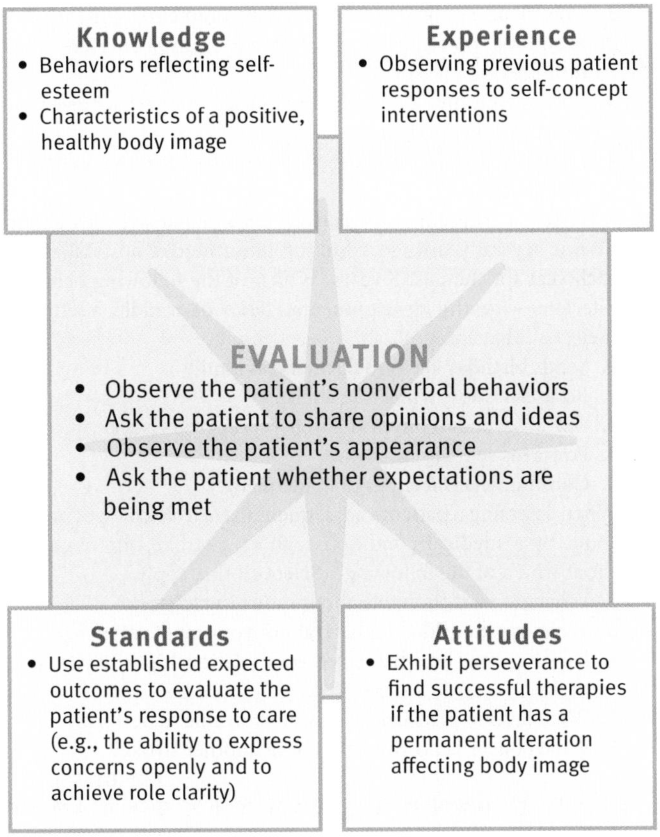

FIG. 33.7 Critical thinking model for self-concept evaluation.

The goals of care sometimes become unrealistic or inappropriate as a patient's condition changes. Revise the plan if needed, reflecting on successful experiences with other patients. Patient adaptation to major changes can take a year or longer, but the fact that this period is long does not suggest problems with adaptation. Look for signs that the patient has reduced some stressors and that some behaviors have become more adaptive. If initial outcomes regarding self-concept are not met, individualize care using the following questions:

- Tell me what you will do if you are not able to return to work (may substitute "school" or "home") as planned.
- Whom will you contact if you are not feeling any better about yourself in 2 weeks?
- What are you doing to actively improve how you view yourself and your perception of how others view you?
- How will you know that your sense of worth is improving?

Changes in self-concept take time. Although change is often slow, care of a patient with a self-concept disturbance is rewarding.

▮ KEY POINTS

- Components of self-concept including identity, body image, and role performance are affected by developmental milestones and life events.
- Self-concept and self-esteem stressors include developmental and relationship changes, illness (particularly chronic illness involving changes in what were normal activities), surgery, accidents, and the responses of other individuals to changes resulting from these events.
- Identity, body image, and role performance change with developmental milestones and the response to those events.

- The nurse influences the self-concept of patients, and the nurse's self-concept is influenced by the practice environment and is positively affected by effective teamwork.
- Planning and implementing nursing interventions for self-concept disturbance involve expanding the patient's self-awareness, encouraging self-exploration, aiding in self-evaluation, helping formulate goals in regard to adaptation, and helping patients achieve these goals.
- Be aware of how cultural variations impact a patient's self-concept and self-esteem and incorporate culturally sensitive interventions.

▮ REFLECTIVE LEARNING

- Reflect on a statement a patient, friend, or family member made about identity, body image, role performance, or self-esteem. How did you respond? How could you have improved your response?
- Describe a situation you encountered recently in which your own self-concept or self-esteem positively influenced the care you provided.
- Describe how you would individualize a self-concept assessment for a patient recovering from a below-the-knee amputation.

▮ REVIEW QUESTIONS

1. A 50-year-old woman is recovering from a bilateral mastectomy. She refuses to eat, discourages visitors, and pays little attention to her appearance. One morning the nurse enters the room to see the patient with her hair combed and makeup applied. Which of the following is the best response from the nurse?
   1. "What's the special occasion?"
   2. "You must be feeling better today."
   3. "This is the first time I've seen you look this good."
   4. "I see that you've combed your hair and put on makeup."
2. A 30-year-old patient diagnosed with major depressive disorder has a nursing diagnosis of *Situational Low Self-Esteem related to negative view of self*. Which of the following are appropriate interventions by the nurse? (Select all that apply.)
   1. Encourage reconnecting with high school friends.
   2. Role-play to increase assertiveness skills.
   3. Focus on identifying strengths and accomplishments.
   4. Provide time for journaling to explore underlying thoughts and feelings.
   5. Explore new job opportunities.
3. A patient who is depressed is crying and verbalizes feelings of low self-esteem and self-worth, such as "I'm such a failure ... I can't do anything right." What is the nurse's best response?
   1. Remain with the patient until he or she validates feeling more stable.
   2. Tell the patient that is not true and that every person has a purpose in life.
   3. Review recent behaviors or accomplishments that demonstrate skill ability.
   4. Reassure the patient that you know how he or she is feeling and that things will get better.
4. A 20-year-old patient diagnosed with an eating disorder has a nursing diagnosis of *Situational Low Self-Esteem*. Which of the following nursing interventions are appropriate to address self-esteem? (Select all that apply.)
   1. Offer independent decision-making opportunities.
   2. Review previously successful coping strategies.
   3. Provide a quiet environment with minimal stimuli.
   4. Support a dependent role throughout treatment.
   5. Increase calorie intake to promote weight stabilization.

5. The nurse can increase a patient's self-awareness and self-concept through which of the following actions? (Select all that apply.)
   1. Helping the patient define personal problems clearly
   2. Allowing the patient to openly explore thoughts and feelings
   3. Reframing the patient's thoughts and feelings in a more positive way
   4. Having family members assume more responsibility during times of stress
   5. Recommending self-help reading materials

6. Which of the following assessment findings suggest an altered self-concept? (Select all that apply.)
   1. Uneven gait
   2. Slumped posture and poor personal hygiene
   3. Avoidance of eye contact when answering a question
   4. Requests for visits from the chaplain
   5. Frequent use of the call light

7. The home health nurse is visiting a 90-year-old man who lives with his 89-year-old wife. He is legally blind and is 3 weeks' post right hip replacement. He ambulates with difficulty with a walker. He comments that he is saddened now that his wife has to do more for him and he is doing less for her. Which of the following is the priority nursing diagnosis?
   1. Impaired Self Toileting
   2. Lack of Knowledge Regarding Resources for the Visually Impaired
   3. Disturbed Body Image
   4. Risk for Situational Low Self-Esteem

8. A nurse is working with an older adult who recently moved to an assisted-living center because of declining physical capabilities associated with the normal aging process. Which nursing interventions are directed at promoting self-esteem in this patient?
   1. Commending the patient's efforts at completing self-care tasks
   2. Assuming that the patient's physical complaints are attention-seeking measures
   3. Minimizing time discussing memories and past achievements spent with the patient
   4. Limiting decision-making opportunities for the patient to reduce stress

9. A nurse is caring for a 40-year-old male diagnosed with Crohn's disease several years ago, resulting in numerous hospitalizations each year for the past 3 years. Which of the following behaviors interfere with the developmental tasks of middle adulthood? (Select all that apply.)
   1. Sends birthday cards to friends and family
   2. Refuses visitors while hospitalized
   3. Self-absorbed in physical and psychological issues
   4. Performs self-care activities
   5. Communicates feelings of inadequacy

10. When assessing a patient's adjustment to the role changes brought about by a medical condition such as a stroke, the nurse asks about which of the following? (Select all that apply.)
    1. What are your thoughts about returning to work?
    2. What questions do you have about your medications?
    3. How has your health affected your relationship with your partner?
    4. What level of physical activity are you able to perform?
    5. What concerns do you have about another stroke?

Answers: 1. 4; **2.** 3, 4; **3.** 1; **4.** 1, 2; **5.** 1, 2, 3; **6.** 2, 3; **7.** 4; **8.** 1; **9.** 2, 3, 5; **10.** 1, 3.

Rationales for Review Questions can be found on the Evolve website.

REFERENCES

American Nurses Association: *Nursing: scope and standards of practice*, ed 3, Silver Spring, MD, 2015, American Nurses Association.

Erikson E: *Childhood and society*, ed 2, New York, 1963, WW Norton.

Halter MJ: *Varcarolis' foundations of psychiatric mental health nursing: a clinical approach*, ed 8, St Louis, 2018, Elsevier.

Hockenberry M, et al.: *Wong's nursing care of infants and children*, ed 11, St Louis, 2019, Mosby.

Kann L, et al.: Youth risk behavior surveillance — United States, 2017, *MMWR Surveill Summ* 67(No. SS-8):1–114, 2018.

Touhy TA, Jett KF: *Ebersole and Hess' toward healthy aging: human needs and nursing response*, ed 9, St Louis, 2016, Elsevier.

Touhy TA, Jett KF: *Ebersole and Hess' Gerontological nursing & healthy aging*, ed 5, St Louis, 2018, Elsevier.

Rosenberg M: *Society and the adolescent self-image*, Princeton, NJ, 1965, Princeton University Press.

RESEARCH REFERENCES

Agrahari SK, Kinra A: A comparative study on self-concept of adolescent boys and girls, *Indian J Posit Psychol* 8(4):519–523, 2017.

Bartsch LA, et al.: Self-esteem and alcohol use among youths, *J Child Adolesc Subst Abuse* 26(5):414–424, 2017.

Benninger E, Savahl S: The children's Delphi: considerations for developing a programme for promoting children's self-concept and well-being, *Child Fam Soc Work* 22(2):1094–1103, 2017.

Bleidorn W, et al.: Age and gender differences in self-esteem—a cross-cultural window, *J Pers Soc Psychol* 111:396–410, 2016.

Crocetti E, et al.: Self-concept clarity in adolescents and parents: a six-wave longitudinal and multi-informant study on development and intergenerational transmission, *J Personal* 84(5):580–593, 2016.

Eleuteri S, et al.: Identity, relationships, sexuality, and risky behaviors of adolescents in the context of social media, *Sex Relation Ther* 32(3-4):354–365, 2017.

Haesler E, et al.: Sexuality, sexual health, and older people: a systematic review of research on the knowledge and attitudes of health professionals, *Nurse Educ Today* 40:57–71, 2016.

Hsu Y, Lu FJH: Older adults' physical exercise and health-related quality of life: the mediating role of physical self-concept, *Educ Gerontol* 44(4):247–254, 2018.

Kerpelman JL, et al.: Engagement in risky sexual behavior: adolescents' perceptions of self and the parent-child relationship matter, *Youth Soc* 48(1):101–125, 2016.

Leão ER, et al.: Stress, self-esteem and well-being among female health professionals: a randomized clinical trial on the impact of a self-care intervention mediated by the senses, *PLoS ONE* 12(2):e0172455, 2017.

Manomenidis G, et al.: Is self-esteem actually the protective factor in nursing burnout? *Int J Caring Sci* 10(3):1348–1359, 2017.

Orth U, et al.: Development of self-esteem from age 4 to 94 years: a meta-analysis of longitudinal studies, *Psychol Bull* 144(10):1045–1080, 2018.

Vartanian LR, et al.: Risk and resiliency factors related to body dissatisfaction and disordered eating: the identity disruption model, *Int J Eat Disord* 51:322–330, 2018.

Smith EM: Suicide risk assessment and prevention, *Nurs Manage* 49(11):22–30, 2018.

Thomaes S, et al.: Why most children think well of themselves, *Child Dev* 88(6):1873–1884, 2017.

Tonsing KN: OwR: Quality of life, self-esteem, and future expectation of adolescent and young adult cancer survivors, *Health & Social Work* 43(1):15, 2018.

White AJ, Taliaferro D: Relationship between postmenopausal women's successful aging, global self-esteem, and sexual quality of life, *Int J Hum Caring* 20(2):102–106, 2016.

Wilkins AC, Miller SA: Secure girls: class, sexuality, and self-esteem, *Sexualities* 20(7):815–834, 2017.

34

Sexuality

OBJECTIVES

- Identify personal attitudes, beliefs, and biases related to sexuality.
- Discuss a nurse's role in maintaining or enhancing a patient's sexual health.
- Describe key concepts of sexual development across the life span.
- Identify causes of sexual dysfunction.
- Assess a patient's sexuality and sexual health.

- Formulate appropriate nursing diagnoses for patients with alterations in sexuality.
- Identify patient risk factors in the area of sexual health.
- Identify and describe nursing interventions to promote sexual health.
- Evaluate patient outcomes related to sexual health needs.
- Use critical thinking skills when helping patients meet their sexual needs.

KEY TERMS

Bisexual, p. 707
Contraception, p. 710
Gay, p. 707
Gender identity, p. 707
Infertility, p. 712

Lesbian, p. 707
Sexual dysfunction, p. 708
Sexual health, p. 705
Sexual identity, p. 707
Sexual orientation, p. 707

Sexuality, p. 705
Sexually transmitted infections (STIs), p. 708
Transgender, p. 707

MEDIA RESOURCES

http://evolve.elsevier.com/Potter/fundamentals/
- Review Questions
- Concept Map Creator
- Case Study with Questions

- Audio Glossary
- Content Updates
- Answers to QSEN Activity and Review Questions

Sexuality is a broad term that refers to all aspects of being sexual, including how you identity yourself sexually and with whom you choose to be intimate. It is a part of who you are as a person and is important for overall health. Sexuality includes a person's thoughts and feelings about the body, a sense of femaleness and maleness, romantic and erotic attachments toward others, and attitudes toward sexual functioning. Our sexual health is based on our ability to form healthy relationships with others. Sex is considered a basic physiological need, and sexual intimacy throughout the life span is equally important for sexual health. Healthy sexuality enables people to develop and maintain their fullest potential.

Sexuality is important for overall health. Even though discussion of sexual topics has increased over the years, individuals of all ages lack knowledge regarding sexuality. Although patients may be hesitant to bring up their concerns, they often share their feelings when a nurse addresses sexuality in a relaxed, matter-of-fact manner. To feel comfortable addressing sexuality, nurses need therapeutic communication skills (see Chapter 24) and must be knowledgeable about all aspects of sexuality, including values and issues surrounding sexuality. Religious teachings, cultural influences on gender roles, beliefs about sexual orientation, and social and environmental climates influence the values systems for both patients and health care providers.

Expression of an individual's sexuality is influenced by interactions among biological, social, psychological, spiritual, religious, economic, political, historical, and cultural factors (World Health Organization [WHO], 2018a). In addition, values, attitudes, and beliefs as well as behaviors and relationships with others influence sexuality.

Sexuality differs from *sexual health*. According to WHO (2018a; 2018b), sexual health is a state of physical, emotional, mental, and social well-being in relation to sexuality and is not merely the absence of disease or dysfunction. Sexual health requires a positive and respectful approach to sexuality and sexual relationships, as well as the possibility of having pleasurable and safe sexual experiences that are free of coercion, discrimination, and violence. People who are sexually healthy have a positive and respectful approach to sexuality and sexual relationships.

SCIENTIFIC KNOWLEDGE BASE

A broad knowledge base allows you to have a holistic view of patients, thus promoting quality patient care that best meets the sexuality and sexual health needs of each patient and family.

A sound scientific knowledge base regarding sexuality provides you with the necessary information to help your patients achieve sexual health. A basic understanding of sexual development, sexual identity and sexual orientation, contraception, and sexually transmitted infections (STIs) is necessary.

Sexual Development

Sexuality changes as a person grows and develops. Each stage of development brings changes in sexual functioning and the role of sexuality in relationships. Sexuality is a complex process that involves many factors. It begins at birth and continues throughout life. Erikson's psychosocial theory of development (1963) helps you understand key tasks that individuals face at various stages of development. Early researchers focused on sexuality from adolescence to middle age, but we now understand that sexuality is already in progress at birth and continues throughout life, including into old age (LeVay et al., 2019).

Infancy and Early Childhood. The first several years of life are crucial in the development of sexuality and gender identity. Commonly, a child identifies with the parent or caregiver of the same sex and develops a complementary relationship with the parent or caregiver of the opposite sex. Children become aware of differences between the sexes, begin to perceive that they identify as male or female, and interpret the behaviors of others as socially consistent with the binary categories of female or male (LeVay et al., 2019).

School-Age Years. During the school years parents, educators, and peer groups serve as role models and teach children how to relate to other people. Preadolescent children often segregate by sex, which minimizes heterosexual activities and facilitates same-sex sexual behaviors. This early sexual behavior is not indicative of sexual orientation (LeVay et al., 2019). School-age children generally have questions regarding the physical and emotional aspects of sex. They need accurate information from home and school about changes in their bodies and emotions during this period and what to expect as they move into puberty. Knowledge about normal emotional and physical changes associated with sexual maturation decreases anxiety as these changes begin to happen.

Puberty/Adolescence. The emotional changes during puberty and adolescence are as dramatic as the physical ones. Pre-adolescence is often marked by increased sexual interest (LeVay et al., 2019). Adolescents function within a powerful peer group, with the almost constant anxiety of "Am I normal?" and "Will I be accepted?" (Fig. 34.1). They face many decisions and need accurate information on topics such as body changes, sexual activity, emotional responses within sexual relationships, STIs, contraception, and pregnancy. The

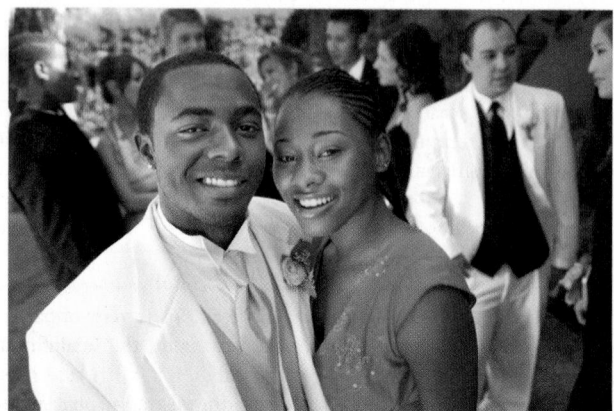

FIG. 34.1 Adolescents function within a powerful network of peers as they explore their sexual identity. (©bikeriderlondon.)

status of sexual health education varies throughout the United States and is insufficient in many areas. In most states, fewer than half of high schools teach all 19 sexual health topics recommended by the Centers for Disease Control and Prevention (CDC). In addition, sex education is not starting early enough; in no state did more than half of middle schools teach all 19 sexual health topics recommended by the CDC. Finally, sex education has been declining over time. The percentage of US schools in which students are required to receive instruction on HIV prevention also significantly decreased (CDC, 2017b).

Adolescence is often a time when individuals explore their sexual identity and primary sexual orientation (LeVay et al., 2019). Adolescents often face significant stress related to sexual identity. They benefit from education about sexuality and sexual health issues, including sexually transmitted infections such as human immunodeficiency virus (HIV) (Strong and Folse, 2015).

In the United States almost 40% of high school students report that they have had sexual intercourse at least one time, and 10% of high school students had had four or more sexual partners (Kann et al., 2018). Social media also impacts adolescent sexuality since it may be the first opportunity to explore their sexuality freely. Social media provides multiple types of sexual experiences, which could include cyberbullying, sexting, and posting of revenge porn (Eleuteri et al., 2017). Adolescents who engage in risky sexual behaviors can experience negative health outcomes such as STIs and unintended pregnancy (LeVay et al., 2019). Some of the highest STI rates are among youth aged 20 to 24, especially youth of color. The presence of another STI greatly increases the likelihood that a person exposed to HIV will become infected (CDC, 2018d).

In addition, the pattern of risk-taking behavior tends to be established and continue throughout life. Parents need to understand the importance of providing factual information, sharing their values, and promoting sound decision-making skills. Adolescents and parents often disagree about whether they talked about sexual issues, which reinforces the need for clear communication (Grossman et al., 2017). Parents and guardians need to know that, even with the best guidance and information, adolescents make their own decisions and need to be held accountable for them. Support from peers, family, school counselors, clergy, nurses, and other health professionals is important during this time.

Young Adulthood. Although young adults have matured physically, they continue to explore and mature emotionally in relationships. Intimacy and sexuality are issues for all young adults whether they are in a sexual relationship, choose to abstain from sex, remain single by choice, or are not in a committed relationship. Sexual activity is often defined as a basic need, and healthy sexual desire is channeled into forms of intimacy throughout a lifetime. At times, young adults require support and education or therapy to achieve satisfying sexual relationships.

Middle Adulthood. Changes in physical appearance in middle adulthood sometimes lead to concerns about sexual attractiveness. In addition, actual physical changes related to aging affect sexual functioning. Decreasing levels of estrogen in perimenopausal woman lead to diminished vaginal lubrication and decreased vaginal elasticity. Both of these changes often lead to dyspareunia, or the occurrence of pain during intercourse. Decreasing levels of estrogen may also result in a decreased desire for sexual activity. As men age they are likely to experience changes such as an increase in the postejaculatory refractory period and delayed ejaculation. Anticipatory guidance regarding these normal changes, using vaginal lubrication, and creating time for caressing and tenderness ease concerns regarding sexual functioning. Some aging adults also need to adjust to the impact of chronic illness, medications, aches, pains, and other health concerns about sexuality. Older adults who report being highly satisfied with their sex lives report moderate to high sexual self-esteem (Santos-Iglesias et al., 2016).

Later in the adult years some individuals have to adjust to the social and emotional changes associated with children moving away from home. This results in either a time of renewed intimacy between partners or a time when formerly intimate partners realize that they no longer care for one another or have common interests. In either case, when children leave home, intimate relationships usually change.

Older Adulthood. Sexuality in older adults is an important aspect of health that often is overlooked by health care providers. Studies show a positive correlation between sexual activity and physical health in older adults (Touhy and Jett, 2018). Research indicates that many older adults are more sexuality active than previously thought and engage in high-risk sexual encounters, resulting in a steady increase of human immunodeficiency virus (HIV) and STI rates (Box 34.1).

Factors that determine sexual activity in older adults include present health status, medications, past and present life satisfaction, and the status of marital or intimate relationships. For example, many older women are widowed or divorced and lack available sexual partners, which accounts for their decline in sexual activity. Nurses working with older adults need to assess the sexuality of their patients, sexual interest and functioning, and plan accordingly (Touhy and Jett, 2016). It is essential to maintain a nonjudgmental attitude and convey that sexual activity is normal in later years. It is important to have adequate knowledge about sexuality across the life span and to be aware of your own attitudes and beliefs while promoting sexual health in elderly patients (Atallah, 2016). Improving health care providers' sexual health knowledge and changing negative attitudes toward the sexuality of the older adult is essential to assure positive patient outcomes (Haesler et al., 2016).

BOX 34.1 FOCUS ON OLDER ADULTS

Sexuality in Older Adults

- Sexuality and continued interest in sex throughout middle and late life are usually associated with good physical health.
- Physiological changes with aging that influence sexual response are multifactorial and related to various factors, including circulation and hormones.
- Issues with the aging sexual response are often related to illnesses and side effects from medications.
- Older adults are often reluctant to discuss sexual problems with health care providers.
- Older adults who live in extended-care facilities often lose their privacy and experience a decline in physical and cognitive abilities that affects their sexual expression. People who live in assisted-living facilities have more privacy and are often able to live as couples.
- As the population ages and remains healthy, increasing numbers of older lesbian, gay, bisexual, and transgendered (LGBTQ+) people remain sexually active.
- Increased availability of treatments for male and female sexual dysfunction contributes to continued sexual activity throughout the life span.
- Older sexually active adults are at risk for contracting sexually transmitted infections. Because the risk of pregnancy is not an issue, older adults often do not recognize the need for protected sex when becoming active with new and/or multiple partners.

Touhy TA, Jett K: *Ebersole & Hess' gerontological nursing and healthy aging*, ed 5, St Louis, 2018, Elsevier.

To be effective in promoting sexual health, you need to understand the normal sexual changes that occur as people age. The excitement phase prolongs in both men and women, and it usually takes longer for them to reach orgasm. The refractory time following orgasm is also longer. Both genders experience a reduced availability of sex hormones. Men often have erections that are less firm and shorter acting. Women usually do not have difficulty maintaining sexual function unless they have a medical condition that impairs their sexual activity. Typically the infrequency of sex in older women is related to the age, health, and sexual function of their partner. Women continue to experience changes related to menopause, and those with problems related to urinary incontinence often experience embarrassment during intercourse. Couples who have physically disabling conditions often need information about which positions are more comfortable when having sexual intercourse (LeVay et al., 2019).

Sexual Identity and Sexual Orientation

Sexual identity is how a person thinks about himself or herself sexually; it includes gender identity, gender role, and sexual orientation. **Gender identity** is a person's private view of maleness and femaleness, and gender role is the feminine and masculine behavior exhibited. Assessing one's **sexual orientation**, defined as a person's sexual identity in relation to the gender to which they are attracted, and gender identity requires you to be accepting of responses that fall within the LGBTQ+ (lesbian, gay, bisexual, transgender, queer, questioning, asexual, and others) continuum (Strong and Folse, 2015).

As a person grows and develops, so does his or her sexuality. Knowledge of sexual development and changes throughout the life span is essential for you as a nurse. An adult has achieved physical maturation but is continuing to explore and define emotional maturation in relationships. Even into adulthood people continue to struggle with questions about who they are, how they want to present themselves, and what type of partners they find most attractive. As a nurse, it helps to have a clear sense of your own sexual identity because it influences your ability to form open relationships, which is needed to support patients' sexual health. You will provide care to individuals whose sexual orientation and sexual identity are heterosexual (attracted to different-sex partners), **lesbian** or **gay** (same-sex partners; women-women and men-men, respectively), **bisexual** (both male and female partners), or **transgender** (people whose gender identity or expression is different from their sex at birth), queer (an umbrella term representing all individuals who fall out of the gender and sexuality binary "norms"), questioning (exploring one's sexual orientation or identity), asexual or aromantic (does not experience sexual or romantic attraction), fluid (fluctuating mix of options), pansexual (sexual attraction to members of all gender identities/expressions), and cisgender (gender identity, gender expression, and biological sex all align), as well as uniquely defined by your patient (VandenBos, 2015). You will also care for patients who are involved in intimate relationships with several partners and for patients whose sexual relationships occur outside of marriage or a committed relationship. You may not learn a great deal about a patient's sexual preferences, even if you ask direct questions. As a caregiver, you must learn to accept a person's sexual orientation and sexual identity and help the individual understand the implications that his or her health condition has on maintaining healthy sexual relationships and on achieving positive health outcomes.

Sexuality Stressors. As a nurse, you work with patients who are making decisions or dealing with issues related to sexuality on a regular basis. For example, people of all ages face reproductive health issues, including contraception, infertility, sexual dysfunction, and sexual satisfaction. Understanding some of the decisions and issues that patients face increases your effectiveness in helping them reach their maximum level of sexual health.

Lesbian, gay, bisexual, or transgender, queer, and other (LGBTQ+) individuals have unique stressors related to their sexual identity and sexual orientation, which is the emotional, romantic, or sexual attraction to others. Peer, family, and social support is often lacking. As nurses, we must increase efforts to ensure a culturally competent and knowledgeable nursing workforce while eliminating health disparities and improving patient outcomes in vulnerable populations, including the LGBTQ+ community. Nurses are in a unique position to support a patient and provide education and resources based on his or her individual needs. Patients who are LGBTQ+ experience barriers to health care that include fear of discrimination, insensitivity, and lack of knowledge about LGBTQ+-specific health needs. This places individuals in this population at high risk for health issues such as sexually transmitted infections, depression, and victimization (Strong and Folse, 2015). Research has also shown that young gay and bisexual men who have sex with older partners are at a greater risk for HIV infection because an older partner is more likely to have had more sexual partners or other risks and is more likely to be infected with HIV (CDC, 2017a).

Health care providers should specifically state it is important to disclose sexual preferences and behaviors since many patients do not make the connection between sexuality and physical health (Fuzzell et al., 2016). Alterations in sexual health occur from a variety of situations such as illness, infertility, trauma, and abuse. Sexual dysfunction involves problems with desire, arousal, or orgasm. Erectile dysfunction is a common problem among older men. It is generally related to chronic diseases such as diabetes, kidney disease, alcohol dependence, depression, neurological disorders, vascular insufficiency, and diseases of the prostate (Touhy and Jett, 2016). In addition, side effects of medications or medical conditions also contribute to sexual dysfunction. Examples of common medications that can cause sexual dysfunction include statins, antihypertensives, antidepressants, antipsychotics, and benzodiazepines. Older adult women can also experience sexual dysfunction. For example, in a study of older women who experienced a stroke, sexuality was affected by negatively impacting self-concept and by limiting the ways in which sexuality could be expressed (Lever and Pryor, 2017). The causes of sexual dysfunction are both physiological and psychological. Sometimes the cause of a dysfunction cannot be identified or is a result of a combination of several factors.

Because sexual dysfunction sometimes results from the use of medications, it is important to include a discussion of sexual side effects in patient teaching. Your patient is more likely to adhere to a treatment plan if you discuss side effects of medications that alter sexual function with both partners and the patient is able to make an informed decision. Our current state of health greatly influences sexual response (from desire to arousal to orgasm). The availability of sexual performance–enhancing medication such as sildenafil and tadalafil has changed the lives of many couples. These medications treat erectile dysfunction but are contraindicated in men with coronary artery disease or those taking common cardiac drugs.

Changing physical appearance and concerns about physical attractiveness affect sexual functioning. Many older adults remain sexually active. Some older adults face health concerns and societal attitudes that make it difficult for them to continue sexual activity. Although declining physical abilities sometimes make sex as they knew it painful or impossible, with intervention older adults are able to experiment with and learn alternative ways of sexual expression.

Hormonally stimulated changes brought on by developmental maturation are also stressors that affect sexuality across the life span. Menarche, the onset of menstrual cycle in girls, is occurring at an earlier age in the United States, and some adolescent girls are unaware that it is normal to grow pubic, underarm, and body hair and deposit more fat on their hips and breasts, all of which also affect body image.

As boys approach puberty, physical changes include nocturnal emissions and ejaculation, increasing sexual desire, and increased hygiene needs. Patient teaching needs to include instruction on breast and testicular self-examinations and prevention of sexually transmitted infections (STIs), which are spread through oral, anal, or vaginal sexual contact. Mutually monogamous relationships, delayed sexual debut, and the consistent use of latex condoms reduce the risk of STIs as well as unplanned pregnancies (Kerpelman et al., 2016). Risky sexual behavior is reduced in adolescents with solid self-esteem; you can support an adolescent's sexual and psychological health by providing health information and reinforcing deliberate sexual decision making (Kerpelman et al., 2016).

Older women experiencing menopause, including the cessation of menstrual periods, experience changes in vaginal lubrication and sexual interest. Most menopausal women recognize the importance of maintaining an active sex life, but many report a reduced sex drive, decreased sexual interest, and mood changes that may require intervention by a health care provider (Touhy and Jett, 2018). High levels of self-esteem and sexual quality of life are associated with successful aging in postmenopausal women (White and Taliaferro, 2016).

Sexual abuse, assault, and rape are also stressors that affect self-concept and sexuality. Be alert to clues that suggest abuse (Table 34.1). In addition, observe the interaction between the patient and partner for additional clues. Controlling behaviors such as speaking for the person or refusing to leave him or her alone with a caregiver are suggestive of emotional and perhaps physical or sexual abuse. If you suspect abuse, interview the patient privately. A patient will probably not admit to problems of abuse with the abuser present. Some of the following questions are useful: "Are you in a relationship in which someone is hurting you?" or "Have you ever been forced to have sex when you didn't want to?" When you recognize or report abuse, mobilize treatment immediately for the victim and the family. The most important factor to consider is the safety of the suspected victim.

REFLECT NOW

Reflect on a statement a patient made recently about sexuality and how you could have improved your response.

NURSING KNOWLEDGE BASE

Use critical thinking skills and basic nursing knowledge when addressing patients' sexual health needs. Draw from the following areas of nursing knowledge: sociocultural dimensions of sexuality, decisional issues, and alterations in sexual health.

Factors Influencing Sexuality

Sociocultural Dimensions of Sexuality. People assign different meanings to sexuality based on their culture, gender, education, socioeconomic status, and religion. Society plays a powerful role in shaping sexual values and attitudes and in supporting specific expression of sexuality in its members.

Each cultural and social group has its own set of rules and norms that guide sexual behavior, sexual health, and the willingness to discuss this private part of life. For example, cultural norms influence how people find partners, whom they choose as partners, how they relate to one another, how often they have sex, and what they do when they have sex. Personal beliefs enable certain practices and prohibit others (Box 34.2).

Impact of Pregnancy and Menstruation on Sexuality. Sexual interest and activity of women and their partners vary during pregnancy and menstruation. Some cultures encourage sexual

TABLE 34.1   Signs and Symptoms That Indicate Possible Current Sexual Abuse or a History of Sexual Abuse

Types of Findings	Symptoms Often Found in Children	Symptoms Often Found in Adults
Injuries and/or physical signs	Bruises, bleeding, soreness, infection, or irritation of external genitalia, anus, mouth, or throat Sexually transmitted infections Recurrent urinary tract infections Unintended pregnancy Chronic pain Difficulty walking or sitting Unusual odor in genital area Penile discharge Torn, stained, or bloody underclothing	Welts, bruising, swelling, scars, burns, or lacerations on arms, legs, breasts, or abdomen Wounds that do not match the patient's "story" Multiple bruises in various stages of healing Vaginal or rectal bleeding Fractures of face, nose, ribs, or arms Trauma to labia, vagina, cervix, or anus Vomiting or abdominal tenderness
Behavior, nonverbal and/or vague somatic complaints	Physical aggression Sexual acting out Excessive masturbation Expressions of low self-esteem Poor school performance Poor peer relationships Sleep disturbances Social withdrawal and excessive daydreaming Running away from home Substance abuse or suicide attempts	Facial grimacing Absence of facial response or flat affect Anxiety Depression Panic attacks Difficulty sleeping Slow, unsteady gait

Data from Hockenberry MJ, Wilson D: *Wong's nursing care of infants and children,* ed 11, St Louis, 2019, Elsevier; Touhy TA, Jett K: *Ebersole & Hess' gerontological nursing and healthy aging,* ed 5, St Louis, 2018, Elsevier.

BOX 34.2   CULTURAL ASPECTS OF CARE

Cultural Factors and Human Immunodeficiency Virus

All sexually active individuals are at risk for HIV; however, some races and cultures have higher infection rates. Black/African American gay and bisexual men account for the largest number of HIV diagnoses, followed by Hispanic/Latino gay and bisexual men, and then white gay and bisexual men. Over time, diagnoses in white gay and bisexual men have decreased, while diagnoses in Latino and black gay and bisexual men have risen (HIV.gov, 2018). African Americans continue to experience the greatest burden of HIV compared with other races and ethnicities. In 2016, African Americans represented 12% of the US population but accounted for 44% of HIV diagnoses. Similarly, Hispanics/Latinos are also disproportionately affected by HIV as they represented about 18% of the US population but accounted for 25% of HIV diagnoses (CDC, 2018a; HIV.gov, 2018).

The most recent data from the Youth Risk Behavior Surveillance System (YRBS), which monitors health risk behaviors that contribute to the leading causes of death and disability among youth, reveal low rates of HIV testing, higher use of substances paired with sexual activity, low rates of condom use, and multiple sexual partners; such behaviors lead to an increased risk of becoming HIV positive. Specifically, only 10% of high school students have been tested for HIV; among male students who had sexual contact with other males, only 21% have ever been tested for HIV. Thirty-two percent of male students who had sexual contact with other males drank alcohol or used drugs before their most recent sexual intercourse, compared with 21% of all students who are currently sexually active. Nationally, 43% of all sexually active high school students and 49% of male students who had sexual contact with other males did not use a condom the last time they had sexual intercourse. One-third (33%) of male students who had sexual contact with other males reported sexual intercourse with 4 or more persons during their lives, compared with 12% of all students who had ever had sexual contact (CDC, 2017a).

Older adults also are a high risk population. People aged 50 and older accounted for 17% of the 39,782 new HIV diagnoses in 2016 in the United States. Among people aged 50 and older, blacks/African Americans accounted for 42% of all new HIV diagnoses. Whites accounted for 37%, Hispanics/Latinos accounted for 18%, and other races/ethnicities accounted for 4%. Among people aged 50 and older, half of new HIV diagnoses were among gay and bisexual men, 15% were among heterosexual men, 24% were among heterosexual women, and 12% were among people who inject drugs. One-third of people aged 50 and older already had late-stage infection (AIDS) when they received an HIV diagnosis, which has implications for inadvertent transmission (CDC, 2018b).

Health care providers need to consider cultural values and their influence on sexual practices when working with the diverse populations. It is important for nurses to develop and implement HIV prevention programs in the communities most affected by HIV. The CDC has committed to funding from 2017 to 2022 for community-based organizations to provide HIV testing to young gay and bisexual men and transgender youth of color, with the goals of identifying previously undiagnosed HIV infections and linking those who have HIV to care and prevention services. CDC grants have also been targeted to deliver effective prevention and evidence-based interventions for antiretroviral therapy adherence for older Americans (Kann et al., 2018).

Implications for Patient-Centered Care

- Establish a therapeutic relationship with a patient/family before discussing sexual health (Halter, 2018).
- Provide both males and females written and verbal information in English and other languages regarding contraception, sexually transmitted infections (STIs), and HIV testing and management options (CDC, 2018a).
- Target adolescents by expanding education on STIs, HIV, and contraception in middle- and high-school curricula (CDC, 2017b).
- Increase HIV testing at community clinics and offer combined laboratory work for STIs and HIV to promote acceptance (CDC, 2018c).
- Promote cultural-specific and bilingual multimedia and community education about HIV risk-reduction strategies (CDC, 2018a).

intercourse or male-female contact during menstruation and pregnancy, but others strictly forbid it. For example, in the Hindu culture a woman avoids worship, cooking, and other members of the family during menstruation. Research has found no physiological contraindication to intercourse during menstruation or during most pregnancies. Female sexual interest tends to fluctuate during pregnancy, with increased interest during the second trimester and often decreased interest during the first and third trimesters. There is often a decrease in libido during the first trimester because of nausea, fatigue, and breast tenderness. During the second trimester blood flow to the pelvic area increases to supply the placenta, resulting in increased sexual enjoyment and libido. During the third trimester the increased abdominal size often makes finding a comfortable position difficult (LeVay et al., 2019).

Discussing Sexual Issues

Sexuality is a significant part of each person's being, yet sexual assessment and interventions are not always included in health care. The area of sexuality is often emotionally charged for nurses and patients. Sometimes nurses avoid discussing sexual issues with patients because they lack information or have different values than their patients. Nurses who have difficulty discussing topics related to sexuality need to explore their discomfort and develop a plan to address it. If you are uncomfortable with topics related to sexuality, the patient is unlikely to share sexual concerns with you. You need to be aware of your personal beliefs before discussing sexuality with your patients.

Decisional Issues

Individuals make many decisions about their sexuality. Some nurses help patients make decisions about contraception and abortion.

Promoting or Preserving Sexual Health

Contraception. Decisions patients make regarding contraception, or the prevention of pregnancy, have far-reaching effects on their lives. Pregnancy, whether planned or unplanned, significantly affects the life of the mother and father and often their support network. Effects are physical, interpersonal, social, financial, and societal. The choice to use contraception is multifaceted and not completely understood. Factors that affect the effectiveness of contraception include the type of method used, the couple's understanding of the method, the consistency of use, and adherence to the requirements of the chosen method. Choice of contraception method varies in relation to the age, ethnicity, marital status, income, education, sexual orientation, and previous pregnancies of the woman. Mobile apps are available to help patients and health professionals monitor reproductive health (e.g., to remind you when to take oral contraceptives, to replace your transdermal patch or vaginal ring, or when your most fertile time is occurring).

Numerous contraceptive options are available to sexually active couples today. They provide varying levels of protection against unwanted pregnancies. Some methods do not require a prescription, whereas others require a prescription or some other type of intervention from a health care provider. Methods that are effective for contraception do not always reduce the risk of STIs. For example, the pill and intrauterine contraceptive device (IUD) are effective as birth control but not for protection from STIs. A latex condom should be used during each act of intercourse to reduce the risk of STIs. Effectiveness varies with each contraceptive method and the consistency of use. Unplanned pregnancies occur because contraceptives are not used, are used inconsistently, or are used improperly. As a nurse, you serve an important role in discussing options with patients. Although reasons for recent declines in teen pregnancy are not totally clear, evidence suggests these declines are due to more teens abstaining from sexual

activity and more teens who are sexually active using birth control than in previous years.

Still, the US teen pregnancy rate is substantially higher than in other Western industrialized nations, and racial/ethnic differences persist (Kann et al., 2018).

Nonprescription Contraceptive Methods. Nonprescription methods for contraception include abstinence, barrier methods, and timing of intercourse with regard to a woman's ovulation cycle. Although abstinence from sexual intercourse is 100% effective in preventing pregnancy, it is often difficult for both men and women to use consistently. Any act of unprotected intercourse potentially results in pregnancy and exposure to STIs.

Barrier methods include over-the-counter spermicidal products and condoms. Spermicidal products (e.g., creams, jellies, foams, and sponges) are put into the vagina before intercourse to create a spermicidal barrier between the uterus and ejaculated sperm. A latex condom is a thin rubber sheath that fits over the penis to prevent entrance of sperm into the vagina. A diaphragm is a barrier method to prevent pregnancy, which must be used with a spermicide with each sexual encounter. Vaginal spermicides and condoms are most effective when instructions are followed carefully; their combined use is more effective in preventing pregnancy than the use of either one alone.

Nonprescription methods of contraception based on the physiological changes of the menstrual cycle include the rhythm, basal body temperature, cervical mucus, and fertility-awareness methods. Couples who use these methods need to understand the reproductive cycle of the woman's body and the subtle signs and signals that her body gives during the cycle. To prevent pregnancy, couples should abstain from sexual intercourse during designated fertile periods.

Contraceptive Methods That Require a Health Care Provider's Intervention. Contraceptive methods that require the intervention of a health care provider include hormonal contraception, IUDs, the diaphragm, the cervical cap, and sterilization. Hormonal contraception is available in several forms: oral contraceptive pills, vaginal contraceptive rings, hormonal injections, subdermal implant, transdermal skin patches, and IUDs. Hormonal contraception alters the hormonal environment to prevent ovulation, thicken cervical mucus, and thin the lining of the uterus.

An IUD is a plastic device inserted by a health care provider into the uterus through the cervical opening. IUDs contain either copper or progesterone, and some contain a progestin hormone called levonorgestrel that is often used in birth control pills. The primary mechanism by which both types of IUDs prevent pregnancy is to stop the sperm from fertilizing an egg. The release of progesterone may also increase cervical mucus thickness and alter the lining of the uterus.

The diaphragm is a round, rubber dome that has a flexible spring around the edge. It is used with a contraceptive cream or jelly and is inserted in the vagina so that it provides a contraceptive barrier over the cervical opening. The woman needs to be refitted after a significant change in weight (10-lb gain or loss) or pregnancy. The cervical cap functions like the diaphragm; however, it covers only the cervix. It may be left in place longer, and some perceive it as more comfortable than the diaphragm.

Sterilization is the most effective contraception method other than abstinence. Female sterilization, or tubal ligation, involves cutting, tying, or otherwise ligating the fallopian tubes. In male sterilization, or vasectomy, the vas deferens, which carries the sperm away from the testicles, is cut and tied. Both a tubal ligation and a vasectomy usually are considered permanent surgical procedures, although reversal is possible and unintended pregnancies have been reported.

Abortion. Nineteen percent of all established pregnancies in the United States end in abortion; it is estimated that 1 in 3 American women will have an abortion by the age of 45. Young single women, low-income women, and minorities are disproportionately represented (LeVay et al., 2019). The most recently reported abortion rates reflect a decline, with women in their twenties accounting for the majority of abortions (Kann et al., 2018). The safety and availability of abortions in the United States improved after the 1973 Supreme Court decision *Roe v Wade*, which established the right of every woman to have an abortion. Abortions are safer and less costly when performed in the early weeks of pregnancy.

Abortion is a hotly debated issue. Women and their partners who face an unwanted pregnancy may consider it as an option. If caring for a patient contemplating abortion, provide an environment in which the patient is able to discuss the issue openly, allowing exploration of various options with an unwanted pregnancy. Discuss religious, social, and personal issues in a nonjudgmental manner with patients. Reasons for choosing an abortion vary and include terminating an unwanted pregnancy or aborting a fetus known to have birth defects. When a woman chooses abortion as a way of dealing with an unwanted pregnancy, the woman and often her partner experience a sense of loss, grief, and/or guilt.

Be aware of personal values related to abortion. As a nurse you are entitled to your personal views. You should not be forced to participate in counseling or procedures contrary to your beliefs and values. It is essential to choose specialties or places of employment where personal values are not compromised and the care of a patient in need of health care is not jeopardized.

Prevention of Sexually Transmitted Infections. Responsible sexual behavior includes knowing one's sexual partner and the partner's sexual history, being able to openly discuss drug-use history with the partner, not allowing drugs or alcohol to influence decision making and sexual practices, and using STI and contraceptive protective devices.

The incidence of STIs continues to increase. Approximately 20 million people in the United States are diagnosed with an STI each year, with the highest incidence occurring in men who have sex with men, bisexual men, and youths between the ages of 15 and 24 (CDC, 2018e). The prevalence of STIs is a major health concern for several reasons. In addition, race, poverty, access to health care, and sexual practices contribute to disparities in the STI rates. Commonly diagnosed STIs include syphilis, gonorrhea, chlamydia, trichomoniasis, and infection with the human papillomavirus (HPV) and herpes simplex virus (HSV) type II (genital warts and genital herpes, respectively).

As the name implies, STIs are transmitted from infected individuals to partners during intimate sexual contact. The site of transmission is usually genital, but sometimes it is oral-genital or anal-genital. People most likely to be infected share one key characteristic: unprotected sex with multiple partners. Gonorrhea, chlamydia, syphilis, and pelvic inflammatory disease (PID) are caused by bacteria and are usually curable with antibiotics. Patients need to take antibiotics for the full course of treatment. However, an emerging concern is that some of these bacterial infections (e.g., gonorrhea and syphilis) are now developing antibiotic-resistant strains. Infections such as HSV types I and II, HPV, and HIV are caused by viruses and cannot be cured.

A major problem in dealing with STIs is finding and treating the people who have them. Some people do not know that they are infected because symptoms are sometimes absent or go unnoticed. Common symptoms of an STI include discharge from the vagina, penis, anus, or throat; pain during sex or when urinating; and unexplained rash or lesions. Because sexual behavior often includes the whole body rather than just the genitalia, many parts of the body are potential sites for an STI. The perineum, anus, and rectum frequently are involved in sexual activity. Furthermore, any contact with another person's body fluids around the head or an open lesion on the skin, anus, or genitalia can transmit an STI (LeVay et al., 2019).

Sometimes people do not seek treatment because they are embarrassed to discuss sexual symptoms or concerns. Often they are hesitant to talk about their sexual behavior if they believe that it is not "normal." Any sexual behavior that embarrasses a patient often hinders the detection of an STI. Develop communication skills and a nonjudgmental attitude to provide effective care for those diagnosed with one. Detect valuable clues about an STI by establishing trust, talking with patients in a matter-of-fact manner, and asking questions in a caring manner. Assess attitudes toward sexuality and adjust the intervention to make it acceptable to the patient's sexual value system.

Human Immunodeficiency Virus Infection. HIV infection is a bloodborne pathogen and is present in most body fluids. It is sometimes spread through sexual contact. Transmission occurs when there is an exchange of body fluid. Primary routes of transmission include contaminated intravenous (IV) needles, anal intercourse, vaginal intercourse, oral-genital sex, and transfusion of blood and blood products.

The natural history of HIV progresses in three stages. The primary infection stage lasts for about a month after contracting the virus. During this time the person often experiences flulike symptoms. Then he or she enters the clinical latency phase; at this time there are no symptoms of infection. HIV antibodies appear in the blood about 6 weeks to 3 months after infection. If left untreated, people who are infected with HIV live about 10 years. The last stage, acquired immunodeficiency syndrome (AIDS), happens when a person begins to show symptoms of the disease. AIDS is a serious, debilitating, and eventually fatal disease. Antiretroviral therapy (ART) or highly active antiretroviral therapy (HAART) and having an experienced HIV clinician greatly increase the survival time of people who live with HIV/AIDS (CDC, 2018c).

Human Papillomavirus Infection. Human papillomavirus (HPV) is the most common sexually transmitted infection in the United States. An estimated 50% to 75% of sexually active men and women acquire HPV at some point in their lives, with 14 million new infections occurring annually. Most HPV infections are asymptomatic and self-limiting; most infected people eventually clear the virus from their bodies and become noninfectious to others in a couple of years (LeVay et al., 2019). However, certain types can cause cervical cancer in women and anogenital cancers and genital warts in both men and women. HPV is spread through direct contact with warts, semen, and other body fluids from others who have the disease. The textured warts often have a cauliflower appearance and are most common on the penis and scrotum in men and the vagina and cervix in women. While there is screening available for cervical cancer for women, there is no screening for the other cancers caused by HPV infection, such as cancers of the mouth/throat, anus/rectum, penis, vagina, or vulva (CDC, 2016).

The HPV vaccination provides safe, effective, and lasting protection against the HPV infections that most commonly cause cancer (CDC, 2016). The Gardasil 9 vaccine is recommended for males and females in early adolescence (ages 11 or 12 years old) to decrease the risk for cancers associated with HPV, including genital warts and cancers of the cervix, vagina, vulva, penis, anus, and throat (CDC, 2016). The greatest benefit occurs when individuals receive the vaccines before sexual activity or exposure to the virus. Two doses of the 9-valent HPV vaccine are recommended for preteens, and 3 doses are advised for older adolescents and young adults. Misinformation remains prevalent and impacts rates of vaccination (Box 34.3).

Barriers Associated With Consenting to the Human Papillomavirus Vaccine

PICOT Question: Does providing education about the human papillomavirus (HPV) vaccine to parents, preteens, and adolescents influence the decision to receive the HPV vaccine?

Evidence Summary

HPV is the most common sexually transmitted infection (STI) in the United States and is associated with development of anogenital cancers and genital warts in males and females (CDC, 2016). The Gardasil-9 vaccine targets 9 types of HPV, including the specific HPVs linked to cancer and warts. It is recommended for all youths ages 11 to 26 years, but vaccination rates in the United States are low. Parental acceptance of the vaccine influences vaccination status, and parents have voiced concern that the vaccine is unsafe or that it will encourage risky sexual behavior despite evidence indicating otherwise (LeVay et al., 2019). Less research has been conducted on male vaccination adherence, but barriers such as lack of knowledge concerning health risks, confusion about the need for vaccination of boys as well as girls, and provider recommendation to parents have all been shown to impact vaccination rates in males. A longitudinal study demonstrated that when administered to adolescents, the Gardasil HPV4 vaccine demonstrated ongoing clinically effective protection and sustained antibody titers over 10 years. Moreover, no new serious adverse effects occurred. Acquisition of new sexual partners among patients 16 years and older averaged 1 per year, which does not support the concern about sexual promiscuity following the vaccine (Ferris et al., 2017). Health care professionals need to consider these findings to encourage vaccine understanding and acceptance among parents and youths.

Application to Nursing Practice
- Vaccine recommendation by health care professionals can increase vaccine acceptance by the public and reduce the incidence of HPV-related cancers.
- Clinicians should recommend HPV vaccination in the same way and on the same day that they recommend other routinely recommended vaccines for preteen patients at age 11 or 12 years (CDC, 2016).
- Nurses need to discuss the benefits of the vaccine with parents and youths ages 11 to 26 years and offer catch-up vaccines as needed.
- Reduce parental concerns by sharing research that indicates that vaccine administration does not increase sexual activity or risk behaviors.
- Continue to teach safe sex practices.

Chlamydia. The bacterium *Chlamydia trachomatis* causes chlamydia. It is the most commonly reported infectious disease in the United States, affecting about 3 million Americans each year (CDC, 2018e). Chlamydia is spread by contact with fluids from the infected site. The infection can be transmitted during the birthing process and cause conjunctivitis and pneumonia in newborns. It frequently infects the cervix and, if left untreated, can cause PID, ectopic pregnancy, and infertility from damage to the female reproductive organs. Most people do not realize that they are infected with chlamydia because it causes few symptoms (CDC, 2018d). Thus, the CDC recommends annual screening for all sexually active women up to age 25. High-risk populations are people who have multiple sex partners or are infected with other STIs and men who have sex with men.

Alterations in Sexual Health

Infertility. Infertility is the inability to conceive after 1 year of unprotected intercourse. A couple who wants to conceive but is unable to has special needs. Some experience a sense of failure and think that their bodies are defective. Sometimes the desire to become pregnant grows until it permeates most waking moments. Some individuals become preoccupied with creating just the right circumstances for conception. With advances in reproductive technology, infertile couples face many choices that involve religious and ethical values and financial limitations.

Choices for the infertile couple include pursuit of adoption, medical assistance with fertilization, or adapting to the probability of remaining childless. Organizations such as RESOLVE: The National Organization of Infertility, a national support group for couples with infertility, or international adoption groups provide couples with support and offer referral sources.

Sexual Abuse. Sexual abuse is a widespread health problem. Abuse crosses all gender, socioeconomic, age, and ethnic groups. Most often it is at the hands of an intimate partner or family member. Sexual abuse has far-ranging effects on physical and psychological functioning. Sometimes it begins, continues, or even intensifies during pregnancy. Cues that raise a question of possible sexual abuse include extreme jealousy and refusal to leave a woman's presence. The overall appearance is sometimes that of a very concerned and caring husband or boyfriend, when the underlying reason for this behavior is very different.

Nurses are in an ideal position to assess occurrences of sexual violence, help patients confront these stressors, and educate individuals regarding community services. Nurses are mandated reporters and must report suspected child and elder abuse to the proper authorities. When you suspect or recognize abuse, mobilize support for the victim and the family. When abuse is suspected, remember to *not* ask the patient about any abusive behaviors in the presence of the suspected abuser. Provide privacy and obtain information in a protective environment. When there is abuse, all family members usually require therapy to promote healthy interactions and relationships.

Patients who have been raped often need to work through the crisis before feeling comfortable with intimate expressions of affection. The partner needs to know how to help and support the patient. Children who have been molested sexually need to understand that they are not at fault for the incident. The parents need to understand that their response is critical to how the child reacts and adapts.

Personal and Emotional Conflicts. Ideally sex is a natural, spontaneous act that passes easily through a number of recognizable physiological stages and ends in one or more orgasms. In reality this sequence of events is more the exception than the rule. You will care for patients who have problems with one or more of the stages of sexual activity, including the feeling of wanting sex, the physiological processes and emotions of having sex, and the feelings experienced after sex. For example, some women and men who are taking antidepressants report that their ability to reach orgasm is affected negatively.

Sexual Dysfunction. Sexual dysfunction, the absence of complete sexual functioning, is common. The incidence of sexual dysfunction in the general population is estimated to be as high as 40% in men and 60% to 80% in women (Touhy and Jett, 2018). It is more prevalent in men and women with poor emotional and physical health (Box 34.4). Sometimes the exact cause cannot be determined.

The incidence of erectile dysfunction (ED) increases with age but can occur in men under 40 (LeVay et al., 2019). Risk factors are similar to those for heart disease (e.g., diabetes mellitus, hyperlipidemia, hypertension, hypothyroidism, chronic renal failure, smoking, obesity, alcohol abuse, and lack of exercise). The etiology of ED is often multifactorial. Neurogenic problems, medications, or endocrine or psychogenic factors can cause it. An age-related decrease in testosterone often results in decreased tone of the erectile tissues.

One of the most common problems affecting women of all ages is hypoactive sexual desire. Biological, organic, or psychosocial factors can contribute to the incidence of HSDD. Chronic medical conditions

BOX 34.4 Illnesses and Medications That Affect the Sexual Health of Men and Women

Illnesses

- Diabetes mellitus
- Cancer (e.g., prostate, breast, colon, ovarian, testicular, rectal)
- Neuropathy
- Spina bifida
- Spinal cord injury
- Heart disease (e.g., unstable angina, uncontrolled hypertension)
- Chronic obstructive pulmonary disease
- Human immunodeficiency virus infection
- Substance abuse
- Depression
- Anxiety

Medications

- Antibiotics and antivirals
- Antihyperlipidemics
- Antihypertensives
- Antiglycemics
- Antiarthritics
- Antiparkinsons
- Analgesics
- Antidepressives
- Anxiolytics
- Antipsychotics
- Diuretics

Data from Touhy TA, Jett K: *Ebersole and Hess' toward healthy aging: human needs and nursing response*, ed 9, St Louis, 2016, Elsevier.

such as breast or gynecological cancers and hormonal fluctuations, pain, or depression and anxiety can contribute to a decreased interest in sexual intimacy (LeVay et al., 2019).

CRITICAL THINKING

Successful critical thinking requires synthesis of knowledge, experience, information gathered from patients, critical thinking attitudes, and intellectual and professional standards. Nurses use clinical judgment to anticipate information needs, analyze assessment data, and make appropriate decisions regarding patient care. Fig. 34.2 shows how to use elements of critical thinking and patient assessment data to develop appropriate nursing diagnoses.

In the case of sexuality, integrate knowledge from nursing and other disciplines. Have a thorough understanding of safe sex practices and the risks and behaviors associated with sexual problems to anticipate how to assess a patient and interpret findings. Use previous experiences to provide care for patients with sexual issues in a more reflective and helpful way. Patients have different customs and values from those of your own. Professional standards require respect for each patient as an individual. Critical thinking attitudes such as integrity require you to recognize when personal opinions and values conflict with those of the patient and to consider how to proceed in a way that is mutually beneficial.

REFLECT NOW

Consider a patient you have cared for who would have benefited from a discussion of sexual health concerns. What factors enhanced or interfered with your ability to discuss those concerns?

❖ NURSING PROCESS

Apply the nursing process and use a critical thinking approach in your care of patients. The nursing process provides a clinical decision-making approach to help you develop and implement an individualized

Knowledge

- Ways to phrase questions about sexuality
- Sexual development and human sexual response patterns
- Impact of self-concept on sexuality
- Sexual orientation
- Effective contraceptive methods
- STIs and associated risk factors
- Safe sex practices
- Behaviors suggestive of current or past sexual abuse
- Diseases and/or medications that affect sexual function
- Interpersonal relationship factors and sexual functioning

Experience

- Communicating with patients and developing rapport
- Working with patients and exploring sexual concerns (e.g., working in OB-GYN setting)
- Personal sexual experience and response

ASSESSMENT

- Assess the patient's developmental stage with regard to sexuality
- Perform physical assessment of urogenital area
- Determine the patient's sexual concerns
- Assess the presence of high-risk behaviors, use of safe sex practices and contraception
- Assess medical conditions and medications that might affect sexual functioning

Standards

- Apply intellectual standards of relevance and plausibility for care to be acceptable to the patient
- Safeguard the patient's right to privacy by judiciously protecting information of a confidential nature
- Demonstrate ethics of care

Attitudes

- Display curiosity; consider why a patient might behave or respond in a particular manner
- Display integrity; your beliefs and values differ from patient's; admit to any inconsistencies between your values and the patient's
- Take risks if necessary to explore both personal sexual issues and concerns and those of the patient

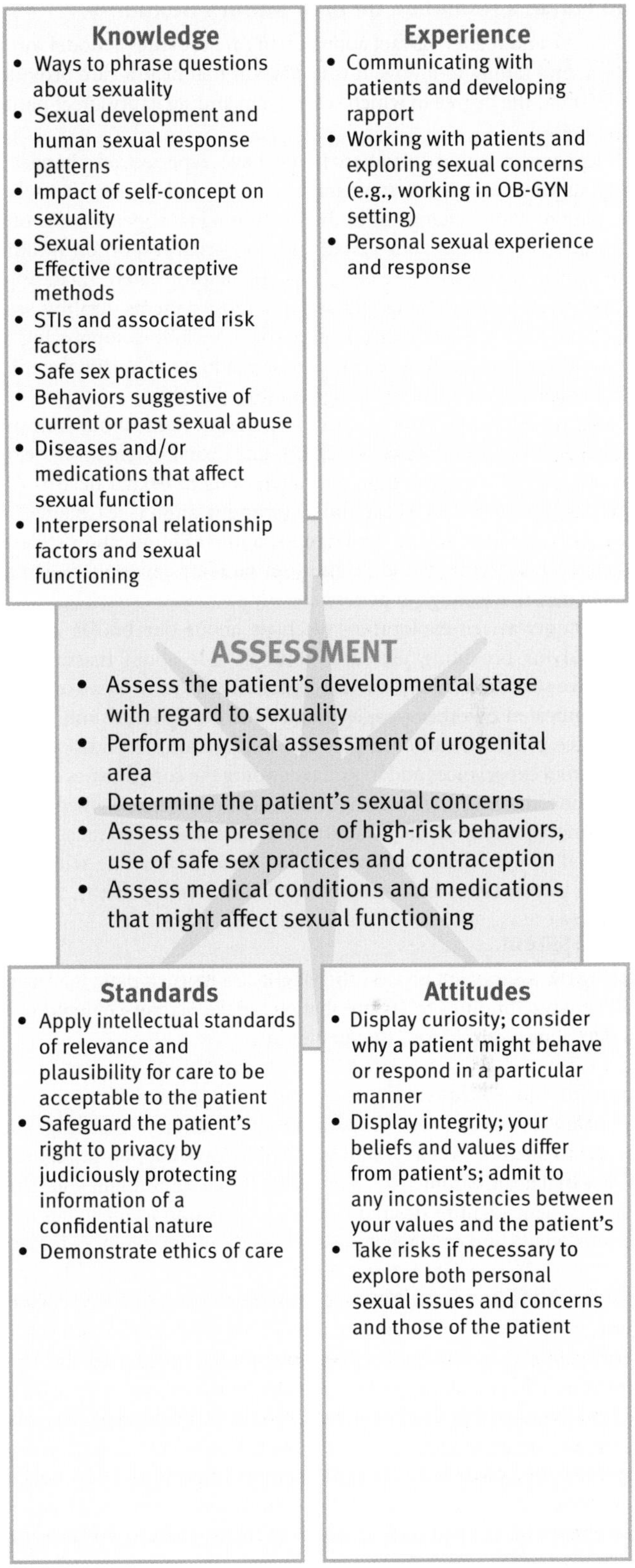

FIG. 34.2 Critical thinking model for sexuality assessment. *OB-GYN,* Obstetric-gynecological; *STI,* sexually transmitted infection.

plan of care. Assess all relevant factors, including physical, psychological, social, and cultural, to determine a patient's sexual well-being. The nursing role in addressing sexual concerns ranges from ongoing assessment to providing information, counseling, and referral. Keep in mind that nurses are not expected to have answers to all identified sexual issues and concerns.

The Nurse's Influence on the Patient's Sexuality

A positive and matter-of-fact approach to care provides a model for the patient and family to follow. It is important that health care providers understand the degree to which self-esteem and sexuality affect patient outcomes.

How you respond to patients who have experienced changes in body appearance sets the stage for how they come to see themselves. The patient with a change in body functioning or appearance is often extremely sensitive to your verbal and nonverbal responses. Building a trusting nurse-patient relationship and appropriately including a patient in decision making will support most patients' healthy sexuality. Sometimes individualized approaches, including supporting the use of alternative healing techniques or methods of spiritual expression, help a patient adapt to changes in sexual health.

When you consider the sexuality of patients, think about your own knowledge regarding sexual development, sexual orientation, sexual response, STIs, contraception, and alterations in sexual health. Also consider your knowledge base about communication (see Chapter 24). Your own sexuality, sexual experiences, and communication style are valuable when trying to understand your patient's experiences. Do not convey negative feelings to patients.

Attempts at self-exploration teach us about our bodies and the potential for providing pleasure. Your attitude about masturbation may have stemmed from personal experience or from values or beliefs communicated by other people. Games such as "doctor" and "nurse" may have provided early sex play and exploration. In addition, your own sexual experiences add to understanding the complexities of a first sexual encounter or the challenges of sexual interactions when you or an intimate partner are ill. In addition to personal experiences related to sexuality, use what you have learned through working with other patients as you assess and develop trust with current patients.

◆ Assessment

During the assessment process thoroughly assess each patient and critically analyze findings to ensure that you make patient-centered clinical decisions required for safe nursing care.

Through the Patient's Eyes. As in any patient assessment, it is important to understand a patient's expectations regarding care. Questions such as "What would you like to have happen in regard to your sexual health problems?" and "What initial steps might you take?" help a patient identify desired outcomes. It is important to set aside personal views and consider a patient's needs and preferences for care.

Factors Affecting Sexuality. In gathering a sexual history consider physical, functional, relationship, lifestyle, developmental, and self-esteem factors that influence sexual functioning. Sexual desire varies among individuals; some people want and enjoy sex every day, whereas others want sex only once a month, and still others have no sexual desire and are quite comfortable with that fact. Sexual desire becomes an issue if the person wants to satisfy it more often, if he or she believes that it is necessary to measure up to some cultural norm, or if there is a discrepancy between the sexual desires of the partners in a relationship.

Ask patients to describe factors that typically influence their sexual desire. Knowing a patient's medical history and probing for information is helpful. For example, minor illness, medications, and fatigue often decrease sexual desire. Lifestyle factors such as the use or abuse of alcohol, lack of sleep, lack of time, or the demands of caring for a new baby are other influencing factors. For example, working parents sometimes feel so overburdened that they perceive sexual advances from a partner as an additional demand on them. Confirm factors that potentially affect sexual desire and determine with the patient the extent to which sexual function is impaired.

BOX 34.5 **PLISSIT Assessment of Sexuality**

Permission to discuss sexuality issues
Limited Information related to sexual health problems being experienced
Specific **S**uggestions—only when the nurse is clear about the problem
Intensive **T**herapy—referral to professional with advanced training if necessary

Modified from Annon JS: The PLISSIT model: a proposed conceptual scheme for the behavioral treatment of sexual problems, *J Sex Educ Ther* 2(2):1, 1976.

BOX 34.6 **Nursing Assessment Questions**

- Are you sexually active?
- With whom do you have sex: men, women, or both?
- How many sexual partners do you have (or have you ever had)?
- How do you feel about the sexual aspects of your life?
- Have you noticed any changes in the way you feel about yourself?
- How has your illness, medication, or surgery affected your sex life?
- It is not unusual for people with your condition to be experiencing some sexual changes. Have you noticed any changes, or do you have any concerns?
- Are you in a relationship in which someone is hurting you?
- Has anyone ever forced you to have sex against your will?
- Tell me what you know about safe sex practices, use of contraceptives, or prevention of sexually transmitted infections.
- Tell me the safe sex practices that you follow.

Self-concept issues (see Chapter 33), including identity, body image, role performance, and self-esteem, affect a patient's sexuality. Consider how these factors relate to a patient's condition. For example, poor body image associated with chronic disease magnifies feelings of rejection. This often results in diminished or absent sexual desire.

Issues in a relationship often affect sexual desire. After the initial glow of a new relationship has faded, some couples find that they have major differences in their values or lifestyles. Ask couples to describe how close they feel to each other and how often they interact on an intimate level. Assess communication patterns between sexual partners to determine sexual satisfaction within a relationship.

Sexual Health History. Most patients want to know how medications, treatments, and surgical procedures influence their sexual relationship even though they often do not ask questions. With experience nurses recognize that most patients welcome the opportunity to talk about their sexuality, especially when they are experiencing difficulties. The classic PLISSIT model (Annon, 1976) provides an approach that nurses can use to assess sexuality in patients (Box 34.5).

Incorporate assessment questions related to sexuality in the nursing history (Box 34.6). Using an opening statement puts a patient at ease when introducing these questions (e.g., "Sex is an important part of life, and a person's health status often affects sexuality. Many people have questions and concerns about their sexual health. What questions or concerns do you have now?"). Use knowledge of developmental stages to determine which areas are likely to be important for your patient. For example, when gathering a sexual history from an older adult, it is important to keep in mind that some have difficulty in discussing intimate details with health care providers.

Nurses who conduct sexual assessments of children and adolescents face special challenges. Use language that is accurate and that the child or adolescent understands. Also promote normal development, avoid minimizing problems, and screen for sexual concerns while making the child or adolescent feel at ease. The sexual counseling of minors raises ethical and legal issues regarding a patient's rights to health care and education on the one hand and a parent's or guardian's right to supervise information on the other. Children and adolescents frequently respond when they know that having questions related to sexuality is normal. Being open, positive, and interested when introducing sexual questions is helpful.

In light of the prevalence of intimate partner violence, questions relating to abusive relationships are important. Address these questions in private. Recognizing both subjective and objective signs and symptoms of abuse in children and adults helps to identify this too-common problem (see Table 34.1).

Some individuals are too embarrassed or do not know how to ask sexual questions directly. Look for clues that a person has questions. For example, a patient expresses concern about how his or her partner will respond now or makes a sexual comment or joke. Observing for and listening to concerns about sexuality take practice. With experience you develop skill in clarifying and paraphrasing to help individuals express sexual concerns. By including sexuality in the nursing history, you acknowledge that it is an important component of health and create an opportunity for a person to discuss sexual concerns.

Sexual Dysfunction. Many illnesses, injuries, medications, and aging changes have a negative effect on sexual health, which results in either temporary or permanent sexual dysfunction. Apply knowledge about conditions and medications that frequently cause sexual dysfunction while assessing a patient's risks (see Box 34.4). Being aware of the possible effects of physical problems, altered self-concept, medications, and the factors addressed thus far on sexual functioning helps you conduct a thorough assessment. Some patients bring up the topic of sexual dysfunction. Other times issues become evident as the patient answers other nursing history questions.

Physical Assessment. The physical examination is important in evaluating the cause of sexual concerns or problems and usually provides the best opportunity to teach an individual about sexuality. In examining a woman's breasts and the external and internal genitalia, a nurse has the opportunity to assess the woman's reaction, answer questions, and provide information about the examination of anatomical and physiological structures. For example, a nurse teaches a woman how to perform breast self-examination during physical assessment. During physical assessment of the genitalia, he or she teaches men how to perform testicular self-examination (see Chapter 30). Knowledge of normal scrotal anatomical structures helps men detect signs of testicular cancer. Instruct both men and women on signs and symptoms of STIs during the examination when patients' histories suggest risks for them.

> ### REFLECT NOW
> Reflect on a statement one of your patients made about sexuality and how you could have improved your response.

◆ Nursing Diagnosis

After completing an assessment, you apply critical thinking to the diagnostic process and select diagnoses applicable to the patient's needs. Assessment findings related to sexuality often include history of surgery of reproductive organs, changes in appearance or body image, a history of or current physical or sexual abuse, chronic illness, or developmental milestones such as puberty or menopause. To make a nursing diagnosis related to sexual dysfunction, consider anatomical, physiological, sociocultural, ethical, and situational issues thoroughly. Possible nursing diagnoses related to sexual functioning are listed here:

BOX 34.7 Nursing Diagnostic Process

Impaired Sexual Functioning

Assessment Activities	Assessment Findings
Review medical and medication history	History of hypertension
	History of uncomplicated myocardial infarction (MI)
	Takes propranolol
Have patient describe sexual problems	Less interested in having intercourse with wife since taking propranolol
	Rarely has sexual intercourse with wife
	Sometimes has trouble having an erection
Patient's fears and concerns	Fearful will have chest pain or another MI while having intercourse

- *Problematic Sexual Behavior*
- *Difficulty Coping*
- *Lack of Knowledge of Contraception*
- *Impaired Sexual Functioning*
- *Risk for Impaired Reproductive Function*

Clarify assessment findings and ensure that the patient perceives a problem or difficulty with sexuality (Box 34.7). Determining the etiological or contributing factors helps you plan effectively and select the appropriate nursing interventions. For example, nursing interventions appropriate for the nursing diagnosis of *Impaired Sexual Functioning* will differ for different etiological factors. *Impaired Sexual Functioning related to misinformation about the risk of sexually transmitted infections* requires counseling and education on how to maintain safe sexual practices. In contrast, patients who experience *Impaired Sexual Functioning related to physical abuse* need counseling and referral to community resources (e.g., crisis services and physical abuse support group).

◆ Planning

Goals and Outcomes. Synthesize information from multiple resources to develop an individualized plan of care (Fig. 34.3). Critical thinking ensures that a patient's plan of care integrates all that a nurse knows about an individual's sexuality. Professional standards are especially important to consider when developing a plan of care. Maintain a patient's dignity and identity at all times. For example, to convey respect for the patient's gender identity preferences, ask the patient about preferred pronouns, and use the patient's preferred pronouns in all interactions.

Develop an individualized plan of care for each nursing diagnosis (see the Nursing Care Plan). Set realistic goals and measurable outcomes with the patient. For example, a patient who has dyspareunia has a nursing diagnosis of *Impaired Sexual Functioning related to decreased sexual desire*. You and your patient develop a goal to report decreased anxiety and greater satisfaction with sexual activity within 1 month. Expected outcomes include that the patient does the following:

- Discusses stressors that contribute to sexual dysfunction with partner within 2 weeks
- Identifies alternative, satisfying, and acceptable sexual practices for self and partner within 4 weeks

A concept map is another method that is useful in organizing patient care (Fig. 34.4). The concept map shows the relationship of a medical diagnosis (decreased libido and depression) to the four nursing diagnoses identified from the patient assessment data. It also shows the links and relationship to the nursing diagnosis and interventions appropriate for each diagnosis. For example, *Difficulty Coping* affects and contributes to *Withdrawn Behavior*, and as long as the patient has difficulty coping, the withdrawn behavior continues or perhaps worsens.

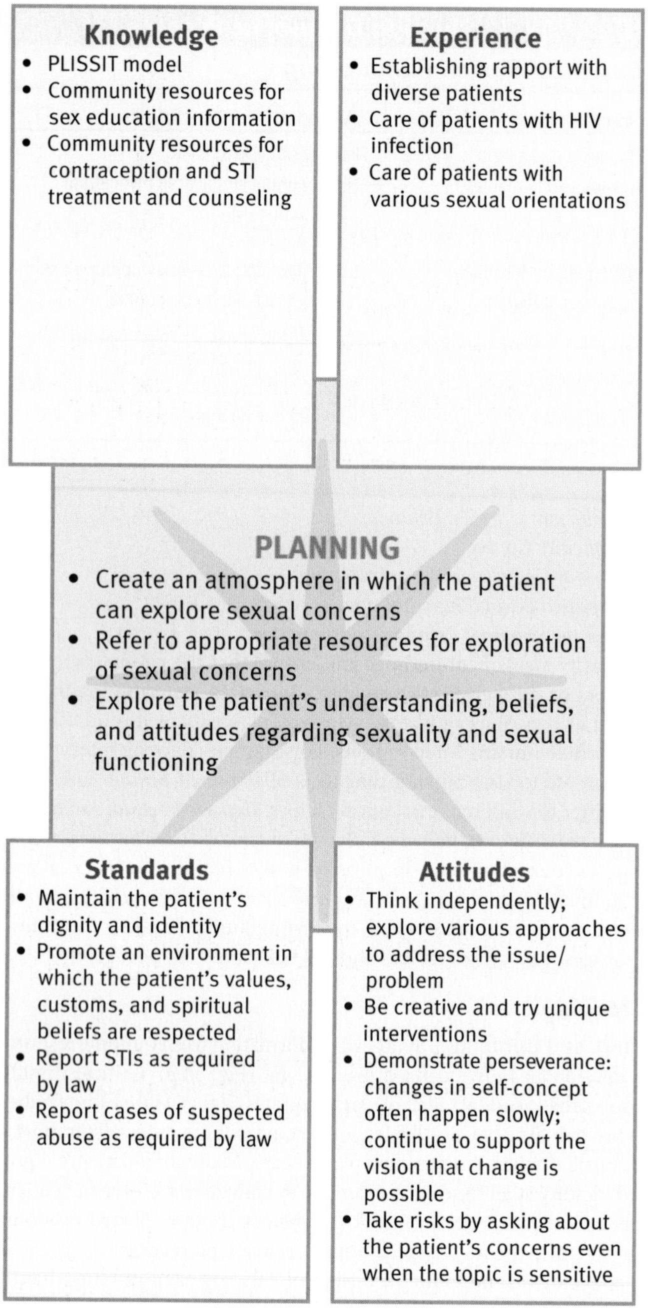

FIG. 34.3 Critical thinking model for sexuality planning. *HIV,* Human immunodeficiency virus; *STI,* sexually transmitted infection.

Setting Priorities. The care plan shows the goals, expected outcomes, and interventions for a patient experiencing impaired sexual functioning. Nursing interventions for patients with sexual concerns focus on supporting a patient's need for intimacy and sexual activity. Patients often feel overwhelmed and hopeless about returning to the level of previous sexual functioning and usually need time to adapt to physical and psychosocial changes that affect their sexuality and sexual health.

The priority in addressing needs related to sexuality includes establishing a therapeutic relationship so that the patient feels comfortable in discussing issues related to sexuality. Look for strengths in both the patient and the family while providing education and access to resources to turn limitations into strengths. Patient teaching communicates the normalcy of feelings following certain situations (e.g., the diagnosis of a chronic illness or the loss of a body part). In collaboration with the patient, you determine a patient's needs and plan accordingly.

A patient's current problems and needs help you determine the priorities related to his or her sexual health. Priorities for sexual health often include resuming sexual activities. For example, if a patient is recovering from a mastectomy and is having problems resuming an intimate relationship with her spouse because of problems related to body image, you help her adapt to and cope with the changes in her body image associated with the mastectomy. Once the patient's issues related to body image are resolved, she is able to restore intimacy with her spouse and address her sexual health needs.

> **QSEN** **Building Competency in Teamwork and Collaboration** Mr. Clements asks what lifestyle changes he will need to make after discharge from the hospital. You know that patients with cardiovascular problems often require an interprofessional approach to achieve optimal recovery, and you arrange for consultation with different health professionals. You inform Mr. Clements that he will work with a team of experts, including cardiologists, physical therapists, dietitians, and counselors. Assure him that you will share your assessment data and plan of care with the team and will recommend nurses who can remain involved in his outpatient care. Discuss how each of these professionals will contribute to Mr. Clements' care during and after hospitalization.
>
> *Answers to QSEN Activities can be found on the Evolve website.*

Teamwork and Collaboration. You often collaborate with other health care providers and make referrals to community resources when planning care for a patient's sexuality (Box 34.8). Nurses generally raise awareness of sexual issues, clarify concerns, and/or provide information. Nurses who have specialized education in sexual functioning and counseling provide more intensive sex therapy. It is necessary to understand the limits of your knowledge base and to include other health care providers, such as sex therapists, clinical psychologists, and social workers as appropriate, to meet patients' needs for sexual health. For example, conflicts in marriage usually require intensive treatment with a mental health professional or certified sex therapist. For the woman who is currently in an abusive relationship, the nurse collaborates with special women's shelters that provide counseling and serve as a safe place for her while further plans are made.

◆ **Implementation**

Promote sexual health as a component of overall health and wellness by identifying patients at increased risk, providing appropriate information, helping individuals gain insight into their problems, and exploring methods to deal with them effectively.

Health Promotion. Helping patients maintain or gain sexual health involves consideration of factors that influence sexual satisfaction. Educate patients about sexual health, including measures for contraception, safe sex practices, and prevention of STIs. Regular breast self-examinations, mammograms, and Papanicolaou (Pap) smears are important sexual health measures for women; testicular self-examinations are important for men. Offer the 9-valent HPV vaccine to males and females who are between 11 and 26 years of age (CDC, 2016). The vaccine is safe for girls as young as 9 years old and is recommended for females ages 11 to 26 if they have not already completed the three required injections. Booster doses currently are not recommended. The vaccine is most effective if administered before sexual activity or exposure.

Exploring an individual's values, discussing levels of satisfaction, and providing sex education require therapeutic communication skills. Structure the environment and timing to provide privacy, comfort, and uninterrupted time. For example, when discussing methods of contraception with a woman, provide education in a private area with the patient fully dressed rather than in the examination room when the patient is only partially clothed.

◎ **NURSING CARE PLAN**

Impaired Sexual Functioning

ASSESSMENT

Mr. Clements is 65 years old and had a myocardial infarction (MI) 3 days ago. He has hypertension, which is being treated with propranolol. Mr. Clements is married and lives with his wife. You know that patients who have had MIs and are taking antihypertensive medications are at risk for experiencing sexual problems. Mrs. Clements expresses a desire to continue having a sexual relationship with her husband.

Assessment Activities	Assessment Findings[a]
Ask Mr. Clements whether his interest in sex has changed since he started to take propranolol.	He responds that he has been **less interested in having sexual intercourse with his wife** since he started to take propranolol.
Ask Mr. Clements whether he has had difficulties with an erection.	He states that since he started to take propranolol, he **sometimes has trouble having an erection.**
Ask Mr. Clements what concerns or fears he has about resuming his sexual relationship with his wife now that he has had an MI.	He states that **he is afraid that after discharge he will have chest pain or another heart attack if he has sexual intercourse** with his wife.

[a]Assessment Findings are shown in bold type.

NURSING DIAGNOSIS: Impaired sexual functioning related to altered body function (side effects of propranolol) and lack of knowledge

PLANNING

Goal	Expected Outcomes (NOC)[b]
Sexual Functioning	
Patient will express satisfaction with sexual relationship with wife within 1 month.	Patient expresses renewed sexual interest within 2 weeks.
	Patient sustains arousal through orgasm within 3 weeks.

[b]Outcome classification labels from Moorhead S, et al: *Nursing Outcomes Classification (NOC): measurement of health outcomes,* ed 6, St Louis, 2018, Elsevier.

INTERVENTIONS (NIC)[c]	RATIONALE
Sexual Counseling	
Establish trust and respect with Mr. Clements. Offer privacy during conversations.	Establishing trust and offering privacy express sense of caring, increasing likelihood of patient's ability to express concerns (Halter, 2018).
Discuss possible effects of MI and propranolol on sexual functioning and resumption of sexual activity.	Discussion enhances understanding about reasons for sexual difficulties and provides safe guidelines for resumption of sexual intercourse following MI.
Include Mrs. Clements in discussions about sexual issues as frequently as possible and when appropriate.	Including partner in the plan of care can enhance personal and intimate relationships and improve health outcomes.
Anxiety Reduction	
Encourage Mr. Clements to express fears about resuming sexual activity, and assure him that others who have had MIs experience similar fears.	Sexual dysfunction sometimes occurs after an MI because of anxiety and/or from side effects of medications. Knowing that feelings and fears are normal helps decrease anxiety and encourages return of sexual activity.

[c]Intervention classification labels from Butcher HK, et al: *Nursing Interventions Classification (NIC),* ed 7, St Louis, 2018, Elsevier.

EVALUATION

Evaluation Activity	Patient Response/Finding	Outcome Status
Ask Mr. Clements whether he and his wife are satisfied with their sexual relationship during return office visit.	Mr. Clements reports that his interest in sex is back to normal and that he is able to have an erection.	Mr. Clements reports sexual interest and function; he and his wife are satisfied with their relationship.

Topics of education vary and often are related to a patient's developmental level. For example, a nurse talks to school-age children regarding the appearance of breast buds or pubic hair. When discussing sexual health with patients of childbearing age, always consider a patient's cultural and religious beliefs regarding contraception. The discussion includes the desire for children, usual sexual practices, and acceptable methods of contraception. Review all methods of contraception to allow patients to make informed decisions.

Major developmental events (e.g., puberty, menopause) prompt education about sexuality. Situational crises such as a life change with pregnancy, illness, divorce, extreme financial stress, placement of a spouse in a nursing home, or loss and grief affect sexuality. Some effects last for days, months, or years and are often minimized when the individual is prepared for possible changes in sexual functioning.

Demonstrate recognition, acceptance, and respect for an older adult's sexuality by displaying a willingness to openly discuss sex and sexuality-related concerns. Strategies that enhance sexual functioning include the following (LeVay et al., 2019).

- Avoid alcohol (in excess) and tobacco.
- Eat well-balanced meals.
- Plan sexual activity for times when the couple feels rested.
- Take pain medication if needed before sexual intercourse.
- Use pillows and alternate positioning to enhance comfort.
- Encourage touch, kissing, hugging, and other tactile stimulation.

CONCEPT MAP

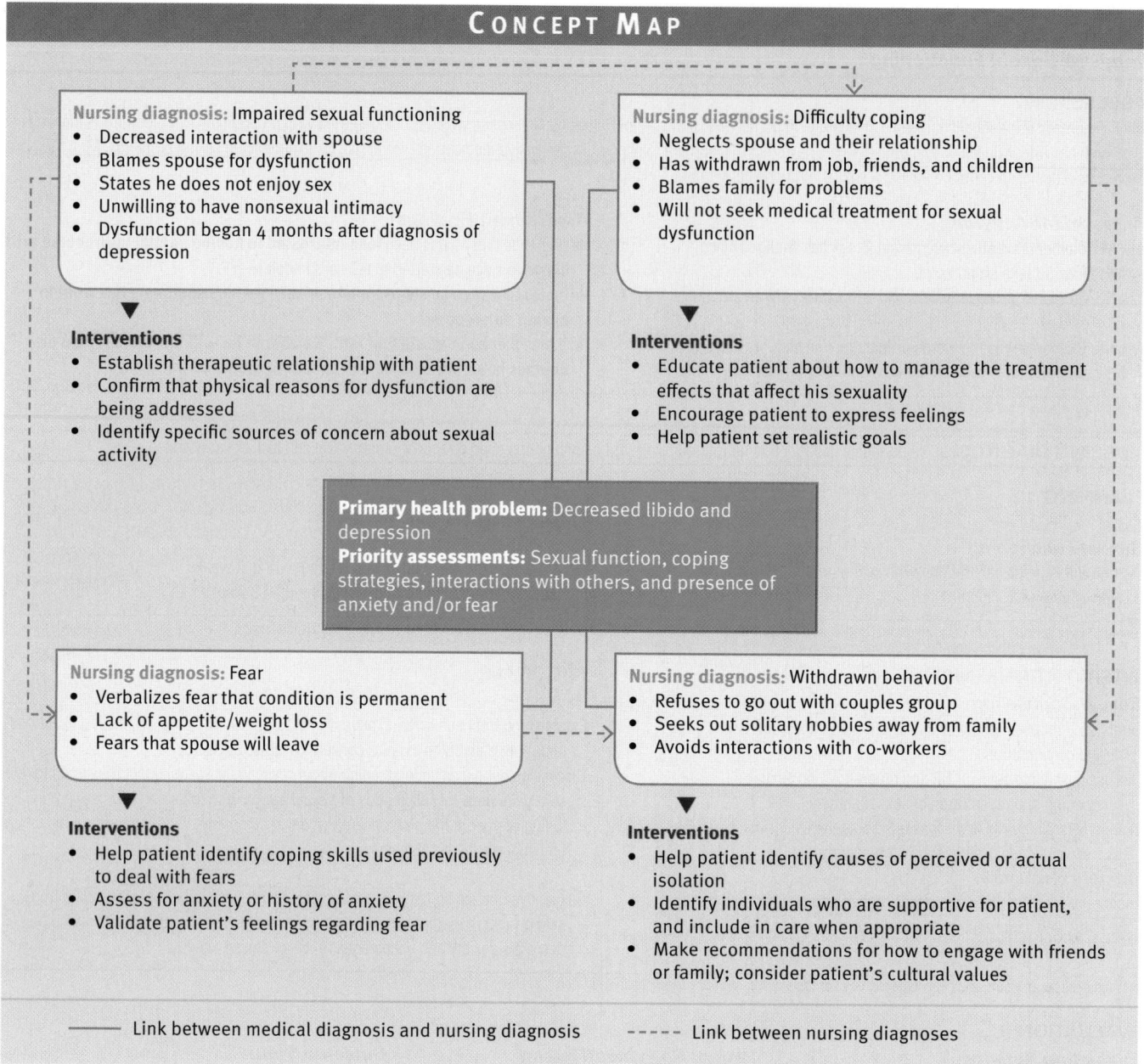

Nursing diagnosis: Impaired sexual functioning
- Decreased interaction with spouse
- Blames spouse for dysfunction
- States he does not enjoy sex
- Unwilling to have nonsexual intimacy
- Dysfunction began 4 months after diagnosis of depression

Interventions
- Establish therapeutic relationship with patient
- Confirm that physical reasons for dysfunction are being addressed
- Identify specific sources of concern about sexual activity

Nursing diagnosis: Difficulty coping
- Neglects spouse and their relationship
- Has withdrawn from job, friends, and children
- Blames family for problems
- Will not seek medical treatment for sexual dysfunction

Interventions
- Educate patient about how to manage the treatment effects that affect his sexuality
- Encourage patient to express feelings
- Help patient set realistic goals

Primary health problem: Decreased libido and depression
Priority assessments: Sexual function, coping strategies, interactions with others, and presence of anxiety and/or fear

Nursing diagnosis: Fear
- Verbalizes fear that condition is permanent
- Lack of appetite/weight loss
- Fears that spouse will leave

Interventions
- Help patient identify coping skills used previously to deal with fears
- Assess for anxiety or history of anxiety
- Validate patient's feelings regarding fear

Nursing diagnosis: Withdrawn behavior
- Refuses to go out with couples group
- Seeks out solitary hobbies away from family
- Avoids interactions with co-workers

Interventions
- Help patient identify causes of perceived or actual isolation
- Identify individuals who are supportive for patient, and include in care when appropriate
- Make recommendations for how to engage with friends or family; consider patient's cultural values

——— Link between medical diagnosis and nursing diagnosis   - - - - - Link between nursing diagnoses

FIG. 34.4 Concept map for Mr. Clements.

BOX 34.8   Examples of Community Resources Relating to Sexuality

- Community and free clinics offering contraceptive information and resources
- Health department (often for both family planning and sexually transmitted infections)
- Groups that provide education/services for those with particular conditions include the following:
  - American Diabetes Association
  - American Heart Association
- Muscular Dystrophy Association
- Muscular Sclerosis Society
- Sexual abuse support groups and hot lines
- Women's shelters (for those who are at risk of continued physical and/or sexual abuse)
- Resolve: The National Infertility Association (http://www.resolve.org)
- North America Menopause Society (http://www.menopause.org)

BOX 34.9 PATIENT TEACHING

Using a Condom Correctly

Objective
- Patient will verbalize correct use of a condom.

Teaching Strategies
- Develop a trusting relationship with patient.
- Explain to patient to always use a latex or rubber condom when having vaginal, oral, or anal sex and to store condoms in a cool, dry place away from sunlight.
- Encourage patient to read the label on the condom package to check the expiration date and ensure that the condom protects against sexually transmitted infections.
- Instruct patient to never reuse a condom or use a damaged condom.
- Explain how to apply the condom correctly (e.g., put it on as soon as the penis is hard and before vaginal, anal, or oral contact; gently squeeze any air out from the tip of the condom, leaving space for semen; unroll the condom to the base of the penis).
- Teach patient to pull out right after ejaculating and hold onto the condom when pulling out.
- Instruct patient to use only water-based lubricants (e.g., K-Y jelly) to prevent the condom from breaking; do not use petroleum jelly, massage oils, body lotions, or cooking oil.

Evaluation
Use the principles of teach-back to evaluate patient/family caregiver learning:
- Ask patient to describe where condoms are stored.
- Ask patient questions that verify understanding of instruction (e.g., What would you do if you noticed that a condom you just opened had an open slit in it?).

- Communicate concerns and fears with partner and health care provider.

Individuals who have more than one sex partner or whose partner has other sexual experiences need to learn about safe sex practices. Provide information about STI symptoms and transmission, use of condoms, and risky sexual activities (e.g., trauma from penile-anal sex). To prevent HIV infection, teach patients to avoid having multiple sex partners and to use condoms correctly to reduce the risk of HIV/AIDS (Box 34.9). Role-playing is useful in helping a person learn to say no or in negotiating with a partner to use a condom. When discussing safe sex, consider patients' physical and emotional health.

Encourage patients to have regular health and screening examinations to maintain sexual health. Often asymptomatic STIs are diagnosed during a physical examination with appropriate laboratory work. Annual health examinations provide an opportunity to discuss contraception and safe sex practices. However, some people do not seek annual health examinations routinely. For example, some women frequently do not have breast examinations, mammograms, and cervical cancer screening because of religious and cultural beliefs about modesty. Develop a therapeutic relationship with patients and provide culturally sensitive education that is written at an appropriate reading level (see Chapter 25). Barriers to reproductive health services include cultural beliefs, access to health care, and low health literacy.

Acute Care. Illness and surgery create situational stressors that often affect a person's sexuality. During periods of illness individuals experience major physical changes, the effects of drugs or treatments, the emotional stress of a prognosis, concern about future functioning, and separation from significant others. Never assume that sexual functioning is not a concern merely because of an individual's age or the severity of prognosis. After identifying concerns, address them in the context of his or her value system.

When a patient identifies sexual concerns, initiate discussion and education appropriately. Refer to appropriate outpatient resources if needed. Help patients anticipate how their illness or disease will change over time and the adjustments that will be necessary to achieve sexual fulfillment.

Restorative and Continuing Care. You need to establish relationships with couples to encourage honest and open discussions about sexual health during restorative or continuing care. Address needs by taking a sexual health history and implementing a basic model such as PLISSIT to provide options for patients (see Box 34.5). Assessment and management of sexual concerns are important when promoting sexual intimacy and providing closeness and closure between partners at the end of life.

In the home environment it is important to provide information on how an illness limits sexual activity and give ideas for adapting or facilitating sexual activity. Interventions range from giving permission for a partner to lie in bed and hold a patient to coordinating nursing care and medications to provide opportunity for privacy and intimacy. Often nurses help individuals create an environment that is comfortable for sexual activity in the home. This sometimes involves making recommendations for ways to arrange the bedroom to accommodate physical limitations. For example, some individuals who are in a wheelchair prefer being able to move the chair close to the side of the bed at an angle that allows for more ease in touching and caressing. Suggestions regarding how to accommodate barriers such as Foley catheters or drainage tubes contribute to sexual activity.

In the long-term care setting facilities need to make proper arrangements for privacy during residents' sexual experiences (LeVay et al., 2019). The ideal situation is to set up a pleasant room that is used for a variety of activities that the resident is able to reserve for private visits with a spouse or partner. If this is not possible, arrange for the roommate of a patient to be somewhere else to allow a couple time alone. Never leave patients alone in a situation in which injury is possible.

◆ Evaluation

Through the Patient's Eyes. Evaluate patients' perceptions of nursing interventions to determine whether their expectations have been met. Critical thinking ensures that you apply what is known about sexuality and a patient's unique situation.

Have follow-up discussions with the patient or partner to determine whether they were satisfied with your approaches. Sexuality is felt more than observed, and sexual expression requires an intimacy that is not amenable to observation.

Patient Outcomes. Evaluate whether your patient achieved outcomes established in the plan of care (Fig. 34.5). Ask patients questions about risk factors, sexual concerns, and their level of satisfaction. Observe behavioral cues such as eye contact, posture, and extraneous hand movements that indicate comfort or suggest continued anxiety or concern as topics are addressed. Anticipate the need to modify expectations with an individual and partner when evaluating outcomes. Sometimes you need to establish more appropriate time frames in which to achieve target goals. Ask patients to define what is acceptable and satisfying while considering the partner's level of sexual satisfaction. When outcomes are not met, begin to ask questions to determine appropriate changes in interventions. Examples of questions include the following:

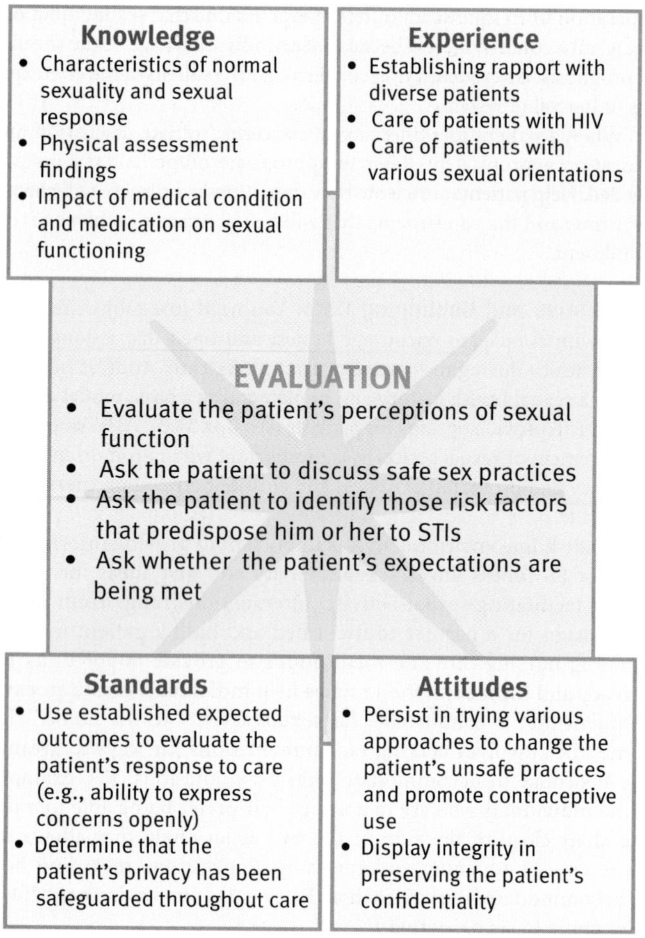

Knowledge
- Characteristics of normal sexuality and sexual response
- Physical assessment findings
- Impact of medical condition and medication on sexual functioning

Experience
- Establishing rapport with diverse patients
- Care of patients with HIV
- Care of patients with various sexual orientations

EVALUATION
- Evaluate the patient's perceptions of sexual function
- Ask the patient to discuss safe sex practices
- Ask the patient to identify those risk factors that predispose him or her to STIs
- Ask whether the patient's expectations are being met

Standards
- Use established expected outcomes to evaluate the patient's response to care (e.g., ability to express concerns openly)
- Determine that the patient's privacy has been safeguarded throughout care

Attitudes
- Persist in trying various approaches to change the patient's unsafe practices and promote contraceptive use
- Display integrity in preserving the patient's confidentiality

FIG. 34.5 Critical thinking model for sexuality evaluation. *HIV,* Human immunodeficiency virus; *STI,* sexually transmitted infection.

- What other questions do you have about your sexual health?
- Did you experience less pain during sexual intercourse after taking your pain medication?
- Which positions did you find most comfortable when you had sexual intercourse? Which positions were most awkward?
- What barriers are preventing you from discussing your feelings and fears with your partner?

KEY POINTS

- Nurses must be knowledgeable about all aspects of sexuality, including how their own values and issues surrounding sexuality impact patient-centered care.
- The nurse is educationally and experientially positioned to take the lead among health care providers to promote sexual health.
- Sexual health involves physical and psychosocial aspects and contributes to an individual's sense of self-worth and positive interpersonal relationships.
- The nurse must thoroughly assess potential causes of sexual dysfunction to promote effective treatment.
- Sexuality is related to all dimensions of health. Therefore, address sexual concerns or problems as a routine part of nursing care.
- Nursing diagnoses related to alterations in sexuality demonstrate the interface between physical and psychological issues.

- Patient risk factors include inadequate sex education and risky behaviors, including low rates of testing, substance use, low condom use, and multiple partners.
- Development and life changes, ethical decisional issues, fertility, personal and emotional conflicts, illness, and hospitalization all affect a patient's sexuality.
- Improved communication with one's partner and establishment or return to a mutually satisfying sex life are important outcomes following alterations in sexual health.
- Expert communication and attention to a patient's nonverbal communication will result in compassionate care surrounding sexuality and sexual health.

REFLECTIVE LEARNING

- State examples of nonjudgmental questions you can ask your patient to determine his or her gender identity.
- How would you establish a therapeutic relationship to put a patient at ease discussing the intimate aspects of his or her life?
- Describe how you would provide patient education to a couple experiencing problems with their sexual functioning. Provide at least three strategies that they could use to enhance their sexual functioning.

REVIEW QUESTIONS

1. A 16-year-old female tells the school nurse that she doesn't need the human papillomavirus (HPV) vaccine since her partner always uses condoms. The best response by the nurse to this statement is:
   1. "Latex condoms are the most effective way to eliminate the risk of HPV transmission."
   2. "Your parents may not want you to receive the HPV vaccine since it has been shown to increase sexual risk taking and sexual activity."
   3. "The HPV 9-valent vaccine is recommended for males and females even if they use condoms because it targets the specific viruses that cause cancer and genital warts."
   4. "You are past the recommended age to receive the vaccine."

2. An adolescent who is pregnant for the first time is at her initial prenatal visit. The women's health nurse practitioner (WHNP) informs the patient that she will be screening her for sexually transmitted infections (STIs). The patient replies, "I know I don't have an STI because I don't have any symptoms." Which responses by the WHNP would be appropriate? (Select all that apply.)
   1. "Untreated STIs can cause serious complications in pregnancy, so we routinely screen pregnant women."
   2. "Bacterial STIs don't usually cause symptoms, or you could have an asymptomatic viral STI."
   3. "Chlamydia screening is recommended for all sexually active women up to age 25 even if asymptomatic."
   4. "People between the ages of 15 and 24 are often asymptomatic and have the highest incidence of STIs."
   5. "There is no need to screen for infection since you aren't having any problems or symptoms."

3. A nurse who recently graduated from nursing school is providing discharge instructions to a patient who suffered a myocardial infarction (MI). The nurse knows that sexual issues are common after an MI but feels uncomfortable bringing up this topic. What is the best way for the nurse to handle this situation? (Select all that apply.)

1. Instruct the patient to discuss any sexual concerns with his or her partner after discharge.
2. Avoid discussing the topic unless the patient brings it up.
3. Ask a more experienced nurse to cover this with the patient and learn from the example.
4. Plan to attend conferences or training soon on how to discuss such issues.
5. Encourage the patient to discuss any personal concerns with the cardiologist.

4. The nurse is gathering a history from a 72-year-old male patient being admitted to a nursing home. The patient requests a private room. The nurse understands that:
   1. The patient cannot be sexually active since he is moving into a nursing home.
   2. The patient may be requesting a private room to facilitate an intimate relationship with his partner.
   3. There is no need to take a sexual history since most older adults are uncomfortable discussing intimate details of their lives.
   4. Older adults in nursing homes usually do not participate in sexual activity.

5. The nurse is providing education on sexually transmitted infections (STIs) to a group of older adults. The nurse knows that further teaching is needed when the participants make which statements? (Select all that apply.)
   1. "I don't need to use condoms since there is no risk for pregnancy."
   2. "I should be screened for an STI each time I'm with a new partner."
   3. "I know I'm not infected because I don't have discharge or sores."
   4. "I was tested for STIs last year, so I know I'm not infected."
   5. "The infection rate in older adults is low because most are not sexually active."

6. The nurse is providing community education about how the sexual response changes with age. Which statement made by one of the adults indicates the need for further information?
   1. "Health problems such as diabetes, chronic obstructive pulmonary disease, and hypertension have little effect on sexual functioning and desire."
   2. "It usually takes longer for both sexes to reach an orgasm."
   3. "Most of the normal changes in function are related to alteration in circulation and hormone levels."
   4. "Many medications can interfere with sexual function."

7. The nurse is gathering a sexual health history on a patient being admitted to the hospital for surgery. Which question demonstrates a nonjudgmental attitude?
   1. Can you tell me your sexual orientation?
   2. How do you and your wife feel about intimacy?

3. Do you have sex with men, women, or both?
4. Do you have sexual intercourse at your age?

8. The nurse reviews the health history of a 48-year-old man and notes that he was started on medications for elevated blood pressure and depression at his last annual physical. He tells the nurse that over the past 6 months he is having difficulty sustaining an erection. The nurse understands that: (Select all that apply.)
   1. Nurses are not expected to discuss sexual issues with male patients and the physician should address this.
   2. Sexual function can be affected by some medications.
   3. Sexually transmitted infections (STIs) can cause complications such as erectile dysfunction and screening should be done.
   4. Some men with health issues experience erectile dysfunction.
   5. Medications used to treat hypertension and depression seldom interfere with sexual function.

9. The school nurse is counseling an adolescent male who is returning to school after attempting suicide. He denies substance abuse and has no history of treatment for depression. He says he has no friends or family who understand him. Critical thinking encourages the nurse to consider all possibilities, including which of the following? (Select all that apply.)
   1. Adolescents often explore their sexual identity and expose themselves to complications such as sexually transmitted infections (STIs) or unplanned pregnancy.
   2. Peer approval and acceptance are not important in this age-group.
   3. Lesbian, gay, bisexual, and transgender (LGBTQ+) youth often experience stress from identification with a sexual minority group.
   4. Knowledge about normal changes associated with puberty and sexuality can decrease stress and anxiety.
   5. Adolescence is a time of emotional stability and self-acceptance.

10. A 53-year-old female being treated for breast cancer tells the nurse that she has no interest in sex since her surgery 2 months ago. The nurse is aware that: (Select all that apply.)
   1. Sexual issues are expected in a woman this age.
   2. Women experience sexual dysfunction more frequently than men.
   3. Hypoactive sexual desire disorder (HSDD) occurs in women over 65 years of age.
   4. Medical conditions such as cancer often contribute to HSDD.
   5. Disturbances in self-concept affect sexual functioning.

Answers: 1. 3; **2.** 1, 3, 4; **3.** 3, 4; **4.** 2; **5.** 1, 3, 4, 5; **6.** 1; **7.** 2; **8.** 2, 4; **9.** 1, 3, 4; **10.** 2, 4, 5.

Rationales for Review Questions can be found on the Evolve website.

REFERENCES

Annon J: The PLISSIT model: a proposed conceptual scheme for the behavioral treatment of sexual problems, *J Sex Educ Ther* 2(2):1, 1976.

Centers for Disease Control and Prevention (CDC): *HPV vaccine information for clinicians*, 2016, https://www.cdc.gov/vaccines/vpd/hpv/hcp/index.html. Accessed November 4, 2018.

Centers for Disease Control and Prevention (CDC): *HIV and youth*, 2017a, https://www.cdc.gov/hiv/group/age/youth/. Accessed November 4, 2018.

Centers for Disease Control and Prevention (CDC): *School health profiles*, 2017b, https://www.cdc.gov/healthyyouth/data/profiles/index.htm. Accessed November 16, 2018.

Centers for Disease Control and Prevention (CDC): Estimated HIV incidence and prevalence in the United States, 2010–2016, *HIV Surveill Supplemental Rep* 24(1), 2018a.

Centers for Disease Control and Prevention (CDC): *HIV among people aged 50 and over*, 2018b, https://www.cdc.gov/hiv/group/age/olderamericans/. Accessed November 4, 2018.

Centers for Disease Control and Prevention (CDC): *HIV/AIDS*, 2018c, https://www.cdc.gov/hiv/basics/index.html. Accessed March 16, 2019.

Centers for Disease Control and Prevention (CDC): *Medical monitoring project*, 2018d, https://www.cdc.gov/hiv/statistics/systems/mmp/index.html. Accessed November 16, 2018.

Centers for Disease Control and Prevention (CDC): *Sexually transmitted disease surveillance 2017*, 2018e, https://www.cdc.gov/std/stats17/default.htm. Accessed November 16, 2018.

Erikson E: *Childhood and society*, ed 2, New York, 1963, WW Norton.

Halter MJ: *Varcarolis' Foundations of psychiatric mental health nursing: a clinical approach*, ed 8, St Louis, 2018, Elsevier.

HIV.gov, *Overview: Data & Trends: U.S. statistics*, 2018, https://www.hiv.gov/hiv-basics/overview/data-and-trends/statistics. Accessed November 16, 2018.

Kann L, et al.: Youth risk behavior surveillance—United States, 2017, *MMWR Surveill Summ* 67(No. SS-8):1–114, 2018.

LeVay S, et al.: *Discovering human sexuality*, ed 4, New York, 2019, Oxford University Press.

Touhy TA, Jett K: *Ebersole and Hess' toward healthy aging: human needs and nursing response*, ed 9, St Louis, 2016, Elsevier.

Touhy TA, Jett KF: *Ebersole and Hess' gerontological nursing & healthy aging*, ed 5, St Louis, 2018, Elsevier.

VandenBos GR: *APA Dictionary of psychology*, Washington, DC, 2015, American Psychological Association.

World Health Organization: *WHO recommendations on adolescent sexual and reproductive health and rights*, Geneva, 2018a, World Health Organization.

World Health Organization: *Defining sexual health*, 2018b, http://www.who.int/reproductivehealth/topics/sexual_health/sh_definitions/en/. Accessed November 2018.

RESEARCH REFERENCES

Atallah S: Cultural aspects in sexual function and dysfunction in the geriatric population: a review of the current literature and clinical overview of clinical interventions with efficacy, *Top Geriatr Rehabil* 32(3):156–166, 2016.

Eleuteri S, et al.: Identity, relationships, sexuality, and risky behaviors of adolescents in the context of social media, *Sex Relation Ther* 32(3/4):354–365, 2017.

Ferris DG, et al.: 4-Valent human papillomavirus (4vHPV) vaccine in preadolescents and adolescents after 10 years, *Pediatrics* 140(6), 2017.

Fuzzell L, et al.: "I just think doctors need to ask more questions": sexual minority and majority adolescents' experiences talking about sexuality with healthcare providers, *Patient Educ Couns* 99(9):1467–1472, 2016.

Grossman JM, et al.: "We talked about sex." "No, we didn't": exploring adolescent and parent agreement about sexuality communication, *Am J Sex Educ* 12(4):343–357, 2017.

Haesler E, et al.: Sexuality, sexual health, and older people: a systematic review of research on the knowledge and attitudes of health professionals, *Nurse Educ Today* 40:57–71, 2016.

Kerpelman JL, et al.: Engagement in risky sexual behavior: adolescents' perceptions of self and the parent-child relationship matter, *Youth Soc* 48(1):101–125, 2016.

Lever S, Pryor J: The impact of stroke on female sexuality, *Disabil Rehabil* 39(20):2011–2020, 2017.

Santos-Iglesias P, et al.: Sexual well-being of older men and women, *Can J Hum Sex* 25(2):86–98, 2016.

Strong K, Folse VN: Assessing undergraduate nursing students' knowledge, attitudes and cultural competence in caring for lesbian, gay, bisexual, and transgender patients, *J Nurs Educ* 54(1):45–49, 2015.

White AJ, Taliaferro D: Relationship between postmenopausal women's successful aging, global self-esteem, and sexual quality of life, *Int J Hum Caring* 20(2):102–106, 2016.

35

Spiritual Health

OBJECTIVES

- Discuss the influence of spirituality on patients' health practices.
- Describe the relationship among faith, hope, and spiritual well-being.
- Compare and contrast the concepts of religion and spirituality.
- Assess a patient's spirituality and spiritual health.
- Explain the importance of establishing caring relationships with patients to provide spiritual care.
- Discuss nursing interventions designed to promote a patient's spiritual health.
- Identify approaches for establishing presence with patients.
- Evaluate patient outcomes related to spiritual health.

KEY TERMS

Agnostic, p. 723
Atheist, p. 723
Connectedness, p. 724
Faith, p. 724
Holistic, p. 734

Hope, p. 724
Self-transcendence, p. 724
Spiritual distress, p. 725
Spirituality, p. 723
Spiritual well-being, p. 724

Transcendence, p. 724
Inner strength and peace, p. 724
Meaning and purpose in life, p. 724

MEDIA RESOURCES

http://evolve.elsevier.com/Potter/fundamentals/
- Review Questions
- Concept Map Creator
- Case Study with Questions

- Audio Glossary
- Content Updates
- Answers to QSEN Activity and Review Questions

The word *spirituality* comes from the Latin word *spiritus,* which refers to breath or wind. The spirit gives life to a person. It signifies whatever is at the center of all aspects of a person's life. Florence Nightingale believed that spirituality was a force that provided energy needed to promote a healthy hospital environment and that caring for a person's spiritual needs was just as essential as caring for his or her physical needs (O'Brien, 2014). Today spirituality is often defined as an awareness of one's inner self and a sense of connection to a higher being, nature, or some purpose greater than oneself (Carson, 2017). It includes personal beliefs that help a person maintain hope and get through difficult situations (March and Caple, 2016). A person's health depends on a balance of physical, psychological, sociological, cultural, developmental, and spiritual factors. Spirituality helps individuals achieve the balance needed to maintain health and well-being and to cope with changes in their health status.

Too often nurses and other health care providers fail to recognize the spiritual dimension of their patients because spirituality is not scientific enough, it has many definitions, and it is difficult to measure. In addition, there are nurses and health care providers who are uncertain about a supreme God or being and uncomfortable with discussing spirituality, while others claim that they do not have time to address patients' spiritual needs (Chen et al., 2017a; Connerton and Moe, 2018). The concepts of spirituality and religion are often interchanged, but spirituality is a much broader and more unifying concept than religion (Dahlkemper, 2016; Carson, 2017). While religion is an organized, institution-related practice that is commonly associated with particular beliefs, spirituality focuses on an individual's connection to a higher being, nature, or some purpose greater than oneself (Caplan, 2017).

The human spirit is powerful, and spirituality has different meanings for different people. Some people do not believe in the existence of God (atheist), or they believe that there is no known ultimate reality (agnostic). Nonetheless spirituality is important regardless of a person's religious beliefs. Atheists search for meaning in life through their work and their relationships with others. Agnostics discover meaning in what they do or how they live, the "here and now," because they find no ultimate meaning for the way things are. They believe that people bring meaning to what they do.

A nurse's personal spiritual health is important to his or her own values and beliefs and can influence attitudes toward spiritual care, professional commitment, and caring (Chiang et al., 2016). You need to be aware of your own spirituality to provide appropriate and relevant spiritual care to others. As a nurse, you need to care for the whole person and accept a patient's beliefs and experiences (Connerton and Moe, 2018). Being able to determine the importance that spirituality holds for patients depends on your ability to develop caring relationships (see Chapter 7).

SCIENTIFIC KNOWLEDGE BASE

The relationship between spirituality and healing is not completely understood. However, an individual's intrinsic spirit seems to be an important factor in healing. Healing often takes place because of believing. For example, research shows that spirituality positively affects and enhances physical and psychological health, quality of life, health promotion behaviors, and disease prevention activities (Heo et al., 2018; Trevino and McConnell, 2015).

Spirituality has a positive impact on the ability to cope with anxiety, stress, and depression in family caregivers (Vitorino et al., 2018), mothers with infants in the neonatal intensive care unit (Alemdar et al., 2018), nursing students (Fabbris et al., 2017), patients living with cancer (Hefner et al., 2017), and patients experiencing infertility (Romeiro et al., 2017). Integrative body-mind techniques that include relaxation, guided imagery, mindfulness training, and music reduce perceptions of pain and anxiety (Fan et al., 2014). A person's inner beliefs and convictions are powerful resources for healing. When you support the spirituality of patients and their families, you help them achieve desirable health outcomes.

> ### REFLECT NOW
>
> What have you observed as patient outcomes when spiritual care was provided to patients?

NURSING KNOWLEDGE BASE

Nursing research shows the association between spirituality and health. For example, spiritual well-being has a potential protective effect against psychosocial distress at the end of life (Bernard et al., 2017). Research also shows that when patients who have cancer participate in religious and spiritual activities, they remain actively engaged socially and continue to have satisfying relationships (Sherman et al., 2015). More research is needed, but the interest in studying the relationship between spirituality and health is greatly contributing to nursing science.

Current Concepts in Spiritual Health

A variety of concepts describing spiritual health are a part of professional nursing practice. To provide meaningful and supportive spiritual care, it is important to understand the concepts of spirituality, spiritual well-being, faith, religion, and hope. Each concept offers direction in understanding the views that individuals have of life and its value.

Spirituality. Spirituality is a complex concept that is unique to each individual; it depends on a person's culture, development, life experiences, beliefs, and ideas about life (Connerton and Moe, 2018). It is an inherent human characteristic that exists in all people, regardless of their religious beliefs. It gives individuals the *energy* needed to discover themselves, cope with difficult situations, and maintain health. Energy generated by spirituality helps patients feel well and guides choices (e.g., type and extent of health care) made throughout life. Spirituality enables a person to love, have faith and hope, seek meaning in life, and nurture relationships with others. Because it is subjective, multidimensional, and personal, researchers and scholars cannot agree on a universal definition of spirituality (Connerton and Moe, 2018). However, five distinct but overlapping constructs define it (Fig. 35.1).

- Self-transcendence—a sense of authentically connecting to one's inner self. This contrasts with transcendence, the belief that a force outside of and greater than the person exists beyond the material world (Hatamipour et al., 2015). Self-transcendence is a positive force. It allows people to have new experiences and develop new perspectives that are beyond ordinary physical boundaries. Examples of transcendent moments include the feeling of awe when holding a new baby or looking at a beautiful sunset.
- Connectedness—being *intrapersonally* connected within oneself; *interpersonally* connected with others and the environment; and *transpersonally* connected with God or an unseen higher power. Through connectedness patients move beyond the stressors of

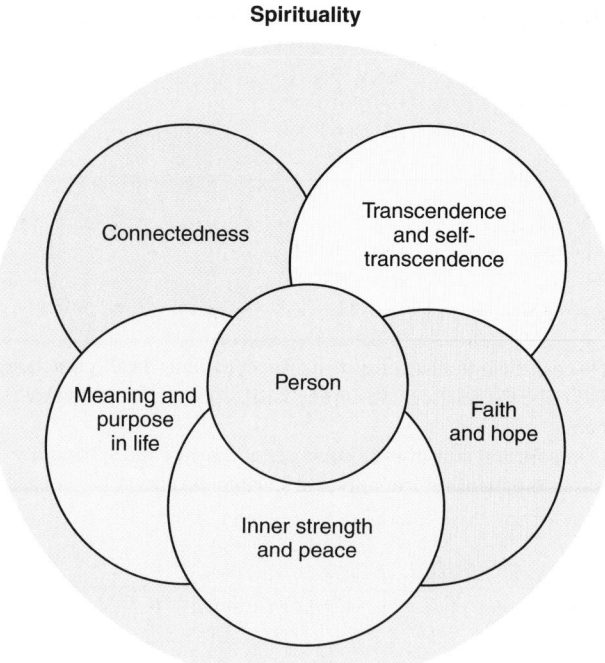

FIG. 35.1 The concept of spirituality has five distinct but overlapping constructs.

everyday life and find comfort, faith, hope, and empowerment (Hakanson and Ohlen, 2016).

- Faith—allows people to have firm beliefs despite lack of physical evidence. Faith enables people to believe in and establish transpersonal connections. Although many people associate faith with religious beliefs, it also exists without them (Christman and Mueller, 2017). For example, one might have faith that all people are good, without being a practitioner of a religion.
- Hope—has several meanings that vary on the basis of how it is being experienced; it usually refers to an energizing source that has an orientation to future goals and outcomes (Griggs and Walker, 2016).
- Inner strength and peace—spirituality gives people the ability to find a dynamic and creative sense of *inner strength* to use when making difficult decisions. This source of energy helps people stay open to change and life challenges, provides confidence in decision making, and promotes connections with others and a positive outlook on life (Boman et al., 2017). *Inner peace* fosters calm, positive, and peaceful feelings despite life experiences of chaos, fear, and uncertainty. These feelings help people feel comforted even in times of great distress (Hatamipour et al., 2015).
- Meaning and purpose in life—spirituality also helps people find meaning and purpose in both positive and negative life events (Dobratz, 2016; Hatamipour et al., 2015).

Spirituality is an integrating theme. A person's concept of spirituality begins in childhood and continues to grow throughout adulthood. It represents the totality of one's being, serving as the overriding perspective that unifies the various aspects of an individual. It spreads through all dimensions of a person's life, whether or not the person acknowledges or develops it.

Spiritual Well-Being. The concept of spiritual well-being has multiple dimensions. The common dimensions of spiritual well-being include meaning and purpose, a sense of peace or fulfillment, and connectedness with others and God or a higher power (Bai et al., 2016). Those who experience spiritual well-being feel connected to others and are able to find meaning or purpose in their lives. Those who are spiritually healthy experience joy, are able to forgive themselves and others, accept hardship and mortality, and report an enhanced quality of life (Haugan et al., 2014; Cottrell, 2016).

Faith. In addition to being a component of spirituality, the concept of faith has other definitions. It is a cultural or institutional religion such as Judaism, Buddhism, Islam, or Christianity. It is also a relationship with a divinity, higher power, or spirit that incorporates a reasoning faith (belief) and a trusting faith (action). Reasoning faith provides confidence in something for which there is no proof. It is an acceptance of what reasoning cannot explain. Sometimes faith involves a belief in a higher power, spirit guide, God, or Allah. It is also the way a person chooses to live. It gives purpose and meaning to an individual's life, allowing for action.

Religion. Religion is associated with the "state of doing," or a specific system of practices associated with a particular denomination, sect, or form of worship. It is a system of organized beliefs and worship that a person practices to outwardly express spirituality. Many people practice a faith or belief in the doctrines and expressions of a specific religion or sect, such as the Lutheran church or Judaism. People from different religions view spirituality differently. For example, a Buddhist believes in Four Noble Truths:

1. Life is suffering.
2. Suffering is caused by karma and disturbing emotions.
3. Suffering can be eliminated by eliminating karma and disturbing emotions.
4. To eliminate karma, disturbing emotions, and suffering, one follows an eightfold path (i.e., right understanding, intention, speech, action, livelihood, effort, mindfulness, and concentration) (Rinpoche, 2017).

A Buddhist turns inward, valuing self-control, whereas a Christian looks to the love of God to provide enlightenment and direction in life.

When providing spiritual care, it is important to understand the differences between religion and spirituality. Many people tend to use the terms interchangeably. Although closely associated, they are not synonymous. Religious practices encompass spirituality, but spirituality does not need to include religious practice. Religious care helps patients maintain their faithfulness to their belief systems and worship practices. Spiritual care helps people identify meaning and purpose in life, look beyond the present, and maintain personal relationships and a relationship with a higher being or life force.

Hope. A spiritual person's faith brings hope. When a person has the attitude of something to live for and look forward to, hope is present. It is a multidimensional concept that provides comfort while people endure life-threatening situations, hardships, and other personal challenges. Hope is closely associated with faith; it is energizing and motivates people to achieve goals, such as adopting healthy behaviors. People express hope in all aspects of their lives to help them deal with life stressors. It is a valuable personal resource whenever someone is facing a loss (see Chapter 36) or a difficult challenge (Griggs and Walker, 2016).

Spiritual Health

People gain spiritual health by finding a balance between their values, goals, and beliefs and their relationships within themselves and others. Throughout life a person often grows more spiritual, becoming increasingly aware of the meaning, purpose, and values of life. In times of stress, illness, loss, or recovery, a person uses previous ways of responding or adjusting to a situation. Often these coping styles lie within a person's spiritual beliefs.

Spiritual beliefs change as patients grow and develop (Table 35.1). Spirituality begins as children learn about themselves and their relationships with others, including a higher power. Nurses who understand a child's spiritual beliefs are able to care for and comfort the child (Johnston Taylor et al., 2015). As children mature into adulthood, they experience spiritual growth by entering into lifelong relationships with people who share similar values and beliefs.

Beliefs among people vary on the basis of cultural factors such as gender, past experience, religion, ethnicity, and economic status. Healthy spirituality in older adults gives peace and acceptance of the self and is often the result of a lifelong connection with a higher power. Illness and loss sometimes threaten and challenge the spiritual developmental process. Older adults often express their spirituality by turning to important relationships and giving of themselves to others (Touhy and Jett, 2018).

Factors Influencing Spirituality

When illness, loss, grief, or a major life change occurs, people either use spiritual resources to help them cope and search for meaning, or spiritual needs and concerns develop. Spiritual distress is "a disruption in the life principle that pervades a person's entire being and transcends the person's biologic and psychosocial nature" (Andrews and Boyle, 2016, p. 399). It causes people to question their identity and feel doubt, loss of faith, and a sense of being alone or abandoned. Individuals often question their spiritual values or the meaning of life, raising questions about their way of life, purpose for living, and source of meaning (Connerton and Moe, 2018). Spiritual distress also occurs when there is conflict between a person's beliefs and prescribed health regimens or the inability to practice usual rituals.

Acute Illness. Sudden, unexpected illness often creates spiritual distress. For example, both a 50-year-old patient who has a heart attack and a 20-year-old patient who is in a motor vehicle accident face crises that threaten spiritual health. The sudden illness or injury creates an unanticipated scramble to integrate and cope with new realities (e.g., disability). People often look for ways to remain faithful to their beliefs and value systems. Some pray, attend religious services more often, or spend time reflecting on the positive aspects of their lives. Often conflicts develop around a person's beliefs and the meaning of life. Anger is common; sometimes patients express it against God or a higher power, their families, themselves, and their nurses or other health care providers. The strength of patients' spirituality influences their ability to cope with and recover from sudden illness or injury. Having a better understanding of your patients' illnesses and conditions helps you spiritually support them (Sweat, 2015). Nurses play a key role in helping patients resolve feelings of spiritual distress. Nurses create a healing environment and maximize recovery by enhancing patients' spiritual well-being (Estores and Frye, 2015)

Chronic Illness. Many chronic illnesses threaten a person's independence, causing fear, anxiety, and spiritual distress. Dependence on others for routine self-care needs often creates feelings of powerlessness. Powerlessness and the loss of a sense of purpose in life impair the ability to cope with alterations in functioning. Spirituality is an important dimension of how patients adapt to and live with chronic illness. Successfully adapting to these changes strengthens a person spiritually, but it sometimes takes a long-term plan to help a patient with a chronic illness achieve spiritual well-being. As a nurse, you are in a unique position to help patients reevaluate their lives and achieve spiritual health (Box 35.1). Successful adaptation provides spiritual growth. Patients who have a sense of spiritual well-being feel connected with a higher power, are able to find meaning and purpose in life, and are

TABLE 35.1 Relationship Between Developmental Stage and Spirituality

Erickson's Developmental Stage	Spiritual Beliefs
Trust vs. Mistrust Birth to 18 months	Spiritual well-being provided by parents Trust provides basis for hope Love, affection, security, and a stimulating environment promote spirituality
Autonomy vs. Shame and Doubt 20-36 months	Fascination with magic and mystery Often believes that illness is related to bad behavior Begins to learn the difference between right and wrong Imitates parents' spiritual or religious actions; recites prayers and sings simple religious songs, but does not understand their meanings Interprets meanings literally
Initiative vs. Guilt 3-6 years	Feels guilty when not acting responsibly Influenced by spiritual and religious stories, examples, moods, and actions Models moral behaviors of parents Begins to ask about God or supreme beings
Industry vs. Inferiority 6-12 years	Wants to learn about spirituality Has a clear picture of God or supreme being, morality, and the difference between right and wrong Sorts fantasy from fact Demands proof of reality and believes literal meanings of spiritual stories
Identity vs. Identity Confusion Adolescence	Reflects on inconsistencies in stories Begins to question spiritual practices, forms own opinions, and occasionally discards parents' beliefs Abstract reasoning leads to exploration of moral issues Spirituality comes from connectedness with family, nature, and God or a supreme being
Intimacy vs. Isolation and Loneliness Young adulthood	Establishes self-identity and world view Forms independent beliefs, attitudes, and lifestyles Uses principles to solve problems when individual's and society's rules conflict
Generativity vs. Stagnation Middle-age adulthood	Develops appreciation of past spiritual experiences Embraces people from different faiths and religions Reviews value system during crisis Values others
Ego identity vs. Despair and Disgust Older adulthood	Values love and interactions with others Focuses on overcoming oppression and violence Beliefs vary based on many factors such as gender, past experiences, religion, economic status, and ethnic background

Data from Edelman CL, Mandle CL: *Health promotion throughout the life span*, ed 8, St Louis, 2014, Elsevier; and Hockenberry MJ, et al: *Wong's nursing care of infants and children*, ed 11, St Louis, 2019, Elsevier.

BOX 35.1   EVIDENCE-BASED PRACTICE

Spiritual Interventions and Patient Outcomes

PICOT Question: Does the use of spiritual care interventions among adults improve patient outcomes?

Evidence Summary

Nursing care for patients needs to focus on mind, body, and spirit. It is important to include spiritual interventions in a patient's plan of care that will help to relieve spiritual distress and enhance spiritual well-being (Ricci-Allegra, 2018). Providing spiritual care to patients helps the patient cope with illness and therapies (Trevino and McConnell, 2015). Researchers have found that the use of spiritual interventions helps to decrease anxiety and reduce depression in patients with cancer and heart failure (Pantuso, 2015; Heo et al., 2018). Both verbal communication and nonverbal communication, such as presence, are useful when providing spiritual care to patients (Minton et al., 2018). The use of a spiritual care board allowing patients to express their feelings helped patients cope with their illnesses and feel at peace (Berning et al., 2016). Before providing spiritual

care to patients, it is important for nurses to assess for patients' cues to respect patient beliefs and autonomy (Ebrahimi et al., 2017).

Application to Nursing Practice

- Use active listening and therapeutic communication to develop rapport with your patients (Bone et al., 2018).
- Offer to pray or read scripture with patients (Minton et al., 2018).
- Turn on a patient's favorite religious music station or television channel (Abuatiq, 2015).
- Conduct a spiritual assessment or history from each of your patients (Pantuso, 2015).
- Be nonjudgmental in your assessment and care of patients, showing respect for each patient's spiritual beliefs (Ebrahimi et al., 2017).
- Offer to contact pastoral care or the chaplain for patients (Bone et al., 2018).

better able to cope with and accept their chronic illness (Carron, 2016). Exploring the meaning of pain and suffering with patients allows you to provide spiritual support during their illnesses (Sweat, 2015).

Terminal Illness. Dying is a holistic process encompassing a patient's physical, social, psychological, and spiritual health (Finocchiaro, 2016). Terminal illness causes fears of physical pain, loss of independence, isolation, the unknown, and dying. It creates an uncertainty about what death means, making patients susceptible to spiritual distress. However, some patients have a spiritual sense of peace that enables them to face death without fear. Spirituality helps these patients find peace in themselves and their death. Individuals experiencing a terminal illness find themselves reviewing life and questioning its meaning. Those who struggle ask common questions, such as "Why is this happening to me?" or "What have I done?" Terminal illness affects family and friends as well. It causes members of the family to ask important questions about its meaning and how it will affect their relationship with the patient (see Chapter 36). When caring for dying patients, help them gain a greater sense of control over their illness, whether they are in a health care setting (e.g., the hospital) or at home.

Near-Death Experience. Some nurses care for patients who have had a near-death experience (NDE). An NDE is a psychological phenomenon of people who either have been close to clinical death or have recovered after being declared dead. It is not associated with a mental disorder. Instead experts agree that NDE describes a powerfully close brush with physical, emotional, and spiritual death. For example, people who have an NDE after cardiopulmonary arrest often tell the same story of feeling themselves rising above their bodies and watching caregivers initiate lifesaving measures. Commonly, patients who have had an NDE describe it as feeling totally at peace, having an out-of-body experience, being pulled into a dark tunnel, seeing bright lights, and meeting people who preceded them in death (Martial et al., 2017). Instead of moving toward the light, they learn that it is not time for them to die, and they return to life (Johnson, 2015; Rawlings and Devery, 2015).

Patients who have an NDE may be reluctant to discuss it, thinking family or caregivers will not understand. A nurse's acceptance and response to the patient's report of the NDE impacts how much the patient shares about the experience (Rawlings and Devery, 2015). NDEs are often transformational and can be either positive or negative experiences (Johnson, 2015). However, individuals experiencing an NDE who discuss it openly with family or caregivers find acceptance and meaning from this powerful experience (Rawlings and Devery, 2015). They are often no longer afraid of death, and they have a decreased desire to achieve material wealth. They also report increased sensitivity to different chemicals such as alcohol and medications. After patients have survived an NDE, promote spiritual well-being by remaining open, giving patients a chance to explore what happened, and supporting them as they share the experience with significant others (Rawlings and Devery, 2015).

CRITICAL THINKING

Successful critical thinking requires a synthesis of knowledge, experience, information gathered from patients, critical thinking attitudes, and intellectual and professional standards. Clinical judgments require you to anticipate information, analyze the data, and make decisions regarding your patient's care. During assessment, consider all elements that build toward making an appropriate nursing diagnosis (Fig. 35.2).

The helping role is important in nursing practice. Patients look to nurses for help that is different from the help they seek from other health

Knowledge
- Therapeutic communication
- Caring practices; presencing, listening
- Loss and grief
- Concepts of spiritual health and religion

Experience
- Caring for patients who exhibit strong spiritual health
- Caring for patients who experience loss
- Personal experience whereby faith and beliefs are challenged or used in coping

ASSESSMENT
- Assess the patient's faith and beliefs
- Review the patient's view of life, self-responsibility, and life satisfaction
- Assess the extent of the patient's fellowship and community
- Review if the patient practices religion and rituals

Standards
- Demonstrate the ethic of care
- Be thorough and ensure that assessment is relevant to the patient's situation
- Follow ANA code of ethics

Attitudes
- Approach assessment with fairness and integrity so as not to let personal beliefs bias conclusions

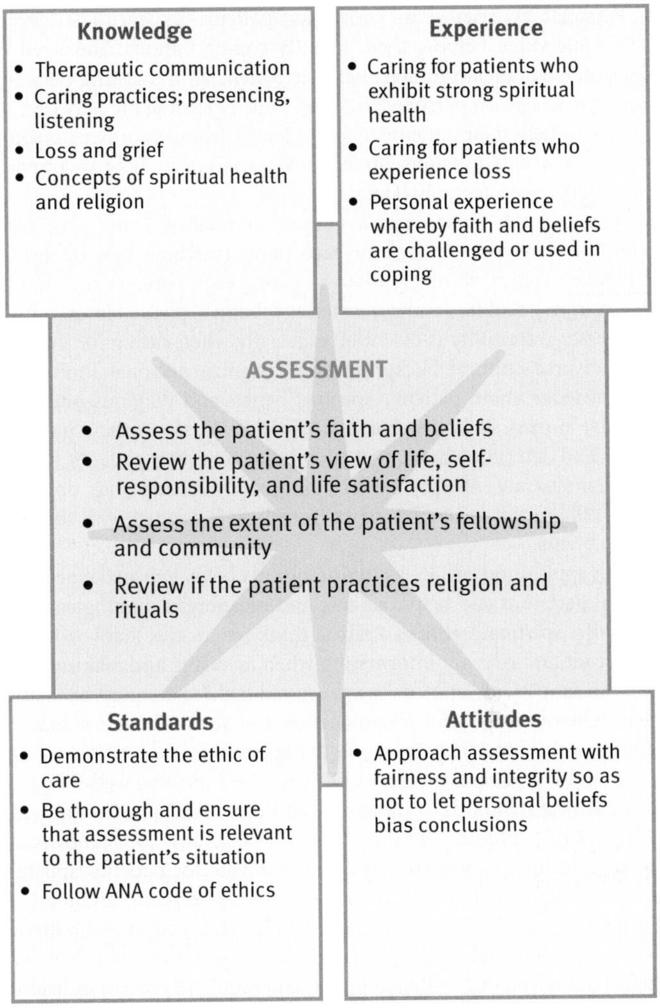

FIG. 35.2 Critical thinking model for spiritual health assessment. *ANA,* American Nurses Association.

care professionals. Expert nurses acquire the ability to anticipate personal issues affecting patients and their spiritual well-being. Critical thinking and the application of knowledge and skills help nurses enhance patients' spiritual well-being and health. Nurses who are comfortable with their own spirituality often are more likely to care for their patients' spiritual needs. Beliefs of a health care provider affect the discussion of treatment options with patients and ultimately their health care choices (Delgado, 2015). There are nurses who feel strongly about providing spiritual care as part of their holistic practice. Nurses who foster their own personal, emotional, and spiritual health become resources for their patients and use their own spirituality as a tool when caring for themselves and their patients.

After becoming comfortable with your own spirituality (e.g., knowing your belief system, following practices that strengthen your meaning and purpose in life), use your nursing knowledge to anticipate your patients' personal issues and the resulting effect on spiritual well-being. Your knowledge about the concept of spirituality, your understanding of ethics (see Chapter 22), and your knowledge of a patient's faith and belief systems help to provide appropriate spiritual care. Knowledge of a patient's values, beliefs, preferences, and needs provides insight into a person's spiritual practices. Application of therapeutic communication principles (see Chapter 24) and caring principles (see Chapter 7) helps you establish therapeutic trust with patients. An individual's spiritual beliefs are very personal. When you integrate patient preferences, values, and beliefs into spiritual care, you provide patient-centered care with sensitivity and respect for the diversity of human experience (QSEN Institute, 2018).

Personal experience in caring for patients in spiritual distress is valuable when helping them identify coping options. You need to determine whether your spirituality is beneficial in assisting patients. Nurses who sense a personal faith and hope regarding life may be better able to help their patients. A nurse learns from his or her personal faith system and previous professional experiences how to provide spiritual care comfortably (Delgado, 2015).

Because each person has a unique spirituality, know your own beliefs so that you can care for each patient without bias (Delgado, 2015). Use critical thinking when assessing each patient's reaction to illness, injury, and loss and determining whether spiritual intervention is necessary. Humility is essential, especially when caring for patients from diverse cultural backgrounds. Recognize personal limitations in knowledge about patients' spiritual beliefs and religious practices. Effective nurses show genuine concern as they assess their patients' beliefs and determine how spirituality influences their patients' health. You demonstrate integrity by refraining from voicing your opinions about religion or spirituality when your beliefs conflict with those of your patients.

The application of intellectual standards helps you make accurate clinical decisions and helps patients find meaningful and logical ways to acquire spiritual wellness. Critical thinking ensures that you obtain significant and relevant information when assessing and making decisions about patients' spiritual needs. Avoid making assumptions about their religion and beliefs. Significance and relevance are standards of critical thinking that allow you to explore the issues that are most meaningful to patients and most likely to affect spiritual well-being.

In setting standards for quality health care, The Joint Commission (TJC) (2017) requires health care organizations to acknowledge patients' rights to spiritual care and to provide for patients' spiritual needs through pastoral care or others who are certified, ordained, or lay individuals. The standards also require that you assess patients' beliefs and spiritual practices. The HealthCare Chaplaincy Network (2016) has developed evidence-based structural and process indicators and outcome metrics for quality spiritual care.

The American Nurses Association *Code of Ethics for Nurses* (2015) requires nurses to practice nursing with compassion and respect for the inherent dignity, worth, and uniqueness of every person. It is essential to promote an environment that respects patients' values, customs, and spiritual beliefs. Routinely implementing standard nursing interventions such as prayer or meditation is coercive and unethical. Therefore, determine which interventions are compatible with your patient's beliefs and values before selecting them based on patient input. An ethic of caring (see Chapter 7) provides a framework for decision making and places the nurse as the patient's advocate.

> ### REFLECT NOW
>
> Consider your own spiritual beliefs and spiritual health. How do your own spiritual beliefs and spiritual health impact the care you provide your patients?

❖ NURSING PROCESS

Apply the nursing process and use a critical thinking approach in your care of patients. The nursing process provides a clinical decision-making approach for you to use to develop and implement an individualized plan of care. Understanding a patient's spirituality and then appropriately identifying the level of support and resources needed require a broad perspective and an open mind. As a nurse you are ethically responsible for meeting the spiritual needs of your patients. People experience the world and find meaning in life differently. Application of the nursing

process from the perspective of a patient's spiritual needs is not simple. It goes beyond assessing his or her religious practices. Caring for your patients' spiritual needs requires you to be compassionate and remove any personal biases or misconceptions. Be willing to share and discover their meaning and purpose in life, illness, and health. Identify common values and respect unique commitments and values with your patients by having quiet conversations, listening effectively, and communicating using presence and touch when appropriate (Delgado, 2015).

◆ Assessment

During the assessment process thoroughly assess each patient and critically analyze findings to ensure that you make patient-centered clinical decisions required for safe nursing care. Because completing a spiritual assessment takes time, conduct an ongoing assessment over the course of a patient's stay in the health care setting if possible. Convey caring in your manner and communication style. Caring is conveyed by knowing your patient's cultural values and beliefs; respecting privacy, diversity and individual needs; and interacting and listening to the patient and his or her family (Darnell and Hickson, 2015). Be open to successfully promoting an honest discussion about each patient's spiritual beliefs. Your spiritual assessment will reveal the patient's beliefs about life, health, and a Supreme Being or power.

Through the Patient's Eyes. It is essential to take the time to assess a patient's viewpoints and establish a trusting relationship. Talking about spirituality with a patient helps build a trusting relationship that often leads to conversations about spirituality and health outcomes (Carson, 2017). As you and your patients reach a point of learning together, spiritual caring occurs. Be sure to discuss what is meaningful and relevant to your patients. Encourage them to discuss their personal beliefs and faith traditions. Explore the meaning that their illnesses have in their lives, based on their faith beliefs. Discover the patients' expectations by asking questions such as "How can we best partner with you to meet your spiritual needs while you are here?" "What is important to you spiritually?" "Are there particular religious or prayer practices that are important for you to continue while you are in the hospital?" "Are there special practices that help you manage your illness or pain?" or "Is there anyone we can call who is a source of strength, support, or comfort for you?" Conducting an assessment is therapeutic for you and your patients because it conveys a level of caring and support from the nurse to the patient (ANA, APA, and ISPN, 2014).

Assessment Tools. Listening to a patient's story is an essential method for obtaining a spiritual assessment. However, you can assess your patients' spiritual health in several different ways, using open-ended questions to prompt them to tell their story or asking them direct questions (Box 35.2). Focus your assessment on aspects of spirituality most likely to be influenced by life experiences, events, and questions in the case of illness and hospitalization. Asking direct questions requires you to feel comfortable in asking others about their spirituality. Some health care agencies and researchers have created assessment tools to clarify patients' values and to assess their level of spirituality. For example, the spiritual well-being (SWB) scale has 20 questions that assess a patient's relationship with God and his or her sense of life purpose and life satisfaction (Life Advance, 2009). The FICA assessment tool (Borneman et al., 2010; Puchalski and Romer, 2000) evaluates spirituality and is closely correlated to quality of life. FICA stands for the following criteria:

F—**Faith or belief**
I—**Importance and Influence**
C—**Community**
A—**Address** (interventions to address)

BOX 35.2 Nursing Assessment Questions

Spirituality and Spiritual Health
- Which experiences in the past have been most difficult for you?
- What gives you hope during those difficult times?
- Which aspects of your spirituality have been most helpful to you?
- Which aspects of your spirituality would you like to discuss?

Faith, Belief, Fellowship, and Community
- To what or whom do you look as a source of strength, hope, or faith in times of difficulty?
- How does your faith help you cope?
- What can I do to support your religious beliefs or faith commitment? Would you like me to pray with you or perhaps read from the Koran or Bible?
- What gives your life meaning?

Life and Self-Responsibility
- How do you feel about the changes this illness has caused?
- How do these changes affect what you now need to do?

Life Satisfaction
- How happy or satisfied are you with your life?
- Which accomplishments help you feel satisfied with your life?
- What is it that makes you feel dissatisfied?

Connectedness
- What feelings do you have after you pray or meditate?
- Who do you feel is the most important person in your life?

Vocation
- How has your illness affected the way you live your life spiritually at home or where you work?
- In what way has your illness affected your ability to express what is important in life to you?

Effective assessment tools such as the SWB scale and FICA help you remember important areas to assess. Patient responses to the assessment items on the tools indicate areas that you need to investigate further. For example, if, after using the FICA tool with a young man who is having difficulty accepting a new diagnosis of prostate cancer, you find out that he does not want you or his pastor to help him address this issue, you need to spend time understanding how the patient plans to manage this new illness. Remember, when using any spiritual assessment tool, do not impose your personal values on your patient. Be careful about making false assumptions about your patients' beliefs based on your personal values and beliefs. When you understand the overall approach to spiritual assessment, you are able to enter into thoughtful discussions with patients, gain a greater awareness of the personal resources they bring to a situation, and incorporate the resources into an effective plan of care.

Faith/Belief. When assessing a patient's faith, first determine his or her beliefs, especially those that influence hope. For example, ask how a patient believes a chemotherapy drug will affect a newly diagnosed form of cancer. Ask the patient whether he or she believes in the skill or competence of his or her physician. Determine which of your patient's beliefs guide him or her to find meaning in life events and to thus make decisions. Ask your patient whether he or she is able to live according to his or her beliefs. Finally, assess to what extent your patient interrelates with self, others, and/or a source of authority. Faith in an authority (such as a health care provider or senior family member) provides a sense of confidence that guides a person in exercising beliefs and

experiencing growth. Assess a person's faith in an authority by asking "To whom do you look to for guidance in life?" The patient's response to an open-ended question such as this is likely to open the door for a meaningful discussion. Listen carefully and explore what is meaningful to the patient.

Determine whether a patient has a religious source of guidance that conflicts with medical treatment plans and affects the options that nurses and other health care providers are able to offer patients. For example, if a patient is a Jehovah's Witness, blood products are not an acceptable form of treatment (Jehovah's Witnesses, 2019). Christian Scientists may refuse any medical intervention, believing that their faith heals them. It is also important to understand a patient's philosophy of life. Your assessment should reveal the basis of the patient's belief system regarding meaning and purpose in life and the patient's spiritual focus. Asking a patient "Describe for me what is most important in your life" or "Tell me what gives your life meaning or purpose" helps to assess the basis of his or her spiritual belief system. This information often reflects the impact that illness, loss, or disability has on a person's life. Considerable religious diversity exists in the United States. A patient's religious faith and practices, views about health, and the response to illness influence how nurses provide support.

Life and Self-Responsibility. Spiritual well-being includes life and self-responsibility. Individuals who accept change in life, make decisions about their lives, and are able to forgive others in times of difficulty have a higher level of spiritual well-being. During illness patients often are unable to accept limitations or do not know how to regain a functional and meaningful life. Their feelings and struggles often reflect spiritual distress. However, they often use their spiritual well-being as a resource for adapting to changes and dealing with limitations. Assess the extent to which a patient understands the limitations or threats posed by an illness (e.g., activity restriction, sexual intimacy with a partner, risk of medical complications) and the manner in which he or she chooses to adjust to them. Ask, "Tell me how you feel about the changes caused by your illness" and "How do these changes affect what you now need to do?"

Connectedness. People who are connected to themselves, others, nature, and God or another Supreme Being usually report higher levels of physical and emotional health (Hakanson and Ohlen, 2016). One way patients remain connected is by praying (Fig. 35.3). Prayer is personal communication with one's higher power that provides a sense of hope, strength, security, and well-being; it is a part of faith. Patients often use prayer when other treatments are ineffective, when they are experiencing fear or anxiety, or when they feel that they have no control over what is happening to them (Christensen et al., 2018; O'Brien, 2014). Help patients become or remain connected by respecting each patient's unique sense of spirituality. Assess a patient's connectedness by asking open-ended questions: "Whom do you believe is the most important person in your life?" "In what way do you stay connected spiritually?" "Is prayer something helpful to you?" or "What feeling do you have after you pray?"

Life Satisfaction. Spiritual well-being is tied to a person's satisfaction with life and what he or she has accomplished, even in the case of children (Dobratz, 2016). When people are satisfied with life and how they are using their abilities, more energy is available to deal with new difficulties and resolve problems. You assess a patient's satisfaction with life by asking questions such as "How happy or satisfied are you with your life?" or "Tell me how satisfied you feel about what you have accomplished in life" or "Describe what makes you feel dissatisfied with your life."

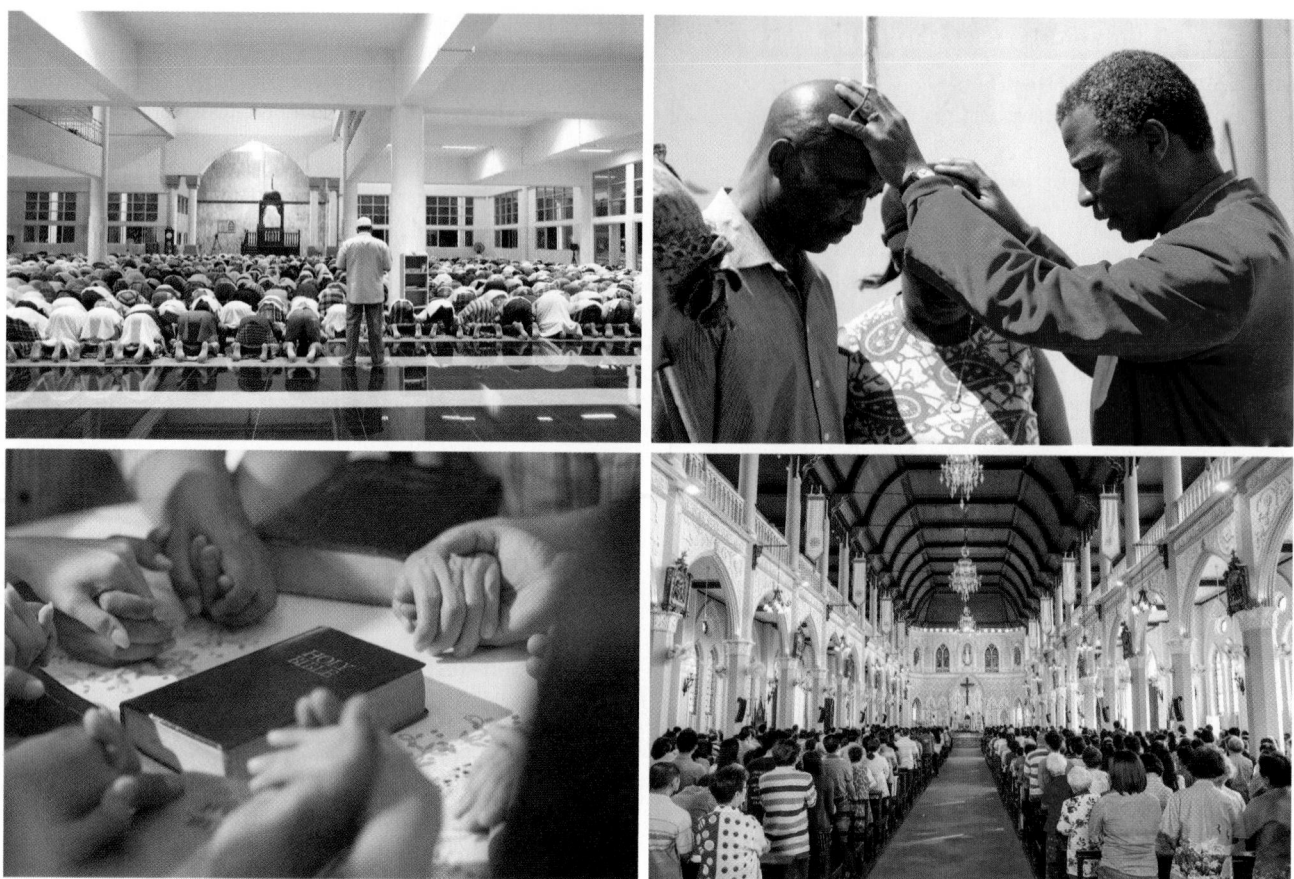

FIG. 35.3 Praying keeps individuals connected to their God. (Copyright © iStock/khunpepe; iStock/Gold-quest; iStock/palidachan; iStock/Sunshine Seeds.)

Culture. Spirituality is a personal experience within a cultural context. It is important to know a patient's cultural background and assess his or her values about the health care problem and impending treatment (see Chapter 9). It is common in many cultures for individuals to believe that they have led a worthwhile and purposeful life. Remaining connected with their cultural heritage often helps patients define their place in the world and express their spirituality. Asking them about their faith and belief systems is a good beginning for understanding the relationship between culture and spirituality (Box 35.3).

Fellowship and Community. Fellowship is one kind of relationship that an individual has with other people, including immediate family, close friends, associates at work or school, fellow members of a place of worship, and neighbors. More specifically, this includes the extent of the community of shared faith between people and their support networks. Many times social support from faith-based groups helps patients cope with illness and participate in health promotion behaviors (Plunkett et al., 2015). To assess a patient's supportive community, ask questions such as "Who do you find to be the greatest source of support in times of difficulty?" or "When you've faced difficult times in the past, who has been your greatest resource?"

Explore the extent and nature of a person's support networks and their relationship with the patient. It is unwise to assume that a given network offers the kind of support that a patient desires. For example, calling a patient's pastor to request a visit is inappropriate if the patient has little fellowship with the pastor or the pastor's faith community.

Does the patient have one significant fellowship or several? What level of support does the community give? Do they visit, say prayers, or support the patient's immediate family? Learn whether openness exists between a patient and the people with whom a fellowship has formed.

Ritual and Practice. Assessing the use of rituals and practices helps you understand a patient's spirituality. Rituals include participation in worship, prayer, sacraments (e.g., baptism, Holy Eucharist), fasting, singing, meditating, scripture reading, and making offerings or sacrifices. Different religions have different rituals for life events. For example, Buddhists practice baptism later in life and find burial or cremation acceptable at death. Followers of Islam practice Salah, the second of the Five Pillars of Islam, requiring all Muslims who have reached puberty to worship five times daily, facing the holy city of Mecca. Orthodox and conservative Jews circumcise their newborn sons 8 days after birth. Determine whether illness or hospitalization has interrupted a patient's ability to follow usual rituals or practices. A ritual often provides the patient with structure and support during difficult times. If rituals are important to a patient, use them as part of nursing intervention.

Vocation. Individuals express their spirituality on a daily basis in life routines, work, play, and relationships. It is often a part of a person's identity and vocation. Determine whether illness, injury, or hospitalization alters the ability to express some aspect of spirituality as it relates to the person's work or daily activities. Expression of spirituality includes showing an appreciation for life in the variety

BOX 35.3 CULTURAL ASPECTS OF CARE

Spirituality and Culture

Spirituality and spiritual health vary among cultures. Remember that a person's culture is defined by his or her age, gender, social position, political association, religion, or other variables such as ethnicity and educational background. One's culture influences religious practices as well as beliefs about health and illness. One way to assess a patient's spirituality through a cultural lens is to first understand his or her definition of health, wellness, and illness. For example, ask questions such as "What do you call your health problem?" "What do you think has caused it?" "What do you think your sickness does to you?" and "How do you find strength to cope with this problem?"

You want to assess how a patient's spirituality is affected by his or her culture. If your focus is on a patient's ethnicity, know the unique characteristics of that ethnic group's spiritual values. Ethnicity impacts culturally significant events such as birth, death, puberty, childbearing, child rearing, and illness and death (Giger, 2018). There are often rituals tied to spirituality and religion for events such as weddings, funerals, and holidays (Giger, 2018). Many cultures have treatments for illness and disease that are rooted in folk medicine, holistic care, or spiritual interventions

Implications for Patient-Centered Care

- Explore the spirituality of patients from different cultural backgrounds; assess the meaning of health and how patients achieve balance, stability, peace, or comfort in their lives.
- Offer a universal and holistic approach when assessing patients' needs (see Chapter 9); demonstrate cultural competence and use therapeutic communication techniques.
- During assessment respect patients' human rights, values, customs, and spiritual beliefs (see Chapter 9).
- Spiritual assessment should be interprofessional. If you feel uncomfortable with religion or spirituality, respectfully identify whether a patient wishes referral to an appropriate professional chaplain or clergy.
- Avoid use of language that alienates or discriminates among different cultures and belief systems.
- Use a professional interpreter if necessary.

BOX 35.4 Nursing Diagnostic Process

Decreased Spiritual Distress

Assessment Activities	Assessment Findings
Ask patient to describe personal source of faith and hope.	Patient expresses inner strength and source of guidance.
Have patient describe level of satisfaction with life.	Life has purpose and meaning; patient finds satisfaction while providing community service as a volunteer.
Determine who provides greatest source of strength and support to patient during times of difficulty.	Patient pursues interactions with friends and family.

REFLECT NOW

Consider how your own spiritual and religious beliefs influence your assessment of your patients' spiritual health. In what ways are you most effective; least effective?

◆ **Nursing Diagnosis**

A spiritual assessment allows a nurse to learn a great deal about a patient and the extent that spirituality plays in his or her life. Exploring a patient's spirituality sometimes reveals responses to health problems that require nursing intervention or the existence of a strong set of resources that allow the patient to cope effectively. Analyze data to find risk factors or patterns of assessment findings, and select appropriate nursing diagnoses (Box 35.4). In identifying diagnoses, recognize the significance that spirituality has for all types of health problems. Ensure that each negative or problem-focused nursing diagnosis has an accurate related factor to guide the selection of individualized, purposeful, and goal-directed interventions (Herdman and Katmisuru, 2018). Examples of nursing diagnoses that apply to spiritual health include the following:

- *Risk for Spiritual Status*
- *Decreased Spiritual Distress*
- *Hopelessness*
- *Powerlessness*
- *Spiritual Distress*

Decreased Spiritual Distress is based on assessment findings that show a person's ability to experience and integrate meaning and purpose in life through connectedness with self and others. A patient with this nursing diagnosis has potential resources on which to draw when faced with illness or a threat to well-being.

The nursing diagnosis *Spiritual Distress* creates a different clinical picture. Assessment findings reveal patterns that reflect a person's actual or potential dispiritedness (e.g., expressing lack of hope, meaning, or purpose in life; expressing anger toward God; or verbalizing conflicts about personal beliefs). Patients likely to experience spiritual distress include those who have poor relationships, have experienced a recent loss, or are suffering some form of mental or physical illness.

Accurate selection of diagnoses requires critical thinking. Review and analyze all concrete data (e.g., religious rituals and sources of fellowship), your assessment of previous patient experiences, your own spirituality, and your appraisal of the patient's spiritual well-being. Commonly patients have multiple nursing diagnoses.

of things people do, living in the moment and not worrying about tomorrow, appreciating nature, expressing love toward others, and being productive. When illness or loss prevents patients from expressing their spirituality, understand the psychological, social, and spiritual implications and provide appropriate guidance and support. Questions to ask include, "How has your illness affected the way you live your life spiritually at home or where you work?" or "How has your illness affected your ability to express what's important in life for you?"

> **QSEN** **Building Competency in Patient-Centered Care** You are caring for Amanda, a 32-year-old who experienced a miscarriage at 14 weeks' gestation. Amanda and her husband have been trying to get pregnant with their second child. They have a 4-year-old son at home. This is the second miscarriage that Amanda has experienced. When you walk into Amanda's room, she is staring out the window and does not turn her head. You can tell that she has been crying. She has a flat affect and states, "I just don't know why God did this to me again. How am I going to go on from here?"
>
> Identify at least three questions you will ask Amanda to assess her spiritual well-being and plan effective, patient-centered care.

Answers to QSEN Activities can be found on the Evolve website.

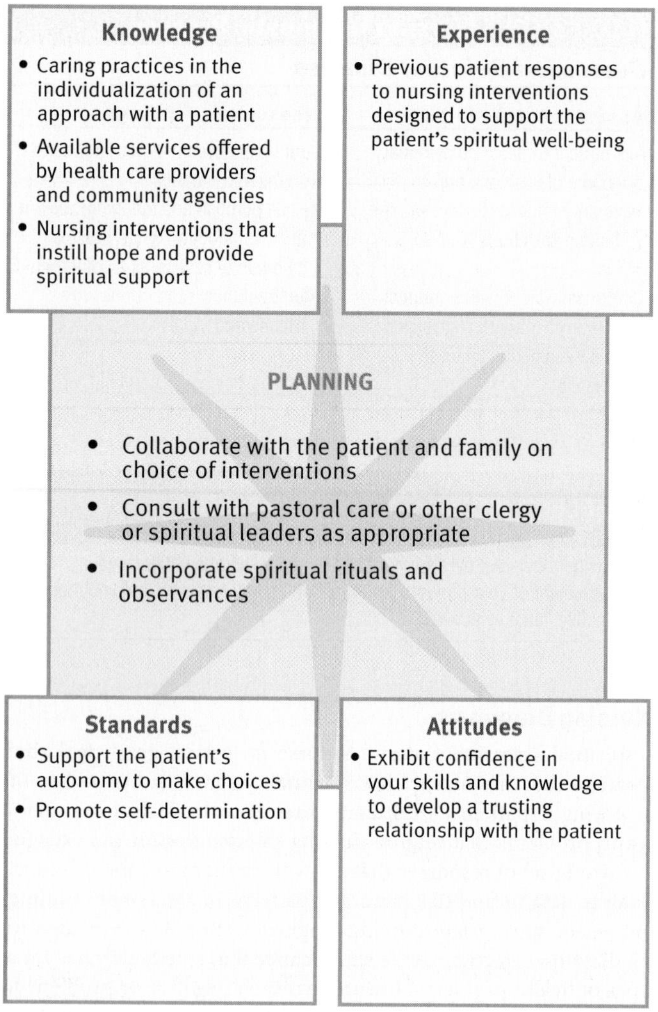

Knowledge	Experience
• Caring practices in the individualization of an approach with a patient • Available services offered by health care providers and community agencies • Nursing interventions that instill hope and provide spiritual support	• Previous patient responses to nursing interventions designed to support the patient's spiritual well-being

PLANNING

• Collaborate with the patient and family on choice of interventions

• Consult with pastoral care or other clergy or spiritual leaders as appropriate

• Incorporate spiritual rituals and observances

Standards	Attitudes
• Support the patient's autonomy to make choices • Promote self-determination	• Exhibit confidence in your skills and knowledge to develop a trusting relationship with the patient

FIG. 35.4 Critical thinking model for spiritual health planning.

◆ Planning

During the planning step of the nursing process, develop a plan of care for each of the patient's nursing diagnoses. Critical thinking at this step is important because you reflect on previous experiences and apply knowledge and critical thinking attitudes and standards in selecting the most appropriate nursing interventions (Fig. 35.4). Prior experience with other patients is valuable when selecting interventions to support spiritual well-being. Integrate assessment data with knowledge about resources and therapies available for spiritual care to develop an individualized plan of care (see the Nursing Care Plan). Match the patient's needs with evidence-based interventions that are supported and recommended in the clinical and research literature. Use a concept map (Fig. 35.5) to organize patient care and show how the patient's medical diagnosis, assessment data, and nursing diagnoses are interrelated.

Confidence, an important critical thinking attitude, builds trust, enabling you and a patient to enter into a healing relationship together. Attempting to meet or support patients' spiritual needs frequently requires the need of additional resources. Because spiritual care is so personal, standards of autonomy and self-determination are critical in supporting the patient's decisions about the plan of care.

Goals and Outcomes. A spiritual care plan includes realistic and individualized goals along with relevant outcomes. Goals for spiritual nursing care focus on helping patients integrate their own religious and spiritual beliefs with their health and illness states to give meaning to their lives (Andrews and Boyle, 2016). It is very important to collaborate closely with patients when setting goals for spiritual support and growth and choosing related interventions. Setting realistic goals requires you to know a patient well. When spiritual care requires helping patients adjust to loss or stressful life situations, goals are long term. However, short-term outcomes such as renewing participation in religious practices help patients progressively reach a more spiritually healthy situation. In establishing a plan of care, an example of a goal and associated outcomes follows:

The patient will improve personal harmony and connections with members of his or her support system.
- The patient expresses an acceptance of illness.
- The patient reports the ability to rely on family members for support.
- The patient initiates social interactions with family and friends.

Setting Priorities. Spiritual care is very personalized. Your relationship with a patient allows you to understand the patient's priorities in the context of his or her spiritual life. When establishing a mutually agreed-on plan with the patient, he or she is able to identify what is most important. Spiritual priorities do not need to be sacrificed for physical care priorities. For example, when a patient is in acute distress, focus care to provide him or her a sense of control to minimize powerlessness. When a patient is terminally ill, spiritual care often is the most important nursing intervention in supporting patients and families in grief (see Chapter 36).

Teamwork and Collaboration. If a patient participates in an organized religion, with permission of the patient, involve members of the clergy or church, temple, mosque, or synagogue in the plan of care when appropriate. In a hospital setting the pastoral care department is a valuable resource. These spiritual care professionals offer insight about how and when to best support patients and their families. Spiritual care providers provide direct support in the form of actively addressing spiritual or religious needs of a patient and family, having discussions about family members' feelings and patient values, and reminiscing with families about a patient (Veloza-Gomez et al., 2017). Significant others such as spouses, siblings, parents, and friends need to be involved in the patient's care as appropriate. This means that you learn from an assessment which individuals or groups have formed a relationship with the patient and which ones the patient desires to involve. These individuals sometimes participate in all levels of the plan of care. They often assist in giving physical care, providing emotional comfort, and sharing spiritual support.

◆ Implementation

After establishing a caring relationship with a patient and an individualized plan of care, you are able to implement a patient-centered care approach. Having a thorough understanding of a patient's spiritual needs enables you to deliver care in a sensitive, creative, and appropriate manner.

Health Promotion. Spiritual care needs to be a central theme in promoting an individual's overall well-being because of its importance in health promotion (Vlasblom et al., 2015). In settings where health promotion activities occur, patients often need information, counseling, and guidance to make the necessary choices to remain healthy.

Establishing Presence. Nurses contribute to a sense of well-being and provide hope for recovery when they spend time with their patients. Establishing presence by sitting with a patient to attentively listen to his or her feelings and situation, talking with the patient, accepting or supporting the patient's need to cry, and simply offering

NURSING CARE PLAN

Decreased Spiritual Distress

ASSESSMENT

Lisa Owens is a 61-year-old female who was diagnosed with stage IV breast cancer over 2 years ago. She has undergone numerous rounds of chemotherapy. Her husband, Richard, is 59 years old and a financial assistant at a local bank. The Owenses have two adult children, with one daughter who is unmarried and lives 2 miles away. The other child, a son, is married; his wife is pregnant, and they live out of town. Lisa has numerous side effects from her advancing disease and chemotherapy. She has ongoing hip pain from the cancer spread to the bone, reduced sensation in her feet, chronic fatigue, and difficulty in sleeping. Her husband provides most of her support at home, but this sometimes interferes with his ability to do the work that he brings home. Lisa is coming to the outpatient chemotherapy infusion center to begin another course of chemotherapy. The nurse who has been seeing Lisa knows that she regularly attends church with her husband.

Assessment Activities	Assessment Findings [a]
Ask Lisa to describe what it is about her cancer that frightens her most.	Lisa explains, "I have found it makes me appreciate what I have with my family. That being said, I worry that I will not see my grandchild born, **but I hope the chemotherapy will give me some time and it will make me feel a bit better.**"
Have Lisa tell you whom she finds to be the greatest source of support since she has been taking chemotherapy.	Lisa has received support from her husband and daughter. **She wants to be able to show them her love, saying, "I still want to be there for them."**
Ask Lisa whether she feels satisfaction with her life.	Lisa responds, "We always want more, don't we? **I have been blessed, but I think God gave me this illness so I can show others what life means**."

[a]**Assessment Findings** are shown in bold type.

NURSING DIAGNOSIS: Decreased Spiritual Distress

PLANNING

Goals	Expected Outcomes (NOC)[b]
	Spiritual Health
Lisa will express a personal sense of spiritual well-being.	Lisa engages in regular prayer and meditation.
	Lisa expresses her feelings through writing.

[b]Outcome classification labels from Moorhead S, et al: *Nursing Outcomes Classification (NOC)*, ed 6, St Louis, 2018, Elsevier.

INTERVENTIONS (NIC)[c]	RATIONALE
Spiritual Growth Facilitation	
Plan discussions with Lisa during treatment and listen, allowing her to sort out concerns she might have about her future. Include Lisa's husband if she desires.	Listening provides support or comfort in spiritual care (Veloza-Gomez et al., 2017). Building a therapeutic relationship is important to providing spiritual care (Minton et al., 2018).
Offer to pray with Lisa as she describes what she hopes for.	Individualized spiritual interventions in patients with cancer can improve spiritual well-being and decrease depression (Pantuso, 2015).
Introduce Lisa to journaling. Encourage her to begin by writing what is meaningful to her about her illness and family	The use of journaling helps individuals facing a crisis deal with the unknown and express their feelings; find meaning and spiritual connection; and physically, emotionally, and spiritually heal (Connerton and Moe, 2018; Neathery, 2018).
Spiritual Support	
Discuss with Lisa the likely times that her chemotherapy will affect her most and how she can schedule involvement in church activities around those times.	Chemotherapy can cause severe fatigue. Faith communities such as a church play an important role in fostering belief systems (Timmins, 2015).
Teach Lisa methods of relaxation, meditation, and guided imagery.	Relaxation methods help promote quality of life and enhance serenity and dignity. Relaxation responses have been associated with improved physiological (blood pressure, exercise capacity, and cardiac symptoms) and psychological (depression and anxiety) outcomes (Heo et al., 2018; Pantuso, 2015).

[c]Intervention classification labels from Butcher HK, et al: *Nursing Interventions Classification (NIC)*, ed 7, St Louis, 2018, Elsevier.

EVALUATION

Evaluation Activity	Patient Response/Finding	Outcome Status
Ask Lisa to describe in what way meditation exercises have helped her.	Lisa reported using meditation daily after being at clinic. She states, "I feel calm. It allows me to connect with God, and know I have my loving family to help me."	Lisa finds meditation to be a helpful way to enhance her spirituality and well-being.
Have Lisa review her discussions with family and/or church members.	Lisa reports, "We have been talking more. My family knows that I see each day as a blessing and that my hope is to see my son's baby. My church really keeps me connected."	Enhanced connectedness is positively affecting sense of spiritual well-being.

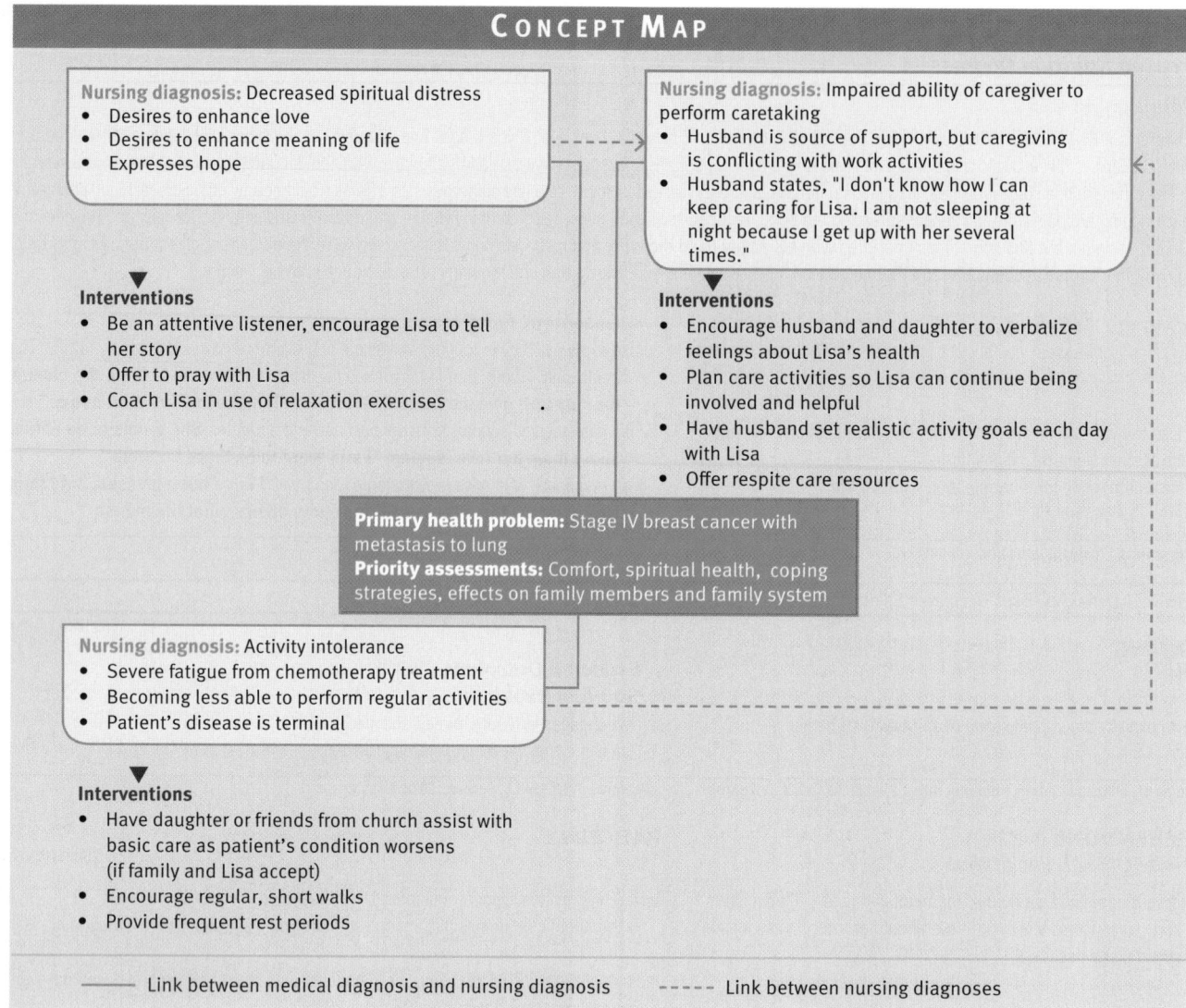

FIG. 35.5 Concept map for Lisa Owens.

time are powerful spiritual care approaches (Carson, 2017). Presence is part of the art of nursing. Benner (1984) explains that presence involves "being with" a patient versus "doing for" a patient. It is being able to offer closeness with a patient physically, psychologically, and spiritually. It helps to prevent emotional and environmental isolation (see Chapter 7).

When health promotion is the focus of care, your presence gives patients the confidence needed to discuss ways to remain healthy. Show your caring presence by listening to patients' concerns; when appropriate, involve family members in discussions about patients' health. Show self-confidence when providing health instruction, and support patients as they make decisions about their health. The patient who seeks health care is often fearful of experiencing an illness that threatens loss of control and looks for someone to offer competent direction. Encouraging words of support and a calm, decisive approach establish a presence that builds trust and well-being.

Supporting a Healing Relationship. Learn to look beyond isolated patient problems and recognize the broader picture of a patient's holistic needs. For example, do not just look at a patient's back pain as a problem to solve with quick remedies; rather look at how the pain influences his or her ability to function and achieve goals established in life. A **holistic** view enables you to establish a helping role and a healing relationship. Three factors are evident when a healing relationship develops between nurse and patient:

1. Realistically mobilizing hope for the nurse and patient
2. Finding an interpretation or understanding of the illness, pain, anxiety, or other stressful emotion that is acceptable to the patient
3. Helping the patient use social, emotional, and spiritual resources (Benner, 1984)

Mobilizing a patient's hope is central to a healing relationship. Hope motivates people to face challenges in life (Broadhurst and Harrington, 2015). Help patients find things for which to hope. For example, help a patient newly diagnosed with diabetes learn how to manage the disease in a way that will allow the patient to continue a productive and satisfying way of life. An adult daughter who has decided to become caregiver to her older adult parent hopes to be able to protect the parent from injury or worsening disability. You instruct the daughter on basic care skills so that her hope can be realistic. Hope is future oriented and helps a patient work toward goals (Yarcheski and Mahon, 2016). Hope helps patients work toward recovery. To help patients achieve hope, work together to find an explanation for their situation that is acceptable to them. Help a patient realistically exercise hope by supporting positive attitudes toward life or the desire to be informed and make decisions.

Remain aware of a patient's spiritual resources and needs. It is always important for patients to be able to express and exercise their beliefs and find spiritual comfort. When life stressors or chronic illness create confusion or uncertainty, recognize the potential effect on a patient's well-being. How do you use and strengthen spiritual resources? Begin by encouraging a patient to discuss the effect that an illness has had on personal beliefs and faith, thus giving the chance to clarify any misconceptions or inaccuracies in information. Having a clear sense of what illness will be like helps an individual apply many resources toward recovery.

Acute Care. Within acute care settings patients experience multiple stressors that threaten their sense of control. Ongoing assessment of spiritual needs is essential because a patient's needs often change rapidly. Support and enhancement of a patient's spiritual well-being are challenges when the focus of health care seems to be on treatment and cure rather than care. Lack of time, lack of education or training, language barriers, confusion over one's own spirituality, lack of family involvement, and patient privacy are other barriers to spiritual care in acute care settings (Chen et al., 2017a; Vlasblom et al., 2015). To meet these challenges, display a soothing presence and supportive touch when providing care. The artful use of hands, encouraging words of support, promotion of connectedness, and a calm and decisive approach establish a nurse presence that builds trust.

Support Systems. Use of support systems is important for patients who are in any health care setting. They provide patients with the greatest sense of well-being during hospitalization and serve as a human link connecting the patient, the nurse, and the patient's lifestyle before an illness. Part of a patient's caregiving environment is the regular presence of supportive family and friends. Provide privacy during visits and plan care with the patient and the patient's support network to promote the interpersonal bonding that is needed for recovery. The support system is a source of faith and hope and an important resource in conducting meaningful religious rituals.

When patients look to family and friends for support, encourage them to visit the patient regularly. Help family members feel comfortable in the health care setting, and use their support and presence to promote the patient's healing. For example, including family members in prayer is a thoughtful gesture if it is appropriate to the patient's religion and if the patient and family members are comfortable with participating together. Having the family bring meaningful spiritual or religious symbols to the patient's bedside offers significant spiritual support.

Other important resources to patients are spiritual advisers and members of the clergy. Collaboration with these individuals fosters an interprofessional approach to patient care (Bone et al., 2018). Professional spiritual care providers, such as chaplains, have expertise in understanding how an illness influences a person's beliefs and how these beliefs influence the patient's responses to illness, recovery, or preparation for death. When members of the clergy are requested by patients or families, keep clergy informed of any physical, psychosocial, or spiritual concerns affecting the patient. A spiritual care provider is especially helpful in discussing patient and family wishes about end-of-life care (Ruth-Sahd et al., 2018) (see Chapter 36). Respect patients' spiritual values and needs by allowing time for pastoral care members to provide spiritual care and facilitating the administration of sacraments, rites, and rituals.

TABLE 35.2 Religious Dietary Regulations Affecting Health Care

Religion	Dietary Practices
Hinduism	Some sects are vegetarians. The belief is not to kill *any* living creature.
Buddhism	Some are vegetarians and do not use alcohol. Many fast on Holy Days.
Islam	Consumption of pork and alcohol is prohibited. Followers fast during the month of Ramadan.
Judaism	Some observe the kosher dietary restrictions (e.g., avoid pork and shellfish, do not prepare and eat milk and meat at same time).
Christianity	Some Baptists, Evangelicals, and Pentecostals discourage use of alcohol and caffeine. Some Roman Catholics fast on Ash Wednesday and Good Friday. Some do not eat meat on Fridays during Lent.
Jehovah's Witnesses	Members avoid food prepared with or containing blood.
Mormonism	Members abstain from alcohol and caffeine.
Russian Orthodox Church	Followers observe fast days and a "no-meat" rule on Wednesdays and Fridays. During Lent all animal products, including dairy products and butter, are forbidden.
Native Americans	Individual tribal beliefs influence food practices.

Diet Therapies. The intake of food satisfies and promotes a sense of comfort. Food and nutrition are important aspects of patient care and often an important component of some religious observances (Table 35.2). Food and the rituals surrounding the preparation and serving of food are sometimes important to a person's spirituality. Consult with a dietitian to integrate patients' dietary preferences into daily care. In the event that a hospital or other health care agency cannot prepare food in the preferred way, ask the family to bring meals that fit into dietary restrictions posed by the patient's condition.

Supporting Rituals. Nurses provide spiritual care by supporting patients' participation in spiritual rituals and activities. Plan care to allow time for religious readings, spiritual visitations, or attendance at religious services. Allow family members to plan a prayer session or an organized reading of scriptures or the Koran on a regular basis. Make arrangements with spiritual care professionals, at the request of the patient, for the patient and family to participate in religious practices (e.g., receiving sacraments). Clergy often visit people who are unable to attend religious services. Taped meditations, classical or religious music, and televised religious services provide other effective options. Always respect the icons, medals, prayer rugs, crosses, or other items that a patient brings to a health care setting, and ensure that they are not accidentally lost, damaged, or misplaced. Supporting spiritual rituals is especially important for older adults (Box 35.5).

Restorative and Continuing Care. For patients who are recovering from a long-term disability or who suffer from chronic or terminal disease, spiritual care becomes especially important. Many of the nursing interventions applicable in health promotion and acute care apply to this level of health care as well.

Prayer. The act of prayer gives an individual the opportunity to renew personal faith and belief in a higher being in a specific, focused way that is either highly ritualized and formal or quite spontaneous and

BOX 35.5 FOCUS ON OLDER ADULTS
Spirituality and Spiritual Health

- There is an association between an older adult's spirituality and his or her ability to adjust or cope with illness and other life stressors (Chen et al., 2017b).
- Older adults achieve spiritual resilience by frequently expressing gratitude (e.g., via prayer, meditation, or discussions with friends) and finding ways to maintain purpose in life (e.g., helping family, volunteering) (Manning, 2014).
- Religious activities, attitudes, and spiritual experiences are very common among older adults. Older adults who experience spiritual well-being have better emotional health, experience a sense of peace that helps them accept life transitions, and experience to some extent improved physical health (Dahlkemper, 2016).
- Enhance connectedness by helping older patients find meaning and purpose in life by listening actively to concerns and being present (Dahlkemper, 2016).
- Beliefs in the afterlife increase as adults age. Offer to coordinate visits from clergy, social workers, lawyers, and financial advisers so that patients feel as though they have completed all unfinished business. Leaving a legacy (e.g., oral history, art, photographs) to loved ones prepares an older adult to leave the world with a sense of meaning and maintains a way to continue connection for the one left behind (Touhy and Jett, 2018).
- Greater social support in older adults positively impacts spiritual well-being (Chen et al., 2017b).

BOX 35.6 PATIENT TEACHING
Meditation Techniques

Objective
- The patient will verbalize feelings of relaxation and self-transcendence after meditation.

Teaching Strategies
- Give patient a brief description of information and a printed teaching guide that describes how to meditate.
- Prepare a space: Simple things such as lighting a candle, turning off a cell phone, or sitting in a special quiet room or place that has minimal interruptions can support meditation practice.
- Set an intention or ask a question: This sets a direction for meditation. Have the patient ask an open-ended question such as "What is my purpose?" or "Who/what am I?"
- Explain that peaceful music or the quiet whirring of a fan also blocks out distractions.
- Teach steps of meditation (i.e., sit in a comfortable position with the back straight; breathe slowly; and focus on a sound, prayer, or image).
- Encourage patient to meditate for 10 to 20 minutes twice a day.
- Answer questions and reinforce information as needed.

Evaluation
Use the principles of teach-back to evaluate patient/family caregiver learning:
- How did you feel after meditating?
- What did you learn about yourself while doing meditation?

informal. For example, a patient may choose to say a prayer just before leaving for a surgical procedure. A patient who is a follower of Islam will want to say daily prayers (Salah) five times a day. Prayer is an effective coping resource for physical and psychological symptoms (deAndrade Alvarenga et al., 2017). Patients pray in private or participate in group prayer with family, friends, or clergy. Muslims must be clean before they pray, so offer hygiene measures according to Islam practices (Islamic Supreme Council of America, 2019). Some pray while listening to music. Be supportive of prayer by giving the patient privacy if desired, learning whether the patient wishes to have you participate, and suggesting prayer when you know that it is a coping resource for the patient. You can also be present with the patient through offering to spend several minutes of silence with the patient (Christensen et al., 2018). Delgado (2015) found that nurses tend to pray for patients rather than with patients; sharing the fact that prayer has been offered gives patients comfort and support. Alternatives include listening to calming music or reading a book, poetry, or inspirational texts selected by the patient.

Meditation. Meditation creates a relaxation response that reduces daily stress. Patients who meditate often state that they have an increased awareness of their spirituality and of the presence of God or a Supreme Being. Meditation improves symptoms and depression in patients and helps patients move from negative to positive thoughts (Heo et al., 2018). Meditation exercises give patients relief from pain, insomnia, anxiety, and depression and increase coping and the ability to relax (Starkweather, 2017). Meditation involves sitting quietly in a comfortable position with eyes closed and repeating a sound, phrase, or sacred word in rhythm with breathing while disregarding intrusive thoughts. Individuals who meditate regularly (twice a day for 10 or 20 minutes) may experience decreased metabolism and heart rate, easier breathing, and slower brain waves (Box 35.6). Chapter 32 addresses relaxation approaches.

Supporting Grief Work. Patients who experience terminal illness or who have suffered permanent loss of body function because of a disabling disease or injury require a nurse's support in grieving and coping with their loss. Your ability to enter into a caring, therapeutic, and spiritual relationship with patients supports them during times of grief (see Chapter 36).

◆ Evaluation

Through the Patient's Eyes. The evaluation of a patient's spiritual care requires you to think critically in determining whether efforts at restoring or maintaining the patient's spiritual health were successful (Fig. 35.6). This requires including the patient by determining whether his or her expectations were met. Ask patients whether you and the health care team met their expectations or whether there was anything else you could have done to enhance their spiritual well-being or to enable them to practice important religious rituals. Additionally, asking a patient "Have you felt comfortable in saying what you feel is important to you spiritually?" will help determine whether you developed an effective healing relationship. In addition, evaluate any other concerns that arise in the course of the patient's spiritual care and support. Apply critical thinking attitudes and use therapeutic communication techniques to ensure sound nursing judgments.

Patient Outcomes. Attaining spiritual health is a lifelong process. In evaluating outcomes established during the planning phase, compare a patient's level of spiritual health with the behaviors and perceptions noted in the nursing assessment. Evaluation data related to spiritual health are usually subjective. For example, if your assessment finds the patient losing hope, the follow-up evaluation involves asking him or her whether feelings of hope have been restored. Include family and friends, as appropriate, when gathering evaluative information. Successful outcomes reveal the patient developing an increased or restored sense of connectedness with family; maintaining, renewing, or reforming a sense of purpose in life; and for some a confidence and

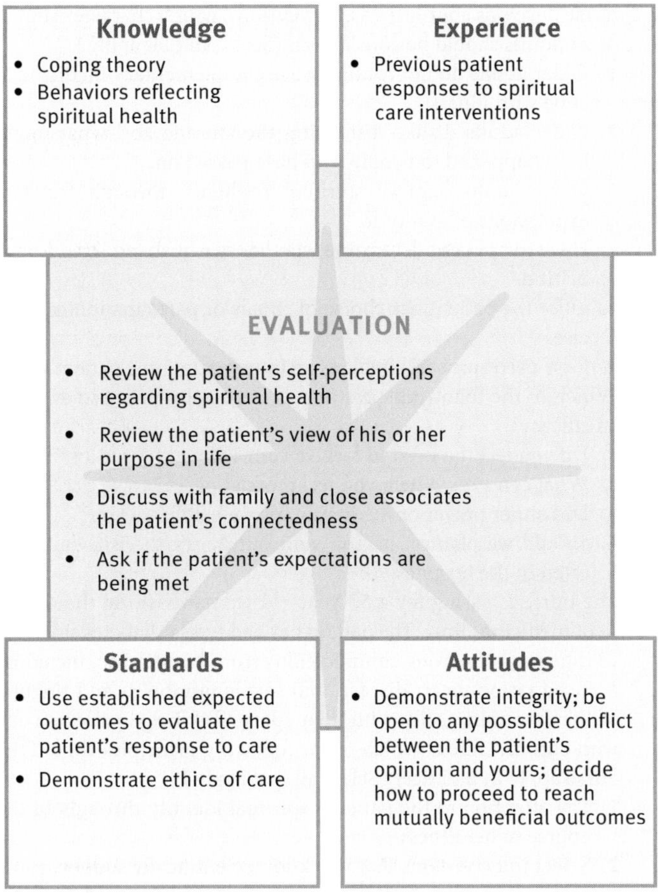

Knowledge
- Coping theory
- Behaviors reflecting spiritual health

Experience
- Previous patient responses to spiritual care interventions

EVALUATION
- Review the patient's self-perceptions regarding spiritual health
- Review the patient's view of his or her purpose in life
- Discuss with family and close associates the patient's connectedness
- Ask if the patient's expectations are being met

Standards
- Use established expected outcomes to evaluate the patient's response to care
- Demonstrate ethics of care

Attitudes
- Demonstrate integrity; be open to any possible conflict between the patient's opinion and yours; decide how to proceed to reach mutually beneficial outcomes

FIG. 35.6 Critical thinking model for spiritual health evaluation.

trust in a Supreme Being or power. When outcomes are not met, ask questions to determine appropriate continuing care. Examples of questions to ask include the following:
- Do you feel the need to forgive someone or to be forgiven by someone?
- Which spiritual activities such as prayer or meditation were helpful to you?
- Would you like for me to ask a friend, family member, or someone from pastoral care to talk with you?
- What can I do to help you feel more at peace?
- Sometimes people need to give themselves permission to feel hope when they experience difficult events. What can you do to allow yourself to feel hope again?

KEY POINTS

- Research shows that spirituality positively affects and enhances physical and psychological health, quality of life, health promotion behaviors, and disease prevention activities.
- Faith and hope are closely linked to a person's spiritual well-being, providing an inner strength for dealing with illness and disability.
- Spirituality is a much broader and more unifying concept than religion, as it is an inherent human characteristic that gives individuals the energy needed to discover themselves, cope with difficult situations, and maintain health.
- Religion differs from spirituality in that it is an organized, institution-related practice that is commonly associated with particular beliefs.

- Nursing assessment of a patient's spiritual needs includes a review of the patient's faith, connectedness, life and self-responsibility, life satisfaction, and fellowship and community.
- An assessment includes patients' cultural backgrounds, including their values about health care problems and impending treatments.
- Learning to practice caring and compassion helps you discover a patient's life values and meaning.
- The personal nature of spirituality requires open communication and the establishment of trust between you and a patient.
- Spiritual care providers provide direct support in the form of actively addressing spiritual or religious needs of a patient and family and having discussions about family members' feelings and patient values.
- Prayer is an evidence-based coping resource for physical and psychological symptoms.
- Common religious rituals include private worship, prayer, singing, use of a rosary, and scripture reading.
- Establishing presence involves attentive listening, talking with patients and answering questions, conveying a sense of trust, and simply offering your time.
- During evaluation successful outcomes reveal a patient developing an increased or restored sense of connectedness with family and maintaining, renewing, or reforming a sense of purpose in life.

REFLECTIVE LEARNING

- Using the FICA assessment tool, complete a personal assessment of your own spirituality.
- Select a patient that you will be assigned to care for during the next week. Assess for and describe the spiritual needs of that patient.
- Discuss the interventions you used to meet the spiritual needs of that patient.

REVIEW QUESTIONS

1. The nurse is caring for a patient who has just had a near-death experience (NDE) following a cardiac arrest. Which intervention by the nurse best promotes the spiritual well-being of the patient after the NDE?
   1. Allowing the patient to discuss the experience
   2. Referring the patient to pastoral care
   3. Having the patient talk to another patient who had an NDE
   4. Offering to pray for the patient
2. The nurse is caring for a patient who is very depressed and decides to complete a spiritual assessment using the FICA tool. Using the FICA assessment tool, match the criteria on the left with the appropriate assessment question on the right.

1. F—Faith ____	a. Tell me if you have a higher power or authority that helps you act on your beliefs
2. I—Importance of spirituality ____	b. Describe which activities give you comfort spiritually
3. C—Community ____	c. To whom do you go for support in times of difficulty?
4. A—Interventions to address spiritual needs ____	d. Your illness has kept you from attending church. Is that a problem for you?

3. Which statement made by a patient who is recovering after recently experiencing third-degree burns shows connectedness?
   1. "My pain medicine helps me feel better."
   2. "I know I will get better if I just keep trying."

3. "I see God's grace and become relaxed when I watch the sun set at night."

4. "I feel so much closer to God after I read my Bible and pray."

4. A nurse is caring for a patient who is Muslim and has diabetes. Which of the following items does the nurse need to remove from the meal tray when it is delivered to the patient?
   1. Small container of vanilla ice cream
   2. A dozen red grapes
   3. Bacon and eggs
   4. Garden salad with ranch dressing

5. A 44-year-old male patient has just been told that his wife and child were killed in an auto accident while coming to visit him in the hospital. Which of the following statements are assessment findings that support a nursing diagnosis of *Spiritual Distress related to loss of family members*? (Select all that apply.)
   1. "I need to call my sister for support."
   2. "I have nothing to live for now."
   3. "Why would my God do this to me?"
   4. "I need to pray for a miracle."
   5. "I want to be more involved in my church."

6. A patient has just learned she has been diagnosed with a malignant brain tumor. She is alone; her family will not be arriving from out of town for an hour. The nurse has been caring for her for only 2 hours but has a good relationship with her. What is the most appropriate intervention for support of her spiritual well-being at this time?
   1. Make a referral to a professional spiritual care adviser.
   2. Sit down and talk with the patient; have her discuss her feelings and listen attentively.
   3. Move the patient's Bible from her bedside cabinet drawer to the top of the over-bed table.
   4. Ask the patient whether she would like to learn more about the implications of having this type of tumor.

7. A nurse is preparing to teach an older adult who has chronic arthritis how to practice meditation. Which of the following strategies are appropriate? (Select all that apply.)
   1. Encourage family members to participate in the exercise.
   2. Have patient identify a quiet room in the home that has minimal interruptions.
   3. Suggest the use of a quiet fan running in the room.
   4. Explain that it is best to meditate about 5 minutes 4 times a day.
   5. Show the patient how to sit comfortably with the limitation of his arthritis and focus on a prayer.

8. A nursing student is developing a plan of care for a 74-year-old-female patient who has spiritual distress over losing a spouse. As the nurse develops appropriate interventions, which characteristics of older adults should be considered? (Select all that apply.)
   1. Older adults do not routinely use complementary medicine to cope with illness.
   2. Older adults dislike discussing the afterlife and what might have happened to people who have passed on.
   3. Older adults achieve spiritual resilience through frequent expressions of gratitude.
   4. Have the patient determine whether her husband left a legacy behind.
   5. Offer the patient her choice of rituals or participation in exercise.

9. A nurse used spiritual rituals as an intervention in a patient's care. Which of the following questions is most appropriate to evaluate its efficacy?
   1. Do you feel the need to forgive your wife over your loss?
   2. What can I do to help you feel more at peace?
   3. Did either prayer or meditation prove helpful to you?
   4. Should we plan on having your family try to visit you more often in the hospital?

10. The nurse is caring for a 50-year-old woman visiting the outpatient medicine clinic. The patient has had type 1 diabetes since age 13. She has numerous complications from her disease, including reduced vision, heart disease, and severe numbness and tingling of the extremities. Knowing that spirituality helps patients cope with chronic illness, which of the following principles should the nurse apply in practice? (Select all that apply.)
   1. Pay attention to the patient's spiritual identity throughout the course of her illness.
   2. Select interventions that you know scientifically support spiritual well-being.
   3. Listen to the patient's story each visit to the clinic, and offer a compassionate presence.
   4. When the patient questions the reason for her long-time suffering, try to provide answers.
   5. Consult with a spiritual care adviser, and have the adviser recommend useful interventions.

Answers: 1. 1; **2.** 1a, 2d, 3c, 4b; **3.** 4; **4.** 3; **5.** 2, 3; **6.** 2; **7.** 2, 3, 5; **8.** 3, 4, 5; **9.** 3; **10.** 1, 3;

Rationales for Review Questions can be found on the Evolve website.

REFERENCES

Abuatiq A: Spiritual care of critical care patients, *Int J Nurs Clin Pract* 2:128, 2015.

American Nurses Association (ANA): *Code of ethics for nurses with interpretive statements*, 2015. https://www.nursingworld.org/coe-view-only. Accessed January 2019.

American Nurses Association (ANA), American Psychiatric Nurses Association (APA), and International Society of Psychiatric–Mental Health Nurses (ISPN): *Psychiatric–mental health nursing: scope and standards of practice*, ed 2, Washington, DC, 2014, ANA.

Andrews MM, Boyle JS: *Transcultural concepts in nursing care*, ed 7, Philadelphia, 2016, Wolters Kluwer.

Benner P: *From novice to expert*, Menlo Park, CA, 1984, Addison-Wesley.

Caplan S: Culture. In Giddens JF, editor: *Concepts for nursing practice*, ed 2, St Louis, 2017, Elsevier.

Carron R: Spirituality. In Larsen PD, editor: *Lubkin's chronic illness: impact and intervention*, ed 9, Burlington, MA, 2016, Jones and Bartlett Learning.

Carson VB: Spirituality. In Giddens JF, editor: *Concepts for nursing practice*, ed 2, St Louis, 2017, Elsevier.

Christensen AR, et al.: How should clinicians respond to requests from patients to participate in prayer? *AMA J Ethics* 20(7):621, 2018.

Christman SK, Mueller JR: Understanding spiritual care: the faith-hope-love model of spiritual wellness, *J Christ Nurs* 34(1):e1, 2017.

Connerton CS, Moe CS: The essence of spiritual care, *Creative Nursing* 24(1):36, 2018.

Dahlkemper TR: *Anderson's caring for older adults holistically*, ed 6, Philadelphia, 2016, FA Davis.

Darnell L, Hickson S: Cultural competent patient-centered nursing care, *Nurs Clin North Am* 50(1):99, 2015.

deAndrade Alvarenga W, et al.: The possibilities and challenges in providing pediatric spiritual care, *J Child Health Care* 21(4):435, 2017.

Dobratz MC: Building a middle-range theory of adaptive spirituality, *Nurs Sci Q* 29(2):146, 2016.

Estores IM, Frye J: Healing environments: integrative medicine and palliative care in acute care settings, *Crit Care Nurs Clin North Am* 27:369, 2015.

Finocchiaro DN: Supporting the patient's spiritual needs at the end of life, *Nursing* 46(5):57, 2016.

Giger JN: In *Transcultural nursing: assessment and intervention*, 7e, St Louis, 2018, Elsevier.

Herdman TH, Kamitsuru S, editors: *NANDA International nursing diagnoses: definitions and classification, 2018-2020*, 11e, New York, 2018, Thieme Publishers.

HealthCare Chaplaincy Network: *What is quality spiritual care in health care and how do you measure it?* 2016. https://www.healthcarechaplaincy.org/docs/research/quality_indicators_document_2_17_16.pdf. Accessed January 2019.

Islamic Supreme Council of America: *Ritual prayer: its meaning and manner*, 2019. http://www.islamicsupremecouncil.org/understanding-islam/legal-rulings/53-ritual-prayer-its-meaning-and-manner.html. Accessed January 2019.

Jehovah's Witnesses: *Why don't Jehovah's Witnesses accept blood transfusions?* 2019. https://www.jw.org/en/jehovahs-witnesses/faq/jehovahs-witnesses-why-no-blood-transfusions/. Accessed January 2019.

Johnson S: Near-death experience in patients on hemodialysis, *Nephrol Nurs J* 42(4):331, 2015.

Life Advance: *The spiritual well-being scale*, 2009. http://www.lifeadvance.com/spiritual-well-being-scale.html. Accessed January 2019.

March P, Caple C: Evidence-based care sheet: spiritual needs of hospitalized patients, *CINAHL Information Systems*, April 29, 2016.

Neathery M: Treatment and spiritual care in mental health recovery as a journey, not a destination, *J Christ Nurs* 35(2):86, 2018.

O'Brien ME: *Spirituality in nursing: standing on holy ground*, ed 5, Washington DC, 2014, Jones and Bartlett.

QSEN Institute: *QSEN competencies*, 2018. http://qsen.org/competencies/pre-licensure-ksas/.

Rinpoche KT: *The Four Noble Truths and the eightfold path*, 2017. http://www.samyeling.org/buddhism-and-meditation/teaching-archive-2/kenchen-thrangu-rinpoche/the-four-noble-truths-and-the-eightfold-path/. Accessed January 2019.

Ruth-Sahd LA, et al.: Collaborating with hospital chaplains to meet the spiritual needs of critical care patients, *Dimens Crit Care Nurs* 37(1):18, 2018.

Starkweather A: Pain. In Giddens JF, editor: *Concepts for nursing practice*, ed 2, St Louis, 2017, Elsevier.

Sweat MT: How do I spiritually support those who are suffering and in pain? *J Christ Nurs* 32(2):123, 2015.

The Joint Commission (TJC): *2018 Comprehensive Accreditation Manual*, Oak Brook, IL, 2017, The Joint Commission.

Touhy TA, Jett KF: In *Ebersole & Hess' gerontological nursing & healthy aging*, ed 5, St Louis, 2018, Elsevier.

RESEARCH REFERENCES

Alemdar DK, et al.: The effect of spiritual care on stress levels of mothers in NICU, *West J Nurs Res* 40(7):997, 2018.

Bai M, et al.: Exploring the individual patterns of spiritual well-being in people newly diagnosed with advanced cancer: a cluster analysis, *Qual Life Res* 25:2765, 2016.

Bernard M, et al.: Relationship between spirituality, meaning in life, psychological distress, wish for hastened death, and their influence on quality of life in palliative care patients, *J Pain Symptom Manage* 54(4):574, 2017.

Berning JN, et al.: A novel picture guide to improve spiritual care and reduce anxiety in mechanically ventilated adults in the intensive care unit, *Ann Am Thorac Soc* 13(8):1333, 2016.

Boman E, et al.: Inner strength and its relationship to health threats in ageing – a cross-sectional study among community-dwelling older women, *J Adv Nurs* 73:2720, 2017.

Bone N, et al.: Critical care nurses' experience with spiritual care: the SPIRIT study, *Am J Crit Care* 27(3):212, 2018.

Borneman T, et al.: Evaluation of the FICA tool for spiritual assessment, *J Pain Symptom Manage* 40(2):163, 2010.

Broadhurst K, Harrington A: A mixed method thematic review: the importance of hope to the dying patient, *J Adv Nurs* 72(1):18, 2015.

Chen SC, et al.: Nurses' perceptions of psychosocial care and barriers to its provision: a qualitative study, *J Nurs Res* 25(6):411, 2017a.

Chen Y, et al.: The relationship of physiopsychosocial factors and spiritual well-being in elderly residents: implications for evidence-based practice, *Worldviews Evid Based Nurs* 14(6):484, 2017b.

Chiang YC, et al.: The impact of nurses' spiritual health on their attitudes toward spiritual care, professional commitment, and caring, *Nurs Outlook* 64(3):215, 2016.

Cottrell L: Joy and happiness: a simultaneous and evolutionary concept analysis, *J Adv Nurs* 72(7):1506, 2016.

Delgado C: Nurses' spiritual care practices: becoming less religious? *J Christ Nurs* 32(2):116, 2015.

Ebrahimi H, et al.: Health care providers' perception of their competence in providing spiritual care for patients, *Indian J Palliat Care* 23(1):57, 2017.

Fabbris JL, et al.: Anxiety and spiritual well-being in nursing students: a cross-sectional study, *J Holist Nurs* 35(3):261, 2017.

Fan Y, et al.: Cortisol level modulated by integrative medication in a dose-dependent fashion, *Stress Health* 30(1):65, 2014.

Griggs S, Walker RK: The role of hope for adolescents with a chronic illness: an integrative review, *J Pediatr Nurs* 31:404, 2016.

Hakanson C, Ohlen J: Connectedness at the end of life among people admitted to inpatient palliative care, *Am J Hospice Palliat Care* 33(1):47, 2016.

Hatamipour K, et al.: Spiritual needs of cancer patients: a qualitative study, *Indian J Palliat Care* 21(1):61, 2015.

Haugan G, et al.: The relationships between self-transcendence and spiritual well-being in cognitively intact nursing home patients, *Int J Older People Nurs* 9(1):65, 2014.

Hefner J, et al.: Adherence and coping strategies in outpatients with chronic myeloid leukemia receiving oral tyrosine kinase inhibitors, *Oncol Nurs Forum* 44(6):e232, 2017.

Heo S, et al.: Testing a holistic meditation intervention to address psychosocial distress in patients with heart failure: a pilot study, *J Cardiovasc Nurs* 33(2):126, 2018.

Manning LK: Enduring as lived experience: exploring the essence of spiritual resilience for women later in life, *J Relig Health* 53(2):352, 2014.

Martial C, et al.: Temporality of features in near-death experience narratives, *Front Hum Neurosci* 11:311, 2017.

Minton ME, et al.: A willingness to go there: nurses and spiritual care, *J Clin Nurs* 27(1/2):173, 2018.

Pantuso T: Spiritual interventions for patients with cancer, *Integr Med Alert* 18(7):79, 2015.

Plunkett R, et al.: Healthy spaces in meaningful places: the rural church and women's health promotion, *J Holist Nurs* 33(2):122, 2015.

Puchalski C, Romer AL: Taking a spiritual history allows clinicians to understand patients more fully, *J Palliat Med* 3(1):129, 2000.

Rawlings D, Devery K: Near death experience and nursing practice: lessons from the palliative care literature, *Aust Nurs Midwifery J* 22(8):26, 2015.

Ricci-Allegra P: Spiritual perspective, mindfulness, and spiritual care practice of hospice and palliative nurses, *J Hosp Palliat Nurs* 20(2):172, 2018.

Romeiro J, et al.: Spiritual aspects of living with infertility: a synthesis of qualitative studies, *J Clin Nurs* 26(23/24):3917, 2017.

Sherman AC, et al.: A meta-analytic review of religious or spiritual involvement and social health among cancer patients, *Cancer* 121(21):3779, 2015.

Taylor EJ: Spirituality and spiritual care of adolescents and young adults with cancer, *Semin Oncol Nurs* 31(3):227, 2015.

Timmins F, et al.: Spiritual dimensions of care: developing an educational package for hospital nurses in the Republic of Ireland, *Holist Nurs Pract* 28(2):106, 2014.

Trevino KM, McConnell TR: Religiosity and spirituality during cardiac rehabilitation: a longitudinal evaluation of patient-reported outcomes and exercise capacity, *J Cardiopulm Rehabil Prev* 35(4):246, 2015.

Veloza-Gomez M, et al.: The importance of spiritual care in nursing practice, *J Holist Nurs* 35(2):118, 2017.

Vitorino LM, et al.: Spiritual/religious coping and depressive symptoms in informal caregivers of hospitalized older adults, *Geriatr Nurs* 39(1):48, 2018.

Vlasblom JP, et al.: Effect of nurses' screening of spiritual needs of hospitalized patients on consultation and perceived nurses' support and patients' spiritual well-being, *Holist Nurs Pract* 29(6):346, 2015.

Yarcheski A, Mahon NE: Meta-analyses of predictors of hope in adolescents, *West J Nurs Res* 38(3):345, 2016.

36

Loss and Grief

OBJECTIVES

- Identify a nurse's role when caring for patients who are experiencing loss, grief, or death.
- Describe the types of loss experienced throughout life.
- Examine grief theories.
- Identify types of grief.
- Describe characteristics of a person experiencing grief.
- Discuss variables that influence a person's response to grief.

- Develop a nursing care plan for a patient and family experiencing loss and grief.
- Identify ways to collaborate with family members and the interprofessional team to provide palliative care.
- Describe interventions for symptom management in patients at the end of life.
- Discuss the criteria for hospice care.
- Describe care of the body after death.

KEY TERMS

Actual loss, p. 741
Ambiguous loss, p. 742
Anticipatory grief, p. 742
Autopsy, p. 755
Bereavement, p. 742
Complicated grief, p. 742
Disenfranchised grief, p. 742

Grief, p. 741
Hope, p. 744
Hospice, p. 751
Maturational loss, p. 741
Mourning, p. 741
Necessary loss, p. 741
Normal (uncomplicated) grief, p. 742

Organ and tissue donation, p. 755
Palliative care, p. 751
Postmortem care, p. 756
Perceived loss, p. 741
Situational loss, p. 741

MEDIA RESOURCES

http://evolve.elsevier.com/Potter/fundamentals/
- Review Questions
- Concept Map Creator
- Case Study with Questions

- Audio Glossary
- Content Updates
- Answers to QSEN Activity and Review Questions

Loss is an inevitable part of life. Accompanying each loss are feelings of grief and sadness. Whether a patient is facing infertility or an amputation, an unwanted diagnosis or impending death, you are in a position to offer both the patient and family support to cope with the loss and comfort when continued life is not possible. Nurses in all practice settings and specialties provide grief support for the majority of dying patients and their families. Like grief, death is as inescapable in practice as it is in life. There is a trend for an increase in palliative and hospice care for patients with serious chronic illness and for patients with terminal diagnoses. Palliative and hospice care can be offered within health care facilities as well as in patients' homes.

Although people agree that death is a part of life, many are hesitant to talk about it because of feelings of fear or uncertainty and not wanting to upset others. Talking openly about death is discouraged in American society (i.e., in our everyday lives, our language, and even our thinking) (Matzo and Sherman, 2015). An example is our avoidance of the word "died" and instead the use of words such as "passed away" or "gone." You need to learn how to become comfortable in discussing such sensitive topics and in providing patients with the opportunity to express their desires for care at the end of life. With the Self-Care Determination Act of 1990 (a law requiring that patients be made aware of their medical decision rights), nurses and other health care providers are starting these conversations earlier, but there is more work left to do. You have the opportunity to advocate for patients and the high quality of care deserved at the end of life.

As a nurse you will learn to provide what patients and families need most at the time of a serious loss as well as at the end of life: compassion, attentiveness, and patient-centered care. As with other nursing situations, the more experience you have in caring for the grieving and the dying, the more confident, courageous, and compassionate you will become when caring for patients and families at this intimate and meaningful time. Your skills and knowledge base will develop quickly if you have the desire and willingness to learn, be present, and seek the help needed to learn how to give excellent care. Whether it is educating patients and families about advance directives, managing patients' symptoms, or simply holding a hand, nurses care for the grieving and dying and their families every day. It is the caring actions of nurses that help a patient and family during these times (see Chapter 7).

SCIENTIFIC KNOWLEDGE BASE

Loss

Life provides each person with multiple opportunities to grieve a loss or change. Sometimes the change is welcomed (marriage, birth of a child), and sometimes not (divorce, loss of a job, death). Changes related to loss can also be expected (child growing older and moving out of parent's home) or unexpected (sudden accident or death). Losses can be of tangible things, such as a body part or function, a pet, or a possession. Or losses can be intangible, such as the loss of self-esteem, a personal relationship, confidence, or a dream.

The experience of loss starts early in life and continues until death. Children develop independence from the adults who raise them, and as they begin and leave school, change friends, begin careers, and form new relationships, loss is a part of their maturation. From birth to death people form attachments and experience loss. Illness can also be a source of loss. It can change a person's functioning and therefore his or her job, family role, income level, and overall quality of life (Table 36.1). How one grieves depends on cultural norms, belief systems, support systems, and personal faith (AACN and CHNMC, 2014).

Life changes are normal, expected, and often positive. As people age, they learn that change always involves a necessary loss. They learn to expect that most necessary losses eventually are replaced by something different or better. However, some losses cause them to undergo permanent changes in their lives that threaten their sense of belonging and security. The death of a loved one, divorce, or loss of independence changes life forever and often significantly disrupts a person's physical, psychological, and spiritual health.

A maturational loss is a form of necessary loss and includes all normally expected life changes across the life span. A toddler experiences separation anxiety from a parent when starting preschool. A grade school child may not want to lose a favorite teacher and classroom. A college student may not want to leave the campus community. Maturational losses associated with normal life transitions help people develop coping skills to use when they experience unplanned, unwanted, or unexpected loss.

Other losses seem unnecessary and are not part of expected maturation experiences. Sudden, unpredictable external events bring about situational loss. For example, a person in an automobile accident sustains an injury with permanent physical changes that make it impossible to return to work or school, leading to loss of function, income, life goals, and self-esteem.

Losses may be actual or perceived. An actual loss occurs when a person can no longer feel, hear, see, or know a person or object. Examples include the loss of a body part, death of a family member, or loss of a job. Lost valued objects include those that wear out or are misplaced, stolen, or ruined. A perceived loss is uniquely defined by the person experiencing the loss and is less obvious to other people. For example, some people perceive rejection by a friend to be a loss, which creates a loss of confidence or changes an individual's status

in the social group. How the individual interprets the meaning of the perceived loss affects the intensity of the grief response. Perceived losses are easy to overlook by others because they are experienced so internally and individually, but they are as painful as an actual loss and grieved in the same way.

Each person responds to loss differently. The type of loss and a person's previous experience with and perception of loss influence the depth and duration of the grief response. For some individuals the loss of an object (e.g., home or treasured gift) generates the same level of distress as the loss of a person, depending on the value the person places on the object. Chronic illnesses, disabilities, and hospitalization produce multiple losses. When entering an institution for care, patients lose access to familiar people and environments, privacy, and control over body functions and daily routines. A chronic illness or disability adds financial hardships for most people and often brings about changes in lifestyle and dependence on others. Even brief illnesses or hospitalizations cause temporary changes in family role functioning, daily activities, and relationships.

Death is the ultimate loss. Although it is an expected part of life, death represents the unknown and can generate anxiety, fear, and uncertainty for many people. It creates a permanent separation of people and can cause fear, sadness, and regret for the dying person, family members, friends, and caregivers. A person's culture, spirituality, personal beliefs, and values; previous experiences with death; and degree of social support influence the way he or she approaches death.

Grief

Grief is a "normal but bewildering cluster of ordinary human emotions arising in response to a significant loss, intensified and complicated by the relationship to the person or the object lost" (Mitchell and Anderson, 1983) (see chapters 9 and 35). The grief experience is not a state but a process (Mughal and Siddiqui, 2019). Grief cannot be prevented. It is very personal. No two people grieve the same loss the same way, nor do they journey through grief in the same way. Grief work is very hard and requires enormous amounts of energy from the griever. It is rarely orderly and predictable. Most individuals recover adequately within a year after a loss; however, some individuals experience an extension of the standard grieving process, described as complicated grief or prolonged grief disorder (Mughal and Siddiqui, 2019). Because objects, memories, and anniversaries can cause a surge in feelings of loss, grief work is never fully completed. However, grief can diminish, and healing can occur when the pain of loss is less (AACN and CHNMC, 2014).

Coping with grief involves a period of mourning, the outward, social expressions of grief and the behavior associated with loss (AACN

TABLE 36.1 **Types of Loss**	
Definition	**Implications of Loss**
Loss of possessions or objects (e.g., theft, deterioration, misplacement, or destruction)	Extent of grieving depends on value of object, sentiment attached to it, or its usefulness.
Loss of known environment (e.g., leaving home, hospitalization, new job, moving out of a rehabilitation unit)	Loss occurs through maturational or situational events or by injury/illness. Loneliness or uncertainty in an unfamiliar setting threatens self-esteem, hopefulness, or belonging.
Loss of a significant other (e.g., divorce, loss of friend, trusted caregiver, or pet)	Close friends, family members, and pets fulfill psychological, safety, love, belonging, and self-esteem needs.
Loss of an aspect of self (e.g., body part, job, psychological or physiological function)	Illness, injury, or developmental changes result in loss of a valued aspect of self, altering personal identity and self-concept.
Loss of life (e.g., death of family member, friend, co-worker, or one's own death)	Those left behind after a death grieve for the loss of life of a loved one. Dying people also feel sadness or fear pain, loss of control, and dependency on others.

and CHNMC, 2014). Most mourning rituals are culturally influenced, learned behaviors. For example, the Jewish mourning ritual of *Shivah* is a time period when normal life activities come to a stop. Those mourning welcome friends into the home as a way of honoring the dead and receive support during the mourning period.

The term bereavement encompasses both grief and mourning and includes the emotional responses and outward behaviors of a person experiencing loss. Allow people experiencing bereavement to talk about their loss. Reassure them that their feelings are normal and encourage them to postpone making major decisions (AACN and CHNMC, 2014). Recognizing that there are different types of grief can help nurses plan and implement appropriate care.

Normal Grief. Normal (uncomplicated) grief is a common and universal reaction characterized by complex emotional, cognitive, social, physical, behavioral, and spiritual responses to loss and death. Some normal feelings of grief are disbelief, yearning, anger, and depression. Although the manner of a person's death (expected, violent, sudden, unexpected) affect a survivor's ability to grieve normally, it does not always determine how an individual will actually grieve. Helpful coping mechanisms for people who are grieving include hardiness and resilience, a personal sense of control, and the ability to make sense of and identify positive possibilities after a loss.

Anticipatory Grief. Often a person experiences anticipatory grief before the actual loss or death occurs, especially in situations of prolonged or predicted loss, such as caring for patients diagnosed with dementia or amyotrophic lateral sclerosis (ALS). Family members often grieve the impending death of a loved one because of the impending loss of companionship, control, and sense of freedom and the mental and physical changes experienced by their loved one. Nurses need to recognize anticipatory grief when it occurs. It is common to misconstrue a patient's symptoms as depression, disrespect, or a dismissive attitude, which is a barrier to providing quality end-of-life care (Moon, 2016).

When grief extends over a long period, people absorb loss gradually and begin to prepare for its inevitability. They may experience intense responses to grief (e.g., shock, denial, and tearfulness) before the actual death occurs and often feel relief when it finally happens. Another way to think about anticipatory grief is that it gives people time to prepare or complete the tasks related to the impending death. Although preparing for death helps some individuals, it increases stress for others, creating an emotional roller coaster of highs and lows.

Disenfranchised Grief. People may experience disenfranchised grief when their relationship to the deceased person is not socially sanctioned, cannot be shared openly, or seems of lesser significance. The person's loss and grief do not meet the norms of grief acknowledged by his or her culture, thereby cutting the grieving person off from social support and the sympathy given to people with more socially acceptable losses. Examples include the death of a former spouse, a married lover, or an incarcerated person, or a terminated pregnancy (AACN and CHNMC, 2014).

Ambiguous Loss. Sometimes people experience losses that are marked by uncertainty. Ambiguous loss, a type of disenfranchised grief, can occur when the person who is lost is physically present but not psychologically available, as in cases of severe dementia or brain injury. Other times the person is gone (e.g., after a kidnapping, when someone is taken as a prisoner of war, when there is no body found after a disaster such as 9/11, or when someone goes missing), but the grieving person maintains an ongoing, intense psychological attachment, never sure of the reality of the situation. Ambiguous losses are particularly difficult to process because of the lack of finality and unknown outcomes (Walter and McCoyd, 2015). Recently, ambiguous loss for parents has become more prevalent as more children identify as transgendered (Coolhart et al., 2018). Nurses also will encounter more refugees and immigrants experiencing ambiguous loss of their homeland (Perez and Arnold-Berkovits, 2018).

Complicated Grief. Some people do not experience a normal grief process. In complicated grief a person has a prolonged or significantly difficult time moving forward after a loss. He or she experiences a chronic and disruptive yearning for the deceased; has trouble accepting the death and trusting others; and/or feels excessively bitter, emotionally numb, or anxious about the future. Complicated grief has prolonged symptoms of painful emotions and sorrow for more than 1 year (Mughal and. Siddiqui, 2019). Complicated grief can also be understood as persistent grief that is so severe that it impacts normal functioning and quality of life (Perng and Renz, 2018). Patients show a preoccupation with the deceased and feel inner emptiness, have no interest in life, and sleep poorly (Mughal and Siddiqui, 2019). Complicated grief occurs more often when a person had a conflicted relationship with the deceased, prior or multiple losses or stressors, mental health issues, or lack of social support. Loss associated with homicide, suicide, sudden accidents, or the death of a child has the potential to become complicated. Specific types of complicated grief include chronic, exaggerated, delayed, and masked grief.

Chronic Grief. A person with chronic grief experiences a normal grief response, except that it extends for a longer period of time. This can include years to decades of intense grieving.

Exaggerated Grief. A person with an exaggerated grief response often exhibits self-destructive or maladaptive behavior, obsessions, or psychiatric disorders. Suicide is a risk for these individuals.

Delayed Grief. In delayed grief a person's grief response is unusually delayed or postponed because the loss is so overwhelming that the person must avoid the full realization of the loss. A delayed grief response is frequently triggered by a second loss, sometimes seemingly not as significant as the first loss—for example, a college student whose parent has died, but the full realization of the loss comes after the family pet dies or the student fails a course.

Masked Grief. Sometimes a grieving person behaves in ways that interfere with normal functioning but is unaware that the disruptive behavior is a result of the loss and ineffective grief resolution (AACN and CHNMC, 2014). Physical symptoms exhibited by the masked grief could be headaches, heartburn, rashes, or tachycardia.

Theories of Grief and Mourning

Knowledge of grief theories and normal responses to loss and bereavement helps you to better understand these complex experiences and how to help a grieving person. Grief theorists describe the physical, psychological, and social reactions to loss. Remember that people who vary from expected norms of grief or theoretical descriptions are not abnormal. The variety of theories supports the complexity and individuality of grief responses. Although most grief theories describe how people cope with death, they also help to understand responses to other significant losses (Table 36.2).

Criticism exists for the stages and task theories because they fail to capture the complexity and diversity of the experience (Hall, 2014). The more recent grief theories take into consideration that human beings construct their own experiences and truths differently and make their own meanings when confronted with loss and death. Differences in social and historical context, family structure and meaning of relationships, and cognitive capacities shape an individual's truths and grief

TABLE 36.2 Theories of Grief and Mourning

Stages of Dying Kübler-Ross (1969)	**Denial** The person cannot accept the fact of the loss. It is a form of psychological protection from a loss that the person cannot yet bear. **Anger** The person expresses resistance or intense anger at God, other people, or the situation. **Bargaining** The person cushions and postpones awareness of the loss by trying to prevent it from happening. **Depression** The person realizes the full impact of the loss. **Acceptance** The person incorporates the loss into life.
Attachment Theory Bowlby (1980)	**Numbing** Protects the person from the full impact of the loss **Yearning and Searching** Emotional outbursts of tearful sobbing and acute distress; common physical symptoms in this stage: tightness in chest and throat, shortness of breath, a feeling of lethargy, insomnia, and loss of appetite **Disorganization and Despair** Endless examination of how and why the loss occurred or expressions of anger at anyone who seems responsible for the loss **Reorganization** Accepts the change, assumes unfamiliar roles, acquires new skills, builds new relationships, and begins to separate himself or herself from the lost relationship without feeling that he or she is lessening its importance
Grief Tasks Model Worden (2008)	Accepts the reality of the loss Experiences the pain of grief Adjusts to a world in which the deceased is missing Emotionally relocates the deceased and moves on with life
Rando's "R" Process Model Rando (1993, 2014)	**Recognize** the loss **React** to the pain of separation **Recollect and re-experience** the relationship with the deceased **Relinquish** old attachments **Readjust** to life after loss **Reinvest** by putting emotional energy into new people
Dual Process Model Stroebe and Schut (1999)	**Loss-Oriented** activities: grief work, dwelling on the loss, breaking connections with the deceased person, and resisting activities to move past the grief **Restoration-Oriented** activities: attending to life changes, finding new roles or relationships, coping with finances, and participating in distractions, which provide balance to the loss-oriented state

experiences. No one's grief follows a predetermined path, nor is it linear. Grief is cyclical, with movement forward and backward. Educating grievers about the cyclical pattern of grief work prepares them for difficult days among the better days. Consider a widow several months after the death of her husband. She may have had several weeks of feeling less sad and depressed. If unprepared for the cyclical nature of

grief, she may be taken off guard by her strong grief reaction to a phone call for her husband or a commercial advertising his favorite candy. Knowing that these feelings will come and go helps the griever to be prepared for them and allows for the necessary self-care.

REFLECT NOW

Reflect on a loss that you experienced. What type of loss was it? How did you experience the cyclical nature of grief related to your loss?

NURSING KNOWLEDGE BASE

Nurses develop plans of care to help patients and family members who are undergoing loss, grief, or death experiences. Nurses implement plans of care in all settings on the basis of nursing research, practice evidence, nursing experience, and patient and family preferences. Extensive nursing education programs support the improvement of end-of-life care. The End-of-Life Nursing Education Consortium (ELNEC) provides nurses with basic and advanced curricula to care for patients and families experiencing loss, grief, death, and bereavement (AACN and CHNMC, 2014). The American Nurses Association (ANA) developed the Scope and Standards of Hospice and Palliative Nursing Practice in conjunction with the Hospice and Palliative Care Nurses Association (ANA, 2014). Professional nursing organizations such as the American Society of Pain Management Nurses and the American Association of Critical Care Nurses offer evidence-based practice guidelines for managing clinical and ethical issues at the end of life in many health care settings.

Factors Influencing Loss and Grief

Multiple factors influence the way a person perceives and responds to loss. They include developmental factors, personal relationships, the nature of the loss, coping strategies, socioeconomic status, and cultural and spiritual influences and beliefs. Nursing research has contributed to this knowledge base.

Human Development. Patient age and stage of development affect the grief response. For example, toddlers cannot understand loss or death but often feel anxiety over the loss of objects and separation from parents. Common expressions of grief include changes in eating and sleeping patterns, bowel and bladder disturbances, and increased fussiness (AACN and CHNMC, 2014). School-age children understand the concepts of permanence and irreversibility but do not always understand the causes of a loss. Some have intense periods of emotional expression and experience changes in eating, sleeping, and level of social engagement (AACN and CHNMC, 2014).

Young adults experience many necessary developmental losses related to their evolving future. Illness or death disrupts the young adult's future dreams and establishment of an autonomous sense of self. Midlife adults also experience major life transitions such as caring for aging parents, dealing with changes in marital status, and adapting to new family roles (Walter and McCoyd, 2015). For older adults the aging process leads to necessary and developmental losses. Some older adults experience age discrimination, especially when they become dependent or are near death, but they show resilience after a loss as a result of their prior experiences and developed coping skills (Box 36.1).

Personal Relationships. When loss involves another person, the quality and meaning of the lost relationship influence the grief response. When a relationship between two people was very rewarding and well connected, the survivor often finds it difficult to move forward after the death. Grief work is hampered by regret and a sense of unfinished business, especially when people are close but did not have a good relationship at the time of death. Social support and the ability to accept help from others are critical variables in recovery from loss and grief. Grievers experience less depression when they have highly satisfying personal relationships and friends to support them in their grief.

Nature of the Loss. Exploring the nature of a loss will help you understand the effect of the loss on a patient's behavior, health, and well-being. Was the loss avoidable? Is it permanent or temporary? Is it actual or imagined? Encouraging patients to share information about their loss will help you better develop appropriate interventions that meet the individualized needs of your patients.

Highly visible losses generally stimulate a helping response from others. For example, the loss of one's home from a tornado often brings community and governmental support. A more private loss such as a miscarriage brings less support from others. A sudden and unexpected death poses challenges different from those of a person in a debilitating chronic illness. When the death is sudden and unexpected, the survivors do not have time to say good-bye. In chronic illness survivors have memories of prolonged suffering, pain, and loss of function. Death by violence or suicide or multiple losses by their very nature complicate the grieving process in unique ways (Walter and McCoyd, 2015).

Coping Strategies. The losses that patients face from the time they were children often influence the coping skills they will use when faced with larger and more painful losses in adulthood. These coping strategies such as talking, journaling, and sharing their emotions with others may be healthy and effective. They may also be unhealthy and ineffective, such as increased use of alcohol, drugs, and violence. Nurses provide support by assessing patients' coping strategies, educating about new and healthy strategies, and encouraging the use of these strategies.

Socioeconomic Status. Socioeconomic status influences a person's grief process in direct and indirect ways. Because of role changes, a newly widowed mother finds herself working several jobs to make ends meet and does not find time to initiate self-care or grieve the loss of her spouse. With limited resources, activities that support healthy grief work such as buying a tree to plant in honor of the deceased or travel to a support group may be unrealistic. Practical implications also exist when there are limited resources. A patient with limited finances is unable to replace a car demolished in an accident and pay for the associated medical expenses.

Culture. During times of loss and grief patients and families draw on the social and spiritual practices of their cultures to find comfort, expression, and meaning in the experience (Walter and McCoyd, 2015). To provide the best care possible, it is necessary for us to ask about cultural beliefs and practices. Patients and families will rarely offer this information without prompting. Expressions of grief in one culture do not always make sense to people from a different culture. Try to understand and appreciate each patient's cultural values related to loss, death, and grieving (see Chapter 9). For example, some cultures hold back their public displays of emotion. In other cultures, behaviors such as public wailing and physical demonstrations of grief, including survivor body mutilation, show respect for the dead. Remember, culture extends beyond the geographic location of a person. Consider the influence of sexual and gender orientation, socioeconomic status, and family makeup (blended versus nuclear) when assessing cultural influence on grief practices and death rituals.

Spiritual and Religious Beliefs. Like cultural influences, spirituality and/or religious practices and beliefs provide a framework to navigate, understand, and heal from loss, death, and grief (see Chapter 35). A person's faith often influences the response to an illness, treatment, advanced life-support options, autopsy, organ donation, and what happens to the body and spirit after death. Patients draw on their spiritual beliefs to provide comfort and seek understanding at times of loss. You must remain open to the varying views and beliefs that are in contrast to your own to best support and care for your patients and their families. To never offend a patient and to offer high-quality care, you must assess your patient's and family's beliefs and practices and encourage expression of them whenever possible. You should encourage patients and families to draw on their spiritual resources (e.g., faith in a higher power, communities of support, friends, a sense of hope and meaning in life, and religious practices). Spirituality affects the patient's and family members' ability to cope with loss as well. Using a holistic approach when caring for a patient and family ensures that you are providing them with the best possible individualized care.

Hope, a multidimensional concept considered to be a component of spirituality, energizes and provides comfort to individuals and families experiencing personal challenges. Hope gives a person the ability to see life as enduring or having meaning or purpose. With hope a patient moves from feelings of weakness and vulnerability to living as fully as possible. Maintaining a sense of hope depends in part on a person having strong relationships and emotional connectedness to others. On the other hand, spiritual distress often arises from a patient's inability to feel hopeful or to foresee any favorable outcomes. Spirituality and hope play a vital role in a patient's adjustment to loss and death (see Chapter 35).

CRITICAL THINKING

Successful critical thinking requires a synthesis of knowledge, experience, information gathered from patients, critical thinking attitudes, and intellectual and professional standards. Clinical judgment requires you to anticipate information, analyze the data, and make decisions regarding your patient's care. During assessment consider all elements that build toward making an appropriate nursing diagnosis (Fig. 36.1).

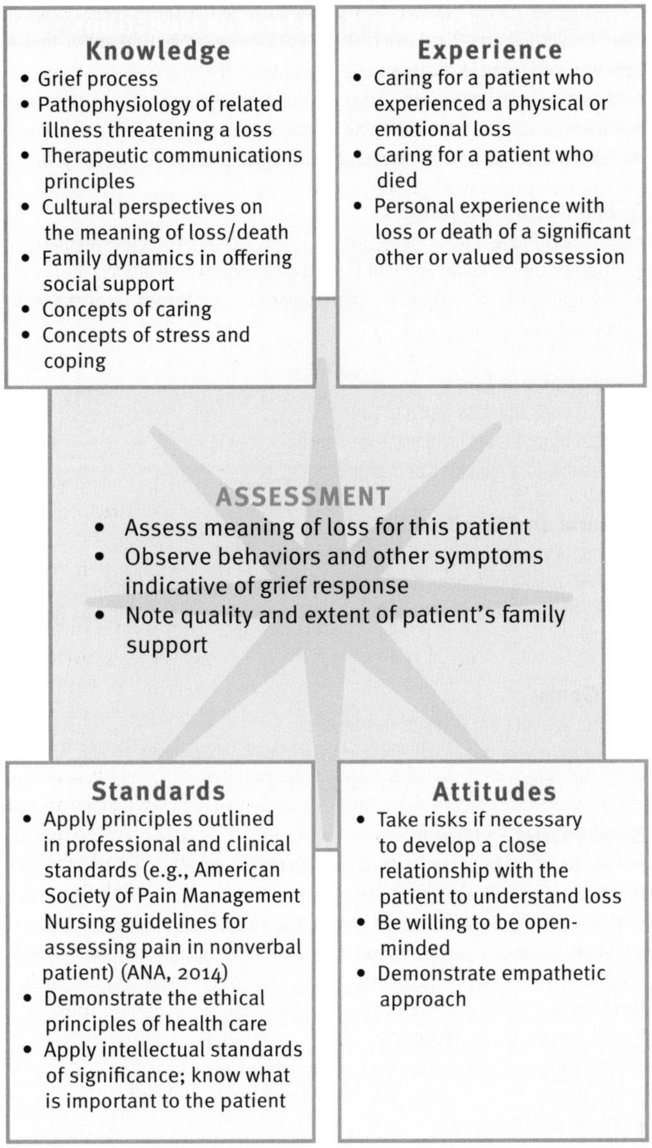

Knowledge
- Grief process
- Pathophysiology of related illness threatening a loss
- Therapeutic communications principles
- Cultural perspectives on the meaning of loss/death
- Family dynamics in offering social support
- Concepts of caring
- Concepts of stress and coping

Experience
- Caring for a patient who experienced a physical or emotional loss
- Caring for a patient who died
- Personal experience with loss or death of a significant other or valued possession

ASSESSMENT
- Assess meaning of loss for this patient
- Observe behaviors and other symptoms indicative of grief response
- Note quality and extent of patient's family support

Standards
- Apply principles outlined in professional and clinical standards (e.g., American Society of Pain Management Nursing guidelines for assessing pain in nonverbal patient) (ANA, 2014)
- Demonstrate the ethical principles of health care
- Apply intellectual standards of significance; know what is important to the patient

Attitudes
- Take risks if necessary to develop a close relationship with the patient to understand loss
- Be willing to be open-minded
- Demonstrate empathetic approach

FIG. 36.1 Critical thinking model for loss, death, and grieving assessment.

BOX 36.2 The Dying Person's Bill of Rights

- I have the right to be treated as a living human until I die.
- I have the right to maintain a sense of hopefulness, however changing its focus may be.
- I have the right to be cared for by those who can maintain a sense of hopefulness, however changing this might be.
- I have the right to express my feelings and emotions about my approaching death in my own way.
- I have the right to participate in decisions concerning my care.
- I have the right to expect continuing medical and nursing attention even though "cure" goals must be changed to "comfort" goals.
- I have the right not to die alone.
- I have the right to be free from pain.
- I have the right to have my questions answered honestly.
- I have the right to retain my individuality and not be judged for my decisions that may be contrary to beliefs of others.
- I have the right to expect that the sanctity of the human body will be respected after death.
- I have the right to be cared for by caring, sensitive, knowledgeable people who will attempt to understand my needs and be able to gain some satisfaction in helping me face my death.

From Betty R. Ferrell, Nessa Coyle: An overview of palliative nursing care, *Am J Nurs* 102(5):26, 2002. © Wolters Kluwer Health, Inc.

REFLECT NOW

Remember how you felt after a loss you experienced. What emotions did you feel and what coping strategies worked for you? How does your family/culture typically respond to death and loss?

❖ NURSING PROCESS

Apply the nursing process and use a critical thinking approach in your care of patients. The nursing process provides a clinical decision-making approach for you to develop and implement an individualized plan of care.

◆ Assessment

During the assessment process thoroughly assess each patient and critically analyze findings to ensure that you make patient-centered clinical decisions required for safe nursing care. A trusting, helping relationship with grieving patients and family members is essential to the assessment process. A caring nurse encourages a patient to tell his or her story. Look for opportunities to invite patients to share their experiences, being aware that attitudes about self-disclosure; sharing of emotions; or talking about illness, fears, and death are shaped by an individual's personality, coping style, and culture. This information is invaluable to understanding the unique and individual needs of each patient.

Through the Patient's Eyes. One of the best things that you can do for patients and families is to be present. By using the skills of active listening, silence, and therapeutic touch, you can establish a trusting relationship with your patients. This trusting relationship will help you explore with patients their unique responses to grief or their preferences for end-of-life care, which may include advance directives. Patient perceptions and expectations influence the prioritization

---

To understand a patient's subjective experiences of loss, form assessment questions on the basis of your theoretical and professional knowledge of grief and loss, but then listen carefully to the patient's perceptions. A culturally competent nurse also uses culture-specific understanding of grief to explore the meaning of loss with a patient.

Being familiar with commonly experienced responses to loss enables you to better understand a patient's emotions and behaviors. Some patients ignore, lash out, plead with, or withdraw from other people as part of a normal response to loss. Instead of "taking things personally," a critically thinking nurse integrates theory, prior experience, appreciation of subjective experiences, and self-knowledge to respond to the patient's emotions with patience and understanding. In designing plans of care, use professional standards, including the Nursing Code of Ethics (see Chapter 22), the dying patient's bill of rights (Box 36.2), the ANA Scope and Standards of Hospice and Palliative Nursing Practice (2014), and the American Society of Pain Management Nursing's position statement for pain management at the end of life (Reynolds et al., 2013).

of nursing diagnoses. To assess patient perceptions, ask, "What is the most important thing I can do for you right now?" You usually gather information from patients first, but with advanced illness and as death approaches, patients often rely on family members to communicate for them. Encourage family members to share their goals and perceptions with you. Most often they provide valuable information about patient preferences and clarify misunderstandings or identify overlooked information. Assess patients' and family members' understanding of treatment options to implement a mutually developed care plan. Assessment of grief responses extends throughout the course of an illness into the bereavement period following a death. During this time, you can work to normalize the grief response (AACN and CHNMC, 2014). Patients with advanced chronic illness and their families eventually face end-of-life care decisions and should discuss the content of any advance directives together. Patients, family members, and the health care team discuss end-of-life care preferences early in the assessment phase of the nursing process. If you feel uncomfortable in assessing a patient's wishes for end-of-life care by yourself, ask a health care provider experienced in discussing these issues to help you. Communicate what you have learned about patient preferences during any registered nurse (RN) hand-off, at health care team conferences, in written care plans, and through ongoing consultation (see Chapter 26).

Speak to patients and family members using honest and open communication, remembering that cultural practices influence how much information the patient shares. Keep an open mind, listen carefully, and observe the patient's verbal and nonverbal responses. Facial expressions, voice tones, and avoided topics often disclose more than words. Anticipate common grief responses but allow patients to describe their experiences in their own words. Open-ended questions such as "What do you understand about your diagnosis?" or "You seem sad today. Can you tell me more?" may open the door to a patient-centered discussion. Many people find it difficult to talk about loss, fear, death, or grief. The use of pauses, gentle questioning, and silence honors the patient's privacy and readiness to talk. Talk to patients and family members in a private, quiet setting, considering the culture normal of the individual. For example, in some cultures, the health care provider will be expected to discuss the information with the husband or father of the female patient, not directly with her, so that the male can pass the filtered information to the female. In other cultures, the patient may want to have family members present so that everyone hears the same thing and has an opportunity to add to the conversation. However, some people want their concerns and questions addressed privately. As you gather assessment data, summarize and validate your impressions with the patient or family member. Information from the medical record and from other members of the health care team, including physicians, social workers, and spiritual care providers, contributes to your assessment data.

Because of the importance of symptom management and priority of comfort in end-of-life care, prioritize your initial assessment to encourage patients to identify any distressing symptoms. Completing a thorough assessment is difficult when patients are in pain, anxious, depressed, or short of breath.

Grief Variables. Conversations about the meaning of loss to a patient often lead to other important areas of assessment, including the patient's coping style, the nature of family relationships, social support systems, the nature of the loss, cultural and spiritual beliefs, life goals, family grief patterns, self-care, and sources of hope (Box 36.3). Use skills appropriate for assessing a patient's culture, family, self-concept, or spiritual beliefs (see Chapters 9, 10, 33, and 35) to gain a deeper understanding of his or her loss.

> **BOX 36.3   Nursing Assessment Questions**
>
> **Nature of Relationships**
> - How long have you known _____ (the deceased person)?
> - What role did (name person) play in your life?
> - Tell me about what your relationship with (name person) meant to you.
>
> **Social Support Systems**
> - In times of loss, who is "there for you"? Absent? Who provides support?
> - What do others do for you that is most meaningful or helpful?
> - Are family/friends available when needed? Which friends or relatives do you wish were here?
>
> **Nature of the Loss**
> - What does this loss mean to you?
> - What other losses have you experienced?
> - Was this loss expected or unexpected?
>
> **Cultural and Spiritual Beliefs**
> - What is your belief about death? Meaning of life?
> - Which rituals/practices are important to you at the end of life?
> - How do members of your culture or religious group respond to this type of loss?
>
> **Life Goals**
> - What are your life goals at this time?
> - How have your goals changed because of this experience?
> - Are you able to see what you will do in the future?
>
> **Family Grief Patterns**
> - How have you/your family dealt with loss in the past?
> - What are your family's strengths?
> - How have family relationships changed as a result of your loss?
> - What role do you assume in your family during stressful situations?
>
> **Self-Care**
> - Tell me how you're feeling.
> - What are you doing to take care of yourself now?
> - What helps you when you feel this sad? What doesn't help?
> - What can I do for you?
>
> **Hope**
> - What do you hope for right now?
> - What helps you to remain hopeful? What causes you to lose hope?

Knowing the commonly experienced reactions to grief and loss and grief theories guides your critical thinking and assessment skills. A single behavior can occur in all types of grief. If a patient who is grieving describes loneliness and difficulty in falling asleep, consider all factors surrounding the loss in context. What was the loss? When did it occur? What was the meaning of the loss to the patient? For example, when your patient exhibits signs of a normal grief reaction, but you learn that the loss occurred 2 years ago, the patient's response most likely indicates a complicated, chronic grief experience. Focus your assessment on how a patient is reacting to loss or grief and not on how *you* believe that patient should be reacting.

Grief Reactions. Use psychological and physical assessment skills to assess a patient's unique grief responses. Most grieving people show some common outward signs and symptoms (Box 36.4). Analyze assessment data and identify possible related causes for the signs and symptoms that you observe. For example, after a significant loss a person may have a sad affect, withdrawn behaviors, headaches, upset stomach, and decreased ability to concentrate. You associate these

BOX 36.4 Symptoms of Normal Grief

Feelings
- Sorrow
- Fear
- Anger
- Guilt or self-reproach
- Anxiety
- Loneliness
- Fatigue
- Helplessness/hopelessness
- Yearning
- Relief

Cognitions (Thought Patterns)
- Disbelief
- Confusion or memory problems
- Problems in making decisions
- Inability to concentrate
- Feeling the presence of the deceased

Physical Sensations
- Headaches
- Nausea and appetite disturbances
- Tightness in the chest and throat
- Insomnia
- Oversensitivity to noise
- Sense of depersonalization ("Nothing seems real")
- Feeling short of breath, choking sensation
- Muscle weakness
- Lack of energy
- Dry mouth

Behaviors
- Crying and frequent sighing
- Distancing from people
- Absentmindedness
- Dreams of the deceased
- Keeping the deceased's room intact
- Loss of interest in regular life events
- Wearing objects that belonged to the deceased

BOX 36.5 Nursing Diagnostic Process

Hopelessness Related to Deteriorating Physiological Condition

Assessment Activities	Assessment Findings
Ask patient to discuss her understanding of her health situation.	Patient sighs and offers a negative view of her future; turns away from health care professionals.
Observe patient's nonverbal behavior.	Patient sighs, keeps eyes closed; decreased verbalization.
Observe patient's responses to care options.	Patient does not want scheduled test. "There is nothing they can do."
Assess activity level.	Patient states that she has no energy and reports pain; can't sleep, wants to stay in bed.
Observe patient's interactions with others.	Patient shows lack of interest, communicates minimally, and does not want to contact daughter yet.

symptoms with several potential causes, including anxiety, gastrointestinal disturbances, medication side effects, or impaired memory. Careful analysis of the symptoms in context leads you to an accurate nursing diagnosis. Ask: How are the symptoms related to one another when they occur? When did they begin? Were they present before the loss? To what does the person attribute them?

Loss takes place in a social context; thus, family assessment is a vital part of your data gathering. If a father of a young family is dying, he will not be able to fulfill certain roles, causing a change in family structure. When a person develops a disability, the patient and family members realign their roles and responsibilities to meet new demands. Family members also experience a variety of physical and psychological symptoms. Assess the family's response to loss and recognize that sometimes they are dealing with their grief at a different pace.

REFLECT NOW

Explore your feelings about entering the sacred space of another's family at the time of an emotionally charged loss. How do you think you would manage your own emotions?

◆ Nursing Diagnosis

Use critical thinking to cluster assessment data cues, identify assessment findings, draw conclusions regarding the patient's actual or potential needs or resources, and identify nursing diagnoses applicable to the patient's situation (Box 36.5). In addition to numerous diagnoses related to physical symptoms at the end of life, additional nursing diagnoses relevant for patients experiencing grief, loss, or death include:

- *Impaired Family Coping*
- *Death Anxiety*
- *Pain (Acute or Chronic)*
- *Dysfunctional Grief*
- *Anticipatory Grief*

You cannot make accurate nursing diagnoses based on just one or two assessment findings. Carefully review your patient's assessment data to consider whether more than one diagnosis applies. For example, a dying patient who cries often, has angry outbursts, and reports nightmares gives evidence of several possible nursing diagnoses: *Pain (Acute or Chronic), Dysfunctional Grief, or Spiritual Distress.* Examine the available data, validate assumptions with the patient, and look for other validating behaviors and symptoms before making a diagnosis.

As part of the diagnostic process, identify the appropriate "related to" factor for each negative or actual nursing diagnosis. Clarification of the related factors ensures that you select appropriate interventions. For example, a nursing diagnosis of *Dysfunctional Grief related to the permanent loss of mobility* requires different interventions than a diagnosis of *Dysfunctional Grief related to infertility after an ectopic pregnancy.*

When identifying nursing diagnoses related to a patient's grief or loss, you sometimes identify other related diagnoses. Some patients experiencing grief or impending death have nursing diagnoses such as *Denial About Illness Severity* or *Impaired Mobility.* A patient entering the phase of active dying often has diagnoses related to physical changes, including *Urinary Incontinence, Bowel Incontinence, Acute Pain, Nausea, Altered Perception,* and *Impaired Breathing.*

◆ Planning

Nurses provide patient-centered holistic care to patients experiencing grief, death, or loss. Fig. 36.2 illustrates the interrelatedness of critical thinking factors during the planning phase of the nursing process. The use of critical thinking ensures a well-designed care plan that supports a patient's self-esteem and autonomy by including him or her in the planning process. A care plan for a patient who is dying focuses on comfort; preserving dignity and quality of life; and providing family members with emotional, social, and spiritual support (see the Nursing Care Plan).

REFLECT NOW

Reflect on your feelings as you plan care for a patient who is terminally ill. How will you feel about engaging in conversations about care while talking about something that causes so many people distress?

◎ NURSING CARE PLAN

Hopelessness

ASSESSMENT

Mrs. Allison, an 80-year-old woman, was brought to the hospital after a neighbor found her lying on the floor, unable to get up after a fall. She lives alone since her husband died 2 years ago. She was admitted to the hospital with low blood pressure, dehydration, severe back pain, and weakness. She reports fatigue, recent weight loss, and loss of appetite. Her diagnostic tests indicate that she has leukemia, for which she needs a bone marrow biopsy for confirmation. The nurse notes that Mrs. Allison appears withdrawn and tearful.

Assessment Activities	*Assessment Findings[a]*
Ask open-ended questions. "It looks as if you're having a difficult time. What do you understand about your situation right now?"	"The doctors say that **I might have leukemia." Shrugging her shoulders,** she states, **"There's nothing they can do. I don't want the bone marrow test."**
Observe Mrs. Allison's behaviors and nonverbal communication.	Mrs. Allison **appears sad and keeps her eyes closed.** She **cries and sighs frequently.**
Assess Mrs. Allison's pain and energy level.	Mrs. Allison's **great toes are swollen and red** and sore to the touch. Reports **constant back pain.** She has **"no energy for anything."**
Observe Mrs. Allison's interactions and interest in others.	Mrs. Allison **does not look at people and does not want to talk to her daughter yet.**
Assess meaning of recent events with Mrs. Allison and invite her to talk about her situation.	Mrs. Allison states, **"I'm done with life and ready to be with my late husband."**

[a]**Assessment findings** are shown in **bold** type.

NURSING DIAGNOSIS: Hopelessness related to declining physical condition

PLANNING

Goals	*Expected Outcomes (NOC)[b]*
	Hope
Mrs. Allison will discuss two care priorities and preferences within 1 day.	Mrs. Allison identifies the concerns causing the greatest amount of suffering or distress.
	Mrs. Allison identifies ways she can live at home with the help of others.

[b]Outcome classification labels from Moorhead S, et al: *Nursing Outcomes Classification (NOC): measurement of health outcomes,* ed 6, St Louis, 2018, Elsevier.

INTERVENTIONS (NIC)[c]	RATIONALE
Hope Inspiration	
Develop an open and caring relationship through active listening and emotional support.	Individuals approaching the end of life often experience fragmented care delivery. Therapeutic communication supports patient- and family-centered care at the end of life and helps to ensure that patient needs are communicated among all health care professionals (Meghani et al., 2015).
Provide frequent conversations with patient and family regarding patient's symptom management and grief.	Frequent conversations with patient and family provide opportunities to discuss end-of-life care values, goals, and preferences (Meghani et al., 2015).
Pain Management	
Provide pharmacological and nonpharmacological relief for chronic back and foot pain.	Anxiety, pain, and suffering are reduced with effective pain management, and quality of life is improved (Paice, 2015).
Grief Work Facilitation	
Help Mrs. Allison identify her personal goals, desires, and priorities. Evaluate effectiveness and promote goal achievement as appropriate.	Allowing the patient to direct care decisions helps the patient and family select priority of care and increases patient and family understanding of current and proposed treatments (Coyle, 2015).
Help Mrs. Allison identify her desires for advance care planning, drawing on available resources in and outside the hospital.	Hope near the end of life can be achieved by having a sense of control over future care (Mattes and Sloane, 2015).
Discuss Mrs. Allison's spiritual beliefs, practices, needs, and resources.	Inclusion of spiritual assessment and spiritual care practices at the end of life increases patient's sense of connectedness and overall quality of life (Dose et al., 2014).

[c]Intervention classification labels from Butcher HK, et al: *Nursing Interventions Classification (NIC),* ed 7, St Louis, 2018, Elsevier.

EVALUATION

Evaluation Activity	*Patient Response/Finding*	*Outcome Status*
Use open-ended question: "Can you tell me what is most distressing or worrisome right now?"	Mrs. Allison explains, "I'm not sure what will happen. I may not be able to take care of myself much longer."	Fear of the unknown is causing the greatest amount of distress.
Ask, "Who has offered to help you when you get home?"	Mrs. Allison states, "Well, my Bible study group will take turns taking me to appointments, and the choir members said they will be happy to bring meals to the house every Tuesday and Thursday."	Identified people who can help provide assistance at home.
Observe Mrs. Allison's planning activities and behavior with her daughter and friends.	Mrs. Allison and daughter discuss what they can do so that she can stay at home longer.	Mrs. Allison is making plans to live at home.

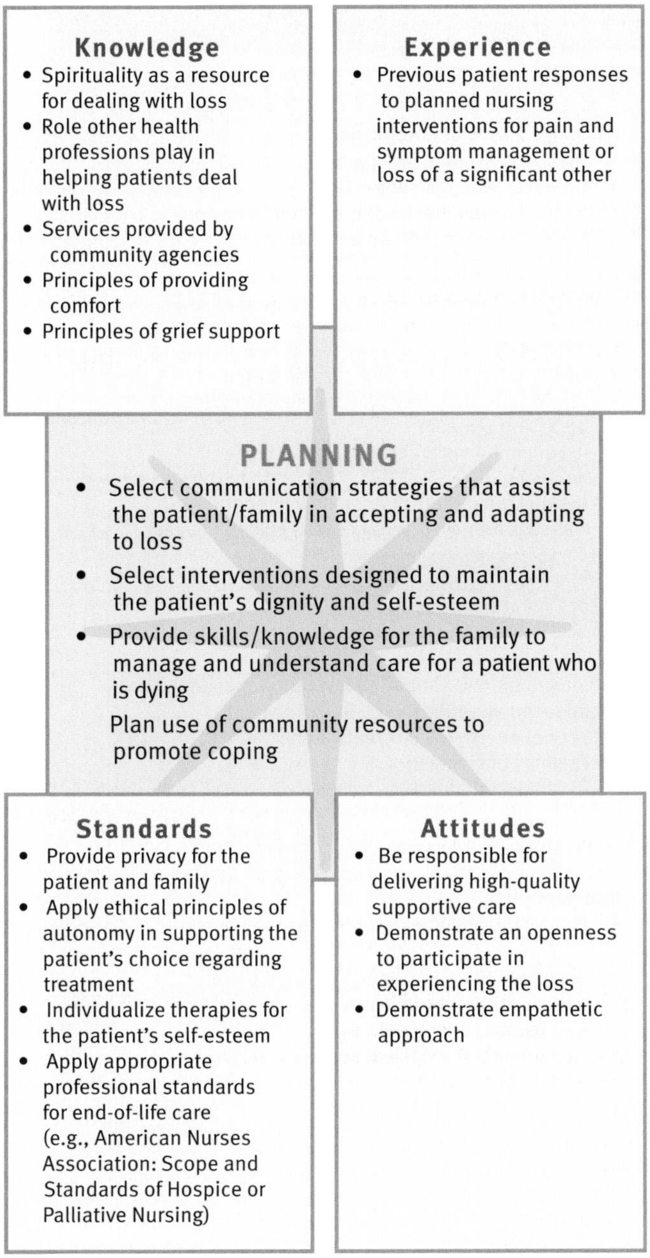

Knowledge

- Spirituality as a resource for dealing with loss
- Role other health professions play in helping patients deal with loss
- Services provided by community agencies
- Principles of providing comfort
- Principles of grief support

Experience

- Previous patient responses to planned nursing interventions for pain and symptom management or loss of a significant other

PLANNING

- Select communication strategies that assist the patient/family in accepting and adapting to loss
- Select interventions designed to maintain the patient's dignity and self-esteem
- Provide skills/knowledge for the family to manage and understand care for a patient who is dying

  Plan use of community resources to promote coping

Standards

- Provide privacy for the patient and family
- Apply ethical principles of autonomy in supporting the patient's choice regarding treatment
- Individualize therapies for the patient's self-esteem
- Apply appropriate professional standards for end-of-life care (e.g., American Nurses Association: Scope and Standards of Hospice or Palliative Nursing)

Attitudes

- Be responsible for delivering high-quality supportive care
- Demonstrate an openness to participate in experiencing the loss
- Demonstrate empathetic approach

FIG. 36.2 Critical thinking model for loss, death, and grieving planning.

Goals and Outcomes. During planning establish realistic goals and expected outcomes on the basis of the nursing diagnoses. Consider a patient's own resources such as physical energy and activity tolerance, family support, and coping style. A nursing diagnosis of *Powerlessness related to experimental cancer therapy* with a goal of "Patient will be able to describe the expected course of disease" is realistic for a patient who frequently asks for clarification about the treatment plan and participates in educational discussions. In contrast, an expected outcome of "Patient will identify a minimum of three effective coping skills" is appropriate for a patient with the same nursing diagnosis who is experiencing depression from feeling powerless about having experimental cancer treatment.

The goals of care for a patient experiencing loss are either short or long term, depending on the nature of the loss and the patient's condition. Some nursing care goals for patients facing loss or death include accommodating grief, accepting the reality of a loss, or maintaining meaningful relationships. A possible goal for a young woman with advanced breast cancer is "Will maintain a sense of control," with the following potential expected outcomes:

- Patient participates in all treatment decisions.
- Patient identifies a minimum of three ways to maintain a parental role in the care of her young child.
- Patient communicates a minimum of three treatment side effects or concerns to the health care team.

Setting Priorities. Encourage patients and family members to share their priorities for care at the end of life. Patients at the end of life or with advanced chronic illness are more likely to want their comfort, social, or spiritual needs met rather than pursuing medical cures. Then as a nurse prioritize a patient's most urgent physical or psychological needs while also considering his or her expectations and priorities. If a patient's goals include pain control and promoting self-esteem at the end of life, pain control takes priority when the patient experiences acute physical discomfort. Many terminal conditions can also influence a patient's ability to breathe. Pharmacological approaches are available to relieve dyspnea. When comfort needs have been met, you address other issues important to the patient and family. When it is realistic for the patient to remain independent, strategies that foster his or her sense of autonomy and ability to function independently take priority. A patient's condition at the end of life often changes quickly; therefore maintain an ongoing assessment to revise the plan of care according to patient needs and preferences.

When a patient has multiple nursing diagnoses, it is not possible to address them all simultaneously. Fig. 36.3 illustrates a concept map developed for Mrs. Allison, an elderly patient with a medical diagnosis of advanced cancer (leukemia). In conjunction with her recent medical diagnosis, she experiences associated health problems identified in the nursing diagnoses *Chronic Pain, Impaired Low Nutritional Intake, Fatigue,* and *Hopelessness.* In such a situation determine which of the four diagnoses should take priority. The chronic pain experienced by the patient is often the first focus. Until her pain is under control, it will not be possible for her to feel more energized, eat well, or regain her sense of hopefulness.

Teamwork and Collaboration. As described previously, grief, loss, and death affect people physically, emotionally, spiritually, and culturally. No one is able to address all of these dimensions alone. A team of nurses, physicians, social workers, spiritual care providers, nutritionists, pharmacists, psychologists, physical and occupational therapists, patients, and family members works together to provide palliative, grief, and end-of-life care. Massage or music/art therapists who provide alternative therapies are sometimes part of the team (see Chapter 32). As a patient's care needs change, team members take a more or less active role, depending on the patient's shifting priorities. Team members communicate with one another on a regular basis to ensure coordination and effectiveness of care.

> **QSEN Building Competency in Teamwork and Collaboration** You are caring for Mrs. Allison, an older patient who has recently been diagnosed with a terminal illness and is preparing for discharge home. She has lost strength as a result of decreased activity, depression, and back pain. Her greatest desire is to be able to attend weekly services at her church, but because of her weakness, pain, and fatigue, she is afraid that she will be unable to do so. She believes that her feelings of depression will improve if she can again participate in church activities. How can you, with the help of the interprofessional team, help Mrs. Allison respond to her spiritual needs and desire to be involved within her faith community?
>
> Answers to QSEN Activities can be found on the Evolve website.

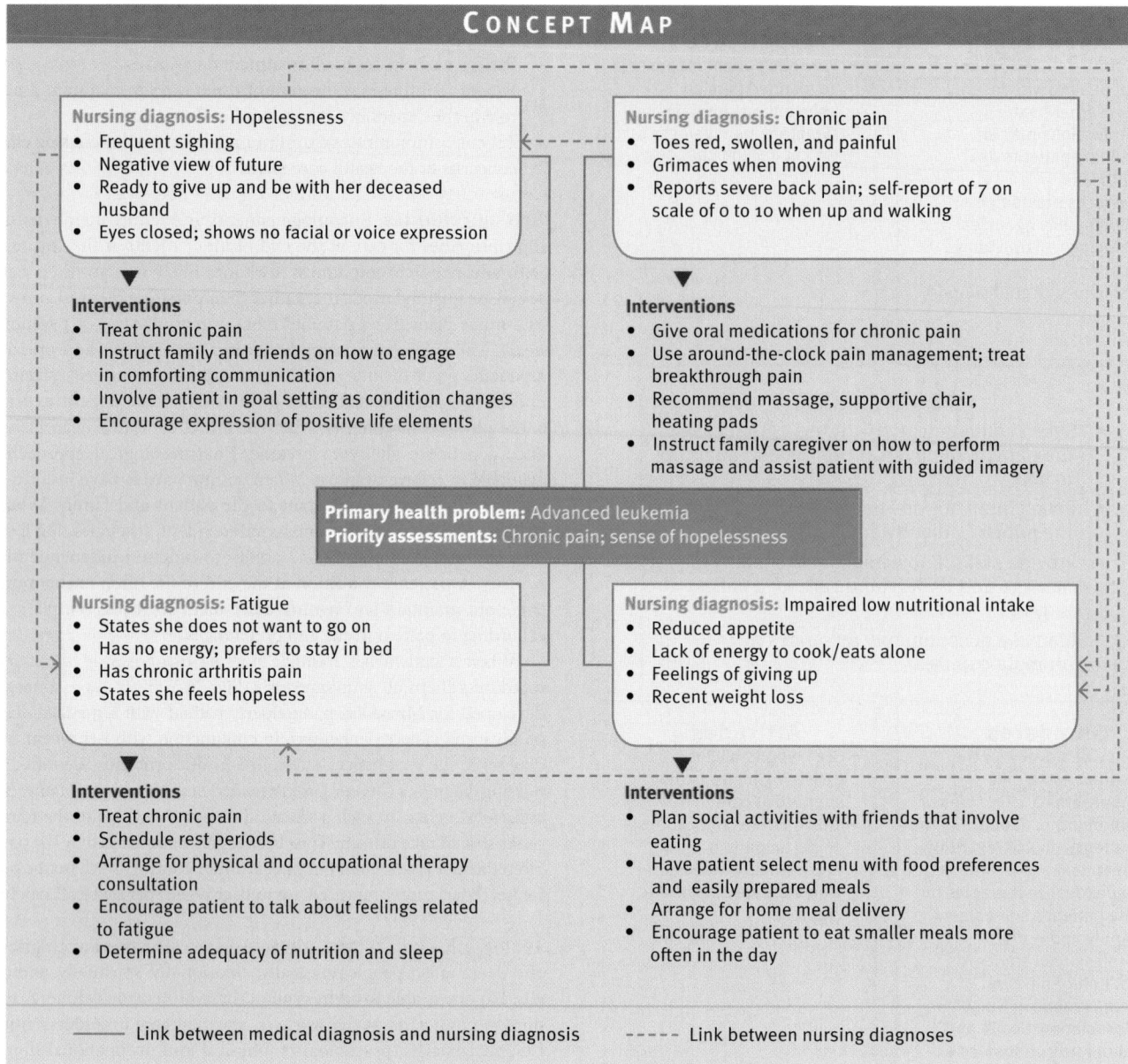

CONCEPT MAP

Nursing diagnosis: Hopelessness
- Frequent sighing
- Negative view of future
- Ready to give up and be with her deceased husband
- Eyes closed; shows no facial or voice expression

Interventions
- Treat chronic pain
- Instruct family and friends on how to engage in comforting communication
- Involve patient in goal setting as condition changes
- Encourage expression of positive life elements

Nursing diagnosis: Chronic pain
- Toes red, swollen, and painful
- Grimaces when moving
- Reports severe back pain; self-report of 7 on scale of 0 to 10 when up and walking

Interventions
- Give oral medications for chronic pain
- Use around-the-clock pain management; treat breakthrough pain
- Recommend massage, supportive chair, heating pads
- Instruct family caregiver on how to perform massage and assist patient with guided imagery

Primary health problem: Advanced leukemia
Priority assessments: Chronic pain; sense of hopelessness

Nursing diagnosis: Fatigue
- States she does not want to go on
- Has no energy; prefers to stay in bed
- Has chronic arthritis pain
- States she feels hopeless

Interventions
- Treat chronic pain
- Schedule rest periods
- Arrange for physical and occupational therapy consultation
- Encourage patient to talk about feelings related to fatigue
- Determine adequacy of nutrition and sleep

Nursing diagnosis: Impaired low nutritional intake
- Reduced appetite
- Lack of energy to cook/eats alone
- Feelings of giving up
- Recent weight loss

Interventions
- Plan social activities with friends that involve eating
- Have patient select menu with food preferences and easily prepared meals
- Arrange for home meal delivery
- Encourage patient to eat smaller meals more often in the day

——— Link between medical diagnosis and nursing diagnosis   - - - - Link between nursing diagnoses

FIG. 36.3 Concept map for Mrs. Allison.

◆ Implementation

Health Promotion. Health promotion in complicated grief, serious chronic illness, or death focuses on facilitating successful coping and optimizing physical, emotional, and spiritual health. Many people continue to look for and find meaning even in difficult life circumstances. They often find personal growth and spiritual insights that they have not previously experienced and need family and nurse support as they strive to maintain a degree of normalcy, live with loss, make health care decisions, prepare for death when applicable, and adjust to disappointments, frustration, and anxieties along the way (Box 36.6).

Assist With End-of-Life Decision Making. Patients and family members often face complex treatment decisions at the end of life. Patients and families must decide which treatments to continue and which to forgo; to enroll in hospice or stay in the hospital; or to transfer to a nursing home, in-patient unit, or home. Even after the decision to enroll in hospice, questions arise about symptom management, artificial nutrition and hydration (e.g., feeding tube or parenteral nutrition), and

the desired location for death. You can support and educate patients and families as they identify, contemplate, and ultimately decide how to best journey to the end of life.

Difficult ethical decisions at the end of life complicate a survivor's grief, create family divisions, or increase family uncertainty at the time of death (see Chapter 22). When ethical decisions are handled well, survivors achieve a sense of control and experience a meaningful conclusion to their loved one's death. Suggest to patients that they clearly communicate their wishes for end-of-life care so that family members are able to act as faithful surrogates when the patient can no longer speak for himself or herself. Some patients and family members rely on the nurse and other members of the health care team to initiate discussions regarding end-of-life care. Nurses often provide options that family members do not know are available and are advocates for patients and family members making decisions at the end of life in the form of an advance directive. When patients sign consent for a DNR (do not resuscitate) order, they have improved autonomy as well as increased quality of end-of-life care (Liang et al., 2016).

BOX 36.6 PATIENT TEACHING

Maintaining Self-Care

Objective
- The patient will participate in activities to manage symptoms.

Teaching Strategies
- Identify ways for patient to achieve personal goals.
- Instruct patient on ways to maintain usual daily routines that provide comfort and sense of normalcy.
- Demonstrate forms of complementary therapy that patient can use for symptom management.
- Discuss ways that patient can maintain a sense of control over end-of-life planning and maintain a realistic outlook (advance directives, funeral planning, and preferred location of death).
- Discuss patient's needs for the presence of particular support people or for solitude.
- Identify methods to facilitate safety and ease in managing activities of daily living as patient's abilities change (assistive devices, in-home caregivers).

Evaluation
Use the principles of teach-back to evaluate patient/family caregiver learning:
- Tell me what symptom-management methods you use and how effective each method is.
- Show me how you perform guided imagery in symptom management.
- Tell me about the changes that you made in your house that improve your safety.

Palliative Care. Patients and families can benefit greatly from the specialized approach of palliative care. This holistic method to prevent and reduce symptoms promotes quality of life and whole-person well-being through care of the mind, body, and spirit.

Palliative care focuses on the prevention, relief, reduction, or soothing of symptoms of disease or disorders throughout the entire course of an illness. It is not simply care of the dying. The primary goal of palliative care is to help patients and families achieve the best possible quality of life (Mariano, 2015). Patients should receive palliative care as soon as possible when chronic or terminal disease starts creating difficult-to-manage symptoms. Palliative care is appropriate for patients of any age, with any diagnosis, at any time, and in any setting.

A large misconception concerning palliative care is that it is used only when curative treatments are no longer pursued. However, it is appropriate both for patients still receiving aggressive treatment with hope of achieving a cure and for patients who have forgone any life-extending treatment (Coyle, 2015). It is important that you help patients and their families understand the distinction because often misunderstanding the purpose of palliative care causes patients to refuse it.

The World Health Organization (2018) summarizes palliative care philosophy as follows:
- Provides relief from pain and other distressing symptoms.
- Affirms life and regards dying as a normal process.
- Intends neither to hasten nor postpone death.
- Integrates the psychological and spiritual aspects of patient care.
- Offers a support system to help patients live as actively as possible until death.
- Offers a support system to help the family cope during the patient's illness and in their own bereavement.
- Uses a team approach to address the needs of patients and their families, including bereavement counseling, if indicated.
- Will enhance the quality of life and may also influence the course of illness.

- Is applicable early in the course of illness in conjunction with other therapies that are intended to prolong life, such as chemotherapy or radiation therapy, and includes those investigations needed to better understand and manage distressing clinical complications.

Because the focus of palliative care is comfort and improved quality of life, it is a valuable approach to caring for patients with a complex illness. A variety of therapies are used to provide patients with a holistic approach to symptom management and ultimately improved quality of life. Complementary therapies using an integrative approach have been shown to have a positive effect on feelings of depression and anxiety (see Chapter 32). For example, fatigue, a common symptom reported by patients receiving palliative care, responds to acupuncture and exercise. Massage has been shown to reduce the symptoms of pain, anxiety, nausea, shortness of breath, and stress and to increase relaxation and peacefulness.

When the goals of care change and cure for illnesses becomes less likely, the focus shifts to more palliative care strategies and ideally transition to hospice care, a more specialized form of palliative care for the dying.

Hospice Care. Hospice care is a philosophy and model for the care of redundant patients and their families at the end of life (Hospice Foundation of America, 2018). It gives priority to managing a patient's pain and other symptoms; comfort; quality of life; and attention to physical, psychological, social, and spiritual needs and resources. Patients accepted into a hospice program usually have less than 6 months to live. Hospice services are available in home, hospital, extended-care, and nursing home settings.

The cornerstone of hospice care is a trusting relationship between the hospice team and the patient and family. Knowing expectations, desired location of care, and family dynamics helps the hospice team provide individualized care at the end of life. Unlike traditional care, patients are active participants in all aspects of hospice care, and caregivers prioritize care according to patient wishes. Patient care goals are mutually set, and all participants fully understand the patient's care preferences and try to honor them. Hospice services provide bereavement visits made by the staff after the death of the patient to help the family move through the grieving process. Hospice programs are built on the following core beliefs and services:
- Patient and family are the unit of care
- Coordinated home care with access to inpatient and nursing home beds when needed
- Symptom management
- Physician-directed services
- Provision of an interprofessional care team
- Medical and nursing services available at all times
- Bereavement follow-up after patient's death
- Use of trained volunteers for visitation and respite support

To be eligible for home hospice services, a patient must have a family caregiver to provide care when the patient is no longer able to function alone. Home care aides offer help with hygienic needs, and a nurse is available to coordinate and manage symptom relief. Nurses providing hospice care use therapeutic communication, offer psychosocial care and expert symptom management, promote patient dignity and self-esteem, maintain a comfortable and peaceful environment, provide spiritual comfort and hope, protect against abandonment or isolation, offer family support, help with ethical decision making, and facilitate mourning. Hospice team members offer 24-hour accessibility and coordinate care between the home and inpatient setting. A patient receiving home hospice care may enter an inpatient hospice unit for stabilization of symptoms or caregiver respite. As a patient's death comes closer, the hospice team provides intensive support to the patient and family (Hospice Foundation of America, 2018).

With the death of a patient, family members benefit from the many resources of the health care team. When the patient chooses to die at home, family members provide direct care, which is often emotionally stressful and physically exhausting. In the home setting family caregivers benefit from respite care. During respite care a patient temporarily receives care from others so that family members are able to get away to rest and relax. Hospice program benefits include some days of respite care. Inform family members of home care, hospice, and community service options so that they can access the best resources for their situation.

Therapeutic Communication Approaches. The heart of nursing care is the establishment of a caring and trusting relationship with your patient. This patient-focused approach allows you to respond to patients rather than react and encourages the sharing of important information. Open-ended questions invite patients to elaborate on their thoughts and encourage them to tell their stories. Patients usually give short answers (yes or no) when you use closed-ended questions, which limit what we can learn about their situation. Use active listening, learn to be comfortable with silence, and use prompts (e.g., "go on," "tell me more") to encourage continued conversation. Empathizing, therapeutic touch, and offering self are also effective ways to therapeutically communicate with patients. Specifically, empathizing allows patients to see that their feelings are normal and that as the nurse you understand. Sometimes questioning a patient feels uncomfortable; thus stating an observation, such as "You look worried" or "You didn't eat much lunch" invites patients to respond without feeling pressure to answer (see Chapter 24).

Feelings of sadness, numbing, or anger make talking about these situations especially difficult. For example, a patient may experience anger during grief and lash out at caregivers. Some patients even become demanding and accusing. Remain supportive by letting patients and family members know that feelings such as anger are normal by saying, "I see that you're upset right now, and that's understandable. I'm here to talk with you if you want." Encourage patients to share the emotions and concerns of greatest importance to them and then acknowledge their feelings and concerns in a nonjudgmental manner. If a patient chooses not to share feelings or concerns, express a willingness to be available at any time. Some patients do not discuss emotions for personal or cultural reasons, and others hesitate to express their emotions for fear that people will abandon or judge them. If you are reassuring and respectful of a patient's privacy, a therapeutic relationship is likely to develop. Sometimes patients need to begin to resolve their grief privately before they discuss their loss with others, especially strangers.

Do not avoid talking about a topic. When you sense that a patient wants to talk about something, make time to do so as soon as possible. This may be very challenging if you are in a busy acute care setting; however, it is a necessary part of quality nursing care and should be made a priority. Above all, remember that a patient's emotions are not something you can "fix." Instead view emotional expressions as an essential part of the patient's adjustment to significant life changes and development of effective coping skills. Help family members access other professional resources. Social workers, psychologists, chaplains, and case managers can offer additional information and support to families and patients in grief.

Provide Psychosocial Care. Patients at the end of life experience a range of psychological symptoms, including anxiety, depression, powerlessness, uncertainty, and isolation. They can experience anguish from the unknown surroundings, treatment options, health status, and the dying process. Worry or fear is common in many patients and often heightens their perception of discomfort and suffering. You can alleviate some of it by providing information to them about their condition, the course of their disease, and the benefits and burdens of treatment options. Most hospitals have health care professionals who can provide counseling.

Manage Symptoms. Managing the multiple symptoms commonly experienced when patients are chronically ill or dying remains a primary goal of palliative care nursing (Table 36.3). Uncontrolled symptoms cause distress, discomfort, and suffering to patients and families, which often complicates the dying experience. Despite the availability of effective treatment options for pain, many patients experience avoidable pain at the end of life because of misconceptions by nurses or family members (see Chapter 44). Maintain an ongoing assessment of a patient's pain and evaluate his or her response to interventions. Reassure the family repeatedly of the need for pain control even if the patient does not appear in pain. Discuss pain control with the family frequently, and dispel any myths regarding dependence on opioids. You are responsible to advocate for change if the patient does not obtain relief from the prescribed regimen. It is imperative that you assess patients' nonverbal cues because they often are unable to communicate their intentions. During the dying process patients' renal and liver function decline, decreasing metabolism and rate of drug clearance, which might require modification to the dosage of medication. Also, be aware that advancing disease pathology, anxiety, or delirium sometimes requires the use of higher doses or different drug therapies.

Remain alert to the potential side effects of opioid administration: constipation, nausea, sedation, respiratory depression, or myoclonus. Family members often worry about potential addiction to opioid medications. Not only is the incidence of true addiction very low, but a patient's need for pain relief at the end of life takes priority. Education is necessary to help families understand the need for appropriate use of opioid medications.

Promote Dignity and Self-Esteem. A patient's sense of dignity depends on a positive self-regard and the ability to find meaning in life and feel valued by others. A sense of dignity is reinforced by respectful treatment from caregivers. Nurses promote a patient's self-esteem and dignity by respecting him or her as a whole person (i.e., as a person with feelings, accomplishments, and passions independent of the illness experience). Respecting and valuing the things that a patient cares about validates the person and at the same time strengthens communication among the patient, family members, and the nurse. Sharing time with patients as they share their life stories helps you know them and facilitates the development of individualized interventions.

Attending to the patient's physical appearance also promotes dignity and self-esteem. Cleanliness, absence of body odors, and clean clothing give patients a sense of worth. When caring for a patient's bodily functions, show patience and respect, especially after the patient becomes dependent on others. Remember that patients are directing care at the end of life. Allow them to make decisions such as how and when to administer personal hygiene, diet preferences, and timing of nursing interventions. Keep the patient and family members informed about daily activities, tests, or therapies; their purposes; and anticipated effects. Provide privacy during nursing care procedures and be sensitive to when the patient and family need time alone together.

Maintain a Comfortable and Peaceful Environment. A comfortable, clean, pleasant environment helps patients relax, promotes good sleep patterns, and minimizes symptom severity. Keep a patient comfortable through frequent repositioning, making sure that bed linens are dry, and controlling extraneous environmental noise and offensive odors. Pictures, cherished objects, and cards or letters from family members and friends create a familiar and comforting environment for the patient dying in an institutional setting. When possible, allow patients to wear their own pajamas or lounging clothes to promote a sense of comfort

TABLE 36.3 Promoting Comfort in the Terminally Ill Patient

Symptoms	Characteristics or Causes	Nursing Implications
Pain	Pain has multiple causes, depending on patient diagnosis.	Collaborate with team members to identify and implement appropriate pharmacological and nonpharmacological interventions to reduce pain and promote comfort (see Chapter 44).
Skin discomfort	Any source of skin irritation increases discomfort.	Keep skin clean, dry, and moisturized. Monitor for incontinence.
Mucous membrane discomfort	Mouth breathing or dehydration leads to dry mucous membranes; tongue and lips become dry or chapped.	Provide oral care at least every 2 to 4 hours. Apply a light film of lip balm for dryness. Apply topical analgesics to oral lesions prn.
Corneal irritation	Blinking reflexes diminish near death, causing drying of cornea.	Optical lubricants or artificial tears reduce corneal drying.
Fatigue	Metabolic demands, stress, disease states, decreased oral intake, and heart function cause weakness and fatigue.	Provide periods of rest and educate patient about energy conservation.
Anxiety	Physical, social, or spiritual distress causes anxiety; causes may be situational or event specific.	Provide opportunity for patient to express feelings though active listening. Provide calm, supportive environment. Consult members of the health care team to determine whether pharmacological interventions are appropriate.
Nausea	Nausea is caused by medications, pain, or decreased intestinal blood flow with impending death.	Determine the cause of nausea and work to reduce nausea triggers such as strong smells. Administer antiemetics or promotility agents. Encourage patients to lie on their right side. Provide oral care at least every 2 to 4 hours.
Constipation	Opioids, other medications, and immobility slow peristalsis. Lack of bulk in diet or reduced fluid is a cause.	Increase fiber in diet if appropriate. Administer stool softeners or laxatives as needed. If possible, encourage increased liquid intake and regular periods of ambulation.
Diarrhea	Disease processes, treatment or medications, and gastrointestinal (GI) infections are causes.	Consult with members of the health care team to determine the cause and make appropriate changes. Provide skin care and easy accessibility to the toilet or bedside commode.
Urinary incontinence	Progressive disease and decreased level of consciousness are causes.	Provide good skin care and frequent assessment for incontinent urine. Place Foley catheter as appropriate.
Altered nutrition	Medications, depression, decreased activity, and decreased blood flow to GI tract are causes. Nausea produces anorexia.	Encourage patient to eat small, frequent meals of preferred foods. Patients should never be forced to eat.
Dehydration	Patient is less willing or able to maintain oral fluid intake; has fever.	Reduce discomfort from dehydration; give mouth care at least every 2 to 4 hours; offer ice chips or moist cloth to lips. Keep lips and tongue moist.
Ineffective breathing patterns (e.g., dyspnea, shortness of breath)	Anxiety; fever; pain; increased oxygen demand; disease processes; and anemia, which reduces oxygen-carrying capacity, are causes.	Treat or control underlying cause. Use nonpharmacological interventions such as elevating the head of the bed to promote lung expansion. Provide oxygen as needed. Keeping the air cool provides ease and comfort for the terminal patient. Using morphine or benzodiazepines to treat tachypnea is sometimes appropriate.
Noisy breathing ("death rattle")	Noisy breathing is the sound of secretions moving in the airway during inspiratory and expiratory phases caused by thick secretions, decreased muscle tone, swallow, and cough.	Elevate head to facilitate postural drainage. Turn patient at least every 2 hours. Provide oral care and maintain hydration as tolerated.

and familiarity. Consider nonpharmacological interventions such as massage therapy to increase patient comfort (Paice, 2015). Family members are often able to provide these interventions, increasing their sense that they are making a positive contribution. Use patient-preferred music in the background, provide guided-imagery exercises, and dim the lights to provide a soothing environment for the patient and family. Patient-preferred forms of complementary therapies offer noninvasive methods to increase comfort and well-being at the end of life (Mariano, 2015) (see Chapter 32).

Promote Spiritual Comfort and Hope. Patients are comforted when they have assurance that some aspect of their lives will transcend death; therefore, helping patients make connections to their spiritual practice or cultural community can be a useful intervention. Draw on the resources of spiritual care providers in an institutional setting or collaborate with the patient's own spiritual or religious leaders and communities. Making an audiotape or videotape for the family, writing letters, or keeping a journal assures patients that something of their essence will survive past their death.

The spiritual concept of hope takes on special significance near the end of life. Nursing strategies that promote hope are often quite simple: be present and provide whole-person care. Patients perceive the love of family and friends, faith, goal setting, positive relationships with professional caregivers, humor, and uplifting memories as hope promoting. Circumstances that hinder the preservation of hope include abandonment or isolation, uncontrolled symptoms, or being devalued as a person. Patients and their families hope for different things over the course of their experience with illness and death. Balancing each perspective is imperative to quality patient care at the end of life. Some hope to live for an anniversary, sit outdoors for a meal, see an important person one last time, gain pain relief, or have a peaceful death. Listen for shifts in patients' hopes and find ways to help them meet their desired goals.

Protect Against Abandonment and Isolation. Many patients with terminal illness fear dying alone. Patients with chronic disease often become socially isolated by choice. However, most patients feel more hopeful when others are near to help them. Nurses in institutional settings need to answer call lights promptly and check on patients often to reassure them that someone is close at hand. If family members always plan to stay with the patient or if you have assessed high privacy needs for the patient and family, a private room is best.

Some family members who have a difficult time accepting a patient's impending death cope by making fewer visits. When family members do visit, inform them of the patient's status and share meaningful insights or encounters that you have had with the patient. Find simple and appropriate care activities for the family to perform, such as offering food, cooling the patient's face, combing hair, or filling out a menu. Nighttime can be particularly lonely for the patient. Suggest that a family member stay through the night if possible. Make exceptions to visiting policies, allowing family members to remain with patients who are dying at any time. Family members appreciate having open access or closeness to their loved one through their experiences at the end of life. Record contact information for them, so you can reach them at any time.

Support the Grieving Family. In palliative and hospice care patients and family members constitute the unit of care. When a patient becomes debilitated or approaches the end of life, family members also suffer. They describe caregiving at the end of life as unpredictable, frightening, and anguishing. Yet many family members find meaning in providing practical and simple care to their loved one. In these extremely intimate and emotionally challenging times, offer holistic, family-centered support, compassion, and education that incorporates the uniqueness of each patient. Often family members face challenging and complex situations long before their loved one is actively dying. Family members caring for people with serious life-limiting illness need attention and support early and consistently throughout the experience of illness and death.

Educate family members in all settings about the symptoms that the patient is likely to experience and the implications for care (see Table 36.3 and Box 36.7). For example, patients in the last days of life often develop anorexia or feel nauseated by food. Illness, excessive respiratory secretions, decreased activity, treatments, and fatigue decrease a patient's caloric needs and appetite. Family members, distressed with the decline, often believe that they need to encourage the patient to eat. Because the goal of palliative care is comfort, do not force the patient to do anything that is causing discomfort. Eating in the last days of life often causes the patient pain and discomfort. In addition, as the body is shutting down, the nutrients in food are not able to be absorbed. Therefore, forcing patients to eat does not benefit the patient. Help families shift their focus to other helping activities during this time.

Family members who have limited experience with death do not know what to expect. They may need personal time with you to share their concerns, ask about treatment options, validate perceived changes in the patient's status, or explore the possible meaning of patient behaviors. Whenever possible, communicate news of a patient's declining condition or impending death when family members are together, so they can support one another. Provide information privately and stay with the family as long as needed or desired. Reduce family member anxiety, stress, or fear by describing what to expect as death approaches. Become familiar with common manifestations of impending death (Box 36.8), remembering that patients usually experience

---

BOX 36.7 **EVIDENCE-BASED PRACTICE**
Managing Opioid-Induced Constipation

PICOT Question: In patients who are terminally ill, what is the effect of pharmacological interventions to reduce opioid-induced constipation compared with nonpharmacological interventions?

Evidence Summary

A majority of patients at the end of life use opioids to control pain and discomfort. A common side effect of opioids is opioid-induced constipation (OIC). This adds to unpleasant and uncomfortable symptoms experienced by the patient. Nurses commonly use nonpharmacological measures such as ambulation and increasing fiber and fluids to help patients with constipation, but these traditional interventions may be inappropriate for patients at the end of life. Besides using laxatives, stimulants, or stool softeners, several new drugs are available. Naloxegol is an oral peripherally acting selective μ-opioid antagonist that has been shown to be safe and effective for the treatment of OIC (Nee et al., 2018). Methylnaltrexone, a derivative of naltrexone, is a subcutaneous drug also with highly positive outcomes (Star and Boland, 2018).

Application to Nursing Practice

- Although there are positive improvements in the treatment of opioid-induced constipation, prevention is key.
- Use the lowest dose possible of the least constipating opioid to control pain—for example, fentanyl instead of oxycodone.
- Try traditional nonpharmacological interventions, if appropriate, and laxatives before trying naloxegol or methylnaltrexone (Star and Boland, 2018).

BOX 36.8 Physical Changes Hours or Days Before Death

- Increased periods of sleeping/unresponsiveness
- Circulatory changes with coolness and color changes in extremities, nose, fingers (cyanosis, pallor, mottling) (see Fig. 36.4)
- Bowel or bladder incontinence
- Decreased urine output; dark-colored urine
- Restlessness, confusion, or disorientation
- Decreased intake of food or fluids; inability to swallow
- Congestion/increased pulmonary secretions; noisy respirations (death rattle)
- Altered breathing (apnea, labored or irregular breathing, Cheyne-Stokes pattern)
- Decreased muscle tone, relaxed jaw muscles, sagging mouth
- Weakness and fatigue

---

some but not all of these changes. Do not try to predict the time of death; instead use your assessments to help family members anticipate what is happening. Be compassionate and sensitive in how you share information. "Mottling is an expected sign as a body begins shutting down" instead of "when a person gets closer to death, we see mottling" (Fig. 36.4). Share your observations and through your role modeling encourage a sense of patience, compassion, and comfort throughout the dying process.

During the dying process check frequently on families, offering support, information, and, if appropriate, encouragement to continue touching and talking with their loved ones. In the time immediately following death determine the family's needs. Some families will want to touch or hold the deceased; others will not. Make the deceased accessible by lowering side rails, leaving hands

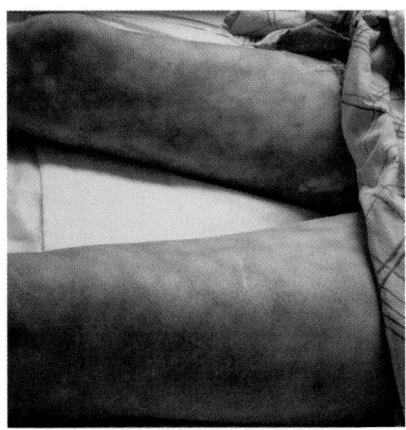

FIG. 36.4 Skin mottling. (From Adams J, et al: *Emergency medicine: clinical essentials,* ed 2, Philadelphia, 2014, Elsevier.)

exposed, and setting a chair close to the bedside. Depending on agency policies, allow the family the necessary time to be with their loved one.

After death help the family make decisions such as notification of a funeral home, transportation of family members, and collection of the patient's belongings. Nurses are a primary source of family support. Remember that, because of differing responses to grief, some family members prefer to be alone at the time of and after the death, whereas others want to be surrounded by a support community. When uncertain about what a family member prefers for support, pose simple questions and offer suggestions for assistance.

Facilitate Mourning. Nurses who work with grieving family members often provide bereavement care after the patient's death. Helpful strategies for assisting grieving persons include the following:

- Help the survivor accept that the loss is real. Discuss how the loss or illness occurred or was discovered, when, under what circumstances, who told him or her about it, and other factual topics to reinforce the reality of the event and put it in perspective.
- Support efforts to adjust to the loss. Use a problem-solving approach. Have survivors make a list of their concerns or needs, help them prioritize, and lead them step-by-step through a discussion of how to proceed. Encourage survivors to ask for help.
- Encourage establishment of new relationships. Reassure people that new relationships do not mean that they are replacing the person who has died. Encourage involvement in nonthreatening group social activities (e.g., volunteer activities or church events).
- Allow time to grieve. "Anniversary reactions" (e.g., renewed grief around the time of the loss in subsequent years) are common, along with renewed grief at holidays. A return to sadness or the pain of grief is often worrisome. Openly acknowledge the loss, provide reassurance that the reaction is normal, and encourage the survivor to reminisce.
- Interpret "normal" behavior. Being distractible, having difficulty sleeping or eating, and thinking that they have heard the deceased's voice are common behaviors for survivors following loss. These symptoms do not mean that an individual has an emotional problem or is becoming ill. Reinforce that these behaviors are normal and will resolve over time.
- Provide continuing support. Following a loss, survivors need the support of a nurse with whom they have bonded for a time, especially in cases of in-home care or hospice nursing. Your goal is to fulfill an important role in the deceased's life and death, helping survivors through some very intimate and memorable times. Attachment for a period of time after the death is appropriate and healing

for both the survivor and you. However, it is imperative that professional boundaries always be maintained.

- Be alert for signs of ineffective, potentially harmful coping mechanisms such as alcohol and substance abuse or excessive use of over-the-counter analgesics or sleep aids.

Care After Death. Federal and state laws require institutions to develop policies and procedures for certain events that occur after death: requesting organ or tissue donation, performing an autopsy, certifying and documenting the occurrence of a death, and providing safe and appropriate postmortem care. In accordance with federal law, a specially trained professional (e.g., transplant coordinator or social worker) makes requests for organ and tissue donation at the time of every death. The person requesting organ or tissue donation provides information about who can give consent legally, which organs or tissues can be donated, associated costs, and how donation affects burial or cremation.

In extremely stressful circumstances created by the loss of a loved one, grieving survivors usually cannot remember all they were told. Nurses provide support and reinforce or clarify explanations. In addition, understanding the physiology of organ donation is often difficult for family members. Even though a patient who is brain dead is legally declared dead, he or she remains on life support to provide the vital organs with blood and oxygen before transplant. The appearance of a live-looking body confuses the family, and they need help to understand that the life support is only preserving the vital organs. Nonvital tissues such as corneas, skin, long bones, and middle ear bones are taken at the time of death without artificially maintaining vital functions. If the deceased has not left behind instructions concerning organ and tissue donation, the family gives or denies consent at the time of death. Review your state organ-retrieval laws and institutional policy and procedure regarding the formal consent process. Be aware that the laws governing whom to approach for organ donation may not be acceptable in other cultures.

Family members give consent for an autopsy (i.e., the surgical dissection of a body after death) to determine the exact cause and circumstances of death or to discover the pathway of a disease (see Chapter 23). In most cases a coroner or medical examiner determines the need to perform an autopsy. Law sometimes requires that an autopsy be performed when death is the result of foul play; homicide; suicide; or accidental causes such as motor vehicle crashes, falls, the ingestion of drugs, or deaths within 24 hours of hospital admission. Follow state and agency requirements regarding removal of lines (e.g., IVs, indwelling urinary catheter) in patients when an autopsy is ordered.

Usually the physician or other designated health care provider asks for autopsy permission while the nurse answers questions and supports the family's choices. Inform family members that an autopsy does not deform the body and that all organs are replaced in the body. Family members are often comforted to know that others may be helped by either the gift of organ and tissue donation or autopsy. Respect and honor family wishes and final decisions.

Documentation of a death provides a legal record of the event. Follow agency policies and procedures carefully to provide an accurate and reliable medical record of all assessments and activities surrounding a death. Physicians or coroners sign some medical forms, such as a request for autopsy, but the nurse gathers and records much of the remaining information surrounding a death. Nurses also usually witness or delegate the signing of forms (e.g., release of body or personal belongings forms). Nursing documentation becomes relevant in risk management or legal investigations into a death, underscoring the importance of accurate, legal reporting. Documentation also validates

BOX 36.9 Documentation of End-of-Life Care

- Time and date of death and all actions taken to respond to the impending death
- Verification of death according to health care agency policy
- Name of health care provider certifying the death
- People notified of the death (e.g., health care providers, family members, organ request team, morgue, funeral home, spiritual care providers) and person who declared the time of death
- Name of person making request for organ or tissue donation
- Special preparations of the body (e.g., desired or required spiritual, religious and cultural rituals)
- Medical tubes, devices, or lines left in or on the body
- Personal articles left on and secured to the body
- Personal items given to the family with description, date, time, to whom given
- Location of body identification tags
- Time of body transfer and destination
- Any other relevant information or family requests that help clarify special circumstances

BOX 36.10 CULTURAL ASPECTS OF CARE

Care of the Body After Death

Loved ones use cultural-specific rituals and mourning practices to achieve a sense of acceptance and inner peace and participate in socially accepted expressions of grief. One's culture greatly influences which behaviors and rituals are expected at the time of death. Institutional guidelines and end-of-life care procedures for patients from all cultures provide standards based on showing compassion, maintaining privacy and dignity, and respecting patients' and family members' cultural beliefs and practices. Expert end-of-life care allows time for patients and their families to make private and public preparations and to complete unfinished communication. Understanding the uniqueness of cultural expectations at the end of life helps you to know which questions to ask. The following cultural or religious practices are not necessarily exclusive to the culture named but are offered to give you an idea of some culture-specific concerns that you may encounter in end-of-life care.

Implications for Patient-Centered Care

Honoring the patient's and the family's cultural and spiritual customs is very important when caring for the dying and the dead. Here are some important things to know (or ask) concerning special ways to care for the body during and after death.

- Will there be large extended-family groups, including the church family, coming to be present at the time of death?
- Will the family be having organs donated or an autopsy completed?
- Do the patient and family believe in an afterlife?
- Should a religious leader be called to the deathbed for a prayer or blessing?
- Does the deceased require special bathing or clothes after death?
- Will family or male members of the religious order need to stay with the deceased while waiting for transport/burial?
- Can only members of the same gender tend to the deceased's body?
- Does the body need to lie with the head facing a certain direction?

success in meeting patient goals or provides justification for changes in treatment or expected outcomes. Box 36.9 lists important documentation elements for end-of-life care.

Family members deserve and expect a clear description of what happened to their loved one, especially in cases of sudden, unusual, or unexpected circumstances. Give *only* factual information in a non-judgmental, objective manner, and avoid sharing your opinions. State law and agency policy govern the sharing of the written medical record information, which usually involves a written request. Follow legal guidelines for documentation and sharing of medical records (see Chapter 23).

When a patient dies in an institutional or home care setting, nurses provide or delegate postmortem care, the care of a body after death. Above all, a deceased person's body deserves the same respect and dignity as that of a living person and needs to be prepared in a manner consistent with the patient's cultural and religious beliefs. Death produces physical changes in the body quite quickly; thus, you need to perform postmortem care as soon as possible to prevent discoloration, tissue damage, or deformities. Many hospitals have a policy for how many hours the body can stay on the unit before being sent to the morgue. This is important as this is the time that family members have to mourn directly after death.

Maintaining the integrity of cultural and religious rituals and mourning practices at the time of death gives survivors a sense of fulfilled obligations and promotes acceptance of the patient's death (Box 36.10). The ability of families to mourn in a manner consistent with cultural values helps survivors experience some predictability and control in an otherwise uncertain and confusing time. Some cultures consider "family" as more than a nuclear biological unit. Health care providers need to understand the makeup of a family network and know which individuals to involve in end-of-life decisions and care.

You will coordinate patient and family care during and after a death. Become familiar with applicable policies and procedures for postmortem care because they vary across settings or institutions. See the procedural guideline (Box 36.11) for standard activities for care of the body after death.

◆ Evaluation

Through the Patient's Eyes. The success of the evaluation process depends partially on the bond that you have formed with the patient and family. Through a trusting relationship, patients are more likely to share personal expectations or their wishes, especially if encouraged through appropriate questioning. The following questions evaluate if patient perceptions have been met:

- What is the most important thing I can do for you at this time?
- Are your needs being addressed in a timely manner?
- Are you getting the care for which you hoped?
- Would you like me to help you in a different way?
- Do you have a specific request that I have not met?

Refer back to the goals and expected outcomes established during the planning phase to determine if the patient and family perceive that goals were met. A patient's responses and perceptions of the effectiveness of nursing interventions help determine whether the existing plan of care is effective or different strategies are necessary. Even when a patient is not seeking care specifically related to a loss, be alert for signs and symptoms of grief. They provide the criteria for evaluating whether a patient is coping with a loss and how he or she is moving through the grief process. Critical thinking ensures that the evaluation process accurately reflects the patient's situation and desired outcomes (Fig. 36.5).

Patient Outcomes. Review the goals and expected outcomes of the plan of care to determine if nursing interventions were successful or if modifications are needed. For example, if the goal is to have the patient communicate a sense of hope to family members, evaluate verbal and nonverbal communication and behaviors for cues related to expressions of hope. If the goal is to achieve a level of comfort, evaluate if the

BOX 36.11 PROCEDURAL GUIDELINES

Care of the Body After Death

Delegation and Collaboration

The skill of care of the body after death can be delegated to assistive personnel (AP). Nurses often find it meaningful to help care for a patient after death and assist the AP whenever possible. Instruct the AP to:

- Contact the nurse for all questions and procedures related to organ/tissue donation and autopsy requests.
- Alert nurse to family members' questions related to manner of death or after-death activities.

Equipment

Bath towels, washcloths, washbasin, scissors, clean disposable gloves, gown (if high risk of exposure to body fluids), shroud kit with name tags, bed linen, documentation forms.

Steps

1. Confirm that the health care provider certified the death and documented the time of death and actions taken.
2. Determine whether the health care provider requested an autopsy. An autopsy is required for deaths that occur under certain circumstances.
3. Validate the status of request for organ or tissue donation. Given the complex and sensitive nature of such requests, only specially trained personnel make the requests. Maintain sensitivity to personal, spiritual, religious, and cultural beliefs in this process.
4. Identify the patient using two identifiers (e.g., name and birthday or name and medical record number according to agency policy).
5. Perform hand hygiene and apply disposable gloves. Apply gown if risk of exposure to body fluids is high.
6. Provide sensitive and dignified nursing care to the patient and family.
   a. Elevate the head of the bed as soon as possible after death to prevent discoloration of the face.
   b. Collect ordered specimens.
   c. Ask whether the family wishes to participate in preparation of the body. Offer to make arrangements for supportive company for the family (patient/family religious leader, spiritual care personnel, or bereavement specialist) during body preparation.
   d. Ask about family requests for body preparation, such as wearing special clothing or religious artifacts. Be aware that personal, religious, or cultural practices determine whether to shave male facial hair. Get permission before shaving a beard.
   e. Remove all equipment, tubes, and indwelling lines. Note that autopsy or organ donation often poses exceptions to removal; thus, consult agency policy in these situations.
   f. Cleanse the body thoroughly, maintaining safety standards for body fluids and contamination when indicated. Remove gloves and gown (if needed) and perform hand hygiene.
   g. Comb patient's hair or apply personal hairpieces.
   h. Cover body with a clean sheet, place head on a pillow, and leave arms outside covers if possible. Close eyes by gently holding them shut; leave dentures in the mouth to maintain facial shape; cover any signs of body trauma.
   i. Prepare and clean the environment, deodorize room if needed, and lower the lights.
   j. Offer family members the option to view the body. Ask whether they want you or other support people to accompany them. Honor and respect individual choices.
   k. Encourage grievers to say goodbye in their own way: words, touch, singing, spiritual or religious rituals, or prayers.
   l. Provide privacy and a quiet, peaceful atmosphere. Assess family members' need or desire for your presence at this time. If you leave, tell them how to reach you.
   k. Determine which personal belongings stay with the body (e.g., wedding ring or religious symbol), and give other personal items to family members. Document time, date, description of the items taken, and who received them. Save any items that are left behind accidentally and contact family for further instructions.
   l. Apply identifying name tags and shroud according to agency policy before transporting the body. Perform hand hygiene.
   m. Complete documentation in the narrative notes section (see Box 36.9).
   n. Maintain privacy and dignity when transporting the body to another location; cover the body or stretcher with a clean sheet.

---

severity of pain has declined and if the patient is able to participate in more self-care activities. Continue to evaluate the patient's progress, the effectiveness of the interventions, and patient and family interactions.

In-home care settings it is critically important to include family members in the evaluation process. The short- and long-term outcomes that signal a family's recovery from a loss guide your evaluation. Short-term outcomes indicating effectiveness of grief interventions include talking about the loss without feeling overwhelmed, improved energy level, normalized sleep and dietary patterns, reorganization of life patterns, improved ability to make decisions, and finding it easier to be around other people. Long-term achievements include the return of a sense of humor and normal life patterns, renewed or new personal relationships, and decrease of inner pain.

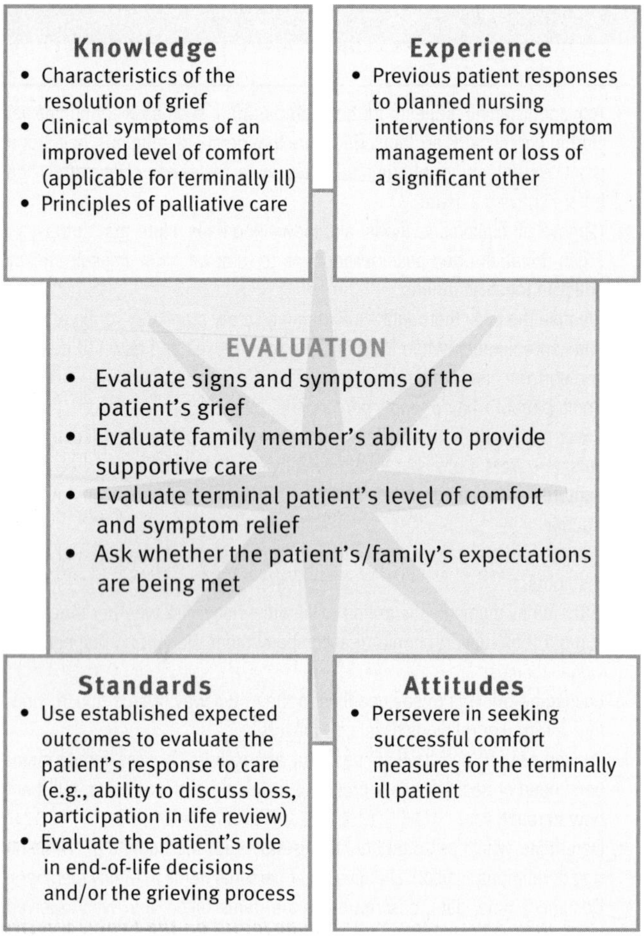

Knowledge
- Characteristics of the resolution of grief
- Clinical symptoms of an improved level of comfort (applicable for terminally ill)
- Principles of palliative care

Experience
- Previous patient responses to planned nursing interventions for symptom management or loss of a significant other

EVALUATION
- Evaluate signs and symptoms of the patient's grief
- Evaluate family member's ability to provide supportive care
- Evaluate terminal patient's level of comfort and symptom relief
- Ask whether the patient's/family's expectations are being met

Standards
- Use established expected outcomes to evaluate the patient's response to care (e.g., ability to discuss loss, participation in life review)
- Evaluate the patient's role in end-of-life decisions and/or the grieving process

Attitudes
- Persevere in seeking successful comfort measures for the terminally ill patient

FIG. 36.5 Critical thinking model for loss, death, and grief evaluation.

KEY POINTS

- When caring for patients who are experiencing loss, facilitate the grief process by helping them feel the loss, express it, and move through their grief.
- Loss comes in many forms, based on the values and priorities learned within a person's sphere of influence (i.e., family, friends, religion, society, and culture) as well as a natural part of maturation.
- Survivors move back and forth through a series of stages or tasks many times, possibly extending over a long period of time.
- Depending on the characteristic and context of the loss, as well as of the griever, there are several types of grief that can be experienced.
- People who are grieving use their own unique history, context, and resources to make meaning out of their loss experiences. Listen as patients share the experience in their own way.
- A person's development, coping strategies, socioeconomic status, personal relationships, nature of loss, and cultural and spiritual beliefs influence the way he or she perceives and responds to grief.
- Assess the wishes of a patient and family for end-of-life care, including the preferred place for death, desired level of intervention, and expectations for pain and symptom management.
- Establish a caring presence and use effective communication strategies to encourage patients to share to the degree they are comfortable. Collaborate with other members of the health care team to provide holistic care for management of symptoms and to provide a variety of support measures to the patient and family.

- Quality end-of-life care focuses on improving quality of life through management of unpleasant symptoms such as pain, anxiety, and nausea.
- Hospice is a philosophy of family-centered, whole-person care for individuals with a life-limiting illness likely to result in death within 6 months.
- After determining that an autopsy will be performed, the body of the deceased is cared for and treated with the same level of care and compassion, respect, and dignity as when the person was alive.

REFLECTIVE LEARNING

- Knowing that you disagree with a patient's choice to not seek further treatment, how do you continue to compassionately support the patient while keeping your personal thoughts and beliefs from influencing your care?
- Think about how, from a cultural or spiritual perspective, you will begin and maintain a conversation about advance directives with your patient and the patient's family.
- Often, we think of death as a form of failure, that somehow health care professionals didn't get it right. However, how can quality end-of-life care embody what it means to truly provide the best for our patients?

REVIEW QUESTIONS

1. To best assist a patient in the grieving process, which factors are most important for the nurse to assess? (Select all that apply.)
   1. Previous experiences with grief and loss
   2. Religious affiliation and denomination
   3. Ethnic background and cultural practices
   4. Current financial status
   5. Current medications
2. Which interventions does a nurse implement to help a patient at the end of life maintain autonomy while in a hospital? (Select all that apply.)
   1. Use therapeutic techniques when communicating with the patient.
   2. Allow the patient to determine timing and scheduling of interventions.
   3. Allow patients to have visitors at any time.
   4. Provide the patient with a private room close to the nurses' station.
   5. Encourage the patient to eat whenever he or she is hungry.
3. The nurse recognizes that which factors influence a person's approach to death? (Select all that apply.)
   1. Culture
   2. Spirituality
   3. Personal beliefs
   4. Previous experiences with death
   5. Gender
   6. Level of education
4. A nurse has the responsibility of managing a patient's postmortem care. What is the proper order for postmortem care when there is no autopsy ordered?
   1. Bathe the body of the deceased.
   2. Collect any needed specimens.
   3. Remove all tubes and indwelling lines.
   4. Position the body for family viewing.
   5. Speak to the family members about their possible participation.

6. Ensure that the request for organ/tissue donation and/or autopsy was completed.

7. Notify support person (e.g., spiritual care provider, bereavement specialist) for the family.

8. Accurately tag the body, including the identity of the deceased and safety issues regarding infection control.

9. Elevate the head of the bed.

5. Which comments to a patient by a new nurse regarding palliative care needs are correct? (Select all that apply.)

1. "Even though you're continuing treatment, palliative care is something we might want to talk about."

2. "Palliative care is appropriate for people with any diagnosis."

3. "Only people who are dying can receive palliative care."

4. "Children are able to receive palliative care."

5. Palliative care is only for people with uncontrolled pain.

6. A patient is receiving palliative care for symptom management related to anxiety and pain. A family member asks whether the patient is dying and now in "hospice." What does the nurse tell the family member about palliative care? (Select all that apply.)

1. Palliative care and hospice are the same thing.

2. Palliative care is for any patient, any time, any disease, in any setting.

3. Palliative care strategies are primarily designed to treat the patient's illness.

4. Palliative care relieves the symptoms of illness and treatment.

5. Palliative care selects home health care services.

7. When planning care for a dying patient, which interventions promote the patient's dignity? (Select all that apply.)

1. Providing respect

2. Viewing the patient as a whole

3. Providing symptom management

4. Showing interest

5. Being present

6. Inserting a straight catheter when the patient has difficulty voiding

8. What are the physical circulatory changes that occur as death approaches?

1. Skin irritation

2. Mottling

3. Increased urine output

4. Weakness

9. When providing postmortem care, which actions are necessary for the nurse to complete?

1. Locating the patient's clothing

2. Calling the funeral home

3. Providing culturally and religiously sensitive care in body preparation

4. Providing postmortem care to protect the family of the deceased from having to view the body

10. Which actions by the nurse help grieving families? (Select all that apply.)

1. Encourage involvement in nonthreatening group social activities.

2. Follow up with the family in their home.

3. Remind them that feelings of sadness or pain can return around anniversaries.

4. Encourage survivors to ask for help.

5. Look for overuse of alcohol, sleeping aids, or street drugs.

Answers: 1. 1, 2, 3; **2.** 2, 3, 5; **3.** 1, 2, 3, 4; **4.** 6, 9, 2, 5, 7, 3, 1, 4, 8; **5.** 1, 2, 4; **6.** 2, 4; **7.** 1, 2, 4, 5; **8.** 2, 4; **9.** 3; **10.** 1, 3, 4, 5.

Rationales for Review Questions can be found on the Evolve website.

REFERENCES

American Association of Colleges of Nursing (AACN) and City of Hope National Medical Center (CHNMC): *End-of-Life Nursing Education Consortium (ELNEC)—core*, Duarte, CA, 2014, The Associations.

American Nurses Association (ANA): *Scope and standards of hospice and palliative nursing practice*, Atlanta, 2014, ANA.

Bowlby J: *Attachment and loss: loss, sadness, and depression*, vol. 3. New York, 1980, Basic Books.

Bruinsma SM, et al.: Risk factors for complicated grief in older adults, *J Palliat Med* 18(5):438–446, 2015.

Coyle N: Introduction to palliative nursing care. In Ferrell B, Coyle N, editors: *Textbook of palliative nursing*, ed 4, New York, 2015, Oxford University Press.

Hall C: Bereavement theory: recent developments in our understanding of grief and bereavement, *Bereavement Care* 33(1):7, 2014.

Hospice Foundation of America: Services. *What is hospice?* 2018, http://hospicefoundation.org/End-of-Life-Support-and-Resources/Coping-with-Terminal-Illness/Hospice-Services. Accessed July 2018.

Kübler-Ross E: *On death and dying*, New York, 1969, Macmillan.

Mariano C: Holistic integrative therapies in palliative care. In Matzo M, Sherman D, editors: *Palliative care nursing: quality care to the end-of-life*, ed 4, New York, 2015, Springer.

Mattes M, Sloane M: Reflections of hope and its implications for end-of-life care, *J Am Geriatr Soc* 63(5):993–996, 2015.

Matzo M, Sherman D: *Palliative care nursing: quality care to the end of life*, ed 4, New York, 2015, Springer.

Meghani S, et al.: Policy brief: the Institute of Medicine report: dying in America: improving quality and honoring individual preferences near the end of life, *Nurs Outlook* 63(1):51, 2015.

Mitchell KR, Anderson H: *All our losses, all our griefs*, Louisville, 1983, Westminster John Know Press.

Moon PJ: Anticipatory grief: a mere concept? *Am J Hosp Palliat Care* 33(5):417–420, 2016.

Mughal S, Siddiqui WJ: Grief reaction, *Stat Pearls*, 2019, https://www.ncbi.nlm.nih.gov/books/NBK507832/. Accessed September 6, 2019.

Paice JA: Pain at the end of life. In Ferrell B, Coyle N, editors: *Textbook of palliative nursing*, ed 4, New York, 2015, Oxford University Press.

Perng A, Renz S: Identifying and treating complicated grief in older adults, *J Nurse Pract* 14(4):289–294, 2018.

Rando T: *Treatment of complicated mourning*, Champaign, IL, 1993, Research Press.

Rando T: *What therapists need to know about traumatic bereavement: what it is and how to approach it*, 2014, http://www.lowcountrymhconference.com/wp-content/uploads/2014/07/drrando_handout.pdf. Accessed September 12, 2019.

Reynolds J, et al.: American Society for Pain Management Nursing position statement: pain management at the end of life, *Pain Manage Nurs* 14(3):172, 2013.

Stroebe M, Schut H: The dual process model of coping with bereavement: rationale and description, *Death Stud* 23(3):197, 1999.

Walter C, McCoyd J: *Grief and loss across the lifespan: a biopsychosocial perspective*, ed 2, New York, 2015, Springer.

Worden JW: *Grief counseling and grief therapy: a handbook for the mental health practitioner*, ed 4, New York, 2008, Springer.

World Health Organization (WHO): *Definition of palliative care*, 2018, http://www.who.int/cancer/palliative/definition/en/. Accessed July 16, 2018.

RESEARCH REFERENCES

Coolhart D, et al.: Experience of ambiguous loss for parents of transgender male youth: a phenomenological exploration, *Contemp Fam Ther* 40:28–41, 2018.

Dose AM, et al.: The meaning of spirituality at the end of life, *J Hop Palliat Nurs* 16(3):138, 2014.

Liang Y, et al.: Do-not-resuscitate consent signed by patients indicates a more favorable quality of end-of-life care for patients with advanced cancer, *Support Care Cancer* 25(2):533–539, 2017.

Nee J, et al.: Efficacy of treatments for opioid-induced constipation: systematic review and meta-analysis, *Clin Gastroenterol Hepatol* 16(10):1569–1584, 2018.

Perez RM, Arnold-Berkovits I: A conceptual framework for understanding Latino immigrant's ambiguous loss of homeland, *Hisp J Behav Sci* 40(2):91–114, 2018.

Star A, Boland JW: Updates in palliative care – recent advancements in the pharmacological management of symptoms, *Clin Med* 18(1):11–16, 2018.

Stress and Coping

OBJECTIVES

- Explain the three stages of the general adaptation syndrome.
- Describe characteristics of post-traumatic stress disorder.
- Discuss the integration of stress theory with nursing theories.
- Identify the effects that compassion fatigue can have in the health care workplace.
- Explain stress-management techniques that help individuals cope with stress.
- Discuss the process of crisis intervention.
- Develop a care plan for patients who are experiencing stress.
- Discuss how stress in the workplace affects nurses.

KEY TERMS

Adventitious crises, p. 764
Alarm stage, p. 762
Allostasis, p. 762
Allostatic load, p. 763
Appraisal, p. 761
Burnout, p. 772
Compassion fatigue , p. 765
Coping, p. 763
Crisis, p. 764
Crisis intervention, p. 773

Developmental crises, p. 764
Ego-defense mechanisms, p. 763
Exhaustion stage, p. 763
Fight-or-flight response, p. 762
Flashbacks, p. 764
General adaptation syndrome (GAS), p. 762
Mindfulness, p. 772
Post-traumatic stress disorder (PTSD), p. 764

Primary appraisal, p. 763
Resistance stage, p. 762
Secondary appraisal, p. 763
Situational crises, p. 764
Stress, p. 761
Stressors, p. 761
Trauma, p. 761

MEDIA RESOURCES

http://evolve.elsevier.com/Potter/fundamentals/
- Review Questions
- Concept Map Creator
- Case Study with Questions

- Audio Glossary
- Content Updates
- Answers to QSEN Activity and Review Questions

Stress can impact the physical and mental well-being of patients as well as their entire families and communities. Nurses need to become familiar with stress and consider its effects when delivering patient care. Equally important, health care professionals also experience stressful events in the course of clinical practice and their own lives. Nurses need to consider their own stress by recognizing burnout, compassion fatigue, and second victim syndrome. It is important for nurses to understand stress-management techniques to aid their own personal coping and to design stress-management interventions for patients and families.

Stress is described as an actual or alleged hazard to the balance of homeostasis. It is often described as a physical, chemical, or emotional factor that produces tension in the body or the mind (Banasik and Copstead, 2019). Such factors are referred to as stressors. Stressors are any physical, psychological, or social stimuli that are capable of producing stress and endangering homeostasis (Banasik and Copstead, 2019). Stressors differ in their scope, strength, and duration. A stressor of less intensity can still have a substantial influence if it continues over time. An important element in the perception of a stressor is appraisal. Appraisal is how a person interprets the impact of the stressor. It is also a personal evaluation of the meaning of the event to what is happening and a consideration of the resources on hand to help manage the stressor. Stress emerges when an individual considers the event as a threat and the ability to respond to the demands placed on the individual by the event to be overwhelming. Thus, stress can lead to personal growth and development or overwhelm a person and lead to illness or worsening of existing acute or chronic illnesses (Liu et al., 2017).

People experience stress as a consequence of daily life events and experiences—such as loss of a loved one, change in job responsibilities, or illness—which stimulates their ability to think clearly and stay alert to the environment. How people react to stress depends on how they view and evaluate the impact of the stressor, its effect on their situation and support at the time of the stress, and their usual coping mechanisms. When stress overwhelms existing coping mechanisms, patients lose emotional balance, and a crisis results. If symptoms of stress persist beyond the duration of the stressor, a person experiences a trauma (Sacks et al., 2017).

SCIENTIFIC KNOWLEDGE BASE

Hans Selye, a Vienna-born endocrinologist, was the first scientist to single out the physical side effects of stress. While conducting experiments related to hormone production, Selye noticed that his subjects showed a similar set of side effects regardless of the type of life-threatening stimulus that researchers presented. Selye termed this collection

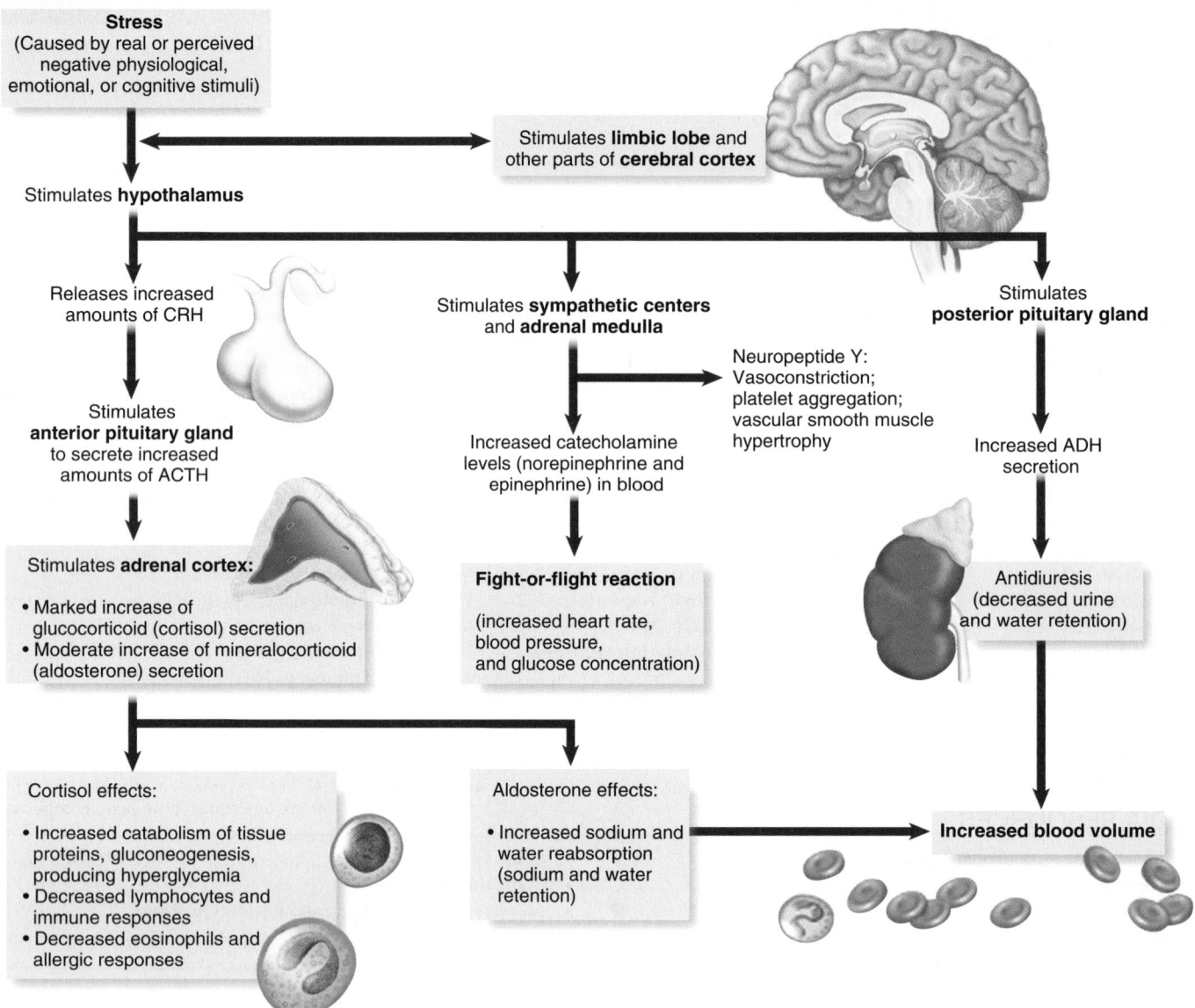

Stress
(Caused by real or perceived negative physiological, emotional, or cognitive stimuli)

Stimulates **limbic lobe** and other parts of **cerebral cortex**

Stimulates **hypothalamus**

Releases increased amounts of CRH

Stimulates **sympathetic centers** and **adrenal medulla**

Stimulates **posterior pituitary gland**

Stimulates **anterior pituitary gland** to secrete increased amounts of ACTH

Neuropeptide Y: Vasoconstriction; platelet aggregation; vascular smooth muscle hypertrophy

Increased catecholamine levels (norepinephrine and epinephrine) in blood

Increased ADH secretion

Stimulates **adrenal cortex:**

• Marked increase of glucocorticoid (cortisol) secretion
• Moderate increase of mineralocorticoid (aldosterone) secretion

Fight-or-flight reaction

(increased heart rate, blood pressure, and glucose concentration)

Antidiuresis (decreased urine and water retention)

Cortisol effects:

• Increased catabolism of tissue proteins, gluconeogenesis, producing hyperglycemia
• Decreased lymphocytes and immune responses
• Decreased eosinophils and allergic responses

Aldosterone effects:

• Increased sodium and water reabsorption (sodium and water retention)

Increased blood volume

FIG. 37.1 Short-term and long-term stress response. Some effects are immediate, such as the sympathetic fight-or-flight reaction, and some effects are longer-term, such as the hormonal effects. *ACTH*, Adrenocorticotropic hormone; *ADH*, antidiuretic hormone; *CRH*, corticotropin-releasing hormone. (From Patton KT: *Anatomy & physiology*, ed 10, St Louis, 2019, Elsevier.)

of responses the general adaptation syndrome (GAS), a three-stage set of physiological processes that prepare, or adapt, the body for danger so that an individual is more likely to survive when faced with a threat (Waude, 2016).

Selye (1993) identified the three stages to the stress response as (1) initial alarm, (2) resistance as a person attempts to compensate for changes induced by the alarm stage, and (3) a state of exhaustion if the person cannot adapt successfully during the stage of resistance or if stress remains unrelieved. When stress reaches chronic and harmful levels, negative consequences follow. Selye's initial theory has evolved as scientists have learned more about the physiological responses to stress.

General Adaptation Syndrome

The general adaptation syndrome (GAS), the three-stage reaction to stress, describes how the body responds physiologically to stressors (Fig. 37.1). The GAS is triggered either directly by a physical event or

indirectly by a psychological event. It involves several body systems, especially the neuroendocrine mechanism, which responds immediately to stress (see Fig. 37.1). When the body encounters a physical demand such as an injury, the pituitary gland initiates the GAS. A fundamental concept underlying this reaction is that the body will attempt to return to a state of balance, a process referred to as allostasis (Banasik and Copstead, 2019).

During the alarm stage the central nervous system is aroused, and body defenses are mobilized; this is the fight-or-flight response. During this stage rising hormone levels result in increased blood volume, blood glucose levels, epinephrine and norepinephrine, heart rate, blood flow to muscles, oxygen intake, and mental alertness. In addition, the pupils of the eyes dilate to produce a greater visual field. If the stressor poses an extreme threat to life or remains for a long time, the person progresses to the second stage, resistance.

The resistance stage also contributes to the fight-or-flight response, and the body stabilizes and responds in an attempt to compensate for the changes induced by the alarm stage (Huether et al., 2017). Hormone levels, heart rate, blood pressure, and cardiac output should return to normal, and the body tries to repair any damage that occurred. However, these compensation attempts consume energy and other bodily resources.

In the exhaustion stage continuous stress causes progressive breakdown of compensatory mechanisms. This occurs when the body is no longer able to resist the effects of the stressor and has depleted the energy necessary to maintain adaptation. The physiological response has intensified, but the person's ability to adapt to the stressor diminishes (Huether et al., 2017). Even in the face of chronic demands, an ongoing state of chronic activation can occur. This chronic arousal with the presence of powerful hormones causes excessive wear and tear on bodily organs and is called allostatic load. A persistent allostatic load can cause long-term physiological problems such as chronic hypertension, depression, sleep deprivation, chronic fatigue syndrome, and autoimmune disorders (Huether et al., 2017).

Immune Response. The physiological interactions between the neuroendocrine stress response and the immune system are complex. The stress response directly influences the immune system (Huether et al., 2017). Stress causes prolonged changes in the immune system, which can result in impaired immune function. As stress increases, the person is more susceptible to changes in health such as increased risk for infection, high blood pressure, diabetes, and cancers (Casey and Tiaki, 2017).

Reaction to Psychological Stress. Each person responds differently to physiological threats. They produce different reactions in different people and indirectly activate the GAS. The intensity and duration of the psychological threat and the number of other stressors that occur at the same time affect the person's response. In addition, whether the person anticipated the stressor influences its effect. It is often more difficult to cope with an unexpected stressor. Personal characteristics that influence the response to a stressor include the level of personal control, presence of a social support system, and feelings of competence.

Stress can be viewed as a transaction between a person and the environment. A person appraises or mentally rates an event in terms of its meaning and then experiences stress only if the event or circumstance is considered significant. Evaluating an event in terms of personal meaning is primary appraisal. Appraisal of an event or circumstance is an ongoing perceptual process. Stress results when a person identifies an event or circumstance as a harm, loss, threat, or challenge. Secondary appraisal, the process by which a person considers possible available coping strategies or resources, occurs at the same time. Stress occurs if the demands placed on the person by the event exceed the ability to cope. Balancing factors contribute to restoring equilibrium. According to crisis theory, because feedback cues lead to reappraisals of the original perception, coping behaviors constantly change as individuals perceive new information. When coping behaviors are ineffective and repeated over and over, a state of stress can result. Stress emerges either when a person views an event as posing a significant risk of harm or when the person is not able to cope with the event's demands.

Coping is a person's cognitive and behavioral efforts to manage a stressor (Can et al., 2017). It is important to physical and psychological health because stress is associated with a range of psychological and health outcomes (Can et al., 2017). The effectiveness of coping strategies is influenced by a variety of factors, such as a person's age, cultural background, individual circumstances, and past use of coping strategies. Thus no single coping strategy works for everyone or for every stressor.

BOX 37.1 Examples of Ego-Defense Mechanisms

- Compensation: Making up for a deficiency in one aspect of self-image by strongly emphasizing a feature considered an asset (e.g., a person who is a poor communicator relies on organizational skills)
- Conversion: Unconsciously repressing an anxiety-producing emotional conflict and transforming it into nonorganic symptoms (e.g., difficulty in sleeping, loss of appetite)
- Denial: Avoiding emotional conflicts by refusing to consciously acknowledge anything that causes intolerable emotional pain (e.g., a person refuses to discuss or acknowledge a personal loss)
- Displacement: Transferring emotions, ideas, or wishes from a stressful situation to a less anxiety-producing substitute (e.g., a person transfers anger over an interpersonal conflict to a malfunctioning computer)
- Identification: Patterning behavior after that of another person and assuming that person's qualities, characteristics, and actions
- Dissociation: Experiencing a subjective sense of numbing and a reduced awareness of one's surroundings
- Regression: Coping with a stressor through actions and behaviors associated with an earlier developmental period

---

In stressful situations most people use a combination of problem- and emotion-focused coping strategies. In other words, when under stress a person obtains information, takes action to change the situation (problem-focused), and regulates emotions tied to the stress (emotion-focused). In some cases, people avoid thinking about the situation or change the way they think about it without changing the actual situation itself.

The type of stress, people's goals, their beliefs about themselves and the world, and personal resources determine how people cope with stress (Enns et al., 2018). Resources include problem-solving skills, financial status, social skills, support from family and friends, physical attractiveness, health and energy, and personal stress-management techniques such as optimism and mindfulness (Desiree et al., 2015).

Coping mechanisms include psychological adaptive behaviors. Such behaviors are often task oriented, involving the use of direct problem-solving techniques to cope with threats. Ego-defense mechanisms regulate emotional distress and thus give a person protection from anxiety and stress. They help a person cope with stress indirectly and offer psychological protection from a stressful event. Everyone uses them unconsciously to protect against feelings of worthlessness and anxiety. Occasionally a defense mechanism becomes distorted and no longer helps the person adapt to a stressor. However, people generally find them very helpful in coping and use them spontaneously (Box 37.1). Frequently short-term stressors activate ego-defense mechanisms. These usually do not result in psychiatric disorders.

Types of Stress

Stress is often caused by work, family, daily hassles, trauma, and crisis. Stress may be acute or chronic. One person looks at a stimulus and sees it as a challenge, leading to mastery and growth. Another sees the same stimulus as a threat, leading to stagnation and loss. The individual with family responsibilities and a full-time job outside the home can experience chronic stress. It occurs in stable conditions and from stressful roles. Living with a long-term illness produces chronic stress. Conversely, time-limited events that threaten a person for a relatively brief period provoke acute stress. Recurrent daily hassles such as commuting to work, maintaining a house, dealing with difficult people, and managing money further complicate chronic or acute stress.

Post-traumatic stress disorder (PTSD) begins when a person experiences or witnesses a traumatic event and responds with intense fear or helplessness. PTSD is common among military personnel and veterans and police, particularly soldiers who have been involved in combat or police involved in violent acts. Soldiers often witness or participate in disturbing events, producing dramatic symptoms. Some other examples of traumatic events that lead to PTSD include motor vehicle crashes, natural disasters, or violent personal assault. Anxiety associated with PTSD is sometimes manifested by nightmares and emotional detachment. Some people with PTSD experience flashbacks, or recurrent and intrusive recollections of the event. Depression and PTSD commonly occur together (Halter, 2018).

Secondary traumatic stress is the trauma a person experiences from witnessing other people's suffering. It is a component of compassion fatigue and is common in health care workers and first responders. Secondary traumatic stress results in intrusive symptoms such as nightmares and anxiety. People with this condition begin to avoid interactions and have difficulties in sleeping and relating to friends or family.

A crisis implies that a person is facing a turning point in life. This means that previous ways of coping are ineffective, and the person must change. There are three types of crises: (1) maturational or developmental crises, (2) situational crises, and (3) disasters or adventitious crises (Halter, 2018). A new developmental stage such as marriage or the birth of a child requires new coping styles. Developmental crises occur as a person moves through the stages of life. External sources such as a job change, a motor vehicle crash, or severe illness provoke situational crises. A major natural disaster, man-made disaster, or crime of violence creates an adventitious crisis.

Patient-centered care offers a context for crisis intervention (Steenkamp, 2015). The view of the person experiencing a crisis is the frame of reference for it. The vital questions for a person in crisis are "What does this mean to you?" and "How is it going to affect your life?" What causes extreme stress for one person is not always stressful to another. The perception of the event, situational supports, and coping mechanisms all influence return of equilibrium. A person either grows or regresses as a result of a crisis, depending on how he or she manages the situation (Halter, 2018).

REFLECT NOW

How would a nurse determine that a patient is moving from the alarm stage to the resistance stage of the general adaptation syndrome?

NURSING KNOWLEDGE BASE

Nurses have proposed theories related to stress and coping. In addition, because nurses commonly assume roles to support patients in stress, research has expanded the knowledge base for the nature of stress and management alternatives.

Nursing Theory and the Role of Stress

Many nursing theories explain and describe stress. For example, explanation of the concepts of stress and reaction to stress are components of the Betty Neuman Systems Model. The Neuman Systems Model uses a systems approach to help you understand the responses of patients, families, and communities to stressors. A systems approach explains that a stressor at one place in a system affects other parts of the system; a system is a person, family, or community. Events are multidimensional and not caused or affected by only one thing. Every person develops a set of responses to stress that constitute the "normal line of defense" (Smith and Parker, 2016; Neuman and Fawcett, 2011). This line of defense maintains health and wellness. Physiological, psychological, sociocultural, developmental, or spiritual influences buffer stress. The Neuman Systems Model of nursing views a patient, family, or community as constantly changing in response to the environment and stressors.

Callista Roy's Adaptation Model describes how an individual can effectively respond to stressors in the environment. According to Roy's theory, a person has the ability to modify external stimuli to allow adaptation to occur. A nurse assists an individual with modifying and regulating peripheral stimuli to promote a supportive healing environment (Cherry and Jacob, 2019).

On the other hand, Pender's Health Promotion Model focuses on promoting health and managing stress (Murdaugh et al., 2015). In this model people are capable of assessing their own abilities and assets and want to live in ways that enable them to be as healthy as possible. Interventions such as increasing physical activity, improving diet and nutrition, and using stress-management strategies help the individual become and remain healthy.

Factors Influencing Stress and Coping

Potential stressors and coping mechanisms vary across the life span (e.g., adolescence, adulthood, and old age bring different stressors). The appraisal of stressors, the amount and type of social support, and coping strategies all depend on previous life experiences and affect how a person reacts to that stressor. Situational and social stressors place people who are vulnerable at higher risk for prolonged stress.

Situational Factors. Situational stressors in the workplace that affect nurses and other health care professionals include high-acuity patient load, job environment, constant distractions, responsibility, conflicting priorities, and intensity of care (e.g., trauma, emergency, or critical care areas) (Mealer et al., 2014; Ueno et al., 2017). In addition, changing shifts increases fatigue and work-related stress.

Some nurses often ease coping with shift work by knowing their own circadian rhythms. People who function best in the morning have the greatest difficulty with night work and changing shifts. As people age, they tend to become more morning oriented. Morning people need to be counseled about the potentially negative effects of night work for them. In general, people doing shift work need to maintain as consistent a sleep and mealtime schedule as possible (Lin et al., 2014; Soloman et al., 2016).

Adjusting to chronic illness is another type of situational stress. The physical limitations posed by a disease state and the uncertainty associated with treatment and illness trigger stress in patients and family caregivers of all ages. Sometimes illness changes how people manage their stress. For example, Antony et al. (2018) found that caregivers of patients with cancer who were receiving palliative care used both negative and positive coping strategies to deal with the stress of caregiving. Having difficulty in paying for treatment and limited access to health care providers also create stress. Although being a family caregiver for someone with a chronic illness such as Alzheimer's disease is stressful, the actions of competent health care providers often help minimize the stress for family caregivers.

Maturational Factors. Stressors vary with life stage. According to Erikson's developmental theory, individuals experience predictable stages of development as particular tasks are accomplished and mastered for each stage. Children who are in the stage of initiative versus guilt identify stressors related to physical appearance, families, friends, and school. During this stage, teaching impulse control and

BOX 37.2 FOCUS ON OLDER ADULTS

Understanding Differences in Stress and Coping Among Older Adults

- Ordinary hassles of day-to-day living create a source of stress; older adults have more hassles with home maintenance and health than do younger people.
- Older adults often use more passive, intrapersonal, emotion-focused forms of coping such as distancing, humor, accepting responsibility, and reappraising the stressor in a positive way.
- Life experiences and perspectives of older adults make most problems seem insignificant, especially when older adults have acquired appropriate stress-management techniques (Jackson et al., 2018).
- Older adults' coping improves based on earlier experience with coping with traumatic situations (Jackson et al., 2018).
- Impaired coping affects overall health in older adults more than in younger adults (Rayens and Reed, 2014).
- Because of the high incidence of depression in older adults, you need to assess for suicidal thoughts and intent.
- When marital or partnership dyads are present, the perceived stress of one member has a greater effect on the other member than occurs with middle or young adults (Rayens and Reed, 2014).

⊕ BOX 37.3 CULTURAL ASPECTS OF CARE

Cultural Variations in Stress Appraisal and Coping Strategies

A patient's culture defines what is stressful to the person and ways of coping with stress (Giger, 2017). Cultural context shapes the types of situations that produce stress. Culture affects how a person leaves the parental home, experiences health crises or chronic illness, cares for the family, or becomes disabled or dependent. Furthermore, how a person appraises stress also depends on his or her culture. What is perceived as a major stressor in one culture is sometimes viewed as a minor problem in another. For example, cultures may address developmental transitions and turning points in life differently.

Coping strategies are also influenced by one's cultural background. Cultures vary in their emotion- and problem-focused coping strategies. Some stress that emotions should be controlled, whereas others believe in expressing emotion. Cultures provide different resources for coping with stress (Giger, 2017). These include the legal system for conflict resolution, advice givers or support groups, and rituals.

Implications for Patient-Centered Care
- Realize that stressors and coping styles vary with different cultures.
- Reflect on your own perceptions of stress and coping in a cultural context.
- Assess the influence of culture on a patient's appraisal of stress.
- Identify the presence of individualized cultural practices related to stress management.
- Determine resources in a patient's culture that facilitate coping.

cooperative behaviors is imperative. Preadolescents experience stress related to self-esteem issues, changing family structure as a result of divorce or death of a parent, or hospitalizations. Erikson asserts that during this stage, they can develop a sense of inferiority without proper support for learning new skills. As adolescents search for identity with peer groups and separate from their families, they also experience stress. In addition, they face stressful questions about sex, jobs, school, career choices, and using mind-altering substances. During this stage of development, stress can occur because of preoccupation with appearance and body image. Adolescents should strive to develop and accept personal identity.

Stress for adults centers around major changes in life circumstances. These include the many milestones of beginning a family and a career, losing parents, seeing children leave home, and accepting physical aging. Social development is important during this stage. In old age stressors include the loss of autonomy and mastery resulting from general frailty or health problems that limit stamina, strength, and cognition (Box 37.2). Nurses and other health care providers need to differentiate signs of stress and crisis in older adults from dementia and acute confusion.

Sociocultural Factors.
Environmental and social stressors often lead to developmental problems. Potential stressors that affect any age-group but that are especially stressful for young people include prolonged poverty and physical disability. Children become vulnerable when they lose parents and caregivers through divorce, imprisonment, or death or when parents have mental illness or substance-abuse disorders. Living under conditions of continuing violence, disintegrated neighborhoods, or homelessness affects people of any age, especially young people (Murdaugh, et al., 2015).

A person's culture also influences stress and coping. Cultural variations produce stress, particularly if a person's values differ from the dominant culture in aspects of gender roles, family relationships, and religious beliefs (Giger, 2017, Shavitt et al., 2016). Other aspects of cultural variations begin with language difference, geographical location, family relationships, time orientation, access to health care programs, and disparities in health care (Box 37.3) (see Chapter 9).

Compassion Fatigue

Compassion fatigue is a term used to describe a state of burnout and secondary traumatic stress. Secondary traumatic stress is the stress that health care providers experience when witnessing and caring for others who are suffering. Examples include an oncology nurse who cares for patients undergoing surgery and chemotherapy over the long term for their cancer or a spouse who witnesses his wife deteriorating over the years from Alzheimer's disease. Burnout occurs when perceived demands outweigh perceived resources (Brown et al., 2018). It is a state of physical and mental fatigue and exhaustion that often affects health care providers because of the nature of their work environment. Perceived inadequate staffing, long work shifts, demands of patient acuity, and dysfunctional relationships (patients and other care providers) serve as triggers for ongoing stress. Over time, giving of oneself in often intense caring environments can result in emotional exhaustion, leaving a nurse feeling irritable, restless, and unable to focus and engage with patients. This condition may be viewed as a failure to cope because it often occurs in situations in which the nurse is unable to practice self-care, social support is lacking, and organizational pressures are influencing staffing levels.

Compassion fatigue is a condition that can overwhelm health care providers and cause physical, mental, and emotional health issues (Hunsaker et al., 2015). The feelings of hopelessness and anxiety from compassion fatigue usually result in feelings of inadequacy and lower self-esteem. These factors can lead to the health care provider lashing out in an attempt to cope with these feelings and stress. This often manifests itself as *lateral violence*, which refers to a deliberate and harmful behavior demonstrated in the workplace by one employee to another. This includes health care providers engaging in bullying and potentially assaultive behaviors toward co-workers (Embree and White, 2010; Christie and Jones, 2013).

Early recognition of the risk for compassion fatigue is essential. A supportive work environment helps guide a nursing unit in designing communication techniques to identify, prevent, and adapt to potential compassion fatigue situations (Hunsaker et al., 2015). For example, a nurse-led program on an oncology unit that included education, exercise and social support was found to be effective in decreasing the nurses' compassion fatigue (Yilmaz et al., 2018).

Second Victim Syndrome

Second victim syndrome affects health care providers when a medical error that results in significant harm to a patient and the patient's family occurs (Hartley, 2018). Often overlooked, nurses who have been involved in such a medical error can sustain complex psychological harm that can lead to detrimental outcomes such as suicide. These fatal errors can haunt nurses throughout their lives, leading to symptoms that are similar to post-traumatic stress disorder. One potential outcome is that nurses "move on" and work on gaining additional knowledge and skills to prevent errors in the future. But in many cases, nurses are reluctant to return to work because of fear of isolation from the organization, loss of confidence, remorse, depression, humiliation, and guilt (Hartley, 2018).

Being aware of the potential for second victim syndrome allows health care agencies to provide support the moment such an event occurs. Health care agencies need to provide support for as long as deemed necessary. Although the care and support of patients and families is a priority, the second victim has a right to be treated with respect and dignity and to be supported by peers and the organization. Proposed rights for second victims include respect, just treatment, understanding and compassion, supportive care, transparency, and the opportunity to contribute (Grissinger, 2014).

CRITICAL THINKING

Successful critical thinking requires a synthesis of knowledge, experience, information gathered from patients, critical thinking attitudes, and intellectual and professional standards. Clinical judgments require you to anticipate information, analyze the data, and make decisions regarding your patient's care. During assessment consider all elements that build toward making an appropriate nursing diagnosis.

Integrate knowledge from nursing and other disciplines, previous experiences, and information gathered from patients to understand stress and its effect on a patient and family. Know the neurophysiological changes that occur in a patient experiencing the alarm reaction, resistance stage, and exhaustion stage of the GAS. In addition, know communication principles that contribute to assessing a patient's behaviors. Give utmost attention to determining the patient's perception of the situation and his or her ability to cope with the stress. If a patient's usual coping skills have not helped or his or her support systems have failed, use crisis intervention counseling.

Experience teaches you to understand the patient's unique perspective and recognize that no two people are exactly alike. Experience with patients also helps you to recognize responses to stress. In addition, personal experiences with stress and coping increase your ability to empathize with a patient temporarily immobilized by stress.

Be confident in the belief that you and your patients can effectively manage stress. Patients who feel overwhelmed and perceive events as beyond their capacity to cope rely on you as an expert. Patients respect your advice and counsel and gain confidence from your belief in their ability to move past the stressful event or illness. Patients overwhelmed by life events are often unable, at least initially, to act on their own behalf and require either direct intervention or guidance. Integrity is an essential attitude that allows you to respect a patient's perception of the stressor. Encourage the patient to explain his or her unique viewpoint and situation.

The practice standards for psychiatric mental health nursing (ANA, 2014) guide assessment of a patient's stress, coping mechanisms, and support system before intervening. Use linguistic and culturally effective communication skills to clearly and precisely understand a patient's perception of stress. Focus on factors relevant to his or her well-being. In addition, the patient expects you to exhibit confidence and integrity when he or she feels vulnerable. Be especially aware of the ethical responsibility in caring for someone who has diminished autonomy as a result of stress.

REFLECT NOW

What questions would you ask a patient to determine whether his or her stress is related to situational, maturational, or sociocultural factors?

❖ NURSING PROCESS

Apply the nursing process and use a critical thinking approach in your care of patients. The nursing process provides a clinical decision-making approach for you to develop and implement an individualized plan of care.

◆ Assessment

During the assessment process, thoroughly assess each patient and critically analyze findings to ensure that you make patient-centered clinical decisions required for safe nursing care.

Through the Patient's Eyes. Assessment of a patient's stress level and coping resources requires that you first establish a trusting nurse-patient relationship because you are asking a patient to share personal and sensitive information. Learn from the patient both by asking questions and by observing nonverbal behavior and the patient's environment. Synthesize the information and adopt a critical thinking attitude while observing and analyzing patient behavior (Fig. 37.2). Often a patient has difficulty in expressing exactly what is most bothersome about a situation until there is an opportunity to discuss it with someone who has time to listen.

Begin your assessment with an open-ended question, such as "What is happening in your life that caused you to come today?" or "What happened in your life that is *different?*" This requires the patient to focus. Next assess the patient's perception of the event, available situational supports, and what he or she usually does when there is an unsolvable problem. Determine whether a person is suicidal or homicidal by asking directly, "Are you thinking of hurting yourself or someone else?" If so, determine in a caring and concerned manner whether the person has a plan and the lethality of the plan (i.e., ingestion of pills versus self-inflicted gunshot wound).

Take time to understand a patient's meaning of the precipitating event and the ways in which stress is affecting his or her life. Allow time for the patient to express priorities for coping with stress. For example, in the case of a woman who has just been told that a breast mass was identified on a routine mammogram, it is important to know what the patient wants and needs most from the nurse. Although some women in this situation identify their need for information about biopsy or mastectomy as their personal priority, others need guidance and support in discussing how to share the news with family members.

Stress also occurs in a family or a community. Stress in a family sometimes arises from a critically ill family member, the sudden loss of a job, a move, or becoming homeless. Community stressors include a natural disaster such as a major flood or the sudden, unexpected death of a beloved teacher or teenager. To develop

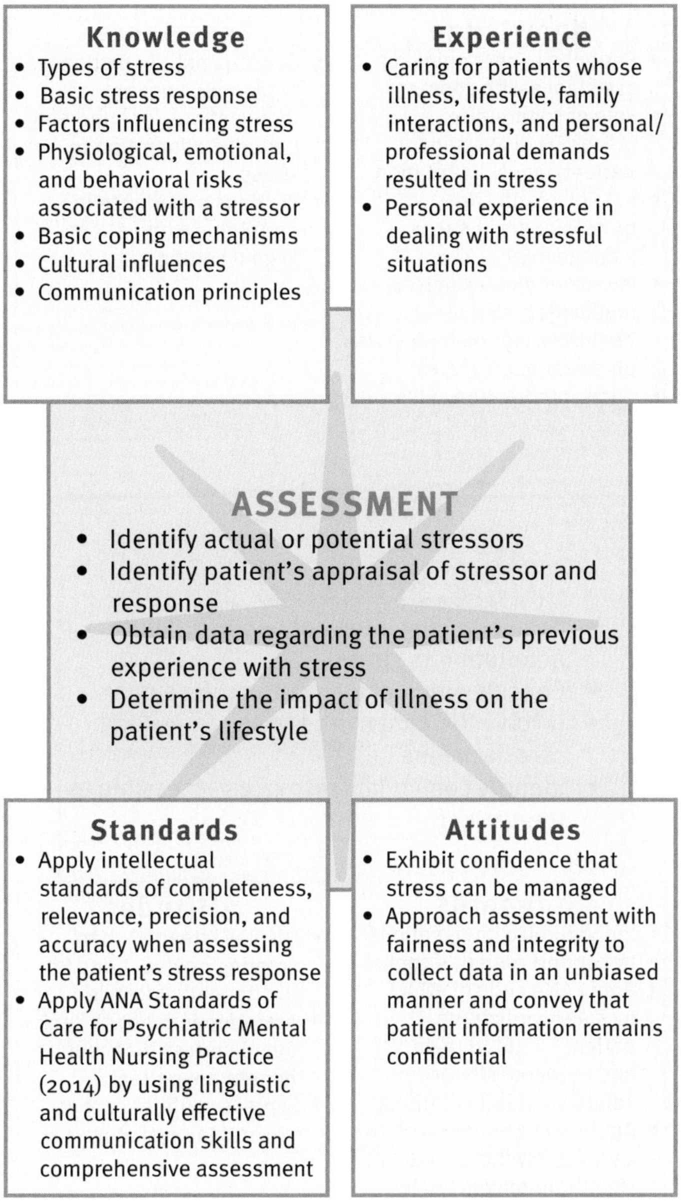

Knowledge
- Types of stress
- Basic stress response
- Factors influencing stress
- Physiological, emotional, and behavioral risks associated with a stressor
- Basic coping mechanisms
- Cultural influences
- Communication principles

Experience
- Caring for patients whose illness, lifestyle, family interactions, and personal/professional demands resulted in stress
- Personal experience in dealing with stressful situations

ASSESSMENT
- Identify actual or potential stressors
- Identify patient's appraisal of stressor and response
- Obtain data regarding the patient's previous experience with stress
- Determine the impact of illness on the patient's lifestyle

Standards
- Apply intellectual standards of completeness, relevance, precision, and accuracy when assessing the patient's stress response
- Apply ANA Standards of Care for Psychiatric Mental Health Nursing Practice (2014) by using linguistic and culturally effective communication skills and comprehensive assessment

Attitudes
- Exhibit confidence that stress can be managed
- Approach assessment with fairness and integrity to collect data in an unbiased manner and convey that patient information remains confidential

FIG. 37.2 Critical thinking model for stress and coping assessment. *ANA,* American Nurses Association.

appropriate and safe nursing care when caring for families or communities, ensure that you understand the meaning stress has for that group.

Subjective Findings. Create a nonthreatening environment when assessing a patient's level of stress and coping resources. Sit at the same height as the patient, arranging the interview environment with the chairs at a 90-degree angle or side by side so that you can maintain or avoid eye contact comfortably (Halter, 2018). Begin to develop a trusting relationship with your patient while you gather information about the patient's health status from his or her perspective. Use the interview to determine the patient's view of the stress, coping resources, any possible maladaptive coping, and adherence to prescribed medical recommendations such as medication or diet (Box 37.4). If the patient is using denial as a coping mechanism, assess if he or she is overlooking necessary information. As in all interactions with the patient, respect the confidentiality and sensitivity of the information shared.

BOX 37.4 Nursing Assessment Questions

Patient Safety
- Are you having difficulty with sleeping? Falling asleep? Staying awake?
- Is there any change in your eating patterns?
- Have you had any accidents at home, in the car, at school, or on the job?
- Do you have any thoughts of harming yourself or others?

Perception of Stressor
- What do you believe is stressing you right now?
- What impact does this stressor have on your lifestyle?
- How does this stressor impact you now? How will it impact you in the future?

Available Coping Resources
- Which strategies have you used in the past to deal with stress?
- Are you able to talk with friends or family?
- What is relaxing for you?

Maladaptive Coping Used
- Have you started using alcohol or tobacco to deal with your stress?
- Do you use any over-the-counter or herbal medications to manage your stress?
- Do you use any street drugs to cope?

Adherence to Healthy Practices
- How long ago did you see your health care provider?
- What is your exercise routine?
- Which type of meals do you eat? Are your meals regular?
- Are you taking your prescribed medications as ordered?

Objective Findings. Obtain objective findings related to stress and coping through observation of the appearance and nonverbal behavior of a patient. Observe grooming and hygiene, gait, characteristics of the handshake, actions while sitting, quality of speech, eye contact, and the attitude of the patient during the interview. Before the interview begins or at the end of the interview, depending on the anxiety level of the patient, obtain basic vital signs to assess for physiological signs of stress such as elevated blood pressure, heart rate, or respiratory rate. Make certain to incorporate cultural components of interpreting the patient's nonverbal communication behaviors.

REFLECT NOW

What is the nurse's priority if a patient expresses thoughts of self-harm?

◆ Nursing Diagnosis

A review of assessment data leads you to cluster data that indicate a potential or actual stressor and the patient's response. Clustering data, along with the application of your knowledge and experiences with patients in stress, leads to individualized nursing diagnoses (Box 37.5).

Nursing diagnoses for people experiencing stress generally focus on coping. Specifically, major assessment findings of *Difficulty Coping* include verbalization of an inability to cope and an inability to ask for help. To gather assessment data, ask the patient what is of most concern at the time of the interview. It is important to allow patients sufficient time to answer. Observe for nonverbal signs of anxiety, fear, anger, irritability, and tension, which may indicate ineffective coping. Other assessment findings include the presence of life stress, an inability to meet role expectations and basic needs, alteration in societal

BOX 37.5   Nursing Diagnostic Process

Difficulty Coping

Assessment Activities	Assessment Findings
Ask patient about change in sleeping patterns.	Sleep disturbance Difficulty falling asleep at night
Ask patient to complete a sleep diary for 2 weeks.	Excessive sleeping Frequent awakenings at night
Observe patient's behavior and response to questions during assessment.	Fatigue Inability to concentrate Inaccurate response to questions Inappropriate laugh or crying
Observe patient's appearance.	Poor grooming Lack of eye contact
Ask patient about changes in eating patterns.	Weight gain or loss Lack of interest in food

participation, self-destructive behavior, change in usual communication patterns, high rate of accidents, excessive food intake, drinking, smoking, and sleep disturbances. Stress or the inability to cope often results in multiple nursing diagnoses. Examples of these diagnoses include but are not limited to the following:

- *Anxiety*
- *Despair*
- *Difficulty Coping*
- *Risk for Post Trauma Response*
- *Stress Overload*

◆ Planning

Goals and Outcomes. Desirable goals for people experiencing stress frequently include effective coping, family coping, and family caregiver emotional health. Examples of outcomes might include the following: patient engages in a support group, family members are able to discuss loss together, or caregiver participates in respite care. A nurse selects interventions for reducing stress and improving coping, such as coping enhancement and crisis intervention. The nurse considers nursing diagnoses and the goals identified mutually with the patient when individualizing interventions and selecting resources available to a patient (Fig. 37.3).

Nursing interventions are designed within the framework of primary, secondary, and tertiary prevention. At the primary level of prevention, you direct nursing activities to identify individuals and populations who may be at risk for stress. Nursing interventions at the secondary level include actions directed at symptoms, such as protecting the patient from self-harm. Tertiary-level interventions help the patient readapt and can include relaxation training and time-management training. The nurse and the patient assess the level and source of the existing stress and determine the appropriate intervention to reduce it (Murdaugh et al., 2015) (see the Nursing Care Plan).

REFLECT NOW

You are planning care for a patient with two school-age children who is also caring for a sick parent in her home. The patient's three siblings who live within a 25-mile radius refuse to help. A diagnosis of *Stress Overload* is included in the plan of care. Identify an appropriate goal and outcome.

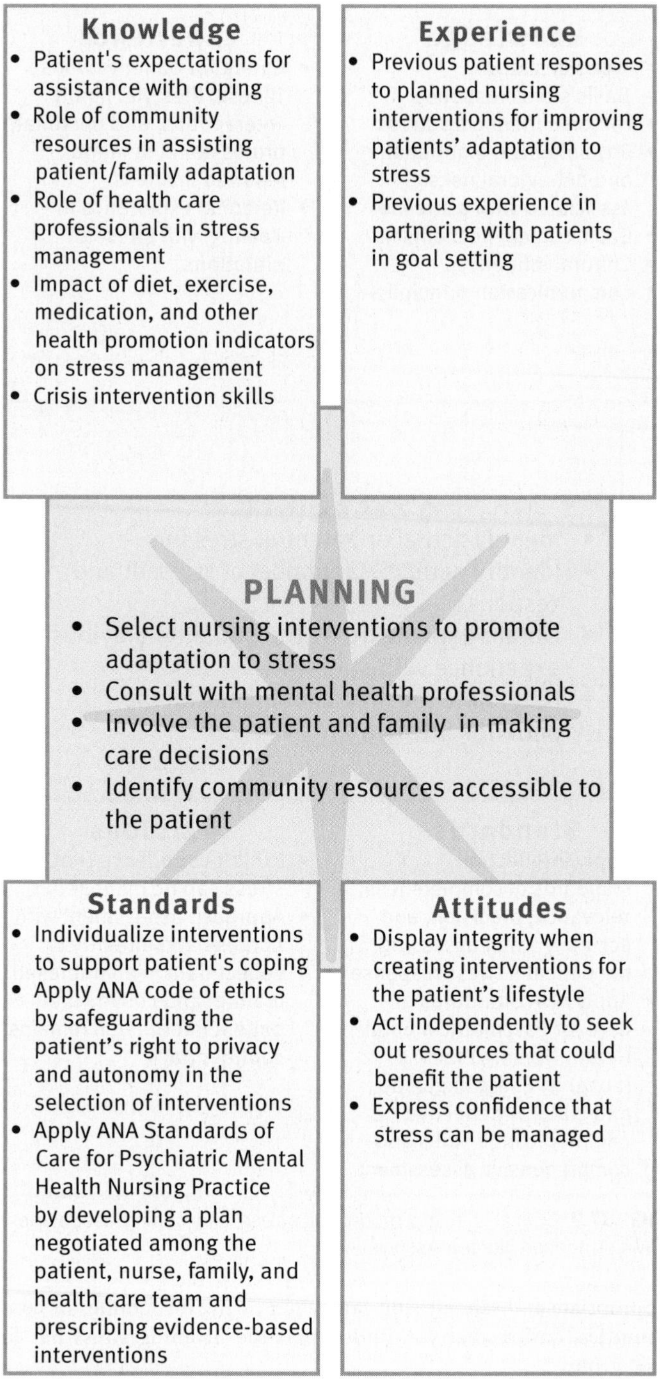

Knowledge
- Patient's expectations for assistance with coping
- Role of community resources in assisting patient/family adaptation
- Role of health care professionals in stress management
- Impact of diet, exercise, medication, and other health promotion indicators on stress management
- Crisis intervention skills

Experience
- Previous patient responses to planned nursing interventions for improving patients' adaptation to stress
- Previous experience in partnering with patients in goal setting

PLANNING
- Select nursing interventions to promote adaptation to stress
- Consult with mental health professionals
- Involve the patient and family in making care decisions
- Identify community resources accessible to the patient

Standards
- Individualize interventions to support patient's coping
- Apply ANA code of ethics by safeguarding the patient's right to privacy and autonomy in the selection of interventions
- Apply ANA Standards of Care for Psychiatric Mental Health Nursing Practice by developing a plan negotiated among the patient, nurse, family, and health care team and prescribing evidence-based interventions

Attitudes
- Display integrity when creating interventions for the patient's lifestyle
- Act independently to seek out resources that could benefit the patient
- Express confidence that stress can be managed

FIG. 37.3 Critical thinking model for stress and coping planning. *ANA,* American Nurses Association.

A tool for planning care is a concept map (Fig. 37.4). Concept maps identify multiple nursing diagnoses for a patient from the assessment database and show how they are related. In this example the nursing diagnoses are linked to the patient's medical diagnosis of depression. In addition, the concept map shows the relationship among the nursing diagnoses *Impaired Low Nutritional Intake: Deficient Food Intake, Difficulty Coping, Anxiety,* and *Powerlessness.* Use of a concept map requires critical thinking skills to organize patient data and helps to plan for patient-centered care.

⊚ NURSING CARE PLAN

Difficulty Coping

ASSESSMENT

Sandra and John have been married 3 years and are both 55 years of age. They both work and are planning their retirement at age 66. Last month, John was diagnosed with stage 3 pancreatic cancer. Presently, John and Sandra are at the Cancer Center to decide on treatment. When you greet the couple, you notice that they both look tired; Sandra is disheveled, and John is clean-shaven and well groomed. John states that he is worried about Sandra as she appears "just worn out," and he expresses fear that she will not be able to help him through this medical crisis.

Assessment Activities	Assessment Findings [a]
Ask Sandra how she feels about John's diagnosis.	Sandra states, **"I don't know how I feel. I know I feel very alone."**
Ask Sandra what she remembers about John's treatment options.	She states, "I really **can't remember anything** but stage 3 pancreatic cancer. I know this is a bad cancer.
Ask John and Sandra about friends and relatives they have for support.	Both are only children and have **no other family**; they moved 1 year ago for new jobs. They both work for the same company but state that they have **few close friends**.
Ask Sandra to identify people she can turn to for help.	Sandra **sobs** and **says that she doesn't have any friends she can rely on.** They are active in their church. On further discussion Sandra mentions a close friend from her hometown.
Ask Sandra about sleep and nutrition patterns.	She **can't get to sleep easily and awakens 3 to 4 times per night.** She states, "My appetite **is poor; I'm just not hungry. I think I've lost weight."**
Assess Sandra's mood and affect by asking how she is feeling.	She states, **"I am so tired and overwhelmed."**

[a]**Assessment findings** are shown in bold type.

NURSING DIAGNOSIS: Difficulty Coping related to insufficient social support

PLANNING

Goals	Expected Outcomes (NOC)[b]
	Social Support
Sandra achieves social support from her community in 1 month.	Sandra identifies at least one person in her community who can help support her in this crisis. Sandra participates in a local support group weekly.

[b]Outcome classification labels from Moorhead S, et al: *Nursing Outcomes Classification (NOC)*, ed 6, St Louis, 2018, Elsevier.

INTERVENTIONS (NIC)[c]	RATIONALE
Support System Enhancement	
Identify community-based cancer support systems for patients and family for Sandra and John.	Support systems for both patient and family are an effective intervention to cope with the stress of a cancer diagnosis and related therapies and decision making (Meiner and Yeager, 2019).
Help Sandra identify a person who is willing to accompany her to some of John's appointments.	Having another person hear some of the treatment options and treatment procedures provides opportunities to clarify the discussion. During high-stress times the patient and family may not hear the material provided by health care providers completely (Doron et al., 2014).
Explore community resources for a short-term educational group for both Sandra and John for self-care tools to reduce stress.	Educational groups help caregivers develop self-care tools to reduce stress, change negative self-talk, communicate more effectively, and make difficult decisions (Oken et al., 2018).

[c]Intervention classification labels from Butcher HK, et al: *Nursing Interventions Classification (NIC)*, ed 7, St Louis, 2018, Elsevier.

EVALUATION

Evaluation Activity	Patient Response/Finding	Outcome Status
Ask Sandra for the name of a person she can call for help during a crisis.	Sandra identified two people in her church community. One is a cancer survivor; the second is the spouse of a patient currently receiving cancer treatment.	Sandra meets with each person in her church at least weekly for coffee or lunch, and she has invited them and their spouses to her home for dinner.
Ask Sandra whether she attended a support group.	Sandra reports she has attended two sessions.	Sandra accepts support from community.

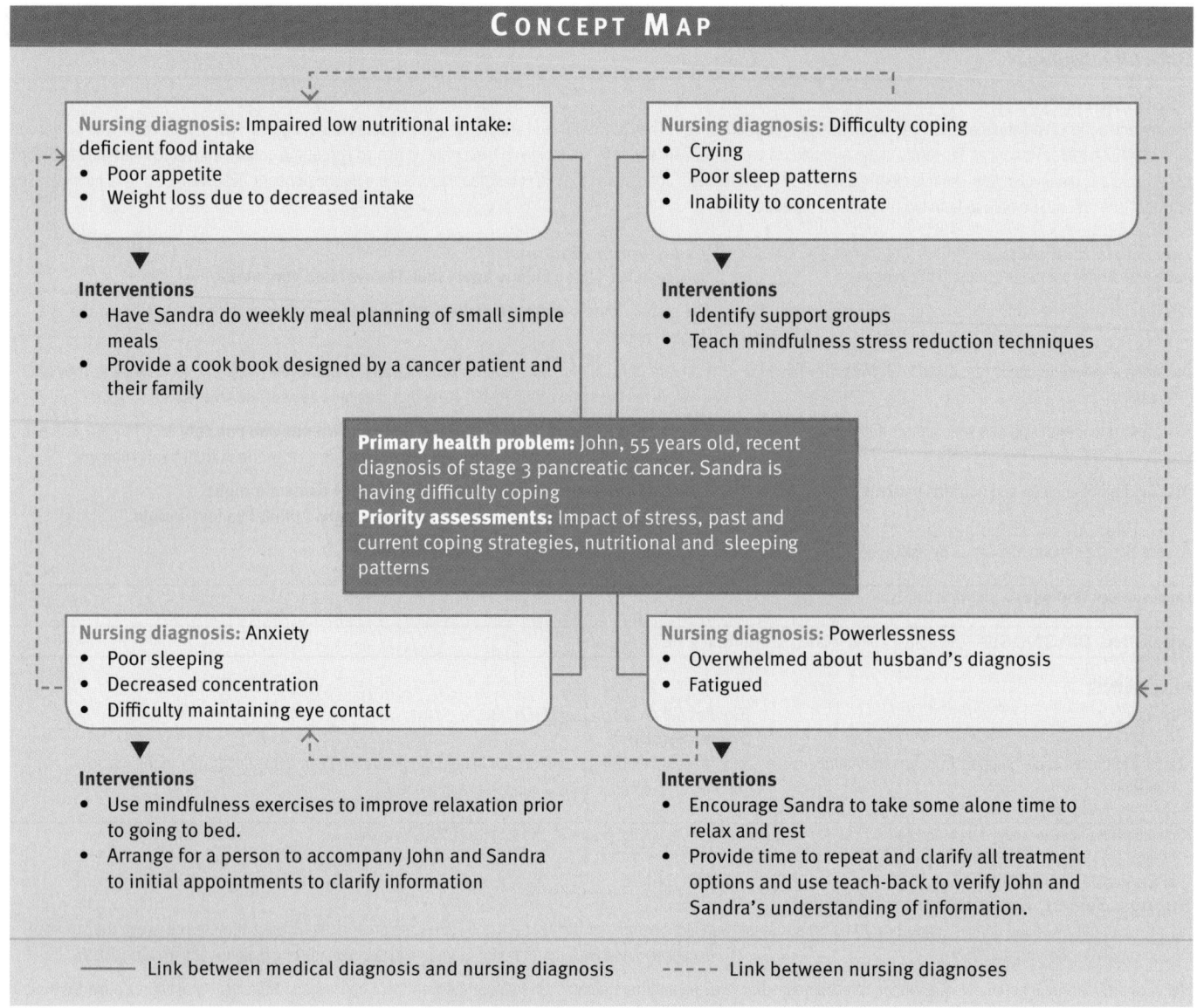

FIG. 37.4 Concept map for Sandra.

Just as the nursing assessment of a patient's stress and coping depends on his or her perception of the problem and coping resources, the interventions focus on a partnership with the patient and support system, usually the family. In the case of a family or community stressor and impaired family or community coping, the view of the situation and resources is broader.

Setting Priorities. Consider the patient's perspective and responses to assessment questions when setting priorities for care (see the Nursing Care Plan). The patient's and family member's physical condition and perception of stressors determine which nursing diagnosis has the greatest priority. As in all areas of nursing, patient safety is the priority.

If suicide or homicide is not an issue, identify if there are potential threats to the safety of vulnerable people who are under the care of the patient. Provide for their temporary care or supervision if necessary. Other potential threats to safety include nutritional deficits; insomnia; self-care deficits; and poor judgment and impulsiveness that may lead to unsafe decisions about sex, drugs, money, or damage to personal relationships that the person might later regret. Determine the degree of work, school, home, and family disruption in the person's life. After you have ensured safety, problem solve with patient in selecting priorities.

Teamwork and Collaboration. Sometimes nursing practice alone does not meet all the patient's and family's needs. To effectively plan individualized care, collaborate with occupational therapists, dietitians, pastoral care professionals, and health care professionals from other clinical specialties, depending on the patient's situation.

Consulting with advanced practice mental health nurses, psychiatrists, psychologists, or psychiatric social workers when a patient is experiencing stress from medical conditions or psychiatric disorders is necessary. An interprofessional approach addresses the holistic needs of the patient. Recognize the need for collaboration and consultation; inform the patient about potential resources; and arrange for interventions such as consultations, group sessions, or therapy as needed. A hospital social worker can share ideas for available resources both within the hospital and in the community. A home care nurse knows community services, support groups, and appropriate contacts.

BOX 37.6 PATIENT TEACHING

Stress Management

Objective
- Patient will report less anxiety, depression, and pain related to chronic health problems.

Teaching Strategies
- Familiarize patient with mind-body therapies that are likely to benefit patient. Refer to a group or specialized practitioner when necessary (Holman et al., 2018; Oken et al., 2018):
  - Meditation
  - Progressive muscle relaxation
  - Guided imagery
  - Hypnosis
  - Yoga
  - Tai Chi
- Teach patient how to incorporate 15-30 minutes of exercise into daily activities (Kravitz, 2019).
- Instruct patient to identify and use relaxation techniques; for example:
  - Listen to music that you enjoy.
  - Keep a journal of your thoughts and feelings.
  - Replace unnecessary time-consuming activities with activities that are pleasurable or interesting.

Evaluation
Use the principles of teach back to evaluate patient/family caregiver learning:
- Tell me how the stress-reduction techniques that we practiced help you to cope.
- Tell me how the mindfulness activities are impacting your anxiety and ability to sleep.
- Show me how you do the progressive muscle relaxation exercises.

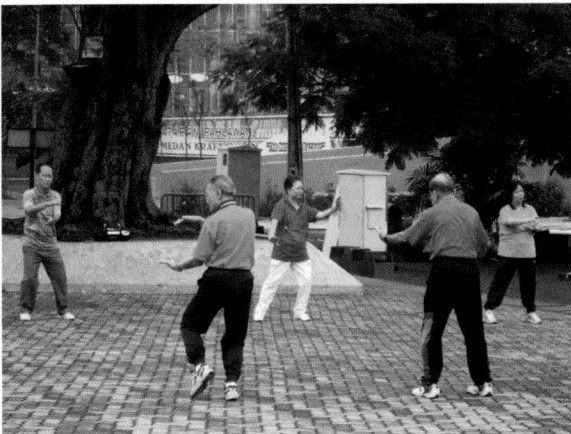

FIG. 37.5 Regular exercise helps to cope with stress. (Courtesy Rudolph A. Furtado.)

QSEN Building Competency in Evidence-Based Practice As a nurse educator in a diabetes management clinic, you recognize the value of exercise for patients with diabetes. However, you know many of your patients have difficulty committing to exercising regularly. You've located current research that supports types of interventions that are effective in promoting physical activity among adults who are chronically ill. Some of these interventions include (1) targeting physical activity exclusively, (2) using behavioral (as opposed to cognitive) strategies, and (3) encouraging self-regulation and monitoring (Park and Iacocca, 2014; Phillips, et al., 2016).

1. Describe the relationship between an individual's beliefs and that person's intentions for engaging in physical activity.
2. Identify possible barriers that prevent patients from initiating or maintaining an exercise plan. How can you help individuals overcome these barriers?

Answers to QSEN Activities can be found on the Evolve website.

In addition to maximizing use of available resources for the patient, collaborative care also benefits the nurse. While working with patients experiencing stress, you gain a broad understanding of the multitude of health care disciplines. Work becomes more satisfying. Contacts with other members of the interprofessional team and the community provide a feeling of contributing to the teamwork of providing holistic care.

◆ Implementation

Health Promotion. Three primary modes of intervention for stress are to decrease stress-producing situations, increase resistance to stress, and learn skills that reduce physiological response to stress (Murdaugh et al., 2015). Educate patients and families about the importance of health promotion (Box 37.6).

Regular Exercise and Rest. A regular exercise program improves muscle tone and posture, controls weight, reduces tension, and promotes relaxation (see Chapter 38). In addition, exercise reduces the risk of cardiovascular disease and improves cardiopulmonary functioning. Patients who have a history of a chronic illness, who are at risk for developing an illness, or are older than 35 years of age should begin a physical exercise program only after discussing the plan with a health care provider (Fig. 37.5).

Regular rest and sleep are also effective in reducing stress and stress-related fatigue. When stressful situations are present, encourage patients and their family members to establish bedtime and sleep routines and try to stick to the schedule (see Chapter 43). Patients and family members who are well rested are able to manage stress, problem solve, and maintain a sense of control over the situation (Kravitz, 2019).

Support Systems. A support system of family, friends, and colleagues who listen, offer advice, and provide emotional support benefits a patient experiencing stress (Sunne and Huntington, 2017). Many support groups are available to individuals (e.g., those sponsored by the American Heart Association, the American Cancer Society, hospitals, churches, and mental health organizations). Recent research shows that cancer survivors who effectively manage their stress make changes in their physical, psychosocial, and preventive health behaviors (Bily, 2017).

Time Management. Time-management techniques include developing lists of prioritized tasks. For example, help patients list tasks that require immediate attention, those that are important, those that can be delayed, and those that are routine and can be accomplished when time becomes available. In many cases setting priorities helps individuals identify tasks that are unnecessary or that can be delegated to someone else.

Guided Imagery and Visualization. Guided imagery is based on the belief that a person significantly reduces stress with imagination. It is a relaxed state in which a person actively uses imagination in a way that allows visualization of a soothing, peaceful setting. Typically, the image created or suggested uses many sensory words to engage the mind and offer distraction and relaxation.

Progressive Muscle Relaxation Therapies. In the presence of anxiety-provoking thoughts and events, a common physiological symptom is muscle tension. Progressive muscular relaxation diminishes physiological tension through a systematic approach to releasing tension in major muscle groups. Typically, an individual achieves a relaxed state through deep breathing. Once the patient is breathing deeply, direct him or her to alternately tighten and relax muscles in specific groupings (Pangotra et al., 2018; Tsitsi et al., 2017).

Assertiveness Training. Assertiveness includes skills for helping individuals communicate effectively regarding their needs and desires. The ability to resolve conflict with others through assertiveness training reduces their stress. Becoming certified in assertiveness training gives you the chance to teach assertiveness in group settings.

Journal Writing. Journal writing is beneficial for enhancing both psychological and physical health (Pavlacic, 2019). For many people keeping a private, personal journal provides a therapeutic outlet for stress. Suggest that patients keep journals, especially during difficult situations. In a private journal, patients can express a full range of emotion and vent their honest feelings without hurting anyone else's feelings and without concern for how they appear to others.

Mindfulness-Based Stress Reduction. Mindfulness is a moment-to-moment present awareness with an attitude on nonjudgment, acceptance, and openness. This technique entails focusing on attentiveness on regular activities and truly enjoying pleasant experiences (Parsons et al., 2017). Mindfulness-based stress reduction (MBSR) meditative practices are effective in reducing psychological and physical symptoms or perceptions. They are effective in stress management and symptom control with certain chronic conditions (Box 37.7). Through mindfulness exercises people learn to self-regulate awareness and attention to feeling and implement effective changes. Patients use cognitive exercises and subjective experiences to process images or feelings (Desiree et al., 2015). Patients evaluate these feelings as pleasant or unpleasant and learn strategies to enhance the pleasant experiences and replace the unpleasant experiences. Through MBSR patients can control their stress response to illnesses and treatments, employees can manage job-related stress, and students can learn to manage stress anxiety.

Stress Management in the Workplace. Stressors such as rapid changes in health care technology, diversity in the workforce, organizational restructuring, and changing work systems place stress on employees. Burnout occurs as a result of chronic stress. In nursing, burnout results when nurses perceive the demands of their work exceed perceived resources. It is manifested as emotional exhaustion, poor decision making, loss of a sense of personal identity, and feelings of failure.

It is important that nurses participate in self-care practices. For example, in oncology settings many nurses experience compassion fatigue. Effective strategies for compassion fatigue and how to help nurses deal with this phenomenon are available (see Chapter 1). Health care facilities use mindfulness exercises, resilience training, staff relationship-building activities, and clinical debriefing to manage job-related stress and reduce burnout and nursing staff turnover (Brown et al., 2018). Recognizing the impact of shift work and changes in schedules enables some managers and nurses to use self-scheduling techniques. This reduces job-related stress and improves sleep quality, collaboration, and teamwork (Lin et al., 2014).

Recognizing the areas over which you have control and can change and those for which you do not have responsibility is a vital insight. Making a clear separation between work and home life is also crucial. Strengthening friendships outside the workplace, participating in creative activities for personal "recharging" of emotional energy, and spending off-duty hours in interesting activities all help reduce compassion fatigue.

REFLECT NOW

Create a personal plan to manage stress in the workplace.

BOX 37.7 EVIDENCE-BASED PRACTICE

Impact of Meditation Therapies on Illness-Related Stressors

PICOT Question: Does the use of a mindfulness-based stress reduction (MBSR) program for adult patients affect their level of anxiety and depression and psychological well-being?

Evidence Summary

Prolonged and recurrent stress is associated with multiple psychological and health outcomes. A person's ability to cope with these stressors impacts physical and psychological health and may result in high rates of morbidity (Greeson et al., 2018; Oken et al., 2018). While conventional medical treatments for common stress-related symptoms may relieve symptoms, they fail to address the underlying causes of stress (Greeson et al., 2018). A participatory medicine approach that incorporates behavioral, self-care practices (e.g., yoga, meditation) with conventional care is often beneficial. For example, patients who practiced yoga were effective in decreasing their anxiety and use of pain medication during a procedure (Kartin et al., 2017). Coping skills training in patients with diabetes decreased symptoms of depression and improved quality of life and metabolic control (Edraki et al., 2018).

Cognitive therapies, such as mindful meditation, have also been shown to improve subjective, patient-reported outcomes, including symptoms of stress, anxiety, depression, pain, fatigue, and quality of life (Oken et al., 2018; Greeson et al., 2018). Mindfulness is marked by a sense of focused attention allowing an individual to consciously act versus automatically react to stress (Greeson et al., 2018).

Cognitive therapies such as meditation and MBSR help patients deal with illness-related stressors. Patients who use these therapies often are better at managing the symptoms and psychological distress associated with their chronic conditions (Grensman et al., 2018). Individualize these therapies to the patient's needs, the ability to learn the therapy, and the concurrent treatment.

Application to Nursing Practice

- Assess a patient's perception of stress and specific coping strategies to help you identify the stressors and the patient's response to them (Lewis et al., 2017; Grensman et al., 2018; Edraki et al., 2018).
- Identify priority coping strategies to improve the patient's quality of life and reduce symptoms (Grensman et al., 2018; Edraki et al., 2018).
- Consider a patient's limitations when discussing specific coping strategies to optimize the patient's experience and increase the chance of success (Greeson et al., 2018; Oken et al., 2018).
- When instructing patients about the use of these techniques, reinforce that these stress-management techniques are to be used in an addition to, not instead of, the patient's current treatment.

Acute Care

Crisis Intervention. Crisis occurs when stress overwhelms a person's usual coping mechanisms and demands mobilization of all available resources. A crisis creates a turning point in a person's life because it changes the direction of his or her life in some way. The precipitating event usually occurs approximately 1 to 2 weeks before the individual seeks help, but sometimes it has occurred within the past 24 hours. Generally, a person resolves the crisis in some way within approximately 6 weeks. Crisis intervention aims to return the person to a precrisis level of functioning and promote growth (Fig. 37.6).

Because an individual's or family's usual coping strategies are ineffective in managing the stress of the precipitating event during crisis, the use of new coping mechanisms is necessary. This experience forces the use of unfamiliar strategies and results in either a heightened

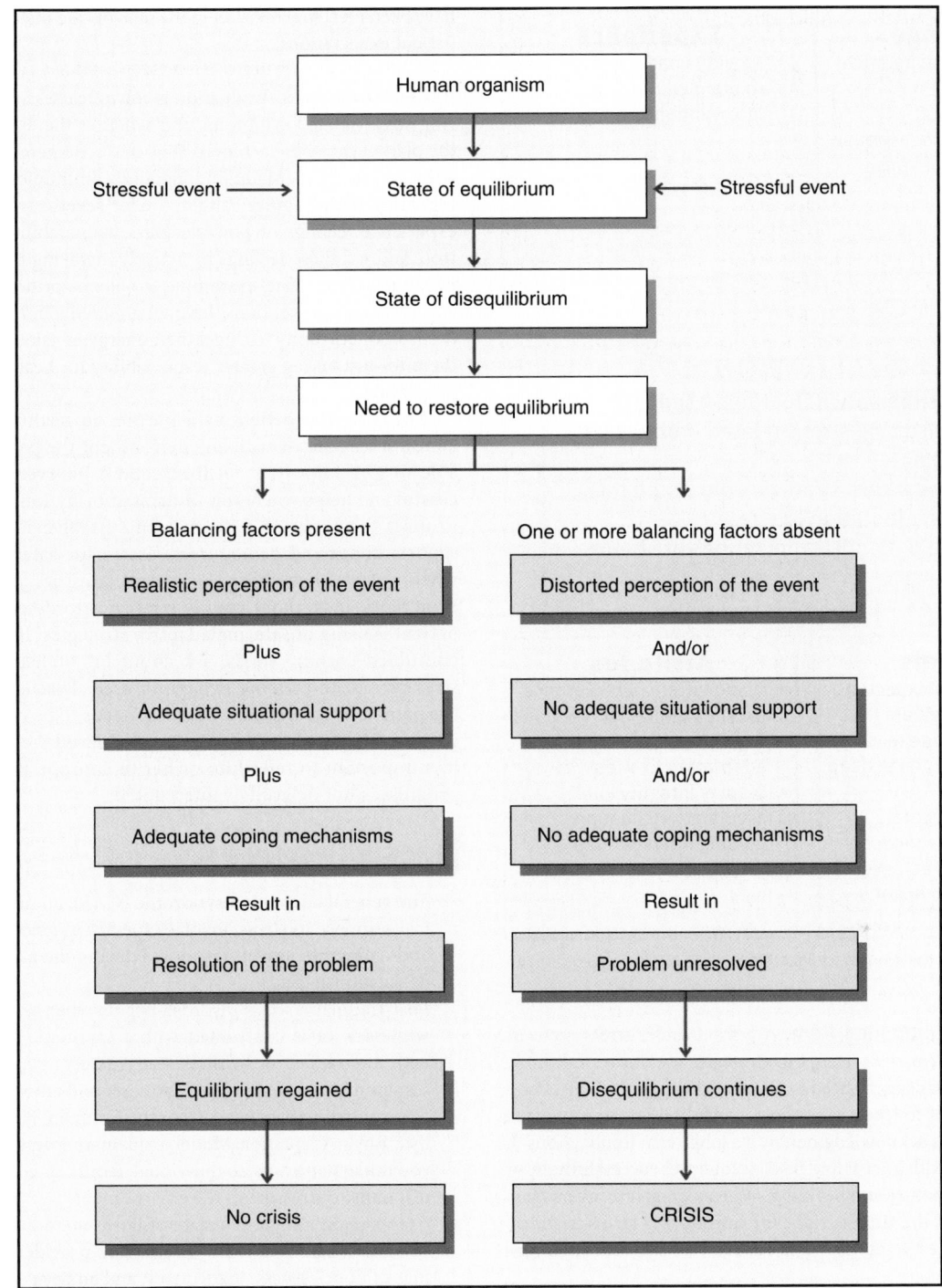

FIG. 37.6 Crisis intervention model. (Redrawn from Aguilera DC: *Crisis intervention: theory and methodology*, ed 8, St Louis, 1998, Mosby.)

awareness of previously unrecognized strengths and resources or deterioration in functioning. Thus, a crisis is often referred to as a situation of both danger and opportunity. Some individuals or families emerge from a crisis state functioning more effectively, whereas others find themselves weakened, and still others are completely dysfunctional.

Crisis intervention is a specific type of brief psychotherapy and has two specific goals. First is patient safety. Use external controls to protect the patient and others if the person is suicidal or homicidal. Second is anxiety reduction using techniques that put a patient's inner resources into effect. It is more directive than traditional psychotherapy or counseling, and any member of the health care team who has been trained in its techniques can use it. The basic approach is problem solving, and it focuses only on the problem presented by the crisis (Halter, 2018).

Help a patient make the mental connection between the stressful event and his or her reaction to it. This is crucial because he or she is sometimes unable to see the whole situation clearly. Help the person explore his or her feelings and emotions such as anger, grief, or guilt to help him or her reduce feelings of tension. In addition, you help the patient explore coping mechanisms, perhaps identifying new methods of coping. Finally, you help the person increase social contacts if he or she has been isolated and overly self-focused.

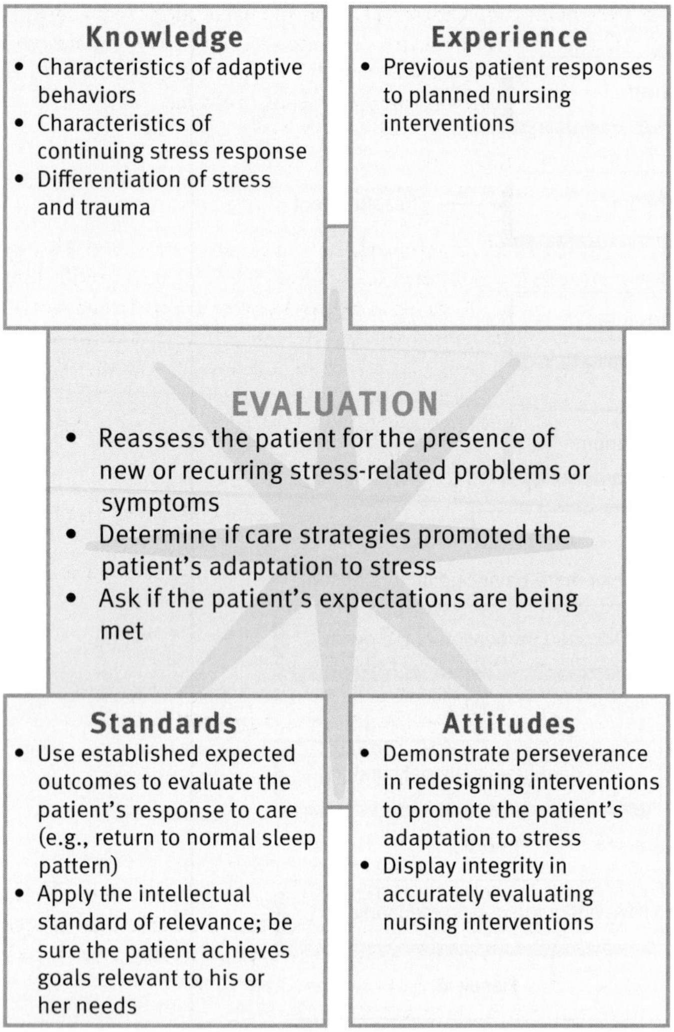

Knowledge	**Experience**
• Characteristics of adaptive behaviors • Characteristics of continuing stress response • Differentiation of stress and trauma	• Previous patient responses to planned nursing interventions

EVALUATION

• Reassess the patient for the presence of new or recurring stress-related problems or symptoms
• Determine if care strategies promoted the patient's adaptation to stress
• Ask if the patient's expectations are being met

Standards	**Attitudes**
• Use established expected outcomes to evaluate the patient's response to care (e.g., return to normal sleep pattern) • Apply the intellectual standard of relevance; be sure the patient achieves goals relevant to his or her needs	• Demonstrate perseverance in redesigning interventions to promote the patient's adaptation to stress • Display integrity in accurately evaluating nursing interventions

FIG. 37.7 Critical thinking model for stress and coping evaluation.

Restorative and Continuing Care. A person under stress recovers when the stress is removed or coping strategies are successful; however, a person who has experienced a crisis has changed, and the effects often last for years or for the rest of the person's life. The final stage of adapting to a crisis is acknowledgment of its long-term implications. If a person has coped with a crisis and its consequences successfully, he or she becomes more mature and healthier. When a person recovers from a stressful situation, the time is right for introducing stress-management skills to reduce the number and intensity of stressful situations in the future.

◆ Evaluation

Through the Patient's Eyes. A patient recovering from acute stress often spontaneously reports feeling better when the stressor is gone. The recovery from chronic stress occurs more gradually as the patient emerges from the strain. Your evaluation must include the patient's perceptions. Ask the patient about sleep patterns, appetite, and ability to concentrate. Ask how the patient feels about coping strategies that are being used, and determine their effectiveness. Ask patients to compare current feelings and behaviors with feelings and behaviors before the patient started experiencing stress (e.g., 6 months ago).

An essential part of the evaluation process is collaborating with patients to determine whether their own expectations from nursing

have been met. Any revision in the plan of care includes steps to address patient expectations.

Patient Outcomes. Evaluation involves reassessing any new or recurring stress-related symptoms and whether the expected outcomes in the plan of care were achieved (Fig. 37.7). Remember that coping with stress takes time. Maintain ongoing communication with patients regarding their coping. Patients under severe stress or trauma often experience feelings of powerlessness, vulnerability, and loss of control. Address these feelings by actively involving patients and families in the processes of re-examining problems, prioritizing, goal setting, and revising interventions. Involving patients in these processes gives them an opportunity to direct their energy in a positive way and moves them toward taking greater responsibility for health maintenance and promotion.

Engaging the patient as a partner in health care creates open communication. In such an environment the patient feels comfortable to give important feedback about interventions that are successful and helps you better understand why some interventions fail to meet the expected outcomes and established goals. If a patient reports continued acute stress, assess for safety by asking about whether there have been any recent stressors at home, in the car, or at work. Ask about coping strategies to determine whether the patient is using unsafe, maladaptive strategies. If the patient reports continued chronic stress, ask about his or her perception of the stressor and the coping behaviors used. Discuss the stressor with the patient to determine whether it needs to be redefined. If contact with a patient ends before you have achieved the resolution of goals, it is important to refer him or her to appropriate resources so that progress is not delayed or interrupted.

■ KEY POINTS

• The general adaptation syndrome (GAS), an immediate physiological response to stress, involves specific autonomic nervous system and endocrine system responses during the alarm, resistance, and exhaustion stages.
• Post-traumatic stress disorder begins when a person experiences, witnesses, or is confronted with a traumatic event and responds with intense fear or helplessness. Anxiety associated with PTSD is sometimes manifested by nightmares and emotional detachment.
• Many nursing theories, such as the Neuman Systems Model or Callista Roy's Adaptation Model, explain and describe stress and help you understand how an individual, family, or community effectively responds to stressors in the environment.
• Compassion fatigue is a state of burnout and secondary traumatic stress that can overwhelm health care providers and result in feelings of hopelessness, inadequacy, and anxiety.
• A regular exercise program improves muscle tone and posture, controls weight, reduces tension, and promotes relaxation.
• An individual whose stress is so severe that he or she is unable to cope using any of the means that have worked before is experiencing a crisis.
• Crisis intervention aims to return the person to a precrisis level of functioning and promote growth.
• Assessment of a patient's stress level and coping resources requires that you first establish a trusting nurse-patient relationship because you are asking a patient to share personal and sensitive information.
• Three primary modes of intervention for stress are to decrease stress-producing situations, increase resistance to stress, and learn skills that reduce physiological responses to stress.

- In nursing, burnout results when nurses perceive that the demands of their work exceed perceived resources. It is manifested as emotional exhaustion, poor decision making, loss of a sense of personal identity, and feelings of failure.

■ REFLECTIVE LEARNING

- Consider the stressors you are experiencing in your own life while you are in your nursing education program. What stress-reducing and coping strategies are you using to manage the stress you are experiencing. What strategy do you find most effective?
- Think about a patient you cared for recently on the clinical unit. How did stress impact the patient's health? Discuss the response of the patient to this stress.
- You are developing a program to help nurses on the clinical unit cope with compassion fatigue. Discuss key points that you will include in the program. What strategies will you teach the nurses to use to combat compassion fatigue?

■ REVIEW QUESTIONS

1. The nurse is interviewing a patient in the community clinic and gathers the following information about her: she is intermittently homeless, a single parent with two children who have developmental delays. She has had asthma since she was a teenager. She does not laugh or smile, does not volunteer any information, and at times appears close to tears. She has no support system and does not work. She is experiencing an allostatic load. As a result, which of the following would be present during complete patient assessment? (Select all that apply.)
   1. Post-traumatic stress disorder
   2. Rising hormone levels
   3. Chronic illness
   4. Insomnia
   5. Depression

2. A patient who is having difficulty managing his diabetes mellitus responds to the news that his hemoglobin A1c, a measure of blood sugar control over the past 90 days, has increased by saying, "The hemoglobin A1c is wrong. My blood sugar levels have been excellent for the last 6 months." Which defense mechanism is the patient using?
   1. Denial
   2. Conversion
   3. Dissociation
   4. Displacement

3. When assessing a young woman who was a victim of a home invasion 3 months earlier, the nurse learns that the woman has vivid images of the event whenever she hears loud yelling or a sudden noise. The nurse recognizes this as _____.

4. While assessing an older woman who is recently widowed, the nurse suspects that this woman is experiencing a developmental crisis. Which questions provide information about the impact of this crisis? (Select all that apply.)
   1. With whom do you talk on a routine basis?
   2. What do you do when you feel lonely?
   3. Tell me what your husband was like.
   4. I know this must be hard for you. Let me tell you what might help.
   5. Have you experienced any changes in lifestyle habits, such as sleeping, eating, smoking, or drinking?

5. The nurse plans care for a 16-year-old male, taking into consideration that stressors experienced most commonly by adolescents include which of the following? (Select all that apply.)
   1. Loss of autonomy caused by health problems
   2. Physical appearance and body image
   3. Accepting one's personal identity
   4. Separation from family
   5. Taking tests in school

6. A 10-year-old girl was playing on a slide at a playground during a summer camp. She fell and broke her arm. The camp notified the parents and took the child to the emergency department according to the camp protocol for injuries. The parents arrive at the emergency department and are stressed and frantic. The 10-year-old is happy in the treatment room, eating a Popsicle and picking out the color of her cast. List in order of priority what the nurse should say to the parents.
   1. "Can I contact someone to help you?"
   2. "Your daughter is happy in the treatment room, eating a Popsicle and picking out the color of her cast."
   3. "I'll have the doctor come out and talk to you as soon as possible."
   4. "I want to be sure you are ok. Let's talk about what your concerns are about your daughter before we go see her."

7. When assessing an older adult who is showing symptoms of anxiety, insomnia, anorexia, and mild confusion, what is the first assessment the nurse conducts?
   1. The amount of family support
   2. A 3-day diet recall
   3. A thorough physical assessment
   4. Threats to safety in her home

8. A 34-year-old single father who is anxious, tearful, and tired from caring for his three young children tells the nurse that he feels depressed and doesn't see how he can go on much longer. Which statement would be the nurse's best response?
   1. "Are you thinking of suicide?"
   2. "You've been doing a good job raising your children. You can do it!"
   3. "Is there someone who can help you during the evenings and weekends?"
   4. "Tell me what you mean when you say you can't go on any longer."

9. The nurse is evaluating how well a patient newly diagnosed with multiple sclerosis and psychomotor impairment is coping. Which statements indicate that the patient is beginning to cope with the diagnosis? (Select all that apply.)
   1. "I'm going to learn to drive a car, so I can be more independent."
   2. "My sister says she feels better when she goes shopping, so I'll go shopping."
   3. "I'm going to let the occupational therapist assess my home to improve efficiency."
   4. "I've always felt better when I go for a long walk. I'll do that when I get home."
   5. "I'm going to attend a support group to learn more about multiple sclerosis."

10. A crisis intervention nurse is working with a mother whose child with Down syndrome has been hospitalized with pneumonia and who has lost her child's disability payment while the child is hospitalized. The mother worries that her daughter will fall behind in her classes during hospitalization. Which strategies are effective in helping this mother cope with these stressors? (Select all that apply.)
    1. Referral to social service process reestablishing the child's disability payment

2. Sending the child home in 72 hours and having the child return to school

3. Coordinating hospital-based and home-based schooling with the child's teacher

4. Teaching the mother signs and symptoms of a respiratory tract infection

5. Telling the mother that the stress will decrease in 6 weeks when everything is back to normal

Answers: 1. 3, 4, 5; **2.** 1; **3.** Post-traumatic stress disorder (PTSD); **4.** 1, 2, 5; **5.** 2, 3, 4, 5; **6.** 2, 4, 3; **7.** 3; **8.** 4; **9.** 3, 5; **10.** 1, 3, 4.

Rationales for Review Questions can be found on the Evolve website.

REFERENCES

American Nurses Association (ANA): *Psychiatric–mental health nursing: scope and standards of practice*, ed 2, Silver Spring, MD, 2014, ANA.

Banasik JL, Copstead LC: *Pathophysiology*, ed 6, St Louis, 2019, Elsevier.

Cherry B, Jacob SR: *Contemporary nursing: issues, trends, & management*, ed 8, St Louis, 2019, Elsevier.

Christie W, Jones S: Lateral violence in nursing and the theory of the nurse as wounded healer, *Online J Issues Nurs* 19(1):5, 2013.

Giger J: *Transcultural nursing*, ed 7, St Louis, 2017, Elsevier.

Halter MJ: *Varcarolis' foundations of psychiatric mental health nursing: a clinical approach*, ed 6, St Louis, 2018, Elsevier.

Holman D, et al.: Stress management interventions: improving subjective psychological well-being in the workplace. In Diener E, et al.: *Handbook of well-being*, Salt Lake City, UT, 2018, DEF Publishers.

Huether SE, et al.: *Understanding pathophysiology*, ed 6, St Louis, 2017, Elsevier.

Kravitz L: Exercise is good for mental health: but keep in mind that overdoing it does more harm than good, *IDEA Fitness Journal* 16(1):12, 2019.

Lewis SL, et al.: *Medical-surgical nursing: assessment and management of clinical problems*, ed 10, St Louis, 2017, Elsevier.

Liu JW, et al.: Re-conceptualizing stress: shifting views on the consequences of stress and its effects on stress reactivity, *PLoS One*, 2017, https://doi.org/10.1371/journal.pone.0173188.

Murdaugh CL, et al.: *Health promotion and nursing practice*, ed 7, Boston, MA, 2015, Pearson.

Neuman B, Fawcett J, editors: *The neuman systems model*, ed 5, Upper Saddle River, NJ, 2011, Pearson.

Sacks SA, et al.: A pilot study of the trauma recovery group for veterans with post traumatic stress disorder and co-occurring serious mental illness, *J Ment Health* 26(3):237, 2017.

Selye H: History of the stress concept. In Goldberger L, Breznitz s, editors: *Handbook of stress: theoretical and clinical aspects*, ed 2, New York, 1993, Free Press.

Smith MC, Parker ME: *Nursing theorists and nursing practice*, ed 4, Philadelphia, PA, 2015, FA Davis.

Waude A, editor: *General adaptation syndrome*, Psychologist World (website), 2016. https://www.ncbi.nlm.nih.gov/pmc/articles/PMC2038162/?page=1. Accessed April 15, 2019.

RESEARCH REFERENCES

Antony L, et al.: Stress, coping, and lived experiences among caregivers of cancer patients on palliative care: a mixed method research, *Indian J Palliat Care* 24(3):313, 2018.

Bily L: Creative therapeutic activities and support groups benefit all those involved in cancer care, *Am Health Drug Benefits* 10(6), 2017.

Brown S, et al.: The impact of resiliency on nurse burnout: an integrative literature review, *Medsurg Nurs* 27(6):349, 2018.

Can G, et al.: The correlation between levels of coping with stress and attitude towards smoking in patients with schizophrenia, *Int J Caring Sci* 10(1), 2017.

Casey G, Tiaki K: Stress and disease, *Nurs N Z* 23:20, 2017.

Desiree GM, et al.: Mindfulness-based stress reduction for lung cancer patients and their partners: results of a mixed methods pilot study, *Palliat Med* 29(7):652, 2015.

Doron J, et al.: Coping profiles, perceived stress and health-related behaviors: a cluster analysis approach, *Health Promot Int* 30(1):88, 2014.

Edraki M, et al.: The effect of coping skills training on depression, anxiety, stress, and self-efficacy in adolescents with diabetes: a randomized controlled trial, *Int J Community Based Nurs Midwifery* 6(4):324–333, 2018.

Embree JL, White AH: Concept analysis nurse-to-nurse lateral violence, *Nurs Forum* 45(3):1266, 2010.

Enns A, et al.: Perceived stress, coping strategies, and emotional intelligence: a cross-sectional study of university students in helping disciplines, *Nurse Educ Today* 68:226, 2018.

Greeson, JM, et al: Mindfulness meditation targets transdiagnostic symptoms implicated in stress-related disorders: understanding relationships between changes in mindfulness, sleep quality, and physical symptoms, *Evid Based Complement Alternat Med (eCAM)* 5/13/2018:1-10, 2018.

Grensman A, et al.: Effect of traditional yoga, mindfulness-based cognitive therapy, and cognitive behavioral therapy, on health related quality of life: a randomized controlled trial on patients on sick leave because of burnout, *BMC Complement Altern Med* 18(1):80, 2018.

Grissinger M: Too many abandon the "second victims" of medical errors, *P T* 39(9):591, 2014.

Hartley H: Concept review: second traumatization and the role of a perioperative advanced practice nurse, *ORNAC J* 36(4):37, 2018.

Hunsaker S, et al.: Factors that influence the development of compassion fatigue, burnout, and compassion satisfaction in emergency department nurses, *J Nurs Scholarsh* 47(2):186, 2015.

Jackson JS, et al.: Social relations, productive activities, and coping with stress in late life. In Stephens MA, et al.: *Stress and coping in later-life families (ebook)*, New York, 2018, Taylor & Francis.

Kartin PT, et al.: The effect of meditation and music listening on the anxiety level, operation tolerance and pain perception in people who were performed colonoscopy, *Int J Caring Sci* 10(3):1587, 2017.

Lin SH, et al.: The impact of shift work on nurses' job stress, sleep quality and self-perceived health status, *J Nurs Manag* 22(5):604, 2014.

Mealer M, et al.: Feasibility and acceptability of a resilience training program for intensive care unit nurses, *Am J Crit Care* 23(6):97, 2014.

Meiner SE, Yeager JJ: *Gerontologic nursing*, ed 6, St Louis, 2019, Elsevier.

Oken BS, et al.: Predictors of improvements in mental health from mindfulness meditation in stressed older adults, *Altern Ther Health Med* 24(1):48, 2018.

Pangotra A, et al.: Effectiveness of progressive muscle relaxation, biofeedback and l-theanine in patients suffering from anxiety disorder, *J Psychosoc Res* 13(1):219, 2018.

Park CL, Iacocca MO: A stress and coping perspective on health behaviors: theoretical and methodological considerations, *Anxiety Stress Coping* 27(2):123, 2014.

Parsons CE, et al.: Home practice in mindfulness-based cognitive therapy and mindfulness-based stress reduction: a systematic review and meta-analysis of participants' mindfulness practice and its association with outcomes, *Behav Res Ther* 95(29), 2017.

Pavlacic J, et al.: A meta-analysis of expressive writing on posttraumatic stress, posttraumatic growth, and quality of life, *Rev Gen Psychol* 23(2):230, 2019. https://journals.sagepub.com/doi/pdf/10.1177/1089268019831645. Accessed April 15, 2019.

Phillips LA, et al.: Self-management of chronic illness: the role of 'habit' versus reflective factors in exercise and medication adherence, *J Behav Med* 39(6):1076, 2016.

Potter P, et al.: Developing a systemic program for compassion fatigue, *Nurs Adm Q* 37(4):326, 2013.

Rayens MK, Reed DB: Predictors of depressive symptoms in older rural couples: the impact of work, stress, and health, *J Rural Health* 30(1):59, 2014.

Shavitt S, et al.: Culture moderates the relation between perceived stress, social support, and mental and physical health, *J Cross Cult Psychol* 47(7):956, 2016.

Solomon D, et al.: Multicenter study of nursing role complexity on environmental stressors and emotional exhaustion, *Appl Nurs Res* 30:52, 2016.

Steenkamp MM: Psychotherapy for military-related PTSD, *JAMA* 314(5):489, 2015.

Sunne R, Huntington MK: The 36 hour day, revisited: implementing a caregiver support system into primary care practice, *S D Med* 70(4):173, 2017.

Tsitsi T, et al.: Effectiveness of a relaxation intervention to reduce anxiety and improve mood of parents of hospitalized children with malignancies, *Eur J Cancer* Suppl 1(72):S143, 2017.

Ueno S, et al.: Occupational stress: stressors referred by the nursing team, *J Nurs* 11(4):1632, 2017.

Yilmaz G, et al.: Effect of a nurse-led intervention programme on professional quality of life and post-traumatic growth in oncology nurses, *Int J Nurs Pract* 24(6):e12687, 2018.

38

Activity and Exercise

OBJECTIVES

- Understand the role of the musculoskeletal and nervous systems in the regulation of activity and exercise.
- Understand the importance of exercise and activity for maintaining and promoting health.
- Apply nursing care interventions for preventing deconditioning in hospitalized inpatients.
- Describe the rationale for the use of safe patient handling techniques when transferring and assisting patients with ambulation.
- Understand factors to consider when planning an exercise program for patients across the life span.

- Describe how to assess patients for level of activity tolerance.
- Identify interventions designed to improve an individual's activity tolerance.
- Discuss the importance of minimal or no-lift policies for patients and health care providers.
- Describe nurses' responsibility in assisting patients to ambulate safely.
- Evaluate the achievement of patient outcomes following use of safe transfer techniques.

KEY TERMS

Activity tolerance, p. 789
Activities of daily living, p. 777
Body alignment, p. 778
Body mechanics, p. 778
Cartilaginous joints, p. 778
Center of gravity, p. 782
Concentric tension, p. 781

Crutch gait, p. 798
Deconditioning, p. 777
Eccentric tension, p. 781
Fibrous joint, p. 778
Isometric contraction, p. 781
Isotonic contraction, p. 781
Muscle tone, p. 782

Proprioception, p. 782
Stretch reflex, p. 781
Synovial joints, p. 778
Unossified, p. 780

MEDIA RESOURCES

http://evolve.elsevier.com/Potter/fundamentals/
- Review Questions
- Video Clips
- Concept Map Creator
- Case Study with Questions

- Audio Glossary
- Content Updates
- Answers to QSEN Activity and Review Questions
- Skills Performance Checklists

Regular physical activity and exercise contribute to individuals' physical and emotional well-being. According to the American Heart Association (2018), physical activity:
- Elevates our mood and attitude.
- Keeps us physically fit.
- Helps one to quit smoking and stay tobacco-free.
- Boosts your energy level so you can get more done.
- Helps in the management of stress.
- Promotes a better quality of sleep.
- Improves your self-image and self-confidence.

Promoting activity and exercise is a principle that you, as a nurse, should apply in the care of patients in all health care settings. When promoting activity it is important to do so in a safe and efficient manner, especially for patients who are functionally impaired and in need of your assistance. Walking, turning, lifting, and carrying all are common actions used in delivering nursing care. These activities also pose risks. Health care workers frequently incur injuries, such as back injuries and overexertion, when moving or lifting patients incorrectly. You will apply safe patient handling standards and principles to reduce the risk of injury to patients and yourself when assisting patients with activities.

Frequently patients experience functional decline (the loss of the ability to perform self-care or activities of daily living). Such decline may result not only directly from illness or adverse treatment effects but also from deconditioning associated with imposed inactivity. The negative effects of deconditioning can be seen after short periods of time. Deconditioning involves physiological changes following a period of inactivity (e.g., bed rest or sedentary lifestyle). It is a particular risk for hospitalized patients who spend most of their time in bed, even when they are able to walk. As a result, nurses play an important role in increasing the overall activity of inpatients routinely to minimize the risk of deconditioning.

A program of regular physical activity and exercise has the potential to enhance all aspects of a patient's health. This chapter provides you with knowledge of exercise and activity as they relate to health promotion, the acute phase of illness, and the restorative and continuing care of patients.

SCIENTIFIC KNOWLEDGE BASE

Regular physical activity and exercise contribute to both physical and emotional well-being. Knowing the physiology and regulation of body mechanics, exercise, and activity helps you to provide individualized patient care.

Nature of Movement

Movement is a complex process that requires coordination between the musculoskeletal and nervous systems. As a nurse you will consider how a patient's physical and psychological conditions affect body movement. Body mechanics is a term that describes the coordinated efforts of the musculoskeletal and nervous systems. Knowing how patients initiate movement and understanding your own movements requires a basic understanding of the physics surrounding body mechanics. The body mechanics applied in the lifting techniques historically used in nursing practice often cause debilitating injuries to nurses and other health care staff (Kanaskie and Snyder, 2018; Noble and Sweeney, 2018). Today nurses use evidence-based information about body alignment, balance, gravity, and friction when implementing nursing interventions such as transferring patients, assisting with ambulation, determining the risk of patient falls, and selecting the safest way to move or transfer patients (AORN, 2018).

Alignment and Balance

The terms body alignment and "posture" are similar and refer to the positioning of the joints, tendons, ligaments, and muscles while standing, sitting, and lying. Body alignment means that an individual's center of gravity is stable. Correct body alignment reduces strain on musculoskeletal structures, aids in maintaining adequate muscle tone, promotes comfort, and contributes to balance and conservation of energy. Without balance control the center of gravity is displaced.

Individuals require balance for maintaining a static position (e.g., sitting) and moving (e.g., transferring or walking). Disease, injury, pain, physical development (e.g., age), and life changes (e.g., pregnancy) compromise the ability to remain balanced. Medications that cause dizziness and prolonged immobility affect balance. Impaired balance is a major threat to mobility and physical safety and contributes to a fear of falling and self-imposed activity restrictions (Dickinson et al., 2018; Musich et al., 2018).

Gravity and Friction

Weight is the force exerted on a body by gravity. The force of weight is always directed downward, which is why an unbalanced object falls. Unsteady patients fall if their center of gravity becomes unbalanced because of the gravitational pull on their weight. To lift safely the lifter has to overcome the weight of the object and know its center of gravity. In symmetrical inanimate objects the center of gravity is at the exact center of the object. However, people are not geometrically perfect;

their centers of gravity are usually at 55% to 57% of standing height and are in the midline, which is why using only the principles of body mechanics in lifting patients often leads to injury of a nurse or other health care professional.

Friction is a force that occurs in a direction to oppose movement. The greater the surface area of the object that is moved, the greater is the friction. A larger object produces greater resistance to movement. In addition, the force exerted against the skin while the skin remains stationary and the bony structures move is called shear. Unfortunately, a common example is when the head of a hospital bed is elevated beyond 60 degrees and gravity pulls a patient so that the bony skeleton moves toward the foot of the bed while the skin remains against the sheets. The blood vessels in the underlying tissue are stretched and damaged, resulting in impeded blood flow to the deep tissues. Ultimately pressure injuries often develop within the undermined tissue; the surface tissue appears less affected (see Chapter 48). To decrease surface area and reduce friction when patients are unable to assist with moving up in bed, nurses use an ergonomic assistive device such as a full-body sling. The sling mechanically lifts a patient off the surface of a bed, thereby preventing friction, tearing, or shearing of the patient's delicate skin; it also protects nurses and other health care staff from injury (Noble and Sweeny, 2018) (see Chapter 39).

Regulation of Movement

Coordinated body movement involves the integrated functioning of the musculoskeletal and nervous systems. Because these systems work together dynamically, they are often considered as a single functional unit.

Skeletal System. The skeletal system provides attachments for muscles and ligaments and the leverage necessary for mobility. Thus the skeleton is the supporting framework of the body and is made up of four types of bones: long, short, flat, and irregular. Bones are important for mobilization because they are firm, rigid, and elastic. The aging process, as well as some nutritional and disease processes, has the potential to change the components of bone, which impacts mobility.

Firmness results from inorganic salts such as calcium and phosphate that are in the bone matrix. It is related to the rigidity of the bone, which is necessary to keep long bones straight, and enables bones to withstand weight-bearing. Elasticity and skeletal flexibility change with age. A newborn has a large amount of cartilage and is highly flexible but is unable to support weight. A toddler's bones are more pliable than those of an older person and are better able to withstand traumatic injury. Older adults, especially women, are more susceptible to bone loss (resorption) and osteoporosis, which increases the risk of fractures.

Joints. The region where two or more bones attach is referred to as a joint. Each joint is classified according to its structure and degree of mobility. There are three classifications of joints: cartilaginous, fibrous, and synovial (McCance and Huether, 2017). Fibrous joints fit closely together and are fixed, permitting little if any movement, such as the syndesmosis between the tibia and fibula (Fig. 38.1A). Cartilaginous joints have little movement but are elastic and use cartilage to unite separate bony surfaces, such as the synchondrosis that attaches the ribs to the costal cartilage. When bone growth is complete, the joints ossify (see Fig. 38.1B). Synovial joints, or true joints, such as the hinge type at the elbow, are freely movable and the most mobile, numerous, and anatomically complex body joints (see Fig. 38.2AB).

Ligaments, Tendons, and Cartilage. Ligaments, tendons, and cartilage support the skeletal system. Ligaments are white, shiny, flexible bands of dense fibrous tissue that bind joints and connect bones and

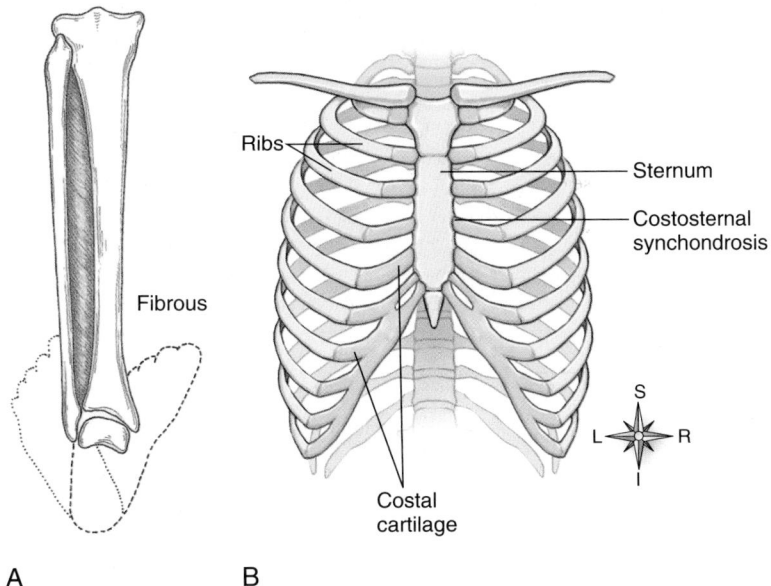

FIG. 38.1 Joint types. **A**, Fibrous. **B**, Cartilaginous. (**B** from Patton KT, Thibodeau GA: *Anatomy & physiology*, ed 10, St Louis, 2019, Elsevier.)

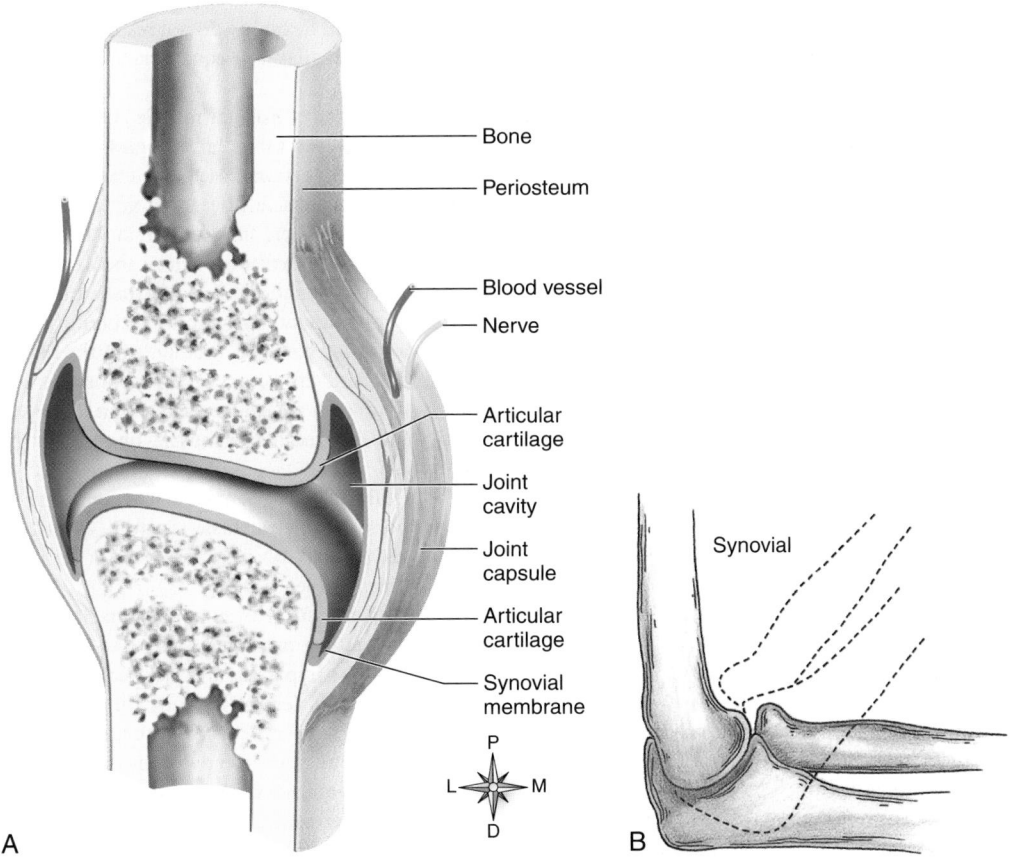

FIG. 38.2 A, Structure of synovial joint. Artist's interpretation (composite drawing of a typical synovial joint). **B**, Synovial joint. (**A** From Patton KT, Thibodeau GA: *Human body in health and disease*, ed 7, St Louis, 2018, Elsevier.)

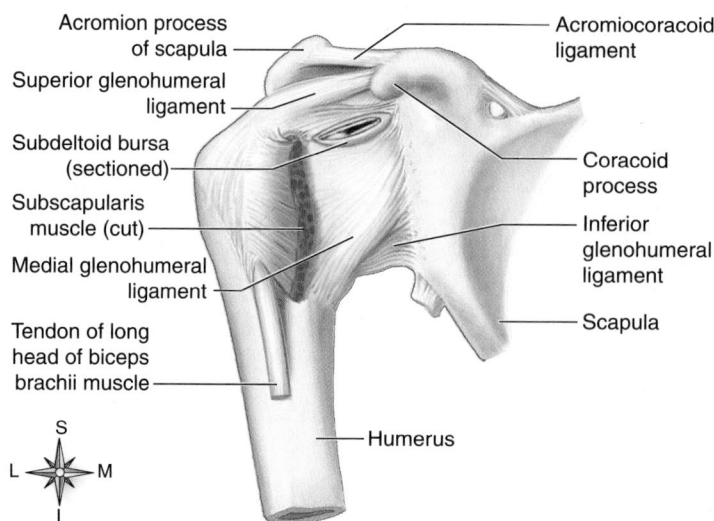

FIG. 38.3 Tendons and ligaments of the shoulder. (B From Patton KT, Thibodeau GA: *Anatomy & physiology,* ed 10, St Louis, 2019, Elsevier.)

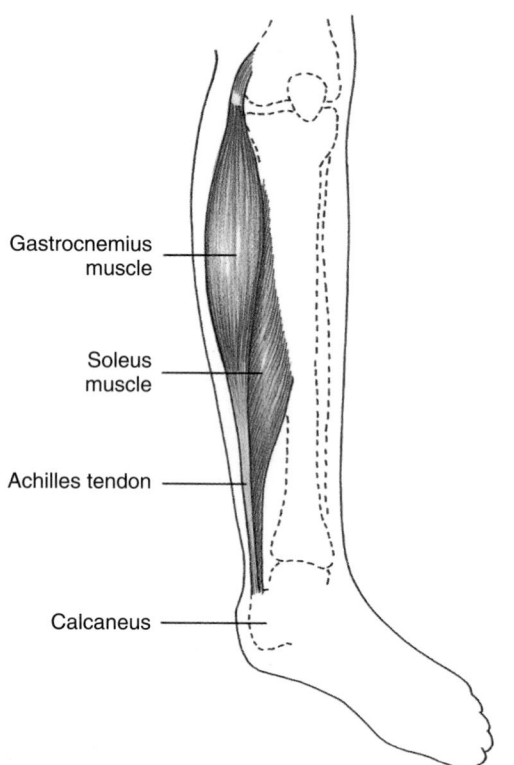

FIG. 38.4 Tendons and muscles of lower leg.

nonvascular (without blood vessels) supporting connective tissue located chiefly in the joints and thorax, trachea, larynx, nose, and ear. It has the flexibility of a firm, plastic material. Because of its gristle-like nature, cartilage sustains weight and serves as a shock absorber between articulating bones. Permanent cartilage is unossified (not hardened), except in advanced age and diseases such as osteoarthritis, which impairs mobility.

Strength and flexibility do not result entirely from joints, ligaments, tendons, and cartilage. Adequate skeletal muscle is also necessary.

Skeletal Muscle. Skeletal muscle cells have the ability to be stimulated, or excited, and thus can respond to regulatory mechanisms such as nerve signals (Patton, 2019). Skeletal muscles are composed of bundles of skeletal muscle fibers that generally extend the entire length of the muscle. Muscle fibers contract when stimulated by an electrochemical impulse that travels from the nerve to the muscle across the neuromuscular junction. The electrochemical impulse causes the filaments (predominantly protein molecules of myosin and actin) within the fiber to slide past one another, with the filaments changing length. Continued and efficient use of adenosine triphosphate (ATP), the energy source for muscular contraction, requires glucose and oxygen. Both nutrients reach the muscle fibers through vascular capillaries (Patton, 2019).

Skeletal muscles contract with varying degrees of strength based on the specific task (Patton, 2019). For example, during prolonged inactivity, muscles usually shrink, a condition called disuse atrophy (see Chapter 39) (Patton, 2019). Active use of muscles during exercise can increase muscle size and lead to hypertrophy. Contraction of skeletal muscles allows people to walk, talk, breathe, or participate in any physical activity. There are more than 600 skeletal muscles in the body. In addition to facilitating movement, these muscles determine the form and contour of our bodies. Most of our muscles span at least one joint and attach to both articulating bones. When contraction occurs, one bone is fixed while the other moves. The origin is the point of attachment that remains still; the insertion is the point that moves when the muscle contracts (Patton, 2019).

The amount of load placed on a muscle influences the strength of a skeletal muscle. Generally, the heavier the load, the stronger the contraction. Imagine lifting your hands with palms up in front of you and placing this textbook in your hand. You will feel your arm muscles contract more strongly as the book is placed in your hand because of the

cartilage. A ligament is one type of collagenous fiber that intertwines in irregular, swirling arrangements to form thick connective tissue (Patton, 2019). Ligaments are predominantly elastic fibers and are thus somewhat elastic in nature (Fig. 38.3). Some ligaments serve a protective function. For example, ligaments between the vertebral bodies and the ligamentum flavum prevent damage to the spinal cord during movement of the back.

Tendons are white, glistening fibrous bands of tissue that occur in various lengths and thicknesses. Tendons connect muscle to bone and are strong, flexible, and inelastic. The Achilles tendon is the thickest and strongest tendon in the body. It begins near the midposterior of the leg and attaches the gastrocnemius and soleus muscles in the calf to the calcaneal bone in the back of the foot (Fig. 38.4). Cartilage is

TABLE 38.1	Functional Classification of Muscle Action	
Term	**Movement**	**Example**
Prime mover	Muscle that directly performs a specific movement.	Brachialis is a prime mover when flexing the elbow.
Antagonist	Muscle that directly when contracting opposes prime mover or agonist. Relaxes while prime mover contracts. Provides precision and control during contraction of prime mover.	The triceps brachii is an extensor that relaxes when brachialis contracts.
Synergists	Muscle that contracts at same time as prime mover. Facilitates prime mover actions to produce more effective movement.	The deltoid contracts when brachialis contracts
Fixators	Muscles that stabilize joints; act as type of synergist. Serve to maintain posture and balance.	The deltoid maintains balance of arm when brachialis contracts.

Adapted from Patton KT: *Anatomy & physiology*, ed 10, St Louis, 2019, Elsevier.

stretch reflex (Patton, 2019). Your arms and hands will try to maintain constancy of muscle length. The body has a negative feedback response when it detects the increased stretch caused by the load of the textbook. The information is relayed back to the central nervous system, which increases its stimulation of the muscle to counteract the stretch (Patton, 2019). The reflex maintains relatively constant muscle length, but when the load becomes too heavy and threatens injury to the muscle, the body ignores the reflex and causes you to relax and drop the textbook (Patton, 2019).

There are two types of muscle contractions, isotonic and isometric. An isotonic or dynamic contraction is mobilizing, causing the body to move (Patton, 2019). In contrast, an isometric contraction is stabilizing, causing the body to hold a stable position (Patton, 2019). Isotonic contractions have two varieties, concentric and eccentric. In concentric tension increased muscle contraction causes muscle shortening, resulting in movement, such as when a patient uses an overhead trapeze to pull up in bed. Eccentric tension causes lengthening of a muscle to control the speed and direction of movement. For example, when using an overhead trapeze, a patient slowly lowers himself to the bed. The lowering is controlled when the antagonistic muscles lengthen. Concentric and eccentric muscle actions are necessary for active movement. Isometric contraction (static contraction) causes an increase in muscle tension or muscle work but no shortening or active movement of the muscle (e.g., instructing a patient to tighten and relax a muscle group, as in quadriceps set exercises or pelvic floor exercises). Voluntary movement is a combination of isotonic and isometric contractions.

Although isometric contractions do not result in muscle shortening, energy expenditure increases. This type of muscle work is comparable to having a car in neutral with the driver continually depressing the accelerator and racing the engine. The driver is not going anywhere but expends a large amount of energy. It is important to understand the energy expenditure (increased respiratory rate and increased work on the heart) associated with isometric exercises because the exercises are sometimes contraindicated in certain patients' illnesses (e.g., myocardial infarction [MI] or chronic obstructive pulmonary disease [COPD]).

Muscles Concerned With Movement. Skeletal muscles usually act in groups, resulting in movement produced by the coordinated action of several muscles (Patton, 2019). Because some muscles contract while

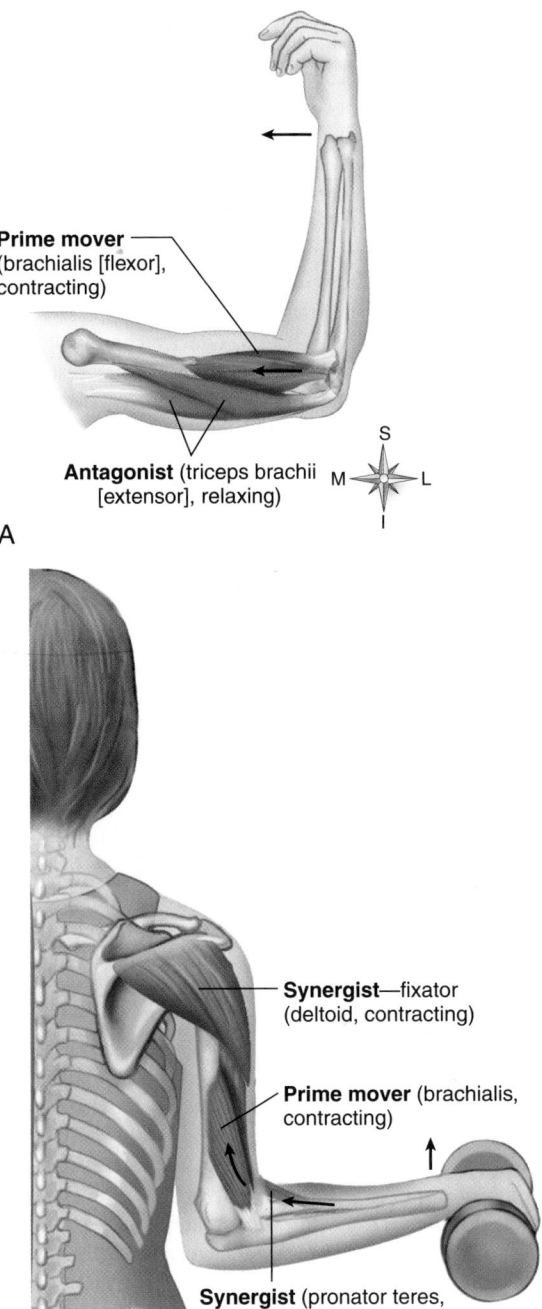

FIG. 38.5 Muscle actions. **A,** The flexor muscle (brachialis) is the prime move in flexing the elbow. The extensor muscle (triceps brachii) is the antagonist, relaxing to permit elbow flexion. The pronator teres muscle acts as a synergist by also flexing the elbow. **B,** The brachialis is the prime mover of flexion of the elbow. The pronator teres muscle acts as a synergist by also flexing the elbow. To prevent the biceps from also moving the shoulder strains against the weight; the posterior portion of the deltoid muscle tenses to stabilize the shoulder, thus acting as a fixator muscle. (From Patton KT, Thibodeau GA: *Anatomy & physiology*, ed 10, St Louis, 2019, Elsevier.)

others relax, there is a functional classification of muscles (Table 38.1). These types of muscle actions are important to understand when you use your own muscles to move patients and when you assist patients in independent movement or exercises (Fig. 38.5). Movement is complex. Most muscles function as all the classifications (Patton, 2019). A prime mover during flexion may be an antagonist during extension or a synergist or fixator in rotation.

When muscles shorten to contract, the type and extent of movement are determined by the load or resistance moved, the attachment of the tendons of the muscle to bone, and the type of joint involved (Patton, 2019). The muscles coordinate movement through a system of levers. The lever system makes the work of moving a weight or load easier. It occurs when specific bones such as the humerus, ulna, and radius and the associated joints such as the elbow act as a lever. Thus the force applied to one end of the bone to lift a weight at another point tends to rotate the bone in the direction opposite that of the applied force. Muscles that attach to bones of leverage provide the necessary strength to move an object.

Muscles Concerned With Posture. Gravity continually pulls on parts of the body; the only way the body is held in position is for muscles to pull on bones in the opposite direction. Muscles accomplish this counterforce by maintaining a low level of sustained contraction. Poor posture places more work on muscles to counteract the force of gravity. This leads to fatigue and eventually interferes with bodily functions and causes deformities.

Posture and movement depend on the skeleton and the shape and development of skeletal muscles. They also contribute to musculoskeletal function and often reflect personality, discomfort, and mood. For example, a person with a dramatic personality gestures with the hands, a person who is tired or depressed may slouch, and a person with abdominal pain may curl into a fetal-like position.

Coordination and regulation of different muscle groups depend on muscle tone and activity of antagonistic, synergistic, and antigravity muscles. Muscle tone, or tonus, is the normal state of balanced muscle tension. The body achieves tension by alternating contraction and relaxation without active movement of neighboring fibers of a specific muscle group. Muscle tone helps maintain functional positions such as sitting or standing without excess muscle fatigue and is maintained through continual use of muscles. Activities of daily living (ADLs) require muscle action and help maintain muscle tone. When a patient is immobile or on prolonged bed rest, activity level, activity tolerance, and muscle tone decrease (see Chapter 39).

Nervous System. The nervous system regulates movement and posture. The precentral gyrus, or motor strip, is the major voluntary motor area and is in the cerebral cortex. A majority of motor fibers descend from the motor strip and cross at the level of the medulla. Transmission of impulses from the nervous system to the musculoskeletal system is an electrochemical event and requires a neurotransmitter. Basically neurotransmitters are chemicals (e.g., acetylcholine) that transfer the electrical impulse from the nerve across the myoneural junction to stimulate the muscle, causing movement. Movement is impaired by disorders that alter neurotransmitter production, transfer of impulses from the nerve to the muscle, or activation of muscle activity. For example, Parkinson's disease alters neurotransmitter production, myasthenia gravis disrupts transfer from the neurotransmitter to the muscle, and multiple sclerosis impairs muscle activity (McCance and Huether, 2017).

Proprioception. Proprioception is a muscle sense that makes us aware of the position of the body and its parts, including body movement, orientation in space, and muscle stretch (Patton, 2019). For example, if you close your eyes and bend your elbow, you will know where your hand and lower arm are even if you cannot see them. Stretch receptors associated with muscles, joint capsules, and tendons are classified as proprioceptors (Patton, 2019). Proprioceptors are located within muscle spindles. Rapidly conducting and slower-conducting nerve fibers encircle an area of the muscle spindle found within skeletal muscles. When a muscle stretches, the afferent impulses from sensory neurons pass to the spinal cord and are relayed to

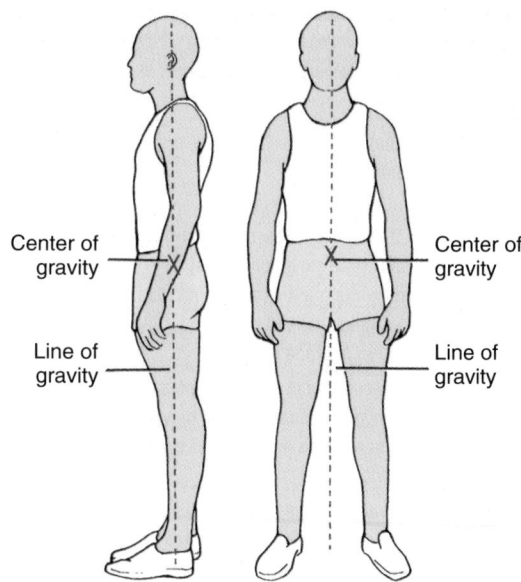

FIG. 38.6 Correct body alignment when standing.

the brain, providing a means to monitor changes in muscle length (Patton, 2019). The nervous system regulates posture, which requires coordination of proprioception and balance. As a person carries out ADLs, proprioceptors monitor muscle activity and body position. For example, the proprioceptors on the soles of the feet contribute to correct posture while standing or walking. In standing, pressure is continuous on the bottom of the feet. The proprioceptors monitor the pressure, communicating this information through the nervous system to the antigravity muscles. The standing person remains upright until deciding to change position. As a person walks, the proprioceptors on the bottom of the feet monitor pressure changes. Thus, when the bottom of the moving foot comes in contact with the walking surface, the individual automatically moves the stationary foot forward.

Balance and Alignment. Body balance occurs when a person is properly aligned with a relatively low center of gravity balanced over a wide, stable base of support. In the case of standing, a vertical line falls from the center of gravity through the base of support (Fig. 38.6). Adequate balance is necessary to stand, walk, turn, lift, or perform ADLs. Proper posture enhances body balance. The term "posture" means maintaining optimal body position or alignment that favors function. It requires the least muscular work to maintain, and places the least strain on muscles, ligaments, and bones (McCance and Huether, 2017). Nurses maintain patient alignment when positioning patients and when turning or moving them (see Chapter 39).

The nervous system controls balance specifically through the inner ear, the cerebellum, and through vision. The inner ear contains specialized mechanoreceptors or hair cells that are stimulated through sound waves, creating nerve impulses perceived in the brain as either sound or balance (Patton, 2019). These sense organs that are involved in balance are located within the vestibule and semicircular canals of the ear. Together the sense organs function in dynamic equilibrium, a function needed to maintain balance when the head or body rotates or suddenly moves (e.g., when turning in circles or bending over) (Patton, 2019). Normal vision aids balance because visual input from the eyes offers feedback as to whether you or the environment around you is moving.

Normal muscle action involves groups of muscles functioning together as a unit. The cerebellum coordinates patterns of muscle movement with the motor control areas of the cerebrum (Patton, 2019). The cerebellum coordinates action of the prime movers, antagonists, synergists and fixator muscles to make normal movement smooth, steady, and precise as to the force, rate, and extent of movement (Patton, 2019). These coordinated patterns of movement, such as the sequence of leg movements needed for walking, are learned and stored in the cerebellum (Patton, 2019).Nurses rely on balance to maintain proper body alignment and posture when providing patient care. This reduces strain on musculoskeletal structures and maintains adequate muscle tone. To achieve balance and alignment follow these steps:

- Widen your base of support by separating the feet to a comfortable distance.
- Bring the center of gravity closer to your base of support to increase balance.
- Bend your knees and flex the hips until squatting, and maintain proper back alignment to keep the trunk erect.

Nurses apply these techniques in a variety of care activities. For example, you raise the height of a hospital bed when performing a procedure such as changing a dressing to prevent bending too far at the waist and shifting the base of support.

Activity and Exercise

Physical activity (PA) is any movement produced by skeletal muscles that results in energy expenditure (e.g., occupational, sports, conditioning, and household activities). Physical exercise is a subset of PA that is planned, structured, and repetitive and has a final or an intermediate objective, such as the improvement or maintenance of physical fitness (Pinto et al., 2018). Sometimes exercise is also a therapeutic measure, as in the case of rehabilitation following surgery. A patient's individualized exercise program depends on the patient's activity tolerance or the type and amount of exercise or activity that the patient is able to perform. Physiological, emotional, and developmental factors influence a patient's activity tolerance (see below).

An active lifestyle is important for maintaining and promoting health and psychological well-being (Covan, 2015; Edelman and Kudzma, 2018). The best program of physical activity is a combination of exercises (isotonic, isometric, and resistive) that produce different physiological and psychological benefits. Isotonic exercises (e.g., walking, swimming, jogging, and bicycling) cause muscle contraction and change in muscle length (isotonic contraction). Isotonic exercises enhance circulatory and respiratory functioning; increase muscle mass, tone, and strength; and promote osteoblastic activity that combats osteoporosis. Isometric exercises (e.g., quadriceps set exercises and contraction of the gluteal muscles) involve tightening or tensing muscles without moving body parts (isometric contraction). This form of exercise is ideal for patients who do not tolerate increased activity, such as a patient who is immobilized in bed (see Chapter 39). The benefits are increased muscle mass, tone, and strength, thus decreasing the potential for muscle wasting; increased circulation to the involved body part; and increased osteoblastic activity.

Resistive isometric exercises are those in which an individual contracts the muscle while pushing against a stationary object or resisting the movement of an object (Kim et al., 2017). A gradual increase in the amount of resistance and the length of time that the muscle contraction is held increases muscle strength and endurance. Examples of resistive isometric exercises are push-ups and hip lifting, in which a patient in a sitting position pushes with the hands against a surface such as a chair seat and raises the hips. Resistive isometric exercises promote muscle strength and provide sufficient stress against bone to promote osteoblastic activity.

Principles for Transfer and Positioning

Transfer and positioning techniques help patients to be more active. For example, transferring a patient from bed to chair enables the

---

BOX 38.1 Principles of Safe Patient Transfer and Positioning

- Use mechanical lifts and lift teams when patients are unable to assist.
- When a patient is able to assist, remember these principles:
  - The wider the base of support, the greater the stability of the nurse.
  - The lower the center of gravity, the greater the stability of the nurse.
  - The equilibrium of an object is maintained as long as the line of gravity passes through its base of support.
  - Facing the direction of movement prevents abnormal twisting of the spine.
  - Dividing balanced activity between arms and legs reduces the risk of back injury.
  - Leverage, rolling, turning, or pivoting requires less work than lifting.
  - When friction is reduced between the object to be moved and the surface on which it is moved, less force is required to move it.

---

patient to be more participative in self-care activities. Using the principles of balance and alignment aids in safe patient transfer and positioning during routine care activities (see Chapter 39). Along with safe patient handling techniques, good balance and alignment decrease work effort and place less strain on musculoskeletal structures (Box 38.1). As a nurse you will teach colleagues and patients' families how to transfer or position patients properly. Teaching a patient's family how to transfer the patient from bed to chair increases and reinforces the family's knowledge about proper transfer and position techniques once the patient returns home. Knowledge of the principles of balance and alignment is crucial. You also incorporate knowledge of physiological and pathological influences on body alignment and mobility.

Pathological Influences on Body Alignment, Mobility, and Activity. Many pathological conditions affect body alignment and mobility. These conditions include congenital defects; disorders of bones, joints, and muscles; central nervous system damage; and musculoskeletal trauma (Table 38.2) (see Chapter 39). In addition, obesity, a chronic public health problem, negatively affects the musculoskeletal system, leading to disability problems. As a nurse, you consider these factors when your goal is to increase patient activity. Patients will have limitations, requiring you to adapt your approaches to care. For example, it is important to understand which type of voluntary and involuntary movement is present after damage to the central nervous system. Does the patient have the ability to move an extremity? Void independently? This information affects the types of interventions you select to maximize your patient's activity level while keeping him or her safe.

Obesity. Obesity deserves special consideration because it is a major international public health problem affecting children and adults. Researchers in the United States have found the obesity prevalence to be 16.9% in the age-group of 2 to 19 years and 8.4% in the age-group of 2 to 5 years (Skinner and Skelton, 2014), with an upward trend of prevalence in children with the severest forms of obesity (Pinto et al., 2016). Risk factors for childhood obesity are numerous; however, poor dietary habits, playing video games with an excess of screen time, and lack of exercise are significant factors. According to the Centers for Disease Control and Prevention (CDC), the prevalence of obesity among adults was 39.8% and affected about 93.3 million of US adults in 2015 to 2016 (CDC, 2018). Adults are more at risk for obesity due to a lack of healthy diet habits and limited physical activity and exercise.

Obesity impairs an individual's musculoskeletal health. Association has been found between obesity and numerous medical conditions, including osteoarthritis, low back pain, osteoporosis, gait disturbances

TABLE 38.2	Pathological Conditions Affecting Body Alignment and Mobility	
Condition	**Pathological Influence**	**Examples**
Congenital defects	Abnormalities affect the efficiency of the musculoskeletal system in regard to alignment, balance, and appearance.	**Osteogenesis imperfecta**—inherited disorder. Causes bones to be porous, short, bowed, and deformed. As a result, children experience curvature of the spine and shortness of stature. **Scoliosis**—a structural curvature of the spine associated with vertebral rotation. Muscles, ligaments, and other soft tissues become shortened, affecting balance and mobility.
Bone, joint, and muscle disorders	Affect integrity of structures.	**Osteoporosis**—reduction of bone density or mass. The bone remains biochemically normal but has difficulty maintaining integrity and support, leading to fractures.
Inflammatory joint diseases	Cause inflammation or destruction of the synovial membrane and articular cartilage and cause systemic signs of inflammation.	**Arthritis**—changes in articular cartilage combined with overgrowth of bone at the articular ends. Degenerative changes commonly affect weight-bearing joints. **Articular disruption**—trauma to the articular capsules and ranges from mild, such as a tear resulting in a sprain, to severe, such as a separation leading to dislocation.
Central nervous system disorder	Damages part of the central nervous system that regulates voluntary movement and causes impaired body alignment and immobility.	**Traumatic head injury**—damage in the motor strip of the cerebrum. The amount of voluntary motor impairment is directly related to the amount of destruction of the motor strip. **Spinal cord injury**—damage to spinal cord results in loss of function (permanent or temporary) below the level of the injury. A patient's loss of function will depend on level of spinal cord affected.
Musculoskeletal trauma	Results in bruises, contusions, sprains, and/or fractures.	**Bone fracture**—simple or complex disruption of bone tissue continuity; often creates need for temporary immobility of affected body part.

(placing more stress on lower extremity joints), and soft tissue problems (e.g., pain in the neck, shoulder, elbow, and wrist/hand) (Anandacoomarasamy et al., 2008). Patients who are obese require adaptations in the approaches used to assist with walking, transfer, and positioning. Obesity directly impacts a patient's quality of life, especially in the ability to perform ADLs effectively.

REFLECT NOW

Consider being assigned to a patient who has a history of arthritis affecting the hips. The patient requires assistance with activities of daily living. Reflect on how musculoskeletal system function might be affected and how it will affect ways for planning patient activity.

NURSING KNOWLEDGE BASE

Application of nursing knowledge about activity and exercise allows you to think critically about the holistic needs of patients and then make sound decisions about the relevant interventions to provide. Nursing knowledge as it pertains to activity and exercise helps you assess, identify, and intervene when patients have decreased activity tolerance or physical limitation that affects their mobility and/or ability to exercise.

Safe Patient Handling and Mobility

Nurses are exposed to overexertion and physical injury from the hazards related to moving and transferring patients. This is true in all patient care settings. Manually lifting and transferring patients has contributed in the past to a high incidence of work-related musculoskeletal problems and back injuries in nurses and other health care staff. Most care activities related to patient handling involve one or more of the following: lifting with extended arms, lifting when near the floor, lifting when sitting or kneeling, lifting with the trunk twisted or the load off to the side of the body, lifting with one hand or in a restricted space, or lifting during a shift lasting longer than eight hours (Waters, 2007). The growing trend

toward injuries in the health care setting led to important nursing research. Research led by Dr. Audrey Nelson and Andrea Baptiste provided standardized methods for determining how to handle, move, and mobilize patients and supported the use of patient handling techniques based on individual patient characteristics and conditions (Nelson and Baptiste, 2006; Martin et al., 2014).

Evidence-based research has shown that safe patient handling and mobility interventions significantly reduce overexertion injuries by replacing manual patient handling with safer methods guided by ergonomic principles (NIOSH, 2016; Matz, 2019). Ergonomics is the design of work tasks to best suit the capabilities of workers. In the case of safe patient handling and mobility (SPHM), it involves improved assessment, the use of mechanical equipment, and safety procedures to lift and move patients. Many states have laws mandating SPHM in health care agencies. Comprehensive SPHM programs include the following (US Department of Veterans Affairs, 2016):

- Standardized assessment tools for identifying a patient's mobility level, such as the Banner Mobility Assessment Tool (BMAT) (Boynton et al., 2014b)
- An ergonomics assessment of patient rooms and health care environments
- Clinical/patient assessment algorithms to select the right equipment and number of staff for each patient handling and mobility task
  - Right equipment includes assistive devices in the form of ceiling lifts made available in patient rooms. Lifts help care providers transfer patients from beds to stretchers or wheelchairs and can be used to assist patients during walking.
  - Portable lifting devices that can be moved from room to room. The lifting equipment uses slings or vests to hold patients securely and reduce the risk of slipping, falling, or being dropped when walking.
- Unit peer leaders who function as safe patient handling experts and staff trainers

- Use of safety huddles to share information among staff members that will keep staff and patients safe
- A minimal-lift policy

The use of SPHM techniques is a standard for best practices in the moving, handling, and transfer of patients. In addition to reducing injuries to health care providers, the use of SPHM techniques improves patient outcomes. OSHA reports that SPHM programs result in patients having fewer falls, skin tears, and pressure injuries (OSHA, 2017).

Factors Influencing Activity and Exercise

Factors influencing activity and exercise include developmental changes, behavioral aspects, environmental issues, family and social support, and cultural and ethnic origin. Consider these areas of knowledge and apply this information in a plan of care whether a patient is seeking health promotion, acute care, or restorative and continuing care.

Developmental Changes. Throughout the life span the appearance and functioning of the body undergo change. Knowledge of growth and development (see Chapters 12 to 14) prepares you to anticipate the types of activities that patients of all ages are capable of performing. For example, the developmental process results in children acquiring independence in daily living by improving their gross motor capacity, as well as manual, intellectual, and communicative functioning (Kim et al., 2017).

A newborn infant's spine is flexed and lacks the anteroposterior curves of an adult. As growth and stability increase, the thoracic spine straightens, and the lumbar spinal curve appears, which allows sitting and standing. As an infant grows, musculoskeletal development permits support of weight for standing and walking, allowing the child to explore its environment. A toddler's posture is awkward because of the slight swayback and protruding abdomen. Toward the end of toddlerhood, posture appears less awkward, curves in the cervical and lumbar vertebrae are accentuated, and foot eversion disappears. From the third year through the beginning of adolescence, the musculoskeletal system continues to grow and develop. Greater coordination enables a child to perform tasks such as washing hands and brushing teeth, which require fine motor skills. Adolescent growth is often sporadic and uneven. As a result, the adolescent appears awkward and uncoordinated. Adolescent girls usually grow and develop earlier than boys. Hips widen, and fat deposits in the upper arms, thighs, and buttocks. The adolescent boy's changes in shape are usually a result of long-bone growth and increased muscle mass.

A middle-age adult should normally have full musculoskeletal function. An adult with correct posture and body alignment feels good, looks good, and generally appears self-confident. A healthy adult also has the necessary musculoskeletal development and coordination to carry out ADLs and physical exercise. However, for people 45 to 64 years of age, the percentage of adults with two or more common chronic conditions increases. Most people with multiple chronic conditions (MCCs) are of working age (Box 38.2). Nurses must consider the burden of MCCs on nonelderly adults, who represent more than 60% of all adults with MCCs (Adams, 2017). Chronic disease significantly affects how to individualize activity and exercise therapy programs.

A progressive loss of total bone mass occurs with older adults. Some of the possible causes of this loss include physical inactivity, hormonal changes, and increased osteoclastic activity (i.e., activity by cells responsible for bone tissue absorption). The effect of bone loss is weaker bones, causing vertebrae to be softer and long shaft bones to be less resistant to bending, making an individual prone to fractures

BOX 38.2 Common Chronic Health Conditions Among Young Adults

- Heart disease
- Stroke
- Asthma
- Arthritis
- Chronic obstructive pulmonary disease
- Cognitive impairment
- Diabetes
- Depression
- Chronic kidney disease
- Cancer other than skin
- Hypertension

Data from Adams ML: *Differences between younger and older US adults with multiple chronic conditions,* Centers for Disease Control and Prevention: Preventing Chronic Disease, Volume 14, September 7, 2017. https://www.cdc.gov/pcd/Issues/2017/16_0613.htm. Accessed April 18, 2019.

and muscle injuries. Older adults may walk more slowly and incorrectly and appear less coordinated. Many are afraid of falling (Lavidan et al., 2018; Tomita et al., 2018) They often take smaller steps and keep their feet closer together, which decreases the base of support and thus alters body balance. Physical exercise can improve endurance, coordination, and muscle stability and reduce the risk for falls and injuries (see Chapter 14).

Behavioral Aspects. It is important to consider your patients' knowledge of exercise and activity, their values and beliefs about exercise and health, barriers to a program of exercise and physical activity, and current exercise behaviors or habits. One barrier to exercise is whether a patient has multiple chronic diseases. Symptoms of one chronic condition (e.g., difficulty in breathing related to asthma) may interfere with another condition (diabetes), preventing the patient from engaging in needed regular exercise. Patients are more open to developing an exercise program if they are at the stage of readiness to change their behavior (Tsang et al., 2015). Patients' decisions to change behavior and include a daily exercise routine in their lives often occur gradually with repeated information individualized to their needs and lifestyle.

Cultural Background. Exercise and physical fitness are beneficial to all people. However, there are cultural differences regarding the extent to which people exercise (Box 38.3). A study has shown that leisure physical activity comprises only about 10% of total nonwork physical activity among adults (Saffer et al., 2013). Individuals with a lower level of education and minority racial/ethnic groups tend to have higher levels of physical activity at work but lower levels of nonwork physical activity. The difference may limit the positive effects of physical activity on an individual's health because nonwork physical activity has a stronger positive association with health relative to work physical activity (Saffer et al., 2013). When developing a physical fitness program for culturally diverse populations, consider their education regarding the value of exercise and learn about what motivates individuals to exercise and which activities are appropriate and enjoyable.

Environmental Issues

Work Site. A common barrier for many individuals to being physically active is the lack of time needed to engage in a daily exercise program. Some work sites help their employees overcome the obstacle of time constraints by offering physical activity opportunities at the work site, reminders, and rewards for those committed to physical fitness. For example, a simple walking path that provides employees with the opportunity to walk at work may address barriers such as not

CULTURAL ASPECTS OF CARE
Physical Inactivity Among Ethnic Groups

The Centers for Disease Control and Prevention (Watson et al., 2016) reports that inactivity prevalence among adults 50 years of age and older was significantly higher among women than men, among Hispanics and non-Hispanic blacks than among non-Hispanic whites, and among adults who reported ever having one or more of seven selected chronic diseases than among those not reporting one. Inactivity prevalence significantly increased with decreasing levels of education and increasing body mass index. Physical activity is identified as having an important role in the prevention and treatment of diseases such as type 2 diabetes (Watson et al., 2016; Scarton et al., 2017).

Implications for Patient-Centered Care

- Physical inactivity is a modifiable risk factor for the development of type 2 diabetes. Prevention and treatment programs need to focus heavily on exercise and be tailored to the activity tolerance of the individual patient.
- Support promotion of physical activity through formal programs in schools, churches, and governmental agencies within black and Native American communities.
- Incorporate motivational factors into exercise programs such as providing a healthy snack or meal for participants and furnishing each patient with a log to monitor weight loss and blood glucose levels.

having time to walk, concerns about their own neighborhood safety, or lack of social support (CDC, 2017). Such activity programs improve worker productivity and morale. Reminders within a work site such as signs that encourage employees to use the stairs instead of elevators are useful. Rewards such as free parking or discounted parking fees are also effective for employees who park in distant lots and walk.

Schools. Children today are less active, resulting in an increase in childhood obesity. Schools are excellent facilitators of physical fitness and exercise. Strategies for physical activity incorporated early into a child's daily routine often provide a foundation for lifetime commitment to exercise and physical fitness.

Community. Creating or modifying environments to make it easier for people to walk, run, or bike is a strategy that not only increases individuals' physical activity, but also makes communities better places to live. Communities designed to support physical activity are often called active communities (CDC, 2019a). Community support of physical fitness is instrumental in promoting the health of its members (e.g., providing walking trails and track facilities in parks, maps to guide access, and physical fitness classes). Success in implementing physical fitness programs depends on collaboration among public health agencies, parks and recreational associations, state and local governmental agencies, health care agencies, and the members of the community.

Family and Social Support. Social support is one motivational tool to encourage and promote exercise and physical fitness. In a systematic review that studied the association between social support and physical activity among older adults, it was found that people with greater social support for physical activity are more likely to do leisure time physical activity, especially when support comes from family members (Smith et al., 2017). This study noted that the physical activity levels of women are more likely than men to be influenced by general social support. A qualitative study identified factors to enable middle-aged women to engage in physical activity included daily structure that incorporated physical activity, anticipated positive feelings associated with physical activity (intrinsic motivator), and accountability to others (psychosocial motivator) (McArthur et al., 2014). An example of social support influencing exercise is having a friend or significant other engage a

patient to participate in a "buddy system" (i.e., they walk together each day at a specified time) or weekly exercise classes. This companionship provides for socialization, increases the enjoyment, and develops a commitment to physical fitness. Parents support their children in engaging in physical activity by providing encouragement, praise, and transportation to sporting events or exercise facilities. Other parents support physical activity by including their children in family outings such as bicycling or a basketball game in the neighborhood schoolyard.

CRITICAL THINKING

Successful critical thinking requires a synthesis of knowledge, experience, information gathered from patients, critical thinking attitudes, and intellectual and professional standards. Clinical judgments require you to anticipate information, analyze the data, and make decisions regarding patient care.

To understand activity tolerance, physical fitness, and the effects on patients, you integrate knowledge from nursing and other disciplines, previous experiences, and information gathered from patients. As you plan patient care, consider the relationship among a variety of concepts to provide the best outcome for your patients. For example, you lay the foundation for planning and decision making by understanding the relationship between the musculoskeletal system and health alterations that may create problems with activity and exercise and transferring and moving patients. Professional standards provide valuable guidelines for exercise and physical fitness. One example is the *Physical Activity Guidelines for Americans* issued by the Department of Health and Human Services (2019); the department's guidelines provide evidence-based recommendations for adults and youth (ages 3 through 17) to safely get the physical activity they need to stay healthy. Another standard is the American Diabetes Association's position statement on physical activity and exercise for individuals with diabetes (Colberg et al., 2016).

Your experiences and critical thinking attitude affect the problem-solving approach with patients and are evaluated with each new patient. Remember that some patients have the capacity for recovery in spite of the loss of some physical function. Restoration of function begins early in the care of patients whose ability to perform self-care is disrupted. Encouragement, support, commitment, and perseverance are important critical thinking attitudes to apply for these patients. Problems with activity and mobility are often prolonged; creativity is necessary when designing interventions for improving patients' activity tolerance and mobility skills.

REFLECT NOW

Think about a patient you cared for; what support systems did he or she have? How did the patient use his or her support system in regard to promoting daily physical activity? How can you incorporate the use of a support system in a patient's exercise program?

❖ NURSING PROCESS

Apply the nursing process and use a critical thinking approach in your care of patients. The nursing process provides a clinical decision-making approach for you to develop and implement an individualized plan of care.

◆ Assessment

An assessment for determining a patient's activity and exercise needs must be comprehensive, considering the patient's physical condition, activity history, socioeconomic resources, and readiness to exercise.

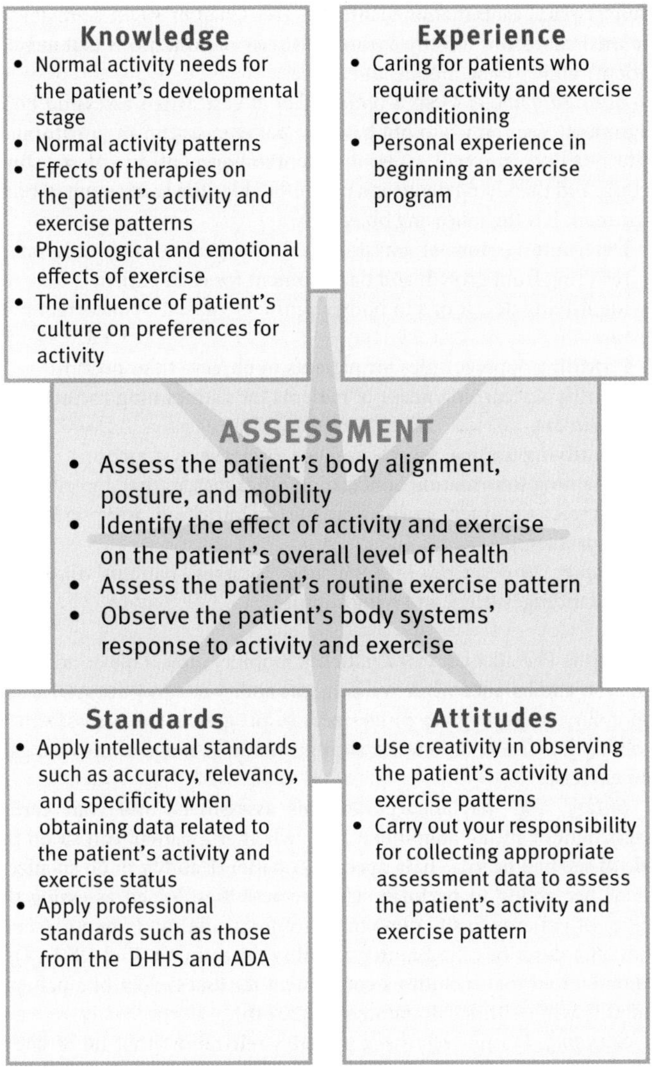

Knowledge
- Normal activity needs for the patient's developmental stage
- Normal activity patterns
- Effects of therapies on the patient's activity and exercise patterns
- Physiological and emotional effects of exercise
- The influence of patient's culture on preferences for activity

Experience
- Caring for patients who require activity and exercise reconditioning
- Personal experience in beginning an exercise program

ASSESSMENT
- Assess the patient's body alignment, posture, and mobility
- Identify the effect of activity and exercise on the patient's overall level of health
- Assess the patient's routine exercise pattern
- Observe the patient's body systems' response to activity and exercise

Standards
- Apply intellectual standards such as accuracy, relevancy, and specificity when obtaining data related to the patient's activity and exercise status
- Apply professional standards such as those from the DHHS and ADA

Attitudes
- Use creativity in observing the patient's activity and exercise patterns
- Carry out your responsibility for collecting appropriate assessment data to assess the patient's activity and exercise pattern

FIG. 38.7 Critical thinking model for activity and exercise assessment. *ADA,* American Diabetes Association; *DHHS,* Department of Health and Human Services.

BOX 38.4 Nursing Assessment Questions

Readiness to Exercise
- To what extent do you enjoy exercising? What is your belief in the ability to exercise?

Nature of the Problem
- Tell me about any problems you are having with staying active and exercising regularly.
- How much do you normally exercise each day? Each week?
- Describe the type of exercise you prefer.
- How long do you exercise at any given time?

Signs and Symptoms
- Tell me about any discomfort you have when you exercise (or after exercising).
- Describe for me the pain or shortness of breath that you feel.
- Do you ever feel chest discomfort or pain during exercise or activity?

Onset and Duration
- Tell me when and how your exercise habits have changed since your illness/injury.
- Which activities cause you to become short of breath/have pain?
- How long does it take to resume normal breathing after exercise or an activity?

Severity
- How far do you walk before the pain in your legs begins?
- On a scale of 0 to 10 (10 being the worst discomfort), rate your leg/back pain.
- Do you describe your shortness of breath as minimal, moderate, or severe after activities and/or exercise?

Barriers to Exercise and Activity
- Tell me what prevents you from exercising regularly each day.
- Do you have any health problems (such as asthma, arthritis) that affect your ability to carry out daily activities such as grocery shopping, washing clothes, or daily walking? Do you have any physical limitations that prevent you from exercising on a daily basis?
- Do you have access to a community walking path and exercise equipment?

Patient Values
- Tell me what you believe about how exercise affects your health.
- How confident are you in being able to perform the exercises your doctor has recommended?

Effect on Patient
- How has the lack of an exercise routine affected your weight?
- Do you feel more tired since you have not been able to exercise routinely?

You critically analyze assessment findings and also determine a patient's personal goals regarding activity to ensure that you make patient-centered clinical decisions required for safe and effective nursing care. During assessment consider normal physiological changes in growth and development and any deviations to expect based on the patient's health condition. Provide opportunities for patients to observe their posture and obtain important information about other factors that contribute to poor alignment, such as inactivity, fatigue, malnutrition, and psychological problems. During assessment (Fig. 38.7) also consider all of the critical thinking elements that help you make appropriate nursing diagnoses.

Through the Patient's Eyes. Your ability to provide patient-centered care requires your patient to be willing and ready to participate in any activity or exercise program you plan. This requires you to assess the patient's expectations, values, and beliefs about how activity and exercise affect his or her health. You will assess the patient's daily activity and exercise routine (Box 38.4), compare with how any illness or injury has changed the routine, and consider the recommendations for exercise made by the patient's health care provider. Discuss with the patient how he or she perceives engaging in activity and exercise at home or in the health care setting. It is also important to assess a patient's perceptions of what is acceptable activity in relationship to any symptoms experienced during exercise. One of the factors affecting physical activity is freedom from pain. When patients experience pain or fatigue following exercise, they often lack commitment to desired interventions. When patients are content with their present physical activity and fitness, they do not perceive a need for improvement.

Readiness to Exercise. Perceived self-efficacy is a judgment of capability and applies to a person's willingness to engage in an activity such as exercise. The outcomes people anticipate, such as from an exercise program, depend on their judgments of how well they will be able to perform in given situations (Bandura, 2006). The Transtheoretical Model (TTM), which incorporates the concept of self-efficacy, can be applied for tailoring interventions to patients' readiness to change and can enhance patient progress and help patients use therapeutic resources more effectively (LaMorte, 2018). However, individualizing an intervention depends on your accurate assessment of a patient's stage of change (SOC).

The TTM is a model of intentional change that focuses on the decision making of an individual regarding changing behavior (e.g., starting to exercise, changing a diet, taking medications correctly). The model operates on the assumption that people do not change behaviors quickly and decisively; instead behavioral change occurs continuously through a cyclical process (LaMorte, 2018). An individual will move back and forth through six stages of change:

- Precontemplation—Individuals do not intend to change their behavior in the next 6 months; they are unaware of the problem behavior or are demoralized by unsuccessful previous attempts to change behavior.
- Contemplation—Individuals are aware they need to change their behavior. They intend to take action within the next 6 months but lack commitment to actually start changing.
- Preparation—Individuals have decided to take action in the immediate future, usually measured as the next month. They often have a concrete plan of action, such as buying an exercise bike, joining a club, or asking family members to walk with them.
- Action —Individuals have made specific overt changes in their lifestyles within the past 6 months.
- Maintenance—People have shown the desired behavior for over 6 months and are working to prevent relapse.

Your assessment of the stage that best describes your patient's readiness to exercise will determine how you plan patient care. Begin by asking the patient to what extent he or she enjoys exercising and his or her belief in the ability to exercise. This is a factor positively associated with adult physical activity (*Healthy People 2020*, 2019). What is the patient's current activity level? If a patient tells you that he or she does not exercise and does not intend to start in the next 6 months, he is in the precontemplation stage. If the patient has been thinking about exercising or has tried to exercise but does so inconsistently, he or she is likely in the contemplation phase. A patient who describes a plan to exercise after discharge from a hospital or rehabilitation center is in the preparation stage. If the patient reports actively being engaged in exercise weekly and for the past several months, the patient is in the action stage. If your patient has been exercising but is facing new obstacles that affect his or her ability to remain active, he or she is in the maintenance stage. Use your assessment findings related to the patient's readiness for change to select the nursing interventions most likely to complement the stage of change and move the patient toward activity engagement.

Socioeconomic Factors. Assess the patient's socioeconomic resources for being able to engage in an activity or exercise plan. Socioeconomic factors will impact a patient's readiness or ability to exercise. For example, does the patient have access to exercise facilities or public parks and walking areas? What time during a typical day does the patient perceive he or she is able to engage in exercise? How many hours in a day does the patient work? Is there social support available to the patient? Studies have shown a correlation between an individual's educational level, income, and ability to pay for fees/equipment with their level of involvement in physical activity (O'Donoghue et al., 2018)

Physical Health. Assess a patient's physical condition to determine readiness to exercise. This includes status of body alignment, muscle strength and coordination, and integrity of joints and other structures

using physical examination techniques (see Chapter 30). Also review in the medical record for any chronic diseases or conditions that affect a patient's ability to be mobile and active.

Body Alignment. Help a patient feel at ease when assessing body alignment. Your aim is to not have the patient assume an unnatural or rigid position. You will assess a patient's alignment during standing, sitting, and then lying down as a patient is able. The assessment of body alignment has the following objectives:

- Determining normal physiological changes in body alignment resulting from growth and development for each patient
- Identifying deviations in body alignment caused by incorrect posture
- Providing opportunities for patients to observe their posture
- Identifying learning needs of patients for maintaining correct body alignment
- Identifying trauma, muscle damage, or nerve dysfunction
- Obtaining information concerning other factors that contribute to incorrect alignment, such as fatigue, malnutrition, and psychological problems

Chapter 39 describes in detail how to assess patients' alignment while standing, sitting, and lying supine.

Mobility. The adequacy of a patient's mobility affects his or her coordination and balance while walking, the ability to carry out ADLs, and the ability to participate in an exercise program. The assessment of mobility has five components: sitting, standing, range of motion, gait, and exercise.

Sitting. You may incorporate this assessment into your earlier assessment of sitting alignment. Note whether a patient can sit on the side of the bed or in a chair upright. A patient's ability to do so affects his or her ability to perform self-care activities. When assessing the ability of patients to sit, allow them to use a side rail (when present). Skill 38.2 describes the Banner Mobility Assessment Tool (BMAT), a validated tool that includes a component for assessment of a patient's mobility while sitting (Boynton et al., 2014b).

Standing. Do not rely on a patient's self-report that he or she is able to stand independently without support or assistance. This commonly occurs when nurses rush to admit or transfer patients, allowing patients to offer simply "yes" or "no" responses to an admission form question. When you assess a patient's ability to stand, it is appropriate to have the patient use an assistive device for support (if one is typically used). The BMAT (Boynton et al., 2014b) includes a measure for assessing a patient while standing. A patient should be able to raise the buttocks off the bed and hold for a count of five (Boynton et al., 2014a,b).The ability to achieve this maneuver indicates good mobility and balance, which are needed to safely stand (see Skill 38.2).

Range of Motion. Observing range of motion (ROM) is one of the first assessment techniques used to determine the degree of limitation or injury to a joint. Assess ROM to clarify the extent of joint stiffness, swelling, pain, limited movement, and unequal movement. Chapter 30 covers a thorough ROM assessment. Limited ROM indicates inflammation such as arthritis, fluid in the joint, altered nerve supply, or contractures. Increased mobility (beyond normal) of a joint indicates connective tissue disorders, ligament tears, and possible joint fractures.

Gait. The term *gait* describes a particular manner or style of walking. It is a coordinated action that requires the integration of sensory function, muscle strength, proprioception, balance, and a properly functioning CNS (vestibular system and cerebellum). A gait cycle begins with the heel strike of one leg and continues to the heel strike of the other leg. Assessing a patient's gait allows you to draw conclusions about balance, posture, and the ability to walk without assistance, all of which affect the risk for falling. Here are a few ways to assess a patient's gait:

1. Observe the patient entering the room, and note speed, stride, and balance.
2. Ask the patient to walk across the room, turn, and come back.
3. Ask the patient to walk heel-to-toe in a straight line. This may be difficult for older patients even in the absence of disease, so stay at the patient's side during the walk.

Exercise. During assessment, determine a patient's preferred form of exercise, level of intensity, and frequency of exercise. Box 38.4 provides examples of questions to ask related to a patient's exercise and activity routines and tolerance. Determine whether a patient participates in sufficient physical activity by comparing your findings with the CDC (2019b) recommendations: Adults need at least 2 hours and 30 minutes (150 minutes) of moderate-intensity aerobic activity) (i.e., brisk walking) every week and muscle-strengthening activities on 2 or more days a week that work all major muscle groups (legs, hips, back, abdomen, chest, shoulders, and arms). The activity can be spread across a week. Your assessment of the patient's activity provides baseline information for both exercise and activity tolerance. In addition, baseline information is beneficial when establishing a patient's exercise and rehabilitation plan following an illness or injury. When a person exercises, physiological changes occur in body systems (Box 38.5).

During exercise you improve muscle tone, strength, and size and cardiopulmonary conditioning. As a result you are able to exercise longer with each strengthening of the muscles. Exercise also enhances joint mobility because the exercise itself requires movement of body parts.

Activity Tolerance. Activity tolerance is the type and amount of exercise or work that a person is able to perform without undue exertion or injury (Box 38.6). Observe patients after ambulation, self-bathing, or sitting in a chair for several hours and assess their verbal report of fatigue and weakness. Do they show difficulty breathing or report being short of breath after exercise? Assess heart rate and blood pressure response to activity by comparing with baseline rates at rest. Both heart rate and blood pressure should increase. When you care for a patient who is relatively healthy and able to exercise regularly, assess what he or she sets as a target heart rate during exercise. Use this finding to determine whether the patient has set an adequate target rate for exercise training (AHA, 2015).

REFLECT NOW

Think about a patient you have cared for who is usually physically active but has been acutely ill. What questions could you ask to assess the patient's current level of physical activity tolerance? What physical assessments would you also measure?

◆ Nursing Diagnosis

A comprehensive patient assessment provides clusters of assessment findings to support a nursing diagnosis. Accuracy is essential when selecting a nursing diagnosis. For example, you consider nursing diagnoses of *Activity Intolerance* or *Fatigue* in a patient who reports being tired and weak. Further review of assessment data (e.g., abnormal heart rate and verbal report of weakness) leads to a definitive diagnosis (*Activity Intolerance*).

When patients have problems with activity and exercise, nursing diagnoses often focus on the ability to move. In the case of negative or problem-focused nursing diagnoses the related factors direct nursing interventions. This requires the correct selection of the related factors. For example, *Activity Intolerance related to excess weight gain* requires very different interventions than if the related factor is prolonged bed rest. Box 38.7 provides an example of how the diagnostic process leads to accurate diagnosis selection. The following are examples of nursing diagnoses related to activity and exercise:

- *Activity Intolerance*
- *Risk for Injury*
- *Impaired Mobility in Bed*
- *Impaired Mobility*
- *Acute or Chronic Pain*

BOX 38.5   Effects of Exercise

Cardiovascular System
- Increased cardiac output
- Improved myocardial contraction, thereby strengthening cardiac muscle
- Decreased resting heart rate
- Improved venous return

Pulmonary System
- Increased respiratory rate and depth followed by a quicker return to resting state
- Improved alveolar ventilation
- Decreased work of breathing
- Improved diaphragmatic excursion

Metabolic System
- Increased basal metabolic rate
- Increased use of glucose and fatty acids
- Increased triglyceride breakdown
- Increased gastric motility
- Increased production of body heat

Musculoskeletal System
- Improved muscle tone
- Increased joint mobility
- Improved muscle tolerance to physical exercise
- Possible increase in muscle mass
- Reduced bone loss

Activity Tolerance
- Improved tolerance
- Decreased fatigue

Psychosocial Factors
- Improved tolerance to stress
- Reports of "feeling better"
- Reports of decrease in illness (e.g., colds, influenza)

Data from McCance KL, Huether SE: *Pathophysiology: the biologic basis for disease in adults and children,* ed 8, St Louis, 2017, Mosby.

BOX 38.6   Factors Influencing Activity Tolerance

Physiological Factors
- Skeletal abnormalities
- Muscular impairments
- Endocrine or metabolic illnesses (e.g., diabetes mellitus, thyroid disease)
- Hypoxemia
- Decreased cardiac function
- Decreased endurance
- Impaired physical stability
- Pain
- Sleep pattern disturbance
- Prior exercise patterns
- Infectious processes and fever

Emotional Factors
- Anxiety
- Depression
- Chemical addictions
- Motivation

Developmental Factors
- Age
- Sex

Pregnancy
- Physical growth and development of muscle and skeletal support

Modified from Lewis SL, et al: *Medical-surgical nursing assessment and management of clinical problems,* ed 10, St Louis, 2017, Mosby.

◆ Planning

During planning synthesize information from multiple resources and involve the patient in decision making (Fig. 38.8). Critical thinking ensures that the patient's plan of care integrates all patient information and is patient centered. Professional standards are especially important to develop a plan that is evidence based. These standards often establish scientifically proven guidelines for selecting effective nursing interventions.

A concept map is a tool to assist in the planning of care. It shows the relationship between multiple nursing diagnoses and planned interventions. Fig. 38.9 shows the relationship between a patient's medical diagnosis of heart failure and the identified nursing diagnoses and related nursing interventions.

Goals and Outcomes. After identifying appropriate nursing diagnoses, you and the patient set goals and expected outcomes to direct interventions. If a goal involves the improvement in a patient's level of activity, integrating the patient's goal is critical to ensure adherence. The plan also includes consideration of any risks for injury to the patient and preexisting health concerns. It is important to have knowledge of the patient's home environment when planning therapies to maintain or improve activity, body alignment, and mobility. Include the patient's family and/or caregiver in the care plan unless the patient prefers no family involvement. Family caregivers play critical roles in the home environment, motivating and coaching patients to stay active. Developing a structured plan for regular exercise has been shown to be beneficial in improving adherence. (McArthur et al., 2014). The general goal related to exercise and activity is to improve or maintain the patient's motor function and independence. The following are examples of outcomes for patients with deficits in activity and exercise:

- Participates in prescribed physical activity while maintaining appropriate heart rate, blood pressure, and breathing rate
- Verbalizes an understanding of the need to gradually increase activity on the basis of tolerance and symptoms
- Explains reason physical condition requires balancing rest and activity

Setting Priorities. Care planning is patient centered, taking into consideration the patient's most immediate needs and preferences. For example, is a patient comfortable enough to participate in exercise, or does the acute occurrence of symptoms require you to delay an exercise session? You determine the immediacy urgency of any problem by its effect on the patient's mental and physical health. Because of the many skills associated with the care of patients who have the diagnoses of *Activity Intolerance* and/or *Impaired Mobility*, such as turning, transferring, and positioning, it is easy to overlook the complications

associated with these health alterations. Therefore be vigilant in monitoring the patient and supervising assistive personnel in carrying out activities to prevent complications and potential injury.

Teamwork and Collaboration. Planning involves understanding the resources needed to maintain a patient's function and independence. For example, it is important to collaborate with health care providers and physical and occupational therapists. Health care providers will prescribe physical and occupational therapy as needed and note any limits or guidelines for activity levels. Physical therapists are best equipped to identify the specific exercises that patients should perform. Occupational therapists assist patients with adaptive devices and techniques to perform ADLs while improving mobility. Sometimes long-term rehabilitation is also necessary. Discharge planning begins when a patient enters the health care system and involves identifying his or her expectations regarding physical activity, readiness to exercise, and what is planned by the health care team. In addition, always individualize a plan of care directed at meeting the actual or potential needs of the patient (see the Nursing Care Plan).

◆ Implementation

Health Promotion. A sedentary lifestyle contributes to the development of many health-related problems. The US Department of Health and Human Services (USDHHS) has developed guidelines recognizing that physical activity is key to improving the health of the nation. The report called *Physical Activity Guidelines for Americans* is based on the latest scientific evidence and is an essential resource for health

---

BOX 38.7 Nursing Diagnostic Process

Impaired Mobility

Assessment Activities	Assessment Findings
Observe patient's gait.	Shuffled gait
	Uncoordinated gait
	Patient report of slower walking speed
Observe patient performing tasks such as feeding, dressing, or recreational activities.	Uncoordinated movements
	Limited fine-motor coordination
Measure range of joint motion.	Reduced joint motion in lower and/or upper extremities
	Stiffness in joints
Measure patient's strength.	Has difficulty rising to sitting position or exiting bed

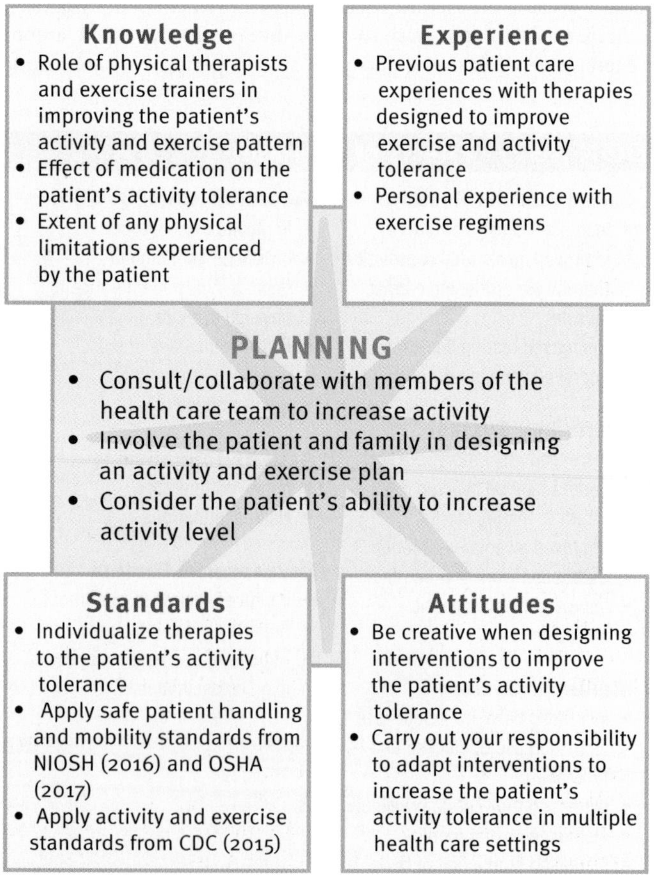

Knowledge
- Role of physical therapists and exercise trainers in improving the patient's activity and exercise pattern
- Effect of medication on the patient's activity tolerance
- Extent of any physical limitations experienced by the patient

Experience
- Previous patient care experiences with therapies designed to improve exercise and activity tolerance
- Personal experience with exercise regimens

PLANNING
- Consult/collaborate with members of the health care team to increase activity
- Involve the patient and family in designing an activity and exercise plan
- Consider the patient's ability to increase activity level

Standards
- Individualize therapies to the patient's activity tolerance
- Apply safe patient handling and mobility standards from NIOSH (2016) and OSHA (2017)
- Apply activity and exercise standards from CDC (2015)

Attitudes
- Be creative when designing interventions to improve the patient's activity tolerance
- Carry out your responsibility to adapt interventions to increase the patient's activity tolerance in multiple health care settings

FIG. 38.8 Critical thinking model for activity and exercise planning. *CDC,* Centers for Disease Control and Prevention; *NIOSH,* National Institute for Occupational Safety and Health; *OSHA,* Occupational Safety and Health Administration.

CONCEPT MAP

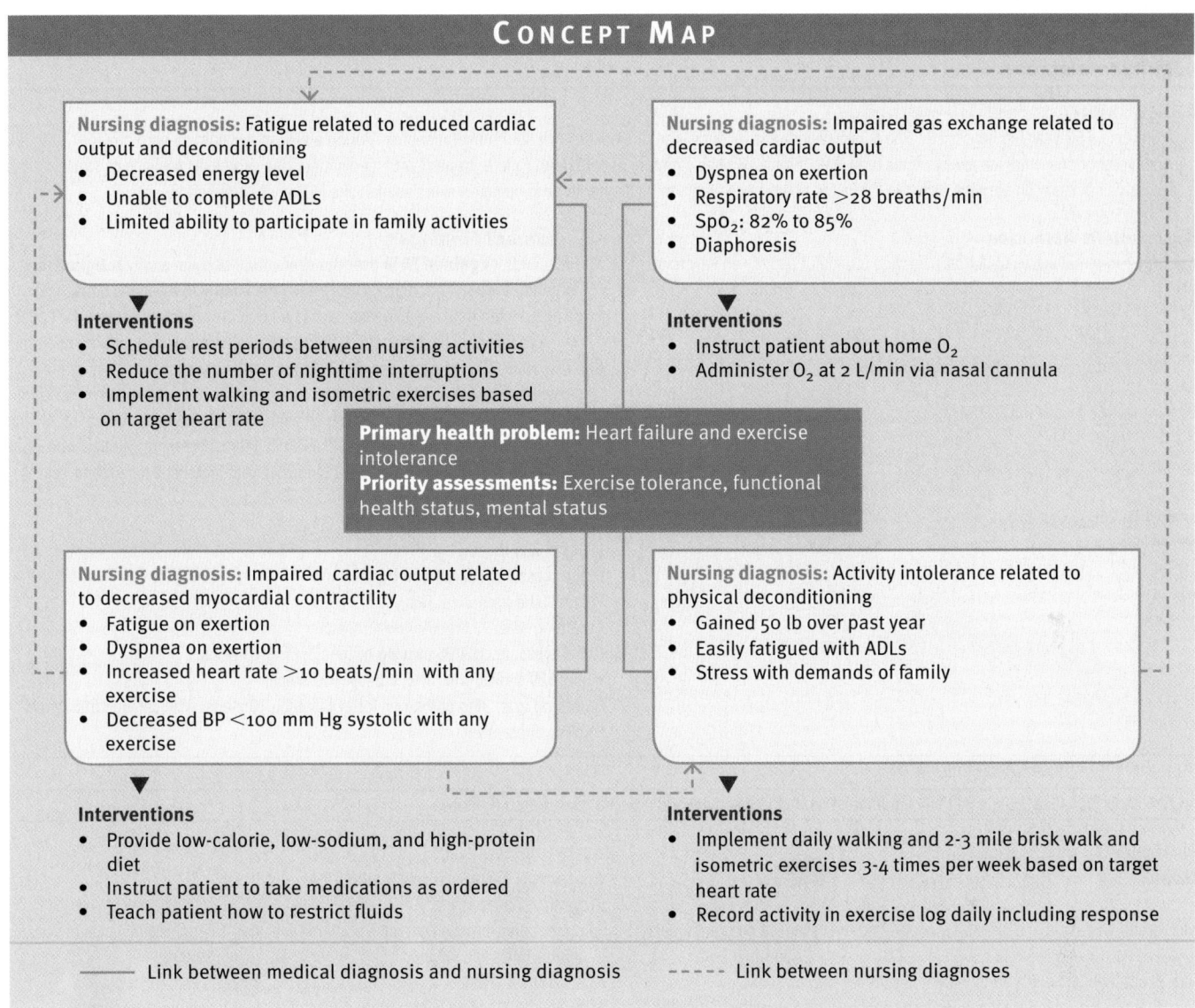

Nursing diagnosis: Fatigue related to reduced cardiac output and deconditioning
- Decreased energy level
- Unable to complete ADLs
- Limited ability to participate in family activities

Interventions
- Schedule rest periods between nursing activities
- Reduce the number of nighttime interruptions
- Implement walking and isometric exercises based on target heart rate

Nursing diagnosis: Impaired gas exchange related to decreased cardiac output
- Dyspnea on exertion
- Respiratory rate >28 breaths/min
- SpO$_2$: 82% to 85%
- Diaphoresis

Interventions
- Instruct patient about home O$_2$
- Administer O$_2$ at 2 L/min via nasal cannula

Primary health problem: Heart failure and exercise intolerance
Priority assessments: Exercise tolerance, functional health status, mental status

Nursing diagnosis: Impaired cardiac output related to decreased myocardial contractility
- Fatigue on exertion
- Dyspnea on exertion
- Increased heart rate >10 beats/min with any exercise
- Decreased BP <100 mm Hg systolic with any exercise

Nursing diagnosis: Activity intolerance related to physical deconditioning
- Gained 50 lb over past year
- Easily fatigued with ADLs
- Stress with demands of family

Interventions
- Provide low-calorie, low-sodium, and high-protein diet
- Instruct patient to take medications as ordered
- Teach patient how to restrict fluids

Interventions
- Implement daily walking and 2-3 mile brisk walk and isometric exercises 3-4 times per week based on target heart rate
- Record activity in exercise log daily including response

———— Link between medical diagnosis and nursing diagnosis   - - - - - Link between nursing diagnoses

FIG. 38.9 Concept map for Mrs. Smith. *ADLs,* Activities of daily living; *BP,* blood pressure.

professionals who make recommendations for how individuals can improve their health through regular physical activity (USDHHS, 2019). There are guidelines for all age-groups, including children, adolescents, adults, older adults, and pregnant women (Box 38.8).

A nurse practicing in a primary care or community setting has a responsibility for partnering with patients to find ways to help them improve their physical activity. For example, community health nurses may work with local governments to find ways to improve access to recreational areas (e.g. parks, walking paths) in a town or city. Participating in health fairs or community walks is a way for nurses to be visible to the community and share information about physical activity with residents.

In primary care a patient-centered approach ensures that individuals set goals for activity that allow them to achieve the benefits they value (USDHHS, 2019). This patient-centered approach helps ensure that an exercise program is relevant and suited to patient preferences and resources (Box 38.9). In setting activity goals, people can consider doing a variety of activities that are both indoor and outdoor. For example, a brisk walk in the neighborhood with friends for 45 minutes on 3 days a week and walking to lunch twice a week may be appropriate for someone who wants to increase both physical activity and socializing

(USDHHS, 2019). Patients who love gardening might plan regular yard work as part of their aerobic activity. Take a holistic approach to develop and implement a plan that enhances the patient's overall physical fitness.

Before starting an exercise program, be sure the patient's health care provider has cleared him or her for regular activity. Then teach patients how to calculate their maximum heart rate:
- First subtract the patient's current age in years from 220.
- Then have the patient calculate his or her target heart rate by taking 60% to 90% of the maximum.

The patient's health care provider should recommend a maximum, or when working with patients, start on the low end and steadily increase the target as exercise tolerance improves.

No matter which exercise prescription is implemented for the patient, warm-up and cool-down periods need to be included in the program (Edelman and Kudzma, 2018). The warm-up period usually lasts about 5 to 10 minutes and frequently includes stretching, calisthenics, and/or the aerobic activity performed at a lower intensity. It prepares the body and decreases the potential for injury. The cool-down period follows the exercise routine and usually lasts about 5 to 10 minutes. It allows the body to readjust gradually to baseline

◎ NURSING CARE PLAN

Activity Intolerance

ASSESSMENT

Mrs. Smith is a 52-year-old housewife. She is overweight and recently was diagnosed with adult-onset diabetes. During a visit to her primary care provider, she tells the nurse practitioner that she always feels tired. Mrs. Smith also has a history of mild heart failure, treated with medication. She expresses feelings of stress caused by excessive demands on her time at work. The nurse practitioner wants to assist her in developing an exercise plan she is likely to adhere to.

Assessment Activities	*Assessment Findings[a]*
Ask Mrs. Smith her views about participating in regular activity and exercise.	She responds, "I **gained 30 lb** over the past year. I become easily **fatigued**, and sometimes when I get home, I don't have the energy to finish my household chores. I used to like to exercise, but now I don't even want to leave the house anymore. I know I have to get healthier, and it's time to do something about it."
Ask Mrs. Smith about her routine exercise habits.	She responds, "I once exercised about 4 days a week, walking in the park just down from my house. About 10 years ago I enjoyed swimming with friends at the Y. But with the recent demands of work, having to do overtime a lot, I have not walked for 2 months. Have not swum in years. I have not felt like walking like I used to. I feel pulled in every direction; that increases my **stress**, and then I want to eat, eat, and eat!"
Perform baseline assessment.	Age: 52 years
	Weight: **225 lb** (102 kg)
	Blood pressure: **152/90 mm Hg** (at rest)
	Pulse: 88 beats/min (at rest)
	Breathing rate: 28 breaths/min (at rest)
	Blood pressure: **164/96 mm Hg** (after climbing 10 steps)
	Pulse: **120 beats/min** (after climbing 10 steps)
	Breathing rate: 36 breaths/min (after climbing 10 steps) with self-reported shortness of breath

[a]**Assessment findings** are shown in bold type.

NURSING DIAGNOSIS: Activity intolerance related to inactivity and reduced cardiovascular fitness

PLANNING

Goals	*Expected Outcomes (NOC)[b]* **Activity Tolerance**
Mrs. Smith will achieve a planned moderate-activity exercise program weekly.	Mrs. Smith performs an exercise plan that includes 150 minutes weekly of walking and swimming combined.
Mrs. Smith will achieve a 30-lb weight loss in 6 months.	Mrs. Smith will follow a DASH diet eating plan of 2000 calories a day.
Mrs. Smith's activity tolerance will improve above baseline within 2 months.	Mrs. Smith will achieve target heart rate of 60% of maximum heart rate (168 beats per min) after 20 min walking – 100 beats/min.
	Mrs. Smith will self-report a reduced sense of shortness of breath following walking at 1 month.

[b]Outcome classification labels from Moorhead S, et al., editors: *Nursing Outcomes Classification (NOC)*, ed 6, St Louis, 2018, Elsevier.

INTERVENTIONS (NIC)[c]

Exercise Promotion

Base Mrs. Smith's instruction about beginning an exercise program on her contemplation phase of readiness. Discuss the physiological benefits of how regular exercise can improve her quality of life.

Develop a progressive exercise plan:

Start with warm-up exercises for 3-5 minutes before walking, and perform cooldown exercises for 3-5 minutes after walking.

Begin walking 20 minutes in neighborhood 2 times a week over the next 2 weeks; then 20 minutes 3-4 times a week in the third and fourth weeks, increasing to 30 minutes, 4 times each week.

Have Mrs. Smith plan a weekly swimming session at the neighborhood Y.

RATIONALE

Regular exercise and physical activity are associated with a significantly lower CVD risk. Long-term studies have shown that increased physical activity is associated with a reduction in all-cause mortality and may modestly increase life expectancy (Nystoriak et al., 2018).

There is a relationship between greater amounts of physical activity and attenuated weight gain in adults, with some evidence to support that this relationship is most pronounced when physical activity exposure is above 150 minutes per week (Office of Disease Prevention and Health Promotion, 2018).

NURSING CARE PLAN—cont'd

INTERVENTIONS (NIC)[c]

Exercise Promotion

Design a DASH eating plan that incorporates the patient's daily meal pattern with food preferences in the following groups:

- Fresh vegetables, fruits, and whole grains
- Fat-free or low-fat dairy products, fish, poultry, beans, nuts, and vegetable oils
- Limiting foods that are high in saturated fat
- Limiting sugar-sweetened beverages and sweets

Schedule routine visits/phone calls with Mrs. Smith for follow-up and review of exercise and dietary log, progress, and barriers.

RATIONALE

DASH is a flexible and balanced eating plan recommended by the National Heart, Lung, and Blood Institute (n.d.a.) It helps create a heart-healthy eating style for life, combining it with other lifestyle changes, such as physical activity, to gain control of blood pressure and LDL-cholesterol levels.

Patients are more likely to increase physical activity and adhere to an exercise program if they are counseled by a health care professional (Edelman and Kudzma, 2018).

[c]Intervention classification labels from Butcher HK, et al., editors: *Interventions Classification (NIC),* ed 7, St Louis, 2018, Elsevier.

EVALUATION

Evaluation Activity	Patient Response/Finding	Outcome Status
Review patient's exercise log.	Patient walked 20 minutes twice the first and second weeks, 20 minutes three times the next week. Went swimming once.	Participation in exercise plan is increasing; achieved 40 to 60 minutes weekly exercise.
Review dietary log and record weight, blood pressure, and pulse.	Weight after 3 weeks, 210 lb; resting heart rate remains between 85 to 90 beats/min; 110 beats/min after walking; blood pressure, 146/86 mm Hg.	15-lb weight loss achieved. Improved exercise tolerance: Resting heart rate is within normal range. Achieved targeted heart rate after walking Blood pressure is lower but not at expected range. Monitor blood pressure as patient continues to lose weight.
Ask Mrs. Smith if she feels short of breath during walking or swimming.	"That first week or so of walking I felt some shortness of breath. I feel it less so now."	Activity tolerance improved with exercise.

---

functioning and provides an opportunity to combine movement such as stretching with relaxation-enhancing mind-body awareness. When caring for older adults, special considerations are needed to adapt an exercise plan that ensures patient safety (Box 38.10).

> **QSEN Building Competency in Quality Improvement** To assess individualized improvement in a patient's tolerance to activity, you need to use quality measures to understand a patient's performance. Determine the optimal cardiopulmonary response(s) to exercise for a patient who is 45 years old and whose health care provider set a desired 80% of maximum heart rate as a target.
>
> Answers to QSEN Activities can be found on the Evolve website.

Many patients find it difficult to incorporate an exercise program into their daily lives because of time constraints or lack of resources (e.g., no open parks or walking paths). For these patients it is beneficial to reinforce that they can use ADLs (e.g., gardening, climbing stairs when doing laundry) to accumulate the recommended 30 minutes or more per day of moderate-intensity physical activity. Other patients benefit from a prescribed exercise and physical fitness program carefully designed to meet their own goals and expectations. A patient-centered exercise program will include a combination of aerobic exercises, stretching and flexibility exercises, and resistance training suited to a patient's home or community environment. Cross-training is recommended for the patient who prefers to exercise every day. For example, the patient runs one day and does yoga the next day.

Stretching and flexibility exercises include active ROM and stretching of all muscle groups and joints. This form of exercise is ideal for warm-up and cool-down periods. Benefits include increased flexibility, improved circulation and posture, and an opportunity for relaxation.

Resistance training increases muscle strength and endurance and is associated with improved performance of ADLs and avoidance of injuries and disability. Formal resistance training includes weight training; but patients can obtain the same benefits by performing ADLs such as pushing a vacuum cleaner, raking leaves, or shoveling snow. Some patients use weight training to bulk up their muscles for the purpose of developing tone and strength and to stimulate and maintain healthy bone.

Acute Care. Because patients in acute care are at risk for deconditioning, the encouragement of early ambulation and performing exercises that involve stretching and active ROM is important. The level of exercise allowed will depend on the patient's physical condition. Physical therapists will collaborate on an exercise plan, including progressive walking, walking with assist devices, and isometric exercises. If needed, provide patients ordered analgesics for pain 30 minutes before exercise. Do not administer an analgesic that makes the patient feel dizzy.

Early Mobility. Recently concerted efforts have been made in hospitals to increase inpatients' activity and mobility levels as soon as possible to prevent deconditioning and other complications of immobilization (see Skill 38.1). The American Association of Critical Care Nurses (AACN) (2013) has developed an early progressive mobility protocol for critical care patients (see agency policy) and similar protocols are being developed for orthopedic (King, 2012), neurosurgery (Walia et al., 2018), and general surgery patients. Use of the protocols has improved patient outcomes (Box 38.11). When patients are transferred out to general nursing units, early mobility protocols should

BOX 38.8 Physical Activity Guidelines for Americans

Adults

- Move more and sit less throughout the day. Some physical activity is better than none. Adults who sit less and do any amount of moderate-to-vigorous physical activity gain some health benefits.
- For substantial health benefits, adults should do at least 150 minutes (2 hours and 30 minutes) to 300 minutes (5 hours) a week of moderate-intensity, or 75 minutes (1 hour and 15 minutes) to 150 minutes (2 hours and 30 minutes) a week of vigorous-intensity aerobic physical activity, or an equivalent combination of moderate- and vigorous-intensity aerobic activity. Preferably, aerobic activity should be spread throughout the week.
- Additional health benefits are gained by engaging in physical activity beyond the equivalent of 300 minutes (5 hours) of moderate-intensity physical activity a week.
- Adults should also do muscle-strengthening activities of moderate or greater intensity and that involve all major muscle groups on 2 or more days a week, as these activities provide additional health benefits.

Older Adults

Key guidelines for adults also apply. In addition, the following key guidelines apply to older adults:

- As part of weekly physical activity, older adults should do multicomponent physical activity that includes balance training as well as aerobic and muscle-strengthening activities.
- Older adults should determine their level of effort for physical activity relative to their level of fitness (e.g., knowing target heart rate).
- Older adults with chronic conditions should understand whether and how their conditions affect their ability to do regular physical activity safely.
- When older adults cannot do 150 minutes of moderate-intensity aerobic activity a week because of chronic conditions, they should be as physically active as their abilities and conditions allow.

From US Department of Health and Human Services: *Physical activity guidelines for Americans*, ed 2, 2018. https://health.gov/paguidelines/second-edition/pdf/Physical_Activity_Guidelines_2nd_edition.pdf. Accessed May 2, 2019.

---

continue. This is often a challenge because staff nurses on general units often have difficulty routinely ambulating patients because of overall patient care demands, access to equipment, or unfamiliarity with transfer skills. Some hospitals have designated special mobility teams or mobility assistants to engage patients in early ambulation and activity. Typical early mobility protocols include specific assessment parameters for each level of mobility, with patients progressing from passive and active assistive ROM exercises to sitting on side of bed, transferring and sitting in a chair, and progressive ambulation (AACN, 2013).

Isometric Exercises. Isometric exercises are prescribed for patients who do not tolerate increased activity (Chapter 39). A physical therapist will typically collaborate with the patient's health care provider in selecting isometric exercises most beneficial for a patient. As a nurse, your role is to support patients in knowing how the exercises are to be performed correctly so that you can observe for any problems or difficulties. For example, an exercise program that includes isometric exercises of the biceps and triceps will prepare a patient for crutch walking. Instruct the patient to stop the activity if pain, fatigue, or discomfort is experienced. Review the patient's chart and collaborate with physical therapy and the health care provider if any clinical changes develop (e.g., increased blood pressure, heart irregularity) that might contraindicate isometric exercise.

During isometrics, a patient tightens or contracts a muscle group for 10 seconds and then completely relaxes for several seconds (Resnick et al., 2012). Repetitions are increased gradually for each muscle group until the isometric exercise is repeated 8 to 10 times. Instruct patients to perform the exercises slowly and to increase repetitions as their physical condition improves. A patient needs to do isometric exercise for quadriceps and gluteal muscle groups, which are used for walking, 4 times a day until the patient is ambulatory.

Range of Motion Exercise. The easiest intervention to maintain or improve joint mobility for patients and one that can be coordinated with other activities is the use of ROM exercises (see Chapter 39). There are three types of range of motion exercise: active, active assisted, and passive. In active range of motion (AROM) exercises patients move specific joints independently based on their muscular weakness and the type of activity that needs strengthening. The exercise moves the joint and soft tissues through the available physiological ranges of

---

BOX 38.9 PROCEDURAL GUIDELINES

Helping Patients to Exercise

Delegation and Collaboration

- The skill of promoting early activity and exercise in the outpatient setting regarding activity and exercise education cannot be delegated.

Equipment

Weights, resistance bands (optional based on physical therapy recommendations)

Steps

1. Identify patient using at least two identifiers (e.g., name and birthday or name and medical record number) according to agency policy.
2. Measure patient's baseline heart rate or have patient/family caregiver do measurement. *Provides baseline for activity tolerance.*
3. Identify patient's activity/exercise history:
   - Which type of regular daily exercise do you perform at home?
   - Do you exercise or play a sport at least 3 times a week?
   - On a scale of 0 to 5 with 0 being no daily exercise and 5 strenuous regular daily exercise, how would you rate yourself?
   - How long have you been exercising regularly?

4. Ask patient to what extent he or she enjoys exercising and what his or her beliefs are about the ability to exercise. Does the patient prefer indoor or outdoor activities?
5. Determine whether patient has social support from peers, family, or spouse.
6. Determine whether patient has access to a fitness center or other area to exercise. Is the neighborhood considered safe?
7. Consider these factors in your assessment: patient's age, income level, time available to exercise, rural resident, overweight, being disabled. *Factors negatively associated with adult participation in activity* (Healthy People 2020, 2019)
8. Have patient rate level of quality of life based on current activity level.
9. Initiate an outpatient exercise program that contains any of the following components:
   - Warm-up (5-10 minutes)—*directs needed blood flow to muscles and prepares body for exercise, helping to prevent injury*
   - Strengthening exercises
   - Endurance exercises

BOX 38.9 PROCEDURAL GUIDELINES—cont'd

Helping Patients to Exercise

- Balance exercises
- Flexibility exercises—*lessen tightness of muscles and improve joint ROM*
- Cool-down exercises (5-10 minutes)—*help body recover from exercises*

Consult with physical therapy to help develop complete exercise program that fits needs of your patient. A good resource is: http://health.gov/paguidelines/guidelines.

10. Recommend strength training for adults to improve strength and bone density in collaboration with physical therapy.
11. Recommend aerobic exercise (see Box 38.8). The US Department of Health and Human Services (2019) recommends aerobic exercises to include moderate and vigorous activities (e.g., climbing stairs; playing sports; or walking, jogging, swimming, or biking). Activities such as dancing, yoga, and yard work are beneficial to older adults who prefer what they perceive as less rigorous forms of exercise.
12. Recommend balance exercises for older adults to decrease risk of falls. Have patient be sure to have something sturdy nearby on which to hold (wall or chair) if he or she becomes unsteady. Perform exercises: standing on one foot, walking heel to toe, balance walking, back leg raises, side leg

raises. Have patient do strength exercises (back leg raises, side leg raises) 2 or more days per week, but not on any 2 days in a row (NIH, n.d.).

13. Recommend that the patient perform a cool-down (5 to 10 minutes) after exercising: quadriceps stretch; hamstring/calf stretch; chest and arm stretch; neck, upper back, and shoulder stretch.
14. Measure heart rate during and after exercise. Compare with baseline. Stop physical activity when:
    - Heart rate (HR) is above targeted heart rate OR
    - HR is more than a 20% decrease from resting value OR
    - HR is less than 40 beats/min
15. **Use Teach-Back:** "We've talked about doing a warm-up and cool-down as part of your exercise plan. Tell me why each is important." Revise your instruction now or develop a plan for revised patient/family caregiver teaching if patient/family caregiver is not able to teach back correctly.
16. Document in outpatient record the exercises recommended. Document patient response if you witness patient exercising.

BOX 38.10 FOCUS ON OLDER ADULTS

Special Considerations for Older Adults in Initiating and Maintaining an Exercise Program

- Encourage older adults to avoid prolonged sitting and get up and stretch. Frequent stretching decreases the risk of developing joint contractures.
- Be sure that the older patient maintains proper body alignment when sitting to minimize joint and muscle stress.
- Teach patients how to use stronger joints or larger muscle groups. Efficient distribution of the workload decreases joint stress and pain.
- Provide resources for planned exercise programs. Weight-bearing exercise, such as tai chi, walking, hiking, jogging, climbing stairs, playing tennis, and dancing, and resistance exercises, such as lifting weights, strengthen bones (NIH, 2018).
- Recommend resistance- and agility-training programs. These forms of exercise reduce fear of falling and increase sense of well-being in older adults (Kwun et al., 2012).

- Have older adults avoid high-impact programs that can lead to bone fractures (NIH, 2018).
- Teach older adults that it is never too late to begin an exercise program (Edelman and Kudzma, 2018). Consult a health care provider before beginning an exercise program, particularly in the presence of heart or lung disease and other chronic illnesses.
- Use assessment data and consult with physical therapy to determine when you need to adjust exercise programs for those in advanced age.
- Encourage older adults who are unable to participate in a formal exercise program to improve joint mobility and enhance circulation by simply stretching and exaggerating movements during the performance of routine activities of daily living.

motion. AROM exercises are used when a patient is able to voluntarily contract, control, and coordinate a movement when such a movement is not contraindicated (Dutton, 2014). As a nurse you should know the contraindications to AROM, including a healing fracture site, a healing surgical site, severe and acute soft tissue trauma, and cardiopulmonary dysfunction (Dutton, 2014). Chapter 39 discusses active assisted and passive ROM exercises.

Walking. Walking increases joint mobility and can be measured by length of time or distance walked, such as down a hospital hallway or actual number of feet walked. Measure distances walked in estimated feet or yards instead of charting "ambulated to nurses' station and back." Some hospital or rehab units will have markers along floorboards designating distances. Illness or trauma usually reduces activity tolerance, resulting in the need for help with walking or the use of assistive devices such as crutches, canes, or walkers. Patients who increase their walking distance before discharge improve their ability to independently perform basic ADLs, increase activity tolerance, and have a faster recovery after surgery (AAN, 2015; Walia et al., 2018).

Helping a Patient Walk. Helping a patient walk requires preparation. Assess the patient's strength, coordination, baseline vital signs,

and balance to determine the type of assistance needed. Also assess his or her orientation and determine whether there are any signs of distress. Postpone walking if you determine that the patient cannot walk safely. Evaluate the environment for safety before ambulation (e.g., removal of obstacles, a clean and dry floor, and the identification of rest points in case the patient's activity tolerance becomes less than expected or if the patient becomes dizzy). Also have the patient wear supportive, nonskid shoes.

Help the patient to a position of sitting at the side of the bed and dangling the legs over the side of the bed for 1 to 2 minutes before standing. Some patients experience orthostatic hypotension (i.e., a drop in systolic pressure by at least 20 mm Hg or a drop in diastolic pressure by at least 10 mm Hg within 3 minutes of rising to an upright position (Shibao et al., 2013; Fedorowski and Melander, 2013). Those at higher risk are patients who are immobilized, patients who are on prolonged bed rest, older adults, and patients with chronic illnesses such as diabetes mellitus and cardiovascular disease. Signs and symptoms of orthostatic hypotension include dizziness, light-headedness, nausea, tachycardia, pallor, and even fainting. Orthostatic hypotension usually stabilizes quickly, but if the patient develops dizziness lasting 60 seconds, return the patient to bed (Myszenski, 2014). Dangling a patient's legs before standing is an intermediate step that

BOX 38.11 EVIDENCE-BASED PRACTICE

Benefits of Early Mobility Protocols

PICOT Question: Do acutely ill hospitalized patients have improved clinical outcomes after participating in early mobility protocols compared with standard postoperative recovery routines?

Evidence Summary

Early mobilization is a complex intervention that requires careful patient assessment and management, as well as interprofessional team cooperation (Hodgson et al., 2018). However, the reported benefits of early mobilization include reduced ICU-acquired weakness, improved functional recovery within the hospital, improved walking distance at hospital discharge, and reduced length of hospital stay (Hashem et al., 2016; Tipping et al., 2017). Outcomes vary depending on patient factors such as physiological instability (hemodynamic, respiratory, neurological), sedation, delirium/agitation, psychological state, and pain (Hodgson et al., 2018). Care team factors can also create barriers to early mobility intervention, including poor work culture, lack of communication, lack of leadership, disengaged team members, and inexperienced staff (Hodgson et al., 2018). Research has shown that unit culture, rather than patient-related factors, may be the main barrier to early mobilization in ICUs (Hodgson et al., 2015).

Application to Nursing Practice

- Having a dedicated mobility team with strong unit leadership facilitates protocol implementation (Hodgson et al., 2018).
- Interprofessional team planning with team meetings and daily goal setting is essential.
- Be knowledgeable of a patient's current condition and the clinical parameters set for early mobility to begin or proceed, and carefully assess patient response to activity.
- The presence of invasive intravenous lines, endotracheal intubation, and feeding tubes do not contraindicate early mobility (Hashem et al., 2016).

allows assessment of the patient before changing positions to maintain safety and prevent injury to the patient. In some instances you need to take the patient's blood pressure while he or she is sitting on the side of the bed.

Several methods are used to help a patient ambulate. For those who can bear weight easily provide support at the waist with a gait belt so that the patient's center of gravity remains midline. The belt helps you to stabilize patients if they lose their balance. A gait belt is *not* to be used in *lifting* or *carrying a patient by the waist*. A gait belt encircles a patient's waist below the belly button, snugly, being sure two fingers fit between the belt and patient's body. Don't place a gait belt over incisions, stitches, tubes, or intravenous lines, and never use one on a pregnant patient When using a gait belt, hold the gait belt behind the patient, with your palms facing up, but avoid trying to lift or catch patients by mistake, causing you a back injury. If the person is unable to walk under his or her own power or has too high a risk of falls, something more protective than a gait belt should be utilized (i.e., motorized sit-to-stand lift, ceiling lift with ambulation sling, or a nonpowered stand-raise aide with ambulation capacity).

If the patient has a fainting (syncope) episode or begins to fall, your natural instinct will be to support or catch the patient. Trying to stop or minimize a fall can cause you injury. However, an approach used by physical therapists involves assuming a wide base of support with one foot in front of the other, thus supporting the patient's body weight (Fig. 38.10A). While holding the gait belt, try to extend one leg, let the patient slide against the leg, and gently lower him or her to the floor, protecting the head (Fig. 38.10BC). Use caution to prevent your own injury, especially if the patient is overweight. When the patient attempts to ambulate again, proceed more slowly, monitoring for reports of dizziness; take the patient's blood pressure before, during, and after ambulation. The key to preventing staff injuries is to focus on reducing the number of preventable patient falls and falls with injury through accurate patient assessments and the use of proper equipment.

Restorative and Continuing Care. Restorative and continuing care involves implementing activity and exercise strategies to help the patient

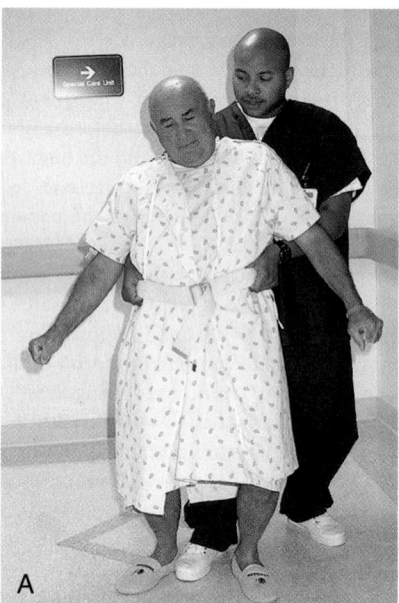
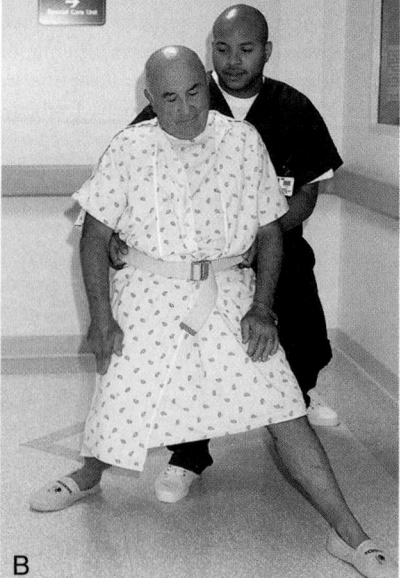
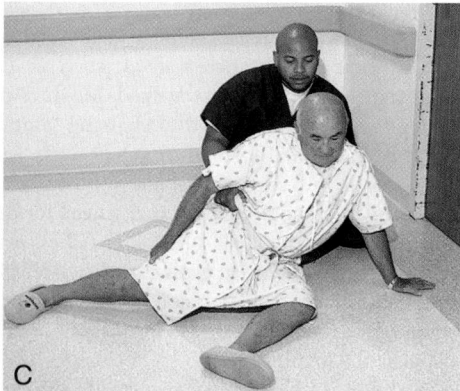

FIG. 38.10 A, Stand with feet apart to provide a broad base of support. **B,** Extend one leg and let patient slide against it to the floor. **C,** Bend knees to lower body as patient slides to the floor.

TABLE 38.3   Types of Assist Devices

Type of Device	Features	Measurement
Canes: lightweight, easily movable devices approximately waist high, made of wood or metal. Two types: single straight-legged and quad (see Fig. 38.12).	Straight canes provide support and balance for patients who have mild balance or strength impairments. Quad canes are often used for patients who have unilateral weakness from a neurological event/disease (i.e., stroke) and require more support than a straight cane. Patient keeps the cane on the stronger side of the body (Fairchild et al., 2018). Nurse stands on the patient's weak side for support (Fairchild et al., 2018).	Have patient stand upright with arms relaxed down with normal bend at the elbow (15 to 30 degrees). The handle of the cane should be close to the patient's wrist crease. Cane handle should fit comfortably in palm of hand.
Crutches: wooden or metal staff. Two types of crutches: the double adjustable Lofstrand or forearm crutch and the axillary wooden or metal crutch.	Use of crutches is usually temporary (e.g., after ligament damage to the knee). Some patients, such as those with paralysis of the lower extremities, need crutches permanently.	Measurements include the patient's height, the angle of elbow flexion, and the distance between the crutch pad and the axilla. Measure standing: Position crutches with crutch tips at 15 cm (6 inches) laterally to side and 15 cm in front of patient's feet (tripod position). Crutch pads should be 3.75–5 cm (1½–2 inches or 2–3 finger widths) under axilla with the elbows slightly flexed (American College of Foot and Ankle Surgeons, 2020; Fairchild et al., 2018). Height of handgrips must be adjusted so that patient's elbow is slightly flexed or grip sits at approximate height of wrist crease. Both height of crutch and handgrip dimensions are adjustable on a well-made crutch.
Walkers: extremely light, movable devices, approximately waist high and made of metal tubing (see Fig. 38.11). They have four widely placed, sturdy legs. They can also have 2–4 wheels.	Has a wide base of support, providing stability and security when walking.	Have patient step inside walker. When patient relaxes arms at side of body and stands up straight, top of walker should line up with crease on inside of wrist). Elbows should flex about 15 to 30 degrees when standing inside walker, with hands on handgrips (American Academy of Orthopaedist Surgeons, 2015; Fairchild et al., 2018).

with ADLs after acute care is no longer needed. Restorative and continuing care also includes activities and exercises that restore and promote optimal functioning in patients with specific chronic illnesses such as coronary heart disease (CHD), hypertension, COPD, and diabetes mellitus.

Assistive Devices for Walking. In collaboration with other health care professionals such as physical therapists, promote activity and exercise by teaching the proper use of canes, walkers, or crutches, depending on the assistive device most appropriate for the patient's condition. Assist devices are recommended for patients unable to bear full weight on one or more joints of the lower extremities. Other indications for use are instability, poor balance, or pain in weight-bearing. An assist device can reduce the risk of fall, decrease pain with mobility, and improve balance (Touhy and Jett, 2018). However, the devices can also be a risk factor for falling if used incorrectly. You will collaborate with a physical therapist in selecting the proper device for a patient (Table 38.3).

Walkers. A walker is a lightweight, movable device that stands about waist high and consists of a metal frame with handgrips, four widely placed sturdy legs, and one open side (Fig. 38.11). A walker can be used by a patient who has lower extremity weakness or has problems with balance. Walkers with wheels are useful for patients who have difficulty lifting and advancing the walker as they walk because of limited balance or endurance. However, the disadvantage is that the walker can roll forward when weight is applied A patient uses a walker correctly by holding the handgrips on the upper bars, taking a step, moving the walker forward, and taking another step. A walker requires a patient to lift the device up and forward. The patient should not lean over the walker or walk behind it; otherwise he or she might lose balance and fall. Walkers should not be used on stairs. Teach patients how to use walkers safely and avoid the risk of falling.

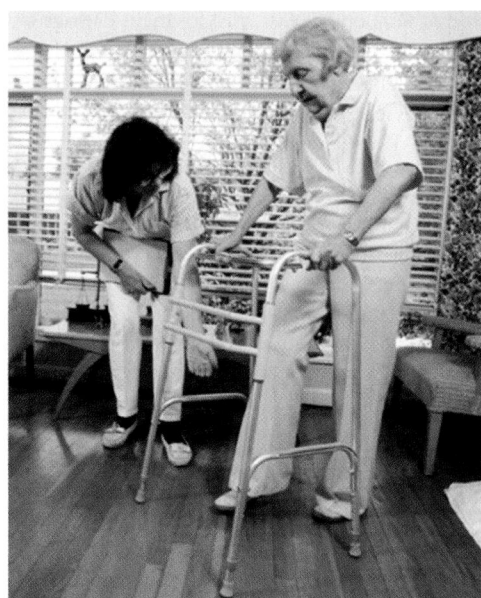

FIG. 38.11 Patient using a walker.

Canes. Canes provide less support than a walker and are less stable. The most common cane is the straight-legged, the length of which should be equal to the distance between the greater trochanter and the floor (Fairchild et al., 2018). Have the patient keep the cane on the stronger side of the body. For maximum support when walking, the patient places the cane forward 15 to 25 cm (6 to 10 inches), keeping body weight on both legs. He or she

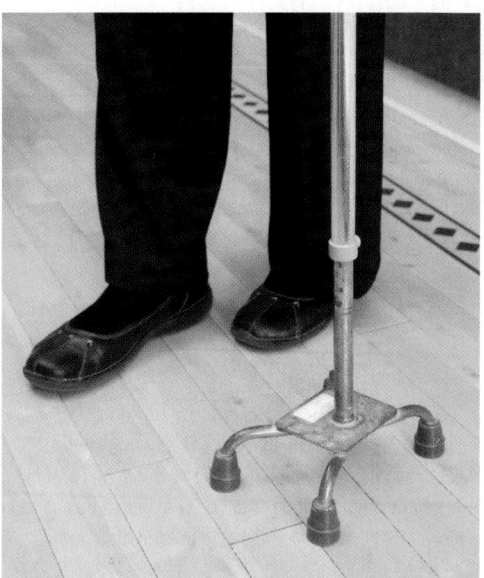

FIG. 38.12 Bottom of quad cane.

moves the weaker leg forward to the cane, so body weight is divided between the cane and the stronger leg. The patient then advances the stronger leg past the cane so the weaker leg and the body weight are supported by the cane and weaker leg. During walking the patient continually repeats these three steps. The patient needs to learn that two points of support such as both feet or one foot and the cane are on the floor at all times.

The quad cane provides the most support and is used when there is partial or complete leg paralysis or some hemiplegia (Fig. 38.12). You teach the patient the same three steps that are used with the straight-legged cane.

Crutches. Crutches are often needed to increase mobility. The use of crutches is often temporary (e.g., after ligament damage to the knee). However, some patients need them permanently. A crutch is a wooden or metal staff. The forearm crutch has a handgrip and a metal band that fits around the patient's forearm. The metal band and the handgrip are adjusted to fit the patient's height. The more common axillary crutch has a padded curved surface at the top, which fits under the axilla. A handgrip in the form of a crossbar is held at the level of the palms to support the body. It is important to measure crutches for the appropriate length and to teach patients how to use their crutches safely to achieve a stable gait, ascend and descend stairs, and rise from a sitting position. Always begin crutch instruction with guidelines for safe use (Box 38.12).

Measuring for Crutches. Measurement for an axillary crutch includes the patient's height, the angle of elbow flexion, and the distance between the crutch pad and the axilla (see Table 38.3). When crutches are fitted, ensure that the length of the crutch is two to three finger widths from the axilla and position the tips approximately 2 inches lateral and 4 to 6 inches anterior to the front of the patient's shoes.

Position the handgrips so that the axillae are not supporting the patient's body weight. Pressure on the axillae increases risk to underlying nerves, which sometimes results in partial paralysis of the arm. Determine correct position of the handgrips with the patient upright, supporting weight by the handgrips with the elbows slightly flexed. Elbow flexion (approximately 15 to 30 degrees) may be verified with a goniometer (Fig. 38.13). When you determine the height and placement of the handgrips, verify that the distance between the crutch pad and the patient's axilla is 1½ to 2 inches (two to three finger widths) (Fig. 38.14).

Crutch Gait. Patients assume a crutch gait by alternately bearing weight on one or both legs and on the crutches. A physical therapist in collaboration with the health care provider will determine the

Crutch Safety

Objective
• Patient will describe and demonstrate safe crutch walking.

Teaching Strategies
• Teach patient not to lean on crutches to support body weight.
• Teach patient with axillary crutches about the dangers of pressure on the axillae, which occurs when patient leans on the crutches to support body weight.
• Explain why patient needs to use only crutches that were measured for him or her.
• Show patient how to routinely inspect crutch tips. Securely attach rubber tips to crutches. Replace worn tips. Rubber crutch tips increase surface friction and help prevent slipping.
• Explain that crutch tips need to remain dry. Water decreases surface friction and increases risk of slipping. Show patient how to dry crutch tips if they become wet; patient may use paper or cloth towels.
• Show patient how to inspect structure of crutches. Cracks in a wooden crutch decrease its ability to support weight. Bends in aluminum crutches alter body alignment.
• Provide patient with list of medical supply companies in the community for obtaining repairs, new rubber tips, handgrips, and crutch pads.
• Instruct patient to have spare crutches and tips readily available.

Evaluation
Use the principles of teach-back to evaluate patient/family caregiver learning:
• Describe four principles of crutch safety that you will use.
• Show me the proper way to use your crutches to walk.
• Describe for me steps you will take to keep your crutches in proper working order.

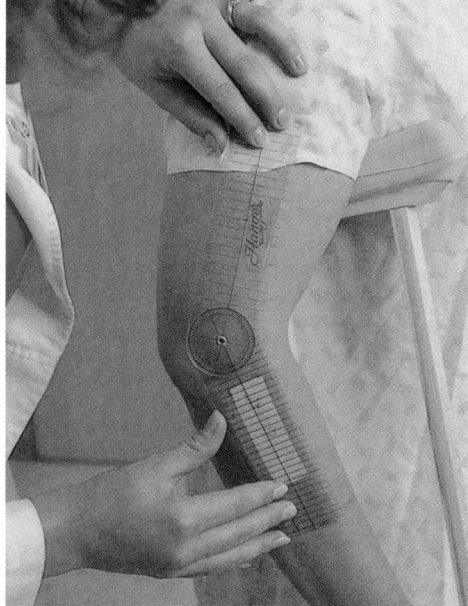

FIG. 38.13 Using the goniometer to verify correct degree of elbow flexion for crutch use.

appropriate gait by assessing the patient's physical and functional abilities and the disease or injury that resulted in the need for crutches. This section summarizes the basic crutch stance and the four standard gaits: four-point alternating gait, three-point alternating gait, two-point gait, and swing-through gait.

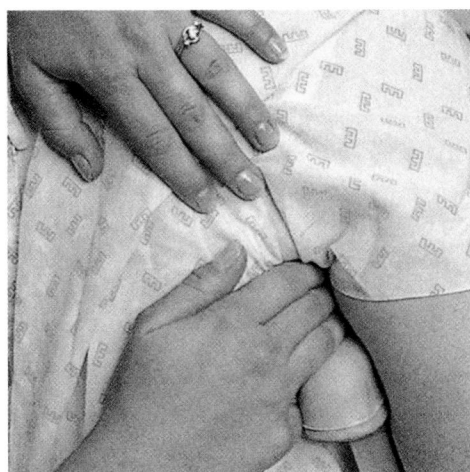

FIG. 38.14 Verifying correct distance between crutch pads and axilla.

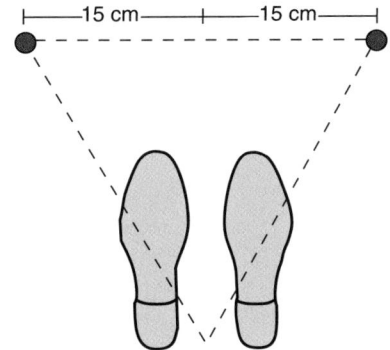

FIG. 38.15 Tripod position, basic crutch stance.

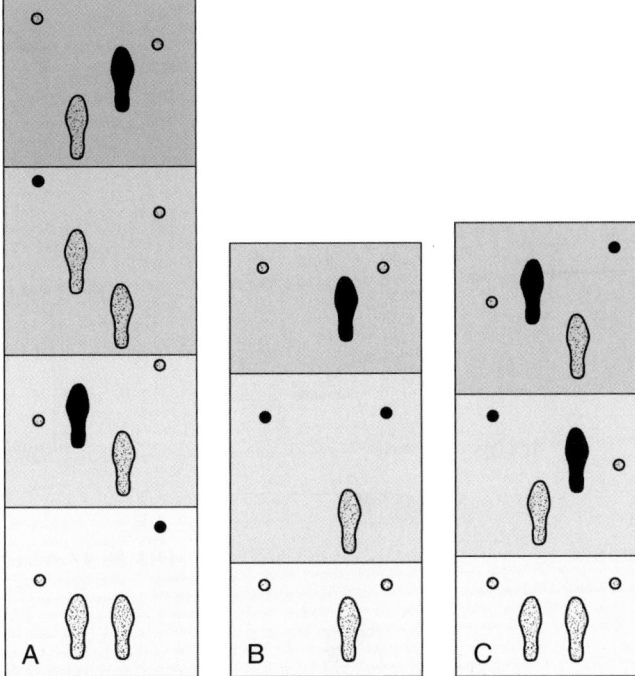

FIG. 38.16 A, Four-point alternating gait. Solid feet and crutch tips show the order of foot and crutch tip movement in each of the four phases. (Read from bottom to top.) B, Three-point gait with weight borne on unaffected leg. Solid foot and crutch tips show weight-bearing in each phase. (Read from bottom to top.) C, Two-point gait with weight borne partially on each foot and each crutch advancing with opposing leg. Solid areas indicate leg and crutch tips bearing weight. (Read from bottom to top.)

The basic crutch stance is the tripod position, formed when the crutches are placed 15 cm (6 inches) in front of and 15 cm (6 inches) to the side of each foot (Fig. 38.15). This position improves the patient's balance by providing a wider base of support. The body alignment of the patient in the tripod position includes an erect head and neck, straight vertebrae, and extended hips and knees. The axillae should not bear any weight. The patient assumes the tripod position before crutch walking.

Four-point alternating, or four-point, gait gives stability to the patient but requires weight-bearing on both legs. Each leg is moved alternately with each opposing crutch so that three points of support are on the floor at all times (Fig. 38.16A).

Three-point alternating, or three-point, gait requires the patient to bear all of the weight on one foot. In a three-point gait the patient bears weight on both crutches and then on the uninvolved leg, repeating the sequence (see Fig. 38.16B). The affected leg does not touch the ground during the early phase of the three-point gait. Gradually the patient progresses to touchdown and full weight-bearing on the affected leg.

The two-point gait requires at least partial weight-bearing on each foot (see Fig. 38.16C). The patient moves a crutch at the same time as the opposing leg, so the crutch movements are similar to arm motion during normal walking.

Individuals with paraplegia who wear weight-supporting braces on their legs frequently use the swing-through gait. With weight placed on the supported legs, the patient places the crutches one stride in front and then swings to or through them while they support his or her weight.

Using Crutches To Ascend and Descend Stairs. Climbing stairs with the use of a railing is the safest way for a patient with crutches to ascend stairs. Be aware that there is a risk for falling using this technique. Your responsibility is to monitor a patient's balance carefully. Be sure there are no obstacles on the stairs, such as stacks of magazines or other items. Have the patient hold the handrail for support with one hand (strong leg next to railing). You carry the crutch positioned next to the handrail as the patient places the other crutch under the axilla of affected side. Have the patient transfer his or her body weight to the crutch while holding the handrail with one hand (Fig. 38.17A). Stay behind the patient, holding on to the gait belt. Then have the patient support his or her weight evenly between the handrail and crutch. Next, the patient places some weight on crutch and then steps up the first step with weight-bearing foot (stronger leg) (Fig. 38.17B). Have patient get his or her balance leaning forward with weight on good leg. Then ask the patient to straighten the good knee, push down on crutches and lift his or her body weight, bringing the affected leg and then the crutch up the stair (Fig. 38.17C). Always make sure the crutch tip is completely on the stair (Washington University Physicians, 2017). Repeat sequence for each step, and instruct patient to climb one stair at a time.

When a patient descends stairs, he or she remains at risk for falling. Assist the patient using extreme caution. Have the patient stand close to the edge of the top step (Fig. 38.18A). Have the patient hold the handrail with one hand (affected leg next to railing). You carry the crutch positioned next to the handrail as the patient places the other crutch under the axilla of the strong side. Stand above the patient while holding the gait belt. For support, have the patient lower the crutch down to the step below and then move his or her affected leg down (Fig. 38.18B) (Washington University Physicians, 2017). The patient then brings the strong leg down the step and supports his or her weight

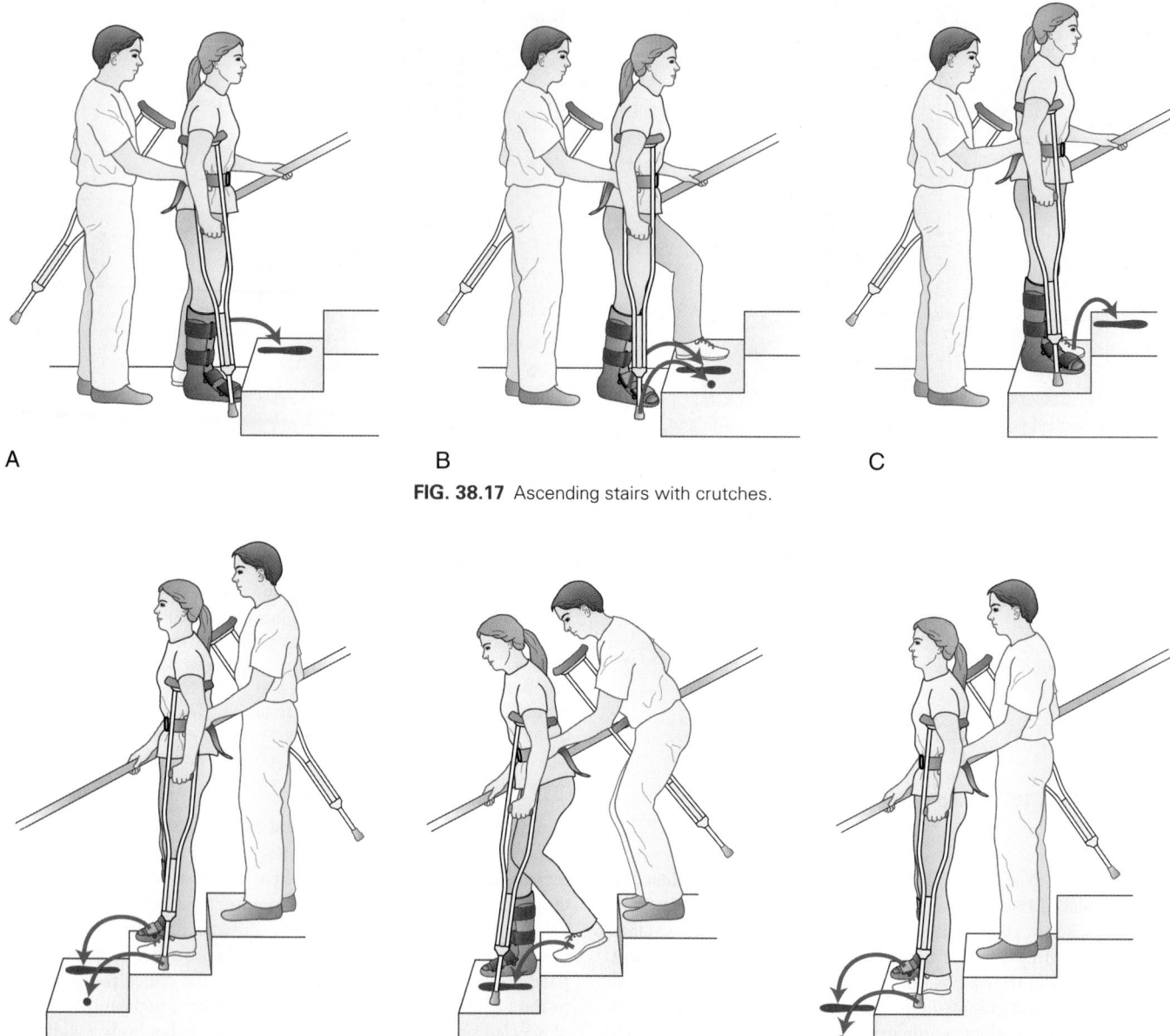

FIG. 38.17 Ascending stairs with crutches.

FIG. 38.18 Descending stairs with crutches.

evenly between handrail, good leg, and crutch (Fig. 38.18C). Be sure that patient has good balance. Always make sure the crutch tip is completely on the stair. Caution patient not to hop.

Remember, when going up stairs, lead with the stronger leg. When going down stairs, lead with the affected leg. Because in most cases patients need to use crutches for some time, they need to be taught to use them on stairs before discharge. Instruction applies to all patients who are dependent on crutches, not just those who have stairs in their homes.

Sitting in a Chair with Crutches. The procedure for sitting in a chair involves phases and requires the patient to transfer weight (Fig. 38.19). First the patient positions himself or herself at the center front of the chair with the posterior aspect of the legs touching the chair. Then the patient holds both crutches in the hand opposite the affected leg. If both legs are affected, as with a person with paraplegia who wears weight-supporting braces, the patient holds the crutches in the hand on his or her stronger side. With both crutches in one

hand, the patient supports body weight on the unaffected leg and the crutches. While still holding the crutches, the patient grasps the arm of the chair with the remaining hand and lowers his or her body into it. To stand the procedure is reversed, and the patient, when fully erect, assumes the tripod position before beginning to walk.

Restoration of Activity and Chronic Illness. Nurses design care plans individualized for increasing activity and exercise in patients with specific disease conditions and chronic illnesses such as coronary artery disease (CAD), hypertension, chronic obstructive pulmonary disease (COPD), and diabetes mellitus.

Coronary Artery Disease. Regular moderate-intensity aerobic exercise has been shown to reduce the risk of sudden cardiac death and acute MI (Bruning and Sturek, 2015). Increasing physical activity is an important modifiable behavior that can reduce the relative risk of CAD events (such as angina and myocardial infarction) because of

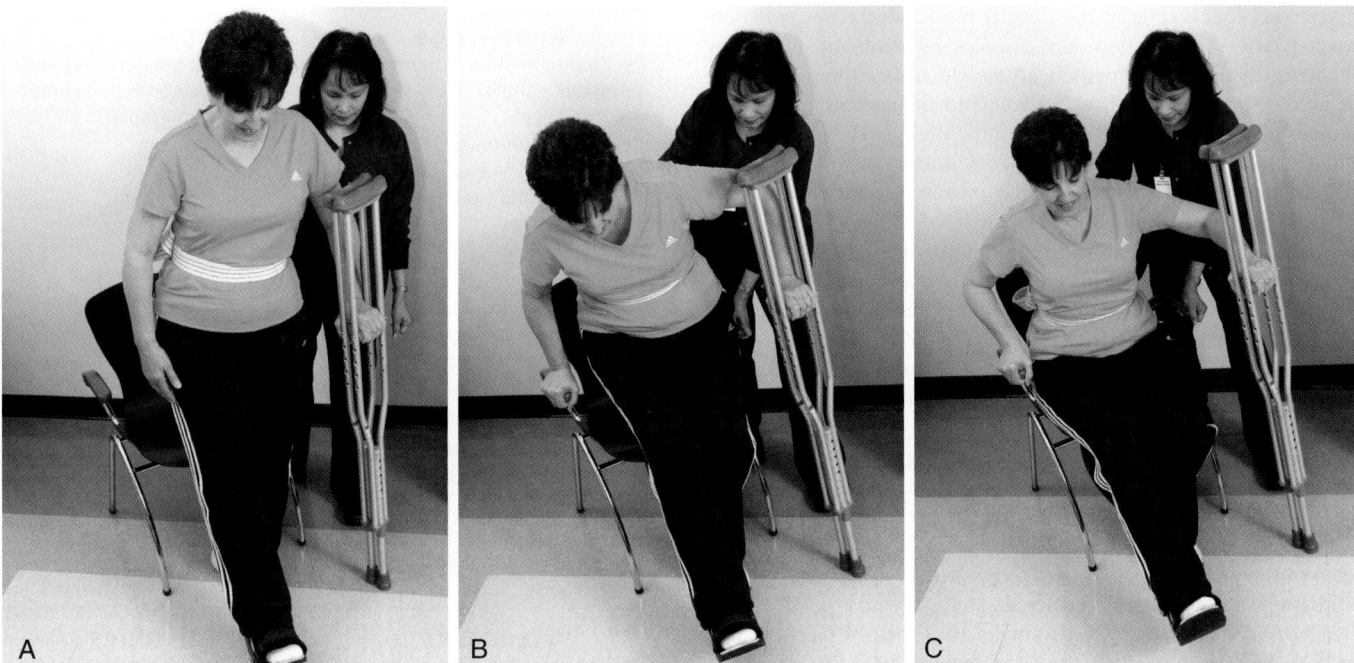

FIG. 38.19 Sitting in a chair. **A,** Both crutches are held in one hand. Patient transfers weight to crutches and unaffected leg. **B,** Patient grasps arm of chair with free hand and begins to lower herself into chair. **C,** Patient completely lowers herself into chair.

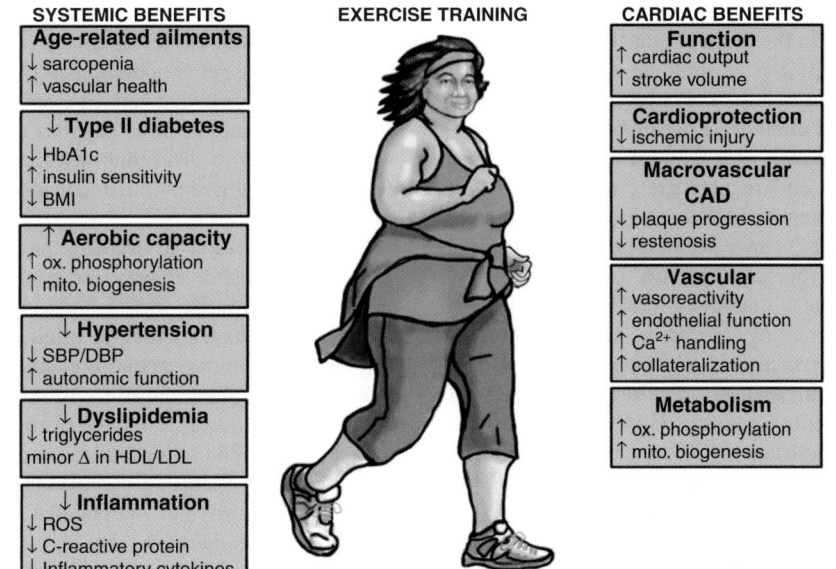

SYSTEMIC BENEFITS

Age-related ailments
↓ sarcopenia
↑ vascular health

↓ Type II diabetes
↓ HbA1c
↑ insulin sensitivity
↓ BMI

↑ Aerobic capacity
↑ ox. phosphorylation
↑ mito. biogenesis

↓ Hypertension
↓ SBP/DBP
↑ autonomic function

↓ Dyslipidemia
↓ triglycerides
minor Δ in HDL/LDL

↓ Inflammation
↓ ROS
↓ C-reactive protein
↓ Inflammatory cytokines

EXERCISE TRAINING

CARDIAC BENEFITS

Function
↑ cardiac output
↑ stroke volume

Cardioprotection
↓ ischemic injury

Macrovascular CAD
↓ plaque progression
↓ restenosis

Vascular
↑ vasoreactivity
↑ endothelial function
↑ Ca^{2+} handling
↑ collateralization

Metabolism
↑ ox. phosphorylation
↑ mito. biogenesis

FIG. 38.20 Systemic benefits of regular moderate-intensity exercise. (From: Prog Cardiovasc Dis. Author manuscript; available in PMC 2016 Mar 1. Published in final edited form as: *Prog Cardiovasc Dis.* 2015 Mar-Apr; 57(5): 443–453.)

its systemic benefits (Fig. 38.20). Regular moderate exercise enhances coronary artery blood flow and reduces incidents of angina by enhancing oxygen delivery to the heart muscle (myocardium) (Bruning and Sturek, 2015). Adherence and access to the necessary resources are often barriers to implementing healthy lifestyle changes in CAD patients (Bruning and Sturek, 2015). As a nurse you will play a role in discussing with patients how regular exercise specifically improves heart function and reduces development of other complications. Collaborate with home health and community nurses to help patients find resources to participate in cardiac rehab programs.

Hypertension. In addition to standard antihypertensive medications, the benefits of physical activity on hypertension and cardiovascular disease have been well demonstrated (Hegde and Solomon, 2015). A number of studies have consistently shown beneficial effects of exercise on hypertension, resulting in reductions in both systolic and diastolic blood pressure with as much as 5 to 7 mm Hg reductions in those with hypertension (Hegde and Solomon, 2015). Encourage patients to participate in low- to moderate-intensity aerobic exercise as it is the most effective in lowering blood pressure. In addition, a tai chi exercise program has demonstrated a significant reduction in systolic and diastolic blood pressures (Lo et al., 2012; Edelman and Kudzma, 2018). Have patients with hypertension measure their BP daily at home and help them learn how reactions to stress can raise BP. Relaxation exercises are useful in reducing stress reactions.

Chronic Obstructive Pulmonary Disease. Pulmonary rehabilitation helps patients reach an optimal level of functioning. Exercise training has been shown to significantly improve health-related quality of life, exercise capacity, respiratory muscle strength, and exertional dyspnea in subjects with COPD and normal exercise capacity. Some patients are fearful of participating in exercise because of the potential of worsening dyspnea (difficulty breathing). This aversion to physical activity sets up a progressive deconditioning in which minimal physical exertion results in dyspnea. Pulmonary rehabilitation can help patients gain strength, reduce symptoms of anxiety or depression, and make it easier to manage routine activities, work, and social activities. Patients may have pulmonary rehabilitation in the hospital or a clinic, or they may learn physical therapy or breathing exercises to do at home (National Heart, Lung and Blood Institute, n.d.b.). Pulmonary rehabilitation provides a safe environment for monitoring patients' progress.

Diabetes Mellitus. Along with diet, glucose monitoring, and medication, physical activity and regular exercise are important components in the care of patients with diabetes mellitus. Moderate to high volumes of aerobic activity have been found to be associated with substantially lower cardiovascular and overall mortality risks in both type 1 and type 2 diabetes (Sluik et al., 2012). In type 1 diabetes, aerobic training increases cardiorespiratory fitness, decreases insulin resistance, and improves lipid levels and endothelial function (Chimen et al., 2012). In individuals with type 2 diabetes, regular training reduces HbA1c, triglycerides, blood pressure, and insulin resistance (Colberg et al., 2016). The recommendations for physical activity and exercise in diabetes from the position statement of the American Diabetes Association (Colberg et al., 2016) can be found at the following website: http://care.diabetesjournals.org/content/39/11/2065. It contains recommendations for reducing sedentary time and the type of physical activity and exercise recommended specifically for patients with type 1 and type 2 diabetes. Such recommendations should be part of your teaching plan for all patients with diabetes.

◆ Evaluation

Through the Patient's Eyes. For activity and exercise you measure the effectiveness of nursing interventions by evaluating whether the

Knowledge
- Characteristics of improved activity and exercise tolerance
- Role of community resources in maintaining activity and exercise

Experience
- Consider previous patient responses to activity and exercise therapies

EVALUATION
- Reassess the patient for signs of improved activity and exercise tolerance
- Ask for the patient's perception of activity and exercise status after interventions
- Ask whether the patient's expectations are being met

Standards
- Use established expected outcomes to evaluate the patient's response to care (e.g., return to resting heart rate within 5 minutes) as standards for evaluation
- Apply goals published by the American College of Sports Medicine to evaluate response to exercise

Attitudes
- Use creativity in redesigning new interventions to improve the patient's activity and exercise tolerance
- Demonstrate perseverance to design interventions to keep the patient motivated to adhere to the activity and exercise plan

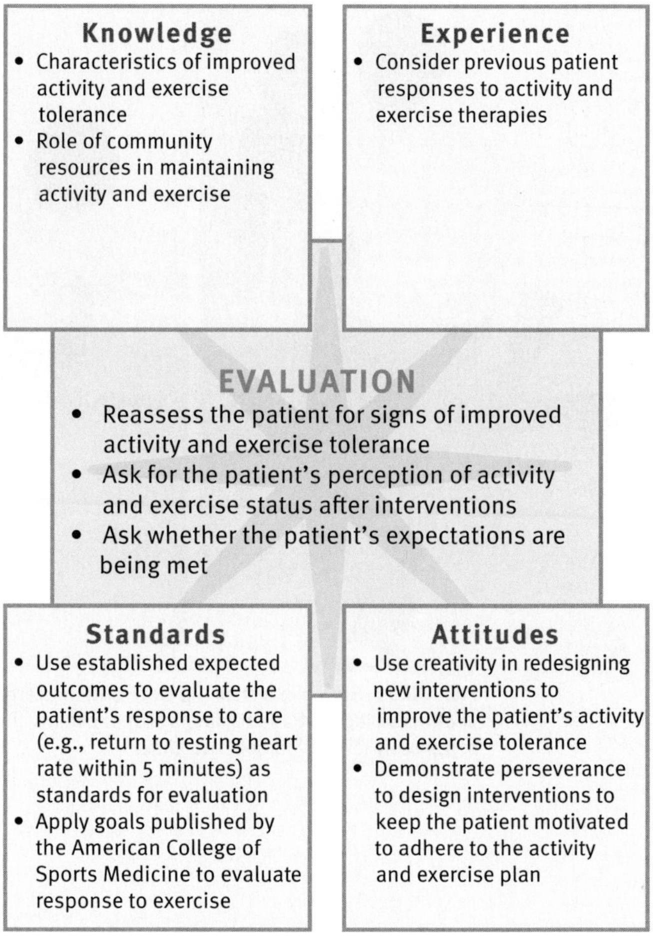

FIG. 38.21 Critical thinking model for activity and exercise evaluation.

patient's expectations and goals of care have been reached. The patient is the only one who knows the effectiveness and benefits of activity and exercise. Ask the patient questions such as "How well did you tolerate walking, and is that what you expected?" and "You have been walking regularly for a month now; how has it made you feel?" Continuous evaluation helps to determine whether new or revised therapies are needed and whether new nursing diagnoses have developed.

Patient Outcomes. To evaluate the effectiveness of nursing interventions to enhance activity and exercise, make comparisons with baseline measures that include pulse, blood pressure, oxygen saturation (when available), strength, fatigue, and psychological well-being (Fig. 38.21). Compare actual outcomes with expected outcomes to determine the patient's health status and progression. Also consider standards for physical activity performance (e.g., ability to reach target heart rate). The following is an example of questions you might ask when your patients do not meet their expected outcomes:

- The last time we met you planned to walk outside for 20 minutes 3 days a week. However, you report that you are able to walk only twice a week right now. Tell me what you think is preventing you from meeting your goal.
- Your weight is the same this month as it was last month. We were hoping that increasing your activity would lead to a decrease in your weight. Help me understand the factors you believe are preventing you from losing weight right now.
- You state that you experience leg pain after walking short distances. Describe your pain. Which pain-relieving measures have you tried?

TABLE 38.4 Preventing Lift Injuries in Health Care Workers

Action	Rationale
When planning to move a patient, arrange for adequate help. If your institution has a lift team, use it as a resource (Lin et al., 2012; OSHA, 2017).	A lift team is properly educated in techniques to prevent musculoskeletal injuries.
Use patient-handling equipment and devices such as height-adjustable beds, ceiling-mounted lifts, friction-reducing slide sheets, and air-assisted devices (OSHA, 2017).	These devices reduce the caregiver's muscular strain during patient handling.
Encourage patient to help as much as possible.	This promotes patient's independence and strength while minimizing workload.
Take position close to patient (or object being lifted).	Keeps object in same plane as lifter and close to caregiver's center of gravity. Reduces horizontal reach and stress on caregiver's back.
Tighten abdominal muscles and keep back, neck, pelvis, and feet aligned. Avoid twisting.	Reduces risk of injury to lumbar vertebrae and muscle groups. Twisting increases risk of injury (Lin et al., 2012).
Bend at knees; keep feet wide apart.	A broad base of support increases stability. Maintains center of gravity.
Use arms and legs (not back).	Leg muscles are stronger, larger muscles capable of greater work without injury.
Slide patient toward your body using pull sheet or slide board. When transferring patient onto a stretcher or bed, a slide board is more appropriate.	Sliding requires less effort than lifting. Pull sheet minimizes shearing forces, which can damage patient's skin.
Person with heaviest load coordinates efforts of team involved by counting to three.	Simultaneous lifting minimizes load for any one lifter.
Perform manual lifting as last resort and only if it does not involve lifting most or all of patient's weight.	Lifting is a high-risk activity that causes significant biochemical and postural stressors.

SAFETY GUIDELINES FOR NURSING SKILLS

Ensuring patient safety is an essential role of the professional nurse. To ensure patient safety, communicate clearly with the members of the health care team, assess and incorporate the patient's priorities of care and preferences, and use the best evidence when making decisions about your patient's care. When performing the skills in this chapter, remember the following points to ensure safe patient handling and individualized patient-centered care.

- Know a patient's level of mobility and strength to determine assistance that is required during ambulation and transferring.
- Assess a patient's physical risks for activity intolerance before beginning early mobility.
- Mentally review the transfer steps before beginning the procedure; this ensures both your safety and that of the patient.

- When assisting orthopedic patients with ambulation, stand on their unaffected side. For patients with neurological deficits stand on the affected side. For all other patients, stand on their affected side.
- Determine the transfer equipment indicated and the number of personnel needed to safely transfer a patient and prevent harm to health care providers (Table 38.4).
- Raise the side rail on the side of the bed opposite of where you are standing to prevent the patient from falling out of bed on that side.
- Arrange equipment (e.g., intravenous lines, feeding tube, indwelling catheter) so that it does not interfere with the transfer process.
- Evaluate the patient for correct body alignment and pressure risks after a transfer.
- Make sure that all personnel understand how the equipment functions before it is used.

SKILL 38.1   ASSISTING WITH AMBULATION (WITHOUT ASSIST DEVICES)

Delegation and Collaboration
The skill of assisting patients with ambulation can be delegated to assistive personnel (AP). The nurse directs the AP to:
- Apply safe patient handling principles when assisting patient out of bed or chair.
- Review steps to ensure patient is not having orthostatic hypotension when rising from a lying position in bed to sitting. Check patient's blood pressure before ambulation.
- Immediately return a patient to the bed or chair if he or she is nauseated, dizzy, pale, or diaphoretic, or if systolic BP has dropped at least 20 mm Hg within

3 minutes of sitting upright (Shibao et al., 2013). Report these signs and symptoms to the nurse immediately.
- Apply safe, nonskid shoes/socks and ensure that the environment is free of clutter and that there is no moisture on the floor before ambulating patient.

Equipment
- Nonskid footwear
- Transfer (gait) belt
- Stethoscope, sphygmomanometer, pulse oximeter (as needed)

Continued

STEPS	RATIONALE
ASSESSMENT	
1. Identify patient using at least two identifiers (e.g., name and birthday or name and medical record number) according to agency policy.	Ensures correct patient. Complies with The Joint Commission standards and improves patient safety (TJC, 2020).
2. Review medical record for patient's most recent activity experience, including distance ambulated, use of assist device, activity tolerance, balance and gait. Note history of orthostatic hypotension and any medications, chronic illnesses, gait alterations, or a history of falling.	Allows you to anticipate precautions to take in ambulating patient. History may reveal factors that will influence patient's ability to ambulate and be at risk for falling
3. Review most recently recorded weight for patient and any report of patient's ability to stand and bear weight.	Determines whether assistance will be required from another health care provider

CLINICAL DECISION: *Use mechanical lift or transfer aid with minimum of two or three caregivers if a patient has partial weight-bearing with upper body strength or caregiver must lift more than 15.9 kg (35 lb) (TVAREF, 2016).*

STEPS	RATIONALE
4. Review health care provider's order for activity; note any mobility, range-of-motion, or weight-bearing restrictions.	Order required for patient to become progressively mobile.
5. Perform hand hygiene. Assess patient's baseline resting heart rate, blood pressure, oxygen saturation (when available), and respirations.	Provides a baseline to compare with assessment data monitored during and after walking to evaluate patient tolerance to exercise.
a. If patient's strength and endurance have been affected by illness or deconditioning, assess range of motion (ROM) and muscle strength (see Chapter 30) of lower extremities while patient in bed. Assess the patient's mobility, including ability to sit up on side of bed or in chair and ability to stand by using the Banner Mobility Assessment Tool (BMAT) (see Skill 38.2) (Boynton et al., 2014b).	Confirms patient's ability to assist with standing and walking. The BMAT is an assessment tool to guide a patient through 4 functional tasks in order to identify the level of mobility the patient can achieve (Boynton et al., 2014b).
6. Assess patient's or family caregiver's knowledge, experience, and health literacy level.	Ensures patient has the capacity to obtain, communicate, process, and understand basic health information (CDC, 2019).
7. Ask whether patient feels excessively tired or is currently experiencing any pain. Determine source and severity of pain (using a 0-to-10 pain-rating scale). Offer an analgesic 30 minutes before ambulation to improve patient's tolerance to exercise.	Pain may delay ambulation.
8. Assess patient's response to commands. Is he or she able to understand instructions and cooperate during ambulation? Is patient willing to ambulate?	Determines how safe it will be to engage patient to ambulate and precautions needed while walking.
9. Assess patient for any hearing or visual deficits (see Chapter 30).	May affect ability to understand instructions.
10. Refer to patient's mobility status and safe-handling algorithm (available in most agencies). Do not start procedure until all required caregivers are available.	Determines whether a lift device or mechanical transfer device is needed and the number of people needed to assist patient to stand.
PLANNING	
1. Determine the best time to ambulate, considering other scheduled activities such as bathing or other medical procedures.	Allows you to lessen likelihood patient will be fatigued at time of ambulation.
2. Provide privacy. Organize and set up any equipment/lift devices.	Ensures more efficiency, safe use of equipment, and safe ambulation.
3. Remove SCD from patient's legs if present (see Chapter 39). Note whether patient wears a mobile compression device; ambulation can occur safely with stockings in place.	Prevents patient from becoming tangled in cords.
4. Explain to patient in simple language how you are going to prepare for ambulation (e.g., gait belt application, distance planned to walk). Discuss benefits of walking and risks that you are adapting for to reduce chance of falling.	Allows patient to cooperate and lessens anxiety.

CLINICAL DECISION: *If patient is on an early progressive mobility protocol, know distance walked during previous ambulation and attempt to increase distance at this time.*

STEPS	RATIONALE
IMPLEMENTATION	
1. If hands became soiled during assessment, perform hand hygiene.	Reduces transfer of microorganisms.
2. Assist patient from supine position to sitting position on edge of bed with bed positioned so that top of mattress is even with your elbows.	Reduces strain on your back.
a. With patient in supine position in bed, raise head of bed 30-45 degrees and place bed in low position, level with your hips. Raise upper side rail on side where patient will exit bed. Apply nonskid shoes or socks. If patient is fully mobile, allow to sit up on side of bed independently, using side rail to raise up.	Reduces strain on back during pivot to side of bed. Nonskid soles decrease risk for slipping during transfer. Always have patient wear nonskid shoes when ambulating; bare feet increase risk for falls.
b. If patient needs assistance to sit on side of bed, turn patient onto his or her side facing you while standing at the side of bed where patient will sit.	Positioning reduces strain on your back.

STEPS	**RATIONALE**

CLINICAL DECISION: *Follow this technique to assist patient to side of bed only if patient has upper body strength and can assist in moving. If patient is uncooperative or has no upper body strength to assist, use a mechanical lift or ceiling lift to move onto side of bed (see Skill 38.2).*

c. Stand opposite patient's hips. Turn diagonally to face patient and far corner of foot of bed.	Maintains straight alignment with patient.
d. Place your feet apart in wide base of support with foot closer to head of bed in front of other foot.	Maintains your balance.
e. Place your arm nearer to head of bed under patient's lower shoulder, supporting his or her head and neck. Place your other arm over and around patient's thighs (see illustration).	Position provides leverage for patient to rise to sitting position.
f. Move patient's lower legs and feet over side of bed as patient uses side rail to push and raise the upper body. Pivot weight onto your rear leg as you allow patient's upper legs to swing downward (see illustration). **Do not lift legs.** At same time, continue to shift weight to your rear leg and guide patient in elevating his/her trunk into upright position	Patient's effort in raising upper body lessens strain on your back. Avoid lifting to prevent accidental injury. Use a mechanical or ceiling lift if it becomes necessary to lift patient.
3. Allow patient to sit on the side of the bed with feet on floor for 2 to 3 minutes. Have patient alternately flex and extend feet, and move lower legs up and down without touching floor. Ask whether patient feels dizzy; if so, check blood pressure. Have patient relax and take a few deep breaths until dizziness subsides and balance is gained. If dizziness lasts more than 60 seconds or if systolic BP has dropped at least 20 mm Hg within 3 minutes of sitting upright, return patient to bed (Shibao et al., 2013; Frith et al., 2014; Mills et al., 2014). Recheck blood pressure.	Allows patient's circulation to equilibrate to reduce chance of orthostatic hypotension. Patient cannot be safely ambulated if dizziness develops.
4. Apply gait belt. Be sure that it completely encircles a patient's waist below the belly button (see illustration). Belt should fit snugly, being sure two fingers fit between the belt and patient's body Avoid placing belt over any intravenous lines, incisions, or drainage tubes.	Gait belt allows you to maintain stability of patient as he/she stands and reduces risk for falling (Degelau et al., 2014; OSHA, 2014).

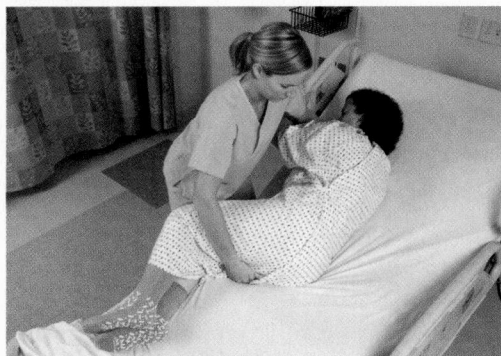

STEP 2e Nurse places arm over patient's thighs, other arm under patient's shoulder as patient raises up.

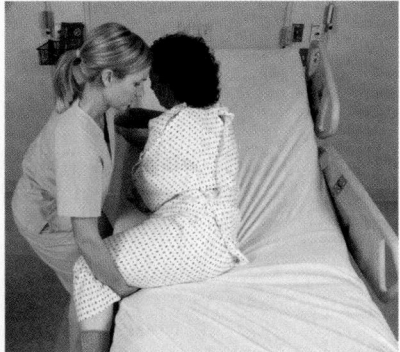

STEP 2f Nurse shifts weight to rear leg and guides patient to raise up to sitting position.

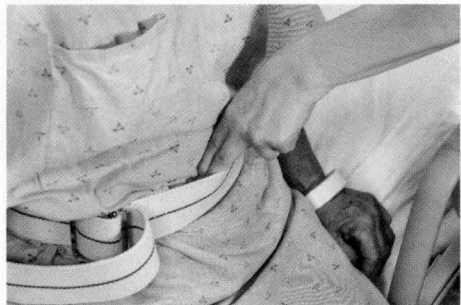

STEP 4 Application of gait/transfer belt.

Continued

SKILL 38.1 — ASSISTING WITH AMBULATION (WITHOUT ASSIST DEVICES)—cont'd

STEPS	RATIONALE
5. If patient is alert and can bear weight and balance while standing, allow him/her to stand independently. Assist by holding gait belt to offer balance assistance.	Patient capable of bearing weight needs assistance to reduce fall risk.
6. If patient cannot bear weight or cannot balance to stand independently and walk, use an ambulation lift or ceiling lift with gait harness (see Skill 38.2). Patient can walk with support of this mechanical device.	Provides needed stability as patient stands and continues to support patient while walking.
7. Confirm with patient the distance to ambulate.	Motivates patient to reach goal.

CLINICAL DECISION: *At any time during ambulation if patient becomes unstable or reports feeling dizzy, seat him or her in chair or return to bed immediately. May need use of mechanical lift (see Skill 38.2). This prevents patient falls.*

STEPS	RATIONALE
8. *Option:* If patient has an IV line, place the IV pole on the same side as the site of infusion and instruct patient where to hold and push the pole while ambulating. It is best if another caregiver can push IV pole.	Prevents accidental pulling on IV catheter. Assist from second caregiver allows patient to focus on walking and may lessen risk of tripping
9. If a Foley catheter is present, carry the bag below the level of the bladder to prevent tension on the tubing.	Prevents reflux of urine from the bag back into bladder.
10. For orthopedic patients stand on patient's unaffected side. For patients with neurological deficits (e.g., stroke) stand on the affected side. For all other patients requiring assistance to maintain balance while weight-bearing, stand on involved side.	Positions provide balance and facilitate lowering patient to the floor if he or she is unable to continue because of weakness or dizziness. Helps support the affected limb of neurological patient (i.e., prevents knee buckling).
11. Grasp belt firmly with palm facing up (see illustration A). Take a few steps, guiding patient with one hand grasping the gait belt and the other hand placed under the elbow of the patient's flexed arm (see illustration B).	Belt used to maintain patient balance.
12. When ambulating in a hallway, position patient between yourself and the wall. Encourage patient to use handrails if available (see illustration B, Step 11).	The wall provides stable support for patients who start to fall away from you.
13. Observe how patient walks (posture, gait, balance), and determine distance patient can safely continue walking. Measure pulse and respirations as needed.	Monitors patient's tolerance to walking.
14. Return patient to bed or chair (independent transfer or use of mechanical lift), and assist patient to assume a comfortable position. Be sure the nurse call system is accessible within patient's reach.	Gives patient sense of well-being. Ensures patient can call for assistance if needed.

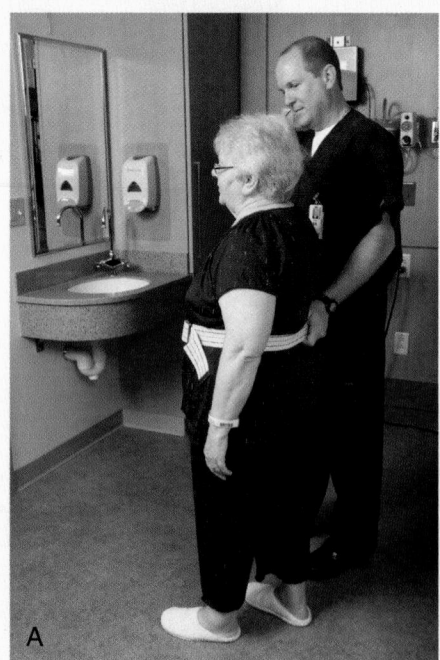 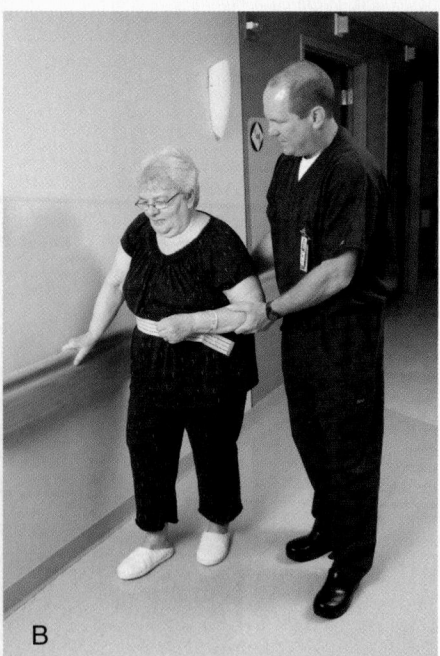

STEP 11 A, Nurse grasps gait belt firmly with palm up. **B,** Nurse guides patient by placing hand on patient's arm.

STEPS	RATIONALE
15. Raise side rails (as appropriate), and lower bed to lowest position. Perform hand hygiene.	Ensures patient safety. Reduces transmission of microorganisms.

EVALUATION

1. Monitor vital signs. Compare HR during ambulation with target HR (if applicable). Ask whether patient feels dizzy or tired. Ask him or her to rate pain on pain scale.	Evaluates patient's response to postural changes and activity.
2. Note patient's behavioral response to walking.	Reveals level of motivation and self-care potential.
3. **Use Teach-Back:** "I want to be sure I explained the importance of increasing your walking distance each day and of continuing to walk once you go home. Tell me why it is important for you to be able to walk farther each day." Revise your instruction now or develop a plan for revised patient/family caregiver teaching if patient/family caregiver is not able to teach back correctly.	Determines patient's/family caregiver's level of understanding of instructional topic.

UNEXPECTED OUTCOMES AND RELATED INTERVENTIONS

1. Patient starts to fall while walking.
   - Grasp patient's gait belt with both hands around his or her waist with palms up.
   - Stand with feet apart for a broad base of support (see Fig. 38.10A).
   - Extend one leg slightly forward, pull patient against you, and let him or her slide down your leg as you ease him or her to the floor (see Fig. 38.10B). *Caution:* If patient is obese, do not risk personal injury. If you extend leg too far, hyperextension could occur.
   - Bend your knees and lower your body as patient slides to floor (see Fig. 38.10C).
   - Stay with patient until help arrives.
2. Patient does not tolerate walking due to fatigue, pain, dizziness, or other symptoms.
   - Return to bed or chair immediately.
   - Measure vital signs.
   - Notify health care provider or nurse in charge.

RECORDING AND REPORTING

- Record procedure and pertinent observations: baseline and postambulatory vital signs, distance walked, patient's tolerance, onset of weakness, fatigue, pain, poor balance or gait.
- Report to health care provider or nurse in charge change in vital signs or patient fall.
- Document evaluation of patient learning.

SKILL 38.2   USING SAFE AND EFFECTIVE TRANSFER TECHNIQUES

Delegation and Collaboration

The skill of effective transfer techniques can be delegated to trained assistive personnel (AP). The nurse is responsible to initially assess patient's readiness and ability to transfer. The nurse directs the AP by:

- Assisting and supervising when moving patients who are transferred for the first time after prolonged bed rest, extensive surgery, critical illness, or spinal cord trauma.
- Explaining the patient's mobility restrictions, changes in blood pressure to look for, or sensory alterations that may affect safe transfer (e.g., medicated or confused).
- Explaining what to observe and report back to the nurse, such as dizziness or the patient's ability/inability to assist.

Equipment

- Gait belt, sling, or lapboard (as needed)
- Nonskid shoes, bath blankets, and pillows
- Chair with arms or wheelchair (position chair at 45- to 60-degree angle to bed, lock brakes, remove footrests, and lock bed brakes)
- Stretcher (position next to bed, lock brakes on stretcher, lock brakes on bed)
- Mechanical/hydraulic lift (use frame, canvas strips or chains, and hammock or canvas strips)
- Stand-assist lift device
- *Option:* Clean gloves (if risk of contacting soiled linen)

STEP	RATIONALE

ASSESSMENT

1. Identify patient using two identifiers (e.g., name and birthday or name and medical record number) according to agency policy. Explain procedure.	Ensures correct patient. Complies with The Joint Commission standards and improves patient safety (TJC, 2020).
2. Refer to medical record for most recent recorded weight and height for patient.	Data determine whether mechanical transfer devices or friction-reducing device is needed for transfer.
3. Review history for previous fall and whether patient has a fear of falling.	Previous fall history is a significant fall risk. Having a fear of falling can alter one's gait and security in walking.
4. Assess medical record for previous mode of transferring to bed or chair (if applicable).	Ensures some consistency in how to assist with transfer.

Continued

SKILL 38.2	USING SAFE AND EFFECTIVE TRANSFER TECHNIQUES—cont'd

STEP	RATIONALE
5. Perform hand hygiene. Assess patient for presence of neuromuscular deficits, motor weakness or incoordination, proprioception (awareness of posture), history of cognitive and visual dysfunction, altered balance (see Chapter 30).	Reduces transmission of microorganisms. Certain conditions increase risk of tripping, falling, or suffering potential injury during fall. Proprioception determines stability of patient's balance for transfer and risk for falls.
6. Assess the patient's mobility, including ability to sit up on side of bed or chair, and ability to stand. *Option:* Administer the Banner Mobility Assessment Tool (BMAT) (Boynton et al., 2014a,b):	The BMAT is a tool that assesses four functional tasks to identify the level of mobility a patient can achieve (Boynton et al., 2014a,b). The assessment aids in determining a patient's level of mobility (e.g., Mobility Level 1) and recommends equipment and tools needed to safely lift, transfer, and mobilize the patient. Findings serve as a communication tool across the continuum of care.
a. Sit and Shake: From a semireclined position, ask patient to sit upright and rotate to a seated position at the side of the bed; patient may use the bed rail. Note patient's ability to maintain bedside position. Ask patient to reach out and grab your hand and shake, making sure patient reaches across his/her midline.	If patient fails to Sit and Shake: use total lift with sling and/or positioning sheet and/or straps, and/or use lateral transfer devices such as rollboard, friction-reducing (slide sheets/tube), or air-assisted device. If patient fails Stretch and Point: use total lift for patient unable to weight-bear on at least one leg; use sit-to-stand lift for patient who can weight-bear on at least one leg. If patient fails to Stand: use nonpowered raising/stand aid (default to powered sit-to-stand lift if no stand aid available) or use total lift with ambulation accessories or use assistive device (cane, walker, crutches). If patient cannot Walk: use nonpowered raising/stand aid (default to powered sit-to-stand lift if no stand aid available) or use total lift with ambulation accessories or use assistive device (cane, walker, crutches).
b. Stretch and Point: With patient in seated position at the side of the bed, have patient place both feet on the floor (or stool) with knees no higher than hips. Ask patient to extend one leg and straighten the knee, then bend the ankle and point the toes. Repeat with the other leg.	
c. Stand: Ask patient to elevate off the bed or chair (seated to standing) using an assistive device (walker, cane, bed rail). Patient should be able to raise buttocks off bed and hold for a count of five. May repeat once.	
d. Walk (march in place and advance step): Ask patient to march in place at bedside, then ask patient to step forward and back with each foot. Patient should display stability while performing tasks. Assess for stability and safety awareness.	

CLINICAL DECISION: *Do not rely on self-report from patient or family caregiver as to patient's ability to sit, stand, or ambulate. An objective assessment is needed to accurately determine a patient's capabilities.*

STEP	RATIONALE
7. While assessing mobility, note any weakness, dizziness, or risk for orthostatic (postural) hypotension (e.g., previously on bed rest, first time arising from supine position after surgical procedure, history of dizziness when arising).	Determines risk of fainting or falling during transfer. Immobilized patients have decreased ability of autonomic nervous system to equalize blood supply, resulting in initial drop of 40 mm Hg systolic or more in blood pressure when rising from sitting position (Frith et al., 2014; Mills et al., 2014).
8. Assess activity tolerance, noting for fatigue during previous sitting and standing.	Determines ability of patient to help with transfer.
9. Assess sensory status, including central and peripheral vision, adequacy of hearing, and presence of peripheral sensation loss.	Visual field loss decreases patients' ability to see in direction of transfer and may impact their balance. Peripheral sensation loss decreases proprioception. Patients with visual and hearing losses need transfer techniques and communication methods adapted to their deficits.

CLINICAL DECISION: *Patients with hemiplegia may "neglect" one side of the body (inattention to or unawareness of one side of body or environment), which distorts perception of the visual field. If patient experiences neglect of one side, instruct him or her to scan all visual fields when transferring.*

STEP	RATIONALE
10. Assess level of comfort (e.g., joint discomfort, muscle spasm), and measure level of pain using scale of 0 to 10. Offer prescribed analgesic 30 minutes before transfer. (**NOTE:** Patient will require assistance when analgesic has been given.)	Pain reduces patient's motivation and ability to be mobile. Pain relief before transfer enhances patient's ability to participate (Schofield, 2014).
11. Assess patient's health literacy and cognitive status, including ability to follow verbal instructions, short-term memory, and recognition of physical deficits and limitations to movement.	Determines patient's ability to follow directions and learn transfer techniques.

CRITICAL DECISION: *Patients with dementia, head trauma, or degenerative neurological disorders may have perceptual cognitive defects that create safety risks. If the patient has difficulty comprehending, simplify instructions by providing one step at a time and maintain consistency.*

STEP	RATIONALE
12. Assess patient's level of motivation, such as eagerness versus unwillingness to be mobile, and perception of value of exercise.	Will affect patient's desire to engage in activity.
13. Assess need for special transfer equipment for home setting and previous mode of transfer (if applicable).	Providing appropriate aids greatly enhances transfer ability at home.
14. Assess patient's vital signs just before transfer.	Baseline measures will determine whether vital sign changes occur during activity, which will indicate activity intolerance. Patient with low blood pressure may not tolerate sudden position change and is at risk for orthostatic hypotension.

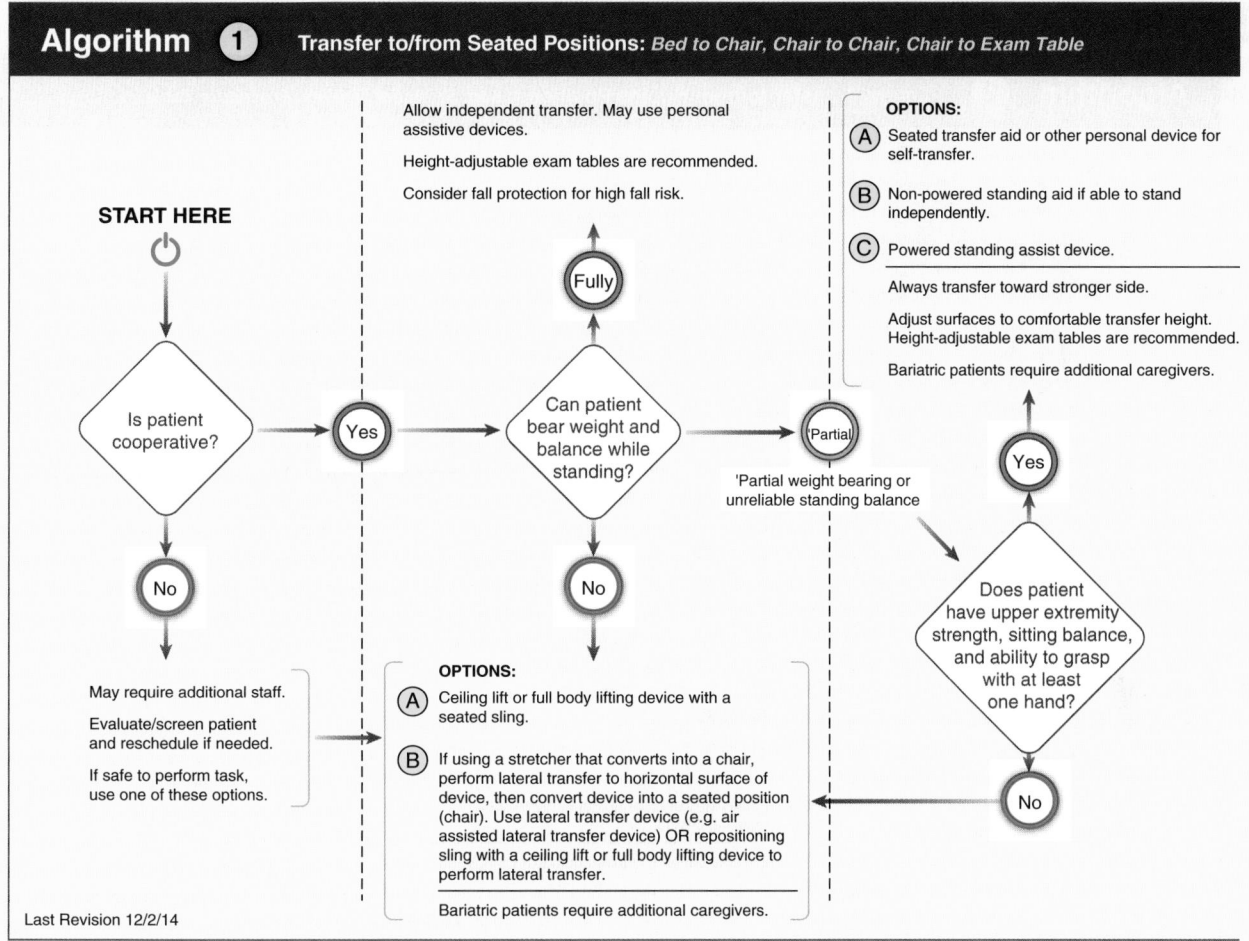

STEP 15 VHA safe patient handling and mobility algorithm 1. (From VHA: *Safe patient handling and mobility algorithms.* 2014 revision. Reprinted with permission of VISN 8 Patient Safety Center of Inquiry, Tampa, FL.)

STEP	RATIONALE
15. Refer to BMAT score or safe-handling algorithm of agency (available in most agencies) to determine whether a lift device or mechanical transfer device is needed and the number of people needed to help with transfer (see illustrations A and B). Do not start procedure until all required caregivers are available.	Ensures safe patient handling, reducing risk of injury to patient and caregivers.
16. Assess patient's or family caregiver's knowledge, experience, and health literacy.	Ensures patient or family caregiver has the capacity to obtain, communicate, process, and understand basic health information (CDC, 2019).

PLANNING

1. Obtain and set up appropriate equipment/lift devices.
2. Provide for patient privacy.
3. Be sure additional caregivers are present to perform transfer.

4. Explain to patient in simple language how you are going to prepare for transfer technique and the safety precautions to be used. Explain benefits and reasons for getting up in a chair, and do so in a way that matches patient's beliefs and values (Shieh et al., 2015).

Organization ensures efficient procedure.
Ensures patient's comfort.
Safe patient handling algorithm determines number of caregivers and type of equipment needed.

IMPLEMENTATION

1. Perform hand hygiene.
2. **Transfer patient from bed to chair.** (*Option:* Apply clean gloves if bed linen soiled.):
    a. Assist patient from supine to sitting position on edge of bed by raising head of bed and helping patient to raise and rotate to edge of bed (see Skill 38.1). Do so with bed positioned so that mattress is at working height. Refer to mobility assessment findings and safe patient handling algorithm to confirm appropriateness to transfer patient and whether other caregivers needed.

Reduces transmission of microorganisms.

Reduces strain on your back.
Assessment findings offer objective measure of readiness for transfer. The use of a safe mobility algorithm aids caregivers in selecting mechanical lifts and transfer devices appropriately for safer transfers (OSHA, 2014; 2017).

Continued

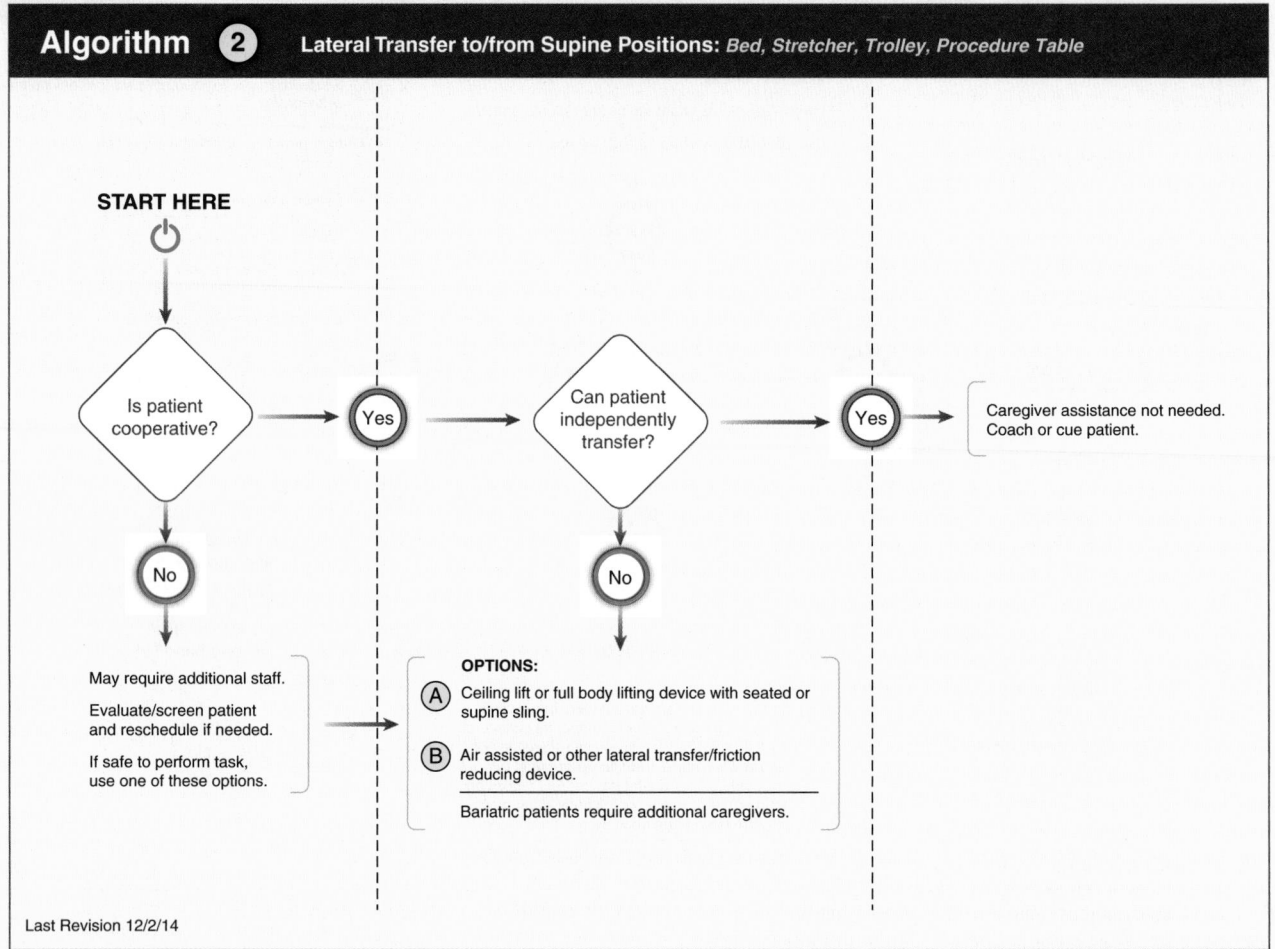

STEP 15 VHA safe patient handling and mobility algorithm 2. (From VHA: *Safe patient handling and mobility algorithms.* 2014 revision. Reprinted with permission of VISN 8 Patient Safety Center of Inquiry, Tampa, FL.)

STEP	RATIONALE
b. Allow patient to sit on the side of the bed for a few minutes. Have patient alternately flex and extend feet, and move lower legs up and down. Ask whether patient feels dizzy; if so, check blood pressure. Have patient relax and take a few deep breaths until dizziness subsides and balance is gained. If dizziness lasts more than 60 seconds, return patient to bed (Frith et al., 2014; Mills et al., 2014). Recheck blood pressure.	Allows patient's circulation to equilibrate to reduce chance of orthostatic hypotension.

CLINICAL DECISION: *Remain in front of patient until he or she regains balance and continue to provide physical support to weak or cognitively impaired patient.*

c. Have a chair in position at 45-degree angle with one side against bed, facing foot of bed. Place bed in low position or to point where patient's feet are comfortably flat on the floor with the hip and knees at a 90-degree angle. Be sure bed brakes are locked.	Positions chair for easy access. Provides patient stability when transferring.

CLINICAL DECISION: *If patient demonstrates weakness or paralysis of one side of the body, place chair on his or her strong side.*

STEP	RATIONALE
d. If patient is cooperative and able to bear weight and balance while standing, allow independent transfer, using stand-and-pivot technique with one caregiver (OSHA, 2017).	Caregiver is providing extra support for balance only, *not* for lifting.

CLINICAL DECISION: *Patient may use assist device during transfer.*

(1) Apply gait/transfer belt (see Skill 38.1).	Transfer belt allows you to maintain stability of patient during transfer and reduces risk for falling (Degelau et al., 2014).
(2) If not already in place, help patient apply stable, nonskid shoes/socks. If patient has a stronger leg, place it forward on floor, with weaker foot back.	Nonskid soles decrease risk for slipping during transfer. Always have patient wear nonskid shoes during transfer; bare feet increase risk for falls.
(3) Spread your feet apart. Flex hips and knees, aligning knees with patient's knees.	Ensures balance with wide base of support. Flexing knees and hips lowers your center of gravity to object that moves; aligning knees with those of patient stabilizes knees when patient stands.
(4) Grasp transfer belt along patient's sides (see illustration).	Transfer belt allows you to help patient move, keeping balance.

CLINICAL DECISION: *Patients should never be lifted with belt or by placing hands under their arms.*

(5) On count of three, instruct patient to stand while straightening hips and legs and keeping knees slightly flexed (see illustration). Make sure that your body weight is moving in the same direction as patient's to ensure that you and patient are moving in same direction simultaneously. Unless contraindicated, patient may be instructed to use hands to push up if applicable.	Coordinated movement allows patient to stand easily as you help to maintain his or her balance.
(6) Maintain patient's balance as you pivot foot farthest from chair and then help patient ease into chair. Have patient hold arm rest for support (see illustration).	Pivoting allows adequate space for patient to move. Ability of patient to stand can be enhanced as you provide assistance with balance.
(7) Assist patient to assume proper alignment in sitting position. Provide support for any weakened upper extremity. You can use a sling or lap board to support an injured or weakened arm.	Prevents injury to patient from poor body alignment.
(i) Proper alignment for sitting position: head is erect, and vertebrae are in straight alignment. Body weight is evenly distributed on buttocks and thighs. Thighs are parallel and in horizontal plane. Both feet are supported flat on floor, and ankles are comfortably flexed. A 2.5- to 5-cm (1- to 2-inch) space is maintained between edge of seat and popliteal space on posterior surface of knee.	Prevents stress on intravertebral joints. Prevents increased pressure over bony prominences and reduces damage to underlying musculoskeletal system.

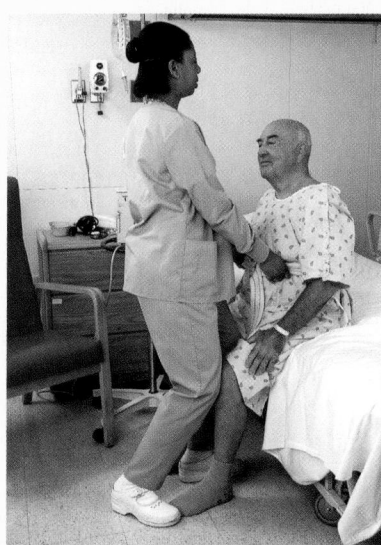 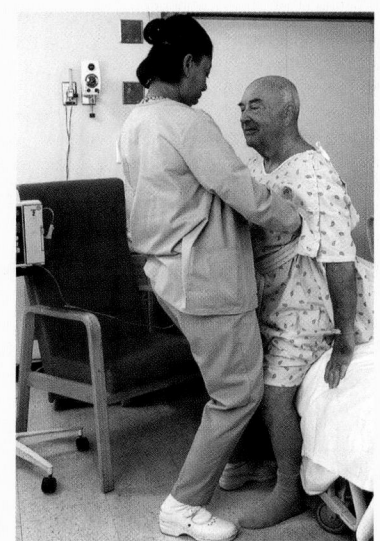 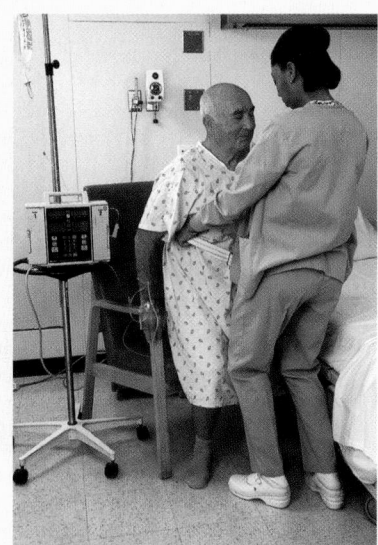

STEP 2d(4) Nurse flexes hips and knees, aligns knees with patient's knee, and grasps transfer belt palms up.

STEP 2d(5) Patient stands up at bedside before pivoting over to chair, bearing weight.

STEP 2d(6) Patient uses armrests to ease into chair.

Continued

SKILL 38.2   USING SAFE AND EFFECTIVE TRANSFER TECHNIQUES—cont'd

STEP	RATIONALE
e. If patient is unable to cooperate (regardless of ability to bear weight) or does not have sufficient upper or lower body strength, use ceiling, hydraulic floor, or power-driven lift (see illustration) to transfer patient from bed to chair (OSHA, 2017). Use a minimum of two to three caregivers. Follow algorithm and manufacturer lift guidelines.	Use of ceiling-mounted lifts is a popular choice because of availability of lift in a patient's room. Power driven mobile lift is especially good for ambulating obese patients for early mobility. The use of mechanical lift devices is strongly recommended to transfer a patient to reduce risk for musculoskeletal injury (Degelau et al., 2014). The use of a safe mobility algorithm aids caregivers in selecting mechanical lifts and transfer devices appropriately for safer transfers (OSHA, 2014, 2017).
(1) Bring mechanical or power mobile lift to bedside or lower the ceiling lift and position properly.	Ensures safe elevation of patient off bed.
(2) Be sure chair is available next to bed for easy access. Allow adequate space to maneuver the lift.	Prepares environment for safe use of lift and subsequent transfer of patient into chair.
(3) Raise bed to high position with mattress flat. Lower side rail on side near chair.	Allows you to use proper body mechanics while positioning patient in hammock.
(4) Have second nurse positioned at opposite side of bed.	Maintains patient safety, preventing fall from bed.
(5) Roll patient on side away from you.	Positions patient for placement of lift sling.
(6) Place the sling or harness on bed so that it aligns correctly with patient's trunk and legs; place it against patient's back.	There are several types of lift slings: hammock sling, commode sling, mesh bath sling, and padded sling with or without head support. Place sling under patient's center of gravity and greatest part of body weight.
(7) Roll patient back toward you as second nurse pulls sling or harness through.	Ensures that sling is in proper position before lift.
(8) Return patient to supine position. Be sure that harness or sling straps are smooth over bed surface. A sling should extend from shoulders to knees (hammock) to support patient's body weight equally.	Completes positioning of patient on mechanical/hydraulic sling.
(9) Remove patient's glasses if appropriate.	Swivel bar is close to patient's head and could break eyeglasses.
(10) Roll the base of floor lift under patient's bed (on side with chair).	Positions lift efficiently and promotes smooth transfer.
(11) Attach lower horizontal bar of ceiling lift to sling level by following manufacturer directions. Lock valve if required.	Positions lift close to patient. Locking valve on hydraulic lift prevents injury to patient.
(12) Attach sling to lift device using sewn-in loop straps, chains, or adjustable straps. Attach hooks on chain to holes in sling. Short chains or straps hook to top holes of sling; longer chains hook to bottom of sling (see manufacturer directions).	Secures hydraulic lift to sling. Be sure any hooks that attach to metal chains face away from patient's skin. Follow manufacturer's instructions for applying sling or harness.
(13) Elevate head of bed to Fowler's position.	Positions patient in sitting position.
(14) Have patient fold arms over chest.	Prevents injury to patient's arms during transfer.

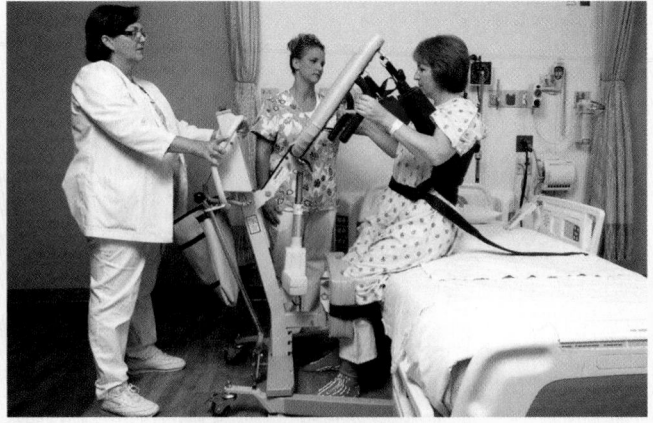

STEP 2e Patient grasps handles as nurse turns on motorized power lift.

STEP	RATIONALE
(15) For ceiling lift turn on control device to raise the patient off the bed (see illustration). If the lift is a nonelectric lift, then pump the hydraulic handle using long, slow, even strokes until patient is raised off bed (see illustration).	Ensures safe support of patient during elevation.
(16) Use lift to raise patient off bed and use steering handle to pull lift from bed as you and another nurse maneuver patient to chair. Have second nurse alongside patient.	Lifts patient off the bed safely; nurse's position reduces any risk of patient falling from sling.
(17) For a hydraulic lift, roll base of lift around chair. Release check valve slowly or push the button down and lower patient into chair (see manufacturer directions) (see illustration).	Positions lift in front of chair into which patient is to be transferred. Safely guides patient into back of chair as seat descends.
(18) Close check valve of hydraulic lift, if needed, as soon as patient is down in chair and straps can be released. Newer lifts may not need this step (see manufacturer's directions).	If valve is left open, boom may continue to lower and injure patient.
(19) For a ceiling lift, steer sling over chair and use power button to lower patient into chair (see manufacturer's directions).	Provides for easy lowering of patient.
(20) Remove lifting device from hammock or sling. Then roll mechanical/hydraulic lift out of patient's path.	Prevents damage to skin and underlying tissues.
(21) Check patient's sitting alignment and correct if necessary.	Prevents injury from poor posture.
3. Perform lateral transfer from bed to stretcher. (*Option:* Apply clean gloves if bed linen soiled.): Assist patient into supine position in bed with head of bed lowered as much as patient can tolerate. Raise bed to working height so that top of mattress is even with your elbows. Refer to mobility assessment findings and safe patient handling algorithm to confirm appropriateness to transfer patient and whether other caregivers are needed.	The three-person lift (using drawsheet) for horizontal transfer from bed to stretcher is no longer recommended and is discouraged (Anderson et al., 2014; OSHA, 2014). Physical stress can be decreased significantly by using slide board or friction-reducing board positioned under drawsheet beneath patient. If available, air lateral transfer devices require less caregiver force to maneuver and are more comfortable for the patient.

CLINICAL DECISION: *Lock brakes on bed and stretcher to prevent accidental patient fall.*

---

a. Can patient assist?	Patient's level of strength and weight determine level of help required for safe transfer. During any patient-transferring task, if any caregiver is required to lift more than 15.9 kg (35 lb) of patient's weight, patient is considered fully dependent, and an assist device is used (OSHA 2014, 2015).
(1) If patient can assist, caregiver is only needed to stand by for safety and coach patient in moving toward stretcher. Keep stretcher and bed locked as patient moves to stretcher.	Promotes patient safety.
(2) If patient is partially or not at all able to assist and is <91 kg (200 lb), use friction-reducing device or lateral transfer board.	Minimizes injury to skin as patient is laterally transferred.
(3) If patient is partially or not at all able to assist and is >91 kg (200 lb), use a ceiling lift with supine sling or a mechanical lateral transfer device with three caregivers.	Prevents need to pull patient if a lateral transfer board or device were to be used.

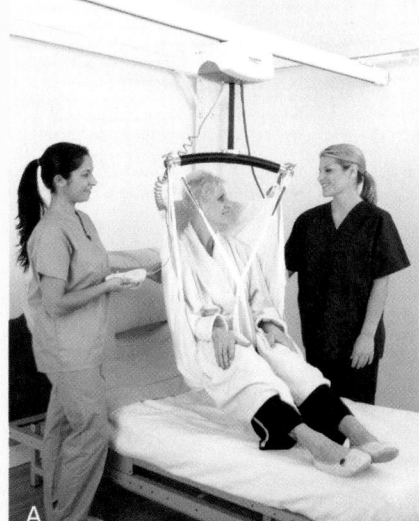
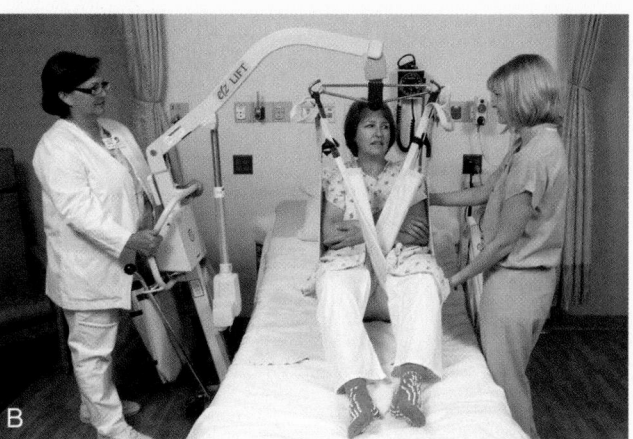

STEP 2e(15) A, Ceiling lift. (Courtesy Waverly Glen Systems, a Prism Medical Co.) **B,** Patient lifted in hydraulic lift above bed.

Continued

SKILL 38.2   **USING SAFE AND EFFECTIVE TRANSFER TECHNIQUES—cont'd**

STEP	RATIONALE
b. Lateral transfer with friction-reducing device—slide board (see illustration) or air assisted device:	Maintains alignment of spinal column. Ensures that bed does not move inadvertently.
(1) Cross patient's arms on chest.	Prevents injury to arms during transfer.
(2) Lower side rails. To place slide board/air-assisted device under patient, position two nurses on side of bed toward which patient will be turned. Position third nurse on other side of bed.	Distributes weight equally between nurses.
(3) Fanfold drawsheet on both sides of patient.	Provides strong handles to grip drawsheet without slipping.
(4) On count of three logroll patient onto side toward the two nurses. Turn patient as one unit with smooth, continuous motion.	Maintains body in alignment, preventing stress on any part.
(5) Place slide board on bed, against patient's back and under drawsheet (see illustration A). *Option:* Apply deflated air-assisted device (see illustration B).	Prevents friction from contact of skin with board.
(6) Gently roll patient back onto slide board/air-assisted device and draw sheet (see illustration A). For an air-assisted device, secure safety straps around patient (see illustration B).	Positions patient for transfer. Safety straps prevent patient fall.
(7) Line up stretcher so that surface is ½ inch lower than bed. Recheck locked brakes on stretcher. Instruct patient not to move.	Eases transfer. Ensures that stretcher does not move inadvertently during transfer.
(8) Two nurses position themselves on side of stretcher while third nurse positions self on side of bed without stretcher. All three nurses place feet widely apart with one foot slightly in front of the other and grasp slide board or friction-reducing device.	Ensures safety and distribution of weight during transfer.

CLINICAL DECISION: *A nurse may also be positioned at the head of patient's bed to protect and support his or her head and neck if patient is weak or unable to help.*

STEP	RATIONALE
(9) Ensure that bed brakes are locked.	Promotes patient comfort and safety.
(10) Holding fan-folded drawsheet and one nurse counting to three, the two nurses pull drawsheet across slide board, positioning patient onto stretcher (see illustration A). The third nurse holds slide board in place. *Option:* Inflate air-assisted device and slide patient across bed onto stretcher (see illustrations B and C).	Slide board remains stationary, provides slippery surface to reduce friction, and allows patient to transfer easily to stretcher.
(11) Position patient in center of stretcher. Raise head of stretcher if not contraindicated. Raise stretcher side rails. Cover patient with blanket.	Provides for patient comfort.
4. After transferring patient to bed or chair, be sure patient is positioned comfortably. Place nurse call system in an accessible location within patient's reach.	Ensures patient safety.
5. Raise side rails (as appropriate) and lower bed to lowest position.	Ensures patient safety.
6. Place nurse call system in accessible location.	Promotes patient safety.
7. Remove and dispose of gloves (if used) and perform hand hygiene.	Reduces transmission of microorganisms.

EVALUATION

1. Monitor vital signs. Ask whether patient feels dizzy or tired. Ask him or her to rate pain on pain scale.	Evaluates patient's response to postural changes and activity.
2. Note patient's behavioral response to transfer.	Reveals level of motivation and self-care potential.

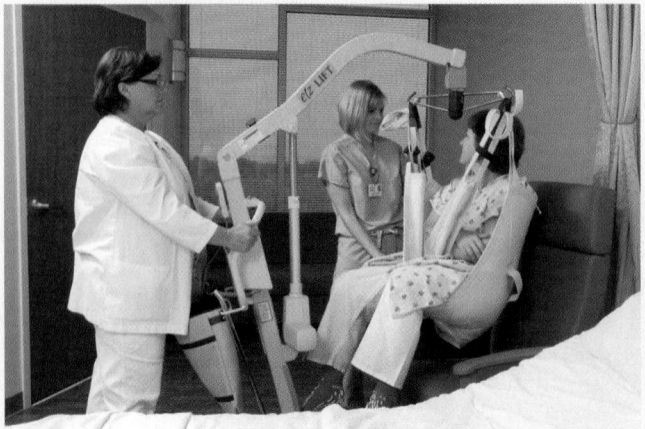

STEP 2e(17) Use of hydraulic lift to lower patient into chair.

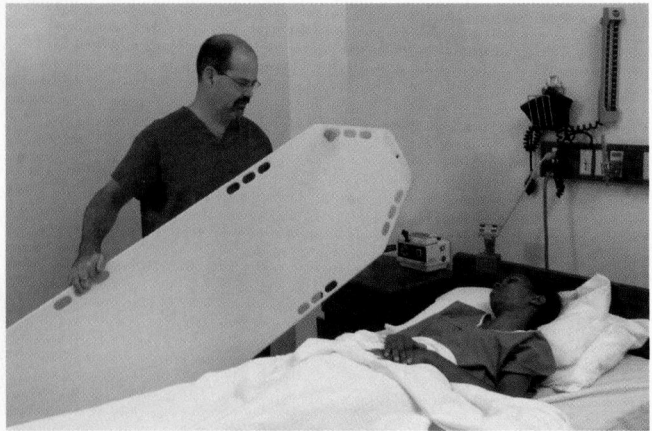

STEP 3b Slide board.

STEP	RATIONALE
3. **Use Teach-Back:** "I want to be sure I explained the steps we are going to use to transfer you to the chair. Tell me the steps you can take to make the transfer safe." Revise your instruction now or develop a plan for revised patient/family caregiver teaching if patient/family caregiver is not able to teach back correctly.	Determines patient's/family caregiver's level of understanding of instructional topic.

UNEXPECTED OUTCOMES AND RELATED INTERVENTIONS

1. Patient is unable to comprehend or is unwilling to follow directions for transfer.
   - Reassess continuity and simplicity of your instruction.
   - If patient is tired or in pain, allow for rest period before transferring.
   - Consider medicating for pain before the next transfer, if indicated.
   - Consider using hydraulic lift.
2. Patient sustains injury on transfer.
   - Evaluate incident that led to injury (e.g., inadequate assessment, change in patient status, improper use of equipment, lack of assistive personnel).
   - Complete incident report according to agency policy.
3. Patient is unable to stand for time required to transfer to chair.
   - Consider use of hydraulic or power lift.

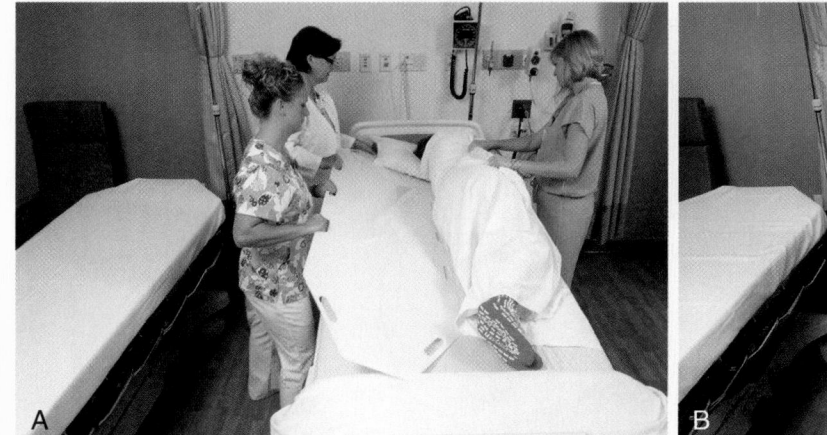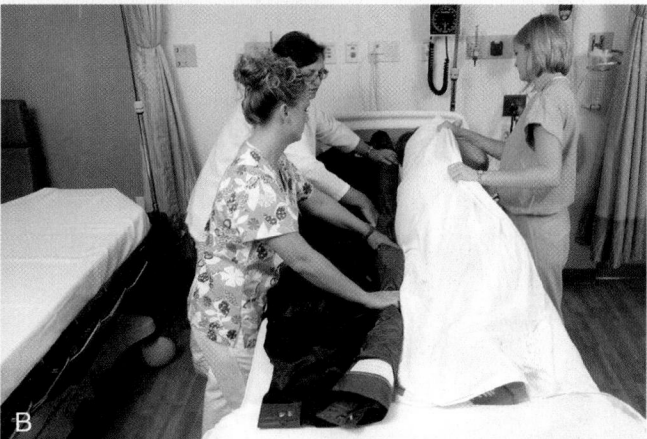

STEP 3b(5) A, Two caregivers placing slide board under drawsheet and patient. **B,** Two caregivers placing air-assisted device under drawsheet and patient.

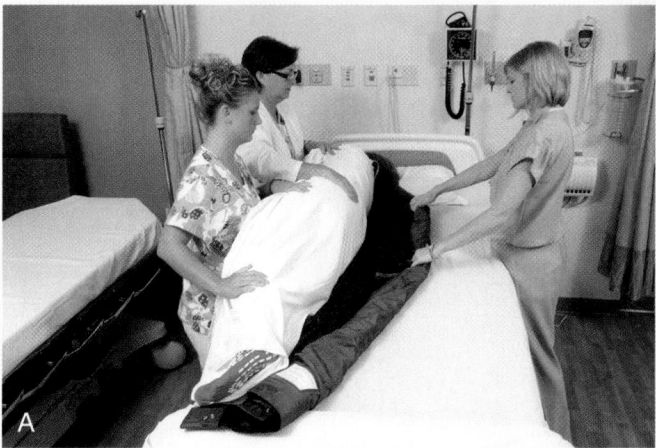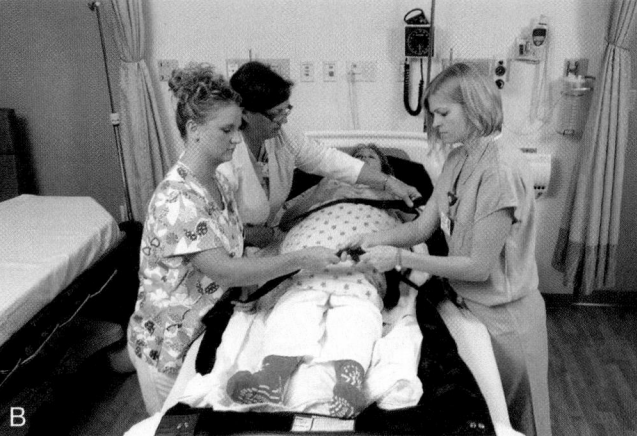

STEP 3b(6) A, Patient rolls to opposite side, while other caregiver unrolls air-assisted device. **B,** Secure safety straps over patient on air-assisted device.

Continued

SKILL 38.2   **USING SAFE AND EFFECTIVE TRANSFER TECHNIQUES—cont'd**

RECORDING AND REPORTING

- Record procedure, including pertinent observations: strength/weakness, ability to follow directions, weight-bearing ability or restrictions, balance, ability to pivot, use of assistive devices or lifts, number of personnel needed to assist, amount of assistance (muscle strength) required, and patient's tolerance to transfer.
- Document your evaluation of patient learning.
- Report transfer ability and assistance needed (including personnel and assist devices) to caregivers on next shift.
- Report progress or remission to rehabilitation staff (physical therapist, occupational therapist).

HOME CARE CONSIDERATIONS

- Teach family how to use safe patient handling equipment if necessary.
- Teach patient and family about the importance of safety while helping patients with mobility.

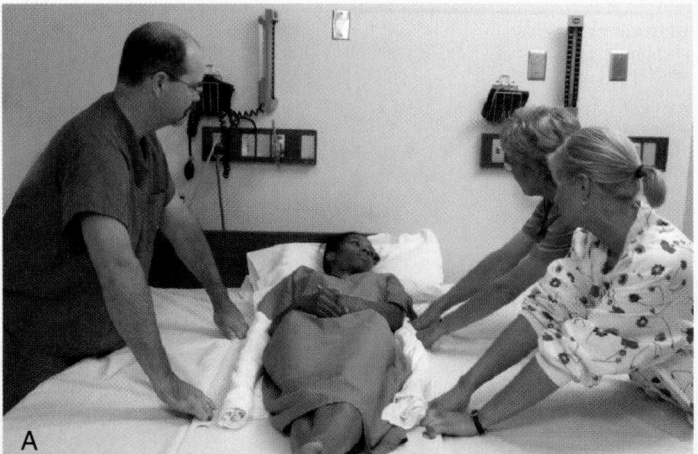

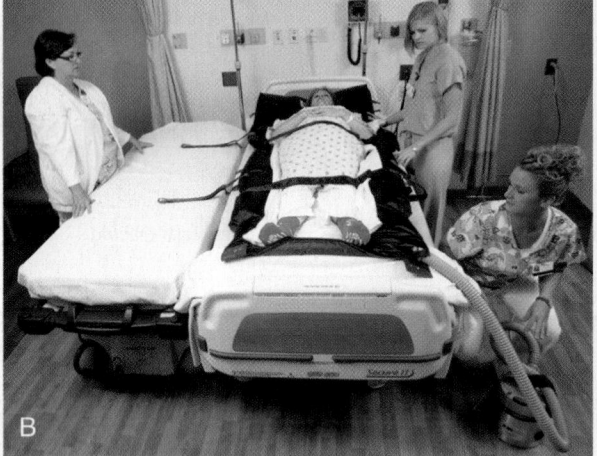
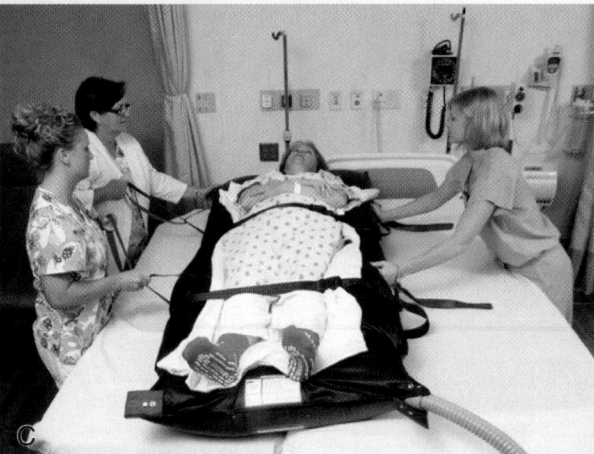

STEP 3b(10) A, Transfer of patient to stretcher using slide board. **B,** Inflating air-assisted transfer device.
C, Transfer of patient using air-assisted transfer device.

KEY POINTS

- The musculoskeletal and nervous systems work in coordination to maintain balance, posture, and body alignment during lifting, bending, moving, and activities of daily living.
- An active lifestyle is important for maintaining and promoting health by enhancing the function of all body systems.
- Nurses intervene to increase inpatients' activity and mobility levels as soon as possible following illness or surgery to prevent deconditioning and other complications, including deep vein thrombosis.
- The use of proper transfer and lift devices and positioning techniques that use a patient's strength as well as proper ergonomics by a health care provider reduces patient injury and work-related injuries involving nurses
- Factors that will influence an exercise program include developmental stages, behavioral aspects, environmental issues, family and social supports, and cultural and ethnic influences.
- Assessment of a patient's verbal report of fatigue and weakness, ability to ambulate, and ability to perform activities of daily living, along with vital signs, determines activity tolerance.
- Helping patients plan for daily exercise, including moderate intensity aerobic activity, improves exercise tolerance.
- Ensuring the use of safe patient handling techniques to minimize manual lifting of patients reduces patient and health care provider injury and improves patient outcomes.
- Ensuring that a patient is safe during assisted ambulation requires you to use a gait belt, to stand on the correct side by the patient, and to monitor the patient's tolerance to walking.
- Comparisons with baseline measures that include pulse, blood pressure, oxygen saturation (when available), strength, fatigue, and psychological well-being determine a patient's response to transferring.

REFLECTIVE LEARNING

- Review your own exercise routines, and compare your activity with what is recommended by the *Physical Activity Guidelines for Americans*. What might you do differently?
- Reflect on a recent patient experience in which a patient needed to perform an activity but was unable to because of voiced complaints of pain. Describe what interventions you implemented.
- Recall any challenges you have recently had in transferring patients to a chair or stretcher, and describe the safe patient handling techniques you applied.

REVIEW QUESTIONS

1. A nurse is instructing a patient who has decreased leg strength on the left side on how to use a cane. Which actions indicate proper cane use by the patient? (Select all that apply.)
   1. The patient keeps the cane on the left side of the body.
   2. The patient slightly leans to one side while walking.
   3. The patient keeps two points of support on the floor at all times.
   4. After the patient places the cane forward, he or she then moves the right leg forward to the cane.
   5. The patient places the cane forward 15 to 25 cm (6 to 10 inches) with each step.
2. A patient is experiencing some problems with joint stability in the right leg. The doctor has prescribed crutches for the patient to use while being allowed to bear weight only on the left leg. Which of the following gaits should the patient be taught to use?

1. Four-point
2. Three-point
3. Two-point
4. Swing-through

3. Which of the following motivates a patient to participate in an exercise program? (Select all that apply.)
   1. Providing a patient with a pamphlet on exercise
   2. Providing information to the patient when he or she is ready to change behavior
   3. Explaining the importance of exercise at the time of diagnosis of a chronic disease
   4. Having a structured daily plan that incorporates physical activity
   5. Having support from significant other to engage in exercise
4. Which of the following is the proper sequence for a four-point crutch gait?

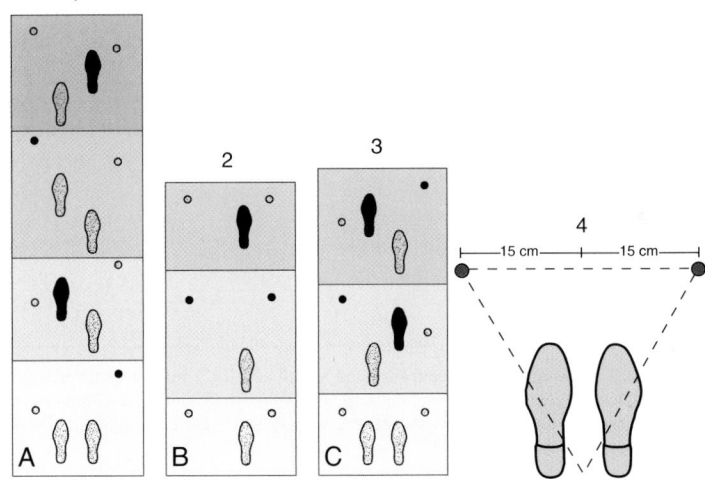

5. The nurse is caring for an older adult in a long-term care setting. The nurse reviews the medical record to find that the patient has progressive loss of total bone mass. The patient's history and tendency to take smaller steps with feet kept closer together will most likely result in which of the following?
   1. Increase the patient's risk for falls and injuries
   2. Result in less stress on the patient's joints
   3. Decrease the amount of work required for patient movement
   4. Allow for mobility in spite of the aging effects on the patient's joints
6. Place in the correct order the steps needed (below) to transfer a patient with sufficient lower body strength to a chair.
   1. On count of three, instruct patient to stand while straightening hips and legs and keeping knees slightly flexed.
   2. Assist patient to assume proper alignment in sitting position.
   3. Help patient apply stable, nonskid shoes/socks.
   4. Spread your feet apart. Flex hips and knees, aligning knees with patient's knees.
   5. Apply gait/transfer belt.
   6. Maintain patient's balance as you pivot foot farthest from chair and then help patient ease into chair.
   7. Grasp transfer belt along patient's sides.
7. Before transferring a patient from the bed to a stretcher, which assessment data does the nurse need to gather? (Select all that apply.)
   1. Patient's weight
   2. Patient's activity tolerance
   3. Patient's level of mobility

4. Recent laboratory values
5. Nutritional intake

8. Which of the following indicates that additional assistance is needed to transfer a patient from the bed to the stretcher? (Select all that apply.)
   1. The patient is 5 feet, 6 inches and weighs 120 lb.
   2. The patient speaks and understands English.
   3. The patient is returning to unit from recovery room after a procedure requiring conscious sedation.
   4. The patient has a history of being able to stand independently.
   5. The patient received analgesia for pain 30 minutes ago.

9. A 51-year-old adult comes to a medical clinic for an annual physical exam. The patient is found to be slightly overweight and reports being inactive, walking only 2 to 3 times a week with his wife after work. He has good muscle strength and coordination of lower extremities. Which of the following recommendations from the *Physical Activity Guidelines for Americans* should the nurse suggest? Choose all that apply
   1. Move more and sit less throughout the day.
   2. Participate in at least 90 minutes a week of moderate-intensity aerobic physical activity.

3. Perform muscle-strengthening activities using light weights on 2 or more days a week.
4. Walk at a vigorous pace with wife at least 150 minutes over five days a week.
5. Focus on balance training.

10. Family members have asked for a meeting with the nursing staff of an assisted-living residential center to discuss the feasibility of their mother using a walker. The family is worried that her health is declining; they wonder whether she can use the walker safely. Which of the following instructions should the nurse give the family after assessing that it is safe for the woman to use a walker? (Select all that apply.)
    1. A walker is useful for patients who have impaired balance.
    2. The patient uses a walker by pushing the device forward.
    3. Leaning over the walker improves the patient's balance.
    4. Walkers should not be used on stairs.
    5. If the patient has difficulty advancing the walker, a walker with wheels is an option.

Answers: 1. 3, 5; **2.** 2, 3; **4.** 2, 4, 5; **4.** 1, 5; **6.** 1, 6, 5; **3.** 4, 7; **1.** 6, 2, 7; **1.** 2, 3; **8.** 3, 5; **9.** 1, 3, 4; **10.** 1, 4, 5.

Rationales for Review Questions can be found on the Evolve website.

REFERENCES

American Academy of Orthopaedist Surgeons: *How to use crutches, canes, and walkers,* 2015. http://orthoinfo.aaos.org/topic.cfm?topic=A00181. Accessed December 2015.

American Association of Critical Care Nurses (AACN): *Early progressive mobility protocol,* 2013. https://www.aacn.org/docs/EventPlanning/WB0007/Mobility-Protocol-szh4mr5a.pdf. http://orthoinfo.aaos.org/topic.cfm?topic=A00181. Accessed May 29, 2019.

American College of Foot & Ankle Surgeons: *Crutch use,* 2020. https://www.foothealthfacts.org/conditions/crutch-use. Accessed January 16, 2020.

American Heart Association (AHA): *Target heart rates,* 2015. http://www.heart.org/HEARTORG/HealthyLiving/PhysicalActivity/FitnessBasics/%3Cbr/%3ETarget-Heart-Rates_UCM_434341_Article.jsp#.XLs9AOTsZPY. Accessed April 20, 2019.

American Heart Association (AHA): *American Heart Association recommendations for physical activity in adults,* 2018. http://www.heart.org/HEARTORG/GettingHealthy/PhysicalActivity/FitnessBasics/American-Heart-Association-Recommendations-for-Physical-Activity-in-Adults_UCM_307976_Article.jsp#.VkjC8aSFOpo. Accessed April 20, 2019.

Anderson MP, et al.: Safe moving and handling of patients: an interprofessional approach, *Nurs Stand* 28(46):37, 2014.

Association of periOperative Registered Nurses (AORN): Guideline summary: prevention of venous thromboembolism, *AORN J* 107(6):750, 2018.

Bandura A: Guide for constructing self-efficacy scales. In Pajares F, Urdan T, editors: *Self-efficacy beliefs of adolescents,* Charlotte, NC, 2006, Information Age Publishing.

Boynton T, et al.: Implementing a mobility assessment tool for nurses: a nurse-driven assessment tool reveals the patient's mobility level and guides SPHM technology choices, *Am Nurse Today* 9(9):13, 2014a. https://americannursetoday.com/wp-content/uploads/2014/09/ant9-Patient-Handling-Supplement-821a_Implementing.pdf. Accessed April 13, 2019.

Centers for Disease Control and Prevention (CDC): What is health literacy?. 2019. https://www.cdc.gov/healthliteracy/learn/index.html. Accessed December 23, 2019.

Centers for Disease Control and Prevention: *Worksite physical activity,* 2017. https://www.cdc.gov/physicalactivity/worksite-pa/index.htm. Accessed April 13, 2019.

Centers for Disease Control and Prevention (CDC): *Adult obesity facts,* 2018. https://www.cdc.gov/obesity/data/adult.html. Accessed April 19, 2019.

Centers for Disease Control and Prevention (CDC): *Physical activity,* 2019a. https://www.cdc.gov/physicalactivity. Accessed September 17, 2019.

Centers for Disease Control and Prevention (CDC): *Physical Activity Basics: How much physical activity do adults need?,* 2019b. https://www.cdc.gov/physicalactivity/basics/adults. Accessed September 17, 2019.

Colberg S, et al.: American Diabetes Association (ADA): Physical activity/exercise and diabetes: a position statement of the American Diabetes Association, *Diabetes Care* 39(11):2065, 2016.

Covan EK: Benefits of exercise for body, mind, and spirit, *Health Care Women Int* 36(3):255, 2015.

Degelau J, et al.: *Institute for Clinical Systems Improvement (ICSI): Prevention of falls (acute care): health care protocol,* Bloomington, MN, 2014, Institute for Clinical Systems Improvement.

Dutton M: *Introduction to physical therapy and patient skills,* New York, 2014, McGraw Hill.

Edelman CL, Kudzma EC: *Health promotion throughout the life span,* ed 9, St Louis, 2018, Mosby.

Fairchild SL, et al.: *Pierson & Fairchild's principles & techniques of patient care,* ed 6, St. Louis, 2018, Elsevier.

Fedorowski A, Melander O: Syndromes of orthostatic intolerance: a hidden danger, *J Intern Med* 273(4):322, 2013.

Frith J, et al.: Measuring and defining orthostatic hypotension in the older person, *Age Aging* 43(2):168, 2014.

Hashem MD, et al.: Early mobilization and rehabilitation in the ICU: moving back to the future, *Respir Care* 61(7):971, 2016.

Hegde SM, Solomon SD: Influence of physical activity on hypertension and cardiac structure and function, *Curr Hypertens Rep* 17(10):77, 2015.

Kanaskie ML, Snyder C: Nurses and nursing assistants decision-making regarding use of safe patient handling and mobility technology: a qualitative study, *Appl Nurs Res* 39:141, 2018.

Kwun S, et al.: Prevention and treatment of postmenopausal osteoporosis, *Obstet Gynaecol* 14:251, 2012.

LaMorte WW: *Behavioral change models: the Transtheoretical Model (stages of change),* Boston University School of Public Health, 20182018. http://sphweb.bumc.bu.edu/otlt/MPH-Modules/SB/BehavioralChangeTheories/BehavioralChangeTheories6.html. Accessed April 20, 2019.

Martin M, et al.: *New and improved VA algorithms,* 2014. http://www.asphp.org/wp-content/uploads/2016/06/New-and-Improved-VA-Algorithms-and-New-SPHM-App-ASPHP-rev-MMM.pptx. Accessed May 25, 2019.

Matz M: Patient handling and mobility assessments, ed 2, The Facility Guidelines Institute, 2019. http://www.fgiguidelines.org/wp-content/uploads/2019/10/FGI-Patient-Handling-and-Mobility-Assessments_191008.pdf. Accessed January 2, 2020.

McCance KL, Huether SE: *Pathophysiology: the biologic basis for disease in adults and children,* ed 8, St Louis, 2017, Mosby.

Mills P, et al.: Five things to know about orthostatic hypotension in the older adult, *J Am Geriatr Soc* 62(9):1822, 2014.

Myszenski A: *The essential role of lab values and vital signs in clinical decision making and patient safety for the acutely ill patient,* 2014. https://www.physicaltherapy.com/articles/essential-role-lab-values-and-3637. Accessed 19 September 2019.

National Heart, lung, and blood institute (NHLBI): *DASH eating plan,* n.d.a., https://www.nhlbi.nih.gov-/health-topics/dash-eating-plan. Accessed May 1, 2019.

National Institutes of Health (NIH): *Osteoporosis and related bone diseases national resource center: exercise for your bone health,* 2018. https://www.bones.nih.gov-/health-info/bone/bone-health/exercise/exercise-your-bone-health. Accessed May 20, 2019.

National Institutes of Health (NIH): *Go for life: improve your strength,* n.d. https://go4life.nia.nih.gov/exercises/strength. Accessed November 16, 2017.

National Institute for Occupational Safety and Health (NIOSH): *Safe patient handling and mobility (SPHM),* 2016. http://www.cdc.gov/niosh/topics/safepatient. Accessed April 17, 2019.

Nelson A, Baptiste AS: Evidence-based practices for safe patient handling and movement, *Orthop Nurs* 25(6): 366, 2006. Manuscript 3.

Nystoriak MA, et al.: Cardiovascular effects and benefits of exercise, *Front Cardiovasc Med* 5:135, 2018.

Noble NL, Sweeney NL: Barriers to the use of assistive devices in patient handling, *Workplace Health Saf* 66(1):41–48, 2018.

Occupational Safety and Health Association (OSHA): *Safe patient handling—preventing musculoskeletal disorders in nursing homes,* OSHA Publication, 2014, p 3708. https://www.osha.gov/Publications/OSHA3708.pdf. Accessed April 29, 2019.

Occupational Safety and Health Administration (OSHA): *Worker safety in hospitals,* OSHA Publication, 2015.

https://www.osha.gov/dsg/hospitals/. Accessed May 26, 2019.

Occupational Safety and Health Administration (OSHA): *Handling with care: practicing safe patient handling,* 2017. https://www.jcrinc.com/assets/1/7/Pages_from_ECN_20_2017_08-2.pdf. Accessed May 25, 2019.

Office of Disease Prevention and Health Promotion: 2018 Physical Activity Guidelines Advisory Committee Scientific Report, Chapter 5: *Cardiometabolic health and prevention of weight gain,* 2018. https://health.gov/paguidelines/second-edition/report/pdf/11_F-5_Cardiometabolic_Health_and_Prevention_of_Weight_Gain.pdf. Accessed May 1, 2019.

Patton KT: *Anatomy & physiology,* ed 10, St Louis, 2019, Elsevier.

Resnick B, et al.: *Restorative care nursing for older adults: a guide for all care settings,* ed 2, New York, 2012, Springer.

Saffer H, et al.: Racial, ethnic, and gender differences in physical activity, *J Hum Cap* 7(4):378, 2013.

Schofield PA: The assessment and management of peri-operative pain in older adults, *Anaesthesia* 69(Suppl 1):54, 2014.

Shibao C, et al.: Evaluation and treatment of orthostatic hypotension, *J Am Soc Hypertens* 7(4):317, 2013.

The Joint Commission (TJC): 2020 *National Patient Safety Goals,* Oakbrook Terrace, IL, 2020, The Commission. https://www.jointcommission.org/en/standards/national-patient-safety-goals/. Accessed January 2, 2020.

Touhy T, Jett K: *Ebersole and Hess' gerontological nursing and healthy aging,* ed 5, St Louis, 2018. Elsevier.

US Department of Health and Human Services (USDHHS): *Physical activity guidelines for Americans,* Office of Disease Prevention and Health Promotion, 2019. https://health.gov/paguidelines/second-edition/. Accessed April 19, 2019.

US Department of Veterans Affairs: *Safe patient handling and mobility,* 2016. https://www.publichealth.va.gov-/employeehealth/patient-handling/index.asp. Accessed April 17, 2019.

Washington University Physicians: *How to fit and use crutches,* Washington University Orthopedics, 20172017. https://www.ortho.wustl.edu/content/Education/3628/Patient-Education/Educational-Materials/How-to-Fit-and-Use-Crutches.aspx. Accessed May 24, 2019.

Waters TR: When is it safe to manually lift a patient? The revised NIOSH lifting equation provides support for recommended weight limits, *Am J Nurs* 107(8):53, 2007.

Watson KB, et al.: Physical inactivity among adults aged 50 years and older — United States, 2014, *MMWR Morb Mortal Wkly Rep* 65(36):954, 2016.

RESEARCH REFERENCES

Adams ML: Differences between younger and older US adults with multiple chronic conditions, *Centers for Disease Control and Prevention: Preventing Chronic Disease* Vol. 14, September 7, 2017. https://www.cdc.gov/pcd/Issues/2017/16_0613.htm. Accessed April 18, 2019.

American Academy of Nursing (AAN): The twenty-five things nurses and patients should question. , http://www.aannet.org/initiatives/choosing-wisely, 2015. Accessed September 15, 2019.

Anandacoomarasamy A, et al.: The impact of obesity on the musculoskeletal system, *Int J Obes* 32(2):211, 2008.

Boynton T, et al.: Banner Mobility Assessment Tool for nurses: instrument validation, *Am J SPHM* 4(3):86, 2014b.

Bruning RS, Sturek M: Benefits of exercise training on coronary blood flow in coronary artery disease patients, *Prog Cardiovasc Dis* 57(5):443, 2015.

Chimen M et al.: What are the health benefits of physical activity in type 1 diabetes mellitus? A literature review, *Diabetologia* 55(3):542, 2012.

Dickinson S, et al.: Integrating a standardized mobility program and safe patient handling, *Crit Care Nurs Q* 41(3):240, 2018.

Healthy People 2020: Physical activity, Office of Disease Prevention and Health Promotion, 2019. http://www.healthypeople.gov/2020/topics-objectives/topic/physical-activity. Accessed April 20, 2019.

Hodgson CL, et al.: Early mobilization and recovery in mechanically ventilated patients in the ICU: a bi-national, multi-centre, prospective cohort study, *Crit Care* 19:81, 2015.

Hodgson CL, et al.: Early mobilization of patients in intensive care: organization, communication and safety factors that influence translation into clinical practice, *Crit Care* 22(1):77, 2018.

Kim K, et al.: Relationship between mobility and self-care activity in children with cerebral palsy, *Ann Rehabil Med* 41(2):266, 2017.

King L: Developing a progressive mobility activity protocol, *Orthop Nurs* 31(5):253, 2012.

Lavidan A, et al.: Fear of falling in community-dwelling older adults: a cause of falls, a consequence, or both? *PLoS One* 13(5):e0197792, 2018. https://journals.plos.org/plosone/article?id=10.1371/journal.pone.0194967. Accessed April 2019.

Lin P, et al.: Prevalence, characteristics, and work-related risk factors of low back pain among hospital nurses in Taiwan: a cross-sectional survey, *Int J Occup Environ Health* 25(1):41, 2012.

Lo HM, et al.: A Tai Chi exercise programme improved exercise behavior and reduced blood pressure in outpatients with hypertension, *Int J Nurs Pract* 18(6):545, 2012.

McArthur D, et al.: Factors influencing adherence to regular exercise in middle-aged women: a qualitative study to inform clinical practice, *BMC Womens Health* 14:49, 2014.

Musich S, et al.: The impact of mobility limitations on health outcomes among older adults, *Geriatr Nurs* 39(2):162, 2018.

National Heart, Lung, and Blood Institute: *Pulmonary rehabilitation,* n.d.b. https://www.nhlbi.nih.gov/health-topics/pulmonary-rehabilitation. Accessed May 24, 2019.

O'Donoghue G, et al.: Socio-economic determinants of physical activity across the life course: a "DEterminants of DIet and Physical ACtivity" (DEDIPAC) umbrella literature review, *PLoS One* 13(1):e0190737, 2018.

Pinto RM, et al.: Basic and genetic aspects of food intake control and obesity: role of dopamine receptor D2 TAQIA polymorphism, *Obes Res Open J* 2:119, 2016.

Pinto RM, et al.: Physical activity: benefits for prevention and treatment of childhood obesity, *J Child Obes* 3(S2-003), 2018. http://childhood-obesity.imedpub.com/physical-activity-benefits-for-prevention-and-treatment-of-childhood-obesity.pdf. Accessed April 19, 2019.

Scarton LJ, et al.: Emotional and behavioral aspects of diabetes in American Indians/Alaska Natives: a systematic literature review, *Health Educ Behav* 44(1):70, 2017.

Shieh C, et al.: Association of self-efficacy and self-regulation with nutrition and exercise behaviors in a community sample of adults, *J Community Health Nurs* 32(4):199, 2015.

Skinner AC, Skelton JA: Prevalence and trends in obesity and severe obesity among children in the United States, 1999-2012, *JAMA Pediatr* 168(6):561, 2014.

Sluik D, et al.: Physical activity and mortality in individuals with diabetes mellitus: a prospective study and meta-analysis, *Arch Intern Med* 172(17):1285, 2012.

Smith GL et al.: The association between social support and physical activity in older adults: a systematic review, *Int J Behav Nutr Phys Act* 14(1):56, 2017.

Tampa VA Research and Education Foundation, Inc. (TVAREF): *VHA safe patient handling and mobility algorithms (2016 revision).* http://www.tampavaref.org/safe-patient-handling.htm.

Tipping CJ, et al.: The effects of active mobilisation and rehabilitation in ICU on mortality and function: a systematic review, *Intensive Care Med* 43:171, 2017.

Tomita Y, et al.: Prevalence of fear of falling and associated factors among Japanese community-dwelling older adults, *Medicine (Baltimore)* 97(4):e9721, 2018.

Tsang M, et al.: Examination of the readiness to learn and the best teaching method regarding health education and promotion within the Chinese elderly population, *Nurs Res* 64(2), 2015.

Walia S, et al.: Early mobilization in the ICU: assessing a standardized early mobility protocol on neurological patients, *Neurology* 90(Suppl 15), 2018.

Immobility

OBJECTIVES

- Discuss physiological and pathological influences on mobility.
- Identify changes in physiological and psychosocial function associated with immobility.
- Assess for correct and impaired body alignment and mobility.
- Formulate appropriate nursing diagnoses for patients with impaired mobility.
- Develop individualized nursing care plans for patients with impaired mobility.
- Describe interventions for improving or maintaining patients' mobility.
- Discuss a nurse's role in the prevention of deep vein thrombosis in patients with reduced mobility.
- Evaluate patient outcomes for improving or maintaining mobility.

KEY TERMS

Activity tolerance p. 830
Atelectasis, p. 823
Bed rest, p. 823
Body alignment, p. 821
Body mechanics, p. 820
Disuse osteoporosis, p. 824
Embolus, p. 832
Footdrop, p. 824
Friction, p. 821
Gait, p. 830
Hemiparesis, p. 846
Hemiplegia, p. 846

Hypostatic pneumonia, p. 824
Immobility, p. 823
Instrumental activities of daily living (IADLs), p. 846
Joint contracture, p. 824
Mobility, p. 823
Muscle atrophy, p. 822
Negative nitrogen balance, p. 823
Orthostatic hypotension, p. 824
Osteoporosis, p. 824
Pathological fractures, p. 821
Pressure injury, p. 825

Range of motion (ROM), p. 826
Renal calculi, p. 825
Shear, p. 821
Thrombus, p. 824
Trapeze bar, p. 844
Trochanter roll, p. 843
Urinary stasis, p. 825
Venous thromboembolism (VTE) p. 832
Virchow's triad, p. 832

MEDIA RESOURCES

http://evolve.elsevier.com/Potter/fundamentals/
- Review Questions
- Video Clips
- Concept Map Creator
- Case Study with Questions

- Audio Glossary
- Content Updates
- Answers to QSEN Activity and Review Questions
- Skills Performance Checklists

Optimized mobility correlates with positive patient outcomes. People are mobile for performing working and leisure tasks and for communicating emotions and nonverbal gestures. Mobility is also essential for self-defense, activities of daily living (ADLs), and recreational activities. Many functions of the body depend on mobility. Intact musculoskeletal and nervous systems are necessary for optimal physical mobility and functioning (see Chapter 38). When patients lose the ability to remain mobile and active, you apply scientific and nursing knowledge and skills to provide appropriate and competent care.

SCIENTIFIC KNOWLEDGE BASE

Nature of Movement

Chapter 38 describes in detail the nature of movement—how muscles, bones, and the nervous system coordinate together to create movement. As a nurse you need to consider how each patient's physical and psychological conditions affect body movement, including balance,

body alignment, posture, and physical activity. Knowing how patients initiate movement and understanding your own movements require a basic understanding of the physics surrounding body mechanics. Body mechanics describes the coordinated efforts of the musculoskeletal and nervous systems. The body mechanics applied in the lifting and positioning techniques historically used in nursing practice often cause debilitating injuries to nurses and other health care staff (Kanaskie and Snyder, 2018; Noble and Sweeney, 2018). Today nurses use evidence-based information about body alignment, balance, gravity, and friction when positioning patients, determining the risk of patient falls, and selecting the safest way to move or transfer patients (AORN, 2018) (see Chapter 38).

Implications of Impaired Mobility. Changes affecting the normal coordination of the musculoskeletal and nervous systems place patients at risk for numerous health-related problems. Understanding the physiology of these changes prepares you to better anticipate problems, implement prevention strategies, and also intervene proactively when problems do develop.

Balance and Alignment. Correct body alignment reduces strain on musculoskeletal structures, aids in maintaining adequate muscle tone, promotes comfort, and contributes to balance and conservation of energy. Without balance control the center of gravity is displaced. Individuals require balance for maintaining a static position (e.g., sitting) and moving (e.g., walking). Disease, injury, pain, physical development (e.g., age), and life changes (e.g., pregnancy) compromise the ability to remain balanced. Medications that cause dizziness and prolonged immobility affect balance. Impaired balance is a major threat to mobility and physical safety and contributes to a fear of falling and self-imposed activity restrictions (Dickinson, et al.,2018; Musich et al., 2018)

Gravity and Friction. Weight is the force exerted on a body by gravity. The force of weight is always directed downward, which is why an unbalanced object falls. Unsteady patients fall if their center of gravity becomes unbalanced because of the gravitational pull on their weight. Patients who are at risk for being unsteady require the use of safe patient-handling techniques (see Chapter 38).

Patient lifting is now discouraged. To lift safely the lifter has to overcome the weight of the object and know its center of gravity. In symmetrical inanimate objects the center of gravity is at the exact center of the object. However, people are not geometrically perfect; their centers of gravity are usually at 55% to 57% of standing height and are in the midline, which is why choosing to use only the principles of body mechanics in lifting patients often leads to injury of a nurse or other health care professional (see Chapter 38).

Friction is a force that occurs in a direction to oppose movement. The greater the surface area of the object that is moved, the greater the friction. A larger object produces greater resistance to movement. In addition, the force exerted against the skin while the skin remains stationary and the bony structures move is called shear. Unfortunately a common example is when the head of a hospital bed is elevated beyond 60 degrees and gravity pulls a patient so that the bony skeleton moves toward the foot of the bed while the skin remains against the sheets. The blood vessels in the underlying tissue are stretched and damaged, resulting in impeded blood flow to the deep tissues. Ultimately pressure injuries often develop within the undermined tissue; the surface tissue appears less affected (see Chapter 48). To decrease surface area and reduce friction when patients are unable to assist with moving up in bed, use ergonomic assistive devices such as a full-body hydraulic lift. The lift moves a patient off the surface of a bed, thereby preventing friction, tearing, or shearing his or her delicate skin, and protects you and other health care staff from injury (Noble and Sweeney, 2018).

Skeletal System. The skeletal system provides attachments for muscles and ligaments and the leverage necessary for mobility. Bones are important for mobilization because they are firm, rigid, and elastic. The aging process, as well as some nutritional and disease processes, has the potential to change the components of bone, which impacts mobility.

Firmness in bones results from inorganic salts such as calcium and phosphate that are in the bone matrix. It is related to the rigidity of the bone, which is necessary to keep long bones straight, and enables bones to withstand weight-bearing. Elasticity and skeletal flexibility change with age. Chapter 38 describes developmental changes in the musculoskeletal system.

The skeletal system protects vital organs (e.g., the skull around the brain and the ribs around the heart and lungs) and aids in calcium regulation. Bones store calcium and release it into the circulation as needed. Patients who have decreased calcium regulation and metabolism and who are immobile are at risk for developing osteoporosis and pathological fractures (fractures caused by weakened bone tissue).

In addition, the internal structure of long bones contains bone marrow, participates in red blood cell (RBC) production, and acts as a reservoir for blood. Patients with altered bone marrow function or diminished RBC production tire easily because of reduced hemoglobin and oxygen-carrying ability. This fatigue decreases their mobility and increases the risk for falling.

Joints. The region where two or more bones attach is referred to as a joint. Each joint is classified according to its structure and degree of mobility (see Chapter 38).

Ligaments, Tendons, and Cartilage. Ligaments are white shiny, flexible bands of fibrous tissue that bind joints together, connect bones and cartilages, and aid joint flexibility and support. Tendons are white, glistening, fibrous bands of tissue that connect muscle to bone and are strong, flexible, and inelastic. Cartilage is nonvascular (without blood vessels) supporting connective tissue located chiefly in the joints and thorax, trachea, larynx, nose, and ear (see Chapter 38). The characteristics of the cartilage change with the aging process.

Skeletal Muscle. Movement of bones and joints involves active processes that are carefully integrated to achieve coordination. Skeletal muscles, because of their ability to contract and relax, are the working elements of movement. Anatomical structure and attachment to the skeleton enhance contractile elements of the skeletal muscle (see Chapter 38).

Nervous System. The nervous system regulates movement and posture. The precentral gyrus, or motor strip, is the major voluntary motor area and is in the cerebral cortex. A majority of motor fibers descend from the motor strip and cross at the level of the medulla. Movement is impaired by disorders that alter neurotransmitter production, transfer of impulses from the nerve to the muscle, or activation of muscle activity.

Pathological Influences on Mobility. Many pathological conditions affect mobility. Although a complete description of each is beyond the scope of this chapter, an overview of five pathological influences is presented.

Postural Abnormalities. Congenital or acquired postural abnormalities affect the efficiency of the musculoskeletal system and body alignment, balance, and appearance. Postural abnormalities can cause pain, impair alignment or mobility, or both. Knowledge about the characteristics, causes, and treatment of common postural abnormalities is necessary for safe lifting, transfer, and positioning (Table 39.1). Some postural abnormalities limit ROM. Nurses intervene to maintain maximum ROM in unaffected joints and often collaborate with physical therapists to design interventions to strengthen affected muscles and joints, improve the patient's posture, and adequately use affected and unaffected muscle groups. Referral to and/or collaboration with a physical therapist enhances your interventions for a patient with postural abnormalities.

Muscle Abnormalities. Diseases lead to numerous alterations in musculoskeletal function. For example, the muscular dystrophies are a group of familial disorders that cause degeneration of skeletal muscle fibers. They are the most prevalent of the muscle diseases in childhood. Patients with muscular dystrophy experience progressive, symmetrical weakness and wasting of skeletal muscle groups, with increasing disability and deformity (McCance and Huether, 2017).

TABLE 39.1   Postural Abnormalities

Abnormality	Description	Cause	Possible Treatments[a] (McCance and Huether, 2017)
Torticollis	Inclining head to affected side, in which sternocleidomastoid muscle is contracted	Congenital or acquired condition	Surgery, heat, support, or immobilization, depending on cause and severity; gentle ROM
Lordosis	Exaggeration of anterior convex curve of lumbar spine	Congenital condition; temporary condition (e.g., pregnancy)	Spine-stretching exercises (based on cause)
Kyphosis	Increased convexity in curvature of thoracic spine	Congenital condition; rickets, osteoporosis; tuberculosis of spine	Spine-stretching exercises, sleeping without pillows, using bed board, bracing, surgical spinal fusion (based on cause and severity)
Scoliosis	Lateral S- or C-shaped spinal column with vertebral rotation, unequal heights of hips and shoulders	Sometimes a consequence of numerous congenital, connective tissue, and neuromuscular disorders	Approximately half of children with scoliosis require surgery Nonsurgical treatment is with braces and exercises
Congenital hip dysplasia	Hip instability with limited abduction of hips and occasionally adduction contractures (head of femur does not articulate with acetabulum because of abnormal shallowness of acetabulum)	Congenital condition (more common with breech deliveries)	Maintenance of continuous abduction of thigh so head of femur presses into center of acetabulum; abduction splints, casting, surgery
Knock-knee (genu valgum)	Legs curved inward so knees come together as person walks	Congenital condition; rickets	Knee braces; surgery if not corrected by growth
Bowlegs (genu varum)	One or both legs bent outward at knee, which is normal until 2 to 3 years of age	Congenital condition; rickets	Slowing rate of curving if not corrected by growth; with rickets, increase of vitamin D, calcium, and phosphorus intake to normal ranges
Clubfoot	*95%:* Medial deviation and plantar flexion of foot (equinovarus) *5%:* Lateral deviation and dorsiflexion (calcaneovalgus)	Congenital condition	Casts, splints such as Denis Browne splint, and surgery (based on degree and rigidity of deformity)
Footdrop	Inability to dorsiflex and invert foot because of peroneal nerve damage	Congenital condition; trauma; improper position of immobilized patient	None (cannot be corrected); prevention through physical therapy; bracing with ankle-foot orthotic (AFO)

ROM, Range of motion.

[a]Severity of condition and cause dictate treatment, which is individualized to the patient's needs.

Damage to the Central Nervous System. Damage to any component of the central nervous system that regulates voluntary movement results in impaired body alignment, balance, and mobility. Trauma from a head injury, ischemia from a stroke (cerebrovascular accident [CVA]), or bacterial infection such as meningitis can damage the cerebellum or the motor strip in the cerebral cortex. Damage to the cerebellum causes problems with balance, and motor impairment is directly related to the amount of destruction of the motor strip. For example, a person with a right-sided cerebral hemorrhage with necrosis has destruction of the right motor strip that results in left-sided hemiplegia. Trauma to the spinal cord also impairs mobility. For example, a complete transection of the spinal cord results in a bilateral loss of voluntary motor control below the level of the trauma because motor fibers are cut. Neurodegenerative disorders also have a negative impact on mobility. For example, symptoms of Parkinson's disease may include rigidity, tremors, and postural instability (Shin et al., 2017).

Direct Trauma to the Musculoskeletal System. Direct trauma to the musculoskeletal system results in bruises, contusions, tears, sprains, and fractures. A fracture is a disruption of bone tissue continuity. Fractures most commonly result from direct external trauma,

but they also occur as a consequence of some deformity of the bone (e.g., pathological fractures of osteoporosis, Paget's disease, metastatic cancer, or osteogenesis imperfecta). Young children are usually able to form new bone more easily than adults and, as a result, have few complications after a fracture. Treatment often includes positioning the fractured bone in proper alignment and immobilizing it to promote healing and restore function. Even this temporary immobilization results in some muscle atrophy, loss of muscle tone, and joint stiffness.

Joint Disease. One of the most common pathological influences on mobility comes in the form of joint disease. As the US population ages, the prevalence of arthritis is expected to increase to 25% of the population by the year 2040 (Hootman et al., 2016). Osteoarthritis, loss of the articular cartilage, is the most common noninflammatory arthritis, while rheumatoid arthritis is an example of a noninfectious inflammatory arthritis (McCance and Huether, 2017). In the acute care setting, nurses may care for patients with a variety of conditions who also have a history of joint disease. In addition, nurses care for medical or surgical admissions related to a specific joint disorder. An example of this is the patient admitted for a total joint replacement.

NURSING KNOWLEDGE BASE

Fully understanding movement and mobility requires more than an overview of movement and the physiology and regulation of movement by the musculoskeletal and nervous systems. You need to know how to apply these scientific principles in the clinical setting to determine the safest way to move patients and to understand the effect of immobility on the physiological, psychosocial, and developmental aspects of patient care.

The Effects of Immobility

To determine how to move patients safely, you will assess their ability to move. Mobility refers to a person's ability to move about freely, and immobility refers to the inability to do so. Think of mobility as a continuum, with mobility on one end, immobility on the other, and varying degrees of partial immobility between the end points. Some patients move back and forth between mobility and immobility, but for others immobility is absolute and continues indefinitely. The terms *bed rest* and *impaired physical mobility* are used frequently when discussing patients on the mobility-immobility continuum.

Bed rest is an intervention that restricts patients to bed for therapeutic reasons and is sometimes prescribed for selected patients. The therapeutic reasons for bed rest include decreasing the oxygen needs of the body, reducing cardiac workload and pain, and allowing a debilitated patient to rest. Bed rest has many different interpretations among health care professionals. The duration of bed rest depends on the illness or injury and a patient's prior state of health.

The effects of muscular deconditioning associated with lack of physical activity are often apparent in a matter of days. The individual of average weight and height without a chronic illness on bed rest loses muscle strength from baseline levels at a rate of 3% a day (McCance and Huether, 2017). Vulnerable populations, such as older adults, are especially at risk for loss of function during acute illness and hospitalization (Wald et al., 2019). Immobility also is associated with cardiovascular, skeletal, and other organ changes. The term *disuse atrophy* describes the tendency of cells and tissue to reduce in size and function in response to prolonged inactivity resulting from bed rest, trauma, casting of a body part, or local nerve damage (McCance and Huether, 2017).

Periods of immobility due to disability or injury or prolonged bed rest during hospitalization cause major physiological, psychological, and social effects. These effects are gradual or immediate and vary from patient to patient. The greater the extent and the longer the duration of immobility, the more pronounced the consequences. The patient with complete mobility restrictions is continually at risk for the hazards of immobility. When possible, it is imperative that patients, especially older adults, have limited bed rest and that their activity is more than bed to chair. Loss of walking independence increases hospital stays, need for rehabilitation services, or nursing home placement. In addition, the deconditioning related to reduced walking increases the risk for patient falls (AAN, 2015; Krupp et al., 2018, Kruschke and Butcher, 2017).

Systemic Effects. All body systems work more efficiently with some form of movement. When there is an alteration in mobility, each body system is at risk for impairment. The severity of the impairment depends on a patient's overall health, degree and length of immobility, and age. For example, older adults with chronic illnesses develop pronounced effects of immobility more quickly than do younger patients with the same immobility problem.

Metabolic Changes. Changes in mobility alter endocrine metabolism, calcium resorption, and functioning of the gastrointestinal (GI) system. The endocrine system, composed of hormone-secreting glands, maintains and regulates vital functions such as (1) response to stress and injury; (2) growth and development; (3) reproduction; (4) maintenance of the internal environment; and (5) energy production, use, and storage.

When injury or stress occurs, the endocrine system triggers a series of responses aimed at maintaining blood pressure and preserving life. It is important in maintaining homeostasis. Tissues and cells live in an internal environment that the endocrine system helps regulate through maintenance of sodium, potassium, water, and acid-base balance. It also regulates energy metabolism. Thyroid hormone increases the basal metabolic rate (BMR), and energy becomes available to cells through the integrated action of GI and pancreatic hormones (McCance and Huether, 2017).

Immobility disrupts normal metabolic processes, decreasing the metabolic rate; altering the metabolism of carbohydrates, fats, and proteins; causing fluid, electrolyte, and calcium imbalances; and causing GI disturbances such as decreased appetite and slowing of peristalsis. However, in the presence of an infectious process, immobilized patients often have an increased BMR as a result of fever or wound healing because these increase cellular oxygen requirements (McCance and Huether, 2017).

A deficiency in calories and protein is characteristic of patients with a decreased appetite secondary to immobility. The body is constantly synthesizing proteins and breaking them down into amino acids to form other proteins (see Chapter 45). When the patient is immobile, his or her body often excretes more nitrogen (the end product of amino acid breakdown) than it ingests in proteins, resulting in negative nitrogen balance. Weight loss, decreased muscle mass, and weakness result from tissue catabolism (tissue breakdown) (McCance and Huether, 2017).

Another metabolic change associated with immobility is calcium resorption (loss) from bones. Immobility causes the release of calcium into the circulation. Normally the kidneys excrete the excess calcium. However, if they are unable to respond appropriately, hypercalcemia results. Pathological fractures may occur if calcium resorption continues as a patient remains on bed rest or continues to be immobile (McCance and Huether, 2017).

Impairments of GI functioning caused by decreased mobility vary. Difficulty in passing stools (constipation) is a common symptom. A condition known as pseudodiarrhea often results from a fecal impaction (accumulation of hardened feces). This finding is not normal diarrhea, but rather liquid stool passing around the area of fecal impaction (see Chapter 47). Left untreated, fecal impaction results in a mechanical bowel obstruction that partly or completely occludes the intestinal lumen, blocking normal propulsion of liquid and gas. The resulting fluid in the intestine produces distention and increases intraluminal pressure. Over time intestinal function becomes depressed, dehydration occurs, absorption ceases, and fluid and electrolyte disturbances worsen.

Respiratory Changes. Lack of movement and exercise places patients at risk for respiratory complications. Patients who are immobile are at high risk for developing pulmonary atelectasis (collapse of alveoli) and

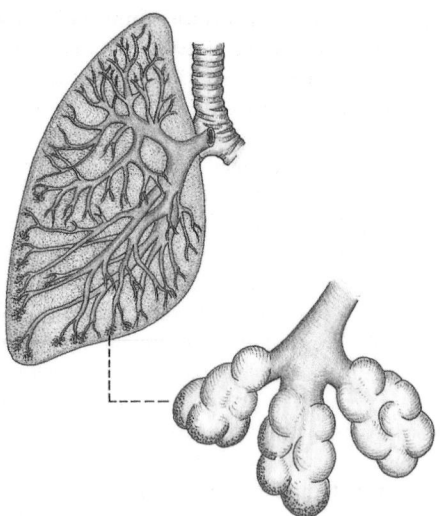

FIG. 39.1 Pooling of secretions in dependent regions of lungs in supine position.

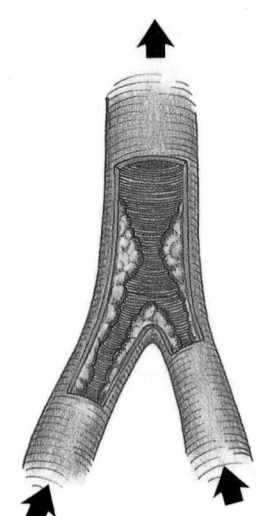

FIG. 39.2 Thrombus formation in a vessel.

hypostatic pneumonia (inflammation of the lung from stasis or pooling of secretions). Both decreased oxygenation and prolonged recovery add to patients' discomfort (Lewis et al., 2017). In atelectasis secretions block a bronchiole or a bronchus, and the distal lung tissue (alveoli) collapses as the existing air is absorbed, producing hypoventilation. The site of the blockage affects the severity of atelectasis. Sometimes an entire lung lobe or a whole lung collapses. At some point in the development of these complications, there is a proportional decline in the patient's ability to cough productively. Ultimately the distribution of mucus in the bronchi increases, particularly when the patient is in the supine, prone, or lateral position. Mucus accumulates in the dependent regions of the airways (Fig. 39.1). Hypostatic pneumonia frequently results because mucus is an excellent place for bacteria to grow.

Cardiovascular Changes. Immobilization also affects the cardiovascular system, frequently resulting in orthostatic hypotension, increased cardiac workload, and thrombus formation. Orthostatic hypotension is a drop in systolic pressure by at least 20 mm Hg or a drop in diastolic pressure by at least 10 mm Hg within 3 minutes of rising to an upright position (Shibao et al., 2013; Ball et al., 2019). Patients also experience symptoms of dizziness, light-headedness, nausea, tachycardia, pallor, or fainting when changing from the supine to standing position (Ball et al., 2019). In the immobilized patient decreased circulating fluid volume, pooling of blood in the lower extremities, and decreased autonomic response occur. These are especially evident in the older adult.

As the workload of the heart increases, so does its oxygen consumption. Therefore the heart works harder and less efficiently during periods of prolonged rest. As immobilization increases, cardiac output falls, further decreasing cardiac efficiency and increasing workload.

Patients who are immobile are also at risk for thrombus formation. A thrombus is an accumulation of platelets, fibrin, clotting factors, and the cellular elements of the blood attached to the interior wall of a vein or artery, which sometimes occludes the lumen of the vessel (Fig. 39.2). Three factors contribute to venous thrombus formation: (1) damage to the vessel wall (e.g., injury during surgical procedures), (2) alterations of blood flow (e.g., slow blood flow in calf veins associated with bed rest), and (3) alterations in blood constituents (e.g., a change in clotting factors or increased platelet activity). These three factors are often referred to as *Virchow's triad* (McCance and Huether, 2017). As a nurse you will practice in numerous situations in which deep vein

thrombosis (DVT) must be prevented, especially during perioperative care (see Chapter 50).

Musculoskeletal Changes. Immobility causes permanent or temporary impairment of musculoskeletal structures. Because of protein breakdown, a patient loses lean body mass during immobility. The reduced muscle mass makes it difficult for patients to sustain activity without increased fatigue. If immobility continues and the patient does not exercise, there is further loss of muscle mass. Prolonged immobility often leads to disuse atrophy. Loss of endurance, decreased muscle mass and strength, and joint instability place patients at risk for falls (see Chapter 27).

Immobilization also causes two skeletal changes: impaired calcium metabolism and joint abnormalities. Because immobilization results in bone resorption, the bone tissue is less dense or atrophied, and disuse osteoporosis results. When disuse osteoporosis occurs, a patient is at risk for pathological fractures.

Osteoporosis is a major health concern in this country. By 2025, it is expected to be responsible for approximately 3 million fractures, with the lifetime risk of an osteoporosis fracture at 50% for women and 20% to 25% for men (Gupta et al., 2018). Although primary osteoporosis is different in origin from the osteoporosis that results from immobility, it is imperative that nurses recognize that immobilized patients are at high risk for accelerated bone loss if they have primary osteoporosis.

Immobility can lead to joint contractures. A joint contracture is an abnormal and possibly permanent condition characterized by fixation of a joint. It is important to note that flexor muscles for joints are stronger than extensor muscles and therefore contribute to the formation of contractures. Disuse, atrophy, and shortening of the muscle fibers cause joint contractures. When a contracture occurs, the joint cannot achieve full ROM. Contractures sometimes leave a joint or joints in a nonfunctional position, as seen in patients who are permanently curled in a fetal position. Early prevention of contractures is essential (Box 39.1) (Meyers, 2017).

One common and debilitating contracture is footdrop (Fig. 39.3). When footdrop occurs, the foot is permanently fixed in plantar flexion. Ambulation is difficult with the foot in this position because the patient cannot dorsiflex the foot. A patient with footdrop is unable to lift the toes off the ground and is at risk of stumbling. Patients who have had CVAs with resulting right- or left-sided paralysis (hemiplegia) are at risk for footdrop.

Urinary Elimination Changes. Immobility alters a patient's urinary elimination. In the upright position urine flows out of the renal pelvis

BOX 39.1 EVIDENCE-BASED PRACTICE

Patient Contractures and Treatments to Reduce Future Contractures for At-Risk Patients

PICOT Question: Can the use of early correct positioning, range-of-motion (ROM) exercises, and mechanical treatment modalities such as dynamic and static splints reduce joint contractures in the lower extremities in patients with at-risk conditions compared with patients who do not have any early intervention?

Evidence Summary

Joint contractures are common preventable disorders that can result in significant long-term morbidity and reduced patient independence. Contracture is the shortening of the connective tissue and is an abnormal and possibly permanent condition characterized by decreased range of joint motion and/or fixation of the joint. Contractures occur following prolonged joint positioning (immobility), neurological disorders, and surgical joint manipulation (Odgaard et al., 2018). Evidence shows that early prevention of contractures is essential (Winterton and Baldwin, 2018). These researchers found nonsurgical approaches such as antispasmodic medications, Botox administration, serial casting, splinting, and physical and occupational therapies such as range-of-motion (ROM) exercises are helpful in preventing and minimizing this complication of impaired mobility.

Application to Nursing Practice

- In conjunction with an interprofessional health care team, develop an early intervention protocol using prescribed positioning, range-of-motion exercises, and/or splints to reduce the risk for contracture formation (Winterton and Baldwin, 2018).
- Health care agencies need to provide equipment (e.g., splints) and appropriate education for staff to reduce the risk of contractures.
- A collaborative plan of care, including a discharge plan, with a contracture prevention and muscle strengthening protocol must be developed on patient admission.
- Use positioning, ROM exercises, and ROM devices according to the individualized need of the patient and as ordered (Winterton and Baldwin, 2018).

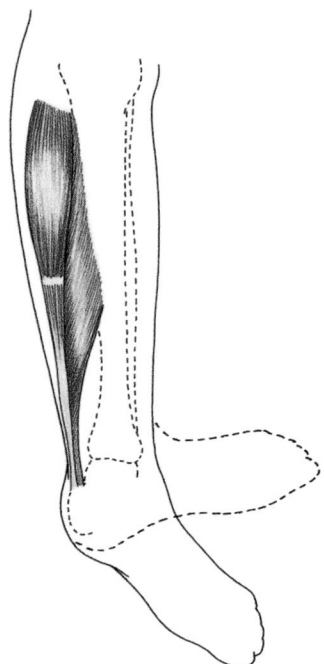

FIG. 39.3 Footdrop. Ankle is fixed in plantar flexion. Normally ankle is able to flex *(dotted line)*, which eases walking.

and into the ureters and bladder because of gravitational forces. When a patient is recumbent or flat, the kidneys and ureters move toward a more level plane. Urine formed by the kidney needs to enter the bladder unaided by gravity. Because the peristaltic contractions of the ureters are insufficient to overcome gravity, the renal pelvis fills before urine enters the ureters. This condition is called **urinary stasis** and increases the risk of urinary tract infection (UTI) and renal calculi (see Chapter 46). **Renal calculi** are calcium stones that lodge in the renal pelvis or pass through the ureters. Immobilized patients are at risk for calculi because they frequently have hypercalcemia (McCance & Huether, 2017).

As the period of immobility continues, fluid intake often diminishes. When combined with other problems such as fever, the risk for dehydration increases. As a result, urinary output declines on or about the fifth or sixth day after immobilization, and the urine becomes concentrated. Concentrated urine increases the risk for calculi formation and infection. Another cause of UTI in immobilized patients is the use of an indwelling urinary catheter (see Chapter 46).

Integumentary Changes. The changes in metabolism that accompany immobility add to the harmful effect of pressure on the skin in immobilized patients. This makes immobility a major risk factor for pressure injuries. Any break in the integrity of the skin is difficult to heal. Preventing a pressure injury is much less expensive than treating one; therefore preventive nursing interventions are imperative (Barnes-Daly, et al, 2018; Zubkoff et al., 2017).

A **pressure injury** is an impairment of the skin as a result of prolonged ischemia (decreased blood supply) in tissues (see Chapter 48). It is characterized initially by inflammation and usually forms over a bony prominence. Ischemia develops when the pressure on the skin is greater than the pressure inside the small peripheral blood vessels supplying blood to the skin (AHRQ, n.d.).

Tissue metabolism depends on the supply of oxygen and nutrients to and the elimination of metabolic wastes from the blood. Pressure affects cellular metabolism by decreasing or totally eliminating tissue circulation. When a patient lies in bed or sits in a chair, the weight of the body is on bony prominences. The longer the pressure is applied, the longer is the period of ischemia and therefore the greater the risk of skin breakdown (Stephens et al., 2018). The prevalence of pressure injuries is highest in long-term care facilities, whereas hospital-acquired pressure injuries are the highest in adult intensive care units (Ayello, 2017).

Psychosocial Effects. Immobilization often leads to emotional and behavioral responses, sensory alterations, and changes in coping. Illnesses that result in limited or impaired mobility can cause social isolation and loneliness (Musich et al., 2018). Every patient responds to immobility differently.

Patients with restricted mobility may have some depression. Depression is an affective disorder characterized by exaggerated feelings of sadness, melancholy, dejection, worthlessness, emptiness, and hopelessness out of proportion to reality. It results from worrying about present and future levels of health, finances, and family needs. Because immobilization removes a patient from a daily routine, he or she has more time to worry about disability. Worrying quickly increases a patient's depression, causing withdrawal. Withdrawn patients often do not want to participate in their own care.

Developmental Changes

Immobility often leads to developmental changes in the very young and in older adults. The immobilized young or middle-age adult who has been healthy experiences few, if any, developmental changes. However, there are exceptions. For example, a mother with complications following birth has to go on bed rest and as a result cannot interact with her newborn as expected.

BOX 39.2   FOCUS ON OLDER ADULTS

Functional Decline in Hospitalized Immobile Older Adults

For many older adults, admission to a hospital often results in functional decline despite the treatment for which they were admitted. Some older adults have problems related to mobility and quickly regress to a dependent state (Chase et al., 2018). Usual aging is associated with decreased muscle strength and aerobic capacity, which become exacerbated if a patient's nutritional state is poor.

- A nutritional assessment needs to be included in the plan of care for the older adult experiencing immobility.
- Anorexia and insufficient assistance with eating lead to malnutrition, which contributes to the known problems associated with immobility.
- Improved nutrition increases patient's ability to perform physical reconditioning exercises (Kruschke and Butcher, 2017).
- There is a direct relationship between the success of older adults' rehabilitation and their nutritional status (Barbour et al., 2017).

Infants, Toddlers, and Preschoolers. As a baby grows, musculoskeletal development permits support of weight for standing and walking. Posture is awkward because the head and upper trunk are carried forward. Because body weight is not distributed evenly along a line of gravity, posture is normally off balance, and falls occur often. When an infant, toddler, or preschooler becomes immobilized, it is usually because of trauma or the need to correct a congenital skeletal abnormality. Prolonged immobilization delays a child's gross motor skills, intellectual development, and musculoskeletal development.

Adolescents. The adolescent stage usually begins with a tremendous increase in growth (see Chapter 12). When the activity level is reduced because of trauma, illness, or surgery, the adolescent is often behind peers in gaining independence and accomplishing certain skills, such as obtaining a driver's license. Social isolation is a concern for this age-group when immobilization occurs.

Adults. An adult who has correct posture and body alignment feels good, looks good, and generally appears self-confident. The healthy adult also has the necessary musculoskeletal development and coordination to carry out ADLs (see Chapter 13). When periods of prolonged immobility occur, all physiological systems are at risk. In addition, the role of the adult often changes with regard to the family or social structure. Some adults lose their jobs, which affects their self-concept (see Chapter 33).

Older Adults. A progressive loss of total bone mass in older adults results from decreased physical activity, hormonal changes, and bone resorption. The effect of bone loss is weaker bones. Older adults often walk more slowly, take smaller steps, and appear less coordinated. Prescribed medications often alter their sense of balance or affect their blood pressure when they change position too quickly, increasing their risk for falls and injuries (see Chapter 27). The outcomes of a fall include not only possible injury but also hospitalization, loss of independence, psychological effects, and quite possibly death (Hallford et al., 2017; Musich et al., 2018; Wald et al., 2019).

Older adults often experience functional status changes secondary to hospitalization and altered mobility status (Box 39.2). Immobilization of older adults increases their physical dependence on others and accelerates functional losses (Chase et al., 2018). Immobilization of some older adults results from degenerative diseases, neurological trauma, or chronic illness. In some it occurs gradually and progressively; in others,

especially those who have had a stroke, it is sudden. When providing nursing care for an older adult, encourage the patient to perform as many self-care activities as possible, thereby maintaining the highest level of mobility. Sometimes nurses inadvertently contribute to a patient's immobility by providing unnecessary help with activities such as bathing and transferring.

REFLECT NOW

Three patients are being admitted to an acute care hospital for surgery on their right hip. Patient #1 is a 9-month-old male, patient #2 is a 44-year-old male, and patient #3 is a 75-year-old female. Using foundational nursing knowledge, compare and contrast developmental needs, effects of immobility, and how their plans of care may differ.

❖ NURSING PROCESS

Apply the nursing process and use a critical thinking approach in your care of patients. The nursing process provides a clinical decision-making approach for you to develop and implement an individualized plan of care. Patients with preexisting mobility impairments and those who are at risk for immobility will greatly benefit from a care plan that improves the patient's functional status, promotes self-care, maintains psychological well-being, and reduces the hazards of immobility.

◆ Assessment

During assessment, consider your patient's normal mobility status, the effects of any diseases or conditions on mobility, and the patient's risks for mobility alterations as a result of treatments (Fig. 39.4). Critically analyze findings to ensure that you make patient-centered clinical decisions required for safe nursing care.

Through the Patient's Eyes. Usually you will assess a patient's degree of mobility and immobility during the history interview and physical examination (Box 39.3). Keep in mind that the patient is a full partner in providing information and designing the plan of care. It is important to understand how any limitations in mobility are perceived by the patient, as well as his or her expectations of care. Does the patient understand whether a particular disease or condition will likely cause permanent disability? Has the patient had a disability for an extended period, and is he or she well adapted to the use of an assist device or even a wheelchair? Is the limitation in mobility sudden and unexpected, causing the patient to be fearful or full of questions? Always convey respect for the patient's preferences, values, and needs during assessment and when designing a plan of care (Ackley and Ladwig, 2017).

Mobility. When unsure of a patient's abilities, begin assessment of mobility with the patient in the most supported position, and move to higher levels according to his or her tolerance. Generally the assessment of movement starts while the patient is lying and proceeds to assessing sitting positions in bed, transfers to chair, and finally walking. This helps to promote the patient's safety.

When a patient is immobile, assessment focuses on the status of the musculoskeletal system and includes ROM, muscle strength, activity tolerance, and posture and alignment. **Range of motion (ROM)** is the maximum amount of movement available at a joint in one of the three planes of the body: sagittal, transverse, or frontal (Fig. 39.5). The sagittal plane is a line that passes through the body from front to back, dividing it into a left and right side. The frontal plane passes through

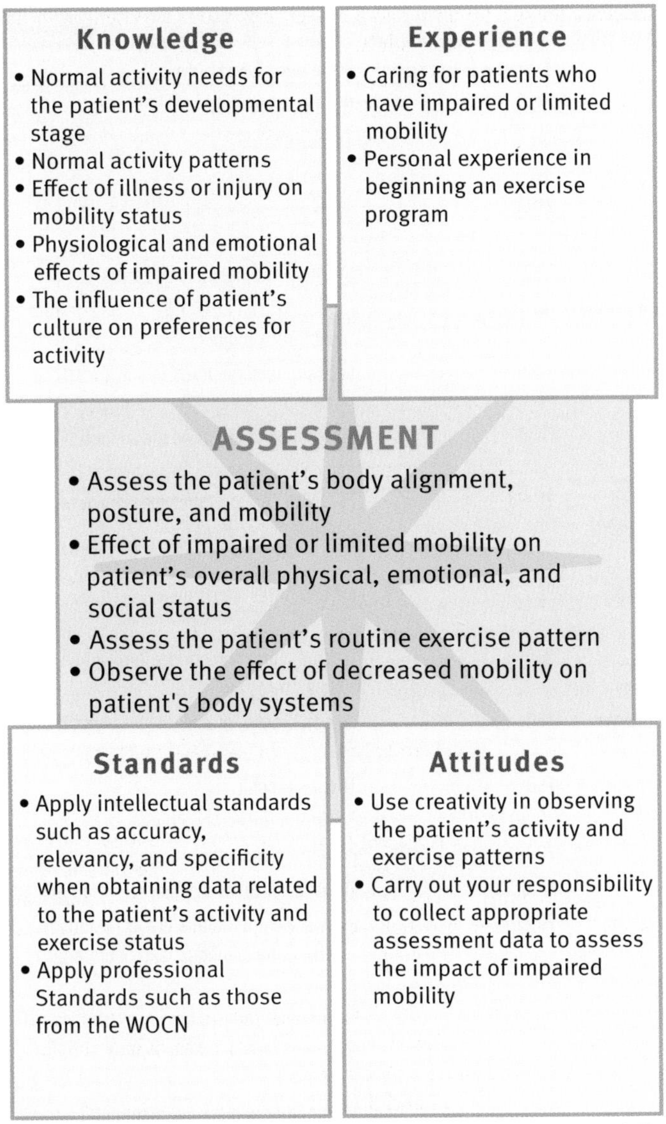

Knowledge

- Normal activity needs for the patient's developmental stage
- Normal activity patterns
- Effect of illness or injury on mobility status
- Physiological and emotional effects of impaired mobility
- The influence of patient's culture on preferences for activity

Experience

- Caring for patients who have impaired or limited mobility
- Personal experience in beginning an exercise program

ASSESSMENT

- Assess the patient's body alignment, posture, and mobility
- Effect of impaired or limited mobility on patient's overall physical, emotional, and social status
- Assess the patient's routine exercise pattern
- Observe the effect of decreased mobility on patient's body systems

Standards

- Apply intellectual standards such as accuracy, relevancy, and specificity when obtaining data related to the patient's activity and exercise status
- Apply professional Standards such as those from the WOCN

Attitudes

- Use creativity in observing the patient's activity and exercise patterns
- Carry out your responsibility to collect appropriate assessment data to assess the impact of impaired mobility

FIG. 39.4 Critical thinking model for assessing impaired mobility. *WOCN, Wound Ostomy and Continent Nurses Society.*

BOX 39.3   Nursing Assessment Questions

Mobility

- Describe any changes you've noticed in your ability to walk and take care of yourself on a daily basis.
- Have you experienced any stiffness, swelling of a joint, muscle or joint pain, or difficulty with moving? If so, describe how this affects your movement and daily activities.
- Have you noticed any shortness of breath; if so, does it worsen when walking?

Immobility

- Describe your normal daily activity. Has this changed recently?
- How have your appetite and diet changed since you've had problems moving around?
- Describe what you eat in a normal day.
- Does your day seem very long?
- Describe for me a typical night's sleep.
- Have you noticed any places on your skin that are reddened or have any open sores?
- Describe any changes you've noticed in urinating and/or having bowel movements.

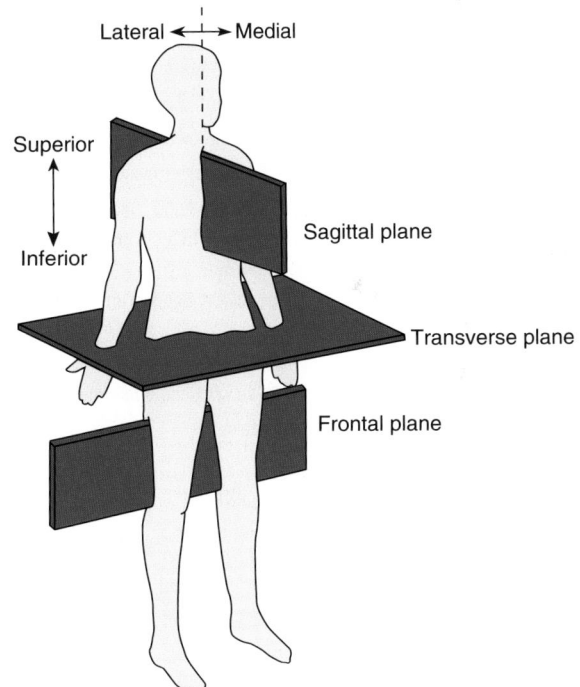

FIG. 39.5 Planes of body.

the body from side to side and divides it into front and back. The transverse plane is a horizontal line that divides the body into upper and lower portions.

Ligaments, muscles, and the nature of the joint limit joint mobility in each of the planes. However, some joint movements are specific to each plane. In the sagittal plane, movements are flexion and extension (e.g., fingers and elbows), dorsiflexion and plantar flexion (feet), and extension (e.g., hip). In the frontal plane, movements are abduction and adduction (e.g., arms and legs) and eversion and inversion (feet). In the transverse plane, movements are pronation and supination (hands) and internal and external rotation (hips).

Assessment of range of motion (ROM) is an important baseline measurement that compares and evaluates whether loss in joint mobility is developing or has occurred. Refer to Table 39.2 for normal joint ROM to compare with findings when you assess a patient's ROM. Be sure to assess all joints in the body. Ask questions about and physically examine a patient for stiffness, swelling, pain, or limited movement, and compare sides for unequal movement (see Chapter 30). If a patient has restricted ROM, your information will help you collaborate with physical therapists to select the type of ROM exercise a patient is able to perform, so you can reduce risk of complications (Table 39.3).

There are three types of range-of-motion exercises: active, active assisted, and passive (see Chapter 38). For example, you might need to provide support for a weak patient and assist while he or she performs most of the joint movement. Some patients are able to move some joints actively, whereas you will passively move others. Ligaments, muscles, and the nature of the joint limit patients' mobility, and some joint movements are specific to their location in the body. Abduction and adduction of the arms and legs are an example of this specific type of movement. Abduction is the movement of an extremity away from the midline of the body, and adduction is the movement of an extremity toward the midline of the body.

TABLE 39.2 Range-of-Motion Exercises

Body Part	Type of Joint	Type of Movement	Range (Degrees)	Primary Muscles
Neck, cervical spine	Pivotal	*Flexion:* Bring chin to rest on chest.	45	Sternocleidomastoid
		Extension: Return head to erect position.	45	Trapezius
		Hyperextension: Bend head back as far as possible.	10	Trapezius
		Lateral flexion: Tilt head as far as possible toward each shoulder.	40-45	Sternocleidomastoid
		Rotation: Turn head as far as possible in circular movement.	180	Sternocleidomastoid, trapezius
Shoulder	Ball and socket	*Flexion:* Raise arm from side position forward to position above head.	45-180	Coracobrachialis, biceps brachii, deltoid, pectoralis major
		Extension: Return arm to position at side of body.	180	Latissimus dorsi, teres major, triceps brachii
		Shoulder extension: Move arm behind body, keeping elbow straight.	0-60	Latissimus dorsi, teres major, deltoid
		Internal rotation: With elbow flexed and shoulder abducted, rotate shoulder by moving arm until thumb is turned inward and toward back.	70-90	Pectoralis major, latissimus dorsi, teres major, subscapularis
		External rotation: With elbow flexed and shoulder abducted, move arm until thumb is upward and lateral to head.	90	Infraspinatus, teres major, deltoid
		Circumduction: Move arm in full circle. (Circumduction is combination of all movements of ball-and-socket joint.)	360	Deltoid, coracobrachialis, latissimus dorsi, teres major
Elbow	Hinge	*Flexion:* Bend elbow so lower arm moves toward its shoulder joint and hand is level with shoulder.	150	Biceps brachii, brachialis, brachioradialis
		Extension: Straighten elbow by lowering hand.	150	Triceps brachii
Forearm	Pivotal	*Supination:* Turn lower arm and hand so palm is up.	70-90	Supinator, biceps brachii
		Pronation: Turn lower arm so palm is down.	70-90	Pronator teres, pronator quadratus
Wrist	Condyloid	*Flexion:* Move palm toward inner aspect of forearm.	80-90	Flexor carpi ulnaris, flexor carpi radialis
		Extension: Move fingers and hand posterior to midline, bring dorsal surface of hand back as far as possible.	70-80	Extensor carpi radialis brevis, extensor carpi radialis longus, extensor carpi ulnaris
		Radial deviation: Bend wrist medially toward thumb.	Up to 30	Flexor carpi radialis brevis, extensor carpi radialis brevis, extensor carpi radialis longus.
		Ulnar deviation: Bend wrist laterally toward fifth finger.	30	Flexor carpi ulnaris, extensor carpi ulnaris
Fingers	Condyloid hinge	*Flexion:* Make fist.	90	Lumbricales, interosseus volaris, interosseus dorsalis
		Extension: Straighten fingers.	90	Extensor digiti quinti proprius, extensor digitorum communis, extensor indicis proprius
		Hyperextension: Bend fingers back as far as possible.	30-60	Extensor digitorum
		Abduction: Spread fingers apart.	30	Interosseus dorsalis
		Adduction: Bring fingers together.	30	Interosseus volaris
Thumb	Saddle	*Flexion:* Move thumb across palmar surface of hand.	90	Flexor pollicis brevis
		Extension: Move thumb straight away from hand.	90	Extensor pollicis longus, extensor pollicis brevis
		Abduction: Extend thumb laterally (usually done when placing fingers in abduction and adduction).	30	Abductor pollicis brevis
		Adduction: Move thumb back toward hand.	30	Adductor pollicis obliquus, adductor pollicis transversus
		Opposition: Touch thumb to each finger of same hand.		Opponens pollicis, opponens digiti minimi

TABLE 39.2   Range-of-Motion Exercises—cont'd

Body Part	Type of Joint	Type of Movement	Range (Degrees)	Primary Muscles
Hip	Ball and socket	*Flexion:* Move leg forward and up.	110-120	Psoas major, iliacus, sartorius
		Extension: Move leg back beside other leg.	90-120	Gluteus maximus, semitendinosus, semimembranosus
		Hyperextension: Move leg behind body as far as possible.	30-50	Gluteus maximus, semitendinosus, semimembranosus
		Abduction: Move leg laterally away from body.	30-50	Gluteus medius, gluteus minimus
		Adduction: Move leg back toward medial position and beyond if possible.	20-30	Adductor longus, adductor brevis, adductor magnus
		Internal rotation: Turn foot and leg toward other leg.	45	Gluteus medius, gluteus minimus, tensor fasciae latae
		External rotation: Turn foot and leg away from other leg.	45	Obturatorius internus, obturatorius externus
		Circumduction: Move leg in circle.		Psoas major, gluteus maximus, gluteus medius, adductor magnus
Knee	Hinge	*Flexion:* Bring heel back toward back of thigh.	120-130	Biceps femoris, semitendinosus, semimembranosus, sartorius
		Extension: Return leg to floor.	120-130	Rectus femoris, vastus lateralis, vastus medialis, vastus intermedius
Ankle	Hinge	*Dorsal flexion:* Move foot so toes are pointed upward.	20-30	Tibialis anterior
		Plantar flexion: Move foot so toes are pointed downward.	45-50	Gastrocnemius, soleus
Foot	Gliding	*Inversion:* Turn sole of foot medially.	35 or less	Tibialis anterior, tibialis posterior
		Eversion: Turn sole of foot laterally.	10 or less	Peroneus longus, peroneus brevis
Toes	Condyloid	*Flexion:* Curl toes downward.	30-60	Flexor digitorum, lumbricalis pedis, flexor hallucis brevis
		Extension: Straighten toes.	30-60	Extensor digitorum longus, extensor digitorum brevis, extensor hallucis longus
		Abduction: Spread toes apart.	15 or less	Abductor hallucis, interosseus dorsalis
		Adduction: Bring toes together.	15 or less	Adductor hallucis, interosseus plantaris

TABLE 39.3   Range-of-Motion Alterations

Body Part	Alteration	Assessment Finding(s)
Neck	Flexion contracture—a patient's neck is permanently flexed with the chin close to or actually touching the chest	Altered body alignment, changes in the visual field, and decreased level of independent functioning
Shoulder	The strongest muscle controlling the shoulder is the deltoid. It is in complete elongation in the normal position, but with alteration there is limited elongation	Difficulty moving the arms
Elbow	Fixed in full extension	Difficulty flexing and using arm for self-care activities
Forearm	Forearm becomes fixed in full supination	Use of hand is limited, unable to perform self-care activities
Wrist	Wrist becomes fixed, slightly flexed	Grasp is weaker
Fingers and thumb	Digits become more flexed; pain with movement	Unable to perform fine motor skills: picking up objects, ADLs, needlework, drawing
Hip	Contractures often fix the hip in positions of deformity. Excessive abduction makes the affected leg appear too short, whereas excessive adduction makes it appear too long	Limited ability to move about; walks with limp. Internal and external rotation contractures cause abnormal and unbalanced gait
Knee	Knees cannot remain stable under weight-bearing conditions unless there is adequate quadriceps power to maintain them in full extension	Knee is stiff. If fixed in full extension, a person needs to sit with leg out in front. If knee is stiffened in flexed position, person limps while walking
Ankle and foot	Joint becomes unstable. When the person relaxes as in sleep or coma, the foot relaxes and assumes a position of plantar flexion. As a result, it becomes fixed in plantar flexion (footdrop)	Abnormal gait. Impaired ability to walk independently
Toes	Excessive flexion of the toes results in clawing. Permanent clawing results in the foot being unable to rest flat on the floor	Abnormal gait

The major musculoskeletal changes expected during assessment of an immobilized patient include decreased muscle strength, loss of muscle tone and mass, and contractures. Patients with musculoskeletal injuries or chronic conditions require careful palpation of joints and extremities to minimize discomfort. Because immobilized patients are weakened, determine whether difficulty in moving joints is the result of fatigue or decreased ROM. Remember that a patient's total musculoskeletal system must be evaluated from the head and neck down to the toes. Any limitation not identified early can result in the patient developing a permanent complication that will impact mobility in the future.

Activity tolerance is the type and amount of exercise or work that a person is able to perform without undue exertion or injury. Many of the patients who have become immobilized may be very limited in their ability to walk or change position in bed. After activity, observe patients for difficulty breathing. Assess heart rate and blood pressure response to activity by comparing with baseline at rest. Both heart rate and blood pressure should increase. Chapter 38 describes how to assess a patient's activity tolerance. Assessment of activity tolerance is necessary when planning activity such as walking, ROM exercises, or ADLs. Activity tolerance assessment includes data from physiological, emotional, and developmental domains.

Observing a patient's posture and alignment while sitting and lying in bed determines the type of assistance the patient requires for safe repositioning (i.e., notice which method the patient uses to push up in bed or whether the patient grabs onto objects to steady himself or herself). Aligning patients properly within their own restrictions helps to reduce discomfort and placement of stress on weakened or injured extremities.

As activity is incorporated into the plan of care, monitor patients' tolerance, and assess for dyspnea, shortness of breath, fatigue, chest pain, and/or a change in heart rate or blood pressure. The weak or acutely ill patient is unable to sustain even slight changes in activity because of the increased demand for energy. Seemingly simple tasks such as eating and moving in bed often result in extreme fatigue. When a patient experiences decreased activity tolerance, carefully assess how much time he or she needs to recover. Decreasing recovery time indicates improving activity tolerance.

Gait. Gait is the manner or style of walking, including rhythm, cadence, length of stride, and speed. Assessing gait allows for conclusions about balance, posture, and the ability to walk without assistance (see Chapter 38). While a patient walks, look for conformity, a regular, smooth rhythm and symmetry in the length of leg swing; smooth swaying related to the gait phase; and a smooth, symmetrical arm swing (Ball et al., 2019). An abnormal gait is a common risk factor for patient falls.

Exercise Pattern. Exercise is physical activity for conditioning the body, improving health, and maintaining fitness. Nurses use it as therapy to correct a deformity or restore the overall body to a maximal state of health. When a person exercises, beneficial physiological changes occur in numerous body systems (see Chapter 38). Assess a patient's exercise history by asking what exercise he or she normally engages in and the normal amount of exercise performed daily and weekly. If a patient does not exercise regularly, you will want to focus on his or her activity tolerance. Chapter 38 describes the approach for assessment of a patient's exercise patterns.

A weak or debilitated patient is unable to sustain even slight changes in activity because of the increased demand for energy. Seemingly simple tasks such as eating and moving in bed often result in extreme fatigue. When the patient experiences decreased activity tolerance, carefully assess how much time he or she needs to recover. Decreasing recovery time indicates improving activity tolerance.

People who are depressed, worried, or anxious are frequently unable to tolerate exercise. Depressed patients tend to withdraw rather than participate. Patients who worry or are frequently anxious expend a tremendous amount of mental energy and often report feeling fatigued. Because of this, they also experience physical and emotional exhaustion.

Body Alignment. The first step in assessing body alignment is to put patients at ease so that they do not assume unnatural or rigid positions. When assessing the body alignment of an immobilized or unconscious patient, remove pillows and positioning supports from the bed and place the patient in the supine position.

Standing. During assessment look for characteristics of correct body alignment for the standing patient:
1. The head is erect and midline.
2. When observed posteriorly, the shoulders and hips are straight and parallel.
3. When observed posteriorly, the vertebral column is straight.
4. When observed laterally, the head is erect, and the spinal curves are aligned in a reversed S pattern. The cervical vertebrae are anteriorly convex, the thoracic vertebrae are posteriorly convex, and the lumbar vertebrae are anteriorly convex.
5. When observed laterally, the abdomen is comfortably tucked in, and the knees and ankles are slightly flexed. The person appears comfortable and does not seem conscious of the flexion of knees or ankles.
6. The arms hang comfortably at the sides.
7. The feet are slightly apart to achieve a base of support, and the toes are pointed forward.
8. When viewing the patient from behind, the center of gravity is in the midline, and the line of gravity is from the middle of the forehead to a midpoint between the feet. Laterally the line of gravity runs vertically from the middle of the skull to the posterior third of the foot (Fig. 39.6).

Sitting. Assessment also includes characteristics of correct alignment of the sitting patient:
1. The head is erect, and the neck and vertebral column are in straight alignment.
2. The body weight is distributed evenly on the buttocks and thighs.
3. The thighs are parallel and in a horizontal plane.

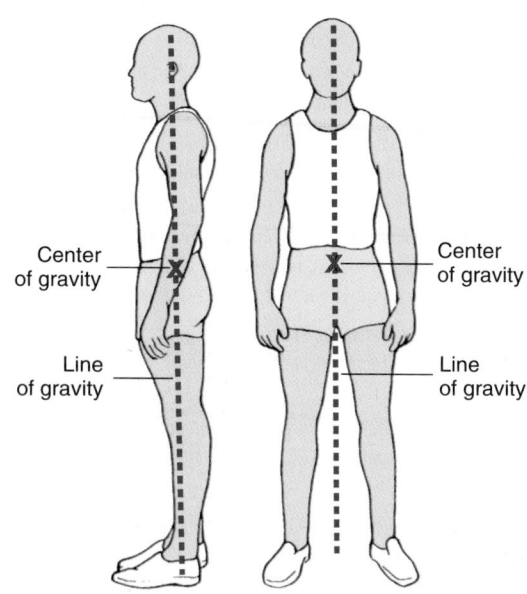

Center of gravity

Center of gravity

Line of gravity

Line of gravity

FIG. 39.6 Correct body alignment when standing.

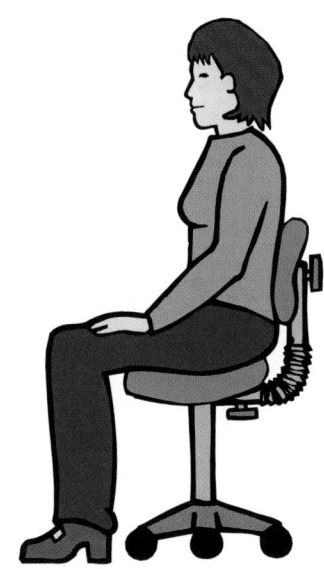

FIG. 39.7 Correct body alignment when sitting.

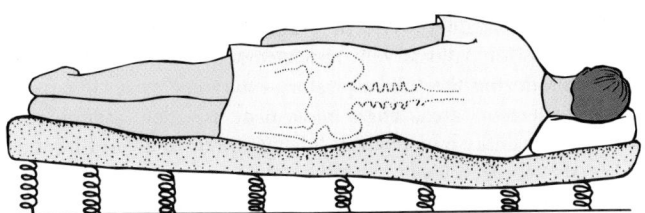

FIG. 39.8 Correct body alignment when lying down.

4. Both feet are supported on the floor (Fig. 39.7), and the ankles are flexed comfortably. With patients of short stature, use a footstool to ensure that ankles are flexed comfortably.
5. A 2.5- to 5-cm (1- to 2-inch) space is maintained between the edge of the seat and the popliteal space on the posterior surface of the knee. This space ensures that there is no pressure on the popliteal artery or nerve to decrease circulation or impair nerve function.
6. The patient's forearms are supported on the armrest, in the lap, or on a table in front of the chair.

It is particularly important to assess alignment when sitting if the patient has muscle weakness, muscle paralysis, or nerve damage. Patients who have these problems have diminished sensation in the affected area and are unable to perceive pressure or decreased circulation. Proper alignment while sitting reduces the risk of musculoskeletal system damage in such a patient. The patient with severe respiratory disease who has orthopnea sometimes assumes a posture of leaning on the table in front of the chair in an attempt to breathe more easily.

Lying. People who are conscious have voluntary muscle control and normal perception of pressure. As a result, they usually assume a position of comfort when lying down. Because their ROM, sensation, and circulation are within normal limits, they change positions when they perceive muscle strain and decreased circulation.

Assess body alignment for a patient who is immobilized or bedridden with the patient in the lateral position (Fig. 39.8). Remove all positioning supports from the bed except for the pillow under the head and support the body with an adequate mattress. This position allows for full view of the spine and back and helps provide other baseline body alignment data such as whether the patient is able to remain positioned without aid. The vertebrae are aligned, and the position does not cause discomfort. Patients with impaired mobility (e.g., traction or arthritis), decreased sensation (e.g., hemiparesis following a CVA), impaired circulation (e.g., diabetes), and lack of voluntary muscle control (e.g., spinal cord injury) are at risk for damage when lying down.

Immobility. Assess the patient for the physiological hazards of immobility while performing a head-to-toe physical assessment (Table 39.4) (see Chapter 30). In addition, focus on the patient's psychosocial and developmental dimensions.

Metabolic System. When assessing metabolic functioning, measures of height and weight figure prominently. Also examine

TABLE 39.4 Assessment of the Physiological Hazards of Immobility

System	Assessment Techniques	Abnormal Findings
Metabolic	Inspection	Slowed wound healing, abnormal laboratory data
	Inspection	Muscle atrophy
	Palpation	Generalized edema
Respiratory	Inspection	Asymmetrical chest wall movement, dyspnea, increased respiratory rate
	Auscultation	Crackles, wheezes
Cardiovascular	Auscultation	Orthostatic hypotension
	Auscultation, palpation	Increased heart rate, third heart sound, weak peripheral pulses, peripheral edema
Musculoskeletal	Inspection	Decreased range of motion, erythema, increased diameter in calf or thigh
	Palpation	Joint contracture, reduced muscle strength
	Inspection	Activity intolerance, muscle atrophy, joint contracture
Skin	Inspection, palpation	Break in skin integrity
Elimination	Inspection	Decreased urine output, cloudy or concentrated urine, decreased frequency of bowel movements
	Palpation	Distended bladder and abdomen
	Auscultation	Decreased bowel sounds

the turgor of the skin. Dehydration and edema increase the rate of skin breakdown in a patient who is immobilized. Review intake and output records for fluid balance. Does intake equal output? Intake and output measurements help to determine whether a fluid imbalance exists (see Chapter 42). Monitoring laboratory data such as levels of electrolytes, serum protein (albumin and total protein), and blood urea nitrogen (BUN) helps you to determine metabolic functioning.

Monitoring food intake and elimination patterns and assessing wound healing help to determine altered GI functioning and potential metabolic problems. If the patient has a wound, the rate of healing is affected by nutritional intake and nutrient absorption. Normal progression of healing indicates that metabolic needs of injured tissues are being met. Anorexia commonly occurs in patients who are immobilized. Assess the patient's food intake before the meal tray is removed to determine the amount eaten. Assess his or her dietary patterns and food preferences at the onset of immobilization to help prevent nutritional imbalances (see Chapter 45).

Respiratory System. Perform a respiratory assessment at least every 2 hours for patients with restricted activity. Inspect chest wall movements during the full inspiratory-expiratory cycle. If a patient has an atelectatic area, chest movement is often asymmetrical. Auscultate the entire lung region to identify diminished breath sounds, crackles, or wheezes. Focus auscultation on the dependent lung fields because pulmonary secretions tend to collect in these lower regions. Assessment findings that indicate pneumonia include productive cough with greenish yellow sputum; fever; pain on breathing; and crackles, wheezes, and dyspnea.

Cardiovascular System. Cardiovascular nursing assessment of a patient who is immobilized includes monitoring blood pressure and heart rate and assessing the arteriovenous system. Because of the risk for orthostatic hypotension, measure blood pressure when a patient moves from lying to a sitting or standing position. Move a patient gradually during position changes, and monitor him or her closely for dizziness while assessing blood pressure in each position. These measurements document the patient's tolerance to postural changes and are vital to know when positioning or transferring patients from one position or location to another. The longer the period of immobility, the greater is the risk of orthostatic hypotension when the patient stands (McCance and Huether, 2017).

Assess heart rate, including the apical pulse. Lying down increases cardiac workload and results in an increased pulse rate. In older adults, the heart rate often does not tolerate the added workload, and a form of cardiac failure may develop. A third heart sound, heard at the apex of the heart, is an early indication of congestive heart failure.

Monitoring peripheral pulses (see Chapter 30) allows you to assess the ability of the heart to pump blood and the condition of the arterial system. Immediately document and report the absence of a peripheral pulse in the lower extremities, especially if the pulse was present previously. Check for capillary refill to determine tissue perfusion. Also note the color of extremities, as changes in venous and arterial function will alter skin color.

Edema sometimes develops in patients who have had tissue injury or whose heart is unable to handle the increased workload of bed rest. Because edema moves to dependent body regions, assessment of the patient experiencing immobility includes inspection of the sacrum, legs, and feet for edema. If the heart is unable to tolerate the increased workload, peripheral body regions such as the hands, feet, nose, and earlobes are colder than central body regions.

Venous thromboembolism (VTE) is a blood clot in a vein. It is related to two life-threatening conditions: deep vein thrombosis (DVT) (a clot in a deep vein, usually the leg) and pulmonary **embolus** (a deep vein clot that breaks free from a vein wall, travels to the lungs, and blocks some or all of the blood supply) (American Heart Association [AHA], 2017). Venous thromboembolism is a hazard of immobility, as well as other medical conditions. Venous emboli that travel to the lungs are sometimes life threatening. More than 90% of all pulmonary emboli begin in the deep veins of the lower extremities (McCance and Huether, 2017).

Common risk factors for VTE include conditions that influence the **Virchow's triad**: *hypercoagulability* (e.g., clotting disorders, fever, dehydration); *venous wall abnormalities* (e.g., orthopedic surgery, varicose veins); and *blood flow stasis* (e.g., immobility, obesity, pregnancy). To assess the venous system for presence of a DVT determine whether the patient is experiencing leg pain by gently palpating under the thighs and along the calves. Note any tenderness or cramping, and look for redness. Gently palpate for presence of edema. Carefully compare findings in both legs; unilateral redness, tenderness, and edema indicate possible DVT. Also consider the patient's risk factors for a DVT

BOX 39.4   Risk Factors for Developing Deep Vein Thrombosis

- Surgery
- Trauma
- Long periods of not moving (bed rest, sitting, long car or airplane trips)
- Cancer and cancer therapy
- Past history of DVT
- Increasing age
- Pregnancy and the 4–6 weeks after giving birth
- Certain illnesses, including heart failure, inflammatory bowel disease, and some kidney disorders
- Hypertension
- Hyperlipidemia
- Nephrotic syndrome
- Autoimmune disease, including systemic lupus erythematosus
- Obesity
- Smoking
- Use of birth control pills
- Varicose veins
- Having a tube in a main vein (sometimes needed to give medications over a period of time)
- Having thrombophilia, one of several diseases in which the blood does not clot correctly

From ACOG: Preventing deep vein thrombosis, August 2011. http://www.acog.org/Patients/FAQs/Preventing-Deep-Vein-Thrombosis Accessed January 18, 2020.

TABLE 39.5   Wells Score for the Prediction of Deep Vein Thrombosis

Parameter	Score
Active cancer (patient receiving treatment for cancer within previous 6 months or currently receiving palliative treatment)	1
Paralysis, paresis, or recent plaster immobilization of lower extremities	1
Recently bedridden for 3 days or more, or major surgery within previous 12 weeks requiring general or regional anesthesia	1
Localized tenderness along distribution of the deep vein system	1
Entire leg swollen	1
Calf swelling at least 3 cm more when compared with asymptomatic leg	1
Pitting edema localized to symptomatic leg	1
Collateral superficial veins	1
Previously documented DVT	1
Alternative diagnosis as likely as or greater than that of DVT	-2

Wells scoring system for DVT: -2 to 0: low probability; 1 to 2 points: moderate probability; 3 to 8 points: high probability.
From *World J Emerg Surg* 11:24, 2016. Published online 2016 Jun 8. https://doi.org/10.1186/s13017-016-0078-1. Accessed January 18, 2020.

(Box 39.4). The Wells score is an objective and widely used measure for determining a patient's risk for a DVT (Table 39.5) (Wells, 1998; Modi, 2016). When you identify clinical indicators of a possible DVT, report to a health care provider immediately, and include the Wells score as appropriate. If a patient has antiembolic stockings or a sequential or mobile compression device (SCD/MCD), remove the stockings or device once every 8 hours or according to agency policy and reassess the calves and thighs.

Measure bilateral calf circumference and record it daily as an alternative assessment for DVT. To do this, mark a point on each calf 10 cm down from the midpatella. Measure the circumference each day, using this mark for placement of the tape measure. Unilateral increases in calf circumference are an early indication of thrombosis (Lewis et al., 2017). If the patient has a history of DVT, measurement of the thighs should also be conducted daily since the upper thigh is a common site for clot formation. Many hospitals now order Doppler ultrasounds to assess blood flow in arteries and veins to detect presence of clots. There is a high prevalence of asymptomatic DVTs, especially among elderly patients.

Musculoskeletal System. Major musculoskeletal abnormalities to identify during nursing assessment include decreased muscle tone and strength, loss of muscle mass, reduced ROM, and contractures. During assessment of ROM (described earlier) you can detect muscle tone by asking the patient to relax and then passively moving each limb at several joints to get a feeling for any resistance or rigidity that may be present. You assess for muscle strength by having the patient assume a stable position and then performing maneuvers to demonstrate strength of the major muscle groups (see Chapter 30).

Physical assessment cannot identify disuse osteoporosis. However, patients on prolonged bed rest, postmenopausal women, patients taking steroids, and people with increased serum and urine calcium levels have a greater risk for bone demineralization. Consider the risk of disuse osteoporosis when planning nursing interventions. Although some falls result in injury, others occur because of pathological fractures secondary to osteoporosis.

Integumentary System. Continually assess a patient's skin for breakdown and color changes such as pallor or redness. Consistently use a standardized assessment tool such as the Braden Scale. The screening tool identifies patients with a high risk for impaired skin integrity or early changes in the condition of patients' skin. Early identification allows for early intervention. Observe the skin often during routine care (e.g., when the patient is turned, during hygiene measures, and when providing for elimination needs). Frequent skin assessment, which can be as often as every hour and is based on patients' mobility, hydration, and physiological status, is essential to promptly identify changes in their skin and underlying tissues (see Chapter 48).

Elimination System. To determine the effects of immobility on elimination, assess the patient's total intake and output each shift and every 24 hours. Compare the amounts over time. Determine that the patient is receiving the correct amount and type of fluids orally or parenterally (see Chapter 42). Inadequate intake and output or fluid and electrolyte imbalances increase the risk for renal system impairment, ranging from recurrent infections to kidney failure. Dehydration also increases the risk for constipation.

Immobility impairs GI peristalsis. Assessment of bowel elimination status includes the adequacy of a patient's dietary choices, bowel sounds, passing of flatus, and the frequency and consistency of bowel movements (see Chapter 47). Accurate assessment enables you to intervene before constipation and fecal impaction occur.

Psychosocial Assessment. Many alterations in developmental functioning are related to immobility. Often these problems are interrelated, and it is imperative that nursing care focus on all dimensions. Often the focus of immobility is on the easily visible physical problems such as skin impairment, but do not overlook its psychosocial and developmental aspects.

Abrupt changes in personality often have a physiological cause such as surgery, a medication reaction, a pulmonary embolus, or an acute infection. For example, the primary symptom of compromised older patients with a UTI or fever is confusion. Identifying confusion is an important component of a nurse's assessment. Acute confusion,

or delirium, is a neuropsychiatric syndrome with alterations in arousal, attention, and cognition (American Psychiatric Association (APA), 2013). Delirium can be triggered by a wide variety of medical or surgical conditions (Mulkey et al., 2018). Delirium in older adults is not normal, especially after surgery or procedures (see Chapter 50). A thorough nursing assessment is the priority (Chase et al., 2018).

Common reactions to immobilization include boredom, anxiety, and feelings of isolation, depression, and anger. These patients often experience an intolerance to exercise. Depressed patients tend to withdraw rather than participate. Observe for changes in a patient's emotional status, and listen carefully to family if they report emotional changes. Examples of change that indicate psychosocial concerns are a cooperative patient who becomes less cooperative or an independent patient who asks for more help than is necessary. Investigate reasons for such alterations. Identifying how a patient usually copes with loss is vital (see Chapters 36 and 37). A change in mobility status, whether permanent or not, causes a grief reaction. Families are a key resource for information about behavioral changes.

Because psychosocial changes usually occur gradually, observe the patient's behavior on a daily basis. If behavioral changes occur, determine the cause(s) and evaluate the changes. Identifying the cause helps you to design appropriate nursing interventions.

Developmental Assessment. Include a developmental assessment of patients who are immobilized. When caring for a young child, determine whether he or she is able to meet developmental tasks and is progressing normally (see Chapter 12). The child's development sometimes regresses or slows because he or she is immobilized

Immobilization of a family member changes family functioning. The family's response to this change often leads to problems, stress, and anxieties. When children see parents who are immobile, they sometimes have difficulty understanding what is occurring and coping. Assess the family's perceptions as to how roles have changed and how they are coping.

Immobility has a significant effect on the older adult's levels of health, independence, and functional status. Focus your assessment on the patient's ability to meet needs independently and to adapt to developmental changes such as declining physical functioning and altered family and peer relationships. A decline in developmental functioning needs prompt investigation to determine why the change occurred and interventions that can return the patient to an optimal level of functioning as soon as possible. Activities that reduce immobility and promote participation in ADLs are vital to preventing functional decline (Hallford et al., 2017; Musich et al., 2018).

QSEN Building Competency in Quality Improvement Ms. Cavallo's skilled care unit is implementing a quality improvement (QI) project focused on prevention of falls. The unit has been experiencing a notable increase in the number of falls over the past several months. A review of the literature notes that the consequences of falls are many, including the need for additional care, psychological effects, and even death. A good starting point is a detailed look at the patients who sustained falls. Did these individuals have risk factors or characteristics in common? Are any of these commonalities related to alterations in mobility? You recognize the need to develop a collaborative plan of care that includes all health care professionals that work on the unit, the patients, and their families. What are the best methods you can use to communicate your findings and strategies for fall prevention to all health care providers and family participating in Ms. Cavallo's care? How do you identify gaps between the unit and best practice? Which measures could you use to evaluate whether change has taken place?

Answers to QSEN Activities can be found on the Evolve website.

BOX 39.5 Nursing Diagnostic Process: Impaired Mobility Related to Left Hip/Leg Pain

Assessment Activities	Assessment Findings
Measure ROM during extension and flexion of the hip.	Patient has limited ROM in left hip/leg.
Observe patient attempt to move her left leg.	Patient unable to lift her left leg off mattress.
Ask patient about perception of pain.	Patient complains of sharp pain (8 on scale of 0 to 10) in hip and leg when she tries to move them.
Ask patient about endurance and activity tolerance.	Patient reports no muscle strength in left leg. "I can't move it by myself."

ROM, Range of motion.

◆ Nursing Diagnosis

A patient who is experiencing an alteration in mobility often has one or more nursing diagnoses. The two diagnoses most directly related to mobility problems are *Impaired Mobility* and *Risk for Disuse Syndrome.* The diagnosis of *Impaired Mobility* applies to the patient who has some limitation but is not completely immobile. The diagnosis of *Risk for Disuse Syndrome* applies to the patient who is immobile and at risk for multisystem problems because of inactivity. Beyond these diagnoses, the list of potential diagnoses is extensive, because immobility affects multiple body systems. Possible nursing diagnoses include the following:

- *Impaired Airway Clearance*
- *Impaired Sleep*
- *Risk for Impaired Skin Integrity*
- *Risk for Constipation*
- *Social Isolation*

Assessment reveals clusters of data that indicate whether a patient is at risk or if a negative or problem-focused diagnosis exists. The clusters of data reveal at-risk factors or assessment findings that are observable assessment cues to support a diagnostic label. In the case of a negative or problem-focused diagnosis, the assessment data will reveal a related factor for the diagnosis. In addition to the accurate clustering of assessment data, an important part of formulating nursing diagnoses is identifying the relevant causative or related factor (when a diagnosis is *negative* or problem focused) or risk factors (when a diagnosis is a risk diagnosis). You choose interventions that treat or modify the related factor or *risk* for the diagnosis to be resolved. Accurate identification of nursing diagnoses is important to planning patient-centered goals and subsequent nursing interventions that will best help the patient.

Impaired Mobility related to reluctance to initiate movement requires slightly different interventions than *Impaired Mobility* related to pain in the left shoulder. Thus it is critical that nursing assessment activities identify and cluster assessment findings that ultimately support the nursing diagnosis selected (Box 39.5). The diagnosis that is related to reluctance to initiate movement requires interventions aimed at keeping the patient as mobile as possible and encouraging him or her to perform self-care and ROM. The diagnosis related to pain requires you to assist the patient with pharmacological and nonpharmacological comfort measures (see Chapter 44) so that he or she is then willing and more able to move. In both situations you would explain how activity enhances healthy body functioning.

Often the physiological dimension is the major focus of nursing care for patients with impaired mobility. Thus the psychosocial and developmental dimensions are neglected. Yet all dimensions are important to health. During immobilization some patients experience decreased social interaction and stimuli. These patients frequently use the nurse's call bell to request minor physical attention when their real need is greater socialization. Nursing diagnoses for health needs in developmental areas reflect changes from the patient's normal activities. Immobility leads to a developmental crisis if the patient is unable to resolve problems and continue to mature.

Immobility also leads to multiple complications (e.g., renal calculi, DVT, pulmonary emboli, or pneumonia). If these conditions develop, collaborate with the health care provider or nurse practitioner for prescribed therapy to intervene. Be alert for and prevent these potential complications when possible.

◆ Planning

During planning, you synthesize information from scientific knowledge, your knowledge of the roles of resources, such as respiratory and physical therapy, and clinical standards, such as skin care guidelines from the Agency for Healthcare Research and Quality (AHRQ, n.d.) and the Wound Ostomy and Continence Nurses Society (WOCN, 2016), and from protocols for patients at risk for falls (AACN, 2014) (Fig. 39.9). You also apply critical thinking attitudes, such as creativity and perseverance, and consider past experiences with immobilized patients. Critical thinking ensures that the patient's plan of care integrates all that you know about the individual patient and key critical thinking elements. Professional standards are especially important to consider when you develop a plan of care. These standards often establish scientifically proven guidelines for selecting effective nursing interventions. Finally, as stated earlier, the patient is a full partner in designing the plan of care, and this input must be reflected when establishing the goals and outcomes.

Impaired mobility affects all physiological symptoms and affects a patient's independence and psychosocial status. Fig. 39.10 shows the relationship between impaired mobility and patient activity.

Goals and Outcomes. Develop an individualized plan of care for each nursing diagnosis (see the Nursing Care Plan). Set realistic expectations for care, and include the patient and family when possible. Set goals that are individualized, realistic, and measurable. The goals focus on preventing problems or risks to impaired body alignment and mobility.

◎ NURSING CARE PLAN

Impaired Mobility

ASSESSMENT

Ms. Carnella Cavallo, a 97-year-old patient, is admitted to a skilled care unit for rehabilitation 6 days after recovering from a surgically repaired fractured left hip. She has a history of smoking but stopped 40 years ago. She has no cardiac problems and no hypertension. She describes having "aches" and "stiffness" when lying still in bed but denies pain. The three small incisions are clean, dry and intact.

Assessment Activities	*Assessment Findings*[a]
Ask Ms. Cavallo to rate her pain on a scale of 0 to 10.	She rates her pain as a 2 on a scale of 0 to 10 at rest, but it **increases to an 8** with any movement of her left leg.
Assess Ms. Cavallo's ability to transfer.	She is **unable to transfer, even** with help from chair to bed.
Ask Ms. Cavallo how her surgery has affected her mobility.	She responds that she wants to get out of bed, but when she moves her left leg, her nonverbal signs (grimacing and groaning) indicate that she is in severe pain. She says that it is a "**sharp, stabbing pain.**"

[a]**Assessment findings** are shown in bold type.

NURSING DIAGNOSIS: Impaired mobility related to musculoskeletal impairment from surgery and pain with movement

PLANNING

Goals	*Expected Outcomes*[b]
	Pain Control
Ms. Cavallo will have reduced pain during activity.	Ms. Cavallo's pain is less than 6 during activity.
	Body positioning will be self-initiated
Ms. Cavallo will be able to transfer with assistive device by discharge.	Ms. Cavallo is able to move from her bed to her chair and back again using her walker and assist ×1 within 3 days.
	Ms. Cavallo is able to transfer from her chair to her bedside commode using her walker within 3 days.
	Ambulation
Ms. Cavallo will walk 300 feet using her walker by discharge.	Ms. Cavallo walks to her door and around her room with her walker within 6 days.
	Ms. Cavallo walks 100 feet at a slow pace using her walker 3 times a day in 14 days at rehab and increases the distance that she walks by 100 feet every day after that.

[b]Nursing outcomes classification from Moorhead S, et al., editors: *Nursing Outcomes Classification (NOC)*, ed 6, St Louis, 2018, Elsevier.

INTERVENTIONS[c]

RATIONALE

Exercise Therapy: Ambulation

Consult with physical therapist on selection of transfer technique.

Instruct Ms. Cavallo on safe transfer and ambulation techniques in an environment with few distractions. Provide written materials and the use of the teach-back method to reinforce verbal instructions.

Establish realistic increments for transferring and increasing distance for ambulation.

Pain Management

Administer pain medication on the basis of your assessment of Ms. Cavallo's needs and on an ATC schedule rather than prn. Consult with health care provider for order to adjust dose if patient exhibits signs of being in pain or complains of pain not relieved with current regimen.

Introduce nonpharmacological modalities such as ice or heat, positioning, mind-body directed therapies, and massage to support pain management.

Observe for signs of pain when patient is moving or attempting exercises from physical therapy (PT) and have prn dose of pain medication ordered if additional pain medication is needed for PT activities.

Ensures safe transfer technique with less risk of patient injury.

Providing instruction in a quiet environment and using the teach-back method enhance learning (Bodenheimer, 2018; Centrella-Nigro and Alexander, 2017).

Physiotherapy exercises, physical activity, and setting realistic goals for ambulation encourage activity in older adults (Kruschke, 2017; Musich et al., 2018).

Obtain order to adjust (increase or decrease dose) on the basis of a patient's report of pain severity or her ability to perform activities of daily living (ADLs) (Bonkowski et al., 2018).

The Joint Commission (TJC) revised its pain mandate to include required addition of evidence-based nonpharmacological therapies for pain as a scorable element of performance (TJC, 2018).

Evidence-based nonpharmacological therapies are safe and effective components in postsurgical pain management and have potential to decrease the use of opioids and the related risk for misuse (Tick et al., 2018).

Have an "as needed" dose of pain medication for patient in case he/she requires a supplemental dose.

[c]Intervention classification labels from Butcher HK, et al., editors: *Nursing Interventions Classification (NIC)*, ed 7, St Louis, 2018, Elsevier.

EVALUATION

Evaluation Activity	*Patient Response/Finding*	*Outcome Status*
Ask Ms. Cavallo to rate her level of pain.	Ms. Cavallo reports pain at 5 during activity.	Ms. Cavallo has achieved improved pain control.
Observe Ms. Cavallo's ability to transfer from bed to chair.	Ms. Cavallo is able to transfer from bed to chair using her walker and stand-by assistance of nurse.	Ms. Cavallo has achieved goal of transferring with walker and assistance.
Assess Ms. Cavallo as she walks in the hall; measure how far she walks.	Ms. Cavallo is able to walk 200 feet in the hall with her walker by day 2 of rehab.	Activity level is improving. Continue interventions and continue to encourage ambulation.

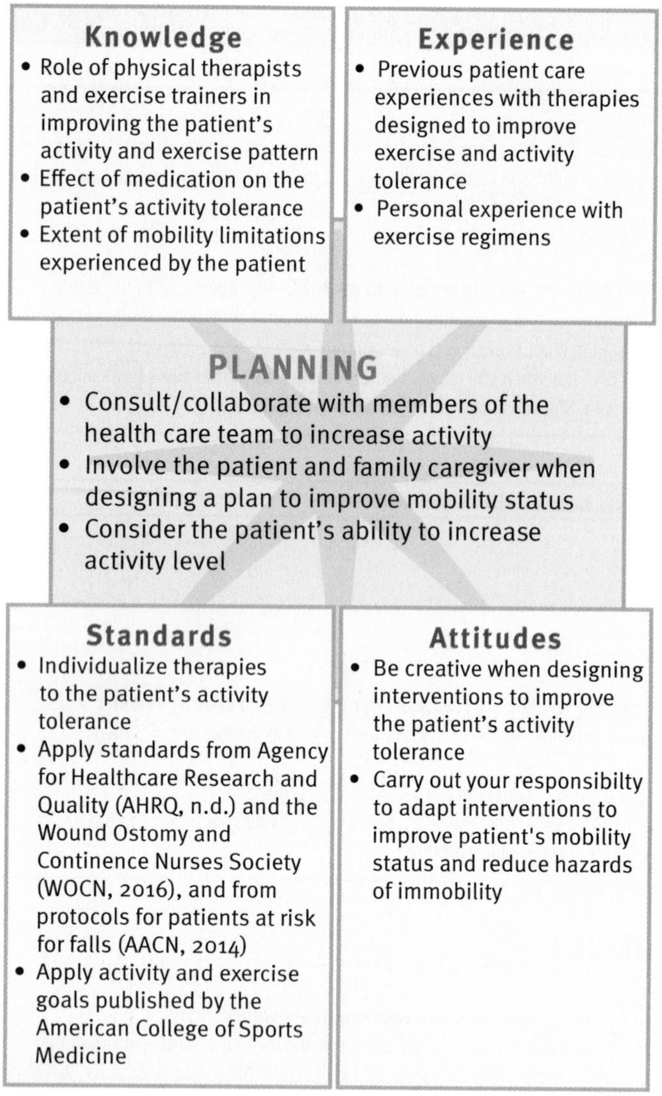

Knowledge

- Role of physical therapists and exercise trainers in improving the patient's activity and exercise pattern
- Effect of medication on the patient's activity tolerance
- Extent of mobility limitations experienced by the patient

Experience

- Previous patient care experiences with therapies designed to improve exercise and activity tolerance
- Personal experience with exercise regimens

PLANNING

- Consult/collaborate with members of the health care team to increase activity
- Involve the patient and family caregiver when designing a plan to improve mobility status
- Consider the patient's ability to increase activity level

Standards

- Individualize therapies to the patient's activity tolerance
- Apply standards from Agency for Healthcare Research and Quality (AHRQ, n.d.) and the Wound Ostomy and Continence Nurses Society (WOCN, 2016), and from protocols for patients at risk for falls (AACN, 2014)
- Apply activity and exercise goals published by the American College of Sports Medicine

Attitudes

- Be creative when designing interventions to improve the patient's activity tolerance
- Carry out your responsibilty to adapt interventions to improve patient's mobility status and reduce hazards of immobility

FIG. 39.9 Critical thinking model for planning for impaired mobility.

Develop goals and expected outcomes to help patients achieve their highest level of mobility and reduce the hazards of immobility. For example, a patient who has left-sided paralysis following a stroke has two long-term goals. The first, directed toward improved mobility, is "Patient will use walker to ambulate safely in the home." A parallel goal directed toward the hazards of immobility is "Patient's skin will remain intact." Both of these goals are essential to restoring the patient's maximal mobility.

Because the patient has impaired sensation, both the patient and caregivers need to be aware of the patient's need to have the skin free of pressure. Expected outcomes for the goal of the skin remaining intact include the following:

- Patient's skin color and temperature return to normal baseline within 20 minutes of position change.
- Patient changes position at least every 2 hours.

Setting Priorities. The effect that problems have on a patient's mental and physical health determines the immediacy of any problem. Set priorities when planning care to ensure that immediate needs are met first. This is particularly important when patients have multiple diagnoses. Plan therapies according to severity of risks to the patient, and individualize the plan according to the patient's developmental stage, level of health, and lifestyle.

It is especially important in priority setting to make sure that you do not overlook potential complications. Many times actual problems such as pressure injuries and disuse syndrome are addressed only after they develop. Therefore monitor the patient often, reinforcing prevention techniques to both the patient and other caregivers and supervising assistive personnel in carrying out activities aimed at preventing complications of impaired mobility.

Teamwork and Collaboration. Care of the patient experiencing alterations in mobility requires a team approach. Nurses often delegate select interventions that are appropriate for assistive personnel (AP) to perform. For example, in the case of postoperative patients who are at risk for respiratory problems from temporary immobility, AP can encourage the patient to do leg exercises, use the incentive spirometer, and cough and deep breathe (see Chapter 50). When patients have limited mobility as a result of paralysis, AP can turn and position patients and apply elastic stockings. They can also help the nurse measure leg circumferences and height and weight.

Collaborate with other health care team members such as physical or occupational therapists when it is essential to consider mobility needs. Understanding the need for and having open communications with other members of the interprofessional care team result in better patient outcomes and hopefully prevent the hazards of immobility. It is through these collaborative efforts and teamwork that patients benefit most. For example, physical therapists are a resource for planning ROM or strengthening exercises, and occupational therapists are a resource for planning new or altered ways to perform ADLs that patients need to learn. Wound care specialists and respiratory therapists are often involved in patient care, especially with patients who are experiencing complications related to their immobility. Consult a registered dietitian when the patient is experiencing nutritional problems; refer him or her to a mental health advanced practice nurse, licensed social worker, or psychologist to assist with coping or other psychosocial issues.

Discharge planning begins when a patient enters the health care system. In anticipation of the patient's discharge from an institution, make appropriate referrals or consult a case manager or a discharge planner to ensure that the patient's needs are met at home. Consider the patient's home environment when planning therapies to maintain or improve body alignment and mobility. Referrals to home care or outpatient therapy are often needed if a patient continues to have mobility limitations when discharged.

◆ Implementation

Health Promotion. Health promotion activities include a variety of interventions such as education, prevention, and early detection. Examples of health promotion activities that address mobility and immobility include prevention of work-related injury, fall prevention measures, exercise, and early detection of scoliosis.

Prevention of Work-Related Musculoskeletal Injuries. The rate of work-related injuries in health care settings has increased in recent years. According to the Department of Labor (USDL, 2017), 59,710 occupational musculoskeletal injuries related to patient handling occurred in 2016. Most of these injuries occurred as a result of overexertion, which resulted in back injuries and other musculoskeletal problems. Back injuries are often the direct result of improper lifting and bending. The most common back injury is strain on the lumbar muscle group, which includes the muscles around the lumbar vertebrae. Injury to these areas affects the ability to bend forward, backward, and from side to side and limits the ability to rotate the hips and lower back. Research has demonstrated that ergonomic programs and safe patient-handling policies in health care facilities reduce costs, injuries to employees, and missed work days (Klein et al., 2018; Noble and Sweeney, 2018).

CONCEPT MAP

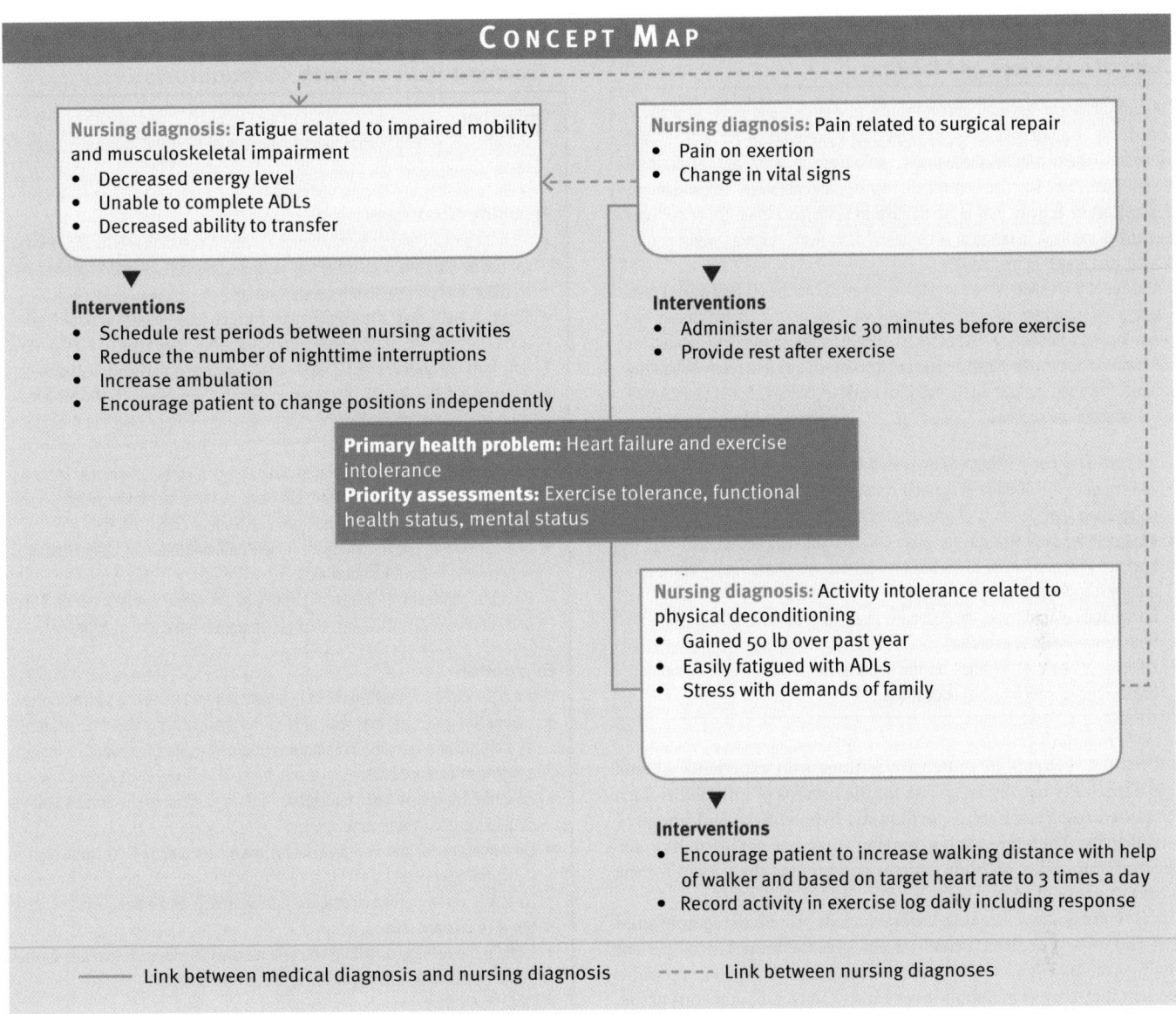

Nursing diagnosis: Fatigue related to impaired mobility and musculoskeletal impairment
- Decreased energy level
- Unable to complete ADLs
- Decreased ability to transfer

Interventions
- Schedule rest periods between nursing activities
- Reduce the number of nighttime interruptions
- Increase ambulation
- Encourage patient to change positions independently

Nursing diagnosis: Pain related to surgical repair
- Pain on exertion
- Change in vital signs

Interventions
- Administer analgesic 30 minutes before exercise
- Provide rest after exercise

Primary health problem: Heart failure and exercise intolerance
Priority assessments: Exercise tolerance, functional health status, mental status

Nursing diagnosis: Activity intolerance related to physical deconditioning
- Gained 50 lb over past year
- Easily fatigued with ADLs
- Stress with demands of family

Interventions
- Encourage patient to increase walking distance with help of walker and based on target heart rate to 3 times a day
- Record activity in exercise log daily including response

———— Link between medical diagnosis and nursing diagnosis   - - - - - Link between nursing diagnoses

FIG 39.10 Concept map for Mrs. Cavallo.

Nurses and other health care staff are especially at risk for injury to lumbar muscles when lifting, transferring, or positioning immobilized patients. Therefore be aware of agency policies and protocols that protect staff and patients from injury. When lifting, assess the weight you will lift and determine the assistance you will need. Current safe patient-handling algorithms support that using mechanical or other ergonomic assistive devices is the safest way to reposition and lift patients who are unable to do these activities themselves. Many agencies have developed special patient lift teams and have instituted a minimal lift policy (see Chapter 38).

Exercise. Although many diseases and physical problems cause or contribute to immobility, it is important to remember that exercise programs enhance feelings of well-being and improve endurance, strength, and health. Exercise reduces the risk of many health problems such as cardiovascular disease, diabetes, and osteoporosis from worsening. It is important to give patients options for how to stay active and how to change their behavior if exercise has not been their routine. The Stanford Medicine (2018) chronic disease self-management program encourages appropriate exercise for maintaining and improving strength, flexibility, and endurance. As a nurse you can encourage all patients to find a type of exercise that meets their lifestyle and particular health-related needs. For example, a patient with severe arthritis of the knees might benefit from aquatic therapy (exercise in a pool) rather than walking. Encourage hospitalized patients to perform stretching, ROM exercises, and light walking within the limits of their condition (see Chapter 38). Take cultural preferences into consideration when helping patients design exercise plans (Box 39.6).

Bone Health in Patients with Osteoporosis. Patients at risk for or diagnosed with osteoporosis have special health promotion needs. Encourage patients at risk to be screened for osteoporosis and assess their diets for calcium and vitamin D intake. Patients who have lactose intolerance need dietary teaching about alternative sources of calcium.

For patients diagnosed with osteoporosis, early evaluation, consultation with, and referral to health care providers, dietitians, and physical therapists are important interventions, especially when they become immobilized. The goal of the patient with osteoporosis is to maintain independence with ADLs. Assistive ambulatory devices, adaptive clothing, and safety bars help patients maintain independence. Patient teaching needs to focus on limiting the severity of the disease through diet and activity (Box 39.7).

BOX 39.6 CULTURAL ASPECTS OF CARE

Cultural Influences on Mobility

Cultural influences have an important role in exercise and physical activity. Specifically, culture influences an individual's preferences for activity and exercise. Certain cultures discourage involvement in organized recreational physical activities such as basketball, running, and aerobics. Ethnic dancing is an effective activity that is acceptable in many countries. Other cultures emphasize exercise in terms of activities of daily living, such as walking, gardening, and prayer or meditation.

A sedentary lifestyle places an individual at risk for being overweight (see Chapter 38). Children from many cultures who live in the United States are becoming more sedentary. Therefore a national health approach is needed for communities to provide social and physical environments that promote healthy choices. From the earliest age preventive health practices should be included in the educational process.

Implications for Patient-Centered Care

- Assess patterns of daily living and culturally prescribed activities before suggesting specific forms of exercise to patients.
- Help patients plan physical activities that are culturally acceptable.
- Exercise programs need to be flexible and accommodate family and community responsibilities of the culture.
- Encourage culturally specific and individually tailored interventions to facilitate commitment to exercise.
- Educate patients of all ages on the importance of exercise in preserving health, and correct any misconceptions.

BOX 39.7 PATIENT TEACHING

Teaching Patients with Osteoporosis

Objective
- Patient will verbalize strategies to prevent or limit the severity of osteoporosis.

Teaching Strategies
- Instruct patient and/or family caregiver about common risk factors and how to modify lifestyle (e.g., smoking, caffeine, alcohol, hormone replacement as recommended by health care provider).
- Teach patient and/or caregiver the current recommended dietary allowances for calcium, and review culturally specific foods high in calcium (e.g., milk fortified with vitamin D, leafy green vegetables, yogurt, and cheese).
- Instruct patient and/or caregiver in appropriate types of weight-bearing exercises as recommended by health care provider or physical therapist to prevent injury or fractures.
- Teach patient and/or caregiver about safety, fall prevention, and strategies to create a safe home environment (e.g., remove scatter rugs; ensure that hallways, steps, and rooms are well lit) (Bodenheimer, 2018).
- Instruct patient and/or caregiver in self-administration of prescribed medication used to treat osteoporosis.
- Promote positive self-image in patient by providing realistic yet optimistic and positive feedback about changes in appearance and mobility.

Evaluation
Use the principles of teach-back to evaluate patient/family caregiver learning:
- I want to make sure that you understand the teaching about osteoporosis. Tell me three lifestyle modifications you can make to prevent or limit the severity of osteoporosis.
- Describe for me at least four foods high in calcium and vitamins that you should include in your diet.
- Demonstrate for me weight-bearing exercises and tell me your plan for doing the exercises.
- Describe three safety strategies that you will implement while you are home to prevent falls.
- Explain the dosage schedule you will follow for your osteoporosis medications and the side effects that you should watch for.
- Describe how the osteoporosis is affecting your lifestyle and activities.

Acute Care. Patients in acute care settings who experience altered physical mobility usually are at risk for the hazards of immobility such as impaired respiratory status, orthostatic hypotension, and impaired skin integrity. Therefore design nursing interventions to reduce the impact of immobility on body systems and prepare the patient for the restorative phase of care.

Metabolic System. Because the body needs protein to repair injured tissue and rebuild depleted protein stores, give the immobilized patient a high-protein, high-calorie diet. A high-calorie intake provides sufficient fuel to meet metabolic needs and replace subcutaneous tissue. Also ensure that the patient is taking vitamin B and C supplements when necessary. Supplementation with vitamin C is needed for skin integrity and wound healing; vitamin B complex assists in energy metabolism.

If the patient is unable to eat, nutrition must be provided parenterally or enterally. Total parenteral nutrition refers to delivery of nutritional supplements through a central or peripheral intravenous catheter. Enteral feedings include delivery through a nasogastric, gastrostomy, or jejunostomy tube of high-protein, high-calorie solutions with complete requirements of vitamins, minerals, and electrolytes (see Chapter 45).

Respiratory System. Patients who are immobilized and have reduced ventilation can benefit from a variety of nursing interventions that promote lung expansion and removal of pulmonary secretions. Patients need to frequently fully expand their lungs to maintain elastic recoil. In addition, secretions accumulate in the dependent areas of the lungs. Often patients with restricted mobility experience weakness, and as this progresses the cough reflex gradually becomes inefficient. All of these factors place patients at risk for developing pneumonia. The stasis of secretions in the lungs is life threatening for an immobilized patient.

Deep-breathing exercises, incentive spirometry, and controlled coughing are among the nursing interventions available to expand the lungs, dislodge and mobilize stagnant secretions, and clear the lungs (see Chapters 41 and 50). All of these interventions help reduce the risk of pneumonia. It is essential to implement pulmonary interventions early in all patients with limited mobility, even those who do not have pneumonia.

Encourage an immobile patient to deep-breathe and cough every 1 to 2 hours. Teach alert patients to deep breathe or yawn every hour or to use an incentive spirometer (when ordered). Controlled coughing, a common therapy for postoperative patients, involves taking in three deep breaths and then coughing with the third exhalation.

Chest physiotherapy (CPT) (percussion and postural drainage) is another method still used by respiratory therapists with the goal of keeping the airways clear (see Chapter 41). It helps the patient drain secretions from specific segments of the bronchi and lungs into the trachea so that he or she is able to cough and expel them. Respiratory assessment findings identify areas of the lungs requiring CPT. While this method is still widely used, high-level evidence for improved patient outcomes has not been seen in existing trials (Strickland et al., 2013).

Ensure that patients who are immobile have an adequate fluid intake. Unless there is a medical contraindication, an adult needs to drink at least 1100 to 1400 mL of noncaffeinated fluids daily. This helps keep mucociliary clearance normal. Expect pulmonary secretions to be removed easily with coughing and appear thin, watery, and clear. Without adequate hydration, pulmonary secretions become thick, tenacious, and difficult to remove. Offering fluids that patients prefer on a regularly timed schedule also helps with bowel and urine elimination and aids in maintaining circulation and skin integrity.

Cardiovascular System. The effects of bed rest or immobilization on the cardiovascular system include orthostatic hypotension, increased cardiac workload, and thrombus formation. Design nursing therapies to minimize or prevent these alterations.

Reducing Orthostatic Hypotension. When patients who are on bed rest or have been immobile move to a sitting or standing position, they often experience orthostatic hypotension. They have an increased pulse rate, a decreased pulse pressure, and a drop in blood pressure. If symptoms become severe enough, the patient can faint (McCance and Huether, 2017). To prevent injury, implement interventions that reduce or eliminate the effects of orthostatic hypotension. It occurs when a normotensive person develops symptoms and a drop in systolic pressure by at least 20 mm Hg or a drop in diastolic pressure by at least 10 mm Hg within 3 minutes of rising to an upright position (Shibao et al., 2013). Mobilize the patient as soon as the physical condition allows, even if this only involves dangling at the bedside or moving to a chair. This activity maintains muscle tone and increases venous return. Isometric exercises (i.e., activities that involve muscle tension without muscle shortening) have no beneficial effect on preventing orthostatic hypotension, but they improve activity tolerance. When getting an immobile patient up for the first time, assess the situation using a safe patient-handling algorithm (US Department of Veterans Affairs, 2018) or another appropriate mobility assessment/screening/scoring system. This is a precautionary step that protects you and the patient from injury and also allows the patient to do as much of the transfer as possible.

Reducing Cardiac Workload. A nursing intervention that reduces cardiac workload involves instructing patients to avoid using a Valsalva maneuver when moving up in bed, defecating, or lifting household objects. During a Valsalva maneuver a patient holds his or her breath and strains, which increases intrathoracic pressure and in turn decreases venous return and cardiac output. When the strain is released, venous return and cardiac output immediately increase, and systolic blood pressure and pulse pressure rise. These pressure changes produce a reflex bradycardia and possible decrease in blood pressure that can result in sudden cardiac death in patients with heart disease. Teach patients to breathe out while defecating, lifting, or moving side-to-side or up in bed and to not hold their breath and strain.

Preventing Thrombus Formation. The Centers for Medicare and Medicaid Services identified 10 "Never Events" in 2008. A Never Event is a hospital-acquired event for which Medicare and other third-party payers will no longer pay hospitals at a higher rate for the increased costs of care. Deep vein thrombosis (DVT) is one of these Never Events. The most cost-effective way to address DVT is through an aggressive program of prophylaxis. Prevention of DVT is critical to reduce the risk of fatal and nonfatal pulmonary embolism. A prophylaxis program begins with identification of patients at risk and continues throughout their immobilization This requires a collaborative role between nurses and health care providers. You will identify patient risk factors from the nursing assessment. There are nursing interventions you can employ to reduce the risk of thrombus formation in immobilized patients. Early ambulation; leg, foot, and ankle exercises; regularly provided fluids; frequent position changes; and patient teaching need to begin when a patient becomes immobile (see Chapter 50).

Prophylaxis also includes anticoagulation, mechanical prevention with graduated compression stockings, intermittent pneumatic compression devices, and foot pumps. Anticoagulation may include the use of aspirin, although this is somewhat controversial. Anticoagulants most often used include unfractionated heparin (UFH) (usually given as 5000 units two or three times daily), low-molecular-weight heparins (LMWHs) (e.g., enoxaparin or dalteparin), vitamin K antagonists (e.g., warfarin, but also acenocoumarol, phenindione, and dicoumarol), and fondaparinux (a selective factor Xa inhibitor) (Cave et al., 2018). Because bleeding is a potential side effect of anticoagulants, continually assess the patient for signs of bleeding, such as hematuria, bruising, coffee ground–like vomitus or GI aspirate, guaiac-positive stools, and bleeding gums.

Sequential compression devices (SCDs) and intermittent pneumatic compression (IPC) are used to prevent blood clots in the lower extremities. Research has shown that IPC significantly reduces the risk of DVT and significantly improves survival in a wide variety of patients who are immobile after stroke (Zhang et al., 2018). The SCD and IPC consist of sleeves or stockings made of fabric or plastic that are wrapped around the leg and secured with Velcro (Box 39.8). Once they are applied, connect the sleeves to a pump that alternately inflates and deflates the stocking around the leg. A typical cycle is inflation for 10 to 15 seconds and deflation for 45 to 60 seconds. Inflation pressures average 40 mm Hg. Use of SCD/IPC on the legs decreases venous stasis by increasing venous return through the deep veins of the legs. For optimal results begin use of SCD/IPC as soon as possible (e.g., immediately after major surgery) and maintain it until the patient becomes fully ambulatory. Increasing numbers of IPC devices allow patients to ambulate with the device in place; this decreases the chances for the device to be removed or turned off during ambulation with a failure to reinitiate in a timely manner (Link, 2018). It is imperative that you take every opportunity to monitor and educate the patient on the importance of mechanical VTE prevention devices.

BOX 39.8 PROCEDURAL GUIDELINES

Applying Sequential Compression Devices and Elastic Stockings

Delegation and Collaboration

The skill of applying and maintaining graduated compression stockings and intermittent SCDs and MCDs may be delegated to assistive personnel (AP). The nurse initially determines the size of elastic stockings and assesses the patient's lower extremities for any signs and symptoms of a DVT or impaired circulation. The nurse directs the AP to:

- Remove SCD sleeves before allowing a patient to get out of bed.
- Report to the nurse if a patient's calf or thigh appears larger than the other or is red, tender, hot, or swollen or if the patient complains of calf pain.

- Report to the nurse if there is redness, itching, or irritation on the legs (signs of allergic reactions to elastic).
- Report to the nurse if the patient is routinely removing the compression device from the legs.

Equipment

Tape measure; powder or cornstarch *(optional)*; graduated compression stockings or Velcro compression device sleeves; SCD/MCD insufflator with air hoses attached; compression device pump; hygiene supplies; *option:* cotton stockinette with MCD

Continued

BOX 39.8   PROCEDURAL GUIDELINES—cont'd

Applying Sequential Compression Devices and Elastic Stockings

Steps

1. Identify patient using at least two patient identifiers (e.g., name and birthday or name and medical record number) according to agency policy (TJC, 2020).

2. Review medical record for order for SCDs/MCDs or graduated compression stocking.

3. Review medical record to assess patient for risk factors for developing DVT (see Box 39.4). *An option is to use The Wells score, an objective and widely used measure for determining a patient's risk for a DVT (Wells, 1998; Modi, 2016) (see Table 39.5).*

4. Perform hand hygiene. Assess for contraindications for use of elastic stockings or compression devices:

   a. Dermatitis or open skin lesions on area to be covered by stockings/sleeves

   b. Recent skin graft to lower leg

   c. Decreased arterial circulation in lower extremities as evidenced by cyanotic, cool extremities and/or gangrenous conditions affecting the lower limb(s)

   d. If signs/symptoms of a DVT are present, *manipulation could cause a clot in vein within the leg to dislodge.*

5. Assess condition of patient's skin and circulation to the legs. Palpate pedal pulses; note any palpable veins, and inspect skin over lower extremities for edema, skin discoloration, warmth, presence of lesions.

6. Assess patient's or family caregiver's knowledge or experience regarding previous use of elastic compression stockings or compression devices. Assess patient's or family caregiver's health literacy.

7. Explain procedure and reason for applying elastic stockings/SCD/MCD to prevent DVT.

8. Close room curtains or door to provide privacy. Position patient in supine position.

9. Perform hand hygiene. Bathe patient's legs as needed. Dry thoroughly. Perform hand hygiene.

10. **Apply graduated compression stocking:**

    a. Use tape measure to measure patient's leg to determine proper elastic stocking size (follow package directions).

    b. *Option:* Apply a small amount of powder or cornstarch to legs provided that patient does not have sensitivity.

    c. Turn elastic stocking inside out: place one hand into stocking, holding heel of stocking. Take other hand and pull stocking inside out until reaching the heel (see illustration).

d. Place patient's toes into foot of elastic stocking up to the heel, making sure that stocking is smooth (see illustration A). Slide remaining portion of stocking over patient's foot, making sure that toes are covered. Make sure that foot fits into toe and heel position of stocking. Stocking will now be right side out (see illustration B).

e. Slide stocking up over patient's calf until sock is completely extended. Be sure that stocking is smooth and that no ridges or wrinkles are present (see illustration).

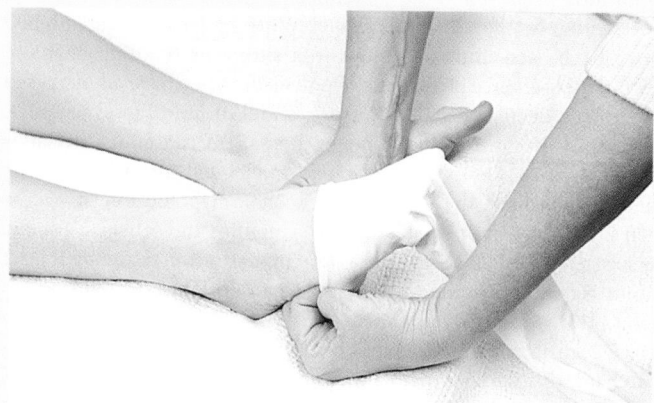

A

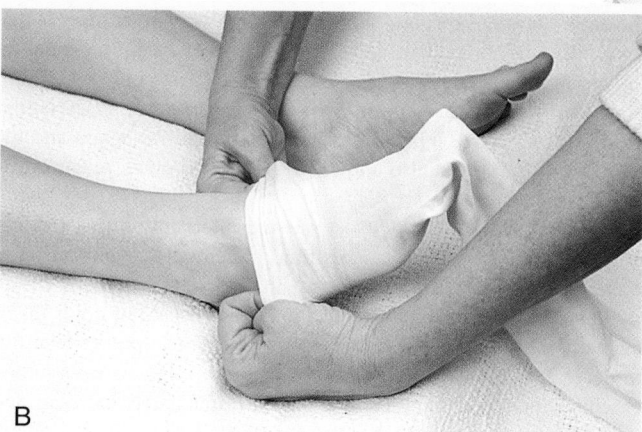

B

STEP 10d A, Place toes into foot of stocking. **B,** Slide remaining part of stocking over foot.

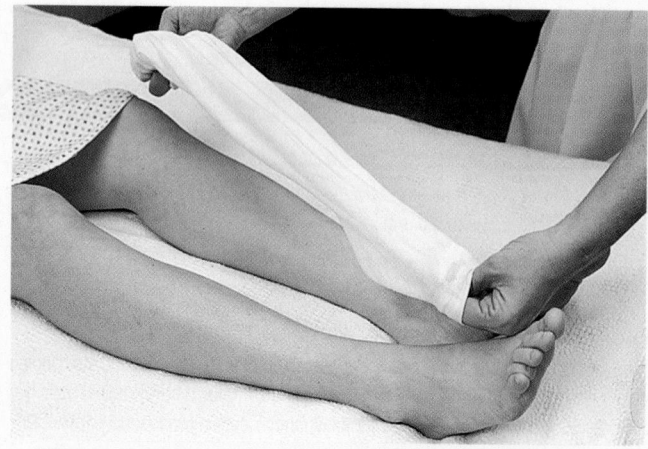

STEP 10c Turn stocking inside out; hold heel and pull through.

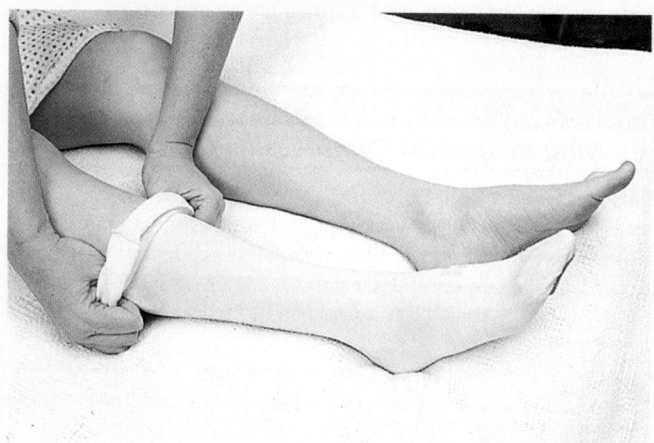

STEP 10e Slide sock up leg until completely extended.

BOX 39.8 PROCEDURAL GUIDELINES—cont'd

Applying Sequential Compression Devices and Elastic Stockings

f. Instruct patient not to roll stockings partially down, to avoid wrinkles, to avoid crossing legs, and to elevate legs while sitting.

11. **Apply SCD sleeve(s):**
    a. Remove SCD sleeves from plastic cover; unfold and flatten onto bed.
    b. Arrange SCD sleeve under patient's leg according to leg position indicated on inner lining of sleeve.
    c. Place patient's leg on SCD sleeve. Back of ankle should line up with ankle marking on inner lining of sleeve.
    d. Position back of knee with popliteal opening on inner sleeve (see illustration).
    e. Wrap SCD sleeve securely around patient's leg. Check fit of SCD sleeve by placing two fingers between patient's leg and sleeve (see illustration).
    f. Attach SCD sleeve connector to plug on mechanical unit. Arrows on connector line up with arrows on plug from mechanical unit (see illustration).

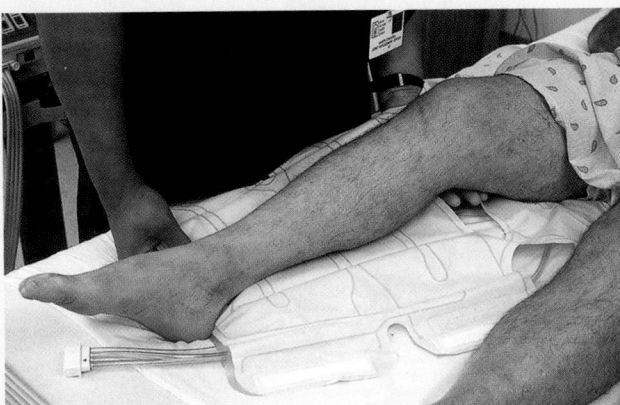

STEP 11d Position back of patient's knee with popliteal opening.

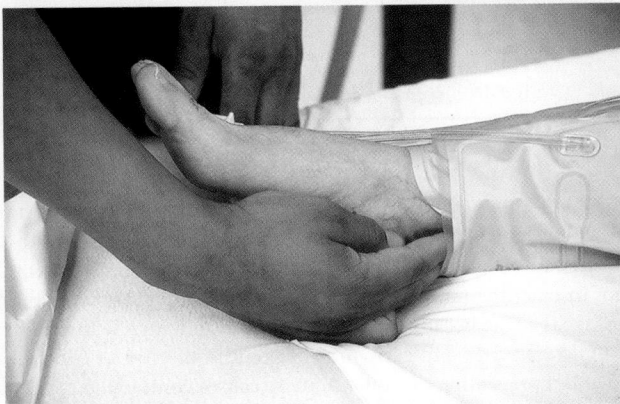

STEP 11e Check fit of SCD sleeve.

g. Turn mechanical unit on. Green light indicates that unit is functioning. Monitor functioning SCD through one full cycle of inflation and deflation.

12. **Apply MCD sleeve** (example: Calf Sleeve ActiveCare+SFT® Application):
    a. A cotton stockinette is provided along with the calf sleeves. Apply over patient's calves.
    b. Wrap the sleeve smoothly around the patient's calf and fasten it, beginning at the top, moving toward the bottom.
    c. Place 2 fingers between patient's calf and sleeve to be sure it is snug but not too tight (see illustration).
    d. The device has two identical extension tubes (see illustration). Use either end of the extension tube to connect to the sleeve or device pump.

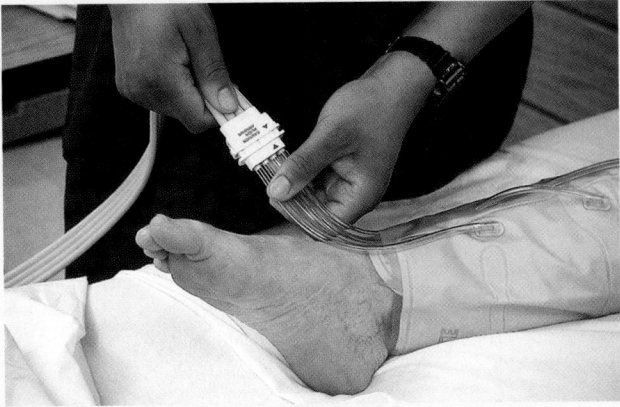

STEP 11f Align arrows when connecting plug to mechanical unit.

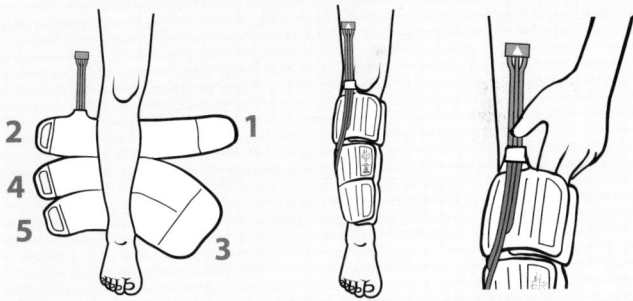

STEP 12c Application of activecare+SFT® MCD to calves. (Courtesy zimmer biomet.)

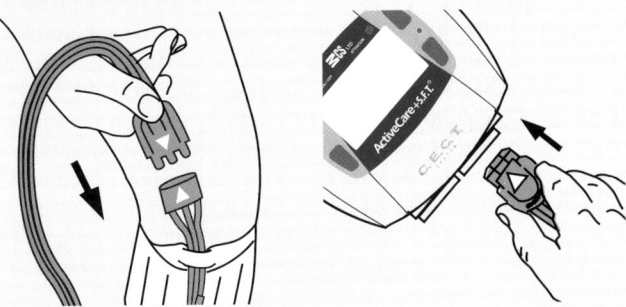

STEP 12d Connection of activecare+SFT® MCD sleeve to extension tube and power source. (Courtesy zimmer biomet.)

Continued

BOX 39.8   PROCEDURAL GUIDELINES—cont'd

Applying Sequential Compression Devices and Elastic Stockings

(1) Connect one end of the extension tube to the sleeve connector. The white arrows should be pointed toward each other.

(2) Connect the other end of the extension tube to the device pump. The white arrow should be facing upward.

e. Press the power switch located at the back of the device to ON position (see illustration). After turning the device on, the Configuration Setup Screen is shown on the LCD screen and the sleeves should immediately start to inflate, from the bottom to the top.

f. Wait 60 seconds for the automatic operation of the device. The device automatically identifies which sleeves are connected, selects the suitable treatment mode, and will display information on the main LCD screen.

13. Position patient comfortably. Then place nurse call system in accessible location within patient's reach.

CLINICAL DECISION: Caution patient not to exit bed and walk with SCDs in place. Have patient call for assistance. The patient may walk with MCD in place (see illustration).

14. Raise side rails (as appropriate) and lower bed to lowest position. Perform hand hygiene.

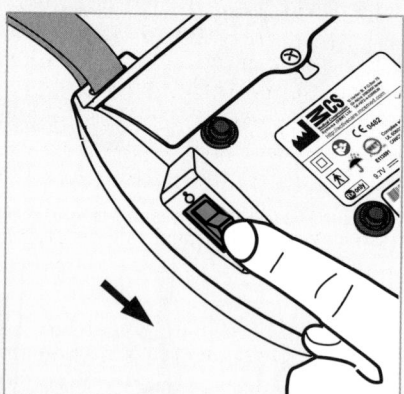

STEP 12e Powering on activecare+SFT® MCD unit. (Courtesy zimmer biomet.)

15. Remove compression stockings or SCD/MCD sleeves at least once per shift (e.g., long enough to inspect skin for irritation or breakdown and to determine patient's comfort level).

16. Evaluate skin integrity and circulation to patient's lower extremities as ordered (see agency policy).

17. **Use Teach-Back:** "We have reviewed the signs and symptoms you might have if a clot forms in your leg. Tell me what those symptoms are." Revise your instruction now or develop a plan for revised patient/family caregiver teaching if patient/family caregiver is not able to teach back correctly.

18. Record condition of lower extremities, application of stockings/SCDs/MCD, patient response to education.

19. Hand-off reporting: Report to health care provider or nurse in charge any signs that may indicate formation of DVT.

⚠ **WARNING:** Extension tubes may become tangled when walking with the **ActiveCare+SFT®** and **ActiveCare+DTx®** Systems. Adjust their length to avoid tripping injury or equipment damage.

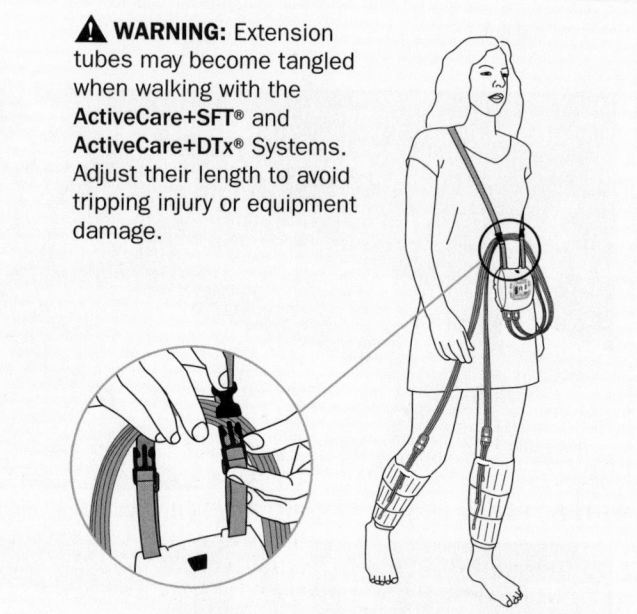

Walking with activecare+SFT® MCD. (Courtesy zimmer biomet.)

Elastic stockings (sometimes called *antiembolitic stockings*) also aid in maintaining external pressure on the muscles of the lower extremities and thus promote venous return (see Box 39.8). To obtain the correct size, measure the patient's calf, thigh, and leg length accurately. When considering applying graded compression stockings, first assess the patient's suitability for wearing them. Do not apply them if he or she has a local condition affecting the leg (e.g., any skin lesion, gangrenous condition, or recent vein ligation) because application compromises circulation. Apply them properly and remove them at least once per shift. Be sure to assess circulation at the toes to ensure that the stockings are not too tight. Another device for preventing DVT is the venous plexus foot pump. It promotes circulation by mimicking the natural action of walking.

Proper positioning reduces a patient's risk of thrombus formation because compression of the leg veins is minimized. Therefore, when positioning patients, use caution to prevent pressure on the posterior knee and deep veins in the lower extremities. Teach patients to avoid the following: crossing the legs, sitting for prolonged periods of time, wearing clothing that constricts the legs or waist, and massaging the legs. Report suspected DVT immediately to the patient's health care provider. Elevate the leg but avoid pressure on the suspected thrombus area. Instruct the family, patient, and all health care personnel not to massage the area because of the danger of dislodging the thrombus.

ROM exercises and early mobility reduce the risk of contractures and aid in preventing thrombi. Activity causes contraction of the skeletal muscles, which in turn exerts pressure on the veins to promote venous return, thereby reducing venous stasis. Specific exercises that help prevent thrombophlebitis are ankle pumps, foot circles, and knee flexion. Ankle pumps, sometimes called *calf pumps,* include alternating plantar flexion and dorsiflexion. Foot circles require the patient to rotate the ankle. Encourage patients to make the letters of the alphabet with their feet every 1 to 2 hours. Knee flexion involves alternately extending and flexing the knee. These exercises are sometimes referred to as *antiembolic exercises* and need to be done hourly while awake.

Maintaining Musculoskeletal Function. Exercises to prevent excessive muscle atrophy and joint contractures help maintain

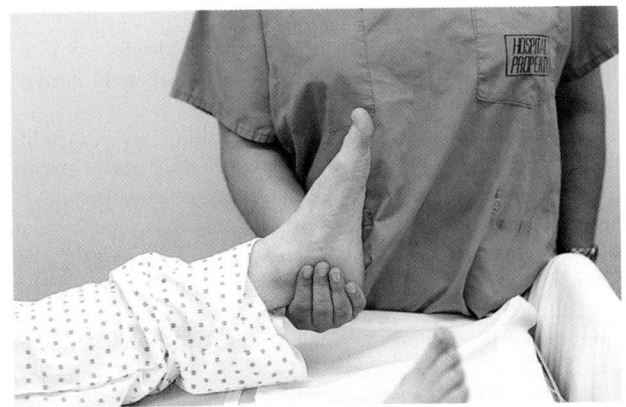

FIG. 39.11 Support joint by holding distal and proximal areas adjacent to joint.

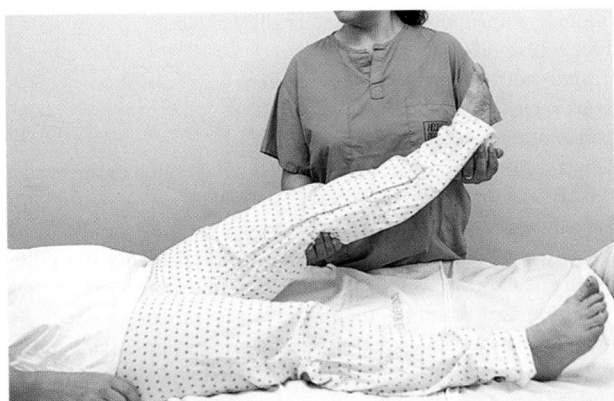

FIG. 39.12 Use cupped hand under joint for support

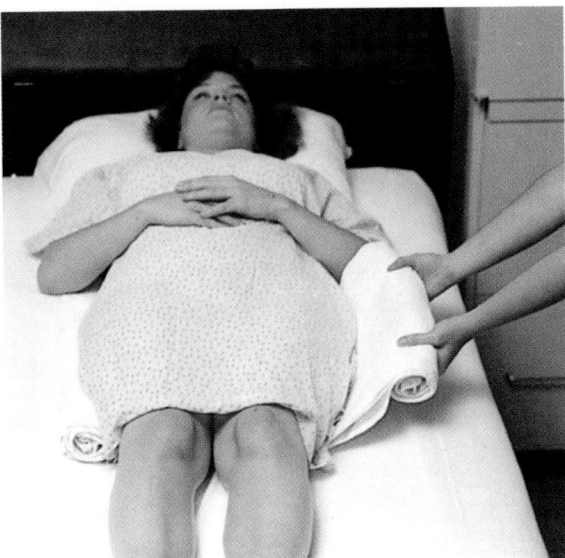

FIG. 39.13 Trochanter roll.

musculoskeletal function. Active ROM should be encouraged for any patient at risk for reduced musculoskeletal strength or functionality by improving joint mobility. When a patient has muscle weakness, fatigue, or pain, active assisted ROM exercises are more appropriate. A patient needs assistance with movement from an external force (e.g., manual support of an extremity, positioning to use the effects of gravity) because of weakness, pain, or changes in muscle tone (Dutton, 2014). Passive ROM exercises are indicated when a patient is not able or permitted to move a body part, as in the case of a paralyzed extremity or healing fracture (Dutton, 2014).

To ensure that patients routinely receive ROM exercises, schedule them at specific times, perhaps during another nursing activity such as the patient's bath. This enables you to systematically reassess mobility while improving the patient's ROM. In addition, bathing usually requires that extremities and joints are put through complete ROM.

Passive ROM exercises begin as soon as a patient's ability to move an extremity or joint is lost. Carry out movements slowly and smoothly, through a prescribed range, just to the point of resistance. ROM exercises should not cause pain. **Never force a joint beyond the point of resistance.** Each joint movement needs to be repeated 5 times during a session, with sessions performed 2 to 3 times a day. When performing passive ROM exercises, stand at the side of the bed closest to the joint being exercised. Use a head-to-toe sequence and move from larger to smaller joints. If an extremity is to be moved or lifted, support the joint by holding distal and proximal areas adjacent to the joint (Fig. 39.11). Use a cupped hand to provide support under the joint (Fig. 39.12). See Table 39.2 for detailed ROM for each joint. Patients on bed rest need to have active ROM exercises incorporated into their daily schedules.

Positioning Techniques. Patients with impaired nervous, skeletal, or muscular system functioning and increased weakness and fatigue often require help from nurses for positioning and maintenance of proper body alignment while in bed or sitting (see Skill 39.1). Several positioning devices are available for maintaining good body alignment for patients. Pillows are positioning aids and are sometimes readily available. Before using a pillow, determine whether it is the proper size. A thick pillow under a patient's head increases cervical flexion, which is not desirable. A thin pillow under bony prominences does not protect skin and tissue from damage caused by pressure. When additional pillows are unavailable or if they are an improper size, use folded sheets, blankets, or towels as positioning aids.

Apply positioning boots to prevent footdrop by maintaining the feet in dorsiflexion. Ankle-foot orthotic (AFO) devices also help maintain dorsiflexion. Patients who wear positioning boots or AFOs need to have these removed periodically (e.g., 2 hours on, 2 hours off).

A trochanter roll prevents external rotation of the hips when a patient is in a supine position. This is especially useful in patients who have lost the ability to move the lower extremities. To form a trochanter roll, fold a cotton bath blanket lengthwise to a width that extends from the greater trochanter of the femur to the lower border of the popliteal space (Fig. 39.13). Place the blanket under the buttocks and roll it counterclockwise until the thigh is in neutral position or inward rotation. When the hip is aligned correctly, the patella faces directly upward. Use sandbags in place of or in addition to trochanter rolls. Sandbags are sand-filled plastic tubes or bags that are shaped to body contours.

Hand rolls maintain the thumb in slight adduction and in opposition to the fingers, which maintain a functional position. Assess the hand roll positioning to make sure that the hand is indeed in a functional position. Hand rolls are most often used with patients whose arms are paralyzed or who are unconscious. Do not use rolled washcloths as hand rolls because they do not keep the thumb well abducted, especially in patients who have a spastic paralysis. Hand-wrist splints are individually molded for a patient to maintain proper alignment of the thumb (slight adduction) and wrist (slight dorsiflexion). Use splints only on the patient for whom they were made and follow the splint schedule (e.g., wear for 2 hours, remove for 2 hours).

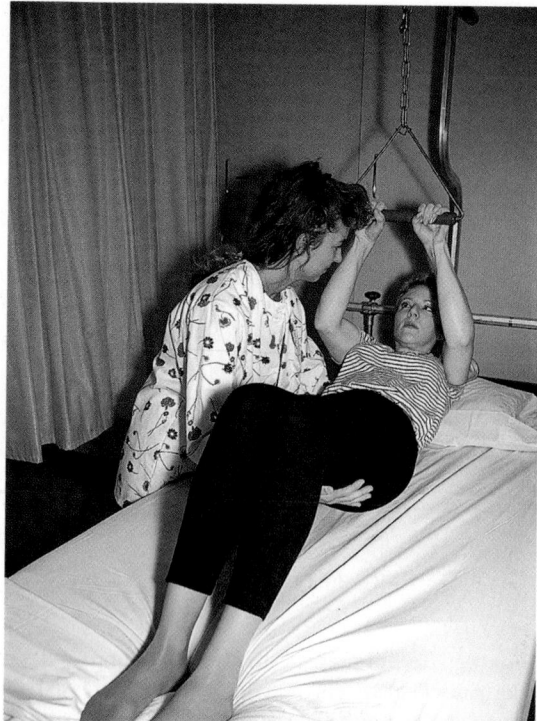

FIG. 39.14 Patient using trapeze bar.

The **trapeze bar** is a triangular device that hangs down from a securely fastened overhead bar that is attached to the bedframe. It allows a patient to pull with the upper extremities to raise the trunk off the bed, assist in transfer from bed to wheelchair, or perform upper-arm exercises (Fig. 39.14). It increases independence, maintains upper-body strength, and decreases the shearing action from sliding across or up and down in bed.

Although each procedure for positioning has specific guidelines, there are universal steps to follow for patients who require positioning assistance. Following the guidelines reduces the risk of injury to the musculoskeletal system when a patient is sitting or lying. When joints are unsupported, their alignment is impaired. Likewise, if joints are not positioned in a slightly flexed position, their mobility is decreased. During positioning also assess for pressure points. When actual or potential pressure areas exist, nursing interventions involve removal of the pressure, thus decreasing the risk for development of pressure injuries and further trauma to the musculoskeletal system. In these patients use the 30-degree lateral position.

Supported Fowler's Position. In the supported Fowler's position the head of the bed is elevated 45 to 60 degrees, and the patient's knees are slightly elevated without pressure to restrict circulation in the lower legs. The patient's illness and overall condition influence the angle of head and knee elevation and the length of time that the patient needs to remain in the supported Fowler's position. Supports need to permit flexion of the hips and knees and proper alignment of the normal curves in the cervical, thoracic, and lumbar vertebrae. The following are common trouble areas for a patient in the supported Fowler's position:

- Increased cervical flexion because the pillow at the head is too thick and the head thrusts forward
- Extension of the knees, allowing the patient to slide to the foot of the bed
- Pressure on the posterior aspect of the knees, decreasing circulation to the feet
- External rotation of the hips
- Arms hanging unsupported at the patient's sides

- Unsupported feet or pressure on the heels
- Unprotected pressure points at the sacrum and heels
- Increased shearing force on the back and heels when the head of the bed is raised greater than 60 degrees

Supine Position. Patients in the supine position rest on their backs. In the supine position the relationship of body parts is essentially the same as in good standing alignment, except that the body is in the horizontal plane. Use pillows, trochanter rolls, and hand rolls or arm splints to increase comfort and reduce injury to the skin or musculoskeletal system. The mattress needs to be firm enough to support the cervical, thoracic, and lumbar vertebrae. Shoulders are supported, and the elbows are slightly flexed to control shoulder rotation. A foot support prevents footdrop and maintains proper alignment. The following are some common trouble areas for patients in the supine position:

- Pillow at the head that is too thick, increasing cervical flexion
- Head flat on the mattress
- Shoulders unsupported and internally rotated
- Elbows extended
- Thumb not in opposition to the fingers
- Hips externally rotated
- Unsupported feet
- Unprotected pressure points at the occipital region of the head, vertebrae, coccyx, elbows, and heels

Prone Position. The patient in the prone position lies face or chest down. Often his or her head is turned to the side, but if a pillow is under the head, it needs to be thin enough to prevent cervical flexion or extension and maintain alignment of the lumbar spine. Placing a pillow under the lower leg permits dorsiflexion of the ankles and some knee flexion, which promote relaxation. If a pillow is unavailable, the ankles need to be in dorsiflexion over the end of the mattress. Although the prone position is seldom used in practice, consider this as an alternative, especially in patients who normally sleep in this position. The prone position also has some benefits in patients with acute respiratory distress syndrome and acute lung injury (Barnes-Daly et al., 2018). Specialty beds that safely position acutely ill patients in the prone position are available. Assess for and correct any of the following potential trouble points with patients in the prone position:

- Neck hyperextension
- Hyperextension of the lumbar spine
- Plantar flexion of the ankles
- Unprotected pressure points at the chin, elbows, female breasts, hips, knees, and toes

Side-Lying Position. In the side-lying (or lateral) position a patient rests on the side with the major portion of body weight on the dependent hip and shoulder. A 30-degree lateral position is recommended for patients at risk for pressure injuries (see Chapter 48). Trunk alignment needs to be the same as in standing. The patient needs to maintain the structural curves of the spine, the head needs to be supported in line with the midline of the trunk, and rotation of the spine needs to be avoided. The following trouble points are common in the side-lying position:

- Lateral flexion of the neck
- Spinal curves out of normal alignment
- Shoulder and hip joints internally rotated, adducted, or unsupported
- Lack of foot support
- Lack of protection for pressure points at the ear, shoulder, anterior iliac spine, trochanter, and ankles
- Excessive lateral flexion of the spine if the patient has large hips and a pillow is not placed superior to the hips at the waist

Sims' Position. Sims' position differs from the side-lying position in the distribution of the patient's weight. In Sims' position the patient places the weight on the anterior ileum, humerus, and clavicle. Trouble points common in Sims' position include the following:

- Lateral flexion of the neck
- Internal rotation, adduction, or lack of support to the shoulders and hips
- Lack of foot support
- Lack of protection for pressure points at the ileum, humerus, clavicle, knees, and ankles

Moving Patients. When moving a patient during repositioning, a safe transfer is the first priority. Patients require various levels of assistance to move up in bed, move to the side-lying position, or sit up at the side of the bed. For example, a young, healthy woman may need minimal support as she sits at the side of the bed for the first time after childbirth, whereas an older man may need help from two or more nurses to do the same task after surgery. Transfer devices are available to assist in patient positioning.

Always ask patients to help to their fullest extent possible during positioning. To determine what a patient is able to do alone and how many people are needed to help with positioning or transferring (see Chapter 38), assess him or her to determine whether the illness contradicts exertion (e.g., cardiovascular disease). Is the patient cooperative and capable of moving? Next determine whether the patient comprehends what is expected. For example, a patient recently medicated for postoperative pain is too lethargic to understand instructions; thus to ensure safety, two nurses are necessary to move him or her. Then determine the patient's comfort level. It is important to assess your personal strength and knowledge of the procedure. Finally determine whether the patient is too heavy or immobile for you to move alone (Kanaskie and Snyder, 2018; Olinsky and Norton, 2017) (see Chapter 38).

Preventing Injury To the Integumentary System. The major risk to the skin from restricted mobility is the formation of pressure injuries. Early identification of high-risk patients helps prevent pressure injuries (see Chapter 48). Interventions aimed at prevention include turning and positioning and the use of therapeutic support surfaces and devices (e.g., low air loss mattresses, heel boots, flotation mattresses) to relieve pressure. Regular skin care (cleansing of soiled areas and use of moisturizers) aims to maintain the condition of the skin. Change the immobilized patient's position according to his or her activity level, perceptual ability, treatment protocols, and daily routines. For example, an obese patient or a very thin patient, both of whom have bowel incontinence, will require more frequent turning than standard practice.

Usually the time that a patient sits uninterrupted in a chair is limited to 1 hour. This interval is shortened in patients who are at very high risk for skin breakdown. Reposition patients frequently because uninterrupted pressure causes skin breakdown. Teach patients to shift their weight in a chair every 15 minutes. Chair-bound patients may benefit from a pressure-relief cushion such as an air, viscous fluid/foam, or gel/foam cushion that reduces pressure.

Elimination System. The nursing interventions for maintaining optimal urinary functioning are directed at keeping the patient well hydrated and preventing urinary stasis, calculi, and infections without causing bladder distention. Normal hydration (e.g., 800 to 2000 mL of noncaffeinated fluids daily) helps prevent renal calculi and UTIs. The well-hydrated patient needs to void large amounts of dilute urine that is approximately equal to fluid intake. Also record the frequency and consistency of bowel movements. Provide a diet rich in fluids, fruits, vegetables, and fiber to facilitate normal peristalsis. If a patient is unable to maintain regular bowel patterns, stool softeners, cathartics, or enemas are sometimes necessary. If the patient is incontinent, modify the care plan to include toileting aids and a hygiene schedule so that the increased urinary output does not cause skin breakdown.

Psychosocial Health. People who have a tendency toward depression or mood swings require nursing interventions that maintain normal development and provide physical and psychosocial stimuli. Anticipate changes in a patient's psychosocial status, and provide routine and informal socialization. Involve family or significant others when appropriate. Observe the patient's ability to cope with restricted mobility. In institutional health care settings try not to schedule nursing care activities between 10:00 PM and 7:00 AM to minimize sleep interruptions. When care is required, combine activities. For example, administer medications, check an IV infusion, and assess vital signs when you enter the room to turn the patient or provide special skin care. If the nursing care plan is not improving coping patterns, consult a clinical nurse specialist, counselor, social worker, spiritual adviser, or other health care professional. Incorporate their recommendations into the care plan.

Nurses provide meaningful stimuli to maintain a patient's orientation. Plan nursing activities so that a patient is able to talk and interact with staff. If possible, place him or her in a room with others who are mobile and interactive. If a private room is required, ask staff members to visit throughout the shift to provide meaningful interaction. A daily newspaper helps the patient keep track of events and time. Bedside conversations at appropriate moments familiarize him or her with nursing activities, meals, and visiting hours. Books help occupy the patient when he or she is alone. The patient can participate in craft activities. Radio, television, iPods, MP3 players, and videotapes provide stimulation and help pass the time.

Involve patients in their care whenever possible. For example, encourage the patient to determine when the bed should be made and when scheduled ambulation is preferred. Some patients rest better during the night when fresh sheets are put on in the evening rather than in the morning. The patient needs to provide as much self-care as possible. Keep hygiene and grooming articles within easy reach. Encourage patients to wear their glasses or artificial teeth and shave or apply makeup. People use these activities to maintain their body image, thus improving their outlook.

Developmental Health. Ideally a patient who is immobilized for a lengthy period is able to maintain normal developmental processes. Nursing care should provide the mental and physical stimulation appropriate to a patient's age and developmental status. In the case of young children, incorporate play activities into the care plan. For example, completing puzzles helps a child to continue developing fine-motor skills, and reading helps him or her develop cognitively. Encourage parents to stay with a child who is hospitalized. Place a child who is immobilized with children of the same age who are not immobilized unless a contagious disease is present. Allow the child to participate in nursing interventions such as dressing changes, cast care, and care of traction. Learn to recognize significant changes from normal behavioral patterns, and consult with a pediatric clinical nurse specialist, counselor, or other health care professional.

Restricted mobility of older patients presents unique nursing problems. Older patients who are frail or have chronic illnesses are often at increased risk for the psychosocial hazards of immobility. Maintaining a calendar and clock with a large dial, conversing about current events and family members, and encouraging visits from significant others reduce the risk of social isolation. Spending time in the room talking and listening to the patient also helps reduce the risk of social isolation.

Encourage older immobilized patients to perform as many ADLs as independently as possible. Patients need to continue to perform personal grooming if they did so before their mobility was restricted. This type of activity preserves the patient's dignity and gives him or her a sense of accomplishment.

Restorative and Continuing Care. The goal of restorative care for the patient who is immobile is to maximize functional mobility and independence and reduce residual functional deficits such as impaired gait and decreased endurance. The focus in restorative care is not only on ADLs that relate to physical self-care but also on instrumental activities of daily living (IADLs). IADLs are activities that are necessary to be independent in society beyond eating, grooming, transferring, and toileting and include such skills as shopping, preparing meals, banking, and taking medications.

Nurses use many of the same interventions as described in the health promotion and acute care sections, but the emphasis is on working collaboratively with patients and their significant others and with other health care professionals to facilitate the patient's return to maximal functional ability in both ADLs and IADLs.

Intensive specialized therapy such as occupational or physical therapy is common. If the patient is in a rehabilitation institution, he or she probably goes to the therapy department 2 to 3 times a day. Your role is to work collaboratively with these professionals and reinforce exercises and teaching. For example, after a stroke, a patient is likely to receive gait training from a physical therapist; speech rehabilitation from a speech therapist; and help from an occupational therapist for household chores or ADLs, such as dressing, bathing, and toileting. The therapy is not always able to restore total functional health, but it often helps the patient adapt to the mobility limitations or complications. Equipment frequently used to help patients adapt to mobility limitations includes walkers, canes, wheelchairs, and assistive devices such as toilet seat extenders, reaching sticks, special silverware, and clothing with Velcro closures.

REFLECT NOW

Mrs. Kline is currently in a rehabilitation facility and uses a walker. Her discharge to home is planned in 2 days. Her husband has participated in her rehabilitation but feels he needs help in the home. Their insurance will provide home physical therapy three times a week for 3 weeks. The first visit will be a home assessment. Think about items in the home that might need modification following a home visit, such as tripping hazards (rugs, floor clutter), and items that need to be relocated to provide a clear walking path, such as an ottoman or coffee table. Think about kitchen items that may need to be relocated to avoid overreaching.

Walking and Exercise. A patient who is receiving restorative care continues to be involved in an exercise program, including progressive walking. Care may also include a continuation of ROM exercises. Chapter 38 describes in detail how to assist a patient to ambulate.

Patients with hemiplegia (one-sided paralysis) or hemiparesis (one-sided weakness) will often need assistance with walking. When an assistive device is used, stand on the patient's affected side and support him or her with a gait belt. Providing support by holding a patient's arm is incorrect because you cannot easily support the patient's weight to lower him or her to the floor if he or she faints or falls. In addition, if the patient falls with the nurse holding an arm, a shoulder joint may be dislocated. Chapter 38 describes how to assist a patient using crutches, walkers, and canes.

Psychotherapy. Recovery from a physical disability is difficult. Psycho-Physical Therapy is one holistic therapeutic approach that acknowledges the importance of addressing the body and spirit as well as the mind during therapeutic work (Good Therapy, 2016). Therapists combine physical movement work and psychotherapy techniques to help patients gain greater awareness of their abilities and how to proceed toward recovery. Rehabilitation psychologists support

Knowledge
- Characteristics of improved mobility
- Role of community resources in maintaining activity and exercise

Experience
- Consider previous patient responses to activity and exercise therapies

EVALUATION
- Reassess patient for improved mobility and activity tolerance
- Ask if the patient's expectations are being met

Standards
- Apply standards from Agency for Healthcare Research and Quality (AHRQ, n.d.) and the Wound, Ostomy and Continence Nurses Society (WOCN, 2016), and from protocols for patients at risk for falls (AACN, 2014)

Attitudes
- Use creativity in designing new interventions to optimize pain control
- Demonstrate perseverance to design interventions to increase walking and activity

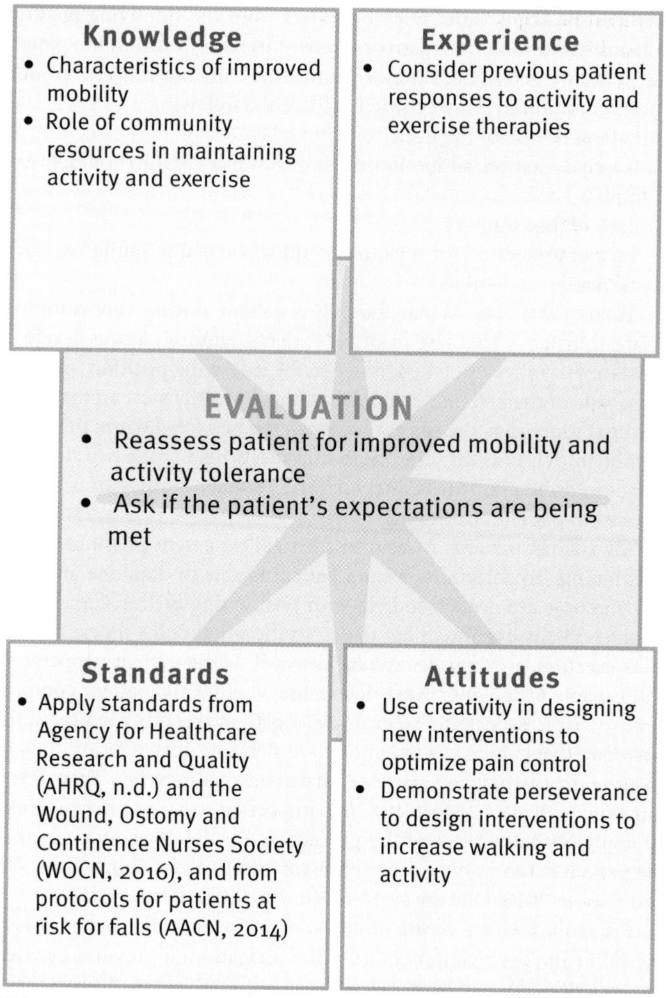

FIG. 39.15 Critical thinking model for evaluation of impaired mobility.

individuals as they cope with the mental and physical challenges their conditions present. They often teach their patients how to adapt and make lifestyle choices that promote good health (APA, 2019). A nurse involved in a patient's rehab collaborates with the patient, family, and therapists to provide continuity in psychological support and patient education.

◆ **Evaluation**

Through the Patient's Eyes. Just as it is important to include the patient during the assessment and planning phase of the care plan, it is essential to have the patient's evaluation of the plan of care (Fig. 39.15). Were the patient's goals or expectations met? Ask the patient to describe his or her perception of recovery from immobilization. Does the patient feel mobility is improving? If not, what factors does the patient perceive are barriers? Determine with the patient and others involved with care whether the goals or outcomes established with and for the patient have indeed been met and whether it is necessary to revise the plan of care. A study involving stroke patients found that patients' intention of becoming independent positively affected their motor recovery, while family members' positive attitudes promoted patient's cognitive improvement (Fang, 2017). Involvement of patient and family is critical.

Patient Outcomes. From your perspective as the nurse, you are to evaluate expected outcomes and a patient's response to nursing care and compare the patient's actual outcomes with the outcomes selected during planning. For example, you evaluate a patient's ability to maintain or improve body alignment, joint mobility, walking, moving, or transferring. Evaluate the effectiveness of specific interventions designed to promote body alignment, improve mobility, and protect the patient from the hazards of immobility. Evaluate the patient's and family's understanding of all teaching provided as well. The continuous nature of evaluation allows you to determine whether new or revised therapies are required and whether new nursing diagnoses have developed.

When outcomes are not met, consider asking the following questions:

- Are there ways we can assist you to increase your activity?
- Which activities are you having trouble completing right now?
- How do you feel about not being able to dress yourself and make your own meals?
- Which exercises do you find most helpful?
- What goals for your activity would you like to set now?

Once these questions have been asked and you have addressed the limited mobility and its associated problems through the patient's eyes, you are prepared to adjust the plan of care to address the remaining clinical problems that your patient is experiencing related to immobility.

SAFETY GUIDELINES FOR NURSING SKILLS

Ensuring patient safety is an essential role of the professional nurse. To ensure patient safety, communicate clearly with the members of the health care team, assess and incorporate the patient's priorities of care and preferences, and use the best evidence when making decisions about your patient's care. When performing the skills in this chapter, remember the following points to ensure safe, individualized patient-centered care.

- Determine the amount and type of assistance required for safe positioning, including any transfer equipment and the number of personnel to safely transfer and prevent harm to patient and health care providers.
- During positioning raise the side rail on the side of the bed opposite of where you are standing to prevent the patient from falling out of bed on that side.
- Arrange equipment (e.g., intravenous lines, feeding tube, indwelling catheter) so that it does not interfere with the positioning process.
- Evaluate the patient for correct body alignment and pressure risks after repositioning.

SKILL 39.1   MOVING AND POSITIONING PATIENTS IN BED

Delegation and Collaboration

The skills of moving and positioning patients in bed and maintaining correct body alignment can be delegated to assistive personnel (AP). The nurse instructs the AP by:

- Explaining any moving and positioning restrictions unique to patient (e.g., avoid prone position, patient has one-sided weakness).
- Designating specific times throughout the shift that AP must reposition patient.
- Providing information about patient's individual needs for body alignment (e.g., patient with spinal cord injury).

Equipment

- Pillows, drawsheet
- Appropriate safe patient-handling assistive devices (e.g., friction-reducing device, ceiling lift, or mechanical floor lift)
- Therapeutic boots/splints *(optional)*
- Trochanter rolls *(optional)*
- Hand rolls *(optional)*
- Clean gloves

STEP	RATIONALE
ASSESSMENT	
1. Identify patient using at least two identifiers (e.g., name and birthday or name and medical record number) according to agency policy.	Ensures correct patient. Complies with The Joint Commission standards and improves patient safety (TJC, 2020).
2. Refer to medical record for most recent recorded weight and height for patient.	Factors help to determine whether mechanical lift, mechanical transfer device, or friction-reducing device is needed for moving patient up in bed.
3. Check health care provider's orders for any restrictions in movement before positioning patient.	Some positions may be contraindicated in situations such as spinal cord injury; hip fracture; respiratory difficulties; neurological conditions; and presence of incisions, drains, or tubing.
4. Perform hand hygiene.	Reduces transmission of microorganisms.
5. Assess patient's or family caregiver's knowledge, experience, and health literacy	Ensures patient or family caregiver has the capacity to obtain, communicate, process, and understand basic health information (CDC, 2019).
6. Assess patient's range of motion (ROM) and current body alignment while patient is lying down.	Provides baseline data for later comparisons. Determines ways to improve position and alignment.
7. Assess for risk factors that contribute to complications of immobility:	Risk factors require patient to be repositioned more frequently.
a. **Reduced sensation:** Cerebrovascular accident (CVA), spinal cord injury, or neuropathy.	With reduced sensation, a patient has difficulty moving, has poor awareness of involved body part, and is unable to position body part and protect it from pressure.
b. **Impaired mobility:** Traction, arthritis, CVA, spinal cord injury, hip fracture, joint surgery, or other contributing disease processes.	Traction, bone fractures, surgery, or arthritic changes result in decreased ROM. Loss of function caused by CVA or spinal injury can lead to contractures.
c. **Impaired circulation:** Arterial insufficiency.	Decreased circulation predisposes patient to pressure injury.
d. **Age:** Very young, older adult.	Premature and young infants require frequent turning because their skin is fragile. Normal physiological changes of aging predispose to greater risks for developing complications of immobility.
8. Assess patient's level of consciousness and ability to cooperate in positioning.	Level of cooperation affects need for special aids or devices and additional caregivers. Patients with altered levels of consciousness may not understand instructions or be able to help during positioning.

Continued

SKILL 39.1 MOVING AND POSITIONING PATIENTS IN BED—cont'd

STEP	RATIONALE
9. Assess patient for presence of pain; rate on scale of 0 to 10 (see Chapter 44).	Pain reduces patient's motivation and ability to be mobile. Pain relief before transfer enhances patient participation.
10. Assess condition of patient's skin, especially over bony prominences (see Chapter 48).	Provides baseline to determine effects of positioning. Routine positioning reduces occurrence of pressure injuries.
11. Assess patient's physical ability to help with moving and positioning. Can patient reposition independently?	Enables you to use patient's existing mobility, strength, and coordination during positioning. Determines need for additional help and assist devices to ensure patient and nurse safety.
12. Assess patient's vision and hearing (see Chapter 30)	Sensory deficits affect patient's ability to cooperate during repositioning.
13. Apply clean gloves (as needed) to assess for presence of drainage tubes, incisions, and equipment (e.g., traction). Empty drainage bags before positioning. Remove and dispose of gloves. Perform hand hygiene.	Alters positioning procedure and affects patient's ability to independently change positions.
14. Assess motivation of patient and ability of family caregivers to participate in moving and positioning if patient to be discharged home.	Indicates level of instruction needed before discharge.

PLANNING

1. Consider all factors applicable to a repositioning algorithm (see illustration) or agency policy, and determine the caregiver resources and positioning equipment needed to perform positioning.	An important element of a safe patient-handling program is patient handling and mobility algorithms (Martin et al., 2014; OSHA, 2017).

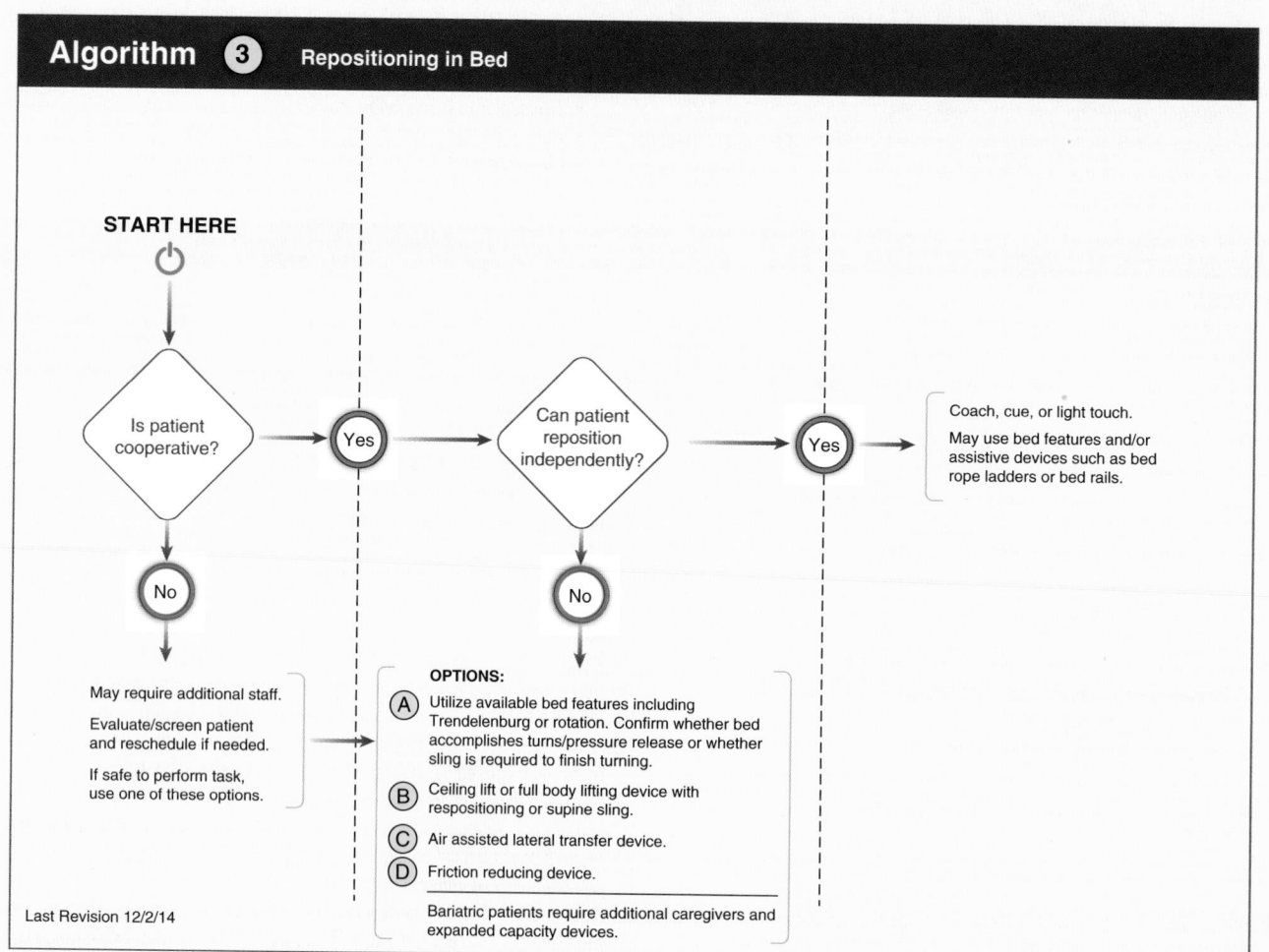

STEP 1 Algorithm for repositioning patients in bed (http://www.asphp.org/Wp-Content/Uploads/2016/06/New-And-Improved-Va-Algorithms-And-New-Sphm-App-Asphp-Rev-Mmm.pptx).

STEP	RATIONALE
2. If patient perceives level of pain to be enough to avoid movement, offer an analgesic (if ordered) 30 minutes before repositioning.	Will lessen discomfort when positioning extremities. **NOTE:** The frequency of an analgesic may not be available as frequently as a patient will require turning.
3. Remove all pillows and devices used in previous position.	Reduces interference during positioning procedure.
4. Explain positioning procedure to patient using plain language.	Helps decrease anxiety and increase cooperation.
5. Close door to room or bedside curtains	Provides for patient privacy.

IMPLEMENTATION

STEP	RATIONALE
1. Perform hand hygiene.	Reduces transmission of microorganisms.
2. Raise level of bed to comfortable working height, level with your elbows. Be sure brakes on bed are locked.	Raises level of work toward nurse's center of gravity and reduces risk for back injuries. Ensures patient safety.
3. **Assist patient to move up in bed:**	This is not a one-person task unless patient can help completely (OSHA, 2014). Pulling patients who have migrated in bed carries an extremely high risk of caregiver injury (Wiggermann, 2014).
a. Determine whether the patient can assist.	Determines degree of risk in repositioning patient and technique required to safely help patient.
(1) *Patient can reposition independently:*	Positioning techniques promote patient independence.
(a) Stand by for safety as needed. Stand at bedside to help with positioning of tubing and equipment as patient moves.	Prevents accidental tube dislodgment.
(b) Have patient place feet flat on mattress, grasp either side rails or overhead trapeze and, on a count of three, lift hips up and push legs so that body moves up in bed.	Patient uses muscles in coordinated way to smoothly move up in bed with hips lifted.
(2) *Patient is unable to reposition independently (see algorithm):*	
(a) Explain to patient how he or she can assist as caregivers use safe handling devices.	Patient cooperation improves efficiency of procedure.
(b) Use any available bed features such as Trendelenburg or rotation to move patient up in bed. Position patient supine with head of bed flat. A nurse stands on each side of bed.	Bed features will minimize amount of effort to reposition patient.
(c) If bed features are unavailable, use friction-reducing device or air-assisted lateral transfer device and three caregivers.	Reduces muscular strain during positioning. Devices avoid injury to patient's skin.
i. Position patient supine with head of bed flat. A nurse stands on each side of bed.	
ii. Remove pillow from under head and shoulders and place it at head of bed.	Provides easy access to move patient upward.
iii. Turn patient side to side to place friction-reducing device under drawsheet on bed, with device extending from shoulders to thighs/ankles. *Option:* Apply deflated air-assisted device.	Ensures device supports patient's full weight.
iv. Return patient to supine position.	
v. Have two caregivers firmly grasp drawsheet (one on each side of bed). Have third nurse hold on to end of friction-reducing device.	Slide board remains stationary, provides slippery surface to reduce friction, and allows patient to move up in bed easily.
vi. Holding fan-folded drawsheet and one nurse counting to three, the two nurses pull drawsheet across slide board, positioning patient up in bed. The third nurse holds slide board in place. *Option:* Inflate air-assisted device and slide patient up in bed	Positions patient smoothly without exerting shear against skin and without risk of injury to nurses.
(d) If patient weighs over 91 kg (200 lb), use appropriate number of caregivers and appropriate safe patient-handling devices (e.g., supine sling with ceiling lift or floor-based lift and two or more caregivers) to move and position patient.	Repositioning patients manually is associated with high risk of musculoskeletal injury (Wiggermann, 2014).

CLINICAL DECISION: *Protect patient's heels from shearing force by having another caregiver lift heels while moving patient up in bed.*

STEP	RATIONALE
4. **Position patient in bed in one of the following positions.** Ensure correct body alignment. Protect pressure areas.	Prevents injury to patient's musculoskeletal system and integument. Even positioning patient side to side requires use of safe patient-handling techniques.
a. Confirm whether patient can cooperate and move independently.	Determines degree of risk in repositioning patient and the technique required to safely help patient.
b. Begin with patient lying supine, and move up in bed following Steps 3a(1)–(2).	

Continued

SKILL 39.1   MOVING AND POSITIONING PATIENTS IN BED—cont'd

STEP	RATIONALE

c. Position patient in supported semi-Fowler's (see illustration) or Fowler's position:

(1) With patient lying supine, elevate head of bed 45 to 60 degrees if not contraindicated.

Increases comfort, improves ventilation, and increases patient's opportunity to socialize or relax.

(2) Rest head against mattress or on small pillow.

Prevents flexion contractures of cervical vertebrae.

(3) Use pillows to support arms and hands if patient does not have voluntary control or use of hands and arms.

Prevents shoulder dislocation from effect of downward pull of unsupported arms, promotes circulation by preventing venous pooling, and prevents flexion contractures of arms and wrists.

(4) Position small pillow at lower back.

Supports lumbar vertebrae and decreases flexion of vertebrae.

(5) Place pillows lengthwise under each leg (midthigh to ankle) to support the knee in slight flexion (avoids hyperextension) and to allow the heels to float.

Prevents hyperextension of knee and occlusion of popliteal artery from pressure from body weight. Heels should not be in contact with bed. Floating heels prevent prolonged pressure of mattress on heels.

d. Position hemiplegic patient in supported semi-Fowler's or Fowler's position:

(1) Elevate head of bed 30 to 60 degrees according to patient's condition. For example, those with increased risk for pressure injury remain at 30-degree angle (see Chapter 48).

Increases comfort, improves ventilation, and increases patient's opportunity to relax.

(2) Position patient in Fowler's position as anatomically straight as possible

Counteracts tendency to slump toward affected side. Improves ventilation and cardiac output; decreases intracranial pressure. Improves patient's ability to swallow and helps prevent aspiration of food, liquids, and gastric secretions.

(3) Position head on small pillow with chin slightly forward. If patient is totally unable to control head movement, avoid hyperextension of neck.

Prevents hyperextension of neck. Too many pillows under head may cause or worsen neck flexion contracture.

(4) Provide support for involved arm and hand by placing arm away from patient's side and supporting elbow with pillow.

Paralyzed muscles do not automatically resist pull of gravity as they do normally. As a result, shoulder subluxation, pain, and edema may occur.

(5) Place rolled blanket (trochanter roll) or pillows firmly alongside patient's legs to help prevent the patient from leaning toward the affected side.

Ensures proper alignment. Prevents external rotation of hips, which contributes to contractures.

(6) Support feet in dorsiflexion with therapeutic boots (see illustration) or splints.

Prevents plantar flexion contractures or footdrop by positioning patient's ankle in neutral dorsiflexion. Positions foot so that heel is aligned in opening of splint to prevent pressure. Other therapeutic boots or splints are manufactured with thick padding to cushion heel and prevent pressure injury.

e. Position patient in supported supine position:

(1) Place patient supine with head of bed flat.

Necessary for properly aligning patient.

(2) Place small rolled towel under lumbar area of back.

Provides support for lumbar spine.

(3) Place pillow under upper shoulders, neck, and head.

Maintains correct alignment and prevents flexion contractures of cervical vertebrae.

(4) Place trochanter rolls or sandbags parallel to lateral surface of patient's thighs.

Reduces external rotation of hip.

(5) Place patient's feet in therapeutic boots or splints.

Maintains feet in dorsiflexion. Prevents plantar flexion contractures or footdrop.

(6) Place pillows under pronated forearms, keeping upper arms parallel to patient's body (see illustration).

Reduces internal rotation of shoulder and prevents extension of elbows. Maintains correct body alignment.

(7) Place hand rolls in patient's hands (see illustration). Consider physical therapy referral for use of hand splints.

Reduces extension of fingers and abduction of thumb. Maintains thumb slightly adducted and in opposition to fingers.

f. Position hemiplegic patient in supine position:

(1) Place head of bed flat.

Necessary for positioning in supine position.

(2) Place folded towel or small pillow under shoulder of affected side.

Decreases possibility of pain, joint contracture, and subluxation. Maintains mobility in muscles around shoulder to permit normal movement patterns.

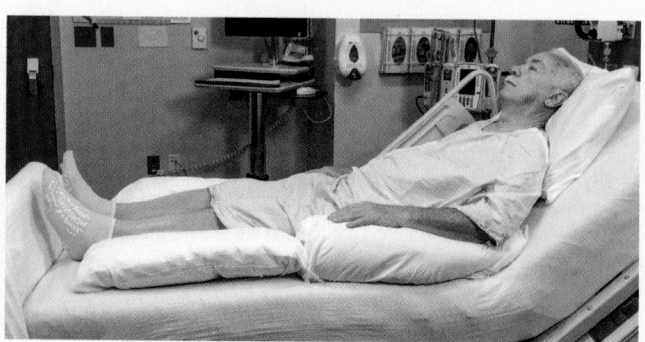

STEP 4c Supported Fowler's position.

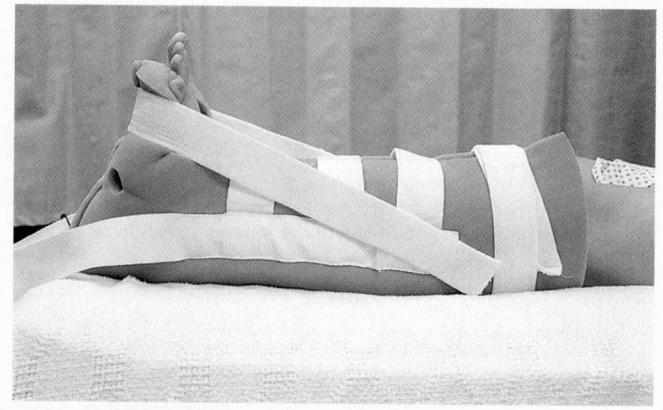

STEP 4d(6) Foot boot with lower leg extension.

STEP	RATIONALE
(3) Keep affected arm away from body with elbow extended and palm up. Position affected hand in one of recommended positions for flaccid or spastic hand. (Alternative is to place arm out to side, with elbow bent and hand toward head of bed.)	Maintains mobility in arm, joints, and shoulder to permit normal movement patterns. (Alternative position counteracts limitation of ability of arm to rotate outward at shoulder [external rotation]. External rotation must be present to raise arm overhead without pain.)
(4) Place folded towel under hip of involved side.	Diminishes effect of spasticity in entire leg by controlling hip position.
(5) Flex affected knee 30 degrees by supporting it on pillow or folded blanket.	Slight flexion breaks up abnormal extension pattern of leg. Extensor spasticity is most severe when patient is supine.
(6) Support feet with soft pillows placed against sole of feet at right angle to leg.	Maintains foot in dorsiflexion and prevents footdrop. Pillows prevent stimulation to ball of foot by hard surface, which has tendency to increase muscle tone in patient with extensor spasticity of lower extremity.

CLINICAL DECISION: *Offer passive range of motion exercises frequently to retain or improve patient's existing ROM.*

---

g. **Position patient in 30-degree lateral (side-lying) position (one nurse):**	This position is recommended to prevent development of pressure injuries by reducing direct contact of trochanter with support surface (see Chapter 48).
(1) Lower head of bed completely or as low as patient can tolerate. Be sure mattress is at your waist level.	Provides position of comfort for patient and removes pressure from bony prominences on back.
(2) Lower side rail and position patient toward side of bed opposite direction toward which patient is to be turned. Place arms under shoulders and move upper trunk toward you first; then place arms under buttocks and upper legs and move lower trunk, supporting hips, toward you.	Provides room for patient to turn to side.
(3) Raise side rail and go to opposite side of bed.	
(4) Lower side rail and flex patient's knee that will not be next to mattress once positioned. Keep foot on mattress. Place one hand on patient's upper bent leg near hip and other hand on patient's shoulder.	Use of leverage makes turning to side easy.
(5) Roll patient onto side toward you.	Rolling decreases trauma to tissues. In addition, patient is positioned so that leverage on hip makes turning easy.
(6) Place pillow under patient's head and neck.	Maintains alignment. Reduces lateral neck flexion. Decreases strain on sternocleidomastoid muscle.
(7) Place your hands under patient's dependent shoulder and bring shoulder blade forward.	Prevents patient's weight from resting directly on shoulder joint.
(8) Position both arms in slightly flexed position. Support upper arm with pillow level with shoulder; other arm, by mattress.	Decreases internal rotation and adduction of shoulder. Supporting both arms in slightly flexed position protects joint. Ventilation improves because chest is able to expand more easily.
(9) Place your hands under patient's dependent hip and bring hip slightly forward so that angle from hip to mattress is approximately 30 degrees.	The 30-degree lateral position reduces pressure on trochanter; designed to prevent pressure injury.
(10) Place small tuck-back pillow behind patient's back. (Make by folding pillow lengthwise. Smooth area is slightly tucked under patient's back.)	Provides support to maintain patient on side.

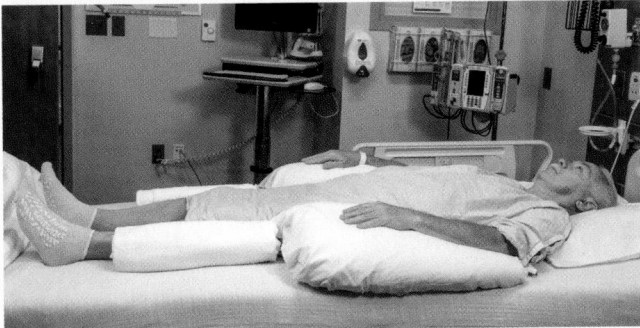

STEP 4e(6) Supported supine position with pillows in place.

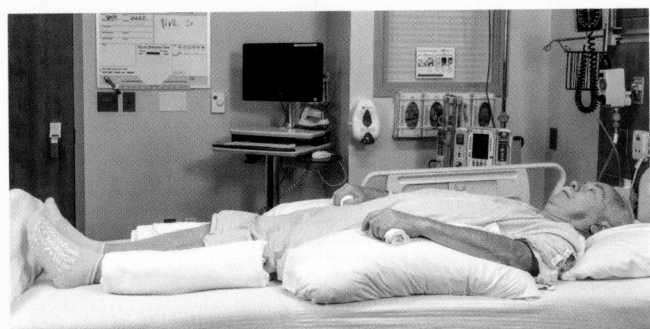

STEP 4e(7) Place hand rolls in patient's hands.

Continued

SKILL 39.1	MOVING AND POSITIONING PATIENTS IN BED—cont'd

STEP	RATIONALE
(11) Place pillow under semiflexed upper leg level at hip from groin to foot (see illustration).	Flexion prevents hyperextension of leg. Maintains leg in correct alignment. Prevents pressure on bony prominences.
Option: Place pillows or sandbags (if available) parallel against plantar surface of dependent foot. May also use ankle-foot orthotic on feet if available.	Maintains dorsiflexion of foot.

h. Position patient in Sims' (semi-prone) position:

(1) Lower head of bed completely. Be sure mattress is at waist level.	Provides for proper body alignment while patient is lying down flat on abdomen. Prepares patient for position change.
(2) Place patient supine on side of bed opposite direction toward which he or she is to be turned. Place your arms under patient's shoulders and move the upper trunk toward you. Next, place arms under buttocks and upper legs to move trunk toward you, supporting the hips.	
(3) Move to other side of bed. Lower side rail and flex patient's knee that will not be next to mattress once positioned. Keep foot on mattress. Place one hand on patient's upper bent leg near hip and other hand on patient's shoulder. Turn patient toward you.	Uses leverage to move patient as a unit onto side.
(4) Position in lateral position with patient lying partially on abdomen. Raise side rail and move to other side of bed. Lower side rail and take your hands to lift patient's dependent shoulder out with arm placed at patient's side (see illustration).	Lifting dependent shoulder avoids pressure on joint.
(5) Place small pillow under patient's head.	Maintains proper alignment and prevents lateral neck flexion.
(6) Place pillow under flexed upper arm, supporting arm level with shoulder.	Prevents internal rotation of shoulder. Maintains alignment.
(7) Place pillow under flexed upper legs, supporting leg level with hip.	Prevents internal rotation of hip and adduction of leg. Flexion prevents hyperextension of leg. Reduces mattress pressure on knees and ankles.
(8) Place sandbag parallel against plantar surface of foot or place both feet in footboots.	Maintains foot in dorsiflexion. Prevents plantar flexion contractures or footdrop.

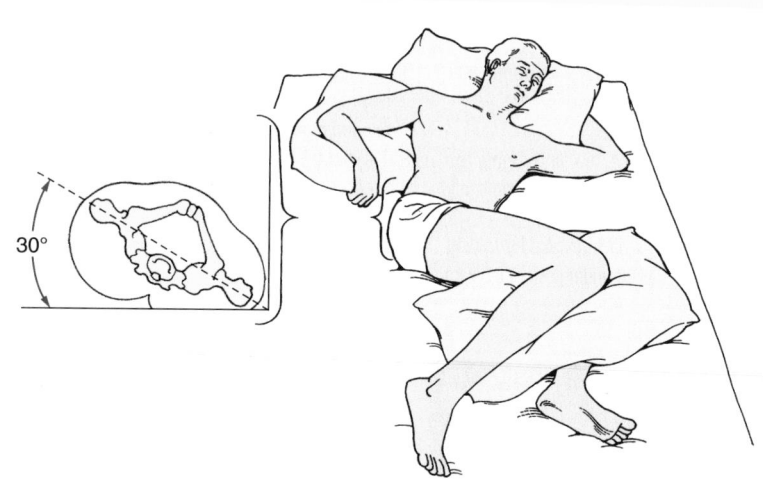

STEP 4g(11) Thirty-degree lateral position with pillows in place.

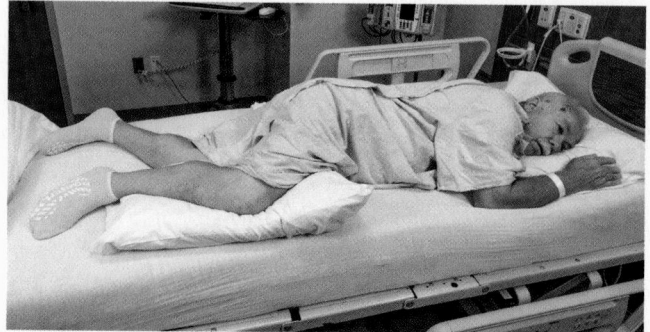

STEP 4h(4) Prone position with pillows supporting lower legs.

STEP	RATIONALE

i. Logroll patient (three nurses):

> **CLINICAL DECISION:** *A registered nurse supervises and helps the AP when there is a health care provider's order to logroll a patient. Patients with spinal cord injuries or who are recovering from neck, back, or spinal surgery need to keep the spinal column in straight alignment to prevent further injury.*

(1) Place small pillow between patient's knees.	Prevents tension on spinal column and adduction of hip.
(2) Cross patient's arms on chest.	Prevents injury to arms.
(3) Position two nurses on side toward which patient is to be turned and one nurse on side where pillows are to be placed behind patient's back(see illustration).	Distributes weight equally among nurses during turning.
(4) Fanfold drawsheet along backside of patient.	Provides strong handles for nurses to grip drawsheet without slipping.
(5) With one nurse grasping drawsheet at lower hips and thighs and the other nurse grasping drawsheet at patient's shoulders and lower back, roll patient as one unit in a smooth, continuous motion on count of three (see illustration).	Maintains proper alignment by moving all body parts at the same time, preventing tension or twisting of spinal column.
(6) Nurse on opposite side of bed places pillows along length of patient for support (see illustration).	Maintains patient in side-lying position.
(7) Gently lean patient, as a unit, back toward pillows for support (see illustration).	Ensures continued straight alignment of spinal column, preventing injury.
5. Be sure patient feels comfortable in new position. Place nurse call system in accessible location within patient's reach.	Gives patient sense of well-being. Ensures patient can call for help if needed.
6. Raise side rails (as appropriate), and lower bed to lowest position.	Ensures patient safety.
7. Perform hand hygiene.	Reduces transmission of microorganisms.

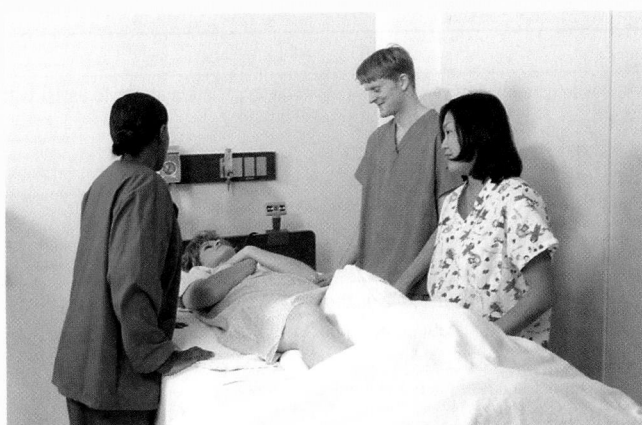

STEP 4i(3) Preparing patient for logroll.

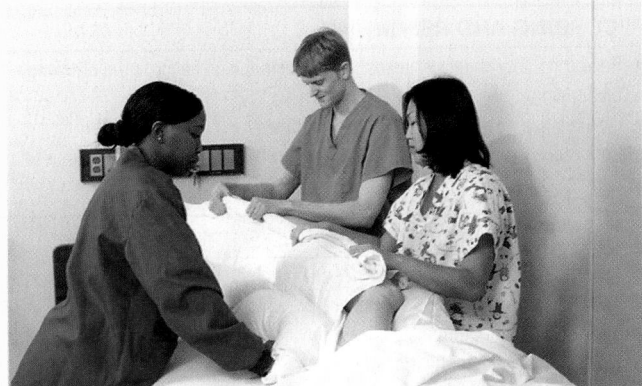

STEP 4i(6) Place pillows along patient's back for support.

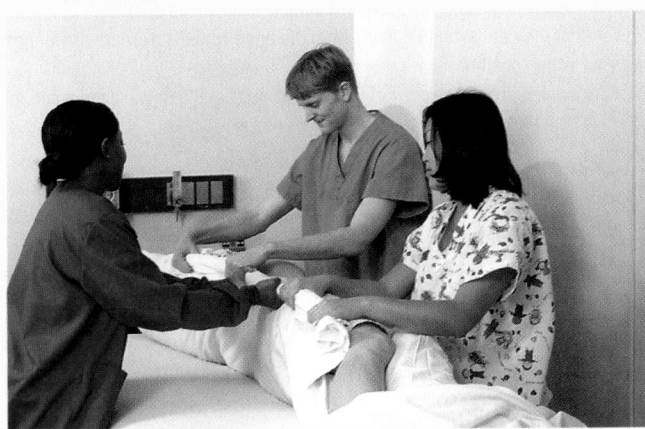

STEP 4i(5) Move patient as a unit, logrolling onto side.

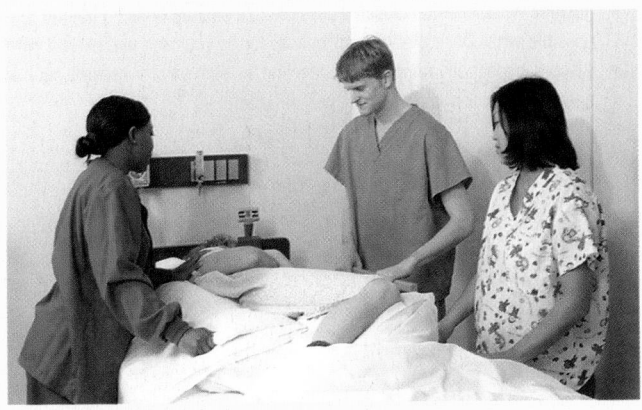

STEP 4i(7) Gently lean patient as a unit against pillows.

Continued

SKILL 39.1	**MOVING AND POSITIONING PATIENTS IN BED—cont'd**
STEP	**RATIONALE**

EVALUATION

1. Assess patient's respiratory status, body alignment, position, and level of comfort. Patient's body should be supported by adequate mattress, and vertebral column should be without observable curves.

2. Measure range of motion (ROM). Assess patient's ability to perform active range of motion and passive range of motion as needed to identify early joint contractures.

3. Observe skin for areas of erythema, blistering, or breakdown. Pay special attention to bony prominences and areas and body regions that may be experiencing extended pressure.

4. **Use Teach-Back:** "I want to be sure I explained the steps we are going to use to move and position you in bed. Please repeat the steps you can follow to help us move you up in bed." Revise your instruction now or develop a plan for revised patient/family caregiver teaching if patient/family caregiver is not able to teach back correctly.

Rationale column:

Determines effectiveness of positioning and patient's tolerance. Additional supports (e.g., pillows, bath blankets) may be added or removed to promote comfort and correct body alignment.

Determines whether joint contracture is developing.

Provides ongoing observation regarding patient's skin and musculoskeletal systems. Indicates complications of immobility or improper positioning of body part.

Determines patient's/family caregiver's level of understanding of instructional topic.

UNEXPECTED OUTCOMES AND RELATED INTERVENTIONS

1. Joint contractures develop or worsen.
   - Increase frequency of ROM exercises to affected and immobilized areas (see Table 39.2).
   - Consider physical therapy consult for different positioning.
2. Skin shows areas of erythema and breakdown.
   - Increase frequency of turning and repositioning.
   - Place turning schedule above patient's bed.
3. Patient avoids moving.
   - Medicate with analgesia as ordered by health care provider to ensure patient's comfort before moving.
   - Allow pain medication to take effect before repositioning.

RECORDING AND REPORTING

- Record on flow sheet or nurses' notes positioning change, time of change, and observations (e.g., condition of skin, joint movement, patient's ability to assist with positioning).
- Document your evaluation of patient learning.
- Report observations of patient's tolerance of position changes to nurse at change of shift.
- Report skin or joint complications to health care provider.

HOME CARE CONSIDERATIONS

- Assess the need for special transfer equipment to be used in the home setting. Assess home environment for hazards (e.g., throw rugs, electrical cords, slippery floors). If wheelchair is used, access must be possible through all doors, and space for transfer must be available in bathroom and bedroom.
- Assess home to determine compatibility of environment with assistive devices (e.g., over-bed trapeze, mechanical lift, hospital bed).
- Assess ability and motivation of patient and family caregivers to participate in moving and positioning patient in bed.
- For patients who use wheelchairs at home, recommend these safety precautions:
  - Always check wheelchair locks, wheels, and footplates for proper functioning before use.
  - Never attempt to reach an object if you must move forward in the wheelchair seat or pick an object up from the floor by reaching between your knees.
  - Position wheelchair as close as possible to a desired object. Position the wheel casters so that they are extended away from the drive wheels to create the longest possible wheelbase. Reach back only as far as your arm will extend without changing your sitting position.
  - Always inspect any ramp, incline, decline, or pathway for hazards such as holes, obstacles, or slippery or uneven surfaces before proceeding. If you cannot see the entire ramp, ask someone to inspect it for you.

KEY POINTS

- Injuries or disease processes that impact coordination and regulation of muscle groups pathologically influence mobility.
- Immobility increases the risk of skin breakdown and is directly related to the development of deep vein thromboses (DVT) and pulmonary emboli (PE).
- Immobility can negatively impact the ability to complete daily activities and can lead to boredom and social isolation.
- The risk of disabilities related to immobilization depends on the extent and duration of immobilization and the patient's overall level of health.
- Observing the appearance of extremities and measuring the range of motion of joints in various body positions assess for correct body alignment.
- The nursing process and critical thinking assist you in identifying nursing diagnoses so that you can individualize care for your patients who are experiencing or are at risk for the adverse effects of impaired body alignment and mobility.
- Patient movement algorithms serve as assessment tools for developing individualized approaches for safe patient handling and movement.
- Patients with impaired body alignment and mobility require the use of correct positioning techniques.
- Working collaboratively with health care providers, a nurse will identify patient risk factors for DVT and employ nursing interventions that reduce risk, such as early ambulation; leg, foot, and ankle exercises; regularly provided fluids; and frequent position changes.
- Careful and continuous evaluation of patient outcomes from both a nursing and patient perspective supports revision of the nursing care plan to continue optimization of mobility.

REFLECTIVE LEARNING

- Reflect on a recent clinical experience in which a patient needed to ambulate but was unable to because of voiced complaints of pain, and describe the interventions you implemented.
- Recall any challenges in patient repositioning experienced during a clinical day, and describe any safe patient-handling techniques you applied.
- Reflect on a patient experience you encountered today, and describe the risks the patient had because of reduced mobility.

REVIEW QUESTIONS

1. A patient has been on bed rest for over 5 days. Which of these findings during the nurse's assessment may indicate a complication of immobility?
   1. Decreased peristalsis
   2. Decreased heart rate
   3. Increased blood pressure
   4. Increased urinary output
2. An older-adult patient has been bedridden for 2 weeks. Which of these complaints by the patient indicates to the nurse that he or she is developing a complication of immobility?
   1. Increase of appetite
   2. Gum soreness
   3. Difficulty in swallowing
   4. Left ankle joint stiffness
3. A patient is receiving 40 mg of enoxaparin subcutaneously every 12 hours while on prolonged bed rest to prevent thrombophlebitis. Because bleeding is a potential side effect of this medication, the nurse should continually assess the patient for what signs of bleeding? (Select all that apply.)
   1. Bruising
   2. Pale yellow urine
   3. Bleeding gums
   4. Coffee ground–like vomitus
   5. Light brown stool
4. Place the following steps in the correct order for positioning a patient in the 30-degree lateral side-lying position.
   1. Raise side rail and go to opposite side of bed.
   2. Lower side rail and flex patient's knee that will not be next to mattress. Keep foot on mattress and place one hand on patient's upper bent leg near hip and other hand on shoulder.
   3. Lower head of bed flat if patient can tolerate it.
   4. Roll patient onto side toward you.
   5. Lower side rail and position patient on side of bed opposite the direction toward which patient is to be turned.
   6. Place hands under patient's dependent shoulder and bring shoulder blade forward.
   7. Place hands under patient's dependent hip and bring hip slightly forward so that angle from hip to mattress is approximately 30 degrees.
5. The effects of immobility on the cardiac system include which of the following? (Select all that apply.)
   1. Thrombus formation
   2. Increased cardiac workload
   3. Weak peripheral pulses
   4. Irregular heartbeat
   5. Orthostatic hypotension
6. A 46-year-old patient is admitted to the emergency department following an automobile accident. The patient has a pelvic fracture and is ordered on bed rest and placed in an immobilization device to limit further injury until the fracture can safely be repaired. Which measures would be appropriate for this patient to prevent complications of bed rest? (Select all that apply.)
   1. Administer intravenous analgesic as ordered.
   2. Have patient perform incentive spirometry.
   3. Support patient in active assistive ROM exercises of upper extremities.
   4. Provide patient a low-calorie diet.
   5. Apply sequential compression devices to legs.
7. A patient has an order for application of compression stockings. Place the following steps for application of the stockings in the correct order:
   1. Place patient's toes into foot of stocking up to the heel; keep smooth.
   2. Use tape measure to measure patient's leg for proper stocking size.
   3. Slide stocking up over patient's calf until sock is completely extended.
   4. Turn elastic stocking inside out, keeping hand inside holding heel. Take other hand and pull stocking inside out until reaching the heel.
   5. Slide remaining portion of stocking over patient's foot, covering toes. Be sure foot fits into toe and heel of stocking.
8. An older-adult patient is admitted following a hip fracture and surgical repair. Before ambulating the patient postoperatively on the evening of surgery, which of the following would be most important to assess? (Select all that apply.)
   1. Patient's usual dietary intake
   2. Time and date of the patient's last bowel movement
   3. Preadmission activity tolerance
   4. Baseline heart rate
   5. Patient's home living situation

9. A nurse is helping a patient perform active assisted range of motion in the right elbow. Which statement describes the correct technique?
   1. Support elbow by holding distal part of extremity.
   2. Grasp joint with fingers to provide support.
   3. Have patient move joint independently.
   4. Move the joint past the point of resistance.
   5. Perform the exercise a few times only, and gradually build up to more.

10. A middle-aged adult patient has limited mobility following a total knee arthroplasty. During assessment, the nurse notes that the patient is having difficulty breathing while lying supine. Which assessment data support a pulmonary issue related to immobility? (Select all that apply.)

1. Oxygen saturation of 89%
2. Irregular radial pulse
3. Diminished breath sounds bilateral bases on auscultation
4. BP: 132/84
5. Pain reported at 3 on scale of 0 to 10 following medication
6. Respiratory rate of 26

Answers: 1. 2; **2.** 4, 3, 1, 3, 4, 5, 1, 2, 4, 6; **3.** 7; **4.** 6; **5.** 1, 2, 5; **6.** 2, 3, 5; **7.** 2, 4, 1, 5, 3; **8.** 3, 5; **9.** 1; **10.** 1, 3, 6.

Rationales for Review Questions can be found on the Evolve website.

REFERENCES

Ackley BJ, Ladwig GB: *Nursing diagnosis handbook: an evidence-based guide to planning care*, ed 11, St Louis, 2017, Elsevier.

American Association of Critical-Care Nurses (AACN): Prevention of falls: applying AACN's healthy work environment standards to a fall campaign, *Crit Care Nurse* 34(5):75, 2014.

American Heart Association: *What is venous thromboembolism (VTE)?* 2017. https://www.heart.org/en/health-topics/venous-thromboembolism/what-is-venous-thromboembolism-vte. Accessed June 10, 2019.

American Psychiatric Association (APA): *Diagnostic and statistical manual of mental disorders*, ed 5, Arlington, VA, 2013, American Psychiatric Publishing.

American Psychological Association (APA): *Understanding rehabilitation psychology*, 2019. https://www.apa.org/action/science/rehabilitation/. Accessed June 7, 2019.

Association of peri/Operative Registered Nurses (AORN): Guideline summary: prevention of venous thromboembolism, *AORN J* 107(6):750–754, 2018.

Ayello EA: CMS MDS 3.0 section M skin conditions in long-term care: pressure ulcers, skin tears, and moisture-associated skin damage data update, *Adv Skin Wound Care* 30(9):415–429, 2017.

Ball JE, et al.: *Seidel's guide to physical examination*, ed 9, St Louis, 2019, Elsevier.

Barbour KE, et al.: Vital signs: prevalence of doctor-diagnosed arthritis and arthritis-attributable activity limitation—United States, 2013–2015, *MMWR Morb Mortal Wkly Rep* 66(9):246–253, 2017.

Barnes-Daly MA, et al.: Improving health care for critically ill patients using an evidence-based collaborative approach to the ABCDEF bundle dissemination and implementation, *Worldviews Evid Based Nurs* 15(3):206–216, 2018.

Bodenheimer T: Teach-back: a simple technique to enhance patients' understanding, *Fam Pract Manag* 25(4):20–22, 2018.

Bonkowski SL, et al.: Evaluation of a pain management education program and operational guideline on nursing practice, attitudes, and pain management, *J Contin Educ Nurs* 49(4):178–185, 2018.

Cave B, et al.: Extended venous thromboembolism prophylaxis in medically ill patients, *Pharmacotherapy* 38(6):597–609, 2018.

Centers for Disease Control and Prevention (CDC): *What is health literacy*, 2019. https://www.cdc.gov/healthliteracy/learn/index.html. Accessed December 23, 2019.

Centrella-Nigro A, Alexander C: Using the teach-back method in patient education to improve patient satisfaction, *J Contin Educ Nurs* 48(1):47–52, 2017.

Dickinson S, et al.: Integrating a standardized mobility program and safe patient handling, *Crit Care Nurs Q* 41(3):240–252, 2018.

Dutton M: *Dutton's introduction to physical therapy and patient skills*, New York, 2014, McGraw Hill.

Good Therapy: *Psycho-physical therapy*, 2016. https://www.goodtherapy.org/learn-about-therapy/types/psycho-physical-therapy. Accessed June 7, 2019.

Gupta MJ, et al.: Rush fracture liaison service for capturing "missed opportunities" to treat osteoporosis in patients with fragility fractures, *Osteoporos Int* 29(8):1861–1874, 2018.

Hallford DJ, et al.: The association between anxiety and falls: a meta-analysis, *J Gerontol B Psychol Sci Soc Sci* 72(5):729–741, 2017.

Hootman JM, et al.: Updated projected prevalence of self-reported doctor-diagnosed arthritis and arthritis-attributable activity limitation among US adults, 2015–2040, *Arthritis Rheum* 68(7):1582–1587, 2016.

Klein LM, et al.: Increasing patient mobility through an individualized goal-centered hospital mobility program: a quasi-experimental quality improvement project, *Nurs Outlook* 66(3):254–262, 2018.

Kruschke C, Butcher HK: Evidence-based practice guideline: fall prevention for older adults, *J Gerontol Nurs* 43(11):15–21, 2017.

Lewis SL, et al.: *Medical-surgical nursing assessment and management of clinical problems*, ed 10, St Louis, 2017, Elsevier.

Link T: Guideline implementation: prevention of venous thromboembolism, *AORN J* 107(6):737–748, 2018.

Martin M, et al.: *New and improved VA algorithms*, 2014. http://www.asphp.org/wp-content/uploads/2016/06/New-and-Improved-VA-Algorithms-and-New-SPHM-App-ASPHP-rev-MMM.pptx. Accessed May 25, 2019.

McCance KL, Huether SE: *Pathophysiology: the biologic basis for disease in adults and children*, ed 8, St Louis, 2017, Elsevier.

Mulkey MA, et al.: Choosing the right delirium assessment tool, *J Neurosci Nurs* 50(6):343–348, 2018.

Musich S, et al.: The impact of mobility limitations on health outcomes among older adults, *Geriatr Nurs* 39(2):162–169, 2018.

Occupational Safety and Health Administration (OSHA): *Safe patient handling: preventing musculoskeletal disorders in nursing homes*, OSHA Publication 3708, 2014. https://www.osha.gov/Publications/OSHA3708.pdf. Accessed June 8, 2019.

Occupational Safety and Health Administration (OSHA): *Handling with care: practicing safe patient handling*,

2017. https://www.jcrinc.com/assets/1/7/Pages_from_ECN_20_2017_08-2.pdf. Accessed May 25, 2019.

Olinsky C, Norton CE: Implementation of a safe patient handling program in a multihospital health system from inception to sustainability, *Workplace Health Saf* 65(11):546–559, 2017.

Shibao C, et al.: Evaluation and treatment of orthostatic hypotension, *J Am Soc Hypertens* 7(4):317, 2013.

Stephens M, et al.: Developing the tissue viability seating guidelines, *J Tissue Viability* 27(1):74–79, 2018.

Strickland SL, et al.: AARC clinical practice guideline: effectiveness of nonpharmacologic airway clearance therapies in hospitalized patients, *Respir Care* 58(12):2187–2193, 2013.

The Joint Commission (TJC): *2020 National Patient Safety Goals*, Oakbrook Terrace, IL, 2020, The Commission. https://www.jointcommission.org/en/standards/national-patient-safety-goals/. Accessed January 2, 2020.

The Joint Commission (TJC): Non-pharmacologic and non-opioid solutions for pain management, *Quick Safety*(issue 44), 2018. https://www.jointcommission.org/assets/1/23/QS_Nonopioid_pain_mgmt_8_15_18_FINAL.pdf. Accessed June 4, 2019.

Tick H, et al.: Evidence-based nonpharmacologic strategies for comprehensive pain care: The Consortium Pain Task Force white paper, *Explore (NY)* 14(3):177–211, 2018.

US Department of Labor (USDL): *Bureau of Labor Statistics*, 2017. https://www.bls.gov/careeroutlook/2017/home.htm. Accessed September 25, 2019.

US Department of Veterans Affairs: *VA National Center for Patient Safety*, 2018. https://www.patientsafety.va.gov. Accessed 4 June 2019.

Wald HL, et al.: The case for mobility assessment in hospitalized older adults: American Geriatric Society white paper executive summary, *J Am Geriatr Soc* 67(1):11, 2019.

Wiggermann N: The sliding patient: how to respond to and prevent migration in bed: migration can cause negative patient outcomes and caregiver injuries related to repositioning, *Am Nurse Today* 9(9):18, 2014.

Winterton MT, Baldwin K: The neuro-orthopedic approach, *Phys Med Rehabil Clin North Am* 29(3):567–591, 2018.

Wound Ostomy and Continence Nurses Society (WOCN): *Guidelines for prevention and management of pressure injuries*, 2016. https://www.ahrq.gov/professionals/systems/hospital/pressureulcertoolkit/index.html. Accessed June 8, 2019.

RESEARCH REFERENCES

Agency for Healthcare Research and Quality (AHRQ): Preventing pressure ulcers in hospitals: a toolkit for improving quality of care, n.d, https://www.ahrq.gov/sites/default/files/publications/files/putoolkit.pdf. Accessed June 3, 2019.

American Academy of Nursing (AAN): *The twenty-five things nurses and patients should question*, 2015. http://www.aannet.org/initiatives/choosing-wisely. Accessed June 7, 2019.

Chase JD, et al.: Identifying factors associated with mobility decline among hospitalized older adults, *Clin Nurs Res* 27(1):81–104, 2018.

Fang Y, et al.: Patient and family member factors influencing outcomes of poststroke inpatient rehabilitation, *Arch Phys Med Rehabil* 98(2), 2017, 249-255.e2.

Kanaskie ML, Snyder C: Nurses and nursing assistants decision-making regarding use of safe patient handling and mobility technology: a qualitative study, *Appl Nurs Res* 39:141–147, 2018.

Krupp A, et al.: A systematic review evaluating the role of nurses and processes for delivering early mobility interventions in the intensive care unit, *Intensive Crit Care Nurs* 47:30–38, 2018.

Meyers T: Prevention of heel pressure injuries and plantar flexion contractures with use of a heel protector in high-risk neurotrauma, medical, and surgical intensive care units: a randomized controlled trial, *J Wound Ostomy Continence Nurs* 44(5):429, 2017.

Modi S, et al.: Wells criteria for DVT is a reliable clinical tool to assess the risk of deep venous thrombosis in trauma patients, *World J Emerg Surg* 11:24, 2016.

Noble NL, Sweeney NL: Barriers to the use of assistive devices in patient handling, *Workplace Health Saf* 66(1):41–48, 2018.

Odgaard L, et al.: Nursing sensitive outcomes after severe traumatic brain injury: a nationwide study, *J Neurosci Nurs* 50(3):149–156, 2018.

Shin JY, et al.: Self-reported symptoms of Parkinson's Disease by sex and disease duration, *West J Nurs Res* 39(11):1412–1428, 2017.

Stanford Medicine: Patient education: chronic disease self-management program. https://www.selfmanagementresource.com/programs/small-group/chronic-pain-self-management, 2018. Accessed August 11, 2018.

Wells PS, et al.: Use of a clinical model for safe management of patients with suspected pulmonary embolism, *Ann Intern Med* 129(12):997–1005, 1998.

Zhang DZ, et al.: Effect of intermittent pneumatic compression on preventing deep vein thrombosis among stroke patients: a systematic review and meta-analysis, *Worldviews Evid Based Nurs* 15(3):189–196, 2018.

Zubkoff L, et al.: Preventing pressure ulcers in the Veterans Health Administration using a virtual breakthrough series collaborative, *J Nurs Care Qual* 32(4):301–308, 2017.

40

Hygiene

OBJECTIVES

- Describe factors that influence personal hygiene practices.
- Discuss how a nurse applies critical thinking when providing hygiene.
- Conduct a comprehensive assessment of a patient's total hygiene needs.
- Discuss conditions that place patients at risk for impaired skin integrity.
- Discuss factors that influence the condition of the nails and feet.
- Explain the importance of foot care for the patient with diabetes.
- Discuss conditions that place patients at risk for impaired oral mucous membranes.
- List common hair and scalp problems and their related interventions.
- Describe how hygiene care for the older adult differs from that for the younger patient.
- Discuss different approaches used in maintaining a patient's comfort and safety during hygiene care.
- Successfully perform hygiene procedures for the care of the skin, perineum, feet and nails, mouth, eyes, ears, and nose.
- Discuss how to adapt hygiene care for a patient who is cognitively impaired.

KEY TERMS

Alopecia, p. 866
Cerumen, p. 866
Cheilitis, p. 866
Complete bed bath, p. 873
Dental caries, p. 860
Edentulous, p. 866

Effleurage, p. 875
Gingivitis, p. 860
Glossitis, p. 866
Halitosis, p. 866
Maceration, p. 875
Mucositis, p. 869

Partial bed bath, p. 874
Pediculosis capitis, p. 866
Perineal care, p. 875
Stomatitis, p. 876
Xerostomia, p. 860

MEDIA RESOURCES

http://evolve.elsevier.com/Potter/fundamentals/

- Review Questions
- Video Clips
- Concept Map Creator
- Case Study with Questions

- Skills Performance Checklists
- Audio Glossary
- Content Updates
- Answers to QSEN Activity and Review Questions

Personal hygiene influences patients' comfort, safety, and well-being. Hygiene includes cleaning and grooming activities that maintain personal body cleanliness and appearance. A variety of personal, social, financial, and cultural factors influence hygiene practices. Because hygiene care requires close contact with your patients, use communication skills (e.g., listening, reflecting, focusing) to promote caring therapeutic relationships (see Chapter 24). When providing hygiene, integrate other nursing activities, including patient assessment and interventions such as range-of-motion (ROM) exercises, application of dressings, or inspection and care of intravenous (IV) sites.

Healthy people are usually able to meet their own hygiene needs. However, physical or cognitive impairments and emotional challenges often cause individuals to need some degree of assistance with hygiene care. In agency and home care settings, assess each patient's ability to perform self–hygiene care according to individual needs and preferences. When making adaptations for hygiene techniques and approaches, always ensure privacy, convey respect, and foster a patient's independence, safety, and comfort.

SCIENTIFIC KNOWLEDGE BASE

Proper hygiene care requires an understanding of the anatomy and physiology of the skin, nails, oral cavity, eyes, ears, and nose. The skin and mucosal cells exchange oxygen, nutrients, and fluids with underlying blood vessels. The cells require adequate nutrition, hydration, and circulation to resist injury and disease. Good hygiene techniques promote the normal structure and function of these tissues.

Apply knowledge of pathophysiology to provide preventive hygiene care. Recognize disease states that create changes in the integument, oral cavity, and sensory organs. For example, diabetes mellitus often results in chronic vascular changes that impair healing of the skin and mucosa. In the early stages of acquired immunodeficiency syndrome (AIDS), fungal infections of the oral cavity are common. Paralysis of the trigeminal nerve (cranial nerve V) eliminates the blink reflex, causing risk of corneal drying. In the presence of conditions such as these, adapt hygiene practices to minimize injury. Use time spent providing hygiene care to assess for and identify abnormalities and initiate appropriate actions to prevent further injury to sensitive tissues.

The Skin

The skin serves several functions, including protection, secretion, excretion, body temperature regulation, and cutaneous sensation (Table 40.1). The layers of the skin include the epidermis, the dermis, and the subcutaneous tissue (also known as the *hypodermis*), which shares some of the protective functions of the skin.

The epidermis (outer layer) shields underlying tissues against water loss and injury, prevents entry of disease-producing microorganisms, and generates new cells to replace the dead cells that are continuously shed from the outer surface of the skin. Bacteria (normal flora) commonly reside on the outer epidermis. The resident normal flora do not cause disease but instead inhibit the multiplication of disease-causing microorganisms (see Chapter 28).

Bundles of collagen and elastic fibers form the thicker dermis that underlies and supports the epidermis. Nerve fibers, blood vessels, sweat glands, sebaceous glands, and hair follicles run through the dermal layers. Sebaceous glands secrete sebum, an oily, odorous fluid, into the hair follicles. Sebum softens and lubricates the skin and slows water loss from the skin when the humidity is low. More important, sebum has bactericidal action.

The subcutaneous tissue functions as a heat insulator, supports upper skin layers in withstanding stresses and pressure, and anchors the skin loosely to underlying structures such as muscle. The subcutaneous tissue layer contains blood vessels, nerves, lymph tissue, and loose connective tissue filled with fat cells. Very little subcutaneous tissue underlies the oral mucosa.

The skin often reflects a change in physical condition by alterations in color, thickness, texture, turgor, temperature, and hydration (see Chapter 30). As long as the skin remains intact and healthy, its physiological function remains optimal. Hygiene practices frequently influence skin status and can have beneficial and negative effects on the skin. For example, too-frequent bathing and use of hot water frequently lead to dry, flaky skin and loss of protective oils.

The Feet, Hands, and Nails

The feet, hands, and nails often require special attention to prevent infection, odor, and injury. The condition of a patient's hands and feet influences the ability to perform hygiene care. Without the ability to bear weight, ambulate, or manipulate the hands, a patient is at risk for losing self-care ability.

A wide range of dexterity exists in the hand because of the movement between the thumb and fingers. Any condition (e.g., arthritis, multiple sclerosis, traumatic hand injury) that interferes with hand movement (e.g., superficial or deep pain or joint inflammation) impairs a patient's self-care abilities. Foot pain often changes a patient's gait, causing strain on different joints and muscle groups. Discomfort while standing or walking limits self-care abilities.

The nails are epithelial tissues that grow from the root of the nail bed, located in the skin at the nail groove hidden by a fold of skin called the *cuticle*. A normal healthy nail appears transparent, smooth, and convex, with a pink nail bed and translucent white tip. Inadequate nutrition and disease cause changes in the shape, thickness, and curvature of the nail (see Chapter 30).

The Oral Cavity

The oral cavity consists of the lips surrounding the opening of the mouth, the cheeks running along the sidewalls of the cavity, the tongue and its muscles, and the hard and soft palate. The mucous membrane, continuous with the skin, lines the oral cavity. The floor of the mouth and the undersurface of the tongue are richly supplied with blood vessels. Normal oral mucosa glistens and is pink, soft,

TABLE 40.1	**Function of the Skin and Implications for Care**
Function/Description	**Implications for Care**
Protection Epidermis is a relatively impermeable layer that prevents entrance of microorganisms. Although microorganisms reside on skin surface and in hair follicles, relative dryness of surface of skin inhibits bacterial growth. Sebum removes bacteria from hair follicles. Acidic pH of skin further retards bacterial growth.	Weakening of the epidermis occurs by scraping or stripping its surface (e.g., use of dry razors, tape removal, improper turning or positioning techniques). Excessive dryness causes cracks and breaks in skin and mucosa that allow bacteria to enter. Emollients soften skin and prevent moisture loss, soaking skin improves moisture retention, and hydrating mucosa prevents dryness. Constant exposure of skin to moisture causes maceration or softening, interrupting dermal integrity and promoting ulcer formation and bacterial growth. Keep bed linen and clothing dry. Misuse of soap, detergents, cosmetics, deodorant, and depilatories causes chemical irritation. Alkaline soaps neutralize the protective acid condition of skin. Cleaning skin removes excess oil, sweat, dead skin cells, and dirt, which promote bacterial growth. Minimize friction to avoid loss of stratum corneum, which increases risk for pressure injuries.
Sensation Skin contains sensory organs for touch, pain, heat, cold, and pressure.	Smooth linen out to remove sources of mechanical irritation. Make sure that bath water is not excessively hot or cold.
Temperature Regulation Radiation, evaporation, conduction, and convection control body temperature.	Factors that interfere with heat loss alter temperature control. Wet bed linen or gowns increase heat loss. Excess blankets or bed coverings conserve heat and interfere with heat loss through radiation and conduction. Coverings promote heat conservation.
Excretion and Secretion Sweat promotes heat loss by evaporation. Sebum lubricates skin and hair.	Perspiration and oil sometimes harbor microorganisms. Bathing removes excess body secretions, but excessive bathing causes dry skin.

moist, smooth, and without lesions. Ulcerations or trauma frequently results in significant bleeding. Several glands within and outside the oral cavity secrete saliva. Saliva cleanses the mouth, dissolves food chemicals to promote taste, moistens food to facilitate bolus formation, and contains enzymes Medications, exposure to radiation, dehydration, and mouth breathing may impair salivary secretion in the mouth, which increases the patient's risk for xerostomia, or dry mouth.

A normal tooth consists of the crown, neck, and root. Healthy teeth appear in a variety of shades of white, smooth, shiny, and aligned. The condition of the oral cavity reflects overall health and indicates oral hygiene needs (see Chapter 30).

Difficulty in chewing develops when surrounding gum tissues become inflamed or infected or when teeth are lost or become loosened. Regular oral hygiene helps to prevent gingivitis (i.e., inflammation of the gums) and dental caries (i.e., tooth decay produced by interaction of food with bacteria).

The Hair

Hair growth, distribution, and pattern indicate a person's general health status. Special hair-care practices focus on care of the scalp, axilla, and pubic areas. Hormonal changes, nutrition, emotional and physical stress, aging, infection, and some illnesses affect hair characteristics. The hair shaft itself is lifeless, and physiological factors do not affect it directly. However, hormonal and nutrient deficiencies of the hair follicle cause changes in hair color or condition.

The Eyes, Ears, and Nose

When providing hygiene, the eyes, ears, and nose require careful attention because of sensitive anatomical structures. For example, the cornea of the eye contains many nerve endings sensitive to irritants such as soap.

The eyes secrete tears, which contain substances to cleanse and lubricate the eye and protect it from bacteria. Specialized glands in the auditory canal secrete cerumen, which traps foreign bodies and repels insects. Cerumen builds up and becomes impacted in some people. Patients with alterations in one or more of the senses often need help to meet their hygiene needs. Chapter 30 describes the structure and function of these organs.

> ### REFLECT NOW
>
> When you were in your anatomy and physiology classes, you learned about the skin and mucous membranes. Think about the impact of sun on the skin. What types of short- or long-term issues can occur on the skin with sun exposure?

NURSING KNOWLEDGE BASE

A number of factors influence personal preferences for hygiene and the ability to maintain hygiene practices. Since no two individuals perform hygiene care in the same manner, you individualize patient care based on learning about his or her unique hygiene practices and preferences. Individualized hygiene care requires knowing the patient and using therapeutic communication skills to promote a trusting therapeutic relationship. Use the opportunities provided during hygiene care to assess a patient's health promotion practices, emotional status, and health care education needs and then offer educational interventions. Be aware that developmental changes influence the need and preferences for types of hygiene care.

Factors Influencing Hygiene

Social Practices. Social groups influence hygiene preferences and practices, including the type of hygiene products used and the nature and frequency of personal care practices. Parents and caregivers perform hygiene care for infants and young children. Family customs play a major role during childhood in determining hygiene practices, such as the frequency of bathing, the time of day bathing is performed, and even whether certain hygiene practices such as brushing the teeth or flossing are performed. As children enter adolescence, peer groups and media often influence hygiene practices, and health education is important. For example, health education impacts adolescent girls' choices related to menstrual hygiene (Kole et al., 2018). Young girls become more interested in their personal appearance and begin to wear makeup. During the adult years, involvement with friends and work groups shapes the expectations that people have about personal appearance. Some individuals' hygiene practices change because of changes in living conditions and available resources. This is common in older adults who have limited finances and in the homeless and people living in poverty.

Personal Preferences. Patients have individual preferences about how and when to perform hygiene and grooming care. Some patients prefer to shower, whereas others prefer to bathe. Patients select different hygiene and grooming products according to personal preferences. Knowing patients' personal preferences promotes individualized care. Culture plays a role in sensitivity to personal space and gender (see Box 40.1 and Chapter 9). Help a patient develop new hygiene practices when indicated by an illness or condition. For example, you may need to teach a patient with diabetes proper foot hygiene or a bariatric patient adaptive bathing methods. Safe and effective patient-centered nursing care improves patient satisfaction and health and reduces costs (Burman et al., 2013).

Body Image. Body image is a person's subjective concept of his or her body, including physical appearance, structure, or function (see Chapter 33). Body image affects the way in which individuals maintain personal hygiene. If a patient maintains a neatly groomed appearance, be sure to consider the details of grooming when planning care, and consult with the patient before making decisions about how to provide hygiene. Patients who appear unkempt or uninterested in hygiene sometimes need education about its importance or further assessment regarding their ability to participate with daily hygiene.

Surgery, illness, or a change in emotional or functional status often affects a patient's body image. Discomfort and pain, emotional stress, and fatigue diminish the ability or desire to perform hygiene self-care and require extra effort to promote hygiene and grooming.

Socioeconomic Status. A person's economic resources influence the type and extent of hygiene practices used. Be sensitive in considering that a patient's economic status influences the ability to regularly maintain hygiene. He or she may not be able to afford desired basic supplies such as deodorant, shampoo, and toothpaste. A patient may need to modify the home environment by adding safety devices such as nonskid surfaces and grab bars in the bath to perform hygiene self-care safely. When patients lack socioeconomic resources, it becomes difficult for them to participate and take responsible roles in health promotion activities such as basic hygiene.

Health Beliefs and Motivation. Knowledge about the importance of hygiene and its implications for well-being influences hygiene practices. However, knowledge alone is not enough. Motivation also plays a

🌐 BOX 40.1 CULTURAL ASPECTS OF CARE

Hygiene Practices

Patients deserve a culturally congruent plan for hygiene care. For many patients, culture influences hygiene practices, and hygiene care may become a potential source of conflict and stress in the caregiving environment (Marion et al., 2017). Patient-centered care mandates that care is aligned with patients' values, needs, practices, and expectations, providing equitable and ethical care, and that care be based on respect for an individual patient's cultural background (Henderson et al., 2018). A nurse must also consider other aspects of culture, such as a patient's educational and developmental levels, extent of any physical disabilities, and geographical location of home when delivering hygiene.

Implications for Patient-Centered Care

- Maintain privacy, especially for women from cultures that value female modesty, and provide gender-congruent caregivers as requested (Giger, 2017).
- Collaborate with community leaders when providing health education for a diverse community (LaFleur et al., 2017).
- Allow family members to participate in care if desired by adapting the schedule of hygiene activities.
- Recognize that some cultures prohibit or restrict touching. Incorporate awareness that people from different cultural backgrounds have differing preferences regarding personal space. In some cases touch is considered magical and healing; others view it as evil or anxiety producing (Giger, 2017).
- Recognize cultural hair practices, and do not cut or shave hair without prior discussion with patient or family (Bowen and O'Brien-Richardson, 2017).
- Be aware that toileting practices vary by culture (Giger, 2017).
- Recognize that different cultures have preferences about hot and cold water and their effects on healing or diseases (Morgan-Consoli and Unzueta, 2018).

---

key role in a patient's hygiene practices. Motivational interviewing can assist you in identifying how a patient perceives benefit in performing hygiene and his or her willingness to change behavior (see Chapter 25). Adapt what you learn about a patient's willingness to change into your patient teaching approach. Provide information that focuses on a patient's personal health-related issues relevant to the desired hygiene care behaviors. Patient perceptions of the benefits of hygiene care and the susceptibility to and seriousness of developing a problem affect the motivation to change behavior. For example, do patients perceive that they are at risk for dental disease, or that dental disease is serious, and that brushing and flossing are effective in reducing risk? When they recognize that there is a risk and that they can take reasonable action without negative consequences, they are more likely to be receptive to modify health behaviors (Broadbent et al., 2016).

Cultural Variables. Cultural beliefs, religious practices, and personal values influence hygiene care (see Box 40.1). People from diverse cultural backgrounds (e.g., level of education, gender preference, geographic location) frequently follow different self-care practices (see Chapter 9). For example, maintaining cleanliness does not hold the same importance for some ethnic or social groups as it does for others (Giger, 2017). In North America many are fortunate to be able to bathe or shower daily and use deodorant to prevent body odors. However, people from some socioeconomic or cultural groups are not sensitive to body odors, prefer to bathe less frequently, and do not use deodorant. Avoid expressing disapproval or forcing changes in hygienic practices

unless the practices affect a patient's health. In these situations, use tact, provide information, and allow choices.

Developmental Stage. The normal process of aging affects the condition of body tissues and structures. Apply your knowledge of physical and psychosocial developmental changes as you assess your patients and plan, implement, and evaluate hygiene care. A patient's developmental stage affects the ability of a patient to perform hygiene care and the type of care needed. Use your knowledge of developmental changes when planning hygiene care.

Skin. The neonate's skin is relatively immature at birth. The epidermis and dermis are bound together loosely, and the skin is very thin. Friction against the skin layers causes bruising. Handle a neonate carefully during bathing. Any break in the skin easily results in an infection.

A toddler's skin layers become more tightly bound together. Thus, the child has a greater resistance to infection and skin irritation. However, because of his or her more active play and the absence of established hygiene habits, parents and caregivers need to provide thorough hygiene and teach good hygiene habits.

During adolescence the growth and maturation of the integument increase. In girls, estrogen secretion causes the skin to become soft, smooth, and thicker with increased vascularity. In boys, male hormones produce an increased thickness of the skin with some darkening in color. Sebaceous glands become more active, predisposing adolescents to acne (i.e., active inflammation of the sebaceous glands accompanied by pimples). Sweat glands become fully functional during puberty. Adolescents usually begin to use antiperspirants. More frequent bathing and shampooing also become necessary to reduce body odors and eliminate oily hair.

The condition of the adult's skin depends on bathing practices and exposure to environmental irritants. Normally the skin is elastic, well hydrated, firm, and smooth. When an adult bathes frequently or is exposed to an environment with low humidity, it becomes dry and flaky. With aging the rate of epidermal cell replacement slows, and the skin thins and loses resiliency. Moisture leaves the skin, increasing the risk for bruising and other types of injury. As the production of lubricating substances from skin glands decreases, the skin becomes dry and itchy (Touhy and Jett, 2018). These changes warrant caution when bathing, turning, and repositioning older adults. Too-frequent bathing and bathing with hot water or harsh soap cause the skin to become excessively dry (American Academy of Dermatology, 2018).

Feet and Nails. Foot health is a key component to a person's mobility, health, and overall well-being. With aging and continued exposure to the trauma of walking and weight-bearing, a patient is more likely to develop chronic foot problems compounded as a result of poor foot care, improper fit of footwear, and local abnormalities and systemic disease (Persaud et al., 2018). For example, Morton's neuroma, a common condition in middle-age women, affects health-related quality of life by causing burning, numbness, and pain of the foot on weight-bearing (Park et al., 2018).

Older adults do not always have the strength, flexibility, visual acuity, or manual dexterity to care for their feet and nails. Foot problems may be overlooked and impact a patient's comfort, mobility, and quality of life (Persaud et al., 2018). Older adults frequently complain of foot pain. They also often have dry feet because of a decrease in sebaceous gland secretion and dehydration of epidermal cells. Common problems of the feet affecting older adults include corns, calluses, bunions, hammertoes, maceration between toes, and fungal infections (Arthritis Foundation, 2017).

The Mouth. At approximately 6 to 8 months of age, infants begin teething. The first permanent (secondary) teeth erupt at about 6 years of age (Hockenberry et al., 2019). From adolescence, when all the permanent teeth are in place, through middle adulthood, the teeth and gums remain healthy if a person follows healthy eating patterns and dental care. Avoiding fermentable carbohydrates and sticky sweets helps to keep the teeth free of dental caries. In addition, regular brushing (twice a day) and flossing reduce caries and periodontal disease.

As a person ages, numerous factors result in poor oral health, including age-related changes of the mouth, changes resulting from chronic disease such as diabetes, physical disabilities involving hand grasp or strength affecting the ability to perform oral care, lack of attention to oral care, and prescribed medications that have oral side effects. Gums lose vascularity and tissue elasticity, which may cause dentures to fit poorly.

Hair. Throughout life, changes in the growth, distribution, and condition of the hair influence hair hygiene. As males reach adolescence, shaving becomes a part of routine grooming. Young girls who reach puberty often begin to shave their legs and axillae. With aging, as scalp hair becomes thinner and drier, shampooing is usually performed less frequently.

Eyes, Ears, and Nose. Chapter 49 addresses changes in hearing, vision, and olfaction across the life span as a result of growth and development. Alterations in sensory function often require modifications in hygiene care. Hygiene of sensory structures must be provided in a way to prevent injury to sensitive tissues such as the cornea of the eye and the internal ear canal.

Physical Condition. Patients with certain types of physical limitations or disabilities associated with disease and injury lack the physical energy and dexterity to perform hygiene self-care safely. A patient whose arm is in a cast or who has an IV line needs help with hygiene care. A weakened grasp resulting from arthritis, stroke, or muscular disorders makes using a toothbrush, washcloth, or hairbrush difficult or ineffective. Sensory deficits not only alter a patient's ability to perform care but also place the patient at risk for injury. Safety is a priority for a patient with a sensory deficit. For example, a patient with paresthesia who is unable to feel that bath water is too hot can incur a burn injury during bathing.

Chronic illnesses such as cardiac, pulmonary, and neurological diseases; cancer; dementia; and some mental health illnesses often exhaust or incapacitate patients. Patients who become tired or short of breath frequently need to have complete hygiene care provided. Include periods of rest during care to allow patients who are tired the opportunity to participate in their care. Pain often accompanies illness and injury, limiting a patient's ability to tolerate hygiene and grooming activities or perform self-care. Pain frequently limits ROM, resulting in impaired use of the arms or hands or limited ability to move about in the environment, impairing the ability to perform hygiene self-care. Sedation and drowsiness associated with analgesics used for pain management also limit a patient's ability to safely participate in care.

Limited mobility caused by a variety of factors (e.g., obesity, physical injury, weakness, surgery, pain, prolonged inactivity, medication effect, and presence of medical devices [e.g., indwelling catheter, feeding tube, or IV line]) decreases a patient's ability to perform hygiene self-care activities safely. Individualized care considers a patient's ability to perform care, the amount of assistance needed, and the need for assistive and safety devices to facilitate safe hygiene care.

Acute and chronic cognitive impairments resulting from conditions such as stroke, brain injury, psychoses, and dementia often result in the inability to perform self-care independently. Patients with dementia often forget to attend to their basic hygiene needs. When people with cognitive impairments are unaware of their hygiene and grooming needs, they may become fearful and agitated during hygiene

Knowledge
- Anatomy and physiology of integument, oral cavity, and sense organs
- Principles of comfort and safety
- Communication principles that convey caring
- Risk factors posing hygiene problems
- Knowledge of cultural variations in hygiene

Experience
- Prior experience caring for patients requiring assistance with hygiene
- Personal hygiene practices

ASSESSMENT
- Observe the patient's physical condition and integrity of integument, oral cavity, and sense organs
- Explore any developmental factors influencing the patient's hygiene needs
- Note the patient's self-care ability and hygiene practices
- Determine the patient's cultural preferences, values, and beliefs regarding hygiene

Standards
- Apply ADA's practice standards for foot care
- Apply WOCN and NPUAP guidelines on prevention and management of pressure injuries
- Assess any skin alterations using accurate and consistent measurements

Attitudes
- Display curiosity; be thorough in assessing the condition of the patient's tissues; changes may indicate signs of disease
- Display humility; hygiene care should be patient centered; know when to learn more about the patient's preferences

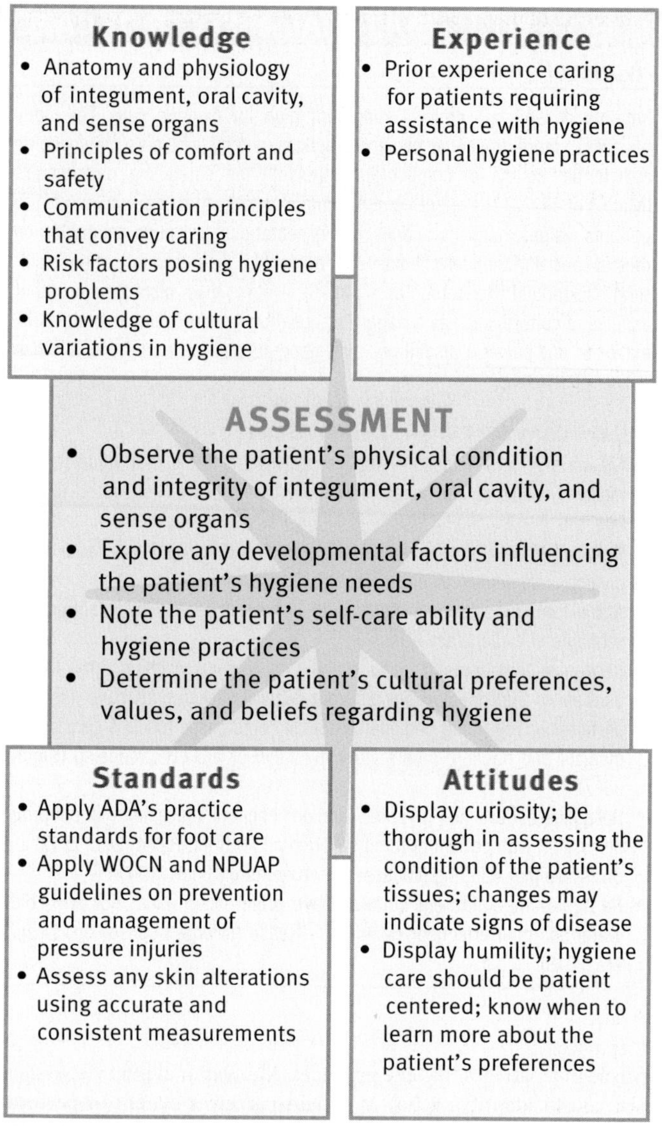

FIG. 40.1 Critical thinking model for hygiene assessment. *ADA,* American Diabetes Association; *NPUAP,* National Pressure Ulcer Advisory Panel; *WOCN,* Wound, Ostomy and Continence Nurses Society.

care, resulting in aggressive behavior (Mendes, 2018). Safe, effective patient-centered care takes the effect of cognitive impairment on personal care into consideration and provides appropriate modifications.

CRITICAL THINKING

Successful critical thinking requires a synthesis of knowledge, experience, information gathered from patients, critical thinking attitudes, and intellectual and professional standards. Clinical judgments require you to anticipate the information, analyze the data, and make decisions regarding your patient's care. During assessment consider all elements that build toward making appropriate nursing diagnoses (Fig. 40.1).

Integrate nursing knowledge with knowledge from other disciplines. For example, a patient with diabetes mellitus has special needs for nail and foot care to prevent injury and infection. Knowledge about the pathophysiology of diabetes and its potential effects on his or her peripheral circulation and sensory status provides the scientific knowledge base needed to implement safe and effective foot care. In addition, integrate knowledge about developmental and cultural influences as you identify and meet hygiene needs.

Be aware of the impact of critical thinking attitudes as you plan and implement care. For example, think creatively to help patients adapt existing hygiene practices or develop new ones when illness, loss of function, or decreased activity tolerance impairs self-care abilities. Be nonjudgmental and confident when providing care. Because of variations in individual patients' physical status and hygiene practices, you need to approach care with an attitude of flexibility. For example, when caring for a patient with decreased activity tolerance, pace activities and plan rest periods during bathing and other hygiene measures.

Draw on your own experiences as you help with your patients' hygiene care. Reflect on times when you helped family members or others close to you with their hygiene. Usually an early clinical experience involves providing or helping with hygiene care for a patient. Finally, rely on professional standards such as those for skin and foot care from the American Diabetes Association (ADA) and specialty nursing groups such as the Wound Ostomy and Continence Nurses Society (WOCN) when planning care to meet a patient's hygiene needs. As your experience and knowledge grow, your comfort and expertise in meeting the individualized hygiene needs of your patients increase.

REFLECT NOW

You know that people and cultures differ in the types and frequencies of hygiene practices. Think about how you might address your own personal biases, so you can provide more patient-centered hygiene care in the future.

❖ NURSING PROCESS

Apply the nursing process and use a critical thinking approach in your care of patients. The nursing process provides a clinical decision-making approach for you to develop and implement an individualized plan of care.

◆ Assessment

Thoroughly assess each patient and critically analyze your findings to ensure you make patient-centered clinical decisions required for safe and effective hygiene. Assessment of a patient's hygiene status and self-care abilities requires you to complete a nursing history and perform a physical assessment (see Chapter 30). You do not assess all body regions routinely before providing hygiene. However, conduct a brief history to determine priority areas (e.g., diabetic patient with foot ulcers, an overweight patient's skinfolds, an immobilized patient's skin condition) and help you plan relevant and individualized hygiene care. Assessment of a patient's ability to provide hygiene self-care helps you decide about the type and amount of hygiene care to provide and how much the patient can be encouraged to participate in care.

Through the Patient's Eyes. Providing safe, quality hygiene care requires a complete awareness of the patient's hygiene preferences and needs. Because patients have varying expectations, you need to avoid making personal hygiene care a simple routine. Complete a nursing history that not only elicits personal preferences but also addresses the patient's cultural or religious customs and beliefs.

Explore a patient's perspective regarding hygiene care by asking him or her about preferred personal hygiene and grooming practices. Ask about personal care products desired and preferences such as frequency, time of day, and amount of assistance needed. Also ask questions such as "To make you most comfortable and feel at home, how can I best perform your bath and personal care?" Determine the patient's awareness of any hygiene-related problems and his or her knowledge and ability to perform hygiene care measures (Box 40.2). Learning a patient's expectations and applying them in practice fosters

---

BOX 40.2 Nursing Assessment Questions

Cultural and/or Religious Practices
- Do you have preferences for how you bathe, shampoo your hair, brush your teeth, or care for your feet?
- How comfortable are you with someone helping you with your bathing?
- In what way can I best help you with your bath, hair care …?

Tolerance of Hygiene Activities
- Tell me about any symptoms, such as shortness of breath, pain, or fatigue, that you have during bathing.
- What can I do to minimize these symptoms?
- Which aspects of bathing, toothbrushing, or foot care cause discomfort or fatigue?

Assistance with Hygiene
- Do you use any aids to help you with your bath such as grab bars in your tub or shower?
- Do you prefer someone of the same gender to help in your hygiene care?
- Which parts of the bath, toothbrushing, and foot care can you do for yourself? With which parts of hygiene care do you need help?

Skin Care
- Which type of bath do you prefer?
- How often and when do you usually bathe?
- What kind of soap and lotion do you use?
- Have you noticed any skin changes or irritation?
- Do you have any known allergies or reactions to soaps, cosmetics, or skin care products?

Mouth Care
- Do you have any mouth pain or toothaches? Have you noticed any sores in your mouth? Do your gums bleed during brushing or flossing?
- Do you wear dentures or a partial plate?

Foot and Nail Care
- How do you usually care for your feet and nails? Do you soak your feet?
- Do you file or trim your own fingernails and toenails?

Hair and Scalp Care
- Have you recently experienced itching of the scalp or noticed flaking or dandruff?
- Have you noticed any changes in the texture or thickness of your hair?

---

a caring relationship. Fully individualizing hygiene care shows your respect for the patient's needs. As you learn what the patient expects, you incorporate this information into a plan of care.

Assessment of Self-Care Ability. Assess a patient's physical ability to perform or assist with hygiene care safely and efficiently; include assessment of the patient's muscle strength, flexibility, balance, visual acuity, and ability to detect thermal and tactile stimuli. Determine your patient's mental status, including orientation and cognitive function (see Chapter 30). A patient with impaired cognitive function may be less able to follow instructions and help with care. Observe the patient performing hygiene care, noting complaints or physical manifestations that suggest activity intolerance. Assess respiratory rate and effort, skin color, and pulse rate. Ask questions to assess the patient for dizziness, weakness, or fatigue. To determine the amount of assistance the patient needs, observe him or her performing care activities such as brushing teeth or combing hair (Fig. 40.2). Patients who have limited upper-extremity mobility and strength, reduced vision, fatigue, or inability to grasp small objects require help. Patients having difficulty with manual dexterity and cognitive function are likely to show deterioration in physical or oral health. Poor oral care increases the risk for aspiration pneumonia in patients recovering from a stroke or who have dementia (Murray and Scholten, 2018). Also note the presence of medical devices such as feeding tubes, IV lines, or urinary catheters. These devices require special hygiene measures.

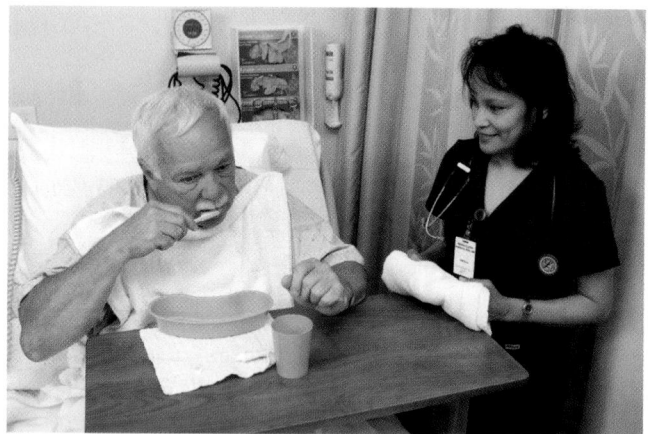

FIG. 40.2 Nurse observes patient brushing teeth. During such observations the nurse can determine how much assistance the patient may need.

When patients have self-care limitations, family may help with care. Work with the family to design patient-centered care. Determine how the family can help the patient, how often they can provide this assistance, and their feelings about being caregivers (Pinkert et al., 2018). In addition, assess the home environment and its influence on the patient's hygiene practices. Are there barriers in the home that affect his or her self-care abilities (e.g., water faucets that are too tight to adjust easily, bathtubs with high sides, a bathroom too small to fit a chair in front of a sink, and lack of adjustable bed or adaptive equipment available for assisting with bathing)?

Assessment of the Skin. Perform an assessment of the skin (see Chapter 30), noting color, texture, thickness, turgor, temperature, and hydration. In the healthy person the skin is smooth, warm, and supple with good turgor. Pay special attention to the presence and condition of any lesions. Note dryness indicated by flaking, redness, scaling, and cracking. Also carefully inspect areas of the skin in contact with any medical device at least daily (e.g., skin under an oxygen cannula or the nasal mucosa under an endotracheal or feeding tube) (NPUAP, 2013) (see Chapter 48). Look for edema under the sites. Discovering manifestations of common skin problems influences how you administer hygiene care (Table 40.2).

TABLE 40.2 Common Skin Problems

Characteristics	Implications	Interventions
Dry Skin Flaky, rough texture on exposed areas such as hands, arms, legs, or face	Skin becomes infected if epidermal layer cracks.	Bathe less frequently. Rinse body of all soap because residue left on skin can cause irritation and breakdown. Add moisture to air with use of humidifier. Increase fluid intake when skin is dry. Use moisturizing cream to aid healing. (Cream forms protective barrier and helps maintain fluid within skin.) Use creams to clean skin that is dry or allergic to soaps and detergents.
Acne Inflammatory, papulopustular skin eruption, usually involving bacterial breakdown of sebum; appears on face, neck, shoulders, and back	Infected material within pustule spreads if area is squeezed or picked. Permanent scarring can result.	Wash hair and skin thoroughly each day with warm water and soap to remove oil. Use cosmetics sparingly. Oily cosmetics or creams accumulate in pores and make condition worse. Implement dietary restrictions if necessary. (Eliminate foods that aggravate condition from diet.) Use prescribed topical antibiotics for severe forms of acne.
Skin Rashes Skin eruptions that result from overexposure to sun or moisture or from allergic reaction (flat or raised, localized or systemic, pruritic or nonpruritic)	If skin is scratched continually, inflammation and infection may occur. Rashes also cause discomfort.	Wash area thoroughly and apply antiseptic spray or lotion to prevent further itching and aid in healing process. Apply warm or cold soaks to relieve inflammation if indicated.
Contact Dermatitis Inflammation of skin characterized by abrupt onset with erythema; pruritus; pain; and appearance of scaly, oozing lesions (seen on face, neck, hands, forearms, and genitalia)	Dermatitis is often difficult to eliminate because person is usually in continual contact with substance causing skin reaction. Substance is often hard to identify.	Avoid causative agents (e.g., cleansers and soaps).
Abrasion Scraping or rubbing away of epidermis that results in localized bleeding and later weeping of serous fluid	Infection occurs easily because of loss of protective skin layer.	Be careful not to scratch patient with jewelry or fingernails. Wash abrasions with mild soap and water; dry thoroughly and gently. Observe dressing or bandage for retained moisture because it increases risk of infection.

TABLE 40.3 Risk Factors for Hygiene Care

Risks	Hygiene Implications
Oral Problems	
Inability to use upper extremities because of paralysis, weakness, or restriction (e.g., cast, dressing)	Patient lacks upper-extremity strength or dexterity needed to brush teeth (Harding et al., 2020).
Dehydration, inability to take fluids or food by mouth (NPO)	Causes excess drying and fragility of mucosa; increases accumulation of secretions on tongue and gums.
Presence of nasogastric or oxygen tubes; mouth breathers	Tubes cause pressure, friction, and drying of mucosa and/or lips.
Chemotherapeutic drugs	Drugs kill rapidly multiplying cells, including normal cells lining oral cavity. Ulcers and inflammation develop.
Lozenges, cough drops, antacids, and chewable over-the-counter vitamins	Medications contain large amounts of sugar. Repeated use increases sugar or acid content in mouth, causing dental caries.
Radiation therapy to head and neck	Reduces salivary flow and lowers pH of saliva; leads to stomatitis and tooth decay (Harding et al., 2020).
Oral surgery, trauma to mouth, placement of oral airway	These cause trauma to oral cavity with swelling, ulcerations, inflammation, and bleeding.
Immunosuppression; altered blood clotting	Predispose to inflammation and bleeding gums.
Diabetes mellitus	Patients are prone to dryness of mouth, gingivitis, periodontal disease, and loss of teeth.
Endotracheal intubation with mechanical ventilation	Potential for ventilator-associated pneumonia (VAP) exists. Chlorhexidine gluconate (CHG) 0.12% is an inexpensive effective agent for reducing VAP, especially in patients who have heart surgery (Nicolosi et al., 2014).
Dialysis	Oral problems commonly found in these patients include halitosis, xerostomia (dry mouth), gingivitis, stomatitis, tooth decay, tooth loss, and jaw problems. Causes may include micronutrient deficiencies, elevated blood sugar, rheumatoid arthritis, weight control, and smoking (Chapple et al., 2017).
Cognitive impairment	Patients are prone to poor oral health and are at risk for aspiration pneumonia (Murray and Scholten, 2017).
Skin Problems	
Immobilization	Dependent body parts are exposed to pressure from underlying surfaces. The inability to turn or change position increases risk for pressure injuries.
Bariatric patient	Patient cannot visualize skin properly and keep it clean and dry. Excessive adipose tissue creates pressure from weight, lack of air circulation, and an increase in moisture with poor tissue perfusion (Dial et al., 2018). Increases risk for pressure injuries.
Reduced sensation caused by stroke, spinal cord injury, diabetes, local nerve damage	Patient unable to sense skin injury. Does not receive normal transmission of nerve impulses when applying excessive heat or cold, pressure, friction, or chemical irritants to skin. Increases risk for pressure injuries.
Altered cognition resulting from dementia, psychological disorders, or temporary delirium	Patient unable to verbalize skin care needs. Does not realize effect of pressure or prolonged contact with excretions or secretions, requiring more vigilant assessment.
Limited protein or caloric intake and reduced hydration (e.g., fever, burns, gastrointestinal alterations, poorly fitting dentures)	Predispose to impaired tissue synthesis. Skin becomes thinner, less elastic, and smoother with loss of subcutaneous tissue. Poor wound healing results. Reduced hydration impairs skin turgor.
Excessive secretions or excretions on skin from perspiration, urine, watery fecal material, and wound drainage	Moisture is medium for bacterial growth and causes local skin irritation, softening of epidermal cells, and skin maceration.
Presence of external medical devices (e.g., cast, restraint, bandage, dressing)	Devices such as casts, cloth restraints, bandages, tubing, and orthopedic devices exert pressure or friction against surface of skin (NPUAP, 2013).
Vascular insufficiency	Arterial blood supply to tissues is inadequate, or venous return is impaired, causing decreased circulation to extremities. Tissue ischemia and breakdown often occur. Risk for infection is high.
Foot Problems	
Patient unable to bend over or has reduced visual acuity	Patient is unable to fully visualize entire surface of each foot, impairing ability to adequately assess condition of skin and nails.
Eye Care Problems	
Reduced dexterity and hand coordination	Physical limitations create inability to safely insert or remove contact lenses.

Determine a patient's level of cleanliness by observing the appearance of the skin and detecting body odors that can indicate inadequate cleansing or excessive perspiration caused by fever or pain. Inspect less obvious or difficult-to-reach skin surfaces such as under the breasts or scrotum, around the female patient's perineum, or in the groin for redness, excessive moisture, and soiling or debris. Separate skinfolds for observation and palpation. It is important to keep these areas dry, especially in patients who are overweight. Cornstarch may be used to decrease friction and absorb moisture (Dial et al., 2018; Cowell and Radley, 2014).

Be attentive to characteristics of skin problems most influenced by hygiene measures. Is the skin dry from too much bathing or from use of hot water or irritating soap? Does the patient have a rash caused by an allergic reaction to a skin care product? Certain conditions place patients at risk for impaired skin integrity (Table 40.3). Because of increased risk be particularly alert when assessing patients with reduced sensation, impaired circulation, nutrition or hydration alterations, body secretions, incontinence, altered cognition, external medical devices, and decreased mobility. Patients may be unaware of skin problems because they are unable to feel pain or pressure or see their skin in some places (e.g., the back or the feet). Carefully assess the skin under orthopedic devices (braces, splints, casts) and beneath items such as antiembolic stockings and tape. Assess the condition and cleanliness of the perineal and anal areas during hygiene care and when the patient requires toileting assistance. When prolonged contact of urine or feces occurs such as with diarrhea or incontinence, skin breakdown often results. Most people consider these areas private; therefore, be sensitive in your approach (Touhy and Jett, 2018).

When caring for patients with dark skin pigmentation, be aware of assessment techniques and skin characteristics unique to highly pigmented skin (Ball et al., 2019). Several skin conditions are more common in persons with skin of color, including certain dermatoses, inflammation of hair follicles, acne keloidalis nuchae, and keloids (Kundu and Patterson, 2013). These conditions require special approaches to skin care. Also be very careful in assessing the skin in dark-skinned patients at risk for pressure injuries (see Chapter 48).

Assessment of the Feet and Nails.
A variety of common foot and nail problems can be caused by inadequate hygiene and are actually detected during hygiene care. Problems sometimes result from abuse or poor care of the feet and hands such as nail biting or trimming nails improperly, exposure to harsh chemicals, and wearing poorly fitting shoes. Question the patient to determine type of footwear and usual foot and nail care practices.

Examine all skin surfaces of the feet, including the areas between the toes and over the entire sole of the foot. Poorly fitting shoes often irritate the heels, soles, and sides of the feet. Inspection of the feet for lesions includes noting areas of dryness, inflammation, or cracking. (Chapman, 2017). Chronic foot problems are common in older adults, who often experience dry feet because of a decrease in sebaceous gland secretion, dehydration, or poor condition of footwear.

People are often unaware of foot or nail problems until pain or discomfort occurs. Assess patients with diseases that affect peripheral circulation and sensation for the adequacy of circulation and sensation of the feet. Diabetic neuropathy and decreased peripheral circulation put people with diabetes at greater risk for foot problems. Daily inspection and preventive foot care help maintain ulcer-free feet (Chapman, 2017). Inspect a patient's shoes and inspect feet for areas of blistering or abrasion from improper shoes or fit (Jeffcoate et al., 2018). Palpate the dorsalis pedis and posterior tibial pulses, and assess for intact sensation to light touch, pinprick, and temperature (Ball et al., 2019).

Observe a patient's gait. Painful foot disorders or decreased sensation cause limping or an unnatural gait. Ask whether the patient has foot discomfort, and determine factors that aggravate the pain. Foot problems sometimes result from bone or muscular alterations or wearing poorly fitting footwear.

Inspect the condition of the fingernails and toenails, looking for lesions, dryness, inflammation, or cracking, which are often associated with a variety of common foot and nail problems (Table 40.4). The cuticle that surrounds the nail can grow over it and become inflamed if nail care is not performed correctly and periodically. Ask women whether they polish their nails and use polish remover frequently because chemicals in these products cause excessive nail dryness. Disease changes the shape and curvature of the nails (Ball et al., 2019). Inflammatory lesions and fungus of the nail bed cause thickened, horny nails that separate from the nail bed.

Assessment of the Oral Cavity.
The condition of the oral cavity reflects overall health and also indicates oral hygiene needs. Inspect all areas of the mouth carefully for color, hydration, texture, and lesions (see Chapter 30). Patients frequently develop common oral problems as a result of inadequate oral care or disease (e.g., oral malignancy) or as a side effect of treatments such as radiation and chemotherapy. These problems include receding gum tissue, inflamed gums (gingivitis), a coated tongue, **glossitis** (inflamed tongue), discolored teeth (particularly along gum margins), **cheilitis** (cracked lips), dental caries, missing teeth, and **halitosis** (foul-smelling breath). Localized pain and infection commonly accompany oral problems.

Apply clean gloves to palpate any tender areas or lesions. Observe for cleanliness and use olfaction to detect halitosis. If you identify any oral problems, notify the patient's health care provider. Early identification of poor oral hygiene practices and common oral problems reduces the risk for gum disease and dental caries (USDHHS, 2018). If the older adult becomes **edentulous** (i.e., without teeth) and wears complete or partial dentures, include an assessment of underlying gums and palate.

Assessment of the Hair.
Assess the condition of a patient's hair and scalp before performing hair care. Findings help determine the frequency and type of care needed. You can anticipate certain patients who might require a more focused assessment, such as a patient who has had head trauma or a homeless patient unable to perform regular hygiene. Normally the hair is clean, shiny, and untangled, and the scalp is clear of lesions. Table 40.5 summarizes hair and scalp problems with implications and interventions.

Observe a patient's ability to perform hair care. A person's appearance and feeling of well-being often are related to the way the hair looks and feels. Illness, disability, and conditions such as arthritis, fatigue, obesity, and the presence of physical barriers (e.g., cast or IV access) alter a patient's ability to maintain daily hair care.

In community health and home care settings it is particularly important to inspect the hair for lice so that you can provide appropriate hygienic treatment. If you suspect **pediculosis capitis** (head lice), guard against self-infestation by hand hygiene and the use of gloves or tongue blades to inspect the patient's hair.

The loss of hair (**alopecia**) results from the effects of chemotherapy medications, hormonal changes, or improper hair care practices. Alopecia often appears as brittle and broken hair in the hair line that progresses to bald patches. If noted, be sure to question the patient about specific hair care practices, especially the use of chemicals and heat application during hair care.

Assessment of the Eyes, Ears, and Nose.
Examine the condition and function of the eyes, ears, and nose (see Chapter 30). The healthy eye is not inflamed and is without drainage. The presence of redness indicates allergic or infectious conjunctivitis, which can be highly contagious. The crusty drainage associated with conjunctivitis easily spreads from one eye to the other. Wear clean gloves to examine the eyes and perform proper hand hygiene before and after the examination. Determine whether a patient wears contact lenses, especially when he or she enters the health care agency in an unresponsive or confused state. To determine whether a contact lens is present, stand to the side of the patient's eyes and observe the corneas for the presence of a soft or rigid lens. Also observe the sclera because the lens may have shifted off the cornea. An undetected contact lens causes corneal injury when left in place too long.

Assessment of the external ear structures includes inspection of the auricle and external ear canal (see Chapter 30). Observe for the presence of accumulated **cerumen** (earwax) or drainage in the ear canal and local inflammation. Question patients about tenderness on palpation or the presence of pain and ask how they usually clean their ears.

TABLE 40.4 Common Foot and Nail Problems

Problem	Characteristics	Implications	Interventions
Callus	Thickened portion of epidermis, consisting of mass of horny, keratotic cells; usually flat and painless; found on undersurface of foot or on palm of hand; caused by local friction or pressure	Foot calluses often cause discomfort when wearing tight-fitting shoes.	Refer patient to podiatrist; do not self-treat. The use of orthotic devices cushions and redistributes weight to relieve pressure on calluses.
Corns From Weston WL, Lane AT: *Color textbook of pediatric dermatology,* ed 4, St Louis, 2007, Mosby.	Keratosis caused by friction and pressure from shoes; mainly on toes, over bony prominence; usually cone shaped, round, and raised; calluses with painful core	Conical shape compresses underlying dermis, making it thin and tender. Tight shoes aggravate pain. Tissue attaches to bone if allowed to grow. Patient may suffer alteration in gait because of pain.	Refer patient to podiatrist. Avoid use of oval corn pads, which increase pressure on toes. Use wider, softer shoes.
Plantar warts From Zitelli BJ, Davis HW: *Atlas of pediatric physical diagnosis,* ed 3, St Louis, 1997, Mosby.	Fungating lesion that appears on sole of foot; caused by papillomavirus	Warts are sometimes contagious, are painful, and make walking difficult.	Refer patient to podiatrist.
Athlete's foot (tinea pedis)	Fungal infection of foot; scaliness and cracking of skin between toes and on soles of feet; small blisters containing fluid appear, apparently induced by constricting footwear (e.g., sneakers)	Athlete's foot can spread to other body parts, especially hands. It is contagious and often recurs.	Feet should be well ventilated. Drying feet well after bathing and applying powder help prevent infection. Wearing clean socks or stockings reduces incidence. Health care provider orders application of griseofulvin, miconazole nitrate, or tolnaftate.
Ingrown nails From Habif TP: *Clinical dermatology: a color guide to diagnosis and therapy,* ed 2, St Louis, 1990, Mosby.	Toenail or fingernail growing inward into soft tissue around nail; results from improper nail trimming, poor shoe fit, or heredity	Ingrown nails cause localized pain in presence of pressure; some become infected.	Treatment is frequent warm soaks *(exception: patient with diabetes or other vascular diseases, such as Berger's disease)* in antiseptic solution and removal of part of nail that has grown into skin. Teach patient proper nail-trimming techniques. Refer to podiatrist.
Paronychia	Inflammation of tissue surrounding nail after hangnail or other injury; occurs in people who frequently have their hands in water; common in patients with diabetes	Area sometimes becomes infected.	Treatment is warm compresses or soaks *(exception: patient with diabetes)* and local application of antibiotic ointments. Paronychia can be prevented by careful manicuring.
Foot odors	Result of excess perspiration promoting microorganism growth; faulty foot hygiene or improper footwear causes foot odor	Odor frequently embarrasses patient.	Frequent washing, use of foot deodorants and powders, and clean footwear prevent or reduce this problem.

TABLE 40.5 Hair and Scalp Problems

Characteristics	Implications	Interventions
Dandruff Scaling of scalp is accompanied by itching. In severe cases dandruff is on eyebrows.	Dandruff causes embarrassment. If it enters eyes, conjunctivitis often develops.	Shampoo regularly with medicated shampoo. In severe cases obtain health care provider's advice.
Ticks Small, gray-brown parasites burrow into skin and suck blood.	Ticks may transmit disease to people, including Rocky Mountain spotted fever, tularemia, and Lyme disease.	Use fine-tipped tweezers to grasp tick as close to the skin's surface as possible. Pull upward with steady, even pressure. Don't twist or jerk the tick; this can cause the mouth-parts to break off and remain in the skin. If this happens, remove the mouth-parts with tweezers. If you are unable to remove the mouth easily with clean tweezers, leave it alone and let the skin heal. After removing the tick, thoroughly clean the bite areas and your hands with rubbing alcohol and iodine scrub, or soap and water. Dispose of a live tick by putting it in alcohol, placing it in a sealed bag/container, wrapping it tightly in tape, or flushing it down the toilet (CDC, 2018). **Follow-up:** If you develop a rash or fever within several weeks of tick removal, contact your health care provider and inform about your tick bite.
Pediculosis (Lice)		
Pediculosis Capitis (Head Lice) Parasite resides on scalp attached to hair strands. Eggs look like oval particles, similar to dandruff. Bites or pustules may be observed behind ears and at hairline.	Head lice are difficult to remove and spread to furniture and other people if not treated. They do not carry disease, cannot fly or jump, and are carried by animals.	Wearing gloves, check entire scalp by using tongue depressor or special lice comb. Use medicated shampoo for eliminating lice. *Caution against use of products containing lindane because the ingredient is toxic and known to cause adverse reactions* (CDC, 2016). Check hair for nits and comb with a nit comb for 2 to 3 days until all lice and nits have been removed. Vacuum infested areas of home.
Pediculosis Corporis (Body Lice) Parasites tend to cling to clothing; thus, they are not always easy to see. Body lice suck blood and lay eggs on clothing and furniture.	Patient itches constantly. Scratches seen on skin become infected. Hemorrhagic spots appear on skin where lice are sucking blood.	Bathe or shower thoroughly. After skin is dried, apply recommended pediculicide lotion. After 12 to 24 hours take another bath or shower. Bag infested clothing or linen until laundered in hot water. Vacuum rooms thoroughly and throw away bag after completion.
Pediculosis Pubis (Crab Lice) Parasites are in pubic hair. Crab lice are gray-white with red legs.	Lice spread through bed linen, clothing, or furniture or between people via sexual contact.	Shave hair off affected area. Clean as for body lice. If lice were sexually transmitted, notify partner.
Hair Loss (Alopecia) Alopecia occurs in all races. Balding patches are in periphery of hair line. Hair becomes brittle and broken.	Patches of uneven hair growth and loss alter patient's appearance.	Stop hair-care practices that damage hair (e.g., teasing hair, hair picks, tight braiding, excessive heat when blow-drying).

Inspect the nares for signs of inflammation, discharge, lesions, edema, and deformity (see Chapter 30). The nasal mucosa is normally pink and clear and has little or no discharge. Allergies cause a clear, watery discharge. If patients have any form of tubing exiting the nose (e.g., nasogastric), observe for edema, skin ulceration, localized tenderness, inflammation, drainage, and bleeding where the tubing comes in contact with the nares.

Use of Sensory Aids.
For patients who wear eyeglasses, contact lenses, artificial eyes, or hearing aids, assess their knowledge and methods used for care, and have them describe the typical approach used in routine care (see Chapter 49). When possible, observe a patient perform care. Compare information gathered from him or her with the proper care technique for these devices. Any difference between a patient's practice and standard practice provides an opportunity for patient education.

Assessment of Hygiene Care Practices. Assessment of hygiene practices reveals a patient's preferences for grooming. For example, a patient chooses to groom the hair in a certain style or trim nails in a certain way. When a patient has a physical disability, special safety precautions are often necessary when grooming. For example, teach patients with loss of sensation to file nails instead of clipping. By observing a patient perform hygiene care, you can detect any needed areas of teaching or assistance while maintaining the patient's maximal level of independence.

Assessment of Cultural Influences. Ask what makes a patient feel most comfortable during a bath or other hygiene measures. Because personal hygiene is very private, this question may help reveal normal cultural practices. Perhaps he or she prefers a partial instead of a full bath from a nurse, with a family member completing the bathing of more private body parts.

Some patients also defer part of hygiene. For example, if you believe that frequent skin care is critical to prevent skin breakdown, take the time to understand the patient's concerns and then offer an explanation that helps him or her accept your intervention. Many institutions are using chlorhexidine gluconate (CHG) for daily bathing. CHG can leave the skin feeling sticky. If patients complain about its use, you need to explain their vulnerability to infection and how CHG helps reduce occurrence of health care–associated infection (HAI). Consider a patient's level of literacy, and be sure that you have adapted your assessment questions to a level the patient can understand.

Patients at Risk for Hygiene Problems. Some patients present risks that require more attentive and rigorous hygiene care (see Table 40.3). These risks may result from side effects of medications or other medical therapy; a lack of knowledge; immobilization; an inability to perform hygiene; or a physical condition that potentially injures the skin, mouth, feet and nails, or hair. Anticipate whether a patient is predisposed to risks and follow through with a complete assessment. For example, if a patient is receiving cancer chemotherapy, there is a risk of the medication producing mouth ulcerations, which are painful and create a risk for infection and impaired nutrition because of reluctance to eat and drink. A patient who receives broad-spectrum antibiotics may develop an opportunistic infection when the normal flora of the mouth is disrupted by the antibiotic. Be thorough and detailed during the oral examination, checking all surfaces of the tongue and mucosa. For a bariatric patient or a patient who is diaphoretic, provide special attention to body areas such as beneath the woman's breasts and in the groin, skinfolds, and perineal area, where moisture collects and irritates skin surfaces (Cowell and Radley, 2014). Assessment should include a review of a patient's medical and surgical history, medications, and the specific risk factors that the patient presents.

REFLECT NOW

Think about how you would modify your nursing assessment to correctly identify a patient's risks for hygiene problems.

◆ Nursing Diagnosis

Data interpretation of your patient's hygiene status and self-care abilities involves recognizing assessment patterns or clusters of data to clearly identify and label the patient's health problems related to hygiene. For example, when caring for an older adult with degenerative arthritis, you observe swollen joints, weakness, and limited ROM in the dominant hand along with a generally unkempt appearance. Closer review of data reveals a pattern that confirms that your patient has difficulty turning and regulating a water faucet and is unable to completely wash body parts. The nursing diagnosis of *Impaired Ability to Bath* becomes part of the plan of care. Accurate selection of nursing diagnoses requires critical thinking to identify actual or potential problems. Be thorough in assessment to reveal all appropriate assessment findings or risk factors so you can make an accurate diagnosis (Box 40.3).

Use a patient's actual alteration (e.g., *Impaired Tissue Integrity*) or one for which the patient is at risk (e.g., *Risk for Infection*) to determine the focus of nursing interventions. A patient with an actual alteration requires extensive hygiene care, often more thorough than routine hygiene. For example, if a patient has the nursing diagnosis *Impaired Tissue Integrity*, initiate care more frequently to keep skin surfaces clean and dry and eliminate factors such as moisture or drainage. Also provide care to promote healing of injured tissue and skin surfaces (see Chapter 48). If a patient is at risk for a problem,

---

BOX 40.3 Nursing Diagnostic Process
Self-Care Deficit: Impaired Ability to Bath

Assessment activities	Assessment findings
Observe patient attempt to bathe self.	Patient is unable to change position in order to wash lower body, back, or perineal area.
Assess patient's upper-extremity strength and range of motion.	Patient has restricted upper-extremity range of motion in elbow and weakness of hand.
	Patient has difficulty turning in bed by self or reaching items needed.
	Patient is unable to turn water faucets on and off without hand pain.
Observe patient's ability to move from bed to bathroom and maneuver in bathroom.	Patient cannot transfer from bed to chair without assistance, cannot ambulate, relies on wheelchair to move around, is unable to maneuver wheelchair in bathroom without help or to transfer to shower seat unassisted. Patient needs lift equipment for transfers.

---

take preventive measures. For example, if a patient is at risk for developing an infection in his or her mouth and has the nursing diagnosis *Risk for Infection,* keep the mucosa well hydrated, minimize foods irritating to tissues, and provide cleaning that soothes and reduces tissue inflammation.

Completing a nursing diagnosis requires identification of the related factor, which will guide your selection of nursing interventions. A diagnosis of *Impaired Oral Mucous Membrane related to malnutrition* and a diagnosis of *Impaired Oral Mucous Membrane related to chemical trauma* require different interventions. When poor nutrition is a causal factor, you need to consult with a registered dietitian for appropriate dietary supplements and incorporate patient education into the plan. When chemotherapy injures the oral mucosa, you follow cancer nursing guidelines regarding care for oral mucositis (i.e., painful inflammation of oral mucous membranes), including frequent gentle brushing with a soft toothbrush, flossing, rinsing with bland rinse, limiting diet to soft foods, and applying water-based moisturizer to lips (USDHHS, 2018). While there are many possible nursing diagnoses for patients in need of supportive hygiene care, the nursing diagnoses in the preceding paragraphs and the following list represent examples of diagnoses commonly associated with hygiene-related problems:

- *Activity Intolerance*
- *Impaired Dressing and Grooming*
- *Impaired Mobility*
- *Impaired Health Maintenance*
- *Impaired Skin Integrity*

◆ Planning

During planning synthesize information from multiple resources (Fig. 40.3). Critical thinking ensures that a patient's plan of care integrates all that is known about the individual patient and key critical thinking elements. In many situations patients present with multiple nursing diagnoses. Use a concept map (Fig. 40.4) to visualize and understand how nursing diagnoses interrelate. Rely on knowledge, experience, and established standards of care when developing a care plan. Remember critical thinking attitudes such as creativity when developing a patient-centered plan for hygiene care. Partner with a

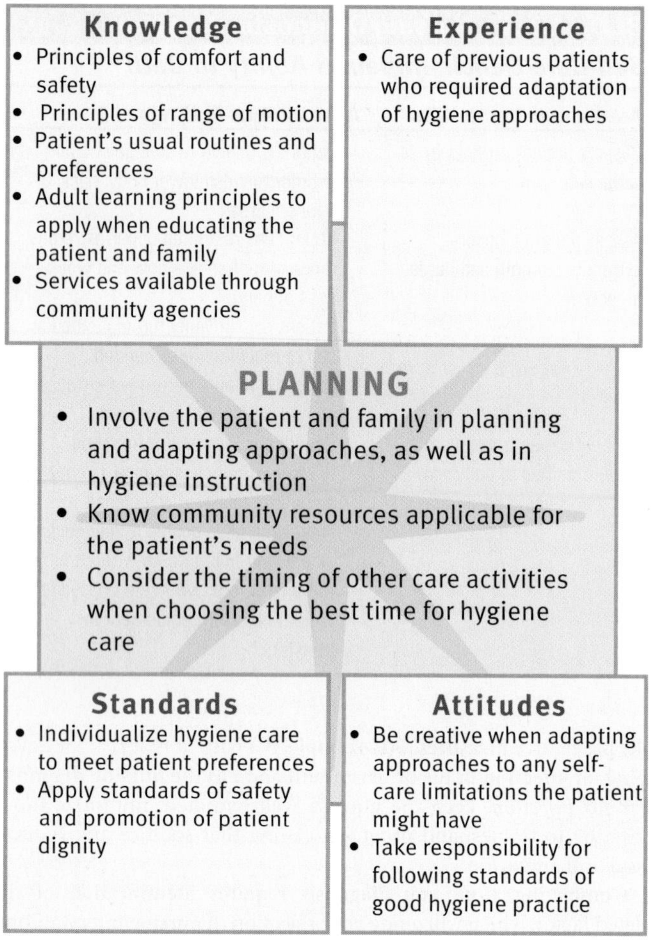

Knowledge	Experience
• Principles of comfort and safety • Principles of range of motion • Patient's usual routines and preferences • Adult learning principles to apply when educating the patient and family • Services available through community agencies	• Care of previous patients who required adaptation of hygiene approaches

PLANNING

- Involve the patient and family in planning and adapting approaches, as well as in hygiene instruction
- Know community resources applicable for the patient's needs
- Consider the timing of other care activities when choosing the best time for hygiene care

Standards	Attitudes
• Individualize hygiene care to meet patient preferences • Apply standards of safety and promotion of patient dignity	• Be creative when adapting approaches to any self-care limitations the patient might have • Take responsibility for following standards of good hygiene practice

FIG. 40.3 Critical thinking model for hygiene planning.

patient to identify patient goals and outcomes, set priorities for care, and select evidence-based interventions. Consider continuity of care and involve other health care team members (e.g., occupational or physical therapy) when developing the plan.

Previous experience with other patients is useful in knowing how to adapt hygiene techniques for special needs. Professional standards guide selection of the most effective nursing interventions. These standards often establish evidence-based guidelines for care.

Goals and Outcomes. Partner with the patient and family to identify goals and expected outcomes to develop a mutually agreed-on plan of care based on the patient's nursing diagnoses (see the Nursing Care Plan). Establish goals that are realistic for the patient's self-care abilities and resources and focus on maintaining or improving the patient's overall hygiene. Make outcomes measurable and achievable within patient limitations. In addition, work with the patient to select individualized hygiene measures. For example, a nurse and a patient who has one-sided paralysis following a cerebral vascular accident develop the following goal: "Patient will be able to groom self (dress and bathe) before discharge." The nurse establishes realistic, individualized expected outcomes to measure the patient's progress toward meeting this goal. These outcomes may include the following:

- Patient is able to bathe in front of sink.
- Patient uses assist devices (bathing mitt and long-handled sponge) for bathing.
- Patient dresses self, using dressing stick and sock aid.

Setting Priorities. A patient's condition influences your priorities for hygiene care. Set priorities based on the necessary assistance required by the patient, the extent of the hygiene-related problems, and the nature of the patient's nursing diagnoses. For example, a seriously ill patient usually needs a daily bath because body secretions accumulate, and the patient is unable to maintain cleanliness independently. Some older patients at home require a visit from a home care aide to help with a tub bath or shower. Patients who are normally inactive during the day and have skin that tends to be dry may need to bathe only twice a week, whereas a patient with urinary and bowel incontinence needs perineal cleaning with each episode of soiling. Plan to help patients who are weakened or possess poor coordination. For example, a patient who is partially paralyzed and has difficulty getting out of a tub needs a tub chair, handrails, or extra personnel available for help.

Timing is also important in planning hygiene care. Being interrupted in the middle of a bath often frustrates and embarrasses a patient. Assess for cultural preferences on time of day or who may help patient with hygiene care.

Teamwork and Collaboration. During hospitalization, know a patient's schedule for therapy or diagnostic procedures and plan hygiene care accordingly. If a patient is hospitalized, plan care before discharge to home, a rehabilitation center, or extended care. Be sure that family caregivers know any physical or cognitive limitations that will affect their ability to provide safe, effective hygiene care. For example, does the patient require assistance to get into a tub or shower, does the patient have reduced sensation making him or her at risk for burns from hot water, and can the patient remember steps to follow for proper foot care? Collaborate with other health team members as indicated (e.g., work with physical and occupational therapy to enhance the patient's independence with self-care activities).

When a patient needs assistance as a result of a self-care limitation and family caregivers are the ones to provide it, proper education and preparation should be included in the plan of care. Give clear directions on how to perform hygiene and how to obtain appropriate equipment and hygiene supplies. Family members also need guidance in providing safety and adapting techniques to fit patient limitations. Be aware of equipment and procedures used in the agency, and support the patient and family to make them knowledgeable about making necessary adaptations. Depending on a patient's limitations, some insurance plans provide home care assistants to help with basic hygiene needs. Explore this option with the patient and family members.

Collaborate with community agencies as needed. For example, the nurse involved in the care of a homeless patient needs to be aware of the location of clothing distribution centers for basic hygiene supplies, a shelter where bathing facilities are available, and any organization that offers free health care or reduced fees. Partner with social workers or staff in local area churches, not-for-profit organizations, and schools to be sure that patients have the resources they need to maintain hygiene.

◆ Implementation

Hygiene is an essential part of basic patient care. When you use caring practices to perform hygiene measures, you reduce the patient's anxiety and promote comfort and relaxation. For example, use a gentle approach when giving patients their baths and changing gowns as you turn and reposition them. A soft, gentle voice when conversing with patients relieves fears or concerns. For patients suffering symptoms such as pain or nausea, administering medications to relieve the symptoms before providing hygiene helps to maintain patient comfort during hygiene procedures.

Consider the stress that hygiene care can cause and be alert for any cues of embarrassment or anxiety. Some patients fear pain or are frightened about falling or sustaining injury when assisting them to a bathroom.

CONCEPT MAP

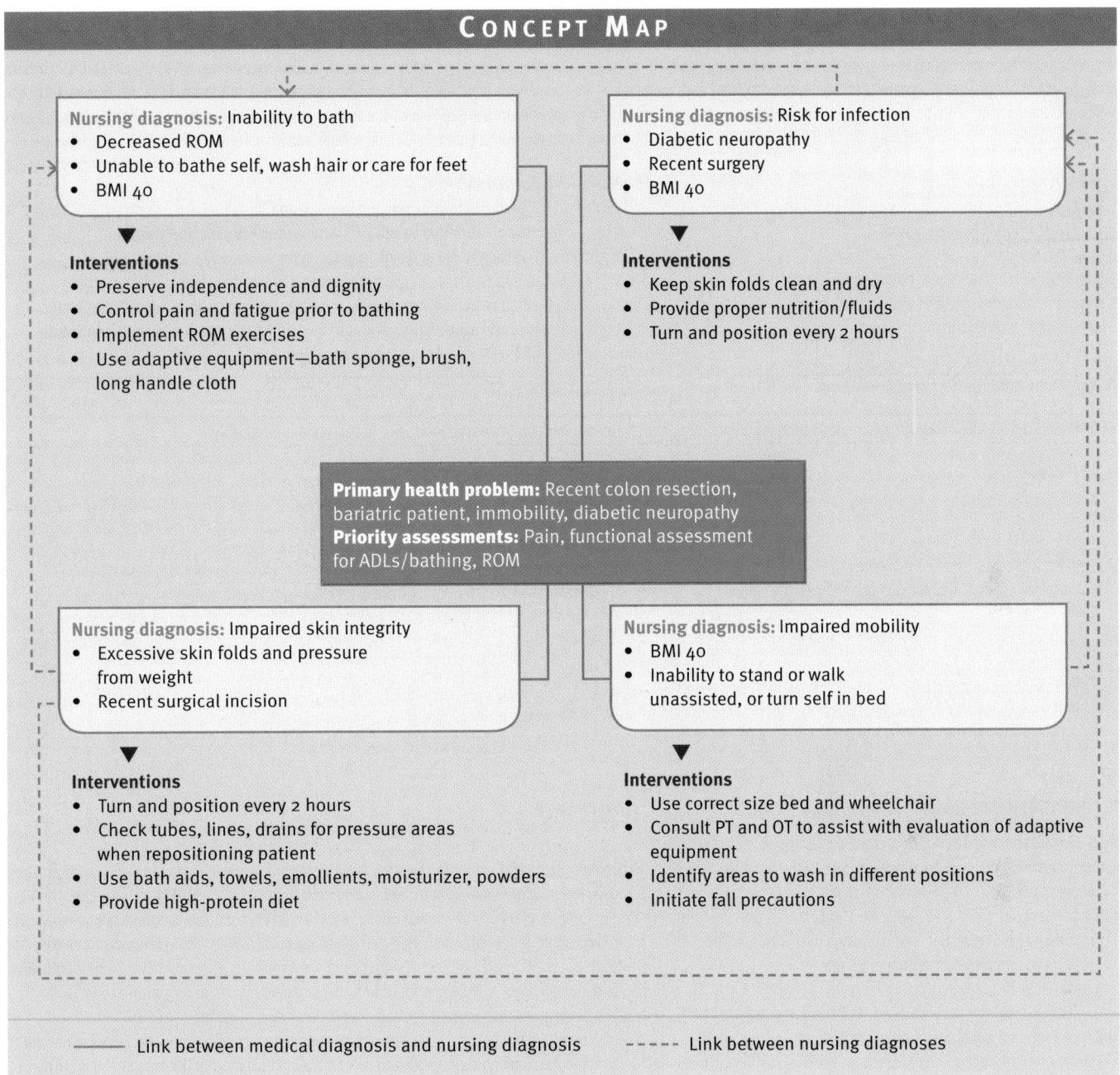

Nursing diagnosis: Inability to bath
- Decreased ROM
- Unable to bathe self, wash hair or care for feet
- BMI 40

Interventions
- Preserve independence and dignity
- Control pain and fatigue prior to bathing
- Implement ROM exercises
- Use adaptive equipment—bath sponge, brush, long handle cloth

Nursing diagnosis: Risk for infection
- Diabetic neuropathy
- Recent surgery
- BMI 40

Interventions
- Keep skin folds clean and dry
- Provide proper nutrition/fluids
- Turn and position every 2 hours

Primary health problem: Recent colon resection, bariatric patient, immobility, diabetic neuropathy
Priority assessments: Pain, functional assessment for ADLs/bathing, ROM

Nursing diagnosis: Impaired skin integrity
- Excessive skin folds and pressure from weight
- Recent surgical incision

Interventions
- Turn and position every 2 hours
- Check tubes, lines, drains for pressure areas when repositioning patient
- Use bath aids, towels, emollients, moisturizer, powders
- Provide high-protein diet

Nursing diagnosis: Impaired mobility
- BMI 40
- Inability to stand or walk unassisted, or turn self in bed

Interventions
- Use correct size bed and wheelchair
- Consult PT and OT to assist with evaluation of adaptive equipment
- Identify areas to wash in different positions
- Initiate fall precautions

——— Link between medical diagnosis and nursing diagnosis   - - - - Link between nursing diagnoses

FIG. 40.4 Concept map for Mrs. White. *ADLs,* Activities of daily living; *BMI,* body mass index; *OT,* occupational therapist; *PT,* physical therapist; *ROM,* range of motion.

Implementation also focuses on assisting and preparing patients to perform much of their hygiene care independently. Discuss any signs and symptoms of hygiene problems. Teach patients proper hygiene techniques and how their use is associated with better health. Inform patients about available resources in the community.

Health Promotion. In primary health care situations educate and counsel patients and family caregivers on why proper hygiene techniques are necessary. For example, a new mother needs to learn how to bathe her newborn to reduce risk of skin irritation and infection, whereas an older adult needs information on the importance of regular ear care to avoid accumulated cerumen and hearing impairment. The hygiene skills described throughout this chapter provide standards for excellent physical care. When caring for patients in primary health

care settings, maintain these standards and incorporate adaptations as needed to meet the patient's lifestyle, functional status, living arrangements, and preferences. Key points when teaching patients about hygiene include the following:
- Make any instruction relevant based on your assessment of the patient's knowledge, motivation, preferences, and health beliefs. For example, when teaching a patient who has diabetes, include risks for impaired foot circulation and how this causes a risk for infection and poor healing, especially when the skin is injured or broken.
- Adapt instruction to a patient's personal bathing facilities and resources. Not all patients have the ideal situation that exists in a health care setting (e.g., easily accessible shower or a bedside table to place over a bed). Adapt available resources so that the patient can reach and use needed items comfortably and safely. For example, a

Self-Care Deficit: Impaired Ability to Bath

ASSESSMENT

Mrs. White is 70 years old and is post-op day 2 after a colon resection. She has diabetes, a history of hypertension, and body mass index of 40. Her mobility is limited because of her abdominal discomfort, although she can walk short distances. She prefers to stay in bed because she states that she feels tired, weak, and sore. She has begun an early mobility protocol and will ambulate this morning. Physical therapy is helping her learn to use a walker. Mrs. White states that her buttocks, thighs, and skinfolds feel inflamed with a pain score of 7/10. She lives alone, but her granddaughter is going to nursing school and has offered to help her at home.

Assessment Activities	*Assessment Findings*[a]
Ask Mrs. White what hygiene care is important this morning.	Mrs. White says, "I want to **feel clean** and **smell good.**"
Assess Mrs. White's skin condition.	Visual inspection reveals **redness at elbows and under breasts and thighs.** The abdominal incision is dry and pink, and the sutures are well approximated.
Assess Mrs. White's ability to bathe, including an assessment of her range of motion (ROM) and upper- and lower-extremity strength.	Mrs. White is unable to gather bath supplies because of her immobility. She can stand and walk to the bathroom sink but is unable to wash her entire body. Mrs. White states that she has **difficulty visualizing areas of her body.** Her **arms are restricted with decreased ROM** and have **decreased sensation.**

[a]**Assessment findings** are shown in bold type.

NURSING DIAGNOSIS: Self-care deficit: Impaired ability to bath related to immobility associated with obesity and limited ROM

PLANNING

Goals	*Expected Outcomes (NOC)*[b]
	Self-Care: Bathing
Mrs. White will remain free of body odor.	Mrs. White self-reports feeling clean and refreshed after bathing each day.
Mrs. White will maintain intact skin during hospitalization.	Skin is clean and dry without skin breakdown between skinfolds.
	Mrs. White describes personal risk factors for impaired skin integrity.
Mrs. White will describe best method to bathe using adaptive devices by discharge.	Mrs. White states two ways to use adaptive equipment during her bath by discharge. She bathes herself, using a bath mitt and mirror.
Mrs. White will accept help from a family caregiver to assist with hygiene care within the next week.	Mrs. White reports satisfaction with assistance in bathing by family caregiver.

[b]Outcome classification labels from Moorhead S, et al: *Nursing Outcomes Classification (NOC),* ed 6, St Louis, 2018, Elsevier.

INTERVENTIONS (NIC)[c]	**RATIONALE**
Self-Care Assistance: Bathing/Hygiene	
Administer prn ordered oral analgesic before bath; begin bath 30 minutes later.	Patient participation in bathing or other self-care activities will improve with pain control. Give prn pain medication before pain is severe (Butcher et al., 2018).
Help patient shower and place her on a shower seat. Demonstrate for patient use of grab bar, and use wash mitt with soap pocket. Stay close by to prevent an accidental fall.	Proper education on use of shower seats, grab bars in showers/baths, and assistive devices reduces the risk for injuries while bathing (King et al., 2018). Using a wash mitt with a soap pocket or a wall-mounted soap dispenser minimizes difficulty of manipulating soap and a washcloth. A shower seat or bath bench makes it easier for patient to focus on washing rather than on balance required for standing (King et al., 2018).
Teach patient and granddaughter (as needed) how to use adaptive equipment for bathing and safe patient-handling skills and how to perform skin assessments. Help Mrs. White plan hygiene schedule with granddaughter.	Family members who are taught methods to meet patient's bathing needs increase patient satisfaction, making the experience safe, easy, and successful (King et al., 2018). Appropriate assistive devices encourage independence.

[c]Intervention classification labels from Butcher HK, et al: *Nursing Interventions Classifications (NIC),* ed 7, St Louis, 2018, Elsevier.

EVALUATION

Evaluation Activity	*Patient Response/Finding*	*Outcome Status*
Ask Mrs. White why it is important for her to inspect skin and have regular bathing.	Mrs. White states that she now knows she is at risk for infection because she is overweight and has diabetes. She also knows her risk for infection is higher in the hospital.	Mrs. White is able to identify her personal risk factors for infection if she does not bathe properly.
Inspect Mrs. White's skin after she bathes in shower and assess for any remaining body odor.	Mrs. White's skin is clear without irritation under breasts and perineum. Had difficulty cleansing back and bottom of feet, but no signs of irritation. No apparent odor. Patient expresses sense of feeling clean. Is able to describe how to use adaptive devices.	Mrs. White requires assistance with bathing in areas of body she could not reach. Will refer to occupational therapy for an appropriate assistive device with long handle.
Observe how the granddaughter assists Mrs. White on to a shower seat; observe their use of adaptive equipment.	Mrs. White and her granddaughter have planned to shower every 3 days in the evening after granddaughter returns from work. Granddaughter is able to explain correct technique for helping patient with walker and transferring to and from shower seat.	Mrs. White has a realistic plan for bathing at home. During a home visit the granddaughter demonstrates knowledge of safe patient handling.

BOX 40.4 Hygiene Care Schedule in Acute and Long-Term Care Settings

Early Morning Care
Nursing personnel on the night shift provide basic hygiene to patients getting ready for breakfast, scheduled tests, or early morning surgery. "AM care" includes offering a bedpan or urinal if the patient is not ambulatory, washing the patient's hands and face, and helping with oral care.

Routine Morning Care
After breakfast help by offering a bedpan or urinal to patients confined to bed; provide a full or partial bath or a shower, including perineal care and oral, foot, nail, and hair care; give a back rub; change a patient's gown or pajamas; change the bed linens; and straighten a patient's bedside unit and room. This is often referred to as "complete AM care."

Afternoon Care
Hospitalized patients often undergo many exhausting diagnostic tests or procedures in the morning. In rehabilitation centers patients participate in physical therapy in the morning. Afternoon hygiene care includes washing the hands and face, helping with oral care, offering a bedpan or urinal, and straightening bed linen.

Evening, or Hour-before-Sleep, Care
Before bedtime offer personal hygiene care that helps patients relax and promotes sleep. "PM care" often includes changing soiled bed linens, gowns, or pajamas; helping patients wash the face and hands; providing oral hygiene; giving a back massage; and offering the bedpan or urinal to nonambulatory patients. Some patients enjoy a beverage such as juice; check diet to determine which beverages are allowed.

BOX 40.5 Types of Baths

Complete bed bath: Bath administered to totally dependent patient in bed (see Skill 40.1).

Partial bed bath: Bed bath that consists of bathing only body parts that would cause discomfort if left unbathed such as the hands, face, axillae, and perineal area. Partial bath may also include washing back and providing back rub. Provide a partial bath to dependent patients in need of partial hygiene or self-sufficient bedridden patients who are unable to reach all body parts.

Sponge bath at the sink: Involves bathing from a bath basin or sink with patient sitting in a chair. Patient is able to perform part of the bath independently. Assistance is needed for hard-to-reach areas.

Tub bath: Involves immersion in a tub of water that allows more thorough washing and rinsing than a bed bath. Commonly used in long-term care. A patient may require the nurse's help. Some institutions have tubs equipped with lifting devices that facilitate positioning dependent patients in the tub.

Shower: Patient sits or stands under a continuous stream of water. The shower provides more thorough cleaning than a bed bath but can cause fatigue.

Bag bath/travel bath: Contains several soft, nonwoven cotton cloths that are premoistened in a solution of no-rinse surfactant cleanser and emollient. The bag bath offers an alternative because of the ease of use, reduced time bathing, and patient comfort.

Chlorhexidine gluconate (CHG) bath: Antimicrobial agent used to reduce incidence of hospital-acquired infections on skin, invasive lines, and catheters (Cassir et al., 2015; Boonyasiri et al., 2016; Shah et al., 2016).

young mother has more room and believes that bathing her infant is safer if she uses her kitchen sink and counter rather than her bathroom sink.

- Teach patients ways to avoid injury. Almost any hygiene procedure poses risks (e.g., cutting a nail too close to the skin or failing to adjust the water temperature of the bath). Include safety risks and tips with all instructions.
- Reinforce infection control practices. Damage to the skin, mucosa, eyes, or other tissues creates an immediate risk for infection. Determine that a patient understands the relationship among healthy and intact skin and tissues, hand hygiene practices, and the prevention of infection (see Chapter 28).

Acute, Restorative, and Continuing Care. Nursing knowledge and skills needed for performing hygiene care are consistent across all health care settings. In addition, some of the skills in this section are applicable in areas of health promotion. The variety, frequency, and timing of hygiene measures vary across health care settings and according to individual patient needs. In the acute care setting factors such as more frequent diagnostic and treatment plans and the need for more extensive hygiene care resulting from acute illness or injury affect scheduling. In extended-care facilities and nursing homes, bathing may be scheduled less frequently.

Bathing and Skin Care. Individualize your care on the basis of the patient's hygiene preferences. The extent, type, and timing or frequency of bathing and the methods used depend on a patient's physical abilities, health problems, and the degree of hygiene required (Boxes 40.4 and 40.5). In addition to cleansing baths, the health care provider may prescribe therapeutic baths, including sitz baths. Medicated baths (e.g., oatmeal, cornstarch, or Aveeno) may be recommended in the

home setting. A sitz bath cleans and reduces pain and inflammation of perineal and anal areas (see Chapter 48). Medicated baths relieve skin irritation and create an antibacterial and drying effect.

If a patient is physically dependent or cognitively impaired, increase the frequency of skin assessment and provide skin care directed toward reducing the risk for skin breakdown. When bathing patients with cognitive impairments, consider their special needs and challenges (Wilson, 2018). These patients easily become afraid. Patients with dementia often refuse, withdraw, or fight during a bath or shower. A person-centered approach can assist in managing their physical limitations and aggressive behaviors (Box 40.6). Use assessment and communication skills to learn possible triggers that affect participation with hygiene care (Yevchak et al., 2017; Konno et al., 2014). For example, unmanaged pain; being cold; feeling frightened, vulnerable, and exposed; feeling embarrassed; feeling a loss of control; or not understanding what is happening often causes aggressive behavior. Adapt your bathing procedures and the environment to reduce the triggers. For example, administer any ordered analgesic 30 minutes before a bath and be gentle in your approach. Keep the patient's body as warm as possible with warm towels, and be sure that the room temperature is comfortable. Reduce fear by making sure that all safety devices (e.g., grab bars in a shower, bath mats) are available. Ask for permission to conduct the bath and give the patient options for making decisions (e.g., choice of soap, timing of when to wash face). Use comforting words during bathing to enhance a patient's relaxation. Collaborate and communicate to teach family members how to communicate with and how to help bathe cognitively impaired patients for optimal outcomes once the patient is discharged (Vaingankar et al., 2016).

Complete Bed Bath. A complete bed bath (see Skill 40.1), tub bath, or shower often exhausts a patient. Turning during a complete bed bath and receiving back care increase oxygen consumption and demand. Getting out of a low tub requires considerable exertion. Assess and be alert for a patient's activity intolerance during hygiene care. Assessing heart rate before, during, and after a bath provides a measure of his or

BOX 40.6   EVIDENCE-BASED PRACTICE

Improving Hygiene Care for Patients with Cognitive Impairments

PICOT Question: Does implementing a person-centered approach for hygiene care improve patient cooperation and nurse satisfaction in adults with cognitive impairments?

Evidence Summary

Noisy and unfamiliar surroundings are very distressing to patients with cognitive impairments, such as confusion or dementia. In addition, this distress is worsened by the patient's physical illness, pain, dehydration, toileting needs, medications, and stimulation from the hospital environment (Mendes, 2018). A person-centered care approach can work with the family caregiver, the patient, and the health care team to design hygiene measures and routines that are congruent with the patient's usual practices (Shelton et al., 2018). Research supports the use of nurse-facilitated person-centered care interventions when caring for patients with cognitive disorders (Yevchak et al., 2017).

Application to Nursing Practice

- Designing person-centered care helps nurses meet the individual needs of their patients and minimize some agency-based constraints on care routines (Pinkert et al., 2018).
- Work with family and patient to determine factors that may trigger anxiety or reduced cooperation. These triggers may vary from person to person and can include (but are not limited to) new nursing staff, a full bladder, the time of day, or too much environmental noise (Hirschman and Hodgson, 2018; Yevchak et al., 2017).
- Avoiding incongruent care preferences between the patient and the agency caregiver reduces patient anxiety (Shelton et al., 2018).
- Whenever possible, involve the patient in the hygiene care plan and maintain prehospital routines (Villar et al., 2018; Mendes, 2018).
- Communicating the patient's preferences related to hygiene and activities of daily living (ADL) with all agency caregivers promotes patient comfort, reduces patient anxiety, and improves nurse satisfaction (Rokstad et al., 2017; Shelton et al., 2018).

her physical tolerance. Provide a **partial bed bath** (see Skill 40.1) to patients who are aging, dependent, in need of only partial hygiene, or bedridden and unable to reach all body parts. Wear gloves when there is a risk of coming in contact with body fluids. Control environmental factors that alter skin integrity, including moisture, heat, and external sources of pressure such as wrinkled bed linen and improperly placed drainage tubing.

Traditionally baths have been given using soap and warm water. The question of whether to use bath basins with soap and water is an issue because bath basins provide a reservoir for bacteria and are a possible source of transmission of hospital-acquired infections (HAIs) (Alserehi et al., 2018; Powers et al., 2012). There is a link between waterborne pathogens and the development of biofilm (multiple colonies of microorganisms attached to a surface such as a bath basin). The formation of a biofilm combined with transmission of organisms through contact with unwashed hands can create a reservoir of bacteria. The bacteria can be transferred to and maintained in a patient's bath basin. In contrast, the use of chlorhexidine gluconate (CHG) 4% solution in place of standard soap and water in washbasins has been shown to decrease bacterial growth in basins (Powers et al., 2012) and reduce critical care unit–acquired methicillin-resistant *Staphylococcus aureus* (MRSA) (Petlin et al., 2014). It is important to air-dry bath basins completely and not to use a basin for storing supplies.

Another option to using CHG in bath basins is the use of CHG 2% in impregnated washcloths. The CHG in the cloths is fast acting, has broad-spectrum microorganism coverage, continues antimicrobial activity up to 24 hours after application, and is rinse free and disposable (AHRQ, 2013). Daily bathing with 2% CHG-impregnated cloths versus nonantimicrobial washcloths reduces cross-contamination and colonization of multidrug-resistant organisms (MDROs) (Ruiz et al., 2017; Climo et al., 2013). Daily bathing with some form of CHG is becoming more of a standard practice across hospitals. Patients often describe their skin as feeling a bit sticky. Be sure to explain to patients the importance of using CHG to protect them against serious infection.

- When using CHG solution in bath water or impregnated cloths, use a clean CHG washcloth/cloth for each area of the body.
  - Do not use above a patient's jawline as it can be irritating to the eyes and ears (AHRQ, 2013).
  - Use a regular washcloth moistened in warm water for the face.
  - Do not rinse the CHG off the body; this interferes with its antibacterial effects.
- There are precautions to follow in using CHG. CHG is safe to use on superficial wounds, abrasions, and rashes (AHRQ, 2013). In the case of open or deep wounds such as stage III or IV pressure injuries, bathe with CHG around a dressing or wound. Do not use CHG on third- or fourth-degree burns (AHRQ, 2013).

Use a tub bath or shower (see Skill 40.1) to give a more thorough bath than a bed bath. CHG 4% solution can be used in showers, but instruct patients to exit the shower after application, and do not rinse the CHG off. Implement safety measures to prevent fall injuries because the surface of a tub or shower stall is slippery. In some settings a health care provider's order for a shower or tub bath is necessary. Place a chair in the shower for patients with weakness or poor balance. Both tubs and showers need to have grab bars for patients to hold during entry and exit and maneuvering during the bath or shower. Patients vary in how much physical assistance they need from care providers. Regardless of the type of bath a patient receives, use the following guidelines:

- *Provide privacy.* Close the door and/or pull room curtains around the bathing area. While bathing a patient, expose only the areas being bathed by using proper draping.
- *Maintain safety.* Keep side rails up when away from a patient's bedside when patients are dependent or unconscious. **NOTE:** When side rails serve as a restraint, you need a health care provider's order (see agency-specific policy for restraint usage) (see Chapter 27). Place the nurse call system in the patient's reach if leaving the bedside even temporarily.
- *Maintain warmth.* Keep the room warm because the patient is partially uncovered and easily chilled. Wet skin causes an excessive loss of heat through evaporation. Control drafts and keep windows closed. Keep the patient covered. Expose only the body part being washed during the bath.
- *Promote independence.* Encourage the patient to participate in as much of the bathing activities as possible. Offer assistance when needed.
- *Anticipate needs.* Bring a new set of clothing and hygiene products to the bedside or bathroom.

Teach patients to follow a few general rules for skin health. Encourage them to routinely inspect their skin for changes in color or texture and report abnormalities to their health care provider. Instruct them to handle the skin gently, avoiding excessive rubbing. Patients with excessively dry skin are predisposed to skin impairment. If patients use bar soap at home, recommend that they choose one that contains emollients to hydrate dry skin. Avoid overly hot water because it can dry the skin by removing natural oils. Lubricate the skin with emollient lotions to reduce dryness.

Good skin health requires patients to eat nutritious foods from all food groups, including those rich in vitamins and minerals, and to consume adequate fluids. Stress safety concerns such as failing to adjust or check the water temperature and slipping on wet surfaces. Ensure that patients understand that healthy and intact skin and tissues protect them from infection. Reinforce infection control practices, including proper hand hygiene.

Perineal Care. Cleansing patients' genital and anal areas is called perineal care. It usually occurs as part of a complete bed bath; however, it must be provided at least once a day and more often (see agency policy) if a patient has a urinary catheter (see Skill 40.1). Patients most in need of perineal care include those at greatest risk for acquiring an infection (e.g., uncircumcised males, patients who have indwelling urinary catheters, or those who are recovering from rectal or genital surgery or childbirth). In addition, women who are having a menstrual period require perineal care. CHG is safe to use on the perineum and external mucosa for thorough cleansing (AHRQ, 2013).

When the patient's condition allows, encourage the patient to perform perineal care. Sometimes you are embarrassed about providing perineal care, particularly to patients of the opposite sex. Similarly, the patient may feel embarrassed. Do not let embarrassment cause you to overlook the patient's hygiene needs. When staffing levels permit, use a gender-congruent caregiver. A professional, dignified, and sensitive approach reduces embarrassment and helps put the patient at ease.

If a patient performs self-care, various problems such as vaginal and urethral discharge, skin irritation, and unpleasant odors often go unnoticed. Stress the importance of perineal care in preventing skin breakdown and infection. Be alert for complaints of burning during urination or localized soreness, excoriation, or pain in the perineum. Inspect vaginal and perineal areas and the patient's bed linen for signs of discharge, and use your sense of smell to detect abnormal odors. Risk factors for skin breakdown in the perineal area include urinary or fecal incontinence, rectal and perineal surgical dressings, indwelling urinary catheters, and morbid obesity.

Back Rub. A back rub or back massage usually follows a patient's bath. It promotes relaxation, relieves muscular tension, and decreases perception of pain. Effleurage (i.e., long, slow, gliding strokes of a massage) is associated with reduced measured anxiety, heart rate, and respiratory rate. Studies show that slow-stroke back massages of 3 minutes and hand massages of 10 minutes significantly improve both physiological and psychological indicators of relaxation in older people (Touhy and Jett, 2018).

When providing a back rub, enhance relaxation by reducing noise and ensuring that the patient is comfortable. It is important to ask whether a patient would like a back rub, because some individuals dislike physical contact. Consult the medical record for any contraindications to a massage (e.g., fractured ribs, burns, heart surgery). Chapter 44 describes steps for back massage.

REFLECT NOW

You had your first clinical experience providing hygiene to a patient with a diagnosis of Alzheimer's disease who became frightened and uncooperative during bathing. Using information in this section and Box 40.6, think about strategies you might use to help make hygiene a more satisfying experience.

Foot and Nail Care. Routine nail and foot care involves soaking the hands and feet to soften cuticles and layers of horny cells, thorough cleaning, drying, and proper nail trimming. The one exception is patients with diabetes mellitus or peripheral vascular disease, who are

---

BOX 40.7 Signs of Peripheral Neuropathy or Vascular Insufficiency

Peripheral Neuropathy	Vascular Insufficiency
• Muscle wasting of lower extremities	• Decreased hair growth on legs and feet
• Foot deformities	• Absent or decreased pulses
• Soft tissue infection in lower extremities	• Infection of the foot
• Abnormal gait	• Poor wound healing
• Absent or decreased deep tendon reflexes and/or response to vibratory, touch, or painful stimuli	• Thickened nails
	• Shiny appearance of the skin
	• Blanching of skin on elevation

Data from Ball J, et al: *Seidel's guide to physical examination*, ed 9, St Louis, 2019, Mosby.

---

at risk for tissue ulceration or infection because soaking causes skin softening or maceration of tissue.

When providing nail care, have the patient remain in bed or sit in a chair (see Skill 40.2). In some settings or with specific patients such as a person with diabetes mellitus, you need a health care provider's order to trim toenails. The risk of accidentally cutting skin around a nail and predisposing a patient to infection is the reason orders are required. Check agency policy to determine whether an order is necessary.

Take time during the procedure to teach the patient and family proper techniques for cleaning and nail trimming. Stress the importance of how thorough nail care prevents infection and promotes good circulation. All patients must learn to protect the feet from injury, never walk barefoot, keep feet clean and dry, and wear footwear that fits properly. Instruct patients in the proper way to inspect all surfaces of the feet and hands for redness, lesions, dryness, or signs of infection. Teach foot care to family caregivers for patients who need regular foot care and have peripheral vascular disease, visual difficulties, physical constraints that prevent movement, or cognitive problems.

Certain conditions place patients with diabetes at increased risk for amputation (ADA, 2016). These factors include peripheral neuropathy, limited joint mobility, bony deformity, peripheral vascular disease, and a history of skin ulcers or previous amputation. Observe for changes that indicate peripheral neuropathy or vascular insufficiency (Box 40.7). Advise patients to use the following guidelines in a routine foot and nail care program (ADA, 2020):

- Inspect the feet daily, including the bottoms and tops, heels, and areas between the toes. Use a mirror to help inspect the feet thoroughly, or ask a family member to check daily.
- Wash feet daily in lukewarm water. Dry thoroughly, especially between the toes. Avoid harsh chemicals or long soaks, which can cause skin softening or maceration of tissue, causing ulceration or infection.
- Wear well-fitting shoes and clean, dry socks at all times; never go barefoot. Check inside shoes before wearing them for rough areas or objects that may rub against the foot.
- Keep skin soft and smooth by applying an emollient lotion over all surfaces of the feet but not between the toes.
- If you can see and reach your toenails, trim them straight across and square file the edges smooth.
- Keep the blood flowing to your feet by putting them up when sitting and wiggling your toes and moving your ankles up and down for 5 minutes, 2 or 3 times a day. Do not cross your legs for long periods and don't smoke.

BOX 40.8   FOCUS ON OLDER ADULTS
Oral Health

- Many older adults are edentulous (without teeth), and the teeth that are present are often diseased or decayed (Touhy and Jett, 2018).
- The periodontal membrane weakens with aging, making it more prone to infection. Periodontal disease predisposes older adults to systemic infection.
- Dentures or partial plates do not always fit properly, causing pain and discomfort, which in turn affects chewing, digestive processes, enjoyment of food, and nutritional status.
- An age-related decline in saliva secretion and some medications (e.g., antihypertensives, diuretics, antiinflammatories, antidepressants) cause dry mouth (Touhy and Jett, 2018).
- Financial limitations and the belief that dentures eliminate the need for routine dental care are some of the reasons why older adults do not seek dental care (Touhy and Jett, 2018).

- Protect the feet from hot and cold. Do not use heating pads or electric blankets and always wear shoes at the beach or on hot pavement.

Oral Hygiene. Regular oral hygiene, including brushing, flossing, and rinsing, prevents and controls plaque-associated oral diseases. Brushing cleans the teeth of food particles, plaque, and bacteria. It also massages the gums and relieves discomfort resulting from unpleasant odors and tastes. Daily flossing removes food particles, plaque, and tartar that collect between teeth and at the gum line. Rinsing removes dislodged food particles and excess toothpaste. Complete oral hygiene enhances well-being and comfort and stimulates the appetite.

When patients become ill, many factors influence their need for oral hygiene, such as their ability to take fluids orally, presence of oral lesions or trauma, and level of consciousness. Patients who are unconscious or have artificial airways, such as tracheostomy or endotracheal tube, have special precautions for oral care because they do not have a gag reflex. Patients in hospitals or long-term care facilities do not always receive the aggressive oral care they need. Base the frequency of care on the condition of the oral cavity, risk for aspiration of saliva, and the patient's level of comfort. Some patients (e.g., stroke, trauma to oral cavity, patient with endotracheal tube) require oral care as often as every 1 to 2 hours.

Brushing. The American Dental Association guidelines (2018) for effective oral hygiene include brushing the teeth at least twice a day with American Dental Association–approved fluoride toothpaste. Fluoride and antimicrobial mouth rinses help prevent tooth decay. Do not use fluoride rinse in children ages 6 or under because of the risk of swallowing the rinse. Use antimicrobial toothpastes and 0.12% CHG oral rinses for patients at increased risk for poor oral hygiene (e.g., older adults and patients with cognitive impairments and who are immunocompromised) (Jenson et al., 2018). The toothbrush needs to have a straight handle and a brush small enough to reach all areas of the mouth. Rounded soft bristles stimulate the gums without causing abrasion and bleeding. Any patient who has decreased dexterity as a result of a medical condition or the aging process requires an enlarged handle with an easier grip (Box 40.8).

Brush all tooth surfaces thoroughly (Box 40.9). Commercially made foam swabs are ineffective in removing plaque. Electric or battery-powered toothbrushes improve the quality of cleaning and may be easier to use than manual brushes when nurses provide care for dependent patients. Do not use lemon-glycerin sponges because they dry mucous membranes and erode tooth enamel.

To prevent cross-contamination, teach patients to avoid sharing toothbrushes with family members or drinking directly from a bottle of mouthwash. Disclosure tablets or drops to stain the plaque that collects at the gum line are useful for showing patients how effectively they brush. Instruct patients to obtain a new toothbrush every 3 months or following a cold or upper respiratory infection to minimize growth of microorganisms on the brush surfaces (American Dental Association, 2018).

Flossing. Dental flossing removes plaque and tartar between teeth. Flossing involves inserting waxed or unwaxed dental floss between all tooth surfaces, one at a time. The seesaw motion used to pull floss between teeth removes plaque and tartar from tooth enamel. Use unwaxed floss and avoid vigorous flossing near the gum line on patients who are receiving chemotherapy, radiation, or anticoagulant therapy to prevent bleeding. If toothpaste is applied to the teeth before flossing, fluoride comes in direct contact with tooth surfaces, aiding in cavity prevention. According to American Dental Association (2018) recommendations, flossing once a day is sufficient. Because it is important to clean all teeth surfaces thoroughly, do not rush to complete flossing. Placing a mirror in front of a patient helps you demonstrate the proper method for holding the floss and cleaning between the teeth. Flossing a patient's teeth is not realistic or appropriate in all care settings.

Patients With Special Needs. Some patients require special oral hygiene methods. For example, patients with diabetes mellitus and who are on chemotherapy frequently experience periodontal disease. Therefore, they need to visit a dentist every 3 to 4 months, clean their teeth up to 4 times a day, and handle oral tissues gently with a minimum of trauma. Xerostomia, bruxism, and dental caries may be present with patients who are methamphetamine users. Cravings for sugary sweets may cause decay and gum disease.

Patients may depend on their caregivers for oral care. Being unconscious or having an artificial airway (e.g., endotracheal or tracheal tubes) increases the susceptibility for patients to have drying of salivary secretions because they are unable to eat or drink, unable to swallow, and frequently breathe through the mouth. Unconscious patients often have a reduced gag reflex, or they cannot swallow salivary secretions that accumulate in the mouth. Pooling of salivary secretions in the back of the throat harbors microorganism growth. These secretions often contain gram-negative bacteria that cause pneumonia if aspirated into the lungs. Proper oral hygiene requires keeping the mucosa moist and removing secretions that contribute to infection. While providing hygiene, protect the patient from choking and aspiration and use topical CHG, especially in ventilated patients (see Skill 40.3). Current evidence shows that use of CHG with oral hygiene reduces the risk for ventilator-associated pneumonia (IHI, 2018; El-Rabbany et al., 2015).

Have two nurses provide the care; turn the patient's head toward you and place the bed in semi-Fowler's position. You can delegate assistive personnel to participate. One nurse does the actual cleaning, and the other caregiver removes secretions with suction equipment. Some agencies use equipment that combines a mouth swab with the suction device; you can use this equipment safely by yourself. While cleansing the oral cavity, use a small oral airway or a padded tongue blade to hold the mouth open. Never use your fingers to hold a patient's mouth open. A human bite contains multiple pathogenic microorganisms. Even though the patient is not awake or alert, explain the steps of mouth care and the sensations that he or she will feel. Also tell the patient when the procedure is completed.

Some treatments such as chemotherapy, immunosuppressive agents, head and neck radiation, and nasogastric intubation place patients at higher risk of experiencing stomatitis or inflammation of the oral mucosa. Stomatitis causes burning, pain, and change in food

BOX 40.9 PROCEDURAL GUIDELINES

Providing Oral Hygiene

Delegation and Collaboration

The skill of oral hygiene (including tooth brushing, flossing, and rinsing) can be delegated to assistive personnel (AP). However, the nurse is responsible for assessing the patient's gag reflex to determine whether the patient is at risk for aspiration. The nurse instructs the AP about:

- Types of changes in oral mucosa (e.g., presence of lesions or open sores) to report to the nurse.
- Positioning the patient to avoid aspiration.
  - Keeping head of bed (HOB) raised 30-45 degrees.
  - Explaining the need to immediately report to the nurse excessive patient coughing or choking during or after oral hygiene.
- Reporting ulcerations, lesions, or bleeding of oral mucosa or gums and patient report of pain.
- Not flossing when the patient has a bleeding tendency.

Equipment

Soft-bristle toothbrush; nonabrasive fluoride toothpaste; dental floss; chlorhexidine gluconate (CHG) solution (*optional; see agency policy*); tongue depressor; water glass with cool water, normal saline, or an antiseptic mouth rinse *(optional depending on patient preference)*; moisturizing lubricant for lips *(optional)*; emesis basin; face towel; paper towels; clean gloves; penlight; linen bag or hamper

Steps

1. Identify patient using at least two identifiers (e.g., name and birthday or name and medical record number) according to agency policy (TJC, 2020).
2. Review medical record and identify presence of common oral hygiene problems.
3. Determine patient's or family caregiver's knowledge, experience, and health literacy
4. Assess patient's oral hygiene practices, such as frequency of brushing and flossing, type of toothpaste and mouthwash used, last and frequency of dental visits.
5. Perform hand hygiene and apply clean gloves.
6. Using tongue depressor and penlight, inspect integrity of lips, teeth, buccal mucosa, gums, palate, and tongue; also assess for gag reflex and ability to swallow (see Chapter 30). Note presence of dental caries—chalky white discoloration of tooth or presence of brown or black discoloration; gingivitis—inflammation of gums; periodontitis—receding gum lines, inflammation, gaps between teeth; halitosis—bad breath; cheilitis—cracked lips; dry, cracked, and coated tongue.
7. Remove and dispose of gloves and perform hand hygiene.
8. Explain procedure to patient, discussing patient's preferences; assess patient's ability to grasp and manipulate toothbrush and willingness to help with oral care.
9. Place paper towels on over-bed table and arrange other equipment within easy reach.
10. Provide privacy by closing room doors and drawing room divider curtain. Raise bed to comfortable working position.
11. Raise head of bed (if allowed) and lower near side rail. Move patient or help him or her move closer to side. Place patient in side-lying position if needed (if aspiration risk). Place towel over patient's chest.
12. Apply clean gloves. Apply enough toothpaste to brush to cover length of bristles. Hold brush over emesis basin. Pour small amount of water over toothpaste.
13. Patient may help with brushing. Hold toothbrush bristles at 45-degree angle to gum line (see illustration A). Be sure that tips of bristles rest against and penetrate under gum line. Brush inner and outer surfaces of upper and lower teeth by brushing from gum to crown of each tooth. Clean biting surfaces of teeth by holding top of bristles parallel with teeth and brushing gently back and forth (see illustration B). Brush sides of teeth by moving bristles back and forth (see illustration C).
14. Have patient hold brush at 45-degree angle and lightly brush over surface and sides of tongue. Avoid initiating gag reflex.
15. Allow patient to rinse mouth thoroughly by taking several sips of cool water, swishing water across all tooth surfaces, and spitting into emesis basin. Use this time to observe patient's brushing technique and teach the importance of regular hygiene (see Fig. 40.2).
16. Have patient rinse mouth with antiseptic rinse for 30 seconds. Then have patient spit rinse into emesis basin. Help wipe patient's mouth.
17. Floss or allow patient to floss between all teeth (see illustration).

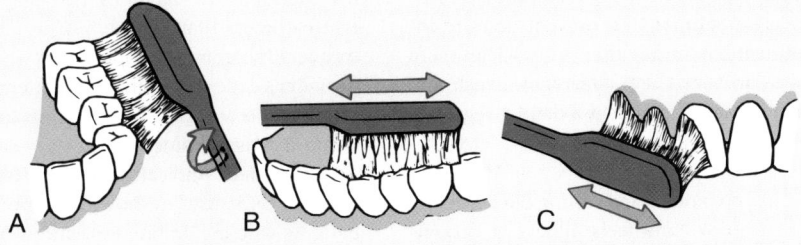

STEP 13 Direction of brushing for tooth brushing.

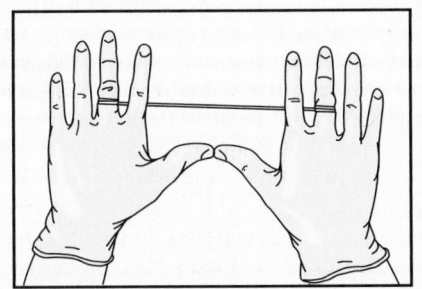 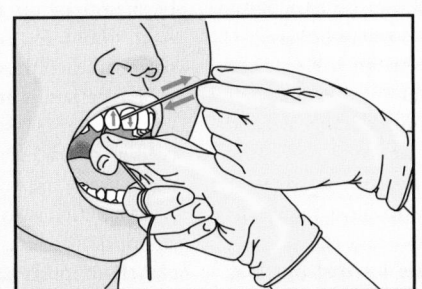 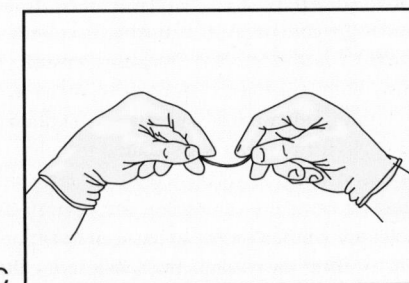

STEP 17 Flossing. **A,** Dental floss is held between middle fingers to floss upper teeth. **B,** Floss is moved in up-and-down motions between teeth. Floss is moved up and down from crown to gum line. **C,** Floss is held with index fingers to floss lower teeth.

Continued

BOX 40.9 PROCEDURAL GUIDELINES—cont'd

Providing Oral Hygiene

18. Allow patient to rinse mouth thoroughly with cool water and spit into emesis basin. Help wipe his or her mouth.
19. Inspect oral cavity to determine effectiveness of oral hygiene and rinsing. Ask patient whether mouth feels clean or if there are any sore or tender areas. Remove towel and place in linen bag.
20. Remove and dispose of gloves and perform hand hygiene. Help patient to comfortable position, raise side rail, and lower bed to original position.

21. **Use Teach-Back:** "I want to be sure you know how often to floss your teeth. Show me how you will floss your teeth." Revise your instruction now or develop a plan for revised patient/family caregiver teaching if patient/family caregiver is not able to teach back correctly.
22. **Record and Report** bleeding, pain, or presence of lesions to nurse in charge or health care provider.

---

and fluid tolerance. When caring for patients with stomatitis, brush with a soft toothbrush and floss gently to prevent bleeding of the gums. In some cases, flossing needs to be omitted temporarily from oral care. Advise patients to avoid alcohol and commercial mouthwash and to stop smoking. Normal saline rinses (approximately 30 mL) on awakening in the morning, after each meal, and at bedtime help clean the oral cavity. Patients can increase the rinses to every 2 hours if necessary. Consult with the health care provider to obtain topical or oral analgesics for pain control.

Denture Care. Encourage patients to clean their dentures on a regular basis to avoid gingival infection and irritation. When patients become disabled, someone else assumes responsibility for denture care (Box 40.10). Dentures are a patient's personal property and must be handled with care because they break easily. They must be removed at night to rest the gums and prevent bacterial buildup. To prevent warping, keep dentures covered in water when they are not worn and always store them in an enclosed, labeled cup with the cup placed on the patient's bedside stand. Discourage patients from removing their dentures and placing them on a napkin or tissue because they could easily be thrown away.

Implement measures to prevent denture-induced stomatitis when caring for patients who wear dentures. Poorly fitting dentures, wearing dentures while sleeping, and poor dental hygiene habits contribute to denture-induced stomatitis (Maciag et al., 2017; Martori et al., 2014). Signs and symptoms range from redness and swelling under the dentures to painful red sores on the roof of the mouth and infection with the yeast *Candida albicans*. Some patients deny pain, and others complain of pain worsened by wearing dentures. To prevent denture-induced stomatitis, rinse the mouth and dentures after meals, clean them carefully and regularly, remove and soak them overnight, brush and floss (if appropriate) any remaining teeth, and visit a dentist regularly for examination (American Dental Association, 2018).

Hair and Scalp Care.
A person's appearance and feeling of well-being often depend on the way the hair looks and feels. Illness or disability often prevents a patient from maintaining daily hair care. When patients are immobilized, their hair soon becomes tangled. Some dressings or diagnostic procedures leave sticky residue on the hair. Basic hair and scalp care includes brushing, combing, and shampooing.

Brushing and Combing. Frequent brushing helps keep hair clean and distributes oil evenly along hair shafts. Combing prevents hair from tangling. Encourage patients to maintain routine hair care and provide help for patients with limited mobility or weakness and those who are confused or weakened by illness. Patients in a hospital or extended-care facility appreciate the opportunity to have their hair brushed and combed before being seen by others.

When caring for patients from different cultures, learn as much as possible from them or their family about preferred hair care practices. For example, the hair of African-Americans tends to be quite dry. Use special lanolin conditioners for conditioning. Cultural preferences also affect how hair is combed and styled and whether it can be cut.

Long hair becomes matted easily when a patient is confined to bed, even for a short period. When lacerations or incisions involve the scalp, blood and topical medications also cause tangling. Frequent brushing and combing keep long hair neatly groomed. Braiding helps to avoid repeated tangles; however, patients need to unbraid hair periodically and comb it to ensure good hygiene. Braids that are too tight lead to bald patches. Obtain permission from the patient before braiding the hair.

To brush hair part it into two sections and separate each section into two more sections. Brushing from the scalp toward the hair ends minimizes pulling. Moistening the hair with water or an alcohol-free detangle product makes it easier to comb. Never cut a patient's hair without consent.

Patients who develop head lice require special considerations in the way combing is performed (Box 40.11). The lice are small, about the size of a sesame seed; thus, you need bright light or natural sunlight to see them. Thorough combing is more effective than use of pediculicidal shampoos, which are often toxic and ineffective against resistant lice.

If a pediculicidal shampoo is ordered, review pertinent information and instruct the patient and caregiver in its proper use. Use with caution because these shampoos may have severe neurological side effects. Make sure to thoroughly rinse shampoo from hair to avoid itching.

Shampooing. Frequency of shampooing depends on a person's daily routines and the condition of the hair. Remind patients in hospitals or extended-care facilities that staying in bed, excess perspiration, or treatments that leave blood or solutions in the hair require more frequent shampooing. In some agencies you need a health care provider's order to shampoo a patient who is dependent or has limited mobility because it is challenging to find ways to shampoo the hair without causing injury.

The patient who can shower or tub bathe usually shampoos the hair without difficulty. A shower or tub chair facilitates shampooing for patients who are ambulatory and weight-bearing and become tired or faint. Handheld shower nozzles allow patients to easily wash the hair in the tub or shower. Some patients allowed to sit in a chair choose to be shampooed in front of a sink or over a washbasin; however, certain conditions (e.g., eye surgery or neck injury) limit bending. In these situations, teach the patient and family the degree of bending allowed.

If a patient is unable to sit but can be moved, transfer him or her to a stretcher for transportation to a sink or shower equipped with a handheld nozzle. Use caution when positioning the patient's head and neck, particularly in patients with any form of head or neck injury.

If a patient is unable to sit in a chair or be transferred to a stretcher, shampoo the hair with him or her in bed (Box 40.12). Position a special shampoo trough under his or her head to catch water and suds. After shampooing, patients like having their hair styled and dried. Most health care centers have portable hair dryers. Dry shampoos that

BOX 40.10 PROCEDURAL GUIDELINES

Care of Dentures

Delegation and Collaboration

The skill of denture care can be delegated to assistive personnel (AP). The nurse instructs the AP to:

- Not use hot or excessively cold water when caring for dentures.
- Inform the nurse if there are cracks in dentures.
- Inform the nurse if the patient has any oral discomfort.

Equipment

Soft-bristled toothbrush or denture toothbrush; denture dentifrice or toothpaste, denture adhesive *(optional)*; glass of water; emesis basin or sink; 4 × 4–inch gauze; washcloth; denture cup (for storage); clean gloves

Steps

1. Identify patient using at least two identifiers (e.g., name and birthday or name and medical record number) according to agency policy (TJC, 2020).
2. Assess environment for safety (e.g., check room for spills; make sure that bed is in locked, low position) (QSEN, 2018).
3. Perform hand hygiene.
4. Determine patient's or family caregiver's knowledge, experience, and health literacy.
5. Ask patient whether dentures fit and whether he or she is experiencing any gum or mucous membrane tenderness or irritation. Ask patient about denture care and product preferences.
6. Determine whether patient has necessary dexterity to clean dentures independently or requires help.
7. Lower side rail. Position patient comfortably sitting up in bed, or help him or her walk from bed to chair placed in front of sink.
8. Fill emesis basin with tepid water. (If using sink, place washcloth in bottom of sink and fill sink with approximately 2.5 cm [1 inch] of water.)
9. Perform hand hygiene again and apply clean gloves.
10. Ask patient to remove dentures. If patient is unable to do this independently, grasp upper plate at front with thumb and index finger wrapped in gauze and pull downward. Gently lift lower denture from jaw and rotate one side downward to remove from patient's mouth. Place dentures in emesis basin or sink lined with washcloth and 2.5 cm (1 inch) of water.
11. Inspect oral cavity, paying attention to gums, tongue, and upper palate. Observe for lesions, plaques, and areas of irritation. Palpate areas as needed.

    CLINICAL DECISION: Oral mucosal lesions are common in older adults, especially those with dentures. These lesions are associated with local and systemic factors, and tongue lesions may be the first to appear (Pedersen et al., 2015).

12. Apply cleaning agent to brush and brush surfaces of dentures (see illustration). Hold dentures close to water. Hold brush horizontally and use back-and-forth motion to clean biting surfaces. Use short strokes from top of denture to biting surfaces to clean outer teeth surfaces. Hold brush vertically and use short strokes to clean inner teeth surfaces. Hold brush horizontally and use back-and-forth motion to clean undersurface of dentures (see Procedural Guideline Box 40.9).

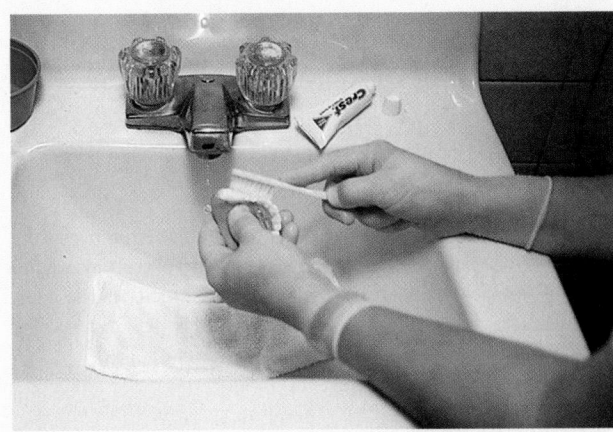

STEP 12 Brushing surface of dentures.

13. Rinse thoroughly in tepid water. If water is too cold, dentures can crack. If it is too hot, dentures can become warped and no longer fit.
14. When necessary, apply a thin layer of denture adhesive to undersurface before inserting.
15. Reinsert dentures as soon as possible. If patient needs help with inserting dentures, moisten upper denture and press firmly to seal it in place. Insert moistened lower denture (if applicable). Ask whether denture(s) feels comfortable. Note: It is common for patients to choose not to wear their dentures during an acute illness.
16. Some patients prefer to store their dentures to give gums a rest and reduce risk for infection. Store in tepid water in enclosed, labeled denture cup. Keep denture cup in a secure place labeled with patient's name to prevent loss when not worn (e.g., at night, during surgery).
17. Dispose of supplies. Remove and discard gloves and perform hand hygiene.
18. Return patient to a comfortable position with bed in low position. Leave nurse call system in reach.
19. Record and report any abnormalities noted involving oral mucosa.

BOX 40.11 Hygiene Care for Head Lice

- Perform hand hygiene and apply disposable gown and gloves.
- Use a grooming comb or hairbrush to remove tangles.
- Divide patient's hair in sections, and fasten off hair that is not being combed.
- Comb out from scalp to the end of the hair (special combs are available in drugstores).
- Dip comb in a cup of water or use a paper towel to remove lice between each passing.
- After combing, look through hair carefully for attached lice; you can catch live lice with a tweezers or comb.
- After combing thoroughly, move to next section of hair.

- Instruct family to clean the comb with an old toothbrush and dental floss. Then boil the comb. The ideal is to discard the comb after each use, but some patients' financial situations prevent the purchase of multiple combs.
- Instruct family to comb and screen for lice daily.
- Instruct family to contain patient's clothes and wash them in hot water.
- Instruct family to vacuum the home and patient's room and immediately empty vacuum bag or bagless collection device.
- Instruct caregivers on how to prevent transmission of lice: Do not share bed linens or hair care products. Avoid placing bare hand on patient's head. Immediately wash hands after providing hair care.

BOX 40.12 PROCEDURAL GUIDELINES

Hair Care: Shampooing and Shaving

Delegation and Collaboration

The skills of combing, shampooing, and shaving can be delegated to assistive personnel (AP). The nurse instructs the AP to:

- Properly position a patient with head or neck mobility restrictions.
- Provide the proper care in cases of head lice, stressing steps to take to prevent transmission to other patients.
- Report how the patient tolerated the procedure and any concerns (e.g., neck pain).
- Use an electric razor for any patient at risk for bleeding tendencies.

Equipment

Hair Care

- Wide-tooth comb and hairbrush

Regular Shampoo

- Washcloth; shampoo, hair conditioner *(optional)*, hydrogen peroxide and saline 50/50 mixture *(optional if blood in hair)*; water pitcher with warm water; plastic shampoo board, washbasin; bath blanket, waterproof pad.

Disposable Shampoo

- Disposable shampoo cap product

Shaving with Razor

- New disposable or electric razor; clean gloves; bath towel(s), mirror, washcloth, washbasin; shaving cream or soap, aftershave lotion (if patient desires and not contraindicated)

Mustache Care

- Scissors, brush or comb; bath towel; gooseneck lamp or overhead light

Steps

1. Identify patient using at least two identifiers (e.g., name and birthday or name and medical record number) according to agency policy (TJC, 2020).
2. Assess whether patient has bleeding tendency. Review medical history, medications, and laboratory values (e.g., platelet count, anticoagulation studies).

   CLINICAL DECISION: Have any patient on anticoagulants or who has low platelets use an electric razor.

3. Review medical record to determine that there are no contraindications to procedure. Check agency policy for health care provider order as needed. Certain medical conditions such as head and neck injuries, spinal cord injuries, and arthritis place patient at risk for injury during shampooing because of positioning and manipulation of patient's head and neck
4. Assess environment for safety (e.g., check room for spills; make sure that bed is in locked, low position) (QSEN, 2018).
5. Perform hand hygiene. Inspect condition of hair and scalp (this can also be done just before starting shampoo or combing). Inspect for presence of any infestation (e.g., pediculosis). Inspect for drainage from any head wounds. NOTE: Apply clean gloves if drainage or infestation is suspected. Apply a gown if infestation is suspected (National Pediculosis Association, 2017).
6. Remove and discard gloves and perform hand hygiene.
7. Determine patient's or family caregiver's knowledge, experience, and health literacy.
8. Assess patient's hair-care and shaving product preferences (e.g., shampoo, aftershave lotion, skin conditioner).
9. Assess patient's ability to manipulate comb, brush, or razor.
10. Gather equipment and supplies at patient's bedside. Explain your intent to provide hair/beard care. Ask patient to explain during procedure the steps that he or she uses to comb hair and/or shave. Ask patient to indicate if he or she becomes uncomfortable during procedure.
11. Position patient sitting in chair or up in bed with head elevated 45 to 90 degrees (as tolerated).
12. Provide privacy; close door or pull curtain. Arrange supplies at bedside table and adjust lighting.
13. Perform hand hygiene.
14. Combing and brushing hair:
    a. Apply clean gloves if necessary. Part hair into two sections and then separate it into two more sections (see illustrations).

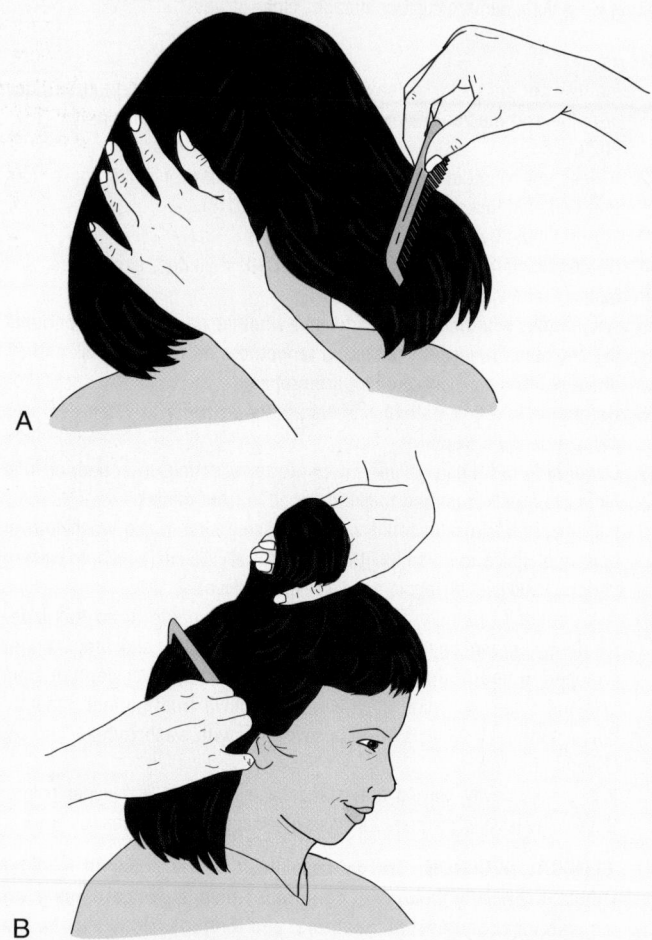

STEP 14a Parting hair. **A,** Part hair down the middle and divide it into two main sections. **B,** Part main section into two smaller sections.

    b. Brush or comb from scalp toward hair ends.
    c. Moisten hair lightly with water, conditioner, or alcohol-free detangle product before combing.
    d. Move fingers through hair to loosen any larger tangles.
    e. Using a wide-tooth comb, start on either side of head and insert comb with teeth upward to hair near scalp. Comb through hair in circular motion by turning wrist while lifting up and out. Continue until all hair is combed through, and comb into place to shape and style.
15. Shampooing bed-bound patient with shampoo board:
    a. Apply clean gloves. Place waterproof pad under patient's shoulders, neck, and head.

BOX 40.12 PROCEDURAL GUIDELINES—cont'd ▶

Hair Care: Shampooing and Shaving

b. Position patient supine with head and shoulders at top edge of bed. Place shampoo board under patient's head and washbasin under end of trough spout (see illustration). Be sure that trough spout extends beyond edge of mattress.

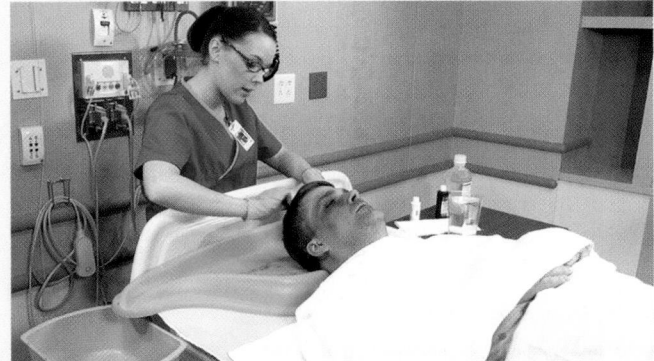

STEP 15b Patient positioned over shampoo board. (Copyright © Mosby's Clinical Skills: Essentials Collection.)

c. Place rolled towel under patient's neck and bath towel over patient's shoulders.

d. Brush and comb patient's hair.

e. Ask patient to hold towel or washcloth over eyes.

f. Test water temperature. Slowly pour water from pitcher over hair until it is completely wet (see illustration). If hair contains matted blood, apply hydrogen peroxide to dissolve clots and rinse with saline. Apply small amount of shampoo.

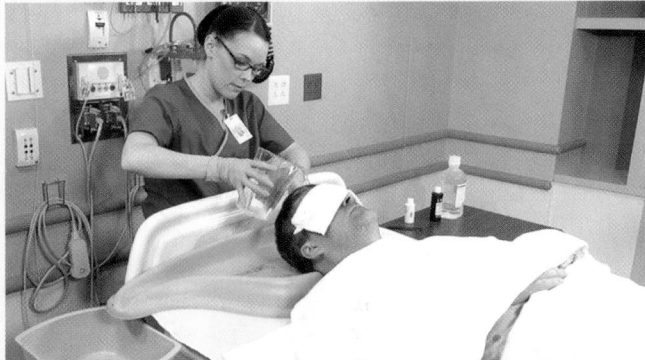

STEP 15f Nurse pouring water over patient's hair. (Copyright © Mosby's Clinical Skills: Essentials Collection.)

g. Work up lather with both hands. Start at hairline and work toward back of neck. Lift head slightly with one hand to wash back of head. Shampoo sides of head. Massage scalp by applying pressure with fingertips.

h. Rinse hair with water. Make sure that water drains into basin. Repeat rinsing until hair is free of soap. (If you need to refill pitcher, raise side rail when leaving bedside.)

i. Apply conditioner or crème rinse if requested, and rinse hair thoroughly.

j. Wrap patient's head in bath towel. Dry face with cloth used to protect eyes. Dry off any moisture along neck or shoulders.

k. Dry patient's hair and scalp. Use second towel if first one becomes saturated.

l. Comb hair to remove tangles and dry with dryer if desired.

m. Apply oil preparation or conditioning product to hair if desired by patient.

n. Variation for patients with coarse, curly hair: Condition hair after washing. To untangle hair, use wide teeth of comb. Beginning at nape of neck, comb small subsections of hair, starting at hair ends. Continue to work through small sections until hair is free of tangles.

16. Shampooing with disposable shampoo product:

a. Patient can be sitting on chair or in bed. Apply clean gloves.

b. Comb hair to remove any tangles or debris (see Step 14 above).

c. Open package, apply cap, and secure all hair beneath cap (see illustration).

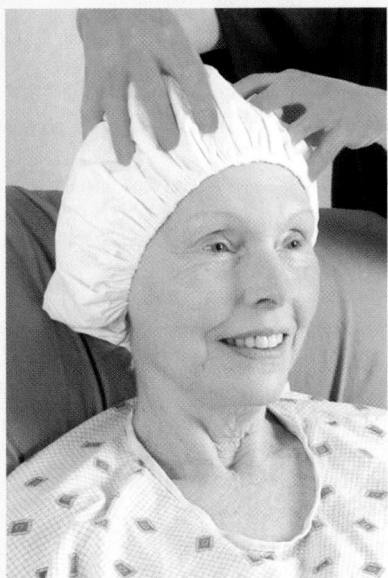

STEP 16c Patient wearing disposable shampoo cap.

d. Massage head through cap. Check fitting around head to maintain correct fit.

e. Massage 2 to 4 minutes according to directions on package; additional time may be required for longer hair or hair matted with blood.

f. Discard cap in trash; do not dispose of in toilet because it may clog plumbing.

g. If patient desires, towel-dry hair. Brush or comb patient's hair.

17. Shaving with disposable razor:

a. Place bath towel over patient's chest and shoulders.

b. Run warm water in washbasin. Check water temperature.

c. Place washcloth in basin and wring out thoroughly. Apply cloth over patient's entire face for several seconds.

d. Apply approximately ¼ inch shaving cream or soap to patient's face. Smooth cream evenly over sides of face, on chin, and under nose.

Continued

BOX 40.12   PROCEDURAL GUIDELINES—cont'd

Hair Care: Shampooing and Shaving

e. Hold razor in dominant hand at 45-degree angle to patient's skin. Begin by shaving across one side of patient's face using short, firm strokes in direction that hair grows (see illustration). Use nondominant hand to gently pull skin taut while shaving. Ask patient whether he feels comfortable.

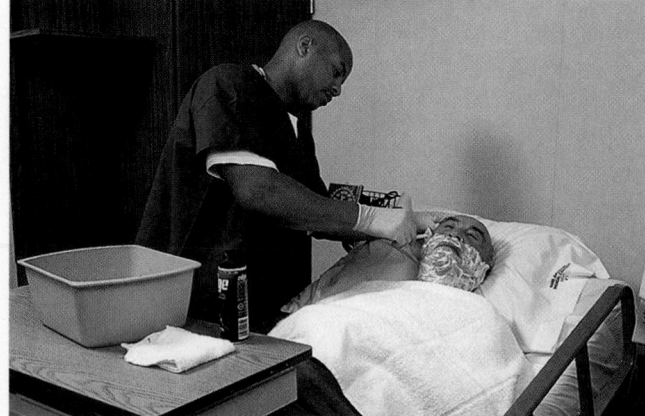

STEP 17e Shaving patient using short, firm strokes.

    f. Dip razor blade in water because shaving cream accumulates on edge of blade.

    g. After all facial hair is shaved, rinse face thoroughly with warm, moistened washcloth.

    h. Dry face thoroughly and apply aftershave lotion if desired. Remove towel.

18. Shaving with electric razor:

    a. Place bath towel over patient's chest and shoulders.

    b. Apply skin conditioner or preshave preparation.

    c. Turn razor on and begin by shaving across side of face. Gently hold skin taut while shaving over surface of skin. Use gentle downward stroke of razor in direction of hair growth.

    d. After completing shave, turn razor off, remove towel and apply aftershave lotion as desired unless contraindicated.

19. Mustache and beard care:

    a. Place bath towel over patient's chest and shoulders.

    b. If necessary, gently comb mustache or beard. Offer option for patient to shampoo beard.

    c. Allow patient to use mirror and direct areas to trim with scissors.

    d. After completing, remove towel.

20. Discard soiled linen in dirty laundry bag. Remove and dispose of gloves. Perform hand hygiene.

21. Help patient to comfortable position with nurse call system in reach, bed in low position.

22. Return reusable equipment to proper place.

23. Inspect condition of hair and scalp, condition of shaved area and skin underneath beard or mustache. Look for areas of localized bleeding from cuts and areas of dryness.

24. Ask patient whether face feels clean and comfortable.

25. **Use Teach-Back:** "Since you are on a blood thinner, I want to be sure I explained to you the risks of using a regular razor at home. What type of razor you should use? Tell me the things to watch for with a bleeding tendency." Revise your instruction now or develop a plan for revised patient/family caregiver teaching if patient/family caregiver is not able to teach back correctly.

26. Record or report any lesions, presence of lice to healthcare provider.

---

reduce the need to wet the patient's hair are also available but are not highly effective. Shampoo caps provide a warm, wet massage to the scalp while cleaning the hair.

Shaving. Shave a patient's facial hair after the bath or shampoo. Some women prefer to shave their legs or axillae while bathing. When helping a patient, take care to avoid cutting him or her with the razor blade. Patients prone to bleeding (e.g., those receiving anticoagulants or high doses of aspirin or those with low platelet counts) need to use their personal electric razor. Before using an electric razor, check for frayed cords or other electrical hazards. Use a razor blade on only one patient because of infection control considerations.

When using a razor blade for shaving, soften the skin to prevent pulling, scraping, or cuts. Moisten the skin with lukewarm water and apply shaving cream. Bar soap may leave a film on the blade, resulting in a poorer-quality shave. You need to shave patients when they are unable to shave themselves independently. To avoid causing discomfort or razor cuts, gently pull the skin taut and use long, firm razor strokes in the direction the hair grows (Fig. 40.5). Short downward strokes work best to remove hair over the upper lip or chin. A patient usually explains the best way to move the razor across the skin.

Facial hair of people of color tends to be curly and becomes ingrown unless shaved close to the skin. However, there are common skin lesions among people of color that require a different shaving technique. An example is the common condition of pseudofolliculitis barbae, commonly referred to as razor bumps and recognized by inflammation of hair follicles and hyperpigmented papules and pustules (Kundu and Patterson, 2013). It typically results from cut hairs penetrating the skin. Use the following techniques for this condition: Avoid a close shave, leaving hair at a length of 0.5 to 3 mm; use clippers, a single-blade razor, or depilatories; if depilatories cause skin irritation,

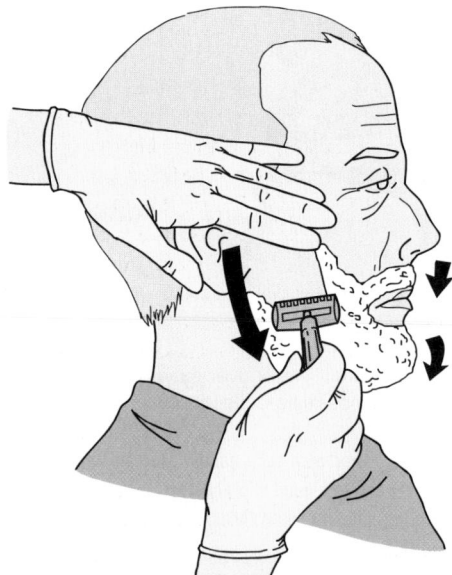

FIG. 40.5 Shave using short, firm strokes in direction of hair growth.

discontinue use, shave in the direction of hair growth, and do not pull the skin taut while shaving (Kundu and Patterson, 2013).

Mustache and Beard Care. Mustaches or beards require daily grooming. including shampooing. Grooming keeps food particles and mucus from collecting in the hair. If a patient is unable to carry out self-care, do so at his or her request. Comb out beards gently, and obtain the patient's permission before trimming or shaving off a mustache or beard.

Care of the Eyes, Ears, and Nose. Give special attention to cleaning the eyes, ears, and nose during a routine bath and when drainage or discharge accumulates. This aspect of hygiene not only makes a patient more comfortable but also improves sensory reception (see Chapter 49). Care focuses on preventing infection and maintaining normal sensory function. In addition, care of the eyes, ears, and nose requires approaches that consider the patient's special needs.

Medical Devices. If a patient has oxygen tubing, a feeding tube, or a nasotracheal tube, it is essential that you care for the area of the skin around the nose or ears underlying the device. The National Pressure Ulcer Advisory Panel (NPUAP, 2013) recommends the following: cushion and protect the skin with dressings in high-risk areas (e.g., nasal bridge) (see Chapter 48), do not place device(s) over sites of prior or existing pressure injury, and be sure to gently cleanse a potential area of irritation that underlies a device at least daily.

Basic Eye Care. Cleaning the eyes involves simply washing with a clean washcloth moistened in water (see Skill 40.1). Soap may cause burning and irritation. Never apply direct pressure over the eyeball because it causes serious injury. When cleaning a patient's eyes, obtain a clean washcloth and clean from inner to outer canthus. Use a different section of the washcloth for each eye. Remember, never use CHG solution or cloths to clean the eyes, ears, or face.

Unconscious patients require more frequent eye care. A complication of sedation and coma is that some patients are unable to maintain effective eye closure, which results in exposure keratopathy. Thus, these patients lose their natural protective mechanisms to protect the cornea. When unprotected, there is an increased risk of corneal dehydration, abrasion, perforation, and infection (Demirel et al., 2014). Normal protective mechanisms include blinking with lubrication of the eye. Blinking provides a mechanical barrier to injury and prevents dehydration. Secretions collect along the lid margins and inner canthus when the blink reflex is absent or when the eye does not close completely. Prompt assessment of impaired blinking is essential to protect your patient's eyes. When an eye does not close completely, you may need to place an eye patch over it to prevent corneal drying and irritation. Apply lubricating eyedrops according to the health care provider's orders (Kocacal et al., 2018).

Eyeglasses. Eyeglasses are expensive. Be careful when cleaning glasses and protect them from breakage or other damage when they are not worn. Put them in a case in a drawer of the bedside table when not in use. Cool water sufficiently cleans glass lenses. Prevent scratching by using a soft cloth for drying; do not use paper towels. Plastic lenses in particular scratch easily; special cleaning solutions and drying tissues are available.

Contact Lenses. A contact lens is a thin, transparent disk that fits directly over the cornea of the eye. Contact lenses correct refractive errors of the eye or abnormalities in the shape of the cornea. In outpatient or home settings instruct patients on the routines to follow for regular cleansing and care (Box 40.13). Explain that all contact lenses must be removed periodically to prevent ocular infection and corneal ulcers or abrasions from infectious agents such as *Pseudomonas aeruginosa* and staphylococci. Pain, tearing, discomfort, and redness of the conjunctivae indicate lens overwear. Encourage patients to report persistence of these symptoms, even after lens removal, to their health care provider.

When patients are admitted to the hospital or agency in an unresponsive or confused state, determine whether they normally wear contact lenses and whether the lenses are in place. If a patient wears contact lenses and no one detects this, severe corneal injury can result. If you find that your patient is wearing contact lenses and cannot remove them, seek help. Once the lenses are removed, document the removal, the condition of the patient's eyes following removal, and the storage of the lenses.

Ear Care. Routine ear care involves cleaning the outer ear with a washcloth and warm water. Cleanse the outer ear canal with the end of a moistened washcloth rotated gently into the canal. Gentle,

---

BOX 40.13 PATIENT TEACHING
Contact Lens Care

Objective
- Patient verbalizes and/or demonstrates proper care for contact lenses and common warning signs of problems associated with contact lens wear.

Teaching Strategies
- Instruct patients on the following:
  - Do not use fingernail on lens to remove dirt or debris.
  - Do not use tap water to clean soft lenses.
  - Follow recommendations of lens manufacturer or eye care practitioner when inserting, cleaning, and disinfecting lenses.
  - Keep lenses moist or wet when not worn.
  - Use fresh solution daily when storing and disinfecting lenses.
  - Thoroughly wash and rinse lens storage case on a daily basis. Clean periodically with soap or liquid detergent, rinse thoroughly with warm water, and air dry.
  - If lens is dropped, moisten finger with cleaning or wetting solution and gently touch lens to pick it up. Then clean, rinse, and disinfect it.
- To avoid mix-up, always start with the same lens when removing or inserting lenses.
- Throw away disposable or planned replacement lenses after prescribed wearing period.
- Encourage patient to remember the acronym RSVP: *R*edness, *S*ensitivity, *V*ision problems, and *P*ain. If one of these problems occurs, remove contact lenses immediately. If problems continue, contact a vision care specialist (Harding et al., 2020).

Evaluation
Use the principles of teach-back to evaluate patient/family caregiver learning:
- Explain to me the warning signs of corneal irritation and eye infection.
- Describe for me the methods of contact lens care that lead to infection.
- I want to make sure that you understand the information on lens cleaning and storage. Show me how you will clean your lenses and store them.

---

downward retraction at the entrance of the ear canal usually causes visible cerumen to loosen and slip out. Instruct patients never to use objects such as bobby pins, toothpicks, paper clips, or cotton-tipped applicators to remove earwax. These objects can injure the ear canal and rupture the tympanic membrane. They may also cause cerumen to become impacted within the ear canal.

Children and older adults commonly have impacted cerumen. You can usually remove excessive or impacted cerumen by irrigation, which requires a health care provider's order. Review the order for type of solution and ear(s) to receive the irrigation. Before irrigation question the patient for history of perforated eardrum and inspect his or her tympanic membrane to be sure that it is intact; a perforated tympanic membrane contradicts performing irrigation. Visually inspect the pinna and external meatus for redness, swelling, drainage, and presence of foreign objects. Also determine the patient's ability to hear in the affected ear before irrigation.

To irrigate the ear, have the patient sit or lie on the side with the affected ear up. For adults and children over 3 years of age, gently pull the pinna up and back. In children 3 years of age or younger, the pinna should be pulled down and back. Using a bulb-irrigating syringe, gently wash the ear canal with warm solution (37°C or 98.6°F), being careful not to occlude the canal, which results in pressure on the tympanic membrane. Direct the fluid slowly and gently toward the superior aspect of the ear canal, maintaining the flow in a steady stream. Periodically during the irrigation ask if the patient is experiencing pain, nausea, or vertigo. These symptoms indicate that the solution is too hot or too cold or is being instilled with too much pressure. After the canal is clear, wipe off any moisture from the ear with cotton balls and inspect the canal for remaining earwax.

Hearing Aid Care. A hearing aid amplifies sounds in a controlled manner; the aid receives normal low-intensity sound inputs and delivers them to a patient's ear as louder outputs. Hearing aids come in a variety of types. The new class of hearing aids reduces background noise interference. Computer chips placed in the aids allow for fine adjustments to the specific patient's hearing needs.

There are several popular types of hearing aids. A completely-in-canal (CIC) aid (Fig. 40.6, *A*) is the newest, smallest, and least visible and fits entirely in the ear canal. It is used for patients with moderately severe hearing loss. It has cosmetic appeal, is easy to manipulate and place in the ear, and does not interfere with wearing eyeglasses or using the telephone. The patient can wear it during most physical exercise. However, it requires adequate ear diameter and depth for proper fit. It does not accommodate progressive hearing loss, and it requires manual dexterity to operate, insert, remove, and change batteries. In addition, cerumen tends to plug this model more than the others.

An in-the-ear (ITE, or intraaural) aid (Fig. 40.6, *B*) fits into the external auditory canal and allows for finer tuning. It is more powerful and stronger and therefore is more useful for mild-to-severe hearing loss than the CIC aid. It is easier to position and adjust and does not interfere with wearing eyeglasses. However, it is more noticeable than the CIC aid and is not for people with moisture or skin problems in the ear canal.

A behind-the-ear (BTE, or postaural) aid (Fig. 40.6, *C*) hooks around and behind the ear. It is connected by a short, clear, hollow plastic tube to an ear mold inserted into the external auditory canal. A BTE aid allows for fine tuning. It is the largest aid and is useful for patients with mild to profound hearing loss or manual dexterity difficulties or for those who find partial ear occlusion intolerable. The larger size of this type of aid can make the use of eyeglasses and phones difficult; it is more difficult to keep in place during physical exercise.

Digital hearing aids (Fig. 40.6, *D*) analyze sounds to remove background noise. This aid is beneficial for people with mild to severe hearing loss. Digital hearing aids program for low-frequency and high-frequency sounds and must be programmed and adjusted by a licensed audiologist. Box 40.14 reviews guidelines for the care and cleaning of hearing aids.

Nasal Care. If a patient cannot remove nasal secretions, help by using a wet washcloth or a cotton-tipped applicator moistened in water or saline. Never insert the applicator beyond the length of the cotton tip. You also can remove excessive nasal secretions through gentle nasal suctioning (see Chapter 41).

When nasogastric, feeding, or endotracheal tubes are inserted through a patient's nose, change the tape anchoring the tube at least once a day. When the tape becomes moist from nasal secretions, the skin and mucosa can easily become macerated (softened by soaking). Friction from a tube causes tissue injury. Anchor tubing correctly with tape or fixative devices to minimize tension or friction on the nares (see Skill 47.2).

Patient's Room Environment. Attempt to make a patient's room as comfortable as the home. It needs to be safe and large enough to allow the patient and visitors to move about freely. Removal of barriers around the bed and along walkways reduces risk of falls. Control room temperature, ventilation, noise, and odors. Keeping the room neat and orderly also contributes to the patient's sense of well-being.

Maintaining Comfort. What makes a comfortable environment depends on a patient's age, severity of illness, and level of normal daily activity. Depending on age and physical condition, maintain the room temperature between 20° and 23°C (68° and 73.4°F). Infants,

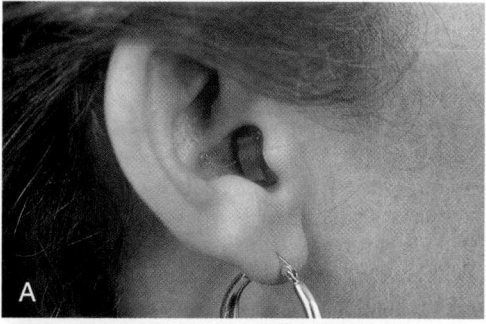
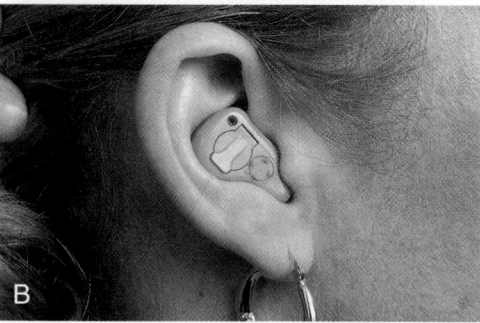
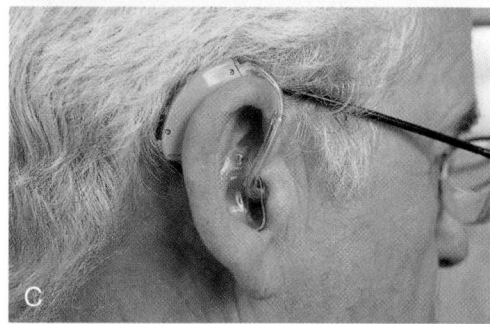
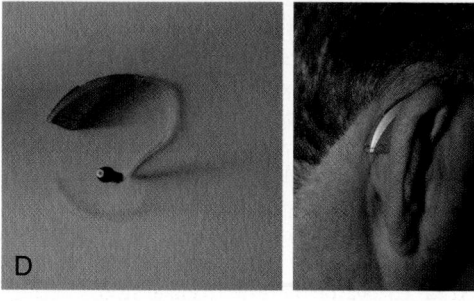

FIG. 40.6 Common types of hearing aids. **A**, Completely-in-canal (CIC) hearing aid. **B**, In-the-ear (ITE) hearing aid. **C**, Behind-the-ear (BTE) hearing aid. **D**, Digital hearing aid.

older adults, and the acutely ill often need a warmer room. However, certain ill patients benefit from cooler room temperatures to lower the metabolic demands of the body.

An effective ventilation system prevents stale air and odors from lingering in the room. Good ventilation reduces lingering odors caused by draining wounds, emesis, bowel movements, and used bedpans and urinals. Always empty and cleanse bedpans and urinals promptly. Room deodorizers help remove many unpleasant odors. Before using room deodorizers, determine that your patient is not allergic or sensitive to the deodorizer itself.

Ill patients seem to be more sensitive to noises and lighting commonly found in health care settings. Try to control the noise level, especially when a patient is trying to sleep. Explain the source of unfamiliar noises such as an IV pump or pulse oximeter alarms.

BOX 40.14 Care and Use of Hearing Aids

- Initially wear hearing aid 15 to 20 minutes; gradually increase time to 10 to 12 hours.
- Once inserted, turn aid slowly to one-third to one-half volume.
- Whistling sound indicates incorrect earmold insertion, improper fit of aid, or buildup of earwax or fluid.
- Adjust volume to comfortable level for talking at distance of 1 yard.
- Do not wear aid under heat lamps or hair dryer or in very wet, cold weather.
- Batteries last 1 week with daily wearing of 10 to 12 hours.
- Remove or disconnect battery when not in use.
- Replace earmolds every 2 or 3 years.
- Routinely check battery compartment: Is it clean? Are batteries inserted properly? Is compartment shut all the way?
- Make sure that dials on hearing aid are clean and easy to rotate, creating no static during adjusting.
- Keep aid clean. See manufacturer instructions. Aids are usually cleaned with a soft cloth.
- Avoid use of hairspray and perfume while wearing hearing aids; residue from spray causes aid to become oily and greasy.
- Do not submerge in water.
- Routinely check cord or tubing (depending on type of aid) for cracking, fraying, and poor connections.
- Routine follow-up with audiologist is recommended to evaluate effectiveness of current aid.

Data from Touhy T, Jett P: *Ebersole and Hess' gerontological nursing & healthy aging*, ed 5, St Louis, 2018, Elsevier.

Proper lighting provides for safety and comfort. A brightly lit room usually stimulates, whereas a darkened room promotes rest and sleep. Adjust room lighting by closing or opening drapes, regulating over-bed and floor lights, and closing or opening room doors. When entering a patient's room at night, refrain from abruptly turning on an overhead light unless necessary.

Room Equipment. Although there are variations across health care settings, a typical hospital room contains the following basic pieces of furniture: over-bed table, bedside stand, chairs, and bed (Fig. 40.7). The over-bed table is an ideal working space for performing procedures. It also serves as a surface for meal trays, toiletry items, and objects that a patient often uses. Clean the top of the over-bed table with an antiseptic cleaner before using it for meals. Do not place a bedpan or urinal on the over-bed table. Use the bedside stand to store a patient's personal possessions and hygiene equipment. Patients often use bedside stands for their telephone, water pitcher, and drinking cup.

Most patient rooms contain a straight-backed chair or an upholstered lounge chair with arms. Armless straight-backed chairs are convenient when temporarily transferring a patient from the bed, such as during bed making. Upholstered lounge chairs or recliners tend to be more comfortable for patients who can sit for longer times.

Each room usually has an over-bed light and floor-level night lighting. Patients need instructions as to how to access to lighting and other controls via their nurse call system (Fig. 40.8). Additional portable or built-in examination lighting provides extra light during bedside procedures.

Other equipment usually found in a patient's room includes the nurses' call system (often integrated into side rails), a television, a wall-mounted blood pressure gauge, oxygen and vacuum wall outlets, and personal care items. Special equipment designed for comfort or positioning patients includes foot boots and special mattresses (see Chapter 48). Whenever you use comfort and positioning equipment, check agency policy and manufacturer directions before application.

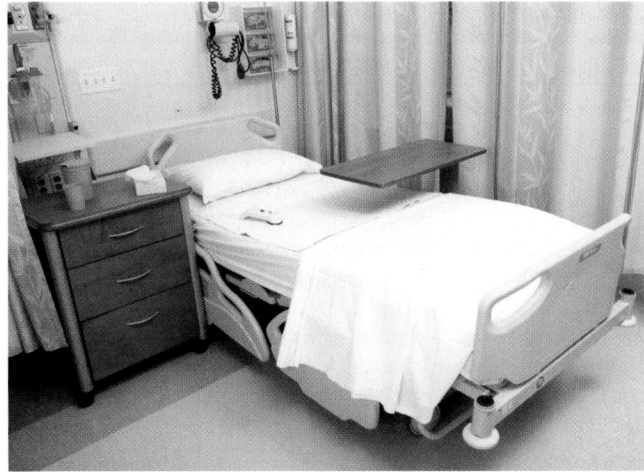

FIG. 40.7 Typical hospital room.

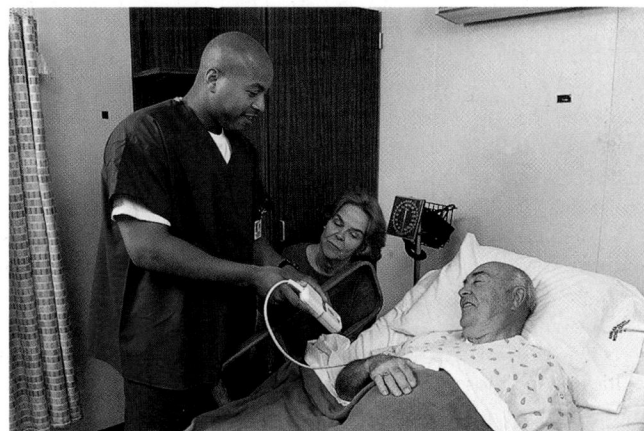

FIG. 40.8 Nurse instructing patient in use of nurse call system and bed controls.

Beds. Seriously ill patients often remain in bed for a long time. Because a bed is the piece of equipment used most by a hospitalized patient, it is designed for comfort, safety, and adaptability for changing positions. A typical hospital bed has a firm mattress on a metal frame that you can raise and lower horizontally. More and more hospitals are converting the standard hospital bed to one in which the mattress surface can be adjusted electronically for safety and comfort. For example, low beds are being used to prevent falls, and beds that regulate pressure in the mattress help to reduce pressure injuries. Different bed positions promote patient comfort, minimize symptoms, promote lung expansion, and improve access during certain procedures (Table 40.6).

You usually change the position of a bed by using electrical controls that are either incorporated into the patient's nurse call system or in a panel on the side or foot of the bed (see Fig. 40.8). Know how to use the bed controls. Ease in raising and lowering a bed and changing position of the head and foot eliminates undue musculoskeletal strain. Also instruct patients and family members in the proper use of controls and caution them against raising the bed to a position that causes the patient harm. Maintain the bed height at the lowest horizontal position when a patient is unattended.

Beds contain safety features such as locks on the wheels or casters. Lock wheels when a bed is stationary to prevent accidental movement. Side rails allow patients to move more easily in bed and prevent accidents. Do not use side rails to restrict a patient from moving in bed. When using side rails as a restraint, you need a health care provider's order (see Chapter 27). You can remove the headboard and footboard

TABLE 40.6 Common Bed Positions

Position	Description	Uses
Fowler's 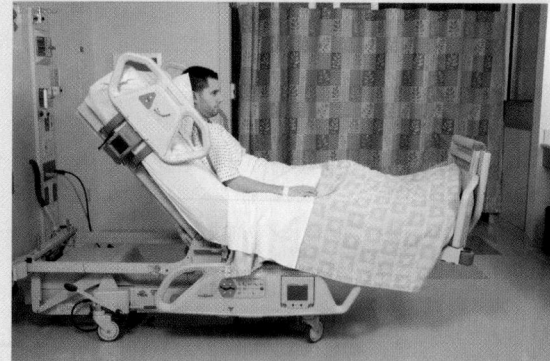	Head of bed raised to angle of 45 to 90 degrees; semi-sitting position; foot of bed may also be raised at knee	While patient is eating During nasogastric tube insertion and nasotracheal suction Promotes lung expansion Eases difficult breathing
Semi-Fowler's 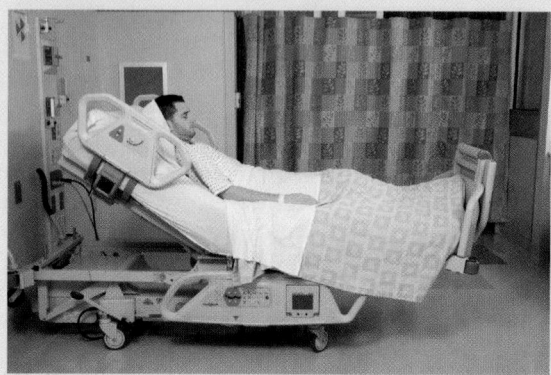	Head of bed raised approximately 30 to 45 degrees; inclination less than Fowler's position; foot of bed may also be raised at knee	Promotes lung expansion, especially with ventilator-assisted patients Used when patients receive oral care and for gastric feedings to reduce regurgitation and risk of aspiration
Trendelenburg's 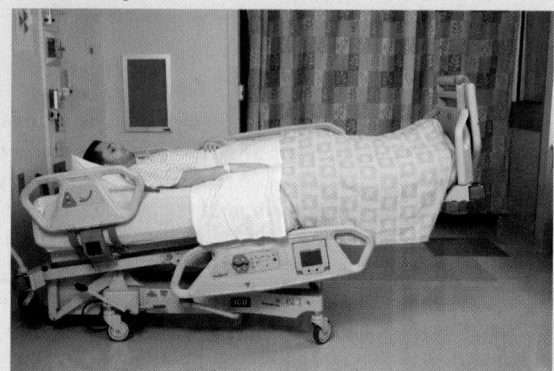	Entire bedframe tilted with head of bed down	Used for postural drainage Facilitates venous return in patients with poor peripheral perfusion
Reverse Trendelenburg's 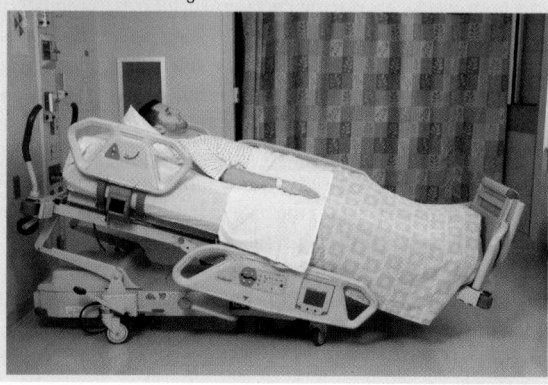	Entire bedframe tilted with foot of bed down	Used infrequently Promotes gastric emptying Prevents esophageal reflux

TABLE 40.6 Common Bed Positions—cont'd

Position	Description	Uses
Flat 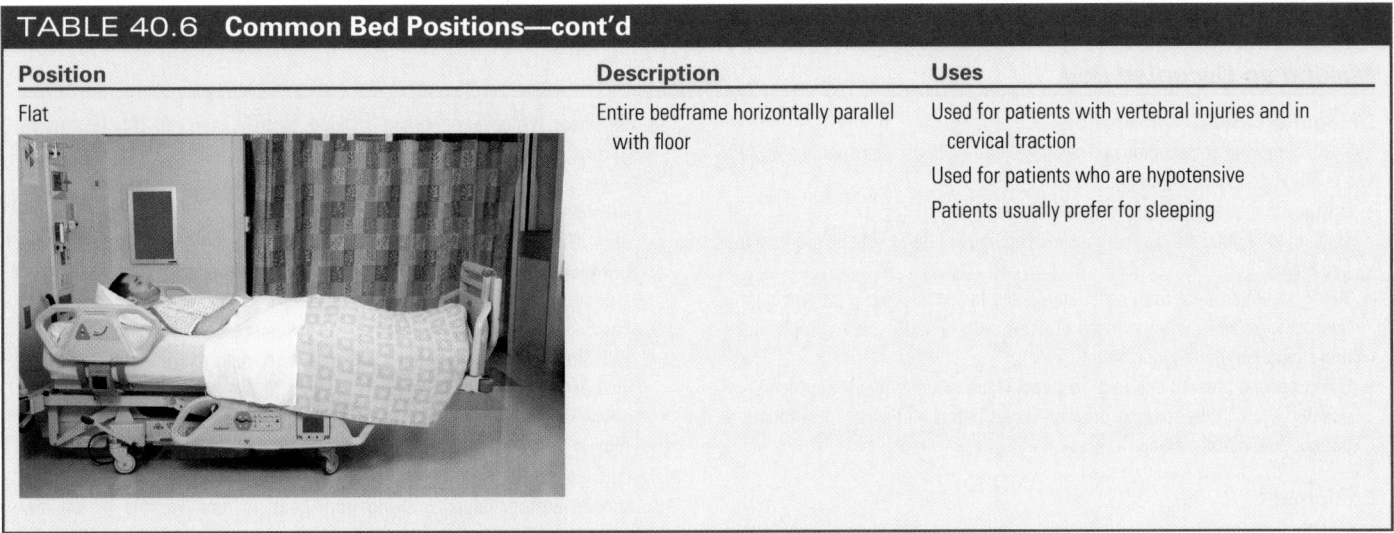	Entire bedframe horizontally parallel with floor	Used for patients with vertebral injuries and in cervical traction Used for patients who are hypotensive Patients usually prefer for sleeping

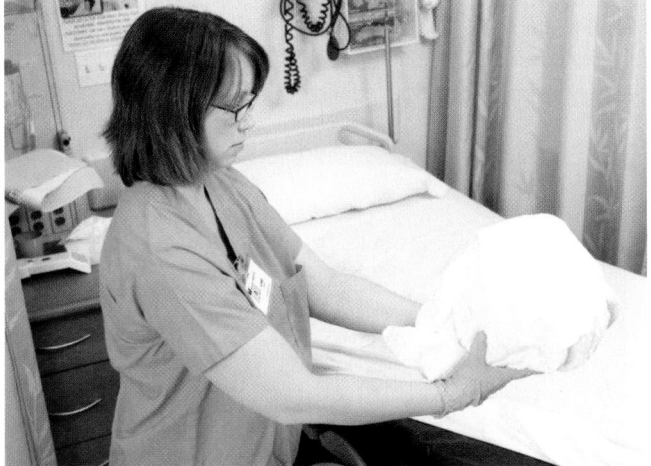

FIG. 40.9 Holding linen away from uniform prevents contact with microorganisms.

from most beds. This is important when the medical team needs to have easy access to the patient such as during cardiopulmonary resuscitation.

Bed Making. Keep a patient's bed clean and comfortable. This requires frequent inspection to be sure that linen is clean, dry, and free of wrinkles. When patients are diaphoretic, have draining wounds, or are incontinent, check more frequently for wet or soiled linen.

Usually you make a bed in the morning after patients bathe or while they bathe at a sink or in a shower, while sitting in a chair eating, or when out of the room for procedures or tests. Throughout the day straighten linen that is loose or wrinkled. Also check the bed linen for food particles after meals and for wetness or soiling. Change any linen that becomes soiled or wet.

When changing bed linen, follow principles of medical asepsis by keeping soiled linen away from your uniform (Fig. 40.9). Place soiled linen in special linen bags before placing in a hamper. To avoid air currents that spread microorganisms, never shake the linen. To avoid transmitting infection, do not place soiled linen on the floor. If clean linen touches the floor or any unclean surface, immediately place it in the dirty-linen container.

During bed making use safe patient-handling procedures (see Chapter 27). Always raise the bed to the appropriate height before changing linen so that you minimize the extent to which you bend or stretch over the mattress. Move back and forth to opposite sides of the bed while applying new linen. Body mechanics and safe handling are important when turning or repositioning a patient in bed.

When patients are confined to bed, you must make an occupied bed. Organize bed-making activities to conserve time and energy (Box 40.15). The patient's privacy, comfort, and safety are all important when making a bed. Using side rails to aid positioning and turning, keeping nurse call systems within the patient's reach, and maintaining the proper bed position help promote comfort and safety. After making a bed, return it to the lowest horizontal position and verify that the wheels are locked to prevent accidental falls when the patient gets in and out of the bed.

When possible, make the bed while it is unoccupied (Box 40.16). Use judgment to determine the best time for a patient to sit in a chair so you can make the bed. When making an unoccupied bed, follow the same basic principles as for occupied bed making.

An unoccupied bed can be made as an open or closed bed. In an open bed the top covers are folded back, so it is easy for a patient to get into bed. Draw up the top sheet, blanket, and bedspread to the head of the mattress and place a pillow at the top to make a closed bed. A closed bed is prepared in a hospital room before a new patient is admitted to that room. A surgical, recovery, or postoperative bed is a modified version of the open bed. The top bed linen is arranged for easy transfer of the patient from a stretcher to the bed. The top sheets and spread are not tucked or mitered at the corners. Instead they are folded to one side or to the bottom third of the bed (Fig. 40.10). This makes patient transfer into the bed easier.

Linens. Many agencies have "nurse servers" either within or just outside a patient's room to store a daily supply of linen. Because of the importance of cost control in health care, avoid bringing excess linen into a patient's room. Once you bring linen into a patient's room, if unused, it must be laundered before being used. Excess linen lying around a patient's room creates clutter and obstacles for patient care activities.

Before making a bed, collect necessary bed linens and the patient's personal items. In this way all equipment is accessible to prepare the bed and room. When fitted sheets are not available, flat sheets usually are pressed with a center crease to be placed down the center of the bed. The linens unfold easily to the sides, with creases often fitting over the mattress edge. Apply clean linens whenever there is soiling.

Handle linen properly to minimize the spread of infection (see Chapter 28). Agency policies provide guidelines for the proper way to bag and dispose of soiled linen. After a patient is discharged, all bed linen goes to the

BOX 40.15 PROCEDURAL GUIDELINE

Making an Occupied Bed

Delegation and Collaboration

The skill of making an occupied bed can be delegated to assistive personnel (AP). The nurse instructs the AP about:

- Any position or activity restrictions that apply.
- Looking for wound drainage or loosened equipment that might be found in the bed linens.
- When to obtain help from other caregivers for positioning a patient during linen change and the importance of using safe patient handling techniques and supporting patient alignment.
- Using special precautions (e.g., aspiration precautions [see Chapter 45] or positioning for tube-feeding infusion [see Chapter 45) when positioning a patient during bed making.

Equipment

Linen bags: mattress pad (change only when soiled); bottom sheet (flat or fitted); draw sheet *(optional)*; top sheet, blanket, bedspread, pillowcases; waterproof pads *(optional)*; clean gloves (if linen is soiled or there is risk of exposure to body fluids); antiseptic cleanser; washcloth

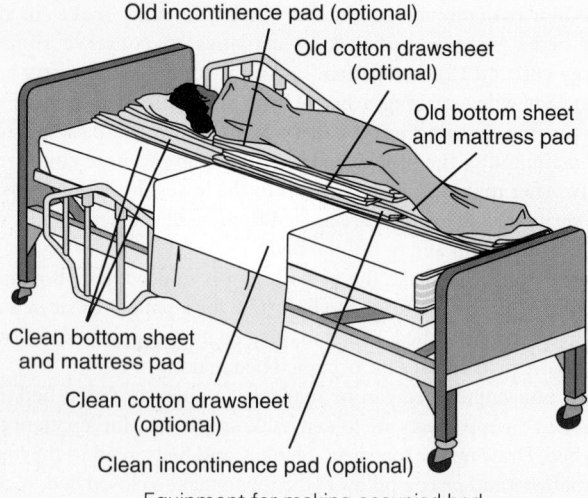

Equipment for making occupied bed.

Steps

1. Review medical record and assess restrictions in mobility/positioning of patient.
2. Organize supplies and close room door or divider curtain to provide privacy.
3. Assess environment for safety (e.g., check room for spills; make sure that equipment is working properly and that bed is in locked position and appropriate number of side rails are raised) (QSEN, 2018).
4. Perform hand hygiene. Apply clean gloves if patient has been incontinent or if drainage is present on linen.
5. Explain procedure to patient, noting that patient will be asked to turn over layers of linen.
6. Raise bed to a comfortable working height; lower head of bed (HOB) as tolerated, keeping patient comfortable. Remove nurse call system (if separate from bed rails).

   CLINICAL DECISION: If patient is on aspiration precautions or receiving tube feeding, keep HOB 30 degrees or higher at all times.

7. Lower side rail on side where you are standing. Loosen all top linen. Remove bedspread and blanket separately, leaving patient covered with top sheet. If blanket or spread is soiled, place in linen bag. If to be reused, fold into square and place over back of chair.
8. Cover patient with clean bath blanket by unfolding it over top sheet. Have patient hold top edge of bath blanket or tuck blanket under shoulders. Grasp top sheet under bath blanket at patient's shoulders and bring sheet down to foot of bed. Remove sheet and discard in dirty laundry bag.
9. Position patient on far side of bed, turned onto side and facing away from you. NOTE: This is when another caregiver can help you by standing at bedside across from you. Encourage patient to use side rail to turn. Adjust pillow under patient's head.
10. Assess to make sure that there is no tension on any external medical devices.
11. Loosen bottom linens, moving from head to foot. Fanfold or roll any cloth incontinence pads, drawsheet (if present), and bottom sheet (in that order) toward patient. Tuck edges of old linen just under patient's buttocks, back, and shoulders (see illustration). Do not fanfold mattress pad (if it is to be reused). Remove any disposable pads and discard in receptacle.

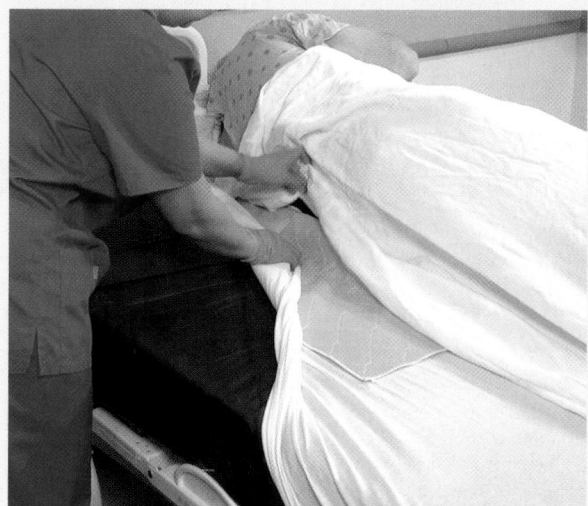

STEP 11 Tuck all soiled linen from one side of bed alongside patient's back.

12. Clean, disinfect, and dry mattress surface if it is soiled or has moisture (see agency policy).
13. Apply clean linens to the exposed half of bed in separate layers. When needed, start with a new mattress pad by placing it lengthwise with center crease in middle of bed. Fanfold pad to center of bed alongside patient. Repeat process with bottom sheet.
14. If bottom sheet is fitted, pull corners of new sheet smoothly over mattress corner at top and bottom of bed. Fold remaining portion of sheet across bed surface, toward patient's back.
15. If bottom sheet is flat, place over mattress. Allow edge of sheet closest to you to hang about 25 cm (10 inches) over mattress edge on side and at head of bed (HOB). Be sure that lower hem of bottom sheet lies seam down along bottom edge of mattress. Spread remaining portion of sheet over mattress toward patient's back.

BOX 40.15 PROCEDURAL GUIDELINE—cont'd

Making an Occupied Bed

16. For a flat sheet, Miter the top corner at HOB.
    a. Face HOB diagonally. Place hand away from HOB under top corner of mattress, near mattress edge, and lift.
    b. With other hand, tuck top edge of bottom sheet smoothly under mattress so that side edges of sheet above and below mattress meet when brought together.
    c. To miter a corner, pick up top edge of sheet at about 45 cm (18 inches) from top end of mattress (see illustration).

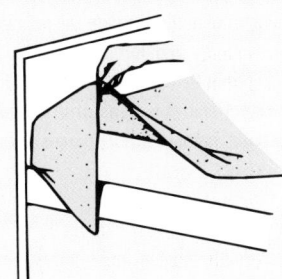

STEP 16c Top edge of sheet picked up.

    d. Lift sheet and lay it on top of mattress to form a neat triangular fold with lower base of triangle even with mattress side edges (see illustration).

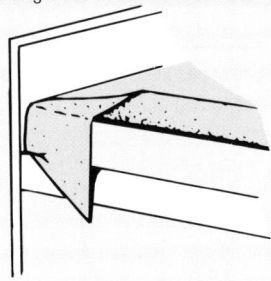

STEP 16d Sheet on top of mattress in a triangular fold.

    e. Tuck lower edge of sheet, which is hanging free below the mattress, under the mattress. Tuck with palms down, without pulling triangular fold.
    f. Hold part of sheet covering side of mattress in place with one hand (see illustrations). With other hand pick up top of triangular linen fold and bring it down over side of mattress. Tuck under mattress with palms down without pulling fold (see illustration).

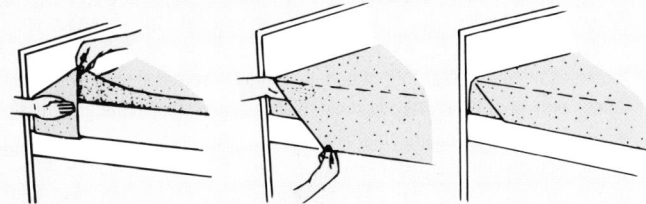

STEP 16f Triangular fold placed over side of mattress; sheet tucked under mattress.

17. Tuck remaining part of sheet under side of mattress, moving toward foot of bed. Keep linen smooth.
18. Place new drawsheet along middle of bed lengthwise. Fanfold or roll drawsheet on top of clean bottom sheet. Tuck under patient's buttocks and torso without touching old linen.

19. Add waterproof pad (absorbent side up) over drawsheet with seam side down. Fanfold toward patient. Continue to keep clean and soiled linen separate. Also keep linen under patient as flat as possible because patient will need to roll over old and new layers of linen when you are ready to make other side of bed.
20. Advise patient that he or she will be rolling over a thick layer of linens. Keeping patient covered, ask him or her to roll toward you slowly over layers of linen and to not raise the hips (see illustration). Stress the need to roll while staying aligned.

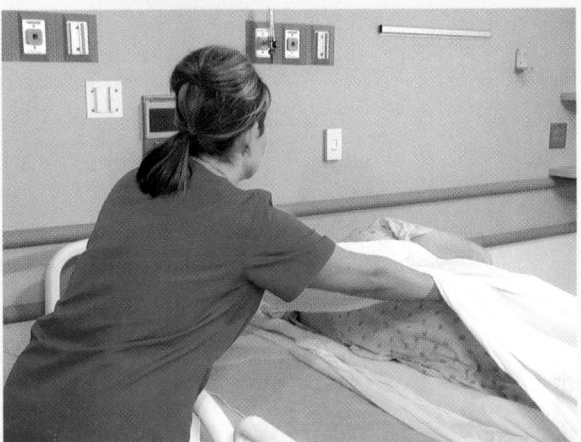

STEP 20 Patient begins rolling over layers of linen.

21. You will now raise side rail and move to opposite side of bed. *Option:* The caregiver helping you will help position patient. Have patient roll away from you toward other side of bed, over all of the folds of linen. Again, have patient keep hips still.
22. Lower side rail. Loosen edges of soiled linen from under mattress. Remove soiled linen by folding into a bundle or square.
23. Hold linen away from your body and place it in laundry bag.
24. Clean, disinfect, and dry other half of mattress as needed.
25. Pull clean, fan-folded or rolled mattress pad; sheet; drawsheet; and incontinence pad out from beneath patient toward you. Smooth all linen out over mattress from head to foot of bed. Help patient roll back to supine position and reposition pillow.
26. If bottom sheet is fitted, pull corners over mattress edges. Smooth out sheet.
27. If flat sheet is used, miter top corner of bottom flat sheet (see Steps 16a–f).
28. Facing side of bed, grasp remaining edge of bottom flat sheet. Lean back slightly, keep back straight, and pull while tucking excess linen under mattress from HOB to foot of bed. Avoid lifting mattress during tucking.
29. Smooth fanfolded drawsheet over bottom sheet (tucking is optional). Smooth waterproof incontinence pads, making sure that bed surface is wrinkle free.
30. Place top sheet over patient with vertical centerfold lengthwise down middle of bed and with seam side of hem facing up. Open sheet out from head to foot and unfold over patient. Be sure that top edge of sheet is even with top edge of mattress.
31. Place clean or reused bed blanket on bed over patient. Make sure that top edge is parallel with top edge of sheet and 15 to 20 cm (6 to 8 inches) from edge of top sheet. Raise side rail.
32. Go to other side of bed. Lower side rail. Spread sheet and blanket out evenly.
33. Have patient hold onto sheet and blanket while you remove bath blanket; discard in linen bag.
34. Make cuff by turning edge of top sheet down over top edge of blanket.
35. Make horizontal toe pleat; stand at foot of bed and fanfold in sheet and blanket 5 to 10 cm (2 to 4 inches) across bed. Pull sheet and blanket up from bottom to make fold approximately 15 cm (6 inches) from bottom edge of mattress.
36. Standing at side of bed, tuck in remaining part of sheet and blanket under foot of mattress. Tuck top sheet and blanket together. Be sure that toe pleats are not pulled out.

Continued

BOX 40.15 PROCEDURAL GUIDELINE—cont'd

Making an Occupied Bed

37. Make modified mitered corner with top sheet and blanket. (Follow Steps 16a–f.) After making triangular fold, do not tuck tip of triangle (see illustration).

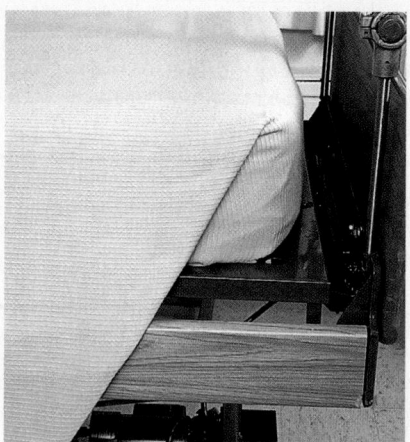

STEP 37 Modified mitered corner.

38. Go to other side of bed. Repeat Steps 35 and 36.
39. Change pillowcase. Have patient raise head. While supporting neck with one hand, remove pillow. Allow patient to lower head. Remove soiled case and place in linen bag. Grasp clean pillowcase at center of closed end. Gather case, turning it inside out over the hand holding it. With the same hand, pick up middle of one end of pillow. Pull pillowcase down over pillow with other hand. Do not hold pillow against your uniform. Be sure that pillow corners fit evenly into corners of case. Reposition pillow under patient's head.
40. Place nurse call system within patient's reach on bedrail or pillow; return bed to locked, low position; and raise side rail (as needed).
41. Place all linen in dirty laundry bag. Remove and dispose of gloves.
42. Arrange and organize patient's room and perform hand hygiene.
43. During procedure inspect skin for areas of irritation. Observe patient for signs of fatigue, dyspnea, pain, or other sources of discomfort.

BOX 40.16 PROCEDURAL GUIDELINES

Making an Unoccupied Bed

Delegation and Collaboration

The skill of making an unoccupied bed can be delegated to assistive personnel (AP).

Equipment

Linen bag, mattress pad (change only when soiled), bottom sheet (flat or fitted), drawsheet *(optional)*, top sheet, blanket, bedspread, waterproof pads *(optional)*, pillowcases, bedside chair or table, clean gloves (if linen is soiled), washcloth or paper towel, and antiseptic cleanser.

Steps

1. Perform hand hygiene. If patient has been incontinent or if excess drainage is on linen, gloves are necessary.
2. Assess activity orders or restrictions in mobility in planning if patient can get out of bed for procedure. Help to bedside chair or recliner.
3. Lower side rails on both sides of bed and raise bed to comfortable working position.
4. Remove soiled linen and place in laundry bag. Avoid shaking or fanning linen.
5. Reposition mattress and wipe off any moisture with a washcloth or paper towel moistened in antiseptic solution. Dry thoroughly.
6. Apply all bottom linen on one side of bed (before moving to opposite side):
   a. To apply a fitted sheet, be sure it is placed smoothly over mattress.
   b. To apply a flat unfitted sheet, allow about 25 cm (10 inches) to hang over sides of mattress edges (along sides and head of bed). Make sure that lower hem of sheet lies seam down, even with bottom edge of mattress. Pull remaining top part of sheet over top edge of mattress.
7. While standing at head of bed, miter top corner of bottom sheet (see Box 40.15, Steps 16a-f).
8. Tuck remaining part of unfitted sheet under mattress from head to foot of bed.
9. *Optional:* Apply drawsheet and waterproof incontinence pad, laying centerfolds along middle of bed lengthwise. Smooth draw sheet and pad over mattress and tuck excess edge of drawsheet under mattress, keeping palms down. Center position of pad over bottom sheet.
10. Move to opposite side of bed and spread bottom sheet smoothly over edge of mattress from head to foot of bed.
11. Apply fitted sheet smoothly over each mattress corner. For an unfitted sheet, miter top corner of bottom sheet (see Step 7), making sure that corner is taut.
12. Grasp remaining edge of unfitted bottom sheet and tuck tightly under mattress while moving from head to foot of bed.
13. Smooth folded drawsheet over bottom sheet and tuck under mattress, first at middle, then at top, and then at bottom.
14. If needed, apply single waterproof pad over bottom sheet or drawsheet.
15. Place top sheet over bed with vertical centerfold lengthwise down middle of bed. Open sheet out from head to foot, being sure that top edge of sheet is even with top edge of mattress.
16. Make horizontal toe pleat: stand at foot of bed and make fanfold in sheet 5 to 10 cm (2 to 4 inches) across bed. Pull sheet up from bottom to make fold approximately 15 cm (6 inches) from bottom edge of mattress.
17. Tuck in remaining part of sheet under foot of mattress. Place blanket over bed with top edge parallel to top edge of sheet and 15 to 20 cm (6 to 8 inches) down from edge of sheet. (*Optional:* Apply additional spread over bed.)
18. Make cuff by turning edge of top sheet down over top edge of blanket and spread.
19. Standing on one side at foot of bed, lift mattress corner slightly with one hand; with other hand tuck top sheet, blanket, and spread under mattress. Be sure that toe pleats are not pulled out.
20. Make modified mitered corner with top sheet, blanket, and spread. After making triangular fold, do not tuck tip of triangle (see Box 40.15, Step 37).
21. Go to other side of bed. Spread sheet, blanket, and spread out evenly. Make cuff with top sheet and blanket. Make modified corner at foot of bed.
22. Apply clean pillowcase.
23. Place nurse call system within patient's reach on bedrail or pillow and return bed to low position allowing for patient transfer. Lock wheels. Help patient to bed.
24. Arrange patient's room. Remove and discard supplies. Perform hand hygiene.

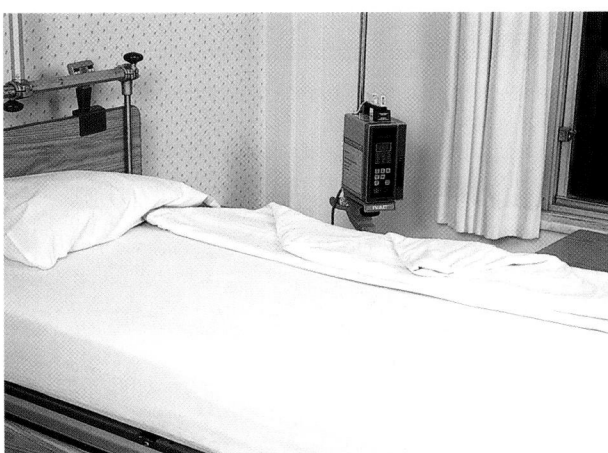

FIG. 40.10 Surgical or recovery bed.

laundry, and housekeeping cleans the mattress and bed before clean linen is applied.

◆ Evaluation

Through the Patient's Eyes. During assessment you collected information about a patient's expectations of care. Both during and after hygiene, determine from the patient whether care is being provided in an acceptable manner (Fig. 40.11). For example, while bathing a patient, encourage him or her to verbalize any discomfort such as too-cool water or discomfort with movement. To evaluate a patient's satisfaction with your care, ask questions, such as "Do you think your bath helped you feel more comfortable?" "Tell me ways we can make you feel less tired during your bath?" "Were you pleased with how we bathed and cleaned your feet?" Being aware of and addressing a patient's expectations and any concerns foster a caring therapeutic relationship.

Patient Outcomes. Evaluate patient responses to hygiene measures both during and after each particular hygiene intervention. For example, while bathing a patient, inspect the skin carefully to see whether soiling or drainage is effectively removed. Once a bath is completed, evaluate whether the patient feels more comfortable by asking him or her to rate the level of comfort using a pain scale (see Chapter 44). Frequently it takes time for hygiene care to result in an improvement in a patient's condition. While the presence of oral lesions, a scalp infestation, or skin excoriation often requires repeated measures and a combination of nursing interventions to fully resolve, you must evaluate these areas following hygiene measures. Your knowledge base and experience provide important perspectives when analyzing ongoing evaluation data about a patient. For example, frequent observation of the skin helps to determine the effectiveness of hygiene practices. Does a rash clear or a pressure injury show signs of healing? Is the patient able to complete hygiene care using adaptive equipment?

To evaluate a patient's or family caregiver's ability to perform self-care hygiene measures use teach-back. For example, say, "I want to be sure you are clear about why foot care is so important for you since you have diabetes. Tell me three things you can do to protect your feet from infection." As another example, say, "We talked about ways to prevent your skin from drying. Describe how you will protect your skin from dryness."

When established outcomes for the care plan are not met, revise it. Continue to apply critical thinking attitudes when considering all

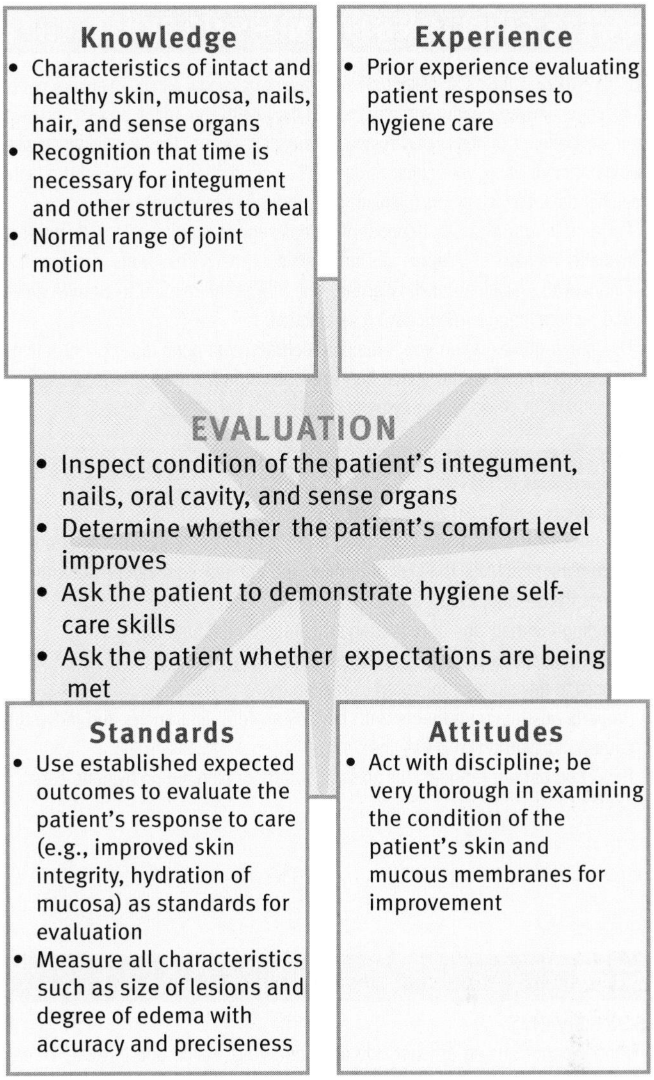

Knowledge
- Characteristics of intact and healthy skin, mucosa, nails, hair, and sense organs
- Recognition that time is necessary for integument and other structures to heal
- Normal range of joint motion

Experience
- Prior experience evaluating patient responses to hygiene care

EVALUATION
- Inspect condition of the patient's integument, nails, oral cavity, and sense organs
- Determine whether the patient's comfort level improves
- Ask the patient to demonstrate hygiene self-care skills
- Ask the patient whether expectations are being met

Standards
- Use established expected outcomes to evaluate the patient's response to care (e.g., improved skin integrity, hydration of mucosa) as standards for evaluation
- Measure all characteristics such as size of lesions and degree of edema with accuracy and preciseness

Attitudes
- Act with discipline; be very thorough in examining the condition of the patient's skin and mucous membranes for improvement

FIG. 40.11 Critical thinking model for hygiene evaluation.

evaluation findings. When outcomes are not met, ask questions by involving the patient to determine appropriate changes in interventions. Examples of questions include:

- What is preventing you from being able to perform your foot care at home?
- Which further measures do you think are necessary to keep your mouth feeling clean?
- What do you think would help you be more independent with your hygiene?

QSEN **Building Competency in Patient Safety** Mrs. White is discharged to her home. Her granddaughter and a home care aide will provide care for her over the next few weeks. During evaluation you note that Mrs. White is making progress using the walker and bath-adaptive equipment that have been ordered for home care. Which assessments should be made for her following discharge from the hospital? What teaching needs to be provided to the family member to perform safe hygiene care for her grandmother?

Answers to QSEN Activities can be found on the Evolve website.

SAFETY GUIDELINES FOR NURSING SKILLS

Ensuring patient safety is an essential role of the professional nurse. To ensure patient safety, communicate clearly with members of the health care team, assess and incorporate the patient's priorities of care and preferences, and use the best evidence when making decisions about your patient's care. When performing the skills in this chapter, remember the following points to ensure safe, individualized patient care.

- Patients who are totally dependent on a caregiver require help with personal hygiene measures. Always perform hygiene measures while moving from cleanest to less clean or dirty areas. This often requires you to change gloves and perform hand hygiene during care activities.
- Use clean gloves when you anticipate contact with nonintact skin or mucous membranes or when there is or may likely be contact with drainage, secretions, excretions, or blood during hygiene care.

- When using water or solutions for hygiene care, be sure to test the temperature to prevent burn injury.
- Use principles of body mechanics and safe patient handling to avoid injury to patient or self when performing hygiene care (QSEN, 2018).
- You are responsible and accountable for the care provided. Give proper direction to AP when delegating hygiene measures.
- Monitor laboratory findings, such as coagulation studies, before administering oral hygiene.
- Determine patient's or family caregiver's knowledge, experience, and health literacy. Ensures patient or family caregiver has the capacity to obtain, communicate, process, and understand basic health information (CDC, 2019).

SKILL 40.1   BATHING AND PERINEAL CARE

Delegation and Collaboration

Assessment of the patient's skin, pain level, and ROM cannot be delegated to assistive personnel (AP). The skill of bathing and perineal care can be delegated to AP. Direct the AP about:

- Avoiding the massage of reddened skin areas during bathing.
- Contraindications to soaking a patient's feet.
- Reporting any signs of impaired skin integrity to the nurse.
- Properly positioning patients with musculoskeletal limitations and indwelling catheters or intravenous (IV) lines.
- Reporting patient fatigue, shortness of breath, or pain during hygiene care.

Equipment

- Washcloths and bath towels
- Bath blanket
- Bar or liquid soap, or 4-oz bottle of 2% to 4% chlorhexidine gluconate (CHG) (dispensed in a single bath-size bottle) (*option:* 2% CHG bathing cloths)
- Toiletry items (deodorant, lotion). NOTE: If using CHG, use a hospital-approved lotion.
- Disposable wipes
- Warm water
- Clean hospital gown or patient's own pajamas or gown
- Laundry bag
- Clean gloves
- Washbasin dedicated for bathing only
- Eye patch/shield and nonallergenic tape (for unconscious patient)

STEP	RATIONALE

ASSESSMENT

1. Identify patient using at least two identifiers (e.g., name and birthday or name and medical record number) according to agency policy.

Ensures correct patient. Complies with The Joint Commission standards and improves patient safety (TJC, 2020).

2. Review medical record for orders for specific precautions concerning patient's movement or positioning and whether there is an order for a therapeutic bath.

Prevents accidental injury to patient during bathing activities. Determines level of help that patient needs.

3. Assess patient's or family caregiver's knowledge, experience, and health literacy.

Ensures patient or family caregiver has the capacity to obtain, communicate, process, and understand basic health information (CDC, 2019).

4. Perform hand hygiene. Assess patient's fall risk status (if partial bathing out of bed or self-bath is to be performed).

Reduces transmission of microorganisms. Allows you to anticipate needed precautions such as having patient sit on chair in front of basin.

5. Assess patient's tolerance for bathing: activity tolerance, comfort level during movement, cognitive function, musculoskeletal function, and presence of shortness of breath (see Chapter 30).

Determines patient's comfort level and ability to perform or tolerate bathing and level of assistance required (e.g., tub bath, partial bed bath).

6. If cognitive level is reduced, assess patient's cognitive (Mini-Mental State Examination) and functional status (e.g., Barthel's index or the index of activities of daily living [ADLs] to measure self-care ability). For patients with suspected dementia, observe behavior, especially after telling patient it is bath time; does he or she become agitated?

Every person entering a long-term care setting should be formally assessed for cognitive and functional status (Hirschman et al., 2018; Shelton et al., 2018). Functional status assesses a patient's capacity for self-bathing and how much supervision/help is needed to accomplish daily ADL tasks. Every attempt should be made to avoid bathing people against their will.

CLINICAL DECISION: *Patients with dementia may become agitated and aggressive during bathing activities. Consider using alternative bathing procedures such as bag wipes with these patients (Villar et al., 2018). Maintain a calm, nonthreatening, quiet environment using therapeutic communication (see Box 40.6).*

STEP	RATIONALE
7. Assess patient's visual status, ability to sit without support, hand grasp, ROM of extremities.	Determines degree of assistance patient needs for bathing. ROM may be delegated to assistive personnel.
8. Assess for presence and position of external medical device/equipment (e.g., intravenous [IV] line, oxygen tubing, Foley catheter).	Affects how you plan bathing activities and positioning. Helps determine how to set up supplies.
9. Assess for allergy or sensitivity to bathing products and CHG.	When allergy or sensitivity is present, select another cleansing solution.
10. Assess patient's bathing preferences: frequency and time of day preferred, type of hygiene products used, and other factors related to patient preferences.	Patient participates in plan of care. Promotes patient's comfort and willingness to cooperate. Incorporates cultural or personal hygiene preferences into care.
11. Ask whether patient has noticed any problems related to condition of skin and genitalia: excess moisture, inflammation, drainage or excretions from lesions or body cavities, rashes or other skin lesions.	Provides you with information to direct physical assessment of skin and genitalia during bathing. Also influences selection of skin care products.
12. Before or during bath assess condition of patient's skin. Note presence of dryness, indicated by flaking, redness, scaling, and cracking.	Provides a baseline for comparison over time in determining whether bathing improves condition of skin.
13. Assess patient's knowledge of skin hygiene in terms of its importance, preventive measures to take, and common problems.	Determines patient's learning needs.

PLANNING

1. Assess room environment for safety (e.g., check room for spills; make sure that equipment is working properly and that bed brakes are locked and bed is in low position).	Identifies safety hazards in patient environment that could cause or potentially lead to harm (QSEN, 2018).
2. Adjust room temperature and ventilation, close room doors and windows, and draw room divider curtain.	Warm room that is free of drafts prevents rapid loss of body heat during bathing. Privacy provides for patient's mental and physical comfort.
3. Prepare equipment and place supplies on bedside table. If it is necessary to leave room, be sure that nurse call system is within patient's reach, bed is in low position, side rails up (as appropriate) and brakes are locked.	Avoids interrupting procedure or leaving patient unattended to retrieve missing equipment. Provides for patient safety.
4. Explain procedure and ask patient for suggestions on how to prepare supplies. If partial bath, ask how much of bath patient wishes to complete. If using CHG, explain benefit of reducing infection and that solution leaves a sticky feeling on the skin.	Promotes patient's cooperation and participation. Patients who prefer using their own bathing supplies may need to discuss benefits of CHG.

IMPLEMENTATION

1. Offer patient bedpan or urinal. Apply clean gloves to help patient as needed. Provide toilet tissue and dispose of any excrement properly. Provide patient towel and moist washcloth. Dispose of gloves if applied and perform hand hygiene.	Patient feels more comfortable after voiding. Prevents interruption of bath. Reduces transmission of microorganisms.
2. Complete or partial bed bath	
a. If patient has nonintact skin or skin is soiled with drainage, excretions, or body secretions, apply clean gloves. Ensure that patient is not allergic to latex.	Prevents allergic reaction if latex gloves are used.
b. Verify that bed is in locked position and raise bed to comfortable working height. Lower side rail closest to you and help patient into comfortable supine position, maintaining body alignment. Bring patient toward side closest to you.	Prevents bed from moving. Helps you reach patient without stretching and reaching across bed, thus minimizing strain on back muscles.
c. Place bath blanket over patient and loosen and remove top covers without exposing him or her. If possible, have patient hold top of bath blanket while you remove linen. Place soiled linen in laundry bag. Take care to not allow linen to touch your uniform. *Optional:* Use top sheet when bath blanket is not available or if patient prefers.	Bath blanket provides warmth and privacy during bath.
d. Remove patient's gown or pajamas.	Provides full exposure of body parts during bathing.
(1) If gown with ties or snaps on sleeves, simply untie or unsnap and remove gown without pulling IV line (if present).	

Continued

SKILL 40.1	BATHING AND PERINEAL CARE—cont'd

STEP	RATIONALE

STEP

(2) If regular gown is used and patient has reduced mobility and IV access, remove gown from *unaffected side first.*

(3) If patient has an IV line and gown with no snaps, remove gown from arm without IV line first. Then remove gown from arm with IV line (see illustration A). Pause IV fluid infusion by pressing appropriate sensor on IV pump. Remove IV tubing from pump; use regulator to slow IV infusion. Remove IV bag from pole (see illustration B) and slide IV bag and tubing through arm of patient's gown (see illustration C). Rehang IV bag (see illustration D), reconnect tubing to pump, open regulator clamp, and restart IV fluid infusion by pressing appropriate sensor on IV pump. If IV fluids are infusing by gravity, check IV flow rate and regulate if necessary. *Do not disconnect IV tubing to remove gown.*

e. Raise side rail. Lower bed temporarily to lowest position. Go and fill washbasin two-thirds full with warm water Place basin and supplies on over-bed table. Raise bed to comfortable working height. Check water temperature and also have patient place fingers in water to test temperature tolerance. Place plastic container of bath lotion in bath water to warm if desired.

f. Lower side rail, remove pillow if tolerated, and raise head of bed 30 to 45 degrees if allowed. Place bath towel under patient's head. Place second bath towel over patient's chest.

g. Wash face.

RATIONALE

Undressing unaffected side first allows easier manipulation of gown over body part with reduced ROM.

Manipulation of IV tubing and container may disrupt flow rate. Do **not** delegate regulation of IV flow rate to AP.

Raising side rail and lowering bed position maintain patient's safety while you leave bedside. Keeping bed at working height during bath prevents back strain. Warm water promotes comfort, relaxes muscles, and prevents unnecessary chilling. CHG is most effective at full strength. Testing temperature prevents accidental burns. Bath water warms lotion for application to patient's skin.

Removal of pillow makes it easier to wash patient's ears and neck. Placing towels prevents bed linen and bath blanket from getting soiled or wet.

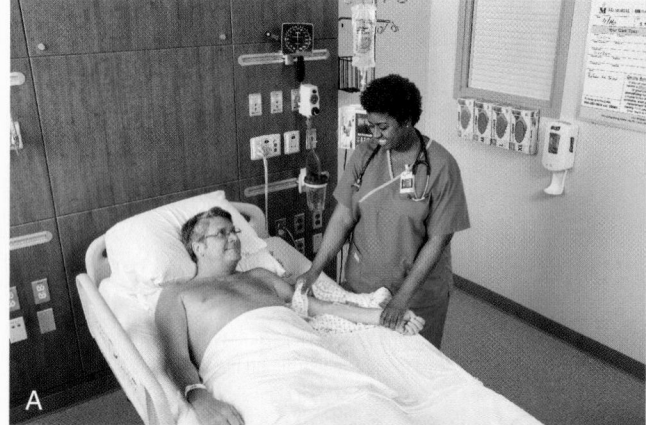
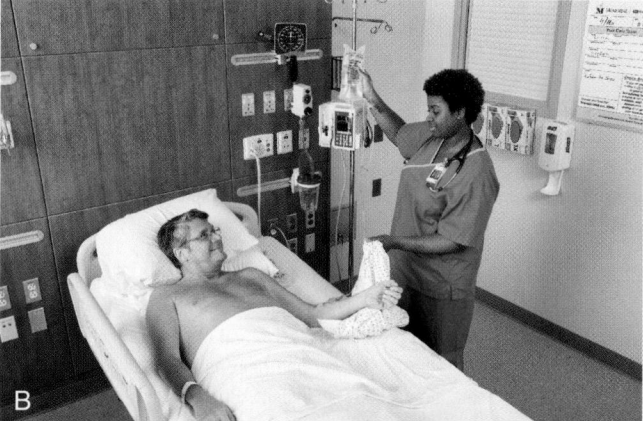
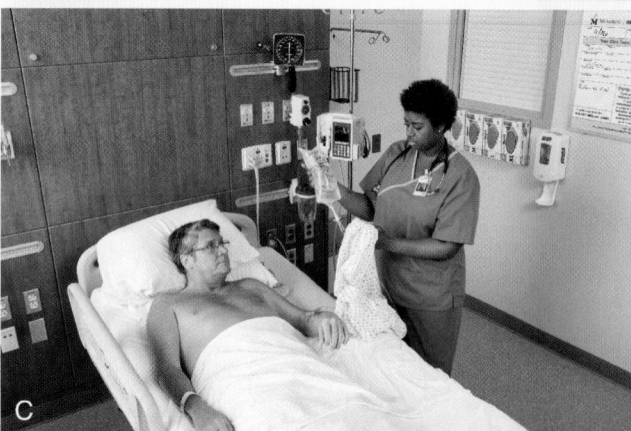
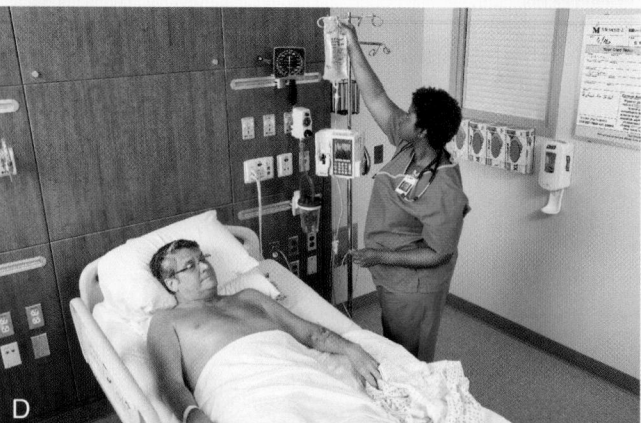

STEP 2d(3) A, Remove patient's gown. **B,** Remove IV tubing from pole. **C,** Slide IV tubing through arm of patient's gown. **D,** Rehang IV bag.

STEP	RATIONALE

CLINICAL DECISION: *Do not use bath water with 4% CHG solution or 2% CHG bathing cloths on the eyes or face. Only use clear water or mild soap and water on the face.*

(1) Ask whether patient is wearing contact lenses. You may choose to remove them at this time.

Prevents accidental injury to eyes.

(2) Fold washcloth around fingers of your hand to form a mitt (see illustration). Immerse mitt in water and wring thoroughly.

Mitt retains water and heat better than loosely held washcloth; keeps cold edges from brushing against patient and prevents splashing.

(3) Wash patient's eyes with plain warm water. Use different section of mitt for each eye. Move mitt from inner to outer canthus (see illustration). Soak any crusts on eyelid for 2 to 3 minutes with damp cloth before attempting removal. Dry eyes thoroughly but gently.

Soap irritates eyes. Use of separate sections of mitt reduces infection transmission. Bathing eye from inner to outer canthus prevents secretions from entering nasolacrimal duct. Pressure can cause internal injury.

(4) Ask whether patient prefers to use soap on face. Otherwise wash, rinse, and dry forehead, cheeks, nose, neck, and ears without using soap. (Men may wish to shave at this point or wait until after bath.)

Soap tends to dry face, which is exposed to air more than other body parts.

(5) Provide eye care for unconscious patient.

Patients who are unconscious have lost the normal protective corneal reflex of blinking, increasing the risk for corneal drying, abrasions, and eye infection (Demirel et al., 2014).

(a) Instill eyedrops or ointment per health care provider's order (see Chapter 31).

Keeps cornea lubricated.

(b) In the absence of blink reflex, keep eyelids closed. Close eye gently, using back of your fingertip, before placing eye patch or shield. Place tape over patch or shield. Do not tape eyelid.

When blink reflex is absent, patient loses a protective mechanism. Keeping eyelids closed maintains eye moisture and prevents injury (Kocacal et al., 2018).

h. Wash trunk and upper extremities.
Option: Change bath water at this time or, if using 4% CHG solution, pour entire 4 ounce single-use container into basin.

Evidence shows that CHG use in daily bathing can reduce incidence of hospital-acquired infections (Martin et al., 2017; Shah et al., 2016). CHG reduces bacteria for up to 24 hours and prevents infection (AHRQ, 2013).

CLINICAL DECISION: *When using CHG in a bath basin of water, use one washcloth for washing each major body part. Then dispose of cloth and use a new cloth for the next body part (Martin et al., 2017). Dipping cloth back into basin contaminates solution and makes CHG less effective. Do not rinse after bathing with CHG solution. Allow CHG to dry on the skin to achieve antimicrobial effects.*

(1) Remove bath blanket from patient's arm that is closest to you. Place bath towel lengthwise under arm. Bathe arm with soap and water using long, firm strokes from distal to proximal areas (fingers to axilla).

Towel prevents soiling of bed. Soap lowers surface tension and facilitates removal of debris and bacteria when friction is applied during washing. Long, firm strokes stimulate circulation; moving distal to proximal promotes venous return.

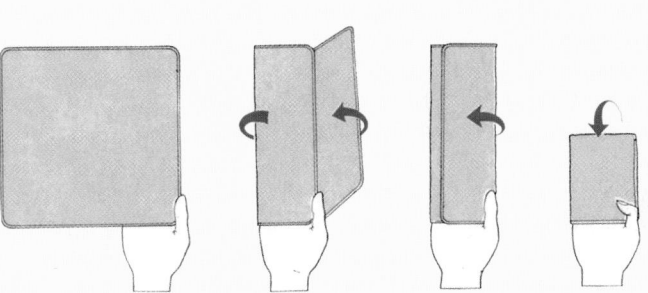

STEP 2g(2) Steps for folding washcloth to form a mitt.

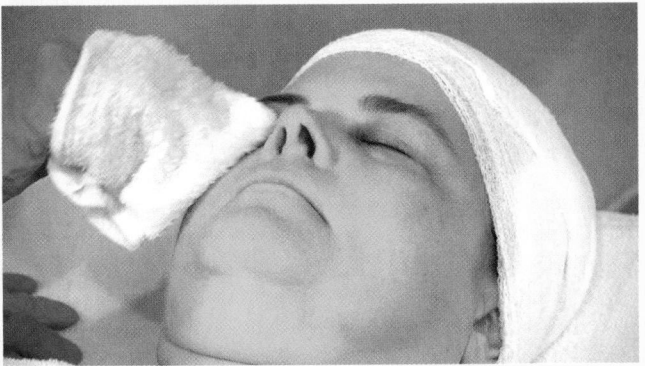

STEP 2g(3) Wash eye from inner to outer canthus. (Copyright © Mosby's Clinical Skills: Essentials Collection.)

Continued

SKILL 40.1	BATHING AND PERINEAL CARE—cont'd

STEP	RATIONALE
(2) Raise and support arm above head (if possible) to wash, rinse, and dry axilla thoroughly (see illustration). Apply deodorant or powder to underarms if desired or needed.	Movement of arm exposes axilla and exercises normal ROM of joint. Alkaline residue from soap discourages growth of normal skin bacteria. Drying prevents excess moisture, which can cause skin maceration or softening. Respect patient's preference for use of hygiene products.
(3) Move to other side of bed and repeat Steps (1) and (2) with other arm.	Provides for better access to patient and helps prevent back strain.
(4) Cover patient's chest with bath towel and fold bath blanket down to umbilicus. Bathe chest with long, firm strokes. Take special care with skin under female patient's breasts, lifting breast upward if necessary while bathing underneath breast. Rinse if using soap and water and dry well.	Draping prevents unnecessary exposure of body parts. Towel maintains warmth and privacy. Secretions and dirt collect easily in areas of tight skinfolds. Skin under breasts is vulnerable to excoriation if not kept clean and dry.
i. Wash hands and nails.	
(1) Fold bath towel in half and lay it on bed beside patient. Place basin on towel. Immerse patient's hand in water. Allow hand to soak for 2 to 3 minutes before washing hand and fingernails. Remove basin and dry hand well. Repeat for other hand.	Soaking softens cuticles and calluses of hand, loosens debris beneath nails, and enhances feeling of cleanliness. Thorough drying removes moisture between fingers.

CLINICAL DECISION: *Do not routinely soak fingers of patient with diabetes mellitus.*

STEP	RATIONALE
j. Check temperature of bath water and change water when cool or soapy. (See agency policy regarding changing water when using CHG solution.)	Warm water maintains patient's comfort. Alkaline soap residue is irritating to skin and can decrease the normal protectiveness of acid pH.

CLINICAL DECISION: *If patient is at risk for falling, be sure that two side rails are up before obtaining fresh water. In addition, lower bed when it is necessary to leave bedside.* NOTE: *Having all side rails raised is considered a restraint. Check agency policy.*

STEP	RATIONALE
k. Wash abdomen.	
(1) Place bath towel lengthwise over chest and abdomen. (Two towels may be needed.) Fold bath blanket down to just above pubic region. With one hand lift bath towel. With mitted hand bathe and rinse abdomen, giving special attention to umbilicus and skinfolds of abdomen and groin. Stroke from side to side. Keep abdomen covered between washing and rinsing. Rinse and dry well.	Draping prevents unnecessary exposure of body parts. Towel maintains warmth and privacy. Keeping skinfolds clean and dry helps prevent odor and skin irritation. Moisture and sediment that collect in skinfolds predispose skin to maceration.
(2) Apply clean gown or pajama top. If an extremity is injured or immobilized, dress affected side first. (This step may be omitted until completion of bath; gown should not become soiled during remainder of bath.)	Maintains patient's warmth and comfort. Dressing affected side first allows easier manipulation of gown over body part with reduced ROM.

CLINICAL DECISION: *If one extremity is injured or immobilized, always dress affected side first.*

STEP	RATIONALE
l. Wash lower extremities.	
(1) Cover chest and abdomen with top of bath blanket. Expose near leg by folding blanket toward midline. Be sure to keep other leg and perineum draped. Place bath towel under leg as you support patient's knee and ankle.	Prevents unnecessary exposure.

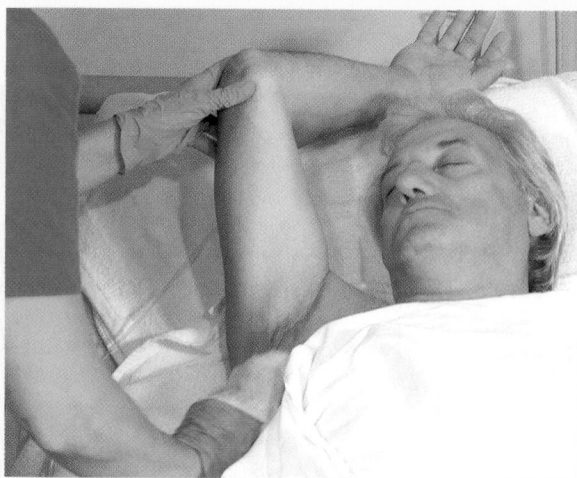

STEP 2h(2) Positioning arm to wash axilla. (Copyright © Mosby's Clinical Skills: Essentials Collection.)

STEP	RATIONALE

(2) Wash leg using long, firm strokes from ankle to knee and from knee to thigh (see illustration). Rinse and dry well. Remove and discard towel.

Promotes circulation and venous return. Excess massage of calf could loosen deep vein thrombus. Secretions and moisture may be present between toes, predisposing patient to maceration and breakdown. **Do Not cut nails of a patient with diabetes.** See agency policy for podiatrist care.

CLINICAL DECISION: *When bathing lower extremities, assess for signs of warmth, redness, swelling, tenderness, and pain in the lower extremities because these might be early signs of deep vein thrombosis (DVT).*

(3) Clean foot, making sure to bathe between toes. Rinse and dry toes and feet completely. Clean and file nails as needed (see Skill 40.2).

(4) Raise side rail, move to opposite side of bed, lower side rail, and repeat Steps (2) and (3) for other leg and foot. If skin is dry, apply moisturizer. When finished, cover patient with bath blanket.

Well-lubricated skin is less at risk for breakdown.

(5) Cover patient with bath blanket, raise side rail for patient's safety, remove and dispose of soiled gloves, and perform hand hygiene. Change bath water and/or CHG solution and water.

Decreased bath water temperature causes chilling. Clean water reduces micro-organism transmission to perineal structures.

m. Provide perineal hygiene.

(1) If patient can maneuver and handle washcloth, allow him or her to clean perineum on own.

Maintains patient's dignity and self-care ability.

CLINICAL DECISION: *CHG is safe to use on the perineum and external mucosa (AHRQ, 2013).*

(2) Female patient

(a) Apply pair of clean gloves. Lower side rail. Help patient into dorsal recumbent position. Note restrictions or limitations in patient's positioning. Place waterproof pad under patient's buttocks. Drape patient with bath blanket placed in shape of a diamond. Lift lower edge of bath blanket to expose perineum (see illustration).

Provides full exposure of female genitalia. If patient is totally dependent, provide assistance to support her in side-lying position and raise leg as perineum is bathed. If position causes patient discomfort, reduce degree of abduction in her hips.

(b) Fold lower corner of bath blanket up between patient's legs onto abdomen. Wash and dry patient's upper thighs.

Keeping patient draped until procedure begins minimizes anxiety. Buildup of perineal secretions soils surrounding skin surfaces.

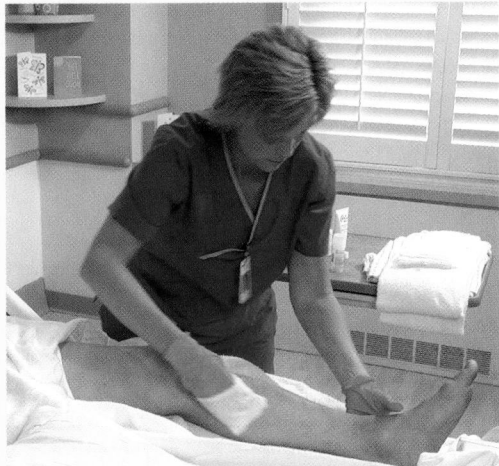

STEP 2l(2) Washing leg. (Copyright © Mosby's Clinical Skills: Essentials Collection.)

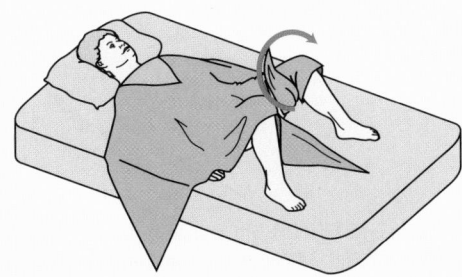

STEP 2m(2)(a) Drape patient for perineal care.

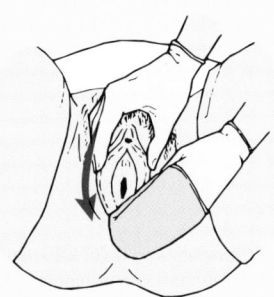

STEP 2m(2)(d) Cleanse from perineum to rectum (front to back).

Continued

SKILL 40.1   BATHING AND PERINEAL CARE—cont'd

STEP	RATIONALE
(c) Wash labia majora. Use nondominant hand to gently retract labia from thigh; with dominant hand wash carefully in skinfolds. Wipe in direction from perineum to rectum. Repeat on opposite side with separate section of washcloth. Rinse and dry area thoroughly.	Perineal care involves thorough cleaning of patient's external genitalia and surrounding skin. Skinfolds may contain body secretions that harbor microorganisms. Wiping front to back reduces chance of transmitting fecal organisms to urinary meatus.
(d) Gently separate labia with nondominant hand to expose urethral meatus and vaginal orifice. With dominant hand, wash downward from pubic area toward rectum in one smooth stroke (see illustration). Wash middle and both sides of perineum. Use separate section of cloth for each stroke. Clean thoroughly around labia minora, clitoris, and vaginal orifice. Avoid placing tension on indwelling catheter if present and clean area around it thoroughly.	Cleansing method reduces transfer of microorganisms to urinary meatus. (For menstruating women or patients with indwelling catheters, clean with cotton balls.)
(e) Provide catheter care as needed per agency requirements (see Chapter 46).	Proper cleansing around periurethral area and catheter reduces the risk for catheter-associated urinary tract infections (CAUTI) (CDC, 2015).
(f) Rinse area thoroughly. May use bedpan and pour warm water over perineal area. Dry thoroughly from front to back.	Rinsing removes soap and microorganisms more effectively than wiping. Retained moisture harbors microorganisms.
(g) Fold lower corner of bath blanket back between patient's legs and over perineum. Ask patient to lower legs and assume comfortable position.	
(3) Male patient	
(a) Apply pair of clean gloves. Lower side rail. Help patient to supine position. Note any restriction in mobility.	Provides full exposure of male genitalia. Position patients who are unable to lie supine on their side.
(b) Fold lower half of bath blanket up to expose upper thighs. Wash and dry thighs.	Buildup of perineal secretions soils surrounding skin surfaces.
(c) Cover thighs with bath towels. Raise bath blanket up to expose genitalia. Gently raise penis and place bath towel underneath. Gently grasp shaft of penis. If patient is uncircumcised, retract foreskin (see illustration). If patient has an erection, defer procedure until later.	Draping minimizes patient anxiety. Towel prevents moisture from collecting in inguinal area. Gentle but firm handling of penis reduces chance of an erection. Secretions capable of harboring microorganisms collect underneath foreskin.
(d) Wash tip of penis at urethral meatus first. Using circular motion, clean from meatus outward (see illustration). Discard washcloth and repeat with clean cloth until penis is clean. Rinse and dry gently.	Direction of cleaning moves from area of least contamination to area of most contamination, preventing microorganisms from entering urethra.
(e) Return foreskin to its natural position. This is extremely important in patients with decreased sensation in their lower extremities.	Tightening of foreskin around shaft of penis causes local edema and discomfort. Patients with reduced sensation do not feel tightening of foreskin.
(f) Gently clean shaft of penis and scrotum by having patient abduct legs. Pay special attention to underlying surface of penis. Lift scrotum carefully and wash underlying skinfolds. Rinse and dry thoroughly.	Vigorous massage of penis may cause an erection. Underlying surface of penis is an area where secretions accumulate. Abduction of legs provides easier access to scrotal tissues. Secretions collect easily between skinfolds.
(g) Avoid placing tension on indwelling catheter if present and clean area around it thoroughly. Provide catheter care (see Chapter 46).	Cleaning along catheter from exit site reduces incidence of nosocomial urinary infection.
(4) Remove soiled gloves and discard in trash; raise side rail before leaving bedside to dispose of water and obtain fresh water.	Prevents transmission of infection. Protects patient from injury.
n. Wash back. (This follows both female and male perineal care.)	
(1) Perform hand hygiene and apply clean pair of gloves. Lower side rail. Help patient into prone or side-lying position (as applicable). Place towel lengthwise along patient's side and keep him or her covered with bath blanket.	Exposes back and buttocks for bathing while limiting exposure.

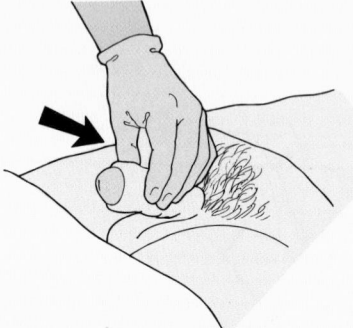

STEP 2m(3)(c) Retract foreskin.

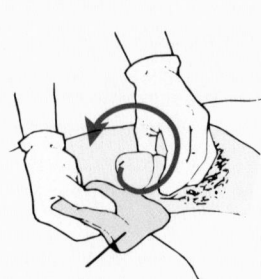

STEP 2m(3)(d) Use circular motion to clean tip of penis.

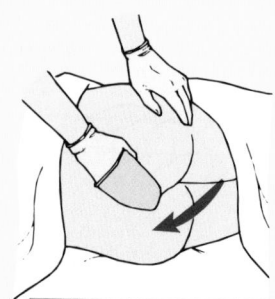

STEP 2n(5) Cleanse buttocks from front to back.

STEP	RATIONALE

(2) Keep patient draped by sliding bath blanket over shoulders and thighs during bathing. Wash, rinse, and dry back from neck to buttocks using long, firm strokes.

Cleaning back before buttocks and anus prevents contamination of water.

(3) Next move from back to buttocks and anus. Have patient remain in prone or side-lying position and keep covered to avoid chilling. Clean anus and buttocks area.

Exposes back and buttocks for bathing while limiting exposure.

(4) If fecal material is present, enclose in fold of underpad or toilet tissue and remove with disposable wipes.

Skinfolds near buttocks and anus may contain fecal secretions that harbor microorganisms.

(5) Clean buttocks and anus, washing front to back (see illustration). Clean, rinse, and dry area thoroughly. If needed, place a clean absorbent pad under patient's buttocks. Remove contaminated gloves. Raise side rail and perform hand hygiene.

Cleaning motion prevents contaminating perineal area with fecal material or microorganisms.

3. Return to bed and lower side rail; give a back rub (see Chapter 44).

Promotes patient relaxation. Make sure that back rub is appropriate for your patient. Back rubs are contraindicated in some cardiac patients.

   a. Apply additional body lotion or oil to patient's skin as needed. When finished, raise side rail.

Moisturizing lotion prevents dry, chapped skin.

4. Remove soiled linen and place in dirty-linen bag. Clean and replace bathing equipment. Perform hand hygiene.

Reduces transmission of microorganisms.

5. Help patient dress. Comb patient's hair. If a woman wants to apply makeup, help as needed.

Promotes patient's body image.

6. Make patient's bed (see Boxes 40.15 and 40.16).

Provides clean, comfortable environment.

7. Check function and position of external devices (e.g., indwelling urethral catheters, nasogastric tubes, IV lines).

Ensures that systems remain functional after bathing activities.

8. Place bed in lowest position. Wheels locked. Side rails up as appropriate.

Maintains patient's safety by decreasing height of bedframe from floor.

9. Replace nurse call system and personal possessions. Leave room as clean and comfortable as possible. Perform hand hygiene.

Prevents transmission of infection. Clean environment promotes patient's comfort. Keeping nurse call system and articles of care within reach promotes patient's safety.

10. **Optional Bathing Methods**

   a. Commercial bag bath or CHG cleansing pack:

     (1) A cleansing pack contains six to eight premoistened towels for cleaning. Warm package contents in microwave following package directions. If you are bathing patient using warm commercial or CHG cloth, check temperature of cloth before use. Gloves diminish sense of heat.

Provides warm, soothing heat. CHG reduces bacteria for up to 24 hours and prevents infection (AHRQ, 2013). Prevents burn to skin.

     (2) Use all six CHG cloths in the following order (see illustration):

Reduces transmission of microorganisms.

- Cloth 1: Neck, shoulders, and chest
- Cloth 2: Both arms, both hands, web spaces, and axilla
- Cloth 3: Abdomen and then groin/perineum
- Cloth 4: Right leg, right foot, and web spaces
- Cloth 5: Left leg, left foot, and web spaces
- Cloth 6: Back of neck, back, and buttocks

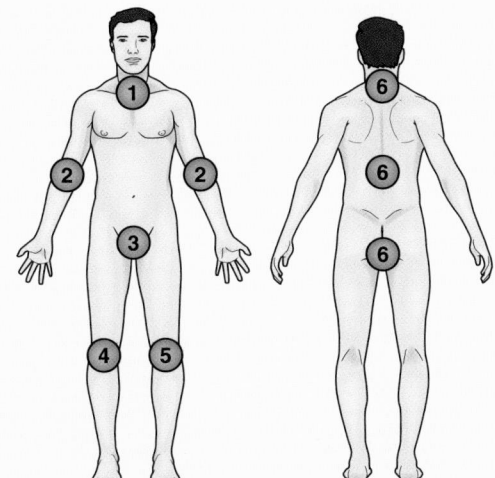

STEP 10a(2) Using CHG bathing cloths. (From Universal ICU decolonization: *An enhanced protocol.* Appendix E: *Training and educational materials,* Rockville, MD, September 2013, Agency for Healthcare Research and Quality.)

Continued

STEP	RATIONALE
(3) Firmly massage skin when using cloth. Allow skin to air-dry for 30 seconds. Do not rinse. It is permissible to lightly cover patient with bath towel to prevent chilling.	Drying skin with towel removes emollient that is left behind after water/cleaner solution evaporates.
(4) **NOTE:** If there is excessive soiling (e.g., in perineal region), use an extra cloth or conventional washcloths, soap, water, and towels.	

b. Tub bath or shower:

STEP	RATIONALE
(1) Consider patient's condition and review orders for precautions concerning his or her movement or positioning.	Prevents accidental injury to patient during bathing.
(2) Schedule use of shower or tub.	Prevents unnecessary waiting, which causes fatigue.
(3) Check tub or shower for cleanliness. Use cleaning techniques outlined in agency policy. Place rubber mat on tub or shower bottom. Place disposable bath mat or towel on floor in front of tub or shower.	Cleaning prevents transmission of microorganisms. Mats prevent slipping and falling.
(4) Collect all hygienic aids, toiletry items, and linens requested by patient. Place within easy reach of tub or shower.	Placing items close at hand prevents possible falls when patient reaches for equipment.
(5) Help patient to bathroom if necessary. Have him or her wear robe and slippers.	Assistance prevents accidental falls. Wearing robe and slippers prevents chilling.
(6) Demonstrate how to use call signal in bathroom for assistance.	Bathrooms are equipped with signaling devices in case patient feels faint or weak or needs immediate assistance. Patients prefer privacy during bath if safety is not jeopardized.
(7) Place "occupied" sign on bathroom door.	Maintains patient's privacy.
(8) Fill bathtub halfway with warm water. Check temperature of bath water, have patient test water, and adjust temperature if water is too warm. Explain which faucet controls hot water. If patient is taking shower, turn shower on and adjust water temperature before he or she enters shower stall. Use shower seat or tub chair if needed (see illustration).	Adjusting water temperature prevents accidental burns. Older adults and patients with neurological alterations (e.g., diabetes, spinal cord injury) are at high risk for burn as a result of reduced sensation. Use of assistive devices facilitates bathing and minimizes physical exertion.
(9) Instruct patient to use safety bars when getting in and out of tub or shower to pull cord to summon assistance (if available). Caution patient against use of bath oil in tub water.	Prevents slipping and falling. Oil causes tub surfaces to become slippery.
(10) Instruct patient not to remain in tub longer than 10 or 15 minutes. Check on him or her every 5 minutes.	Prolonged exposure to warm water causes vasodilation and pooling of blood in some patients, leading to light-headedness or dizziness.
(11) Return to bathroom when patient signals and knock before entering.	Provides privacy.
(12) For patient who is unsteady, drain tub of water before he or she tries to get out. Place bath towel over patient's shoulders. Help patient out of tub as needed and help with drying.	Prevents accidental falls. Patient may become chilled as water drains.

CLINICAL DECISION: *Weak or unstable patients need extra assistance in getting out of a tub. Planning for additional personnel is essential before attempting to help the patient. Lift equipment may be used for transfer. See agency policy.*

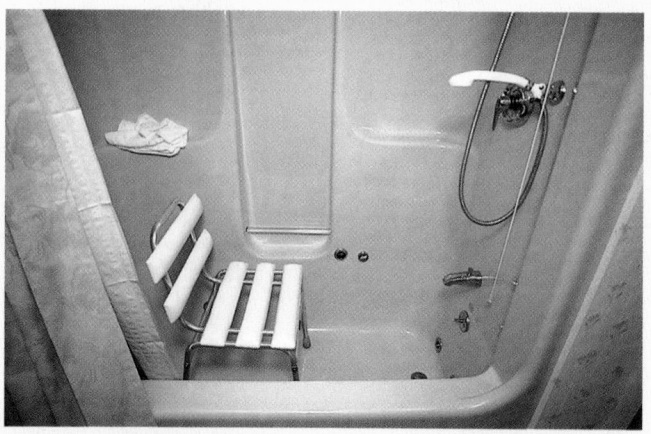

STEP 10b(8) Shower seat for patient safety.

STEP	RATIONALE
c. Help patient as needed with getting dressed in clean gown or pajamas, slippers, and robe. (In home setting patient may put on regular clothing.)	Maintains warmth to prevent chilling.
d. Help patient to room and comfortable position in bed or chair.	Maintains relaxation gained from bathing.
e. Clean tub or shower according to agency policy.	Prevents transmission of infection through soiled linen and moisture.
f. Remove soiled linen and place in dirty-linen bag. Discard disposable equipment in proper receptacle. Place "unoccupied" sign on bathroom door. Return supplies to storage area.	Reduces transmission of infection.
g. Perform hand hygiene.	Reduces transfer of microorganisms.

EVALUATION

1. Observe skin, paying particular attention to areas previously soiled, reddened, dry, or showing early signs of pressure or pressure injuries.	Techniques used during bathing leave skin clean and clear. Over time dry skin diminishes. If patient shows areas of redness, use Braden scale to measure risk for pressure injury (see Chapter 48).
2. Observe ROM during bath.	Measures joint mobility.
3. Ask patient to rate level of comfort (on a scale of 0-10).	Determines patient's tolerance of bathing activities.
4. Ask patient to rate level of fatigue (on a scale of 0-10).	Determines patient's tolerance of bathing activities.
5. **Use Teach-Back:** "We talked about the importance of keeping your skin clean with these special bathing cloths. Explain to me why we are using bathing cloths for your bath." Revise your instruction now or develop a plan for revised patient/family caregiver teaching if patient/family caregiver is not able to teach back correctly.	Determines patient's/family caregiver's level of understanding of instructional topic.

UNEXPECTED OUTCOMES AND RELATED INTERVENTIONS

1. Areas of excessive dryness, rashes, or pressure injuries appear on skin.
   - Complete pressure injury assessment (see Chapter 48).
   - Apply moisturizing lotions or topical skin applications per agency policy.
   - Limit frequency of complete baths. It may become necessary (if patient has a sensitivity to CHG) to switch to plain soap and water.
   - Obtain special bed surface if patient is at risk for skin breakdown.
2. Patient becomes excessively tired or unable to cooperate or participate in bathing.
   - Reschedule bathing to a time when patient is more rested.
   - Provide pillow or elevate head of bed during bath for patient with breathing difficulties.
   - Notify health care provider if this is a change in patient's fatigue level.
   - Perform hygiene measures in stages between scheduled rest periods.
3. The rectum, perineum, or genital area is inflamed or swollen or has foul-smelling odor.
   - Bathe perineal area frequently enough to keep clean and dry.
   - Obtain an order for a sitz bath.
   - Apply protective barrier ointment or anti-inflammatory cream.
   - Report findings to health care provider.

RECORDING AND REPORTING

- Record procedure, amount of assistance provided, patient's participation in care, condition of skin, and any significant findings (e.g., reddened areas, breaks in skin, inflammation, ulcerations).
- Document your evaluation of patient learning.
- Report any skin irritations, breaks in skin, or ulcerations to nurse in charge or health care provider. These are serious in patients with altered circulation to the lower extremities.
- Report intolerance of activity to patient's oncoming nurse.

HOME CARE CONSIDERATIONS

- Assess patient's tub and shower area for need for safety devices (e.g., grab bars, shower chair, handheld shower).
- Assess patient for the need for assistive bathing devices (e.g., long-handle sponge, mirrors, or lift equipment).

Continued

SKILL 40.2   PERFORMING NAIL AND FOOT CARE

Delegation and Collaboration

The skill of nail and foot care of patients *without diabetes mellitus* or *peripheral vascular disease* can be delegated to assistive personnel (AP). The nurse instructs the AP about:

- Not trimming patient's nails (unless permitted by agency or health care provider).
- Special considerations for patient positioning.
- Reporting any breaks in skin, redness, numbness, swelling, or pain to the nurse.

Equipment

- Washbasin
- Emesis basin
- Washcloth and towel
- Nail clippers (check agency policy)
- Soft nail or cuticle brush
- Plastic applicator stick
- Emery board or nail file
- Body lotion
- Disposable bath mat
- Clean gloves

STEP	RATIONALE
ASSESSMENT	
1. Identify patient using at least two identifiers (e.g., name and birthday or name and medical record number) according to agency policy.	Ensures correct patient. Complies with The Joint Commission standards and improves patient safety (TJC, 2020).
2. Verify health care provider's order for cutting nails (check agency policy).	Patients with diabetes or reduced peripheral circulation are more at risk for infection. Accidental cutting of skin increases risk for infection.
3. Perform hand hygiene. Apply clean gloves if drainage is present. Inspect all surfaces of fingers, toes, feet, and nails. Pay particular attention to areas of dryness, inflammation, or cracking. Also inspect areas between toes, heels, and soles of feet.	Integrity of feet and nails determines frequency and level of hygiene required. Heels, soles, and sides of feet are prone to irritation from ill-fitting shoes.

CLINICAL DECISION: *Patients with peripheral vascular diseases or diabetes mellitus, older adults, and patients whose immune system is suppressed often require nail care from a specialist to reduce the risk of tissue injury and infection. Defer care other than washing the feet in these cases until patient has been evaluated.*

STEP	RATIONALE
4. Assess color and temperature of toes, feet, and fingers. Assess capillary refill of nails. Palpate radial and ulnar pulse of each hand and dorsalis pedis pulse of each foot; note character of pulses (see Chapter 30). Remove and dispose of gloves. Perform hand hygiene.	Assesses adequacy of blood flow to extremities. Circulatory alterations often change integrity of nails and increase patient's chance of localized infection when break in skin integrity occurs.
5. Assess patient's or family caregiver's knowledge, experience, and health literacy.	Ensures patient or family caregiver has the capacity to obtain, communicate, process, and understand basic health information (CDC, 2019).
6. Assess type of footwear worn by patients, including type and cleanliness of socks worn, type and fit of shoes, and whether restrictive garters or knee-high hose are worn.	Types of shoes and footwear predispose patient to foot and nail problems (e.g., infection, areas of friction, ulcerations). These conditions decrease mobility and increase risk for amputation in patient with diabetes (Chapman, 2017).
7. If possible, observe patients walking to assess their gait.	Alterations in bony structures of the foot or sores cause pain, imbalance, and unsteady gait.
8. Ask female patients whether they use nail polish and polish remover frequently.	Chemicals in these products cause excessive dryness.
9. Identify patients at risk for foot or nail problems.	Certain conditions increase risk for foot or nail problems.
a. Older adult	Normal physiological changes such as poor vision, lack of coordination, or inability to bend over contribute to difficulty in performing foot and nail care (Touhy and Jett, 2018).
b. Diabetes mellitus, peripheral vascular disease	Vascular changes associated with diabetes mellitus reduce blood flow to peripheral tissues. Break in skin integrity places patient with diabetes at high risk for skin infection.
c. Heart failure, renal disease	Both conditions increase tissue edema, particularly in dependent areas (e.g., feet). Edema reduces blood flow to neighboring tissues.
d. Cerebrovascular accident (stroke)	Presence of residual foot or leg weakness or paralysis results in altered walking patterns. Altered gait pattern causes increased friction and pressure on feet.
10. Assess type of home remedies that patient or family caregiver uses for existing foot problems (use this time for instruction):	Certain preparations or applications cause more injury to soft tissue than initial foot problem.
a. Over-the-counter liquid preparations to remove corns	Liquid preparations cause burns and ulcerations.
b. Cutting corns or calluses with razor blade or scissors	Cutting corns or calluses sometimes results in infection caused by a break in skin integrity. The patient with diabetes or any patient with decreased peripheral circulation has an increased risk for infection secondary to a break in skin integrity.

STEP	RATIONALE
c. Use of oval corn pads	Oval pads exert pressure on toes, thereby decreasing circulation to surrounding tissues.
d. Application of adhesive tape	Skin of older adult is thin and delicate and prone to tearing when adhesive tape is removed.
11. Assess patient's ability to care for nails or feet: visual alterations, fatigue, and musculoskeletal weakness.	Determines patient's ability to perform self-care and degree of assistance required from nurse.
12. Assess patient's knowledge of foot and nail care practices.	Ensures patient has the capability to obtain, communicate, process, and understand basic health information (CDC, 2019).

PLANNING

1. Assess environment for spills on floor and make sure that bed brakes are locked and bed is in low position.	Ensures patient safety.
2. Collect appropriate equipment and arrange on over-bed table.	Provides each access to equipment and promotes an organized procedure.
3. Close room door or pull curtain around patient's bed.	Provides privacy.
4. Explain procedure, including need to soak feet, which requires several minutes.	Patient needs to be able to place fingers and feet in basin for 10 to 20 minutes. Some patients may become tired.

IMPLEMENTATION

1. Assist ambulatory patient to seated position in bedside chair. Help bed-bound patient to supine position with head of bed elevated. Place disposable bath mat or towel on floor under patient's feet, or place towel on bed.	Sitting in chair facilitates immersion of feet in basin. Bath mat or towel protects feet from exposure to soil or microorganisms on floor; towel lessens chance of splashing water on floor or bed.

CLINICAL DECISION: *Soaking the feet of patients with diabetes mellitus or peripheral vascular disease is not recommended. Soaking may lead to maceration (excessive softening of the skin) and drying of the skin (ADA, 2020), leading to tissue breakdown and infection.*

2. Adjust over-bed table to low position and place it over patient's lap. (Patient sits in chair or lies in bed.)	Easy access prevents accidental spills.
3. Fill washbasin with warm water. Test water temperature. Place basin on floor and lower side rail or place basin on waterproof pad on the mattress. Assist patient to immerse feet.	Warm water softens nails and thickened epidermal cells, reduces inflammation of skin, and promotes local circulation. Proper water temperature prevents burns.
4. Instruct patient to place fingers in emesis basin and arms in comfortable position.	Prolonged positioning causes discomfort unless normal anatomical alignment is maintained.
5. Allow patient's feet and fingernails to soak for 10 to 20 minutes. Rewarm water after 10 minutes. **NOTE:** If patient is diabetic or has peripheral vascular disease, skip this step.	Softening corns, calluses, and cuticles ensures easy removal of dead cells and easy manipulation of cuticle. *Do not soak if patient has diabetes.*
6. Perform hand hygiene and apply clean gloves. Clean gently under nails with plastic applicator stick or soft brush while immersing fingers (see illustration).	Removes debris under nails that harbors microorganisms.
7. Use soft cuticle brush or nail brush to clean around cuticles to decrease overgrowth.	Nail brush helps prevent inflammation and injury to cuticles. The cuticle grows slowly over the nail and must be pushed back with a soft nail brush regularly.

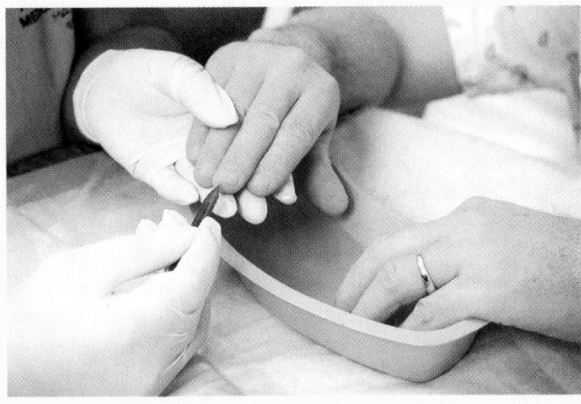

STEP 6 Clean under fingernails.

Continued

SKILL 40.2	PERFORMING NAIL AND FOOT CARE—cont'd

STEP	RATIONALE

CLINICAL DECISION: *Check agency policy regarding appropriate nail care for cleaning under nail and trimming. Do not use orange stick or end of cotton swab.*

STEP	RATIONALE
8. Remove hands from basin and dry thoroughly.	Thorough drying impedes fungal nail growth and prevents maceration of tissues.
9. File fingernails straight across and even with tops of fingers. If permitted by agency policy, use nail clippers and clip fingernails straight across and even with tops of fingers (see illustration); then smooth nail, using file. Remove and dispose of gloves and perform hand hygiene.	Reduces tearing or splitting of nails. Shaping corners of nails can damage tissues.
10. Move over-bed table away from patient and begin foot care. Apply clean gloves and scrub callused areas of feet with washcloth.	Provides easier access to patient's feet. Friction removes dead skin layers. Gloves prevent transmission of fungal infection.
11. Clean between toes with washcloth.	Areas between toes harbor debris.
12. Dry feet thoroughly and clean under nails (see Step 6).	Nails harbor debris and dirt and are a source of potential infection from poor care habits (Ball et al., 2019).
13. Trim toenails using procedures in Step 9. Do not file corners of toenails. Check agency policy for trimming patient's nails.	Shaping corners of toenails damages tissues, which increases the risk for infection (Jeffcoate et al., 2018).
14. Apply lotion to hands and feet. Rub in thoroughly. Do not leave excess lotion between toes.	Lotion lubricates dry skin by helping to retain moisture.
15. Assist patient back to bed or into a comfortable chair.	
16. Be sure nurse call system is within reach and patient knows how to use it.	Ensures patient can ask for assistance if needed.
17. Sanitize equipment according to agency policy. Dispose of used equipment, remove and dispose of gloves and perform hand hygiene.	Reduces transmission of infection.

CLINICAL DECISION: *Instruct patients to report any of the following to their health care provider: abnormalities or changes in the nail, including changes in nail shape or color; bleeding around the nails; thinning or thickening of the nails; and redness, swelling, or pain around the nails.*

EVALUATION

1. Inspect nails, cuticles, and areas between fingers and toes and surrounding skin surfaces.	Inspection enables you to evaluate condition of skin and nails. Allows you to note any remaining rough nail edges.
2. When possible, observe patient walking after foot and nail care.	Evaluates level of comfort and whether nail care removed excess skin or uneven nail surfaces that caused discomfort or problems with mobility.
3. **Use Teach-Back:** "I want to be sure you know what problems you can have if you do not trim your nails correctly. Show me how to properly trim your toenails." Revise your instruction now or develop a plan for revised patient/family caregiver teaching if patient/family caregiver is not able to teach back correctly.	Determines patient's/family caregiver's level of understanding of instructional topic.

UNEXPECTED OUTCOMES AND RELATED INTERVENTIONS

1. Cuticles and surrounding tissues are inflamed and tender to touch.
   - Repeated soakings are necessary to relieve inflammation and loosen layers of skin cells.
   - Patients with peripheral vascular disease or diabetes often require referral to a podiatrist.
   - Evaluate need for antifungal cream.

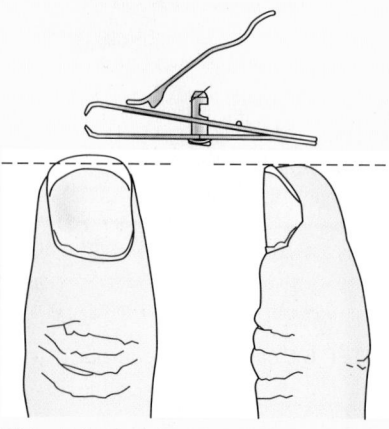

STEP 9 Trim nails straight across when using nail clipper.

2. Localized areas of tenderness occur on feet with calluses or corns at point of friction.
   - Recommend a change in footwear if necessary.
   - Refer to a podiatrist or nurse in charge.
3. Tissue injury appears between toes or other pressure areas in foot.
   - Notify physician or nurse in charge.
   - Implement appropriate pressure injury interventions (see Chapter 48).

RECORDING AND REPORTING

- Record procedure and observations of integument (e.g., breaks in skin, inflammation, ulcerations).
- Report any breaks in skin or ulcerations to nurse in charge or physician. These are serious in patients with peripheral vascular disease and illnesses in which patient's circulation is impaired. Special foot-care treatments are often necessary.
- Document your evaluation of patient learning.

HOME CARE CONSIDERATIONS

- Instruct family and patient to remove foot hazards from the home, e.g., throw rugs, objects that block pathways, or uneven flooring.
- Alternative therapies: moleskin applied to areas of feet that are under friction is less likely to cause pressure to tissues; wrapping small pieces of lamb's wool around toes reduces irritation of soft corns between toes.
- Provide contact information for a podiatrist; this is especially important for patients with diabetes or peripheral vascular disease.

SKILL 40.3   PERFORMING MOUTH CARE FOR AN UNCONSCIOUS OR DEBILITATED PATIENT

Delegation and Collaboration

The skill of providing oral hygiene to an unconscious or debilitated patient can be delegated to assistive personnel (AP). The nurse is responsible for assessing a patient's gag reflex. The nurse instructs the AP to:

- Have another AP assist and properly position patient for mouth care.
- Be aware of aspiration precautions.
- Use an oral suction catheter for clearing oral secretions (see Chapter 41, Skill 41.1).
- Report any lesions or bleeding of mucosa or gums, excessive coughing, or choking to the nurse.

Equipment

- Small pediatric, soft-bristled toothbrush, toothette sponges, or suction toothbrushes for patients for whom brushing is contraindicated
- Antibacterial solution per agency policy (e.g., chlorhexidine gluconate [CHG] 0.12%)
- Fluoride toothpaste
- Water-based mouth moisturizer
- Tongue blade
- Penlight
- Oral suction equipment
- Oral airway (uncooperative patient or patient who shows bite reflex)
- Water-soluble lip lubricant
- Water glass with cool water
- Face and bath towel
- Emesis basin
- Clean gloves

STEP	RATIONALE
ASSESSMENT	
1. Identify patient using at least two identifiers (e.g., name and birthday or name and medical record number) according to agency policy.	Ensures correct patient. Complies with The Joint Commission standards and improves patient safety (TJC, 2020).
2. Assess patient's risk for oral hygiene problems (see Procedural Guideline 40.9).	Certain conditions increase likelihood of alterations in integrity of oral cavity mucosa and structures, necessitating more frequent care.
3. Perform hand hygiene and apply clean gloves.	Reduces transmission of microorganisms in blood or saliva.
4. Assess for presence of gag reflex by placing tongue blade on back half of tongue.	Helps in determining aspiration risk.

> **CLINICAL DECISION:** *Patients with impaired gag reflex are unable to clear airway secretions and often accumulate secretions in the back of the oral cavity and have a higher risk for aspiration. Keep suction equipment available when caring for patients who are at risk for aspiration.*

5. Inspect condition of oral cavity. Inspect lips, teeth, gums, buccal mucosa, palate, and tongue using tongue depressor and penlight if necessary (see Chapter 30). Observe for color, moisture, lesions, injury or ulcers, and condition of teeth or dentures.	Determines condition of oral cavity and need for hygiene. Establishes baseline to show improvement following oral care.

> **CLINICAL DECISION:** *The critically ill patient with an artificial airway and who is on mechanical ventilation is at risk for ventilator-associated pneumonia (VAP). Once intubated, the artificial airway causes a bypass of normal airway defenses, which also causes a rapid change in the normal oral flora (IHI, 2018; Klompas et al., 2014). Some patients require mouth care as often as every 1 to 2 hours until the mucosa returns to normal.*

6. Assess patient's respirations or oxygen saturation.	Assists in early recognition of aspiration.
7. Remove and dispose of gloves. Perform hand hygiene.	Prevents transmission of infection.

Continued

SKILL 40.3	PERFORMING MOUTH CARE FOR AN UNCONSCIOUS OR DEBILITATED PATIENT—cont'd

STEP	RATIONALE

PLANNING

1. Assess environment for safety (e.g., check the room for spills, make sure that suction equipment is working properly, and check that bed is in locked, low position).
2. Gather equipment and supplies at bedside.

3. Close room door or pull curtain around bed
4. Explain procedure to patient or family caregiver if present.

Identifies safety hazards in patient environment that could cause or potentially lead to harm (QSEN, 2018).
Avoids interrupting procedure or leaving patient unattended to retrieve missing equipment.
Provides privacy
Even debilitated or intubated patients are usually able to hear. Explanation can reduce anxiety.

IMPLEMENTATION

1. Perform hand hygiene and apply clean gloves.
2. Raise bed to appropriate working height; lower side rail.
3. Unless contraindicated (e.g., head injury, neck trauma), position patient in Sims' or side-lying position. Turn patient's head toward mattress in dependent position with HOB elevated at least 30 degrees.
4. Place towel on over-bed table and arrange equipment. If needed, turn on suction machine and connect tubing to suction catheter.
5. Place second towel under patient's head and emesis basin under chin.
6. Remove dentures or partial plates if present.
7. If patient is uncooperative or having difficulty keeping mouth open, insert an oral airway. Insert upside down and turn airway sideways and over tongue to keep teeth apart. Insert when patient is relaxed if possible. Do not use force.

Reduces transfer of microorganisms.
Promotes good body mechanics for caregiver.
Position promotes drainage of secretions from mouth instead of collecting in back of pharynx. Prevents aspiration.

Prevents soiling of tabletop. Equipment prepared in advance ensures smooth, safe procedure. Supplies within reach create organized workspace.
Prevents soiling of bed linen.
Allows for thorough cleaning of prosthetics later. Provides clearer access to oral cavity.
Prevents patient from biting down on nurse's fingers and provides access to oral cavity.

CLINICAL DECISION: *Never place fingers into the mouth of an unconscious or debilitated patient. This could occlude the airway. Also, the normal patient response is to bite down.*

---

8. Clean mouth using brush moistened in water. Apply toothpaste or use antibacterial solution first to loosen crusts. Hold toothbrush bristles at 45-degree angle to gum line. Be sure that tips of bristles rest against and penetrate under gum line. Brush inner and outer surfaces of upper and lower teeth by brushing from gum to crown of each tooth; then clean biting surfaces of teeth by holding top of bristles parallel with teeth and brushing gently back and forth (see Box 40.9 Procedural Guidelines). Brush sides of teeth by moving bristles back and forth. Use a toothette sponge if patient has a bleeding tendency or if use of toothbrush is contraindicated (see illustration). Suction any accumulated secretions. Moisten brush with clear water or CHG solution to rinse. Use brush or toothette to clean roof of mouth, gums, and inside cheeks. Gently brush tongue, but avoid stimulating gag reflex (if present). Repeat rinsing several times and use suction to remove secretions. Use towel to dry off lips.
9. Apply thin layer of water-soluble moisturizer to lips (see illustration).

Brushing action removes food particles between teeth and along chewing surfaces and removes crusts and secretions from mucosa.
The use of a chlorhexidine gluconate (CHG) oral hygiene protocol as part of daily oral care reduces the incidence of ventilator-associated pneumonia (VAP) (Villar et al., 2015; de Lacerda Vidal et al., 2017). The Institute for Healthcare Improvement (2018) recommends the use of 0.12% chlorhexidine gluconate (CHG) as part of daily oral care in critically ill patients.
Repeated rinsing removes all debris and aids in moistening mucosa. Suction removes secretions and fluids that collect in posterior pharynx, thus reducing aspiration risk.

Lubricates lips to prevent drying and cracking.

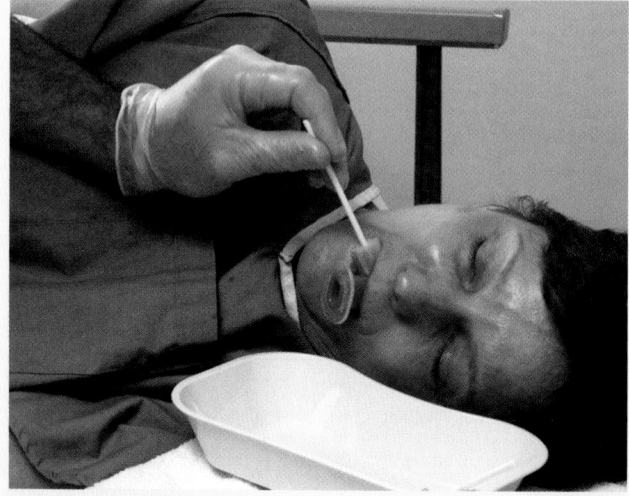

STEP 8 Cleaning lips and mucosa around oral airway with toothette.

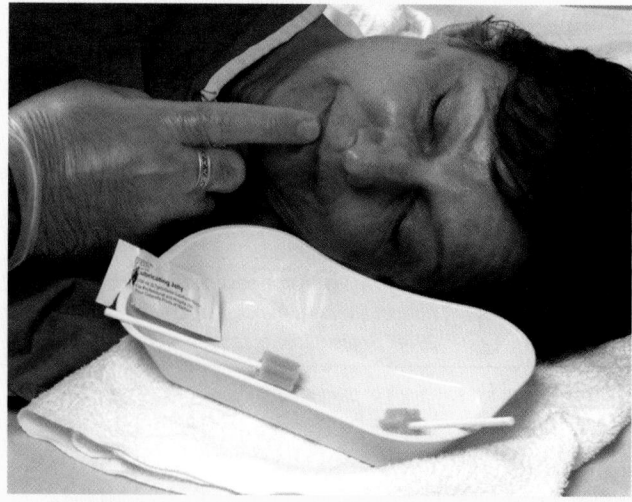

STEP 9 Application of water-soluble moisturizer to lips.

STEP	RATIONALE
10. Inform patient that procedure is completed. Return him or her to comfortable and safe position.	Provides meaningful stimulation to unconscious or less-responsive patient.
11. Raise side rails as appropriate and return bed to locked, low position. Leave nurse call system within reach.	Reduces risk of falls from bed.
12. Clean equipment and return to its proper place. Place soiled linen in dirty laundry bag.	Proper disposal of soiled equipment prevents spread of infection.
13. Remove and dispose of gloves in proper receptacle and perform hand hygiene.	Reduces transmission of microorganisms.

EVALUATION

1. Apply clean gloves and use tongue blade and penlight to inspect oral cavity.	Determines efficacy of cleaning. Once thick secretions are removed, underlying inflammation or lesions may be revealed.
2. Ask debilitated patient if mouth feels clean.	Evaluates level of comfort.
3. **Use Teach-Back:** "I explained what is needed to reduce your husband's risk of choking on secretions in his throat. Tell me the ways to prevent him from choking." Revise your instruction now or develop a plan for revised patient/family caregiver teaching if family caregiver is not able to teach back correctly.	Determines patient's/family caregiver's level of understanding of instructional topic.

UNEXPECTED OUTCOMES AND RELATED INTERVENTIONS

1. Secretions or crusts remain on mucosa, tongue, or gums.
   - Provide more frequent oral hygiene.
2. Localized inflammation or bleeding of gums or mucosa is present.
   - Provide more frequent oral hygiene with toothette sponges.
   - Apply a water-based mouth moisturizer to provide moisture and maintain integrity of oral mucosa.
   - Chemotherapy and radiation can cause mucositis (inflammation of mucous membranes in mouth) because of sloughing of epithelial tissue. Room temperature saline rinses, bicarbonate and sterile water rinses, and oral care with a soft-bristled toothbrush decrease severity and duration of mucositis.
3. Lips are cracked or inflamed.
   - Apply moisturizing gel or water-soluble lubricant to lips more often.
4. Patient aspirates secretions.
   - Suction oral airway to maintain airway patency (see Chapter 41).
   - Elevate patient's HOB to facilitate breathing.
   - If aspiration is suspected, notify health care provider immediately. Prepare patient for chest x-ray examination.

RECORDING AND REPORTING

- Record procedure, appearance of oral cavity before and after procedure, presence of gag reflex, and patient's response to procedure.
- Document your evaluation of patient/family caregiver learning.
- Use agency's standardized hand-off communication to communicate specific patient risks for aspiration and dry mouth. Discuss patient-specific interventions taken.
- Report any unusual findings (e.g., bleeding, ulceration, lesions, choking response) to nurse in charge or health care provider.
- Report immediately to the health care provider if patient aspirates.

HOME CARE CONSIDERATIONS

- Irrigate oral cavity with bulb syringe; patient can use a gravy baster to remove secretions.
- Give mouth care at least twice a day.
- Have caregivers demonstrate positioning patient to prevent aspiration.

KEY POINTS

- Various health beliefs, personal, sociocultural, economic, and developmental factors influence patients' hygiene preferences and practices.
- Hygiene needs, preferences, and the ability to participate in care change as people get older.
- Assess a patient's skin, feet and nails, oral mucosa, hair, and eyes and ears to obtain a complete assessment of the patient's hygiene needs.
- Assess a patient's physical and cognitive ability to perform basic hygiene measures.
- Vascular insufficiency and reduced mobility, cognition, and sensation increase a patient's risk for impaired skin integrity.
- Diabetes and peripheral vascular diseases increase the patient's risk for foot and nail problems.

- Critically thinking about a patient's hygiene preferences, needs, and ability to participate in care results in patient-centered hygiene care matching the patient's needs and preferences.
- Administering therapies to relieve symptoms such as pain or nausea before hygiene better prepares patients for any procedure.
- Position patients and make suction available to reduce the risk for aspiration when providing oral care to unconscious patients.
- A patient's environment needs to be comfortable, safe, and large enough to provide care and allow the patient and visitors to move about freely.
- Evaluation of hygiene procedures is based on outcomes of care; a patient's sense of comfort, relaxation, and well-being; and a patient's understanding of hygiene techniques.

REFLECTIVE LEARNING

- Your patient has diabetes and needs foot care. She asks why foot care is important. What would you tell her about why foot care is important and her associated risks?
- You have been assigned to your first comatose patient, and you notice 0.12% chlorhexidine gluconate (CHG) solution is ordered. Why is this necessary? What is the benefit to the patient?

- Your female patient has a Foley catheter in place. What are the necessary modifications in perineal care to reduce the risks of catheter-associated urinary tract infection (CAUTI)?

REVIEW QUESTIONS

1. What is the proper position to use for an unresponsive patient during oral care to prevent aspiration? (Select all that apply.)
   1. Prone position
   2. Sims' position
   3. Semi-Fowler's position with head to side
   4. Trendelenburg position
   5. Supine position
2. The student nurse is teaching a family member the importance of foot care for his or her mother, who has diabetes. Which safety precautions are important for the family member to know to prevent infection? (Select all that apply.)
   1. Cut nails frequently.
   2. Assess skin for redness, abrasions, and open areas daily.
   3. Soak feet in water at least 10 minutes before nail care.
   4. Apply lotion to feet daily.
   5. Clean between toes after bathing.
3. Integrity of the oral mucosa depends on salivary secretion. Which of the following factors impairs salivary secretion? (Select all that apply.)
   1. Use of cough drops
   2. Immunosuppression
   3. Radiation therapy
   4. Dehydration
   5. Presence of oral airway
4. A nurse is assigned to care for the following patients. Which patient is most at risk for developing skin problems and thus requiring thorough bathing and skin care?
   1. A 44-year-old female patient who has had removal of a breast lesion and is having her menstrual period
   2. A 56-year-old male patient who is homeless and admitted to the emergency department with malnutrition and dehydration and who has an intravenous line
   3. A 60-year-old female patient who experienced a stroke with right-sided paralysis and has an orthopedic brace applied to the left leg

4. A 70-year-old patient who has diabetes and dementia and has been incontinent of stool
5. When the nurse is assigned to a patient who has a reduced level of consciousness and requires mouth care, which physical assessment techniques should the nurse perform before the procedure? (Select all that apply.)
   1. Oxygen saturation
   2. Heart rate
   3. Respirations
   4. Gag reflex
   5. Response to painful stimulus
6. The American Dental Association suggests that patients who are at risk for poor hygiene use the following interventions for oral care: (Select all that apply.)
   1. Use antimicrobial toothpaste.
   2. Brush teeth 4 times a day.
   3. Use 0.12% chlorhexidine gluconate (CHG) oral rinses.
   4. Use a soft toothbrush for oral care.
   5. Avoid cleaning the gums and tongue.
7. While planning morning care, which of the following patients would have the highest priority to receive his or her bath first?
   1. A patient who just returned to the nursing unit from a diagnostic test
   2. A patient who prefers a bath in the evening when his wife visits and can help him
   3. A patient who is experiencing frequent incontinent diarrheal stools and urine
   4. A patient who has been awake all night because of pain 8/10
8. A patient with a malignant brain tumor requires oral care. The patient's level of consciousness has declined, with the patient only being able to respond to voice commands. Place the following steps in the correct order for administration of oral care.
   1. If patient is uncooperative or having difficulty keeping mouth open, insert an oral airway.

2. Raise bed, lower side rail, and position patient close to side of bed with head of bed raised up to 30 degrees.

3. Using a brush moistened with chlorhexidine paste, clean chewing and inner tooth surfaces first.

4. For patients without teeth, use a toothette moistened in chlorhexidine rinse to clean oral cavity.

5. Remove partial plate or dentures if present.

6. Gently brush tongue, but avoid stimulating gag reflex.

9. The nurse delegates needed hygiene care for an alert elderly patient who had a stroke. Which intervention would be appropriate for the assistive personnel to accomplish during the bath? (Select all that apply)

1. Checking distal pulses

2. Providing range-of-motion (ROM) exercises to extremities

3. Determining type of treatment for stage 1 pressure injury

4. Changing the dressing over an intravenous site

5. Providing special skin care

10. The nurse observes an adult Middle Eastern patient attempting to bathe himself with only his left hand. The nurse recognizes that this behavior likely relates to:

1. Obsessive-compulsive behavior.

2. Personal preferences.

3. The patient's cultural norm.

4. Controlling behaviors.

Answers: 1. 2, 3; **2.** 2, 4, 5; **3.** 3, 4, 4, 5; **4.** 6; **5.** 1, 3, 4; **7.** 3; **8.** 2, 5, 1, 3, 6, 4; **9.** 2, 5; **10.** 3.

Rationales for Review Questions can be found on the Evolve website.

REFERENCES

Agency for Healthcare Research and Quality (AHRQ): *Universal ICU decolonization: an enhanced protocol*, 2013, https://www.ahrq.gov/professionals/systems/hospital/universal_icu_decolonization/universal-icu-overvw.html. Accessed December 2018.

American Academy of Dermatology: *Dermatologists' top tips for relieving dry skin*, 2018, https://www.aad.org/public/skin-hair-nails/skin-care/dry-skin. Accessed July 2018.

American Dental Association: *Mouth healthy: brushing your teeth*, 2018, http://www.mouthhealthy.org/en/az-topics/b/brushing-your-teeth.aspx. Accessed July 28, 2018.

American Diabetes Association (ADA): Foot complications, 1995-2020, https://www.diabetes.org/diabetes/complications/foot-complications Accessed January 30, 2020.

American Diabetes Association (ADA): *Foot complications/neuropathy*, 2016, http://www.diabetes.org/living-with-diabetes/complications/foot-complications/. Accessed July 2018.

Arthritis Foundation: Foot pain, *Arthritis Today* 31(2):36, 2017.

Ball J, et al.: *Seidel's guide to physical examination*, ed 8, St Louis, 2019, Elsevier.

Bowen F, O'Brien-Richardson P: Cultural hair practices, physical activity, and obesity among urban African-American girls, *J Am Assoc Nurse Pract* 29(12):754, 2017.

Broadbent JM, et al.: Oral health-related beliefs, behaviors, and outcomes through life course, *J Dent Res* 95(7):808, 2016.

Butcher HK, et al.: *Nursing Interventions Classification (NIC)*, ed 7, St Louis, 2018, Elsevier.

Burman M, et al.: Linking evidenced-based nursing practice and patient-centered care through patient preferences, *Nurs Adm Q* 37(3):231, 2013.

Centers for Disease Control and Prevention (CDC): Catheter-associated urinary tract infections (CAUTI): guidelines for prevention of *CAUTI 2009*, 2015. https://www.cdc.gov/hai/ca_uti/uti.html Accessed September 30, 2019.

Centers for Disease Control and Prevention (CDC): *Parasites-lice-head lice*, 2016, http://www.cdc.gov/parasites/lice/head/treatment.html. Accessed July 2018.

Centers for Disease Control and Prevention (CDC): *Tick removal*, 2018. https://www.cdc.gov/lyme/removal/index.html. Accessed July 2018.

Centers for Disease Control and Prevention (CDC): *What is health literacy*, 2019. https://www.cdc.gov/healthliteracy/learn/index.html. Accessed December 23, 2019.

Chapman S: Foot care for people with diabetes: prevention of complications and treatment, *Br J Community Nurs* 22(5):226, 2017.

Cowell F, Radley K: What do we know about skin-hygiene care for patients with bariatric needs? Implications for nursing practice, *J Adv Nurs* 70(3):543, 2014.

Giger J: *Transcultural nursing: assessment and intervention*, ed 7, St Louis, 2017, Elsevier.

Harding MM, et al.: *Lewis's medical-surgical nursing: assessment and managment of clinical problems*, ed 11, St Louis, 2020, Elsevier.

Hockenberry ML, et al.: *Wong's nursing care of infants and children*, ed 11, St Louis, 2019, Mosby.

Institute for Healthcare Improvement (IHI): *How-to guide: prevent ventilator-associated pneumonia*, Modified, 2018. http://www.ihi.org/resources/Pages/Tools/HowtoGuidePreventVAP.aspx. Accessed July 2018.

Jeffcoate WJ, et al.: Current challenges and opportunities in the prevention and management of diabetic foot ulcers, *Diabetes Care* 41(4):645, 2018.

King EC, et al.: Care challenges in the bathroom: the views of professional care providers working in clients' homes, *J Appl Gerontol* 37(4):493, 2018.

Marion L, et al.: Implementing the new ANA Standard 8: culturally congruent practice, *Online J Issues Nurs* 22(1):1, 2017.

Mendes A: Meeting the care needs of a person with dementia who is distressed, *Br J Nurs* 27(4):219, 2018.

Morgan-Consoli M, Unzueta E: Female Mexican immigrants in the United States: cultural knowledge and healing, *Women Ther* 41(2):165, 2018.

National Pediculosis Association: *Welcome to headlice.org*. 2017, http://www.headlice.org/index.html. Accessed July 2018.

National Pressure Ulcer Advisory Panel (NPUAP): *Best practices for prevention of medical device pressure injuries*, updated, 2013, https://www.medlineuniversity.com/HigherLogic/System/DownloadDocumentFile.ashx?DocumentFileKey=cf6fe74b-3aed-2df9-731a-19c206016203&forceDialog=0. Accessed December 2018.

Pedersen L, et al.: Oral mucosal lesions in older people: relation to salivary secretion, systemic diseases and medications, *Oral Dis* 21(6):721, 2015.

Quality Safety Education for Nurses (QSEN): QSEN competencies, 2018, update, http://qsen.org/competencies/pre-licensure-ksas/. Accessed July 2018.

The Joint Commission (TJC): *2020 National patient safety goals*, Oakbrook Terrace, IL, 2020, The Commission, https://www.jointcommission.org/en/standards/national-patient-safety-goals/. Accessed January 2, 2020.

Touhy T, Jett P: *Ebersole & Hess' Gerontological nursing & healthy aging*, ed 5, St Louis, 2018, Elsevier.

US Department of Health and Human Services (USDHHS): *Oral health*, 2018. http://www.healthypeople.gov/2020/topics-objectives/topic/oral-health. Accessed July 2018.

Wilson M: Skin care for older people living with dementia, *Nurs Resid Care* 20(3):151, 2018.

RESEARCH REFERENCES

Alserehi H, et al.: Chlorhexidine gluconate bathing practices and skin concentrations in intensive care unit patients, *Am J Infect Cont* 46(2):226, 2018.

Boonyasiri A, et al.: Effectiveness of chlorhexidine wipes for the prevention of multidrug-resistant bacterial colonization and hospital-acquired infections in intensive care unit patients: a randomized trial in Thailand, *Infect Control Hosp Epidemiol* 37(3):245, 2016.

Cassir N, et al.: Chlorhexidine daily bathing: impact on health care-associated infections caused by gram-negative bacteria, *Am J Infect Control* 43(6):640, 2015.

Climo M, et al.: Effect of daily chlorhexidine bathing on hospital-acquired infection, *N Engl J Med* 368(6):533, 2013.

Chapple ILC, et al.: Interaction of lifestyle, behaviour or systemic diseases with dental caries and periodontal diseases: consensus report of group2 of the joint EFP/ORCA workshop on the boundaries between caries and periodontal diseases, *J Clinical Peridontol* 44(Suppl 18):S39, 2017.

de Lacerda Vidal CF, et al.: Impact of oral hygiene involving toothbrushing versus chlorhexidine irrigation in the prevention of ventilator-associated pneumonia: a randomized study, *BMC Infect Dis* 17(1):112, 2017.

Demirel S, et al.: Effective management of exposure keratopathy developed in intensive care units: the impact of an evidence based eye care education programme, *Intensive Crit Care Nurs* 30(1):38, 2014.

Dial M, et al.: "I do the best I can:" Personal care preferences of patients of size, *App Nurs Res* 39:259, 2018.

El-Rabbany M, et al.: Prophylactic oral health procedures to prevent hospital-acquired ventilator-associated pneumonia: a systematic review, *Int J Nurs Stud* 52(1):452, 2015.

Henderson S, et al.: Cultural competence in healthcare in the community: a concept analysis, *Health Soc Care Community* 26(4):590, 2018.

Hirschman KB, Hodgson NA: Evidence-based interventions for transitions in care for individuals living with dementia, *Gerontol* 58(Suppl 1):S129, 2018.

Jenson H, et al.: Improving oral care in hospitalized non-ventilated patients: standardizing products and protocol, *Medsurg Nurs* 27(1):38, 2018.

Klompas M, et al.: Strategies to prevent ventilator-associated pneumonia in acute care hospitals: 2014 update, *Infect Control Hosp Epidemiol* 35(8):915, 2014.

Kocacal G, et al.: Nurses can play an active role in the early diagnosis of exposure keratopathy in intensive care patients, *Crit Care Nurs* 15(1):31, 2018.

Kole U, et al.: Knowledge in practice regarding menstrual hygiene among female students in selected schools, *Int J Nurs Educ* 10(2):85, 2018.

Konno R, et al.: A best-evidence review of intervention studies for minimizing resistance-to-care behaviours for older adults with dementia in nursing homes, *J Adv Nurs* 70(10):2167, 2014.

Kundu RV, Patterson S: Dermatologic conditions in skin of color: Part II. Disorders occurring predominantly in skin of color, *Am Fam Physician* 87(12):859, 2013.

LaFleur RC, et al.: Improving culturally congruent health care for children with disabilities: stakeholder perspectives of cultural competence training in an interdisciplinary training program, *J Transcult Nurs* 29(1):101, 2017.

Maciag J, et al.: The effects of treatment of denture-related stomatitis on peripheral T cells and monocytes, *Oral Health Prev Dent* 15(3):259, 2017.

Martin ET, et al.: Bathing hospitalized dependent patients with prepackaged disposable washcloths instead of traditional bath basins: a case crossover study, *Am J Infect Control* 45(9):990, 2017.

Martori E, et al.: Risk factors for denture-related oral mucosal lesions in a geriatric population, *J Prosthet Dent* 111(4):273, 2014.

Murray J, Scholten I: An oral hygiene protocol improves oral health for patients in inpatient stroke rehabilitation, *Gerodontology* 35(1):18, 2018.

Nicolosi L, et al.: Effect of oral hygiene and 0.12% chlorhexidine gluconate oral rinse in preventing ventilator-associated pneumonia after cardiovascular surgery, *Respir Care* 59(4):504, 2014.

Park YH, et al.: Risk factors and the associated cutoff values for failure of corticosteroid injection in treatment of Morton's neuroma, *Int Orthop* 42(2):323, 2018.

Persaud R, et al.: Validation of the healthy foot screen: a novel assessment tool for common clinical abnormalities, *Adv Skin Wound Care* 31(4):154, 2018.

Petlin A, et al.: Chlorhexidine gluconate bathing to reduce methicillin-resistant Staphylococcus aureus acquisition, *Crit Care Nurse* 34(5):17, 2014.

Pinkert C, et al.: Experiences of nurses with care of patients with dementia in acute hospitals: a secondary analysis, *J Clin Nurs* 27:163, 2018.

Powers J, et al.: Chlorhexidine bathing and microbial contamination in patients' bath basins, *Am J Crit Care* 21(5):338, 2012.

Rokstad AMM, et al.: The impact of the Dementia ABC educational programme on competence in person-centred dementia care and job satisfaction of care staff, *Int J Older People Nurs* 12(2): n/a N.PAG, 2017.

Ruiz J, et al.: Daily bathing strategies and cross-contamination of multidrug-resistant organisms: impact of chlorhexidine-impregnated wipes in a multidrug-resistant gram-negative bacteria endemic intensive care unit, *Am J Infect Control* 45(10):1069, 2017.

Shah H, et al.: Bathing with 2% chlorhexidine gluconate, *Crit Care Nurs Q* 39(1):42, 2016.

Shelton EG, et al.: Does it matter if we disagree? The impact of incongruent care preferences on persons with dementia and their care partners, *Gerontol* 58(3):556, 2018.

Vaingankar JA: Care participation and burden among informal caregivers of older adults with care needs and associations with dementia, *Int Psychogeriatr* 28(2):221, 2016.

Villar A, et al.: Diagnosis and management of xerostomia and hyposalivation, *Ther Clin Risk Manag* 11:45, 2015.

Villar F, et al.: Involving institutionalised people with dementia in their care-planning meetings: lessons learnt by staff, *Scand J Caring Sci* 32(2):567, 2018.

Yevchak A, et al.: Implementing nurse-facilitated person-centered care approaches for patient with delirium superimposed on dementia in the acute care setting, *J Gerontol Nurs* 43(12):21, 2017.

41

Oxygenation

OBJECTIVES

- Describe the structure and function of the cardiopulmonary system.
- Describe the physiological processes of ventilation, perfusion, and exchange of respiratory gases.
- Differentiate among the physiological processes of cardiac output, myocardial blood flow, and systemic circulation.
- Describe the relationship of cardiac output (preload, afterload, contractility, and heart rate) to the process of oxygenation.
- Identify the potential clinical outcomes occurring as a result of hyperventilation, hypoventilation, and/or hypoxemia.
- Identify the potential clinical outcomes occurring as a result of disturbances in conduction, altered cardiac output, impaired valvular function, myocardial ischemia, and/or impaired tissue perfusion.

- Describe the effect of a patient's level of health, age, lifestyle, and environment on oxygenation.
- Describe how to assess for the risk factors affecting a patient's oxygenation.
- Describe how to assess for the physical manifestations that occur with alterations in oxygenation.
- Develop a plan of care for a patient with altered oxygenation.
- Describe nursing care interventions used to promote oxygenation in the primary care, acute care, and restorative and continuing care settings.
- Describe strategies to use to maintain a patient's airway.
- Evaluate a patient's responses to oxygenation therapies.

KEY TERMS

Acute coronary syndrome (ACS), p. 918
Afterload, p. 914
Angina pectoris, p. 918
Bilevel positive airway pressure (BiPAP), p. 938
Bronchoscopy, p. 922
Capnography, p. 921
Cardiac output, p. 914
Cardiopulmonary rehabilitation, p. 944
Cardiopulmonary resuscitation (CPR), p. 944
Chest physiotherapy (CPT), p. 933
Chest tube, p. 939
Cheyne-Stokes respiration, p. 924
Continuous positive airway pressure (CPAP), p. 938
Diaphragmatic breathing, p. 944

Diffusion, p. 912
Electrocardiogram (ECG), p. 915
Endotracheal (ET) tube, p. 937
Hematemesis, p. 922
Hemoptysis, p. 922
Hemothorax, p. 939
Humidification, p. 932
Hyperventilation, p. 917
Hypoventilation, p. 916
Hypovolemia, p. 916
Hypoxia, p. 917
Incentive spirometry, p. 935
Invasive mechanical ventilation, p. 937
Kussmaul respiration, p. 924
Myocardial infarction (MI), p. 918
Myocardial ischemia, p. 918
Nasal cannula, p. 943

Nebulization, p. 932
Noninvasive positive-pressure ventilation (NPPV), p. 937
Orthopnea, p. 922
Perfusion, p. 912
Pneumothorax, p. 939
Postural drainage, p. 933
Preload, p. 914
Pursed-lip breathing, p. 944
Stroke volume, p. 913
Tracheostomy, p. 937
Ventilation, p. 912
Ventilator-associated pneumonia (VAP), p. 937
Ventricular fibrillation, p. 917
Ventricular tachycardia, p. 917

MEDIA RESOURCES

http://evolve.elsevier.com/Potter/fundamentals/
- Review Questions
- Video Clips
- Concept Map Creator
- Case Study with Questions

- Skills Performance Checklists
- Audio Glossary
- Content Updates
- Answers to QSEN Activity and Review Questions

Disturbances in oxygenation often result from ineffective gas exchange (lungs) or an ineffective pump (heart). You will learn about the physiology of the cardiopulmonary system and how the heart and the lungs work together to provide oxygen to the tissues of the body. This chapter describes how to assess and care for a patient with a disturbance in oxygenation.

SCIENTIFIC KNOWLEDGE BASE

Oxygen is a basic human need. The cardiac and respiratory systems work together to supply the body with oxygen necessary for carrying out the respiratory and metabolic processes needed to sustain life. Blood is oxygenated through the mechanisms of ventilation, perfusion, and transport of respiratory gases. Neural and chemical regulators control the rate and depth of respiration in response to changing tissue oxygen demands. The cardiovascular system provides the transport mechanisms to distribute oxygen to cells and tissues of the body (McCance and Huether, 2019).

Respiratory Physiology

Respiration is the exchange of oxygen and carbon dioxide during cellular metabolism. It is commonly confused as the act of air moving in and out of the lungs, which is actually ventilation. The airways of the lung transfer oxygen from the atmosphere to the alveoli, where the oxygen is exchanged for carbon dioxide (CO_2). Through the alveolar capillary membrane, oxygen transfers to the blood, and CO_2 transfers from the blood to the alveoli. There are three steps in the process of oxygenation: ventilation, perfusion, and diffusion (McCance and Huether, 2019).

Structure and Function.
The respiratory muscles, pleural space, lungs, and alveoli are essential for ventilation, perfusion, and exchange of respiratory gases. Gases move into and out of the lungs through pressure changes. Intrapleural pressure is negative, or less than atmospheric pressure, which is 760 mm Hg at sea level. For air to flow into the lungs, intrapleural pressure becomes more negative, setting up a pressure gradient between the atmosphere and the alveoli. The diaphragm and external intercostal muscles contract (move downward and outward) to create a negative pleural pressure and increase the size of the thorax for inspiration. Relaxation of the diaphragm and contraction of the internal intercostal muscles allow air to escape from the lungs (Cedar, 2018; McCance and Huether, 2019).

Ventilation is the process of moving gases into and out of the lungs with air flowing into the lungs during inhalation (inspiration) and out of the lungs during exhalation (expiration). It requires coordination of the muscular and elastic properties of the lungs and thorax. The major inspiratory muscle of respiration is the diaphragm. It is innervated by the phrenic nerve, which exits the spinal cord at the fourth cervical vertebra. Perfusion relates to the ability of the cardiovascular system to pump oxygenated blood to the tissues and return deoxygenated blood to the lungs. Finally, diffusion is responsible for moving the respiratory gases from one area to another by concentration gradients. For the exchange of respiratory gases to occur, the organs, nerves, and muscles of respiration need to be intact and the central nervous system needs to be able to regulate the respiratory cycle (Cedar, 2018; McCance and Huether, 2019).

Conditions or diseases that change the structure and function of the pulmonary system alter respiration. Some of these conditions include chronic obstructive pulmonary disease (COPD), asthma, lung cancer, and cystic fibrosis. In these conditions, you could find increased respiratory rate, decreased oxygen saturation levels, or adventitious lung sounds (McCance and Huether, 2019).

Work of Breathing.
Work of breathing (WOB) is the effort required to expand and contract the lungs. In the healthy individual breathing is quiet and accomplished with minimal effort. The amount of energy expended on breathing depends on the rate and depth of breathing, the ease in which the lungs can be expanded (compliance), and airway resistance (McCance and Huether, 2019).

Inspiration is an active process, stimulated by chemical receptors in the aorta. Expiration is a passive process that depends on the elastic recoil properties of the lungs, requiring little or no muscle work. Surfactant is a chemical produced in the lungs to maintain the surface tension of the alveoli and keep them from collapsing. Patients with advanced COPD lose the elastic recoil of the lungs and thorax. As a result, the patient's work of breathing increases. In addition, patients with certain pulmonary diseases have decreased surfactant production

and sometimes develop atelectasis. Atelectasis is a collapse of the alveoli that prevents normal exchange of oxygen and carbon dioxide (McCance and Huether, 2019).

Accessory muscles of respiration (the intercostal muscles in the rib cage and abdominal muscles) can increase lung volume during inspiration. Patients with COPD, especially emphysema, frequently use these muscles to increase lung volume. Prolonged use of the accessory muscles does not promote effective ventilation and eventually causes fatigue. During assessment a patient's clavicles may elevate during inspiration, which can indicate ventilatory fatigue, air hunger, or decreased lung expansion (McCance and Huether, 2019).

Compliance is the ability of the lungs to distend or expand in response to increased intra-alveolar pressure. Compliance decreases in diseases such as pulmonary edema, interstitial and pleural fibrosis, and congenital or traumatic structural abnormalities such as kyphosis or fractured ribs (McCance and Huether, 2019).

Airway resistance is the increase in pressure that occurs as the diameter of the airways decreases from mouth/nose to alveoli. Any further decrease in airway diameter by bronchoconstriction or the presences of excess mucus can increase airway resistance. Diseases causing airway obstruction, such as asthma, tracheal edema, or COPD, increase airway resistance. When airway resistance increases, the amount of oxygen delivered to the alveoli decreases (McCance and Huether, 2019).

Decreased lung compliance, increased airway resistance, and the increased use of accessory muscles increase the WOB, resulting in increased energy expenditure. Therefore, the body increases its metabolic rate and the need for more oxygen. The need for elimination of carbon dioxide also increases. This sequence is a vicious cycle for a patient with impaired ventilation, causing further deterioration of respiratory status and the ability to oxygenate adequately (McCance and Huether, 2019).

Lung Volumes.
The normal lung volumes are determined by age, gender, and height. Tidal volume is the amount of air exhaled following a normal inspiration. Residual volume is the amount of air left in the alveoli after a full expiration. Forced vital capacity is the maximum amount of air that can be removed from the lungs during forced expiration (McCance and Huether, 2019). Variations in tidal volume and other lung volumes are associated with alterations in patients' health status or activity, such as pregnancy, exercise, obesity, or obstructive and restrictive conditions of the lungs.

Pulmonary Circulation.
The primary function of pulmonary circulation is to move blood to and from the alveolar capillary membrane for gas exchange. Pulmonary circulation begins at the pulmonary artery, which receives poorly oxygenated mixed venous blood from the right ventricle. Blood flow through this system depends on the pumping ability of the right ventricle. The flow continues from the pulmonary artery through the pulmonary arterioles to the pulmonary capillaries, where blood comes in contact with the alveolar capillary membrane and the exchange of respiratory gases occurs. The oxygen-rich blood then circulates through the pulmonary venules and pulmonary veins, returning to the left atrium (McCance and Huether, 2019).

Respiratory Gas Exchange.
Diffusion is the process for the exchange of respiratory gases in the alveoli of the lungs and the capillaries of the body tissues. Diffusion of respiratory gases occurs at the alveolar capillary membrane (Fig. 41.1). The thickness of the membrane affects the rate of diffusion. Increased thickness of the membrane impedes diffusion because gases take longer to transfer across the membrane. Patients with pulmonary edema, pulmonary infiltrates, or pulmonary effusion have a thickened membrane, resulting in slow diffusion, slow exchange

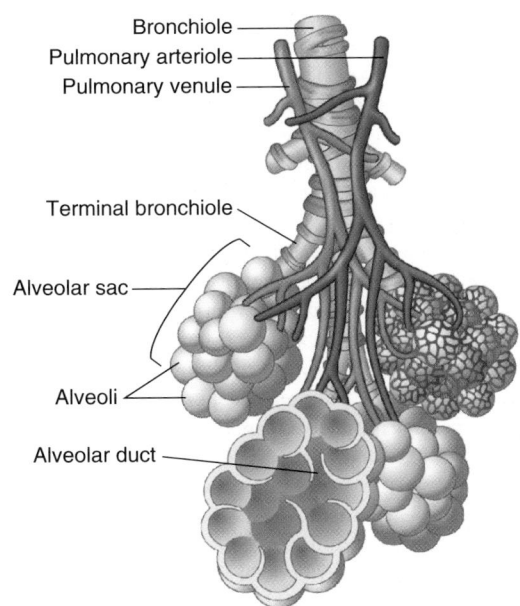

FIG. 41.1 Alveoli at terminal end of lower airway. (From Patton KT, Thibodeau GA: *Human body in health and disease,* ed 7, St Louis, 2018, Elsevier.)

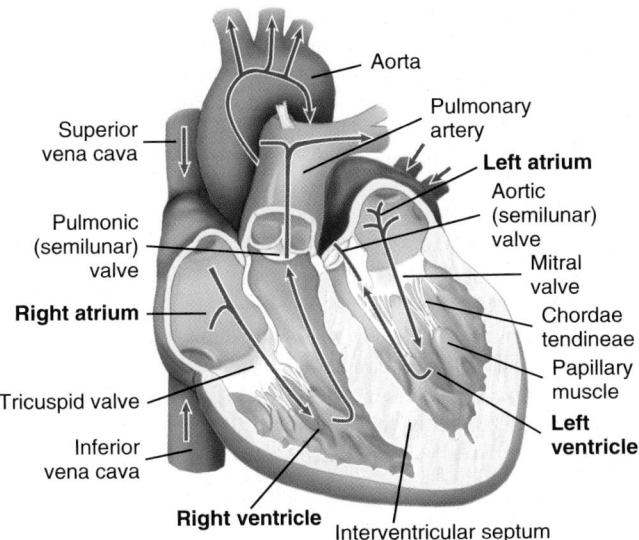

FIG. 41.2 Schematic representation of blood flow through the heart. *Arrows* indicate direction of flow and pulmonary circulation. (Modified from Lewis SM, et al: *Medical surgical nursing: assessment and management of clinical problems,* ed 10, St Louis, 2017, Mosby.)

of respiratory gases, and decreased delivery of oxygen to tissues. Chronic diseases (e.g., emphysema), acute diseases (e.g., pneumothorax), and surgical processes (e.g., lobectomy) often alter the amount of alveolar capillary membrane surface area (McCance and Huether, 2019).

Oxygen Transport. The oxygen-transport system consists of the lungs and cardiovascular system. Delivery depends on the amount of oxygen entering the lungs (ventilation), blood flow to the lungs and tissues (perfusion), rate of diffusion, and oxygen-carrying capacity. Three things influence the capacity of the blood to carry oxygen: the amount of dissolved oxygen in the plasma, the amount of hemoglobin, and the ability of hemoglobin to bind with oxygen. Hemoglobin, which is a carrier for oxygen and carbon dioxide, transports most oxygen (approximately 97%). The hemoglobin molecule combines with oxygen to form oxyhemoglobin. The formation of oxyhemoglobin is easily reversible, allowing hemoglobin and oxygen to dissociate (deoxyhemoglobin), which frees oxygen to enter tissues. Patients who are acidotic (pH less than 7.35; seen in patients with sepsis or diabetic ketoacidosis), hypercapnic (elevated $PaCO_2$ levels; seen in patients with COPD), or who have low hemoglobin levels (seen in patients with anemia or excess blood loss) have decreased ability to carry oxygen and therefore to deliver oxygen to the tissues (McCance and Huether, 2019).

Carbon Dioxide Transport. Carbon dioxide, a product of cellular metabolism, diffuses into red blood cells and is rapidly hydrated into carbonic acid (H_2CO_3). The carbonic acid then dissociates into hydrogen (H) and bicarbonate (HCO_3^-) ions. Hemoglobin buffers the hydrogen ion, and the HCO_3^- diffuses into the plasma. Reduced hemoglobin (deoxyhemoglobin) combines with carbon dioxide, and the venous blood transports the majority of carbon dioxide back to the lungs to be exhaled (McCance and Huether, 2019).

Regulation of Ventilation. Regulation of ventilation is necessary to ensure sufficient oxygen intake and carbon dioxide elimination to meet the demands of the body (e.g., during exercise, infection, or pregnancy). Neural and chemical regulators control the process of ventilation. Neural regulation includes the CNS control of respiratory rate, depth, and rhythm. The cerebral cortex regulates the voluntary control of respiration by delivering impulses to the respiratory motor neurons by way of the spinal cord. Chemical regulation maintains the appropriate rate and depth of respirations based on changes in the carbon dioxide (CO_2), oxygen (O_2), and hydrogen ion (H^+) concentration (pH) in the blood. Changes in levels of O_2, CO_2, and H^+ (pH) stimulate the chemoreceptors located in the medulla, aortic body, and carotid body, which in turn stimulate neural regulators to adjust the rate and depth of ventilation to maintain normal arterial blood gas levels (McCance and Huether, 2019).

Cardiovascular Physiology

Cardiopulmonary physiology involves delivery of deoxygenated blood (blood high in carbon dioxide and low in oxygen) to the right side of the heart and then to the lungs, where it is oxygenated. Oxygenated blood (blood high in oxygen and low in carbon dioxide) then travels from the lungs to the left side of the heart and the tissues. The cardiac system delivers oxygen, nutrients, and other substances to the tissues and facilitates the removal of cellular metabolism waste products by way of blood flow through other body systems such as respiratory, digestive, and renal (McCance and Huether, 2019).

Structure and Function. The right ventricle pumps deoxygenated blood through the pulmonary circulation (Fig. 41.2). The left ventricle pumps oxygenated blood through the systemic circulation. As blood passes through the circulatory system, there is an exchange of respiratory gases, nutrients, and waste products between the blood and the tissues. Alterations in structure and function of the heart can lead to a variety of symptoms, including but not limited to dyspnea, edema, and weak pulses. Nurses hear abnormal heart sounds, such as murmurs or rubs, when the structure of the heart is altered (McCance and Huether, 2019).

Myocardial Pump. The pumping action of the heart is essential to oxygen delivery. There are four cardiac chambers: two atria and two ventricles. The ventricles fill with blood during diastole and empty during systole. The volume of blood ejected from the ventricles during systole is the **stroke volume**. Hemorrhage and dehydration cause a decrease in circulating blood volume and a decrease in stroke volume (McCance and Huether, 2019).

Myocardial fibers have contractile properties that allow them to stretch during cardiac filling. In a healthy heart this stretch is proportionally related to the strength of contraction. As the myocardium stretches, the strength of the subsequent contraction increases; this is known as the *Frank-Starling (Starling's) law of the heart.* In the diseased heart (cardiomyopathy), Starling's law does not apply because the increased stretch of the myocardium is beyond the physiological limits of the heart. The subsequent contractile response results in insufficient stroke volume, and blood begins to "back up" in the pulmonary (left heart failure) or systemic (right heart failure) circulation (McCance and Huether, 2019).

Myocardial Blood Flow. To maintain adequate blood flow to the pulmonary and systemic circulation, myocardial blood flow must supply sufficient oxygen and nutrients to the myocardium itself. Blood flow through the heart is unidirectional. The four heart valves ensure this forward blood flow (see Fig. 41.2). During ventricular diastole the atrioventricular (mitral and tricuspid) valves open, and blood flows from the higher-pressure atria into the relaxed ventricles. As systole begins, ventricular pressure rises and the mitral and tricuspid valves close. Valve closure causes the first heart sound (S_1) (McCance and Huether, 2019) (see Chapter 30).

During the systolic phase the semilunar (aortic and pulmonic) valves open, and blood flows from the ventricles into the aorta and pulmonary artery. The mitral and tricuspid valves stay closed during systole, so all of the blood is moved forward into the pulmonary artery and aorta. As the ventricles empty, the ventricular pressures decrease, allowing closure of the aortic and pulmonic valves. Valve closure causes the second heart sound (S_2). Some patients with valvular disease have backflow or regurgitation of blood through the incompetent valve, causing a murmur that you can hear on auscultation (see Chapter 30) (McCance and Huether, 2019).

Coronary Artery Circulation. The coronary circulation is the branch of the systemic circulation that supplies the myocardium with oxygen and nutrients and removes waste. The coronary arteries fill during ventricular diastole. The left coronary artery has the most abundant blood supply and feeds the more muscular left ventricular myocardium, which does most of the work of the heart (McCance and Huether, 2019).

Systemic Circulation. The arteries of the systemic circulation deliver nutrients and oxygen to tissues, and the veins remove waste from tissues. Oxygenated blood flows from the left ventricle through the aorta and into large systemic arteries. These arteries branch into smaller arteries; then arterioles; and finally, the smallest vessels, the capillaries. The exchange of respiratory gases occurs at the capillary level, where the tissues are oxygenated. The waste products exit the capillary network through venules that join to form veins. These veins become larger and form the vena cava, which carry deoxygenated blood back to the right side of the heart, where it then returns to the pulmonary circulation (McCance and Huether, 2019).

Blood Flow Regulation. The amount of blood ejected from the left ventricle each minute is the cardiac output. The normal cardiac output is 4 to 8 L/min in the healthy adult at rest. The circulating volume of blood changes according to the oxygen and metabolic needs of the body. For example, cardiac output increases during exercise, pregnancy, and fever but decreases during sleep. The following formula represents cardiac output:

Cardiac output (CO) = Stroke volume (SV) × Heart rate (HR)

Stroke volume is the amount of blood ejected from the ventricle with each contraction. The normal range for a healthy adult is 50 to 75 mL per contraction. Preload, afterload, and myocardial contractility all affect stroke volume. Preload is the amount of blood in the left ventricle at the end of diastole, before the next contraction. It is often referred to as end-diastolic volume. The ventricles stretch when filling with blood. The more stretch on the ventricular muscle, the greater the contraction and the greater the stroke volume (Starling's law). In certain clinical situations, medical treatment alters preload and subsequent stroke volumes by changing the amount of circulating blood volume. For example, when treating a patient who is hemorrhaging, increased fluid therapy and replacement of blood increase circulating volume, thus increasing the preload and stroke volume, which in turn increases cardiac output. If volume is not replaced, preload, stroke volume, and the subsequent cardiac output decrease (McCance and Huether, 2019).

Afterload is the resistance to the ejection of blood from the left ventricle. The heart works harder to overcome the resistance so that blood can be ejected from the left ventricle. The diastolic aortic pressure is a good clinical measure of afterload. In hypertension, the afterload increases, causing an increase in cardiac workload (McCance and Huether, 2019).

Myocardial contractility is the ability of the heart to squeeze blood from the ventricles. It also affects stroke volume and cardiac output. Poor ventricular contraction decreases the amount of blood ejected. Injury to the myocardial muscle, such as an acute MI, causes a decrease in myocardial contractility (McCance and Huether, 2019). The myocardium in some older adults is stiffer with a slower ventricular filling rate and prolonged contraction time (Touhy and Jett, 2018).

Heart rate affects blood flow because of the relationship between heart rate and diastolic filling time. For example, a sustained heart rate greater than 160 beats/min decreases diastolic filling time, which decreases stroke volume and cardiac output (McCance and Huether, 2019). The heart rate of the older adult is slow to increase under stress, but studies have found that this may be caused more by lack of conditioning than age. Exercise is beneficial in maintaining function at any age (Touhy and Jett, 2018).

Conduction System. The rhythmic relaxation and contraction of the atria and ventricles depend on continuous, organized transmission of electrical impulses. The cardiac conduction system generates and transmits these impulses (Fig. 41.3).

The conduction system of the heart generates the impulses needed to initiate the electrical chain of events for a normal heartbeat. The autonomic nervous system influences the rate of impulse generation and the speed of transmission through the conductive pathway and the strength of atrial and ventricular contractions. Sympathetic and parasympathetic nerve fibers innervate all parts of the atria and ventricles and the sinoatrial (SA) and atrioventricular (AV) nodes. Sympathetic fibers increase the rate of impulse generation and speed of transmission. The parasympathetic fibers originating from the vagus nerve decrease the rate (McCance and Huether, 2019).

The conduction system originates with the SA node, the "pacemaker" of the heart. The SA node is in the right atrium next to the entrance of the superior vena cava. Impulses are initiated at the SA node at an intrinsic rate of 60 to 100 cardiac action potentials per minute in an adult at rest. The electrical impulses are transmitted through the atria along intraatrial and internodal pathways to the AV node. The AV node mediates impulses between the atria and the ventricles. It assists atrial emptying by delaying the impulse before transmitting it through the bundle of His and the ventricular Purkinje network. A normal sinus rhythm is necessary to ensure optimal perfusion of the tissues in the body (McCance and Huether, 2019).

An electrocardiogram (ECG) is a measurement of the electrical activity of the conduction system. An ECG monitors the regularity and path of the electrical impulse through the conduction system; however, it does not reflect the muscular work of the heart. The normal sequence on the ECG is called the normal sinus rhythm (NSR) (see Fig. 41.3) (Urden et al., 2020).

NSR implies that the impulse originates at the SA node and follows the normal sequence through the conduction system. The P wave (atrial depolarization) represents the electrical conduction through both atria. Atrial contraction follows the P wave. The PR interval represents the impulse travel time from the SA node through the AV node, through the bundle of His, and to the Purkinje fibers. The normal length for the PR interval is 0.12 to 0.2 seconds. An increase in the time greater than 0.2 seconds indicates a block in the impulse transmission through the AV node, whereas a decrease, less than 0.12 seconds, indicates the initiation of the electrical impulse from a source other than the SA node (Urden et al., 2020).

The QRS complex (ventricular depolarization) indicates that the electrical impulse traveled through the ventricles. Normal QRS duration is 0.06 to 0.1 seconds. An increase in QRS duration indicates a delay in conduction time through the ventricles. Ventricular contraction usually follows the QRS complex (Urden et al., 2020).

The QT interval represents the time needed for ventricular depolarization and repolarization. The normal QT interval is 0.12 to 0.42 seconds. This interval varies inversely with changes in heart rate. Changes in electrolyte values, such as hypocalcemia or hypomagnesemia, or therapy with medications (disopyramide, amiodarone, haloperidol, and azithromycin are examples) increases the QT interval. An increased QT interval increases the person's risk for lethal dysrhythmias (Urden et al., 2020).

Factors Affecting Oxygenation

Four factors influence adequacy of circulation, ventilation, perfusion, and transport of respiratory gases to the tissues: (1) physiological, (2) developmental, (3) lifestyle, and (4) environmental. The physiological factors are discussed here, and the others are discussed in the Nursing Knowledge Base section that follows.

Physiological Factors. Any condition affecting cardiopulmonary functioning directly affects the ability of the body to meet oxygen demands. Respiratory disorders include hyperventilation, hypoventilation, and hypoxia. Cardiac disorders include disturbances in conduction, impaired valvular function, myocardial hypoxia, cardiomyopathy conditions, and peripheral tissue hypoxia. Other physiological processes affecting a patient's oxygenation include alterations affecting the oxygen-carrying capacity of blood (anemia), decreased inspired oxygen concentration, increases in the metabolic demand of the body (fever), and alterations affecting chest wall movement caused by musculoskeletal abnormalities or neuromuscular alterations (muscular dystrophy) (McCance and Huether, 2019; Urden et al., 2020).

Decreased Oxygen-Carrying Capacity. Hemoglobin carries the majority of oxygen to tissues. Anemia and inhalation of toxic substances decrease the oxygen-carrying capacity of blood by reducing the amount of available hemoglobin to transport oxygen. Anemia (e.g., a lower-than-normal hemoglobin level) is a result of decreased hemoglobin production, increased red blood cell destruction, and/or blood loss. Patients have fatigue, decreased activity tolerance, increased breathlessness, increased heart rate, and pallor (especially seen in the conjunctiva of the eye). Oxygenation decreases as a secondary effect with anemia. The physiological response to chronic hypoxemia is the development of increased red blood cells (polycythemia). This is the adaptive response of the body to increase the amount of hemoglobin and the available oxygen-binding sites (Lewis et al., 2017; McCance and Huether, 2019).

Carbon monoxide (CO) is a colorless, odorless gas that causes decreased oxygen-carrying capacity of blood. In CO toxicity, hemoglobin strongly binds with CO, creating a functional anemia. Because of the strength of the bond, CO does not easily dissociate

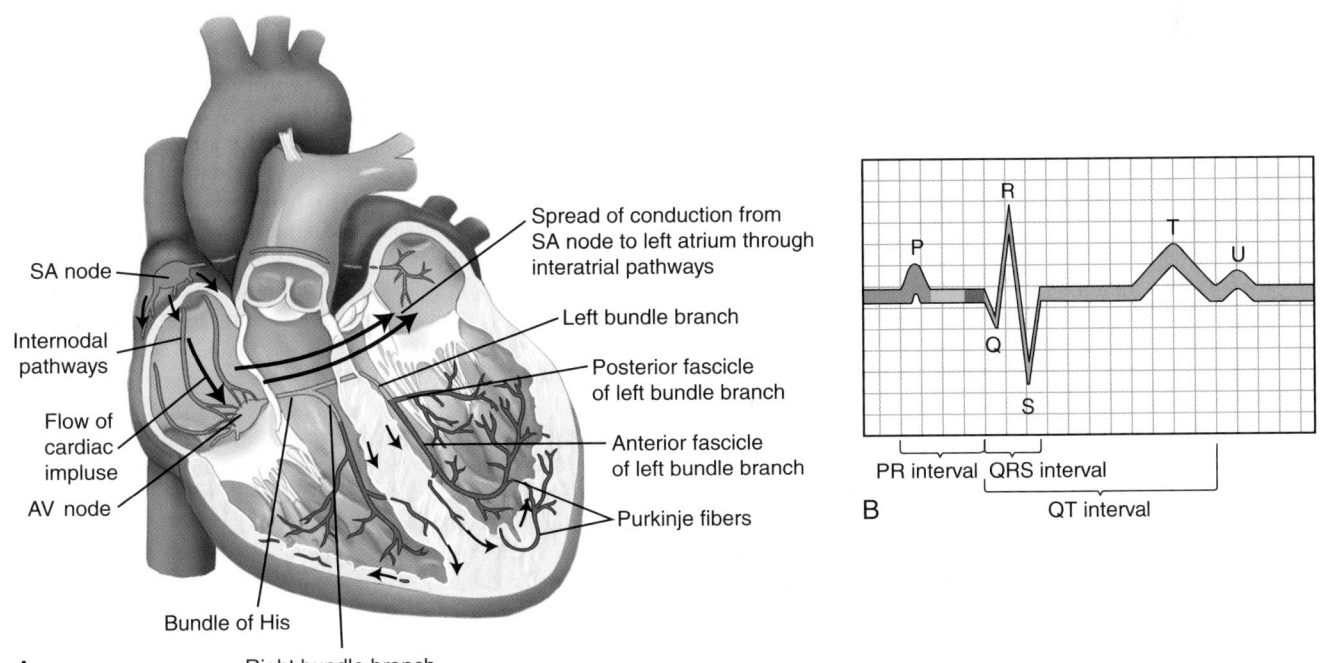

FIG. 41.3 Conduction system of the heart. *AV,* Atrioventricular; *SA,* sinoatrial. (From Lewis SL et al: *Medical-surgical nursing: assessment and management of clinical problems,* ed 10, St Louis, 2017, Mosby.)

from hemoglobin, making hemoglobin unavailable for oxygen transport. People with CO poisoning are often unaware of their exposure to this gas, and the symptoms of CO poisoning (headache, dizziness, nausea, vomiting, and dyspnea) mimic other illnesses (Urden et al., 2020).

Hypovolemia. Conditions such as shock and severe dehydration cause extracellular fluid loss and reduced circulating blood volume, or hypovolemia. Decreased circulating blood volume results in hypoxia to body tissues. With significant fluid loss, the body tries to adapt by peripheral vasoconstriction and by increasing the heart rate to increase the volume of blood returned to the heart, thus increasing the cardiac output (McCance and Huether, 2019).

Decreased Inspired Oxygen Concentration. With the decline of the concentration of inspired oxygen, the oxygen-carrying capacity of the blood decreases. Decreases in the fraction of inspired oxygen concentration (FiO_2) are caused by upper or lower airway obstruction, which limits delivery of inspired oxygen to alveoli; decreased environmental oxygen (at high altitudes); or hypoventilation (occurs in opiate overdoses) (Lewis et al., 2017).

Increased Metabolic Rate. Increased metabolic activity increases oxygen demand. The level of oxygenation declines when body systems are unable to meet this demand. An increased metabolic rate is normal in pregnancy, wound healing, and exercise because the body is using energy for building tissue. Most people are able to meet the increased oxygen demand and do not display signs of oxygen deprivation. Fever increases the tissues' need for oxygen; as a result, carbon dioxide production increases. When fever persists, the metabolic rate remains high, and the body begins to break down protein stores. This causes muscle wasting and decreased muscle mass, including respiratory muscles such as the diaphragm and intercostal muscles. The body attempts to adapt to the increased carbon dioxide levels by increasing the rate and depth of respiration. The patient's WOB increases, and the patient eventually displays signs and symptoms of hypoxemia. Patients with pulmonary diseases are at greater risk for hypoxemia (McCance and Huether, 2019).

Conditions Affecting Chest Wall Movement. Any condition reducing chest wall movement results in decreased ventilation. If the diaphragm does not fully descend with breathing, the volume of inspired air decreases, delivering less oxygen to the alveoli and tissues (McCance and Huether, 2019).

Pregnancy. As the fetus grows during pregnancy, the enlarging uterus pushes abdominal contents upward against the diaphragm. In the last trimester of pregnancy, the inspiratory capacity declines, resulting in dyspnea on exertion and increased fatigue (Ball et al., 2019).

Obesity. Patients who are morbidly obese have reduced lung volumes from the heavy lower thorax and abdomen, particularly when in the recumbent and supine positions. Many morbidly obese patients suffer from obstructive sleep apnea. Morbidly obese patients have a reduction in lung and chest wall compliance as a result of encroachment of the abdomen into the chest, increased WOB, and decreased lung volumes. In some patients an obesity-hypoventilation syndrome develops in which oxygenation is decreased and carbon dioxide is retained. The obese patient is also susceptible to atelectasis or pneumonia after surgery because the lungs do not expand fully and the lower lobes retain pulmonary secretions (McCance and Huether, 2019).

Musculoskeletal Abnormalities. Musculoskeletal impairments in the thoracic region reduce oxygenation. Such impairments result from abnormal structural configurations, trauma, muscular diseases, and diseases of the central nervous system. Abnormal structural configurations impairing oxygenation include those affecting the rib cage, such as pectus excavatum, and the vertebral column, such as kyphosis, lordosis, or scoliosis (Ball et al., 2019; McCance and Huether, 2019).

Trauma. Flail chest is a condition in which multiple rib fractures cause chest wall instability. This instability allows the lung under the injured area to contract on inspiration and bulge on expiration, resulting in hypoxia. Patients with thoracic or upper abdominal surgical incisions use shallow respirations to avoid pain, which also decreases chest wall movement. Opioids used to treat pain depress the respiratory center, further decreasing respiratory rate and chest wall expansion (Urden et al., 2020).

Neuromuscular Diseases. Neuromuscular diseases affect tissue oxygenation by decreasing a patient's ability to expand and contract the chest wall. Ventilation is impaired, resulting in atelectasis, hypercapnia, and hypoxemia. Examples of conditions causing hypoventilation include myasthenia gravis and Guillain-Barré syndrome (McCance and Huether, 2019).

Central Nervous System Alterations. Diseases or trauma of the medulla oblongata and/or spinal cord result in impaired ventilation. When the medulla oblongata is affected, neural regulation of ventilation is impaired, and abnormal breathing patterns develop. Cervical trauma at C3 to C5 usually results in paralysis of the phrenic nerve. When the phrenic nerve is damaged, the diaphragm does not descend properly, thus reducing inspiratory lung volumes and causing hypoxemia. Spinal cord trauma below the C5 vertebra usually leaves the phrenic nerve intact but damages nerves that innervate the intercostal muscles, preventing anteroposterior chest expansion.

Influences of Chronic Lung Disease. Oxygenation decreases as a direct consequence of chronic lung disease. Changes in the anteroposterior diameter of the chest wall (barrel chest) occur because of overuse of accessory muscles and air trapping in COPD or cystic fibrosis. Chronic lung disease often results in varying degrees of dyspnea, tachypnea, hypoxemia and/or hypercapnia (Ball et al., 2019; Lewis et al., 2017; McCance and Huether, 2019).

Alterations in Respiratory Functioning

Illnesses and conditions affecting ventilation or oxygen transport alter respiratory functioning. The three primary alterations are hypoventilation, hyperventilation, and hypoxia.

The goal of ventilation is to produce a normal arterial carbon dioxide tension ($PaCO_2$) between 35 and 45 mm Hg and a normal arterial oxygen tension (PaO_2) between 80 and 100 mm Hg. Hypoventilation and hyperventilation are often determined by arterial blood gas analysis (McCance and Huether, 2019). Hypoxemia refers to a decrease in the amount of arterial oxygen. Nurses monitor arterial oxygen saturation (SpO_2) using a pulse oximeter, a noninvasive oxygen saturation monitor. Normally SpO_2 is greater than or equal to 95% (see Chapter 30).

Hypoventilation. Hypoventilation occurs when alveolar ventilation is inadequate to meet the oxygen demand of the body or eliminate sufficient carbon dioxide. As alveolar ventilation decreases, the body retains carbon dioxide. For example, atelectasis, a collapse of the alveoli, prevents normal exchange of oxygen and carbon dioxide. As more alveoli collapse, less of the lung is ventilated, and hypoventilation occurs.

In patients with COPD, the administration of excessive oxygen results in hypoventilation. These patients have adapted to a high carbon dioxide level, so their carbon dioxide–sensitive chemoreceptors do not function normally. Their peripheral chemoreceptors of the aortic arch and carotid bodies are primarily sensitive to lower oxygen levels, causing increased ventilation. Because the stimulus to breathe is a decreased arterial oxygen (PaO_2) level (hypoxic drive to breathe), administration of oxygen greater than 24% to 28% (1 to 3 L/min) prevents the PaO_2 from falling to a level (60 mm Hg) that stimulates the peripheral receptors, thus destroying the stimulus to breathe. The resulting hypoventilation causes excessive retention of carbon dioxide, which can lead to respiratory acidosis and respiratory arrest. Signs and symptoms of hypoventilation include mental status changes, dysrhythmias, and potential cardiac arrest. If untreated, the patient's status rapidly declines, leading to convulsions, unconsciousness, and death (McCance and Huether, 2019).

Hyperventilation. Hyperventilation is a state of ventilation in which the lungs remove carbon dioxide faster than it is produced by cellular metabolism. Severe anxiety, infection, drugs, or an acid-base imbalance induces hyperventilation (see Chapter 42). Acute anxiety leads to hyperventilation and exhalation of excessive amounts of carbon dioxide. Increased body temperature (fever) increases the metabolic rate, thereby increasing carbon dioxide production. The increased carbon dioxide level stimulates an increase in the patient's rate and depth of respiration, causing hyperventilation (McCance and Huether, 2019).

Hyperventilation is sometimes chemically induced. For example, salicylate (aspirin) poisoning and amphetamine use result in excess carbon dioxide production, stimulating the respiratory center to compensate by increasing the rate and depth of respiration. It also occurs as the body tries to compensate for metabolic acidosis. For example, the patient with diabetes in ketoacidosis produces large amounts of metabolic acids. The respiratory system tries to correct the acid-base balance by overbreathing. Ventilation increases to reduce the amount of carbon dioxide available to form carbonic acid (see Chapter 42). This can also result in the patient developing respiratory alkalosis. Signs and symptoms of hyperventilation include rapid respirations, sighing breaths, numbness and tingling of hands/feet, light-headedness, and loss of consciousness (McCance and Huether, 2019).

Hypoxia. Hypoxia is inadequate tissue oxygenation at the cellular level. It results from a deficiency in oxygen delivery or oxygen use at the cellular level. It is a life-threatening condition. Untreated, it has the potential to produce fatal cardiac dysrhythmias (McCance and Huether, 2019).

Causes of hypoxia include (1) a decreased hemoglobin level and lowered oxygen-carrying capacity of the blood; (2) a diminished concentration of inspired oxygen, which occurs at high altitudes; (3) the inability of the tissues to extract oxygen from the blood, as with cyanide poisoning; (4) decreased diffusion of oxygen from the alveoli to the blood, as in pneumonia; (5) poor tissue perfusion with oxygenated blood, as with shock; and (6) impaired ventilation, as with multiple rib fractures or chest trauma (McCance and Huether, 2019).

The clinical signs and symptoms of hypoxia include apprehension, restlessness (often an early sign), inability to concentrate, decreased level of consciousness, dizziness, and behavioral changes. The patient with hypoxia is unable to lie flat and appears both fatigued and agitated. Vital sign changes include an increased pulse rate and increased rate and depth of respiration. During early stages of hypoxia the blood pressure is elevated unless the condition is caused by shock. As the hypoxia worsens, the respiratory rate declines as a result of respiratory muscle fatigue (Lewis et al., 2017).

Cyanosis, blue discoloration of the skin and mucous membranes caused by the presence of desaturated hemoglobin in capillaries, is a late sign of hypoxia. The presence or absence of cyanosis is not a reliable measure of oxygen status. Central cyanosis, observed in the tongue, soft palate, and conjunctiva of the eye where blood flow is high, indicates hypoxemia. Peripheral cyanosis, seen in the extremities, nail beds, and earlobes, is often a result of vasoconstriction and stagnant blood flow (Ball et al., 2019; Lewis et al., 2017).

Alterations in Cardiac Functioning

Illnesses and conditions affecting cardiac rhythm, strength of contraction, blood flow through the heart or to the heart muscle, and decreased peripheral circulation alter cardiac function. Older adults have structural changes in the heart, including vascular and valve stiffening, increased left ventricular wall thickness, and fibrosis. In addition, there are changes in the conduction system. Fat accumulates around the SA node, sometimes creating a partial or complete separation of the node from the atrial tissue. A pronounced decline in the number of pacemaker cells occurs after 60 years of age (Strait and Lakatta, 2012; Touhy and Jett, 2018).

Disturbances in Conduction. Electrical impulses that do not originate from the SA node cause conduction disturbances. These rhythm disturbances are called dysrhythmias, meaning a deviation from the normal sinus heart rhythm. Dysrhythmias occur as a primary conduction disturbance such as in response to ischemia; valvular abnormality; anxiety; drug toxicity; caffeine, alcohol, or tobacco use; or a complication of acid-base or electrolyte imbalance (see Chapter 42).

Dysrhythmias are classified by cardiac response and site of impulse origin. Cardiac response is tachycardia (greater than 100 beats/min), bradycardia (less than 60 beats/min), a premature (early) beat, or a blocked (delayed or absent) beat. Tachydysrhythmias and bradydysrhythmias lower cardiac output and blood pressure. Tachydysrhythmias reduce cardiac output by decreasing diastolic filling time. Bradydysrhythmias lower cardiac output because of the decreased heart rate (McCance and Huether, 2019; Urden et al., 2020).

Atrial fibrillation is a common dysrhythmia in older adults. The electrical impulse in the atria is chaotic and originates from multiple sites. The rhythm is irregular because of the multiple pacemaker sites and the unpredictable conduction to the ventricles. The QRS complex is normal; however, it occurs at irregular intervals. Atrial fibrillation is often described as an irregularly irregular rhythm. It decreases cardiac output by altering preload and contractility (Hartjes, 2018; McCance and Huether, 2019; Urden et al., 2020).

Abnormal impulses originating above the ventricles are supraventricular dysrhythmias. The abnormality on the waveform is the configuration and placement of the P wave. Ventricular conduction usually remains normal, and there is a normal QRS complex. Paroxysmal supraventricular tachycardia is a sudden, rapid onset of tachycardia originating above the AV node. It often begins and ends spontaneously. Sometimes excitement, fatigue, caffeine, smoking, or alcohol use precipitates paroxysmal supraventricular tachycardia (McCance and Huether, 2019; Urden et al., 2020).

Ventricular dysrhythmias represent an ectopic site of impulse formation within the ventricles. It is ectopic in that the impulse originates in the ventricle, not the SA node. The configuration of the QRS complex is usually widened and bizarre. P waves are not always present; often they are buried in the QRS complex. Ventricular tachycardia and ventricular fibrillation are life-threatening rhythms that require immediate intervention. Ventricular tachycardia is a life-threatening dysrhythmia because of the decreased cardiac output and the potential to deteriorate into ventricular fibrillation or sudden cardiac death (Hartjes, 2018; Urden et al., 2020).

Altered Cardiac Output. Failure of the myocardium to eject sufficient volume to the systemic and pulmonary circulations occurs in heart failure. Primary coronary artery disease, cardiomyopathy, valvular disorders, and pulmonary disease lead to myocardial pump failure (McCance and Huether, 2019; Urden et al., 2020).

Left-Sided Heart Failure. Left-sided heart failure is an abnormal condition characterized by decreased functioning of the left ventricle. If left ventricular failure is significant, the amount of blood ejected from the left ventricle drops greatly, resulting in decreased cardiac output. Signs and symptoms include fatigue, breathlessness, dizziness, and confusion as a result of tissue hypoxia from the diminished cardiac output. As the left ventricle continues to fail, blood begins to pool in the pulmonary circulation, causing pulmonary congestion. Clinical findings include crackles in the bases of the lungs on auscultation, hypoxia, shortness of breath on exertion, cough, and paroxysmal nocturnal dyspnea (Hartjes, 2018; McCance and Huether, 2019).

Right-Sided Heart Failure. Right-sided heart failure results from impaired functioning of the right ventricle. It more commonly results from pulmonary disease or as a result of long-term left-sided failure. The primary pathological factor in right-sided failure is elevated pulmonary vascular resistance (PVR). As the PVR continues to rise, the right ventricle works harder, and the oxygen demand of the heart increases. As the failure continues, the amount of blood ejected from the right ventricle declines, and blood begins to "back up" in the systemic circulation. Clinically the patient has systemic symptoms, such as weight gain, distended neck veins, hepatomegaly and splenomegaly, and dependent peripheral edema (Hartjes, 2018; McCance and Huether, 2019).

Impaired Valvular Function. Valvular heart disease is an acquired or congenital disorder of a cardiac valve that causes either hardening (stenosis) or impaired closure (regurgitation) of the valves. When stenosis occurs, the flow of blood through the valves is obstructed. For example, when stenosis occurs in the semilunar valves (aortic and pulmonic valves), the adjacent ventricles have to work harder to move the ventricular blood volume beyond the stenotic valve. Over time the stenosis causes the ventricle to hypertrophy (enlarge), and if the condition is untreated, left- or right-sided heart failure occurs. When regurgitation occurs, there is a backflow of blood into an adjacent chamber. For example, in mitral regurgitation the mitral leaflets do not close completely. When the ventricles contract, blood escapes back into the atria, causing a murmur, or "whooshing" sound (see Chapter 30) (Hartjes, 2018; McCance and Huether, 2019).

Myocardial Ischemia. Myocardial ischemia results when the supply of blood to the myocardium from the coronary arteries is insufficient to meet myocardial oxygen demands. Two common outcomes of this ischemia are angina pectoris and myocardial infarction (Hartjes, 2018; McCance and Huether, 2019).

Angina. Angina pectoris is a transient imbalance between myocardial oxygen supply and demand. The condition results in chest pain that is aching, sharp, tingling, or burning or that feels like pressure. Typically, chest pain is left sided or substernal and often radiates to the left or both arms, the jaw, neck, and back. In some patients, angina pain does not radiate. It usually lasts from 3 to 5 minutes. Patients report that it is often precipitated by activities that increase myocardial oxygen demand (e.g., eating heavy meals, exercise, or stress). It is usually relieved with rest and coronary vasodilators, the most common being a nitroglycerin preparation (McCance and Huether, 2019).

Myocardial Infarction. Myocardial infarction (MI) or acute coronary syndrome (ACS) results from sudden decreases in coronary blood flow or an increase in myocardial oxygen demand without

adequate coronary perfusion. Infarction occurs because ischemia is not reversed. Cellular death occurs after 20 minutes of myocardial ischemia (McCance and Huether, 2019).

Chest pain associated with MI in men is usually described as crushing, squeezing, or stabbing. The pain is often in the left chest and sternal area; may be felt in the back; and radiates down the left arm to the neck, jaws, teeth, epigastric area, and back. It occurs at rest or exertion and lasts more than 20 minutes. Rest, position change, or sublingual nitroglycerin administration does not relieve the pain (Hartjes, 2018; McCance and Huether, 2019).

There are differences between men and women in relation to coronary artery disease. As women get older, their risk of heart disease begins to rise, making it the leading cause of death for women in the United States. Women on average have greater blood cholesterol and triglyceride levels than men. Obesity in women is more prevalent, which also increases risk for diabetes and cardiac disease. Women's symptoms differ from those of men. The most common initial symptom in women is angina, but they also present with atypical symptoms such as fatigue, indigestion, shortness of breath, and back or jaw pain. Women have twice the risk of dying within the first year after a heart attack than men (CDC, 2019a; 2017 Ball et al., 2019; Lewis et al.,).

REFLECT NOW

You are caring for a patient who was recently told he has decreased cardiac output due to atrial fibrillation. How would you describe cardiac output, the conduction system, and this dysrhythmia to the patient?

NURSING KNOWLEDGE BASE

Factors Influencing Oxygenation

In addition to physiological factors, multiple developmental, lifestyle, and environmental factors affect patients' oxygenation status. It is important to recognize these as possible risks or factors that impact their health care goals.

Developmental Factors. The developmental stage of a patient and the normal aging process affect tissue oxygenation.

Infants and Toddlers. Healthy full-term infants younger than 3 months of age are presumed to have a lower infection rate because of the protective function of maternal antibodies. The infection rate increases in infants from 3 to 6 months of age. Infants and toddlers are at risk for upper respiratory tract infections, especially when they are exposed to secondhand smoke or other children. Upper respiratory tract infections are usually not dangerous, and infants and toddlers recover with little difficulty. Infants and toddlers are also at risk for airway obstruction because of their anatomically smaller airways and their tendency to place foreign objects in their mouths (Hockenberry et al., 2019).

School-Age Children and Adolescents. School-age children and adolescents are exposed to respiratory infections and respiratory risk factors such as cigarette smoking or secondhand smoke. This age-group is also at risk for experimenting with cigarette smoking and other recreational inhalants. A healthy child usually does not have adverse pulmonary effects from respiratory infections. The CDC (2018b) reported that 5.6% of middle school–age children and 19.6% of high school–age children use tobacco products, with electronic cigarettes being the most commonly used tobacco product among these age-groups. However, current cigarette smoking among middle school– and high school–age children has declined (CDC, 2018b). School-age children and adolescents possess other cardiopulmonary disease risk factors such as obesity, inactive lifestyles, unhealthy diets, and excessive use of caffeinated beverages or other energy drinks (Hockenberry et al., 2019).

Young and Middle-Age Adults. Young and middle-age adults are exposed to multiple cardiopulmonary risk factors: an unhealthy diet, lack of exercise, stress, over-the-counter and prescription drugs not used as intended, illegal substances, and smoking. Reducing these modifiable factors decreases a patient's risk for cardiac or pulmonary diseases. This is also the time when individuals establish lifelong habits and lifestyles. It is important to help your patients make good choices and informed decisions about their health care practices. The increased cost of cigarettes plus the states' smoke-free air policies, laws that reduce smoking in public places, and access to cessation programs and medications have proven to be helpful in smoking cessation (CDC, 2018a).

Older Adults. The cardiac and respiratory systems undergo changes throughout the aging process (Box 41.1). The changes are associated with calcification of the heart valves, vascular stiffening and increased left ventricular wall thickness, fewer SA nodes, and costal cartilage stiffening. The arterial system develops atherosclerotic plaques.

Osteoporosis leads to changes in the size and shape of the thorax. The trachea and large bronchi become enlarged from calcification of the airways. The alveoli enlarge, decreasing the surface area available for gas exchange. The number of functional cilia is reduced, causing a decrease in the effectiveness of the cough mechanism, putting the older adult at increased risk for respiratory infections (Touhy and Jett, 2018).

BOX 41.1 FOCUS ON OLDER ADULTS

Cardiopulmonary Implication in Older Adults

- The tuberculin skin test is an unreliable indicator of tuberculosis in older patients. They frequently display false-positive or false-negative skin test reactions.
- Older patients are at an increased risk for reactivation of dormant organisms that were present for decades as a result of age-related changes in the immune system.
- The standard 5-TU Mantoux test is given and repeated or repeated with the 250-TU strength to create a booster effect. If the older patient has a positive reaction, a complete history is necessary to determine any risk factors.
- Cardiac problems differ from other chronic conditions in that when they become acute, symptoms worsen rapidly and necessitate hospitalization, whereas other chronic conditions can be managed in the home (Touhy and Jett, 2018).
- Controlling blood pressure in older adults results in 30% fewer strokes, 64% less heart failure, 23% fewer fatal cardiac events, and 21% fewer cardiac-related deaths (Touhy and Jett, 2018).
- Mental status changes are often the first signs of cardiac and/or respiratory problems and often include forgetfulness and irritability.
- Changes in the older adult's cough mechanism lead to retention of pulmonary secretions, airway plugging, and atelectasis if patients do not use cough suppressants with caution.
- Age-related changes in the immune system lead to a decline of both cell-mediated and humoral immunity, resulting in an increased risk of respiratory infections (McCance and Huether, 2019).
- Changes in the thorax that occur from ossification of costal cartilage, decreased space between vertebrae, and diminished respiratory muscle strength lead to problems with chest expansion and oxygenation (Touhy and Jett, 2018).

Lifestyle Factors. Lifestyle modifications are difficult for patients because they often have to change an enjoyable habit such as cigarette smoking or eating certain foods. Risk-factor modification is important and includes smoking cessation, weight reduction, a low-cholesterol and low-sodium diet, management of hypertension, and moderate exercise (see Chapter 6). Although it is difficult to change long-term behavior, helping patients acquire healthy behaviors reduces the risk for or slows or halts the progression of cardiopulmonary diseases.

Nutrition. Good nutrition affects cardiopulmonary function by supporting normal metabolic functions. A poor diet leads to risk factors affecting the heart and lungs. Without essential nutrients, a patient may experience respiratory muscle wasting, resulting in decreased muscle strength and respiratory excursion. Cough efficiency is reduced secondary to respiratory muscle weakness, putting a patient at risk for retention of pulmonary secretions. A patient with chronic lung disease often requires a diet higher in calories and smaller, more frequent meals due to the increased work of breathing. A diet with a moderate amount of carbohydrates is recommended to prevent an increase in carbon dioxide production. Obesity affects the respiratory and cardiovascular systems. It can lead to a decrease in lung expansion and an increase in oxygen demand to meet metabolic demands (Lewis et al., 2017).

Dietary practices also influence the prevalence of cardiovascular diseases (see Chapter 45). Patients with nutritional alterations are at risk for anemia, which reduces the oxygen-carrying capacity of the blood and can alter cardiac output. Cardioprotective nutrition includes diets rich in fiber; whole grains; fresh fruits and vegetables; nuts; antioxidants; lean meats, fish, and chicken; and omega-3 fatty acids. A diet of fruits, vegetables, and low-fat dairy foods that are high in fiber, potassium, calcium, and magnesium and low in saturated and total fat helps prevent and reduce the effects of hypertension (Lewis et al., 2017).

Hydration. Fluid intake is essential for cellular health. Fluid volume overload may lead to vascular congestion in patients with heart, kidney, or lung diseases and impair the body's ability to deliver oxygen to the tissues. Dehydration or fluid volume deficit may result in dizziness, fainting, hypotension, or a thickening of respiratory secretions, which makes it difficult for a patient to expectorate secretions (Lewis et al., 2017).

Exercise. Exercise increases the metabolic activity and oxygen demand of the body. The rate and depth of respiration increase, enabling the person to inhale more oxygen and exhale excess carbon dioxide. A physical exercise program has many benefits (see Chapter 38). People who exercise for 30 to 60 minutes daily have a lower pulse rate and blood pressure, decreased cholesterol level, increased blood flow, and greater oxygen extraction by working muscles (Lewis et al., 2017).

Smoking. Cigarette smoking and secondhand smoke are associated with a number of diseases, including heart disease, COPD, and lung cancer. Cigarette smoking worsens peripheral vascular and coronary artery diseases. Inhaled nicotine causes vasoconstriction of peripheral and coronary blood vessels, increasing blood pressure and decreasing blood flow to peripheral vessels (McCance and Huether, 2019).

Women who take birth control pills and smoke cigarettes have an increased risk for thrombophlebitis and pulmonary emboli. Smoking during pregnancy can result in low-birth-weight babies, preterm delivery, and babies with reduced lung function (CDC, 2018c).

Smoking accounts for approximately 30% of all cancer deaths in the United States, including 80% of all lung cancer deaths. Smoking has been linked to the development of other cancers, including mouth, esophagus, liver, bladder, kidney, cervix, and myeloid leukemia (ACS, 2018). Nicotine patches, gum, and lozenges are available over the counter, and nicotine nasal spray and inhalers can be obtained by prescription. Prescription drugs such as bupropion and varenicline are also available to help people quit smoking (ACS, 2017).

Exposure to environmental tobacco smoke (secondhand smoke) increases the risk of lung cancer and cardiovascular disease in the nonsmoker. Children with parents who smoke have a higher incidence of asthma, pneumonia, and ear infections. Infants exposed to secondhand smoke are at higher risk for sudden infant death syndrome (NCI, 2018).

Substance Abuse. Excessive use of alcohol and other illicit drugs impairs tissue oxygenation in two ways. First, the person who chronically abuses substances often has a poor nutritional intake. With the resultant decrease in intake of iron-rich foods, hemoglobin production declines. Second, excessive use of alcohol and certain other drugs depresses the respiratory center, reducing the rate and depth of respiration and the amount of inhaled oxygen. Substance abuse by either smoking or inhaling substances such as crack cocaine or fumes from paint or glue cans causes direct injury to lung tissue that leads to permanent lung damage (McCance and Huether, 2019). The report on inhalant abuse (huffing) by teenagers to get a euphoric effect includes use of a wide variety of substances such as paint thinner, nail polish remover, glue, spray paint, nitrous oxide, and other common household products. Sudden death can occur from cardiac arrhythmias, or chronic abuse can cause damage to heart, lungs, and kidneys (NIDA, 2017).

Stress. Stress is a perceived threat that results in sympathetic stimulation. Continuous stress adversely affects a patient's health and well-being (see Chapter 37). A continuous state of stress increases the metabolic rate and oxygen demand of the body. The body responds to stress with an increased rate and depth of respiration and increased cardiac output. Stress causes an increased release of cortisol, which affects the metabolism of fat and creates a risk for CAD and hypertension. Stressors can be a trigger for asthma exacerbations. Patients with chronic illnesses or life-threatening illnesses cannot tolerate the oxygen demands associated with stress (Huether and McCance, 2017).

Environmental Factors. The environment influences oxygenation. The prevalence of COPD is higher in rural areas versus those who live in urban areas (CDC, 2018f). In addition, a patient's workplace sometimes increases the risk for pulmonary disease. Occupational pollutants include asbestos, talcum powder, dust, and airborne fibers. For example, farm workers in dry regions of the southwestern United States are at risk for coccidioidomycosis, a fungal disease caused by inhalation of spores of the airborne bacterium *Coccidioides immitis* (CDC, 2019b). Asbestosis is an occupational lung disease that develops after exposure to asbestos. The lung with asbestosis often has diffuse interstitial fibrosis, creating a restrictive lung disease. Patients exposed to asbestos are at risk for developing lung cancer, and this risk increases with exposure to tobacco smoke (McCance and Huether, 2019).

CRITICAL THINKING

Successful critical thinking requires a synthesis of knowledge, experience, information gathered from patients, critical thinking attitudes, and intellectual and professional standards. Clinical judgments require you to anticipate information, analyze the data, and make

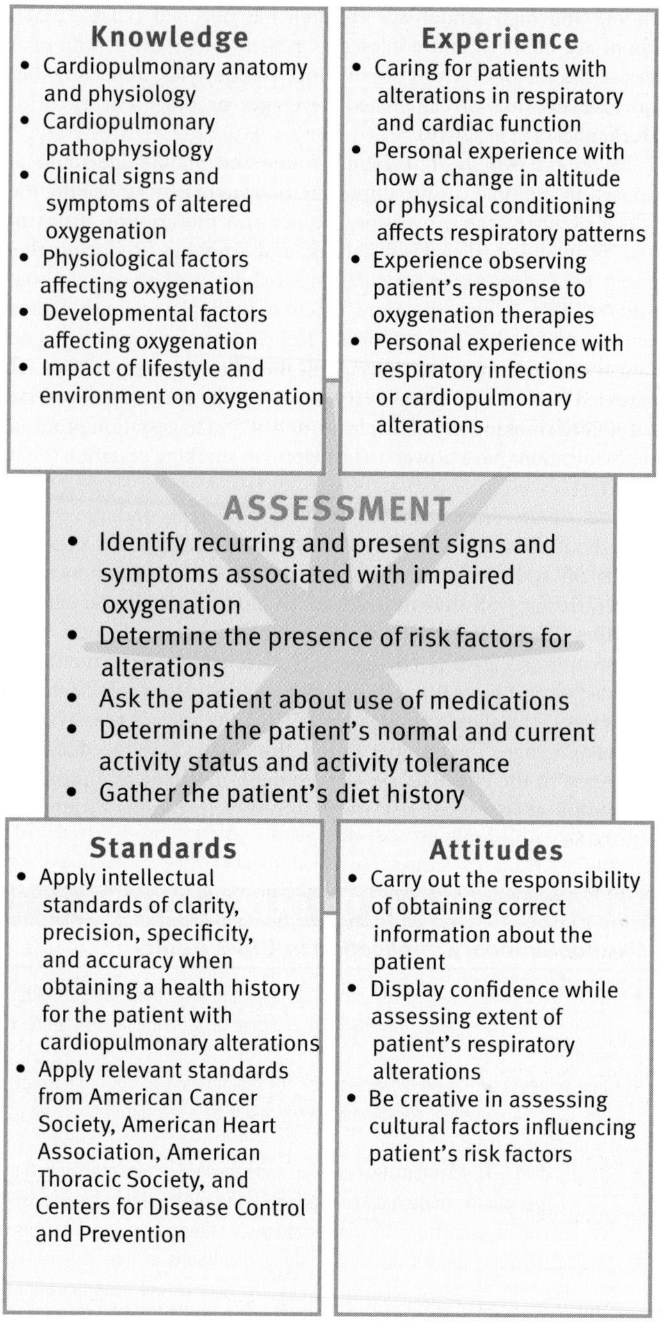

FIG. 41.4 Critical thinking model for oxygenation assessment.

decisions regarding your patient's care. During assessment consider all elements that build toward making an appropriate nursing diagnosis (Fig. 41.4).

To understand how alterations in oxygenation affect patients and your selection of appropriate interventions, you need to integrate knowledge from nursing and other disciplines and information gathered from patients. Critical thinking attitudes ensure that you approach patient care in a methodical and logical way. The use of professional standards such as The American Association for Respiratory Care (AARC) and the American Nurses Association (ANA) provide valuable guidelines for care and management of patients (see Fig. 41.4).

❖ NURSING PROCESS

Apply the nursing process and use a critical thinking approach in your care of patients. The nursing process provides a clinical decision-making approach for you to develop and implement an individualized plan of care.

◆ Assessment

During the assessment process, thoroughly assess each patient and critically analyze findings to ensure that you make patient-centered clinical decisions required for safe nursing care. Nursing assessment of cardiopulmonary functioning includes an in-depth history of a patient's normal and present cardiopulmonary function, past impairments in circulatory or respiratory functioning, and methods that a patient uses to optimize oxygenation. The nursing history includes a review of drug, food, and other allergies. Physical examination of a patient's cardiopulmonary status reveals the extent of existing signs and symptoms (Ball et al., 2019) (see Chapter 30). Utilizing assessment values of pulse oximetry and capnography aids in the assessment of patients with spontaneous breathing, intubated patients, and patients requiring oxygen therapy or mechanical ventilation. Pulse oximetry provides an instant feedback about the patient's level of oxygenation. Capnography, also known as *end-tidal CO_2 monitoring*, provides instant information about the patient's ventilation (how effectively CO_2 is being eliminated by the pulmonary system), perfusion (how effectively CO_2 is being transported through the vascular system), and how effectively CO_2 is produced by cellular metabolism (Hartjes, 2018; Urden et al., 2020). Capnography is measured near the end of exhalation. Finally, a review of laboratory and diagnostic test results provides valuable assessment data.

Through the Patient's Eyes. Ask patients about their priorities and what they expect from their health care visit. Identifying their expectations regarding their health, symptoms, and treatment plan involves patients in the decision-making process and helps them participate in their care. For example, planning a smoking-cessation program for a patient who is not ready for the change is frustrating for both the patient and you. Establish realistic, short-term outcomes that build to a larger goal. For example, tobacco-cessation treatments are effective, but a patient needs to be willing to participate in the program and may need to use several strategies to be successful. Educating the patient on the opportunities for individual, group, or telephone counseling and identifying a social support system give more individual choices when developing the cessation plan. After this is determined, the various nicotine and non-nicotine medications for treatment of tobacco dependence can be discussed to find one that may fit the patient's lifestyle. A combination of counseling and medication is more effective than either one alone (CDC, 2017a).

BOX 41.2 Nursing Assessment Questions

Nature of the Cardiopulmonary Problem
- Describe the problem that you're having with your heart.
- Does the problem (e.g., chest pain, rapid heart rate) occur at a specific time of the day, during or after exercise, or all the time?
- Do you notice abnormal beats?
- If you have chest pain, what relieves or makes the pain worse?

Questions to Ask Associated With Breathing
- Describe the breathing problems you are having.
- How has your breathing pattern changed?
- Do you have a cough? Is the coughing increasing? Is it worse at a certain time of day?
- Describe your cough. Is it dry or moist? Do you have sputum with coughing? Is this different in color, volume, or thickness?
- On a scale of 0 to 10, with 10 being the most severe, rate your shortness of breath. What helps your shortness of breath?

Questions to Ask Related to Chest Pain
- If you are having chest pain, what causes the pain and how long does it last? Is this a different type of pain? Can you show me where the pain is located?
- Does the chest pain occur with coughing?
- On a scale of 0 to 10, with 0 being no pain and 10 being the most severe pain, rate your chest pain at its worst. Is the pain different today?

Questions to Ask Regarding Predisposing Factors
- Have you been exposed to a cold or flu or other respiratory illnesses?
- Tell me the medications you are taking. Are you taking over-the-counter medications or supplements? If so, what are they?
- Do you smoke? Have you been exposed to secondhand smoke?
- Have you been doing any unusual exercises?

Questions to Ask Regarding Effect of Symptoms
- Describe for me a typical daily diet.
- Tell me how your symptoms affect daily activities, your appetite, sleeping, and exercise routine.

Remember that your goals and expectations do not always coincide with those of your patient. By addressing a patient's concerns and expectations, you establish a relationship that addresses other health care goals and expected outcomes. Knowing your patients' mind-sets and respecting their wishes go a long way in helping them make significant beneficial lifestyle changes.

Nursing History. The nursing history focuses on the patient's ability to meet oxygen needs and maintain cardiorespiratory health. The nursing history for respiratory function includes the presence of a cough, shortness of breath, dyspnea, wheezing, pain, environmental exposures, frequency of respiratory tract infections, pulmonary risk factors, past respiratory problems, current medication use, and smoking history or secondhand smoke exposure. The nursing history for cardiac function includes pain and characteristics of pain, fatigue, peripheral circulation, cardiac risk factors, diet, and the presence of past or concurrent cardiac conditions. Ask specific questions related to cardiopulmonary disease (Box 41.2).

Health Risks. Determine familial risk factors such as a family history of lung cancer or cardiovascular disease. Documentation includes blood relatives who had cardiopulmonary disease and their present level of health or age at time of death. Assess for an exposure to infectious organisms, such as tuberculosis (TB). Occupational and environment risk factors (e.g., asbestos exposure) should also be addressed (Ball et al., 2019; McCance and Huether, 2019).

Pain. The presence of chest pain requires an immediate thorough assessment, including location, duration, radiation, and frequency. In addition, it is important to note any other symptoms associated with chest pain, such as nausea, diaphoresis, extreme fatigue, or weakness. Cardiac pain does not occur with respiratory variations. Chest pain in men is most often on the left side of the chest and radiates to the left arm. Chest pain in women is much less definitive and is often a sensation of breathlessness, jaw or back pain, nausea, and/or fatigue (CDC, 2019a). Pericardial pain results from inflammation of the pericardial sac, occurs on inspiration, and does not usually radiate (Ball et al., 2019).

Pleuritic chest pain results from inflammation of the pleural space of the lungs; the pain is peripheral and radiates to the scapular regions. Inspiratory maneuvers such as coughing, yawning, and sighing worsen pleuritic chest pain. Patients usually describe it as knifelike, lasting from a minute to hours and always in association with inspiration. Musculoskeletal pain is often present following exercise, rib trauma, and prolonged coughing episodes. Inspiration worsens this pain, and patients often confuse it with pleuritic chest pain (Ball et al., 2019).

Fatigue. Fatigue is a subjective sensation in which a patient reports a loss of endurance. Fatigue in the patient with cardiopulmonary alterations is often an early sign of a worsening of the chronic underlying process. To provide an objective measure of fatigue, ask the patient to rate it on a scale of 0 to 10, with 10 being the worst level and 0 representing no fatigue. Ask your patients when they noticed the fatigue, what makes it better or worse, if the onset was sudden or gradual, if it is worse in the morning or later in the day, and how the fatigue affects what they want to do (Ball et al., 2019; Lewis et al., 2017).

Dyspnea. Dyspnea is associated with hypoxia. It is the subjective sensation of difficult or uncomfortable breathing or observed labored breathing with shortness of breath. Dyspnea is usually associated with exercise or excitement, but in some patients, it is present without any relation to activity or exercise. It is associated with many conditions, such as pulmonary diseases, cardiovascular diseases, neuromuscular conditions, and anemia. In addition, it occurs in the pregnant woman in the final months of pregnancy. Finally, environmental factors such as pollution, cold air, and smoking also cause or worsen dyspnea (Ball et al., 2019).

When gathering information about a patient's sensation of dyspnea, ask the patient when the dyspnea occurs (such as with exertion, stress, or respiratory tract infection) and what improves the dyspnea (e.g., rest, inhaled medication, or position change). Determine whether the patient's dyspnea affects the ability to lie flat. Orthopnea is an abnormal condition in which a patient uses multiple pillows when reclining to breathe easier or sits leaning forward with arms elevated. The number of pillows used usually helps to quantify the orthopnea (e.g., two- or three-pillow orthopnea). Also ask whether the patient must sleep in a recliner chair to breathe easier. Paroxysmal nocturnal dyspnea (PND) occurs when a patient is sleeping. The patient often awakens in a panic, feels as if he or she is suffocating, and has a strong need to sit up to relieve the breathlessness (Ball et al., 2019).

Cough. Coughing is a protective reflex to clear the trachea, bronchi, and lungs of irritants and secretions. Patients with a chronic cough tend to deny, underestimate, or minimize their coughing, often because they are so accustomed to it that they are unaware of its frequency (Ball et al., 2019).

If a patient has a cough, determine the onset of the cough, how frequently it occurs, and whether it is productive or nonproductive. Chronic coughs are often a sign of chronic lung disease, whereas acute coughs can be a sign of infection or an inhaled irritant. A nonproductive cough is often associated with allergies or gastroesophageal reflux disease. A productive cough results in sputum production (e.g., material coughed up from the lungs that a patient swallows or expectorates). Sputum contains mucus, cellular debris, microorganisms, and sometimes pus or blood. Collect data about the type and quantity of sputum. Instruct patients to try to cough up some sputum and not to simply clear the throat, which produces only saliva. Have the patient cough into a specimen cup. Inspect the sputum for color (such as green or blood tinged), consistency (such as thin or thick), odor (none or foul), and amount in tablespoons or milliliters (Ball et al., 2019).

If hemoptysis (bloody sputum) is present, determine whether it is associated with coughing and bleeding from the upper respiratory tract, sinus drainage, or the gastrointestinal tract (hematemesis). Hemoptysis has an alkaline pH, and hematemesis has an acidic pH; thus, pH testing of the specimen may help to determine the source (McCance and Huether, 2019). Describe hemoptysis according to amount and color and whether it is mixed with sputum. Note whether the patient is on anticoagulant therapy. When there is bloody or blood-tinged sputum, health care providers frequently perform diagnostic tests such as examination of sputum specimens, chest x-ray examinations, bronchoscopy, and other scans.

Environmental and Occupational Exposures. Environmental exposure to inhaled substances, such as smog, dust, silicon, mold, cockroaches, pet dander, and asbestos, is closely linked with respiratory disease. Investigate exposures in the patient's home, workplace, and recent travel. In addition, determine whether a patient who is a nonsmoker is exposed to secondhand smoke (ATSDR, 2016; McCance and Huether, 2019).

Carbon monoxide (CO) poisoning often results from an improperly vented furnace flue or fireplace. The patient will have vague complaints of general malaise, flulike symptoms, and excessive sleepiness. Patients are particularly at risk in the late fall when they turn the furnace on or begin to use the fireplace again (CDC, 2018d). Ask whether there is a CO detector in the home.

Radon gas is a radioactive substance from the breakdown of uranium in soil, rock, and water that enters homes through the ground or well water. When homes are poorly ventilated, this gas is unable to escape and becomes trapped. If a patient who smokes also lives in a home with a high radon level, the risk for lung cancer is very high (EPA, 2016). Ask whether the patient has any radon detectors in the home.

Smoking. It is important to determine a patient's direct and secondary exposure to tobacco. Ask about any history of smoking; include the number of years smoked and the number of packages smoked per day. This is recorded as pack-year history (packages per day × years smoked). For example, if a patient smoked two packs a day for 20 years, the patient has a 40 pack-year history. Determine exposure to secondhand smoke, because any form of tobacco exposure increases a patient's risk for cardiopulmonary diseases (ALA, 2019a).

Respiratory Infections. Obtain information about a patient's frequency and duration of respiratory tract infections. Although everyone occasionally has a cold, for some people it results in bronchitis or pneumonia. On average, patients have four colds per year. Determine if and when a patient has had a pneumococcal or influenza (flu) vaccine. This is especially important when assessing older adults because of their increased risk for respiratory disease (Touhy and Jett, 2018). Ask about any known exposure to tuberculosis (TB) and the date and results of the last tuberculin skin test.

Determine a patient's risk for human immunodeficiency virus (HIV) infection. Patients with a history of intravenous (IV) drug use and multiple unprotected sex partners are at risk of developing HIV infection. Patients do not always display symptoms of HIV infection until they present with *Pneumocystis* or *Mycoplasma* pneumonia. Patients with HIV/AIDS (acquired immunodeficiency syndrome) or other immunocompromised states are at increased risk for respiratory infections (McCance and Huether, 2019).

Allergies. Inquire about your patient's exposure to airborne allergens (e.g., pet dander, pollen, or mold). The allergic response is often watery eyes, sneezing, runny nose, or respiratory symptoms such as cough or wheezing. When obtaining information from the patient, ask specific questions about the type of allergens, response to these allergens, and successful and unsuccessful relief measures. In addition, determine the effect of environmental air quality and secondhand smoke exposure on the patient's allergy and symptoms. Safe nursing practice also includes obtaining information about food, drug, or insect sting allergies on the initial history and physical. However, always double-check this information with the patient on any subsequent assessment, especially concerning respiratory allergens (Ball et al., 2019).

Medications. Another component of the nursing history includes determining all the medications that a patient is using. These include prescribed medications, over-the-counter medications, folk medicine, herbal medicines, alternative therapies, and illicit drugs and substances. Some of these preparations have adverse effects by themselves or because of interactions with other drugs (Ball et al., 2019). For example, a person using a prescribed bronchodilator drug may choose to use an over-the-counter inhalant as well. Many of these contain ephedrine or *ma huang*, a natural ephedrine, which acts like epinephrine. This product reacts with the prescribed medication by potentiating or decreasing the effect of the prescribed medication. Patients taking warfarin (Coumadin) for blood thinning prolong the prothrombin time (PT)/international normalized ratio (INR) results if they are taking ginkgo biloba, garlic, or ginseng with the anticoagulant. The drug interaction can precipitate a life-threatening bleed (Lewis et al., 2017).

It is important to determine whether a patient uses illicit drugs. Inhaled opioids, which are often diluted with talcum powder, cause pulmonary disorders resulting from the irritant effect of the powder on lung tissues. Marijuana is usually smoked in the form of a joint or pipe. Marijuana smoke is an irritant to the lungs, putting users at higher risk for respiratory illnesses (NIDA, 2018a). Cocaine is snorted through the nose, placed on the gums, smoked, or injected. Cocaine abusers can have acute cardiovascular changes such as constricted blood vessels and increased heart rate and blood pressure. People who use the inhaled form of cocaine often develop respiratory infections such as pneumonia. Cocaine deaths are often caused by heart attack or stroke (NIDA, 2018b).

As with all medications, assess the patient's knowledge and ability to self-administer medications correctly (see Chapter 31). Of particular importance is the assessment that the patient understands the potential side effects of medications. Patients need to recognize adverse reactions and be aware of the dangers in combining prescribed medications with over-the-counter drugs.

TABLE 41.1 Effects of Aging on Cardiopulmonary Assessment Findings

Function	Pathophysiological Change	Key Clinical Findings
Heart		
Muscle contraction	Thickening of the ventricular wall, increased collagen and decreased elastin in the heart muscle	Decreased cardiac output (edema, dyspnea, activity intolerance, inability to lie flat for extended time)
Blood flow	Heart valves become thicker and stiffer, more often in the mitral and aortic valves	Systolic ejection murmur
Conduction system	SA node becomes fibrotic from calcification; decrease in number of pacemaker cells in SA node	Increased P-R, QRS, and Q-T intervals, decreased amplitude of QRS complex; tachycardia more poorly tolerated
Arterial vessel compliance	Calcified vessels, loss of arterial distensibility, decreased elastin in vessel walls, more tortuous vessels	Hypertension with an increase in systolic blood pressure.
Lungs		
Breathing mechanics	Decreased chest wall compliance, loss of elastic recoil Decreased respiratory muscle mass/strength	Prolonged exhalation phase Decreased vital capacity Activity intolerance
Oxygenation	Decreased alveolar surface area Decreased carbon dioxide diffusion capacity	Decreased PaO_2 Slightly increased $PaCO_2$
Breathing control/ breathing pattern	Decreased responsiveness of central and peripheral chemoreceptors to hypoxemia and hypercapnia	Increased respiratory rate Decreased tidal volume
Lung defense mechanisms	Decreased number of cilia Decreased IgA production and humoral and cellular immunity Drier mucus membranes	Decreased airway clearance Diminished cough reflex Increased risk for infection
Sleep and breathing	Decreased respiratory drive Decreased tone of upper airway muscles	Increased risk of aspiration and respiratory infection Snoring, obstructive sleep apnea

IgA, Immunoglobulin A; *PaCO₂,* arterial carbon dioxide tension; *PaO₂,* arterial oxygen tension; *SA,* sinoatrial. (Data from Ball J, et al: *Seidel's guide to physical examination,* ed 9, St Louis, 2019, Elsevier, and Touhy T, Jett K: *Gerontological nursing and healthy aging,* ed 5, St Louis, 2018, Elsevier.)

Physical Examination. The physical examination includes assessment of the cardiopulmonary system (see Chapter 30). Give special consideration when assessing an older adult patient for changes that occur with the aging process (Table 41.1). These changes affect

TABLE 41.2   Inspection of Cardiopulmonary Status

Abnormality	Cause
Eyes	
Xanthelasma (yellow lipid lesions on eyelids)	Hyperlipidemia
Pale conjunctivae	Anemia
Cyanotic conjunctivae	Hypoxemia
Petechiae on conjunctivae	Fat embolus or bacterial endocarditis
Nose	
Flaring nares	Air hunger, dyspnea
Mouth and Lips	
Cyanotic mucous membranes	Decreased oxygenation (hypoxia)
Pursed-lip breathing	Associated with chronic lung disease
Pallor	Anemia
Neck Veins	
Distention	Associated with right-sided heart failure
Chest	
Retractions	Increased work of breathing, dyspnea
Asymmetry	Chest wall injury
Barrel chest	COPD; may be normal in some older adults.
Fingertips and Nail Beds	
Cyanosis	Decreased cardiac output or hypoxia
Splinter hemorrhages	Infective endocarditis
Clubbing of nail beds	Chronic hypoxemia
Skin	
Peripheral cyanosis	Vasoconstriction and diminished blood flow; cold environment
Central cyanosis	Hypoxemia
Decreased skin turgor	Dehydration (normal finding in older adults as a result of decreased skin elasticity)
Dependent edema	Associated with right- and left-sided heart failure
Periorbital edema	Associated with kidney disease

From Ball JW et al: *Seidel's Physical examination handbook*, ed 9, St Louis, 2019, Elsevier; and Lewis, S, et al: *Medical-surgical nursing assessment and management of clinical problems*, ed 9, St Louis, 2017, Mosby.

the patient's activity tolerance and level of fatigue or cause transient changes in vital signs and are not always associated with a specific cardiopulmonary disease.

Inspection. Using inspection techniques, perform a head-to-toe observation of the patient for skin and mucous membrane color, general appearance, level of consciousness, adequacy of systemic circulation, breathing patterns, and chest wall movement (Table 41.2). Investigate any abnormalities further during palpation, percussion, and auscultation.

Inspection includes observations of the nails for clubbing (see Chapter 30). Clubbed nails often occur in patients with chronic oxygen deficiency, such as cystic fibrosis and congenital heart defects.

Also note the shape of the chest wall. Conditions such as advancing age and chronic obstructive pulmonary disease (COPD) cause the chest to assume a rounded "barrel" shape (Ball et al., 2019; Lewis et al., 2017).

Observe chest wall movement for retraction (e.g., sinking in of soft tissues of the chest between the intercostal spaces) and use of accessory muscles. Elevation of a patient's clavicles at rest reveals increased work of breathing. Also observe the patient's breathing pattern and assess for paradoxical breathing (the chest wall contracts during inspiration and expands during exhalation) or asynchronous breathing. At rest the normal adult respiratory rate is 12 to 20 breaths/min. Bradypnea is less than 12 breaths/min, and tachypnea is greater than 20 breaths/min (see Chapter 29). In some conditions, such as metabolic acidosis, the acidic pH stimulates an increase in rate, usually greater than 35 breaths/min, and depth of respirations (Kussmaul respiration) to compensate by decreasing carbon dioxide levels. Apnea is the absence of respirations for 15 to 20 seconds or longer. Cheyne-Stokes respiration occurs when there is decreased blood flow or injury to the brainstem. This type of breathing is an abnormal respiratory pattern, with periods of apnea followed by periods of deep breathing and then shallow breathing followed by more apnea (Huether and McCance, 2020; Lewis et al., 2017).

Palpation. Palpation of the chest provides assessment data in several areas. It documents the type and amount of thoracic excursion; elicits any areas of tenderness; and helps to identify tactile fremitus, thrills, heaves, and the cardiac point of maximal impulse (PMI). Palpation of the extremities provides data about the peripheral circulation (e.g., the presence and quality of peripheral pulses, skin temperature, color, and capillary refill) (see Chapter 30).

Palpation of the feet and legs determines the presence or absence of peripheral edema. Patients with alterations in cardiac function, such as those with heart failure or hypertension, often have pedal or lower-extremity edema. Edema is graded from 1+ to 4+, depending on the depth of visible indentation after firm finger pressure (see Chapter 30).

Palpate the pulses in the neck and extremities to assess arterial blood flow (see Chapter 30). Use a scale of 0 (absent pulse) to 4+ (full, bounding pulse) to describe what you feel. The normal pulse is 2+; a weak, thready pulse is 1+. Never palpate both carotid arteries at the same time as doing so may cause the patient to lose consciousness (Ball et al., 2019).

Percussion. Percussion detects the presence of abnormal fluid or air in the lungs. It also determines diaphragmatic excursion (see Chapter 30).

Auscultation. Auscultation helps identify normal and abnormal heart and lung sounds (see Chapter 30). Auscultation of the cardiovascular system includes assessing for normal S_1 and S_2 sounds and the presence of abnormal S_3 and S_4 sounds (gallops), murmurs, or rubs. Identify the location, intensity, pitch, and quality of a murmur. Auscultation also identifies any bruits over the carotid, abdominal aorta, and femoral arteries (Ball et al., 2019).

"Adventitious breath sounds" is another term for abnormal breath sounds. They include wheezing, crackles, and rhonchi. Wheezing is a continuous, high-pitched musical sound caused by high-velocity movement of air through a narrowed airway. It is associated with asthma, acute bronchitis, or pneumonia. It occurs during inspiration, expiration, or both. Determine whether there are any precipitating factors, such as respiratory infection, allergens, exercise, or stress. Crackles are discontinuous sounds of various pitch most often heard during inspiration. They are a result of the disruption of the small respiratory passages and cannot be cleared by coughing. They are often heard in patients with pneumonia or emphysema or chronic bronchitis. Rhonchi, or sonorous wheezes, are deeper sounding in pitch than crackles and are often heard during expiration. They reflect the presence of thick secretions or muscle spasms in the airway. Rhonchi can often be cleared by coughing and are most commonly heard in patients with asthma or pneumonia (Ball et al., 2019).

Diagnostic Tests. A variety of diagnostic tests are used to monitor and assess cardiopulmonary function. Some of these tests are noninvasive, while others are more invasive. Diagnostic testing used in the assessment and evaluation of the patient with cardiopulmonary alterations is summarized in Tables 41.3 through 41.5. When reviewing results of pulmonary function studies, be aware of expected variations in patients from different cultures (Box 41.3).

One screening test is TB Mantoux skin testing (Box 41.4). This is a simple test and is recommended for health care workers who care for patients at increased risk for TB disease. Those patients at greater risk include people from countries where TB disease is common (most countries in Latin America, Africa, and Asia, for example), prisoners and correctional facility employees, and residents of long-term care facilities (CDC, 2016a).

Invasive diagnostic tests, such as a thoracentesis, are painful. How painful a diagnostic procedure is depends on the patient's tolerance for

TABLE 41.3 Cardiopulmonary Diagnostic Blood Studies

Test and Normal Values	Interpretation
Complete Blood Count Normal values for a complete blood count (CBC) vary with age and gender	A CBC determines the number and type of red and white blood cells per cubic millimeter of blood. White blood cells assess for presence of infection. Red blood cells and hemoglobin assess for presence of anemia and ability of the blood to carry oxygen to the tissues.
Cardiac Enzymes *Creatine kinase (CK-MB):* Cardio specific enzyme released from cells when myocardial tissue is damaged. If greater than 4%-6% of total CK, then highly indicative of MI; levels increase within 4-6 hours of MI	Providers use cardiac enzymes, along with troponin, to diagnose acute myocardial infarcts.
Cardiac Troponins Plasma cardiac troponin I <0.03 ng/mL	Value elevates as early as 3 hours after myocardial injury.
Plasma cardiac troponin T <0.1 ng/mL	Value often remains elevated for 10-14 days.
Serum Electrolytes Potassium (K+) 3.5-5 mEq/L or 3.5-5 mmol/L	Patients on diuretic therapy are at risk for hypokalemia (low potassium). Patients receiving angiotensin-converting enzyme (ACE) inhibitors are at risk for hyperkalemia (elevated potassium). Since potassium has an effect on cardiac rhythm, it is important to keep this value as close to normal as possible.
Cholesterol Fasting cholesterol less than 200 mg/dL or less than 5.2 mmol/L (SI units)	Contributing factors include sedentary lifestyle with intake of saturated fatty acids, familial hypercholesterolemia.
Low-density lipoproteins (LDLs) (bad cholesterol) <130 mg/dL Very low–density lipoproteins (VLDLs) 7-32 mg/dl	High LDL cholesterol (hypercholesterolemia) is caused by excessive intake of saturated fatty acids, dietary cholesterol intake, and obesity. Familial hypercholesterolemia and hyperlipidemia, hypothyroidism, nephrotic syndrome, and diabetes mellitus are also contributing factors. VLDLs are predominant carriers of triglycerides and can be converted to LDL by lipoprotein lipase. Levels in excess of 25%-50% indicate increased risk of cardiac disease.
High-density lipoproteins (HDLs) (good cholesterol) Male: >45 mg/dL; female: >55 mg/dL	Factors such as cigarette smoking, obesity, lack of regular exercise, beta-adrenergic blocking agents, genetic disorders of HDL metabolism, hypertriglyceridemia, and type 2 diabetes cause low HDL cholesterol.
Triglycerides Male: 40-160 mg/dL; female: 35-135 mg/dL	Obesity, excessive alcohol intake, diabetes mellitus, beta-adrenergic blocking agents, and familial hypertriglyceridemia cause hypertriglyceridemia.
Additional Tests Brain natriuretic peptide <100 pg/mL	Increased levels may be used to help determine severity of congestive heart failure.
C-reactive protein <0.1/dL or <10 mg/L	Test used by clinicians to detect inflammation if there is a high suspicion of tissue injury or infection somewhere in the body. It can also be used to evaluate a patient's risk of developing coronary artery disease and stroke. Used to help evaluate patient for sepsis.

Data from Pagana KD et al: *Mosby's diagnostic and laboratory test reference,* ed 14, St Louis, 2019, Mosby.

TABLE 41.4   Cardiac Function Diagnostic Tests

Test	Significance
Holter monitor	Portable ECG worn by a patient at home or work or school. The test produces a continuous ECG tracing over a period of time. Patients keep a diary of activity, noting when they experience rapid heartbeats or dizziness. Evaluation of the ECG recording along with the diary provides information about the electrical activity of the heart during activities of daily living.
ECG exercise stress test	ECG is monitored while a patient walks on a treadmill at a specified speed and duration of time. Test evaluates the cardiac response to physical stress. It is not a valuable tool for evaluation of cardiac response in women because of an increased false-positive finding.
Thallium stress test	ECG stress test with the addition of thallium-201 injected intravenously. It determines coronary blood flow changes with increased activity. Often used for people who cannot walk on the treadmill.
Electrophysiological study (EPS)	EPS is an invasive measure of intracardiac electrical pathways. It provides more specific information about difficult-to-treat dysrhythmias and assesses adequacy of antidysrhythmic medication.
Transthoracic echocardiography	This is a noninvasive measure of heart structure and heart wall motion. It graphically demonstrates overall cardiac performance.
Scintigraphy	Scintigraphy is radionuclide angiography; used to evaluate cardiac structure, myocardial perfusion, and contractility.
Cardiac catheterization and angiography	These are used to visualize cardiac chambers, valves, the great vessels, and coronary arteries. Pressures and volumes within the four chambers of the heart are also measured.

ECG, Electrocardiogram.
Data from Pagana KD, et al: *Mosby's diagnostic and laboratory test reference,* ed 14, St Louis, 2019, Mosby.

TABLE 41.5   Ventilation and Oxygenation Diagnostic Studies

Measurement and Normal Values	Interpretation/Purpose
Arterial Blood Gases pH 7.35-7.45 PCO_2 35-45 mm Hg HCO_3 21-28 mEq/L PO_2 80-100 mm Hg SaO_2 saturation 95%-100% Older adult: 95% Base excess 0 ± 2 mEq/L	Provides important information for assessment of patient's respiratory and metabolic acid/base balance and adequacy of oxygenation (see Chapter 42)
Pulmonary Function Tests Basic ventilation studies (Pulmonary functions vary by ethnic group.)	Determines ability of the lungs to efficiently exchange oxygen and carbon dioxide Used to differentiate pulmonary obstructive from restrictive disease
Peak Expiratory Flow Rate (PEFR) The point of highest flow during maximal expiration (Normal in adults is based on age and body weight.)	Reflects changes in large airway sizes; an excellent predictor of overall airway resistance in a patient with asthma Daily measurement for early detection of asthma exacerbations
Bronchoscopy Normal airways without masses, pus, or foreign bodies	Visual examination of the tracheobronchial tree through a narrow, flexible fiberoptic bronchoscope Performed to obtain fluid, sputum, or biopsy samples; remove mucus plugs or foreign bodies
Lung Scan Normal lung structure without masses	Nuclear scanning test used to identify abnormal masses by size and location Identification of masses used in planning therapy and treatments Also used to find a blood clot preventing normal perfusion or ventilation ($\dot{V}/\dot{Q}$ scan)
Thoracentesis Surgical perforation of chest wall and pleural space with a needle to aspirate fluid for diagnostic or therapeutic purposes or to remove a specimen for biopsy; performed using aseptic technique and local anesthetic (Patient usually sits upright with the anterior thorax supported by pillows or an over-bed table.)	Specimen of pleural fluid obtained for cytological examination Results may indicate an infection or neoplastic disease Identification of infection or a type of cancer important in determining a plan of care

TABLE 41.5   Ventilation and Oxygenation Diagnostic Studies—cont'd

Measurement and Normal Values	Interpretation/Purpose
Sputum specimens	Nasal aspirate/swabs for respiratory syncytial virus, influenza; sometimes are obtained while patient expectorates into specimen container; true sputum cultures are obtained via airway suctioning or through bronchoscopy
• Normal: negative	
• Sputum culture and sensitivity	Obtained to identify a specific microorganism or organism growing in sputum Identifies drug resistance and sensitivities to determine appropriate antibiotic therapy
• Sputum for acid-fast bacillus (AFB)	Screens for presence of AFB for detection of tuberculosis by early-morning specimens on 3 consecutive days
• Sputum for cytology	Obtained to identify lung cancer Differentiates type of cancer cells (small cell, oat cell, large cell)

Data from Pagana KD, et al: *Mosby's diagnostic and laboratory test reference,* ed 14, St Louis, 2019, Mosby.

pain (see Chapter 44). Reduce the patient's anxiety by explaining the procedure and telling him or her what to expect. Be sure that he or she understands the importance of following instructions related to the procedure. For example, a patient undergoing a thoracentesis will need to understand the importance of not coughing during the procedure. Provide appropriate pain management 30 to 60 minutes before procedures, as ordered, to reduce the perception of pain. After any procedure monitor the patient for signs of changes in cardiopulmonary functioning such as sudden shortness of breath, pain, oxygen desaturation, and anxiety.

> **REFLECT NOW**
>
> You are preparing to assess a patient with COPD. What would be important questions to ask this patient when gathering a health history? What are your expected physical assessment findings? What diagnostic tests would you expect the health care provider to order for this patient?

◆ Nursing Diagnosis

Based upon your assessment findings, you develop nursing diagnoses (see Chapter 17) for patients with oxygenation problems by clustering specific assessment findings and identifying the related etiology (Box 41.5). The assessment findings for diagnoses related to oxygenation can be similar. For example, both *Impaired Gas Exchange* and *Impaired Breathing* have dyspnea and nasal flaring. A closer review of assessment findings, as well as an analysis of the patient's history, will help you clarify and select the correct diagnosis. For example, a trauma patient who has rib pain and is showing an increased respiratory rate is more likely to have *Impaired Breathing*. The clustered assessment findings and related factors support a problem or negative nursing diagnosis. If assessment results in the clustering of risk factors, a risk nursing diagnosis will be made.

These additional nursing diagnosis examples may apply when planning care for the patient with alterations in oxygenation:

- *Impaired Cardiac Output*
- *Acute Pain*
- *Activity Intolerance*
- *Risk for Activity Intolerance*
- *Impaired Airway Clearance*

◆ Planning

During planning, use critical thinking skills to synthesize information from multiple sources (Fig. 41.5). Critical thinking ensures that your plan of care integrates individualized patient needs. Professional standards are especially important to consider when developing a plan of care. These standards often establish scientifically proven guidelines for selecting effective nursing interventions.

Goals and Outcomes. Develop an individualized plan of care for each nursing diagnosis (see the Nursing Care Plan). Together, with your patient, set realistic expectations, relevant goals, and measurable outcomes of care.

Patients with impaired oxygenation require a nursing care plan directed toward meeting actual or potential oxygenation needs. Allow patients to collaborate with you. Develop individual outcomes based on patient-centered goals. For example, for the goal of an improved breathing pattern, select specific expected outcomes, such as the following:

- Patient's respiratory rate is between 12 and 20 breaths/minute.
- Patient achieves bilateral lung expansion.
- Patient breathes without the use of accessory muscles.

Often a patient with cardiopulmonary disease has multiple nursing diagnoses (Fig. 41.6). In this case, identify when goals or outcomes apply to more than one diagnosis. The presence of multiple diagnoses also makes priority setting a critical activity.

Setting Priorities. A patient's level of health, age, lifestyle, and environmental risk factors affect tissue oxygenation. Patients with severe impairments in oxygenation frequently require nursing interventions in multiple areas. Consider which goal/outcome is the most important to achieve while the patient is in the hospital or primary care setting. For example, in an acute care setting, maintaining a patent airway has a higher priority than improving the patient's exercise tolerance. The need for a patent airway is immediate; as the patient's level of oxygen improves, activity tolerance increases (Urden et al., 2020). In a second example, when caring for a patient who has an abdominal incision, pain control is a priority. In this situation, controlling the patient's pain facilitates coughing and deep breathing and activity (Lewis et al., 2017).

However, in a community-based or primary care setting, priorities often focus on primary or tertiary health promotion activities, such as smoking cessation, exercise, and/or diet modifications. Both you and the patient need to focus on the same goal and expected outcomes. In addition to individualizing each goal, be sure that the goals are realistic, have reasonable time frames, and are attainable for the patient. In addition, be sure to respect the patient's preferences for his or her degree of active engagement in the care process. Some will choose to be very active and desire to make day-to-day decisions. Others may choose to assume a more passive role, preferring you to choose a course of action while keeping them informed (Lewis et al., 2017).

BOX 41.3 CULTURAL ASPECTS OF CARE

Cultural Impact on Pulmonary Diseases

The impact of pulmonary diseases on patients and their families varies among cultures. It is important to understand these variations in terms of assessing for and providing care in patients with lung diseases. In 2018, approximately two-thirds of the new cases of TB diagnosed in the United States occurred in people who were not born in the United States. The countries where these patients were most likely to be born were Mexico, the Philippines, India, Vietnam, and China (CDC, 2019c).

The cigarette smoking rate in the United States is highest in American Indian/Alaskan Natives (24.6%), followed by Caucasians (15.3%), African-Americans (15.1%), Hispanics (9.9%), and Asians (7.0%). Smoking rates are also highest in those who have less than a high school education (22%) than in those who have a baccalaureate degree or higher (5.8%). Smoking increases the risk for a number of cancer types, chronic obstructive pulmonary disease (COPD), and heart disease (ALA, 2019b).

People of certain ethnic or cultural backgrounds tend to live in the same area, which can affect their exposure to certain environmental pollutants or triggers of respiratory exacerbations. Their location of living can also affect their socioeconomic status and their access to health care, which can also have a great impact on their pulmonary health (Celedon et al., 2017).

While ethnic and cultural differences can contribute to overall health, it should be noted that in today's globalization, health care providers should look more at acculturation (cultural exchange of beliefs, values, or behaviors as a result of interacting with people of other cultures) as an influence on a person's or a family's health. For example, smoking rates are higher in females of Mexican descent who have lived in the United States (Celedon et al., 2017).

The American Thoracic Society and the National Heart, Lung, and Blood Institute recommend looking more at the individual person and less at the person's race or ethnicity when trying to develop a plan of care. There is discussion about looking at a person's genetic makeup to develop a plan of care as genetic testing could help determine actual risk of disease and which medications would work best for that particular patient (Celedon et al., 2017).

Implications for Patient-Centered Care

- If your patients are foreign born, ask whether they have had the bacille Calmette-Guérin (BCG) vaccine, which can cause a positive reaction to the TB skin test. Also assess their exposure to people with known TB or other pulmonary infectious diseases (CDC, 2019c).
- Immunization clinics should concentrate on the underserved urban communities, especially those with large numbers of older adults. Provide TB skin testing, flu vaccines, and pneumonia vaccines as needed.
- Community health departments need to target at-risk populations for flu and pneumonia vaccine clinics.
- Public health programs for those at highest risk for pulmonary diseases should focus on pollution prevention, immunizations, and smoking-cessation programs.

BOX 41.4 Tuberculosis Skin Testing

- Skin testing determines whether a person is infected with *Mycobacterium tuberculosis*.
- Tuberculosis (TB) skin testing (TST) is performed by an intradermal injection of 0.1 mL of tuberculin purified protein derivative (PPD) on the inner surface of the forearm (see Chapter 31). The injection produces a pale elevation of the skin (a wheal) 6 to 10 mm in diameter. Afterward the injection site is circled, and the patient is instructed not to wash the circle off.
- Read tuberculin skin tests between 48 and 72 hours after the test. If the site is not read within 72 hours, a patient must have another skin test.
- *Positive results:* A palpable elevated, hardened area around the injection site, caused by edema and inflammation from the antigen-antibody reaction, measured in millimeters. (See Chapter 31 for evaluation of positive results by millimeters.)
- People born outside the United States may have had bacille Calmette-Guérin (BCG) vaccine for TB disease, which results in a positive reaction to the TST and may complicate the treatment plan. The positive skin reaction does not indicate that the BCG vaccine provided protection against the disease (CDC, 2016a, b).
- Reddened flat areas are *not* positive reactions and are not measured.
- TST is less reliable in older adults (see Box 41.1) and in those with an altered immune function, such as a human immunodeficiency virus (HIV)–positive patient or someone receiving chemotherapy.

BOX 41.5 Nursing Diagnostic Process

Impaired Gas Exchange Related to Decreased Lung Expansion

Assessment Activities	Assessment Findings
Ask patient or family about patient's mood, attentiveness, memory, and activity level.	Confusion Decreased activity Fatigue Irritability Restlessness Sleepiness
Observe patient's respirations for rate, rhythm, depth.	Dyspnea Nasal flaring Tachypnea Use of accessory muscles
Inspect skin and mucous membranes.	Diaphoresis Pallor Cyanosis
Auscultate chest.	Decreased respiratory excursion Abnormal, distant lung sounds

Teamwork and Collaboration. The time spent with a patient in any setting is limited. Therefore, collaborate with family members, colleagues, and other health care specialists to achieve the established goals and expected outcomes. Some patients need to improve their exercise and activity tolerance; for other patients, continuing care involves participating in a community-based cardiopulmonary rehabilitation program. Some patients need home physical therapy.

Collaboration with physical therapists, nutritionists, respiratory therapists, and community-based nurses is valuable for patients with heart failure or chronic lung conditions. These professionals work with patients and their caregivers using resources in the community to assist them in attaining and maintaining the highest possible level of wellness. In addition, professionals identify community resources and support systems to help prevent and manage symptoms related to cardiopulmonary diseases. Communication among everyone on the patient's health care team and recognition of everyone's contributions in achieving the health care goals for the patient are imperative.

◆ Implementation

There are interventions for promoting and maintaining adequate oxygenation across the continuum of care. As a nurse, you will be responsible for independent interventions such as positioning, coughing techniques, and health education for disease prevention. In addition, you will provide physician-initiated interventions such as oxygen therapy, lung inflation techniques, and chest physiotherapy.

Health Promotion. Maintaining a patient's optimal level of health reduces the number and/or severity of respiratory symptoms.

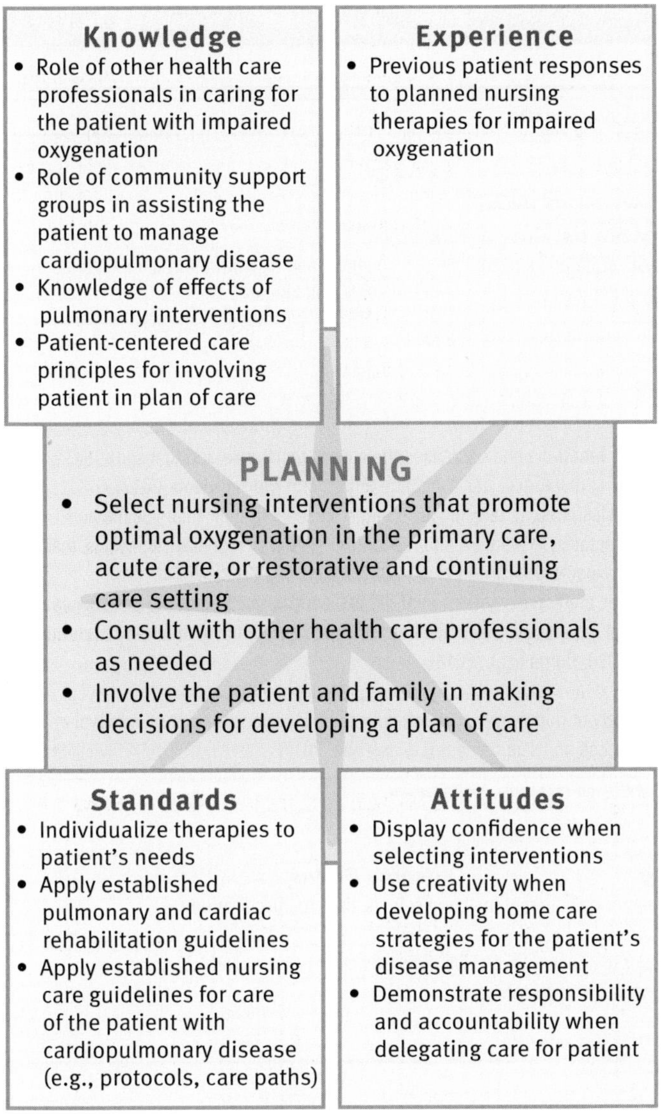

Knowledge
- Role of other health care professionals in caring for the patient with impaired oxygenation
- Role of community support groups in assisting the patient to manage cardiopulmonary disease
- Knowledge of effects of pulmonary interventions
- Patient-centered care principles for involving patient in plan of care

Experience
- Previous patient responses to planned nursing therapies for impaired oxygenation

PLANNING
- Select nursing interventions that promote optimal oxygenation in the primary care, acute care, or restorative and continuing care setting
- Consult with other health care professionals as needed
- Involve the patient and family in making decisions for developing a plan of care

Standards
- Individualize therapies to patient's needs
- Apply established pulmonary and cardiac rehabilitation guidelines
- Apply established nursing care guidelines for care of the patient with cardiopulmonary disease (e.g., protocols, care paths)

Attitudes
- Display confidence when selecting interventions
- Use creativity when developing home care strategies for the patient's disease management
- Demonstrate responsibility and accountability when delegating care for patient

FIG. 41.5 Critical thinking model for oxygenation planning.

Prevention of respiratory infections is foremost in maintaining optimal health (Box 41.6). Providing cardiopulmonary-related health information is an important nursing responsibility.

The health information that your patients and their families bring to the situation varies. Some patients have a lot of exposure to health care information and understand their treatment plans. Other families might have a lot of exposure to health care information but are unable to understand and follow treatment plans. Last, you might encounter families who are experiencing their first exposure to health care information and are very unsure of their interpretation of the information. When providing health information, be sure to assess a patient's health literacy level and then individualize findings into an individualized education session (see Chapter 25).

Vaccinations. Seasonal flu vaccine protects against influenza viruses that research indicates will be the most common during that year. The vaccines are formulated annually based on worldwide surveillance data. Annual flu vaccines are recommended for all people 6 months and older. Patients with chronic illnesses (heart, lung, kidney, or immunocompromised), infants, older adults, and pregnant women can get very sick; thus, they should be immunized (CDC, 2018e). The vaccine is also recommended for people in close or frequent contact with anyone in the high-risk groups, including infants and health care workers. It is effective in reducing the severity of illness and the risk of serious complications and death. It is important to assess a patient's allergies and any allergic response to vaccines or any components. People with a known hypersensitivity to eggs or other components of the vaccine should consult their physician before being vaccinated (CDC, 2018e). Adults with an acute febrile illness should schedule the vaccination after they have recovered. The live, attenuated nasal spray vaccine is given to healthy people from 2 through 49 years of age if they are not pregnant. The live vaccine is also not indicated in people who are immunocompromised or have certain chronic health conditions such as asthma or heart disease (CDC, 2018e).

Pneumococcal vaccine (PCV13) is routinely given to children younger than 2 years of age and is recommended for patients with certain medical conditions (such as heart disease) that are at risk of complications from pneumococcal disease. Adults over 65 years of age and any adult who smokes may receive the pneumococcal polysaccharide vaccine (PPSV23). These vaccines should not be administered if the patient has had an allergic reaction to the vaccine in

---

◎ NURSING CARE PLAN

Impaired Airway Clearance

ASSESSMENT

Mr. Edwards is a 75-year-old currently lying in a semi-Fowler's position in bed, talking with his wife. He is admitted with community-acquired right upper lobe pneumonia and has a 2-year history of COPD. He has an intermittent productive cough with occasional thick, yellow sputum. Lying flat makes the cough worse.

Assessment Activities	Assessment Findings[a]
Ask Mr. Edwards how long he has had this cough and how frequently he coughs.	He replies, "I have a morning **cough** every day, but this cough is different. It started about a week ago. It is **worse when I lie flat**."
Ask Mr. Edwards what is different about this cough.	He replies, "It is difficult to cough up anything, my **mouth** is **dry**, and I have become more **fatigued**. My ribs are starting to get sore."
Assess Mr. Edwards' respiratory rate, work of breathing, and whether he is using accessory muscles.	There is **minor use of abdominal muscles** while breathing. He replies, "I feel **short of breath** when I walk."
Obtain vital signs.	Temperature: 101.4 F (38.5 C); pulse 102 beats/min; respirations 30 breaths/min; BP 130/90 mm Hg, and SpO$_2$ 84%. He states he has a pain score of 4 out of 10 on visual analog scale.
Auscultate lung fields.	**Abnormal lung sounds** (crackles) are heard in the right upper lobe and left and right lower lobes.
Ask Mr. Edwards to produce a sputum sample.	Sputum is **thick** and **discolored** yellow to yellow-green and difficult to cough up and expectorate.

[a]**Assessment findings** are shown in **bold** type.

Continued

◎ **NURSING CARE PLAN—cont'd**

Impaired Airway Clearance

NURSING DIAGNOSIS: Impaired airway clearance related to retained thick pulmonary secretions

PLANNING

Goals	Expected Outcomes (NOC)[b]
	Respiratory Status: Airway Patency
Mr. Edwards will be able to effectively clear secretions by discharge.	Mr. Edwards will state an increased ease in coughing and expectorating within 48 hours.
	Lung sounds will improve with fewer crackles within 48 hours.

[b]Outcome classification labels from Moorhead S, et al.: *Nursing Outcomes Classification (NOC),* ed 6, St Louis, 2018, Elsevier.

INTERVENTIONS (NIC)[c]	RATIONALE
Airway Management	
Position Mr. Edwards with head elevated at least 30-45 degrees.	Increases depth of breathing and decreases the airway resistance during inspiration, thereby improving respiratory gas exchange (Elliott and Morrell-Scott, 2017).
Ambulate in room or hall progressively as tolerated at least 2 times a day. If unable to ambulate, reposition from side to side every 2 hours or more.	Body movement helps patients take bigger breaths, increasing their tidal volume and preventing atelectasis. Movement and repositioning help to mobilize secretions, making them easier to expectorate (Urden et al., 2020; Atkins and Kautz, 2014).
Have Mr. Edwards deep-breathe and cough every hour. Teach him to take a deep breath, hold it for several seconds, open his mouth, tighten his abdominal muscles, and cough 2 to 3 times with his mouth open.	Retained secretions predispose patient to atelectasis and worsening of the pneumonia. Controlled coughing improves effectiveness of cough and removal of airway secretions (Urden et al., 2020; Borge et al., 2014).
Increase fluids to 2500 mL in 24 hours if not contraindicated by cardiac or renal status. Offer fluids Mr. Edwards prefers.	Fluids help to liquefy or thin the sputum, which may help promote secretion removal and relieve oral mucosa and skin dryness (Lewis et al., 2017).

[c]Intervention classification labels from Butcher HK, et al: *Nursing Interventions Classification (NIC),* ed 7, St Louis, 2018, Elsevier.

EVALUATION

Evaluation Activity	Patient Response/Finding	Outcome Status
Auscultate the lungs.	Lung sounds are clear in left lung, crackles present in right lower lobe.	Lung sounds clear to auscultation.
Ask Mr. Edwards whether he can cough and expectorate sputum; observe him perform this action.	Mr. Edwards reports that it is easier to cough up his secretions; Mr. Edwards is observed expectorating thin, pale yellow sputum.	Mr. Edwards clears airway with coughing.

---

the past or while the patient is recovering from a febrile illness. Women should not receive the vaccine while pregnant; instead, they should try to receive the vaccine before pregnancy (CDC, 2017b).

Healthy Lifestyle. Identification and elimination of risk factors for cardiopulmonary disease are important parts of primary care. The risk factors for cardiac disease are lower when total cholesterol levels are less than 200 mg/dL, high-density lipoprotein (HDL) levels are greater than 40 mg/dL in men and 50 mg/dL in women, and low-density lipoprotein (LDL) levels are less than 160 mg/dL (Lewis et al., 2017). Encourage patients to eat a healthy low-fat, high-fiber diet and maintain a body weight in proportion to their height (see Chapter 45). The Dietary Approaches to Stop Hypertension (DASH) diet, along with exercise, stress reduction, and limiting alcohol intake, has been shown to decrease a patient's risk of hypertension (NHLBI, n.d.a). Eliminating cigarettes and other tobacco and adequately hydrating are additional healthy behaviors. Encourage patients to examine their habits and make appropriate changes. Patients with cardiopulmonary alterations need to minimize their risk for infection, especially during the winter months (see Box 41.6).

Exercise is a key factor in promoting and maintaining a healthy heart and lungs. Encourage patients to have at least 150 minutes a week of moderate intensity exercise and at least 2 days a week of muscle strengthening activity (USDHHS, 2018). Aerobic exercise is necessary to improve lung and heart function and strengthen muscles. Walking is an efficient way to achieve a good aerobic workout.

Many shopping malls have programs allowing people to walk in the enclosed mall before the shops open. During the hot summer months, teach patients to limit activities to early in the day or late in the evening, when temperatures are lower. In addition, teach the importance of maintaining adequate hydration and sodium intake, especially if they are taking diuretics. Patients with known cardiac disease and those with multiple risk factors are cautioned to avoid exertion in cold weather. Shoveling snow is especially risky and often precipitates a cardiac event. Other activities, such as hanging holiday lights and decorations in the extreme cold, can precipitate chest pain and bronchospasm. Please refer to Chapter 38 for further discussion on activity and exercise.

Environmental Pollutants. Avoiding exposure to secondhand smoke is essential to maintaining optimal cardiopulmonary function. Most public places, such as businesses or restaurants, ban smoking or have separate areas designated as smoking areas. Provide counseling and support so that a patient who lives with secondhand smoke in the home understands its effects. If the patient is a smoker who wants to quit smoking, the patient's family should be told to encourage and support the patient in the attempt to quit.

Patients should try to avoid environmental hazards in their home or work environments. For example, patients who know that pollen triggers an asthma exacerbation should be taught to keep windows closed and use air filters when air pollen counts are high (Hockenberry et al.,

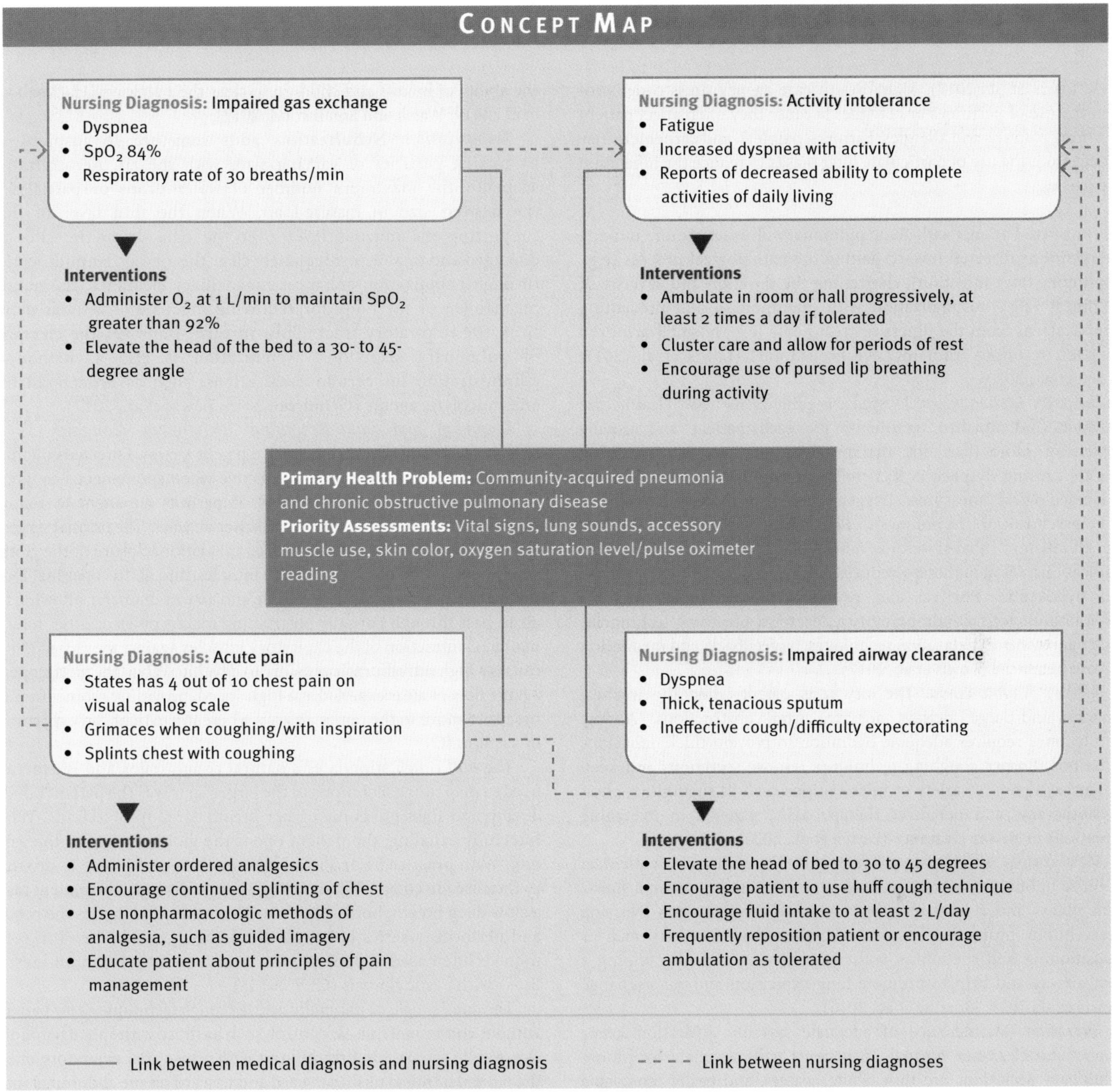

CONCEPT MAP

Nursing Diagnosis: Impaired gas exchange
- Dyspnea
- SpO$_2$ 84%
- Respiratory rate of 30 breaths/min

Interventions
- Administer O$_2$ at 1 L/min to maintain SpO$_2$ greater than 92%
- Elevate the head of the bed to a 30- to 45-degree angle

Nursing Diagnosis: Activity intolerance
- Fatigue
- Increased dyspnea with activity
- Reports of decreased ability to complete activities of daily living

Interventions
- Ambulate in room or hall progressively, at least 2 times a day if tolerated
- Cluster care and allow for periods of rest
- Encourage use of pursed lip breathing during activity

Primary Health Problem: Community-acquired pneumonia and chronic obstructive pulmonary disease
Priority Assessments: Vital signs, lung sounds, accessory muscle use, skin color, oxygen saturation level/pulse oximeter reading

Nursing Diagnosis: Acute pain
- States has 4 out of 10 chest pain on visual analog scale
- Grimaces when coughing/with inspiration
- Splints chest with coughing

Interventions
- Administer ordered analgesics
- Encourage continued splinting of chest
- Use nonpharmacologic methods of analgesia, such as guided imagery
- Educate patient about principles of pain management

Nursing Diagnosis: Impaired airway clearance
- Dyspnea
- Thick, tenacious sputum
- Ineffective cough/difficulty expectorating

Interventions
- Elevate the head of bed to 30 to 45 degrees
- Encourage patient to use huff cough technique
- Encourage fluid intake to at least 2 L/day
- Frequently reposition patient or encourage ambulation as tolerated

——— Link between medical diagnosis and nursing diagnosis   - - - - Link between nursing diagnoses

FIG. 41.6 Concept map for Mr. Edwards.

BOX 41.6 PATIENT TEACHING

Prevention of Recurrent Respiratory Infections

Objective
- The patient will be able to describe how to reduce the risk factors for recurring respiratory infections.

Teaching Strategies
- Adapt teaching strategies to the patient's health literacy, educational background, reading level, and cultural preferences (CDC, 2019c).
- Communicate with patient and family to identify collaborative goals for reducing risk factors.
- Explain the link between smoking and increased risk for respiratory infections (CDC, 2018a; McCance and Huether, 2019).
- Refer to smoking cessation programs and discuss appropriate medication to support smoking cessation from the primary health provider (ACS, 2017).
- If a patient does not smoke, teach the importance of avoiding secondhand smoke and areas of high air pollution.

- Instruct patient and family about appropriate hand hygiene techniques to reduce transmission of microorganisms.
- Explain to patient and family why annual influenza vaccines and appropriate pneumonia vaccines are needed (CDC, 2018e; CDC, 2017b).
- Instruct patient and family about signs and symptoms of respiratory infection that should be reported to health care provider, such as increased coughing, shortness of breath, change of color of sputum, fever, and fatigue.

Evaluation
Use the principles of teach-back to evaluate patient/family caregiver learning:
- Ask patient to state benefits of smoking cessation and the risks for secondhand smoke.
- Ask patient about plans for flu and pneumonia vaccines.
- Ask patient to describe in simple terms the symptoms of respiratory infection and when to call the health care provider.

2019; Lewis et al., 2017). Many health care agency dress codes prohibit the use of perfumes or colognes because they often affect patient breathing patterns and allergies. Farmers, painters, and carpenters may benefit from the use of particulate filter masks to reduce the inhalation of particles.

Acute Care. Patients with acute pulmonary illnesses require nursing interventions directed toward halting the pathological process (e.g., respiratory tract infection), shortening the duration and severity of an illness (e.g., hospitalization with pneumonia), and preventing complications from the illness or treatments (e.g., hospital-acquired infection resulting from invasive procedures) (Lewis et al., 2017; Urden et al., 2020).

Dyspnea Management. Dyspnea is difficult to treat. Health care providers individualize treatments for each patient and usually implement more than one therapy. Treatment of the underlying process causing dyspnea is then followed with other therapies (e.g., pharmacological measures, oxygen therapy, physical techniques, and psychosocial techniques). Pharmacological agents include bronchodilators, inhaled steroids, mucolytics, and low-dose antianxiety medications. Oxygen therapy reduces dyspnea associated with exercise and hypoxemia. Physical and psychological techniques such as cardiopulmonary reconditioning (e.g., exercise, breathing techniques, and cough control), relaxation techniques, biofeedback, and meditation are also beneficial (Lewis et al., 2017).

Airway Maintenance. The airway is patent when the trachea, bronchi, and large airways are free from obstructions. Airway maintenance requires adequate hydration to prevent thick, tenacious secretions. Proper coughing techniques remove secretions and keep the airway open. A variety of interventions such as suctioning, chest physiotherapy, and nebulizer therapy assist patients in managing alterations in airway clearance (Urden et al., 2020).

Mobilization of Pulmonary Secretions. The ability of a patient to mobilize pulmonary secretions makes the difference between a short-term illness and a long recovery involving complications. Nursing interventions promoting removal of pulmonary secretions such as repositioning and suctioning assist in achieving and maintaining a clear airway and help to promote lung expansion and gas exchange (Lewis et al., 2017; Morrow et al., 2016).

Hydration. Maintenance of adequate systemic hydration keeps mucociliary clearance normal. In patients with adequate hydration, pulmonary secretions are thin, white, watery, and easily removable with minimal coughing. Excessive coughing to clear thick, tenacious secretions is fatiguing and energy depleting. It can also cause pain in the chest muscles and ribs, which further decreases the patient's ability to cough and clear secretions. The best way to maintain thin secretions is to provide a fluid intake of 1500 to 2500 mL/day unless contraindicated by cardiac or renal status. The color, consistency, and ease of mucus expectoration determines adequacy of hydration (Lewis et al., 2017).

Humidification. Humidification is the process of adding water to gas to keep airways moist. It is necessary for patients receiving oxygen therapy at high flow rates, typically greater than 4 L/minute (see agency protocols). Oxygen humidification via nasal cannula or face mask is achieved by bubbling oxygen through sterile water (see Skill 41.4). Sterile water should be used to decrease the risk of hospital-acquired infection; agency protocols must be followed for changing the solution (Wen et al., 2017).

When caring for pediatric patients, humidity may be applied to all oxygen devices, regardless of flow rates. Infants and children have smaller airways than adults, and secretions are more likely to obstruct airways in the younger population. Humidity is added to help ease the ability of infants and children to clear their airways (Hockenberry et al., 2019; Walsh and Smallwood, 2017).

Nebulization. Nebulization adds moisture to inspired air by mixing particles of varying sizes with the air. Aerosolization suspends the maximum number of water drops or particles of the desired size in inspired air. When the thin layer of fluid supporting the mucous layer over the cilia dries, the cilia are damaged and unable to adequately clear the airway. Humidification through nebulization enhances mucociliary clearance, the natural mechanism of the body for removing mucus and cellular debris from the respiratory tract. This, in turn, improves the clearance of pulmonary secretions. Nebulization is also a method of administration for certain medications, such as bronchodilators and mucolytic agents (Grindrod, 2015; Lewis et al., 2017).

Coughing and Deep-Breathing Techniques. Coughing is an effective technique for maintaining a patent airway. Directed coughing is a deliberate maneuver that is effective when spontaneous coughing is inadequate (Borge et al., 2014). It permits a patient to remove secretions from both the upper and lower airways. The normal series of events in the directed cough are deep inhalation, closure of the glottis, active contraction of the expiratory muscles, and glottis opening. Deep inhalation increases the lung volume and airway diameter, allowing the air to pass through partially obstructing mucus plugs or other foreign matter. Contraction of the expiratory muscles against the closed glottis causes a high intrathoracic pressure to develop. When the glottis opens, a large flow of air is expelled at a high speed, providing momentum for mucus to move to the upper airways where the patient can expectorate or swallow it.

The *huff cough* stimulates a natural cough reflex and is generally used to help move secretions to the larger airways. The patient inhales deeply and then holds his or her breath for 2 to 3 seconds. While forcefully exhaling, the patient opens the glottis by saying the word *huff*. With practice he or she inhales more air and is able to progress to the cascade cough. When using a cascade cough, the patient takes a slow deep breath, holds it for 1 to 2 seconds, then opens the mouth and performs a series of coughs throughout exhalation. This technique is often used in patients with large amounts of sputum, such as those with cystic fibrosis (CFF, 2015a).

The *quad cough,* or *manually assisted cough* technique, is for patients without abdominal muscle control, such as those with spinal cord injuries. While the patient breathes out with a maximal expiratory effort, the patient or nurse pushes inward and upward on the abdominal muscles toward the diaphragm, causing the cough (Chatwin et al., 2018).

Diaphragmatic breathing is a technique that encourages deep breathing to increase air to the lower lungs. The diaphragm descends (belly moves out) when breathing in and ascends (belly sinks in) when breathing out. This technique has been shown to decrease dyspnea for a short period of time, particularly in patients with COPD, by increasing diaphragmatic excursion and reducing accessory muscle use (Morrow et al., 2016).

Evaluate the effectiveness of coughing by the patient's ability to expectorate sputum, the patient's report of swallowed sputum, or clearing of adventitious sounds by auscultation. Encourage patients with chronic pulmonary diseases, upper respiratory tract infections, and lower respiratory tract infections to deep breathe and cough at least every 2 hours while awake. Encourage patients with a large amount of sputum to cough every hour while awake. After some surgeries, it is recommended that patients perform deep breathing and coughing techniques every 2 to 4 hours while awake to prevent accumulation of secretions. Offer postoperative patients support devices (folded blanket, pillow, or palmed hands) to splint an abdominal or thoracic incision to minimize pain during directed

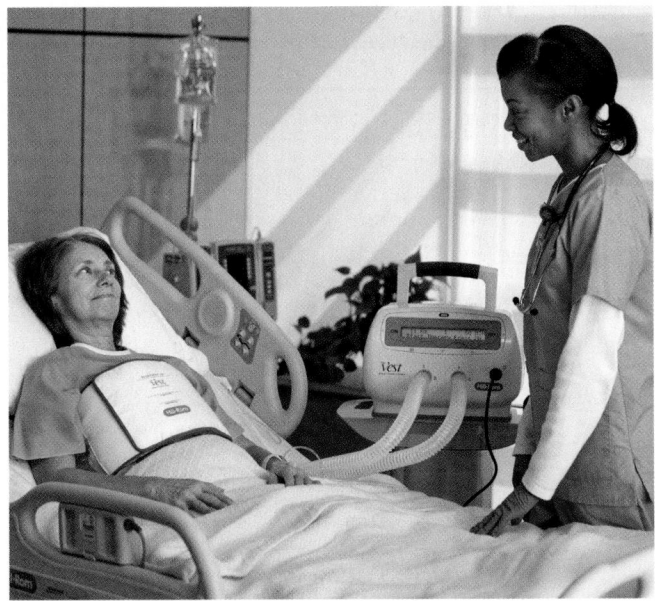

FIG. 41.7 High-frequency chest wall compression (HFCWC). (Copyright © 2019 Hill-Rom Services, Inc. Reprinted with permission. All rights reserved.)

BOX 41.7 Guidelines for Chest Physiotherapy

Nursing and respiratory therapy collaborate with the health care provider to determine whether chest physiotherapy (CPT) is best for a patient. The following guidelines help in physical assessment and subsequent decision making:

- Conduct a complete respiratory assessment to confirm need for CPT, including sputum production, effectiveness of cough, history of pulmonary problems successfully relieved with CPT, abnormal lung sounds, and documented conditions such as atelectasis, complicated pneumonia, vital signs, or changes in oxygenation status (Lewis et al., 2017; Strickland, 2013).
- Know the patient's medications. Certain medications, particularly diuretics and antihypertensives, cause fluid and hemodynamic changes. These decrease a patient's tolerance to positional changes and postural drainage. Long-term steroid use increases a patient's risk of pathological rib fractures and often contraindicates vibration.
- Know the patient's medical history. Certain conditions such as increased intracranial pressure, spinal cord injuries, and abdominal aneurysm resection contraindicate the positional changes of postural drainage. Thoracic trauma or surgery contraindicates percussion and vibration.
- Know the patient's level of cognitive function. Participation in controlled coughing techniques requires him or her to follow instructions. Congenital or acquired cognitive limitations alter a patient's ability to learn and participate in these techniques.
- Be aware of the patient's exercise tolerance. CPT maneuvers are fatiguing (Strickland, 2015).

---

coughing. Cough is a source of droplet transmission of pulmonary pathogens; thus, the health care provider should follow Standard Precautions (Lewis et al., 2017).

Chest Physiotherapy. Chest physiotherapy (CPT) is external chest wall manipulation using percussion, vibration, or high-frequency chest wall compression (HFCWC) (Fig. 41.7). It is often used in conjunction with postural drainage and can help mobilize pulmonary secretions in a select group of patients. Box 41.7 describes the guidelines to determine whether CPT is indicated. The American Association for Respiratory Care (AARC) does not support the routine use of CPT

with all patients. There is no evidence to support its routine use in all patient populations, instead reserving its use for patients with retained secretions who cannot expectorate those secretions, such as patients with cystic fibrosis (CF) (Strickland, 2015; Strickland et al., 2013).

Postural drainage is a component of pulmonary hygiene; it consists of drainage, positioning, and turning and is sometimes accompanied by chest percussion and vibration. It aids in improving secretion clearance and oxygenation. Positioning involves draining affected lung segments (Table 41.6) and helps to drain secretions from those segments of the lungs and bronchi into the trachea. Some patients do not require postural drainage of all lung segments, and clinical assessment is crucial in identifying specific lung segments requiring it. For example, patients with left lower lobe atelectasis require postural drainage of only the affected region, whereas a child with CF often requires postural drainage of all lung segments (CFF, n.d.; Hockenberry et al., 2019; Lewis et al., 2017).

Manual chest percussion involves rhythmically clapping on the chest wall over the area being drained to force secretions into larger airways for expectoration (Strickland et al., 2013). It is commonly performed by respiratory therapists in larger health care settings. Position your hand so that the fingers and thumb touch and the hands are cupped. The cupping makes the hand conform to the chest wall while trapping a cushion of air to soften the intensity of the clapping. The procedure should produce a hollow sound and should not be painful. Perform chest percussion by vigorously striking the chest wall alternately with cupped hands (Fig. 41.8). Perform percussion over a single layer of clothing, not over buttons, snaps, or zippers. The single layer of clothing prevents slapping the patient's skin. Thicker or multiple layers of material dampen the vibrations. Percussion is contraindicated in patients with bleeding disorders, osteoporosis, or fractured ribs. Avoid percussion over burns, open wounds, or skin infections of the thorax. Take caution to percuss the lung fields under the ribs and not over the spine, breastbone, stomach, or lower back or trauma can occur to the spleen, liver, or kidneys. Commercial devices that are shaped similar to cups are also available to use to perform manual chest percussion (CFF, n.d.).

Vibration is a gentle shaking pressure applied to the chest wall only during exhalation to shake secretions into larger airways. This pressure can be applied either manually or with a commercially available device. Vibration may be tolerated better than percussion. You use vibration most often with patients with CF (CFF, n.d.).

High-frequency chest wall compression (HFCWC) consists of an inflatable vest that is attached to an air-pulse generator (Fig. 41.9). HFCWC loosens and removes secretions from the airway by delivering high-frequency, small-volume expiratory pulses to a patient's external chest wall. The vest can be worn over clothes. This therapy is beneficial for patients with neuromuscular diseases and for patients with chronic lung diseases with thick sputum, such as CF (Strickland, 2014; Strickland et al., 2013).

Positive Expiratory Pressure. Positive expiratory pressure (PEP) is an airway clearance technique that can be used with and without oscillation. Its use is typically reserved for patients with CF or other lung diseases in which sputum is retained (Franks et al., 2019; Strickland, 2015). The Acapella and Flutter devices are commonly used PEP devices (Fig. 41.10). PEP allows air to be inhaled easily but forces the patient to exhale against resistance. This action helps air get behind the mucus, which then makes it easier to expectorate the mucus (CFF, 2015b; Franks et al., 2019). The patient must be physically capable of maintaining a seal with their mouth around the device.

Maintenance and Promotion of Lung Expansion. Nursing interventions to maintain or promote lung expansion include noninvasive techniques such as ambulation, positioning, incentive

TABLE 41.6   Positions for Postural Drainage

Lung Segment	Position of Patient	Lung Segment	Position of Patient

Adult – Make sure to assess patient prior to positioning. Some patients, such as those with head injuries, heart failure, or pulmonary embolus, should not be placed in the Trendelenburg position (Lewis et al., 2017).

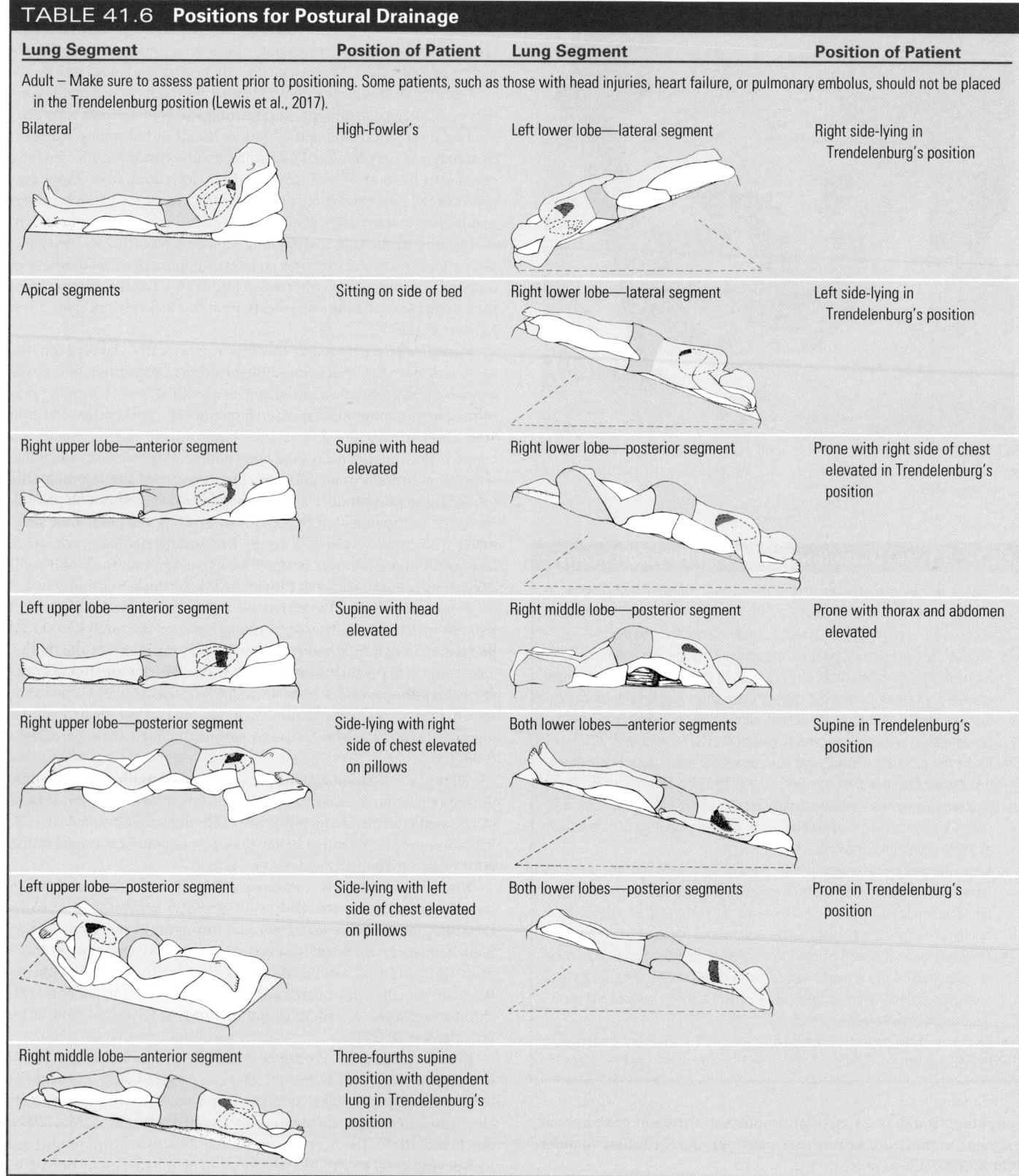

Lung Segment	Position of Patient	Lung Segment	Position of Patient
Bilateral	High-Fowler's	Left lower lobe—lateral segment	Right side-lying in Trendelenburg's position
Apical segments	Sitting on side of bed	Right lower lobe—lateral segment	Left side-lying in Trendelenburg's position
Right upper lobe—anterior segment	Supine with head elevated	Right lower lobe—posterior segment	Prone with right side of chest elevated in Trendelenburg's position
Left upper lobe—anterior segment	Supine with head elevated	Right middle lobe—posterior segment	Prone with thorax and abdomen elevated
Right upper lobe—posterior segment	Side-lying with right side of chest elevated on pillows	Both lower lobes—anterior segments	Supine in Trendelenburg's position
Left upper lobe—posterior segment	Side-lying with left side of chest elevated on pillows	Both lower lobes—posterior segments	Prone in Trendelenburg's position
Right middle lobe—anterior segment	Three-fourths supine position with dependent lung in Trendelenburg's position		

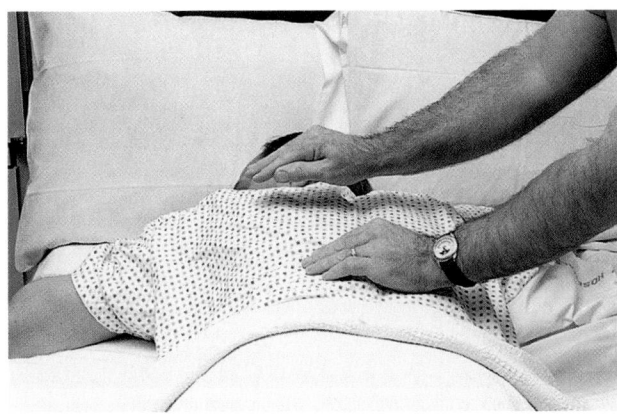

FIG. 41.8 Chest wall percussion, alternating hand clapping against patient's chest wall.

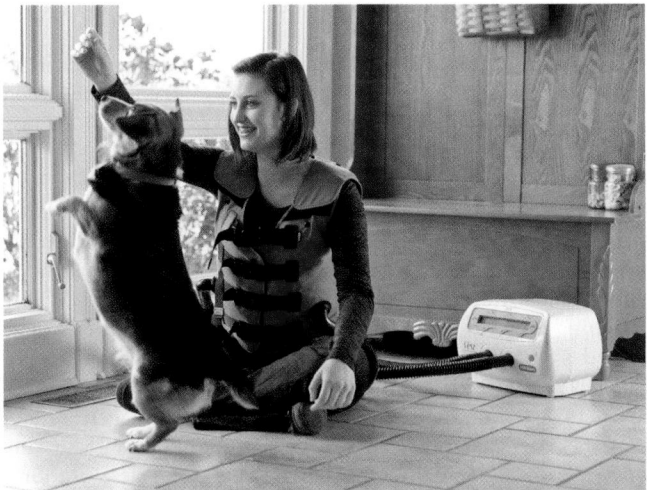

FIG. 41.9 High-frequency chest wall oscillation vest for home use. (Copyright © 2012 Hill-Rom Services, Inc. Reprinted with permission. All rights reserved.)

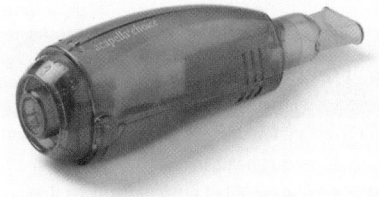

FIG. 41.10 Acapella airway clearance device. (Courtesy Smiths Medical North America.)

spirometry, and noninvasive ventilation. Invasive medical interventions, such as chest tube insertion and management, assist in restoring lung expansion.

Ambulation. Immobility is a major factor in developing atelectasis, ventilator-associated pneumonia (VAP), and functional limitations, including muscle weakness and fatigue (Nuwi and Irwan, 2018). This decline in status is often referred to as deconditioning. Early ambulation studies indicate that the therapeutic benefits of activity include an increase in general strength and lung expansion. Even the patient who requires invasive mechanical ventilation benefits by an early mobility program. Such mobility programs should include input from both respiratory and physical therapists in the treatment plan. Progressive mobilization from dangling the legs to standing and then

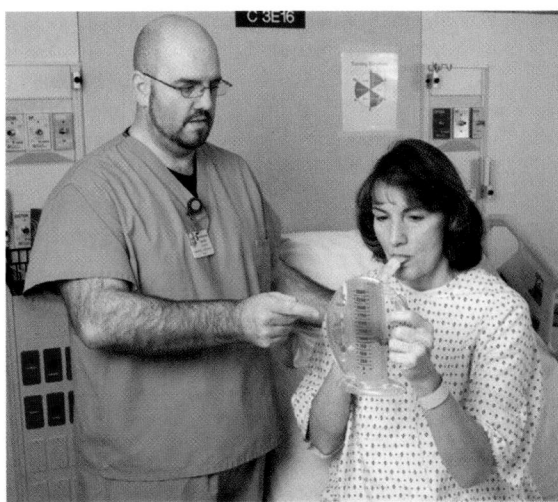

FIG. 41.11 Volume-oriented incentive spirometer.

walking is safe for intubated patients (Atkins and Kautz, 2014; Hartjes, 2018) (see Chapter 38).

Positioning. The healthy, completely mobile person maintains adequate ventilation and oxygenation by frequent position changes during daily activities. However, when a person's illness or injury restricts mobility, the risk for respiratory impairment is increased. Frequent changes of position are simple and cost-effective methods for reducing stasis of pulmonary secretions and decreased chest wall expansion, both of which increase the risk of pneumonia.

The 45-degree semi-Fowler's is the most effective position to promote lung expansion and reduce pressure from the abdomen on the diaphragm. When a patient is in this position, be sure that he or she does not slide down in bed, which can reduce lung expansion. Sliding also increases the risk of pressure injuries. A patient with unilateral lung disease, such as pneumothorax, atelectasis, or pneumonia of one lung, should be positioned in a manner to promote perfusion of the healthy lung and improve oxygenation. In most cases, position the patient with the good lung down. In the presence of pulmonary abscess or hemorrhage, position the patient with the affected lung down to prevent drainage toward the healthy lung. For bilateral lung disease, the best position depends on the severity of the disease (Lewis et al., 2017; Urden et al., 2020).

Incentive Spirometry. Incentive spirometry encourages voluntary deep breathing by providing visual feedback to patients about inspiratory volume. It is a commonly used intervention that promotes deep breathing and is thought to prevent or treat atelectasis in the postoperative patient. Recent evidence suggests that the use of the incentive spirometer is not as effective at preventing postoperative pulmonary complications as it once was thought to be. The AARC recommends that its use be reserved for patients with existing atelectasis or those with risk factors for developing atelectasis, such as those who have undergone thoracic or abdominal surgery, patients with prolonged bed rest, or patients with neuromuscular disease or spinal cord injuries (AARC, 2011; Eltorai et al., 2018).

There are two types of incentive spirometers. Flow-oriented incentive spirometers consist of one or more plastic chambers that contain freely moving colored balls. A patient inhales slowly and with an even flow to elevate the balls and keep them floating as long as possible to ensure a maximally sustained inhalation. Volume-oriented incentive spirometry devices have a bellows that is raised to a predetermined volume by an inhaled breath (Fig. 41.11). An achievement light or counter provides visual feedback. Some devices are constructed so the light does not turn on unless the bellows is held at a minimum desired volume for a specified period to enhance lung expansion (see Chapter 50).

The AARC guidelines (2011) recommend 5 to 10 breaths per session every hour while awake. Administration of pain medications before incentive spirometry helps a patient achieve deep breathing by reducing pain and splinting. Use incentive spirometry in combination with other pulmonary measures, such as deep breathing and coughing and early mobilization in patients who are at risk for atelectasis (do Nascimento et al., 2014).

Suctioning Techniques. Suctioning is necessary when patients are unable to clear respiratory secretions from the airways by coughing or other less invasive procedures. Suctioning techniques include oropharyngeal and nasopharyngeal suctioning, orotracheal and nasotracheal suctioning, and suctioning an artificial airway.

In most cases, use sterile technique for suctioning because the oropharynx and trachea are considered sterile. The mouth is considered clean, so it only requires clean technique. When suctioning both the oral pharynx and the trachea, always suction the nasotracheal and/or trachea (sterile) before the oral pharynx (clean) (AARC, 2004, 2010a; Wiegand, 2017).

Each type of suctioning requires the use of a round-tipped, flexible catheter with holes on the sides and end of the catheter. When suctioning, you apply negative pressures (100-150 mm Hg for adults) during withdrawal of the catheter and **never** on insertion (Myatt, 2015; Wiegand, 2017). Patient assessment determines the frequency of suctioning. It is indicated when rhonchi, gurgling breath sounds, and diminished breath sounds are audible on auscultation or visible secretions are present after other methods to remove airway secretions have failed. You may also use suctioning to obtain a sputum specimen for culture or cytology if the patient is unable to cough productively. There is no evidence to support suctioning on a scheduled basis. Too-frequent suctioning puts patients at risk for development of hypoxemia, hypotension, arrhythmias, and possible trauma to the mucosa of the lungs (Myatt, 2015; Wiegand, 2017).

Oropharyngeal and Nasopharyngeal Suctioning. Perform oropharyngeal or nasopharyngeal suctioning when a patient is able to cough effectively but is unable to clear secretions by expectorating. Apply suction after a patient has coughed (see Skill 41.1). Once the pulmonary secretions decrease and a patient is less fatigued, he or she is then able to expectorate or swallow the mucus, and suctioning is no longer necessary.

Orotracheal and Nasotracheal Suctioning. Perform orotracheal or nasotracheal suctioning is necessary when a patient with pulmonary secretions is unable to manage secretions by coughing and does not have an artificial airway present (see Skill 41.1). You pass a sterile catheter through the mouth or nose into the trachea. The nose is the preferred route because stimulation of the gag reflex is minimal. The procedure is similar to nasopharyngeal suctioning, but you advance the catheter tip farther into the patient's trachea. The entire procedure from catheter passage to its removal is done quickly, lasting no longer than 10 seconds (AARC, 2010a; Wiegand, 2017). Allow the patient to rest between passes of the catheter. If the patient develops respiratory distress, stop suctioning unless the collection of secretions is causing distress. If the patient is using supplemental oxygen, replace the oxygen cannula or mask during rest periods.

Tracheal Suctioning. Perform tracheal suctioning through an artificial airway such as an endotracheal (ET) or tracheostomy tube. The size of a catheter should be as small as possible but large enough to remove secretions. Never apply suction pressure while inserting the catheter to avoid traumatizing the lung mucosa. Once you insert a catheter the necessary distance, maintain suction pressure between 80 and 120 mm Hg (Wiegand, 2017) as you withdraw. Apply suction

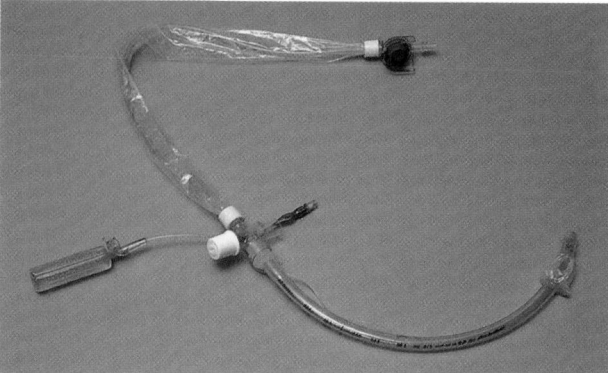

FIG. 41.12 Ballard tracheal care, closed suction catheter.

intermittently only while withdrawing the catheter. Rotating the catheter enhances removal of secretions that have adhered to the sides of the airway.

The practice of normal saline instillation (NSI) into artificial airways to improve secretion removal may be harmful and is not recommended. Clinical studies comparing the results of suctioning following NSI with standard suctioning have not shown any clinical or significant results (AARC, 2010a; Wang et al., 2017).

The two current methods of suctioning are the open and closed methods. Open suctioning involves using a new sterile catheter for each suction session (Wiegand, 2017). Wear sterile gloves and follow Standard Precautions during the suction procedure. Closed suctioning involves using a reusable sterile suction catheter that is encased in a plastic sheath to protect it between suction sessions (Fig. 41.12). Closed suctioning is most often used on patients who require invasive mechanical ventilation to support their respiratory efforts because it permits continuous delivery of oxygen while suction is performed and reduces the risk of oxygen desaturation. It is also associated with a decrease in the development of late-onset ventilator-associated pneumonia (Letchford and Bench, 2018). Although sterile gloves are not used in this procedure, nonsterile gloves are recommended to prevent contact with splashes from body fluids (see Skill 41.1).

REFLECT NOW

You are caring for a patient with cystic fibrosis. When entering the room, you note the patient to be in a supine position and complaining of a frequent, nonproductive cough. What are interventions that you can perform to help increase the patient's ability to expectorate the sputum?

Artificial Airways. An artificial airway is for a patient with a decreased level of consciousness or airway obstruction or who is in need of prolonged ventilatory support and aids in removal of tracheobronchial secretions and maintaining a patent airway. The presence of an artificial airway places a patient at high risk for infection and airway injury. Use clean technique for oral airways, but use sterile technique in caring for and maintaining endotracheal and tracheal airways to prevent health care–associated infections (HAIs). Artificial airways need to stay in the correct position to prevent airway damage (Higginson et al., 2016; Wiegand, 2017) (see Skill 41.2).

Oral Airway. The oral airway, the simplest type of artificial airway, prevents obstruction of the trachea by displacement of the tongue into the oropharynx (Fig. 41.13). The oral airway extends from the teeth to the oropharynx, maintaining the tongue in the normal position.

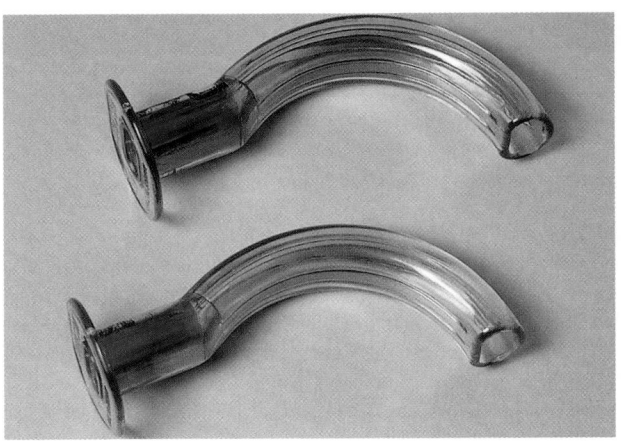

FIG. 41.13 Artificial oral airways.

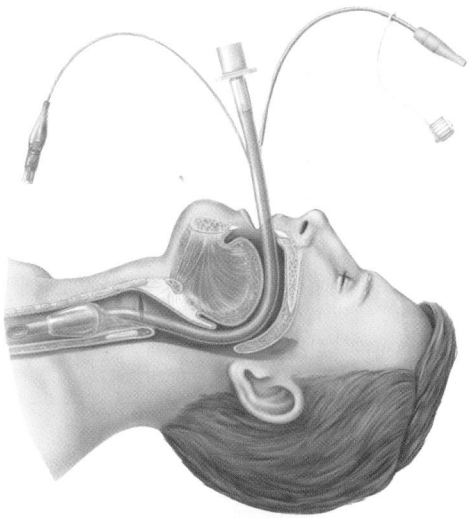

FIG. 41.14 Endotracheal tube inserted into trachea. Cuff inflated to maintain position. (Copyright © 2015 Medtronic. All rights reserved. Used with the permission of Medtronic.)

Determine the proper oral airway size by measuring the distance from the corner of the mouth to the angle of the jaw just below the ear. The length is equal to the distance from the flange of the airway to the tip. Use only the correct size airway. If the airway is too small, the tongue does not stay in the anterior portion of the mouth; if the airway is too large, it forces the tongue toward the epiglottis and obstructs the airway (Wiegand, 2017).

Insert the airway upside down, then turn the curve of the airway toward the cheek and place it over the tongue. When the airway is in the oropharynx, turn it so that the opening points downward. Correctly placed, the airway moves the tongue forward away from the oropharynx, and the flange (e.g., the flat portion of the airway) rests against the patient's teeth. Incorrect insertion merely forces the tongue back into the oropharynx (Wiegand, 2017).

Endotracheal and Tracheal Airways. An endotracheal (ET) tube is a short-term artificial airway used to administer invasive mechanical ventilation, relieve upper airway obstruction, protect against aspiration, or clear secretions. A physician or specially trained clinician inserts the ET tube. The tube is passed through the patient's mouth, past the pharynx, and into the trachea (Fig. 41.14). It is generally removed within 14 days; however, it is sometimes used for a longer period of time if the patient is still showing progress toward weaning from invasive mechanical ventilation and extubation (removal of the endotracheal tube) (Urden et al., 2020; Wiegand, 2017).

If a patient requires long-term assistance from an artificial airway, a tracheostomy is considered. A surgical incision is made into the inferior border of the cricoid cartilage of the trachea, and a short tracheostomy tube is inserted. Most tracheostomies have a small plastic inner tube that fits inside a larger one (the inner cannula). The most common complication of a tracheostomy tube is partial or total airway obstruction caused by buildup of respiratory secretions. If this occurs, the inner tube can be removed and cleaned or replaced with a temporary spare inner tube that should be kept at the patient's bedside. Keep tracheal dilators at the bedside to have available for emergency tube replacement or reinsertion. Humidification from air humidifiers or humidified oxygen tracheostomy collars can help prevent drying of secretions that cause occlusion. Tracheostomy suctioning should be done as necessary to clear secretions. The majority of patients with a tracheostomy tube cannot speak because the tube is inserted below the vocal cords. It is important to use written or nonverbal communication (lipreading) strategies to help patients communicate. Be sure to assess patients for anxiety caused by the inability to speak. Care and cleaning of the tracheostomy tube is discussed in Skill 41.2 (Urden et al., 2020; Wiegand, 2017).

Invasive Mechanical Ventilation. Invasive mechanical ventilation, also referred to as positive-pressure ventilation, is a lifesaving technique used with artificial airways (ET or tracheostomy) for various physiological and clinical indications. Physiological indications for invasive mechanical ventilation include supporting cardiopulmonary gas exchange (alveolar ventilation and arterial oxygenation), increasing lung volume, and reducing the work of breathing (Urden et al., 2020). Clinical indications for invasive mechanical ventilation include reversing hypoxia and acute respiratory acidosis; relieving respiratory distress; preventing or reversing atelectasis and respiratory muscle fatigue; allowing for sedation and/or other neuromuscular blockade, thereby decreasing oxygen consumption; and stabilizing the chest wall (Urden et al., 2020). It can be used to either fully or partially replace spontaneous breathing, depending on the need of the patient. Invasive mechanical ventilation also redistributes oxygen demand from working respiratory muscles to other vital organs.

Ventilator-associated pneumonia (VAP) is a significant potential complication because the artificial airway tube bypasses many of the airway's and lung's normal defense mechanisms. Ventilator associated pneumonia (VAP) is a health care–acquired infection (HAI) that develops 48 hours or more after endotracheal intubation and mechanical ventilation (Letchford and Bench, 2018). It is a potentially serious complication in patients who are already critically ill. VAP mortality rates range from 10% to 55% among ventilated patients; VAP increases patient time in the ICU by 4 to 6 days and is estimated to add an additional $40,000 to the cost of a hospital admission (Chahoud et al., 2015; Larrow and Klich-Heartt, 2016) (Box 41.8). Hospitals are not reimbursed for costs associated with VAP.

Noninvasive Ventilation. Noninvasive positive-pressure ventilation (NPPV), a form of noninvasive ventilation (NIV), maintains positive airway pressure and improves alveolar ventilation without the need for an artificial airway. It is used for the treatment of obstructive sleep apnea, in patients with respiratory failure, and following extubation of an ET tube (Gale et al., 2015). This alternative to invasive ventilation reduces and reverses atelectasis; improves oxygenation; reduces pulmonary edema; and improves cardiac function. Positive-pressure ventilation keeps the alveoli partially inflated, reducing the risk of atelectasis. Because the alveoli remain partially inflated, there is a continuous exchange of respiratory gas, which leads to improved oxygenation. In patients with obstructive sleep apnea, the NPPV helps to keep the airway open (Hortal et al., 2016; Xu et al., 2015). Goals of this type of ventilation include improved gas exchange, improved

BOX 41.8 EVIDENCE-BASED PRACTICE

Adherence to a Ventilator Care Bundle on Reducing Ventilator-Associated Pneumonia

PICOT Question: In patients requiring invasive mechanical ventilation, does adhering to an evidenced-based ventilator care bundle contribute to a reduction of ventilator-associated pneumonia (VAP)?

Evidence Summary

Ventilator associated pneumonia (VAP) is a health care–acquired infection (HAI) that develops in a person requiring invasive mechanical ventilation (via endotracheal intubation or tracheostomy tube) for at least 48 hours (Bassi et al., 2017). *Pseudomonas, Acinetobacter,* and methicillin-resistant *Staphylococcus aureus* are frequent bacterial causes of VAP (Chacko et al., 2017). Patients with VAP have fever, increased secretions, and pulmonary infiltrates seen on chest radiograph. Over time these infiltrates progressively increase, and the patient's lung functions decline. VAP increases length of stay in the intensive care unit, is associated with increased morbidity and mortality, and increases the patient's cost of hospitalization (Chacko et al., 2017; Larrow and Klich-Heartt, 2016).

In 2012, the Institute for Healthcare Improvement published an evidence-based how-to guide for the prevention of VAP (IHI, 2012). This guide was the beginning of a series of evidenced-based interventions related to ventilator care that, when implemented together, achieve significantly better outcomes than when implemented individually (Bassi et al., 2017). The key components of the VAP bundle include:

- Elevation of the head of the bed (HOB) greater than 30 degrees
- Daily "sedation vacations" and assessment of readiness to extubate
- Peptic ulcer disease prophylaxis
- Venous thromboembolism prophylaxis
- Daily oral care with chlorhexidine (Hua et al., 2016)
- Delirium monitoring

- Early mobilization (Bassi et al., 2017; Larrow and Klich-Heartt, 2016)

The use of the bundle (known as the VAP bundle or the ABCDE bundle) has been known to decrease rates of VAP (Kram et al., 2015; AACN, 2017a,b).

Application to Nursing Practice

- Implement the VAP bundle when mechanical ventilation is initiated (Anand et al., 2018).
- Avoid prolonged supine positioning. Pulmonary aspiration is increased by supine positioning and pooling of secretions above the ET tube cuff (AACN, 2018).
- Position with HOB elevation to 45 degrees or higher significantly reduces gastric reflux and VAP.
- Orotracheal and orogastric tubes are preferred over nasal devices to reduce the risk of VAP (Rouzé et al., 2017).
- Suction frequently to remove oropharyngeal and subglottic secretions to reduce the risk of early-onset VAP. Utilize subglottic suctioning to decrease the amount of secretions that pool in the oropharyngeal cavity (Bassi et al., 2017; Li et al., 2017) .
- Perform endotracheal and tracheostomy tube suctioning only when indicated by patient assessment findings and not on a scheduled basis.
- Monitor cuff pressure of the endotracheal and tracheostomy tubes frequently to ensure that there is an adequate seal to prevent aspiration of secretions.
- Always drain ventilator circuit condensation away from patient and into the appropriate receptacle. Drain the tubing hourly to prevent accumulation.
- Assess for and treat delirium.
- Change ventilator circuits only when visibly soiled.
- Ensure that humidity is added to the ventilator circuit.

---

sleep, enhanced quality of life, reduction of morbidity, and improved physical function. The most common modes of NPPV are **continuous positive airway pressure (CPAP)** and **bilevel positive airway pressure (BiPAP)**.

CPAP maintains a steady stream of pressure throughout a patient's breathing cycle. It benefits patients with obstructive sleep apnea (OSA), patients with heart failure, and preterm infants with underdeveloped lungs. In obstructive sleep apnea (OSA), the upper airway collapses, causing obstruction that leads to shallow or absent breathing. Any air moving past the obstruction results in loud snoring. An overnight sleep study may be needed to determine the need and the correct settings for a CPAP machine (see Chapter 43). Equipment includes a mask (Fig. 41.15) that fits over the nose or both nose and mouth and a CPAP machine that delivers air to the mask (Hortal et al., 2016). The smallest mask with the proper fit is the most effective. It must be tight enough to form a seal on the face so that the air does not escape but not so tight as to cause pressure injury formation or necrosis where the mask is against the face (Schallom et al., 2015).

BiPAP works by providing assistance during inspiration and preventing alveolar closure during expiration. It provides both inspiratory positive airway pressure (IPAP) and expiratory airway pressure (EPAP), also known as *positive end-expiratory pressure (PEEP)*. During inhalation the positive pressure increases the patient's tidal volume and alveolar ventilation. The pressure support decreases when the patient exhales, allowing for easier exhalation. The overall result of BiPAP is an increased amount of air in the lungs at the end of expiration (functional residual capacity), reduced airway closure, expansion of areas of atelectasis, and improved oxygenation (Hartjes, 2018; Urden et al., 2020).

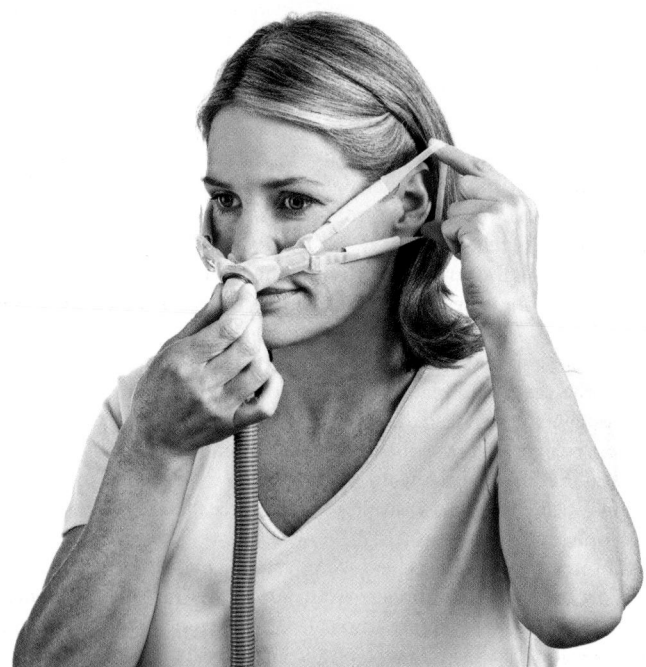

FIG. 41.15 CPAP mask. (Courtesy ResMed.)

Complications of noninvasive ventilation include facial and nasal injury and skin breakdown, dry mucous membranes and thick secretions, and aspiration of gastric contents if vomiting occurs (AACN,

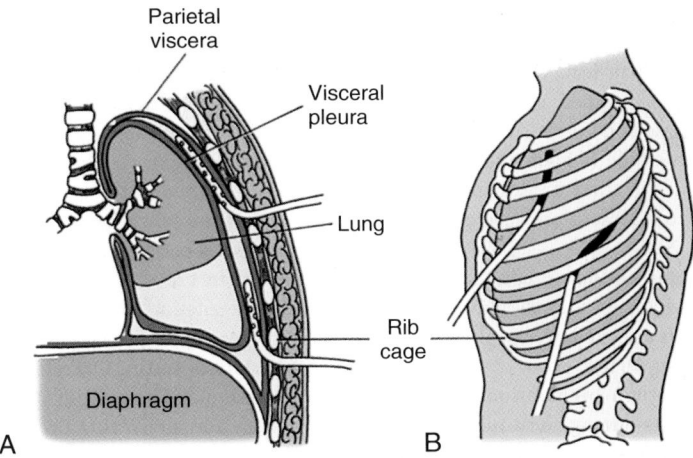

FIG. 41.16 Diagram of sites for chest tube placement. **A,** Anatomical drawing of upper tube placement for removal of air and lower tube placement for blood and fluid. **B,** View of tubes exiting through intracostal sites.

2018). Complications avoided by noninvasive ventilation are VAP, sinusitis, and the effects of large-dose sedative agents. Use of noninvasive ventilation results in shorter intensive care unit (ICU) and hospital stays (Gale et al., 2015; Schallom et al., 2015). Perform good oral hygiene every few hours while a patient is on NPPV to relieve dryness.

Chest Tubes. A chest tube (Fig. 41.16) is a catheter inserted through the rib cage into the pleural space to remove air, fluids, or blood; to prevent air or fluid from reentering the pleural space; or to reestablish normal intrapleural and intrapulmonic pressures after trauma or surgery (Chotai and Mosenifar, 2018). Chest tubes are common after chest surgery and chest trauma and are used for treatment of pneumothorax or hemothorax to promote lung reexpansion (see Skill 41.3).

A pneumothorax is a collection of air in the pleural space. The loss of negative intrapleural pressure causes the lung to collapse. There are a variety of causes for a pneumothorax. A pneumothorax can occur as a result of chest trauma (e.g., stabbing, gunshot wound, or rib fracture). Other causes of pneumothorax are the rupture of an emphysematous bleb on the surface of the lung (the destruction caused by emphysema), tearing of the pleura from an invasive procedure such as surgery, insertion of a subclavian IV line, and invasive mechanical ventilation, including PEEP. Spontaneous pneumothorax occurs due to the rupture of small blebs (air-filled sacs). A spontaneous pneumothorax can occur in young, healthy individuals or in patients with a history of lung disease such as COPD or CF (Lewis et al., 2017). A patient with a pneumothorax usually feels sharp pain that is pleuritic and worsens on inspiration. Dyspnea is common and worsens as the size of the pneumothorax increases.

A tension pneumothorax is a life-threatening condition in which air enters the pleural space and cannot escape. The accumulation of air eventually leads to compression of the affected lung and pressure on the heart, causing the heart and great vessels to shift to the unaffected side. This shift then leads to compression of the unaffected lung, leading to decreased oxygenation and decreased cardiac output. Clinical manifestations include dyspnea, tachycardia, tracheal deviation laterally, and absent breath sounds on the affected side. A tension pneumothorax is a medical emergency and requires immediate intervention, including needle decompression and chest tube placement (Zardo et al., 2015; Urden et al., 2020).

A hemothorax is an accumulation of blood and fluid in the pleural space, usually as a result of trauma. It produces a counter pressure and prevents the lung from full expansion. A rupture of small blood vessels

from inflammatory processes such as pneumonia or TB can cause a hemothorax, as can trauma. In addition to pain and dyspnea, signs and symptoms of shock develop if blood loss is severe (Lewis et al., 2017; Urden et al., 2020).

A variety of chest tubes are available to drain air or excess fluid from the pleural space to relieve respiratory distress. Typically, a small-bore chest tube (12 to 20 Fr) is used to remove a small amount of air, and a larger-bore chest tube (greater than 20 Fr) is used to remove large amounts of fluid or blood (Zardo et al., 2015).

After a chest tube is inserted, it is attached to a drainage system. A traditional chest drainage unit (CDU) has three chambers for collection of drainage, water seal, and suction control. This unit can drain a large amount of both fluid and air. Disposable chest drainage systems, such as the Codman, Pleur-evac, or Atrium, allow for more mobility than previous bottle systems and are now more commonly used. The disposable systems also allow for increased ability to maintain sterility of the system (Chotai and Mosenifar, 2018). Nonventilated patients and patients who had thoracoscopic lung surgery or minimally invasive cardiac surgery do well with these mobile chest drains.

Special Considerations. Keep a chest tube drainage system closed and below the chest (see Skill 41.3). The chest tube should be secured to the chest wall. Watch for slow, steady bubbling in the water seal chamber and keep it filled with sterile water at the prescribed level. A constant or intermittent bubbling in the water-seal chamber, or new more vigorous bubbling, indicates a leak in the drainage system or another pneumothorax, and you must assess the system and the patient to accurately identify the source of the leak. Watch for fluctuation (tailing) of the fluid level to ensure that the chest tube and system are working. Mark the level on the outside of the collection chambers every shift. Report any unexpected cloudy or bloody drainage. Avoid kinks and dependent loops in the tubing. Ideally, it should lie horizontally across the bed or chair before dropping vertically into the drainage device. Encourage your patient to cough, breathe deeply, and use the incentive spirometer. Make sure that he or she is in a semi-Fowler or high-Fowler (45-90 degrees) position and is ambulated if not contraindicated. Routinely evaluate respiratory rate, breath sounds, SpO_2 levels, and the insertion site for subcutaneous emphysema (Chotai and Mosenifar, 2018). Subcutaneous emphysema is the presence of air under the skin, and crepitus is palpated in the area where it is located (Hartjes, 2018).

Clamping a chest tube is contraindicated when ambulating or transporting a patient. Clamping can result in a tension pneumothorax. Air pressure builds in the pleural space, collapsing the lung and creating a life-threatening event. A chest tube is clamped only when replacing the chest drainage system, assessing for an air leak, or as a trial before removal to assess whether the air leak has stopped. Stripping or milking chest tubes to keep them patent is based on nursing assessment and may be necessary to remove clots in the tube (Chotai and Mosenifar, 2018). Routine milking or stripping of the chest tubes is not recommended as it can cause increased intrathoracic pressure and tissue damage (Wiegand, 2017; Makic et al., 2015).

Handle the chest drainage unit carefully, and maintain the drainage device below the patient's chest. The drainage unit should always be maintained in an upright position. If it is knocked over, replacement of the unit is needed (Chotai and Mosenifar, 2018).

Removal of chest tubes requires patient preparation. The most frequent sensations reported by patients during chest tube removal include burning, pain, and a pulling sensation. Make sure that the patient is given pain medication at least 30 minutes before removal. The nurse assists the health care provider in removing the chest tube and monitors the dressing placed over the insertion site and the patient's respiratory status after tube removal (Wiegand, 2017). An unplanned removal of the chest tube, such as the tube being accidentally removed while repositioning the patient, requires the nurse to cover the site with a gloved hand and ask for help in retrieving supplies to cover the site. Petrolatum gauze, dry gauze, and tape will be needed to dress the site. If the chest tube becomes disconnected from the drainage system, clamp the tubing with the shodded hemostat or crimp the tubing with a gloved hand to prevent air from entering the pleural space. Ask for someone to get a new chest drainage system and attach it to the chest tube in a sterile manner. Regardless of how the tube comes out, monitor the patient for signs of respiratory distress and auscultate lung sounds (Muzzy and Butler, 2015).

Maintenance and Promotion of Oxygenation. Promotion of lung expansion, mobilization of secretions, and maintenance of a patent airway assist patients in meeting their oxygenation needs. However, some patients also require oxygen therapy to keep a healthy level of tissue oxygenation.

Oxygen Therapy. Oxygen therapy is widely available and used in a variety of settings to relieve or prevent hypoxia, which can lead to hypoxemia. The goal of oxygen therapy is to prevent or relieve hypoxemia by delivering the lowest amount of oxygen possible and achieve adequate tissue oxygenation (Walsh and Smallwood, 2017). The dosage or concentration of oxygen is monitored continuously. Routinely check the health care provider's orders to verify that the patient is receiving the prescribed oxygen concentration. The seven rights of medication administration also pertain to oxygen administration (see Chapter 31).

Supplemental oxygen therapy offers many benefits to patients with acute and/or chronic cardiopulmonary diseases. This therapy reduces mortality, increases exercise tolerance, decreases pulmonary hypertension, and improves a patient's quality of life (Franchini et al., 2016; Wen et al., 2017). It is important to reinforce to your patients why they may

---

BOX 41.9 PROCEDURAL GUIDELINES

Applying a Nasal Cannula or Oxygen Mask

Delegation and Collaboration

The skill of applying a nasal cannula or oxygen mask can be delegated to assistive personnel (AP) after the method of delivery and percentage of oxygen needed by a patient is determined. The nurse is responsible for assessing the patient's respiratory system and the response to oxygen therapy. The nurse, in some agencies, may collaborate with the respiratory therapist in the setup of oxygen therapy, including adjustment of oxygen flow rate. The nurse instructs the AP to:

- Safely adjust the device (e.g., loosening the strap on the oxygen cannula or mask) and clarify its correct placement and positioning.
- Inform the nurse immediately about any changes in vital signs; changes in pulse oximetry (SpO_2); changes in level of consciousness (LOC); skin irritation from the cannula, mask, or straps; or patient complaints of pain or shortness of breath.
- Provide extra skin care around patient's ears and nose or other parts of the patient's body that might be irritated by the device.

Equipment

(**Note:** If device is used in the home, the home care equipment vendor provides the equipment.)

Oxygen delivery device as ordered by health care provider; oxygen tubing (consider extension tubing as needed); humidifier, if indicated; sterile water for humidifier; oxygen source; oxygen flowmeter; "oxygen in use" sign; pulse oximeter; stethoscope; clean gloves; face shield, if risk of splash from secretions is present

Steps

1. Identify patient using at least two identifiers (e.g., name and birthday or name and medical record number) according to agency policy. Compare identifiers with information on patient's MAR or medical record.

2. Review accuracy of health care provider's order for oxygen, noting delivery method, flow rate, duration of oxygen therapy, and parameters for titration of oxygen settings.

3. Obtain data from patient's electronic health record (vital signs, pulse oximetry, arterial blood gas values).

4. Perform hand hygiene and apply gloves. Perform respiratory assessment, including symmetry of chest wall expansion, chest wall abnormalities (e.g., kyphosis), temporary conditions (e.g., pregnancy, trauma) affecting ventilation, respiratory rate and depth, sputum production, lung sounds, and signs and symptoms associated with hypoxia.

5. Observe for cognitive and/or behavioral changes (e.g., apprehension, anxiety, confusion, decreased ability to concentrate, decreased LOC, fatigue, and dizziness).

CLINICAL DECISION: Patients with sudden changes in their vital signs, LOC, or behavior may be experiencing profound hypoxia. Patients who demonstrate subtle changes over time may have worsening of a chronic or existing condition or a new medical condition (Lewis et al., 2017).

6. Assess airway patency and remove airway secretions by having patient cough and expectorate mucus or by suctioning (see Skill 41.1). **Note:** Continue wearing gloves. However, remove and dispose of gloves and perform hand hygiene if there is contact with mucus. Then reapply gloves if contact with mucus is likely.

CLINICAL DECISION: Excessive amounts of secretions, signs of respiratory distress (increased work of breathing, increased respiratory rate), presence of rhonchi on auscultation, excessive coughing, or decrease in patient pulse oximeter indicate need for suctioning.

7. Inspect condition of skin around nose and ears.

BOX 41.9 PROCEDURAL GUIDELINES—cont'd

Applying a Nasal Cannula or Oxygen Mask

8. Assess patient's or family caregiver's knowledge, experience, and health literacy level.
9. Apply face shield if risk of exposure to splashing mucus exists.
10. Attach oxygen-delivery device (e.g., cannula, mask) to oxygen tubing and attach end of tubing to humidified oxygen source adjusted to prescribed flow rate (see illustration).
11. Apply oxygen device:
    a. Place tips of the cannula into patient's nares. If tips are curved, they should point downward inside nostrils. Then loop cannula tubing up and over patient's ears. Adjust lanyard so that cannula fits snugly but not too tight and without pressure to patient nares and ears (see illustration).
    b. Apply a mask by placing it over patient's mouth and nose. Then bring straps over patient's head and adjust to form a comfortable but tight seal.

c. Maintain sufficient slack on oxygen tubing and secure to patient's clothes.
12. Observe for proper function of oxygen-delivery device:
    a. *Nasal cannula:* Cannula is positioned properly in nares; oxygen flows through tips.
    b. *Partial nonrebreather mask:* Mask seals tightly around mouth. Reservoir fills on exhalation and almost collapses on inspiration. Reservoir should not collapse completely (see illustration).
    c. *Oxygen-conserving cannula (Oxymizer):* Fit as for nasal cannula. Reservoir is located under patient's nose or worn as a pendant.
    d. *Nonrebreather mask:* Apply as regular mask. Contains one-way valves with reservoir; exhaled air does not enter reservoir bag. Can be combined with nasal cannula to provide higher inspired oxygen concentration (FiO_2).
    e. *Simple face mask:* Select appropriate flow rate (see illustration).

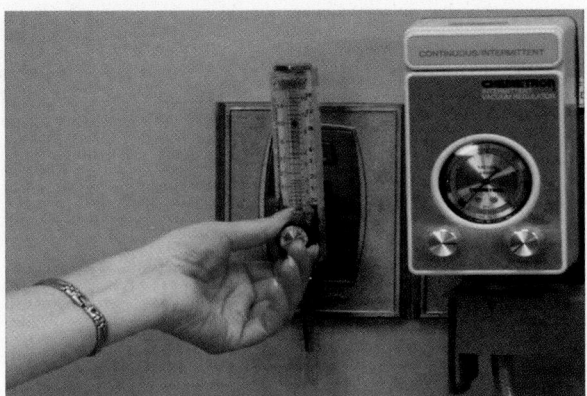

STEP 10 Flowmeter attached to oxygen source.

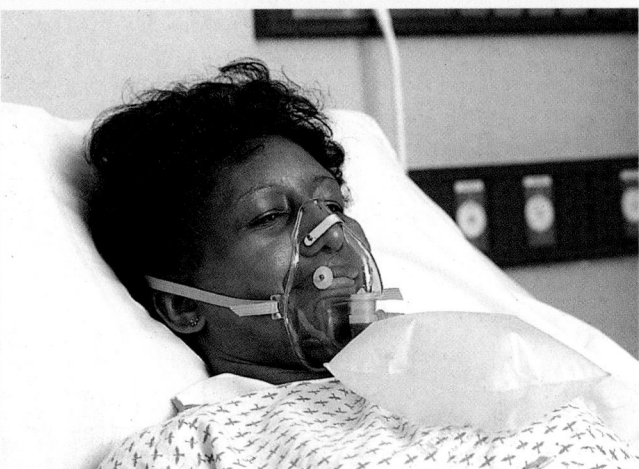

STEP 12b Plastic face mask with reservoir bag.

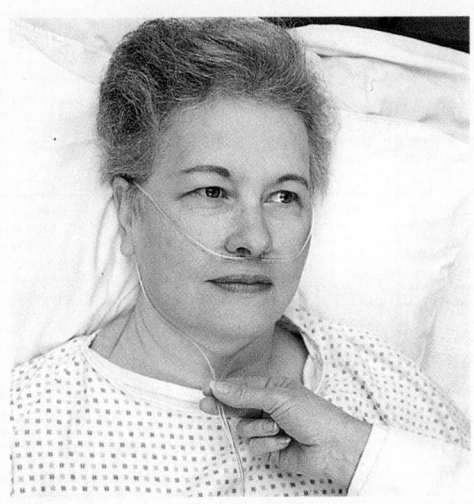

STEP 11a Nasal cannula adjusted for proper fit.

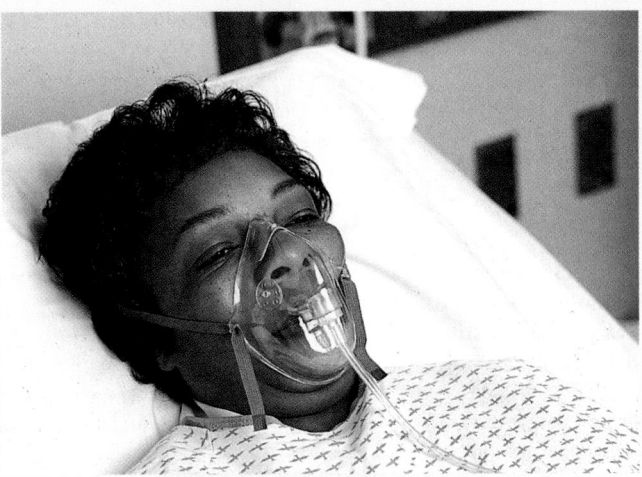

STEP 12e Simple face mask.

Continued

BOX 41.9   PROCEDURAL GUIDELINES—cont'd

Applying a Nasal Cannula or Oxygen Mask

f. *Venturi* mask (see illustration): Apply as regular mask. Select appropriate flow rate (see Table 41.7).

g. *High-flow nasal cannula* (see illustration).

13. Verify setting on flowmeter and oxygen source for proper setup and prescribed flow rate.

14. Check cannula/mask every 8 hours or as agency policy indicates. Keep humidification container filled at all times.

15. Post "Oxygen in use" signs on wall behind bed and at entrance to room.

16. Properly dispose of gloves (if used) and perform hand hygiene.

17. Be sure nurse call system is accessible and within patient's reach. Instruct the patient on its use.

18. Monitor patient's response to changes in oxygen flow rate with SpO_2.
NOTE: Monitor ABGs when ordered; however, obtaining ABG measurement is an invasive procedure, and ABGs are not measured frequently.

19. Perform physical assessment, auscultating lung sounds; palpating chest excursion; inspecting color and condition of skin; and observing for decreased anxiety, improved LOC and cognitive abilities, decreased fatigue, and absence of dizziness. Measure vital signs.

20. Assess adequacy of oxygen flow each shift or as agency policy dictates.

21. Observe patient's external ears, bridge of nose, nares, and nasal mucous membranes for evidence of skin breakdown.

22. **Use Teach-Back:** "I want to be sure I explained how oxygen will help you. Tell me why oxygen is beneficial for you." Revise your instruction now or develop a plan for revised patient/family caregiver teaching if patient/family caregiver is not able to teach back correctly.

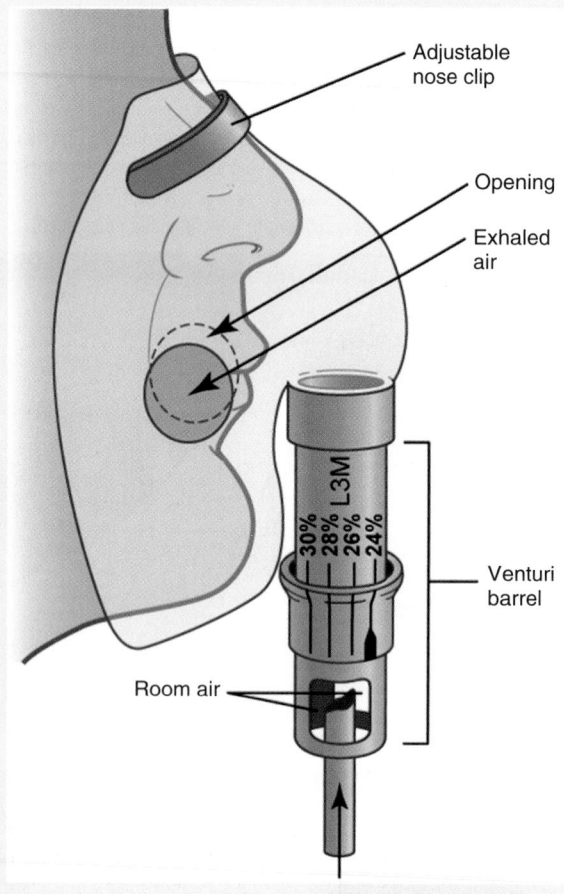

STEP 12f Venturi mask.

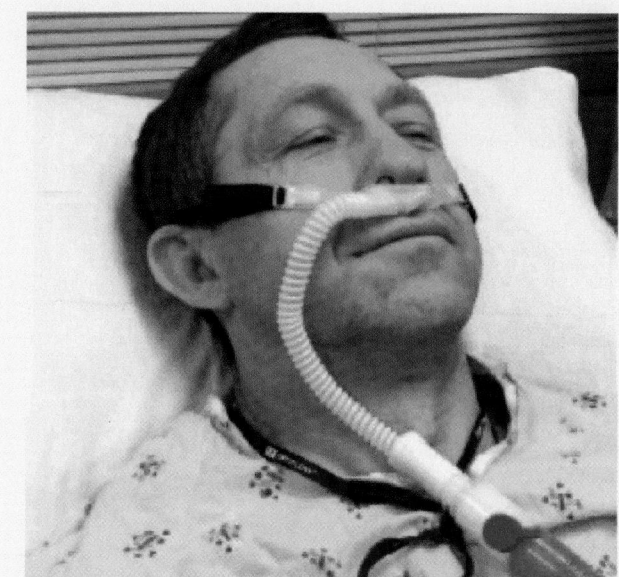

STEP 12g High-flow nasal cannula. (Courtesy Fischer & Paykel Healthcare.)

require supplemental oxygen in the acute care setting, as well as possible home use (Box 41.9).

Safety Precautions. Oxygen is a highly combustible gas. Although it does not burn spontaneously or cause an explosion, it can easily cause a fire in a patient's room if it contacts a spark from an open flame or electrical equipment. With increasing use of home oxygen therapy, patients and health care professionals need to be aware of the dangers of combustion (AARC, 2007). Be cognizant of agency procedures for managing a fire or know the local emergency response phone number (often 911) in case of a fire at a patient's home.

Follow these oxygen safety precautions:

- Oxygen is a therapeutic gas and must be prescribed and adjusted only with a health care provider's order. Distribution must be in accordance with federal, state, and local regulations (Jacobs et al., 2018).

- Keep oxygen-delivery systems 10 feet from any open flames.

- Oxygen is a combustible substance. Determine that all electrical equipment in the room is functioning correctly and properly grounded (see Chapter 27). An electrical spark in the presence of oxygen can result in a serious fire as oxygen supports combustion.

- When using oxygen cylinders, secure them so that they do not fall over. Store them upright and either chained or secured in appropriate holders.

- Check the oxygen level of portable tanks before transporting a patient to ensure that there is enough oxygen in the tank.

- Ensure that patients have adequate oxygen tubing to safely move around their agency or home environment.

TABLE 41.7 Oxygen Delivery Systems

Delivery System	FiO$_2$ Delivered	Advantages	Disadvantages
Low-Flow Delivery Devices			
Nasal cannula	1-6 L/min: 24%-44%	Safe and simple Easily tolerated Effective for low concentrations Does not impede eating or talking Inexpensive, disposable	Unable to use with nasal obstruction Drying to mucous membranes Can dislodge easily May cause skin irritation or breakdown around ears or nares Patient's breathing pattern (mouth or nasal) affects exact FiO$_2$
Oxygen-conserving cannula *(Oxymizer)*	8 L/min: up to 30%-50%	Indicated for long-term O$_2$ use in the home Allows increased O$_2$ concentration and lower flow	Cannula cannot be cleaned More expensive than standard cannula
Simple face mask	6-12 L/min: 35%-50%	Useful for short periods such as patient transportation	Contraindicated for patients who retain CO$_2$ May induce feelings of claustrophobia Therapy interrupted with eating and drinking Increased risk of aspiration
Partial and nonrebreather masks (**NOTE:** Reservoir bag should always remain partially inflated.)	10-15 L/min: 60%-90%	Useful for short periods Delivers increased FiO$_2$ Easily humidifies O$_2$ Does not dry mucous membranes	Hot and confining; may irritate skin; tight seal necessary Interferes with eating and talking Bag may twist or kink; should not totally deflate
High-Flow Delivery Devices			
Venturi mask	24%-50%	Provides specific amount of oxygen with humidity added Administers low, constant O$_2$	Mask and added humidity may irritate skin Therapy interrupted with eating and drinking Specific flow rate must be followed
High-flow nasal cannula	Adjustable FiO$_2$ (0.21-1) with modifiable flow (up to 60 L/min)	Wide range of FiO$_2$ Can use on adults, children, and infants	FiO$_2$ dependent on patient respiratory pattern and input flow Risk for infection (Urden et al., 2020)
Noninvasive Ventilation			
Continuous positive airway pressure (CPAP) and bilevel positive airway pressure (BiPAP)	21%-100%	Avoids the use of an artificial airway in some patients with acute respiratory distress, postextubation respiratory failure, or neuromuscular disorders Successfully treats obstructive sleep apnea	Nasal pillows/face masks can cause skin breakdown May cause claustrophobia in some patients

CO$_2$, Carbon dioxide; *FiO$_2$,* fraction of inspired oxygen concentration. *FiO$_2$* delivered may differ by manufacturer; check manufacturer's guidelines. Data for high-flow cannula: Walsh BK, Smallwood CD: Pediatric oxygen therapy: a review and update, *Respir Care* 62(6):645, 2017. Source for noninvasive ventilation: Wiegand D: *AACN procedure manual for high acuity, progressive, and critical care,* ed 7, St Louis, 2017, Elsevier.

Supply of Oxygen. Oxygen is supplied to a patient's bedside either by oxygen tanks or through a permanent wall-piped system. Oxygen tanks are transported on wide-based carriers that allow the tank to be placed upright at the bedside. Regulators control the amount of oxygen delivered. One common type is an upright flowmeter with a flow adjustment valve at the top. A second type is a cylinder indicator with a flow adjustment handle.

Methods of Oxygen Delivery. The nasal cannula and oxygen masks are the most common devices to deliver oxygen to patients. These devices deliver different levels of oxygen to patients (see Box 41.9; Table 41.7).

Nasal Cannula. A nasal cannula has two nasal prongs that are slightly curved and inserted in a patient's nostrils. To keep the nasal prongs in place, fit the attached tubing over the patient's ears and secure it under the chin using the sliding connector. Be alert for skin breakdown over the ears and in the nostrils from too tight an application. Attach the nasal cannula to an oxygen source with a flow rate of 1 to 6 L/min (24% to 44% oxygen). Flow rates equal to or greater than 4 L/min have a drying effect on the mucosa and thus need to be humidified (AARC, 2007; Hartjes, 2018). Know which flow rate produces a given percentage of inspired oxygen concentration (FiO$_2$).

High-Flow Nasal Cannula. High-flow nasal cannula (HFNC) is a relatively new method of oxygen delivery. It provides heated, humidified oxygen through a nasal cannula at flow rates as high as 60 L/minute while an air-oxygen blender allows for the titration of the FiO$_2$. The cannula is typically larger in diameter than the standard nasal cannula. HFNC is used to treat respiratory failure, and early evidence indicates that there is less need for invasive ventilation in patients who are initially treated with HFNC (Walsh and Smallwood, 2017; Xu et al., 2018).

Oxygen Masks. An oxygen mask is a plastic device that fits snugly over the mouth and nose and is secured in place with a strap. It delivers oxygen as the patient breathes through either the mouth or nose by way of a plastic tubing at the base of the mask that is attached to an oxygen source. An adjustable elastic band is attached to either side of the mask that slides over the head to above the ears to hold the mask in place. There are two primary types of oxygen masks: those delivering low concentrations of oxygen and those delivering high concentrations.

The simple face mask is used for short-term oxygen therapy. It fits loosely and delivers oxygen concentrations from 6 to 12 L/min (35% to 50% oxygen). The mask is contraindicated for patients with carbon dioxide retention because retention can be worsened, leading to decreased levels of consciousness. Flow rates should be 6 L or more to avoid rebreathing exhaled carbon dioxide retained in the mask. Be alert to skin breakdown under the mask with long-term use (Hartjes, 2018).

Partial rebreather and nonrebreather masks are simple masks with a reservoir bag that are capable of delivering higher concentrations of oxygen for a short period of time (60% to 90% oxygen at a flow rate of 10 to 15 L/min). Frequently inspect the reservoir bag to make sure that it is inflated. If it is deflated, the patient is breathing large amounts of exhaled carbon dioxide. (Hartjes, 2018; Lewis et al., 2017).

The Venturi mask delivers high flow, more precise oxygen concentrations of 24% to 60% and usually requires oxygen flow rates of 4 to 12 L/min, depending on the flow-control meter selected. Its use is typically reserved for patients with COPD who need low, constant oxygen concentrations (Hartjes, 2018; Lewis et al., 2017).

> **QSEN** **Building Competency in Safety** Mr. Edwards, a 75-year-old man with COPD, is receiving oxygen therapy via nasal cannula. What are ways you can prevent complications from this type of oxygen delivery device?
>
> Answers to QSEN Activities can be found on the Evolve website.

Restoration of Cardiopulmonary Functioning.
If a patient's hypoxia is severe and prolonged, cardiac arrest results. A cardiac arrest is a sudden cessation of cardiac output and circulation. When this occurs, oxygen is not delivered to tissues, carbon dioxide is not transported from tissues, tissue metabolism becomes anaerobic, and metabolic and respiratory acidosis occur. Permanent damage to the heart, brain, and other tissue occurs within 4 to 6 minutes.

Cardiopulmonary Resuscitation. During cardiac arrest there is an absence of pulse and respiration. Patients in cardiac arrest require immediate cardiopulmonary resuscitation (CPR), a basic emergency procedure of artificial respiration and manual external cardiac massage. The sequence for CPR is C-A-B: chest compression, early defibrillation, establishing an airway, and rescue breathing (Link et al., 2015).

The American Heart Association (AHA, 2015) continues to research cardiac arrest treatment and outcomes. In adults (the majority of cardiac arrests) the critical initial elements found to be essential for survival were adequate chest compressions and early defibrillation. Adequate compressions in adults need to occur at a rate of 100 to 120/minute with a depth of at least 2 inches and allowance for time for the chest to recoil. Passive ventilation is no longer recommended in patients undergoing conventional CPR in the community setting, although it may be used in emergency medical service settings (Neumar et al., 2015).

Defibrillation delivers an electrical current to the myocardium that stops all electrical activity and allows the heart's normal pacemaker to resume its normal activity (Wiegand, 2017). It is recommended that defibrillation occur within 5 minutes for an out-of-hospital sudden cardiac arrest and within 3 minutes for a patient in a hospital. An automated external defibrillator (AED) (Box 41.10), available in many public places, such as schools, airports, and workplaces, can be used by health care providers and lay individuals alike to defibrillate people with cardiac arrest (AHA, 2018; Neumar et al., 2015).

If a person is choking and has an obstructed airway, perform abdominal thrusts until the person is able to speak and breathe unassisted or becomes unconscious. Then you perform CPR. You may sweep the mouth and remove the foreign body if you can see it (AHA, 2015).

Restorative and Continuing Care.
Restorative and continuing care emphasizes cardiopulmonary reconditioning as a structured rehabilitation program. Cardiopulmonary rehabilitation helps patients achieve and maintain an optimal level of health through controlled

> **BOX 41.10** **Automated External Defibrillator**
> - The automated external defibrillator (AED) is a device used to administer an electrical shock through the chest wall to the heart to stop the abnormal rhythm and restore a normal heart rhythm.
> - The AED has built-in computers that assess a patient's heart rhythm and determine whether defibrillation is necessary. New technology has made them user friendly, with audio and visual cues telling users what to do when using them. The AED delivers a shock to the patient after announcing, "Everyone stand clear of patient." A shock is delivered only if the patient needs it (NHLBI, n.d.b).
> - Lay rescuer AED programs train lay personnel on the use of the AED (AHA, 2018).
> - The AED is used to strengthen the chain of survival. Patients who received a shock from an AED available in the public had a higher survival rate and rate of discharge from the hospital than those who did not (AHA, 2018).
> - For witnessed ventricular fibrillation, early cardiopulmonary resuscitation with defibrillation within the first 3 to 5 minutes results in greater survival rates (Lewis et al., 2017).

physical exercise, nutritional counseling, relaxation and stress-management techniques, and prescribed medications and oxygen. As physical reconditioning occurs, a patient's complaints of dyspnea, chest pain, fatigue, and activity intolerance decrease. In addition, the patient's anxiety, depression, or somatic concerns often decrease. The patient and the rehabilitation team define the goals of rehabilitation.

Respiratory Muscle Training.
Respiratory muscle training improves muscle strength and endurance, resulting in improved activity tolerance. It typically consists of repetitive breathing exercises performed against some external force or load. Respiratory muscle training prevents respiratory failure in patients with COPD. There are several devices and methods available for this type of training. One method for respiratory muscle training is the incentive spirometer (Ahmadi et al., 2016; Menzes et al., 2018).

Breathing Exercises.
Breathing exercises include techniques to improve ventilation and oxygenation. The three basic techniques are deep-breathing and coughing exercises, pursed-lip breathing, and diaphragmatic breathing. Deep-breathing and coughing exercises, previously discussed, are routine interventions used by postoperative patients (see Chapter 50).

Pursed-Lip Breathing. Pursed-lip breathing involves deep inspiration and prolonged expiration through pursed lips to prevent alveolar collapse. While sitting up, instruct the patient to take a deep breath and exhale slowly through pursed lips as if blowing out a candle. Patients need to gain control of the exhalation phase so that it is longer than inhalation. The patient is usually able to perfect this technique by counting the inhalation time and gradually increasing the count during exhalation (COPD Foundation, 2019). In studies using pursed-lip breathing as a method to improve exercise tolerance in patients with COPD, patients were able to demonstrate increases in their exercise tolerance, breathing pattern, and arterial oxygen saturation (Cabral et al., 2015).

Diaphragmatic Breathing. Diaphragmatic breathing is useful for patients with pulmonary disease and dyspnea secondary to heart failure. This type of breathing increases tidal volume and decreases respiratory rate, which leads to an overall improved breathing pattern and quality of life (Morrow et al., 2016; Seo et al., 2016).

Diaphragmatic breathing is more difficult than other breathing methods because it requires a patient to relax intercostal and accessory respiratory muscles while taking deep inspirations,

TABLE 41.8 Home Oxygen Storage Systems

Primary Use	Advantages	Disadvantages
Compressed Gas Cylinders Stationary and portable systems designed for intermittent therapy such as for exercise or sleep or as a backup system for a concentrator only.	100% oxygen stored in steel or aluminum cylinders; relatively inexpensive, no loss of gas during storage, relatively portable, delivery of up to 15 L/min; does not require electrical source; smaller tanks available for portability.	Bulky and heavy; must be secured safely to prevent them from falling over; frequent refilling necessary with continuous use; patient must know how to read regulator and understand when to call supplier; portable cylinders weigh 15 lb.
Liquid Oxygen Systems Stationary and portable system of choice for high-volume users and active patients.	100% oxygen; more oxygen occupies a smaller space; patient carries convenient ambulatory units refilled at home as shoulder bag, backpack, or wheeled luggage cart; delivery of up to 6 L/min; they come with a battery pack or electrical connections for cars; patient can safely refill ambulatory units from larger reservoir; quiet and easy operation; minimal maintenance; does not require electricity for operation; requires relatively fewer deliveries of oxygen.	Evaporates, especially in warmer temperatures and when not in use; potential for connections to freeze together or form frost at connections if tight connection not maintained during filling; costly setup and delivery fees. The liquid oxygen is very cold and can harm the skin instantly upon contact.
Oxygen Concentrators Stationary system; cost-effective for patients requiring low-flow continuous oxygen and patients with limited mobility inside or outside the home.	Provide a large source of oxygen, inexpensive, fixed monthly costs; most units with delivery of 1 to 5 L/min; good choice for people who do not leave their homes frequently; no cylinders or tanks to refill; delivery up to 10 L/min with specific makes and models. They must be placed in an open, well-ventilated area away from heat and flames. They work by removing nitrogen from room air to make the air 94% to 98% oxygen. They can be small and can weigh from 22 to 70 lb.	Oxygen concentration decreases as liter flow increases; power supply needed; increased electric costs; is not an ambulatory unit; therefore, it requires second system for portability; requires regular maintenance and backup system.
Compressed Gas Small cylinders with compressed gas that allow for portability.	Different models allow from 1 to 5 hours of portable oxygen. Cylinders can be easily wheeled on a cart or a stroller. Smaller tanks can be carried in backpacks, fanny packs, or shoulder bags. Each cylinder is fitted with a regulator used for adjusting the flow rate. At a rate of 2 L/min, they last only a few hours. The most common cylinder used is the E-cylinder; it lasts about 5 hours at a rate of 2 L/min.	They last only a few hours. E-cylinders are not appropriate as a sole source of oxygen for continuous, long-term therapy.

American Thoracic Society (ATS): *Oxygen therapy,* updated 2016, http://www.thoracic.org/patients/patient-resources/resources/oxygen-therapy.pdf, accessed May 2019, and McCoy RW: Options for home oxygen therapy equipment: storage and metering of oxygen in the home, *Resp Care* 58(1):65, 2013.

which takes practice. The patient places one hand flat below the breastbone (upper hand) and the other hand (lower hand) flat on the abdomen. Ask him or her to inhale slowly, making the abdomen push out (as the diaphragm flattens, the abdomen should extend out) and moving the lower hand outward. When the patient exhales, the abdomen goes in (the diaphragm ascends and pushes on lungs to help expel trapped air). The patient practices these exercises initially in the supine position and then while sitting and standing. The exercise is often used with the pursed-lip breathing technique.

Home Oxygen Therapy. Indications for home oxygen therapy include an arterial partial pressure (PaO_2) of 55 mm Hg or less or an arterial oxygen saturation (SaO_2) of 88% or less on room air at rest, on exertion, or with exercise (CMS, 2017). Home oxygen therapy is administered via nasal cannula or face mask. Patients with permanent tracheostomies use either a T tube or tracheostomy collar (AARC, 2007; Wiegand, 2017). Home oxygen therapy has beneficial effects for patients with chronic cardiopulmonary diseases. This therapy improves patients' exercise tolerance and fatigue levels and, in some situations, assists in the management of dyspnea (see Skill 41.4).

There are three types of oxygen-delivery systems: compressed gas cylinders, liquid oxygen, and oxygen concentrators. Before placing a certain delivery system in a home, assess the advantages and disadvantages (Table 41.8) of each type, along with the patient's needs and community resources. In the home the major consideration is the oxygen-delivery source.

Patients and their family caregivers need extensive teaching to be able to manage oxygen therapy efficiently and safely (see Skill 41.4). Teach the patient and family about home oxygen delivery (e.g., oxygen safety, regulation of the amount of oxygen, and how to use the prescribed home oxygen-delivery system) to ensure their ability to maintain the oxygen-delivery system. The home health nurse coordinates the efforts of the patient and family, home respiratory therapist, and home oxygen equipment vendor. The social worker usually assists initially with arranging for the home care nurse and oxygen vendor.

◆ Evaluation

Evaluate nursing interventions and therapies by evaluating whether patient expectations have been met and by comparing the patient's progress with the goals and expected outcomes of the nursing care plan (Fig. 41.17).

Through the Patient's Eyes. It is important to determine a patient's perceptions of his or her care. Does the home care patient feel that

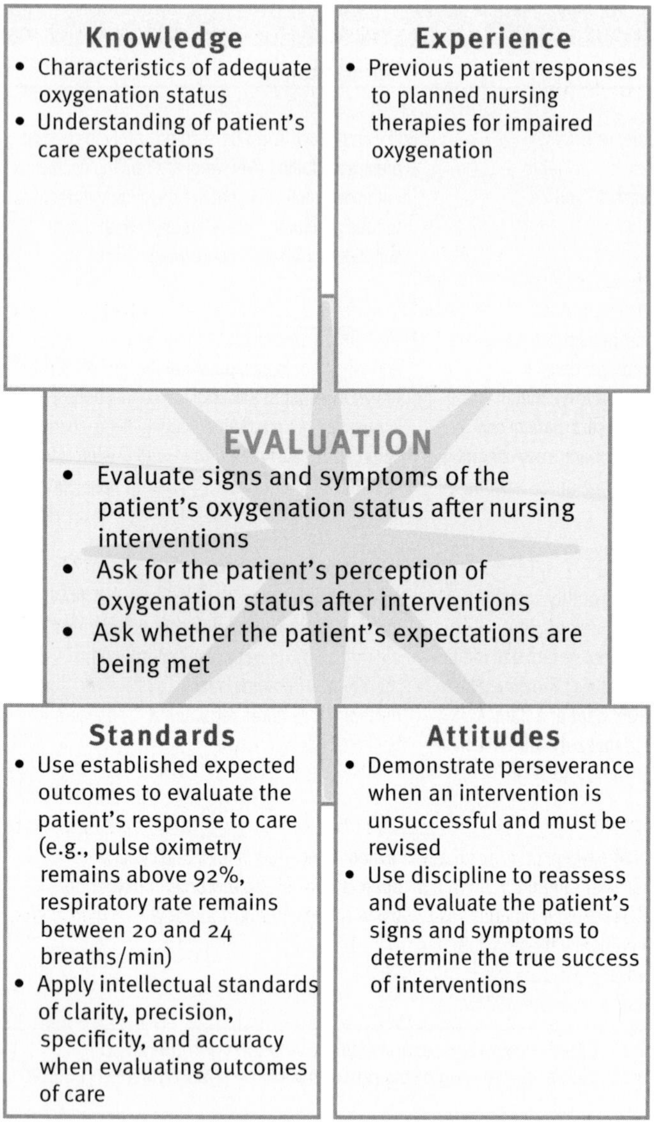

Knowledge
- Characteristics of adequate oxygenation status
- Understanding of patient's care expectations

Experience
- Previous patient responses to planned nursing therapies for impaired oxygenation

EVALUATION
- Evaluate signs and symptoms of the patient's oxygenation status after nursing interventions
- Ask for the patient's perception of oxygenation status after interventions
- Ask whether the patient's expectations are being met

Standards
- Use established expected outcomes to evaluate the patient's response to care (e.g., pulse oximetry remains above 92%, respiratory rate remains between 20 and 24 breaths/min)
- Apply intellectual standards of clarity, precision, specificity, and accuracy when evaluating outcomes of care

Attitudes
- Demonstrate perseverance when an intervention is unsuccessful and must be revised
- Use discipline to reassess and evaluate the patient's signs and symptoms to determine the true success of interventions

FIG. 41.17 Critical thinking model for oxygenation evaluation.

interventions have improved the ability to maintain a more normal lifestyle? Does the acute care patient feel more at ease breathing? Focus on evaluating how a disease is affecting day-to-day activities and the patient's perceived response to treatment. Patients who have chronic heart and lung problems often must be motivated to participate in necessary therapies. Evaluate the patient's motivation and emotional readiness to adhere to treatments provided. Be aware of the need to change a treatment plan to be culturally sensitive to improve adherence. Determine whether the patient and family caregiver feel more in control of their health situation after you have provided instruction. There are a considerable number of surveys that health care team members can utilize to determine the patient's quality of life.

Patient Outcomes. Compare the patient's actual progress with the goals and expected outcomes of the nursing care plan to determine his or her health status. If the nursing measures used are unsuccessful in improving oxygenation, modify the care plan and reevaluate. Continuous evaluation helps to determine whether new or revised therapies are required and whether new nursing diagnoses have developed and require a new plan of care. Do not hesitate to notify the health care provider about a patient's deteriorating oxygenation status. Prompt notification helps avoid an emergency situation or even the need for CPR. Examples of evaluative measures include:

- Ask the patient about his or her degree of breathlessness. Observe respiratory rate before, during, and after any activity or procedure.
- Ask the patient about fatigue during ambulation. Monitor pulse oximetry and pulse rate before, during, and after any activity or procedure.
- Ask the patient to rate breathlessness on a scale of 0 to 10, with 0 being no shortness of breath and 10 being severe shortness of breath.
- Ask the patient which interventions help reduce dyspnea.
- Ask the patient about frequency of cough and sputum production, and assess any sputum produced.
- Auscultate lung sounds for improvement in adventitious sounds.
- When needed, monitor arterial blood gas levels, pulmonary function tests, chest x-ray films, ECG tracings, and physical assessment data to provide objective measurement of the success of therapies and treatments.

SAFETY GUIDELINES FOR NURSING SKILLS

Ensuring patient safety is an essential role of the professional nurse. To ensure patient safety, communicate clearly with members of the health care team, assess and incorporate the patient's priorities of care and preferences, and use the best evidence when making decisions about your patient's care. When performing the skills in this chapter, remember the following points to ensure safe, individualized patient care.

- Know a patient's baseline range of vital signs. Patients with sudden changes in their vital signs, level of consciousness, or behavior are possibly experiencing profound hypoxemia. Patients who demonstrate subtle changes over time have worsening of a chronic or existing condition or a new medical condition. (Hartjes, 2018).
- Limit the introduction of the catheter to 2 times with each suctioning procedure (Wiegand, 2017).
- Perform tracheal suctioning before pharyngeal suctioning whenever possible. The mouth and pharynx contain more bacteria than the trachea. If there is an abundance of oral secretions present before beginning the procedure, suction mouth with separate oral suction device.

- Use caution when suctioning patients with a head injury. Suctioning elevates the intracranial pressure (ICP). Reduce this risk by hyperventilating on a ventilator prior to suctioning. This results in hypocarbia that in turn induces vasoconstriction. Vasoconstriction reduces the potential increase in ICP.
- The routine use of normal saline instillation (NSI) into the airway before endotracheal and tracheostomy suctioning is not recommended. Use of NSI is associated with the adverse effects of excessive coughing, bronchospasm, spread of organisms to the lower respiratory tract, and decreased oxygen saturation (AARC, 2010b, Wang et al., 2017). In certain circumstances, if it is necessary to stimulate a cough, normal saline may be indicated. This requires collaboration with the health care team.
- Review institutional policy before stripping or milking chest tubes. Most institutions have stopped using this practice because stripping the tube greatly increases intrapleural pressure, which can damage the pleural tissue and cause pneumothorax or worsen an existing pneumothorax.
- The most serious tracheostomy complication is airway obstruction, which can result in cardiac arrest. Most tracheostomy tubes are designed with a small

plastic inner tube/cannula that sits inside the larger one. If the airway becomes occluded, the smaller one can be removed and replaced with a temporary spare. It is important to always have a spare at the bedside for emergency replacement.

- Patients with COPD who are breathing spontaneously should cautiously receive high levels of oxygen therapy because it results in a decreased stimulus to breathe (Grindrod, 2015).

SKILL 41.1   SUITIONING

Delegation and Collaboration

The skill of artificial airway suctioning of newly inserted artificial airways cannot be delegated to assistive personnel (AP). However, when a patient has been assessed by the nurse as stable, oropharyngeal and well-established tracheostomy tube suctioning can be delegated. The nurse directs the AP about:

- Any modifications of the skill such as the need for supplemental oxygen.
- Appropriate suction limits for suctioning nasotracheally and for suctioning ETTs and TTs and risks of applying excessive or inadequate suction pressure.
- Reporting any changes in patient's respiratory status, level of consciousness, restlessness, secretion color and amount, and unresolved coughing or gagging.
- Reporting any changes in patient's color, vital signs, or complaints of pain.

The nurse may need to collaborate with the respiratory therapist as respiratory therapists are also allowed to perform this procedure at certain health care agencies.

Equipment
Oropharyngeal Suctioning
- Clean, nonsterile suction catheter or Yankauer suction tip catheter
- Clean gloves
- Clean towel or paper drape
- Mask, goggles, or face shield if indicated; gown if isolation procedures dictate
- Disposable cup or basin
- Tap water or normal saline (about 100 mL)
- Suction machine or wall suction device with regulator
- Connecting tubing (6 feet)
- Stethoscope
- Pulse oximeter
- Oral airway (if indicated)
- Washcloth
- Manual self-inflating resuscitation bag (bag-valve-mask) with oxygen connecting tubing

Nasotracheal Suctioning
- Sterile suction catheter (12 to 16 Fr) (smallest diameter that effectively removes secretions)
- Two sterile gloves or one sterile and one clean glove
- Sterile basin (e.g., sterile disposable cup)

- Sterile water or normal saline (about 100 mL)
- Clean towel or paper drape
- Mask, goggles, or face shield if indicated; gown if isolation procedures dictate
- Stethoscope
- Pulse oximeter
- Suction machine or wall suction device with regulator
- Connecting tubing (6 feet)
- Manual self-inflating resuscitation bag (bag-valve-mask) with oxygen connecting tubing

Endotracheal or Tracheostomy Suctioning
- Appropriate-size suction catheter, usually 12 to 16 Fr (smallest diameter that will remove secretions effectively, preferably one that is no more than half of the internal diameter of the artificial airway to minimize decrease in PaO_2) (AARC, 2010a; Branson et al., 2014)
- Suction machine or wall suction device with regulator
- Two sterile gloves or one sterile and one clean glove
- Sterile basin
- Sterile normal saline (about 100 mL)
- Clean towel or sterile drape
- Mask, goggles, or face shield, if indicated; gown if isolation procedures dictate
- Small Y-adapter (if catheter does not have a suction control port)
- Pulse oximeter, stethoscope and end-tidal CO_2 detector
- Manual self-inflating resuscitation bag (bag-valve-mask) with oxygen connecting tubing
- PEEP valve for resuscitation bag

Closed-System on In-Line Suctioning
- Closed-system or in-line suction catheter
- 5- to 10-mL normal saline in syringe or vials
- Two clean gloves
- Suction machine or wall suction device with regulator
- Connecting tubing (6 feet)
- Oral suction kit/supplies for oropharyngeal suctioning
- Mask, goggles, or face shield if indicated; gown if isolation procedures dictate
- Pulse oximeter and stethoscope
- Manual self-inflating resuscitation bag (bag-valve-mask) with oxygen connecting tubing, while not necessary for the procedure, is safe to have on hand.

STEP	RATIONALE
ASSESSMENT	
1. Identify patient using at least two identifiers (e.g., name and birthday or name and account number) according to agency policy. Compare identifiers with information on patient's MAR or medical record.	Ensures correct patient. Complies with The Joint Commission standards and improves patient safety (TJC, 2020).
2. Review medical record to identify contraindications to nasotracheal suctioning: occluded nasal passages; nasal bleeding; epiglottitis or croup; acute head, facial, or neck injury or surgery; coagulopathy or bleeding disorder; irritable airway; laryngospasm or bronchospasm; gastric surgery with high anastomosis; myocardial infarction (AARC, 2004; Hockenberry et al., 2019; Wiegand, 2017).	These conditions are contraindicated because passage of suction catheter through nasal route causes trauma to existing facial trauma/surgery, increases nasal bleeding, or causes severe bleeding in presence of coagulopathy or bleeding disorders. In presence of epiglottitis or croup, laryngospasm, or irritable airway, passage of suction catheter through nose causes intractable coughing, hypoxemia, and severe bronchospasm, necessitating emergency intubation or tracheostomy. Hypoxemia could worsen cardiac damage in myocardial infarction (AARC, 2004; Hockenberry et al., 2019; Wiegand, 2017).

Continued

SKILL 41.1   **SUCTIONING—cont'd**

STEP	RATIONALE
3. Review sputum microbiology data in laboratory report.	Certain bacteria are easier to transmit or require isolation because of virulence or antibiotic resistance.
4. Perform hand hygiene and apply gloves. Assess for signs and symptoms of upper and lower airway obstruction requiring suctioning: abnormal respiratory rate, adventitious lung sounds, nasal secretions, gurgling, drooling, restlessness, gastric secretions or vomitus in mouth, and coughing without clearing airway secretions and/or improving adventitious lung sounds.	Physical signs and symptoms result from secretions in upper and lower airways and decreased oxygen to the tissues. Presuction assessment provides baseline data to identify need for suctioning and measures the effectiveness of suction procedures (Wiegand, 2017; Branson et al., 2014).
5. Assess vital signs and signs and symptoms associated with hypoxia and hypercapnia: decreased pulse oximetry (SpO$_2$), increased pulse and blood pressure, apprehension, anxiety, lack of concentration, lethargy, decreased level of consciousness, confusion, dizziness, behavioral changes (e.g., irritability), irregular heart pulse, pallor, and cyanosis (a very late sign of hypoxia). Keep pulse oximeter on patient.	Physical signs and symptoms resulting from decreased tissue oxygenation. Provides presuction baseline to measure patient tolerance to suctioning and effectiveness of suctioning on SpO$_2$ levels.
6. Assess for risk factors for upper and lower airway obstruction, including chronic obstructive pulmonary disease, impaired mobility, decreased level of consciousness, nasal feeding tube, decreased cough or gag reflex, and decreased swallowing ability.	Risk factors can impair patient's ability to clear secretions from airway, increase risk for retaining secretions, and necessitate nasopharyngeal or nasotracheal suctioning (Urden et al., 2020).
7. Identify patients with an increased risk for ineffective airway clearance (e.g., patients with decreased level of consciousness, neuromuscular or neurological impairment, or anatomical factors that influence upper or lower airway function, such as recent surgery; head, chest, or neck trauma; tumors).	Changes in neurological status and neuromuscular impairment increase likelihood that patient is unable to clear respiratory secretions. Abnormal anatomy or head and neck surgery/trauma and tumors in and around lower airway impair normal secretion clearance. Accumulating pulmonary secretions impede patient's ability to effectively clear airway through cough mechanism (Urden et al., 2020).
8. Assess for excessive amounts of secretions or secretions visible in the oral cavity or artificial airway, signs of respiratory distress (increased work of breathing, increased respiratory rate), presence of rhonchi on auscultation, excessive coughing, increased peak inspiratory pressures (if on mechanical ventilator), sawtooth pattern on ventilator monitor, or changes in capnography waveform (if patient on mechanical ventilator) or decrease in patient pulse oximeter (Branson et al., 2014; Sole et al., 2015).	Suctioning should be performed only as patient condition indicates and not in a scheduled fashion such as hourly (Lewis et al., 2017; Myatt, 2015).
9. Assess patency of ETT (if present) with capnography/end-tidal carbon dioxide (CO$_2$) detector.	ETT may become displaced or blocked by secretions. Capnography allows for the detection of secretions by visualizing the sawtooth pattern on the capnography monitor (Sole et al., 2015; Wiegand, 2017).
10. Assess factors that may affect volume and consistency of secretions.	Thickened or copious secretions increase risk for airway obstruction.
a. Fluid balance	Fluid overload increases amount of secretions. Dehydration can cause thicker secretions.
b. Lack of humidity	Environment influences secretion formation and gas exchange. Lack of humidity, particularly in patients with artificial airways, can lead to atelectasis or airway obstruction (Hanlon, 2016).
c. Infection (e.g., pneumonia)	Patients with respiratory infections are prone to increased secretions that are thicker and sometimes more difficult to expectorate.
11. For endotracheal suctioning, assess patient's peak inspiratory pressure when on volume-controlled ventilation or tidal volume during pressure-controlled ventilation. Remove gloves and perform hand hygiene.	Increased peak inspiratory pressure or decreased tidal volume may indicate airway obstruction (Urden et al., 2020). Prevents transmission of microorganisms.

CLINICAL DECISION: *The patient's vital signs, pulse oximetry, end-tidal CO$_2$, and respiratory status will be assessed before and continuously throughout the procedure (Wiegand, 2017).*

STEP	RATIONALE
12. Determine presence of apprehension, anxiety, decreased ability to concentrate, lethargy, decreased level of consciousness (especially acute), increased fatigue, dizziness, behavioral changes (especially irritability), pallor, cyanosis, dyspnea, or use of accessory muscles.	These are signs and symptoms of hypoxia and/or hypercapnia, which can indicate need for suction. These signs can also help to identify patient's ability to cooperate with procedure.
13. Assess patient's or family caregiver's knowledge, experience, and health literacy.	Ensures patient or family caregiver has the capacity to obtain, communicate, process, and understand basic health information (CDC, 2019c).
14. Assess for patient's understanding of procedure and presence of any apprehension.	Reveals need for instruction or psychosocial support.

STEP	RATIONALE

PLANNING

1. Provide privacy and assist patient to comfortable position, typically semi-Fowler's or high Fowler's.

Reduces stimulation of gag reflex, promotes patient comfort and secretion drainage, and prevents aspiration.

2. If not already present, place pulse oximeter on patient's finger. Take reading and leave oximeter in place.

Provides continuous SpO_2 value to determine patient's response to suctioning.

3. Prepare and organize equipment. Place towel across patient's chest.

Ensures that you have the necessary equipment in place to complete procedure.

4. Explain to patient how procedure will help clear airway and relieve some breathing difficulty. Explain that temporary coughing, sneezing, gagging, or shortness of breath is normal during procedure.

Encourages cooperation and minimizes anxiety and pain of procedure.

IMPLEMENTATION

1. Perform hand hygiene and apply appropriate personal protective equipment (mask with face shield or goggles; gown if necessary).

Reduces transmission of microorganisms.

2. Adjust bed to appropriate height (if not already done) and lower side rail on side nearest you. Check locks on bed wheel.

Minimizes caregiver's muscle strain and prevents injury. Prevents bed from moving.

3. Connect one end of connecting tubing to wall suction device and place other end in convenient location near patient. Turn suction device on and set suction pressure to as low a level as possible and yet able to effectively clear secretions. This value is typically between 80 and 120 mm Hg in adults (between 60 and 100 mm Hg in neonates) (AARC, 2010a). Suction pressure should not exceed 180 mm Hg (Branson et al., 2014). Occlude end of suction tubing to check pressure.

Ensures equipment function. Excessive negative pressure damages tracheal mucosa and induces greater hypoxia (Wiegand, 2017).

4. Prepare suction catheter for all types of open suctioning.

  a. Onetime use catheter (open suction technique).

    (1) Using aseptic technique, open suction kit or catheter package. If sterile drape is available, place it across patient's chest or on bedside table. Do not allow suction catheter to touch any nonsterile surfaces. **Note**: When performing oropharyngeal suction only, there is no need to place a sterile drape; it is a clean procedure, not sterile.

Prepares catheter, maintains asepsis, and reduces transmission of microorganisms. Provides sterile surface on which to lay catheter between passes.

    (2) Unwrap or open sterile basin and place on bedside table. Be careful not to touch inside of basin. Fill with about 100 mL sterile normal saline solution or water (see illustration).

Saline or water is used to clean tubing after each suction pass.

    (3) If performing nasotracheal suctioning, open packet of water-soluble lubricant and apply small amount (about 1 inch) along catheter tip. **Note**: *Lubricant is not necessary for artificial airway suctioning.*

Water-soluble lubricant helps avoid lipid aspiration pneumonia. Excessive amount of lubricant occludes catheter.

5. Apply gloves: Note that oropharyngeal suctioning is a clean technique and clean gloves are appropriate. For nasotracheal, endotracheal tube, or tracheal tube suctioning, sterile gloves are required. When this is the case, apply sterile gloves to each hand or nonsterile glove to nondominant hand and sterile glove to dominant hand.

Reduces transmission of microorganisms and maintains sterility of suction catheter.

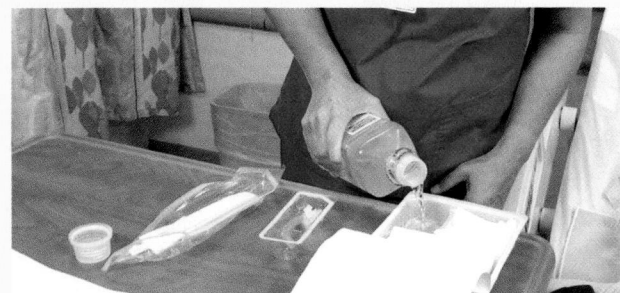

STEP 4a(2) Pouring sterile saline into tray. (Copyright © Mosby's Clinical Skills: Essentials Collection.)

Continued

STEP	RATIONALE
6. Pick up suction catheter with dominant hand without touching nonsterile surfaces. Pick up connecting tubing with nondominant hand. Secure catheter to tubing (see illustration).	Maintains catheter sterility. Connects catheter to suction.

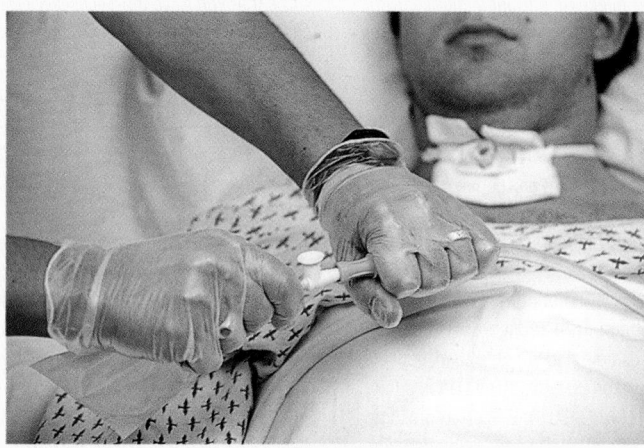

STEP 6 Attaching suction catheter to suction tubing.

STEP	RATIONALE
7. Place tip of catheter into sterile basin and suction small amount of normal saline solution from basin by occluding suction vent.	Ensures equipment function. Lubricates internal catheter and tubing.
8. Suction airway.	
a. Nasopharyngeal and nasotracheal suctioning:	
(1) Have patient take deep breaths, if able, or increase oxygen flow rate with delivery device through cannula or mask (if ordered).	May help to decrease risks of hypoxemia.
(2) Lightly coat distal 6 to 8 cm (2–3 inches) of catheter with water-soluble lubricant.	Lubricates catheter for easier insertion.
(3) Remove oxygen-delivery device, if applicable, with nondominant hand.	Allows access to nares and catheter.

CLINICAL DECISION: *Be sure to insert catheter during patient inhalation, especially if inserting it into trachea, because epiglottis is open. Do not insert during swallowing or catheter will most likely enter esophagus.* **Never apply suction during insertion.** *Patient should cough. If patient gags or becomes nauseated, catheter is most likely in esophagus, and you need to remove it.*

STEP	RATIONALE
(4) Apply suction.	
(a) *Nasopharyngeal* (without applying suction): As patient takes deep breath, insert catheter following natural course of naris; slightly slant catheter downward and advance to back of pharynx. Do not force through nares. In adults insert catheter approximately 16 cm (6.5 inches); in older children, 8–12 cm (3–5 inches); in infants and young children, 4–7.5 cm (1.5–3 inches). Rule of thumb is to insert catheter distance from tip of nose (or mouth) to angle of mandible.	Ensure that catheter tip reaches pharynx for suctioning.

CLINICAL DECISION: *If resistance is met during insertion, you may need to try the other naris. Do not force the catheter up the nares because this will cause mucosal damage.*

STEP	RATIONALE
i. Apply intermittent suction for no more than 10 seconds by placing and releasing nondominant thumb over catheter vent (Wiegand, 2017). Slowly withdraw catheter while rotating it back and forth between thumb and forefinger.	Intermittent suction up to 10 seconds safely removes pharyngeal secretions. Suction time greater than 10 seconds increases risk for suction-induced hypoxemia (AARC, 2010a; Branson et al., 2014; Wiegand, 2017).

STEP	RATIONALE

(b) *Nasotracheal* (without applying suction): As patient takes deep breath, advance catheter following natural course of naris. Advance catheter slightly slanted and downward to just above entrance into larynx and then trachea. While patient takes deep breath, quickly insert catheter: for adults insert approximately 16–20 cm (6–8 inches) into trachea (see illustration). Patient will begin to cough; then pull back catheter 1–2 cm (½ inch) before applying suction. **NOTE**: In older children, 16–20 cm (6–8 inches); in infants and young children, 8–14 cm (3–5½ inches).

Ensure that catheter tip reaches trachea for suctioning.

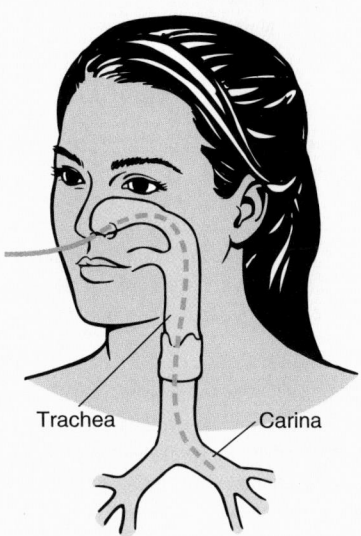

Trachea Carina

STEP 8a(4)(b) Distance of insertion of nasotracheal catheter.

CLINICAL DECISION: *When using the nasal approach, perform tracheal suctioning before pharyngeal suctioning whenever possible. The mouth and pharynx contain more bacteria than the trachea.*

CLINICAL DECISION: *When there is difficulty passing the catheter, ask patient to cough or say "ahh" or try to advance the catheter during inspiration. Both measures help to open the glottis to permit passage of the catheter into the trachea.*

(c) *Positioning option:* In some instances, turning patient's head helps you suction more effectively. If you feel resistance after insertion of catheter, use caution; it has probably hit the carina. Pull catheter back 1–2 cm (0.4–0.8 inches) before applying suction (AARC, 2004; Wiegand, 2017).

Turning patient's head to side elevates bronchial passage on opposite side. Turning head to right helps with suctioning of left mainstem bronchus; turning head to left helps you suction right mainstem bronchus. Suctioning too deep may cause tracheal mucosa trauma.

   i. Apply intermittent suction for no more than 10 seconds by placing and releasing nondominant thumb over catheter vent (Wiegand, 2017). Slowly withdraw catheter while rotating it back and forth between thumb and forefinger.

Suction time greater than 15 seconds increases risk for suction-induced hypoxemia (AARC, 2010a; Branson et al., 2014; Wiegand, 2017). Intermittent suction and rotation of catheter prevents injury to tracheal mucosa. If catheter "grabs" mucosa, remove thumb to release suction.

CLINICAL DECISION: *Monitor patient's vital signs and oxygen saturation throughout suctioning process. Stop suctioning if there is a 20 beats/min change (increase or decrease) in pulse rate or if SpO$_2$ falls below 90% or 5% from baseline.*

(5) Reapply oxygen-delivery device and encourage patient to take some deep breaths, if able.

Helps to decrease risk of hypoxia. Increases patient comfort.

(6) Rinse catheter and connecting tubing with normal saline or water until cleared.

Secretions that remain in suction catheter or connecting tubing decrease suctioning efficiency.

(7) Assess for need to repeat suctioning. Do not perform more than two passes with catheter. Allow patient to rest at least 1 minute (AARC, 2010a; Wiegand, 2017). Ask patient to deep breathe and cough.

Observe for alterations in cardiopulmonary status. Suctioning induces hypoxemia, irregular pulse, laryngospasm, and bronchospasm (AARC, 2010a; Wiegand, 2017). Hyperoxygenation is recommended before, during, and after open suctioning to reduce suction-induced hypoxemia (Galbiati and Paola, 2015).

Continued

SKILL 41.1   **SUCTIONING—cont'd**

STEP	RATIONALE

b. Artificial airway:

(1) When patient has an artificial airway, hyperoxygenate him or her with 100% oxygen for at least 30 to 60 seconds before suctioning by (1) pressing suction hyperoxygenation button on ventilator **OR** (2) increasing baseline fraction of inspired oxygen (FiO_2) level on mechanical ventilator **OR** (3) disconnecting ventilator, attaching self-inflating resuscitation bag-valve device to tube with nondominant hand (or have assistant do this), and administering 5–6 breaths over 30 seconds (or have assistant do this) (Wiegand, 2017). **NOTE:** Some mechanical ventilators have a button that, when pushed, delivers 100% oxygen for a few minutes and then resets to previous setting.

Preoxygenation decreases risk of decreased arterial oxygen levels while ventilation or oxygenation is interrupted and volume is lost during suctioning. Some models of resuscitation bags do not deliver 100% oxygen; therefore, this is not the best way to oxygenate patient (Wiegand, 2017).

(2) If patient is receiving mechanical ventilation, open swivel adapter or, if necessary, remove oxygen- or humidity-delivery device with nondominant hand.

Exposes artificial airway.

CLINICAL DECISION: *Suctioning can cause elevations in intracranial pressure (ICP) in patients with head injuries. Reduce this risk by presuction hyperoxygenation, which results in hypocarbia, which in turn induces vasoconstriction. Vasoconstriction reduces the potential for an increase in ICP (Urden et al., 2020).*

---

(3) Advise patient that you are about to begin suctioning. Without applying suction, gently but quickly insert catheter into artificial airway using dominant thumb and forefinger (it is best to try to time catheter insertion into artificial airway with inspiration) (see illustration). Advance catheter until you meet resistance or patient coughs; then pull back 1 cm (0.4 inch) (Wiegand, 2017).

Application of suction pressure while introducing catheter into trachea increases risk for damage to tracheal mucosa and increased hypoxia. Pulling back stimulates cough and removes catheter from mucosal wall so that catheter is not resting against tracheal mucosa during suctioning. Shallow suctioning is recommended to prevent tracheal mucosa trauma (AARC, 2010a; Wiegand, 2017).

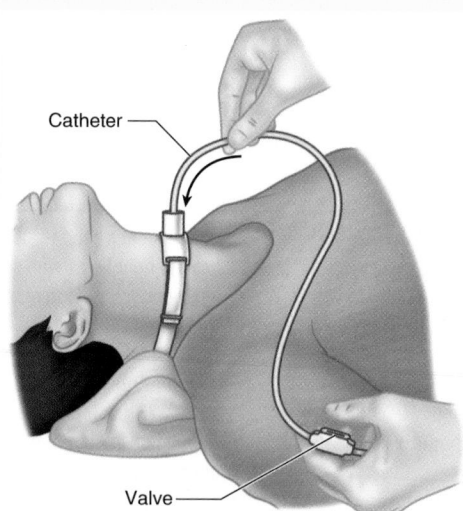

Catheter

Valve

STEP 8b(3) Suctioning tracheostomy.

CLINICAL DECISION: *If unable to insert catheter past the end of the ETT, the catheter is probably caught in the Murphy eye (i.e., side hole at the distal end of the ETT that allows for collateral airflow in the event of tracheal mainstem intubation). If this happens, rotate the catheter to reposition it away from the Murphy eye or withdraw it slightly and reinsert with the next inhalation. Usually the catheter meets resistance at the carina. One indication that the catheter is at the carina is acute onset of coughing because the carina contains many cough receptors. Pull the catheter back 1 cm (½ inch).*

STEP	RATIONALE
(4) Apply intermittent suction for 10 seconds (AARC, 2010a; Wiegand, 2017). Place and release nondominant thumb over vent of catheter; slowly withdraw catheter while rotating it back and forth between dominant thumb and forefinger. Do not use suction for greater than 15 seconds. Encourage patient to cough. Watch for respiratory distress.	Suction time greater than 10 seconds increases risk for suction-induced hypoxemia (AARC, 2010a; Branson et al., 2014; Wiegand, 2017). Intermittent suction and rotation of catheter prevent injury to tracheal mucosa. If catheter "grabs" mucosa, remove thumb to release suction.

CLINICAL DECISION: *If patient develops respiratory distress during the suction procedure, immediately withdraw catheter and supply additional oxygen and breaths as needed. In an emergency administer oxygen directly through the catheter. Disconnect suction and attach oxygen at prescribed flow rate through the catheter. If the patient does not tolerate the suctioning procedure, you may need to consider switching to closed (in-line) suctioning or allowing longer recovery times. Notify health care provider if patient develops significant cardiopulmonary compromise during suctioning (Urden et al., 2020; Wiegand, 2017).*

STEP	RATIONALE
(5) If patient is receiving mechanical ventilation, close swivel adapter or replace oxygen-delivery device. Hyperoxygenate patient for 30–60 seconds.	Reestablishes artificial airway. Helps to decrease risks of hypoxia.
(6) Rinse catheter and connecting tubing with normal saline until clear. Use continuous suction.	Removes catheter secretions. Secretions left in tubing decrease suctioning efficiency and provide environment for microorganism growth.
(7) Assess patient's vital signs, cardiopulmonary status, and ventilator measures for secretion clearance. Repeat Steps (1) through (6) once or twice more to clear secretions. Unless the patient is in respiratory distress, allow adequate time (at least 1 full minute) between suction passes (Wiegand, 2017).	Suctioning can induce dysrhythmias, hypoxia, and bronchospasm and impair cerebral circulation or adversely affect hemodynamic stability (Wiegand, 2017).

CLINICAL DECISION: *The number of suction passes should be based on patient assessment and presence of secretions. If secretions persist after two passes, reapply oxygen source and allow patient more time to rest and recover from these procedures (Wiegand, 2017).*

STEP	RATIONALE
(8) When pharynx and trachea are sufficiently cleared of secretions, perform oropharyngeal suctioning (see Step 8d) to clear mouth of secretions. Do not suction nose again after suctioning mouth.	Removes upper airway secretions. More microorganisms generally are present in mouth. Upper airway is considered "clean," and lower airway is considered "sterile." You can use same catheter to suction from sterile to clean areas (e.g., tracheal suctioning to oropharyngeal suctioning) but not from clean to sterile areas.
c. Artificial airway using in-line or closed suctioning	
(1) Open suction catheter package using aseptic technique and attach closed suction catheter unit to ventilator circuit. In many agencies, a respiratory therapist attaches the catheter to the mechanical ventilator circuit.	Attaches the suction catheter to the ETT or tracheostomy tube in order to perform in-line or closed suctioning.
(2) Connect one end of connecting tubing to suction machine; connect other end to the end of the closed-system or in-line suction catheter. Turn suction device on, set vacuum regulator to appropriate negative pressure, and check pressure.	Prepares the system for suction.
(3) When patient has an artificial airway, hyperoxygenate with 100% oxygen for at least 30 seconds before suctioning by (1) pressing suction hyperoxygenation button on ventilator **OR** (2) increasing baseline fraction of inspired oxygen (FiO$_2$) level on mechanical ventilator. **NOTE:** Some mechanical ventilators have a button that, when pushed, delivers 100% oxygen for a few minutes and then resets to previous setting.	Preoxygenation decreases risk of decreased arterial oxygen levels while ventilation or oxygenation is interrupted and volume is lost during suctioning (AARC, 2010a; Wiegand, 2020).

CLINICAL DECISION: *Suctioning can cause elevations in intracranial pressure (ICP) in patients with head injuries. Reduce this risk by presuction hyperoxygenation, which results in hypocarbia, which in turn induces vasoconstriction. Vasoconstriction reduces the potential for an increase in ICP (Urden et al., 2020).*

STEP	RATIONALE
(4) Unlock suction control mechanism, if required by manufacturer. Open saline port and attach saline syringe or vial.	Allows for suctioning and prepares the saline that is used to rinse the catheter between suction attempts.
(5) Pick up suction catheter enclosed in plastic sleeve with dominant hand.	
(6) Advise patient that you are about to begin suctioning. Without applying suction, gently but quickly insert catheter into artificial airway using dominant thumb and forefinger (it is best to try to time catheter insertion into artificial airway with inspiration). Advance catheter until you meet resistance or patient coughs; then pull back 1 cm (0.4 inch) (Wiegand, 2017).	Application of suction pressure while introducing catheter into trachea increases risk for damage to tracheal mucosa and increased hypoxia. Pulling back stimulates cough and removes catheter from mucosal wall so that catheter is not resting against tracheal mucosa during suctioning. Shallow suctioning is recommended to prevent tracheal mucosa trauma (AARC, 2010a; Wiegand, 2017).

Continued

STEP	RATIONALE
(7) Encourage patient to cough, and apply suction by squeezing on suction control mechanism while withdrawing catheter. Be sure to withdraw catheter completely into plastic sheath and past the tip of the airway so that it does not obstruct airflow.	

CLINICAL DECISION: *It is difficult to apply intermittent pulses of suction and nearly impossible to rotate the catheter compared to the standard catheter. Apply continuous suction for 10 seconds but no longer as you remove the suction catheter (AARC, 2010a; Branson et al., 2014; Wiegand, 2017).*

STEP	RATIONALE
(8) Assess patient's vital signs, cardiopulmonary status, and ventilator measures for secretion clearance. Repeat Steps (1) through (7) once or twice more to clear secretions. Allow adequate time (at least 1 full minute) between suction passes.	Suctioning can induce dysrhythmias, hypoxia, and bronchospasm and impair cerebral circulation or adversely affect hemodynamic stability (Wiegand, 2017).
(9) When airway is clear, withdraw catheter completely into sheath. Be sure that colored indicator line on catheter is visible in the sheath. Squeeze saline vial or push syringe while applying suction to rinse inner lumen of catheter. Use at least 5 to 10 mL of saline to rinse the catheter until it is clear of retained secretions.	Cleans the suction catheter, thereby reducing risk of bacterial growth and infection.
(10) Lock the suction mechanism, if applicable. Perform oropharyngeal suctioning if patient requires.	Prevents migration of the suction catheter into the airway, which could lead to obstruction.
d. Oropharyngeal suctioning	In patients who require sterile suctioning of the airways, oropharyngeal suction is performed ***after*** the sterile suctioning to prevent contamination of the suction catheters or tubing with bacteria present in the oral cavity (Wiegand, 2017). If the patient does not require sterile suctioning, use oropharyngeal suctioning to remove oral secretions.
(1) Apply clean gloves.	Reduces transmission of microorganisms.
(2) Connect the Yankauer suction catheter to the connecting tubing.	Prepares the suction apparatus.
(3) Remove patient's oxygen mask, if present, but keep it close. Nasal cannula may remain in place.	Allows access to mouth. Reduces chance of hypoxia.

CLINICAL DECISION: *If patient has been suctioned prior to oropharyngeal suctioning, they may require some recovery from the suctioning procedure before oropharyngeal suctioning is performed. Allow for that recovery to happen by reapplying the oxygen mask until just before oropharyngeal suctioning.*

STEP	RATIONALE
(4) Insert catheter into mouth along gum line to pharynx. Move catheter around mouth until secretions have cleared. Encourage patient to cough. Replace oxygen mask.	Movement of catheter prevents suction tip from invaginating oral mucosal surfaces and causing trauma. Coughing moves secretions from lower airway into mouth and upper airway.

CLINICAL DECISION: *If ETT is present, be careful when moving the catheter so as not to dislodge the ETT. Be careful when suctioning a patient who had recent oral or head/neck surgery. Aggressive suctioning and excessive coughing should not be used or encouraged in patients who have undergone throat surgery, such as a tonsillectomy. Aggressive suctioning in these patient populations can aggravate the operative site, increasing the risk of bleeding or infection (Urden, 2020).*

STEP	RATIONALE
(5) Rinse catheter with water or normal saline in cup or basin until connecting tubing is cleared of secretions. Turn off suction. Place catheter in clean, dry area.	Rinses catheter and reduces probability of transmission of microorganisms. Clean suction tubing enhances delivery of set suction pressure. Catheter may be reused.
9. When suctioning is complete, disconnect catheter from connecting tubing. Roll catheter around fingers of dominant hand. Pull off other glove over first glove in same way. Discard in appropriate receptacle.	Seals contaminants in gloves. Reduces transmission of microorganisms.
10. Remove towel, place in laundry or appropriate receptacle, and reposition patient.	Reduces transmission of microorganisms.
11. If oxygen level was changed during procedure, readjust oxygen to original ordered level because patient's blood oxygen level should have returned to baseline.	Prevents absorption atelectasis (i.e., tendency for airways to collapse if proximally obstructed by secretions). Prevents oxygen toxicity while allowing patient time to reoxygenate blood.
12. Apply clean gloves to continue personal care, such as washing the patient's face or performing oral hygiene.	Promotes comfort.
13. Discard remainder of normal saline into appropriate receptacle. If basin is disposable, discard into appropriate receptacle. If basin is reusable, rinse it out and place it in soiled utility room.	Reduces transmission of microorganisms.

STEP	RATIONALE
14. Remove personal protective equipment and discard into appropriate receptacle. Perform hand hygiene.	Reduces transmission of microorganisms.
15. Place unopened suction kit on suction machine table or at head of bed.	Provides immediate access to suction catheter for next procedure.
16. Help patient to comfortable position and provide oral hygiene as needed.	
17. Raise side rails (as appropriate), lower bed to lowest position. Place nurse call system in an accessible location within patient's reach.	Ensures patient safety and patient's ability to call for assistance.

EVALUATION

1. Compare patient's vital signs, cardiopulmonary assessments, E_tCO_2 and SpO_2 values before and after suctioning. If on ventilator, compare FiO_2 and tidal volumes and peak inspiratory pressures.	Identifies physiological effects of suction procedure to restore airway patency.
2. Ask patient whether breathing is easier and congestion is decreased.	Provides subjective confirmation that suctioning procedure has relieved airway.
3. Auscultate lungs and compare patient's respiratory assessment before and after suctioning.	Provides objective information about any change in lung sounds.
4. Observe character of airway secretions.	Provides data to document presence or absence of respiratory tract infection or thickened secretions.
5. **Use Teach-Back:** "I need to suction your father, and I want to be sure that I explained the suctioning procedure and when I need to do it. Please tell me in your own words why suctioning is beneficial." Revise your instruction now or develop a plan for revised patient/family caregiver teaching if patient/family caregiver is not able to teach back correctly.	Determines patient's/family caregiver's level of understanding of instructional topic.

UNEXPECTED OUTCOMES AND RELATED INTERVENTIONS

1. Patient has decrease in overall cardiopulmonary status as evidenced by decreased SpO_2, increased E_tCO_2, continued tachypnea, continued increased work of breathing, and cardiac dysrhythmias.
   - Limit length of suctioning.
   - Determine need for more frequent suctioning, possibly of shorter duration.
   - Determine need for supplemental or increase in supplemental oxygen. Supply oxygen between suctioning passes.
   - Notify health care provider.
2. Bloody secretions are returned after suctioning.
   - Determine amount of suction pressure used. May need to be decreased.
   - Ensure that suction is completed correctly using intermittent suction and catheter rotation. Do not apply suction until after catheter has been pulled back 1 cm (0.4 inches) to prevent applying suction while catheter is touching carina.
   - Evaluate suctioning frequency.
   - Provide more frequent oral hygiene.
3. Inability to obtain secretions during suction procedure
   - Evaluate patient's fluid status and adequacy of humidification on oxygen-delivery device.
   - Assess for signs of infection.
   - Determine need for chest physiotherapy.

RECORDING AND REPORTING

- Respiratory assessments before and after suctioning; size of catheter used; suctioning route; amount, consistency, and color of secretions obtained; frequency of suctioning; patient tolerance of suctioning procedure, including changes in vital signs, pulse oximetry values, and E_tCO_2 values (if applicable), and oxygen requirement after procedure.
- Note which naris was used/should be used and why for nasopharyngeal/tracheal suctioning.
- Quantity and quality of sputum obtained during suction procedure, including whether blood was present.
- Document your evaluation of patient learning.

HOME CARE CONSIDERATIONS

- Adhere to best practices for infection control while weighing cost-effectiveness in the presence of a chronic situation. If a patient has an established tracheostomy or requires long-term nasotracheal suctioning and infection is not present, clean suction technique may be deemed appropriate.
- Although most patients with airway clearance problems at home have a tracheostomy, some also require nasal pharyngeal suctioning. Catheters are often used for a 24-hour period and then cleaned and disinfected, or they are cleaned with soapy water after each use and discarded after 24 hours.
- Stress to family caregivers the importance of brief intervals of applying suction pressure. Instruct those performing suction to hold their breath during the application of negative suction pressure to help them remember to not suction too long.
- Instruct patient and family caregiver about infection control practices (e.g., to clean and disinfect or change the secretion collection container every 24 hours according to home care or institutional protocol and to avoid splash when emptying the suction container jar in the toilet). Instruct caregiver to apply mask (shield if available) and gloves and bring the jar as close to the toilet bowl as possible to decrease the risk of splash.
- Power companies should be notified of homes in which there are patients receiving home suction or ventilation. In the event of a power outage, these homes would be the priority for receiving power.

Continued

Delegation and Collaboration

This skill of performing ETT care cannot be delegated to assistive personnel (AP). AP may assist the nurse with ETT care. Often, the nurse collaborates with a respiratory therapist in performing this care. In some settings, the skill of TT care for patients with a well-established TT can be delegated to AP. The nurse directs the AP to:

- Immediately report any signs of respiratory problems or increased airway secretions.
- Immediately report if the ETT or TT appears to have moved or become obstructed or dislodged.
- Immediately report changes in patient's mood, level of consciousness, irritability, vital signs, decreased pulse oximetry value, or changes in end-tidal CO_2 values.
- Immediately report abnormal color of the tracheal stoma and drainage.

Equipment

- Towel
- Stethoscope
- Pulse oximeter and end-tidal CO_2 detector
- Personal protective equipment: goggles/mask/face shield; gloves; gown
- Oral and artificial airway suction supplies
- Oxygen source
- Self-inflating manual resuscitation bag-valve device and appropriate-size mask
- Oral hygiene supplies (e.g., pediatric-size toothbrush, sponge toothette for edentulous patients, toothpaste, cleaning solution, and nonalcohol-based mouthwash)
- Communication device—*optional* (letter or picture board, tablet, pen and paper)
- Reintubation equipment should be available at bedside in case of accidental tube dislodgment

Endotracheal Tube Care

- Additional health care team member (two people are needed to safely complete some of the ETT care steps)
- ETT and oropharyngeal suction equipment

- 1- to 1½-inch adhesive or waterproof tape (not paper tape) or commercial ETT stabilizer (follow manufacturer's or health care agencies' instructions for securing the ETT)
- Two pairs of clean gloves
- Adhesive remover swab
- Face cleanser (e.g., wet washcloth, towel, soap, shaving supplies)
- Clean 2 × 2–inch gauze
- Tincture of benzoin or liquid adhesive
- Oral airway or bite block
- Tongue blade *(optional)*

Tracheostomy Care

- Additional health care team member (two people are needed to safely complete some of the TT care steps)
- Sterile tracheostomy care kit, if available, or:
  - Three sterile 4 × 4–inch gauze pads
  - Sterile cotton-tipped applicators
  - Sterile tracheostomy dressing
  - Sterile basin
  - Small sterile brush (or disposable cannula)
  - Tracheostomy ties (e.g., twill tape, manufactured tracheostomy ties, Velcro tracheostomy ties)
- Sterile normal saline or water
- TT and oropharyngeal suction equipment
- Scissors
- Pair of sterile and clean gloves
- Disposable inner cannula, if patient has one
- Extra sterile tracheostomy kit
- Cuff pressure manometer

STEP	**RATIONALE**

ASSESSMENT

1. Identify patient using at least two identifiers (e.g., name and birthday or name and account number) according to agency policy. Compare identifiers with information on patient's MAR or medical record.

Ensures correct patient. Complies with The Joint Commission standards and improves patient safety (TJC, 2020).

2. Review medical record to assess patient's hydration status, humidity delivered to airway/ventilator circuit, status of any existing infection, patient's nutritional status, and ability to cough.

Determines factors that affect amount and consistency of secretions in ETT/TT and patient's ability to clear airway.

3. Perform hand hygiene, apply gloves, and perform complete assessment of patient's cardiopulmonary status, including lung sounds, pulse oximetry, E_tCO_2, vital signs, and level of consciousness. Keep pulse oximeter in place.

Provides baseline to determine status of ventilation and patient response to and tolerance of therapy.

4. Observe condition of tissues surrounding ETT/TT for impaired skin integrity (e.g., blistering, abrasions, pressure injuries) on nares, lips, cheeks, corner of mouth, or neck; excess nasal or oral secretions; patient moving tube with tongue or biting tube or tongue; or foul-smelling mouth.

Increased risk for developing pressure areas around ETT or TT from impaired circulation as tube is pulled or pressed against mucosal tissues (Pittman et al., 2015). Presence of ETT or TT impairs ability of patient to swallow oral secretions.

5. Observe patency of airway: excess peristomal, intratracheal, or endotracheal secretions; diminished airflow; or signs and symptoms of airway obstruction.

Buildup of secretions in ETT/TT impairs oxygen delivery and subsequent tissue oxygenation. Excess secretions in the artificial airways may indicate need for suctioning before performing any other airway care.

6. Observe for signs and symptoms of gurgling on expiration, decreased exhaled tidal volume (mechanically ventilated patient), signs and symptoms of inadequate ventilation (rising end-tidal carbon dioxide concentration [E_tCO_2], patient-ventilator desynchrony, or dyspnea), spasmodic coughing, tense test balloon on tube, flaccid test balloon on tube, and ability to speak or vocalize.

Cuff underinflation increases risk for aspiration, allows secretions to enter the trachea, and permits vocalization. Cuff overinflation may cause ischemia or necrosis of tracheal tissue from obstruction of capillary bed, resulting in tracheomalacia or tracheoesophageal fistula (Myatt, 2015; Rouzé et al., 2017). End-tidal carbon dioxide concentration [E_tCO_2] validates the correct placement of the ETT by analyzing the exhaled gas for carbon dioxide levels (Wiegand, 2017).

CLINICAL DECISION: *For possible overinflation or underinflation of ETT/TT cuff, notify respiratory therapy and follow agency policy for correcting cuff pressures. Most sources agree that 20 cm H_2O is the lowest accepted pressure, but some sources recommend that the highest pressure to maintain the cuff is 25 cm H_2O (Myatt, 2015).*

STEP	**RATIONALE**
7. Observe for factors that increase risk for complications from ETT/TT: type and size of tube, movement of tube up and down trachea (in and out), duration of tube placement, presence of facial trauma, malnutrition, and neck or thoracic radiation.	Tube pressure can cause medical device–related pressure injuries. Tube can become dislodged from lower airway (incidental extubation), or it can enter right mainstem bronchus.
8. **FOR ETT:** Determine proper ETT depth as noted by centimeters at lip or gum line. This line is marked on tube and recorded in patient's record at time of intubation and every shift. Remove and dispose of gloves. Perform hand hygiene.	Ensures that tube is at proper depth to adequately ventilate both lungs and that it is not too high, which causes vocal cord damage, or too low, which results in right mainstem intubation, in which only the right lung is ventilated. Reduces transmission of microorganisms.
9. Determine when oral and airway care were last performed. Know the health care agency protocols and procedures, but be aware of patient-specific needs for more frequent care.	Oral care is performed every 2-4 hours. TT care is performed every 4-8 hours (Wiegand, 2017).
10. Assess patient's or family caregiver's knowledge of procedure, literacy level, and ability to provide own care, as allowed.	Ensures patient or caregiver has the capacity to obtain, communicate process, and understand basic health information (CDC, 2019c).

PLANNING

1. Gather equipment/supplies and arrange at bedside. Close room curtain or door.	Ensures the necessary equipment is available to implement all interventions that should be completed for the patient. Ensures patient privacy.
2. Obtain assistance from available staff.	Reduces risk for accidental extubation of ETT or dislodgment of the TT.
3. Assist patient in assuming comfortable position for both patient and staff. Elevate patient's head to at least 30 degrees, unless contraindicated.	Provides access to site and facilitates completion of procedure. Prepares patient for any suctioning that may be required. Position may decrease risk of aspiration (AACN, 2018).
4. Explain procedure and patient's need to participate, including not biting or moving ETT with tongue, trying not to cough when tape or holder is off ETT/TT, keeping hands down, and not pulling on tubing.	Reduces anxiety, encourages cooperation, and reduces risk of accidental extubation or tube dislodgment.

CLINICAL DECISION: *For patients with TT: at some agencies, it is standard practice to have an extra TT that is the same size as the patient's current TT and a TT one size smaller at the bedside at all times in case there is an emergent need to replace the TT because of obstruction or dislodgment.*

IMPLEMENTATION

1. Perform hand hygiene. Apply clean gloves and mask, goggles, or face shield if indicated. Have assistant do so as well.	Reduces transmission of microorganisms.
2. Place clean towel across patient's chest.	Reduces soiling of bedclothes and linen.
3. Perform airway suctioning if indicated.	Removes secretions. Diminishes patient's need to cough during procedure.
4. Perform ETT care	
a. Connect Yankauer suction catheter to suction source and have it ready to use. Ensure that suction source/machine for oral suctioning is on and functioning properly.	Need to have functioning equipment to perform oral care appropriately. Prepares suction apparatus.
b. Remove oral airway or bite block, if present, and place on towel.	Provides access to and complete observation of patient's oral cavity.

CLINICAL DECISION: *If patient is biting the tube, do not remove bite block until absolutely necessary. This prevents obstruction of the ETT and occlusion of the artificial airway.*

c. Brush teeth with soft toothbrush, using solution or toothpaste that helps to break down plaque buildup on teeth. Suction oropharyngeal secretions as necessary.	There may be need for pediatric toothbrush, depending on size of patient's oral cavity. It is recommended to brush teeth at least twice a day (AACN, 2017a; Wiegand, 2017).
d. Use chlorhexidine solution and oral swabs to clean mouth. Suction oropharyngeal secretions as necessary. Apply mouth moisturizer to oral mucosa and lips after each cleaning.	This step should be completed every 2 to 4 hours (AACN, 2017a; Wiegand, 2017). The swabs, solution, and moisturizer may come in a prepackaged kit from manufacturer. The use of chlorhexidine mouthwash or gel is effective in reducing VAP (AACN, 2017b; Hua et al., 2016; Munro and Ruggiero, 2014).

Continued

STEP	RATIONALE

e. Prepare ETT securement options:

(1) *Tape method:* Prepare tape by cutting piece of tape long enough to go completely around patient's head from naris to naris plus 15 cm (6 inches). This is typically 30–60 cm (12–24 inches) in total length. Lay tape adhesive-side up on bedside table. Cut and lay 8–15 cm (3–6 inches) of second piece of tape, adhesive sides together, in center of the long strip to prevent tape from sticking to hair. Smaller strip of tape should cover area between ears around back of head (see illustration).

Preparing tape ahead decreases amount of time one must manually hold ETT throughout procedure, therefore decreasing risk of tube dislodgment. Adhesive tape needs to encircle head below ears with sufficient tape left to wrap around tube.

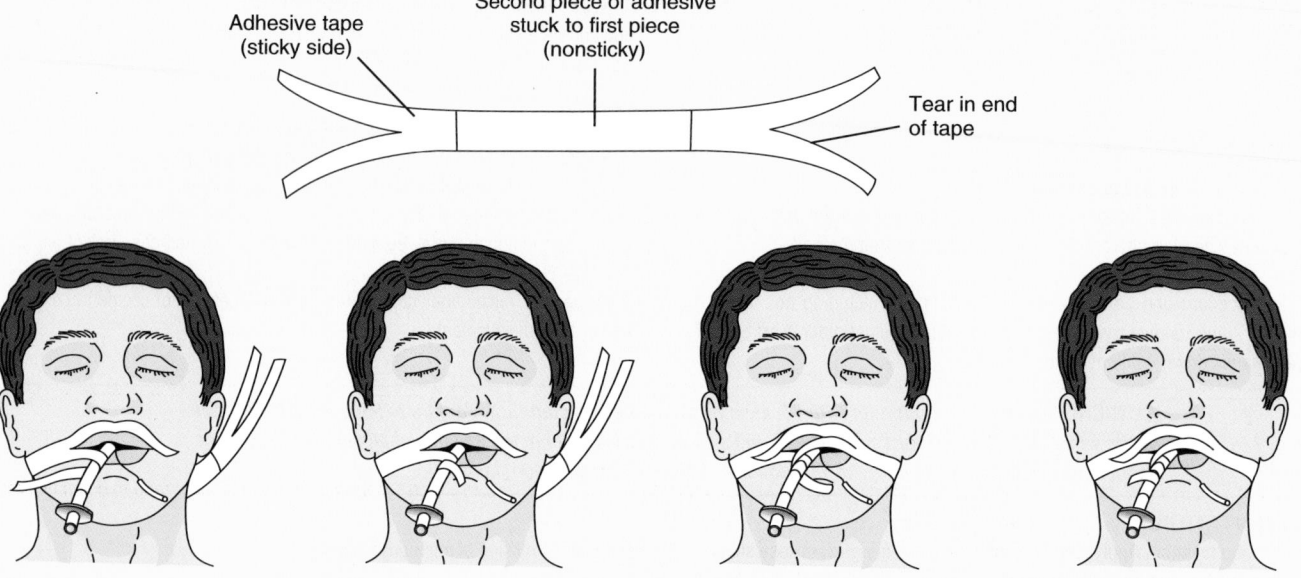

STEP 4e(1) Methods of securing adhesive tape. (From *Wiegand's AACN procedure manual for high acuity, progressive and acuity care*, St Louis, 2017, Elsevier.)

(2) *Commercially available ET holder:* Open package per manufacturer's instructions. Set *device* aside with head guard in place and Velcro strips open.

Commercial devices are latex free, fast, convenient, and disposable.

CLINICAL DECISION: *It is a nursing decision whether to use tape or a commercially available ET holder. There are advantages and disadvantages to both. The commercial tube holders allow for less slippage of the ETT and easier access for oral care but have an increased risk of the formation of pressure injuries (Branson et al., 2014; Smith and Pietrantonio, 2016).*

f. Remove old tape or device.

(1) *Tape:* While one person is holding and stabilizing ETT, the other person should remove tape from patient, using adhesive tape remover. The tape will also need to be removed from ETT itself.

Provides access to skin under tape for assessment and hygiene. Adhesive tape remover ensures easier, less traumatic removal of the tape.

CLINICAL DECISION: *Clean outside of ETT tube with soap and water or saline as needed. Do not apply adhesive tape remover to the ETT itself. This action will make it nearly impossible for the new tape to appropriately stick to the ETT, which increases risk of tube dislodgment. Do not allow assistant to hold the tube away from the lips or nares. Doing so allows too much movement in the tube and increases the risk for tube movement and accidental extubation. Never let go of the ETT because it could become dislodged (Lewis et al., 2017; Wiegand, 2017).*

(2) *Commercially available device:* Remove Velcro strips from ETT and remove ETT holder from patient.

Velcro adhesive strips hold ETT in place and provide marker to measure distance to patient's lips or gums. These devices all permit access to patient's mouth and lips for ease in oropharyngeal suctioning and oral hygiene.

STEP	RATIONALE

g. Remove excess secretions or adhesive from patient's face. Clean facial skin with mild soap and water and dry thoroughly. May need to apply tape adherence product such as tincture of benzoin to face. **NOTE:** Determine if patient needs face shaved and complete before re-taping ET tube.

Application of tape adherence product allows for new tape or device to stay on patient's face (Wiegand, 2017).

CLINICAL DECISION: *When shaving patients, take great care to keep the cuff inflation port away from the razor. The razor can inadvertently cut or nick the tubing, causing air loss from the cuff and the possible need for reintubation.*

CLINICAL DECISION: *Do not remove oral airway or bite block if patient is still actively biting. Wait until the new tape or commercial device is partially or completely secured to ETT.*

---

h. Note level of ETT by looking at mark or noting centimeter value on tube itself. Move oral ETT to other side of mouth and ensure that tube marking at lip is unchanged. Perform oral care as needed on side where tube was initially positioned. Clean oral airway or bite block with warm soapy water and rinse well. Reinsert as necessary.

Changing sides of ETT removes pressure and decreases risk of breakdown at corners of mouth and oral mucosa (Pittman et al., 2015; Wiegand, 2017).

CLINICAL DECISION: *The patient may cough excessively when the tube is being moved. The person who is holding the tube in place should be prepared for this and take extra caution while holding. In some instances, the ETT may need to be secured with the tape before the rest of the oral care is performed. In some cases, the patient may need to be administered a dose of an antianxiety or sedating medication.*
The cuff of the ETT may need to be deflated before changing its position. If cuff deflation is necessary, perform deep oral suctioning before deflation of the cuff, then provide oral care after the cuff is properly reinflated (Wiegand, 2017).

---

i. Secure tube (assistant continues to hold ET tube).
  (1) Tape method:
   (a) Slip tape under patient's head and neck, adhesive side up. Take care not to twist tape or catch hair. Do not allow tape to stick to itself. It helps to gently stick end of tape to a tongue blade, which serves as guide. Then slide tongue blade under patient's neck. Center tape so double-faced tape extends around back of neck from ear to ear.

Positions tape to secure ETT in proper position. Don't allow tape to go on or over earlobe.

   (b) On one side of face secure tape from ear to naris (nasal ETT) or over lip to ETT (oral ETT). Tear remaining tape in half lengthwise, forming two pieces that are 1–1.5 cm (0.4–0.6 inch) wide. Secure bottom half of tape across upper lip (oral ETT) or across top of nose (nasal ETT) to opposite ear (see illustration A). Wrap top half of tape around tube and up from bottom (see illustration B). Tape should encircle tube at least 2 times for security.

Secures tape to face. Using top tape to wrap prevents downward drag on ETT.

   (c) Gently pull other side of tape firmly to pick up slack and secure to opposite side of face and ETT same as first piece. **NOTE:** ETT is secured. Assistant can release hold. Check depth mark at lips or gum line.

Secures tape to face and tube. ETT should be at same depth at lips or gum line. Check earlier assessment for verification of tube depth in centimeters.

  (2) Commercially available ETT tube securement device:

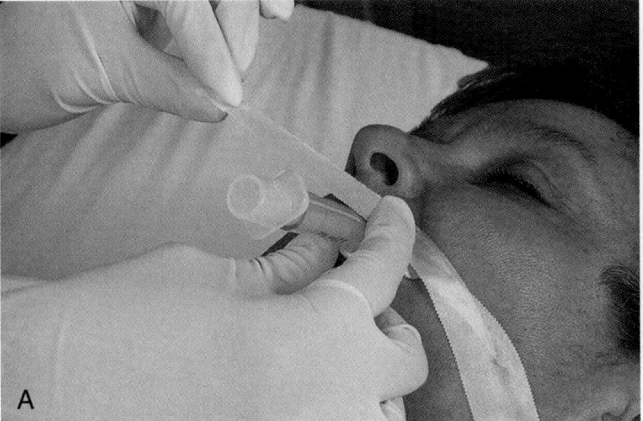 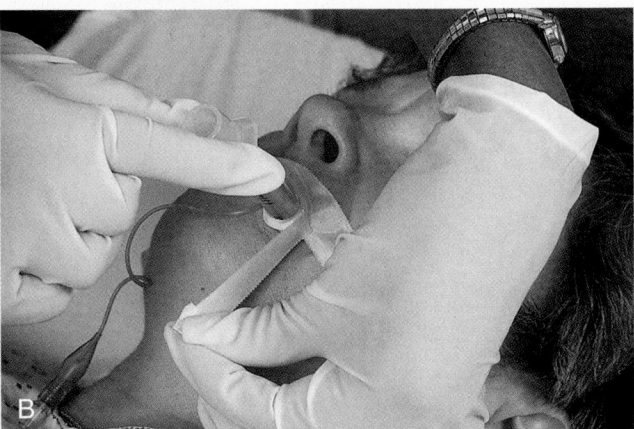

STEP 4i(1)(b) A, Securing bottom half of tape across patient's upper lip. **B,** Securing top half of tape around tube.

Continued

CLINICAL DECISION: *This step will only need to be completed if the device is visibly soiled and cannot be cleaned or if it is no longer adhering to the face and keeping the ETT secure.*

(a) Thread ETT through opening designed to secure it. Be sure that pilot balloon is accessible.	Commercially available holders have a slit in front of holder designed to secure ETT.
(b) Place strips of ETT holder under patient at occipital region of head.	
(c) Verify that ETT is at established depth using lip or gum line marker as guide.	Ensures that ETT remains at correct depth as determined during assessment.
(d) Attach Velcro strips at base of patient's head. Leave 1 cm (0.4 inch) slack in strips.	
(e) Verify that tube is secure, that it does not move forward from patient's mouth or backward down into patient's throat, and that there are no pressure areas on oral mucosa or occipital region of head (see illustration).	Tube must be secure, so it remains at correct depth. It can be secured without being tight and causing pressure.
j. For unconscious patient, reinsert oral airway without pushing tongue into oropharynx, and secure with tape.	Prevents patient from biting ETT and allows access for oropharyngeal suctioning. An oral airway is not used in a conscious, cooperative patient because it causes excessive gagging and pressure areas to mouth and tongue.
k. Clean rest of face and neck with soapy washcloth, rinse, and dry. Shave male patient as necessary.	Moisture and beard growth prevent adhesive tape adherence.

CLINICAL DECISION: *If a nasotracheal tube is in place, all the preceding steps will be completed, except that the tube will not be moved, nor its position changed. It is out of the scope of nurse practice to move the ETT from one naris to another and could cause great harm to the patient.*

5. Perform tracheostomy tube care:

a. Preoxygenate patient for 30 seconds or ask patient to take 5 to 6 deep breaths. Then suction tracheostomy (see Skill 41.1). Before removing gloves, remove soiled tracheostomy dressing and discard in glove with coiled catheter.	Removes secretions to avoid occluding outer cannula while inner cannula is removed. Reduces need for patient to cough.
b. Perform hand hygiene. Open sterile tracheostomy kit (if available). Open two 4 × 4–inch gauze packages using aseptic technique and pour normal saline on one package. Leave second package dry. Open two cotton-tipped swab packages and pour normal saline on one package. Do not recap normal saline.	Decreases risk of infection. Prepares equipment and allows for smooth, organized completion of tracheostomy care. Tracheostomy care should be performed every 4 to 8 hours or per agency protocol (Wiegand, 2017).
c. Open sterile tracheostomy dressing package.	

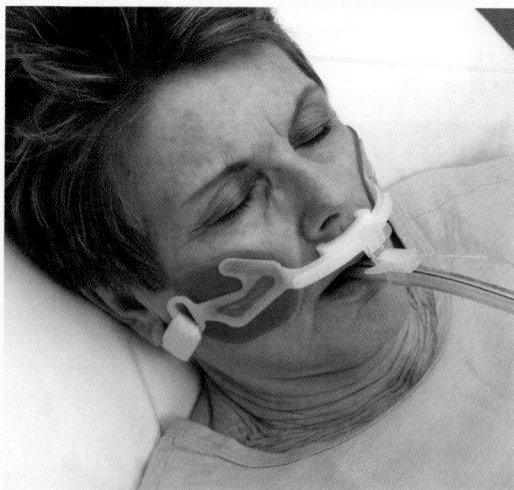

STEP 4i(2)(e) Commercial endotracheal tube holder. (Modified from Sills JR: *Entry-level respiratory therapist exam guide,* St Louis, 2000, Mosby.)

STEP	RATIONALE

d. Unwrap sterile basin and pour about 0.5–2 cm (0.2–1 inch) of normal saline into it.

e. Prepare TT fixation device.

  (1) If using twill tape: Prepare length of twill tape long enough to go around patient's neck 2 times, about 60–75 cm (24–30 inches) for an adult. Cut ends on diagonal. Lay aside in dry area.   *Cutting ends of tie on diagonal aids in inserting tie through eyelet.*

  (2) If using commercially available TT holder, open package according to manufacturer's directions.

f. Open inner cannula package (if new one is to be inserted such as with disposable inner cannulas or if patient does not tolerate being disconnected from oxygen source while cleaning reusable inner cannula).

g. Apply sterile gloves. Keep dominant hand sterile throughout procedure.   *Reduces transmission of microorganisms.*

h. Remove oxygen source if present.

CLINICAL DECISION: *It is always important to stabilize TT during tracheostomy care to prevent injury, unnecessary discomfort, or accidental dislodgment. Have an assistant such as an AP, nurse, or respiratory therapist help during the procedure. Instruct assistant to apply clean gloves.*

---

i. Care of tracheostomy with reusable inner cannula:

  (1) While touching only outer aspect of tube, unlock and remove inner cannula with nondominant hand following line of tracheostomy. Drop inner cannula into normal saline basin.   *Removes inner cannula for cleaning. Normal saline loosens secretions from inner cannula.*

CLINICAL DECISION: *If patient is receiving mechanical ventilation, you may want the person assisting you to hold the TT stable and remove the ventilator tube from the connection while you remove the inner cannula. This action helps to ensure that the TT itself is not removed accidentally if difficulties removing the ventilator from the TT or removing the inner cannula from the TT occur.*

---

  (2) Place tracheostomy collar, T tube, or ventilator oxygen source over outer cannula. (**NOTE:** May not be able to attach T tube and ventilator oxygen devices to all outer cannulas when inner cannula is removed.)   *Maintains supply of oxygen to patient as needed.*

CLINICAL DECISION: *If patient is unable to tolerate being disconnected from the ventilator, replace the inner cannula with a clean new one and reattach the ventilator to the tracheostomy. Then proceed with cleaning the original inner cannula as described in the next steps and store it in a sterile container until the next inner cannula change (Wiegand, 2017).*

---

  (3) To prevent oxygen desaturation if patient is affected, quickly pick up inner cannula and use small brush to remove secretions inside and outside inner cannula (see illustration).   *Tracheostomy brush provides mechanical force to remove thick or dried secretions.*

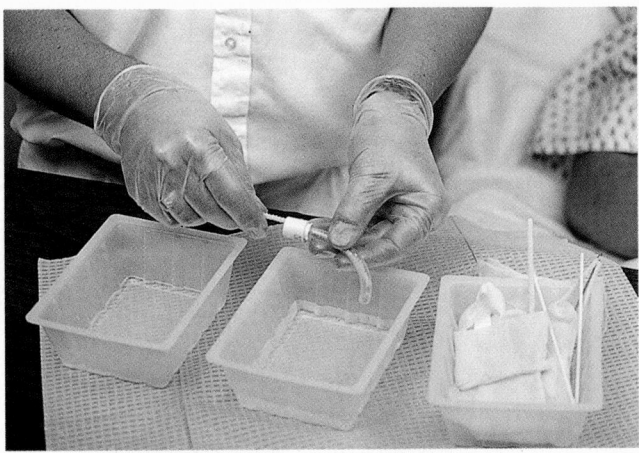

STEP 5i(3) Cleaning tracheostomy inner cannula.

Continued

SKILL 41.2	CARE OF AN ARTIFICIAL AIRWAY—cont'd

STEP	RATIONALE
(4) Hold inner cannula over basin and rinse with sterile normal saline, using nondominant (clean) hand to pour normal saline.	Removes secretions and normal saline from inner cannula.
(5) Remove oxygen source, replace inner cannula (see illustration), and secure "locking" mechanism. Reapply ventilator, tracheostomy collar, or T tube. Hyperoxygenate patient if needed.	Secures inner cannula and reestablishes oxygen supply.
j. Tracheostomy with disposable inner cannula:	
(1) Remove new cannula from manufacturer packaging.	Prepares you for change of inner cannula.
(2) While touching only outer aspect of tube, withdraw inner cannula and replace with new cannula by inserting it at a 90-degree angle then rotate downward. Lock into position.	Provides clean, sterile inner cannula for patient.

CLINICAL DECISION: *If patient is receiving mechanical ventilation, you may want the person assisting you to hold the TT stable and remove the ventilator tube from the connection while you remove the inner cannula. This action helps to ensure that the TT itself is not accidentally removed if difficulties removing the ventilator or the inner cannula from the TT occur.*

STEP	RATIONALE
(3) Dispose of contaminated cannula in appropriate receptacle and reconnect to ventilator or oxygen supply.	Prevents transmission of infection. Restores oxygen delivery.
k. Using normal saline-saturated cotton-tipped swabs and 4 × 4–inch gauze, clean exposed outer cannula surfaces and stoma under faceplate extending 5–10 cm (2–4 inches) in all directions from stoma (see illustration). Clean in circular motion from stoma site outward with dominant hand to handle sterile supplies. Do not go over previously cleaned area.	Aseptically removes secretions from stoma site. Moving in outward circle pulls mucus and other contaminants from stoma to periphery.
l. Using dry 4 × 4–inch gauze, pat lightly at skin and exposed outer cannula surfaces.	Dry surfaces prohibit formation of moist environment for microorganism growth and skin excoriation (Wiegand, 2017).
m. Secure tracheostomy.	

CLINICAL DECISION: *Some agencies do not recommend changing the securement device for the first 72 hours after insertion of the TT because of risk of stoma closure if the tube were to become dislodged accidentally (Wiegand, 2017).*

STEP	RATIONALE
(1) Tracheostomy tie method:	
(a) Instruct assistant, if available, to apply clean gloves and securely hold TT in place. With assistant holding TT, cut old ties. **Do not cut pilot balloon of cuff.**	Prevents transmission of infection. Secures TT to prevent incidental dislodgment. If pilot balloon is cut, there is no ability to inflate cuff (Wiegand, 2017).

CLINICAL DECISION: *Assistant must not release hold on TT until new ties are firmly tied. If working without an assistant, do not cut old ties until new ties are in place and securely tied (Lewis et al., 2017). When ties are off, this is a good time to clean the back of the patient's neck and assess patient's skin under TT flange and under the ties or tube holder, making sure that skin is intact, free of pressure, and dry before applying securement device.*

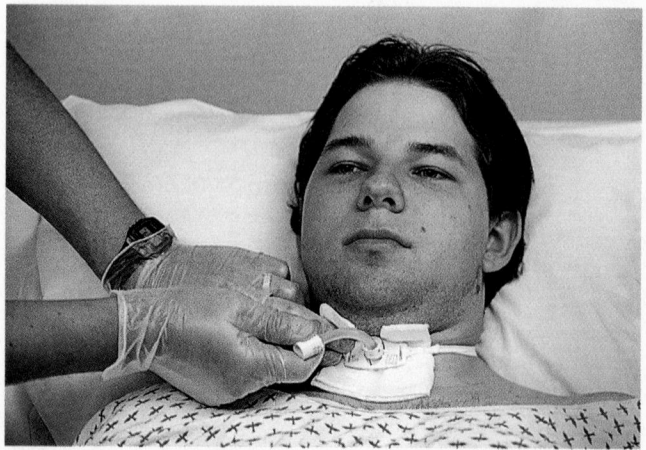

STEP 5i(5) Reinserting inner cannula.

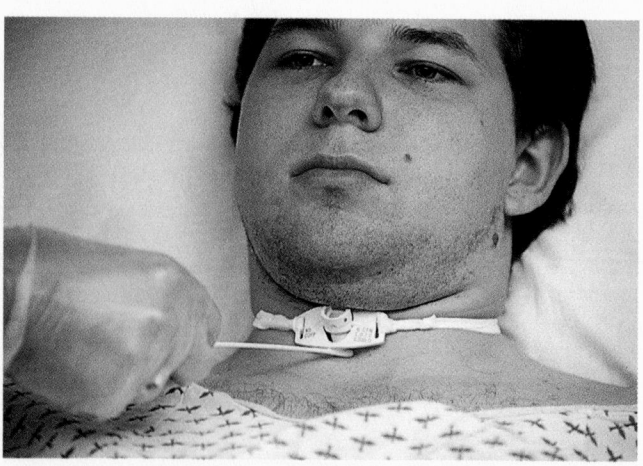

STEP 5k Cleaning around stoma.

STEP	RATIONALE
(b) Take prepared twill tape, insert one end of tie through faceplate eyelet, and pull ends even (see illustration).	Diagonal cuts ensure ease of threading end of tie through holes of eyelet (Wiegand, 2017).
(c) Slide both ends of tie behind head and around neck to other eyelet and insert one tie through second eyelet.	
(d) Pull snugly	Secures TT.
(e) Tie ends securely in double square knot, allowing space for insertion of only one loose or two snug finger widths between tie and neck (see illustration).	One finger width of slack prevents ties from being too tight when tracheostomy dressing is in place and prevents movement of tracheostomy tube into lower airway (Wiegand, 2017).
(f) Insert fresh 4 × 4–inch tracheostomy dressing under clean ties and faceplate (see illustration).	Absorbs drainage. Dressing prevents pressure on clavicle heads (Wiegand, 2017).

CLINICAL DECISION: *Never cut a 2 × 2–inch or 4 × 4–inch gauze pad because the cut edges fray and increase the risk of infection (Wiegand, 2017).*

STEP	RATIONALE
(2) Tracheostomy tube holder method:	
(a) Instruct assistant, if available, to apply clean gloves and securely hold TT in place. When an assistant is unavailable, leave old TT holder in place until new device is secure.	Ensures that tracheostomy stays in correct position. Prevents incidental dislodgment of tube.
(b) Align strap under patient's neck. Be sure that Velcro attachments are on either side of TT.	Ensures proper securement of TT.
(c) Place narrow end of ties under and through faceplate eyelets. Pull ends even and secure with Velcro closures (see illustration).	
(d) Verify that there is space for only one loose or two snug finger widths to be inserted under neck strap.	Ensures proper securement of TT without securement device being too tight.
n. Discard soiled items in appropriate receptacle. Remove towel and place in laundry.	Reduces transmission of microorganisms.
o. Perform oral care with toothbrush or oral swabs and chlorhexidine rinse.	Use of chlorhexidine may decrease patient risk of developing a ventilator-associated event (VAE)/ventilator-associated pneumonia (VAP) and promotes patient comfort (AACN, 2017b; Hua et al., 2016).
p. Measure TT cuff pressure.	Cuff pressures should be measured every 8 hours and following any tracheostomy-related intervention or after the patient has been repositioned (Intensive Care Society [ICS], 2018).
(1) Attach a commercial pressure gauge/manometer to the tracheal cuff.	Allows for measurement of the pressure of TT cuff.

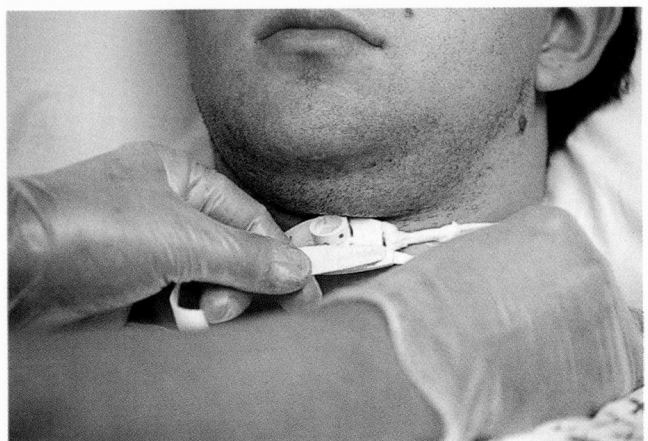

STEP 5m(1)(b) Replacing tracheostomy ties. Do not remove old tracheostomy ties until new ones are secure.

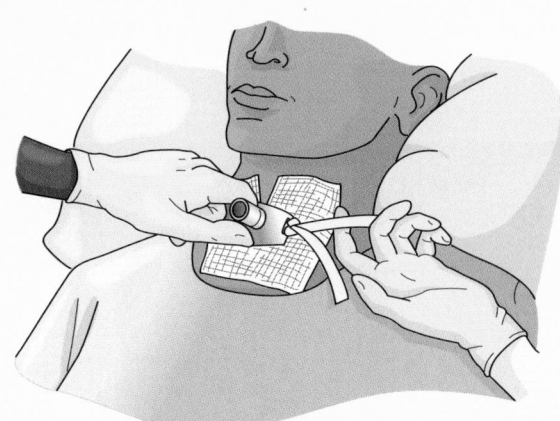

STEP 5m(1)(e) Tracheostomy ties properly placed. (From Sorrentino SA: *Mosby's textbook for nursing assistants*, ed 8, St Louis, 2013, Mosby.)

Continued

SKILL 41.2 **CARE OF AN ARTIFICIAL AIRWAY—cont'd**

STEP	RATIONALE
(2) Read the measurement. If the cuff pressure is greater than 25 cm H2O, then release some air from the cuff (using the pressure gauge on the manometer) until the pressure reaches between 20 and 25 cm H2O. If the pressure is less than 20 cm H2O, add air by squeezing the bulb on the manometer until the pressure is between 20 and 25 cm H2O.	Overinflated cuffs can lead to tracheal stenosis, necrosis, tracheomalacia, and fistula formation. Underinflated cuffs can lead to ineffective mechanical ventilation and increase risk of aspiration (Myatt, 2015; Wiegand, 2017)
6. Discard soiled items in appropriate receptacle; remove towel and place in laundry. Remove gloves and mask, goggles, or face shield or gown; discard in receptacle; and perform hand hygiene. (Assistant performs same steps.) Place clean items (e.g., tincture of benzoin, oral care solution, excess swabs) in place of storage.	Reduces transmission of microorganisms. Ensures that contaminated gloves and hands do not touch clean items.
7. Reposition patient and ask him or her what else he or she needs.	Promotes comfort; gives patients opportunity to communicate their needs.
8. Be sure nurse call system is in an accessible location within patient's reach.	Ensures patient can call for assistance if needed.
9. Raise side rails (as appropriate) and lower bed to lowest position.	Ensures patient safety.
10. Be sure that oxygen and/or humidification delivery sources are in place and set at correct levels.	Humidification helps prevent airway obstruction and atelectasis (Hanlon, 2016).

EVALUATION

1. Compare respiratory assessments before and after ETT/TT care.	Identifies any physiological changes, including presence and quality of breath sounds after procedure.
2. Observe depth and position of ETT according to health care provider recommendation.	Position of ETT should not be altered.
3. Assess security of tape by *gently* tugging at tube.	Tape should remain attached to face. Patient may cough during tugging.
4. Assess skin around mouth, oral mucous membranes, and/or tracheal stoma for intactness and pressure sores.	Tape should not tear skin. Pressure areas should be absent.
5. Compare pulse oximeter and E_tCO_2 values from before and after ETT/TT care.	Changes in oxygen saturation and E_tCO_2 can help identify displacement or dislodgment of ETT/TT.
6. Observe for excessive phonation or presence of gastric secretions in airway secretions.	Occurs with inadequate or excessive cuff inflation.
7. **Use Teach-Back:** "I want to be sure I explained why we need to clean your breathing tube routinely. Tell me why the cleaning of your tube is important for your breathing." Revise your instruction now or develop plan for patient/family caregiver teaching if patient/family caregiver is not able to teach back correctly.	Determines patient's/family caregiver's level of understanding of instructional topic.

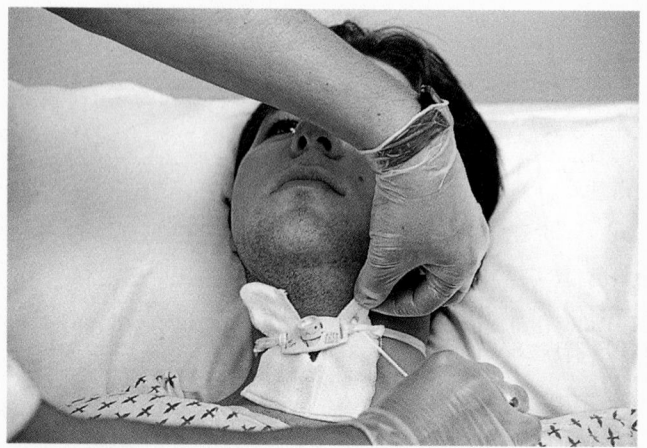

STEP 5m(1)(f) Applying tracheostomy dressing.

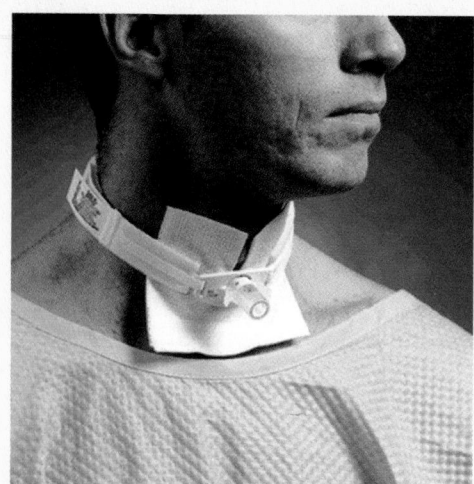

STEP 5m(2)(c) Tracheostomy tube holder in place. (Courtesy Dale Medical Products, Plainville, MA.)

STEP	**RATIONALE**

UNEXPECTED OUTCOMES AND RELATED INTERVENTIONS

1. Tube is dislodged or misplaced accidentally, including extubation.
- Remain with patient while calling for help.
- Ventilate with bag-valve-mask as needed.
- Assess patient for airway patency, spontaneous breathing, and vital signs.
- Prepare for retaping or securing procedure or reintubation.

2. Patient has pressure injury in mouth, lips, nares, or tracheal stoma.
- Increase frequency of ETT care.
- Apply antimicrobial ointment per agency protocol.
- Align oxygen and humidity supply tubing so that they do not pull ETT, creating pressure sores.
- Monitor for infection. If skin tear is present on cheeks or over nose or upper lip, apply protective barrier such as stoma adhesive patch or hydrocolloid dressing and apply tape to it.

3. Cuff leak develops.
- Verify position of tube, notify respiratory therapy, and follow agency policy.

RECORDING AND REPORTING

- Record respiratory assessments before and after tube care, depth of ETT or type and size of tracheostomy tube, frequency and extent of care, patient tolerance, and any complications related to presence of the tube.
- Document your evaluation of patient learning.
- Report signs of infection or displacement of ETT or tracheostomy tube immediately.
- Report time of care and patient tolerance, including vital sign changes or any changes in pulse oximeter, E_tCO_2, or respiratory status, and presence of any areas of impaired skin integrity on face or neck, in the mouth, or around the nares or tracheal stoma.

HOME CARE CONSIDERATIONS

- Instruct family caregivers in how to obtain supplies. Routine tracheostomy care should be done at least once a day after discharge from hospital. At home, clean technique with nonsterile gloves is usually used.
- Patients with tracheostomies may need to communicate with others by writing or use of computer. Ensure that they have communication devices that meet their needs.
- Instruct family caregivers in signs and symptoms of respiratory distress, tube dysfunction, and respiratory and stoma infections. Call health care provider if patient feels pain or discomfort longer than a week after insertion, if breathing does not improve after usual method of clearing secretions, or if secretions become thick or mucus plugs are present.
- When outside, use tracheostomy covers to protect from dust or cold air.
- Never remove the outer cannula unless instructed by health care provider to do so.

SKILL 41.3	**CARE OF PATIENTS WITH CHEST TUBES**

Delegation and Collaboration

The skill of chest tube management cannot be delegated to assistive personnel (AP). The nurse directs the AP about:
- Proper positioning of the patient with chest tubes to facilitate chest tube drainage and optimal functioning of the system, including maintaining the drainage system at a level lower than the insertion site and not lying on tubing.
- Ambulating and transferring patient with chest drainage.
- Reporting changes in vital signs, complaints of chest pain or sudden shortness of breath, or excessive bubbling in water-seal chamber to the nurse immediately.
- Danger of any disconnection of drainage system, change in type and amount of drainage, sudden bleeding, or sudden cessation of bubbling.

Equipment
- Local anesthetic, if not an emergent procedure
- Prescribed chest drainage system
- Water-seal system versus waterless system: sterile water or normal saline per manufacturer's directions
- Clean gloves
- Suction source and setup
- Sterile skin preparation solution (povidone-iodine or chlorhexidine solutions)
- Chest tube tray (all items are sterile), typically: knife handle, clamps, small sponge forceps, needle holder, knife blade No. 10, 3-0 silk sutures, sterile drape, two clamps, 4 × 4–inch sponges, suture scissors, and sterile gloves
- Dressings: Petroleum or Xeroform gauze, large dressing of choice, split chest tube dressing, additional 4 × 4–inch dressings, 4-inch tape or elastic bandage
- Two rubber-tipped hemostats (shodded) for each chest tube
- 1-inch waterproof adhesive tape for taping connections
- Face mask, face shield, or head cover
- Sterile gloves
- 1-inch adhesive tape or zip tie for securing connections
- Stethoscope, sphygmomanometer, and pulse oximeter

Continued

SKILL 41.3   CARE OF PATIENTS WITH CHEST TUBES—cont'd

STEP	RATIONALE

ASSESSMENT

1. Identify patient using at least two identifiers (e.g., name and birthday or name and account number) according to agency policy. Compare identifiers with information on the patient's MAR or medical record.

Ensures correct patient. Complies with a recommended National Patient Safety Goal (TJC, 2020).

2. Review health care provider's order for chest tube placement.

Insertion of chest tube requires health care provider order.

3. Review patient's medication record for anticoagulant therapy, including aspirin, warfarin, heparin, or platelet aggregation inhibitors such as ticlopidine or dipyridamole.

Anticoagulation therapy can increase procedure-related blood loss.

4. Review patient's hemoglobin and hematocrit levels.

Parameters reflect whether blood loss is occurring, which may affect oxygenation.

5. Assess patient's or family caregiver's knowledge, experience, and health literacy.

Ensures patient or family caregiver has the capacity to obtain, communicate, process, and understand basic health information (CDC, 2019c).

6. Assess patient for known allergies. Ask patient whether he or she has had a problem with medications, latex, or anything applied to skin.

Povidone-iodine or chlorhexidine are antiseptic solutions often used to clean skin before tube insertion. Lidocaine is a local anesthetic administered to reduce pain. The chest tube will be held in place with tape and sutures (Wiegand, 2017).

7. Perform hand hygiene and perform a complete respiratory assessment, baseline vital signs, and pulse oximetry (SpO$_2$).

Baseline assessment and vital signs are essential for any invasive procedure. Chest tube insertion often relieves respiratory distress.

   a. Assess for signs and symptoms of increased respiratory distress and hypoxia (e.g., decreased breath sounds over affected and unaffected lungs, marked cyanosis, asymmetrical chest movements, displaced trachea, shortness of breath, and confusion).

Signs and symptoms associated with respiratory distress are related to type and size of pneumothorax, hemothorax, or preexisting illness. Signs of hypoxia are related to inadequate oxygen to tissues.

   b. Assess for sharp, stabbing chest pain or chest pain on inspiration, hypotension, and tachycardia. If possible, ask patient to rate level of comfort on a scale of 0 to 10.

Sharp, stabbing chest pain with or without decreased blood pressure and increased heart rate may indicate tension pneumothorax. Presence of pneumothorax or hemothorax is painful, frequently causing sharp inspiratory pain. In addition, discomfort is associated with presence of a chest tube, not just with its insertion. Adequate pain control promotes better patient participation in activity (Chotai and Monsenifar, 2018).

8. For patients who have existing chest tubes, observe:

   a. Chest tube dressing and site surrounding tube insertion.

Ensures that dressing is intact and occlusive seal remains without air or fluid leaks and that area surrounding insertion site is free of drainage or skin irritation (Chotai and Mosenifar, 2018).

   b. Tubing for kinks, dependent loops, or clots.

Maintains a patent, freely draining system, preventing fluid accumulation in chest cavity. When tubing is coiled, looped, or clotted, drainage is impeded, and there is an increased risk for tension pneumothorax or surgical emphysema (Chotai and Mosenifar, 2018).

   c. Chest drainage system should remain upright and below level of tube insertion.

An upright drainage system facilitates drainage and maintains water seal.

9. Remove and dispose of gloves. Perform hand hygiene.

10. Assess patient's comfort level on a scale of 0 to 10.

Provides a baseline to compare after chest tube insertion.

11. Determine patient's knowledge of procedure.

Encourages cooperation, minimizes risks and anxiety. Identifies teaching needs.

PLANNING

1. Gather equipment/supplies and arrange at bedside. Close room curtain or door.

Ensures the necessary equipment is available to implement all interventions that should be completed for the patient. Ensures patient privacy.

2. Assist patient in assuming appropriate position for insertion of the chest tube, or a position of optimal comfort during other chest tube care.

Appropriate positioning is important for the proper insertion of the chest tube. Position of optimal comfort, once tube is inserted, will allow for increase in physical activity, including deep breathing, coughing, and use of the incentive spirometer.

3. Be available while provider explains insertion procedure to the patient. Once tube is inserted and during normal management, explain the care that you will be providing.

Reduces anxiety and encourages cooperation.

IMPLEMENTATION

1. Check agency policy and determine whether informed consent is needed. Complete "Time Out" procedure.

Invasive medical procedures typically require informed consent. "Time Out" is completed to determine right patient, procedure, and location of insertion or incision site (Wiegand, 2017).

2. Perform hand hygiene.

Reduces transmission of microorganisms.

STEP	RATIONALE
3. Set up water-seal system (or dry system with suction); see manufacturer guidelines.	The water-seal system contains two or three compartments or chambers (see illustration. Fluid drains into the first chamber. The second chamber contains the water seal, which allows air to escape because of the force of expiration but not to reenter on inspiration. If suction is needed, a third chamber is used.
a. Obtain chest drainage system. Remove wrappers and prepare to set up two- or three-chamber system.	Maintains sterility of system for use under sterile operating room conditions.
b. While maintaining sterility of drainage tubing, stand system upright and add sterile water or normal saline (NS) to appropriate compartments.	Reduces possibility of contamination.
(1) *Two-chamber system (without suction):* Add sterile solution to water-seal chamber (second chamber), bringing fluid to required level as indicated.	Water-seal chamber acts as one-way valve, so air cannot enter pleural space (Chotai and Mosenifar, 2018).
(2) *Three-chamber system (with suction):* Add sterile solution to water-seal chamber (second chamber). Add amount of sterile solution prescribed by health care provider to suction-control chamber (third chamber), usually 20 cm H_2O pressure. Connect tubing from suction-control chamber to suction source. Tailor length of drainage tube to patient. **NOTE:** Suction control chamber vent must not be occluded when using suction (see illustration).	Depth of fluid level dictates highest amount of negative pressure that can be present within system. For example, 20 cm of water is approximately 20 cm of water pressure. After chest tube is inserted, turn up the wall or portable suction device until water in suction-control bottle exhibits continuous, gentle bubbling.

CLINICAL DECISION: *When increasing suction, remember that increased bubbling does not result in more suction to the chest cavity, but only serves to evaporate the water more quickly. The suction pressure should not exceed -20 cm H_2O because lung tissue damage may occur (Chotai and Mosenifar, 2018).*

---

(3) *Dry suction system:* Fill water-seal chamber with sterile solution. Adjust suction-control dial to prescribed level of suction; suction ranges from –10 to –40 cm of water pressure. Suction-control chamber vent is never occluded when suction is used. **NOTE:** On dry suction system, *DO NOT* obstruct positive-pressure relief valve. This allows air to escape.	Automatic control valve on dry suction-control device adjusts to changes in patient air leaks and fluctuation in suction source and vacuum to deliver prescribed amount of suction.

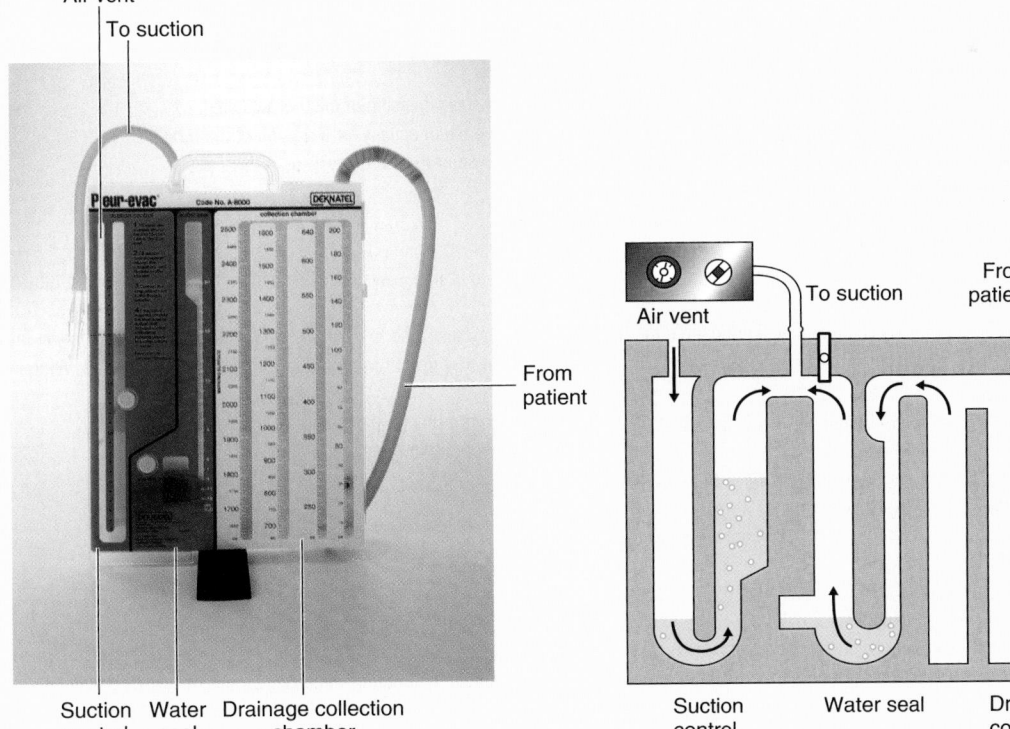

STEP 3b(2) *Left*, Pleur-Evac three-chamber drainage system. *Right*, Schematic of drainage device.

Continued

SKILL 41.3	CARE OF PATIENTS WITH CHEST TUBES—cont'd

STEP	RATIONALE
4. Set up waterless system (see manufacturer guidelines).	A waterless system is like a water seal system except that sterile water is not required for suction. The suction-control chamber is replaced by a one-way valve located near the top of the system. The suction-control chamber contains a suction-control float ball that is set by a suction-control dial (between −10 and −40 cm H_2O after the suction is connected and turned on) (Zisis et al., 2015).
a. Remove sterile wrappers and prepare to set up.	Maintains sterility of system for use under sterile operating room conditions.
b. For two-chamber system (without suction), nothing is added or needs to be done to system.	Waterless two-chamber system is ready for connecting to patient's chest tube after opening wrappers.
c. For three-chamber system (with suction), connect tubing from suction-control chamber to suction source.	Suction source provides additional negative pressure to system.
d. Instill 15 mL of sterile water or NS into diagnostic indicator injection port located on top of system.	Allows observation of rise and fall of water in diagnostic air leak window. Constant left-to-right bubbling or rocking is abnormal and indicates air leak. This is not necessary for mediastinal drainage because there is no tidaling. In an emergency, system *does not* require water for setup.
5. Secure all tubing connections with tape applied in double-spiral fashion using 2.5-cm (1-inch) adhesive tape or zip ties (nylon cable) with a clamp. Check system for patency by:	Prevents atmospheric air from leaking into system and patient's intrapleural space. Provides chance to ensure airtight system before connection to patient.
a. Clamping drainage tubing that will connect to patient's chest tube.	
b. Connecting tubing from float ball chamber to suction source.	
c. Turning on suction to prescribed level.	
6. Turn off suction source and unclamp drainage tubing before connecting patient to system. Suction source is turned on again after patient is connected.	Having patient connected to suction when it is initiated could damage pleural tissues from sudden increase in negative pressure. Tubing that is coiled or looped prevents adequate drainage and may cause tension pneumothorax (Wiegand, 2017).
7. Administer procedure medications such as sedatives or analgesics as ordered. (Give medications 30 minutes before procedure.)	Reduces patient anxiety and pain during procedure.

CLINICAL DECISION: *During procedure, carefully monitor patient for changes in level of sedation.*

STEP	RATIONALE
8. Provide psychological support to patient.	
a. Reinforce preprocedure explanation.	Reduces patient anxiety and helps complete procedure efficiently.
b. Coach and support patient throughout procedure.	
9. Perform hand hygiene and apply clean gloves. Position patient for tube insertion so that side in which tube is to be inserted is accessible to health care provider.	Reduces transmission of microorganisms. Allows ease of access for insertion of the tube.
10. Assist health care provider with chest tube insertion by providing needed equipment and local analgesic. Health care provider anesthetizes skin over insertion site, makes small skin incision, inserts clamped tube, sutures it in place, and applies occlusive dressing.	Ensures smooth insertion.
11. Help health care provider attach drainage tube to chest tube; remove clamp. Turn on suction to prescribed level.	Connects drainage system and suction (if ordered) to chest tube.
12. Tape or zip-tie all connections between chest tube and drainage tube. (**NOTE:** Chest tube is usually taped by health care provider at time of tube placement; check agency policy.)	Secures chest tube to drainage system and reduces risk for air leak that causes breaks in airtight system (Chotai and Mosenifar, 2018; Wiegand, 2017).
13. Check systems for proper functioning. Health care provider orders chest x-ray film.	Verifies intrapleural placement of tube.
14. After tube placement position patient:	Permits optimum drainage of fluid and/or air.
a. Semi-Fowler's or high-Fowler's position to evacuate air (pneumothorax) (Chotai and Mosenifar, 2018)	
b. High-Fowler's position to drain fluid (hemothorax) (Chotai and Mosenifar, 2018)	
15. Check patency of air vents in system.	
a. Water-seal vent must have no occlusion.	Permits displaced air to pass into atmosphere.
b. Suction-control chamber vent is not occluded when suction is used.	Provides safety factor of releasing excess negative pressure into atmosphere.
c. Waterless systems have relief valves without caps.	Provides safety factor of releasing excess negative pressure.
16. Position excess tubing horizontally on mattress next to patient. Secure with clamp provided so that it does not obstruct tubing.	Prevents excess tubing from hanging over edge of mattress in dependent loop. Drainage collected in loop can occlude drainage system, which predisposes patient to tension pneumothorax (Wiegand, 2017).
17. Adjust tubing to hang in straight line from chest tube to drainage chamber.	Promotes drainage and prevents fluid or blood from accumulating in pleural cavity.

STEP	RATIONALE

CLINICAL DECISION: *Gentle lifting of the drainage tubing allows gravity to help blood and other viscous material to move to the drainage bottle and avoid stasis in the tubing, which can lead to obstruction of the system and increased pressure in the thoracic cavity. Patients with recent chest surgery or trauma may need to have the chest drain tubing lifted more frequently, based on assessment of the amount of drainage (Wiegand, 2017).*

18. Place two rubber-tipped hemostats (for each chest tube) in easily accessible position (e.g., taped to top of patient's headboard). These should remain with patient when ambulating.	Chest tubes are double clamped under specific circumstances: (1) to assess for air leak, (2) to empty or quickly change disposable systems, (3) to assess whether patient is ready to have tube removed, or (4) if chest tube becomes accidentally disconnected from drainage system (Muzzy and Butler, 2015).

CLINICAL DECISION: *In the event of a chest tube disconnection or if the drainage system breaks, submerge the distal part of the tube 2 to 4 cm (1 to 2 inches) below the surface of a 250-mL bottle of sterile water or NS until a new chest tube unit can be set up (Lewis et al., 2017; Muzzy and Butler, 2015).*

19. Dispose of sharps in proper container, dispose of used supplies, and perform hand hygiene.	Reduces transmission of microorganisms.
20. Care of patient after chest tube insertion/existing chest tube:	
a. Perform hand hygiene and apply clean gloves. Assess vital signs; oxygen saturation; skin color; breath sounds; rate, depth, and ease of respirations; and insertion site every 15 minutes for first 2 hours, and then at least every shift (see agency policy).	Provides immediate information about procedure-related complications such as respiratory distress and leakage. Provides information about status of patient with existing chest tube.
b. Monitor color, consistency, and amount of chest tube drainage every 15 minutes for first 2 hours after insertion. Indicate level of drainage fluid, date, and time on write-on surface of chamber.	Provides baseline for continuous assessment of type and quantity of drainage. Ensures early detection of complications.
(1) From mediastinal tube, expect less than 100 mL/hr immediately after surgery and no more than 500 mL in first 24 hours.	Sudden gush of drainage may result from coughing or changing patient's position (i.e., releasing pooled/collected blood rather than indicating active bleeding). Acute bleeding indicates hemorrhage. Health care provider should be notified if there is more than 100–200 mL of bloody drainage in an hour (Lewis et al., 2017; Wiegand, 2017).
(2) Expect little or no output from anterior chest tube that is inserted for a pneumothorax (Wiegand, 2017).	

CLINICAL DECISION: *Routine stripping or milking of the chest tube is not a recommended practice. Doing so can result in increased pressure in the thoracic cavity, causing damage to the lungs or the pleural tissues. If there is a visible clot in the tubing, gentle milking of the tubing (manual squeezing and releasing of parts of the tubing) may be indicated, but only if the patient is at risk of further harm from the clot, such as the development of a tension pneumothorax (Makic et al., 2015; Wiegand, 2017).*

c. Observe chest dressing for drainage and determine whether it is still occlusive.	Drainage around tube may indicate blockage of the tube. Many health care agencies require the chest tube dressings to be occlusive in nature.

CLINICAL DECISION: *If the dressing is not occlusive or is saturated with drainage, it may need to be changed. There is no standard for how chest tube dressings should be performed, such as sterile versus a nonsterile dressing change. Know the health care agency standards for this procedure. Some health care agencies require the use of petrolatum gauze around the chest tube while others do not (Gross et al., 2016).*

d. Palpate around tube for swelling and crepitus (subcutaneous emphysema) as noted by crackling.	Indicates presence of air trapping in subcutaneous tissues. Small amounts are commonly absorbed. Large amounts are potentially dangerous. Most occurrences of crepitus are minor (Mao et al., 2015).

CLINICAL DECISION: *Some patients may develop subcutaneous emphysema (i.e., a collection of air under the skin after chest tube placement), which can occur if tubing is blocked or kinked. When this occurs, a crepitus (a crackling sensation) is felt with tactile fremitus on palpation.*

e. Check tubing to ensure that it is free of kinks and dependent loops.	Promotes drainage and prevents the development of a tension pneumothorax.

Continued

SKILL 41.3	CARE OF PATIENTS WITH CHEST TUBES—cont'd

STEP	RATIONALE

f. Observe for fluctuation of water-seal chamber and drainage in tubing during inspiration and expiration. Observe for clots or debris in tubing.	If fluctuation or tidaling stops, it means that either the lung is fully expanded or system is obstructed (Wiegand, 2017). In spontaneously breathing patient, fluid rises in water-seal or diagnostic indicator (waterless system) with inspiration and falls with expiration. The opposite occurs in patient who is mechanically ventilated. This indicates that system is functioning properly (Atrium, 2015).
g. Keep drainage system upright and below level of patient's chest.	Promotes gravity drainage and prevents backflow of fluid and air into pleural space.
h. Check for air leaks by monitoring bubbling in water-seal chamber. Intermittent bubbling is normal during expiration when air is being evacuated from pleural cavity, but continuous bubbling during both inspiration and expiration indicates leak in system.	Absence of bubbling may indicate that lung is fully expanded in patient with pneumothorax. Check all connections and locate sources of air leak.
i. Remove and dispose of gloves and dispose of used soiled equipment in appropriate biohazard container. Perform hand hygiene.	Prevents accidents involving contaminated equipment.
21. Instruct patient how to regularly take deep breaths, and reposition as often as possible.	Facilitates and maintains lung expansion.
22. Be sure nurse call system is in an accessible location within patient's reach.	Ensures patient can call for assistance if needed.
23. Raise side rails (as appropriate) and lower bed to lowest position.	Ensures patient safety.

EVALUATION

1. Evaluate patient for decreased respiratory distress and chest pain. Auscultate patient's lungs and observe chest expansion.	Determines status of lung expansion.
2. Monitor vital signs and SpO$_2$.	Determines whether level of oxygenation has improved.
3. Reassess patient's level of comfort on scale of 0 to 10, comparing level with comfort before chest tube insertion and/or pain medication administration.	Indicates need for analgesia. Patient with chest tube discomfort hesitates to take deep breaths and as a result is at risk for pneumonia and atelectasis.
4. Evaluate patient's ability to use deep-breathing exercises and reposition self while maintaining comfort.	Indicates patient's ability to promote lung expansion and prevent complications. Patients need to be repositioned every 2 hours when a chest tube is in place (Wiegand, 2017).
5. Monitor continued functioning of system as indicated by reduction in amount of drainage, resolution of air leak, and complete reexpansion of the lung.	Detects early signs of system complications or indicates possible removal of chest tube.
6. Use Teach-Back: "I want to be sure I explained why you have a chest tube. Explain to me why you have this tube and what we are doing to keep the system functioning." Revise your instruction now or develop a plan for revised patient/family caregiver teaching if patient/family caregiver is not able to teach back correctly.	Determines patient's/family caregiver's level of understanding of instructional topic.

UNEXPECTED OUTCOMES AND RELATED INTERVENTIONS

1. Patient develops respiratory distress. Chest pain, decrease in breath sounds over affected and unaffected lungs, marked cyanosis, asymmetrical chest movements, presence of subcutaneous emphysema around tube insertion site or neck, hypotension, tachycardia, and/or mediastinal shift are critical and indicate severe change in patient status, such as excessive blood loss or tension pneumothorax.
   - Notify health care provider immediately.
   - Collect set of vital signs and SpO$_2$.
   - Prepare for chest x-ray film.
   - Provide oxygen as ordered.
   - Be sure patient has head of bed elevated.
2. Air leak is unrelated to patient's respirations.
   - Locate leak by clamping chest tube with two rubber-shodded or toothless clamps close to the chest wall. If bubbling stops, air leak is inside patient's thorax or at the insertion site, and the health care provider should be notified.
   - If bubbling continues with the clamps near the chest wall, gradually move one clamp at a time down the drainage tubing away from the patient and toward the drainage chamber. When the bubbling stops, the leak is in the section of the tubing between the 2 clamps. If the leak occurs when the clamps are near the drainage system, then the leak is in the drainage system itself. If there is a leak in the tubing or the drainage system, the nurse can replace the tubing or the drainage system (Muzzy and Butler, 2015).
3. Chest tube is disconnected/dislodged.
   - Check connections and reattach using sterile technique (Chotai and Mosenifar, 2018).
   - Immediately apply dressing and/or pressure over chest tube insertion site (Muzzy and Butler, 2015).
   - Notify health care provider.

RECORDING AND REPORTING

- Record and report respiratory assessment; amount of suction, if used; amount of drainage since the previous assessment; type and amount of drainage in chest tubing; and presence or absence of an air leak, including amount if present, and patient comfort level.
- Record integrity of dressing and presence of drainage on dressing.
- Document your evaluation of patient learning.
- Record and report patient tolerance to new chest tube insertion; comfort level and any analgesia; respiratory assessment before and after insertion; quantity and quality of chest tube drainage.

HOME CARE CONSIDERATIONS

- Patients with chronic conditions (e.g., uncomplicated pneumothorax, effusions, empyema) that require long-term chest tube therapy may be discharged with smaller mobile drains. These systems do not have a suction-control chamber and use a mechanical one-way valve instead of a water-seal chamber.
- Instruct patient in how to ambulate and remain active with a mobile chest tube drainage system.
- Provide patient with information as to when to contact health care professionals regarding changes in health status or drainage system (e.g., chest pain, breathlessness, change in drainage).

SKILL 41.4	USING HOME OXYGEN EQUIPMENT

Delegation and Collaboration

The skill of administering home oxygen equipment cannot be delegated to assistive personnel (AP). Instruct the AP about:

- The unique needs of patient (e.g., amount of assistance in applying nasal cannula or mask) and any assistance needed in filling liquid canisters.
- The type of equipment patient should have in the home and the oxygen flow rate.
- Immediately reporting to the nurse increased rate of breathing, decreased level of consciousness, increased confusion, and pain.

Equipment

- Nasal cannula equipment (see Procedural Guideline, Box 41.9, for required equipment)
- Humidification device if oxygen delivery greater than 4 L/min
- Oxygen tubing available in lengths of 50 feet
- Home low-flow oxygen-delivery system with appropriate equipment

---

STEP	RATIONALE

ASSESSMENT

1. Identify patient using at least two identifiers (e.g., name and birthday or name and account number) according to agency policy. Compare identifiers with information on patient's MAR or medical record.

Ensures correct patient. Complies with The Joint Commission Standards and improves patient safety (TJC, 2020).

2. Review health care provider's order for home oxygen equipment.

A health care provider's order is required for home oxygen use.

3. Assess patient's or family caregiver's knowledge, experience, and health literacy.

Ensures patient or family caregiver has the capacity to obtain, communicate, process, and understand basic health information (CDC, 2019c).

4. While patient is still in the hospital, determine patient's or family caregiver's ability to use oxygen equipment correctly. In home setting, reassess for access to and appropriate use of equipment.

Physical or cognitive impairments necessitate instructing family member or significant other how to operate home oxygen equipment. Ongoing assessment enables you to determine specific components of skill that patient or family can complete easily.

5. Inform the patient/family caregiver that the home oxygen vendor will assess home environment for adequate electrical service if oxygen concentrator is ordered.

Oxygen concentrators require electricity to work. Continuous oxygen therapy must not be interrupted.

6. Assess patient's and family's knowledge of home oxygen use, their ability to understand safety precautions, and their ability to observe for signs and symptoms of hypoxia: apprehension, anxiety, decreased ability to concentrate, decreased level of consciousness, increased fatigue, dizziness, behavioral changes, increased pulse, increased respiratory rate, pallor, or cyanosis of the mucous membranes.

Hypoxia occurs at home despite use of oxygen therapy. Worsening of patient's physical condition or another underlying condition such as a change in the respiratory status can cause hypoxia.

PLANNING

1. Explain need for and use of home oxygen therapy.

Improves adherence to the treatment regimen. Decreases anxiety and the need for home oxygen.

2. Determine appropriate resources in community for equipment and assistance, including maintenance and repair services and medical equipment supplier.

Ensures readily available assistance for patients with home oxygen systems. Delivery and setup with basic instruction on how to use and maintain home oxygen equipment must be in accordance with federal, state, and local laws (CMS, 2017; Jacobs, 2018).

Continued

SKILL 41.4	USING HOME OXYGEN EQUIPMENT—cont'd

STEP	RATIONALE
3. Provide family resources to investigate municipal requirements for home medical equipment, especially oxygen.	Many municipalities require that patients with home oxygen equipment notify emergency medical service (EMS) before bringing equipment home. When there is a power outage, EMS calls the home, and in some cases the home is on a priority list for power restoration.
4. Obtain appropriate referrals to determine whether patient meets standards for third-party reimbursement.	Indications for home oxygen therapy include (1) a PaO_2 less than or equal to 55 mm Hg or SaO_2 less than or equal to 88% breathing room air; (2) PaO_2 less than or equal to 56-59 mm Hg or SaO_2 less than or equal to 89% with conditions such as cor pulmonale, heart failure, or hematocrit greater than 56%; or (3) oxygen therapy is needed during activities that cause hypoxia such as ambulation, sleep, or exercise causing an SaO_2 of less than or equal to 88% (CMS, 2017). Providing evidence of inclusion criteria is often necessary for third-party reimbursement.

IMPLEMENTATION

1. Perform hand hygiene.	Reduces transmission of infection.
2. Place oxygen-delivery system in clutter-free environment that is well ventilated; away from walls, drapes, bedding, and combustible materials; and at least 8 feet from heat source.	Prevents injury from improper placement of oxygen equipment (ATS, 2016).
3. Demonstrate each step for preparation and completion of oxygen therapy.	Teaches psychomotor skills and enables patient to ask questions. When patients and family caregivers are adequately informed about supplemental oxygen therapy, the patient's consistent use of the therapy is enhanced (Lewis et al., 2017).
a. **Compressed oxygen system**—available in large cylinders as stationary units or smaller, lightweight cylinders in carrying bags and/or wheel carts.	Smaller units are used for ambulation and as a backup of stationary unit if there is power failure or equipment malfunction (ATS, 2016).
(1) Turn cylinder valve counterclockwise two or three turns with wrench. Store wrench with oxygen tank.	Turns on oxygen. Keeps wrench available.
(2) Check cylinders by reading amount on pressure gauge. Store wrench in a safe place near the system.	Verifies adequate oxygen supply for patient use.
b. **Oxygen concentrator system**—available as stationary unit or portable device.	Extracts oxygen from other gases in atmospheric air (ATS, 2016).
(1) Plug concentrator into appropriate outlet.	Provides power source. Make sure that it is in an open area and never in a closet or other closed space
(2) Turn on power switch.	Starts concentrator motor.
(3) Alarm sounds for a few seconds.	Alarm turns off when desired pressure inside concentrator is reached.
c. **Liquid oxygen systems**—available in large-reservoir canisters that can be used to refill a smaller portable unit (ATS, 2016). Portable unit weighs around 11 pounds and can be carried with a shoulder strap or pulled on a cart.	When liquid oxygen is warmed, it goes from liquid to gas. More oxygen can be stored as a liquid than gas.
(1) Check liquid system by depressing button, often located in lower right corner, and reading dial on stationary oxygen reservoir or ambulatory tank.	Verifies amount of oxygen supply for patient use.
(2) Collaborate with durable medical equipment (DME) vendor to provide instruction in refilling ambulatory tank.	Ensures continuation of home oxygen therapy.
(3) Refill oxygen tank.	
(a) Wipe both filling connectors with clean, dry, lint-free cloth.	Removes dust and moisture from system.
(b) Turn off flow selector of ambulatory unit.	

STEP	**RATIONALE**
(c) Attach ambulatory unit to stationary reservoir by inserting adapter from ambulatory tank into adapter of stationary reservoir (see illustration).	
(d) Open fill valve on ambulatory tank and apply firm pressure to top of stationary reservoir. Stay with unit while it is filling. You will hear a loud hissing noise. Tank fills in about 2 minutes) (see illustration).	Prevents leaking of oxygen during filling process. If oxygen leaks during filling process, connection between ambulatory tank and reservoir ices up and valves stick together.
(e) Disconnect ambulatory unit from stationary reservoir when hissing noise changes and vapor cloud begins to form from stationary unit.	Overfilling causes ambulatory unit to malfunction, caused by high pressure in tank.

CLINICAL DECISION: *If ambulatory unit does not separate easily, valves from reservoir and ambulatory unit may be frozen together. Wait until valves warm to disengage (about 5 to 10 minutes). Do not touch any frosted areas because contact with skin causes skin damage from frostbite.*

STEP	**RATIONALE**
(f) Wipe both filling connectors with clean, dry, lint-free cloth.	Ice sometimes forms during filling. Removes moisture from oxygen system.
4. Connect oxygen-delivery device to oxygen system. (see illustration).	Connects oxygen source to delivery system.
5. Adjust to prescribed flow rate (L/min).	Ensures appropriate oxygen prescription.
6. Have patient or family caregiver apply oxygen-delivery device. Ensure that patient knows to have two sets of oxygen-delivery devices and tubing.	Verifies that patient or family caregiver can apply device. Extra set of equipment is necessary for cleaning or in case of equipment malfunction.
7. Instruct patient and family caregiver not to change oxygen flow rate.	Exceeding prescribed amount of oxygen is harmful in some patients, such as those with chronic obstructive pulmonary disease (COPD).
8. Guide patient and family caregiver as they perform each step. Provide written material for reinforcement and review.	Allows you to correct for errors in technique and discuss their implications.
9. Instruct patient and family caregiver to notify health care provider if signs or symptoms of hypoxia or respiratory tract infection (e.g., fever, increased sputum, change in color of sputum, or odor) occur.	Respiratory tract infections increase oxygen demand and affect oxygen transfer from lungs to blood. Can create severe exacerbation of patient's pulmonary disease.

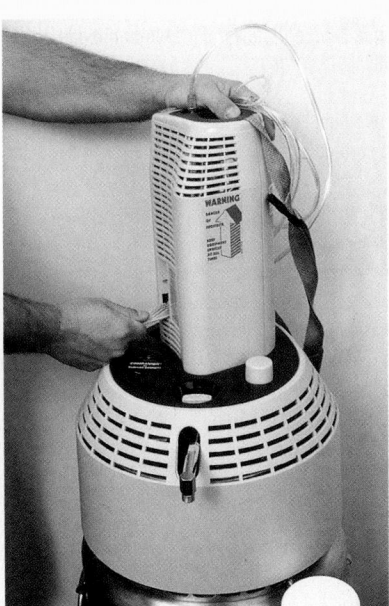
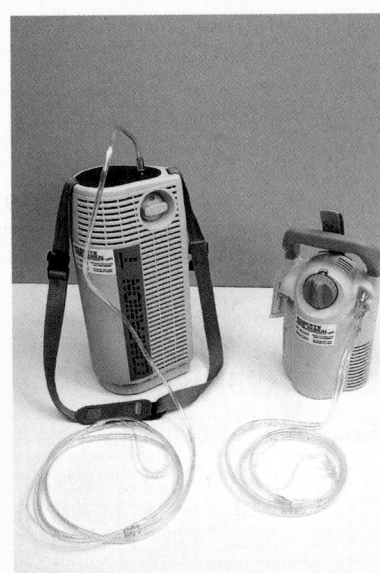

STEP 3c(3)(c) Top view of stationary reservoir.

STEP 3c(3)(d) Fill valve on ambulatory tank is opened while applying firm pressure to top of ambulatory unit.

STEP 4 Oxygen delivery device (nasal cannulas) and tubing attached to ambulatory oxygen tanks.

Ambulatory unit

Continued

SKILL 41.4 **USING HOME OXYGEN EQUIPMENT—cont'd**

STEP	RATIONALE
10. Discuss emergency plan for power loss, natural disaster, and acute respiratory distress. Have patient or family caregiver call 911 and notify health care provider and home care agency.	Ensures appropriate response and prevents worsening of patient's condition. Power companies will often work to supply power to houses requiring oxygen therapy first.
11. Instruct patient and family caregiver in safe home oxygen practices, including not allowing smoking in the house, keeping oxygen tanks away from open flame, and storing tanks upright.	Ensures safe use of oxygen in the home and prevents injury to patient and family.
12. Instruct patient and family caregiver that home oxygen-delivery equipment must be maintained and serviced routinely according to manufacturer's guidelines (CMS, 2017).	Routine maintenance ensures proper function of equipment.

EVALUATION

1. During each home visit monitor oxygen delivery rate.	Verifies whether patient or family caregiver is using oxygen at prescribed rate.
2. Ask patient and family caregiver about any problems or concerns with the home oxygen equipment.	Determines whether patient and family caregivers are able to safely use the equipment and solve minor problems.
3. Ask patient and family about ease of administering or any problems with the home oxygen delivery system.	Determines ability of patient and family to deal with stressors associated with home oxygen use.
4. Ask patient and family caregiver to state safety guidelines, emergency precautions, and emergency plan.	Determines patient's knowledge of what to do if power fails, if equipment fails, or if patient's status worsens.
5. **Use Teach-Back:** "I want to be sure I explained how to administer and use the home oxygen equipment. Show me how to apply your nasal cannula and regulate the oxygen source." Revise your instruction now or develop a plan for revised patient/family caregiver teaching if patient/family caregiver is not able to teach back correctly.	Determines patient's/family caregiver's level of understanding of instructional topic.

UNEXPECTED OUTCOMES AND RELATED INTERVENTIONS

1. Patient reports no oxygen flow.
   - Check tank pressure gauge. If level of oxygen is low, refill tank if portable or provide alternate source of oxygen such as concentrator.
   - Notify home oxygen supplier of need for refill.
   - Reassure patient and family.
2. Patient or family caregiver is unable to fill portable liquid oxygen from main source.
   - Check to see that portable tank is connected correctly.
   - Determine whether valve is frozen.
   - Contact home oxygen supplier for service visit.
   - Provide alternate oxygen source if necessary.

RECORDING AND REPORTING

- Record teaching plan and describe patient's and family caregiver's ability to safely use home oxygen equipment.
- Record type of home oxygen equipment being used and oxygen flow rate, knowledge of safety guidelines, how to use equipment, unexpected outcomes to observe, and ability to return demonstrate proper use of oxygen-delivery device.

HOME CARE CONSIDERATIONS

- Ensure emergency numbers are programmed into a phone or are readily available for use in case of an emergency. These numbers include health care provider, supplier of medical equipment, and utility company.
- Power companies should be notified of homes in which there are patients receiving home oxygen. In the event of a power outage, these homes would be the priority for receiving power.

KEY POINTS

- Cardiopulmonary system consists of heart, lungs, airways, and blood vessels. They function to provide and deliver oxygen to the tissues and to remove carbon dioxide from the body.
- Ventilation, diffusion, respiration, and perfusion are processes for providing adequate oxygenation from the alveoli to the blood.
- Cardiac output is determined by the patient's heart rate, strength of contraction, amount of blood in the ventricle, and amount of resistance the heart has to overcome to eject the blood.
- Myocardial blood flow is the path the blood takes to perfuse the muscles of the heart.
- Systemic circulation allows for the perfusion of tissues, delivering oxygen to the tissues and taking carbon dioxide and other waste substances away from the tissues.
- Patients with decreased cardiac output have difficulties in delivering oxygen to the tissues.
- Patients who are hypoxic are at risk for decreased cardiac output.
- Altered level of consciousness, tachypnea, dyspnea, and anxiety are all signs of hypoxemia.
- Electrical disturbances, dysrhythmias, and mechanical dysfunction of the heart (impaired valve function) can lead to decreased cardiac output, leading to decreased delivery of oxygen to the tissues.
- Myocardial ischemia can damage the cardiac muscle, thereby decreasing cardiac output, which leads to decreased oxygen delivery to the tissues.
- Decreased hemoglobin levels, seen in patients with anemia or blood loss, alter a patient's ability to transport oxygen, causing disturbances in oxygenation.
- Age (both young and the elderly), nutritional intake, hydration status, level of exercise, exposure to smoke or other environmental pollutants, and stress can all have a negative impact on a patient's oxygenation status.

- Nurses and health care providers should ask patients about their risk factors for altered oxygenation, such as smoking history, substance abuse, exposure to pollutants and environmental substances, exercise patterns, diet patterns, and other chronic illnesses.
- Nursing assessment includes respiratory rate and pattern, presence of cough and/or secretions, fatigue, dyspnea, wheezing, chest pain, oxygen saturation, VS, and signs of respiratory infection.
- Assess for signs of chronic hypoxemia, such as clubbed fingers or barrel chest.
- Nursing plan of care should include positioning, medication administration, oxygen administration, respiratory muscle training, and airway suctioning.
- Oxygen therapy, either by nasal cannula, mask or mechanical ventilation, helps to improve tissue oxygenation by increasing the amount of oxygen available to the patient.
- Breathing exercises, such as diaphragmatic breathing and pursed-lip breathing, benefit patients with chronic pulmonary disease.
- Chest physiotherapy is reserved for use in patients with thick secretions to help them mobilize those secretions.
- Vaccinations, smoking-cessation programs, exercise programs, and nutritional support are health promotion strategies to utilize when working with patients and their families.
- Mobilization of secretions through positioning and adequate hydration helps to maintain the airway.
- Suctioning may be necessary to maintain airway patency in patients who have difficulties in maintaining their own airway.
- Artificial airways may be used in patients who cannot maintain their own airway.
- Assess breath sounds, SpO_2 levels, breathing rate and patterns, activity tolerance, level of fatigue, and ability to maintain airway to determine a patient's response to therapies.

REFLECTIVE LEARNING

- Consider a patient experience you have had. What clinical assessments did you find that indicated the patient had a disturbance in oxygenation?
- Reflect upon past clinical experiences in which your patient was receiving therapy for a disturbance in oxygenation. What therapies were the health care providers prescribing for that patient, and how did the patient respond to the therapies?

- Think about a patient with a disturbance in oxygenation that you have cared for during your clinical experience. How did you know that your interventions were working and that the patient was progressing toward meeting his or her expected outcomes? What would you have done if the patient were not making progress toward those outcomes?

REVIEW QUESTIONS

1. The nurse is preparing to perform nasotracheal suctioning on a patient. Arrange the steps in order.
   1. Apply suction.
   2. Assist patient to semi-Fowler's or high Fowler's position, if able.
   3. Advance catheter through nares and into trachea.
   4. Have patient take deep breaths.
   5. Lubricate catheter with water-soluble lubricant.
   6. Apply sterile gloves.
   7. Perform hand hygiene.
   8. Withdraw catheter.
2. Which skills can the nurse delegate to assistive personnel (AP)? (Select all that apply.)

   1. Initiate oxygen therapy via nasal cannula.
   2. Perform nasotracheal suctioning of a patient.
   3. Educate the patient about the use of an incentive spirometer.
   4. Assist with care of an established tracheostomy tube.
   5. Reposition a patient with a chest tube.
3. The nurse is caring for a patient with pneumonia. On entering the room, the nurse finds the patient lying in bed, coughing, and unable to clear secretions. What should the nurse do first?
   1. Start oxygen at 2 L/min via nasal cannula.
   2. Elevate the head of the bed to 45 degrees.
   3. Encourage the patient to use the incentive spirometer.
   4. Notify the health care provider.

4. The nurse is performing discharge teaching for a patient with chronic obstructive pulmonary disease (COPD). What statement, made by the patient, indicates the need for further teaching?
   1. "Pursed-lip breathing is like exercise for my lungs and will help me strengthen my breathing muscles."
   2. "When I am sick, I should limit the amount of fluids I drink so that I don't produce excess mucus."
   3. "I will ensure that I receive an influenza vaccine every year, preferably in the fall."
   4. "I will look for a smoking-cessation support group in my neighborhood."

5. Which assessment findings indicate that the patient is experiencing an acute disturbance in oxygenation and requires immediate intervention? (Select all that apply.)
   1. SpO_2 value of 95%
   2. Retractions
   3. Respiratory rate of 28 breaths per minute
   4. Nasal flaring
   5. Clubbing of fingers

6. The nurse is caring for a patient with an artificial airway. What are reasons to suction the patient? (Select all that apply.)
   1. The patient has visible secretions in the airway.
   2. There is a sawtooth pattern on the patient's E_tCO_2 monitor.
   3. The patient has clear breath sounds.
   4. It has been 3 hours since the patient was last suctioned.
   5. The patient has excessive coughing.

7. The nurse is caring for a patient with a chest tube for treatment of a right pneumothorax. Which assessment finding necessitates immediate notification of the health care provider?
   1. New, vigorous bubbling in the water seal chamber.
   2. Scant amount of sanguineous drainage noted on the dressing.
   3. Clear but slightly diminished breath sounds on the right side of the chest.
   4. Pain score of 2 one hour after the administration of the prescribed analgesic.

8. The nurse has just witnessed her patient go into cardiac arrest. What priority interventions should the nurse perform at this time? (Select all that apply.)
   1. Perform chest compressions.

2. Ask someone to bring the defibrillator to the room for immediate defibrillation.
   3. Apply oxygen via nasal cannula.
   4. Place the patient in the high Fowler's position.
   5. Educate the family about the need for CPR.

9. The nurse is performing tracheostomy care on a patient. What finding would indicate that the tracheostomy tube has become dislodged?
   1. Clear breath sounds
   2. Patient speaking to nurse
   3. SpO_2 reading of 96%
   4. Respiratory rate of 18 breaths/minute

10. Which number corresponds to the spot where you would assess for an air leak in the patient with a chest tube?

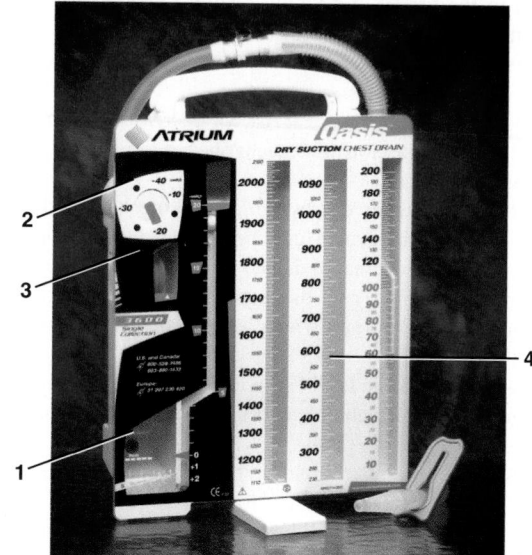

(Courtesy Atrium Medical Corp.)

Rationales for Review Questions can be found on the Evolve website.

REFERENCES

Agency for Toxic Substances and Disease Registry (ATSDR): *Environmental triggers of asthma*, 2016. https://www.atsdr.cdc.gov/csem/csem.asp?csem=32&po=6. Accessed June 21, 2019.

Ahmadi SH, et al.: Comparing the effect of resistive inspiratory muscle training and incentive spirometry on respiratory pattern of COPD patients, *Evid Based Care* 6(3):45, 2016.

American Association of Critical Care Nurses (AACN): *AACN practice alert: prevention of aspiration*, update 2018. http://www.aacn.org/wd/practice/content/practicealerts/aspiration-practice-alert.pcms?menu=practice. Accessed June 21, 2019.

American Association of Critical Care Nurses (AACN): AACN practice alert: oral care for acutely and critically ill patients, *Crit Care Nurse* 37(3):e19, 2017a.

American Association of Critical Care Nurses (AACN): *AACN practice alert: prevention of ventilator-associated pneumonia in adults*, 2017b. https://www.aacn.org/clinical-resources/practice-alerts/ventilator-associated-pneumonia-vap. Accessed January 2019.

American Association of Respiratory Care (AARC): AARC clinical practice guideline, nasotracheal suctioning—2004 revision and update, *Respir Care* 49:1080, 2004.

American Association of Respiratory Care (AARC): AARC clinical practice guideline, oxygen therapy in the home or alternate site health care facility—2007 revision and update, *Respir Care* 52(1):1063, 2007.

American Association of Respiratory Care (AARC): AARC clinical practice guideline, endotracheal suctioning of mechanically ventilated patients with artificial airways—2010 update, *Respir Care* 55(60):758, 2010a.

American Association of Respiratory Care (AARC): AARC clinical practice guideline, providing patient and caregiver training—2010, *Respir Care* 55:765, 2010b.

American Association of Respiratory Care (AARC): Clinical practice guideline: incentive spirometry, *Respir Care* 56(10):1600, 2011.

American Cancer Society (ACS): *Prescription drugs to help you quit tobacco*, 2017. https://www.cancer.org/healthy/stay-away-from-tobacco/guide-quitting-smoking/prescription-drugs-to-help-you-quit-smoking.html. Accessed June 21, 2019.

American Cancer Society (ACS): *Health risks of smoking tobacco*, 2018. https://www.cancer.org/cancer/cancer-causes/tobacco-and-cancer/health-risks-of-smoking-tobacco.html. Accessed June 21, 2019.

American Heart Association (AHA): *Cardiac arrest survival greatly increases when bystanders use an automated external defibrillator*, 2018. http://newsroom.heart.org/news/cardiac-arrest-survival-greatly-increases-when-bystanders-use-an-automated-external-defibrillator. Accessed June 21, 2019.

American Heart Association (AHA): *Highlights of the 2015 American heart association guidelines update for CPR and ECC*, 2015. http://eccguidelines.heart.org/wp-content/uploads/2015/10/2015-AHA-Guidelines-Highlights-English.pdf. Accessed June 21, 2019.

American Lung Association (ALA): *Health effects of secondhand smoke*, 2019a. https://www.lung.org/stop-smoking/smoking-facts/health-effects-of-secondhand-smoke.html. Accessed June 21, 2019.

American Lung Association (ALA): *Current cigarette smoking comparisons and disparities*, 2019b. https://www.lung.org/our-initiatives/research/monitoring-trends-in-lung-disease/tobacco-trend-brief/current-smoking-comparisons.html. Accessed June 21, 2019.

American Thoracic Society (ATS): *Oxygen therapy*, update 2016. http://www.thoracic.org/patients/patient-resources/resources/oxygen-therapy.pdf. Accessed June 21, 2019.

Atkins JR, Kautz DD: Move to improve: progressive mobility in the intensive care unit, *Dimens Crit Care Nurs* 33(5):275, 2014.

Atrium: *Evidence-based care of patients with chest tubes*, NH, 2015, Hudson. http://www.atriummed.com/EN/chest_drainage/Documents/NTI-2015Evidence-BasedCareofPatientswithChestTubes.pdf. Accessed June 21, 2019.

Ball J, et al.: *Seidel's guide to physical examination*, ed 9, St Louis, 2019, Elsevier.

Branson RD, et al.: Management of the artificial airway, *Respir Care* 59(6):974, 2014.

Cedar SH: Every breath you take: the process of breathing explained, *Nurs Times* 114(1):47, 2018.

Centers for Disease Control and Prevention (CDC): *Women and heart disease*, 2019a. https://www.cdc.gov/heartdisease/women.htm. Accessed June 21, 2019.

Centers for Disease Control and Prevention (CDC): *Valley fever: coccidiomycosis*, 2019b. https://www.cdc.gov/fungal/diseases/coccidioidomycosis/index.html. Accessed June 21, 2019.

Centers for Disease Control and Prevention (CDC): *What is health literacy*, 2019c. https://www.cdc.gov/healthliteracy/learn/index.html. Accessed December 23, 2019.

Centers for Disease Control and Prevention (CDC): Tuberculosis – United States, 2018, *MMWR Morb Mortal Wkly Rep* 68(11):257, 2019c.

Centers for Disease Control and Prevention (CDC): Quitting smoking among adults – 2000-2015, *MMWR Morb Mortal Wkly Rep* 65(52):1457, 2017a.

Centers for Disease Control and Prevention (CDC): *Pneumococcal vaccination: what everyone should know*, 2017b. https://www.cdc.gov/vaccines/vpd/pneumo/public/index.html. Accessed January 2019.

Centers for Disease Control and Prevention (CDC): Current cigarette smoking among adults — United States, 2016, *MMWR Morb Mortal Wkly Rep* 67(2):53, 2018a.

Centers for Disease Control and Prevention (CDC): Tobacco product use among middle and high school students — United States, 2011–2017, *MMWR Morb Mortal Wkly Rep* 67(22):893, 2018b.

Centers for Disease Control and Prevention (CDC): *How does smoking during pregnancy harm my health and my baby?* 2018c. https://www.cdc.gov/reproductivehealth/maternalinfanthealth/tobaccousepregnancy/index.htm. Accessed June 21, 2019.

Centers for Disease Control and Prevention (CDC): *Carbon monoxide poisoning*, 2018d. https://www.cdc.gov/co/faqs.htm. Accessed June 21, 2019.

Centers for Disease Control and Prevention (CDC): *Vaccinations: who should do it, who should not, and who should take precautions*, 2018e. https://www.cdc.gov/flu/protect/whoshouldvax.htm. Accessed June 21, 2019.

Centers for Disease Control and Prevention (CDC): *Urban-rural differences in chronic obstructive pulmonary disease (COPD)*, 2018f. https://www.cdc.gov/ruralhealth/copd/index.html. Accessed June 21, 2019.

Centers for Disease Control and Prevention (CDC): *Tuberculosis: who should be tested*, 2016a. https://www.cdc.gov/tb/topic/testing/whobetested.htm. Accessed June 21, 2019.

Centers for Disease Control and Prevention (CDC): *Tuberculosis*, 2016b. https://www.cdc.gov/tb/topic/basics/default.htm. Accessed June 21, 2019.

Centers for Medicare and Medicaid Services (CMS): *Home oxygen therapy*, 2017. https://www.cms.gov/Outreach-and-Education/Medicare-Learning-Network-MLN/MLNProducts/Downloads/Home-Oxygen-Therapy-Text-Only.pdf. Accessed June 21, 2019.

Chotai P, Mosenifar Z: *Tube thoracostomy management*, 2018. https://emedicine.medscape.com/article/1503275-overview. Accessed June 21, 2019.

COPD Foundation: *Breathing exercises and techniques*, 2019. https://www.copdfoundation.org/Learn-More/I-am-a-Person-with-COPD/Breathing-Techniques.aspx. Accessed June 21, 2019.

Cystic Fibrosis Foundation (CFF): *Basics of postural drainage and percussion*, n.d. https://www.cff.org/Life-With-CF/Treatments-and-Therapies/Airway-Clearance/Basics-of-Postural-Drainage-and-Percussion/. Accessed June 21, 2019.

Cystic Fibrosis Foundation (CFF): *Coughing and huffing*, 2015a. https://www.cff.org/Life-With-CF/Treatments-and-Therapies/Airway-Clearance/Coughing-and-Huffing/. Accessed June 21, 2019.

Cystic Fibrosis Foundation (CFF): *Positive expiratory pressure*, 2015b. https://www.cff.org/Life-With-CF/Treatments-and-Therapies/Airway-Clearance/Positive-Expiratory-Pressure/. Accessed June 21, 2019.

do Nascimento P, et al.: Incentive spirometry for prevention of post-operative pulmonary complication in upper abdominal surgery, *Cochrane Database Syst Rev* 2:CD006058, 2014.

Environmental Protection Agency (EPA): *A citizen's guide to radon: the guide to protecting yourself and your family*, 2016. https://www.epa.gov/sites/production/files/2016-12/documents/2016_a_citizens_guide_to_radon.pdf. Accessed June 21, 2019.

Franks LJ, et al.: Comparing the performance characteristics of different positive expiratory pressure devices, *Respir Care* 64(4):434, 2019.

Galbiati G, Paola C: Effects of open and closed endotracheal suctioning on intracranial pressure and cerebral perfusion pressure in adult patients with severe brain injury: a literature review, *J Neurosci Nurs* 47(4):239, 2015.

Grindrod K: Management of stable chronic obstructive pulmonary disease, *Br J Community Nurs* 20(2):58, 2015.

Gross SL, et al.: Comparison of three practices for dressing chest tube insertion sites: a randomized controlled trial, *MedSurg Nurs* 25(4):229, 2016.

Hanlon P: *Physiological effects of humidification*, 2016. http://www.rtmagazine.com/2016/04/physiological-effects-humidification. Accessed June 21, 2019.

Hartjes TM: *AACN core curriculum for high acuity, progressive, and critical care nursing*, ed 7, St Louis, 2018, Elsevier.

Higginson R, et al.: Airway management in the hospital environment, *Br J Nurs* 25(2):94, 2016.

Hockenberry MJ, et al.: *Wong's nursing care of infants and children*, ed 11, St Louis, 2019, Elsevier.

Intensive Care Society (ICS): *Standards for the care of adult patients with a temporary tracheostomy*, 2018. http://ics.ac.uk/GuidelinesAndStandards/ICSuidelines.aspx. Accessed September 2019.

Jacobs SS, et al.: Optimizing home oxygen therapy: an official American Thoracic Society workshop report, *Ann Am Thorac Soc* 15(12):1369, 2018.

Larrow V, Klich-Heartt EI: Prevention of ventilator-associated pneumonia in the intensive care unit: beyond the basics, *J Neurosci Nurs* 48(3):160, 2016.

Letchford E, Bench S: Ventilator-associated pneumonia and suction: a review of the literature, *Br J Nurs* 27(1):13, 2018.

Lewis SL, et al.: *Medical surgical nursing, assessment and management of clinical problems*, ed 10, St Louis, 2017, Mosby.

Link M, et al.: Part 7: Adult advanced cardiovascular life support: 2015 American Heart Association guidelines update for cardiopulmonary resuscitation and emergency cardiovascular care, *Circulation* 132(18 Suppl 2):s444, 2015.

Makic MBF, et al.: Continuing to challenge practice to be evidence based, *Crit Care Nurse* 35(2):39, 2015.

Mao M, et al.: Complications of chest tubes: a focused clinical synopsis, *Curr Opin Pulm Med* 21(4):376, 2015.

McCance KL, Huether SE: *Pathophysiology: the biologic basis for disease in adults and children*, ed 8, St Louis, 2019, Mosby Elsevier.

Menzes KKP, et al.: A review on respiratory muscle training devices, *J Pulm Respir Med* 8(2):451, 2018.

Munro N, Ruggiero M: Ventilator-associated pneumonia bundle reconstruction for best care, *AACN Adv Crit Care* 25(2):163, 2014.

Muzzy AC, Butler AK: Managing chest tubes: air leaks and unplanned tube removal, *American Nurse Today* 10(5), 2015. https://www.americannursetoday.com/managing-chest-tubes-air-leaks-unplanned-tube-removal/. Accessed June 21, 2019.

Myatt R: Nursing care of patient with a temporary tracheostomy, *Nurs Stand* 29(26):42, 2015.

National Cancer Institute (NCI): *Secondhand smoke and cancer*, 2018. https://www.cancer.gov/about-cancer/causes-prevention/risk/tobacco/second-hand-smoke-fact-sheet. Accessed June 21, 2019.

National Heart Lung and Blood Institute (NHLBI): *DASH eating plan*, n.d.a National Institutes of Health. https://www.nhlbi.nih.gov/health-topics/dash-eating-plan. Accessed June 21, 2019.

National Heart Lung and Blood Institute (NHLBI): *Defibrillators*, n.d.b National Institutes of Health. https://www.nhlbi.nih.gov/health-topics/defibrillators. Accessed June 21, 2019.

National Institute on Drug Abuse (NIDA): *DrugFacts: marijuana*, National Institutes of Health, 2018a. http://www.drugabuse.gov/publications/drugfacts/marijuana. Accessed June 21, 2019.

National Institute on Drug Abuse (NIDA): *DrugFacts: cocaine*, National Institutes of Health, 2018b. http://www.drugabuse.gov/publications/drugfacts/cocaine. Accessed June 21, 2019.

National Institute on Drug Abuse (NIDA): *DrugFacts: inhalants*, National Institutes of Health, 2017. https://www.drugabuse.gov/publications/drugfacts/inhalants. Accessed June 21, 2019.

Neumar RW, et al.: Part 1: Executive summary 2015 American Heart Association guidelines update for cardiopulmonary resuscitation and emergency cardiovascular care, *Circulation* 132(18 Suppl 2):S315, 2015.

Pittman J, et al.: Medical device-related hospital-acquired pressure ulcers, *J Wound Ostomy Continence Nurs* 42(2):151, 2015.

Rouzé A, et al.: Tracheal tube design and ventilator-associated pneumonia, *Respir Care* 62(10):1316, 2017.

Seo Y, et al.: A home-based diaphragmatic breathing retraining in rural patients with heart failure, *West J Nurs Res* 38(3):270, 2016.

Smith SG, Pietrantonio T: Best method for securing an endotracheal tube, *Crit Care Nurs* 36(2):78, 2016.

Sole ML, et al.: Clinical indicators for endotracheal suctioning in adult patients receiving mechanical ventilation, *Am J Crit Care* 24(4):318, 2015.

Strait JB, Lakatta EG: Aging-associated cardiovascular changes and their relationship to heart failure, *Heart Fail Clin*, 8(1):143, 2012.

Strickland SL: Year in review 2014: Airway clearance, *Respir Care* 60(4):603, 2015.

Strickland SL, et al.: AARC clinical practice guideline: effectiveness of nonpharmacologic airway clearance techniques in hospitalized patients, *Respir Care* 58(12):2187, 2013.

The Joint Commission (TJC): *2020 National Patient Safety Goals*, Oakbrook Terrace, IL, 2020, The Commission. http://www.jointcommission.org/en/standards/national-patient-safety-goals/. Accessed January 2, 2020.

Touhy T, Jett K: *Gerontological nursing and healthy aging*, ed 5, St Louis, 2018, Elsevier.

US Department of Health and Human Services (USDHHS): *Physical activity guidelines for Americans*, ed 2, 2018. https://health.gov/paguidelines/second-edition/pdf/Physical_Activity_Guidelines_2nd_edition.pdf. Accessed June 21, 2019.

Urden LD, et al.: *Priorities in critical care nursing*, ed 8, St Louis, 2020, Elsevier.

Walsh BK, Smallwood CD: Pediatric oxygen therapy: a review and update, *Resp Care* 62(6):645, 2017.

Wiegand D: *AACN procedure manual for high acuity, progressive, and critical care*, ed 7, St Louis, 2017, Elsevier.

Zardo P, et al.: Chest tube management: state of the art, *Curr Opin Anesthesiol* 28(1):45, 2015.

Zisis C, et al.: Chest drainage systems in use, *Ann Transl Med* 3(3):43, 2015.

RESEARCH REFERENCES

Anand T, et al.: Results from a quality improvement project to decrease infection-related ventilator events in trauma patients at a community teaching hospital, *Am Surg* 84(10):1701, 2018.

Bassi GL, et al.: Prevention of ventilator-associated pneumonia, *Curr Opin Infect Dis* 30(2):214, 2017.

Borge CR, et al.: Effects of controlled breathing exercises and respiratory muscle training in people with chronic obstructive pulmonary disease: results from evaluating the quality of evidence in systematic reviews, *BMC Pulm Med* 14:184, 2014.

Cabral LF, et al.: Pursed lip breathing improves exercise tolerance in COPD: a randomized crossover study, *Eur J Phys Rehabil Med* 51(1):79, 2015.

Celedon JC, et al.: An American Thoracic Society/National Heart, Lung, and Blood Institute workshop report: addressing respiratory health equality in the United States, *Ann Am Thorac Soc* 14(5):814, 2017.

Chacko R, et al.: Oral decontamination techniques and ventilator-associated pneumonia, *Br J Nurs* 26(11):594, 2017.

Chahoud J, et al.: Ventilator-associated events prevention, learning lessons from the past: a systematic review, *Heart Lung* 44(3):251, 2015.

Chatwin M, et al.: Airway clearance techniques in neuromuscular disorders: a state of the art review, *Respir Med* 136:98, 2018.

Elliott S, Morrell-Scott N: Care of patients undergoing weaning from mechanical ventilation in critical care, *Nurs Stand* 32(13):41, 2017.

Eltorai AE, et al.: Perspectives on incentive spirometry utility and patient protocols, *Respir Care* 63(5):519, 2018.

Franchini ML, et al.: Oxygen with cold bubble humidification is no better than dry oxygen in preventing mucus dehydration, decreased mucociliary clearance, and decline in pulmonary function, *Chest* 150(2):407, 2016.

Gale NK, et al.: Adapting to domiciliary non-invasive ventilation in chronic obstructive pulmonary disease: a qualitative interview study, *Palliat Med* 29(3):268, 2015.

Hortal MCR, et al.: Non-invasive ventilation as airway clearance technique in cystic fibrosis, *Physiother Res Int* 22(2017):e1667, 2016.

Hua F, et al: Oral hygiene care for critically ill patients to prevent ventilator-associated pneumonia, *Cochrane Database Syst Rev* (8):CD008367, update 2016. https://www.cochranelibrary.com/cdsr/doi/10.1002/14651858.CD008367.pub3/full. Accessed June 21, 2019.

Institute for Healthcare Improvement (IHI): *Implement the IHI ventilator bundle*, 2012. http://www.ihi.org/resources/Pages/Tools/HowtoGuidePreventVAP.aspx. Accessed June 21, 2019.

Kram SL, et al.: Implementation of the ABCDE bundle to improve patient outcomes in the intensive care unit in a rural community hospital, *Dimens Crit Care Nurs* 34(5):250, 2015.

Li J, et al.: Evaluation of the safety and effectiveness of the rapid flow expulsion maneuver to clear subglottic secretions in vitro and in vivo, *Resp Care* 62(8):1007, 2017.

Morrow B, et al.: The effect of positioning and diaphragmatic breathing exercises on respiratory muscle activity in people with chronic obstructive pulmonary disease, *S Afr J Physiother* 72(1):315, 2016.

Nuwi D, Irwan AM: Effect of active mobilization on patients in the intensive care unit: a systematic review, *Int J Caring Sci* 11(3):1942, 2018.

Schallom M, et al.: Pressure ulcer incidence in patients wearing nasal-oral versus full-face noninvasive ventilation masks, *Am J Crit Care* 24(4):349, 2015.

Wang CH, et al.: Normal saline instillation before suctioning: a meta-analysis of randomized controlled trials, *Aust Crit Care* 30(5):260, 2017.

Wen Z, et al.: Is humidified better than non-humidified low-flow oxygen therapy? A systematic review and meta-analysis, *J Adv Nurs* 73(11):2522, 2017.

Xu H, et al.: Effect of CPAP on endothelial function in subjects with obstructive sleep apnea: a meta-analysis, *Resp Care* 60(5):749, 2015.

Xu Z, et al.: High-flow nasal cannula in adults with acute respiratory failure and after extubation: a systematic review and meta-analysis, *Respir Res* 19(1):202, 2018.

Fluid, Electrolyte, and Acid-Base Balance

OBJECTIVES

- Describe processes that regulate fluid distribution, extracellular fluid volume, and body fluid osmolality.
- Describe processes that regulate electrolyte balance.
- Describe processes that regulate acid-base balance.
- Describe common fluid, electrolyte, and acid-base imbalances.
- Identify risk factors for fluid, electrolyte, and acid-base imbalances.
- Apply the nursing process when caring for patients with fluid, electrolyte, and acid-base imbalances.
- Choose appropriate clinical assessments for specific fluid, electrolyte, and acid-base imbalances.
- Describe purpose and procedures for measuring and recording daily weights and fluid intake and output.
- Explain rationale and procedures for initiating an intravenous line; maintaining the system; changing intravenous solution containers, tubing, and dressings; and discontinuing peripheral venous access.
- Describe potential complications of intravenous therapy and what to do if they occur.
- Discuss the procedure for initiating and monitoring a blood transfusion and the appropriate nursing actions to take if transfusion reactions occur.
- Identify how to evaluate the outcomes of care of patients with fluid, electrolyte, and acid-base imbalances.

KEY TERMS

Acidosis, p. 989
Alkalosis, p. 989
Anion gap, p. 989
Arterial blood gases (ABGs), p. 988
Autologous transfusion, p. 1008
Buffers, p. 988
Colloid osmotic pressure, p. 981
Colloids, p. 981
Crystalloids, p. 999
Extracellular fluid (ECF), p. 980
Extracellular volume deficit (ECV deficit), p. 984
Extracellular volume excess (ECV excess), p. 984
Extravasation, p. 1005
Filtration, p. 981

Fluid, p. 980
Hydrostatic pressure, p. 981
Hypercalcemia, p. 986
Hyperkalemia, p. 986
Hypermagnesemia, p. 986
Hypernatremia, p. 984
Hypertonic, p. 980
Hypocalcemia, p. 986
Hypokalemia, p. 985
Hypomagnesemia, p. 986
Hyponatremia, p. 984
Hypotonic, p. 980
Hypovolemia, p. 984
Infiltration, p. 1005
Interstitial fluid, p. 980
Intracellular fluid (ICF), p. 980

Intravascular fluid, p. 980
Isotonic, p. 980
Metabolic acidosis, p. 989
Metabolic alkalosis, p. 989
Oncotic pressure, p. 981
Osmolality, p. 980
Osmosis, p. 981
Osmotic pressure, p. 981
Phlebitis, p. 1005
Respiratory acidosis, p. 989
Respiratory alkalosis, p. 989
Transfusion reaction, p. 1007
Vascular access devices (VADs), p. 1001
Venipuncture, p. 1002

MEDIA RESOURCES

http://evolve.elsevier.com/Potter/fundamentals/
- Review Questions
- Video Clips
- Case Study with Questions
- Skills Performance Checklists

- Audio Glossary
- Butterfield's Fluids and Electrolytes Tutorial
- Content Updates
- Answers to QSEN Activity and Review Questions

Fluid is inside and surrounds all the cells in the body. Cellular fluids contain electrolytes such as sodium and potassium and also have a degree of acidity. Fluid, electrolyte, and acid-base balances within the body maintain the health and function of all body systems. The characteristics of body fluids influence body system function because of their effects on cell function. These characteristics include the fluid amount (volume), concentration (osmolality), composition (electrolyte concentration), and degree of acidity (pH). All of these characteristics have regulatory mechanisms that keep them in balance for normal cellular function. It is important to understand how the body normally maintains fluid, electrolyte, and acid-base balance. You also need to understand how imbalances develop; how various fluid, electrolyte, and acid-base imbalances affect patients; and ways to help patients maintain or restore balance safely.

SCIENTIFIC KNOWLEDGE BASE

This section provides the foundation of scientific knowledge for your critical thinking regarding patients who have or are at risk of having fluid, electrolyte, or acid-base imbalances.

Location and Movement of Water and Electrolytes

Water is a substantial proportion of body weight. In fact, about 60% of the body weight of an adult man is water. This proportion decreases with age; approximately 50% of an older man's weight is water. Women typically have less water content than men. People who are obese have less water in their bodies than people who are lean because fat contains less water than muscle (Hall, 2016). The term fluid means water that contains dissolved or suspended substances such as glucose, mineral salts, and proteins.

Fluid Distribution. Body fluids are located in two distinct compartments: extracellular fluid (ECF) outside the cells and intracellular fluid (ICF) inside the cells (Fig. 42.1). In adults ICF is approximately two-thirds of total body water. ECF is approximately one-third of total body water. ECF has two major divisions (intravascular fluid and interstitial fluid) and a minor division (transcellular fluids). Intravascular fluid is the liquid part of the blood (i.e., the plasma). Interstitial fluid is located between the cells and outside the blood vessels. Transcellular fluids such as cerebrospinal, pleural, peritoneal, and synovial fluids are secreted by epithelial cells (Hall, 2016).

Composition of Body Fluids. Fluid in the body compartments contains mineral salts known technically as electrolytes. An electrolyte is a compound that separates into ions (charged particles) when it dissolves in water. Ions that are positively charged are called cations; ions that are negatively charged are called anions. Cations in body fluids are sodium (Na^+), potassium (K^+), calcium (Ca^{2+}), and magnesium ions (Mg^{2+}). Anions in body fluids are chloride (Cl^-) and bicarbonate (HCO_3^-). Anions and cations combine to make salts. If you put table salt (NaCl)

in water, it separates into Na^+ and Cl^-. Other combinations of anions and cations do the same. Clinical laboratories usually report electrolyte measurements in milliequivalents per liter (mEq/L) or millimoles per liter (mmol/L), which are two different units of concentration (Table 42.1). Millimoles per liter represent the number of milligrams of the electrolyte divided by its molecular weight that are contained in a liter of the fluid being measured (usually blood plasma or serum). Milliequivalents per liter are the millimoles per liter multiplied by the electrolyte charge (e.g., 1 for Na^+, 2 for Ca^{2+}). One milliequivalent of one electrolyte can combine with one milliequivalent of another electrolyte, which is why this measurement unit is used.

Fluid that contains a large number of dissolved particles is more concentrated than the same amount of fluid that contains only a few particles. Osmolality of a fluid is a measure of the number of particles per kilogram of water. Some particles (e.g., urea) pass easily through cell membranes; others such as Na^+ cannot cross easily. The particles that cannot cross cell membranes easily determine the tonicity (effective concentration) of a fluid. A fluid with the same tonicity as normal blood is called isotonic. A hypotonic solution is more dilute than the blood, and a hypertonic solution is more concentrated than normal blood (Fig. 42.2).

Movement of Water and Electrolytes. Active transport, diffusion, osmosis, and filtration are processes that move water and electrolytes between body compartments. These processes maintain equal osmolality in all compartments while allowing for different electrolyte concentrations.

Active Transport. Fluids in different body compartments have different concentrations of electrolytes that are necessary for normal function. For example, concentrations of Na^+, Cl^-, and HCO_3^- are higher

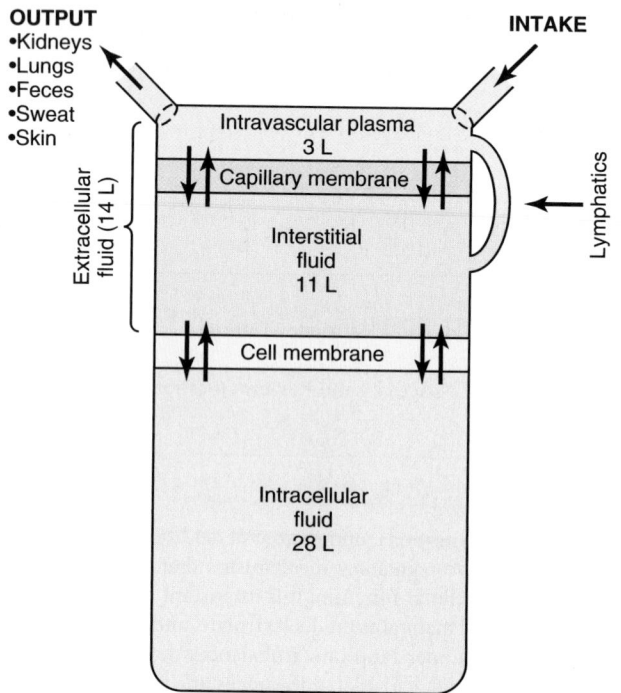

FIG. 42.1 Body fluid compartments. (From Hall JE: *Guyton and Hall textbook of medical physiology*, ed 13, Philadelphia, 2016, Saunders.)

TABLE 42.1	Normal Laboratory Values for Adults
Item Measured	**Normal Value in Serum or Blood**
Osmolality	285-295 mOsm/kg H_2O (285-295 mmol/kg H_2O)
Electrolytes	
Sodium (Na^+)	136-145 mEq/L (136-145 mmol/L)
Potassium (K^+)	3.5-5.0 mEq/L (3.5-5 mmol/L)
Chloride (Cl^-)	98-106 mEq/L (98-106 mmol/L)
Total CO_2 (CO_2 total content)	22-30 mEq/L (22-30 mmol/L)
Bicarbonate (HCO_3^-)	Arterial 21-28 mEq/L (21-28 mmol/L)
	Venous 24-30 mEq/L (24-30 mmol/L)
Total calcium (Ca^{2+})	9.0-10.5 mg/dL (2.25-2.62 mmol/L)
Ionized calcium (Ca^{2+})	4.5-5.6 mg/dL (1.05-1.3 mmol/L)
Magnesium (Mg^{2+})	1.3-2.1 mEq/L (0.65-1.05 mmol/L)
Phosphate	3.0-4.5 mg/dL (0.97-1.45 mmol/L)
Anion gap	6 +/- 4 mEq/L (6 +/-4 mmol/L)
Arterial Blood Gases	
pH	7.35-7.45
$PaCO_2$	35-45 mm Hg (4.7-6 kPa)
PaO_2	80-100 mm Hg (10.7-13.3 kPa)
O_2 saturation	95%-100% (0.95-1.00)
Base excess	−2 to +2 mm Eq/L (mmol/L)

in the ECF, whereas the concentrations of K^+, Mg^{2+}, and phosphate are higher in the ICF. Cells maintain their high intracellular electrolyte concentration by active transport. Active transport requires energy in the form of adenosine triphosphate (ATP) to move electrolytes across cell membranes against the concentration gradient (from areas of lower concentration to areas of higher concentration). One example of active transport is the sodium-potassium pump, which moves Na^+ out of a cell and K^+ into it, keeping ICF lower in Na^+ and higher in K^+ than the ECF.

Diffusion. Diffusion is passive movement of electrolytes or other particles down a concentration gradient (from areas of higher concentration to areas of lower concentration). Within a body compartment electrolytes diffuse easily by random movements until the concentration is the same in all areas. However, diffusion of electrolytes across cell membranes requires proteins that serve as ion channels. For example, when a sodium channel in a cell membrane is open, Na^+ diffuses passively across the cell membrane into the ICF because concentration is lower in the ICF. Opening of ion channels is tightly controlled and plays an important part in muscle and nerve function.

Osmosis. Water moves across cell membranes by osmosis, a process by which water moves through a membrane that separates fluids with different particle concentrations (Fig. 42.3). Cell membranes are semipermeable, which means that water crosses them easily but they are not freely permeable to many types of particles, including electrolytes such as sodium and potassium. These semipermeable cell membranes separate interstitial fluid from ICF. The fluid in each of these compartments exerts osmotic pressure, an inward-pulling force caused by particles in the fluid. The particles already inside the cell exert ICF osmotic pressure, which tends to pull water into the cell. The particles in the interstitial fluid exert interstitial fluid osmotic pressure, which tends to pull water out of the cell. Water moves into the compartment that has a higher osmotic pressure (inward-pulling force) until the particle concentration is equal in the two compartments.

If the particle concentration in the interstitial compartment changes, osmosis occurs rapidly and moves water into or out of cells to equalize the osmotic pressures. For example, when a hypotonic solution (more dilute than normal body fluids) is administered intravenously, it dilutes the interstitial fluid, decreasing its osmotic pressure below intracellular osmotic pressure. Water moves rapidly into cells until the two osmotic pressures are equal again. On the other hand, infusion of a hypertonic intravenous (IV) solution (more concentrated than normal body fluids) causes water to leave cells by osmosis to equalize the osmolality between interstitial and intracellular compartments.

Filtration. Fluid moves into and out of capillaries (between the vascular and interstitial compartments) by the process of filtration (Fig. 42.4). Filtration is the net effect of four forces, two that tend to move fluid out of capillaries and small venules and two that tend to move fluid back into them. Hydrostatic pressure is the force of the fluid pressing outward against a surface. Similarly, capillary hydrostatic pressure is a relatively strong outward-pushing force that helps move fluid from capillaries into the interstitial area. Interstitial fluid hydrostatic pressure is a weaker opposing force that tends to push fluid back into capillaries (Hall, 2016).

Blood contains albumin and other proteins known as colloids. These proteins are much larger than electrolytes, glucose, and other molecules that dissolve easily. Most colloids are too large to leave capillaries in the fluid that is filtered; thus they remain in the blood. Because they are particles, colloids exert osmotic pressure. Blood colloid osmotic pressure, also called oncotic pressure, is an inward-pulling force caused by blood proteins that helps move fluid from the interstitial area back into capillaries. Interstitial fluid colloid osmotic pressure normally is a very small opposing force.

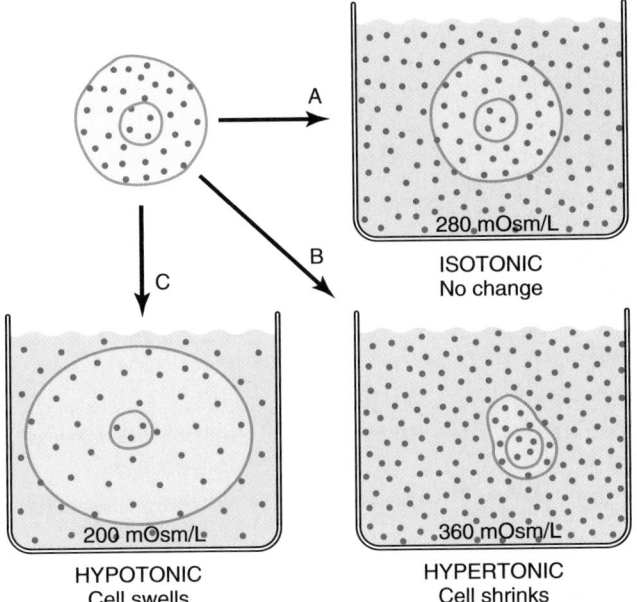

FIG. 42.2 Effects of isotonic, hypotonic, and hypertonic solutions. (From Hall JE: *Guyton and Hall textbook of medical physiology*, ed 13, Philadelphia, 2016, Saunders.)

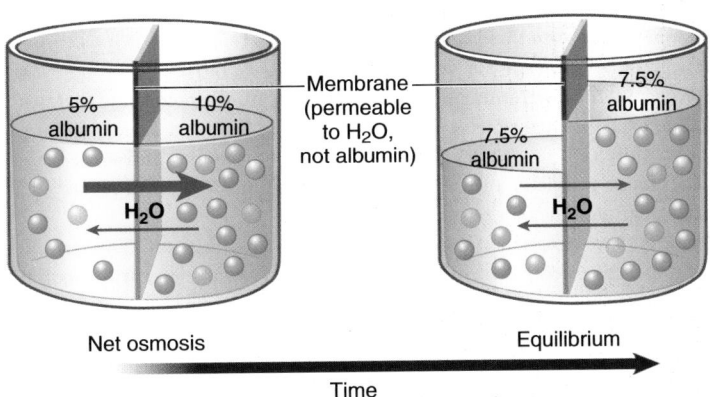

FIG. 42.3 Osmosis moves water through semipermeable membrane. (From Patton KT, Thibodeau GA: *The human body in health and disease*, ed 7, St Louis, 2018, Elsevier.)

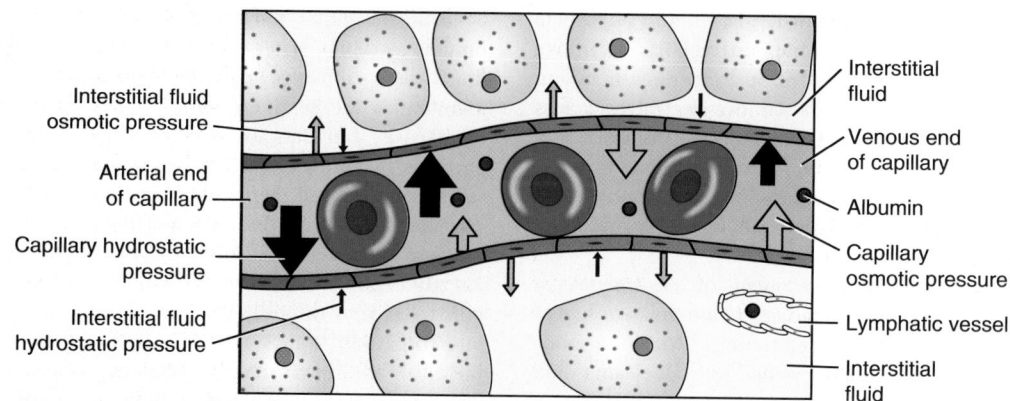

FIG. 42.4 Capillary filtration moves fluid between vascular and interstitial compartments. (From Banasik JL, Copstead LC: *Pathophysiology*, ed 6, St Louis, 2019, Saunders.)

Capillary hydrostatic pressure is strongest at the arterial end of a normal capillary. Fluid moves from the capillary into the interstitial area, bringing nutrients to cells. At the venous end capillary hydrostatic pressure is weaker, and the colloid osmotic pressure of the blood is stronger. Thus fluid moves into the capillary at the venous end, removing waste products from cellular metabolism. Lymph vessels remove any extra fluid and proteins that have leaked into the interstitial fluid.

Disease processes and other factors that alter these forces may cause accumulation of excess fluid in the interstitial space, known as *edema*. For example, people with heart failure often develop edema. In this situation, venous congestion from a weakened heart that no longer pumps effectively increases capillary hydrostatic pressure, causing edema by moving excessive fluid into the interstitial space. Inflammation is another cause of edema. It increases capillary blood flow and allows capillaries to leak colloids into the interstitial space. The resulting increased capillary hydrostatic pressure and increased interstitial colloid osmotic pressure produce localized edema in the inflamed tissues.

Fluid Balance

Fluid homeostasis is the dynamic interplay of three processes: fluid intake and absorption, fluid distribution, and fluid output (Felver, 2019d). To maintain fluid balance, fluid intake must equal output. Because some of the normal daily fluid output (e.g., urine, sweat) is a hypotonic salt solution, people must have an equivalent fluid intake of hypotonic sodium-containing fluid (or water plus foods with some salt) to maintain fluid balance (intake equal to output).

Fluid Intake. Fluid intake occurs orally through drinking but also through eating because most foods contain some water. Food metabolism creates additional water. Average fluid intake from these routes for healthy adults is about 2300 mL, although this amount can vary widely, depending on exercise habits, preferences, and the environment (Table 42.2). Other routes of fluid intake include IV, rectal (e.g., enemas), and irrigation of body cavities that can absorb fluid.

Although you might think that the major regulator of oral fluid intake is thirst, habit and social reasons also play major roles in fluid intake. Thirst, the conscious desire for water, is an important regulator of fluid intake when plasma osmolality increases (osmoreceptor-mediated thirst) or the blood volume decreases (baroreceptor-mediated thirst and angiotensin II– and III–mediated thirst) (Gizowski and Bourgue, 2018). The thirst-control mechanism is located within the hypothalamus in the brain (Fig. 42.5). Osmoreceptors continually monitor plasma osmolality; when it increases, they cause thirst by stimulating neurons in the hypothalamus. People who are alert can

TABLE 42.2 **Healthy Adult Average Fluid Intake and Output**		
	Normal (per Day)	**Prolonged Heavy Exercise (per Hour)**
Fluid Intake		
Fluids Ingested		
Oral	1100-1400 mL	280-1100 mL/hr
Foods	800-1000 mL	Highly variable
Metabolism	300 mL	16-50 mL/hr
TOTAL	2200-2700 mL	300-1150 mL/hr
Fluid Output		
Skin (insensible and sweat)	500-600 mL	300-2100 mL/hr
Insensible lungs	400 mL	20 mL/hr
Gastrointestinal	100-200 mL	Negligible, unless diarrhea during exercise
Urine	1200-1500 mL	20-1000 mL/hr, depending on hydration status
TOTAL	2200-2700 mL	340-3120 mL/hr Rehydration with Na+-containing fluid necessary after prolonged vigorous exercise

Data from Hall JE: *Guyton and Hall textbook of medical physiology*, ed 13, Philadelphia, 2016, Saunders.

obtain fluid or communicate their thirst to others, and fluid intake restores fluid balance. Infants, patients with neurological or psychological problems, and some older adults who are unable to perceive or communicate their thirst are at risk for dehydration.

Fluid Distribution. The term *fluid distribution* means the movement of fluid among its various compartments. Fluid distribution between the extracellular and intracellular compartments occurs by osmosis. Fluid distribution between the vascular and interstitial parts of the ECF occurs by filtration.

Fluid Output. Fluid output normally occurs through four organs: the skin, lungs, gastrointestinal (GI) tract, and kidneys. Examples of abnormal fluid output include vomiting, wound drainage, or hemorrhage (Felver, 2019d). Table 42.2 shows average amounts of fluid excretion for healthy adults, although urine output varies greatly, depending on fluid intake. Insensible (not visible) water loss through the skin and lungs is continuous. It increases when a person has a fever or a recent burn to the skin (Kamel and Halperin, 2017). Sweat, which is visible and contains sodium, occurs intermittently and increases fluid output substantially. The GI tract plays a vital role in fluid balance. Approximately 3 to 6 L of fluid moves into the GI tract daily and returns to the ECF. The average adult normally excretes only 100 mL of fluid each day through feces. However, diarrhea causes a large fluid output from the GI tract (Kear, 2017).

The kidneys are the major regulator of fluid output because they respond to hormones that influence urine production. When healthy

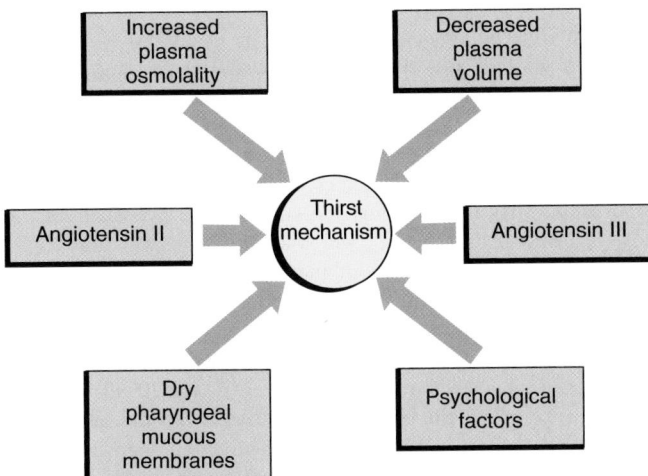

FIG. 42.5 Stimuli affecting thirst mechanism.

adults drink more water, they increase urine production to maintain fluid balance. If they drink less water, sweat a lot, or lose fluid by vomiting, their urine volume decreases to maintain fluid balance. These adjustments primarily are caused by the actions of antidiuretic hormone (ADH), the renin-angiotensin-aldosterone system (RAAS), and atrial natriuretic peptides (ANPs) (Hall, 2016) (Fig. 42.6).

Antidiuretic Hormone. ADH regulates the osmolality of the body fluids by influencing how much water is excreted in urine. It is synthesized by neurons in the hypothalamus that release it from the posterior pituitary gland. ADH circulates in the blood to the kidneys, where it acts on the collecting ducts (Hall, 2016). Its name—antidiuretic hormone—tells you what it does. It causes renal cells to resorb water, taking water from the renal tubular fluid and putting it back in the blood. This action decreases urine volume, concentrating the urine while diluting the blood by adding water to it (see Fig. 42.6A).

People normally have some ADH release to maintain fluid balance. More ADH is released if body fluids become more concentrated. Factors that increase ADH levels include severely decreased blood volume (e.g., dehydration, hemorrhage), pain, stressors, and some medications.

ADH levels decrease if body fluids become too dilute. This allows more water to be excreted in urine, creating a larger volume of dilute urine and concentrating the body fluids back to normal osmolality. For example, ethyl alcohol decreases ADH release, which causes people to urinate frequently when they drink alcoholic beverages (Hall, 2016).

Renin-Angiotensin-Aldosterone System. The renin-angiotensin-aldosterone system (RAAS) regulates ECF volume by influencing how much sodium and water are excreted in urine. It also contributes to regulation of blood pressure. Specialized cells in the kidneys release the enzyme renin, which acts on angiotensinogen, an inactive protein secreted by the liver that circulates in the blood. Renin converts angiotensinogen to angiotensin I, which is converted to angiotensin II by other enzymes in the lung capillaries (Hall, 2016). Angiotensin II

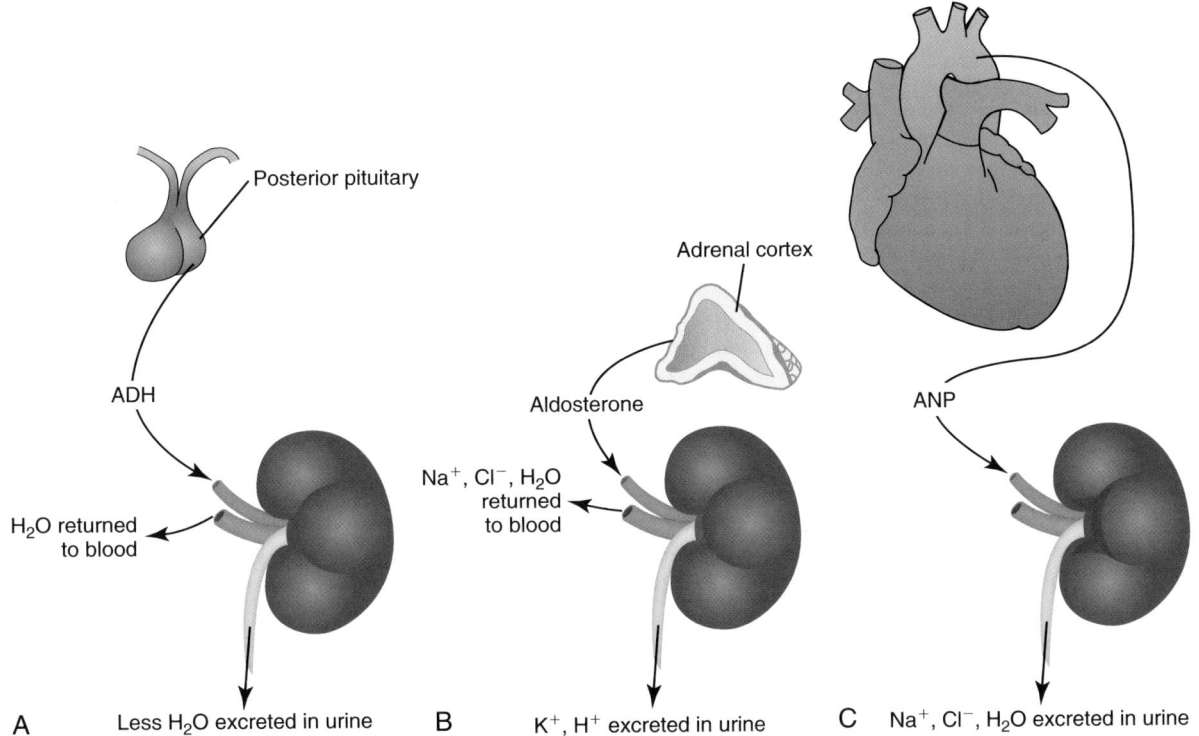

FIG. 42.6 Major hormones that influence renal fluid excretion. **A,** Antidiuretic hormone (ADH). **B,** Aldosterone. **C,** Atrial natriuretic peptide (ANP).

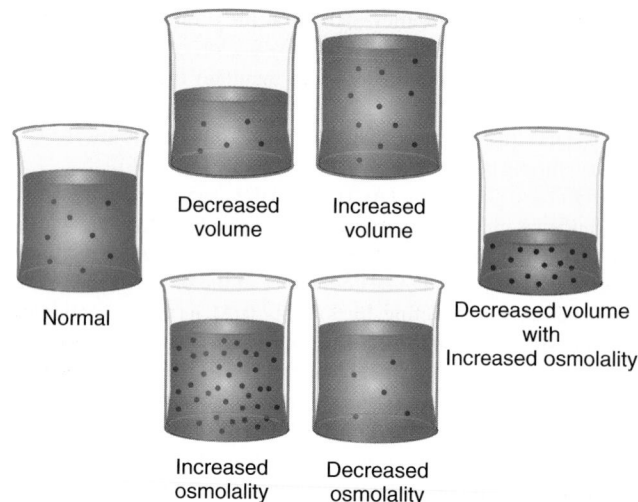

Normal

Decreased volume

Increased volume

Decreased volume with Increased osmolality

Increased osmolality

Decreased osmolality

FIG. 42.7 Fluid volume and osmolality imbalances. (From Banasik JL, Copstead LC: *Pathophysiology online for pathophysiology*, ed 6, St Louis, 2019, Mosby.)

has several functions, one of which is vasoconstriction in some vascular beds. The important fluid homeostasis functions of angiotensin II include stimulation of aldosterone release from the adrenal cortex.

Aldosterone circulates to the kidneys, where it causes resorption of sodium and water in isotonic proportion in the distal renal tubules. Removing sodium and water from the renal tubules and returning it to the blood increases the volume of the ECF (see Fig. 42.6B). Aldosterone also contributes to electrolyte and acid-base balance by increasing urinary excretion of potassium and hydrogen ions.

To maintain fluid balance, normally some action of the RAAS occurs. Certain stimuli increase or decrease the activity of this system to restore fluid balance. For example, if hemorrhage or vomiting decreases the extracellular fluid volume (ECV), blood flow decreases through the renal arteries, and more renin is released. This increased RAAS activity causes more sodium and water retention, helping to restore ECV.

Atrial Natriuretic Peptide. ANP also regulates ECV by influencing how much sodium and water are excreted in urine. Cells in the atria of the heart release ANP when they are stretched (e.g., by an increased ECV). ANP is a weak hormone that increases the loss of sodium and water in the urine (see Fig. 42.6C). Thus ANP opposes the effect of aldosterone (Hall, 2016).

Fluid Imbalances

If disease processes, medications, or other factors disrupt fluid intake or output, imbalances sometimes occur (Felver, 2019d). For example, with diarrhea there is an increase in fluid output, and a fluid imbalance (dehydration) occurs if fluid intake does not increase appropriately. There are two major types of fluid imbalances: volume imbalances and osmolality imbalances (Fig. 42.7). Volume imbalances are disturbances of the *amount of fluid in the extracellular compartment*. Osmolality imbalances are disturbances of the *concentration of body fluids*. Volume and osmolality imbalances occur separately or in combination.

Extracellular Fluid Volume Imbalances.
In an ECV imbalance there is either too little (ECV deficit) or too much (ECV excess) isotonic fluid. Extracellular volume deficit is present when there is insufficient isotonic fluid in the extracellular compartment. Remember that there is a lot of sodium in normal ECF. With ECV deficit, output of isotonic fluid exceeds intake of sodium-containing fluid. Because ECF

is both vascular and interstitial, signs and symptoms arise from lack of volume in both of these compartments. Table 42.3 lists specific causes and signs and symptoms of ECV deficit. The term hypovolemia means decreased vascular volume and often is used when discussing ECV deficit (Kamel and Halperin, 2017).

Extracellular volume excess occurs when there is too much isotonic fluid in the extracellular compartment. Intake of sodium-containing isotonic fluid has exceeded fluid output. For example, when you eat more salty foods than usual and drink water, you may notice that your ankles swell or rings on your fingers feel tight and you gain 2 lb (1 kg) or more overnight. These are manifestations of mild ECV excess. See Table 42.3 for other specific causes and signs and symptoms.

Osmolality Imbalances. In an osmolality imbalance body fluids become hypertonic or hypotonic, which causes osmotic shifts of water across cell membranes. The osmolality imbalances are called *hypernatremia* and *hyponatremia*.

Hypernatremia, also called *water deficit*, is a hypertonic condition. Two general causes make body fluids too concentrated: loss of relatively more water than salt or gain of relatively more salt than water (Felver, 2019d). Table 42.3 lists specific causes under these categories. When the interstitial fluid becomes hypertonic, water leaves cells by osmosis, and they shrivel. Signs and symptoms of hypernatremia are those of cerebral dysfunction, which arise when brain cells shrivel. Hypernatremia may occur in combination with ECV deficit; this combined disorder is called clinical dehydration.

Hyponatremia, also called *water excess* or *water intoxication*, is a hypotonic condition. It arises from gain of relatively more water than salt or loss of relatively more salt than water (Felver, 2019d) (see Table 42.3). The excessively dilute condition of interstitial fluid causes water to enter cells by osmosis, causing the cells to swell. Signs and symptoms of cerebral dysfunction occur when brain cells swell (Hoorn et al., 2017).

Clinical Dehydration. ECV deficit and hypernatremia often occur at the same time; this combination is called *clinical dehydration*. The ECV is too low, and the body fluids are too concentrated. Clinical dehydration is common with gastroenteritis or other causes of severe vomiting and diarrhea when people are unable to replace their fluid output with enough intake of dilute sodium-containing fluids. Signs and symptoms of clinical dehydration are those of both ECV deficit and hypernatremia (see Table 42.3).

Electrolyte Balance

You can best understand electrolyte balance by considering the three processes involved in electrolyte homeostasis: electrolyte intake and absorption, electrolyte distribution, and electrolyte output (Table 42.4) (Felver, 2019d). Although sodium is an electrolyte, it is not included here because serum sodium imbalances are the osmolality imbalances discussed previously.

Electrolyte distribution is an important issue. Plasma concentrations of K^+, Ca^{2+}, Mg^{2+}, and phosphate are very low compared with their concentrations in cells and bone (Hall, 2016). These concentration differences are necessary for normal muscle and nerve function. The electrolyte values that you review from laboratory reports are measured in blood serum and do not measure intracellular levels.

Electrolyte output occurs through normal excretion in urine, feces, and sweat. Output also occurs through vomiting, drainage tubes, or fistulas. When electrolyte output increases, electrolyte intake must increase to maintain electrolyte balance. Similarly, if electrolyte output decreases such as with oliguria, electrolyte intake must also decrease to maintain balance (Felver, 2019c).

TABLE 42.3 Fluid Imbalances

Imbalance and Related Causes	Signs and Symptoms
Isotonic Imbalances—Water and Sodium Lost or Gained in Equal or Isotonic Proportions	
Extracellular Fluid Volume Deficit—Body Fluids Have Decreased Volume but Normal Osmolality	
Sodium and Water Intake Less Than Output, Causing Isotonic Loss: Severely decreased oral intake of water and salt Increased GI output: vomiting, diarrhea, laxative overuse, drainage from fistulas or tubes Increased renal output: use of diuretics, adrenal insufficiency (deficit of cortisol and aldosterone) Loss of blood or plasma: hemorrhage, burns Massive sweating without water and salt intake	*Physical examination:* Sudden weight loss (overnight), postural hypotension, tachycardia, thready pulse, dry mucous membranes, poor skin turgor, slow vein filling, flat neck veins when supine, dark yellow urine If severe: thirst, restlessness, confusion, hypotension; oliguria (urine output ***below*** 30 mL/hr); cold, clammy skin; hypovolemic shock *Laboratory findings:* Increased hematocrit; increased BUN ***above*** 20 mg/dL (7.1 mmol/L) (hemoconcentration); urine specific gravity usually ***above*** 1.030, unless renal cause
Extracellular Fluid Volume Excess—Body Fluids Have Increased Volume but Normal Osmolality	
Sodium and Water Intake Greater Than Output, Causing Isotonic Gain: Excessive administration of Na⁺-containing isotonic IV fluids or oral intake of salty foods and water Renal retention of Na⁺ and water: heart failure, cirrhosis, aldosterone or glucocorticoid excess, acute or chronic oliguric renal disease	*Physical examination:* Sudden weight gain (overnight), edema (especially in dependent areas), full neck veins when upright or semi-upright, crackles in lungs If severe: confusion, pulmonary edema *Laboratory findings:* Decreased hematocrit, decreased BUN ***below*** 10 mg/dL (3.6 mmol/L) (hemodilution)
Osmolality Imbalances	
Hypernatremia (Water Deficit; Hyperosmolar Imbalance)—Body Fluids Too Concentrated	
Loss of Relatively More Water Than Salt: Diabetes insipidus (ADH deficiency) Osmotic diuresis Large insensible perspiration and respiratory water output without increased water intake **Gain of Relatively More Salt Than Water:** Administration of tube feedings, hypertonic parenteral fluids, or salt tablets Lack of access to water, deliberate water deprivation, inability to respond to thirst (e.g., immobility, aphasia) Dysfunction of osmoreceptor-driven thirst drive	*Physical examination:* Decreased level of consciousness (confusion, lethargy, coma), perhaps thirst, seizures if develops rapidly or is very severe *Laboratory findings:* Serum Na⁺ level ***above*** 145 mEq/L (145 mmol/L), serum osmolality ***above*** 295 mOsm/kg (295 mmol/kg)
Hyponatremia (Water Excess; Water Intoxication; Hypoosmolar Imbalance)—Body Fluids Too Dilute	
Gain of Relatively More Water Than Salt: Excessive ADH (SIADH) Psychogenic polydipsia or forced excessive water intake Excessive IV administration of D₅W Use of hypotonic irrigating solutions Tap-water enemas **Loss of Relatively More Salt Than Water:** Replacement of large body fluid output (e.g., diarrhea, vomiting) with water but no salt	*Physical examination:* Decreased level of consciousness (confusion, lethargy, coma), seizures if develops rapidly or is very severe *Laboratory findings:* Serum Na⁺ level ***below*** 136 mEq/L (136 mmol/L), serum osmolality ***below*** 285 mOsm/kg (285 mmol/kg)
Combined Volume and Osmolality Imbalance	
Clinical Dehydration (ECV Deficit plus Hypernatremia)—Body Fluids Have Decreased Volume and Are Too Concentrated	
Sodium and Water Intake Less Than Output, With Loss of Relatively More Water Than Salt: All of the causes of ECV deficit (see previous causes) plus poor or no water intake, often with fever causing increased insensible water output	*Physical examination and laboratory findings:* Combination of those for ECV deficit plus those for hypernatremia (see previous signs)

ADH, Antidiuretic hormone; *BUN,* blood urea nitrogen; *ECV,* extracellular fluid volume; *GI,* gastrointestinal; *D₅W,* 5% dextrose in water; *IV,* intravenous; *SIADH,* syndrome of inappropriate secretion of antidiuretic hormone.

Electrolyte Imbalances

Factors such as diarrhea, endocrine disorders, and medications that disrupt electrolyte homeostasis cause electrolyte imbalances. Electrolyte intake greater than electrolyte output or a shift of electrolytes from cells or bone into the ECF causes plasma electrolyte excess. Electrolyte intake less than electrolyte output or shift of electrolyte from the ECF into cells or bone causes plasma electrolyte deficit (Felver, 2019c).

Potassium Imbalances. Hypokalemia is abnormally low potassium concentration in the blood. It results from decreased potassium intake and absorption, a shift of potassium from the ECF into cells, and an

TABLE 42.4   Electrolyte Intake and Absorption, Distribution, and Output

Electrolyte	Intake and Absorption	Distribution	Output/Loss	Important Function
Potassium (K^+)	Fruits Potatoes Instant coffee Molasses Brazil nuts Absorbs easily	Low in ECF, high in ICF. Insulin, epinephrine, and alkalosis shift K^+ into cells. Some types of acidosis shift K^+ out of cells.	Aldosterone, black licorice, hypomagnesemia, and polyuria increase renal excretion; oliguria decreases renal excretion. Acute or chronic diarrhea increases fecal excretion.	Maintains resting membrane potential of skeletal, smooth, and cardiac muscle, allowing normal muscle function
Calcium (Ca^{2+})	Dairy products Canned fish with bones Broccoli Oranges Requires vitamin D for best absorption Undigested fat prevents absorption	Ca^{2+} is low in ECF, mostly in bones and intracellular. Some Ca^{2+} in blood is bound and inactive; only ionized Ca^{2+} is active. Parathyroid hormone shifts Ca^{2+} out of bone; calcitonin shifts Ca^{2+} into bone. Ca^{2+} decreases in blood if phosphate rises and vice versa.	Thiazide diuretics decrease renal excretion. Chronic diarrhea and undigested fat increase fecal excretion.	Influences excitability of nerve and muscle cells; necessary for muscle contraction
Magnesium (Mg^{2+})	Dark green leafy vegetables Whole grains Mg^{2+}-containing laxatives and antacids Undigested fat prevents absorption	Mg^{2+} is low in ECF, mostly in bones and intracellular. Some Mg^{2+} in blood is bound and inactive; only free Mg^{2+} is active.	Rising blood ethanol increases renal excretion; oliguria decreases renal excretion. Chronic diarrhea and undigested fat increase fecal excretion.	Influences function of neuromuscular junctions; is a cofactor for numerous enzymes
Phosphate	Milk Processed foods Aluminum antacids prevent absorption	Phosphate is low in ECF; it is higher in ICF and in bones. Insulin and epinephrine shift phosphate into cells. Decreases in blood if calcium rises and vice versa.	Oliguria and elevated fibroblast growth factor 23 (FGF-23) decrease renal excretion.	Necessary for production of ATP, the energy source for cellular metabolism

ATP, Adenosine triphosphate; *ECF,* extracellular fluid volume; *ICF,* intracellular fluid.

increased potassium output (Table 42.5). Common causes of hypokalemia from increased potassium output include diarrhea, repeated vomiting, and use of potassium-wasting diuretics (Kovesdy et al., 2017). People who have these conditions need to increase their potassium intake to reduce their risk of hypokalemia. Hypokalemia causes muscle weakness, which becomes life threatening if it includes respiratory muscles. It can also cause potentially life-threatening cardiac dysrhythmias.

Hyperkalemia is abnormally high potassium ion concentration in the blood. Its general causes are increased potassium intake and absorption, shift of potassium from cells into the ECF, and decreased potassium output (see Table 42.5). People who have oliguria (decreased urine output) are at high risk of hyperkalemia from the resultant decreased potassium output unless their potassium intake also decreases substantially. Understanding this principle helps you remember to check urine output before you administer IV solutions containing potassium. Hyperkalemia can cause muscle weakness, potentially life-threatening cardiac dysrhythmias, and cardiac arrest (Heckle et al., 2018).

Calcium Imbalances.
Hypocalcemia is abnormally low calcium concentration in the blood (see Table 42.5). The physiologically active form of calcium in the blood is ionized calcium. Total blood calcium also contains inactive forms that are bound to plasma proteins and small anions such as citrate. Factors that cause too much ionized calcium to shift to the bound forms cause symptomatic *ionized hypocalcemia* (Kyle et al., 2018). People who have acute pancreatitis frequently develop hypocalcemia because calcium binds to undigested fat in their feces and is excreted. This process decreases absorption of dietary calcium and also increases calcium output by preventing reabsorption of calcium contained in GI fluids. Hypocalcemia increases neuromuscular excitability, the basis for its signs and symptoms.

Hypercalcemia is abnormally high calcium concentration in the blood. Hypercalcemia results from increased calcium intake and absorption, shift of calcium from bones into the ECF, and decreased calcium output (see Table 42.5). Patients with some types of cancers such as lung and breast cancers often develop hypercalcemia because some cancer cells secrete chemicals into the blood that are related to parathyroid hormone. When these chemicals reach the bones, they cause shift of calcium from bones into the ECF. This weakens bones, and the person sometimes develops pathological fractures (i.e., bone breakage caused by forces that would not break a healthy bone). Hypercalcemia decreases neuromuscular excitability, the basis for its other signs and symptoms, the most common of which is lethargy (Turner, 2017).

Magnesium Imbalances.
Hypomagnesemia is abnormally low magnesium concentration in the blood. Its general causes are decreased magnesium intake and absorption, shift of plasma magnesium to its inactive bound form, and increased magnesium output (see Table 42.5). Signs and symptoms are similar to those of hypocalcemia because hypomagnesemia also increases neuromuscular excitability (Eberhard et al., 2017).

Hypermagnesemia is abnormally high magnesium concentration in the blood (see Table 42.5). End-stage renal disease causes hypermagnesemia unless the person decreases magnesium intake to match the decreased output. Signs and symptoms are caused by decreased neuromuscular excitability, with lethargy and decreased deep tendon reflexes being most common (Kala and Abudayyeh, 2017).

TABLE 42.5   Electrolyte Imbalances

Imbalance and Related Causes	Signs and Symptoms
Hypokalemia—Low Serum Potassium (K⁺) Concentration **Decreased K⁺ Intake:** Excessive use of K⁺-free IV solutions **Shift of K⁺ into Cells:** Alkalosis; treatment of diabetic ketoacidosis with insulin **Increased K⁺ Output:** Acute or chronic diarrhea; vomiting; other GI losses (e.g., nasogastric or fistula drainage); use of potassium-wasting diuretics; aldosterone excess; polyuria; glucocorticoid therapy	*Physical examination:* Bilateral muscle weakness that begins in quadriceps and may ascend to respiratory muscles, abdominal distention, decreased bowel sounds, constipation, dysrhythmias *Laboratory findings:* Serum K⁺ level ***below*** 3.5 mEq/L (3.5 mmol/L); ECG abnormalities: U waves, flattened or inverted T waves; ST segment depression
Hyperkalemia—High Serum Potassium (K⁺) Concentration **Increased K⁺ Intake:** Iatrogenic administration of large amounts of IV K⁺; rapid infusion of stored blood; excess ingestion of K⁺ salt substitutes **Shift of K⁺ out of Cells:** Massive cellular damage (e.g., crushing trauma, cytotoxic chemotherapy); insufficient insulin (e.g., diabetic ketoacidosis); some types of acidosis **Decreased K⁺ Output:** Acute or chronic oliguria (e.g., severe ECV deficit, end-stage renal disease); use of potassium-sparing diuretics; adrenal insufficiency (deficit of cortisol and aldosterone)	*Physical examination:* Bilateral muscle weakness in quadriceps, transient abdominal cramps, diarrhea, dysrhythmias, cardiac arrest if severe *Laboratory findings:* Serum K⁺ level ***above*** 5 mEq/L (5 mmol/L); ECG abnormalities: peaked T waves; widened QRS complex; PR prolongation; terminal sine-wave pattern
Hypocalcemia—Low Serum Calcium (Ca²⁺) Concentration **Decreased Ca²⁺ Intake and Absorption**: Calcium-deficient diet; vitamin D deficiency (includes end-stage renal disease); chronic diarrhea; laxative misuse; steatorrhea **Shift of Ca²⁺ into Bone or Inactive Form:** Hypoparathyroidism; rapid administration of citrated blood; hypoalbuminemia; alkalosis; pancreatitis; hyperphosphatemia (includes end-stage renal disease) **Increased Ca²⁺ Output:** Chronic diarrhea; steatorrhea	*Physical examination:* Numbness and tingling of fingers, toes, and circumoral (around mouth) region, positive Chvostek's sign (contraction of facial muscles when facial nerve is tapped), hyperactive reflexes, muscle twitching and cramping; carpal and pedal spasms, tetany, seizures, laryngospasm, dysrhythmias *Laboratory findings:* Total serum Ca²⁺ level ***below*** 9.0 mg/dL (2.25 mmol/L) or serum ionized Ca²⁺ level ***below*** 4.5 mg/dL (1.05 mmol/L); ECG abnormalities: prolonged ST segments
Hypercalcemia—High Serum Calcium (Ca²⁺) Concentration **Increased Ca²⁺ Intake and Absorption:** Milk-alkali syndrome **Shift of Ca²⁺ out of Bone:** Prolonged immobilization; hyperparathyroidism; bone tumors; nonosseous cancers that secrete bone-resorbing factors **Decreased Ca²⁺ Output:** Use of thiazide diuretics	*Physical examination:* Anorexia, nausea and vomiting, constipation, fatigue, diminished reflexes, lethargy, decreased level of consciousness, confusion, personality change, cardiac arrest if severe *Laboratory findings:* Total serum Ca²⁺ level ***above*** 10.5 mg/dL (2.62 mmol/L) or serum ionized Ca²⁺ level ***above*** 5.6 mg/dL (1.3 mmol/L); ECG abnormalities: heart block, shortened ST segments
Hypomagnesemia—Low Serum Magnesium (Mg²⁺) Concentration **Decreased Mg²⁺ Intake and Absorption:** Malnutrition; chronic alcoholism; chronic diarrhea; laxative misuse; steatorrhea **Shift of Mg²⁺ Into Inactive Form:** Rapid administration of citrated blood **Increased Mg²⁺ Output:** Chronic diarrhea; steatorrhea; other GI losses (e.g., vomiting, nasogastric or fistula drainage); use of thiazide or loop diuretics; aldosterone excess	*Physical examination:* Positive Chvostek's sign, hyperactive deep tendon reflexes, muscle cramps and twitching, grimacing, dysphagia, tetany, seizures, insomnia, tachycardia, hypertension, dysrhythmias *Laboratory findings:* Serum Mg²⁺ level ***below*** 1.3 mEq/L (0.65 mmol/L); ECG abnormalities: prolonged QT interval
Hypermagnesemia—High Serum Magnesium (Mg²⁺) Concentration **Increased Mg²⁺ Intake and Absorption:** Excessive use of Mg²⁺-containing laxatives and antacids; parenteral overload of magnesium **Decreased Mg²⁺ Output:** Oliguric end-stage renal disease; adrenal insufficiency	*Physical examination:* Lethargy, hypoactive deep tendon reflexes, bradycardia, hypotension Acute elevation in Mg²⁺ levels: Flushing, sensation of warmth Severe acute hypermagnesemia: Decreased rate and depth of respirations, dysrhythmias, cardiac arrest *Laboratory findings:* Serum Mg²⁺ level ***above*** 2.1 mEq/L (1.05 mmol/L); ECG abnormalities: prolonged PR interval

ECG, Electrocardiogram, *ECV*, extracellular fluid volume, *GI*, gastrointestinal, *IV*, intravenous.
Data from Felver L: Fluid and electrolyte homeostasis and imbalances. In Banasik JL, Copstead LC, editors: *Pathophysiology*, ed 6, St Louis, 2019, Saunders.

Acid-Base Balance

For optimal cell function the body maintains a balance between acids and bases. Acid-base homeostasis is the dynamic interplay of three processes: acid production, acid buffering, and acid excretion (Felver, 2019a). Normal acid-base balance is maintained with acid excretion equal to acid production. Acids release hydrogen (H⁺) ions; bases (alkaline substances) take up H⁺ ions. The more H⁺ ions that are present, the more acidic is a solution.

The degree of acidity in blood and other body fluids is reported from the clinical laboratory as pH. The pH scale goes from 1.0 (very acid) to

TABLE 42.6   Arterial Blood Gas Measures

Laboratory Measure	Normal Range in Adult Arterial Blood	Definition and Interpretation
pH	7.35-7.45	pH is a negative logarithm of the free H^+ concentration, a measure of the blood's acidity or alkalinity. Values below 7.35 indicate abnormally acid; above 7.45 they indicate abnormally alkaline. Small changes in pH denote large changes in H^+ concentration and are clinically important.
$PaCO_2$	35-45 mm Hg (4.7-6 kPa)	$PaCO_2$ is partial pressure of carbon dioxide (CO_2), a measure of how well the lungs are excreting CO_2 produced by cells. Increased $PaCO_2$ indicates CO_2 accumulation in blood (more carbonic acid) caused by hypoventilation; decreased $PaCO_2$ indicates excessive CO_2 excretion (less carbonic acid) through hyperventilation.
HCO_3^-	21-28 mEq/L (21-28 mmol/L)	HCO_3^- is concentration of the base (alkaline substance) bicarbonate, a measure of how well the kidneys are excreting metabolic acids. Increased HCO_3^- indicates that the blood has too few metabolic acids; decreased HCO_3^- indicates that the blood has too many metabolic acids.
PaO_2	80-100 mm Hg (10.7-13.3 kPa)	PaO_2 is partial pressure of oxygen (O_2), a measure of how well gas exchange is occurring in the alveoli of the lungs. Values below normal indicate poor oxygenation of the blood.
SaO_2	95%-100%	SaO_2 is oxygen saturation, the percentage of hemoglobin that is carrying as much O_2 as possible. It is influenced by pH, $PaCO_2$, and body temperature. It drops rapidly when PaO_2 falls below 60 mm Hg (8 kPa).
Base excess	−2 to +2 mEq/L (mmol/L)	Base excess is observed buffering capacity minus the normal buffering capacity, a measure of how well the blood buffers are managing metabolic acids. Values below −2 (negative base excess) indicate excessive metabolic acids; values above +2 indicate excessive amounts of bicarbonate.

14.0 (very alkaline; basic). A pH of 7.0 is considered neutral. The normal pH range of adult arterial blood is 7.35 to 7.45. Maintaining pH within this normal range is very important for optimal cell function. If the pH goes outside the normal range, enzymes within cells do not function properly, hemoglobin does not manage oxygen properly, and serious physiological problems occur, including death. Laboratory tests of a sample of arterial blood called arterial blood gases (ABGs) are used to monitor a patient's acid-base balance (Felver, 2019a) (Table 42.6).

Acid Production. Cellular metabolism constantly creates two types of acids: carbonic acid and metabolic acids (Fig. 42.8).

Reviewing the formula below, cells produce carbon dioxide (CO_2), which combine with water to produce carbonic acid (H_2CO_3). The carbonic acid (H_2CO_3) can then separate to a hydrogen ion (H^+) and a bicarbonate ion (HCO_3^-):

$$CO_2 + H_2O \leftrightarrow H_2CO_3 \leftrightarrow H^+ + HCO_3^-$$

Carbon dioxide + Water ↔ Carbonic acid ↔ Hydrogen ion + Bicarbonate

Metabolic acids are any acids that are not carbonic acid. They include citric acid, lactic acid, and many others.

Acid Buffering. Buffers are pairs of chemicals that work together to maintain normal pH of body fluids. If there are too many free H^+ ions, a buffer takes them up so that they no longer are free. If there are too few, a buffer can release H^+ ions to prevent an acid-base imbalance. Buffers work rapidly, within seconds.

All body fluids contain buffers. The major buffer in the ECF is the bicarbonate (HCO_3^-) buffer system, which buffers metabolic acids. It consists of a lot of bicarbonate and a small amount of carbonic acid (normally a 20 to 1 ratio). Addition of H^+ released by a metabolic acid to a bicarbonate ion makes more carbonic acid. Now the H^+ is no longer free and will not decrease the blood pH:

$$HCO_3^- + H^+ \leftrightarrow H_2CO_3$$

Bicarbonate ion + Hydrogen ion ↔ Carbonic acid

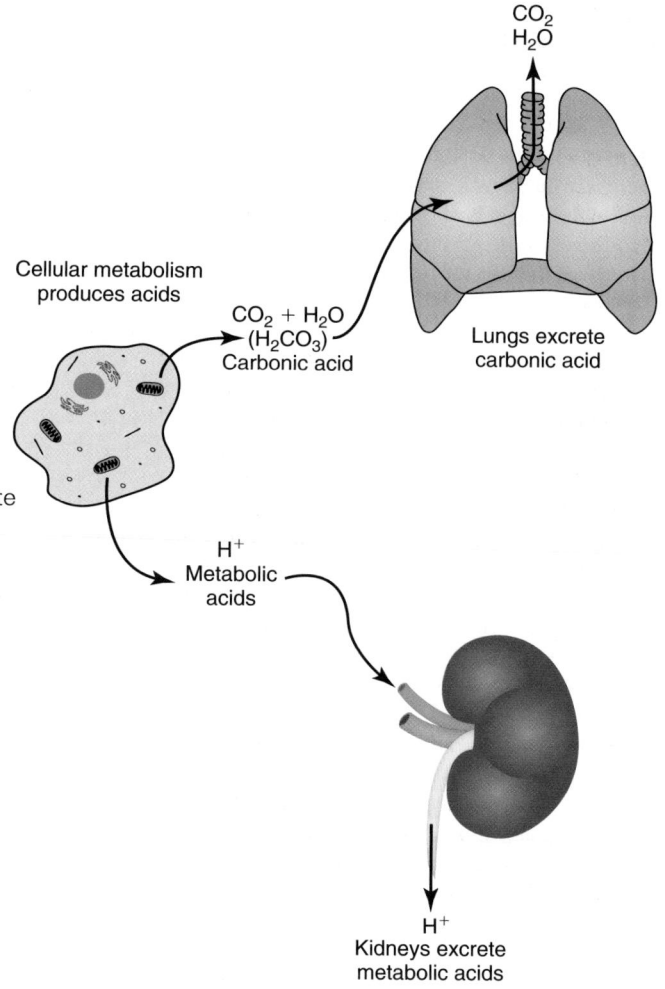

FIG. 42.8 Acid production and excretion.

If there are too few H^+ ions, the carbonic acid part of the buffer pair releases some, increasing the bicarbonate, again returning pH to normal.

$$H_2CO_3 \leftrightarrow HCO_3^- + H^+$$

Carbonic acid $\leftrightarrow$ Bicarbonate ion + Hydrogen ion

Other buffers include hemoglobin, protein buffers, and phosphate buffers. Cellular and bone buffers also contribute to acid-base balance. Buffers normally keep the blood from becoming too acid when acids that are produced by cells circulate to the lungs and kidneys for excretion.

Acid Excretion. The body has two acid-excretion systems: lungs and kidneys. The lungs excrete carbonic acid; the kidneys excrete metabolic acids (see Fig. 42.8).

Excretion of Carbonic Acid. When you exhale, you excrete carbonic acid in the form of CO_2 and water. If the $PaCO_2$ (i.e., level of CO_2 in the blood) rises, the chemoreceptors trigger faster and deeper respirations to excrete the excess. If the $PaCO_2$ falls, the chemoreceptors trigger slower and shallower respirations so that more of the CO_2 produced by cells remains in the blood and makes up the deficit. These alterations in respiratory rate and depth maintain the carbonic acid part of acid-base balance (Kamel and Halperin, 2017). People who have respiratory disease may be unable to excrete enough carbonic acid, which causes the blood to become more acidic and blood CO_2 to increase. If an increased respiratory rate is unable to correct the problem, the kidneys begin some compensatory excretion of metabolic acid.

Excretion of Metabolic Acids. The kidneys excrete all acids except carbonic acid. They secrete H^+ into the renal tubular fluid, putting HCO_3^- back into the blood at the same time. If there are too many H^+ ions in the blood, renal cells move more H^+ ions into the renal tubules for excretion, retaining more HCO_3^- in the process. If there are too few H^+ ions in the blood, renal cells secrete fewer H^+ ions.

Phosphate buffers in the renal tubular fluid keep the urine from becoming too acidic when the kidneys excrete H^+ ions. If the kidneys need to excrete a lot of H^+, renal tubular cells secrete ammonia, which combines with the H^+ ions in the tubules to make NH_4^+, ammonium ions. Buffering by phosphate and the creation of NH_4^+ turn free H^+ ions into other molecules in the renal tubular fluid (Kamel and Halperin, 2017). This process enables metabolic acid excretion in urine without making urine too acidic. People who have oliguric kidney disease often are unable to excrete metabolic acids normally, and these acids accumulate, making the blood too acidic (Nagami and Hamm, 2017). If the kidneys are unable to correct this problem, respiratory rate and depth increase, causing compensatory excretion of carbonic acid.

Acid-Base Imbalances

People develop acid-base imbalances when their normal homeostatic mechanisms are dysfunctional or overwhelmed. The term acidosis describes a condition that tends to make the blood relatively too acidic. Because our cells produce two types of acid, there are two different types of acidosis: respiratory acidosis and metabolic acidosis. The term alkalosis describes a condition that tends to make the blood relatively too basic (alkaline). There are two types of alkalosis: respiratory alkalosis and metabolic alkalosis.

The body has compensatory mechanisms that limit the extent of pH change with acid-base imbalances (Kamel and Halperin, 2017). Compensation involves physiological changes that help normalize the pH but do not correct the cause of the problem. If the problem is a respiratory acid-base imbalance, only the lungs can correct the problem, but the kidneys can compensate by changing the amount of metabolic acid in the blood. If the problem is a metabolic acid-base imbalance, only the kidneys can correct the problem, but the lungs can compensate by changing the amount of carbonic acid in the blood. Thus the kidneys compensate for respiratory acid-base imbalances; the respiratory system compensates for metabolic acid-base imbalances. These compensatory mechanisms do not correct the problem, but they help the body survive by moving the blood pH toward normal. However, if the underlying condition is not corrected, these compensatory mechanisms eventually will fail.

Respiratory Acidosis. Respiratory acidosis arises from alveolar hypoventilation; the lungs are unable to excrete enough CO_2. The $PaCO_2$ rises, creating an excess of carbonic acid in the blood, which decreases pH (Table 42.7). The kidneys compensate by increasing excretion of metabolic acids in the urine, which increases blood bicarbonate. This compensatory process is slow, often taking 24 hours to show clinical effect and 3 to 5 days to reach steady state. Decreased cerebrospinal fluid (CSF) pH and intracellular pH of brain cells cause decreased level of consciousness.

Respiratory Alkalosis. Respiratory alkalosis arises from alveolar hyperventilation; the lungs excrete too much carbonic acid (CO_2 and water). The $PaCO_2$ falls, creating a deficit of carbonic acid in the blood, which increases pH (see Table 42.7). Respiratory alkalosis usually is short lived; thus the kidneys do not have time to compensate. When the pH of blood, CSF, and ICF increases acutely, cell membrane excitability also increases, which can cause neurological symptoms such as excitement, confusion, and paresthesia. If the pH rises high enough, central nervous system (CNS) depression can occur.

Metabolic Acidosis. Metabolic acidosis occurs from an increase of metabolic acid or a decrease of base (bicarbonate). The kidneys are unable to excrete enough metabolic acids, which accumulate in the blood, or bicarbonate is removed from the body directly as with diarrhea (see Table 42.7). In either case the blood HCO_3^- decreases, and the pH falls (Ferrari et al., 2017). With an increase of metabolic acids, blood HCO_3^- decreases because it is used to buffer metabolic acids. Similarly, when patients have conditions that cause the removal of HCO_3^-, the amount of HCO_3^- in the blood decreases. To help identify the specific cause, health care providers and the laboratory calculate the anion gap, a reflection of unmeasured anions in plasma. You calculate anion gap by subtracting the sum of plasma concentrations of the anions Cl^- and HCO_3^- from the plasma concentration of the cation Na^+ (Kamel and Halperin, 2017). When reviewing laboratory reports, check the reference values from the laboratory that measured the electrolyte concentrations (Table 42.8).

The abnormally low pH in metabolic acidosis stimulates the chemoreceptors, so the respiratory system compensates for the acidosis by hyperventilation. Compensatory hyperventilation begins in a few minutes and removes carbonic acid from the body. This process does not correct the problem, but it helps limit the pH decrease. Metabolic acidosis decreases a person's level of consciousness (see Table 42.7).

Metabolic Alkalosis. Metabolic alkalosis occurs from a direct increase of base HCO_3^- or a decrease of metabolic acid, which increases blood HCO_3^- by releasing it from its buffering function. Common causes include vomiting and gastric suction (see Table 42.7). The respiratory compensation for metabolic alkalosis is hypoventilation. The decreased rate and depth of respiration allow carbonic acid to increase in the blood, as seen by an increased $PaCO_2$. The need for oxygen may limit the degree of respiratory compensation for metabolic alkalosis.

TABLE 42.7   Acid-Base Imbalances

Imbalance and Related Causes	Signs and Symptoms
Respiratory Acidosis—Excessive Carbonic Acid Caused by Alveolar Hypoventilation	
Impaired Gas Exchange:	*Physical examination:* Headache, light-headedness, decreased level of
Type B COPD (chronic bronchitis) or end-stage type A COPD (emphysema)	consciousness (confusion, lethargy, coma), dysrhythmias
Bacterial pneumonia	*Laboratory findings:* Arterial blood gas alterations: pH ***below*** 7.35, PaCO$_2$ ***above***
Airway obstruction	45 mm Hg (6 kPa), HCO$_3^-$ level normal if uncompensated or ***above*** 28 mEq/L (28
Extensive atelectasis (collapsed alveoli)	mmol/L) if compensated
Severe acute asthma episode	
Impaired Neuromuscular Function:	
Respiratory muscle weakness or paralysis from hypokalemia or neurological dysfunction	
Respiratory muscle fatigue, respiratory failure	
Chest wall injury or surgery causing pain with respiration	
Dysfunction of Brainstem Respiratory Control:	
Drug overdose with a respiratory depressant	
Some types of head injury	
Respiratory Alkalosis—Deficient Carbonic Acid Caused by Alveolar Hyperventilation	
Hypoxemia from any cause (e.g., initial part of asthma episode, pneumonia)	*Physical examination:* Light-headedness, numbness and tingling of fingers, toes,
Acute pain	and circumoral region, increased rate and depth of respirations, excitement and
Anxiety, psychological distress, sobbing	confusion possibly followed by decreased level of consciousness, dysrhythmias
Inappropriate mechanical ventilator settings	*Laboratory findings:* Arterial blood gas alterations: pH ***above*** 7.45, PaCO$_2$ ***below***
Stimulation of brainstem respiratory control (e.g., meningitis, gram-negative sepsis, head injury, aspirin overdose)	35 mm Hg (4.7 kPa), HCO$_3^-$ level normal if short lived or uncompensated or ***below*** 21 mEq/L (21 mmol/L) if compensated
Metabolic Acidosis—Excessive Metabolic Acids	
Increase of Metabolic Acids (High Anion Gap):	*Physical examination:* Decreased level of consciousness (lethargy, confusion,
Ketoacidosis (diabetes, starvation, alcoholism)	coma), abdominal pain, dysrhythmias, increased rate and depth of respirations
Hypermetabolic state (severe hyperthyroidism, burns, severe infection)	(compensatory hyperventilation)
Oliguric renal disease (acute kidney injury, end-stage renal disease)	*Laboratory findings:* Arterial blood gas alterations: pH ***below*** 7.35, PaCO$_2$ normal
Circulatory shock (lactic acidosis)	if uncompensated or ***below*** 35 mm Hg (4.7 kPa) if compensated, HCO$_3^-$ level
Ingestion of acid or acid precursors (e.g., methanol, ethylene glycol, boric acid)	***below*** 21 mEq/L (21 mmol/L)
Loss of Bicarbonate (Normal Anion Gap):	
Diarrhea	
Pancreatic fistula or intestinal decompression	
Renal tubular acidosis	
Metabolic Alkalosis—Deficient Metabolic Acids	
Increase of Bicarbonate:	*Physical examination:* Light-headedness, numbness and tingling of fingers, toes,
Excessive administration of sodium bicarbonate	and circumoral region; muscle cramps; possible excitement and confusion
Massive blood transfusion (liver converts citrate to HCO$_3^-$ Mild or moderate ECV deficit (contraction alkalosis)	followed by decreased level of consciousness, dysrhythmias (may be caused by concurrent hypokalemia)
Loss of Metabolic Acid:	*Laboratory findings:* Arterial blood gas alterations: pH ***above*** 7.45, PaCO$_2$ normal
Excessive vomiting or gastric suctioning	if uncompensated or ***above*** 45 mm Hg (6.0 kPa) if compensated, HCO$_3^-$ ***above***
Hypokalemia	28 mEq/L (28 mmol/L)
Excess aldosterone	

COPD, Chronic obstructive pulmonary disease, *ECV,* extracellular fluid volume.
Data from Felver L: Acid-base homeostasis and imbalances. In Banasik JL, Copstead LC, editors: *Pathophysiology,* ed 6, St Louis, 2019, Saunders.

Because HCO$_3^-$ crosses the blood-brain barrier with difficulty, neurological signs and symptoms are less severe or even absent with metabolic alkalosis (Kamel and Halperin, 2017).

REFLECT NOW

Think about the risk for specific fluid, electrolyte, and acid-base imbalance when caring for a patient with chronic diarrhea. What types of imbalances is the patient likely to have?

NURSING KNOWLEDGE BASE

You will apply knowledge about fluid, electrolyte, and acid-base imbalance in many clinical settings. In addition to scientific knowledge, there is a nursing knowledge base established from research and nursing practice, such as the Infusion Nurses Society standards of practice. Nursing knowledge also includes risk factors for fluid imbalances. For example, incorporate this knowledge along with physiology of normal aging when assessing older adults, knowing that this age-group has high risk of fluid imbalances (Touhy and Jett, 2016). Your nursing knowledge helps you formulate assessment

TABLE 42.8	Anion Gap in Metabolic Acidosis	
Anion Gap Type	**Values (Without K+)**	**Causes**
Normal anion gap	6 +/- 4 mEq/L (6 +/- 4 mmol/L) Varies, depending on laboratory	*Excess output of bicarbonate:* Diarrhea, pancreatic fistula, intestinal decompression, renal tubular acidosis Increase of chloride-containing acid: Parenteral HCl therapy
High anion gap	Greater than 5 mEq/L (5 mmol/L) above the laboratory reference range	*Increase of any acid except HCl:* Ketoacids (DKA, starvation, alcoholism), lactic acid (circulatory shock, extreme exercise), excessive normal metabolic acids (oliguric acute kidney injury, end-stage renal disease, severe hyperthyroidism, burns, severe infection), unusual organic acids (salicylate overdose, acids metabolized from methanol, ethylene glycol, paraldehyde)

DKA, Diabetic ketoacidosis.
Data from Kamel K, Halperin M: *Fluid, electrolyte, and acid–base physiology,* ed 5, St Louis, 2017, Elsevier.

questions to determine patients' risk factors for fluid, electrolyte, and acid-base imbalance; assess for signs and symptoms of these imbalances; and implement nursing and collaborative interventions to maintain or restore fluid and electrolyte and acid-base balance (Felver, 2019a,b,c). Skills and techniques for safe IV therapy are a vital area of the nursing knowledge base and the focus of nursing research to support evidence-based practice.

CRITICAL THINKING

Successful critical thinking requires a synthesis of knowledge, experience, information gathered from patients, critical thinking attitudes, and intellectual and professional standards. Clinical judgments require you to anticipate the information necessary to analyze the data and make decisions regarding patient care. During assessment consider all elements that build toward making an appropriate nursing diagnosis (Fig. 42.9).

In the case of fluid, electrolyte, and acid-base balance, you integrate knowledge of physiology, pathophysiology, and pharmacology and previous experiences and information gathered from patients. Critical analysis of data enables an understanding of how fluid, electrolyte, and acid-base imbalances affect a specific patient and his or her family. In addition, critical thinking attitudes such as accountability, discipline, and integrity, applied during assessment, help you identify appropriate nursing diagnoses and plan successful interventions. Professional standards such as the Infusion Nurses Society (INS) standards of practice (INS, 2016a) provide valuable guidance for appropriate assessment.

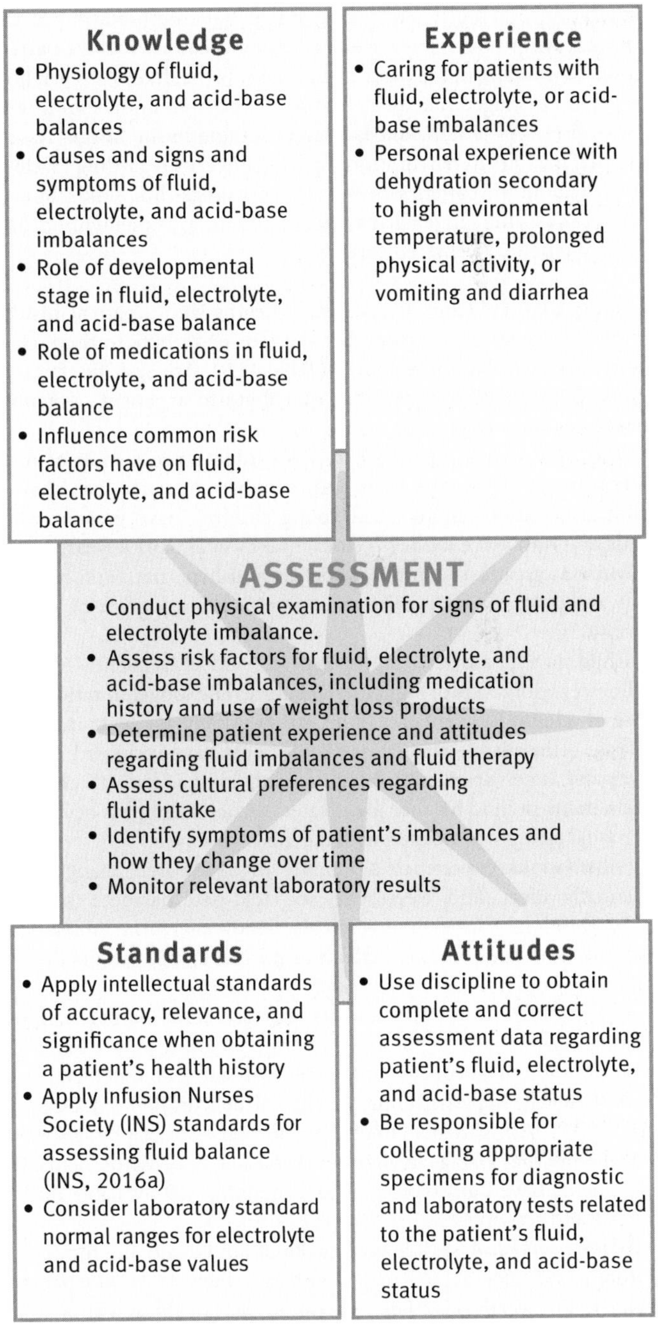

REFLECT NOW

You are preparing to care for a patient with dehydration. What scientific concepts and standards will guide you in obtaining accurate assessment data regarding a patient's fluid, electrolyte, and acid-base status?

❖ NURSING PROCESS

Apply the nursing process and use a critical thinking approach in your care of patients. The nursing process provides a clinical decision-making approach for you to develop and implement an individualized plan of care. For patients at high risk for fluid, electrolyte, and/or acid-base imbalances or those who already have these imbalances, an individualized approach is the foundation for safe and effective patient-centered nursing care.

Knowledge
- Physiology of fluid, electrolyte, and acid-base balances
- Causes and signs and symptoms of fluid, electrolyte, and acid-base imbalances
- Role of developmental stage in fluid, electrolyte, and acid-base balance
- Role of medications in fluid, electrolyte, and acid-base balance
- Influence common risk factors have on fluid, electrolyte, and acid-base balance

Experience
- Caring for patients with fluid, electrolyte, or acid-base imbalances
- Personal experience with dehydration secondary to high environmental temperature, prolonged physical activity, or vomiting and diarrhea

ASSESSMENT
- Conduct physical examination for signs of fluid and electrolyte imbalance.
- Assess risk factors for fluid, electrolyte, and acid-base imbalances, including medication history and use of weight loss products
- Determine patient experience and attitudes regarding fluid imbalances and fluid therapy
- Assess cultural preferences regarding fluid intake
- Identify symptoms of patient's imbalances and how they change over time
- Monitor relevant laboratory results

Standards
- Apply intellectual standards of accuracy, relevance, and significance when obtaining a patient's health history
- Apply Infusion Nurses Society (INS) standards for assessing fluid balance (INS, 2016a)
- Consider laboratory standard normal ranges for electrolyte and acid-base values

Attitudes
- Use discipline to obtain complete and correct assessment data regarding patient's fluid, electrolyte, and acid-base status
- Be responsible for collecting appropriate specimens for diagnostic and laboratory tests related to the patient's fluid, electrolyte, and acid-base status

FIG. 42.9 Critical thinking model for fluid, electrolyte, and acid-base balance assessment.

◆ Assessment

During the assessment process thoroughly assess each patient and critically analyze findings to ensure that you make patient-centered clinical decisions required for safe nursing care. Using a systematic approach in assessment enables you to help patients maintain or restore fluid, electrolyte, and acid-base balances safely (see Fig. 42.9).

Through the Patient's Eyes. A patient's fluid, electrolyte, or acid-base imbalance is sometimes so severe that it is difficult to determine a patient's needs, values, and preferences. However, when a patient is alert enough to discuss care, be sure to conduct a thorough patient-centered assessment. Focus on the patient's experience with fluid, electrolyte, or acid-base alterations and his or her perceptions of the illness. For example, for a patient who is hospitalized for clinical dehydration from diarrhea, ask whether he or she has experienced dehydration previously, and assess his or her interpretation of the signs and symptoms experienced and possible causes. Did the patient require IV therapy in the past? If so, what was that like? Also ask how the person managed diarrhea at home to assess an understanding of how to prevent the imbalances from occurring in the future. Assess potential barriers to rehydration, such as concerns regarding IV therapy. Ask about the patient's greatest concerns regarding fluid status to build the basis for active partnership in planning, implementing, and evaluating patient-centered care.

Nursing History. Clinical assessment begins with a patient history designed to reveal risk factors that cause or contribute to fluid, electrolyte, and acid-base imbalances (Table 42.9). Ask specific, focused questions to identify factors that contribute to a patient's potential imbalances (Box 42.1).

Age. First assess a patient's age. An infant's proportion of total body water (70% to 80% total body weight) is greater than that of children or adults. Infants and young children have greater water needs and immature kidneys (Hockenberry et al., 2019; Kear, 2017). They are at greater risk for ECV deficit and hypernatremia because body water loss is proportionately greater per kilogram of weight (Box 42.2).

Children who are between the ages of 2 and 12 frequently respond to illnesses with fevers of higher temperatures and longer duration than those of adults (Hockenberry et al., 2019). At any age fever increases the rate of insensible water loss. Adolescents have increased metabolism and water production because of their rapid growth changes. Fluctuations in fluid balance are greater in adolescent girls because of hormonal changes associated with the menstrual cycle.

Older adults experience a number of age-related changes that potentially affect fluid, electrolyte, and acid-base balances (see Box 42.2). They often have more difficulty recovering from imbalances resulting from the combined effects of normal aging, various disease conditions, and multiple medications (Kear, 2017).

Environment. Hot environments increase fluid output through sweating. Sweat is a hypotonic sodium-containing fluid. Excessive sweating without adequate replacement of salt and water can lead to ECV deficit, hypernatremia, or clinical dehydration (McDermott et al., 2017). Ask patients about their normal level of physical work and whether they engage in vigorous exercise in hot environments. Do the patients have fluid replacements containing salt available during exercise and activity?

Dietary Intake. Assess dietary intake of fluids; salt; and foods rich in potassium, calcium, and magnesium (see Table 42.4). Ask patients if they follow weight-loss diets. Starvation diets or those with high fat and no carbohydrate content often lead to metabolic acidosis (see Table 42.7). In addition, assess a patient's ability to chew and swallow, which,

TABLE 42.9	Risk Factors for Fluid, Electrolyte, and Acid-Base Imbalances
Age	*Very young:* ECV deficit, osmolality imbalances, clinical dehydration *Very old:* ECV excess or deficit, osmolality imbalances
Environment	*Sodium-rich diet:* ECV excess *Electrolyte-poor diet:* Electrolyte deficits *Hot weather:* Clinical dehydration
Gastrointestinal output	*Diarrhea:* ECV deficit, clinical dehydration, hypokalemia, hypocalcemia (if chronic), hypomagnesemia (if chronic), metabolic acidosis *Drainage (e.g., nasogastric suctioning, fistulas):* ECV deficit, hypokalemia; metabolic acidosis if intestinal or pancreatic drainage *Vomiting:* ECV deficit, clinical dehydration, hypokalemia, hypomagnesemia, metabolic alkalosis
Chronic diseases	*Cancer:* Hypercalcemia; with tumor lysis syndrome: hyperkalemia, hypocalcemia, hyperphosphatemia; other imbalances, depending on side effects of therapy *Chronic obstructive pulmonary disease:* Respiratory acidosis *Cirrhosis:* ECV excess, hypokalemia *Heart failure:* ECV excess; other imbalances, depending on therapy *Oliguric renal disease:* ECV excess, hyperkalemia, hypermagnesemia, hyperphosphatemia, metabolic acidosis
Trauma	*Burns:* ECV deficit, metabolic acidosis *Crush injuries:* Hyperkalemia *Head injuries:* Hyponatremia or hypernatremia, depending on ADH response *Hemorrhage:* ECV deficit, hyperkalemia if circulatory shock
Therapies	*Diuretics and other medications* (see Box 42.3) *IV therapy:* ECV excess, osmolality imbalances, electrolyte excesses *PN:* Any fluid or electrolyte imbalance, depending on components of solution

ADH, Antidiuretic hormone; *ECV,* extracellular fluid volume; *IV,* intravenous; *PN,* parenteral nutrition.

if altered, interferes with adequate intake of electrolyte-rich foods and fluids.

Lifestyle. Assess your patient's alcohol intake. How many days does a person have an alcoholic drink each week, and how many drinks does he or she have at any one time? Chronic alcohol abuse commonly causes hypomagnesemia, in part because it increases renal magnesium excretion (Palmer and Clegg, 2017).

Medications. Obtain a complete list of your patient's current medications, including over-the-counter (OTC) and herbal preparations, to assess the risk for fluid, electrolyte, and acid-base imbalances (Box 42.3). Use a drug reference book or reputable online database to check the potential effects of other medications. Ask specifically about the use of baking soda as an antacid, which can cause ECV excess because of its high sodium content that holds water in the extracellular compartments. For an individual who uses laxatives, ask about the type of laxative, the frequency of use, and the consistency and frequency of stools. Multiple loose stools remove fluid and electrolytes from the body, thus causing numerous imbalances.

BOX 42.1 Nursing Assessment Questions

Environment
- Do you work or exercise in a hot environment?
- If so, which type of fluid do you drink during that time?

Dietary Intake
- About how many glasses of fluids do you usually drink every day? Which type of fluids do you normally drink?
- Tell me what you usually eat in a day.
- In the past month, was there any day when you went hungry because you did not have enough money for food?
- Which snacks do you usually eat?
- Are you on a special diet because of a medical problem? How does that work for you?
- Are you following any weight-loss program?
- Do you use a salt substitute?
- Do you take calcium, magnesium, or potassium supplements? If so, how often?
- Do you have any difficulties chewing or swallowing?

Lifestyle
- How much alcohol do you drink in a typical week?

Gastrointestinal Output
- Have you had recent vomiting or diarrhea? If so, for how long? How many times per day?

Medications and Other Therapies
- Which medicines/herbal remedies do you use regularly? Occasionally?
- Do you take diuretics? Drugs for high blood pressure?
- Do you use antacids? If so, which ones? How often? Do you ever use baking soda as an antacid? Do you use fizzy (effervescent) medications for colds?
- Do you use laxatives? If so, how often? Which type of stool do you get when you use them?
- What do you use for an upset stomach?

Signs and Symptoms
- If you weigh yourself every day, how has your weight changed over the past few days?
- Do you get light-headed when you stand up?
- Do you feel thirsty, have a dry mouth, or notice a lack of tears?
- Have you noticed a change in your urine output: decreased volume, dark color, or concentrated appearance?
- Are you experiencing swelling of your fingers, feet, or ankles?
- Do you have difficulty breathing when you lie down at night?
- Are you having difficulty concentrating, or do you feel confused? What is normal for you?
- Are you having more difficulty than usual standing up from a sofa or soft chair? Do your legs feel unusually heavy when you climb stairs? Do you have muscle weakness that is unusual for you?
- Have you noticed any muscle cramps or unusual sensations such as numbness or tingling fingers?

BOX 42.2 FOCUS ON OLDER ADULTS

Factors Affecting Fluid, Electrolyte, and Acid-Base Balance

- During aging, body composition changes, causing a decreased percentage of body weight as water (50%), which increases risk of extracellular fluid volume (ECV) deficit and dehydration (Felver, 2019d).
- The combined effects of age (neonates, infants, and older adults), chronic diseases, and multiple medications often pose challenges to maintaining fluid and electrolyte balance.
- Patients with impaired mobility or bladder control issues may restrict fluid intake, which increases the risk of hypernatremia and ECV deficit.
- Decreased thirst sensation increases risk of hypernatremia and dehydration; do not rely on thirst to assess hypernatremia, ECV deficit, or dehydration in patients who are confused, patients with altered level of consciousness, the very young, and older adults.
- Severe dehydration can result in postural hypotension; have patients, especially older adults, arise slowly when you take orthostatic blood pressure measurements.
- Cardiovascular illnesses can decrease the body's ability to adapt to a sudden increase in vascular volume, increasing risk of pulmonary edema with rapid infusion of isotonic intravenous fluids.
- Chronic renal disease results in a decrease in the kidneys' ability to concentrate urine, thus increasing the risk for hypernatremia, ECV deficit, and dehydration.
- Kidney changes of normal aging make it more difficult to excrete a large acid load, increasing the risk of metabolic acidosis (Touhy and Jett, 2016).

BOX 42.3 Commonly Used Medications That Cause Fluid, Electrolyte, and Acid-Base Imbalances

- *ACE inhibitors (e.g., captopril) and angiotensin II receptor blockers (e.g., losartan):* Hyperkalemia
- *Antidepressants, SSRI (e.g., fluoxetine [Prozac]):* Hyponatremia
- *Calcium carbonate antacids:* Hypercalcemia, mild metabolic alkalosis
- *Corticosteroids (e.g., prednisone):* Hypokalemia, metabolic alkalosis
- *Diuretics, potassium-wasting (e.g., furosemide [Lasix], thiazides):* ECV deficit, hyponatremia (thiazides), hypokalemia, hypomagnesemia, mild metabolic alkalosis
- *Diuretics, potassium-sparing (e.g., spironolactone):* Hyperkalemia, mild metabolic acidosis
- *Effervescent* (fizzy) *antacids and cold medications (high Na⁺ content):* ECV excess
- *Laxatives:* ECV deficit, hypokalemia, hypocalcemia, hypomagnesemia, metabolic acidosis
- *Magnesium hydroxide (e.g., Milk of Magnesia):* Hypermagnesemia
- *Nonsteroidal antiinflammatory drugs (e.g., ibuprofen):* Mild ECV excess, hyponatremia
- *Penicillins, high-dose (e.g., carbenicillin):* Hypokalemia, metabolic alkalosis; hyperkalemia with penicillin G (contains K⁺)

ACE, Angiotensin-converting enzyme; *ECV,* extracellular fluid volume; *SSRI,* selective serotonin reuptake inhibitor.
Data from Burchum JR, Rosenthal LD: *Lehne's pharmacology for nursing care,* ed 10, St Louis, 2019, Elsevier.

Medical History

Recent Surgery. Surgery causes a physiological stress response, which increases with extensive surgery and blood loss. In the first 24 to 48 hours after surgery, increased secretion of aldosterone, glucocorticoids, and ADH cause increased ECV, decreased osmolality, and increased potassium excretion (Lewis et al., 2017). In otherwise healthy patients these imbalances resolve without difficulty, but patients who have preexisting illnesses or additional risk factors often need treatment during this period.

Gastrointestinal Output. Increased output of fluid through the GI tract is a common and important cause of fluid, electrolyte, and acid-base imbalances that requires careful assessment. Vomiting and diarrhea, either acute or chronic, can cause ECV deficit, hypernatremia, clinical dehydration, and hypokalemia by increasing the output of fluid,

Na^+, and K^+. In addition, chronic diarrhea can cause hypocalcemia and hypomagnesemia by decreasing electrolyte absorption. Removal of gastric acid from the body through vomiting or nasogastric suction can cause metabolic alkalosis. In contrast, removal of the bicarbonate-rich intestinal or pancreatic fluids through diarrhea, intestinal suction, or fistula can cause metabolic acidosis (Ferrari et al., 2017).

Acute Illness or Trauma. Acute conditions that place patients at high risk for fluid, electrolyte, and acid-base alterations include respiratory diseases, burns, trauma, GI alterations, and acute oliguric renal disease.

Respiratory Disorders. Many acute respiratory disorders predispose patients to respiratory acidosis. For example, bacterial pneumonia causes alveoli to fill with exudate that impairs gas exchange, causing the patient to retain carbon dioxide, which leads to increased $PaCO_2$ and respiratory acidosis.

Burns. Burns place patients at high risk for ECV deficit from numerous mechanisms, including plasma-to-interstitial fluid shift and increased evaporative and exudate output. Fluid loss increases with the percentage of body surface burned (Lewis et al., 2017). Patients with burns have cellular damage that releases potassium into the blood, and they may become hyperkalemic. In addition, these patients often develop metabolic acidosis because of greatly increased cellular metabolism, which produces more metabolic acids than their kidneys are able to excrete.

Trauma. Hemorrhage from any type of trauma causes ECV deficit from blood loss. Some types of trauma create additional risks. For example, crush injuries destroy cellular structure, causing hyperkalemia by massive release of intracellular K^+ into the blood.

Head injury typically alters ADH secretion. It may cause diabetes insipidus (deficit of ADH), in which patients excrete large volumes of very dilute urine and develop hypernatremia. In contrast, head injury may cause the syndrome of inappropriate antidiuretic hormone (SIADH), in which excess secretion of ADH causes hyponatremia by retaining too much water and concentrating the urine (Lewis et al., 2017).

Chronic Illness. Many chronic diseases create ongoing risk of fluid, electrolyte, and acid-base imbalances. For example, type B chronic obstructive pulmonary disease (COPD) often causes chronic respiratory acidosis. In addition, the treatment regimens for chronic disease often cause imbalances. Assess patients for the presence of these conditions (see Box 42.2).

Cancer. The specific fluid and electrolyte imbalances that occur with cancer depend on the type and progression of the cancer and the treatment regimen. Many patients with cancer develop hypercalcemia when their cancer cells secrete chemicals that circulate to bones and cause calcium to enter the blood. Other fluid and electrolyte imbalances occur in cancer because some types of tumors cause metabolic and endocrine abnormalities (Wagner and Arora, 2017). In addition, patients with cancer are at risk for fluid and electrolyte imbalances as a result of the side effects (e.g., anorexia, diarrhea) of chemotherapy, biological response modifiers, or radiation (Lewis et al., 2017).

Heart Failure. Patients who have chronic heart failure have diminished cardiac output, which reduces kidney perfusion and activates the RAAS. The action of aldosterone on the kidneys causes ECV excess and risk of hypokalemia. Most diuretics used to treat heart failure increase the risk of hypokalemia while reducing the ECV excess. Dietary sodium restriction is important with heart failure because Na^+ holds water in the ECF, making the ECV excess worse. In severe heart failure a restriction of both fluid and sodium may be prescribed to decrease the workload of the heart by reducing excess circulating fluid volume (Lewis et al., 2017).

Oliguric Renal Disease. Oliguria occurs when the kidneys have a reduced capacity to make urine. Some conditions such as acute nephritis cause sudden onset of oliguria, whereas other problems such as chronic kidney disease lead to chronic oliguria. Oliguric renal disease prevents normal excretion of fluid, electrolytes, and metabolic acids, resulting in ECV excess, hyperkalemia, hypermagnesemia, hyperphosphatemia, and metabolic acidosis. The severity of these imbalances is proportional to the degree of renal failure. Although chronic kidney disease is progressive, successful management of imbalances is possible with dietary restriction of sodium and other electrolytes, fluid restriction in severe cases, and eventually dialysis or renal transplant (Lewis et al., 2017).

Physical Assessment. Data gathered through a focused physical assessment validates and extends the information collected in the patient history. Table 42.10 summarizes focused assessments for patients with fluid, electrolyte, and acid-base imbalances. Focus your assessment on the areas pertinent to each patient situation. For example, for patients at risk of fluid imbalances, focus your assessment on body weight changes, clinical markers of vascular and interstitial volume, thirst, behavioral changes, and level of consciousness. Additional focused assessments for patients at high risk of electrolyte and acid-base imbalances include specific cardiac, respiratory, neuromuscular, and GI markers. Grouping your assessments under these categories helps you know which assessments to prioritize and enables you to assess effectively.

Daily Weights and Fluid Intake and Output Measurement. Daily weights are an important indicator of fluid status (Felver, 2019c). Each kilogram (2.2 lb) of weight gained or lost overnight is equal to 1 L of fluid retained or lost. These fluid gains or losses indicate changes in the amount of total body fluid, usually ECF, but do not indicate shift between body compartments. Weigh patients with heart failure and those who are at high risk for or actually have ECV excess daily. Daily weights are also useful for patients with clinical dehydration or other causes or risks for ECV deficit. Weigh the patient at the same time each day with the same scale after a patient voids. Calibrate the scale each day or routinely. The patient needs to wear the same clothes or clothes that weigh the same; if using a bed scale, use the same number of sheets on the scale with each weighing. Compare the weight of each day with that of the previous day to determine fluid gains or losses. Look at the weights over several days to recognize trends. Interpretation of daily weights guides medical therapy and nursing care.

Teach patients with heart failure to take and record their daily weights at home and to contact their health care provider if their weight increases suddenly by a set amount (obtain parameters from their health care providers). Recognizing trends in daily weights taken at home is important (Park et al., 2017). Patients who are hospitalized for decompensated heart failure often experience steady increases in daily weights during the week before hospitalization.

Measuring and recording all liquid intake and output (I&O) during a 24-hour period is an important aspect of fluid balance assessment. Compare a patient's 24-hour intake with his or her 24-hour output. The two measures should be approximately equal if the person has normal fluid balance (Felver, 2019c). To interpret situations in which I&O are substantially different, consider the individual patient. For example, if intake is substantially greater than output, there are two possibilities: the patient may be gaining excessive fluid or returning to normal fluid status by replacing fluid lost previously from the body. Similarly, if intake is substantially smaller than output, there are also two possibilities: the patient may be losing needed fluid from the body and developing ECV deficit and/or hypernatremia or returning to normal fluid status by excreting excessive fluid gained previously.

TABLE 42.10 Focused Nursing Assessments for Patients with Fluid, Electrolyte, and Acid-Base Imbalances

Assessment	Imbalances
Body Weight Changes from Previous Day	
Loss of 2.2 lb (1 kg) or more in 24 hours for adults	ECV deficit
Gain of 2.2 lb (1 kg) or more in 24 hours for adults	ECV excess
Clinical Markers of Vascular Volume	
Blood pressure:	
Hypotension or orthostatic hypotension	ECV deficit
Light-headedness on sitting upright or standing	ECV deficit
Pulse rate and character:	
Rapid, thready	ECV deficit
Bounding	ECV excess
Fullness of neck veins:	
Flat or collapsing with inhalation when supine	ECV deficit
Full or distended when upright or semi-upright	ECV excess
Other assessments of vascular volume:	
Capillary refill: Sluggish	ECV deficit
Lung auscultation, dependent lobe: Crackles or rhonchi with progressive dyspnea	ECV excess
Urine output: Small volume of dark yellow urine	ECV deficit
Clinical Markers of Interstitial Volume	
Inspection and Palpation	
Presence of edema: Present in dependent areas (ankles or sacrum) and possibly fingers or around eyes	ECV excess
Mucous membranes: Dry between cheek and gum, decreased or absent tearing	ECV deficit
Skin turgor: Pinched skin fails to return to normal position within 3 seconds	ECV deficit
Presence of thirst: Thirst present	Hypernatremia, severe ECV deficit
Behavior and level of consciousness	
Restlessness and mild confusion	Severe ECV deficit
Decreased level of consciousness (lethargy, confusion, coma)	Hyponatremia, hypernatremia, hypercalcemia, acid-base imbalances
Cardiac and Respiratory Signs of Electrolyte or Acid-Base Imbalances	
Pulse rhythm and ECG: Irregular pulse and ECG changes	K^+, Ca^{2+}, Mg^{2+}, and/or acid-base imbalances
Rate and depth of respirations:	
Increased rate and depth	Metabolic acidosis (compensatory mechanism); respiratory alkalosis (cause)
Decreased rate and depth	Metabolic alkalosis (compensatory mechanism); respiratory acidosis (cause)
Neuromuscular Markers of Electrolyte or Acid-Base Imbalances	
Muscle strength bilaterally, especially quadriceps muscles:	
Muscle weakness	Hypokalemia, hyperkalemia
Reflexes and sensations:	
Decreased deep tendon reflexes	Hypercalcemia, hypermagnesemia
Hyperactive reflexes, muscle twitching and cramps, tetany	Hypocalcemia, hypomagnesemia
Numbness, tingling in fingertips, around mouth	Hypocalcemia, hypomagnesemia, respiratory alkalosis
Muscle cramps, tetany	Hypocalcemia, hypomagnesemia, respiratory alkalosis
Tremors	Hypomagnesemia
Gastrointestinal Signs of Electrolyte Imbalances	
Inspection and auscultation:	
Abdominal distention	Hypokalemia, third-spacing of fluid
Decreased bowel sounds	Hypokalemia
Motility: Constipation	Hypokalemia, hypercalcemia

ECG, Electrocardiogram; *ECV,* extracellular fluid volume.

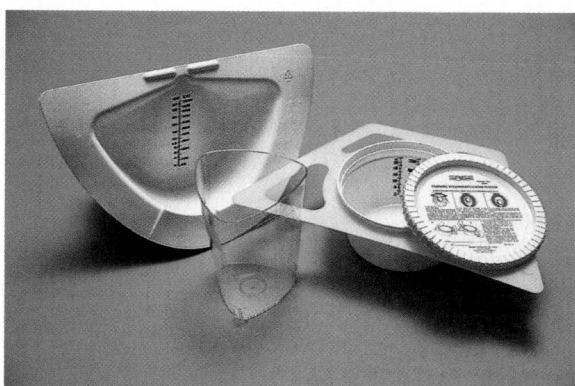

FIG. 42.10 Containers for measuring urine output.

In most health care settings I&O measurement is a nursing assessment. Some agencies require a health care provider's order for I&O. If you want to measure I&O for a patient with compromised fluid status, check your agency policies to determine whether you can set it up or if you need a health care provider's order.

Fluid intake includes all liquids that a person eats (e.g., gelatin, ice cream, soup), drinks (e.g., water, coffee, juice), or receives through nasogastric or jejunostomy feeding tubes (see Chapter 45). IV fluids (continuous infusions and intermittent IV piggybacks) and blood components also are sources of intake. Water swallowed while taking pills and liquid medications counts as intake. A patient receiving tube feedings often receives numerous liquid medications, and water is used to flush the tube before and/or after medications. Over a 24-hour period these liquids amount to significant intake and always are recorded on the I&O record. Ask patients who are alert and oriented to help with measuring their oral intake and explain to families why they should not drink or eat from the patient's meal trays or water pitcher.

Fluid output includes urine, diarrhea, vomitus, gastric suction, and drainage from postsurgical wounds or other tubes (see Chapter 50). Record a patient's urinary output after each voiding. Instruct patients who are alert, oriented, and ambulatory to save their urine in a urinal or a calibrated insert, which attaches to the rim of the toilet bowl (Fig. 42.10). Teach patients and families the purpose of I&O measurements. Also teach them to notify the nurse or assistive personnel (AP) to empty any container with voided fluid or how to measure and empty the container themselves and report the result appropriately. Patients need to have good vision and motor skills to perform these measurements. Active involvement of patient and family is an aspect of patient-centered care that is essential to maintaining accurate I&O measurements. When a patient has an indwelling urinary catheter, drainage tube, or suction, record output (e.g., at the end of each nursing shift or every hour) as the patient's condition requires.

You can delegate parts of I&O measurement and recording to AP with competent skills in measurement. Actual measurement of fluid volumes is more accurate than visual estimates. In many institutions AP record oral intake but not intake through feeding or IV tubes, which are nursing responsibilities. Similarly AP often record urine, diarrhea, and vomitus output but not drainage through tubes. The responsible registered nurse (RN) or licensed practical nurse/licensed vocational nurse (LPN/LVN) and the AP work as a team to record measurements in the designated location in the electronic health record (EHR), often on a flow sheet with other information. The EHR program usually calculates the 24-hour totals. If an EHR is not used, record I&O on paper forms attached to the bedside chart or room door. You or the AP calculates the 24-hour totals (see agency policy). Accurate I&O facilitates ongoing evaluation of a patient's hydration status.

Laboratory Values. Review the patient's laboratory test results and compare them with the normal ranges to obtain further objective data about fluid, electrolyte, and acid-base balances. Normal and abnormal test results are summarized in Tables 42.1, 42.3, and 42.5 to 42.7. The frequency of electrolyte level measurements depends on the severity of a patient's illness. Analyzing a patient's laboratory results requires you to be thorough and to apply extensive scientific and nursing knowledge, especially if a person develops an acute imbalance while also having a chronic disease. Serum electrolyte tests usually are performed routinely on patients entering a hospital to screen for imbalances and serve as a baseline for future comparisons.

> **REFLECT NOW**
>
> How would your assessments related to fluid, electrolyte, and acid-base imbalances differ between patients with acute illness and patients with chronic illnesses?

◆ Nursing Diagnosis

When caring for patients with suspected fluid, electrolyte, and acid-base imbalances, it is particularly important to use critical thinking to formulate nursing diagnoses. The assessment data that establish the risk for or the actual presence of a nursing diagnosis in these areas may be subtle, and patterns and trends emerge only when there has been astute assessment. Multiple body systems often are involved; careful clustering of assessment findings leads to selection of the appropriate diagnoses (Box 42.4).

In addition to the accurate clustering of assessment data, an important part of formulating nursing diagnoses is identifying the relevant causative or related factor (when a diagnosis is negative or problem focused) or risk factors (when a diagnosis is a risk diagnosis). You choose interventions that treat or modify the related factor or risk for the diagnosis to be resolved. For example, *Dehydration related to loss of GI fluids from vomiting* requires therapies that manage the patients' emesis and restore fluid volume with IV therapy. In contrast, the diagnosis of *Fluid Imbalance related to elevated body temperature* requires therapies to lower the patient's body temperature and replace lost body fluids through oral fluid replacement or possibly IV therapy. Possible nursing diagnoses for patients with fluid, electrolyte, and acid-base alterations include the following:

- *Fluid Imbalance*
- *Dehydration*
- *Electrolyte Imbalance*
- *Acid Base Imbalance*
- *Lack of Knowledge of Fluid Regimen*

◆ Planning

During the planning process use critical thinking to synthesize information from multiple resources (Fig. 42.11). Ensure that a patient's plan of care integrates both scientific and nursing knowledge and all of the information that you collected about the individual patient.

BOX 42.4 Nursing Diagnostic Process

Dehydration Related to Loss of Gastrointestinal Fluids via Vomiting

Assessment Activities	Assessment Findings
Assess postural blood pressure and pulse.	Patient has postural hypotension with increased heart rate; pulse is weak.
Inspect oral mucous membranes for degree of moisture.	Oral mucous membranes between cheek and gum are dry.
Obtain daily weight measurements.	Adult patient loses 2.2 lb (1 kg) or more in 24 hours.
Measure urine output and observe color; if available, measure specific gravity of urine.	Patient produces small volume of dark yellow urine; urine specific gravity is increased.
Test skin turgor (not reliable for older adults).	Decreased skin turgor noted.

Goals and Outcomes. Establish an individual patient plan of care for each nursing diagnosis (see the Nursing Care Plan) that includes mutually established patient goals for each diagnosis. Collaborate with and inform patients as you individualize goals with realistic, measurable outcomes. For example, with a nursing diagnosis of *Dehydration*, the following related outcomes might be established for the goal "The patient achieves normal hydration status at discharge":

- The patient is free of complications associated with the IV device throughout the duration of IV therapy.
- The patient demonstrates balanced I&O measurements within 48 hours.

Setting Priorities. The patient's clinical condition determines which of the nursing diagnoses takes the greatest priority. Many nursing diagnoses in the area of fluid, electrolyte, and acid-base balances are of highest priority because the consequences for the patient can be serious or even life threatening. For example, in the concept map (Fig. 42.12) for Mrs. Mendoza, the occurrence of vomiting and diarrhea created a high-priority nursing diagnosis of *Dehydration*. The priority for Mrs. Mendoza is to restore her fluid balance. To achieve this priority, her vomiting and diarrhea must be controlled and resolved, and her fluid volume replaced. If these goals are unmet, Mrs. Mendoza's fluid imbalance is likely to worsen.

Teamwork and Collaboration. Consultation with a patient's health care provider helps to set realistic time frames for the goals of care, particularly when a patient's physiological status is unstable. Ongoing communication and consultation are important because the patient's condition can change quickly. Collaboration with the patient and family and other members of the interprofessional health care team such as IV therapists and pharmacists helps in achieving patient outcomes. Patients and family members are very helpful in identifying approaches for successful therapies such as ways to increase fluid intake. Incorporate patient preferences and resources into the plan of care. Do not delegate administration of IV fluid and hemodynamic assessment to AP. When the patient is stable, you can delegate daily weights, I&O, and direct physical care to AP (INS, 2016a).

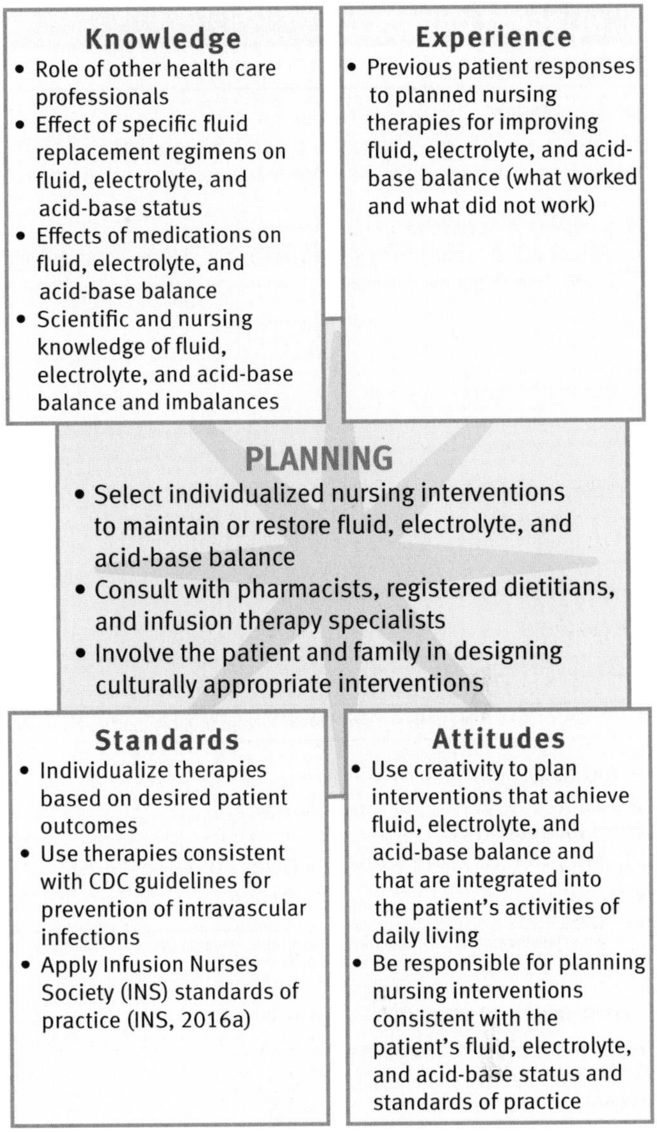

Knowledge
- Role of other health care professionals
- Effect of specific fluid replacement regimens on fluid, electrolyte, and acid-base status
- Effects of medications on fluid, electrolyte, and acid-base balance
- Scientific and nursing knowledge of fluid, electrolyte, and acid-base balance and imbalances

Experience
- Previous patient responses to planned nursing therapies for improving fluid, electrolyte, and acid-base balance (what worked and what did not work)

PLANNING
- Select individualized nursing interventions to maintain or restore fluid, electrolyte, and acid-base balance
- Consult with pharmacists, registered dietitians, and infusion therapy specialists
- Involve the patient and family in designing culturally appropriate interventions

Standards
- Individualize therapies based on desired patient outcomes
- Use therapies consistent with CDC guidelines for prevention of intravascular infections
- Apply Infusion Nurses Society (INS) standards of practice (INS, 2016a)

Attitudes
- Use creativity to plan interventions that achieve fluid, electrolyte, and acid-base balance and that are integrated into the patient's activities of daily living
- Be responsible for planning nursing interventions consistent with the patient's fluid, electrolyte, and acid-base status and standards of practice

FIG. 42.11 Critical thinking model for fluid, electrolyte, and acid-base balance planning. *CDC,* Centers for Disease Control and Prevention.

Begin discharge planning early for patients with acute or chronic fluid and electrolyte disturbances by anticipating the needs of the patient and family as they transition to another setting. In the hospital collaboration with other members of the health care team ensures that care will continue in the home or long-term care setting with few disruptions. You ensure that therapeutic regimens established in one setting continue through completion at the next setting. For example, for a patient who is discharged on IV therapy, you assess the knowledge and skills of the family member or friend who will assume caregiving responsibilities and initiate a referral to home IV therapy as soon as possible. Close collaboration with members of the health care team such as the patient's health care provider, registered dietitian, and pharmacist is essential to ensure positive patient outcomes. A registered dietitian is a valuable resource in recommending food sources to increase or reduce intake of specific electrolytes, incorporating the patient's preferences when possible (see Chapter 45). A pharmacist helps identify medications or combinations of medications likely to cause electrolyte or acid-base disturbances and offers information regarding patient education

◎ **NURSING CARE PLAN**

Dehydration

ASSESSMENT

Mrs.Mendoza, age 77, fell at home after having vomiting and diarrhea for 24 hours. She was admitted to the hospital for oral and intravenous (IV) fluid therapy after x-rays indicated no broken bones. Mrs. Mendoza lives alone in an apartment and has no chronic illnesses except osteoarthritis of her hands.

Assessment Activities	*Assessment Findings*[a]
Ask Mrs. Mendoza to describe when her vomiting and diarrhea began and any accompanying signs and symptoms.	Gastrointestinal (GI) problems began suddenly yesterday. Reports **getting weak and light-headed when she stands or sits upright.**
Ask her about current status of vomiting and diarrhea.	Says she was vomiting earlier this morning but not in the past 3 hours. Had three episodes of watery diarrhea this morning and more than six yesterday.
Assess Mrs. Mendoza's vital signs.	**Heart rate 110** beats/min; regular, **weak pulse; supine blood pressure (BP) 90/58 mm Hg.** Temperature and respirations within normal limits. Postural BP measurement omitted for patient safety.
Evaluate physical signs of extracellular fluid volume (ECV).	**Neck veins flat when supine; 100 mL of dark yellow urine** in past 4 hours; **dry mucous membranes between cheek and gum; prolonged capillary refill time** of 5 seconds.
Weigh Mrs. Mendoza using a bed scale.	Weight 120 lb (54.5 kg). States usual weight at home is 127 lb (46.27 kg) **(7-lb [3.17-kg] weight loss).**

[a]**Assessment findings** are shown in **bold** type.

NURSING DIAGNOSIS: Dehydration related to prolonged vomiting and diarrhea

PLANNING

Goals	*Expected Outcomes (NOC)*[b]
Fluid Balance	
Mrs. Mendoza's fluid volume will return to normal by hospital discharge.	Denies light-headedness when sitting or standing within 24 hours.
	Daily output of light yellow urine equals intake of at least 1500 mL by discharge.

[b]Outcome classification labels from Moorhead S, et al: *Nursing Outcomes Classification (NOC)*, ed 6, St Louis, 2018, Elsevier.

INTERVENTIONS[c] **(NIC)**	**RATIONALE**
Fluid/Electrolyte Management	
Provide Mrs. Mendoza's favorite fluids at her preferred temperature.	Patient-centered care takes individual preferences into account; types and temperature of oral fluids can influence oral intake (Giger, 2017; Rong et al., 2017).
Provide pitcher and glass of water at Mrs. Mendoza's preferred temperature at her bedside; ensure that she can access and pour from it easily; provide straw if she wishes.	Chronic disease such as osteoarthritis of hands may make it difficult to manipulate a full water pitcher. Make fluid available in form that is easy for patient to access (Felver, 2019c).
Administer IV therapy as prescribed, monitoring closely for early side effects of complications.	IV fluid replacement augments oral replacement when ECV deficit exists. Age-appropriate care is needed because of older adult's anatomical and physiological changes that affect volume delivery (INS, 2016a).

[c]Intervention classification labels from Butcher HK, et al.: *Nursing Interventions Classification (NIC)*, ed 7, St Louis, 2018, Elsevier.

EVALUATION

Evaluation Activity	*Patient Response/Finding*	*Outcome Status*
Monitor vital signs, intake and output (I&O), daily weight, and postural BP when no longer light-headed.	T 37° C (98.6° F), RR 10, HR 72 beats/min, BP 120/78 sitting, 122/78 standing, denies light-headedness	Symptoms of fluid volume deficit are resolving.
Assess intake and output and mucous membranes.	Intake 2000 mL, output 2000 mL of light yellow urine Today's weight 129 lb (58.5 kg) Mucous membranes moist	Patient showing resolution of dehydration.

about side effects to anticipate for prescribed drugs. The patient's health care provider directs the treatment of fluid, electrolyte, or acid-base imbalances.

◆ Implementation

Health Promotion. Health promotion activities focus primarily on patient education, which you provide based on a patient's and family's health literacy. Use plain language to teach patients and caregivers to recognize risk factors for developing imbalances and implement appropriate preventive measures. For example, parents of infants need to understand that GI losses quickly lead to serious imbalances; therefore, when vomiting or diarrhea occurs in an infant, they need to promptly rehydrate with sodium-containing fluid or seek health care to restore normal balance. People of any age need to learn to replace body fluid losses with sodium-containing fluid and water.

Patients with chronic health alterations often are at risk for developing fluid, electrolyte, and acid-base imbalances. They need to understand their own risk factors and the measures they need to take to avoid imbalances. For example, patients with end-stage renal disease often need to restrict intake of fluid, sodium, potassium, magnesium, and phosphate (Norton et al., 2017). Through diet education these patients learn the types of foods to avoid and the suitable volume of fluid that they are permitted daily (see Chapter 45). Teach patients with chronic diseases and their family caregivers the early signs and symptoms of the fluid, electrolyte, and acid-base imbalances for which they are at risk and what to do if these occur.

REFLECT NOW

What should you teach an older adult who has frequent diarrhea about how to replace fluids to avoid dehydration?

Acute Care. Although fluid, electrolyte, and/or acid-base imbalances occur in all settings, they are common in acute care. Acute care nurses administer medications and oral and IV fluids to replace fluid and electrolyte deficits or maintain normal homeostasis; they also help with restricting intake as part of therapy for fluid excesses.

Enteral Replacement of Fluids. Oral replacement of fluids and electrolytes is appropriate as long as the patient is not so physiologically unstable that they cannot be replaced rapidly enough (Carson et al., 2017). Oral replacement of fluids is contraindicated when a patient has a mechanical obstruction of the GI tract, severe nausea, is at high risk for aspiration, or has impaired swallowing. Some patients unable to tolerate solid foods are still able to ingest fluids. Strategies to encourage fluid intake include offering frequent small sips of fluid, popsicles, and ice chips. Record one-half the volume of the ice chips in I&O measurement. For example, if a patient ingests 240 mL of ice chips, you record 120 mL of intake. Encourage patients to keep their own record of intake to involve them actively. Family members who are properly instructed can also help. Pay attention to each patient's preferred temperature of oral fluids. Cultural beliefs regarding appropriate fluids and fluid temperature may become a barrier to achieving adequate fluid intake unless the fluid with the preferred temperature is available (Box 42.5).

When replacing fluids by mouth in a patient with ECV deficit, choose fluids that contain sodium (e.g., Pedialyte and Gastrolyte).

Liquids that contain lactose or have low-sodium content are inappropriate when a patient has diarrhea.

A feeding tube is appropriate when a patient's GI tract is healthy, but he or she cannot ingest fluids (e.g., after oral surgery or with impaired swallowing). Options for administering fluids include gastrostomy or jejunostomy instillations or infusions through small-bore nasogastric feeding tubes (see Chapter 45).

Restriction of Fluids. Patients who have hyponatremia usually require restricted water intake. Patients who have very severe ECV excess sometimes have both sodium and fluid restrictions. Fluid restriction often is difficult for patients, particularly if they take medications that dry the oral mucous membranes or if they are mouth breathers. Explain the reason that fluids are restricted. Make sure that the patient, family, and visitors know the amount of fluid permitted orally and understand that ice chips, gelatin, and ice cream are fluids. Help the patient decide the amount of fluid to drink with each meal, between meals, before bed, and with medications. It is important to allow patients to choose preferred fluids unless contraindicated. Frequently patients on fluid restriction can swallow a number of pills with as little as 1 oz (30 mL) of liquid.

In acute care settings fluid restrictions usually allot half the total oral fluids between 7 AM and 3 PM (i.e., the period when patients are more active, receive two meals, and take most of their oral medications). Offer the remainder of the fluids during the evening and night shifts. Patients on fluid restriction need frequent mouth care to moisten mucous membranes, decrease the chance of mucosal drying and cracking, and maintain comfort (see Chapter 40).

Parenteral Replacement of Fluids and Electrolytes. Fluid and electrolytes may be replaced through infusion of fluids directly into veins (intravenously) rather than via the digestive system. Parenteral replacement includes parenteral nutrition (PN), IV fluid and electrolyte therapy (crystalloids), and blood and blood component (colloids) administration. IV devices are called *peripheral IVs* when the catheter tip lies in a vein in one of the extremities; they are called *central venous catheters (CVCs) or IVs* when the catheter tip lies in the central circulatory system (e.g., in the vena cava close to the right atrium of the heart) (Fig. 42.13).

Practice standard body fluid precautions when preparing and administering parenteral fluids (see Chapter 28) to minimize your own risk for exposure to bloodborne pathogens. Read and understand the policy and procedures for parenteral infusions at the agency for which you work.

Parenteral Nutrition. Parenteral nutrition (PN), also called *total PN (TPN)*, is IV administration of a complex, highly concentrated solution containing nutrients and electrolytes that is formulated to meet a patient's needs. Depending on their osmolality, PN solutions are administered through a CVC in cases of high osmolality or through a peripheral intravenous (IV) line for lower osmolality solutions. Safe administration depends on appropriate assessment of nutrition needs, meticulous management of the CVC or IV to prevent infection, and careful monitoring to prevent metabolic complications. Chapter 45 reviews principles and guidelines for PN administration, which is used when patients are unable to receive enough nutrition orally or through enteral feeding.

Intravenous Therapy (Crystalloids). The goal of IV fluid administration is to correct or prevent fluid and electrolyte disturbances. It allows for direct access to the vascular system, permitting the continuous infusion of fluids over a period of time. IV therapy requires a health care provider's order for type, amount, and speed of administration of a solution. You regulate IV fluid

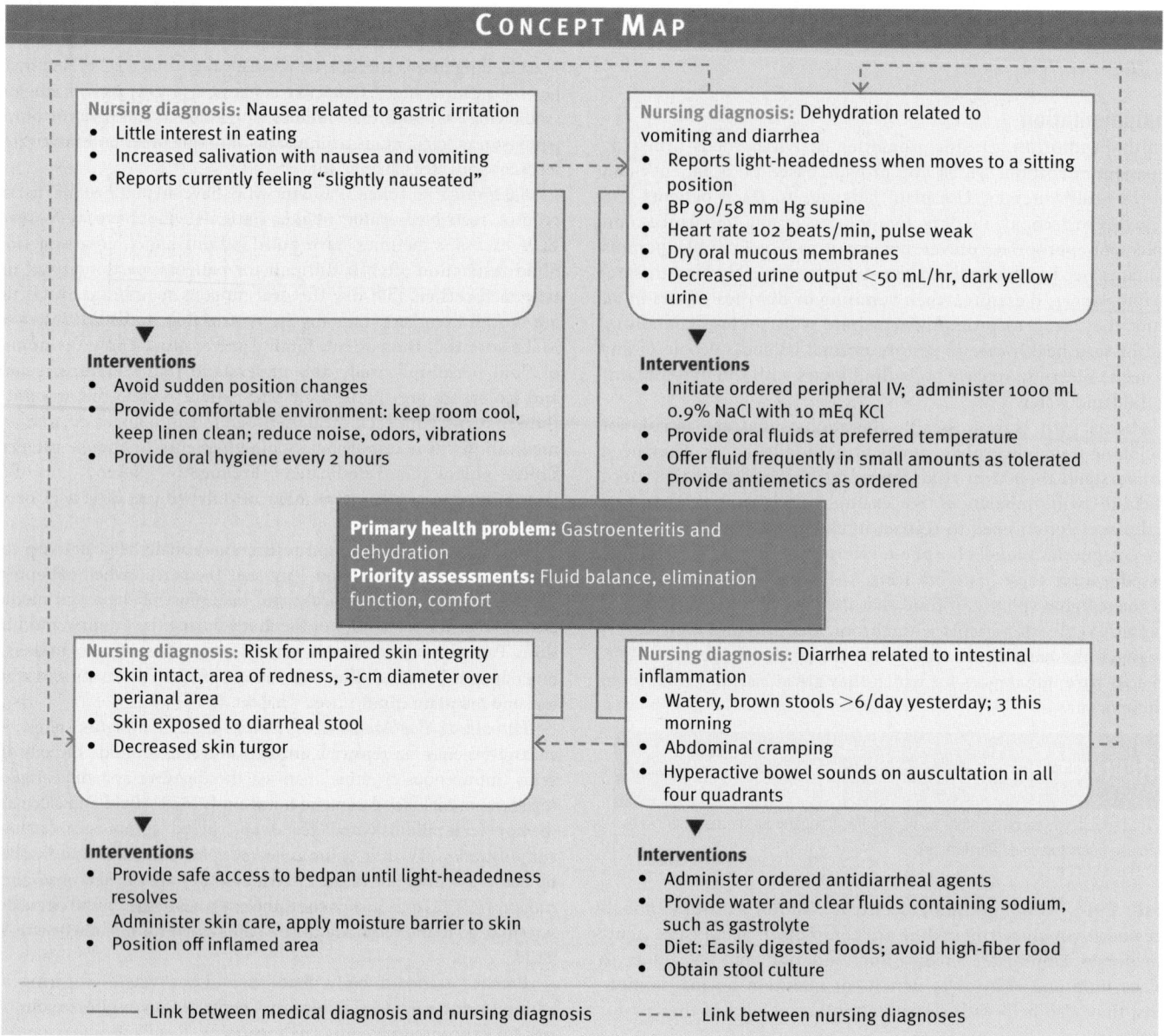

CONCEPT MAP

Nursing diagnosis: Nausea related to gastric irritation
- Little interest in eating
- Increased salivation with nausea and vomiting
- Reports currently feeling "slightly nauseated"

Interventions
- Avoid sudden position changes
- Provide comfortable environment: keep room cool, keep linen clean; reduce noise, odors, vibrations
- Provide oral hygiene every 2 hours

Nursing diagnosis: Dehydration related to vomiting and diarrhea
- Reports light-headedness when moves to a sitting position
- BP 90/58 mm Hg supine
- Heart rate 102 beats/min, pulse weak
- Dry oral mucous membranes
- Decreased urine output <50 mL/hr, dark yellow urine

Interventions
- Initiate ordered peripheral IV; administer 1000 mL 0.9% NaCl with 10 mEq KCl
- Provide oral fluids at preferred temperature
- Offer fluid frequently in small amounts as tolerated
- Provide antiemetics as ordered

Primary health problem: Gastroenteritis and dehydration
Priority assessments: Fluid balance, elimination function, comfort

Nursing diagnosis: Risk for impaired skin integrity
- Skin intact, area of redness, 3-cm diameter over perianal area
- Skin exposed to diarrheal stool
- Decreased skin turgor

Interventions
- Provide safe access to bedpan until light-headedness resolves
- Administer skin care, apply moisture barrier to skin
- Position off inflamed area

Nursing diagnosis: Diarrhea related to intestinal inflammation
- Watery, brown stools >6/day yesterday; 3 this morning
- Abdominal cramping
- Hyperactive bowel sounds on auscultation in all four quadrants

Interventions
- Administer ordered antidiarrheal agents
- Provide water and clear fluids containing sodium, such as gastrolyte
- Diet: Easily digested foods; avoid high-fiber food
- Obtain stool culture

——— Link between medical diagnosis and nursing diagnosis   - - - - Link between nursing diagnoses

FIG. 42.12 Concept map for Mrs. Mendoza.

therapy continuously because of ongoing changes in a patient's fluid and electrolyte balance. To provide safe and appropriate therapy to patients who require IV fluids, you need knowledge of the correct ordered solution, the reason the solution was ordered, the equipment needed, the procedures required to initiate an infusion, how to regulate the infusion rate and maintain the system, how to identify and correct problems, and how to discontinue the infusion.

Types of Solutions. Many prepared IV solutions are available for use (Table 42.11). An IV solution is isotonic, hypotonic, or hypertonic. Isotonic solutions have the same effective osmolality as body fluids. Sodium-containing isotonic solutions such as normal saline are indicated for ECV replacement to prevent or treat ECV deficit. Hypotonic solutions have an effective osmolality less than body fluids, thus decreasing osmolality by diluting body fluids and moving water into cells. Hypertonic solutions have an effective osmolality greater than body fluids. If they are hypertonic sodium-containing solutions, they increase osmolality rapidly and pull

water out of cells, causing them to shrivel (Hall, 2016). The decision to use a hypotonic or hypertonic solution is made on the basis of a patient's specific fluid and electrolyte imbalance. For example, a patient with hypernatremia that cannot be treated with oral water generally receives a hypotonic IV solution to dilute the ECF and rehydrate cells. Too-rapid or excessive infusion of any IV fluid has the potential to cause serious patient problems.

Additives such as potassium chloride (KCl) are common in IV solutions (e.g., 1000 mL D_5 ½ NS with 20 mEq KCl at 125 mL/hr). Administer KCl carefully because hyperkalemia can cause fatal cardiac dysrhythmias. **Under no circumstances should KCl be administered by IV push (directly through a port in IV tubing).** Verify that a patient has adequate kidney function and urine output before administering an IV solution containing potassium. Patients with normal renal function who are receiving nothing by mouth should have potassium added to IV solutions. The body cannot conserve potassium, and the kidneys continue to excrete it even when the plasma level falls. Without potassium intake, hypokalemia develops quickly.

Fluid Therapy

Cultural and religious beliefs influence how you manage fluid therapy and how patients communicate their needs. For example, a family elder may be the person who receives explanations and makes health care decisions rather than the patient. A person may refuse therapies because of cultural and religious beliefs. For example, hot-cold beliefs cause some patients to refuse cold oral fluids when they have certain illnesses because they believe that hot fluids are needed to restore balance (Giger, 2017). Religious practices may require modifications of intravenous (IV) tubing length (e.g., when patients need to kneel on the floor and pray several times daily).

Implications for Patient-Centered Care

- Establish communication. If appropriate, determine who makes decisions for the patient and explain fluid restriction or IV therapy procedures.
- Elicit patient/family values and preferences in your clinical interview. Ask specifically about preferred temperature of oral fluids and provide (if oral intake is allowed).
- Determine needed length of IV tubing and incorporate one or more segments of long extension tubing into the IV setup if patient kneels on the floor to pray.
- Determine acceptance of or abstinence from therapeutic regimens and respect patient/family choices regarding therapy (Boucher et al., 2017).
- Know patient's beliefs regarding blood therapy. Although some patients refuse whole blood or packed red blood cells because of religious or personal beliefs, they may accept other blood products or alternatives (Tingle, 2017).

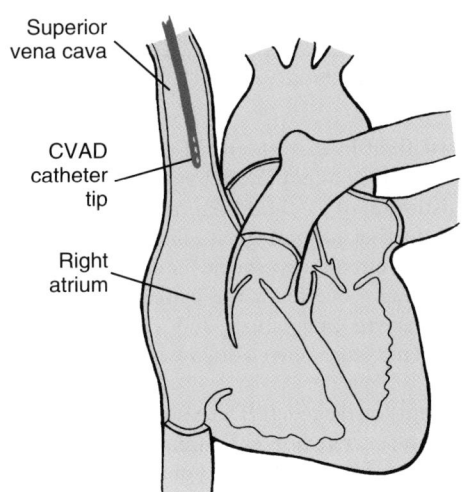

FIG. 42.13 Central venous lines deliver intravenous fluid into superior vena cava near heart. *CVAD,* Central venous access device.

Vascular Access Devices. Vascular access devices (VADs) are catheters or infusion ports designed for repeated access to the vascular system. Peripheral catheters are for short-term use (e.g., fluid restoration after surgery and short-term antibiotic administration). Devices for long-term use include central catheters and implanted ports, which empty into a central vein. Remember that the term *central* applies to the location of the catheter tip, not to the insertion site. Peripherally inserted central catheters (PICC lines) enter a peripheral arm vein and extend through the venous system to the superior vena cava, where they terminate. Other central lines enter a central vein such as the subclavian or jugular vein or are tunneled through subcutaneous tissue before entering a central vein. Central lines are more effective than peripheral catheters for administering large volumes of fluid, PN, and medications or fluids that irritate veins. Proper care of central line insertion sites is critical for the prevention of central line–associated bloodstream infection (CLABSI) (Box 42.6) (CDC, 2017; INS, 2016a). Nurses and health care providers must have specialized education regarding care of CVCs and implanted infusion ports (TJC, 2018). Nursing responsibilities for central lines include careful monitoring, flushing to keep the line patent, and site care and dressing changes to prevent CLABSIs (INS, 2016a).

Equipment. Correct selection and preparation of IV equipment helps in safe and rapid placement of an IV line. Because fluids infuse directly into the bloodstream, sterile technique is necessary. Organize all equipment at the bedside for an efficient insertion. IV equipment includes VADs; tourniquet; clean gloves; dressings; IV fluid containers; various types of tubing; and electronic infusion devices (EIDs), also called *infusion pumps.* VADs that are short peripheral IV catheters are available in a variety of gauges, such as the commonly used 20 and 22 gauges. A larger gauge indicates a smaller-diameter catheter. A peripheral VAD is called an over-the-needle catheter; it consists of a small plastic tube or catheter threaded over a sharp stylet (needle). Once you insert a stylet and advance the catheter into the vein, you withdraw the stylet, leaving the catheter in place. These devices have a safety mechanism that covers the sharp stylet when withdrawing it to reduce the risk of needlestick injury (Fig. 42.14). Needleless systems allow you to make connections without using needles, which reduces needlestick injuries.

The main IV fluid used in a continuous infusion flows through tubing called the *primary line.* The primary line connects to the IV catheter. Injectable medications such as antibiotics are usually added to a small IV solution bag and "piggybacked" as a secondary set into the primary line or as a primary intermittent infusion to be administered over a 30- to 60-minute period (Thoele et al., 2018). The type and amount of solution are prescribed by the patient's health care provider and depend on the medication added and the patient's physiological status. If an IV infusion is connected to an EID, use the tubing designated for that EID. For gravity-flow IVs (not using an EID), select tubing as described in the equipment list of Skill 42.1. Add IV extension tubing to increase the length of the primary line, which reduces pulling of the tubing and increases a patient's mobility when changing positions.

Inserting the Intravenous Line. After you collect the equipment at the patient's bedside, prepare to insert the IV line by assessing the patient for a venipuncture site (see Skill 42.1). The most common IV sites are on the inner arm (Fig. 42.15). Do not use hand veins on older adults or patients who are ambulatory. IV insertion in a foot vein is common with children but avoid these sites in adults because of the increased risk of thrombophlebitis (INS, 2016a).

As you assess a patient for potential venipuncture sites, consider conditions that exclude certain sites. Venipuncture is contraindicated in a site that has signs of infection, infiltration, or thrombosis. An infected site is red, tender, swollen, and possibly warm to the touch. Exudate may be present. Do not use an infected site because of the danger of introducing bacteria from the skin surface into the bloodstream. Avoid using an extremity with a vascular (dialysis) graft/fistula or on the same side as a mastectomy. Avoid areas of flexion if possible and choose the most distal appropriate site (INS, 2016a). Using a distal

TABLE 42.11 Intravenous Solutions

Solution	Concentration in IV Container and at Tip of VAD	Effective Concentration in Body	Comments
Dextrose (Glucose) in Water Solutions			
Dextrose 5% in water (D₅W)	Isotonic	Hypotonic	Isotonic when first enters vein; dextrose enters cells rapidly, leaving free water, which dilutes ECF; most of the water then enters cells by osmosis.
Dextrose 10% in water (D₁₀W)	Hypertonic	Hypotonic	Hypertonic when first enters vein; dextrose enters cells rapidly, leaving free water, which dilutes ECF; most of the water then enters cells by osmosis.
Saline (Sodium Chloride [NaCl] in Water) Solutions			
0.225% NaCl (quarter NS; ¼NS)	Hypotonic	Hypotonic	Expands ECV (vascular and interstitial) and rehydrates cells.
0.45% NaCl (half NS; ½NS)	Hypotonic	Hypotonic	Expands ECV (vascular and interstitial) and rehydrates cells.
0.9% NaCl (NS)	Isotonic	Isotonic	Expands ECV (vascular and interstitial); does not enter cells.
3% or 5% NaCl (hypertonic saline; 3% or 5% NaCl)	Hypertonic	Hypertonic	Draws water from cells into ECF by osmosis.
Dextrose in Saline Solutions			
Dextrose 5% in 0.45% NaCl (½NS; D₅ 0.45% NaCl)	Hypertonic	Hypotonic	Dextrose enters cells rapidly, leaving 0.45% NaCl.
Dextrose 5% in 0.9% NaCl (D₅NS; D₅ 0.9% NaCl)	Hypertonic	Isotonic	Dextrose enters cells rapidly, leaving 0.9% NaCl.
Multiple Electrolyte Solutions			
Lactated Ringer's (LR) solution	Isotonic	Isotonic	LR contains Na⁺, K⁺, Ca²⁺, Cl⁻, and lactate, which liver metabolizes to HCO₃⁻; expands ECV (vascular and interstitial); does not enter cells.
Dextrose 5% in LR (D₅LR)	Hypertonic	Isotonic	Dextrose enters cells rapidly, leaving LR.

ECF, Extracellular fluid; *ECV,* extracellular fluid volume; *NS,* normal saline; *VAD,* vascular access device.

site first allows for the use of proximal sites later if the patient needs a venipuncture site change.

Venipuncture is a technique in which a vein is punctured through the skin by a sharp rigid stylet (e.g., metal needle). The stylet is partially covered either with a plastic catheter or a needle attached to a syringe. General purposes of venipuncture are to collect a blood specimen, start an IV infusion, provide vascular access for later use, instill a medication, or inject a radiopaque or other tracer for special diagnostic examinations. Skill 42.1 describes venipuncture for peripheral IV fluid infusion, incorporating INS standards of practice (INS, 2016a). It takes practice to become proficient in venipuncture. Only experienced practitioners should perform it for patients whose veins are fragile or collapse easily such as older adults. Box 42.7 describes principles to follow for venipuncture in older adults.

Nurses require specialized knowledge and education to place PICCs. Some central lines and implanted ports require insertion by physicians or advanced practice nurses. Both types of central catheters require close monitoring and maintenance. This chapter focuses on peripheral catheters.

Regulating the Infusion Flow Rate. After initiating a peripheral IV infusion and checking it for patency, regulate the rate of infusion according to the health care provider's orders (see Skill 42.2). For patient safety avoid uncontrolled flow of IV fluid into a patient. You are responsible for calculating the flow rate (mL/hr) that

delivers the IV fluid in the prescribed time frame. The correct IV infusion rate ensures patient safety by preventing too-slow or too-rapid administration of IV fluids. An infusion rate that is too slow often leads to further physiological compromise in a patient who is dehydrated, in circulatory shock, or critically ill. An infusion rate that is too rapid overloads the patient with IV fluid, causing fluid and electrolyte imbalances and cardiac complications in vulnerable patients (e.g., older adults or patients with preexisting heart disease).

Electronic infusion devices (EIDs), also called *IV pumps* or *infusion pumps,* deliver an accurate hourly IV infusion rate. EIDs use positive pressure to deliver a measured amount of fluid during a specified unit of time (e.g., 125 mL/hr). Familiarize yourself with the brand of EID in use at your agency so that you are able to set the flow rate accurately. Many EIDs have capabilities that allow for single- and multiple-solution infusions at different rates. Electronic detectors and alarms respond to air in IV lines, occlusion, completion of infusion, high and low pressure, and low battery power.

When you open a roller clamp or other type of clamp on an infusion tubing that is not yet properly inserted in an EID or on a gravity-flow IV system, the IV fluid infuses very rapidly. Nonelectronic volume-control devices are used occasionally with an IV solution infused by gravity to prevent accidental infusion of a large fluid volume. These devices hang between the IV bag and the patient and hold only a small volume of fluid that can infuse into the patient.

BOX 42.6 EVIDENCE-BASED PRACTICE

Preventing Central Line–Associated Bloodstream Infections (CLABSI)

PICOT Question: In patients who are hospitalized, do bundled interventions compared with routine central line site care alone prevent central line–associated bloodstream infection (CLABSI)?

Evidence Summary

CLABSI is a serious complication of intravenous (IV) therapy that increases morbidity, hospital length of stay, and health care costs. Research shows that effective strategies for prevention of CLABSI include the use of several evidence-based practices together as a multicomponent "bundle" (Biasucci et al., 2018). Such bundles are effective in reducing CLABSIs at the time of insertion of central lines and also during their maintenance (Biasucci et al., 2018). The Infusion Nursing Standards of Practice (INS, 2016a) and the Centers for Disease Control and Prevention (CDC, 2017) specify a central line bundle: hand hygiene; maximum sterile barrier precautions; chlorhexidine skin antisepsis using chlorhexidine (>0.5%) in alcohol; avoidance of the femoral vein for central venous access for adults; and placement under planned controlled conditions. For the most effective reduction of CLABSIs, The Joint Commission (2018) requires ongoing staff education to promote consistent adherence to bundle components and attention to institutional support and culture in addition to the use of bundled central line insertion and maintenance practices (Hawes and Lee, 2018; Grover, 2015). Units with a higher proportion of Critical Care Registered Nurse (CCRN) certifications have been shown to have lower rates of CLABSI (Boev et al., 2015).

Application to Nursing Practice

- Verify and use all of the components of the CLABSI prevention bundle (Biasucci et al., 2018; Hawes and Lee, 2018).
- Work with a practice or infection control committee to perform an audit of adherence to CLABSI prevention practices in your unit (INS, 2016a; CDC, 2017).
- If your agency does not have a multidisciplinary CLABSI prevention program, collaborate with infection control personnel and medical and nursing administration to establish one that includes institutional support for education, competency demonstration, use of insertion and maintenance bundles, and daily line audits with feedback to nurses (TJC, 2018; INS, 2016a).

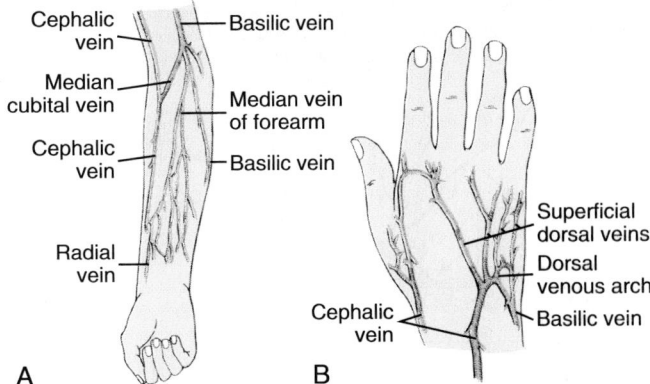

FIG. 42.15 Cephalic, basilic, and median cubital veins are best for IV placement in adults.

BOX 42.7 FOCUS ON OLDER ADULTS

Protection of Skin and Veins During Intravenous Therapy

- Use the smallest-gauge catheter or needle possible (e.g., 22 to 24 gauge). Veins are very fragile, and a smaller gauge allows better blood flow to provide increased hemodilution of the intravenous (IV) fluids or medications (INS, 2016a).
- Avoid the back of the hand, which may compromise a patient's need for independence and mobility.
- Avoid placement of an IV line in veins that are easily bumped because older adults have less subcutaneous support tissue (Touhy and Jett, 2016).
- Avoid vigorous friction while cleaning a site to prevent tearing fragile skin.
- If a patient has fragile skin and veins, use minimal or no tourniquet pressure (INS, 2016a).
- If using a tourniquet, place it over the patient's sleeve or use a blood pressure cuff.
- With loss of supportive tissue, veins tend to lie more superficially; lower the insertion angle for venipuncture to 10 to 15 degrees after penetrating the skin.
- Veins roll away from the needle easily because of loss of subcutaneous tissue. To stabilize a vein, apply traction to the skin below the projected insertion site.
- Secure IV site with a catheter stabilization device, avoiding excessive use of tape on fragile skin; consider covering the site additionally with surgical stretch mesh.
- Numerous medications and supplements (e.g., anticoagulants, antibiotics, glucocorticoids, and garlic) increase the likelihood of bruising and bleeding (Burchum et al., 2019).

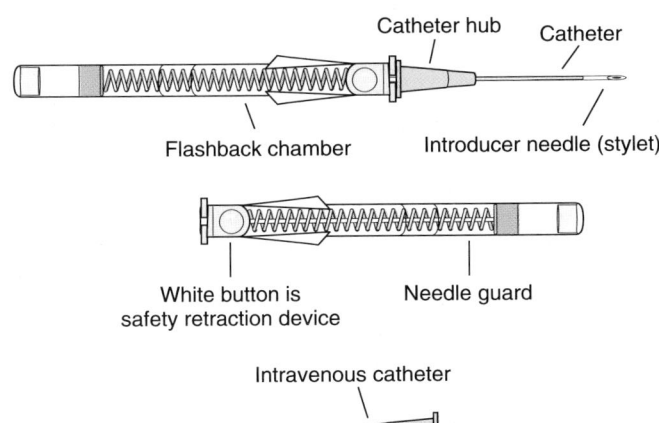

FIG. 42.14 Over-the-needle catheter for venipuncture.

Regardless of the device in use, monitor the patient regularly to verify correct infusion of IV fluids.

Patency of an IV catheter means that IV fluid flows easily through it. For patency there must be no clots at the tip of the catheter, and the catheter tip must not be against the vein wall. A blocked catheter slows or stops the rate of infusion of the IV fluids. IV flow rate also can be slowed by infiltration, vasospasm, a knot or kink in the tubing, external pressure on the tubing, and position changes of the patient's extremity. If the flow decreases or stops and the EID is working correctly, inspect the tubing. Sometimes the patient is lying or sitting on it. The tubing may be kinked or caught in or under equipment. Also inspect the area around the insertion site for anything that obstructs the flow of IV fluids. For gravity flow, the height of the container influences flow rate. Raising the container usually increases the rate because of increased driving pressure.

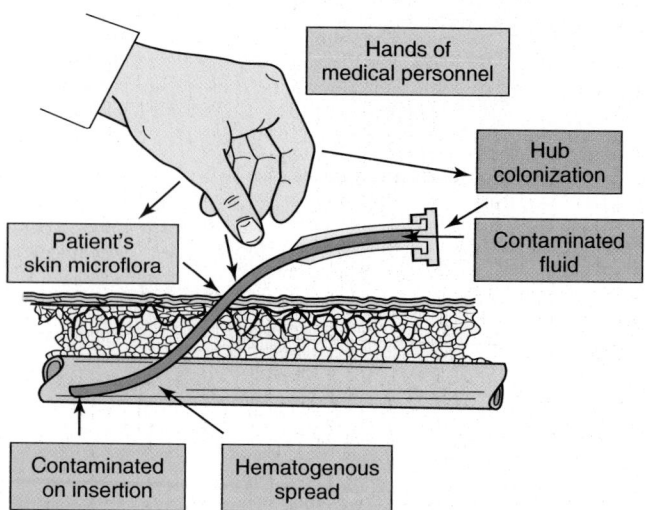

FIG. 42.16 Potential sites for contamination of vascular access device.

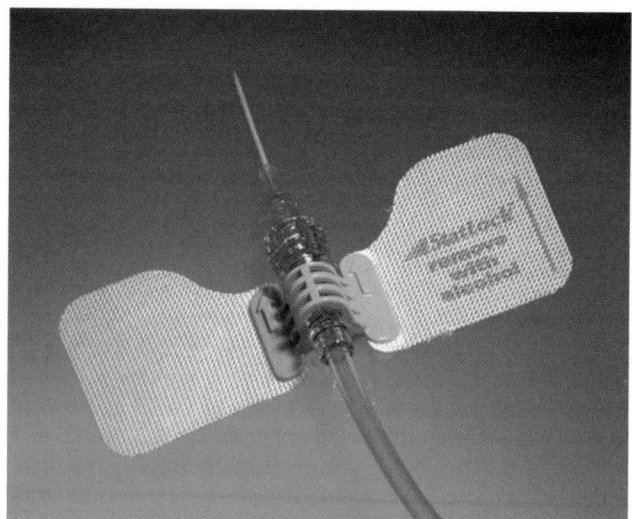

FIG. 42.17 Catheter stabilization device. (Copyright © C.R. Bard, Inc. Used with permission.)

Flexion of an extremity, particularly at the hand and wrist or elbow, can decrease IV flow rate by compressing the vein. Although VAD placement in areas of flexion is discouraged, occasionally it becomes necessary. In that case INS standards specify use of a hand or arm joint stabilization device to protect the IV site by keeping the joint extended (INS, 2016a). Use padding with arm boards because they may cause skin or nerve damage from pressure. Starting an infusion in a new location rather than relying on a site that causes problems may be more comfortable for a patient. Before discontinuing the current infusion, choose another site and start the infusion to verify that the patient has other accessible veins.

Maintaining the System. After placing an IV line and regulating the flow rate, maintain the IV system. Line maintenance involves (1) keeping the system sterile and intact; (2) changing IV fluid containers, tubing, and contaminated site dressings; (3) helping a patient with self-care activities so as not to disrupt the system; and (4) monitoring for complications of IV therapy. The frequency and options for maintaining the system are identified in agency policies.

An important component of patient care is maintaining the integrity of an IV line to prevent infection. Potential sites for contamination of a VAD are shown in Fig. 42.16. Inserting an IV line under appropriate aseptic technique reduces the chances of contamination from a patient's skin. After insertion, prevent infection by the conscientious use of infection control principles such as thorough hand hygiene before and after handling any part of the IV system and maintaining sterility of the system during tubing and fluid container changes.

Always maintain the integrity of an IV system. Never disconnect tubing because it becomes tangled or it might seem more convenient for positioning or moving a patient or applying a gown. If a patient needs more room to maneuver, use aseptic technique to add extension tubing to an IV line. However, keep the use of extension tubing to a minimum because each connection of tubing provides opportunity for contamination. *Never let IV tubing touch the floor.* Do not use stopcocks for connecting more than one solution to a single IV site because they are sources of contamination (Hadaway, 2018; INS, 2016a). IV tubing contains needleless injection ports through which syringes or other adaptors can be inserted for medication administration. Clean an injection port thoroughly with 2% chlorhexidine (preferred), 70% alcohol, or

povidone-iodine solution and let it dry before accessing the system (INS, 2016a).

Protective devices designed to prevent movement or accidental dislodgment of a VAD are called *catheter stabilization devices* (Fig. 42.17). These devices are available in many hospitals, and nurses decide whether to use them when starting an IV line. This is a patient safety issue. Movement of the VAD in a vein can cause phlebitis and infiltration; VAD dislodgment requires using another VAD at a new IV infusion site. INS standards indicate that use of these devices is preferable over taping when feasible (INS, 2016a).

Changing Intravenous Fluid Containers, Tubing, and Dressings. Patients receiving IV therapy over several days require periodic changes of IV fluid containers (Skill 42.3). It is important to organize tasks so that you can change containers rapidly before a thrombus forms in a catheter.

Recommended frequency of IV tubing change depends on whether it is used for continuous or intermittent infusion. INS standards (INS, 2016a) specify that continuous infusion tubing changes occur *no more frequently* than every 96 hours unless the tubing has been compromised or become contaminated, which requires immediate tubing change. In contrast, change tubing for *intermittent* infusion every 24 hours because of the increased risk of contamination from opening the IV system (INS, 2016a). Blood, blood components, and lipids are likely to promote bacterial growth in tubing. INS standards (INS, 2016a) specify tubing changes every 4 hours for blood and blood components and every 24 hours for continuous IV lipids. For lipids use tubing that is free of diethylhexyl-phthalate (DEHP), a toxin that leaches into lipid solutions (INS, 2016a). Whenever possible, schedule tubing changes when it is time to hang a new IV container to decrease risk of infection. To prevent entry of bacteria into the bloodstream, maintain sterility during tubing and IV fluid container changes (INS, 2016a).

A sterile dressing over an IV site reduces the entrance of bacteria into the insertion site. Transparent dressings, the most common type, help secure the VAD, allow continuous visual inspection of the IV site, and are less easily soiled or moistened than gauze dressings. Leave transparent dressings in place until the IV tubing is replaced (INS, 2016a). If a gauze dressing is used, change it every 48 hours (INS, 2016a). Both types of dressings must be changed when the IV device is removed or replaced or when the dressing becomes damp, loosened, or soiled (INS, 2016a) (see Skill 42.4).

Helping Patients to Protect Intravenous Integrity. To prevent the accidental disruption of an IV system, a patient often needs help with hygiene, comfort measures, meals, and ambulation. Changing gowns is difficult for a patient with an IV in the arm. Teach AP and patients that they must not break the integrity of an IV line to change a gown because it leads to contamination. It helps to use a gown with snaps along the top sleeve seam to facilitate changing the gown without disturbing the venipuncture site. Change regular gowns by following these steps for maximum speed and arm mobility (see also Skill 40.1 for photos):

1. *To remove a gown,* remove the sleeve of the gown from the arm without the IV line, maintaining the patient's privacy.
2. Remove the sleeve of the gown from the arm with the IV line.
3. Remove the IV solution container from its stand and pass it and the tubing through the sleeve. (If this involves removing the tubing from an EID, use the roller clamp to slow the infusion to prevent the accidental infusion of a large volume of solution or medication).
4. *To apply a gown,* place the IV solution container and tubing through the sleeve of the clean gown and hang it on its stand. (If the IV line is controlled by an EID, reassemble, turn on the pump, and open the roller clamp.)
5. Place the arm with the IV line through the gown sleeve.
6. Place the arm without the IV line through the other gown sleeve.

A patient with an arm or a hand infusion is able to walk unless contraindicated. Offer a rolling IV pole on wheels. Help the patient get out of bed and place the IV pole next to the involved arm. Teach him or her to hold the pole with the involved hand and push it while walking. Check that the IV container is at the proper height, there is no tension on the tubing, and the flow rate is correct. Infusion pumps connect to IV poles and can be used during ambulation because they will function on battery power during the time the patient walks. Instruct the patient to report any blood in the tubing, a stoppage in the flow, or increased discomfort. Once patient returns to a bed or chair, plug in the infusion pump.

Complications of Intravenous Therapy. Carefully assess and monitor your patient's response to IV therapy (Table 42.12). A severe complication is circulatory overload, which occurs when a patient receives too-rapid administration or an excessive amount of fluids. Assessment findings depend on the type of IV solution that infuses in excess. The signs and symptoms of circulatory overload and other complications often arise rapidly, which highlights the importance of frequent assessment of patients receiving IV therapy.

QSEN Building Competency in Safety A patient who has a peripheral intravenous (IV) infusion wants to wear a special shirt rather than a hospital gown when family members come to celebrate a birthday later today. How can you assist the patient while maintaining patient safety in this situation?

Answers to QSEN Activities can be found on the Evolve website.

Infiltration occurs when an IV catheter becomes dislodged or a vein ruptures and IV fluids inadvertently enter subcutaneous tissue around the venipuncture site (Major and Huey, 2016). When the IV fluid contains additives that damage tissue, extravasation occurs (Matsui et al., 2017). Infiltration and extravasation cause coolness, paleness, and swelling of the area. When infiltration occurs, immediately assess for any additives in the infiltrated fluid

to determine the type of action necessary to prevent local tissue damage and sloughing. Vasoconstrictors, high-dose potassium, and other IV additives in subcutaneous tissue need different treatments from those needed for an infiltrated additive-free IV (see Table 42.12). Although the INS does not include an infiltration scale for adults in its 2016 standards, the society does recommend using a scale. Table 42.13 has an infiltration scale, which is commonly used.

Phlebitis (i.e., inflammation of a vein) results from chemical, mechanical, or bacterial causes. Risk factors for phlebitis include acidic or hypertonic IV solutions; rapid IV rate; IV drugs such as KCl, vancomycin, and penicillin; VAD inserted in area of flexion; poorly secured catheter; poor hand hygiene; and lack of aseptic technique. The typical signs of inflammation (i.e., heat, erythema [redness], tenderness) occur along the course of a vein. Table 42.14 offers a validated scale for assessing severity of phlebitis. When a patient has dark skin, these signs may be less obvious; assess carefully for subtle color changes at the vascular access device site that might indicate phlebitis.

Phlebitis is dangerous because the inflammation of the vein wall can lead to associated blood clots (thrombophlebitis). Clots form along the vein and in some cases cause emboli, which can break off and enter the circulation. This may permanently damage veins. Routine changes of peripheral IV catheters to reduce infection are not recommended (Helton et al., 2016). The INS Standards of Practice (INS, 2016a) recommend avoiding routine replacement of peripheral IV catheters in infants and children and replacement of a peripheral IV catheter in adults only if clinically indicated. The standards provide these guidelines for how frequently to assess a peripheral VAD site to see if its replacement is clinically indicated:

- At least every 4 hours for alert, oriented adults who are able to report problems at the VAD site and are not receiving vesicant (tissue-damaging) infusions
- At least every 1 to 2 hours for adults who are critically ill or sedated or who are cognitively impaired
- At least every hour for neonates and children
- Several times per hour during infusions of vesicants or vasoconstrictors
- During every home or outpatient visit

In the absence of phlebitis, local infection at the venipuncture site is usually caused by poor aseptic technique during catheter insertion, daily monitoring, or catheter removal. Early recognition of local infection and treatment is important to prevent bacteria from entering the bloodstream (see Table 42.12). Bloodstream infections may arise from short peripheral IV catheter sites.

Air embolism occurs when air is present inside syringes, IV tubing is not primed with fluid, or connectors are not removed before use and cause air to enter a patient's vein. It also can occur if the VAD is not clamped before changing the tubing or if the IV tubing is punctured inadvertently (INS, 2016a; Mattox, 2017).

Bleeding can occur around the venipuncture site during the infusion or through the catheter or tubing if these become disconnected inadvertently (see Table 42.12). Bleeding is more common in patients who receive heparin or other anticoagulants or who have a bleeding disorder (e.g., hemophilia or thrombocytopenia).

Discontinuing Peripheral Intravenous Access. Discontinue IV access after infusion of the prescribed amount of fluid; when infiltration, phlebitis, or local infection occurs; or if the IV infusion slows or stops, indicating the catheter has developed a thrombus at its tip. Skill 42.3 presents the steps for discontinuing peripheral IV access. Help patients

TABLE 42.12   Complications of Intravenous Therapy with Nursing Interventions

Complication	Description	Assessment Findings	Nursing Interventions
Circulatory overload of IV solution	IV solution infused too rapidly or in too great an amount	Depends on type of solution ECV excess with Na⁺-containing isotonic fluid (crackles in dependent parts of lungs, shortness of breath, dependent edema) Hyponatremia with hypotonic fluid (confusion, seizures) Hypernatremia with Na⁺-containing hypertonic fluid (confusion, seizures) Hyperkalemia from K⁺-containing fluid (cardiac dysrhythmias, muscle weakness, abdominal distention)	If symptoms appear, reduce IV flow rate and notify patient's health care provider. With ECV excess raise head of bed; administer oxygen and diuretics if ordered. Monitor vital signs and laboratory reports of serum levels. Health care provider may adjust additives in IV solution or type of IV fluid; watch for and implement order.
Infiltration and extravasation	IV fluid entering subcutaneous tissue around venipuncture site Extravasation: technical term used when a vesicant (tissue-damaging) drug (e.g., chemotherapy) enters tissues	Skin around catheter site taut, blanched, cool to touch, edematous; may be painful as infiltration or extravasation increases; infusion may slow or stop	Stop infusion. Discontinue IV infusion if no vesicant drug (see Skill 42.3). If vesicant drug, disconnect IV tubing and aspirate drug from catheter. Agency policy and procedures may require delivery of antidote through catheter before removal. Elevate affected extremity. Avoid applying pressure over site; can force solution into contact with more tissue. Contact health care provider if solution contained KCl, a vasoconstrictor, or other potential vesicant. Apply warm, moist or cold compress according to procedure for type of solution infiltrated. Start new IV line in other extremity. Use standard scale for assessing and documenting infiltration (INS, 2016a).
Phlebitis	Inflammation of inner layer of a vein	Redness, tenderness, pain, warmth along course of vein starting at access site; possible red streak and/or palpable cord along vein	Stop infusion and discontinue IV line (see Skill 42.3). Start new IV line in other extremity or proximal to previous insertion site if continued IV therapy is necessary. Apply warm, moist compress or contact IV therapy team or health care provider if area needs additional treatment. Elevate affected extremity. Document phlebitis using a standardized scale, including nursing interventions per agency policy and procedure.
Local infection	Infection at catheter-skin entry point during infusion or after removal of IV catheter	Redness, heat, swelling at catheter-skin entry point; possible purulent drainage	Culture any drainage (if ordered). Clean skin with alcohol; remove catheter and save for culture; apply sterile dressing. Notify health care provider. Start new IV line in other extremity. Initiate appropriate wound care (see Chapter 48) if needed.
Air embolism	Air in the vein from unpurged syringe or tubing.	Sudden onset of dyspnea, coughing, chest pain, hypotension, tachycardia, decreased level of consciousness, possible signs of stroke	Prevent further air from entering the system by clamping or covering the leak. Place patient on left side, preferably with head of bed raised, to trap air in the lower portion of the left ventricle. Call emergency support team and notify patient's health care provider.
Bleeding at venipuncture site	Oozing or slow, continuous seepage of blood from venipuncture site	Fresh blood evident at venipuncture site, sometimes pooling under extremity	Assess whether IV system is intact. If catheter is within vein, apply pressure dressing over site or change dressing. Start new IV line in other extremity or proximal to previous insertion site if VAD is dislodged, IV is disconnected, or bleeding from site does not stop.

ECV, Extracellular volume; *IV,* intravenous; *VAD,* vascular access device.

TABLE 42.13 Infiltration Scale

Grade	Clinical Criteria
0	No symptoms
1	Skin blanched Edema <2.54 cm (1 inch) in any direction Cool to touch With or without pain
2	Skin blanched Edema 2.54-15.2 cm (1-6 inches) in any direction Cool to touch With or without pain
3	Skin blanched, translucent Gross edema >15.2 cm (6 inches) in any direction Cool to touch Mild-moderate pain Possible numbness
4	Skin blanched, translucent Skin tight, leaking Skin discolored, bruised, swollen Gross edema >15.2 cm (6 inches) in any direction Deep pitting tissue edema Circulatory impairment Moderate-to-severe pain Infiltration of any amount of blood product, irritant, or vesicant

From Groll D, et al: Evaluation of the psychometric properties of the phlebitis and infiltration scales for the assessment of complications of peripheral vascular access devices, *J Infus Nurs* 33(6):385, 2010.

TABLE 42.14 Phlebitis Scale

Grade	Clinical Criteria
0	No symptoms
1	Erythema at access site with or without pain
2	Pain at access site with erythema and/or edema
3	Pain at access site with erythema and/or edema; streak formation; palpable venous cord
4	Pain at access site with erythema and/or edema; streak formation; palpable venous cord >2.54 cm (1 inch) in length; purulent drainage

From Infusion Nurses Society (INS): Infusion therapy standards of practice. *J Infus Nurs,* 39(1 Suppl):S1, 2016a.

TABLE 42.15 ABO Compatibilities for Transfusion Therapy

Component	Compatibilities	
Whole blood	**Give type-specific blood only**	
Packed red cells (stored, washed, or frozen/ washed)	**Donor**	**Recipient**
	0	0, A, B, AB
	A	A, AB
	B	B, AB
	AB	AB
Fresh-frozen plasma	**Donor**	**Recipient**
	0	0
	A	A, 0
	B	B, 0
	AB	AB, B, A, 0
Platelets	RBC: ABO and Rh compatible *preferred*	
	Donor	**Recipient**
	0	0, A, B, AB
	A	A, AB
	B	B, AB
	AB	AB

ABO, Blood group consisting of groups A, AB, B, and O.
Data from Alexander M et al: *Core curriculum for infusion nursing,* ed 4, Philadelphia, 2014, Lippincott, Williams & Wilkins.

and families understand that moving from IV infusion to oral fluid intake is a sign of progress toward recovery.

Blood Transfusion. Blood transfusion, or blood component therapy, is the IV administration of whole blood or a blood component such as packed red blood cells (RBCs), platelets, or plasma. Objectives for administering blood transfusions include (1) increasing circulating blood volume after surgery, trauma, or hemorrhage; (2) increasing the number of RBCs and maintaining hemoglobin levels in patients with severe anemia; and (3) providing selected cellular components as replacement therapy (e.g., clotting factors, platelets, albumin).

Caring for patients receiving blood or blood-product transfusion is a nursing responsibility. You must be thorough in patient assessment, checking the blood product against prescriber's orders, checking it against patient identifiers, and monitoring for any adverse reactions. Blood transfusions are never regarded as routine; overlooking any minor detail can have dangerous and life-threatening events for a patient (AABB, 2017, 2018).

Blood Groups and Types. Blood transfusions must be matched to each patient to avoid incompatibility. RBCs have antigens in their membranes; the plasma contains antibodies against specific RBC antigens. If incompatible blood is transfused (i.e., a patient's RBC antigens differ from those transfused), the patient's antibodies trigger RBC destruction in a potentially dangerous **transfusion reaction** (i.e., an immune response to the transfused blood components).

The most important grouping for transfusion purposes is the ABO system, which identifies A, B, O, and AB blood types. Determination of blood type is made on the basis of the presence or absence of A and B RBC antigens. Individuals with type A blood have A antigens on their RBCs and anti-B antibodies in their plasma. Individuals with type B blood have B antigens on their RBCs and anti-A antibodies in their plasma. A person who has type AB blood has both A and B antigens on the RBCs and no antibodies against either antigen in the plasma. A type O individual has neither A nor B antigens on RBCs but has both anti-A and anti-B antibodies in the plasma (Alexander et al., 2014). Table 42.15 shows the compatibilities between blood types of donors and recipients. People with type O-negative blood are considered universal blood donors because they can donate packed RBCs and platelets to people with any ABO blood type. People with type AB-positive blood are called *universal blood recipients* because they can receive packed RBCs and platelets of any ABO type.

Another consideration when matching blood components for transfusions is the Rh factor, which refers to another antigen in RBC membranes. Most people have this antigen and are Rh positive; a person without it is Rh negative. People who are Rh negative receive only Rh-negative blood components.

Autologous Transfusion. Autologous transfusion (autotransfusion) is the collection and reinfusion of a patient's own blood. Blood for an autologous transfusion most commonly is obtained by preoperative donation up to 6 weeks before a scheduled surgery (e.g., heart, orthopedic, plastic, or gynecological). A patient can donate several units of blood, depending on the type of surgery and his or her ability to maintain an acceptable hematocrit. Blood for autologous transfusion is also obtained at the time of surgery or through blood salvage (e.g., during surgery for liver transplantation, trauma, or vascular and orthopedic conditions). After surgery blood is salvaged from drainage from chest tubes or joint cavities. Autologous transfusions are safer for patients because they decrease the risk of mismatched blood and exposure to bloodborne infectious agents (Alexander et al., 2014).

Transfusing Blood. Transfusion of blood or blood components is a nursing procedure that requires an order from a health care provider. Patient safety is a nursing priority, and patient assessment, verification of the health care provider's order, and verification of correct blood products for the correct patient are imperative (AABB, 2017, 2018).

Perform a thorough patient assessment before initiating a transfusion, and monitor carefully during and after the transfusion. Assessment is critical because of the risk of transfusion reactions. Pretransfusion assessment includes establishing whether a patient knows the reason for the blood transfusion and whether he or she has ever had a previous transfusion or transfusion reaction. A patient who has had a transfusion reaction is usually at no greater risk for a reaction with a subsequent transfusion. However, he or she may be anxious about the transfusion, requiring nursing intervention. Before beginning a transfusion, explain the procedure and instruct the patient (if alert) to report any side effects (e.g., chills, dizziness, or fever) once the transfusion begins. Have a professional translator available if the patient does not speak English. Ensure that he or she has signed an informed consent. Patients with certain cultural or religious backgrounds may refuse blood transfusions (see Box 42.5).

Because of the danger of transfusion reactions, your pretransfusion assessment always includes the patient's baseline vital signs. These data allow you to identify when vital sign changes occur as a result of a transfusion reaction.

Always follow agency policy and procedures before initiating any blood therapy. For patient safety always verify three things: (1) that blood components delivered are the ones that were ordered, (2) that blood delivered to a patient is compatible with the blood type listed in the medical record, and (3) that the right patient receives the blood. Together two RNs or one RN and an LPN (check agency policy and procedures) must check the label on the blood product against the medical record and the patient's identification number, blood group, and complete name. If even a minor discrepancy exists, do not give the blood; notify the blood bank immediately to prevent infusion errors.

When administering a transfusion, you need an appropriate-size IV catheter and blood administration tubing that has a special in-line filter (Fig. 42.18). Adults require a large catheter (e.g., 18- or 20-gauge) because blood is more viscous than crystalloid IV fluids. Children with small veins need a smaller catheter. Prime the tubing with 0.9% sodium chloride (normal saline) to prevent hemolysis or breakdown of RBCs. Initiate a transfusion slowly to allow for the early detection of a transfusion reaction. Always have a second IV infusion bag containing 0.9% sodium chloride on standby in case it becomes necessary to stop the blood infusion. Maintain the ordered blood infusion rate, monitor for side effects, assess vital signs, and promptly record all findings. It is important to stay with the patient during the first 15 minutes because this is the time when a reaction

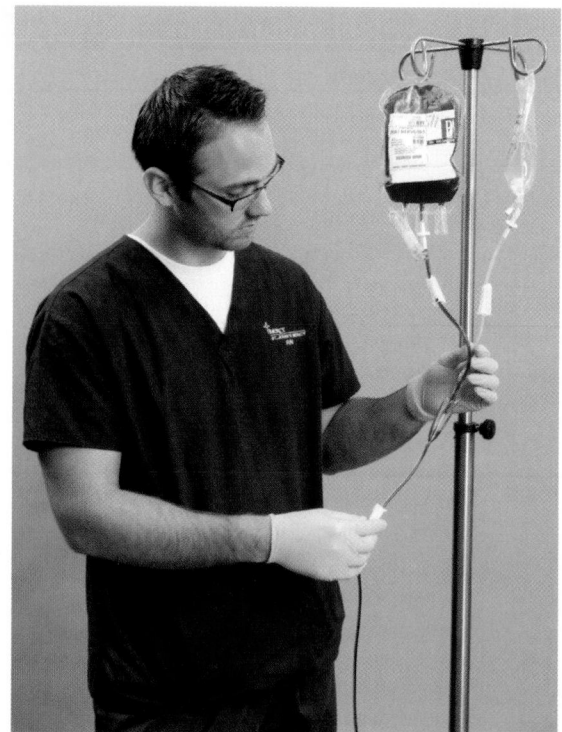

FIG. 42.18 Blood administration set primed with normal saline.

is most likely to occur (DeLisle, 2018). After the initial time period, continue to monitor the patient and obtain vital signs periodically during the transfusion as directed by agency policy. If a transfusion reaction is anticipated or suspected, obtain vital signs more frequently (Table 42.16).

The transfusion rate usually is specified in the health care provider's orders. Ideally a unit of whole blood or packed RBCs is transfused in 2 hours. This time can be lengthened to 4 hours if the patient is at risk for ECV excess. Beyond 4 hours there is a risk for bacterial contamination of the blood.

When patients have a severe blood loss such as with hemorrhage, they often receive rapid transfusions through a central venous catheter. A blood-warming device often is necessary because the tip of the central venous catheter lies in the superior vena cava, above the right atrium. Rapid administration of cold blood can cause cardiac dysrhythmias. Patients who receive large-volume transfusion of citrated blood have a high risk of hyperkalemia, hypocalcemia, hypomagnesemia, and metabolic alkalosis; therefore they need careful monitoring (Lim et al., 2017).

Transfusion Reactions. A transfusion reaction is an adverse event that occurs from transfusion of a blood product (DeLisle, 2018). Many transfusion reactions involve immune system reaction to the transfusion that ranges from a mild response to severe anaphylactic shock or acute intravascular hemolysis, both of which can be fatal. Table 42.16 presents the causes, manifestations, management, and prevention of the most common acute transfusion reactions. Prompt intervention when a transfusion reaction occurs maintains or restores a patient's physiological stability. When you suspect acute intravascular hemolysis, do the following (Alexander et al., 2014; DeLisle, 2018):

- Stop the transfusion immediately.
- Keep the IV line open by replacing the IV tubing down to the catheter hub with new tubing and running 0.9% sodium chloride (normal saline) at a slow rate.
- ***Do not*** turn off the blood and simply turn on the 0.9% sodium chloride (normal saline) that is connected to the Y-tubing infusion set.

TABLE 42.16 Acute Adverse Effects of Transfusions

Adverse Effect	Cause	Clinical Manifestations	Management	Prevention
Caused by Immune Response to Blood Components				
Acute intravascular hemolytic reaction	Infusion of ABO-incompatible whole blood, RBCs, or components containing 10 mL or more of RBCs Antibodies in recipient's plasma attach to antigens on transfused RBCs, causing RBC destruction	Chills, fever, low back pain, flushing, tachycardia, tachypnea, hypotension, hemoglobinuria, hemoglobinemia, sudden oliguria (acute kidney injury), circulatory shock, cardiac arrest, death	Stop transfusion and save blood bag and administration set for follow-up. Keep IV site open with normal saline infused through new tubing. Maintain BP and treat shock as ordered, if present. Obtain blood samples **slowly** to avoid hemolysis; send for serological testing. Send urine specimen to laboratory. Give diuretics as prescribed to maintain urine flow. Insert indwelling urinary catheter or measure each voiding to monitor hourly urine output. Dialysis may be required if acute kidney injury occurs. *Patient safety alert:* Do not transfuse additional RBC-containing components until transfusion service provides newly cross-matched units.	Meticulously verify and document patient identification from sample collection to component infusion.
Febrile nonhemolytic reaction (most common)	Antibodies against donor white blood cells	Sudden shaking chills (rigors), fever (rise in temperature 0.5°C [1°F] or more from start), headache, flushing, anxiety, muscle pain	Stop transfusion. Give antipyretics as prescribed; avoid aspirin in thrombocytopenic patients. *Patient safety alert:* Do not restart transfusion.	Consider leukocyte-poor blood products (filtered, washed, or frozen). Pretreat with antipyretics if prior history.
Mild allergic reaction	Antibodies against donor plasma proteins	Flushing, itching, urticaria (hives)	Stop transfusion temporarily. Give antihistamine as directed. If symptoms are mild and transient, restart transfusion slowly. *Patient safety alert:* Do not restart transfusion if fever, pulmonary symptoms, or hypotension develop.	Treat prophylactically with antihistamines.
Anaphylactic reaction	Antibodies to donor plasma, especially anti-IgA	Anxiety, urticaria, dyspnea, wheezing, progressing to cyanosis, severe hypotension, circulatory shock, possible cardiac arrest	Stop transfusion. Have epinephrine ready for injection (0.4 mL of 1:1000 solution subcutaneously or 0.1 mL of 1:1000 solution diluted to 10 mL with saline for IV use). Provide blood pressure support as ordered. Initiate CPR if indicated. *Patient safety alert:* Do not restart transfusion.	Transfuse extensively washed RBC products from which all plasma has been removed. Alternately use blood from IgA-deficient donor.
Not Caused by Immune Response				
Transfusion-associated circulatory overload (TACO)	Blood administered faster than circulation can accommodate	*Dyspnea*, cough, crackles, or rales in dependent lobes of lungs; distended neck veins when upright	Turn down transfusion rate or stop transfusion. Place patient upright with feet in dependent position. Administer prescribed diuretics, oxygen, morphine. Phlebotomy may be indicated.	Adjust transfusion volume and flow rate on basis of patient size and clinical status. Have transfusion service divide unit into smaller aliquots for better spacing of fluid input.
Sepsis	Bacterial contamination of transfused blood components	Rapid onset of chills, high fever, severe hypotension, and circulatory shock *May occur:* Vomiting, diarrhea, sudden oliguria (acute kidney injury), disseminated intravascular coagulation (DIC)	Stop transfusion. Obtain culture of patient's blood and send bag with remaining blood to transfusion service for further study. Treat as ordered: antibiotics, IV fluids, vasopressors, glucocorticoids.	Collect, process, store, and transfuse blood products according to blood-banking standards and infuse within 4 hours of starting time.

ABO, Blood group consisting of groups A, AB, B, and O; *BP*, blood pressure; *CPR*, cardiopulmonary resuscitation; *DIC*, disseminated intravascular coagulation; *IgA*, immunoglobulin A; *IV*, intravenous; *RBC*, red blood cell.
Data from Alexander M, et al: *Core curriculum for infusion nursing*, ed 4, Philadelphia, 2014, Lippincott, Williams & Wilkins; DeLisle J: Is this a blood transfusion reaction? Don't hesitate; check it out, *J Infus Nurs* 41(1):42, 2018.

This would cause blood remaining in the IV tubing to infuse into the patient. Even a small amount of additional blood can make the situation worse. **You must change out all the IV tubing.**

- Immediately notify the health care provider or emergency response team.
- Remain with the patient, observing signs and symptoms and monitoring vital signs as often as every 5 minutes.
- Prepare to administer emergency drugs such as antihistamines, vasopressors, fluids, and corticosteroids per health care provider order or protocol.
- Prepare to perform cardiopulmonary resuscitation.
- Save the blood container, tubing, attached labels, and transfusion record for return to the blood bank.
- Obtain blood and urine specimens per health care provider order or protocol.

Acute transfusion reactions that do not involve an immune response to the blood components also can occur (see Table 42.16). Transfusion-associated circulatory overload (TACO) is a risk when a patient receives massive whole blood or packed RBC transfusions for massive hemorrhagic shock or when a patient with normal blood volume receives blood. Patients particularly at risk for circulatory overload are older adults and those with cardiopulmonary diseases. Transfusion of blood components that are contaminated with bacteria, especially gram-negative bacteria, can cause sepsis.

Blood from infected donors who are asymptomatic can transmit diseases. Symptoms of these conditions may arise long after a transfusion. Diseases transmitted through transfusions include hepatitis B and C, human immunodeficiency virus (HIV) infection and acquired immunodeficiency syndrome (AIDS), Chagas disease, and cytomegalovirus infection. In the United States all units of blood for blood banks undergo screening for HIV, hepatitis B and C viruses, syphilis, and West Nile virus, which reduces the risk of acquiring these bloodborne infections (CDC, 2019a).

Interventions for Electrolyte Imbalances. In addition to the administration of prescribed medical therapies, nursing interventions preserve or restore electrolyte imbalance (Felver, 2019c). For example, people who have hypokalemia or hypercalcemia often need bowel management for constipation. Patient safety interventions to prevent falls are vital for patients who become lethargic from hypercalcemia and those with muscle weakness. Patients who have hypercalcemia need an increased fluid intake to prevent renal damage; nurses can help them meet the oral fluid intake goals. Teach patients the reasons for their therapies and the importance of balancing electrolyte I&O to prevent imbalances in the future.

Interventions for Acid-Base Imbalances. Nursing interventions to promote acid-base balance support prescribed medical therapies and aim at reversing the existing acid-base imbalance while providing for patient safety (Felver, 2019b). When these imbalances are life threatening, they require rapid treatment. Maintain a functional IV line and check the health care provider's orders frequently for new medications or fluids. Give fluid and electrolyte replacement and prescribed drugs such as insulin promptly. In addition, monitor patients closely for changes in their status. Use protective measures such as side rails for patients with decreased level of consciousness. Support compensatory hyperventilation for patients with metabolic acidosis by keeping their oral mucous membranes moist and positioning them to facilitate chest expansion. Chapter 41 reviews appropriate therapies for patients with respiratory acidosis. Patients with acid-base imbalances often require repeated ABG analysis.

Arterial Blood Gases. Determination of a patient's acid-base status requires obtaining a sample of arterial blood for laboratory testing. ABG analysis reveals acid-base status and the adequacy of ventilation and oxygenation. A qualified RN or other health care provider draws arterial blood from a peripheral artery (usually the radial) or from an existing arterial line (see agency policy and procedures). Before an arterial blood draw, perform an Allen test, which assesses arterial circulation in the hand (Pagana et al., 2018). When performing the Allen test, apply pressure to both the ulnar and radial arteries in the selected hand. The fingers to the hand should be pale and blanched, indicating a lack of arterial blood flow. Release the pressure on the ulnar artery and observe for color to return to the fingers and hand, which indicates that there is adequate circulation to the hand and fingers via the ulnar artery. The Allen test ensures that a patient will have adequate blood flow to the hand if the radial artery is damaged. If color does not return, do not perform radial artery puncture on that arm. After the ABG puncture, apply pressure to the puncture site for at least 5 minutes to reduce the risk of hematoma formation. A longer time is necessary if the patient takes anticoagulant medications. Reassess the radial pulse after removing the pressure. After obtaining the specimen, take care to prevent air from entering the syringe because this alters the blood gas values. To reduce oxygen usage by blood cells, submerge the syringe in crushed ice and transport it immediately to the laboratory.

Restorative Care. After experiencing acute alterations in fluid, electrolyte, or acid-base balance, patients often require ongoing maintenance to prevent a recurrence of health alterations. Older adults require special considerations to prevent complications from developing (see Box 42.2).

Home Intravenous Therapy. IV therapy often continues in the home setting for patients requiring long-term hydration, PN, or long-term medication administration. Initiate patient referral for discharge planning to social services, counselors, or a home care coordinator for assessment of patient and community resources. A home IV therapy nurse works closely with a patient to ensure that a sterile IV system is maintained and that complications can be avoided or recognized promptly. Box 42.8 summarizes patient education guidelines for home IV therapy.

Nutritional Support. Most patients who have had electrolyte disorders or metabolic acid-base imbalances require ongoing nutritional support. Depending on the type of disorder, fluid or food intake may be encouraged or restricted (see Chapter 45). Patients or family members who are responsible for meal preparation need to learn to understand nutritional content of foods and read the labels of commercially prepared foods.

Medication Safety. Numerous medications, OTC drugs, and herbal preparations contain components or create potential side effects that can alter fluid and electrolyte balance. Patients with chronic disease who are receiving multiple medications and those with renal disorders are at significant risk for imbalances. Once patients return to restorative care settings, whether in the home, long-term care, or other setting, drug safety is very important. Patient and family education regarding potential side effects and drug interactions that can alter fluid, electrolyte, or acid-base balance is essential. Review all medications with patients and encourage them to consult with their local pharmacist, especially if they wish to try a new OTC drug or herbal preparation (Chapter 32).

◆ Evaluation

Through the Patient's Eyes. Review with patients how well their major concerns and expectations regarding fluid, electrolyte, or acid-base management were alleviated or addressed. For example, ask a person admitted with dehydration who was concerned about falling because of light-headedness, "Tell me if you feel we took the precautions necessary to reduce your risk of falling." If the patient's concern was feeling uncomfortable with a very dry mouth, ask, "How does your mouth feel now? Do you feel we made you comfortable?" If the patient's concerns involved having a better understanding of a chronic problem, focus the evaluation on the patient's view of his or her understanding after patient education was provided. A patient's perspectives

BOX 42.8 PATIENT TEACHING

Home Intravenous Therapy

Objective

- The patient and/or family caregiver will demonstrate competence with administering intravenous (IV) therapy safely in the home.

Teaching Strategies

- Explain the importance of IV therapy in maintaining hydration and access for the delivery of medications.
- Emphasize the risks involved when the IV system is not kept sterile.
- Be sure that the patient and/or family caregiver is able to manipulate the required equipment.
- Instruct in aseptic technique and hand hygiene in the handling of all IV equipment.
- Teach how to change IV solutions, tubing, and dressing when they become soiled or dislodged (INS, 2016a). (NOTE: As the home care nurse, you may be able to visit frequently enough to perform scheduled tubing changes.)
- Teach procedures for safe disposal in appropriate containers of all sharps and IV materials exposed to blood. Check with the patient's local trash removal services or health department to see which disposal methods are available in the community (US Food and Drug Administration, 2018). Keep sharps containers away from children (see Chapter 28).
- Instruct to apply pressure with sterile gauze if catheter falls out and, if patient is on anticoagulants, to tape pieces of sterile gauze in place for at least 20 minutes with pressure or until bleeding stops.
- Instruct about signs and symptoms of infiltration, phlebitis, and infection and the need to report symptoms immediately.
- Instruct patient and/or family caregiver to report if the infusion slows or stops or if blood is seen in the tubing.
- Teach patient with family caregiver's assistance how to ambulate, perform hygiene, and participate in other activities of daily living without dislodging or disconnecting catheter and tubing:
  - For showering, protect the IV site and dressing from getting wet by covering it completely with plastic. If using an electronic infusion device, unplug around water.
  - Wear clothes that avoid pressure on the IV site, and avoid trauma to the site when changing clothes.
  - Have patient avoid strenuous exercise of the arm with the IV line.

Evaluation

Use the principles of teach-back to evaluate patient/family caregiver learning:

- I want to be sure I explained how to care for your IV correctly. Please tell and/or show me how you will start and stop your infusion, and change the IV container, tubing and dressing.
- Describe what you would do if your IV infusion stops flowing.
- What would you see if your IV site developed an infection? What would you do next?

Knowledge
- Characteristics of fluid, electrolyte, and acid-base imbalances
- Effects of pathophysiology on fluid, electrolyte, and acid-base balances
- Effects of nursing and medical interventions on fluid, electrolyte, and acid-base balances

Experience
- Previous patient responses to planned nursing therapies for improving fluid, electrolyte, and acid-base balance (what worked and what did not work)

EVALUATION
- Reassess signs and symptoms of the patient's fluid, electrolyte, and acid-base imbalance
- Ask the patient for perceptions of fluid balance after interventions
- Ask how well patient's expectations have been addressed
- Observe the most current laboratory results

Standards
- Use established expected outcomes to evaluate the patient's response to care (e.g., oral mucous membranes will be moist, postural hypotension and tachycardia will not occur upon standing)

Attitudes
- Display integrity when identifying those interventions that were not successful
- Be independent when redesigning successful hospital-based interventions for the home care setting

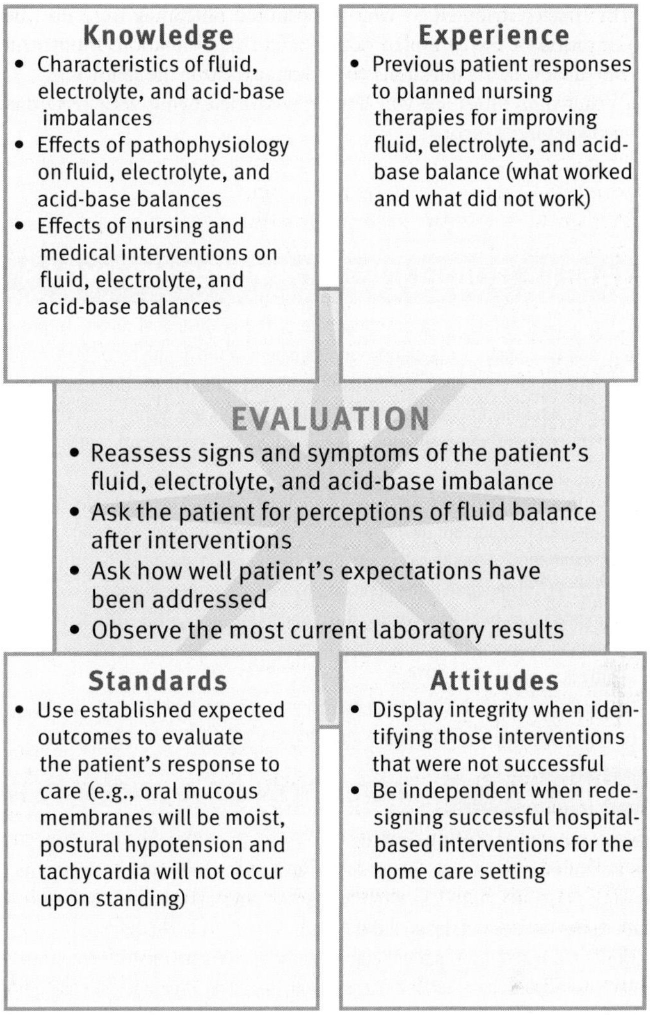

FIG. 42.19 Critical thinking model for fluid, electrolyte, and acid-base balances evaluation.

potential causative agent. For evaluation, apply knowledge of how various pathophysiological conditions affect fluid, electrolyte, and acid-base balance; the effects of medications and fluids; and the patient's presenting clinical status when making clinical decisions (Fig. 42.19).

Compare your current evaluation findings with the previous patient assessment. For example, a patient's hypokalemia demonstrates improvement when the serum potassium is increasing toward normal and the physical signs and symptoms of hypokalemia begin to disappear or lessen in intensity. Specifically, the patient's quadriceps muscles become stronger, normal bowel function returns, and heart rhythm becomes more regular.

For patients with less acute alterations, evaluation is likely to occur over a longer period. In this situation evaluation may be more focused on behavioral changes (e.g., the patient's adherence to dietary restrictions and medication schedules). Another important element of evaluation is the family's ability to anticipate alterations and prevent a recurrence of problems.

The patient's level of progress determines whether the plan of care needs to continue or be revised. If goals are not met, you may need to consult a health care provider to discuss additional methods, such as increasing the frequency of an intervention (e.g., providing more fluids to a patient experiencing dehydration), introducing a new therapy (e.g., initiating insertion of an IV line), or discontinuing a therapy. Once outcomes are met, the nursing diagnosis is resolved and you are able to focus on other priorities, including maintaining normal fluid, electrolyte, and acid-base balance. If established outcomes are not achieved, explore

regarding care often depend in part on involvement of family and friends. If patients have concerns about returning home or to a different care setting, it is important to evaluate how well prepared they feel for the transition from acute care.

Patient Outcomes. Evaluate the effectiveness of interventions using the goals and outcomes established for the patient's nursing diagnoses. Evaluation of a patient's clinical status is especially important if acute fluid, electrolyte, and/or acid-base imbalances exist. A patient's condition can change very quickly, and it is important to recognize impending problems by integrating information about his or her presenting risk factors, clinical status, effects of the present treatment regimen, and factors that contributed to why the planned outcomes were not met. Modification of the care plan occurs after this evaluation. If outcomes are not achieved, the questions you ask may include the following:

- "What difficulties are you having with measuring your I&O daily and keeping a record?"

- "What barriers are preventing you from obtaining the potassium-rich foods you need?"
- "Are you continuing to have frequent loose stools or diarrhea?"
- "Have you purchased an antacid, or are you still using baking soda as an antacid?"

SAFETY GUIDELINES FOR NURSING SKILLS

Ensuring patient safety is an essential role of the professional nurse. To ensure patient safety, communicate clearly with members of the health care team, assess and incorporate the patient's priorities of care and preferences, and use the best evidence when making decisions about your patient's care. When performing the skills in this chapter, remember the following points to ensure safe, individualized patient care:

- Check that you have the necessary information, a health care provider's order if required, and equipment available for the procedure before beginning.
- Before initiation of therapy, check patient identification using two patient identifiers (TJC, 2020) and assess the appropriate route and rate of infusion and potential incompatibilities between infusing fluids and medications (INS, 2016a).
- Determine whether the patient has a latex allergy and use nonlatex items if allergy is present (INS, 2016a).
- Conduct a complete history and physical assessment, including vital signs, and review laboratory findings before initiating any solutions or medications.

- Know the indications for prescribed therapy before initiating IV therapy. Obtain and review health care provider's order to ensure appropriateness of the prescribed solution of medications (INS, 2016a).
- Use special designated tubing for the brand of EID and for blood transfusions and some medications.
- Review the steps of the procedure mentally before entering a patient's room (i.e., consider modifications that you may need to make for this specific patient and verify that the type of IV solution is appropriate for this patient).
- Maintain strict aseptic and sterile techniques when required and sterility and integrity of the IV system to prevent bloodstream infections (INS, 2016a).
- If you contaminate a sterile object during the procedure, do not use it. Use a new sterile one.
- Use standard body fluid precautions during procedures and place all disposable blood-contaminated items and sharp items in designated puncture-resistant biohazard containers (INS, 2016a).

SKILL 42.1   INSERTION OF A SHORT-PERIPHERAL INTRAVENOUS DEVICE

Delegation and Collaboration

The skill of inserting a short-peripheral IV access device cannot be delegated to assistive personnel (AP). Delegation to licensed practical nurses (LPNs) varies by State Nurse Practice Act. Instruct the AP to:

- Notify the nurse if the patient complains of any IV site–related complications such as redness, pain, tenderness, swelling, bleeding, drainage, or leaking from under dressing.
- Notify the nurse if the patient's IV dressing becomes wet or loose.
- Notify the nurse if the level of fluid in the IV bag is low or the electronic infusion device (EID) is alarming.

Equipment

- Short-peripheral IV start kit supplies (available in some agencies): single-use tourniquet, tape, transparent semipermeable membrane (TSM) dressing or sterile gauze and sterile tape, antiseptic solution (alcoholic chlorhexidine solution preferred, 70% alcohol, povidone-iodine, or tincture of iodine), 2 × 2–inch gauze pads, and label
- Appropriate short-peripheral IV catheter with safety mechanism for venipuncture; for adults select 20- to 24- gauge catheter; for neonates, children, and older adults 22- to 24-gauge; for rapid fluid replacement 16- to 20-gauge; based on vein size for blood transfusion 20- to 24- gauge; and for short-term therapy or a single dose, steel-winged device (INS, 2016a)
- Clean gloves (latex free for patients with latex allergy); sterile gloves are needed if palpating the site after skin antisepsis (INS, 2016a)
- Single-use hair clippers or scissors for hair removal if indicated
- Short extension tubing with fused needleless connector or separate needleless connector (also called *injection cap, saline lock, heparin lock, IV plug, buff cap, buffalo cap, or PRN adapter*)
- 10-mL syringe prefilled with preservative-free 0.9% sodium chloride (normal saline [NS]) (INS, 2016a)
- Antiseptic swabs
- Engineered catheter stabilization device (if available) and polymer-based skin protectant swab
- *Option:* IV site protection device
- Prescribed IV solution or medication
- IV administration set (IV tubing), either macrodrip or microdrip , depending on prescribed rate; if using EID, appropriate administration set
- 0.2-micron filter for nonlipid (fat emulsions) solutions (may be incorporated into the infusion set)
- Personal protective equipment: goggles and mask (*optional* based on agency policy)
- Electronic infusion device (EID) and IV pole
- Vein visualization device (*optional* based on agency policy)
- Stethoscope
- Watch with second hand to calculate drip rate
- Special patient gown with snaps at shoulder seams if available
- Needle disposal container (*sharps container* or *biohazard container*)
- *Option:* Hand or arm joint stabilization device

STEP	RATIONALE

ASSESSMENT

1. Review accuracy of health care provider's order: date and time, IV solution, route of administration, volume, rate, duration, and signature of ordering health care provider (Gorski, 2018). Follow the seven rights of medication administration.

Before IV therapy, an order from a health care provider is needed (INS, 2016a). Verification that order is complete prevents medication errors.

   a. Check approved online database, drug reference book, or pharmacist about IV solution composition, purpose, potential incompatibilities, adverse reactions, and side effects.

Ensures safe and correct administration of IV therapy and appropriate selection of VAD.

2. Obtain data from patient's electronic health record of clinical factors/conditions that will respond to or be affected by administration of IV solutions.

Provides baseline to determine effectiveness of prescribed therapy. A systems approach is recommended to assess for fluid and electrolyte imbalances (Gorski, 2018).

   a. Body weight

Changes in body weight can be an indication of fluid loss or gain (Gorski, 2018).

   b. Clinical markers of vascular volume:

     (1) Urine output (decreased, dark yellow)

Kidneys respond to extracellular volume (ECV) deficit by reducing urine production and concentrating urine. Kidney disease can also cause oliguria.

     (2) Vital signs: blood pressure, respirations, pulse, temperature

Changes in blood pressure may be associated with fluid volume status (fluid volume deficit [FVD]) seen in postural hypotension.

Respirations can be altered in presence of acid-base imbalances.

Temperature elevations increase need for fluid requirements (temperature of 38.3°C [101°F] to 39.4°C [103°F] require at least 500 mL of fluid replacement within a 24-hr period) (Gorski, 2018).

     (3) Distended neck veins (normally veins are full when person is supine and flat when person is upright)

Indicator of fluid volume status: flat or collapsing with inhalation when supine with ECV deficit; full when upright or semi-upright with ECV excess.

     (4) Auscultation of lungs

Crackles or rhonchi in dependent parts of lung may signal fluid buildup caused by ECV excess.

     (5) Capillary refill

Indirect measure of tissue perfusion (sluggish with ECV deficit).

   c. Clinical markers of interstitial volume:

     (1) Skin turgor (pinch skin over sternum or inside of forearm)

Failure of skin to return to normal position after several seconds indicates FVD (Alexander et al., 2014).

     (2) Dependent edema (pitting or nonpitting)

Edema is not usually apparent until 4.4–8.8 lb (2–4 kg) of fluid is retained. A weight gain of 2.2 lb (1 kg) is equivalent to the retention of 1 L of body water (Gorski, 2018).

     (3) Oral mucous membrane between cheek and gum

More reliable indicator than dry lips or skin. Dry between cheek and gums indicates ECV deficit.

   d. Thirst

Occurs with hypernatremia and severe ECV deficit. Not a reliable indicator for older adults (Kear, 2017).

   e. Behavior and level of consciousness

     (1) Restlessness and mild confusion

Occurs with FVD or acid-base imbalance.

     (2) Decreased level of consciousness (lethargy, confusion, coma)

Occurs with severe ECV deficit. May occur with osmolality, fluid and electrolyte, and acid-base imbalances.

3. Determine whether patient is to undergo any planned surgeries or procedures.

Allows anticipation and placement of appropriate VAD for infusion and avoids placement in an area that will interfere with medical procedures (INS, 2016a).

4. Assess available laboratory data (e.g., hematocrit, serum electrolytes, arterial blood gases, and kidney functions [blood urea nitrogen, urine specific gravity, and urine osmolality]).

Helps determine priority assessments and establishes baseline for determining whether therapy is effective. Laboratory values are an assessment of hydration status (Alexander et al., 2014).

5. Assess patient's or family caregiver's knowledge, experience, and health literacy regarding IV therapy.

Ensures patient or family caregiver has the capacity to obtain, communicate, process, and understand basic health information (Centers for Disease Control and Prevention [CDC], 2019).

6. Assess patient's history of allergies, especially to iodine, adhesive, or latex.

Equipment used during VAD insertion may contain substances to which patient is allergic. When a patient has a latex allergy, health care providers will need to use latex-free gloves.

7. Assess patient's arm preference for placement of IV.

Provides patient-centered care by determining level of emotional support and instruction needed.

PLANNING

1. Close room door or bedside curtains. Remove clutter from the over-bed or bedside table.

Providing privacy and preparing the environment ensures patient comfort and organizes procedure.

2. Perform hand hygiene. Collect and organize equipment on clean bedside table. Verify that you have the correct infusion set for the EID that will be used.

Reduces transmission of microorganisms. Easy access to equipment improves efficiency. Ensures patient safety.

Continued

SKILL 42.1	INSERTION OF A SHORT-PERIPHERAL INTRAVENOUS DEVICE—cont'd

STEP	RATIONALE
3. Select appropriate-sized catheter; open and prepare sterile packages using sterile aseptic technique (see Chapter 28).	Use smallest-gauge peripheral catheter that will accommodate prescribed therapy and patient needs (INS, 2016a).
4. Help patient to comfortable sitting or supine position. Change patient's gown to one more easily removed with snaps at shoulder if available. Provide adequate lighting.	Promotes comfort and relaxation for patient. Use of this type of gown decreases risk of accidental dislodgment of catheter or administration set. Aids in successful vein location.
5. Explain/instruct patient about rationale for infusion, including solution and medications ordered, procedure for IV insertion, and signs and symptoms of complications (e.g. bleeding, tenderness and swelling) to watch out for.	Provides patient with information about procedure and promotes adherence (INS, 2016a). May minimize anxiety.

IMPLEMENTATION

STEP	RATIONALE
1. Identify patient using at least two identifiers (e.g., name and birthday or name and medical record number) according to agency policy. Compare identifiers with information on patient's MAR or medical record.	Ensures correct patient. Complies with a recommended National Patient Safety Goal (TJC, 2020).
2. Perform hand hygiene. Prepare short extension tubing with fused needleless connector or separate needleless connector (injection cap) to attach to catheter hub.	Needleless connectors protect health care workers by eliminating needles and potential for needlestick injuries when accessing VAD (INS, 2016a).
a. Remove protective cap from needleless connector and attach syringe with 1 to 3 mL 0.9% sodium chloride (normal saline), maintaining sterility. Slowly inject enough saline to prime (fill) short extension tubing and connector, removing all air. Leave syringe attached to tubing.	Replaces air with normal saline, preventing air from entering patient's vein later during VAD insertion.
b. Maintain sterility of end of connector by reapplying end caps and set aside for attaching to catheter hub after successful venipuncture. Do not overtighten end caps.	Prevents touch contamination, which allows microorganisms to enter infusion equipment and bloodstream. Overtightening end caps will make it difficult to remove them.

CLINICAL DECISION: *Short extension sets may be used on short-peripheral catheters. Reduces catheter manipulation. For patient safety, all connections should be of Luer-Lok type (INS, 2016a). Luer-Lok connections should be used to prevent accidental disconnection (INS, 2016a). Many agencies use short extension tubing for continuous infusions and stand-alone saline locks (capped catheters).*

3. Prepare IV tubing and solution for continuous infusion.

STEP	RATIONALE
a. Check IV solution using seven rights of medication administration (see Chapter 31) and review label for name and concentration of solution, type and concentration of any additives, volume, beyond-use and expiration dates, and sterility state. If using bar code, scan code on patient's wristband and then on IV fluid container. Be sure that prescribed additives such as potassium and vitamins have been added. Check solution for color and clarity. Check bag for leaks.	Reviewing label for accuracy reduces risk for medication errors (INS, 2016a). Risk for medication errors can be reduced with safe medication practices, including (INS, 2016a): • Do not add medications to infusing containers of IV solutions (INS, 2016a). • Do not use IV solutions that are discolored, contain precipitates, or are expired.
b. Open IV infusion set, maintaining sterility. Note: EIDs sometimes have a dedicated administration set; follow manufacturer's instructions.	Prevents touch contamination, which allows microorganisms to enter infusion equipment and bloodstream.
c. Place roller clamp (see illustration A) about 2 to 5 cm (1 to 2 inches) below drip chamber and move roller clamp to "off" position (see illustration B).	Close proximity of roller clamp to drip chamber allows more accurate regulation of flow rate. Moving clamp to "off" prevents accidental spillage of IV solution during priming.

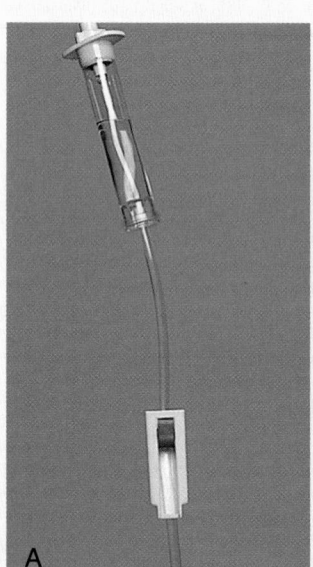 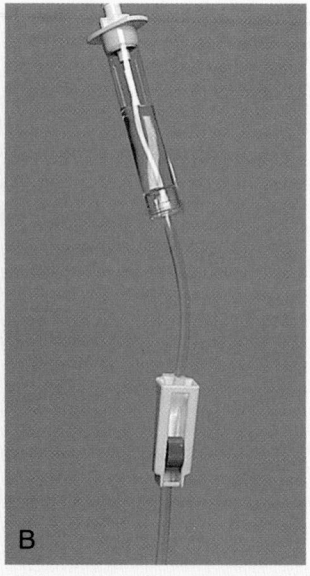 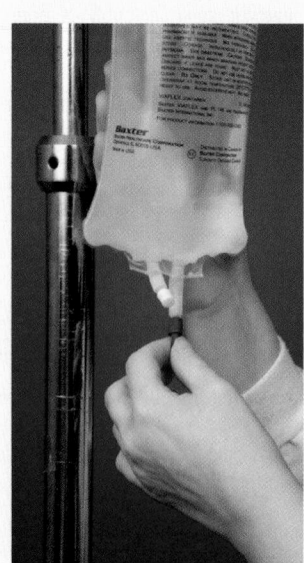 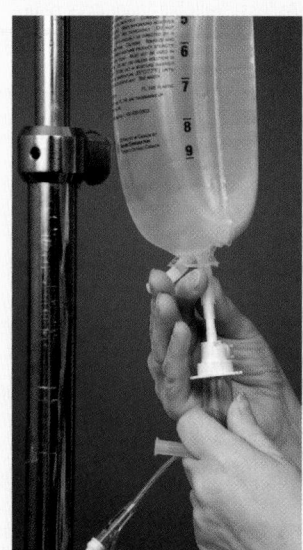

STEP 3c A, Roller clamp in open position. B, Roller clamp in closed position.

STEP 3d Removing protective sheath from IV tubing port.

STEP 3e Inserting spike into IV bag.

STEP	RATIONALE
d. Remove protective sheath over IV tubing port on plastic IV solution bag (see illustration) or top of IV solution bottle while maintaining sterility.	Provides access for insertion of IV tubing spike into solution using sterile technique.
e. Remove protective cover from IV tubing spike while maintaining sterility of spike. Insert spike into port of IV bag using a twisting motion (see illustration). If solution container is glass bottle, clean rubber stopper on glass-bottled solution with antiseptic swab and insert spike into rubber stopper of IV bottle. Bottles require vented tubing.	Flat surface on top of bottled solution may contain contaminants, whereas opening to plastic bag is recessed. Prevents contamination of bottled solution during insertion of spike. If sterility of spike is compromised, discard IV tubing and obtain new one.
f. Compress drip chamber and release, allowing it to fill one-third to one-half full (see illustration).	Compression creates suction effect; fluid enters drip chamber to prevent air from entering tubing.
g. Prime air out of IV tubing by filling with IV solution: Remove protective cover on end of IV tubing (some tubing can be primed without removing protective cover) and slowly open roller clamp to allow fluid to flow from drip chamber to distal end of IV tubing. If tubing has a Y connector, invert Y connector when fluid reaches it to displace air. Return roller clamp to "off" position after priming tubing (filled with IV fluid). Replace protective cover on distal end of tubing. Label IV tubing with date according to agency policy and procedure.	Priming ensures that IV tubing is clear of air and filled with IV solution before connecting to VAD. Slowly filling tubing decreases turbulence and chance of bubble formation. Closing clamp prevents accidental loss of fluid. Maintains sterility. Labeling IV tubing allows for recognition of length of time that tubing has been in use and when to change it.
h. Be certain that IV tubing is clear of air and air bubbles. To remove small air bubbles, firmly tap tubing where they are located. Air bubbles will ascend to drip chamber. Check entire length of tubing to ensure that all air bubbles are removed (see illustration).	Large air bubbles act as emboli and should be avoided (Mattox, 2017).
i. If using optional long extension tubing, remove protective cover and attach it to distal end of IV tubing, maintaining sterility. Then prime long extension tubing with IV solution. Insert IV tubing into EID with power off.	Priming removes air from long extension tubing so that it does not enter patient's vascular system. Facilitates starting infusion as soon as IV site is ready.
4. Perform hand hygiene.	Decreases potential risk of microbial contamination and cross-contamination (INS, 2016a).

CLINICAL DECISION: *Gloves are not necessary to locate vein but must be applied for VAD insertion using a no-touch technique where the site is not palpated after skin antisepsis (INS, 2016a, 2016b).*

---

5. Apply tourniquet around upper arm about 10 to 15 cm (4 to 6 inches) above proposed insertion site (see illustration). Do not apply tourniquet too tightly. Check for presence of pulse distal to tourniquet.	Tourniquet should be tight enough to impede venous flow while maintaining arterial circulation (INS, 2016a, 2016b). If patient has fragile veins or bruises easily, tourniquet should be applied loosely or not at all to prevent damage to veins and bruising (INS, 2016a).
Option A: Apply tourniquet on top of thin layer of clothing such as gown sleeve to protect fragile or hairy skin.	
Option B: Blood pressure cuff may be used in place of tourniquet: activate cuff and hold at approximately 50 mm Hg.	Reduces trauma to skin.

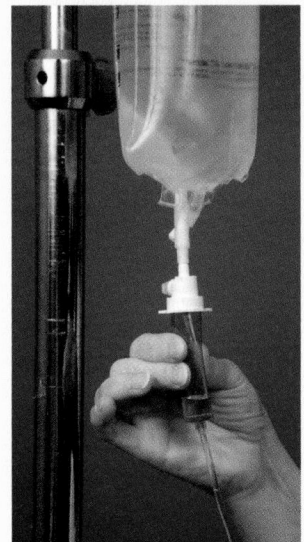

STEP 3f Squeezing drip chamber to fill with fluid one-third to one-half full.

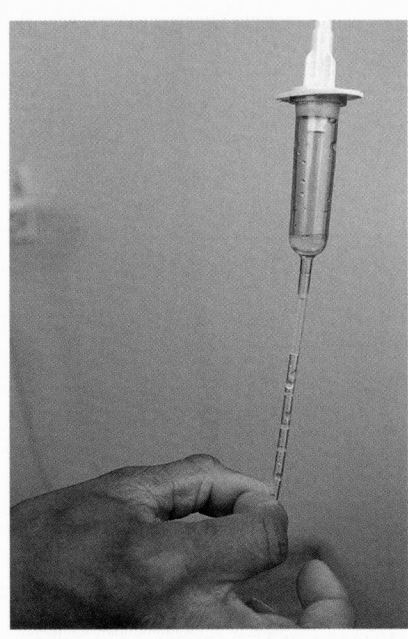

STEP 3h Removing air bubbles from tubing.

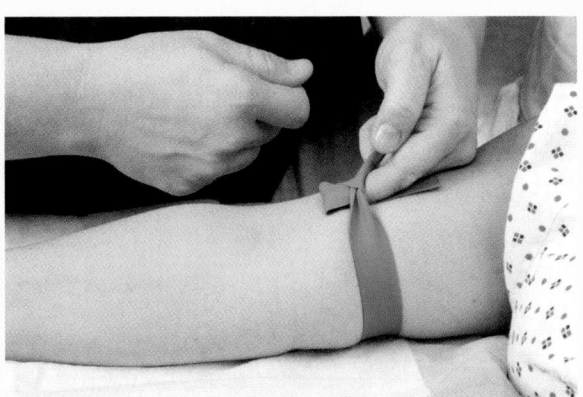

STEP 5 Tourniquet placed on arm for initial vein selection.

Continued

SKILL 42.1   INSERTION OF A SHORT-PERIPHERAL INTRAVENOUS DEVICE—cont'd

STEP	RATIONALE
6. Select vein for VAD insertion (see Fig. 42.15). Veins on dorsal and ventral surfaces of arms (e.g., metacarpal, cephalic, basilic, or median) are preferred in adults.	Ensures adequate vein that is easy to puncture and less likely to rupture.
a. Use most distal site in nondominant arm if possible.	Patients with VAD placement in their dominant hand have decreased ability to perform self-care.
b. With your fingertip, palpate vein at intended insertion site by pressing downward. Note resilient, soft, bouncy feeling while releasing pressure (see illustration).	Fingertip is more sensitive and better for assessing vein location and condition.
c. Select well-dilated vein. Methods to improve vascular distention:	Increased volume of blood in vein at venipuncture site makes vein more visible.
(1) Position extremity lower than heart, have patient open and close fist slowly, and lightly stroke vein downward.	Use of gravity promotes vascular distention (INS, 2016a).
(2) Apply dry heat to extremity for several minutes.	Dry heat has been found to promote vein dilation and increase successful peripheral catheter insertion (INS, 2016a).

CLINICAL DECISION: *Vigorous friction, slapping or hard tapping of a vein, especially in older adults, can cause venous constriction and/or bruising and hematoma (Gorski, 2018).*

7. When selecting a vein:	
a. Avoid vein selection in:	
(1) Areas with pain on palpation, compromised areas, sites distal to compromised areas (e.g., open wounds, bruising, infection, infiltration, and extravasation) (INS, 2016a).	It would be difficult to assess for any signs or symptoms of complications if an IV device were inserted in an area already compromised.
(2) Upper extremity on side of breast surgery with axillary node dissection or lymphedema or after radiation, arteriovenous (AV) fistulas/grafts; or affected extremity from cerebrovascular accident (CVA) (INS, 2016a).	Increases risk for complications such as infection, lymphedema, or vessel damage.
(3) Site distal to previous venipuncture site, sclerosed or hardened veins, previous infiltrations or extravasations, areas of venous valves, or phlebitic vessels.	Such sites cause infiltration around newly placed VAD site and vessel damage.
(4) Fragile dorsal hand veins in older adults, veins in lower extremities, and veins in an extremity with poor circulation.	Veins have increased risk for infiltration, tissue damage, and thrombophlebitis (INS, 2016a).
(5) Areas of flexion such as wrist or antecubital area (INS, 2016a).	Veins have increased risk for occlusion, infiltration, phlebitis, or dislodgment.
(6) Ventral surface of wrist (10–12.5 cm [4–5 inches])	Venipuncture in ventral surface of wrist is painful and has potential for nerve damage (INS, 2016a).
b. Choose site that will not interfere with patient's activities of daily living (ADLs), use of assist devices, or planned procedures.	Keeps patient as mobile as possible.
8. Release tourniquet temporarily.	Restores blood flow and prevents venospasm when preparing for venipuncture.

CLINICAL DECISION: *If hair removal is needed, do not shave area with a razor. Shaving may increase risk of infection (INS, 2016a). Clip hair with scissors or hair clippers to prepare area for application of transparent semipermeable membrane (TSM) dressing if necessary (explain to patient).*

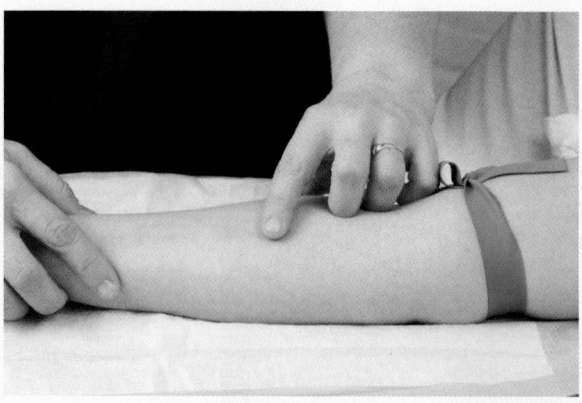

STEP 6b Palpate vein.

STEP	RATIONALE

CLINICAL DECISION: *Local anesthetic reduces discomfort associated with insertion of a VAD. Both topical and injectable drugs can reduce pain and require a health care provider's order. You may apply topical local anesthetic to intended IV site 30 minutes before procedure. Follow manufacturer recommendations and monitor for allergic reaction (Alexander et al., 2014; INS, 2016a).*

9. Perform hand hygiene and apply clean gloves. Wear eye protection and mask (see agency policy) if splash or spray of blood is possible.
10. Place adapter end of short extension set (prepared in Step 2) or needleless connector (injection cap) for saline lock nearby in sterile package.
11. If area of insertion is visibly soiled, clean site with antiseptic soap and water first and dry. Perform skin antisepsis with alcoholic chlorhexidine solution using friction in back-and-forth motion (see illustration) for 30 seconds and allow to dry completely. If using plain alcohol or povidone-iodine, clean in concentric circle, moving from insertion site outward with swab. Allow drying time between agents if agents are used in combination (alcohol and povidone-iodine).

Decreases potential risk of microbial contamination and cross-contamination (INS, 2016a).
Permits smooth, quick connection of infusion to short-peripheral catheter once vein is accessed.
Mechanical friction in this pattern allows penetration of antiseptic solution to epidermal layer of skin (Alexander et al., 2014). Reduces incidence of catheter-related infections (Alexander et al., 2014).
Allow any skin antiseptic agent to fully dry for complete antisepsis—alcoholic chlorhexidine solutions for at least 30 seconds, iodophors for at least 1.5 to 2 minutes (INS, 2016a).

CLINICAL DECISION: *If vein palpation is necessary after performing skin antisepsis, use sterile gloves for palpation or perform skin antisepsis again because touching cleaned area introduces microorganisms from your finger to site (INS, 2016a, 2016b).*

12. Reapply tourniquet 10 to 15 cm (4 to 6 inches) above anticipated insertion site. Check for presence of pulse distal to tourniquet.
13. Perform venipuncture. Anchor vein below anticipated insertion site by placing thumb over vein 4 to 5 cm (1½ to 2 inches) distal to site (see illustration) and gently stretching skin against direction of insertion. Instruct patient to relax hand.

    a. Warn patient of a sharp stick.
    b. Hold VAD with needle bevel up. Align catheter on top of vein at 10- to 30-degree angle. Puncture skin and anterior vein wall (see illustration).

Pressure of tourniquet promotes vein distention. Diminished arterial flow prevents venous filling.
Stabilizes vein for needle insertion, prevents vein from rolling, and stretches skin taut, decreasing drag during insertion. Some devices require loosening needle (stylet) from catheter before venipuncture. Follow manufacturer directions for use.
Accessing vein at an angle reduces risk of puncturing posterior vein wall. Superficial veins require smaller angle. Deeper veins require greater angle.

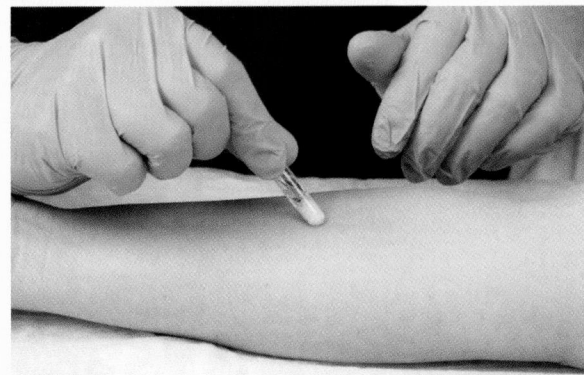

STEP 11 Clean site with antiseptic swab (alcoholic chlorhexidine solution preferred, 70% alcohol, or povidone-iodine).

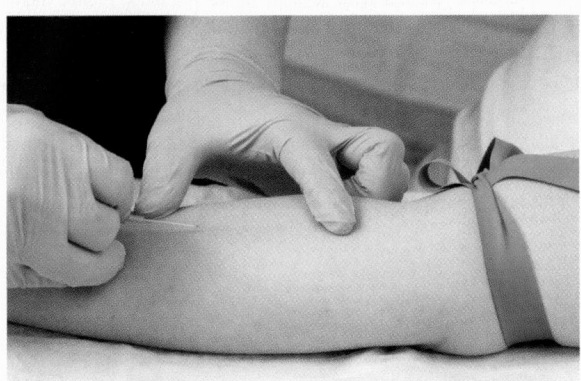

STEP 13 Stabilize vein below insertion site.

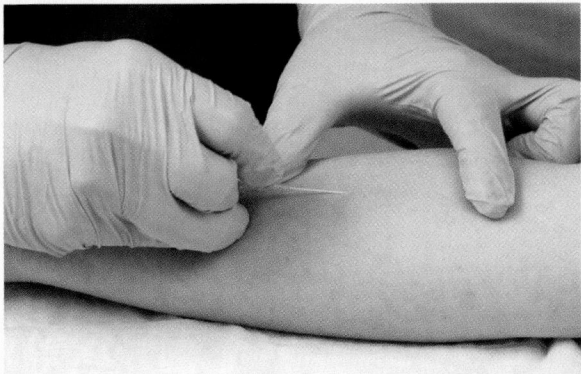

STEP 13b Puncture skin with catheter at 10- to 30-degree angle.

Continued

SKILL 42.1	INSERTION OF A SHORT-PERIPHERAL INTRAVENOUS DEVICE—cont'd
STEP	**RATIONALE**

CLINICAL DECISION: *Use each catheter only once for each insertion attempt.*

14. Observe for blood return in catheter or flashback chamber of catheter, indicating that bevel of needle has entered vein (see illustration A). Advance VAD approximately ¼ inch (0.6 cm) into vein and loosen stylet (needle) of ONC. Continue to hold skin taut while stabilizing VAD and, with index finger on push-off tab of VAD, advance catheter off needle into vein until hub rests at venipuncture site (see illustration B). *Do not reinsert stylet into catheter once catheter has been advanced into vein.* Advance catheter while safety device automatically retracts stylet (techniques for retracting stylet vary with different VADs). Place stylet directly into sharps container.

Increased venous pressure from tourniquet causes backflow of blood into catheter and/or flashback chamber. Some VADs have a notch in the stylet, allowing flash of blood into catheter. Stabilizing VAD allows for placement of catheter into vein and advancement of catheter off stylet.

Advancing entire stylet into vein may penetrate wall of vein, resulting in hematoma.

Advancing catheter with finger on open hub causes contamination (INS, 2016a).

Reinsertion of stylet can cause catheter to shear off and embolize into vein. Devices with safety mechanisms and proper sharps disposal prevent needle-stick injuries (OSHA, 2012).

CLINICAL DECISION: *A single clinician should not make more than two attempts at initiating IV access and limit total attempts to no more than 4 (INS, 2016a).*

15. Stabilize VAD with nondominant hand and release tourniquet or blood pressure cuff with other. Apply gentle but firm pressure with middle finger of nondominant hand 3 cm (1¼ inches) above insertion site. Keep catheter stable with index finger.

Permits venous flow and reduces backflow of blood.

Digital pressure minimizes blood loss and allows attachment of extension set or needleless connector (INS, 2016b).

16. Quickly connect Luer-Lok end of short extension tubing with needleless connector to end of catheter hub. Secure connection. Avoid touching sterile connection ends.
    Option: IV tubing can be attached directly to catheter hub in place of short extension tubing or needleless connector.

Prompt connection maintains patency of vein, minimizes blood loss, and prevents risk of exposure to blood. Maintains sterility.

17. Take the previously attached 10-mL prefilled syringe that contains 0.9% sodium chloride (normal saline [NS]) and is connected to short extension set. Aspirate by pulling back on syringe to remove air and assess blood return. Then, slowly inject NS from syringe into VAD (see illustration A). Remove syringe and discard.
    Option: To begin primary infusion, swab needleless connector with antiseptic swab and attach Luer-Lok end of IV tubing to needleless connector (see illustration B). Open roller clamp of IV tubing, turn on EID, and program it. Begin infusion at correct rate. If using gravity flow instead of EID, begin infusion by slowly opening roller clamp to regulate rate.

Aspirating air prevents air embolism. Blood return that is color and consistency of whole blood confirms placement of catheter in vein (INS, 2016a).

Flushing prevents reflux of blood into catheter and occlusion (INS, 2016b).

Initiates flow of fluid through IV catheter, preventing clotting of device.

Swelling indicates infiltration, and catheter would need to be removed.

Initiates flow of fluid through IV catheter, preventing clotting of VAD.

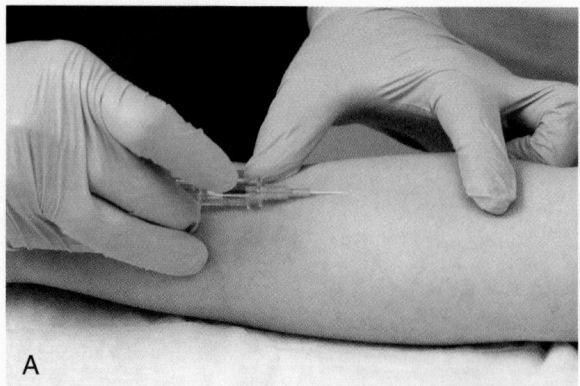
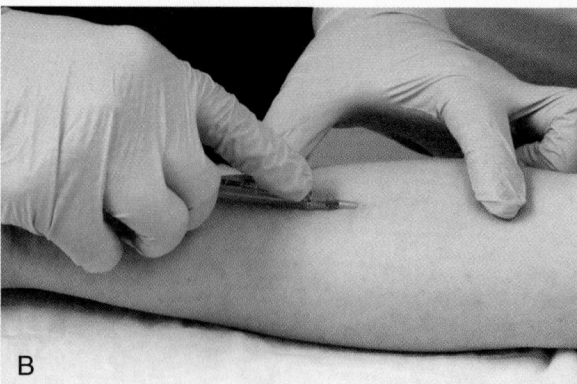

STEP 14 A, Observe for blood return in catheter and/or flashback chamber. **B,** Advance catheter into vein until hub rests at venipuncture site.

STEP	RATIONALE

CLINICAL DECISION: *Needleless connectors protect health care workers and decrease risk for needlestick injuries. They have different internal mechanisms for fluid displacement and vary in the flush-clamp-disconnect sequence to prevent reflux of blood into catheter on disconnection (INS, 2016a). The sequence depends on the type of internal mechanism (Gorski, 2018):*
- *Neutral displacement devices do not have a specified flush-clamp-disconnect sequence.*
- *For negative-pressure displacement devices, flush, clamp catheter, then disconnect syringe.*
- *For positive-pressure displacement, flush, disconnect syringe, then clamp catheter.*

18. Observe insertion site for swelling.

19. Apply sterile dressing over site.

  a. **Transparent semipermeable membrane (TSM) dressing:**

   (1) Continue to secure catheter with nondominant hand. Remove adherent backing. Apply one edge of dressing and gently smooth remaining dressing over IV insertion site, leaving Luer-Lok connection between tubing and catheter hub uncovered. Gently press dressing to adhere to skin. Remove outer covering and smooth dressing gently over site (see illustration).

   (2) Place 2.5 cm (2-inch) piece of tape over Luer-Lok connection (see illustration). Do not apply tape on top of TSM dressing.

  b. **Sterile gauze dressing:**

   (1) Place 5-cm (2-inch) piece of sterile tape over catheter hub (see illustration).

   (2) Place 2 × 2–inch gauze pad over insertion site and edge of catheter hub. Secure all edges with tape. Do not place tape over insertion site. Do not cover connection between IV tubing and catheter hub (see illustration).

Swelling indicates infiltration, which requires immediate catheter removal.

Protects catheter insertion site and minimizes risk for infection (Gorski, 2018). Allows visualization of insertion site and surrounding area for complications (INS, 2016a). Access to Luer-Lok connection between tubing and catheter hub facilitates changing tubing if necessary.

Removal of tape from TSM dressing can tear dressing and cause catheter dislodgement.
Tape on top of TSM dressing prevents moisture from being carried away from skin.

Stabilizes catheter under gauze dressing.
Use gauze dressings for site drainage, excessive perspiration, or sensitivity/allergic reactions to TSM dressings (INS, 2016a; Gorski, 2018).

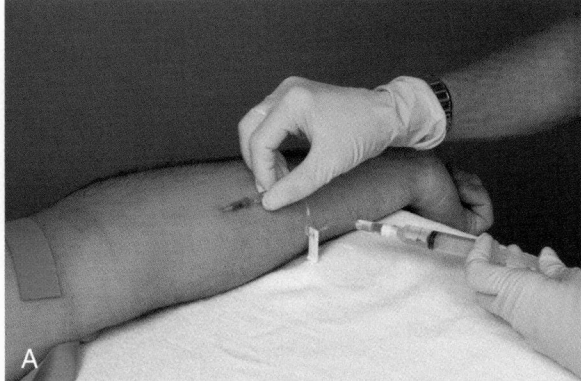

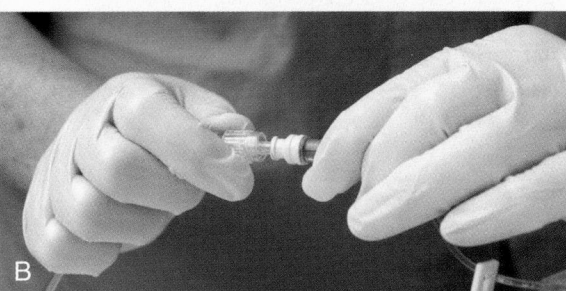

STEP 17 A, Flush short extension set after aspirating air and assessing blood return. **B,** Connect IV tubing to the short extension set that is attached to the catheter.

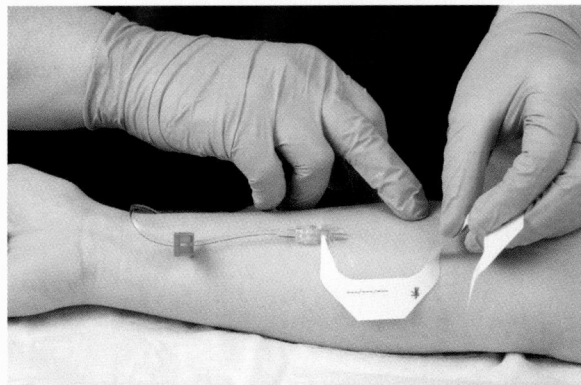

STEP 19a(1) Apply transparent semipermeable membrane (TSM) dressing.

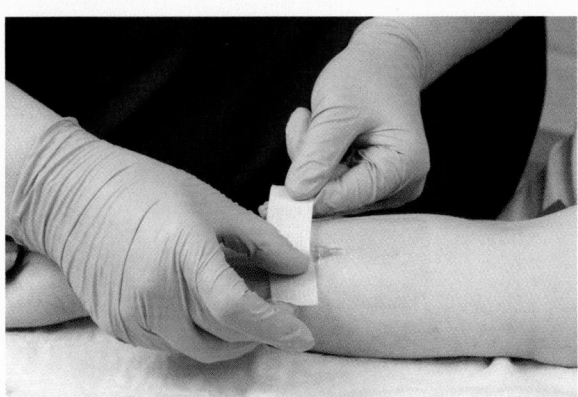

STEP 19a(2) Place tape over administration set tubing.

Continued

SKILL 42.1   **INSERTION OF A SHORT-PERIPHERAL INTRAVENOUS DEVICE—cont'd**

STEP	RATIONALE
(3) Fold 2 × 2–inch gauze in half and cover with 1 inch–wide tape so about an inch extends on each side. Place under Luer-Lok connection (see illustration). Secure Luer-Lok connection and tubing to tape on folded gauze with 2.5-cm (1-inch) piece of tape. Avoid applying tape or gauze around arm. Do not use rolled bandages with or without elastic to secure VAD. Taping Luer-Lok connection can be eliminated if engineered stabilization device is to be used.	Tape on top of gauze makes it easier to access hub/tubing junction. Gauze pad elevates hub off skin to prevent pressure area. Prevents back-and-forth motion of catheter. Rolled bandages do not secure VAD adequately, can impair circulation or flow of infusion, and obscure visualization for complications (INS, 2016a).
20. *Option:* Secure IV catheter using engineered stabilization device (follow manufacturer directions and agency policy).	Use of engineered stabilization devices that allow visual inspection of insertion site can reduce risk of VAD complications (i.e., phlebitis, infection, migration) and unintentional loss of access (INS, 2016a).
a. Apply polymer-based skin protectant to area of skin around IV site and allow to dry completely.	Risk for medical adhesive–related skin injury (MARSI) is increased as result of age, joint movement, and edema; use of skin protectant can decrease risk (INS, 2016a).
(1) Align anchoring pads with directional arrow pointing to insertion site. Press device retainer over top of Luer-Lok connection while supporting underneath connection.	
(2) Stabilize catheter and peel off one side of liner and press to adhere to skin. Repeat on other side (see illustration).	
(3) Monitor for medical adhesive–related skin injury (MARSI).	
21. *Option:* Apply site protection device (e.g., I.V. House UltraDressing®).	Reduces risk of VAD dislodgement (INS, 2016a).
22. Loop extension or IV tubing alongside dressing on arm and secure with second piece of tape directly over tubing (see illustration).	Securing tubing reduces risk for dislodging catheter if IV tubing is pulled (i.e., loop comes apart before catheter dislodges).
23. For continuous infusion, verify ordered rate of infusion and be sure EID is programmed correctly. If infusing by gravity drip, adjust flow rate to correct drops per minute.	Ensures prescribed rate of infusion.
24. Label dressing per agency policy. Include date and time of IV insertion, VAD gauge size and length, and your initials (see illustration).	Allows for recognition of type of device and length of time that device has been in place.
25. Dispose of any remaining sharps in appropriate sharps container. Discard supplies.	Prevents accidental needlestick injuries (OSHA, 2012).
26. Remove and dispose of gloves and perform hand hygiene.	Reduces risk of contamination (INS, 2016b).

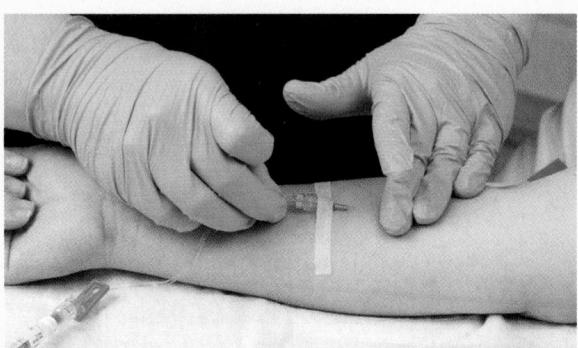

STEP 19b(1) Place sterile tape over catheter hub.

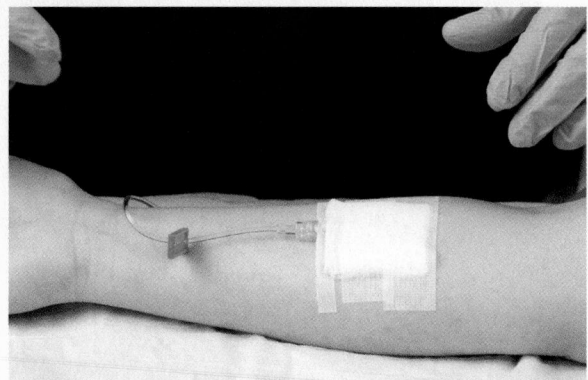

STEP 19b(2) Place 2 × 2–inch gauze over insertion site and catheter hub.

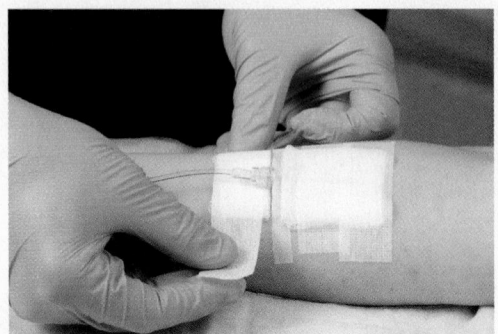

STEP 19b(3) Apply 2 × 2–inch gauze dressing under tubing junction.

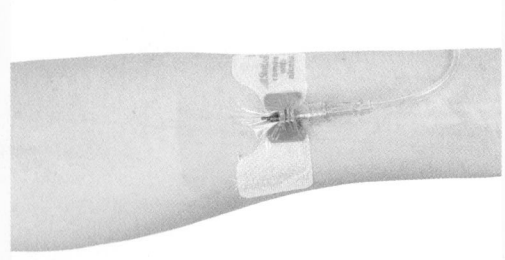

STEP 20a(2) Catheter stabilization device in place. (Image Courtesy C.R. Bard, Inc. All rights reserved.)

STEP	RATIONALE
27. Assist patient to a comfortable position and instruct how to move and turn without dislodging VAD.	Prevents accidental dislodgment of catheter and minimizes risk for falls.
28. Raise bed rails (as appropriate) and lower bed to lowest position.	Minimizes risks for falls and injury
29. Be sure nurse call system is in an accessible location within patient's reach. Instruct patient in its use.	Ensures patient can call for assistance if needed.

EVALUATION

(1) Observe patient every 1 to 2 hours, or at established intervals per agency policy and procedure for function, intactness, and patency of IV system and for correct infusion rate and accurate type/amount of IV solution infused by observing level in IV container.	Ensures delivery of prescribed volume over prescribed time and decreases risk for fluid and electrolyte imbalance.
(2) Evaluate patient to determine response to therapy (e.g., laboratory values, input and output [I&O], weights, vital signs, postprocedure assessments).	Early recognition of complications leads to prompt treatment.
(3) Evaluate patient with a short-peripheral IV at least every 4 hours, or every 1 to 2 hours for patients that are critically ill, sedated, or have cognitive deficits (INS, 2016a), or at established intervals per agency policy and procedure for signs and symptoms of catheter-related complications. Assess the VAD catheter-skin junction site and surrounding area by visually inspecting and palpating through the intact dressing for redness, tenderness, swelling, and drainage.	Identifies complications that compromise integrity of VAD or cause inaccurate IV solution flow rate.

CLINICAL DECISION: *If IV is positional, fluid will run slowly or stop, depending on position of patient's arm; if this continues, you may have to restart IV line.*

4. **Use Teach-Back:** "I want to make sure that I explained the problems that can happen with your IV. Tell me the signs or symptoms that you should tell me or the other nurses about." Revise your instruction now or develop a plan for revised patient/family caregiver teaching if patient/family caregiver is not able to teach back correctly.	Determines patient's/family caregiver's level of understanding of instructional topic.

UNEXPECTED OUTCOMES AND RELATED INTERVENTIONS

1. Fluid and electrolyte imbalances, including FVD, FVE, and abnormal serum electrolyte levels.
   - Notify health care provider.
   - Readjust infusion rate based on health care provider order.
   - Adjust additives in type of IV fluid as ordered.
2. IV-related complications including infiltration, phlebitis, local infection, air embolus and bleeding.
   - See Table 42.12
3. Catheter occlusion can occur from bent catheter, positional catheter (catheter resting against catheter wall), kink or knot in infusion tubing, clot formation, or precipitate formation from administration of incompatible medications or solutions (Gorski, 2018).
   - Determine cause and consider catheter removal.
   - Positional catheters can be repositioned to improve IV flow.
   - Remove occluded IV catheter. Occluded catheters should not be flushed because an embolus can result from dislodging a clot (Gorski, 2018).
4. Catheter-related infection can present as redness, swelling around or above IV site, pain, purulent drainage at insertion site, and body temperature elevations (INS, 2016a).
   - Notify health care provider. Obtain order to culture drainage (INS, 2016a).
   - Remove IV catheter and culture purulent drainage from around IV site (see Chapter 48) (INS, 2016a).

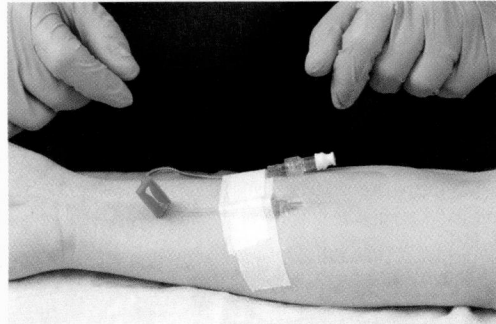

STEP 22 Loop and secure tubing.

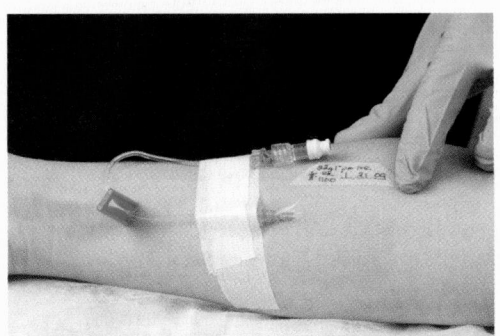

STEP 24 Label IV dressing.

Continued

SKILL 42.1	INSERTION OF A SHORT-PERIPHERAL INTRAVENOUS DEVICE—cont'd

RECORDING AND REPORTING

- Record number of attempts at insertion; date and time of insertion; type of solution and additives infusing; precise description of insertion site; catheter gauge, type, length and brand; rate and method of infusion (e.g., gravity or name of EID); purpose of infusion; patient's response to insertion (e.g., what he or she reports); and when infusion was started. Always complete entry with full signature and credentials.
- After each shift, document patient's status, IV fluid infusing, amount infused, and integrity and patency of system.
- Record and report signs or symptoms of observed or patient-reported IV-related complications (e.g. redness, tenderness, swelling, drainage, leaking from under dressing, change in flow rate, or infection).
- Document your evaluation of patient learning.
- Report to health care provider any adverse events occurring upon VAD placement (e.g., persistent pain or suspected nerve damage, hematoma formation, or arterial puncture).
- Report to health care provider any signs or symptoms of complications.

HOME CARE CONSIDERATIONS

- Ensure that patient is able and willing to self-administer IV therapy or that a reliable family caregiver will provide IV therapy at home.
- Teach patient and family caregiver information needed to administer IV therapy safely (see Box 42.8). Consider their cultural norms (e.g., health beliefs and comfort with caregivers using touch).

SKILL 42.2	REGULATING INTRAVENOUS FLOW RATE

Delegation and Collaboration

The skill of regulating IV flow rates cannot be delegated to assistive personnel (AP). Delegation to licensed practical nurses (LPNs) varies by state Nurse Practice Act. The nurse instructs the AP to:

- Inform the nurse when the EID alarm signals.
- Inform the nurse when the fluid container is near completion.
- Report any patient complaints of discomfort related to infusion such as pain, burning, bleeding, or swelling.

Equipment

- Watch with a second hand
- Calculator, paper, and pencil/pen
- Label
- IV solution bag and appropriate administration set
- EID, IV regulating device
- Clean gloves

STEP	RATIONALE

ASSESSMENT

1. Review accuracy and completeness of health care provider order in patient's medical record for patient name, type and volume of IV fluid, additives, infusion rate, and duration of IV therapy. Follow seven rights of medication administration.

Ensures administration of correct IV fluid at proper rate. IV fluids are medications. The seven rights prevent medication administration error.

2. Review medical record and identify patient risk for fluid and electrolyte imbalance given type of IV solution (e.g., neonate, history of cardiac or renal disease).

Helps prioritize assessments. Volume control needs to be strict. Guides choice of infusion device.

3. Perform hand hygiene and apply clean gloves.

Reduces risk of contamination (INS, 2016b).

4. Check infusion system from solution container down to vascular access device (VAD) insertion site for integrity.

Identifies complications that can compromise integrity of VAD and patient safety.

   a. Assess IV container for discoloration, cloudiness, leakage, and expiration date.

Incompatibility of solutions or medications compromises integrity of VAD and patient safety (Gorski, 2018).

   b. Assess IV tubing for puncture, contamination, or occlusion.

Compromised tubing results in fluid leakage and bacterial contamination.

5. Assess the integrity, patency, and functioning of the existing VAD (according to agency policy). Assess the VAD catheter-skin junction site and surrounding area for catheter-related complications by visually inspecting and palpating through the intact dressing for redness, tenderness, swelling, and drainage.

Identifies complications that compromise integrity of VAD and necessitate replacement of VAD.

6. Remove and dispose of gloves and perform hand hygiene.

Reduces risk of contamination (INS, 2016b).

7. Assess patient's and family caregiver's knowledge, experience, and health literacy regarding how positioning of IV site affects flow rate.

Ensures patient or family caregiver has the capacity to obtain, communicate, process, and understand basic health information (CDC, 2019b).

PLANNING

1. Prepare and organize equipment

   a. Gather paper and pencil or calculator to calculate flow rate.

Calculating hourly flow rates ensures that the prescribed amount of fluid to be infused over the prescribed time frame is correct.

   b. Check medical order to see how long each liter of fluid should infuse. If hourly rate (mL/hr) is not provided in order, calculate it by dividing volume by hours. For example:

Basis of calculation to ensure infusion of solution over prescribed hourly rate.

$$mL/hr = \frac{Total\ infusion\ volume\ (mL)}{Hours\ of\ infusion}$$

$$1000\ mL/8\ hr = 125\ mL/hr$$

or if 3 L is ordered for 24 hours,

$$3000\ mL/24\ hr = 125\ mL/hr$$

STEP	**RATIONALE**

CLINICAL DECISION: *It is common for health care providers to write an abbreviated IV order such as "D₅W with 20 mEq KCl 125 mL/hr continuous." This order implies that IV infusion should be maintained at this rate until an order has been written for IV infusion to be discontinued or changed to another order.*

c. If keep-vein-open (KVO) rate is ordered, check agency policy regarding flow rate.	Prevents catheter clotting, thus preserving venous access while infusing a minimal amount of fluid. An order for KVO rate must specify an infusion rate as required by the seven rights of medication administration (see Chapter 31). Rates may vary from 0.5 mL/hr to 30 mL/hr based of type of VAD, patient-specific therapy, and method of infusion (gravity or EID).
d. Use hourly rate to program EID (see Implementation) or, if gravity-flow infusion, use minute flow rate (drops per minute; gtt/min).	EID automatically delivers correct minute flow rate. Gravity infusion requires calculation of gtt/min.
e. Know calibration (drop factor), in drops per milliliter (gtt/mL) of infusion set used by agency.	Drop factor for macrodrip tubing varies with manufacturer.
(1) Microdrip: 60 gtt/mL: used to deliver rates less than 100 mL/hr.	Microdrip tubing universally delivers 60 gtt/mL. Used when small or precise volumes are ordered.
(2) *Macrodrip:* 10 or 15 gtt/mL: used to deliver rates greater than 100 mL/hr.	These are different commercial parenteral administration sets for macrodrip tubing. Used when large volumes or fast rates are necessary. **Know drip factor for tubing being used.**
f. Select one of the following formulas to calculate minute flow rate (drops/min) based on drop factor of infusion set:	Formulas compute correct flow rate over 1 minute.

(1) mL/hr/60 min = mL/min

Drop factor × mL/min = gtt/min

Or

(2) mL/hr × drop factor/60 min = gtt/min

g. Calculate minute flow rate for a bag of 1000 mL with 20 mEq of KCl at 125 mL/hr:	Once you determine hourly rate, these formulas compute the correct flow rate. When using microdrip, mL/hr always equals gtt/min.

Microdrip:

125 mL/hr × 60 gtt/mL = 7500 gtt/hr

7500 gtt ÷ 60 minutes = 125 gtt/min

Macrodrip:

125 mL/hr × 15 gtt/mL = 1875 gtt/hr

1875 gtt ÷ 60 minutes = 31–32 gtt/min

Multiply hourly rate (mL/hr) by drop factor and divide product by 60 to convert hours to minutes.

2. Explain/instruct patient and family caregiver on reasons for ongoing IV therapy.	Provides patient and family caregiver with information about procedure and promotes adherence (INS, 2016a).

IMPLEMENTATION

1. Identify patient using at least two identifiers (e.g., name and birthday or name and medical record number) according to agency policy. Compare identifiers with information on patient's MAR or medical record.	Ensures correct patient. Complies with a recommended National Patient Safety Goal (TJC, 2020).

CLINICAL DECISION: *Manual and mechanical flow-control devices may be used for infusions that do not require strict rate control (INS, 2016b). Fluids run by gravity are adjusted through use of a flow control/regulator. Manual flow regulators (i.e., roller clamp, dial, or barrel-shaped) are not recommended for use in infants and children because accuracy cannot be guaranteed (Alexander et al., 2014; Gorski, 2018) and can be affected by mechanical and patient factors. A calibrated chamber is a volume-controlled flow regulator that uses gravity to deliver only a limited amount of solution. It is placed between the IV container and the insertion spike and drip chamber of an administration set. Mechanical infusion devices (i.e., elastomeric devices, piston-driven pumps) regulate infusion rates with no outside power source (Alexander et al., 2014).*

2. Regulate gravity infusion.

a. Ensure that IV container is at least 76.2 cm (30 inches) above IV site for adults and increase height for more viscous fluids (Alexander et al., 2014).	Pressure caused by gravity is necessary to overcome venous pressure and resistance from tubing and catheter.

Continued

SKILL 42.2	REGULATING INTRAVENOUS FLOW RATE—cont'd

STEP	RATIONALE
b. Slowly open roller clamp on tubing until you can see drops in drip chamber. Hold a watch with second hand at same level as drip chamber and count drip rate for 1 minute (see illustration). Adjust roller clamp to increase or decrease rate of infusion.	Regulates flow to prescribed rate.
c. Monitor drip rate at least hourly.	Many factors influence drip rate; frequent monitoring ensures IV fluid administration as prescribed.

CLINICAL DECISION: *An electronic infusion device (EID) uses positive pressure to maintain correct flow rates and catheter patency to deliver a measured amount of fluid over a prescribed period of time (e.g., 100 mL/hr). Infusion pumps are needed for patients requiring low hourly rates, at risk for volume overload, with impaired renal function, or receiving solutions or medications that require a specific hourly volume.*
EIDs use an electronic sensor and an alarm that signals if pressure in the system changes and the desired flow rate changes. Many EIDs have operating and programming capabilities that allow for infusions of single or multiple solutions at different rates. Various detectors and alarms respond to air in IV lines, completion of infusion, high and low pressure, low battery power, occlusion, and the inability to deliver at a preset rate. The use of an EID still requires you to check to ensure that the pump is functioning and infusing at the prescribed rate.

STEP	RATIONALE
3. Regulate EID (infusion pump or smart pump): Follow manufacturer guidelines for setup of EID. Be sure you are using infusion tubing compatible with EID.	Smart pumps with medication safety software are designed for administration of IV fluids that contain medications.
a. Close roller clamp on primed IV infusion tubing. Roller clamp on IV tubing goes between EID and patient.	Prevents fluid leakage.
b. Insert infusion tubing into chamber of control mechanism (see manufacturer directions) (see illustration).	Most EIDs use positive pressure to infuse. Infusion pumps propel fluid through tubing by compressing and milking IV tubing.
c. Secure part of IV tubing through "air in line" alarm system. Close door (see illustration A) and turn on power button, select required drops per minute or volume per hour, close door to control chamber, and press start button (see illustration B). If infusing medication, access the smart pump drug library of medications and set appropriate rate and dose limits. If smart pump alarms immediately and shuts down, your settings were outside unit parameters.	Ensures safe administration of ordered flow rate or medication dose. Smart pumps require additional information such as patient unit and medication. Computer matches pump setting against a drug database and dose error reduction systems (DERSs) provide a means for decreasing IV medication administration errors (Wolf, 2018).

CLINICAL DECISION: *An anti–free-flow safeguard (preventing bolus infusion in the event of machine malfunction or when tubing is removed from machine) is an important element of an EID and is required. Always check and follow manufacturer recommendations for specific device features (Alexander et al., 2014; Gorski, 2018).*

STEP	RATIONALE
d. Open roller clamp on infusion tubing to wide open while EID is in use.	Ensures that pump freely regulates infusion rate.
e. Monitor infusion rate and IV site for complications according to agency policy. Use watch to verify rate of infusion, even when using EID.	Flow controllers and pumps do not replace frequent, accurate nursing evaluation. EIDs can continue to infuse IV solutions after a complication has developed (INS, 2016a).
f. Assess IV system from container to VAD insertion site when alarm signals.	Alarm indicates situation that requires attention. Empty solution container, tubing kinks, closed clamp, infiltration, clotted catheter, air in tubing, and/or low battery can trigger EID alarm.

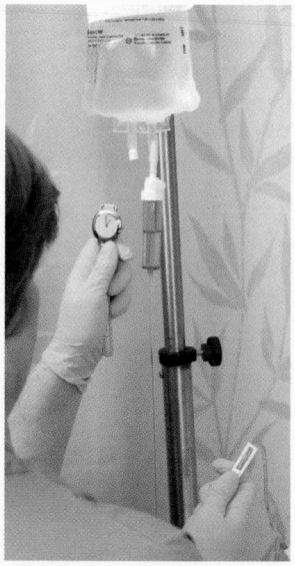

STEP 2b Nurse counting drip rate on gravity infusion.

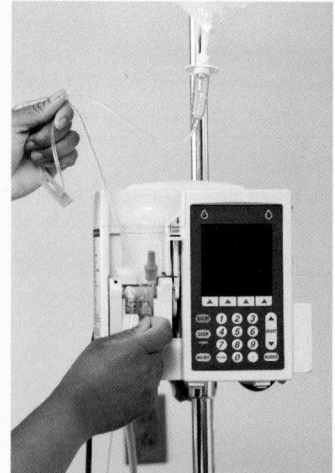

STEP 3b Insert IV tubing into chamber of control mechanism.

STEP	RATIONALE
4. Attach label to IV solution container with date and time container is changed (check agency policy).	Provides reference to determine next time for container change, especially with keep vein open (KVO) rate that contains a specific infusion rate as ordered by health care provider.
5. Teach patient purpose of EID if infusion therapy is delivered by EID, purpose of alarms, to avoid raising hand or arm that affects flow rate, and to avoid touching control clamp.	Information allows patient to protect IV site and informs him or her about rationale for not altering control rate.
6. Dispose of any used supplies. Remove and dispose of gloves and perform hand hygiene.	Reduces risk of contamination (INS, 2016b).
7. Assist patient to a comfortable position and instruct how to move and turn without dislodging VAD.	Prevents accidental dislodgment of catheter and minimizes risk for falls.
8. Raise bed rails (as appropriate) and lower bed to lowest position.	Minimizes risk for falls and injury.
9. Be sure nurse call system is in an accessible location within patient's reach. Instruct patient in its use.	Ensures patient can call for assistance if needed.

EVALUATION

1. Observe patient every 1 to 2 hours (see agency policy), noting volume of IV fluid infused, rate of infusion.	Ensures delivery of prescribed volume over prescribed time and decreases risk for fluid and electrolyte imbalance.
2. Evaluate patient's response to therapy (e.g., laboratory values, input and output [I&O], weights, vital signs, postprocedure assessments).	Provides ongoing evaluation of patient's fluid status, including monitoring for FVE or FVD. Early recognition of complications leads to prompt treatment.
3. Evaluate patient with a short-peripheral IV at least every 4 hours, or every 1 to 2 hours for patients who are critically ill, sedated, or have cognitive deficits (INS, 2016a), or at established intervals per agency policy and procedure. Evaluate IV site for signs and symptoms of IV-related complications.	Prevents complications that compromise integrity of VAD or cause inaccurate IV solution flow rate.
4. **Use Teach-Back:** "I want to be sure that I explained the importance of your IV fluids running on time at the rate ordered. Tell me what you think may cause the pump to alarm and what you would do." Revise your instruction now or develop a plan for revised patient/family caregiver teaching if patient/family caregiver is not able to teach back correctly.	Determines patient's/family caregiver's level of understanding of instructional topic.

UNEXPECTED OUTCOMES AND RELATED INTERVENTIONS

1. Solution does not infuse at prescribed rate.
   a. Sudden infusion of large volume of solution occurs; patient develops dyspnea, crackles in lung, dependent edema (edema in legs), and increased urine output, indicating FVE.
   - Slow infusion rate: KVO rates must have specific rate ordered by health care provider.
   - Notify health care provider immediately.
   - Place patient in high-Fowler's position.
   - Anticipate new IV orders.
   - Anticipate administration of oxygen per order.
   - Administer diuretics if ordered.

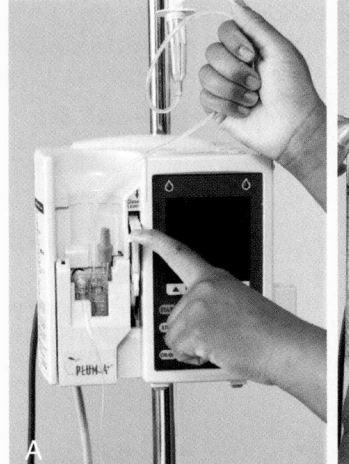 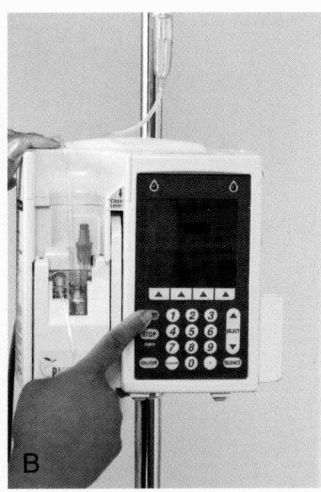

STEP 3c A, Close door of control mechanism. **B,** Select rate and volume to be infused and press start button.

Continued

SKILL 42.2	REGULATING INTRAVENOUS FLOW RATE—cont'd

STEP	RATIONALE

b. IV solution runs slower than ordered.

- Check for positional change that affects rate, height of IV container, kinking of tubing, or obstruction.
- Check VAD site for complications.
- Consult health care provider for new order to provide necessary fluid volume.

2. IV is no longer patent.

- Discontinue present IV infusion and restart new short-peripheral catheter in new site.

RECORDING AND REPORTING

- Record type and rate of infusion in milliliters per hour (drops per minute in gravity flow) in patient's medical record and any ordered change in fluid rates, rate of infusion, and volume left in infusion. Document use of EID.
- Document your evaluation of patient learning.
- Report at end of shift current IV flow rate and status of IV site.
- Report to provider any signs or symptoms of IV rate–related complication (e.g., fluid and electrolyte imbalances).

HOME CARE CONSIDERATIONS

- Ensure that patient or family caregiver is able and willing to operate infusion pump and administer IV therapy. Assess for any visual or physical limitations with ability to connect and disconnect infusion therapy and problem solve infusion pump malfunction (Alexander et al., 2014).
- Home care nurse should be in the home during initiation of infusion therapy to ensure correct pump settings for solution, rate, time, and alarms. The nurse ensures that EID functions properly before use and that patient's electrical outlets are properly grounded.
- Provide a 24-hour access telephone number for patient to call for assistance.

SKILL 42.3	MAINTENANCE OF INTRAVENOUS SYSTEM

Delegation and Collaboration

The skill of changing an IV fluid container and tubing cannot be delegated to assistive personnel (AP). Delegation to licensed practical nurses (LPNs) varies by state Nurse Practice Act. Instruct the AP to:

- Inform the nurse when an IV container is near completion.
- Report any cloudiness or precipitate in the IV solution.
- Report any alarm sounding on electronic infusion device (EID).
- Report any patient complaints of discomfort related to infusion such as pain, burning, bleeding, or swelling.
- Report any leakage from or around the IV tubing.
- Report if tubing has become contaminated (lying on the floor).
- Protect the IV dressing during hygiene and activities of daily living (ADL)

Equipment

- Handheld bar code scanner if using bar code system to charge supplies.

Changing Intravenous Container

- Correct volume and type of solution (with additives if indicated) as ordered by health care provider
- Time tape
- Pen

Changing Infusion Tubing

- Clean gloves
- Antiseptic swabs (alcoholic chlorhexidine solution preferred, 70% alcohol, or povidone-iodine)
- Tubing label
- Sterile 2 × 2–inch gauze pads *(optional)*

Continuous IV Infusion

- Microdrip or macrodrip administration set as appropriate
- Add-on device as necessary (e.g., filters, extension set, needleless connector)

Intermittent Extension Set

- Syringe prefilled with preservative-free 0.9% sodium chloride (normal saline [NS]) (INS, 2016a)
- Short extension tubing (if necessary), injection cap

Discontinuing Peripheral IV Access

- Clean gloves
- Sterile 2 × 2– or 4 × 4–inch gauze pad
- Antiseptic swab (alcoholic chlorhexidine solution preferred) (INS, 2016a)
- Tape

STEP	**RATIONALE**

ASSESSMENT

1. Review accuracy and completeness of health care provider's order in patient's medical record for patient name and correct solution: type, volume, additives, rate, and duration of IV therapy. Follow seven rights of medication administration.

Ensures delivery of correct IV solution and prescribed volume over prescribed time (INS, 2016a).

2. Check medical record for pertinent laboratory data such as potassium level.

Compare data with baseline to determine ongoing response to IV solution administration.

3. Determine compatibility of all IV solutions and additives by consulting approved online database, drug reference, or pharmacist.

Incompatibilities cause physical, chemical, and therapeutic changes with adverse patient outcomes (Alexander et al., 2014).

4. Perform hand hygiene and apply clean gloves.

Reduces risk of contamination and cross-contamination (INS, 2016b).

5. Note labels on tubing for date and time when IV tubing were last changed.

Ensures correct timing of tubing changes. Decreases risk for infection.

6. Check infusion system from solution container down to vascular access device (VAD) insertion site for integrity.

Identifies complications that can compromise integrity of VAD and patient safety.

  a. Assess IV container for discoloration, cloudiness, leakage, and expiration date.

Incompatibility of solutions or medications compromises integrity of VAD and patient safety (Gorski, 2018).

  b. Assess IV tubing for puncture, contamination, or occlusion.

Compromised tubing results in fluid leakage and bacterial contamination.

CLINICAL DECISION: *If the tubing and/or IV bag becomes damaged, is leaking, or becomes contaminated, it must be changed, regardless of the tubing change schedule. If there has been a break in the integrity of the solution container, a new container is needed (Gorski, 2018).*

7. Determine when dressing on VAD was last changed. Ensure label includes date and time applied, size and type of VAD, and insertion date.

Provides information regarding length of time dressing has been in place and allows planning for dressing change (see Skill 42.4).

8. Assess the integrity, patency and functioning of the existing VAD (check agency policy). Assess the VAD catheter-skin junction site and surrounding area for catheter-related complications by visually inspecting and palpating through the intact dressing for redness, tenderness, swelling, and drainage.

Identifies complications that compromise integrity of VAD and necessitate replacement of VAD.

9. Remove and dispose of gloves and perform hand hygiene.

Reduces risk of contamination (INS, 2016b).

10. Assess patient's and family caregiver's knowledge, experience and health literacy regarding protection of IV site, need to change tubing, or reason for discontinuing IV.

Ensures patient and family caregiver have the capacity to obtain, communicate, process, and understand basic health information (CDC, 2019b).

PLANNING

1. Close room door or bedside curtains. Remove clutter from the over-bed or bedside table.

Provides privacy. Prepares the setting for the procedure.

2. Perform hand hygiene. Collect and organize equipment on clean, over-bed or bedside table.

Reduces transmission of microorganisms. Keeps procedure organized and provides patient safety.

  a. Have next solution prepared at least 1 hour before needed. If prepared in pharmacy, ensure that it has been delivered to patient care unit. Check that solution is correct and properly labeled. Allow solution to warm to room temperature if refrigerated. Follow seven rights of medication administration and verify solution expiration date. Observe for precipitate, discoloration, and leakage.

Adequate planning for changing solution reduces risk of clot formation at catheter tip caused by lack of flow from an empty IV container. Checking that a solution is correct prevents medication error (INS, 2016a).

  b. Verify correct administration set for the type of infusion and the electronic infusion device (EID). Coordinate IV tubing changes with solution changes when possible.

Ensures patient safety. Decreasing the number of times the system is open reduces the transmission of infection and contamination of equipment (INS, 2016a).

3. Assist patient to a comfortable position.

Promotes comfort and relaxation.

4. Explain to patient/family member procedure, its purpose, and what is expected of patient.

For discontinuing peripheral IV access: Explain that patient must hold extremity still; that he or she may feel burning sensation when you remove catheter; and that procedure will take about 5 minutes.

Provides patient and family caregiver with information about procedure and promotes adherence (INS, 2016a). May also minimize anxiety.

IMPLEMENTATION

1. Identify patient using at least two identifiers (e.g., name and birthday or name and medical record number) according to agency policy. Compare identifiers with information on patient's MAR or medical record.

Ensures correct patient. Complies with a recommended National Patient Safety Goal (TJC, 2020).

2. **Changing IV fluid container**

Patients receiving intravenous therapy periodically require changes of IV solutions or containers depending on the rate of infusion, volume in the container, and stability of the solution or medication (INS, 2016b). It becomes clinically appropriate to change the type of solution, depending on a patient's fluid and electrolyte balance, response to therapy (e.g., therapeutic drug monitoring), and goals of therapy.

Continued

SKILL 42.3	MAINTENANCE OF INTRAVENOUS SYSTEM—cont'd

STEP	RATIONALE
a. Change solution when fluid remains only in neck of container (about 50 mL) or when new type of solution has been ordered.	A container is changed when there is an order for a new solution or when it becomes time to add a sequential container to avoid exceeding hang time (Alexander et al., 2014). Prevents waste of solution.

CLINICAL DECISION: *The maximum hang time for routine replacement of IV containers is established by agency policy and procedure. Maximum hang time is based upon factors such as the use of strict aseptic technique, whether the system remains closed without injection ports or add-on tubing, stability of the solution or medication being infused, and how long the solution in the IV container will last (Gorski, 2018). It is recommended that each container be changed within 24 hours after the administration set is added (INS, 2016b). Solution and medication containers on ambulatory infusion devices may remain longer than 24 hours if aseptic technique is used, the system remains closed without injection ports or add-on tubing, and the medication is stable for the anticipated infusion time (Gorski, 2018).*

STEP	RATIONALE
b. Perform hand hygiene.	Reduces transmission of microorganisms.
c. Prepare new solution for changing. If using plastic bag, hang on IV pole and remove protective cover from IV tubing port. If using glass bottle, remove metal cap and metal and rubber disks.	Solution and medication containers include plastic bags, plastic bottles, and glass bottles. Permits quick, smooth, organized change from old to new container.
d. Close roller clamp on existing solution to stop flow rate. Remove IV tubing from EID (if used). Then remove old IV solution container from IV pole. Hold container with tubing port pointing upward.	Prevents solution remaining in drip chamber from emptying while changing solutions. Prevents solution in bag from spilling.
e. Quickly remove spike from old solution container and, without touching tip, insert spike into new container (see illustrations).	Reduces risk for solution in drip chamber becoming empty and maintains sterility.

CLINICAL DECISION: *If spike becomes contaminated by touching an unsterile object, you will need a new IV tubing set.*

STEP	RATIONALE
f. Hang new container of solution on IV pole.	Gravity helps with delivery of fluid into drip chamber.
g. Check for air in IV tubing. If air bubbles have formed, remove them by closing roller clamp, stretching tubing downward, and tapping tubing with finger (bubbles rise in fluid to drip chamber) (see Skill 42-1, Step 3h).	Reduces risk of air entering tubing. Use of an air-eliminating filter also reduces risk.
h. Make sure that drip chamber is one-third to one-half full. If drip chamber is too full, level can be decreased by removing bag from IV pole, pinching off IV tubing below drip chamber, inverting container, squeezing drip chamber (see illustration), releasing and turning solution container upright, and releasing pinch on tubing.	Reduces risk for air entering IV tubing. If chamber is filled, you cannot observe or regulate drip rate.
i. Regulate flow to ordered rate by opening and adjusting roller clamp on IV tubing or by opening roller clamp and programming and turning on EID.	Maintains measures to restore fluid balance and deliver IV solution as ordered.
j. Place time label on side of container and label with time hung, time of completion, and appropriate intervals. If using plastic bags, mark only on label and not container.	Provides visual comparison of volume infused compared with prescribed rate of infusion.
k. Instruct patient on purpose of new IV solution, additives, flow rate, potential side effects, how to avoid occluding tubing, and what to report.	Information informs patient about purpose for continued IV therapy and what to report and protects VAD patency.

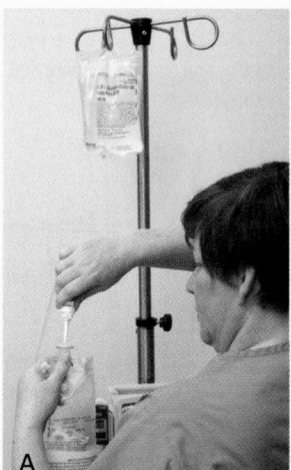 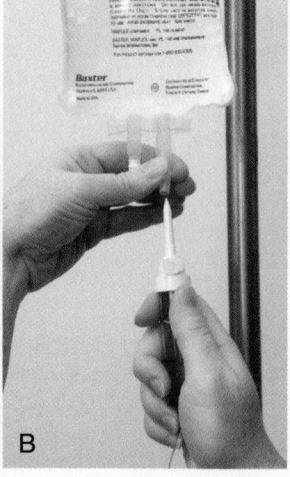

STEP 2e A, Remove spike from old solution container. **B,** Without touching tip, insert spike into new container.

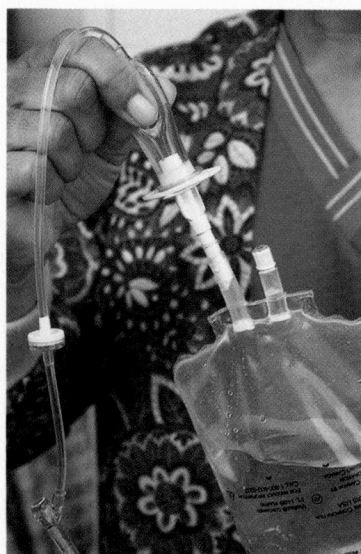

STEP 2h Squeeze drip chamber to fill with fluid. Be sure to leave chamber one-third to one-half full.

STEP	RATIONALE

3. Changing infusion tubing

CLINICAL DECISION: *Administration sets are the primary method to carry a solution or medication to a patient. These administration sets are considered the primary set. In addition, patients may have add-on devices (e.g., filters, extension sets), which you connect to the primary set as indicated by the prescribed therapy. Secondary sets may be used as a method to administer additional medications in conjunction with the primary infusion (e.g., antibiotics). Follow agency policy and procedures for specific requirements.*

a. Perform hand hygiene. Open new infusion set and connect add-on pieces (e.g., filters, extension tubing) using aseptic technique. Keep protective coverings over infusion spike and distal adapter. Place roller clamp about 2–2.5 cm (1–2 inches) below drip chamber and move roller clamp to "off" position. Secure all connections.

Close proximity of roller clamp to drip chamber allows more accurate regulation of flow rate. Securing connections reduces risk later of air emboli and infection. Protective covers reduce entrance of microorganisms. All connections should be of Luer-Lok type (INS, 2016a).

b. Apply clean gloves. If patient's IV cannula hub is not visible, remove IV dressing as described in Skill 42.4. **Do not** remove tape securing cannula to skin.

Cannula hub must be visible to provide smooth transition when removing old and inserting new tubing.

c. To prepare IV tubing with new IV infusion bag (see Skill 42.1, Step 3). Use sterile technique.

d. Prepare IV tubing with existing continuous IV infusion bag.
  (1) Move roller clamp on new IV tubing to "off" position.
  (2) Slow rate of infusion through old tubing to keep vein open (KVO) rate using EID or roller clamp.
  (3) Compress and fill drip chamber of old tubing.
  (4) Invert container and remove old tubing. Keep spike sterile and upright.
  (5) Insert spike of new infusion tubing into solution container. Hang solution bag on IV pole, compress drip chamber on new tubing, and release, allowing it to fill one-third to one-half full.
  (6) Prime air out of IV tubing by filling with IV solution: Remove protective cover on end of tubing and slowly open roller clamp to allow solution to flow from drip chamber to distal end of IV tubing. If tubing has Y connector, invert Y connector when solution reaches it to displace air. Return roller clamp to "off" position after priming tubing (filled with IV solution). Replace protective cover on end of IV tubing. Place end of adapter near patient's IV site.
  (7) Stop EID or turn roller clamp on old tubing to "off" position.

e. Prepare tubing with extension set or saline lock.

Prevents fluid spillage.
Prevents occlusion of VAD.

Ensures that drip chamber remains full until new tubing is changed.
Solution in drip chamber will continue to run and maintain catheter patency.
Permits drip chamber to fill and promotes rapid, smooth flow of solution through tubing.

Priming ensures that IV tubing is clear of air before connection with VAD and filled with IV solution. Slow fill of tubing decreases turbulence and chance of bubble formation. Closing clamp prevents accidental loss of fluid.
Maintains sterility. Equipment is positioned for quick connection of new tubing.

Prevents fluid spillage. Prepares EID for insertion of new tubing.
Placement of a short extension tubing or loop between a catheter hub and injection cap allows manipulation of the injection cap without moving the catheter.

CLINICAL DECISION: *The extension tubing remains attached to the short-peripheral catheter and is changed when the catheter is changed.*

  (1) If short extension tubing is needed, use sterile technique to connect new injection cap to new extension set or IV tubing.
  (2) Scrub injection cap with antiseptic swab for at least 15 seconds and allow to dry completely. Attach syringe with 3 to 5 mL of NS flush solution and inject through injection cap into extension set.

f. Reestablish infusion.
  (1) Gently disconnect old tubing from extension tubing (or from IV catheter hub) and quickly insert Luer-Lok end of new tubing or saline lock into extension tubing connection (or IV catheter hub) (see illustrations for example of connecting tubing to short extension set).

Prepares extension set for connecting with IV.

Ensures effective disinfection (INS, 2016a). Maintains patency of catheter.

Allows smooth transition from old to new tubing, minimizing time that system is open.

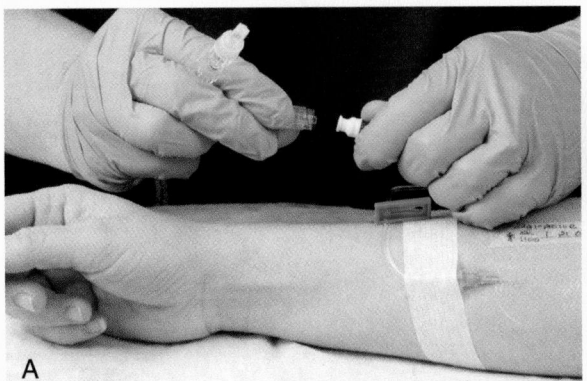
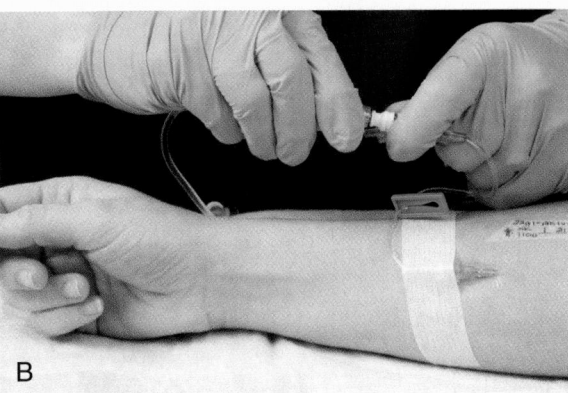

STEP 3f(1) A, Disconnect old tubing. **B,** Insert adapter of new tubing.

Continued

SKILL 41.3 **MAINTENANCE OF INTRAVENOUS SYSTEM—cont'd**

STEP	RATIONALE
(2) For continuous infusion, open roller clamp on new tubing and regulate drip rate using roller clamp, or insert tubing into EID, program to desired rate, and push the power button on.	Ensures catheter patency and prevents occlusion.
(3) Attach piece of tape or preprinted label with date and time of IV tubing change onto tubing below drip chamber.	Provides reference to determine next time for tubing change.
(4) Form loop of tubing and secure it to patient's arm with strip of tape.	Avoids accidental pulling against site and stabilizes catheter.
(5) If necessary, apply new dressing (Skill 42.4).	Maintains integrity of VAD site.

CLINICAL DECISION: *You may need to assist patients with many aspects of hygiene (e.g., gown changes, bathing) while patients are receiving IV therapy. Never disconnect infusion tubing to change a gown or any article of clothing. Coordinate care so that bathing or hygiene activities are done after discontinuing an IV site and before another venipuncture is performed. If infusion cannot be discontinued, use special "IV gowns" if available.*

---

4. Discontinuing peripheral IV access

STEP	RATIONALE
a. Perform hand hygiene. Apply clean gloves.	Reduces transmission of microorganisms.
b. Observe existing IV site for signs and symptoms of IV-related complications (redness, pain, tenderness, swelling, bleeding, drainage, or leaking from under dressing). Palpate catheter site through intact dressing.	Identifies the need for postprocedure interventions, such as warm compress to site.
c. Assess whether patient is receiving an anticoagulant or has a history of a coagulopathy.	Requires an increase in the time needed to apply pressure to puncture site following catheter removal.
d. Turn off EID and close roller clamp or, if no EID, close roller clamp that controls rate.	Prevents spillage of IV fluid.
e. Remove IV site dressing and catheter engineered stabilization device (see Skill 42.4). Do not use scissors. Avoid tearing patient's skin.	Exposes catheter with minimal discomfort. Scissors might accidentally damage catheter or injure patient (INS, 2016a).
f. Stabilize IV catheter hub and clean site with antiseptic swab. Allow to dry completely.	Removes secretions around skin puncture site.
g. Place clean sterile gauze above insertion site and, using dominant hand, withdraw catheter using a slow, steady motion, keeping the hub parallel to the skin (see illustration). Do not raise or lift catheter before it is completely out of vein. Inspect end of catheter, being sure it is intact after removal.	Dry pad causes less irritation to puncture site. Removal technique avoids trauma to vein or hematoma formation. Inspection determines whether catheter tip is intact. Tip of catheter can break off and embolize, which is an emergency situation.
h. Keep gauze in place and apply continuous pressure to site for 30 seconds or until bleeding has stopped.	Controls bleeding and hematoma formation. Pressure should be applied until hemostasis occurs (INS, 2016a).

CLINICAL DECISION: *If patient receives anticoagulants or platelet inhibitors (e.g., low-dose aspirin, warfarin sodium [Coumadin], heparin) or has a low platelet count, apply steady pressure longer (for 5 to 10 minutes) and assess bleeding.*

STEP	RATIONALE
i. Apply sterile folded gauze dressing over insertion site and secure with tape.	Maintains pressure to prevent bleeding and reduces bacterial entry into puncture site.
5. Dispose of any used supplies. Remove and dispose of gloves and perform hand hygiene.	Reduces transmission of microorganisms (INS, 2016a).
6. Assist patient to a comfortable position and instruct how to move and turn properly with VAD.	Prevents accidental dislodgment of IV catheter.
7. Raise bed rails (as appropriate) and lower bed to lowest position.	Minimizes risk for falls and injury.
8. Be sure nurse call system is in an accessible location within patient's reach. Instruct patient in its use.	Ensures patient can call for assistance if needed.

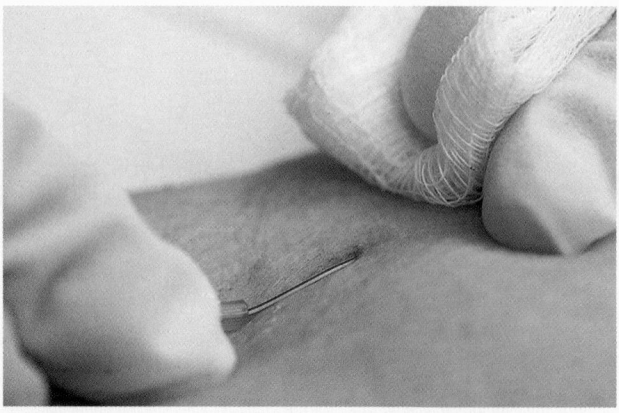

STEP 4g Remove IV catheter slowly, keeping catheter parallel to vein.

STEP	RATIONALE

EVALUATION

1. Observe patient with a short-peripheral IV at least every 4 hours, or every 1 to 2 hours for patients who are critically ill, sedated, or have cognitive deficits (INS, 2016a), or at established intervals per agency policy and procedure for:
   Ensures delivery of infusion therapy as ordered.

   a. Correct type and amount of solution infused
   Ensures delivery of prescribed volume over prescribed time and decreases risk for fluid and electrolyte imbalance.

   b. Leaking at connection sites
   Minimizes risk of infection caused by breach in system integrity.

   c. Function, intactness, and patency of IV system
   Validates that IV line is patent and functioning correctly. Manipulation of catheter and tubing may affect rate of infusion.

   d. IV-related complications by visually inspecting and gently palpating skin around and above IV site through the intact dressing
   Identifies complications that compromise integrity of VAD or cause inaccurate IV solution flow rate.

2. Evaluate patient to determine response to therapy (e.g., laboratory values, input and output [I&O], weights, vital signs, postprocedure assessments).
   Provides ongoing evaluation of patient's fluid status.

3. Monitor patient for signs of ECV excess, ECV deficit, or signs and symptoms of electrolyte imbalances.
   Early recognition of complications leads to prompt treatment.

4. **Use Teach-Back:** "We talked about the importance of your IV solutions running as prescribed. I want to be sure I explained this clearly. Tell me in your own words what you should do if you notice that the IV is not dripping or you notice leaking." Revise your instruction now or develop a plan for revised patient/family caregiver teaching if patient/family caregiver is not able to teach back correctly.
   Determines patient's/family caregiver's level of understanding of instructional topic.

5. *For discontinuing short-peripheral IV access:*

   a. Observe site for bleeding soon after procedure and redness, tenderness, drainage, or swelling during a later evaluation.
   Detects bleeding after catheter removal.
   Detects local infection or postinfusion phlebitis (INS, 2016a).

   b. **Use Teach-Back**: "I want to be sure I explained why I removed the IV. Please tell me why you no longer need an IV." Revise your instruction now or develop a plan for revised patient/family caregiver teaching if patient/family caregiver is not able to teach back correctly.
   Determines patient's/family caregiver's level of understanding of instructional topic.

UNEXPECTED OUTCOMES AND RELATED INTERVENTIONS

1. Flow rate is incorrect; patient receives too little or too much solution.
   - Notify health care provider if patient's anticipated infusion is 100 to 200 mL less than or greater than anticipated (per agency policy and procedure).
   - Evaluate patient for signs and symptoms of adverse effects of infusion (e.g., ECV excess or deficit).
   - Consult health care provider for new order to provide necessary fluid volume.
   - Check for positional IV site and reposition catheter; apply new dressing if necessary.
   - Check IV catheter for loss of patency or dislodgment; catheter may require replacement.
   - Check VAD site for complications.
2. Leaking occurs at IV connection.
   - Determine site of leaking and secure connection.
   - Apply new dressing if necessary (see Skill 42.4).

Continued

MAINTENANCE OF INTRAVENOUS SYSTEM—cont'd

3. IV catheter is removed or dislodged accidentally.
   - Restart new short-peripheral IV line in other extremity or above previous insertion site if continued therapy is necessary (see Skill 42.1).
4. Catheter tip is missing after withdrawal.
   - Apply tourniquet high on extremity to restrict mobility of catheter embolus.
   - Immediately notify health care provider.

RECORDING AND REPORTING

- Record solution and tubing changes, type of infusion solution including any additives, volume of container, and rate of infusion. Record time of discontinuing solution or IV medication.
- Record time that peripheral IV access was discontinued, site assessment information, and status of catheter, including gauge, length, and catheter tip integrity.
- Document your evaluation of patient learning.
- Report details of tubing and or equipment change or discontinuing of IV. Report any complications, treatments; report any changes in IV catheter, tubing, and IV fluid type and rate.

HOME CARE CONSIDERATIONS

- Ensure that patient is able and willing to self-manage IV therapy (including changing IV containers) or that reliable family caregiver is at home to provide IV care.
- Instruct patient or family caregiver in procedure for performing an IV solution and tubing change. Consider their cultural norms (e.g., health beliefs and comfort with caregivers using touch).
- Instruct patient or caregiver to notify health care provider if bleeding or drainage is noted at insertion site or if pain or tenderness occurs up to 4 days after catheter removal.

CHANGING A SHORT-PERIPHERAL INTRAVENOUS DRESSING

Delegation and Collaboration

The skill of changing a short-peripheral intravenous (IV) dressing cannot be delegated to assistive personnel (AP). Delegation to licensed practical nurses (LPNs) varies by state Nurse Practice Act. Instruct the AP to:

- Report to the nurse if a patient indicates moistness or loosening of an IV dressing.
- Protect the IV dressing during hygiene and activities of daily living (ADLs).

Equipment

- Antiseptic swabs (alcoholic chlorhexidine solution preferred [INS, 2016a], 70% alcohol, or povidone-iodine)
- Adhesive remover *(optional)*
- Polymer-based skin protectant swab *(optional)*
- Clean gloves
- Engineered catheter stabilization device if available or precut strips of sterile nonallergic tape
- Commercially available IV site protector device (see Step 8, *optional*)
- Sterile transparent semipermeable membrane (TSM) dressing or sterile 2 × 2–inch gauze pads and tape

STEP	RATIONALE

ASSESSMENT

1. Identify patient using at least two identifiers (e.g., name and birthday or name and medical record number) according to agency policy. Compare identifiers with information on patient's MAR or medical record.

Ensures correct patient. Complies with a recommended National Patient Safety Goal (TJC, 2020).

2. Determine agency policy regarding peripheral IV dressing changes. Transparent (TSM) dressings usually remain in place until IV site is changed unless dressing becomes wet, visibly soiled, or loose, and at least every 5-7 days. Gauze dressings may be changed every 2 days.

Dressing change increases risk of catheter displacement and is performed only if dressing is compromised or every 5-7 days for transparent dressings or every 2 days for gauze dressings (INS, 2016a).

3. Perform hand hygiene. Observe present dressing for moisture and intactness. Determine whether moisture is from site leakage or external source.

Moisture is a medium for bacterial growth and contaminates dressing. Loose dressing increases risk for bacterial contamination of venipuncture site or displacement of vascular access device (VAD).

STEP	RATIONALE
4. Observe IV system for proper functioning or complications (see Skill 42.3). Apply clean gloves if dressing is moist. Palpate VAD site through intact dressing, assessing for pain or burning.	Unexplained decrease in flow rate requires investigating VAD placement and patency. Pain is associated with both phlebitis and infiltration.
5. Assess patient's and family caregiver's knowledge, experience and health literacy regarding the needed for continued IV therapy.	Ensures patient and family caregiver has the capacity to obtain, communicate, process, and understand basic health information (CDC, 2019b).

PLANNING

1. Close room curtains or door. Prepare environment by removing clutter from bedside and overbed table.	Provides privacy. Prepares environment for efficient procedure.
2. Perform hand hygiene. Collect and organize equipment on clean over-bed or bedside table.	Reduces transmission of microorganisms. Keeps procedure organized and provides patient safety.
3. Explain procedure and purpose to patient and family. Explain that patient must hold affected extremity still and how long procedure will take.	Decreases anxiety, promotes cooperation, and gives patient time frame around which to plan personal activities.

IMPLEMENTATION

1. Perform hand hygiene and apply clean gloves.	Reduces transmission of microorganisms.
2. Remove existing dressing.	
a. For TSM dressing: Stabilize catheter with nondominant hand (see illustration). Use alcohol swab on edges of TSM dressing next to patient's skin. Remove dressing by pulling up one corner and gently pulling straight out and parallel to skin. Repeat on all sides until dressing has been removed.	Prevents accidental displacement of VAD. Technique minimizes discomfort during removal. Use of alcohol swab loosens dressing.
b. For gauze dressing: Stabilize catheter hub while loosening tape and removing old dressing one layer at a time by pulling toward insertion site. Be cautious if tubing becomes tangled between two layers of dressing.	
3. Assess VAD insertion site for signs and symptoms of IV-related complications (Tables 42.12 to 42.14). If complication exists, determine whether VAD requires removal. Remove catheter if ordered by health care provider (see Skill 42.3).	Presence of complication may require VAD removal.
4. If catheter is to remain in place, assess integrity of engineered stabilization device. Continue to stabilize catheter and remove as recommended by manufacturer directions for use. Inspect for adhesive residue or signs of adhesive-related skin injury from adhesive-based engineered stabilization devices.	Removing stabilization device allows for appropriate skin antisepsis before applying dressing and new stabilization device (INS, 2016a).
NOTE: Some stabilization devices are designed to remain in place for length of time VAD is in as long as adequate stabilization is evident.	

CLINICAL DECISION: *Keep one finger stabilizing VAD at all times until dressing secures catheter hub. This requires careful planning regarding placing and opening supplies and how to work with one hand. If patient is restless or uncooperative, it is helpful to have another staff member help with procedure.*

5. While stabilizing IV line, use adhesive remover to remove adhesive residue if needed. Then perform skin antisepsis to insertion site with antiseptic wipe using friction in back-and-forth motion for 30 seconds; allow to dry completely. If using alcohol or povidone-iodine, clean in concentric circle, moving from insertion site outward with the swab (see illustration). Allow antiseptic solution to dry completely.	Adhesive residue decreases ability of new tape to adhere securely to skin. Skin antisepsis reduces incidence of catheter-related infections (Alexander, et al., 2014). Allow any skin antiseptic agent to fully dry for complete antisepsis (INS, 2016a).
6. *Option:* Apply skin protectant to area where you will apply tape, dressing, or engineered stabilization device. Allow to dry.	Coats skin with protective solution to maintain skin integrity, prevents irritation from adhesive, and promotes adherence of dressing.
7. While stabilizing VAD, apply new sterile dressing over site (procedures differ; follow agency policy).	Prevents accidental dislodgment of catheter and protects site from infection (INS, 2016a).

CLINICAL DECISION: *Because adhesive Band-Aids are not occlusive and nonsterile tape increases the risk for insertion site infection, do not use either over catheter insertion points.*

a. *TSM dressing:* Apply as directed in Skill 42.1, Step 19a.	Occlusive dressing protects site from bacterial contamination (INS, 2016a).
b. *Gauze dressing:* Apply as directed in Skill 42.1, Step 19b.	Less frequently used than transparent dressing.

Continued

STEP	RATIONALE
8. *Option:* Apply polymer-based site protection device (e.g., I.V. House UltraDressing®) or other protective device over area if patient may pick at or bump dressing (see illustration).	Site-protection devices include vented plastic or stretch netting coverings and mitts for hands. Designed to reduce risk of phlebitis, infiltration, or catheter displacement from mechanical motion.
9. Anchor extension tubing or IV tubing alongside dressing on arm, and secure with tape directly over tubing. When using TSM dressing, avoid placing tape over dressing.	Prevents accidental dislodgment of VAD or tubing. More frequent dressing changes due to dislodgment are associated with greater risk of infection (INS, 2016a).
10. Label dressing per agency policy. Label information should include date and time of original IV insertion, VAD gauge and length, and your initials.	Communicates type of device and time interval for dressing change.
11. Dispose of any used supplies. Remove and dispose of gloves and perform hand hygiene.	Reduces transmission of microorganisms (INS, 2016a).
12. Assist patient to a comfortable position and instruct how to move and turn properly with VAD.	Prevents accidental dislodgment of IV catheter.
13. Raise bed rails (as appropriate) and lower bed to lowest position.	Minimizes risk for falls and injury.
14. Be sure nurse call system is in an accessible location within patient's reach. Instruct patient in its use.	Ensures patient can call for assistance if needed.

EVALUATION

1. Observe new dressing to be sure that it is applied, taped, and labeled properly.

   Validates quality of completed dressing change.

2. Ensure that flow rate is accurate.

   Validates that IV line is patent and functioning correctly. Manipulation of catheter and tubing may affect rate of infusion.

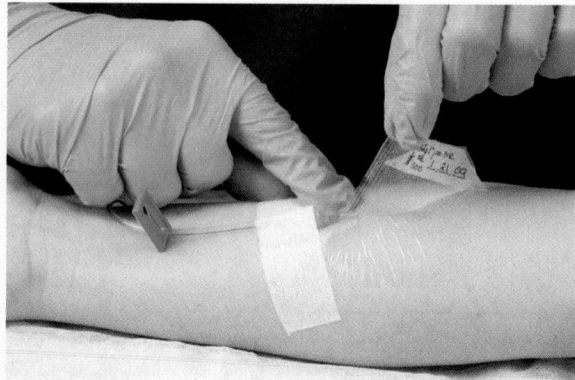

STEP 2a Remove transparent semipermeable membrane (TSM) dressing by pulling side laterally.

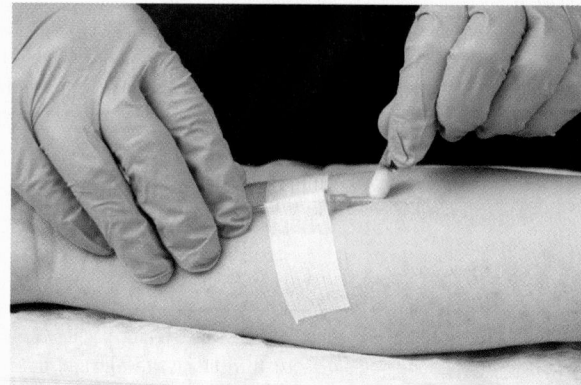

STEP 5 Cleanse peripheral insertion site with antiseptic swab.

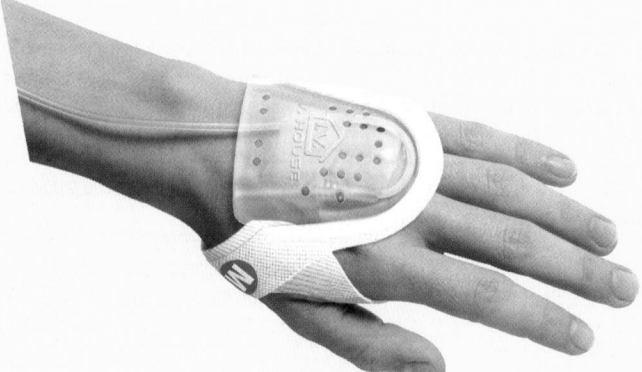

STEP 8 I.V. House protective device. (Courtesy I.V. House, St. Louis, MO)

STEP	RATIONALE
3. **Use Teach-Back**: "I want to be sure I explained why I changed your IV dressing. Tell me why I needed to change your dressing." Revise your instruction now or develop a plan for revised patient/family caregiver teaching if patient/family caregiver is not able to teach back correctly.	Determines patient's/family caregiver's level of understanding of instructional topic.

UNEXPECTED OUTCOMES AND RELATED INTERVENTIONS

1. VAD is accidentally dislodged or removed.
   - Start new IV line in other extremity or proximal to previous insertion site if continued therapy is necessary.
2. IV site develops infiltration, phlebitis, and local infection.
   - See Table 42.12.

RECORDING AND REPORTING

- Record time that peripheral dressing was changed, reason for change, type of dressing material used, patency of system and IV infusion rate, and description of venipuncture site.
- Document any complication of VAD.
- Document your evaluation of patient learning.
- Report to charge nurse or oncoming nursing shift that dressing was changed and any significant information about integrity of system.
- Report any complications to health care provider.

KEY POINTS

- Body fluids containing water, Na^+, and other electrolytes are distributed between ECF and ICF compartments.
- The interplay of fluid intake (thirst, habit, social aspects, nonoral routes), fluid distribution (filtration and osmosis), and fluid output (skin, lungs, GI tract, kidneys) determines the location, volume, and osmolality of body fluid.
- Fluid moves between blood vessels and interstitial fluid by filtration; water moves between ECF and ICF by osmosis.
- The relationship of electrolyte intake and absorption; electrolyte distribution between plasma, cells, and bones; and electrolyte output determines the plasma concentrations of potassium, calcium, magnesium, and phosphate ions.
- Acid production is a product of cellular metabolism. Acid-base imbalances are excesses or deficits of carbonic or metabolic acids.
- ECV deficit and excess are abnormal *volumes* of isotonic fluid in the vascular and interstitial compartments.
- Plasma electrolyte imbalances (e.g., potassium, sodium, calcium, and magnesium) affect body electrolyte content and/or abnormal distribution of electrolytes.
- Risk factors for fluid, electrolyte, and acid-base imbalances include factors that alter the regulatory mechanisms, such as age (very young or very old), environmental factors, increases in gastrointestinal output, chronic diseases, trauma, and therapies such as medications or IV infusions.
- Clinical assessments for ECV imbalances include sudden changes in body weight and markers of vascular and interstitial volume.
- The osmolality imbalances hyponatremia and hypernatremia manifest as decreased level of consciousness and abnormal serum Na^+ levels.
- Potassium imbalances manifest as bilateral muscle weakness, cardiac dysrhythmias, and abnormal serum K^+ levels.
- Calcium and magnesium imbalances manifest as altered neuromuscular excitability and abnormal serum Ca^{++} or Mg^{++} levels.
- Acid-base imbalances manifest as changes in level of consciousness, abnormal breathing patterns, and abnormalities of $PaCO_2$, HCO_3^-, and pH.
- During initiation and maintenance of intravenous therapy, nurses maintain sterility and patency of the system by following safety guidelines and making clinical decisions regarding assessment, organized planning with appropriate equipment, skillful implementation of procedural steps, evaluation of outcomes, and careful recording and reporting.
- Nurses monitor vigilantly and take immediate appropriate action for complications of intravenous therapy, which include circulatory overload of the IV solution, infiltration and extravasation, phlebitis, local infection, air embolism, and bleeding at the insertion site.
- Blood and blood products must be matched to each patient to avoid incompatibility. Administration involves patient safety steps and use of special equipment, careful monitoring, and rapid knowledgeable action in case of transfusion reaction or other acute adverse events.
- Evaluation of interventions for specific fluid, electrolyte, and acid-base imbalances requires comparison of current clinical signs and symptoms and laboratory status with previous findings, discussion of patient concerns and expectations, and evaluation of patient learning about prevention and treatment of their fluid, electrolyte, or acid-base imbalances.

REFLECTIVE LEARNING

- Consider a patient experience and describe concepts of fluid, electrolyte, and acid-base homeostasis and imbalances that you applied.
- Think about a recent patient and describe that person's risk factors for fluid, electrolyte, and acid-base imbalances.
- Given your clinical setting, what environmental, organizational, or other factors did you see that influence patient intake or output of fluid and electrolytes?

REVIEW QUESTIONS

1. An intravenous (IV) fluid is infusing slower than ordered. The infusion pump is set correctly. Which factors could cause this slowing? (Select all that apply.)
   1. Infiltration at vascular access device (VAD) site
   2. Patient lying on tubing
   3. Roller clamp wide open
   4. Tubing kinked in bedrails
   5. Circulatory overload

2. The nurse assesses pain and redness at a vascular access device (VAD) site. Which action is taken first?
   1. Apply a warm, moist compress.
   2. Aspirate the infusing fluid from the VAD.
   3. Report the situation to the health care provider.
   4. Discontinue the intravenous infusion.

3. When delegating input and output (I&O) measurement to assistive personnel, the nurse instructs them to record what information for ice chips?
   1. Two-thirds of the volume
   2. One-half of the volume
   3. One-quarter of the volume
   4. Two times the volume

4. What assessments does a nurse make before hanging an intravenous (IV) fluid that contains potassium? (Select all that apply.)
   1. Urine output
   2. Arterial blood gases
   3. Fullness of neck veins
   4. Serum potassium laboratory value in EHR
   5. Level of consciousness

5. The health care provider's order is 500 mL 0.9% NaCl intravenously over 4 hours. Which rate does the nurse program into the infusion pump?
   1. 100 mL/hr
   2. 125 mL/hr
   3. 167 mL/hr
   4. 200 mL/hr

6. An older-adult patient is receiving intravenous (IV) 0.9% NaCl. The nurse detects new onset of crackles in the lung bases. What is the priority action?
   1. Notify a health care provider.
   2. Decrease the IV flow rate.
   3. Lower the head of the bed.
   4. Discontinue the IV site.

7. Place the following steps for discontinuing intravenous (IV) access in the correct order:
   1. Perform hand hygiene and apply gloves.
   2. Explain procedure to patient.
   3. Remove IV site dressing and tape.
   4. Use two identifiers to ensure correct patient.
   5. Stop the infusion and clamp the tubing.
   6. Carefully check the health care provider's order.
   7. Clean the site, withdraw the catheter, and apply pressure.

8. A patient has hypokalemia with stable cardiac function. What are the priority nursing interventions? (Select all that apply.)
   1. Fall prevention interventions
   2. Teaching regarding sodium restriction
   3. Encouraging increased fluid intake
   4. Monitoring for constipation
   5. Explaining how to take daily weights

9. A patient is admitted to the hospital with severe dyspnea and wheezing. Arterial blood gas levels on admission are pH 7.26; $PaCO_2$, 55 mm Hg; PaO_2, 68 mm Hg; and HCO_3^-, 24. How does the nurse interpret these laboratory values?
   1. Metabolic acidosis
   2. Metabolic alkalosis
   3. Respiratory acidosis
   4. Respiratory alkalosis

10. Which assessment does the nurse use as a clinical marker of vascular volume in a patient at high risk of extracellular fluid volume (ECV) deficit?
    1. Dryness of mucous membranes
    2. Skin turgor
    3. Fullness of neck veins when supine
    4. Fullness of neck veins when upright

Answers: 1. 1, 2, 4; **2.** 4; **3.** 2; **4.** 1, 4, 5; **5.** 2; **6.** 2; **7.** 6, 4, 2, 1, 5, 3, 7; **8.** 1, 4; **9.** 3; **10.** 3.

Rationales for Review Questions can be found on the Evolve website.

REFERENCES

Alexander M, et al.: *Core curriculum for infusion nursing*, ed 4, Philadelphia, 2014, Lippincott, Williams & Wilkins.

American Association of Blood Banks (AABB): *Technical manual*, ed 19, Bethesda, MD, 2017, AABB.

American Association of Blood Banks (AABB): *Standards for blood banks and transfusion services*, ed 31, Bethesda, 2018, MD, AABB.

Boucher, et al.: Supporting Muslim patients during advanced illness, *Perm J* 21:16, 2017.

Burchum JR, Rosenthal LD: *Lehne's pharmacology for nursing care*, ed 10, St Louis, 2019, Elsevier.

Centers for Disease Control and Prevention (CDC): *Blood safety basics*, 2019a. https://www.cdc.gov/bloodsafety/basics.html. Accessed March 3, 2019.

Centers for Disease Control and Prevention (CDC): *What is health literacy*, 2019b. https://www.cdc.gov/healthliteracy/learn/index.html. Accessed December 23, 2019.

Centers for Disease Control and Prevention: *Updated recommendations on the use of chlorhexidine-impregnated dressings for prevention of intravascular catheter-related infections*, 2017. https://www.cdc.gov/infectioncontrol/guidelines/bsi/updates.html. Accessed March 3, 2019.

DeLisle J: Is this a blood transfusion reaction? Don't hesitate; check it out, *J Infus Nurs* 41(1):42, 2018.

Felver L: Acid-base balance. In Giddens JF, editor: *Concepts for nursing practice*, ed 3, St Louis, 2019a, Mosby.

Felver L: Acid-base homeostasis and imbalances. In Banasik JL, Copstead LC, editors: *Pathophysiology*, ed 6, St Louis, 2019b, Saunders.

Felver L: Fluid and electrolyte balance. In Giddens JF, editor: *Concepts for nursing practice*, ed 3, St Louis, 2019c, Mosby.

Felver L: Fluid and electrolyte homeostasis and imbalances. In Banasik JL, Copstead LC, editors: *Pathophysiology*, ed 6, St Louis, 2019d, Saunders.

Ferrari MC, et al.: Watery stools and metabolic acidosis, *Intern Emerg Med* 12(4):487, 2017.

Giger JN: *Transcultural nursing: assessment and intervention*, ed 7, St Louis, 2017, Mosby.

Gizowski C, Bourgue CW: The neural basis of homeostatic and anticipatory thirst, *Nat Rev Nephrol* 14(1):11, 2018.

Gorski L: *Manual of IV therapeutics: evidence-based practice for infusion therapy*, ed 7, Philadelphia, 2018, FA Davis.

Hadaway L: Stopcocks for infusion therapy: evidence and experience, *J Infus Nurs* 41(1):24, 2018.

Hall JE: *Guyton and Hall textbook of medical physiology*, ed 13, Philadelphia, 2016, Saunders.

Heckle M, et al.: ST elevations in the setting of hyperkalemia, *JAMA Internal Med* 178:133, 2018.

Hockenberry MJ, et al.: *Wong's nursing care of infants and children*, ed 11, St Louis, 2019, Mosby.

Hoorn EJ, et al.: Diagnosis and treatment of hyponatremia: compilation of the guidelines, *J Am Soc Nephrol* 28(5):1340, 2017.

Infusion Nurses Society (INS): Infusion therapy standards of practice, *J Infus Nurs* 39(1 Suppl.):S1, 2016a.

Infusion Nurses Society (INS): *Policy and procedures for infusion therapy*, ed 5, Norwood, MA, 2016b, Author.

Kala J, Abudayyeh A: Magnesium: an overlooked electrolyte, *J Emerg Med* 52(5):741, 2017.

Kamel K, Halperin M: *Fluid, electrolyte, and acid–base physiology*, ed 5, St. Louis, 2017, Elsevier.

Kear TM: Fluid and electrolyte management across the age continuum, *Nephrol Nurs J* 44(6):491, 2017.

Kovesdy CP, et al.: Potassium homeostasis in health and disease: a scientific workshop cosponsored by the national kidney foundation and the American Society of Hypertension, *Am J Kidney Dis* 70:844, 2017.

Lewis SL, et al.: *Medical-surgical nursing: assessment and management of clinical problems*, ed 10, St Louis, 2017, Mosby.

Lim F, et al.: Managing hypocalcemia in massive blood transfusion, *Nursing* 47(5):26, 2017.

Mattox EA: Complications of peripheral venous access devices: prevention, detection, and recovery strategies, *Crit Care Nurs* 37(2):e1, 2017.

McDermott BP, et al.: National athletic trainers' association position statement: fluid replacement for the physically active, *J Athl Train* 52(9):877, 2017.

Nagami GT, Hamm LL: Regulation of acid-base balance in chronic kidney disease, *Adv Chronic Kidney Dis* 24(5):274, 2017.

Norton JM, et al.: Improving outcomes for patients with chronic kidney disease: part 1, *Am J Nurs* 117(2):22, 2017.

Occupational Safety and Health Administration (OSHA): *Bloodborne pathogens standard*, US Department of Labor, last amended April 3 2012, https://www.osha.gov/laws-regs/regulations/standardnumber/1910/1910.1030. Accessed March 3, 2019.

Pagana KD, et al.: *Mosby's manual of diagnostic and laboratory tests*, ed 6, St Louis, 2018, Mosby.

Palmer BF, Clegg DJ: Electrolyte disturbances in patients with chronic alcohol-use disorder, *N Engl J Med* 377(14):1368, 2017.

Rong X, et al.: Cultural factors influencing dietary and fluid restriction behaviour: perceptions of older Chinese patients with heart failure, *J Clin Nurs* 26(5/6):717, 2017.

The Joint Commission (TJC): 2020 National Patient Safety Goals, Oakbrook Terrace, IL, 2019, The Commission. https://www.jointcommission.org/en/standards/national-patient-safety-goals/.

The Joint Commission (TJC): *Changes for National Patient Safety Goal 7 on Health Care Associated infections*, 2018. https://www.jointcommission.org/assets/1/6/Changes_NPSG_7_hai.pdf. Accessed October 9, 2019.

Tingle J: Patient consent and conscientious objection, *Brit J Nurs* 26(2):118, 2017.

Touhy TA, Jett KF: *Ebersole and Hess' toward healthy aging*, ed 9, St Louis, 2016, Mosby.

Turner JJP: Hypercalcemia – presentation and management, *Clin Med* 17(3):270, 2017.

US Food and Drug Administration: Best way to get rid of used needles and other sharps, 2018, https://www.fda.gov/medical-devices/safely-using-sharps-needles-and-syringes-home-work-and-travel/best-way-get-rid-used-needles-and-other-sharps. Accessed October 26, 2019.

Wagner J, Arora S: Oncologic metabolic emergencies, *Hematol Oncol Clin North Am* 31:941, 2017.

Wolf ZR: Strategies to reduce patient harm from infusion-related medication errors, *J Infus Nurs* 41(1):58, 2018.

RESEARCH REFERENCES

Biasucci DG, et al.: Targeting zero catheter-related bloodstream infections in pediatric intensive care unit: a retrospective matched case-control study, *J Vasc Access* 19(2):119, 2018.

Boev C, et al.: Nursing job satisfaction, certification and healthcare-associated infections in critical care, *Intensive Crit Care Nurs* 31(5):276, 2015.

Carson RA, et al.: Evaluation of a nurse-initiated acute gastroenteritis pathway in the pediatric emergency department, *J Emerg Nurs* 43(5):406, 2017.

Grover TR, et al.: Interdisciplinary teamwork and the power of a quality improvement collaborative in tertiary neonatal intensive care units, *J Perinat Neonatal Nurs* 29(2):179, 2015.

Hawes JA, Lee KS: Reduction in central line-associated bloodstream infections in a NICU: practical lessons for its achievement and sustainability, *J Neonat Network* 37(2):105, 2018.

Helton J, et al.: Peripheral IV site rotation based on clinical assessment vs. length of time since insertion, *Medsurg Nurs* 25(1):44, 2016.

Kyle T, et al.: Ionised calcium levels in major trauma patients who received blood en route to a military medical treatment facility, *Emerg Med J* 35(3):176, 2018.

Major TW, Huey TK: Decreasing IV infiltrates in the pediatric patient—system-based improvement project, *Pediatr Nurs* 42(1):14, 2016.

Matsui Y, et al.: Evaluation of the predictive validity of thermography in identifying extravasation with intravenous chemotherapy infusions, *J Infus Nurs* 40(6):367, 2017.

Park LG, et al.: Symptom diary use and improved survival for patients with heart failure, *Circ Heart Fail* 10:e003874, 2017.

Thoele K, et al.: Optimizing drug delivery of small-volume infusions, *J Infus Nurs* 41(2):113, 2018.

43

Sleep

OBJECTIVES

- Explain the effects that the 24-hour sleep-wake cycle has on biological function.
- Discuss mechanisms that regulate sleep.
- Explain the stages of a normal sleep cycle.
- Explain the functions of sleep.
- Compare and contrast the sleep requirements of different age-groups.

- Identify factors that normally promote and disrupt sleep.
- Discuss characteristics of common sleep disorders.
- Conduct a sleep history for a patient.
- Identify nursing interventions designed to promote normal sleep cycles for patients of all ages.
- Explain ways to evaluate the effects of sleep therapies.

KEY TERMS

Biological clocks, p. 1038
Cataplexy, p. 1042
Circadian rhythm, p. 1038
Excessive daytime sleepiness (EDS), p. 1042
Hypersomnolence, p. 1041
Hypnotics, p. 1056
Insomnia, p. 1041

Narcolepsy, p. 1042
Nocturia, p. 1040
Nonrapid eye movement (NREM) sleep, p. 1039
Polysomnogram, p. 1041
Rapid eye movement (REM) sleep, p. 1039
Rest, p. 1043

Sedatives, p. 1056
Sleep, p. 1038
Sleep apnea, p. 1042
Sleep deprivation, p. 1042
Sleep hygiene, p. 1042

MEDIA RESOURCES

- Review Questions
- Concept Map Creator
- Case Study with Questions

- Audio Glossary
- Content Updates
- Answers to QSEN Activity and Review Questions

Proper rest and sleep are as important to health as good nutrition and adequate exercise. Physical and emotional health depend on the ability to fulfill these basic human needs. Individuals need different amounts of sleep and rest. Without proper amounts, the ability to concentrate, make judgments, and participate in daily activities decreases, and irritability increases.

Identifying and treating patients' sleep pattern disturbances are important goals. To help patients you need to understand the nature of sleep, the factors influencing it, and patients' sleep habits. Patients require individualized approaches based on their personal habits, patterns of sleep, and the particular problem influencing sleep. Nursing interventions are often effective in resolving short- and long-term sleep disturbances.

Sleep provides healing and restoration (Huether et al., 2017). Achieving the best possible sleep quality is important for the promotion of good health and recovery from illness. Patients who are ill often require more sleep and rest than patients who are healthy. However, the nature of illness often prevents some patients from getting adequate rest and sleep. The environment of a hospital or long-term care facility and the activities of health care personnel often make sleep difficult. Some patients have preexisting sleep disturbances; others develop sleep problems because of an illness or hospitalization.

SCIENTIFIC KNOWLEDGE BASE

Physiology of Sleep

Sleep is a cyclical physiological process that alternates with longer periods of wakefulness. The sleep-wake cycle influences and regulates physiological function and behavioral responses.

Circadian Rhythms. People experience cyclical rhythms as part of their everyday lives. The most familiar rhythm is the 24-hour, day-night cycle known as the diurnal or circadian rhythm (derived from Latin: *circa,* "about," and *dies,* "day"). The suprachiasmatic nucleus (SCN) nerve cells in the hypothalamus control the rhythm of the sleep-wake cycle and coordinate this cycle with other circadian rhythms (Huether et al., 2017). Circadian rhythms influence the pattern of major biological and behavioral functions. The predictable changing of body temperature, heart rate, blood pressure, hormone secretion, sensory acuity, and mood depend on the maintenance of the 24-hour circadian cycle (Kryger et al., 2017).

Factors such as light, temperature, social activities, and work routines affect circadian rhythms and daily sleep-wake cycles. All people have biological clocks that synchronize their sleep cycles. This explains why some people fall asleep at 8 PM, whereas others go to bed at midnight or early in the morning. Different people also function best at different times of the day.

Hospitals or extended-care centers usually do not adapt care to an individual's sleep-wake cycle preferences. Typical hospital routines interrupt sleep or prevent patients from falling asleep at their usual time. Poor quality of sleep results when a person's sleep-wake cycle changes. Reversals in the sleep-wake cycle, such as when a person who is normally awake during the day falls asleep during the day, sometimes indicate a serious illness.

The biological rhythm of sleep frequently becomes synchronized with other body functions. For example, changes in body temperature correlate with sleep patterns. Normally body temperature peaks in the afternoon, decreases gradually, and drops sharply after a person falls asleep. When the sleep-wake cycle becomes disrupted (e.g., by working rotating shifts), other physiological functions usually change as well. For example, a new nurse who starts working the night shift experiences a decreased appetite and loses weight. Anxiety, restlessness, irritability, and impaired judgment are other common symptoms of sleep cycle disturbances. Failure to maintain an individual's usual sleep-wake cycle negatively influences a patient's overall health.

Sleep Regulation. Sleep involves a sequence of physiological states maintained by highly integrated central nervous system (CNS) activity. It is associated with changes in the peripheral nervous, endocrine, cardiovascular, respiratory, and muscular systems (Huether et al., 2017). Specific physiological responses and patterns of brain activity identify each sequence. Instruments such as the electroencephalogram (EEG), which measures electrical activity in the cerebral cortex; the electromyogram (EMG), which measures muscle tone; and the electrooculogram (EOG), which measures eye movements provide information about some structural physiological aspects of sleep.

The major sleep center in the body is the hypothalamus. It secretes hypocretins (orexins) that promote wakefulness and rapid eye movement (REM) sleep. Prostaglandin D_2, L-tryptophan, and growth factors control sleep (Huether et al., 2017).

Researchers believe that the ascending reticular activating system (RAS) located in the upper brainstem contains special cells that maintain alertness and wakefulness. The RAS receives visual, auditory, pain, and tactile sensory stimuli. Activity from the cerebral cortex (e.g., emotions or thought processes) also stimulates the RAS. Arousal, wakefulness, and maintenance of consciousness result from neurons in the RAS releasing catecholamines such as norepinephrine (Kryger et al., 2017).

Current evidence suggests two processes help to regulate sleep/wake cycles. The homeostatic process (Process S), which primarily regulates the length and depth of sleep; and the circadian rhythms (Process C: "biological time clocks"), which influence the internal organization of sleep and the timing and duration of sleep-wake cycles, operate simultaneously to regulate sleep and wakefulness (Kryger et al., 2017). Time of wake up is defined by the intersection of Process S and Process C (Fig. 43.1).

Stages of Sleep. There are two sleep phases: **nonrapid eye movement (NREM) sleep** and **rapid eye movement (REM) sleep** (Box 43.1). In the classical definition of NREM sleep, people progress through four stages during a typical 90-minute sleep cycle. The American Academy of Sleep Medicine defines three stages in NREM sleep, combining stages 3 and 4 (Kryger et al., 2017). The quality of sleep from stage 1 through stage 4 becomes increasingly deep. Lighter sleep is characteristic of stages 1 and 2, when a person is more easily arousable. Combined stages 3 and 4 involve a deeper sleep called slow-wave sleep, from which a person is more difficult to arouse (Kryger et al., 2017). REM sleep is the phase at the end of each 90-minute sleep cycle. During REM sleep there is increased brain activity associated with rapid eye movements and muscle atonia.

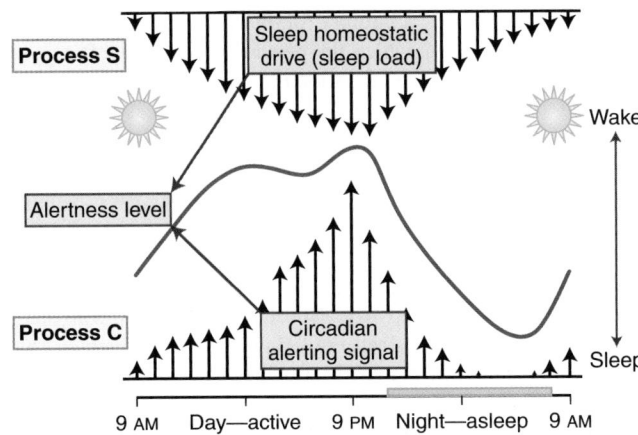

FIG. 43.1 Two-process model of sleep regulation shows the time course of the homeostatic process (Process S) and the circadian process (Process C). Process S rises during waking and declines during sleep. The intersection of Process S and Process C defines the time of wake-up. (From Daroff RB, et al: *Bradley's neurology in clinical practice*, ed 7, Philadelphia, 2016, Elsevier.)

BOX 43.1 Stages of the Sleep Cycle

NREM (75% of Night)

N1 (Formerly Stage 1)
- Stage of lightest level of sleep, lasting a few minutes.
- Decreased physiological activity begins with gradual fall in vital signs and metabolism.
- Sensory stimuli such as noise easily arouse sleeper.
- If awakened, person feels as though daydreaming has occurred.

N2 (Formerly Stage 2)
- Stage of sound sleep during which relaxation progresses.
- Arousal is still relatively easy.
- Brain and muscle activity continue to slow.

N3 (Formerly Stages 3 and 4)
- Called slow-wave sleep.
- Deepest stage of sleep.
- Sleeper is difficult to arouse and rarely moves.
- Brain and muscle activity are significantly decreased.
- Vital signs are lower than during waking hours.

REM Sleep (25% of Night)
- Vivid, full-color dreaming occurs.
- Stage usually begins about 90 minutes after sleep has begun.
- Stage is typified by autonomic response of rapidly moving eyes, fluctuating heart and respiratory rates, and increased or fluctuating blood pressure.
- Loss of skeletal muscle tone occurs.
- Gastric secretions increase.
- It is very difficult to arouse sleeper.
- Duration of REM sleep increases with each cycle and averages 20 minutes.

NREM, Nonrapid eye movement; *REM,* rapid eye movement.
Data from American Sleep Association: *What is sleep?* 2017, https://sleepassociation.org/patients-general-public/what-is-sleep, accessed July 29, 2018.; Kryger M, et al: *Principles and practice of sleep medicine,* 6e, St Louis, 2017, Elsevier; National Sleep Foundation: *What happens when you sleep?* 2018, https://sleepfoundation.org/how-sleep-works/what-happens-when-you-sleep, accessed July 29, 2018.

Sleep Cycle. Normally an adult's routine sleep pattern begins with a presleep period during which the person is aware only of a gradually developing sleepiness. This period normally lasts 10 to 30 minutes. Individuals who have trouble falling asleep often remain in this stage for an hour or more. Once asleep a person usually passes through four to six complete sleep cycles, each cycle consisting of three stages of NREM sleep and a period of REM sleep, for a total of 90 to 110 minutes (Huether et al., 2017).

With each successive cycle, stage 3 (combined 3 and 4) of NREM sleep shortens, and REM sleep lengthens. REM sleep lasts up to 60 minutes during the last sleep cycle. Not all people progress consistently through the usual stages of sleep. For example, a sleeper fluctuates back and forth for short intervals between NREM stages 2, and 3 before entering REM sleep. The amount of time spent in each stage varies. The number of sleep cycles depends on the total amount of time that the person spends sleeping.

Functions of Sleep

Sleep functions as a time of restoration, memory consolidation, and preparation for the next period of wakefulness (Huether et al., 2017). During NREM sleep biological functions slow. A healthy adult's heart rate decreases from a normal average of 70 to 80 beats/min to 60 beats/min or less during sleep, thus preserving cardiac function. Other biological functions that decrease during sleep are respirations, temperature, blood pressure, and muscle tone (Kryger et al., 2017).

Sleep restores biological processes. During NREM stage 3 sleep, the body releases human growth hormone for the repair and renewal of epithelial and specialized cells such as brain cells (Huether et al., 2017). Protein synthesis and cell division for the renewal of tissues also occur during rest and sleep. The basal metabolic rate lowers during sleep, which conserves the energy supply of the body (Huether et al., 2017).

REM sleep appears to be important for early brain development, cognition, and memory. Researchers associate REM sleep with changes in the brain, including cerebral blood flow and increased cortical activity. In addition, there is increased oxygen consumption and epinephrine release. These changes are associated with memory storage and learning (Huether et al., 2017).

The benefits of sleep often go unnoticed until a person develops a problem resulting from sleep deprivation. Current estimates show that 50 million to 70 million adults in the United States have some type of sleep-wake problem (American Sleep Association, 2018). Sleep deprivation affects immune function, metabolism, nitrogen balance, and protein catabolism. A loss of REM sleep often leads to confusion and suspicion. Prolonged sleep loss alters various body functions (e.g., mood, motor performance, memory, equilibrium) (National Sleep Foundation, 2018b). Individuals with sleep problems are also more likely to have chronic diseases such as hypertension, diabetes, and obesity. They sometimes also experience poorer quality of life and productivity (Kohansieh and Makaryus, 2015). Millions of health care dollars are spent on indirect costs related to sleep deprivation, such as motor vehicle and industrial accidents, litigation, property damage, hospitalization, medical errors, and death (Liu et al., 2016).

Dreams. Although dreams occur during both NREM and REM sleep, the dreams of REM sleep are more vivid and elaborate, and some believe that they are functionally important to learning, memory processing, and adaptation to stress (Kryger et al., 2017). REM dreams progress in content throughout the night from dreams about current events to emotional dreams of childhood or the past. Personality influences the quality of dreams (e.g., a creative person has elaborate and complex dreams, whereas a depressed person dreams of helplessness).

Most people dream about immediate concerns such as an argument with a spouse or worries over work. Sometimes a person is unaware of fears represented in bizarre dreams. Clinical psychologists try to analyze the symbolic nature of dreams as part of a patient's psychotherapy. The ability to describe a dream and interpret its significance sometimes helps resolve personal concerns or fears.

Another theory suggests that dreams erase certain fantasies or nonsensical memories. Because most people forget their dreams, few have dream recall or do not believe they dream at all. To remember a dream, a person has to consciously think about it on awakening. People who recall dreams vividly usually awake just after a period of REM sleep.

Physical Illness

Any illness that causes pain, physical discomfort, or mood problems such as anxiety or depression often results in sleep problems. People with such alterations frequently have trouble falling or staying asleep. Illnesses also force patients to sleep in unfamiliar positions. For example, it is difficult for a patient with an arm or leg in traction to rest comfortably.

Respiratory disease also interferes with sleep. Patients with chronic lung disease such as emphysema are short of breath and frequently cannot sleep without two or three pillows to raise their heads. Asthma, bronchitis, and allergic rhinitis alter the rhythm of breathing and disturb sleep. A person with a common cold has nasal congestion, sinus drainage, and a sore throat, which impair breathing and the ability to relax.

Connections among heart disease, sleep, and sleep disorders exist. Sleep-related breathing disorders are linked to increased incidence of nocturnal angina (chest pain), increased heart rate, electrocardiogram changes, high blood pressure, and risk of heart diseases and stroke (Huether et al., 2017). Hypertension often causes early-morning awakening and fatigue. Research also identifies an increased risk of sudden cardiac death in the first hours after awakening. Sleep disruptions and frequent arousals occur in people with heart failure because of the apnea, hypercapnia, and hypoxemia that develop as the disease progresses (Kryger et al., 2017). Hypothyroidism decreases the last sleep stage, whereas hyperthyroidism causes people to take more time to fall asleep.

Nocturia, or urination during the night, disrupts sleep and the sleep cycle. After repeated awakenings to urinate, returning to sleep is difficult, and the sleep cycle is incomplete. Although this condition is most common in older people with reduced bladder tone or people with cardiac disease, diabetes, urethritis, or prostatic disease, it also occurs in a significant number of younger people (Madhu et al., 2015).

Many people experience restless legs syndrome (RLS), which occurs before sleep onset. More common in women, older people, and those with iron deficiency anemia, RLS symptoms include recurrent, rhythmical movements of the feet and legs. Patients feel an itching sensation deep in the muscles. Relief comes only from moving the legs, which prevents relaxation and subsequent sleep. RLS is sometimes a relatively benign condition, depending on how severely sleep is disrupted. Primary RLS is a CNS disorder. Researchers associate secondary RLS with lower levels of iron, pregnancy, renal failure, stress, diet, Parkinson's disease, or a side effect of drugs (Rizek and Kumar, 2017).

Researchers have found a relationship between sleep and gastrointestinal diseases. People with peptic ulcer disease often awaken in the middle of the night. Studies showing a relationship between gastric acid secretion and stages of sleep are conflicting. One consistent finding is that people with duodenal ulcers fail to suppress acid secretion in the first 2 hours of sleep (Kryger et al., 2017). The challenge to researchers is to determine whether sleep disruption impacts gastrointestinal problems such as gastroesophageal reflux and irritable bowel disease or if the diseases disrupt the sleep cycle (Parekh et al., 2018).

Sleep Disorders

Sleep disorders are conditions that, if untreated, generally cause disturbed nighttime sleep that results in one of three problems: insomnia, abnormal movements or sensation during sleep or when waking up at night, or excessive daytime sleepiness (EDS) (Kryger et al., 2017). Many adults in the United States have significant sleep problems from inadequacies in either the quantity or quality of their nighttime sleep and experience hypersomnolence daily (National Sleep Foundation, 2018d). Sleep disorders are more common in children and adolescents with either neurologic conditions or neurodevelopmental disabilities (Maski and Owens, 2018). The American Academy of Sleep Medicine developed the International Classification of Sleep Disorders version 2 (ICSD-2), which classifies sleep disorders into eight major categories (Box 43.2).

Insomnia disorders are related to difficulty falling asleep, frequently awaking from sleep, short periods of sleep, or sleep that is nonrestorative (Kryger et al., 2017). Individuals with sleep-related breathing disorders have changes in respirations during sleep. Hypersomnias are sleep disturbances that result in daytime sleepiness and are not caused by disturbed sleep or alterations in circadian rhythms (Kryger et al., 2017). The circadian rhythm sleep disorders are caused by a misalignment between the timing of sleep and individual desires or the societal norm. The parasomnias are undesirable behaviors that occur usually during sleep. Sleep and wake disturbances are associated with many medical and psychiatric sleep disorders, including psychiatric, neurological, or other medical disorders. In sleep-related movement disorders the person experiences simple stereotyped movements that disturb sleep. The category of "isolated symptoms, apparently normal variants, and unresolved issues" includes sleep-related symptoms that fall between normal and abnormal sleep. The "other sleep disorders" category contains sleep problems that do not fit into other categories.

Sleep laboratory studies diagnose a sleep disorder. A polysomnogram involves the use of EEG, EMG, and EOG to monitor stages of sleep and wakefulness during nighttime sleep. The Multiple Sleep Latency Test (MSLT) provides objective information about sleepiness and selected aspects of sleep structure by measuring eye movements, muscle-tone changes, and brain electrical activity during at least four napping opportunities spread throughout the day. The MSLT takes 8 to 10 hours to complete. Patients wear an Actigraph device on the wrist to measure sleep-wake patterns over an extended period of time such as one week. Actigraphy data provide information about sleep time, sleep efficiency, number and duration of awakenings, and levels of activity and rest. An increasingly popular alternative, particularly among younger adults, is the use of technology in the form of sleep apps for smartphones (Adams et al., 2017). Further study of these sleep apps needs to be conducted to validate the accuracy of measurement of sleep (Lorenz and Williams, 2017).

Insomnia. Insomnia is a symptom that patients experience when they have chronic difficulty in falling asleep, frequent awakenings from sleep, and/or a short sleep or nonrestorative sleep (Kryger et al., 2017). It is the most common sleep-related complaint, with up to 30% of adults suffering from the problem (Haynes et al., 2018). It is commonly experienced by individuals diagnosed with depression (Trauer et al., 2015). People with insomnia experience EDS and insufficient sleep quantity and quality. However, frequently a patient gets more sleep than he or she realizes. Insomnia often signals an underlying physical or psychological disorder. It occurs more frequently in and is the most common sleep problem for women.

People experience transient insomnia because of situational stresses such as family, work, or school problems; jet lag; illness; or loss of a loved one. Insomnia sometimes recurs, but between episodes a patient is able to sleep well. However, a temporary case of insomnia caused by a stressful situation can lead to chronic difficulty in getting enough sleep, perhaps because of the worry and anxiety that develop about getting it.

Insomnia is often associated with poor sleep hygiene, or practices that a patient associates with sleep (Badin et al., 2016). If the condition continues, the fear of not being able to sleep is enough to cause wakefulness. During the day people with chronic insomnia feel sleepy, fatigued, depressed, and anxious. Treatment is symptomatic, including improved sleep-hygiene measures, biofeedback, cognitive techniques, and relaxation techniques (Chung et al., 2017). Behavioral and cognitive therapies have few adverse effects and show evidence of sustained improvement in sleep over time (Haynes et al., 2018).

Sleep Apnea. Sleep apnea is a disorder in which an individual is unable to breathe and sleep at the same time. There is a lack of airflow through the nose and mouth for periods from 10 seconds to 1 to 2 minutes in length. There are three types of sleep apnea: obstructive; central; and mixed apnea, which has both an obstructive and a central component.

The most common form is obstructive sleep apnea (OSA), which is a cessation or stopping of airflow despite the effort to breathe. It occurs when muscles or soft structures of the oral cavity or throat relax during sleep. The upper airway becomes partially or completely blocked, and nasal airflow diminishes (hypopnea) or stops (apnea). The person tries to breathe because chest and abdominal movements continue, which often results in loud snoring sounds. When breathing is partially or completely diminished, the person becomes sufficiently hypoxic and must awaken to breathe. Structural abnormalities such as a deviated septum, nasal polyps, narrow lower jaw, or enlarged tonsils sometimes predispose a patient to OSA. It is estimated that 10% to 17% of adults in the United States are affected by OSA (Qaseem et al., 2014). However, a large majority of people are undiagnosed and untreated (Kryger et al., 2017).

Obesity and hypertension are major factors in OSA. Smoking, increasing age (greater than 65 years old), heart failure, alcohol, nasopharyngeal structural abnormalities, large neck circumferences, and menopause are increased risks for OSA (Qaseem et al., 2014; Schub, 2016). Some research indicates that there may be a link between OSA and occupations in which the individual is exposed to and breathes in solvents (Schwartz et al., 2017). The risk for OSA is similar among African Americans, Asians, and Caucasians (Kryger et al., 2017).

Central sleep apnea (CSA) involves dysfunction in the respiratory control center of the brain. The impulse to breathe fails temporarily, and nasal airflow and chest wall movement cease. The oxygen saturation of the blood falls. The condition is common in patients with brainstem injury, stroke, obesity, muscular dystrophy, and encephalitis. Less than 10% of sleep apnea is predominantly central in origin. People with CSA tend to awaken during sleep and therefore complain of insomnia and EDS. Mild and intermittent snoring is also present.

Excessive daytime sleepiness (EDS) is a common complaint in people experiencing OSA and CSA. Other common symptoms of OSA include fatigue, morning headaches, irritability, depression, difficulty concentrating, and a decrease in sex drive (Kryger et al., 2017). Untreated sleep apnea increases the risk of hypertension, diabetes, heart disease, and heart failure. Lifestyle changes, including a weight-reduction program in people who are obese, improved sleep hygiene, bilevel positive airway pressure (BPAP or BiPAP), continuous positive airway pressure (CPAP), surgery, and oral repositioning devices for the jaw and tongue, are treatment options for OSA (Rotenberg et al., 2016; Schub, 2016).

OSA causes a serious decline in arterial oxygen saturation level. Patients are at risk for cardiac dysrhythmias, right heart failure, pulmonary hypertension, angina attacks, stroke, and hypertension.

Patients with sleep apnea rarely achieve deep sleep. In addition to complaints of EDS, sleep attacks, fatigue, morning headaches, irritability, depression, difficulty concentrating, and a decrease in sex drive are common (Kryger et al., 2017). OSA affects quality-of-life issues such as marital relationships and interactions within and outside the family and often is an embarrassment to a patient (Campos-Rodriguez et al., 2016). Treatment includes therapy for underlying cardiac or respiratory complications and any emotional problems that occur as a result of the symptoms of this disorder.

Narcolepsy. Narcolepsy is a dysfunction of the processes that regulate sleep and wake states. Excessive daytime sleepiness is the most common complaint associated with this disorder. During the day a person suddenly feels an overwhelming wave of sleepiness and falls asleep; REM sleep occurs within 15 minutes of falling asleep. Cataplexy, or sudden muscle weakness during intense emotions such as anger, sadness, or laughter that occurs at any time during the day, is a symptom of narcolepsy type 1, differentiating it from narcolepsy type 2 (Dauvilliers and Barateau, 2017; Maski and Owens, 2018). Cataplexy usually lasts only a few seconds, but if the cataplectic attack is severe, a patient loses voluntary muscle control and falls to the floor (Maski and Owens, 2018). A person with narcolepsy often has vivid dreams that occur as he or she is falling asleep. These dreams are difficult to distinguish from reality. Sleep paralysis, or the feeling of being unable to move or talk just before waking or falling asleep, is another symptom. Some studies show a genetic link for narcolepsy (Dauvilliers and Barateau, 2017).

A person with narcolepsy falls asleep uncontrollably at inappropriate times. When individuals do not understand this disorder, a sleep attack is easily mistaken for laziness, lack of interest in activities, or drunkenness. Typically, the symptoms first begin to appear in adolescence and are often confused with the EDS that commonly occurs in teens. Patients diagnosed with narcolepsy are treated with stimulants or wakefulness-promoting agents such as modafinil, armodafinil, methylphenidate, or sodium oxybate, which only partially increase wakefulness and reduce sleep attacks (Dauvilliers and Barateau, 2017; Maski and Owens, 2018). Patients also receive antidepressant medications that suppress cataplexy and the other REM-related symptoms. Brief daytime naps no longer than 20 minutes help reduce subjective feelings of sleepiness. Other management methods that help are following a regular exercise program, practicing good sleep habits, avoiding shifts in sleep, strategically timing daytime naps if possible, eating light meals high in protein, practicing deep breathing, chewing gum, and taking vitamins (Kryger et al., 2017). Patients with narcolepsy need to avoid factors that increase drowsiness (e.g., alcohol, heavy meals, exhausting activities, long-distance driving, and long periods of sitting in hot, stuffy rooms).

Sleep Deprivation. Many patients experience sleep deprivation because of a sleep disorder. It can be acute or chronic and results from insufficient or disrupted sleep. Causes include illness (e.g., fever, difficulty breathing, or pain), emotional stress, medications, environmental disturbances (e.g., frequent interruptions in sleep during nursing care, noisy neighbors or pets), and variability in the timing of sleep as a result of shift work. Sleep disorders such as sleep apnea or insomnia can cause sleep deprivation.

With sleep deprivation, there is a decrease in the quantity or quality of sleep and/or an inconsistency in the timing of sleep. When sleep becomes interrupted or fragmented, changes in the normal sequencing of the sleep cycles occur. Cumulative sleep deprivation develops over time.

Individuals respond to sleep deprivation differently. Patients experience a variety of physiological and psychological symptoms (Box 43.3). The severity of symptoms is often related to the duration of sleep deprivation. The most effective treatment for sleep deprivation is elimination or correction of environmental factors and patient care activities that disrupt the sleep pattern. Nurses play an important role in identifying treatable sleep-deprivation problems. Evidence suggests that chronic sleep deprivation is associated with obesity, type 2 diabetes, poor memory, depression, digestive problems, and the development of cardiovascular disease (Kohansieh and Makaryus, 2015).

Parasomnias. The parasomnias are sleep problems that are more common in children than adults and occur during non-REM or REM sleep (Maski and Owens, 2018). Some have hypothesized that sudden infant death syndrome (SIDS) is thought to be related to apnea, hypoxia, and cardiac arrhythmias caused by abnormalities in the autonomic nervous system that are manifested during sleep (Kryger et al., 2017). Because of an association between the prone position and the occurrence of SIDS, the American Academy of Pediatrics (AAP) recommends that parents place apparently healthy infants in the supine position during sleep to reduce the risk of sudden infant death syndrome (AAP, 2016).

Parasomnias that occur among older children include confusional arousals, somnambulism (sleepwalking), night terrors, nightmares, nocturnal enuresis (bed-wetting), body rocking, and bruxism (teeth grinding). Parasomnias in children are usually benign and the child will "outgrow" the problem (Maski and Owens, 2018). When adults have these problems, it often indicates more serious disorders. Specific treatment varies. However, in all cases it is important to support patients and maintain their safety.

REFLECT NOW

Interview a patient with chronic respiratory, renal, or cardiac disease. Discuss how the disease affects their ability to sleep.

NURSING KNOWLEDGE BASE

Sleep and Rest

When people are at **rest**, they usually feel mentally relaxed, free from anxiety, and physically calm. Rest does not imply inactivity, although everyone often thinks of it as settling down in a comfortable chair or lying in bed. When people are at rest, they are in a state of mental,

---

BOX 43.3 Sleep-Deprivation Symptoms

Physiological Symptoms	Psychological Symptoms
• Ptosis, blurred vision	• Confused and disoriented
• Fine-motor clumsiness	• Increased sensitivity to pain
• Decreased reflexes	• Irritable, withdrawn, apathetic
• Slowed response time	• Agitated
• Decreased reasoning and judgment	• Hyperactive
• Decreased auditory and visual alertness	• Decreased motivation
• Cardiac arrhythmias	• Excessive sleepiness

---

physical, and spiritual activity that leaves them feeling refreshed, rejuvenated, and ready to resume the activities of the day. People have their own habits for obtaining rest and can find ways to adjust to new environments or conditions that affect the ability to rest. They rest by reading a book, practicing a relaxation exercise, listening to music, taking a long walk, or sitting quietly.

Illness and unfamiliar health care routines easily affect the usual rest and sleep patterns of people entering a hospital or other health care setting. Nurses frequently care for patients who are on bed rest to reduce physical and psychological demands on the body in a variety of health care settings. However, patients on bed rest do not necessarily feel rested. Some experience emotional distress that prevents complete relaxation. For example, concern over physical limitations or a fear of being unable to return to their usual lifestyle causes such patients to feel stressed and unable to relax. You must always be aware of a patient's need for rest. A lack of rest for long periods causes illness or worsening of existing illness.

Normal Sleep Requirements and Patterns

Sleep duration and quality vary among people of all age-groups. For example, one person feels adequately rested with 4 hours of sleep, whereas another requires 10 hours. Nurses play an important role in identifying treatable sleep-deprivation problems.

Neonates. The neonate up to the age of 3 months averages about 16 hours of sleep a day, sleeping almost constantly during the first week. The sleep cycle is generally 40 to 50 minutes with wakening occurring after one to two sleep cycles. Approximately 50% of this sleep is REM sleep, which stimulates the higher brain centers. This is essential for development because the neonate is not awake long enough for significant external stimulation.

Infants. Infants usually develop a nighttime pattern of sleep by 3 months of age. The infant normally takes several naps during the day but usually sleeps an average of 8 to 10 hours during the night for a total daily sleep time of 15 hours. About 30% of sleep time is in the REM cycle. Awakening commonly occurs early in the morning, although it is not unusual for an infant to wake up during the night.

Toddlers. By the age of 2 children usually sleep through the night and take daily naps. Total sleep averages 12 hours a day. After 3 years of age children often give up daytime naps (Hockenberry and Wilson, 2019). It is common for toddlers to awaken during the night. The percentage of REM sleep continues to fall. During this period toddlers may be unwilling to go to bed at night because they need autonomy or fear separation from their parents.

Preschoolers. On average a preschooler sleeps about 12 hours a night (about 20% is REM). By the age of 5 he or she rarely takes daytime naps except in cultures in which a siesta is the custom (Hockenberry and Wilson, 2019). The preschooler usually has difficulty relaxing or quieting down after long, active days and has bedtime fears, awakens during the night, or has nightmares. Partial awakening followed by normal return to sleep is frequent (Hockenberry and Wilson, 2019). In the awake period the child exhibits brief crying, walking around, unintelligible speech, sleepwalking, or bed-wetting.

School-Age Children. The amount of sleep needed varies during the school years. A 6-year-old averages 11 to 12 hours of sleep nightly, whereas an 11-year-old sleeps about 9 to 10 hours (Hockenberry and Wilson, 2019). The 6- or 7-year-old usually goes to bed with some encouragement or by doing quiet activities. The older child often resists sleeping because he or she is unaware of fatigue or has a need to be independent.

Adolescents.
On average the majority of teenagers get about 7 hours or less of sleep per night, although the recommended requirement is 8 to 10 hours (Hirschkowitz et al., 2015; National Sleep Foundation, 2018c). The typical adolescent is subject to many changes, such as school demands, after-school social activities, and part-time jobs, which reduce the time spent sleeping (Bruce et al., 2017). Adolescents typically have electronic devices such as televisions, computers, smartphones, or video games in their rooms, which further contribute to sleep disruption, poor sleep quality, and decreased amount of sleep (Bruce et al., 2017; Shimura et al., 2018). Shortened sleep time often results in EDS, which frequently leads to reduced performance in school, vulnerability to accidents, behavioral and mood problems, and increased use of alcohol (Wiggins and Freeman, 2014).

Young Adults.
Most young adults average 6 to 8½ hours of sleep a night. Approximately 20% of sleep time is REM sleep, which remains consistent throughout life. It is common for the stresses of jobs, family relationships, and social activities to frequently lead to insomnia, and some may use medication to help them sleep. Daytime sleepiness contributes to an increased number of accidents, decreased productivity, and interpersonal problems in this age-group.

Pregnancy increases the need for sleep and rest. However, a majority of pregnant women describe variations in sleep habits (Erwin, 2017). Sleep disruption occurs due to pregnancy-related hormone changes and the anatomic and physiological changes that occur in the body to maintain the pregnancy (Erwin, 2017). First-trimester sleep disturbances include a reduction in overall sleep time and quality. Daytime drowsiness, insomnia, and nighttime awakenings also increase because of frequent nocturnal voiding. These disturbances level off in the second trimester. Insomnia, periodic limb movements, RLS, and sleep-disordered breathing are common problems during the third trimester of pregnancy (Kryger et al., 2017).

Middle Adults.
The recommended sleep requirement for adults is 7 to 9 hours per night (Hirschkowitz et al., 2015). During middle adulthood the total time spent sleeping at night begins to decline. The amount of stage 4 sleep begins to fall, a decline that continues with advancing age. Insomnia is particularly common, probably because of the changes and stresses of middle age. Anxiety, depression, or certain physical illnesses cause sleep disturbances. Women experiencing menopausal symptoms often experience insomnia.

Older Adults.
Sleeping difficulties increase with age. Approximately 40% of older adults report problems with sleep (Kryger et al., 2017; National Sleep Foundation, 2018a). Older adults spend more time in stage 1 and less time in stages 3 and 4 (NREM sleep); some older adults have almost no NREM stage 4 or deep sleep. Episodes of REM sleep tend to shorten. Older adults experience fewer episodes of deep sleep and more episodes of lighter sleep. They tend to awaken more often during the night, and it takes more time for them to fall asleep. To compensate they increase the number of naps taken during the day.

Older adults who have a chronic illness often experience sleep disturbances. For example, an older adult with arthritis frequently has difficulty sleeping because of painful joints. Changes in sleep pattern are often caused by changes in the CNS that affect the regulation of sleep. Many older adults with insomnia have co-morbid psychiatric illness

or medical conditions, take medications that disrupt sleep patterns, or use drugs or alcohol. Sensory impairment reduces an older person's sensitivity to time cues that maintain circadian rhythms.

Factors Influencing Sleep

Many factors affect the quantity and quality of sleep. Often a single factor is not the only cause for a sleep problem. Physiological, psychological, and environmental factors frequently alter the quality and quantity of sleep.

Drugs and Substances.
Sleepiness, insomnia, and fatigue often result as a direct effect of commonly prescribed medications (Box 43.4). These medications alter sleep and weaken daytime alertness, which is problematic (Kryger et al., 2017). Medications prescribed for sleep often cause more problems than benefits. Older adults take a variety of drugs to control or treat chronic illness, and the combined effects of their drugs often seriously disrupt sleep. Some substances such as L-tryptophan, a natural protein found in foods such as milk, cheese, and meats, promote sleep.

Lifestyle.
A person's daily routine influences sleep patterns. An individual working a rotating shift (e.g., 2 weeks of days followed by a week of nights) often has difficulty adjusting to the altered sleep schedule. For example, the body's internal clock is set at 11 PM, but the work schedule forces sleep at 9 AM instead. The individual is able to sleep only 3 or 4 hours because his or her body clock perceives that it is time to be awake and active. Difficulties maintaining alertness during work time result in decreased and even hazardous performance. After several

---

BOX 43.4 Drugs and Their Effects on Sleep

Hypnotics
- Interfere with reaching deeper sleep stages
- Provide only temporary (1-week) increase in quantity of sleep
- Eventually cause "hangover" during day; excess drowsiness, confusion, decreased energy
- Sometimes worsen sleep apnea in older adults

Antidepressants and Stimulants
- Suppress REM sleep
- Decrease total sleep time

Alcohol
- Speeds onset of sleep
- Reduces REM sleep
- Awakens person during night and causes difficulty returning to sleep

Caffeine
- Prevents person from falling asleep
- Causes person to awaken during night
- Interferes with REM sleep

Diuretics
- Nighttime awakenings caused by nocturia

Beta-Adrenergic Blockers
- Cause nightmares
- Cause insomnia
- Cause awakening from sleep

Benzodiazepines
- Alter REM sleep
- Increase sleep time
- Increase daytime sleepiness

Nicotine
- Decreases total sleep time
- Decreases REM sleep time
- Causes awakening from sleep
- Causes difficulty staying asleep

Opiates
- Suppress REM sleep
- Cause increased daytime drowsiness

Anticonvulsants
- Decrease REM sleep time
- Cause daytime drowsiness

REM, Rapid eye movement.

weeks of working a night shift, a person's biological clock usually does adjust. Other alterations in routines that disrupt sleep patterns include performing unaccustomed heavy work, engaging in late-night social activities, and changing evening mealtime.

Usual Sleep Patterns. In the past century the amount of sleep obtained nightly by US citizens has decreased, causing many Americans to be sleep deprived and to experience excessive sleepiness during the day. Sleepiness becomes pathological when it occurs at times when individuals need or want to be awake. People who experience temporary sleep deprivation as a result of an active social evening or lengthened work schedule usually feel sleepy the next day. However, they are able to overcome these feelings even though they have difficulty performing tasks and remaining attentive. Chronic lack of sleep is much more serious and causes serious alterations in the ability to perform daily functions. Sleepiness tends to be most difficult to overcome during sedentary (inactive) tasks such as driving. An increasingly common contributor to EDS is the use of technology close to bedtime, such as watching television, talking or texting on a cellphone, or reading information on electronic devices.

Emotional Stress. Worry over personal problems or a situation frequently disrupts sleep. Emotional stress causes a person to be tense and often leads to frustration when sleep does not occur. Stress also causes a person to try too hard to fall asleep, to awaken frequently during the sleep cycle, or to oversleep. Continued stress causes poor sleep habits.

Older patients frequently experience losses that lead to emotional stress such as retirement, physical impairment, or the death of a loved one. Older adults and other individuals who experience depressive mood problems experience delays in falling asleep, earlier appearance of REM sleep, frequent or early waking, feelings of sleeping poorly, and daytime sleepiness.

Environment. The physical environment in which a person sleeps significantly influences the ability to fall and remain asleep. Good ventilation is essential for restful sleep. The size, firmness, and position of the bed affect the quality of sleep. If a person usually sleeps with another individual, sleeping alone often causes wakefulness. On the other hand, sleeping with a restless or snoring bed partner disrupts sleep.

In hospitals and other inpatient facilities, noise creates a problem for patients. Noise in hospitals is usually new or strange and often loud. Thus patients wake easily. This problem is greatest the first night of hospitalization, when patients often experience increased total wake time, increased awakenings, and decreased REM sleep and total sleep time. People-induced noises (e.g., nursing activities) are sources of increased sound levels. ICUs are sources of high noise levels because of staff, monitor alarms, and equipment. Close proximity of patients, noise from confused and ill patients, ringing alarm systems and telephones, and disturbances caused by emergencies make the environment unpleasant. Noise causes increased agitation, delayed healing, impaired immune function, and increased blood pressure, heart rate, and stress (Patel et al., 2018).

Light levels affect the ability to fall asleep. Some patients prefer a dark room, whereas others such as children or older adults prefer keeping a soft light on during sleep. Patients also have trouble sleeping because of the room temperature. A room that is too warm or too cold often causes a patient to become restless.

Exercise and Fatigue. A person who is moderately fatigued usually achieves restful sleep, especially if the fatigue is the result of enjoyable work or exercise. Exercising 2 hours or more before bedtime allows the body to cool down and maintain a state of fatigue that promotes relaxation. However, excess fatigue resulting from exhausting or stressful

work makes falling asleep difficult. This is often seen in grade-school children and adolescents who keep long, stressful schedules because of school, social activities, and work.

Food and Caloric Intake. Following good eating habits is important for proper sleep. Eating a large, heavy, and/or spicy meal at night often results in indigestion that interferes with sleep. Caffeine, alcohol, and nicotine consumed in the evening produce insomnia. Coffee, tea, cola, and chocolate contain caffeine and xanthines that cause sleeplessness. Thus drastically reducing or avoiding these substances can improve sleep. Some food allergies cause insomnia. A milk allergy sometimes causes nighttime waking and crying or colic in infants.

Weight loss or gain influences sleep patterns. Weight gain contributes to OSA because of increased size of the soft tissue structures in the upper airway (Kryger et al., 2017). Weight loss caused by semi-starvation diets sometimes causes sleep disorders such as reduced sleep and insomnia.

CRITICAL THINKING

Successful critical thinking requires a synthesis of knowledge, experience, information gathered from patients, critical thinking attitudes, and intellectual and professional standards. Clinical judgments require you to anticipate the information necessary, analyze the data, and make decisions regarding patient care. During assessment consider all elements to build toward making an appropriate nursing diagnosis.

In the case of sleep, integrate knowledge from nursing and other disciplines such as pharmacology and psychology. Personal experience with a sleep problem and experience with patients prepares you to know effective forms of sleep therapies. You use critical thinking attitudes such as perseverance, confidence, and discipline to complete a comprehensive assessment and develop a plan of care to provide successful management of the sleep problem. Professional standards such as the *Nursing Scope and Standards of Practice* (American Nurses Association, 2015), *Clinical Practice Guidelines for the Pharmacologic Treatment of Chronic Insomnia in Adults: An American Academy of Sleep Medicine Clinical Practice Guideline* (Sateia et al., 2017), and "Excessive Sleepiness" in *Evidence-based Geriatrics Nursing Protocols for Best Practice* (Chasens and Umlauf, 2012) provide valuable guidelines to assess and address the needs of patients with sleep disorders.

REFLECT NOW

Consider your lifestyle choices. What factors contribute to promoting or disrupting your sleep. What changes can you make that will improve your sleep?

❖ NURSING PROCESS

Apply the nursing process and use a critical thinking approach in your care of patients. The nursing process provides a clinical decision-making approach for you to develop and implement an individualized plan of care.

◆ Assessment

During the assessment process thoroughly assess each patient and critically analyze findings to ensure that you make patient-centered clinical decisions required for safe nursing care (Fig. 43.2).

Through the Patient's Eyes. Sleep is a subjective experience. Only the patient is able to report whether it is sufficient and restful. If the patient is satisfied with the quantity and quality of sleep received,

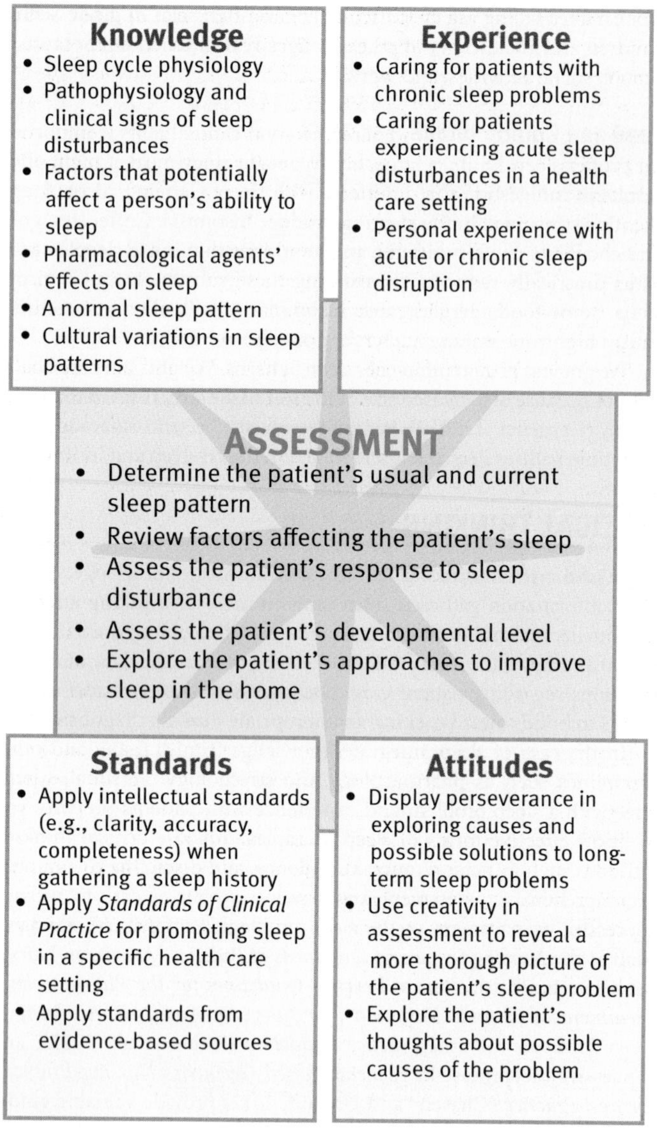

Knowledge
- Sleep cycle physiology
- Pathophysiology and clinical signs of sleep disturbances
- Factors that potentially affect a person's ability to sleep
- Pharmacological agents' effects on sleep
- A normal sleep pattern
- Cultural variations in sleep patterns

Experience
- Caring for patients with chronic sleep problems
- Caring for patients experiencing acute sleep disturbances in a health care setting
- Personal experience with acute or chronic sleep disruption

ASSESSMENT
- Determine the patient's usual and current sleep pattern
- Review factors affecting the patient's sleep
- Assess the patient's response to sleep disturbance
- Assess the patient's developmental level
- Explore the patient's approaches to improve sleep in the home

Standards
- Apply intellectual standards (e.g., clarity, accuracy, completeness) when gathering a sleep history
- Apply *Standards of Clinical Practice* for promoting sleep in a specific health care setting
- Apply standards from evidence-based sources

Attitudes
- Display perseverance in exploring causes and possible solutions to long-term sleep problems
- Use creativity in assessment to reveal a more thorough picture of the patient's sleep problem
- Explore the patient's thoughts about possible causes of the problem

FIG. 43.2 Critical thinking model for sleep assessment.

you consider it normal, and the nursing history that you will collect is brief. If a patient admits to or suspects a sleep problem, you will need a detailed history and assessment. If a patient has an obvious sleep problem, consider asking whether his or her sleep partner can be approached for further assessment data.

A poor night's sleep for a patient often starts a vicious cycle of anticipatory anxiety. The patient fears that sleep will again be disturbed while trying harder and harder to sleep. Use a skilled and caring approach to assess the patient's sleep needs. A caring nurse individualizes care for each patient. Always ask patients what they expect regarding sleep. This includes asking about the interventions that they currently use and how successful they are. It is important to understand patients' expectations regarding their sleep pattern. When they ask for help because of sleep disturbances, they typically expect a nurse to respond promptly to help them improve the quantity and quality of their sleep.

Sleep Assessment. Most people are able to provide a reasonably accurate estimate of their sleep patterns, particularly if any changes have occurred. Aim your assessment at first understanding the characteristics of the patient's sleep problem and usual sleep habits so that you incorporate ways for promoting sleep into nursing care. For example,

if the nursing history reveals that a patient always reads before falling asleep, it makes sense to offer reading material at bedtime.

Sources for Sleep Assessment. Usually patients are the best resource for describing sleep problems and how they are a change from their usual sleep and waking patterns. Often the patient knows the cause for sleep problems, such as a noisy environment or worry over a relationship.

In addition, bed partners are able to provide information about patients' sleep patterns that help reveal the nature of certain sleep disorders. For example, partners of patients with sleep apnea often complain that the patients' snoring disturbs their sleep. Ask bed partners (if the patient agrees) whether patients have breathing pauses during sleep and how frequently the apneic attacks occur. Some partners mention becoming fearful when patients apparently stop breathing for periods.

When caring for children, seek information about sleep patterns from parents or guardians because they are usually a reliable source of information. Hunger, excessive warmth, and separation anxiety often contribute to an infant's difficulty in going to sleep or frequent awakenings during the night. Parents of infants need to keep a 24-hour log of their infant's waking and sleeping behavior for several days to determine the cause of the problem. Describing the infant's eating pattern and sleeping environment in the log will help identify which factors are influencing the baby's sleeping behavior. Older children often are able to relate fears or worries that inhibit their ability to fall asleep. If children frequently awaken in the middle of bad dreams, parents are able to identify the problem but perhaps do not understand the meaning of the dreams. Ask parents to describe the typical behavior patterns that foster or impair sleep. For example, excessive stimulation from active play or visiting friends predictably impairs sleep. With chronic sleep problems, parents need to relate the duration of the problem, its progression, and children's responses.

Tools for Sleep Assessment. Two effective subjective measures of sleep are the Epworth Sleepiness Scale and the Pittsburgh Sleep Quality Index. The Epworth Sleepiness Scale contains eight questions about the likeliness of a patient being sleepy during certain activities (e.g., watching television, reading, sitting and talking with someone) on a scale of 0 (would never doze or sleep) to 3 (high chance of dozing or sleeping). A score of 0 to 5 indicates lower normal daytime sleepiness; 6 to 10 is considered higher than normal daytime sleepiness; a score of 11 or 12 is mild excessive daytime sleepiness; 13 to 15 is moderate excessive daytime sleepiness; and a score of 16 to 24 is severe excessive daytime sleepiness (Johns, n.d.). The scale is available at http://epworthsleepinessscale.com/about-the-ess/. The second tool, the Pittsburgh Sleep Quality Index assesses sleep quality and patterns (Mollayeva et al., 2016). This scale is available at https://consultgeri.org/try-this/general-assessment/issue-6.1.pdf.

Another brief, effective method for assessing sleep quality is the use of a visual analog scale. Draw a straight horizontal line 100 mm (4 inches) long. Opposing statements such as "best night's sleep" and "worst night's sleep" are at opposite ends of the line. Ask patients to place a mark on the horizontal line at the point corresponding to their perceptions of the previous night's sleep. Measuring the distances of the mark along the line in millimeters offers a numerical value for satisfaction with sleep. Use the scale repeatedly to show change over time. Such a scale is useful to assess an individual patient, not to compare patients.

Another brief, subjective method to assess sleep is a numeric scale with a 0-to-10 sleep rating. Ask individuals to separately rate the quantity and quality of their sleep on the scale. Instruct them to indicate with a number between 0 and 10 their sleep quantity and then their quality of sleep, with 0 being the worst sleep and 10 being the best.

Sleep History. When you suspect a patient has a sleep problem, assess the quality and characteristics of sleep in greater depth by asking the patient to describe the problem. This includes recent changes in sleep pattern, sleep symptoms experienced during waking hours, the use of prescribed or over-the-counter sleep medications, diet and intake of substances such as caffeine or alcohol that influence sleep, and recent life events that have affected the patient's mental and emotional status.

Description of Sleeping Problems. Conduct a more detailed history when a patient has a persistent or what appears to be a serious sleep problem. Open-ended questions help a patient describe a problem more fully. A general description of the problem followed by more focused questions usually reveals specific characteristics that are useful in planning therapies. To begin, you need to understand the nature of the sleep problem, its signs and symptoms, its onset and duration, its severity, any predisposing factors or causes, and the overall effect on the patient. Ask specific questions related to the sleep problem (Box 43.5).

Proper questioning helps to determine the type of sleep disturbance and the nature of the problem. Box 43.6 gives examples of additional questions for you to ask a patient when you suspect specific sleep disorders. The STOP-BANG sleep assessment tool is a reliable evidence-based tool used to screen for OSA and is frequently used in preanesthesia and/or preoperative assessments (see Chapter 50) (Chung et al., 2016). The questions help to select specific sleep therapies and the best time for implementation.

To add to the sleep history, have the patient and bed partner keep a sleep-wake log for 1 to 4 weeks. The patient completes the sleep-wake log daily to provide information on day-to-day variations in sleep-wake patterns over extended periods. Entries in the log often include 24-hour information about various waking and sleeping health behaviors such as physical activities, mealtimes, type and amount of intake (alcohol and caffeine), time and length of daytime naps, evening and bedtime routines, the time the patient tries to fall asleep, nighttime awakenings, and the time of morning awakening. A partner helps record the estimated times the patient falls asleep or awakens. Although the log is helpful, the patient needs to be motivated to participate in its completion.

Usual Sleep Pattern. Normal sleep is difficult to define because individuals vary in their perception of adequate quantity and quality of sleep. However, it is important to have patients describe their usual sleep pattern to determine the significance of the changes caused by a sleep disorder. Knowing a patient's usual, preferred sleep pattern allows you to try to match sleeping conditions in the health care setting with those in the home. Ask the following questions to determine a patient's sleep pattern:

1. What time do you usually get in bed each night?
2. How much time does it usually take to fall asleep? Do you do anything special to help you fall asleep?
3. How many times do you wake up during the night? What do you think is the cause?
4. What time do you typically wake up in the morning?

BOX 43.5 Nursing Assessment Questions

Nature of the Problem
- Describe the type of sleep problem you're having.
- Why do you think you're not getting enough sleep?
- Describe a recent night's sleep. How is this sleep different from your usual sleep?

Signs and Symptoms
- Do you have difficulty falling asleep, staying asleep, or waking up?
- Have you been told that you snore loudly?
- Do you have headaches when awakening?

Onset and Duration of Signs and Symptoms
- When did you notice the problem?
- What do you do to relieve the symptom?
- How long has this problem lasted?

Severity
- How long does it take you to fall asleep?
- How often during the week do you have trouble falling asleep?
- On average, how many hours of sleep a night did you get this week?
- How does this compare to your usual amount of sleep?
- What do you do when you awaken during the night or too early in the morning?

Predisposing Factors
- What do you do just before you go to bed?
- Have you recently had any changes at work or at home?
- How is your mood? Have you noticed any changes recently?
- Which medications or recreational drugs do you take on a regular basis?
- Are you taking any new prescriptions or over-the-counter medications?
- Do you eat food (spicy or greasy foods) or drink substances (alcohol or caffeinated beverages) that affect your sleep?
- Do you have a physical illness that affects your sleep?
- Does anyone in your family have a history of sleep problems?

Effect on Patient
- How has the loss of sleep affected you?
- Do you feel excessively sleepy or irritable or have trouble concentrating during waking hours?
- Do you have trouble staying awake? Have you fallen asleep at the wrong times (e.g., while driving, sitting quietly in a meeting)?

BOX 43.6 Questions to Ask to Assess for Specific Sleep Disorders

Impaired Sleep
- How easily do you fall asleep?
- Do you fall asleep and have difficulty staying asleep? How many times do you awaken?
- What time do you awaken in the morning? What causes you to awaken early?
- What do you do to prepare for sleep? To improve your sleep?
- What do you think about as you try to fall asleep?
- How often do you have trouble sleeping?

Sleep Apnea
- Do you snore loudly? Does anyone else in your family snore loudly?
- Has anyone ever told you that you often stop breathing for short periods during sleep? (Spouse or bed partner/roommate may report this.)
- Do you experience headaches after awakening?
- Do you have difficulty staying awake during the day?

Narcolepsy
- Do you fall asleep at the wrong times? (Friends or relatives may report this.)
- Do you have episodes of losing muscle control or falling to the floor?
- Have you ever had the feeling of being unable to move or talk just before waking or falling asleep?
- Do you have vivid, lifelike dreams when going to sleep or awakening?

Compare patient data with their pattern before the sleep problem or with the predominant pattern usually found for other patients of the same age. Use this comparison to assess for identifiable patterns such as insomnia. Patients with sleep problems frequently report sleep patterns that are drastically different from their normal patterns, or sometimes the change is relatively minor. Patients in the hospital usually need or want more sleep as a result of illness. However, some require less sleep because they are less active. Some patients who are ill think that it is important to try to sleep more than usual, eventually making sleeping difficult.

Physical and Psychological Illness. Determine whether the patient has any preexisting health problems that interfere with sleep. Chronic diseases such as chronic obstructive pulmonary disease and painful disorders such as arthritis interfere with sleep. Also assess the patient's medication history, including a description of over-the-counter and prescribed drugs. A history of psychiatric problems also makes a difference. For example, a patient who is living with bipolar disorder sleeps more when depressed than when manic. A patient who is depressed often experiences an inadequate amount of fragmented sleep. If a patient takes medications to aid sleep, gather information about the type and amount of medication and the frequency of its use. Also assess the patient's daily caffeine intake.

If the patient has recently undergone surgery with general anesthesia, expect him or her to experience some sleep disturbance. Patients usually awaken frequently during the first night after surgery and receive little deep or REM sleep. Depending on the type of anesthesia, it takes several days to months for a normal sleep cycle to return.

Current Life Events. In your assessment learn whether the patient is experiencing any changes in lifestyle that disrupt sleep. A person's occupation often offers a clue to the nature of the sleep problem. Changes in job responsibilities, rotating shifts, or long hours contribute to a sleep disturbance. Questions about social activities, recent travel, or mealtime schedules help clarify the assessment.

Emotional and Mental Status. A patient's emotions and mental status affect the ability to sleep. For example, if a patient is experiencing anxiety, emotional stress related to illness, or situational crises such as loss of job or a loved one, he or she often experiences insomnia. When a sleep disturbance is related to an emotional problem, the key is to treat the primary problem; its resolution often improves sleep (Murawski et al., 2017). Patients with mental illnesses may need mild sedation for adequate rest. Assess the effectiveness of any medication and its effect on daytime function.

Bedtime Routines. Ask patients what they do to prepare for sleep. For example, some patients drink a glass of milk, take a sleeping pill, eat a snack, or watch television. Assess habits that are beneficial compared with those that disturb sleep. For example, watching television promotes sleep for one person, whereas it stimulates another to stay awake. Sometimes pointing out that a habit is interfering with sleep helps patients find ways to change or eliminate habits that are disrupting sleep.

Pay special attention to a child's bedtime rituals. For example, the parents need to report whether it is necessary to read a bedtime story, rock the child to sleep, or engage in quiet play. Some young children need a special blanket or stuffed animal when going to sleep.

Bedtime Environment. During assessment ask the patient to describe preferred bedroom conditions, including preferences for lighting in the room, music or television in the background, or needing to have the door open versus closed. Include questions about the presence of electronic devices in the bedroom (e.g., phones, televisions), all of which have small lights that remain on or have a light that blinks when the battery is low. Patients are often surprised how many of these devices are in the sleeping environment.

In addition, some children need the company of a parent to fall asleep. Environmental distractions in a health care setting such as a roommate's television, an electronic monitor in the hallway, a noisy nurses' station, or another patient who cries out at night often interfere with sleep. Modify the environment whenever possible to promote sleep.

Behaviors of Sleep Deprivation. Some patients are unaware of how their sleep problems affect their behavior. Observe for behaviors such as irritability, disorientation (similar to a drunken state), frequent yawning, and slurred speech. If sleep deprivation has lasted a long time, psychotic behavior such as delusions and paranoia sometimes develops. For example, a patient reports seeing strange objects or colors in the room, or he or she acts afraid when the nurse enters the room.

REFLECT NOW

Take either the Epworth Sleepiness Scale or Pittsburgh Sleep Quality Index. After analyzing your results, what does the instrument tell you about your sleep quality?

◆ **Nursing Diagnosis**

Review your assessment data, looking for clusters that include assessment findings of a sleep pattern disturbance or other health problem. If you identify a sleep problem, specify the condition, such as insomnia or sleep deprivation. By specifying the sleep disturbance diagnosis, you are able to design more effective interventions. For example, you choose different therapies for patients with insomnia who are unable to fall asleep than for those with sleep deprivation. Box 43.7 demonstrates how to use nursing assessment activities to identify and cluster assessment findings to make an accurate nursing diagnosis.

Assessment also identifies the related factor or probable cause of a sleep disturbance such as a noisy environment or a high intake of caffeinated beverages in the evening. These causes become the focus of interventions for minimizing or eliminating a negative or problem-focused diagnosis. For example, if a patient is experiencing insomnia as a result of a noisy health care environment, offer some basic recommendations for helping sleep, such as controlling the noise of hospital equipment, reducing interruptions, or keeping doors closed. If

---

BOX 43.7 Nursing Diagnostic Process

Impaired Sleep

Assessment Activities	Assessment Findings
Ask patient to explain nature of sleep problem.	Patient reports difficulty falling asleep, taking up to 1 hour. Patient reports waking up two to three times nightly with difficulty returning to sleep.
Observe patient's behavior and ask spouse whether patient is experiencing behavioral changes.	Patient admits to not feeling well rested. Spouse describes times when patient was lethargic and irritable.
Determine whether patient has had recent lifestyle changes.	Spouse reports that patient recently lost job and is concerned about finding new position.

the insomnia is related to anxiety or stress over a threatened marital separation, introduce coping strategies and create an environment for sleep. If you incorrectly define the probable cause or related factors, the patient does not benefit from care.

Sleep problems affect patients in other ways. For example, you find that a patient with sleep apnea has problems with a spouse who is tired and frustrated over the patient's snoring. In addition, the spouse is concerned that the patient is breathing improperly and thus is in danger. Examples of nursing diagnoses for patients with sleep problems include the following:

- *Adequate Sleep*
- *Fatigue*
- *Impaired Sleep*
- *Impaired Alertness*
- *Sleep Deprivation*

◆ Planning

Goals and Outcomes. During planning you again synthesize information from multiple resources to develop an individualized plan of care (Fig. 43.3) (see the Nursing Care Plan). Professional standards are especially important to consider in developing a care plan. These standards often offer evidence-based guidelines for effective nursing interventions. For example, in *Evidence-Based Geriatrics Nursing Protocols for Best Practice,* the chapter titled "Excessive Sleepiness" (Chasens and Umlauf, 2012) recommends individualized nursing interventions that maintain and support an older adult's normal sleep pattern and bedtime ritual. It is important for a plan of care for sleep promotion

to include strategies appropriate to the patient's sleep routines, living environment, and lifestyle.

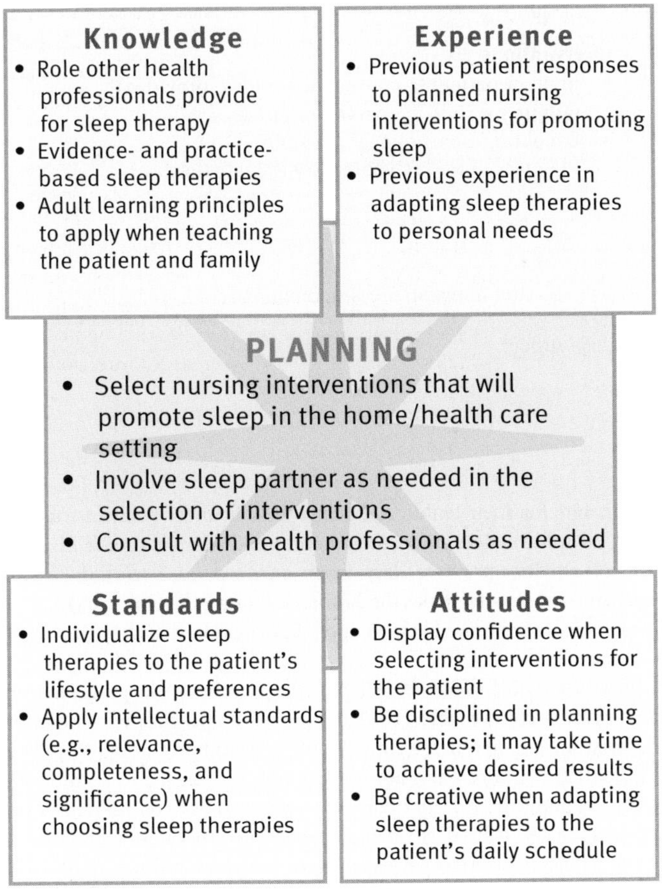

As you plan care for a patient with sleep disturbances, creation of a concept map is another method for developing holistic patient-centered care (Fig. 43.4). Create the map after identifying relevant nursing diagnoses from the assessment database. In this example the nursing diagnoses are linked to the patient's medical diagnosis of depression and situational stress. The concept map shows the relationships among the nursing diagnoses *Impaired Sleep, Caregiver Stress, Fatigue,* and *Impaired Health Maintenance.* This approach to planning care helps you recognize relationships among planned interventions. For this patient, interventions and successful outcomes for one nursing diagnosis affect the resolution of another. When developing goals and outcomes, it is important for you to collaborate with your patients. As a result, you are more likely to set realistic goals and measurable outcomes with your patients. An effective plan includes outcomes established over a realistic time frame that focus on the goal of improving the quantity and quality of sleep in the home. Often family members are very helpful in contributing to the plan. A sleep-promotion plan frequently requires many weeks to accomplish.

Setting Priorities. Work with patients to establish priority outcomes and interventions. Frequently sleep disturbances are the result of other health problems. For example, when physical symptoms interfere with sleep, managing the symptoms is your first priority. After symptoms are relieved, focus on sleep therapies. Patients are a helpful resource in determining which interventions hold priority. For example, once patients understand the factors that disrupt sleep, they make choices about the types of changes they would like to make in their lifestyle or sleeping environment.

Teamwork and Collaboration. Partner closely with the patient and sleep partner to ensure that any therapies such as a change in the sleep schedule or changes to the bedroom environment are realistic and achievable. In a health care setting, plan treatments or routines so that the patient is able to rest. For example, in the ICU use available electronic monitors to track trends in vital signs without waking a patient each hour. Other staff members need to be aware of the care plan so that they can cluster activities at certain times to reduce awakenings. In a nursing home the focus of the plan involves better planning of rest periods around the activities of the other residents. Roommates often have very different schedules.

When patients have chronic sleep problems, the initial referral for a patient is often to a comprehensive sleep center for assessment of the problem. The nature of the sleep disturbance then determines whether referrals to additional health care providers are necessary. For example, if a sleep problem is related to a situational crisis or emotional problem, refer the patient to a mental health clinical nurse specialist or clinical psychologist for counseling. If the nurse works in an inpatient setting and the patient needs a referral for continued care after discharge, offering information about the sleep problem is useful to the home care nurse. The success of sleep therapy depends on an approach that fits the patient's lifestyle and the nature of the sleep disorder.

Knowledge
- Role other health professionals provide for sleep therapy
- Evidence- and practice-based sleep therapies
- Adult learning principles to apply when teaching the patient and family

Experience
- Previous patient responses to planned nursing interventions for promoting sleep
- Previous experience in adapting sleep therapies to personal needs

PLANNING
- Select nursing interventions that will promote sleep in the home/health care setting
- Involve sleep partner as needed in the selection of interventions
- Consult with health professionals as needed

Standards
- Individualize sleep therapies to the patient's lifestyle and preferences
- Apply intellectual standards (e.g., relevance, completeness, and significance) when choosing sleep therapies

Attitudes
- Display confidence when selecting interventions for the patient
- Be disciplined in planning therapies; it may take time to achieve desired results
- Be creative when adapting sleep therapies to the patient's daily schedule

FIG. 43.3 Critical thinking model for sleep planning.

REFLECT NOW

Analyze the results of your sleep quality using one of the instruments described in the assessment section. Based on the results, develop one goal and two outcomes for yourself that focus on improving your sleep quality or sleep hygiene habits.

CONCEPT MAP

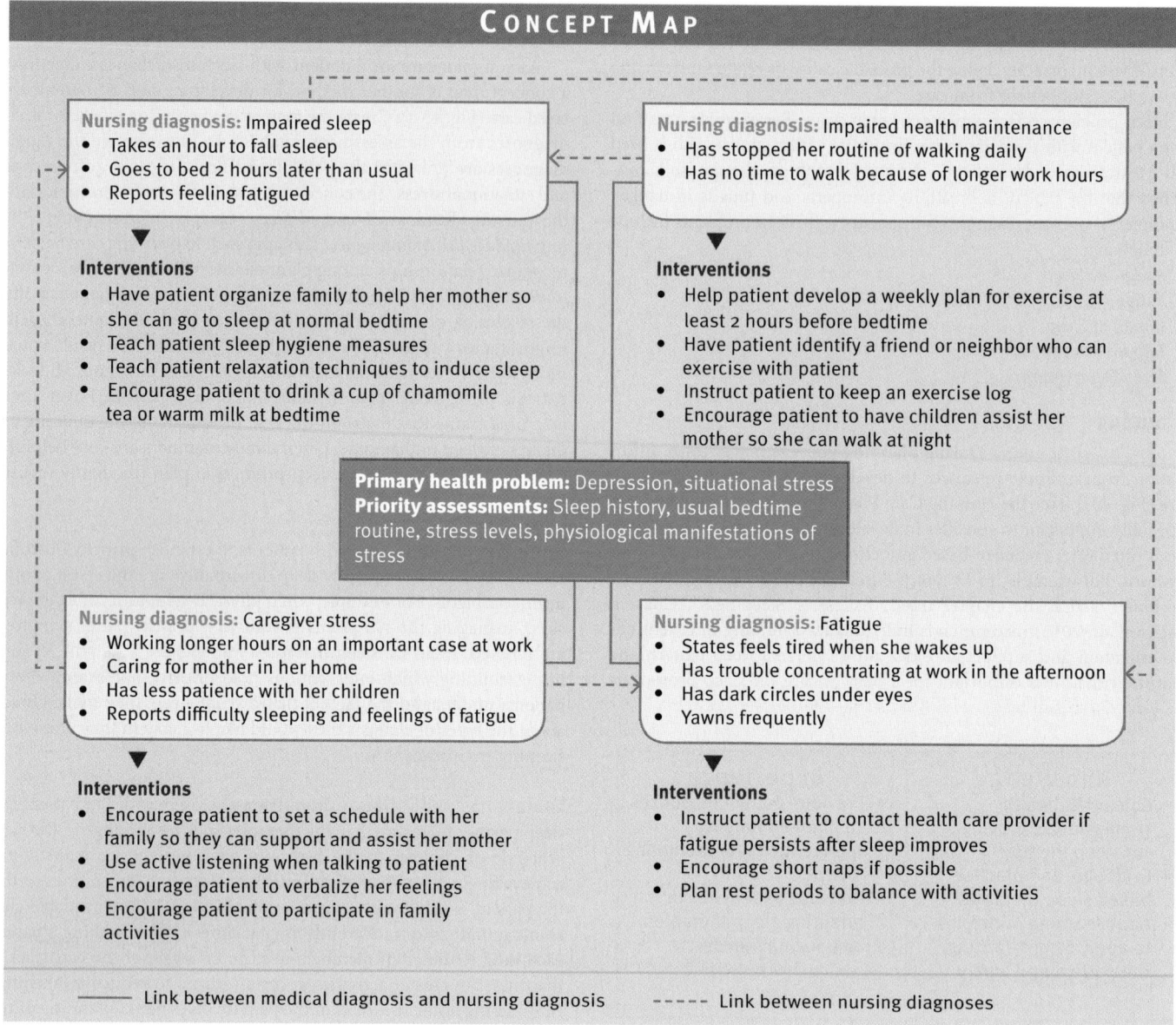

Nursing diagnosis: Impaired sleep
- Takes an hour to fall asleep
- Goes to bed 2 hours later than usual
- Reports feeling fatigued

Interventions
- Have patient organize family to help her mother so she can go to sleep at normal bedtime
- Teach patient sleep hygiene measures
- Teach patient relaxation techniques to induce sleep
- Encourage patient to drink a cup of chamomile tea or warm milk at bedtime

Nursing diagnosis: Impaired health maintenance
- Has stopped her routine of walking daily
- Has no time to walk because of longer work hours

Interventions
- Help patient develop a weekly plan for exercise at least 2 hours before bedtime
- Have patient identify a friend or neighbor who can exercise with patient
- Instruct patient to keep an exercise log
- Encourage patient to have children assist her mother so she can walk at night

Primary health problem: Depression, situational stress
Priority assessments: Sleep history, usual bedtime routine, stress levels, physiological manifestations of stress

Nursing diagnosis: Caregiver stress
- Working longer hours on an important case at work
- Caring for mother in her home
- Has less patience with her children
- Reports difficulty sleeping and feelings of fatigue

Interventions
- Encourage patient to set a schedule with her family so they can support and assist her mother
- Use active listening when talking to patient
- Encourage patient to verbalize her feelings
- Encourage patient to participate in family activities

Nursing diagnosis: Fatigue
- States feels tired when she wakes up
- Has trouble concentrating at work in the afternoon
- Has dark circles under eyes
- Yawns frequently

Interventions
- Instruct patient to contact health care provider if fatigue persists after sleep improves
- Encourage short naps if possible
- Plan rest periods to balance with activities

—— Link between medical diagnosis and nursing diagnosis   - - - - Link between nursing diagnoses

FIG. 43.4 Concept map for Julie Arnold.

◆ Implementation

Nursing interventions designed to improve the quality of a person's rest and sleep are largely focused on health promotion. Patients need adequate sleep and rest to maintain active and productive lifestyles. During times of illness, rest and sleep promotion are important for recovery. Nursing care in an acute, restorative, or continuing care setting differs from that provided in a patient's home. The primary differences are in the environment and the nurse's ability to support normal rest and sleep habits. A patient's age also influences the types of therapies that are most effective. Box 43.8 provides principles for promoting sleep in older patients.

Health Promotion. In community health and home settings help patients develop behaviors conducive to rest and relaxation. To develop good sleep habits at home, patients and their bed partners need to learn techniques that promote sleep and the conditions that interfere with it (Kryger et al., 2017) (Box 43.9). Parents also learn how to promote good

sleep habits for their children. Patients benefit most from instructions based on information about their homes and lifestyles, such as which types of activities promote sleep when a person must work during the night shift or how to make the home environment more conducive to sleep. Patients are more likely to apply information that they find useful and valuable.

Environmental Controls. All patients require a sleeping environment with a comfortable room temperature and proper ventilation, minimal sources of noise, a comfortable bed, and proper lighting (Patel et al., 2018). Children and adults vary more in regard to comfortable room temperature. Instruct parents to place infants on matresses that are covered by a fitted sheet that meets current safety standards; to clothe babies in sleepers for warmth; to not place pillows, quilts, toys, or anything in cribs; and to position cribs away from open windows or drafts (AAP, 2016; Gaw et al., 2017). Older adults often require extra blankets or covers.

NURSING CARE PLAN

Impaired Sleep

ASSESSMENT

Julie Arnold, a 43-year old attorney, is the first patient of the morning at the neighborhood health clinic where you work. When you ask her how she's doing, she tells you that she's having difficulty sleeping. Her health care provider has diagnosed that she's suffering from depression. Julie is married and has two school-age children. She also tells you that she is caring for her mother, who is staying with them after she was discharged from the hospital following an exacerbation of her heart failure.

Assessment Activities	Assessment Findings[a]
Ask Julie to explain the nature of her sleep problem.	Julie explains that she **wakes up once or twice a night.** She states, **"I feel tired when I wake up, and I have trouble concentrating at work in the afternoon."**
Ask Julie if there have been any recent changes in her life.	Julie reports that, because of her heavy work schedule, she has stopped her routine of walking 1 to 2 miles daily. She reports that she has no time for any exercise when she gets home because **she needs to take care of her mother and the children.**
Ask Julie to describe her bedtime routine.	Julie responds that she is **going to bed** between 12 AM and 1 AM, which is **2 hours later than her usual bedtime. It takes her an hour to fall asleep.** She says that she used to get 7 to 8 hours of sleep a night and now **it is more like 5 to 6 hours.** She drinks two to three cups of coffee after dinner while she is working on her case before bedtime.
Assess Julie for physical signs of sleep problems.	During the examination you note that Julie has dark circles under her eyes; she shifts her position in the chair multiple times and yawns frequently. She admits to **fatigue.**

[a]**Assessment findings** are shown in bold type.

NURSING DIAGNOSIS: Impaired Sleep

PLANNING

Goals	Expected Outcomes (NOC)[b] Sleep
Patient will achieve an improved sense of adequate sleep within 4 weeks.	Patient reports waking up less frequently during the night and feeling rested within 4 weeks. Patient verbalizes adherence to a regular bedtime routine within 4 weeks.

[b]Outcome classification labels from Moorhead S, et al: *Nursing outcomes classification (NOC)*, ed 6, St Louis, 2018, Elsevier.

INTERVENTIONS (NIC)[c] *Sleep Enhancement*	RATIONALE
Encourage patient to establish a bedtime routine and a regular sleep pattern.	Maintaining a consistent schedule helps induce sleep (Avidan and Neubauer, 2017).
Instruct patient to avoid caffeine and nicotine before bedtime.	Caffeine and nicotine are stimulants and cause difficulty in falling asleep.
Help patient identify ways to eliminate stressful concerns about work before bedtime (e.g., taking time before actual sleep to read a light novel).	Excess worry and intense activities before bedtime stimulate patient and prevent sleep (Taylor et al., 2017).
Adjust environment; have patient control noise, temperature, and light in the bedroom.	Creates an environment conducive to sleep (Patel et al., 2018).
Relaxation Therapy	
Teach patient how to perform muscle relaxation before bedtime; include demonstration.	Relaxation reduces anxiety, which interferes with sleep (National Sleep Foundation, 2018b; Patel et al., 2018).

[c]Intervention classification labels from Butcher HK, et al: *Nursing interventions classification (NIC)*, ed 7, St Louis, 2018, Elsevier.

EVALUATION

Evaluation Activity	Patient Response/Finding	Outcome Status
Ask Julie whether she is able to fall asleep and stay asleep.	Julie responds, "It usually takes 15 to 20 minutes to fall asleep; last week, on two separate nights, I only woke up once each night."	Julie reports fewer awakenings during night and falling asleep within 30 minutes.
Ask Julie to describe her waking behaviors at work and home during the day.	Julie responds that she has completed her case at work and feels less pressure. She has restarted her walking routine and is better able to cope with her children. She can concentrate at work more.	Julie reports feeling more rested.
Observe Julie's waking nonverbal expressions and behavior.	Julie sits in the chair without shifting position. She does not yawn during the conversation. The dark circles under her eyes are almost gone.	Julie's nonverbal behaviors are consistent with improved sleep.

BOX 43.8 FOCUS ON OLDER ADULTS
Promoting Sleep

Sleep-Wake Pattern
- Maintain a regular bedtime and wake-up schedule (Taylor et al., 2017).
- Eliminate naps unless they are a routine part of the schedule.
- If naps are taken, limit to 20 minutes or less twice a day (Touhy and Jett, 2018).
- Go to bed when sleepy.
- Use warm bath and relaxation techniques (Touhy and Jett, 2018).
- If unable to sleep in 15 to 30 minutes, do a relaxing activity such as reading (Haynes et al., 2018).
- Avoid stimulating activities such as exercise or watching television before bedtime (Chasens and Umlauf, 2012).

Environment
- Sleep where you sleep best.
- Keep noise to a minimum; use soft music to mask it if necessary.
- Use night-light and keep path to bathroom free of obstacles.
- Set room temperature to preference; use socks to promote warmth.
- Listen to relaxing music (Touhy and Jett, 2018).
- Sit in natural sunlight for two hours each morning if possible (Duzgun and Akyol, 2017).

Medications
- Use sedatives and hypnotics with caution as last resort and then only short term if absolutely necessary (Kryger et al., 2017).
- Adjust medications being taken for other conditions and assess for drug interactions that may cause insomnia or excessive daytime sleepiness.

Diet
- Limit alcohol, caffeine, and nicotine in late afternoon and evening (Touhy and Jett, 2018).
- Consume carbohydrates or milk as a light snack before bedtime (Touhy and Jett, 2018).
- Decrease fluids 2 to 4 hours before sleep (Touhy and Jett, 2018).

Physiological/Illness Factors
- Elevate head of bed and provide extra pillows as preferred.
- Use analgesics 30 minutes before bed to ease aches and pains.
- Use therapeutics to control symptoms of chronic conditions as prescribed (Chasens and Umlauf, 2012).

BOX 43.9 PATIENT TEACHING
Sleep-Hygiene Habits

Objective
- Patient will follow proper sleep-hygiene habits at home.

Teaching Strategies
- Instruct patient to try to exercise daily, preferably in the morning or afternoon, and to avoid vigorous exercise in the evening within 2 hours of bedtime.
- Caution patient against sleeping long hours during weekends or holidays to prevent disturbance of normal sleep-wake cycle.
- Explain that, if possible, patients should not use the bedroom for intensive studying, snacking, television watching, or other nonsleep activity besides sex.
- Encourage patients to try to avoid worrisome thinking when going to bed and to use relaxation exercises.
- If patient does not fall asleep within 30 minutes of going to bed, advise him or her to get out of bed and do some quiet activity until feeling sleepy enough to go back to bed.
- Recommend that patients limit caffeine to morning coffee and limit alcohol intake (more than one to two drinks a day interrupts sleep cycle).
- Recommend that patients discontinue use of electronic devices about 30 minutes before going to bed.
- Ask patient to examine environment. Instruct that use of earplugs and eye-shades may be helpful.
- Instruct patient to avoid heavy meals 3 hours before bedtime; a light snack may help.

Evaluation
Use the principles of teach-back to evaluate patient/family caregiver learning:
- "I want to be sure I explained the important information you need to include in your sleep-wake log. Explain the information you are going to include in your log for the next week."
- "Tell me about three of the approaches we planned to help you sleep at home."

and prevents falls when walking to the bathroom. If streetlights shine through windows or when patients nap during the day, heavy shades, drapes, or slatted blinds are helpful.

Avoid excessive use of smart phones, tablets, and computers in the bedroom. Electronic devices and some smart televisions emit a blue light that affects sleep and circadian rhythms in some patients (Gronil et al., 2016). These devices increase sleep deprivation in all age-groups, with the greatest impact in children and adolescents (Glauser, 2018). Encourage patients to not use their electronic devices in bed and, whenever possible, to discontinue use about 30 minutes before sleep.

Promoting Bedtime Routines. Bedtime routines and sleep-hygiene measures relax patients in preparation for sleep. It is always important for people to go to sleep when they feel tired or sleepy. Going to bed while fully awake and thinking about other things often causes insomnia and interferes with the bed as a stimulus for sleep. Newborns and infants sleep through so much of the day that a specific routine is hardly necessary. However, quiet activities such as holding them snugly in blankets, singing or talking softly, and gentle rocking help them fall asleep.

A bedtime routine (e.g., same hour for bedtime, snack, or quiet activity) used consistently helps young children avoid delaying sleep. Parents need to reinforce patterns of preparing for bedtime. Quiet activities such as reading stories, coloring, allowing children to sit in a parent's lap while listening to music or listening to a prayer are routines that are often associated with preparing for bed.

Eliminate distracting noise, so the bedroom is as quiet as possible. In the home the television, telephone, or intermittent chiming of a clock often disrupts a patient's sleep. Involve the family in identifying approaches for reducing noise in the home, especially if there are several family members, all with different sleep schedules. It is also important to remember that some patients sleep with familiar inside noises such as the hum of a fan. Some patients benefit from using commercial products that produce a soothing noise, such as the sounds of ocean waves or rainfall, to create an environment for sleep.

A bed and mattress need to provide support and comfortable firmness. Bed boards placed under mattresses add support. Sometimes extra pillows are important to help a person position comfortably in bed. The position of the bed in the room also makes a difference for some patients.

Patients vary in regard to the amount of light that they prefer at night. Infants and older adults sleep best in softly lit rooms. Light should not shine directly on their eyes. Small table lamps prevent total darkness. For older adults, light reduces the chance of confusion

Adults need to avoid excessive mental stimulation just before bedtime. Reading a light novel or listening to music helps a person relax. Relaxation exercises such as slow, deep breathing for 1 or 2 minutes relieve tension and prepare the body for rest (see Chapter 44). Guided imagery and praying also promote sleep for some patients.

At home discourage patients from trying to finish office work or resolve family problems before bedtime. The bedroom is not a place to work, and patients need to always associate it with sleep. Working toward a consistent time for sleep and awakening helps most patients gain a healthy sleep pattern and strengthens the rhythm of the sleep-wake cycle.

Promoting Safety. For any patient prone to confusion or falls, safety is critical. A small night-light helps a patient orient to the room environment before going to the bathroom. Beds set lower to the floor can lessen the chance of a person falling when first standing. Instruct patients to remove clutter and throw rugs from the path used to walk from the bed to the bathroom. If a patient needs help to ambulate from a bed to the bathroom, place a small bell at the bedside to call family members. Sleepwalkers are unaware of their surroundings and are slow to react, increasing the risk of falls. Do not startle sleepwalkers but instead gently wake them and lead them back to beds.

Infants' beds need to be safe. To reduce the chance of suffocation, do not place pillows, stuffed toys, or the ends of loose blankets in cribs (AAP, 2016). Loose-fitting plastic mattress covers are dangerous because infants pull them over their faces and suffocate.

Promoting Comfort. People fall asleep only after feeling comfortable and relaxed. Minor irritants often keep patients awake. Soft cotton nightclothes keep infants or small children warm and comfortable. Instruct patients to wear loose-fitting nightwear. An extra blanket is sometimes all that is necessary to prevent a person from feeling chilled and being unable to fall asleep. Patients need to void before going to bed so they are not kept awake by a full bladder.

Promoting Activity. In the home encourage patients to stay physically active during the day so that they are more likely to sleep at night. Increasing daytime activity lessens problems with falling asleep. Always plan rigorous exercise at least 2 to 3 hours before bedtime because exercise just before bed acts as a stimulant (Markwald et al., 2018). Research indicates that exercise is beneficial, particularly for older adults, to improve nighttime sleep. General recommendations include increasing daytime activity or exercise (Meiner and Yeager, 2019). However, older adults with chronic diseases that influence their functional abilities are likely to have limited activity (Touhy and Jett, 2018). Recommend activities that are safe for older patients to perform. Walking, swimming, wheelchair propulsion, and cycling on a stationary bike are excellent for patients with limited physical impairment. Weight lifting using light weights (e.g., 2 to 5 lb) builds upper body strength and endurance. Activity and exercise often prove to be beneficial by improving activity endurance, mobility, and sense of well-being.

Stress Reduction. The inability to sleep because of emotional stress also makes a person feel irritable and tense. When patients are emotionally upset, encourage them to try not to force sleep. Otherwise, insomnia frequently develops, and soon bedtime is associated with the inability to relax. Encourage a patient who has difficulty in falling asleep to get up and pursue a relaxing activity such as sewing or reading rather than staying in bed and thinking about sleep.

Preschoolers have bedtime fears (fear of the dark or strange noises), awaken during the night, or have nightmares. After nightmares encourage the parent to enter the child's room immediately and talk to the child briefly about fears to provide a cooling-down period. One approach is to comfort children and leave them in their own beds so that their fears are not used as excuses to delay bedtime. Keeping a light on in the room also helps some children. Cultural tradition causes

---

🌐 BOX 43.10 CULTURAL ASPECTS OF CARE

Co-sleeping/Bed-sharing

Practices and patterns of sleep and rest vary among cultures. Culture and biology influence the development of sleep problems in children. Sleep patterns, bedtime routines, sleep aids, and sleep arrangements are components of cultural practices related to the use of space and interaction distances (Giger, 2018). Traditionally experts recommend having infants and children sleep in their own beds. Co-sleeping or bed-sharing, in which infants and children sleep with their parents, is a culturally preferred habit that varies among cultures (Mileva-Seitz et al., 2016). In the United States, bed-sharing is more common in younger, less-educated, minority/ethnic mothers (Bombard et al., 2018). Reasons for bed-sharing practices relate to breastfeeding, comfort, tradition, better or more sleep, and protection for an infant (i.e., to protect against the cold) (Mileva-Seitz et al., 2016). Health care providers in the United States discourage it because of safety issues. One belief is that co-sleeping does not promote independence (Mileva-Seitz et al., 2016). Research results indicate that co-sleeping or bed-sharing is a risk factor for sudden infant death syndrome (SIDS) (Carlin and Moon, 2017). Research does not show that using a device to make bed-sharing safe reduces infant suffocation or SIDS (AAP, 2016). Bed-sharing is not recommended for infants who were born prematurely or with parents who use alcohol or drugs or smoke because of the increased risk for SIDS (Mitchell et al., 20107; Carlin and Moon, 2017). Bed-sharing is often related to infant sleep problems such as frequent awakenings, nighttime crying, increased time spent awake at night and less nighttime sleep (Mileva-Seitz et al., 2016; Mindell et al., 2017). As a nurse, be culturally sensitive when discussing co-sleeping practices with parents and developing sleeping plans for children.

Implications for Patient-Centered Care

- Complete a thorough sleep assessment of the child and family.
- Discuss the risks of co-sleeping with parents. During the discussion remain culturally sensitive and respectful of the parents' views (Mileva-Seitz et al., 2016).
- Instruct parents who practice co-sleeping to avoid using alcohol or drugs that impair arousal. Decreased arousal prevents the parents from waking if the child is having problems (Mitchell et al., 2017).
- Recommend to parents that they share a room but not the bed with their infant (Bombard et al., 2018).
- Encourage parents to use light sleeping clothes, to keep room temperature comfortable, and to avoid bundling the child tightly or in too many clothes.
- Remove pillows and blankets from the infant's bed (Gaw et al., 2017).

---

families to approach sleep practices differently (Box 43.10). Always respect those practices that differ from traditional recommendations.

Bedtime Snacks. Some people enjoy bedtime snacks, whereas others cannot sleep after eating. A dairy product such as warm milk or cocoa that contains L-tryptophan is often helpful in promoting sleep. A full meal before bedtime often causes gastrointestinal upset or reflux and interferes with the ability to fall asleep.

Warn patients against drinking or eating foods high in sugar or with caffeine before bedtime. Coffee, tea, colas, and chocolate act as stimulants, causing a person to stay awake or to awaken throughout the night. Caffeinated foods and liquids and alcohol act as diuretics and cause a person to awaken in the night to void.

Infants require special measures to minimize nighttime awakenings for feeding. It is common for children to need middle-of-the-night bottle-feeding or breastfeeding. Hockenberry and Wilson (2019) recommend offering the last feeding as late as possible. Tell parents not to give infants bottles in bed.

QSEN **Building Competency in Evidence-Based Practice** At her annual checkup, Julie Arnold tells you that she continues to have trouble falling asleep, so she drinks 1 to 2 glasses of wine before bedtime to make her sleepy. Based on the current evidence, what is your best response?

Answers to QSEN Activities can be found on the Evolve website.

Pharmacological Approaches. Melatonin is a neurohormone produced in the brain that helps control circadian rhythms and promote sleep (Kryger et al., 2017). It is a popular nutritional supplement that is found to be helpful in improving sleep efficiency and decreasing nighttime awakenings. The recommended dose is 0.3 to 3 mg taken 2 hours before bedtime. Older adults who have decreased levels of melatonin find it beneficial as a sleep aid (Kryger et al., 2017). Short-term use of melatonin has been found to be safe, with mild side effects of nausea, headache, and dizziness being infrequent. A melatonin receptor agonist, such as ramelteon or tasimelteon, is well tolerated and appears to be effective in improving sleep by improving the circadian rhythm and shortening the time needed for sleep onset (Avidan and Neubauer, 2017; Patel et al., 2018). It is safe for long- and short-term use, particularly in older adults. Common side effects include diarrhea, drowsiness, tiredness and dizziness.

Several other herbal products help in sleep. Valerian is effective in mild insomnia and RLS. It affects the release of neurotransmitters and produces very mild sedation (WebMD, 2017). Lavender essential oil may improve sleep quality (O'Malley, 2017). Passionflower (maypop) has mild sedative effects and is used as a natural sleep aid (WebMD, 2017). Chamomile, an herbal tea, has a mild sedative effect that may be beneficial in promoting sleep (MacMillan, 2017). Caution patients about the dosage and use of herbal compounds because the US Food and Drug Administration (FDA) does not regulate them. Herbal compounds may interact with prescribed medications, and patients need to avoid using these together (Meiner and Yeager, 2019).

The use of nonprescription sleeping medications is inadvisable. Patients need to learn the risks of such drugs. Over the long term these drugs lead to further sleep disruption, even when they initially seemed effective. Caution older adults about using over-the-counter antihistamines because of their long duration of action, which can cause confusion, constipation, urinary retention, and an increased risk of falls (Avidan and Neubauer, 2017). Help patients use behavioral and proper sleep-hygiene measures to establish sleep patterns that do not require the use of drugs.

Acute Care.
Patients in acute care settings have their normal rest and sleep routine disrupted, which generally leads to sleep problems. In this setting nursing interventions focus on controlling factors in the environment that disrupt sleep, relieving physiological or psychological disruptions to sleep, and providing for uninterrupted rest and sleep periods for patients. "Excessive Sleepiness" in the *Evidence-based Geriatric Nursing Protocols for Best Practice* is based on the principle that nurses need to individualize an effective strategy based on patient needs and that sleep medications are a last-resort intervention (Chasens and Umlauf, 2012).

Environmental Controls. In a hospital you control the environment in several ways (Box 43.11). Close the curtains between patients in semiprivate rooms. Dim lights on a hospital nursing unit at night. One of the biggest problems for patients in the hospital is noise. Important ways to reduce noise are to conduct conversations and reports in a private area away from patient rooms and to keep necessary conversations to a minimum, especially at night (Flynn Makic et al., 2014). Provide patients with ear plugs or eye masks to decrease noise and light stimulation (Caple and March, 2016; Litton et al., 2016). Additional ways to control noise in the hospital are listed in Box 43.12.

BOX 43.11 EVIDENCE-BASED PRACTICE
Sleep Hygiene in Hospitalized Patients

PICOT Question: Does the use of a sleep-hygiene protocol versus routine care in patients in the intensive care unit decrease delirium related to decreased sleep?

Evidence Summary

Sleep disruption commonly occurs in patients in the intensive care unit because of disruption of normal routines, anxiety and stress, noise, pain, medical treatments, and environmental factors (Martinez et al., 2017; Owens et al., 2017). Sleep deprivation impacts physical and psychological healing and often causes delirium (Flannery et al., 2016). Implementation of nurse-driven sleep-hygiene protocols has been shown to be effective in improving sleep in patients in the intensive care unit (Martinez et al., 2017; Smithburger et al., 2017). Effective strategies in the protocols focused on education of staff nurses on protocol and interventions to decrease environmental stimuli and limit patient disruptions, pain management, avoidance of the use of restraints, early mobility, and family involvement (Martinez et al., 2017; Smithburger et al., 2017). Implementing these strategies improved patient sleep and decreased delirium (Flannery et al., 2016; Martinez et al., 2017).

Application to Nursing Practice

- Work with nurses on the unit to develop a sleep-hygiene protocol.
- Cluster nursing activities to provide uninterrupted periods of sleep (Martinez et al., 2017).
- Provide early physical therapy and mobility for patients (Hayhurst et al., 2016; Martinez et al., 2017).
- Reduce lighting, telephone volumes, and staff conversations in the halls during quiet time and nighttime (Martinez et al., 2017).
- Use sleep-hygiene measures with patients such as personal hygiene, adjusting room temperature, and relaxation methods.
- Educate and involve family in implementing strategies (Smithburger et al., 2017).

Promoting Comfort. Make the patient more comfortable by providing personal hygiene before bedtime. A warm bath or shower is very relaxing. Offer patients restricted to bed the opportunity to wash their face and hands. Tooth brushing and care of dentures also help to prepare the patient for sleep. Have patients void before going to bed so that they are not kept awake by a full bladder. While a patient prepares for bed, help to position him or her off any potential pressure sites (Fig. 43.5). Offering a back rub or massage helps relax the patient.

Removal of irritating stimuli is another way to improve the patient's comfort for a restful sleep. Changing or removing moist dressings, repositioning drainage tubing, reapplying wrinkled thromboembolic hose, and changing tape on nasogastric tubes eliminate constant irritants to the patient's skin. Cleanse the perineal or anal area thoroughly for patients who are incontinent. Patients who are diaphoretic benefit from a cool bath and dry clothes or linens.

Establishing Periods of Rest and Sleep. In a hospital or extended-care setting it is difficult to provide patients with the time needed to rest and sleep. The most effective treatment for sleep disturbances is to eliminate factors that disrupt the sleep pattern. You need to plan care to avoid waking patients for nonessential tasks. Do this by scheduling assessments, treatments, procedures, and routines for times when patients are awake. For example, if a patient's physical condition has been stable, avoid waking him or her to check vital signs, unless ordered. Allowing patients to determine the timing and methods of delivery of basic care measures promotes rest. Do not give baths and routine hygiene measures during the night for nursing convenience.

BOX 43.12 Control of Noise in the Hospital

- Close doors to patients' room when possible.
- Keep doors to work areas on unit closed when in use.
- Reduce volume of nearby telephone and paging equipment.
- Wear rubber-soled shoes. Avoid clogs.
- Turn off bedside oxygen and other equipment that is not in use.
- Turn down alarms and beeps on bedside monitoring equipment.
- Turn off room television and radio unless patient prefers soft music.
- Avoid abrupt loud noise such as flushing a toilet or moving a bed.
- Keep necessary conversations at low levels, particularly at night.
- Designate a time period during the day for "quiet time" for patients.

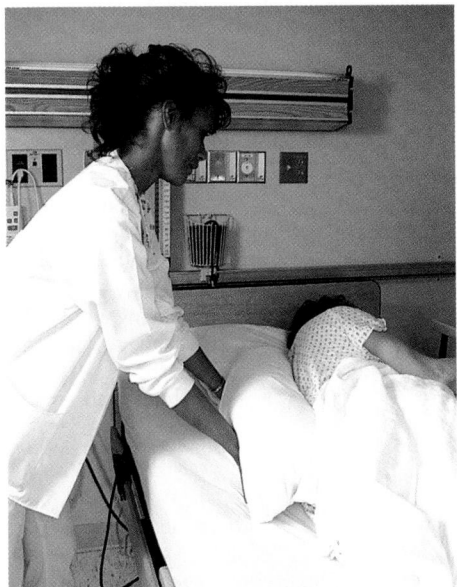

FIG. 43.5 Positioning patient for sleep.

Draw blood samples at a time when the patient is awake. Unless maintaining the therapeutic blood level of a drug is essential, give medications during waking hours. Work with the radiology department and other support services to schedule diagnostic studies and therapies at intervals that allow patients time for rest. Always try to provide the patient with 2 to 3 hours of uninterrupted sleep during the night.

When the patient's condition demands more frequent monitoring, plan activities to allow extended rest periods. A nurse instructs assistive personnel in the coordination of patient care to reduce patient disturbances. This means planning activities so that the patient has as long as an hour or more to rest quietly rather than having a nurse or other personnel return to the room every few minutes. For example, if a patient needs frequent dressing changes, is receiving intravenous therapy, and has drainage tubes from several sites, do not make a separate trip into the room to check each problem. Instead use a single visit to perform all three tasks. Become the patient's advocate for promoting optimal sleep. This means becoming a gatekeeper by postponing or rescheduling visits by family or by questioning the frequency of certain procedures.

Promoting Safety. Patients with OSA are at risk for complications while in the hospital. Surgery and anesthesia disrupt normal sleep patterns (see Chapter 50). After surgery patients reach deep levels of REM sleep. This deep sleep causes muscle relaxation that leads to OSA. Patients with OSA who are given opioid analgesics after surgery have an increased risk of developing airway obstruction because the medications suppress normal arousal mechanisms. These patients often need ventilator support in the postoperative period because of the increased risk of respiratory complications. Monitor the patient's airway, respiratory rate and depth, and breath sounds frequently after surgery.

Recommend lifestyle changes to patients with OSA, changes such as sleep hygiene, alcohol moderation, smoking cessation, and a weight-loss program (McNicholas, 2017). Teach the patient to elevate the head of the bed and use a side or prone position for sleep. Use pillows to prevent a supine position.

If patients normally use a continuous positive airway pressure (CPAP) machine at home because of sleep apnea, it is important that they bring their home equipment with them to the hospital and use it every night. Check to make sure the mask fits snugly and is put on correctly so that the positive pressure is maintained (Schub, 2016). In patients with sleep apnea who have surgery and receive general anesthesia, the anesthesia in combination with pain medications used after surgery reduces the patient's defenses against airway obstruction. After surgery the patient achieves very deep levels of REM sleep that lead to muscle relaxation and airway obstruction. Use pain medication carefully in these patients. These patients need ventilator support in the postoperative period because OSA is linked to increased postoperative respiratory complications. Monitor the patient's breathing and oxygen saturation levels regularly (see Chapter 29). Notify the health care provider right away if the patient is difficult to arouse or is having trouble breathing.

Patients who experience EDS can fall asleep while sitting up in a chair or wheelchair. Position patients so that they do not fall out of the chair when sleeping. Elevating their feet on an ottoman or small bench may help to position them safely. A pillow placed in the patient's lap offers some support. If a patient enjoys leaning over an over-bed table while sitting in a chair, be sure that the table is locked and secure. Do not use safety belts because they are considered restraints (see Chapter 27).

Stress Reduction. Patients who are hospitalized for extensive diagnostic testing often have difficulty resting or sleeping because of uncertainty about their health. Giving patients control over their health care minimizes uncertainty and anxiety. Providing information about the purpose of procedures and routines and answering questions gives patients the peace of mind needed to rest or fall asleep. Take time to sit and talk with your patients who are unable to sleep to determine the factors keeping them awake. Providing comfort measures such as back rubs also help patients relax more thoroughly. If a sedative is indicated, confer with the patient's health care provider to be sure that the lowest dose is used initially. Discontinuing a sedative as soon as possible prevents a dependence that seriously disrupts the normal sleep cycle. Older adults' metabolism of drugs is slow, making them more vulnerable to the side effects of sedatives, hypnotics, antianxiety drugs, or analgesics.

Restorative or Continuing Care. The nursing interventions implemented in the acute care setting are also used in the restorative or continuing care environment. Controlling the environment, especially noise; establishing periods of rest and sleep; and promoting comfort are important considerations. Nursing interventions related to stress reduction and controlling physiological disturbances are also implemented in these settings. Helping a patient achieve restful sleep in this environment sometimes takes time.

Maintaining Activity. Limit the time residents spend in bed whenever possible. In long-term care settings, serve meals in the resident dining area. Make sure residents are up in a chair for meals and for personal hygiene activities. It is also important to keep the residents involved in planned social activities (e.g., card playing or arts and crafts). Regular exercise keeps people active and stimulated. It is also ideal to limit daytime napping to 30 minutes or less. Short naps taken in the midafternoon increase alertness and cognitive ability. Research has shown that exposure to natural sunlight for 2 hours a day improved the sleep quality of residents in a nursing home (Duzgun and Akyol, 2017).

Residents with dementia often have disrupted sleep-wake cycles. They often become easily fatigued and experience periods of insomnia (Meiner and Yeager, 2019). In this situation shorten activities and visits to allow patients to maintain an adequate energy level. If a patient wakes up during the night, keeping the lights at a low level and using soothing techniques such as quiet music or a back rub promote returning to sleep.

Controlling Physiological Disturbances. As a nurse you learn to control symptoms of physical illness that disrupt sleep. For example, a patient with respiratory abnormalities sleeps with two pillows or in a semi-sitting position to ease the effort to breathe. He or she benefits from taking prescribed bronchodilators before sleep to prevent airway obstruction. A patient with a hiatal hernia also needs special care. After meals he or she often experiences a burning sensation as a result of gastric reflux. To prevent sleep disturbances, have the patient eat a small meal several hours before bedtime and sleep in a semi-sitting position. Time medications to relieve pain, nausea, or other recurrent symptoms so that the drug takes effect at bedtime. Remove or change any irritants against the patient's skin such as moist dressings or drainage tubes.

Pharmacological Approaches. The liberal use of drugs to manage insomnia is quite common in American culture. CNS stimulants such as amphetamines, caffeine, nicotine, terbutaline, theophylline, and modafinil need to be used sparingly and under medical management (Burchum and Rosenthal, 2019). In addition, withdrawal from CNS depressants such as alcohol, barbiturates, tricyclic antidepressants (amitriptyline, imipramine, and doxepin), and triazolam causes insomnia. Consult with pharmacists and health care providers about managing doses.

Medications that induce sleep are called **hypnotics**. **Sedatives** are medications that produce a calming or soothing effect (Burchum and Rosenthal, 2019). A patient who takes sleep medications needs to know about their proper use and their risks and possible side effects. Long-term use of antianxiety, sedative, or hypnotic agents disrupts sleep and leads to more serious problems. The FDA requires that the product labels of all sleep medications contain safety information related to the potential adverse effects of severe allergic reactions; severe facial swelling; and complex sleep behaviors such as sleep-driving, making phone calls, and preparing and eating food while asleep (USFDA, 2018).

Benzodiazepines and benzodiazepine-like drugs are commonly used to treat sleep problems and are intended for short-term use (Avidan and Neubauer, 2017). The benzodiazepine-like drugs are the treatment of choice for insomnia because of improved efficacy and safety of use (Burchum and Rosenthal, 2019). Experts recommend a low dose of a short-acting medication such as zolpidem (Ambien) for short-term use (no longer than 2 to 3 weeks) (Burchum and Rosenthal, 2019). These drugs cause fewer problems with dependence and abuse and fewer rebound insomnia and hangover effects than benzodiazepines.

The benzodiazepines cause relaxation, antianxiety, and hypnotic effects by facilitating the action of neurons in the CNS that suppress responsiveness to stimulation, thereby decreasing levels of arousal (Burchum and Rosenthal, 2019). Short-acting benzodiazepines (e.g., oxazepam, lorazepam, or temazepam) at the lowest possible dose for short-term treatment of insomnia are recommended. Initial doses are small, and increments are added gradually, based on patient response, for a limited time. Warn patients not to take more than the prescribed dose, especially if the medication seems to become less effective after initial use. The use of benzodiazepines in older adults is potentially dangerous because of the tendency of the drugs to remain active in the body for a longer time. As a result, they also cause respiratory depression; next-day sedation; amnesia; rebound insomnia; and impaired motor functioning and coordination, which leads to an increased risk

Knowledge	Experience
• Characteristics of desirable sleep pattern • Behaviors reflecting adequate sleep	• Previous patient responses to planned nursing interventions for promoting sleep • Previous experience in adapting sleep therapies to personal needs

EVALUATION
• Evaluate signs and symptoms of the patient's sleep disturbance
• Review the patient's sleep pattern
• Ask the patient's sleep partner to report the patient's response to sleep therapies
• Ask the patient whether expectations of care are being met

Standards	Attitudes
• Use established expected outcomes to evaluate the patient's response to care (e.g., improved duration of sleep, fewer awakenings)	• Demonstrate humility if an intervention is unsuccessful; rethink your approach • Display perseverance in staying with a plan or in trying new approaches in the case of chronic sleep problems

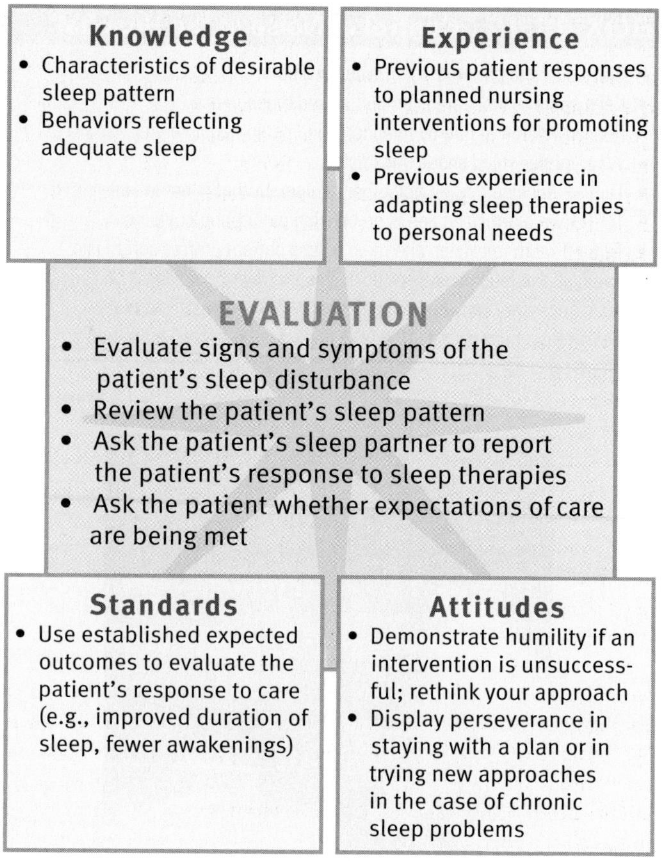

FIG. 43.6 Critical thinking model for sleep evaluation.

of falls (Picton et al., 2018). If older patients who were recently continent, ambulatory, and alert become incontinent or confused and/or demonstrate impaired mobility, the use of benzodiazepines needs to be considered as a possible cause.

Administer benzodiazepines cautiously to children under 12 years of age. These medications are contraindicated in infants less than 6 months old. Patients who are pregnant need to avoid them because their use is associated with risk of congenital anomalies. Mothers who are breastfeeding do not receive the drugs because they are excreted in breast milk. Raise these issues with patients' health care providers if you are concerned about the safety of a prescribed medication.

Trazodone is a serotonin antagonist and reuptake inhibitor (SARI) antidepressant often used in patients with depression or anxiety and insomnia. The most common side effects are daytime grogginess and orthostatic hypotension. Low-dose trazodone is often used as an alternative to benzodiazepines, especially in older patients.

Regular use of any sleep medication often leads to tolerance and withdrawal. Rebound insomnia is a problem after stopping a medication, particularly the benzodiazepines (Avidan and Neubauer, 2017). Immediately administering a sleeping medication when a hospitalized patient complains of being unable to sleep does the patient more harm than good. Consider alternative approaches to promote sleep first. Routine monitoring of patient response to sleeping medications is important.

◆ **Evaluation**

Through the Patient's Eyes. The patient is the source for evaluating whether expectations about sleep are met. Each patient has a unique need for sleep and rest. He or she is the only one who knows whether sleep problems are improved and which interventions or therapies are most successful in promoting sleep (Fig. 43.6). It is important to ask the patient if his or her sleep needs have been met. For example, ask the patient, "Are you feeling more rested?" or "Can you tell me if you believe that we've done all we can to help improve your sleep?" or "Which interventions have been most effective in helping you sleep?" If expectations have not been met, you need to spend more time trying to understand the patient's needs and preferences. Working closely with the patient and bed partner enables you to redefine expectations that can be met realistically within the limits of the patient's condition and treatment.

Patient Outcomes. To evaluate the effectiveness of your nursing care, make comparisons with baseline assessment data to evaluate whether your patient's sleep has improved. Determine whether expected outcomes have been met. Use evaluative measures shortly after a therapy has been implemented (e.g., observing whether a patient falls asleep after reducing noise and darkening a room). Use other evaluative measures after a patient wakes from sleep (e.g., asking him or her to describe the number of awakenings during the previous night). The patient and bed partner usually provide accurate evaluative information. Over longer periods use assessment tools such as the visual analog or sleep-rating scale to determine whether sleep has progressively improved or changed.

Also evaluate the level of understanding that patients or family caregivers gain after receiving instruction in sleep habits. You measure adherence to these practices during a home visit, when you are able to observe the environment. When expected outcomes are not met, revise the nursing measures or expected outcomes based on the patient's needs or preferences. When outcomes are not met, ask questions such as:

- Are you able to fall asleep within 20 minutes of getting in bed?
- Describe how well you sleep when you exercise.
- Does the use of quiet music at bedtime help you to relax?
- Do you feel rested when you wake up?

If you have successfully developed a good relationship with a patient and a therapeutic plan of care, subtle behaviors often indicate the level of the patient's satisfaction. Note the absence of signs of sleep problems such as lethargy, frequent yawning, or position changes in the patient. You are effective in promoting rest and sleep if the patient's goals and expectations are met.

KEY POINTS

- The 24-hour sleep-wake cycle is a circadian rhythm that influences physiological function and behavior.
- The control and regulation of sleep depend on a balance among regulators within the CNS.
- During a typical night's sleep, a person passes through four to five complete sleep cycles. Each sleep cycle contains three NREM stages of sleep and a period of REM sleep; time in each stage varies.
- Sleep provides physiological and psychological restoration.
- Sleep requirements vary by age, with neonates sleeping on average 16 hours a day and older adults needing 7 to 8 hours of sleep a night.
- The hectic pace of a person's lifestyle, emotional and psychological stress, and alcohol ingestion frequently disrupt the sleep pattern.
- An environment with a darkened room, reduced noise, comfortable bed, and good ventilation promotes sleep.
- A regular bedtime routine of relaxing activities prepares a person physically and mentally for sleep.
- The most common type of sleep disorder is insomnia. Characteristics of insomnia include the inability to fall asleep, to remain asleep during the night, or to go back to sleep after waking up earlier than desired.

- If a patient's sleep is adequate, assess his or her usual bedtime, normal bedtime ritual, preferred environment for sleeping, and usual preferred rising time.
- When planning interventions to promote sleep, consider the usual characteristics of the patient's home environment and normal lifestyle.
- Important nursing interventions for promoting sleep in the hospitalized patient are to establish periods for uninterrupted sleep and rest and to control noise levels.
- Use your patient's self-report to determine whether sleep was restful.

REFLECTIVE LEARNING

- Reflect on your own sleep hygiene practices. What changes can you make to improve your sleep practices?
- Ask your patient about his or her sleep quality since being in the hospital. How has your patient's sleep been affected?
- Working with two to three of your peers, develop a program on improving sleep for students in college. Offer the program on your campus.

REVIEW QUESTIONS

1. A nurse is developing a plan for a patient who was diagnosed with narcolepsy. Which interventions should the nurse include on the plan? (Select all that apply.)
   1. Take brief, 20-minute naps no more than twice a day.
   2. Drink a glass of wine with dinner.
   3. Eat a large meal at lunch rather than dinner.
   4. Establish a regular exercise program.
   5. Teach the patient about the side effects of modafinil.
2. Which statements from a patient indicate an understanding of behaviors that will promote sleep? (Select all that apply.)
   1. "I will not watch television in bed."
   2. "I will not drink caffeine later in the day."
   3. "A short nap late in the evening will lead to a more restful night of sleep."
   4. "I am going to start eating dinner closer to my bedtime"
   5. "I will start to exercise regularly during the day."
3. A 72-year-old patient asks the nurse about using an over-the-counter antihistamine as a sleeping pill to help her get to sleep. What is the nurse's best response?
   1. "Antihistamines are better than prescription medications because prescription medications can cause a lot of problems."
   2. "Antihistamines should not be used because they can cause confusion and increase your risk of falls."
   3. "Antihistamines are effective sleep aids because they do not have many side effects."
   4. "Over-the-counter medications when combined with sleep-hygiene measures are a good plan for sleep."
4. Which nursing intervention(s) best promote(s) effective sleep in an older adult? (Select all that apply.)
   1. Limit fluids 2 to 4 hours before sleep.
   2. Ensure that the room is completely dark.
   3. Ensure that the room temperature is comfortably cool.
   4. Provide warm covers.
   5. Encourage walking an hour before going to bed.
5. Which statement made by the patient indicates an understanding of sleep-hygiene practices?
   1. "I usually drink a cup of warm milk in the evening to help me sleep."

2. "If I exercise right before bedtime, I will be tired and fall asleep faster."

3. "I know it does not matter what time I go to bed as long as I am tired."

4. "If I use hypnotics for a long time, my insomnia will be cured."

6. Which nursing interventions are appropriate to include in a plan of care to promote sleep for patients who are hospitalized? (Select all that apply.)

1. Give patients a cup of coffee 1 hour before bedtime.
2. Plan vital signs to be taken before the patients are asleep.
3. Turn television on 15 minutes before bedtime.
4. Have patients follow at-home bedtime schedule.
5. Close the door to patients' rooms at bedtime.

7. The nurse is contacting the health care provider about a patient's sleep problem. Place the steps of the SBAR (situation, background, assessment, recommendation) in the correct order.

1. Mrs. Dodd, 46 years old, was admitted 3 days ago following a motor vehicle accident. She is in balanced skeletal traction for a fractured left femur. She is having difficulty falling asleep.

2. "Dr. Smithson, this is Pam, the nurse caring for Mrs. Dodd. I'm calling because Mrs. Dodd is having difficulty sleeping."

3. "I'm calling to ask if you would order a hypnotic such as zolpidem to use on a prn basis."

4. Mrs. Dodd is taking her pain medication every 4 hours as ordered and rates her pain as 2 out of 10. Last night she was still awake at 0100. She states that she is comfortable but just can't fall asleep. Her vital signs are BP 124/76, P 78, R 12 and T 37.1°C (98.8°F).

8. Which statement made by a mother being discharged to home with her newborn infant indicates that she understands the discharge teaching related to best sleep practices?

1. "I'll give the baby a bottle to help her fall asleep."
2. "We'll place the baby on her back to sleep."
3. "We put the baby's stuffed animals in the crib to make her feel safe."
4. "I know the baby will not need to be fed until morning."

9. A nurse is taking a sleep history from a patient. Which statement made by the patient needs further follow-up?

1. "I feel refreshed when I wake up in the morning."
2. "I use soft music at night to help me relax."
3. "It takes me about 45 to 60 minutes to fall asleep."
4. "I take the pain medication for my leg pain about 30 minutes before I go to bed."

10. Which sleep-hygiene actions at bedtime can the nurse delegate to assistive personnel? (Select all that apply.)

1. Giving the patient a back rub
2. Turning on quiet music
3. Dimming the lights in the patient's room
4. Giving a patient a cup of coffee
5. Monitoring for the effect of the sleeping medication that was given

Answers: 1. 1, 4, 5; **2.** 1, 2, 5; **3.** 2, 4; **4.** 1, 3, 4, 5; **5.** 1; **6.** 2, 4, 5; **7.** 2, 1, 4, 3; **8.** 2; **9.** 3; **10.** 1, 2, 3.

Rationales for Review Questions can be found on the Evolve website.

REFERENCES

Adams SK, et al.: Technology as a tool to encourage young adults to sleep and eat healthy, *ACSM's Health Fit J* 21(4):4, 2017.

American Academy of Pediatrics: *SIDS and other sleep-related infant deaths: updated 2016 recommendations for a safe infant sleeping environment*, 2016. http://pediatrics.aappublications.org/content/138/5/e20162938. Accessed July 29, 2018.

American Nurses Association: *Nursing scope and standards of practice*, Washington, DC, 2015, American Nurses Association.

American Sleep Association: *Sleep and sleep disorder statistics*, 2018. https://www.sleepassociation.org/about-sleep/sleep-statistics/. Accessed July 29, 2018.

Avidan AY, Neubauer DN: Chronic insomnia disorder, *Continuum (Minneap Minn)* 23(4):1064, 2017.

Badin E, et al.: Insomnia: the sleeping giant of pediatric public health, *Curr Psychiatry Rep* 18(5):47, 2016.

Bruce ES, et al.: Sleep in adolescents and young adults, *Clin Med (Lond)* 17(5):424, 2017.

Burchum JR, Rosenthal LD: *Lehne's pharmacology for nurses*, ed 10, St Louis, 2019, Elsevier.

Caple C, March P: *Evidence-based care sheet: sleep and hospitalization*, CINAHL Nursing Guide, Cinahl Information Systems, May 20, 2016.

Chasens ER, Umlauf MG: Excessive sleepiness. In Boltz M, et al.: *Evidence-based geriatric nursing protocols for best practice*, ed 4, New York, 2012, Springer.

Dauvilliers Y, Brateau L: Narcolepsy and other central hypersomnias, *Continuum (Minneap Minn)* 23(4):989, 2017.

Erwin AM: Sleep during pregnancy, *Nursing made incredibly easy!* 15(1):15, 2017.

Giger JN: *Transcultural nursing: assessment and intervention*, ed 7, St Louis, 2018, Elsevier.

Glauser W: Overscheduled and glued to screens: children are sleeping less than ever before, *CMAJ* 190(48):E1428, 2018.

Hayhurst CJ, et al.: Intensive care unit delirium: a review of diagnosis, prevention, and treatment, *Anesthesiology* 125(6):1229, 2016.

Haynes J, et al.: Cognitive behavioral therapy in the treatment of insomnia, *South Med J* 111(20):75, 2018.

Hockenberry MJ, Wilson D: *Wong's nursing care of infants and children*, ed 11, St Louis, 2019, Elsevier.

Huether SE, et al.: *Understanding pathophysiology*, ed 6, St Louis, 2017, Elsevier.

Johns M: About the ESS, *n.d.* http://epworthsleepinessscale.com/about-the-ess/. Accessed July 29, 2018.

Kryger MH, et al.: *Principles and practice of sleep medicine*, ed 6, St Louis, 2017, Elsevier.

Liu Y, et al.: Prevalence of healthy sleep duration among adults: United States, 2014, *MMWR* 65(6):1, 2016.

Lorenz CP, Williams AJ: Sleep apps: what role do they play in clinical medicine? *Curr Opin Pulm Med* 23(6):512, 2017.

MacMillan A: *6 science-backed sleep remedies*, 2017. http://time.com/4732464/natural-sleep-remedies-insomnia/. Accessed July 29, 2018.

Markwald RR, et al.: Behavioral strategies, including exercise, for addressing insomnia, *ACSM's Health Fit J* 22(2):23, 2018.

Maski K, Owens J: Pediatric sleep disorders, *Continuum (Minneap Minn)* 24(1):210, 2018.

Meiner SE, Yeager JJ: *Gerontologic nursing*, ed 6, St Louis, 2019, Mosby.

National Sleep Foundation: *Aging and sleep*, 2018a, Washington, DC. http://www.sleepfoundation.org/article/sleep-topics/aging-and-sleep. Accessed July 29, 2018.

National Sleep Foundation: *Depression and sleep*, 2018b. https://www.sleepfoundation.org/articles/depression-and-sleep. Accessed July 29, 2018.

National Sleep Foundation: *National Sleep Foundation's 2018 Sleep in America® poll shows Americans failing to prioritize sleep*, 2018c, Washington, DC. https://www.sleepfoundation.org/media-center/press-release/2018-sleep-in-america-poll-shows. Accessed July 29, 2018.

National Sleep Foundation: *How much sleep do we really need?*, 2018d, Washington, DC. https://www.sleepfoundation.org/articles/how-much-sleep-do-we-really-need. Accessed July 29, 2018.

O'Malley PA: Lavender for sleep, rest, and pain: evidence for practice and research, *Clin Nurse Spec* 31(2):74, 2017.

Owens RL, et al.: Sleep in the intensive care unit in a model of family-centered care, *AACN Adv Crit Care* 28(2):171, 2017.

Parekh PJ, et al.: The effects of sleep on the commensal microbiota: eyes wide open? *J Clin Gastroenterol* 52(3):204, 2018.

Picton JD, et al.: Benzodiazepine use and cognitive decline in the elderly, *Am J Health Syst Pharm* 75(1):e6, 2018.

Rizek P, Kumar J: Restless legs syndrome, *CMAJ* 189(6):E245, 2017.

Sateia MJ, et al.: Clinical practice guideline for the pharmacologic treatment of chronic insomnia in adults: an American Academy of Sleep Medicine clinical practice guideline, *J Clin Sleep Med* 13(2):307, 2017.

Schub T: *Obstructive sleep apnea in adults*, CINAHL Nursing Guide, Cinahl Information Systems, June 3, 2016.

Taylor K, et al.: A nonpharmacologic approach to managing insomnia in primary care, *JAAPA* 30(11):10, 2017.

Touhy TA, Jett KF: *Ebersole and Hess' gerontological nursing healthy aging*, ed 5, St Louis, 2018, Elsevier.

Trauer JM, et al.: Cognitive behavioral therapy for chronic insomnia, *Ann Intern Med* 163(3):191, 2015.

US Food and Drug Administration (USFDA): *Sleep problems*, 2018. https://www.fda.gov/forconsumers/b-
yaudience/forwomen/ucm118563.htm. Accessed July 29, 2018.

WebMD: *Natural sleep aids and remedies*, 2017. https://www.webmd.com/women/natural-sleep-remedies#1. Accessed July 29, 2018.

RESEARCH REFERENCES

Bombard JM, et al.: Vital signs: trends and disparities in infant safe sleep practices, United States, 2009-2015, *MMWR Morb Mortal Wkly Rep* 67(1):39, 2018.

Carlin RF, Moon RY: Risk factors, protective factors, and current recommendations to reduce sudden infant death syndrome: a review, *JAMA Pediatr* 171(2):175, 2017.

Campos-Rodriguez F, et al.: Continuous positive airway pressure improves quality of life in women with obstructive sleep apnea: a randomized controlled trial, *Am J Respir Crit Care Med* 194(10):1286, 2016.

Chung F, et al.: STOP-Bang questionnaire: a practical approach to screen for obstructive sleep apnea, *Chest* 149(3):631, 2016.

Chung KF, et al.: Sleep hygiene education as a treatment of insomnia: a systematic review and meta-analysis, *Fam Pract* 35(4):1, 2017.

Duzgun G, Akyol AD: Effect of natural sunlight on sleep problems and sleep quality of the elderly staying in the nursing home, *Holist Nurs Pract* 31(5):295, 2017.

Flannery AH, et al.: The impact of interventions to improve sleep on delirium in the ICU: a systematic review and research framework, *Crit Care Med* 44(12):2231, 2016.

Flynn Makic MB, et al.: Examining the evidence to guide practice: challenging practice habits, *Crit Care Nurse* 34(2):28, 2014.

Gaw CE, et al.: Types of objects in the sleep environment associated with infant suffocation and strangulation, *Acad Pediatr* 17(8):893, 2017.

Gronli J, et al.: Reading from an iPad or book in bed: the impact on human sleep. A randomized crossover trial, *Sleep Medicine* 21(May):86, 2016.

Hirschkowitz M, et al.: National Sleep Foundation sleep time duration recommendations: methodology and results summary, *Sleep Health* 1(1):40, 2015.

Kohansieh M, Makaryus AN: Sleep deficiency and deprivation leading to cardiovascular disease, *Int J Hypertens* 1:2015, 2015.

Litton E, et al.: The efficacy of earplugs as a sleep hygiene strategy for reducing delirium in the ICU: a systematic review and meta-analysis, *Crit Care Med* 44(5):992, 2016.

Madhu C, et al.: Nocturia: risk factors and associated comorbidities; findings from the EpiLUTS study, *Int J Clin Pract* 69(12):1508, 2015.

Martinez F, et al.: Implementing a multicomponent intervention to prevent delirium among critically ill patients, *Crit Care Nurse* 37(6):36, 2017.

McNicholas WT: Obstructive sleep apnoea of mild severity: should it be treated? *Curr Opin Pulm Med* 23(6):506, 2017.

Mileva-Seitz VR, et al.: Parent-child bed-sharing: the good, the bad, and the burden of evidence, *Sleep Med Rev* March 1, 2016.

Mindell JA, et al.: Sleep location and parent-perceived sleep outcomes in older infants, *Sleep Med* 39(1), 2017.

Mitchell EA, et al.: The combination of bed sharing and maternal smoking leads to a greatly increased risk of sudden unexpected death in infancy: the New Zealand SUDI Nationwide Case Control Study, *N Z Med J* 130(1456):52, 2017.

Mollayeva T, et al.: The Pittsburgh sleep quality index as a screening tool for sleep dysfunction in clinical and non-clinical samples: a systematic review and meta-analysis, *Sleep Med Rev* 25:52, 2016.

Murawski B, et al.: A systematic review and meta-analysis of cognitive and behavioral interventions to improve sleep health in adults without sleep disorders, *Sleep Med Rev*, 2017. https://doi.org/10.1016/j.smrv.2017.12.003. Accessed July 29, 2018.

Patel R, et al.: Innovations in insomnia management: a review of current approaches and novel targets including orexin receptor antagonists, *Am J Ther* 25:e28, 2018.

Qaseem A, et al.: Diagnosis of obstructive sleep apnea in adults: a clinical practice guideline from the American College of Physicians, *Ann Intern Med* 161(3):210, 2014.

Rotenberg BW, et al.: Reconsidering first-line treatment for obstructive sleep apnea: a systematic review of the literature, *J Otolaryngol Head Neck Surg* 45:23, 2016.

Schwartz DA, et al.: Occupation and obstructive sleep apnea: a meta-analysis, *J Occup Environ Med* 59(6):502, 2017.

Shimura A, et al.: Comprehensive assessment of the impact of life habits on sleep disturbance, chronotype, and daytime sleepiness among high-school students, *Sleep Med* 44(12), 2018.

Smithburger PL, et al.: Perceptions of family members, nurses, and physicians on involving patients' families in delirium prevention, *Crit Care Nurse* 37(6):48, 2017.

Wiggins SA, Freeman JL: Understanding sleep during adolescence, *Pediatr Nurs* 40(2):91, 2014.

44

Pain Management

OBJECTIVES

- Describe the physiology of nociceptive pain.
- List the characteristics used to differentiate categories of pain.
- Identify the various factors that influence pain.
- Explain how cultural factors influence the pain experience.
- Demonstrate how to assess a patient experiencing pain.
- Contrast the characteristics of acute pain with those of chronic pain

- Explain the nursing guidelines for administering analgesics safely
- Explain various nonpharmacological and pharmacological approaches to treating pain.
- Identify barriers to effective pain management.
- Evaluate a patient's response to pain interventions.

KEY TERMS

Acupressure, p. 1081
Acute pain, p. 1063
Addiction, p. 1091
Adjuvants, p. 1082
Analgesics, p. 1082
Biofeedback, p. 1079
Breakthrough cancer pain, p. 1089
Chronic pain, p. 1064
Cutaneous stimulation, p. 1080
Drug tolerance, p. 1091
Epidural analgesia, p. 1087

Guided imagery, p. 1079
Idiopathic pain, p. 1064
Local anesthesia, p. 1087
Modulation, p. 1062
Multimodal analgesia, p. 1084
Nociception, p. 1061
Opioids, p. 1082
Pain threshold, p. 1066
Pain tolerance, p. 1063
Patient-controlled analgesia (PCA), p. 1086
Perineural infusions, p. 1087

Physical dependence, p. 1091
Placebos, p. 1091
Pseudoaddiction, p. 1091
Regional anesthesia, p. 1087
Relaxation, p. 1079
Transcutaneous electrical nerve stimulation (TENS), p. 1080
Transduction, p. 1061
Transmission, p. 1061

MEDIA RESOURCES

http://evolve.elsevier.com/Potter/fundamentals/
- Review Questions
- Video Clips
- Concept Map Creator
- Case Study with Questions

- Skills Performance Checklists
- Audio Glossary
- Content Updates
- Answers to QSEN Activity and Review Questions

Pain is a universal but individual experience and a condition that nurses encounter among patients in all settings. It is the most common reason for seeking health care, yet it is often underrecognized, misunderstood, and inadequately treated. A person in pain often feels distress or suffering and seeks relief. One of the major challenges of pain is that as a nurse you cannot see or feel a patient's pain. It is purely subjective. No two people experience pain in the same way, and no two painful events create identical responses or feelings in a person. The International Association for the Study of Pain (IASP) defines it as "an unpleasant, subjective sensory *and* emotional experience associated with actual or potential tissue damage, or described in terms of such damage" (IASP, 2017). In the "Declaration of Montreal," the IASP declared that access to pain management is a fundamental human right (IASP, 2018a).

Nurses are legally and ethically responsible for assessing and managing pain (American Nurses Association, 2018). Recently there has been a call for increased coordination of pain research and pain management across the United States in response to various

deficiencies in pain care identified in the Institute of Medicine's 2011 report, *Relieving Pain in America*. The opioid crisis added another dimension to the urgency in identifying ways to effectively reduce pain while protecting patients from harm (CDC, 2016). With the aim of enhancing pain research efforts and promoting collaboration across governmental agencies, a federal advisory committee, the Interagency Pain Research Coordinating Committee (IPRCC), was commissioned by the Department of Health and Human Services (DHHS, 2016). In 2016, the IPRCC and DHHS published the National Pain Strategy, a broad-ranging plan to change how the nation perceives and manages pain (DHHS, 2016). Following this report, the IPRCC published the Federal Pain Research Strategy, which provides a long-term strategic plan to guide federal agencies that support pain research and advance the science to better understand pain and improve pain care (IPRCC, 2018). Many of the recommendations directly address the need to improve systems of care for pain management and increase resources to prevent and treat substance use disorders, which disproportionately affect patients with chronic pain conditions.

Pain management needs to be patient centered, with nurses practicing patient advocacy, empowerment, compassion, and respect. Caring for patients in pain requires recognition that pain can and should be relieved. Effective communication among the patient, family, and professional caregivers is essential to achieve adequate pain management. Recognition of the subjective nature of pain and respect for the patient in pain are demonstrated when a nurse accepts McCaffery's classic definition: "Pain is whatever the experiencing person says it is, existing whenever he says it does" (Pasero and McCaffery, 2011). Effective pain management improves quality of life, reduces physical discomfort, promotes earlier mobilization and return to previous baseline functional activity levels, results in fewer hospital and clinic visits, and decreases hospital lengths of stay, resulting in lower health care costs.

SCIENTIFIC KNOWLEDGE BASE

Nature of Pain

The pain experience is complex, involving more than a single physiological sensation caused by a specific stimulus. It has physical, emotional, and cognitive components. It is subjective and highly individualized. It depletes a person's energy and may contribute to chronic fatigue. It interferes with interpersonal relationships and influences the meaning of life. Left untreated, it may lead to serious physical, psychological, social, and financial consequences. Pain itself cannot be measured objectively. Only the patient knows whether pain is present and how the experience feels. However, careful assessment is critical as you assess the behaviors and physiological changes associated with pain. It is not the responsibility of a patient to prove that he or she is in pain; it is your responsibility to assess a patient's condition and accept his or her subjective report.

Physiology of Pain

In contrast to pain being a first-person, subjective perception, **nociception** is defined as an observable activity in the nervous system in response to an adequate stimulus (third-person perspective) (Treede, 2018). Normal or nociceptive pain is the protective physiologic series of events that bring awareness of actual or potential tissue damage. There are four physiological processes of nociception: transduction, transmission, perception, and modulation (Das, 2015). A patient in pain cannot discriminate among the processes. Understanding each process helps you recognize factors that cause pain, symptoms that accompany it, and the rationale for selected therapies.

Transduction. Thermal, chemical, or mechanical stimuli can cause nociceptive pain when the amount of stimuli is strong enough to meet the activation threshold of nociceptors, which are specialized nerve endings distributed throughout the skin, muscles, joints, and viscera. Nociceptors are classified by the type of stimuli they respond to, and some nociceptors respond to multiple types of stimuli (polymodal nociceptors). Transduction is the process whereby an activated nociceptor converts energy produced by these stimuli (e.g., exposure to pressure or a hot surface) into an action potential. Once transduction is complete, transmission of the nociceptive impulse begins.

Inflammation caused by disease processes or cellular damage resulting from thermal, mechanical, or chemical stimuli cause the release of vasoactive and pro-nociceptive mediators such as prostaglandins, bradykinin, substance P, and histamine (Box 44.1). These substances directly affect the nerve fibers, lowering the threshold required to activate nociceptors and generating action potentials across the synaptic cleft, a process known as peripheral sensitization (Starkweather et al., 2016) (Fig. 44.1). Peripheral sensitization, which lowers the threshold for causing an action potential within the peripheral afferent neurons, can also result from changes in receptors, ion channels, and the amount neurotransmitters released.

BOX 44.1 Neurophysiology of Pain: Neuroregulators

Neurotransmitters (Excitatory)

Prostaglandins
- Generated from the breakdown of phospholipids in cell membranes
- Thought to increase sensitivity to pain

Bradykinin
- Released from plasma that leaks from surrounding blood vessels at the site of tissue injury
- Binds to receptors on peripheral nerves, increasing pain stimuli
- Binds to cells that cause the chain reaction producing prostaglandins

Substance P
- Found in pain neurons of dorsal horn (excitatory peptide)
- Needed to transmit pain impulses from periphery to higher brain centers
- Causes vasodilation and edema

Histamine
- Produced by mast cells, causing capillary dilation and increased capillary permeability

Serotonin
- Released from the brainstem and dorsal horn to inhibit pain transmission

Neuromodulators (Inhibitory)
- Are the natural supply of morphinelike substances in the body
- Activated by stress and pain
- Located within the brain, spinal cord, and gastrointestinal tract
- Cause analgesia when they attach to opiate receptors in the brain
- Present in higher levels in people who have less pain than others with a similar injury

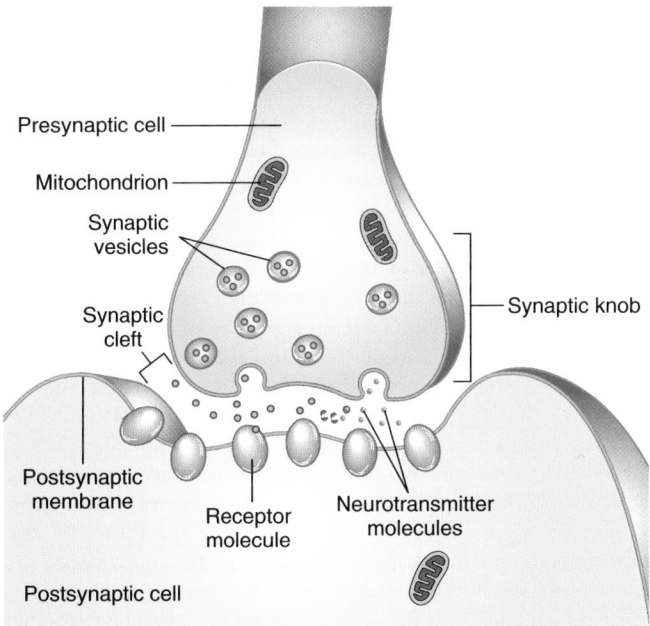

FIG. 44.1 Chemical synapses involve transmitter chemicals (neurotransmitters) that signal postsynaptic cells. (From Patton KT, Thibodeau GA: *Anatomy & physiology*, ed 9, St Louis, 2016, Mosby.)

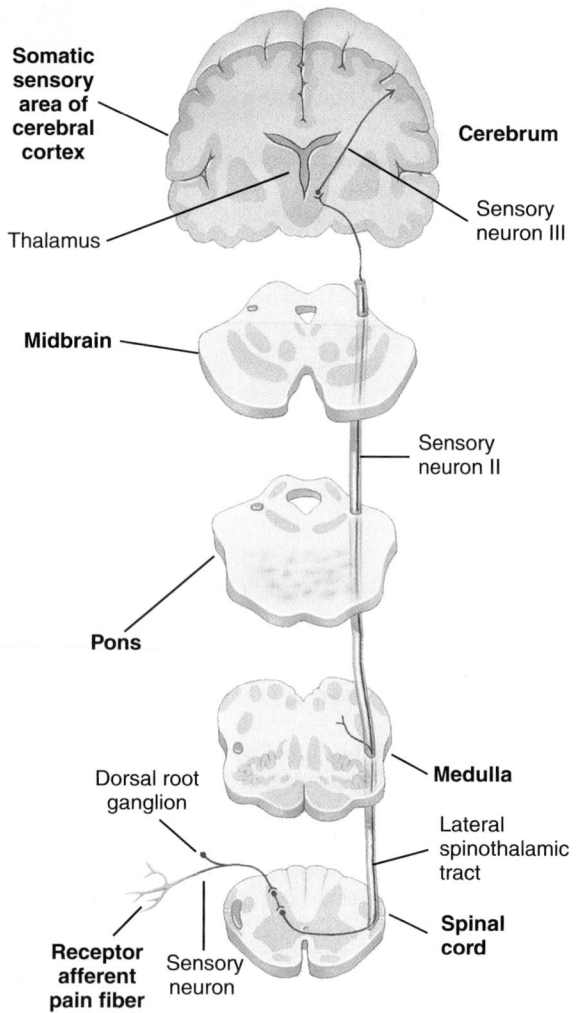

FIG. 44.2 Spinothalamic pathway that conducts pain stimuli to the brain.

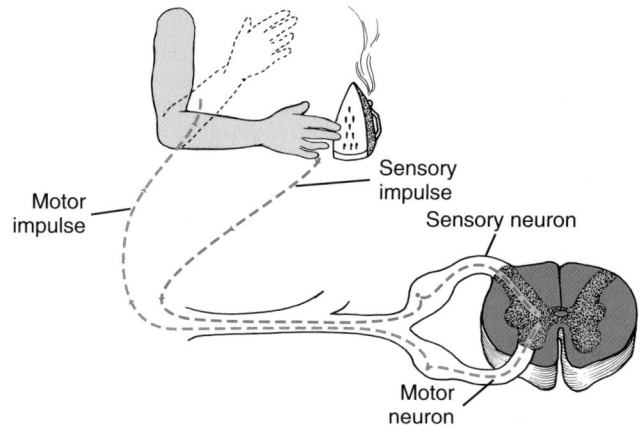

FIG. 44.3 Protective reflex to pain stimulus.

Transmission. Each nociceptor has an axon composed of peripheral afferent nerve fibers that are either myelinated (A-delta fibers) or unmyelinated (C fibers). The nociceptive impulses are transmitted from the periphery to the spinal cord via the peripheral afferent fibers to the dorsal root ganglia and the superficial lamina I/II of the dorsal horn of the spinal cord. The fast-transmitting myelinated A-delta fibers transmit sharp, localized nociceptive information, whereas the smaller-diameter unmyelinated C fibers relay impulses that are dull, achy, and poorly localized. For example, after stepping on a nail, a person initially feels a sharp, localized pain, which is a result of A-fiber transmission, or first pain. Within a few seconds the whole foot aches from C-fiber transmission, or second pain (Steeds, 2016).

The A-delta fibers transmit nociceptive impulses from the dorsal horn to the interior deeper laminae (III-IV) of the spinal cord and higher centers of the brain by way of the spinothalamic tracts (Fig. 44.2). Dorsal horn neurons carrying nociceptive input include projection neurons, local interneurons, and propriospinal neurons. Many of the projection neurons have axons that cross the midline and ascend to multiple areas of the brain, including the thalamus, gray matter of the cerebral cortex, the pons, and parts of the medullary reticular formation. It is through this cellular system of communication (action potentials carrying nociceptive input) that pain, arising from any area of the body including the nerve or areas of the brain itself, can be perceived by the individual.

Perception. Once a pain stimulus reaches the cerebral cortex, the brain interprets the quality of the pain and processes information from past experience, knowledge, and cultural associations in the perception of the pain (Fenton et al., 2015). Perception is the point at which a person is aware of nociceptive impulses and perceives pain. The somatosensory cortex identifies the location and intensity of pain, whereas the association cortex, primarily the limbic system, determines how a person feels about it. There is no single pain center.

As a person becomes aware of pain, a complex reaction occurs. Psychological and cognitive factors interact with neurophysiological ones. Perception gives awareness and meaning to pain, resulting in a reaction. The reaction to pain includes the physiological and behavioral responses that occur after an individual perceives pain.

Modulation. Projection neurons activate endogenous descending inhibitory mediators (see Box 44.1), such as endorphins (endogenous opioids), serotonin, norepinephrine, and gamma-aminobutyric acid (GABA), that aid in producing an analgesic effect. These mediators hinder the transmission of nociceptive impulses in the dorsal horn neurons. This inhibition of the pain impulse is the fourth and last phase of the normal pain process known as *modulation* (Pasero and McCaffery, 2011). Modulation can also occur through peripheral and/or central sensitization, resulting in increased perception of pain (Bourne et al., 2014). Afferent nerve fibers sensitized by vasoactive and pronociceptive mediators lower the threshold of activation and result in continuous nociceptive input to dorsal horn neurons and central sensitization. Clinical manifestations of central sensitization include expansion of the pain beyond the initial location, exaggerated response to noxious stimuli known as hyperalgesia, and pain in response to normally non-noxious stimuli, also called allodynia.

A protective reflex response also occurs with pain (Fig. 44.3). A-delta fibers send sensory impulses to the spinal cord, where they synapse with spinal motor neurons. The motor impulses travel via a reflex arc along efferent (motor) nerve fibers back to a peripheral muscle near the site of stimulation, thus bypassing the brain. Contraction of the muscle leads to a protective withdrawal from the source of pain. For example, when you accidentally touch a hot iron, you feel a burning sensation, but your hand also reflexively withdraws from the surface of the iron. Pain perception requires consciousness and an intact central nervous system. Common factors that disrupt the pain process include trauma, drugs, tumor growth, and metabolic disorders.

Gate-Control Theory of Pain

Melzack and Wall's gate-control theory (1965) was the first to suggest that pain has emotional and cognitive components in addition to

TABLE 44.1 Physiological Reactions to Pain

Response	Cause or Effect
Sympathetic Stimulation[a]	
Dilation of bronchial tubes and increased respiratory rate	Provides increased oxygen intake
Increased heart rate	Provides increased oxygen transport
Peripheral vasoconstriction (pallor, elevation in blood pressure)	Elevates blood pressure with shift of blood supply from periphery and viscera to skeletal muscles and brain
Increased blood glucose level	Provides additional energy
Increased cortisol level (short term)	Heightened memory functions, a burst of increased immunity, and lower sensitivity to pain
Diaphoresis	Controls body temperature during stress
Increased muscle tension	Prepares muscles for action
Dilation of pupils	Affords better vision
Decreased gastrointestinal motility	Frees energy for more immediate activity
Parasympathetic Stimulation[b]	
Pallor	Causes blood supply to shift away from periphery
Nausea and vomiting	Vagus nerve sends impulses to chemoreceptor trigger zone in the brain
Decreased heart rate and blood pressure	Results from vagal stimulation
Rapid, irregular breathing	Causes body defenses to fail under prolonged stress of pain

[a]Pain of low-to-moderate intensity and superficial pain.
[b]Severe or deep pain.

physical sensations. The theory explains how rubbing an injured area can reduce pain. The small-diameter fibers activated by noxious stimuli open the gate to pain transmission, and the large-diameter fibers have inhibitory effects to shut the gate. Rubbing the injured area promotes proprioceptive large-diameter fiber input and therefore inhibits further transmission of pain signals from small-diameter nerves to the brain. Melzack (1999) later proposed the neuromatrix theory of pain, postulating that each individual possesses a genetically determined neural matrix that develops and is modulated by sensory input, making pain perception unique to each individual.

Physiological Responses. As pain impulses ascend the spinal cord toward the brainstem and thalamus, the stress response stimulates the autonomic nervous system (ANS). Pain of low-to-moderate intensity and superficial pain elicit the fight-or-flight reaction of the general adaptation syndrome (see Chapter 37). Stimulation of the sympathetic branch of the ANS results in physiological responses (Table 44.1). Continuous, severe, or deep pain typically involving the visceral organs (e.g., with a myocardial infarction or colic from gallbladder or renal stones) activates the parasympathetic nervous system. Except in cases of severe traumatic pain, which cause a person to go into shock, most people adapt to their pain reflexively, and their physical signs return to normal baseline. Note that normal is not the same for each individual. Thus patients in pain do *not* always have changes in their vital signs. Changes in vital signs more often indicate problems other than pain (Manocha and Taneja, 2016).

Behavioral Responses. The pain response is complex, influenced by a person's culture, pain experiences, perception of pain, and ability to manage stress. If left untreated or unrelieved, pain significantly alters quality of life with physical and psychological consequences; this phenomenon is referred to as high-impact pain (Dahlhamer et al., 2018). The widespread effects of pain support why effective pain management is essential. Some patients choose not to report pain if they believe that it inconveniences others or if it signals loss of self-control.

Others endure severe pain without asking for assistance. Clenching the teeth, facial grimacing, holding or guarding the painful part, and bent posture are common indications of acute pain. Chronic pain can affect a patient's activity (eating, sleeping, socialization), thinking (confusion, forgetfulness), emotions (anger, depression, irritability), quality of life, and productivity (IOM, 2011). You soon learn to recognize patterns of behavior that reflect pain even when patients offer no verbal report, especially those with dementia or other cognitive changes.

Recognizing a patient's unique response to pain allows you to assess the success of pain-management therapies. Encourage your patients to accept pain-relieving measures so that they remain active and continue to maintain daily activities. A patient's ability to tolerate pain significantly influences your perceptions of the degree of his or her discomfort. Patients who have a low **pain tolerance** (level of pain a person is willing to accept) are sometimes inaccurately perceived as complainers. Teach patients the importance of reporting their pain sooner rather than later to facilitate better control and optimal functional status.

Acute and Chronic Pain

Pain is categorized by duration (acute or chronic) or pathological condition (e.g., cancer or neuropathic). The two types of pain that you observe in patients are acute (transient) and chronic (persistent), which includes cancer and noncancer pain.

Acute/Transient Pain. Acute pain is protective, usually has an identifiable cause, is of short duration, and has limited tissue damage and emotional response. It is common after acute injury, disease, or surgery. Acute pain warns people of injury or disease; thus it is protective. It eventually resolves, with or without treatment, after an injured area heals. Patients in acute pain are frightened and anxious and expect relief quickly. It is self-limiting; therefore a patient knows that an end is in sight. Because acute pain has a predictable ending (healing) and an identifiable cause, health team members are usually willing to treat it aggressively.

Acute pain seriously threatens a patient's recovery by hampering his or her ability to become active and involved in self-care. This results in prolonged hospitalization from complications such as physical and emotional exhaustion, immobility, sleep deprivation, and pulmonary complications. Physical and psychological progress is delayed as long as acute pain persists because a patient focuses all energy on pain relief. Efforts aimed at teaching and motivating a patient toward self-care can be hindered until the pain is managed successfully. Complete pain relief is not always achievable, but reducing pain to a tolerable level is a realistic goal. A primary nursing goal is to provide pain relief that allows patients to participate in their recovery, prevent complications, and improve functional status. Unrelieved acute pain can progress to chronic pain.

Chronic/Persistent Noncancer Pain. Chronic pain affects more than 50 million American adults, and among those affected, nearly 20 million live with high-impact chronic pain (Dahlhamer et al., 2018). Unlike acute pain, chronic pain is not protective and thus serves no purpose, but it has a dramatic effect on a person's quality of life. Chronic noncancer pain is ongoing or recurrent pain that lasts beyond the usual course of an acute illness or the healing of an injury (more than 3 to 6 months) and that adversely affects an individual's well-being (ACPA, 2018). It does not always have an identifiable cause and leads to great personal suffering. Examples of chronic noncancer pain include arthritis, low back pain, headache, fibromyalgia, and peripheral neuropathy. It may result from an initial injury such as a back sprain, or there may be an ongoing cause such as illness. Chronic noncancer pain may be viewed as a disease since it has a distinct pathology that causes changes throughout the nervous system that may worsen over time. It has significant psychological and cognitive effects and can constitute a serious, separate disease entity itself. Chronic noncancer pain is usually non–life threatening. In some cases an injured area healed long ago, yet the pain is ongoing and does not respond to treatment.

The possible unknown cause of chronic pain, combined with ineffective treatments and the unrelenting nature and uncertainty of its duration, frustrates a patient, frequently leading to psychological depression and even suicide. Chronic pain is a major cause of psychological and physical disability, leading to problems such as job loss, inability to perform simple daily activities, sexual dysfunction, and social isolation. The goal of treating chronic noncancer pain is to improve functional status with a multimodality plan.

The person with chronic noncancer pain often experiences pain that may not have the same physiological response as acute pain; however, the subjective reports and interference with activities of daily living (ADLs), socialization, and ability to perform work duties is very real. Patients often suffer more with time because of physical and mental exhaustion. Associated symptoms of chronic pain include fatigue, insomnia, anorexia, weight loss, apathy, hopelessness, depression, and anger. Chronic pain creates the uncertainty of how one will feel from day to day. A person with chronic noncancer pain often does not show obvious symptoms and does not adapt to the pain. Often a person with chronic pain who consults with numerous health care providers is labeled a drug seeker when he or she is actually seeking adequate pain relief. Nurses need to discourage patients from having multiple health care providers for treating pain and encourage the use of both pharmacological and nonpharmacological management. Pain centers specialize in diagnostic testing and in noninvasive and invasive treatments that patients may be able to obtain from their general health care providers.

Chronic Episodic Pain. Pain that occurs sporadically over an extended period of time is episodic pain. Pain episodes last for hours, days, or weeks. An example of chronic episodic pain is the migraine headache that occurs up to 14 days per month compared with chronic migraine, which occurs more than 15 days per month (Katsarava et al., 2012).

Cancer Pain. Not all patients with cancer experience pain. Cancer pain can be relieved often with simple interventions in 90% of patients (Burchum and Rosenthal, 2019). Some patients with cancer experience acute and/or chronic pain. The pain is normal (nociceptive), resulting from stimulus of an undamaged nerve, and/or neuropathic, arising from abnormal or damaged pain nerves (Table 44.2). Cancer pain is usually caused by tumor progression and related pathological processes, invasive procedures, toxicities of chemotherapy, and infection. A patient senses pain at the actual site of the tumor or distant to the site, called *referred pain*. Always completely assess reports of new pain by a patient with existing pain. Despite the availability and wide use of effective therapies and updated guidelines from reliable leading professional societies, the undertreatment of cancer pain is still frequent (Burchum and Rosenthal, 2019). Research shows that approximately one-third of patients who receive treatment for pain still do not receive pain medication proportional to their pain intensity (Greco et al., 2014).

Idiopathic Pain. Idiopathic pain is chronic pain in the absence of an identifiable physical or psychological cause or pain perceived as excessive for the extent of an organic pathological condition. An example of idiopathic pain is complex regional pain syndrome (CRPS). Research is needed to better identify the causes of idiopathic pain to identify more effective treatments.

REFLECT NOW

A nurse is caring for one patient who is experiencing acute abdominal pain related to appendicitis and another patient who is experiencing abdominal pain related to ovarian cancer. Compare the pain of these two patients. How might the patients' pain be similar? How might they be different?

NURSING KNOWLEDGE BASE

Nursing knowledge of pain mechanisms and interventions continues to grow through nursing research. This section explores factors that influence the pain experience.

Knowledge, Attitudes, and Beliefs

Attitudes of nurses and other health care providers affect pain management. The traditional medical model of illness generates attitudes about pain. This model suggests that physical problems result from physical causes. Thus pain is a physical response to organic dysfunction. When there is no obvious source of pain (e.g., the patient with chronic low back pain or neuropathies), health care providers sometimes stereotype patients with pain as malingerers, complainers, or difficult patients.

Studies of nurses' attitudes regarding pain management show that a nurse's personal opinion about a patient's self-report of pain affects pain assessment and titration of medication doses. It has been shown that nurses' assessment of pain intensity often underestimates patients' pain reports (Goulet et al., 2013; Desai et al, 2014). Also, nurses may infer cues on pain severity solely from how pain is treated and then use

TABLE 44.2 Classification of Pain By Inferred Pathology

Nociceptive Pain	Neuropathic Pain

I. *Nociceptive pain:* Normal stimulation of special peripheral nerve endings—called *nociceptors;* usually responsive to nonopioids and/or opioids.
  A. *Somatic pain:* Comes from bone, joint, muscle, skin, or connective tissue; is usually aching or throbbing in quality and well localized
  B. *Visceral pain:* Arises from visceral organs such as the gastrointestinal tract and pancreas; is sometimes subdivided:
    1. Tumor involvement of organ capsule that causes aching and fairly well-localized pain.
    2. Obstruction of hollow viscus, which causes intermittent cramping and poorly localized pain.
	II. *Neuropathic pain:* Pain caused by a lesion or disease of the somatosensory nervous system; treatment usually includes adjuvant analgesics.
	  A. Centrally generated pain
	    1. *Deafferentation pain:* Injury to either the peripheral or central nervous system.
	    Examples: Phantom pain indicates injury to the peripheral nervous system; burning pain below the level of a spinal cord lesion reflects injury to the central nervous system.
	    2. *Sympathetically maintained pain:* Associated with impaired regulation of the autonomic nervous system.
	    Examples: Pain is associated with complex regional pain syndrome, type I, type II.
	  B. Peripherally generated pain
	    1. *Painful polyneuropathies:* Pain felt along the distribution of many peripheral nerves.
	    Examples: Diabetic neuropathy, alcohol-nutritional neuropathy, and Guillain-Barré syndrome.
	    2. *Painful mononeuropathies:* Usually associated with a known peripheral nerve injury; pain is felt at least partly along the distribution of the damaged nerve.
	    Examples: Nerve root compression, nerve entrapment, trigeminal neuralgia.

From Pasero C, McCaffery M: *Pain assessment and pharmacologic management,* St Louis, 2011, Mosby.

the cues when making symptom judgments, often leading to underestimation and overestimation of pain (Dekel et al., 2016). Patients with a high self-report of pain, even when nurses are aware of their pain experience and analgesic treatment, are vulnerable to underestimation and hence to pain undertreatment (Dekel et al., 2016). Also, patients with a low self-report of pain are subject to overestimation and thus are exposed to overtreatment with potential treatment hazards. A number of nurse and patient variables, including cultural (e.g., gender, age, education), knowledge, and patient diagnosis, contribute to the differences in pain ratings. A study showed that patients treated by nurses who have postgraduate training and/or attend continuous education programs and who have greater autonomy in modifying pain treatment protocols experience better quality of care (Tomaszek and Debska, 2018).

Nurses' assumptions about patients in pain seriously limit their ability to offer pain relief. Biases based on culture, education, and experience influence everyone. Too often nurses allow misconceptions about pain (Box 44.2) to affect their willingness to intervene. Clinical practices can also play a role. For example, when there are conditions of symptom uncertainty and ambiguous clinical judgment, nurses may incorrectly use medical evidence cues alone and follow established clinical protocols or pathways that may simplify clinical decisions but will bias pain estimation (Dekel et al., 2016). Some nurses avoid acknowledging a patient's pain because of their own fear and denial. They do not believe a patient's report of pain if he or she does not appear to be in pain. A nurse is entitled to personal beliefs; however, he or she must *accept* a patient's report of pain, act according to professional guidelines, standards, and position statements, and individualize appropriate policies and procedures, protocols, and evidence-based research findings (American Nurses Association, 2018).

To help a patient gain pain relief, it is important to view the experience through the patient's eyes. Acknowledging a personal prejudice or misconception helps to address patient problems more professionally. When one becomes an active, knowledgeable observer of a patient in pain, it is possible to more objectively analyze the pain experience. The

BOX 44.2 Common Biases and Misconceptions About Pain

The following statements are *false:*
- Patients who abuse substances (e.g., use drugs or alcohol) overreact to discomforts.
- Patients with minor illnesses have less pain than those with severe physical alteration.
- Administering analgesics regularly leads to drug addiction.
- The amount of tissue damage in an injury accurately indicates pain intensity.
- Health care personnel are the best authorities on the nature of a patient's pain.
- Psychogenic pain is not real.
- Chronic pain is psychological.
- Patients who are hospitalized experience pain.
- Patients who cannot speak do not feel pain.

patient makes the diagnosis that pain is present, and the nurse provides interventions that ultimately offer relief.

Factors Influencing Pain

Pain is a complex process, involving physiological, social, spiritual, psychological, and cultural influences. Thus each individual's pain experience is different. Consider all factors that affect a patient in pain to ensure a holistic approach to the assessment and care of the patient. Some of these factors are modifiable, things that can change, while others are nonmodifiable, such as age. Nursing interventions target the modifiable factors, such as attention, fear, and anxiety, by providing patients and families with the knowledge and skills to cope with pain.

Physiological Factors

Age. Age influences the pain experience. It is important to consider how a painful event affects a patient developmentally. For example pain may prevent an adolescent from engaging socially with friends. A middle-aged adult may be unable to continue work in cases when pain is severe. It is particularly important to recognize how developmental differences affect how infants and older adults react to pain. Young children have trouble understanding pain, its meaning, and the procedures that cause it. If they have not developed full vocabularies, they have difficulty with verbally describing and expressing pain to parents or caregivers. Toddlers and preschoolers are unable to recall explanations about pain or to associate it with experiences that may be unrelated to the painful condition. With these developmental considerations in mind, it is necessary to adapt approaches for assessing a child's pain (e.g., what to ask, including what to ask parents) and to learn which behaviors to observe and how to prepare a child for a painful medical procedure.

Pain is not an inevitable part of aging. Likewise pain perception does not decrease with age. However, older adults have a greater likelihood of developing pathological conditions, which are accompanied by acute and chronic pain. Persistent pain may be associated with impaired physical function, falls, diminished appetite, dysmobility, impaired sleep, depression, anxiety, agitation and delirium, as well as more subtle decrements in cognitive function (Galicia-Castillo and Weiner, 2019). In addition, age-related changes and increased frailty may lead to a less predictable response to analgesics, increased sensitivity to medications, and potentially harmful drug effects (O'Sullivan et al., 2017). Serious impairment of functional status often accompanies pain in older patients. It potentially reduces mobility, ADLs, involvement in social activities and physical activity, and activity tolerance. The presence of pain in an older adult requires aggressive assessment, diagnosis, and management (Box 44.3).

The ability of older patients to interpret pain is sometimes complicated. They often suffer from multiple diseases with symptoms that affect similar parts of the body. This requires you to make detailed assessments when the source of pain is unclear. Different diseases sometimes cause similar symptoms. For example, chest pain does not always indicate a heart attack; it also is a symptom of arthritis of the spine or an abdominal disorder. When older adults experience cognitive impairment and confusion, they have difficulty in recalling pain experiences and in providing detailed explanations of their pain (Pasero and McCaffery, 2011). It is necessary to address misconceptions about pain management in the very young and in older adults before intervening for a patient (Tables 44.3 and 44.4).

Fatigue. Fatigue heightens the perception of pain and decreases coping abilities. If it occurs along with sleeplessness, the perception of pain is even greater. Pain is often experienced less after a restful sleep than at the end of a long day.

Genes. Research on healthy human subjects suggests that genetic information passed on by parents possibly increases or decreases a person's sensitivity to pain and determines pain threshold or tolerance. Recent advances in the study of genetics and pain have shown that even slight changes in deoxyribonucleic acid (DNA) or expression of genes could partly explain individual differences in pain. Numerous genetic risk factors have been identified for pain in musculoskeletal, neuropathic, and vascular conditions, as well as migraine (Zorina-Lichtenwalter et al., 2016) Genetic influences have been shown to play

BOX 44.3 FOCUS ON OLDER ADULTS
Factors Influencing Pain in Older Adults

- With aging, muscle mass decreases, body fat increases, and percentage of body water decreases. This increases the concentration of water-soluble drugs such as morphine given in normal doses. The volume of distribution for fat-soluble drugs such as fentanyl increases (Burchum and Rosenthal, 2019).
- Older adults frequently eat poorly, resulting in low serum albumin levels. Many analgesics are highly protein bound. In the presence of low serum albumin, more free drug (active form) is available, thus increasing the risk for side effects or toxic effects (Burchum and Rosenthal, 2019; Tracy and Sean Morrison, 2013).
- A decline of liver and renal function naturally occurs with aging. This results in reduced metabolism and excretion of drugs. Thus, older adults often experience a greater peak effect and longer duration of analgesics (Abdulla, 2013).
- Pain is common in the advanced stages of many chronic diseases, including heart failure, end-stage renal disease, and chronic obstructive pulmonary disease. In addition, millions of joint repair and replacement surgeries are performed annually in the United States, and an important minority of patients undergoing these procedures report chronic pain despite surgery (Reid et al., 2015).
- Age-related changes in the skin such as thinning and loss of elasticity affect the absorption rate of topical analgesics.

TABLE 44.3 Pain in Infants

Misconception	Correction
Infants cannot feel pain.	Infants have the anatomical and functional requirements for pain processing by mid- to late gestation.
Infants are less sensitive to pain than older children and adults.	Term neonates have the same sensitivity to pain as older infants and children. Preterm neonates have a greater sensitivity to pain than term neonates or older children.
Infants cannot express pain.	Although infants cannot verbalize pain, they respond with behavioral cues and physiological indicators that are observable.
Infants must learn about pain from previous painful experiences.	Pain requires no prior experience; infants do not need to learn it from earlier painful experience. It occurs with the first insult.
You cannot accurately assess pain in infants.	You use behavioral cues (e.g., facial expressions, cry, body movements) and physiological indicators of pain (e.g., changes in vital signs) to reliably and validly assess pain in infants.
You cannot safely give analgesics and anesthetics to infants and neonates because of their immature capacity to metabolize and eliminate drugs and their sensitivity to opioid-induced respiratory depression.	Infants are very sensitive to drugs. Response to drugs is often intense and prolonged. Absorption is faster than expected. Dosages of drugs excreted by the kidneys need to be reduced (Burchum and Rosenthal, 2019). Prescribers carefully select the medication, dosage, administration route, and time. Nurses monitor frequently for desired and undesired effects. They also follow medication orders to titrate and wean medications to minimize adverse effects.

TABLE 44.4 Misconceptions About Pain in Older Adults

Misconception	Correction
Pain is a natural outcome of growing old.	Older adults are at greater risk (as much as twofold) than younger adults for many painful conditions; however, pain is not an inevitable result of aging.
Pain perception, or sensitivity, decreases with age.	This assumption is unsafe. Although there is evidence that emotional suffering specifically related to pain may be less in older than in younger patients, no scientific basis exists for the claim that a decrease in perception of pain occurs with age or that age dulls sensitivity to pain.
If the older patient does not report pain, he or she does not have pain.	Older patients commonly underreport pain. Reasons include expecting to have pain with increasing age; not wanting to alarm loved ones; being fearful of losing their independence; not wanting to distract, anger, or bother caregivers; and believing that caregivers know they have pain and are doing all they can to relieve it. The absence of a report of pain does not mean the absence of pain.
If an older patient appears to be occupied, asleep, or otherwise distracted from pain, he or she does not have pain.	Older patients often believe that it is unacceptable to show pain and have learned to use a variety of ways to cope with it (e.g., many patients use distraction successfully for short periods of time). Sleeping is sometimes a coping strategy; alternately, it indicates exhaustion, not pain relief. Do not make assumptions about the presence or absence of pain solely on the basis of a patient's behavior.
The potential side effects of opioids make them too dangerous to use to relieve pain in older adults.	In most cases nonopioids are preferred to opioids for noncancer pain, but opioids can be used safely for older adults with moderate-to-severe cancer pain. Although the opioid-naïve older adult is usually more sensitive to opioids, this does not justify withholding their use in pain management. Analgesics should be initiated at the lowest effective dose and titrated to achieve pain control with minimal adverse effects; this requires frequent reassessment of patients for pain relief and side effects as doses are adjusted (Galicia-Castillo and Weiner, 2019).
Patients with Alzheimer's disease and other cognitive impairments do not feel pain, and their reports of pain are most likely invalid.	No evidence exists that older adults who are cognitively impaired experience less pain or that their reports of pain are less valid than those of individuals with intact cognitive function (Horgas, 2018). Patients with dementia or other deficits of cognition most likely suffer significant unrelieved pain and discomfort. The best approach to assessment is to accept a patient's report of pain and use relevant pain assessment tools.
Older patients report more pain as they age.	Even though older patients experience a higher incidence of painful conditions such as arthritis, osteoporosis, peripheral vascular disease, and cancer than younger patients, studies show that they underreport pain. Many older adults grew up valuing the ability to "grin and bear it" (Pasero and McCaffery, 2011).

a role in sensitivity, perception, and expression of pain in a variety of conditions (James, 2013). As a nurse you may encourage patients who have persistent pain syndromes to seek genetic counseling.

Neurological Function. A patient's neurological function influences the pain experience. Any factor that interrupts or influences normal pain reception or perception (e.g., spinal cord injury, peripheral neuropathy, or neurological disease) affects a patient's awareness of and response to pain. Some pharmacological agents (analgesics, sedatives, and anesthetics) influence pain perception and response because of the manner in which they affect the nervous system.

Social Factors

Previous Experience. Each person learns from painful experiences. Prior experience does not mean that a person accepts pain more easily in the future. Previous frequent episodes of pain without relief or bouts of severe pain cause anxiety or fear. In contrast, if a person repeatedly experiences the same type of pain that was relieved successfully in the past, he or she finds it easier to interpret the pain sensation. As a result, the patient is better prepared to take necessary actions to relieve the pain.

When a patient has no experience with a painful condition, the first perception of pain often impairs the ability to cope. For example, after abdominal surgery patients often experience severe incisional pain for several days. Unless a patient knows that this is a common occurrence following surgery, the onset of pain seems like a serious complication. Rather than participate actively in postoperative breathing exercises (see Chapter 50), the patient lies immobile in bed and breathes shallowly because of fear that something is not right. In the preoperative and anticipatory phase of the pain experience, you need to prepare a patient with a clear explanation of the type of pain to expect and methods to reduce it. This usually results in a reduced perception of pain.

Family and Social Network. People in pain often depend on family members or close friends for support, assistance, or protection. Although pain still exists, the presence of family or friends can often make the experience less stressful. Conversation with family is a useful distraction. The presence of parents is especially important for children experiencing pain.

Spiritual Factors. Spirituality is an active search for meaning in situations (see Chapter 35). Spiritual beliefs affect the way patients view or cope with pain. Research has shown accumulating evidence that interventions that address spirituality have benefits for individuals' physical and emotional health, including the relief of pain (Siddall et al., 2015).

Patients often ask spiritually based questions, such as "Why has this happened to me?" or "Why am I suffering?" Spiritual pain goes beyond what we can see. "Why has God done this to me?" "Is this suffering teaching me something?" Other spiritual concerns include loss of independence and becoming a burden to family. Recall that pain is an experience that has physical *and* emotional components. Patients who deal with persistent pain using positive spiritual coping practices such as looking to a higher being for strength and support adjust better to pain and have significantly better mental health (Siddall et al., 2015). Providing support for patients to utilize their spiritual practices is essential for pain management.

Psychological Factors

Attention. The degree to which a patient focuses attention on pain influences his or her perception. Increased attention is associated with increased pain, whereas distraction is associated with a diminished pain response. This concept is one that nurses apply in various pain-relief interventions such as relaxation, guided imagery, and massage. By focusing patients' attention and concentration on other stimuli, their perception of pain declines (see Chapter 32).

Anxiety and Fear. A person perceives pain differently if it suggests a threat, loss, punishment, or challenge. For example, a woman in labor perceives pain differently than a woman with a history of cancer who is experiencing a new pain and fearing recurrence. In addition, the degree and quality of pain perceived by a patient influence its meaning. The relationship between pain and anxiety and fear is complex. Both emotions often increase the perception of pain, and pain causes feelings of anxiety and fear. It is difficult to separate the two sensations.

Critically ill or injured patients who perceive a lack of control over their environment and their care have high anxiety levels. This anxiety leads to serious pain-management problems. Pharmacological and nonpharmacological approaches to the management of anxiety are appropriate; however, anxiolytic medications are not a substitute for analgesia (Pasero and McCaffery, 2011).

Coping Style. Pain is a lonely experience that often causes patients to feel a loss of control. Coping style influences the ability to deal with it (see Chapter 37). People with internal loci of control perceive themselves as having control over events in their lives and the outcomes such as pain. They ask questions, desire information, and make choices about treatment. In contrast, people with external loci of control perceive that other factors in their lives, such as nurses, are responsible for the outcome of events. These patients follow directions and are more passive in managing their pain. Learn to understand patients' coping resources during painful experiences so that you can incorporate these into your plan of care. For example, a patient who does not ask for pain medication but shows behavioral signs of discomfort might require you to be more responsive in offering prn medications on time.

Cultural Factors. The meaning that a person associates with pain affects the experience of pain and how one adapts to it. This is often closely associated with a person's cultural background, including age, education, race, and familial factors. Cultural beliefs and values affect how individuals cope with pain. They learn what is expected and accepted by their culture, including how to react to pain.

An example comes from a qualitative study conducted among members of a South African culture. The study found gender differences among members of the groups interviewed; the expression or acknowledgment of pain could almost be described as a cultural taboo associated with weakness and a lack of honor and courage among men (Nortje and Albertyn, 2015). Historical folklore, songs, and poems describing the stories of fallen heroes and ancestors were often used to train African children to deal with pain in a stoic and resilient manner.

A study has shown that cultural values regarding work and family play a large role in Hispanic Americans' pain behaviors (Hollingshead et al., 2016). In that study, Mexican-American men reported enduring pain in order to support and provide for their families, whereas Mexican-American women reported enduring pain to care for and nurture their families. When pain threatens an individual's family or work role, an individual may not necessarily seek pain care but instead attempt to endure the discomfort to stay independent and productive.

Health care providers often mistakenly assume that everyone responds to pain in the same way. Different meanings and attitudes are associated with pain across various cultural groups. An understanding of the cultural meaning of pain helps you design culturally sensitive care for people with pain.

⊕ BOX 44.4   CULTURAL ASPECTS OF CARE

Assessing Pain in Culturally Diverse Patients

Pain is a biopsychosocial phenomenon. Culture shapes the experience of pain, including its expression and a patient's behaviors, or coping responses. For example, an individual from a higher socioeconomic group has more resources for managing pain and is more likely to adapt behaviors that will lessen pain. Several research studies have shown that people in the lowest as compared with the highest socioeconomic class are more likely to feel disabled through pain (Dahlhamer et al., 2018). A recent literature review demonstrated that Hispanic Americans face numerous barriers to seeking and receiving pain care, including financial limitations, lack of insurance, language barriers, and immigration status (Hollingshead et al., 2016). Culture also affects a person's choice of lay remedies, help-seeking activities, and receptivity to medical treatment. Some health care providers undertreat pain because they do not understand the cultural effects on the perception of pain intensity. Nurses care for patients with pain from a variety of cultural backgrounds; thus you need to develop strategies to assess and manage pain in culturally diverse patients.

Implications for Patient-Centered Care

- Use culturally appropriate assessment tools, such as tools written in the patient's native language, to assess pain (CDC, 2019).
- Assess a patient's health literacy level because this affects your ability to provide appropriate education about pain management and therapies (CDC, 2019). Spanish-speaking Hispanic-American patients report difficulty in describing their pain experiences to providers and report better pain control when a Spanish-language translator is present (Hollingshead et al., 2016).
- Recognize variations in subjective responses to pain. Undertreatment or overtreatment might occur if members of the health care team are unaware of the cultural norms associated with pain and pain expression, since pain is subjective (Nortjé and Albertyn, 2015).
- Be sensitive to variations in communication styles. Some cultures believe that nonverbal expression of pain is sufficient to describe the pain experience, whereas others assume that if pain medication is appropriate, the nurse will bring it; thus asking is inappropriate.
- Understand that expression of pain is unacceptable within certain cultures. Some patients believe that asking for help indicates a lack of respect, whereas others believe acknowledging pain is a sign of weakness.
- Pain is personal and related to religious beliefs. Some cultures consider suffering a part of life to be endured to enter heaven.
- Use knowledge of biological variations of pain. Significant differences in drug metabolism, dosing requirements, therapeutic response, and adverse effects occur in cultural groups. A wide range of responses is also possible within this group. Therefore assess each patient's response to pain medication carefully.
- Develop a personal awareness of your own values and beliefs that affect your responses to patients' reports of pain.

Culture affects pain expression. Some people believe that it is natural to be demonstrative about pain. Others tend to be more introverted. When a person moves to another country, it is important to know to what extent the individual has assimilated into his or her new home. For example, if several generations of a Hispanic patient's family have lived in the United States, the influence of the Spanish culture may be limited, whereas newly immigrated patients still often embrace their cultural norms.

As a nurse, explore the impact of cultural differences on a patient's pain experience and make adjustments to the plan of care (Box 44.4). Ask whether the patient has had previous bad experiences with pain management. Work with a patient and family to learn their cultural beliefs, values, and preferences to adequately assess and manage pain (see Chapter 9). Find a culturally appropriate assessment tool, and communicate the use of that tool to other health care providers in an effort to provide culturally competent care.

Factors Impacted By Pain

Quality of Life. Pain affects a patient's daily activities and quality of life. Pain affects an individual's ability to provide self-care, work, perform at school, and interact socially with friends and family. Chronic pain is a major public health problem, producing significant economic and social burdens that affect the patient, family, and social circles (Dueñas et al., 2016). The biopsychosocial model for chronic pain offers a valuable framework for understanding how a variety of factors can contribute to chronic pain and ultimately the quality of an individual's life.

Self-Care. Pain can readily limit how a person is able to perform the activities of self-care, including activities of daily living (ADLs) and instrumental activities of daily living (IADLs) (e.g., shopping and house cleaning). Pain is often debilitating. Research shows a strong correlation between chronic pain and reduced physical activity (Lerman et al., 2015). In addition, most individuals who experienced chronic pain in one study suffered different limitations affecting the ability to perform intense physical exercise, walk, perform domestic chores, participate in social activities, and maintain an independent lifestyle (Dueñas et al., 2016).

Work. Pain, both acute and chronic, affects how a person performs at work or in the case of students, school. Research has shown that patients who are affected by pain present problems of absenteeism. Not only must individuals often change their occupational duties or positions, but they may also end up losing their jobs as a result of their pain symptoms (Dueñas et al., 2016).When a person is unable to perform as he or she expects, the threatened loss can result in loss of sleep, change in eating habits, depression, and fear of loss of independence.

Social Support. Support from family and friends is critical for a patient who is experiencing pain. But when a person has pain, the members of the family are also affected. Pain will restrict an individual's leisure activities and social contacts. Social isolation becomes a common problem. The negative emotions, irritability, and feelings of anger that affect patients in pain have a negative impact on interpersonal relationships and the levels of stress in families and social connections. When a family caregiver becomes involved in the care of a patient with chronic pain, the quality of the caregiver's life can decline (Dueñas et al., 2016).

REFLECT NOW

Modifiable and nonmodifiable factors can influence pain. Helping the patient and the patient's family to understand that mood, coping strategies, and the social environment can all have positive and negative influences on pain and functional outcomes is important. What type of modifiable and nonmodifiable factors that affect pain can you identify in a family member you know who had pain or a patient for whom you have provided care?

CRITICAL THINKING

Successful critical thinking requires a synthesis of knowledge, experience, information gathered from patients, critical thinking attitudes, and intellectual and professional standards. To make clinical judgments, you anticipate the information you need, analyze the data, and make decisions regarding patient care. A patient's condition or situation is always changing. During assessment consider all critical thinking elements that lead to appropriate nursing diagnoses.

Knowledge of pain physiology and the many factors that influence pain help you manage a patient's pain. Previous experience in caring for patients with pain sharpens your assessment skills and ability to choose effective therapies. Critical thinking attitudes and intellectual standards ensure the aggressive assessment, creative planning, and thorough evaluation needed to obtain an acceptable level of patient pain relief while balancing treatment benefits with treatment-associated risks. Successful pain management does not necessarily mean pain elimination but rather attainment of a mutually agreed-on pain-relief goal that allows patients to control their pain instead of the pain controlling them.

❖ NURSING PROCESS

Apply the nursing process and use a critical thinking approach in your care of patients. The nursing process provides a clinical decision-making approach for you to develop and implement an individualized plan of care. Nurses approach pain management systematically to understand and treat a patient's pain. Successful management of pain depends on establishing a relationship of trust among health care providers, patient, and family. Pain management extends beyond relief, encompassing ways to improve or maintain a patient's quality of life and ability to work productively, enjoy recreation, and function normally in the family and society.

The American Nurses Association (ANA, 2018) upholds that pain assessment and pain management are within the scope of every nurse's practice. Thus the ANA offers a certification examination in pain management to staff nurses (http://www.aspmn.org/certification). Several clinical guidelines are available for managing pain in specific disorders. Guidelines are available through the American Pain Society (APS) on the management of pain in the primary care setting; sickle cell pain; cancer pain in adults and children; and pain in osteoarthritis, rheumatoid arthritis, and juvenile chronic arthritis. Sigma Theta Tau International offers guidelines for the older adult on its website (www.geriatricpain.org). In addition, the American Academy of Pain Medicine (http://www.painmed.org/library/clinical-guidelines/) and Centers for Disease Control and Prevention (https://www.cdc.gov/drugoverdose/prescribing/guideline.html) post a variety of pain-management guidelines.

◆ Assessment

During the assessment process, thoroughly assess each patient and critically analyze findings to ensure that you make patient-centered clinical decisions required for safe nursing care. A comprehensive assessment of pain aims to gather information about the cause of a person's pain and determine its effect on his or her ability to function.

Through the Patient's Eyes. Many people view pain as a part of life. Some patients experience it for hours or days before seeking health care assistance. They often expect and even accept a certain amount of pain while being hospitalized. It is important to learn a patient's own values and beliefs about the management of pain and recognize that patient expectations will influence your ability to achieve outcomes in its management (QSEN, 2019). Asking a patient about his or her tolerable pain level is a first step in helping a patient to regain control. Assessing previous pain experiences and effective home interventions provides a foundation on which you can build. Patients expect nurses to accept their reports of pain and be prompt in meeting their pain needs.

When assessing pain, be sensitive to the level of discomfort and determine which level will allow your patient to function. For example, when caring for a patient with pain, ask, "Which level of pain will allow you to walk down the hall?" The patient answers that walking is possible when pain is at a level of 2 on a scale of 0 to 10, with 0 being no pain and 10 being worst pain imaginable. You then plan therapies to decrease the patient's pain to that level. Be sure that he or she is a partner in making decisions about the best approaches for managing pain.

Another aspect of assessing pain through the patient's eyes is to determine his or her health literacy. People who struggle to find a range of words to talk about their pain lack the ability to use language for symptom relief. Psychologists suggest that having a wide vocabulary with which to describe pain symptoms helps equip a person to better manage pain and reduce distress. Many agencies have assessment tools that allow you to get a more accurate measure of a patient's literacy skills.

If pain is acute or severe, it is unlikely that a patient is able to provide a detailed description of the entire experience. During an episode of acute pain, streamline your assessment and assess its location, severity, and quality. Collect a more detailed acute pain assessment when a patient is more comfortable (Box 44.5). For patients with chronic pain, a thorough pain assessment includes affective, cognitive, behavioral, spiritual, and social dimensions. In the home care setting family members can assess pain by using the ABCs of pain assessment and management (Box 44.6).

Because pain is dynamic, accurate assessment requires you to monitor it on a regular basis along with other vital signs. Some institutions treat it as the fifth vital sign. Pain assessment is *not* simply a number. Relying solely on a number fails to capture the multidimensionality of pain and may be unsafe, particularly when the number fails to reflect the entire pain experience or when a patient does not understand the use of the selected pain-rating scale. Pain assessment is a nursing responsibility. However, assistive personnel (AP), physical therapists, social workers, and others also screen for pain by asking patients whether they are uncomfortable or in pain. When pain is noted by any care provider, it is essential that a nurse be informed immediately so that he or she can make a thorough assessment to confirm the patient's discomfort and provide appropriate treatment.

The ability to establish a nursing diagnosis, decide on appropriate interventions, and evaluate a patient's response (outcomes) to interventions depends on the fundamental activity of a factual, timely, accurate pain assessment (Fig. 44.4). The core of this complex activity is the exploration of the pain experience through the eyes of the patient. Nurses use a variety of tools to assess nociceptive and neuropathic pain. In selecting a tool to be used with a patient, be aware of the clinical usefulness, reliability, and validity of the tool in that specific patient population. For example, a tool that has been validated for use with preverbal children may not have validity or reliability for use with adults. Assessment tools (or scales) are available for use with a number of different patient populations, including critically ill adults, young children, or adults with advanced dementia. The goal in using these tools is to identify how much pain exists, not to identify how much pain the patient tolerates.

It is necessary to be aware of possible errors in pain assessment (Box 44.7). Using the right tools and methods helps to avoid errors and ensures the selection of the right pain interventions. Failure

---

BOX 44.5 Nursing Assessment Questions

Current Pain: (Modify Assessment for Patient's Age, Cognitive Ability, Culture, Language, and Other Factors)

Palliative or Provocative factors: What makes your pain worse? What makes it better?

Quality: Describe your pain for me.

Relief measures: What do you take at home to gain pain relief? What makes your pain go away?

Region (location): Show me where you hurt.

Severity: On a scale of 0 to 10, how bad is your pain now?
- What is the worst pain you have had in the past 24 hours?
- What is the average pain you have had in the past 24 hours?

Timing: Do you have pain all of the time, only at certain times, or only on certain days?

U: Effect of pain: What are you not able to do because of your pain?
- With whom do you live, and how do they help you when you have pain?

Current Medications
- Which medications/herbs are you taking now?
- Tell me how these medications and herbs affect your pain?
- What approaches other than medications have you tried to relieve the pain?
- Have you ever used recreational drugs or alcohol to alleviate pain?

Activity
- What level of daily exercise can you maintain with your pain?
- Which type of movement increases or relieves your pain?
- Which type of activities do you now avoid because of your pain?

BOX 44.6 Routine Clinical Approach to Pain Assessment and Management: ABCDE

A: ***Ask*** about pain regularly. Assess pain systematically.

B: ***Believe*** patient and family in their report of pain and what relieves it.

C: ***Choose*** pain control options appropriate for the patient, family, and setting.

D: ***Deliver*** interventions in a timely, logical, and coordinated fashion.

E: ***Empower*** patients and their families. Enable them to control their course to the greatest extent possible.

From Jacox A, et al: *Management of cancer pain,* Clinical Practice Guideline No. 9, AHCPR Publication No. 94-0592, Rockville, MD, 1994, Agency for Health Care Policy and Research, Public Health Service, US Department of Health and Human Services.

---

of clinicians to accurately assess a patient's pain, accept the findings, and treat the report is a common cause of unrelieved pain and suffering.

Patient's Expression of Pain. A patient's self-report of pain is the single most reliable indicator of its existence and intensity (Pasero and McCaffery, 2011). Pain is individualistic. Many patients fail to report or discuss discomfort. At the same time many nurses believe that patients report pain if they have it. If patients sense that you doubt their pain exists, they share little information about their pain experience or minimize their report. Establish a caring therapeutic relationship with the patient to promote open communication. Simple measures, such as sitting when talking to patients about pain, let them know that you are sincerely concerned about their pain.

Patients unable to communicate effectively often require special attention during assessment. Infants and children, people who are developmentally delayed, patients who are psychotic, a patient who is

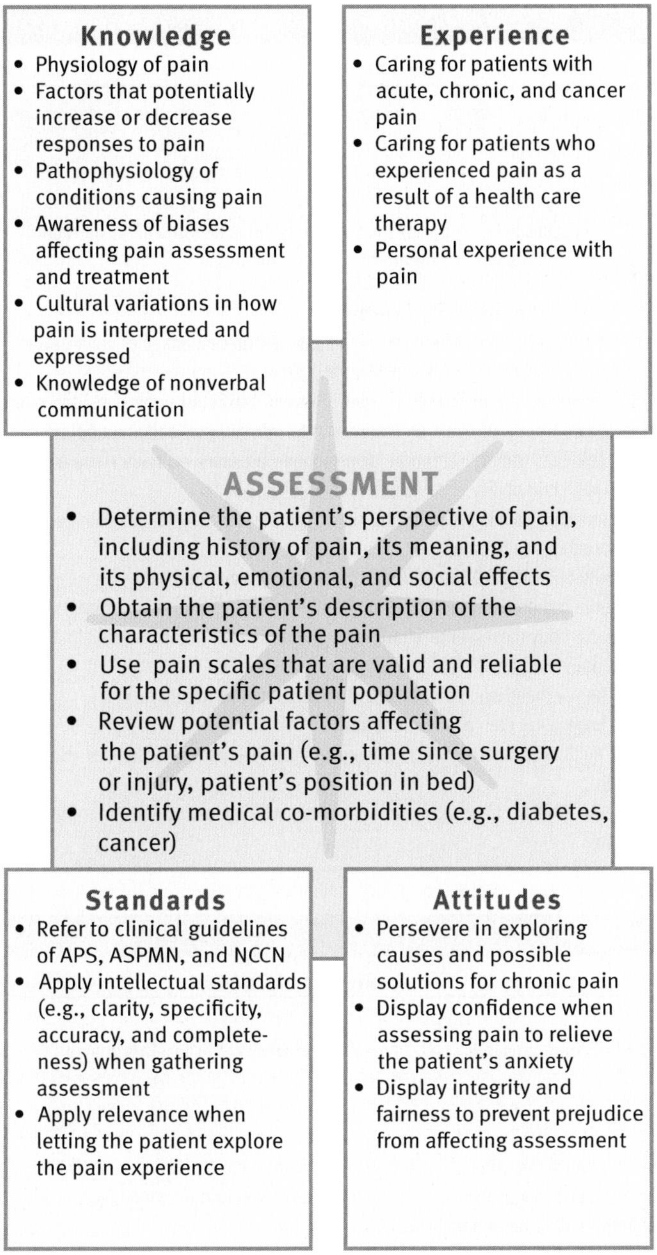

Knowledge
- Physiology of pain
- Factors that potentially increase or decrease responses to pain
- Pathophysiology of conditions causing pain
- Awareness of biases affecting pain assessment and treatment
- Cultural variations in how pain is interpreted and expressed
- Knowledge of nonverbal communication

Experience
- Caring for patients with acute, chronic, and cancer pain
- Caring for patients who experienced pain as a result of a health care therapy
- Personal experience with pain

ASSESSMENT
- Determine the patient's perspective of pain, including history of pain, its meaning, and its physical, emotional, and social effects
- Obtain the patient's description of the characteristics of the pain
- Use pain scales that are valid and reliable for the specific patient population
- Review potential factors affecting the patient's pain (e.g., time since surgery or injury, patient's position in bed)
- Identify medical co-morbidities (e.g., diabetes, cancer)

Standards
- Refer to clinical guidelines of APS, ASPMN, and NCCN
- Apply intellectual standards (e.g., clarity, specificity, accuracy, and completeness) when gathering assessment
- Apply relevance when letting the patient explore the pain experience

Attitudes
- Persevere in exploring causes and possible solutions for chronic pain
- Display confidence when assessing pain to relieve the patient's anxiety
- Display integrity and fairness to prevent prejudice from affecting assessment

FIG. 44.4 Critical thinking model for pain assessment. *APS,* American Pain Society; *ASPMN,* American Society for Pain Management Nursing; *NCCN,* National Comprehensive Cancer Network.

BOX 44.7 Possible Sources for Error in Pain Assessment

- Bias, which causes nurses to consistently overestimate or underestimate the pain that patients experience
- Vague, closed-ended, or unclear assessment questions, which lead to unreliable assessment data
- Use of pain assessment tools that are not evidence based or validated for a particular patient population
- Use of medical terms that patients with low health literacy cannot understand
- Patients who do not always provide complete, relevant, and accurate pain information
- Patients who are cognitively impaired and unable to use pain scales

---

critically ill or at end of life, patients with dementia, and patients who are aphasic or do not speak English all require different approaches. Clinical practice recommendations have been developed for the use of behavior-assessment pain tools with patients who are cognitively impaired (Box 44.8). However, you need to understand that the number obtained when using a pain-behavior scale is a behavior score, not a pain-intensity rating (Pasero and McCaffery, 2011). These tools identify the presence of pain but do not determine its intensity.

Patients with cognitive impairments require insightful assessment approaches involving close observation of vocal response, facial movements (e.g., grimacing, clenched teeth), and body movements (e.g., restlessness, pacing). Also assess social interaction (e.g., does the patient avoid conversation?). Patients who are critically ill and have a clouded sensorium or the presence of nasogastric tubes or artificial airways require specific questions that they can answer with a nod of the head or by writing out a response. If a patient speaks a different language, pain assessment is difficult and requires the assistance of a professional interpreter.

Physical Examination. When a patient is in pain, conduct a focused physical and neurological examination and observe for nonverbal responses to pain (e.g., grimacing, rigid body posture, limping, frowning, or crying) (see Chapter 30). Examine the affected painful area to see whether palpation or manipulation of the site increases pain. Assess the patient's cognitive status and ability to respond appropriately to questions. Also assess a patient's mobility/balance, especially in older adults with persistent pain. Mobility assessment is critical because of the potential impact of pain and some analgesics on the risk for falling (Galicia-Castillo and Weiner, 2019).

Characteristics of Pain. Assessment of the characteristics of pain allows you to understand the type of pain, its pattern, and the types of interventions that bring relief. Use of assessment tools to quantify the extent and degree of pain depends on a patient being cognitively alert enough to be able to understand and follow instructions.

Timing (Onset, Duration, and Pattern). Ask questions to determine the onset, duration, and time sequence of pain. When did it begin? How long has it lasted? Does it occur at the same time each day? Is it intermittent, constant, or a combination? How often does it recur? It is sometimes easier to diagnose the nature of pain by identifying time factors. Knowing the time cycle or pattern of pain helps you intervene before the pain occurs or worsens (see Box 44.5).

Location. Ask a patient to describe or point to all areas of discomfort to assess pain location. To localize the pain specifically, have him or her trace the area from the most severe point outward. This is difficult to do if pain is diffuse or involves several sites or parts of the body. Do not assume that your patient's pain always occurs in the same location. When describing pain location to other health care providers, use anatomical landmarks and descriptive terminology. The statement "Pain is localized in the upper right abdominal quadrant" is more specific than "The patient states the pain is in the abdomen." Pain classified by location can be further classified as superficial or cutaneous, deep or visceral, referred, or radiating (Table 44.5).

Severity. One of the most subjective and therefore most useful characteristics for reporting pain is its severity. Nurses teach patients how to use pain scales to help them communicate pain severity or intensity. Many scales are available in several languages to aid nurses when a professional interpreter is not present. The purpose of using a pain scale is to identify a patient's perception of pain intensity over time so that the effectiveness of interventions can be evaluated (Pasero and McCaffery, 2011). It is important

BOX 44.8 EVIDENCE-BASED PRACTICE

Pain Assessment in the Nonverbal Patient

PICOT Question: In elderly nonverbal patients, which pain-assessment tool is most effective in determining presence of pain?

Evidence Summary

A common misconception is that individuals who are nonverbal as a result of dementia or cognitive impairments do not experience pain. These patients often present with atypical manifestations of pain caused by pathophysiological changes in the brain. Manifestations often include fearful expressions, combativeness, and resistance to care (Atee et al., 2017). An evidence-based position statement and clinical practice recommendations for pain assessment in patients who are nonverbal was developed by the Hartford Institute for Geriatric Nursing and the Alzheimer's Association (Horgas, 2018). No single assessment strategy, such as interpretation of behaviors, pathology, or estimates of pain by others, is sufficient by itself in determining the presence of pain in a patient who is unable to communicate. However, initial assessment can be performed by using self-assessment with a numeric rating scale or verbal descriptor scale (Horgas, 2017).

A number of tools have been developed to assess for the presence of pain in adults who are cognitively impaired. Although research studies have demonstrated that these tools can be used to determine the presence of pain, there has been little evidence to determine whether they can be used to identify pain intensity. Commonly used instruments include the Abbey Pain Scale, Pain Assessment in Advanced Dementia Scale (PAINAD), and Noncommunicative Patient's Pain Assessment Instrument (NOPPAIN) to recognize the presence or absence of pain and provide a rating of pain severity in older people with impaired cognition. An electronic pain assessment tool (ePAT) app was recently developed to provide

point-of-care facial recognition technology for detecting facial micro-expression indicative of pain, as well as the presence of pain-related behaviors under five additional domains (voice, movement, behavior, activity, and body) (Atee, 2017). An analysis revealed a sensitivity of 96.1% and accuracy of 95% (Hoti et al., 2018). This assessment supports the clinical usefulness of the ePAT for identifying pain in patients with moderate to severe dementia.

Application to Nursing Practice

- Attempt a self-report of pain using simple yes/no responses or vocalizations or a numerical rating scale (Chow et al., 2016).
- Search for potential causes of pain (Horgas, 2018). Examples include pain associated with intravenous insertion site infiltrations, abdominal cramping and fullness, urinary retention, or prolonged pressure on body parts associated with immobility.
- Assume that pain is present after ruling out other problems (infection, constipation) that cause pain.
- Identify pathological conditions or procedures that cause pain.
- Observe patient behaviors and list behaviors (e.g., facial expressions, vocalizations, body movements, changes in interactions or mental status) that indicate pain (Horgas, 2018).
- Ask family members, parents, or caregivers for a surrogate report.
- Use behavioral pain assessment tools.
- Use evidence-based tools to ensure appropriate pain assessment (Horgas, 2018).
- Use the PAINAD to assess pain in patients with advanced dementia (Horgas, 2018).

TABLE 44.5 Classification of Pain By Location

Location	Characteristics	Examples of Causes
Superficial or Cutaneous		
Pain resulting from stimulation of skin	Pain is of short duration and localized. It usually is a sharp sensation.	Needlestick; small cut or laceration
Deep or Visceral		
Pain resulting from stimulation of internal organs	Pain is diffuse and radiates in several directions. Duration varies, but it usually lasts longer than superficial pain. Pain is sharp, dull, or unique to organ involved.	Crushing sensation (e.g., angina pectoris); burning sensation (e.g., gastric ulcer)
Referred		
Common in visceral pain because many organs themselves have no pain receptors (The entrance of sensory neurons from affected organ into same spinal cord segment as neurons from areas where individual feels pain causes perception of pain in unaffected areas.)	Pain is in part of body separate from source of pain and assumes any characteristic.	Myocardial infarction, which causes referred pain to the jaw, left arm, and left shoulder; kidney stones, which refer pain to groin
Radiating		
Sensation of pain extending from initial site of injury to another body part	Pain feels as though it travels down or along body part. It is intermittent or constant.	Low back pain from ruptured intravertebral disk accompanied by pain radiating down leg from sciatic nerve irritation

to select the scale that is appropriate for a patient's age, language, condition, and ability and to ensure that the patient understands how to use it.

Pain Scales. A numerical rating scale (NRS) requires patients to rate pain on an 11-point line of 0 to 10, with 0 representing no pain and 10 representing the worst pain the patient can imagine (Fig. 44.5A). The scale has been found to be very effective in many populations, including youth with disabilities (Miró et al., 2016). This scale is also used to assess pain intensity before and after therapeutic interventions. A verbal descriptive scale (VDS) consists of a line with two- to six-word descriptors equally spaced along the line (Fig. 44.5B). Show a patient the scale and ask him or her to choose the descriptor that best represents the severity of pain. A visual analog scale (VAS) consists of a straight line without labeled subdivisions (Fig. 44.5C). The straight line shows a continuum of intensity and has labeled end points. A patient indicates pain by marking the appropriate point on the line. Use a scale to measure the current severity of a patient's pain. Also ask patients to rate their average pain and the worst pain they have had in the past 24 hours. This information allows you to see trends in pain severity.

Another pain scale, originally developed for children to assess pain, is now used worldwide with people ages 3 and older (Faces of Pain Care, 2016). The Wong-Baker Faces Pain Rating Scale (FPS-revised) provides a pictorial representation of pain intensity (Fig. 44.6) (Wong and Baker, 1988; IASP, 2018b). Young children do not always know what the word *pain* means; therefore assessment requires you to use words such as *owie, boo-boo,* or *hurt.* However, the "faces" scale has been shown through research to be very reliable and valid in measuring pain severity. Also, a recent study among adults from a developing country showed the "faces" scale to be preferred over the NRS (Pathak et al., 2018). Such self-report measures of pain are most often used for children older than 3 to 4 years, but even 2-year-olds can report pain (Hockenberry and Wilson, 2019). As children develop, newer cognitive skills such as measurement and classification mature so that school-age children can use the NRS to assess pain (Hockenberry and Wilson,

2019). Another popular pain scale shown to be valid and reliable is the Oucher pain scale (0-10) (Beyer et al., 1992). It uses a series of photographic images of faces in varying degrees of distress (Fig. 44.7). A child points to a face on the tool, thus simplifying the task of describing the pain. Different forms of the Oucher pain scale have been developed for specific ethnic groups, including Asian, Hispanic, and African American. A good pain scale is easy to use, understandable, and not time consuming. If a patient is able to read and understand a scale easily, the pain description is more accurate. If patients use a hearing aid or glasses, be sure that they are using them when answering pain-assessment questions or marking a pain scale. Once you select a scale that works for a patient, be sure to use it consistently. Do not use a pain scale to compare the pain of one patient with that of another.

Quality. There is no common or specific pain vocabulary in general use. Patients describe pain in their own way. A study conducted in 1990 showed that Hispanics, American Indians, blacks, and whites all rated *pain* as the most intense term, followed by *hurt; ache* was the least intense (Gaston-Johansson et al., 1990). The research is dated, but it shows the importance of not assuming that one patient perceives pain differently from another only on the basis of cultural background. Assess the terms that patients use to describe their discomfort; then use these words consistently to obtain an accurate report. For example, say, "Tell me what your discomfort feels like. What do you call it?" The patient may describe the pain as crushing, throbbing, sharp, or dull. For example, if it is dull, when you return to the patient, ask if it is still "dull." It is always more accurate to have patients describe the pain in their own words whenever possible.

There is some consistency in the way people describe certain types of pain. The pain associated with a myocardial infarction is often described as crushing or viselike, whereas the pain of a surgical incision is often described as dull, aching, and throbbing, indicating nociceptive pain. Neuropathic pain is usually pricking pain, burning, electric-like, or numbness (Colloca et al, 2017). When a patient's descriptions fit the pattern forming in the assessment, you then make a clearer analysis of the nature and type of pain. This leads to more appropriate pain management because you treat nociceptive and neuropathic pain differently.

Aggravating and Precipitating Factors. Various factors or conditions precipitate or aggravate pain. Ask a patient to describe activities that cause or aggravate pain, such as physical movement, positions, drinking coffee or alcohol, urination, swallowing, eating food, or psychological stress. Also ask them to demonstrate actions that cause a painful response, such as coughing or turning a certain way. Some symptoms (depression, anxiety, fatigue, sedation, anorexia, sleep disruption, spiritual distress, and guilt) cause a worsening of pain or may be aggravated by it. Assess for these associated symptoms and evaluate their effects on the

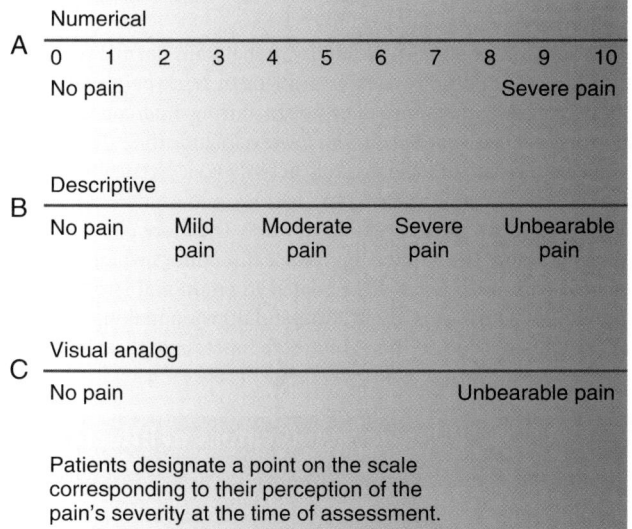

FIG. 44.5 Sample pain scales. **A,** Numerical. **B,** Verbal descriptive. **C,** Visual analog.

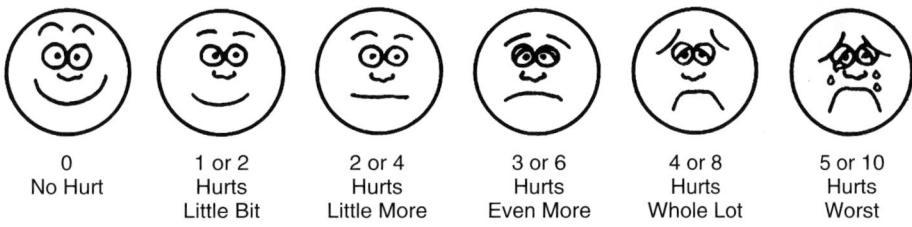

Brief word instructions: Point to each face using the words to describe the pain intensity. Ask the child to choose face that best describes own pain and record the appropriate number.

FIG. 44.6 Wong-Baker Faces Pain Scale-Revised. (From Hockenberry MJ, et al: *Wong's nursing care of infants and children,* ed 11, St Louis, 2019, Elsevier.)

patient's pain perception. After identifying specific aggravating or precipitating factors, it is easier to plan interventions to avoid worsening the pain.

Relief Measures. Ask patients how they relieve their pain, such as changing position, using ritualistic behavior (pacing, rocking, or rubbing), eating, meditating, praying, or applying heat or cold to a painful site. Encourage patients to continue using their own pain-relieving measures if they are effective and appropriate to the cause of pain. Patients gain trust when they know that nurses are willing to try their relief measures, especially in the home setting. Patients gain a sense of control over the pain instead of the pain controlling them. Identify all the patient's health care providers (e.g., internist, orthopedist, acupuncturist, chiropractor, or dentist) in addition to assessing relief measures.

Effects of Pain on the Patient. Pain alters a person's lifestyle and psychological well-being. For example, chronic/persistent pain causes suffering, loss of control, loneliness, exhaustion, and an impaired quality of life. To understand a pain experience, ask the patient what the pain prevents him or her from doing.

Behavioral Effects. When a patient has pain, assess verbalization, vocal response, facial and body movements, and social interaction. A verbal report of pain is a vital part of assessment. You need to be willing to listen and understand. When a patient is unable to communicate

pain, it is especially important for you to be alert for behaviors that indicate it (Box 44.9).

The nonverbal expression of pain either supports or contradicts other information about it. If a woman in labor reports that her labor pains are occurring more frequently and if she begins to massage her abdomen more often, this confirms her report. If a patient reports severe abdominal pain but continues to grasp the chest, a more detailed assessment is probably needed.

Influence on Activities of Daily Living. Patients who live with daily pain or have prolonged pain during a hospitalization are less able to participate in routine activities, which results in physical deconditioning. This deconditioning can slow a patient's recovery (see Chapter 38). Assessment of these changes reveals the extent of a patients' disabilities and adjustments necessary to help them participate in self-care. The primary goal of the nurse is to improve patient function.

Ask a patient whether pain interferes with sleep. Some patients experience difficulty in falling asleep and/or staying asleep. The pain may awaken the patient during the night and make it hard to fall back to sleep.

Depending on the location of the pain, some patients have difficulty independently performing ADLs. For example, some pain restricts mobility to the point at which a patient is no longer able to bathe in a bathtub or dress himself or herself. Some patients with severe arthritis find it painful to grasp eating utensils or lower themselves to a toilet seat. Assess the patient's need for help with self-care activities, determine whether a family caregiver provides assistance at home, and collaborate with members of the health care team (e.g., physical and occupational therapy).

Pain sometimes impairs the ability to maintain normal sexual relations. Physical conditions such as arthritis or back pain may prevent patients from assuming usual positions during intercourse. Pain or fatigue may reduce a patient's desire for sex. Include the extent to which pain affects the patient's usual sexual activity (i.e., physically unable or reduced desire) in your assessment.

Pain threatens a person's ability to work. The more physical activity required in a job, the greater the risk of discomfort when the pain is associated with movement. Pain related to emotional stress increases in individuals whose jobs involve stressful decision making. Assess the work that patients do and their abilities to function in their jobs. Assess

Oucher®

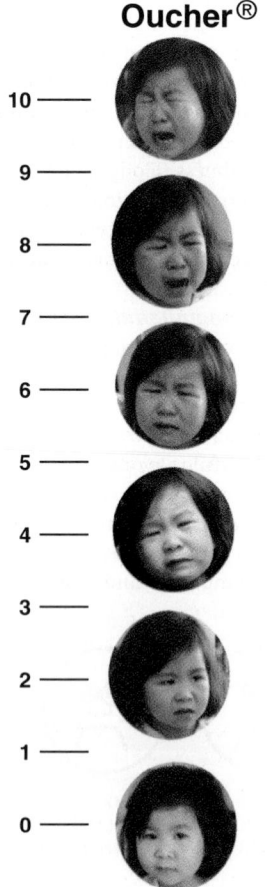

10 ——
9 ——
8 ——
7 ——
6 ——
5 ——
4 ——
3 ——
2 ——
1 ——
0 ——

FIG. 44.7 Asian girl version of the Oucher pain scale. (The Asian versions of the Oucher scale [male and female] were developed and copyrighted in 2003 by CH Yeh [University of Pittsburgh] and CH Wang, Taiwan.)

BOX 44.9	Behavioral Indicators of Effects of Pain

Vocalizations
- Moaning
- Crying
- Gasping
- Grunting

Facial Expressions
- Grimace
- Clenched teeth
- Wrinkled forehead
- Tightly closed or widely opened eyes or mouth
- Lip biting

Body Movement
- Restlessness
- Immobilization

- Muscle tension
- Increased hand and finger movements
- Pacing activities
- Rhythmic or rubbing motions
- Protective movement of body parts
- Grabbing or holding a body part

Social Interaction
- Avoidance of conversation
- Focus only on activities for pain relief
- Avoidance of social contacts
- Reduced attention span
- Reduced interaction with environment

the daily chores of homemakers in the same manner as the duties involved in jobs outside the home. Also assess whether it is necessary for patients to stop activity occasionally because of pain, and help them select ways to minimize or control it so that they are able to remain productive.

Include an assessment of the effect of pain on social activities. Some pain is so debilitating that the patient becomes too exhausted to socialize. Identify a patient's normal social activities, the extent to which activities have been disrupted, and the desire to participate in these activities.

Concomitant Symptoms. Concomitant symptoms occur with pain and usually increase a patient's pain severity. Examples include nausea, headache, dizziness, urge to urinate, constipation, depression, and restlessness. Certain types of pain have predictable concomitant symptoms. For example, severe rectal pain often leads to constipation. These symptoms are as much a problem to a patient as the pain itself.

REFLECT NOW

Consider a patient you recently cared for in a clinical experience or consider a time when you experienced a painful condition. In what way did pain limit your daily activities/the activities of the patient? How did you or the patient adapt to those limitations?

◆ Nursing Diagnosis

An accurate nursing diagnosis may be made only after you perform a complete assessment. The development of accurate nursing diagnoses for a patient in pain results from thorough data collection and analysis (Box 44.10). Careful assessment reveals the presence or a potential for pain. Be sure that your assessment includes the patient's history of recent procedures or preexisting painful conditions.

The nursing diagnosis focuses on the specific nature of a patient's pain to identify the most relevant types of interventions for alleviating it and improving the patient's function. *Acute Pain related to physical trauma* and *Acute Pain related to natural childbirth processes* require very different nursing interventions. Accurate identification of related factors for problem-focused or negative nursing diagnoses helps you choose appropriate nursing interventions. You will sometimes use this information to identify interventions that treat or modify the related factor *or risk* for the diagnosis to be resolved. For example, interventions for *Acute Pain related to physical trauma* usually require pharmacological intervention, whereas *Acute Pain related to natural childbirth processes* is sometimes managed more appropriately with nonpharmacological interventions, such as controlled breathing techniques.

A pain assessment often directs you to identify additional diagnoses other than that of *Acute* or *Chronic Pain*. The extent to which pain affects a patient's function and general state of health determines whether other nursing diagnoses are relevant. For example, your assessment reveals that a patient reports having pain of the hands and shoulders and has difficulty removing or fastening necessary items of clothing. The patient has had osteoarthritis for over 3 years with persistent discomfort and weakness of the upper extremities. The nursing diagnoses for this patient are *Self-Care Deficit; Impaired Ability to Dress* and *Chronic Pain*. The diagnosis of *Self-Care Deficit; Impaired Ability to Dress* requires involvement by members of the interprofessional health care team to provide the

---

BOX 44.10 Nursing Diagnostic Process

Chronic Pain

Assessment Activities	Assessment Findings
Have patient describe pain intensity.	Pain is constant; patient verbally reports 5 on a scale of 0 to 10
Assess onset and location of pain.	Present for 7 months in lower lumbar area
Observe patient behaviors.	Grimaces and grunts when sitting, rubs flanks frequently; reduced movement in upper trunk and legs
Assess effect of pain on activities of daily living (ADLs).	Appetite poor; gets little sleep; difficulty dressing
Review medical history.	Previous trauma; effectiveness of past pain-control measures

---

patient with assistive devices for performing self-care. Examples of other diagnoses that may be related to pain follow:

- *Difficulty Coping*
- *Fatigue*
- *Impaired Mobility*
- *Impaired Sleep*
- *Social Isolation*

◆ Planning

During the planning step of the nursing process, analyze information from multiple sources, including the patient, family, and other health care providers. Critical thinking ensures that a patient's plan of care (see the Nursing Care Plan) integrates all that is known about the individual and key critical thinking elements (Fig. 44.8). Professional standards are especially important to consider when developing a plan of care. These standards establish evidence-based guidelines for selecting effective nursing interventions. Professional standards of care regarding pain management are available as agency policies or through professional organizations such as the American Society for Pain Management Nursing (ASPMN).

Another strategy for planning care is using a concept map. Patients who are in pain frequently have interrelated problems. As one problem gets worse, other aspects of a patient's level of health also change. A concept map helps you determine how the nursing diagnoses are interrelated with one another and linked to the patient's medical diagnosis. This eventually allows you to also see how interventions are related for different diagnoses. See the example for Mrs. Mays' plan of care (Fig. 44.9). Identifying the relationships between diagnoses and interventions helps you develop a holistic and patient-centered plan of care.

Goals and Outcomes. Because the pain experience is so closely connected to a patient's perceptions, beliefs, and attitudes, it is essential that your plan include goals of care accepted by the patient. A patient-centered plan will more likely promote the patient's optimal function. Partner with the patient to determine relevant and realistic expectations for pain relief. Decide on a mutually acceptable level of pain that allows return of function. Make sure that the patient understands that complete pain relief may not be possible but that every effort will be made to allow him or her to safely reach a pain level that allows for maximum function.

NURSING CARE PLAN

Acute Pain

ASSESSMENT

Mrs. Mays, 72 years old, was diagnosed with a cancerous tumor in her left lung 2 months ago. She takes ibuprofen on an as-needed (prn) basis to manage her arthritis pain. She is admitted to the hospital with uncontrollable pain in her chest, shortness of breath, and possible pneumonia.

Assessment Activities	*Assessment Findings*[a]
Ask Mrs. Mays what she did at home to control her pain.	Her **pain rapidly escalated** over several hours from a 3 to a 10 on a scale of 0 to 10, so she doubled her ibuprofen and went to bed, but this did not help.
Ask Mrs. Mays to describe the pain she is having now.	She is having sharp, stabbing constant pain on the lower left side of her chest.
Ask Mrs. Mays to rate her pain on a scale of 0 to 10.	She **rates her pain at a 7.**
Ask Mrs. Mays what has helped and worsened her pain.	She responds that her pain decreases when she stays still and takes shallow breaths. It is worsened by activity (e.g., walking, completing ADLS), deeper breaths, and coughing.
Observe Mrs. Mays' nonverbal behavior.	She is **restless,** is **unable to stay focused,** her **muscles tense, and** she is **frowning** during the history taking.

[a]**Assessment findings** are shown in bold type.

NURSING DIAGNOSIS: Acute pain related to abrupt onset of pulmonary inflammation

PLANNING

Goals	*Expected Outcomes (NOC)*[b]
	Pain Control
Mrs. Mays will perceive a tolerable level of pain before discharge.	Mrs. Mays reports chest pain at target goal of 3 or below.
	Mrs. Mays demonstrates use of nonpharmacologic therapies.
	Pain: Disruptive Effects
Mrs. Mays will actively participate in activities of daily living (ADLs).	Mrs. Mays reports sleeping for 5 to 6 hours without interruption from pain.
	Mrs. Mays completes her own hygiene with minimal assistance.
	Mrs. Mays walks the hallway with her husband every 4 hours for 15 minutes.

[b]Outcome classification labels from Moorhead S, et al: *Nursing Outcomes Classification (NOC),* ed 6, St Louis, 2018, Elsevier.

INTERVENTIONS (NIC)[c]	RATIONALE
Pain Management: Acute	
Begin around-the-clock (ATC) prescribed dose of opioid and co-analgesic.	Severe acute pain requires immediate-release opioid (US Dept of Veterans Affairs, 2017). Most opioids may be given around the clock (ATC) for continuous pain. ATC dosing is recommended after an optimal dose is established by dose titration (National Pharmaceutical Council, 2001)
Consult with health care provider for providing a multimodal pharmacological regimen	Combining analgesics with at least two different mechanisms of action can optimize pain control.
Have patient select nonpharmacological interventions that have relieved her pain in the past (e.g., distraction, music, simple relaxation therapy) or that are acceptable to her.	Nonpharmacological approaches augment pharmacological therapy and help patients improve quality of life and decrease anxiety and depression (Tick et al., 2018).
Teach spouse how to perform slow-stroke back massage when pain has lessened.	Slow-stroke back massage is easy to do, takes a short time, and induces relaxation (Tick et al., 2018). Not likely effective during most acute pain.

[c]Intervention classification labels from Bulechek GM, et al: *Nursing Interventions Classification (NIC),* ed 7, St Louis, 2018, Elsevier.

EVALUATION

Evaluation Activity	*Patient Response/Finding*	*Outcome Status*
Ask Mrs. Mays if she has attained her pain-relief goal most of the time.	She responds, "My pain usually runs around a 3, except when I start coughing or walking."	Mrs. Mays reports an acceptable level of pain.
Observe Mrs. Mays performing ADLs, walking, and during sleep.	Mrs. Mays is dressed for breakfast, walking the hallway every 4 hours with her husband. The night nurse's notes indicate that she slept through the night.	Ability to perform ADLs and sleep has improved. Continue to monitor.
Ask Mr. Mays if he was able to give his wife a back rub.	Mr. Mays reported that she did not want a back rub but preferred to have her feet rubbed, which he was happy to do. "She said it made her feel more relaxed."	Nonpharmacological intervention was successful but needs to be changed from back rub to foot rub in the nursing care plan.

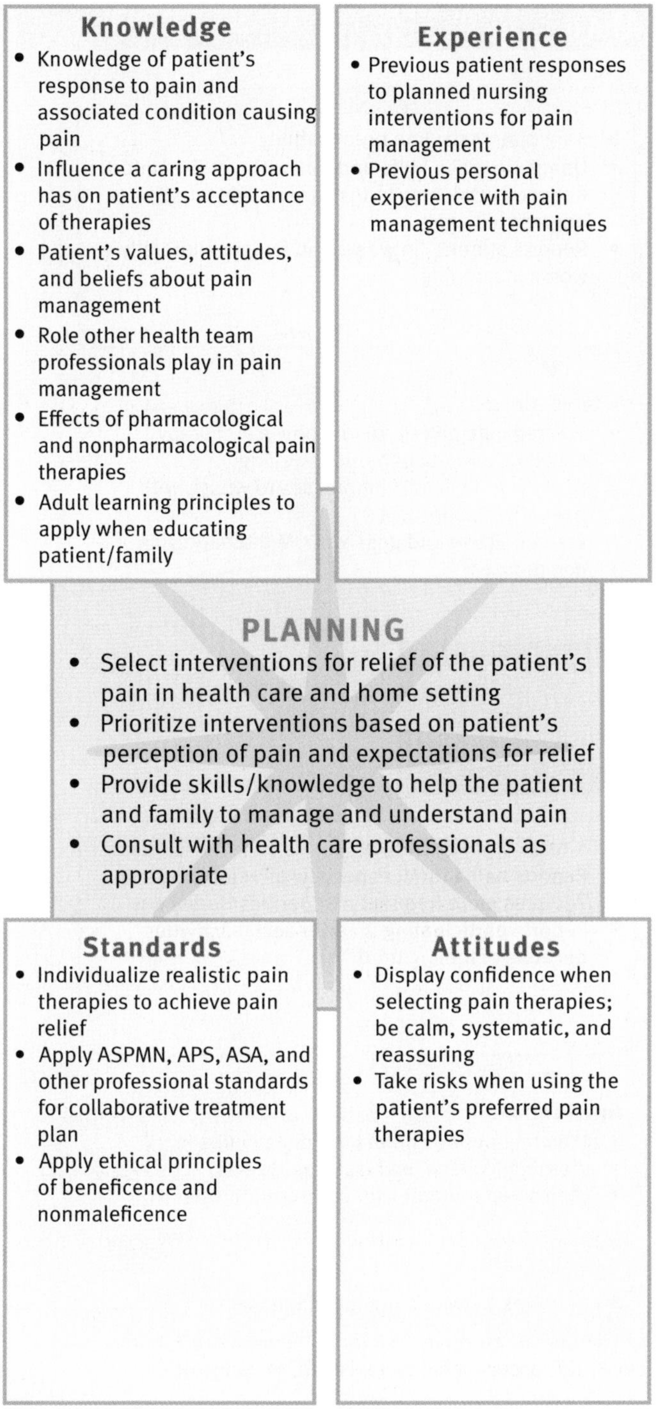

Knowledge

- Knowledge of patient's response to pain and associated condition causing pain
- Influence a caring approach has on patient's acceptance of therapies
- Patient's values, attitudes, and beliefs about pain management
- Role other health team professionals play in pain management
- Effects of pharmacological and nonpharmacological pain therapies
- Adult learning principles to apply when educating patient/family

Experience

- Previous patient responses to planned nursing interventions for pain management
- Previous personal experience with pain management techniques

PLANNING

- Select interventions for relief of the patient's pain in health care and home setting
- Prioritize interventions based on patient's perception of pain and expectations for relief
- Provide skills/knowledge to help the patient and family to manage and understand pain
- Consult with health care professionals as appropriate

Standards

- Individualize realistic pain therapies to achieve pain relief
- Apply ASPMN, APS, ASA, and other professional standards for collaborative treatment plan
- Apply ethical principles of beneficence and nonmaleficence

Attitudes

- Display confidence when selecting pain therapies; be calm, systematic, and reassuring
- Take risks when using the patient's preferred pain therapies

FIG. 44.8 Critical thinking model for pain management planning. *APS,* American Pain Society; *ASPMN,* American Society Pain Management Nursing; *ASA,* American Society of Anesthesiologists.

It is important to remember that a successful plan of care requires a therapeutic relationship with a patient and family to focus on a relevant education plan. Helping patients learn how to manage their pain is always a goal of care. You help best by listening to the patient's concerns, needs, and understanding of available pain-relief measures. A patient knows the most about his or her pain and is an important partner in selecting successful pain therapies.

An indication of the success of a plan of care is determined through attainment of goals and outcomes. For example, for the goal "the patient will achieve a satisfactory level of pain relief within 24 hours," the following are possible outcomes:

- Reports that pain is a 3 or less on a scale of 0 to 10
- Avoids factors that intensify pain
- Uses pain-relief measures safely
- Is able to dress self

REFLECT NOW

In addition to goals for reducing pain intensity, goals should be set with patients concerning their physiological, affective, cognitive, behavioral, spiritual, and social functioning with the use of pharmacological and nonpharmacological management strategies. Why is it important to address these other domains of pain rather than just focusing on reducing pain intensity?

Setting Priorities. When setting priorities in pain management, consider the type of pain the patient is experiencing and the effect that it has on function and quality of life. The primary goal often is to decrease pain to help the patient improve function. Any episode of acute pain is a priority because of its potential effects on physical and psychological function. In addition, acute pain may cause the interruption or delay of other important therapies (e.g., ambulation, physical therapy, or a planned diagnostic procedure). For less acute pain, work with the patient to select interventions that are appropriate and relevant. For example, if an analgesic is relieving acute pain, turn your attention to how the pain is affecting the patient's activity, appetite, and sleep. What other therapies can you provide? Priorities change as a patient's pain experience changes.

Teamwork and Collaboration. A comprehensive plan includes the collaboration of a variety of members from the health care team, including advanced practice nurses, doctors of pharmacology (PharmDs), physical therapists, occupational therapists, physicians, social workers, psychologists, and clergy. An oncology or pain clinical nurse specialist is very familiar with pharmacological and nonpharmacological interventions that are most effective for chronic/persistent pain. PharmDs are knowledgeable about pharmacological treatments of pain. Physical therapists plan exercises that strengthen muscle groups and lessen pain in affected areas. Occupational therapists devise splints to support painful body parts and plan approaches for performing ADLs. Physicians are familiar with pharmacological interventions, and some are skilled in interventional pain procedures such as nerve blocks and spinal cord stimulator implantations. Social workers and psychologists may offer cognitive behavioral therapy or mindfulness training for pain relief. Clergy members help patients focus on spiritual health by helping patients find the meaning of their pain. It is important to also involve family caregivers in the plan of care. They will often administer care in the home after discharge. If the pain-management plan is unsuccessful in achieving the identified pain-relief goal(s), talk with the patient's health care provider about revising it. Consultation with a pain expert is sometimes necessary.

◆ Implementation

Pain therapy requires an individualized approach, perhaps more so than any other patient problem. The nurse, patient, and frequently the family are partners in pain management. You are responsible for administering and monitoring therapies ordered by health care

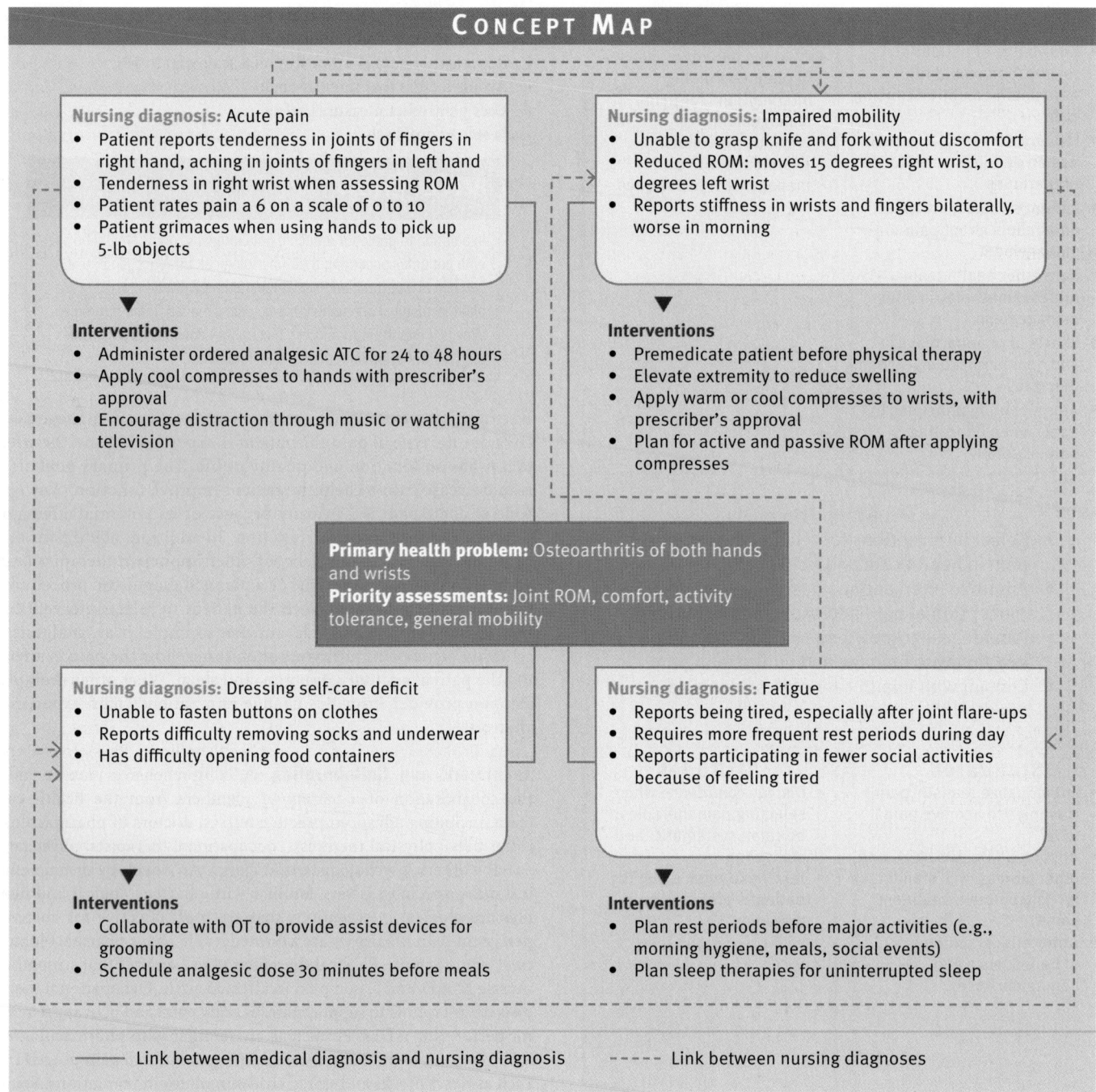

CONCEPT MAP

Nursing diagnosis: Acute pain
- Patient reports tenderness in joints of fingers in right hand, aching in joints of fingers in left hand
- Tenderness in right wrist when assessing ROM
- Patient rates pain a 6 on a scale of 0 to 10
- Patient grimaces when using hands to pick up 5-lb objects

Interventions
- Administer ordered analgesic ATC for 24 to 48 hours
- Apply cool compresses to hands with prescriber's approval
- Encourage distraction through music or watching television

Nursing diagnosis: Impaired mobility
- Unable to grasp knife and fork without discomfort
- Reduced ROM: moves 15 degrees right wrist, 10 degrees left wrist
- Reports stiffness in wrists and fingers bilaterally, worse in morning

Interventions
- Premedicate patient before physical therapy
- Elevate extremity to reduce swelling
- Apply warm or cool compresses to wrists, with prescriber's approval
- Plan for active and passive ROM after applying compresses

Primary health problem: Osteoarthritis of both hands and wrists
Priority assessments: Joint ROM, comfort, activity tolerance, general mobility

Nursing diagnosis: Dressing self-care deficit
- Unable to fasten buttons on clothes
- Reports difficulty removing socks and underwear
- Has difficulty opening food containers

Nursing diagnosis: Fatigue
- Reports being tired, especially after joint flare-ups
- Requires more frequent rest periods during day
- Reports participating in fewer social activities because of feeling tired

Interventions
- Collaborate with OT to provide assist devices for grooming
- Schedule analgesic dose 30 minutes before meals

Interventions
- Plan rest periods before major activities (e.g., morning hygiene, meals, social events)
- Plan sleep therapies for uninterrupted sleep

——— Link between medical diagnosis and nursing diagnosis   - - - - Link between nursing diagnoses

FIG. 44.9 Concept map for Mrs. Mays. *ATC,* Around the clock; *OT,* occupational therapist; *ROM,* range of motion.

providers for pain relief and independently providing measures that complement those prescribed. Generally try the least invasive or safest therapy first along with previously used successful patient remedies. If you question a medical therapy, consult with the health care provider.

Your ability to show compassionate care toward patients has the potential for maximizing their pain control. You can help a patient minimize pain through caring behaviors such as listening, offering a gentle touch, and responding promptly to a pain request.

Health Promotion. When providing pain-relief measures, apply these guidelines for individualizing pain therapy:

- Use different types of pain-relief measures. Persistent pain is multifactorial, requiring an approach that addresses a variety of etiologies and includes pharmacological and nonpharmacological strategies (Galicia-Castillo and Weiner, 2019).
- Be willing to use more than one type of pain relief measure as appropriate.
- Use measures that the patient believes are effective.
- Keep an open mind about ways to relieve pain.
- Keep trying. When efforts at pain relief fail, do not abandon the patient but reassess the situation. Persistent pain is treatable, with improvement anticipated, but it is not curable (Galicia-Castillo and Weiner, 2019).

- Although pain may not be totally eliminated, substantial improvement in function is realistic (Galicia-Castillo and Weiner, 2019).

Maintaining Wellness. Patients are better prepared to handle almost any situation when they understand it. The experience of pain and its related therapies is no exception. However, patients with moderate-to-severe pain are not always able to participate in decision making until the pain is controlled at an acceptable level. Once you accomplish this, you can begin teaching.

Pain often affects a patient's ability to sleep and remain asleep. Consider consulting with a health care provider on appropriate medications for the patient, and try nonpharmacological interventions to promote sleep (see Chapter 43). Instruct patients not to use medications that promote sleep as a substitute for pain relief.

Health literacy significantly affects a patient's pain experience and understanding of pain-management strategies. Low health literacy poses significant barriers to optimal pain management. In a study of patients with chronic pain, patients with low health literacy were found to have low overall pain medication knowledge and did not know where to find health care professionals to help them with their pain (Devraj et al., 2013). The patients in the study also lacked knowledge about nonpharmacological approaches to pain management and did not know which nonprescription pain medications could provide pain relief. In another study Spanish-speaking Hispanic Americans commonly reported difficulties in describing their pain experience and problems in understanding clinical recommendations from non–Spanish-speaking health care providers (Hollingshead et al., 2016).

Research conducted with patients with chronic back pain and other patient groups provides evidence for why educational materials and approaches must be adapted so that they are suited for patients with low health literacy. In addition, combat any cultural norms that may stop patients from talking about pain at all. Stoicism (suffering without verbalizing complaint) not only potentially obscures dangerous signs about which you should know, but also denies people the opportunity to use labels as a tool to cope with pain. Help patients find words to describe their pain when they are experiencing difficulty explaining it on their own (Pasero and McCaffery, 2011). Because pain affects physical and mental functioning, holistic health approaches are important interventions. Holistic health is an ongoing state of wellness that involves taking care of the whole person: body, mind, spirit, and emotions. To achieve optimal health and well-being, it is necessary to have balance of all of the interdependent elements of the whole person (Matthews-Kozanecka, 2014).

Patients actively participate in their own well-being whenever possible. Common holistic health approaches include wellness education, regular exercise, rest, relaxation techniques (see Chapter 32), attention to good hygiene practices and nutrition, and management of interpersonal relationships. When a person develops pain, offer nonpharmacological strategies. Several nonpharmacological interventions are nurse initiated.

Nonpharmacological Pain-Relief Interventions. Nonpharmacological interventions can be used alone or in combination with pharmacological measures. However, in the case of moderate to severe acute pain, nonpharmacological therapies should not be used in place of pharmacological therapies. A number of nonpharmacological interventions are available for lessening pain. Evidence-based therapies include acupuncture and massage, osteopathic and chiropractic manipulation, cognitive-behavioral intervention, meditative movement and mind-body interventions, and dietary and self-management approaches to pain management (see Chapter 32) (Tick et al., 2018).

Researchers suggest that these evidence-based nonpharmacological interventions should be used routinely to provide a comprehensive plan for pain management, although the effectiveness may vary depending on the type of pain that the patient is experiencing and the patient's belief in the therapy. Both active (physical movement) and passive nonpharmacological strategies can target different pathways for pain relief while increasing physical functioning. For example, cognitive-behavioral interventions change patients' perceptions of pain, alter pain behavior, and provide patients with a greater sense of control. Distraction, prayer, mindfulness, relaxation, guided imagery, music, and biofeedback are examples of therapies frequently initiated by nurses (US Department of Veterans Affairs, 2017).

Physical approaches aim to provide pain relief, correct physical dysfunction, alter physiological responses, and reduce fear associated with pain-related immobility. Complementary and alternative medicine (CAM) therapies such as therapeutic touch and mindfulness meditation help to alleviate pain in some patients (see Chapter 32). An evidence-based practice protocol for pain management in older adults recommends these guidelines for nonpharmacological therapies (Abdulla et al., 2013):

- Tailor nonpharmacological techniques to the individual.
- Cognitive behavioral strategies may be inappropriate for the cognitively impaired.
- Physical pain-relief strategies (e.g., heat, cold, transcutaneous electrical nerve stimulation [TENS]) focus on promoting comfort and altering physiological responses to pain and are generally safe and effective.

Relaxation and Guided Imagery. Relaxation and guided imagery allow patients to alter affective-motivational and cognitive pain perception. Relaxation is mental and physical freedom from tension or stress that provides individuals a sense of self-control. You use relaxation techniques at any phase of health or illness. Physiological and behavioral changes associated with relaxation include decreased pulse, blood pressure, and respirations; heightened awareness; decreased oxygen consumption; a sense of peace; and decreased muscle tension and metabolic rate (Tick et al., 2018). Relaxation techniques include meditation, yoga, Zen, guided imagery, and progressive relaxation exercises (see Chapter 32). For effective relaxation, teach techniques only when a patient is not distracted by acute discomfort. Sometimes a combination of these techniques is needed to achieve optimal pain relief. With practice the patient performs relaxation exercises independently.

Distraction. The reticular activating system inhibits painful stimuli if a person receives sufficient or excessive sensory input. With sufficient sensory stimuli, a person ignores or becomes unaware of pain. People who are bored or in isolation have only their pain to think about and thus perceive it more acutely. Distraction directs a patient's attention to something other than pain and thus reduces awareness of it. A disadvantage of distraction is that, if it works, health care providers or family members may question the existence or severity of the pain. Distraction works best for short, intense pain lasting a few minutes such as during an invasive procedure or while waiting for an analgesic to work. Use activities enjoyed by the patient as distractions (e.g., singing, praying, listening to music, or playing games).

Music. Music therapy may be useful in treating acute or chronic pain, stress, anxiety, fatigue, and depression (Korhan et al., 2014; American Music Therapy Association [AMTA], 2019). It diverts a person's attention away from the pain and creates a relaxation response. Specifically, music therapy can result in physiological changes, including improved respiration, lower blood pressure, improved cardiac output, reduced heart rate, and reduced muscle tension (AMTA, 2019).

Music creates positive changes in mood and emotional states and allows patients to actively participate in treatment. It can be used with relaxation to help patients cue positive visual imagery. Music therapy uses all kinds of music. It is important to let patients select the types of music they prefer. Music produces an altered state of consciousness through sound, silence, space, and time. Therapeutic sessions usually last 20 to 30 minutes (Tick et al., 2018). Patients may use earphones to enhance their concentration on the music. This allows them to adjust the volume without interrupting other patients or staff. Evidence shows that music contributes to the pain relief of hospitalized patients and may decrease the use of analgesics in some postoperative patients (Cole and LoBiondo-Wood, 2014; Tick et al., 2018).

Cutaneous Stimulation. Stimulation of the skin through a massage, warm bath, cold application, or transcutaneous electrical nerve stimulation (TENS) may reduce pain perception. How cutaneous stimulation works is unclear. One suggestion is that it causes release of endorphins, thus blocking the transmission of painful stimuli. The gate-control theory suggests that cutaneous stimulation activates larger, faster-transmitting A-beta sensory nerve fibers. This closes the gate, thus decreasing pain transmission through small-diameter C fibers (Melzack and Wall, 1965).

Cutaneous stimulation gives patients and families some control over pain symptoms and treatment in the home. Using it properly helps to reduce muscle tension, resulting in less pain. When using cutaneous stimulation, eliminate sources of environmental noise, help the patient to assume a comfortable position, and explain the purpose of the therapy. Do not use it directly on sensitive skin areas (e.g., burns, bruises, skin rashes, inflammation, and underlying bone fractures).

Massage produces physical and mental relaxation, reduces pain, and enhances the effectiveness of pain medication. Massaging the back, shoulders, hands, and/or feet for 3 to 5 minutes relaxes muscles and

---

BOX 44.11   PROCEDURAL GUIDELINES

Massage

Delegation and Collaboration

Assessment of a patient's pain cannot be delegated to assistive personnel (AP). The skill of massage can be delegated to AP. The nurse directs the AP by:

- Identifying and explaining when massage can work best for a patient.
- Explaining how to adapt use of massage to patient restrictions (e.g., massage in side-lying versus prone position).
- Instructing to report worsening of a patient's pain.

Equipment

Lotion or oil (consider lavender aromatherapy lotion [non–alcohol-based]), sheet, bath towel

Steps

1. Identify patient using at least two identifiers (e.g., name and birthday or name and medical record number) according to agency policy.
2. Perform hand hygiene. Perform complete pain assessment.
3. Assess character of patient's respirations.
4. Review health care provider's orders for pain relief (if required by agency).
5. Review medical record for any restrictions in patient's mobility or positioning.
6. Assess patient's and/or family caregiver's knowledge, experience, and health literacy level.
7. Assess patient's language level and values he or she has regarding alternative pain-relief approaches. Identify descriptive terms that you will use when guiding patient through relaxation during massage.
8. Dim room lights and/or turn on soft music according to patient preference.

CLINICAL DECISION: *Massage is contraindicated in cases of muscle, bone, or joint injury; bruised, swollen, or inflamed areas.*

9. Place patient in comfortable position such as prone or side-lying. Have patients with difficulty breathing lie on side of bed with head of bed elevated.
10. Adjust bed to comfortable position for you; lower upper side rail on side where you are standing. Drape patient to expose only area that you will massage.
11. Ensure that patient is not allergic to lotion. Warm lotion in hands or place bottle in basin of warm water. **N**ote: If you massage head and scalp, delay use of lotion until completed.
12. Choose stroke technique based on desired effect or body part.

CLINICAL DECISION: *Use very gentle massage with patients who are unable to communicate, and monitor nonverbal behavior because they cannot tell you if massage becomes uncomfortable.*

  a. Effleurage: massaging upward and outward from vertebral column and back again (see illustration). Smooths and extends muscles; improves lymph and venous circulation.
  b. Pétrissage: kneading tense muscle groups (see illustration). Promotes relaxation and stimulates local circulation.
  c. Friction: strong circular strokes bring blood to skin surface. Increases local circulation and loosens tight muscles.
13. Encourage patient to breathe deeply and relax during massage.
14. Standing behind patient, stimulate scalp and temples.

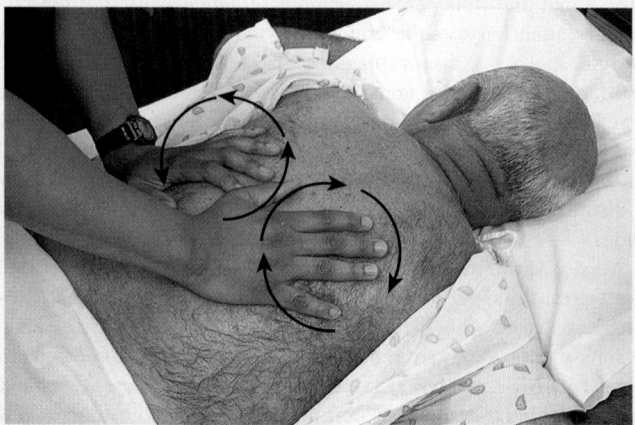

STEP 12a Effleurage.

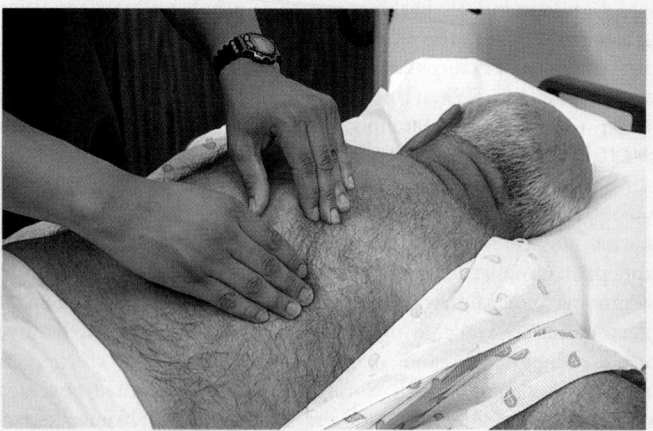

STEP 12b Pétrissage.

Continued

BOX 44.11 PROCEDURAL GUIDELINES—cont'd

Massage

15. Supporting patient's head, use friction to rub muscles at base of head.
16. Reposition if needed. With patient in supine position, massage hands and arms as appropriate.
    a. Support hand and apply friction to palm using both thumbs.
    b. Support base of finger and work each finger in corkscrew-like motion.
    c. Complete hand massage using effleurage strokes from fingertips to wrist.
    d. Knead muscles of forearm and upper arm between thumb and forefinger.
17. After determining that patient has no neck injury or condition that contraindicates neck manipulation, massage neck as appropriate:
    a. Place patient prone unless contraindicated.
    b. Knead each neck muscle between thumb and forefinger.
    c. Gently stretch neck by placing one hand on top of shoulders and other at base of head. Gently move hands away from one another.
18. Massage back as appropriate:
    a. Assist patient to prone position unless contraindicated; side-lying position is an option.
    b. Do not allow hands to leave patient's skin.

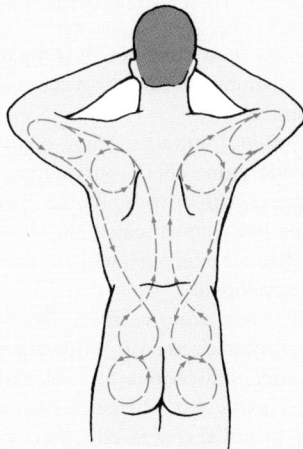

STEP 18C Circular massage of the back.

c. Apply hands first to sacral area; massage in circular motion. Stroke upward from buttocks to shoulders. Massage over scapulae with smooth, firm stroke. Continue in one smooth stroke to upper arms and laterally along sides of back down to iliac crest (see illustration). Continue massage pattern for 3 minutes.
    d. Use effleurage along muscles of spine in upward and outward motion.
    e. Use pétrissage on muscles of each shoulder toward front of patient.
    f. Use palms in upward and outward circular motion from lower buttocks to neck.
    g. Knead muscles of upper back and shoulder between thumb and forefinger.
    h. Use both hands to knead muscles up one side of back and then the other.
    i. End massage with long, stroking effleurage movements.
19. Massage feet as appropriate:
    a. Place patient in supine position.
    b. Hold foot firmly. Support ankle with one hand or support sides of foot with each hand while performing massage.
    c. Make circular motions with thumb and fingers around bones of ankle and top of foot.
    d. Trace space between tendons with firm finger pressure, moving from toe to ankle.
    e. Massage sides and top of each toe.
    f. Use top of fist to make circular motions on bottom of foot.
    g. Knead sides of foot between index finger and thumb.
    h. Conclude with firm, sweeping motions over top and bottom of foot.
20. Tell patient that you are ending massage.
21. When procedure is complete, instruct patient to relax and inhale deeply and exhale slowly. Caution him or her to move slowly after resting a few minutes.
22. Wipe excess lotion or oil from patient's body with bath towel.
23. Observe character of respirations, body position, facial expression, tone of voice, mood, mannerisms, verbalization of discomfort.
24. Ask patient to use pain rating scale to rate comfort level; compare with patient's goal.
25. Observe patient perform pain-control measures.
26. Perform teach-back: "I want to ensure you know how to perform massage for your husband. Show me how you would massage his back and feet."
27. Record in EHR or printed record patient's response to massage.

promotes sleep and comfort (Tick et al., 2018). Massages communicate caring and are easy for family members or other health care personnel to learn (Box 44.11).

Cold and heat applications (see Chapter 48) relieve pain and promote healing. The selection of heat-versus-cold interventions varies with patients' conditions (Tick et al., 2018). For example, moist heat helps to relieve the pain from a tension headache, and cold applications reduce the acute pain from inflamed joints. When using any form of heat or cold application, instruct the patient to avoid injury to the skin by checking the temperature and not applying cold or heat directly to the skin. Especially at risk for injury are patients with diabetic neuropathies, spinal cord or other neurological disorders, older adults, and patients who are confused.

Ice massage is effective for acute pain relief. It involves the use of a large ice cube or a small paper cup filled with water and frozen (water rises out of the cup as it freezes to create a smooth surface of ice for massage). A nurse or the patient applies the ice with firm pressure to the skin, which is covered with a lightweight cloth. Then use a slow, steady circular massage over the area. Apply cold within a 6-inch circular area near the pain site or on the opposite side of the body corresponding to the pain site. Limit application to 5 minutes or until the patient feels numbness. Application near the actual site of pain tends to work best, and it can be applied several times each hour to help reduce pain (Tick et al., 2018). Cold is effective for tooth or mouth pain when you place the ice on the web of the hand between the thumb and index finger. This point on the hand is an **acupressure** point that influences nerve pathways to the face and head. Cold applications are also effective before vaccine injections (Taddio et al., 2015).

Heat application is more effective for patients with chronic pain. Chapter 48 discusses in detail the types of heat devices (e.g., warm compresses and commercial heat packs) that are safe to use. Never place a heat application in a microwave unless it is directed by the manufacturer. Then follow directions carefully. Teach patients to check the temperature of a compress carefully and not to lie on the heating element because burning can occur.

Another form of cutaneous stimulation is TENS, involving stimulation of the skin with a mild electrical current passed through external electrodes. A TENS unit consists of a battery-powered transmitter, lead wires, and electrodes. TENS works both peripherally and centrally: centrally it acts by activating sites in the spinal cord and brainstem that use opioid and serotonin receptors; peripherally neuroreceptors at the site of the TENS application produce analgesia (Tick et al., 2018). It can be applied at various frequencies (<10 Hz to >50 Hz) and intensity (sensory versus motor). Stimulation intensity has been shown to be the critical factor in TENS efficacy. A TENS unit requires a health care provider's order that identifies the site for the TENS electrode placement. Remove any hair or skin preparations before attaching the electrodes. Then place the electrodes directly over or near the pain site. Turn the transmitter on to the ordered level when the patient feels pain. The TENS creates a buzzing or tingling sensation. After assessing the patient's tolerance, he or she can then turn on the transmitter and adjust the intensity and quality of skin stimulation until pain relief occurs. TENS is effective for acute, emergent, and postsurgical and procedural pain control (Tick et al., 2018).

Herbals. Many patients use herbals and dietary supplements such as echinacea, ginseng, ginkgo biloba, and garlic despite conflicting research evidence supporting their use in pain relief. Significant attention has been paid to the potential benefits of glucosamine and chondroitin in the treatment of pain from osteoarthritis, but the evidence suggests that chondroitin isn't helpful for pain from osteoarthritis of the knee or hip, and it is unclear whether glucosamine helps with osteoarthritis knee pain or whether either supplement lessens osteoarthritis pain in other joints (NIH, 2014). Herbal supplements may interact with prescribed analgesics and condition-specific medications. For example, glucosamine and chondroitin supplements may interact with the anticoagulant drug warfarin and increase the risk of bleeding (NIH, 2014). Thus it is important to ask patients to report to their health care provider all of the substances taken to relieve pain (see Chapter 32).

Reducing Pain Perception and Reception. One simple way to promote comfort is to remove or prevent painful stimuli (Box 44.12). This is especially important for patients who are immobilized or who have difficulty expressing themselves. For example, your patient becomes constipated and has abdominal distention and cramping. You intervene to ensure that the normal elimination process continues: increasing fluids, ambulating the patient, and/or requesting stool softeners or laxatives. Another example involves reducing pain perception during procedures using techniques such as proper patient positioning and coaching to perform progressive muscle relaxation. Always consider the patient's condition, aspects of the procedure that are uncomfortable, and techniques to avoid causing pain. In a patient with severe arthritic knee pain who has severe discomfort during any extreme flexion of the knee, take precautions before walking the patient to the bathroom. Use an elevated toilet seat to allow him or her to sit and rise with minimal discomfort.

Acute Care. Nurses often care for patients who have acute pain resulting from invasive procedures (e.g., surgery) or trauma. Many professional organizations such as the APS, American Society of Anesthesiologists (ASA, 2010), and the ASPMN and ANA (2016) have published guidelines and position papers related to acute pain management. The key to success is ongoing pain assessment and evaluation of the efficacy of interventions. Does the patient feel relief? Are there any

---

BOX 44.12   Controlling Painful Stimuli in Patient's Environment

- Tighten and smooth wrinkled bed linen.
- Reposition patient anatomically to relieve any pressure points according to individual preferences or requirements.
- Reposition patient to avoid lying on tubing (e.g., intravenous tubing, chest tubes).
- Loosen constricting bandages (unless specifically applied as a pressure dressing).
- Change wet dressings and linens.
- Check temperature of hot or cold applications, including bath water.
- Lift patient in bed—do not pull. Use safe patient-handling lift devices and techniques.
- Position patient correctly on a bedpan.
- Avoid exposing skin or mucous membranes to irritants (e.g., urine, stool, wound drainage).
- Keep patients clean, dry, and turned if needed. Use urinary incontinence pads if indicated.
- Prevent urinary retention by keeping Foley catheters patent and free flowing if in use, while also monitoring urinary output.
- Prevent constipation with fluids, diet, exercise, and stimulant laxatives if needed.

---

unacceptable side effects from therapies? It is the responsibility of the health care team to collaborate to find the combination of therapy that works best for a patient.

Pharmacological Pain Therapies. Many pharmacological agents are available to provide pain relief. Your judgment in the use and management of analgesics with or without other pain therapies ensures the best pain relief possible. Unfortunately the ideal analgesic (i.e., one that provides highly effective pain relief without significant risks or side effects) has yet to be developed.

Analgesics. Analgesics are the most common and effective method of pain relief. Nurses need to understand the medications available for pain relief, indications for use and pharmacological effects, and risks for addiction. Reassure patients that treatment of pain is necessary to aid recovery and that nonpharmacological strategies can be used to augment the effectiveness of analgesics, healing, and pain relief.

There are three types of analgesics: (1) nonopioids, including acetaminophen and nonsteroidal antiinflammatory drugs (NSAIDs); (2) opioids (traditionally called *narcotics*); and (3) adjuvants or co-analgesics, a variety of medications that enhance analgesics or have analgesic properties (US Department of Veterans Affairs, 2017).

Nonopioids. Acetaminophen (Tylenol), considered one of the most tolerated and safest analgesics available, is available in a variety of over-the-counter (OTC) oral medications (e.g., cold and flu remedies) or rectal forms and in an intravenous (IV) preparation (Ofirmev). The analgesic effect of acetaminophen is not entirely clear, but it is believed to have a direct effect on the central nervous system by selectively inhibiting cyclooxygenase, an enzyme needed to make prostaglandins (Burchum and Rosenthal, 2019). It has limited effects on the peripheral nervous system. Acetaminophen has analgesic and antipyretic properties but no antiinflammatory effects (Burchum and Rosenthal, 2019). IV acetaminophen (Ofirmev) is effective because it crosses the blood-brain barrier rapidly, thus providing nonopioid analgesia for patients after surgery, especially those who cannot take oral medications. The maximum 24-hour dose is 4 g (the same limitation as aspirin). Acetaminophen is often combined with opioids (e.g., oxycodone, hydrocodone, tramadol) because it reduces the dose of opioid needed to achieve successful pain control. When acetaminophen is combined with an opioid in these products, it is important to recognize the abbreviations that describe the contents of the product. The order and package label often state "name of opioid/acetaminophen (abbreviated as APAP) 5/325" which means that the opioid is 5 mg and the acetaminophen (APAP) is 325 mg per tablet. For example, oxycodone/APAP 5/325 indicates that each tablet contains 5 mg of oxycodone and 325 mg of acetaminophen. Similar abbreviations are used for combination products of hydrocodone and tramadol.

The major adverse effect of acetaminophen is hepatotoxicity; and, because the drug is so widely used, the Food and Drug Administration (USFDA, 2014) issued an order to limit the amount of acetaminophen in prescription combination products to 325 mg per tablet, capsule, or other dosage unit. Instructions for acetaminophen-containing products such as 1 to 2 tablets every 4 to 6 hours, were not required to change in the order. Higher dosing units continue to be available in OTC products, but the products are required to include dosage labeling information about safety risks, including liver injury and the risks of serious skin rashes. Although some manufacturers have voluntarily reduced the maximum daily acetaminophen dose labeling on their OTC products, the FDA has not reduced the maximum daily dose limit of 4 g for adults. Reduced doses are necessary for inadequate liver function and are recommended to prevent accidental overdose in the outpatient setting. It is important to read and understand these warning labels. Dangerous hepatotoxic overdoses of acetaminophen are treated with acetylcysteine (Burchum and Rosenthal, 2019).

Nonselective NSAIDs such as aspirin, ibuprofen, and naproxen relieve mild-to-moderate acute intermittent pain such as that from headache or muscle strain. Treatment of mild-to-moderate postoperative pain begins with an NSAID unless contraindicated (Chou et al., 2015). NSAIDs act by inhibiting cyclooxygenase (COX), the enzyme that synthesizes prostaglandins and related compounds (Burchum and Rosenthal, 2019). The drugs inhibit cellular responses to inflammation. Most NSAIDs act on peripheral nerve receptors to reduce transmission of pain stimuli and inflammation. Unlike opioids, NSAIDs do not depress the central nervous system, nor do they interfere with bowel or bladder function. However, NSAIDs do increase gastrointestinal irritation because COX normally synthesizes the prostaglandins that protect gastric mucosa. NSAIDs may reduce renal blood flow since COX causes vasodilation to maintain renal blood flow (Burchum and Rosenthal, 2019). Thus NSAID use in the older patient is not recommended because it is associated with more frequent adverse effects (gastrointestinal bleeding as well as renal insufficiency) (American Geriatrics Society Beers Criteria Expert Panel, 2015). Mild-to-moderate musculoskeletal pain in older adults is managed effectively with acetaminophen (Abdulla et al., 2013). Some patients with asthma or an allergy to aspirin are also allergic to NSAIDs (Morales et al., 2015). As with all OTC medications, patients should be advised to discuss their use of NSAIDs and their pain with their health care provider.

Opioids. Opioid or opioid-like analgesics are prescribed for moderate-to-severe pain. In any acute pain situation, opioids are not always necessary, but with severe trauma and immediately postoperatively, short-term use of opioid medications (3-5 days) is rarely a problem although side effects are most problematic when initiating treatment (ACPA, 2018). The misuse and improper prescribing of opioids has led to a crisis in the United States. Among patients who use opioids for more than 8 days, 13.5% will be on opioids at 1 year; in addition, 30% of persons taking opioids for more than 31

days remain on them at 1 year (ACPA, 2018). Nurses play a key role in monitoring patient response early when opioids are being used and in detecting potential misuse or prolonged unnecessary use. Long-term use can lead to problems with tolerance, loss of benefit from prescribed dosage with time, and escalating usage despite decreases in function and increases in side effects in some individuals (ACPA, 2018). Opioids, however, do play an important role in pain management. Be knowledgeable of the effects of opioids and implications for patient monitoring and management.

Opiates act on higher centers of the brain and spinal cord by binding with opiate receptors to modify perceptions of pain. Examples of opioids include morphine, codeine, hydromorphone, fentanyl, oxycodone, and hydrocodone. Some are available in IV and oral preparations (morphine and hydromorphone), whereas others are available only in oral formulations (oxycodone and hydrocodone). Most are available in a short-acting form, which provides relief for about 4 hours; some are also available in longer-acting preparations (oral morphine, oxycodone, hydromorphone, and a transdermal fentanyl patch).

One out of every two patients taking oral opioids experiences at least one adverse event/effect (Box 44.13). The most common side effects of opioids include nausea, vomiting, constipation, and memory and thought changes (ACPA, 2018). Except for constipation and

---

BOX 44.13 Common Opioid Side Effects

Central Nervous System (CNS) Toxicity
- Thought and memory impairment
- Drowsiness, sedation, and sleep disturbance
- Confusion
- Hallucinations, potential for diminished psychomotor performance
- Delirium
- Depression
- Dizziness and seizures

Ocular
- Pupil constriction

Respiratory
- Bradypnea
- Hypoventilation

Cardiac
- Hypotension
- Bradycardia
- Peripheral edema

Gastrointestinal
- Constipation
- Nausea and vomiting
- Delayed gastric emptying

Genitourinary
- Urinary retention

Endocrine
- Hormonal and sexual dysfunction
- Hypoglycemia—reported with tramadol and methadone

Skin
- Pruritus

Immunological
- Immune system impairment possible with chronic use

Musculoskeletal
- Muscle rigidity and contractions
- Osteoporosis

Pregnancy and Breastfeeding
- When at all possible, avoid opioid use during pregnancy to prevent fetal risks

Tolerance
- Over time, increased doses needed to obtain analgesic effect

Withdrawal Syndrome
- Rapid or sudden cessation or marked dose reduction may cause rhinitis, chills, pupil dilation, diarrhea, "gooseflesh"

Adapted from American Chronic Pain Association (ACPA): *ACPA resource guide to chronic pain medication & treatment,* 2018 edition, 2018, https://www.theacpa.org/wp-content/uploads/2018/03/ACPA_Resource_Guide_2018-Final-v2.pdf. Accessed March 27, 2019.

central nervous system changes, patients usually become tolerant to many of the opioid side effects. To reduce side effects, patients should take the lowest dose of an opioid needed to manage pain. For example, if the prescriber initially ordered oxycodone 10 mg PO every 4 hours and the patient has nausea and is very drowsy, the nurse might suggest that the prescriber reduce the dose to 5 mg. After administration, reassess a patient for the effect of the lowered dose on pain level and side effects. If reducing a dose does not relieve a side effect, confer with the prescriber about a change in the type of opioid. If side effects persist, it may be necessary to prevent or treat them by administering other medications (antihistamines, antiemetics, stimulants). Constipation should always be anticipated and prevented through diet, hydration, and the use of stool softeners and stimulants as needed.

An adverse effect of opioids in opioid-naïve patients (patients who have used opioid around the clock [ATC] *less* than approximately 1 week), as well as in patients on high-dose opioids or who are taking opioids with benzodiazepine medications, is respiratory depression. Sedation always occurs before respiratory depression. Closely monitor for sedation in opioid-naïve patients. Respiratory depression is clinically significant only if there is a decrease in the rate and depth of respirations from a patient's baseline assessment (Pasero and McCaffery, 2011). It is important for nurses to obtain a complete opioid medication history, including dose, frequency, and duration of use, to determine whether patients are opioid naïve or tolerant. All patients who receive opioids are at risk. However, patients who are opioid naïve (new or restarting opioids), who have a history or show signs of obstructive sleep disorder, who are on high-dose opioids, or who are taking opioids with other sedative medications are at greater risk (US Department of Veterans Affairs, 2017). If an adult patient experiences respiratory depression, administer naloxone (0.4 mg diluted with 9 mL saline) IV push (IVP) at a rate prescribed by health care provider. For initial treatment, IV administration is recommended, and once respiratory depression has been reversed, IM or subcutaneous routes can be used (Burchum and Rosenthal, 2019). Administering naloxone faster than recommended may cause severe pain and serious complications such as hypotension and hypertension, cardiac arrhythmias, dyspnea, and pulmonary edema (Pasero and McCaffery, 2011). Evaluate patients who receive naloxone every 15 minutes for 2 hours following drug administration because its duration may be less than that of the opioid, and respiratory depression sometimes returns.

One way to maximize pain relief while potentially decreasing opioid use is to administer analgesics around the clock (ATC) or at scheduled times rather than a prn basis. This approach ensures a more constant therapeutic blood level of an analgesic. There are also a variety of extended- or controlled-release oral opioid formulations (dosing intervals of 8, 10, 12, or 24 hours) and transdermal patches (72 hours). These formulations maintain constant serum opioid concentration, minimizing toxic and subtherapeutic concentrations (Burchum and Rosenthal, 2019). An ATC medication lessens the severity of end-of-dose pain, allowing a patient to sleep through the night and reduce "clock watching" for the next dose.

Careful assessment and critical thinking are required to safely administer analgesics (Box 44.14). The current pharmacological approach to acute and chronic pain management is to provide mul-timodal analgesia. Multimodal analgesia combines drugs with at least two different mechanisms of action to optimize pain control. Medications are combined to target different sites in the peripheral or central pain pathways (Fig. 44.10). The use of different agents allows for lower-than-usual doses of each medication, which is a benefit of multimodal analgesia. A multimodal regimen lowers the risk of side effects while providing pain relief that is as good as or even better than could be obtained from each of the medications alone.

BOX 44.14 Nursing Principles for Administering Analgesics

Know Patient's Previous Response to Analgesics
- Determine whether patient has sensitivities or allergies.
- Know whether patient is at risk for using NSAIDs (e.g., history of GI bleeding or renal insufficiency) or opioids (e.g., history of obstructive or central sleep apnea).
- Identify previous doses and routes of analgesic administration to avoid undertreatment.
- Determine whether patient obtained relief.
- Ask whether a nonopioid was as effective as an opioid.

Select Proper Medications When More Than One Is Ordered
- Consult with health care provider to use nonopioid analgesics or opioid combination drugs for mild-to-moderate pain.
- Recommend opioids with nonopioids to provide a multimodal analgesia approach.
- Avoid using multiple opioids with the same duration and mechanism of action.
- Intravenous medications act more quickly and usually relieve severe, acute pain within 1 hour, whereas oral medications take as long as 2 hours to relieve pain.
- Avoid intramuscular analgesics, especially in older adults.
- Recommend use of an opioid with a nonopioid analgesic for severe pain because such combinations treat pain peripherally and centrally.
- For chronic pain give sustained-release oral formulations ATC.

Know Accurate Dosage
- Recall that 4 g is considered the maximum 24-hour dosage for acetaminophen and acetylsalicylic acid (ASA); 3200 mg for ibuprofen.
- Adjust doses as appropriate for children and older patients.
- Large doses of opioids are acceptable in opioid-tolerant patients but not in opioid-naïve patients.
- When titrating an opioid, it is important to titrate to effect or to uncontrollable side effects.

Assess Right Time and Interval for Administration
- Administer analgesics as soon as pain occurs and before it increases in severity.
- An ATC administration schedule is usually best.
- Give analgesics before pain-producing procedures or activities.
- Know the average duration of action for a drug and the time of administration so that the peak effect occurs when the pain is most intense.
- Use extended-release opioid formulations to treat chronic pain.
- Avoid stopping opioids abruptly in patients who are opioid tolerant.

ATC, Around the clock; *GI,* gastrointestinal; *NSAIDs,* nonsteroidal antiinflammatory drugs.
Modified from Centers for Disease Control and Prevention: CDC guideline for prescribing opioids for chronic pain—United States, 2016, *MMWR* 65(1):1-49, 2016.

A person's response to an analgesic is highly individualized. If the pain is caused by inflammation, an NSAID is sometimes as effective as, or more effective than, an opioid. An orally administered analgesic usually has a longer onset and duration of action than an injectable form. In addition, for pain that persists for most of the day, controlled- or extended-release opioid formulations (morphine sulfate extended release, oxycodone sustained/extended release, and methadone) are available for administration every 8 to 12 hours ATC; they are not ordered prn.

When you convert a patient from an IV to an oral form of the same opioid, understand that the dose of the oral opioid is usually much

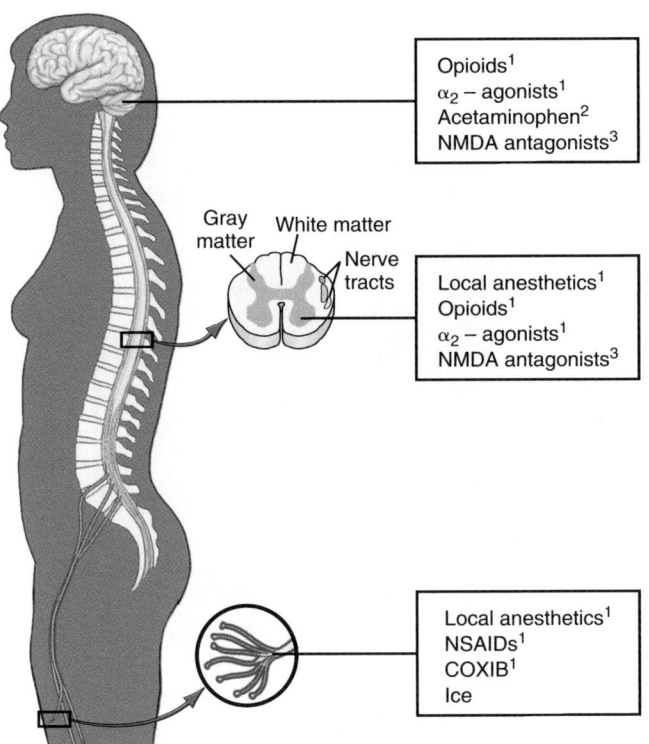

FIG. 44.10 Multimodal analgesia sites of action. (© Elsevier collections.) *COXIB,* Cox-2 inhibitor; *NMDA, N*-methyl-d-aspartate; *NSAID,* nonsteroidal antiinflammatory drug. 1. Gottschalk A, Smith DS. New concepts in acute pain therapy: preemptive analgesia. *Am Fam Physician* 63(10):1979-1984, 2001. (http://www.aafp.org/afp/2001/0515/p19 79.html). 2. Smith HS. Potential analgesic mechanisms of acetaminophen. *Pain Physician* 12:269-280, 2009. (http://www.painphysicianjournal.com/current/pdf?article=MTE4NA%3D%3D&journal=47). 3. Sinatra RS, Jahr JS, editors. *The essence of analgesia and analgesics.* New York, 2011, Cambridge University Press.

higher than the IV dose because of the first-pass effect. Morphine is inactivated by hepatic metabolism; thus, when taken orally, the drug must pass through the liver on its way to systemic circulation. Much of an oral dose is inactivated during this first pass through the liver. A drug can be completely inactivated on its first pass through the liver, with minimal or no therapeutic effects (Burchum and Rosenthal, 2019). As a result oral doses need to be substantially larger than parenteral doses to achieve equivalent analgesic effects (Burchum and Rosenthal, 2019). Know the comparative potencies of analgesics in oral and injectable form. In addition, know the route of administration most effective for a patient so that controlled, sustained pain relief is achieved. The intramuscular (IM) and subcutaneous routes are painful; absorption is unreliable and thus are generally avoided (Burchum and Rosenthal, 2019). When comparing opioids, equianalgesic charts (i.e., charts converting one opioid to another or parenteral forms of opioids [e.g., morphine to hydromorphone] to oral forms [or vice versa]) should be available on nursing units or by contacting pharmacy staff. There are "smartphone apps" for opioid dosing conversions, but check with the pharmacy staff and agency policies to ensure accuracy before using these electronic conversion tools.

Opioids are usually necessary and effective for acute pain and cancer pain of moderate or severe intensity. The goal of opioid therapy is a reduction in pain intensity to a level of acceptable comfort. In both types of pain, progress toward pain relief is measured by changes in pain-intensity scores. Opioid doses often need to be adjusted up or

down according to individual patient circumstances and conditions. A prescriber must carefully individualize drug selection, dosing, and schedule. Many patients are at higher risk for opioid-related adverse drug events (Box 44.15). In addition, morphine-like drugs can interact unfavorably with a number of other medications. For example, morphine-like drugs can interact adversely with CNS depressants, anticholinergic drugs, hypotensives, and monoamine oxidase inhibitors (Burchum and Rosenthal, 2019).

Opioid administration in older adults should follow a "start-low" (dose) and "go-slow" (upward dose titration) philosophy (Abdulla et al., 2013). Careful use of multiple drugs together can be seen as potentially helpful. Combining smaller doses of more than one medication may minimize the dose-limiting adverse effects of using a particular single drug (ACPA, 2018). The elderly require special consideration because age-related changes and increased frailty lead to less predictable drug responses, including increased drug sensitivity and severity of side effects (Abdulla et al., 2013). Opioids may place the elderly at increased risk for falls and other injuries. Many elderly patients have multiple co-morbidities and require various medications, placing them at risk for polypharmacy and drug-drug interactions. Dizziness, confusion, and changes in vision are opioid-related side effects that pose increased safety risks for the elderly; special care must be taken to ensure that the environment is safe and patients are educated about the need for caution. Avoid unintentional medication overdoses by helping an older adult with memory problems receive assistance in creating a safe plan for taking medication (ACPA, 2018). Appropriate interventions may include help from family caregivers, home care medication reconciliation, or using time-of-day labeled pillboxes (that are also kept in a locked safe).

Despite these concerns, elderly patients should receive opioid therapy when needed to treat pain. Carefully selected opioids and doses for all patients, along with patient education and monitoring, are important in providing safe and effective pain management. Box 44.16 offers key steps for the safe use of opioids.

Because there is such a wide variability in patient response to analgesics, as-needed (prn) range orders for opioids (e.g., "morphine 2 to 6 mg IV q2h prn for pain") are commonly used to provide flexibility in dosing to meet individual patients' needs (Drew et al., 2018). The Joint Commission requires health care agencies, where permissible, to have range-order policies in place to guide nurses in selecting the most appropriate dose of a medication. Range orders are medication orders in which a dose varies over a prescribed range to provide flexibility

BOX 44.16 Key Steps for Safe Opioid Use

- Only fill opioid prescriptions from one health care provider.
- Notify all health care providers about your opioid use. Alert your opioid prescriber about any new medications.
- Inform your health care provider about current/past history of alcohol or substance abuse.
- Follow directions for taking opioids carefully. Do not crush, break, or dissolve pills.
- Reduce the risk of drug interactions. Do not mix opioids with alcohol, antihistamines, barbiturates, benzodiazepines, other sedatives, or muscle relaxants.
- Prevent theft, diversion, and child access to opioids. Keep opioids in a locked box.
- Keep track of when refills are needed to prevent going without medications, which can lead to withdrawal.

Adapted from American Chronic Pain Association (ACPA): *ACPA Resource Guide to Chronic Pain Management*, 2018. https://www.theacpa.org/wp-content/uploads/2018/03/ACPA_Resource_Guide_2018-Final-v2.pdf. Accessed March 28, 2019.

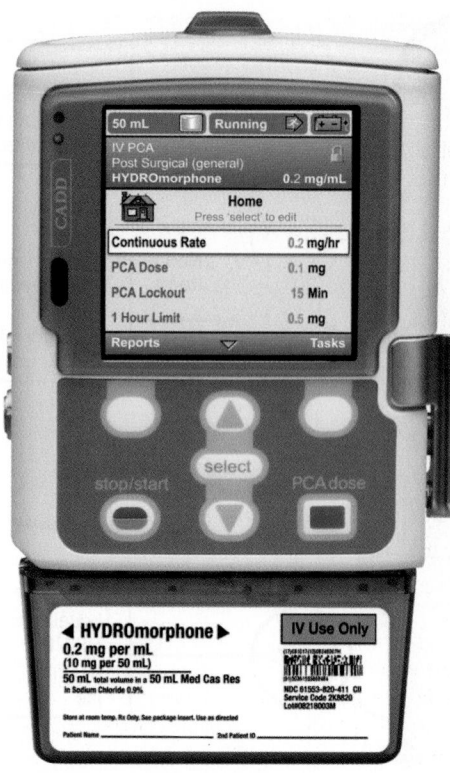

FIG. 44.11 Patient-controlled analgesia pump with cassette. (Courtesy Smiths Medical ASD, Inc., St Paul, MN.)

in dosing depending on a patient's condition or situation (Drew et al., 2014). Chapter 31 describes principles of range orders. A proper range order offers specifics (e.g., a patient's pain severity score) for when a range of doses can be given and gives nurses the flexibility needed to treat patients' pain in a timely way while allowing for differences in patient response to pain and analgesia. Nurses base decisions about the administration of range orders on a thorough pain assessment and knowledge of the drug to be administered (Drew et al., 2018). Safe and effective range orders consider the patient's age, pain intensity, pain tolerance, pharmacogenetic profile, renal and liver function, and co-morbidities and prescribe a maximum dose that ranges to 2 to 3 times the lower or minimum dose (Coluzzi, et al., 2016; Drew et al., 2018).

Adjuvants. Co-analgesics or adjuvants are drugs originally developed to treat conditions other than pain but that also have analgesic properties. For example, tricyclic antidepressants (e.g., nortriptyline), anticonvulsants (e.g., gabapentin), and infusional lidocaine successfully treat chronic pain, especially neuropathic pain. Corticosteroids relieve the pain from inflammation and bone metastasis. Other examples of co-analgesics are bisphosphonates and calcitonin for bone pain. Adjuvants have analgesic properties, enhance pain control, or relieve other symptoms associated with neuropathic pain. You give adjuvants alone or with analgesics. Sedatives, antianxiety agents, and muscle relaxants have *no* analgesic effect, although they may be effective for their specific indications.

Patient-Controlled Analgesia. When patients depend on nurses for prn analgesia, an erratic cycle of alternating pain and analgesia often occurs. A patient feels pain and asks for medication, but the patient first must be assessed, and then the medication must be obtained and prepared. Under this circumstance analgesia finally occurs in about an hour, but pain relief may last only 30 minutes. Gradually the patient again feels discomfort, and the cycle begins again. The patient is constantly going in and out of analgesic therapeutic range.

A drug delivery system called **patient-controlled analgesia (PCA)** is a method for pain management that many patients prefer (see Skill 44.1). It is a drug delivery system that allows patients to self-administer opioids (usually morphine, hydromorphone, or fentanyl) with minimal risk of overdose. The goal is to maintain a constant plasma level of analgesic to avoid the problems of prn dosing. Systemic PCA traditionally involves IV or subcutaneous drug administration; however, a controlled analgesia device for oral medications is available. This device allows patients access to their own oral prn mediations,

including opioids and other analgesics, antiemetics, and anxiolytics, at the bedside.

PCA infusion pumps are portable and computerized and contain a chamber for a syringe or bag that delivers a small, preset dose of opioid (Fig. 44.11). To receive a demand dose, a patient pushes a button attached to the PCA device. The PCA infusion pumps are designed to deliver a specific dose, which is programmed to be available at specific time intervals (usually in the range of 8 to 15 minutes) when the patient activates the delivery button. A limit on the number of doses per hour or a 4-hour interval may also be set. In opioid-naïve patients, do not increase demand or basal dose *and* shorten the interval time simultaneously because this increases the risk for oversedation and respiratory depression. PCA basal doses are also *not* recommended for opioid-naïve patients following surgery because of the possibility for respiratory depression.

Most pumps have locked safety systems that prevent tampering by patients or family members and are generally safe to be managed in the home. For opioid-tolerant patients such as those with cancer pain, a low-dose continuous infusion (basal rate) is sometimes programmed to deliver a steady dose of continuous medication (Pasero and McCaffery, 2011).

There are many benefits to PCA use. The patient gains control over pain, and pain relief does not depend on nurse availability. Patients also have access to medication when they need it. This decreases anxiety and leads to decreased medication use. Small doses of medications are delivered at short intervals, stabilizing serum drug concentrations for sustained pain relief.

Patient preparation and teaching are critical to the safe and effective use of PCA devices (Box 44.17). A patient needs to understand the PCA and be physically able to locate and press the button to deliver a dose. Family members and visitors must be instructed not to "push the button" for the patient (a dangerous action known as "PCA by proxy"), as this bypasses the safety feature of PCA, which requires an awake

BOX 44.17 PATIENT TEACHING

Patient-Controlled Analgesia

Objective
- Patient will achieve pain control with proper use of the patient-controlled analgesia (PCA) device.

Teaching Strategies
- Teach how to use the PCA before procedures so that patient understands how to use it after awakening from anesthesia or sedation. Include demonstration of use of pump.
- Instruct patient in the purpose of PCA, emphasizing that patient controls medication delivery.
- Explain that the pump reduces risk of overdose.
- Reinforce instruction as needed with teach-back.

Evaluation
Use the principles of teach-back to evaluate patient/family caregiver learning:
- Please describe why you are using the PCA device.
- When are you planning on pushing the button?

patient to activate the device. In particular situations, when patients are unable to activate the PCA device, a carefully selected family member or nurse may be authorized to activate the device based on specific criteria. Authorized agent–controlled analgesia (AACA) guidelines should be used to guide this practice when appropriate (Cooney et al., 2013).

Programming the settings usually requires independent verification by two nurses to ensure accuracy. Even though patients control administration of analgesics, a nurse's diligence is needed to prevent errors related to programmable PCA devices. Document drug dosages and track medication wastes according to agency policy.

Topical and Transdermal Analgesics. Topical analgesics include prescription and OTC creams, gels, sprays, liquids, patches, or rubs applied on the skin over painful muscles or joints and for peripheral neuropathy (ACPA, 2018) Commonly used topical agents include NSAID products (ketoprofen patch) and capsaicin and local anesthetics such as lidocaine, prilocaine and diclofenac (ACPA, 2018). The medications are effective in chronic pain management. Topical agents work locally, have few side effects, and must be applied directly over the painful area.

Transdermal drugs are also applied directly to the skin but have systemic effects and work when applied away from the area of pain (ACPA, 2018). Transdermal medication in a patch is absorbed through the skin by the bloodstream over a period of time. Examples of analgesic transdermal medications are fentanyl, buprenorphine, and clonidine. Chapter 31 describes the administration of topical and transdermal medications.

The Lidoderm patch is a topical analgesic effective for cutaneous neuropathic pain such as postherpetic neuralgia in adults. Place three patches, cut to size, on and around the pain site using a 12-hour on, 12-hour off schedule (Pasero and McCaffery, 2011). Products such as ELA-Max/LMX and eutectic mixture of local anesthetics (EMLA) are available for children. Apply EMLA via a disk or thick cream to the skin 30 to 60 minutes before minor procedures (e.g., IV start, intramuscular injection) or anesthetic infiltration of soft tissue.

Do not place topical or transdermal analgesics on wounds, damaged skin, or the face. Pruritus or burning of the skin or a localized rash is common after topical applications. Application of a topical analgesic to vascular mucous membranes increases the chance of systemic effects such as a change in heart rate. Wear disposable gloves when removing

and applying transdermal patches. Lastly, after application, wash your hands thoroughly to avoid getting these products in sensitive areas such as the eyes (ACPA, 2018).

Local Anesthesia via Injection. Local anesthesia is the local infiltration of an anesthetic medication to induce loss of sensation to a body part. Health care providers often use local anesthesia during brief surgical procedures such as removing a skin lesion or suturing a wound by applying local anesthetics topically on skin and mucous membranes or injecting them subcutaneously or intradermally to anesthetize a body part. Regional anesthesia is the injection or infusion of local anesthetics to block a group of sensory nerve fibers. The anesthetics produce temporary loss of sensation by inhibiting nerve conduction. Local anesthetics also block motor and autonomic functions, depending on the amount used and the location and depth of administration. Smaller sensory nerve fibers are more sensitive to local anesthetics than are large motor fibers. As a result, the patient loses sensation before losing motor function; conversely, motor activity returns before sensation.

Perineural Local Anesthetic Infusion. A type of regional anesthesia is the use of perineural injections and infusions of local anesthetic agents to relieve pain. This technique is used for a variety of inpatient and outpatient adult and pediatric surgical procedures. A surgeon places the tip of an unsutured catheter near a nerve or groups of nerves, and the catheter exits from the surgical wound. Infusions of local anesthetics (bupivacaine or ropivacaine) may be run on a pump similar to those used for IV infusions, on ambulatory pumps, or on disposable systems (e.g., On-Q). The pump may be set on demand or continuous mode, and the catheter is usually left in place for 48 hours. Some patients have pump systems that are left in place even after discharge. Patients learn how to discontinue the pump at home and bring the catheter to the next health care provider visit. Some patients still need oral analgesics, but perineural infusions often reduce the total dosage (Chou et al., 2016).

Local anesthetics cause side effects, depending on their absorption into the circulation. The use of local anesthetics in peripheral nerve and epidural infusions (see following paragraph) may block both motor nerves and sensory nerves. This effect resolves within hours of the reduction or discontinuation of an infusion.

Epidural Analgesia. Another pain therapy that often involves the administration of anesthetic agents is epidural analgesia, a form of regional anesthesia. Preservative-free opioids are often administered as single agents or in combination with local anesthetics into a patient's epidural space. Epidural analgesia effectively treats acute postoperative pain, rib fracture pain, labor and delivery pain, and chronic cancer pain. Research has shown that adults having surgery under general anesthesia experience fewer postoperative cardiovascular, respiratory, and gastrointestinal complications when receiving epidural analgesia compared with patients receiving systemic analgesia (IV analgesics) (Pöpping et al., 2014). Epidural analgesia controls or reduces severe pain and reduces a patient's overall opioid requirement, thus minimizing adverse effects. It is short or long term, depending on a patient's condition and life expectancy.

The health care provider administers epidural analgesia into the spinal epidural space (Fig. 44.12) by inserting a blunt-tip needle into the level of the vertebral interspace nearest to the area requiring analgesia. He or she advances the catheter into the epidural space, removes the needle, and secures the remainder of the catheter with a dressing while ensuring that the catheter is taped securely. The end of the catheter is capped, or if a continuous infusion is prescribed, it is connected to special tubing and an infusion pump that is designated for epidural infusion. Nurse anesthetists, anesthesiologists, and certified nurses control epidural analgesia, depending on agency policy. Some patients

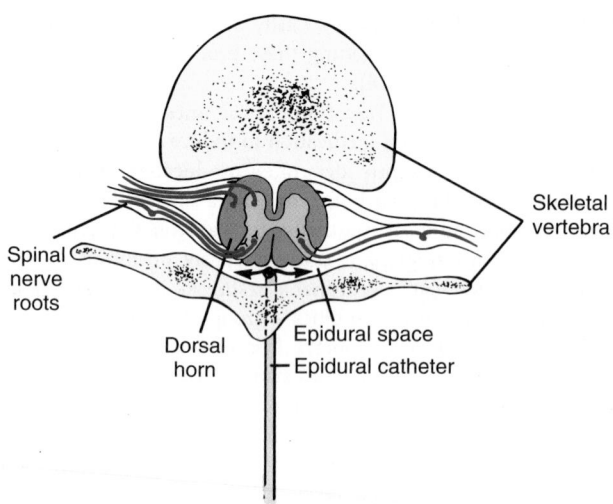

FIG. 44.12 Anatomical drawing of epidural space.

are able to use a technique known as *patient-controlled epidural analgesia (PCEA),* which allows them to self-administer demand doses of epidural solution when connected to a special administration pump (Chou et al., 2016).

One of the concerns related to the use of peripheral and epidural anesthetic techniques is the risk of bleeding and subsequent hematoma formation near the injection/insertion site. Although relatively uncommon, the risk is increased when patients receive anticoagulant or antiplatelet medications. Safe placement or removal of these injections and catheters is made on the basis of knowledge of the patients' coagulation status and the timing of administration of anticoagulant or antiplatelet medications. Guidelines for the use of anticoagulation in patients with regional anesthesia are available (Narouze et al., 2015) Because the epidural space is a highly vascular area, patients with epidural catheters are at risk for the development of epidural hematomas, which may lead to ischemia of the spinal cord and if unaddressed, serious neurological complications.

Nursing Implications for Local and Regional Anesthesia. Provide emotional support to patients receiving local or regional anesthesia by explaining the insertion technique and warning patients that they will temporarily lose sensory function within minutes of injection. Motor and autonomic (bowel and bladder control) function may also be lost quickly, depending on the area anesthetized. It is common for patients to fear paralysis because epidural and spinal injections come close to the spinal cord. To reassure the patient, explain that numbness, tingling, and coldness are common. Catheter insertion should be comfortable because the health care provider should first numb the injection site. Prepare patients for possible discomfort. Before a patient receives an analgesic, check for allergies. Also check to be sure that the drugs (e.g., morphine injection and fentanyl citrate) administered via the epidural catheter are free of potentially neurotoxic substances such as preservatives and additives. Assess vital signs to monitor systemic effects.

After administration of a local or regional anesthetic, protect the patient from injury until full sensory and motor function return. Patients are at risk for injuring an anesthetized body part without knowing it. For patients with topical anesthesia, do not apply heat or cold to numb areas. After an injection into the knee joint, warn the patient to avoid standing without assistance because there is a high risk of falling. With peripheral nerve or epidural local anesthetics, patients may experience sensory loss along with significant motor weakness. Assess patients for sensory and motor nerve blockade, and notify the

prescriber when motor blockade is unintended. Protect patients from injury and educate about necessary precautions until full sensory and motor function return. During and after epidural anesthesia a patient stays in bed until motor function returns. Help the patient the first time he or she tries to get out of bed.

When managing epidural infusions, if agency policy allows, connect the catheter to an infusion pump, a port, or a reservoir or cap it off for bolus injections. To reduce the risk of accidental epidural injection of drugs intended for IV use, clearly label the catheter *epidural catheter.* Always administer continuous infusions through appropriately labeled electronic infusion devices for proper control. Because of the catheter location, use surgical asepsis to prevent a serious and potentially fatal infection. Notify a patient's health care provider immediately of any signs or symptoms of infection or pain at the insertion site. Thorough hygiene is necessary during nursing procedures to keep the catheter system clean and dry. Maintain a closed system and prevent catheter disconnection by ensuring tight connections.

Nursing implications for managing epidural analgesia are numerous (Table 44.6). Do not administer supplemental doses of opioids or sedative/hypnotics because of possible additive central nervous system adverse effects. Monitoring for effects of medications differs, depending on the medication being administered and whether infusions are intermittent or continuous. Complications of epidural opioid use include nausea and vomiting, hypotension, urinary retention, constipation, respiratory depression, and pruritus (Pasero and McCaffery, 2011). When patients receive epidural analgesia, initially monitor them as often as every 15 minutes, including assessment of vital signs, respiratory effort, and skin color. Once stabilized, monitoring occurs every hour in the first 12 to 24 hours and then with less frequency if the patient is stable (refer to agency policy).

To minimize bleeding risks and the potential for hematoma formation, do not administer anticoagulant and antiplatelet medications until a pain specialist can verify safe use. To detect development of a possible epidural hematoma, notify the health care provider or pain specialist if the patient develops severe pain at the epidural insertion site or unexplained sensory or motor loss. Also notify the provider who performs the procedure when patients with peripheral nerve injections/catheter have similar signs and symptoms.

Provide thorough patient education about epidural analgesia in terms of the action of the medication and its advantages and disadvantages. Instruct patients about the potential for side effects and advise them to notify you if side effects develop. If the patient requires long-term epidural use, the health care provider tunnels a permanent catheter through the skin. The catheter exits at the patient's side. Teach a patient on long-term therapy how to safely administer home infusions with minimal ongoing nursing intervention, which signs and symptoms need to be reported to the health care provider, and to coordinate with the case manager or social worker to ensure that appropriate home care services are provided.

Invasive Interventions for Pain Relief. When severe pain persists despite medical treatment, available invasive interventions include intrathecal implantable pumps or injections, spinal cord and deep brain stimulation, neuroablative procedures (cordotomy, rhizotomy), trigger point injections, cryoablation, and intraspinal medications (e.g., opioids, steroids, local anesthetics). These techniques are useful for chronic pain. It is unacceptable to tell a patient with severe unrelieved pain that there is "nothing more we can do for you." Refer patients with severe chronic pain to comprehensive pain-management programs whenever possible. These programs offer many different interventional strategies, pharmacological options, physical medicine, and rehabilitation therapies to address the complex needs of patients with chronic pain. When comprehensive pain programs are unavailable, refer patients to a chronic pain-management program.

TABLE 44.6 Nursing Care for Patients With Epidural Infusions

Goal	Actions
Prevent catheter displacement.	Secure catheter (if not connected to implanted reservoir) carefully to outside skin.
Maintain catheter function.	Check external dressing around catheter site for dampness or discharge. (Leakage of epidural solution may occur if catheter is dislodged.) Use transparent dressing to secure catheter and aid inspection. Inspect catheter for breaks.
Prevent infection.	Use strict aseptic technique when caring for catheter (see Chapter 28). Do not change dressing routinely over site. Inspect insertions site for signs of infection. Follow institutional policies for tubing change.
Monitor for respiratory depression.	Monitor vital signs, especially respirations, and level of consciousness per policy. Use pulse oximetry, end-tidal carbon dioxide, and apnea monitoring.
Prevent undesirable complications.	Assess for hypotension: • Ensure adequate hydration and administer prescribed intravenous fluids. • Notify prescriber if significant change in vital signs occurs, and reduce or stop epidural infusion. • Anticipate need for change in epidural solution. Assess for pruritus (itching) and nausea and vomiting associated with use of epidural opioids: • Notify prescriber for dose reduction or epidural solution change. • Administer antihistamines and antiemetics as ordered. Assess sensation and motor strength; notify health care provider if deviation from baseline.
Maintain urinary and bowel function.	Monitor intake and output. Assess for bladder and bowel distention. Assess for discomfort, frequency, and urgency.

BOX 44.18 Types of Breakthrough Pain and Treatment

Types of Breakthrough Pain

Incident pain: Pain that is predictable and elicited by specific behaviors or triggers, such as a voluntary act (walking), involuntary act (coughing), or treatments (e.g., wound dressing changes)

End-of-dose failure pain: Pain that occurs toward the end of the usual dosing interval of a regularly scheduled analgesic

Spontaneous pain: Pain that is unpredictable and not associated with any activity or event

Treatment
- Lifestyle changes
- Management of reversible causes
- Modification of pathological processes
- Nonpharmacological management
- Pharmacological management—rescue dose of medication
- Interventional techniques

From Scarborough BM, Smith CB: Optimal pain management for patients with cancer in the modern era, *CA Cancer J Clin* 68(3):182-196, 2018.

Pain Management for Procedures. Diagnostic and treatment procedures potentially produce pain and anxiety, both of which should be assessed and treated before a procedure begins. Barriers to successful pain control include numerous patient-specific factors, but perhaps more influential is the lack of acknowledgment by health care providers that pain may occur during or after a procedure. Without this acknowledgment, the necessary anticipation, prevention, and management of potential or actual procedural pain cannot occur (Lee et al., 2014). Many types of routine procedures can cause pain, especially in patients who are critically ill, including turning, wound drain removal, femoral catheter removal, placement of a central line or feeding tube, and changing wound dressings. Common pharmacological agents for managing procedural comfort include local anesthetics, NSAIDs, acetaminophen, opioids, anxiolytics, and sedatives (Lee et al., 2014). Premedicating patients before painful procedures allows them to cooperate more fully and reduces the experience of pain. Using nonpharmacological therapies such as relaxation techniques, meditation, imagery, and music, in addition to medications, has

also been effective in select situations (Lee et al., 2014). When you premedicate a patient before a procedure, keep in mind how long it takes for the onset and peak effect of the analgesic to occur so you can properly time the beginning of the painful procedure to coincide with the medication's peak effect.

Cancer Pain and Chronic Noncancer Pain Management. Cancer pain varies among patients and can be either chronic or acute. A review of research spanning 40 years shows the prevalence of pain ranges from 64% in patients with metastatic, advanced, or terminal phases of the disease; to 59% in patients on anticancer treatment; and up to 40% in patients after curative treatment (Paice et al., 2016). Organizations such as the APS and the National Comprehensive Cancer Network (NCCN) have published guidelines for assessing and treating cancer-related pain. The guidelines support comprehensive and aggressive treatment, including many options for pain relief. The best choice of pain treatment often changes as a patient's condition and the characteristics of pain change. Use multimodal pharmacological strategies and nonpharmacological interventions to optimize pain management (ACPA, 2018).

Many patients with cancer experience breakthrough cancer pain (BTCP), a transitory increase in pain in someone who has relatively stable and an adequately controlled level of baseline pain (ACPA, 2018). It occurs either spontaneously or in relation to a specific predictable or unpredictable trigger (Scarborough and Smith, 2018). BTCP is a challenging aspect of cancer because, even though it is self-limiting in nature, its presence has a significant, negative impact on the quality of life of patients and family caregivers (Scarborough and Smith, 2018). Individualized assessment is critical for understanding how BTCP affects a patient's life. A holistic approach to care is often needed (Box 44.18).

In all pain management cases opioids should be used judiciously. The ACPA (2018) reports that the benefits from use of opioids for chronic pain are measured by an increase in the person's level of functioning, a reduction or elimination of pain complaints, a more positive, hopeful attitude, and by minimal or controllable side effects. The use of opioid therapy in patients with chronic pain requires careful patient selection and consideration of the risks and benefits of opioids. For example, to determine whether opioids are beneficial for a patient,

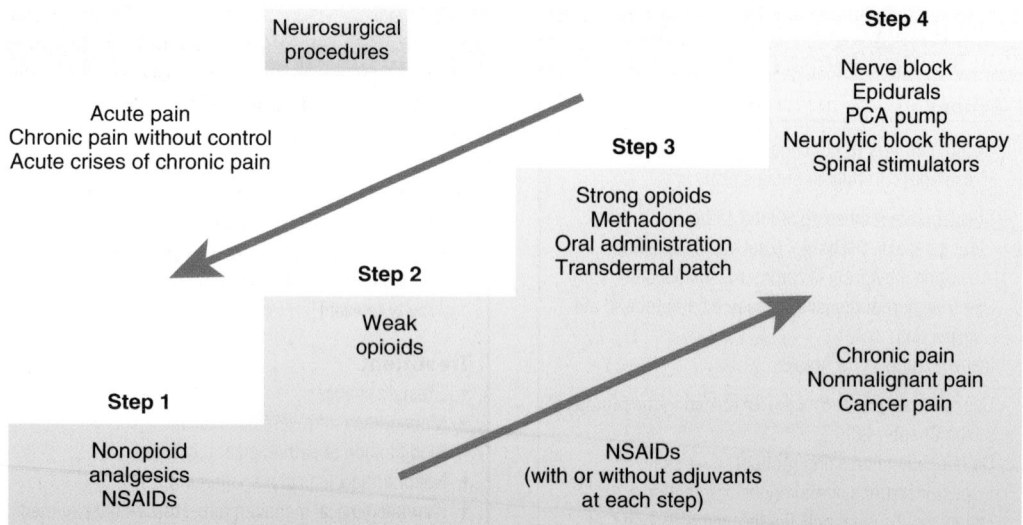

FIG. 44.13 Adaptation of the WHO analgesic ladder. *NSAID,* Nonsteroidal antiinflammatory drug; *PCA,* patient-controlled analgesia. (From Vargas-Schaffer G: Is the WHO analgesic ladder still valid?: twenty-four years of experience, *Can Fam Physician* 56:514, 2010.)

it is necessary to assess his or her opioid addiction risk, level of participation in ADLs, physical therapy, family activities, and work-related functions (CDC, 2016). Family members are often included in office visits to provide input about a patient's functional level. Research has not yet provided clear evidence to support or guide the use of chronic opioid therapy for patients with chronic noncancer pain (Chou et al., 2015). Use of opioids can increase adverse events and lead to polypharmacy when medications are added to treat side effects of the opioids (ACPA, 2018). It is recommended that each person with chronic noncancer pain be medically managed individually; medication use should be determined by weighing benefit compared with other alternatives, cost, potential side effects, and the person's other medical problems (ACPA, 2018).

The World Health Organization (WHO) in 1986 introduced the WHO three-step analgesic ladder as a recommended approach for the slow introduction and upward titration of analgesics for managing pain. This approach has been used worldwide and has been praised for its simplicity and ease of use. However, the ladder has been the object of criticism because of the absence of nonpharmacological therapies in providing analgesia, with modifications suggested in subsequent iterations (US Department of Veterans Affairs, 2017) (Fig. 44.13). The original three-step approach recommended that therapy begin at the first step with the use of nonopioid analgesics and/or adjuvants and progress to the next higher step, using opioids as pain intensity increases.

Modification of the steps aims to facilitate use of the ladder for different pain presentations. A bidirectional approach has been suggested, which adds a step-down approach to the original step-up approach for patients with intense acute pain, uncontrolled cancer pain, and breakthrough pain (Thapa et al., 2011). With this modification, therapy would begin at the third step with the strong opioids and descend down the ladder with improvement in pain. Another modification includes the addition of a fourth step, which recommends neurosurgical and other invasive procedures and also includes management of pediatric and acute pain in emergency departments and postoperative situations (Vargas-Schaffer, 2010). The fourth step is recommended for the treatment of crises of chronic pain.

Long-acting or controlled-release medications may provide relief for cancer pain, but are not recommended for the treatment of noncancer pain (CDC, 2016). These controlled-release medications (e.g., morphine sulfate extended release and oxycodone HCl) relieve pain for 8 to 12 hours. Long-acting or sustained-release opioids are dosed on a scheduled basis, not prn or "as needed." Transdermal fentanyl, which is 100 times more potent than morphine, is available for opioid-tolerant patients with cancer or chronic pain. It delivers predetermined doses that provide analgesia for up to 72 hours. The transdermal route is useful when patients are unable to take drugs orally. Patients find the transdermal patch easy to use because it allows for continuous opioid administration without needles or pumps. Self-adhesive patches release the medication slowly over time, achieving effective analgesia. Transdermal fentanyl is not for adult patients who weigh less than 100 lb (too little subcutaneous tissue for absorption) or who are hyperthermic (increases drug absorption). *Do not place heating pads over a patch and never cut a patch.* To dispose of a patch, fold in half, adhesive side onto itself, and flush down the toilet.

All patients on chronic opioid therapy require monitoring and follow-up. Side effects should be anticipated, prevented when possible, and treated when necessary. Over time, patients develop tolerance to the analgesic effect of opioids, requiring higher doses to achieve pain relief. The higher opioid dose is usually not lethal because patients also develop a tolerance to respiratory depression. Less commonly, chronic opioid use may lead to hyperalgesia (increased pain sensitivity). Especially in the case of noncancer pain, monitor patients closely for signs of aberrant opioid-related behaviors such as misuse, abuse, and addiction.

A transmucosal fentanyl "unit" treats breakthrough pain in opioid-tolerant patients. Patients take the medication by placing an opened transmucosal package in their mouth between the buccal mucosa and gums and actively sucking on the medicine. Patients need to let it dissolve in the mouth. Teach patients to not chew it and to allow it to absorb over a 15-minute period, delay swallowing as long as possible, and avoid drinking water or other liquid. A patient should not use more than 1 unit of oral transmucosal fentanyl citrate at a time and no more than 2 units of oral transmucosal fentanyl citrate during each episode of breakthrough cancer pain. If a patient has more than four episodes of breakthrough cancer pain per day, he or she should contact the health care provider.

Many patients, family members, and health care providers have concerns about the risks of addiction associated with opioid use. The estimated prevalence of prescription opioid abuse and opioid use disorders ranges from less than 1% to 40% due to the limited availability of uniform definitions of what constitutes misuse, abuse, and addiction (Cheatle, 2015). Patients who consult with numerous health care providers may be labeled as drug seekers when they actually may be seeking adequate pain relief. This situation may be associated with behaviors that are indicative of pseudoaddiction. Nurses need to discourage patients from "doctor shopping" and having multiple health care providers for treating pain and refer them to pain specialists when effective management cannot be obtained through their general health care providers.

As with constant acute pain, it is necessary to give patients with chronic pain required analgesics on a regular basis. The oral route of administration of analgesic drugs should be used as the first choice (CDC, 2016). The patient with chronic pain may need to take an analgesic ATC, as regular administration maintains therapeutic drug blood levels for ongoing pain control. However, the need for continuation of analgesics should be assessed routinely by the health care provider (CDC, 2016).

Administer analgesics rectally when patients are unable to swallow, have nausea or vomiting, or are near death. This route is contraindicated for patients with diarrhea or cancerous lesions involving the anus or rectum. Morphine, hydromorphone, and oxymorphone are available in suppositories.

Some patients use PCA devices to treat severe cancer pain in the home. PCA devices provide improved, uniform pain control with fewer peaks and valleys in plasma concentration, more effective drug action, and lower drug dosages overall. Patients who usually benefit from continuous infusions include those with severe pain for whom oral and injectable medications provide minimal relief, those with severe nausea and vomiting, and those unable to swallow oral medications.

When a patient receives continuous-drip opioids, ensure the IV access is patent and without complications (see Chapter 42). A central venous catheter, an implanted venous access port, or a peripherally inserted central catheter is usually best for long-term IV infusion. When IV access is poor, the subcutaneous route with a concentrated dose is possible. When an infusion begins, monitor a patient's sedation level and respiratory status closely during the first 24 hours and with any increases in the infusion rate (follow agency policy). Patients who are placed on continuous analgesic infusions are opioid tolerant; thus respiratory depression is rare.

QSEN Building Competency in Patient-Centered Care You are assigned to make home visits to a 68-year-old female patient who was discharged from the hospital a day ago. The patient has diabetes and underwent a wound debridement of the left leg during hospitalization. When you arrive, the patient describes the pain around the wound as "throbbing" and "never gets much better." The patient tells you that the NSAID prescribed for wound pain has not worked very well. She states, "I have been taking this medication that I had left over from my surgery last year to help with my pain since this new medication isn't working." You note that the medication the patient has been taking is hydrocodone, an oral opioid. What options do you have in helping this patient achieve a realistic and effective approach to managing her pain?

Answers to QSEN Activities can be found on the Evolve website.

Barriers to Effective Pain Management. Barriers to effective pain management are complex and often involve the patient, the patient's family caregivers, health care providers, and the health care system (Box 44.19). Lack of knowledge and misconceptions about pain and appropriate pain management present significant barriers. Various cultural beliefs about the meaning of pain and pain interventions also pose challenges to effective pain management. Controversy among health care providers exists related to the use of opioid therapy, particularly for the treatment of patients with chronic noncancer pain.

Patients and health care providers often do not understand the differences among physical dependence, addiction, and drug tolerance (Box 44.20). Experiencing a physical dependency does not imply addiction, and drug tolerance in and of itself is not the same as addiction. That is not to say that addiction does not occur or that patients who suffer from addiction should not be treated for pain. Patients with addiction and pain should be treated with the same amount of dignity and respect as all other patients, although safety and monitoring are priority concerns. An interprofessional team approach ensures a more effective pain-management plan for a patient with acute pain who also suffers from addiction. Nurses and health care providers need to avoid labeling patients as *drug seeking* because this term is poorly defined and can cause bias and prejudice. If there are concerns that a patient is abusing opioids, they should be voiced to the patient, and the patient's health care provider should be advised of the concerns. Many patients on long-term opioid medications enter into "pain contracts" that state the expected responsibilities of both the patient and health care provider. If the agreement is violated or other assessments dictate, additional resources may be identified to aid the patient in addressing the addictive illness.

Placebos. There are many different definitions and interpretations of the terms *placebo* and *placebo effect*. It is generally accepted that placebos are pharmacologically inactive preparations or procedures that produce no beneficial or therapeutic effect. Many professional organizations discourage the use of placebos to treat pain. The ethics of therapeutic placebo use is highly controversial; however, evidence suggests that health care providers frequently use placebo treatments, and patients may be open to these interventions under certain situations (Kisaalita et al., 2016). A study involving a patient-centered approach surveyed patients with chronic musculoskeletal pain about their knowledge and acceptability of placebo analgesic use across different clinical contexts. The survey assessed the role of deception and placebo effectiveness on mood and provider trust. Results showed that participants' acceptability was dependent on the context of an intervention, as placebo treatments were considered acceptable when used as complementary/adjunct treatments and when no other established treatments were available. When there was no other established treatment for pain relief and patients were involved in deciding the use of placebos, the intervention was more acceptable than when deceptive placebos were used (Kisaalita et al., 2016). Deceptive placebo use jeopardizes the trust between patients and their caregivers. If a placebo is ordered without a patient's understanding of its purpose, question the order. Many health care agencies have policies that limit the use of placebos to only research.

Restorative and Continuing Care

Pain Clinics, Palliative Care, and Hospices. Health professionals recognize pain as a significant health problem. The growth of pain centers, palliative care departments, and hospices designed to manage pain and suffering has increased. The Commission on Accreditation

---

BOX 44.19 Barriers to Effective Pain Management

Patient Barriers
- Fear of addiction
- Worry about side effects
- Fear of tolerance (won't be there when I need it)
- Takes too many pills already
- Concern about not being a "good" patient
- Doesn't want to worry family and friends
- May need more tests
- Suffering in silence is expected and needs to suffer to be cured
- Inadequate education
- Reluctance to discuss pain
- Pain inevitable
- Pain part of aging
- Fear of disease progression
- Believes health care providers and nurses are doing all they can
- Just forgets to take analgesics
- Fear of distracting health care providers from treating illness
- Believes health care providers have more important or sicker patients to see

Health Care Provider Barriers
- Inadequate pain-assessment skills
- Concern with addiction or accidental overdose
- Concern with co-morbid mental health conditions

- Opiophobia, fear of opioids
- Fear of legal repercussions
- Patient shows no visible cause of pain
- Belief that patients need to learn to live with pain
- Reluctance to deal with side effects of analgesics
- Not believing patient's report of pain
- Fear that giving a dose will kill patient
- Time constraints
- Inadequate reimbursement
- Belief that opioids "mask" symptoms
- Belief that pain is part of aging
- Overestimation of rates of respiratory depression

Health Care System Barriers
- Concern with creating "addicts"
- Difficulty in filling prescriptions
- Absolute dollar restriction on amount reimbursed for prescriptions
- Mail-order pharmacy restrictions
- Advanced practice nurses not used efficiently
- Poor pain policies and procedures regarding pain management
- Inadequate access to pain clinics
- Poor understanding of economic impact of unrelieved pain

BOX 44.20 Definitions Related to the Use of Opioids in Pain Treatment[a]

Physical Dependence

A state of adaptation that is manifested by a drug class–specific withdrawal syndrome produced by abrupt cessation, rapid dose reduction, decreasing blood level of the drug, and/or administration of an antagonist. Common symptoms of opioid withdrawal include shaking, chills, abdominal cramps, excessive yawning, and joint pain.

Addiction

A primary chronic neurobiological disease with genetic, psychosocial, and environmental factors influencing its development and manifestations. Addictive behaviors include one or more of the following: impaired control over drug use, compulsive use, continued use despite harm, and craving.

Drug Tolerance

A state of adaptation in which exposure to a drug induces changes that result in a diminution of one or more effects of the drug over time.

[a]Approved by the Boards of Directors of the American Academy of Pain Medicine, the American Pain Society, and the American Society of Addiction Medicine, February 2001 (American Pain Society, 2011).

of Rehabilitation Facilities (CARF) accredits chronic pain treatment programs and sets standards for chronic pain management. A comprehensive pain center treats people on an inpatient or outpatient basis. Staff members representing all health care disciplines work with patients to find the most effective pain-relief measures. A comprehensive clinic provides diverse therapies and research into new treatments and training for professionals.

Many hospitals have palliative-care departments to help patients and their family members successfully manage their life-limiting conditions. The goal of palliative care is to help patients manage disease-related symptoms while living life fully with an incurable condition (see Chapter 36). Patients and their family members need ongoing

assistance in managing pain at home. Teaching pain management during discharge and ensuring the continuation of pain management after discharge are essential.

Hospices are programs that care for patients at the end of life (see Chapter 36). Hospice provides support and care for people in the last stages of incurable disease, with an emphasis on enhancing the quality of remaining life (Cherny et al., 2014). It helps patients who are nearing the end of life to continue to live at home or in a health care setting in comfort and privacy. Pain control is a priority for hospices. Under the guidance of hospice nurses, families learn to monitor patients' symptoms and become the primary caregivers. Some hospice patients become hospitalized such as in the event of a brief acute care crisis or family problem.

Hospice program practices help nurses overcome their fears of contributing to a patient's death when administering large doses of opioids. The ANA supports aggressive treatment of pain and suffering even if it hastens a patient's death (Fowler, 2015). The ANA position is supported by the ethical principle of double effect, which, when applied to pain at end of life, supports the use of opioids for the purpose of pain relief, despite the risk that a secondary effect may be the hastening of the patient's death from respiratory depression.

◆ Evaluation

Through the Patient's Eyes. Evaluate patients' perceptions of the effectiveness of interventions used to relieve pain. Patients help decide the best times to attempt pain treatments. Essentially they are the best judge of whether a pain-relief intervention works. Often the family is another valuable resource, particularly in the case of a patient with pain who is unable to express discomfort. For patients with chronic pain, consider the effect of the pain intervention on the patient's function when evaluating the patient's perception of his or her response to treatment. You view the pain intervention positively if the intervention results in the patient feeling an improvement in the participation in self-care or activities such as physical therapy.

Also ask patients about tolerance to therapy and the overall amount of relief obtained. If patients state that an intervention is unhelpful or even aggravates the discomfort, stop it immediately and seek an alternative. Time and patience are necessary to maximize the effectiveness of pain management. Educate patients about what to expect. For a patient in acute pain, reassure him or her that you will check back frequently to assess for changes in pain level. Continually assess if the character of the patient's pain changes and whether individual interventions are effective.

Patient Outcomes. Evaluation of pain is one of many nursing responsibilities that require effective critical thinking (Fig. 44.14). Evaluate your success in achieving the outcomes of the plan of care. A patient's behavioral responses to pain-relief interventions are not always obvious. Evaluating the effectiveness of a pain intervention requires you to evaluate for change in the severity and quality of the pain. Also be sure to evaluate after an appropriate period of time. For instance, oral medications usually peak in about 1 hour, whereas IVP medications peak in 15 to 30 minutes. Ask a patient whether a medication alleviates the pain when the medication's effect is peaking. Do not expect the patient to volunteer the information. Evaluate psychological and physiological responses to pain (e.g., check for changes in vital signs and ask questions such as "Tell me how you feel since we gave you your pain medicine.") It is also important to evaluate whether the patient has any adverse effects from pain therapies.

If a patient continues to have discomfort after an intervention, try a different approach. For example, if an analgesic provides only partial relief, add massage or guided-imagery exercises. Consult with the patient's health care provider about increasing the dose, decreasing the interval between doses, or trying different analgesics. If patient outcomes are not met, ask the patient:

- What is your current pain level?
- How far away is your pain level from your goal?
- Which side effects are you experiencing from your pain medication?
- What have you done to help manage your pain?
- Describe limitations in function that you are experiencing related to uncontrolled pain.
- How is your pain limiting or altering your rest and sleep?

Effective communication of the evaluation of a patient's pain and the response to intervention is facilitated by accurate and thorough documentation. This communication needs to happen from nurse to nurse, shift to shift, and nurse to other health care providers. The nurse caring for the patient has a professional responsibility to report the effectiveness of interventions for managing the patient's pain and

evaluation of patient care goals and outcomes. A variety of tools such as a pain flow sheet or diary help centralize information about pain management. The patient expects you to be sensitive to his or her pain and to be attentive in attempts to manage that pain. Effectively communicating with colleagues helps you achieve optimal pain relief for patients. For example, during a hand-off report communicate this information: (1) the patient's current pain rating, (2) the period of time at that level of pain, and (3) what pain rating is acceptable to the patient. Evaluation of pain management requires a patient-centered approach.

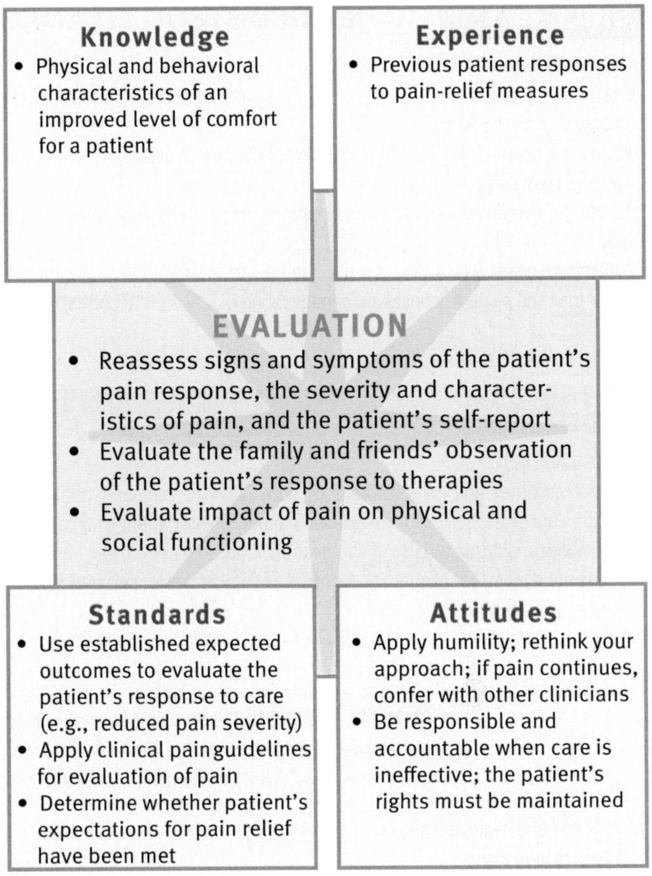

Knowledge
- Physical and behavioral characteristics of an improved level of comfort for a patient

Experience
- Previous patient responses to pain-relief measures

EVALUATION
- Reassess signs and symptoms of the patient's pain response, the severity and characteristics of pain, and the patient's self-report
- Evaluate the family and friends' observation of the patient's response to therapies
- Evaluate impact of pain on physical and social functioning

Standards
- Use established expected outcomes to evaluate the patient's response to care (e.g., reduced pain severity)
- Apply clinical pain guidelines for evaluation of pain
- Determine whether patient's expectations for pain relief have been met

Attitudes
- Apply humility; rethink your approach; if pain continues, confer with other clinicians
- Be responsible and accountable when care is ineffective; the patient's rights must be maintained

FIG. 44.14 Critical thinking model for pain-management evaluation.

SAFETY GUIDELINES FOR NURSING SKILLS

Ensuring patient safety is an essential role of the professional nurse. To ensure patient safety, communicate clearly with members of the health care team, assess and incorporate the patient's priorities of care and preferences, and use the best evidence when making decisions about the patient's care. When performing the skills in this chapter, remember the following points to ensure safe, individualized patient care:

- The patient is the only person who should press a PCA button to administer the pain medication.
- Monitor the patient for signs and symptoms of oversedation and respiratory depression.
- Monitor for potential side effects of opioid analgesics.

SKILL 44.1   PATIENT-CONTROLLED ANALGESIA

Delegation and Collaboration

The skill of PCA administration cannot be delegated to assistive personnel (AP). The nurse directs the AP to:

- Notify the nurse if the patient complains of change in status, including unrelieved pain or difficulty awakening.
- Notify the nurse if the patient has questions about the PCA process or equipment.
- Never administer a PCA dose for the patient and to notify the nurse if anyone other than the patient is observed administering a dose for the patient.

Equipment

- PCA pump system and tubing
- Analgesic cartridge or syringe with identification label and time tape (may already be attached and completed by pharmacy)
- Needleless connector
- Antiseptic swab
- Adhesive tape
- Clean gloves (when applicable)
- Opioid reversal agent (e.g., naloxone)
- Equipment for vital signs, pulse oximetry, and capnography
- Medication administration record (MAR)

STEP	RATIONALE

ASSESSMENT

1. Check accuracy and completeness of each MAR or computer printout with health care provider's written medication order. Check patient's name, medication name and dosage, route of administration, lockout period, and frequency of medication (demand, continuous, or both). Recopy or reprint any portion of MAR that is difficult to read.

   The order sheet is the most reliable source and only legal record of medications that patient is to receive. Ensures that patient receives the correct medications (Mandrack et al., 2012). Illegible MARs are a source of medication errors.

2. Assess patient's medical and medication history, including drug allergies.

   Determines need for medication or possible contraindications for medication administration.

CLINICAL DECISION: *When assessing allergies, be aware that nausea is not an allergic reaction and that it can be treated; pruritus alone is not an allergic reaction and is common with opioid use. Pruritus is treatable and does not contraindicate the use of PCA (Masato et al., 2017).*

---

3. Perform hand hygiene. Perform a complete assessment of character of pain, and measure vital signs.

   Reduces transmission of microorganisms. Provides baseline for type and nature of pain condition for determination of efficacy of PCA.

4. Review medication information in drug reference manual or consult with pharmacist if uncertain about any PCA medications to be administered.

   Understanding medications before administering them prevents medication errors (Pasero et al., 2015).

5. Assess environment for factors that could contribute to pain (e.g., noise, room temperature).

   Elimination of irritating stimuli may help to reduce pain perception.

6. Assess for conditions that predispose patients to unwanted effects from opioids. For example, assess for obstructive sleep apnea syndrome (OSAS) before surgery by anesthesia using the STOP-BANG questionnaire (see Chapter 50) (Gokay et al., 2016) (see agency policy).

   Use assessment data to prevent unwanted effects from opioids. For example, known, untreated, or unknown OSAS poses a significant risk for respiratory depression, especially when receiving anesthesia (Gokay et al., 2016). Identification allows treatment teams (surgeon, respiratory therapy, anesthesia) to take appropriate precautions such as making continuous positive airway pressure or bi-level positive airway pressure ventilation devices available.

7. Apply clean gloves. Assess patency of intravenous (IV) access and surrounding tissue for inflammation or swelling (see Chapter 42).

   IV line needs to be patent for safe administration of pain medication. Confirmation of placement of IV catheter and integrity of surrounding tissues ensures that medication is safely administered.

8. If patient has had surgery, inspect incision, continuing to wear clean gloves. Gently palpate around area for tenderness. Use sterile gloves if necessary to place hand directly on incision. Remove and dispose of gloves and perform hand hygiene.

   Unusual incisional pain, swelling, redness, and/or discharge may indicate infection. Reduces transmission of infection.

9. Assess patient's or family caregiver's knowledge, experience, and health literacy level.

   Ensures patient has the capacity to obtain, communicate, process, and understand basic health information (CDC, 2019).

10. Assess patient's ability to manipulate PCA control and cognitive status for ability to understand purpose of PCA and how to use control device.

    Determines patient's competency and ability to use PCA safely and correctly.

11. Assess patient's knowledge and perceived effectiveness of previous pain-management strategies, especially previous PCA use.

    Response to pain-control strategies helps identify learning needs and affects patient's willingness to try therapy.

PLANNING

1. Provide privacy and prepare bedside environment for patient safety.

   Maintains patient comfort and removes barriers that may interfere with procedure.

2. Collect and bring appropriate supplies to the patient's bedside.

   Ensures an organized approach.

3. Assist patient into a comfortable position.

IMPLEMENTATION

1. Perform hand hygiene.

   Reduces transmission of microorganisms.

2. Follow "seven rights" for administration of medications (see Chapter 31). Obtain PCA analgesic in module prepared by pharmacy. Check label of medication 2 times—when removed from storage and when preparing for assembly.

   Ensures safe and appropriate medication administration. *This is the first and second check for accuracy.*

STEP	**RATIONALE**
3. At bedside identify patient using at least two identifiers (e.g., name and birthday or name and medical record number) according to agency policy. Compare identifiers with information on patient's MAR or medical record.	Ensures correct patient. Complies with The Joint Commission standards and improves patient safety (TJC, 2020).
4. At bedside compare MAR or computer printout with name of medication on drug cartridge. Have second registered nurse (RN) confirm health care provider's order and correct setup of PCA. Second RN should check order and the device independently and not just look at existing setup.	Ensures that correct patient receives right medication. *This is the third check for accuracy.*
5. Before initiating analgesia, demonstrate function of PCA to patient and family caregiver. This includes education about the use of PCA and verbal and written instruction warning against anyone other than the patient pressing the PCA button (Cooney et al., 2013; Pasero, 2015)	It is important that the patient and family members understand how to use PCA safely. Allows for patient-centered care and improved patient outcomes with pain control (Shindul-Rothschild, 2017).
a. Explain type of medication in device.	Informs patient of therapy to be received.

CLINICAL DECISION: *Background basal infusion opioids have been associated with increased risk of nausea, vomiting, and respiratory depression. However, in patients with opioid tolerance, a background basal infusion may be necessary due to the potential for undertreatment and possible opioid withdrawal (Chou et al., 2016).*

STEP	**RATIONALE**
b. If a background basal rate is used, explain that device safely administers continuous medication; however, self-initiated small but frequent amounts of medication can be administered for unrelieved pain by using the PCA button.	A background basal infusion delivers a continuous dose of analgesic medication. The PCA pump is programmed to allow additional patient-controlled doses for pain that is not relieved by the continuous infusion (breakthrough pain) (Pasero, 2015).
c. Explain that self-dosing aids in repositioning, walking, coughing, and deep breathing.	Promotes patient's participation in care.
d. Explain that device is programmed to deliver ordered type and dose of pain medication, lockout interval, and 1- to 4-hour dosage limits. Explain how lockout time prevents overdose.	Relieves anxiety in patients who might be concerned about overdosing.
e. Demonstrate to patient how to push medication demand button (see illustration). Instruct family caregiver not to push PCA button to give medication.	Administration by proxy is not recommended in adults (Chou et al., 2016; TJC, 2017).
f. Instruct patient to notify a nurse for possible side effects, problems in gaining pain relief, changes in severity or location of pain, alarm sounding, or questions.	Engages patient as partner in care.
6. Apply clean gloves. Check infuser and patient-control module for accurate labeling or evidence of leaking.	Avoids medication error and injury to patient.
7. Reposition patient to be sure that venipuncture or central line site is accessible.	Ensures unimpeded flow of infusion.
8. Insert drug cartridge into infusion device (see illustration) and prime tubing.	Locks system and prevents air from infusing into IV tubing.

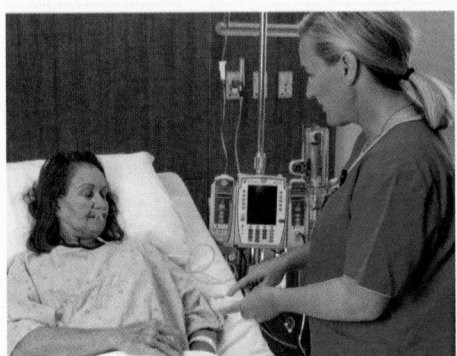
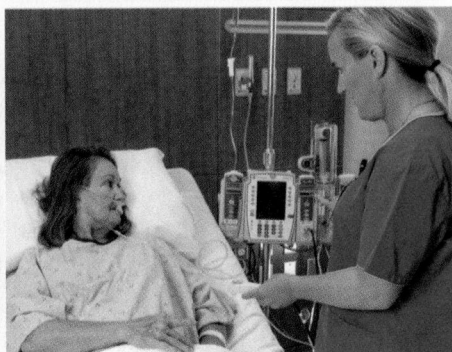

STEP 5e Patient learns how to press PCA device button.

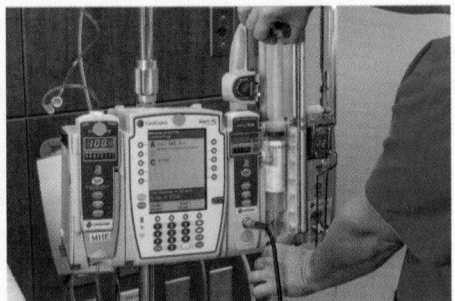

STEP 8 Nurse inserting drug cartridge into PCA device.

Continued

SKILL 44.1   **PATIENT-CONTROLLED ANALGESIA—cont'd**

STEP	RATIONALE
9. Attach needleless adapter to tubing adapter of patient-controlled module.	Needed to connect with IV line.
10. Wipe injection port of maintenance IV line vigorously with antiseptic swab for 15 seconds and allow to dry.	Minimizes entry of surface microorganisms during needle insertion, reducing risk of catheter-related bloodstream infection.
11. Insert needleless adapter into injection port nearest patient (at Y-site of peripheral IV or central line or connect to its own IV site). There should not be a chance to use PCA tubing for administering IV push with another drug.	Establishes route for medication to enter main IV line. Needleless systems prevent needlestick injuries. Prevents medication interaction and incompatibility.
12. Secure connection and anchor PCA tubing with tape. Label PCA tubing.	Prevents dislodging of needleless adapter from port. Facilitates patient's ability to ambulate. Label prevents error from connecting tubing from different device to PCA.
13. Program computerized PCA pump as ordered to deliver prescribed medication dose and lockout interval. Have second nurse check setting. (**NOTE:** Recheck with oncoming RN during shift hand-off to ensure line reconciliation.)	Ensures safe, therapeutic drug administration. With appropriate dose intervals (e.g., 10 min), patient usually experiences an analgesic effect and/or mild sedation before being able to access the next dose; thus, there is lower chance for oversedation and respiratory depression. A second nurse check reduces risk for medication error (Kane-Gill et al., 2017).
14. Administer loading dose of analgesia as prescribed. Manually give 1-time dose or turn on pump and program dose into pump.	Establishes initial level of analgesia.
15. Remove and discard gloves and used supplies in appropriate containers. Dispose of empty cassette or syringe to adhere to institutional policy. Perform hand hygiene.	Reduces transmission of microorganisms. The Federal Controlled Substances Act regulates control and dispensation of opioids for all institutions.
16. If experiencing pain, have patient demonstrate use of PCA system; if not, have patient repeat instructions given earlier.	Repeating instructions reinforces learning. Checking a patient's understanding through return demonstration helps you determine patient's level of understanding and ability to manipulate device.
17. Be sure that venipuncture or central line site is protected and recheck infusion rate before leaving patient.	Ensures patency of IV line.
18. Assist patient into comfortable position.	Patient comfort.
19. Raise side rails (as appropriate) and lower bed to lowest position.	Patient safety precaution.
20. Place nurse call system within patient's reach and instruct patient in its use.	Patient safety precaution.
21. **To discontinue PCA:**	
a. Check health care provider order for discontinuation. Obtain necessary PCA information from pump for documentation; note date, time, amount infused and amount of drug wasted, and reason for wastage.	Ensures correct documentation of a schedule II drug. Two RNs must witness wastage of opioids (narcotics) and sign record to meet requirements of the Controlled Substances Act for scheduled drugs.
b. Perform hand hygiene and apply clean gloves. Turn off pump. Disconnect PCA tubing from primary IV line, but maintain IV access.	Reduces transmission of microorganisms. Follow health care provider order for maintenance of IV site.
c. Dispose of empty cartridge, tubing and gloves according to agency policy. Remove and dispose of gloves and perform hand hygiene.	Reduces transmission of microorganisms.
d. Follow steps 18-20.	Promotes patient comfort.

EVALUATION

1. Use pain rating scale to evaluate patient's pain intensity following treatments and procedures according to agency policy.

   Determines response to PCA dosing. Documenting "PCA in use" or "PCA effective" is not an adequate record of patient's pain level.

2. Observe patient for nausea or pruritus.

   Common treatable side effects of opioids.

3. Monitor patient's level of sedation. It is recommended that the Pasero Opioid Sedation Scale (POSS) be used to monitor for unintended patient sedation (Davis et al., 2017; TJC, 2017). Use vital signs, pulse oximetry, and capnography for monitoring. Study findings report nurse observation and administration of the POSS as superior in earlier identification of respiratory depression and oversedation (Chou et al., 2016). Monitoring should be frequent per agency policy and health care provider order (e.g., every 1 to 2 hours for first 12 hours for the first 24-hour period after surgery. Monitor more often at start, during first 24 hours, and at night when hypoventilation and hypoxia tend to occur during sleep.

   Patient is at highest risk for oversedation and respiratory distress (OSRD) during the first 24 hours of PCA administration. Although there is low sensitivity for detecting hypoventilation with pulse oximetry when supplemental oxygen is used and evidence is insufficient to firmly recommend capnography (Chou et al., 2016), these interventions are used in monitoring for OSRD and provide important clinical information in your assessment. Excess sedation (difficult to arouse) precedes respiratory depression. Differences in ventilation are observed between wakefulness and sleep, which correlates with states of brain arousal. Opioid-induced respiratory depression is also regulated by sleep-wake mechanisms (Nagappa et al., 2017).

STEP	RATIONALE
4. Have patient demonstrate dose delivery.	Evaluates skill in use of PCA.
5. According to agency policy, evaluate number of attempts (number of times patient pushed button), delivery of demand doses (number of times drug actually given and total amount of medication delivered in particular time frame), and basal dose if ordered.	Helps to evaluate effectiveness of PCA dose and frequency in relieving pain. Maintains compliance with Controlled Substances Act.
6. Observe patient initiate self-care.	Demonstrates pain relief.
7. **Use Teach-Back:** "I want to be sure I explained how the PCA will help with your pain and how you should use the device. Tell me the steps you will use to activate the PCA." Revise your instruction now or develop a plan for revised patient/family caregiver teaching if patient/family caregiver is not able to teach back correctly.	Determines patient's/family caregiver's level of understanding of instructional topic.

UNEXPECTED OUTCOMES AND RELATED INTERVENTIONS

1. Patient verbalizes continued or worsening discomfort or displays nonverbal behaviors indicative of pain, suggesting that underlying condition has changed or that patient is undermedicated.
   - Perform complete pain reassessment.
   - Assess for possible complications.
   - Inspect IV site for possible catheter occlusion or infiltration.
   - Evaluate number of attempts and deliveries initiated by patient.
   - Check that maintenance of IV fluid is running continuously.
   - Evaluate pump for operational problems.
   - Consult with health care provider.
2. Patient is sedated and not easily aroused.
   - Stop PCA. Notify health care provider immediately.
   - Elevate head of bed 30 degrees unless contraindicated.
   - Instruct patient to take deep breaths.
   - Apply oxygen at 2 L/min per nasal cannula (if ordered).
   - Assess vital signs, oxygen saturation, and/or capnography. Monitor frequently.
   - Evaluate amount of opioid delivered within the past 4 to 8 hours.
   - Ask family members if they pressed button without patient's knowledge.
   - Review MAR for other possible sedating drugs.
   - Prepare to administer naloxone if signs or symptoms of respiratory depression are noted.
3. Patient unable to manipulate PCA device to maintain pain control.
   - Consult with health care provider regarding alternative medication route or possibly a basal (continuous) dose.

RECORDING AND REPORTING

- Record appropriate drug, concentration, dose (basal and demand), time started, lockout time, and amount of solution infused and remaining per agency policy. Many agencies have a separate flow sheet for PCA documentation.
- Record assessment of patient's response to analgesic on PCA medication form, narrative notes, or patient assessment flow sheet (see agency policy), including vital signs, oximetry and capnography results, sedation status, pain rating, and status of vascular access device.
- Calculate infused dose: add demand and continuous dose together.
- Document your evaluation of patient learning.
- During hand-off report, the oncoming and outgoing nurses should inspect and agree with PCA pump programming as a means of medication reconciliation (Kane-Gill, 2017).
- Hand-off report should include detailed information regarding vital signs, pulse oximetry and capnography, pain assessment scores, STOP-BANG score for OSAS if done, POSS sedation scores, level of consciousness, anxiety level, and activity level (Chou et al., 2016; Cooney, 2016; Meisenberg et al., 2017).
- Nursing research has been reported on the benefit of "safety priming" during hand-off report, such as using words to activate a mental construct, prompting nursing safety-oriented behavior (Groves et al., 2017). An example of safety priming during hand-off report may include the nurse's words to express concern of what may happen (e.g., excess opioid infusion) because of certain behaviors, instead of reporting only factual information.

KEY POINTS

- There are four physiological processes of nociceptive pain: transduction, transmission, perception, and modulation.
- Pain is characterized by its duration, location, cause, intensity, and impact on the individual.
- Individual, physiological, psychological, social, cultural, and environment factors influence pain.
- Cultural beliefs affect how individuals cope with pain as they learn what is expected and accepted by their culture, including how to react to pain.
- The assessment of pain incorporates a patient's physiological, affective, cognitive, behavioral, spiritual, and social dimensions.
- Acute pain is protective, usually has an identifiable cause, is of short duration, and has limited tissue damage and emotional response. In contrast, chronic pain is not protective and thus serves no purpose, but it has a dramatic effect on a person's quality of life.
- Active and passive nonpharmacological measures can be used along with analgesics (nonopioid or opioid) and adjuvant medications for the treatment of pain.
- When administering analgesics, consider that opioids given with nonopioids provide a multimodal analgesia approach, but always avoid using multiple opioids with the same duration and mechanism of action.
- Lack of knowledge and misconceptions about pain and appropriate pain management are significant barriers to pain management.
- Evaluation of the response to pain should include pain intensity, as well as side effects, behavior, and functional outcomes.

REFLECTIVE LEARNING

- Think about a patient you cared for who experienced pain. Was your assessment comprehensive?
- What pain medications were ordered for your patient, and how did you ensure the seven rights of medication administration before administering them?
- Describe the monitoring you did and the side effects you observed for with the ordered medications. How did you determine if the patient's pain management plan was effective?

REVIEW QUESTIONS

1. Which of the following signs or symptoms in a patient who is opioid-naïve is of greatest concern to the nurse when assessing the patient 1 hour after administering an opioid?
   1. Oxygen saturation of 95%
   2. Difficulty arousing the patient
   3. Respiratory rate of 12 breaths/min
   4. Pain intensity rating of 5 on a scale of 0 to 10
2. A health care provider writes the following order for a patient who is opioid-naïve who returned from the operating room following a total hip replacement: "Fentanyl patch 100 mcg, change every 3 days." On the basis of this order, the nurse takes the following action:
   1. Calls the health care provider and questions the order
   2. Applies the patch the third postoperative day
   3. Applies the patch as soon as the patient reports pain
   4. Places the patch as close to the hip dressing as possible

3. A patient is being discharged home on an around-the-clock (ATC) opioid for postoperative pain. Because of this order, the nurse anticipates an additional order for which class of medication?
   1. Opioid antagonists
   2. Antiemetics
   3. Stool softeners
   4. Muscle relaxants
4. A new medical resident writes an order for oxycodone CR 10 mg PO q2h prn. Which part of the order does the nurse question?
   1. The drug
   2. The time interval
   3. The dose
   4. The route
5. The nurse reviews a patient's medical administration record (MAR) and finds that the patient has received oxycodone/acetaminophen (5/325), two tablets PO every 3 hours for the past 3 days. What concerns the nurse the most?
   1. The patient's level of pain
   2. The potential for addiction
   3. The amount of daily acetaminophen
   4. The risk for gastrointestinal bleeding
6. When using ice massage for pain relief, which of the following is correct? (Select all that apply.)
   1. Apply ice using firm pressure over the skin.
   2. Apply ice for 5 minutes or until numbness occurs.
   3. Apply ice no more than 3 times a day.
   4. Limit application of ice to no longer than 10 minutes.
   5. Use a slow, circular steady massage.
7. A patient with a 3-day history of a stroke that left her confused and unable to communicate returns from interventional radiology following placement of a gastrostomy tube. The patient had been taking hydrocodone/APAP 5/325 up to four tablets/day before her stroke for the past year to manage her arthritic pain. The health care provider's order reads as follows: "Hydrocodone/APAP 5/325 1 tab, per gastrostomy tube, q4h, prn." Which action by the nurse is most appropriate?
   1. No action is required by the nurse because the order is appropriate.
   2. Request to have the order changed to around the clock (ATC) for the first 48 hours.
   3. Ask for a change of medication to meperidine (Demerol) 50 mg IVP, q3h, prn.
   4. Begin the hydrocodone/APAP when the patient shows nonverbal symptoms of pain.
8. Place the following steps in the correct order for administration of patient-controlled analgesia:
   1. Insert drug cartridge into infusion device and prime tubing.
   2. Wipe injection port of maintenance IV line vigorously with antiseptic swab for 15 seconds and allow to dry.
   3. Demonstrate to patient how to push medication demand button.
   4. Secure connection and anchor PCA tubing with tape.
   5. Instruct patient to notify a nurse for possible side effects or changes in the severity or location of pain.
   6. Insert needleless adapter into injection port nearest patient.
   7. Apply clean gloves. Check infuser and patient-control module for accurate labeling or evidence of leaking.
   8. Program computerized PCA pump as ordered to deliver prescribed medication dose and lockout interval.

9. Attach needleless adapter to tubing adapter of patient-controlled module.

9. When teaching a patient about transcutaneous electrical nerve stimulation (TENS), which of the following represent an accurate description of the nonpharmacological therapy? (Select all that apply.)

   1. Turn TENS on before patient feels discomfort.
   2. TENS works peripherally and centrally on nerve receptors.
   3. TENS does not require a health care provider order.
   4. Remove any skin preparations before attaching TENS electrodes.
   5. Placing electrodes directly over or near the pain site works best.

10. Match the characteristics on the left with the appropriate pain category on the right.

	Acute Pain	Chronic Pain

A. Has a protective effect

B. Lasts more than 3 to 6 months

C. Usually has identifiable cause

D. Dramatically affects quality of life

E. Viewed as a disease

F. Eventually resolves with or without treatment

Answers: 1. 2; **2.** 1; **3.** 4; **4.** 2; **5.** 3; **6.** 1, 2, 5; **7.** 2, 8; **8.** 3, 5, 7, 1, 9, 2, 6, 4, 8; **9.** 2, 4, 5; **10.** Acute pain: A, C, F; Chronic pain: B, D, E.

Rationales for Review Questions can be found on the Evolve website.

REFERENCES

Abdulla A, et al.: Evidence-based clinical practice guidelines on management of pain in older people, *Age Ageing* 42(2):151–153, 2013.

American Chronic Pain Association (ACPA): *ACPA resource guide to chronic pain medication & treatment*, 2018 edition. https://www.theacpa.org/wp-content/uploads/2018/03/ACPA_Resource_Guide_2018-Final-v2.pdf. Accessed November 24, 2019.

American Geriatrics Society Beers Criteria Update Expert Panel: American Geriatrics Society 2015 updated beers criteria for potentially inappropriate medication use in older adults, *J Am Geriatr Soc* 63(11):2227–2246, 2015.

American Music Therapy Association (AMTA): *Music therapy and music-based interventions in the treatment and management of pain: selected references and key findings*, 2019. https://www.musictherapy.org/research/factsheets/. Accessed May 11, 2019.

American Nurses Association (ANA): *The ethical responsibility to manage pain and the suffering it causes*, Silver Spring, MD, 2018, The Association.

American Nurses Association *(ANA) and American Society for Pain Management Nursing (ASPMN): Scope and standards of practice: pain management nursing*, ed 2, Silver Spring, MD, 2016, The Association.

American Society of Anesthesiologists (ASA): Practice guidelines for chronic pain management, *Anesthesiology* 112:1, 2010.

Atee M, et al.: Pain assessment in dementia: evaluation of a point-of-care technological solution, *J Alzheimers Dis* 60(1):137–150, 2017.

Bourne SL, et al.: Basic anatomy and physiology of pain pathways, *Neurosurg Clin N Am* 25(4):629, 2014.

Burchum JR, Rosenthal LD: *Lehne's pharmacology for nursing care*, ed 10, St Louis, 2019, Elsevier.

Centers for Disease Control and Prevention: CDC guideline for prescribing opioids for chronic pain – United States, *MMWR* 65(1):1–49, 2016.

Centers for Disease Control and Prevention (CDC): *What is health literacy*, 2019, https://www.cdc.gov/healthliteracy/learn/index.html. Accessed December 23, 2019.

Cheatle MD: Prescription opioid misuse, abuse, morbidity, and mortality: balancing effective pain management and safety, *Pain Med* 16(Suppl 1):S3–S8, 2015.

Cherny NI, ESMO Guidelines Working Group: ESMO clinical practice guidelines for the management of refracto-

ry symptoms at the end of life and the use of palliative sedation, *Ann Oncol* 25(Suppl 3):iii143–iii152, 2014.

Chou R, et al.: Management of postoperative pain: a clinical practice guideline from the American Pain Society, the American Society of Regional Anesthesia and Pain Medicine, and the American Society of Anesthesiologists' Committee on Regional Anesthesia, Executive Committee, and Administrative Council, *J Pain* 17(2):131, 2016.

Chow S, et al.: Pain assessment tools for older adults with dementia in long-term care facilities: a systematic review, *Neurodegener Dis Manag* 6(6):525–538, 2016.

Colloca L, et al.: Neuropathic pain, *Nar Rev Dis Primers* 16(3):17002, 2017. https://doi.org/10.1038/nrdp.2017.2.

Coluzzi F, et al.: Good clinical practice guide for opioids in pain management: the three Ts–titration (trial), tweaking (tailoring), transition (tapering), *Revista Brasilieira de Anestesiologia* 66(3):310, 2016.

Cooney MF: Postoperative pain management: clinical practice guidelines, *J PeriAnesth Nurs* 31(5):445, 2016.

Cooney MF, et al.: American Society for Pain Management Nursing position statement with clinical practice guidelines: authorized agent–controlled analgesia, *Pain Manag Nurs* 14(3):178, 2013.

Dahlhamer J, et al.: Prevalence of chronic pain and high-impact chronic pain among adults—United States, *MMWR Morb Mortal Wkly Rep* 67(36):1001–1006, 2018.

Das V: An introduction to pain pathways and pain "targets, *Prog Mol Biol Transl Sci* 131:1–30, 2015.

Davis C, et al.: A multisite retrospective study evaluating the implementation of the Pasero Opioid-Induced Sedation Scale (POSS) and its effect on patient safety outcomes, *Pain Manag Nurs* 18(4):193, 2017.

Department of Health and Human Services: National pain strategy. 2016, https://iprcc.nih.gov/sites/default/files/HHSNational_Pain_Strategy_508C.pdf. Accessed April 27, 2019.

Devraj R, et al.: Pain awareness and medication knowledge: a health literacy evaluation, *J Pain Palliat Care Pharmacother* 27(1):19, 2013.

Drew DJ, et al.: The use of "as-needed" range orders for opioid analgesics in the management of pain: a consensus statement of the American Society for Pain Management Nursing and the American Pain Society, *Pain Manag Nurs* 15(2):551, 2014.

Drew DJ, et al.: "As-needed" range orders for opioid analgesics in the management of pain: a consensus statement of the American Society for Pain Management Nursing and the American Pain Society, *Pain Manag Nurs* 19(3):207–210, 2018.

Faces of Pain Care: *Wong-baker faces® pain rating scale*, 2016. https://wongbakerfaces.org/. Accessed March 25, 2019.

Fenton BW, et al.: The neurobiology of pain perception in normal and persistent pain, *Pain Manag* 5(4):297–317, 2015.

Fowler MDM: *Guide to the code of ethics for nurses with interpretive statements*, ed 2, Silver Spring, MD, 2015, American Nurses Association.

Galicia-Castillo C, Weiner DK: Treatment of persistent pain in older adults, *UpToDate*, 2019. https://www.uptodate.com/contents/treatment-of-persistent-pain-in-older-adults. Accessed May 8, 2019.

Gokay P, et al.: Is there a difference between the STOP-BANG and the Berlin Obstructive Sleep Apnoea Syndrome questionnaires for determining respiratory complications during the perioperative period? *J Clin Nurs* 25(9/10):1238–1252, 2016.

Hockenberry MJ, Wilson D: *Wong's nursing care of infants and children*, ed 11, St Louis, 2019, Mosby.

Horgas A: *Assessing pain in older adults with dementia. Try this: best practices in nursing care to older adults with dementia*, 2018. https://consultgeri.org/try-this/dementia/issue-d2.pdf. Accessed October 31, 2018.

Horgas AL: Pain assessment in older adults, *Nurs Clin North Am* 52(3):375–385, 2017.

Hoti K, et al.: Clinimetric properties of the electronic Pain Assessment Tool (ePAT) for aged-care residents with moderate to severe dementia, *J Pain Res* 11:1037–1044, 2018.

Institute of Medicine (IOM): *Relieving pain in America: a blueprint for transforming prevention, care, education, and research*, Washington, DC, 2011, National Academies Press.

Interagency Pain Research Coordinating Committee (IPRCC): *Federal Pain Research Strategy overview*, 2018. https://iprcc.nih.gov/Federal-Pain-Research-Strategy/Overview.

International Association for the Study of Pain (IASP): *IASP terminology*, 2017. https://www.iasp-pain.org/Education/Content.aspx?ItemNumber=1698#Pain. Accessed March 23, 2019.

International Association for the Study of Pain (IASP): *Declaration of montreal*, 2018a. http://www.iasp-pain.org/DeclarationofMontreal. Accessed May 5, 2019.

International Association for the Study of Pain (IASP): *Faces pain scale—revised home*, 2018b. http://www.iasp-pain.org/Education/Content.aspx?ItemNumber=1519. Accessed March 23, 2019.

James S: Human pain and genetics: some basics, *Br J Pain* 7(4):171, 2013.

Kane-Gill S, et al.: Clinical practice guideline: safe medication use in the ICU, *Crit Care Med* 45(9):e877, 2017.

Katsarava Z, et al.: Defining the differences between episodic migraine and chronic migraine, *Curr Pain Headache Rep* 16(1):86, 2012.

Lee GY, et al.: Pediatric clinical practice guidelines for acute procedural pain: a systematic review, *Pediatrics* 133(3):500–515, 2014.

Mandrack M, et al.: Nursing best practices using automated dispensing cabinets: nurses' key role in improving medication safety, *Medsurg Nurs* 21(3):134, 2012.

Manocha S, Taneja N: Assessment of paediatric pain: a critical review, *J Basic Clin Physiol Pharmacol* 27(4):1–10, 2016.

Masato H, et al.: Prophylactic pentazocine reduces the incidence of pruritus after cesarean delivery under spinal anesthesia with opioids: a prospective randomized clinical trial, *Anesth Analg* 124(6):1930, 2017.

Matthews-Kozanecka M: Holistic approach to treatment in the context of bioethics, *Dev Period Med* 18(1):13, 2014.

Meisenberg B, et al.: Implementation of solutions to reduce opioid-induced oversedation and respiratory depression, *Am J Health Syst Pharm* 74(3):162, 2017.

Melzack R: From the gate to the neuromatrix, *Pain* 6(Suppl):S121–S126, 1999.

Melzack R, Wall PD: Pain mechanisms: a new theory, *Science* 150:971, 1965.

Nagappa M, et al.: Opioids, respiratory depression, and sleep-disordered breathing, *Best Pract Res Clin Anaesthesiol* 31(4):469–485, 2017.

Narouze S, et al.: Interventional spine and pain procedures in patients on antiplatelet and anticoagulant medications: guidelines from The American Society of Regional Anesthesia and Pain Medicine, The European Society of Regional Anaesthesia and Pain Therapy, The American Academy of Pain Medicine, The International Neuromodulation Society, The North American Neuromodulation Society, and The World Institute of Pain, *Reg Anesth Pain Med* 40(3):182, 2015.

National Institutes of Health: *National center for complementary and integrative health: glucosamine and chondroitin for osteoarthritis*, 2014. https://nccih.nih.gov/health/glucosaminechondroitin. Accessed March 27, 2019.

National Pharmaceutical Council: *Pain: current understanding of assessment, management, and treatments – section III: types of treatments*. 2001, https://www.npcnow.org/system/files/research/download/Pain-Current-Understanding-of-Assessment-Management-and-Treatments.pdf. Accessed November 24, 2019.

O'Sullivan K, et al.: Understanding pain among older persons: part 1 – the development of novel pain profiles and their association with disability and quality of life, *Age Ageing* 46(1):46–51, 2017.

Paice JA, et al.: Management of chronic pain in survivors of adult cancers: ASCO clinical practice guideline summary, *J Oncol Pract* 12(8):757–762, 2016.

Pasero C: Unconventional use of a PCA pump: nurse-activated dosing, *J Perianesth Nurs* 30(1):68, 2015.

Pasero C, McCaffery M: *Pain assessment and pharmacologic management*, St Louis, 2011, Mosby.

QSEN Institute: Pre-licensure KSAS. 2019, http://qsen.org/competencies/pre-licensure-ksas/. Accessed March 25, 2019.

Reid MC, et al.: Management of chronic pain in older adults, *BMJ* 350:h532, 2015.

Scarborough BM, Smith CB: Optimal pain management for patients with cancer in the modern era, *CA Cancer J Clin* 68(3):182–196, 2018.

Shindul-Rothschild J, et al.: Beyond the pain scale: provider communication and staffing predictive of patients' satisfaction with pain control, *Pain Manag Nurs* 18(6):401, 2017.

Starkweather AR, et al.: Methods to measure peripheral and central sensitization using quantitative sensory testing: a focus on individuals with low back pain, *Appl Nurs Res* 29:237–241, 2016.

Steeds CE: The anatomy and physiology of pain, *Surgery* 34(2):55–59, 2016.

Taddio A, et al.: Reducing pain during vaccine injections: clinical practice guideline, *CMAJ* 187(13):975–982, 2015.

Thapa D, et al.: Cancer pain management-current status, *J Anaesthesiol Clin Pharmacol* 27(2):162, 2011.

The Joint Commission (TJC): *Prepublication standards—standards revisions related to pain assessment and management*, Oakbrook Terrace, IL, 2017, Author. https://www.jointcommission.org/standards_information/prepublication_standards.aspx. Accessed April 27, 2019.

The Joint Commission (TJC): *2020 National patient safety goals*, Oakbrook Terrace, IL, 2020. The Commission. https://www.jointcommission.org/en/standards/national-patient-safety-goals/. Accessed January 2, 2020.

Treede RD: The International association for the study of pain definition of pain: as valid in 2018 as in 1979, but in need of regularly updated footnotes, *Pain Rep* 3(2):e643, 2018.

US Food and Drug Administration (USFDA): *FDA drug safety communication: prescription acetaminophen products to be limited to 325 mg per dosage unit; boxed warning will highlight potential for severe liver failure*. 2014, http://www.fda.gov/Drugs/DrugSafety/ucm239821.htm. Accessed May 11, 2019.

Vargas-Schaffer G: Is the WHO analgesic ladder still valid? *Can Fam Physician* 56(6):514, 2010.

Wong DL, Baker CM: Pain in children: comparison of assessment scales, *Okla Nurse* 33(1):8, 1988.

Zorina-Lichtenwalter K, et al.: Genetic predictors of human chronic pain conditions, *Neuroscience* 338:36–62, 2016.

RESEARCH REFERENCES

Beyer JE, et al.: The creation, validation, and continuing development of the Oucher: a measure of pain intensity in children, *J Pediatr Nurs* 7(5):335, 1992.

Chou R, et al.: The effectiveness and risks of long-term opioid therapy for chronic pain: a systematic review for a National Institutes of Health Pathways to Prevention Workshop, *Ann Intern Med* 162(4):276, 2015.

Cole LC, LoBiondo-Wood G: Music as an adjuvant therapy in control of pain and symptoms in hospitalized adults: a systematic review, *Pain Manag Nurs* 15(1):406, 2014.

Dekel BGS, et al.: Medical evidence influence on inpatients and nurses pain ratings agreement, *Pain Res Manag* 2016:9267536, 2016. https://www.hindawi.com/journals/prm/2016/9267536/. Accessed May 8, 2019.

Desai G, et al.: Does pain behavior influence assessment of pain severity? *Indian J Palliat Care* 20(2):134–136, 2014.

Dueñas M, et al.: A review of chronic pain impact on patients, their social environment and the health care system, *J Pain Res* 9:457–467, 2016.

Gaston-Johansson F, et al.: Similarities in pain descriptions of four different ethnic-culture groups, *J Pain Symptom Manage* 5(2):94, 1990.

Goulet JL, et al.: Agreement between electronic medical-based and self-administered pain numeric rating scale: clinical and research implications, *Med Care* 51(3):245, 2013.

Greco TM, et al: Quality of cancer pain management: an update of a systematic review of undertreatment of patients with cancer, *J Clin Oncol* epub November 17, 2014. http://jco.ascopubs.org/content/early/2014/11/20/JCO.2014.56.0383.full. Accessed April 27, 2019.

Groves PS, et al.: Priming patient safety through nursing handoff communication: a simulation pilot study, *Western Journal of Nursing Research* 39(11):1394–1411, 2017.

Hollingshead NA, et al.: The pain experience of Hispanic Americans: a critical literature review and conceptual model, *J Pain* 17(5):513–528, 2016.

Kisaalita N, et al.: Placebo use in pain management: a mechanism-based educational intervention enhances placebo treatment acceptability, *J Pain* 17(2):257–269, 2016.

Korhan E, et al.: The effects of music therapy on pain in patients with neuropathic pain, *Pain Manag Nurs* 15(1):306, 2014.

Lerman SF, et al.: Longitudinal associations between depression, anxiety, pain, and pain-related disability in chronic pain patients, *Psychosom Med* 77(3):333–341, 2015.

Miró J, et al.: Validity of three rating scales for measuring pain intensity in youths with physical disabilities, *Eur J Pain* 20(1):130–137, 2016.

Morales DR, et al.: NSAID-exacerbated respiratory disease: a meta-analysis evaluating prevalence, mean provocative dose of aspirin and increased asthma morbidity, *Allergy* 70(7):828, 2015.

Nortjé N, Albertyn R: The cultural language of pain: a South African study, *S Afr Family Pract* 57(1), 2015. https://www.tandfonline.com/doi/full/10.1080/20786190.2014.977034. Accessed May 9, 2019.

Pathak A, et al.: The utility and validity of pain intensity rating scales for use in developing countries, *Pain Rep* 3(5):e672, 2018.

Pöpping DM, et al.: Impact of epidural analgesia on mortality and morbidity after surgery: systematic review and meta-analysis of randomized controlled trials, *Ann Surg* 259(6):1056, 2014.

Siddall PJ, et al.: Spirituality: what is its role in pain medicine? *Pain Med* 16(1):51–60, 2015.

Tick H, et al.: Pain Task Force of the Academic Consortium for Integrative Medicine and Health: Evidence-based nonpharmacologic strategies for comprehensive pain care: The Consortium Pain Task Force White Paper, *Explore* 14(3):177–211, 2018.

Tomaszek L, Dębska G: Knowledge, compliance with good clinical practices and barriers to effective control of postoperative pain among nurses from hospitals with and without a "Hospital without Pain" certificate, *J Clin Nurs* 27(7-8):1641–1652, 2018.

Tracy B, Sean Morrison R: Pain management in older adults, *Clin Ther* 35(11):1659, 2013.

US Department of Veterans Affairs: *Acute pain management: meeting the challenges*, P#96864, July 2017. https://www.pbm.va.gov/PBM/AcademicDetailingService/Documents/Academic_Detailing_Educational_Material_Catalog/Pain_Provider_AcutePainProvider-EducationalGuide_IB10998.pdf. Accessed May 11, 2019.

45

Nutrition

OBJECTIVES

- Explain the effects of a well-balanced diet on the body throughout the life span.
- Discuss the process of digestion and absorption.
- Explain the ChooseMyPlate and discuss its value in planning meals for healthy nutrition.
- List the current dietary guidelines for the general population.
- Explain the variance in nutritional requirements throughout the life span.
- Discuss the major methods of nutritional assessment.
- Correctly perform the procedure for initiation and management of enteral feedings.
- Explain the nursing management of enteral feedings.
- Critique the approaches for how to avoid complications of parenteral nutrition.
- Discuss medical nutrition therapy in relation to three medical conditions.
- Discuss how to implement diet counseling and patient teaching in relation to patient expectations.

KEY TERMS

Albumin, p. 1102
Anabolism, p. 1105
Anorexia nervosa, p. 1107
Anthropometry, p. 1111
Basal metabolic rate (BMR), p. 1102
Body mass index (BMI), p. 1112
Bulimia nervosa, p. 1107
Carbohydrates, p. 1102
Catabolism, p. 1105
Chyme, p. 1105
Daily values, p. 1106
Dietary reference intakes (DRIs), p. 1105
Dispensable amino acids, p. 1102
Dysphagia, p. 1114
Enteral nutrition (EN), p. 1120

Fat-soluble vitamins, p. 1103
Fiber, p. 1102
Food security, p. 1101
Hypervitaminosis, p. 1103
Ideal body weight (IBW), p. 1112
Indispensable amino acids, p. 1102
Insulin, p. 1102
Intravenous fat emulsions, p. 1124
Ketones, p. 1105
Kilocalories (kcal), p. 1102
Lipids, p. 1103
Macrominerals, p. 1103
Malabsorption, p. 1128
Malnutrition, p. 1111
Medical nutrition therapy (MNT), p. 1128

Metabolism, p. 1105
Minerals, p. 1103
Nitrogen balance, p. 1103
Nutrient density, p. 1102
Nutrients, p. 1102
Parenteral nutrition (PN), p. 1124
Peristalsis, p. 1104
Resting energy expenditure (REE), p. 1102
Simple carbohydrate, p. 1102
Trace elements, p. 1103
Triglycerides, p. 1103
Vegetarianism, p. 1110
Vitamins, p. 1103
Water-soluble vitamins, p. 1103

MEDIA RESOURCES

http://evolve.elsevier.com/Potter/fundamentals/
- Review Questions
- Video Clips
- Concept Map Creator
- Case Study with Questions

- Skills Performance Checklists
- Audio Glossary
- Content Updates
- Answers to QSEN Activity and Review Questions

Nutrition is a basic component of health and is essential for normal growth and development, tissue maintenance and repair, cellular metabolism, and organ function. Adequate access to nutrition is imperative to attain and maintain this component of health. In 2015, nearly 42.2 million Americans lived in a household that lacked access to proper nutrition (Swinburne et al., 2017). **Food security** is critical for all members of a household. This term means that all household members have access to sufficient, safe, and nutritious food to maintain a healthy lifestyle. Household members should have sufficient food available on a consistent basis and the resources to obtain appropriate food for a nutritious diet. The importance of food security is supported by the US Department of Agriculture, which found that many children in this country live in a home that lacks the access to enough quality food to maintain an active healthy life (Huang and Barnidge, 2016). Decreased food security or access to healthy nutrition can result in poor patient outcomes such as longer hospital admissions due to delayed healing or adverse effects on health conditions (Giddens, 2017). Therefore, nutrition and health are interrelated and represent an important concept in nursing practice.

Medical nutrition therapy (MNT) uses nutrition therapy and counseling to manage diseases (American Dietetic Association, 2019). In some illnesses such as type 1 diabetes mellitus (DM) or mild hypertension, diet therapy is often the major treatment for disease control (ADA, 2019). Other conditions such as severe inflammatory bowel disease require specialized nutrition support such as enteral nutrition (EN) or parenteral nutrition (PN). Current standards of care promote optimal nutrition in all patients, including a low-fat diet and limiting red meat specifically (ACS, 2019; AHA, 2018).

The US Department of Health and Human Services (USDHHS) and the Public Health Service established nutritional goals and objectives for *Healthy People 2020* (USDHHS, 2019). *Healthy People 2020* is the United States' contribution to the "Health for All" strategy of the World Health Organization (WHO, 2019). *Healthy People 2020* (Box 45.1) continues the objectives initiated in *Healthy People 2000* and *Healthy People 2010,* with overall goals of promoting health and reducing chronic disease. All nutrition-related objectives include baseline data from which progress is measured. The challenge remains to motivate consumers to put these dietary recommendations into practice.

SCIENTIFIC KNOWLEDGE BASE

Nutrients: The Biochemical Units of Nutrition

The body requires fuel to provide energy for cellular metabolism and repair, organ function, growth, and body movement. The basal metabolic rate (BMR) is the energy needed at rest to maintain life-sustaining activities (breathing, circulation, heart rate, and temperature) for a specific amount of time. Factors such as age, body mass, gender, fever, starvation, menstruation, illness, injury, infection, activity level, and thyroid function affect energy requirements. The resting energy expenditure (REE), or resting metabolic rate, is the amount of energy you need to consume over a 24-hour period for your body to maintain all of its internal working activities while at rest. Factors that affect metabolism include illness, pregnancy, lactation, and activity level.

When the kilocalories (kcal) of the food we eat meet our energy requirements, our weight does not change (Nix, 2017). When the kilocalories ingested exceed our energy demands, we gain weight. Likewise, if the kilocalories ingested fail to meet our energy requirements, we lose weight.

Nutrients are the elements necessary for the normal function of numerous body processes. We meet energy needs through the intake of a variety of nutrients: carbohydrates, proteins, fats, water, vitamins, and minerals. The nutrient density of food refers to the proportion of essential nutrients to the number of kilocalories. High–nutrient dense foods such as fruits and vegetables provide a large number of nutrients in relationship to kilocalories. Low–nutrient dense foods such as alcohol or sugar are high in kilocalories but nutrient poor.

Carbohydrates. Carbohydrates, composed of carbon, hydrogen, and oxygen, are the main source of energy in the diet. Each gram of carbohydrate produces 4 kcal/g and serves as the main source of fuel (glucose) for the brain, skeletal muscles during exercise, erythrocyte and leukocyte production, and cell function of the renal medulla. We obtain carbohydrates primarily from plant foods, except for lactose (milk sugar). Carbohydrate classification occurs according to their carbohydrate units, or saccharides.

Monosaccharides such as glucose (dextrose) or fructose do not break down into a more basic carbohydrate unit. Disaccharides such as sucrose, lactose, and maltose are composed of two monosaccharides and water. Simple carbohydrate is the classification for both monosaccharides and disaccharides; they are found primarily in sugars. Polysaccharides such as glycogen make up carbohydrate units too (i.e., complex carbohydrates). They are insoluble in water and digested to varying degrees. Starches are polysaccharides.

The body is unable to digest some polysaccharides because we do not have enzymes capable of breaking them down. Fiber, a polysaccharide, is the structural part of plants that is not broken down by our digestive enzymes. The inability to break down fiber means that it does not contribute calories to the diet. Therefore, insoluble fibers, including cellulose, hemicellulose, and lignin, are not digestible. Soluble fibers dissolve in water and include barley, cereal grains, cornmeal, and oats.

Proteins. Proteins provide a source of energy (4 kcal/g); they are essential for the growth, maintenance, and repair of body tissue. Collagen, hormones, enzymes, immune cells, deoxyribonucleic acid (DNA), and ribonucleic acid (RNA) are all made of protein. In addition, blood clotting, fluid regulation, and acid-base balance require proteins. Proteins transport nutrients and many drugs in the blood. Ingestion of proteins maintains nitrogen balance.

The simplest form of protein is the amino acid, consisting of hydrogen, oxygen, carbon, and nitrogen. Because the body does not synthesize indispensable amino acids, we need these to be provided in our diet. Examples of indispensable amino acids are histidine, lysine, and phenylalanine. The body synthesizes dispensable amino acids. Examples of amino acids synthesized in the body are alanine, asparagine, and glutamic acid. Amino acids can link together. Albumin and insulin are simple proteins because they contain only amino acids or their derivatives. The combination of a simple protein with a nonprotein substance produces a complex protein such as lipoprotein, formed by a combination of a lipid and a simple protein.

A complete protein, also called a *high-quality protein,* contains all essential amino acids in sufficient quantity to support growth and maintain nitrogen balance. Most complete proteins come from animal sources, such as fish, poultry, beef, milk, cheese, and eggs, but they can also come from plant sources, such as soy. Incomplete proteins are missing one or more of the nine indispensable amino acids and include grains, seeds and nuts, legumes, and vegetables. Complementary proteins are pairs of incomplete proteins that, when combined, supply the total amount of protein provided by complete protein sources.

Nitrogen is a byproduct of protein catabolism. Achieving nitrogen balance means that the intake and output of nitrogen are equal. When the intake of nitrogen is greater than the output, the body is in positive nitrogen balance. Positive nitrogen balance is required for growth, normal pregnancy, maintenance of lean muscle mass and vital organs, and wound healing. The body uses nitrogen to build, repair, and replace body tissues. Negative nitrogen balance occurs when the body loses more nitrogen than it gains (e.g., with infection, burns, fever, starvation, head injury, and trauma). The increased nitrogen loss is the result of body tissue destruction or loss of nitrogen-containing body fluids. Nutrition during this period needs to provide nutrients to put patients into positive balance for healing.

Protein provides energy, but because its essential role is to promote growth, maintenance, and repair, a diet needs to provide adequate kilocalories from nonprotein sources. When there is sufficient carbohydrate in the diet to meet the energy needs of the body, protein is spared as an energy source.

Fats. Fats (lipids) are the most calorie-dense nutrient, providing 9 kcal/g. Fats are composed of triglycerides and fatty acids. Triglycerides circulate in the blood and are composed of three fatty acids attached to a glycerol. Fatty acids are composed of chains of carbon and hydrogen atoms with an acid group on one end of the chain and a methyl group at the other. Fatty acids can be *saturated,* in which each carbon in the chain has two attached hydrogen atoms, or *unsaturated,* in which an unequal number of hydrogen atoms are attached and the carbon atoms attach to one another with a double bond. Monounsaturated fatty acids have one double bond, whereas polyunsaturated fatty acids have two or more double carbon bonds. The various types of fatty acids referred to in the dietary guidelines have significance for health and the incidence of disease.

Fatty acids are also classified as essential or nonessential. Linoleic acid, an unsaturated fatty acid, is the only essential fatty acid in humans. Linolenic acid and arachidonic acid, other types of unsaturated fatty acids, are important for metabolic processes. The body manufactures them when linoleic acid is available. Deficiency occurs when fat intake falls below 10% of daily nutrition. Most animal fats have high proportions of saturated fatty acids, whereas vegetable fats have higher amounts of unsaturated and polyunsaturated fatty acids.

Water. Water is critical because cell function depends on a fluid environment. Water makes up 60% to 70% of total body weight. People who are lean have a greater percent of total body water than those who are obese because muscle contains more water than any other tissue except blood. Infants have the greatest percentage of total body water because of greater surface area, and older people have the least. When deprived of water, a person usually cannot survive for more than a few days.

We meet our fluid needs by drinking liquids and eating solid foods high in water content such as fresh fruits and vegetables. Digestion produces fluid during food oxidation. In a healthy individual fluid intake from all sources equals fluid output through elimination, respiration, and sweating (see Chapters 41 and 46). An ill person has an increased need for fluid (e.g., with fever or gastrointestinal [GI] losses).

By contrast, he or she also has a decreased ability to excrete fluid (e.g., with cardiopulmonary or renal disease), which often leads to the need for fluid restriction.

Vitamins. Vitamins are organic substances present in small amounts in foods that are essential to normal metabolism. They are chemicals that act as catalysts in biochemical reactions. When there is enough of any specific vitamin to meet the catalytic demands of the body, the rest of the vitamin supply acts as a free chemical and is often toxic to the body. Certain vitamins are currently of interest in their role as antioxidants. These vitamins neutralize substances called *free radicals,* which produce oxidative damage to body cells and tissues. Researchers think that oxidative damage increases a person's risk for various cancers. Antioxidant vitamins include beta-carotene and vitamins A, C, and E (Nix, 2017).

The body is unable to synthesize vitamins in the required amounts. Vitamin synthesis depends on dietary intake. Vitamin content is usually highest in fresh foods that have minimal exposure to heat, air, or water before their use. Vitamin classifications include fat soluble or water soluble.

Fat-Soluble Vitamins. The fat-soluble vitamins (A, D, E, and K) are stored in the fatty compartments of the body. People acquire vitamins primarily through dietary intake, although vitamin D also comes from the sun. The body has a high storage capacity for fat-soluble vitamins. As a result, toxicity is possible when a person takes large doses of them. Hypervitaminosis of fat-soluble vitamins results from megadoses (intentional or unintentional) of supplemental vitamins, excessive amounts in fortified food, and large intake of fish oils.

Water-Soluble Vitamins. The water-soluble vitamins are vitamin C and the B complex (which is eight vitamins). The body does not store water-soluble vitamins; thus, we need them provided in our daily food intake. Water-soluble vitamins absorb easily from the GI tract. Although they are not stored, toxicity can still occur.

Minerals. Minerals are inorganic elements essential to the body as catalysts in biochemical reactions. They are classified as macrominerals when the daily requirement is 100 mg or more and microminerals or trace elements when less than 100 mg is needed daily. Macrominerals help to balance the pH of the body, and specific amounts are necessary in the blood and cells to promote acid-base balance. Interactions occur among trace minerals. For example, excess of one trace mineral sometimes causes deficiency of another. Selenium is a trace element that also has antioxidant properties. Silicon, vanadium, nickel, tin, cadmium, arsenic, aluminum, and boron are trace elements. Arsenic, aluminum, and cadmium can have toxic effects.

Anatomy and Physiology of the Digestive System

Digestion. Digestion of food is the mechanical breakdown that results from chewing, churning, and mixing with fluid and chemical reactions in which food reduces to its simplest form (Grodner, 2020). Each part of the GI system has an important digestive or absorptive function (Fig. 45.1). Enzymes are the protein-like substances that act as catalysts to speed up chemical reactions. They are an essential part of the chemistry of digestion.

Most enzymes have one specific function. Each enzyme works best at a specific pH. For example, the enzyme amylase in the saliva breaks down starches into sugars. The secretions of the GI tract have very different pH levels. Saliva is relatively neutral, gastric juice is highly acidic, and the secretions of the small intestine are alkaline.

The mechanical, chemical, and hormonal activities of digestion are interdependent. Enzyme activity depends on the mechanical breakdown of food to increase its surface area for chemical action.

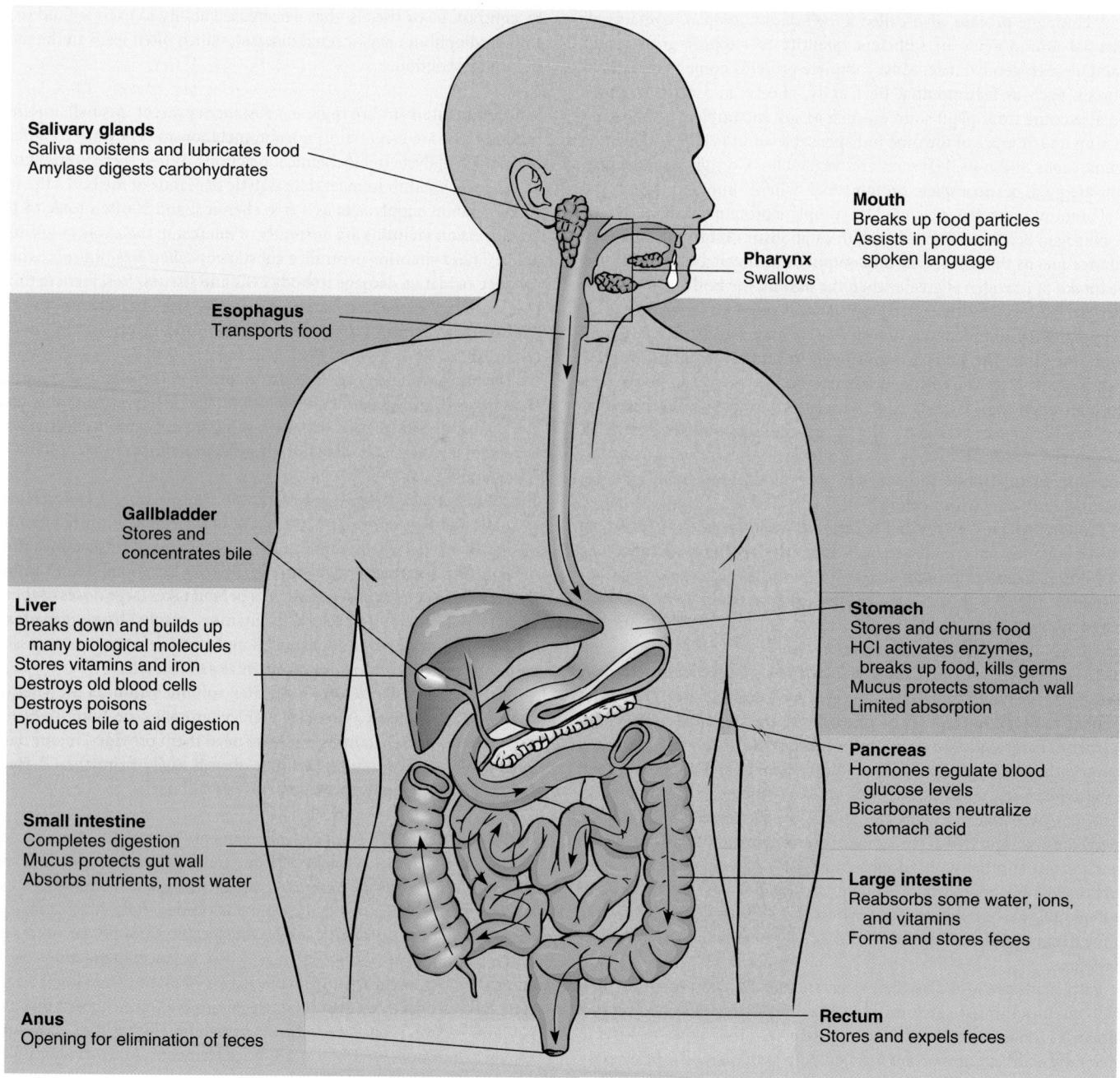

Salivary glands
Saliva moistens and lubricates food
Amylase digests carbohydrates

Mouth
Breaks up food particles
Assists in producing
  spoken language

Pharynx
Swallows

Esophagus
Transports food

Gallbladder
Stores and
concentrates bile

Liver
Breaks down and builds up
  many biological molecules
Stores vitamins and iron
Destroys old blood cells
Destroys poisons
Produces bile to aid digestion

Stomach
Stores and churns food
HCl activates enzymes,
  breaks up food, kills germs
Mucus protects stomach wall
Limited absorption

Pancreas
Hormones regulate blood
  glucose levels
Bicarbonates neutralize
  stomach acid

Small intestine
Completes digestion
Mucus protects gut wall
Absorbs nutrients, most water

Large intestine
Reabsorbs some water, ions,
  and vitamins
Forms and stores feces

Anus
Opening for elimination of feces

Rectum
Stores and expels feces

FIG. 45.1 Summary of digestive system anatomy/organ function. *HCl,* Hydrochloric acid.

Hormones regulate the flow of digestive secretions needed for enzyme supply. Physical, chemical, and hormonal factors regulate the secretion of digestive juices and the motility of the GI tract. Nerve stimulation from the parasympathetic nervous system (e.g., the vagus nerve) increases GI tract action (Grodner, 2020).

Digestion begins in the mouth, where chewing mechanically breaks down food. The food mixes with saliva, which contains ptyalin (salivary amylase), an enzyme that acts on cooked starch to begin its conversion to maltose. The longer an individual chews food, the more starch digestion occurs in the mouth. Proteins and fats are broken down physically, but remain unchanged chemically because enzymes in the mouth do not react with these nutrients. Chewing reduces food particles to a size suitable for swallowing, and saliva provides lubrication to ease swallowing of the food. The epiglottis is a flap of skin that closes over the trachea as a person swallows to prevent aspiration. Swallowed food enters the

esophagus, and wavelike muscular contractions (**peristalsis**) move the food to the base of the esophagus, above the cardiac sphincter. Pressure from a bolus of food at the cardiac sphincter causes it to relax, allowing the food to enter the fundus, or uppermost part, of the stomach.

The chief cells in the stomach secrete pepsinogen, and the pyloric glands secrete gastrin, a hormone that triggers parietal cells to secrete hydrochloric acid (HCl). The parietal cells also secrete HCl and intrinsic factor (IF), which is necessary for absorption of vitamin B_{12} in the ileum. HCl turns pepsinogen into pepsin, a protein-splitting enzyme. The body produces gastric lipase and amylase to begin fat and starch digestion, respectively. A thick layer of mucus protects the lining of the stomach from autodigestion. Alcohol and aspirin are two substances directly absorbed through the lining of the stomach. The stomach acts as a reservoir where food remains for approximately 3 hours, with a range of 1 to 7 hours.

TABLE 45.1 Mechanisms for Intestinal Absorption of Nutrients

Mechanism	Definition
Active transport	An energy-dependent process whereby particles move from an area of greater concentration to an area of lesser concentration. A special "carrier" moves the particle across the cell membrane.
Passive diffusion	The force by which particles move outward from an area of greater concentration to one of lesser concentration. The particles do not need a special "carrier" to move outward in all directions.
Osmosis	Movement of water through a semipermeable membrane that separates solutions of different concentrations. Water moves to equalize the concentration pressures on both sides of the membrane.
Pinocytosis	Engulfing of large molecules of nutrients by the absorbing cell when the molecule attaches to the absorbing cell membrane.

Data from Nix S: *Williams' basic nutrition and diet therapy*, ed 15, St Louis, 2017, Mosby.

Food leaves the antrum, or distal stomach, through the pyloric sphincter and enters the duodenum. Food is now an acidic, liquefied mass called chyme. Chyme flows into the duodenum and quickly mixes with bile, intestinal juices, and pancreatic secretions. The small intestine secretes the hormones secretin and cholecystokinin (CCK). Secretin activates release of bicarbonate from the pancreas, raising the pH of chyme. CCK inhibits further gastrin secretion and initiates release of additional digestive enzymes from the pancreas and gallbladder.

Bile, manufactured in the liver, is then concentrated and stored in the gallbladder. It acts as a detergent because it emulsifies fat to permit enzyme action while suspending fatty acids in solution. Pancreatic secretions contain six enzymes: amylase to digest starch; lipase to break down emulsified fats; and trypsin, elastase, chymotrypsin, and carboxypeptidase to break down proteins.

Peristalsis continues in the small intestine, mixing the secretions with chyme. The mixture becomes increasingly alkaline, inhibiting the action of the gastric enzymes and promoting the action of the duodenal secretions. Epithelial cells in the small intestinal villi secrete enzymes (e.g., sucrase, lactase, maltase, lipase, and peptidase) to facilitate digestion. The major part of digestion occurs in the small intestine, producing glucose, fructose, and galactose from carbohydrates; amino acids and dipeptides from proteins; and fatty acids, glycerides, and glycerol from lipids. Peristalsis usually takes approximately 5 hours to pass food through the small intestine.

Absorption. The small intestine, lined with fingerlike projections called *villi*, is the primary absorption site for nutrients. Villi increase the surface area available for absorption. The body absorbs nutrients by means of passive diffusion, osmosis, active transport, and pinocytosis (Table 45.1).

Absorption of carbohydrates, protein, minerals, and water-soluble vitamins occurs in the small intestine. Then the nutrients are processed in the liver and released into the portal vein circulation. Fatty acids are absorbed in the lymphatic circulatory systems through lacteal ducts at the center of each microvilli in the small intestine.

Approximately 85% to 90% of water is absorbed in the small intestine (McCance et al., 2019). The GI tract manages approximately 8.5 L of GI secretions and 1.5 L of oral intake daily. The small intestine resorbs 9.5 L, and the colon absorbs approximately 0.4 L. Elimination of the remaining 0.1 L occurs via feces. In addition, electrolytes and minerals are absorbed in the colon, and bacteria synthesize vitamin K and some B-complex vitamins. Finally, feces form for elimination.

Metabolism and Storage of Nutrients. Metabolism refers to all the biochemical reactions within the cells of the body. Metabolic processes are anabolic (building) or catabolic (breaking down). Anabolism is the building of more complex biochemical substances by synthesis of nutrients. It occurs when an individual adds lean muscle through diet and exercise. Amino acids are anabolized into tissues, hormones, and enzymes. Normal metabolism and anabolism are physiologically possible when the body is in positive nitrogen balance. Catabolism is the breakdown of biochemical substances into simpler substances and occurs during physiological states of negative nitrogen balance. Starvation is an example of catabolism when wasting of body tissues occurs.

Nutrients absorbed in the intestines, including water, transport through the circulatory system to the body tissues. Through the chemical changes of metabolism, the body converts nutrients into a number of required substances. Carbohydrates, protein, and fat metabolism produce chemical energy and maintain a balance between anabolism and catabolism. To carry out the work of the body, the chemical energy produced by metabolism converts to other types of energy by different tissues. Muscle contraction involves mechanical energy, nervous system function involves electrical energy, and the mechanisms of heat production involve thermal energy.

Some of the nutrients required by the body are stored in tissues. The major form of body reserve energy is fat, stored as adipose tissue. Protein is stored in muscle mass. When the energy requirements of the body exceed the energy supplied by ingested nutrients, stored energy is used. Monoglycerides from the digested part of fats convert to glucose by gluconeogenesis. Amino acids are also converted to fat and stored or catabolized into energy through gluconeogenesis. All body cells except red blood cells and neurons oxidize fatty acids into ketones for energy when dietary carbohydrates (glucose) are not adequate. Glycogen, synthesized from glucose, provides energy during brief periods of fasting (e.g., during sleep). It is stored in small reserves in liver and muscle tissue. Nutrient metabolism consists of three main processes:

1. Catabolism of glycogen into glucose, carbon dioxide, and water (glycogenolysis)
2. Anabolism of glucose into glycogen for storage (glycogenesis)
3. Catabolism of amino acids and glycerol into glucose for energy (gluconeogenesis)

Elimination. Chyme moves by peristaltic action through the ileocecal valve into the large intestine, where it becomes feces (see Chapter 47). Water absorbs in the mucosa as feces move toward the rectum. The longer the material stays in the large intestine, the more water is absorbed, causing the feces to become firmer. Exercise and fiber stimulate peristalsis, and water maintains consistency. Feces contain cellulose and similar indigestible substances, sloughed epithelial cells from the GI tract, digestive secretions, water, and microbes.

Dietary Guidelines

Dietary Reference Intakes. Dietary reference intakes (DRIs) present evidence-based criteria for an acceptable range of amounts of vitamins and nutrients for each gender and age-group (National Academies of Sciences Engineering Medicine Health and Medicine Division, 2019).

BOX 45.2   2015-2020 Dietary Guidelines for Americans: Key Recommendations for the General Population

- Adopt a healthful eating pattern at an appropriate calorie level with a variety of nutrient-dense foods and beverages among all the food groups.
- Maintain body weight in a healthy range.
- Encourage physical activity and decrease sedentary activities.
- Encourage fruits, vegetables, whole-grain products, seafood, and fat-free or low-fat milk.
- Eat a variety of proteins, including lean meats, seafood, poultry, eggs, legumes, nuts, seeds, and soy products.
- Limit saturated fats and trans fats, consuming less than 10% of calories per day from saturated fats.
- Limit added sugar or sweeteners so that less than 10% of calories comes from added sugars.
- Consume less than 2300 milligrams (mg) of sodium per day.
- Choose and prepare foods with little salt, and eat potassium-rich foods.
- Limit intake of alcohol to moderate use (i.e., one drink daily for women and two drinks daily for men).
- Practice food safety to prevent bacterial foodborne illness. Use food-safety principles of Clean, Separate, Cook, and Chill.

Data from US Department of Health and Human Services and US Department of Agriculture: *Dietary guidelines for Americans 2015-2020*, 8e, http://health.gov/dietaryguidelines/2015/guidelines. Accessed June 26, 2019.

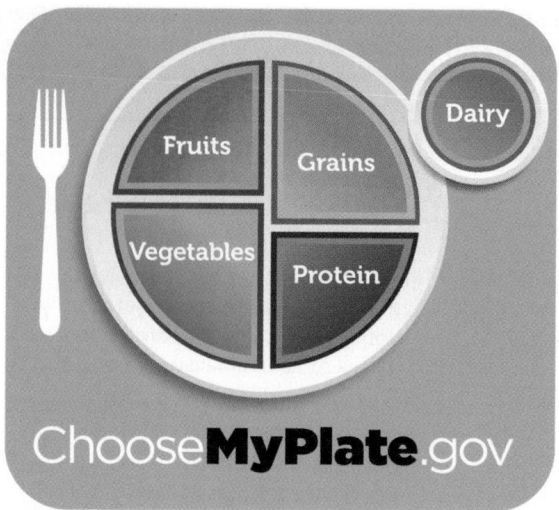

FIG. 45.2 ChooseMyPlate. (From US Department of Agriculture: ChooseMyPlate, 2011, http://www.choosemyplate.gov).

There are four components to the DRIs. The estimated average requirement (EAR) is the recommended amount of a nutrient that appears sufficient to maintain a specific body function for 50% of the population on the basis of age and gender. The recommended dietary allowance (RDA) represents the average needs of 98% of the population, not the exact needs of the individual. The adequate intake (AI) is the suggested intake for individuals based on observed or experimentally determined estimates of nutrient intakes and is used when there is not enough evidence to set the RDA. The tolerable upper intake level (UL) is the highest level that likely poses no risk of adverse health events. It is not a recommended level of intake (NIH, n.d.)

Food Guidelines. The US Department of Health and Human Services (USDHHS) and the US Department of Agriculture (USDA) published the *Dietary Guidelines for Americans 2015-2020* and provide average daily consumption guidelines for the five food groups: grains, vegetables, fruits, dairy products, and meats (Box 45.2). These guidelines are for Americans over the age of 2 years. As a nurse, consider the food preferences of patients from different cultural groups, vegetarians, and others when planning diets. The USDA developed the *ChooseMyPlate* program to replace the *My Food Pyramid* program. *ChooseMyPlate* provides a basic guide for making food choices for a healthy lifestyle (Fig. 45.2). It includes guidelines for balancing calories; decreasing portion size; increasing healthy foods; increasing water consumption; and decreasing fats, sodium, and sugars (USDA, 2017a).

Daily Values. The US Food and Drug Administration (FDA) created daily values for food labels in response to the 1990 Nutrition Labeling and Education Act (NLEA). The FDA first established two sets of reference values. The referenced daily intakes (RDIs) are the first set, comprising protein, vitamins, and minerals based on the RDA. The daily reference values (DRVs) make up the second set and consist of nutrients such as total fat, saturated fat, cholesterol, carbohydrates, fiber,

sodium, and potassium. Combined, both sets make up the daily values used on food labels. Daily values did not replace RDAs but provided a separate, more understandable format for the public. Daily values are based on percentages of a diet consisting of 2000 kcal/day for adults and children 4 years or older.

REFLECT NOW

In your geographic area, identify a population at risk for poor nutrition. What is the population, and what nutritional deficiencies do you believe they are most at risk for having and why?

NURSING KNOWLEDGE BASE

There are many sociological and psychological factors associated with eating and drinking in all societies. We celebrate holidays and events with food, bring it to those who are grieving, and use it for medicinal purposes. We incorporate food into family traditions and rituals and often associate food with eating behaviors. You need to understand patients' values, beliefs, and attitudes about food and how these values affect food purchase, preparation, and intake to affect eating patterns.

Nutritional requirements depend on many factors. Individual caloric and nutrient requirements vary by stage of development, body composition, activity levels, pregnancy and lactation, and the presence of disease. Registered dietitians (RDs) use predictive equations that take into account some of these factors to estimate patients' nutritional requirements.

Factors Influencing Nutrition

Environmental Factors. Environmental factors beyond the control of individuals contribute to the development of obesity. Obesity is an epidemic in the United States. Presently 68.7% of Americans are overweight or obese (CDC, 2019). Overweight is defined as having a BMI of 25 to 29, while obesity is defined as a BMI of 30 or greater (CDC, 2019). Obesity is often associated with a number of factors, such as sedentary lifestyle, overeating, and genetics (Giddens, 2017). Environmental factors can limit a person's likelihood of healthy eating and participation in exercise or other activities of healthy living. Lack of access to full-service grocery stores, high cost of healthy food, widespread availability of less healthy foods in fast-food restaurants, widespread advertising of less healthy food, and lack of access to safe places to play and exercise are environmental factors that contribute to obesity (Haung and Barnidge, 2016).

Developmental Needs

Infants Through School-Age. Rapid growth and high protein, vitamin, mineral, and energy requirements mark the developmental stage of infancy. The average birth weight of an American baby is 7 to 7½ lb. (3.2 to 3.4 kg). An infant usually doubles birth weight at 4 to 5 months and triples it at 1 year. Infants need an energy intake of approximately 90 to 110 kcal/kg of body weight per day, with premature infants needing 105 to 130 kcal/kg per day (Nix, 2017). Commercial formulas and human breast milk both provide approximately 20 kcal/oz. A full-term newborn is able to digest and absorb simple carbohydrates, proteins, and a moderate amount of emulsified fat. Infants need about 100 to 120 mL/kg/day of fluid because a large part of total body weight is water.

Breastfeeding. The American Academy of Pediatrics strongly supports breastfeeding for the first 6 months of life and breastfeeding with complementary foods from 6 to 12 months (AAP, 2017). Breastfeeding has multiple benefits for both infant and mother, including fewer food allergies and intolerances; fewer infant infections; easier digestion; convenience, availability, and freshness; temperature always correct; economical because it is less expensive than formula; and increased time for mother and infant interaction.

Formula. Infant formulas contain the approximate nutrient composition of human milk. Protein in the formula is typically whey, soy, cow's milk base, casein hydrolysate, or elemental amino acids. Infants with allergies or an intolerance to cow's milk should consume soy protein–based formulas instead (Nix, 2017).

Infants should not have regular cow's milk during the first year of life. It is too concentrated for an infant's kidneys to manage, increases the risk of milk-product allergies, and is a poor source of iron and vitamins C and E (Nix, 2017). Furthermore, children under 1 year of age should never ingest honey and corn syrup products because they are potential sources of the botulism toxin, which increases the risk of infant death.

Introduction to Solid Food. Breast milk or formula provides sufficient nutrition for the first 4 to 6 months of life. The development of fine-motor skills of the hand and fingers parallels an infant's interest in food and self-feeding. Iron-fortified cereals are typically the first semisolid food to be introduced. For infants 4 to 11 months, cereals are the most important nonmilk source of protein (Hockenberry et al., 2019).

Adding foods to an infant's diet depends on the infant's nutrient needs, physical readiness to handle different forms of foods, and the need to detect and control allergic reactions. Introducing foods that have a high incidence of causing allergic reactions such as wheat, egg white, nuts, citrus juice, and chocolate should happen later in the infant's life (Nix, 2017). In addition, caregivers should introduce new foods one at a time, approximately 4 to 7 days apart, to identify allergies. It is best to introduce new foods before milk or other foods to avoid satiety (Hockenberry et al., 2019).

The growth rate slows during toddler years (1 to 3 years). A toddler needs fewer kilocalories but an increased amount of protein in relation to body weight; consequently, appetite often decreases at 18 months of age. Toddlers exhibit strong food preferences and become picky eaters. Small, frequent meals consisting of breakfast, lunch, and dinner with three interspersed high nutrient–dense snacks help improve nutritional intake (Hockenberry et al., 2019). Calcium and phosphorus are important for healthy bone growth.

Toddlers who consume more than 24 ounces of milk daily in place of other foods sometimes develop milk anemia because milk is a poor source of iron. Toddlers need to drink whole milk until the age of 2 years to make sure that there is adequate intake of fatty acids necessary for brain and neurological development. Avoid certain foods such as hot dogs, hard candy, nuts, grapes, raw vegetables, and popcorn because they present a choking hazard. Dietary requirements for preschoolers (3 to 5 years) are similar to those for toddlers. They consume slightly more than toddlers, and nutrient density is more important than quantity.

School-age children, 6 to 12 years old, grow at a slower and steadier rate, with a gradual decline in energy requirements per unit of body weight. Despite better appetites and more varied food intake, you need to assess school-age children's diets carefully for adequate protein and vitamins A and C. They often fail to eat a proper breakfast and have unsupervised intake at school. Diets high in fat, sugar, and salt result from too-liberal intake of snack foods. Physical activity level decreases consistently, and consumption of high-calorie, readily available food increases, leading to an increase in childhood obesity (Haung and Barnidge, 2016).

In the past 10 years, obesity rates have reached a plateau in children and adolescents, although extreme obesity has increased (Ogden et al., 2016). A combination of factors contributes to the problem, including a diet rich in high-calorie foods, food advertising targeting children, inactivity, genetic predisposition, use of food as a coping mechanism for stress or boredom or as a reward or celebration, and family and socioeconomic factors (Hockenberry et al., 2019). Childhood obesity contributes to medical problems related to the cardiovascular system, endocrine system, and mental health. With the increase in obesity, the incidence of type 2 diabetes in children is also increasing. Prevention of childhood obesity is critical because of its long-term effects. Family education is an important component in decreasing the prevalence of this problem. Promote healthy food choices and eating in moderation along with increased physical activity.

Adolescents. During adolescence physiological age is a better guide to nutritional needs than chronological age. Energy needs increase to meet greater metabolic demands of growth. Daily requirement of protein also increases. Calcium is essential for the rapid bone growth of adolescence, and girls need a continuous source of iron to replace menstrual losses. Boys also need adequate iron for muscle development. Iodine supports increased thyroid activity, and the use of iodized table salt ensures availability. B-complex vitamins are necessary to support heightened metabolic activity.

Many factors other than nutritional needs influence the adolescent's diet, including concern about body image and appearance, desire for independence, eating at fast-food restaurants, peer pressure, and fad diets. Nutritional deficiencies often occur in adolescent girls because of dieting and use of oral contraceptives. An adolescent boy's diet is often inadequate in total kilocalories, protein, iron, folic acid, B vitamins, and iodine. Snacks provide approximately 25% of a teenager's total dietary intake. Fast food, particularly value-size or super-size meals, is common and adds extra salt, fat, and kilocalories. Skipping meals or eating meals with unhealthy choices of snacks contributes to nutrient deficiency and obesity (Hockenberry et al., 2019). Furthermore, research on public school lunch programs demonstrates that adolescents have higher BMIs than students enrolled in private school lunch programs (Bogart et al., 2016).

Fortified foods (nutrients added) are important sources of vitamins and minerals. Snack food from the dairy, fruit, and vegetable groups are good choices. To counter obesity, increasing physical activity is often more important than curbing intake. The onset of eating disorders such as anorexia nervosa or bulimia nervosa often occurs during adolescence. Recognition of eating disorders is essential for early intervention (Box 45.3).

BOX 45.3 Diagnostic Criteria for Eating Disorders

Anorexia Nervosa

- Restriction of energy intake relative to requirements, leading to a significantly low body weight in relation to age, sex, developmental trajectory, and physical health
- Intense fear of gaining weight or of becoming fat, or persistent behavior that interferes with weight gain, even though at a significantly low weight
- Disturbance in the way in which one's body weight, size, or shape is experienced; undue influence of body weight or shape on self-evaluation; or persistent lack of recognition of the seriousness of the current low body weight (e.g., the person claims to "feel fat" even when emaciated, believes that one area of the body is "too fat" even when obviously underweight)

Bulimia Nervosa

- Recurrent episodes of binge eating (rapid consumption of a large amount of food in a discrete period of time)
- A feeling of lack of control over eating behavior during eating binges
- Recurrent inappropriate compensatory behaviors to prevent weight gain, such as self-induced vomiting, use of laxatives or diuretics, strict dieting or fasting, or vigorous exercise
- Binge eating and inappropriate compensatory behaviors that both occur, on average, at least once a week for 3 months
- Self-evaluation unduly influenced by body shape and weight

Reprinted with permission from the *Diagnostic and Statistical Manual of Mental Disorders*, Fifth Edition, Text Revision (Copyright ©2013), American Psychiatric Association.

Sports and regular moderate-to-intense exercise necessitate dietary modification to meet increased energy needs for adolescents. Carbohydrates, both simple and complex, are the main source of energy, providing 55% to 60% of total daily kilocalories. Protein needs increase to 1 to 1.5 g/kg/day. Fat needs do not increase. Adequate hydration is very important. Adolescents need to ingest water before and after exercise to prevent dehydration, especially in hot, humid environments. Vitamin and mineral supplements are not required, but intake of iron-rich foods is required to prevent anemia.

Parents have more influence on adolescents' diets than they believe. Effective strategies include limiting the amount of unhealthy food choices kept at home; encouraging smart snacks such as fruits, vegetables, or string cheese; and enhancing the appearance and taste of healthy foods (Mayo Clinic, 2019). Some ways to promote healthy eating include making healthful food choices more convenient at home and at fast-food restaurants and discouraging adolescents from eating while watching television or using the computer.

Pregnancy occurring within 4 years of menarche places a mother and fetus at risk because of anatomical and physiological immaturity. Malnutrition at the time of conception increases risk to the adolescent and her fetus. Most teenage girls do not want to gain weight. Counseling related to nutritional needs of pregnancy is often difficult, and teens tolerate suggestions better than rigid directions. The diet of pregnant adolescents is often deficient in calcium, iron, and vitamins A and C. The American College of Obstetricians and Gynecologists recommends prenatal vitamin and mineral supplements.

Young and Middle Adults. There is a reduction in nutrient demands as the growth period ends. Mature adults need nutrients for energy, maintenance, and repair. Energy needs usually decline over the years. Obesity becomes a problem because of decreased physical exercise, dining out more often, and increased ability to afford more luxury foods. Adult women who use oral contraceptives often need extra vitamins. Iron and calcium intake continue to be important.

BOX 45.4 FOCUS ON OLDER ADULTS

Factors Affecting Nutritional Status

- Age-related gastrointestinal changes that affect digestion of food and maintenance of nutrition include changes in the teeth and gums, reduced saliva production, atrophy of oral mucosal epithelial cells, increased taste threshold, decreased thirst sensation, reduced gag reflex, and decreased esophageal and colonic peristalsis (Touhy and Jett, 2018).
- The presence of chronic illnesses (e.g., diabetes mellitus, end-stage renal disease, cancer) often affects nutrition intake.
- Adequate nutrition in older adults is affected by multiple causes, such as lifelong eating habits, culture, socialization, income, educational level, physical functional level to meet activities of daily living (ADLs), loss, dentition, and transportation (Touhy and Jett, 2018).
- Adverse effects of medications cause problems such as anorexia, gastrointestinal bleeding, xerostomia, early satiety, and impaired smell and taste perception (Burchum and Rosenthal, 2019).
- Cognitive impairments such as delirium, dementia, and depression affect ability to obtain, prepare, and eat healthy foods.

Pregnancy. Poor nutrition during pregnancy causes low birth weight in infants and decreases chances of survival. Generally, meeting the needs of a fetus is at the expense of the mother. However, if nutrient sources are unavailable, both suffer. The nutritional status of the mother at the time of conception is important. Significant aspects of fetal growth and development often occur before the mother suspects the pregnancy. The energy requirements of pregnancy relate to the mother's body weight and activity. The quality of nutrition during pregnancy is important, and food intake in the first trimester includes balanced parts of essential nutrients with emphasis on quality. Protein intake throughout pregnancy needs to increase to 60 g daily. Calcium intake is especially critical in the third trimester, when fetal bones mineralize. Providing iron supplements to meet the mother's increased blood volume, fetal blood storage, and blood loss during delivery is important.

Folic acid intake is particularly important for DNA synthesis and the growth of red blood cells. Inadequate intake can lead to fetal neural tube defects, anencephaly, or maternal megaloblastic anemia (Nix, 2017). Women of childbearing age need to consume 400 mcg of folic acid daily, increasing to 600 mcg daily during pregnancy. Prenatal care usually includes vitamin and mineral supplementation to ensure daily intakes; however, pregnant women should not take additional supplements beyond prescribed amounts.

Lactation. Women who are lactating need 500 kcal/day above the usual allowance because the production of milk increases energy requirements. Protein requirements during lactation are greater than those required during pregnancy. The need for calcium remains the same as during pregnancy. There is an increased need for vitamins A and C. Daily intake of water-soluble vitamins (B and C) is necessary to ensure adequate levels in breast milk. Fluid intake needs to be adequate but not excessive. Excretion of caffeine, alcohol, and drugs occurs through breast milk. Therefore mothers who are lactating need to avoid their ingestion.

Older Adults. Adults 65 years and older have a decreased need for energy because their metabolic rate slows with age. However, vitamin and mineral requirements remain unchanged from middle adulthood. Numerous factors influence the nutritional status of the older adult (Box 45.4). Age-related changes in appetite, taste, smell, and the digestive system affect nutrition (Touhy and Jett, 2018). For example, older adults often experience a decrease in taste cells that alters food flavor and may decrease intake. Multiple factors contribute to the risk of food insecurity in the older adult. Income is significant because living on a fixed income often reduces the amount of money available to buy food. Health is another important influence that affects a person's desire and ability to eat. Lack of transportation or ability to get to the grocery store because of mobility problems contributes to inability to purchase adequate and nutritious food. Often availability of nutritionally adequate and safe foods is limited or uncertain.

Maintaining good oral health is significant throughout adulthood, particularly as an individual ages. Difficulty in chewing, missing teeth, having teeth in poor condition, and oral pain result from poor oral health. These often contribute to malnutrition and dehydration in

older adults (Touhy and Jett, 2018). Poor oral hygiene and periodontal disease are potential risk factors for systemic diseases such as joint infections, ischemic stroke, cardiovascular disease, DM, and aspiration pneumonia (Touhy and Jett, 2018).

The older adult is often on a therapeutic diet; has difficulty eating because of physical symptoms, lack of teeth, or dentures; or is at risk for drug-nutrient interactions (Table 45.2). Caution older adults to avoid grapefruit and grapefruit juice because they alter absorption of many drugs. Thirst sensation diminishes, leading to inadequate fluid intake

TABLE 45.2 Sample of Drug-Nutrient Interactions[a]

Drug	Effect	Drug	Effect
Analgesic		Fluoxetine (Prozac) (selective serotonin reuptake inhibitors [SSRIs])	Taste alteration, anorexia
Acetaminophen	Decreased drug absorption with food; overdose associated with liver failure	**Antihypertensive**	
		Captopril (Capoten)	Taste alteration, anorexia
Aspirin	Absorbed directly through stomach; decreased drug absorption with food; decreased folic acid, vitamins C and K, and iron absorption	Hydralazine	Enhanced drug absorption with food, decreased vitamin B_6
		Labetalol (Normodyne)	Taste alteration (weight gain for all beta blockers)
Antacid		Methyldopa	Decreased vitamin B_{12}, folic acid, iron
Aluminum hydroxide	Decreased phosphate absorption	**Antiinflammatory**	
Sodium bicarbonate	Decreased folic acid absorption	All steroids	Increased appetite and weight, increased folic acid, decreased calcium (osteoporosis with long-term use); promotes gluconeogenesis of protein
Antiarrhythmic			
Amiodarone (Cordarone)	Taste alteration		
Digitalis	Anorexia, decreased renal clearance in older people		
		Antiparkinson	
Antibiotic		Levodopa (Dopar)	Taste alteration, decreased vitamin B_6 and drug absorption with food
Penicillin	Decreased drug absorption with food, taste alteration		
		Antipsychotic	
Cephalosporin	Decreased vitamin K	Chlorpromazine	Increased appetite
Rifampin (Rifadin)	Decreased vitamin B_6, niacin, vitamin D	Thiothixene	Decreased riboflavin, increased need
Tetracycline	Decreased drug absorption with milk and antacids; decreased nutrient absorption of calcium, riboflavin, vitamin C caused by binding	**Bronchodilator**	
		Albuterol sulfate	Appetite stimulant
		Theophylline	Anorexia
		Cholesterol Lowering	
Trimethoprim/ sulfamethoxazole	Decreased folic acid	Cholestyramine (Prevalite)	Decreased fat-soluble vitamins (A, D, E, K), vitamin B_{12}, iron
Anticoagulant		**Diuretic**	
Warfarin (Coumadin)	Acts as antagonist to vitamin K	Furosemide (Lasix)	Decreased drug absorption with food
		Spironolactone (Aldactone)	Increased drug absorption with food
Anticonvulsant		Thiazides	Decreased magnesium, zinc, and potassium
Carbamazepine (Tegretol)	Increased drug absorption with food	**Laxative**	
Phenytoin (Dilantin)	Decreased calcium absorption; decreased vitamins D and K and folic acid; taste alteration; decreased drug absorption with food	Mineral oil	Decreased absorption of fat-soluble vitamins (A, D, E, K), carotene
		Platelet Aggregate Inhibitor	
		Dipyridamole (Persantine)	Decreased drug absorption with food
Antidepressant		**Potassium Replacement**	
Amitriptyline	Appetite stimulant	Potassium chloride	Decreased vitamin B_{12}
Clomipramine (Anafranil)	Taste alteration, appetite stimulant	**Tranquilizer**	
		Benzodiazepines	Increased appetite

[a]Not intended to be an exhaustive or all-inclusive list. Always check pharmacology references before administering medications.
Data from Hermann J: *Nutrient and drug interactions,* http://pods.dasnr.okstate.edu/docushare/dsweb/Get/Document-2458/T-3120web.pdf. Accessed August 20, 2014; Burcham and Rosenthal: *Lehne's pharmacology for nursing care,* ed 9, St Louis, 2016, Elsevier.

or dehydration (see Chapter 42). Symptoms of dehydration in older adults include confusion; weakness; hot, dry skin; furrowed tongue; rapid pulse; and high urinary sodium. Some older adults avoid meats because of cost or because they are difficult to chew. Cream soups and meat-based vegetable soups are nutrient-dense sources of protein. Cheese, eggs, and peanut butter are also useful high-protein alternatives. Foods rich in calcium, such as dairy products, green leafy vegetables, soy, nuts, fish (canned sardines and salmon with bones), and fortified grains, help protect against osteoporosis (a decrease of bone mass density) (NOF, 2019). Screening and treatment are necessary for both older men and women. Vitamin D supplements are important for improving strength and balance, strengthening bone health, and preventing bone fractures and falls. The diet of older adults needs to contain choices from all food groups and often requires a vitamin and mineral supplement. MyPlate for Older Adults addresses the specific nutritional needs for older adults and encourages physical activity (USDA, 2017).

The USDHHS Administration on Aging (AOA) requires states to provide nutritional screening services to older adults who benefit from home-delivered or congregate meal services. This program requires meals to provide at least one-third of the DRI for an older adult and meet the Dietary Guidelines for Americans (American Dietetic Association, 2019). Homebound older adults with chronic illnesses have additional nutritional risks. They frequently live alone with little or no social or financial resources to help obtain or prepare nutritionally sound meals, contributing to the risk for food insecurity. Approximately 19% of older adults experience some degree of food insecurity resulting from low income or poverty (American Dietetic Association, 2019). Increased nutritional screening by nurses results in early recognition and treatment of nutritional deficiencies. Undernourishment of older adults often results in health problems that lead to admission to acute care hospitals or long-term care facilities.

Alternative Food Patterns

Long before the FDA issued recommended allowances and guidelines, many people followed special patterns of food intake on the basis of religion (Table 45.3), cultural background (Box 45.5), health beliefs, personal preference, or concern for the efficient use of land to produce food. Such special diets are not necessarily more or less nutritious than diets based on the MyPlate or other nutritional guidelines because good nutrition depends on a balanced intake of all required nutrients.

Vegetarian Diet. A common alternative dietary pattern is the vegetarian diet. Vegetarianism is the consumption of a diet consisting predominantly of plant foods. Some vegetarians are ovolactovegetarian (avoid meat, fish, and poultry but eat eggs and milk), lactovegetarians (drink milk but avoid eggs), or vegans (consume only plant foods). Through careful selection of foods, individuals following a vegetarian diet can meet recommendations for proteins and essential nutrients (Nix, 2017). Children who follow a vegetarian diet are especially at risk for protein and vitamin deficiencies, such as a lack of vitamin B_{12}. Careful planning helps to ensure a balanced, healthy diet.

CRITICAL THINKING

Successful critical thinking requires a synthesis of knowledge, experience, information gathered from patients, critical thinking attitudes, and intellectual and professional standards. Clinical judgments require you to anticipate information, analyze the data, and make decisions regarding your patient's care. During assessment consider all elements that build toward making an appropriate nursing diagnosis (Fig. 45.3).

Integrate knowledge from nursing and other disciplines, previous experiences, and information gathered from patients and families regarding customary food preferences and recent diet history. Use of professional standards such as the DRIs, the USDA MyPlate dietary guidelines, and *Healthy People 2020* objectives provide guidelines to assess and maintain patients' nutritional status. Other professional standards by the AHA (2018), the American Diabetes Association (ADA, 2019), the ACS (2019), and the American Society for Parenteral and Enteral Guidelines (2019) are available. These standards are evidence based and regularly updated for optimal patient care.

REFLECT NOW

What assessment findings in an adolescent child would be indicative of altered nutrition? What are risk factors that lead to altered nutritional status in this age-group?

TABLE 45.3 Religious Dietary Restrictions

Muslim	Christianity	Hinduism	Judaism	Church of Jesus Christ of Latter-Day Saints (Mormons)	Seventh-Day Adventists Church
Pork	Some faiths such as	All meats	Pork	Alcohol	Pork
Alcohol	Baptists have minimal or	Fish, shellfish	Predatory fowl	Tobacco	Shellfish
Caffeine	no alcohol	with some	Shellfish (eat only fish with scales)	Caffeine such as teas,	Fish
Ramadan fasting	Some meatless days may	restrictions	Rare meats	coffees, and sodas	Alcohol
sunrise to sunset	be observed during the	Alcohol	Blood (e.g., blood sausage)		Caffeine
for a month	calendar year, commonly		Mixing of milk or dairy products with		Vegetarian or ovolac-
Ritualized methods	during Lent		meat dishes		tovegetarian diets
of animal slaughter			Must adhere to kosher food prepara-		encouraged
required for meat			tion methods		
ingestion			24 hr of fasting on Yom Kippur, a day		
			of atonement		
			No leavened bread eaten during Pass-		
			over (8 days)		
			No cooking on the Sabbath from sun-		
			down Friday to sundown Saturday		

⊕ BOX 45.5 CULTURAL ASPECTS OF CARE

Nutrition

Food patterns developed as a child, habits, and culture interact to influence food intake. Culture also influences the meaning of food not related to nutrition. Eating is associated with sentiments and feelings such as "good" and "bad." For example, children are often rewarded for "being good" with a treat such as candy. They then associate candy with "being good." Food frequently enhances interpersonal relationships and demonstrates love and caring.

Sometimes certain ethnic groups develop genetically related conditions. For example, lactose intolerance, a deficiency of the intestinal enzyme lactase, can be found among Asian-Pacific, African and African American, Native American, Mexican American, Middle Eastern, and Caucasians. Lactose intolerance affects nutrient absorption. Calcium deficiency often results, causing decreased bone mass density.

The theory of hot and cold foods predominates in many cultures. The origin appears to be from Hippocratic beliefs concerning health and the four humors. Arabs were keepers of this knowledge during the Dark Ages and later influenced the Spanish to adopt this belief system in the later Middle Ages. The foundation of the theory is keeping harmony with nature by balancing "cold," "hot," "wet," and "dry." Some cultures believe that hot is warmth, strength, and reassurance, whereas cold is menacing and weak. Classification has nothing to do with spiciness but is a symbolic representation of temperature (Giger, 2016). Different cultures also have beliefs about food and special dishes that should be eaten when sick (e.g., chicken soup during illness).

Implications for Patient-Centered Care
- Ask patient or family caregiver to identify the meaning that types of food have for each patient.
- Lactose and other food intolerances unique to specific cultures require diet adaptation to meet nutrient, mineral, and vitamin daily intake requirements.
- When patients use hot and cold foods as part of their cultural health practices, dietary modifications are necessary. Hot foods include rice, grain cereals, alcohol, beef, lamb, chili peppers, chocolate, cheese, temperate zone fruits, eggs, peas, goat's milk, cornhusks, oils, onions, pork, radishes, and tamales. By contrast, cold foods are beans, citrus fruits, tropical fruits, dairy products, most vegetables, honey, raisins, chicken, fish, and goat.
- Ask patient or family caregiver if there are:
  - Specific conditions such as menstruation, cancer, pneumonia, earache, colds, paralysis, headache, or rheumatism, which are cold illnesses and require hot foods.
  - Other conditions such as pregnancy, fever, infections, diarrhea, rashes, ulcers, liver problems, constipation, kidney problems, or sore throats, which are hot conditions and require cold foods.

❖ NURSING PROCESS

Apply the nursing process and use a critical thinking approach in your care of patients. The nursing process provides a clinical decision-making approach for you to develop and implement an individualized plan of care.

◆ Assessment

During the assessment process thoroughly assess each patient and critically analyze findings to ensure that you make patient-centered clinical decisions required for safe nursing care. Early recognition of patients who are malnourished or at risk has a strong positive influence on both short- and long-term health outcomes. Studies demonstrate a link between malnutrition in adult hospitalized patients and readmission rates, higher mortality rates, and increased cost (Reed Mangels, 2018). Patients who are malnourished on admission are at greater risk of significant complications such as arrhythmia, skin breakdown, sepsis, or hemorrhage during hospitalization.

Through the Patient's Eyes. Close contact with patients and their families enables you to observe physical status, food intake, food preferences, weight changes, and cultural practices in eating. Always ask patients about their food preferences, values regarding nutrition, and expectations from nutritional therapy. For example, does a patient want to learn about a diet? In attempting to affect eating patterns, you need to understand patients' values, beliefs, and attitudes about food. Assess family traditions and rituals related to food, cultural values and beliefs, and nutritional needs. Determine how these factors affect food purchase, preparation, and intake.

Screening. Assess patients' nutritional status by using the nursing history to gather information about factors that usually influence nutrition. You are in an excellent position to recognize signs of poor nutrition and take steps to initiate change. Nutrition screening is an essential part of an initial assessment. Screening a patient is a quick method of identifying malnutrition or risk of malnutrition using simple tools (McEvilly, 2017). Nutrition screening tools gather data on the current condition and typically include objective measures such as height, weight, weight change, primary diagnosis, and the presence of other co-morbidities (McEvilly, 2017). Combine multiple objective measures with subjective measures related to nutrition to adequately screen for nutritional problems. Identification of risk factors such as unintentional weight loss, presence of a modified diet, or the presence of altered nutritional symptoms (i.e., nausea, vomiting, diarrhea, and constipation) requires nutritional consultation.

Several standardized nutritional screening tools are available for use in outpatient and inpatient settings. The Subjective Global Assessment (SGA) uses the patient history, weight, and physical assessment data to assess nutritional status (Wittenaar and Ottery, 2017). The SGA is a simple, inexpensive technique that is able to predict nutrition-related complications. The Mini Nutritional Assessment (MNA) (Fig. 45.4) screens older adults in home care programs, nursing homes, and hospitals. The tool has 18 items divided into screening and assessment. If a patient scores 11 or less on the screening part, the health care provider completes the assessment part. A total score of less than 17 indicates protein-energy malnutrition (Agarwalla et al., 2015). Malnutrition screening tools (MSTs) are an effective way to measure nutritional problems for patients in a variety of health care settings.

Assess patients for malnutrition when they have conditions that interfere with their ability to ingest, digest, or absorb adequate nutrients. Use standardized tools to assess nutritional risks when possible. Congenital anomalies and surgical revisions of the GI tract interfere with normal function. Patients receiving only an IV infusion of 5% or 10% dextrose are at risk for nutritional deficiencies. Chronic diseases or increased metabolic requirements are risk factors for development of nutritional problems. Infants and older adults are at greatest risk.

Anthropometry. Anthropometry is a systematic method of measuring the size and makeup of the body. Nurses obtain height and weight for each patient on hospital admission or entry into any health care setting. If you are unable to measure height with the patient standing, position him or her lying flat in bed as straight as possible with arms folded on the chest and measure him or her lengthwise. Serial measures of weight over time provide more useful information than one

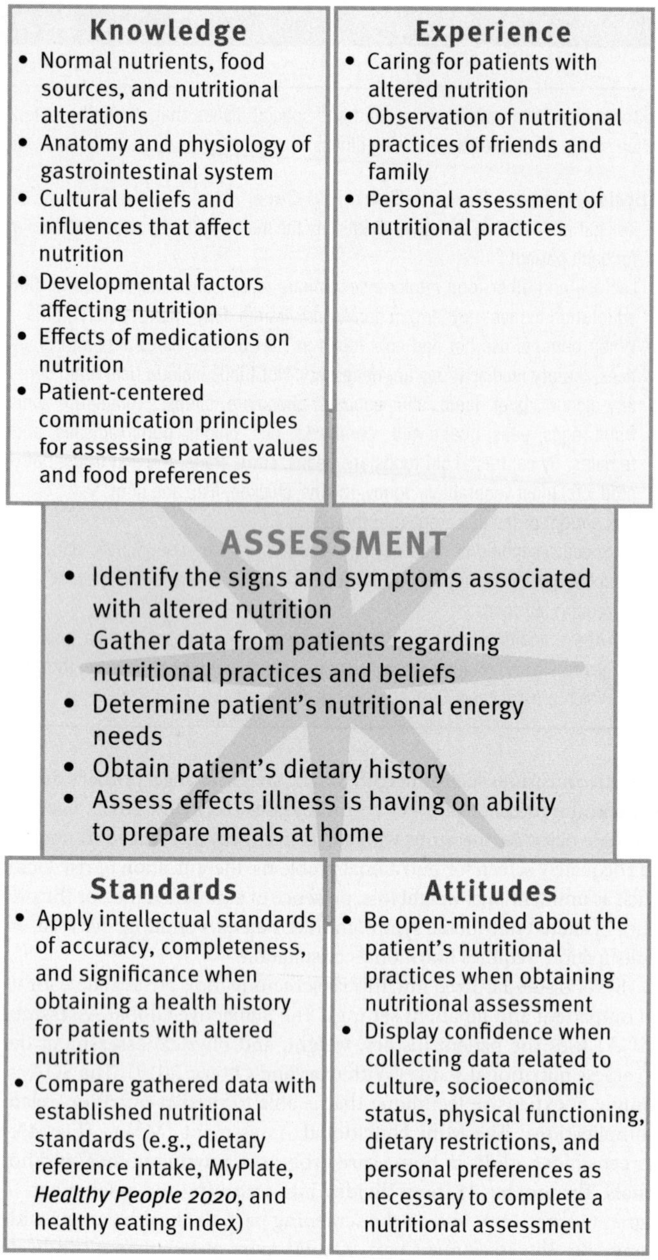

Knowledge

- Normal nutrients, food sources, and nutritional alterations
- Anatomy and physiology of gastrointestinal system
- Cultural beliefs and influences that affect nutrition
- Developmental factors affecting nutrition
- Effects of medications on nutrition
- Patient-centered communication principles for assessing patient values and food preferences

Experience

- Caring for patients with altered nutrition
- Observation of nutritional practices of friends and family
- Personal assessment of nutritional practices

ASSESSMENT

- Identify the signs and symptoms associated with altered nutrition
- Gather data from patients regarding nutritional practices and beliefs
- Determine patient's nutritional energy needs
- Obtain patient's dietary history
- Assess effects illness is having on ability to prepare meals at home

Standards

- Apply intellectual standards of accuracy, completeness, and significance when obtaining a health history for patients with altered nutrition
- Compare gathered data with established nutritional standards (e.g., dietary reference intake, MyPlate, *Healthy People 2020*, and healthy eating index)

Attitudes

- Be open-minded about the patient's nutritional practices when obtaining nutritional assessment
- Display confidence when collecting data related to culture, socioeconomic status, physical functioning, dietary restrictions, and personal preferences as necessary to complete a nutritional assessment

FIG. 45.3 Critical thinking model for nutrition assessment.

measurement. Weigh the patient at the same time each day, on the same scale, and with the same type of clothing or linen. Document the patient's actual weight and compare height and weight with standards for height-weight relationships. An **ideal body weight (IBW)** provides an estimate of what a person should weigh.

Rapid weight gain or loss is important to note because it usually reflects fluid shifts. One pint or 500 mL of fluid equals 1 lb (0.45 kg). For example, for a patient with renal failure, a weight increase of 2 lb (0.90 kg) in 24 hours is significant because it usually indicates that the patient has retained 1 L (1000 mL) of fluid.

Other anthropometric measurements often obtained by RDs help identify nutritional problems. These include the ratio of height-to-wrist circumference, mid–upper arm circumference (MAC), triceps skinfold (TSF), and mid–upper arm muscle circumference (MAMC). An RD compares values for MAC, TSF, and MAMC to standards and calculates them as a percentage of the standard. Changes in values for an individual over weeks to months are of greater significance than isolated measurements (Nix, 2017).

Body mass index (BMI) measures weight corrected for height and serves as an alternative to traditional height-weight relationships. Calculate BMI by dividing a patient's weight in kilograms by height in meters squared: weight (kg) divided by height^2 (m^2). For example, a patient who weighs 165 lb (75 kg) and is 1.8 m (5 feet, 9 inches) tall has a BMI of 23.15 (75 ÷ 1.8^2 = 23.15). The website for the National Heart, Lung, and Blood Institute (https://www.nhlbi.nih.gov/health/educational/lose_wt/BMI/bmicalc.htm) provides an easy way to calculate BMI. A patient is overweight if his or her BMI is 25 to 30. Obesity, defined by a BMI of greater than 30, places a patient at higher medical risk of coronary heart disease, some cancers, DM, and hypertension.

Laboratory and Biochemical Tests. No single laboratory or biochemical test is diagnostic for malnutrition. Factors that frequently alter test results include fluid balance, liver function, kidney function, and the presence of disease. Common laboratory tests used to study nutritional status include measures of plasma proteins such as albumin, transferrin, prealbumin, retinol-binding protein, total iron-binding capacity, and hemoglobin. After feeding, the response time for changes in these proteins ranges from hours to weeks. The metabolic half-life of albumin is 21 days, transferrin is 8 days, prealbumin is 2 days, and retinol-binding protein is 12 hours. Use this information to determine the most effective measure of plasma proteins for your patients. Factors that affect serum albumin levels include hydration; hemorrhage; renal or hepatic disease; large amounts of drainage from wounds, drains, burns, or the GI tract; steroid administration; exogenous albumin infusions; age; and trauma, burns, stress, or surgery. Albumin level is a better indicator for chronic illnesses, whereas prealbumin level is preferred for acute conditions (Bharadwaj et al., 2016).

Nitrogen balance is important in determining serum protein status (see discussion of protein in this chapter). Calculate nitrogen balance by dividing 6.25 into the total grams of protein ingested in a day (24 hours). Use laboratory analysis of a 24-hour urine urea nitrogen (UUN) to determine nitrogen output. For patients with diarrhea or fistula drainage, estimate a further addition of 2 to 4 g of nitrogen output. Calculate nitrogen balance by subtracting the nitrogen output from the nitrogen intake. A positive 2- to 3-g nitrogen balance is necessary for anabolism. By contrast, negative nitrogen balance is present when catabolic states exist.

Diet History and Health History. In addition to the general nursing history, use data from a more specific diet history to assess a patient's actual or potential nutritional needs. Box 45.6 lists some specific assessment questions to ask in the diet history. The diet history focuses on a patient's habitual intake of foods and liquids and includes information about preferences, allergies, and other relevant areas such as the patient's ability to obtain food. Gather information about the patient's illness/activity level to determine energy needs and compare food intake. Your nursing assessment of nutrition includes health status; age; cultural background (see Box 45.5); religious food patterns (see Table 45.3); socioeconomic status; personal food preferences; psychological factors; use of alcohol or illegal drugs; use of vitamin, mineral, or herbal supplements; prescription or over-the-counter (OTC) drugs (see Table 45.2); and the patient's general nutrition knowledge.

In an outpatient setting, have a patient keep a 3- to 7-day food diary. This allows you to calculate nutritional intake and to compare it with DRI to see whether the patient's dietary habits are adequate. Use food questionnaires to establish patterns over time. In a health care setting nurses collaborate with RDs to complete calorie counts for patients.

Physical Examination. The physical examination is one of the most important aspects of a nutritional assessment. Because improper

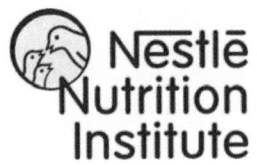

Nestlé Nutrition Institute

Mini Nutritional Assessment
MNA®

Last name: _____   First name: _____

Sex: _____   Age: _____   Weight, kg: _____   Height, cm: _____   Date: _____

Complete the screen by filling in the boxes with the appropriate numbers. Total the numbers for the final screening score.

Screening

A Has food intake declined over the past 3 months due to loss of appetite, digestive problems, chewing or swallowing difficulties?
0 = severe decrease in food intake
1 = moderate decrease in food intake
2 = no decrease in food intake   ☐

B Weight loss during the last 3 months
0 = weight loss greater than 3 kg (6.6 lbs)
1 = does not know
2 = weight loss between 1 and 3 kg (2.2 and 6.6 lbs)
3 = no weight loss   ☐

C Mobility
0 = bed or chair bound
1 = able to get out of bed / chair but does not go out
2 = goes out   ☐

D Has suffered psychological stress or acute disease in the past 3 months?
0 = yes   2 = no   ☐

E Neuropsychological problems
0 = severe dementia or depression
1 = mild dementia
2 = no psychological problems   ☐

F1 Body Mass Index (BMI) (weight in kg) / (height in m^2)
0 = BMI less than 19
1 = BMI 19 to less than 21
2 = BMI 21 to less than 23
3 = BMI 23 or greater   ☐

IF BMI IS NOT AVAILABLE, REPLACE QUESTION F1 WITH QUESTION F2.
DO NOT ANSWER QUESTION F2 IF QUESTION F1 IS ALREADY COMPLETED.

F2 Calf circumference (CC) in cm
0 = CC less than 31
3 = CC 31 or greater   ☐

Screening score   ☐☐
(max. 14 points)

12-14 points: Normal nutritional status
8-11 points: At risk of malnutrition
0-7 points: Malnourished

Ref.   Vellas B, Villars H, Abellan G, et al. *Overview of the MNA® - Its History and Challenges.* J Nutr Health Aging 2006;10:456-465.

Rubenstein LZ, Harker JO, Salva A, Guigoz Y, Vellas B. *Screening for Undernutrition in Geriatric Practice: Developing the Short-Form Mini Nutritional Assessment (MNA-SF).* J. Geront 2001;56A: M366-377.

Guigoz Y. *The Mini-Nutritional Assessment (MNA®) Review of the Literature - What does it tell us?* J Nutr Health Aging 2006; 10:466-487.

Kaiser MJ, Bauer JM, Ramsch C, et al. *Validation of the Mini Nutritional Assessment Short-Form (MNA®-SF): A practical tool for identification of nutritional status.* J Nutr Health Aging 2009; 13:782-788.

® Société des Produits Nestlé, S.A., Vevey, Switzerland, Trademark Owners

© Nestlé, 1994, Revision 2009. N67200 12/99 10M

For more information: www.mna-elderly.com

FIG. 45.4 Mini Nutritional Assessment (MNA). (Copyright ©Nestlé, 1994, Revision 2009. N67200 12/99 10M.)

BOX 45.6 Nursing Assessment Questions

Dietary Intake and Food Preferences
- What type of food do you like?
- How many meals a day do you eat?
- What times do you normally eat meals and snacks?
- What portion sizes do you eat at each meal?
- Are you on a special diet because of a medical problem?
- Tell me about your dietary religious or cultural food preferences.
- Who prepares the food at home?
- Who purchases the food?
- How do you cook your food (e.g., fried, broiled, baked, grilled)?

Unpleasant Symptoms
- Which foods cause indigestion, gas, or heartburn?
- How often does this occur?
- What relieves the symptoms?

Allergies
- Are you allergic to any foods?
- Which types of problems do you have with these foods?
- How are these food allergies treated (e.g., EpiPen, oral antihistamines)?

Taste, Chewing, and Swallowing
- Have you noticed any changes in taste?
- Did these changes occur with medications or following an illness?
- Do you wear dentures? Are the dentures comfortable?
- Do you have any mouth pain or sores (e.g., cold sore, canker sores)?
- Do you have difficulty swallowing?
- Do you cough or gag when you swallow?

Appetite and Weight
- Tell me about any recent change in appetite.
- Tell me about any recent change in your weight.
- Was this change anticipated (e.g., were you on a weight-reduction diet)?

Use of Medications
- Which medications do you take?
- Do you take any over-the-counter medications that your doctor does not prescribe?
- Do you take any nutritional or herbal supplements?

TABLE 45.4 Physical Signs of Nutritional Status

Body Area	Indicators of Malnutrition
General appearance	Easily fatigued, no energy, falls asleep easily; looks tired, apathetic, cachectic
Weight	Overweight, obese, or underweight (special concern for underweight); unplanned weight loss over period of time
Posture	Poor posture, sagging shoulders, sunken chest, humped back
Muscles	Flaccid, weak, poor tone, tender; "wasted" appearance; impaired mobility
Mental status	Inattentive, irritable, confused
Neurological function	Burning and tingling of hands and feet (paresthesia), loss of position and vibratory sense, decrease or loss of ankle and knee reflexes
Gastrointestinal function	Anorexia, indigestion, constipation or diarrhea, symptoms of malabsorption, liver or spleen enlargement, abdominal distention
Cardiovascular function	Tachycardia, abnormal rhythm, elevated blood pressure
Hair	Stringy, dull, brittle, dry, thin and sparse, depigmented
Skin (general)	Rough, dry, scaly, pale, pigmented, irritated, bruises, petechiae
Face and neck	Swollen, skin dark over cheeks and under eyes
Lips	Dry, scaly, swollen; redness and swelling at the corners of the mouth (cheilosis); angular lesions at corners of mouth, fissures, or scars (stomatitis)
Mouth, oral mucous membranes	Swollen, deep red oral mucous membranes; oral lesions
Gums	Spongy, bleed easily, inflamed, receding
Tongue	Swelling, scarlet and raw, magenta color, beefy (glossitis)
Teeth	Missing teeth, broken teeth
Eyes	Eye membranes pale (pale conjunctivae), redness of membrane (conjunctival injection), dryness or infection
Nails	Spoon-shaped (koilonychia), brittle, ridged
Legs and feet	Edema, tender calf, tingling, weakness, lesions
Skeleton	Bowlegs, knock-knees, chest deformity at diaphragm, beaded ribs, prominent scapulas

Data from Jelliffe DB: The assessment of the nutritional status of the community, WHO Monograph No. 53, Geneva, 1966; Clinical assessment of nutritional status, *Am J Public Health* 63(11 Suppl):18, 1973, http://ajph.aphapublications.org/doi/pdf/10.2105/AJPH.63.11_Suppl.18; and Williams SR: Nutritional assessment and guidance in prenatal care. In Worthington-Roberts BS, Williams SR: *Nutrition in pregnancy and lactation*, ed 5, New York, 1993, McGraw-Hill.

nutrition affects all body systems, observe for malnutrition during physical assessment (see Chapter 30). Complete the general physical assessment of body systems and recheck relevant areas to evaluate a patient's nutritional status. The clinical signs of nutritional status (Table 45.4) serve as guidelines for observation during physical assessment.

Dysphagia. Dysphagia refers to difficulty swallowing. There are a variety of causes and complications of dysphagia (Box 45.7). Complications include aspiration pneumonia, dehydration, decreased nutritional status, and weight loss. Dysphagia leads to disability or decreased functional status, increased length of stay and health care costs, increased likelihood of discharge to institutionalized care, and increased mortality (Yang et al., 2017).

Be aware of warning signs for dysphagia. They include cough during eating; change in voice tone or quality after swallowing; abnormal movements of the mouth, tongue, or lips; and slow, weak, imprecise, or uncoordinated speech. Abnormal gag, delayed swallowing, incomplete oral clearance or pocketing, regurgitation, pharyngeal pooling, delayed or absent trigger of swallow, and inability to speak consistently are other signs of dysphagia. Patients with dysphagia often do not show overt signs such as coughing when food enters the airway. *Silent aspiration* is aspiration that occurs in patients with neurological problems that leads to decreased sensation. It often occurs without a cough, and symptoms (for example, adventitious breath sounds, slight fever) usually do not appear for 24 hours. Silent aspiration is common in patients with dysphagia following stroke (Yang et al., 2017).

Dysphagia often leads to an inadequate amount of food intake, which results in malnutrition. Frequently patients with dysphagia

BOX 45.7 Causes of Dysphagia

Myogenic
- Myasthenia gravis
- Aging
- Muscular dystrophy
- Polymyositis

Neurogenic
- Stroke
- Cerebral palsy
- Guillain-Barré syndrome
- Multiple sclerosis
- Amyotrophic lateral sclerosis (Lou Gehrig disease)
- Diabetic neuropathy
- Parkinson's disease

Obstructive
- Benign peptic stricture
- Lower esophageal ring
- Candidiasis
- Head and neck cancer
- Inflammatory masses
- Trauma/surgical resection
- Anterior mediastinal masses
- Cervical spondylosis

Other
- Gastrointestinal or esophageal resection
- Rheumatological disorders
- Connective tissue disorders
- Vagotomy

BOX 45.8 Nursing Diagnostic Process

Impaired Low Nutrition Intake

Assessment Activities	Assessment Findings
Body mass index (BMI)	Body mass index (BMI) = 17
Obtain weight	68-year-old woman
	24-lb (10.8-kg) weight loss
	Weight is 20% below her ideal body weight
Obtain 24-hour food and fluid history	Lack of satiety
	Lack of interest in food
	Fluid intake is juice and coffee
	Eats sandwich in afternoon
Physical assessment	Poor muscle tone
	Fatigue
	Hair loss
	Dry, scaly skin
	Pale conjunctiva and mucous membranes
Medication	Takes sertraline for depression
Social	Husband died 6 months ago
	Has quit attending monthly quilting club
	Started counseling 3 months ago

become frustrated with eating and show changes in skinfold thickness and albumin. During the rehabilitation period patients experience longer adjustment periods regarding new dietary restrictions. Furthermore, malnutrition significantly slows swallowing recovery and may increase mortality (Bharadwaj et al., 2016).

Dysphagia screening quickly identifies problems with swallowing and helps you initiate referrals for more in-depth assessment by an RD or a speech-language pathologist (SLP) (see Skill 45.1). Early and ongoing assessment of patients with dysphagia using a valid dysphagia-screening tool increases quality of care and decreases incidence of aspiration pneumonia. Dysphagia screening includes medical record review; observation of a patient at a meal for change in voice quality, posture, and head control; percentage of meal consumed; eating time; drooling or leakage of liquids and solids; cough during/after a swallow; facial or tongue weakness; palatal movement; difficulty with secretions; pocketing; choking; and a spontaneous dry cough. Several validated screening tools are available such as the Bedside Swallowing Assessment, Burke Dysphagia Screening Test, Acute Stroke Dysphagia Screen, and Standardized Swallowing Assessment (Dong et al., 2016). The Acute Stroke Dysphagia Screen is an easily administered and reliable tool for health care professionals who are not speech-language pathologists (SLPs). Screening for and treatment of dysphagia requires an interprofessional team approach of nurses, RDs, health care providers, and SLPs (ASHA 019).

REFLECT NOW

Consider a patient you recently cared for during a clinical experience and who had risks for nutritional alterations. What assessments did you make of his or her nutritional status? What are some risk factors that potentially put your patient at risk for malnutrition?

◆ Nursing Diagnosis

Cluster all assessment data to identify appropriate nursing diagnoses (Box 45.8). A nutritional problem occurs when overall intake is significantly decreased or increased or when one or more nutrients are not ingested, completely digested, or completely absorbed. When identifying a negative or problem-focused nursing diagnosis, you select the appropriate related factors (e.g., inability to digest food or reduced daily activity). Related factors need to be accurate, so you select the right

interventions. For example, *Impaired Low Nutritional Intake* related to economic disadvantage will require very different interventions than *Impaired Low Nutritional Intake* related to an inability to ingest food.

A patient will have a risk nursing diagnosis when assessment reveals risk factors. For example, *Risk for Nutritional Excess* can be identified by the presence of risk factors such as excessive alcohol consumption or high frequency of eating restaurant food and adult BMI approaching 25 kg/m². Be specific so that you can direct interventions toward risk factors.

Assessment findings may also point to a health promotion diagnosis such as *Health Seeking Behavior*. The following are examples of nursing diagnoses applicable to nutritional problems:

- *Risk for Aspiration*
- *Overweight*
- *Impaired Low Nutritional Intake*
- *Impaired Self Feeding*
- *Impaired Swallowing*

In addition, there are clinical situations in which patients have multiple related nursing diagnoses. The concept map in Fig. 45.5 shows the relationship of nursing diagnoses for Mrs. Cooper.

◆ Planning

Planning to maintain patients' optimal nutritional status requires a higher level of care than simply correcting nutritional problems. Often there is a need for patients to make long-term changes for nutrition to improve. Synthesis of patient information from multiple sources is necessary to create an individualized approach of care that is relevant to a patient's needs and situation (Fig. 45.6). Apply critical thinking to ensure that you consider all data sources in developing a patient's plan of care. The accurate identification of nursing diagnoses related to patients' nutritional problems results in a care plan that is relevant and appropriate (see the Nursing Care Plan). Referring to professional standards for nutrition is especially important during this step, because scientific findings support current published standards.

Goals and Outcomes. Goals and outcomes of care reflect a patient's physiological, therapeutic, and individualized needs. Nutritional education and counseling are important to prevent disease and promote health. Plan to educate your patients about any therapeutic

Impaired Low Nutrition Intake

ASSESSMENT

A nurse practitioner (NP) at a senior center is seeing Mrs. Cooper, who is 68 years old and has a history of heart failure. Recently Mrs. Cooper experienced an unexpected 15% weight loss. Three months ago, she started taking sertraline (Zoloft) for depression related to the loss of her husband earlier in the year. She no longer participates in her monthly quilting club. Mrs. Cooper started counseling 3 months ago for help with her grief and depression. When the NP inquires about her financial situation, Mrs. Cooper responds by saying that it is tight living on a small pension and Social Security but that she is able to manage.

Assessment Activities	*Assessment Findings[a]*
Ask Mrs. Cooper about her food intake during the past 2 days.	She responds that she drinks some juice in the morning and two or three cups of coffee. In addition, she often has a sandwich in the late afternoon. She often **skips dinner.** "**I'm just not interested in food.** It has no taste."
Ask Mrs. Cooper about social interaction.	Mrs. Cooper **complains of loneliness** and says that she does not get out much. Her friends at church call her to come back to meetings, but she is just not ready. She says that she **tires easily** and no longer attends the monthly meetings of her quilt club.
Weigh patient and assess posture.	Her **weight is 20% below her ideal body weight (IBW)** and her body mass index (BMI) is 17. This weight loss has happened over the past 6 months, and she has **lost 24 lb.** Stooped posture
Observe Mrs. Cooper for signs of poor nutrition.	**Hair loss** **Sore oral mucous membranes** **Pale mucous membranes**

[a]**Assessment findings** are shown in bold type.

NURSING DIAGNOSIS: Impaired Low Nutrition Intake related to a decreased ability to ingest food as a result of depression and insufficient intake

---

PLANNING
Goals

Mrs. Cooper will progressively gain weight.

Expected Outcomes (NOC)[b]
Weight Gain Behavior

Mrs. Cooper gains 1 to 2 lb per month until reaching a goal of 130 lb.

Physical assessment findings are within normal limits.

[b]Outcome classification labels from Moorhead S, et al: *Nursing Outcomes Classification (NOC)*, ed 6, St Louis, 2018, Elsevier.

INTERVENTIONS (NIC)[c] *Nutritional Counseling*	RATIONALE
Coordinate plan of care with health care provider, psychologist, Mrs. Cooper, and registered dietitian.	Successful nutrition care planning is a multidisciplinary approach throughout the continuum of care (Phelps et al., 2017).
Individualize menu plans according to Mrs. Cooper's preferences.	Incorporating her food preferences into the meal plans encourages the patient to eat (Phelps et al., 2017).
Teach Mrs. Cooper about MyPlate for Older Adults.	MyPlate for Older Adults is adapted to meet the nutritional requirements for older adults (USDA, 2017a).
Nutritional Management	
Encourage Mrs. Cooper to eat small nutritious meals and snacks and to increase dietary intake to help offset anorexia secondary to sertraline.	Sertraline is a selective serotonin reuptake inhibitor (SSRI) antidepressant medication that causes diminished taste and anorexia. Frequent small nutritious meals and snacks help to reduce anorexia-associated weight loss.
Encourage fluid intake to eight 8-oz glasses daily.	Older adults need eight 8-oz (240 mL) glasses per day of fluid from beverage and food sources. Concentrating intake in the morning and early afternoon is acceptable to prevent nocturia (Meiner and Yeager, 2019).
Encourage fiber intake.	Prevents constipation and enhances appetite.
Encourage Mrs. Cooper to eat lunch at the senior center 5 times per week.	Eating with others encourages good nutrition and promotes socialization with peers (American Dietetic Association, 2019; Nix, 2017).

[c]Intervention classification labels from Butcher HK, et al: *Nursing Interventions Classification (NIC)*, ed 7, St Louis, 2018, Elsevier.

EVALUATION

Evaluation Activity	*Patient Response/Finding*	*Outcome Status*
Monitor Mrs. Cooper monthly for weight gain, anemia, serum albumin level, and transferrin levels.	After 2 weeks Mrs. Cooper has gained 3 lb, and her hemoglobin B level is 12.	Mrs. Cooper is making progress with weight gain; her hemoglobin level still reflects mild anemia.
Observe Mrs. Cooper's physical appearance.	At 2 weeks her mucous membranes are less pale, and her hair appears to be in better condition and styled.	Mrs. Cooper has improved physical parameters of nutrition; still needs follow-up.
Ask Mrs. Cooper about appetite and energy level.	Mrs. Cooper responds that on days that she eats at the senior center her appetite seems better and she "wants to do more things." She notes that weekends are very lonely.	Weekday support for nutritional status appears effective; need to increase patient's activity status and nutritional intake during weekends.

CONCEPT MAP

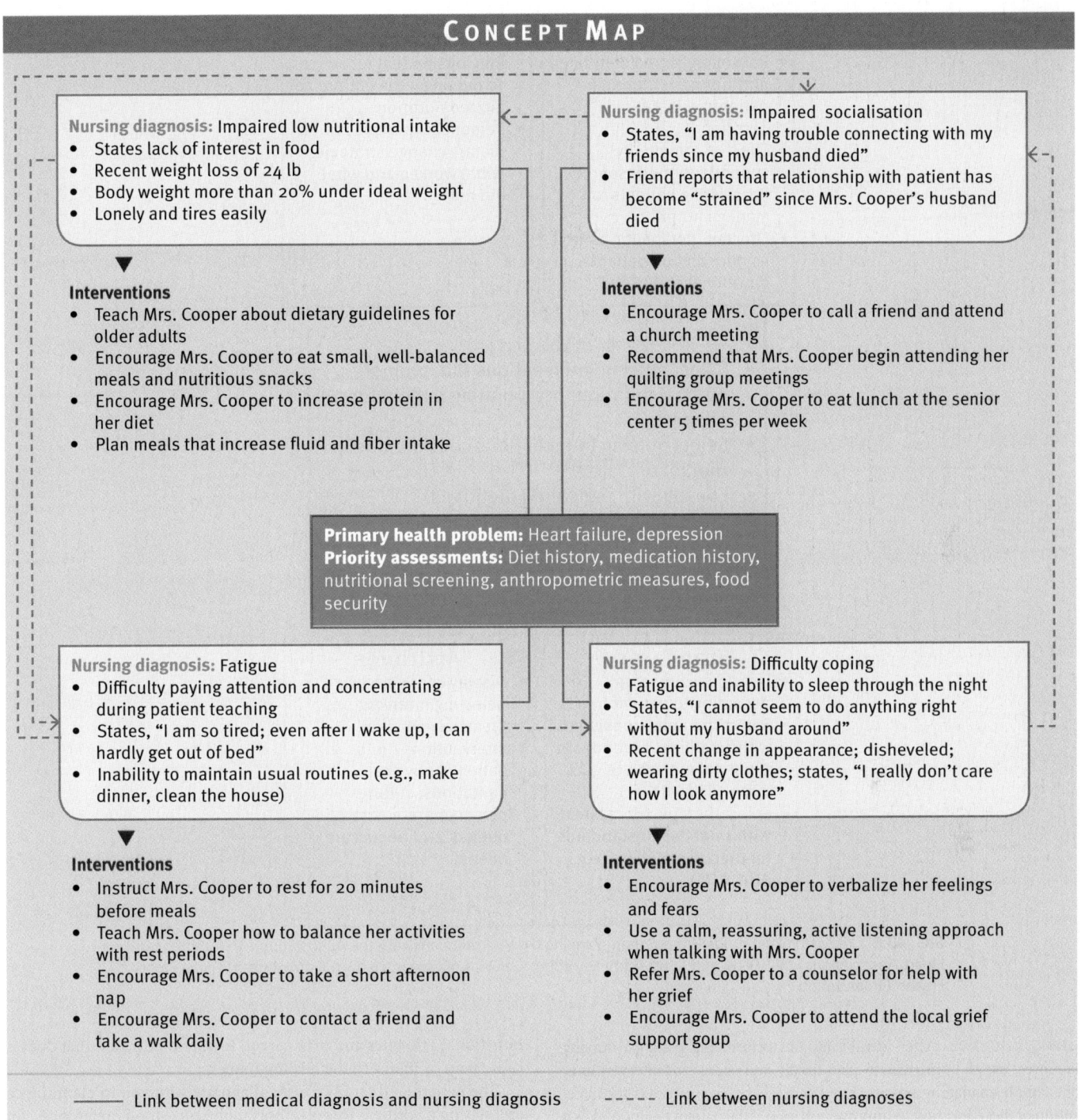

Nursing diagnosis: Impaired low nutritional intake
- States lack of interest in food
- Recent weight loss of 24 lb
- Body weight more than 20% under ideal weight
- Lonely and tires easily

Interventions
- Teach Mrs. Cooper about dietary guidelines for older adults
- Encourage Mrs. Cooper to eat small, well-balanced meals and nutritious snacks
- Encourage Mrs. Cooper to increase protein in her diet
- Plan meals that increase fluid and fiber intake

Nursing diagnosis: Impaired socialisation
- States, "I am having trouble connecting with my friends since my husband died"
- Friend reports that relationship with patient has become "strained" since Mrs. Cooper's husband died

Interventions
- Encourage Mrs. Cooper to call a friend and attend a church meeting
- Recommend that Mrs. Cooper begin attending her quilting group meetings
- Encourage Mrs. Cooper to eat lunch at the senior center 5 times per week

Primary health problem: Heart failure, depression
Priority assessments: Diet history, medication history, nutritional screening, anthropometric measures, food security

Nursing diagnosis: Fatigue
- Difficulty paying attention and concentrating during patient teaching
- States, "I am so tired; even after I wake up, I can hardly get out of bed"
- Inability to maintain usual routines (e.g., make dinner, clean the house)

Interventions
- Instruct Mrs. Cooper to rest for 20 minutes before meals
- Teach Mrs. Cooper how to balance her activities with rest periods
- Encourage Mrs. Cooper to take a short afternoon nap
- Encourage Mrs. Cooper to contact a friend and take a walk daily

Nursing diagnosis: Difficulty coping
- Fatigue and inability to sleep through the night
- States, "I cannot seem to do anything right without my husband around"
- Recent change in appearance; disheveled; wearing dirty clothes; states, "I really don't care how I look anymore"

Interventions
- Encourage Mrs. Cooper to verbalize her feelings and fears
- Use a calm, reassuring, active listening approach when talking with Mrs. Cooper
- Refer Mrs. Cooper to a counselor for help with her grief
- Encourage Mrs. Cooper to attend the local grief support goup

——— Link between medical diagnosis and nursing diagnosis   - - - - Link between nursing diagnoses

FIG. 45.5 Concept map for Mrs. Cooper.

diets prescribed, specifically how diets control their illnesses and whether there are any implications. When planning care, be aware of all factors that influence a patient's food intake. For example, patients with heart failure often experience decreased hunger, dietary restrictions, fatigue, shortness of breath, and sadness, which influence their food intake.

Individualized planning is essential. Incorporate what you learned about a patients' feelings about food, their weight, diet, and medical condition to set realistic and achievable goals. Mutually planned goals negotiated among the patient, RD, health care provider, and nurse ensure success. For the patient with heart failure described previously, an overall goal is "Patient will achieve appropriate BMI height-weight

range or be within 10% of IBW." The following outcomes help to achieve this goal:
- Patient's daily nutritional intake meets the minimal DRIs.
- Patient will eat well-balanced meals and healthy snacks every day.
- Patient will increase daily protein intake.

Meeting nutritional goals requires input from the patient and the interprofessional team. Knowledge of the role of each discipline in providing nutritional support is necessary to maximize nutritional outcomes. For example, collaboration with an RD helps develop appropriate nutritional treatment plans. Calorie counts are frequently ordered, and help is necessary to obtain accurate data. An effective plan of care requires accurate exchange of information among disciplines.

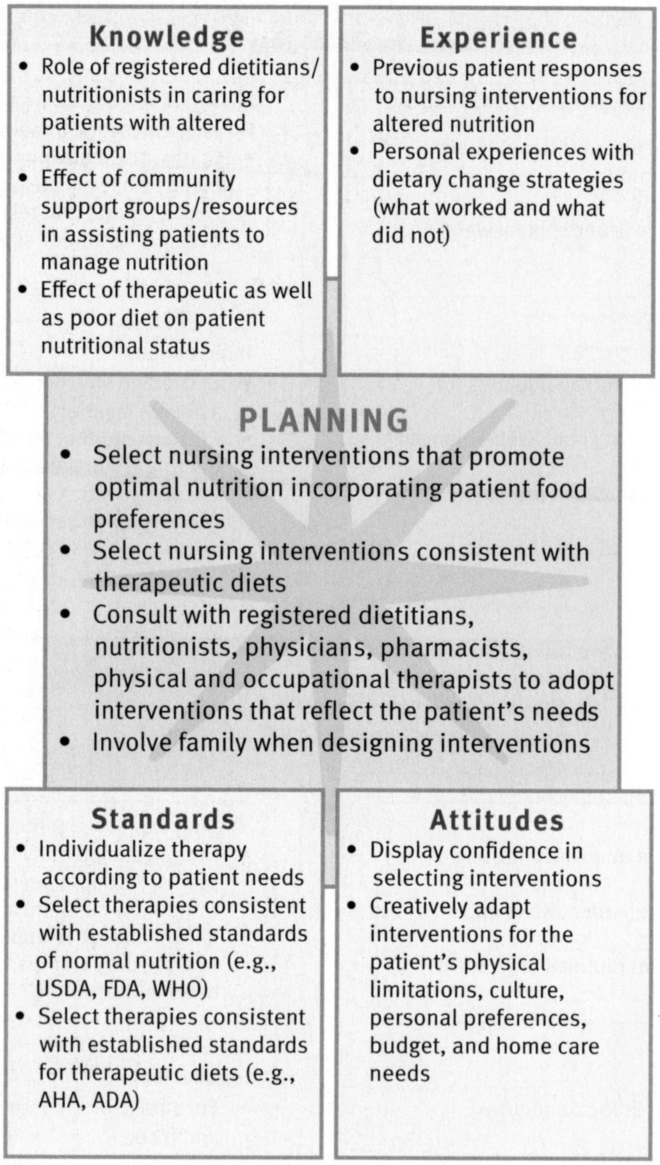

FIG. 45.6 Critical thinking model for nutrition planning. *ADA,* American Diabetes Association; *AHA,* American Heart Association; *FDA,* Food and Drug Administration; *USDA,* US Department of Agriculture; *WHO,* World Health Organization.

Setting Priorities. After identifying and prioritizing patients' nursing diagnoses, use the priorities to plan timely and successful interventions. For example, managing a patient's oral pain will be a priority over the intervention of diet education to improve nutrition if the patient's paint makes it difficult to swallow and maintain adequate food intake. *Lack of Knowledge* regarding diet therapy will become a priority if it is necessary to promote long-term and effective weight loss for a patient being discharged from a hospital.

During acute illness and surgery, food intake varies in the perioperative period. The priority of care is to provide optimal preoperative nutritional support in patients with malnutrition. The priority for the resumption of food intake after surgery depends on the return of bowel function, the extent of the surgical procedure, and the presence of any complications (see Chapter 50). For example, when patients have oral and throat surgery, they chew and swallow food in the presence of excision sites, sutures, or tissue manipulated during surgery. The priority of care is to first provide comfort and pain control. Then address

nutritional priorities and plan care to maintain nutrition that does not cause pain or injury to the healing tissues.

The patient and family must collaborate with you in planning care and setting priorities. This is important because food preferences, food purchases, and preparation involve the entire family. The plan of care cannot succeed without their commitment to, involvement in, and understanding of the nutritional priorities.

Teamwork and Collaboration. The care of a patient often extends beyond the acute hospital setting, requiring continued collaboration among members of the health care team. It is important that discharge planning include nutritional interventions as patients return to their homes or extended-care settings. Communication of patient goals and planned interventions to all team members helps to achieve expected patient outcomes. In addition, consult with an SLP, RD, pharmacist, and/or occupational therapist about patients with dysphagia and those who need ongoing nutritional assessment and interventions to meet their nutritional needs.

When patients have difficulty in feeding themselves, occupational therapists work with patients and their families to identify assistive devices. Devices such as utensils with large handles and plates with elevated sides help a patient with self-feeding. An SLP helps a patient with swallowing exercises and techniques to reduce the risk of aspiration. Occupational therapists also help patients maintain function in the home setting by rearranging food preparation areas in an effort to maximize a patient's functional capacity.

REFLECT NOW

Identify nursing interventions that you would use on clinical to assist a patient with dysphagia to improve his or her nutritional status.

◆ Implementation

Diet therapies are numerous and chosen on the basis of a patient's overall health status, ability to eat and digest normally, and long-term nutritional needs. The focus of health promotion is to educate patients and family caregivers about balanced nutrition and to help them obtain resources to eat high-quality meals. In acute care your role as a nurse is to manage acute conditions that alter patients' nutritional status and to help in ways that promote their appetite and ability to take in nutrients. Patients who are ill or debilitated often have poor appetites (anorexia). Anorexia has many causes (e.g., pain, fatigue, and the effects of medications). Help patients understand the factors that cause anorexia and use creative approaches to stimulate appetite. In the restorative care setting you help patients learn how to follow the therapeutic diets necessary for recovery and treatment of chronic health conditions.

Health Promotion. As a nurse you are in a key position to educate patients about healthful diet choices and good nutrition. Incorporating knowledge of nutrition into patients' lifestyles serves to prevent the development of many diseases. Outpatient and community-based settings are optimal locations for nursing assessment of nutritional practices and status. Early identification of potential or actual problems is the best way to avoid serious problems. Similarly, in other health care settings patients with nutritional problems such as obesity often require help in menu planning and adherence strategies. Your role as educator includes reassessing a patient's and family's health literacy (i.e., how much do they understand regarding their nutritional need) and providing nutritional education and information about community resources. Telephone numbers of an RD or nurse for follow-up questions are always a part of counseling.

Meal planning considers a family's budget and different preferences of family members. Choose specific foods on the basis of the dietary prescription and recommended food groups. For families on limited budgets, use substitutes. For example, bean or cheese dishes often replace meat in a meal, and the use of evaporated milk or dry skim milk when cooking is a low-cost nutritional supplement. Have patients modify the method of preparation when it is necessary to minimize certain substances. For example, baking rather than frying reduces fat intake, and patients can use lemon juice or spices to add flavor to low-sodium diets.

Planning menus a week in advance has several benefits. It helps ensure good nutrition or adherence to a specific diet and helps families stay within their allotted budgets. Nurses or RDs need to check menus for content. Often a simple tip is helpful in meal planning, such as avoiding grocery shopping when hungry, which can lead to impulsive purchases

of more expensive or less nutritious foods that are not included in meal plans. The US Department of Agriculture (USDA, 2017b) pr ovides sample weekly meal-planning services for a range of budgets on its website.

Support individuals who are interested in losing weight. A high percentage of those who attempt to lose weight are unsuccessful, regaining lost weight over time. Adherence to diet and exercise affect success with weight loss. Information on weight loss is available from multiple sources. Help patients develop a successful weight-loss plan that considers their preferences and resources and includes awareness of portion sizes and knowledge of energy content of food (AHA, 2018).

Food safety is an important public health issue. Foodborne bacteria can occur from improper food cleaning, preparation, or poor hygiene practices of food workers. Health care professionals not only need to be aware of the factors related to food safety but also should provide patient education to reduce the risks for foodborne illnesses (Table 45.5; Box 45.9).

QSEN **Building Competency in Teamwork and Collaboration** You are the nurse in charge of developing an interprofessional team to help patients with Crohn's disease, an inflammatory bowel disease, manage their diets at home. Knowing that patients with Crohn's disease must adhere to a diet that is low in fiber and high in calories and protein, you bring your nursing knowledge to the team. What strengths and limitations do you bring to the team? What other members of the team would you need to help prepare the plan of care for patients with Crohn's disease? How would you promote effective teamwork?

Answers to QSEN Activities can be found on the Evolve website.

Acute Care. The nutritional care of patients who are acutely ill requires you to consider a variety of factors that influence nutritional intake. Diagnostic testing and procedures in the acute care setting disrupt food intake. Often a patient must refrain from eating or drinking anything by mouth (NPO) as he or she prepares for or recovers from a diagnostic test. Frequent interruptions during mealtimes occur in the health care setting, or patients have poor appetites. Patients often are too tired or uncomfortable to eat. It is important to assess a patient's nutritional status continuously and to adopt interventions that promote normal intake, digestion, and metabolism of nutrients. Patients who are NPO and receive only standard IV fluids for more than 5 to 7 days are at high nutritional risk.

Advancing Diets. Acute and chronic conditions affect a patient's immune system and nutritional status. Patients with decreased immune function (e.g., from cancer, chemotherapy, human immunodeficiency virus/acquired immunodeficiency syndrome [HIV/AIDS], or organ transplants) require special diets that decrease exposure to microorganisms and are higher in selected nutrients. Table 45.6 provides an overview of the immune system, the impact of malnutrition, and beneficial nutrients. In addition, patients who are ill, who have had surgical procedures, or who were NPO for an extended time have specialized dietary needs. Health care providers order a gradual progression of dietary intake or therapeutic diet to manage patients' illness (Box 45.10).

Promoting Appetite. Providing an environment that promotes nutritional intake includes keeping a patient's environment free of odors, providing oral hygiene as needed to remove unpleasant tastes, and maintaining patient comfort. Offering smaller, more frequent meals often helps. In addition, certain medications affect dietary intake and nutrient use. For example, medications such as insulin, glucocorticoids, and thyroid hormones affect metabolism. Other medications such as antifungal agents frequently affect taste. Some of the psychotropic medications affect appetite, cause nausea, and alter taste. You and the RD help patients select foods that reduce the altered taste sensations or nausea. Consult with an RD regarding using seasonings that improve food taste.

TABLE 45.5 Food Safety

Foodborne Disease	Organism	Food Source	Symptoms[a]
Botulism	*Clostridium botulinum*	Improperly home-canned foods, smoked and salted fish, ham, sausage, shellfish	Symptoms vary from mild discomfort to death in 24 hours; initially nausea, vomiting, dizziness, and weakness progressing to motor (respiratory) paralysis
Escherichia coli	*E. coli*	Undercooked meat (ground beef)	Severe cramps, nausea, vomiting, diarrhea (may be bloody), renal failure; appears 1-8 days after eating; lasts 1-7 days
Listeriosis	*Listeria* *L. monocytogenes*	Soft cheese, meat (hot dogs, pâté, lunch meats), unpasteurized milk, poultry, seafood	Severe diarrhea, fever, headache, pneumonia, meningitis, endocarditis; appears 3-21 days after infection
Perfringens enteritis	*Clostridium* *C. perfringens*	Cooked meats, meat dishes held at room or warm temperature	Mild diarrhea, vomiting; appears 8-24 hours after eating; lasts 1-2 days
Salmonellosis	*Salmonella* *S. typhi* *S. paratyphi*	Milk, custards, egg dishes, salad dressings, sandwich fillings, polluted shellfish	Mild-to-severe diarrhea, cramps, vomiting; appears up to 72 hours after ingestion; lasts 4-7 days
Shigellosis	*Shigella* *S. dysenteriae*	Milk, milk products, seafood, salads	Cramps, diarrhea to fatal dysentery; appears 12-50 hours after ingestion; lasts 3-14 days
Staphylococcus	*Staphylococcus* *S. aureus*	Custards, cream fillings, processed meats, ham, cheese, ice cream, potato salad, sauces, casseroles	Severe abdominal cramps, pain, vomiting, diarrhea, perspiration, headache, fever, prostration; appears 1-6 hours after ingestion; lasts 1-2 days

[a]Symptoms are generally most severe for youngest and oldest age-groups.
From Nix S: *Williams' basic nutrition and diet therapy*, ed 15, St Louis, 2017, Mosby.

In other situations, medications need to be changed. Assessing patients for the need for pharmacological agents to stimulate appetite such as cyproheptadine, megestrol, or dronabinol or to manage symptoms that interfere with nutrition requires health care provider consultation.

Mealtime is usually a social activity. If appropriate, encourage visitors to eat with a patient. When patients experience anorexia, encourage other nurses or care providers to converse and engage them in conversation. Mealtime is also an excellent opportunity for any patient education topic. Instruct a patient about any therapeutic diets, medications, energy conservation measures, or adaptive devices to help with independent feeding.

Assisting Patients With Oral Feeding. When a patient needs help, it is important to protect his or her safety, independence, and dignity. Clear the table or over-bed tray of clutter. Assess his or her risk of aspiration (see Skill 45.1). Patients at high risk for aspiration have decreased level of alertness, decreased gag and/or cough reflexes, and difficulty managing saliva (see Assessment section of this chapter).

Patients with dysphagia are at risk for aspiration and need more help with feeding and swallowing. An SLP identifies patients at risk and provides recommendations for therapy (Pietsch et al., 2018). Provide a 30-minute rest period before eating and position the patient in an upright, seated position in a chair or raise the head of the bed to 90 degrees. Have the patient flex the head slightly to a chin-down position to help prevent aspiration. If the patient has unilateral weakness, teach him or her and the caregiver to place food in the stronger side of the mouth. With the help of an SLP, determine the viscosity of foods that the patient tolerates best using trials of different consistencies of foods and fluids. Thicker fluids are generally easier to swallow. According to the American Speech-Language-Hearing Association (ASHA, 2019), there are four levels of diet: dysphagia puree, dysphagia mechanically altered, dysphagia advanced, and regular. The four levels of liquid include thin liquids (low viscosity), nectarlike liquids (medium viscosity), honeylike liquids (viscosity of honey), and spoon-thick liquids (viscosity of pudding).

Feed a patient with dysphagia slowly, providing smaller-size bites. Allow him or her to chew thoroughly and swallow the bite before taking another. More frequent chewing and swallowing assessments throughout the meal are necessary. Allow the patient time to empty the mouth after each spoonful, matching the speed of feeding to the patient's readiness (see Skill 45.1). If he or she begins to cough or choke, remove the food immediately. Sometimes it is necessary to have oral suction equipment available at the patient's bedside.

Provide opportunities for patients to direct the order in which they want to eat the food items and how fast they wish to eat. Determine a patient's food preferences and, unless contraindicated, try to have these items included on his or her dietary tray. Ask the patient whether the food is the right temperature. These seem like small acts, but they go a long way in maintaining the patient's sense of independence.

Patients with visual deficits also need special assistance. Patients with decreased vision are able to feed themselves when given adequate information. For example, identify the food location on a meal plate as if it were a clock (e.g., meat at 9 o'clock and vegetable at 3 o'clock). Tell the patient where the beverages are located in relation to the plate. Be sure that other care providers set the meal tray and plate in the same manner. Patients with impaired vision and those with decreased motor skills are more independent during mealtimes with the use of large-handled adaptive utensils (Fig. 45.7). These are easier to grip and manipulate.

Enteral Tube Feeding. Enteral nutrition (EN) provides nutrients into the GI tract. It is the preferred method of meeting nutritional needs if a patient is unable to swallow or take in nutrients orally yet has a functioning GI tract. EN provides physiological, safe, and economical nutritional support. Patients with enteral feedings receive formula via nasogastric, jejunal, or gastric tubes. Patients with a low risk of gastric reflux receive gastric feedings; however, if there is a risk of gastric reflux, which leads to aspiration, jejunal feeding is preferred. Box 45.11 lists indications for tube feeding. Either a nurse or a family caregiver can easily give enteral tube feedings in the home setting. After insertion of an enteral tube, it is initially necessary to verify tube placement by x-ray film examination. Confirmation of placement is needed before a patient receives the first enteral feeding (see Skill 45.2).

An enteral formula is usually one of four types. Polymeric (1 to 2 kcal/mL) includes milk-based blenderized foods prepared by hospital

BOX 45.9 PATIENT TEACHING

Food Safety

Objective

- Patient is able to verbalize measures to protect from foodborne illness.

Teaching Strategies

- Explain that food safety is an important public health issue. Populations particularly at risk are older and younger people and immunosuppressed individuals.
- Instruct patients using the following four principles:

1. CLEAN
   - Wash hands with warm, soapy water before touching or eating food.
   - Wash fresh fruits and vegetables thoroughly.
   - Clean the inside of refrigerator and microwave regularly to prevent microbial growth.
   - Clean cutting surfaces after each use.
   - When possible, use separate surfaces for fruit, meat, poultry, fish

2. SEPARATE
   - Wash cooking utensils and cutting boards with hot, soapy water.
   - Wash hands after handling foods, especially meats, poultry, and eggs.
   - Clean vegetables and lettuce used in salads thoroughly.
   - Wash dishrags, towels, and sponges regularly or use paper towels.

3. COOK
   - Use a food thermometer to verify that meat, poultry, and fish are cooked properly.
   - Do not eat raw meats or unpasteurized milk.

4. CHILL
   - Keep foods properly refrigerated at 40° F (4.4° C) and frozen at 0° F (−17.8° C).
   - Do not save leftovers for more than 2 days in refrigerator.

Evaluation

Use the principles of teach-back to evaluate patient/family caregiver learning:

- Tell me what you do to prevent foodborne illnesses while you are preparing meals.
- Please show me what you do while cooking to ensure safe food-preparation practices.

Data from US Department of Agriculture: 10 tips: be food safe, n.d., https://www.choosemyplate.gov/ten-tips-be-food-safe.

dietary staff or in a patient's home. The polymeric classification also includes commercially prepared whole-nutrient formulas. For this type of formula to be effective, a patient's GI tract needs to be able to absorb whole nutrients. The second type, modular formulas (3.8 to 4 kcal/mL), consists of single macronutrient (e.g., protein, glucose, polymers, or lipids) preparations and is not nutritionally complete. You can add this type of formula to other foods to meet your patient's individual nutritional needs. The third type, elemental formulas (1 to 3 kcal/mL), contains predigested nutrients that are easier for a partially dysfunctional GI tract to absorb. Finally, specialty formulas (1 to 2 kcal/mL) are designed to meet specific nutritional needs in certain illnesses (e.g., liver failure, pulmonary disease, or HIV infection).

Typically tube feedings start at full strength at slow rates (see Skill 45.3; Box 45.12). Increase the hourly rate every 8 to 12 hours per health care provider's order if no signs of intolerance appear (high gastric residuals, nausea, cramping, vomiting, or diarrhea). Implement evidence-based guidelines when caring for patients receiving tube feedings (Box 45.13). Studies have demonstrated a beneficial effect of enteral feedings compared with PN. Feeding by the enteral route reduces sepsis, minimizes the hypermetabolic response to trauma, decreases hospital mortality, and maintains intestinal structure and function (Lewis et al., 2017). EN is successful within 24 to 48 hours after surgery or trauma to provide fluids, electrolytes, and nutritional support. If the patient develops a gastric ileus, it prevents instituting nasogastric feedings. Nasointestinal or jejunal tubes allow successful postpyloric feeding because the formula instills directly into the small intestine or jejunum or beyond the pyloric sphincter of the stomach (Lewis et al., 2017).

A serious complication associated with enteral feedings is aspiration of formula into the tracheobronchial tree. Aspiration of enteral formula into the lungs irritates the bronchial mucosa, resulting in decreased blood supply to affected pulmonary tissue (McCance, 2019). This leads to necrotizing infection, pneumonia, and potential abscess formation. The high glucose content of a feeding serves as a bacterial medium for growth, promoting infection. Acute respiratory distress syndrome (ARDS) is also an outcome frequently associated with pulmonary aspiration. Some of the common conditions that increase the risk of aspiration include coughing, gastroesophageal reflux disease (GERD), cerebral vascular accident (CVA), Parkinson's disease, nasotracheal suctioning, an artificial airway, decreased level of consciousness, and lying flat. Prokinetic medications such as metoclopramide, erythromycin, or cisapride promote gastric emptying and decrease

TABLE 45.6 Nutrition and the Immune System

Immune/Physiological Component	Malnutrition Effect	Vital Nutrient
Antibodies	Decreased amount	Protein, vitamins A, B_6, B_{12}, C, folic acid, thiamin, biotin, riboflavin, niacin
GI tract	Systemic movement of bacteria	Arginine, glutamine, omega-3 fatty acids
Granulocytes and macrocytes	Longer time for phagocytosis kill time and lymphocyte activation	Protein, vitamins A, B_6, B_{12}, C, folic acid, thiamin, riboflavin, niacin, zinc, iron
Mucus	Flat microvilli in GI tract, decreased antibody secretion	Vitamins B_6, B_{12}, C, biotin
Skin	Integrity compromised, density reduced, wound healing slowed	Protein, vitamins A, B_{12}, C, niacin, copper, zinc
T-lymphocytes	Depressed T-cell distribution	Protein, arginine, iron, zinc, omega-3 fatty acids, vitamins A, B_6, B_{12}, folic acid, thiamin, riboflavin, niacin, pantothenic acid

GI, Gastrointestinal.

Modified from Grodner M, et al: *Foundations and clinical applications of nutrition: a nursing approach,* ed 7, St Louis, 2020, Elsevier.

BOX 45.10 Diet Progression and Therapeutic Diets

Clear Liquid

Clear fat-free broth, bouillon, coffee, tea, carbonated beverages, clear fruit juices, gelatin, fruit ices, popsicles

Full Liquid

As for clear liquid, with addition of smooth-textured dairy products (e.g., ice cream), strained or blended cream soups, custards, refined cooked cereals, vegetable juice, pureed vegetables, all fruit juices, sherbets, puddings, frozen yogurt

Dysphagia Stages, Thickened Liquids, Pureed

As for clear and full liquid, with addition of scrambled eggs; pureed meats, vegetables, and fruits; mashed potatoes and gravy

Mechanical Soft

As for clear and full liquid and pureed, with addition of all cream soups, ground or finely diced meats, flaked fish, cottage cheese, cheese, rice, potatoes, pancakes, light breads, cooked vegetables, cooked or canned fruits, bananas, soups, peanut butter, eggs (not fried)

Soft/Low Residue

Addition of low-fiber, easily digested foods such as pastas, casseroles, moist tender meats, and canned cooked fruits and vegetables; desserts, cakes, and cookies without nuts or coconut

High Fiber

Addition of fresh uncooked fruits, steamed vegetables, bran, oatmeal, and dried fruits

Low Sodium

4-g (no added salt), 2-g, 1-g, or 500-mg sodium diets; vary from no-added-salt to severe sodium restriction (500-mg sodium diet), which requires selective food purchases

Low Cholesterol

300 mg/day cholesterol, in keeping with American Heart Association guidelines for serum lipid reduction

Diabetic

Nutrition recommendations by the American Diabetes Association: focus on total energy, nutrient and food distribution; include a balanced intake of carbohydrates, fats, and proteins; varied caloric recommendations to accommodate patient's metabolic demands

Gluten Free

Eliminates wheat, oats, rye, barley, and their derivatives

Regular

No restrictions unless specified

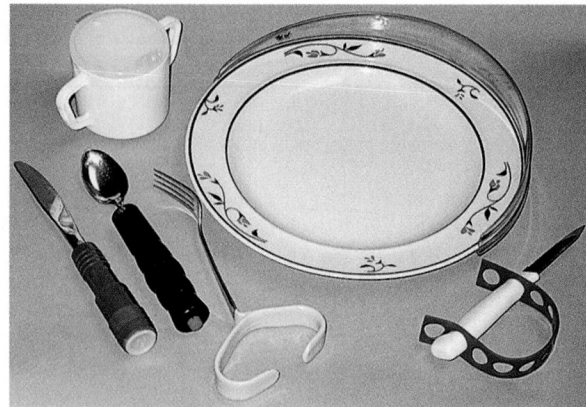

FIG. 45.7 Adaptive equipment. Clockwise from upper left: Two-handled cup with lid, plate with plate guard, utensils with splints, and utensils with enlarged handles.

BOX 45.11 Indications for Enteral and Parenteral Nutrition

Enteral Nutrition
(Used with patients who have a functional gastrointestinal tract)

- Cancer
  - Head and neck
  - Upper GI
- Critical illness/trauma
- Neurological and muscular disorders
  - Brain neoplasm
  - Cerebrovascular accident
  - Dementia
  - Myopathy
  - Parkinson's disease
- GI disorders
  - Enterocutaneous fistula
  - Inflammatory bowel disease
  - Mild pancreatitis
- Respiratory failure with prolonged intubation
- Inadequate oral intake
  - Anorexia nervosa
  - Difficulty chewing, swallowing
- Severe depression

Parenteral Nutrition

- Nonfunctional GI tract
  - Massive small bowel resection/GI surgery/massive GI bleed
  - Paralytic ileus
  - Intestinal obstruction
  - Trauma to abdomen, head, or neck
  - Severe malabsorption
  - Intolerance to enteral feeding (established by trial)
  - Chemotherapy, radiation therapy, bone marrow transplantation
- Extended bowel rest
  - Enterocutaneous fistula
  - Inflammatory bowel disease exacerbation
  - Severe diarrhea
  - Moderate-to-severe pancreatitis
- Preoperative total parenteral nutrition
  - Preoperative bowel rest
  - Treatment for co-morbid severe malnutrition in patients with nonfunctional GI tracts
- Severely catabolic patients when GI tract not usable for more than 4 to 5 days

GI, Gastrointestinal.

the risk of aspiration (McCuiston et al., 2018). Keep the head of the bed elevated a minimum of 30 degrees, preferably 45 degrees, unless medically contraindicated, during feedings and for 30 to 60 minutes after feeding (Lewis et al., 2017). You need to measure gastric residual volumes (GRVs) every 4 to 6 hours in patients receiving continuous feedings and immediately before the feeding in patients receiving intermittent feedings (Lewis et al., 2017). Delayed gastric emptying is a concern if 250 mL or more remains in a patient's stomach on two consecutive assessments (1 hour apart) or if a single GRV measurement exceeds 500 mL (Stewart, 2014). A gastric residual volume of between 250 and 500 mL should lead to implementation of measures to reduce

the risk of aspiration (Boullata et al., 2017). The North American Summit on Aspiration in the Critically Ill Patient recommends the following: (1) stop feedings immediately if aspiration occurs; (2) withhold feedings and reassess patient tolerance to feedings if GRV is over 500 mL; (3) routinely evaluate the patient for aspiration; and (4) use nursing measures to reduce the risk of aspiration if GRV is between 250 and 500 mL (Boullata et al., 2017).

Enteral Access Tubes. Enteral tube feedings are used with patients who are unable to ingest food but maintain the ability to digest and absorb nutrients. Feeding tubes are inserted through the nose (nasogastric or nasointestinal), surgically (gastrostomy

BOX 45.12 Advancing the Rate of Tube Feeding

Protocols for advancing tube feedings are commonly institution specific. There does not appear to be a benefit to slow initiation of enteral nutrition over days. Most patients are able to tolerate feeding 24 to 48 hours after initiation. Do not dilute formulas with water; this increases the risk of bacterial contamination (Lewis, 2017). The common delivery options for enteral feedings are continuous, intermittent via a pump or gravity, and cyclical. Usually patients who are more critically ill receive continuous feedings (Lewis, 2017). Patients who are stable or are getting feedings in the home frequently receive intermittent feedings (Lewis, 2017). Cyclical feedings are used when patients begin to eat a normal diet but still need additional nutritional support (Lewis, 2017).

Intermittent

1. Start formula at full strength for isotonic formulas (300 to 400 mOsm) or at ordered concentration.
2. Infuse bolus of formula over at least 20 to 30 minutes via syringe or feeding container.
3. Begin feedings with a volume of 2.5 to 5 mL/kg 5 to 8 times per day. Increase by 60 to 120 mL per feeding every 8 to 12 hours to achieve needed volume and calories in four to six feedings (Stewart, 2014).

Continuous

1. Start formula at full strength for isotonic formulas (300 to 400 mOsm) or at ordered concentration.
2. Begin infusion rate at designated rate typically at 10 to 40 mL/hr (Stewart, 2014).
3. Advance rate slowly (e.g., 10 to 20 mL/hr every 8 to 12 hours) to target rate if tolerated (tolerance indicated by absence of nausea and diarrhea and low gastric residuals) (Stewart, 2014).

BOX 45.13 EVIDENCE-BASED PRACTICE

Reducing Malnutrition and Risk of Aspiration with Enteral Feedings

PICOT Question: In adult patients who are receiving tube feedings, does regular nutritional assessment reduce malnutrition and the risk of aspiration?

Evidence Summary

Enteral feedings provide calories, preserve the client's immune system, preserve the integrity of the gut, and reduce the severity of disease (VanBlarcom and McCoy, 2018). It is essential is to perform a nutritional assessment regularly in adult patients who are receiving tube feedings. According to ASPEN (2019), clients are considered malnourished if they exhibit two of the following six characteristics: insufficient protein intake, weight loss, loss of muscle mass, loss of subcutaneous fat, localized or generalized fluid accumulation, and diminished functional status measured by handgrip strength.

In collaboration with the dietitian, the nurse will work to prevent undernutrition and aspiration, two common complications associated with tube feedings that can lead to pneumonia. According to VanBlarcom and McCoy (2018), one cause of undernutrition in patients in critical care units is interrupted enteral feedings. Each time the head of the bed is lowered below 30 degrees (e.g., for hygiene care, dressing changes, moving the patient), the nurse pauses a patient's feeding to prevent aspiration. However, this interruption in tube feedings can contribute to poor nutrition.

To reduce the risk for aspiration, nurses follow several practices, such as keeping the head of bed elevated at 30 to 45 degrees, reducing the use of sedatives, assessing placement of the enteral access device and tolerance to the enteral feeding every 4 hours, and ensuring adequate bowel function (VanBlarcom and McCoy, 2018). Patients diagnosed with pancreatitis, gastric outlet obstruction, gastroparesis, and a history of aspiration are at an increased risk for aspiration with an enteral feeding and may benefit from a small-bore feeding tube placed into the duodenum (VanBlarcomm and McCoy, 2018).

In addition to reducing the risk of aspiration, the nurse needs to assess a patient's tolerance to enteral feedings. New guidelines from ASPEN (2019) limit the use of measuring gastric residual volumes as an assessment tool to determine the patient's tolerance to enteral feeding. The current literature indicates that there is no correlation between gastric residual volumes and gastric emptying and that these are poor indicators of intolerance to enteral feedings (VanBlarcom and McCoy, 2018). Additionally, measuring gastric residual volumes may lead to a clogged enteral access device and inappropriate cessation of the enteral feeding, which also places the client at an increased risk for undernutrition. Implementing an evidence-based nutrition bundle is effective in reducing malnutrition and the risk of aspiration (VanBlarcom and McCoy, 2018).

Application to Nursing Practice

- Implement an evidence-based nutrition bundle to reduce malnutrition and reduce the risk of aspiration, such as the one created by ASPEN in conjunction with the Society of Critical Care Medicine (VanBlarcom and McCoy, 2018).
- Assess patients for malnutrition by using the gold standard of indirect calorimetry to estimate protein/energy needs (ASPEN, 2019).
- Initiate and maintain enteral feedings appropriately.
- Implement enteral feeding institution-specific protocols.
- Initiate parenteral feeding when enteral nutrition cannot be initiated.
- Administer a prokinetic agent, especially in patients with high gastric residual volumes, as ordered to reduce the risk of aspiration (VanBlarcom and McCoy, 2018).

---

or jejunostomy), or endoscopically (percutaneous endoscopic gastrostomy or jejunostomy [PEG or PEJ]). Nasogastric or nasojejunal feeding tubes may be used if a patient is expected to need EN therapy for less than 4 weeks. Surgically or endoscopically placed tubes are preferred for long-term feeding (more than 6 weeks) to reduce the discomfort of a nasal tube and provide a more secure, reliable access (Lewis et al., 2017). Some patients such as those with gastroparesis (decreased or absent innervation to the stomach that results in delayed gastric emptying), esophageal reflux, or a history of aspiration pneumonia require placement of tubes beyond the stomach into the intestine (Lewis et al., 2017).

Most health care settings use small-bore feeding tubes because they create less discomfort for a patient (Fig. 45.8, *A*). Adult patients typically have an 8- to 12-Fr tube that is 36 to 44 inches (90 to 110 cm) long. These flexible tubes come with a stylet, which makes the tube stiffer and is used when the tube is inserted. The stylet is removed after correct tube location is confirmed and before feedings are started. **Never reinsert the stylet in the tube.** It is now standard to use an enteral-only connector (ENFit) designed for the specific enteral tube. Standardization of connector tubing improves patient safety (Fig. 45.8, *B*). Tubing standards are designed to reduce tubing misconnections that result in patient injury (TJC, 2018). Skill 45.3 describes the procedure for initiating nasogastric, gastrostomy, and jejunostomy enteral feedings.

Historically nurses confirmed placement of feeding tubes by injecting air into the tube while auscultating the stomach for a bubbling or gurgling sound or by asking the patient to speak. Current evidence shows these methods are ineffective in verifying tube placement. Currently, the most accurate method for verification of tube placement is x-ray film examination. At the bedside, nurses test the pH of

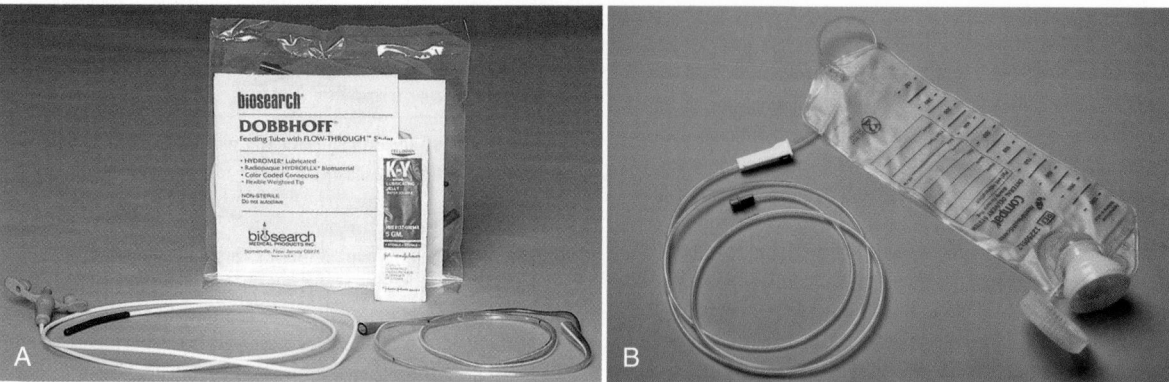

FIG. 45.8 A, Enteral tubes, small-bore. **B,** Enteral-only connector (ENFit) designed to fit the specific enteral tube.

secretions withdrawn from the feeding tube to confirm tube location on an ongoing basis (Box 45.14).

Table 45.7 outlines major complications of EN. Of special note, patients who are severely malnourished are at risk for electrolyte disturbances from refeeding syndrome during EN or PN therapy. In refeeding syndrome, potassium, magnesium, and phosphate move intracellularly, resulting in low serum (extracellular) levels and edema. These changes may cause cardiac dysrhythmias, heart failure, respiratory distress, convulsions, coma, or death.

Parenteral Nutrition. Parenteral nutrition (PN) is a form of specialized nutritional support provided intravenously. Patients who are unable to digest or absorb EN benefit from PN. Patients in highly stressed physiological states such as sepsis, head injury, or burns are candidates for PN therapy (see Box 45.11). A basic PN formula is a combination of crystalline amino acids, hypertonic dextrose, electrolytes, vitamins, and trace elements. Total PN (TPN), administered through a central line, is a 2-in-1 formula in which administration of fat emulsions occurs separately from the protein and dextrose solution (Lewis et al., 2017). Safe administration depends on appropriate assessment of nutritional needs, meticulous management of the central venous catheter (CVC), and careful monitoring to prevent or treat metabolic complications. Administration of PN happens in a variety of settings, including a patient's home. Regardless of the setting, adhere to principles of asepsis and infusion management to ensure safe nutritional support.

PN therapy requires clinical and laboratory monitoring by an interprofessional team. Consistent reevaluation for the continuation of PN is required. The goal to move toward use of the GI tract is constant (Lewis et al., 2017). Disuse of the GI tract has been associated with villus atrophy and generalized cell shrinkage. Furthermore, the disuse of the GI tract may cause bacteria to move from the unused gut into the bloodstream, resulting in gram-negative septicemia.

Sometimes adding intravenous fat emulsions to PN supports the patient's need for supplemental kilocalories to prevent essential fatty-acid deficiencies and help control hyperglycemia during periods of stress (Phillips, 2018). Administer these emulsions through a separate peripheral line, through the central line by using Y-connector tubing (see Chapter 42), or as an admixture to the PN solution. The addition of fat emulsion to a PN solution is called a *3-in-1 admixture* or *total nutrient admixture*. The patient receives it over a 24-hour period. Do not use the admixture if you observe oil droplets or an oily or creamy layer on the surface of the admixture. This observation indicates that the emulsion has broken into large lipid droplets that cause fat emboli if administered. IV fat emulsions are white and opaque. Take care to avoid confusing enteral formula with parenteral lipids.

Initiating Parenteral Nutrition. Patients with short-term nutritional needs often receive IV solutions of less than 10% dextrose via a peripheral vein in combination with amino acids and lipids. TPN is more calorically dense than peripheral solutions; therefore, peripheral solutions are usually temporary. PN with greater than 10% dextrose requires a CVC that a health care provider places into a high-flow central vein such as the superior vena cava under sterile conditions (see Chapter 42). If you are using a CVC that has multiple lumens, use a port exclusively dedicated for the TPN. Label the port for TPN and do not infuse other solutions or medications through it (Lewis et al., 2018). Nurses with special training insert peripherally inserted central catheters (PICCs) that start in a vein of the arm and then thread into the subclavian or superior vena cava vein.

After catheter placement wait to flush and use the catheter until position confirmation by radiology. The health care provider secures the CVC with a securement device and covers the site with a sterile bio-occlusive dressing. Before applying the sterile dressing, stabilize the PICC with sterile strips of tape, and follow the institution's central line infection prevention protocol (Lewis et al., 2017).

Before beginning any PN infusion, verify the health care provider's order and inspect the solution for particulate matter or a break in the fat emulsion. Always use an infusion pump to deliver a constant rate. The initial rate delivers no more than 50% of estimated needs for the first 24 to 48 hours and gradually increases the rate until a patient's complete nutritional needs are supplied. Patients receiving PN at home frequently administer the entire daily solution over 12 hours at night. This allows the patient to disconnect from the infusion each morning, flush the central line, and have independent mobility during the day.

Preventing Complications. Complications of PN include catheter-related problems and metabolic alterations (Table 45.8). Pneumothorax results from an initial puncture during catheter insertion, resulting in the accumulation of air in the pleural cavity with subsequent collapse of the lung and impaired breathing. The clinical symptoms of a pneumothorax include sudden sharp chest pain, dyspnea, and coughing. In relation to PN, pneumothorax most often occurs during CVC placement. Monitor a patient with a CVC for the first 24 hours for signs and symptoms of pulmonary distress.

An air embolus possibly occurs during insertion of the catheter or when changing the tubing or cap. Turn the patient into a left lateral decubitus position and have him or her perform a Valsalva maneuver (holding the breath and "bearing down") during catheter insertion to help prevent air embolus. The increased venous pressure created by the maneuver prevents air from entering the bloodstream. Maintaining integrity of the closed IV system also helps prevent air embolus.

BOX 45.14 PROCEDURAL GUIDELINES

Obtaining Gastrointestinal Aspirate for pH Measurement, Large-Bore, and Small-Bore Feeding Tubes: Intermittent and Continuous Feeding

Delegation and Collaboration

The skill of verifying tube placement and irrigating a feeding tube is the responsibility of the nurse and cannot be delegated to assistive personnel (AP). The nurse directs the AP to:

- Immediately inform the nurse if patient's respirations change or patient complains of shortness of breath, coughing, or choking.
- Immediately inform the nurse if the patient vomits or the AP notices vomitus in patient's mouth during oral hygiene.
- Immediately inform the nurse if nasal skin irritation or excoriation is present.
- Immediately inform the nurse if a change in the external length of the tube occurs, which could indicate displacement of the tube.
- Report when a continuous tube feeding stops infusing.

Equipment

60-mL ENFit syringe; water (tap water or sterile [see agency policy], dated and initialed container at patient's bedside); towel; stethoscope; clean gloves; pH indicator strip (scale of 1.0 to 11.0); small medication cup; measuring tape/device; pulse oximeter

Steps

1. Review agency policy and procedures for frequency of irrigation and frequency and method of checking tube placement. **Do not insufflate air into tube to check placement.**
2. Identify patient using at least two identifiers (e.g., name and birthday or name and medical record number) according to agency policy (TJC, 2020).
3. Review patient's medication record for orders for enteral feeding, a gastric acid inhibitor (e.g., ranitidine, famotidine, nizatidine), or a proton pump inhibitor (e.g., omeprazole).
4. Review patient's medical record for history of prior tube displacement.
5. Observe for signs and symptoms of respiratory distress during feeding: coughing, choking, or reduced oxygen saturation.
6. Identify conditions that increase risk for spontaneous tube migration or dislocation: altered level of consciousness, agitation; retching, vomiting; nasotracheal suction.
7. Perform hand hygiene. Assess bowel sounds and perform abdominal exam.
8. Obtain pulse oximetry reading.
9. Note ease with which previous tube feedings infuse through tubing. Monitor volume of continuous enteral formula administered during shift and compare with ordered amount.
10. Assess patient's or family caregiver's knowledge, experience, and health literacy level. Perform hand hygiene and apply clean gloves. Be sure pulse oximeter is in place.
11. Verify tube placement.

CLINICAL DECISION: Listening for insufflated air instilled through tube to check tube tip position is unreliable (Boullata et al., 2017; Fan et al., 2017).

- a. Check tube placement at following times
  - (1) For patients receiving intermittent tube feedings, test placement immediately before each feeding (usually a period of at least 4 hours will have elapsed since previous feeding) and before medications.
  - (2) Follow agency policy regarding when to test pH for patients receiving continuous tube feedings. AACN (2016) recommends stopping continuous feedings for several hours to obtain reliable pH readings. However this is not always appropriate for a patient's therapeutic plan of care.
  - (3) Wait to verify placement at least 1 hour after medication administration by tube or mouth.
  - (4) Measure length of tube extending from nare.
- b. If tube feeding is infusing, turn off or place tube feeding on hold. Clamp or kink feeding tube and disconnect from end of infusion bag tubing. For intermittent feedings, remove plug at end of feeding tube. Draw up 30 mL of air into a 60-mL ENFit syringe. Place tip of syringe into end of gastric or small bowel feeding tube. Flush with air before attempting to aspirate fluid. Repositioning patient from side to side is helpful. In some cases more than one bolus of air is necessary.
- c. Draw back on syringe slowly and obtain 5 to 10 mL of gastric aspirate (see illustration). Observe appearance of aspirate. Aspirates from gastric tubes of patients receiving continuous tube feedings often look like curdled enteral formula. Gastric aspirates from patients receiving intermittent feedings typically are not bile stained (unless intestinal fluid has refluxed into stomach) (AACN, 2016).

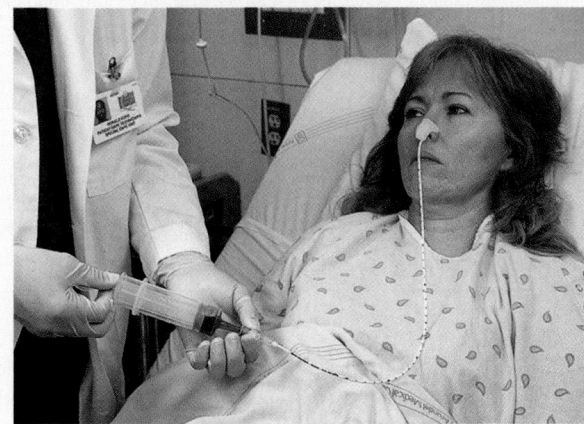

STEP 11c Obtain gastric aspirate.

- d. Gently mix aspirate in syringe. Expel few drops into clean medicine cup. Note color of aspirate. Measure pH of aspirated GI contents by dipping pH strip into fluid or applying few drops of fluid to strip. Compare color of strip with color on chart (see illustration) provided by manufacturer.

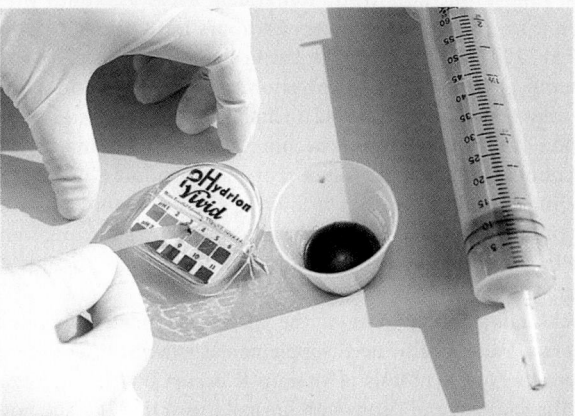

STEP 11d Compare color on test strip with color on pH chart.

Continued

BOX 45.14 PROCEDURAL GUIDELINES—cont'd

Obtaining Gastrointestinal Aspirate for pH Measurement, Large-Bore, and Small-Bore Feeding Tubes: Intermittent and Continuous Feeding

(1) Gastric fluid from patient who has fasted for at least 4 hours usually has pH range of 5.0 or less.

(2) Fluid from tube in small intestine of patient who is fasting usually has pH greater than 6.0 (Bourgault et al., 2015).

(3) The pH of pleural fluid from the tracheobronchial tree is generally greater than 6.0.

12. If after repeated attempts it is not possible to aspirate fluid from tube that was confirmed by x-ray film to be in desired position and if (1) there are no risk factors for tube dislocation, (2) tube has remained in original taped position, (3) patient is not in respiratory distress, assume that tube is correctly placed. Continue with irrigation (AACN, 2016; Bourgault et al., 2015; Fan et al., 2017).

13. Irrigate tube.

a. Irrigate routinely before, between, and after final medication (before feedings are reinstituted), and before an intermittent feeding is administered.

b. Draw up 30 mL of water in ENFit syringe. Do not use irrigation fluids from bottles that are used on other patients. Patient should have individual bottle of solution.

CLINICAL DECISION: Do not use cola or fruit juices for flushing tubing as these liquids can clog tube.

c. Change irrigation bottle every 24 hours. Irrigation trays, which hold both irrigation fluid and syringe, are considered open systems and may be more easily contaminated than sterile water bottles. Note: Be sure that syringe in tray has ENFit adapter.

d. Kink feeding tube while disconnecting it from infusion tubing (continuous feeding) or while removing plug at end of tube (intermittent feeding).

e. Insert tip of ENFit syringe into end of feeding tube. Release kink and slowly instill irrigation solution.

f. If unable to instill fluid, reposition patient on left side and try again.

g. When water or sterile saline has been instilled, remove syringe. Reinstitute tube feeding or administer medication as ordered. Then flush each medication completely through tube (see Chapter 31).

14. Help patient assume comfortable position. Raise side rails as appropriate and lower bed to lowest position. Remove and discard gloves; dispose of supplies in appropriate receptacle and perform hand hygiene.

15. Place nurse call system in an accessible location within patient's reach. Instruct patient in its use.

16. Observe patient for respiratory distress: persistent gagging, paroxysms of coughing, drop in oxygen (O_2) saturation, or respiratory patterns (e.g., rate and depth) that are inconsistent with baseline measures.

17. Verify that external length of tube, pH, and appearance of aspirate are consistent with initial tube placement.

18. Observe ease with which tube feeding instills through tubing.

19. Monitor patient's caloric intake.

20. **Use Teach-Back:** "I want to go over what I explained earlier. Tell me why it is important for me to test the gastric pH and the color of the gastric secretions in your stomach before feedings." Revise your instruction now or develop a plan for revised patient/family caregiver teaching if patient/family caregiver is not able to teach back correctly.

Catheter occlusion is present when there is sluggish or no flow through the catheter. Temporarily stop the infusion and flush with saline or per protocol orders. If this is unsuccessful, attempt to aspirate a clot. If still unsuccessful, follow institution protocol for use of a thrombolytic agent (e.g., urokinase).

Suspect catheter sepsis if a patient develops fever, chills, or glucose intolerance and has a positive blood culture. To prevent infection, change the TPN infusion tubing every 24 hours. Do not hang a single container of PN for more than 24 hours or lipids more than 12 hours. Change the administration system every 72 hours when infusing a 2-in-1 solution and every 24 hours for a 3-in-1 solution (Lewis et al., 2017). During CVC dressing changes always use a sterile mask and gloves and assess insertion sites for signs and symptoms of infection (see Chapter 42). Change the CVC dressing per institution policy and any time it becomes wet or contaminated. Use either alcohol or an alcoholic solution of chlorhexidine gluconate to clean the injection port or catheter hub 15 seconds before and after each time it is used. Use a 1.2-micron filter for 3-in-1 formulas and an inline 0.22-micron filter for PN solutions that do not include IV fat emulsions.

PN solutions contain most of the major electrolytes, vitamins, and minerals. Patients also need supplemental vitamin K as ordered throughout therapy. Synthesis of vitamin K occurs by the microflora found in the jejunum and ileum with normal use of the GI tract; however, because PN circumvents GI use, patients need to receive exogenous vitamin K.

Electrolyte and mineral imbalances often occur. Administration of concentrated glucose accompanies an increase in endogenous insulin production, which causes cations (potassium, magnesium, and phosphorus) to move intracellularly. Monitor blood glucose levels every 6 hours to assess for hyperglycemia, and administer supplemental insulin as ordered (Lewis et al., 2017) (see Skill 45.4).

Too-rapid administration of hypertonic dextrose can result in an osmotic diuresis and dehydration (see Chapter 42). If an infusion falls behind schedule, do not increase the rate in an attempt to catch up. Sudden discontinuation of a solution can cause hypoglycemia. Usually it is recommended to infuse 10% dextrose when discontinuing PN solution suddenly. Patients with diabetes are more at risk.

The goal is to move patients from PN to EN and/or oral feeding. Once patients are meeting one-third to one-half of their kilocalorie needs per day, health care providers usually decrease PN by half the original volume and increase EN feedings to meet the patient's nutritional needs. Patients who make the transition from PN to oral feedings typically have early satiety and decreased appetite. Consult with RD about decreasing PN in response to increased oral intake. If oral intake is inadequate, small frequent meals are helpful. Recommend calorie/protein counts when patients begin taking soft foods. When meeting 75% of nutritional needs by enteral feedings or reliable dietary intake, it is usually safe to discontinue PN therapy. Discontinuation of PN may also happen if complications occur or the health care provider determines that it is not benefiting the patient (Lewis et al., 2017).

Restorative and Continuing Care. Patients discharged from a hospital with diet prescriptions often need dietary education to plan meals that meet specific therapeutic requirements. Restorative care includes both immediate postsurgical care and routine medical care and therefore includes patients in the hospital and at home. The following

TABLE 45.7 Enteral Tube-Feeding Complications

Problem	Possible Cause	Intervention[a]
Pulmonary aspiration	Regurgitation of formula	Verify tube placement. Place patient in high-Fowler's position or elevate head of bed a minimum of 30 (preferably 45) degrees during feedings and for 2 hours afterward.
	Feeding tube displaced	Reposition tube and verify tube placement by ordered x-ray.
	Deficient gag reflex	Reassess for return of normal gag reflex; until then place patient on aspiration precautions and in semi-Fowler's position.
	Delayed gastric emptying	See delayed gastric emptying below.
Diarrhea	Hyperosmolar formula or medications	Deliver formula continuously, lower rate, dilute, or change to isotonic enteral nutrition.
	Antibiotic therapy	Antibiotics destroy normal intestinal flora; consult with health care provider to consider changing medication; treat symptoms with antidiarrheal agents; culture stool for *Clostridium difficile*.
	Bacterial contamination	Do not hang formula longer than 4-8 hours in bag, wash bag out well when refilling, change tube-feeding bags and tubing q24h, and use aseptic practices. Check expiration dates.
	Malabsorption	Check for pancreatic insufficiency; use low-fat, lactose-free formula and continuous feedings.
Constipation	Lack of fiber	Consult with a dietitian to select a formula containing fiber.
	Lack of free water	Add water during tube flushes.[a]
	Inactivity	Monitor patient's ability to ambulate; collaborate with health care provider and/or physical therapist for activity order.
Tube occlusion	Pulverized medications given per tube	Irrigate with 30 mL of water before and after each medication per tube.[a] Use liquid medications when available. Completely dissolve crushed medications in liquid if liquid medication is unavailable.
	Sedimentation of formula	Shake cans well before administering (read label).
	Reaction of incompatible medications or formula	Read pharmacological information on compatibility of drugs and formula.
Tube displacement	Coughing, vomiting	Replace tube and confirm placement before restarting tube feeding.
	Not taped securely	With placement verification check that tape is secure (nasoenteric).
Abdominal cramping, nausea/vomiting	High osmolality of formula	Suggest an isotonic formula or dilution of current formula to health care provider.
	Rapid increase in rate/volume	Lower rate of delivery to increase tolerance. Maintain head of bed at least 45 degrees.
	Lactose intolerance	Suggest use of lactose-free formula.
	Intestinal obstruction	Stop feeding with GI obstruction.
	High-fat formula used	Use greater proportion of carbohydrate.
	Cold formula used	Warm formula to room temperature.
Delayed gastric emptying	Diabetic gastroparesis	Consult with health care provider regarding prokinetic medication for increasing gastric motility.
	Serious illnesses	Consult health care provider regarding advancing tube to intestinal placement.
	Inactivity	Monitor medications and pathological conditions that affect GI motility.
Serum electrolyte imbalance	Excess GI losses Dehydration Presence of disease states such as cirrhosis, renal insufficiency, heart failure, or diabetes mellitus	Monitor serum electrolyte levels daily. Provide free water per registered dietitian recommendation.
Fluid overload	Refeeding syndrome in malnutrition	Restrict fluids if necessary and use either a specialized formula or a diluted enteral formula at first.
	Excess free water or diluted (hypotonic) formula	Monitor levels of serum proteins and electrolytes. Use more concentrated formula with fluid volume excess without risk of refeeding syndrome.
Hyperosmolar dehydration	Hypertonic formula with insufficient free water	Slow rate of delivery, dilute, or change to isotonic formula.

[a]First, check for fluid-restricted conditions that affect how much water can be given safely.
GI, Gastrointestinal.

TABLE 45.8 Metabolic Complications of Parenteral Nutrition

Problem	Signs/Symptoms	Intervention
Electrolyte imbalance	See Chapter 42 for signs of deficiency/toxicity	Check TPN for supplemental electrolyte levels. Notify health care provider of imbalances. Maintain steady rate of infusion. Monitor intake and output.
Hypercapnia	Increased oxygen consumption, CO_2, respiratory quotient (>1), and minute ventilation	Patients who are dependent on a ventilator are at risk; provide 30% to 60% of energy requirements per health care provider's order.
Hypoglycemia	Diaphoresis, shakiness, confusion, loss of consciousness	To prevent hypoglycemia, do not abruptly discontinue TPN but taper rate down to within 10% of infusion rate 1 to 2 hours before stopping. If you suspect hypoglycemia, test blood glucose and administer IV bolus of 50% dextrose or glucagon per order or protocol if necessary.
Hyperglycemia	Thirst, headache, lethargy, increased urination	Monitor blood glucose level every 6 hours. Initiate TPN slowly and taper up to maximal infusion rate to prevent hyperglycemia. Additional insulin may be required during therapy if problem persists or patient has diabetes mellitus.
Hyperglycemic hyperosmolar nonketotic coma (HHNKC) or hyperosmolar hyperglycemic nonketotic syndrome (HHNS)	Hyperglycemia (>500 mg/dL), glycosuria, serum osmolarity >350 mOsm/L, confusion, azotemia, headache, severe signs of dehydration (see Chapter 42), hypernatremia, metabolic acidosis, convulsions, coma	Monitor blood glucose, BUN, serum osmolarity, glucose in urine, and fluid losses; administer insulin as ordered; replace fluids as ordered; maintain constant infusion rate; and provide 30% of daily energy needs as fat. Patients at risk are those receiving steroids; older adults diagnosed with diabetes who have impaired renal or pancreatic function or increased metabolism or who are septic.

BUN, Blood urea nitrogen; *IV,* intravenous; *TPN,* total parenteral nutrition.

sections address nutritional interventions for some common disease states.

Medical Nutrition Therapy. Optimal nutrition is just as important in illness as it is in health. As a result, dietary modifications and intake are often needed to maintain the nutritional requirements of patients with certain illnesses. Medical nutrition therapy (MNT) is the use of specific nutritional therapies to treat an illness, injury, or condition. It is necessary to help the body metabolize certain nutrients, correct nutritional deficiencies related to a disease, and eliminate foods that may exacerbate disease symptoms. It is most effective using a team approach that promotes collaboration between the health care team and an RD (American Dietetic Association, 2019).

Gastrointestinal Diseases. Control peptic ulcers with regular meals and ordered medications such as histamine receptor antagonists that block secretion of HCl or proton pump inhibitors. *Helicobacter pylori* was indentified in 1984. *H. pylori,* a bacterium that causes up to 85% of peptic ulcers, is confirmed by laboratory tests or a biopsy during endoscopy (Nix, 2017). Antibiotics treat and control the bacterial infection. Stress and overproduction of gastric HCl also irritate a preexisting ulcer. Encourage patients to avoid foods that increase stomach acidity and pain such as caffeine, decaffeinated coffee, frequent milk intake, citric acid juices, and certain seasonings (hot chili peppers, chili powder, black pepper). Discourage smoking, alcohol, aspirin, and nonsteroidal antiinflammatory drugs (NSAIDs). Teach patients to eat a well-balanced, healthy diet; avoid eating large meals; and eat three regular meals (or several small meals) without snacks, especially at bedtime (Nix, 2017). Family members of the patient with *H. pylori* infection also need to be tested and, if indicated, treated.

Inflammatory bowel disease includes Crohn's disease and idiopathic ulcerative colitis. Treatment of acute inflammatory bowel disease includes elemental diets (formula with the nutrients in their simplest form ready for absorption) or PN when symptoms such as diarrhea and weight loss are prevalent. In the chronic stage of the disease, a regular highly nourishing diet is appropriate. Vitamins and iron supplements are often required to correct or prevent anemia. Patients manage inflammatory bowel syndrome by decreasing fiber, reducing fat, avoiding large meals, and avoiding lactose or sorbitol-containing foods for susceptible individuals.

The treatment of malabsorption syndromes such as celiac disease includes a gluten-free diet. Gluten is present in wheat, rye, and barley. Short-bowel syndrome results from extensive resection of the bowel, after which patients suffer from malabsorption caused by lack of intestinal surface area. These patients require lifetime feeding with either elemental enteral formulas or PN.

Diverticulitis is a condition that results from an inflammation of diverticula, which are abnormal but common pouchlike herniations that occur in the bowel lining. Nutritional treatment for diverticulitis includes a moderate- or low-residue diet until the infection subsides. Afterward, prescribing a high-fiber diet for chronic diverticula problems ensues.

Diabetes Mellitus. Type 1 DM requires both insulin and dietary management for optimal control, with treatment beginning at diagnosis (ADA, 2019). By contrast, patients often control type 2 DM initially with exercise and diet therapy. If these measures prove ineffective, it is common to add oral medications. Insulin injections often follow if type 2 DM worsens or fails to respond to these initial interventions.

Individualize the diet according to a patient's age, build, weight, and activity level. Maintaining a prescribed carbohydrate intake is the key in diabetes management. The ADA recommends a diet that includes carbohydrates from fruits, vegetables, whole grains, legumes, and low-fat milk (American Dietetic Association, 2019). Monitoring carbohydrate consumption is a key strategy in achieving glycemic control (ADA, 2019). Limit saturated fat to less than 7% of the total calories and cholesterol intake to less than 200 mg/day. In addition, varieties of foods containing fiber are recommended. Patients are able to substitute sucrose-containing foods for carbohydrates but need to make sure to avoid excess energy intake. Patients with diabetes can eat sugar alcohols and nonnutritive sweeteners as long as they follow the recommended daily intake level (ADA, 2019). Patients with diabetes and normal renal function should continue to consume usual amounts of protein (15% to 20% of energy) (ADA, 2019).

The goal of MNT treatment is to have glycemic levels that are normal or as close to normal as safely possible; lipid and lipoprotein profiles that decrease the risk of microvascular (e.g., renal and eye disease), cardiovascular, neurological, and peripheral vascular complications; and blood pressure in the normal or near-normal range (ADA, 2019). Be aware of signs and symptoms of hypoglycemia and hyperglycemia.

Cardiovascular Diseases. The goal of the American Heart Association (AHA) dietary guidelines (AHA, 2018) is to reduce risk factors for the development of hypertension and coronary artery disease. Diet therapy for reducing the risk of cardiovascular disease includes balancing calorie intake with exercise to maintain a healthy body weight; eating a diet high in fruits, vegetables, and whole-grain high-fiber foods; eating fish at least 2 times per week; and limiting food and beverages that are high in added sugar and salt. The AHA guidelines also recommend limiting saturated fat to less than 7%, trans fat to less than 1%, and cholesterol to less than 300 mg/day. To accomplish this goal, patients choose lean meats and vegetables, use fat-free dairy products, and limit intake of fats and sodium (Nix, 2017).

Cancer and Cancer Treatment. Malignant cells compete with normal cells for nutrients, increasing a patient's metabolic needs. Most cancer treatments cause nutritional problems. Patients with cancer often experience anorexia, nausea, vomiting, and taste distortions. The goal of nutritional therapy is to meet the increased metabolic needs of a patient (Nix, 2017). Malnutrition in cancer is associated with increased morbidity and mortality. Enhanced nutritional status often improves a patient's quality of life.

Radiation therapy destroys rapidly dividing malignant cells; however, normal rapidly dividing cells such as the epithelial lining of the GI tract are often affected. Radiation therapy causes anorexia, stomatitis, severe diarrhea, strictures of the intestine, and pain. Radiation treatment of the head and neck region causes taste and smell disturbances, decreased salivation, and dysphagia. Nutritional management of a patient with cancer focuses on maximizing intake of nutrients and fluids. Individualize diet choices to a patient's needs, symptoms, and situation (Nix, 2017). Use creative approaches to manage alterations in taste and smell. For example, patients with altered taste often prefer chilled foods or foods that are spicy. Encourage patients to eat small frequent meals and snacks that are nutritious and easy to digest.

Human Immunodeficiency Virus/Acquired Immunodeficiency Syndrome. Patients with HIV/AIDS typically experience body wasting and severe weight loss related to anorexia, stomatitis, oral thrush infection, nausea, or recurrent vomiting, all resulting in inadequate intake. Factors associated with weight loss and malnutrition include severe diarrhea, GI malabsorption, and altered metabolism of nutrients. Systemic infection results in hypermetabolism from cytokine elevation. The medications that treat HIV infection often cause side effects that alter patients' nutritional status.

Restorative care of malnutrition resulting from AIDS focuses on maximizing kilocalories and nutrients. Address each cause of nutritional depletion in the care plan. The progression of individually tailored nutritional support begins with administering oral, to enteral, and finally to parenteral nutrition. Good hand hygiene and food safety are essential because of a patient's reduced resistance to infection. For example, minimization of exposure to *Cryptosporidium* in drinking water, lakes, or swimming pools is important. Small, frequent, nutrient-dense meals that limit fatty and overly sweet foods are easier to tolerate. Patients benefit from eating cold foods and drier or saltier foods with fluid in between (Nix, 2017).

◆ Evaluation

Through the Patient's Eyes. Patients expect competent, timely, and accurate care. Patients also expect nurses to determine when nutritional therapies do not result in successful outcomes and alter the plan of care accordingly. Expectations and health care values held by nurses frequently differ from those held by patients. Successful interventions and outcomes require nurses to know what patients expect in addition to nursing knowledge and skill. Work closely with patients to confirm their expectations and talk with them about their concerns if their expectations are not realistic. Consider the limits of your patients' conditions and treatment, their dietary preferences, and their cultural beliefs when evaluating outcomes.

Patient Outcomes. Care plans need to reflect achievable goals and outcomes. Evaluate the actual outcomes of nursing actions and compare them with expected outcomes to determine whether the goals were met (Fig. 45.9). Interprofessional collaboration remains essential in providing nutritional support. Nutritional therapy does not always produce rapid results. You need to evaluate a patient's current weight in comparison with his or her baseline weight, serum albumin or prealbumin, and protein and kilocalorie intake routinely. If your patient does not gain weight gradually or continues to lose weight, evaluate the

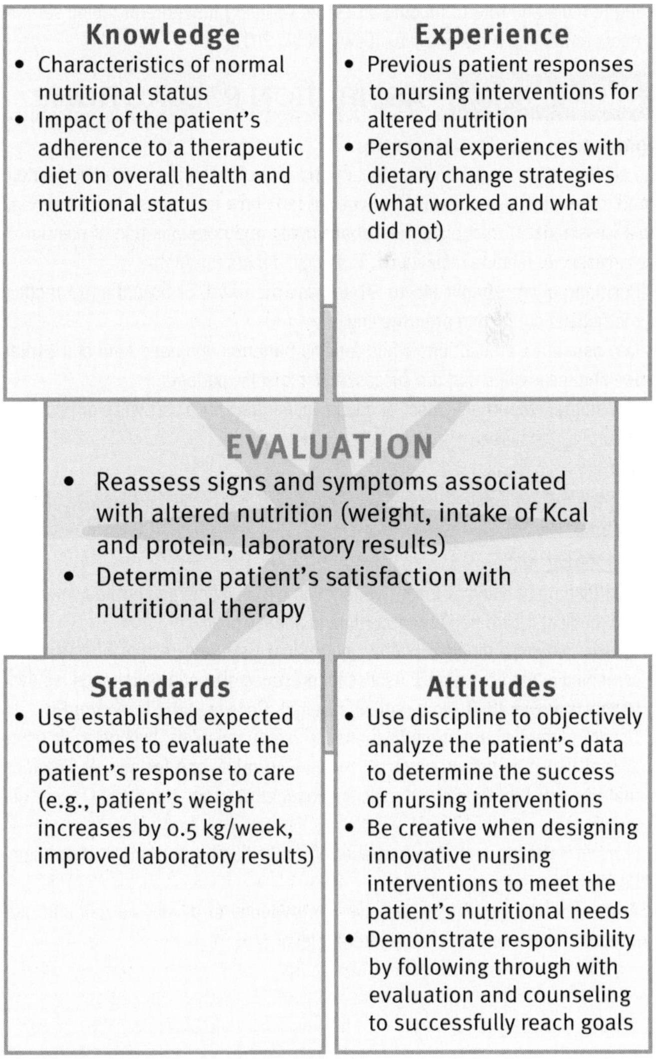

Knowledge	Experience
• Characteristics of normal nutritional status • Impact of the patient's adherence to a therapeutic diet on overall health and nutritional status	• Previous patient responses to nursing interventions for altered nutrition • Personal experiences with dietary change strategies (what worked and what did not)

EVALUATION
- Reassess signs and symptoms associated with altered nutrition (weight, intake of Kcal and protein, laboratory results)
- Determine patient's satisfaction with nutritional therapy

Standards	Attitudes
• Use established expected outcomes to evaluate the patient's response to care (e.g., patient's weight increases by 0.5 kg/week, improved laboratory results)	• Use discipline to objectively analyze the patient's data to determine the success of nursing interventions • Be creative when designing innovative nursing interventions to meet the patient's nutritional needs • Demonstrate responsibility by following through with evaluation and counseling to successfully reach goals

FIG. 45.9 Critical thinking model for nutrition evaluation.

dietary EN prescription and determine whether the patient is experiencing any adverse effects from medications that are affecting his or her nutritional status. Changes in condition also indicate a need to change the nutritional plan of care. Consult with all members of the health care team in an effort to better individualize this plan. The patient is an active participant whenever possible. In the end a patient's ability to incorporate dietary changes into his or her lifestyle with the least

amount of stress or disruption facilitates attainment of outcome measures. Failing to meet expected outcomes requires revising the nursing interventions or expected outcomes on the basis of the patient's most current nursing diagnoses. When outcomes are unmet, ask questions such as "How has your appetite been?" "Have you noticed a change in your weight?" "How much would you like to weigh?" or "Have you changed your exercise pattern?"

SAFETY GUIDELINES FOR NURSING SKILLS

Ensuring patient safety is an essential role of the professional nurse. To ensure patient safety, communicate clearly with members of the health care team, assess and incorporate a patient's priorities of care and preferences, and use the best evidence when making decisions about your patient's care. When performing the skills in this chapter, remember the following points to ensure safe, individualized patient care.

- Verify that the appropriate ENFit connector is attached to the enteral tube when administering tube feedings (TJC, 2018).
- Use aseptic technique when preparing and delivering enteral feedings. Check agency policy for wearing gloves when handling feedings (Lewis et al., 2017).
- Label enteral equipment with patient name and room number; formula name, rate, and date and time of initiation; and nurse initials (Lewis et al., 2017).
- Practice "right patient, right formula, right tube, right ENFit adapter" by matching formula and rate to feeding order and verifying that enteral tubing set connects formula to a feeding tube (Lewis et al., 2017).

- Position the patient upright or elevate the head of the bed a minimum of 30 (preferably 45) degrees unless medically contraindicated for patients receiving enteral feedings (Lewis et al., 2017).
- Trace all lines and tubing back to the patient to ensure only enteral-to-enteral connections (Lewis et al., 2017).
- Do not add food coloring or dye to EN because the use of dye has been linked to hypotension, metabolic acidosis, and death (Lewis et al., 2017).
- Refer to manufacturer guidelines to determine hang time for enteral feedings. Maximum hang time for formula is 8 hours in an open system and 24 to 48 hours in a closed, ready-to-hang system (if it remains closed). There is increased risk of bacterial growth in feedings that exceed the recommended hang time.
- Always use an infusion pump for continuous enteral feedings and PN.
- Be alert for signs of aspiration during oral feedings as well as when EN is administered.

SKILL 45.1   ASPIRATION PRECAUTIONS

Delegation and Collaboration

The skill of following aspiration precautions while feeding a patient can be delegated to assistive personnel (AP). However, the nurse is responsible for the ongoing assessment of a patient's risk for aspiration and determination of positioning and any special feeding techniques. The nurse directs the AP to:

- Position patient upright (45 to 90 degrees preferred) or according to medical restrictions during and after feeding.
- Use aspiration precautions while feeding patients who need help and explain feeding techniques that are successful for specific patients.
- Immediately report any onset of coughing, gagging, or a wet voice or pocketing of food to the nurse.

Equipment

- Chair or bed that allows patient to sit upright
- Thickening agents as ordered by SLP (rice, cereal, yogurt, gelatin, commercial thickener)
- Tongue blade
- Penlight
- Oral hygiene supplies (see Chapter 40)
- Suction equipment (see Chapter 41)
- Clean gloves
- *Option:* Pulse oximeter

STEP	RATIONALE
ASSESSMENT	
1. Identify patient using at least two identifiers (e.g., name and birthday or name and medical record number) according to agency policy.	Ensures correct patient. Complies with The Joint Commission standards and improves patient safety (TJC, 2020).
2. Review patient's medical history, nutritional risks and results of nutritional screening in medical record. Assess for presence of conditions that cause dysphagia (see Box 45.7). Note patient's weight. Consult with SLP and/or RD.	Reveals patient risk patterns for altered nutrition and dysphagia. Weight provides baseline for determining change in nutritional status.
3. Assess patient's current medications for use of sedatives, hypnotics, or other agents that may impair cough or swallowing reflex and for any medications that dry oral secretions (e.g., calcium channel blockers, diuretics) (Tan et al., 2018).	Medication side effects may increase risk of developing dysphagia.
4. Perform hand hygiene. Assess patient for signs and symptoms of dysphagia. Consult with SLP.	Patient symptoms aid in determining whether further swallow evaluation is needed and approach to feeding.
5. Assess patient's or family caregiver's knowledge of dysphagia risk and diet options, experience, and health literacy level.	Ensures patient has the capacity to obtain, communicate, process, and understand basic health information (CDC, 2016).

STEP	RATIONALE
6. Assess patient's mental status: alertness, orientation, and ability to follow simple commands (e.g., open your mouth; stick out your tongue).	Disorientation and inability to follow commands present higher risk for dysphagia.
7. Apply gloves. Assess patient's oral cavity, level of dental hygiene, missing teeth, or poorly fitting dentures. Remove and dispose of gloves.	Poorly fitting dentures and absence of teeth can cause chewing and swallowing difficulties, increasing aspiration risk. Poor oral hygiene and periodontal disease can result in growth of bacteria in oropharynx, which if aspirated, can lead to pneumonia (Liantonio et al., 2014). Findings indicate level of oral hygiene needed and diet selection needed.
8. *Option:* Obtain baseline assessment oxygen saturation. A decline in SpO_2 ≥2% has been regarded as a possible marker of aspiration (Marian et al., 2017). Perform hand hygiene.	Despite its clinical use, research findings question whether oximetry can reliably detect aspiration (American Speech-Language-Hearing Association [ASHA], 2016; Lancaster, 2015; Marian et al., 2017).
9. Prepare to observe patient during mealtime for signs of dysphagia. Observe patient attempt to feed self; note type of food consistencies and liquids able to swallow. Note during and at end of meal if patient tires.	Detects abnormal eating patterns such as frequent clearing of throat or prolonged eating time. Chewing and sitting up for feeding bring on onset of fatigue (Meiner and Yeager, 2019). Provides data for future planning of meal assistance.
10. Indicate in patient's health record that dysphagia/aspiration risk is present. *Option:* Some agencies use different-colored meal trays to signify patients at risk for aspiration.	Identifying patients with dysphagia reduces risk that they will receive improperly prepared oral nutrition without supervision.

PLANNING

1. Provide patient rest time before meals.	Some practitioners recommend rest time before meals (Metheny, 2012). Muscle weakness and fatigue may increase risk of aspiration.
2. Explain to patient why you are observing him or her while eating.	Signs or symptoms associated with aspiration indicate need for further swallowing evaluation such as fluoroscopic examination.
3. Explain to patient and family caregiver about the aspiration precautions you are implementing.	Increases patient cooperation and prepares family caregiver for being able to assist.

IMPLEMENTATION

1. Perform hand hygiene and have patient or family caregiver (if going to help with feeding) perform hand hygiene.	Prevents transmission of microorganisms. Educates patient and family caregiver about need to maintain infection control practices.
2. Apply clean gloves. Use penlight and tongue blade to gently inspect mouth for pockets of food.	Pockets of food found inside cheeks occur when patient has difficulty moving food from mouth into pharynx; may lead to aspiration (Zupec-Kania and O'Flaherty, 2017). Patient is usually unaware of pocketing.
3. Provide thorough oral hygiene, including brushing tongue, before meal (see Chapter 40). Remove and dispose of gloves, perform hand hygiene.	Risk for aspiration pneumonia has been associated with poor oral hygiene (Liantonio et al., 2014).
4. Position patient upright (90 degrees) in chair or elevate head of patient's bed to a 90-degree angle or highest position allowed by medical condition during meal.	Position facilitates safe swallowing and enhances esophageal motility (Liantonio et al., 2014; Metheny and Frantz, 2013). Side-lying position is an option if patient cannot have head elevated.
5. *Option:* Apply pulse oximeter to patient's finger; monitor during feeding.	Pulse oximetry continues to be used in many agencies in an effort to predict aspiration, but recent research questions its efficacy (ASHA, 2016; Marian et al., 2017)
6. Provide appropriate thickness of liquids per SLP and RD assessment (International Dysphagia Diet Standardisation Initiative, 2016). Encourage patient to feed self.	Thin liquids are difficult to control in mouth and pharynx and are more easily aspirated.
7. Have patient assume chin-down position. Remind patient to not tilt head backward when eating or while drinking.	Chin-down position may help reduce aspiration (Kagaya et al., 2011; Liantonio et al., 2014). One study suggests a head-turn-plus-chin-down maneuver may be more successful (Nagy et al., 2016).
8. Adjust the rate of feeding and size of bites to match the patient's tolerance. If patient unable to feed self, place ½ to 1 teaspoon of food on unaffected side of mouth, allowing utensil to touch mouth or tongue (Liantonio et al., 2014).	Small bites help patient swallow (Liantonio et al., 2014). Provides tactile cue to food being eaten; avoids pocketing of food on weaker side.
9. Provide verbal coaching: remind patient to chew and think about swallowing with comments such as the ones that follow. Open your mouth. Feel the food in your mouth. Chew and taste the food. Raise your tongue to the roof of your mouth. Think about swallowing. Close your mouth and swallow. Swallow again. Cough to clear your airway.	Verbal cueing keeps patient focused on normal swallowing (Metheny, 2012). Positive reinforcement enhances patient's confidence in ability to swallow.
10. Avoid mixing food of different textures in same mouthful. Alternate liquids and bites of food (Liantonio et al., 2014). Refer to RD for next meal if patient has difficulty with particular consistency.	Gradual increase in types and textures combined with constant monitoring helps patient to eat more safely. Single textures are easier to swallow than multiple textures. Alternating solids with liquids removes food residue in mouth.

Continued

SKILL 45.1	ASPIRATION PRECAUTIONS—cont'd

STEP	RATIONALE
11. During the meal explain to patient and family caregiver the techniques being used to promote swallowing.	Enhances patient and family caregiver's ability to use techniques in the home.
12. Monitor swallowing and observe for any respiratory difficulty. Observe for throat clearing, coughing, choking, gagging, and drooling of food; suction airway as needed (see Chapter 41).	These are indications that suggest dysphagia and thus pose risk for aspiration (National Stroke Association, 2017).
13. Minimize distractions, do not talk, and do not rush patient (Liantonio et al., 2014). Allow time for adequate chewing and swallowing. Provide rest periods as needed during meal.	Environmental distractions and conversations during mealtime increase risk for aspiration. Avoiding fatigue reduces aspiration risk.

CLINICAL DECISION: *If patient remains stable without difficulty, this is good time to delegate continued feeding to AP so that you can attend to other patients and assigned priorities.*

STEP	RATIONALE
14. Use sauces, condiments, and gravies (if part of dysphagia diet) to facilitate cohesive food bolus formation.	Cohesive food bolus helps to prevent pocketing or small food particles from entering the airway.
15. Ask patient to remain sitting upright for at least 30 to 60 minutes after a meal. Provide nurse call system to patient and instruct patient to utilize if needed	Remaining upright after meals or snack reduces chance of aspiration by allowing food particles remaining in pharynx to clear (Metheny, 2012). Promotes patient safety.
16. Apply gloves. Provide thorough oral hygiene after meal (see Chapter 40).	Rigorous oral hygiene reduces plaque and secretions containing bacteria, with studies showing reduction in incidence of pneumonia (Liantonio et al., 2014).
17. Return patient's tray to appropriate place. Remove and dispose of gloves.	Reduces spread of microorganisms.
18. Raise side rails (as appropriate) and lower bed to lowest position. Perform hand hygiene	Promotes patient safety. Reduces transmission of microorganisms.

EVALUATION

1. Observe patient's ability to swallow food and fluids of various textures and thickness without choking.	Indicates whether there is ease with swallowing and absence of signs related to aspiration.
2. Monitor pulse oximetry readings (if ordered) for high-risk patients during eating.	Deteriorating oxygen saturation levels may indicate aspiration, but current research questions predictive accuracy of oximetry.
3. Monitor patient's intake and output (I&O), calorie count, and food intake.	Helps to detect malnutrition and dehydration resulting from dysphagia.
4. Weigh patient daily or weekly.	Determines whether weight is stable and reflects nutritional status.
5. Observe patient's oral cavity after meal.	Determines presence of food pockets after meal that has included foods of various textures.
6. **Use Teach-Back:** "We talked about why your husband is at risk to aspirate his food. Tell me the things to observe for that will tell you if he is having trouble swallowing. What should you do if these things happen during a meal?" Revise your instruction now or develop a plan for revised patient/family caregiver teaching if patient/family caregiver is not able to teach back correctly.	Determines patient's/family caregiver's level of understanding of instructional topic.

UNEXPECTED OUTCOMES AND RELATED INTERVENTIONS

1. Patient coughs, gags, complains of food "stuck in throat," and has wet quality to voice when eating.
   - Stop feeding immediately and place patient on NPO.
   - Notify health care provider and suction as needed (see Chapter 41).
   - Anticipate consultation with SLP for swallowing exercises and techniques to improve swallowing.
2. Patient experiences weight loss over next several days/weeks.
   - Discuss findings with health care provider and RD. Determine whether increasing frequency or quality of foods is needed.
   - Nutritional supplements may be needed.

RECORDING AND REPORTING

- Record patient's diet, tolerance of liquids and food textures, amount of assistance required, response to instruction, position during meal, absence or presence of any symptoms of dysphagia, fluid intake, and amount of food eaten.
- Document your evaluation of patient learning.
- Report patient's tolerance to diet and degree of assistance required during hand-off report.
- Report any coughing, gagging, choking, or swallowing difficulties to nurse in charge or health care provider immediately.

HOME CARE CONSIDERATIONS

- Teach the patient and family the importance of frequent small meals with small bites and balancing with MNT.
- Teach patient and family how to recognize problems in swallowing.
- Teach patient and family about when to seek medical attention and what to report to the health care provider.

SKILL 45.2 — INSERTING AND REMOVING A SMALL-BORE NASOENTERIC TUBE FOR ENTERAL FEEDINGS

Delegation and Collaboration

The skill of feeding tube insertion cannot be delegated to assistive personnel (AP). However, AP may help with patient positioning and comfort measures during tube insertion.

Equipment (Insertion)

- Small-bore feeding tube with or without stylet (select the smallest diameter possible to enhance patient comfort)
- 60-mL ENFit syringe
- Stethoscope, pulse oximeter, capnography *(optional)*
- Hypoallergenic tape, semipermeable (transparent) dressing, or tube fixation device
- Tincture of benzoin or other skin barrier protectant
- pH indicator strip (scale 1.0 to 11.0)
- Cup of water and straw or ice chips (for patients able to swallow)
- Water-soluble lubricant
- Emesis basin
- Towel or disposable pad
- Facial tissues
- Clean gloves
- Suction equipment in case of aspiration
- Penlight to check placement in nasopharynx
- Tongue blade
- Oral hygiene supplies
- Measuring tape

Equipment (Removal)

- Disposable pad
- Tissues
- Clean gloves
- Disposable plastic bag
- Towel

STEP	RATIONALE

ASSESSMENT

1. Verify health care provider's order for type of tube and EN feeding schedule. Also check order to determine whether health care provider wants prokinetic agent (e.g., metoclopramide) given before tube placement.

   Health care provider's order is needed to insert feeding tube. Prokinetic agent given before tube placement may help advance tube (if it is to be advanced into intestine).

2. Identify patient using at least two identifiers (e.g., name and birthday or name and medical record number) according to agency policy.

   Ensures correct patient. Complies with The Joint Commission standards and improves patient safety (TJC, 2020).

3. Review patient's medical history (e.g., for basilar skull fracture, nasal problems, nosebleeds, facial trauma, nasal-facial surgery, deviated septum, anticoagulant therapy, coagulopathy).

   History of these problems may require you to consult with health care provider to change route of nutritional support. Passage of tube intracranially can cause neurological injury.

CLINICAL DECISION: *If a patient is at risk for intracranial passage of the tube, avoid the nasal route. Oral placement or placement under medical supervision using fluoroscopic direct visualization is preferable. Insertion of a gastrostomy or jejunostomy tube is another alternative.*

---

4. Assess patient's height, weight, hydration status, electrolyte balance, caloric needs and intake and output (I&O).

   Provides baseline information to measure nutritional improvement after enteral feedings.

5. Perform hand hygiene. Have patient close each nostril alternately and breathe. Examine each naris for patency and skin breakdown (apply clean gloves if drainage present). If patient previously had NG tube, check for medical device related pressure injury (see illustration).

   Reduces transmission of microorganisms. Nares can sometimes be obstructed or irritated, or septal defect or facial fractures are present. Place tube in most patent naris.

6. Perform physical assessment of abdomen (see Chapter 30). Remove and dispose of gloves (if worn). Perform hand hygiene.

   Absent bowel sounds, abdominal pain, tenderness, or distention may indicate medical problem contraindicating feedings. Reduces transmission of microorganisms.

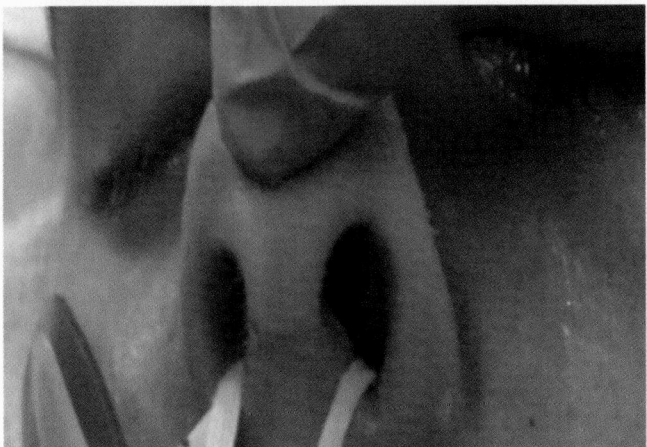

STEP 5 Medical device–related pressure injury under nose.

Continued

SKILL 45.2 **INSERTING AND REMOVING A SMALL-BORE NASOENTERIC TUBE FOR ENTERAL FEEDINGS—cont'd**

STEP	RATIONALE
7. Assess patient's knowledge and health literacy level.	Ensures patient has the capacity to obtain, communicate, process, and understand basic health information (CDC, 2019).
8. Assess patient's mental status (ability to cooperate with procedure, level of sedation), presence of cough and gag reflex, ability to swallow, critical illness, and presence of artificial airway.	These are risk factors for inadvertent tube placement into tracheobronchial tree (Metheny, 2012). Sedation impairs the ability of the patient to clear contents in the pharynx, thus increasing the risk of aspiration (Boullata et al., 2017).
9. Assess patient's experience with procedure and expectations.	Provides data to determine level of instruction needed.

CLINICAL DECISION: *Recognize situations in which blind placement of a feeding tube poses an unacceptable risk for placement. Devices designed to detect pulmonary intubation such as CO_2 sensors or electromagnetic tracking devices enhance patient safety. Alternatively, to avoid insertion complications from blind placement in high-risk situations, clinicians trained in the use of visualization or imaging techniques should place tubes (Metheny and Meert, 2017; Milsom et al., 2015).*

PLANNING

1. Provide privacy and prepare bedside environment for patient safety.	Promotes patient comfort and safety.
2. Prepare and organize equipment needed for insertion of NG feeding tube.	Ensures an organized approach for insertion of NG feeding tube.
3. Explain procedure to patient, including sensations anticipated during insertion (burning in nasal passages) and to raise index finger to indicate gagging or discomfort during insertion	Reduces anxiety and helps patient assist in insertion.

IMPLEMENTATION

1. Perform hand hygiene. Stand on same side of bed as naris chosen for insertion and position patient upright in high-Fowler's position (unless contraindicated). If patient is comatose, raise head of bed as tolerated in semi-Fowler's position with head tipped forward, using a pillow chin to chest. If necessary have an AP help with positioning of confused or comatose patients. If patient is forced to lie supine, place in reverse Trendelenburg's position.	Reduces transmission of microorganisms. Allows for easier manipulation of tube. Fowler's position reduces risk of aspiration and promotes effective swallowing. Forward head position helps with closure of airway and passage of tube into esophagus.
2. Apply pulse oximeter/capnograph and measure vital signs. Maintain oximetry or capnography continuously.	Provides baseline for objective assessment of respiratory status during tube insertion and throughout time a tube is in place. Lowered oxygen saturation or increased end-tidal CO_2 can indicate tube being misplaced into the lungs or moving out of the stomach into lungs (Holland et al., 2013).

CLINICAL DECISION: *If patient has increase in end-tidal carbon dioxide or decrease in oxygen saturation, tube should not be inserted until you determine patient stability.*

3. Place bath towel over patient's chest. Keep facial tissues within reach.	Prevents soiling of gown. Insertion of tube frequently produces tearing.
4. Determine length of tube to be inserted and mark location with tape or indelible ink. Some tubes have centimeter markings.	Ensures organized procedure and estimation of the proper length of tube to insert into patient.
a. *Option, Adult:* Measure distance from tip of nose to earlobe to xyphoid process (NEX) of sternum (see illustration). Mark this distance on tube with tape.	Most traditional method. Length approximates distance from nose to stomach. Research has shown this method may be least effective compared with others, though more research is needed (Santos et al., 2016).

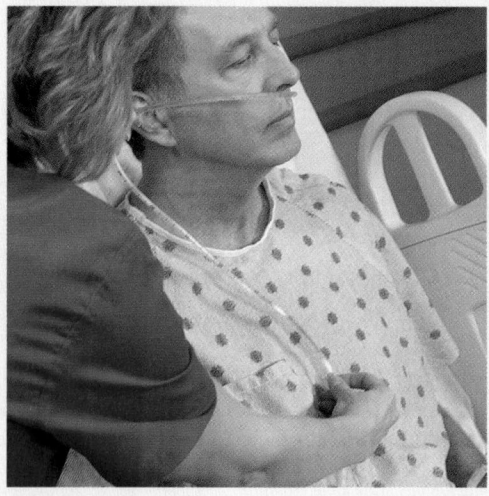

STEP 4a Measure to determine length of tube to insert. (Copyright © Mosby's Clinical Skills: Essentials Collection.)

STEP	RATIONALE

b. *Option, Adult:* A nose to earlobe to mid-umbilicus (NEMU) method to estimate appropriate nasogastric tube placement has been recommended.

Promotes placement of the tube end holes in or closer to the gastric fluid pool (Boullata et al., 2017).

c. *Option, Adult:* Measure distance from xyphoid process to earlobe to nose (XEN) + 10 cm (Taylor et al., 2014).

Shown to be more accurate than NEX (Taylor et al., 2014).

d. *Option, Children:* Use NEMU option.

Estimates proper length of tube insertion for pediatric patient.

e. Add 20 to 30 cm (8 to 12 inches) for post-pyloric tubes.

Length approximates distance from nose to jejunum.

CLINICAL DECISION: *Tip of pre-pyloric tubes must reach stomach to avoid the risk for pulmonary aspiration, which occurs when tubes end instead in the esophagus. Research has mixed findings regarding the best technique for estimating tube length (Santos et al., 2016). Confirmation of placement via x-ray immediately after completed insertion is still needed.*

---

5. Prepare tube for intubation.

NOTE: Do not ice tubes.

Iced tube becomes stiff and inflexible, causing trauma to nasal mucosa.

a. Obtain order for stylet tube and check agency policy for trained clinician to insert tube.

The practice of inserting a tube requires great care and attention to practice guidelines.

b. If tube has guidewire or stylet, inject 10 mL of water from ENFit syringe into tube.

Aids in guidewire or stylet removal. Activates lubrication of tube for easier passage and ensures that tube is patent. ENFit devices are not compatible with Luer connection or any other type of small-bore medical connector, thus preventing misadministration of an enteral feeding (ISMP, 2015).

c. If using stylet, make certain that it is positioned securely within tube. Inject 10 mL of water from ENFit syringe into tube.

Promotes smooth passage of tube into gastrointestinal (GI) tract. Improperly positioned stylet can cause tube to kink or injure patient. Ensures that tube is patent and aids in stylet removal. Once tube insertion is confirmed, have trained clinician remove stylet.

6. Prepare tube fixation materials. Cut hypoallergenic tape 10 cm (4 inches) long or prepare membrane dressing or other tube fixation device (e.g., bridle).

Used to secure tubing after insertion. Fixation devices allow tube to float free of nares, thus reducing pressure on nares, preventing device-related pressure injury (DRPI).

7. Apply clean gloves.

Reduces transmission of microorganisms.

8. *Option:* Dip tube with surface lubricant into glass of room-temperature water or apply water-soluble lubricant (see manufacturer directions).

Activates lubricant to facilitate passage of tube into naris and GI tract.

9. Offer an patient a cup of water with straw (if alert and able to swallow).

Patient is asked to swallow water to facilitate tube passage.

10. Explain next steps and gently insert tube through nostril to back of throat (posterior nasopharynx). This may cause patient to gag. Aim back and down toward ear (see illustration).

Natural contours facilitate passage of tube into GI tract.

11. Have patient take deep breath, relax, and flex head toward chest after tube has passed through nasopharynx.

Closes off glottis and reduces risk for tube entering trachea.

12. Encourage patient to swallow small sips of water. Advance tube as patient swallows. Rotate tube gently 180 degrees while inserting.

Swallowing water lubricates and facilitates passage of tube into esophagus. Distinct tug may be felt as patient swallows, indicating that tube is following expected path. Tube rotation redirects the tip of tube away from glottis.

13. Emphasize need to mouth breathe and swallow during insertion.

Helps facilitate passage of tube and alleviates patient's fears during procedure.

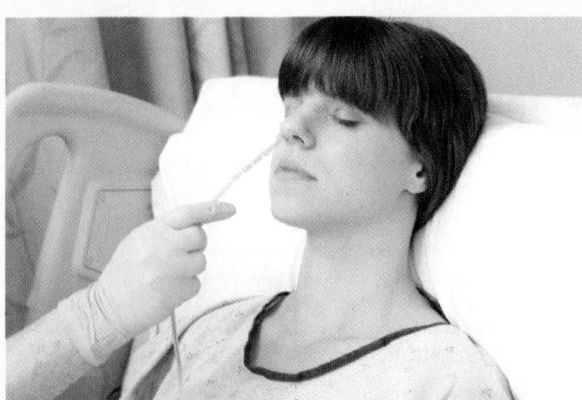

STEP 10 Insert tube through nostril to back of throat.

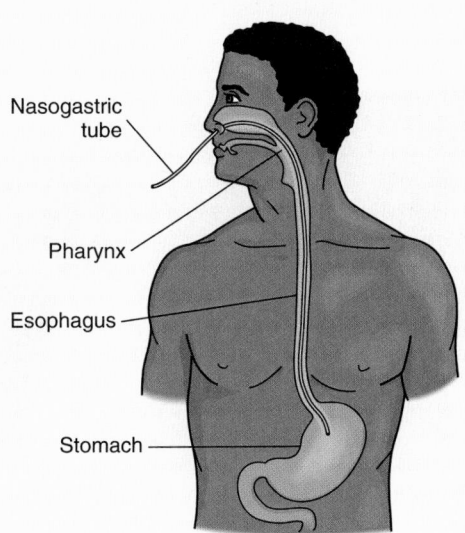

STEP 15 NG tube inserted through nasopharynx and esophagus into stomach.

Continued

STEP	RATIONALE
14. Do not advance tube during inspiration or coughing because it is more likely to enter respiratory tract. Monitor oximetry and capnography at this time.	Can cause tube to inadvertently enter patient's airway, which will be reflected in changes in oxygen saturation and/or capnography.
15. Advance tube each time patient swallows until desired length has been reached (see illustration).	Reduces discomfort and trauma to patient. Helps facilitate tube passage.

CLINICAL DECISION: *Do not force the tube or push against resistance. If patient starts to cough, experiences a drop in oxygen saturation, rise in end-tidal CO_2, or shows other signs of respiratory distress, withdraw the tube into the posterior nasopharynx until normal breathing resumes.*

STEP	RATIONALE
16. Check for position of tube in back of throat using penlight and tongue blade.	Tube may be coiled, kinked, or entering trachea.
17. Temporarily anchor tube to nose with small piece of tape.	Movement of tube stimulates gagging. Assesses general position before anchoring tube more securely.
18. Keep tube secure and check its placement by aspirating stomach contents to measure gastric pH (see Box 45.14). Also measure amount, color, and quality of return.	Provides baseline for appearance and pH of aspirate at initial location before x-ray confirmatiion.

CLINICAL DECISION: *Insufflation of air into tube while auscultating abdomen is not a reliable means to determine position of feeding tube tip (Bourgault et al., 2015).*

STEP	RATIONALE
19. Anchor tube to patient's nose, avoiding pressure on nares. Mark exit site on tube with indelible ink. Select one of the following options for anchoring:	Marking tube can alert nurses to possible displacement of tube. Properly secured tube allows patient more mobility and prevents trauma to nasal mucosa (Matheny, 2016).
a. Apply membrane dressing or tube fixation device:	Permits longer securement without need to change dressing.
(1) Membrane dressing:	Allows membrane to adhere to skin.
(a) Apply tincture of benzoin or other skin protector to patient's cheek and area of tube to be secured.	Used to protect the skin from irritation and infection.
(b) Place tube against patient's cheek and secure tube with membrane dressing, out of patient's line of vision.	Eliminates application of tape around naris. Decreases risk for patient's inadvertent extubation.
(2) Tube fixation device:	Secures tube and reduces friction on naris.
(a) Apply wide end of patch to bridge of nose (see illustration).	
(b) Slip connector around feeding tube as it exits nose (see illustration).	
b. Apply tape:	Prevents pulling of tube. May require frequent change if tape becomes soiled.
(1) Apply tincture of benzoin or other skin adhesive on tip of patient's nose and allow it to become "tacky."	Helps tape adhere better. Protects skin from breakdown.
(2) Remove gloves and tear two horizontal slits on each side of tape at ⅓ and ⅔ length. Do not split tape. Fold middle sections forward.	Creates a gap in tape that once secured will allow tube to float and exert less pressure on naris.
(3) Tear vertical strip at bottom of tape. Print date and time on nasal part of tape.	Secures tube firmly and provides date of insertion.

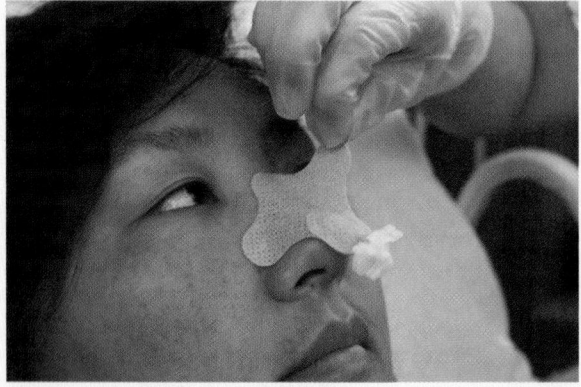

STEP 19a(2)(a) Apply tube fixation device to bridge of nose.

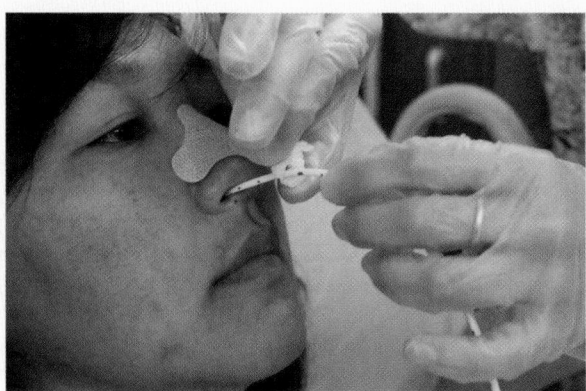

STEP 19a(2)(b) Slip connector around feeding tube.

STEP	RATIONALE
(4) Place intact end of tape over bridge of patient's nose. Wrap each strip around tube as it exits (see illustration).	Tube is free floating in the naris with this taping method, resulting in movement of tube in pharynx. Securing tape to naris in this method reduces pressure on naris and risk for medical device–related pressure injury (Markowitz et al., 2013).
20. Fasten end of tube to patient's gown using clip (see illustration) or piece of tape. Do not use safety pins to secure tube to gown.	Reduces traction on naris if tube moves, which can cause medical device–related pressure injury. Safety pins become unfastened and cause injury to patients.
21. Help patient to comfortable position but keep head of the bed elevated at least 30 degrees (preferably 45 degrees) unless contraindicated (Schallom et al., 2015).	Promotes patient comfort and lowers risk of aspiration should patient receive tube feeding.
22. Remove gloves and perform hand hygiene.	Reduces transmission of microorganisms.

CLINICAL DECISION: *Leave stylet in place until correct position is verified by x-ray film. Never reinsert a partially or fully removed stylet while feeding tube is in place. This can cause perforation of tube and injure patient. Contact the health care provider if problems arise with feeding tube.*

STEP	RATIONALE
23. Contact radiology to obtain x-ray film of chest/abdomen.	Radiographic examination is most accurate method to determine feeding-tube placement (Milsom et al., 2015).
24. Perform hand hygiene. Apply clean gloves and administer oral hygiene (see Chapter 40). Clean tubing at nostril with washcloth dampened in mild soap and water.	Promotes patient comfort and integrity of oral mucous membranes. Reduces transmission of microorganisms.
25. Remove and dispose of equipment, remove and dispose of gloves, and perform hand hygiene.	Reduces transmission of microorganisms.
26. Place nurse call system in an accessible location within patient's reach. Instruct patient in its use.	Promotes patient safety.
27. Raise side rails as appropriate and lower bed to lowest position.	Promotes patient safety.
28. Tube Removal	
a. Verify health care provider's order for tube removal.	Health care provider's order is needed to remove feeding tube.
b. Gather equipment.	Ensures organized procedure.
c Explain procedure to patient.	Encourages cooperation, reduces anxiety, and minimizes risks. Identifies teaching needs.
d. Perform hand hygiene. Apply clean gloves.	Reduces transmission of microorganisms.
e. Position patient in high-Fowler's position unless contraindicated.	Reduces risk for pulmonary aspiration in event patient should vomit.
f. Place disposable pad or towel over patient's chest.	Prevents mucus and gastric secretions from soiling patient's clothing.
g. Disconnect tube from feeding administration set (if present), and clamp or cap end.	Prevents formula from spilling from tube as it is removed.

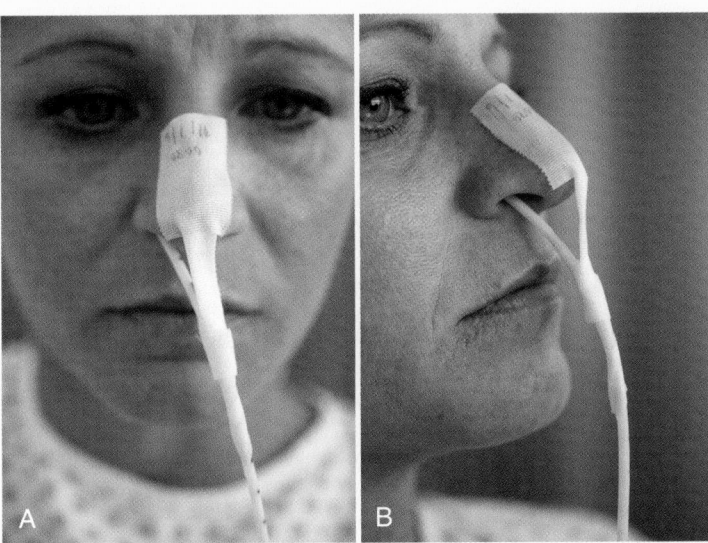

STEP 19b(4) A, Applying tape to anchor nasoenteral tube. **B,** Naris is free of pressure from tape and tube.

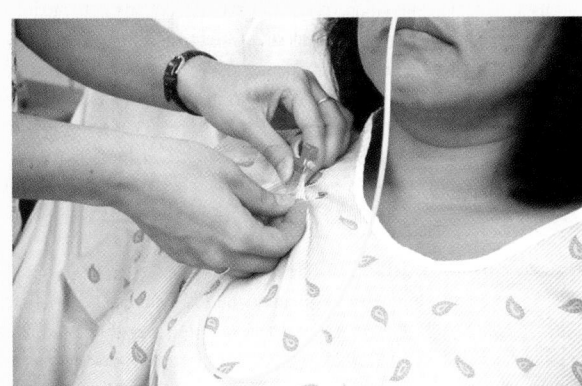

STEP 20 Fasten feeding tube to patient's gown.

Continued

SKILL 45.2	INSERTING AND REMOVING A SMALL-BORE NASOENTERIC TUBE FOR ENTERAL FEEDINGS—cont'd

STEP	RATIONALE
h. Remove tape or tube fixation device from patient's nose. Unclip tube from patient's gown.	Allows tube to be removed easily.
i. Instruct patient to take deep breath and hold it. Then as you kink end of tube securely (folding it over on itself), completely withdraw tube by pulling it out steadily and smoothly onto towel or disposable bag. Dispose of it into appropriate receptacle.	Prevents inadvertent aspiration of gastric contents while tube is removed. Kinking prevents leakage of fluid from tube. Promotes patient comfort. Reduces transmission of microorganisms.
j. Offer tissues to patient to blow nose.	Clears nasal passages of remaining secretions.
k. Offer mouth care.	Promotes patient's comfort.
l. Remove and dispose of gloves; perform hand hygiene.	Reduces transmission of microorganisms.

EVALUATION

1. Observe patient's response to tube placement. Assess lung sounds; have patient speak; check vital signs; note any coughing, dyspnea, cyanosis, or decrease in oxygen saturation or increase in end-tidal CO_2.	Symptoms may indicate placement in respiratory tract. Auscultation of crackles, wheezes, dyspnea, or fever may be delayed response to aspiration. Lowered oxygen saturation or increased end-tidal CO_2 may detect tip of tube is in trachea or lung.
2. Confirm radiographic film results with health care provider.	Verifies position of tube before initiating enteral feeding.
3. Remove stylet after x-ray film verification of correct placement. Review agency policy regarding requirement of trained clinician for insertion.	If placement needs adjustment, stylet is still in place and contact health care provider.
4. Check condition of nares, location of external exit site marking on tube, and color and pH of fluid aspirated from tube per agency policy.	Routine evaluation ensures no formation of medical device–related pressure injury and correct placement of tube.
5. Assess patient's level of comfort after removal.	Provides for continued comfort of patient.
6. **Use Teach-Back:** "I want to be sure that I explained to you what you can do during insertion of the nasogastric tube so that you can communicate with me. Tell me how you are going to communicate with me during tube insertion." Revise your instruction now or develop a plan for revised patient/family caregiver teaching if patient/family caregiver is not able to teach back correctly.	Determines patient's/family caregiver's level of understanding of instructional topic.

UNEXPECTED OUTCOMES AND RELATED INTERVENTIONS

1. Aspiration of stomach contents into respiratory tract (delayed response or small-volume aspiration), evidenced by auscultation of crackles or wheezes, dyspnea, or fever
   - Report change in patient condition to health care provider immediately; if there has not been a recent chest x-ray film, suggest ordering one.
   - Position patient on side to protect airway.
   - Suction nasotracheally and orotracheally (Chapter 41).
   - Prepare for possible initiation of antibiotics.
2. Displacement of feeding tube to another site (e.g., from duodenum to stomach) possibly occurs when patient coughs or vomits.
   - Aspirate GI contents and measure pH.
   - Remove displaced tube and insert and verify placement of new tube.
   - If there is question of aspiration, obtain chest x-ray film.

RECORDING AND REPORTING

- Tube insertion: Record procedure and report type and size of tube placed; location of distal tip of tube; patient's tolerance of procedure; confirmation of tube position by x-ray film examination; length of tube that extends from nostril; color, pH, and amount of aspirate; securing device.
- Tube removal: Record procedure and patient's level of comfort and condition of naris.
- Report any type of unexpected outcome and the interventions performed to health care provider.
- Report during hand-off tube placement, when confirmation of placement was received, condition of patient's nares.

SKILL 45.3	ADMINISTERING ENTERAL FEEDINGS VIA NASOENTERIC, GASTROSTOMY, OR JEJUNOSTOMY TUBES

Delegation and Collaboration

The skill of administration of nasoenteric tube feeding can be delegated to assistive personnel (AP) (refer to agency policy). A registered nurse (RN) or licensed practical nurse (LPN) must first verify tube placement and patency. The nurse directs the AP to:

- Elevate head of bed to 30 to 45 degrees or sit patient up in bed or a chair unless contraindicated.
- Not adjust feeding rate; infuse the feeding as ordered.
- Report any difficulty in infusing the feeding or any discomfort voiced by the patient.
- Report any gagging, vomiting, paroxysms of coughing, or choking.
- Provide frequent oral hygiene.

Equipment

- Disposable feeding bag, tubing, or ready-to-hang system
- 60-mL or larger ENFit syringe
- Stethoscope
- Enteral infusion pump for continuous feedings
- pH indicator strip (scale 1.0 to 11.0)
- Water for flushing tube; sterile or purified water as indicated
- Prescribed enteral formula (standard polymeric or high protein) (McClave et al., 2016)
- Clean gloves
- ENFit connector

STEP	**RATIONALE**

ASSESSMENT

1. Verify health care provider's order for type of tube feeding formula, rate, route, and frequency.

   Ensures that correct formula will be administered in appropriate volume. Enteral formulas are not interchangeable.

2. Identify patient using at least two identifiers (e.g., name and birthday or name and medical record number) according to agency policy.

   Ensures correct patient. Complies with The Joint Commission standards and improves patient safety (TJC,2020).

3. Review medical record for risk factors of malnutrition and current clinical characteristics of malnutrition (see Table 45.4). Consult with nutritional support team and health care provider.

   Determines patient's risk for malnutrition and potential need for early initiation of EN (McClave et al., 2016; Meehan et al., 2016; White et al., 2012).

4. Assess patient for factors that increase risk for aspiration: sedation, mechanical ventilation, nasotracheal suctioning, neurological compromise, lying flat, and sepsis (Eglseer et al., 2018).

   Identifies patients at high risk for aspiration so that decision may be made based on safety of gastric versus intestinal feeding (McClave et al., 2016).

5. Perform hand hygiene. Perform physical assessment of abdomen, including auscultation for bowel sounds, before feeding (see Chapter 30).

   Objective measures for assessing tolerance include changes in bowel sounds, expanding girth, tenderness and firmness on palpation, increasing nasogastric (NG) output, and vomiting (McCarthy and Martindale, 2015). Report findings to health care provider to determine whether tube feeding can proceed safely.

6. Obtain baseline weight and review serum electrolytes and blood glucose measurement (see Skill 45.4). Assess patient for fluid volume excess or deficit, electrolyte abnormalities, and metabolic abnormalities (e.g., hyperglycemia).

   Enteral feedings should restore or maintain patient's nutritional status. Measures provide objective data and baseline to determine selection of formula and measure effectiveness of feedings.

7. Collaborate with RD for determination of patient's caloric and protein requirements. Then set goal for delivery of EN (McClave et al., 2016).

   Sets objective measure for determining percent of prescribed calories and protein delivered.

8. Assess patient's or family caregiver's knowledge, experience and health literacy level.

   Ensures patient has the capacity to obtain, communicate, process, and understand basic health information (CDC, 2019).

PLANNING

1. Provide privacy and prepare bedside environment for patient safety.

   Promotes patient's comfort and safety.

2. Prepare and organize equipment for enteral feeding administration.

   Ensures organized approach for administration of feedings.

3. Explain enteral feeding administration procedure to patient and/or caregiver.

   Decreases patient anxiety. Promotes patient cooperation and increases adherence.

IMPLEMENTATION

1. Perform hand hygiene. Apply clean gloves.

   Reduces transmission of microorganisms and potential contamination of enteral formula.

2. Reverify correct formula and check expiration date; note integrity of container and appearance of formula.

   Ensures that correct therapy is to be administered and checks integrity of formula.

   a. Prepare formula for administration, following manufacturer guidelines.

CLINICAL DECISION: *Discard unused reconstituted and refrigerated formulas within 24 hours of preparation (Boullata et al., 2017).*

---

b. Have formula at room temperature.

   Cold formula causes gastric cramping and discomfort because liquid is not warmed by mouth and esophagus.

c. Use aseptic technique to connect administration set tubing to container as needed. Use proper ENFit connecter and avoid handling feeding system or touching can tops, container openings, spike, and spike port.

   Bag, connections, and tubing must be free of contamination to prevent bacterial growth. The use of a closed system lowers the risk of infections due to bacterial contamination (Boullata et al., 2017).

d. Shake formula container well. Clean top of canned formula with alcohol swab before opening it.

   Ensures integrity of formula; prevents transmission of microorganisms.

Continued

| SKILL 45.3 | ADMINISTERING ENTERAL FEEDINGS VIA NASOENTERIC, GASTROSTOMY, OR JEJUNOSTOMY TUBES—cont'd |

STEP	RATIONALE
e. For closed systems connect administration tubing to container. If using open system, pour formula from brick pack or can into administration bag (see illustration).	Formulas are available in closed-system containers that contain a 24- to 48-hour supply of formula or in an open system, in which formula must be transferred from brick packs or cans to a bag before administration.
4. Open roller clamp and allow administration tubing to fill. Clamp off tubing with roller clamp. Hang container on intravenous (IV) pole.	Prevents introduction of air into stomach once feeding begins.
5. Keep patient in high-Fowler's position or elevate head of bed at least 30 degrees (45 degrees recommended). For patient forced to remain supine, place in reverse Trendelenburg's position, which raises head.	Elevation of head of bed helps prevent pulmonary aspiration (Boullata et al., 2017). Researchers recommend HOB elevation of 45 degrees for patients receiving EN who require mechanical ventilation or are heavily sedated, but lowering the head to 30 degrees might be done periodically for patient comfort and in patients at risk of developing pressure injury (Schallom et al., 2015).
6. Verify tube placement (see Skill 45.2). Observe appearance of aspirate, measure the length of the tube extending from the nares and compare to the insertion length, and note pH.	Verifies whether tip of tube is in stomach, intestine, or lung based on pH value (<5.0) (Fan et al., 2017; Ni et al., 2017).
a. *Nasoenteric and gastrostomy tube:* Attach ENFit syringe to end of enteral feeding tube and aspirate gastric or intestinal contents.	Gastric fluid for patient who has fasted for at least 4 hours usually has pH of 1.0 to 4.0 (if not receiving gastric acid inhibitor, then pH of <5.0) (Fan et al., 2017). If continuous feedings into stomach or intestine, check pH if feedings held for at least 1 hour for diagnostic reason (stomach pH <5.0; intestinal pH >6.0) (Fan et al., 2017).
b. *Jejunostomy tube:* Attach ENFit syringe to end of tube and aspirate intestinal secretions. Observe appearance; if significant amounts are returned or resemble gastric secretions, check pH.	Presence of intestinal fluid at pH greater than 6.0 indicates that end of tube is in small intestine. If fluid tests acidic on pH test or looks like gastric fluid, tube may be displaced into stomach.
7. Check gastric residual volume (GRV) per agency policy. Routine use is no longer recommended (Boullata et al., 2017) and should not be used as a single measure of tolerance.	GRV has poor correlation with pneumonia, regurgitation and aspiration. Frequent checking may delay feeding. However, if other signs of intolerance (e.g., abdominal distention, vomiting, or pain) are present, GRV of 250 to 500 mL may indicate the need to take measures to prevent aspiration or hold feeding completely (Boullata et al., 2017). Intestinal residual is usually very small. If residual volume is greater than 10 mL, displacement of intestinal tube into stomach may have occurred.

CLINICAL DECISION: *Limit gastric residual checks to recommended standard intervals as acidic gastric contents may cause protein in enteral formulas to precipitate within the lumen of the tube, creating risk for obstruction (Boullata et al., 2017). Use of GRVs leads to increased EAD clogging, inappropriate cessation of EN, consumption of nursing time, and allocation of health care resources and may adversely affect outcome through reduced volume of EN delivered (Boullata et al., 2017).*

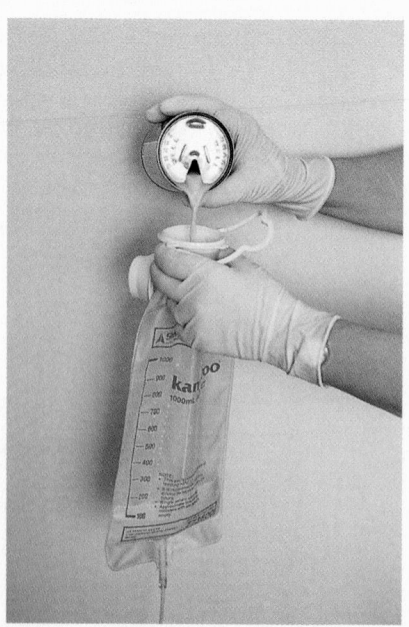

STEP 3e Pour formula into open feeding container.

STEP	RATIONALE
a. Draw up 10 to 30 mL air into ENFit syringe and connect to end of feeding tube. Inject air slowly into tube. Pull back slowly and aspirate total amount of gastric contents you can aspirate.	GRV may not be easy to obtain from small-bore feeding tube. A 60-mL syringe prevents gastric tube collapse.
b. Return aspirated contents to stomach slowly. Refer to agency policy for any cutoff to hold aspirated contents instead (McCarthy and Martindale, 2015).	Prevents loss of nutrients and electrolytes in discarded fluid. Some questions exist regarding safety of returning high volumes of fluid into stomach.
c. GRVs in range of 200 to 500 mL may raise concern and lead to implementation of measures to reduce risk of aspiration. Automatic cessation of feeding shouldn't occur for GRV less than 500 mL in absence of other signs of intolerance (Boullata et al., 2017, McClave et al., 2016).	Raising cutoff value for GRV from lower number to higher number doesn't increase risk for regurgitation, aspiration, or pneumonia (Boullata et al., 2017).
d. Flush feeding tube with 30 mL water.	Prevents clogging of tubing and ensures that complete feeding is administered.

CLINICAL DECISION: *Minimize the use of sedatives in patients receiving continuous feeding because airway clearance is reduced in sedated patients (Boullata et al., 2017).*

---

8. Intermittent feeding (administered at certain times during the day):	
a. Pinch proximal end of feeding tube and remove cap. Connect distal end of administration set tubing to ENFit device on feeding tube and release tubing.	Prevents excessive air from entering patient's stomach and leakage of gastric contents. Ensures that feeding will be administered into correct tubing (Boullata et al., 2017).
b. Set rate by adjusting roller clamp on tubing or attach tubing to feeding pump (see illustration). Allow bag to empty gradually over 30 to 45 minutes (length of time of a comfortable meal). Bag label should include: patient identifiers, formula type, enteral delivery site (route and access), administration method and type, and volume and frequency of water flushes (Boullata et al., 2017). Also include a label with date, time, and initials when hanging a feeding.	Gradual emptying of tube feeding reduces risk for abdominal discomfort, vomiting, or diarrhea induced by bolus or too-rapid infusion of tube feedings. Critical elements for an EN order should be on EN label (Boullata et al., 2017). Labeling indicates when to change administration set and confirms that right patient is receiving feeding.

CLINICAL DECISION: *Use pumps designated for tube feeding, not IV fluids.*

---

c. Immediately follow feeding with prescribed amount of water (per health care provider's orders or agency policy). Cover end of feeding tube with cap when not in use. Keep bag as clean as possible. Change administration set every 24 hours.	Prevents tube from clogging. Prevents air from entering stomach between feedings and limits microbial contamination of system.
9. Continuous infusion method:	Method delivers prescribed hourly rate of feeding and reduces risk for abdominal discomfort.
a. Remove cap on tubing and connect distal end of administration set tubing to feeding tube using ENFit connector as in Step 8a.	Prevents excess air from entering patient's stomach and leakage of gastric contents.

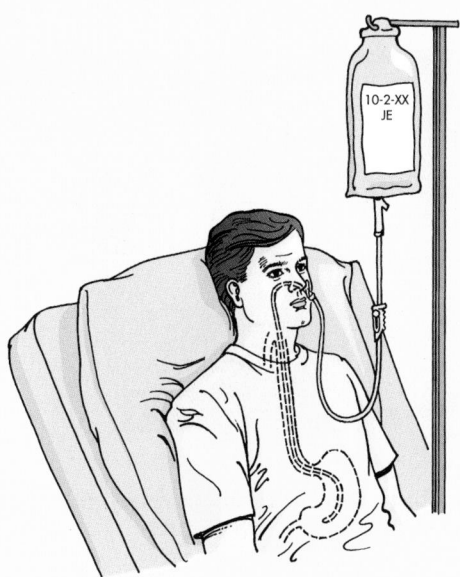

STEP 8b Administer intermittent feeding.

Continued

SKILL 45.3 **ADMINISTERING ENTERAL FEEDINGS VIA NASOENTERIC, GASTROSTOMY, OR JEJUNOSTOMY TUBES—cont'd**

STEP	RATIONALE
b. Thread tubing through feeding pump; set rate on pump and turn on (see illustration).	Delivers continuous feeding at steady rate and pressure. Feeding pump alarms for increased resistance.
c. Advance rate of tube feeding (and concentration of feeding) gradually, as ordered.	Tube feeding can usually begin with full-strength formula. Conservative initiation and advancement of EN nutrition depend on patient's age, medical condition, nutritional status, and expected patient tolerance (Kozeniecki and Fritzshall, 2015).

CLINICAL DECISION: *Limit infusion time for open EN feeding systems to 4 to 8 hours maximum (12 hours in the home setting) (Boullata et al., 2017). Follow the manufacturer's recommendations for duration of infusion through an intact closed delivery device (Boullata et al., 2017).*

STEP	RATIONALE
10. After feeding, flush tubing with 30 mL water every 4 hours during continuous feeding (see agency policy) or before and after an intermittent feeding. Have RD recommend total free-water requirement per day and obtain health care provider's order.	Provides patient with source of water to help maintain fluid and electrolyte balance. Clears tubing of formula and helps maintain tube patency.
11. Rinse bag and tubing with warm water whenever feedings are interrupted. Use new administration set every 24 hours.	Rinsing bag and tubing with warm water clears old tube feedings and reduces bacterial growth.
12. Dispose of supplies and perform hand hygiene.	Reduces transmission of microorganisms.
13. Be sure patient is comfortable and remains in position with head of elevated 30 to 45 degrees. Provide nurse call bell system to patient, and instruct patient to use if needed.	Reduces risk of aspiration. Call system summons nurse to patient bedside if assistance required.
14. Raise side rails (as appropriate) and lower bed to lowest position.	Promotes patient safety.

EVALUATION

1. Monitor patient's tolerance to feeding by assessing for abdominal distention, firmness, feeling of fullness, or nausea (Boullata et al., 2017). GRV checks should be limited and done per policy.	Symptoms are warnings that patient may have gastric reflux, leading to aspiration. Bowel sounds indicate whether peristalsis is present.
2. Monitor intake and output at least every 8 hours, and calculate daily totals every 24 hours.	Intake and output are indications of fluid balance, which can indicate fluid volume excess or deficit.
3. Weigh patient daily until maximum administration rate is reached and maintained for 24 hours; then weigh patient 3 times per week.	Slow weight gain is indicator of improved nutritional status; however, sudden gain of more than 2 lb (0.9 kg) in 24 hours usually indicates fluid retention.

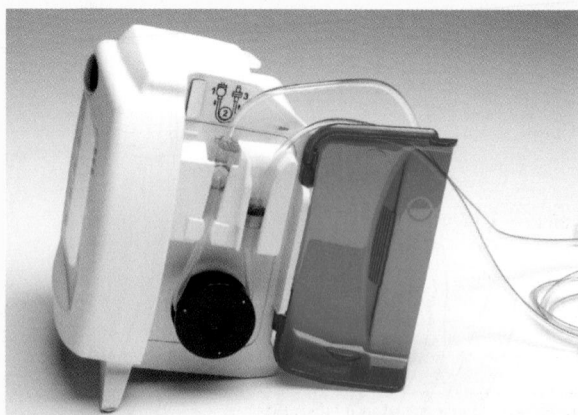

STEP 9b Connect tubing through infusion pump. (Kangaroo™ ePump © 2018 Courtesy of Cardinal Health UK Ltd.)

STEP	RATIONALE
4. Monitor patient for appropriate feeding tube placement at least every 4 hours or per agency protocol. Monitor visible length of tubing or marking at tube exit site (naris or stoma); check placement when a deviation is noted (Boullata et al., 2017).	Accidental displacement of tip of tube could lead to aspiration.
5. Monitor laboratory values as ordered by health care provider.	Determines correct administration of formula rate and strength.
6. Observe patient's respiratory status for coughing, dyspnea, tachypnea, change in oxygen saturation, hoarseness, crackles in lungs.	Change in respiratory status may indicate aspiration of tube feeding into respiratory tract.
7. Inspect site of gastrostomy or jejunostomy tube for signs of impaired skin integrity and symptoms of infection, injury, or tightness of tube.	Enteral tubes often cause pressure and excoriation at insertion site.
8. Observe nasoenteral tube insertion site at least daily (see agency policy). Note skin integrity and look for edema under device, excoriation, or presence of injury.	Allows for early detection of excoriation that can progress to a medical device–related pressure injury.
9. **Use Teach-Back:** "I want to be sure that I explained to you what you need to look for that may tell us you're not tolerating your tube feeding. Tell me two things that may tell us that you are not tolerating your tube feedings." Revise your instruction now or develop a plan for revised patient/family caregiver teaching if patient/family caregiver is not able to teach back correctly.	Determines patient's/family caregiver's level of understanding of instructional topic.

UNEXPECTED OUTCOMES AND RELATED INTERVENTIONS

1. Feeding tube becomes clogged.
   - Attempt to flush tube with water.
   - Special products are available for unclogging feeding tubes; **do not** use carbonated beverages and juices.
   - Hold feeding and notify health care provider.
   - Maintain patient in semi-Fowler's position.
   - Contact pharmacist to change medications to liquid form and flush before and after intermittent feedings and medications (Kozeniecki and Fritzshall, 2015).
2. Patient develops large amount of diarrhea (more than three loose stools in 24 hours).
   - Notify health care provider.
   - Consult dietitian about need to change formula to prevent malabsorption.
   - Identify and treat underlying medical/surgical issues and infections (Kozeniecki and Fritzshall, 2015).
   - Provide perianal skin care after each stool.
   - Determine other causes of diarrhea (e.g., *Clostridium difficile* infection, contaminated tube feeding, medication containing sorbitol).
3. Patient has an enteral tube misconnection (e.g., connecting an enteral tube to an intravenous [IV] site or ventilator in-line suction catheter).
   - Infusion of enteral feeding into vein or directly into lung is a medical emergency.
   - **Call health care provider and rapid response team immediately.**
4. Patient aspirates formula indicated by sudden appearance of respiratory symptoms (such as severe coughing, dyspnea, and cyanosis) associated with eating, drinking, or regurgitation of gastric contents. Auscultation of lungs reveals crackles or wheezes.
   - Immediately position patient on side with head of bed elevated.
   - Report change in condition to health care provider.
   - Suction nasotracheally or orotracheally.

> **CLINICAL DECISION:** *Small-volume aspirations that produce no overt symptoms are common and are often not discovered until the condition progresses to aspiration pneumonia (Eglseer et al., 2018).*

RECORDING AND REPORTING

- Record placement checks (length of tube, GRV type, pH, and amount), findings on abdominal assessment, amount and type of feeding, infusion rate (continuous feeding) or time for infusion (bolus method), patient's response to tube feeding, patency of tube, and condition of skin at tube site.
- Document your evaluation of patient learning.
- Record volume of formula and any additional water on I&O form.
- Report adverse outcomes to health care provider.
- During a hand-off report note the type of feeding, infusion rate and volume infused during shift, status of feeding tube placement, and patient's tolerance, and trace the administration set tubing to the enteral tube connection point to ensure the feeding is being infused enterally (Boullata et al., 2017).

HOME CARE CONSIDERATIONS

- Teach patient or family caregiver how to determine correct placement of feeding tube.
- Inform patient or family caregiver of signs associated with pulmonary aspiration, delayed gastric emptying.
- Reinforce signs and symptoms associated with feeding tube complications and when to call health care provider.
- Explain and demonstrate how to do skin care around gastrostomy or jejunostomy tube, and explain signs and symptoms of infection at the insertion site.

| SKILL 45.4 | BLOOD GLUCOSE MONITORING |

Delegation and Collaboration

During an acute illness assessment of a patient's blood glucose cannot be delegated to assistive personnel (AP). When the patient's condition is stable, the skill of obtaining and testing for blood glucose level can be delegated to AP. The nurse informs the AP by:

- Explaining appropriate sites to use for puncture and when to obtain glucose levels.
- Instructing AP to report all glucose levels to RN.

Equipment

- Antiseptic swab
- Cotton ball
- Lancet device, either self-activating or button activated
- Blood glucose meter (e.g., Accucheck III, OneTouch) (Fig. 45.10)
- Blood glucose test strips appropriate for meter brand used
- Clean gloves
- Paper towel

| STEP | RATIONALE |

ASSESSMENT

1. Identify patient using at least two identifiers (e.g., name and birthday or name and medical record number) according to agency policy. Compare identifiers with information on patient's MAR or medical record.

   Ensures correct patient. Complies with The Joint Commission standards and improves patient safety (TJC, 2020).

2. Review health care provider's order for time or frequency of measurement.

   Health care provider determines test schedule on basis of patient's physiological status and risk for glucose imbalance.

> **CLINICAL DECISION:** *For some critically ill patients, handheld point-of-care glucometers yield inconsistent results when the patient has low hematocrit levels or is hypotensive; in the presence of vasopressors, ascorbic acid, or other medications; or in the use of capillary blood specimens as opposed to arterial or venous blood samples. These factors can potentially lead to incorrect insulin dosing (Isbell, 2017).*

3. Determine whether specific conditions need to be met before or after sample collection (e.g., fasting, postprandial, after certain medications, before insulin doses).

   Dietary intake of carbohydrates and ingestion of concentrated glucose preparations alter blood glucose levels.

4. Determine whether risks exist for performing skin puncture (e.g., low platelet count, anticoagulant therapy, bleeding disorders).

   Abnormal clotting mechanisms increase risk for local ecchymosis and bleeding.

5. Perform hand hygiene. Assess area of skin to be used as puncture site. Inspect fingers or forearms for edema, inflammation, cuts, or sores. Avoid areas of bruising, recently punctured areas, and open lesions. Avoid using hand on side of mastectomy. Sides of fingers are commonly selected because they have fewer nerve endings.

   Recently punctured sites are avoided because these factors cause increased interstitial fluid and blood to mix and increase risk for infection.

6. Assess patient's or family caregiver's health literacy.

   Ensures patient or family caregiver has the capacity to obtain, communicate, process, and understand basic health information (CDC, 2019).

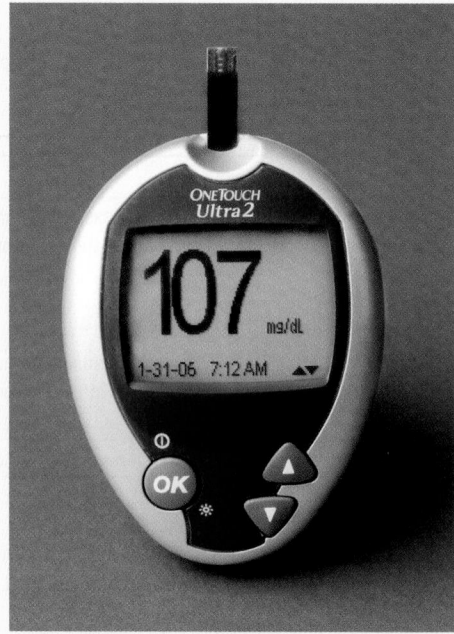

FIG. 45.10 Blood glucose monitor. (Courtesy LifeScan, Inc., Milpitas, CA.)

STEP	**RATIONALE**
7. Assess patient's understanding of procedure, purpose of blood glucose monitoring, ability to perform test, and its importance in glucose control.	Provides baseline for developing teaching plan. Patient's physical health may change (e.g., vision disturbance, fatigue, pain, disease process) and affect him or her when performing test.

PLANNING

1. Provide privacy and prepare bedside environment for patient safety.	Promotes patient comfort and safety.
2. Prepare and organize equipment needed for blood glucose monitoring.	Ensures an organized approach for the procedure.
3. Explain procedure and purpose to patient and family. Offer patient and family opportunity to practice testing procedure. Provide resources and teaching aids for patient and family.	Promotes understanding of the procedure and cooperation.

IMPLEMENTATION

1. Perform hand hygiene. Instruct adult to perform hand hygiene, including forearm (if applicable), with soap and warm water. Rinse and dry.	Promotes skin cleansing and vasodilation at selected puncture site. Reduces transmission of microorganisms.
2. Remove reagent strip from vial and tightly seal cap. Check code on test strip vial. Use only test strips recommended for glucose meter. Some newer meters do not require code and/or have disk or drum with 10 or more test strips.	Protects strips from accidental discoloration caused by exposure to air or light. Code on test strip vial must match code entered into glucose meter.
3. Insert strip into meter (refer to manufacturer directions (see illustration). Do not bend strip. Meter turns on automatically.	Some machines must be calibrated; others require zeroing of timer. Each meter is adjusted differently.
4. Remove unused reagent strip from meter and place on paper towel or clean, dry surface with test pad facing up (see manufacturer directions).	Moisture on strip can alter accuracy of final test results.
5. Meter displays code on screen that must match code from test strip vial. Press proper button on meter to confirm matching codes. Meter is ready for use.	Codes must match for meter to operate. Meters have different messages that confirm that meter is ready for testing and blood can be applied.
6. Perform hand hygiene and apply clean gloves. Prepare single-use lancet or multiple-use lancet device. **NOTE:** Some meters recommend that this step be completed before preparing test strip. Remove cap from lancet device; insert new lancet. Some lancet devices have disk or cylinder that rotates to new lancet.	Reduces transmission of microorganisms. Never reuse a lancet because of risk of infection.
a. Twist off protective cover on tip of lancet. Replace cap of lancet device.	
b. Cock lancet device, adjusting for proper puncture depth.	Each patient varies as to depth of insertion needed for lancet to produce blood drop.
7. Obtain blood sample.	
a. Wipe patient's finger or forearm lightly with antiseptic swab and allow to dry. Choose vascular area for puncture site. In stable adults select lateral side of finger. Avoid central tip of finger, which has denser nerve supply (Pagana et al., 2019).	Removes microorganisms from skin surface. Side of finger is less sensitive to pain.
b. Hold area to be punctured in dependent position. Do not milk or massage finger site.	Increases blood flow to area before puncture. Milking may hemolyze specimen and introduce excess tissue fluid (Pagana et al., 2019).
c. Hold tip of lancet device against area of skin chosen for test site (see illustration). Press release button on device. Some devices allow you to see blood sample forming. Remove device.	Placement ensures that lancet enters skin properly.
d. With some devices, a blood sample begins to appear. Otherwise gently squeeze or massage fingertip until round drop of blood forms (see illustration).	Adequate-size blood sample is needed to test glucose.

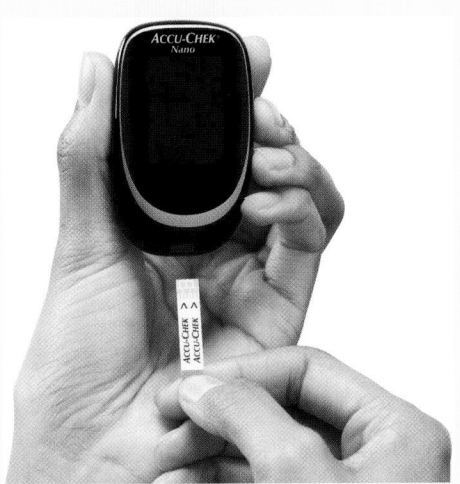

STEP 3 Load test strip into meter. (Courtesy Accucheck Glucometer.)

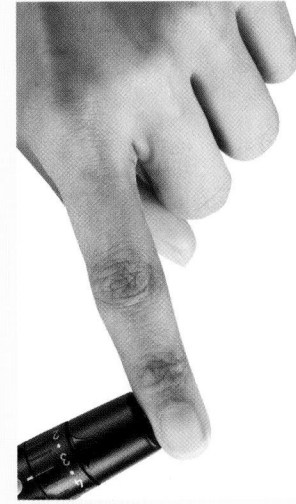

STEP 7c Prick side of finger with lancet. (Courtesy Accucheck Glucometer.)

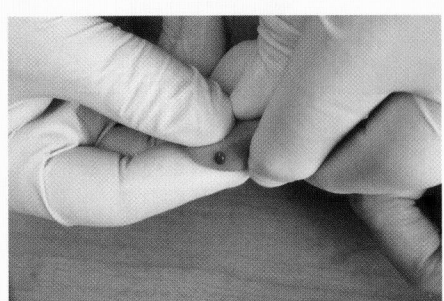

STEP 7d Gently squeeze puncture site until drop of blood forms.

Continued

STEP	RATIONALE
8. Obtain test results.	Exposure of blood to test strip for prescribed time ensures proper results.
a. Be sure that meter is still on. Bring test strip in meter to drop of blood. Blood will be wicked onto test strip (see illustration). Follow specific meter instructions to be sure that you obtain adequate sample.	Blood enters strip, and glucose device shows message on screen to signal that enough blood is obtained.

CLINICAL DECISION: *Do not scrape blood onto the test strips or apply it to wrong side of test strip. This results in an inaccurate glucose measurement.*

b. Blood glucose test result will appear on screen (see illustration). Some devices "beep" when completed.	
9. Turn meter off. Some meters turn off automatically. Dispose of test strip, lancet, and gloves in proper receptacles.	Meter is battery powered. Proper disposal reduces risk for needlestick injury and spread of infection.

CLINICAL DECISION: *Point-of-care (POC) blood glucose testing meters must be cleaned and disinfected after each patient use.*

10. Remove and dispose of gloves and perform hand hygiene.	Reduces transmission of microorganisms.
11. Discuss test results with patient and encourage questions and eventual participation in care if this is a new diabetes mellitus diagnosis.	Promotes participation and adherence to therapy.

EVALUATION

1. Inspect puncture site for bleeding or tissue injury.	Site can be source of discomfort and infection.
2. Compare glucose meter reading with normal blood glucose levels and previous test results.	Determines whether glucose level is normal.
3. **Use Teach-Back:** "I want to be sure I explained the way to obtain a blood glucose reading. Show me the steps you will use to obtain your blood glucose measurement." Revise your instruction now or develop a plan for revised patient/family caregiver teaching if patient/family caregiver is not able to teach back correctly.	Determines patient's/family caregiver's level of understanding of instructional topic.

UNEXPECTED OUTCOMES AND RELATED INTERVENTIONS

1. Puncture site is bruised or continues to bleed.
- Apply pressure.
- Notify health care provider if bleeding continues.

2. Blood glucose level is above or below target range.
- Continue to monitor patient.
- Check for any medication orders for deviations in glucose level.
- Notify health care provider.
- Administer insulin or carbohydrate source as ordered, depending on glucose level.

3. Glucose meter malfunctions.
- Review instructions for troubleshooting glucose meter.
- Repeat test.

RECORDING AND REPORTING

- Record glucose results on appropriate flow sheet and describe response, including presence or absence of pain or excessive oozing of blood at puncture site.
- Document your evaluation of patient learning
- Report blood glucose levels out of target range and the action taken for hypoglycemia or hyperglycemia.
- Report patient response to treatment for out-of-range blood glucose levels.

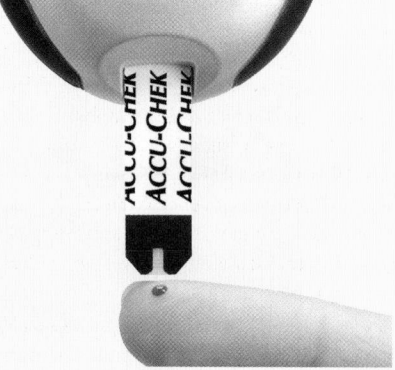

STEP 8a Touch test strip to blood drop. Blood wicks into test strip. (Courtesy Accucheck Glucometer.)

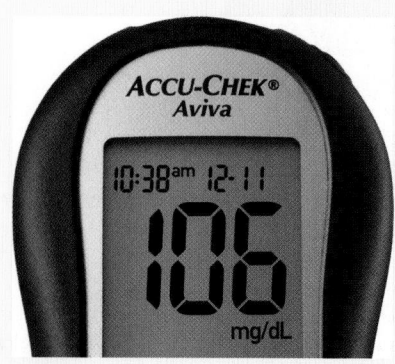

STEP 8b Results appear on meter screen. (Courtesy Accucheck Glucometer.)

KEY POINTS

- Ingestion of a diet balanced with carbohydrates, fats, proteins, and vitamins and minerals provides the essential nutrients to carry out the normal physiological functioning of the body across the life span.
- Through digestion food is broken down into its simplest form for absorption. Digestion and absorption occur mainly in the small intestine.
- The ChooseMyPlate program provides guidelines for a heart-healthy lifestyle.
- Guidelines for dietary change recommend reduced fat, saturated fats, sodium, refined sugar, and cholesterol and increased intake of complex carbohydrates and fiber.
- Patients with alterations in chewing and swallowing are at risk for aspiration.
- Improper nutrition impacts all body systems; nutritional assessment includes a review of physical assessment.
- Enteral feedings are for patients who are unable to ingest food but who have a functioning GI tract.
- One of the most important responsibilities of a nurse administering enteral feedings is to take precautions to prevent patients from aspirating the feeding.
- The most important responsibility of the nurse monitoring parenteral nutrition is to take precautions to prevent patients from developing a catheter-related infection, hyperglycemia, or fluid overload.
- MNT is a recognized treatment modality for both acute and chronic disease states.
- Special diets alter the composition, texture, digestibility, and residue of foods to suit the patient's needs.

REFLECTIVE LEARNING

- You are providing nursing care to a patient with cardiovascular disease. What assessment data would you need to gather to help you develop an MNT plan for the patient? What points would you include in your teaching plan?
- Consider a patient that you cared for on the clinical unit who was having nutritional problems. What strategies did you find most effective to help this patient? Why were the strategies effective?
- Using your knowledge of enteral feedings, develop a discharge teaching plan for a patient who will be going home with enteral feedings.

REVIEW QUESTIONS

1. The nurse is caring for a client with pneumonia, who has severe malnutrition. The nurse should assess the patient for which of the following assessment findings? (Select all that apply.)
   1. Heart disease
   2. Sepsis
   3. Hemorrhage
   4. Skin breakdown
   5. Diarrhea
2. The nurse is evaluating the recent lab results for a patient. Which labs are the best indicators for malnutrition? (Select all that apply.)
   1. Serum total protein
   2. Potassium
   3. Lipids
   4. Albumin
   5. Serum BUN
3. The nurse is caring for a client with dysphagia and is feeding her a pureed chicken diet when she begins to choke. What is the priority nursing intervention?
   1. Suction her mouth and throat.

2. Turn her on her side.
   3. Put on oxygen at 2 L nasal cannula.
   4. Stop feeding her.
4. A client who is receiving parenteral nutrition (PN) through a central venous catheter (CVC) has an air embolus. What should be the nurse's priority action?
   1. Have the patient turn on the left side and perform a Valsalva maneuver.
   2. Clamp the intravenous (IV) tubing to prevent more air from entering the line.
   3. Have the patient take a deep breath and hold it.
   4. Notify the health care provider immediately.
5. A patient is receiving both parenteral (PN) and enteral nutrition (EN). When would the nurse collaborate with the health care provider and request a discontinuation of parenteral nutrition?
   1. When 25% of the patient's nutritional needs are met by the tube feedings
   2. When bowel sounds return
   3. When the central line has been in for 10 days
   4. When 75% of the patient's nutritional needs are met by the tube feedings
6. A client is receiving an enteral feeding at 65 mL/hr. The gastric residual volume in 4 hours was 125 mL. What is the priority nursing intervention?
   1. Assess bowel sounds.
   2. Raise the head of the bed to at least 45 degrees.
   3. Continue the feedings; this is normal gastric residual for this feeding.
   4. Hold the feeding until you talk to the primary care provider.
7. Which action can a nurse delegate to assistive personnel (AP)?
   1. Performing glucose monitoring every 6 hours on a patient
   2. Teaching the client about the need for enteral feeding
   3. Administering enteral feeding bolus after tube placement has been verified
   4. Evaluating the client's tolerance of the enteral feeding
8. Which statement made by the parents of a 2-month-old infant requires further education by the nurse?
   1. "I'll continue to use formula for the baby until he is at least a year old."
   2. "I'll make sure that I purchase iron-fortified formula."
   3. "I'll start feeding the baby cereal at 4 months."
   4. "I'm going to alternate formula with whole milk, starting next month."
9. A nurse sees an assistive personnel (AP) perform the following intervention for a patient receiving continuous enteral feedings. Which action would require immediate attention by the nurse?
   1. Fastening tube to the gown with new tape
   2. Placing client supine while giving a bath
   3. Monitoring the client's weight as ordered
   4. Ambulating patient with enteral feedings still infusing
10. A patient is receiving total parenteral nutrition (TPN). What are the primary interventions the nurse should follow to prevent a central line infection? (Select all that apply.)
    1. Change the dressing using sterile technique.
    2. Change TPN containers every 48 hours.
    3. Change the TPN tubing every 24 hours.
    4. Monitor glucose levels to watch and assess for glucose intolerance.
    5. Elevate head of the bed 45 degrees to prevent aspiration.

Answers: 1. 2, 3, 4; **2.** 1, 5; **3.** 4; **4.** 1; **5.** 4; **6.** 3; **7.** 1; **8.** 4; **9.** 2; **10.** 1, 3.

Rationales for Review Questions can be found on the Evolve website.

REFERENCES

American Academy of Pediatrics (AAP): Policy statement: breast feeding and the use of human milk, *Pediatrics* 129(3):496, 2017.

American Association of Critical-Care Nurses (AACN): *AACN practice alerts: initial and ongoing verification of feeding tube placement in adults*, 2016. https://ccn.aacn-journals.org/content/36/2/e8.full.pdf+html.

American Cancer Society (ACS): *American Cancer Society guidelines on nutrition and physical activity for cancer prevention*, 2019. http://www.cancer.org/healthy/eathealthygetactive/acsguidelinesonnutritionphysicalactivityforcancerprevention/acs-guidelines-on-nutrition-and-physical-activity-for-cancer-prevention-intro.

American Diabetes Association (ADA): Management of hyperglycemia in type 2 diabetes: a patient-centered approach, *Diabetes Care* 35(6):1364, 2019.

American Dietetic Association: *Medical nutrition therapy*, 2019. https://www.diet.com.

American Heart Association (AHA): *Diet and lifestyle recommendations revision*, 2018. http://www.heart.org/HEARTORG/GettingHealthy/Diet-and-Lifestyle-Recommendations_UCM_305855_Article.jsp.

American Society for Parenteral and Enteral Nutrition (ASPEN): *Clinical guidelines*, 2019. https://www.nutritioncare.org/Guidelines_and_Clinical_Resources.

Boullata J, et al.: ASPEN safe practices for enteral nutrition therapy, *JPEN J Parenter Enteral Nutr* 41(1):15, 2017.

Bourgault A, et al.: Methods used by critical care nurses to verify feeding tube placement in clinical practice, *Crit Care Nurse* 35(1):e1, 2015.

Burchum JR, Rosenthal LD: *Lehne's pharmacology for nursing care*, ed 10, St Louis, 2019, Elsevier.

Centers for Disease Control and Prevention (CDC): *Childhood obesity facts*, 2019. https://www.cdc.gov/obesity/data/childhood.html.

Centers for Disease Control and Prevention (CDC): *What is health literacy*, 2019. https://www.cdc.gov/healthliteracy/learn/index.html. Accessed December 23, 2019.

Eglseer D, et al.: Dysphagia in hospitalized older patients: associated factors and nutritional interventions, *J Nutr Health Aging* 22(1):103, 2018.

Fan EMP, et al.: Nasogastric tube placement confirmation: where we are and where we should be heading, *Proc Singapore Healthc* 26(3):189, 2017.

Giddens J: *Concepts for nursing practice*, ed 2, St Louis, 2017, Elsevier.

Giger JN: *Transcultural nursing: assessment and intervention*, ed 7, St Louis, 2016, Elsevier.

Grodner M, et al.: *Nutritional foundations and clinical applications: a nursing approach*, ed 7, St Louis, 2020, Elsevier.

Hockenberry MJ, et al.: *Wong's nursing care of infants and children*, ed 11, St Louis, 2019, Elsevier.

Huang J, Barnidge E: Low-income children's participation in the National School Lunch Program and household food insufficiency, *Soc Sci Med* 150:8–14, 2016.

Institute for Safe Medication Practices (ISMP): *ISMP Medication Safety Alert: ENFit enteral devices are on their way…Important safety considerations for hospitals*, 2015. https://www.ismp.org/resources/enfit-enteral-devices-are-their-wayimportant-safety-considerations-hospitals. Accessed December 8, 2019.

International Dysphagia Diet Standardisation Initiative: *IDDSI framework*, 2016. http://iddsi.org/resources/framework. Accessed December 8, 2019.

Isbell TS: Bedside blood glucose testing in critically ill patients, *Med Lib Observ* 49(4):8, 2017.

Kagaya H, et al.: Body positions and functional training to reduce aspiration in patients with dysphagia, *Japan Med Assoc J* 54(1):35–38, 2011.

Kozeniecki M, Fritzshall R: Enteral nutrition for adults in the hospital setting, *Nutr Clin Pract* 30(5):634, 2015.

Lancaster J: Dysphagia: its nature, assessment and management, *Br J Community Nurs* S28, 2015.

Lewis S, et al.: *Medical-surgical nursing: assessment and management of clinical problems*, ed 10, St Louis, 2017, Elsevier.

Liantonio J, et al.: Preventing aspiration pneumonia by addressing three key risk factors: dysphagia, poor oral hygiene, and medication use, *Ann Longterm Care* 22(1):42, 2014.

Markowitz J, et al.: *American Association of Critical-Care Nurses (AACN)/Clinical Scene Investigator (CSI) academy: device-related pressure ulcers*, 2013. http://www.aacn.org/wd/csi/docs/FinalProjects/IU%20Methodist%20ACC%20-%20Power%20Point%20Presentation.pdf.

Matheny N: AACN practice alert: initial and ongoing verification of feeding tube placement in adults, *Crit Care Nurse* 36(2):e8–e13, 2016.

Metheny N: Preventing aspiration in older adults with dysphagia, *Try This: Best Practices in Nursing Care to Older Adults Issue No 20*, 2012. https://consultgeri.org/try-this/general-assessment/issue-20.pdf.

Metheny NA, Meert KL: Update on effectiveness of an electromagnetic feeding tube-placement device in detecting respiratory placements, *Am J Crit Care* 26(2):157, 2017.

Mayo Clinic: *Childhood obesity*, 2019. https://www.mayoclinic.org/diseases-conditions/childhood-obesity/symptoms-causes/syc-20354827. Accessed December 8, 2019.

McCance KL, et al.: *Pathophysiology: the biologic basis for disease in adults and children*, ed 8, St Louis, 2019, Elsevier.

McCarthy MS, Martindale RG: What's on the menu? Delivering evidence-based nutritional therapy, *Nursing* 45(8):36, 2015.

McClave SA, et al.: ACG clinical guidelines: nutrition therapy in the adult hospitalized patient, *Am J Gastroenterol* 111(3):315–334, 2016.

McCuistion LE, et al: *Pharmacology: A patient-centered nursing process approach*, ed 9, St. Louis, 2018, Elsevier.

McEvilly A: Causes of malnutrition in older adults and what can be done to prevent it, *Brit J Community Nurs* 22(10):474–476, 2017.

Meehan A, et al.: Health system quality improvement: impact of prompt nutrition care on patient outcomes and health care costs, *J Nurs Care Qual* 31(3):217, 2016.

Meiner SE, Yeager JJ: *Gerontologic nursing*, ed 6, St Louis, 2019, Elsevier.

National Academies of Sciences: *Engineering, and medicine: health and medicine division: food and nutrition*, 2019. www.nationalacademies.org/hmd/Global/Topics/Food-Nutrition.aspx.

National Institutes of Health: *Tolerable upper-level intake*, n.d. http://ods.od.nih.gov/pubs/conferences/tolerable_upper_intake.pdf.

National Osteoporosis Foundation (NOF): *Nutrition: food and your bones – osteoporosis nutrition guidelines*, 2019. https://www.nof.org/patients/treatment/nutrition/.

National Stroke Association: *Dysphagia*, 2017. http://www.stroke.org/we-can-help/survivors/stroke-recovery/post-stroke-conditions/physical/dysphagia.

Nix S: *Williams' basic nutrition and diet therapy*, ed 15, St Louis, 2017, Mosby.

Pagana KD, et al.: *Mosby's diagnostic and laboratory test reference*, ed 14, St Louis, 2019, Elsevier.

Phelps L, et al.: *Sparks & Taylor's nursing diagnosis reference manual*, ed 10, Philadelphia, PA, 2017, Lippincott Williams, and Wilkins.

Phillips LD: *Manual of IV therapeutics: evidence-based practice for infusion therapy*, ed 7, Philadelphia, 2018, FA Davis.

Pietsch K, et al.: Rehabilitation in patients with dysphonia. Speech Language Pathology Rehabilitation, *Med Clin* 102(6):1121–1134, 2018.

Swinburne M, et al.: Reducing hospital readmissions: addressing the impact of food security and nutrition, *J Law Med Ethics* 45(Suppl 1):86–89, 2017.

Taylor SJ, et al.: Nasogastric tube depth: the 'NEX' guideline is incorrect, *Br J Nurs* 23(12):641, 2014.

The Joint Commission (TJC): *Sentinel alert event: managing risk during transition to new ISO tubing connector standards*, 2018. http://www.jointcommission.org/assets/1/6/SEA_53_Connectors_8_19_14_final.pdf.

The Joint Commission (TJC): *2020 National Patient Safety Goals*, Oakbrook Terrace, IL, 2020, The Commission. https://www.jointcommission.org/en/standards/national-patient-safety-goals/. Accessed January 2, 2020.

Touhy TA, Jett KF: *Ebersole and Hess' gerontological nursing healthy aging*, ed 5, St Louis, 2018, Elsevier.

US Department of Agriculture (USDA): *ChooseMyPlate*, 2017a. http://www.choosemyplate.gov. Accessed December 8, 2019.

US Department of Agriculture (USDA): *Economic research service*, 2017b. https://www.ers.usda.gov.

US Department of Health and Human Services (USDHHS): *Healthy People 2020*, 2019. http://www.healthypeople.gov/.

VanBlarcom A, McCoy MA: New nutrition guidelines: promoting enteral nutrition via a nutrition bundle, *Crit Care Nurse* 38(3):46–52, 2018, https://doi.org/10.4037/ccn2018617.

White JW, et al.: Consensus statement of the academy of nutrition and dietetics/American society for parenteral and enteral nutrition: characteristics recommended for the identification and documentation of adult malnutrition, *JPEN J Parenter Enteral Nutr* 112(5):730, 2012.

World Health Organization (WHO): *Food security*, 2019. http://www.emro.who.int/nutrition/food-security/. Accessed December 8, 2019.

Zupec-Kania B, O'Flaherty T: Medical nutrition therapy for neurologic disorders. In Mahan LK, Raymond JL, editors: *Krause's food nutrition and the nutrition care process*, ed 14, Philadelphia, 2017, Elsevier.

RESEARCH REFERENCES

Agarwalla R, et al.: Assessment of the nutritional status of the elderly and its correlates, *J Family Community Med* 22(1):39, 2015.

American Speech-Language-Hearing Association (ASHA): *Pediatric dysphagia: causes*, 2016. http://www.asha.org/PRPSpecificTopic.aspx?folderid=8589934965&section=Causes.

American Speech-Language-Hearing Association (ASHA): *Dysphagia diets*, 2019. https://www.asha.org/SLP/clinical/dysphagia/Dysphagia-Diets/.

Bharadwaj S, et al.: Malnutrition: laboratory markers vs nutritional assessment, *Gastroenterol Rep (Oxf)* 4(4):272–280, 2016.

Bogart LM, et al.: Two-year BMI outcomes from a school-based intervention for nutrition and exercise: a randomized trial, *Pediatrics* 137(5), 2016, https://doi.org/10.1542/peds.2015-2493.

Dong Y, et al.: Clinical application of ICF key codes to evaluate patients with dysphagia following stroke, *Medicine* 95(38):e4479, 2016.

Holland A, et al.: Carbon dioxide detection for testing nasogastric tube placement in adults, *Cochrane Database Syst Rev* 10:CD010773, 2013. http://onlinelibrary.wiley.com/doi/10.1002/14651858.CD010773/full.

Marian T, et al.: Measurement of oxygen desaturation is not useful for the detection of aspiration in dysphagic stroke patients, *Cerebrovasc Dis Extra* 7(1):44, 2017.

Metheny NA, Frantz RA: Head-of-bed elevation in critically ill patients: a review, *Crit Care Nurse* 33(3):53, 2013.

Milsom SA, et al.: Naso-enteric tube placement: a review of methods to confirm tip location, global applicability and requirements, *World J Surg* 39(9):2243, 2015.

Nagy A, et al.: The effectiveness of the head-turn-plus-chin-down maneuver for eliminating vallecular residue, *Codas* 28(2):113, 2016.

Ni MA, et al.: Selecting pH cut-offs for the safe verification of nasogastric feeding tube placement: a decision analytical modelling approach, *BMJ Open* 7(11):e018128, 2017.

Ogden C, et al.: Trends in obesity prevalence among children and adolescents in the United States, 1988-1994 through 2013-2014, *JAMA* 315(21):2292–2299, 2016, 2016, https://doi.org/10.1001/jama.2016.6361.

Reed Mangels A: Malnutrition in older adults: an evidence-based review of risk factors, assessment, and intervention, *Am J Nurs* 118(3):34–43, 2018.

Santos SC, et al.: Methods to determine the internal length of nasogastric feeding tubes: an integrative review, *Int J Nurs Stud* 61:95, 2016.

Schallom M, et al.: Head-of-bed elevation and early outcomes of gastric reflux, aspiration and pressure ulcers: a feasibility study, *Am J Crit Care* 24(1):57, 2015.

Stewart ML: Interruptions in enteral nutrition delivery in the critically ill patients and recommendations for clinical practice, *Crit Care Nurse* 34(4):14, 2014.

Tan ECK, et al.: Medications that cause dry mouth as an adverse effect in older people: a systematic review and meta-analysis, *J Am Geriatr Soc* 66(1):76, 2018.

Wittenaar H, Ottery F: Assessing nutritional status in cancer: role of the Patient-Generated Subjective Global Assessment, *Curr Opin Clin Nutr Metab Care* 20(5):322–329, 2017.

Yang W, et al.: Research progress on nurses' ability to identify and manage dysphagia in stroke patients, *Chin Nurs Res* 31(36):4602–4604, 2017, https://doi.org/10.3969/j.issn.1009-6493.2017.36.004.

46

Urinary Elimination

OBJECTIVES

- Explain the function and role of urinary system structures in urine formation and elimination.
- Identify factors that commonly impact urinary elimination.
- Compare and contrast common alterations associated with urinary elimination.
- Obtain a nursing history from a patient with an alteration in urinary elimination.
- Perform a physical assessment focused on urinary elimination.
- Interpret features of normal and abnormal urine.

- Appraise nursing implications of common diagnostic tests of the urinary system.
- Select nursing diagnoses associated with alterations in urinary elimination.
- Discuss nursing interventions to promote normal urinary elimination.
- Discuss nursing interventions to reduce risk for urinary tract infections.
- Perform safely skills associated with assessment and promotion of urinary elimination.

KEY TERMS

Bacteremia, p. 1152
Bacteriuria, p. 1152
Catheter-associated urinary tract infection (CAUTI), p. 1154
Catheterization, p. 1166
Cystitis, p. 1152
Dysuria, p. 1152

Hematuria, p. 1151
Micturition, p. 1150
Nephrostomy, p. 1155
Pelvic floor muscle training, p. 1173
Postvoid residual (PVR), p. 1152
Proteinuria, p. 1151
Pyelonephritis, p. 1152

Suprapubic catheter, p. 1171
Urinary incontinence (UI), p. 1154
Urinary retention, p. 1152
Ureterostomy, p. 1155

MEDIA RESOURCES

http://evolve.elsevier.com/Potter/fundamentals/

- Review Questions
- Video Clips
- Concept Map Creator
- Case Study with Questions

- Skills Performance Checklists
- Audio Glossary
- Content Updates
- Answers to QSEN Activity and Review Questions

A basic human function is urinary elimination. This function can be compromised by a variety of illnesses and conditions. Nurses are key members of the health care team when treating patients with urinary problems. It is your role to assess patients' urinary tract functions and provide support for bladder emptying. During acute illness a patient may require urinary catheterization for close monitoring of urine output or to facilitate bladder emptying when bladder function is compromised. Some patients require long-term indwelling urethral or suprapubic catheters, when the bladder fails to empty effectively. You also implement measures to minimize risk for infection when bladder function is impaired or urinary drainage tubes are required. Nurses in all health care settings play an important role in teaching patients about bladder health and in supporting them to improve or obtain continence.

SCIENTIFIC KNOWLEDGE BASE

Urinary elimination is the last step in the removal and elimination of excess water and by-products of body metabolism. Adequate elimination depends on the coordinated function of the kidneys, ureters, bladder, and urethra (Fig. 46.1). The kidneys filter waste products of metabolism from the blood. The ureters transport urine from the kidneys to the bladder. The bladder holds urine until the volume in the bladder triggers a sensation of urge, indicating the need to pass urine. Micturition occurs when the brain gives the bladder permission to empty, the bladder contracts, the urinary sphincter relaxes, and urine leaves the body through the urethra.

Kidneys

The kidneys lie retroperitoneal on either side of the vertebral column behind the peritoneum and against the deep muscles of the back. Normally the left kidney is higher than the right because of the anatomical position of the liver.

Nephrons, the functional unit of the kidneys, remove waste products from the blood and play a major role in the regulation of fluid and electrolyte balance. Each nephron contains a cluster of capillaries called the *glomerulus*. The glomerulus filters water, glucose, amino acids, urea, uric acid, creatinine, and major electrolytes. Large proteins and

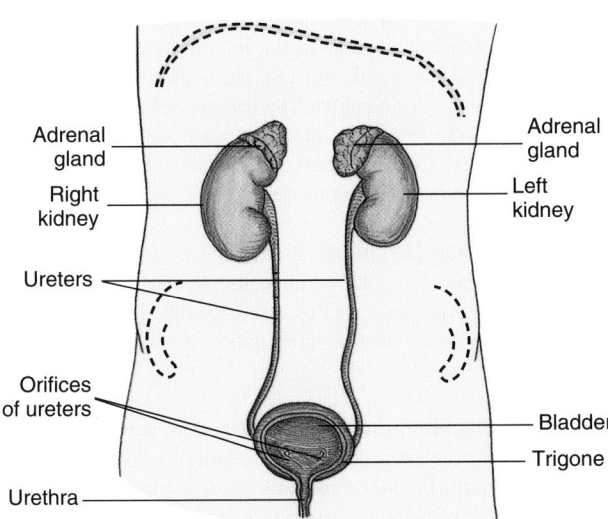

FIG. 46.1 Organs of urinary system.

blood cells do not normally filter through the glomerulus. When protein (**proteinuria**) or blood (**hematuria**) is found in the urine, glomerular injury is suspected.

Not all glomerular filtrate is excreted as urine. Approximately 99% is resorbed into the plasma by the proximal convoluted tubule of the nephron, the loop of Henle, and the distal tubule. The remaining 1% is excreted as urine. It is in the resorption process that the delicate balance of fluid and electrolytes is maintained. The normal range of urine production is 1 to 2 L/day (Huether and McCance, 2017). Many factors can influence the production of urine such as fluid intake and body temperature (Box 46.1).

The kidneys have essential functions other than elimination of body wastes. Erythropoietin, produced by the kidneys, stimulates red blood cell production and maturation in bone marrow. Patients with chronic kidney conditions cannot produce sufficient quantities of this hormone; therefore, they are prone to anemia. The kidneys play a major role in blood pressure control via the renin-angiotensin system (i.e., release of aldosterone and prostacyclin) (Huether and McCance, 2017). In times of renal ischemia (decreased blood supply), renin is released from juxtaglomerular cells. Renin functions as an enzyme to convert

---

BOX 46.1   Factors Influencing Urinary Elimination

Growth and Development
- Children cannot voluntarily control voiding until 18 to 24 months.
- Readiness for toilet training includes the ability to recognize the feeling of bladder fullness, hold urine for 1 to 2 hours, and communicate the sense of urgency.
- Older adults may experience a decrease in bladder capacity, increased bladder irritability, and an increased frequency of bladder contractions during bladder filling.
- In older adults the ability to hold urine between the initial desire to void and an urgent need to void decreases.
- Older adults are at increased risk for urinary incontinence because of chronic illnesses and factors that interfere with mobility, cognition, and manual dexterity.

Sociocultural Factors
- Cultural and gender norms vary. Some cultures expect toilet facilities to be private, whereas some cultures accept communal toilet facilities.
- Religious or cultural norms may dictate who is acceptable to help with elimination practices.
- Social expectations (e.g., school recesses, work breaks) can interfere with timely voiding.

Psychological Factors
- Anxiety and stress sometimes affect a sense of urgency and increase the frequency of voiding.
- Anxiety can impact bladder emptying because of inadequate relaxation of the pelvic floor muscles and urinary sphincter.
- Depression can decrease the desire for urinary continence.

Personal Habits
- The need for privacy and adequate time to void can influence the ability to empty the bladder adequately.

Fluid Intake
- If fluids, electrolytes, and solutes are balanced, increased fluid intake increases urine production.
- Alcohol decreases the release of antidiuretic hormones, thus increasing urine production.

- Fluids containing caffeine and other bladder irritants can prompt unsolicited bladder contractions, resulting in frequency, urgency, and incontinence.

Pathological Conditions
- Diabetes mellitus, multiple sclerosis, and stroke can alter bladder contractility and the ability to sense bladder filling. Patients experience either bladder overactivity or deficient bladder emptying.
- Arthritis, Parkinson's disease, dementia, and chronic pain syndromes can interfere with timely access to a toilet.
- Spinal cord injury or intervertebral disk disease (above S1) can cause the loss of urine control because of bladder overactivity and impaired coordination between the contracting bladder and urinary sphincter.
- Prostatic enlargement (e.g., benign prostatic hyperplasia [BPH]) can cause obstruction of the bladder outlet, causing urinary retention.

Surgical Procedures
- Local trauma during lower abdominal and pelvic surgery sometimes obstructs urine flow, requiring temporary use of an indwelling urinary catheter.
- Urinary retention in the postoperative period has two main causes—one is mechanical obstruction of the lower urinary tract; the other is altered neural control of the bladder and detrusor mechanism, most commonly due to analgesic drugs (Akkoc et al., 2016).

Medications
- Diuretics increase urinary output by preventing resorption of water and certain electrolytes.
- Some drugs change the color of urine (e.g., phenazopyridine-orange, riboflavin–intense yellow).
- Anticholinergics (e.g., atropine, overactive agents) may increase the risk for urinary retention by inhibiting bladder contractility (Burchum and Rosenthal, 2019).
- Hypnotics and sedatives (e.g., analgesics, antianxiety agents) may reduce the ability to recognize and act on the urge to void.

Diagnostic Examinations
- Cystoscopy may cause localized trauma of the urethra, resulting in transient (1 to 2 days) dysuria and hematuria.
- Whenever the sterile urinary tract is catheterized, there is a risk for infection.

angiotensinogen (a substance synthesized by the liver) into angiotensin I. Angiotensin I is converted to angiotensin II in the lungs. Angiotensin II causes vasoconstriction and stimulates aldosterone release from the adrenal cortex. Aldosterone causes retention of water, which increases blood volume. The kidneys also produce prostaglandin E_2 and prostacyclin, which help maintain renal blood flow through vasodilation. These mechanisms increase arterial blood pressure and renal blood flow (Huether and McCance, 2017).

The kidneys affect calcium and phosphate regulation by producing a substance that converts vitamin D into its active form. Patients with kidney impairment can have problems such as anemia, hypertension, and electrolyte imbalances.

Ureters

A ureter is attached to each kidney pelvis and carries urinary waste to the bladder. Urine draining from the ureters to the bladder is sterile. Peristaltic waves cause the urine to enter the bladder in spurts rather than steadily. Contractions of the bladder during micturition compress the lower part of the ureters to prevent urine from backflowing into the ureters (Huether and McCance, 2017). Obstruction of urine flow through the ureters such as by a kidney stone can cause a backflow of urine (urinary reflux) into the ureters and pelvis of the kidney, causing distention (hydroureter/hydronephrosis) and in some cases permanent damage to sensitive kidney structures and function.

Bladder

The urinary bladder is a hollow, distensible, muscular organ that holds urine. When empty, the bladder lies in the pelvic cavity behind the symphysis pubis. In males the bladder rests against the rectum, and in females it rests against the anterior wall of the uterus and vagina. The bladder has two parts, a fixed base called the *trigone* and a distensible body called the *detrusor*. The bladder expands as it fills with urine. Normally the pressure in the bladder during filling remains low, and this prevents the dangerous backward flow of urine into the ureters and kidneys. Backflow can cause infection. In a pregnant woman the developing fetus pushes against the bladder, reducing capacity and causing a feeling of fullness.

Urethra

Urine travels from the bladder through the urethra and passes to the outside of the body through the urethral meatus. The urethra passes through a thick layer of skeletal muscles called the *pelvic floor muscles.* These muscles stabilize the urethra and contribute to urinary continence. The external urethral sphincter, made up of striated muscles, contributes to voluntary control over the flow of urine. The female urethra is approximately 3 to 4 cm (1 to 1.5 inches) long, and the male urethra is about 18 to 20 cm (7 to 8 inches) long. The shorter length of the female urethra increases risk for urinary tract infection (UTI) because of close access to the bacteria-contaminated perineal area (Huether and McCance, 2017).

Act of Urination

Urination, micturition, and voiding are all terms that describe the process of bladder emptying. Micturition is a complex interaction among the bladder, urinary sphincter, and central nervous system. Several areas in the brain are involved in bladder control: cerebral cortex, thalamus, hypothalamus, and brainstem. There are two micturition centers in the spinal cord: one coordinates inhibition of bladder contraction; the other coordinates bladder contractility. As the bladder fills and stretches, bladder contractions are inhibited by sympathetic stimulation from the thoracic micturition center. When the bladder fills to approximately 400 to 600 mL, most people experience a strong sensation of urgency. When in the appropriate place to void, the central nervous system sends a message to the micturition centers, stopping sympathetic stimulation and starting parasympathetic stimulation from the sacral micturition center. The urinary sphincter relaxes, and the bladder contracts. When the time and place are inappropriate, the brain sends messages to the micturition centers to contract the urinary sphincter and relax the bladder muscle.

Factors Influencing Urination. Physiological factors, psychosocial conditions, and diagnostic or treatment-induced factors can all affect normal urinary elimination (see Box 46.1). Knowledge of these factors enables you to anticipate possible elimination problems and intervene when problems develop.

Common Urinary Elimination Problems. The most common urinary elimination problems involve the inability to store urine or fully empty urine from the bladder. Problems can result from infection; irritable or overactive bladder; obstruction of urine flow; impaired bladder contractility; or issues that impair innervation to the bladder, resulting in sensory or motor dysfunction.

Urinary Retention. Urinary retention is the inability to partially or completely empty the bladder. Acute or rapid-onset urinary retention stretches the bladder, causing feelings of pressure, discomfort/pain, tenderness over the symphysis pubis, restlessness, and sometimes diaphoresis. Patients may have no urine output over several hours and in some cases experience frequency, urgency, small-volume voiding, or incontinence of small volumes of urine. Chronic urinary retention has a slow, gradual onset during which patients may experience a decrease in voiding volumes, straining to void, frequency, urgency, incontinence, and sensations of incomplete emptying. Postvoid residual (PVR) is the amount of urine left in the bladder after voiding and is measured either by ultrasound or straight catheterization. Incontinence caused by urinary retention is called *overflow incontinence* or *incontinence associated with chronic retention of urine.* The pressure in the bladder exceeds the ability of the sphincter to prevent the passage of urine, and the patient will dribble urine (Table 46.1).

Urinary Tract Infections (UTIs). UTIs are the fourth most common type of health care–associated infection, virtually all caused by instrumentation of the urinary tract (CDC, 2019). *Escherichia coli,* a bacterium commonly found in the colon, is the most common causative pathogen (Nicolle, 2014). The risk for a UTI increases in the presence of an indwelling catheter, any instrumentation of the urinary tract, urinary retention, urinary and fecal incontinence, and poor perineal hygiene practices.

UTIs are characterized by location (i.e., upper urinary tract [kidney] or lower urinary tract [bladder, urethra]) and have signs and symptoms of infection. Bacteriuria, or bacteria in the urine, does not always mean that there is a UTI. In the absence of symptoms, the presence of bacteria in the urine as found on a urine culture is called *asymptomatic bacteriuria* and is not considered an infection and should not be treated with antibiotics (Duncan, 2019). Symptomatic infection of the bladder can lead to a serious upper UTI (pyelonephritis) and life-threatening bloodstream infection (bacteremia or urosepsis) and should be treated with antibiotics. Symptoms of a lower UTI (bladder) can include burning or pain with urination (dysuria); irritation of the bladder (cystitis) characterized by urgency, frequency, incontinence, or suprapubic tenderness; and foul-smelling cloudy urine. Elderly people with infections, including UTIs, often have nonspecific symptoms such as delirium, confusion, fatigue, loss of appetite, decline in function, mental status changes, incontinence, falls, or subnormal temperature. (Touhy and Jett, 2018).

TABLE 46.1   Urinary Incontinence

Definition	Characteristics	Selected Nursing Interventions
Transient Incontinence		
Incontinence caused by medical conditions that in many cases are treatable and reversible	Common reversible causes include: • Delirium and/or acute confusion • Inflammation (e.g., urinary tract infection [UTI], urethritis) • Medications (e.g., diuretics) (Burchum and Rosenthal, 2019) • Excessive urine output (e.g., hyperglycemia, congestive heart failure) • Mobility impairment from any cause • Fecal impaction • Depression • Acute urinary retention	With new-onset or increased incontinence, look for reversible causes. Notify health care provider of any suspected reversible causes.
Functional Incontinence		
Loss of continence because of causes outside the urinary tract Usually related to functional deficits such as altered mobility and manual dexterity, cognitive impairment, poor motivation, or environmental barriers Direct result of caregivers not responding in a timely manner to requests for help with toileting	Toilet access restricted by: • Sensory impairments (e.g., vision) • Cognitive impairments (e.g., delirium, dementia, severe retardation) • Altered mobility (e.g., hip fracture, arthritis, chronic pain, spastic paralysis associated with multiple sclerosis, slow movements associated with Parkinson's disease, hemiparesis) • Altered manual dexterity (e.g., arthritis, upper extremity fracture) • Environmental barriers (e.g., caregiver not available to help with transfers, pathway to bathroom not maneuverable with a walker, tight clothing that is difficult to remove, incontinence briefs)	Adequate lighting in the bathroom Individualized toileting program designed for the degree of cognitive impairment: habit training program, scheduled toileting program, prompted voiding program Mobility aides (e.g., raised toilet seats, toilet grab bars) Toilet area cleared to allow access for a walker or wheelchair Elastic-waist pants without buttons or zippers Nurse call system always within reach Use of incontinence containment product patient can easily remove such as a pull-up–type pant or a pad that can be moved aside easily for voiding
Urinary Incontinence Associated with Chronic Retention of Urine (Overflow Urinary Incontinence)		
Involuntary loss of urine caused by an overdistended bladder often related to bladder outlet obstruction or poor bladder emptying because of weak or absent bladder contractions	Distended bladder on palpation High postvoid residual Frequency Involuntary leakage of small volumes of urine Nocturia	Interventions are individualized related to the severity of the urinary retention, ability of bladder to contract, existing kidney damage. Mild retention with some bladder function: • Timed voiding • Double voiding • Monitor postvoid residual per health care provider's direction • Intermittent catheterization Severe retention, no bladder function: • Intermittent catheterization • Indwelling catheterization
Stress Urinary Incontinence		
Involuntary leakage of small volumes of urine associated with increased intraabdominal pressure related to either urethral hypermobility or an incompetent urinary sphincter (e.g., weak pelvic floor muscles, trauma after childbirth, radical prostatectomy) Result of weakness or injury to the urinary sphincter or pelvic floor muscles Underlying result: urethra cannot stay closed as pressure increases in the bladder as a result of increased abdominal pressure (e.g., a sneeze or cough)	Small-volume loss of urine with coughing, laughing, exercise, walking, getting up from a chair Usually does not leak urine at night when sleeping	As directed by the health care provider, instruct patient in pelvic muscle exercises.

Continued

TABLE 46.1	Urinary Incontinence—cont'd	
Definition	**Characteristics**	**Selected Nursing Interventions**
Urge or Urgency Urinary Incontinence		
Involuntary passage of urine often associated with strong sense of urgency related to an overactive bladder caused by neurological problems, bladder inflammation, or bladder outlet obstruction In many cases bladder overactivity is idiopathic; cause is not known Caused by involuntary contractions of the bladder associated with an urge to void that causes leakage of urine	May experience one or all of the following symptoms: • Urgency • Frequency • Nocturia • Difficulty or inability to hold urine once the urge to void occurs • Leaks on the way to the bathroom • Leaks larger volumes of urine, sometimes enough to wet outer clothing • Dribbles small amounts on the way to the bathroom • Strong urge/leaks when one hears water running, washes hands, drinks fluids	Ask patient about symptoms of a UTI. Avoid bladder irritants (e.g., caffeine, artificial sweeteners, alcohol). As directed by the health care provider, instruct patient in pelvic muscle exercises, in urge-inhibition exercises, and/or in bladder training. If ordered by the health care provider, monitor patient symptoms and for the presence of side effects of antimuscarinic medications.
Reflex Urinary Incontinence		
Involuntary loss of urine occurring at somewhat predictable intervals when patient reaches specific bladder volume related to spinal cord damage between C1 and S2	Diminished or absent awareness of bladder filling and the urge to void Leakage of urine without awareness May not completely empty the bladder because of dyssynergia of the urinary sphincter—inappropriate contraction of the sphincter when the bladder contracts, causing obstruction to urine flow **CAUTION:** At risk for developing autonomic dysreflexia, a life-threatening condition that causes severe elevation of blood pressure and pulse rate and diaphoresis	Follow the prescribed schedule for emptying the bladder either through voiding or by intermittent catheterization. Supply urine-containment products: condom catheter, undergarments, pads, briefs. Monitor for signs and symptoms of urinary retention and UTI. Monitor for autonomic dysreflexia; this is a medical emergency requiring immediate intervention. Notify the health care provider immediately.

Urinary tract infections are the most common hospital-acquired infection, accounting for up to 40% of infections reported by acute care hospitals. The major risk factors for catheter-associated urinary tract infection (CAUTI) are the presence of an indwelling urinary catheter and the length of its use. Because a CAUTI is common, costly, and believed to be reasonably preventable, as of October 1, 2008, the Centers for Medicare and Medicaid Services (CMS) chose it as one of the complications for which hospitals no longer receive additional payment to compensate for the extra cost of treatment. Consequently there has been a shift in clinical care practices from the traditional focus on early recognition and prompt treatment to one of prevention. Effective prevention strategies that must be implemented to reduce the risk of CAUTIs include training and education of health care providers and increasing their awareness regarding basic infection control knowledge of optimal hand hygiene practices and methods for handling indwelling catheter and urine collecting systems appropriately, securing catheters properly, and maintaining unobstructed urine flow and closed sterile drainage system using sterile technique properly (CDC, 2015; Assadi, 2018).

Urinary Incontinence. Urinary incontinence (UI) is defined as the "complaint of any involuntary loss of urine" (Wilson, 2016; Vethanayagam et al., 2017) (see Table 46.1). UI is a common problem, affecting 27% of men and 43% women over the age of 40, 20% to 40% of older adults, and over 70% of elderly nursing home patients (Testa, 2015; Coyne and Wein, 2014). Common forms of UI are urge or urgency UI (involuntary leakage associated with urgency) and stress UI (involuntary loss of urine associated with effort or exertion on sneezing or coughing (Bardsley, 2016). Mixed UI is when stress- and urgency-type symptoms are both present. Overactive bladder is defined as urinary urgency, often accompanied by increased urinary frequency and nocturia that may or may not be associated with urgency incontinence and is present without obvious bladder pathology or infection. UI associated with chronic retention of urine (formally called *overflow UI*) is urine leakage caused by an overfull bladder. Functional UI is caused by factors that prohibit or interfere with a patient's access to the toilet or other acceptable receptacle for urine. In most cases there is no bladder pathology. It is a significant problem for older adults who experience problems with mobility or the dexterity to manage their clothing and toileting behaviors. Patients with other types of incontinence can also have a functional aspect to their incontinence (Seshan et al., 2016). A recently added category of incontinence is identified as multifactorial incontinence. This describes incontinence that has multiple interacting risk factors, some within the urinary tract and others not, such as multiple chronic illnesses, medications, age-related factors, and environmental factors (Saito et al., 2017).

Urinary Diversions. Patients who have had the bladder removed (cystectomy) because of cancer or significant bladder dysfunction related to radiation injury or neurogenic dysfunction with frequent UTI require surgical procedures that divert urine to the outside of the body through an opening in the abdominal wall called a *stoma*. Urinary diversions are constructed from a section of intestine to create a storage reservoir or conduit for urine. Diversions can be temporary or permanent, continent or incontinent.

There are two types of continent urinary diversions. The first is called a *continent urinary reservoir* (Fig. 46.2, *A*), which is created from a distal part of the ileum and proximal part of the colon. The ureters are embedded into the reservoir. This reservoir is situated under the abdominal wall and has a narrow ileal segment brought out through the abdominal wall to form a small stoma. The ileocecal valve creates a one-way valve in the pouch through which a catheter is inserted through the

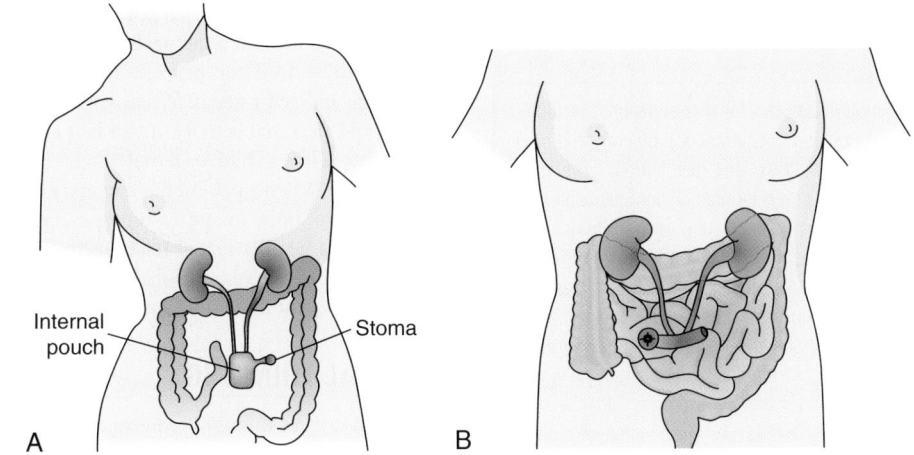

FIG. 46.2 Types of urinary diversions. **A,** Continent urinary reservoir. **B,** Ureterostomy (ileal conduit).

stoma to empty the urine from the pouch. Patients must be willing and able to catheterize the pouch 4 to 6 times a day for the rest of their lives.

The second type of continent urinary diversion is called an *orthotopic neobladder,* which uses an ileal pouch to replace the bladder. Anatomically the pouch is in the same position as the bladder was before removal, allowing a patient to void through the urethra using a Valsalva technique.

A **ureterostomy** or ileal conduit is a permanent incontinent urinary diversion created by transplanting the ureters into a closed-off part of the intestinal ileum and bringing the other end out onto the abdominal wall, forming a stoma (Fig. 46.2, *B*). The patient has no sensation or control over the continuous flow of urine through the ileal conduit, requiring the effluent (drainage) to be collected in a pouch.

Nephrostomy tubes are small tubes that are tunneled through the skin into the renal pelvis. These tubes are placed to drain the renal pelvis when the ureter is obstructed. Patients do go home with these tubes and need careful teaching about site care and signs of infection (Fig. 46.3).

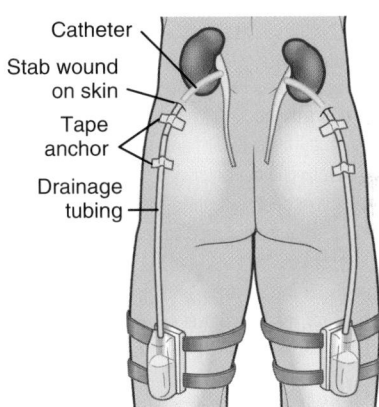

Bilateral nephrostomy tubes inserted into renal pelvis; catheters exit through an incision on each flank, or there may be just one kidney

FIG. 46.3 Nephrostomy tubes. (From Lewis SL, et al: *Medical-surgical nursing,* ed 10, St Louis, 2017, Elsevier.)

> **REFLECT NOW**
>
> You recently cared for a young woman with recurrent urinary tract infections (UTIs). Think about how these affect her lifestyle.

NURSING KNOWLEDGE BASE

Urinary elimination is a basic body function and carries with it a variety of psychological and physiological needs. When illness or disability interferes with meeting these needs, nursing care that addresses both the physiological and the psychological needs is essential. You need an understanding beyond anatomy and physiology of the urinary system to give appropriate care.

Infection Control and Hygiene

The urinary tract is sterile. Use infection control principles to help prevent the development and spread of UTIs. You need to follow the principles of medical and surgical asepsis when carrying out procedures involving the urinary tract or external genitalia. Perineal hygiene is an essential component of care (see Chapter 40) when there is an alteration in the usual pattern of urinary elimination. Perineal care or examination of the genitalia requires medical asepsis, including proper hand hygiene. Any invasive procedure such as catheterization requires sterile aseptic technique.

Growth and Development

It is important to apply knowledge of normal growth and development when caring for the patient with urinary problems. A patient's ability to control micturition changes during the life span. The neurological system is not well developed until 2 to 3 years of age. Until this stage of development, the small child is unable to associate the sensation of filling and urge with urination. When the child recognizes feelings of urge, can hold urine for 1 to 2 hours, and is able to communicate his or her needs, toilet training becomes successful. Continence starts during daytime hours. Children who wet the bed at night without waking from sleep have what is called *nocturnal enuresis.* In some cases they can experience this nighttime incontinence until late in childhood. Infants and young children cannot effectively concentrate urine. Their urine appears light yellow or clear. In relation to their small body size, infants and children excrete large volumes of urine. For example, a 6-month-old infant who weighs 13 to 18 lb (6 to 8 kg) excretes 400 to 500 mL of urine daily.

BOX 46.2 FOCUS ON OLDER ADULTS

Urinary Incontinence

Urinary incontinence is due to anatomical and functional deficits, including inappropriately functioning lower urinary tract, physical problems, cognitive decline, functional impairment co-morbidities, and medications. The most common type of urinary incontinence is urgency urinary incontinence in both elderly men and women. The most common reasons for urgency urinary incontinence in men and women are prostate hypertrophy and atrophic urethral mucosa, respectively. Age-related urinary incontinence often remains untreated in the elderly because the condition is considered a part of normal aging (Eshkoor et al., 2017). Older adults have a decreased ability to delay voiding, an increased incidence of overactive bladder, and potentially a loss of bladder contractility, increasing the risk for urinary retention. Older women have a decrease in estrogenization of perineal tissue, which increases the risk of urinary tract infection (Seshan et al., 2016). The use of multiple medications, called *polypharmacy*, is more common in older adults (Touhy and Jett, 2018). Many of these medications have the potential to impact normal elimination by affecting the ability of the bladder to hold urine or adequately empty (antihypertensives, cholinesterase inhibitors, antidepressants, sedatives) (Burchum and Rosenthal, 2019).

Implications for Practice

- Older adults with cognitive impairment may need to be reminded to void more frequently to improve continence.
- Evaluate all possible causes of new-onset incontinence, which should include taking note of any new medications that might impact cognition, alertness, mobility, or voiding.
- Older adults newly started on an antimuscarinic medication should be assessed carefully for mental status changes. This class of medications has the potential to cause cognitive impairment in older adults (American Geriatrics Society, 2018).
- Older adults with impaired mobility and incontinence should have interventions put in place to maximize self-care and continence (e.g., toileting program, mobility aids, help with hygiene).
- Teach older women with stress incontinence about pelvic muscle exercises. There is no age limit on their effectiveness.
- The sensation of thirst decreases with aging. Adequate hydration promotes bladder health. Older adults may need to be reminded to drink adequate amounts of water (Touhy and Jett, 2018).
- To decrease nocturia, instruct patients to restrict fluid intake for the 2 hours before bedtime.
- Older men with voiding pattern changes (e.g., urgency, frequency, slow stream, decreased output, dribbling) should be assessed for urinary retention because of age-related prostate enlargement.

Pregnancy causes many changes in the body, including the urinary tract. In early and late pregnancy urinary frequency is common. Hormonal changes and the pressure of the growing fetus on the bladder cause increased urine production and shrinking bladder capacity.

Normal aging causes changes in the urinary tract and the rest of the body. These changes are not the cause of bladder dysfunction, but age does increase risk and incidence (Box 46.2).

Psychosocial Implications

Self-concept, culture, and sexuality are all closely related concepts that are affected when patients have elimination problems. Self-concept changes over one's life span and includes body image, self-esteem, roles, and identity (see Chapters 33 and 34). When children begin to achieve bladder control and learn the appropriate toileting skills, they sometimes resist urinating on the toilet and associate their urine and feces as

extensions of self and thus do not want to flush them away. The process of micturition is often a culturally private event and requires you to be sensitive to a need for privacy. Incontinence can be devastating to self-image and self-esteem. When your patient asks for help for such a private and personal activity, it can be perceived as embarrassing or as being treated like a child, or it may threaten the patient's sense of self-determination. When a patient has a urinary diversion, it will influence his or her sense of body image, resulting in a perceived threat in being able to maintain a healthy sexual relationship with a partner. As a nurse, be aware of how elimination disorders affect patients psychosocially so that you can understand the full impact of the patient's elimination problem.

CRITICAL THINKING

Successful critical thinking requires synthesis of knowledge, experience, information gathered from patients, critical thinking attitudes, and intellectual and professional standards. Clinical judgments require you to anticipate and collect necessary information, analyze the data, and make decisions regarding your patient's care. During assessment consider all elements that build toward making an appropriate nursing diagnosis (Fig. 46.4).

When applying the nursing process, take into consideration the knowledge you have learned about the urinary system. Integrate the knowledge from nursing and other disciplines, previous experiences, and patients to understand the process of urinary elimination and the impact on a patient and family. The urinary system is affected by many factors, both as part of and outside the urinary tract. As a result you are able to identify the unique impact of these problems on patients and families. For example, men after prostate cancer surgery may experience stress UI because of trauma to the urinary sphincter, people with high caffeine intake or those who take a diuretic may experience increased urinary urgency and frequency, and patients who are normally continent and become immobile may become incontinent.

Urinary elimination problems are common in all health care settings. Reflect on previous and personal experiences to help you determine a patient's elimination needs. If you have personally had a UTI, the experience helps you to understand a patient's frustration and embarrassment as a result of frequency, urgency, and dysuria. Caring for other older adults with functional disabilities helps you to anticipate patient needs related to toileting.

In addition, use critical thinking attitudes such as perseverance to find a plan of care to provide successful management of urinary elimination problems. Professional standards also provide valuable directions. You are in a key position to serve as a patient advocate by suggesting noninvasive alternatives to catheterization use (e.g., the use of a bladder scanner to evaluate urine volume without invasive instrumentation or implementation of a voiding schedule for the incontinent patient).

Practice standards and guidelines prepared by nursing specialty organizations and those developed by national and international professional organizations are valuable tools to use when critically assessing patient problems and developing a plan of care. Box 46.3 lists some of these resources. The professional nurse incorporates such evidence-based guidelines into the plan of care.

REFLECT NOW

You have received shift report and your patient assignment includes a 65-year-old male with an indwelling catheter. How can you reduce the risk for a CAUTI?

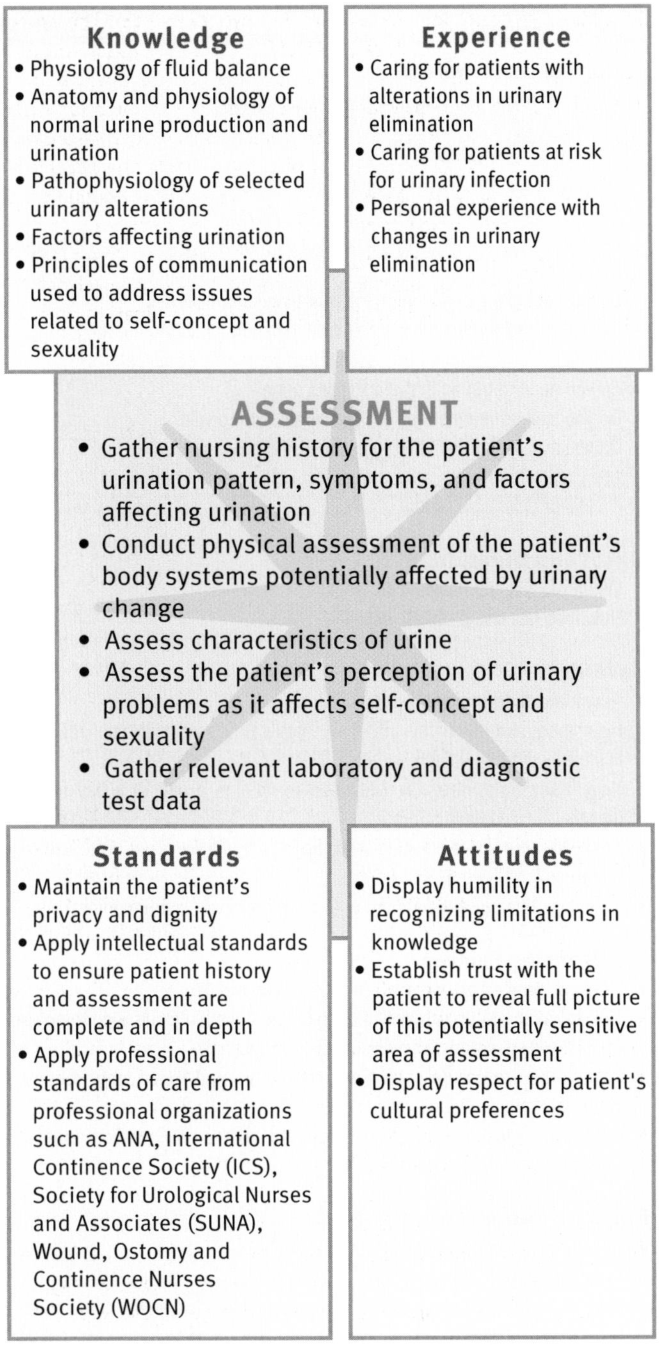

Knowledge

- Physiology of fluid balance
- Anatomy and physiology of normal urine production and urination
- Pathophysiology of selected urinary alterations
- Factors affecting urination
- Principles of communication used to address issues related to self-concept and sexuality

Experience

- Caring for patients with alterations in urinary elimination
- Caring for patients at risk for urinary infection
- Personal experience with changes in urinary elimination

ASSESSMENT

- Gather nursing history for the patient's urination pattern, symptoms, and factors affecting urination
- Conduct physical assessment of the patient's body systems potentially affected by urinary change
- Assess characteristics of urine
- Assess the patient's perception of urinary problems as it affects self-concept and sexuality
- Gather relevant laboratory and diagnostic test data

Standards

- Maintain the patient's privacy and dignity
- Apply intellectual standards to ensure patient history and assessment are complete and in depth
- Apply professional standards of care from professional organizations such as ANA, International Continence Society (ICS), Society for Urological Nurses and Associates (SUNA), Wound, Ostomy and Continence Nurses Society (WOCN)

Attitudes

- Display humility in recognizing limitations in knowledge
- Establish trust with the patient to reveal full picture of this potentially sensitive area of assessment
- Display respect for patient's cultural preferences

FIG. 46.4 Critical thinking model for urinary elimination assessment. *ANA*, American Nurses Association.

❖ NURSING PROCESS

Apply the nursing process and use a critical thinking approach in the care of patients. The nursing process provides a clinical decision-making approach for you to develop and implement an individualized plan of care.

◆ Assessment

During the assessment process, thoroughly assess each patient and critically analyze assessment findings to ensure that you make patient-centered clinical decisions required for safe nursing care.

BOX 46.3 Resources for Urology/Continence Nurses

- Centers for Disease Control and Prevention (CDC, 2019): Catheter-associated urinary tract infection (CAUTI) and non–catheter-associated urinary tract infection (UTI) and other urinary system infection (USI) events, https://www.cdc.gov/nhsn/PDFs/pscManual/7pscCAUTIcurrent.pdf
- Centers for Disease Control and Prevention (CDC, 2015): Health care–associated infections (HAIs); catheter-associated urinary tract infections (CAUTI), http://www.cdc.gov/HAI/ca_uti/uti.html
- European Association of Urology Nurses (EAUN): http://www.uroweb.org/nurses/nursing-guidelines/
- International Continence Society (ICS): http://www.ics.org/
- National Association For Continence (NAFC): http://www.nafc.org/
- Society of Urologic Nurses and Associates (SUNA): https://www.suna.org/
- The Simon Foundation for Continence: http://www.simonfoundation.org/index.html
- The Wound, Ostomy and Continence Nurses Society™ (WOCN): http://www.wocn.org/

Through the Patient's Eyes. Throughout the nursing assessment it is important for you to consider a patient's frame of reference related to his or her illness or urinary problem. Assess the patient's understanding of the urinary problem and expectations of treatment. Because urination is a private matter, some patients find it difficult to talk about urinary incontinence or their voiding habits. Approach patients in a professional manner and assure them that their problems will be kept confidential. Postoperative patients or patients receiving medications that affect bladder function may become concerned that something is wrong when you assess voiding amount and frequency. Patients receiving intravenous (IV) fluids do not always realize that they have an increased need for urination. Sensitivity to patient misconceptions will allow you to quickly identify areas for patient education. Always ask what he or she expects from care. For example, does the patient expect that the UTI will be resolved? Does the patient expect the ureterostomy to be only temporary?

Self-Care Ability. It is very important to thoroughly assess patients' ability to perform necessary behaviors associated with voiding. Investigate their expectations of how nurses will assist them and what they can do independently. Do not assume that because a patient has a diagnosis of cognitive impairment that he or she cannot understand or participate in care. Balancing patient safety and supporting self-care are sometimes challenges and should be discussed with the patient. For example, a patient with poor balance will need assistance with transfers to a toilet and may need continued supervision while on the toilet, something the patient may find embarrassing or demeaning.

Cultural Considerations. Assess cultural and gender differences related to the very private act of voiding and how they affect nursing assessment and care. Be sensitive and ask questions in a straightforward manner. Be aware of gender preferences in positioning for urination: most men stand to void, whereas women sit. This makes a difference in how you will assist patients unable to use a bathroom. There are gender-linked urinary alterations such as prostate

⊕ BOX 46.4 CULTURAL ASPECTS OF CARE

Urinary Elimination

Urinary elimination is private. It is important when caring for patients from diverse cultures and religions to incorporate into the plan of care sensitivity and awareness of factors that may impact care when dealing with urinary elimination problems. Some cultures may have specific beliefs and practices related to elimination, privacy, and gender-specific care. Because of the personal nature and cultural practices surrounding elimination, urinary problems such as incontinence often are not discussed with medical professionals (Wang et al., 2014; Lai et al., 2017). Variations within a cultural group are common; thus each patient must be assessed and cared for as an individual.

Implications for Patient-Centered Care

- Each patient is unique. As a professional nurse you must determine the extent to which a patient's cultural background, such as age-group, geographic location, ethnicity, or race, affects individual elimination problems.
- Whenever possible, provide for a same-gender caregiver for individuals whose cultural preferences emphasize female modesty and prohibit non-related males and females from touching (Jarvis, 2016).
- Privacy is important in many cultures; thus careful attention to closing doors, bedside curtains, and draping is important (Lai et al., 2017).
- Pay special attention that the patient understands instructions and patient education when English is not the primary language. If available, provide written materials in patient's primary language. Provide a professional interpreter as needed.
- Certain cultures may observe meticulous hygiene practices that designate the left hand to perform unclean procedures, such as genitourinary hygiene. Ask patient or family caregivers their practice preferences.
- Some cultures may continue to practice female genital circumcision, leaving only a small opening for urine and menses (Clarke, 2016; Malik et al., 2018). Long-term consequences include recurrent urinary tract infections, incontinence, pelvic infections, fistulas, scarring, and sexual dysfunction (Malik et al., 2018).
- Cultural practices dictate the level of involvement of family in a patient's care. This source of strength is important to the health of the patient, and family must be included in the plan of care.

BOX 46.5 Nursing Assessment Questions

Nature of the Problem
- Which problems are you having with passing urine?

Signs and Symptoms
- Does it hurt or burn when you pass your urine?
- Are you having abdominal pain/flank pain/fevers/chills?
- Has there been a change in the color or odor of your urine? Please describe that change.
- Do you feel like you are emptying your bladder completely?
- Are you passing urine more frequently than normal during the day?
- Do you need to strain and/or wait before your urine stream starts?
- Do you need to get up at night to pass urine?
- Do you leak urine when feeling a strong desire to void?
- Do you ever leak urine when you cough, sneeze, and/or exercise?
- Are you ever wet with urine and do not know when it happened?
- Do you dribble urine before you void, after you void, or at other times?

Onset and Duration
- When did you first notice a problem?
- How long has this problem lasted?

Severity
- How many times a day do you pass urine?
- How many times a day and how many times at night do you leak urine?
- How many times are you wet/need to change a pad in a day and at night?
- How often are you awakened with the urge to void and get up to use the bathroom?
- How does this pattern compare with the pattern you last remember?

Predisposing Factors
- Have you noticed any patterns to your urinary problem?
- Tell me what you usually eat/drink in a day. Does it include such things as caffeinated beverages, chocolate, citrus, or alcohol?
- Which medicines do you take routinely, and have any recently changed?
- Have you been hospitalized or diagnosed with a new medical problem recently?

Effect on Patient
- How have these symptoms affected your life?
- Tell me how your urinary problem affects any of your usual activities.
- Have you ever tried any treatment for this problem (self-help, complementary therapies, over-the-counter remedies, medical professional, or specialist)?

enlargement in men and pelvic organ prolapse in women. Culture often dictates gender-specific roles when it comes to care of elimination issues. It may be inappropriate for a male to touch or even talk about elimination matters with a woman (Box 46.4).

Nursing History. Before gathering a history, assess your patient's health literacy to be sure you communicate clearly and can understand patient's problems. The nursing history includes a review of the patient's elimination patterns, symptoms of urinary alterations, and assessment of factors that are affecting the ability to urinate normally. Box 46.5 lists nursing history questions that will help direct the patient to focus on urinary problems.

Pattern of Urination. Ask the patient about daily voiding patterns, including frequency and times of day, normal volume at each voiding, and history of recent changes. Frequency of voiding varies among individuals depending on fluid intake, medications such as diuretics, and the intake of bladder irritants such as caffeine or other caffeinated beverages. The common times for urination are on awakening, after meals, and before bedtime. Most people void an average of 5 or more times a day. Be sure to ask whether the patient is awakened from

sleep with an urge to void and how many times this occurs. It is normal for patients who wake at night because of noise, pain, or nighttime treatments to experience an urge to void. Information about the pattern of urination is necessary to establish a baseline for comparison.

Symptoms of Urinary Alterations. Certain symptoms specific to urinary alterations may occur in more than one type of disorder. During assessment ask the patient about the presence of symptoms related to urination (Table 46.2). Also determine whether the patient is aware of conditions or factors that precipitate or aggravate the

TABLE 46.2   Common Symptoms of Urinary Alterations

Description	Common Causes	Description	Common Causes
Urgency An immediate and strong desire to void that is not easily deferred	Full bladder Urinary tract infection Inflammation or irritation of the bladder Overactive bladder	**Nocturia** Awakened from sleep because of the urge to void	Excess intake of fluids (especially coffee or alcohol before bedtime) Bladder outlet obstruction (e.g., prostate enlargement) Overactive bladder Medications (e.g., diuretic taken in the evening) Cardiovascular disease (e.g., hypertension) Urinary tract infection
Dysuria Pain or discomfort associated with voiding	Urinary tract infection Inflammation of the prostate Urethritis Trauma to the lower urinary tract Urinary tract tumors	**Dribbling** Leakage of small amounts of urine despite voluntary control of micturition	Bladder outlet obstruction (e.g., prostatic enlargement) Incomplete bladder emptying Stress incontinence
Frequency Voiding more than 8 times during waking hours and/or at decreased intervals, such as less than every 2 hours	High volumes of fluid intake Bladder irritants (e.g., caffeine) Urinary tract infection Increased pressure on bladder (e.g., pregnancy) Bladder outlet obstruction (e.g., prostate enlargement, pelvic organ prolapse) Overactive bladder	**Hematuria** Presence of blood in urine Gross hematuria (blood is easily seen in urine) Microscopic hematuria (blood not visualized but measured on urinalysis)	Tumors (e.g., kidney, bladder) Infection (e.g., glomerular nephritis, cystitis) Urinary tract calculi Trauma to the urinary tract
Hesitancy Delay in start of urinary stream when voiding	Anxiety (e.g., voiding in public restroom) Bladder outlet obstruction (e.g., prostate enlargement, urethral stricture)	**Retention** Acute retention: Suddenly unable to void when bladder is adequately full or overfull Chronic retention: Bladder does not empty completely during voiding, and urine is retained in the bladder	Bladder outlet obstruction (e.g., prostatic enlargement, urethral obstruction) Absent or weak bladder contractility (e.g., neurological dysfunction such as caused by diabetes, multiple sclerosis, lower spinal cord injury) Side effects of certain medications (e.g., anesthesia, anticholinergics, antispasmodics, antidepressants)
Polyuria Voiding excessive amounts of urine	High volumes of fluid intake Uncontrolled diabetes mellitus Diabetes insipidus Diuretic therapy		
Oliguria Diminished urinary output in relation to fluid intake	Fluid and electrolyte imbalance (e.g., dehydration) Kidney dysfunction or failure Increased secretion of antidiuretic hormone (ADH) Urinary tract obstruction		

symptoms and determine what he or she does if any of these symptoms occur.

Physical Assessment. A physical examination (see Chapter 30) provides you with data to determine the presence and severity of urinary elimination problems. The primary areas to assess include the kidneys, bladder, external genitalia, urethral meatus, and perineal skin. Fluid intake, voiding pattern, and amounts provide additional objective data.

Kidneys. When the kidneys become infected or inflamed, they can become tender, resulting in flank pain. You assess for tenderness by gently percussing the costovertebral angle (the angle formed by the spine and twelfth rib). Auscultation with the bell of the stethoscope is sometimes performed to detect the presence of a renal artery bruit (sound resulting from turbulent blood flow through a narrowed artery), but this skill is usually performed by an advanced practice nurse.

Bladder. In adults the bladder rests below the symphysis pubis. When distended with urine, the bladder will rise above the symphysis pubis along the midline of the abdomen. A very full bladder can extend as far as the umbilicus. On inspection you may observe a swelling or convex curvature of the lower abdomen. On gentle palpation of the lower abdomen, a full bladder may be felt as a smooth and rounded mass. When a full bladder is palpated, patients report a sensation of urinary urge tenderness or even pain. If an overfull bladder is suspected, further assessment with an ultrasound device or a bladder scanner is recommended if available.

External Genitalia and Urethral Meatus. Careful and sensitive inspection of the external genitalia and urethral meatus yields important data that may indicate inflammation and infection. Normally there should be no drainage or inflammation. To best examine the female patient, position her in the dorsal recumbent position to provide full exposure of the genitalia. Observe the labia majora for swelling, redness, tenderness, rashes, lesions, or evidence of scratching. Using a gloved hand, retract the labial folds. The labia minora is normally pink and moist. The urethral meatus will appear as an irregular or slitlike opening below the clitoris and above the vaginal opening. Look for drainage and lesions, and ask the patient whether there is discomfort. If there is drainage, note the color and consistency and any odor. The vaginal tissue of a postmenopausal woman may be drier and less pink than that of younger women.

For the male patient, examine the penis. Look for any redness or irritation. If the man is uncircumcised, retract the foreskin or ask the patient to do so. The foreskin should move back easily to expose the glans penis. In some cases the foreskin will become tight and cannot be retracted (phimosis), increasing risk for inflammation and infection. The urethral meatus is a slitlike opening just below the tip of the penis. Inspect the glans penis and meatus for discharge, lesions, and inflammation. Following inspection, return the foreskin to the unretracted position. Retracted foreskins can cause dangerous swelling (paraphimosis) of the penis (Ball et al., 2019).

All patients with an indwelling catheter should have the urinary meatus assessed for catheter-related damage and for the presence of inflammation and discharge that can indicate infection. Pulling and traction on catheters can damage the urinary meatus by creating pressure on the urethra and meatus. In some severe cases the catheter will erode through the meatus to the vagina or in men through the glans and shaft of the penis. Early detection of trauma means that a plan for prevention for further damage can be implemented.

Perineal Skin. Assessment of skin exposed to moisture, especially urine, needs to occur at least daily (and more often if incontinence is ongoing) to pick up early signs of skin damage related to the moisture. Observe for erythema in areas exposed to moisture, skin erosion, and patient complaints of a burning, itching pain.

Assessment of Urine. The assessment of urine includes measuring the patient's fluid intake and urinary output (I&O) and observing the characteristics of the urine.

Intake and Output. Assessment of I&O is a way to evaluate bladder emptying, renal function, and fluid and electrolyte balance. Although often written as part of a health care provider's order, placing a patient on I&O is also a nursing judgment. Obtaining accurate I&O measurement often requires cooperation and assistance from the patient and family. Intake measurements need to include all oral liquids and semiliquids, enteral feedings, and any parenteral fluids (see Chapter 42). Output measurement includes not only urine but any fluid that leaves the body that can be measured such as vomitus, gastric drainage tubes, and wound drains.

Urinary output is a key indicator of kidney and bladder function. A change in urine volume can be a significant indicator of fluid imbalance, kidney dysfunction, or decreased blood volume. For example, a postoperative catheterized patient's hourly urinary output provides an indirect measure of circulating blood volume. If the urinary output falls below 30 mL/hr, the nurse should immediately assess for signs of blood loss and notify the health care provider. Urinary output is also an indicator of bladder function. Patients who have not voided for longer than 3 to 6 hours and have had fluid intake recorded should be evaluated for urinary retention. Just helping some patients to a normal position to void prompts voiding. Assess for any extreme increase or decrease in urine volume. Urine output of less than 30 mL per hour for more than 2 consecutive hours or excessive urine output (polyuria) is a cause for concern and should prompt further assessment and notification of the health care provider.

Urine volume is measured using receptacles with volume-measurement markings. After a patient voids in a bedside commode, bedpan, or urinal, or when urine is emptied from a catheter drainage bag, urine can be measured using a graduated measuring

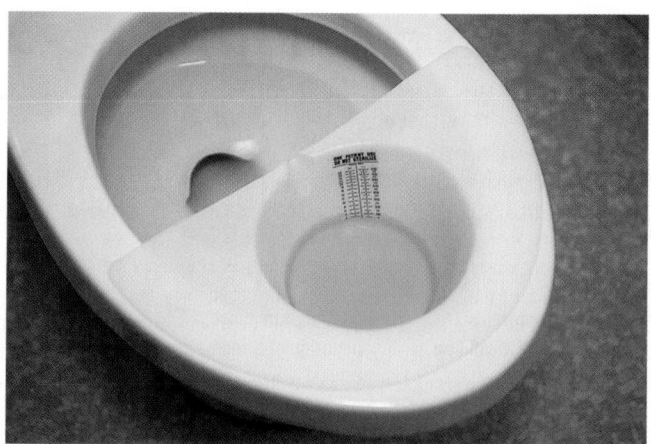

FIG. 46.5 Urine hat.

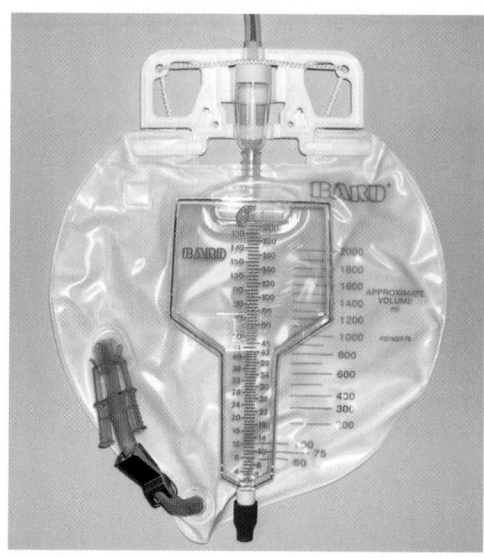

FIG. 46.6 Urometer. (Courtesy Michael Gallagher, RN, BSN, OSF Saint Francis Medical Center, Peoria, IL.)

container. For patients who void in a toilet, a urine hat (Fig. 46.5) collects urine, allowing for patient privacy in the bathroom. Catheterized patients may have a specialized drainage bag with a urometer (Fig. 46.6) attached between the drainage tubing and drainage bag that allows for accurate hourly urine measurement. When emptying catheter drainage bags, follow Standard Precautions (Chapter 28), and make sure that the drainage tube is reclamped and secured. Each patient needs to have a graduated receptacle for individual use to prevent potential cross-contamination. Label each container with the patient's name or other identifiers according to agency policy. The container needs to be rinsed after each use to minimize odor and bacterial growth.

Characteristics of Urine. Inspect the patient's urine for color, clarity, and odor. Monitor and document any changes.

Color. Normal urine ranges in color from a pale straw to amber, depending on its concentration. Urine is usually more concentrated in the morning or with fluid volume deficits. As the patient drinks more fluids, urine becomes less concentrated, and the color lightens. Patients taking diuretics commonly void dilute urine while the medication is active.

Blood in the urine (hematuria) is never a normal finding. Bleeding from the kidneys or ureters usually causes urine to become dark red; bleeding from the bladder or urethra usually causes bright red urine. Hematuria and blood clots are a common cause of urinary catheter blockage.

Various medications and foods change the color of the urine. For example, patients taking phenazopyridine, a urinary analgesic, void urine that is bright orange. Eating beets, rhubarb, and blackberries causes red urine. The kidneys excrete special dyes used in IV diagnostic studies, and this discolors the urine. Dark amber urine is the result of high concentrations of bilirubin (urobilinogen) in patients with liver disease. Report unexpected color changes to the health care provider.

Clarity. Normal urine appears transparent at the time of voiding. Urine that stands several minutes in a container becomes cloudy. In patients with renal disease, freshly voided urine appears cloudy because of protein concentration. Urine may also appear thick and cloudy as a result of bacteria and white blood cells. Early-morning voided urine may be cloudy because of urine held in the bladder overnight but will be clear on the next voiding.

Odor. Urine has a characteristic ammonia odor. The more concentrated the urine, the stronger the odor. As urine remains standing (e.g., in a collection device), more ammonia breakdown occurs, and the odor becomes stronger. A foul odor may indicate a UTI. Some foods such as asparagus and garlic can change the odor of urine.

Laboratory and Diagnostic Testing. You are often responsible for collecting urine specimens for laboratory testing. The type of test determines the method of collection. Label all specimens with the patient's name, date, time, and type of collection. Most urine specimens need to reach the laboratory within 2 hours of collection or must be preserved according to the laboratory protocol (Pagana et al., 2019). Urine that stands in a container at room temperature without the required preservative will grow bacteria resulting in changes that will affect the accuracy of the test. Agency infection control policies require adherence to Standard Precautions during the handling of urine specimens (see Chapter 28). To obtain urine that is fresh or new, you need to ask the patient to double void. The second voided specimen is the one sent to the laboratory. To obtain urine as free of bacterial contamination as possible, a midstream clean-catch urine specimen may be required. Table 46.3 describes nursing considerations for a variety of common tests. Table 46.4 describes the components of the most common of the urinary tests, urinalysis.

Diagnostic Examinations. The urinary system is one of the few organ systems accessible to accurate diagnostic study by radiographic techniques. Studies can be simple and noninvasive or complex and invasive. See Table 46.5 for a review of some common diagnostic testing of the urinary tract.

Many of the nursing responsibilities related to diagnostic testing of the urinary tract are common to most studies. Those responsibilities before testing include the following:
- Ensure that a signed consent is completed (check agency policy).
- Assess the patient for any iodinated dye allergies and whether he or she has experienced a previous reaction to a contrast agent (Pagana et al., 2019).
- Administer agency bowel-cleansing protocol to ensure kidneys can be visualized (check agency policy).
- Ensure that the patient adheres to the appropriate pretest diet (clear liquids) or nothing by mouth (NPO).
- Responsibilities after testing include:
  - Assessing I&O.
  - Assessing voiding and urine (color, clarity, presence of blood, dysuria, problems with emptying).
  - Encouraging fluid intake, especially if using radiopaque dye.

> **REFLECT NOW**
>
> In providing care for a patient with urinary incontinence, what are some physical assessment findings to expect?

◆ Nursing Diagnosis

A thorough assessment of a patient's urinary elimination function reveals patterns of data that allow a nurse to make relevant and accurate nursing diagnoses. Use critical thinking to reflect on knowledge of previous patients, apply knowledge of urinary function and the effects of disorders, review assessment findings, and make a specific nursing diagnosis. Data from questions about the urinary system are important in identifying nursing diagnoses. The diagnosis focuses on a specific urinary elimination alteration or an associated problem such as *Impaired Tissue Integrity related to urinary incontinence*. Identification of assessment findings leads to selection of an appropriate negative or problem-focused diagnosis. Identification of risk factors leads to selection of a risk diagnosis (see Chapter 17).

An important part of formulating negative or problem-focused nursing diagnoses lies in identifying the relevant causative or related factor. In the case of risk diagnoses, you select correct risk factors. You will choose interventions that treat or modify the related factor or risk factor for the diagnosis to be resolved. Specifying related factors for a diagnosis allows selection of individualized nursing interventions. For example, *Impaired Self Toileting related to an impaired ability to transfer* status guides the selection of nursing interventions that remove barriers to toilet access. *Impaired Self Toileting related to cognitive impairment* guides the selection of nursing interventions such as a prompted voiding program or habit training program. Box 46.6 provides an example of diagnostic reasoning. Some nursing diagnoses common to patients with urinary elimination problems include the following:
- *Urinary Incontinence: Functional; Overflow; Reflex; Stress; Urge*
- *Infection*
- *Impaired Self Toileting*
- *Impaired Skin Integrity*
- *Urinary Retention*

◆ Planning

During planning integrate the knowledge from assessment and information about available resources and therapies to develop an individualized plan of care (see the Nursing Care Plan). Match the patient's needs with clinical and professional standards recommended in the literature (Fig. 46.7). Building a relationship of trust with patients is important because the implementation of care involves interaction of a very personal nature.

Goals and Outcomes. The plan of care for urinary elimination alterations must include realistic and individualized goals along with relevant outcomes. The nurse and the patient need to collaborate in setting goals and outcomes and ultimately in choosing nursing interventions. A general goal is often normal urinary elimination, but sometimes the individual goal differs, depending on the problem. The goals are short term or long term.

For example, a realistic short-term goal for a patient with *Impaired Self Toileting related to impaired mobility status* would be that the patient will be able to independently use the toilet. An appropriate outcome would be that the "patient is observed to safely transfer to the

TABLE 46.3 Urine Testing

Collection Type/Use of Specimen	Nursing Considerations
Random (routine urinalysis) Includes a number of tests that are used for screening and are diagnostic for fluid and electrolyte disturbances, urinary tract infection, presence of blood and other metabolic problems	Collect during normal voiding or from an indwelling catheter or urinary diversion collection bag. Do not collect from an indwelling catheter drainage bag (urine is not freshly voided). Use a clean specimen cup. In some health care settings you may be responsible for testing urine with reagent strips. Follow manufacturer instructions when performing and reading the strips. Dip the reagent strip into fresh urine, then observe color changes on the strip. Compare the color on the strip with the color chart on the reagent strip container. Each color is examined at the exact time indicated on the container.
Clean-voided or midstream (culture and sensitivity)	Urine may be collected by the patient after detailed instruction on proper cleansing and collection technique (see Skill 46.1). Always use a sterile specimen cup.
Sterile specimen for culture and sensitivity Determines the presence of bacteria and to which antibiotic the bacteria are sensitive	If the patient has an indwelling catheter, collect a specimen by using sterile aseptic technique through the special sampling port (see Fig. 46.12) found on the side of the catheter. Never collect the specimen from the drainage bag. Clamp the tubing below the port, allowing fresh, uncontaminated urine to collect in the tube. After wiping the port with an antimicrobial swab, insert a sterile syringe hub and withdraw at least 3 to 5 mL of urine (check agency policy). Using sterile aseptic technique, transfer the urine to a sterile container (see Chapter 28). Patients with a urinary diversion need to have the stoma catheterized to obtain an accurate specimen. A preliminary report will be available in 24 hours, but usually 48 to 72 hours is needed for bacterial growth and sensitivity testing.
Timed urine specimens Measure bodily substances that may be excreted at higher levels at specific times of the day or over a specific time period	Requires urine collection and testing either at specific time of day or urine collected over a specific time period (e.g., 2-, 12-, or 24-hour collections). The timed period begins after the patient urinates and ends with a final voiding at the end of the time period. In most 24-hour specimen collections discard the first voided specimen and then start collecting urine. Patient voids into a clean receptacle, and the urine is transferred to the special collection container, which often contains special preservatives. Depending on the test, the urine container may need to be kept cool by setting it in a container of ice. Each specimen must be free of feces and toilet tissue. Missed specimens make the whole collection inaccurate. Check with agency policy and the laboratory for specific instructions. Patients' education should include an explanation of the test, an emphasis on the need to collect all urine voided during the prescribed time period, and urine collection procedure.

TABLE 46.4 Routine Urinalysis

Measurement (Normal Value)	Interpretation
pH (4.6 to 8.0)	pH level indicates acid-base balance. Acid pH helps protect against bacterial growth. Urine that stands for several hours becomes alkaline from bacterial growth.
Protein (up to 8 mg/100 mL)	Protein is normally not present in urine. The presence of protein is a very sensitive indicator of kidney function. Damage to the glomerular membrane (such as in glomerulonephritis) allows for the filtration of larger molecules such as protein to seep through.
Glucose (not normally present)	Patients with poorly controlled diabetes have glucose in the urine because of inability of tubules to resorb high serum glucose concentrations (>180 mg/100 mL). Ingestion of high concentrations of glucose causes some to appear in urine of healthy people.
Ketones (not normally present)	With poor control of diabetes, patients experience breakdown of fatty acids. End products of fatty acid metabolism are ketones. Patients with dehydration, starvation, or excessive aspirin ingestion also have ketonuria.
Specific gravity (1.005 to 1.030)	Specific gravity tests measure concentration of particles in urine. High specific gravity reflects concentrated urine, and low specific gravity reflects diluted urine. Dehydration, reduced renal blood flow, and increase in ADH secretion elevate specific gravity. Overhydration, early renal disease, and inadequate ADH secretion reduce specific gravity.
Microscopic examination RBC (up to 2)	Damage to glomeruli or tubules allows RBCs to enter the urine. Trauma, disease, presence of urethral catheters, or surgery of the lower urinary tract also causes RBCs to be present.
WBCs (0-4 per low-power field)	Elevated numbers indicate inflammation or infection.
Bacteria (not normally present)	Bacteria in the urine can mean infection or colonization (if the patient shows no symptoms).
Casts (cylindrical bodies not normally present, the shapes of which take on the likeness of objects within the renal tubule)	Types include hyaline, WBCs, RBCs, granular cells, and epithelial cells. Their presence indicates renal disease.
Crystals (not normally present)	Crystals indicate increased risk for the development of renal calculi (stone). Patients with high uric acid levels (gout) may develop uric acid crystals.

ADH, Antidiuretic hormone; *RBC*, red blood cell; *WBC*, white blood cell.
Data from Pagana KD, et al: *Mosby's diagnostic and laboratory test reference*, ed 14, St Louis, 2019, Elsevier.

TABLE 46.5 Common Diagnostic Tests of Urinary Tract

Procedure	Description	Special Nursing Considerations
Noninvasive Procedures		
Abdominal roentgenogram (plain film; kidney, ureter, bladder [KUB] or flat plate)	X-ray film of the abdomen to determine the size, shape, symmetry, and location of the structures of the lower urinary tract. Common uses: Detect and measure the size of urinary calculi	No special preparation
Computed tomography of abdomen and pelvis (CT)	Detailed imagery of the abdominal structures provided by computerized reconstruction of cross-sectional images. Common uses: Identify anatomical abnormalities, renal tumors and cysts, calculi, and obstruction of the ureters	Preparation: Explain procedure to patient Assess for presence of any allergies and previous reaction to contrast iodinated dye. All patients with allergies are at increased risk for anaphylactoid reactions to radiocontrast. NPO: Restrict food and fluid up to 4 hours before test (see agency or health care provider protocol). After procedure: Encourage fluids to promote dye excretion. Assess for delayed hypersensitivity reaction to the contrast media. Patient teaching: Explain that he or she will be placed on a special bed that will move through a tunnel-like imaging chamber. He or she will need to lie still when instructed by the technician; some patients may feel claustrophobic.
Intravenous pyelogram (IVP)	Imaging of the urinary tract that views the collecting ducts and renal pelvis and outlines the ureters, bladder, and urethra. (After intravenous injection of contrast media [iodine based that converts to a dye], a series of x-ray films are taken to observe the passage of urine from the renal pelvis to the bladder.) Common uses: Detect and measure urinary calculi, tumors, hematuria, obstruction of the urinary tract	Preparation: Assess for allergies to iodinated dyes. Assess for dehydration. Follow agency bowel cleansing protocol. Follow agency food and fluid restriction protocol. After procedure: Assess for delayed hypersensitivity to the contrast media. Encourage fluids after the test to dilute and flush dye from the patient. Assess urine output. Less than 30 mL/hr increases risk for contrast-induced nephropathy. Patient teaching: Facial flushing is a normal response during dye injection, and patients may feel dizzy or warm or feel some nausea.
Ultrasound: Renal bladder	Imaging of the kidneys, ureters, and bladder using sound waves. Identifies gross structural abnormalities and estimates the volume of urine in the bladder. Common uses: Detect masses, obstruction, presence of hydronephrosis or hydroureter, abnormalities of the bladder wall, and calculi; measure postvoid residual	Patients may be instructed to void before scan or come with a full bladder; verify preprocedure order for patient. Do not schedule within 24 hours after intravenous pyelogram.
Invasive Procedures		
Cystoscopy	Introduction of a cystoscope through the urethra into the bladder to provide direct visualization, specimen collection, and/or treatment of the bladder and urethra. (In most cases the procedure is performed using local anesthesia, but under certain circumstances general anesthesia or conscious sedation may be used.) Common uses: Microscopic hematuria, detect bladder tumors and obstruction of the bladder outlet and urethra	Follow agency bowel cleansing protocol. Patients may be requested to drink fluids before procedure. Patient teaching: Urine may be pink tinged after the test; signs and symptoms of urinary tract infection.

Data from Pagana KD, et al: *Mosby's diagnostic and laboratory test reference*, ed 14, St Louis, 2019, Elsevier.

toilet." To achieve this outcome you identify a number of interventions, such as ensuring that the nurse call system is within reach, providing assistive devices such as a raised toilet seat, and providing easy access to the urinal when in bed. Conversely, the patient with stress incontinence often has a long-term goal that depends on weeks of pelvic floor muscle exercise to improve urinary control: Patient will experience normal continence. An outcome for this goal would be to "decrease the number of incontinence pads by 1 to 2 within 8 weeks." Interventions will include daily Kegel exercises. Make sure that goals and outcomes are reasonably achievable and relevant to the patient's situation (see Box 46.8).

Setting Priorities. It is important to establish priorities of care on the basis of a patient's immediate physical and safety needs, patient

---

BOX 46.6   Nursing Diagnostic Process

Urge Urinary Incontinence Related to Bladder Infection

Assessment Activities	Assessment Findings
Ask patient to describe voiding problems/incontinence.	Patient complains of urine leakage associated with a strong urge to void.
Assess patient's voiding pattern.	Bladder record shows episodes of urinary incontinence.
	Patient describes or is observed to leak urine on the way to or at the toilet.
	Patient describes or is observed to rush or hurry to the toilet.

---

expectations, and readiness to perform some self-care activities. Establish a relationship with the patient that allows discussion and intervention. While you are collaborating with the patient, priorities become apparent, enhancing patient understanding of all the goals. When a patient has multiple nursing diagnoses (Fig. 46.8), it is important to recognize the primary health problem and its influence on other problems. For example, a patient with a long-term indwelling catheter is admitted to acute care with a severe UTI. The patient expects to resume self-care of the catheter. However, because of the severity of the infection and the patient's condition, the nurse needs to perform all care for the patient's catheter. In this case the priorities are to treat the infection, prevent reinfection, and teach the patient how to resume care of the catheter using techniques to prevent infection.

Teamwork and Collaboration. When planning individualized care, it is essential to use the expertise of the health care team and incorporate them into the plan. For example, when planning care for a patient with urge UI, incorporate the expertise of a continence nurse specialist to help the patient learn techniques to inhibit the urinary urge, strengthen pelvic floor muscles, and learn fluid and food modifications. Have the occupational therapist help the patient learn efficient and safe toilet transfers; the physical therapist help with strengthening exercises of the lower extremities; and the social worker facilitate obtaining assistive devices in the home that are covered by insurance. The family caregiver is included in planning when applicable. When a patient requires an indwelling urinary catheter because of acute illness and a need to measure accurate urinary output, the nurse is a key member of the team by monitoring patient progress and ensuring that the catheter is removed in a timely manner. Your active and thoughtful role in planning these interventions will result in the patient's progress toward improved urinary elimination.

◆ Implementation

Complete independent and collaborative interventions to help the patient achieve the desired outcomes and goals. The independent activities are those in which nurses use their own judgment. An example of this is teaching self-care activities to the patient. Collaborative activities are those prescribed by the health care provider and carried out by the nurse, such as medication administration.

Health Promotion. Health promotion helps the patient understand and participate in self-care practices to preserve and protect healthy urinary system function (Box 46.7). You can achieve this focus using several means.

Patient Education. Success of therapies aimed at eliminating or minimizing urinary elimination problems depends in part on successful patient education (see Box 46.7). Although many patients need to learn about all aspects of healthy urinary elimination, it is best to focus on a specific elimination problem first. For example, a patient who presents with a UTI would greatly benefit from learning about symptoms of UTI and preventive measures in order to potentially prevent recurring UTIs. You can easily incorporate teaching when giving nursing care. For example, teach about common bladder irritants such as caffeine when preparing a clinic patient for discharge. Include in any teaching an awareness of the patient's health literacy. Pictures are helpful when teaching about urinary tract anatomy and the relationship with UTI. If a patient speaks a different language, involve a professional interpreter.

Promoting Normal Micturition. Maintaining normal urinary micturition helps to prevent many problems. Many measures that promote normal voiding are independent nursing interventions.

Maintaining Elimination Habits. Many patients follow routines to promote normal voiding. When in a hospital or long-term care setting, institutional routines often conflict with those of the patient. Integrating the patient's habits into the care plan fosters a more normal voiding pattern. Elimination is a very private act. Create as much privacy as possible by closing the door and bedside curtain; asking visitors to leave a room when a bedside commode, bedpan, or urinal is used; and masking the sounds of voiding with running water. Respond to requests for help with toileting as quickly as possible. Embarrassing accidents are easily avoided when help comes in time. Avoid the use of incontinence-containment products unless needed for uncontrolled urine leakage. Some containment products may be difficult to remove and interfere with prompt toilet access.

Maintaining Adequate Fluid Intake. A simple method to promote normal micturition is to maintain optimal fluid intake. A patient with normal renal function who does not have heart disease or alterations requiring fluid restriction should have approximately 2300 mL of fluid in a 24-hour period. Adequate fluid intake will help flush out solutes or particles that collect in the urinary system and decrease bladder irritability. Help patients change their fluid intake by teaching the importance of adequate hydration. If a patient needs to increase fluid intake, set a schedule for drinking extra fluids, identify fluid preferences, increase high fluid foods such as fruits, and encourage fluid intake in small volumes frequently. Excessive fluid intake should be avoided. To prevent nocturia, suggest that the patient avoid drinking fluids 2 hours before bedtime.

Promoting Complete Bladder Emptying. It is normal for a small volume of urine to remain in the bladder after micturition. When the bladder does not empty completely and residual urine volumes are high, there is risk for incontinence and dangerous urinary retention. Urinary retention increases the risk for UTI and damage to the kidneys. Adequate bladder emptying depends on feeling an urge to urinate, contraction of the bladder, and the ability to relax the urethral sphincter. A strategy to promote relaxation and stimulate bladder contractions is to help patients assume the normal position for voiding. The normal anatomical position for female voiding is in the squatting position. Women empty the bladder better when sitting on the toilet or bedside commode with the feet on the floor. If the patient cannot use a toilet, position her on a bedpan (see Chapter 47). After bedpan use help the patient perform perineal hygiene (see Chapter 40). A man voids more easily in the standing position. If the patient is unable to reach a toilet, have him stand at the bedside and void into a urinal (a plastic or metal receptacle for urine) (Fig. 46.9, *A*). Always assess mobility status

Stress Incontinence of Urine

ASSESSMENT

Mrs. Grayson is 65 years old and the mother of five adult children. She was widowed 6 months ago; before her husband's death she was his primary caregiver for 4 years. She is preparing for retirement and would like to travel. For the past 2 years she noticed an increase in urine incontinence when she sneezes, laughs, or coughs. She recently noted incontinence when exercising. She feels the weight she gained while caring for her husband made the incontinence worse.

Assessment Activities	*Assessment Findings*[a]
Ask Mrs. Grayson about the effects of her urinary symptoms on her daily life.	She responds, "I find myself being embarrassed and frustrated for **losing control. I dribble** when I'm on the way to the bathroom. I'm afraid to cough, sneeze, or laugh because I **leak urine.** I don't go places and try to avoid being close to other people because I'm afraid I might have an odor."
Ask her about any interventions she has tried to help with the incontinence.	She states, "I've been **wearing a pad and will go to the bathroom** every hour just in case. I try to limit the amount of water I drink, so I will not have to go to the bathroom."
Ask Mrs. Grayson about any other effects caused by her leakage.	She begins to cry and states, "I don't even like to go to the movies or visit my grandchildren. It's safer to stay home."
Observe Mrs. Grayson's behavior.	She appears **anxious and sad**.
Conduct a focused nursing history addressing urinary leakage and other lower urinary tract symptoms.	Mrs. Grayson's report of **urine leakage on physical exertion, sneezing, coughing, and laughing** and leakage on the way to the bathroom increases the likelihood of a diagnosis of mixed incontinence. Her risk factors for this condition include **five pregnancies,** being **postmenopausal,** and being **overweight.** The history helps to define the proper interventions.

[a]**Assessment findings** are shown in bold type.

NURSING DIAGNOSIS: Stress incontinence of urine related to weakened pelvic musculature

Goals	*Expected Outcomes (NOC)*[b] *Urinary Continence*
Mrs. Grayson will have reduced episodes of urine leakage (incontinence) between voiding within 6 to 8 weeks.	Patient reports fewer than two episodes of daily incontinence. Patient reports less incontinence during coughing or sneezing. Patient states decreased anxiety about her incontinence.

[b]Outcome classification labels from Moorhead S, et al: *Nursing Outcomes Classification (NOC)*, ed 6, St Louis, 2018, Elsevier.

## INTERVENTIONS (NIC)[c]	## RATIONALE
### Urinary Incontinence Care	
Teach Mrs. Grayson measures to reduce intraabdominal pressure by: • Losing weight. • Avoiding heavy lifting.	These measures reduce intraabdominal and bladder pressure, which increase leakage.
Teach Mrs. Grayson about how to keep her bladder healthy (see Box 46.7): • Avoid bladder irritants (e.g., caffeine) • Drink adequate amounts of water; avoid drinking large amounts at one time.	Fluids that contain caffeine and other irritants can prompt unwanted bladder contractions, resulting in frequency, urgency, and incontinence.
### Pelvic Muscle Exercise	
Teach Mrs. Grayson how to perform pelvic muscle exercises (see Box 46.8): • Instruct her how to identify and contract the muscle. • Help her set up a daily schedule for performing the exercises.	Pelvic muscle training is effective in treating stress urinary incontinence (Shivkumar et al., 2015).
Bladder retraining (behavioral therapy) • Instruct her how to inhibit strong sensations of urinary urgency by taking slow and deep breaths to relax and performing 5 to 6 quick, strong pelvic muscle exercises (flicks) in quick succession, followed by focusing the attention away from the bladder sensations. • Once successful with inhibiting the urge to void and avoiding incontinence, instruct her to gradually increase the time period between trips to the bathroom.	Bladder training and pelvic floor muscle exercises progressively re-establish voluntary control over micturition (Shivkumar et al., 2015).

[c]Intervention classification labels from Butcher HK, et al: *Nursing Interventions Classifications (NIC)*, ed 7, St Louis, 2018, Elsevier.

EVALUATION

Evaluation Activity	*Patient Response/Finding*	*Outcome Status*
Ask Mrs. Grayson about frequency of incontinence.	She responds, "I'm dry most of the time now. I'm now babysitting my grandchildren and have returned to my volunteer job."	Mrs. Grayson is experiencing reduced episodes of urine leakage (incontinence).
Ask Mrs. Grayson to keep a 3-day bladder diary.	Bladder diary revealed one small-volume loss of urine with a strong cough and voiding every 3 to 4 hours.	Mrs. Grayson is experiencing reduced episodes of urine leakage during stressful event.

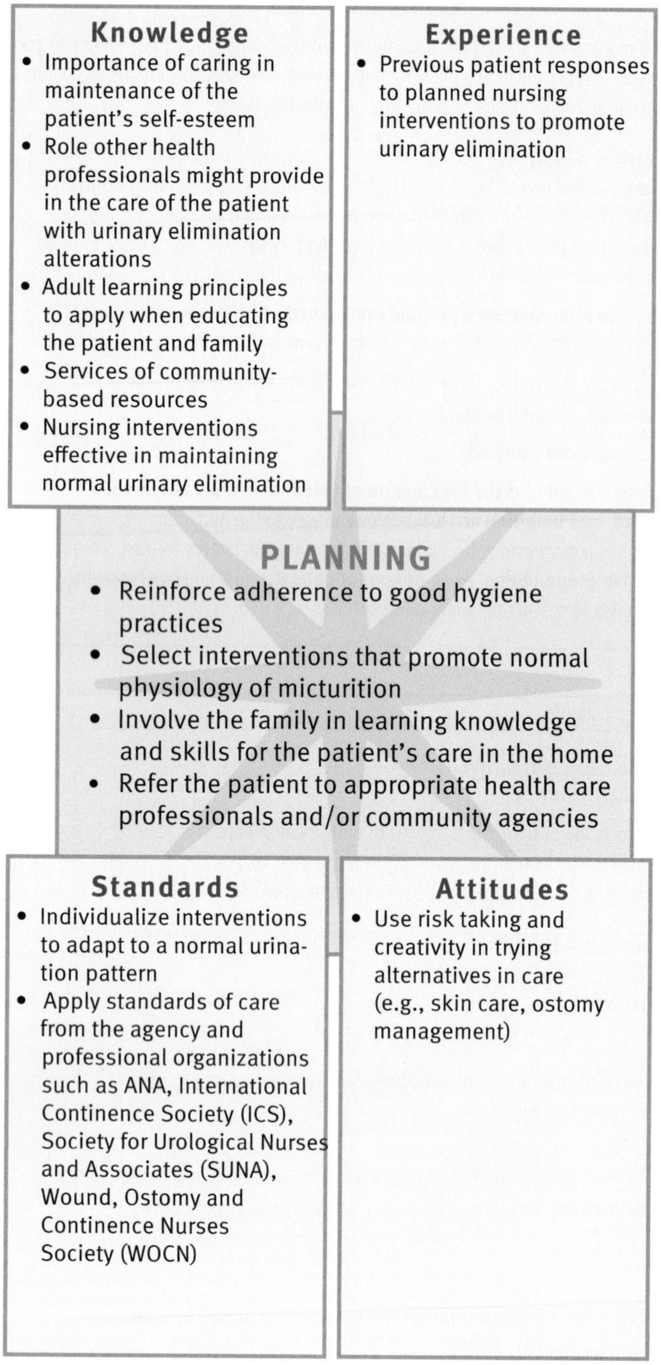

Knowledge
- Importance of caring in maintenance of the patient's self-esteem
- Role other health professionals might provide in the care of the patient with urinary elimination alterations
- Adult learning principles to apply when educating the patient and family
- Services of community-based resources
- Nursing interventions effective in maintaining normal urinary elimination

Experience
- Previous patient responses to planned nursing interventions to promote urinary elimination

PLANNING
- Reinforce adherence to good hygiene practices
- Select interventions that promote normal physiology of micturition
- Involve the family in learning knowledge and skills for the patient's care in the home
- Refer the patient to appropriate health care professionals and/or community agencies

Standards
- Individualize interventions to adapt to a normal urination pattern
- Apply standards of care from the agency and professional organizations such as ANA, International Continence Society (ICS), Society for Urological Nurses and Associates (SUNA), Wound, Ostomy and Continence Nurses Society (WOCN)

Attitudes
- Use risk taking and creativity in trying alternatives in care (e.g., skin care, ostomy management)

FIG. 46.7 Critical thinking model for urinary elimination planning. *ANA*, American Nurses Association.

and determine whether he can stand safely. At times it is necessary for one or more nurses to help a male patient stand. If the patient is unable to stand at the bedside, you will need to help him use the urinal in bed. Some patients need the nurse to position the penis completely within the urinal and hold the urinal in place or help them hold the urinal. Once the patient has finished voiding,

carefully remove the urinal and perform perineal hygiene (see Chapter 40).

There are specially designed urinals for women (see Fig. 46.9, *B*). The female urinal has a larger opening at the top with a defined rim, which helps position the urinal closely against the genitalia.

There are other measures that improve bladder emptying. To promote relaxation and stimulate bladder contractions, use sensory stimuli (e.g., turning on running water, putting a patient's hand in a pan of warm water) and provide privacy. In addition, bladder exercises help to improve pelvic muscles, which reduces stress incontinence and improves bladder emptying (Box 46.8).

To improve bladder emptying, encourage patients to wait until the urine flow completely stops when voiding and encourage them to attempt a second void (double voiding). Timed voiding is voiding according to the clock, not the urge to void, and is a helpful strategy when the bladder does not fully empty. The Credé method or manual compression of the bladder (i.e., placing the hands over the bladder and compressing it to help in emptying) should not be implemented until consultation with the health care provider. In the presence of high PVRs or a complete inability of the bladder to empty, urinary catheterization, either intermittent or indwelling, is needed.

Preventing Infection. UTIs are the fourth most common type of health care–associated infection (CDC, 2019). It is important to implement evidence-based practices to avoid this common and potentially dangerous infection. Some key interventions include promoting adequate fluid intake, promoting perineal hygiene, and having patients void at regular intervals. Encourage women to wipe front to back after voiding and defecation and teach them to avoid perfumed perineal washes and sprays, bubble baths, and tight clothing. If a patient has a problem with urine leakage, hygiene should be especially stressed. Patients should use containment products that are designed for urine and wick wetness away from the body. Prolonged periods of urine wetness should be avoided.

REFLECT NOW

Think about health promotion for your next assigned patient. What strategies would improve this patient's elimination?

Acute Care. Patients with acute illness, surgery, or impaired function of the urinary tract may require more invasive interventions that support urinary elimination.

Catheterization. Urinary catheterization is the placement of a tube through the urethra into the bladder to drain urine (see Skill 46.2). There is a risk for catheter-associated urinary tract infections (CAUTIs), which are the fourth leading cause of health care–associated infections in acute care hospitals (Ferguson, 2018). The ANA developed an evidenced-based tool, the *ANA CAUTI Prevention Tool*, to guide the decision making of the health care team regarding indwelling catheter insertion and care, maintenance of sterile technique, and best practices for timely catheter removal (Panchisin, 2016).

CONCEPT MAP

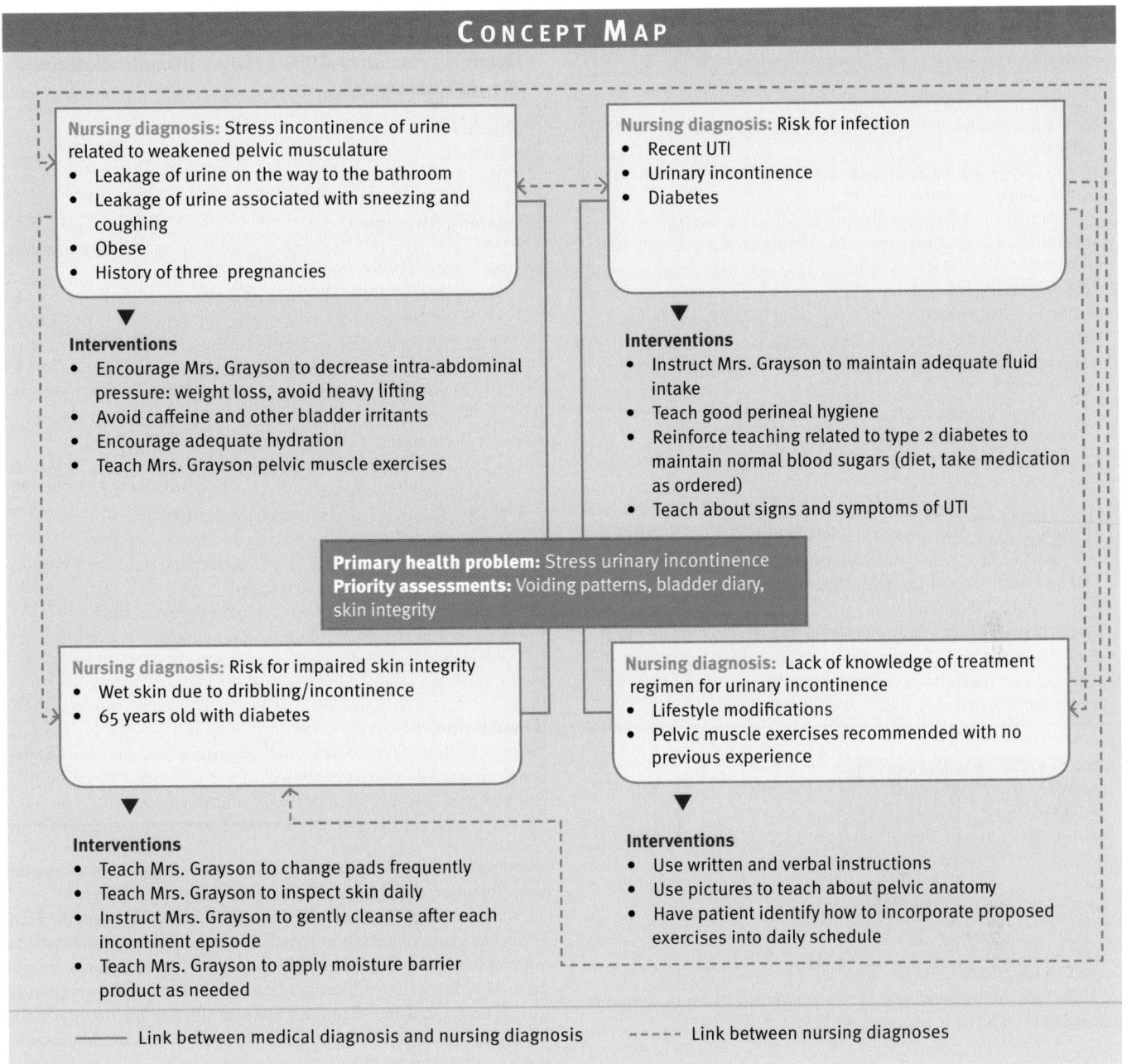

Nursing diagnosis: Stress incontinence of urine related to weakened pelvic musculature
- Leakage of urine on the way to the bathroom
- Leakage of urine associated with sneezing and coughing
- Obese
- History of three pregnancies

Interventions
- Encourage Mrs. Grayson to decrease intra-abdominal pressure: weight loss, avoid heavy lifting
- Avoid caffeine and other bladder irritants
- Encourage adequate hydration
- Teach Mrs. Grayson pelvic muscle exercises

Nursing diagnosis: Risk for infection
- Recent UTI
- Urinary incontinence
- Diabetes

Interventions
- Instruct Mrs. Grayson to maintain adequate fluid intake
- Teach good perineal hygiene
- Reinforce teaching related to type 2 diabetes to maintain normal blood sugars (diet, take medication as ordered)
- Teach about signs and symptoms of UTI

Primary health problem: Stress urinary incontinence
Priority assessments: Voiding patterns, bladder diary, skin integrity

Nursing diagnosis: Risk for impaired skin integrity
- Wet skin due to dribbling/incontinence
- 65 years old with diabetes

Interventions
- Teach Mrs. Grayson to change pads frequently
- Teach Mrs. Grayson to inspect skin daily
- Instruct Mrs. Grayson to gently cleanse after each incontinent episode
- Teach Mrs. Grayson to apply moisture barrier product as needed

Nursing diagnosis: Lack of knowledge of treatment regimen for urinary incontinence
- Lifestyle modifications
- Pelvic muscle exercises recommended with no previous experience

Interventions
- Use written and verbal instructions
- Use pictures to teach about pelvic anatomy
- Have patient identify how to incorporate proposed exercises into daily schedule

——— Link between medical diagnosis and nursing diagnosis   - - - - - Link between nursing diagnoses

FIG. 46.8 Concept map for Mrs. Grayson.

Urinary catheterization can be intermittent (one-time catheterization for bladder emptying) or indwelling (remains in place over a period of time). Indwelling catheterization may be short term (2 weeks or less) or long term (more than 1 month) (Taylor, 2018; Yates, 2016). Conditions requiring the use of a short- or long-term urinary catheter include the need for accurate monitoring of urine output either perioperative or postoperative after urological or gynecological procedures, or when the bladder inadequately empties because of obstruction or a neurological condition. Excessive accumulation of urine in the bladder is painful for a patient, increases the risk for UTI, and can cause backward flow of urine up the ureters, increasing risk for kidney damage. For some patients, the only

method of managing their bladder dysfunction is through a catheter (Davey, 2015). Intermittent catheterization is used to measure PVR when ultrasound or a bladder scanner is unavailable or as a way to manage chronic urinary retention.

Types of Catheters. The difference among urinary catheters is related to the number of catheter lumens, the presence of a balloon to keep the indwelling catheter in place, the shape of the catheter, and a closed drainage system. Urinary catheters are made with one to three lumens. Single-lumen catheters (see Fig. 46.10A) are used for intermittent/straight catheterization. Double-lumen catheters, designed for indwelling catheters, provide one lumen for urinary drainage while a second lumen is used to inflate a balloon that keeps

BOX 46.7 Health Promotion/Restoration: Patient Education for a Healthy Bladder

1. Maintain adequate hydration.
   - Drink six to eight glasses of water a day. Spread it out evenly throughout the day.
   - Avoid or limit drinking beverages that contain caffeine (coffee, tea, chocolate drinks, soft drinks).
   - To decrease nocturia, avoid drinking fluids 2 hours before bedtime.
   - Do not limit fluids if you experience incontinence. Concentrated urine may irritate the bladder and increase bladder symptoms.
2. Keep good voiding habits.
   - Women: Sit well back on the toilet seat, avoid "hovering over the toilet," and make sure that the feet are flat on the floor.
   - Void at regular intervals, usually every 3 to 4 hours, depending on fluid intake.
   - Avoid straining when voiding or moving the bowels.
   - Take enough time to empty the bladder completely.
3. Keep the bowels regular. A rectum full of stool may irritate the bladder, causing urgency and frequency.
4. Prevent urinary tract infections.
   - Women: Cleanse the perineum from front to back after each voiding and bowel movement; wear cotton undergarments.
   - Drink enough water to pass pale yellow urine.
   - Shower or bathe regularly.
5. Stop smoking to reduce your risk for bladder cancer and reduce the risk of developing a cough, which can contribute to stress urinary incontinence.
6. Report to your health care provider any changes in bladder habits, frequency, urgency, pain when voiding, or blood in the urine.

BOX 46.8 Patient Teaching

Teaching Patients About Pelvic Muscle Exercises (Kegel Exercises)

Objective
- Patient will verbalize and/or demonstrate how to perform pelvic muscle exercises (Kegel exercises).

Teaching Strategies
- Use pictures and plain language to teach the patient pelvic anatomy and the location of the pelvic muscles (see Fig. 46.16).
- Teach patient how to identify and contract the correct muscle.
  - Women: Instruct the patient to squeeze the anus as if to hold in gas or to insert a finger into the vagina and feel the muscle squeeze around her finger. The woman can also observe the perineum pulling in by using a mirror.
  - Men: Instruct the patient to stand in front of a mirror, squeeze the anus as if to hold in gas, and watch to see if the penis moves up and down as he contracts the pelvic floor muscles.
  - Instruct to not contract the abdomen, buttocks, or thighs when contracting the pelvic muscles.
- Teach patients pelvic muscle contraction exercises.
  - Quick flicks: Squeeze the muscle for 2 to 3 seconds and relax.
  - Sustained contractions: Squeeze the muscle for 10 seconds and relax after each contraction for 10 seconds.
  - Counting out loud prevents breath holding during exercises.
- Teach patient to maintain a daily exercise schedule.
  - Perform three to five quick flicks followed by 10 sustained contractions.
  - Do these exercises 3 to 4 times a day.

Evaluation
Use the principles of teach-back to evaluate patient/family caregiver learning:
- Describe how you would correctly identify the pelvic floor muscles.
- Explain how you would perform pelvic muscle exercises.

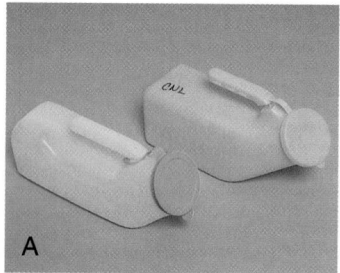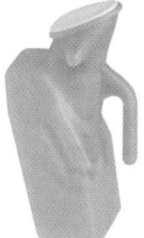

A   **B**

FIG. 46.9 Types of male (A) and female (B) urinals. (B courtesy Briggs Medical Service Co.)

the catheter in place (see Fig. 46.10B). Triple-lumen catheters (see Fig. 46.10C) are used for continuous bladder irrigation (CBI) or when it becomes necessary to instill medications into the bladder. One lumen drains the bladder, a second lumen is used to inflate the balloon, and a third lumen delivers irrigation fluid into the bladder.

A health care provider chooses a catheter on the basis of factors such as latex allergy, history of catheter encrustation, anatomical factors, and susceptibility to infection. Indwelling catheters are made of latex or silicone. Latex catheters with special coatings reduce urethral irritation (Yates, 2016). All silicone catheters have a larger internal diameter and may be helpful in patients who require frequent catheter changes as a result of encrustation. Intermittent/straight catheters are made of rubber (softer and more flexible) or polyvinyl chloride (PVC). Patients who self-catheterize have a large selection of catheters, some with special coatings that do not require lubrication and others that are self-contained systems consisting of a prelubricated catheter and packaged with a preconnected drainage bag. Catheter shape can differ; shape chosen is based on anatomical differences in patients. One such catheter is a Coudé-tip catheter. This catheter has a curvature at the end that helps it

maneuver through the prostatic urethra in the presence of a large prostate. Nurses need special training to use this type of catheter.

Catheter Sizes. The size of a urinary catheter is based on the French (Fr) scale, which reflects the internal diameter of the catheter. Most adults with an indwelling catheter should use a size 10 to 12 Fr for women and 12 to 14 Fr for men to minimize trauma and risk for infection (Bardsley, 2015). Larger catheter diameters increase the risk for urethral trauma (Yates, 2016). However, larger sizes are used in special circumstances, such as after urological surgery or in the presence of gross hematuria. Smaller sizes are needed for children, such as a 5 to 6 Fr for infants, 8 to 10 Fr for children, and 12 Fr for young girls.

Indwelling catheters come in a variety of balloon sizes—from 3 mL (for a child) to 30 mL for CBI. The size of the balloon is usually printed on the catheter port (Fig. 46.11). The recommended balloon size for an adult is a 10-mL balloon (the balloon is 5 mL and requires 10 mL to fill completely) (Yates, 2016). Long-term use of larger balloons (30 mL) has been associated with increased patient discomfort, irritation and trauma to the urethra, increased risk of catheter expulsion, and incomplete emptying of the bladder resulting from urine that pools below the level of the catheter drainage eyes.

Catheter Changes. Use clinical indicators, such as obstruction, prior treatment of a symptomatic infection, malfunction of the catheter, or compromise of the closed system to determine when to change long-term indwelling catheters and drainage bags (Gesmundo, 2016a,b). When long-term catheterization is required, the catheter will need to be changed every 4 to 6 weeks. Whenever possible, avoid the use of long-term catheterization due to the increased risk for CAUTI.

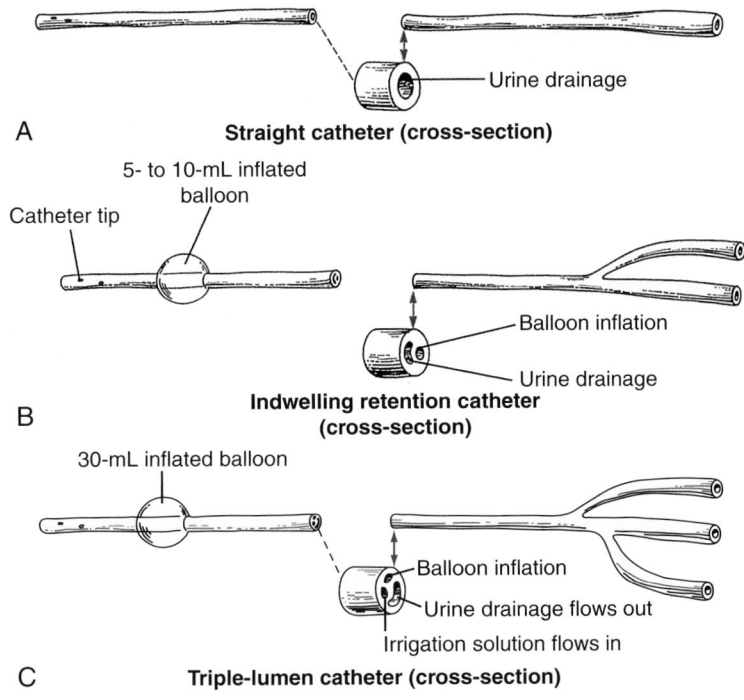

FIG. 46.10 A, Straight catheter (cross-section). B, Indwelling (Foley) retention catheter (cross-section). C, Triple-lumen catheter (cross-section).

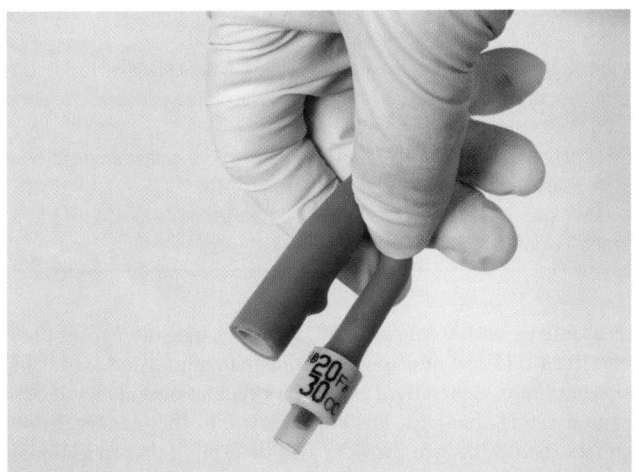

FIG. 46.11 Size of catheter and balloon printed on catheter.

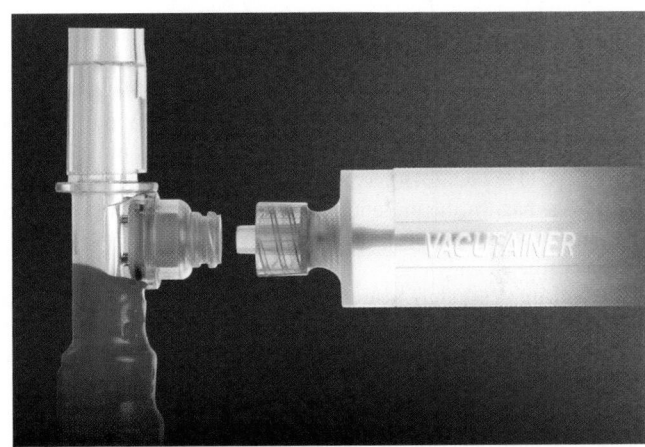

FIG. 46.12 Urine specimen collection: aspiration from a collection port in drainage tubing of indwelling catheter (needleless technique). (Courtesy and © Becton, Dickinson and Company.)

Closed Drainage Systems. An indwelling catheter is attached to a urinary drainage bag to collect the continuous flow of urine. This is a closed drainage system and tubing connections should not be separated to avoid introducing pathogens. In patients with indwelling catheters specimens are collected without opening the drainage system by using a special port in the tubing (Fig. 46.12). Always hang the drainage bag below the level of the bladder on the bedframe or a chair so that urine will drain down out of the bladder. The bag should never touch the floor to prevent accidental contamination during emptying. When a patient ambulates, carry the bag below the level of the patient's bladder. Ambulatory patients may use a leg bag. This is a bag that attaches to the leg with straps.

Leg bags are usually worn during the day and replaced at night with a standard drainage bag. The only drainage bag that does not need to be kept dependent to the bladder is a specially designed drainage bag (belly bag) that is worn across the abdomen. A one-way valve prevents the back flow of urine into the bladder. To keep the drainage system patent, check for kinks or bends in the tubing, avoid positioning the patient on drainage tubing, prevent tubing from becoming dependent, and observe for clots or sediment that may block the catheter or tubing.

Routine Catheter Care. Patients with indwelling catheters require regular perineal hygiene, especially after a bowel movement, to reduce the risk for CAUTI (CDC, 2019; Lo et al., 2014). In many institutions

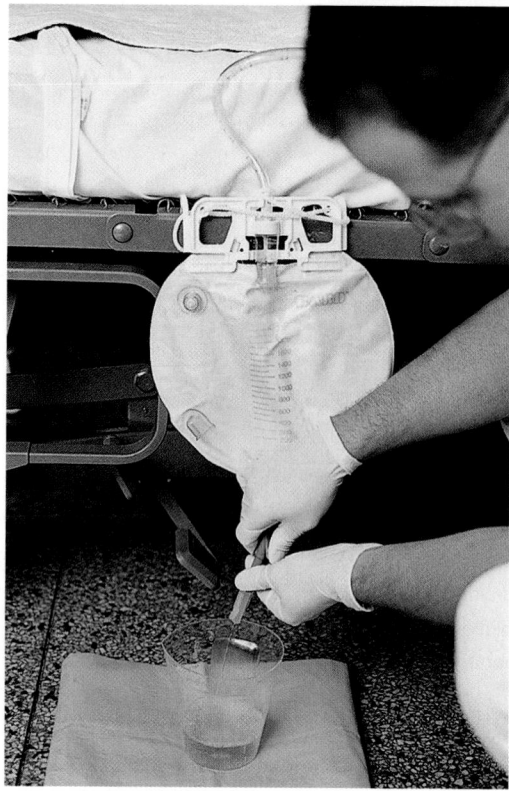

FIG. 46.13 Urine drainage bag.

patients receive catheter care every 8 hours as the minimal standard of care. See Chapter 40 for routine perineal care and Skill 46.3 for catheter care. Empty drainage bags when they are half full (Fig. 46.13). An overfull drainage bag can create tension and pull on the catheter, resulting in trauma to the urethra and/or urinary meatus and increasing risk for CAUTI (CDC, 2019). Expect continuous drainage of urine into the drainage bag. In the presence of no urine drainage, first check to make sure that there are no kinks or obvious occlusion of the drainage tubing or catheter.

Preventing Catheter-Associated Infection. A critical part of routine catheter care is reducing the risk for CAUTI (Box 46.9). In addition, there are specific CDC (2019) guidelines and interventions (Box 46.10). A key intervention to prevent infection is to maintain a closed urinary drainage system. Portals for entry of bacteria into the system are illustrated in Fig. 46.14. Another key intervention is prevention of urine backflow from the tubing and bag into the bladder. Many urine drainage systems are equipped with an antireflux valve, but you should monitor the system to prevent pooling of urine within the tubing and to keep the drainage bag below the level of the bladder.

QSEN **Building Competency in Evidence-Based Practice** A nursing unit is experiencing an increase in catheter-associated urinary tract infections (CAUTIs). A team of staff nurses is investigating this problem and discovers that some nurses are resistant to implementing new evidence-based practice (EBP) guidelines in CAUTI prevention. What can you do to decrease resistance and enhance EBP care on this unit?

Answers to QSEN Activities can be found on the Evolve website.

Catheter Irrigations and Instillations. To maintain the patency of indwelling urinary catheters, it is sometimes necessary to irrigate or

---

BOX 46.9 EVIDENCE-BASED PRACTICE

Factors to Decrease Catheter-Associated Urinary Tract Infection (CAUTI)

PICOT Question: Does the use of evidence-based nursing protocols reduce the occurrence of catheter-associated urinary tract infection (CAUTI) in hospitalized patients with an indwelling catheter?

Evidence Summary

Approximately 12% to 16% of adult hospital inpatients will have an indwelling urinary catheter at some time during their hospitalization, and each day the indwelling urinary catheter remains, a patient has a 3% to 7% increased risk of acquiring a catheter-associated urinary tract infection (CAUTI) (CDC, 2019). A systematic review and meta-analysis of studies regarding measures to use to reduce catheter use and decrease CAUTI showed that CAUTI rates can be reduced when reminders to evaluate catheter need and stop orders are in place (Meddings et al., 2014). Measures to reduce CAUTI are organized into five areas: appropriate catheter use, proper insertion and maintenance techniques, quality improvement programs, ongoing surveillance for CAUTI, and related causative factors (CDC, 2019). Nurse-led interventions reduced the duration of indwelling catheter use and incidence of CAUTI (Scanlon et al., 2017; Dy et al., 2016). In addition, a hospital-wide strategy that included reeducation of nurses about CAUTI prevention and infusing best practice into current-practice nursing care also decreased CAUTI rates (McNeil, 2017; Cartwright, 2018). Best practices, staff education, data reporting, and the use of an icon in the electronic health record as a catheter reminder decreased the CAUTI rates (Ferguson, 2018; Purvis et al., 2014).

Application to Nursing Practice
- Become familiar with guidelines related to CAUTI prevention and care (see Box 46.10). (Galiczweski, 2016).
- Be aware of indications for catheter insertion and be prepared to advocate for the patient if the indications do not meet accepted guidelines (Ferguson, 2018; Bardsley, 2015).
- Collaborate with health care providers to remove catheters early when medical indications no longer exist (Dy et al., 2016).
- Develop or use evidence-based nurse-driven protocols for CAUTI prevention (Ferguson, 2018; Dy et al., 2016).

---

flush a catheter with sterile solution. However, irrigation poses the risk of causing a UTI and thus must be done maintaining a closed urinary drainage system. Generally, if a catheter becomes occluded, it is best to change it rather than risk flushing debris into the bladder. In some instances the health care provider will determine that irrigations are needed to keep a catheter patent such as after genitourinary surgery when there is high risk for catheter occlusion from blood clots. Bladder instillations are used to instill medication into the bladder. Refer to specific instructions for these medications in terms of how long the medication needs to stay in the bladder.

Closed catheter irrigation provides intermittent or continuous irrigation of a urinary catheter without disrupting the sterile connection between the catheter and the drainage system (see Skill 46.4). CBI is an example of a continuous infusion of a sterile solution into the bladder, usually using a three-way irrigation closed system with a triple-lumen catheter. CBI is frequently used following genitourinary surgery to keep the bladder clear and free of blood clots or sediment.

Removal of Indwelling Catheter. The Centers for Medicare and Medicaid Services (CMS) identified CAUTI as a never event (Galiczewski, 2016; CDC, 2019). Prompt removal of an indwelling catheter after it is no longer needed is a key intervention that has proven to decrease the incidence and prevalence of hospital-acquired

UTIs (HAUTIs) (see Skill 46.2). Monitor patient's voiding after catheter removal for at least 24 to 48 hours by using a voiding record or bladder diary. The bladder diary should record the time and amount of each voiding, including any incontinence. The use of ultrasound or a bladder scanner can monitor bladder function by measuring postvoid residual (PVR) volume (Box 46.11). The first few times a patient voids after catheter removal may be accompanied by some discomfort, but continued complaints of painful urination indicate possible infection. Abdominal pain and distention, a sensation of incomplete emptying, incontinence, constant dribbling of urine, and voiding in very small amounts can indicate inadequate bladder emptying requiring intervention.

Alternative to Urethral Catheterization. To avoid the risks associated with urethral catheters, two alternatives are available for urinary drainage.

Suprapubic Catheterization. A suprapubic catheter is a urinary drainage tube inserted surgically into the bladder through the abdominal wall above the symphysis pubis (Fig. 46.15). The catheter may be sutured to the skin, secured with an adhesive material, or retained in the bladder with a fluid-filled balloon similar to an indwelling catheter. Suprapubic catheters are placed when there is blockage of the urethra (e.g., enlarged prostate, urethral stricture, after urological surgery) and in situations in which a long-term urethral catheter causes irritation or discomfort or interferes with sexual functioning.

Care of a suprapubic catheter involves daily cleansing of the insertion site and catheter. The same care for the tubing and drainage bag for a urethral catheter applies to a suprapubic catheter. The insertion site should be assessed for signs of inflammation and the growth of over-granulation tissue. If insertion is new, slight inflammation may be expected as part of normal wound healing, but it can also indicate infection. Overgranulation tissue can develop at the insertion site as a reaction to the catheter. In some instances intervention may be needed. Site care applies the principles of applying a dry dressing; institutional policy will indicate whether aseptic or sterile technique is required (see Chapter 48).

External Catheter. The external catheter, also called a *condom catheter* or *penile sheath,* is a soft, pliable condom-like sheath that fits over the penis, providing a safe and noninvasive way to contain urine. Most external catheters are made of soft silicone that aids in reducing friction and are clear to allow for easy visualization of skin under the catheter. Latex catheters are still available and used by some patients. It is important to verify that a patient does not have a latex allergy before applying this type of catheter. Condom-type external catheters are held in place by an adhesive coating of the internal lining of the sheath, a double-sided self-adhesive strip, brush-on adhesive applied to the penile shaft, or in rare cases an external strap or tape. They may be attached to a small-volume (leg) drainage bag or a large-volume (bedside) urinary drainage bag, both of which need to be kept lower than the level of the bladder. The condom-type external catheter is suitable for incontinent patients who have complete and spontaneous bladder emptying. Condom-type external catheters come in a variety of styles and sizes. For the best fit and correct application it is important to refer to manufacturer guidelines. See Box 46.12 for the steps in applying a condom catheter. Condom-type external catheters are associated with less risk for UTI than indwelling catheters; thus they are an excellent option for the male with UI. For men who cannot be fitted for a condom-type external catheter, there are other externally applied catheters.

Urinary Diversions. Immediately after surgery the patient with an incontinent urinary diversion must wear a pouch to collect the effluent (drainage). The pouch will keep the patient clean and dry, protect the skin from damage, and provide a barrier against odor. Urinary pouches with an antireflux flap can be opaque or clear, drainable one-piece or

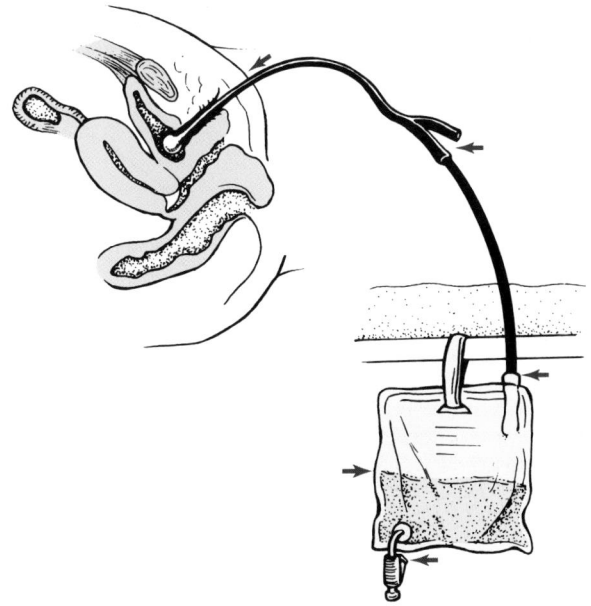

FIG. 46.14 Potential sites for introduction of infectious organisms into urinary drainage system.

BOX 46.11   PROCEDURAL GUIDELINES

Using a Bladder Scanner to Measure Postvoid Residual

Delegation and Collaboration

The skill of measuring bladder volume by bladder scan can be delegated to assistive personnel (AP). The nurse must first determine the timing and frequency of the bladder scan measurement and interpret the measurements obtained. The nurse also assesses the patient's ability to toilet before measuring postvoid residual (PVR) and the abdomen for distention if urinary retention is suspected. The nurse directs the AP to:

- Follow manufacturer recommendations for the use of the device.
- Measure PVR volumes within 5 to 15 minutes after helping the patient to void.
- Report and record bladder scan volumes.

Equipment

Bladder scanner, ultrasound gel, cleansing agent (e.g. alcohol pad) for scanner head, urethral catheterization tray for single-use catheter/intermittent (see Skill 46.2), paper towel or washcloth

Steps

1. Identify patient using at least two identifiers (e.g., name and birthday or name and medical record number) according to agency policy (TJC, 2020).
2. Assess intake and output (I&O) record to determine urine output trends and whether patient has voided since surgery; check the plan of care to verify correct timing of the bladder scan measurement.
3. Assess patient's health literacy to determine approach for teaching about procedure.
4. Provide privacy by closing room door and bedside curtain.
5. Help patient to supine position with head slightly elevated. Raise bed to appropriate working height. If side rails are raised, lower side rail on working side.
6. Perform hand hygiene and apply clean gloves.
7. Discuss procedure with patient. If measurement is for PVR, ask patient to void and measure volume retained in bladder with scanner within 5 to 15 minutes of voiding:
   a. Pull back sheet to expose patient's lower abdomen.
   b. Turn on scanner per manufacturer guidelines.
   c. Set gender designation per manufacturer guidelines. Women who have had a hysterectomy should be designated as male.
   d. Wipe scanner head with alcohol pad or other cleaner and allow to air-dry.
   e. Palpate patient's symphysis pubis (pubic bone). Apply generous amount of ultrasound gel (or if available a bladder scan gel pad) to midline abdomen 2.5 to 4 cm (1 to 1.5 inches) above symphysis pubis.
   f. Place scanner head on gel, ensuring that scanner head is oriented per manufacturer guidelines.
   g. Apply light pressure, keep scanner head steady, and point it slightly downward toward bladder. Press and release the scan button (see illustration).
   h. Verify accurate aim (refer to manufacturer guidelines). Complete scan and print image (if needed).

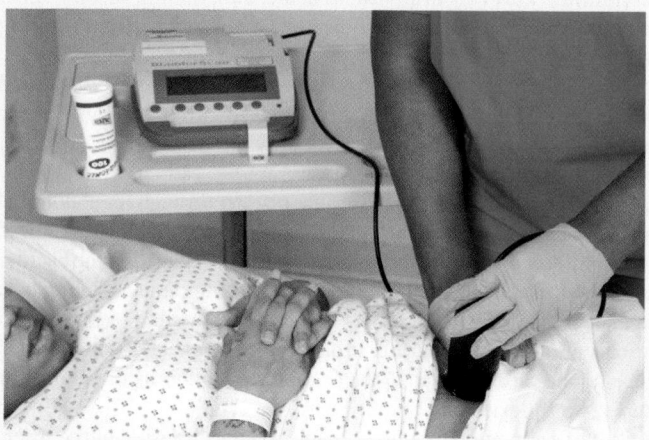

STEP 7g Placement of bladder scan head.

8. Remove ultrasound gel from patient's abdomen with paper towel or moist cloth.
9. Remove ultrasound gel from scanner head and wipe with alcohol pad or other cleaner; allow to air-dry.
10. Help patient to comfortable position. Raise side rails (as appropriate) and lower bed to lowest position. Be sure nurse call system is in an accessible location within patient's reach.
11. Remove and dispose of gloves and perform hand hygiene.
12. Compare PVR results with prevoiding scan (if available); urine volume should be less. Or if first-time scan, PVR should be <100 mL urine.
13. Review health care provider's order to determine how often to assess residual urine or if catheterization is ordered.
14. Review I&O record to determine urine output trends.
15. Record findings of scan, PVR, and patient tolerance of procedure.

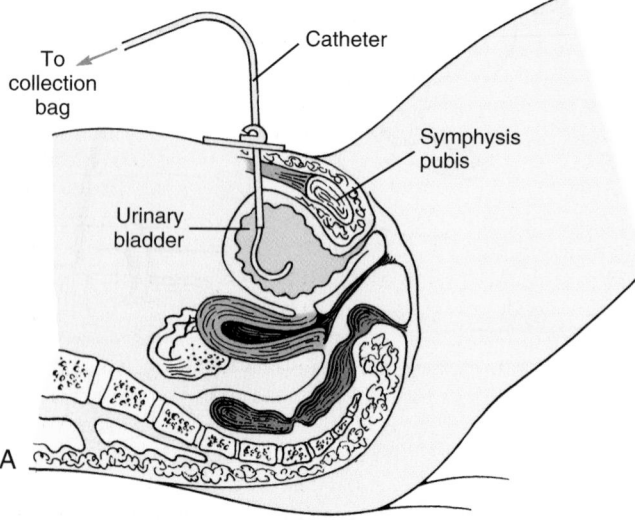

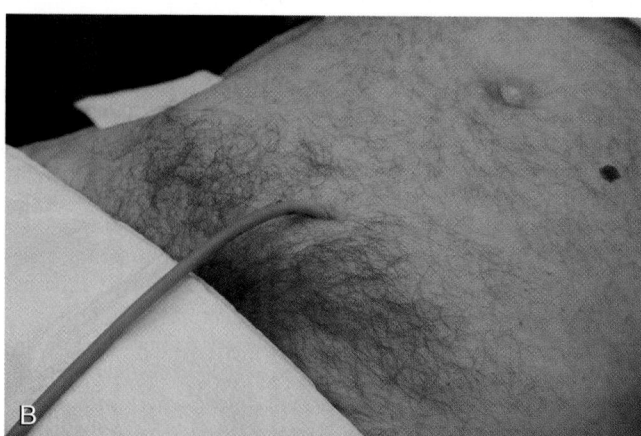

FIG. 46.15 A, Placement of suprapubic catheter above symphysis pubis. B, Suprapubic catheter without a dressing.

two-piece pouches, with cut-to-fit or precut wafers. The pouch should be changed every 4 to 6 days. Each pouch may be connected to a bedside drainage bag for use at night.

When changing a pouch, gently cleanse the skin surrounding the stoma with warm tap water using a washcloth and pat dry. Do not use soap because it can leave a residue on the skin. Measure the stoma and cut the opening in the pouch. Then apply the pouch after removing the protective backing from the adhesive surface. Press firmly into place over the stoma. Observe the appearance of the stoma and surrounding skin. The stoma is normally red and moist and is located in the right lower quadrant of the abdomen. It is important for the patient to have the correct type and fit of an ostomy pouch. A specialty ostomy nurse is an essential resource when selecting the right appliance so that the pouch fits snugly against the surface of the skin around the stoma, preventing damaging leakage of urine (see Chapter 47).

Patients with continent urinary diversions do not have to wear an external pouch. However, if the patient has a continent urinary reservoir, he or she must be taught how to intermittently catheterize the pouch. Patients need to be able and willing to do this 4 to 6 times a day for the rest of their lives. After creation of an orthotopic neobladder, patients will have frequent episodes of incontinence until the neobladder slowly stretches and the urinary sphincter is strong enough to contain the urine. To achieve continence the patient will need to follow a bladder-training schedule and perform pelvic muscle exercises (Shivkumar et al., 2015). The postoperative care of patients having continent urinary diversions varies widely with the surgical techniques used; it is important to learn the surgeon's preferred routine or health care agency procedures before caring for these patients.

Medications. A small number of medications, antimuscarinics (e.g., oxybutynin and trospium), are used to treat urinary urgency. Another medication, mirabegron, is in a class of medications called beta-3 adrenergic agonists. It relaxes the bladder muscles to prevent urgent, or uncontrolled, urination. The most common adverse effects of antimuscarinics are dry mouth, constipation, and blurred vision. In some cases these medications can cause a change in mental status in older adults (Burchum and Rosenthal, 2019). Patients taking mirabegron should have their blood pressure monitored because of possible increases. There are no medications, other than off-label use of vaginal estrogen in postmenopausal women, to treat stress urinary incontinence (Lukacz et al., 2017). Urinary retention is sometimes treated with bethanechol, and men with outlet obstruction caused by an enlarged prostate are treated with agents that relax the smooth muscle of the prostatic urethra, such as tamsulosin and silodosin and agents that shrink the prostate, such as finasteride and dutasteride. Know the medications and indications for all medications your patient is taking.

When a patient is newly started on an antimuscarinic, monitor for effectiveness, including a decrease in urgency, frequency, and incontinence episodes. A bladder diary is one of the best ways to do this. In addition, regularly assess the patient for side effects such as constipation by monitoring the bowel movement record. Watch for a decrease in bowel movement frequency, straining at bowel movements, and changes in stool consistency.

UTIs are treated with antibiotics. Patients with painful urination are sometimes prescribed urinary analgesics that act on the urethral and bladder mucosa (e.g., phenazopyridine). Patients taking drugs with phenazopyridine need to be aware that their urine will be orange. They must drink large amounts of fluids to prevent toxicity from the sulfonamides and maintain optimal flow through the urinary system (Burchum and Rosenthal, 2019).

Continuing and Restorative Care. There are techniques that can improve control over bladder emptying and restore some degree of urinary continence. These techniques are commonly referred to as behavioral therapy and are considered first-line treatment for stress, urge, and mixed incontinence (Lukacz et al., 2017). They include lifestyle changes, pelvic floor muscle training (PFMT), bladder retraining, and a variety of toileting schedules (see Table 46.1). In some cases, when the bladder does not empty, patients or caregivers learn to intermittently catheterize. Whenever there is a risk for urine leakage, skin care is an essential component of the plan of care. Adequate urine containment and skin protection promote patient comfort and dignity.

Lifestyle Changes. A number of lifestyle modifications can improve bladder function and decrease incontinence. In addition to interventions listed earlier in this chapter under health promotion and in Box 46.7, you can teach patients about foods and fluids that cause bladder irritation and increase symptoms, such as frequency, urgency, and incontinence. Teach patients to avoid common irritants such as artificial sweeteners, spicy foods, citrus products, and especially caffeine (Bykoviene et al., 2018). Discourage patients from drinking large volumes of fluid at one time. Constipation can also impact bladder symptoms, and measures to promote bowel regularity should be implemented (see Chapter 47). Encourage patients with edema to elevate the feet for a minimum of a few hours in the afternoon to help diminish nighttime voiding frequency.

Pelvic Floor Muscle Training. Evidence has shown that patients with urgency, stress, and mixed UI experience improvement and can eventually achieve continence when treated with pelvic floor muscle training (Lukacz et al., 2017; Bykoviene et al., 2018). Pelvic floor muscle training involves teaching patients how to identify and contract the pelvic floor muscles in a structured exercise program. This exercise program is commonly called *Kegel exercises* and is based on therapy first developed by obstetrician gynecologist Dr. Arnold Kegel in the 1940s. The exercises work by increasing the pressure within the urethra by strengthening the pelvic floor muscles and inhibiting unwanted bladder contractions (Fig. 46.16). Many patients benefit from verbal instructions on how to do the exercises (see Box 46.8). Patients who have difficulty correctly identifying and contracting the pelvic floor muscles can be sent to a continence specialist for biofeedback. Biofeedback involves intensive instruction augmented by computerized measurement of muscle activity that is displayed on a monitor. The visual feedback helps the patient learn to contract the muscles correctly.

Bladder Retraining. Bladder retraining is a behavioral therapy designed to help patients control bothersome urinary urgency and frequency. Patients are taught about their bladder and techniques to suppress urgency. They are given a schedule of toileting on the basis of their diary of voiding and leaking; the schedule is designed to slowly increase the interval between voiding. Successful bladder retraining requires that patients get regular support and positive reinforcement. Patients are taught to inhibit the urge to void by taking slow, deep breaths to relax, performing five to six quick, strong pelvic muscle exercises (flicks) in quick succession, followed by distracting attention from bladder sensations. When the urge to void becomes less severe or subsides, only then should the patient start his or her trip to the bathroom. Only highly motivated and cognitively intact patients are candidates for this therapy. If a patient is in such a program, you can support him or her by reinforcing the schedule and providing emotional encouragement.

Toileting Schedules. A key component to any treatment plan for urinary incontinence is regular toilet access. Toileting schedules should be individualized based on the type of incontinence and functional

BOX 46.12 **PROCEDURAL GUIDELINES**

Applying a Male Incontinence Device

Delegation and Collaboration

Assessment of the skin of a patient's penile shaft and determination of a latex allergy are done by a nurse before catheter application. The skill of applying a condom catheter can be delegated to assistive personnel (AP), depending on agency policy. The nurse directs the AP to:

- Follow manufacturer directions for applying the condom catheter and securing device.
- Monitor intake and output (I&O) and record if applicable.
- Immediately report any redness, swelling, or skin irritation or breakdown of glans penis or penile shaft.

Equipment

- Condom catheter kit—condom sheath of appropriate size, securing device (internal adhesive, strap), skin preparation solution (per manufacturer's recommendations); *Option:* hydrocolloid incontinence device; urinary collection bag with drainage tubing or leg bag and straps; basin with warm water and soap; towels, washcloth, bath blanket; clean gloves; scissors, hair guard, or paper towel

Steps

1. Identify patient using at least two identifiers (e.g., name and birthday or name and medical record number) according to agency policy (TJC, 2020).
2. Review electronic health record (EHR), and assess urinary pattern, ability to empty bladder effectively, and degree of urinary continence.
3. Assess patient's or family caregiver's knowledge, experience, and health literacy.
4. Review EHR for history of allergy to rubber or latex. Confirm with patient if possible. Check patient's allergy wristband.
5. Assess patient's or family caregiver's mental status, knowledge of and experience with condom-type catheter, and ability to apply device.
6. Perform hand hygiene. Assess integrity of penile tissue. Verify patient's size and type of condom catheter from plan of care, or use manufacturer measuring guide to measure length and diameter of penis in flaccid state (apply gloves for measurement). Perform hand hygiene.

CLINICAL DECISION: Apply condom catheters only when the skin on the penile surface is intact.

7. Provide privacy by closing room door or curtain. Organize and set up equipment needed.
8. Raise bed to appropriate working height. Lower side rail on working side.
9. Explain procedure to patient.
10. Perform hand hygiene.
11. Prepare urinary drainage collection bag and tubing (large-volume drainage bag or leg bag). Clamp off drainage bag port. Place nearby ready to attach to condom after applied.
12. Help patient to supine or sitting position.
13. Place bath blanket over upper torso. Fold sheets so that only penis is exposed.
14. Apply clean gloves. Provide perineal care (see Chapter 40). Dry thoroughly before applying device. In uncircumcised male, ensure that foreskin has been replaced to normal position before applying condom catheter. Do not apply barrier cream.
15. Remove and dispose of gloves. Perform hand hygiene.
16. Apply clean gloves. Assess skin of penis for rashes, erythema, and/or open areas.
17. Clip hair at base of penis as necessary before application of condom sheath. Some manufacturers provide hair guard that is placed over penis before applying device. Remove hair guard after applying catheter. An alternative to hair guard is to tear a hole in a paper towel, place it over penis, and remove after application of device.

CLINICAL DECISION: The pubic area should not be shaved because any microabrasions in skin increase risk for skin irritation and infection.

18. Apply incontinence device
    a. **Condom catheter.** With nondominant hand, grasp penis along shaft. With dominant hand, hold rolled condom sheath at tip of penis with head

of penis in cone. Smoothly roll sheath onto penis. Allow 2.5 to 5 cm (1 to 2 inches) of space between tip of glans penis and end of condom catheter (see illustration).

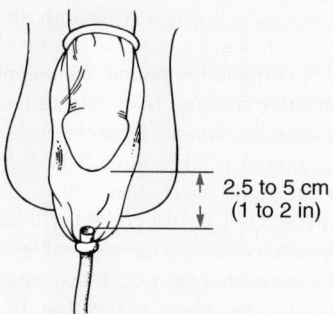

STEP 18a Condom catheter.

   b. **Hydrocolloid device.** One size fits all. Place the device onto the tip of the penis, not the shaft (see manufacturer's directions, see Step 19c):
19. Apply appropriate securement device as indicated in manufacturer guidelines.
    a. Self-adhesive condom catheters: After application apply gentle pressure on penile shaft for 10 to 15 seconds.
    b. Outer securing strip-type condom catheters: Spiral wrap penile shaft with strip of supplied elastic adhesive. Strip should not overlap itself. Elastic strip should be snug, not tight (see illustration).

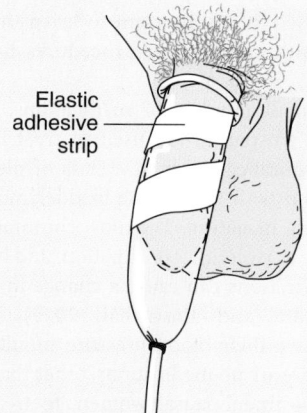

Elastic adhesive strip

STEP 19b Spiral application of adhesive strip.

   c. Hydrocolloid incontinence device: Remove release papers from adhesive on faceplate of device. Center faceplate over opening of urinary meatus. Smooth hydrocolloid adhesive backing strips onto tip of penis. Then cover with hydrocolloid seal (see illustration).

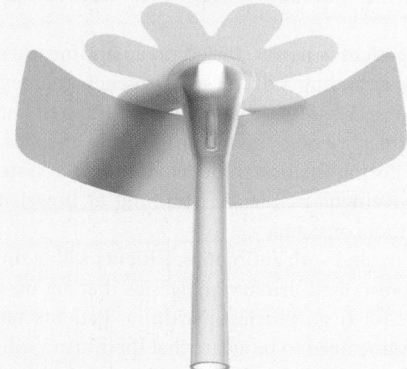

STEP 19c Men's Liberty acute male incontinence device. (Courtesy BioDerm, Inc. Largo, Florida.)

BOX 46.12 Procedural Guidelines—cont'd

Applying a Male Incontinence Device

CLINICAL DECISION: Never use regular adhesive tape to secure a condom catheter. Constriction from tape can reduce blood flow to tissues.

20. Remove hair guard or paper towel (if used). Connect drainage tubing to end of incontinence device. Be sure that a condom catheter is not twisted. If using large drainage bag, place excess tubing on bed and secure to bottom sheet.
21. Help patient to safe, comfortable position. Raise side rails (as appropriate) and lower bed to lowest position.
22. Be sure nurse call system is in an accessible location within patient's reach.
23. Dispose of contaminated supplies, remove and dispose of gloves, and perform hand hygiene.
24. Remove and reapply daily following the previous steps unless an extended-wear device is used. To remove condom, wash penis with warm, soapy water and gently roll sheath and adhesive off penile shaft

25. Observe urinary drainage.
26. Inspect penis with condom catheter in place within 15 to 30 minutes after application. Assess for swelling and discoloration, and ask patient whether there is any discomfort.
27. Inspect skin on penile shaft for signs of breakdown or irritation at least daily, when performing hygiene, and before reapplying condom or incontinence device.
28. Record condition of penis, type of external device applied, patient's response to procedure, and patient's level of understanding of purpose of device.

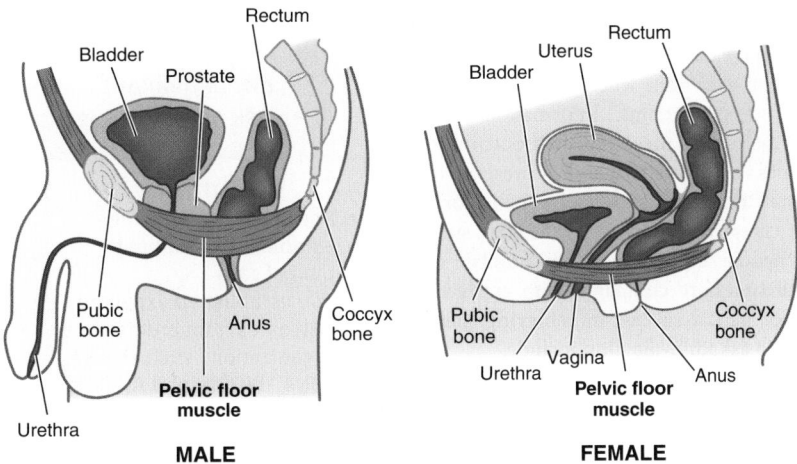

FIG. 46.16 Pelvic floor muscles. (From Lewis S, et al: *Medical-surgical nursing: assessment and management of clinical problems*, ed 10, St Louis, 2017, Elsevier.)

disability (e.g., cognitive impairment). Toileting can be implemented in any care setting and should be the first plan of action when you assess a patient to be incontinent. Timed voiding or scheduled toileting is toileting based on a fixed schedule, not the patient's urge to void. The schedule may be set by a time interval, such as every 2 to 3 hours, or at times of day, such as before and after meals. It is very successful with moderate-to-severe cognitively and mobility-impaired adults. Habit training is a toileting schedule based on the patient's usual voiding pattern. Using a bladder diary, the usual times a patient voids are identified. It is at these times that the patient is then toileted. Prompted voiding is a program of toileting designed for patients with mild or moderate cognitive impairment. Patients are toileted based on their usual voiding pattern. Caregivers ask the patient if he or she is wet or dry, give positive feedback for dryness, prompt the patient to toilet, and reward the patient for desired behavior. This is a very successful toileting program; but it does require a consistent and motivated caregiver, a cooperative patient, and evidence that the patient will void when toileted at least 50% of the time or more.

Intermittent Catheterization. Some patients experience chronic inability to completely empty the bladder as a result of neuromuscular damage related to multiple sclerosis, diabetes, spinal cord injury, and urinary retention caused by outlet obstruction. To minimize the risk of UTI, patients or family caregivers are taught to catheterize the bladder. It is important they follow the principles of asepsis as discussed earlier in the chapter. Teach patients and caregivers about the importance of adequate fluid intake, signs of infection, and their individualized catheterization schedule. The goal for intermittent catheterization is drainage of 400 mL of urine with the schedule individualized to meet this goal.

Skin Care. Incontinence-associated dermatitis (IAD) presents as inflammation of the skin and can also cause blistering and swelling to the affected area (Paulin and Dowling-Castronovo, 2017). IAD is a multifaceted condition and should be treated as such. However, the main cause is moisture from incontinence, so preventing incontinence or having a good management plan when a patient is incontinent is imperative. The *do's* for effective management include identification and treatment, use of skin risk assessment tools, use of appropriate barrier products, and ensuring adequate hydration. The *don'ts* include only using traditional soap and water for cleaning, double padding the bed, leaving soiled pads in contact with the skin, and assuming incontinence is inevitable (Yates, 2018).

REFLECT NOW

Complementary approaches to care can often resolve incontinency. What are interventions that you would choose for an older adult to promote urinary continence and comfort?

◆ **Evaluation**

Through the Patient's Eyes. The patient is the best source of evaluation of outcomes and responses to nursing care. Include patients in the revision of the care plan based on their perception of its success. It is important to remember that urinary problems impact the patient not only physically but emotionally, psychologically, spiritually, and socially. Carefully assess the patient's self-image, social interactions, sexuality, and emotional status as impacted by the urinary problem (Fig. 46.17).

Patient Outcomes. To evaluate the care plan use the expected outcomes developed during planning to determine whether interventions were effective. This evaluation process is dynamic. Information gathered is used to modify the plan of care to meet expected outcomes. Evaluate for changes in the patient's voiding pattern and/or presence of symptoms such as dysuria, urinary retention, and UI. If a behavioral plan is in effect, evaluate patient/caregiver adherence to the plan, such as toileting according to the schedule, or determine the number of incontinent episodes. Actual outcomes are compared with expected outcomes to determine success or partial success in achieving these outcomes. Examples of questions to ask for evaluation include:

- "Tell me, how frequently are you voiding now?" "How many times are you awakened from sleep with a strong urge to void?"
- "Do you continue to experience that sensation of urgency or need to rush to the toilet?"
- "How many episodes of urine leakage have you experienced over the past week?"
- "Do you have pain or burning when you pass urine?

The effectiveness of an intervention may take place within a day or two, or it may take weeks or months to fully evaluate effectiveness. Evaluate initial adherence to dietary changes, understanding of instructions for pelvic muscle exercise, or effectiveness of antibiotic treatment for UTI in 1 to 2 days. Evaluation of the effectiveness of pelvic muscle exercises in decreasing urgency and incontinence will need to be weeks or months after therapy is started. Continuous evaluation, when possible, allows you to determine progress toward goals, encourage adherence, and revise the diagnosis and/or plan as needed.

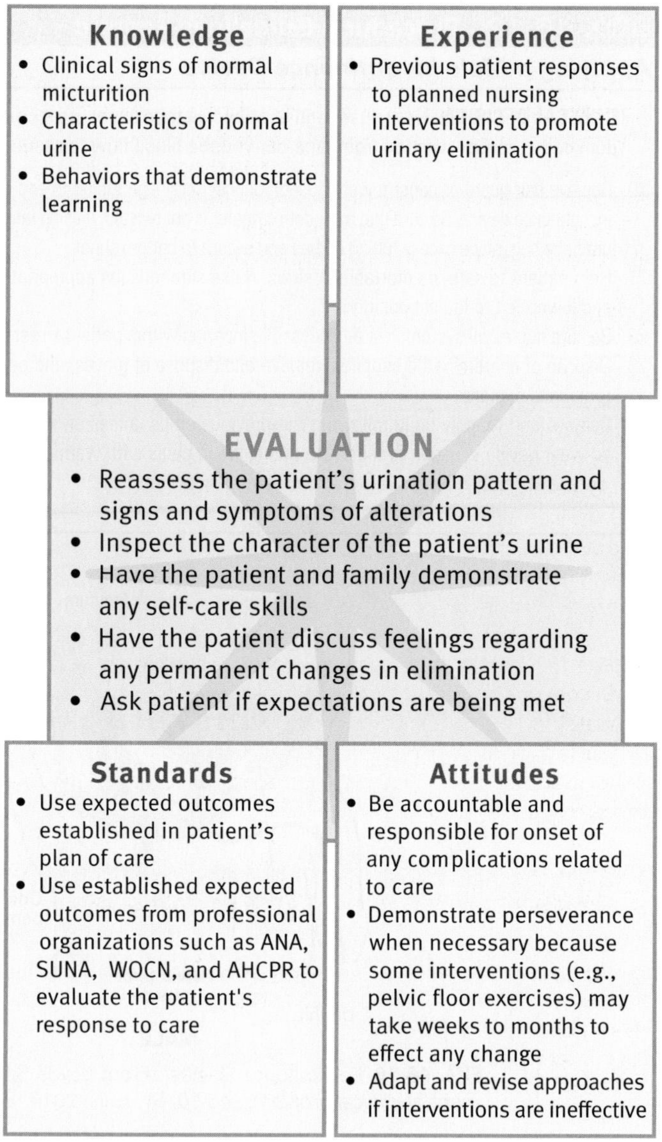

Knowledge
- Clinical signs of normal micturition
- Characteristics of normal urine
- Behaviors that demonstrate learning

Experience
- Previous patient responses to planned nursing interventions to promote urinary elimination

EVALUATION
- Reassess the patient's urination pattern and signs and symptoms of alterations
- Inspect the character of the patient's urine
- Have the patient and family demonstrate any self-care skills
- Have the patient discuss feelings regarding any permanent changes in elimination
- Ask patient if expectations are being met

Standards
- Use expected outcomes established in patient's plan of care
- Use established expected outcomes from professional organizations such as ANA, SUNA, WOCN, and AHCPR to evaluate the patient's response to care

Attitudes
- Be accountable and responsible for onset of any complications related to care
- Demonstrate perseverance when necessary because some interventions (e.g., pelvic floor exercises) may take weeks to months to effect any change
- Adapt and revise approaches if interventions are ineffective

FIG. 46.17 Critical thinking model for urinary elimination evaluation. *AHCPR*, Agency for Health Care Policy and Research; *ANA*, American Nurses Association, *SUNA*, Society of Urologic Nurses and Associates; *WOCN*, Wound, Ostomy and Continence Nurses Society.

SAFETY GUIDELINES FOR NURSING SKILLS

Ensuring patient safety is an essential role of the professional nurse. To ensure patient safety, communicate clearly with members of the health care team, assess and incorporate a patient's priorities of care and preferences, and use the best evidence when making decisions about your patient's care. When performing the skills in this chapter, remember to follow points to ensure safe, individualized care:

- Follow principles of surgical and medical asepsis as indicated when performing catheterizations, handling urine specimens, or helping patients with their toileting needs.

- Identify patients at risk for latex allergies (i.e., patient history of hay fever; asthma; and allergies to certain foods such as bananas, grapes, apricots, kiwifruit, and hazelnuts).
- Identify patients with allergies to povidone-iodine. Provide alternatives such as chlorhexidine.

SKILL 46.1 COLLECTING MIDSTREAM (CLEAN-VOIDED) URINE SPECIMEN

Delegation and Collaboration

The skill of collecting urine specimens can be delegated to assistive personnel (AP). The nurse instructs the AP to:

- Obtain the specimens at a specified time when appropriate.
- Position patient as necessary when mobility restrictions are present.
- Report to the nurse if the urine is not clear (e.g., contains blood, cloudiness, or excess sediment).
- Report to the nurse when a patient is unable to initiate a stream or has pain or burning on urination.

Equipment

- Completed identification labels with appropriate patient identifiers
- Completed laboratory requisition, including patient identification, date, time, name of test, and source of culture
- Biohazard bag or container for delivery of specimen to laboratory (as specified by agency)

Clean-Voided Urine Specimen

- Commercial kit (Fig. 46.18) for clean-voided urine, containing:
  - Sterile cotton balls or antiseptic towelettes
  - Antiseptic solution (chlorhexidine or povidone-iodine solution)
  - Sterile water or normal saline
  - Sterile specimen container
  - Urine cup
- Clean gloves
- Soap, water, washcloth, and towel
- Bedpan (for nonambulatory patient), specimen hat (for ambulatory patient)

Sterile Urine Specimen From Urinary Catheter

- 20-mL Luer-Lok for routine urinalysis or 3-mL safety Luer-Lok syringe for culture
- Alcohol, chlorhexidine, or other disinfectant swab
- Clamp or rubber band
- Specimen container (nonsterile for routine urinalysis; sterile for culture)
- Clean gloves

STEP	RATIONALE

ASSESSMENT

1. Identify patient using at least two identifiers (e.g., name and birthday or name and medical record number) according to agency policy.
2. Review health care provider's order.
3. Refer to agency procedures for specimen collection methods.
4. Assess patient's or family caregiver's knowledge, experience, and health literacy.
5. Assess patient's ability to help with urine specimen collection; able to position self and hold container.
6. Assess for signs and symptoms of UTI (frequency, urgency, dysuria, hematuria, flank pain, fever; cloudy malodorous urine).
7. Assess patient's or family caregiver's understanding of purpose of test and method of collection.

Ensures correct patient. Complies with The Joint Commission standards and improves patient safety (TJC, 2020).
Ensures accurate testing of specimen; order is needed to perform test.
Agency policies may vary regarding collection and/or handling of specimens.
Ensures patient or family caregiver has the capacity to obtain, communicate, process, and understand basic health information (CDC, 2019).
Determines degree of help patient requires.

May indicate need for health care provider intervention.

Allows you to clarify misunderstanding; promotes patient cooperation.

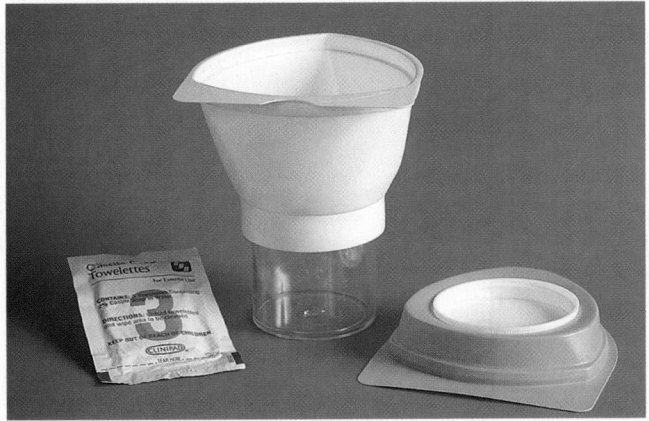

FIG. 46.18 Commercial midstream urine collection kit.

Continued

| **SKILL 46.1** | **COLLECTING MIDSTREAM (CLEAN-VOIDED) URINE SPECIMEN—cont'd** | |

| **STEP** | **RATIONALE** |

PLANNING

1. Perform hand hygiene. Close room door or bedside curtains around bed.
2. Organize equipment needed for procedure (see Fig. 46.18).
3. Explain the procedure and what is required of the patient. **NOTE:** Mobile patients may be able to collect a clean-voided specimen in the bathroom.

Reduces transmission of microorganisms. Provides privacy.
Facilitates organized completion of procedure.
Patients often prefer to obtain their own clean voided specimen but need appropriate education to correctly collect the sample.

IMPLEMENTATION

1. Check labels and verify complete laboratory requisition for specimen container.
2. **Collect clean-voided urine specimen.**
   a. Perform hand hygiene and apply clean gloves. Give patient cleaning towelette or towel, washcloth, and soap to clean perineum or help with cleaning perineum. Help bedridden patient onto bedpan to facilitate access to perineum. Remove and dispose of gloves and perform hand hygiene.

   b. Using aseptic technique, open outer package of commercial specimen kit.
   c. Apply clean gloves.
   d. Pour antiseptic solution over cotton balls (unless kit contains prepared antiseptic towelettes).

   e. Open specimen container, maintaining sterility of inside specimen container, and place cap with sterile inside up. Do not touch inside of cap or container.
   f. Use aseptic technique to help patient or allow patient to independently clean perineum and collect specimen. Amount of help needed varies with each patient. Inform patient that antiseptic solution will feel cold.
      (1) *Male:*
         (a) Hold penis with one hand; using circular motion and antiseptic towelette, clean meatus, moving from center to outside 3 times with 3 different towelettes (see illustration). Have uncircumcised male patient retract foreskin for effective cleaning of urinary meatus and keep retracted during voiding. Return foreskin when done.

         (b) If agency procedure indicates, rinse area with sterile water and dry with cotton balls or gauze pad.
         (c) After patient initiates urine stream into toilet, urinal, or bedpan, have him pass urine specimen container into stream and collect 90 to 120 mL of urine (Pagana et al., 2019) (see illustration).

      (2) *Female:*
         (a) Either nurse or patient spreads labia minora with fingers of nondominant hand.

Organizes procedure.

Reduces transfer of microorganisms. Patients prefer to wash their own perineal areas when possible. Cleaning prevents contamination of specimen from skin and surface bacteria after urine passes from urethra.

Maintains sterility of equipment.
Prevents contact of microorganisms on your hands.
Cotton ball or towelette is used to clean perineum.

Contaminated specimen is most frequent reason for inaccurate reporting of urine C&S.
Maintains patient's dignity and comfort.

Reduces number of microorganisms at urethral meatus and moves from areas of least to most contamination. Return of foreskin prevents stricture of penis.

Prevents contamination of specimen with antiseptic solution.

Initial urine flushes out microorganisms that normally accumulate at urinary meatus and prevents transfer into specimen.

Provides access to urethral meatus.

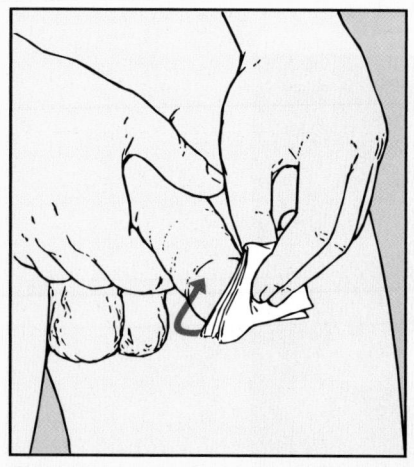

STEP 2f(1)(a) Cleaning technique (male).

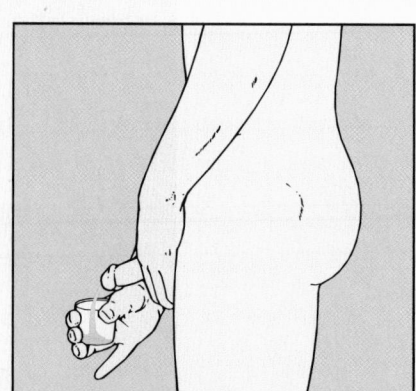

STEP 2f(1)(c) Collecting midstream urine specimen (male).

STEP	**RATIONALE**

(b) With dominant hand clean urethral area with antiseptic swab (cotton ball or gauze). Move from front (above urethral orifice) to back (toward anus). Use fresh swab each time; clean 3 times; begin with labial fold farthest from you, then labial fold closest, and then down center (see illustration).

Prevents contamination of urinary meatus with fecal material. Cleaning down center last decreases contamination from labia.

(c) If agency procedure indicates, rinse area with sterile water and dry with cotton ball.

Prevents contamination of specimen with antiseptic solution.

(d) While continuing to hold labia apart, patient initiates urine stream into toilet or bedpan; after stream is achieved, pass specimen container into stream and collect 90 to 120 mL of urine (Pagana et al., 2019) (see illustration).

Initial stream flushes out resident microorganisms that accumulate at urethral meatus and prevents transfer into specimen.

g. Remove specimen container before flow of urine stops and before releasing labia or penis. Patient finishes voiding into bedpan or toilet. Offer to help with personal hygiene as appropriate.

Prevents contamination of specimen with skin flora. Prevents sediment from bladder getting into specimen.

h. Replace cap securely on specimen container, touching only outside.

Retains sterility of inside of container and prevents spillage of urine.

i. Clean urine from exterior surface of container.

Prevents transfer of microorganisms to others.

3. Collect urine from indwelling urinary catheter.

a. Explain that you will use syringe without needle to remove urine through catheter port and that patient will not experience any discomfort.

Minimizes anxiety when you manipulate catheter and aspirate urine with syringe from catheter port.

b. Explain that you will need to clamp catheter for 10 to 15 minutes before obtaining urine specimen and that urine cannot be obtained from drainage bag.

Allows urine to accumulate in catheter. Urine in drainage bag is not considered sterile.

c. Perform hand hygiene and apply clean gloves. Clamp drainage tubing with clamp or rubber band for as long as 15 minutes below site chosen for withdrawal (see illustration).

Permits collection of fresh sterile urine in catheter tubing rather than draining into bag.

d. After 15 minutes, position patient so that catheter sampling port is easily accessible. Location of port is where catheter attaches to drainage bag tube (see Fig. 46-12).Clean port for 15 seconds with disinfectant swab and allow to dry.

Prevents entry of microorganisms into catheter.

e. Attach needleless Luer-Lok syringe to built-in catheter sampling port (see illustration). Some needleless ports use blunt plastic valve or slip-tip syringe inserted into port diaphragm.

Guideline recommends use of Luer-Lok needleless system. Needleless system prevents injury by needlestick.

f. Withdraw 3 mL for culture or 20 mL for routine urinalysis.

Allows collection of urine without contamination. Proper volume is needed to perform test.

g. Transfer urine from syringe into clean urine container for routine urinalysis or into sterile urine container for culture.

Prevents contamination of urine during transfer procedure.

h. Place lid tightly on container.

Prevents contamination of specimen by air and loss by spillage.

i. Unclamp catheter and allow urine to flow into drainage bag. Ensure that urine flows freely.

Allows urine to drain by gravity and prevents stasis of urine in bladder.

4. Securely attach label to container (not lid). If patient is female, indicate if she is menstruating. In presence of patient, complete label (two identifiers, specimen source, collection date and time) and attach to container. Attach completed laboratory requisition to container. Enclose specimen in a biohazard bag and send immediately to laboratory.

Incorrect patient identification could lead to diagnostic or therapeutic error (TJC, 2020). Bacteria multiply quickly. Specimen should be analyzed promptly for accurate results.

5. Dispose of soiled supplies. Remove and dispose of gloves and perform hand hygiene.

Prevents transmission of microorganisms.

6. Offer patient hand hygiene or provide time to wash hands.

Reduces transmission of microorganisms

7. Assist patient to comfortable position.

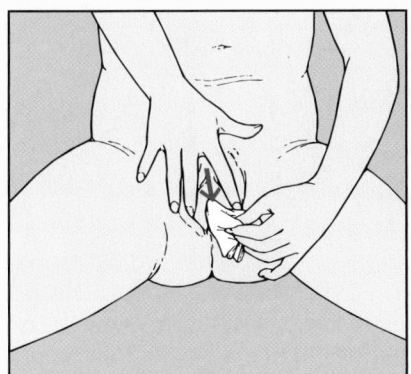

STEP 2f(2)(b) Clean from front to back, holding labia apart.

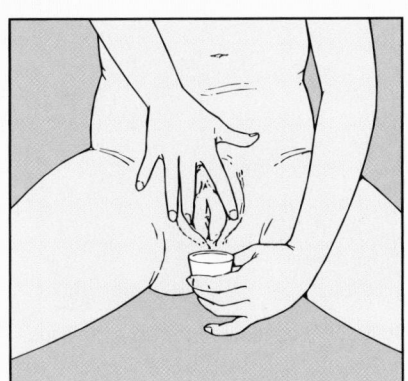

STEP 2f(2)(d) Collecting midstream urine specimen (female).

Continued

STEP	RATIONALE
8. Ensure that the nurse call system is in an accessible location and within patient's reach, and instruct patient in its use.	Provides for patient safety.
9. Send specimen and completed requisition to laboratory within 20 minutes. Refrigerate specimen if delay cannot be avoided.	Delay of analysis may significantly alter test results (Pagana et al., 2019).

EVALUATION

1. Inspect clean-voided specimen for contamination with toilet paper or stool.	Contaminants prevent specimen from being used.
2. Evaluate patient's urine C&S report for bacterial growth.	Routine cultures identify organism(s), and sensitivity study identifies antimicrobial medications that may be effective against pathogen.
3. Observe urinary drainage system in catheterized patient to ensure that it is intact and patent.	System must remain closed to remain sterile.
4. **Use Teach-Back:** "I want to be sure I explained the way to obtain a clean-voided specimen. Please repeat the steps back to me." Revise your instruction now or develop a plan for revised patient/family caregiver teaching if patient/family caregiver is not able to teach back correctly.	Determines patient's/family caregiver's level of understanding of instructional topic.

UNEXPECTED OUTCOMES AND RELATED INTERVENTIONS

1. Urine specimen is contaminated with stool or toilet paper.
   - Repeat patient instruction and specimen collection. If unable to obtain specimen through clean voiding, patient may need catheterization (see Skill 46.2).
2. Urine culture reveals bacterial growth (determined by colony count of more than 10,000 organisms per milliliter).
   - Report findings to health care provider.
   - Administer medications as ordered.
   - Monitor patient for fever and dysuria.
3. Lumen leading to balloon that holds catheter in place is punctured.
   - Notify health care provider.
   - Prepare for removal of existing catheter and insertion of new catheter.

RECORDING AND REPORTING

- Record method used to obtain specimen, date and time collected, type of test ordered, laboratory receiving specimen, characteristics of specimen, and patient's tolerance to procedure of specimen collection.
- Document your evaluation of patient learning.
- Report any abnormal findings to health care provider, the type of urinalysis, and when specimen was sent to laboratory.

HOME CARE CONSIDERATIONS

- If patient is to collect specimen as outpatient, a clean technique may be used. Provide instruction for collection and appropriate equipment.
- Provide information about storing specimen until time for delivery to health care provider's office or hospital laboratory.

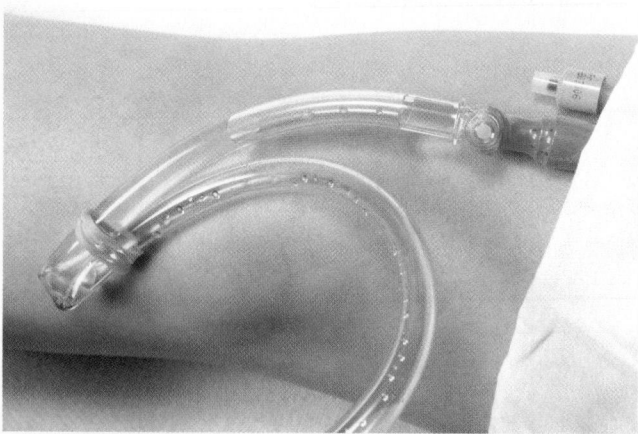

STEP 3c Rubber band used to clamp drainage tube.

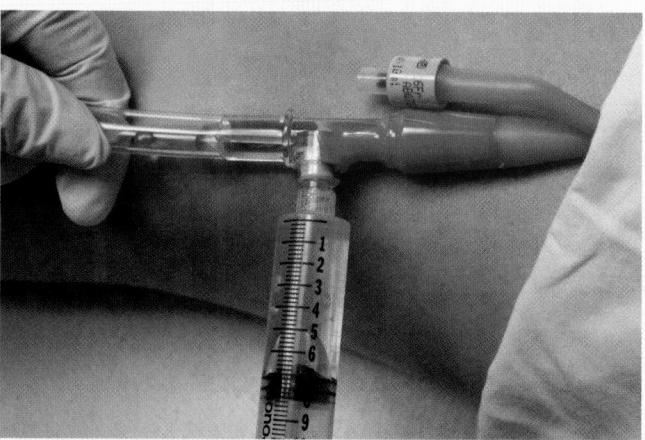

STEP 3e Access urinary catheter port with Luer-Lok syringe or syringe with blunt plastic valve.

SKILL 46.2	INSERTING AND REMOVING A STRAIGHT (INTERMITTENT) OR INDWELLING CATHETER

Delegation and Collaboration

The skill of inserting a straight or indwelling urinary catheter cannot be delegated to assistive personnel (AP). The nurse directs the AP to:

- Assist the nurse with patient positioning, focus lighting for the procedure, maintain privacy, empty urine from collection bag, and help with perineal care.
- Report postprocedure patient discomfort or fever to the nurse.
- Report abnormal color, odor, or amount of urine in drainage bag and whether the catheter is leaking or causes pain.

Equipment

- Catheter kit containing sterile items (**Note:** Catheter kits vary.)
  - Straight catheterization kit: single-lumen catheter (12 to 14 Fr), drapes (one fenestrated—has an opening in the center), sterile gloves, lubricant, cleansing solution incorporated in an applicator or to be added to cotton balls, and specimen container and label.

- Indwelling catheterization kit (see Fig. 46.11: double-lumen catheter, drapes (one fenestrated—has an opening in the center), sterile gloves, lubricant, antiseptic cleansing solution incorporated in an applicator or to be added to cotton balls, specimen container and label, and a prefilled syringe with sterile water or normal saline (to inflate balloon). **Note:** Some kits contain a catheter with attached drainage bag; others contain only a catheter; others have no catheter.
- Sterile drainage tubing and bag (if not included in indwelling catheter insertion kit)
- Device to secure catheter (catheter strap or other device)
- Extra sterile gloves and catheter *(optional)*
- Clean gloves
- Basin with warm water, washcloth, towel, and soap for perineal care
- Flashlight or other additional light source
- Bath blanket, waterproof absorbent pad
- Measuring container for urine

STEP	RATIONALE

ASSESSMENT

1. Identify patient using at least two identifiers (e.g., name and birthday or name and medical record number) according to agency policy. Compare identifiers with information on patient's MAR or medical record.

2. Review patient's EHR, including health care provider's order and nurses' notes. Note previous catheterization, including catheter size, response of patient, and time of catheterization.

3. Review EHR for any pathological conditions that may impair passage of catheter (e.g., enlarged prostate gland in men, urethral strictures).

4. Assess patient's gender and age.

5. Assess patient's or family caregiver's knowledge, experience, and health literacy.

6. Ask patient and check EHR for history of allergies. Check allergy bracelet.

7. Perform hand hygiene. Assess patient's weight, level of consciousness, developmental level, ability to cooperate, and mobility.

8. Assess for pain and bladder fullness. Palpate bladder over symphysis pubis or use bladder scanner (if available) (see Box 46.11).

9. Apply clean gloves. Inspect perineal region, observing for perineal anatomical landmarks, erythema, drainage or discharge, and odor. Remove and dispose of gloves and perform hand hygiene.

10. Assess patient's knowledge, prior experience with catheterization, and feelings about procedure.

Ensures correct patient. Complies with The Joint Commission standards and improves patient safety (TJC, 2020).

Identifies purpose of inserting catheter (such as for measurement of PVR, preparation for surgery, or specimen collection) and potential difficulty with catheter insertion.

Obstruction of urethra may prevent passage of catheter into bladder.

Assists with selection of catheter size.

Ensures patient or family caregiver has the capacity to obtain, communicate, process, and understand basic health information (CDC, 2019).

Catheter made of different material is needed if patient has latex allergy.

Determines positioning to use for catheterization; indicates how much help is needed to properly position patient, ability of patient to cooperate during procedure, and level of explanation needed.

Palpation of full bladder causes pain and/or urge to void, indicating full or overfull bladder.

Assessment of perineum (especially female perineal landmarks) improves accuracy and speed of catheter insertion. Reduces transmission of microorganisms.

Reveals need for patient instruction and/or support.

PLANNING

1. Close room door or curtains around bed.
2. Organize and set up any equipment needed to perform the procedure.

Provides privacy.
Organization ensures efficiency in completing the skill.

CLINICAL DECISION: *Some patients may be unable to assume positioning independently. Arrange for extra assistance before initiating the procedure.*

---

3. Explain procedure to patient.

Reduces patient anxiety and promotes cooperation.

Continued

SKILL 46.2	INSERTING AND REMOVING A STRAIGHT (INTERMITTENT) OR INDWELLING CATHETER—cont'd

STEP	RATIONALE

IMPLEMENTATION

1. Check patient's plan of care for size and type of catheter (if this is a rein-sertion). Use smallest-size catheter possible. Size 14 to 16 Fr most common for adults; older adults (12 to 14 Fr); larger sizes (20 to 22 Fr) are needed in special circumstances, such as after urological surgery or in the presence of gross hematuria.

Ensures that patient receives correct size and type of catheter. Larger catheter diameters increase the risk for urethral trauma. Small catheter allows for adequate drainage of periurethral glands.

2. Perform hand hygiene.

Reduces transmission of microorganisms.

3. Raise bed to appropriate working height. If side rails in use, raise side rail on opposite side of bed and lower side rail on working side.

Promotes good body mechanics. Use of side rails in this manner promotes patient safety.

4. Place waterproof pad under patient.

Prevents soiling bed linen.

CLINICAL DECISION: *Obtain help to position and support patients who are weak, frail, obese, or confused.*

---

5. Position patient:
   a. **Female patient:**
      (1) Help to dorsal recumbent position (on back with knees flexed). Ask patient to relax thighs so that you can rotate hips.

   Exposes perineum and allows hip joints to be externally rotated.

      (2) Alternate female position: Position side-lying (Sims') position with upper leg flexed at knee and hip. Support patient with pillows if necessary to maintain position.

   Alternate position is more comfortable if patient cannot abduct leg at hip joint (e.g., patient has arthritic joints or contractures).

   b. **Male patient:**
      (1) Position supine with legs extended and thighs slightly abducted.

   Comfortable position for patient and aids in visualization of penis.

6. **Drape patient**
   a. Female
      (1) Drape with bath blanket. Place blanket diamond fashion over patient, with one corner at patient's midsections, side corners over each thigh and abdomen, and last corner over perineum (see illustration).

   b. Male
      (1) Drape patient by covering upper part of body with small sheet or towel; drape with separate sheet or bath blanket so that only perineum is exposed (see illustration).

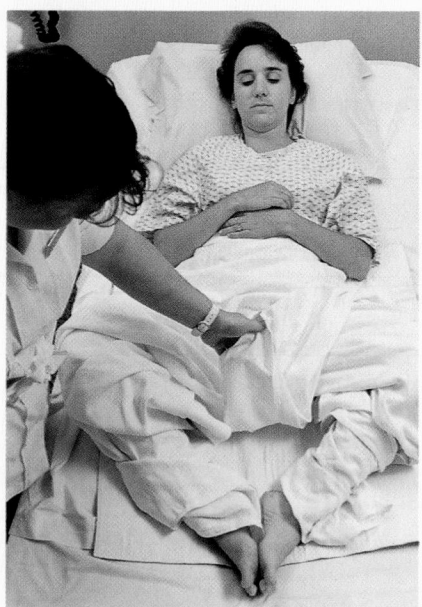

STEP 6a(1) Female patient draped and in dorsal recumbent position.

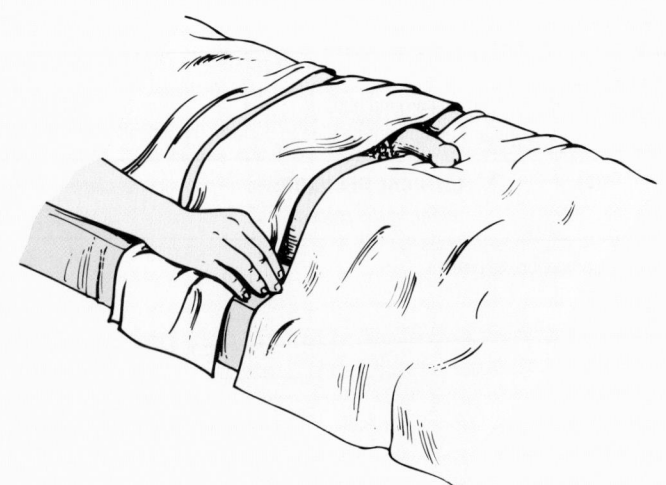

STEP 6b(1) Drape male patient with blankets.

STEP	**RATIONALE**
7. Apply clean gloves. Clean perineal area with soap and water, rinse, and dry (see Chapter 40). Use gloves to examine patient and identify urinary meatus. Remove and discard gloves. Perform hand hygiene.	Hygiene before initiating aseptic catheter insertion removes secretions, urine, and feces that could contaminate sterile field and increase risk for catheter-associated urinary tract infection (CAUTI). Perform hand hygiene immediately before catheter insertion (Gould et al., 2017).
8. Position portable light to illuminate genitals or have assistant available to hold light.	Adequate visualization of urinary meatus assists with accuracy of catheter insertion.
9. Open outer wrapping of catheterization kit. Place inner wrapped catheter kit tray on clean, accessible surface such as bedside table or, if possible, between patient's open legs. Patient size and positioning dictate exact placement.	Provides easy access to supplies during catheter insertion.
10. Open inner sterile wrap covering tray containing catheterization supplies using sterile technique (see Chapter 28). Fold back each flap of sterile covering with first flap opened away from you, next two flaps open to each side one at a time, and last flap opened toward patient.	Sterile wrap serves as sterile field. Sequence prevents you from reaching over sterile field.
a. Indwelling catheterization open system: Open separate package containing drainage bag, check to make sure that clamp on drainage port is closed, and place drainage bag and tubing in easily accessible location. Open outer package of sterile catheter, maintaining sterility of inner wrapper (see Chapter 28).	Open drainage bag systems have separate sterile packaging for sterile catheter, drainage bag and tubing, and insertion kit.
b. Indwelling catheterization closed system: All supplies are in sterile tray and arranged in sequence of use.	Closed drainage bag systems have catheter preattached to drainage tubing and bag.
c. Straight catheterization: All needed supplies are in sterile tray that contains supplies and can be used for urine collection.	
11. Apply sterile gloves.	Maintains surgical asepsis.
12. *Option:* Apply sterile drape with ungloved hands when drape is packed as first item. Touch only 1-inch edges of drape. Then apply sterile gloves.	Maintains surgical asepsis.
13. Drape perineum, keeping gloves and working surface of drape sterile.	Sterile drapes provide sterile field over which you will work during catheterization.
a. Drape female:	
(1) Pick up square sterile drape touching only edges (2.5 cm [1 inch]).	
(2) Allow drape to unfold without touching unsterile surfaces. Allow top edge of drape (2.5 to 5 cm [1 to 2 inches]) to form cuff over both hands.	When creating cuff over sterile gloved hands, sterility of gloves and workspace is maintained.
(3) Place drape with shiny side down on bed between patient's thighs. Slip cuffed edge just under buttocks as you ask patient to lift hips. Take care not to touch contaminated surfaces or patient's thighs with sterile gloves. If gloves are contaminated, remove and apply new pair.	
(4) Pick up fenestrated sterile drape out of tray. Allow drape to unfold without touching unsterile surfaces. Allow top edge of drape to form cuff over both hands. Apply drape over perineum so that opening is over exposed labia (see illustration).	Opening in drape creates sterile field around labia.

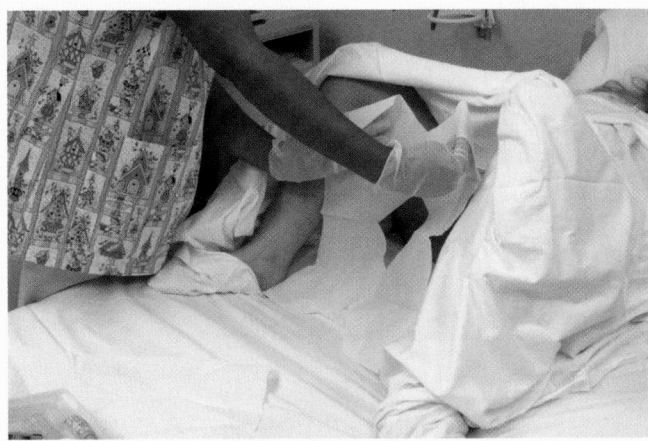

STEP 13a(4) Place sterile fenestrated drape (with opening in center) over female's perineum.

Continued

SKILL 46.2	INSERTING AND REMOVING A STRAIGHT (INTERMITTENT) OR INDWELLING CATHETER—cont'd

STEP	RATIONALE

b. Drape Male:

    (1) Use of square drape is optional; you may apply fenestrated drape instead.

    (2) Pick up edges of square drape and allow to unfold without touching unsterile surfaces. Place over thighs, with shiny side down, just below penis. Take care not to touch contaminated surfaces with sterile gloves.

    (3) Place fenestrated drape with opening centered over penis (see illustration).

14. Move tray closer to patient. Arrange remaining supplies on sterile field, maintaining sterility of gloves. Place sterile tray with cleaning solution (premoistened swab sticks or cotton balls, forceps, and solution), lubricant, catheter, and prefilled syringe for inflating balloon (indwelling catheterization only) on sterile drape.

    Provides easy access to supplies during catheter insertion and helps to maintain aseptic technique. Appropriate placement is determined by size of patient and position during catheterization.

    a. If kit contains sterile cotton balls, open package of sterile antiseptic solution and pour over cotton balls. Some kits contain package of premoistened swab sticks. Open end of package for easy access (see illustration).

    Use of sterile supplies and antiseptic solution reduces risk of CAUTI (Gould et al., 2017)

    b. Open sterile specimen container if specimen is to be obtained (see Skill 46.1).

    Makes container accessible to receive urine from catheter if specimen is needed.

    c. For indwelling catheterization, open sterile inner wrapper of catheter and leave catheter on sterile field. If part of closed system kit, remove tray with catheter and preattached drainage bag and place on sterile drape. Make sure that clamp on drainage port of bag is closed. If needed and if part of sterile tray, attach catheter to drainage tubing.

    Indwelling catheterization trays vary. Some have preattached catheters; others need to be attached but are part of the sterile tray; others do not have catheter or drainage system as part of tray.

    d. Open packet of lubricant and squeeze out on sterile field. Lubricate catheter tip by dipping it into water-soluble gel 2.5 to 5 cm (1 to 2 inches) for women and 12.5 to 17.5 cm (5 to 7 inches) for men (see illustration).

    Lubrication minimizes trauma to urethra and discomfort during catheter insertion. Male catheter needs enough lubricant to cover length of catheter inserted.

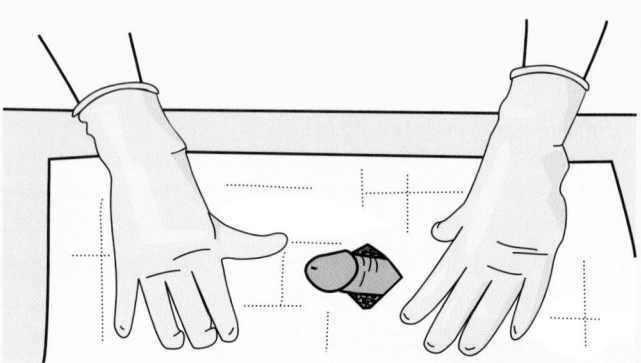

STEP 13b(3) Drape male with fenestrated drape.

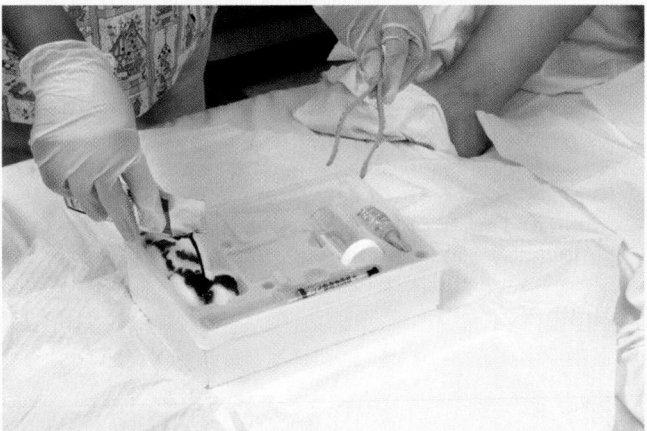

STEP 14a Sterile kit includes antiseptic swabs.

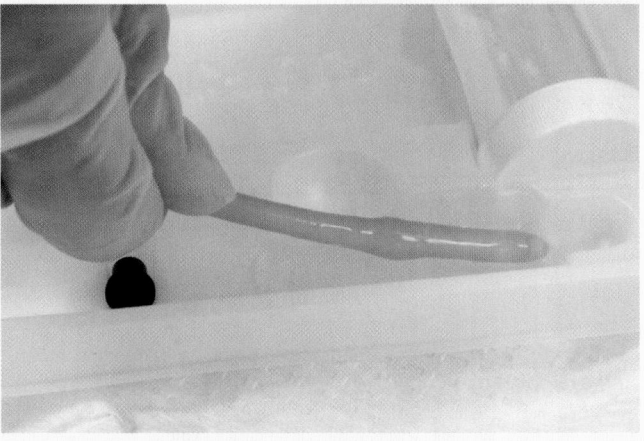

STEP 14d Lubricate catheter.

STEP	RATIONALE

CLINICAL DECISION: *Pretesting a balloon on an indwelling catheter by injecting fluid from the prefilled sterile normal saline syringe into the balloon port is* **no longer recommended**. *Testing the balloon may distort and stretch it and lead to damage, causing increased trauma on insertion.*

15. Clean urethral meatus:
    a. **Female patient:**
       (1) Separate labia with fingers of nondominant hand (now contaminated) to fully expose urethral meatus.
       (2) Maintain position of nondominant hand throughout procedure.

       (3) Holding forceps in dominant hand, pick up one moistened cotton ball or pick up one swab stick at a time. Clean labia and urinary meatus from clitoris toward anus. Use new cotton ball or swab for each area that you clean. Clean by wiping far labial fold, near labial fold, and last, directly over center of urethral meatus (see illustration).

    b. **Male patient:**
       (1) With nondominant hand (now contaminated) retract foreskin (if uncircumcised) and gently grasp penis at shaft just below glans. Hold shaft of penis at right angle to body. This hand remains in this position for remainder of procedure.
       (2) Using uncontaminated dominant hand, clean meatus with cotton balls/swab sticks, using circular strokes, beginning at meatus and working outward in spiral motion.
       (3) Repeat cleaning 3 times using clean cotton ball/swab stick each time (see illustration).
16. Pick up and hold catheter 7.5 to 10 cm (3 to 4 inches) from catheter tip with catheter loosely coiled in palm of hand. If catheter is not attached to drainage bag, make sure to position urine tray so that end of catheter can be placed there once insertion begins.

Optimal visualization of urethral meatus is possible.

Closure of labia during cleaning means that area is contaminated and requires cleaning procedure to be repeated.
Front-to-back cleaning moves from area of least contamination toward highly contaminated area. Follows principles of medical asepsis (see Chapter 28). Dominant gloved hand remains sterile.

When grasping shaft of penis, avoid pressure on dorsal surface to prevent compression of urethra.
Losing grasp during cleaning means that area is contaminated and requires cleaning procedure to be repeated.
Circular cleaning pattern follows principles of medical asepsis (see Chapter 28).

Holding catheter near tip allows for its easier manipulation during insertion.
Coiling catheter in palm prevents distal end from striking nonsterile surface.

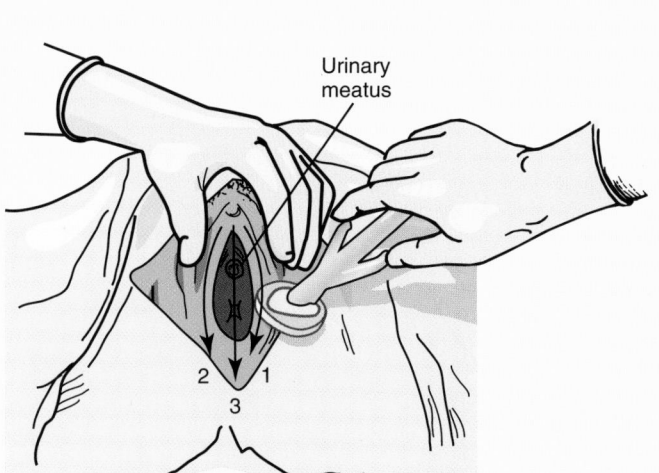

STEP 15a(3) Clean female perineum.

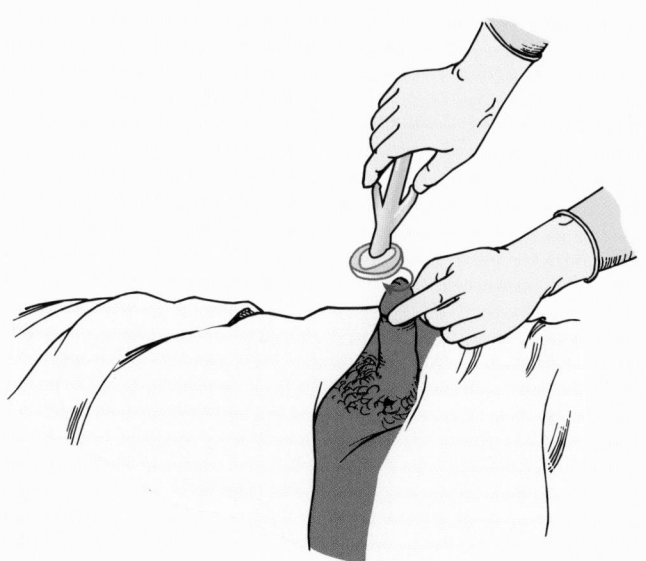

STEP 15b(3) Clean male urinary meatus.

Continued

STEP	**RATIONALE**

17. Insert catheter. Explain to patient that feeling of discomfort or pressure may be experienced as catheter is inserted into urethra. This sensation is normal and will go away quickly.

Helps to minimize patient anxiety.

a. Female patient:

  (1) Ask patient to bear down gently and slowly insert catheter through urethral meatus (see illustration).

Bearing down may help visualize urinary meatus and promotes relaxation of external urinary sphincter, aiding in catheter insertion.

  (2) Advance catheter total of 5 to 7.5 cm (2 to 3 inches) or until urine flows out of catheter. When urine appears, advance catheter another 2.5 to 5 cm (1 to 2 inches). Do not use force to insert catheter.

Urine flow indicates that catheter tip is in bladder or lower urethra.

  (3) Release labia and hold catheter securely with nondominant hand.

Prevents accidental expulsion of catheter from the patient's bladder.

b. Male patient

  (1) Lift penis to position perpendicular (90 degrees) to patient's body and apply gentle upward traction.

Straightens urethra to ease catheter insertion.

  (2) Ask patient to bear down as if to void, and slowly insert catheter through urethral meatus (see illustration).

Relaxation of external sphincter aids in insertion of catheter.

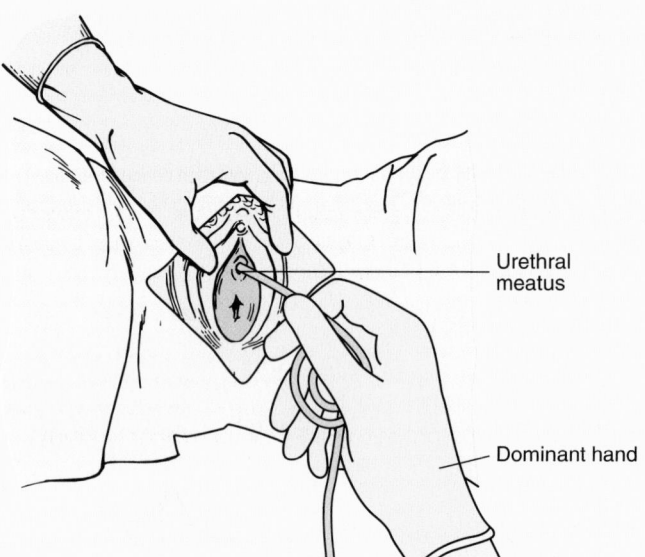

Urethral meatus

Dominant hand

STEP 17a(1) Insert catheter into female urinary meatus.

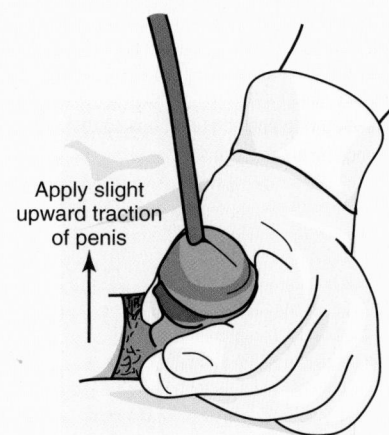

Apply slight upward traction of penis

STEP 17b(2) Insert catheter into male urinary meatus.

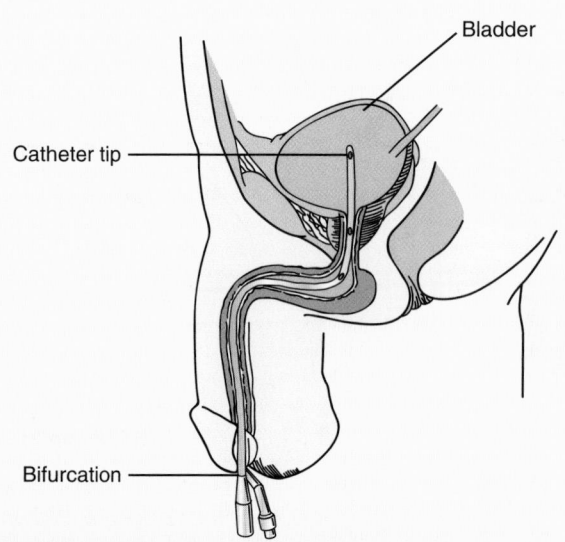

Bladder

Catheter tip

Bifurcation

STEP 17b(4) Male anatomy with correct catheter insertion to bifurcation.

STEP	**RATIONALE**
(3) Advance catheter 17 to 22.5 cm (7 to 9 inches) or until urine flows out end of catheter.	Length of male urethra varies. Flow of urine indicates that tip of catheter is in bladder or urethra but not necessarily that balloon part of indwelling catheter is in bladder.
(4) Stop advancing with straight catheter. When urine appears in indwelling catheter, advance it to bifurcation (inflation and deflation ports exposed) (see illustration).	Further advancement of catheter to bifurcation of drainage and balloon inflation port ensures that balloon part of catheter is not still in prostatic urethra.
(5) Lower penis and hold catheter securely in nondominant hand.	Prevents accidental expulsion of catheter from the patient's bladder.
18. Allow bladder to empty fully unless agency policy restricts maximum volume of urine drained (see agency policy).	There is no definitive evidence regarding whether there is benefit in limiting maximal volume drained.
19. Collect urine specimen as needed (see Skill 46.1). Fill specimen container to 20 to 30 mL by holding end of catheter over cup. Set aside. Keep end of catheter sterile.	Sterile specimen for culture analysis can be obtained.
20. *Option for straight* catheterization: When urine stops flowing, withdraw catheter slowly and smoothly until removed.	Minimizes trauma to urethra.
21. Inflate indwelling catheter balloon with amount of fluid designated by manufacturer.	Indwelling catheter balloon should not be underinflated. Underinflation causes balloon distortion and potential bladder damage.
a. Continue to hold catheter with nondominant hand.	Holding on to catheter before inflating balloon prevents expulsion of catheter from urethra.
b. With free dominant hand, connect prefilled syringe to injection port at end of catheter.	
c. Slowly inject total amount of solution (see illustration).	Full amount of solution needed to inflate balloon properly.

CLINICAL DECISION: *If patient reports sudden pain during inflation of a catheter balloon or when resistance is felt when inflating the balloon, stop inflation, allow the fluid from the balloon to flow back into the syringe, advance catheter farther, and reinflate balloon. The balloon may have been inflating in the urethra. If pain continues, remove catheter and notify the health care provider.*

STEP	**RATIONALE**
d. After inflating catheter balloon, release catheter from nondominant hand. *Gently* pull catheter until resistance is felt. Then advance catheter slightly.	By moving catheter slightly back into bladder, pressure on bladder neck is avoided.
e. Connect drainage tubing to catheter if it is not already preconnected.	
22. Secure indwelling catheter with catheter strap or other securement device. Leave enough slack to allow leg movement. Attach securement device at tubing just above catheter bifurcation.	Securing catheter reduces risk of movement, urethral erosion, CAUTI, or accidental catheter removal (Gould et al., 2017; McNeill, 2017). Attachment of securement device at catheter bifurcation prevents occlusion of catheter.
a. Female patient	
(1) Secure catheter tubing to inner thigh, allowing enough slack to prevent tension (see illustration).	
b. Male patient	
(1) Secure catheter tubing to upper thigh (see illustration) or lower abdomen (with penis directed toward chest). Allow slack in catheter so that movement does not create tension on catheter.	Anchoring catheter reduces traction on urethra and minimizes urethral injury (Gould et al., 2017; McNeill, 2017).
(2) If retracted, replace foreskin over glans penis.	Leaving foreskin retracted can cause discomfort and dangerous edema.

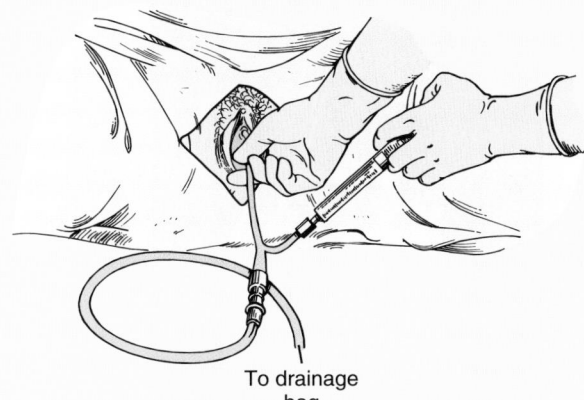

To drainage bag

STEP 21c Inflate balloon (indwelling catheter).

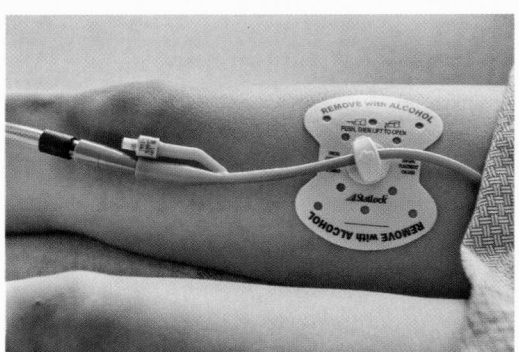

STEP 22a(1) Secure indwelling catheter on female with adhesive securement device.

Continued

SKILL 46.2   INSERTING AND REMOVING A STRAIGHT (INTERMITTENT) OR INDWELLING CATHETER—cont'd

STEP	RATIONALE
23. Clip drainage tubing to edge of mattress. Position drainage bag below level of bladder by attaching to bedframe (Gould et al., 2017). Do not attach to side rails of bed, and do not rest on floor (see illustration).	Keeping the collection bag below the level of the bladder at all times prevents backflow into bladder, which can cause risk for CAUTI (Gould et al., 2017). Bags attached to movable objects such as side rail increase risk for urethral trauma because of pulling or accidental dislodgment.
24. Check to ensure that there is no obstruction to urine flow. Coil excess tubing on bed and fasten to bottom sheet with clip or other securement device.	Keeping the catheter and collecting tube free from kinking may reduce risk of CAUTI (Gould et al., 2017).
25. Provide perineal hygiene as needed. Help patient to comfortable position.	Promotes patient comfort
26. Dispose of supplies in appropriate receptacles.	Reduces transmission of microorganisms.
27. If ordered, label and bag specimen according to agency policy. Label specimen in front of patient. Send to laboratory as soon as possible.	Fresh urine specimen ensures more accurate findings. Labeling ensures that diagnostic results will be connected to correct patient (TJC, 2020).
28. Measure urine and record.	Provides baseline for urine output.
29. Remove and dispose of gloves and perform hand hygiene.	Reduces transmission of infection.
30. Raise side rails (as appropriate) and lower bed to lowest position. Be sure nurse call system is in an accessible location within patient's reach.	Promotes patient comfort and safety. Ensures patient can call for assistance if needed.

EVALUATION

1. Palpate bladder for distention or use bladder scan (see Box 46.11) as per agency protocol.	Determines whether distention is relieved.
2. Ask patient to describe level of comfort.	Determines whether patient's sensation of discomfort or fullness has been relieved.
3. Indwelling catheter: Observe character and amount of urine in drainage system.	Determines whether urine is flowing adequately.
4. Indwelling catheter: Determine that there is no urine leaking from catheter or tubing connections.	Prevents injury to patient's skin and ensures closed sterile system.
5. **Use Teach-Back:** "I want to be sure I explained clearly about your urinary catheter and some things you can do to ensure the urine flows out of the catheter. Tell me what you can do to keep the urine flowing." Revise your instruction now or develop a plan for revised patient/family caregiver teaching if patient/family caregiver is not able to teach back correctly.	Determines patient's/family caregiver's level of understanding of instructional topic.

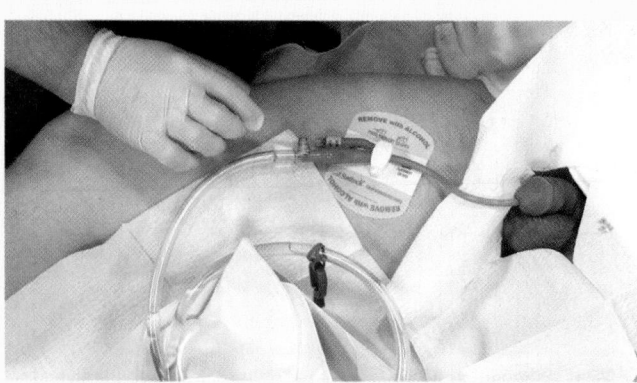

STEP 22b(1) Secure indwelling catheter on male.

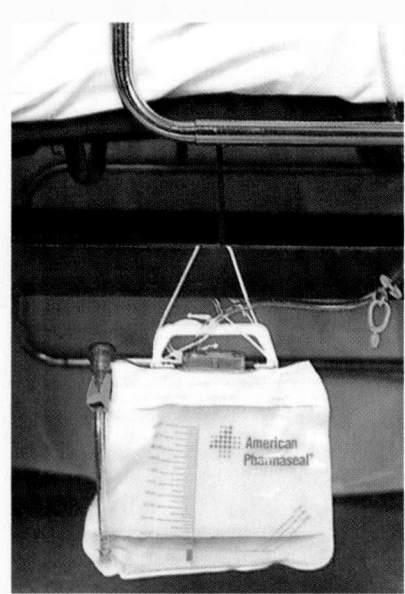

STEP 23 Drainage Bag below level of bladder.

STEP	RATIONALE

UNEXPECTED OUTCOMES AND RELATED INTERVENTIONS

1. Catheter goes into vagina.
- Leave first catheter in vagina so that you can correctly identify the urinary meatus.
- Clean urinary meatus again. Using **another** catheter kit, reinsert sterile catheter into meatus (check agency policy). **NOTE:** If gloves become contaminated, start procedure again.
- Remove first catheter that was left in vagina after successful insertion of second catheter.

2. Sterility is broken during catheterization by nurse or patient.
- Replace gloves if contaminated and start over.
- If patient touches sterile field but equipment and supplies remain sterile, avoid touching that part of sterile field.
- If equipment and/or supplies become contaminated, replace with sterile items or start over with new sterile kit.

3. Patient reports bladder discomfort, and catheter is patent as evidenced by adequate urine flow.
- Check catheter to ensure that there is no traction on it.
- Notify health care provider. Patient may be experiencing bladder spasms or symptoms of UTI.
- Monitor catheter output for color, clarity, odor, and amount.

RECORDING AND RECORDING

- Record reason for catheterization, type and size of catheter inserted, amount of fluid used to inflate balloon, specimen collection (if applicable), characteristics and amount of urine, patient's response to procedure, and evaluation of patient learning.
- Record I&O on flow sheet record.
- Report at change of shift reason for catheterization, type and size of catheter inserted, amount of fluid used to inflate balloon, specimen collection (if applicable), characteristics and amount of urine, patient's response to procedure, and any education.
- Report to health care provider persistent catheter-related pain and discomfort.

HOME CARE CONSIDERATIONS

- Patients who are at home may use a leg bag during the day and switch to a larger-volume bag at night. If a patient changes from a large-volume bag to a leg bag, instruct in the importance of handwashing and cleansing the connection ports with alcohol before changing bags.
- Teach patients and family caregivers how to properly position the drainage bag, empty a urinary drainage bag, and observe urine color, clarity, odor, and amount.
- Educate patients and/or caregivers about the signs of UTI and troubleshooting techniques for a leaking catheter.
- Arrange for home delivery of catheter supplies, always ensuring that there is at least one extra catheter, insertion kit, and drainage bag in the home.

SKILL 46.3   CARE AND REMOVAL OF AN INDWELLING CATHETER

Delegation and Collaboration

The skill of performing routine catheter care can be delegated to assistive personnel (AP). Depending on agency policy, the skill of removing an indwelling catheter may be delegated to AP; however, a nurse must first assess a patient's status and verify the order. The nurse directs the AP to:

- Report characteristics of the urine (color, clarity, odor, and amount) before and after removal.
- Report the condition of the patient's genital area (e.g., color, rashes, open areas, odor, soiling from fecal incontinence, trauma to tissues around urinary meatus).
- If allowed to remove catheter per agency policy, check size of balloon and syringe needed to deflate balloon; report if balloon does not deflate and if there is bleeding after removal.
- Report time and amount of first voiding after catheter is removed.
- Report if patient experiences fever, chills, change in mental status, burning, flank or back pain, and/or hematuria (signs of UTI); dysuria after catheter removal.

Equipment

Catheter Care
- Clean gloves
- Waterproof pad
- Bath blanket
- Basin with warm water, washcloth, towel, and soap for perineal care

Catheter Removal
- Clean gloves
- 10-mL syringe or larger without a needle (size depends on volume of solution used to inflate the balloon)
- Graduated cylinder to measure urine
- Waterproof pad
- Toilet, bedside commode, urine "hat," urinal, or bedpan
- Bladder scanner (as indicated)

Continued

SKILL 46.3	CARE AND REMOVAL OF AN INDWELLING CATHETER—cont'd

STEP	RATIONALE

ASSESSMENT

1. Identify patient using at least two identifiers (e.g., name and birthday or name and medical record number) according to agency policy.

2. Perform hand hygiene. Apply clean gloves.

3. **Assess need for catheter care:**

    a. Observe urinary output and urine characteristics.

    b. Assess for history or presence of bowel incontinence.

    c. Position patient, retract labia or foreskin to observe for any discharge, redness, bleeding, or presence of tissue trauma around urethral meatus (this may be deferred until catheter care).

    d. Remove and dispose of gloves; perform hand hygiene.

4. **Assess need for catheter removal:**

    a. Review patient's electronic health record (EHR), including health care provider's order and nurses' notes. Note length of time catheter has been in place.

    b. Perform hand hygiene and apply clean gloves. Assess urine color, clarity, odor, and amount. Note any urethral discharge, irritation of genital region, or trauma to urinary meatus (this may be deferred until just before removal). Remove and dispose of gloves. Perform hand hygiene.

    c. Determine size of catheter inflation balloon by looking at balloon inflation valve.

5. Assess patient's or family caregiver's knowledge, health literacy, and prior experience with catheter care and/or catheter removal.

Rationale column:

Ensures correct patient. Complies with The Joint Commission standards and improves patient safety (TJC, 2020).
Reduces transmission of microorganisms.

Sudden decrease in urine output may indicate occlusion of catheter. Cloudy, foul-smelling urine associated with other systemic symptoms may indicate CAUTI.
Most common bacteria to cause CAUTI are *Escherichia coli,* a major colonizer of the bowel; thus, fecal incontinence increases risk for CAUTI (Fekete, 2018).
Indicates inflammatory process, possible infection, or erosion of catheter through urethra.

Reduces transmission of microorganisms.

Catheters in place for more than a few days cause higher risk for catheter encrustation and UTI.

May be indicator of inflammation or UTI and source of discomfort during catheter removal. Reduces transmission of microorganisms.

Determines size of syringe needed to deflate balloon and amount of fluid expected in syringe after deflation.
Ensures patient has the capacity to obtain, communicate, process and understand basic health information (CDC, 2019).

PLANNING

1. Close room door and bedside curtain

2. Obtain and organize equipment for perineal care/catheter removal at bedside.

3. Explain procedure to patient. Discuss signs and symptoms of UTI. If applicable, teach patient or family caregiver how to perform catheter hygiene.

Rationale column:

Provides privacy.
Ensures more efficient procedure.

Reduces anxiety and promotes cooperation. Self-care supports patient's sense of autonomy.

IMPLEMENTATION

1. Perform hand hygiene.

2. Raise bed to appropriate working height. If side rails are raised, lower side rail on working side.

3. Position patient with waterproof pad under buttocks and cover with bath blanket, exposing only genital area and catheter (see Skill 46.2).

    a. Female in dorsal recumbent position.

    b. Male in supine position.

4. Apply clean gloves.

5. Remove catheter securement device while maintaining connection with drainage tubing.

6. **Catheter care:**

    a. *Female:* Use nondominant hand to gently separate labia to fully expose urethral meatus and catheter. Maintain position of hand throughout procedure.

    b. *Male:* Use nondominant hand to retract foreskin if not circumcised and hold penis at shaft just below glans. Maintain hand position throughout procedure.

    c. Grasp catheter with two fingers of nondominant hand to stabilize it.

Rationale column:

Reduces transmission of microorganisms.
Promotes use of proper body mechanics.

Shows respect for patient dignity by exposing only genital area and catheter.

Reduces transmission of microorganisms.
Provides ability to easily clean around catheter and to remove it.

Provides full visualization of urethral meatus. Full separation of labia prevents contamination of meatus during cleaning.
Retraction of foreskin provides full visualization of urethral meatus.

Prevents unnecessary traction on catheter.
Pulling on catheter is cause of discomfort for patient and can damage urethra and bladder neck.

STEP	RATIONALE
d. If not performed earlier, assess urethral meatus and surrounding tissues for inflammation, swelling, discharge, or tissue trauma, and ask patient if burning or discomfort is present.	Determines frequency and type of ongoing care required. Indicates possibility of CAUTI or catheter erosion through urethra.
e. Provide perineal hygiene using mild soap and warm water (see Chapter 40). *Option:* Use chlorhexidine gluconate (CHG) 2% cloth.	Antiseptic cleaners have not been shown to definitively decrease CAUTI; mild soap and water are appropriate (McNeill, 2017). Although chlorhexidine 2% cloth can be used, there is no clear scientific evidence for use of antiseptics versus nonantiseptics to reduce rates of CAUTI (Fasugba et al., 2017).
f. Using clean washcloth or CHG cloth, clean catheter.	
(1) Starting close to urinary meatus, clean catheter in circular motion along its length for about 10 cm (4 inches), moving away from body (see illustration). Remove all traces of soap. *For male patients:* Reduce or reposition foreskin after care.	Reduces presence of secretions or drainage on outside catheter surface.
g. Reapply catheter securement device. Allow slack in catheter so that movement does not create tension on it.	Securing indwelling catheter reduces risk of urethral trauma, urethral erosion, CAUTI, or accidental removal (Gould et al., 2017; McNeill, 2017).
7. Routinely check drainage tubing and bag.	
a. Catheter is secured to upper thigh.	Maintains unobstructed flow of urine out of bladder (Gould et al., 2017; McNeill, 2017).
b. Tubing is coiled and secured onto bed linen.	
c. Tubing is not looped or positioned above level of bladder.	
d. Tubing is not kinked or clamped.	
e. Drainage bag is positioned below level of bladder with urine flowing freely into bag.	
f. Drainage bag is not overfull. Empty drainage bag when ½ full.	Overfull drainage bag creates tension and pulls on catheter, resulting in trauma to urethra and/or urinary meatus. Facilitates unobstructed flow of urine (Gould et al., 2017).

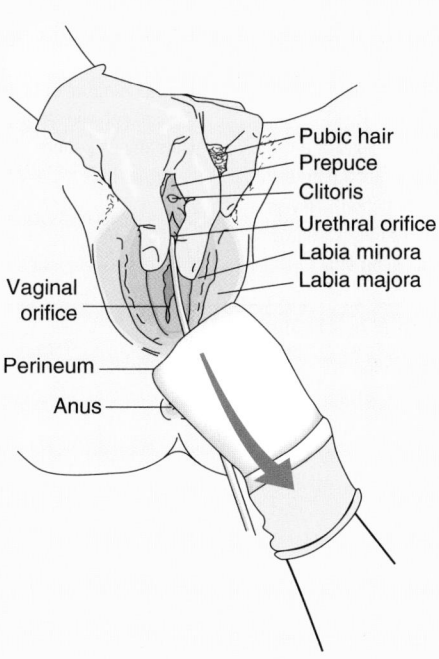

Pubic hair
Prepuce
Clitoris
Urethral orifice
Labia minora
Labia majora

Vaginal orifice

Perineum

Anus

STEP 6f(1) Clean Catheter starting at meatus and moving downward while holding it securely.

Continued

SKILL 46.3 CARE AND REMOVAL OF AN INDWELLING CATHETER—cont'd

STEP	RATIONALE
8. **Catheter removal:** (Perform catheter care; see Step 6 before catheter removal.)	
a. With clean gloves still on, move syringe plunger up and down to loosen and then pull it back to 0.5 mL. Insert hub of syringe into inflation valve (balloon port). Allow balloon fluid to drain into syringe automatically by itself. Syringe should fill. Make sure that entire amount of fluid is removed by comparing removed amount to volume needed for inflation.	Partially inflated balloon can traumatize urethral wall during removal. Passive drainage of catheter balloon prevents formation of ridges in balloon. These ridges can cause discomfort or trauma during removal.
b. Pull catheter out smoothly and slowly. Examine it to ensure that it is whole. Catheter should slide out easily. Do not use force. If you note any resistance, repeat Step 8a to remove remaining inflation fluid.	A nonwhole catheter means that pieces of catheter may still be in bladder. Notify health care provider immediately.
c. Wrap contaminated catheter in waterproof pad. Unhook collection bag and drainage tubing from bed.	Promotes safety and reduces the risk for transmission of microorganisms.
d. Empty, measure, and record urine present in drainage bag.	Documents urinary output.
e. Encourage patient to maintain or increase fluid intake (unless contraindicated by restrictions).	Maintains normal urine output.
f. Initiate voiding record or bladder diary. Instruct patient to tell you when need to empty bladder occurs, and that all urine needs to be measured. Make sure that patient understands how to use collection container.	Evaluates bladder function.
g. Explain that many patients experience mild burning, discomfort, or small-volume voiding with first voiding, which soon subsides.	Burning results from urethral irritation.
h. Measure PVR volume (if ordered) (see Box 46.11) within 5 to 15 minutes after helping the patient to void.	Provides the most reliable PVR reading (Huether and McCance, 2017).
i. Inform patient to report any signs of UTI.	Promotes patient safety.
j. Ensure easy access to toilet, commode, bedpan, or urinal. Place urine "hat" on toilet seat if patient is using toilet. Place nurse call system within easy reach.	Reduces incidence of falls during toileting. Urine hat collects first voided urine.
9. Provide patient personal hygiene as needed. Dispose of all contaminated supplies in appropriate receptacle, remove and dispose of gloves, and perform hand hygiene.	Promotes patient comfort and safety. Reduces transmission of microorganisms.
10. Help patient to comfortable position. Raise side rails (as appropriate) and lower bed to lowest position. Be sure nurse call system is in an accessible location within patient's reach.	Promotes patient comfort and safety. Ensures patient can call for assistance if needed.

EVALUATION

1. Inspect catheter and genital area for soiling, irritation, and skin breakdown. Ask patient about discomfort.	Determines whether area is cleaned properly and/or if patient has any irritation.
2. Observe time and measure amount of first voiding after catheter removal.	Indicates return of bladder function after catheter removal.
3. Evaluate patient for signs and symptoms of UTI.	Any patient who has a catheter or has had a catheter removed recently is at risk for UTI.
4. **Use Teach-Back:** "I want to be sure I explained clearly the signs of a urinary tract infection and some things you should do to prevent infection. Tell me some ways in which you can prevent a urinary tract infection." Revise your instruction now or develop plan for revised patient/family caregiver teaching if patient/family caregiver is not able to teach back correctly.	Determines patient's/family caregiver's level of understanding of instructional topic.

UNEXPECTED OUTCOMES AND RELATED INTERVENTIONS

1. Normal saline from inflation balloon does not return into syringe.
   - Reposition patient; ensure that catheter is not pinched or kinked.
   - Remove syringe. Attach new syringe and allow enough time for passive emptying.
   - Attempt to empty balloon by gently pulling back on syringe plunger.
   - If catheter balloon does not deflate, *do not* cut balloon inflation valve to drain fluid. Notify health care provider.
2. Patient has cloudy foul-smelling urine, fever, chills, dysuria, flank pain, back pain, hematuria, urgency, frequency, lower abdominal pain, change in mental status, and lethargy.
   - Assess for bladder distention and tenderness.
   - Monitor vital signs and urine output.
   - Report findings to health care provider; signs and symptoms may indicate UTI.
   - Consult with health care provider for order to remove catheter.
3. Patient is unable to void within 6 to 8 hours after catheter removal, has sensation of not emptying, strains to void, or experiences small voiding amounts with increasing frequency.
   - Assess for bladder distention. Perform bladder scan (see Box 46.11)
   - Help to normal position for voiding and provide privacy.
   - If patient is unable to void within 6 to 8 hours of catheter removal and/or experiences abdominal pain, notify health care provider.

STEP	RATIONALE

RECORDING AND REPORTING

- Record time catheter was removed; teaching related to increasing fluid intake and signs and symptoms of UTI; and time, amount, and characteristics of first voiding.
- Record intake and voiding times and amounts on voiding record or bladder diary as indicated.
- Record patient symptoms experienced upon and after catheter removal.
- Document your evaluation of patient learning.
- Report hematuria, dysuria, inability or difficulty voiding, and any new incontinence after a catheter is removed to health care provider.

HOME CARE CONSIDERATIONS

- If patient is discharged with indwelling catheter, teach patient and family catheter care and signs and symptoms to report to nurse or health care provider.

SKILL 46.4   CLOSED CATHETER IRRIGATION

Delegation and Collaboration

The skill of catheter irrigation cannot be delegated to assistive personnel (AP). The nurse directs the AP to:

- Report if the patient has concerns of pain, discomfort, or leakage of fluid around the catheter.
- Monitor and record intake and output (I&O) and to report immediately any decrease in urine output to the nurse.
- Report any change in the color of the urine, especially if blood clots are noted.

Equipment

- Clean gloves
- Antiseptic swabs

- Container of sterile irrigation solution at room temperature as prescribed
- Intravenous (IV) pole (closed continuous or intermittent)

Closed Intermittent Irrigation

- Sterile 50-mL syringe to access system: Luer-Lok syringe for needleless access port (per manufacturer's instructions)
- Screw clamp or rubber band (used to occlude catheter temporarily as irrigant is instilled)

Closed Continuous Irrigation

- Sterile irrigation tubing with clamp to regulate irrigation flow rate
- Y connector (optional) to connect irrigation tubing to triple-lumen catheter

STEP	RATIONALE

ASSESSMENT

1. Identify patient using at least two identifiers (e.g., name and birthday or name and medical record number), according to agency policy. Compare identifiers with information on patient's MAR or medical record.

   Ensures correct patient. Complies with The Joint Commission standards and improves patient safety (TJC, 2020).

2. Verify in electronic health record (EHR):

   a. Order for irrigation method (continuous or intermittent), solution type (sterile saline or medicated solution), and amount of irrigant.

   Health care provider's order is required to initiate therapy. Frequency and volume of solution used for irrigation may be in the order or standardized as part of agency policy.

   b. Type of catheter in place (see Fig. 46.10).

   Triple-lumen catheters are used for intermittent and continuous closed irrigation.

3. Perform hand hygiene. Palpate bladder for distention and tenderness or use bladder scan (see Box 46.11).

   Reduces transmission of microorganisms. Bladder distention indicates that flow of urine may be blocked from draining.

4. Assess patient for abdominal pain or spasms, sensation of bladder fullness, or catheter bypassing (leaking). (Wear clean gloves if risk of contacting urine).

   May indicate overdistention of bladder caused by catheter blockage. Offers baseline to determine whether therapy is successful.

5. Observe urine for color, amount, clarity, and presence of mucus, clots, or sediment. Remove and dispose of gloves (if worn), perform hand hygiene.

   Indicates if patient is bleeding or sloughing tissue, which would require increased irrigation rate or frequency of catheter irrigation.

6. Monitor I&O. If continuous bladder irrigation (CBI) is being used, amount of fluid draining from bladder should exceed amount of fluid infused into bladder.

   If output does not exceed irrigant infused, catheter obstruction (i.e., blood clots, kinked tubing) should be suspected, irrigation stopped, and prescriber notified (Ignatavicius et al., 2018).

7. Assess patient's or family caregiver's knowledge, experience, and health literacy.

   Ensures patient has the capacity to obtain, communicate, process, and understand basic health information (CDC, 2019).

PLANNING

1. Close room door and bedside curtains.

   Provides privacy.

2. Obtain supplies and set up at bedside.

   Ensures efficient procedure.

3. Raise bed to an appropriate working height. If side rails are raised, lower side rail on working side.

   Promotes good body mechanics. Position provides access to catheter.

4. Explain procedure to patient.

   Reduces anxiety and promotes cooperation.

IMPLEMENTATION

1. Perform hand hygiene.

   Reduces transmission of microorganisms.

2. Position patient supine and expose catheter junctions (catheter and drainage tubing).

   Position provides access to catheter and promotes patient dignity as much as possible.

Continued

STEP	**RATIONALE**
3. Remove catheter securement device.	Eases access to catheter parts.
4. Organize supplies according to type of irrigation prescribed. Apply clean gloves.	Ensures an efficient procedure.
5. **Closed continuous irrigation:**	
a. Close clamp on new irrigation tubing and hang bag of irrigating solution on IV pole. Insert (spike) tip of sterile irrigation tubing into designated port of irrigation solution bag using aseptic technique (see illustration).	Prevents air from entering tubing. Air can cause bladder spasms. Technique prevents transmission of microorganisms.
b. Fill drip chamber half full by squeezing chamber. Remove cap at end of tubing, and then open clamp and allow solution to flow (prime) through tubing, keeping end of tubing sterile. Once fluid has completely filled tubing, close clamp and recap end of tubing.	Priming tubing with fluid prevents introduction of air into bladder.
c. Using aseptic technique, remove cap and connect end of tubing securely to port for infusing irrigation fluid into double/triple–lumen catheter.	Reduces transmission of microorganisms.
d. Adjust clamp on irrigation tubing to begin flow of solution into bladder. If set volume rate is ordered, calculate drip rate and adjust rate at roller clamp (see Chapter 42). If urine is bright red or has clots, increase irrigation rate until drainage appears pink (according to ordered rate or agency protocol).	Continuous drainage is expected. It helps to prevent clotting in presence of active bleeding in bladder and flushes clots out of bladder.
e. Observe for outflow of fluid into drainage bag. Empty catheter drainage bag as needed.	Discomfort, bladder distention, and possible injury can occur from overdistention of bladder when bladder irrigant cannot adequately flow from bladder. Bag will fill rapidly and may need to be emptied every 1 to 2 hours.
6. **Closed intermittent irrigation:**	Fluid is instilled through catheter in a bolus, flushing system. Fluid drains out after irrigation is complete.
a. Pour prescribed sterile irrigation solution into sterile container.	
b. Draw prescribed volume of irrigant (usually 30 to 50 mL) into sterile syringe, using aseptic technique. Place sterile cap on tip of needleless syringe.	Ensures sterility of irrigating fluid.
c. Clamp catheter tubing below soft injection port with screw clamp (or fold catheter tubing onto itself and secure with rubber band).	Occluding catheter tubing below point of injection allows irrigating solution to enter catheter and flow into bladder.

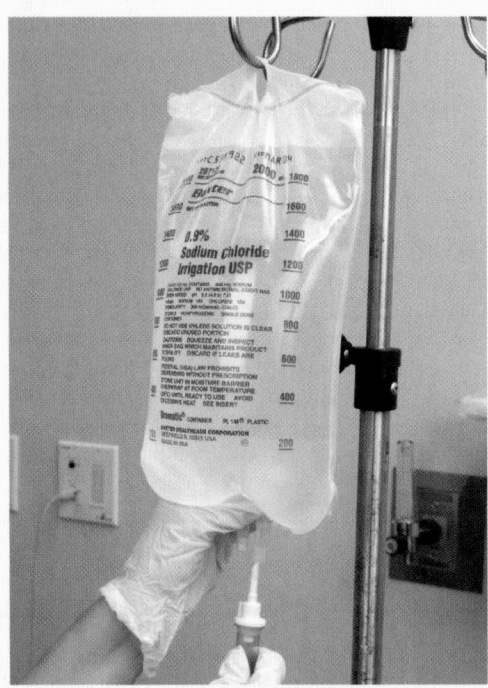

STEP 5a Spiking bag of sterile irrigation solution for continuous bladder irrigation.

STEP	RATIONALE
d. Using circular motion, clean catheter port (specimen port) with antiseptic swab. Allow to dry.	Reduces transmission of microorganisms.
e. Insert tip of needleless syringe using twisting motion into port.	Ensures that catheter tip enters lumen of catheter.
f. Inject solution using slow, even pressure.	Gentle instillation of solution minimizes trauma to bladder mucosa.
g. Remove syringe and clamp (or rubber band), allowing solution to drain into urinary drainage bag. (**NOTE:** Some medicated irrigants may need to dwell in bladder for prescribed period, requiring catheter to be clamped temporarily before being allowed to drain.)	Allows drainage to flow out by gravity. Medications must be instilled long enough to be absorbed by lining of bladder. Clamped drainage tubing and bag should not be left unattended.
7. Anchor catheter with catheter securement device (see Skill 46.2).	Prevents trauma to urethral tissue caused by pulling catheter.
8. Help patient to safe and comfortable position. Lower bed and place side rails accordingly. Place nurse call light in reach and instruct patient in its use.	Promotes patient comfort and safety.
9. Dispose of all contaminated supplies in appropriate receptacle, remove and dispose of gloves, and perform hand hygiene.	Reduces transmission of microorganisms.

EVALUATION

1. Measure actual urine output by subtracting total amount of irrigation fluid infused from total volume drained into collection bag or basin.	Determines accurate urinary output.
2. Review I&O flow sheet to verify that hourly output into drainage bag is in appropriate proportion to irrigating solution entering bladder. Expect more output than fluid instilled because of urine production.	Determines urinary output in relation to irrigation.
3. Inspect urine for blood clots and sediment, and be sure that tubing is not kinked or occluded.	Decrease in blood clots means that therapy is successful in maintaining catheter patency. System is patent.
4. Evaluate patient's comfort level.	Indicates catheter patency by absence of symptoms of bladder distention.
5. Monitor for signs and symptoms of infection.	Patients with indwelling catheters remain at risk for infection.
6. Use Teach-Back: "I want to be sure I explained clearly about why we are irrigating your catheter. Tell me in your own words the reason we are doing the irrigation." Revise your instruction now or develop plan for revised patient/family caregiver teaching if patient/family caregiver is not able to teach back correctly.	Determines patient's/family caregiver's level of understanding of instructional topic.

UNEXPECTED OUTCOMES AND RELATED INTERVENTIONS

1. Drainage output is less than amount of irrigation solution infused.
   - Examine drainage tubing for clots, sediment, or kinks.
   - Inspect urine for presence of or increase in blood clots and sediment.
   - Evaluate patient for pain and distended bladder.
   - Notify health care provider.
2. Bright-red bleeding with the irrigation (CBI) infusion wide open.
   - Assess for hypovolemic shock (vital signs, skin color and moisture, anxiety level).
   - Leave irrigation infusion wide open and notify health care provider.
3. Patient experiences pain with irrigation.
   - Examine drainage tubing for clots, sediment, or kinks.
   - Evaluate urine for presence of or increase in blood clots and sediment.
   - Evaluate for distended bladder.
   - Notify health care provider.

RECORDING AND REPORTING

- Record irrigation method, amount of and type of irrigation solution, amount returned as drainage, characteristics of output, and urine output.
- Record I&O.
- Document your evaluation of patient learning.
- Report catheter occlusion, sudden bleeding, infection, or increased pain.

HOME CARE CONSIDERATIONS

- Patients and/or family caregivers can be taught to perform catheter irrigations with adequate support, demonstration/return demonstration, and written instructions.
- Teach patients and/or family caregivers to observe urine color, clarity, odor, and amount and to observe for signs of catheter obstruction and UTI.
- Arrange for home delivery and storage of catheter/irrigation supplies.

KEY POINTS

- Micturition involves complex interactions between the central nervous system, bladder, and urinary sphincter.
- Common urinary tract symptoms include urgency, dysuria, frequency, hesitancy, polyuria, oliguria, nocturia, dribbling, hematuria, and urinary retention.
- Nursing care for patients with urinary dysfunction needs to take into account multiple factors that affect urinary function such as fluid intake, medications, functional ability, environment, medical problems outside the urinary tract, and dysfunction within the urinary tract.
- The presence or recent history of an indwelling catheter increases risk for a UTI.
- Prevention of catheter-associated urinary tract infection (CAUTI) requires use of an evidence-based "bundle" to perform all elements of care at one time.
- To minimize the risk for infection when caring for a patient with a closed bladder drainage system, nursing care must include careful attention to aseptic technique.
- Planning care for an incontinent patient requires selecting interventions specific to the type of incontinence.
- A key intervention when caring for an incontinent patient is to ensure regular toilet access.

REFLECTIVE LEARNING

- At the end of your clinical practice day, your instructor asks how you promoted urinary elimination for a confused older adult. What would be your answer?
- Consider a moment in which you actively prevented infection during the shift. What did you do that was successful in preventing infection?
- Think of some ways to best promote comfort when assessing the urinary system. What would be the biggest barriers to these care components?

REVIEW QUESTIONS

1. A patient is scheduled to have an intravenous pyelogram (IVP) the next morning. Which nursing measures should be implemented before the test? (Select all that apply.)
   1. Ask the patient about any allergies and reactions.
   2. Instruct the patient that a full bladder is required for the test.
   3. Instruct the patient to save all urine in a special container.
   4. Ensure that informed consent has been obtained.
   5. Instruct the patient that facial flushing can occur when the contrast media is given.
2. What is a critical step when inserting an indwelling catheter into a male patient?
   1. Slowly inflate the catheter balloon with sterile saline.
   2. Secure the catheter drainage tubing to the bedsheets.
   3. Advance the catheter to the bifurcation of the drainage and balloon ports.
   4. Advance the catheter until urine flows, then insert ¼ inch more.
3. Which instruction should the nurse give the assistive personnel (AP) concerning a patient who has had an indwelling urinary catheter removed that day?
   1. Limit oral fluid intake to avoid possible urinary incontinence.
   2. Expect patient complaints of suprapubic fullness and discomfort.
   3. Report the time and amount of first voiding.
   4. Instruct patient to stay in bed and use a urinal or bedpan.

4. A postoperative patient with a three-way indwelling urinary catheter and continuous bladder irrigation (CBI) complains of lower abdominal pain and distention. What should be the nurse's *initial* intervention(s)? (Select all that apply.)
   1. Increase the rate of the CBI.
   2. Assess the patency of the drainage system.
   3. Measure urine output.
   4. Assess vital signs.
   5. Administer ordered pain medication.
5. An ambulatory elderly woman with dementia is incontinent of urine. She has poor short-term memory and has not been seen toileting independently. What is the *best* nursing intervention for this patient?
   1. Recommend that she be evaluated for an overactive bladder (OAB) medication.
   2. Establish a toileting schedule.
   3. Recommend that she be evaluated for an indwelling catheter.
   4. Start a bladder-retraining program.
6. What should the nurse teach a young woman with a history of urinary tract infections (UTIs) about UTI prevention? (Select all that apply.)
   1. Maintain regular bowel elimination.
   2. Limit water intake to 1 to 2 glasses a day.
   3. Wear cotton underwear.
   4. Cleanse the perineum from front to back.
   5. Practice pelvic muscle exercise (Kegel) daily.
7. Place the following steps for insertion of an indwelling catheter in a female patient in appropriate order.
   1. Insert and advance catheter.
   2. Lubricate catheter.
   3. Inflate catheter balloon.
   4. Cleanse urethral meatus with antiseptic solution.
   5. Drape patient with the sterile square and fenestrated drapes.
   6. When urine appears, advance another 2.5 to 5 cm.
   7. Prepare sterile field and supplies.
   8. Gently pull catheter until resistance is felt.
   9. Attach drainage tubing.
8. Which nursing interventions should a nurse implement when removing an indwelling urinary catheter in an adult patient? (Select all that apply.)
   1. Attach a 3-mL syringe to the inflation port.
   2. Allow the balloon to drain into the syringe by gravity.
   3. Initiate a voiding record/bladder diary.
   4. Pull the catheter quickly.
   5. Clamp the catheter before removal.
9. Which nursing intervention decreases the risk for catheter-associated urinary tract infection (CAUTI)?
   1. Cleansing the urinary meatus 3 to 4 times daily with antiseptic solution
   2. Hanging the urinary drainage bag below the level of the bladder
   3. Emptying the urinary drainage bag daily
   4. Irrigating the urinary catheter with sterile water
10. There is no urine when a catheter is inserted 3 inches into a female's urethra. What should the nurse do next?
    1. Remove the catheter and start all over with a new kit and catheter.
    2. Leave the catheter there and start over with a new catheter.
    3. Pull the catheter back and reinsert at a different angle.
    4. Ask the patient to bear down and insert the catheter farther.

Answers: 1. 1, 4, 5; 2. 3, 3; 3. 4, 3; 4. 2, 3; 5. 2; 6. 1, 3, 4; 7. 7, 5, 2, 4, 1, 6, 3, 8, 9, 8, 2, 3; 9. 2; 10. 2.

Answers to Review Questions can be found on the Evolve website.

REFERENCES

AACN Clinical Practice Alert: Prevention of catheter-associated urinary tract infections in adults, *Crit Care Nurs* 38(1):84, 2018.

Akkoc A, et al.: Prophylactic effects of alpha-blockers, Tamsulosin and Alfuzosin, on postoperative urinary retention in male patients undergoing urologic surgery under spinal anesthesia, *Int Braz J Urol* 42(3):578, 2016.

American Geriatrics Society: Updated Beers Criteria for potentially inappropriate medication use in older adults, 2018, https://www.americangeriatrics.org/media-center/news/draft-ags-updated-2018-beers-criteriar-potentially-inappropriate-medication-use. Accessed October 30, 2019.

Assadi F: Strategies for preventing catheter-associated urinary tract Infection, *Int J Prev Med* 9 50:2–3, 2018.

Ball JW, et al.: *Seidel's Guide to physical examination*, ed 9, St Louis, 2019, Elsevier.

Bardsley A: Safe and effective catheterization for patients in the community, *Br J Community Nurs* 20(4):116, 2015.

Bardsley A: An overview of urinary incontinence, *Br J Nurs* 25(18):S14, 2016.

Burchum JR, Rosenthal LD: *Lehne's Pharmacology for nursing care*, ed 10, St Louis, 2019, Elsevier.

Bykoviene L, et al.: Pelvic floor muscle training with or without tibial nerve stimulation and lifestyle changes have comparable effects on the overactive bladder: a randomized clinical trial, *Urol J* 15(4):186, 2018.

Cartwright A: Reducing catheter-associated urinary infections: standardizing practice, *Br J Nurs* 27(1):7–12, 2018.

Centers for Disease Control and Prevention (CDC): *Catheter-associated urinary tract infection (CAUTI) toolkit*, 2015. http://www.cdc.gov/HAI/prevent/prevention_tools.html. Accessed December 6, 2015.

Centers for Disease Control and Prevention (CDC): *What is health literacy*, 2019. https://www.cdc.gov/healthliteracy/learn/index.html. Accessed December 23, 2019.

Centers for Disease Control and Prevention (CDC): *Urinary tract infection (catheter-associated urinary tract infection [CAUTI] and non-catheter-associated urinary tract infection [UTI]) and other urinary system infection [USI] events*, 2019. http://www.cdc.gov/nhsn/PDF/pscManual/7pscCAUTIcurrent.pdf. Accessed October 30, 2019.

Clarke E: Female genital mutilation: a urology focus, *Br J Nurs* 25(18):1022, 2016.

Davey G: Troubleshooting indwelling catheter problems in the community, *J Community Nurs* 29(4):67, 2015.

Duncan D: Alternative to antibiotics for managing asymptomatic and non-symptomatic bacteriuria in older persons: a review, *Br J Community Nurs* 24(3):116–119, 2019.

Dy S, et al.: A nurse-driven protocol for removal of indwelling urinary catheters across a multi- hospital academic healthcare system, *Urol Nurs* 36(5):243, 2016.

Eshkoor S, et al.: Factors related to urinary incontinence among the Malaysian elderly, *J Nutr Health Aging* 21(2):220, 2017.

Fekete T: Catheter-associated urinary tract infection in adults, 2018, https://www.uptodate.com/contents/catheter-associated-urinary-tract-infection-in-adults. Accessed February 28, 2019.

Gesmundo M: Managing indwelling urinary catheters, *Nurs N Z* 22(6):14, 2016a.

Gould CV, et al.: *Guideline for prevention of catheter-associated urinary tract infections 2009, Healthcare Infection Control Practices Advisory Committee, Centers for Disease Control and Prevention*, 2017, updated February, https://www.cdc.gov/infectioncontrol/pdf/guidelines/cauti-guidelines-H.pdf. Accessed October 27, 2019.

Huether SE, McCance KL: *Understanding pathophysiology*, ed 6, St Louis, 2017, Mosby.

Ignatavicius D, et al.: *Medical-surgical nursing: concepts for interprofessional collaborative care*, ed 9, St Louis, 2018, Elsevier.

Jarvis C: *Physical examination & health assessment*, St Louis, 2016, Elsevier.

Lai D, et al.: Mediating effect of social participation on the relationship between incontinence and depressive symptoms in older Chinese women, *Health Soc Work* 42(2):e94, 2017.

Malik Y, et al.: Mandatory reporting of female genital mutilation in children in the UK, *Br J Nurs* 26(6):377, 2018.

Lukacz ES, et al.: Urinary incontinence in women: a review, *JAMA* 318(16):1592, 2017.

McNeill L: Back to basics: how evidence-based nursing practice can prevent catheter-associated urinary tract infections, *Urol Nurs* 37(4):204, 2017.

Nicolle LE: Catheter-associated urinary tract infections, *Antimicrob Resist Infect Control* 3:23, 2014.

Pagana KD, et al.: *Mosby's diagnostic and laboratory test reference*, ed 14, St Louis, 2019, Elsevier.

Panchisin T: Improving outcomes with the ANA CAUTI Prevention Tool, *Nursing* 46(3):55, 2016.

Paulin R, Dowling-Castronovo A: Incontinence-associated dermatitis - it is not a pressure injury, *Urol Nurs* 37(6):304–309, 2017.

Saito M, et al.: No association of caffeinated beverage or caffeine intake with prevalence of urinary incontinence among middle-aged Japanese women: a multicenter cross-sectional study, *J Womens Health* 26(8):860–869, 2017.

Scanlon K, et al.: Saving lives and reducing harm: a CAUTI reduction program, *Nurs Econ* 35(3):134, 2017.

Shivkumar R, et al.: Effects of bladder training and pelvic floor muscle exercise in urinary stress incontinence during postpartum period, *Indian J Physiother Occup Ther* 9(4):194, 2015.

Taylor J: Reducing the incidence of inappropriate indwelling urinary catheterisation, *J Community Nurs* 32(3):50, 2018.

Testa A: Understanding urinary incontinence in adults, *Urol Nurs* 35(2):82, 2015.

The Joint Commission (TJC): *2020 National Patient Safety Goals*, Oakbrook Terrace, IL, 2020, The Commission. https://www.jointcommission.org/en/standards/national-patient-safety-goals/. Accessed January 2, 2020.

Touhy TA, Jett KF: *Ebersole and Hess' Gerontological nursing and healthy aging*, ed 5, St Louis, 2018, Elsevier.

Vethanayagam N, et al.: Understanding help-seeking in older people with urinary incontinence: an interview study, *Health Soc Care Community* 25(3):1061–1069, 2017.

Wang C, et al.: Effects of stigma on Chinese women's attitudes towards seeking treatment for urinary incontinence, *J Clin Nurs* 24(7/8) 1112, 2014.

Wilson M: Urinary incontinence: considering the physical and psychological implications, *Br J Community Nurs* 21(5):222, 2016.

Yates A: Incontinence-associated dermatitis in older people: prevention and management, *Br J Community Nurs* 23(5):218, 2018.

Yates A: Indwelling urinary catheterisation: what is best practice? *Br J Nurs* 25(9):S4, 2016.

RESEARCH REFERENCES

Coyne KS, Wein A: Economic burden of urgency urinary incontinence in the United States: a systemic review, *J Manag Care Pharm* 20(2):130, 2014.

Fasugba O, et al.: Systematic review and meta-analysis of the effectiveness of antiseptic agents for meatal cleaning in the prevention of catheter-associated urinary tract infections, *J Hosp Infect* 95(3):233, 2017.

Ferguson A: Implementing a CAUTI prevention program in an acute care hospital setting, *Urol Nurs* 38(6):273, 2018.

Galiczweski JM: Interventions for the prevention of catheter associated urinary tract infections in intensive care units: an integrative review, *Intensive Crit Care Nurs* 32:1, 2016.

Galiczweski JM, Shurpin KM: An intervention to improve the catheter associated urinary tract infection rate in a medical intensive care unit: direct observation of catheter insertion procedure, *Intensive Crit Care Nurs* 40:26, 2017.

Gesmundo M: Enhancing nurses' knowledge on catheter-associated urinary tract infection (CAUTI) prevention, *Kai Tiaki Nurs Res* 7(1):32, 2016b.

Lo E, et al.: Strategies to prevent catheter-associated urinary tract infections in acute care hospitals, *Infect Control Hosp Epidemiol* 35(5):464, 2014.

Meddings J, et al.: Reducing unnecessary urinary catheter use and other strategies to prevent catheter-associated urinary tract infection: an integrative review, *BMJ Qual Saf* 23(4):277, 2014.

Purvis S, et al.: Catheter-associated urinary tract infection: a successful prevention effort employing a multipronged initiative at an academic medical center, *J Nurs Care Qual* 29(2):141, 2014.

Seshan V, et al.: Risk factors of urinary incontinence in women: a literature review, *Int J Urol Nurs* 10(3):118, 2016.

47

Bowel Elimination

OBJECTIVES

- Discuss the role of gastrointestinal organs and their physiological function in digestion and elimination.
- Discuss how psychological and physiological factors may alter the elimination process.
- Assess a patient's elimination pattern.
- Describe nursing implications for common diagnostic examinations of the gastrointestinal tract.

- List nursing interventions that promote normal elimination.
- Discuss nursing care measures required for patients with an intestinal diversion.
- Describe nursing procedures related to bowel elimination.
- Explain how critical thinking is important in providing care to patients with alterations in bowel elimination.

KEY TERMS

Bowel training, p. 1218
Cathartics, p. 1200
Chyme, p. 1199
Clostridium difficile, p. 1201
Colonoscopy, p. 1205
Colostomy, p. 1202
Constipation, p. 1199
Diarrhea, p. 1201
Effluent, p. 1202

Endoscopy, p. 1208
Enemas, p. 1200
Fecal occult blood test (FOBT), p. 1205
Fecal immunochemical test (FIT), p. 1205
Flatulence, p. 1202
Hemorrhoid, p. 1199
Ileostomy, p. 1202
Ileus, p. 1200
Impaction, p. 1201

Incontinence, p. 1201
Laxatives, p. 1200
Peristalsis, p. 1198
Polyps, p. 1209
Stoma, p. 1202
Wound, ostomy, and continence nurse (WOCN), p. 1217

MEDIA RESOURCES

http://evolve.elsevier.com/Potter/fundamentals/

- Review Questions
- Video Clips
- Concept Map Creator
- Case Study with Questions

- Skills Performance Checklists
- Audio Glossary
- Content Updates
- Answers to QSEN Activity and Review Questions

Regular elimination of bowel waste products is essential for normal body functioning. Alterations in bowel elimination are often early signs or symptoms of problems within either the gastrointestinal (GI) tract or other body systems. Because bowel function depends on the balance of several factors, elimination patterns and habits vary among individuals.

Understanding normal bowel elimination and factors that promote, impede, or cause alterations in elimination help a nurse manage patients' elimination problems. Supportive nursing care respects a patient's privacy and emotional needs. Measures designed to promote normal elimination also need to minimize a patient's discomfort and embarrassment.

SCIENTIFIC KNOWLEDGE BASE

The GI tract consists of the alimentary canal and its accessory organs. The alimentary canal is a single tube that extends from the mouth to the anus and includes the mouth, esophagus, stomach, and intestines. The accessory organs are the teeth, tongue, salivary glands, liver, pancreas, and gallbladder. These organs absorb fluid and nutrients, prepare food for absorption and use by body cells, and provide for temporary storage of feces (Fig. 47.1). The GI tract absorbs high volumes of fluids, making fluid and electrolyte balance a key function of the GI system. In addition to ingested fluids and foods, the GI tract also receives secretions from the gallbladder and pancreas.

Mouth

The mouth mechanically and chemically breaks down nutrients into usable size and form. The teeth chew food, breaking it down into a size suitable for swallowing. Saliva, produced by the salivary glands in the mouth, dilutes and softens the food in the mouth for easier swallowing.

Esophagus

As food enters the upper esophagus, it passes through the upper esophageal sphincter, a circular muscle that prevents air from entering the esophagus and food from refluxing into the throat. The bolus of food travels down the esophagus with the aid of peristalsis, which is a contraction that propels food through the length of the GI tract. The food moves down the esophagus and reaches the cardiac sphincter, which lies between the esophagus and the upper end of the stomach. The sphincter prevents reflux of stomach contents back into the esophagus.

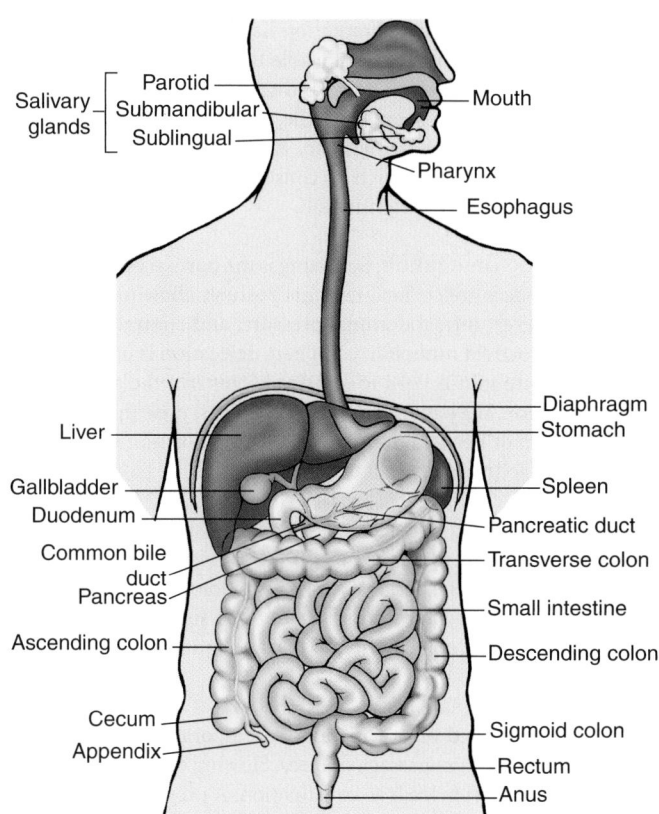

FIG. 47.1 Organs of gastrointestinal tract. (From Monahan FD, Neighbors M: *Medical-surgical nursing,* ed 2, Philadelphia, 1998, Saunders.)

Stomach

The stomach performs three tasks: storage of swallowed food and liquid, mixing of food with digestive juices into a substance called chyme, and regulated emptying of its contents into the small intestine. The stomach produces and secretes hydrochloric acid (HCl), mucus, the enzyme pepsin, and intrinsic factor. Pepsin and HCl help to digest protein. Mucus protects the stomach mucosa from acidity and enzyme activity. Intrinsic factor is essential in the absorption of vitamin B_{12}.

Small Intestine

Movement within the small intestine, occurring by peristalsis, facilitates both digestion and absorption. Chyme comes into the small intestine as a liquid material and mixes with digestive enzymes. Resorption in the small intestine is so efficient that, by the time the fluid reaches the end of the small intestine, it is a thick liquid with some semisolid particles. The small intestine is divided into three sections: the duodenum, the jejunum, and the ileum.

The duodenum is approximately 20 to 28 cm (8 to 11 inches) long and continues to process fluid from the stomach. The second section, the jejunum, is approximately 2.5 m (8 feet) long and absorbs carbohydrates and proteins. The ileum is approximately 3.7 m (12 feet) long and absorbs water, fats, and bile salts. The duodenum and jejunum absorb most nutrients and electrolytes in the small intestine. The ileum absorbs certain vitamins, iron, and bile salts. Digestive enzymes and bile enter the small intestine from the pancreas and the liver to further break down nutrients into a form usable by the body.

The digestive process is greatly altered when small intestine function is impaired. Conditions such as inflammation, infection, surgical resection, or obstruction disrupt peristalsis, reduce absorption, or block the passage of fluid, resulting in electrolyte and nutrient deficiencies.

Large Intestine

The lower GI tract is called the *large intestine* or *colon* because it is larger in diameter than the small intestine. However, its length, 1.5 to 1.8 m (5 to 6 feet), is much shorter. The large intestine is divided into the cecum, ascending colon, transverse colon, descending colon, sigmoid colon, and rectum. The large intestine is the primary organ of bowel elimination.

Digestive fluid enters the large intestine by waves of peristalsis through the ileocecal valve (i.e., a circular muscle layer that prevents regurgitation back into the small intestine). The muscular tissue of the colon allows it to accommodate and eliminate large quantities of waste and gas (flatus). The colon has three functions: absorption, secretion, and elimination. The colon resorbs a large volume of water (up to 1.5 L) and significant amounts of sodium and chloride daily. The amount of water absorbed depends on the speed at which colonic contents move. Normally the fecal matter becomes a soft, formed solid or semisolid mass. If peristalsis is abnormally fast, there is less time for water to be absorbed, and the stool will be watery. If peristaltic contractions slow down, water continues to be absorbed, and a hard mass of stool forms, resulting in constipation.

Peristaltic contractions move contents through the colon. Mass peristalsis pushes undigested food toward the rectum. These mass movements occur only 3 or 4 times daily, with the strongest during the hour after mealtime.

The rectum is the final part of the large intestine. Normally the rectum is empty of fecal matter until just before defecation. It contains vertical and transverse folds of tissue that help to control expulsion of fecal contents during defecation. Each fold contains veins that can become distended from pressure during straining. This distention results in hemorrhoid formation.

Anus

The body expels feces and flatus from the rectum through the anus. Contraction and relaxation of the internal and external sphincters, which are innervated by sympathetic and parasympathetic nerves, aid in the control of defecation. The anal canal contains a rich supply of sensory nerves that allow people to tell when there is solid, liquid, or gas that needs to be expelled and aids in maintaining continence.

Defecation

The physiological factors essential to bowel function and defecation include normal GI tract function, sensory awareness of rectal distention and rectal contents, voluntary sphincter control, and adequate rectal capacity and compliance. Normal defecation begins with movement in the left colon, moving stool toward the anus. When stool reaches the rectum, the distention causes relaxation of the internal sphincter and an awareness of the need to defecate. At the time of defecation, the external sphincter relaxes, and abdominal muscles contract, increasing intrarectal pressure and forcing the stool out. Normally defecation is painless, resulting in passage of soft, formed stool. Straining while having a bowel movement indicates that the patient may need changes in diet or fluid intake or that there is an underlying disorder in GI function.

REFLECT NOW

The digestive system is a complex group of organs that allow the body to transport and digest food and fluids and eliminate waste products. Each part of the system plays an important role, yet illness or surgery can cause significant changes in digestive function. Consider symptoms patients may experience as a result of these changes and how their quality of life may be affected.

NURSING KNOWLEDGE BASE

Factors Influencing Bowel Elimination

Many factors influence the process of bowel elimination. Knowledge of these factors helps to anticipate measures required to maintain a normal elimination pattern.

Age. Infants have a smaller stomach capacity, less secretion of digestive enzymes, and more rapid intestinal peristalsis. The ability to control defecation does not occur until 2 to 3 years of age. Adolescents experience rapid growth and increased metabolic rate. There is also rapid growth of the large intestine and increased secretion of gastric acids to digest food fibers and act as a bactericide against swallowed organisms. Older adults may have decreased chewing ability. Partially chewed food is not digested as easily. Peristalsis declines, and esophageal emptying slows. This impairs absorption by the intestinal mucosa. Muscle tone in the perineal floor and anal sphincter weakens, which sometimes causes difficulty in controlling defecation (NIH, 2018a).

Diet. Regular daily food intake helps maintain a regular pattern of peristalsis in the colon. Fiber in the diet provides the bulk in the fecal material. Bulk-forming foods such as whole grains, fresh fruits, and vegetables help remove the fats and waste products from the body with more efficiency. Some of these foods such as cabbage, broccoli, or beans may also produce gas, which distends the intestinal walls and increases colonic motility. The bowel walls stretch, creating peristalsis and initiating the defecation reflex.

Fluid Intake. Although individual fluid needs vary with the person, a fluid intake of 3.7 L per day for men and 2.7 L per day for women is recommended (Mayo Clinic, 2017). Some fluid needs are met by drinking fluids, but there is also fluid in foods that are ingested such as fruits. An inadequate fluid intake or disturbances resulting in fluid loss (such as vomiting) affect the character of feces. Fluid liquefies intestinal contents by absorbing into the fiber from the diet and creating a larger, softer stool mass. This increases peristalsis and promotes movement of stool through the colon. Reduced fluid and fiber intake slows the passage of food through the intestine and results in hardening of stool contents, causing constipation.

Physical Activity. Physical activity promotes peristalsis, whereas immobilization depresses it. Encourage early ambulation as illness begins to resolve or as soon as possible after surgery to promote maintenance of peristalsis and normal elimination. Maintaining tone of skeletal muscles used during defecation is important. Weakened abdominal and pelvic floor muscles impair the ability to increase intraabdominal pressure and control the external sphincter. Muscle tone is sometimes weakened or lost as a result of long-term illness, spinal cord injury, or neurological diseases that impair nerve transmission. As a result of these changes in the abdominal and pelvic floor muscles, there is an increased risk for constipation.

Psychological Factors. Prolonged emotional stress impairs the function of almost all body systems (see Chapter 37). During emotional stress the digestive process is accelerated, and peristalsis is increased. Side effects of increased peristalsis include diarrhea and gaseous distention. Several diseases of the GI tract are exacerbated by stress, including ulcerative colitis, irritable bowel syndrome, certain gastric and duodenal ulcers, and Crohn's disease. If a person becomes depressed, the autonomic nervous system may slow impulses that decrease peristalsis, resulting in constipation.

Personal Habits. Personal elimination habits influence bowel function. Most people benefit from being able to use their own toilet facilities at a time that is most effective and convenient for them. A busy work schedule sometimes prevents the individual from responding appropriately to the urge to defecate, disrupting regular habits and causing possible alterations such as constipation. Individuals need to recognize the best time for elimination.

Position During Defecation. Squatting is the normal position during defecation. Modern toilets facilitate this posture, allowing a person to lean forward, exert intraabdominal pressure, and contract the gluteal muscles. For a patient immobilized in bed, defecation is often difficult. In a supine position it is hard to effectively contract the muscles used during defecation. If a patient's condition permits, raise the head of the bed to help him or her to a more normal sitting position on a bedpan, enhancing the ability to defecate.

Pain. Normally the act of defecation is painless. However, several conditions such as hemorrhoids; rectal surgery; anal fissures, which are painful linear splits in the perianal area; and abdominal surgery result in discomfort. In these instances, the patient often suppresses the urge to defecate to avoid pain, contributing to the development of constipation.

Pregnancy. As pregnancy advances, the size of the fetus increases, and pressure is exerted on the rectum. A temporary obstruction created by the fetus impairs passage of feces. Slowing of peristalsis during the third trimester often leads to constipation. A pregnant woman's frequent straining during defecation or delivery may result in formation of hemorrhoids.

Surgery and Anesthesia. General anesthetic agents used during surgery cause temporary cessation of peristalsis (see Chapter 50). Inhaled anesthetic agents block parasympathetic impulses to the intestinal musculature. The action of the anesthetic slows or stops peristaltic waves. A patient who receives a local or regional anesthetic is less at risk for elimination alterations because this type of anesthesia generally affects bowel activity minimally or not at all.

Any surgery that involves direct manipulation of the bowel temporarily stops peristalsis. This condition, called an **ileus**, usually lasts about 24 to 48 hours. If a patient remains inactive or is unable to eat after surgery, return of normal bowel elimination is further delayed.

Medications. Many medications prescribed for acute and chronic conditions have secondary effects on a patient's bowel elimination patterns. For example, opioid analgesics slow peristalsis and contractions, often resulting in constipation; and antibiotics decrease intestinal bacterial flora, often resulting in diarrhea (Burchum and Rosenthal, 2019). It is important for the nurse and patient to be aware of these possible side effects and use appropriate measures to promote healthy bowel elimination. Some medications are used primarily for their action on the bowel and will promote defecation, such as **laxatives** or **cathartics**, or control diarrhea. If laxatives are needed for regular evacuation of the rectum, a fiber laxative is the first type used. If this is not enough to relieve constipation, the next one tried should be an osmotic laxative. Patients need to avoid regular use of a stimulant laxative because the intestine often becomes dependent on it.

Diagnostic Tests. Diagnostic examinations involving visualization of GI structures often require a prescribed bowel preparation (e.g., laxatives and/or **enemas**) to ensure that the bowel is empty. Usually patients cannot eat or drink several hours before examinations such as an endoscopy, colonoscopy, or other testing that requires visualization

---

BOX 47.1   Common Causes of Constipation

- Irregular bowel habits and ignoring the urge to defecate
- Chronic illnesses (e.g., Parkinson's disease, multiple sclerosis, rheumatoid arthritis, chronic bowel diseases, depression, eating disorders)
- Low-fiber diet high in animal fats (e.g., meats and carbohydrates); low fluid intake
- Stress (e.g., illness of a family member, death of a loved one, divorce)
- Physical inactivity
- Medications, especially use of opiates
- Changes in life or routine, such as pregnancy, aging, and travel
- Neurological conditions that block nerve impulses to the colon (e.g., stroke, spinal cord injury, tumor)
- Chronic bowel dysfunction (e.g., colonic inertia, irritable bowel)

BOX 47.2   Signs of Dehydration

- Signs of dehydration in adults include:
  - Thirst
  - Less frequent urination than usual
  - Dark-colored urine
  - Dry skin
  - Fatigue
  - Dizziness
  - Light-headedness
- Signs of dehydration in infants and young children include:
  - Dry mouth and tongue
  - No tears when crying
  - No wet diapers for 3 hours or more
  - Sunken eyes or cheeks or soft spot in the skull
  - High fever
  - Listlessness or irritability

---

of the GI tract. Following the diagnostic procedure, changes in elimination such as increased gas or loose stools often occur until the patient resumes a normal eating pattern.

Common Bowel Elimination Problems

You will frequently care for patients who have or are at risk for elimination problems because of physiological changes in the GI tract, such as abdominal surgery, inflammatory diseases, medications, emotional stress, environmental factors, or disorders impairing defecation.

Constipation. Constipation is a symptom, not a disease, and there are many possible causes (Box 47.1). Improper diet, reduced fluid intake, lack of exercise, and certain medications can cause constipation. For example, patients receiving opioids for pain after surgery often require a stool softener or laxative to prevent constipation. A research study of the bowel function of men and women revealed that female gender and older age were the highest risk factors for constipation (Uduak et al., 2016). Signs of constipation include infrequent bowel movements (less than three per week) and hard, dry stools that are difficult to pass (NIH, 2018a.). When intestinal motility slows, the fecal mass becomes exposed to the intestinal walls over time, and most of the fecal water content is absorbed. Little water is left to soften and lubricate the stool. Passage of a dry, hard stool often causes rectal pain. Constipation is a significant source of discomfort. Assess the need for intervention before defecation becomes painful or the stool is impacted.

Impaction. Fecal impaction results when a patient has unrelieved constipation and is unable to expel the hardened feces retained in the rectum. In cases of severe impaction, the mass extends up into the sigmoid colon. If not resolved or removed, severe impaction results in intestinal obstruction. Patients who are debilitated, confused, or unconscious are most at risk for impaction. They are dehydrated or too weak or unaware of the need to defecate, and the stool becomes too hard and dry to pass.

An obvious sign of impaction is the inability to pass a stool for several days, despite the repeated urge to defecate. Suspect an impaction when a continuous oozing of liquid stool occurs. The liquid part of feces located higher in the colon seeps around the impacted mass. Loss of appetite (anorexia), nausea and/or vomiting, abdominal distention and cramping, and rectal pain may accompany the condition. If you suspect an impaction, gently perform a digital examination of the rectum and palpate for the impacted mass (Hussain et al., 2014).

Diarrhea. Diarrhea is an increase in the number of stools and the passage of liquid, unformed feces. It is associated with disorders affecting digestion, absorption, and secretion in the GI tract. Intestinal contents pass through the small and large intestine too quickly to allow for the usual absorption of fluid and nutrients. Irritation within the colon results in increased mucus secretion. As a result, feces become watery, and the patient often has difficulty controlling the urge to defecate.

Excess loss of colonic fluid results in dehydration (Box 47.2) with fluid and electrolyte or acid-base imbalances if the fluid is not replaced. Infants and older adults are particularly susceptible to associated complications (see Chapter 42). Because repeated passage of diarrhea stools exposes the skin of the perineum and buttocks to irritating intestinal contents, meticulous skin care and containment of fecal drainage is necessary to prevent skin breakdown (see Chapter 48).

Incontinence. Fecal incontinence is the inability to control passage of feces and gas from the anus. Incontinence harms a patient's body image (see Chapter 33). The embarrassment of soiling clothes often leads to social isolation. Physical conditions that impair anal sphincter function or large-volume liquid stools cause incontinence. Impaired cognitive function often leads to incontinence of both urine and stool.

Many conditions cause fecal incontinence or diarrhea. You need to identify precipitating conditions and refer patients to health care providers for medication management. Antibiotic use alters the normal flora in the GI tract. A common causative agent of diarrhea is *Clostridium difficile* (*C. difficile*), which produces symptoms ranging from mild diarrhea to severe colitis. The Infectious Diseases Society of America (IDSA) has identified *C. difficile* as the most common health care–related infection in America. Patients acquire *C. difficile* infection in one of two ways: by antibiotic therapy that causes an overgrowth of *C. difficile* and by contact with the *C. difficile* organism. Patients are exposed to the organism from a health care worker's hands or direct contact with environmental surfaces contaminated with it. Only hand hygiene with soap and water is effective to physically remove *C. difficile* spores from the hands. New tests have been developed for detecting the infection in the stool, and the 2017 IDSA guidelines recommend an NAAT (nucleic acid amplification test). Research is ongoing to determine the most sensitive and accurate diagnostic test and the most effective treatment regimen (McDonald et al., 2018). Elderly patients are especially vulnerable to *C. difficile* infection when exposed to antibiotics, and higher mortality and morbidity are observed in this age-group (McDonald et al., 2018). To decrease the spread of infection, patients with *C. difficile* are placed on contact/enteric isolation precautions.

Communicable foodborne pathogens also cause diarrhea. Hand hygiene following the use of the bathroom, before and after preparing foods, and when cleaning and storing fresh produce and meats greatly reduces the risk of foodborne illnesses. When diarrhea results from

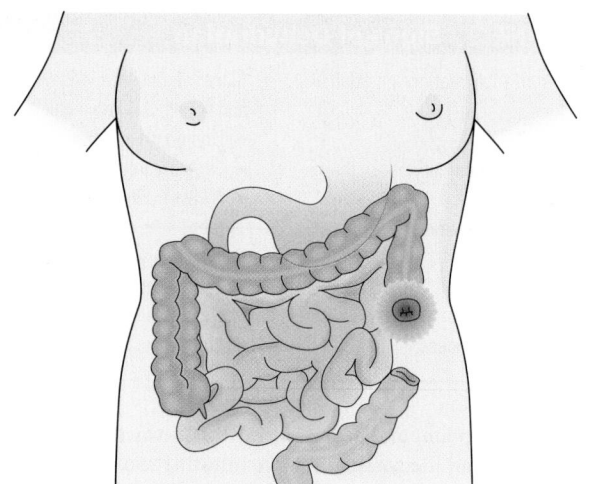

FIG. 47.2 Sigmoid colostomy.

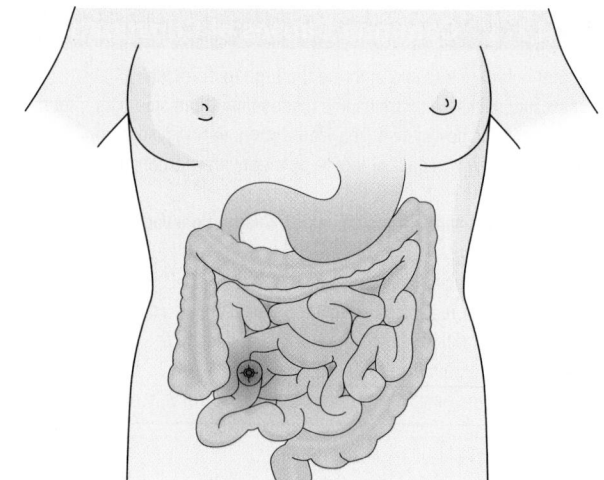

FIG. 47.3 Ileostomy.

a foodborne pathogen, the goal usually is to rid the GI system of the pathogen rather than slow peristalsis.

Surgeries or diagnostic testing of the lower GI tract may also cause diarrhea. Patients receiving enteral nutrition are also at risk for diarrhea and need a dietary consult to find the right formula for the feeding (see Chapter 45). Food intolerances can increase peristalsis and cause diarrhea. Food intolerance is not an allergy; rather, a particular food causes the body distress within a few hours of ingestion. The result is diarrhea, cramps, or flatulence. For example, people who drink cow's milk and have these symptoms are not allergic to milk but lack the enzyme needed to digest the milk sugar lactase and therefore are lactose intolerant. Another condition called *celiac disease* is a syndrome in which a patient has a hypersensitivity to protein in certain cereal grains and gluten. Food allergies are less common but do occur, and people with these allergies need to know how to read labels on foods carefully. True food allergies may be life threatening and lead to anaphylaxis (USFDA, 2018).

Flatulence. As gas accumulates in the lumen of the intestines, the bowel wall stretches and distends. Flatulence is a common cause of abdominal fullness, pain, and cramping. Normally intestinal gas escapes through the mouth (belching) or the anus (passing of flatus). However, flatulence causes abdominal distention and severe, sharp pain if intestinal motility is reduced because of opiates, general anesthetics, abdominal surgery, or immobilization.

Hemorrhoids. Hemorrhoids are dilated, engorged veins in the lining of the rectum. They are either external or internal. External hemorrhoids are clearly visible as protrusions of skin. There is usually a purplish discoloration (thrombosis) if the underlying vein is hardened. This causes increased pain and sometimes requires excision. Internal hemorrhoids occur in the anal canal and may be inflamed and distended. Increased venous pressure from straining at defecation, pregnancy, heart failure, and chronic liver disease causes hemorrhoids.

Bowel Diversions

Certain diseases or surgical alterations make the normal passage of intestinal contents throughout the small and large intestine difficult or inadvisable. When these conditions are present, a temporary or permanent opening (stoma) is created surgically by bringing part of the intestine out through the abdominal wall. These surgical openings are called an ileostomy or colostomy, depending on which part of the intestinal tract is used to create the stoma (Figs. 47.2 and 47.3). Newer surgical techniques allow more patients to have parts of their small and large

intestine removed and the remaining parts reconnected, so they will continue to defecate through the anal canal.

Ostomies. The location of an ostomy determines stool consistency. A person with a sigmoid colostomy will have a more formed stool. The output from a transverse colostomy will be thick liquid to soft consistency. These ostomies are the easiest to perform surgically and are done as a temporary means to divert stool from an area of trauma or perianal wounds. They may also be a palliative diversion if obstruction from a tumor is present. With an ileostomy the fecal effluent leaves the body before it enters the colon, creating frequent, liquid stools.

Loop colostomies are reversible stomas that a surgeon constructs in the ileum or the colon. The surgeon pulls a loop of intestine onto the abdomen and often places a plastic rod, bridge, or rubber catheter temporarily under the bowel loop to keep it from slipping back. The surgeon then opens the bowel and sutures it to the skin of the abdomen. The loop ostomy has two openings through the stoma. The proximal end drains fecal effluent, and the distal part drains mucus.

The end colostomy consists of a stoma formed by bringing a piece of intestine out through a surgically created opening in the abdominal wall, turning it down like a turtleneck and suturing it to the abdominal wall. The intestine distal to the stoma is either removed or sewn closed (called *Hartmann's pouch;* see Fig. 47.2) and left in the abdominal cavity. End ostomies are permanent or reversible. The rectum is either left intact or removed.

Other Procedures

Ileoanal Pouch Anastomosis. The ileoanal pouch anastomosis is a surgical procedure for patients who need to have a colectomy for treatment of ulcerative colitis or familial adenopolyposis (FAP) (Goldberg et al., 2017). In this procedure the surgeon removes the colon, creates a pouch from the end of the small intestine, and attaches the pouch to the patient's anus (Fig. 47.4). This pouch provides for the collection of fecal material, which simulates the function of the rectum. The patient is continent of stool because stool is evacuated via the anus. When the ileal pouch is created, the patient has a temporary ileostomy to divert the effluent and allow the suture lines in the pouch to heal.

A continent ileostomy involves creating a pouch from the small intestine. The pouch has a continent stoma on the abdomen created with a valve that can be drained only when the patient places a large catheter into the stoma. The patient empties the pouch several times a day. This procedure is rarely performed now.

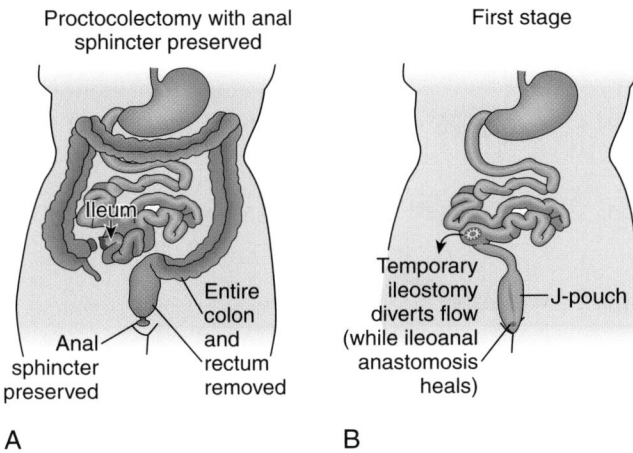

FIG. 47.4 Ileoanal pouch anastomosis.

Children with fecal soiling associated with neuropathic or structural abnormalities of the anal sphincter sometimes have an antegrade continence enema (ACE) procedure. The surgeon creates a continence valve with an opening on to the abdomen in the intestine, so the patient or caregiver can insert a tube and give himself or herself an enema that comes out through the anus. Colonic evacuation begins about 10 to 20 minutes after a patient receives the enema fluid.

CRITICAL THINKING

Successful critical thinking requires a synthesis of knowledge, experience, information gathered from patients, critical thinking attitudes, and intellectual and professional standards. Clinical judgments require you to anticipate the information necessary, analyze the data, and make decisions regarding your patient's care. During assessment consider all elements that build toward making an appropriate nursing diagnosis (Fig. 47.5).

In the case of bowel elimination, integrate knowledge from nursing and other disciplines to understand a patient's response to bowel elimination alterations. Experience in caring for patients with elimination alterations helps you provide an appropriate plan of care. Use critical thinking attitudes such as fairness, confidence, and discipline when listening to and exploring a patient's nursing history. Apply relevant standards of practice when selecting nursing measures.

> ### REFLECT NOW
>
> Consider the social stigma of impaired bowel function and try to understand your personal attitudes toward caring for a patient who may suffer from odor, soiling, and embarrassment when he or she loses control of this important bodily function.

❖ NURSING PROCESS

Apply the nursing process and use a critical thinking approach in your care of patients. The nursing process provides a clinical decision-making approach for you to develop and implement an individualized plan of care.

◆ Assessment

Assessment for bowel elimination patterns and abnormalities includes a nursing history, physical assessment of the abdomen, inspection of fecal characteristics, and review of relevant test results. In addition,

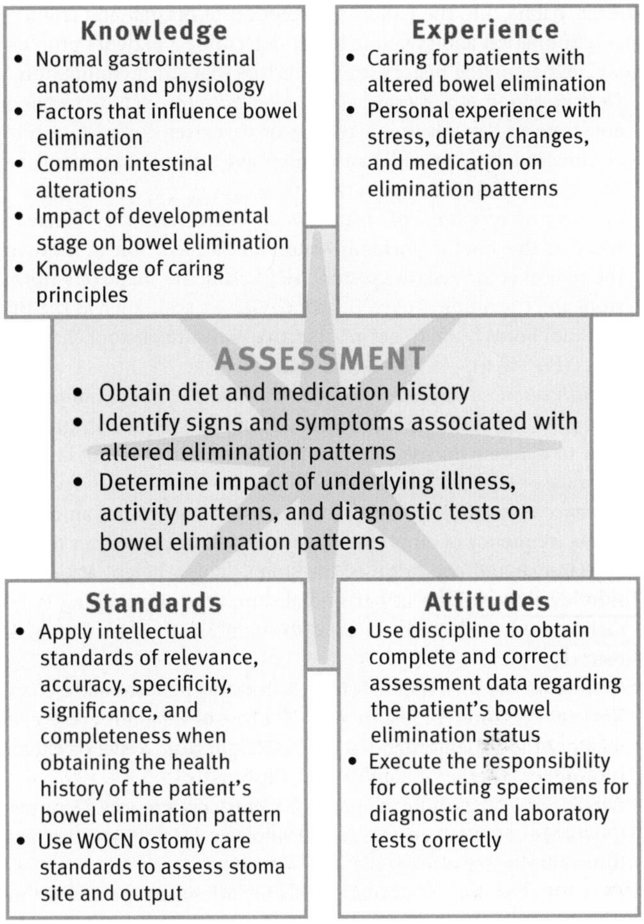

Knowledge
- Normal gastrointestinal anatomy and physiology
- Factors that influence bowel elimination
- Common intestinal alterations
- Impact of developmental stage on bowel elimination
- Knowledge of caring principles

Experience
- Caring for patients with altered bowel elimination
- Personal experience with stress, dietary changes, and medication on elimination patterns

ASSESSMENT
- Obtain diet and medication history
- Identify signs and symptoms associated with altered elimination patterns
- Determine impact of underlying illness, activity patterns, and diagnostic tests on bowel elimination patterns

Standards
- Apply intellectual standards of relevance, accuracy, specificity, significance, and completeness when obtaining the health history of the patient's bowel elimination pattern
- Use WOCN ostomy care standards to assess stoma site and output

Attitudes
- Use discipline to obtain complete and correct assessment data regarding the patient's bowel elimination status
- Execute the responsibility for collecting specimens for diagnostic and laboratory tests correctly

FIG. 47.5 Critical thinking model for elimination assessment. *WOCN,* Wound, Ostomy and Continence Nurses Society.

determine the patient's medical history, pattern and types of fluid and food intake, mobility, chewing ability, medications, recent illnesses and/or stressors, and environmental situation.

Through the Patient's Eyes. Patients expect nurses to answer all of their questions regarding diagnostic tests and the preparation for these tests. They are concerned about discomfort and exposure of their perineal area. Bowel problems are often a source of discomfort and embarrassment for patients and their families. Fecal and urinary incontinence in older people is often a reason for admission to a long-term care agency, and the rate of development of both fecal and urinary incontinence after admission to a long-term care facility is 28% at 6 months, 42% at 1 year, and 61% 2 years after admission (Bliss, 2017). Some older patients who fail to recognize their elimination needs require monitoring for elimination patterns so that negative consequences do not occur. Remember that each patient has a unique situation and a perception of what is "right" for him or her. Patients expect a knowledgeable nurse with the ability to teach methods of promoting and maintaining normal bowel elimination patterns or means of managing altered elimination. Encourage the patient and/or caregiver to describe cultural practices and use this information when providing care to enhance the patient's comfort.

Nursing History. The nursing history provides information about a patient's usual bowel pattern and habits. What a patient describes as normal or abnormal is often different from factors and conditions that tend to promote normal elimination. Identifying normal and abnormal patterns, habits, and the patient's perception of normal and abnormal bowel elimination allows you to better determine a patient's problems. Organize the nursing history around factors that affect elimination.

- *Determination of the usual elimination pattern:* Include frequency and time of day. Having a patient or caregiver complete a bowel elimination diary provides an accurate assessment of a patient's current bowel elimination pattern.
- *Patient's description of usual stool characteristics:* Determine whether the stool is normally watery or formed, soft or hard, and the typical color. Ask the patient to describe the shape of a normal stool and the number of stools per day. Use a scale such as the Bristol Stool Form Scale to get an objective measure of stool characteristics (Fig. 47.6).
- *Identification of routines followed to promote bowel elimination:* Examples are drinking hot liquids, eating specific foods, or taking time to defecate during a certain part of the day or use of laxatives, enemas, or bulk-forming fiber additives.
- *Presence and status of bowel diversions:* If a patient has an ostomy, assess frequency of emptying the ostomy pouch, character of feces, appearance and condition of the stoma (color, height at or above skin level), condition of peristomal skin, type of pouching system device used, and methods used to maintain the function of the ostomy.
- *Changes in appetite:* Include changes in eating patterns and a change in weight (amount of loss or gain). If a loss of weight is present, ask whether the patient intended to lose weight (e.g., a diet or exercise routine) or whether it happened unexpectedly.
- *Diet history:* Determine the patient's dietary preferences. Determine the intake of fruits, vegetables, and whole grains and whether mealtimes are regular or irregular.
- *Description of daily fluid intake:* This includes the type and amount of fluid. Patients often estimate the amount using common household measurements.
- *History of surgery or illnesses affecting the GI tract:* This information helps explain symptoms, the potential for maintaining or restoring normal bowel elimination pattern, and whether there is a family history of GI cancer.
- *Medication history:* Ask patients for a list of all the medications they take, and assess whether they take medications such as laxatives, antacids, iron supplements, and analgesics that alter defecation or fecal characteristics.
- *Emotional state:* A patient's emotional status may alter frequency of defecation. Ask the patient whether he or she has experienced unusual stress and if so, whether he or she thinks that this may have caused a change in bowel movements.
- *History of exercise:* Ask the patient to specifically describe the type and amount of daily exercise.
- *History of pain or discomfort:* Ask the patient whether there is a history of abdominal or anal pain. The type, frequency, and location of pain help identify the source of the problem. For instance, cramping pain, nausea, and the absence of bowel movements sometimes indicate there is an intestinal obstruction.
- *Social history:* Patients have many different living arrangements. Where patients live affects their toileting habits. If the patient lives with other people, ask how many bathrooms there are. Find out whether the patient must share a bathroom, creating a need to adjust the time that he or she uses the bathroom to accommodate others. If the patient lives alone, can he or she ambulate to the toilet safely? When patients are not independent in bowel management, determine who helps them and how.
- *Mobility and dexterity:* Evaluate patients' mobility and dexterity to determine whether they need assistive devices or help from personnel

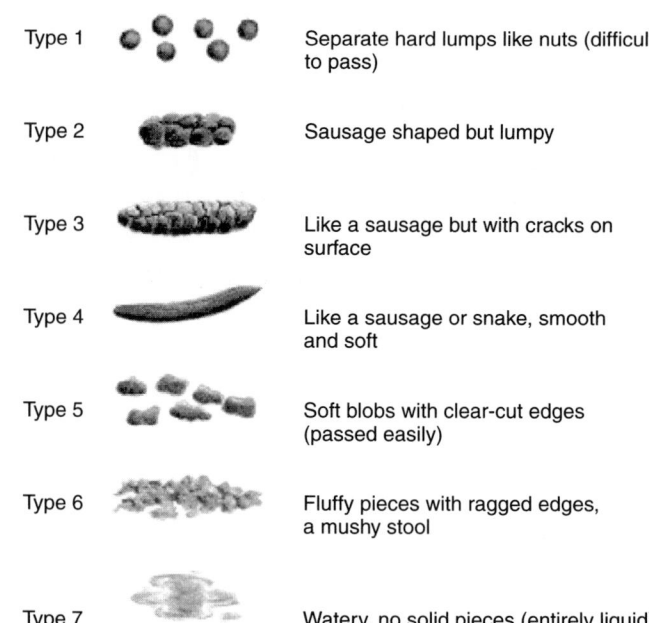

Type 1	Separate hard lumps like nuts (difficult to pass)
Type 2	Sausage shaped but lumpy
Type 3	Like a sausage but with cracks on surface
Type 4	Like a sausage or snake, smooth and soft
Type 5	Soft blobs with clear-cut edges (passed easily)
Type 6	Fluffy pieces with ragged edges, a mushy stool
Type 7	Watery, no solid pieces (entirely liquid)

FIG. 47.6 Bristol Stool Form Scale. (Used with permission. Bristol Stool Form Guideline. https://www.webmd.com/digestive-disorders/poop-chart-bristol-stool-scale.)

See Box 47.3 for a summary of the types of assessment questions to use for gathering a detailed nursing history.

Physical Assessment. Conduct a physical assessment of body systems and functions likely to be influenced by the presence of elimination problems (see Chapter 30).

Mouth. Inspect the patient's teeth, tongue, and gums. Poor dentition or poorly fitting dentures influence the ability to chew. Sores in the mouth make eating not only difficult but also painful.

Abdomen. Inspect all four abdominal quadrants for contour, shape, symmetry, and skin color. Note masses, peristaltic waves, scars, venous patterns, stomas, and lesions. Normally you do not see peristaltic waves. Observable peristalsis is often a sign of intestinal obstruction

Abdominal distention appears as an overall outward protuberance of the abdomen. Intestinal gas, large tumors, or fluid in the peritoneal cavity causes distention. A distended abdomen feels tight like a drum; the skin is taut and appears stretched.

Normal bowel sounds occur every 5 to 15 seconds and last a second to several seconds. Absent (no auscultated bowel sounds) or hypoactive sounds occur with an ileus such as after abdominal surgery but may also mean that you did not capture the bowel sounds when you were assessing them. High-pitched and hyperactive bowel sounds occur with small intestine obstruction and inflammatory disorders. Although auscultating bowel sounds during assessment is standard nursing practice, some current research questions its validity.

Auscultation of the abdomen is done with a stethoscope, but the validity and reliability of this practice has come into question. A 2018 systematic review of the literature on bowel sound auscultation in ICU patients concluded that there is a low sensitivity, low positive predictive value, and poor inter- and intra-observer agreement in auscultating bowel sounds. The authors stated that bowel sounds were not sufficiently accurate for clinical decision making and questioned the usefulness of the practice (Van Bree et al., 2018).

Percussion identifies underlying abdominal structures and detects lesions, fluid, or gas within the abdomen. Gas or flatulence creates a tympanic note. Masses, tumors, and fluid are dull to percussion.

BOX 47.3 Nursing Assessment Questions

Signs and Symptoms
Nausea or Vomiting: Onset, Duration, Associated Symptoms, Character, Exposures
- When did the nausea/vomiting start?
- Is it related to particular stimuli (odors, after eating specific food)?
- How does the emesis look (mucus, blood, coffee-ground appearance, undigested food), and what is the color?
- Do you have other symptoms such as fever, dizziness, headaches, abdominal pain, or weight loss?
- Do you have family members who are experiencing the same symptoms?

Indigestion: Onset, Character, Location, Associated Symptoms, Alleviating Factors
- Is the indigestion related to meals, types or quantity of food, time of day or night?
- Does the discomfort from indigestion radiate to the shoulders or arms?
- Do you feel bloated after eating?
- Do you have any other symptoms (vomiting, headaches, diarrhea, belching, flatulence, heartburn, or pain)?
- Does the indigestion respond to antacids or other self-care measures?

Diarrhea: Onset, Duration, Character, Associated Symptoms, Alleviating Factors, Exposure
- When did the diarrhea start? Was it gradual or sudden?
- How many stools do you have per day? Is it watery or explosive? What is the color and consistency?
- Have you had fever, chills, weight loss, or abdominal pain?
- Have you taken antibiotics recently?

- Have you been under stress?
- What have you used to try to alleviate the diarrhea? Was it successful?
- Have you been out of the country recently?

Constipation: Onset, Character, Symptoms, Alleviating Factors
- When was your last bowel movement? How many bowel movements do you have in a typical week?
- Is this a recent occurrence or a long-standing problem?
- Describe your bowel movements.
- Do you have to strain to have a bowel movement?
- Do you have abdominal or rectal pain when you have a bowel movement?
- Do you feel as though your bowel movements are incomplete?
- Have you recently changed your diet or fluid intake?
- Do you use stool softeners, laxatives, or enemas?
- Has it ever been necessary to manually remove the bowel movements?

Medical History
- Do you have a previous history of gastrointestinal problems or disease? If yes, explain.
- Have you had abdominal surgery or trauma?
- Do you have a history of major illnesses such as cancer; arthritis; or respiratory, kidney, or cardiac disease?
- Which medications do you take?

Effect on the Patient
- How do these symptoms affect you?
- Have you missed work or social engagements because of these symptoms?

Gently palpate the abdomen for masses or areas of tenderness. It is important for your patient to relax. Tensing abdominal muscles interferes with palpating underlying organs or masses.

Rectum. Inspect the area around the anus for lesions, discoloration, inflammation, and hemorrhoids. Pain results when hemorrhoid tissues are irritated. The primary goal for a patient with hemorrhoids is to have soft-formed, painless bowel movements. Proper diet, fluids, and regular exercise improve the likelihood of stools being soft. If the patient becomes constipated, passage of hard stools causes bleeding and irritation. An ice pack or a warm sitz bath (see Chapter 48) provides temporary relief of swollen hemorrhoids. A health care provider sometimes prescribes topical medication to relieve the swelling and pain.

Laboratory Tests. There are no blood tests to specifically diagnose most GI disorders, but hemoglobin and hematocrit help determine whether anemia from GI bleeding is present. Other laboratory tests often ordered by the health care provider include liver function tests, serum amylase, and serum lipase, which are used to assess for hepatobiliary diseases and pancreatitis.

Fecal Specimens. You need to ensure that specimens are obtained accurately, labeled properly in appropriate containers, and transported to the laboratory on time. Laboratories provide special containers for fecal specimens. Some tests require that specimens are placed in chemical preservatives, and some require that they are refrigerated or placed on ice after collection and before delivery to the laboratory. Use medical aseptic technique during collection of stool specimens (see Chapter 28).

Hand hygiene is necessary for anyone who comes in contact with the specimen. Often the patient is able to obtain the specimen if properly instructed. Teach the patient to avoid mixing feces with urine or

water. He or she defecates into a clean, dry bedpan or a special container under the toilet seat. Observe the stool characteristics when collecting a specimen (Table 47.1).

Tests performed by the laboratory for occult (microscopic) blood in the stool and stool cultures require only a small sample. Collect about a 3-cm (1-inch) mass of formed stool or 15 to 30 mL of liquid stool. Tests for measuring the output of fecal fat require a 3- to 5-day collection of stool. You need to save all fecal material throughout the test period.

After obtaining a specimen, label and tightly seal the container and complete all laboratory requisition forms. Record specimen collections in the patient's medical record. It is important to avoid delays in sending specimens to the laboratory. Some tests such as measurement for ova and parasites require the stool to be warm. When stool specimens remain at room temperature, bacteriological changes that alter test results occur.

A common stool test is the fecal occult blood test (FOBT), which measures microscopic amounts of blood in the feces. It is a useful screening test for colon cancer as recommended by the American Cancer Society. There are two types of tests, the guaiac fecal occult blood test (gFOBT) and the fecal immunochemical test (FIT). The FIT test requires no preparation or dietary restrictions and is a more sensitive test, but it is more expensive; thus, the gFOBT is more commonly used. The nurse or the patient needs to repeat the test at least 3 times on three separate bowel movements. The FOBT is done in a patient's home or health care provider's office (Box 47.4). All positive tests are followed up with flexible sigmoidoscopy or colonoscopy (ACS, 2018).

When your patients are going to have a gFOBT, it is important to instruct them to avoid eating red meat for 3 days before testing. If there are no contraindications and it is approved by the health care provider,

TABLE 47.1   Fecal Characteristics

Characteristic	Normal	Abnormal	Abnormal Cause
Color	Infant: yellow; adult: brown	White or clay	Absence of bile
		Black or tarry (melena)	Iron ingestion or gastrointestinal (GI) bleeding
		Red	GI bleeding, hemorrhoids, ingestion of beets
		Pale and oily	Malabsorption of fat
Odor	Malodorous; may be affected by certain foods	Noxious change	Blood in feces or infection
Consistency	Soft, formed	Liquid	Diarrhea, reduced absorption
		Hard	Constipation
Frequency	Varies: infant 4 to 6 times daily (breastfed) or 1 to 3 times daily (bottle-fed); adult twice daily to 3 times a week	Infant more than 6 times daily or less than once every 1 to 2 days; adult more than 3 times a day or less than once a week	Hypermotility or hypomotility
Shape	Resembles diameter of rectum	Narrow, pencil shaped	Obstruction, increased peristalsis
Constituents	Undigested food, dead bacteria, fat, bile pigment, cells lining intestinal mucosa, water	Blood, pus, foreign bodies, mucus, worms	Internal bleeding, infection, swallowed objects, irritation, inflammation, infestation of parasites
		Oily stool	Malabsorption syndrome, enteritis, pancreatic disease, surgical resection of intestine
		Mucus	Intestinal irritation, inflammation, infection, or injury

instruct your patient to stop taking aspirin, ibuprofen, naproxen, or other nonsteroidal antiinflammatory drugs for 7 days because these could cause a false-positive test result. Patients also need to avoid vitamin C supplements and citrus fruits and juices for 3 days before the test because they can cause a false-negative result (ACS, 2018).

Diagnostic Examinations. For patients experiencing alterations in the GI system, various radiological and diagnostic examinations such as a colonoscopy require bowel preparation (bowel prep) for the test to be completed successfully. A bowel-cleansing program is sometimes difficult or unpleasant for patients. You provide education and support to ensure an optimal test result (Box 47.5).

REFLECT NOW

The assessment of the body and fecal matter related to bowel elimination requires questions and procedures that are very private to many patients. What actions can you take while conducting this assessment that promote patients' comfort and decrease their embarrassment?

◆ Nursing Diagnosis

Nursing assessment of a patient's bowel function sometimes reveals data that indicate an actual or potential elimination problem or a problem resulting from elimination alterations. In the examples discussed in the Nursing Care Plan, a patient has constipation as a result of pain medications and decreased fiber intake. Examples of diagnoses that apply to patients with elimination problems include the following:

- *Bowel Incontinence*
- *Constipation*
- *Risk for Constipation*
- *Lack of Knowledge of Dietary Regime*

Associated problems such as age, body-image changes, or skin breakdown require interventions unrelated to bowel function impairment. It

is important to establish the correct "related to" factor for a diagnosis. This depends on the thoroughness of your assessment and your recognition of the assessment findings and factors that impair elimination (Box 47.6). For example, with the diagnosis of *Constipation* you distinguish between related factors of *nutritional imbalance, exercise, medications,* and *emotional problems.* Selection of the correct related factors for each diagnosis ensures that you will implement the appropriate nursing interventions.

◆ Planning

When planning care, synthesize information from multiple resources (Fig. 47.7). Critical thinking ensures that the plan of care integrates everything known about a patient and current clinical problem. Rely on professional standards when possible—for example, the *American College of Gastroenterology Rome IV Criteria for Colorectal Disorders* (Simren et al., 2017). For the patient with a fecal diversion, referring to *Clinical Guideline: Management of the Adult with a Fecal or Urinary Ostomy* (WOCN, 2017), may be helpful.

Goals and Outcomes. Help patients establish goals and outcomes by incorporating their elimination habits or routines as much as possible and reinforcing the routines that promote health (see the Nursing Care Plan). In addition, consider preexisting health concerns. For example, if a patient's diet, activity, and irregular bowel habits caused the elimination problem, help him or her learn to make lifestyle changes to improve bowel function. The overall goal of returning a patient to a normal bowel elimination pattern includes the following outcomes:

- Patient establishes a regular defecation schedule
- Patient lists proper fluid and food intake needed to soften stool and promote regular bowel elimination
- Patient implements a regular exercise program
- Patient reports daily passage of soft, formed brown stool
- Patient does not report straining or discomfort associated with defecation

Constipation

ASSESSMENT

The home health nurse is visiting Mr. Johnson, age 76, at his home, where he lives alone. Mr. Johnson has two grown children who live in another state. They came to visit him and help him get settled back in his home after being hospitalized. Mr. Johnson had surgery 10 days ago for a total knee replacement after suffering from osteoarthritis for many years. He tells the nurse that he is trying to follow the exercise program that the physical therapist has recommended but is having difficulty because of pain. He is taking the prescribed pain medication because of the continued pain. His history includes hypertension, which has been controlled with medication for the past 10 years. He had some edema of both feet in the hospital and took a mild diuretic for 5 days for relief. The nurse knows that immobility from the surgery, recent use of a diuretic, and opioid pain medication are factors that can cause constipation.

Assessment Activities	Assessment Findings[a]
Ask Mr. Johnson about his bowel elimination patterns since his surgery.	Mr. Johnson tells the nurse that **he had one small, hard bowel movement in the hospital but has not had one in the 7 days since he has been home.**
Review patient's medication.	Mr. Johnson says he is taking his blood pressure medication, a daily multivitamin with **iron**, a stool softener once a day, and 1 or 2 **oxycodone** 4 times a day (Burchum and Rosenthal, 2019).
Review dietary and fluid intake over last day.	Diet included **whole-grain cereal**, a banana, and toast for breakfast; a sandwich for lunch; and a frozen dinner in the evening, which has a small serving of meat, potatoes or rice, and corn or green beans. He says he is **trying to drink fluids but has started feeling a little nauseated when he drinks very much.** He also isn't sure if too much fluid would make his feet swell again. He has a cup of coffee and a small glass of orange juice in the morning. He drinks a small glass of iced tea with lunch and dinner.
Assess which foods and fluids Mr. Johnson likes, can obtain, and will prepare.	He reports that a friend will shop for him for groceries. Occasionally a friend brings him dinner, but he relies on frozen dinners because they are easy to get and to heat. **He hates prune juice but will drink apple or orange juice. He agrees that he can drink more water but prefers iced tea with sugar. He likes lettuce and tomato salads; most fruits; and frozen peas, corn, or green beans. He'll try whole-grain bread but prefers white bread.**
Ask about any nausea or vomiting.	Complains of **mild nausea** when he eats and a constant **feeling of fullness** but no vomiting.
Palpate abdomen.	While the nurse is palpating Mr. Johnson's abdomen, Mr. Johnson says, "It really feels full," and he winces with very little pressure applied. Abdomen feels taut and mildly distended.

[a]**Assessment findings** are shown in bold type.

NURSING DIAGNOSIS: Constipation related to opiate-containing pain medication, decreased mobility, and decreased food and fluid intake

PLANNING

Goals	Expected Outcomes (NOC)[b]
	Bowel Elimination
Mr. Johnson will establish normal defecation.	Mr. Johnson reports passage of soft, formed stool without straining in next 24 hours.
	Nutritional Status: Food and Fluid Intake
Mr. Johnson will make changes to his diet to prevent constipation.	Mr. Johnson drinks at least 1500 mL of fluid over the next 24 hours.
	Mr. Johnson increases the fiber content of his diet by eating an apple with his breakfast, lettuce and tomato on his sandwich, and some carrots with his dinner.

[b]Outcome classification labels from Moorhead S, et al: *Nursing Outcomes Classification (NOC)*, ed 6, St Louis, 2018, Elsevier.

INTERVENTIONS (NIC)[c]	RATIONALE
Constipation/Impaction Management	
Encourage fluid intake of appropriate fluids, fruit juice, and water.	At least 1500 mL fluid intake daily will help to soften the stool (Mayo Clinic, 2017).
Encourage activity within patient's mobility regimen.	Minimal activity (such as leg lifts) increases peristalsis (Harding et al, 2020).
Instruct Mr. Johnson to eat more fruits and vegetables and have a bran cereal for breakfast.	Added fiber in food relieves constipation (NIH, 2018a).
Provide stimulant laxative and stool softeners as ordered.	Stimulant laxatives increase peristalsis and are an effective way to relieve constipation and promote normal bowel function when used on a short-term basis (Burchum and Rosenthal, 2019).
Encourage Mr. Johnson to try to have a bowel movement at the same time each day.	A regular time for bowel movements encourages normal bowel function (Harding et al, 2020).

[c]Intervention classification labels from Butcher HK, et al: *Nursing Interventions Classification (NIC)*, ed 7, St Louis, 2018, Elsevier.

EVALUATION

Evaluation Activity	Patient Response/Finding	Outcome Status
Ask Mr. Johnson to identify foods high in fiber and fluid intake.	Able to state appropriate foods and fluids but still has little appetite and feels full soon after eating.	Mr. Johnson verbalizes understanding of teaching.
Get medication history for past 2 days.	Patient has taken a stimulant laxative and stool softener twice a day for last 2 days.	Patient has not had a bowel movement.
Ask Mr. Johnson about physical activity.	Mr. Johnson states that he has not changed his activity pattern because of the pain from surgery.	Mr. Johnson did not increase activity pattern and needs to continue to work on this intervention. Revise care plan.
Inquire about bowel movements.	Mr. Johnson still has not had a bowel movement.	Mr. Johnson did not achieve passage of regular, formed stool. Revise care plan.

BOX 47.4 PROCEDURAL GUIDELINES

Performing a Guaiac Fecal Occult Blood Test

Delegation and Collaboration

The skill of fecal occult blood test (FOBT) can be delegated to assistive personnel (AP). However, the nurse is responsible for assessing the significance of the findings. You may need to send the specimen to the laboratory. Refer to your agency policies. The nurse instructs the AP to:

- Notify the nurse if frank bleeding occurs after obtaining the sample.

Equipment

Hemoccult test paper, Hemoccult developer, wooden applicator, and clean gloves (Check the expiration dates on the developer and the test paper before using.)

Steps

1. Identify patient using at least two identifiers (e.g., name and birthday or name and account number) according to agency policy.
2. Explain purpose of test and ways patient can help. Patient can collect own specimen if possible.
3. Perform hand hygiene and apply clean gloves.
4. Use tip of wooden applicator (see illustration) to obtain a small part of stool specimen. Be sure that specimen is free of toilet paper and not contaminated with urine.

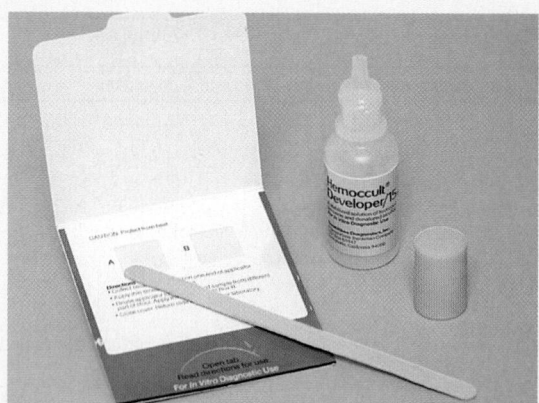

STEP 4 Equipment needed for fecal occult blood testing.

5. Perform Hemoccult slide test:
   a. Open flap of slide and, using a wooden applicator, thinly smear stool in first box of the guaiac paper. Apply a second fecal specimen from a different part of the stool to second box of slide (see illustration).

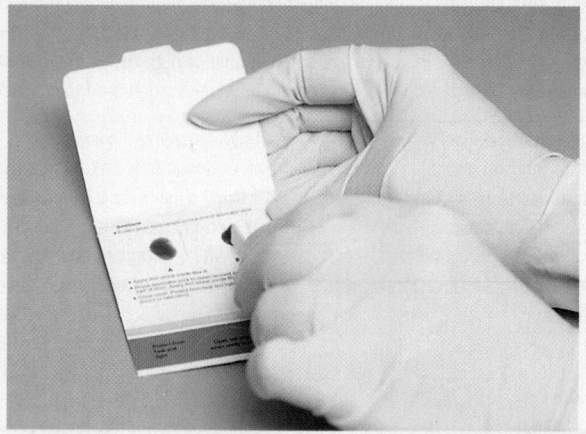

STEP 5a Application of fecal specimen on guaiac paper.

   b. Close slide cover and turn the packet over to reverse side (see illustration). After waiting 3 to 5 minutes, open cardboard flap and apply 2 drops of developing solution on each box of guaiac paper. A blue color indicates a positive guaiac or presence of fecal occult blood.

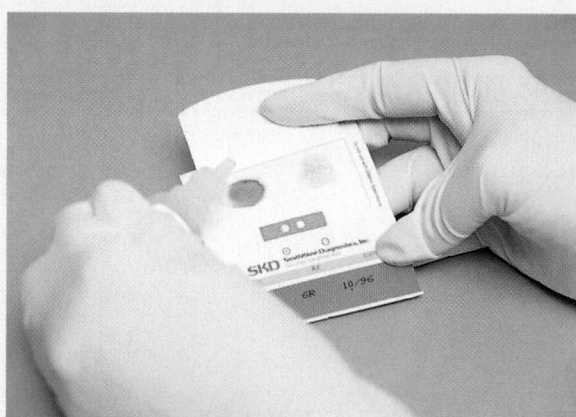

STEP 5b Application of Hemoccult developing solution on guaiac paper on reverse side of test kit.

   c. Interpret the color of the guaiac paper after 30 to 60 seconds.
   d. After determining whether the patient's specimen is positive or negative, apply 1 drop of developer to the quality control section and interpret within 10 seconds.
   e. Dispose of test slide in proper receptacle.
6. Wrap wooden applicator in paper towel, remove gloves, and discard in proper receptacle.
7. Perform hand hygiene.
8. Record results of test; note any unusual fecal characteristics. (Submit only one sample per day.)

BOX 47.5 Radiological and Diagnostic Tests

Direct Visualization

Endoscopy

- Examinations such as a gastroscopy or colonoscopy use a lighted fiberoptic tube to gain direct visualization of the upper gastrointestinal (GI) tract (upper endoscopy) or large intestine (colonoscopy). The fiberoptic tube contains a lens, forceps, and brushes for biopsy. If an endoscopy identifies a lesion such as a polyp, the polyp can be removed, and a biopsy will be done.

- These tests are done under sedation, usually in outpatient centers.
- Patients receive instruction about the preparation needed for the tests at the time they are scheduled for the procedure. Patients are usually on a clear liquid diet the day before the test. Bowel preparation is necessary before a colonoscopy can be performed successfully.

BOX 47.5 Radiological and Diagnostic Tests—Cont'd

Indirect Visualization

Anorectal Manometry

- Measures the pressure activity of internal and external anal sphincters and reflexes during rectal distention, relaxation during straining, and rectal sensation.

Plain Film of Abdomen/Kidneys, Ureter, Bladder (KUB)

- A simple x-ray film of the abdomen requiring no preparation.

Barium Swallow/Enema

- An x-ray film examination using an opaque contrast medium (barium, which is swallowed) to examine the structure and motility of the upper GI tract, including pharynx, esophagus, and stomach. Barium instilled through the anal opening via an enema provides visualization of the structures of the lower GI tract.
- Preparation required varies by physician and agency doing the procedure but usually includes a clear liquid diet, laxatives the day before the procedure, and in some instances enemas to empty out any remaining stool particles.

Ultrasound Imaging

- A technique that uses high-frequency sound waves to echo off body organs, creating a picture of the GI tract

Computed Tomography Scan (Virtual Colonoscopy)

- An x-ray examination of the body from many angles using a scanner analyzed by a computer. An oral contrast solution for the patient to drink may be ordered before the test. Intravenous contrast solution may be injected during the test to improve visualization. If contrast is used, patient should not have food or fluids for 4 to 6 hours before the examination.
- Virtual colonoscopy or computerized tomography (CT) colonography requires bowel preparation before the test. This does not replace the colonoscopy because it does not allow for removal of **polyps** and for biopsies to be obtained.

Colonic Transit Study

- The patient swallows a capsule containing radiopaque markers.
- The patient maintains his or her normal diet and fluid intake for 5 days and refrains from medications that affect bowel function. On the fifth day x-ray film examination is performed.

Magnetic Resonance Imaging

- A noninvasive examination that uses magnet and radio waves to produce a picture of the inside of the body.
- Preparation is NPO 4 to 6 hours before examination.
- The patient needs to lie very still. If claustrophobia is a problem, light sedation may be ordered.
- No metallic objects, including metal objects on clothes, are allowed in the room. If the patient has a pacemaker or a metal implanted in his or her body, he or she may not be able to have magnetic resonance imaging (MRI).

BOX 47.6 Nursing Diagnostic Process: Constipation

Assessment Activities	Assessment Findings
Ask patient about bowel elimination patterns.	Patient reports no bowel movement for 4 days.
Ask patient about other gastrointestinal symptoms.	Patient denies any feeling of nausea, abdominal cramping, or loss of appetite.
Ask patient to describe recent food and fluid intake.	Patient reports drinking two cups of coffee and one glass of iced tea each day; eating one serving of cooked vegetables and a banana every other day; having peanut butter and jelly sandwiches, meat, potatoes, and white bread every day.
Palpate abdomen.	Patient reports feeling of fullness. Left lower quadrant is firm.

QSEN **Building Competency in Patient-Centered Care** Mr. Johnson started taking a stimulant laxative every day to avoid constipation after he had a fecal impaction removed. He drank more fluids, especially water, and began to add more fruits and vegetables to his diet. On the day after the impaction was removed, he had a formed, firm bowel movement with some straining required. Then he began to have daily bowel movements with soft, formed stool. Now it is 1 month later, and he is still taking laxatives but not continuing with the fluid and dietary modifications that were recommended for him. The physical therapist is ready to discharge him from home care but asks the nurse to make another visit when Mr. Johnson states he is having trouble moving his bowels. Which assessment questions and teaching strategies, approaches, and tools does the nurse use to enhance Mr. Johnson's learning and ability to prevent constipation?

Answers to QSEN Activities can be found on the Evolve website.

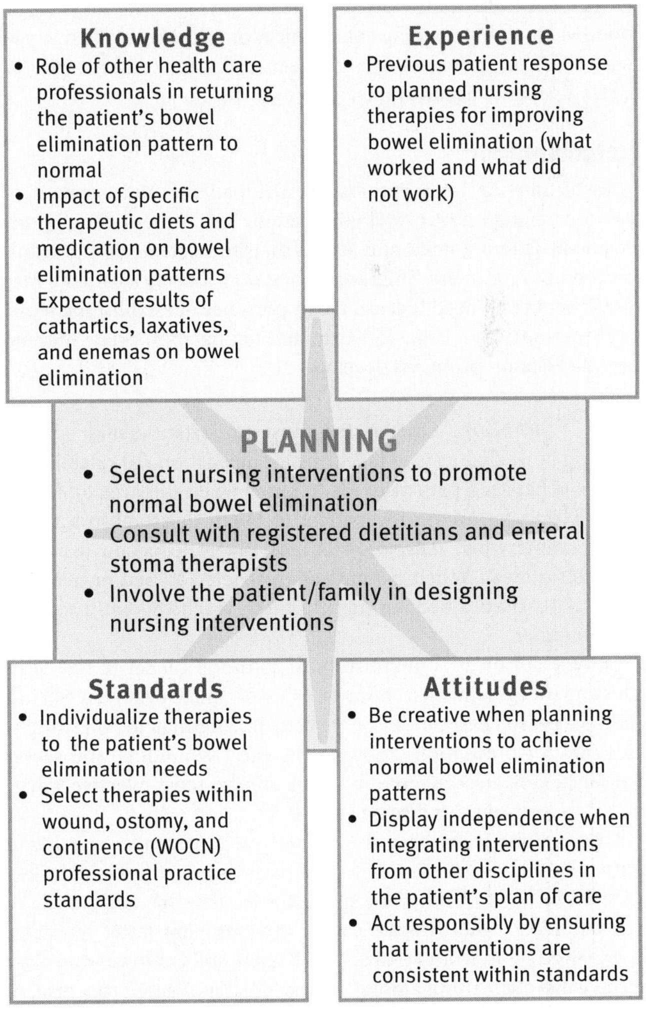

Knowledge

- Role of other health care professionals in returning the patient's bowel elimination pattern to normal
- Impact of specific therapeutic diets and medication on bowel elimination patterns
- Expected results of cathartics, laxatives, and enemas on bowel elimination

Experience

- Previous patient response to planned nursing therapies for improving bowel elimination (what worked and what did not work)

PLANNING

- Select nursing interventions to promote normal bowel elimination
- Consult with registered dietitians and enteral stoma therapists
- Involve the patient/family in designing nursing interventions

Standards

- Individualize therapies to the patient's bowel elimination needs
- Select therapies within wound, ostomy, and continence (WOCN) professional practice standards

Attitudes

- Be creative when planning interventions to achieve normal bowel elimination patterns
- Display independence when integrating interventions from other disciplines in the patient's plan of care
- Act responsibly by ensuring that interventions are consistent within standards

FIG. 47.7 Critical thinking model for elimination planning.

Setting Priorities. Defecation patterns vary among individuals. For this reason, a nurse and patient work together closely to plan effective interventions. Patients often have multiple diagnoses. The concept map (Fig. 47.8) shows an example of how the nursing diagnosis of constipation is related to three other diagnoses and their respective interventions. A realistic time frame to establish a normal defecation pattern for one patient is sometimes very different for another. In a patient with recent abdominal surgery, the priorities of pain management and the avoidance of constipation through increasing fluids in the diet and encouraging early ambulation help in the recovery process.

Teamwork and Collaboration. When patients are disabled or debilitated by illness, you need to include the family in the plan of care. In some situations, family members have the same ineffective elimination habits as the patient. Thus, patient and family teaching is an important part of the care plan. Other health team members such as registered dietitians and WOCNs are often valuable resources. You coordinate activities of the interprofessional health care team.

A patient with alterations in bowel elimination sometimes requires intervention from several members of the health care team. Certain tasks such as assisting patients onto the bedpan or bedside commode are appropriate to delegate to assistive personnel (AP). It is important to remind the AP to report any abnormal findings or difficulties encountered during the elimination process. Many of the diagnostic tests for evaluation of the GI system are performed by nonnursing personnel. Maintaining ongoing communication with these caregivers will ensure that you provide safe and effective patient-centered care and address a patient's needs, wants, and concerns.

◆ Implementation

Successful nursing interventions improve patients' and family members' understanding of bowel elimination. Teach them about proper diet, adequate fluid intake, and factors that stimulate or slow peristalsis such as emotional stress. This is often best done during a patient's mealtime. Patients also need to learn the importance of establishing regular bowel routines, exercising regularly, and taking appropriate measures when elimination problems develop.

Health Promotion. One of the most important habits to teach regarding bowel habits is to take time for defecation. To establish regular bowel habits, a patient needs to know when the urge to defecate normally occurs. Advise the patient to begin to establish a routine during a time when defecation is most likely to occur, usually an hour after a meal. When patients are restricted to bed or need help to ambulate, offer a bedpan or help them reach the bathroom in a timely manner.

Colorectal cancer is the third most common cancer in the United States and the second most common cause of cancer death (ACS, 2018). When diagnosed early, it can be treated and eliminated. Following the guidelines for prevention, knowing the early symptoms, and seeking medical help if these symptoms occur are the most effective ways to prevent death from this disease (Box 47.7).

African Americans have the highest rates of cancer and highest death rates from cancer of any cultural group in the United States. However, for the first time, one study showed that the death rates from lung, colorectal, and prostate cancer are dropping faster in African Americans than in whites (ACS, 2019). There still is a lower rate of colorectal cancer screening among Africian Americans, but this disparity is decreasing (Box 47.8).

Promotion of Normal Defecation. A number of interventions stimulate the defecation reflex, affect the character of feces, or increase peristalsis to help patients evacuate bowel contents normally and without discomfort.

Sitting Position. Help patients who have difficulty sitting because of muscular weakness and mobility problems. Place an elevated seat on the toilet or a bedside commode when patients are unable to lower themselves to a sitting position because of pain or weakness. These seats require patients to use less effort to sit or stand.

Positioning on Bedpan. Patients restricted to bed use bedpans for defecation. Women use bedpans to pass both urine and feces, whereas men use bedpans only for defecation. Sitting on a bedpan is often uncomfortable. Help position patients comfortably. Two types of bedpans are available (Fig. 47.9). The regular bedpan, made of plastic, has a curved smooth upper end and a sharper-edged lower end and is about 5 cm (2 inches) deep. The smaller fracture pan, designed for patients with lower-extremity fractures, has a shallow upper end about 2.5 cm (1 inch) deep. The shallow end of the pan fits under the buttocks toward the sacrum; the deeper end, which has a handle, goes just under the upper thighs. The pan needs to be high enough that feces enter it.

When positioning a patient, it is important to prevent muscle strain and discomfort. Never try to lift a patient onto a bedpan. Never place a patient on a bedpan and then leave with the bed flat unless activity restrictions demand it because it forces the patient to hyperextend the back to lift the hips on the pan. The proper position for the patient on a bedpan is with the head of the bed elevated 30 to 45 degrees (Figs. 47.10 and 47.11). When patients are immobile or it is unsafe to allow them to raise their hips, it is safest for both caregivers and patients to roll them on to the bedpan (Box 47.9). Always wear gloves when handling a bedpan.

Acute Care. With some acute illnesses the GI system becomes affected. Changes in a patient's fluid status, mobility patterns, nutrition, and sleep cycle affect regular bowel habits. Surgical interventions on the GI tract obviously affect bowel elimination. However, surgery on other systems (e.g., the musculoskeletal and cardiovascular systems) sometimes also affects it.

Chronically ill and hospitalized patients are not always able to maintain privacy during defecation. In a hospital or extended-care setting, patients sometimes share bathroom facilities with a roommate. In addition, chronic illness may limit a patient's mobility and activity tolerance and require the use of a bedpan or bedside commode. The sights, sounds, and odors associated with sharing toilet facilities or using bedpans are often embarrassing. This embarrassment often causes patients to ignore the urge to defecate, which leads to constipation and discomfort. Remain sensitive to patients' elimination needs, and intervene to help them maintain bowel elimination habits that are as normal as possible.

Cathartics and Laxatives. Some medications initiate and facilitate stool passage. Laxatives and cathartics have the short-term action of emptying the bowel. These agents are also used to cleanse the bowel for patients undergoing GI tests and abdominal surgery. Although the terms *laxative* and *cathartic* are often used interchangeably, cathartics generally have a stronger and more rapid effect on the intestines. Teach patients about the potential harmful effects of overuse of laxatives such as impaired bowel motility and decreased response to sensory stimulus. Make sure patients understand that laxatives are not to be used long term for maintenance of bowel function.

Although patients usually take medications orally, laxatives prepared as suppositories may act more quickly because of their stimulant

CONCEPT MAP

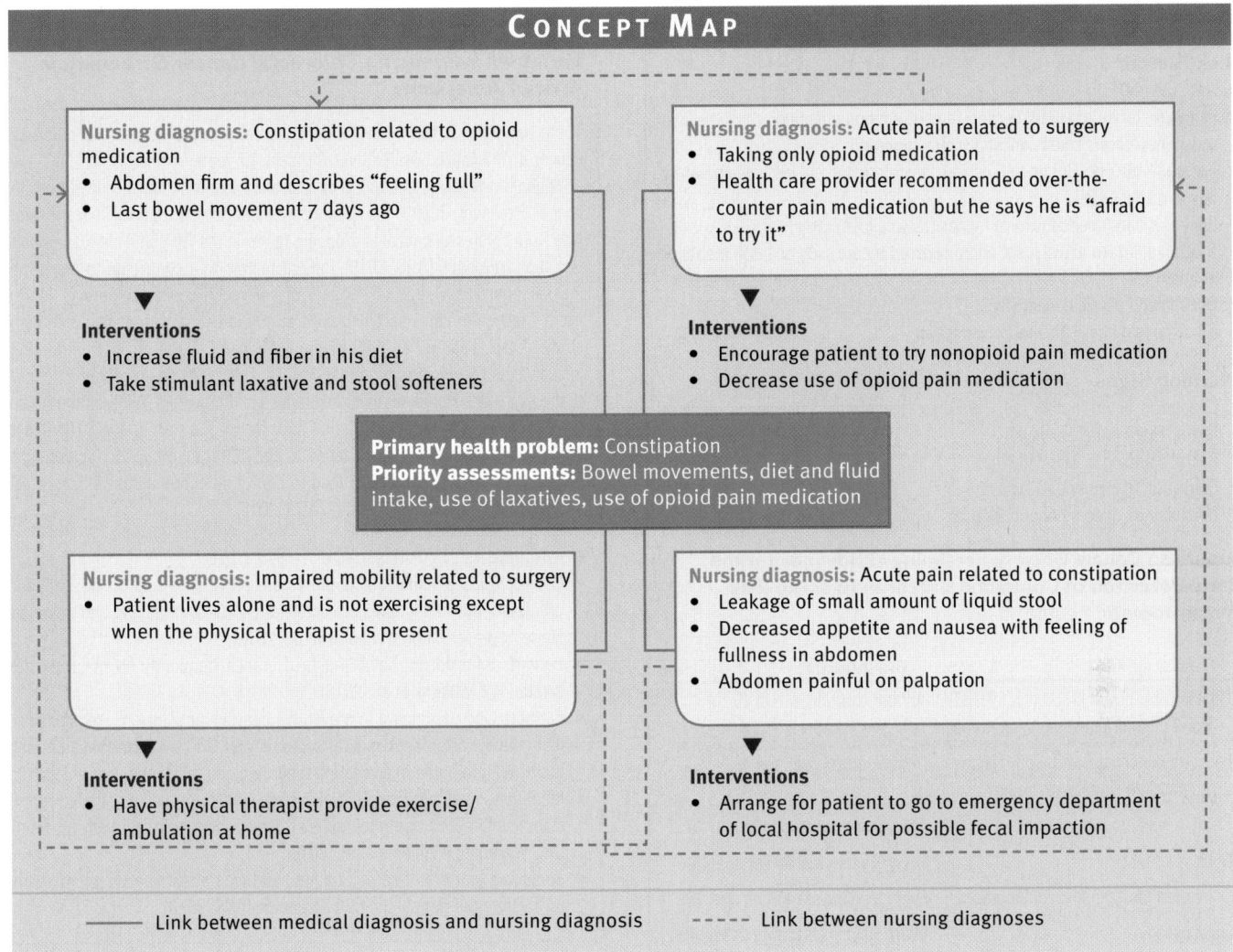

Nursing diagnosis: Constipation related to opioid medication
- Abdomen firm and describes "feeling full"
- Last bowel movement 7 days ago

Interventions
- Increase fluid and fiber in his diet
- Take stimulant laxative and stool softeners

Nursing diagnosis: Acute pain related to surgery
- Taking only opioid medication
- Health care provider recommended over-the-counter pain medication but he says he is "afraid to try it"

Interventions
- Encourage patient to try nonopioid pain medication
- Decrease use of opioid pain medication

Primary health problem: Constipation
Priority assessments: Bowel movements, diet and fluid intake, use of laxatives, use of opioid pain medication

Nursing diagnosis: Impaired mobility related to surgery
- Patient lives alone and is not exercising except when the physical therapist is present

Interventions
- Have physical therapist provide exercise/ambulation at home

Nursing diagnosis: Acute pain related to constipation
- Leakage of small amount of liquid stool
- Decreased appetite and nausea with feeling of fullness in abdomen
- Abdomen painful on palpation

Interventions
- Arrange for patient to go to emergency department of local hospital for possible fecal impaction

——— Link between medical diagnosis and nursing diagnosis   - - - - - Link between nursing diagnoses

FIG. 47.8 Concept map for Mr. Johnson.

effect on the rectal mucosa. Suppositories such as bisacodyl act within 30 minutes. Give the suppository shortly before a patient's usual time to defecate or immediately after a meal.

Laxatives are classified by the method by which the agent promotes defecation (Table 47.2). Some newer drugs are being used now for chronic constipation or motility disorders. It is too soon to tell whether these medications will be effective and safe for long-term treatment, but they are not used for the relief of occasional constipation.

Antidiarrheal Agents. Antidiarrheal agents decrease intestinal muscle tone to slow the passage of feces. As a result, the body absorbs more water through the intestinal walls. However, the cause of diarrhea must be determined before effective treatment can be ordered by a health care provider. For example, if an infection is the causative factor, an antibiotic may be used for treatment; if inflammation is the cause, steroids may be given. The most commonly used antidiarrheal agents are loperamide or diphenoxylate with atropine. Codeine or tincture of opium may be used for management of chronic severe diarrhea in patients with diseases such as Crohn's disease, ulcerative colitis, and acquired immunodeficiency syndrome (AIDS). Patients need to use antidiarrheal agents that contain opiates with caution because opiates are habit forming.

Enemas. An enema is the instillation of a solution into the rectum and sigmoid colon. The primary reason for an enema is to promote defecation by stimulating peristalsis. The volume of fluid instilled breaks up the fecal mass, stretches the rectal wall, and initiates the defecation reflex. Enemas are also a vehicle for medications that exert a local effect on rectal mucosa. They are used most commonly for the immediate relief of constipation, emptying the bowel before diagnostic tests or surgery, and beginning a program of bowel training.

Cleansing Enemas. Cleansing enemas promote the complete evacuation of feces from the colon. They act by stimulating peristalsis through the infusion of a large volume of solution or through local irritation of the mucosa of the colon. They include tap water, normal saline, soapsuds solution, and low-volume hypertonic saline. Each solution has a different osmotic effect, influencing the movement of fluids between the colon and interstitial spaces beyond the intestinal wall. Infants and children receive only normal saline because they are at greater risk for fluid imbalance.

Tap Water. Tap water is hypotonic and exerts an osmotic pressure lower than fluid in interstitial spaces. After infusion into the colon, tap water escapes from the bowel lumen into interstitial spaces. The net movement of water is low. The infused volume stimulates defecation before large amounts of water leave the bowel. Use caution if ordered to repeat tap-water enemas because water toxicity or circulatory overload develops if the body absorbs large amounts of water.

BOX 47.7   Screening for Colorectal Cancer

Risk Factors
- Age: Over 50
- Family history: Colorectal cancer, familial adenomatous polyposis, hereditary nonpolyposis colon cancer (Lynch syndrome)
- Personal history: Colorectal cancer or colorectal polyps, inflammatory bowel disease (IBD)
- Race: African Americans have highest colon cancer rates
- Diet: High intake of red meat and processed meats such as lunch meats or hot dogs
- Obesity and physical inactivity
- Smoking and heavy alcohol consumption

Warning Signs
- Change in bowel habits (e.g., diarrhea, constipation, narrowing of stool lasting more than few days)
- Rectal bleeding or blood in stool
- Sensation of incomplete evacuation
- Unexplained abdominal or back pain

American Cancer Society Screening Guidelines for the Early Detection of Colorectal Cancer in Average-Risk Asymptomatic People

Test	Frequency
Guaiac fecal occult blood test (gFOBT) done on multiple samples at home	Annual, starting at age 45
Fecal immunochemical test (FIT) done on multiple samples at home	Annual, starting at age 45
Flexible sigmoidoscopy	Every 5 years, starting at age 45
DNA stool test	Every 3 years starting at age 45
Computed tomography, colonography	Every 5 years, starting at age 45
Colonoscopy	Every 10 years, starting at age 45

These procedures will be ordered by a health care provider, depending on availability of resources and patient needs. If positive findings result from the flexible sigmoidoscopy or colonography, follow-up with a colonoscopy should be done. Those with higher risk of colorectal cancer due to personal or family history may be advised to have earlier or more frequent screening.

Data from American Cancer Society, 2018, www.cancer.gov.

🌐 BOX 47.8   CULTURAL ASPECTS OF CARE

Variables Influencing Colorectal Cancer Screening in African Americans

There has been a decline in the incidence and mortality rates for colorectal cancer in the United States over the past 10 years. African Americans have a higher incidence of colorectal cancer and have a higher of death from the cancer. However, in 2019 the American Cancer Society reported that the death rate from colorectal cancer is dropping faster in the African-American population than in whites (ACS, 2019). Patient factors that contribute to disparities include poor knowledge of benefits of colorectal cancer screening, limited access to health care, and insurance status, along with fear and anxiety. A study of this disparity in 2005 by the American College of Gastroenterology included the recommendation that African Americans begin cancer screening at the age of 45. However, most insurances and providers followed the American Cancer Society recommendation for screening to start at age 50 (Williams et al., 2016). With the recent change to age 45 for all groups for screening to begin, it is hoped that this will lead to earlier detection across all racial and ethnic groups in the United States (ACS, 2018).

Implications for Patient-Centered Care
- Lack of routine visits to a primary care provider is one of the strongest predictors for inadequate colorectal cancer (CRC) screening and advanced stage at presentation (Williams et al., 2016).
- Patients who do not have health insurance frequently do not seek CRC screening (Williams et al., 2016).
- Patients who participate in preventive health practices (e.g., regular physical activity) often seek regular screening for CRC because these patients are often interested in promoting their own health (Williams et al., 2016).
- Identification of additional social system predictors such as family support, church affiliation, and geographical access also help in receiving timely CRC screening (Williams et al., 2016).
- Removing barriers of safety, quality, and cost-effectiveness improves the involvement of patients in CRC screening (ACS, 2018).

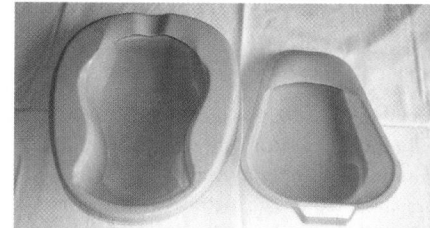

FIG. 47.9 Types of bedpans. From left, regular bedpan and fracture bedpan.

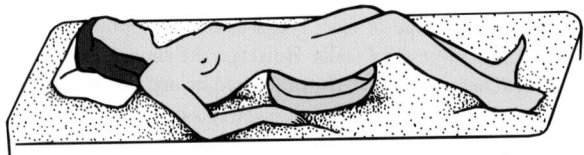

FIG. 47.10 Improper positioning of patient on bedpan.

Normal Saline. Physiologically normal saline is the safest solution to use because it exerts the same osmotic pressure as fluids in interstitial spaces surrounding the bowel. The volume of infused saline stimulates peristalsis. Giving saline enemas lessens the danger of excess fluid absorption.

Hypertonic Solutions. Hypertonic solutions infused into the bowel exert osmotic pressure that pulls fluids out of interstitial spaces. The colon fills with fluid, and the resultant distention promotes defecation. Patients unable to tolerate large volumes of fluid benefit most from this type of enema, which is by design low volume. This type of enema is contraindicated for patients who are dehydrated and young infants. A hypertonic solution of 120 to 180 mL (4 to 6 ounces) is usually effective. The commercially prepared Fleet enema is the most common.

Soapsuds. You add soapsuds to tap water or saline to create the effect of intestinal irritation to stimulate peristalsis. Use only pure castile soap that comes in a liquid form, included in most soapsuds enema kits. Use soapsuds enemas with caution in pregnant women and older adults because they could cause electrolyte imbalance or damage to the intestinal mucosa.

A health care provider sometimes orders a high- or low-cleansing enema. The terms *high* and *low* refer to the height from which, and hence the pressure with which, the fluid is delivered. High enemas

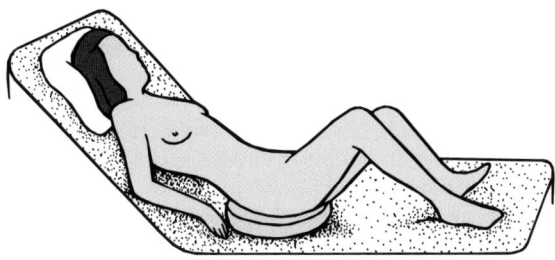

FIG. 47.11 Proper position reduces patient's back strain.

cleanse more of the colon. After the enema is infused, ask the patient to turn from the left lateral to the dorsal recumbent, over to the right lateral position. The position change ensures that fluid reaches the large intestine. A low enema cleanses only the rectum and sigmoid colon.

Oil Retention. Oil-retention enemas lubricate the feces in the rectum and colon. The feces absorb the oil and become softer and easier to pass. To enhance action of the oil, the patient retains the enema for several hours if possible.

Other Types of Enemas. Carminative enemas provide relief from gaseous distention. They improve the ability to pass flatus. An example

---

BOX 47.9 PROCEDURAL GUIDELINES

Assisting Patient On and Off a Bedpan

Delegation and Collaboration

The skill of providing a bedpan can be delegated to assistive personnel (AP). The nurse instructs the AP to:

- Correctly position patients with mobility restrictions or those who have therapeutic equipment such as wound drains, intravenous (IV) catheters, or traction.
- Provide perineal and hand hygiene for patient as necessary after using a bedpan.

Equipment

Clean gloves; bedpan (regular or fracture) (Fig. 47.9); bedpan cover; toilet tissue or premoisturized perineal wipes; specimen container (if necessary); plastic bag clearly labeled with date, patient's name, and identification number; basin; washcloths; towels; soap; waterproof, absorbent pads (if necessary); clean drawsheet (if necessary); stethoscope.

Steps

1. Assess patient's normal bowel elimination habits: routine pattern, character of stool, effect of certain foods/fluids and eating habits on bowel elimination patterns, effect of stress and level of activity on normal bowel elimination patterns, current medications, and normal fluid intake.
2. Determine need for stool specimen before bedpan use
3. Perform hand hygiene

CLINICAL DECISION: If patient is postoperative or has a gastrointestinal illness, auscultate for bowel sounds and palpate abdomen for distention.

4. Assess patient to determine level of mobility, including ability to sit upright and lift hips or turn.
5. Assess patient's level of comfort. Ask about presence of rectal or abdominal pain, presence of hemorrhoids, or irritation of skin surrounding anus.
6. Apply clean gloves. Inspect condition of perianal and perineal skin. Remove and dispose of gloves and perform hand hygiene.
7. For patient comfort prepare metal bedpan by running warm water over it for a few minutes.

CLINICAL DECISION: Use a fracture pan if the patient had a total hip replacement. An abduction pillow must be placed between the legs when turning patient to prevent dislocation of new joint.

8. Provide privacy by closing curtains around bed or door of room.
9. Raise side rail on opposite side of bed.
10. Raise bed horizontally according to your height.
11. Assist patient to the supine position.
12. Place patient who can assist on bedpan.
    a. Perform hand hygiene and apply clean gloves. Raise head of patient's bed 30 to 60 degrees.
    b. Remove upper bed linens so that they are out of the way but do not expose patient.
    c. Have patient flex knees and lift hips upward.

d. Place hand closest to patient's head palm up under patient's sacrum to help lift. Ask patient to bend knees and raise hips. As patient raises hips, use other hand to slip bedpan under him or her (see illustration). Be sure that open rim of bedpan is facing toward foot of bed. Do not force pan under patient's hips (see Fig. 47.11). (*Optional:* Have patient use overhead trapeze frame to raise hips.)

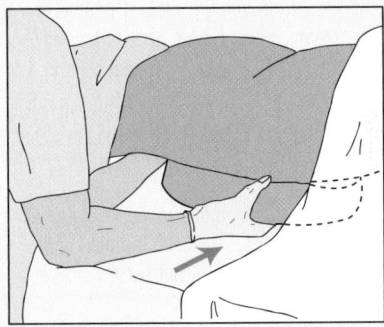

STEP 12d Placing bedpan under patient's hips.

e. *Optional:* If using fracture pan, slip it under patient as hips are raised (see illustration). Be sure that deep, open, lower end of bedpan is facing toward foot of bed.

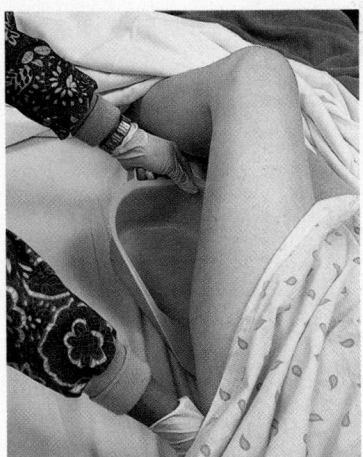

STEP 12e Patient lifts hips as fracture pan is positioned.

13. Place patient who is immobile or has mobility restrictions on bedpan.
    a. Perform hand hygiene and apply clean gloves. Lower head of bed flat or raise head slightly (if tolerated by medical condition).
    b. Remove top linens as necessary to turn patient while minimizing exposure.
    c. Assist patient to roll onto side with back toward you. Place bedpan firmly against patient's buttocks and down into mattress. Be sure that open rim of bedpan is facing toward foot of bed (see illustrations).

Continued

BOX 47.9   PROCEDURAL GUIDELINES—cont'd

Assisting Patient On and Off a Bedpan

   d. Keep one hand against bedpan; place other around far hip of patient. Assist patient to roll back onto bedpan, flat in bed. Do not force pan under patient.

   e. Raise patient's head 30 degrees or to a comfortable level (unless contraindicated).

   f. Have patient bend knees (unless contraindicated).

14. Maintain patient's comfort, privacy, and safety. Cover patient for warmth. Place small pillow or rolled towel under lumbar curve of back. Leave room but stay close by.

15. Place nurse call system and toilet tissue within reach for patient.

16. Ensure that bed is in lowest position and raise upper side rails.

17. Remove and discard gloves and perform hand hygiene.

18. Allow patient to be alone, but monitor status and respond promptly.

19. Perform hand hygiene and apply clean gloves.

20. Remove bedpan:

   a. Perform hand hygiene and apply clean gloves. Place patient's bedside chair close to working side of bed.

   b. Maintain privacy; determine if patient is able to wipe own perineal area. If you clean perineal area, apply clean gloves and use several layers of toilet tissue or disposable washcloths. For female patients clean from mons pubis toward rectal area.

   c. Deposit contaminated tissue in bedpan if no specimen or intake and output (I&O) is needed. Remove and dispose of gloves and perform hand hygiene.

   d. **For mobile patient:** Ask patient to flex knees, placing body weight on lower legs, feet, and upper torso; lift buttocks up from bedpan. At same time place hand farthest from patient on side of bedpan to support

it (prevent spillage) and place other hand (closest to patient) under sacrum to help lift. Have patient lift and remove bedpan. Place bedpan on draped bedside chair and cover.

   e. **For immobile patient:** Apply clean gloves. Lower head of bed. Help patient roll onto side away from you and off bedpan. Hold bedpan flat and steady while patient is rolling off; otherwise spillage will occur. Place bedpan on draped bedside chair and cover.

   f. Assist patient with hand and perineal hygiene as needed.

21. Change soiled linens, remove and dispose of gloves, and return patient to comfortable position.

22. Place bed in its lowest position. Ensure that nurse call system, drinking water, and desired personal items (e.g., books) are within easy access *Option:* Obtain stool specimen as ordered. Wear clean gloves when emptying contents of bedpan into toilet or in special receptacle in utility room. Use spray faucet attached to most institution toilets to rinse bedpan thoroughly. Use disinfectant if required by agency; store pan. Remove and dispose of gloves.

23. Perform hand hygiene and apply clean gloves. Assess characteristics of stool. Note color, odor, consistency, frequency, amount, shape, and constituents. Assess characteristics of urine if patient voided in bedpan.

24. Evaluate patient's ability to use bedpan.

25. Inspect patient's perianal area and surrounding skin while removing bedpan.

26. **Use Teach-Back:** "Since your leg is immobilized, I want to make sure you're comfortable getting off and on the bedpan by using the trapeze to pull your torso off the bed. Show me how you use the trapeze to move your torso." Revise your instruction now or develop a plan for revised patient/family caregiver teaching if patient/family caregiver is not able to teach back correctly.

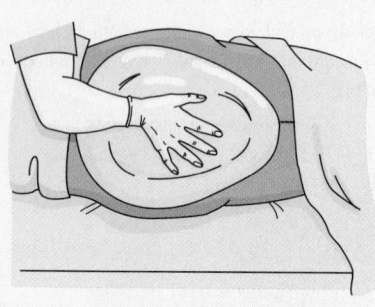
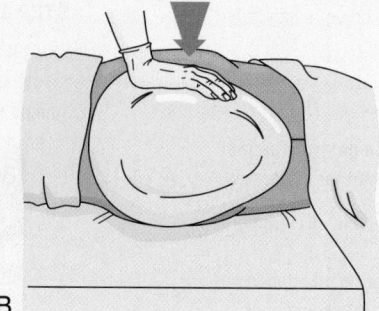
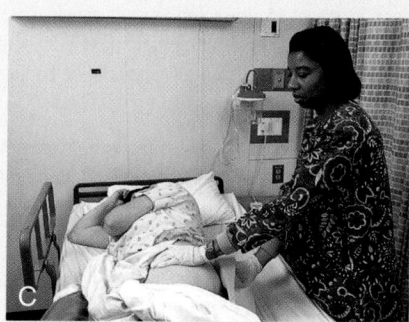

STEP 13c A, Position patient on one side and place bedpan firmly against buttocks. B, Push down on bedpan and toward patient. C, Nurse places bedpan in position. (A and B from Sorrentino SA, Remmert LA: *Mosby's textbook for nursing assistants*, ed 9, St Louis, 2017, Elsevier.)

of a carminative enema is MGW solution, which contains 30 mL of magnesium, 60 mL of glycerin, and 90 mL of water.

   Medicated enemas contain drugs. An example is sodium polystyrene sulfonate (Kayexalate), used to treat patients with dangerously high serum potassium levels. This drug contains a resin that exchanges sodium ions for potassium ions in the large intestine. Another medicated enema is neomycin solution, an antibiotic used to reduce bacteria

in the colon before bowel surgery. An enema containing steroid medication may be used for acute inflammation in the lower colon.

   Enema Administration. Enemas are available in commercially packaged, disposable units or with reusable equipment prepared before use. Sterile technique is unnecessary because the colon normally contains bacteria. However, wear gloves to prevent the transmission of fecal microorganisms.

TABLE 47.2 Common Types of Laxatives and Cathartics

Agent/Brand Name	Action	Indications	Risks
Bulk Forming Methylcellulose (Citrucel) Psyllium (Metamucil, Naturacil) Polycarbophil (Fibercon)	High-fiber content absorbs water and increases solid intestinal bulk, which will stretch intestinal wall to stimulate peristalsis. Passage of stool will occur in 12 to 24 hours. These agents must be taken with water and should be used with patients who have an adequate food and fluid intake. Patients may note increased gas formation and flatus when they first start taking these laxatives, but this will abate after 4-5 days.	Agents are least irritating, most natural, and safest type of laxatives. Agents are drugs of choice for chronic constipation (e.g., pregnancy, low-residue diet). They also relieve mild diarrhea. If treating diarrhea, administer less water.	Agents that are in powder form could cause constipation if not mixed with at least 240 mL of water or juice and swallowed quickly. Caution is necessary with bulk-forming laxatives that also contain stimulants. Agents are not for patients for whom large fluid intake is contraindicated.
Emollient or Wetting Docusate sodium (Colace) Docusate calcium (Surfak) Docusate potassium (Dialose)	Stool softeners are detergents that lower surface tension of feces, allowing water and fat to penetrate. They increase secretion of water by intestine.	Agents are for short-term therapy to relieve straining on defecation (e.g., hemorrhoids, perianal surgery, pregnancy, recovery from myocardial infarction).	Agents are of little value for treatment of chronic constipation.
Osmotic Saline-based Magnesium citrate or citrate of magnesia Magnesium hydroxide (Milk of Magnesia) Sodium phosphate (Fleet Phospho-Soda) Polyethylene glycol, lactulose, sorbitol based, Lactulose, Miralax	Osmotic effect increases pressure in bowel to act as stimulant for peristalsis. Osmotic laxatives are any agents that pull fluid into the bowel to soften the stool and distend the bowel to stimulate peristalsis.	Saline-based agents are only for acute emptying of bowel (e.g., endoscopic examination, suspected poisoning, acute constipation). Agents may be used to treat chronic constipation.	Saline-based agents are not for long-term management of constipation or for patients with kidney dysfunction. They may cause toxic buildup of magnesium. Phosphate salts are not recommended for patients on fluid restriction.
Stimulant Cathartics Bisacodyl (Dulcolax) Castor oil Casanthranol (Peri-Colace) Correctol Senna (Ex-Lax, Senokot)	Agents cause local irritation to the intestinal mucosa, increase intestinal motility, and inhibit resorption of water in the large intestine. The rapid movement of feces causes retention of water in the stool. The drugs cause formation of a soft-to-liquid stool in 6 to 8 hours and usually contain bisacodyl or senna. These laxatives should be used occasionally because regular use of a stimulant laxative can lead to dependence on the stimulus for defecation.	Agents prepare bowel for diagnostic procedures or may be needed for those with constipation from frequent opioid use	Agents cause severe cramping. Agents are not for long-term use. Chronic use could cause fluid and electrolyte imbalances.

Explain the procedure, including the position to assume, precautions to take to avoid discomfort, and length of time necessary to retain the solution before defecation. If a patient needs to take the enema at home, explain the procedure to a family member.

Giving an enema to a patient who is unable to contract the external sphincter poses difficulties. Give the enema with the patient positioned on the bedpan. Giving the enema with a patient sitting on the toilet is unsafe because the position of the rectal tubing could injure the rectal wall. Skill 47.1 outlines the steps for an enema administration.

Digital Removal of Stool. For a patient with an impaction, the fecal mass is sometimes too large to pass voluntarily. If a digital rectal examination reveals a hard stool mass in the rectum, it may be necessary to manually remove it by breaking it up and bringing out a section at a time. Digital removal is the last resort in the management of severe constipation, but it may be necessary if the fecal mass is too large to pass through the anal canal. The procedure (Box 47.10) is very uncomfortable

for the patient. Excess rectal manipulation causes irritation to the mucosa, bleeding, and stimulation of the vagus nerve, which sometimes results in a reflex slowing of the heart rate (Hussain et al., 2014).

Inserting and Maintaining a Nasogastric Tube. A patient's condition or situation sometimes requires special interventions to decompress the GI tract. Such conditions include surgery (see Chapter 50), obstruction of the GI tract often caused by tumors, trauma to the GI tract, and conditions in which peristalsis is absent.

A nasogastric (NG) tube is a pliable hollow tube that is inserted through the patient's nasopharynx into the stomach. NG intubation has several purposes (Table 47.3). There are two main categories of NG tubes: fine- or small-bore tubes and large-bore tubes. Small-bore tubes are frequently used for medication administration and enteral feedings (see Chapter 45 for enteral feedings). Large-bore tubes, 12-Fr and above, are usually used for gastric decompression or removal of gastric secretions. The Levin and Salem sump tubes are the most common for

BOX 47.10   PROCEDURAL GUIDELINES

Digital Removal of Stool

Delegation and Collaboration

The skill of digitally removing stool cannot be delegated to assistive personnel (AP). In some institutions only health care providers perform this procedure. The nurse instructs the AP:

- To provide perineal care and other necessary hygiene following each bowel movement.
- To observe any evacuated stool for color and consistency.

Equipment

Bedpan, waterproof pad, water-soluble lubricant, washcloths, towels, soap, and clean gloves

Steps

1. Identify patient using at least two identifiers (e.g., name and birthday or name and medical record number) according to agency policy.
2. Perform hand hygiene, pull curtains around bed, obtain patient's baseline vital signs and assess level of comfort, auscultate bowel sounds, and palpate for abdominal distention before the procedure.
3. Explain the procedure and help patient lie on left side in Sims' position with knees flexed and back toward you.
4. Drape trunk and lower extremities with a bath blanket and place a waterproof pad under buttocks. Keep a bedpan next to patient.
5. Perform hand hygiene and apply clean gloves; lubricate index finger of dominant hand with water-soluble lubricant.
6. Instruct patient to take slow, deep breaths. Gradually and gently insert index finger into the rectum and advance the finger slowly along the rectal wall.
7. Gently loosen the fecal mass by massaging around it. Work the finger into the hardened mass.
8. Work the feces downward toward the end of the rectum. Remove small pieces one at a time and discard into bedpan.
9. Periodically reassess patient's pulse and level of comfort and look for signs of fatigue. Stop the procedure if pulse rate drops significantly (check agency policy) or rhythm changes.
10. Continue to clear rectum of feces and allow patient to rest at intervals.
11. After completion, wash and dry buttocks and anal area.
12. Remove bedpan; inspect feces for color and consistency. Dispose of feces. Remove gloves by turning them inside out and then discard.
13. Help patient to toilet or on a bedpan if urge to defecate develops.
14. Perform hand hygiene. Record results of procedure by describing fecal characteristics and amount.
15. Follow procedure with enemas or cathartics as ordered by health care provider.
16. Reassess patient's vital signs and level of comfort, auscultate bowel sounds, and observe status of abdominal distention.

stomach decompression. The Levin tube is a single-lumen tube with holes near the tip. It is connected to a drainage bag or an intermittent suction device to drain stomach secretions.

The Salem sump tube is preferable for stomach decompression. The tube has two lumina: one for removal of gastric contents and one to provide an air vent. A blue "pigtail" is the air vent that connects with the second lumen. When the main lumen of the sump tube is connected to suction, the air vent permits free, continuous drainage of secretions. Do not clamp off the air vent if the tube is connected to suction.

NG tube insertion does not require sterile technique. Instead you use clean technique. The procedure is uncomfortable. Patients experience a burning sensation as the tube passes through the sensitive nasal mucosa. When it reaches the back of the pharynx, patients sometimes begin to gag. Help them relax to make tube insertion easier. Some institutions allow the use of Xylocaine jelly or atomized lidocaine when inserting the tube because it decreases patient discomfort during the procedure. The procedure for inserting an NG tube is described in Skill 47.2.

One of the greatest problems in caring for a patient with a NG tube is to maintain comfort. Because the tube irritates the nasal and pharyngeal mucosa, you assess the condition of the patient's nares and throat for inflammation. The tape or fixation device used to anchor the tube often becomes soiled or loosened. Change it as needed to prevent migration of the tube. Frequent lubrication of the nares may minimize discomfort. With one nostril occluded, the patient breathes through the mouth. Frequent mouth care helps minimize discomfort from a dry mouth. Water-moistened swabs or lozenges for the patient to suck may provide some relief of mouth and throat dryness. Often patients complain of a sore throat. A health care provider may order gargles with topical Xylocaine jelly to minimize the irritation.

After you insert the tube, you need to maintain its patency. Sometimes the tip of the tubing rests against the stomach wall, or the tube becomes blocked with thick secretions. Flushing the tube regularly with a catheter-tipped syringe filled with normal saline or warm water helps to prevent blockage of the tube. If an NG tube does not drain properly after flushing, reposition it by advancing or withdrawing it slightly. A change in tube position could require physician-ordered imaging to verify correct placement in the patient's GI tract. Consult agency policy and/or provider preferences as necessary.

Continuing and Restorative Care. Regular elimination patterns should begin before a patient goes home or to an extended-care setting. With a new ostomy, a patient or a caregiver needs to learn to manage the care that is required (Box 47.11). Other patients require bowel retraining. It is important to remember that you initiate ostomy care and bowel retraining in acute care settings. However, because these are long-term care needs, teaching usually continues in restorative care or home settings.

Care of Ostomies. Patients with temporary or permanent bowel diversions have unique elimination needs. An individual with an ostomy wears a pouch to collect effluent or output from the stoma. The pouches are odor-proof and have a protective skin barrier surrounding the stoma. Empty the pouch when it is one-third to one-half full. Change the pouching system approximately every 3 to 7 days, depending on a patient's individual needs (Goldberg et al., 2017). Assess the stoma color. It should be pink or red. You observe the skin at each pouch change for signs of irritation or skin breakdown. Skin protection is important because the effluent has digestive enzymes that cause irritant dermatitis if there is leakage on the peristomal skin. Other peristomal skin problems are fungal rashes, folliculitis, or ulcerations. Refer patients with these problems to an ostomy care nurse (Goldberg et al., 2017) (Box 47.12).

Irrigating a Colostomy. Although this practice is not as common because of improved odor-proof pouches, some patients irrigate their sigmoid colostomies to regulate colon emptying. This process takes about an hour a day to complete but usually means that a patient wears only a mini-pouch afterward to absorb mucus from the stoma and contain gas. Specific equipment designed for ostomies is used. The equipment has a silicone cone attached by plastic tubing to a bag that will hold the irrigation fluid, which is usually warm water. Follow the routine that the patient has established for this care. Occasionally a patient with a colostomy who has constipation will have an irrigation or enema ordered. Use equipment that is designed specifically for the irrigation rather than an enema administration set used by patients without a stoma.

TABLE 47.3 Purposes of Nasogastric Intubation

Purpose	Description	Type of Tube
Decompression	Removal of secretions and gaseous substances from gastrointestinal (GI) tract; prevention or relief of abdominal distention (Harding et al., 2017)	Salem sump, Levin, Miller-Abbott
Enteral feeding (see Chapter 45)	Instillation of liquid nutritional supplements or feedings into stomach or small intestine for patients with impaired swallowing (Harding et al., 2017)	Duo, Dobhoff, Levin
Compression	Internal application of pressure by means of inflated balloon to prevent internal esophageal or GI hemorrhage (Harding et al., 2017)	Sengstaken-Blakemore
Lavage	Irrigation of stomach in cases of active bleeding, poisoning, or gastric dilation (Harding et al., 2017)	Levin, Ewald, Salem sump

---

BOX 47.11 PATIENT TEACHING
Teaching Patients How to Provide Ostomy Care

Objective
- Patient/caregiver will demonstrate how to empty and change an ostomy pouch.

Teaching Strategies
- Provide a comprehensive list of the products needed to care for the ostomy (Prinz et al., 2015)
- Provide patient/caregiver with supplies to last 1 to 2 weeks and the contact number information for a medical supply company (Prinz et al., 2015).
- Show patient/caregiver the step-by-step approach for changing an ostomy pouch.
- Provide at least one opportunity for patient/caregiver to empty and change the ostomy pouch while patient is in the hospital (Prinz et al., 2015).
- Provide detailed instructions for diet and fluids; peristomal skin care; restrictions on lifting; resuming exercise and intimacy; and when to contact the health care provider (Prinz et al., 2015).
- Arrange follow-up with an ostomy nurse if possible.

Evaluation
Use the principles of teach-back to evaluate patient/family caregiver learning:
- Show me how you change your ostomy pouch.
- Tell me three important points about your diet and fluid intake that you need to follow now that you have an ostomy.

BOX 47.12 EVIDENCE-BASED PRACTICE
Recognition of Peristomal Skin Problems

PICOT Question: In patients with ostomies, what is the effect of patient education and knowledge on the prevention of peristomal skin breakdown?

Evidence Summary
Patients with an ostomy are at risk for development of peristomal skin problems. Studies show that 23% to 45% of persons with ileostomies and 7% to 20% of persons with colostomies will develop peristomal skin complications (Steinhagen et al., 2017). Maintenance of healthy peristomal skin, with the skin around the stoma being clean, dry, and intact, is a priority following ostomy surgery (Goldberg et al., 2017). The most common cause of peristomal skin disorders is effluent, which causes skin irritation, ulceration, or erosion. Reasons for effluent leakage include poor-fitting stoma pouches, poor adhesive adherence, peristomal hernia, and surgical complications (Burch, 2017). With shorter postoperative hospital stays, it is challenging for nurses to provide the extensive patient education on pouching systems, ostomy care, and problem-solving techniques needed to prevent peristomal skin problems (Goldberg et al., 2017). Patients often failed to recognize early signs of skin irritation and did not report a skin problem (Steinhagen et al., 2017). This lack of knowledge resulted in delays in patients seeking health care to treat the skin problem. Patient education is an important factor in preventing complications following ostomy surgery. Nurses need to provide education to patients before discharge and follow up with them after discharge to prevent peristomal skin problems (Prinz et al., 2015).

Application to Nursing Practice
- Evaluate patients' knowledge and ability to assess their peristomal skin changes for early recognition and treatment of skin disorders.
- Provide patient education about signs and symptoms of skin disorders to ensure early identification of skin problems.
- Refer patients to an ostomy nurse if assistance is needed to manage the ostomy (Goldberg et al., 2017).

Pouching Ostomies. An ostomy requires a pouch to collect fecal material. An effective pouching system protects the skin, contains fecal material, remains odor free, and is comfortable and inconspicuous. A person wearing a pouch needs to feel secure enough to participate in any activity (Goldberg et al., 2017).

Many pouching systems are available. To ensure that a pouch fits well and meets a patient's needs, consider the location of the ostomy, type and size of the stoma, type and amount of ostomy drainage, size and contour of the abdomen, condition of the skin around the stoma, physical activities of the patient, patient's personal preference, age and dexterity, and cost of equipment. A **wound, ostomy, and continence nurse (WOCN)** is a nurse specially educated to care for ostomy patients. A WOCN collaborates with staff nurses and patients to be sure that the patients have the best pouching system for their individual needs. A pouching system consists of a pouch and skin barrier (Fig. 47.12). Pouches come in one- and two-piece systems and are flat or convex. Some pouches have the opening precut by the manufacturer; others require the stoma opening to be custom cut to a patient's specific stoma size. Newer pouches have an integrated closure; older ones use a clip to close the pouch. One of the first skills to teach a patient with a new ostomy is how to open and close the pouch. Skill 47.3 describes steps for applying an ostomy pouch.

Nutritional Considerations. After surgery it usually takes a few days for patients with new ostomies to feel that their appetite has returned

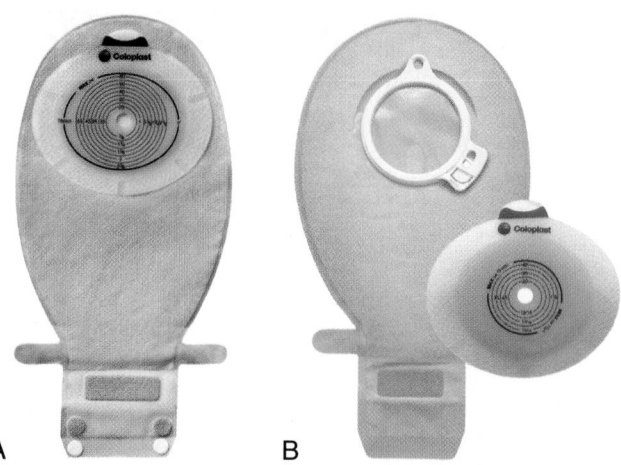

FIG. 47.12 Ostomy pouches and skin barriers. **A**, One-piece pouch with Velcro closure. **B**, Two-piece pouching system with separate skin barrier and attachable pouch. **NOTE:** Skin barriers need to be custom cut according to stoma size. (Courtesy Coloplast, Minneapolis, MN.)

to normal. Small servings of soft foods are typically more appetizing, as they would be for any patient who has had an abdominal surgery.

Patients with colostomies have no diet restrictions other than the diet discussed for normal healthy bowel function, with adequate fiber and fluid to keep the stool softly formed. Patients with ileostomies digest their food completely but lose both fluid and salt through their stoma and need to be sure to replace this to avoid dehydration. A good reminder for patients is to encourage drinking an 8-ounce glass of fluid when they empty their pouch. This helps them remember that they have greater fluid needs than they did before having an ileostomy. A condition that occurs infrequently with people with ileostomies is called a *food blockage*. Foods with indigestible fiber such as sweet corn, popcorn, raw mushrooms, fresh pineapple, and Chinese cabbage can cause this problem. However, if patients eat these foods in small quantities, drink fluids with the food, and chew it well, they are unlikely to experience any difficulty.

Psychological Considerations. After ostomy surgery patients face a variety of anxieties and concerns, from learning how to manage their stoma to coping with conflicts of self-esteem, body image, and sexuality. Provide emotional support before and after surgery (Goldberg et al., 2017). Adjustment to a stoma takes time and is a very individual matter. A study of patients with colorectal cancer and a colostomy showed that the lowest quality of life after ostomy surgery occurred at 2 months, with improvement at 6 months and return to almost preoperative levels at 12 months (Goldberg et al., 2017). Important factors affecting adjustment to the stoma include the ability to successfully assume care of the ostomy, including emptying the pouch and changing the pouching system so that unexpected odor and leakage of stool does not occur. Inability to resume self-care sometimes causes a loss of self-esteem. The aging process often affects the ability to manage stomas, even in people who have had them for years. You need to recognize and intervene when problems resulting from advanced age such as skin changes, weight loss or gain, visual impairments, or changes in diet occur. If possible, consult with an ostomy nurse. The Wound, Ostomy and Continence Nurses Society (http://www.wocn.org) provides information and helps patients locate a WOCN. Consider referral to local ostomy groups such as those affiliated with the United Ostomy Associations of America at http://www.ostomy.org.

BOX 47.13   FOCUS ON OLDER ADULTS
Bowel Retraining

- Older age is a risk factor for having constipation. Constipation affects people living in nursing homes, and between 50% and 74% of residents use laxatives (Blekken et al, 2016).
- Increase fiber in diet with whole grains, legumes, fruits, and vegetables.
- A minimum of 1500 mL of fluid per day reduces the risk of constipation, with increased fluid needs during summer months and for those on diuretics with stable cardiovascular status.
- If holding a drinking cup is a problem, consider using a lighter plastic cup and filling half full, refilling frequently.
- Encourage regular exercise within the limitations imposed by other conditions.
- Patients need to feel at ease during elimination. Lack of privacy leads a patient to ignore the urge to defecate.
- Review all medications with a patient's health care provider to substitute medications that are less likely to cause constipation whenever possible.
- Behavioral interventions such as timed toileting help establish a scheduled time for bowel elimination. Try to maintain the same schedule each day for toileting.

Bowel Training. A patient with chronic constipation or fecal incontinence secondary to cognitive impairment may benefit from bowel training, also called *habit training*. (NIH, 2018b) The training program involves setting up a daily routine. By attempting to defecate at the same time each day and using measures that promote defecation, a patient may establish a normal defecation pattern. The program requires time, patience, and consistency. A patient with cognitive impairment needs to have a caregiver able to devote the time to the training program. A successful program includes the following:

- Assessing the normal elimination pattern and recording times when a patient is incontinent
- Incorporating principles of gerontological nursing when providing bowel retraining programs for an older adult (Box 47.13)
- Choosing a time based on the patient's pattern to initiate defecation-control measures
- Offering a hot drink (hot tea) or fruit juice (prune juice) (or whatever fluids normally stimulate peristalsis for the patient) before the defecation time
- Helping the patient to the toilet at the designated time
- Providing privacy
- Instructing the patient to lean forward at the hips while sitting on the toilet, apply manual pressure with the hands over the abdomen, and bear down but not strain to stimulate colon emptying
- An unhurried environment and a nonjudgmental caregiver
- Maintaining normal exercise within the patient's physical ability

Maintenance of Proper Fluid and Food Intake. In choosing a diet for promoting normal elimination, consider the frequency of defecation, characteristics of feces, and types of foods that impair or promote defecation. A well-balanced diet with whole grains, legumes, fresh fruits, and vegetables eaten regularly promotes normal elimination. Fiber adds bulk to the stool, eliminates excess fluids, and promotes more frequent and regular movements. With increasing fiber, it is important to drink enough fluids. If fluid intake is inadequate, the stool becomes hard because less water is retained in the large intestine to soften it. The amount of fiber and fluids necessary for optimal bowel function varies among individuals. Consulting a registered dietitian may be helpful if a patient has chronic problems with constipation.

When a patient has diarrhea, low-residue foods such as white rice, potatoes, bread, bananas, and cooked cereals are recommended until the diarrhea is controlled. Discourage foods that typically cause gastric upset or abdominal cramping. Diarrhea caused by illness is sometimes debilitating. If the patient cannot tolerate foods or liquids orally, intravenous therapy with electrolyte replacement is necessary. The patient returns to a normal diet slowly, often beginning with fluids.

Promotion of Regular Exercise. A daily exercise program helps prevent elimination problems. Walking, riding a stationary bicycle, or swimming stimulates peristalsis. It is recommended by the American Heart Association and the Centers for Disease Control and Prevention that adults get at least 150 minutes of exercise each week.

For a patient temporarily immobilized, attempt ambulation as soon as possible. If the condition permits, help the patient walk to a chair on the evening of the day of surgery and encourage him or her to walk a little more each day.

Management of the Patient With Fecal Incontinence or Diarrhea. You may apply a fecal collector around the anal opening if the skin is intact. These can be difficult to apply when there is a deep fold between the buttocks and there is hair in the area, but it may be considered if a patient is having very frequent liquid stools. There are also fecal-management systems available for short-term use with high-volume diarrhea. They are intended for use primarily in acute care settings. The devices have an intra-anal soft silicone catheter with a retention balloon much like a Foley catheter for insertion into the rectal vault to divert liquid stool away from the skin in immobilized patients. The catheter is connected to a drainage bag for collection of the liquid fecal effluent. Refer to package insertion instructions and agency policies for appropriate use.

Maintenance of Skin Integrity. A patient with diarrhea, fecal incontinence, or an ileostomy is at risk for skin breakdown when fecal contents remain on the skin. Liquid stool usually contains digestive enzymes, which causes rapid skin breakdown. Irritation from repeated wiping with toilet tissue or frequent ostomy pouch changes further irritate the skin. Meticulous perianal skin care and frequent removal of fecal drainage is necessary to prevent skin breakdown (see Chapter 48). Clean the skin with a no-rinse cleanser and apply a barrier ointment after each episode of diarrhea. If a patient is incontinent, check on the patient frequently and change absorbent products immediately after providing thorough but gentle skin cleansing. Patients with ostomies are often unaware of the skin irritation under their ostomy wafer or think that this is a normal part of having an ostomy. Education about skin breakdown and its management are important roles for the ostomy nurse (see Box 47.12).

◆ Evaluation

Through the Patient's Eyes. The effectiveness of care depends on success in meeting the expected outcomes of self-care. Optimally a

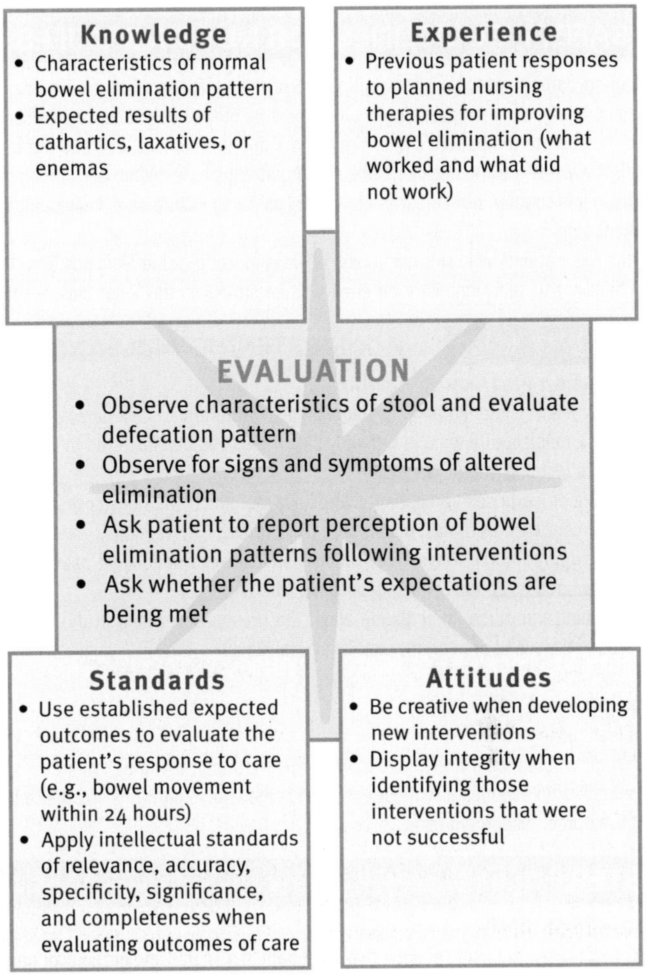

FIG. 47.13 Critical thinking model for elimination evaluation.

patient will be able to have regular, pain-free defecation of soft-formed stools. The patient or caregiver is the only one able to determine whether the bowel elimination problems have been relieved and which therapies were the most effective (Fig. 47.13).

Patient Outcomes. When you establish a therapeutic relationship with a patient, the patient feels comfortable to discuss the intimate details often associated with bowel elimination. Patients are less embarrassed as you help them with elimination needs. Patients relate feelings of comfort and freedom from pain as elimination needs are met within the limits of their condition and treatment. Evaluate a patient's level of knowledge regarding establishing a normal elimination pattern, caring for an ostomy, and promoting skin integrity. Also determine the extent to which the patient accomplishes normal defecation. Ask the patient to describe changes in diet, fluid intake, and activity to promote bowel health. Ask the following questions when the patient's expected outcome has not been achieved:

- Do you use medications such as laxatives or enemas to help you defecate? How often?
- Which barriers prevent you from eating a diet high in fiber and participating in regular exercise?
- How much fluid do you drink in a typical day? Which types of fluids do you normally drink?
- What challenges do you encounter when you change your ostomy pouch?

SAFETY GUIDELINES FOR NURSING SKILLS

Ensuring patient safety is an essential role of the professional nurse. To ensure patient safety, communicate clearly with members of the health care team, assess and incorporate the patient's priorities of care and preferences, and use the best evidence when making decisions about your patient's care. When performing the skills in this chapter, remember the following points to ensure safe, individualized, patient care:

- Instruct patients who self-administer enemas to use the side-lying position. Tell them not to self-administer an enema while sitting on the toilet because this position results in the rectal tubing causing friction that could injure the rectal wall

- If a patient has cardiac disease or is taking cardiac or hypertensive medication, obtain a pulse rate, because manipulation of rectal tissue stimulates the vagus nerve and sometimes causes a sudden decline in pulse rate, which increases the patient's risk of fainting while on the bedpan, bedside commode, or toilet

SKILL 47.1   ADMINISTERING A CLEANSING ENEMA

Delegation and Collaboration

The skill of administering an enema can be delegated to assistive personnel (AP). NOTE: If a medicated enema is ordered, then it must be administered by a nurse. The nurse instructs the AP about:

- How to properly position patients who have mobility restrictions or therapeutic equipment such as drains, intravenous (IV) catheters, or traction.
- Informing the nurse immediately about patient's new abdominal pain (*exception:* a patient reports cramping) or rectal bleeding.
- Informing the nurse immediately about the presence of blood in the stool or around the rectal area or any change in vital signs.

Equipment

- Clean gloves
- Water-soluble local anesthetic lubricant (NOTE: Some facilities require use of water-soluble lubricant without anesthetic when nurse performs procedure.)
- Waterproof, absorbent pads

- Bedpan
- Bedpan cover *(optional if available)*
- Bath blanket
- Washbasin, washcloths, towels, and soap
- Stethoscope

Enema Bag Administration

- Enema container
- IV pole
- Tubing and clamp (if not already attached to container)
- Appropriate-size rectal tube (adult, 22 to 30 Fr; child, 12 to 18 Fr)
- Correct volume of warmed (tepid) solution (adult, 750 to 1000 mL; adolescent, 500 to 700 mL; school-age child, 300 to 500 mL; toddler, 250 to 350 mL; infant, 150 to 250 mL)

Prepackaged Enema

- Prepackaged enema container with lubricated rectal tip (Fig. 47.14)

STEP	RATIONALE
ASSESSMENT	
1. Identify patient using at least two identifiers (e.g., name and birthday or name and medical record number) according to agency policy.	Ensures correct patient. Complies with The Joint Commission standards and improves patient safety (TJC, 2020).
2. Review health care provider's order for enema and clarify reason for administration.	Order by health care provider is usually required for hospitalized patient. Order states which type of enema patient will receive.
3. Review medical record and assess last bowel movement, normal versus most recent bowel pattern, presence of hemorrhoids, and presence of abdominal pain or cramping.	Determines need for enema and type of enema used. Also establishes baseline for bowel function. Hemorrhoids may obscure rectal opening and cause discomfort or bleeding during evacuation.
4. Assess patient's mobility and ability to turn and position on side.	Determines whether assistance is needed for positioning patient.
5. Assess patient for allergy to any active ingredients of Fleet enema.	Reduces risk for allergic reaction.
6. Perform hand hygiene.	Reduces transmission of microorganisms.

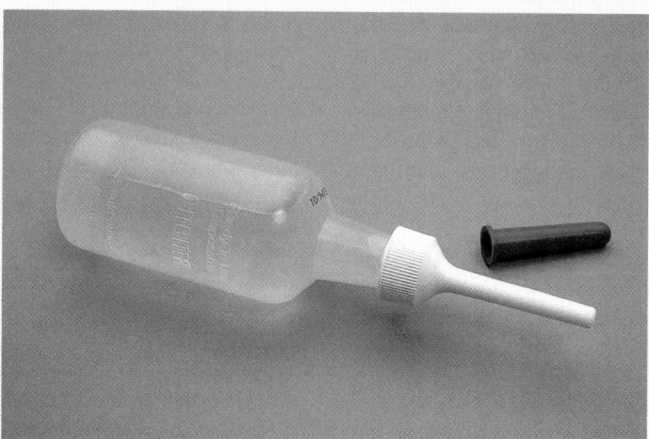

FIG. 47.14 Prepackaged enema container with rectal tip.

STEP	RATIONALE
7. Inspect and palpate abdomen for presence of distention, and auscultate for bowel sounds.	Establishes assessment baseline before enema administration.
8. Assess patient's or family caregiver's knowledge, experience, and health literacy.	Ensures patient or family caregiver has the capacity to obtain, communicate, process, and understand basic health information (CDC, 2019).

CLINICAL DECISION: *When "enemas until clear" is ordered, the water expelled may be tinted but should not contain solid fecal material. It is essential to observe contents of solution passed. Check agency policy, but a patient should receive only three consecutive enemas to prevent fluid and electrolyte imbalance.*

PLANNING

1. Provide privacy by closing curtains around bed or closing door, and prepare bedside environment for patient safety.	Respects patient right to privacy. Preparing the environment helps the nurse think about the steps needed; removing clutter from over-bed table removes barriers to completing procedure.
2. Prepare and organize enema equipment at bedside.	Ensures organized approach to enema administration.
3. Place bedpan or bedside commode in easily accessible position. If patient will be expelling contents in toilet, ensure that the toilet is available and place patient's nonskid slippers and bathrobe in easily accessible position.	Bedpan is used if patient is unable to get out of bed. Nonskid slippers help to prevent falls when moving from bed to bathroom.
4. Explain enema administration procedure to patient and/or caregiver.	Decreases patient anxiety and promotes patient cooperation.

IMPLEMENTATION

1. Check accuracy and completeness of each medication administration record (MAR) with health care provider's written order. Check patient's name, type of enema, and time for administration. Compare MAR with label of enema solution. **NOTE:** If enema is medicated, the skill may not be delegated to AP (see agency policy).	The health care provider's order is the most reliable source and only legal record of drugs or procedure that patient is to receive. Ensures that patient receives correct enema.
2. Perform hand hygiene.	Reduces transmission of microorganisms.
3. With side rail raised on patient's right side and bed raised to appropriate working height, help patient turn onto left side-lying (Sims') position with right knee flexed. Determine that patient is comfortable and encourage patient to remain in position until procedure is complete. **NOTE:** Place a child in the dorsal recumbent position.	Allows enema solution to flow downward by gravity along natural curve of sigmoid colon and rectum, thus improving retention of solution.

CLINICAL DECISION: *Patients with poor sphincter control require placement of a bedpan under the buttocks. Administering enema with patient sitting on toilet is unsafe because curved rectal tubing can abrade rectal wall.*

---

4. Apply clean gloves and place waterproof pad, absorbent side up, under hips and buttocks. Cover patient with bath blanket, exposing only rectal area, clearly visualizing anus.	Pad prevents soiling of linen. Blanket provides warmth, reduces exposure of body parts, and allows patient to feel more relaxed and comfortable.
5. Separate buttocks and examine perianal region for abnormalities, including hemorrhoids, anal fissure, and rectal prolapse.	Findings influence approach for inserting enema tip. Prolapse contraindicates enema.
6. Administer enema.	
a. Administer prepackaged disposable enema:	
(1) Remove plastic cap from tip of container. Tip may already be lubricated. Apply more water-soluble lubricant as needed. (see Fig. 47.14).	Lubrication provides for smooth insertion of rectal tube without causing rectal irritation or trauma. With presence of hemorrhoids, extra lubricant provides added comfort.
(2) Gently separate buttocks and locate anus. Instruct patient to relax by breathing out slowly through mouth.	Breathing out promotes relaxation of external rectal sphincter.
(3) Hold container upright and expel any air from enema container.	Introducing air into colon causes further distention and discomfort.
(4) Insert lubricated tip of container gently into anal canal toward umbilicus (see illustration). *Adult:* 7.5–10 cm (3–4 inches) *Adolescent:* 7.5 cm–10 cm (3–4 inches) *Child:* 5–7.5 cm (2–3 inches) *Infant:* 2.5–3.75 cm (1–1½ inches)	Gentle insertion prevents trauma to rectal mucosa.

CLINICAL DECISION: *If pain occurs or you feel resistance at any time during procedure, stop and discuss with health care provider. Do not force insertion.*

---

(5) Squeeze and roll plastic bottle from bottom to tip until all of solution has entered rectum and colon. Instruct patient to retain solution until urge to defecate occurs, usually 2 to 5 minutes.	Prevents instillation of air into colon and ensures that all content enters rectum. Hypertonic solutions require only small volumes to stimulate defecation.

Continued

SKILL 47.1   **ADMINISTERING A CLEANSING ENEMA—cont'd**

STEP	RATIONALE
b. Administer enema in standard enema bag:	
(1) Add warmed prescribed type of solution and amount to enema bag. Warm tap water as it flows from faucet. Place saline container in basin of warm water before adding saline to enema bag. Check temperature of solution by pouring small amount of solution over inner wrist.	Hot water burns intestinal mucosa. Cold water causes abdominal cramping and is difficult to retain.
(2) If soapsuds enema (SSE) is ordered, add castile soap after water.	Reduces suds in enema bag.
(3) Raise container, release clamp, and allow solution to flow long enough to fill tubing.	Removes air from tubing.
(4) Reclamp tubing.	Prevents further loss of solution.
(5) Lubricate 6–8 cm (2½ -3 inches) of tip of rectal tube with lubricant.	Allows smooth insertion of rectal tube without risk for irritation or trauma to mucosa.
(6) Gently separate buttocks and locate anus. Instruct patient to relax by breathing out slowly through mouth. Touch patient's skin next to anus with tip of rectal tube.	Breathing out and touching skin with tube promotes relaxation of external anal sphincter.
(7) Insert tip of rectal tube slowly by pointing it in direction of patient's umbilicus. Length of insertion varies (see Step 6a [4]).	Careful insertion prevents trauma to rectal mucosa from accidental lodging of tube against rectal wall. Insertion beyond proper limit can cause bowel perforation.

CLINICAL DECISION: *If tube does not pass easily, do not force. Consider allowing a small amount of fluid to infuse and then try to reinsert the tube slowly. The instillation of fluid relaxes the sphincter and provides additional lubrication. If fecal impaction is present, remove it before administering the enema.*

(8) Hold tubing in rectum constantly until end of fluid instillation.	Prevents expulsion of rectal tube during bowel contractions.
(9) Open regulating clamp and allow solution to enter slowly with container at patient's hip level.	Rapid infusion stimulates evacuation of tubing and can cause cramping.
(10) Raise height of enema container slowly to appropriate level: 12 inches above anus and 18 inches above mattress. (see illustration). Instillation time varies with volume of solution administered (e.g., 1 L may take 10 minutes). You may use an IV pole to hold an enema bag once you establish a slow flow of fluid.	Allows for continuous, slow instillation of solution. Raising container too high causes rapid instillation and possible painful distention of colon. High pressure can result in bowel rupture.

CLINICAL DECISION: *Temporary cessation of infusion minimizes cramping and promotes ability to retain solution. Lower container or clamp tubing if patient complains of cramping or if fluid escapes around rectal tube.*

(11) Instill all solution and clamp tubing. Tell patient that procedure is completed and that you will remove tubing.	Prevents entrance of air into rectum. Patients may misinterpret sensation of removing tube as loss of control.
7. Place layers of toilet tissue around tube at anus and gently withdraw rectal tube and tip.	Provides for patient's comfort and cleanliness.

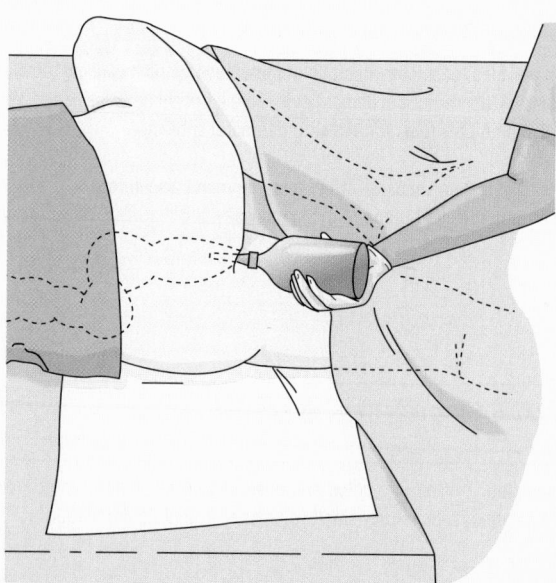

STEP 6a(4) With patient in left lateral sims' position, insert tip of commercial enema into rectum. (From Sorrentino SA, Remmert LA: *Mosby's textbook for nursing assistants*, ed 9, St Louis, 2017, Elsevier.)

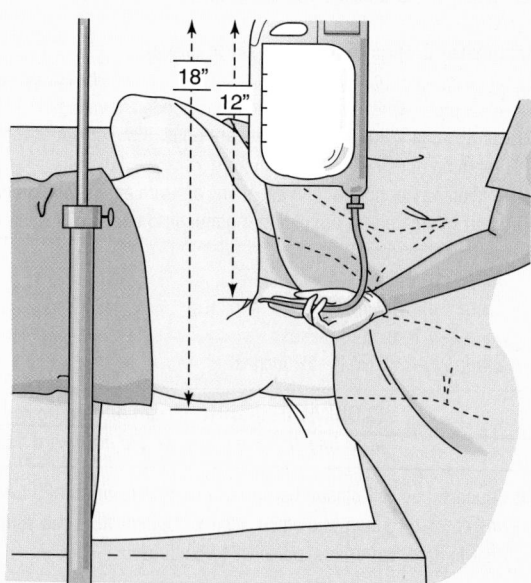

STEP 6b(10) IV pole is positioned so that the enema bag is 12 inches above the anus and 18 inches above the mattress. (From Sorrentino SA, Remmert LA: *Mosby's textbook for nursing assistants*, ed 9, St Louis, 2017, Elsevier.)

STEP	RATIONALE
8. Explain to patient that some distention and abdominal cramping are normal. Ask the patient to retain solution as long as possible until urge to defecate occurs. This usually takes a few minutes. Stay at bedside. Have patient lie quietly in bed if possible. (For infant or young child gently hold buttocks together for few minutes.)	Solution distends bowel. Length of retention varies with type of enema and patient's ability to contract rectal sphincter. Longer retention promotes stimulation of peristalsis and defecation.
9. Discard enema container or disposable bag and tubing in proper receptacle. Remove and dispose of gloves and perform hand hygiene.	Reduces transmission and growth of microorganisms.
10. Help patient to bathroom or commode if possible. If using bedpan, apply clean gloves and help patient to as near a normal position for evacuation as possible (see Box 47.9).	Normal squatting position promotes defecation.
11. Observe character of stool and solution (instruct patient not to flush toilet before inspection).	Determines whether enema was effective.
12. Help patient as needed to wash anal area with warm soap and water (use gloves for perineal care).	Fecal contents irritate skin. Hygiene promotes patient's comfort.
13. Remove and discard gloves and perform hand hygiene.	Reduces transmission of microorganisms.

EVALUATION

1. Inspect color, consistency, and amount of stool; odor; and fluid passed.	Determines whether stool is evacuated or fluid is retained. Note abnormalities such as presence of blood or mucus.
2. Palpate for abdominal distention.	Determines whether distention is relieved.
3. **Use Teach-Back:** "I want to be sure I explained clearly how to position yourself in bed if you need to self-administer a Fleet enema. Show me how you would position yourself." Revise your instruction now or develop a plan for revised patient/family caregiver teaching if patient/family caregiver is not able to teach back correctly.	Determines patient's/family caregiver's level of understanding of instructional topic.

UNEXPECTED OUTCOMES AND RELATED INTERVENTIONS

1. Severe abdominal cramping, bleeding, or sudden abdominal pain develops and is unrelieved by temporarily stopping or slowing flow of solution.
   - Stop enema.
   - Notify health care provider.
   - Obtain vital signs.
2. Patient is unable to hold enema solution.
   - If this occurs during installation, slow rate of infusion.

RECORDING AND REPORTING

- Record the time, type, and volume of enema administered; patient's signs and symptoms; response to enema; and results, including color, amount, and appearance of stool.
- Report failure of patient to defecate or any adverse reactions to health care provider.

HOME CARE CONSIDERATIONS

- For patients who require enemas at home, instruct family not to exceed recommended fluid volume levels or number of enemas. Instruct family about need for slow administration of warmed fluid.
- Place waterproof padding on the bed.
- Instruct family members not to give the enema on the toilet.

Continued

Delegation and Collaboration

The skill of inserting and maintaining an NG tube cannot be delegated to assistive personnel (AP). The nurse instructs the AP to:

- Measure and record the drainage from an NG tube.
- Provide oral and nasal hygiene measures.
- Perform selected comfort measures such as positioning or offering ice chips if allowed.
- Anchor the tube to patient's gown during routine care to prevent accidental displacement.
- Immediately report to the nurse any patient complaints of burning or signs of redness or irritation to nares.

Equipment

- 14 Fr or 16 Fr NG tube (smaller-lumen catheters are not used for decompression in adults because they must be able to remove thick secretions)
- Water-soluble lubricating jelly
- pH test strips 1.0 to 11.0 or higher (measure gastric aspirate acidity)
- Tongue blade
- Clean gloves
- Flashlight
- Emesis basin
- Asepto bulb or catheter-tipped syringe
- Commercial fixation device or 2.5 cm (1 inch)–wide hypoallergenic tape (*option:* Bridle nasal tube system)
- Rubber band and plastic clip to attach tube to gown
- Clamp, drainage bag, or suction machine or pressure gauge if wall suction is to be used
- Towel
- Glass of water with straw
- Facial tissues
- Normal saline
- Tincture of benzoin *(optional)*
- Gastric suction equipment
- Stethoscope
- Pulse oximeter

STEP	RATIONALE

ASSESSMENT

1. Identify patient using at least two identifiers (e.g., name and birthday or name and medical record number) according to agency policy.

Ensures correct patient. Complies with The Joint Commission standards and improves patient safety (TJC, 2020).

2. Verify health care provider order for type of NG tube to be placed and whether tube is to be attached to suction or drainage bag.

Requires order from health care provider. Adequate decompression depends on NG suction.

3. Perform hand hygiene (apply clean gloves if risk of body fluid exposure). Inspect condition of skin integrity around patient's nares and nasal and oral cavity.

Provides baseline data on the condition of the patient's skin before NG tube insertion. All patients with any medical device are at risk for pressure injury (Delmore and Ayello, 2017).

4. Assess patient's or caregiver's knowledge, experience, and health literacy.

Ensures patient or family caregiver has the capacity to obtain, communicate, process, and understand basic health information (CDC, 2019).

5. Ask whether patient has history of nasal surgery or congestion and allergies, and note whether deviated nasal septum is present.

Alerts nurse to potential obstruction. Insert tube into uninvolved nasal passage. Procedure may be contraindicated if surgery is recent.

6. Auscultate for bowel sounds. Palpate patient's abdomen for distention, pain, and rigidity. Remove and discard gloves if applied and perform hand hygiene.

In presence of diminished or absent bowel sounds, auscultate abdomen in all four quadrants (Ball et al., 2019). Documents baseline for any abdominal distention, gastrointestinal (GI) ileus, and general GI function, which later serves as comparison once tube is inserted.

7. Assess patient's level of consciousness and ability to follow instructions.

Determines patient's ability to help in procedure.

CLINICAL DECISION: *If patient is confused, disoriented, or unable to follow commands, get help from another staff member to insert the tube.*

---

8. Determine whether patient had previous NG tube, and if so, which naris was used.

Patient's previous experience complements any explanations and prepares patient for NG tube placement.

PLANNING

1. Provide privacy by closing curtains around bed or closing door, and prepare bedside environment for patient safety.

Respects patient's right to privacy. Preparing the environment helps the nurse think about the steps needed; removing clutter from over-bed table removes barriers to completing procedure.

2. Prepare and organize NG tube equipment at bedside.

Ensures organized approach to NG tube insertion.

3. Explain NG tube insertion procedure to patient and/or caregiver. Inform patient that procedure may cause gagging and that there may be a burning sensation in nasopharynx as tube is passed. Develop hand signal with patient if too much discomfort occurs.

Decreases patient anxiety and promotes patient cooperation. If patient is too uncomfortable or unable to tolerate procedure, the use of a hand signal will alert the nurse.

IMPLEMENTATION

1. Raise the bed to working height. Position patient upright in high-Fowler's position unless contraindicated. If patient is comatose, raise head of bed as tolerated in semi-Fowler's position with head tipped forward, chin to chest.

Promotes patient's ability to swallow during procedure. Good body mechanics prevent injury to you or patient.

2. Perform hand hygiene and place bath towel over patient's chest; give facial tissues to patient. Allow to blow nose if necessary. Place emesis basin within reach.

Prevents soiling of patient's gown. Tube insertion through nasal passages may cause tearing and coughing with increased salivation.

3. Wash bridge of nose with soap and water or alcohol swab. Dry thoroughly.

Removes oils from nose to allow fixation devices to adhere completely.

STEP	**RATIONALE**
4. Stand on patient's right side if right-handed, left side if left-handed. Lower side rail.	Allows easiest manipulation of tubing.
5. Instruct patient to relax and breathe normally while occluding one naris. Then repeat this action for other naris. Select nostril with greater airflow.	Tube passes more easily through naris that is more patent.

CLINICAL DECISION: *Insertion of a nasogastric tube is a painful procedure. Research provides evidence that in some instances, topical lidocaine, either as a gel or spray, significantly reduces pain (Solomon and Jurica, 2017).*

6. Determine length of tube to be inserted, and mark location with tape or indelible ink.	Ensures organized procedure and estimation of the proper length of tube to insert into patient.
a. *Option for adults:* Measure distance from tip of nose to earlobe to xyphoid process (NEX) of sternum (see illustration). Mark this distance on tube with tape.	Most traditional method. Length approximates distance from nose to stomach. Research has shown this method may be least effective compared with others, though more research is needed (Santos et al., 2016).
b. *Option for adults:* Measure distance from tip of nose to earlobe to mid-umbilicus (NEMU); also used for pediatric patients.	Promotes placement of the tube end holes in or closer to the gastric fluid pool (Boullata et al., 2017).
c. *Option for adults:* Measure distance from xyphoid process to earlobe to nose (XEN) + 10 cm (Taylor et al., 2014).	Shown to be more accurate than NEX (Taylor et al., 2014).
d. *Option for children:* Use the NEMU method (Hockenberry et al., 2019).	Estimates proper length of tube insertion for the pediatric patient.

CLINICAL DECISION: *Tip of NG tube must reach stomach to avoid the risk for pulmonary aspiration, which occurs when tubes terminate in the esophagus. Research has mixed findings in regard to the best technique for estimating tube length (Santos et al., 2016). Confirmation of placement via x-ray immediately after completed insertion is still needed.*

7. With small piece of tape placed around tube, mark length that will be inserted.	Indicates length of tube you will insert.
8. Prepare materials for tube fixation. Tear off a 7.5- to 10-cm (3- to 4-inch) length of hypoallergenic tape or open membrane dressing or another fixation device (see Step 22a[2]).	Fixation devices allow tube to float free of nares, thus reducing pressure on nares and preventing medical device–related pressure injuries (MDRPI) (Pittman et al., 2015).
9. Perform hand hygiene and apply clean gloves.	Reduces transmission of infection.
10. Apply pulse oximetry/capnography device and measure vital signs. Monitor oximetry/capnography during insertion.	Provides objective assessment of respiratory status before and during tube insertion.
11. *Option:* Dip tube with surface lubricant into glass of room temperature water or lubricate 7.5 to 10 cm (3-4 inches) of end of tube with water-soluble lubricant (see manufacturer directions).	Water activates lubricant, minimizes friction against nasal mucosa, and aids in insertion of tube. Water-soluble lubricant is less toxic than oil-based lubricant if aspirated.
12. Hand an alert patient a cup of water if able to hold cup and swallow. Explain that you are about to insert tube.	Swallowing water facilitates tube passage. Explanation decreases patient anxiety and increases patient cooperation.
13. Explain next steps. Insert tube gently and slowly through naris to back of throat (posterior nasopharynx). Aim back and down toward patient's ear.	Natural contour facilitates passage of tube into GI tract and reduces gagging.
14. Have patient relax and flex head toward chest after tube is passed through nasopharynx.	Closes off glottis and reduces risk of tube entering trachea.
15. Encourage patient to swallow by taking small sips of water when possible. Advance tube as patient swallows. Rotate tube gently 180 degrees while inserting.	Swallowing facilitates passage of tube past oropharynx. A tug may be felt as patient swallows, indicating that tube is following desired path.
16. Emphasize need to mouth breathe during procedure.	Helps facilitate passage of tube and alleviates patient's anxiety and fear during procedure.

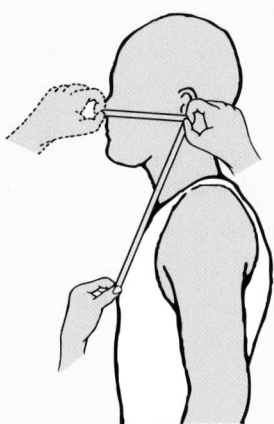

STEP 6a Determine length of tube to be inserted.

Continued

SKILL 47.2	INSERTING AND MAINTAINING A NASOGASTRIC TUBE FOR GASTRIC DECOMPRESSION—cont'd

STEP	RATIONALE
17. Do not advance tube during inspiration or coughing because it is likely to enter respiratory tract. Monitor oximetry/capnography.	When tube inadvertently enters airway, changes in oxygen saturation or end-tidal CO_2 (capnography) occur.
18. Advance tube each time patient swallows until you reach desired length.	Reduces discomfort and trauma to patient.

CLINICAL DECISION: *Do not force NG tube. If patient starts to cough or has a drop in O_2 saturation or an increased CO_2, withdraw tube into the posterior nasopharynx until normal breathing resumes.*

STEP	RATIONALE
19. Using penlight and tongue blade, check to be sure that tube is not positioned or coiled in back of throat.	Tube could become coiled, kinked, or enter trachea.
20. Temporarily anchor tube to nose with small piece of tape.	Securing tube prevents movement of tube and subsequent gagging. Allows for verification of tube placement.
21. Verify tube placement. Check agency policy for recommended methods of checking tube placement.	
a. Follow order for bedside x-ray film and notify radiology for examination of chest and abdomen.	Radiography remains the gold standard for verification of initial placement of tube (McFarland, 2017; Mordiffi et al., 2016). This must be done before any medication or liquid is administered (ENA, 2015).
b. While waiting for x-ray film to be performed, follow these procedures: Attach Asepto or catheter-tipped syringe to end of tube. Aspirate gently back on syringe to obtain gastric contents, observing amount, color, and quality of return.	Observation of gastric contents is useful to determine initial tube placement. Gastric contents are usually green but are sometimes off-white, tan, bloody, or brown in color. Other common aspirate colors include yellow or bile stained (duodenal placement) or possibly saliva-appearing (esophagus) (Mordiffi et al., 2016).
c. Use pH test paper to measure aspirate for pH with color-coded pH paper. Be sure that paper range of pH is at least from 1.0 to 11.0 (see illustration).	Evidence supports pH test to be used as indicator for placement (McFarland, 2017; Tho et al., 2011). A pH of 1.0 to 4.0 is a good indicator of gastric placement.
22. After tube is properly inserted and positioned, either clamp end or connect it to drainage bag or suction source. Anchor tube with a fixation device, avoiding pressure on the nares. Select one of the following fixation methods.	Drainage bag is used for gravity drainage. Intermittent low suction is most effective for decompression. Proper anchoring and marking of tube helps prevent migration of tube and pressure injury formation.
a. Apply tape.	
(1) Apply tincture of benzoin or other skin adhesive on bridge of patient's nose and allow it to become "tacky."	Helps tape adhere better. Protects underlying skin.
(2) Tear small horizontal slits at one-third and two-thirds length of tape without splitting tape (see illustration). Fold middle sections toward one another to form a closed strip.	The strip holds tubing to lessen rubbing against soft palate and naris.
(3) Print date and time on tape and place top end of tape over bridge of patient's nose.	
(4) Wrap bottom end of tape around tube as it exits nose (see illustration).	
b. Apply tube fixation device using shaped adhesive patch (see manufacturer directions).	Secures tube and reduces friction on nares, and decreases risk for MDRPI (Delmore and Ayello, 2017).
(1) Apply wide end of patch to bridge of nose (see illustration).	
(2) Slip connector around tube as it exits nose (see illustration).	

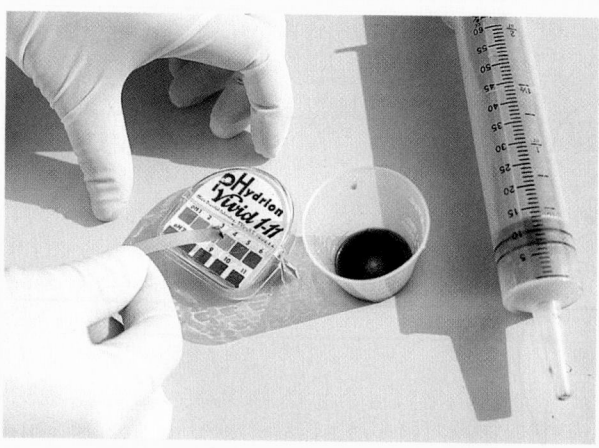

STEP 21c Checking pH of gastric aspirate.

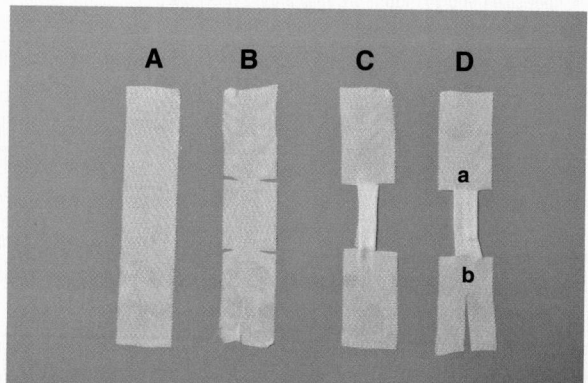

STEP 22a(2) Taping method. **A,** Start with piece of tape. **B,** Make two slits on both sides of tape. **C,** Fold middle section inward. **D,** Tear a new slit in bottom of tape. Top part (A) should attach to patient's nose; bottom part (B) should be wrapped around tube.

STEP	RATIONALE

CLINICAL DECISION: *Assess at least twice daily the condition of the naris and mucosa for inflammation, blistering, excoriation, or any type of skin or tissue injury. Injury can develop for many reasons: rigidity of device rubbing against mucosa, difficulty in securing or adjusting the device to the body, increased moisture surrounding the tubing, tight securement of the device, and poor positioning or fixation of the device (Delmore and Ayello, 2017).*

23. Fasten end of nasogastric tube to patient's gown with piece of tape (see illustration). Do not use safety pins to fasten tube to gown.

Anchors tubing to prevent pulling on nose.

24. Keep head of bed elevated 30 to 45 degrees (preferably 45 degrees) unless contraindicated (AACN, 2017).

Patients receiving nasogastric tube feedings have an increased risk for aspiration (AACN, 2017). Head-of-bed elevation reduces risk for aspiration of stomach contents (Metheny, 2016).

CLINICAL DECISION: *If inserting a Salem sump tube, keep the blue "pigtail" of the tube above level of the stomach. This prevents a siphoning action that clogs the tube. The blue "pigtail" is the air vent that connects with the second lumen When the main lumen of the sump tube is connected to suction, the air vent permits free, continuous drainage of secretions. Never clamp off the air vent, connect to suction, or use for irrigation.*

25. Assist radiology as needed in obtaining ordered x-ray film of chest and abdomen.

X-ray verification is the gold standard for NG tube verification (ENA, 2018; McFarland, 2017; Mordiffi et al., 2016).

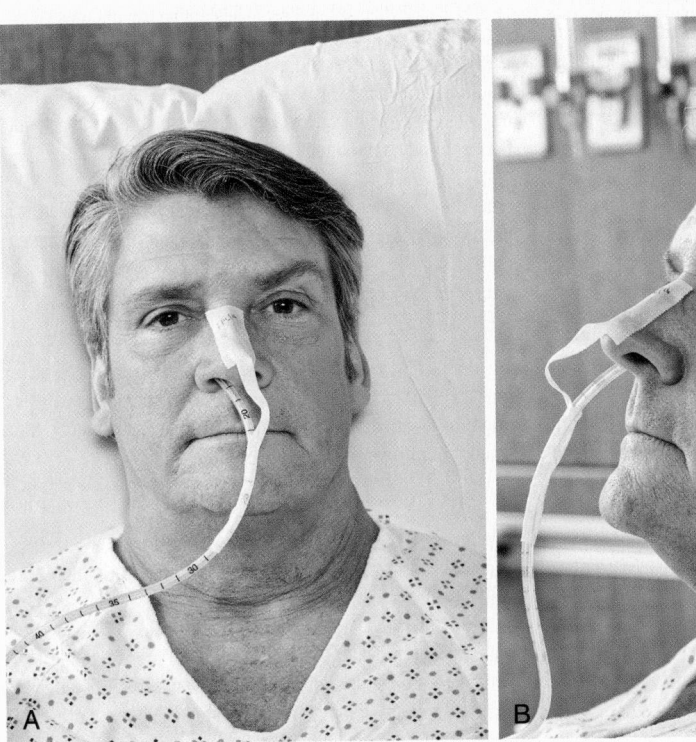 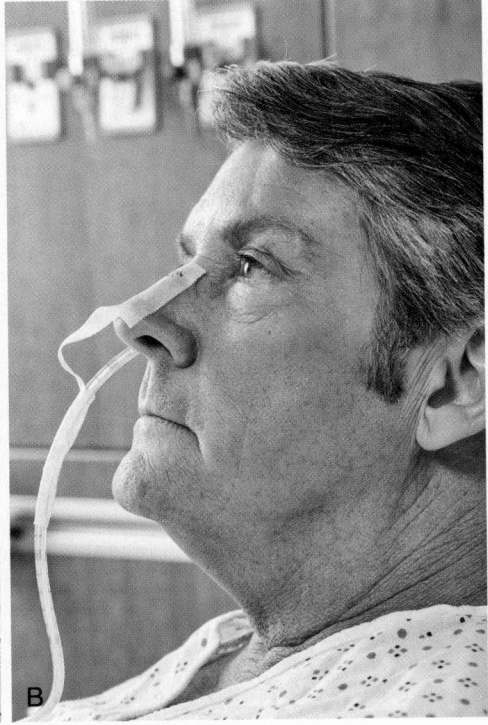

STEP 22a(4) A, Tape applied to anchor nasogastric tube. **B,** Nares are free of pressure from tape and tube.

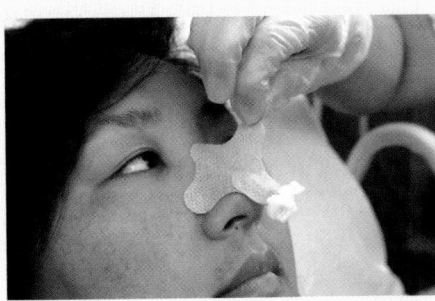 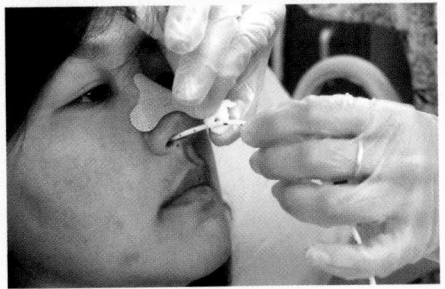 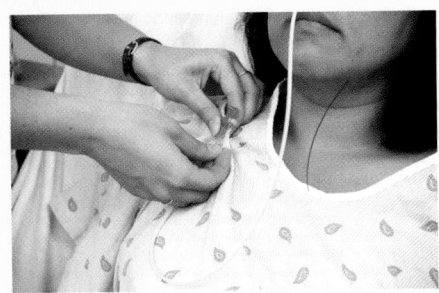

STEP 22b(1) Apply patch to bridge of nose.   **STEP 22b(2)** Slip connector around nasogastric tube.   **STEP 23** Fasten nasogastric tube to patient gown.

Continued

SKILL 47.2	INSERTING AND MAINTAINING A NASOGASTRIC TUBE FOR GASTRIC DECOMPRESSION—cont'd

STEP	RATIONALE
26. Remove and dispose of gloves, perform hand hygiene, and help patient to comfortable position.	Reduces transmission of microorganisms.
27. Once placement is confirmed, measure amount of tube that is external and mark exit of tube at nares with indelible marker as guide for any tube displacement. Record this information in nurses' notes in electronic health record (EHR) or chart.	The mark alerts nurses and other health care providers to possible tube displacement, which will require confirmation of tube placement.

CLINICAL DECISION: *Never reposition an NG tube of a gastric surgical patient since positioning can rupture the suture line.*

28. Attach NG tube to suction as ordered.	Suction setting is usually ordered low intermittent, which decreases gastric irritation from NG tube.

CLINICAL DECISION: *If lumen of tube is narrow and secretions are thick, NG will not drain as desired. Irrigate tube (see Step 29). Consult with health care provider for higher suction setting if unable to irrigate tube because of thick secretions.*

29. NG tube irrigation:	
a. Perform hand hygiene and apply clean gloves.	Reduces transmission of microorganisms.
b. Verify tube placement in stomach by disconnecting NG tube, connecting irrigating syringe, and aspirating contents (see Step 21b). Temporarily clamp NG tube or reconnect to connecting tube and remove syringe.	pH of gastric aspirate must measure between 1.0 and 4.0 to ensure that NG tube is in the stomach (McFarland, 2017). Prevents accidental entrance of irrigating solution into lungs.
c. Empty syringe of aspirate and use it to draw up 30 mL of normal saline.	Use of saline minimizes loss of electrolytes from stomach fluids.
d. Disconnect NG from connecting tubing and lay end of connection tubing on towel.	Reduces soiling of patient's gown and bed linen.
e. Insert tip of irrigating syringe into end of NG tube. Remove clamp. Hold syringe with tip pointed at floor, and inject saline slowly and evenly. Do not force solution.	Position of syringe prevents introduction of air into vent tubing, which causes gastric distention. Solution introduced under pressure causes gastric trauma.

CLINICAL DECISION: *Do not introduce saline through blue "pigtail" air vent of Salem sump tube.*

f. If resistance occurs, check for kinks in tubing. Turn patient onto left side. Repeated resistance should be reported to health care provider.	Tip of tube may lie against stomach lining. Repositioning on left side may dislodge tube away from stomach lining. Buildup of secretions causes distention.
g. After instilling saline, immediately aspirate or pull back slowly on syringe to withdraw fluid. If amount aspirated is greater than amount instilled, record difference as output. If amount aspirated is less than amount instilled, record difference as intake.	Irrigation clears tubing, so stomach should remain empty. Measure and document amount of irrigant fluid inserted in tube as intake.
h. Use an Asepto syringe to place 10 mL of air into blue pigtail.	Ensures patency of air vent.
i. Reconnect NG tube to drainage or suction. (Repeat irrigation if solution does not return.)	Reestablishes drainage collection; may repeat irrigation or repositioning of tube until NG tube drains properly.
30. Removal of NG tube:	
a. Verify order to remove NG tube.	A health care provider order is required for procedure.
b. Per agency policy, auscultate abdomen for presence of bowel sounds or clamp the tube for a short period of time, assessing for nausea or discomfort.	Verifies return of peristalsis. Early removal of the NG tube helps to restore normal anatomy and physiology of the GI system (Goudar et al., 2017).
c. Explain procedure to patient and reassure that removal is less distressing than insertion.	Minimizes anxiety and increases cooperation. Tube passes out smoothly.
d. Perform hand hygiene and apply clean gloves.	Reduces transmission of microorganisms.
e. Turn off suction and disconnect NG tube from drainage bag or suction. With irrigating syringe, insert 20 mL of air into lumen of NG tube. Remove tape or fixation device from bridge of nose and patient's gown.	Have tube free of connections before removal. Clears gastric fluids from tube to prevent aspiration of contents or soiling of clothing and bedding.
f. Hand patient facial tissue; place clean towel across chest. Instruct patient to take and hold breath as tube is removed.	Some patients wish to blow nose after tube is removed. Towel keeps gown from soiling. Temporary airway obstruction occurs during tube removal.

STEP	RATIONALE
g. Clamp or kink tubing securely and pull tube out steadily and smoothly into towel held in other hand while patient holds breath.	Clamping prevents tube contents from draining into oropharynx. Reduces trauma to mucosa and minimizes patient's discomfort. Towel covers tube, which is an unpleasant sight. Holding breath helps to prevent aspiration.
h. Inspect intactness of tube.	
i. Measure amount of drainage and note character of content. Dispose of tube and drainage equipment into proper container.	Provides accurate measure of fluid output. Reduces transfer of microorganisms.
j. Clean nares and provide mouth care.	Promotes comfort.
k. Position patient comfortably and explain procedure for drinking fluids if not contraindicated. Instruct patient to notify you if nausea occurs.	Sometimes patients are not allowed anything by mouth (NPO) for up to 24 hours. When fluids are allowed, orders usually begin with small amount of ice chips each hour and increase as patient is able to tolerate more.
31. For all procedures, clean equipment and return to proper place. Place soiled linen in utility room or proper receptacle.	Proper disposal of equipment prevents spread of microorganisms and ensures proper exchange procedures.
32. Remove and discard gloves and perform hand hygiene.	Reduces transmission of microorganisms.

EVALUATION

1. Observe amount and character of contents draining from NG tube. Ask if patient feels nauseated.	Determines if tube is decompressing stomach of contents.
2. Auscultate for presence of bowel sounds. Turn off suction while auscultating. Assess for nausea and patient discomfort if tube is clamped for short trial period.	Sound of suction apparatus is sometimes misinterpreted as bowel sounds. Nausea and discomfort will occur if peristalsis is not returned.
3. Palpate patient's abdomen periodically. Note any distention, pain, and rigidity.	Determines success of abdominal decompression and return of peristalsis.
4. Inspect condition of nares, nose, and all skin and tissue around NG tubing.	Evaluates onset of skin and tissue irritation.
5. Observe position of tubing.	Prevents tension applied to nasal structures.
6. Explain that it is normal if patient feels sore throat or irritation in pharynx.	Result of tube irritation.
7. **Use Teach-Back:** "I need to be sure I explained the importance of letting me know if you are nauseated. Tell me why it is important for me to know if you feel nauseated." Revise your instruction now or develop a plan for revised patient/family caregiver teaching if patient/family caregiver is not able to teach back correctly.	Determines patient's/family caregiver's level of understanding of instructional topic.

UNEXPECTED OUTCOMES AND RELATED INTERVENTIONS

1. Patient complains of nausea, or patient's abdomen is distended and painful.
   - Assess patency of tube. NG tube may be occluded or no longer in stomach.
   - Irrigate tube.
   - Verify that suction is on as ordered.
   - Notify health care provider if distention is unrelieved.
2. Patient develops irritation or erosion of skin around naris.
   - Provide frequent skin care to area.
   - Use taping method designed to reduce MDRPI (see taping methods, Step 22).
   - Consider switching tube to other naris.
3. Patient develops signs and symptoms of pulmonary aspiration: fever, shortness of breath, or pulmonary congestion.
   - Perform complete respiratory assessment.
   - Notify health care provider.
   - Obtain chest x-ray film examination as ordered.

RECORDING AND REPORTING

- Record length, size, type of gastric tube inserted, and naris in which tube was introduced. Also record patient's tolerance of procedure, confirmation of tube placement, character and pH of gastric contents, results of x-ray film, whether the tube is clamped or connected to drainage bag or to suction, and amount of suction supplied.
- Document your evaluation of patient learning.
- When irrigating NG tube, record difference between amount of normal saline instilled and amount of gastric aspirate removed on I&O sheet. Record amount and character of contents draining from NG tube every shift in nurses' notes or flow sheet.
- Record removal of tube "intact," patient's tolerance to procedure, and final amount and character of drainage.
- Report occurrence of abdominal distention, unexpected increase or sudden stoppage in gastric drainage, and patient complaining of gastric distress to health care provider.

| SKILL 47.3 | POUCHING AN OSTOMY |

Delegation and Collaboration

The skill of pouching a new ostomy should not be delegated to assistive personnel (AP). In some agencies care of an established ostomy (4 to 6 weeks or more after surgery) can be delegated to AP. The nurse directs the AP about:

- The expected amount, color, and consistency of drainage from an ostomy
- The expected appearance of the stoma
- Special equipment needed to complete a particular patient's pouching
- The changes in a patient's stoma and surrounding skin integrity that should be reported

Equipment

- Pouch: drainable one-piece or two-piece, cut-to-fit, precut size, or moldable
- Pouch closure device, such as a clip, if needed
- Measuring guide
- Adhesive releaser *(optional)*
- Clean gloves
- Washcloth
- Towel or disposable waterproof barrier
- Basin with warm tap water
- Scissors
- Waterproof bag for disposal of pouch
- Gown and goggles (if there is a risk of splashing when emptying the pouch)

| STEP | RATIONALE |

ASSESSMENT

1. Identify patient using at least two identifiers (e.g., name and birthday or name and medical record number) according to agency policy.	Ensures correct patient. Complies with The Joint Commission standards and improves patient safety (TJC, 2020).
2. Perform hand hygiene and apply clean gloves.	Reduces transmission of microorganisms.
3. Observe existing skin barrier and pouch for leakage and length of time in place. Pouch should be changed every 3 to 7 days, not daily (Carmel et al., 2016). If an opaque pouch is being used, remove it to fully observe stoma. Dispose of such a pouch in proper receptacle.	Assesses effectiveness of pouching system and detects potential for problems. To minimize skin irritation, avoid unnecessary changing of entire pouching system. When pouch leaks, skin damage from effluent causes more skin trauma than early removal of wafer.

> **CLINICAL DECISION:** *Repeated leaking may indicate need for different type of pouch or addition of accessory products such as rings, seals, or paste. If the pouch is leaking, change it. Taping or patching it to contain effluent leaves the skin exposed to chemical or enzymatic irritation.*

4. Remove used pouch and skin barrier gently, and observe amount of effluent. Empty the effluent if it is more than one-third to one-half full by opening the pouch and draining it into a container for measurement of output. Note consistency of effluent, and record intake and output.	Weight of pouch may disrupt seal of adhesive on skin. Monitors fluid balance and bowel function after surgery. Normal colostomy effluent is soft or formed stool, whereas normal ileostomy effluent is liquid.
5. Observe stoma for type, location, color, swelling, presence of sutures, trauma, and healing or irritation of peristomal skin (see illustrations).	Stoma characteristics influence selection of an appropriate pouching system. Convexity in skin barrier is often necessary with a flush or retracted stoma.
6. Observe placement of stoma in relation to abdominal contours and presence of scars or incisions. Remove and dispose of gloves; perform hand hygiene.	Determines whether current pouching system is effective or new selection is needed. Abdominal contours, scars, or incisions affect type of system and adhesion to skin surface. Reduces transmission of microorganisms.
7. Assess patient's or family caregiver's knowledge, experience, and health literacy.	Ensures patient or family caregiver has the capacity to obtain, communicate, process, and understand basic health information (CDC, 2019).
8. Explore patient's attitudes, perceptions, knowledge, and acceptance of stoma; discuss interest in learning self-care. Identify others who will be helping patient after leaving hospital.	Determines patient's willingness to learn. Facilitates teaching plan and timing of care to coincide with availability of family caregivers.

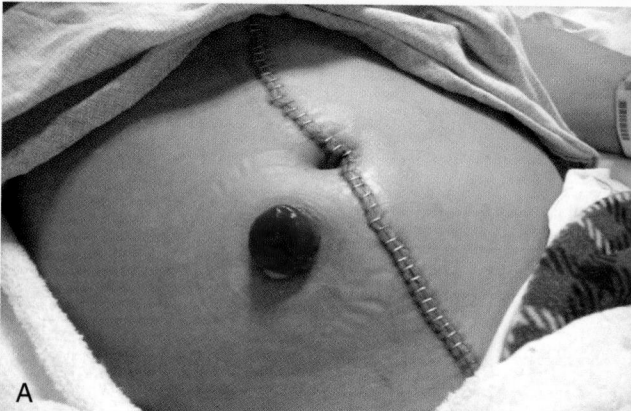 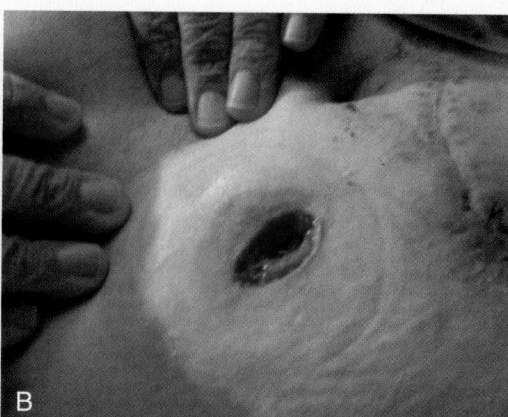

STEP 5 A, Budded stoma. **B,** Retracted stoma. (Courtesy Jane Fellows.)

STEP	RATIONALE

PLANNING

1. Provide privacy by closing curtains around bed or closing door, and prepare bedside environment for patient safety.

Respects patient right to privacy. Preparing the environment helps the nurse think about the steps needed; removing clutter from over-bed table removes barriers to completing procedure.

2. Prepare and organize ostomy pouching equipment at bedside.

Ensures organized approach to changing the ostomy pouch.

3. Explain ostomy pouching procedure to patient and/or caregiver.

Decreases patient anxiety and promotes patient cooperation.

IMPLEMENTATION

1. Have patient assume semi-reclining or supine position (same position assumed during assessment and pouching). (**NOTE:** Some patients with established ostomies prefer to stand.) If possible, provide patient with mirror for observation.

When patient is semi-reclining, there are fewer skinfolds, which allows for ease of application of pouching system.

2. Perform hand hygiene and apply clean gloves.

Reduces transmission of microorganisms.

3. Place towel or disposable waterproof barrier under patient and across patient's lower abdomen.

Protects bed linen; maintains patient's dignity.

4. If not done during assessment, remove used pouch and skin barrier gently by pushing skin away from barrier. Use adhesive releaser to facilitate removal of skin barrier. Empty pouch and dispose of it in an appropriate receptacle. Measure output if needed. **NOTE:** There may be no output at time of first pouch change.

Reduces skin trauma. Improper removal of pouch and barrier can cause peristomal skin irritation or breakdown.

5. Clean peristomal skin gently with warm tap water using washcloth; do not scrub skin. If you touch stoma, minor bleeding is normal. Pat skin dry. Have washcloth handy for additional cleaning if there is output from the stoma while preparing pouch.

Soap leaves residue on skin, which may irritate skin. Pouch does not adhere to wet skin.
Ileostomies have frequent output, especially after eating.

6. Measure stoma (see illustration). Expect size of stoma to change for first 4 to 6 weeks after surgery.

Allows for proper fit of pouch that will protect peristomal skin.

7. Trace pattern of stoma measurement on pouch backing or skin barrier (see illustration).

Prepares for cutting opening in pouch.

8. Cut opening on backing or skin barrier wafer (see illustration). If using moldable or shape to fit barrier, use fingers to mold shape to fit stoma.

Customizes pouch to provide appropriate fit over stoma.

9. Remove protective backing from adhesive backing or wafer (see illustration).

Prepares skin barrier for placement.

10. Apply pouch over stoma (see illustration). Press firmly into place around stoma and outside edges. Have patient hold hand over pouch to apply heat to secure seal.

Pouch adhesives are heat and pressure sensitive and hold more securely at body temperature.

11. Close end of pouch with clip or integrated closure. Remove drape from patient. Help patient to assume comfortable position.

Ensures that pouch is secure. Contains effluent. Gives patient sense of well-being.

12. Be sure nurse call system is in an accessible location within patient's reach.

Ensures patient can call for assistance if needed.

13. Raise side rails (as appropriate) and lower bed to lowest position.

Ensures patient safety.

14. Remove and dispose of gloves and other disposables. Perform hand hygiene.

Reduces transmission of microorganisms.

EVALUATION

1. Observe condition of skin barrier and adherence of pouch to abdominal surface

Determines presence of leaks.

2. Observe appearance of stoma, peristomal skin, abdominal contours, suture line, and presence of any flatus during pouch change.

Determines condition of stoma and peristomal skin and progress of wound healing.

3. Note whether there is presence of any flatus during pouch change.

Determines whether peristalsis is returning.

4. Observe patient's and family caregiver's willingness to view stoma and ask questions about procedure.

Determines level of adjustment and understanding of stoma care and pouch application. Allows planning for future education needs and progress toward acceptance of altered body image.

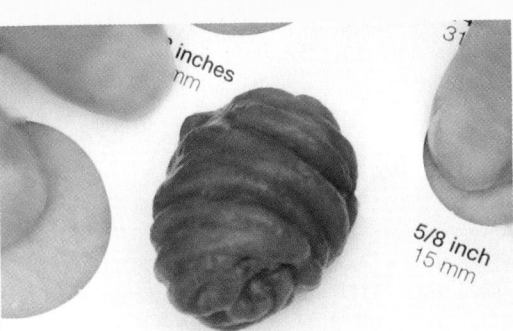

STEP 6 Measure stoma. (Courtesy Coloplast, Minneapolis, MN.)

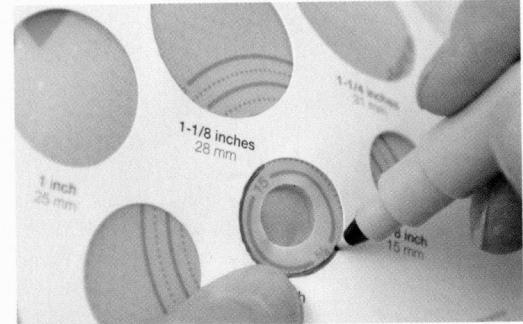

STEP 7 Trace measurement on skin barrier. (Courtesy Coloplast, Minneapolis, MN.)

Continued

SKILL 47.3 **POUCHING AN OSTOMY—cont'd**

STEP	RATIONALE
5. Use Teach-Back: "I want to be sure you understand what is involved in changing your ostomy pouch. Tell me what you should do to prevent your skin from becoming irritated and the frequency with which you should empty your pouch." Revise your instruction now or develop a plan for revised patient/family caregiver teaching if patient/family caregiver is not able to teach back correctly.	Determines patient's/family caregiver's level of understanding of instructional topic.

UNEXPECTED OUTCOMES AND RELATED INTERVENTIONS

1. Skin around stoma is irritated, blistered, or bleeding or a rash is noted. May be caused by undermining of pouch seal by fecal contents, causing irritant dermatitis, or by adhesive removal causing skin stripping or fungal or other skin eruption.
   - Remove pouch more carefully.
   - Change pouch more frequently or use different type of pouching system.
   - Consult ostomy care nurse.
2. Necrotic stoma is manifested by purple or black color, dry instead of moist texture, failure to bleed when washed gently, or tissue sloughing.
   - Report to nurse in charge or health care provider.
   - Document appearance.
3. Patient refuses to view stoma or participate in care.
   - Obtain referral for ostomy care nurse.
   - Allow patient to express feelings.
   - Encourage family support.

RECORDING AND REPORTING

- Record type of pouch and skin barrier applied, amount and appearance of effluent in pouch, size and appearance of stoma, and condition of peristomal skin. Record what patient and family caregivers are able to demonstrate and level of participation.
- Document your evaluation of patient learning.
- Record abnormal appearance of stoma, suture line, or peristomal skin or change in volume, consistency, or color of output.
- Record whether pouch change was done.
- Record patient's response to pouch change and participation in process.

HOME CARE CONSIDERATIONS

- Evaluate patient's home toileting facilities and help patient develop an ostomy care routine that is compatible with available facilities. Ostomy pouches are not flushable.
- Encourage patient to stand in front of a mirror when changing pouch to increase visibility and avoid abdominal creases that might be present in the sitting position.

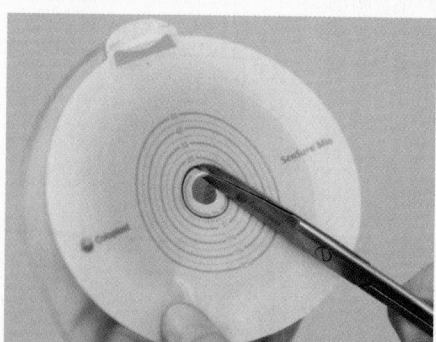
STEP 8 Cut opening in wafer. (Courtesy Coloplast, Minneapolis, MN.)

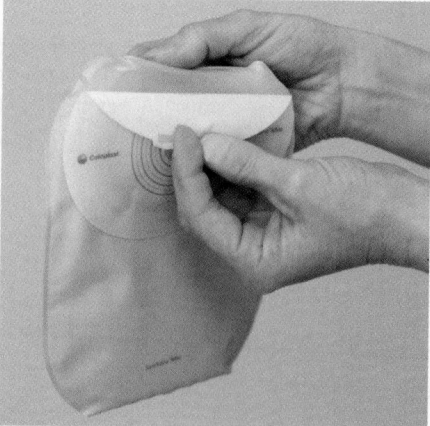
STEP 9 Remove protective backing. (Courtesy Coloplast, Minneapolis, MN.)

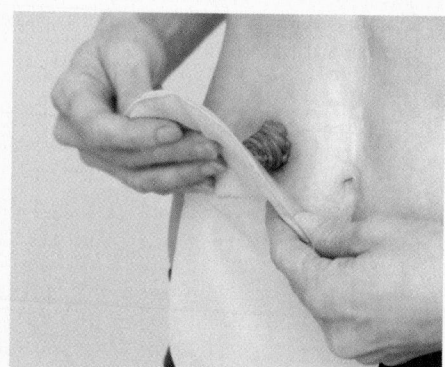
STEP 10 Apply pouch over stoma. (Courtesy Coloplast, Minneapolis, MN.)

KEY POINTS

- To effectively manage symptoms of altered or impaired digestive function, a knowledge of how the various organs work together to transport and utilize nutrients and eliminate waste is essential.
- There are many factors both simple and complex to consider when a patient presents with symptoms related to digestion and elimination.
- Listening carefully to patient or caregiver reporting and thorough physical assessment are necessary steps to determine the appropriate plan of care for a patient with alterations in his or her usual pattern of elimination.
- Knowledge of diagnostic and screening testing for gastrointestinal evaluation is important for the nurse to know so that appropriate patient education can be provided.
- Nursing interventions to promote normal bowel elimination include lifestyle changes, medications, and procedures that patients need to learn to improve bodily function and quality of life.
- A patient with a new ostomy needs both physical and emotional support from the nurse and should be referred to a nurse with specialized ostomy training whenever available.
- Nurses need to be proficient in the skills needed to relieve physical and psychological discomfort from altered bowel elimination.
- Every patient has bowel elimination needs regardless of age, care setting, diagnosis and co-morbid conditions. Critical thinking is essential in promoting normal bowel elimination and in providing care to patients with altered bowel elimination.

REFLECTIVE LEARNING

- A single young person with Crohn's disease is facing life with an ileostomy. The patient is relieved not to have the chronic pain he or she has been experiencing for years, but now the patient must navigate dating and intimacy issues with an ostomy. Think about how you would feel in the same situation and what would be helpful in discussing this patient's concerns.
- Most people with bowel elimination problems that require the assistance of health care personnel experience embarrassment. How can you treat them in a way that increases their comfort in both discussion of their bowel function and the performance of procedures related to bowel function?
- Often solutions to chronic constipation require lifestyle changes. What are some ways to motivate people to make these changes?

REVIEW QUESTIONS

1. Which nursing actions do you take when placing a bedpan under an immobilized patient? (Select all that apply.)
   1. Lift the patient's hips off the bed and slide the bedpan under the patient.
   2. After positioning the patient on the bedpan, elevate the head of the bed to a 45-degree angle.
   3. Adjust the head of the bed so that it is lower than the feet, and use gentle but firm pressure to push the bedpan under the patient.
   4. Have the patient stand beside the bed, and then have him or her sit on the bedpan on the edge of the bed.
   5. Make sure the patient has a nurse call system in reach to notify the nurse when he or she is ready to have the bedpan removed.

2. During the administration of a warm tap-water enema, a patient complains of cramping abdominal pain that he rates 6 out of 10. What nursing intervention should the nurse do first?
   1. Stop the instillation.
   2. Ask the patient to take deep breaths to decrease the pain.
   3. Tell the patient to bear down as he would when having a bowel movement.
   4. Continue the instillation; then administer a pain medication.

3. Which instructions do you include when educating a person with chronic constipation? (Select all that apply.)
   1. Increase fiber and fluids in the diet.
   2. Use a low-volume enema daily.
   3. Avoid gluten in the diet.
   4. Take laxatives twice a day.
   5. Exercise for 30 minutes every day.
   6. Schedule time to use the toilet at the same time every day.
   7. Take probiotics 5 times a week.

4. Which skills does the nurse teach a patient with a new colostomy before discharge from the hospital? (Select all that apply.)
   1. How to change the pouch
   2. How to empty the pouch
   3. How to open and close the pouch
   4. How to irrigate the colostomy
   5. How to determine whether the ostomy is healing appropriately

5. Place the steps for an ileostomy pouch change in the correct order.
   1. Close the end of the pouch.
   2. Measure the stoma.
   3. Cut the hole in the wafer to fit around the stoma and not leave skin exposed to the effluent.
   4. Press the pouch in place over the stoma.
   5. Remove the old pouch.
   6. Trace the correct measurement onto the back of the wafer.
   7. Assess the stoma and the skin around it.
   8. Cleanse and dry the peristomal skin.

6. Which symptoms are warning signs of possible colorectal cancer according to the American Cancer Society guidelines? (Select all that apply.)
   1. Change in bowel habits
   2. Blood in the stool
   3. A larger-than-normal bowel movement
   4. Fecal impaction
   5. Muscle aches
   6. Incomplete emptying of the colon
   7. Food particles in the stool
   8. Unexplained abdominal or back pain

7. A nurse is teaching a patient to obtain a specimen for fecal occult blood testing using fecal immunochemical testing (FIT) at home. How does the nurse instruct the patient to collect the specimen?
   1. Get three fecal smears from one bowel movement.
   2. Obtain one fecal smear from an early-morning bowel movement.
   3. Collect one fecal smear from three separate bowel movements.
   4. Get three fecal smears when you see blood in your bowel movement.

8. What should the nurse teach family caregivers when a patient has fecal incontinence because of cognitive impairment?
   1. Cleanse the skin with antibacterial soap, and apply talcum powder to the buttocks.
   2. Initiate bowel or habit training program to promote continence.
   3. Help the patient to toilet once every hour.
   4. Use sanitary pads in the patient's underwear.

9. The patient states, "I have diarrhea and cramping every time I have ice cream. I am sure this is because the food is cold." Based on this assessment data, which health problem does the nurse suspect?
   1. A food allergy
   2. Irritable bowel syndrome
   3. Increased peristalsis
   4. Lactose intolerance

10. A nurse is taking a health history of a newly admitted patient with a diagnosis of possible fecal impaction. Which question is the priority to ask the patient or caregiver?
    1. Have you eaten more high-fiber foods lately?
    2. Have you taken antibiotics recently?
    3. Do you have gluten intolerance?
    4. Have you experienced frequent, small liquid stools recently?

Answers: 1. 2, 5; **2.** 1; **3.** 1, 5, 6; **4.** 1, 2, 3, 5; **5.** 5; **6.** 3, 4; **7.** 2, 6, 3, 4, 1; **6.** 1, 2, 6, **8.** 7, 3, 8, 2, 9, 4; **10.** 4

Rationales for Review Questions can be found on the Evolve website.

REFERENCES

American Association of Critical-Care Nurses (AACN): AACN practice alert: prevention of aspiration in adults, *Crit Care Nurse* 37(3):88, 2017.

American Cancer Society (ACS): *Colorectal cancer*, 2018. http://www.cancer.org/Cancer/ColonandRectumCancer/DetailedGuide/index. Accessed September 3, 2018.

American Cancer Society (ACS): *Gap in cancer death rates narrows*, 2019. https://www.cancer.org/latest-news/gap-in-cancer-death-rates-between-blacks-and-whites-narrows.html. Accessed March 4, 2019.

Ball J, et al.: *Seidel's guide to physical examination*, ed 9, St Louis, 2019, Elsevier.

Blekken LE, et al.: Constipation and laxative use among nursing home patients: prevalence and associations derived from the Residents Assessment Instrument for Long-Term Care Facilities (interRAI LTCF), *Gastroenterol Res Pract* 2016:1215746, 2016.

Boullata J, et al.: ASPEN safe practices for enteral nutrition therapy, *J Parenter Enteral Nutr* 41(1):15, 2017.

Burchum JR, Rosenthal LD: *Lehne's pharmacology for nursing care*, ed 10, St Louis, 2019, Elsevier.

Carmel JE, et al.: *Wound, ostomy, and continence nurses Society: core curriculum ostomy management*, Philadelphia, 2016, Wolters Kluwer.

Centers for Disease Control and Prevention (CDC): *What is health literacy*, 2019, https://www.cdc.gov/healthliteracy/learn/index.html. Accessed December 23, 2019.

Delmore BA, Ayello EA: Pressure injuries caused by medical devices and other objects: a clinical update, *Am J Nurs* 117(12):36, 2017.

Emergency Nurses Association (ENA): *Clinical practice guideline: gastric tube placement verification*, 2018. https://www.ena.org/docs/default-source/resource-library/practice-resources/cpg/gastric-tubecpg7b5530b71c1e49e8b155b6cca1870adc.pdf?sfvrsn=a8e9dd7a_8. Accessed October 28 2019.

Goldberg M, et al.: *Clinical guideline: management of the adult patient with a fecal or urinary stoma*, Mount Laurel, NJ, 2017, Wound, Ostomy and Continence Nurses Society.

Harding MM, et al.: *Lewis's Medical-surgical nursing: assessment and management of clinical problems*, ed 11, St Louis, 2020, Elsevier.

Hockenberry ML, et al.: *Wong's nursing care of infants and children*, ed 11, Sr. Louis, 2019, Elsevier.

Hussain Z, et al.: Fecal impaction, *Curr Gastroenterol Rep* 16(9):404, 2014.

Mayo Clinic: *Water: how much should you drink every day?* 2017. http://www.mayoclinic.org/healthy-living/nutrition-and-healthy-eating/in-depth/water/art-20044256. Accessed September 3, 2018.

McDonald L, et al.: Clinical practice guidelines for *Clostridium difficile* infection in adults and children, *Clin Infect Dis* 66(7):1–48, 2018.

Metheny NA: AACN practice alert: prevention of aspiration in adults, *Crit Care Nurse* 36(1):e20, 2016.

National Institutes of Health (NIH): *National Institute of Diabetes and digestive kidney diseases: constipation*, 2018a. https://www.niddk.nih.gov/health-information/digestive-diseases/constipation/eating-diet-nutrition. Accessed September 3, 2018.

National Institutes of Health (NIH): *National Institute of Diabetes and digestive kidney diseases: fecal incontinence*, 2018b. https://www.niddk.nih.gov/health-information/digestive-diseases/bowel-control-problems-fecal-incontinence/treatment. Accessed September 3, 2018.

Pittman J, et al.: Medical device-related hospital-acquired pressure ulcers, *J Wound Ostomy Continence Nurs* 42(2):151, 2015.

Prinz A, et al.: Discharge planning for a patient with a new ostomy: best practice for clinicians, *J Wound Ostomy Continence Nurs* 42(1):79, 2015.

Simren M, et al.: Update on Rome IV Criteria for colorectal disorders: implications for clinical practice, *Curr Gastroenterol Rep* 19(4):L 15, 2017, 2017.

Solomon R, Jurica K: Closing the research-practice gap: increasing evidence-based practice for nasogastric tube insertion using education and an electronic order set, *J Emerg Nurs* 43(2):133, 2017.

The Joint Commission: *2020 National Patient Safety Goals*, Oakbrook Terrace, IL, 2020, The Commission, 2019 https://www.jointcommission.org/en/standards/national-patient-safety-goals/. Accessed January 2, 2020.

Uduak UA, et al.: Shared risk factors for constipation, fecal incontinence, and combined symptoms in older U.S. adults, *J Am Geriatr Soc* 64(11):e183, 2016.

US Food and Drug Administration (USFDA): *Food allergies: what you need to know*, 2018. https://www.fda.gov/Food/IngredientsPackagingLabeling/FoodAllergens/ucm079311.htm. Accessed September 3, 2018.

Williams R, et al.: Colorectal cancer in African Americans: an update prepared by the Committee on Minority Affairs and cultural diversity, American College of Gastroenterology, *Clin Transl Gastroenterol* 7(7):185–194, 2016.

Wound, Ostomy and Continence Nurses Society (WOCN): *Guideline for prevention and management of pressure ulcers (injuries)*, WOCN Clinical Practice Guideline Series, Mount Laurel, NJ, 2016, The Society.

RESEARCH REFERENCES

Bliss D, et al.: Time to and predictors of dual incontinence in older nursing home admissions, *Neurourol Urodyn* 37(1):229–236, 2017.

Burch J: Maintaining peristomal skin integrity, *Br J Community Nurs* 23(1):30–33, 2017.

Goudar BV, et al.: Early removal versus conventional removal of nasogastric tube after abdominal surgery: a prospective randomized controlled study, *Int Surg J* 4(1):229, 2017.

McFarland A: A cost utility analysis of the clinical algorithm for nasogastric tube placement confirmation in adult hospital patients, *J Adv Nurs* 73(1):201, 2017.

Mordiffi SZ, et al.: Confirming nasogastric tube placement: is the colorimeter as sensitive and specific as x-ray? A diagnostic accuracy study, *Int J Nurs Stud* 61:248, 2016.

Santos SCV, et al.: Methods to determine internal length of nasogastric feeding tubes: an integrative review, *Int J Nurs Stud* 61:95, 2016.

Steinhagen E, et al.: Intestinal stomas—postoperative stoma care and peristomal skin complications, *Clin Colon Rectal Surg* 30(3):184–192, 2017.

Taylor SJ, et al.: Nasogastric tube depth: the 'NEX' guideline is incorrect, *Br J Nurs* 23(12):641, 2014.

Tho PC, et al.: Implementation of the evidence-review on best practice for confirming the correct placement of nasogastric tube in patients in an acute care hospital, *Int J Evid Based Healthc* 9(1):51, 2011.

Van Bree SHW, et al.: Auscultation for bowel sounds in patients with ileus: an outdated practice in the ICU? *Netherlands J Crit Care* 26(4):142, 2018.

48

Skin Integrity and Wound Care

OBJECTIVES

- Discuss the risk factors that contribute to pressure injury formation.
- Describe the pressure injury staging system.
- Discuss the normal process of wound healing.
- Describe the differences in wound healing by primary and secondary intention.
- Explain the factors that impede or promote wound healing.
- Describe the differences in nursing care with acute and chronic wounds.
- Complete an assessment for a patient with impaired skin integrity.
- Develop a nursing care plan for a patient with impaired skin integrity.
- Apply critical thinking when providing care to patients at risk for or with actual impaired skin integrity.

KEY TERMS

Abrasion, p. 1249
Approximated, p. 1241
Blanching, p. 1237
Blanchable hyperemia, p. 1237
Debridement, p. 1258
Dehiscence, p. 1242
Drainage evacuators, p. 1266
Epithelialization, p. 1242
Eschar, p. 1248
Evisceration, p. 1242
Exudate, p. 1248
Fluctuance, p. 1238

Friction, p. 1238
Granulation tissue, p. 1248
Hemostasis, p. 1241
Induration, p. 1248
Laceration, p. 1249
Negative-pressure wound therapy, p. 1263
Nonblanchable erythema, p. 1237
Pressure injury, p. 1236
Primary intention, p. 1241
Puncture wound, p. 1249
Purulent, p. 1242
Reactive hyperemia, p. 1255

Sanguineous, p. 1243
Secondary intention, p. 1241
Serosanguineous, p. 1243
Serous, p. 1241
Shearing force, p. 1255
Slough, p. 1248
Tissue ischemia, p. 1237
Vacuum-assisted closure, p. 1263
Wound, p. 1239

MEDIA RESOURCES

http://evolve.elsevier.com/Potter/fundamentals/
- Review Questions
- Video Clips
- Concept Map Creator
- Case Study with Questions

- Skills Performance Checklists
- Audio Glossary
- Content Updates
- Answers to QSEN Activity and Review Questions

Skin, the largest organ in the body, is a protective barrier against disease-causing organisms and a sensory organ for pain, temperature, and touch; it also synthesizes vitamin D (Wysocki, 2016). Injury to the skin poses risks to an individual's safety and triggers a complex healing response. Your most important responsibilities include assessing and monitoring skin integrity, identifying patient risks for skin problems, identifying actual problems, and planning, implementing, and evaluating interventions to maintain skin integrity. Once a wound occurs, it is critical to know the process of normal wound healing to identify and implement the appropriate nursing interventions.

SCIENTIFIC KNOWLEDGE BASE

Skin

The skin has two layers: the epidermis and the dermis (Fig. 48.1). They are separated by a membrane, often referred to as the *dermal-epidermal junction*. The epidermis, or the top layer, has several layers. The stratum corneum is the thin outermost layer of the epidermis. It consists of flattened, dead, keratinized cells. The cells originate from the innermost epidermal layer, commonly called the *basal layer*. Cells in the basal layer divide, proliferate, and migrate toward the epidermal surface. After they reach the stratum corneum, they flatten and die. This constant movement ensures replacement of surface cells sloughed during normal desquamation or shedding. The thin stratum corneum protects underlying cells and tissues from dehydration and prevents entrance of certain chemical agents. The stratum corneum allows evaporation of water from the skin and permits absorption of certain topical medications.

The dermis, the inner layer of the skin, provides tensile strength; mechanical support; and protection for the underlying muscles, bones, and organs. It differs from the epidermis in that it contains mostly connective tissue and few skin cells. Collagen (a tough, fibrous protein), blood vessels, and nerves are found in the dermal layer. Fibroblasts, which are responsible for collagen formation, are the only distinctive cell type within the dermis.

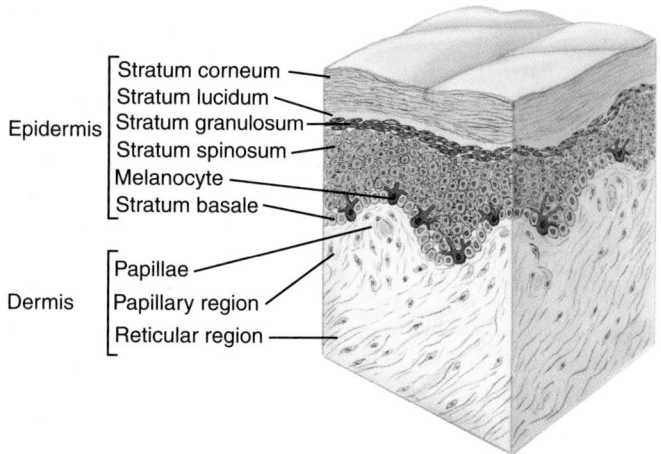

FIG. 48.1 Layers of skin. (From Applegate E: *The anatomy and physiology learning system*, ed 4, St Louis, 2011, Saunders.)

Epidermis
- Stratum corneum
- Stratum lucidum
- Stratum granulosum
- Stratum spinosum
- Melanocyte
- Stratum basale

Dermis
- Papillae
- Papillary region
- Reticular region

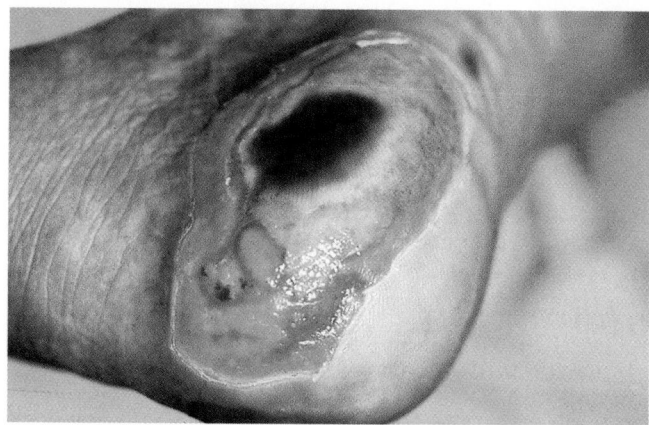

FIG. 48.2 Pressure injury with tissue necrosis.

BOX 48.1 FOCUS ON OLDER ADULTS

Skin-Associated Issues

When caring for the older adult there are several skin-related issues to consider when assessing skin and risk for skin breakdown. Age-related changes such as reduced skin elasticity, decreased collagen, and thinning of underlying muscle and tissues cause the older adult's skin to be easily torn in response to mechanical trauma, especially shearing forces (Wysocki, 2016). The attachment between the epidermis and dermis becomes flattened in older adults, allowing the skin to be easily torn in response to mechanical trauma (e.g., tape removal). Existing medical conditions and polypharmacy are factors that interfere with wound healing. Aging causes a diminished inflammatory response, resulting in slow epithelialization and wound healing (Doughty and Sparks, 2016).

Implications for Practice
- There is a decreased barrier function and less protection from excessive moisture, shear, friction, and pressure.
- Aging skin has decreased epidermal turnover, and healing requires more time.
- When removing any adhesive dressings or tapes, gently release the skin from the tape; do not pull the tape away from the skin. Release the skin from the adhesive by gently pushing the skin from the adhesive.
- Decreased subcutaneous tissue reduces padding protection over bony prominences.
- There is a decrease in subcutaneous padding over bony prominences, where impaired skin integrity and injury to other tissues are most likely to occur (Wysocki, 2016).

Understanding skin structure helps you understand the risks for impaired skin integrity and promote wound healing. Intact skin protects the patient from chemical and mechanical injury. When the skin is injured, the epidermis functions to resurface the wound and restore the barrier against invading organisms, and the dermis responds to restore the structural integrity (collagen) and the physical properties of the skin. The normal aging process alters skin characteristics and makes skin more vulnerable to damage (see Box 48.1).

Pressure Injuries

Pressure injury, pressure ulcer, decubitus ulcer, and *bedsore* are terms used to describe impaired skin integrity related to unrelieved, prolonged pressure. The most current terminology is pressure injury (Fig. 48.2), which is consistent with the recommendations of the National Pressure Ulcer Advisory Panel (Edsberg et al., 2016). A pressure injury is localized damage to the skin and underlying soft tissue, usually over a bony prominence or related to a medical device or other device. The injury can present as intact skin, a blister, or an open ulcer and may be painful. The injury occurs as a result of intense and/or prolonged pressure or pressure in combination with shear (Edsberg et al., 2016). The tolerance of soft tissue for pressure and shear may also be affected by microclimate, nutrition, perfusion, co-morbidities, and condition of the soft tissue.

A number of contributing factors are associated with pressure injuries; the significance of these factors is not yet clear (EPUAP, NPIAP, PPPIA, 2019a). Any patient experiencing decreased mobility, decreased sensory perception, fecal or urinary incontinence, and/or poor nutrition is at risk for pressure injury development. Examples of patients who are at risk for the development of pressure injuries include the following:
- Older adults, those who have experienced trauma
- Those with spinal-cord injuries (SCI)
- Those who have sustained a fractured hip
- Those in long-term homes or community care, the acutely ill, or those in a hospice setting
- Individuals with diabetes
- Patients in critical care settings (EPUAP, NPIAP, PPPIA, 2019a)

Pressure is a major cause of injury. Tissue receives oxygen and nutrients and eliminates metabolic wastes via the blood. Pressure or other factors that interfere with blood flow in turn interfere with cellular metabolism and the function or life of the cells. Prolonged, intense pressure affects cellular metabolism by decreasing or obliterating blood flow, resulting in tissue ischemia and ultimately tissue death.

Pathogenesis of Pressure Injuries. Pressure is the major element in the cause of pressure injuries. Current theory suggests that skin and soft tissue damage can begin at the surface and progress inward or begin at the muscle and progress outward, depending on causation (WOCN, 2016). Top-down damage (superficial) is thought to be caused by superficial shear or friction, presenting as red skin (stage 1 pressure injury). Bottom-up (deep) damage is believed to be caused by several pressure-related factors: (1) pressure intensity, (2) pressure duration, and (3) tissue tolerance.

Pressure Intensity. A classic research study identified capillary closing pressure as the minimal amount of pressure required to collapse a capillary (e.g., when the pressure exceeds the normal capillary pressure range of 15 to 32 mm Hg) (Burton and Yamada, 1951). Therefore, when the pressure applied over a capillary exceeds the normal capillary pressure and the vessel is occluded for a prolonged

🌐 BOX 48.2 CULTURAL ASPECTS OF CARE

Impact of Skin Color

Detecting cyanosis and other changes in skin color in patients is an important clinical skill. However, this detection becomes a challenge in patients with darkly pigmented skin (EPUAP, NPIAP, PPPIA, 2019a; Henderson et al., 1997). Color differentiation of cyanosis varies according to skin pigmentation. In patients with darkly pigmented skin, you need to know the individual's baseline skin tone. For example, do not confuse the normal hyperpigmentation of Mongolian spots that are seen on the sacrum of African, Native American, and Asian patients with cyanosis.

Implications for Patient-Centered Care

- Patients with darkly pigmented skin cannot be assessed for pressure injury risk by examining only skin color (EPUAP, NPIAP, PPPIA, 2019a).
- Use natural lighting but note that visual inspection techniques to identify pressure injuries are ineffective in darkly pigmented skin. Assess for changes in sensation, temperature, or tissue consistency, which may precede visual skin changes (Ratliff et al., 2017; WOCN, 2016).
- Examine body sites with the least melanin such as under the arm for underlying color identification (Nix, 2016).
- Assess pressure areas and localized skin color changes. Any of the following may appear (WOCN, 2016):
  - Color remains unchanged when pressure is applied.
  - Color changes occur at site of pressure, which differ from patient's usual skin color.
  - If patient previously had a pressure injury, that area of skin may be lighter than original color.
  - Localized area of skin may be purple/blue or violet instead of red. Purple or maroon discoloration may indicate deep tissue injury.
- Palpate surrounding tissues to identify any changes in temperature, edema, or tissue consistency between area of injury or suspected injury and normal tissue (EPUAP, NPIAP, PPPIA, 2019a; Nix, 2016).
- Circumscribed area of intact skin may be warm to touch. As tissue changes color, intact skin will feel cool to touch. NOTE: Gloves may decrease sensitivity to changes in skin temperature.
- Localized heat (inflammation) is detected by making comparisons to surrounding skin. Localized area of warmth eventually will be replaced by area of coolness, which is a sign of tissue devitalization.
- Edema may occur with induration of more than 15 mm in diameter, and skin may appear taut and shiny (Nix, 2016).

---

boggy [less than normal stiffness or mushy] when palpated), sensation (pain), edema, and warmer or cooler temperature (EPUAP, NPIAP, PPPIA, 2019a,b; Bryant and Nix, 2016a).

Pressure Duration. Low pressure over a prolonged period and high-intensity pressure over a short period are two concerns related to duration of pressure. Both types of pressure cause tissue damage. Extended pressure occludes blood flow and nutrients and contributes to cell death (Pieper, 2016). Clinical implications of pressure duration include evaluating the amount of pressure (checking skin for nonblanching hyperemia) and determining the amount of time that a patient tolerates pressure (checking to be sure after relieving pressure that the affected area blanches).

Tissue Tolerance. The ability of tissue to endure pressure depends on the integrity of the tissue and the supporting structures. The extrinsic factors of shear, friction, and moisture affect the ability of the skin to tolerate pressure: the greater the degree to which the factors of shear, friction, and moisture are present, the more susceptible the skin will be to damage from pressure. The second factor related to tissue tolerance is the ability of the underlying skin structures (blood vessels, collagen) to help redistribute pressure. Systemic factors such as poor nutrition, aging, hydration status, and low blood pressure affect the tolerance of the tissue to externally applied pressure.

Risk Factors for Pressure Injury Development. A variety of factors predispose a patient to pressure injury formation. These factors may be related to a disease (e.g., reduced peripheral circulation from diabetes), or they may be secondary to an illness (e.g., decreased sensation following a cerebrovascular accident).

Impaired Sensory Perception. Patients with altered sensory perception for pain and pressure are more at risk for impaired skin integrity. They are unable to feel when a part of their body undergoes increased, prolonged pressure or pain. Thus a patient who can't feel or sense that there is pain or pressure is at risk for the development of pressure injuries.

Impaired Mobility. Patients who are unable to independently change positions are at risk for pressure injury. For example, a patient who is seriously ill will be weakened and less likely to turn independently. Patients with spinal cord injuries have decreased or absent motor and sensory function and are unable to reposition off bony prominences.

Alteration in Level of Consciousness. Patients who are comatose, confused or disoriented; those who have expressive aphasia or the inability to verbalize; and those with changing levels of consciousness are unable to protect themselves from pressure injury. Also patients who are confused or disoriented may be able to feel pressure but are not always able to understand how to relieve it or communicate their discomfort. A patient in a coma cannot perceive pressure and is unable to move voluntarily to relieve pressure.

Shear. Shear force is the sliding movement of skin and subcutaneous tissue while the underlying muscle and bone are stationary (Bryant, 2016). Shear force occurs when the head of the bed is elevated and the sliding of the skeleton starts but the skin is fixed because of friction with the bed (Fig. 48.3). It also occurs when transferring a patient from bed to stretcher when a patient's skin is pulled across the bed. (This can be avoided using safe patient handling techniques.) When shear is present, the skin and subcutaneous layers adhere to the surface of the bed, and the layers of muscle and the bones slide in the direction of body movement. The damage that shear causes occurs at the deeper fascial level of the tissues over the bony prominence (Pieper, 2016). The underlying tissue capillaries are stretched and angulated by the shear force. As a result, necrosis occurs deep within the tissue layers. The tissue damage is deep in the tissues and causes undermining of the dermis and is a cause of pressure injury development.

---

period of time, tissue ischemia can occur. If the patient has reduced sensation and cannot respond to the discomfort of the ischemia, tissue ischemia and tissue death result.

The clinical presentation of obstructed blood flow occurs when evaluating areas of pressure. After a period of tissue ischemia, if the pressure is relieved and the blood flow returns, the skin turns red. The effect of this redness is vasodilation (blood vessel expansion), called *hyperemia* (redness). You assess an area of hyperemia by pressing a finger over the affected area. If it blanches (turns lighter in color) and the erythema returns when you remove your finger, the hyperemia is transient and is an attempt to overcome the ischemic episode, thus called blanchable hyperemia. However, if the erythematous area does not blanch (nonblanchable erythema) when you apply pressure, deep tissue damage is probable.

Blanching occurs when the normal red tones of the light-skinned patient are absent. When checking for pressure injuries in patients with darkly pigmented skin, dark skin may not show the blanch response. Inspect suspected pressure-related skin alterations with an adjacent or opposite area of the body for comparison (Box 48.2). Skin inspection should include assessment of changes in skin tissue, consistency (firm vs.

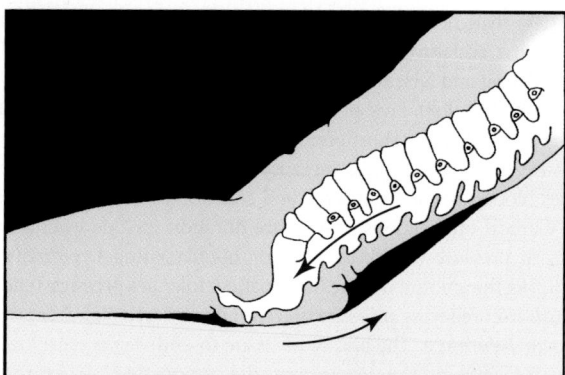

FIG. 48.3 Shear exerted in sacral area.

Friction. The force of two surfaces moving across one another such as the mechanical force exerted when skin is dragged across a coarse surface such as bed linens is called friction (WOCN, 2016). Unlike shear injuries, friction injuries affect the epidermis or top layer of the skin (superficial skin loss). The denuded skin appears red and painful and is sometimes referred to as a *sheet burn.* A friction injury occurs in patients who are restless, in those who have uncontrollable movements such as spastic conditions, and in those whose skin is dragged rather than lifted from the bed surface during position changes or transfer to a stretcher. This type of injury should not be classified as a pressure injury (EPUAP, NPIAP, PPPIA, 2019b). Friction leads to pressure injury formation only when it causes harmful shear stress and strain (Brienza et al., 2015).

Moisture. The presence and duration of moisture on the skin increases the risk of pressure injury. Moisture reduces the resistance of the skin to other physical factors such as pressure, friction, or shear. Prolonged moisture softens skin, making it more susceptible to damage. The term moisture-associated skin damage (MASD) is defined as inflammation and erosion to the skin caused by prolonged exposure to various sources of moisture, including wound drainage, urine or stool, perspiration, wound exudate, mucus or saliva (Colwell et al., 2011).

Classification of Pressure Injuries

A staging system classifies pressure injuries. Accurate staging requires knowledge of the skin layers. A major drawback of a staging system is that you cannot stage an injury when it is covered with necrotic tissue because the necrotic tissue is covering the depth of the injury. In serious wounds with necrotic tissue, the wound must be debrided or removed (if appropriate to the overall treatment plan) to expose the wound base to allow for assessment.

Pressure injury staging describes the pressure injury depth at the point of assessment. Thus, once you have staged the pressure injury, this stage endures even as it heals. Pressure injuries do not progress from a stage 3 to a stage 1; rather, a stage 3 injury demonstrating signs of healing is described as a healing stage 3 pressure injury (Pieper, 2016). In 2016, the National Pressure Advisory Panel developed the following classification/staging system (EPUAP, NPIAP, PPPIA, 2019b; Edsberg et al., 2016):

- **Stage 1 Pressure Injury:** Nonblanchable erythema of intact skin
  Intact skin with a localized area of nonblanchable erythema, which may appear differently in darkly pigmented skin (Fig. 48.4A). Presence of blanchable erythema or changes in sensation, temperature, or firmness may precede visual changes. Color changes do not include purple or maroon discoloration; these may indicate deep tissue pressure injury.
- **Stage 2 Pressure Injury:** Partial-thickness skin loss with exposed dermis
  Partial-thickness loss of skin with exposed dermis (see Fig. 48.4B). The wound bed is viable, pink or red, and moist and may also present as an intact or ruptured serum-filled blister. Adipose (fat) is not visible, and deeper tissues are not visible. Granulation tissue, slough, and eschar are not present. These injuries commonly result from adverse microclimate and shear in the skin over the pelvis and shear in the heel. This stage should not be used to describe moisture-associated skin damage (MASD), including incontinence-associated dermatitis (IAD), intertriginous dermatitis (ITD), medical adhesive–related skin injury (MARSI), or traumatic wounds (skin tears, burns, abrasions).
- **Stage 3 Pressure Injury:** Full-thickness skin loss
  Full-thickness loss of skin, in which adipose (fat) is visible in the ulcer and granulation tissue and epibole (rolled wound edges) are often present (see Fig. 48.4C). Slough and/or eschar may be visible. The depth of tissue damage varies by anatomical location; areas of significant adiposity can develop in deep wounds. Undermining and tunneling may occur. Fascia, muscle, tendon, ligament, cartilage, and/or bone are not exposed. If slough or eschar obscures the extent of tissue loss, this is an Unstageable Pressure Injury.
- **Stage 4 Pressure Injury:** Full-thickness skin and tissue loss
  Full-thickness skin and tissue loss with exposed or directly palpable fascia, muscle, tendon, ligament, cartilage, or bone in the ulcer (see Fig. 48.4D). Slough and/or eschar may be visible. Epibole (rolled edges), undermining, and/or tunneling often occur. Depth varies by anatomical location. If slough or eschar obscures the extent of tissue loss this is an Unstageable Pressure Injury.
- **Deep-Tissue Pressure Injury:** Persistent nonblanchable deep red, maroon, or purple discoloration
  Intact or nonintact skin with localized area of persistent nonblanchable deep red, maroon, purple discoloration or epidermal separation revealing a dark wound bed or blood-filled blister (see Fig. 48.4E). Pain and temperature change often precede skin color changes. Discoloration may appear differently in darkly pigmented skin. This injury results from intense and/or prolonged pressure and shear forces at the bone-muscle interface. The wound may evolve rapidly to reveal the actual extent of tissue injury or may resolve without tissue loss. If necrotic tissue, subcutaneous tissue, granulation tissue, fascia, muscle or other underlying structures are visible, this indicates a full-thickness pressure injury (Unstageable, Stage 3, or Stage 4). Do not use Deep-Tissue Pressure Injury to describe vascular, traumatic, neuropathic, or dermatologic conditions.
- **Unstageable Pressure Injury:** Obscured full-thickness skin and tissue loss
  Full-thickness skin and tissue loss in which the extent of tissue damage within the ulcer cannot be confirmed because it is obscured by slough or eschar (see Fig. 48.4F). If slough or eschar is removed, a Stage 3 or Stage 4 pressure injury will be revealed. Stable eschar (i.e., dry, adherent, intact without erythema or fluctuance) on the heel or ischemic limb should not be softened or removed.

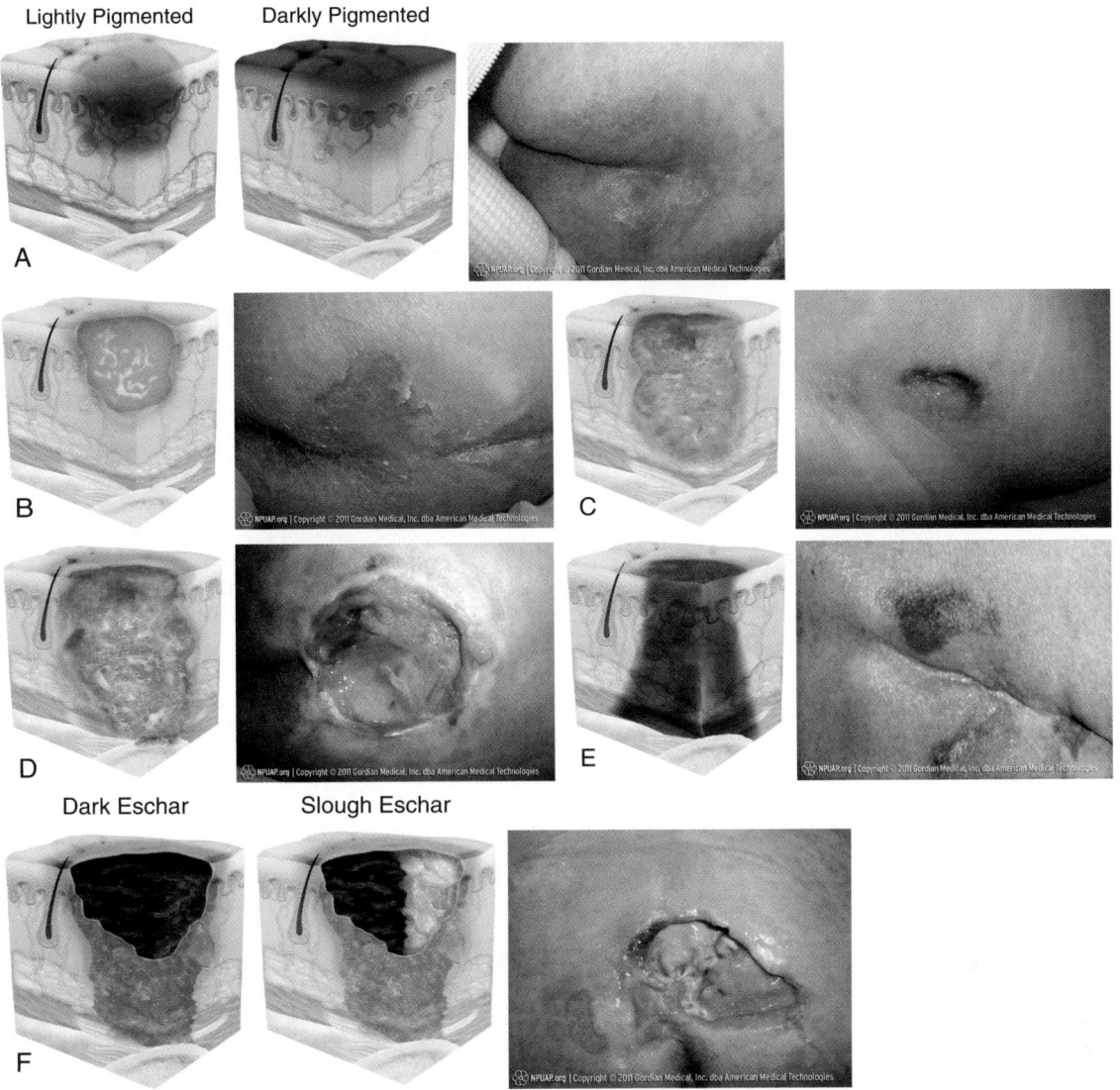

FIG. 48.4 Diagram of Pressure Injury Stages. **A,** Stage 1 pressure injury. **B,** Stage 2 pressure injury. **C,** Stage 3 pressure injury. **D,** Stage 4 pressure injury. **E,** Deep tissue injury. **F,** Unstageable pressure injury. (Used with permission of the European Pressure Ulcer Advisory Panel [EPUAP] and National Pressure Injury Advisory Panel [NPIAP], and Pan Pacific Pressure Injury Alliance: Treatment of pressure ulcers/injuries: Quick Reference Guide, Emily Haesler (Ed.). EPUAP/NPIAP/PPPIA, 2019.)

The EPUAP, NPIAP, PPPIA (2019 a, b) guidelines suggest that when conducting a skin assessment on an individual with darkly pigmented skin, carefully inspect any discoloration over pressure areas, and surrounding skin should be assessed more closely for temperature changes, edema, and changes in tissue consistency and pain . For additional aspects of assessing darkly pigmented skin, see Box 48.2.

Wound Classifications

A wound is a disruption of the integrity and function of tissues in the body (Baranoski et al., 2016).

All wounds require careful evaluation and treatment based on a thorough assessment, the patient's overall condition, and the goal of treatment. Understanding the etiology of a wound is important because the treatment will vary depending on the underlying disease process.

There are many ways to classify surgical and traumatic wounds. Wound classification systems describe onset and duration of healing process (e.g., the status of skin integrity, cause of the wound, or severity or extent of tissue injury or damage) (Table 48.1) and descriptive qualities of the pressure injury or wound tissue such as color (Fig. 48.5). Wound classification enables a nurse to understand the risks associated with a wound and implications for healing.

Process of Wound Healing. Wound healing involves integrated physiological processes. The tissue layers involved and their capacity

TABLE 48.1   Wound Classification

Description	Causes	Implications for Healing
Onset and Duration		
Acute		
Wound that proceeds through an orderly and timely reparative process that results in sustained restoration of anatomical and functional integrity	Trauma Surgical incision	Wound edges are clean and intact.
Chronic		
Wound that fails to proceed through an orderly and timely process to produce anatomical and functional integrity	Vascular compromise, chronic inflammation, or repetitive insults to tissue (Doughty and Sparks, 2016)	Continued exposure to insult impedes wound healing.
Healing Process		
Primary Intention		
Wound that is closed	Surgical incision Wound that is sutured or stapled	Healing occurs by epithelialization; heals quickly with minimal scar formation.
Secondary Intention		
Wound edges not approximated	Surgical wounds that have tissue loss or contamination	Wound heals by granulation tissue formation, wound contraction, and epithelialization.
Tertiary Intention		
Wound that is left open for several days; then wound edges are approximated (see Fig. 48.4,*C*)	Wounds that are contaminated and require observation for signs of inflammation	Closure of wound is delayed until risk of infection is resolved (Doughty and Sparks, 2016).

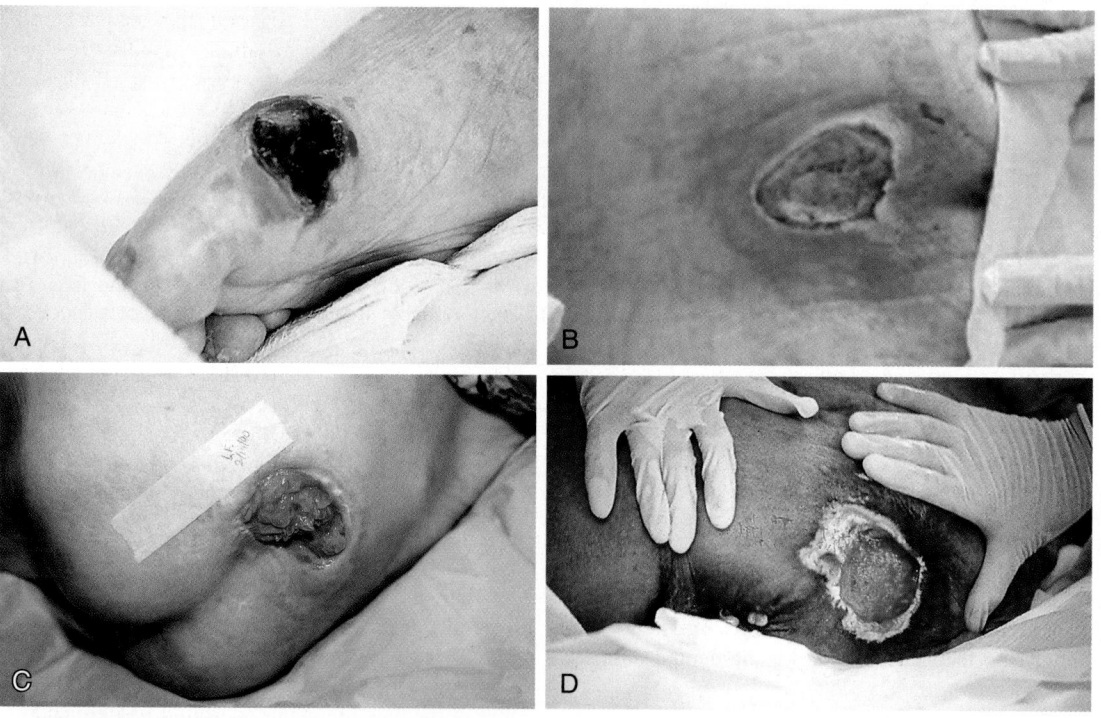

FIG. 48.5 Wounds classified by color assessment. **A**, Black wound. **B**, Yellow wound. **C**, Red wound. **D**, Mixed-color wound. (**A** and **D** Courtesy Scott Health Care—A Mölnlycke Company, Philadelphia, PA; **B** and **C** from Bryant RA, Nix DP, editors: *Acute and chronic wounds: current management concepts*, ed 5, St Louis, 2016, Elsevier.)

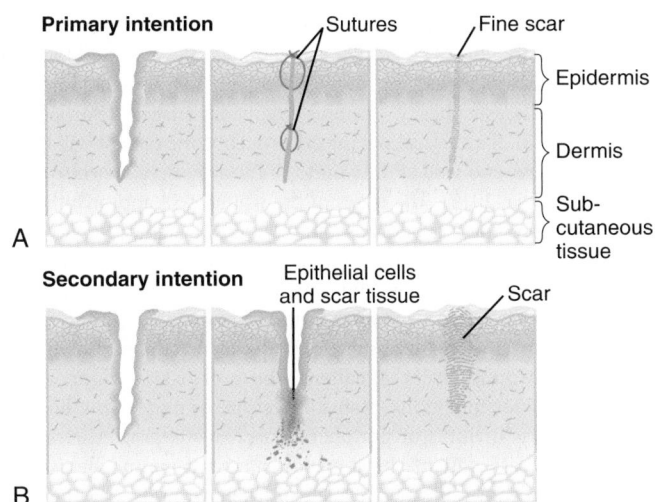

FIG. 48.6 A, Wound healing by primary intention such as a surgical incision. Wound healing edges are pulled together and approximated with sutures or staples, and healing occurs by connective tissue deposition. B, Wound healing by secondary intention. Wound edges are not approximated, and healing occurs by granulation tissue formation and contraction of the wound edges. (From Black JM, Hawks JH: *Medical-surgical nursing: clinical management for positive outcomes,* ed 8, St Louis, 2009, Mosby.)

for regeneration determine the mechanism for repair for any wound (Doughty and Sparks, 2016). Table 48.1 reviews the classification of wounds by onset and duration and healing process. Wounds can also be classified by the extent of tissue loss: partial-thickness wounds that involve only a partial loss of skin layers (the epidermis and superficial dermal layers) and full-thickness wounds that involve total loss of the skin layers (epidermis and dermis) (Doughty and Sparks, 2016). Partial-thickness wounds are shallow in depth, moist, and painful, and the wound base generally appears red. A full-thickness wound extends into the subcutaneous layer, can be painful, and the depth and tissue type varies, depending on body location. The significance of determining whether an injury is a partial- or full-thickness wound lies in the mechanism of healing. A partial-thickness wound heals by regeneration, and a full-thickness wound heals by forming new tissue, a process that can take longer than the healing of a partial-thickness wound.

A clean surgical incision is an example of a wound with little tissue loss. The surgical incision heals by primary intention (Fig. 48.6A). The skin edges are approximated, or closed, and the risk of infection is low. Healing occurs quickly, with minimal scar formation, as long as infection and secondary breakdown are prevented (Doughty and Sparks, 2016). In contrast, a wound involving loss of tissue such as a burn, stage II pressure injury, or severe laceration heals by secondary intention. The wound is left open until it becomes filled by scar tissue. It takes longer for a wound to heal by secondary intention; thus the chance of infection is greater. If scarring from secondary intention is severe, loss of tissue function is often permanent (see Fig. 48.6B).

Wound Repair. Partial-thickness wounds are shallow, involving loss of epidermis and possible loss of dermis. These wounds heal by regeneration because epidermis regenerates. An example of a partial-thickness wound is a scrape or an abrasion. Full-thickness wounds extend into the dermis and heal by scar formation because deeper structures do not regenerate. Stage III and IV pressure injuries are examples of full-thickness wounds.

Partial-Thickness Wound Repair. Three components are involved in the healing process of a partial-thickness wound: inflammatory response, epithelial proliferation (reproduction) and migration, and reestablishment of the epidermal layers.

Tissue trauma causes the *inflammatory response,* which in turn causes redness and swelling to the area with a moderate amount of serous exudate. This response generally is limited to the first 24 hours after wounding. The epithelial cells begin to regenerate, providing new cells to replace the lost cells. The *epithelial proliferation and migration* start at both the wound edges and the epidermal cells lining the epidermal appendages, allowing for quick resurfacing. Epithelial cells begin to migrate across a wound bed soon after the wound occurs. A wound that is kept moist can resurface in 4 days, whereas one left open to air can resurface within 6 to 7 days. The difference in the healing rate is related to the fact that epidermal cells only migrate across a moist surface. In a dry wound the cells migrate down into a moist level before migration can occur (Doughty and Sparks, 2016). New epithelium is only a few cells thick and must undergo *reestablishment of the epidermal layers.* The cells slowly reestablish normal thickness and appear as dry pink tissue.

Full-Thickness Wound Repair. The four phases involved in the healing process of a full-thickness wound are hemostasis, inflammatory, proliferative, and maturation.

Hemostasis. A series of physiological events designed to control blood loss, establish bacterial control, and seal the defect occurs when there is an injury. During hemostasis injured blood vessels constrict, and platelets gather to stop bleeding. Clots form a fibrin matrix that later provides a framework for cellular repair.

Inflammatory Phase. In the inflammatory stage damaged tissue and mast cells secrete histamine, resulting in vasodilation of surrounding capillaries and movement/migration of serum and white blood cells into the damaged tissues. This results in localized redness, edema, warmth, and throbbing. The inflammatory response is beneficial, and there is no value in attempting to cool the area or reduce the swelling unless the swelling occurs within a closed compartment (e.g., spinal cord injury, ankle, or neck) (Kelechi et al., 2017).

Leukocytes (white blood cells) reach a wound within a few hours. The primary-acting white blood cell is the neutrophil, which begins to ingest bacteria and small debris. The second important leukocyte is the monocyte, which transforms into macrophages. The macrophages are the "garbage cells" that clean a wound of bacteria, dead cells, and debris by phagocytosis. Macrophages continue the process of clearing a wound of debris and release growth factors that attract fibroblasts, the cells that synthesize collagen (connective tissue). Collagen appears as early as the second day and is the main component of scar tissue.

In a clean wound the inflammatory phase establishes a clean wound bed. The inflammatory phase is prolonged if too little inflammation occurs, as in a debilitating disease such as cancer or after administration of steroids. Too much inflammation also prolongs healing because arriving cells compete for available nutrients. An example is a wound infection in which the increased metabolic energy requirements present in an infected wound compete for the available calorie intake.

Proliferative Phase. With the appearance of new blood vessels as reconstruction progresses, the proliferative phase begins and lasts from 3 to 24 days. The main activities during this phase are the filling of a wound with granulation tissue, wound contraction, and wound resurfacing by epithelialization. Fibroblasts are present in this phase and are the cells that synthesize collagen, providing the matrix for granulation. Collagen mixes with the granulation tissue to form a matrix that supports the reepithelialization. Collagen provides strength and structural integrity to a wound. During this period a wound contracts to reduce the area that requires healing. Finally the epithelial cells migrate from the wound edges to resurface. In a clean wound the proliferative phase accomplishes the following: the vascular bed is reestablished (granulation tissue), the area is filled with replacement tissue (collagen, contraction, and granulation tissue), and the surface is repaired (epithelialization). Impairment of healing during this stage usually results from systemic factors such as age, anemia, hypoprotein-emia, and zinc deficiency.

Maturation. Maturation, the final stage of healing, sometimes takes place for more than a year, depending on the depth and extent of the wound. The collagen scar continues to reorganize and gain strength for several months. However, a healed wound usually does not have the tensile strength of the tissue it replaces. Collagen fibers undergo remodeling or reorganization before assuming their normal appearance. Usually scar tissue contains fewer pigmented cells (melanocytes) and has a lighter color than normal skin. In individuals with darkly pigmented skin, the scar tissue may be more highly pigmented than surrounding skin.

Complications of Wound Healing

Hemorrhage. Hemorrhage, or bleeding from a wound site, is normal during and immediately after initial trauma. However hemostasis occurs within several minutes unless large blood vessels are involved or a patient has poor clotting function. Hemorrhage occurring after hemostasis indicates a dislodged surgical suture, a clot, infection, or erosion of a blood vessel by a foreign object (e.g., a drain). Hemorrhage may occur externally or internally. For example, if a surgical suture is dislodged from a blood vessel, bleeding occurs internally within the tissues, and there may not be visible signs of blood unless a surgical drain is present. A surgical drain may be inserted into tissues beneath a wound to remove fluid that collects in underlying tissues.

You detect internal hemorrhaging by looking for distention or swelling of the affected body part, a change in the type and amount of drainage from a surgical drain, or signs of hypovolemic shock. A hematoma is a localized collection of blood underneath the tissues. It appears as swelling, change in color, sensation, or warmth that often takes on a bluish discoloration. A hematoma near a major artery or vein is dangerous because pressure from the expanding hematoma obstructs blood flow.

External hemorrhaging is obvious. You observe dressings covering a wound for bloody drainage, and you observe for blood underneath the body. If bleeding is extensive, the dressing soon becomes saturated, and frequently blood drains from under the dressing and pools beneath the patient. Observe all wounds closely, particularly surgical wounds, in which the risk of hemorrhage is great during the first 24 to 48 hours after surgery or injury.

Infection. Wound infection is the second most common health care–associated infection (see Chapter 28). All wounds have some level of bacterial burden; few wounds are infected (Stotts, 2016b). Wound infection is present when the microorganisms invade the wound tissues. The local clinical signs of wound infection can include erythema; increased amount of wound drainage; change in appearance of the wound drainage (thick, color change, presence of odor); and periwound warmth, pain, or edema. A patient may have a fever and an increase in white blood cell count. Laboratory tests such as a wound culture or tissue biopsy can be done to evaluate the wound for infection.

Some contaminated or traumatic wounds show signs of infection early, within 2 to 3 days. Surgical site infections occur within 30 days of surgery; risk factors include hyperglycemia, smoking, untreated peripheral vascular disease, obesity, age, and emergency surgery (Burden and Thornton, 2018). If a surgical site infection occurs, the patient will have a fever, tenderness, and pain at the wound site and an elevated white blood cell count (Stryja, 2018). The edges of the wound will appear inflamed. If drainage is present, it is odorous and purulent, which causes a yellow, green, or brown color, depending on the causative organism (Table 48.2).

Dehiscence. When an incision fails to heal properly, the layers of skin and tissue separate. This most commonly occurs before collagen formation (3 to 11 days after injury). Dehiscence is the partial or total separation of wound layers. A patient who is at risk for poor wound healing (e.g., poor nutritional status, infection, or underlying diseases such as diabetes mellitus or peripheral vascular disease) is at risk for dehiscence. Obese patients have a higher risk of wound dehiscence because of the constant strain placed on their wounds and the poor healing qualities of fat tissue (Pierpont et al., 2014). Dehiscence can happen in abdominal surgical wounds and occurs after a sudden strain such as coughing, vomiting, or sitting up in bed. Patients often report feeling as though something has given way. When there is an increase in serosanguineous drainage from a wound in the first few days after surgery, be alert for the potential for dehiscence.

Evisceration. With total separation of wound layers, evisceration (protrusion of visceral organs through a wound opening) occurs. The condition is an emergency that requires surgical repair. When evisceration occurs, place sterile gauze soaked in sterile saline over the extruding tissues to reduce chances of bacterial invasion and drying of the tissues. If the organs protrude through the wound, blood supply to the tissues can be compromised. Then contact the surgical team, do not allow the patient anything by mouth (NPO), observe for signs and symptoms of shock, and prepare the patient for emergency surgery.

REFLECT NOW

Consider a patient you recently cared for. What were the patient's risk factors for pressure injuries and in what way did those risk factors affect the condition of the skin?

NURSING KNOWLEDGE BASE

Prediction and Prevention of Pressure Injuries

Preventing pressure injuries is a priority and is not limited to patients with restrictions in mobility. Impaired skin integrity usually is not a problem in healthy individuals but is a serious and potentially devastating problem in ill or debilitated patients (WOCN, 2016). Consistent, planned skin-care interventions are critical to ensuring high-quality care. Whenever you are in direct contact with a patient, observe the skin for impaired skin integrity and/or pressure injury.

Risk Assessment. Several tools are available for assessing patients who are at risk for developing a pressure injury. By identifying at-risk patients, you are able to put preventive interventions into place and also spare those low-risk patients unnecessary and sometimes costly preventive treatments.

The incidence of pressure injuries in a health care agency is an important indicator of quality of care. Evidence exists that a program of prevention guided by risk assessment simultaneously reduces the institutional incidence of pressure injuries by as much as 60% and brings

TABLE 48.2   Types of Wound Drainage

Type	Appearance
Serous	Clear, watery plasma
	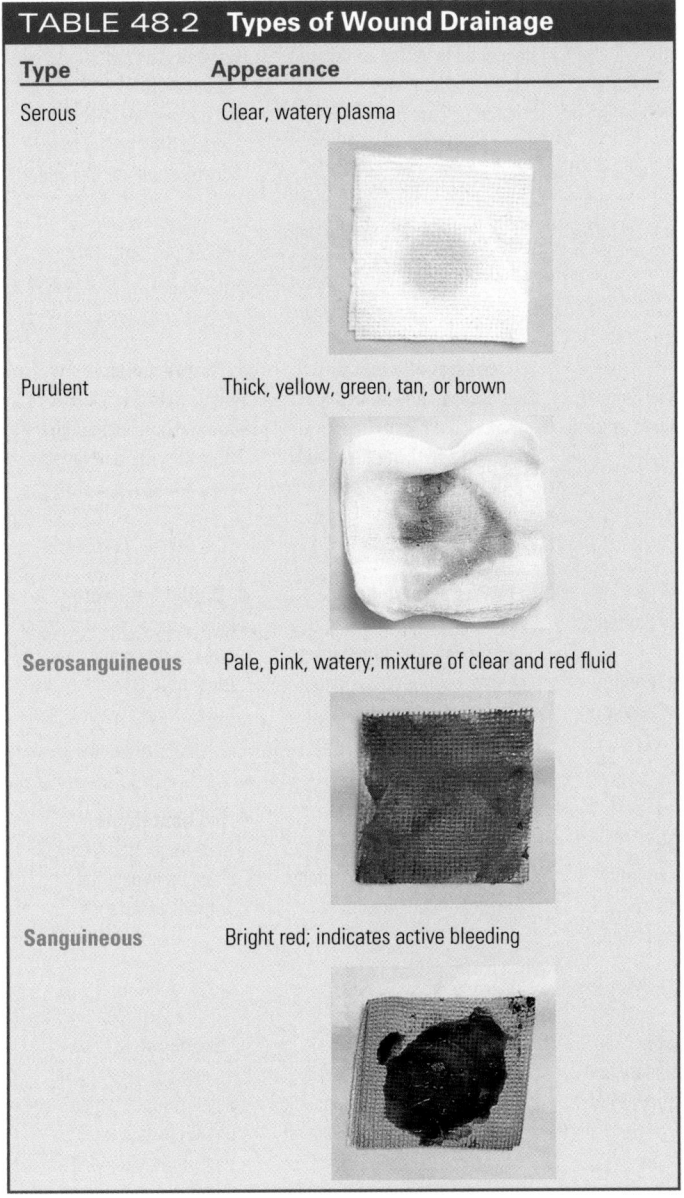
Purulent	Thick, yellow, green, tan, or brown
Serosanguineous	Pale, pink, watery; mixture of clear and red fluid
Sanguineous	Bright red; indicates active bleeding

down the costs of prevention at the same time (Martin et al., 2017). Several risk-assessment scales developed by nurses enable systematic risk assessment of patients. The Braden Scale is the most widely used risk-assessment tool for pressure injuries and is in the WOCN guidelines (2016) as being a valid tool to use for pressure injury risk assessment. The Braden Scale (Table 48.3) was developed on the basis of risk factors in a nursing home population (Braden and Bergstrom, 1994) and is widely used on general patient care units in hospitals. However, the Braden Scale has shown insufficient predictive validity and poor accuracy in discriminating intensive care patients at risk for developing pressure injuries (Han et al., 2018; Hyun et al., 2013). Research involving critical care patients continues. The Braden Scale contains six subscales: sensory perception, moisture, activity, mobility, nutrition, and friction/shear. The total score ranges from 6 to 23; a lower total score indicates a higher risk for pressure injury development (Braden and Bergstrom, 1989). The cutoff score for patients not at risk for pressure injury in the general adult population is 18 (Ayello et al., 2016). Research has shown that the cutoff score for onset of risk in intensive care patients is 13 (Hyun et al., 2013).

Economic Consequences of Pressure Injuries. Pressure injuries are a continual problem in acute and restorative care settings, especially in patients 65 years and older (WOCN, 2016). Paralysis and spinal cord injury are common preexisting conditions among younger adults with primary diagnosis of pressure injuries. Older adults admitted to acute and long-term facilities are a vulnerable population. Although the cost to provide pressure injury prevention to patients at risk can impact health care services' budgets, the costs to treat a severe pressure injury are substantially higher (Demarré et al., 2015).

When a pressure injury occurs, the length of stay in a hospital and the overall cost of health care increase. These injuries are also costly to patients in terms of disability, pain, and suffering. About 1.6 million patients each year in acute care settings develop pressure injuries, representing a cost of $11 billion to $17.2 billion to the US health care system (Pieper, 2016). The Centers for Medicare and Medicaid Services (CMS) implemented a policy effective October 1, 2008, whereby hospitals no longer receive reimbursement for care related to stage 3 and 4 pressure injuries that occur during a hospitalization. Guidelines such as the WOCN Guidelines (WOCN, 2016) help reduce or eliminate the occurrence of pressure injuries and prevent the expenses that will not be reimbursed.

Factors Influencing Pressure Injury Formation and Wound Healing

In addition to previously discussed risk factors of impaired sensation, impaired mobility, shear, friction, and moisture, a patient's nutrition, tissue perfusion, infection, or age may increase the risk for pressure injury and poor wound healing.

Nutrition. Normal wound healing requires proper nutrition (Table 48.4). Deficiencies in any of the nutrients result in impaired or delayed healing (Stotts, 2016a). Physiological processes of wound healing depend on the availability of protein, vitamins (especially A and C), and the trace minerals zinc and copper. Collagen is a protein formed from amino acids acquired by fibroblasts from protein ingested in food. Vitamin C is necessary for synthesis of collagen. Vitamin A reduces the negative effects of steroids on wound healing. Trace elements are also necessary (i.e., zinc for epithelialization and collagen synthesis and copper for collagen fiber linking).

Calories provide the energy source needed to support the cellular activity of wound healing. Protein needs especially are increased and are essential for tissue repair and growth. A balanced intake of various nutrients (i.e., protein, fat, carbohydrates, vitamins, and minerals) is critical to support wound healing. Consult with a nutritional team for dietary prescriptions individualized for the caloric needs of patients who are assessed as being at risk of malnutrition (EPUAP, NPIAP, PPPIA, 2019a).

Serum proteins are biochemical indicators of malnutrition (Stotts, 2016a). Serum albumin is probably the most frequently measured of these laboratory parameters. Albumin alone is not sensitive to rapid changes in nutritional status. The best measure of nutritional status is prealbumin because it reflects not only what the patient has recently ingested but also what the body has absorbed, digested, and metabolized (Stotts, 2016a).

Tissue Perfusion. Oxygen fuels the cellular functions essential to the healing process; therefore the ability to perfuse the tissues with adequate amounts of oxygenated blood is critical to wound healing (Doughty and Sparks, 2016). Patients with diabetes and peripheral vascular disease are at risk for poor tissue perfusion because of poor circulation. Oxygen requirements depend on the phase of wound healing (e.g., chronic tissue hypoxia is associated with impaired collagen synthesis and reduced tissue resistance to infection).

TABLE 48.3 Braden Scale for Predicting Pressure Ulcer Risk

Sensory Perception
Ability to respond appropriately to pressure-related discomfort

1. Completely limited:
Unresponsive (does not moan, flinch, or grasp) to painful stimuli caused by diminished level of consciousness or sedation
or
Limited ability to feel pain over most of body surface

2. Very limited:
Responds only to painful stimuli. Cannot communicate discomfort except by moaning or restlessness
or
Has sensory impairment that limits ability to feel pain or discomfort over half of body

3. Slightly limited:
Responds to verbal commands but cannot always communicate discomfort or need to be turned
or
Has some sensory impairment that limits ability to feel pain or discomfort in one or two extremities

4. No impairment:
Responds to verbal commands
Has no sensory deficit that would limit ability to feel or voice pain or discomfort

Moisture
Degree to which skin is exposed to moisture

1. Constantly moist:
Skin kept moist almost constantly by bodily elimination such as perspiration or urine
Dampness detected every time patient is moved or turned

2. Very moist:
Skin often, but not always, moist
Necessary to change linen at least once a shift

3. Occasionally moist:
Skin occasionally moist, requiring an extra linen change approximately once a day

4. Rarely moist:
Skin usually dry
Required linen changing only at routine intervals

Activity
Degree of physical activity

1. Bedfast:
Confined to bed

2. Chairfast:
Ability to walk severely limited or nonexistent
Cannot bear own weight and/or must be helped into chair or wheelchair

3. Walks occasionally:
Walks occasionally during day but for very short distances, with or without assistance
Spends majority of each shift in bed or chair

4. Walks frequently:
Walks outside room at least twice a day and inside room at least once every 2 hours during waking hours

Mobility
Ability to change and control body position

1. Completely immobile:
Does not make even slight changes in body or extremity position without assistance

2. Very limited:
Makes occasional slight changes in body or extremity position but unable to make frequent or significant changes independently

3. Slightly limited:
Makes frequent, though slight, changes in body or extremity position independently

4. No limitations:
Makes major and frequent changes in position without assistance

Nutrition
Usual food intake pattern

1. Very poor:
Never eats a complete meal; rarely eats more than one-third of any food offered; eats two servings or less of protein (meat or dairy products) per day
Takes fluids poorly
Does not take a liquid dietary supplement
or
Is NPO and/or maintained on clear liquids or IV for more than 5 days

2. Probably inadequate:
Rarely eats a complete meal and generally eats only about ½ of any food offered
Protein intake includes only 3 servings of meat or dairy products per day
Occasionally takes a dietary supplement
or
Receives less than optimum amount of liquid diet or tube feeding

3. Adequate:
Eats over half of most meals
Eats a total of four servings of protein (meat, dairy products) each day
Occasionally refuses a meal but usually takes a supplement if offered
or
Is on tube feeding or TPN regimen that probably meets most of nutritional needs

4. Excellent:
Eats most of every meal; never refuses a meal; usually eats a total of four or more servings of meat and dairy products
Occasionally eats between meals
Does not require supplementation

Friction and Shear

1. Problem:
Requires moderate-to-maximum help to move; complete lifting without sliding against sheets impossible
Frequently slides down in bed or chair, requiring frequent repositioning with maximum assistance
Spasticity, contractures, or agitation leads to almost constant friction

2. Potential problem:
Moves feebly or requires minimum assistance; during a move skin probably slides to some extent against sheets, chair, restraints, or other devices
Maintains relatively good position in chair or bed most of the time but occasionally slides down

3. No apparent problem:
Moves in bed and in chair independently and has sufficient muscle strength to sit up completely during move
Maintains good position in bed or chair at all times

TOTAL SCORE

NPO, nothing by mouth.; *TPN,* total parenteral nutrition.

Instructions: Score patient in each of the six subscales for overall score. Level of risk: *Not at risk,* greater than 18; *mild risk,* 15-18; *moderate risk,* 13-14; *high risk,* 10-12; and *very high risk,* less than 9.

TABLE 48.4 Role of Selected Nutrients in Wound Healing

Nutrient	Role in Healing	Recommendations	Sources
Calories	Fuel for cell energy "Protein protection"	30-35 kcal/kg/day (Individuals who are underweight or have significant unintentional weight loss may need additional calories.)	Protein smoothies, whole milk, nuts, beans, salmon
Protein	Fibroplasia, angiogenesis, collagen formation and wound remodeling, immune function	1.25-1.5 g protein/kg body weight	Poultry, fish, eggs, beef, milk
Vitamin C (ascorbic acid)	Collagen synthesis, capillary wall integrity, fibroblast function, immunological function, antioxidant	1000 mg/day	Citrus fruits, tomatoes, potatoes, fortified fruit juices
Vitamin A	Epithelialization, wound closure, inflammatory response, angiogenesis, collagen formation Can reverse steroid effects on skin and delayed healing	1600-2000 retinol equivalents per day	Green leafy vegetables (spinach), broccoli, carrots, sweet potatoes, liver
Zinc	Collagen formation, protein synthesis, cell membrane and host defenses	15-30 mg Correct deficiencies No improvement in wound healing with supplementation unless zinc deficient Use with caution—large doses can be toxic May inhibit copper metabolism and impair immune function	Vegetables, meats, legumes
Fluid	Essential fluid environment for all cell function	30-35 mL/kg/day	Use noncaffeinated, nonalcoholic fluids without sugar Water is best—6-8 glasses/day

Adapted from Stotts NA: Nutritional assessment and support. In Bryant RA, Nix DP, editors: *Acute and chronic wounds: current management concepts*, ed 5, St Louis, 2016a, Elsevier.

Infection. Wound infection prolongs the inflammatory phase; delays collagen synthesis; prevents epithelialization; and increases the production of proinflammatory cytokines, which leads to additional tissue destruction (Stotts, 2016b). Indications that a wound infection is present include the presence of purulent drainage; change in odor, volume, or character of wound drainage; redness in the surrounding tissue; fever; or pain.

Age. The physiological changes associated with aging affect all phases of wound healing. A decrease in the functioning of macrophages leads to a delayed inflammatory response, delayed collagen synthesis, and slower epithelialization.

Psychosocial Impact of Wounds. The psychosocial impact of wounds on the physiological process of healing is unknown. Body image changes often impose a great stress on a patient's adaptive mechanisms. They also influence self-concept (see Chapter 33) and sexuality (see Chapter 34). Factors that affect a patient's perception of a wound include: location, the presence of scars, stitches, drains (often needed for weeks or months), odor from drainage, and temporary or permanent prosthetic devices.

CRITICAL THINKING

Successful critical thinking requires a synthesis of knowledge, experience, information gathered from patients, critical thinking attitudes, and intellectual and professional standards. Clinical judgments require a nurse to anticipate the information necessary, analyze the data, and make decisions regarding patient care. Critical thinking is always changing. During assessment (Fig. 48.7) consider all elements that build toward making appropriate nursing diagnoses.

When caring for patients who have impaired skin integrity and chronic wounds, integrate knowledge from nursing and other disciplines, previous experiences, practice standards, and information gathered from patients to understand the risk to skin integrity and wound healing. Knowledge of normal musculoskeletal physiology, the pathogenesis of pressure injuries, pressure injury stages, normal wound healing, and the pathophysiology of underlying diseases enables you to have a scientific basis for care. The WOCN (2016) has guidelines for assessment of risk for impaired skin integrity, prevention measures, interventions to promote wound healing, and other standards of practice, which you should use in planning care. Past experience with patients at risk for impaired skin integrity or patients with wounds increases the experiential knowledge base, helping you to identify interventions. Finally you need to be disciplined during assessment to obtain comprehensive and correct data. You also need to be creative. Because chronic wounds are difficult to heal, be diligent in evaluating nursing interventions and in determining which interventions are effective and which need modification.

> ### REFLECT NOW
> Think about the information in the Braden Scale. How will this impact your knowledge about identifying risks for pressure injuries and potential interventions?

❖ NURSING PROCESS

Apply the nursing process and use a critical thinking approach in your care of patients. The nursing process provides a clinical decision-making approach for you to develop and implement an individualized plan of care.

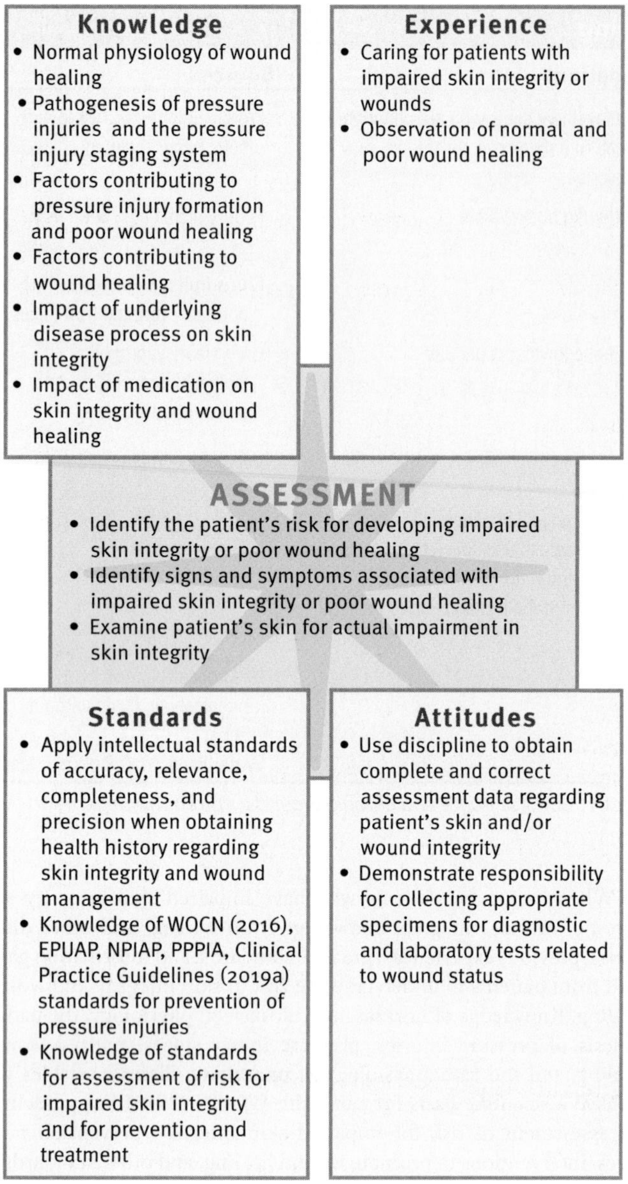

Knowledge

- Normal physiology of wound healing
- Pathogenesis of pressure injuries and the pressure injury staging system
- Factors contributing to pressure injury formation and poor wound healing
- Factors contributing to wound healing
- Impact of underlying disease process on skin integrity
- Impact of medication on skin integrity and wound healing

Experience

- Caring for patients with impaired skin integrity or wounds
- Observation of normal and poor wound healing

ASSESSMENT

- Identify the patient's risk for developing impaired skin integrity or poor wound healing
- Identify signs and symptoms associated with impaired skin integrity or poor wound healing
- Examine patient's skin for actual impairment in skin integrity

Standards

- Apply intellectual standards of accuracy, relevance, completeness, and precision when obtaining health history regarding skin integrity and wound management
- Knowledge of WOCN (2016), EPUAP, NPIAP, PPPIA, Clinical Practice Guidelines (2019a) standards for prevention of pressure injuries
- Knowledge of standards for assessment of risk for impaired skin integrity and for prevention and treatment

Attitudes

- Use discipline to obtain complete and correct assessment data regarding patient's skin and/or wound integrity
- Demonstrate responsibility for collecting appropriate specimens for diagnostic and laboratory tests related to wound status

FIG. 48.7 Critical thinking model for skin integrity and wound-care assessment. *WOCN,* Wound, Ostomy and Continence Nurses Society.

BOX 48.3 Nursing Assessment Questions

Sensation

- Do you have tingling, decreased feeling, or absent feeling in your extremities?
- Can you feel pressure when sitting or lying down?
- When preparing a bath is your skin sensitive to heat or cold?

Mobility

- Do you have any physical limitations, injury, or paralysis that limits your ability to move on your own?
- Can you change your position easily?
- Tell me about any pain you have when you walk, sit down, or move about your home.

Continence

- Do you have any problems or accidents leaking urine or stool?
- What help do you need when using the toilet? In what way?
- How often do you need to use the toilet? During the day? At night?

Presence of Wound

- What do you believe caused your wound?
- When did the wound occur? Where is it located?
- When did you receive a tetanus shot?
- What has happened to this wound since it occurred? What were the changes and what caused them?
- What have you done to treat the wound? Which treatments, activities, or care have slowed or helped the wound to heal?
- Do you have any pain, itching, or other symptoms with the wound? How are you managing the itching, and what works best for you?
- Who helps you care for your wound?

◆ Assessment

During the assessment process, thoroughly assess each patient and critically analyze findings to ensure that you make patient-centered clinical decisions required for safe nursing care. Baseline and continual assessment data provide critical information about a patient's skin integrity and the increased risk for pressure injury development. Focusing on specific elements such as a patient's level of sensation, movement, and continence status helps guide the skin assessment (Box 48.3).

Through the Patient's Eyes. When patients have acute surgical or traumatic wounds, the wounds sometimes heal promptly and without complications. However, when pressure injuries or chronic wounds develop, the course of treatments can be lengthy and costly. Because a patient and family need to be involved with wound-care management, it is important to know a patient's expectations. Does the patient

expect to have home care? Is there the expectation the patient will heal to allow a quick return to work? A patient who has realistic goals and is informed about the length of time for wound healing is more likely to adhere to the specific therapies designed to promote healing and prevent further skin breakdown. Therefore assess each patient's perception of proposed wound treatment and what is occurring once wound-healing interventions begin. For example, why are certain dressings being used and how do they work? You want to determine a patient's and family's understanding of wound assessment; wound interventions; and supportive interventions such as positioning, nutrition, and ambulation.

Skin. Perform skin assessment of a patient when you initiate care and then at a minimum of once a shift (see agency policies). Inspect the skin for signs of skin breakdown and/or injury development (see Skill 48.1). High-risk patients—including those who are neurologically impaired, chronically ill in long-term care, or have altered mental status; those in the intensive care unit (ICU), oncology units, hospice, or orthopedic units; and patients with medical devices—need more frequent skin assessments, such as every 4 hours.

Assessment for tissue pressure damage includes visual and tactile inspection of the skin. Perform a baseline assessment to determine a patient's normal skin characteristics and any actual or potential areas of breakdown (Nix, 2016). Individualize assessment characteristics of a patient's skin, depending on his or her skin tone (EPUAP, NPIAP, PPPIA, 2019a,b). Accurate assessment of patients with darker skin pigmentation is an essential skill for all health care providers (see Boxes 48.2 and 48.3).

TABLE 48.5   Strategies to Prevent Medical and Immobilization Device–Related Pressure Injuries

Device	Pressure Areas	Prevention Strategies[a]
Feeding tubes and nasogastric tubes	Nares Skin on nasal bridge	Secure tube using pressure-relieving techniques, which direct the pressure from the tube away from the nares (see Chapters 45 and 47). Reposition tube.
Endotracheal tubes	Lips Tongue	Remove securing device daily and inspect for pressure injury (Branson et al., 2014) (see Chapter 41). Rotate tube every shift or more often.
Nasotracheal tube	Nose/nasal bridge Nares	Remove securing device daily and inspect for pressure injury (Branson et al., 2014) (see Chapter 41). Reposition.
Tracheostomy tubes	Front of neck and stoma site	Remove securing device daily. Increase stoma care (Chapter 41).
Oxygen cannula and tubing	Ears Nose	Apply dressing to external ear. Periodically remove cannula to relieve pressure and inspect for pressure injury (Schallom et al., 2015) (Chapter 41).
Noninvasive positive-pressure ventilation (NIPPV)/bi-level positive airway pressure (BiPAP)	Forehead Nose/nasal bridge	Apply protective dressing or liquid skin barrier to bridge of nose or forehead before application of device. If appropriate, remove mask periodically for a few minutes.
Drainage tubing	Area immediately next to drainage tube Adjacent area during patient position changes	Apply appropriate dressing around drainage tube insertion site. Check tubing placement with each position change. Instruct patient not to lie on the tubing (Pittman et al., 2015).
Indwelling urinary catheter	Thighs Female: urethra, labia Male: tip of penis	Provide meticulous perineal care (see Chapter 40). Anchor and secure catheter to reduce pressure (see Chapter 46).
Orthopedic devices	All areas where device (e.g., cast or brace) comes in contact with patient's skin and tissues	When possible and not contraindicated, inspect under the device.
Neck collar	Neck and occipital region Scalp	Remove hard collars as soon as possible and replace with softer collar (Black et al., 2015). Inspect scalp daily.
Compression stockings	Calf Behind knee Heel Toes	Verify proper fit. To reduce pressure and risk of injury to skin and underlying tissue, remove stockings twice daily for at least 1 hour (Black et al., 2015) (Chapter 39).
Immobilization devices	Wrists Ankles	Apply dressing between immobilizer and patient's skin (Black et al., 2015). Verify that there is some space between immobilizer and patient's skin. With assistive personnel present, remove restraints one at a time to inspect skin (see Chapter 27).

[a]In addition to routine inspection and cleaning of skin under and around medical device.

Medical device–related pressure injuries (MDRPIs) are injuries that result from the use of devices designed and applied for diagnostic or therapeutic purposes (Kayser et al., 2018). Upon assessment, the resultant pressure injury generally closely conforms to the pattern or shape of the device (EPUAP, NPIAP, PPPIA, 2019b; Pittman et al., 2015). Pay particular attention to areas located over bony prominences; next to and around medical devices; and under casts, traction, splints, braces, collars, or other orthopedic devices (Table 48.5). The frequency of pressure checks depends on the response of the skin to the external pressure (Fig. 48.8). Consider adults with medical devices (e.g., tubes, drainage systems, and oxygen devices) to be at risk for pressure injuries (Black et al., 2010; Black and Kalowes, 2016).

Medical adhesive–related pressure injury is an occurrence in which erythema and/or other manifestation of cutaneous abnormality (including but not limited to vesicle, bulla, erosion, or skin tear) persists 30 minutes or more after removal of the adhesive. Skin stripping, or tape burns, from adhesives is the most commonly reported injury;

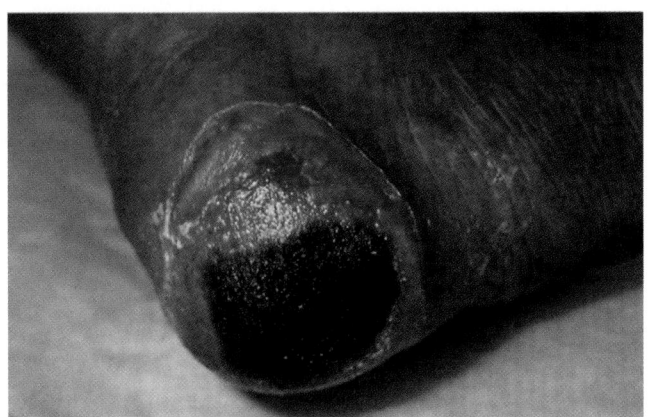

FIG. 48.8 Formation of pressure injury on heel resulting from external pressure from bed mattress. (Courtesy Janice Colwell, RN, MS, CWOCN, FAAN, Clinical Nurse Specialist, University of Chicago Medicine.)

thus a careful assessment of skin exposed to adhesive tape or other adhesive devices should be routinely done (McNichol et al., 2013).

When you note hyperemia of the skin, gently palpate the reddened tissue; differentiate whether the skin redness is blanchable or nonblanchable. Blanchable erythema is visible skin redness that becomes pale or white when pressure is applied and reddens when pressure is relieved. It may result from normal reactive hyperemia that should disappear within several hours or from inflammatory erythema with an intact capillary bed. Nonblanchable erythema is visible skin redness that persists with the application of pressure. It indicates structural damage to the capillary bed/microcirculation. This is an indication for a stage 1 pressure injury (EPUAP, NPIAP, PPPIA, 2019a).

Use visual and tactile inspection over the body areas most frequently at risk for pressure injury development (Fig. 48.9). For example, when a patient lies in bed or sits in a chair, he or she places body weight heavily on certain bony prominences. Turn the patient in bed to inspect the skin and, once you return a patient to bed from a chair, look at all areas exposed to pressure. Body surfaces subjected to the greatest weight or pressure are at greatest risk for pressure injury formation.

Wounds and Pressure Injuries. When you identify the presence of a skin wound or pressure injury, closer assessment is required. Assess the type of tissue in the wound base so that you can plan appropriate interventions. The assessment includes the amount (percentage) and appearance (color) of viable and nonviable tissue. Granulation tissue is red, moist tissue composed of new blood vessels, the presence of which indicates progression toward healing. Soft yellow or white tissue is characteristic of slough (stringy substance attached to wound bed), and it must eventually be removed by a qualified clinician or by an appropriate wound dressing before the wound is able to heal. Black, brown, tan or necrotic tissue is eschar, which also needs to be removed before healing can occur.

Measurement of the wound size provides information on overall changes in dimensions, which is an indicator for wound healing

progress (Nix, 2016). This includes measuring the length and width of a wound, as well as determining its depth (see Skill 48.2). Use a disposable wound-measuring device to measure wound width and length. This approach offers a uniform, consistent method for measuring meaningful comparisons of wound status across time (EPUAP, NPIAP, PPPIA, 2019b). Measure depth by using a cotton-tipped applicator in the wound bed (see Skill 48.2). Note that if a deep laceration exists it will likely require suturing by a qualified clinician.

Assessment of wound exudate should describe the amount, color, consistency, and odor of wound drainage. Excessive exudate indicates the presence of infection. Wound pain, including the location, distribution, type, quality and intensity, and any aggravating or relieving factors, also should be assessed (Krasner, 2016). Examine the skin around the wound (periwound) for redness, warmth, and signs of maceration, and palpate the area for signs of pain or induration. The presence of any of these factors on the periwound skin indicates wound deterioration.

Predictive Measures. On admission to acute care, rehabilitation hospitals, nursing homes, home care, and other health care facilities, patients are assessed for risk of pressure injury development (WOCN, 2016). Assessment for pressure injury risk includes using an appropriate predictive measure and assessing a patient's mobility, nutrition, presence of body fluids, and comfort level (see Skill 48.1). Perform pressure injury risk assessment systematically (WOCN, 2016) using an assessment tool such as the Braden Scale (see Table 48.3) or a tool preferred by your agency. The interpretation of the meaning of the total numerical scores differs with each risk-assessment scale relevant to the population being assessed by the agency. Lower numerical scores on the Braden Scale indicate that the patient is at high risk for skin breakdown. A benefit of the predictive instruments is to increase a nurse's early detection of patients at greater risk for injury development (WOCN, 2016). Perform reassessment for pressure injury risk on a scheduled basis (see agency policy).

Mobility. Assessment includes documenting the baseline level of mobility and the potential effects of impaired mobility on skin integrity.

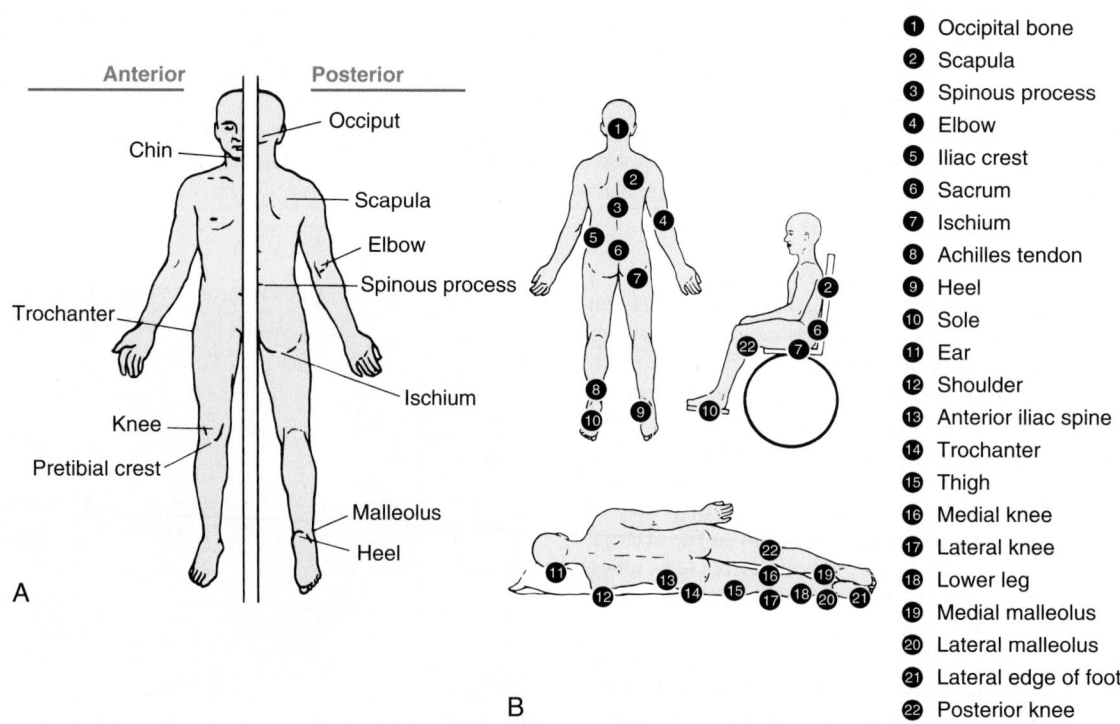

FIG. 48.9 **A,** Bony prominences most frequently underlying pressure injury. **B,** Pressure injury sites. (Modified from Trelease CC: Developing standards for wound care, *Ostomy Wound Manage* 20:46, 1988.)

Documenting assessment of mobility includes obtaining data regarding the quality of muscle tone and strength. For example, determine whether the patient is able to lift his or her weight off the sacral area and roll the body to a side-lying position. Some patients have inadequate range of motion to move independently into a more protective position. Finally, assess a patient's activity tolerance to determine whether the patient can be transferred to a chair or ambulated more often to relieve pressure from lying down (see Chapter 39).

Nutritional Status. An assessment of a patient's nutritional status is an integral part of the initial assessment data for any patient, especially one at risk for impaired skin integrity (Stotts, 2016a). The Joint Commission (2019) recommends nutritional assessment within 24 hours of admission. Weigh the patient and perform this measure more often for at-risk patients. A loss of 5% of usual weight, weight less than 90% of ideal body weight, and a decrease of 10 lb in a brief period are all signs of actual or potential nutritional problems (Stotts, 2016a). Assess the patient's mouth and teeth for oral sores and ill-fitting dentures that impact nutritional intake (see Chapter 45).

Body Fluids. It is important to prevent and reduce the patient's exposure to body fluids; when exposure occurs, provide meticulous hygiene and skin care. Continual exposure of the skin to body fluids increases a patient's risk for skin breakdown and pressure injury formation. Some body fluids such as saliva and serosanguineous drainage are not as caustic, and the risk of skin breakdown from exposure to these fluids is low. However, exposure to urine, bile, stool, ascitic fluid, and purulent wound exudate carries a moderate risk for skin breakdown, especially in patients who have other risk factors such as chronic illness or poor nutrition. Frequent exposure to urine and fecal contents increases patients' risk for incontinence-associated dermatitis (IAD) (McNichol et al., 2018). Additionally, exposure to gastric and pancreatic drainage has the highest risk for skin breakdown. These fluids have digestive qualities that can irritate and break down the skin quickly.

Pain. Significant research has been conducted in the study of pain in surgical patients with wounds. The routine assessment of pain in surgical patients is critical to selecting appropriate pain management therapies and to determine a patient's ability to progress toward recovery. The WOCN (2016) has recommended that assessment and management of pain also be included in the care of patients with pressure injuries (EPUAP, NPIAP, PPPIA, 2019b). Use standard pain assessment tools to measure pain acuity, and be thorough in assessing the character of a patient's pain (see Chapter 44). Maintaining adequate pain control and patient comfort increases the patient's willingness and ability to increase mobility, which in turn reduces pressure injury risk.

Surgical and Traumatic Wounds.
Assess wounds at the time of injury, during wound care, when a patient's overall condition changes, and on a regularly scheduled basis. Regardless of the setting, it is important that you initially obtain information regarding the cause and history of the wound, treatment of the wound, wound description (location, dimensions, quality of the wound base tissue, and presence of odor, warmth, or redness on the periwound skin), and response to therapy.

Emergency Setting. You see wounds in any setting, including clinics, emergency departments, youth camps, or your own backyard. The type of wound determines the criteria for inspection. For example, you do not need to inspect for signs of internal bleeding after an abrasion, but you should inspect in the event of a puncture wound.

After a traumatic wound, when you judge a patient's condition to be stable because of the presence of spontaneous breathing, a clear airway, and a strong carotid pulse (see Chapters 30 and 41), inspect the wound for bleeding. An **abrasion** is superficial with little bleeding and

is considered a partial-thickness wound. The wound often appears "weepy" because of plasma leakage from damaged capillaries. A **laceration** sometimes may bleed more profusely (especially if the patient is taking anticoagulants or other blood thinners), depending on the depth and location of the wound. For example, minor scalp lacerations tend to bleed profusely because of the rich blood supply to the scalp. Lacerations greater than 5 cm (2 inches) long or 2.5 cm (1 inch) deep cause serious bleeding. **Puncture wounds** bleed in relation to the depth, size, and location of the wound (e.g., a nail puncture does not cause as much bleeding as a knife wound). A puncture wound is usually a small, circular wound with the edges coming together toward the center. The primary dangers of puncture wounds are internal bleeding and infection.

Inspect traumatic wounds for foreign bodies or contaminant material. Most traumatic wounds are dirty. Soil, broken glass, shreds of cloth, and foreign substances clinging to penetrating objects sometimes become embedded in a wound. Next, assess the size and depth of a wound (see Skill 48.2).

When an injury is a result of trauma from a dirty penetrating object, determine when the patient last received a tetanus toxoid injection. Tetanus bacteria reside in soil and in the gut of humans and animals.

Stable Setting. When a patient's condition is stabilized (e.g., after surgery or treatment), assess the wound to determine progress toward healing. If the wound is covered by a dressing and the health care provider has not ordered it changed, do not inspect it directly unless you suspect serious complications such as a large volume of bright red bleeding, excessive odor, or severe pain under the dressing. In such a situation inspect only the dressing and any external drains. If the health care provider prefers to change the dressing, he or she should assess the wound at least daily. When removing dressings, remove one dressing layer at a time to avoid accidental removal or displacement of underlying drains. Because removal of dressings can be painful, consider giving an analgesic at least 30 minutes before exposing a wound.

Wound Appearance. A surgical incision healing by primary intention should have clean, well-approximated edges. There may be some redness at the edges of the incision that can be present for the first few days after surgery. Crusts often form along wound edges from exudate. If a wound is open, the edges are separated, and you inspect the condition of tissue at the wound base. The outer edges of a wound normally appear inflamed for the first 2 to 3 days, but this slowly disappears. Within 7 to 10 days a normally healing wound resurfaces with epithelial cells, and edges close. Table 48.6 lists assessment characteristics for abnormal wound healing in

TABLE 48.6 Assessment of Abnormal Healing in Primary- and Secondary-Intention Wounds

Primary Intention Wounds	Secondary Intention Wounds
Incision line poorly approximated	Pale or fragile granulation tissue, hypergranulation tissue present
Drainage present more than 3 days after closure	Wound exudate is purulent
Inflammation increased in first 3-5 days after injury	Nonviable tissues such as necrotic or slough in wound base
No healing ridge by day 9	Fruity, earthy, or putrid odor present after wound base is cleansed
	Presence of fistula(s), tunneling, undermining

Modified from Nix D: Skin and wound inspection and assessment. In Bryant RA, Nix DP, editors: *Acute and chronic wounds: current management concepts*, ed 5, St Louis, 2016, Elsevier.

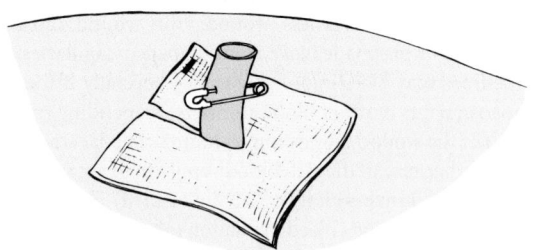

FIG. 48.10 Penrose drain with dressing.

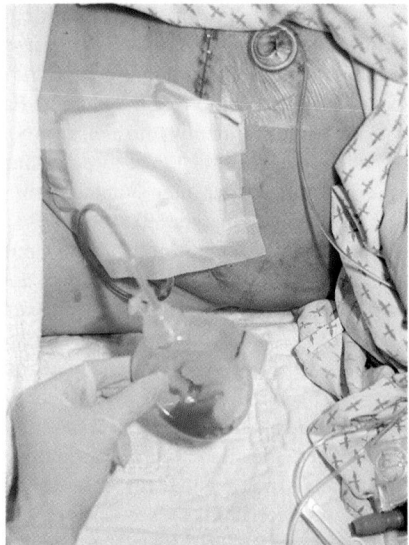

FIG. 48.11 Jackson-Pratt drainage device. Drainage tube and reservoir.

primary and secondary wounds. If infection develops, the area directly surrounding the wound becomes brightly inflamed and swollen.

Skin discoloration usually results from bruising of interstitial tissues or hematoma formation. Blood collecting beneath the skin first takes on a bluish or purplish appearance. Gradually, as the clotted blood is broken down, shades of brown and yellow appear.

Character of Wound Drainage. Note the amount, color, odor, and consistency of wound drainage (see Table 48.2). The amount of drainage depends on the type of wound. For example, drainage is minimal after a simple appendectomy. In contrast, it is moderate for 1 to 2 days after drainage of a large abscess. When you need an accurate measurement of the amount of drainage within a dressing, weigh the dressing and compare it with the weight of the same dressing that is clean and dry. The general rule is that 1 g of drainage equals 1 mL of volume of drainage. Another method of quantifying wound drainage is to chart the number of dressings used and the frequency of change. An increase or decrease in the number or frequency of dressings indicates a relative increase or decrease in wound drainage. If the drainage has a pungent or strong odor, you should suspect an infection. Describe the appearance of the wound according to characteristics observed, the type of closures used, and the dressing changes performed.

Drains. Drains provide a means for fluid or blood that accumulates within a wound bed to drain out of the body. A surgeon inserts a drain into or near a surgical wound if there is a large amount of drainage. A drain can also be placed by the interventional radiologist to drain an area found after or before surgery. Some drains are sutured in place. Exercise caution when changing a dressing around drains that are not sutured in place to prevent accidental removal. A Penrose drain lies under a dressing; at the time of placement a pin or clip is placed through the drain to prevent it from slipping farther into a wound (Fig. 48.10). One dressing is split and placed around the drain and another over the drain to collect drainage. When removing the dressings remove one dressing at a time to prevent accidental dislodgement of the drain. It is usually the health care provider's responsibility to pull or advance the drain as drainage decreases to permit healing deep within the drain site. The wound will heal from the inside out.

Assess the number and type of drains, drain placement, character of drainage, and condition of collecting equipment. Observe the security of the drain and its location with respect to the wound. Next note the character of drainage. If there is a collecting device, measure the drainage volume. Because a drainage system needs to be patent, look for drainage flow through and around the tubing. A sudden decrease in drainage through the tubing may indicate a blocked drain, and you need to notify the health care provider. When a drain is connected to suction, assess the system to be sure that the pressure ordered is being exerted. Evacuator units such as a Hemovac or Jackson-Pratt (Fig. 48.11) exert a constant low pressure as long as the suction device (bladder or container) is fully compressed. When the evacuator device is unable to maintain a vacuum on its own, notify the surgeon, who then orders a secondary vacuum system (such as wall suction). If fluid accumulates within the tissues, wound healing does not progress at an optimal rate, and this increases the risk of infection.

Wound Closures. Surgical wounds are closed with staples, sutures, or wound adhesives. A frequent skin closure is the stainless-steel staple. The staple provides more strength than nylon or silk sutures and tends to cause less irritation to tissue. Look for irritation with redness around staple or suture sites and note whether closures are intact. Normally for the first 2 to 3 days after surgery the skin around sutures or staples is edematous because of the normal inflammatory response.

Dermabond is a liquid tissue adhesive that forms a strong bond across approximated wound edges, allowing normal healing to occur below. It can be used to replace small sutures for incisional repair. A vial containing the Dermabond solution is used to apply the product to approximated tissue. The wound edges are held together until the solution dries, providing an adhesive closure. Tissue adhesives take less time to apply, have lower risk of infection, have tensile strength comparable to sutures, and also provide less pain and anxiety (Januchowski and Ferguson, 2014).

Palpation of Wound. When inspecting a wound, observe for swelling or separation of wound edges. While wearing clean gloves, lightly press the wound edges, detecting localized areas of tenderness or drainage collection. If pressure causes fluid to be expressed, note the characteristics of the drainage. The patient is normally sensitive to palpation of wound edges. Extreme tenderness indicates infection.

Wound Cultures. If you detect purulent or suspicious-looking drainage, report to the health care provider because a specimen of the drainage may need to be obtained for culture. Never collect a wound culture sample from old drainage. Resident colonies of bacteria flora from the skin grow within exudate and are not always the true causative organisms of a wound infection. Clean a wound first with normal saline to remove skin flora. Aerobic organisms grow in superficial wounds exposed to the air, and anaerobic organisms tend to grow within body cavities. Use a different method of specimen collection for each type of organism per agency policy (Box 48.4).

Gram stains of drainage are often performed as well. This test allows the health care provider to order appropriate treatment earlier than when only cultures are done. No additional specimens are usually required. The microbiology laboratory needs only to be notified to perform the additional test.

The gold standard of wound culture is tissue biopsy. A health care provider or wound-care specialist with special training obtains the biopsy (Stotts, 2016b).

BOX 48.4 Recommendations for Standardized Techniques for Wound Cultures[a]

Needle Aspiration Procedure (Anaerobic Organisms)

- Clean intact skin with povidone iodine and allow to dry for 60 seconds to remove skin flora. Then wipe the skin with alcohol and allow to dry, which reduces the possibility that the specimen will be altered by the iodine on the skin surface.
- Use a sterile 10-mL disposable syringe with a 22-gauge needle, pulling 0.5 mL of air into the syringe.
- Insert the needle through intact skin next to the wound; withdraw plunger and apply suction to the 10-mL mark.
- Move the needle back and forward at different angles for two to four explorations. The plunger is then released back to the 0.5 mL mark, the needle is withdrawn, and the syringe is capped and sent to the lab (Weir and Schultz, 2016).

Quantitative Swab Procedure (Aerobic Organisms)

- Clean the wound surface with an antiseptic solution. Allow to dry.
- Use a sterile swab from a culturette tube (Fig. 48.12).
- Identify a 1-cm area of the wound that is free from necrotic tissue. Rotate the swab while applying pressure sufficient to express fluid from the wound tissue (Weir and Schultz, 2016).
- Insert the tip of the swab into the appropriate sterile container, label, and transport to the laboratory.

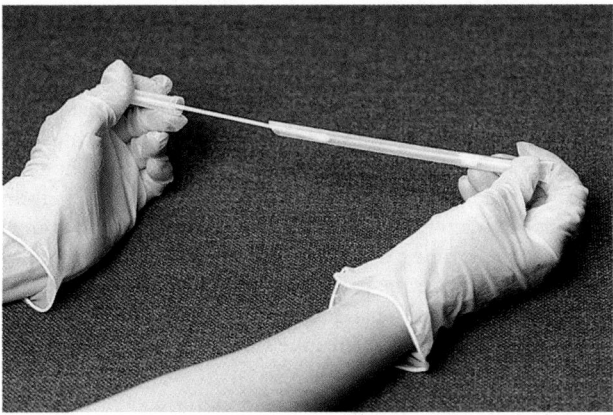

FIG. 48.12 Wound culturette tube.

Psychosocial. Assess how a wound is influencing a patient's self-perception and socialization. Ask the patient to describe how the wound affects his or her view of self. Does the patient have unwarranted fears that the wound will not heal? Does a chronic wound interfere with the patient's willingness to participate in social activities at home? Does it affect the patient's ability to continue working? Make sure that the patient's personal and social resources for adaptation are a part of your assessment. Is there a family caregiver who is able to assist with wound care in the home?

REFLECT NOW

Think about a patient you have recently cared for and who had a medical device, such as a urinary catheter, oxygen mask, or feeding tube. What were the patient's risks for skin breakdown? How did you assess the patient for medical device pressure injury?

BOX 48.5 Nursing Diagnostic Process

Impaired Skin Integrity Related to Infection

Assessment Activities	Assessment Findings
Inspect surface of wound and periwound skin.	Break in skin integrity Yellow, foul-smelling drainage from wound Edges of wound red and warm, not approximated Macerated periwound area
Inspect wound for signs of healing.	Brown-red or beige drainage 5 days after surgery Edges of wound not approximated
Palpate wound and ask patient if there is tenderness.	Patient expresses pain on palpation; rates pain as a 5 on scale of 0 to 10 Periwound edema
Obtain patient's temperature, heart rate, white blood cell count.	Patient febrile, heart rate 125 beats/min, leukocyte (white blood cell) count 12,000/mm^3

◆ Nursing Diagnosis

Assessment reveals clusters of data to indicate whether a problem-focused or negative diagnosis of *Impaired Skin Integrity* or a risk diagnosis of *Risk for Impaired Skin Integrity* exists. In addition, the assessment data provide information about the related factor. For example, a postoperative patient has purulent drainage from a surgical wound and reports tenderness around the area of the wound. These data support a nursing diagnosis of *Impaired Skin Integrity* related to infection (Box 48.5). After completing an assessment of a patient's wound, the nurse identifies nursing diagnoses that direct the interventions that will be needed to support wound healing and prevent complications. Additional nursing diagnoses associated with impaired skin integrity and wounds:

- *Risk for Infection*
- *Acute or Chronic Pain*
- *Impaired Mobility*
- *Impaired Peripheral Tissue Perfusion*

Some patients are at risk for poor wound healing because of the presence of previously defined conditions that impair healing. Thus, even though a patient's wound appears normal, the nurse identifies nursing diagnoses such as *Impaired Nutritional Intake* or *Ineffective Tissue Perfusion* that direct nursing care toward support of wound repair.

The nature of a wound can cause problems unrelated to wound healing. An alteration in comfort with the diagnosis of *Acute Pain* and *Impaired Mobility* have implications for a patient's eventual recovery. For example, a large abdominal incision causes enough pain to interfere with the patient's ability to turn in bed effectively, making him or her at risk for impaired skin integrity.

◆ Planning

After identifying nursing diagnoses, develop a plan of care for a patient so that interventions promote wound healing and prevent complications of any existing wounds. During planning synthesize information from multiple resources (Fig. 48.13). Critical thinking ensures that a patient's plan of care integrates all that you know about the individual and key critical thinking elements. Professional standards are especially important to consider when you develop a plan of care. Practice standards will ensure your use of appropriate wound therapies.

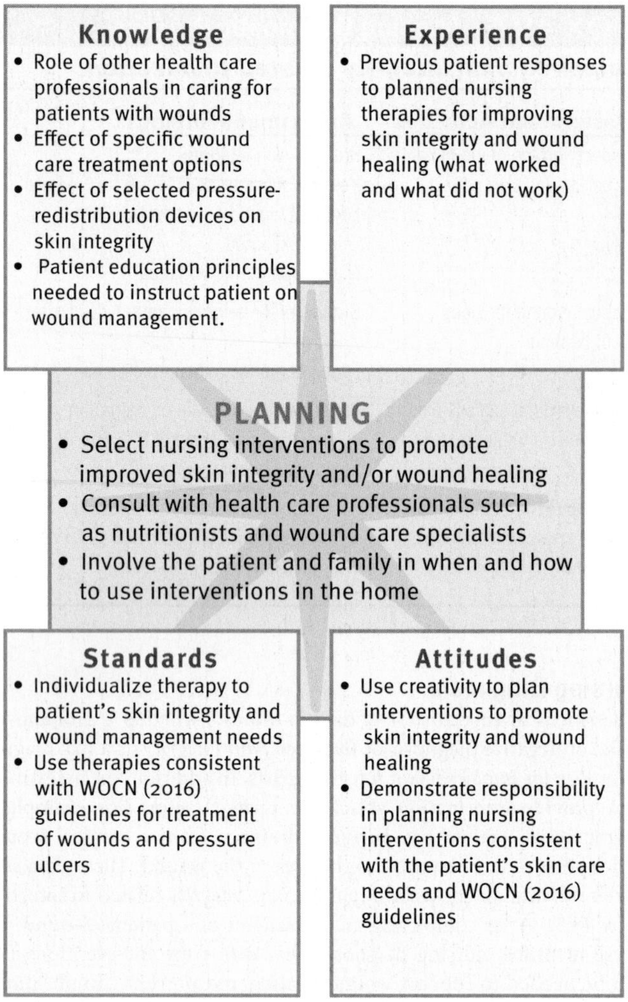

Knowledge
- Role of other health care professionals in caring for patients with wounds
- Effect of specific wound care treatment options
- Effect of selected pressure-redistribution devices on skin integrity
- Patient education principles needed to instruct patient on wound management.

Experience
- Previous patient responses to planned nursing therapies for improving skin integrity and wound healing (what worked and what did not work)

PLANNING
- Select nursing interventions to promote improved skin integrity and/or wound healing
- Consult with health care professionals such as nutritionists and wound care specialists
- Involve the patient and family in when and how to use interventions in the home

Standards
- Individualize therapy to patient's skin integrity and wound management needs
- Use therapies consistent with WOCN (2016) guidelines for treatment of wounds and pressure ulcers

Attitudes
- Use creativity to plan interventions to promote skin integrity and wound healing
- Demonstrate responsibility in planning nursing interventions consistent with the patient's skin care needs and WOCN (2016) guidelines

FIG. 48.13 Critical thinking model for skin integrity and wound-care planning. *WOCN,* Wound, Ostomy and Continence Nurses Society.

Patients who have large chronic wounds or infected wounds have multiple nursing care needs. A concept map helps to individualize care for a patient who has multiple health problems and related nursing diagnoses (Fig. 48.14). This map helps you use critical thinking skills to organize complex patient assessment data into related nursing diagnoses with the patient's chief medical diagnosis. As you identify links between the nursing diagnoses and the chief medical diagnosis, the concept map also links potential interventions that apply to the patient's multiple health care needs.

Goals and Outcomes. Nursing care is based on a patient's identified needs and priorities. You establish goals and expected outcomes, and from the goals you plan interventions according to the risk for pressure injuries or the type and severity of the wound and the presence of any complications such as infection, poor nutrition, peripheral vascular diseases, or immunosuppression that can affect wound healing (see the Nursing Care Plan). A goal frequently identified when working with a patient with a wound is to see the wound progressing toward healing within a 2-week period. The outcomes of this goal can include the following:

- Increase in the percentage of granulation tissue in the wound base
- No further skin breakdown
- Increase in caloric intake by 10%

These outcomes are reasonable if the overall goal for the patient is to heal the wound. Plan therapies according to the severity and type of wound and the presence of any complicating conditions (e.g., infection, poor nutrition, immunosuppression, and diabetes) that affect wound healing. Other goals of care for patients with wounds include the following: promoting wound hemostasis, preventing infection, promoting wound healing, maintaining skin integrity, gaining comfort, and promoting health.

Setting Priorities. Establish nursing care priorities in wound care on the basis of the comprehensive patient assessment and goals and established outcomes. These priorities also depend on whether the patient's condition is stable or emergent. When there is a risk for pressure injury development, preventive interventions such as skin-care practices, elimination of risks, and positioning are high priorities. An acute wound needs immediate intervention, whereas in the presence of a chronic, stable wound, the patient's hygiene and education on wound care are more important. Promotion of wound healing and the type of wound care administered depend on the type, size, and location of the wound and overall treatment goals.

Other patient factors to consider when establishing priorities include patient preferences, daily activities, and family factors. These factors are important, regardless of the setting for health care. The priorities of care may not vary from outpatient, home, acute care, or restorative care settings.

Teamwork and Collaboration. With early discharge from health care settings, it is important to consider a patient's plan for discharge as soon as a patient is admitted to a facility. Anticipating the patient's discharge wound-care needs and related equipment and health care resources such as referral to a home care agency or outpatient wound-care clinic helps to improve not only wound healing but also the patient's level of independence. Patients and their family caregivers often need to continue the objectives of wound management after discharge. Carefully consider the ability of a family caregiver and the amount of time needed to change a particular dressing when selecting a dressing for the patient to use after discharge. For example, in the home setting a patient's spouse may choose more expensive dressing materials to reduce the frequency of dressing changes (Box 48.6).

◆ Implementation

Health Promotion. Prompt identification of patients at high risk for pressure injuries or for impaired wound healing require timely and appropriate preventive measures.

Nutrition. Patients with existing wounds or those at risk for pressure injury will need extra protein, calories, and nutrients. The Cleveland Clinic (2017) recommends these daily nutrients to improve and promote wound healing:

- Protein (5 to 8 servings daily). Eat the protein portion of your meals first in case you become too full.
- Whole grains for higher protein content (5 servings daily)
- Vegetables (2 servings daily). Add to fruit smoothies for an extra boost without a bitter taste.
- Fruit (3 servings daily). Use as toppings for cooked cereals, yogurt, and ice cream. Choose fruit for dessert.
- Dairy (3 servings daily). Substitute milk for water in recipes; add powdered milk or yogurt to shakes, smoothies, and cooked cereals. Top soups with cheese or Greek yogurt.

Prevention of Pressure Injuries. Nursing interventions for patients who are immobile or have other risk factors for pressure injuries focus on prevention (Table 48.7). Prevention minimizes the impact that risk

Impaired Skin Integrity

ASSESSMENT

Mrs. Stein, an 86-year-old patient, fell at home and fractured her left hip. She had a hip replacement 2 days ago and has been hesitant to move due to pain and fear of falling. When asked to participate in repositioning, she slides her body up and down in bed while protecting her hip. She does not like the staff to use a lift sheet to reposition her in bed. She becomes slightly diaphoretic when moving, causing her to sweat upon movement. You note drainage on her gown over the area of the hip.

Assessment Activities	*Assessment Findings[a]*
Ask Mrs. Stein about her mobility.	She relates that her hip always aches, **limiting movement,** and that her lower leg is sore and the pain increases on movement. She tells you that she prefers to **keep the hip and leg immobile** to keep the pain level down. Position of comfort is supine, and Mrs. Stein resists position changes.
Assess sacral area.	There is a partial-thickness injury directly over the sacral area. Patient has **nonblanchable erythema** around the open sacral area. Incontinent of urine.
Assess left hip, surgical incision.	Small openings between staples oozing tan, foul-smelling fluid. Periwound area red and warm.

[a]**Assessment Findings** are shown in bold type.

NURSING DIAGNOSIS: Impaired Skin Integrity related to pressure, friction, and shearing forces over sacral bony prominence and infectious drainage from surgical site

PLANNING

Goals	*Expected Outcomes (NOC)[b]* *Tissue Integrity: Skin and Mucous Membranes*
Injury to Mrs. Stein's skin and underlying tissue resulting from pressure, friction, and shear over the bony prominence will be reduced within 2 to 4 weeks.	Intact skin integrity in the area of nonblanching erythema. Sacral injury shows signs of healing. Intact skin over other pressure points.

[b]Outcome classification labels from Moorhead S, et al: *Nursing Outcomes Classification (NOC)*, ed 6, St Louis, 2018, Elsevier.

INTERVENTIONS (NIC)[c]	**RATIONALE**
Skin Surveillance	
Place an order for a pressure reduction mattress per agency's protocol and place on bed.	Reduces the duration and magnitude of pressure over vulnerable areas of the body and contributes to comfort, hygiene, dignity, and functional ability (Bryant and Nix, 2016a).
Assist with repositioning every 90 minutes as her condition allows. Use a drawsheet when helping to reposition.	Repositioning is still required for pressure redistribution and comfort when a support surface is in use. A lift or transfer sheet minimizes friction and/or shear (EPUAP, NPIAP, PPPIA, 2019a).
Elevate head of bed no more than 30 degrees (EPUAP, NPIAP, PPPIA, 2019a,b). **Note:** Some hip replacement patients may not be allowed to turn in to 30-degree lateral position.	A slouched position places pressure and shear on the sacrum and coccyx (EPUAP, NPIAP, PPPIA, 2019a).
Keep skin dry and clean; avoid rubbing or massaging around the open area (McNichol et al., 2018).	The presence of skin damage from moisture/maceration contributes to the development of pressure injuries (Colwell et al., 2011; EPUAP, NPIAP, PPPIA, 2019a). Rubbing or massaging areas of nonblanching erythema can cause further tissue damage (WOCN, 2016).
Use moisture barrier ointment over the injury at least 3 times a day to decrease friction and provide moisture to the open tissue.	An ointment covers the area, providing base of ulcer with moisture, which encourages healing. Ointment prevents sheets from rubbing on area, thus decreasing the friction (Bryant and Nix, 2016a).
Wound Care	
Irrigate wound with saline solution twice a day per wound-care provider's order.	Cleanse wound and surrounding area of wound debris and exudate.
Apply dressing (i.e., gauze moistened with solution twice a day after irrigation) according to wound-care provider's order.	Provides appropriate topical therapy to wound, placing wound in best environment for healing (Bryant and Nix, 2016b).
Evaluate patient's pain level at least every 2 hours and offer pain medication as indicated by assessment.	Provides patient with pain reduction/relief, allowing for greater mobility and comfort (Krasner, 2016).

[c]Intervention classification labels from Butcher HK, et al: *Nursing Interventions Classification (NIC)*, ed 7, St Louis, 2018, Elsevier.

EVALUATION

Evaluation Activity	*Patient Response/Findings*	*Outcome Status*
Perform daily total body skin and wound assessments.	Skin intact in area of nonblanching erythema.	Intact skin integrity in the area of nonblanching erythema. Intact skin over other pressure points.
	Decreased redness at the sacral area. Presence of reepithelialization in sacral area.	Injury in sacral region improving.
Palpate reddened area around sacrum.	Sacral area begins to show signs of reactive hyperemia and blanching following palpation; no new break in epidermis.	Intact skin over other pressure points. Sacral area improving. Reactive hyperemia with blanching occurring.

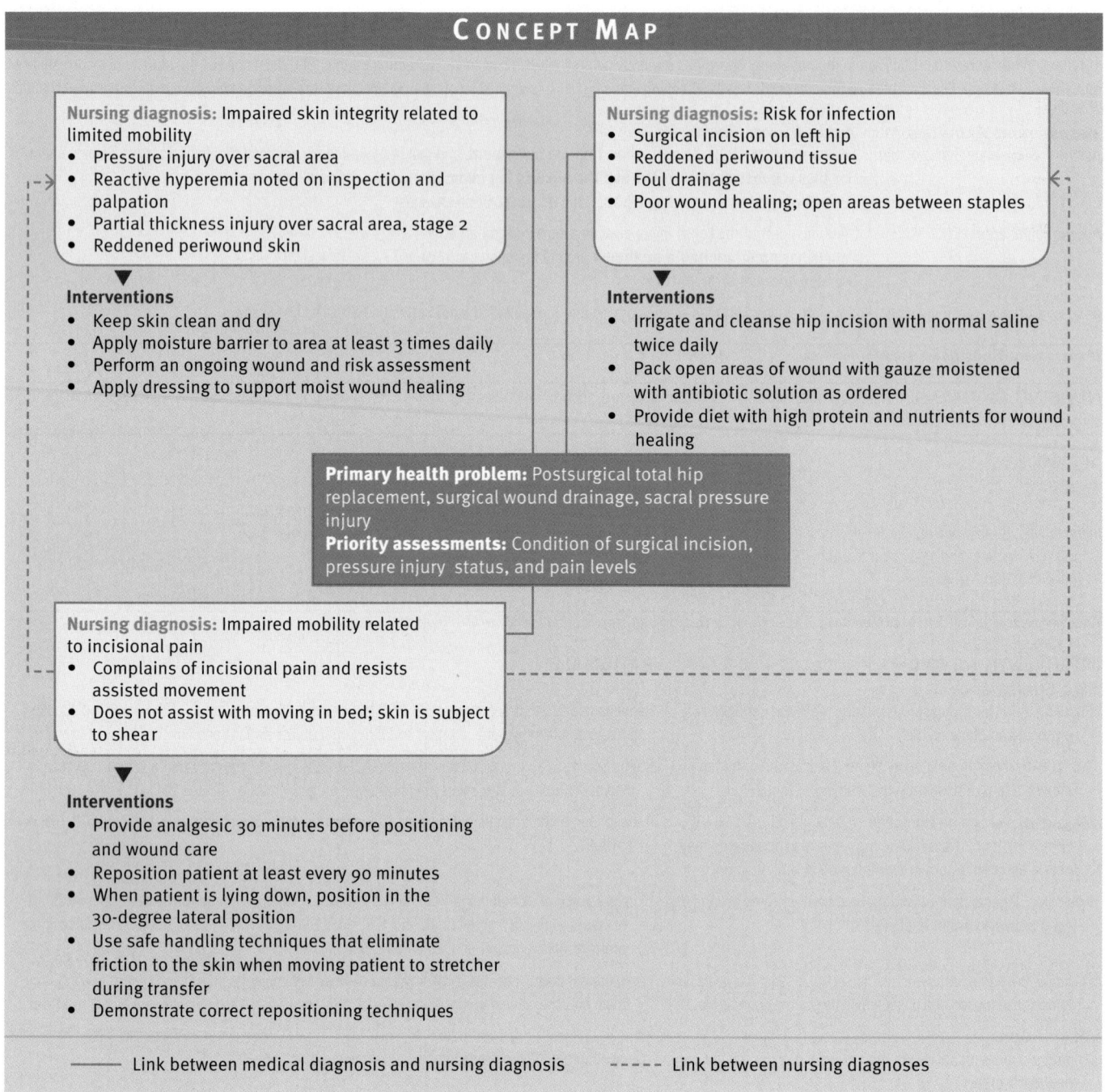

CONCEPT MAP

Nursing diagnosis: Impaired skin integrity related to limited mobility
- Pressure injury over sacral area
- Reactive hyperemia noted on inspection and palpation
- Partial thickness injury over sacral area, stage 2
- Reddened periwound skin

Interventions
- Keep skin clean and dry
- Apply moisture barrier to area at least 3 times daily
- Perform an ongoing wound and risk assessment
- Apply dressing to support moist wound healing

Nursing diagnosis: Risk for infection
- Surgical incision on left hip
- Reddened periwound tissue
- Foul drainage
- Poor wound healing; open areas between staples

Interventions
- Irrigate and cleanse hip incision with normal saline twice daily
- Pack open areas of wound with gauze moistened with antibiotic solution as ordered
- Provide diet with high protein and nutrients for wound healing

Primary health problem: Postsurgical total hip replacement, surgical wound drainage, sacral pressure injury
Priority assessments: Condition of surgical incision, pressure injury status, and pain levels

Nursing diagnosis: Impaired mobility related to incisional pain
- Complains of incisional pain and resists assisted movement
- Does not assist with moving in bed; skin is subject to shear

Interventions
- Provide analgesic 30 minutes before positioning and wound care
- Reposition patient at least every 90 minutes
- When patient is lying down, position in the 30-degree lateral position
- Use safe handling techniques that eliminate friction to the skin when moving patient to stretcher during transfer
- Demonstrate correct repositioning techniques

——— Link between medical diagnosis and nursing diagnosis   - - - - Link between nursing diagnoses

FIG. 48.14 Concept map for Mrs. Stein.

factors or contributing factors have on pressure injury development. Three major areas of nursing interventions for prevention of pressure injuries are (1) skin care and management of incontinence; (2) mechanical loading and support devices, which include proper positioning and the use of therapeutic surfaces; and (3) education (WOCN, 2016).

Topical Skin Care and Incontinence Management. When you clean the skin, avoid soap and hot water. Use cleaners with nonionic surfactants that are gentle to the skin (WOCN, 2016). Many types of products are available for skin care, and you need to match their use to the specific needs of the patient. After you clean the skin and make sure that it is completely dry, apply moisturizer to keep the epidermis well lubricated but not oversaturated.

Make an effort to control, contain, or correct incontinence, perspiration, or wound drainage (see Chapters 46 and 47). Patients who have fecal incontinence and who are also receiving enteral tube feeding provide a management challenge. Often the feedings can result in diarrhea. When patients have an incontinent episode, gently clean the area, dry, and apply a thick layer of moisture barrier to the exposed areas. A moisture barrier protects the skin from excessive moisture and from bacteria found in the urine or stool (McNichol et al., 2018).

It is helpful to use the expertise of an advanced practice nurse with a focus on wound care or management of incontinence while caring for at-risk patients. Methods for controlling or containing incontinence vary. Bowel incontinence can sometimes be better managed with proper diet and medications. Urinary incontinence is treated with

BOX 48.6 Home Care Recommendations

Injury/Wound Assessment

Assessment and documentation of a pressure injury/wound needs to occur at least weekly unless there is evidence of deterioration, in which case the nurse needs to reassess both the pressure injury and the patient's overall management immediately. In the home setting this requires the help of the patient and family because weekly assessment is not always feasible. Wound assessment in the home is the same as in a health care agency; see Skills 48.1 and 48.2 for specific assessment parameters.

Injury Care Dressings

- Consider family caregiver time and ability when selecting a dressing.
- In the home setting some family caregivers choose dressing materials manufactured to reduce the frequency of dressing changes.

Infection Control

- Clean dressings, as opposed to sterile ones, are recommended for home use until research demonstrates otherwise. This recommendation is in keeping with principles regarding nosocomial infections and with past success of clean urinary catheterization in the home setting, and it takes into account the expense of sterile dressings and the dexterity required for application. The family caregiver can use the "no-touch" technique for dressing changes. This technique is a method of changing surface dressings without touching the wound or the surface of any dressing that might be in contact with the wound. Adherent dressings should be grasped by the corner and removed slowly, whereas gauze dressings can be pinched in the center and lifted off.
- Contaminated dressings in the home should be disposed of in a manner consistent with local regulations. The Environmental Protection Agency recommends placing soiled dressings in securely fastened plastic bags before adding them to other household trash. However, local regulations vary, and home care agencies and patients need to follow procedures that are consistent with local laws.

Modified from Agency for Health Care Policy and Research, Panel for the Treatment of Pressure Ulcers in Adults: *Treatment of pressure ulcers,* Clinical Practice Guideline No. 15, AHCPR Pub No. 95-0653, Rockville, MD, 1994, Agency for Health Care Policy and Research, Public Health Service, US Department of Health and Human Services.

TABLE 48.7 Quick Guide to Pressure Injury Prevention

Risk Factor	Nursing Interventions
Decreased sensory perception	Provide pressure-redistribution surface (Gruccio and Ashton, 2018).
Medical device	Protect pressure points from medical devices such as oxygen tubing, feeding tubes, and casts (Kayser et al., 2018; Black et al., 2015).
Moisture	Following each incontinent episode, clean area with no-rinse perineal cleaner and protect skin with moisture-barrier ointment (Bryant and Nix, 2016a). Keep skin dry and free of maceration (Collier, 2016; Colwell et al., 2011).
Friction and shear	Reposition patient using drawsheet or a transfer board surface. Provide trapeze to facilitate movement in bed. Position patient at a 30-degree lateral turn and limit head elevation to 30 degrees (see Fig. 48.15).
Decreased activity/ mobility	Establish and post individualized turning schedule. Turn patient off at-risk areas often.
Poor nutrition	Provide adequate nutritional and fluid intake; help with intake as necessary (Stotts, 2016a). Consult dietitian for nutritional assessment and recommended nutrients.

position changes without tissue injury. When repositioning, use positioning devices to protect bony prominences (WOCN, 2016). The WOCN guidelines (2016) recommend a 30-degree lateral position (Fig. 48.15), which should prevent positioning directly over the bony prominence. To prevent shear and friction injuries, use a transfer device to lift rather than drag the patient when changing positions (see Chapter 39).

QSEN Building Competency in Evidence-Based Practice

The nurses on a neurology unit are concerned about patients who develop skin breakdown after recovery from a stroke. The nurses would like to implement a new evidence-based positioning protocol using safe patient handling with the goal of preventing pressure injury development. What is the nurses' PICOT question, and what topics should the nurses include in the evidence-based literature review?

Answers to QSEN Activities can be found on the Evolve website.

---

behavioral techniques, medication, and surgery. Behavioral techniques help patients learn ways to control their bladder and sphincter muscles.

Consider using absorbent pads and garments only after trying these measures. Although controversial, absorbent products such as absorptive underpads and garments are sometimes part of the treatment plan for an incontinent patient. Use only products that wick moisture away from the patient's skin (WOCN, 2016).

Positioning. Repositioning (turning) patients is a consistent element of evidence-based pressure injury prevention (EPUAP, NPIAP, PPPIA, 2019a). The twofold aim of repositioning should be to reduce or relieve pressure at the interface between bony prominence and support surface (bed or chair) and to limit the amount of time the tissue is exposed to pressure (Maklebust and Magnan, 2016). Elevating the head of the bed to 30 degrees or less decreases the chance of pressure injury development from shearing forces (WOCN, 2016). Change the immobilized patient's position according to tissue tolerance, level of activity and mobility, general medical condition, overall treatment objectives, skin condition, and comfort (EPUAP, NPIAP, PPPIA, 2019a). A standard turning interval of 1.5 to 2 hours does not always prevent pressure injury development; repositioning intervals are based on patient assessment. Some patients may need more frequent position changes, while other patients can tolerate every-2-hour

For patients at risk for skin breakdown who are able to sit in a chair, limit the amount of time they sit to 2 hours or less at any given time. In the sitting position the pressure on the ischial tuberosities is greater than in the supine position. In addition, teach the patient to shift weight every 15 minutes while sitting (WOCN, 2016). Shifting weight provides short-term relief on the ischial tuberosities. Also have him or her sit on foam, gel, or an air cushion to redistribute weight away from the ischial areas. Rigid and donut-shaped cushions are contraindicated because they reduce blood supply to the area, resulting in wider areas of ischemia (WOCN, 2016).

After repositioning the patient, reassess the skin. Remember to use caution when evaluating early signs of tissue ischemia in darkly pigmented skin. For patients with light-toned skin, observe for reactive hyperemia and blanching. Never massage reddened areas. Massaging reddened areas increases the breakdown of the capillaries in the underlying tissues and leads to the risk of tissue injury and pressure injury formation (WOCN, 2016).

Support Surfaces (Therapeutic Beds and Mattresses). Support surfaces are "specialized devices for pressure redistribution designed for management of tissue loads, microclimate, and/or other therapeutic functions (i.e., any mattress, integrated bed system, mattress replacement, overlay, seat cushion, or seat cushion overlay)" (EPUAP, NPIAP, PPPIA, 2019a). Support surfaces redistribute tissue loads by immersion (depth of penetration or sinking into the support surface by the patient's body) and envelopment (deformment around the body), thus evenly distributing pressure across the entire body surface (Jordan and Phipps, 2019; Maklebust and Magnan, 2016). Support surfaces reduce the hazards of immobility to the skin and musculoskeletal system. However, none eliminates the need for meticulous skin assessment and skin care. No single device completely eliminates the effects of pressure on the skin.

When selecting support surfaces, consider a patient's unique needs. Knowledge about support-surface characteristics (Table 48.8) helps you in clinical decision making. In selecting a support surface, know

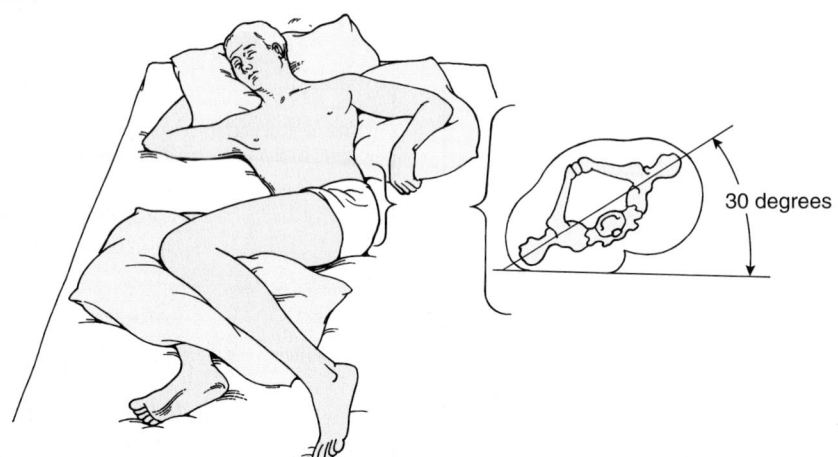

FIG. 48.15 Thirty-degree lateral position at which pressure points are avoided. (Adapted from Bryant RA, Nix DP, editors: *Acute and chronic wounds: current management concepts,* ed 5, St Louis, 2016, Elsevier.)

TABLE 48.8 Support Surfaces

Category and Mechanism of Action	Indications for Use	Advantages	Disadvantages
Support Surfaces and Overlays			
Foam Overlay (Available as an Overlay or in a Full Mattress)			
Reduces pressure; the cover (top) can reduce friction and shear. Base height of 7.5-10 cm (3-4 inches); see manufacturer guidelines regarding amount of body weight supported	Use for moderate- to high-risk patients	Onetime charge No setup fee Cannot be punctured Available in various sizes (e.g., bed, chair, operating room table) Little maintenance Does not need electricity	Elevated body temperature Hot and may trap moisture Limited life span Plastic protective sheet needed for incontinent patients or patients with draining wounds Not indicated for those with existing stage 3 or 4 pressure injuries
Water Overlay (Available as an Overlay or in a Full Mattress)			
Redistributes pressure and pressure points because surface provides flotation by redistributing patient's weight evenly over entire support surface	Use for high-risk patients	Readily available Some control over motion sensations Easy to clean	Easily punctured Heavy Fluid motion may make procedures (e.g., dressing changes, CPR) difficult Maintenance needed to prevent microorganism growth Patient transfers out of bed are difficult. Difficult to raise and lower head of bed
Gel Overlay			
Redistributes pressure because surface provides flotation by redistributing patient's weight evenly over entire support surface	Use for moderate- to high-risk patients Use for patients who are wheelchair dependent	Low maintenance Easy to clean Multiple-patient use Impermeable to needle punctures	Heavy Expensive Lacks airflow for moisture control Variable friction control

TABLE 48.8 Support Surfaces—cont'd

Category and Mechanism of Action	Indications for Use	Advantages	Disadvantages
Nonpowered Air-Filled Overlay Redistributes pressure by lowering mean interface pressure between patient's tissue and overlay	Use for moderate- to high-risk patients Use for patients who can reposition themselves	Easy to clean Multiple-patient use Low maintenance Potential repair of some air-filled products Durable	Damaged by punctures from needles and sharps Requires routine monitoring to determine adequate inflation pressure Patient transfers out of bed can be difficult
Low-Air-Loss Overlay (Available as an Overlay or in a Full Mattress) Maintains constant and slight air movement against patient's skin; redistributes pressure, assists in managing the heat and humidity (microclimate) of the skin	Use for moderate- to high-risk patients	Easy to clean Maintains constant inflation Deflates to facilitate transfer and CPR Moisture control Fabric covering overlay is air permeable, bacteria impermeable, and waterproof Reduces shear and friction Setup provided by manufacturer	Damaged by needles and sharps Can be noisy Requires electricity, some are available with short backup battery In home may need to purchase backup generator in case of loss of electrical power
Specialty Beds **Air-Fluidized Bed** Bedframe contains silicone-coated beads and provides pressure redistribution by the fluidlike medium that is created by forcing air through beads, resulting in immersion and envelopment of the patient.	Use for high-risk patients Use for patients with stage 3 or 4 pressure injuries or burns	Less frequent turning or repositioning Improved patient comfort Becomes firm for CPR or other treatments when device is turned "off" Reduces shear, friction, and edema to site May facilitate management of copious wound drainage or incontinence Setup provided by manufacturer	Continuous circulation of warm, dry air may increase patient risk for dehydration Possible increase in room temperature Patient may experience disorientation Patient transfer difficult Heavy Expensive May not be wide enough for use with obese patients or patients with contractures Patient cannot lie prone because of risk of suffocation
Low-Air-Loss Bed Bedframe with series of connected air-filled pillows. The flow of air controls the amount of pressure in each pillow and assists in managing the heat and humidity (microclimate) of the patient's skin. Redistributes pressure.	Use for patients who need pressure redistribution, those who cannot be repositioned frequently, or those who have skin breakdown on more than one surface Contraindicated in patients with unstable spinal column	Can raise and lower head and foot of bed Easy transfer in and out of bed Setup provided by manufacturer	Portable motor can be noisy Bed surface material slippery; patients can easily slide down mattress or out of bed when being transferred
Kinetic Therapy Provides continuous passive motion to promote mobilization of pulmonary secretions and low air loss and provides pressure redistribution	Used primarily to facilitate pulmonary hygiene in patients with acute respiratory conditions Should not be used when the patient is hemodynamically unstable	Reduces pulmonary complications associated with restricted mobility	Does not reduce shear or moisture Cannot be used with cervical or skeletal traction Possible motion sickness initially

CPR, Cardiopulmonary resuscitation.
Data from Doughty D, McNichol L: *Wound, Ostomy and Continence Nurses Society (WOCN): Core curriculum: wound management,* Philadelphia, 2016, Wound, Ostomy, and Continence Society; Wound, Ostomy and Continence Nurses Society (WOCN): *Guideline for prevention and management of pressure ulcers, WOCN clinical practice guideline series,* ed 2, Mt. Laurel, NJ, 2016, Author.

BOX 48.7   PATIENT TEACHING

Pressure-Redistribution Surfaces

Objective
- Patient and family caregiver will describe understanding of the purposes and basic operations of the pressure-redistribution surface.

Teaching Strategies
- Explain the reasons for the pressure-redistribution surface.
- Explain the need to maintain proper body mechanics while using the pressure-redistribution surface. Demonstrate technique.
- Discuss possible patient sensations associated with the device.
- Instruct that minimal layers of linens should be placed over the pressure-redistribution surface.
- Educate in the use and care of the pressure-redistribution surface (based on manufacturer guidelines).

- Explain common errors in the use of support surfaces.
- Explain additional pressure-redistribution measures (e.g., safe patient handling during turning, avoidance of friction, 30-degree lateral position (WOCN, 2016).

Evaluation
Use the principles of teach-back to evaluate patient/family caregiver learning:
- Now that we have discussed the use of the pressure-redistribution surface, explain to me the purpose for using the device.
- Describe to me the possible sensations that you might experience while using the support surface.
- Show me how you will correctly position yourself on the pressure-redistribution surface.

---

the patient's risks and the purpose for the support surface; a flow chart is often helpful. If your agency has a wound care clinical nurse specialist, consult with him or her on choice of support surface. Teach patients and families the reason for and proper use of the devices (Box 48.7). Some common errors with support surfaces are placing the wrong side of the support surface toward the patient, not plugging powered support surfaces into the electrical source, not turning on the power source for powered support surfaces, failing to place a hand between the metal bedframe and the mattress to determine whether the patient sinks to the point of touching the bedframe for some support surfaces, using several layers of sheets and pads between the patient and the surface, and improperly inflating some support surfaces. When used correctly, these support surfaces help redistribute pressure to the skin of patients who are at risk for or have skin breakdown.

Acute Care

Management of Pressure Injuries. Treatment of patients with pressure injuries requires a holistic approach that uses interprofessional expertise (WOCN, 2016). In addition to the nurse, the health care provider, wound-care nurse specialist, physical therapist, occupational therapist, nutritionist, and pharmacist are involved. Aspects of pressure injury treatment include local care of the wound and supportive measures such as adequate nutrients and redistribution of pressure (see Skill 48.2).

Before treating a pressure injury, reassess the wound for location, stage, size, tissue type and amount, exudate, and surrounding skin condition (see Skill 48.1) (Nix, 2016). Acute wounds require close monitoring (every 4-8 hours; check agency policy). Chronic wound assessment occurs less frequently. Depending on the topical management system, evaluate the wound with every dressing change, usually not more than once a day.

The use and documentation of a systematic approach to monitor progress of an actual pressure injury leads to better decision making and optimal outcomes (Nix, 2016). Several healing and documentation tools are available to document wound assessments over time. Using a tool helps link assessment to outcomes so that an evaluation of the plan of care follows objective criteria (Nix, 2016). For example, the Bates-Jensen Wound Assessment Tool (BWAT) (Bates-Jensen, 2016) addresses 15 wound characteristics. You score individual items and calculate the sum total, providing an overall indication of wound status. The scoring helps to evaluate whether the goals of the wound management are effective.

Wound Management. Maintenance of a physiological local wound environment is the goal of effective wound management (Bryant and

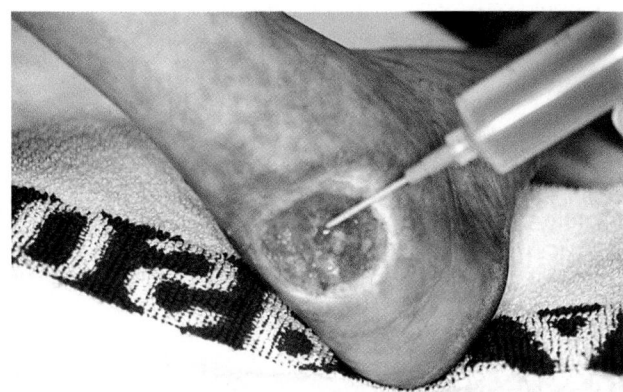

FIG. 48.16 Wound irrigation.

Nix, 2016b). To maintain a healthy wound environment, you need to address the following objectives: prevent and manage infection, clean the wound, remove nonviable tissue, maintain the wound in a moist environment, eliminate dead space, control odor, eliminate or minimize pain, and protect the wound and periwound skin (Ramundo, 2016).

A wound does not move through the phases of healing if infected. Preventing wound infection includes cleaning and removing nonviable tissue. Clean pressure injuries *only with noncytotoxic wound cleaners* such as normal saline or commercial wound cleaners. Noncytotoxic cleaners do not damage or kill fibroblasts and healing tissue (Bryant and Nix, 2016b). Some commonly used cytotoxic solutions are Dakin's solution (sodium hypochlorite solution), acetic acid, and povidone-iodine. These are not to be used in clean, granulating wounds.

Irrigation is a common method of delivering a wound-cleansing solution to the wound. Wound irrigation cleans and debrides necrotic tissue with pressure that can remove debris from the wound bed without damaging healthy tissue (Ramundo, 2016). One method to ensure an irrigation pressure within the correct range is to use a 19-gauge angiocatheter and a 35-mL syringe, which delivers saline to a pressure injury at 8 psi (Fig. 48.16).

Debridement is the removal of nonviable, necrotic tissue. Removal of necrotic tissue is necessary to rid the wound of a source of infection, enable visualization of the wound bed, and provide a clean base necessary for healing.

The method of debridement depends on which is most appropriate for a patient's condition and goals of care (WOCN, 2016). It is important to remember that during the debridement process some normal wound observations include an increase in wound exudate, odor, and size. You need to assess and prevent or effectively manage pain that occurs with debridement (WOCN, 2016). Plan to administer an ordered analgesic 30 minutes before debridement.

Methods of debridement include mechanical, autolytic, chemical, and sharp/surgical. Autolytic debridement is the removal of dead tissue via lysis of necrotic tissue by the white blood cells and natural enzymes of the body (Ramundo, 2016). You accomplish this by using dressings that support moisture at the wound surface. If the wound base is dry, use a dressing that adds moisture; if there is excessive exudate, use a dressing that absorbs the excessive moisture while maintaining moisture at the wound bed. Some examples of these dressings are transparent film and hydrocolloid dressings.

You can accomplish chemical debridement with the use of a topical enzyme preparation, Dakin's solution, or sterile maggots. Topical enzymes induce changes in the substrate, resulting in the breakdown of necrotic tissue (Ramundo, 2016). Depending on the type of enzyme used, the preparation either digests or dissolves the tissue. These preparations require a health care provider's order. Dakin's solution breaks down and loosens dead tissue in a wound. Apply the solution to gauze and apply to the wound. Sterile maggots are used in a wound because it is thought that they ingest the dead tissue.

Surgical debridement is the removal of devitalized tissue with a scalpel, scissors, or other sharp instrument. Physicians and, in some states, trained advanced practice nurses perform surgical debridement of an injury or wound. Nurses should check the Nurse Practice Act for their state to see whether surgical debridement is a nursing function. It is the quickest method of debridement. It is usually indicated when the patient has signs of cellulitis or sepsis. Other methods of mechanical debridement are wound irrigation (high-pressure irrigation and pulsatile high-pressure lavage) and whirlpool treatments (Ramundo, 2016).

A moist environment supports the movement of epithelial cells and facilitates wound closure. A wound that has excessive exudate (drainage) provides an environment that supports bacterial growth, macerates the periwound skin, and slows the healing process. If excessive wound exudate is present, evaluate the volume, consistency, and odor of the drainage to determine whether an infection is present.

Remember, the wound will not heal unless the contributory factors are controlled or eliminated. Therefore it is critically important for you to address the causative factors (e.g., shear, friction, pressure, and moisture), or it is unlikely that the wound will heal despite topical therapy (Bryant and Nix, 2016b).

The treatment plan needs to be altered as a wound heals. For example, a transparent film dressing is used initially to autolytically debride (liquefy the tissue using body moisture) a necrotic wound. Once the wound is cleaned of necrotic tissue, discontinue the transparent film dressing; and, on the basis of the wound base characteristics, choose a new dressing. A wound with excessive drainage requires a dressing with a high absorptive capacity. Continued reassessment is key to supporting the wound as it moves through the phases of wound healing.

Protection. Protecting a wound from further injury is a priority. A strategy to prevent surgical wound dehiscence is to place a folded thin blanket or pillow over an abdominal wound so that a patient can splint the area during coughing (see Chapter 50). Because coughing increases the intraabdominal pressure, the patient applies light but firm pressure over the wound when coughing to support the healing tissue. A patient may also wear an abdominal binder to make movement less uncomfortable and to provide support for the abdomen and surgical site. Teach the patient this technique and keep the splint within hand's reach.

Education. Education of the patient and family caregivers is an important nursing function (Bryant and Nix, 2016a). A variety of educational tools, including videos and written materials, are available for you to use when teaching patients and family caregivers how to prevent and treat pressure injuries and care for wounds. The US National Library of Medicine (2019) has an excellent website with information on the prevention of pressure injuries (https://www.nlm.nih.gov/medlineplus/ency/patientinstructions/000147.htm).

Understanding and assessing the experience of the patient and support person are also important dimensions in the treatment of people with wounds and pressure injuries (WOCN, 2016). Clinicians are only just now exploring through research the caregiver's perspective of the concerns and issues faced by frail older spouses caring for their loved ones with pressure injuries. Plan interventions to meet the identified psychosocial needs of patients and their support people (WOCN, 2016).

Nutritional Status. Nutritional support of a patient with a wound is based on the appreciation that nutrition is fundamental to normal cellular integrity and tissue repair (Stotts, 2016a). Early intervention is necessary to correct inadequate nutrition and support healing. Refer patients with pressure injuries to a registered dietitian for early intervention involving therapeutic diets or enteral or parenteral nutrition (see Chapter 45). Your patient will need 30 to 35 calories/kg of body weight if a pressure injury is present and he or she is assessed to be at risk for malnutrition. Increased caloric intake helps replace subcutaneous tissue. Patients will also receive vitamin and mineral supplements if suspected or known deficiencies exist. Vitamin C promotes collagen synthesis, capillary wall integrity, fibroblast function, and immunological function.

Patients with pressure injuries who are underweight or losing weight need enhanced protein supplementation (WOCN, 2016). A patient can lose as much as 50 g of protein per day from an open, high exudative pressure injury. Although the recommended intake of protein for adults is 0.8 g/kg/day, a higher intake up to 1.8 g/kg/day is necessary for healing. Increased protein intake helps rebuild epidermal tissue (EPUAP, NPIAP, PPPIA, 2019a). Evaluation of weight, laboratory values, and skin parameters reflect changes in status and effects of nutritional interventions (Stotts, 2016a).

First Aid for Wounds. Use first-aid measures for wound protection and management in an emergency situation. Under stable conditions a variety of interventions ensure wound healing. When a patient suffers a traumatic wound, first-aid interventions include stabilizing cardiopulmonary function (see Chapter 41), promoting hemostasis, cleaning the wound, and protecting it from further injury.

Hemostasis. After assessing the type and extent of a wound, control bleeding by applying direct pressure with a sterile or clean dressing such as a washcloth. After bleeding subsides, an adhesive bandage or gauze dressing taped over the laceration allows skin edges to close and a blood clot to form. If a dressing becomes saturated with blood, add another layer of dressing, continue to apply pressure, and elevate the affected part. Avoid further disruption of skin layers. Serious lacerations need to be sutured by a health care provider. Pressure dressings used during the first 24 to 48 hours after trauma help maintain hemostasis.

Normally allow a puncture wound to bleed to remove dirt and other contaminants such as saliva from a dog bite. When a penetrating object such as a knife blade is present, *do not remove the object.* The presence of the object provides pressure and controls some bleeding. Removal causes massive, uncontrolled bleeding. Except for skull injuries, apply pressure around the penetrating object but not on it, and transport the patient to an emergency department.

Cleaning. The process of cleaning a wound involves selecting an appropriate cleaning solution and using a mechanical means of delivering that solution without causing injury to the healing wound tissue (WOCN, 2016). Gently cleaning a wound removes contaminants that serve as sources of infection. However, vigorous cleaning using a method with too much mechanical force causes bleeding or further injury. For abrasions, minor lacerations, and small puncture wounds, first rinse the wound with normal saline and lightly cover the area with a dressing. When a laceration is bleeding profusely, only brush away surface contaminants and concentrate on hemostasis until the patient can be cared for in a clinic or hospital.

According to the WOCN guidelines (2016), normal saline is the preferred cleaning agent. It is physiologically neutral and does not harm tissue. Normal saline keeps the wound surface moist to promote the development and migration of epithelial tissue. Gentle cleansing with normal saline and application of moist saline dressings are commonly used for healing wounds.

Protection. Regardless of whether bleeding has stopped, protect a traumatic wound from further injury by applying sterile or clean dressings and immobilizing the body part. A light dressing applied over minor wounds prevents entrance of microorganisms.

Dressings. The use of dressings requires an understanding of wound healing. A variety of dressing materials are available commercially. The correct dressing selection facilitates wound healing (Bryant and Nix, 2016b). The dressing type depends on the assessment of the wound and the phase of wound healing. When you identify the objectives for the wound care, the dressing choice becomes clear. A wound that requires infection management requires a different set of dressings than one requiring the removal of nonviable tissue.

The more extensive a wound, the larger the dressing required. For example, a bulky dressing applied with pressure minimizes movement of underlying tissues and helps immobilize the entire body part. A bandage or cloth wrapped around a penetrating object should immobilize it adequately.

Alternative dressings are available to cover and protect certain types of wounds such as large wounds, wounds with drainage tubes or suction catheters in the wound, and wounds that need frequent changing because of excessive drainage. In the home setting a clean towel or diaper is often the best secondary dressing. Pouches or special wound collection systems cover wounds with excessive drainage and collect the drainage. Some of the collection systems have a plastic window on the front of the wound pouch, allowing you to change the packing without removing the pouch from the skin.

Many surgical wounds no longer have dressings (see Chapter 50). However, when a surgical wound has a dressing, its purpose is to promote wound healing by primary intention. Thus it is common to remove surgical dressings as soon as drainage stops. In contrast, when dressing a wound healing by secondary intention, the dressing material becomes a means for providing moisture to the wound or helping in debridement.

Purposes of Dressings. A dressing serves several purposes:
- Protects a wound from microorganism contamination
- Aids in hemostasis
- Promotes healing by absorbing drainage and debriding a wound
- Supports or splints a wound site
- Promotes thermal insulation of a wound surface
- Provides a moist environment

When the skin is broken, a dressing helps reduce exposure to microorganisms. However, when drainage is minimal, the healing process forms a natural fibrin seal that eliminates the need for a dressing. Wounds with extensive tissue loss always need a dressing.

Pressure dressings promote hemostasis. Applied with elastic bandages, a pressure dressing exerts localized downward pressure over an actual or potential bleeding site. It eliminates dead space in underlying tissues so that wound healing progresses normally. Check pressure dressings to be sure that they do not interfere with circulation to a body part. Assess skin color, pulses in distal extremities, the patient's comfort, and changes in sensation. Pressure dressings are not removed routinely.

The functions of a dressing on a healing wound are to provide protection, deliver medication, and absorb drainage. Gauze dressings come in various types, including gauze sponges, used to pack wounds with depth and drainage; gauze placed over a shallow healing wound as a topper dressing; or gauze placed over a wound to wick the wound drainage. Gauze dressings are available in several sizes, frequently 2 × 2–inch or 4 × 4–inch squares. A problem occurs if wound drainage dries, causing the dressing to stick to the suture line. Improperly removing a dressing disrupts the healing epidermal surface. If a gauze dressing sticks to a surgical incision, lightly moisten it with saline solution before removal. This saturates the dressing and loosens it from the incisional area, thus preventing trauma to the incisional area during removal.

The dressing technique varies, depending on the goal of the treatment plan for a wound. For example, if the goal is to maintain a moist environment to promote wound healing, it is important to not let the saline-moistened gauze dressing become dry and stick to the wound. This is in direct contrast to the dressing technique that you use if the goal of care is to mechanically debride the wound using a saline moist-to-dry dressing. When wounds such as a necrotic wound require debriding, a moist-to-dry dressing technique can be considered. You place the moist dressing (contact dressing) over the wound bed, cover with a clean gauze, and allow the contact layer to dry. In this case the contact dressing is allowed to dry so that it sticks to underlying tissue and debrides the wound during removal. This type of debridement is nonselective and can remove viable tissue; it is recommended for debridement in a necrotic wound (Ramundo, 2016).

Dressings applied to a draining wound require frequent changing to prevent microorganism growth and skin breakdown. Bacteria grow readily in the dark, warm, moist environment under a dressing. The periwound area can become macerated and irritated. Minimize periwound skin breakdown by keeping the skin clean and dry and reducing the use of tape. The absorbent dressing inner layer serves as a reservoir for secretions. The wicking action of woven gauze dressings pulls excess drainage into the dressing and away from the wound. The final outer layer of the dressing (usually an ABD pad that has an outer layer that prevents strike-through) helps prevent bacteria and other external contaminants from reaching the wound surface. Apply adhesives to this layer to secure the dressings.

A dressing needs to support a moist wound environment if the wound is healing by secondary intention. A moist wound base facilitates the movement of epithelialization, thus allowing the wound to resurface as quickly as possible.

Types of Dressings. Dressings vary by type of material and mode of application (moist or dry) (see Skill 48.3). They need to be easy to apply, comfortable, and made of materials that promote wound healing. The WOCN guidelines (2016) are helpful when selecting dressings based on the goal of wound treatment (Box 48.8). To avoid causing damage to the periwound skin, it is important that the dressing technique that you use to treat pressure injuries and other wounds is not excessively moist (Box 48.9).

Most pressure injuries require dressings. The type of dressing is usually based on the stage of the pressure injury, the type of tissue in the wound, and the function of the dressing (Table 48.9). Before placing a dressing on a pressure injury, it is important, based on the nursing diagnosis, to understand the goal of the treatment, the mechanism of action of the dressing, and principles of wound care.

Gauze sponges are the oldest and most common dressing. They are absorbent and are especially useful in wounds to wick away wound

BOX 48.8 Dressing Considerations

- Clean the wound and periwound area at each dressing change, minimizing trauma to the wound (WOCN, 2016).
- Use a dressing that continuously provides a moist environment.
- Perform wound care using topical dressings as determined by a thorough assessment.
- No specific studies have proven an optimal dressing type for pressure injuries (WOCN, 2016).
- Choose a dressing that keeps the periwound skin dry while keeping the injury bed moist.
- Choose a dressing that controls exudate but does not desiccate the injury bed.
- The type of dressing may change over time as the pressure injury heals or deteriorates. The wound should be monitored at every dressing change and regularly assessed to determine whether modifications in the dressing type are needed (WOCN, 2016).
- Consider caregiver time, ease of use, availability, and cost when selecting a dressing.

BOX 48.9 EVIDENCE-BASED PRACTICE

Moisture-Associated Skin Damage

PICOT Question: In hospitalized patients, which interventions prevent or reduce the risk of medical device–related pressure injuries?

Evidence Summary

Medical device–related (MDR) pressure injuries are becoming more common (Kayser et al., 2018; Black and Kalowes, 2016). In 2016, the NPUAP defined a medical device–related pressure injury (MDRPI) as arising "from the use of devices designed and applied for diagnostic or therapeutic purposes. The resultant pressure injury generally conforms to the pattern or shape of the device" (EPUAP, NPIAP, PPPIA, 2019a). Critically ill patients and neonates are particularly vulnerable to MDR pressure injuries (Maklebust and Magnan, 2016). Because MDRPIs form faster than non-MDRPIs, timely proactive assessment and prevention measures are critical. Most MDRPIs occur at the face and head region, and the ears specifically (Kayser et al., 2018). The most common devices linked with MDRPIs are oxygen tubing and masks. Devices include nasal cannulas, cervical collars, Foley catheter and bedside collection tubing, braces, endotracheal tubes, and pulse oximetry devices (see also Table 48.5). It is important to be aware of devices that are used for patient care that could damage edematous tissue and to plan care to cushion or redistribute pressure away from susceptible skin.

Application to Nursing Practice

- Choose the correct size of medical device(s) to fit the individual, especially endotracheal tubes and oxygen equipment.
- Cushion and protect the skin with dressings in high-risk areas (e.g., nasal bridge).
- Remove or move removable devices to assess skin at least daily.
- Avoid placement of device(s) over sites of prior or existing pressure injury.
- Assess skin underneath device for edema, risks for potential for skin breakdown, and early signs of skin breakdown
- Assessment under, around, and at the edges of medical devices is critical for prevention and early intervention of these injuries. It is important that intervention such as foam padding be considered to reduce or eliminate the pressure injury (Black and Kalowes, 2016).
- Confirm that devices are not placed directly under an individual who is bedridden or immobile.

exudate. Gauze is available in different textures and various lengths and sizes; the 4 × 4 is the most common size. Gauze can be saturated with solutions and used to clean and pack a wound. When used to pack a wound, the gauze is saturated with the solution (usually normal saline), wrung out (leaving the gauze only moist), unfolded, and lightly packed into the wound. Unfolding the dressing allows easy wicking action. The purpose of this type of dressing is to provide moisture to the wound yet to allow wound drainage to be wicked into the dry cover gauze pad.

Another type of dressing is a self-adhesive, transparent film that traps moisture over a wound, providing a moist environment to encourage epithelial cell growth (Fig. 48.17). A transparent dressing adheres to undamaged skin, does not need a secondary dressing, and permits viewing of the wound. It is ideal for small superficial wounds such as a stage 1 pressure injury or a partial-thickness wound. Use a film dressing as a secondary dressing and for autolytic debridement of small wounds. It serves as a barrier to external fluids and bacteria but still allows the wound surface to "breathe" because oxygen passes through the transparent dressing (McNichol et al., 2018). This dressing promotes a moist environment to encourage epithelial cell growth. It adheres to undamaged skin, does not need a secondary dressing, and permits viewing of the wound.

Hydrocolloid dressings are dressings with complex formulations of colloids and adhesive components. They are adhesive and occlusive. The wound contact layer of this dressing forms a gel as wound exudate is absorbed and maintains a moist healing environment. Hydrocolloids support healing in clean granulating wounds and autolytically debride necrotic wounds; they are available in a variety of sizes and shapes. This type of dressing absorbs drainage through the use of exudate absorbers in the dressing; maintains wound moisture; slowly liquefies necrotic debris; and can be left in place for 3 to 5 days. In addition, hydrocolloid dressings are impermeable to bacteria and other contaminants, act as a preventive dressing for high-risk friction areas, and are self-adhesive and mold to the wound.

The hydrocolloid dressing is useful on shallow-to–moderately deep dermal injuries. Hydrocolloid dressings cannot absorb drainage from heavily draining wounds, and some are contraindicated for use in full-thickness and infected wounds. Most hydrocolloids leave a residue in the wound bed that is easy to confuse with purulent drainage.

Hydrogel dressings are gauze or sheet dressings impregnated with water or glycerin-based amorphous gel. This type of dressing hydrates wounds and absorbs small amounts of exudate. Hydrogel dressings are indicated for use in partial-thickness and full-thickness wounds, deep wounds with some exudate, necrotic wounds, burns, and radiation-damaged skin. They debride necrotic tissue by softening the necrotic area. They can be very useful in painful wounds because they are very soothing to a patient and do not adhere to the wound bed and thus cause little pain during removal. A disadvantage is that some hydrogels require a secondary dressing and you must take care to prevent periwound maceration. Hydrogels also come in a tube; thus you are able to squirt the gel directly into the wound base.

Many other types of dressings are available. Foam and alginate dressings are for wounds with large amounts of exudate and those that need packing. Foam dressings are also used around drainage tubes to absorb drainage. Calcium alginate dressings are manufactured from seaweed and come in sheet and rope form. The alginate forms a soft gel when in contact with wound fluid. These highly absorbent dressings are for wounds with an excessive amount of drainage and do not cause trauma when removed from the wound. *Do not use these in dry wounds, and they require a secondary dressing.* Several manufacturers produce composite dressings, which combine two different dressing types into one dressing. Research is ongoing regarding which type of dressing is best for which type of wound.

TABLE 48.9   Dressings By Pressure Injury Stage

Pressure Injury Stage	Pressure Injury Status	Dressing	Comments[a]	Expected Change	Adjuvants
1	Intact	None Transparent dressing Hydrocolloid	Allows visual assessment. Protects from shear. Do not use transparent dressing in presence of excessive moisture. Hydrocolloid does not allow visual assessment.	Resolves slowly without epidermal loss over 7 to 14 days	Turning schedule. Support hydration. Nutritional support. Use pressure-redistribution bed or chair cushion.
2	Clean	Composite film Hydrocolloid Hydrogel covered with foam or gauze dressing.	Limits shear. Change when seal of dressing breaks; maximal wear time 7 days. Provides moist environment.	Heals through re-epithelialization	See previous stage. Manage incontinence.
3	Clean	Hydrocolloid Hydrogel covered with foam dressing Calcium alginate Gauze	Change when seal of dressing breaks; maximum wear time 7 days. Apply over wound to protect and absorb moisture. Use when there is significant exudate. Cover with secondary dressing. Use with normal saline or other prescribed solution. Wring out excess solution; unfold to make contact with wound. Cover with dry dressing tape in place.	Heals through granulation and reepithelialization	See previous stages. Evaluate pressure-redistribution needs.
4	Clean	Hydrogel covered with foam dressing Calcium alginate Gauze	See stage 3: clean. Used with significant exudate; must cover with secondary dressing See stage 3: clean.	Heals through granulation, scar tissue development, and reepithelialization	Surgical consultation may be necessary for closure. See stages 1, 2, and 3.
Unstageable	Wound covered with eschar	Adherent film Gauze plus ordered solution Enzymes None	Facilitates softening of eschar. Delivers solution and may soften the eschar. Breaks down eschar, providing debridement. If eschar is dry and intact and debridement is not part of the plan of care, no dressing is used, allowing eschar to act as physiological cover.	Eschar lifts at edges as healing progresses Eschar loosens over time.	See previous stages. Surgical consultation may be considered for debridement. May be considered for slow debridement.

[a]As with *all* occlusive dressings, wounds should not be clinically infected.

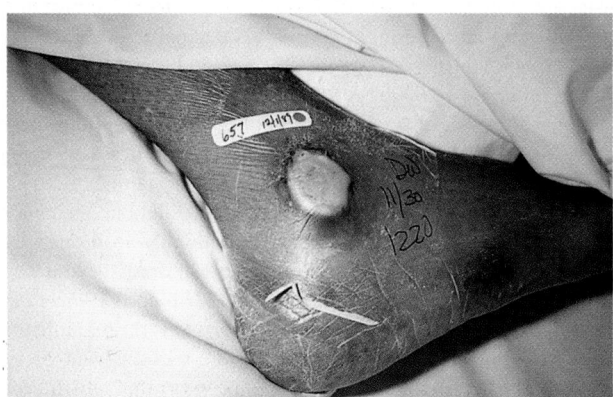

FIG. 48.17 Transparent film dressing.

Changing Dressings. A health care provider's order for wound care indicates the dressing type, the frequency of changing, and any solutions or ointments to be applied to the wound. An order to "reinforce dressing prn" (add dressings without removing the original one) is common right after surgery, when the health care provider does not want accidental disruption of the suture line or bleeding. The medical or operating room record usually indicates whether drains are present and from which body cavity they drain.

Always know the type of wound and dressing, the presence of underlying drains or tubing, and the type of supplies needed for wound care. Poor preparation causes a break in aseptic technique (see Chapter 28) or accidental pulling of wound tissue or dislodgement of a drain. Your judgment in modifying a dressing-change procedure is important during wound care, particularly if the character of a wound changes. Notifying the health care provider of any change is essential.

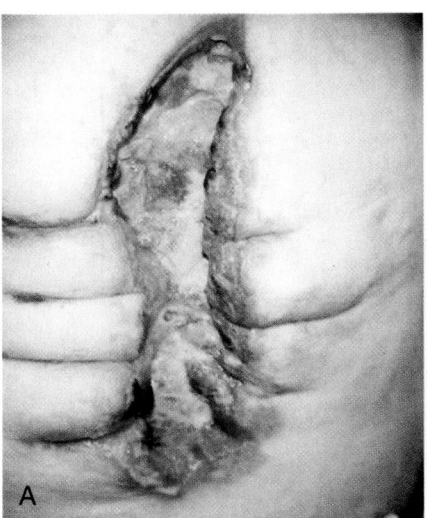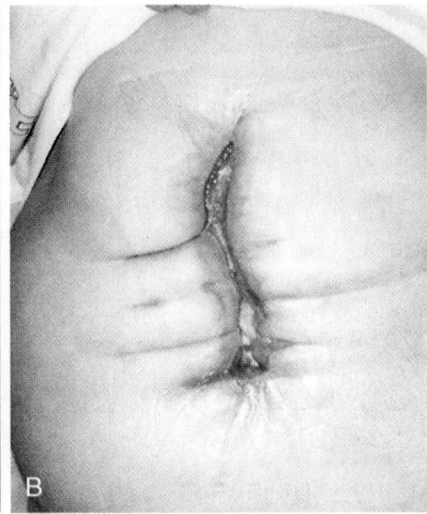

FIG. 48.18 A, Dehisced wound before wound V.A.C. therapy. B, Dehisced wound after wound V.A.C. therapy. *V.A.C.*, Vacuum-assisted closure. (Courtesy Kinetic Concepts [KCI], San Antonio, TX.)

Sometimes (e.g., with chronic nonsurgical wounds) you will use clean medical aseptic technique for a dressing change. The clean technique refers to the fact that the nurse maintains medical versus sterile asepsis (see Chapter 28). You will wear clean gloves, but the dressing materials are in sterile packages and are carefully placed over the wound. Deep wounds that require irrigation are usually irrigated with a sterile solution. A complete patient and wound history is essential in determining when a clean dressing technique is appropriate. For example, chronic pressure injury wounds use clean technique. On the other hand, a fresh surgical wound may require sterile technique, which requires the use of sterile gloves to prevent the introduction of microorganisms into a healing wound. After the first dressing change, describe the location of drains and the type of dressing materials and solutions to use in the patient's care plan.

Often it is necessary to teach patients how to change dressings in preparation for home care. In this situation, demonstrate dressing changes to a patient or family caregiver, and provide an opportunity for practice. Usually wound healing has progressed to the point that risks of complications such as dehiscence or evisceration are minimal. A patient needs to be able to change a dressing independently or with help from a family caregiver before discharge. Contaminated dressings in the home should be disposed of in a manner consistent with local regulations. Skill 48.3 outlines the steps for changing dry and moist dressings.

Packing a Wound. The first step in packing a wound is to assess its size, depth, and shape. These characteristics are important in determining the size and type of dressing used to pack a wound. The dressing needs to be flexible and in contact with the entire wound surface. Make sure that the type of material used to pack the wound is appropriate. If gauze is the appropriate dressing material, saturate with the ordered solution, wring out, unfold, and lightly pack into the wound. The entire wound surface needs to be in contact with part of the moist gauze dressing (see Skill 48.3).

It is important to remember not to pack a wound too tightly. Overpacking causes pressure on the wound bed tissue. Pack the wound only until the packing material reaches the surface of the wound; there should never be so much packing material that it extends higher than the wound surface. Packing that overlaps onto the wound edges causes maceration of the skin surrounding the wound.

One treatment modality for wounds is negative-pressure wound therapy (NPWT) or vacuum-assisted closure (one brand name is V.A.C.). NPWT is the application of subatmospheric (negative)

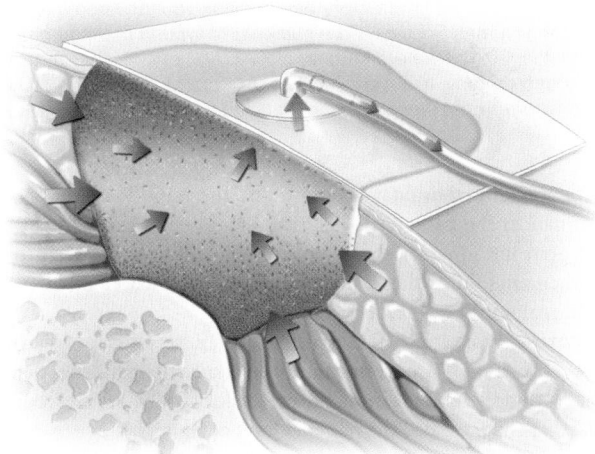

FIG. 48.19 V.A.C. system using negative pressure to remove fluid from area surrounding wound, reducing edema and improving circulation to area. *V.A.C.*, Vacuum-assisted closure. (Courtesy Kinetic Concepts [KCI], San Antonio, TX.)

pressure to a wound through suction to facilitate healing and collect wound fluid (Netsch et al., 2016). The vacuum-assisted closure (V.A.C.) is a device that helps in wound closure by applying localized negative pressure to draw the edges of a wound together (Fig. 48.18A-B). NPWT supports wound healing by reduction of edema and fluid removal, macro deformation and wound contraction, and micro deformation and mechanical stretch perfusion (see Skill 48.4). Secondary effects include angiogenesis, granulation tissue formation, and reduction in bacterial bioburden (Netsch et al., 2016) (Fig. 48.19). The V.A.C. Instill system allows intermittent instillation of fluids into a wound and liquefies infectious material and wound debris, especially in wounds not responding to traditional NPWT (Fernandez et al., 2019).

NPWT treats acute and chronic wounds, and the schedule for changing NPWT dressings varies, depending on the type of wound and amount of drainage. Wear time for the dressing is anywhere from 24 hours to 5 days. As a wound heals, granulation tissue lines its surface. The wound has a stippled or granulated appearance. The surface area sometimes increases or decreases, depending on wound location

BOX 48.10   Negative-Pressure Wound Therapy: Maintaining an Airtight Seal

To avoid loss of suction (negative pressure), the wound and dressing must stay sealed after therapy is initiated. Problem seal areas include wounds around joints; near skin creases and folds; and near moisture such as diaphoresis, wound drainage, and urine or stool. The following points may help to maintain an airtight seal:

- Clip hair on skin around wound (check agency policy).
- Fill uneven skin surfaces with a skin-barrier product such as paste or strips.
- Make sure that periwound skin surface is dry.
- Cut transparent film to extend 2.5 to 5 cm (1 to 2 inches) beyond wound perimeter.
- Frame periwound area with liquid skin barrier, solid skin barrier, or hydrocolloid dressing.
- Cut transparent dressing to fit wound.
- Avoid wrinkles when applying transparent film.
- Identify any air leaks with a stethoscope and repair them with the transparent dressing.
- Use only one or two additional layers for large leaks. Multiple layers reduce moisture vapor transmission and cause maceration of wound.

Data from Netsch DS: Refractory wounds. In Wound Ostomy and Continence Nurses Society: *Core curriculum: wound management*, Philadelphia, 2016, Wolters Kluwer; Netsch DS, et al: Negative-pressure wound therapy. In Bryant RA, Nix DP, editors: *Acute and chronic wounds: current management concepts*, ed 5, St Louis, 2016, Mosby.

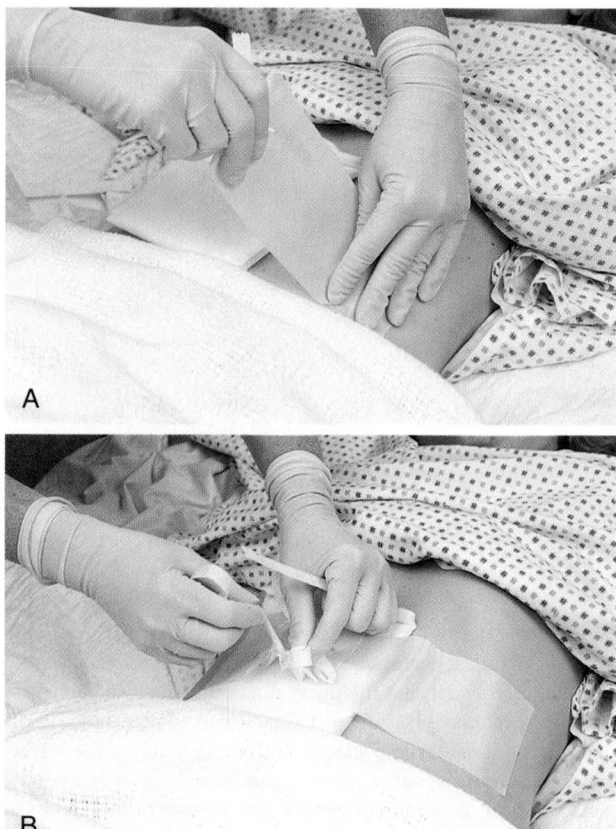

FIG. 48.20 Montgomery ties. **A,** Each tie is placed at side of dressing. **B,** Securing ties encloses dressing.

and the amount of drainage removed by the NPWT system. NPWT also enhances the adherence of split-thickness skin grafts. It is placed over a graft intraoperatively, decreasing the ability of the graft to shift and evacuating fluids that build up under it (Netsch et al., 2016). An airtight seal must be maintained (Box 48.10).

Securing Dressings. Use tape, ties, or a secondary dressing to secure a dressing over a wound site. The choice of anchoring depends on the wound size and location, the presence of drainage, the frequency of dressing changes, and the patient's level of activity.

You will most often use strips of tape to secure dressings. Nonallergenic paper and silicone tapes minimize skin reactions. Common adhesive tape adheres well to the surface of the skin, whereas elastic adhesive tape compresses closely around pressure bandages and permits more movement of a body part. Skin sensitive to adhesive tape becomes severely inflamed and denuded and, in some cases, even sloughs when the tape is removed. It is important to assess the condition of the skin under tape at each dressing change.

Tape is available in various widths such as 1.3, 2.5, 5, and 7.5 cm (½, 1, 2, and 3 inches). Choose the size that secures a dressing sufficiently. For example, a large abdominal wound dressing needs to remain secure over a large area despite frequent stress from movement, respiratory effort, and possibly abdominal distention. Strips of 7.5-cm (3-inch) adhesive stabilize such a large dressing, so it does not continually slip off. When applying tape, ensure that it adheres to several inches of skin on both sides of the dressing and that it is placed across the middle of the dressing. When securing a dressing, press the tape gently to the skin and the topper dressing. Never apply tape over irritated or broken skin. Protect irritated skin by using a solid skin barrier and applying the tape over the barrier.

To remove tape safely, loosen the ends and gently pull the outer end parallel with the skin surface toward the wound. Gently push the skin away from the wound as the tape is loosened and removed. Adhesive remover also loosens the tape from the skin. If tape covers an area of hair growth, a patient experiences less discomfort if you pull the tape in the direction of the hair growth.

To avoid repeated removal of tape from sensitive skin, secure dressings with pairs of reusable Montgomery ties (Fig. 48.20). Each section consists of a long strip; half contains an adhesive backing to apply to the skin, and the other half folds back and contains a cloth tie or a safety pin/rubber band combination that you fasten across a dressing and untie at dressing changes. A large, bulky dressing often requires two or more sets of Montgomery ties. Another method to protect the surrounding skin on wounds that need frequent dressing changes is to place strips of hydrocolloid dressings on either side of the wound edges, cover the wound with a dressing, and apply the tape to the dressing. To provide even support to a wound and immobilize a body part, apply elastic gauze, elastic stretch net, or binders over a dressing.

Comfort Measures. A wound is often painful, depending on the extent of tissue injury, and wound care often requires the use of well-timed analgesia before any wound procedure (Krasner, 2016). Administer analgesic medications 30 to 60 minutes before dressing changes, depending on the time of peak action of a drug. In addition, several techniques are useful in minimizing discomfort during wound care. Carefully removing tape, gently cleaning wound edges, and carefully manipulating dressings and drains minimize stress on sensitive tissues. Careful turning and positioning also reduce strain on a wound.

Cleaning Skin and Drain Sites. Although a moderate amount of wound exudate promotes epithelial cell growth, some health care providers order cleaning a wound or drain site if a dressing does not absorb drainage properly or if an open drain deposits drainage onto the skin. Wound cleaning requires good hand hygiene and aseptic techniques (see Chapter 28). You can use irrigation to remove debris from a wound.

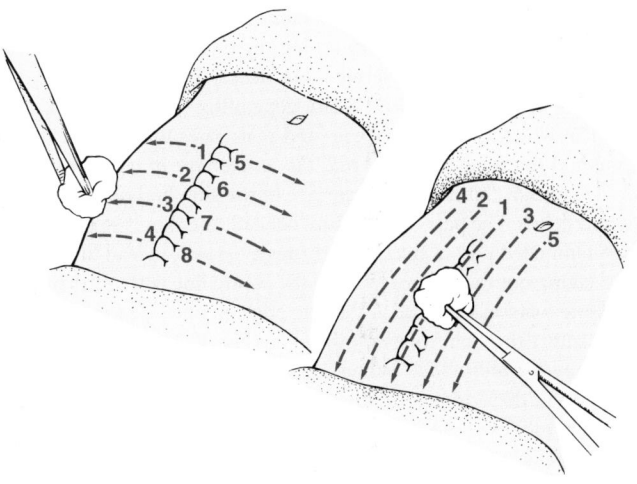

FIG. 48.21 Methods for cleaning wound site.

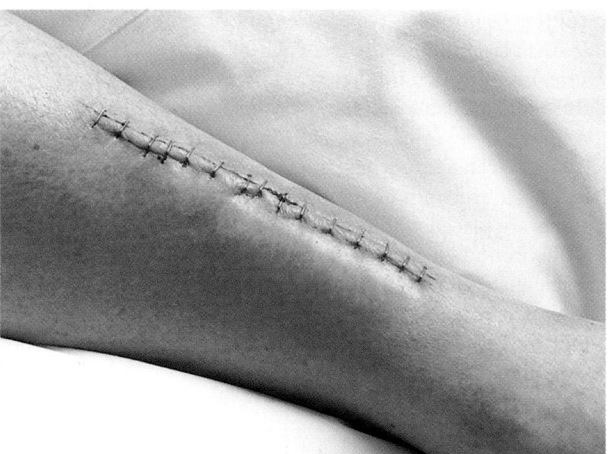

FIG. 48.23 Incision closed with metal staples.

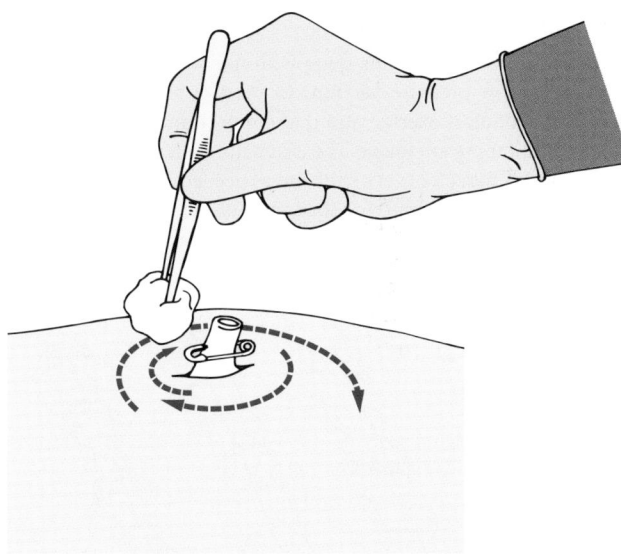

FIG. 48.22 Cleaning drain site.

REFLECT NOW

A patient has a draining wound and requires dressing changes every 4 hours. Think about what types of dressings are effective and how to secure the dressings without further injury to a patient's skin.

Basic Skin Cleaning. Clean surgical or traumatic wounds by applying noncytotoxic solutions with sterile gauze or by irrigation. The following three principles are important when cleaning an incision or the area surrounding a drain:

1. Clean in a direction from the least contaminated area, such as from a wound or incision to the surrounding skin (Fig. 48.21) or from an isolated drain site to the surrounding skin (Fig. 48.22).
2. Use gentle friction when applying solutions locally to the skin.
3. When irrigating, allow the solution to flow from the least to most contaminated area (see Skill 48.5).

After applying a solution to sterile gauze, clean away from the wound. Never use the same piece of gauze to clean across an incision or wound twice.

Drain sites are a source of contamination because moist drainage harbors microorganisms. If a wound has a dry incisional area and a moist drain site, cleaning moves from the incisional area toward the drain. Use two separate swabs or gauze pads, one to clean from the top of the incision toward the drain and one to clean from the bottom of the incision toward the drain. To clean the area of an isolated drain site, clean around the drain, moving in circular rotations outward from a point closest to the drain. In this situation the skin near the site is more contaminated than the site itself. To clean circular wounds, use the same technique as in cleaning around a drain.

Irrigation. Irrigation is a way of cleaning wounds. Use an irrigation syringe to flush the wound with a constant low-pressure flow of solution. The gentle washing action of the irrigation cleanses a wound of exudate and debris. Irrigation is particularly useful for open, deep wounds; wounds involving an inaccessible body part such as the ear canal; or when cleaning sensitive body parts such as the conjunctival lining of the eye.

Irrigation of an open wound requires sterile technique. Use a 35-mL syringe with a 19-gauge soft angiocatheter (Ramundo, 2016) to deliver the solution. This irrigation system has a safe pressure and does not damage healing wound tissue. It is important to never occlude a wound opening with a syringe because this results in the introduction of irrigating fluid into a closed space. The pressure of the fluid causes tissue damage and discomfort and possibly forces infection or debris into the wound bed. Always irrigate a wound with the syringe tip over but not in the drainage site. Make sure that fluid flows directly into the wound and not over a contaminated area before entering the wound (see Skill 48.5).

Skin Glue and Suture Care. A surgeon closes a wound by bringing the wound edges as close together as possible to reduce scar formation. Proper wound closure involves minimal trauma and tension to tissues with control of bleeding.

Skin glue is a clear gel or paste applied to the edges of clean small wounds to hold the edges of the wound together. It takes only a few minutes for the glue to set, and it usually peels off in 5 to 7 days (NHS, 2018). Patients will go home with the skin glue in place. Instruct them to avoid touching the glue for 24 hours, to try to keep the wound dry for the first 5 days, that showers are preferable to baths to avoid soaking the wound, to use a shower cap if the wound is on the head, and to pat (not rub) the wound dry if it gets wet (NHS, 2018). Skin glue is not used over joints, the hand, or the groin area. A systematic review of the use of glue compared with traditional sutures showed that medical glues appear to be a viable alternative to staples in select types of surgeries and often are associated with lower pain when compared to staples (CADTH, 2017).

Sutures are threads or metal used to sew body tissues together (Fig. 48.23). A patient's history of wound healing, the site of surgery, the tissues involved, and the purpose of the sutures determine the suture material used. For example, if a patient has had repeated surgery for an abdominal hernia, the health care provider can choose wire sutures to provide greater strength for wound closure. In contrast, a small laceration of the face calls for the use of very fine Dacron (polyester) sutures to minimize scar formation.

Sutures are available in a variety of materials, including silk, steel, cotton, linen, wire, nylon, and Dacron. Sutures such as PDS, Vicryl, and Monocryl can be absorbed; others, such as nylon, silk and steel, are nonabsorbable and must be removed.

Sutures are placed within tissue layers in deep wounds and superficially for wound closure. Deep sutures are usually composed of an absorbable material that disappears over time. Sutures are foreign bodies and thus are capable of causing local inflammation. A surgeon tries to minimize tissue injury by using the finest suture possible and the smallest number necessary.

Policies vary within institutions as to who is able to remove sutures. If it is appropriate that the nurse remove them, a health care provider's order is required. An order for suture removal is not written until the health care provider believes that the wound has closed (usually in 7 days). Special scissors with curved cutting tips, scissors and pickups from a sterile suture removal kit, or special staple removers slide under the skin closures for suture removal. The health care provider usually specifies the number of sutures or staples to remove. If the suture line appears to be healing in certain locations better than in others, some health care providers choose to have only some sutures removed (e.g., every other one).

To remove staples, insert the tips of the staple remover under each wire staple. While slowly closing the ends of the staple remover together, squeeze the center of the staple with the tips, freeing it from the skin, and gently lift up and out of the skin (Fig. 48.24).

To remove sutures, first check the type of suturing used (Fig. 48.25). With intermittent suturing the surgeon ties each individual suture made in the skin. Continuous suturing, as the name implies, is a series of sutures with only two knots, one at the beginning and one at the end of the suture line. Retention sutures are placed more deeply than skin sutures, and nurses may or may not remove them, depending on agency policy. The manner in which the suture crosses and penetrates the skin determines the method for removal. *Never pull the visible part of a suture through underlying tissue.* Sutures on the surface of the skin harbor microorganisms and debris. The part of the suture beneath the skin is sterile. Pulling the contaminated part of the suture through tissues can lead to infection. Before taking out the sutures, cleanse the suture line with normal saline. Clip suture materials as close to the skin edge on one side as possible and pull the suture through from the other side (Fig. 48.26).

Drainage Evacuation. When drainage interferes with healing, evacuation of the drainage is achieved by using either a drain alone or a drainage tube with continuous suction. You may apply special skin barriers, including hydrocolloid dressings similar to those used with ostomies (see Chapter 47), around drain sites with significant drainage for skin protection. The skin barriers are soft material applied to the skin with adhesive. Drainage flows on the barrier but not directly on the skin. **Drainage evacuators** (Fig. 48.27) are convenient portable units that connect to tubular drains lying within a wound bed and exert a safe, constant low-pressure vacuum to remove and collect drainage. Ensure that suction is exerted and that connection points between the evacuator and tubing are intact. The evacuator collects drainage. Assess for volume and character every shift and as needed. When the evacuator fills, measure output by emptying the contents into a graduated cylinder, immediately reset the evacuator to apply suction, and record the output.

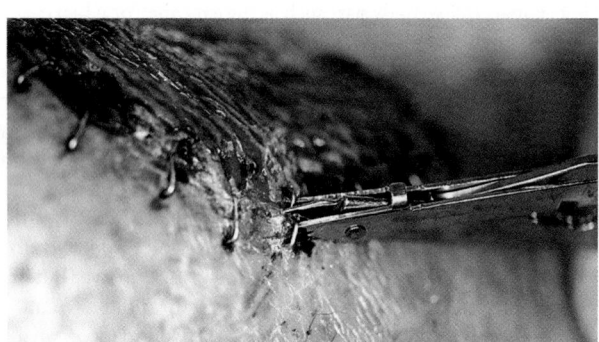

FIG. 48.24 Staple remover.

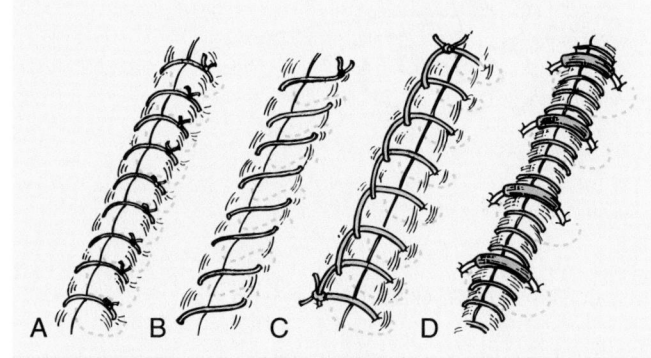

FIG. 48.25 Examples of suturing methods. **A,** Intermittent. **B,** Continuous. **C,** Blanket continuous. **D,** Retention.

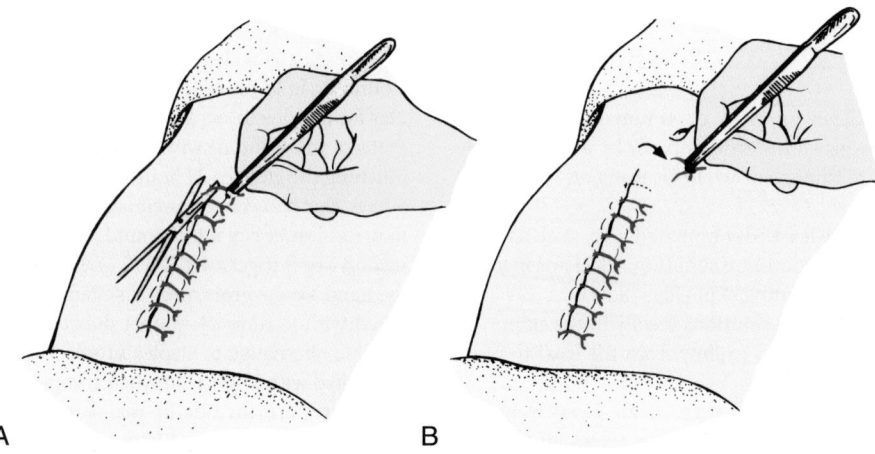

FIG. 48.26 Removal of intermittent suture. **A,** Cut suture as close to skin as possible, away from knot. **B,** Remove suture and never pull contaminated stitch through tissues.

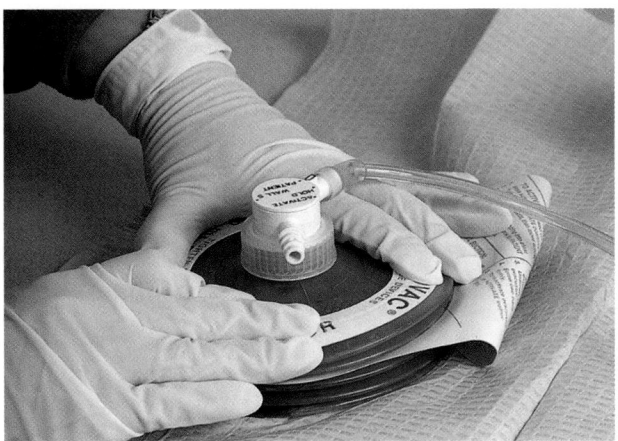

FIG. 48.27 Setting suction on drainage evacuator. *1*, With drainage port open, raise level on diaphragm. *2*, Push straight down on lever to lower diaphragm. *3*, Closure of port prevents escape of air and creates vacuum pressure.

Bandages, Binders, and Slings. A simple gauze dressing is often not enough to immobilize or provide support to a wound and a larger dressing or bandage is required. Binders are bandages that are made of large pieces of material, usually elastic or cotton, to fit a specific body part (Box 48.11). The most common type is an abdominal binder, which supports large abdominal incisions that are vulnerable to tension or stress as a patient moves or coughs (Fig. 48.28).

A systematic review of studies examining the efficacy of abdominal binders found that they reduce postoperative psychological distress, but their effect on postoperative pain after abdominal laparotomy and seroma formation after ventral hernia repair was unclear (Rothman et al., 2014). A more recent study involving patients who underwent major abdominal surgery found that an abdominal binder increased patient mobility soon after surgery, and there was a measurable reduction in pain in patients who used an abdominal binder after any exercise or activity (Arici et al., 2016). Giller and colleagues (2016) found that abdominal binders provide a noninvasive intervention for enhancing recovery of walk performance, controlling pain, and reducing stress on abdominal muscles following caesarean section. The quality

---

BOX 48.11 PROCEDURAL GUIDELINES

Applying a Binder

Delegation and Collaboration

The skill of applying a binder can be delegated to assistive personnel (AP). However, the nurse must first assess the condition of any incision, the skin, and patient's ability to breathe before binder application. The nurse directs the AP about:

- How to modify the skill, such as special wrapping or manner of securing the binder.
- Reporting patient's complaint of pain, numbness, tingling, or difficulty breathing after applying abdominal binder or any changes in patient's skin color or temperature.

Equipment

Clean gloves if wound drainage present; gauze bandage as needed; correct type and size of binder; closures for cloth binder

Steps

1. Identify patient using at least two identifiers (e.g., name and birthday or name and medical record number) according to agency policy.
2. Review medical record for order for binder (check agency policy).
3. Observe patient who needs support of thorax or abdomen; observe ability to breathe deeply, cough effectively, and turn or move independently.
4. Perform hand hygiene; apply clean gloves as needed. Inspect skin for actual or potential alterations in integrity. Observe for irritation, abrasion, and skin surfaces that rub against one another.
5. Inspect any surgical dressing for intactness, presence of drainage, and coverage of incision. Change any soiled dressing before applying binder (using clean gloves).
6. Determine patient's level of comfort using scale of 0 to 10. When necessary, administer prescribed analgesic 30 minutes before dressing change.
7. Gather necessary data regarding size of patient and appropriate binder to use (see manufacturer guidelines) to ensure proper fit.
8. Assess patient's or family caregiver's knowledge, experience, and health literacy.
9. Close curtains or room door.
10. Perform hand hygiene and apply clean gloves (if likely to contact wound drainage).
11. Apply abdominal binder:
    a. Position patient in supine position with head slightly elevated and knees slightly flexed.
    b. Fanfold far side of binder toward midline of binder so that patient can roll over with minimal effort.

c. Help patient roll on side away from you toward raised side rail while firmly supporting abdominal incision and dressing with hands.
d. Place fanfolded ends of binder under patient.
e. Instruct patient or help him or her roll over folded binder. For overweight patients consider asking nurse colleague to help.
f. Unfold and stretch ends out smoothly on far side of bed. Then stretch out ends on near side of bed.
g. Instruct patient to roll back into supine position.
h. Adjust binder so supine patient is centered over binder, using symphysis pubis and costal margins as lower and upper landmarks.
i. If patient is very thin, pad iliac prominences with gauze bandage.
j. Close binder. Pull one end of binder over center of patient's abdomen. While maintaining tension on that end of binder, pull opposite end of binder over center and secure with Velcro closure tabs or metal fasteners. Provides continuous wound support and comfort.

CLINICAL DECISION: After binder is in place, assess patient's ability to deep breathe and cough effectively. When applied correctly, an abdominal binder over midline abdominal incisions should not affect the patient's pulmonary function.

12. Assess patient's comfort level and adjust binder as necessary. Ask patient to rate pain on scale of 0 to 10.
13. Remove and dispose of gloves and perform hand hygiene.
14. Help patient to a comfortable position.
15. Be sure nurse call system is in an accessible location within patient's reach.
16. Raise side rail (as appropriate), and lower bed to lowest position.
17. Remove binder and surgical dressing to assess skin and wound characteristics at least every 8 hours.
18. Evaluate patient's ability to ventilate properly, including deep breathing and coughing, every 4 hours to determine presence of impaired ventilation and potential pulmonary complications.
19. Document baseline and postbinder condition of skin, circulation, integrity of underlying dressing, and patient's comfort level in nurses' notes in the electronic health record (EHR) or chart. Also record type of bandage applied.
20. Report any complications (e.g., pain, skin irritation, impaired ventilation). Report reduced ventilation (e.g., pulse oximetry, pulmonary function tests), change in incision, or change in drainage to health care provider immediately.

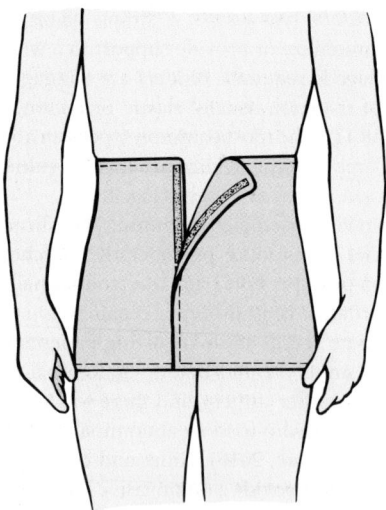

FIG. 48.28 Securing abdominal binder with Velcro.

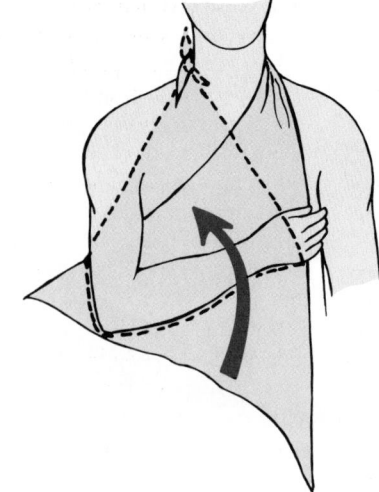

FIG. 48.29 Application of sling.

of scientific evidence regarding the benefits of binders is limited, but binders are still used by many clinicians.

Binders and bandages applied over or around dressings provide extra protection and therapeutic benefits by the following:

1. Creating pressure over a body part (e.g., an elastic pressure bandage applied over an arterial puncture site)
2. Immobilizing a body part (e.g., an elastic bandage applied around a sprained ankle)
3. Supporting a wound (e.g., an abdominal binder applied over a large abdominal incision and dressing)
4. Reducing or preventing edema (e.g., a stretch pressure bandage applied to the lower leg)
5. Securing a splint (e.g., a bandage applied around hand splints for correction of deformities)
6. Securing dressings (e.g., elastic webbing applied around leg dressings after a vein stripping)

Bandages are available in rolls of various widths and materials, including gauze, elasticized knit, elastic webbing, flannel, and muslin. Gauze bandages are lightweight and inexpensive, mold easily around contours of the body, and permit air circulation to prevent skin maceration. Elastic bandages conform well to body parts but are also for exerting pressure.

Binders are bandages that are made of large pieces of material to fit a specific body part. Most binders are made of elastic or cotton. An abdominal binder and a breast binder are examples.

Principles for Applying Bandages and Binders. Correctly applied bandages and binders do not cause injury to underlying and nearby body parts or create discomfort for a patient. For example, a chest binder should not be so tight as to restrict chest wall expansion. Before applying a bandage or binder, a nurse's responsibilities include the following:

- Inspecting the skin for abrasions, edema, discoloration, or exposed wound edges
- Covering exposed wounds or open abrasions with a dressing
- Assessing the condition of underlying dressings and changing if soiled
- Assessing the skin of underlying areas that will be distal to the bandage for signs of circulatory impairment (coolness, pallor or cyanosis, diminished or absent pulses, swelling, numbness, and tingling) to provide a means for comparing changes in circulation after bandage application

After applying a bandage or binder , the nurse assesses, documents, and immediately reports changes in circulation, skin integrity, comfort level, and body function (e.g., ventilation or movement). The nurse who applies a bandage or binder loosens or readjusts it as necessary. A health care provider's order is necessary before loosening or removing

a bandage applied by the health care provider. The nurse explains to the patient that any bandage or binder feels relatively firm or tight. Carefully assess a bandage to be sure that it is applied properly and providing therapeutic benefit and replace any soiled bandages.

Slings. Slings support arms with muscular sprains or fractures. A commercially manufactured sling consists of a long sleeve that extends above the elbow with a strap that fits around the neck. In the home patients can use a large triangular piece of cloth. The patient sits or lies supine during sling application (Fig. 48.29). Instruct him or her to bend the affected arm, bringing the forearm straight across the chest. The open sling fits under the patient's arm and over the chest, with the base of the triangle under the wrist and the point of the triangle at his or her elbow. One end of the sling fits around the back of the patient's neck. Bring the other end up and over the affected arm while supporting the extremity. Tie the two ends at the side of the neck so that the knot does not press against the cervical spine. Fold the loose material at the elbow evenly around the elbow and then pin to secure. Always support the lower arm and hand at a level above the elbow to prevent the formation of dependent edema.

Roll Bandage Application. Rolls of bandage secure or support dressings over irregularly shaped body parts. Each roll has a free outer end and a terminal end at the center of the roll. The rolled part of the bandage is its body, and its outer surface is placed against the patient's skin or dressing. Use a variety of bandage turns, depending on the body part to be bandaged (see Skill 48.6).

Heat and Cold Therapy. Moist heat applications are therapeutically beneficial in increasing muscle and ligament flexibility; promoting relaxation and healing; and relieving spasm, joint stiffness, and pain. Moist heat has many indications; however, it is most commonly used following the acute phase of a musculoskeletal injury and during and after childbirth, surgery, and superficial thrombophlebitis (Petrofsky et al., 2017; Szekeres et al., 2017). Moist heat applications include warm compresses and commercial moist heat packs, warm baths, soaks, and sitz baths. Dry heat is also used to reduce pain and increase healing by increasing blood flow in tissues and can be used at a low level for a longer period with little chance of tissue injury (Petrofsky et al., 2016).

Cold therapy refers to the superficial application of cold to the surface of the skin, with or without compression and with or without a mechanical recirculating device to maintain cold temperatures (Chou et al, 2016). Cold therapy is designed to treat the localized inflammatory response of an injured body part that presents as edema, hemorrhage, muscle spasm, or pain. Improvement to joint mobility following cold therapy is related to reducing pain and swelling, inhibiting muscle spasm, and reducing muscle tension (Chatterjee, 2017; Quinlan et al., 2017). Cold therapy most commonly is used immediately after soft tissue and musculoskeletal injuries such as sprains or strains; however, it has been used in the postoperative setting with patients who have undergone orthopedic surgeries, spinal fusion, and lumbar discectomy (Quinlan et al., 2017). Research trials of cold therapy have been inconsistent and frequently found no differences compared with no cold therapy in postoperative pain or analgesic use (Chou et al., 2016).

Assessment for Temperature Tolerance. Before applying heat or cold therapies, assess a patient's physical condition for signs of potential intolerance to heat and cold. First observe the area to be treated. Assess the skin, looking for any open areas such as alterations in skin integrity (e.g., abrasions, open wounds, edema, bruising, bleeding, or localized areas of inflammation) that increase a patient's risk for injury. Because a health care provider commonly orders heat and cold applications for traumatized areas, the baseline skin assessment provides a guide for evaluating skin changes that can occur during therapy. Assess neurological function, testing for sensation to light touch, pinprick, and mild temperature variations (see Chapter 30). Sensory status reveals the ability of a patient to recognize when heat or cold becomes excessive. Assess a patient's mental status to be sure that he or she can correctly communicate any issues with the hot or cold therapy. Level of consciousness influences the ability to perceive heat, cold, and pain. If a patient is confused or unresponsive, the nurse needs to make frequent observations of skin integrity after therapy begins.

Assess for conditions that contraindicate heat or cold therapy. Do not cover an active area of bleeding with a warm application because bleeding will continue. Warm applications are contraindicated when a patient has an acute, localized inflammation such as appendicitis because the heat could cause the appendix to rupture. If a patient has cardiovascular problems, it is unwise to apply heat to large parts of the body because the resulting massive vasodilation disrupts blood supply to vital organs.

Cold is contraindicated if the site of injury is already edematous. It further retards circulation to the area and prevents absorption of the interstitial fluid. If a patient has impaired circulation (e.g., arteriosclerosis), it further reduces blood supply to the affected area. Cold therapy is also contraindicated in the presence of neuropathy, because the patient is unable to perceive temperature change and damage resulting from temperature extremes. One other contraindication for cold therapy is shivering. Cold applications sometimes intensify shivering and dangerously increase body temperature.

If a patient has peripheral vascular disease, pay particular attention to the integrity of extremities. For example, if the health care provider's order is to apply a cold compress to a lower extremity, assess circulation to the leg by assessing for capillary refill; observing skin color; and palpating skin temperatures, distal pulses, and edematous areas. If

signs of circulatory inadequacy are present, it is important for you to question the order.

When applying heat or cold pads, check electrical equipment for cracked cords, frayed wires, damaged insulation, and exposed heating components. Make sure that equipment containing circulating fluids does not have leaks. Check equipment for evenness of temperature distribution.

Bodily Responses to Heat and Cold. Exposure to heat and cold causes systemic and local responses. Systemic responses occur through heat-loss mechanisms (sweating and vasodilation) or mechanisms promoting heat conservation (vasoconstriction and piloerection) and heat production (shivering) (see Chapter 30). Local responses to heat and cold occur through stimulation of temperature-sensitive nerve endings within the skin. This stimulation sends impulses from the periphery to the hypothalamus, which becomes aware of local temperature sensations and triggers adaptive responses for maintenance of normal body temperature. If alterations occur along temperature sensation pathways, the reception and eventual perception of stimuli are altered.

The body is able to tolerate wide variations in temperature. The normal temperature of the surface of the skin is 34°C (93.2°F), but temperature receptors usually adapt quickly to local temperatures between 15° and 45°C (59° and 113°F). Pain develops when local temperatures exceed this range. Excessive heat causes a burning sensation. Cold produces a numbing sensation before pain.

The adaptive ability of the body creates the major problem in protecting patients from injury resulting from temperature extremes. A person initially feels an extreme change in temperature but within a short time hardly notices it. This is dangerous because a person insensitive to heat and cold extremes can suffer serious tissue injury. You need to recognize patients most at risk for injuries from heat and cold applications (Table 48.10).

Local Effects of Heat and Cold Applications. Heat and cold stimuli create different physiological responses. The choice of heat or cold therapy depends on local responses desired for wound healing (Table 48.11).

Effects of Heat Application. Generally heat is quite therapeutic, improving blood flow to an injured part. However, if it is applied for 1 hour or more, the body reduces blood flow by a reflex vasoconstriction to control heat loss from the area. Periodic removal and reapplication of local heat restores vasodilation. Continuous exposure to heat damages epithelial cells, causing redness, localized tenderness, and even blistering.

Effects of Cold Application. The application of cold initially diminishes swelling and pain. Prolonged exposure of the skin to cold results in a reflex vasodilation. The inability of the cells to receive adequate blood flow and nutrients results in tissue ischemia. The skin initially takes on a reddened appearance, followed by a bluish-purple

TABLE 48.10	Conditions That Increase Risk of Injury From Heat and Cold Application	
Condition	**Risk Factors**
Very young or older patients	Thinner skin layers in children increase risk of burns. Older patients have reduced sensitivity to pain and may not perceive any pain associated with heat or cold applications.
Open wounds, broken skin, stomas	Subcutaneous and visceral tissues are more sensitive to temperature variations. They also contain no temperature and fewer pain receptors.
Areas of edema or scar formation	Reduced sensation to temperature stimuli occurs because of thickening of skin layers from fluid buildup or scar formation.
Peripheral vascular disease (e.g., diabetes, arteriosclerosis)	As a result of decreased peripheral circulation, extremities are less sensitive to temperature and pain stimuli because of circulatory impairment and local tissue injury. Cold application further compromises blood flow.
Confusion or unconsciousness	Reduced perception of sensory or painful stimuli. Patient may be unable to move away from or to indicate discomfort from the heat or cold application.
Spinal cord injury	Alterations in nerve pathways prevent reception of sensory or painful stimuli.
Abscessed tooth or appendix	Infection is highly localized. Application of heat causes rupture, with spread of microorganisms systemically.

TABLE 48.11 Therapeutic Effects of Heat and Cold Applications

Physiological Response	Therapeutic Benefit	Examples of Conditions Treated
Heat Therapy		
Vasodilation	Improve blood flow to injured body part	Arthritis or degenerative joint disease
Reduced blood viscosity	Promote delivery of nutrients and removal of wastes	Localized joint pain or muscle strains
Reduced muscle tension	Improve delivery of leukocytes and antibiotics to wound site	Low back pain
Increased tissue metabolism	Promote muscle relaxation	Menstrual cramping
Increased capillary permeability	Reduce pain from spasm or stiffness	Hemorrhoid, perianal, and vaginal inflammation
	Increase blood flow	Local skin abscesses
	Provide local warmth	
	Promote movement of waste products and nutrients	
Cold Therapy		
Vasoconstriction	Reduce blood flow to injured site, preventing edema formation	Immediately after direct trauma (e.g., sprains, strains, fractures, muscle spasms)
Local anesthesia	Reduce inflammation	Superficial laceration or puncture wound
Reduced cell metabolism	Reduce localized pain	Minor burn
Increased blood viscosity	Reduce oxygen needs of tissues	After injections
Decreased muscle tension	Promote blood coagulation at injury site	Chronic pain from arthritis, joint trauma, or delayed-onset muscle soreness; inflammation
	Relieve pain	

mottling, with numbness and a burning type of pain. Skin tissues freeze from exposure to extreme cold.

Factors Influencing Heat and Cold Tolerance. The response of the body to heat and cold therapies depends on the following factors:

- A person is better able to tolerate short exposure to temperature extremes than prolonged exposure.
- Exposed skin layers and certain areas of the skin (e.g., the neck, inner aspect of the wrist and forearm, and perineal region) are more sensitive to temperature variations. The foot and palm of the hand are less sensitive.
- The body responds best to minor temperature adjustments. If a body part is cool and a hot stimulus touches the skin, the response is greater than if the skin were already warm.
- A person has less tolerance to temperature changes to which a large area of the body is exposed.
- Tolerance to temperature variations changes with age. Patients who are very young or old are most sensitive to heat and cold.
- If a patient's physical condition reduces the reception or perception of sensory stimuli, tolerance to temperature extremes is high, but the risk of injury is also high.
- Uneven temperature distribution suggests that the equipment is functioning improperly.

Application of Heat and Cold Therapies. A prerequisite to using any heat or cold application is a health care provider's order, which includes the body site to be treated and the type, frequency, and duration of application. Safety guidelines for the use of heat and cold are summarized in Box 48.12. Consult agency procedure manual for correct temperatures to use.

You can administer heat and cold applications in dry or moist forms. The type of wound or injury, the location of the body part, and the presence of drainage or inflammation are factors to consider in selecting dry or moist applications. Box 48.13 summarizes advantages and disadvantages of both.

Warm, Moist Compresses. Warm, moist compresses improve circulation, relieve edema, and promote consolidation of purulent drainage. A compress is a piece of gauze dressing moistened in a prescribed warmed solution.

Heat from warm compresses dissipates quickly. To maintain a constant temperature, you need to change the compress often. You can use a layer of plastic wrap or a dry towel to insulate the compress and retain

BOX 48.12 Safety Suggestions for Applying Heat or Cold Therapy

- *Explain* to patient sensations to be felt during the procedure.
- *Prevention:* Injuries from heat and cold therapies are preventable (NQF, 2011).
- *Instruct* patient that exposed layers of skin are more sensitive to heat and cold application than intact skin. Therefore instruct patient and family to protect skin when applying heat or cold therapy.
- *Instruct* patient to report changes in sensation or discomfort immediately.
- *Provide* a timer, clock, or watch so that patient can help the nurse time the application.
- *Check* patient and skin frequently every 20 minutes during therapy. Observe for excess redness, pain, tingling.
- *Keep* the nurse call system within patient's reach.
- *Refer* to the policy and procedure manual of the institution for safe temperatures.
- *Do not* allow patient to adjust temperature settings.
- *Do not* allow patient to move an application or place hands on the wound site.
- *Do not* place patient in a position that prevents movement away from the temperature source.
- *Do not* leave unattended a patient who is unable to sense temperature changes or move from the temperature source.

heat. Moist heat promotes vasodilation and evaporation of heat from the surface of the skin. For this reason a patient can feel chilly. Always try to control drafts within the room, and keep the patient covered with a blanket or robe.

Warm Soaks. Immersion of a body part in a warmed solution promotes circulation, lessens edema, increases muscle relaxation, and provides a means to apply medicated solution. Sometimes a soak is also accompanied by wrapping the body part in dressings and saturating them with the warmed solution.

Position the patient comfortably, place waterproof pads under the area to be treated, and heat the solution to about 40.5° to 43°C (105° to 110°F). Pour solution into a clean or sterile basin or container, then immerse the body part. Cover the container and extremity with a towel to reduce heat loss. It is usually necessary to remove the cooled solution and add heated solution after about 10 minutes. The challenge is to keep the solution at a constant temperature. Never add a hotter

BOX 48.13 Choice of Dry or Moist Applications

Advantages

Moist Applications

- Moist application reduces drying of skin and softens wound exudate.
- Moist compresses conform well to most body areas.
- Moist heat penetrates deeply into tissue layers.
- Warm, moist heat does not promote sweating and insensible fluid loss.

Dry Applications

- Dry heat has less risk of burns to skin than moist applications.
- Dry application does not cause skin maceration.
- Dry heat retains temperature longer because evaporation does not occur.

Disadvantages

Moist Applications

- Prolonged exposure causes maceration of skin.
- Moist heat cools rapidly because of moisture evaporation.
- Moist heat creates greater risk for burns to skin because moisture conducts heat.

Dry Applications

- Dry heat increases body fluid loss through sweating.
- Dry applications do not penetrate deep into tissues.
- Dry heat causes increased drying of skin.

solution while the body part remains immersed. After any soak dry the body part thoroughly to prevent maceration.

Sitz Baths. A patient who has had rectal surgery, an episiotomy during childbirth, painful hemorrhoids, or vaginal inflammation benefits from a sitz bath, a bath in which only the pelvic area is immersed in warm or, in some situations, cool fluid. The patient sits in a special tub or chair or a basin that fits on the toilet seat so the legs and feet remain out of the water. Immersing the entire body causes widespread vasodilation and nullifies the effect of local heat application to the pelvic area.

The desired temperature for a sitz bath depends on whether the purpose is to promote relaxation or to clean a wound. It is often necessary to add warm or cool water during the procedure, which normally lasts 20 minutes, to maintain a constant temperature. Agency procedure manuals recommend safe water temperatures. A disposable sitz basin contains an attachment resembling an enema bag that allows gradual introduction of additional water.

Prevent overexposure of patients by draping bath blankets around their shoulders and thighs and controlling drafts. A patient should be able to sit in the basin or tub with feet flat on the floor and without pressure on the sacrum or thighs. Because exposure of a large part of the body to heat causes extensive vasodilation, assess the pulse and facial color and ask whether the patient feels light-headed or nauseated.

Commercial Hot and Cold Packs. Commercially prepared disposable hot packs apply warm, dry heat to an injured area. The chemicals mix and release heat when you strike, knead, or squeeze the pack. Package directions recommend the time for heat application.

Commercially prepared cold packs that are similar to the disposable hot packs for dry applications are available. They come in various shapes and sizes to fit different body parts. When using cold compresses, observe for adverse reactions such as burning or numbness, mottling of the skin, redness, extreme paleness, and a bluish skin discoloration.

Cold, Moist, and Dry Compresses. The procedure for applying cold, moist compresses is the same as that for warm compresses. Apply cold compresses for 20 minutes at a temperature of 15°C (59°F) to relieve inflammation and swelling. You can use clean or sterile compresses.

Cold Soaks. The procedure for preparing cold soaks and immersing a body part is the same as for warm soaks. The desired temperature for a 20-minute cold soak is 15°C (59°F). Control drafts and use outer coverings to protect the patient from chilling. It is often necessary to add cold water during the procedure to maintain a constant temperature.

Ice Bags or Collars. For a patient who has a muscle sprain, localized hemorrhage, or hematoma or who has undergone dental surgery, an ice bag is ideal to prevent edema formation, control bleeding, and anesthetize the body part. Proper use of the bag requires the following steps:

1. Fill the bag with water, secure the cap, invert to check for leaks, and pour out the water.
2. Fill the bag two-thirds full with crushed ice, so you are able to easily mold it over a body part.
3. Release any air from the bag by squeezing its sides before securing the cap because excess air interferes with conduction of cold.
4. Wipe off excess moisture.
5. Cover the bag with a flannel cover, towel, or pillowcase.
6. Apply the bag to the injury site for 30 minutes; you can reapply the bag in an hour.

◆ Evaluation

You evaluate the effectiveness of nursing interventions for reducing and treating pressure injuries and other wounds by determining the patient's response to nursing therapies, determining outcomes, and evaluating whether he or she achieved each goal. The optimal outcomes are to prevent injury to the skin, to reduce injury to the skin and underlying tissues, and possible wound healing with restoration of skin integrity.

Through the Patient's Eyes. It is important to include the patient and family caregiver in the evaluation process. Review whether their expectations of care were met. For example, is the patient satisfied with the level of comfort achieved during wound care? Chronic wounds such as pressure injuries take time to heal, so home care is likely. Do the patient and family caregiver feel comfortable or confident in being able to perform wound care at home? Does the family caregiver feel he or she has the information needed to know when to report a problem with a wound? If patient and family caregiver expectations are unmet, revise your plan of care to select the best ways to support and re-educate.

Patient Outcomes. The outcomes selected for a patient in the plan of care are the milestones you hope to achieve to meet the goals of care. Each patient will have unique outcomes depending on whether he or she has an actual wound or is at risk to develop a wound. Evaluate nursing interventions for reducing and treating pressure injuries by determining the patient's response and comparing with expected outcomes to determine whether he or she achieved each goal (Fig. 48.30).

You will evaluate patients with impaired skin integrity on an ongoing basis for factors that contribute to skin breakdown and wound status. For example, during direct patient contact, if a patient continues to be diaphoretic or incontinent, apply wound assessment skills to determine the condition of the skin and decide whether additional therapies are needed to treat a patient's skin moisture. Use a validated wound assessment tool when appropriate. Evaluation provides information regarding the patient's progress toward wound healing or maintenance of skin integrity.

If the identified outcomes are not met for a patient with impaired skin integrity, questions to ask include the following:

- Was the etiology of the skin impairment addressed? Were the pressure, friction, shear, and moisture components identified, and did the plan of care decrease the contribution of each of these components?
- Was wound healing supported by providing the wound with a moist protected environment?
- Was nutrition assessed and a plan of care developed that provided the patient with the calories to support healing?

Finally evaluate the need for additional referrals to other experts in wound care and pressure injuries, such as nurses certified in wound care. Care of patients with a pressure injury or wound requires an interprofessional team approach.

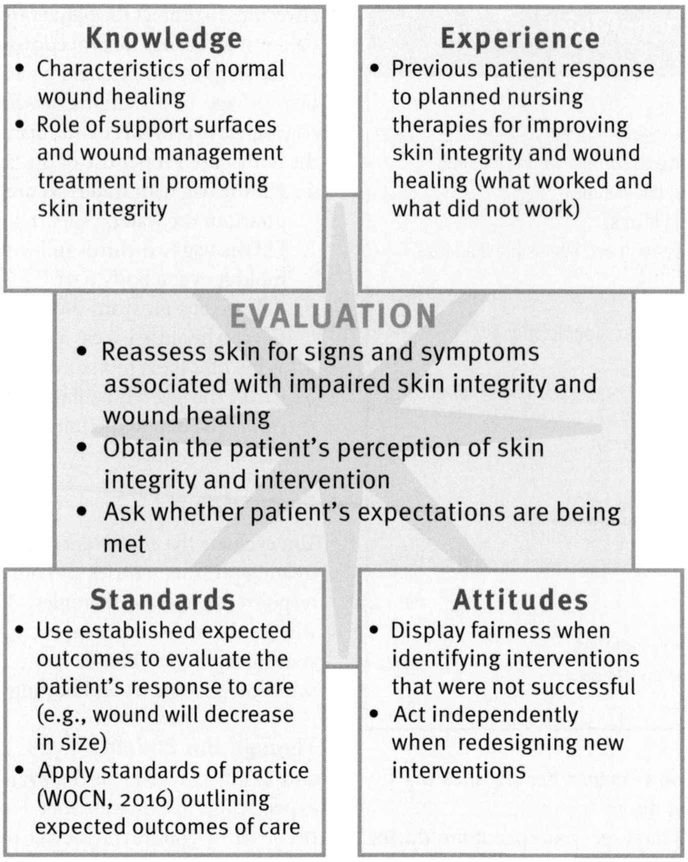

Knowledge
- Characteristics of normal wound healing
- Role of support surfaces and wound management treatment in promoting skin integrity

Experience
- Previous patient response to planned nursing therapies for improving skin integrity and wound healing (what worked and what did not work)

EVALUATION
- Reassess skin for signs and symptoms associated with impaired skin integrity and wound healing
- Obtain the patient's perception of skin integrity and intervention
- Ask whether patient's expectations are being met

Standards
- Use established expected outcomes to evaluate the patient's response to care (e.g., wound will decrease in size)
- Apply standards of practice (WOCN, 2016) outlining expected outcomes of care

Attitudes
- Display fairness when identifying interventions that were not successful
- Act independently when redesigning new interventions

FIG. 48.30 Critical thinking model for skin integrity and wound-care evaluation.

SAFETY GUIDELINES FOR NURSING SKILLS

Ensuring patient safety is an essential role of the professional nurse. To ensure patient safety, communicate clearly with members of the health care team, assess and incorporate the patient's priorities of care and preferences, and use the best evidence when making decisions about your patient's care. When performing the skills in this chapter, remember the following points to ensure safe, individualized patient care.

- When changing wound dressings, follow proper aseptic technique. Keep a plastic bag within reach to discard dressing and prevent cross-contamination. Keep extra gloves within reach in case of contamination or additional wound assessment.
- Perform pressure injury risk assessment on all patients who have one or more risk factors when admitted to an acute care setting, home care, hospice, or extended-care facility (EPUAP, NPIAP, PPPIA, 2019b, WOCN, 2016). Use a risk assessment tool; the Braden Scale is one of the most widely used and researched scales (Bryant and Nix, 2016a).

- Inspect skin at least daily or according to agency policy, and note and document all pressure points. Modify frequency of skin and wound assessment and frequency of skin care practices based on patient's risk factors and/or wound condition.
- Use approaches to minimize friction and shear. Use lift sheets when repositioning patients to reduce rubbing skin against sheets. Raise the head of the bed no more than 30 degrees (unless medically contraindicated) to prevent sliding and shear injury (WOCN, 2016).
- When a patient has a previous history of pressure injury or skin damage, the healed area presents a greater risk for skin breakdown than healthy, unwounded skin.
- Chronic diseases, especially vascular disease and diabetes, increase a patient's risk for pressure injury development and impede wound healing.

SKILL 48.1   ASSESSMENT AND PREVENTION STRATEGIES FOR PRESSURE INJURY DEVELOPMENT

Delegation and Collaboration

The skill of pressure injury risk assessment cannot be delegated to assistive personnel (AP). Instruct the AP to:
- Frequently change patient's position and specific positions individualized for the patient.
- Keep patient's skin dry, and provide hygiene following fecal or urinary incontinence or exposure of skin to wound drainage.
- Report any changes in patient's skin, such as redness or break in the patient's skin.
- Report any redness and/or abrasion from medical devices.

Equipment
- Risk assessment tool (see agency policy)
- Pressure redistribution mattresses, bed, or chair cushion as needed
- Positioning aids
- Clean gloves

STEP	RATIONALE

ASSESSMENT

1. Identify patient using at least two identifiers (e.g., name and birthday or name and account number) according to agency policy.

Ensures correct patient. Complies with The Joint Commission standards and improves patient safety (TJC, 2020).

2. Review medical record to assess patient's risk for pressure injury formation:

Determines need to administer preventive care and identifies specific factors that place patient at risk (Haesler, 2017; EPUAP, NPIAP, PPPIA, 2019b).

  a. Paralysis or immobilization caused by restrictive devices.

Patient is unable to turn or reposition independently to relieve pressure.

  b. Presence of medical device such as nasogastric (NG) tube, oxygen equipment, artificial airways, drainage tubing, or mechanical devices (Doughty and McNichol, 2016).

Medical devices have potential to exert pressure on patient's nares or ears or on tissue adjacent to devices such as artificial airways and drainage tubes (Pittman et al., 2015).

    (1) If not medically contraindicated, remove medical device to observe and palpate skin and tissues under and around each medical device.

Pressure area assumes same configuration as medical device (WOCN, 2016; Schallom et al., 2015).

  c. Sensory loss (e.g., hemiplegia, spinal cord injury).

Patient is unable to feel discomfort from pressure and does not independently change position.

  d. Circulatory disorders (e.g., peripheral vascular diseases, vascular changes from diabetes mellitus, neuropathy).

Reduce perfusion of tissue layers of skin.

  e. Fever.

Increases metabolic demands of tissues. Accompanying diaphoresis leaves skin moist.

  f. Anemia.

Decreased hemoglobin level reduces oxygen-carrying capacity of blood and amount of oxygen available to tissues.

  g. Malnutrition: weight loss, loss of muscle mass and or subcutaneous fat.

Inadequate nutrition leads to weight loss, muscle atrophy, and reduced tissue mass. Nutrient deficiencies result in impaired or delayed healing (Stotts, 2016a).

  h. Fecal or urinary incontinence.

Skin becomes exposed to moist environment that contains bacteria. Excessive moisture macerates skin (McNichol et al., 2018; Ayello, 2017).

  i. Heavy sedation and anesthesia.

Sedation alters sensory perception and patient does not perceive pressure and change position.

  j. Age.

Neonates and very young children are at high risk, with the head being most common site of pressure injury occurrence (WOCN, 2016).

There is loss of dermal thickness in older adults, impairing ability to distribute pressure (Pieper, 2016).

  k. Dehydration.

Results in decreased skin elasticity and turgor.

  l. Edema.

Edematous tissues are less tolerant of pressure, friction, and shear.

  m. Existing pressure injuries.

Limit surfaces available for position changes, placing available tissues at increased risk.

  n. History of pressure injury.

Tensile strength of skin from previously healed pressure injury is 80% or less; therefore, this area cannot tolerate pressure as much as undamaged skin (Doughty and Sparks, 2016).

3. Select agency-approved risk assessment tool such as the Braden Scale or Norton Scale. Perform risk assessment when patient enters health care setting and repeat on regularly scheduled basis or when there is significant change in patient's condition (see agency policy) (WOCN, 2016).

Valid and reliable risk-assessment tools evaluate patient's risk for developing a pressure injury. Identifying risk factors that contribute to the potential for skin breakdown allows you to target specific interventions for decreasing risk.

CLINICAL DECISION: *In acute care settings, perform initial assessment within 8 hours of admission and reassess every 24 hours or as patient condition changes; in critical care areas perform assessment on admission and reassess every 24 hours or as patient condition changes; and in long-term and home care settings perform assessment on admission. In long-term care settings reassess weekly and then according to agency standards or when patient condition changes. In home care setting reassess every registered nurse visit.*

4. Obtain risk score (see Table 48.3) and evaluate its meaning based on patient's unique characteristics. When using the Braden scale there are risk scores identified for specific patient populations: Intensive care patients ≤14; older adults ≤14 (Alderden et al., 2017).

Risk cutoff score depends on instrument used. Score involves identifying risk factors that contributed to it and minimizing these specific deficits (Alderden et al., 2017; Ayello, 2017).

5. Close room or pull curtains around bed.

Maintains patient privacy.

6. Perform hand hygiene. Assess condition of patient's skin, focusing on pressure points (see Fig. 48.9). Apply gloves as needed with open and/or draining wounds.

Body weight against bony prominences places underlying skin at risk for the development of skin injuries.

Continued

SKILL 48.1	ASSESSMENT AND PREVENTION STRATEGIES FOR PRESSURE INJURY DEVELOPMENT—cont'd

STEP	RATIONALE
a. Inspect for skin discoloration (see Box 48.2) for patients with darkly pigmented skin) and tissue consistency (firm or boggy feel) and/or palpate for abnormal sensations (Nix, 2016).	Indicates that tissue was under pressure; hyperemia is a normal physiological response to hypoxemia in tissues.
b. Palpate discolored area on skin and under and around medical devices, release your fingertip, and look for blanching. If on palpation an area of redness blanches (lightens in color), this indicates normal reactive hyperemia; tissue is not at risk for the development of an injury. If area does not blanch, suspect tissue injury and recheck in 1 hour.	Tissue that does not blanch when palpated indicates abnormal reactive hyperemia, an indication of possible ischemic injury.
c. Inspect for pallor and mottling.	Persistent hypoxia in tissues that were under pressure, an abnormal physiological response.
d. Inspect for absence of superficial skin layers.	Represents early pressure injury formation; usually a partial-thickness wound that may have resulted from friction and/or shear.
e. Inspect for changes in skin temperature, edema, and tissue consistency, especially in individuals with darkly pigmented skin (EPAUP, NPIAP, PPPIA, 2019a).	Localized heat, edema, and induration have been identified as warning signs for pressure injury development. Because it is not always possible to observe changes in skin color on darkly pigmented skin, these additional signs should be considered in assessment (EPAUP, NPIAP, PPPIA, 2019a).
f. Inspect for wound drainage.	Wound drainage increases risk for skin breakdown because it is caustic to skin and underlying tissues.
7. Assess skin and tissue around and beneath medical devices every nursing shift for additional areas of potential pressure injury resulting from medical devices (Black and Kalowes, 2016; Black et al., 2015) (Table 48.5). NOTE: Pressure area assumes same configuration as medical device (WOCN, 2016; Schallom et al., 2015).	Patients at high risk have multiple sites for pressure necrosis from medical devices in areas other than bony prominences (Chaboyer et al., 2017; Makic, 2015). Pressure points around medical devices can cause pressure injury to underlying tissue and become full-thickness pressure injuries (Kayser et al., 2018; Black et al., 2015; Schallom et al., 2015).
a. Nares: NG tube, feeding tube, oxygen cannula.	Pressure to nares occurs from tape and other materials used to secure NG tube.
b. Ears: oxygen cannula, pillow.	Oxygen equipment is a significant risk for pressure injuries (Padula et al., 2017). Patients' ears and tips of nares are at risk for pressure injuries from nasal cannula (Black et al., 2015; Schallom et al., 2015).
c. Tongue and lips: oral airway, endotracheal (ET) tube.	Pressure can result from artificial airway and materials used to secure airway (Padula et al., 2017; Black et al., 2015).
d. Forehead: pulse oximetry device.	Adhesive can cause skin blistering.
e. Drainage or other tubing.	Stress and pressure against tissue at exit site or from tubing lying under any part of patient's body can cause skin injury (Black et al., 2015).
f. Indwelling urethral (Foley) catheter.	For female patients catheter can place pressure on labia, especially when edematous. For male patients pressure from catheter not properly anchored can put pressure on tip of penis and urethra (Black et al., 2015).
g. Orthopedic and positioning devices such as casts, neck collars, splints.	Applied devices have potential to cause pressure to underlying and adjacent skin and tissue (Black et al., 2015).
h. Compression stockings.	Compression stockings have potential to cause pressure, especially if they fit poorly or are rolled down (Black et al., 2015).
i. Immobilization device and restraints.	Pressure points can occur if the device is too tight or poorly placed or if the patient strains against the device.
8. Observe patient for preferred positions when in bed or chair.	Preferred positions result in weight of body being placed on certain bony prominences. Presence of contractures may result in pressure exerted in unexpected places.
9. Observe ability of patient to initiate and help with position changes.	Potential for pressure, friction, and shear increases when patient is completely dependent on others for position changes.
10. Assess patient's/family caregiver's knowledge, experience, and health literacy level.	Ensures patient has the capacity to obtain, communicate, process, and understand basic health information (CDC, 2019).
11. Assess patient's and family caregiver's understanding of what a pressure injury is and the individual risks for patient to develop pressure injuries.	Determines baseline knowledge for pressure injury risk and identifies areas for patient teaching.

PLANNING

1. Explain procedure to patient before starting.	Reduces anxiety and provides opportunity for patient/family caregiver education.
2. Lower side rails. Position patient comfortably in bed in anatomical position.	Facilitates ability to perform prevention strategies.

STEP	RATIONALE

IMPLEMENTATION

1. Perform hand hygiene. If patient has open, draining wounds, apply clean gloves.
2. Implement prevention guidelines adapted from WOCN Society *Guideline for Prevention and Management of Pressure Ulcers* (2016).
3. Following initial assessment, continue to inspect skin at least once a day as per agency policy.

Use of Standard Precautions prevents accidental exposure to body fluids. Reduces patient's risk for developing pressure injury.

CLINICAL DECISION: *Do not massage reddened areas because doing so may cause additional tissue trauma. Reddened areas indicate blood vessel damage, and massaging can further damage the vessel (Bryant and Nix, 2016a).*

---

   a. If patient has darkly pigmented skin, look for color changes that differ from his or her normal skin color.

Darkly pigmented skin may not blanch. A change in color may occur at the site of pressure; this change in color differs from patient's usual skin color (EPUAP, NPIAP, PPPIA, 2019a,b) (see Box 48.2).

4. Each shift, check all medical treatment and assistive devices for potential pressure points.

   a. Verify that device is correctly sized, positioned, and secured.

Pressure from these devices increases risk on bony prominences and other areas. Incorrect size, placement, and securing of medical device can cause excessive pressure and rubbing by device on underlying skin (Makic, 2015).

   b. Consider protecting underlying at-risk skin with a protective dressing (silicone, hydrocolloid).

Dressings absorb moisture from body and reduce pressure to underlying skin (Black et al., 2015; Makic, 2015).

CLINICAL DECISION: *Inspect skin around and beneath orthopedic devices (e.g., cervical collar, braces, or cast). Note any abrasions or warmth in areas where devices can rub against the skin (Pittman et al., 2015; Schallom et al., 2015).*

---

5. Remove and dispose of gloves; perform hand hygiene. Reapply gloves if exposure to body fluids is anticipated during interventions.

Reduces transmission of microorganisms.

6. Review patient's pressure injury risk assessment score. Adapt interventions based on those risks (WOCN, 2016).

Risk scores aid in identifying interventions to lessen or eliminate present risk factors.

7. If immobility, inactivity, or poor sensory perception is a risk factor for patient, consider one of the following interventions (WOCN, 2016):

Immobility and inactivity reduce patient's ability or desire to independently change position. Poor sensory perception decreases patient's ability to feel sensation of pressure or discomfort.

   a. Educate patient and family regarding specific pressure injury risk factors and prevention.

Helps patients and family understand and adhere to interventions designed to reduce pressure injury risk (Berlowitz, 2018).

   b. When patient is in side-lying position in bed, use 30-degree lateral position (see Fig. 48.15). Avoid 90-degree lateral position.

Reduces direct contact of trochanter with support surface.

   c. Place patient (when lying in bed) on pressure-redistribution surface.

Reduces amount of pressure exerted on tissues.

   d. Place patient (when in chair) on pressure-redistribution device and shift points under pressure at least every hour (WOCN, 2016).

Reduces amount of pressure on sacral and ischial areas.

8. If friction and shear are identified as risk factors, consider the following interventions:

Friction and shear damage underlying skin.

   a. Use safe patient-handling guidelines to reposition patient. For example, use slide board to transfer patient from bed to stretcher.

Proper repositioning of patient prevents creating shear from dragging patient along sheets. Slide board provides slippery surface to reduce friction. Use lift team when appropriate.

   b. Ensure that heels are free from surface of bed by using a pillow under calves to elevate heels, or use a heel-suspension device; knees should be in 5- to 10-degree flexion (WOCN, 2016; Baath et al., 2015).

"Floating" heels from bed surface offload the heel completely and redistribute the weight of the leg along the calf without applying pressure on the Achilles tendon (Baath et al., 2015).

   c. Maintain head of the bed at 30 degrees or lower or at the lowest degree of elevation consistent with patient's condition (do not lower HOB if patient is at risk for aspiration) (WOCN, 2016).

Decreases potential for patient to slide toward foot of bed and incur shear injury.

9. If patient receives low score on moisture subscale, consider one of the following interventions:

Continual exposure of body fluids on patient's skin increases risk for skin breakdown and pressure injury development.

   a. Apply clean gloves. Clean and dry the skin as soon as possible after each incontinent episode (WOCN, 2016). Then apply moisture barrier ointment to perineum and surrounding skin.

Protects skin from fecal or urinary incontinence. Friction and shear are enhanced in the presence of moisture (McNichol et al., 2018).

   b. If skin is denuded, use protective barrier paste after each incontinent episode.

Provides barrier between skin and stool/urine, allowing for healing.

   c. If moisture source is from wound drainage, consider more frequent dressing changes, skin protection with protective barriers, or collection devices.

Removes frequent exposure to wound drainage from skin.

10. If friction and shear are risk factors and patient is chair bound:

Relief of pressure by changing from lying to sitting position is insufficient if sitting lasts a prolonged time. The maximum amount of time a patient can sit before there is a need to reposition is unknown (WOCN, 2016).

   a. Tilt patient's chair seat to prevent sliding forward, and support arms, legs, and feet to maintain proper posture (EPUAP, NPIAP, PPPIA, 2019a).

   b. Limit amount of time patient spends in a chair without pressure redistribution (EPUAP, NPIAP, PPPIA, 2019a).

Relieves pressure on ischial tuberosities and sacrum.

   c. For patients who can reposition themselves while sitting, encourage pressure redistribution every 15 minutes using chair push-ups, forward lean, or side to side (WOCN, 2016).

Continued

SKILL 48.1 ASSESSMENT AND PREVENTION STRATEGIES FOR PRESSURE INJURY DEVELOPMENT—cont'd

STEP	RATIONALE
11. Educate patient and family caregiver regarding pressure injury risk and prevention strategies (WOCN, 2016).	Helps to adhere to interventions to reduce pressure injury risk.
12. Remove gloves and discard in appropriate receptacle. Perform hand hygiene.	Reduces transmission of microorganisms.
13. Assist patient to a comfortable position.	Enhances patient comfort and relaxation.
14. Raise side rails (as appropriate) and lower bed to lowest position	Provides for patient safety and reduces the risk for falls.
15. Place call nurse call system within reach; instruct patient in use.	Assists patient or family member in calling for assistance.

EVALUATION

1. Continually observe patient's skin for areas at risk for tissue damage, noting change in color, appearance, or texture.	Enables you to evaluate success of prevention techniques.
2. Observe tolerance of patient for position change by measuring level of comfort on pain scale.	Position changes sometimes interfere with patient's sleep and rest pattern.
3. Compare subsequent risk-assessment scores and skin assessments.	Provides ongoing comparison of patient's risk level to facilitate appropriateness of plan of care.
4. **Use Teach-Back:** "I want you to understand why we need to assess your skin on an ongoing basis. Tell me in your own words why we will be checking your skin on a regular basis." Revise your instruction now or develop a plan for revised patient/family caregiver teaching if patient/family caregiver is not able to teach back correctly.	Determines patient's/family caregiver's level of understanding of instructional topic.

UNEXPECTED OUTCOMES AND RELATED INTERVENTIONS

1. Skin becomes mottled, reddened, purplish, or bluish.
   - Refer patient to wound, ostomy, and continence (WOC) nurse; registered dietitian; clinical nurse specialist (CNS); nurse practitioner (NP); and/or physical therapist as necessary. Reevaluate position changes and bed surface.
2. Areas under pressure develop persistent discoloration, induration, or temperature changes.
   - Refer patient to WOC nurse, registered dietitian, CNS, NP, and/or physical therapist as necessary.
   - Modify patient's positioning and turning schedule.

RECORDING AND REPORTING

- Record patient's risk score and skin assessments, turning intervals, pressure-redistribution support surface, care of medical devices, and moisture protection interventions in electronic health record (EHR) or chart.
- Report need for additional consultations (if indicated) for high-risk patient.
- Document your evaluation of patient learning.

HOME CARE CONSIDERATIONS

- Instruct family caregiver in use of the 30-degree lateral position and how to assist patient into the position. This position prolongs the time between position changes, resulting in fewer sleep interruptions for patient and caregiver.
- Individualize pressure-redistribution maneuvers for patient needs and home environment.
- Provide family with community resources for hospital equipment.

SKILL 48.2 TREATING PRESSURE INJURIES AND WOUNDS

Delegation and Collaboration

The skill of treating pressure injuries and wounds cannot be delegated to assistive personnel (AP). Instruct the AP to:

- Report immediately to the nurse pain, fever, or any wound drainage.
- Report immediately to the nurse any change in skin integrity.
- Report any potential contamination to existing dressing, such as patient incontinence or dislodgement of the dressing.

Equipment

- Clean gloves
- Sterile gloves *(optional)*
- Goggles, mask, and cover gown (if splash is a risk)
- Biohazard bag for dressing disposal
- Wound-measuring device
- Cotton-tipped applicators
- Normal saline or cleansing agent (as ordered)
- Topical agent or solution (as ordered)
- Dressings
- Hypoallergenic tape if needed
- Irrigating syringe *(optional)*

STEP	RATIONALE

ASSESSMENT

1. Identify patient using at least two identifiers (e.g., name and birthday or name and account number) according to agency policy. Compare identifiers with information on patient's MAR or medical record.

   Ensures correct patient. Complies with The Joint Commission standards and improves patient safety (TJC, 2020).

2. Review medical orders for type of dressing. Review previous nurses' notes in electronic health record (EHR) or chart for type of dressing applied.

   Ensures administration of proper medication and treatment.

CLINICAL DECISION: *Verify that the order is consistent with established wound care guidelines and outcomes for a patient. If the order is inconsistent with guidelines or varies from the identified outcome for a patient, review with the health care team.*

---

3. Assess patient's/family caregiver's knowledge, experience, and health literacy level.

   Ensures patient/family caregiver has the capacity to obtain, communicate, process, and understand basic health information (CDC, 2019).

4. Assess patient's level of comfort on pain scale of 0 to 10. If patient is in pain, determine whether prn pain medication has been ordered and administer30 minutes before dressing change. .

   Dressing change should not be traumatic for patient; evaluate wound pain before, during, and after wound-care management (Hopf et al, 2016).

5. Determine whether patient has allergies to topical agents.

   Topical agents could contain elements that cause localized skin reactions.

6. Close room door or bedside curtains.

   Provides privacy.

7. Position patient to allow dressing removal and position biohazard bag for dressing disposal. **NOTE:** This step can also be done during implementation, just before dressing change.

   Provides an accessible area for dressing change. Proper disposal of old dressing promotes proper handling of contaminated waste.

8. Perform hand hygiene and apply clean gloves. Remove and discard old dressing.

   Reduces transmission of microorganisms and prevents accidental exposure to body fluids.

9. Assess patient's wounds using wound parameters and continue ongoing wound assessment per agency policy. **NOTE:** This may be done during wound care procedure.

   Provides baseline or comparison with previous dressing changes for condition of wound and effectiveness of wound care (WOCN, 2016).

   a. *Wound location:* Describe body site where wound is located.

   b. *Stage/classification of wound:* Describe extent of tissue destruction using wound classification for surgical and traumatic wounds and stage of a pressure injury

   Staging is way to assess a pressure injury based on depth of tissue destruction (Edsberg et al., 2016). Classification of a wound provides guideline for type of dressing to apply.

   c. *Wound size:* Measure length, width, and depth of wound per agency protocol. Use disposable measuring guide for length and width. Use cotton-tipped applicator to assess depth (see illustration).

   Injury size changes as healing progresses; therefore, longest and widest areas of wound change over time. Measuring width and length by measuring consistent areas provides consistent measurement (Nix, 2016).

   d. *Presence of undermining, sinus tracts, or tunnels:* Use sterile cotton-tipped applicator to measure depth and, if needed, a gloved finger to examine wound edges.

   Wound depth determines amount of tissue loss.

   e. *Condition of wound bed:* Describe type and percentage of tissue in wound bed. Approximate percentage of each type of tissue in wound provides critical information on progress of wound healing and choice of dressing

   Approximate percentage of each type of wound provides critical information of progress of wound healing and choice of dressing. Wound with high percentage of black tissue requires debridement; yellow tissue or slough tissue may indicate presence of infection or colonization; and granulation tissue indicates that wound is moving toward healing.

   f. *Volume of exudate:* Describe amount, characteristics, odor, and color.

   Amount and type of drainage or exudate may indicate type and frequency of dressing changes (Bates-Jensen, 2016).

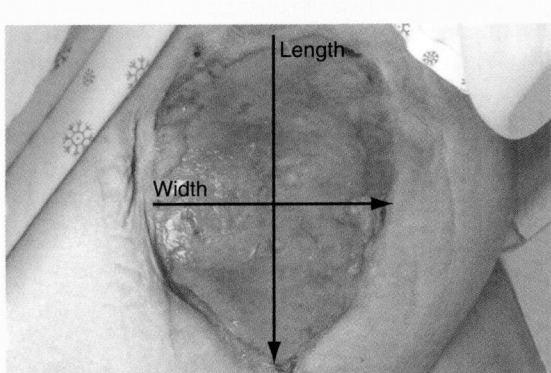
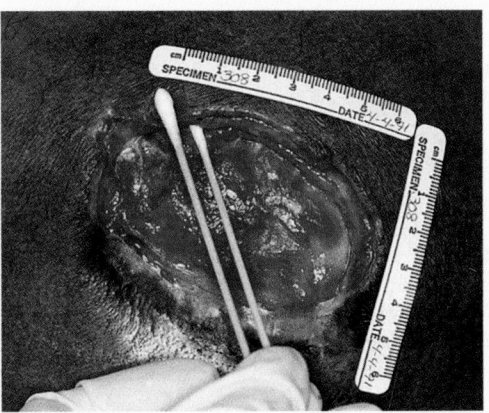

STEP 9c Measuring wound width, length, and undermining of skin. (Left image from Bryant RA, Nix DP, editors: *Acute and chronic wounds: current management concepts*, ed 5, St Louis, 2016, Elsevier.)

Continued

SKILL 48.2	TREATING PRESSURE INJURIES AND WOUNDS—cont'd

STEP	RATIONALE
g. *Condition of periwound skin:* Examine skin for breaks, dryness, maceration, and presence of rash, swelling, redness, or warmth. Modify assessment based on patient's skin color (see Box 48.2).	Impaired skin condition at edge of a wound or pressure injury indicates progressive tissue damage. Maceration on periwound skin shows need to alter choice of wound dressing.
h. *Wound edges:* Examine edges for condition of tissue.	Provides information regarding epithelialization, chronicity, and etiology.
10. Remove gloves and discard in appropriate receptacle. Perform hand hygiene.	Reduces transmission of microorganisms.

CLINICAL DECISION: *Repeated hand hygiene will be necessary as you assess other wounds or pressure areas. Different organisms contaminate different wounds.*

11. Assess for factors affecting wound healing: poor perfusion, immunosuppression, or preexisting infection.	Factors affect treatment and wound healing.
12. Assess patient's nutritional status (see Chapter 45). Clinically significant malnutrition is present if (1) serum albumin level is less than 3.5 g/dL, (2) lymphocyte count is less than 1800/mm^3, or (3) body weight decreases more than 15% (WOCN, 2016).	Delayed wound healing occurs in poorly nourished patients.

CLINICAL DECISION: *When you suspect malnutrition, obtain a nutritional consultation to modify patient's diet to promote wound healing.*

13. Assess patient's/family caregiver's understanding of wound condition, treatment plan, and complications of planned treatments.	Patient/family caregiver need to partner with health care providers to provide wound care at home as needed to prevent further skin breakdown.

PLANNING

1. Provide privacy by pulling the curtain around the patient, and position the patient so that only the area currently being examined is exposed; use sheet to cover rest of the body. Instruct patient not to touch wound or sterile supplies.	Providing privacy and preparing equipment before the procedure helps to ensure a clean and distraction-free area for organizing procedure-related equipment. Prevents accidental contamination of sterile supplies.
2. Explain procedure to patient before starting.	Reduces anxiety and provides opportunity for patient/family caregiver education.
3. Organize and prepare the following equipment and supplies.	
a. Normal saline or other wound-cleaning agent in sterile solution container	Cleanses injury surface before applying topical agents and new dressing.
b. Prescribed topical agent	
(1) Enzyme debriding agents. (Follow specific manufacturer directions for frequency of application.)	Enzymes debride dead tissue to clean injury surface. Enzymes are not applied to healthy tissue.
(2) Topical antibiotics	Topical antibiotics decrease bioburden of wound and should be considered for use if no healing is noted after 2 to 4 weeks of optimal care (WOCN, 2016).
c. Select appropriate dressing based on pressure injury characteristics, principles of wound management, and patient care setting. Dressing options include (see Table 48.9):	Dressing should maintain moist environment for wound while keeping surrounding skin dry (Bryant & Nix, 2016b).
(1) Gauze—Apply as moist dressing, as a dry cover dressing over clean surgical wound, as a dry cover dressing when using enzymes or topical antibiotics, or as a means to deliver solution to wound.	Gauze delivers moisture to wound and is absorptive.
(2) Transparent film dressing—Apply over superficial injuries with minimal or no exudate and skin subjected to friction.	Maintains moist environment and offers intact skin protection.
(3) Hydrocolloid dressing	Maintains moist environment to facilitate wound healing while protecting wound base.
(4) Hydrogel—available in sheet or in tube	Maintains moist environment to facilitate wound healing.
(5) Calcium alginate	Highly absorbent of wound exudate in heavily draining wounds.
(6) Foam dressings	Protective and prevents wound dehydration; also absorbs moderate-to-large amounts of drainage.
(7) Silver-impregnated dressings/gels	Controls bacterial burden in wound.
(8) Wound fillers	Fills shallow wounds, hydrates, and absorbs.
d. Hypoallergenic tape or adhesive dressing	Used to secure nonadherent dressing. Prevents skin irritation and tearing.

IMPLEMENTATION

1. Assemble supplies at bedside.	Ensures organized procedure.
2. Perform hand hygiene and apply clean gloves. Open sterile packages and topical solution containers (see Chapter 28). Keep dressings sterile. Wear goggles, mask, and moisture-proof cover gown if potential for contamination from spray exists when cleaning wound.	Reduces transmission of microorganisms.
3. Remove bed linen and arrange patient's gown to expose wound and surrounding skin. Keep remaining body parts draped.	Prevents unnecessary exposure of body parts.

STEP	RATIONALE
4. Moisten gauze in cleaning solution. Clean wound thoroughly with normal saline or prescribed wound-cleaning agent from least contaminated to most contaminated area. For deep injuries or wounds, clean with saline delivered with irrigating syringe as ordered (see Skill 48.5). Dry skin around wound thoroughly using clean gauze. Remove gloves and discard.	Cleaning wound removes wound exudate and/or dressing residue and reduces surface bacteria.
5. Perform hand hygiene and apply clean or sterile gloves. (Refer to agency policy.)	Maintains aseptic technique during cleaning, measuring, and applying dressings.
6. Apply topical agents to wound using cotton-tipped applicators or gauze as ordered:	
a. Enzymes	Follow manufacturer directions for method and frequency of application. Be aware of which solutions inactivate enzymes and avoid their use in wound cleaning.
(1) Apply small amount of enzyme debridement ointment directly to necrotic areas in the pressure injury. *Do not apply enzyme to surrounding healthy skin.*	Thin layer absorbs and acts more effectively than thick layer. Excess medication irritates surrounding healthy skin (Bryant and Nix, 2016b). Proper distribution of ointment ensures effective action.

CLINICAL DECISION: *If using an enzymatic debriding agent, do not use wound-cleaning agents with metals.*

STEP	RATIONALE
(2) Place moist gauze dressing directly over wound followed by a dry dressing. Follow specific manufacturer recommendation for type of dressing material to use to cover a pressure injury when using enzymes. Tape dressing in place.	Protects wound and prevents removal of ointment during turning or repositioning.
b. **Antibacterials** (e.g., bacitracin, metronidazole, and silver sulfadiazine). Apply evenly over wound surface.	Reduces bacterial growth.
7. Apply prescribed wound dressing:	
a. Apply gauze dressing as described in Skill 48.3	Gauze is applied dry or as a damp-to-dry dressing, common for poorly healing surgical wounds and traumatic wounds.
b. **Hydrogel:**	Hydrogel dressings are designed to hydrate and brings moisture to wound (Bryant and Nix, 2016b).
(1) Cover surface of wound with thick layer of amorphous hydrogel or cut sheet to fit wound base.	Provides moist environment to facilitate wound healing.
(2) Apply secondary dressing such as dry gauze; tape in place.	Holds hydrogel against wound surface because amorphous hydrogel (in tube) or sheet form does not adhere to wound and requires secondary dressing to hold it in place.
(3) If using impregnated gauze, pack loosely into wound; cover with secondary gauze dressing and tape.	A loosely packed dressing delivers gel to wound base and allows any wound debris to be trapped in gauze.
c. **Calcium alginate:**	Alginate dressings absorb serous fluid or exudate, forming a nonadhesive hydrophilic gel, which conforms to shape of wound (Bryant and Nix, 2016b). Use in heavily draining wounds.
(1) Lightly pack wound with alginate using sterile cotton-tipped applicator or gloved finger.	The dressing swells and increases in size; tight packing can compromise blood flow to the tissues.
(2) Apply secondary dressing and tape in place.	
d. **Transparent film dressing:**	
(1) Be sure skin around wound is thoroughly dry.	Moisture prevents transparent dressing from adhering.
(2) Remove paper backing, taking care not to allow adhesive areas to touch one another. **Do not stretch a film dressing and avoid wrinkles.**	Ensures smooth application.
(3) Place film smoothly over wound and use your fingers to smooth and adhere dressing over skin.	Ensures occlusive application.
(4) Label dressing with date, your initials, and time of dressing change.	Provides guideline for timing of next dressing change.

CLINICAL DECISION: *Use transparent dressings for minor cuts or abrasions and for autolytic debridement of noninfected superficial pressure injuries. A hydrocolloid dressing protects skin from friction and/or provides moisture to a wound. Some brands have custom shapes available for specific anatomical parts such as heels, elbows, and sacrum.*

STEP	RATIONALE
e. **Hydrocolloid dressing:**	
(1) Select proper size wafer, allowing dressing to extend onto intact periwound skin at least 2.5 cm (1 inch). **Do not stretch dressing and avoid wrinkles**.	Dressing prevents shear and friction from loosening edges and circumvents need for tape along dressing borders (Bryant and Nix, 2016b).
(2) For deep wounds, apply hydrocolloid granules, impregnated gauze, or paste before the wafer.	Functions as filler material to ensure contact with all wound surfaces. Cushions wound for pain reduction and protection.

Continued

SKILL 48.2   TREATING PRESSURE INJURIES AND WOUNDS—cont'd

STEP	RATIONALE
(3) Remove paper backing from adhesive side and place over wound. Do not stretch, and avoid wrinkles or tenting. Hold dressing in place for 30 to 60 seconds after application.	Molds dressing at body temperature (Bryant and Nix, 2016b).
(4) If cut from large piece of wafer, tape edges with nonallergenic tape.	Avoids rolling of edges of dressing or adherence to clothing.
f. Foam dressing:	
(1) Refer to manufacturer guidelines for removal and application characteristics of specific foam dressing brand.	Foam dressings collect moderate to heavy wound exudate; however, some contain an antimicrobial substance to reduce risk for bacterial colonization in wounds.
(2) Apply a skin barrier wipe to surrounding skin that will come in contact with the thin foam dressing adhesive.	Protects skin from maceration or irritation of adhesive.
(3) Cut foam sheet to extend 2.5 cm (1 inch) out onto intact periwound skin. (Verify which side of foam dressing should be placed toward wound bed and which side should face away from it; see product instructions)	Ensures proper absorption and keeps wound exudate away from wound (Bryant and Nix, 2016b).
(4) Cover with secondary dressing as needed.	Protects dressing.
8. Reposition patient comfortably off pressure injury.	Prevents pressure to injury.
9. Remove and dispose of gloves. Dispose of soiled supplies in appropriate receptacle. Perform hand hygiene.	Reduces transmission of microorganisms.
10. Assist patient to comfortable position.	Enhances patient comfort and relaxation.
11. Raise side rails (as appropriate) and lower bed to lowest position	Provides for patient safety and reduces the risk for falls.
12. Place nurse call system within reach; instruct patient in use.	Assists patient or family member in calling for assistance.

EVALUATION

1. Observe skin surrounding injury for inflammation, edema, and tenderness.	Determines progress of wound healing.
2. Compare observations of the wound with previous assessments : observing for drainage, wound size, foul odor, and tissue necrosis. Monitor patient for signs and symptoms of infection: fever and elevated white blood cell (WBC) count.	Injuries can become infected.
3. Compare subsequent injury measurements, using one of the scales designed to measure wound healing such as PUSH Tool or BWAT Assessment.	Allows comparison of serial measurements to evaluate wound healing. Provides standard method of data collection that demonstrates injury progress or lack thereof.
4. **Use Teach-Back:** "I want to be sure that you understand why we measure and assess your pressure injury on an ongoing basis. Tell me why we measure the injury and look at the tissue type and surrounding skin." Revise your instruction now or develop a plan for revised patient/family caregiver teaching if patient/family caregiver is not able to teach back correctly.	Determines patient's/family caregiver's level of understanding of instructional topic.

UNEXPECTED OUTCOMES AND RELATED INTERVENTIONS

1. Skin surrounding injury becomes macerated.
   - Reduce exposure of surrounding skin to topical agents and moisture.
   - Select dressing that has increased moisture-absorbing capacity.
2. Wound becomes deeper with increased drainage and/or development of necrotic tissue.
   Cover with secondary dressing as needed.
   - Review current wound-care management.
   - Consult with interprofessional team regarding changes in wound-care regimen.
   - Obtain wound cultures.
3. Pressure injury extends beyond original margins.
   - Monitor for systemic signs and symptoms of poor wound healing such as abnormal laboratory results (WBC count, levels of hemoglobin/hematocrit, serum albumin, serum prealbumin, total proteins), weight loss, and fluid imbalances.
   - Assess and revise current turning schedule.
   - Consider alternate pressure-redistribution devices.

RECORDING AND REPORTING

- Record appearance and condition of the wound/pressure injury, type of topical agent or dressing used, presence of pain and how treated, and patient's response in electronic health record (EHR) or chart.
- Document your evaluation of patient learning.
- Report any deterioration in wound appearance.
- Describe the location of the wound; type and percentage of wound tissue; presence or absence of wound drainage, odor; type and quantity of dressings used and the location of the dressings (for the next dressing change); and patient's response.

HOME CARE CONSIDERATIONS

- Clean dressings are often used in the home setting.
- Patients need to dispose of contaminated dressings in the home in a manner consistent with local regulations for contaminated waste.
- Teach patient and family caregiver about the signs of wound infection.

SKILL 48.3	APPLYING DRY AND MOIST DRESSINGS

Delegation and Collaboration

The skill of applying dry and damp-to-dry dressings can be delegated to assistive personnel (AP) if the wound is chronic (see agency policy and Nurse Practice Act). However, the nurse must first assess the wound and is responsible for the care of acute new wounds, wound care requiring sterile technique, and evaluation of wound healing. Direct the AP about:

- Any unique modifications of the dressing change such as the need for use of special tape or taping techniques to secure the dressing.
- Reporting pain, fever, bleeding, or wound drainage to the nurse immediately.
- Reporting any potential contamination to existing dressing (e.g., patient incontinence or other body fluids, a dressing that becomes dislodged).

Equipment

- Clean and sterile gloves
- Sterile dressing set including scissors and forceps (check agency policy)
- Sterile drape (optional)
- Necessary dressings: fine-mesh gauze, 4 × 4–inch gauze, abdominal pads (ABDs)
- Sterile basin (optional)
- Antiseptic ointment (as prescribed)
- Wound cleanser (as prescribed)
- Sterile normal saline (or prescribed solution)
- Débriding gel as ordered
- Tape (include nonallergenic tape as necessary), Montgomery ties, or bandages as needed
- Skin barrier (optional if using Montgomery ties)
- Measuring device: cotton-tipped applicator, measuring guide, camera
- Adhesive remover, scissors, or hair clipper (optional)
- Protective waterproof underpad
- Biohazard bag
- Personal protective equipment (PPE) (i.e., gown, goggles, mask) if needed
- Additional lighting if needed (e.g., flashlight, treatment light)

STEP	RATIONALE

ASSESSMENT

1. Identify patient using at least two identifiers (e.g., name and birthday or name and account number) according to agency policy. Compare identifiers with information on patient's MAR or medical record.

Ensures correct patient. Complies with The Joint Commission standards and improves patient safety (TJC, 2020).

2. Assess patient's/family caregiver's knowledge, experience, and health literacy level.

Ensures patient/family caregiver have the capacity to obtain, communicate, and understand basic health information (CDC, 2019).

3. Assess patient for allergies, especially to antiseptics, tape, or latex.

Reduces risk for localized or systemic allergic reactions to these supplies.

4. Ask patient to rate level of pain using a pain scale of 0 to 10 and to assess character of pain. Administer prescribed analgesic as needed 30 minutes before dressing change.

Superficial wounds with multiple exposed nerves may be intensely painful, whereas deeper wounds with destruction of dermis should be less painful (Krasner, 2016). A comfortable patient is less likely to move suddenly, causing contamination to wound or supplies. Serves as baseline to measure response to dressing therapy.

5. Review medical orders for type of dressing. Review previous nurses' notes in electronic health record (EHR) or chart.

Indicates types of dressing supplies needed.

6. Review medical record to identify patient's risk for wound-healing problems, including aging, premature infant, obesity, diabetes mellitus, circulation disorders, nutritional deficit, immunosuppression, radiation therapy, high levels of stress, and use of steroids.

Physiological changes resulting from aging, chronic illness, poor nutrition, medications that affect wound healing, and cancer treatments have potential to affect wound healing (Doughty and Sparks, 2016).

7. Perform hand hygiene and apply gloves as needed.

Reduces transmission of microorganisms.

8. Assess condition of skin around wound and existing dressing (see Skill 48.2). Remove and dispose of gloves if worn and perform hand hygiene.

Provides baseline or comparison with previous dressing changes for condition of skin around wound. Helps to plan for proper dressing type and securement of supplies needed and for whether help is needed during dressing procedure.

9. Assess need, readiness, and willingness for patient or family caregiver to participate in dressing wound.

Identifies areas for patient education to prepare patient or family caregiver if dressing must be changed at home.

PLANNING

1. Close room door or bedside curtains. Gather all necessary supplies.

Provides privacy and ensures organized procedure.

2. Position patient comfortably and drape to expose only wound site. Instruct patient not to touch wound or sterile supplies.

Draping provides access to wound while minimizing exposure. Dressing supplies become contaminated when touched by patient's hand.

3. Organize workspace at bedside.

Facilitates a smooth and organized dressing change.

Continued

SKILL 48.3	APPLYING DRY AND MOIST DRESSINGS—cont'd

STEP	RATIONALE
4. Place disposable biohazard bag within reach of work area (see illustration). Perform hand hygiene and apply clean gloves. Apply gown, goggles, and mask if risk for splashing exists.	Ensures easy disposal of soiled dressings. Use of PPE reduces transmission of microorganisms.
5. Explain procedure to patient and/or family caregiver.	Decreases patient's anxiety.

IMPLEMENTATION

STEP	RATIONALE
1. Perform hand hygiene and gently remove tape, bandages, or ties from existing dressing. Use nondominant hand to support dressing and with your dominant hand pull tape parallel to skin and toward dressing. If dressing is over hairy area, remove in direction of hair growth. Get patient permission to clip or shave area (check agency policy). Remove any adhesive from skin.	Pulling tape toward dressing reduces stress on suture line or wound edges, irritation, and discomfort.
2. With gloved hand or forceps remove dressing one layer at a time, observing appearance and drainage of dressing. Carefully remove outer secondary dressing first; then remove inner primary dressing that is in contact with wound bed. If drains are present, slowly and carefully remove dressings (see Fig. 48.10) and avoid tension on any drainage devices. Keep soiled undersurface from patient's sight.	Purpose of primary dressing is to remove necrotic tissue and exudate. Appearance of drainage may be upsetting to patient. Avoids accidental removal of drain.
a. If bottom layer of damp-to-dry dressing adheres to wound and debridement of tissue is the goal, gently free dressing and alert patient of discomfort.	Damp-to-dry dressing should debride wound (WOCN, 2016; Wysocki, 2016).
b. If dry dressing adheres to wound that is not to be debrided, moisten with normal saline, wait 1 to 2 minutes, and remove.	Prevents injury to wound surface and periwound during dressing removal.
3. Inspect wound and periwound for appearance, color, size (length, width, and depth), drainage, edema, presence and condition of drains, approximation (wound edges are together), granulation tissue, or odor. Use measuring guide or ruler to measure size of wound (see Skill 48.2). Gently palpate wound edges for bogginess or patient report of increased pain.	Assesses wound and periwound condition. Indicates status of healing.
4. Fold dressings with drainage contained inside and remove gloves inside out. With small dressings remove gloves inside out over dressing (see illustrations). Dispose of gloves and soiled dressing according to agency policy. Cover wound lightly with sterile gauze pad and perform hand hygiene.	Contains soiled dressings, prevents contact of nurse's hands with drainage, and reduces cross-contamination and transmission of microorganisms.

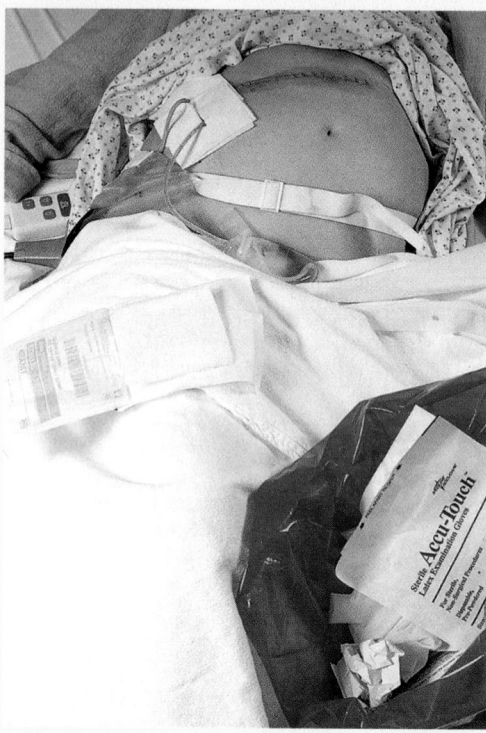

STEP 4 Disposable waterproof bag placed near dressing site.

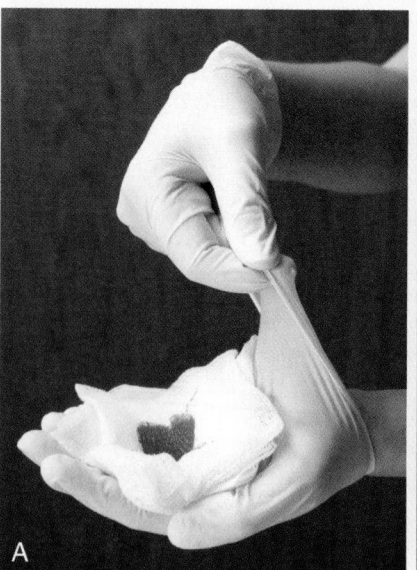
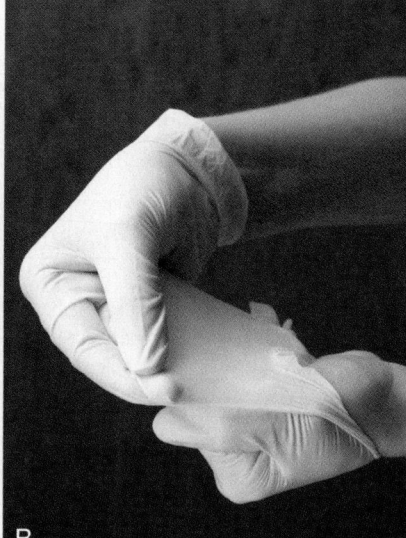

STEP 4 A and **B,** dispose of soiled dressings by placing in gloved hand and pulling glove off over dressing and then off hand.

STEP	RATIONALE

5. Describe appearance of wound and any indicators of wound healing to patient.

6. Create sterile field with sterile dressing tray or individually wrapped sterile supplies on over-bed table (see Chapter 28). Pour any prescribed solution into sterile basin.

7. Clean wound
   a. Perform hand hygiene and apply clean gloves. Use gauze or cotton ball moistened in saline or antiseptic swab (per health care provider order) for each cleaning stroke, or spray wound surface with wound cleaner.
   b. Clean from least to most contaminated area (see Fig. 48.21).
   c. Clean around any drain (if present), using circular strokes starting near drain and moving outward and away from insertion site (see Fig. 48.22).

8. Use sterile dry gauze to blot wound bed in same manner as in Step 7.

9. Apply antiseptic ointment (if ordered) with sterile cotton-tipped applicator or gauze, using same technique to apply as for cleaning. Remove and dispose of gloves. Perform hand hygiene.

10. Apply dressing (see agency policy):
    a. Dry sterile dressing:

Rationale:
Wounds may be unsettling and frightening to patients. It helps patient to know that wound appearance is as expected and whether healing is taking place.
Sterile dressings remain sterile while on or within sterile surface. Preparation of all supplies before dressing change prevents break in technique during dressing change.

Prevents transfer of organisms from previously cleaned area.

Cleaning in this direction prevents introduction of organisms into wound.
Correct aseptic technique in cleaning prevents contamination.

Drying reduces excess moisture, which could eventually harbor microorganisms.
Helps reduce growth of microorganisms.

CLINICAL DECISION: *Dry dressings are inappropriate for debriding wounds. In the presence of drainage, a dry dressing may adhere to the wound bed and surrounding tissue, causing pain and trauma on removal. Dry dressings have the disadvantage of moisture evaporating quickly, which can cause a dressing to dry out. As a result, frequent dressing changes are usually needed, and there is an increase in infection rate when compared with semi-occlusive dressings (Bryant and Nix, 2016b).*

(1) Apply clean gloves (see agency policy).
(2) Apply loose woven gauze as contact layer (see illustration).
(3) If drain is present, apply precut, split 4 × 4–inch gauze around drain.
(4) Apply additional layers of gauze as needed.
(5) Apply thicker woven pad (e.g., Surgipad, abdominal [ABD] pad) (see illustration).
b. A damp-to-dry dressing.

Some agencies or condition of wounds may require sterile gloves.
Promotes proper absorption of drainage.
Secures drain and promotes drainage absorption at site.
Ensures proper coverage and optimal absorption.
This dressing is used on postoperative wounds when there is excessive drainage.
A damp-to-dry dressing is a moist primary dressing that brings moisture to the wound surface. The moistened gauze increases the absorptive ability of the dressing to collect exudate and wound debris while providing the wound base with moisture to facilitate healing.

(1) Apply sterile gloves (see agency policy).
(2) Place fine-mesh or loose 4 × 4–inch gauze in container of prescribed sterile solution. Wring out excess solution.

Reduces transmission of infection.
Damp gauze absorbs drainage and, when allowed to dry, traps debris.

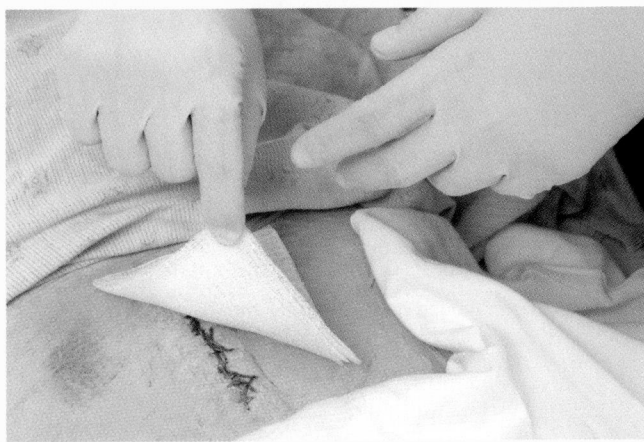
STEP 10a(2) Placing dry gauze dressing over simple wound.

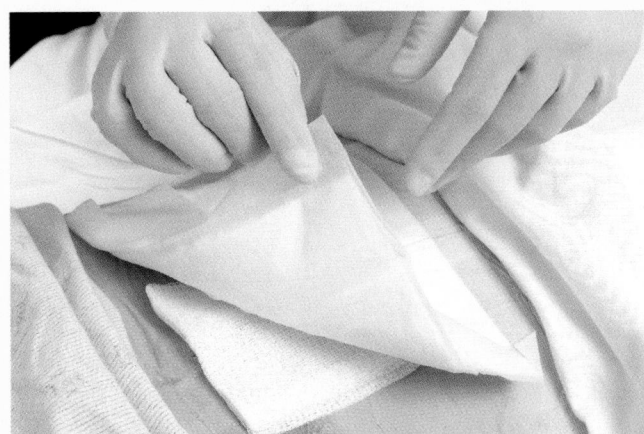
STEP 10a(5) Placing abdominal pad over gauze dressing.

Continued

SKILL 48.3   APPLYING DRY AND MOIST DRESSINGS—cont'd

STEP	RATIONALE

CLINICAL DECISION: *If using "packing strips," use sterile scissors to cut the amount of dressing that you will use to pack the wound. Do not let the packing strip touch the side of the bottle. Place packing strip in container of prescribed sterile solution. Wring out excess solution.*

(3) Apply damp fine-mesh or open-weave gauze as single layer directly onto wound surface. If wound is deep, gently pack gauze into wound with sterile gloved hand or forceps until all wound surfaces are in contact with moist gauze, including dead spaces from sinus tracts, tunnels, and undermining (see illustration A). Be sure that gauze does not touch periwound skin (see illustration B).

Inner gauze should be damp, not dripping wet, to absorb drainage and adhere to debris. When packing a wound, gauze should conform to base and side of wound (Bryant and Nix, 2016b). Wound is loosely packed to facilitate wicking of drainage into absorbent outer layer of dressing. Moisture that escapes dressing often macerates the periwound area.

CLINICAL DECISION: *Be sure to count how many pieces of gauze are packed in the wound, especially deep wounds. This ensures that all gauze from previous dressing change is removed from the wound.*

CLINICAL DECISION: *When packing the wound, do not overpack or underpack (Bryant and Nix, 2016b). Packing should fill the wound but should not be above the level of the skin.*

(4) Apply dry sterile 4 × 4–inch gauze over moist gauze.

Dry layer pulls moisture from wound.

(5) Cover with ABD pad, Surgipad, or gauze.

Protects wound from entrance of microorganisms.

11. Secure dressing.

    a. *Tape:* Apply tape 2.5 to 5 cm (1 to 2 inches) beyond dressing. Use nonallergenic tape when necessary.

Supports wound and ensures placement and stability of dressing.

    b. Montgomery ties (see Fig. 48.20).

Prevents skin irritation. Ties allow for repeated dressing changes without removal of tape.

    (1) Be sure that skin is clean. Application of skin barrier is recommended.

Skin barrier (a hydrocolloid) protects intact skin from stretch and tension of adhesive tape.

    (2) Expose adhesive surface of tape ends.

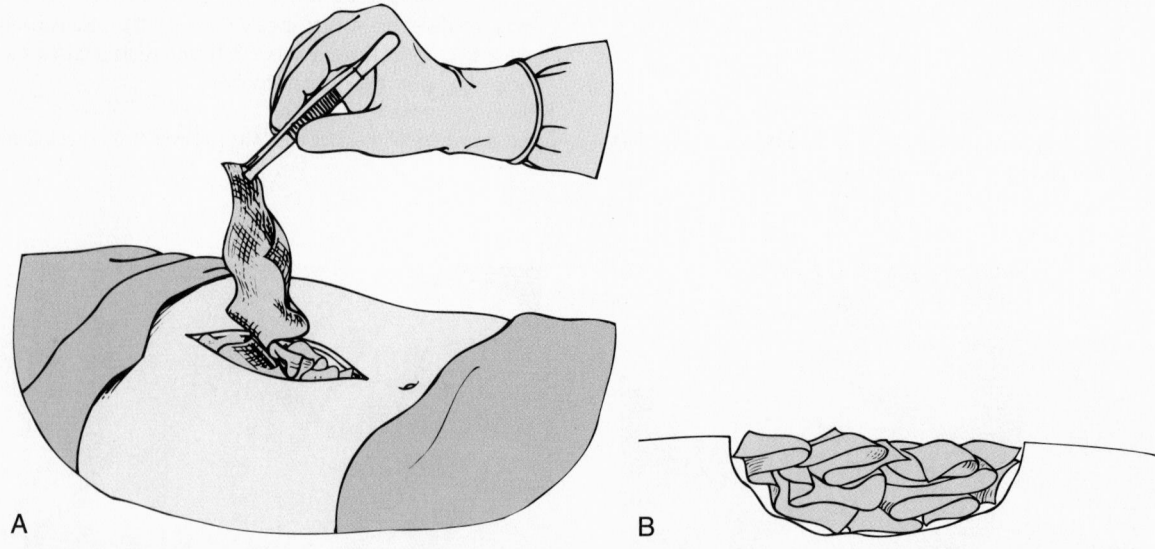

A

B

STEP 10b(3)   A, Packing wound with fine-mesh gauze. **B,** Cross-section of deep wound packed loosely with gauze roll.

STEP	RATIONALE

(3) Place ties on opposite sides of dressing over skin or skin barrier.

(4) Secure dressing by lacing ties across dressing snugly enough to hold it secure but without placing pressure on skin.

c. For protective window:

A protective window is an alternative to Montgomery ties for smaller wounds. There is less skin irritation by placing tape on window strips.

(1) Cut strip of a hydrocolloid pad into 1-cm (½-inch) strips.

(2) Use skin barrier to wipe areas of skin where strips will be applied.

(3) Apply hydrocolloid dressing strips to frame a "window" around the wound using four strips, one on each side, one on the top, and one on the bottom of the dressing material (see illustrations).

(4) Apply dressing; secure tape ends to adhesive strips (see illustration).

d. For dressing extremity, secure with roller gauze (see illustration) or elastic net.

Roller gauze conforms to contour of foot or hand.

12. Dispose of all dressing supplies. Remove cover gown and goggles; remove gloves inside out; dispose of them according to agency policy. Perform hand hygiene.

Reduces transmission of microorganisms. Clean environment enhances patient comfort.

13. Label tape over dressing with your initials and date dressing is changed.

Provides timeline for when next dressing change is to be scheduled.

14. Help patient to comfortable position.

Promotes patient's sense of well-being.

15. Be sure nurse call system is in an accessible location within patient's reach.

Ensures patient can call for assistance if needed.

16. Raise side rails (as appropriate) and lower bed to lowest position.

Ensures patient safety.

EVALUATION

1. Compare observations of the wound with previous assessment and observe appearance of wound for healing: measure size of wound; observe amount, color, and type of drainage and periwound erythema or swelling.

Determines rate of healing.

2. Ask patient to rate pain using a scale of 0 to 10.

Increased pain is often indication of wound complications such as infection or result of dressing pulling tissue.

3. Inspect condition of dressing at least every shift.

Determines status of wound drainage.

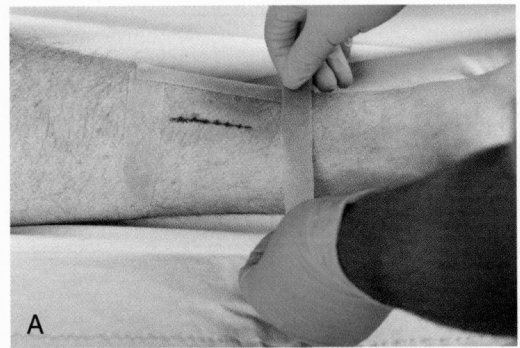
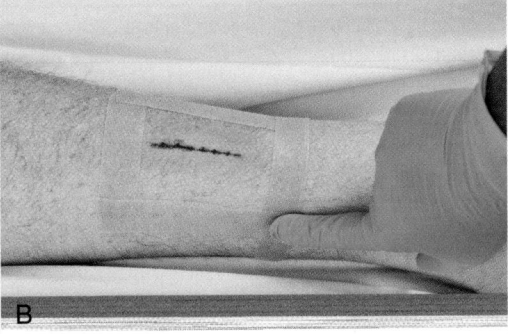

STEP 11c(3) Apply adhesive strips to frame a "window" around wound using four strips.

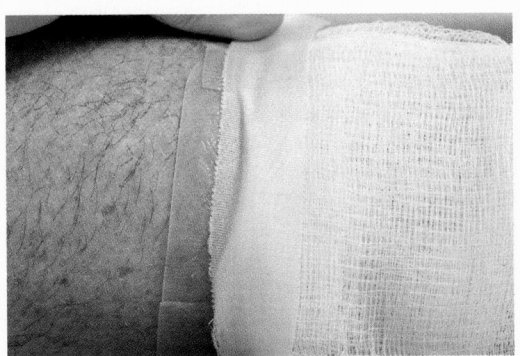

STEP 11c(4) Apply dressing; secure tape ends to adhesive strips.

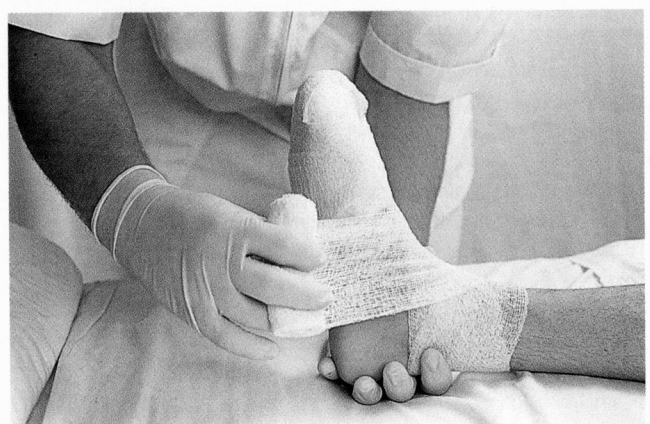

STEP 11d Wrap roller gauze around extremity to secure dressing.

Continued

SKILL 48.3	APPLYING DRY AND MOIST DRESSINGS—cont'd

STEP	RATIONALE
4. **Use Teach-Back:** "I want to be sure I explained why and how often you need to continue these dressing changes when you go home tomorrow. Tell me why it is important to change your dressing and how often you will do this." Revise your instruction now or develop a plan for revised patient/family caregiver teaching if patient/family caregiver is not able to teach back correctly.	Determines patient's/family caregiver's level of understanding of instructional topic.

UNEXPECTED OUTCOMES AND RELATED INTERVENTIONS

1. Wound appears inflamed and tender, drainage is evident, and/or odor is present.
   - Monitor patient for signs of infection (e.g., fever, increased white blood cell count).
   - Notify health care provider.
   - Obtain wound cultures as ordered.
   - If there is yellow, tan, or brown necrotic tissue, notify health care provider to determine need for debridement (see Table 48.2).
2. Wound bleeds during dressing change.
   - Observe color and amount of bloody drainage. If excessive, may need to apply direct dressing.
   - Inspect area along dressing and directly underneath patient to determine amount of bleeding.
   - Obtain vital signs as needed.
   - Notify health care provider.
3. Patient reports sensation that "something has given way under the dressing."
   - Observe wound for increased drainage or dehiscence (partial or total separation of wound layers) or evisceration (total separation of wound layers and protrusion of viscera through wound opening).
   - If dehiscence or evisceration occurs, protect wound. Cover with sterile saline moistened dressing.
   - If evisceration, do not move patient. Transfer patient to surgery in patient's bed.
   - Instruct patient to lie still.
   - Stay with patient to monitor vital signs.
   - Notify health care provider.

RECORDING AND REPORTING

- Record size and appearance of wound, characteristics of drainage, presence of necrotic tissue, type of dressings applied, response to dressing change, and level of comfort in electronic health record (EHR) or chart.
- Document your evaluation of patient learning.
- Report any unexpected appearance of wound drainage or bright red bleeding.
- Report any change in wound integrity (e.g., dehiscence or evisceration).

HOME CARE CONSIDERATIONS

- More expensive specialty dressings are sometimes used because they decrease the frequency of dressing changes.
- Clean dressings may also be used in the home setting.
- Patients need to dispose of contaminated dressings in the home in a manner consistent with local regulations.
- Be sure patient has a family caregiver able to assist with and/or apply dressing, and instruct caregiver on dressing procedure, signs of infection, and when to notify physician.

SKILL 48.4	IMPLEMENTATION OF NEGATIVE-PRESSURE WOUND THERAPY (NPWT)

Delegation and Collaboration

The skill of NPWT cannot be delegated to assistive personnel (AP). Direct the AP to:
- Use caution in positioning or turning patient to avoid tubing displacement.
- Report any change in dressing shape or integrity to the nurse.
- Report any change in patient's temperature or comfort level to the nurse.
- Report any wound fluid leakage around the edges of the adhesive drape.

Equipment
- NPWT unit (requires health care provider's order)
- NPWT dressing (gauze or foam, depending on manufacturer's recommendations; transparent dressing, adhesive drape)
- NPWT suction device
- Supplies for irrigation (see Skill 48.5)
- Tubing for connection between NPWT unit and NPWT dressing
- 3 pairs gloves, clean and sterile
- Sterile scissors
- Skin preparation/skin barrier protectant/hydrocolloid dressing/skin barrier
- Personal protective equipment (PPE): gown, mask, and goggles if splashing is a risk
- Waterproof, disposable trash biohazard bag

STEP	**RATIONALE**

ASSESSMENT

1. Identify patient using at least two identifiers (e.g., name and birthday or name and account number) according to agency policy. Compare identifiers with information on patient's MAR or medical record.

Ensures correct patient. Complies with The Joint Commission standards and improves patient safety (TJC, 2020).

2. Review health care provider's orders for frequency of dressing change, amount of negative pressure, type of foam or gauze to use, and pressure cycle (intermittent or continuous).

Determines frequency of dressing change, negative-pressure setting, and special instructions. Health care provider's order is also necessary for reimbursement.

3. Review medical record for signs and symptoms related to condition of patient's wound.

Provides baseline to compare your findings with previous dressing change assessments and reflects wound-healing progress.

4. Assess patient's/family caregiver's knowledge, experience, and health literacy level.

Ensures that patient has the capacity to obtain, communicate, process, and understand basic health information (CDC, 2019).

5. Assess patient's level of comfort on pain scale of 0 to 10.

Serves as baseline to measure patient's level of comfort during and after wound therapy

6. Perform hand hygiene. Apply clean gloves. Assess condition of wound and status of NPWT dressing (see Skill 48.2). Remove and dispose of gloves. Perform hand hygiene.

Provides information regarding condition of skin around wound and existing dressing, presence of complications, and proper type of supplies and help needed.

7. Assess patient's and family caregiver's knowledge of purpose of dressing and whether they will participate in dressing wound.

Identifies patient's learning needs. Prepares patient and family caregivers if dressing will need to be changed at home.

PLANNING

1. Close room door or bed curtains. Position the patient so that only the area currently being examined is exposed; use sheet to cover rest of the body.

Provides privacy and comfort.

2. Administer prescribed analgesic as needed 30 minutes before dressing change.

Comfortable patient will be less likely to move suddenly, causing contamination to wound or supplies.

3. Organize dressing supplies as bedside.

Facilitates a smooth and organized procedure.

4. Explain procedure to patient and family caregiver, instructing not to touch wound or sterile supplies.

Relieves anxiety and promotes understanding of healing process. Prevents contamination of sterile supplies.

IMPLEMENTATION

1. Cuff top of disposable waterproof biohazard bag and place within reach of work area.

Cuff prevents accidental contamination of top of outer bag.

2. Perform hand hygiene and apply clean gloves. If risk for spray exists, apply protective gown, goggles, and mask.

Reduces transmission of microorganisms from soiled dressings to nurse's hands.

3. Follow manufacturer directions for removal and replacement because each NPWT unit varies slightly with approach. Turn off NPWT unit by pushing therapy on/off button.

Deactivates therapy and allows for proper drainage of fluid in drainage tubing.

   a. Keeping tube connectors attached to NPWT unit, raise tubing connectors; disconnect tubes from one another and drain fluids into drainage collector.

Prevents backflow of any drainage in tubing back into wound.

   b. Before draining, tighten clamp on canister tube and disconnect canister and dressing tubing at connection points.

Prevents drainage from exiting tubing when removed.

4. Remove transparent film by gently stretching, and slowly pull away from skin.

Prevents injury to wound tissue.
Protects periwound skin breakdown from transparent adhesive.

5. Remove old dressing one layer at a time and discard in bag. Observe drainage on dressing. Use caution to avoid tension on any drains that are present near the wound or surrounding area. Remove and dispose of gloves.

Determines type and amount of dressings needed for replacement. Prevents accidental removal of drains.

6. Perform hand hygiene and conduct a wound assessment. Observe surface area and tissue type, color, odor, and drainage within wound. Measure length, width, and depth of wound as ordered (see Skill 48.2).

Measurement of wound is necessary to assess wound healing progression and to justify continuation of NPWT for third-party payers (Netsch et al., 2016).
Determines condition of wound and need for replacement of dressing.

CLINICAL DECISION: *This is a time when a wound-care nurse or physician might debride the wound. Debridement of eschar or slough, if present, should be performed for removal of devitalized tissue to prepare the wound bed (Netsch et al., 2016).*

7. Remove and discard gloves bag and perform hand hygiene. Avoid having patient see old dressing because sight of wound drainage may be upsetting.

Reduces transmission of microorganisms. Lessens patient anxiety during procedure.

8. Clean wound.

   a. Perform hand hygiene and apply sterile or clean gloves, depending on agency policy and wound status.

Cleaning periwound is essential for airtight seal.

   b. If ordered, irrigate wound with normal saline or other solution ordered by health care provider (see Skill 48.5). Gently blot periwound with gauze to dry thoroughly.

Irrigation removes wound debris and cleans wound bed. Cleaning and removal of infectious material showed reduced infection and improved healing (Fernandez et al., 2019).

Continued

SKILL 48.4   IMPLEMENTATION OF NEGATIVE-PRESSURE WOUND THERAPY (NPWT)—cont'd

STEP	RATIONALE

CLINICAL DECISION: *Health care providers may order wound cultures routinely. However, obtain wound culture when drainage is more copious, looks purulent, or has a foul odor. This may be an indication that NPWT may need to be discontinued.*

9. Apply skin protectant, barrier film, solid skin barrier sheet, or hydrocolloid dressing to periwound skin.	Maintains airtight seal needed for NPWT wound therapy. Protects periwound skin from moisture-associated skin damage (Netsch et al., 2016).
10. Fill any uneven skin surfaces (e.g., creases, scars, and skinfolds) with skin-barrier product (e.g., paste, strip).	Further helps to maintain airtight seal (Netsch et al., 2016).
11. Remove and discard gloves. Perform hand hygiene.	Prevents transmission of microorganisms.
12. Depending on type of wound, apply sterile or new clean gloves (see agency policy).	Fresh sterile wounds require sterile gloves. Chronic wounds require clean technique (WOCN, 2016).
13. Apply NPWT.	
a. Prepare NPWT filler dressing. Consult with wound-care expert for appropriate type.	Filler dressing depends on NPWT used and can include foam or gauze dressings with or without antimicrobials such as silver. Type of dressing may be adjusted based on undermining, tunneling, or sinus tracts present (Netsch et al., 2016).
(1) Measure wound and select appropriate-size dressing.	Black polyurethane (PU) foam has larger pores and is most effective in stimulating granulation tissue and wound contraction. White soft foam is denser with smaller pores and used when growth of granulation tissue needs to be restricted (Netsch et al., 2016).
(2) Using sterile scissors, cut filler gauze dressing or foam to wound size, making sure to fit exact size and shape of wound, including tunnels and undermined areas.	Proper size of dressing maintains negative pressure to entire wound (Netsch et al., 2016).

CLINICAL DECISION: *In some instances, an antimicrobial product such as silver-impregnated gauze or topical antibiotic is in order. These products help reduce the bioburden of the wound.*

b. Place filler dressing in wound following manufacturer instructions. Be sure that filler dressing is in contact with entire wound base, margins, and tunneled and undermined areas. Count number of filler dressings, and document in patient's chart.	Maintains negative pressure to entire wound. Edges of dressing must be in direct contact with patient's skin. Dressing count provides the number of filler dressings that should be removed at the next dressing change.
c. Place suction device per manufacturer instructions.	
d. Apply NPWT transparent dressing over foam or gauze filler dressing.	
(1) Trim dressing to cover wound and dressing, so it will extend onto periwound skin approximately 2.5 to 5 cm (1 to 2 inches).	Prepares dressing for appropriate size of the wound.
(2) Apply transparent dressing, keeping it airtight and wrinkle-free (see illustration).	Dressing should be airtight with no wrinkles or tunnels to maintain a negative-pressure environment. A snug and tight application of the dressing must be applied to ensure an airtight seal (Box 48.10).
(3) Secure tubing to transparent film, aligning drainage holes to ensure occlusive seal. Do not apply tension.	Excessive tension may compress foam dressing and impede wound healing. It also produces shear force on periwound area (Netsch et al., 2016).
(4) Secure tubing several centimeters away from dressing, avoiding pressure points.	Drainage tubes over bony pressure prominences can cause medical device–related pressure injuries (Netsch et al., 2016; Pittman et al., 2015).
14. After wound is completely covered, connect tubing from dressing to tubing from canister and NPWT unit and set at ordered suction level.	Intermittent or continuous negative pressure varies from −75 mm Hg to −125 mm Hg, depending on the device and the characteristics of the wound (Netsch et al., 2016; WOCN, 2016).
a. Remove canister from sterile packing and push unit until you hear click. **NOTE:** An alarm sounds if canister is not properly engaged.	

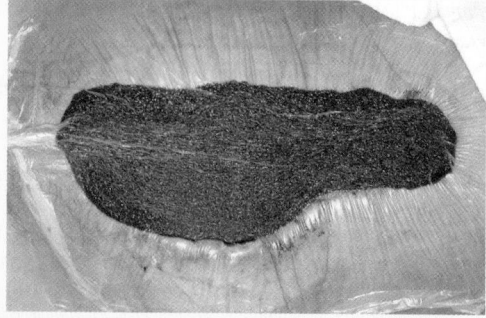

STEP 13d(2) Foam wound filler; transparent dressing over existing wound. (Courtesy Kinetic Concepts, Inc [KCI], San Antonio, Texas.)

STEP	RATIONALE

b. Connect dressing tubing to canister tubing (follow manufacturers' instructions). Make sure that both clamps are open.

c. Place on level surface or hang from foot of bed. **NOTE:** Unit alarms and deactivates therapy if it is tilted beyond 45 degrees.

d. Press power button (commonly this is a green-lit button) and set pressure as ordered.

15. Remove and dispose of gloves. Perform hand hygiene. — Reduces transmission of microorganisms.

16. Inspect NPWT system.

    a. Verify that the system is on. This is different for each type of NPWT unit. For example, on some units the display screen shows "Therapy On." Check agency policy and procedure for specific information.

    b. Verify that all clamps are open and that all tubing is patent.

    c. Examine system to be sure that seal is intact and therapy is working. — Negative pressure is achieved when a tight seal is present (Netsch et al., 2016).

    d. If a leak is present, perform hand hygiene and apply gloves. Use strips of transparent dressing to patch areas around edges of wound.

17. Record initials, date, and time on new dressing. — Provides reference for next dressing change.

18. Discard gloves and dispose of any dressing material. Perform hand hygiene. — Prevents transmission of microorganisms.

19. Help patient to comfortable position. Patients may ambulate with NPWT. — Enhances patient comfort and relaxation.

20. Raise side rails (as appropriate) and lower bed to lowest position. — Provides for patient safety and reduces the risk for falls.

21. Place call nurse call system within reach; instruct patient in use. — Provides patient or family member a resource to call for assistance.

EVALUATION

1. Inspect condition of wound and wound bed on an ongoing basis; note drainage and odor. — Determines status of wound healing.

2. Ask patient to rate pain using scale of 0 to 10. — Determines patient's level of comfort following procedure.

3. Verify airtight dressing seal and correct negative-pressure setting. — Determines effective negative pressure being applied.

4. Measure wound drainage output in canister on regular basis. — Monitors fluid balance and wound drainage.

5. **Use Teach-Back:** "Before you are discharged, I want to be sure I have explained clearly what your wound should look like as it is healing and the signs of infection. Explain to me what your wound will look like as it begins to heal." Revise your instruction now or develop a plan for revised patient/family caregiver teaching if patient/family caregiver is not able to teach back correctly. — Determines patient's/family caregiver's level of understanding of instructional topic.

UNEXPECTED OUTCOMES AND RELATED INTERVENTIONS

1. Wound appears inflamed and tender, wound hemorrhages, drainage has increased, and odor is present.
- Notify health care provider.
- Obtain wound culture.
- May need to stop NPWT.

2. Patient reports increase in pain.
- Consult with health care provider about changing analgesia.
- Instill normal saline to moisten filler dressings to allow loosening from granulation tissue.
- Decrease pressure setting.
- Change from intermittent to continuous cycling.
- Change type of NPWT system.

3. Negative-pressure seal has broken.
- Take preventive measures (Box 48.10).

RECORDING AND REPORTING

- Record appearance of wound (characteristics of wound bed and drainage), placement of NPWT, negative pressure setting, and patient's response in electronic health record (EHR) or chart.
- Report brisk, bright bleeding; evidence of poor wound healing; and possible wound infection to health care provider.
- Report on location of NPWT, time of dressing change if done, and any interventions, such as reinforcement of dressing.
- Discuss whether the patient or caregiver is participating in changing the NPWT dressing.
- Document your evaluation of patient learning

HOME CARE CONSIDERATIONS

- Be sure that patient and family members understand the importance of maintaining a seal on the NPWT dressing and that they have been educated on how to seal the dressing and know whom to call if the alarm alerts them to a leak of the system and they are unable to seal.
- Review how to attach the device to a wall outlet to recharge the battery.
- Instruct the patient and family members on the schedule for the NPWT change.

SKILL 48.5   PERFORMING WOUND IRRIGATION

Delegation and Collaboration

The skill of wound irrigation cannot be delegated to assistive personnel (AP) unless it is a chronic wound (see agency policy). It is the nurse's responsibility to assess and document wound characteristics. Direct the AP to:

- Notify the nurse when the wound is exposed, so an assessment can be completed.
- Report to the nurse the patient's pain, presence of blood, drainage.

Equipment

- Irrigation/cleansing solution per order (volume 1.5 to 2 times the estimated wound volume)
- Irrigation delivery system (per order), depending on amount of desired pressure: sterile irrigation 35-mL syringe with sterile soft angiocatheter or 19-gauge needle (WOCN, 2016) or handheld shower.
- Personal protective equipment (PPE): sterile gloves, gown, and goggles if splash or spray risk exists
- Waterproof underpad if needed
- Dressing supplies (see Skills 48.2 and 48.3)
- Disposable waterproof biohazard bag
- Wound assessment supplies (see Skill 48.2)

STEP	RATIONALE

ASSESSMENT

1. Identify patient using at least two identifiers (e.g., name and birthday or name and account number) according to agency policy. Compare identifiers with information on patient's MAR or medical record.

Ensures correct patient. Complies with The Joint Commission standards and improves patient safety (TJC, 2020).

2. Review health care provider's order for irrigation of open wound and type of solution to be used.

Open-wound irrigation requires medical order, including type of solution(s) to use.

3. Review medical record for signs and symptoms related to patient's open wound.

Provides ongoing data to indicate change in wound status (Nix, 2016).

   a. Extent of impairment of skin integrity, including size of wound

   b. Verify number of drains present.

Awareness of drain position facilitates safe dressing removal and determines need for special dressings.

   c. Drainage, including amount, color, consistency, and any odor noted

Ongoing data; drainage should decrease in healing wound. When drainage increases, it is often related to infection (Doughty and Sparks et al., 2016).

   d. Wound tissue color

Color represents type of tissue present in the wound; red tissue indicates healthy tissue; white, brown, or black tissue is devitalized tissue. Proper selection of wound-care products on basis of wound color facilitates removal of necrotic tissue and promotes new tissue growth (Nix, 2016).

   e. Culture reports. Infected wound is colonized with bacteria.

Culture reports identify type of bacteria and proper treatment. Ongoing wound cultures document resolution of infectious process (Stotts, 2016b).

4. Assess patient's/family caregiver's knowledge, experience, and health literacy level.

Ensures patient has the capacity to obtain, communicate, process, and understand basic health information (CDC, 2019).

5. Assess patient's level of comfort using pain scale of 0 to 10.

Serves as baseline to measure patient's level of comfort before wound irrigation.

6. Assess patient for history of allergies to antiseptics, solutions, medications, tapes, or dressing material.

Known allergies suggest applying sample of prescribed wound treatment as skin test before flushing wound with large volume of solution or selecting different tape or dressing material.

7. Assess patient's and family caregiver's understanding of need for irrigation and of signs of wound infection.

Determines extent of instruction required.

PLANNING

1. Perform hand hygiene and administer prescribed analgesic as needed 30 minutes before dressing change.

Comfortable patient will be less likely to move suddenly, causing contamination of wound or supplies.

2. Gather appropriate supplies for wound irrigation and dressing.

Ensures an organized procedure.

3. Explain procedure to patient and family caregiver, instructing not to touch wound or sterile supplies.

Relieves anxiety and promotes understanding of healing process. Prevents contamination of sterile supplies.

4. Close room door or bedside curtains, perform hand hygiene, and position patient.

Maintains privacy.

   a. Position patient comfortably to permit gravitational flow of irrigating solution over wound and into collection receptacle (see illustration).

Directing solution from top to bottom of wound and from cleanest to contaminated area prevents further infection. Position also avoids fluid retention in the wound as the flow of the irrigant moves away from the wound.

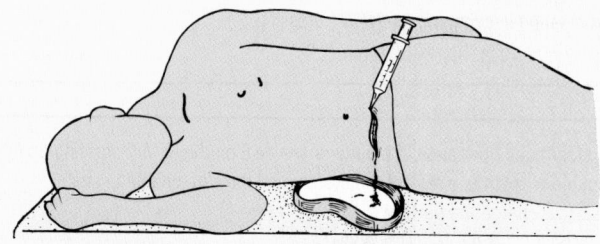

STEP 4a Patient position for wound irrigation.

STEP	RATIONALE
b. Ensure that irrigant is at room temperature, and position patient so that wound is vertical to collection basin.	Room temperature solution increases comfort and reduces vasoconstriction response in tissues
c. Place padding or extra towel on bed under area where irrigation will take place.	Protects bedding from becoming wet.

IMPLEMENTATION

STEP	RATIONALE
1. Perform hand hygiene.	Reduces transmission of microorganisms.
2. Form cuff on waterproof biohazard bag and place near bed.	Cuffing helps to maintain large opening, thereby permitting placement of contaminated dressings without touching bag itself.
3. Apply gown, mask, goggles as indicated; apply clean gloves and remove old dressing. Clean wound (see Skill 48.2).	Reduces transmission of microorganisms. Protects from splashes or sprays of blood and body fluids. While cleaning wound, use meticulous hand hygiene and proper infection control procedures before and after removing soiled dressings to limit risk for health care–acquired infection (Jaszarowski and Murphree, 2016).
4. Discard old dressing and gloves in biohazard bag. Perform hand hygiene.	Reduces transmission of microorganisms.
5. Apply clean or sterile gloves (check agency policy). Perform wound assessment (see Skill 48.2) and examine recent charted assessment of patient's open wound.	Provides ongoing wound-healing data. Use sterile precautions when sterile gloves are needed.
6. Expose area near wound only.	Provides privacy and prevents chilling of patient.
7. Irrigate wound with wide opening:	The cleansing solution is introduced directly into the wound with a syringe, a syringe and catheter, or a pulsed lavage device.
a. Fill 35-mL syringe with irrigation solution.	Irrigating wound uses mechanical force, which helps with separation and removal of necrotic debris and surface bacteria (Jaszarowski and Murphree, 2016). Flushing wound helps remove debris and facilitates healing by secondary intention.
b. Attach 19-gauge angiocatheter.	Catheter lumen delivers ideal pressure for cleaning and removing debris with minimal risk for tissue injury (Ramundo, 2016). Mechanical debridement is achieved with irrigation pressures delivered between 4 and 15 psi (WOCN, 2016).

> **CLINICAL DECISION:** *Pulsatile high-pressure lavage is an alternative to using the 35-mL syringe and the 19-gauge angiocatheter. A pulsatile lavage machine combines intermittent high-pressure lavage with suction to loosen necrotic tissue and facilitate removal by other methods of debridement (Ramundo, 2016).*

STEP	RATIONALE
c. Hold syringe tip 2.5 cm (1 inch) above upper end of wound and over area being cleaned.	Prevents syringe contamination. Careful placement of syringe prevents unsafe pressure of flowing solution.
d. Using continuous pressure, flush wound; repeat Steps 7a to 7d until solution draining into basin is clear.	Flushing wound helps to remove debris; clear solution indicates removal of all debris.
8. Irrigate deep wound with very small opening:	
a. Attach soft catheter to filled irrigation syringe.	Catheter permits direct flow of irrigant into wound. Expect wound to take longer to empty when opening is small.
b. Gently insert tip of catheter into opening about 1.3 cm (0.5 inch).	Prevents tip from touching fragile inner wall of wound.

> **CLINICAL DECISION:** *Do not force catheter into the wound because this will cause tissue damage.*

STEP	RATIONALE
c. Using slow, continuous pressure, flush wound.	Use of slow mechanical force of stream of solution loosens particulate matter on wound surface and promotes healing (Ramundo, 2016).

> **CLINICAL DECISION:** *Pulsatile high-pressure lavage is often the irrigation of choice for necrotic wounds. Pressure settings should be set per provider order, usually between 4 and 15 psi, and should not be used on skin grafts, exposed blood vessels, muscle, tendon, or bone. Use with caution if patient has coagulation disorder or is taking anticoagulants (Ramundo, 2016).*

STEP	RATIONALE
d. While keeping catheter in place, pinch it off just below syringe.	Avoids contamination of sterile solution.
e. Remove and refill syringe. Reconnect to catheter and repeat until solution draining into basin is clear.	
9. Clean wound with handheld shower:	
a. With patient seated comfortably in shower chair or standing if condition allows, adjust spray to gentle flow; make sure that water is warm.	Useful for patients able to shower with help or independently. May be accomplished at home.
b. Shower for 5 to 10 minutes with shower head 30 cm (12 inches) from wound.	Ensures that wound is cleaned thoroughly.
10. When indicated, obtain cultures after cleaning with nonbacteriostatic saline.	WOCN (2016) recommends using quantitative bacterial cultures (tissue biopsy or swab cultures). The most common types of wound cultures are swab technique, aspirated wound fluid, or tissue biopsy.

Continued

SKILL 48.5	PERFORMING WOUND IRRIGATION—cont'd
STEP	**RATIONALE**

CLINICAL DECISION: *Obtain a wound culture if indicated by the presence of inflammation around the wound, purulent odor or drainage, new drainage, or a febrile patient.*

STEP	RATIONALE
11. Dry wound edges with gauze; dry patient after shower.	Prevents maceration of surrounding tissue from excess moisture.
12. Remove and dispose of gloves. Perform hand hygiene. Apply clean or sterile gloves (see agency policy). Apply appropriate dressing and label with time, date, and nurse's initials.	Reduces transmission of microorganisms. Maintains protective barrier and healing environment for wound.
13. Remove mask, goggles, and gown.	Prevents transfer of microorganisms.
14. Dispose of equipment and soiled supplies; remove and dispose of gloves. Perform hand hygiene.	Reduces transmission of microorganisms.
15. Help patient to comfortable position.	
16. Raise side rails (as appropriate) and lower bed to lowest position.	Provides for patient safety and reduces the risk for falls.
17. Place nurse call system within reach; instruct patient in use.	Assists patient or family member in calling for assistance.

EVALUATION

1. Have patient rate level of comfort on scale of 0 to 10.	Patient's pain should not increase as a result of wound irrigation.
2. Monitor type of tissue in wound bed.	Identifies wound healing progress and determines type of wound cleaning and dressing needed.
3. Inspect dressing periodically (see agency policy).	Determines patient's response to wound irrigation and need to modify plan of care.
4. Evaluate periwound skin integrity.	Determines whether extension of wound has occurred or signs of infection are present (warm red periwound skin).
5. Observe for presence of retained irrigant.	Retained irrigant is medium for bacterial growth and subsequent infection.
6. **Use Teach-Back:** "I want to be sure that I explained how to irrigate your wound. You are going to be doing this at home; please show me how you will irrigate the wound with this syringe." Revise your instruction now or develop a plan for revised patient/family caregiver teaching if patient/family caregiver is not able to teach back correctly.	Determines patient's/family caregiver's level of understanding of instructional topic.

UNEXPECTED OUTCOMES AND RELATED INTERVENTIONS

1. Bleeding or serosanguineous drainage appears.
   - Flush wound during next irrigation using less pressure.
   - Notify health care provider of bleeding.
2. Increased pain or discomfort occurs.
   - Decrease force of pressure during wound irrigation.
   - Assess patient for need for additional analgesia before wound care.
3. Suture line opening extends.
   - Notify health care provider.
   - Reevaluate amount of pressure to use for next wound irrigation.

RECORDING AND REPORTING

- Record wound assessment before and after irrigation, amount and type of solution used, irrigation device used, patient tolerance of the procedure, and type of dressing applied after irrigation in electronic health record (EHR) or chart.
- Document your evaluation of patient learning.
- Report the location of the wound irrigated; discuss the type of solution used, the quality of the return irrigation, and the last time the wound was irrigated.
- Immediately report to the attending health care provider any evidence of fresh bleeding, sharp increase in pain, retention of irrigant, or signs of shock.

HOME CARE CONSIDERATIONS

- Teach the patient and family caregiver how to make normal saline, especially if cost is an issue. You make normal saline by using 8 tsp of salt in 1 gallon of distilled water.
- Instruct the family caregiver on irrigation technique, and have the caregiver demonstrate.
- Be sure the patient and family know signs of infection and when to notify the health care provider.

| SKILL 48.6 | APPLYING GAUZE OR ELASTIC BANDAGE |

Delegation and Collaboration

The skill of applying a gauze or an elastic bandage for compression cannot be delegated to assistive personnel (AP). A nurse assesses the condition of any wound or dressing before applying a bandage. The skill of applying bandages to secure nonsterile dressings can be delegated to AP (refer to agency policy). Direct the AP about:

- Modifying the bandage application, such as with special taping.
- Reviewing what to observe and report back to the nurse (e.g., patient's complaint of pain, numbness, or tingling after application or changes in patient's skin color or temperature).

Equipment

- Correct width and number of gauze or elastic bandages
- Clips or adhesive tape
- Clean gloves if wound drainage is present
- *Option:* Pillow

STEP	RATIONALE

ASSESSMENT

1. Identify patient using at least two identifiers (e.g., name and birthday or name and account number) according to agency policy. Compare identifiers with information on patient's MAR or medical record.	Ensures correct patient. Complies with The Joint Commission standards and improves patient safety (TJC, 2020).
2. Review patient's medical record for specific orders related to application of gauze or elastic bandage. Note area to be covered, type of bandage required, frequency of change, and previous response to treatment.	Ensures use of correct products.
3. Assess patient's/family caregiver's knowledge, experience, and health literacy level.	Ensures patient/family caregiver has the capacity to obtain, communicate, process, and understand basic health information (CDC, 2019).
4. Assess patient's level of comfort (pain scale of 0 to 10).	Serves as baseline to measure patient's level of comfort when dressing change is performed.
5. Perform hand hygiene. Observe adequacy of circulation to extremity by palpating temperature of skin and pulses, presence of edema, and sensation (distal to area to be bandaged). Observe skin color and movement of body part to be wrapped.	Assesses status of circulation to extremity. Impaired circulation from constricting bandage may delay wound healing. Detection of change to circulation requires frequent observation.

> **CLINICAL DECISION**: *Impaired circulation may result in pain, coolness to touch when compared with the opposite side of the body, cyanosis or pallor of skin, diminished or absent pulses, edema or localized pooling, and numbness and/or tingling of body part.*

6. Apply clean gloves (if drainage or break in skin is present). Inspect skin of area to be bandaged for alterations in integrity as indicated by presence of abrasion, discoloration, or chafing. Pay close attention to areas over bony prominences and areas around medical devices.	It is important to determine whether any new skin alterations are present so that the plan of care can be altered as needed. Bony prominences and pressure areas from medical devices are areas at high risk for skin injury.
7. Inspect the condition of any wound for appearance, size, and presence and character of drainage, and be sure that it is covered with a proper dressing. If not, reapply dressing (check agency policy for type of gloves to use). Remove and dispose of gloves and perform hand hygiene.	An ongoing wound assessment is necessary to judge the progress or lack of progress of the wound toward healing and to plan the appropriate interventions.
8. Assess for size of bandage:	
a. *Gauze or basic elastic bandage to secure a dressing:* Assess size of area to be covered. Each successive roll of gauze/elastic should overlap previous layer. Use smaller widths for upper extremities, larger widths for lower extremities.	A bandage too small or too large for the area may not provide the necessary support to stabilize underlying dressings.
b. Elastic bandage to provide simple *compression:* Assess circumference of lower extremity before or shortly after patient gets out of bed in the morning or after patient has been in bed for at least 15 minutes. Select width that will cover and overlap without bulkiness.	An elastic bandage that is too large may not provide sufficient support to immobilize and protect an injured extremity. An elastic bandage that is too small may compromise circulation to the distal extremity.
9. Assess patient's and family caregiver's knowledge of purpose of dressing and whether they will participate in dressing wound.	Identifies patient's learning needs. Prepares patient and family caregivers if dressing will need to be changed at home.

PLANNING

1. Close room door and pull curtain around the patient's bed. Position patient so that only the affected wound or extremity is exposed; use sheet to cover rest of the body.	Provides privacy and places patient in a position of comfort.
2. Perform hand hygiene and administer prescribed analgesic as needed 30 minutes before applying bandage.	Comfortable patient will be less likely to move suddenly, causing wound or supply contamination or extremity pain.
3. Gather and organize equipment at bedside.	Ensures a clean and distraction-free procedure.
4. Explain procedure to patient before starting.	Reduces anxiety and provides opportunity for patient/family caregiver education.

Continued

SKILL 48.6   APPLYING GAUZE OR ELASTIC BANDAGE—cont'd

STEP	RATIONALE

IMPLEMENTATION

1. Perform hand hygiene and apply clean gloves if drainage is present.

   Reduces transmission of microorganisms.

2. Apply gauze or elastic bandage to secure dressings:

   a. Make sure that primary dressing over wound is securely in place.

   Wound needs to remain protected once bandage in place.

   b. Hold roll of bandage in your dominant hand and use other hand to lightly hold beginning layer.

   Maintains appropriate and consistent bandage tension.

   c. Apply bandage from distal point toward proximal boundary, using appropriate turns to cover various shapes of body parts.

   Bandage is applied in this manner so that it conforms evenly to body part and promotes venous return.

   (1) Spiral dressing is often used to cover cylindrical body parts, such as a wrist. Roll gauze, overlapping each layer by one-half to two-thirds the width of the bandage (see illustration)

   (2) Use figure-eight dressing to cover joint because a snug fit provides support and immobilization to an injured joint. To apply overlap turns, alternate ascending and descending over bandaged part, each turn crossing previous one to form a figure-eight.

CLINICAL DECISION: *Double-check your tension and ensure that bandage is snug but not tight and that primary dressing or splint is positioned correctly. A tight bandage may cause numbness and tingling from impaired circulation and/or pressure on peripheral nerves.*

---

   (3) Unroll and very slightly stretch bandage.

   Maintains bandage tension.

   (4) Overlap turns by one-half to two-thirds width of bandage roll.

   Prevents uneven bandage tension and circulatory impairment.

   (5) Secure bandage with clip before applying additional rolls.

   (6) End bandage with two circular turns; secure end of gauze or elastic bandage to outside layer of bandage, not skin, with tape or clips (see illustration).

CLINICAL DECISION: *Keep toes or fingertips uncovered and visible for follow-up circulatory assessment, except in cases in which toes or fingers are treated because of wounds.*

---

3. Apply elastic bandage over amputated stump (see illustrations):

   Elevation promotes venous return. Bandage turns are designed for uniform bandage tension.

   a. Elevate stump with pillow or support it with the help of another person.

   b. Secure bandage by wrapping it twice around proximal end of stump or person's waist (depending on size of stump)

   c. Make half turn with bandage perpendicular to its edge.

   d. Bring body of bandage over distal end of stump.

   e. Continue to fold bandage over stump, wrapping from distal to proximal points.

   f. Secure with metal clips, Velcro if provided, or tape,

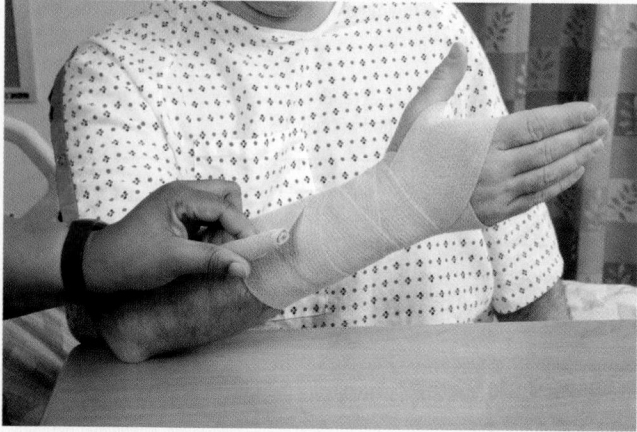

STEP 2c(1) Apply bandage from distal to proximal.

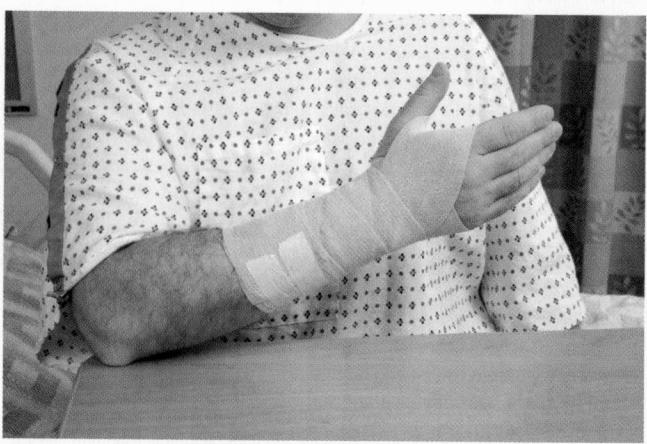

STEP 2c(6) Secure with tape or closure device.

STEP	RATIONALE
4. Remove and dispose of gloves if worn and perform hand hygiene.	Reduces transmission of microorganisms.
5. Help patient to comfortable position.	
6. Raise side rails (as appropriate) and lower bed to lowest position.	Provides for patient safety and reduces the risk for falls.
7. Place nurse call system within reach; instruct patient in use.	Assists patient or family member in calling for assistance.

EVALUATION

1. Assess degree of tightness of bandage and presence of wrinkles, looseness, and of drainage.	Identifies any pressure areas that may cause tissue injury.
2. When bandage application is complete, at least twice during next 8 hours, and then at least every shift assess distal extremity circulation.	Early detection of circulatory impairment promotes neurovascular functioning.
a. Observe skin color for pallor or cyanosis and palpate skin for warmth.	Pallor and cyanosis and cool skin as compared to other extremity indicate diminished blood flow.
b. Palpate distal pulses and compare bilaterally.	Documents status of circulatory flow.
c. Ask patient to rate any pain on scale of 0 to 10 and to describe any numbness, tingling, or other discomfort to evaluate for neurological and vascular changes.	Signs of neurovascular changes that indicate impaired venous return.
3. Observe mobility of extremity.	Determines whether bandage is too tight, which restricts movement, or if joint immobilization is attained.
4. **Use Teach-Back:** "I want to be sure I explained how to apply the elastic roll to your sprained ankle. Show me how you would apply this elastic roll to your ankle." Revise your instruction now or develop a plan for revised patient/family caregiver teaching if patient/family caregiver is not able to teach back correctly.	Determines patient's/family's level of understanding of instructional topic.

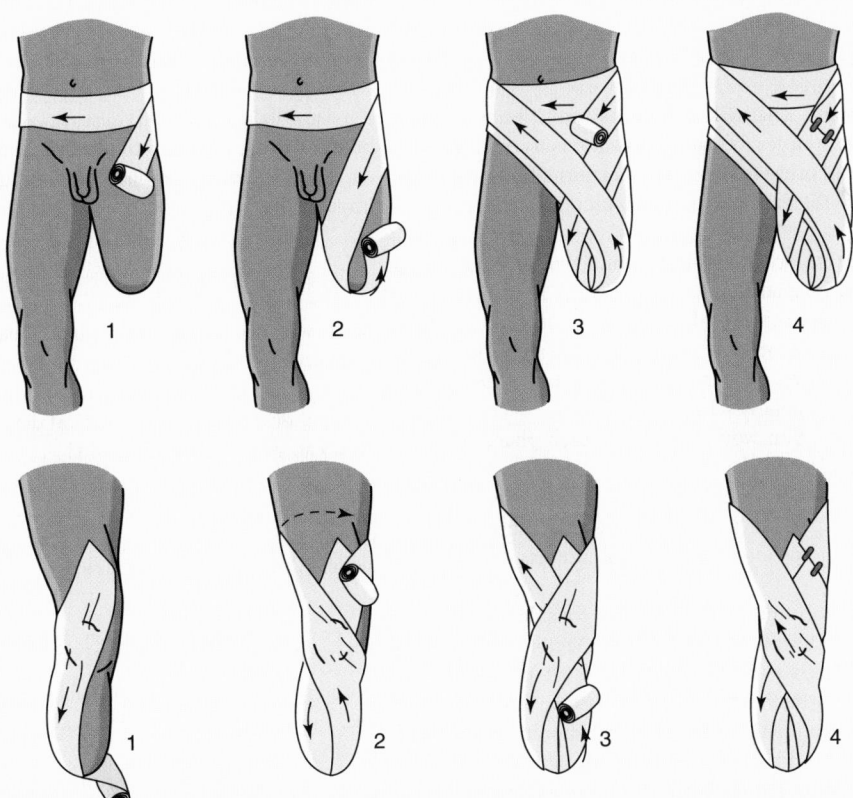

STEP 3 *Top,* correct method for bandaging midthigh amputation stump. Note that bandage must be anchored around patient's waist. *Bottom,* correct method for bandaging midcalf amputation stump. Note that bandage need not be anchored around waist. (From Monahan F et al: *Phipps' medical-surgical nursing: health and illness perspectives,* ed 8, St Louis, 2006, Mosby.)

Continued

| **SKILL 48.6** | **APPLYING GAUZE OR ELASTIC BANDAGE—cont'd** |

UNEXPECTED OUTCOMES AND RELATED INTERVENTIONS

1. Impaired circulation distal to elastic bandage
   - Release bandage
   - Palpate extremity and assess pulse, temperature, and capillary refill. **NOTE:** If abnormal, notify health care provider.
   - Reapply bandage with less pressure.
2. Patient complains of pain or numbness in extremity.
   - Unwrap bandage, check extremity temperature, note color of tissue, compare to other extremity, and check pulse.
   - Rewrap with less tension and assess patient's response. **NOTE:** If same complaint is present, notify health care provider.

RECORDING AND REPORTING

- Record patient's level of comfort, circulation status, type of bandage applied, presence of swelling, and range of motion at baseline and after bandage application on flow sheet in nurses' notes in electronic health record (EHR) or chart.
- Document your evaluation of patient learning.
- Report any changes in neurological or circulatory status to health care provider.

HOME CARE CONSIDERATIONS

- Demonstrate to patient or family caregiver how to correctly apply bandage so that it is not too tight.
- Instruct patient or family caregiver about the signs of impaired circulation.
- Elastic bandages that reduce swelling are best applied to the feet and ankles in the morning, before getting out of bed.
- Instruct patient and family caregiver to remove an elastic bandage daily and inspect skin beneath it twice daily.

▌KEY POINTS

- It is important to understand what risk factors may contribute to pressure injury formation in order to plan interventions to reduce or eliminate risk factors and prevent pressure injury formation.
- Pressure injury stages describe the depth of tissue injury, which will guide treatment.
- Most wounds heal in a normal trajectory, but chronic wounds may fail to heal; an overview of normal wound healing is key to understanding how to assess and plan care for the patient with a wound.
- Valid and reliable risk-assessment tools assess a patient's risk for developing a pressure injury and are completed on admission to a health care agency and on a regularly scheduled basis.
- Primary and secondary intention wounds differ in each phase of wound healing, which impacts the plan of care.
- Assessment of the patient with a wound will include the systemic and local complications that affect wound healing and must be addressed with the appropriate interventions that address those complications.
- Many factors that affect wound healing need to be considered in managing the patient with a wound. The negative factors, such as diabetes and smoking, need to be addressed, and the positive effects, such as an adequate protein intake, need to be supported.
- Acute wounds are usually traumatic or surgical and should move predictably through the wound healing process. Chronic wounds are caused by vascular compromise, reinjury, or chronic inflammation and fail to close or heal in a timely fashion.
- A wound assessment provides the foundation for developing a care plan, including selection of the correct treatment or dressing.

- Perform wound irrigation in a manner that avoids further injury to tissue.
- Exposure to heat and cold causes normal systemic and local responses but can also cause injury to the skin if applied too long or incorrectly.
- An elastic bandage applied too tightly can result in circulatory impairment.

▌REFLECTIVE LEARNING

- What will you include in a plan of care for impaired sacral skin integrity?
- During postclinical conference you discuss skin impairment from medical devices. How do medical devices create pressure injuries? How can you reduce these risks?
- A patient has a foul-smelling tan-colored drainage from a recent hip incision; the staples were removed, and an order was written for moist saline gauze dressing to the area 3 times a day. What are the critical wound assessment factors?

▌REVIEW QUESTIONS

1. When repositioning an immobile patient, the nurse notices redness over the hip bone. What is indicated when a reddened area blanches on fingertip touch?
   1. A local skin infection requiring antibiotics
   2. Sensitive skin that requires special bed linen
   3. A stage 3 pressure injury needing the appropriate dressing
   4. Blanching hyperemia, indicating the attempt by the body to overcome the ischemic episode

2. Match the pressure injury stages with the correct definition.

1. Stage 1 **a.** Partial-thickness loss of skin with exposed dermis.
2. Stage 2   The wound bed is viable, pink or red, moist, and
3. Stage 3   may also present as an intact or ruptured serum-
4. Stage 4   filled blister. Adipose (fat) is not visible, and
      deeper tissues are not visible. Granulation tissue,
      slough, and eschar are not present. These injuries
      commonly result from adverse microclimate and
      shear in the skin over the pelvis and shear in the
      heel. This stage should not be used to describe
      moisture-associated skin damage (MASD), includ-
      ing incontinence-associated dermatitis (IAD),
      intertriginous dermatitis (ITD), medical adhesive–
      related skin injury (MARSI), or traumatic wounds
      (skin tears, burns, abrasions).

    b. Intact skin with a localized area of nonblanchable
      erythema, which may appear differently in darkly
      pigmented skin. Presence of blanchable erythema
      or changes in sensation, temperature, or firmness
      may precede visual changes. Color changes do
      not include purple or maroon discoloration;
      these may indicate deep tissue pressure injury.

    c. Full-thickness skin and tissue loss with exposed
      or directly palpable fascia, muscle, tendon, liga-
      ment, cartilage, or bone in the ulcer. Slough and/
      or eschar may be visible. Epibole (rolled edges),
      undermining, and/or tunneling often occurs.
      Depth varies by anatomical location. If slough or
      eschar obscures the extent of tissue loss, this is an
      Unstageable Pressure Injury.

    d. Full-thickness loss of skin, in which adipose (fat)
      is visible in the ulcer and granulation tissue and
      epibole (rolled wound edges) are often present.
      Slough and/or eschar may be visible. The depth
      of tissue damage varies by anatomical location;
      areas of significant adiposity can develop deep
      wounds. Undermining and tunneling may occur.
      Fascia, muscle, tendon, ligament, cartilage, and/
      or bone are not exposed. If slough or eschar
      obscures the extent of tissue loss, this is an
      Unstageable Pressure Injury.

3. After surgery the patient with a closed abdominal wound reports a sudden "pop" after coughing. When the nurse examines the surgical wound site, the sutures are open, and pieces of small bowel are noted at the bottom of the now-opened wound. Which are the priority nursing interventions? (Select all that apply.)
   1. Notify the health care provider.
   2. Allow the area to be exposed to air until all drainage has stopped.
   3. Place several cold packs over the area, protecting the skin around the wound.
   4. Cover the area with sterile, saline-soaked towels immediately.
   5. Cover the area with sterile gauze and apply an abdominal binder.

4. What is the correct sequence of steps when performing wound irrigation to a large open wound?
   1. Use slow, continuous pressure to irrigate wound.
   2. Attach 19-gauge angiocatheter to syringe.
   3. Fill syringe with irrigation fluid.
   4. Place biohazard bag near bed.
   5. Position angiocatheter over wound.

5. Which skin-care measures are used to manage a patient who is experiencing fecal and/or urinary incontinence? (Select all that apply.)
   1. Frequent position changes
   2. Keeping the buttocks exposed to air at all times
   3. Using a large absorbent diaper, changing when saturated
   4. Using an incontinence cleaner
   5. Applying a moisture barrier ointment

6. Which of the following describes a hydrocolloid dressing?
   1. A seaweed derivative that is highly absorptive
   2. Premoistened gauze placed over a granulating wound
   3. A debriding enzyme that is used to remove necrotic tissue
   4. A dressing that forms a gel that interacts with the wound surface

7. Which of the following is an indication for a binder to be placed around a surgical patient with a new abdominal wound? (Select all that apply.)
   1. Collection of wound drainage
   2. Providing support to abdominal tissues when coughing or walking
   3. Reduction of abdominal swelling
   4. Reduction of stress on the abdominal incision
   5. Stimulation of peristalsis (return of bowel function) from direct pressure

8. When is the application of a warm compress to an ankle muscle sprain indicated? (Select all that apply.)
   1. To relieve edema
   2. To reduce shivering
   3. To improve blood flow to an injured part
   4. To protect bony prominences from pressure injuries
   5. To immobilize area

9. What is the removal of devitalized tissue from a wound called?
   1. Debridement
   2. Pressure distribution
   3. Negative-pressure wound therapy
   4. Sanitization

10. Which of the following are measures to reduce tissue damage from shear? (Select all that apply.)
    1. Use a transfer device (e.g., transfer board)
    2. Have head of bed elevated when transferring patient
    3. Have head of bed flat when repositioning patient
    4. Raise head of bed 60 degrees when patient positioned supine
    5. Raise head of bed 30 degrees when patient positioned supine

Answers: 1. 4; **2.** Stage 1 is *b*, stage 2 is *a*, stage 3 is *d*, and stage 4 is *c*; **3.** 1, 4; **4.** 4, 3, 2, 5, 1; **5.** 1, 4; **6.** 4; **7.** 2, 4; **8.** 1, 3; **9.** 1; **10.** 1, 3, 5.

Rationales for Review Questions can be found on the Evolve website.

REFERENCES

Ayello EA, et al: Pressure ulcers. In Baranoski S, Ayello AE, editors: *Wound care essentials: practice principles*, ed 4, Philadelphia, 2016, Lippincott Williams & Wilkins.

Ayello EA: CMS MDS 3.0 Section M Skin Conditions in long-term care: pressure ulcers, skin tears, and moisture-associated skin damage data update, *Adv Skin Wound Care* 30(9):415, 2017.

Baranoski S, et al: Wound assessment. In Baranoski S, Ayello AE, editors: *Wound care essentials: practice principles*, ed 4, Philadelphia, 2016, Lippincott, Williams & Wilkins.

Bates-Jensen BM: Assessment of the patient with a wound. In *Core curriculum: wound management*, Philadelphia, PA, 2016, Wolters Kluwer.

Berlowitz D: *Epidemiology, pathogenesis, and risk assessment of pressure-induced skin and soft tissue injury*, UpToDate, 2018. https://uptodate.com/contents/epidemiology-pathogenesis-and-risk-assessment-of-pressure-induced-skin-and-soft-tissue-injury. .

Black J, et al: Use of wound dressings to enhance prevention of pressure ulcers caused by medical devices, *Int Wound J* 12:322, 2015.

Branson RD, et al: Management of the artifical airway, *Respir Care* 59(6):974, 2014.

Brienza D, et al: Friction-induced skin injuries—are they pressure ulcers? An updated NPUAP White Paper, *J Wound Ostomy Continence Nurs* 42(1):62, 2015.

Bryant RA: Types of skin damage and differential diagnosis. In Bryant RA, Nix DP, editors: *Acute and chronic wounds: current management concepts*, ed 5, St Louis, 2016, Elsevier.

Bryant RA, Nix DP: Developing and maintaining a pressure ulcer prevention program. In Bryant RA, Nix DP, editors: *Acute and chronic wounds: current management concepts*, ed 5, St Louis, 2016a, Elsevier.

Bryant RA, Nix DP: Principles of wound healing and topical management. In Bryant RA, Nix DP, editors: *Acute and chronic wounds: current management concepts*, ed 5, St Louis, 2016b, Elsevier.

Burden M, Thornton M: Reducing the risks of surgical site infection: the importance of the multidisciplinary team, *Br J Nurs* 27(17):976, 2018.

Canadian Agency for Drugs and Technologies in Health (CADTH): *CADTH rapid response report: summary of abstracts - The Use of Medical Glue to Close Surgical Wounds: Clinical Effectiveness and Guidelines*, 2017. https://www.cadth.ca/sites/default/files/pdf/htis/2017/RB1133%20-%20Medical%20Glue%20Final.pdf. Accessed November 24, 2019.

Centers for Disease Control and Prevention (CDC): *What is health literacy*, 2019. https://www.cdc.gov/healthliteracy/learn/index.html. Accessed December 23, 2019.

Chaboyer W, et al: Adherence to evidence-based pressure injury prevention guidelines in routine clinical practice: a longitudinal study, *Int Wound J* 14(6):1290, 2017.

Chatterjee R: Elbow pain: the 10-minute assessment, *Co-Kinetic Journal* 73:18, 2017.

Chou R, et al: Management of postoperative pain: a clinical practice guideline from the American Pain Society, the American Society of Regional Anesthesia and Pain Medicine, and the American Society of Anesthesiologists' Committee on Regional Anesthesia, Executive Committee, and Administrative Council, *J Pain* 17(2):131, 2016.

Collier M: Protecting vulnerable skin from moisture-associated skin damage, *Br J Nurs* 25(20):S26, 2016.

Colwell JC, et al: MASD part 3: peristomal moisture–associated dermatitis and periwound moisture–associated dermatitis: a consensus, *J Wound Ostomy Continence Nurs* 38(5):541, 2011.

Demarré L, et al: The cost of prevention and treatment of pressure ulcers: a systematic review, *Int J Nurs Stud* 52(11):1754, 2015.

Doughty D, McNichol L: In *Wound, Ostomy and Continence Nurses Society (WOCN) Core curriculum: wound management*, Philadelphia, 2016, Wound, Ostomy and Continence Nurses Society.

Doughty DB, Sparks B: Wound-healing physiology and factors that affect the repair process. In Bryant RA, Nix DP, editors: *Acute and chronic wounds: current management concepts*, ed 6, St Louis, 2016, Elsevier.

Edsberg LE, et al: Revised National Pressure Ulcer Advisory Panel pressure injury staging system, *J Wound Ostomy Continence Nurs* 43(6):585, 2016.

European Pressure Ulcer Advisory Panel (EPUAP) and National Pressure injury Advisory Panel (NPIAP), and Pan Pacific Pressure Injury Alliance: Treatment of pressure ulcers/injuries: Clinical Practice Guideline. The International Guideline, Emily Haesler (ED). EPUAP/NPIAP/PPPIA, 2019a.

European Pressure Ulcer Advisory Panel (EPUAP) and National Pressure injury Advisory Panel (NPIAP), and Pan Pacific Pressure Injury Alliance: Treatment of pressure ulcers/injuries: Quick Reference Guide, Emily Haesler (ED). EPUAP/NPIAP/PPPIA, 2019b.

Gruccio P, Ashton K: Support surface technology: an essential component of pressure injury prevention, *J Leg Nurse Consult* 29(1):30, 2018.

Haesler E: Evidence summary: pressure injuries: preventing medical device related pressure injuries, *Wound Pract Res* 25(4):214, 2017.

Henderson CT, et al: Draft definition of stage I pressure ulcers: inclusion of persons with darkly pigmented skin, *Adv Wound Care* 10(5):16, 1997.

Hopf H, et al: Managing wound pain. In Bryant RA, Nix DP, editors: *Acute and chronic wounds: current management concepts*, ed 5, St Louis, 2016, Elsevier.

Jaszarowski KA, Murphree RW: Wound cleansing and dressing selection. In Wound, Ostomy and Continence Nurses Society, editor: *Core curriculum: wound management*, Philadelphia, 2016, Wolters Kluwer.

Jordan RS, Phipps S: Understanding therapeutic support surfaces, *Wound Care Advisor*, 2019. https://woundcareadvisor.com/support-surfaces/. Accessed November 24, 2019.

Krasner DL: Wound pain: impact and assessment. In Bryant RA, Nix DP, editors: *Acute and chronic wounds: nursing management*, ed 5, St Louis, 2016, Elsevier.

Makic MB: Medical device–related pressure ulcers and intensive care, *J Perianesth Nurs* 30(4):336, 2015.

Maklebust J, Magnan MA: Pressure ulcer prevention: specific measures and agency-wide strategies. In Doughty DB, McNichol LL, editors: *Core curriculum wound management*, Philadelphia, 2016, Wolters Kluwer.

McNichol L, et al: Medical adhesives and patient safety: state of the science: consensus statements for the assessment, prevention, and treatment of adhesive-related skin injuries, *J Wound Ostomy Continence Nurs* 40(4):365, 2013.

National Health Service (United Kingdom): *How do I care for a wound treated with skin glue?* 2018. https://www.nhs.uk/common-health-questions/accidents-first-aid-and-treatments/how-do-i-care-for-a-wound-treated-with-skin-glue/. Accessed November 24 2019.

National Quality Forum (NQF): *National Voluntary Consensus Standards for Public Reporting of Patient Safety Event Information*, 2011. http://www.qualityforum.org/Publications/2011/02/National_Voluntary_Consensus_Standards_for_Public_Reporting_of_Patient_Safety_Event_Information.aspx. Accessed March 2019.

Netsch DS, et al: Negative-pressure wound therapy. In Bryant RA, Nix DP, editors: *Acute and chronic wounds: current management concepts*, ed 5, St Louis, 2016, Elsevier.

Nix D: Skin and wound inspection and assessment. In Bryant RA, Nix DP, editors: *Acute and chronic wounds: current management concepts*, ed 5, St Louis, 2016, Elsevier.

Padula CA, et al: Prevention of medical device-related pressure injuries associated with respiratory equipment use in a critical care unit, *J Wound Ostomy Continence Nurs* 44(2):138, 2017.

Pieper B: Pressure ulcers: impact, etiology, and classification. In Bryant RA, Nix DP, editors: *Acute and chronic wounds: current management concepts*, ed 5, St Louis, 2016, Elsevier.

Pittman J, et al: Medical device–related hospital-acquired pressure ulcers, *J Wound Ostomy Continence Nurs* 42(2):151, 2015.

Ramundo JM: Wound debridement. In Bryant RA, Nix DP, editors: *Acute and chronic wounds: current management concepts*, ed 5, St Louis, 2016, Elsevier.

Ratliff CR, et al: WOCN 2016 guidelines for prevention and management of pressure injuries (ulcers): an executive summary, *J Wound Ostomy Continence Nurs* 44(3):241, 2017.

Schallom M, et al: Pressure ulcer incidence in patients wearing nasal-oral versus full-face noninvasive ventilation masks, *Am J Crit Care* 24(4):349, 2015.

Stotts NA: Nutritional assessment and support. In Bryant RA, Nix DP, editors: *Acute and chronic wounds: current management concepts*, ed 5, St Louis, 2016a, Elsevier.

Stotts NA: Wound infection: diagnosis and management. In Bryant RA, Nix DP, editors: *Acute and chronic wounds: current management concepts*, ed 5, St Louis, 2016b, Elsevier.

Stryja J: Ten top tips: prevention of surgical site infections, *Wounds Int* 9(2):16, 2018.

The Joint Commission (TJC): *Nutritional, functional and pain assessments and screens*, 2019, update https://www.jointcommission.org/standardsnational-patient-safety-goals/.aspx?StandardsFaqId=1604&ProgramId=46. Accessed January 2019.

The Joint Commission (TJC): *2020 National patient safety goals*, Oakbrook Terrace, IL, 2020, The Commission. https://www.jointcommission.org/en/standards/national-patient-safety-goals/. Accessed January 2, 2020.

US National Library of Medicine: *Preventing pressure ulcers*, 2019. https://medlineplus.gov/ency/patientinstructions/000147.htm. Accessed March 2019.

Weir D, Schultz G: Assessment and management of wound-related infection. In Doughty DB, McNichol LL, editors: *Core curriculum wound management*, Philadelphia, 2016, Walters Kluwer.

Wound Ostomy, Continence Nurses Society (WOCN): *Guideline for prevention and management of pressure ulcers (injuries), WOCN clinical practice guideline series*, Mount Laurel, NJ, 2016, The Society.

Wysocki AB: Wound-healing physiology. In Bryant RA, Nix DP, editors: *Acute and chronic wounds: current management concepts*, ed 5, St Louis, 2016, Elsevier.

RESEARCH REFERENCES

Alderden J, et al: Midrange Braden subscale scores are associated with increased risk for pressure injury development among critical care patients, *J Wound Ostomy Continence Nurs* 44(5):420, 2017.

Arici A, et al: The effect of using an abdominal binder on postoperative gastrointestinal function, mobilization, pulmonary function, and pain in patients undergoing major abdominal surgery: a randomized controlled trial, *Int J Nurs Stud* 62:108, 2016.

Baath C, et al: Prevention of heel pressure ulcers among older patients--from ambulance care to hospital discharge: a multi-centre randomized controlled trial, *Appl Nurs Res* 30:170, 2015.

Black JM, et al: Medical device related pressure ulcers in hospitalized patients, *Int Wound J* 7(5):358, 2010.

Black J, Kalowes P: Medical device-related pressure ulcers, *Chronic Wound Care Manag Res* 3:91, 2016.

Black JM, et al: Use of wound dressings to enhance prevention of pressure ulcers caused by medical devices, *Int Wound J* 12(3):322, 2015.

Braden BJ, Bergstrom N: Clinical utility of the Braden Scale for predicting pressure sore risk, *Decubitus* 2(3):50, 1989.

Braden BJ, Bergstrom N: Predictive validity of the Braden Scale for pressure sore risk in a nursing home population, *Res Nurs Health* 17(6):459, 1994.

Burton AC, Yamada S: Relation between blood pressure and flow in the human forearm, *J Appl Physiol* 4(5):329, 1951.

Fernandez L, et al: Use of negative pressure wound therapy with instillation in the management of complex wounds in critically ill patients, *Wounds* 31(1):E1, 2019.

Giller CM, et al: A randomized controlled trial of abdominal binders for the management of postoperative pain and distress after cesarean delivery, *Int J Gynaecol Obstet* 133(2):188, 2016.

Han Y, et al: Usefulness of the Braden Scale in intensive care units: a study based on electronic health record data, *J Nurs Care Qual* 33(3):238, 2018.

Hyun S, et al: Predictive validity of the Braden Scale for patients in intensive care units, *Am J Crit Care* 22(6):514, 2013.

Januchowski R, Ferguson WJ: The clinical use of tissue adhesives: a review of the literature, *Osteopath Fam Physician* 6(2):25, 2014.

Kayser SA, et al: Prevalence and analysis of medical device-related pressure injuries: results from the international pressure prevalence survey, *Adv Skin Wound Care* 31(6):276, 2018.

Kelechi TJ, et al: Does cryotherapy improve circulation compared with compression and elevation in preventing venous leg ulcers, *Int Wound J* 14(4):641, 2017.

Martin D, et al: Healthy skin wins: a glowing pressure ulcer prevention program that can guide evidence-based practice, *Worldviews Evid Based Nurs* 14(6):473, 2017.

McNichol LL, et al: Incontinence-associated dermatitis: state of the science and knowledge translation, *Adv Skin Wound Care* 31(11):502, 2018.

Petrofsky J, et al: Use of low level of continuous heat as an adjunct to physical therapy improves knee pain recovery and the compliance for home exercise in patients with chronic knee pain: a randomized controlled trial, *J Strength Cond Res* 30(11):3107, 2016.

Petrofsky J, et al: The efficacy of sustained heat treatment on delayed-onset muscle soreness, *Clin J Sport Med* 27(4):329, 2017.

Pierpont VN, et al: Obesity and surgical wound healing: a current review, *ISRN Obes*, 2014, https://doi.org/10.1155/2014/638936.

Quinlan P, et al: Effects of localized cold therapy on pain in postoperative spinal fusion patients: a randomized control trial, *Orthop Nurs* 36(5):344, 2017.

Rothman JP, et al: Abdominal binders may reduce pain and improve physical function after major abdominal surgery - a systematic review, *Dan Med J* 61(11):A4941, 2014.

Szekeres M et al: The short-term effects of hot packs vs therapeutic whirlpool on active wrist range of motion for patients with distal radius fracture: a randomized controlled trial, *J Hand Ther*, published online September 8, 2017.

49

Sensory Alterations

OBJECTIVES

- Differentiate among the processes of reception, perception, and reaction to sensory stimuli.
- Compare and contrast sensory deprivation and sensory overload.
- Discuss factors influencing sensory function.
- Discuss how sensory function affects an individual's level of wellness.
- Discuss the components that make up assessment of the sensory system.
- Assess patients for signs and symptoms of sensory alterations.
- Identify nursing diagnoses and outcomes relevant to patients with sensory alterations.
- Discuss health promotion strategies for normal sensory function.
- Plan and implement nursing interventions for patients with sensory deficits, sensory deprivation, and sensory overload.
- Discuss strategies to maintain a safe environment for patients with altered sensation.

KEY TERMS

Aphasia, p. 1306
Auditory, p. 1300
Conductive hearing loss, p. 1313
Expressive aphasia, p. 1306
Gustatory, p. 1300
Hyperesthesia, p. 1313
Kinesthetic, p. 1300

Olfactory, p. 1300
Otolaryngologist, p. 1304
Ototoxic, p. 1307
Proprioceptive, p. 1303
Receptive aphasia, p. 1306
Refractive error, p. 1309
Sensory deficit, p. 1301

Sensory deprivation, p. 1301
Sensory overload, p. 1302
Stereognosis, p. 1300
Strabismus, p. 1309
Tactile, p. 1300

MEDIA RESOURCES

http://evolve.elsevier.com/Potter/fundamentals/
- Review Questions
- Concept Map Creator
- Case Study with Questions
- Audio Glossary
- Content Updates
- Answers to QSEN Activity and Review Questions

Imagine the world without sight, hearing, the ability to feel objects, or the ability to sense aromas around you. People rely on a variety of sensory stimuli to give meaning and order to events occurring in their environment. The senses form the perceptual base of our world. Stimulation comes from many sources in and outside the body, particularly through the senses of sight (visual), hearing (auditory), touch (tactile), smell (olfactory), and taste (gustatory). The body also has a kinesthetic sense that enables a person to be aware of the position and movement of body parts without seeing them. Stereognosis is a sense that allows a person to recognize the size, shape, and texture of an object. Although the ability to speak is not a sense, it is similar because sometimes patients lose the ability to interact meaningfully with other human beings. Meaningful stimuli allow a person to learn about the environment and are necessary for healthy functioning and normal development. When sensory function is altered, a person's ability to relate to and function within the environment changes drastically.

Many patients seeking health care have preexisting sensory alterations. Others develop them because of medical treatment (e.g., hearing loss from antibiotic use or hearing or visual loss from brain tumor removal) or hospitalization. The health care environment is a place of unfamiliar sights, sounds, and smells and minimal contact with family and friends. If patients feel depersonalized and are unable to receive meaningful stimuli, serious sensory alterations sometimes develop.

As a nurse you meet the needs of patients with existing sensory alterations and recognize those most at risk for developing sensory problems. You also help patients who have partial or complete loss of a major sense to find alternate ways to function safely within their environment.

SCIENTIFIC KNOWLEDGE BASE

Normal Sensation

The nervous system continually receives thousands of stimuli from sensory nerve organs, relays the information through appropriate neurological channels, and integrates the information into a meaningful response. Sensory stimuli reach the sensory organs to elicit an immediate reaction or store information in the brain for future use. The nervous system must be intact for sensory stimuli to reach appropriate brain centers and for an individual to perceive the sensation. After interpreting the significance of a sensation, the person is then able to react to the stimulus. Table 49.1 summarizes normal hearing and vision.

TABLE 49.1	**Normal Hearing and Vision**
Function	**Anatomy and Physiology**
Ear	
Transmits to brain a pattern of all sounds received from the environment, the relative intensity of these sounds, and the direction from which they originate	Two ears provide stereophonic hearing to judge sound direction.
	The external ear canal shelters the eardrum and maintains relatively constant temperature and humidity to maintain elasticity.
	The middle ear is an air-containing space between the eardrum and oval window. It contains three small bones (ossicles).
	The eardrum and ossicles transfer sound to the fluid-filled inner ear.
	Movement of the stapes in the oval window creates vibrations in the fluid that bathes the membranous labyrinth, which contains the end organs of hearing and balance.
	The union of the vestibular (balance) and cochlear (hearing) parts of the labyrinth explains the combination of hearing and balance symptoms that occur with inner ear disorders.
	Vibration of the eardrum transmits through the bony ossicles. Vibrations at the oval window transmit in perilymph within the inner ear to stimulate hair cells that send impulses along the eighth cranial nerve to the brain.
Eye	
Transmits a pattern of light to the brain that is reflected from solid objects in the environment and becomes transformed into color and hue	Light rays enter the convex cornea and begin to converge.
	An adjustment of light rays occurs as they pass through the pupil and lens.
	Change in the shape of the lens focuses light on the retina.
	The retina has a pigmented layer of cells to enhance visual acuity.
	The sensory retina contains the rods and cones (i.e., photoreceptor cells sensitive to stimulation from light).
	Photoreceptor cells send electrical potentials by way of the optic nerve to the brain.

Reception, perception, and reaction are the three components of any sensory experience. Reception begins with stimulation of a nerve cell called a *receptor,* which is usually for only one type of stimulus such as light, touch, taste, or sound. In the case of special senses, the receptors are grouped close together or located in specialized organs such as the taste buds of the tongue or the retina of the eye. When a nerve impulse is created, it travels along pathways to the spinal cord or directly to the brain. For example, sound waves stimulate hair cell receptors within the organ of Corti in the ear, which causes impulses to travel along the eighth cranial nerve to the acoustic area of the temporal lobe. Sensory nerve pathways usually cross over to send stimuli to opposite sides of the brain.

The actual perception or awareness of unique sensations depends on the receiving region of the cerebral cortex, where specialized neurons interpret the quality and nature of sensory stimuli. When a person becomes conscious of a stimulus and receives the information, perception takes place. Perception includes integration and interpretation of stimuli based on a person's experiences. A person's level of consciousness influences perception and interpretation of stimuli. Any factors lowering consciousness impair sensory perception. If sensation is incomplete, such as blurred vision, or if past experience is inadequate for understanding stimuli such as pain, the person can react inappropriately to the sensory stimulus.

It is impossible to react to all stimuli entering the nervous system. The brain prevents sensory bombardment by discarding or storing sensory information. A person usually reacts to stimuli that are most meaningful or significant at the time. After continued reception of the same stimulus, a person stops responding, and the sensory experience goes unnoticed. For example, a person concentrating on reading a good book is not aware of background music. This adaptability phenomenon occurs with most sensory stimuli except for those of pain.

The balance between sensory stimuli entering the brain and those actually reaching a person's conscious awareness maintains a person's well-being. Sensory alterations occur when an individual attempts to react to every stimulus within the environment or if the variety and quality of stimuli are insufficient.

Sensory Alterations

The most common sensory alterations are sensory deficits, sensory deprivation, and sensory overload. A patient's ability to function and relate effectively within the environment is seriously impaired when the patient has more than one sensory alteration.

Sensory Deficits. A deficit in the normal function of sensory reception and perception is a sensory deficit. When a person loses visual or hearing acuity, he or she withdraws by avoiding communication or socialization with others to cope with the sensory loss. It becomes difficult for the person to interact safely with the environment until he or she learns new skills. When a deficit develops gradually or when considerable time has passed since the onset of an acute sensory loss, a person learns to rely on unaffected senses. Some senses may even become more acute to compensate for an alteration. For example, a patient who is blind develops an acute sense of hearing to compensate for visual loss.

Patients with sensory deficits often change behavior in adaptive or maladaptive ways. For example, a patient with a hearing impairment turns the unaffected ear toward the speaker to hear better, whereas another patient avoids people because he or she is embarrassed about not being able to understand what other people say. Box 49.1 summarizes common sensory deficits and their influence on those affected.

Sensory Deprivation. The reticular activating system in the brainstem mediates all sensory stimuli to the cerebral cortex; thus patients are able to receive stimuli even while sleeping deeply. Sensory stimulation must be of sufficient quality and quantity to maintain a person's awareness. Three types of sensory deprivation are reduced sensory input (sensory deficit from visual or hearing loss), the elimination of patterns or meaning from input (e.g., exposure to strange environments), and restrictive environments (e.g., bed rest) that produce monotony and boredom (Touhy and Jett, 2018).

There are many effects of sensory deprivation (Box 49.2). In adults the symptoms are similar to those of psychological illness, confusion,

---

BOX 49.1   Common Sensory Deficits

Visual Deficits

Presbyopia: A gradual decline in the ability of the lens to accommodate or focus on close objects. Individual is unable to see near objects clearly.

Cataract: Cloudy or opaque areas in part of the lens or the entire lens that interfere with passage of light through the lens, causing problems with glare and blurred vision. Cataracts usually develop gradually, without pain, redness, or tearing in the eye.

Computer vision syndrome or digital eye strain: Describes a group of eye and vision-related problems that result from prolonged computer, tablet, e-reader, and cell phone use. Most commonly causes eye strain, headaches, blurred vision, and dry eyes.

Dry eyes: Result when tear glands produce too few tears, resulting in itching, burning, or even reduced vision.

Glaucoma: A slowly progressive increase in intraocular pressure that, if left untreated, causes progressive pressure against the optic nerve, resulting in peripheral visual loss, decreased visual acuity with difficulty adapting to darkness, and a halo effect around lights.

Diabetic retinopathy: Pathological changes occur in the blood vessels of the retina, resulting in decreased vision or vision loss caused by hemorrhage and macular edema.

Macular degeneration: Condition in which the macula (specialized part of the retina responsible for central vision) loses its ability to function efficiently. First signs include blurring of reading matter, distortion or loss of central vision, and distortion of vertical lines.

Hearing Deficits

Presbycusis: A common progressive hearing disorder in older adults.

Cerumen accumulation: Buildup of earwax in the external auditory canal. Cerumen becomes hard and collects in the canal and causes conduction deafness.

Balance Deficit

Dizziness and disequilibrium: Common condition in older adulthood, usually resulting from vestibular dysfunction. Frequently a change in position of the head precipitates an episode of vertigo or disequilibrium.

Taste Deficit

Xerostomia: Decrease in salivary production that leads to thicker mucus and a dry mouth. Often interferes with the ability to eat and leads to appetite and nutritional problems.

Neurological Deficits

Peripheral neuropathy: Disorder of the peripheral nervous system, characterized by symptoms that include numbness and tingling of the affected area and stumbling gait.

Stroke: Cerebrovascular accident caused by clot, hemorrhage, or emboli disrupting blood flow to the brain. Creates altered proprioception with marked incoordination and imbalance. Loss of sensation and motor function in extremities controlled by the affected area of the brain also occurs. A stroke affecting the left hemisphere of the brain results in symptoms on the right side, such as difficulty with speech. A stroke on the right hemisphere has symptoms on the left side, which may include visual spatial alterations, such as loss of half of a visual field or inattention and neglect, especially to the left side.

BOX 49.2   Effects of Sensory Deprivation

Cognitive
- Reduced capacity to learn
- Inability to think or problem solve
- Poor task performance
- Disorientation/confusion
- Bizarre thinking
- Increased need for socialization, altered mechanisms of attention

Affective
- Boredom
- Restlessness
- Increased anxiety

- Emotional lability
- Panic
- Increased need for physical stimulation

Perceptual
- Changes in visual/motor coordination
- Reduced color perception
- Less tactile accuracy
- Changes in ability to perceive size and shape
- Changes in spatial and time judgment

---

severe electrolyte imbalance, or the influence of psychotropic drugs. Therefore, always be aware of a patient's existing sensory function and the quality of stimuli within the environment.

Sensory Overload. When a person receives multiple sensory stimuli and cannot perceptually disregard or selectively ignore some stimuli, sensory overload occurs. Excessive sensory stimulation prevents the brain from responding appropriately to or ignoring certain stimuli. Because of the multitude of stimuli leading to overload, a person no longer perceives the environment in a way that makes sense. Overload prevents meaningful response by the brain; the patient's thoughts race, attention scatters in many directions, and anxiety and

restlessness occur. As a result, overload causes a state similar to sensory deprivation. However, in contrast to deprivation, overload is individualized. The amount of stimuli necessary for healthy function varies with each individual. People are often subject to environmental overload more at one time than another. A person's tolerance to sensory overload varies with level of fatigue, attitude, and emotional and physical well-being.

A patient who is acutely ill, especially one in a critical care unit, easily experiences sensory overload. A patient in constant pain or who requires frequent monitoring of vital signs is also at risk. Multiple stimuli combine to cause overload even if you offer a comforting word or provide a gentle back rub. Some patients do not benefit from nursing intervention because their attention and energy are focused on more stressful stimuli. In a critical care unit where the activity is constant, the lights are frequently on. Patients can hear sounds from monitoring equipment, staff conversations, equipment alarms, and the activities of people entering the unit.

It is easy to confuse the behavioral changes associated with sensory overload with mood swings or simple disorientation. Look for symptoms such as racing thoughts, scattered attention, restlessness, and anxiety. Patients in intensive care units (ICUs) sometimes constantly play with tubes and dressings. Constant reorientation and control of excessive stimuli become an important part of a patient's care.

REFLECT NOW

Compare and contrast the symptoms of patients who have sensory deprivation with those of patients who experience sensory overload.

NURSING KNOWLEDGE BASE

Factors Influencing Sensory Function

Many factors influence the capacity to receive or perceive stimuli. You will consider the influence these conditions or factors have on patients' sensation when delivering patient care.

Age. Infants and children are at risk for visual and hearing impairment because of several genetic, prenatal, and postnatal conditions. Early intense visual and auditory stimulation can adversely affect visual and auditory pathways and alter the developmental course of other sensory organs in high-risk neonates (Hockenberry et al., 2019). Visual changes during adulthood include presbyopia and the need for glasses for reading. These changes usually occur from ages 40 to 50. In addition, the cornea, which assists with light refraction to the retina, becomes flatter and thicker, which often leads to astigmatism. Pigment is lost from the iris, and collagen fibers build up in the anterior chamber, which increases the risk of glaucoma by decreasing the resorption of intraocular fluid. Other normal visual changes associated with aging include reduced visual fields, increased glare sensitivity, impaired night vision, reduced depth perception, and reduced color discrimination.

Hearing changes begin at the age of 30. Changes associated with aging include decreased hearing acuity, speech intelligibility, and pitch discrimination. Low-pitched sounds are easiest to hear, but it is difficult to hear conversation over background noise. It is also difficult to discriminate the consonants *(z, t, f, g)* and high-frequency sounds *(s, sh, ph, k)*. Vowels that have a low pitch are easiest to hear. Speech sounds are distorted, and there is a delayed reception and reaction to speech. A concern with normal age-related sensory changes is that older adults with a deficit are sometimes inappropriately diagnosed with dementia (Touhy and Jett, 2018).

Gustatory and olfactory changes begin around age 50 and include a decrease in the number of taste buds and sensory cells in the nasal lining. Reduced taste discrimination and sensitivity to odors are common.

Proprioceptive changes common after age 60 include increased difficulty with balance, spatial orientation, and coordination. The person cannot avoid obstacles as quickly, and the automatic response to protect and brace oneself when falling is slower. There are also tactile changes, including declining sensitivity to pain, pressure, and temperature secondary to peripheral vascular disease and neuropathies.

Meaningful Stimuli. Meaningful stimuli reduce the incidence of sensory deprivation. In the home meaningful stimuli include pets, music, television, pictures of family members, and a calendar and clock. The same stimuli need to be present in health care settings. Note whether patients have roommates or visitors. The presence of others offers positive stimulation. However, a roommate who constantly watches television, persistently tries to talk, or continuously keeps lights on contributes to sensory overload. The presence or absence of meaningful stimuli influences alertness and the ability to participate in care.

Amount of Stimuli. Excessive stimuli in an environment cause sensory overload. The frequency of observations and the number of procedures performed in an acute health care setting are often stressful. If a patient is in pain or restricted by a cast or traction, overstimulation frequently is a problem. In addition, a room that is near repetitive or loud noises (e.g., an elevator, stairwell, or nurses' station) contributes to sensory overload.

Social Interaction. The amount and quality of social contact with supportive family members and significant others influence sensory function. The absence of visitors during hospitalization or residency in an extended-care facility influences the degree of isolation a patient feels. This is a common problem in hospital intensive care settings, where visiting is often restricted. The ability to discuss concerns with loved ones is an important coping mechanism for most people. Therefore the absence of meaningful conversation results in feelings of isolation, loneliness, anxiety, and depression for a patient. Often this is not apparent until behavioral changes occur.

Environmental Factors. A person's occupation places him or her at risk for hearing, visual, and peripheral nerve alterations. Individuals who have occupations involving exposure to high noise levels (e.g., factory or airport workers) are at risk for noise-induced hearing loss and need to be screened for hearing impairments. Hazardous loud noise is common in work settings and recreational activities. Noisy recreational activities that weaken hearing ability include target shooting and hunting, woodworking, and listening to loud music. Individuals who have occupations involving risk of exposure to chemicals or flying objects (e.g., welders) are at risk for eye injuries and need to be screened for visual impairments. Sports activities and consumer fireworks also place individuals at risk for eye injuries. Occupations that involve repetitive wrist or finger movements (e.g., heavy assembly line work, long periods of computer use) cause pressure on the median nerve, which runs from the forearm into the palm of the hand, resulting in carpal tunnel syndrome. Carpal tunnel syndrome alters tactile sensation and is one of the most common industrial or work-related injuries.

A patient who is hospitalized is sometimes at risk for sensory alterations because of exposure to environmental stimuli or a change in sensory input. Patients who are immobilized by bed rest or who have a chronic disability are unable to experience all the normal sensations of free movement. Another group at risk includes patients isolated in a health care setting or at home because of conditions such as bone marrow transplant or active tuberculosis (see Chapter 28). These patients stay in private rooms and are often unable to enjoy normal interactions with visitors.

Cultural Factors. Some sensory alterations occur more commonly in select cultural groups. Analysis of data from the National Health Interview Survey (NHIS), Centers for Disease Control and Prevention (CDC), and National Center for Health Statistics showed that African Americans had a higher prevalence of visual impairment due to glaucoma than Hispanics and non-Hispanic whites. African-American children and adolescents also have higher rates of blindness and visual impairment than other ethnicities (USDHHS, 2018b). Cultural disparities in vision impairment are significant, in part because vision impairment is associated with a decrease in physical and mental health and quality of life (Box 49.3) (Tseng, YC et al., 2018). Changes in hearing and visual acuity also impact a person's health literacy and his or her ability to understand medications, procedures, and restorative and home care interventions, which are further complicated when English is a second language.

CRITICAL THINKING

Successful critical thinking requires a synthesis of knowledge and information gathered from patients, experience, critical thinking attitudes, and intellectual and professional standards. Clinical judgments require you to anticipate the information necessary, analyze the data, and make decisions regarding patient care. Patients' conditions are always changing. During assessment consider all critical thinking elements that help you make appropriate nursing diagnoses (Fig. 49.1). In the case of sensory alterations, integrate knowledge of the pathophysiology of sensory deficits, factors that affect sensory function, and therapeutic communication principles. This knowledge enables you to conduct appropriate assessments, anticipate what to recognize when a patient describes a

🌐 BOX 49.3 CULTURAL ASPECTS OF CARE

Disparities in Eye Care

By the year 2050, non-Hispanic white individuals, women, and older adults will experience the highest rate of visual impairments and blindness. Data also suggest that Hispanic individuals will have the highest prevalence of visual impairment among minorities. This change from African Americans to Hispanics is related to the growing population of Hispanic individuals (Varma et al., 2016). Unfortunately, some individuals do not receive the vision services necessary to improve their quality of life. Findings from the National Health and Aging Trends Survey reveal that Medicare beneficiaries who are older and nonwhite are less likely to report the use of eyeglasses. People with lower socioeconomic and educational levels are also less likely to report the use of eyeglasses (Otte et al., 2018). A disparity also exists between patients with Medicaid and those with private health care insurance. Individuals with Medicaid have been found to be less successful in obtaining eye care appointments (Yoon et al., 2018). These findings are critical since the early diagnosis of visual impairments allows for early intervention to help prevent irreversible causes of vision loss (Umfress et al., 2016).

Implications for Patient-Centered Care

- Encourage patients to discuss changes in visually acuity or other eye or vision issues by asking a few focused questions.
- Educate patients on age-related eye diseases and conditions, eye care services, and the importance of taking care of their eyes (Umfress et al., 2016).
- Collaborate with the interprofessional team to help improve access to eye care services.
- Follow up with patients to reiterate important points and to check on their progress.
- Provide written eye care instructions in type that uses large fonts (14-point type or larger) and sharp contrast to improve readability (Umfress et al., 2016).

sensory problem, and make judgments of abnormalities. For example, knowing the typical symptoms caused by a cataract helps you recognize the pattern of visual changes that a patient with cataracts reports.

Previous experiences in caring for patients with sensory deficits help you recognize limitations in a patient's functioning and how these limitations affect the ability to carry out daily activities. For example, after caring for one patient with a hearing impairment, you are able to conduct a more effective assessment of the next patient by using previously successful approaches that promote the patient's ability to hear your questions.

When you apply critical thinking attitudes and standards during assessment, you establish a thorough and accurate database from which to make decisions. For example, perseverance is necessary to learn details about how visual changes influence a patient's ability to socialize. Evidence-based standards of care and practice such as those from the American Academy of Ophthalmology and the American Speech-Language-Hearing Association provide criteria for screening sensory problems and establishing standards for competent, safe, effective care and practice. Use critical thinking to conduct a thorough assessment; then plan, implement, and evaluate care that enables a patient to function safely and effectively.

REFLECT NOW

The parents of a toddler share with you their plan to take the toddler to a fireworks show. What recommendations would you share with the parents, and why?

❖ NURSING PROCESS

Apply the nursing process and use a critical thinking approach in your care of patients. The nursing process provides a clinical decision-making approach for you to develop and implement an individualized plan of care.

◆ Assessment

During the assessment process, thoroughly assess each patient and critically analyze findings to ensure that you make appropriate and relevant nursing diagnoses and patient-centered clinical decisions required for safe nursing care.

Through the Patient's Eyes. When conducting an assessment, value the patient as a full partner. This will ensure a more thorough database so that you can plan, implement, and evaluate care. Patients are often hesitant to admit sensory losses. Therefore start gathering information by establishing a therapeutic rapport with the patient. Elicit his or her values, preferences, and expectations regarding his or her sensory impairment. Many patients have a definite plan as to how they want their care delivered. Some patients expect caregivers to recognize and appropriately manage and adjust their environment to meet their sensory needs. This includes helping the family and patient ultimately learn and adapt to a changed lifestyle based on the specific sensory impairment. Determine from the patient which interventions if any were helpful in the past in managing limitations. Assess the patient's expertise with his or her own health and symptoms. Always remember that patients with sensory alterations have strengthened their other senses and expect caregivers to anticipate their needs (e.g., for safety and security).

When assessing a patient with or at risk for sensory alteration, first consider the pathophysiology of existing deficits and the factors influencing sensory function to anticipate how to approach his or her assessment. For example, if a patient has a hearing disorder, adjust your communication style and focus your assessment on relevant criteria related to hearing deficits. Collect a history that also assesses the patient's current sensory status and the degree to which a sensory deficit affects the patient's lifestyle, psychosocial adjustment, developmental status, self-care ability, health promotion habits, and safety. Also focus the assessment on the quality and quantity of stimuli within the patient's environment.

People at Risk. Determine if your patient is at risk for a sensory alteration. Older adults are a high-risk group because of normal physiological changes involving sensory organs. However, be careful not to automatically assume that a patient's sensory problem is related to advancing age. For example, adult sensorineural hearing loss is often caused by exposure to excess and prolonged noise or metabolic, vascular, and other systemic alterations. Some patients benefit from a referral to an audiologist or otolaryngologist when serious hearing problems are identified during assessment.

Other individuals at risk for sensory alterations include those living in a confined environment such as a nursing home. For example, an individual with poor hearing who is confined to a wheelchair, has decreased energy, and avoids contact with others is at significant risk for sensory deprivation. Quality nursing homes or centers offer meaningful stimulation through group activities, environmental design, and mealtime gatherings to better manage sensory alterations in their residents.

Patients who are acutely ill are also at risk because of an unfamiliar and unresponsive environment. This does not mean that all patients in the hospital have sensory alterations. However, you need

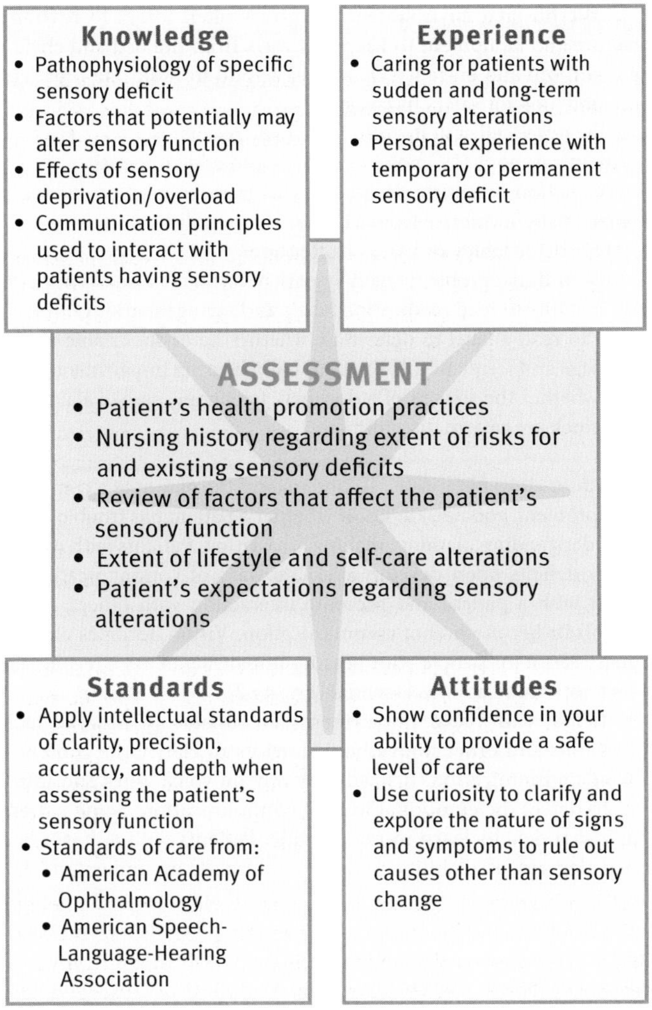

Knowledge
- Pathophysiology of specific sensory deficit
- Factors that potentially may alter sensory function
- Effects of sensory deprivation/overload
- Communication principles used to interact with patients having sensory deficits

Experience
- Caring for patients with sudden and long-term sensory alterations
- Personal experience with temporary or permanent sensory deficit

ASSESSMENT
- Patient's health promotion practices
- Nursing history regarding extent of risks for and existing sensory deficits
- Review of factors that affect the patient's sensory function
- Extent of lifestyle and self-care alterations
- Patient's expectations regarding sensory alterations

Standards
- Apply intellectual standards of clarity, precision, accuracy, and depth when assessing the patient's sensory function
- Standards of care from:
  - American Academy of Ophthalmology
  - American Speech-Language-Hearing Association

Attitudes
- Show confidence in your ability to provide a safe level of care
- Use curiosity to clarify and explore the nature of signs and symptoms to rule out causes other than sensory change

FIG. 49.1 Critical thinking model for sensory alterations assessment.

to carefully assess patients exposed to continued sensory stimulation (e.g., ICU settings, long-term hospitalization, or multiple therapies). Assess a patient's environment within both the health care setting and the home, looking for factors that pose risks or need adjustment to provide safety and more appropriate sensory stimulation.

Sensory Alterations History. The nursing history includes assessment of the nature and characteristics of sensory alterations or any problem related to an alteration (Box 49.4). When taking the history, consider the ethnic or cultural background of the patient because certain alterations are higher in some cultural groups.

During the history it is useful to have a patient self-rate his or her sensory deficit by asking, "Rate your hearing as excellent, good, fair, poor, or bad." Then, based on the patient's self-rating, explore his or her perception of a sensory loss more fully. This provides an in-depth look at how the sensory loss influences the patient's quality of life. In the case of hearing problems, a screening tool such as the Hearing Handicap Inventory for the Elderly (HHIE-S) effectively identifies patients needing audiological intervention (Servidoni et al., 2018). The HHIE-S is a 5-minute, 10-item questionnaire that assesses how an individual perceives the social and emotional effects of hearing loss. The higher the HHIE-S score, the greater the handicapping effect of a hearing impairment.

A nursing history also reveals any recent changes in a patient's behavior. Frequently friends or family are the best resources for this information. Ask the family the following questions:
- Has your family member shown any recent mood swings (e.g., outbursts of anger, nervousness, fear, or irritability)?
- Have you noticed the family member avoiding social activities?

Mental Status. Assessment of mental status is valuable when you suspect sensory deprivation or overload. Observation of a patient during history taking, during the physical examination (see Chapter 30), and while providing nursing care offers valuable data about a patient's behaviors and mental status. Observe the patient's physical appearance and behavior, measure cognitive ability, and assess his or her emotional status. Use the Mini-Mental State Examination (MMSE) to measure disorientation, change in problem-solving abilities, and altered conceptualization and abstract thinking (see Chapter 30). For example, a patient with severe sensory deprivation is not always able to carry on a conversation, remain attentive, or display recent or past memory. An important step toward preventing cognition-related disability is education by nurses about disease process, available services, and assistive devices.

Physical Assessment. To identify sensory deficits and their severity, use physical assessment techniques to assess vision; hearing; olfaction; taste; and the ability to discriminate light touch, temperature, pain, and position (see Chapter 30). Table 49.2 summarizes specific assessment techniques for identifying sensory deficits. You gather more accurate data when the examination room is private, quiet, and comfortable for the patient. In addition, rely on personal observation to detect sensory alterations. Patients with a hearing impairment may seem inattentive to others, respond with inappropriate anger when spoken to, believe people are talking about them, answer questions inappropriately, have trouble following clear directions, and have monotonous voice quality or speak unusually loud or soft.

Ability to Perform Self-Care. Assess patients' functional abilities in their home environment or health care setting, including the ability to perform feeding, dressing, grooming, and toileting activities. For example, assess whether a patient with altered vision is able to find items on a meal tray and read directions on a prescription. Can a patient recovering from a stroke manipulate buttons or zippers for dressing? Also determine a patient's ability to perform instrumental activities of daily living (IADLs) such as reading bills and writing checks, differentiating money denominations, and driving a vehicle at night. If a patient seems to have a sensory deficit, does he or she show concern for grooming? Does a patient's loss of balance prevent rising from a toilet seat safely? If a sensory alteration impairs a patient's functional ability, providing resources within the home is a necessary part of discharge planning. Your findings may indicate the need for an occupational therapy consultation.

Health Promotion Habits. Assess the daily routines that patients follow to maintain sensory function. Which type of eye and ear care is a part of a patient's daily hygiene? For individuals who participate in sports (e.g., ice hockey, lacrosse) or recreational activities (e.g., motorcycle riding) or who work in a setting in which ear or eye injury is a possibility (e.g., chemical exposure, welding, glass or stone polishing, or constant exposure to loud noise), determine whether they wear safety glasses or hearing-protective devices (HPDs).

It is also important to assess a patient's adherence to routine health screening. When was the last time the patient had an eye examination or hearing evaluation? For adults routine screening of visual and

BOX 49.4   Nursing Assessment Questions

Nature of the Problem

- Describe the problem you are having with your vision/hearing.
- What have you tried to correct the vision/hearing difficulty?
- Do you use any devices to improve your vision/hearing?
- How effective are your glasses or hearing aids? If you are having problems, describe them for me.

Signs and Symptoms

- Ask a patient with visual alterations: Do you require books with large print or on audiotape? Are you able to prepare a meal or write a check? Do you notice any eye irritation or drainage?
- Ask a patient with hearing alterations: Which types of sounds or tones do you have difficulty hearing? Do people tell you that they have to "shout" for you to hear them? Do people ask you not to talk so loud? Do you have a ringing, crackling, or buzzing in your ears? Is there pain: sharp, dull, burning, itching? Have you noticed any redness, swelling, or drainage?

Onset and Duration

- When did you notice the problem? How long has it lasted?
- Does it come and go, or is it constant?
- What makes the problem better or worse?

Predisposing Factors

- Do you work or participate in any activities that have the potential for vision/hearing injury? If so, how do you protect your hearing and vision?
- Do you have a family history of cataracts, glaucoma, macular degeneration, or hearing loss?
- When was your last vision/hearing examination?

Effect on Patient

- What effect has your vision/hearing problem had on your work, family, or social life?
- Have changes in your vision/hearing affected your feelings of independence?
- How does your vision/hearing problem make you feel about yourself?
- Do you have problems with routine care of glasses, contact lenses, or hearing aids?

hearing function is imperative to detect problems early. This is especially true in the case of glaucoma, which, if undetected, leads to permanent vision loss. Recommended screening guidelines usually occur based on age. When a patient begins to show a hearing deficit, incorporate routine screening in regular examinations.

Environmental Hazards. Patients with sensory alterations are at risk for injury if their living environments are unsafe. For example, a patient with reduced vision cannot see potential hazards clearly. A patient with proprioceptive problems loses balance easily. A patient with reduced sensation cannot perceive hot-versus-cold temperatures. The condition of the home, the rooms, and the front and back entrances is often problematic to the patient with sensory alterations. Assess his or her home for common hazards, including the following:

- Uneven, cracked walkways leading to front/back door
- Extension and phone cords in the main route of walking traffic
- Loose area rugs and runners placed over carpeting
- Bathrooms without shower or tub grab bars
- Water faucets unmarked to designate hot and cold
- Unlit stairways, lack of handrails
- Poor lighting in stairways, halls, and entrance doors

In the hospital environment caregivers often forget to rearrange furniture and equipment to keep pathways from the bed and chair to the bathroom and entrance clear. It is helpful to walk into a patient's room and look for safety hazards:

- Is the nurse call system within easy, safe reach?
- Are intravenous (IV) poles on wheels and easy to move?
- Are suction machines, IV pumps, or drainage bags positioned so that a patient can rise from a bed or chair easily?
- Are bedside tables and areas clutter free?

An additional problem faced by patients who are visually impaired is the inability to read medication labels and syringe markings. Ask the patient to read a label to determine whether he or she is able to read the dosage and frequency. If a patient has a hearing impairment, check to see whether the sounds of a doorbell, telephone, smoke alarm, and alarm clock are easy to discriminate.

Communication Methods. To understand the nature of a communication problem, you need to know whether a patient has trouble speaking, understanding, naming, reading, or writing. Patients with existing sensory deficits often develop alternate ways of communicating. To interact with a patient and promote interaction with others, understand his or her method of communication. Vision becomes almost a primary sense for people with hearing impairments. As a result, face-to-face communication is essential (Fig. 49.2).

Patients with visual impairments are unable to observe facial expressions and other nonverbal behaviors to clarify the content of spoken communication. Instead they rely on voice tones and inflections to detect the emotional tone of communication. Some patients with visual deficits learn to read Braille. Patients with aphasia have varied degrees of inability to speak, interpret, or understand language. Expressive aphasia, a motor type of aphasia, is the inability to name common objects or express simple ideas in words or writing. For example, a patient understands a question but is unable to express an answer. Sensory or receptive aphasia is the inability to understand written or spoken language. A patient is able to express words but is unable to understand the questions or comments of others. Global aphasia is the inability to understand language or communicate orally.

The temporary or permanent loss of the ability to speak is extremely traumatic to an individual. Assess for alternate communication methods and whether they cause anxiety. Patients who have undergone laryngectomies often write notes, use communication boards or laptop computers, speak with mechanical vibrators, or use esophageal speech. Patients with endotracheal or tracheostomy tubes have a temporary loss of speech. Most use a notepad to write their questions and requests. However, some patients are unable to write messages. Determine whether the patient has developed a sign-language system or symbols to communicate needs.

Social Support. Determine whether a patient lives alone and how often family or friends visit. Assess the patient's social skills and level of satisfaction with the support given by family and friends. Is the patient satisfied with the support available? Is he or she able to solve problems with family members? Is there a family caregiver who offers support when the patient requires assistance because of a sensory loss? The long-term effects of sensory alterations influence family dynamics and a patient's willingness to remain active in society.

Use of Assistive Devices. Assess the use of assistive devices (e.g., use of a hearing aid or glasses) and whether they currently are in working order. Assess whether the patient thinks that these devices

TABLE 49.2   Assessment of Sensory Function

Assessment Activities	Behavior Indicating Deficit (Children)	Behavior Indicating Deficit (Adults)
Vision Ask patient to read newspaper, magazine, or lettering on menu. Ask patient to identify colors on color chart or crayons. Observe patients performing ADLs.	Self-stimulation, including eye rubbing, body rocking, sniffing or smelling, arm twirling; hitching (using legs to propel while in sitting position) instead of crawling	Poor coordination, squinting, underreaching or overreaching for objects, persistent repositioning of objects, impaired night vision, accidental falls
Hearing Assess patient's hearing acuity (see Chapter 30) using spoken word and tuning fork tests. Assess for history of tinnitus. Observe patient conversing with others. Inspect ear canal for hardened cerumen. Observe patient behaviors in a group.	Frightened when unfamiliar people approach, no reflex or purposeful response to sounds, failure to be awakened by loud noise, slow or absent development of speech, greater response to movement than to sound, avoidance of social interaction with other children	Blank looks, decreased attention span, lack of reaction to loud noises, increased volume of speech, positioning of head toward sound, smiling and nodding of head in approval when someone speaks, use of other means of communication such as lip-reading or writing, complaints of ringing in ears
Touch Check patient's ability to discriminate between sharp and dull stimuli. Assess whether patient is able to distinguish objects (coin or safety pin) in the hand with eyes closed. Ask whether patient feels unusual sensations. Assess patients at risk for carpal tunnel syndrome for numbness, tingling, weakness, and pain in hands.	Inability to perform developmental tasks related to grasping objects or drawing, repeated injury from handling of harmful objects (e.g., hot stove, sharp knife)	Clumsiness, overreaction or underreaction to painful stimulus, failure to respond when touched, avoidance of touch, sensation of pins and needles, numbness Unable to identify object placed in hand Decreased grip strength may make it difficult to form a fist, grasp small objects, or perform other manual tasks. Usually starts gradually, with frequent burning, tingling, or itching numbness in the palm of the hand and the fingers, especially the thumb and the index and middle fingers (NINDS, 2019)
Smell Have patient close eyes and identify several nonirritating odors (e.g., coffee, vanilla).	Difficulty in discriminating noxious odors; difficult to assess until child is 6 or 7 years old	Failure to react to noxious or strong odor, increased body odor, decreased sensitivity to odors
Taste Ask patient to sample and distinguish different tastes (e.g., lemon, sugar, salt). (Have patient drink or sip water and wait 1 minute between each taste.)	Inability to tell whether food is salty or sweet; possible ingestion of strange-tasting things	Change in appetite, excessive use of seasoning and sugar, complaints about taste of food, weight change

ADLs, Activities of daily living.

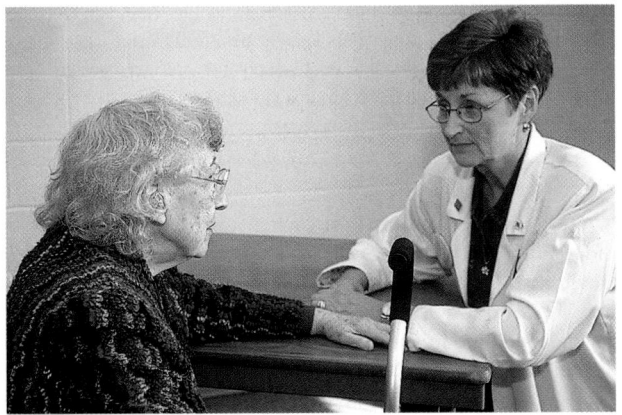

FIG. 49.2 Nurse sits at eye level so that patient with hearing impairment can communicate.

the individual has a device, it does not mean that it works or that the patient uses it or benefits from it.

Other Factors Affecting Perception. Factors other than sensory deprivation or overload cause impaired perception (e.g., medications or pain). Assess the patient's medication history, which includes prescribed and over-the-counter medications and herbal products. Also gather information regarding the frequency, dose, method of administration, and last time the patient took the medications. Some antibiotics (e.g., streptomycin, gentamicin, and tobramycin) are *ototoxic* and permanently damage the auditory nerve, whereas chloramphenicol sometimes irritates the optic nerve. Opioid analgesics, sedatives, and antidepressant medications often alter the perception of stimuli. Conduct a thorough pain assessment when you suspect that pain is causing perceptual problems (see Chapter 44).

are beneficial. This includes learning how often the patient uses the devices, the patient's or family caregiver's method of caring for and cleaning the devices routinely (see Chapter 40), and the patient's knowledge of what to do when a problem develops. When you identify that a patient has an assistive device, remember that just because

REFLECT NOW

How would you assess a patient who recently became confused and is having hallucinations for sensory alterations?

BOX 49.5   Nursing Diagnostic Process

Risk for Injury

Assessment Activities	Assessment Findings
Assess patient's visual acuity.	Reduced ability to see objects clearly; needs brighter light to read; has trouble distinguishing edges of stairs
Visit home setting and inspect for hazards that pose risks to patient.	Lighting in rooms, hallways, and stairwells very dim; carpet in living room old, edges curled up; steps leading up to front entrance of home
Review medical record from clinic visit.	Bilateral cataracts

◆ Nursing Diagnosis

After assessment review all available data and look critically for patterns and trends suggestive of a nursing diagnosis or health problem relating to sensory alterations (e.g., visual problems [Box 49.5]). Validate findings to ensure accuracy of a diagnosis. Determine the factor that likely caused or is creating a patient's health problem. The etiology or related factor of a nursing diagnosis is a condition that nursing interventions can affect. The etiology needs to be accurate; otherwise nursing therapies are ineffective.

Some patients have health care problems for which sensory alteration is the etiology, such as with the diagnosis of *Risk for Injury*. You select nursing diagnoses by recognizing the way in which sensory alterations affect a patient's ability to function (e.g., *Self Care Deficit*). In addition, most patients present themselves to health care professionals with multiple diagnoses (Fig. 49.3). In the concept map example, a patient with a cataract has the nursing diagnoses of *Risk for Injury, Anxiety, Fear,* and *Risk for Fall*. The sensory alteration caused by the cataract is an etiology for both risk for injury and risk for falls. Furthermore, fear occurs as a response to a perceived risk of falling. You need to recognize patterns of data that reveal health problems created by a patient's sensory alteration. Examples of nursing diagnoses that apply to patients with sensory alterations include the following:

- *Risk for Injury*
- *Risk for Fall*
- *Impaired Verbal Communication*
- *Impaired Socialisation*
- *Impaired Mobility*

◆ Planning

During planning synthesize information from multiple resources (Fig. 49.4). Reflect on knowledge gained from the assessment and knowledge of how sensory deficits affect normal functioning. In this way you are able to recognize the extent of a patient's deficit and know the types of interventions most likely to be helpful. Also consider the role that health professionals play in planning care and the available community resources that will be useful. Previous experience in caring for patients with sensory alterations is invaluable.

When applying critical thinking to planning care, professional standards are particularly useful. These standards recommend evidence-based interventions for the patient's condition. For example, patients who have visual deficits and are hospitalized are often placed on a fall-prevention protocol that incorporates research-based precautions to ensure patient safety.

Goals and Outcomes. During planning develop an individualized plan of care for each nursing diagnosis (see the Nursing Care Plan). Partner with your patient to develop a realistic plan that incorporates what you know about his or her sensory problems and the extent to which he or she can maintain or improve sensory function. Goals and outcomes need to be realistic and measurable. An example of a goal of care for a patient with an actual or potential sensory alteration is "The patient will achieve improvement in hearing acuity within 2 weeks." Associated outcomes for this goal include the following:

- The patient and family report using communication techniques to send and receive messages within 2 days.
- The patient successfully demonstrates correct technique for cleaning a hearing aid within 1 week.
- The patient self-reports improved hearing acuity.

Setting Priorities. Consider the type and extent of sensory alteration affecting a patient when determining priorities of care. For example, a patient who enters the emergency department after experiencing eye trauma has priorities of reducing anxiety and preventing further injury to the eye. In contrast, a patient who is being discharged from an outpatient surgery department following cataract removal has the priority of learning about self-care restrictions. Safety is always a top priority. The patient also helps prioritize aspects of care—for example, a patient might wish to learn ways to communicate more effectively or to participate in favorite hobbies given his or her limitation.

Some sensory alterations are short term (e.g., a patient experiencing sensory overload in an ICU). Thus appropriate interventions are likely to be temporary (e.g., frequent reorientation or introduction of pleasant stimuli such as a back rub). Some sensory alterations such as permanent visual loss require long-term goals of care for patients to adapt. Patients who have sensory alterations at the time of entering a health care setting are usually most informed about how to adapt interventions to their lifestyles. For example, allow patients who are blind to control whichever parts of their care they can. Sometimes it becomes necessary for a patient to make major changes in self-care activities, communication, and socialization to ensure safe and effective nursing care.

QSEN QSEN: Building Competency in Safety Ms. Long's church asks you to provide a presentation on fall prevention for older adult members of the congregation. Many members also have impaired vision. How will you develop a program to educate this elderly population and communicate observations or concerns related to fall hazards to them?

Answers to QSEN Activities can be found on the Evolve website.

Teamwork and Collaboration. When developing a plan of care, consider all resources available to patients. The family plays a key role in providing meaningful stimulation and in learning ways to help the patient adjust to any limitations. Engaging the family or designated surrogate is a fundamental skill of patient-centered care (Institute for Patient- and Family-Centered Care, 2016). You also refer patients to other health care professionals when appropriate. For example, if a patient has a major loss of sensory function and is also unable to manage medical needs such as medication self-administration or dressing changes, you make a referral to home care. Valuing interprofessional collaboration is an essential nurse competency that results in better patient health outcomes and greater patient and family satisfaction (Interprofessional Education Collaborative Expert Panel, 2016). Numerous community-based resources (e.g., local chapter of the Society for the Blind and Visually Impaired and the Area Agency

CONCEPT MAP

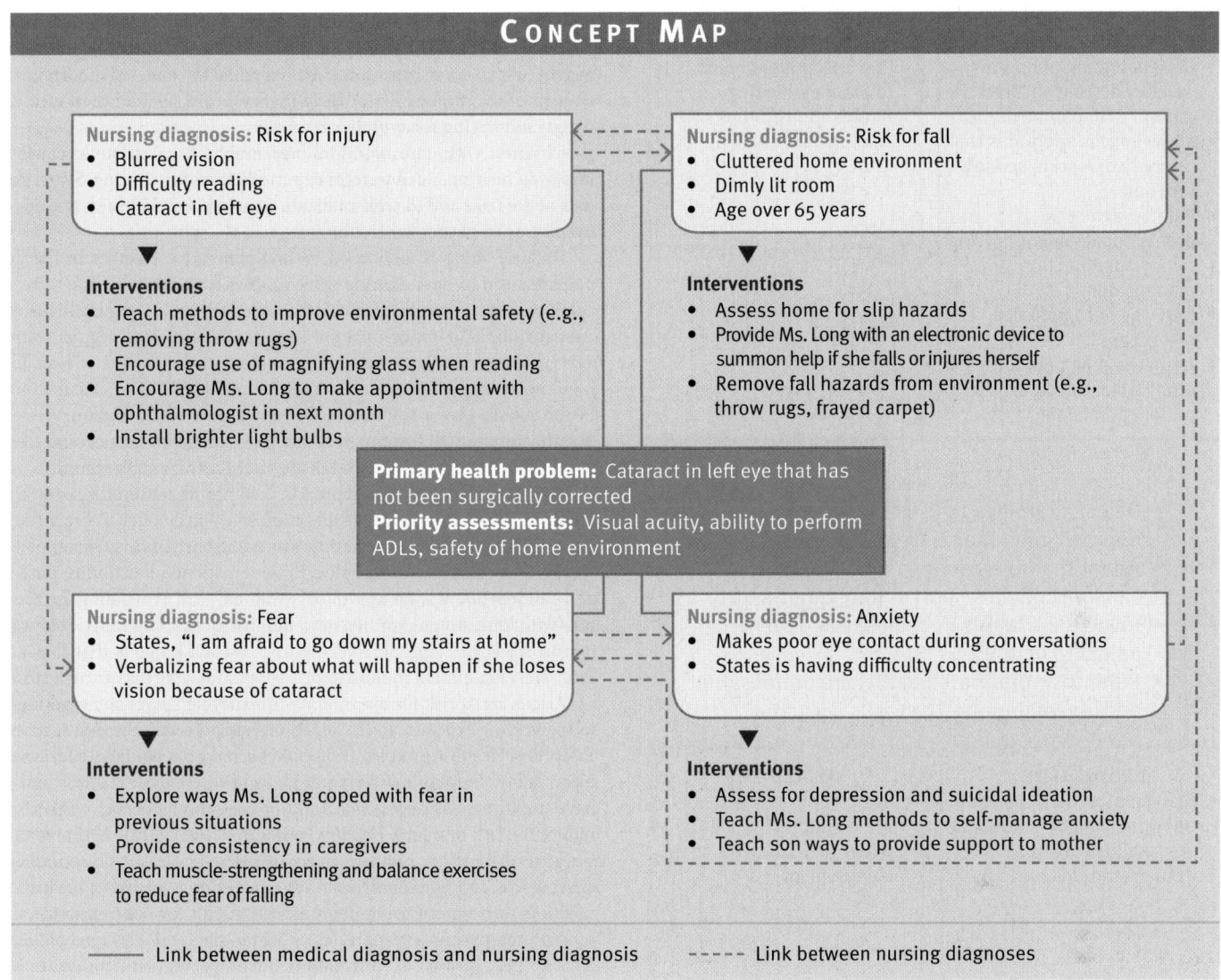

Nursing diagnosis: Risk for injury
- Blurred vision
- Difficulty reading
- Cataract in left eye

Interventions
- Teach methods to improve environmental safety (e.g., removing throw rugs)
- Encourage use of magnifying glass when reading
- Encourage Ms. Long to make appointment with ophthalmologist in next month
- Install brighter light bulbs

Nursing diagnosis: Risk for fall
- Cluttered home environment
- Dimly lit room
- Age over 65 years

Interventions
- Assess home for slip hazards
- Provide Ms. Long with an electronic device to summon help if she falls or injures herself
- Remove fall hazards from environment (e.g., throw rugs, frayed carpet)

Primary health problem: Cataract in left eye that has not been surgically corrected
Priority assessments: Visual acuity, ability to perform ADLs, safety of home environment

Nursing diagnosis: Fear
- States, "I am afraid to go down my stairs at home"
- Verbalizing fear about what will happen if she loses vision because of cataract

Interventions
- Explore ways Ms. Long coped with fear in previous situations
- Provide consistency in caregivers
- Teach muscle-strengthening and balance exercises to reduce fear of falling

Nursing diagnosis: Anxiety
- Makes poor eye contact during conversations
- States is having difficulty concentrating

Interventions
- Assess for depression and suicidal ideation
- Teach Ms. Long methods to self-manage anxiety
- Teach son ways to provide support to mother

——— Link between medical diagnosis and nursing diagnosis   - - - - Link between nursing diagnoses

FIG. 49.3 Concept map for Ms. Long.

on Aging) are also available. Try to arrange for a volunteer to visit a patient or have printed materials made available that describe ways to cope with sensory problems.

◆ Implementation

Nursing interventions involve patients and their families so that patients are able to maintain a safe, pleasant, and stimulating sensory environments. The most effective interventions enable a patient with sensory alterations to function safely with existing deficits and continue a normal lifestyle. Patients can learn to adjust to sensory impairments at any age with the proper support and resources. Use measures to maintain a patient's sensory function at the highest level possible.

Health Promotion. Good sensory function begins with prevention. When a patient seeks health care, provide education about interventions that reduce the risk for sensory losses. Also recommend relevant visual and hearing guidelines. Remember to assess a patient's capacity to process and understand the health information to ensure that the patient makes appropriate decisions regarding his or her health.

Screening. An estimated 4.2 million adults in the world have uncorrectable vision impairment, including blindness. By the year 2050, this number is expected to more than double (Varma et al.,

2016). This raises questions about the etiology of vision impairments, as well as strategies to improve access to early screening programs. Preventable blindness is a worldwide health issue that begins with children and requires appropriate screening. Four recommended interventions are: (1) screening for rubella, syphilis, chlamydia, and gonorrhea in women who are considering pregnancy; (2) advocating for adequate prenatal care to prevent premature birth (with the danger of exposure of the infant to excessive oxygen); (3) administering eye prophylaxis in the form of erythromycin ointment approximately 1 hour after an infant's birth; and (4) periodic screening of all children, especially newborns through preschoolers, for congenital blindness and visual impairment caused by refractive errors and strabismus (Hockenberry et al., 2019).

Visual impairments are common during childhood. The most common visual problem is a refractive error such as nearsightedness. The nurse's role is one of detection, education, and referral. Parents need to know the signs of visual impairment (e.g., failure to react to light and reduced eye contact from the infant). Instruct parents to report these signs to their health care provider immediately. When follow-up is available, vision screening of school-age children and adolescents can detect early visual impairments (Rodriguez et al., 2018). School nurses are usually responsible for vision testing.

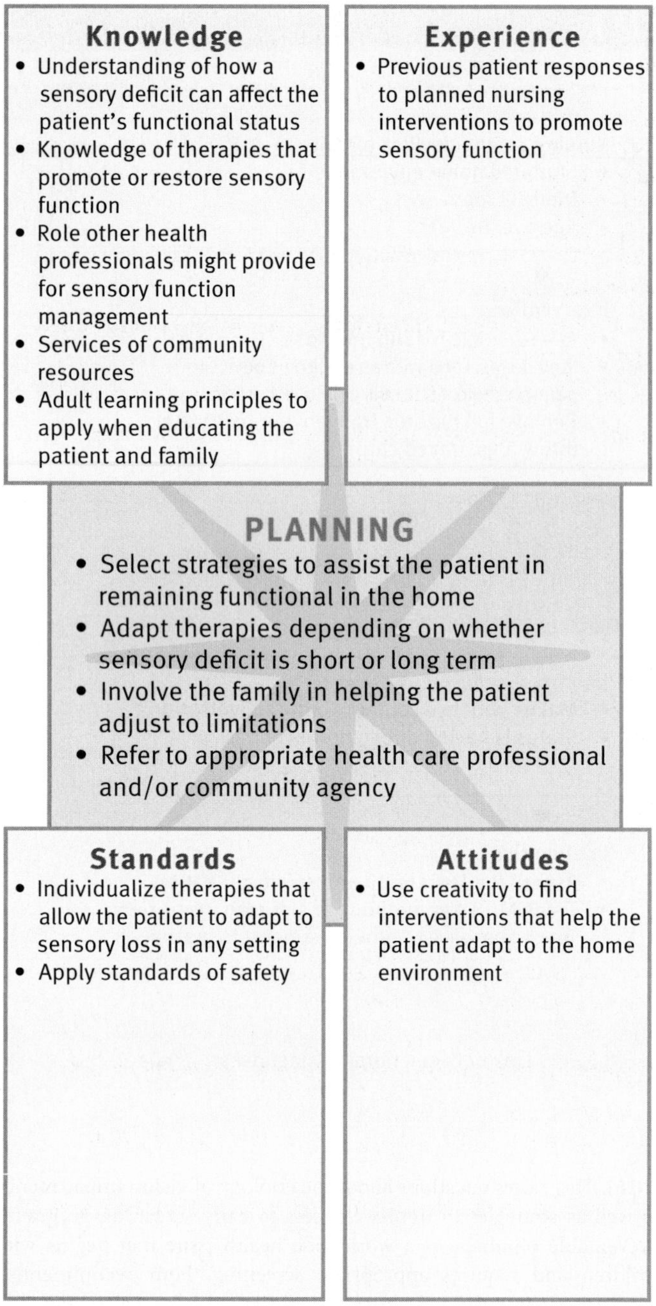

Knowledge
- Understanding of how a sensory deficit can affect the patient's functional status
- Knowledge of therapies that promote or restore sensory function
- Role other health professionals might provide for sensory function management
- Services of community resources
- Adult learning principles to apply when educating the patient and family

Experience
- Previous patient responses to planned nursing interventions to promote sensory function

PLANNING
- Select strategies to assist the patient in remaining functional in the home
- Adapt therapies depending on whether sensory deficit is short or long term
- Involve the family in helping the patient adjust to limitations
- Refer to appropriate health care professional and/or community agency

Standards
- Individualize therapies that allow the patient to adapt to sensory loss in any setting
- Apply standards of safety

Attitudes
- Use creativity to find interventions that help the patient adapt to the home environment

FIG. 49.4 Critical thinking model for sensory alterations planning.

In the United States glaucoma is the second leading cause of blindness in the general population and the primary cause of blindness in African Americans. If left undetected and untreated, it leads to permanent vision loss. The CDC (2018) recommends that people with diabetes have a dilated eye exam every year. Individuals who are at a higher risk for glaucoma should have a dilated eye exam every two years. Individuals at a higher risk include the following: African Americans 40 years and older and all adults older than 60, especially Mexican Americans and people with a family history of glaucoma. Individuals who have had eye surgery or who have other health concerns or conditions are also at risk for the development of vision problems.

Hearing impairment is one of the most common disabilities in the United States. The prevalence of hearing loss is nearly 50% in those older than 75 years of age (NIDCD, 2018). Deafness or hearing impairment affects not only older adults but also children. Children at risk include those with a family history of childhood hearing impairment, perinatal infection (rubella, herpes, or cytomegalovirus), low birth weight, chronic ear infection, and Down syndrome. Advise pregnant women of the importance of early prenatal care, avoidance of ototoxic drugs, and testing for syphilis or rubella.

Children with chronic middle ear infections, a common cause of impaired hearing, need to receive periodic auditory testing. Warn parents of the risks and to seek medical care when a child has symptoms of earache or respiratory infection.

Because aging is associated with degenerative changes in the ear, patients need to have hearing screenings at least every decade through age 50 and every 3 years thereafter (American Speech-Language-Hearing Association, n.d.). Once a patient reports a hearing loss, regular testing also becomes necessary. In addition, a patient who works or lives in a high–noise level environment requires annual screening. Occupational health nurses play a key role in the assessment of the auditory system and the initiation of prompt referrals. The early identification and treatment of problems help older adults be more active and healthier.

Preventive Measures. Trauma is a common cause of blindness in children. Penetrating injury from propulsive objects such as firecrackers or slingshots or from penetrating wounds from sticks, scissors, or toy weapons are just a few examples. Provide patient education to parents and children about ways to avoid eye trauma, such as avoiding the use of toys with long, pointed projections and instructing children not to walk or run while carrying pointed objects. Instruct patients that they can find safety equipment in most sports shops and large department stores.

Adults are at risk for eye injury while playing sports and working in jobs involving exposure to chemicals or flying objects. The Occupational Safety and Health Administration (OSHA, n.d.) has guidelines for workplace safety. Employers are required to have eyewash stations and to have employees wear eye goggles and/or use equipment such as HPDs to reduce the risk of injury. *Healthy People 2020* (USDHHS, 2018a) identifies goals that include reducing new cases of work-related, noise-induced hearing loss. Occupational health nurses reinforce the use of devices. In addition, nurses need to routinely assess patients for noise exposure and provide hearing conservation classes for teachers, students, and patients.

Another means of prevention involves regular immunization of children against diseases capable of causing hearing loss (e.g., rubella, mumps, and measles). Nurses who work in health care providers' offices, schools, and community clinics instruct patients about the importance of early and timely immunization. Use caution when administering ototoxic drugs in all populations.

The average American worker spends 7 hours a day on the computer either in the office or working from home. To help prevent or alleviate digital eye strain, the American Optometric Association (2019) recommends following the 20-20-20 rule; take a 20-second break to view something 20 feet away every 20 minutes. Educate patients at risk for computer eye strain to adopt preventive eye care and computer viewing practices (Box 49.6).

Use of Assistive Devices. Patients who wear corrective contact lenses, eyeglasses, or hearing aids need to make sure that they are clean, accessible, and functional (see Chapter 40). It is helpful to have a family member or friend who also knows how to care for and clean an assistive aid. A contact lens wearer must clean lenses frequently (see Chapter 40) and use the appropriate solutions for cleaning and disinfection. Contact lens wearers are subject to serious eye infections caused by infrequent lens disinfection, contamination of lens storage cases or contact lens solutions, and use of homemade saline. Swimming while wearing lenses also creates a serious risk of infection. Reinforce proper lens care in any health maintenance discussion.

Older adults are often reluctant to use hearing aids. Reasons cited most often include cost, appearance, insufficient knowledge about

⊙ **NURSING CARE PLAN**

Risk for Injury

ASSESSMENT

Ms. Long is a 70-year-old retired widow who lives in a one-level home with her son. Their home has a walkout basement. Ms. Long enjoys reading and sewing, but she is experiencing reduced vision, which is affecting her ability to participate in these activities. She is fearful of falling and visited an ophthalmologist a year ago.

Assessment Activities	*Assessment Findings*[a]
Ask Ms. Long to describe her visual acuity and vision changes.	Ms. Long states, "My left eye has a film over it that makes my **vision blurred.** I am having **difficulty reading and driving at night."**
Ask Ms. Long to describe life changes that have occurred since the change in vision.	Ms. Long states, "I can no longer drive at night. **I'm afraid to use the stairs at home because I can't judge steps clearly.**"
Ask Ms. Long the results of the visit to the ophthalmologist.	Ms. Long states, "I was told I had a **cataract of the left eye,** and surgery was recommended."
Conduct a home hazard assessment.	There is **clutter in the home, dim lighting,** and stairs with **poor lighting and a broken handrail.**

[a]**Assessment Findings** are shown in bold type.

NURSING DIAGNOSIS: Risk for injury

PLANNING

Goal	*Expected Outcomes (NOC)[b]* *Safe Home Environment*
Ms. Long will maintain independence in a safe home environment.	Ms. Long and her son make recommended changes in lighting, repair the broken handrail, and reduce clutter in the home environment within 4 weeks.
	Ms. Long reports an increased sense of home safety and independence within 4 weeks.

[b]Outcome classification labels from Moorhead S, et al: *Nursing Outcomes Classification (NOC),* ed 6, St Louis, 2018, Elsevier.

INTERVENTIONS (NIC)[c]	RATIONALE
Environmental Management	
Teach Ms. Long and her son methods to improve environmental safety, such as installing handrails along stairs, raising toilet seats, removing throw rugs, and painting stairs.	Home environmental and health-related factors place a patient at risk for falls. Environmental safety modifications reduce the risk of falls and injury (Powell-Cope et al., 2018).
Teach Ms. Long to use a light over the shoulder for reading and sewing.	Warm incandescent lighting helps reduce eye strain and increase enjoyment (Touhy and Jett, 2016).
Explain use of a pocket magnifier, and offer list of locations where Ms. Long can purchase one.	Magnifier enlarges visual images when reading or doing close work (Touhy and Jett, 2016).
Have Ms. Long make appointment with ophthalmologist within the next 4 weeks.	Adults over the age of 60 need a routine eye examination yearly (American Optometric Association, 2018).
Emotional Support	
Encourage Ms. Long to discuss with family and friends how a loss of vision affects her independence and lifestyle.	Visual impairments are associated with mobility and activity limitations, social restrictions, and reduced quality of life (Nael et al., 2017; Ya-Chuan et al., 2018).

[c]Intervention classification labels from Butcher HK, et al: *Nursing Interventions Classification (NIC),* ed 7, St Louis, 2018, Elsevier.

EVALUATION

Evaluation Activity	*Patient Response/Finding*	*Outcome Status*
Ask Ms. Long to describe the changes made in the home to reduce environmental hazards.	Ms. Long responds that she removed the clutter and placed handrails at the entryway. She also placed lighting behind her chair, and there are 100-watt lights in the living room. She has a specific craft light that provides additional "over-the-shoulder" lighting.	Ms. Long and her son made recommended changes in the home environment, resulting in improved home safety.
Ask Ms. Long whether she is able to maintain a degree of independence with the environmental and lifestyle modifications.	Ms. Long states, "I'm more independent at home, and I am able to enjoy my hobbies. Until surgery I don't mind having someone drive for me."	Ms. Long reported an increased sense of home safety and independence.

BOX 49.6 Preventing Computer or Digital Eye Strain

Eye Care

- Encourage patients to ask their optometrist or ophthalmologist if they might benefit from glasses prescribed specifically for computer use.
- Persons already wearing glasses may find their current prescription does not provide optimal vision for viewing a computer.
- Special lens designs, lens powers, or lens tints/coatings may help to maximize visual abilities and comfort.
- Vision therapy may be needed. Vision therapy, also called visual training, is a prescribed program of visual activities to improve visual abilities. It trains the eyes and brain to work together more effectively.

Computer Viewing

- Improve the conditions for using computers.
- Optimally, a computer screen should be located 15 to 20 degrees below eye level (about 4 or 5 inches) as measured from the center of the screen and 20 to 28 inches from the eyes.
- Reference materials should be placed above the keyboard and below the monitor. If such placement is not possible, a document holder can be used next to the monitor.
- Position the computer screen to avoid glare, particularly from overhead lighting or windows. Use blinds or drapes on windows and use lower wattage light bulbs in desk lamps.
- If there is no way to minimize glare from light sources, consider using an antiglare screen filter.
- Chairs should be comfortably padded and conform to the body. Chair height should be adjusted so that the feet rest flat on the floor. If a chair has arms, adjust armrests to provide support while typing. The wrists should not rest on the keyboard.
- Rest the eyes when using the computer for long periods—15 minutes for every 2 hours of continuous computer use. In addition, for every 20 minutes of computer viewing, look into the distance for 20 seconds to allow the eyes to refocus.

Adapted from American Optometric Association: Computer Vision Syndrome, 2019, https://www.aoa.org/patients-and-public/caring-for-your-vision/protecting-your-vision/computer-vision-syndrome

BOX 49.7 PATIENT TEACHING
Effective Use of a Hearing Aid

Objective

- Patient and family member will describe the steps to take for correct care and use of a hearing aid.

Teaching Strategies

- Show patient and family member locations on hearing aid device where damage (e.g., cracks, fraying) is likely to occur: earmold or case, earphone, dials, cord, and connection plugs.
- Instruct patient and family on how to assess the integrity of the aid each day.
- Demonstrate battery replacement: Have an extra set of unused batteries available.
- Instruct patient to store batteries in a dry, secure place away from pets and children.
- Instruct patient to clean ear canal daily.
- Instruct patient not to use hair spray or other hair products when hearing aid is in place.
- Review method to check volume: Turn dial to maximum gain and check. Is voice clear?
- Review factors to report to hearing aid laboratory: static, distortion of sound, poor volume quality.

Evaluation

Use the principles of teach-back to evaluate patient/family caregiver learning:

- Tell me what we discussed about storage of your hearing aid.
- Tell me how you check the volume of your hearing aid.
- Tell me what we discussed about ways to clean and protect your hearing aid.
- Tell me what we discussed about battery removal and cleaning of your hearing aid.

hearing aids, amplification of competing noise, and unrealistic expectations. Neuromuscular changes in the older adult such as stiff fingers, enlarged joints, and decreased sensory perception also make the handling and care of a hearing aid difficult. Fortunately today there are a wide variety of aids that not only enhance a person's hearing but also are cosmetically acceptable and useful for people with manual dexterity issues. Chapter 40 summarizes the types of hearing aids available and tips for proper care and use.

Acknowledging a need to improve hearing is a person's first step. Give patients useful information on the benefits of hearing aid use. A person who understands the need for good hearing will likely be influenced to wear hearing aids. It is also important to have a significant other available to assist with hearing aid adjustment (Box 49.7). Federal regulations require prospective hearing aid users younger than 18 years of age to have a medical examination before hearing aids are purchased. Prospective hearing aid users 18 years of age and older need a medical evaluation by a licensed physician (US Food and Drug Administration, 2018a). Hearing aid dispensers should have prospective users consult their health care provider or an otolaryngologist for the following conditions: visible congenital or traumatic deformity of the ear, active drainage in the last 90 days, sudden or progressive hearing loss within the last 90 days, acute or chronic dizziness, unilateral sudden hearing loss within the last 90 days, visible cerumen accumulation or a foreign body in the ear canal, pain or discomfort in the ear, or an audiometric air-bone gap of 15 decibels or greater (US Food and Drug Administration, 2018b).

Promoting Meaningful Stimulation. Life becomes more enriching and satisfying when meaningful and pleasant stimuli exist within the environment. You can help patients adjust to their environment in many ways to make it more stimulating. You do this best by considering the normal physiological changes that accompany sensory deficits.

Vision. The pupil's ability to adjust to light diminishes as a result of the normal changes of aging; thus older adults are often very sensitive to glare. Suggest the use of yellow or amber lenses and shades or blinds on windows to minimize glare. Wearing sunglasses outside obviously reduces the glare of direct sunlight. Other interventions to enhance vision for patients with visual impairment include warm incandescent lighting and colors with sharp contrast and intensity.

The ability to read is important. Therefore allow patients to use their glasses whenever possible (e.g., during procedures and instruction). Some patients with reduced visual acuity need more than corrective lenses. A pocket magnifier helps a patient read most printed material. Telescopic-lens eyeglasses are smaller, easier to focus, and have a greater range. Many books and other publications are available in large-print formats. If a patient has a legal document or other important document that he or she wishes to read, standard copying machines have enlarging capabilities. Software is also available that converts text into artificial voice output (Touhy and Jett, 2016).

With aging a person experiences a change in color perception. Perception of the colors blue, violet, and green usually declines. Brighter colors such as red, orange, and yellow are easier to see. Offer suggestions of ways to decorate a room and paint hallways or stairwells so the patient is able to differentiate surfaces and objects in a room.

Hearing. To maximize residual hearing function, work closely with a patient to suggest ways to modify the environment. For example, patients can amplify the sound of telephones and televisions. An innovative way to enrich the lives of patients with hearing impairments is recorded music. Some patients with severe hearing loss are able to hear music recorded in the low-frequency sound cycles.

One way to help an individual with a hearing loss is to ensure that the problem is not impacted cerumen. With aging cerumen thickens and builds up in the ear canal. Excessive cerumen occluding the ear canal causes conductive hearing loss. Wax-removal medication, such as carbamide peroxide (Debrox Earwax Removal Kit, Murine Ear Wax Removal System) can be effective. Because these drops can irritate the delicate skin of the eardrum and ear canal, use them only as directed (Mayo Clinic, 2019). In the home setting, suggest patients use an eyedropper to apply a few drops of baby oil, mineral oil, glycerin, or hydrogen peroxide in the ear canal to soften the cerumen (Mayo Clinic, 2019).

Taste and Smell. Promote the sense of taste by using measures to enhance remaining taste perception. Good oral hygiene keeps the taste buds well hydrated. Well-seasoned, differently textured food eaten separately heightens taste perception. Flavored vinegar or lemon juice adds tartness to food. Always ask a patient which foods are most appealing. Improving taste perception improves food intake and appetite as well.

Stimulation of the sense of smell with aromas such as brewed coffee, cooked garlic, and baked bread heightens taste sensation. Patients need to avoid blending or mixing foods because these actions make it difficult to identify tastes. Older people need to chew food thoroughly to allow more food to contact remaining taste buds.

Improve smell by strengthening pleasant olfactory stimulation. Make a patient's environment more pleasant with smells such as cologne, mild room deodorizers, fragrant flowers, and sachets. Consult with patients to find out which scents they can tolerate. The removal of unpleasant odors (e.g., bedpans or soiled dressings) also improves the quality of a patient's environment.

Touch. Patients with reduced tactile sensation usually have the impairment over a limited part of their bodies. Providing touch therapy stimulates existing function. If a patient is willing to be touched, hair brushing and combing, a back rub, and touching the arms or shoulders are ways to increase tactile contact. When sensation is reduced, a firm pressure is often necessary for a patient to feel a nurse's hand. Turning and repositioning also improve the quality of tactile sensation.

If a patient is overly sensitive to tactile stimuli (hyperesthesia), minimize irritating stimuli. Keeping bed linens loose to minimize direct contact with a patient and protecting the skin from exposure to irritants are helpful measures. Physical therapists can recommend special wrist splints for patients to wear to dorsiflex their wrists and relieve nerve pressure when they have numbness and tingling or pain in the hands, as with carpal tunnel syndrome. For patients who use computers, special keyboards and wrist pads are available to decrease the pressure on the median nerve, aid in pain relief, and promote healing.

Establishing Safe Environments. When sensory function becomes impaired, individuals become less secure within their home and workplace. Security is necessary for a person to feel independent. Make recommendations for improving safety within a patient's living environment without restricting independence. During a home visit or while completing an examination in the clinic, offer several useful suggestions for home safety. The nature of the actual or potential sensory loss determines the safety precautions you take.

Adaptations for Visual Loss. When a patient experiences a decrease in visual acuity, peripheral vision, adaptation to the dark, or depth perception, safety is a concern. With reduced peripheral vision a patient cannot see panoramically because the outer visual field is less discrete. With reduced depth perception a person is unable to judge how far away objects are located. This is a special danger when he or she walks down stairs or over uneven surfaces.

Driving is a particular safety hazard for older adults with visual alterations. Reduced peripheral vision prevents a driver from seeing a car in an adjacent lane. A sensitivity to glare creates a problem for driving at night with headlights. Vision is a primary consideration for safety, but there are other factors as well. In the case of older adults, decreased reaction time, reduced hearing, and decreased strength in the legs and arms further compromise driving skills. Some safety tips to share with those who continue to drive include the following: drive in familiar areas, do not drive during rush hour, avoid interstate highways for local drives, drive defensively, use rear-view and side-view mirrors when changing lanes, avoid driving at dusk or night, go slow but not too slow, keep the car in good working condition, and carry a preprogrammed cellular phone.

The presence of visual alterations makes it difficult for a person to conduct normal activities of daily living within the home. Because of reduced depth perception, patients can trip on throw rugs, runners, or the edge of stairs. Teach patients and family members to keep all flooring in good condition, and advise them to use low-pile carpeting. Thresholds between rooms need to be level with the floor. Recommend the removal of clutter to ensure clear pathways for walking, and arrange furniture so that a patient can move about easily without fear of tripping or running into objects. Suggest that stairwells have a securely fastened banister or handrail extending the full length of the stairs.

Front and back entrances to the home, work areas, and stairwells need to be lighted properly. Light fixtures need high-wattage bulbs with wider illumination. Stairwells need a light switch at both the top and bottom of the stairs. It is also important to be sure that lighting on the stairs does not cast shadows. Have a family member paint the edge of steps so that the patient can see each step, especially the first and last, clearly. When possible, have patients replace steps inside and outside the home with ramps.

An added consideration is to administer eye medications safely (see Chapter 31). Patients need to closely adhere to regular medication schedules for conditions such as glaucoma. Labels on medication containers need to be in large print. Make sure that a friend or spouse is familiar with dosage schedules in case a patient is unable to self-administer a medication. Patients with visual impairments often have difficulty manipulating eyedroppers.

Adaptations for Reduced Hearing. Patients hear important environmental sounds (e.g., doorbells and alarm clocks) best if they are amplified or changed to a lower-pitched, buzzerlike sound. Lamps designed to turn on in response to sounds such as doorbells, burglar alarms, smoke detectors, and babies crying are also available. Family members or anyone else who calls the patient regularly needs to learn to let the phone ring for a longer period. Amplified receivers for telephones and telephone communication devices (TCDs) are available that use a computer and printer to transfer words over the telephone for the hearing impaired. Both sender and receiver need to have the special device to complete a call.

Adaptations for Reduced Olfaction. The patient with a reduced sensitivity to odors is often unable to smell leaking gas, a smoldering cigarette, fire, or spoiled food. Advise patients to use smoke detectors and take precautions such as checking ashtrays or placing cigarette butts in water. In addition, teach patients to check food package dates, inspect the appearance of food, and keep leftovers in labeled containers with the preparation date. Pilot gas flames need to be checked visually.

Adaptations for Reduced Tactile Sensation. When patients have reduced sensation in their extremities, they are at risk for impaired skin integrity and injury from exposure to temperature extremes. Always caution these patients about the use of heating and cooling devices (see Chapter 48). The temperature setting on the home water heater should be no higher than 48.8° C (120° F). If a patient also has a visual impairment, it is important to be sure that water faucets are clearly marked "hot" and "cold" or use color codes (i.e., red for hot and blue for cold). Discourage the use of heating pads in this population.

Communication. A sensory deficit often causes a person to feel isolated because of an inability to communicate with others. It is important for individuals to be able to interact with people around them. The nature of the sensory loss influences the methods and styles of communication that nurses use during interactions with patients (Box 49.8). You also teach communication methods to family members and significant others. For patients with visual deficits or blindness, speak normally, not from a distance, and be sure to have sufficient lighting.

The patient with a hearing impairment is often able to speak normally. To more clearly hear what a person communicates, family and friends need to learn to move away from background noise, rephrase rather than repeat sentences, be positive, and have patience. In a group setting it is better to form a semicircle in front of the patient so that he or she can see who is speaking next; this helps foster group involvement. On the other hand, some patients who are deaf have serious speech alterations. Some use sign language or lipreading, wear special hearing aids, write with a pad and pencil, or learn to use a computer for communication. Special communication boards that contain common terms (e.g., *pain, bathroom, dizzy,* or *walk*) help patients express their needs.

Patient education is one aspect of communication. Teaching booklets are available in large print for patients with visual loss. The patient who is blind often requires more frequent and detailed verbal descriptions of information. This is particularly true if there are no instructional booklets written in Braille. Patients with visual impairments can also learn by listening to audiotapes or the sound part of a televised teaching session. Patients with hearing impairments often benefit from written instructional materials and visual teaching aids (e.g., posters and graphs). Demonstrations by the nurse are very useful. Hospitals are required to make professional interpreters available to read sign language for patients who are deaf.

Acute Care. When patients enter acute care settings for therapeutic management of sensory deficits or as a result of traumatic injury, use different approaches to maximize sensory function existing at the time. Safety is an obvious priority until a patient's sensory status is either stabilized or improved. For example, patients with sensory deficits have a high risk for falls in the acute care environment. It is very important to know the extent of any existing sensory impairment before the acute episode of illness so that you are able to reinforce what the patient already knows about self-care or to plan for more instruction before and after discharge.

Orientation to the Environment. A patient with a sensory impairment requires a complete orientation to the immediate environment. Provide reorientation as needed to the institutional environment by ensuring

---

BOX 49.8 Communication Methods

Patients With Aphasia
- Listen to patient and provide sufficient time for him or her to communicate.
- Do not shout or speak loudly (hearing loss is not the problem).
- If patient has problems with comprehension, use simple, short questions and facial gestures to give additional clues.
- Speak of things familiar and of interest to patient.
- If patient has problems speaking, ask questions that require simple yes or no answers or blinking of the eyes. Offer pictures or a communication board so patient can point.
- Speak slowly and give patient time to understand; be calm and patient; do not pressure or tire him or her.
- Avoid patronizing and childish phrases.

Patients With an Artificial Airway
- Use pictures, objects, or word cards so patient can point.
- Offer a pad and pencil or Magic Slate for patient to write messages.
- Do not shout or speak loudly.
- Give patient time to write messages because patients tire easily.
- Provide an artificial voice box (vibrator) for patient with a laryngectomy to use to speak.

Patients With Hearing Impairment
- Get patient's attention. Do not startle him or her when entering the room. Do not approach patient from behind. Be sure that he or she knows that you want to speak.
- Face patient and stand or sit on the same level. Be sure that your face and lips are illuminated to promote lipreading. Keep hands away from mouth.
- Be sure that the environment is not noisy.
- Be sure that patients keep eyeglasses clean, so they are able to see your gestures and face.
- If patient wears a hearing aid, make sure that it is in place and working.
- Speak slowly and articulate clearly. Sometimes people with hearing loss take longer to process verbal messages.
- Use a normal tone of voice and inflections of speech. Do not speak with something in your mouth.
- When you are not understood, rephrase rather than repeat the conversation.
- Use visible expressions. Speak with your hands, face, and eyes.
- Do not shout. Loud sounds are usually higher pitched and often impede hearing by accentuating vowel sounds and concealing consonants. If you need to raise your voice, speak in lower tones.
- Talk toward patient's best or normal ear.
- Use written information to enhance the spoken word.
- Do not restrict the hands of patient who is deaf. Never have intravenous lines in both of patient's hands if the preferred method of communication is sign language.
- Avoid eating, chewing, or smoking while speaking.
- Avoid speaking from another room or while walking away.

---

that name tags on uniforms are visible, addressing the patient by name, explaining where the patient is (especially if patients are transported to different areas for treatment), and using conversational cues to time or location. Reduce the tendency for patients to become confused by offering short, simple, repeated explanations and reassurance. Encourage family members and visitors to help orient patients to the hospital surroundings.

Patients with serious visual impairment need to feel comfortable in knowing the boundaries of the immediate environment. Normally people see physical boundaries within a room. Patients who are blind or severely visually impaired often touch the boundaries or objects to gain a sense of their surroundings. The patient needs to walk through a room and feel the walls to establish a sense of direction. Help patients by explaining objects within the hospital room such as furniture or equipment. It takes time for a patient to absorb room arrangement. He or she often needs to reorient again as you explain the location of key items (e.g., nurse call system, telephone, and chair). Remember to approach the patient from the front to avoid startling him or her.

It is important to keep all objects in the same position and place. After an object is moved even a short distance, it no longer exists for a person who is blind. Simply moving a chair creates a safety hazard. Ask the patient whether any item needs to be rearranged to make ambulation easier. Clear traffic patterns to the bathroom. Give the patient extra time to perform tasks. He or she moves slowly to remain safe and needs a detailed description of how to perform an activity. .

Patients confined to bed are at risk for sensory deprivation. Normally, movement gives an awareness of self through vestibular and tactile stimulation. Movement patterns influence sensory perception. The limited movement of bed rest changes how a person interprets the environment; surroundings seem different, and objects seem to assume shapes different from normal. A person who is on bed rest requires routine stimulation through range-of-motion exercises, positioning, and participation in self-care activities (as appropriate). Comfort measures, such as washing the face and hands and providing back rubs, improve the quality of stimulation and lessen the chance of sensory deprivation. Planning time to talk with patients is also essential. Explain unfamiliar environmental noises and sensations. A calm, unhurried approach gives you quality time to help reorient and familiarize the patient with care activities. The patient who is well enough to read will benefit from a variety of reading materials.

Communication. The most common language disorder following a stroke is aphasia. Depending on the type of aphasia, the inability to communicate is often frustrating and frightening (see Box 49.8). Initially you need to establish very basic communication and recognize that it does not indicate intellectual impairment or degeneration of personality. Explain situations and treatments that are pertinent to the patient because he or she is able to understand the speaker's words. Because a stroke often causes partial or complete paralysis of one side of a patient's body, the patient needs special assistive devices. A variety of communication boards for different levels of disability are available. Sensitive pressure switches activated by the touch of an ear, nose, or chin control electronic communication boards (Touhy and Jett, 2018). Make referrals to speech therapists to develop appropriate rehabilitation plans.

In acute care hospitals or long-term care facilities, nurses often care for patients with artificial airways (such as an endotracheal tube) (see Chapter 41). The placement of an endotracheal tube prevents a patient from speaking. In this case the nurse uses special communication methods to facilitate the patient's ability to express needs. The patient is sometimes completely alert and able to hear and see the nurse normally. Giving him or her time to convey any needs or requests is very important. Use creative communication techniques (e.g., a communication board or electronic tablet) to foster and strengthen the patient's interactions with health care personnel, family, and friends.

Controlling Sensory Stimuli. Patients need time for rest and freedom from stress caused by frequent monitoring and repeated tests. Reduce sensory overload by organizing the patient's plan of care. Combine activities such as dressing changes, bathing, and vital sign measurement in one visit to conserve a patient's energy and prevent fatigue. A patient also needs scheduled time for rest and quiet. Planning for rest periods often requires cooperation from family, visitors, and health care colleagues. Coordination with laboratory and radiology departments minimizes the number of interruptions for procedures. A creative solution to decrease excessive environmental stimuli that prevents restful, healing sleep is to institute "quiet time" in ICUs. Quiet time means dimming the lights throughout the unit, closing the shades, and shutting the doors. Data collected from one hospital that implemented a quiet time protocol found decreased sleep disorders of the patients hospitalized in the ICU and improved sleep quality (Chamanzari et al., 2016) (Box 49.9).

When patients experience sensory overload or deprivation, their behavior is often difficult for family or friends to accept. Encourage the family not to argue with or contradict the patient but to calmly explain location, identity, and time of day. Engaging a patient in a normal discussion about familiar topics helps in reorientation. Anticipating patient needs such as voiding helps reduce uncomfortable stimuli.

Try to control extraneous noise in and around a patient's room. It is often necessary to ask a roommate to lower the volume on a television or to move the patient to a quieter room. Keep equipment noise to a minimum. Turn off bedside equipment not in use such as suction and oxygen equipment. Avoid making abrupt loud noises such as dropping objects or causing the over-bed table to suddenly adjust to the lowest level. Nursing staff also need to control laughter or conversation outside the patients' rooms. Allow patients to close their room doors.

When a patient leaves an acute care setting for the home environment, communicate with colleagues in the home care setting about the patient's existing sensory deficits and the interventions that helped the patient adapt to sensory problems. You achieve continuity of care when the patient has to make only minimal changes in the home setting.

Safety Measures. A patient with recent visual impairment often requires help with walking. The presence of an eye patch, frequently instilled eyedrops, and the swelling of eyelid structures following surgery are just a few factors that cause a patient to need more help than usual. A sighted guide gives confidence to patients with visual impairments and ensures safe mobility. Bosma Enterprises (n.d.) lists several suggestions for a sighted guide:

1. Ask the patient if he or she wants a "sighted guide." If assistance is accepted, offer your arm. Tap the back of your hand against his or her hand. The person will then grasp your arm directly above the elbow (Fig. 49.5).
2. Relax and walk at a comfortable pace. Walk one step ahead of the person you are guiding, except at the top and bottom of stairs and streets. At these places pause and stand alongside the person. Be sure that the person has a strong grasp on your arm.
3. While walking with a patient, describe the surroundings and ensure that obstacles have been removed. Never leave a patient with a visual impairment standing alone in an unfamiliar area.
4. To guide a person to a seat, place his or her hand on the back of the seat. The person you are guiding will find the seat by following along your arm.

It is important to teach family members techniques for helping with ambulation. Nursing staff also need to ensure that the patient knows where the nurse call system is before leaving him or her alone. Place necessary objects in front of the patient to prevent falls caused by reaching over the bedside. Appropriate use of side rails is also an option.

Nurses often rely on patients in health care settings to report unusual sounds such as a suction apparatus running improperly or an IV pump alarm. However, a patient with a hearing loss does not always hear these sounds and thus requires more frequent visits by nurses. The patient also benefits from learning to use vision to discover sources of danger. It is wise to note on the intercom system at the nurse's station and in the medical record if the patient is deaf and/or blind. A patient

BOX 49.9 EVIDENCE-BASED PRACTICE

Quiet Time and Improved Patient Well-Being

PICOT Question: Does a "quiet time" intervention compared with routine intensive care unit practices improve sleep quality and satisfaction with care in hospitalized patients?

Evidence Summary

A quiet environment promotes rest and healing, but many factors contribute to a noisy hospital environment. The number of patient rooms and design of the unit, as well as admissions and discharges throughout the day, influence noise levels in health care settings. One strategy suggested to reduce noise to recommended levels is a "quiet time" intervention. "Quiet time" is observed in a number of different ways, but Goeren et al. (2018) found that limiting conversations, eliminating environmental noise, and dimming the lights are strategies that can be implemented to reduce noise. While it can be challenging to create a daily period without distractions, current evidence shows "quiet time" interventions have improved patients' well-being, as well as satisfaction with care (Applebaum et al., 2016; McGough et al., 2018). "Quiet time" interventions have also been found to improve patients' sleep quality and improve restfulness (Lim, 2018).

Application to Nursing Practice

- Encourage visitors to take breaks to allow their loved ones time to rest.
- Designate areas away from patient rooms for phone conversations and for the health care team to conduct student teaching sessions (Goeren et al., 2018).
- Collaborate with the interprofessional team to provide "quiet time" for patients (Goeren et al., 2018).
- Review alarm parameters and adjust the default settings as appropriate (Goeren et al., 2018).
- Modify your workflow to establish a restful environment for patients during "quiet time."

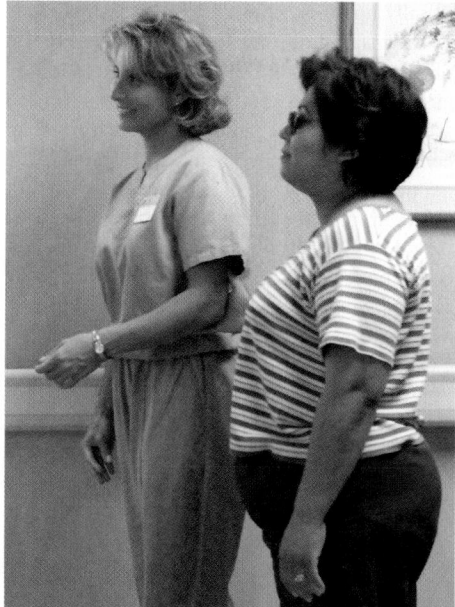

FIG. 49.5 Nurse helps to ambulate patient with visual impairment. (From Sorrentino SA, Remmert LN: *Mosby's essentials for nursing assistants*, ed 6, St Louis, 2019, Elsevier.)

lacking the ability to speak cannot call out for assistance. Patients need to have message boards and nurse call system close at hand.

Patients with reduced tactile sensation risk injury when their conditions confine them to bed because they are unable to sense pressure on bony prominences or the need to change position. These patients rely on nurses for timely repositioning, moving tubes or devices on which the patient is lying, and turning to avoid skin breakdown. When a patient is less able to sense temperature variations, use extra caution in applying heat and cold therapies (see Chapter 48) and preparing bathwater. Check the condition of the patient's skin frequently.

Restorative and Continuing Care

Maintaining Healthy Lifestyles. After a patient has experienced a sensory loss, it becomes important to understand the implications of the loss and make adjustments needed to continue a normal lifestyle. Sensory impairments need not prevent a person from leading an active, rewarding life. Many of the interventions applicable to health promotion such as adapting the home environment are useful after a patient leaves an acute care setting.

Understanding Sensory Loss. Patients who have experienced a recent sensory loss need to understand how to adapt so that their living environments are safe and appropriately stimulating. All family members need to understand how a patient's sensory impairment affects normal daily activities. Family and friends are more supportive when they understand sensory deficits and factors that worsen or lessen sensory problems. For example, they need to learn how to communicate with someone who has a hearing loss. Community

resources are available to provide information to help patients with personal management needs. The American Foundation for the Blind, American Red Cross, and National Association for Speech and Hearing offer resource materials and product information.

Socialization. The ability to communicate is gratifying. It tests a person's intellect, opens opportunities, and allows him or her to exchange the feelings that he or she has about others. When sensory alterations hinder interactions, a person feels ineffective and loses self-esteem. When patients feel socially unaccepted, they perceive sensory losses as seriously impairing their quality of life.

Interacting with others becomes a burden for many patients with sensory alterations. They lose the motivation to engage in social situations, resulting in a deep sense of loneliness. Use therapies to reduce loneliness, particularly in older adults (Box 49.10). These principles support the *Healthy People 2020* objective to increase the proportion of adults with disabilities reporting sufficient emotional support. In addition, family members need to learn to focus on a person's ability to interact rather than on his or her disability. For example, do not assume that a person who is hard of hearing does not want to speak. A person who is blind can still enjoy a walk through a park with a companion describing the sights around them.

Promoting Self-Care. The ability to perform self-care is essential for self-esteem. Frequently family members and nurses believe that people with sensory impairments require assistance, when in fact they are able to help themselves. To help with meals, arrange food on the plate and condiments, salad, or drinks according to numbers on the face of a clock (Fig. 49.6). A patient can also use this method to place personal care items on the bedside or on the bathroom vanity. It is easy for a patient to become oriented to the items after a nurse or family member explains the location of each item.

Help patients reach toilet facilities safely. Safety bars need to be installed near the toilet. It is often helpful to have the bar a different color than the wall for easier visibility. Never place towels on a safety bar because they interfere with a person's grasp. Toilet paper needs to be within easy reach. Sharply contrasting colors within the room help the partially sighted and promote functional independence. General

BOX 49.10 FOCUS ON OLDER ADULTS

Principles for Reducing Loneliness in Patients with Sensory Impairments

- Spend time with a person in silence or conversation.
- When it is culturally appropriate, use physical contact (e.g., holding a hand, embracing a shoulder) to convey caring.
- Recommend alterations in living arrangements if physical isolation is a factor.
- Help patients keep contact with people important to them.
- Provide information about support groups or groups that provide assistive services.
- Arrange for security escort services as needed.
- Introduce the idea of bringing a companion such as a pet into the home when appropriate.
- Link a person with organizations attuned to the social needs of older adults.

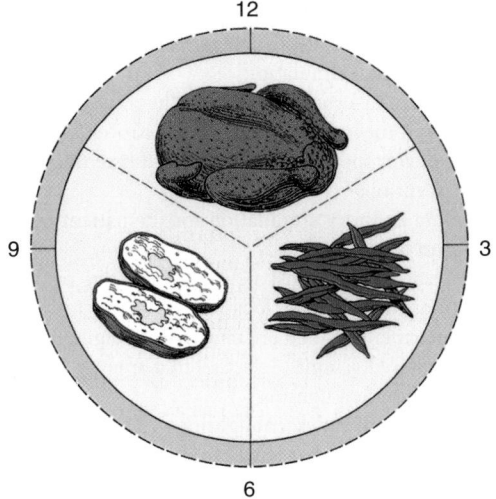

FIG. 49.6 Location of food using clock as frame of reference.

principles for promoting self-care in older adults also include the assurance of adequate lighting and the control of glare by using shades and blinds (Touhy and Jett, 2016).

If the sense of touch is diminished, a patient can dress more easily with zippers or Velcro strips, pullover sweaters or blouses, and elasticized waists. If a patient has partial paralysis and reduced sensation, he or she dresses the affected side first. Encourage family members responsible for selecting clothing for patients with visual impairments to follow the patient's preferences. Any sensory impairment has a significant influence on body image, and it is important for a patient to feel well groomed and attractive. Some patients need assistance with basic grooming such as brushing, combing, and shampooing hair. Others need assistance with medication administration, clothing identification, and learning to manage routine procedures such as blood pressure and glucose monitoring. An assortment of low-vision devices is now available. It is important for you to make appropriate referrals to allow patients to maintain a maximum degree of independence.

Patients with proprioceptive problems often lose their balance easily. Make sure that bathrooms have nonskid surfaces in the tub and shower. Install grab bars either vertically or horizontally in tubs and showers, depending on how a patient is able to grasp or hold onto the bar. Instruct family members to supervise ambulation and sitting, make frequent checks to prevent falls, and caution the patient against leaning forward.

◆ Evaluation

Through the Patient's Eyes. It is important to evaluate whether patients perceive that care measures maintained or improved their ability to interact and function within the environment. The patient is the source for evaluating whether their expectations were met. He or she is the only one who knows whether sensory abilities are improved and which specific interventions or therapies are most successful in facilitating a change in his or her performance. Ask patients for example, "Have we been able to meet your expectation of keeping you safe given your vision losses?" or "Tell me how we can improve ways to communicate with you."

If you have developed a positive relationship with a patient successfully, notice that subtle behaviors often indicate the level of his or her satisfaction. You may notice that the patient responds appropriately, such as by smiling. However, it is important for you to ask the patient whether his or her sensory needs have been met. For example, ask, "Have we done all we can do to help improve your ability to hear?" If the patient's expectations have not been met, ask, "How can the health care team better meet your needs?" Working closely with the patient and family enables you to redefine expectations that can be met realistically within the limits of the patient's condition and therapies. You have been effective when the patient's goals and expectations have been met.

Patient Outcomes. To evaluate the effectiveness of specific nursing interventions, use critical thinking and make comparisons with baseline sensory assessment data to evaluate if sensory alterations have changed (Fig. 49.7). It is your responsibility to determine whether expected outcomes have been met. For example, use evaluative data to determine whether care measures improve or at least maintain a patient's ability to interact and function within the environment. The nature of a patient's sensory alterations influences how you evaluate the outcome of care. When caring for a patient with a hearing deficit, use proper communication techniques and then evaluate whether he or she has gained the ability to hear or interact more effectively. When expected outcomes have not been achieved, there is a need to change interventions or alter the patient's environment. If outcomes are unmet, it is important to ask questions such as "How are you feeling emotionally?" or "Do you feel that you are at risk for injury?" Collaborate with family members to determine whether a patient's ability to function within the home has improved.

If you have directed nursing care at improving or maintaining sensory acuity, evaluate the integrity of the sensory organs and the patient's ability to perceive stimuli. Evaluate interventions designed to relieve problems associated with sensory alterations on the basis of a patient's ability to function normally without injury. When you directly or indirectly (through education) alter a patient's environment, evaluate by observing whether the patient makes environmental changes. When designing patient teaching to improve sensory function, it is important to determine whether the patient is following recommended therapies and meeting mutually set goals. Asking a patient to explain or demonstrate self-care skills is an effective evaluative measure. It is often necessary to reinforce previous instruction if learning has not taken place. If outcomes are unmet, these are examples of questions to ask:

- "How often do you wear your hearing aids/corrective lenses?"
- "Are you able to participate in a small group discussion?"
- "Are you able to read the newspaper without squinting?"

The results of your evaluation will determine whether to continue the existing plan of care, make modifications, or end the use of select interventions.

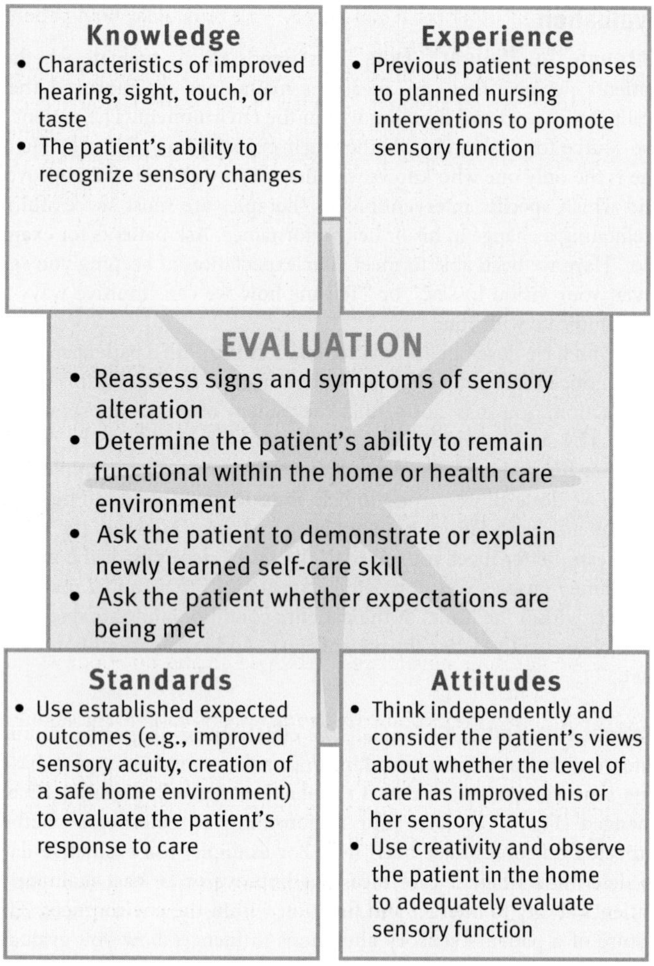

Knowledge	Experience
• Characteristics of improved hearing, sight, touch, or taste • The patient's ability to recognize sensory changes	• Previous patient responses to planned nursing interventions to promote sensory function

EVALUATION
- Reassess signs and symptoms of sensory alteration
- Determine the patient's ability to remain functional within the home or health care environment
- Ask the patient to demonstrate or explain newly learned self-care skill
- Ask the patient whether expectations are being met

Standards	Attitudes
• Use established expected outcomes (e.g., improved sensory acuity, creation of a safe home environment) to evaluate the patient's response to care	• Think independently and consider the patient's views about whether the level of care has improved his or her sensory status • Use creativity and observe the patient in the home to adequately evaluate sensory function

FIG. 49.7 Critical thinking model for sensory alterations evaluation.

KEY POINTS

- Your senses receive information from your environment. Sensory information is converted into nerve signals that travel to the brain and are turned into meaningful sensations.
- Sensory alterations occur when external stimuli are meaningless or deficient (sensory deprivation) or when there is excessive stimulation (sensory overload).
- Many factors affect sensory function. Aging results in a gradual decline of acuity in all senses.
- Sensory alterations can limit a patient's ability to interact and function within the environment.
- A thorough assessment of the sensory system allows for the development and implementation of an individualized plan of care.
- When conducting an assessment, gather information by establishing a therapeutic rapport with the patient.
- Nursing diagnoses are selected by recognizing the way that sensory alterations affect a person's ability to function.
- Preventive actions and the early identification of sensory alterations require periodic health screenings.
- Individualized plans of care with both patient and family involvement influence the quality of sensory experiences.
- An assessment of hazards in the environment is important to reduce the risk of injury among patients with sensory deficits. Proper support and resources are necessary for a person to adjust to a sensory impairment.

REFLECTIVE LEARNING

- Consider a patient experience you have encountered and describe three strategies that you implemented to minimize sensory overload.
- Consider a patient experience you provided to a patient with a sensory alteration. What could you do differently next time to better support and encourage the same patient or a different one?
- Consider a patient experience you provided to a patient with a hearing impairment. What were some of the most challenging moments? What were your limitations, if any?

REVIEW QUESTIONS

1. A patient has been on contact isolation for 4 days because of a hospital-acquired infection. He has had few visitors and few opportunities to leave his room. His ambulation is also still limited. Which are the correct nursing interventions to reduce sensory deprivation? (Select all that apply.)
   1. Teaching how activities such as reading and using crossword puzzles provide stimulation
   2. Moving him to a room away from the nurses' station
   3. Turning on the lights and opening the room blinds
   4. Sitting down, speaking, touching, and listening to his feelings and perceptions
   5. Providing auditory stimulation for the patient by keeping the television on continuously

2. The home care nurse is instructing an assistive personnel about interventions to facilitate location of items for patients with vision impairment. Which are effective strategies for enhancing a patient's impaired vision? (Select all that apply.)
   1. Use of fluorescent lighting
   2. Use of warm incandescent lighting
   3. Use of yellow or amber lenses to decrease glare
   4. Use of adjustable blinds, sheer curtains, or draperies
   5. Indirect lighting to reduce glare

3. An older adult patient with bilateral hearing loss wears a hearing aid in her left ear. Which of the following approaches best facilitates communication with her? (Select all that apply.)
   1. Talk to the patient at a distance so he or she may read your lips.
   2. Keep your arms at your side; speak directly into the patient's left ear.
   3. Face the patient when speaking; demonstrate ideas you wish to convey.
   4. Position the patient so that the light is on his or her face when speaking.
   5. Verify that the information that has been given has been clearly understood.

4. A patient is returning to an assisted-living apartment following a diagnosis of declining, progressive visual loss. Although she is familiar with her apartment and residence, she reports feeling a little uncertain about walking alone. There is one step into her apartment. Her children are scheduling themselves to be available to their mom for the next 2 weeks. Which of the following approaches will you teach the children to assist ambulation? (Select all that apply.)
   1. Walk one-half step behind and slightly to her side.
   2. Have her grasp your arm just above the elbow and walk at a comfortable pace.
   3. Stand next to your mom at the top and bottom of stairs.
   4. Stand one step ahead of mom at the top of the stairs.

5. Place yourself alongside your mom and hold onto her waist.

5. A new nurse is going to help a patient walk down the corridor and sit in a chair. The patient has an eye patch over the left eye and poor vision in the right eye. What is the correct order of steps to help the patient safely walk down the hall and sit in the chair?
   1. Tell patient when you are approaching the chair.
   2. Walk at a relaxed pace.
   3. Guide patient's hand to nurse's arm, resting just above the elbow.
   4. Position yourself one-half step in front of patient.
   5. Position patient's hand on back of chair.

6. A patient with progressive vision impairments had to surrender his driver's license 6 months ago. He comes to the medical clinic for a routine checkup. He is accompanied by his son. His wife died 2 years ago, and he admits to feeling lonely much of the time. Which of the following interventions reduce loneliness? (Select all that apply.)
   1. Sharing information about senior transportation services
   2. Reassuring the patient that loneliness is a normal part of aging
   3. Maintaining distance while talking to avoid overstimulating the patient
   4. Providing information about local social groups in the patient's neighborhood
   5. Recommending that the patient consider making living arrangements that will put him closer to family or friends

7. A nurse is performing an assessment on a patient admitted to the unit following treatment in the emergency department for severe bilateral eye trauma. During patient admission the nurse's priority interventions include which of the following? (Select all that apply.)
   1. Conducting a home-safety assessment and identifying hazards in the patient's living environment
   2. Reinforcing eye safety at work and in activities that place the patient at risk for eye injury
   3. Placing necessary objects such as the nurse call system and water in front of the patient to prevent falls caused by reaching
   4. Orienting the patient to the environment to reduce anxiety and prevent further injury to the eye

5. Alerting other nurses and health care providers about patient's visual status during hand-off reports

8. An older adult is admitted from a skilled nursing home to a medical unit with pneumonia. A review of the medical record reveals that he had a stroke affecting the right hemisphere of the brain 6 months ago and was placed in the skilled nursing home because he was unable to care for himself. Which of these assessment findings does the nurse expect to find? (Select all that apply.)
   1. Slow, cautious behavioral style
   2. Inattention and neglect, especially to the left side
   3. Cloudy or opaque areas in part of the lens or the entire lens
   4. Visual spatial alterations such as loss of half of a visual field
   5. Loss of sensation and motor function on the right side of the body

9. A nurse is performing a home care assessment on a patient with a hearing impairment. The patient reports, "I think my hearing aid is broken. I can't hear anything." After determining that the patient's hearing aid works and that the patient is having trouble managing the hearing aid at home, which of the following teaching strategies does the nurse implement? (Select all that apply.)
   1. Demonstrate hearing aid battery replacement.
   2. Review method to check volume on hearing aid.
   3. Demonstrate how to wash the earmold and microphone with hot water.
   4. Discuss the importance of having wax buildup in the ear canal removed.
   5. Recommend a chemical cleaner to remove difficult buildup.

10. Identify the measures to ensure safety for a patient who has no sensation on one side of the body.

Answers: 1. 1, 3, 4; **2.** 2, 3, 4; **3.** 5, 4, 2, 3; **4.** 2, 3, 5; **5.** 4, 2, 1, 5; **6.** 1, 4, 5; **7.** 3, 4, 5; **8.** 2, 4; **9.** 1, 2, 4; **10.** *See Evolve.*

Rationales for Review Questions can be found on the Evolve website.

REFERENCES

American Optometric Association: Adult vision: over 60 years of age, 2018, https://www.aoa.org/patients-and-public/good-vision-throughout-life/adult-vision-19-to-40-years-of-age/adult-vision-over-60-years-of-age. Accessed October 23, 2018.

American Optometric Association: Computer vision syndrome, 2019, https://www.aoa.org/patients-and-public/caring-for-your-vision/protecting-your-vision/computer-vision-syndrome. Accessed November 19, 2019.

American Speech-Language-Hearing Association: *Hearing screening*, n.d., https://www.asha.org/public/hearing/Hearing-Screening/. Accessed September 28, 2018.

Bosma Enterprises: *Human guide techniques*, n.d., https://www.bosma.org/Navigating-Blindness/Sighted-Guide-Techniques.

Centers for Disease Control and Prevention (CDC): *Keep an eye on your vision health*, 2018, https://www.cdc.gov/features/healthyvision/index.html. Accessed September 28, 2018.

Hockenberry MJ, et al.: *Wong's nursing care of infants and children*, ed 11, St Louis, 2019, Elsevier.

Institute for Patient- and Family-Centered Care: *Advancing the practice of patient- and family-centered care in primary care and other ambulatory settings*, 2016, http://www.ipfcc.org/resources/GettingStarted-AmbulatoryCare.pdf. Accessed October 23, 2018.

Interprofessional Education Collaborative Expert Panel: *Core competencies for interprofessional collaborative practice: 2016 update*, 2016, https://nebula.wsimg.com/2f68a39520b03336b41038c370497473?AccessKeyId=DC06780E69ED19E2B3A5&disposition=0&alloworigin=1. Accessed October 23, 2018.

Mayo Clinic: Earwax blockage, 2019, https://www.mayoclinic.org/diseases-conditions/earwax-blockage/diagnosis-treatment/drc-20353007. Accessed November 19, 2019.

National Institute on Deafness and other Communication Disorders (NIDCD): *Hearing loss and older adults*, 2018, https://www.nidcd.nih.gov/health/hearing-loss-older-adults, 2018. Accessed September 28, 2018.

National Institute of Neurological disorders and stroke (NINDS): Carpal tunnel syndrome fact sheet, 2019, https://www.ninds.nih.gov/Disorders/Patient-Caregiver-Education/Fact-Sheets/Carpal-Tunnel-Syndrome-Fact-Sheet. Accessed November 19, 2019.

Occupational Safety and Health Administration (OSHA): *Eye and face protection*, n.d., https://www.osha.gov/SLTC/eyefaceprotection/standards.html. Accessed September 28, 2018.

Powell-Cope G, et al.: Preventing falls and fall-related injuries at home, *Am J Nurs* 118(1):58, 2018.

Touhy T, Jett P: *Ebersole and Hess' gerontological nursing & healthy aging*, ed 5, St Louis, 2018, Elsevier.

Touhy T, Jett P: *Ebersole and Hess' toward healthy aging: human needs & nursing response*, ed 9, St Louis, 2016, Elsevier.

Umfress A, et al.: Eye care disparities and health related consequences in elderly patients with age-related eye disease, *Semin Ophthalmol* 31(4):432, 2016.

US Food and Drug Administration: *How to get hearing aids*, 2018a, http://www.fda.gov/MedicalDevices/ProductsandMedicalProcedures/HomeHealthandConsumer/ConsumerProducts/HearingAids/ucm181479.htm. Accessed October 24, 2018.

US Food and Drug Administration: *CFR code of federal regulations title 21*, 2018b, http://www.accessdata.fda.gov/scripts/cdrh/cfdocs/cfcfr/CFRSearch.cfm?fr=801.420, 2018b. Accessed October 24, 2018.

US Department of Health and Human Services (USDHHS): *Healthy people 2020, occupational safety and health*, 2018a, http://www.healthypeople.gov/2020/topics-objectives/topic/occupational-safety-and-health. Accessed September 28, 2018.

US Department of Health and Human Services (USDHHS): *Vision*, 2018b, https://www.healthypeople.gov/2020/topics-objectives/topic/vision/national-snapshot. Accessed October 23, 2018.

RESEARCH REFERENCES

Applebaum D, et al.: Implementation of a quiet time for noise reduction on a medical-surgical unit, *J Nurs Admin* 46(12):669, 2016.

Chamanzari H, et al.: Effects of a quiet time protocol on the sleep quality of patients admitted in the intensive care unit, *Medsurg Nurs* 5(1):43, 2016.

Goeren D, et al.: Quiet time: a noise reduction initiative in a neurosurgical intensive care unit, *Crit Care Nurse* 38(4):38, 2018.

Lim R: Benefits of quiet time interventions in the intensive care unit: a literature review, *Nurs Stand* 32(30):41, 2018.

McGough N, et al.: Noise reduction in progressive care units, *J Nurs Care Qual* 33(2):166, 2018.

Nael V, et al.: Visual impairment, uncorrected refractive errors, and activity limitations in older adults: findings from the three-city Alienor study, *Invest Ophthalmol Vis Sci* 58(4):2359, 2017.

Otte B, et al.: Self-reported eyeglass use by US Medicare beneficiaries aged 65 years or older, *JAMA Ophthalmol* 136(9):1047, 2018.

Rodriguez E, et al.: Increasing screening follow-up for vulnerable children: a partnership with schools, *Int J Environ Res Public Health* 15(8):1572, 2018.

Servidoni AB, et al.: Hearing loss in the elderly: is the hearing handicap inventory for the elderly: screening version effective in diagnosis when compared to the audiometric test? *Int Arch Otorhinolaryngol* 22(1):1, 2018.

Tseng YC, et al.: Quality of life in older adults with sensory impairments: a systematic review, *Qual Life Res* 27(8):1957, 2018.

Varma R, et al.: Visual impairment and blindness in adults in the united states: demographic and geographic variations from 2015 to 2050, *JAMA Ophthalmol* 134(7):802, 2016.

Yoon H, et al.: Comparison of access to eye care appointments between patients with medicaid and those with private insurance, *JAMA Ophthalmol* 136(6):622, 2018.

50

Perioperative Nursing Care

OBJECTIVES

- Describe the three phases of perioperative nursing.
- Explain the rationale for a nursing assessment of a patient's surgical risk factors.
- Identify co-morbid conditions that increase patient risks for postoperative complications.
- Explain the approach for assessing a patient's potential psychological response to impending surgery.
- Explain the influence a preoperative teaching plan can have on a patient's surgical recovery.
- Explain the rationale for postoperative exercises and early ambulation.
- Describe how a nurse's intraoperative assessment promotes patient safety
- Explain the differences between intraoperative phases.
- Describe the components of SBAR communication for perioperative hand-off.
- Identify nursing care priorities for postoperative patients.
- Describe the principles for providing education to surgical patients during the restorative phase of recovery

KEY TERMS

Ambulatory surgery, p. 1331
American Society of Anesthesiologists (ASA), p. 1322
American Society of PeriAnesthesia Nurses (ASPAN), p. 1327
Association of periOperative Registered Nurses (AORN), p. 1327
Atelectasis, p. 1325
Bariatric, p. 1325
Circulating nurse, p. 1343
Co-morbid, p. 1325

Conscious sedation, p. 1345
General anesthesia, p. 1344
Intermittent pneumatic compression (IPC) stockings, p. 1341
Informed consent, p. 1337
Laparoscopy, p. 1339
Latex sensitivity, p. 1344
Local anesthesia, p. 1344
Malignant hyperthermia, p. 1349
Moribund, p. 1323
Never event, p. 1326

Obstructive sleep apnea (OSA), p. 1325
Oxygen desaturation, p. 1325
Paralytic ileus, p. 1350
Perioperative nursing, p. 1321
Postanesthesia recovery score (PARS), p. 1347
Preanesthesia care unit (PCU), p. 1343
Preoperative teaching plan, p. 1335
Regional anesthesia, p. 1344
Scrub nurse, p. 1343

MEDIA RESOURCES

http://evolve.elsevier.com/Potter/fundamentals/
- Review Questions
- Video Clips
- Concept Map Creator
- Case Study with Questions

- Skills Performance Checklists
- Audio Glossary
- Content Updates
- Answers to QSEN Activity and Review Questions

Perioperative nursing includes a registered nurse's planned patient-centered approach in providing care to patients preoperatively, intraoperatively, and postoperatively. Through the application of national practice standards, the registered nurse's role in providing quality patient care before, during, and after surgery is crucial in maintaining patient safety. The perioperative nurse utilizes the nursing process to guide the delivery of care to patients in hospitals, surgical centers, and/or health care providers' offices. Nursing goals in the preoperative area are based on the following:
- Quality improvement and evidence-based practices through the application of current research and the generation of ideas for new research knowledge
- Patient safety through high-quality care
- Teamwork and collaboration

- Effective communication and interactions with a patient, the patient's family members, and the surgical team, fostering shared decision making
- The nursing process to deliver timely assessment and interventions in all phases of surgery
- Advocacy for a patient and the patient's family
- Cost containment

Perioperative nursing includes multiple intersecting processes guided by theoretical knowledge, ethical principles, ongoing research, specialized clinical skills, and caring practices (Association of periOperative Registered Nurses, 2018a). A nurse working within the perioperative setting responds to complex and fluctuating clinical needs during a crucial period of a patient's surgical experience. A nurse who works in any perioperative setting relies on clinical reasoning skills

TABLE 50.1   Classification of Surgical Procedures

Classification Type	Description	Example
Seriousness		
Major	Involves extensive reconstruction or alteration in body parts; poses great risks to well-being	Coronary artery bypass, colon resection, removal of larynx, resection of lung lobe
Minor	Involves minimal alteration in body parts; designed to correct deformities; involves minimal risks to well-being.	Cataract extraction, facial plastic surgery, tooth extraction
Urgency		
Elective	Performed on basis of patient's choice; is not essential and is not always necessary for health	Bunionectomy; facial plastic surgery; hernia repair; breast reconstruction
Urgent	Necessary for patient's health; often prevents development of additional problems (e.g., tissue destruction or impaired organ function); not necessarily emergency	Excision of cancerous tumor; removal of gallbladder for stones; vascular repair for obstructed artery (e.g., coronary artery bypass)
Emergency	Must be done immediately to save life or preserve function of body part	Repair of perforated appendix or traumatic amputation; control of internal hemorrhaging
Purpose		
Diagnostic	Surgical exploration performed to confirm diagnosis; often involves removal of tissue for further diagnostic testing	Exploratory laparotomy (incision into peritoneal cavity to inspect abdominal organs); breast mass biopsy
Ablative	Excision or removal of diseased body part	Amputation; removal of appendix or an organ such as gallbladder (cholecystectomy)
Palliative	Relieves or reduces intensity of disease symptoms; does not produce cure	Colostomy; debridement of necrotic tissue; resection of nerve roots
Reconstructive/restorative	Restores function or appearance to traumatized or malfunctioning tissues	Internal fixation of fractures; scar revision
Procurement for transplant	Removal of organs and/or tissues from a person pronounced brain dead or from living donors for transplantation into another person	Kidney, heart, or liver transplant
Constructive	Restores function lost or reduced as result of congenital anomalies	Repair of cleft palate; closure of atrial septal defect in heart
Cosmetic	Performed to improve personal appearance	Blepharoplasty for eyelid deformities; rhinoplasty to reshape nose

to maintain surgical asepsis, communicate effectively with members of the surgical team, and emphasize patient safety in each phase of surgery. Effective teaching and discharge planning involving patients and their family members prevent or minimize complications and contribute to quality outcomes. The nursing process provides a basis for perioperative nursing, allowing nurses to individualize patient care strategies throughout the perioperative period. A patient's smooth transition from admission into the health care system through recovery is the aim of quality perioperative care.

Care of a patient having surgery has shifted from a hospital- to home-based focus. Often recovery occurs in the home or in rehabilitation settings within long-term care centers. When care is in the home, responsibility shifts to the patient and/or family caregiver. As the length of hospital stay decreases, the educational needs of a patient undergoing a surgical procedure increase. Patients return home with complex medical/surgical conditions that require education and follow-up. Proper patient and family education is essential to ensuring positive surgical outcomes.

SCIENTIFIC KNOWLEDGE BASE

Classification of Surgery

The types of surgical procedures are classified according to seriousness, urgency, and purpose (Table 50.1). Although surgeries are classified as major or minor, any procedure can be considered major from the perspective of the patient and/or the family. Some procedures fall into more than one classification. For example, a colon resection to remove a malignant tumor is major in seriousness, urgent in urgency, and ablative in purpose. In many instances, the classifications intersect. Urgent procedures are major in seriousness. Frequently, the same procedure is performed for different reasons on different patients. For example, a gastrectomy may be performed as an emergency procedure to resect a bleeding ulcer or as an urgent procedure to remove a malignant tumor. Knowing the classifications assists in planning appropriate perioperative care.

The surgical classification describes the condition of a patient facing impending surgery. The American Society of Anesthesiologists (ASA) assigns classification on the basis of a patient's physiological condition independent of the proposed surgical procedure (Table 50.2). The classification is a risk assessment that allows surgeons and anesthesia providers to consider factors that influence how surgery will be performed. Anesthesia involves risks even in healthy patients; however, some patients, including but not limited to those with metabolic and cardiac dysfunction, are at higher risk.

Surgical Risk Factors

Numerous factors create risks for patients planning surgery. Risk factors can affect patients in any phase of the perioperative experience. One common risk factor for all patients is the surgical stress response.

TABLE 50.2 ASA Physical Status (PS) Classification

Asa Ps Class	Definition	Characteristics
ASA I	A normal healthy patient	No physiological, biological, organic disturbance; healthy, nonsmoking; no or minimal alcohol use
ASA II	A patient with mild systemic disease	Mild diseases only without substantive functional changes (e.g., current smoker, social alcohol drinker, pregnancy, obesity [BMI 30-39], well-controlled DM/HTN, mild lung disease)
ASA III	A patient with severe systemic disease	Substantive functional changes with one or more moderate-to-severe diseases (e.g., poorly controlled DM or HTN, COPD, morbid obesity [BMI 40 or greater], active hepatitis, alcohol dependence or abuse, implanted pacemaker, or moderate reduction of cardiac ejection fraction)
ASA IV	A patient with severe systemic disease that is a constant threat to life	Examples include recent (less than 3 months) MI, CVA, TIA, ongoing cardiac ischemia or severe valve dysfunction, sepsis, disseminated intravascular coagulation, end-stage renal disease not undergoing regularly scheduled dialysis
ASA V	A moribund patient who is not expected to survive without the operation	Examples include ruptured abdominal/thoracic aneurysm, massive trauma, intracranial bleed with mass effect, ischemic bowel with significant cardiac pathology
ASA VI	A patient declared brain dead whose organs are being removed for donor purpose	Wide variety of dysfunctions that are being managed to optimize blood flow to the heart and organs (e.g., aggressive fluid replacement and blood pressure medications)

Modified from American Society of Anesthesiologists: *ASA Physical Status Classification System,* October 15, 2014, http://www.asahq.org/resources/clinical-information/asa-physical-status-classification-system. Accessed July 15, 2018.

Understanding the physiology of the stress response (Chapter 37) and risk factors that affect patients' responses to surgery is necessary to anticipate patient needs and the types of preparation required preoperatively.

Smoking. Surgical patients who smoke are at a higher risk for developing pneumonia, atelectasis, and delayed wound healing (Wechter et al., 2016). Chronic smoking increases the amount and thickness of airway secretions, thus increasing the risk of aspiration. After surgery, a patient who smokes has greater difficulty clearing the airways of mucus, thus contributing to the development of pneumonia. Smoking decreases the amount of oxygen that reaches the cells in the surgical wound. As a result, the wound may heal more slowly and is more likely to become infected (Wechter et al., 2016). Further, current research suggests that surgical patients who use electronic cigarettes, also known as "vaping," are at risk for delayed wound healing and vascular necrosis (Fracol et al., 2017). Although decades of research correlate cigarette smoking to poor patient outcomes in all phases of the perioperative experience, some preoperative patients are unaware of the surgical risks associated with smoking. Recent studies suggest the need for health care providers to implement systematic and planned measures targeted at educating preoperative patients on the surgical risks of smoking all forms of cigarettes (Fracol et al., 2017).

Age. Very young and older patients are at greater surgical risk as a result of an immature or a declining physiological status (Mistry et al., 2017; Linnaus and Ostlie, 2016). Both populations often present problems in temperature control during surgery. General anesthetics inhibit shivering and cause vasodilation, which results in heat loss. These anesthetic changes coupled with age-related physiological factors increase the risk for unintended hypothermia. Infants also have difficulty in maintaining normal circulatory blood volume, causing risks for dehydration and overhydration.

Older adults account for the majority of surgeries performed in the United States (Lin et al., 2016). Their risks are significant. Among persons age 65 and over, chronic health conditions (co-morbidities) such as hypertension, heart disease, cancer, and diabetes are surgical risk factors (National Center for Health Statistics, 2017). Older patients often experience diminished cardiac, pulmonary, and renal function,

which decreases older adults' ability to maintain homeostasis perioperatively (Table 50.3). Baroreceptor function, which regulates blood pressure, may be insufficient and cause postural hypotension and dizziness, increasing fall risks. Decreased respiratory function, impaired functional reserve of the pulmonary system, and decreased cough reflex increase the risk for aspiration, infection, and bronchospasm. Further, dehydration and fluid imbalance (common in nursing home residents) require a need for hydration if the patient is unable to drink before surgery (Nicholas, 2014).

Nutrition. Tissue repair and resistance to infection depend on adequate nutrition. Surgery increases the need for nutrients (Weimann et al., 2017). Patients who are thin or obese are often deficient in protein and vitamins, putting them at greater risk for complications following surgery (Lewis et al., 2017). After surgery, a patient requires at least 1500 kcal/day to maintain energy reserves. This intake is difficult to attain when a patient's food and/or fluid intake is limited after surgery or if a patient experiences postoperative nausea and vomiting (PONV). Postoperatively, patients gradually increase their dietary intake (once gastrointestinal activity returns) over 1 to 2 days 3 to 5 days after surgery until they can tolerate normal meals. Patients who enter surgery malnourished are more likely to have poor tolerance for anesthesia, negative nitrogen balance, delayed postoperative recovery, infection, and delayed wound healing. Current recommendations suggest replacing iron, vitamin B_{12}, and folate at least 28 days before scheduled elective surgery (Weimann et al., 2017). Some studies indicate that recovery can also be enhanced by regulating the metabolic status of a patient before surgery (e.g., minimizing metabolic stress and insulin resistance by giving carbohydrate-based drinks and fluid loading) and after surgery (e.g., early oral feeding and giving prokinetic medications to enhance gastric motility, resulting in improved enteral feeding tolerance) (Weimann et al., 2017).

Obesity. Patients who are morbidly obese typically live up to 14 years less than their average-weight counterparts (Hales et al., 2017). According to the National Center for Health Statistics (2017), the prevalence of obesity among US adults was 39.8%. Approximately 18.5% of America's youth were obese in 2015–2016 (Hales et al., 2017). As a patient's weight increases, his or her ventilatory and cardiac function

TABLE 50.3   Physiological Factors That Place the Older Adult at Risk During Surgery

Alterations	Risks	Nursing Implications
Cardiovascular System		
Degenerative change in myocardium and valves	Decreased cardiac reserve puts older adults at risk for decreased cardiac output, especially during times of stress (AORN, 2015)	Assess baseline vital signs for tachycardia, fatigue, and arrhythmias (AORN, 2015).
Rigidity of arterial walls and reduction in sympathetic and parasympathetic innervation to the heart	Alterations predispose patient to postoperative hemorrhage and rise in systolic and diastolic blood pressure	Maintain adequate fluid balance to minimize stress to the heart. Ensure that blood pressure level is adequate to meet circulatory demands.
Increased calcium and cholesterol deposits within small arteries; thickened arterial walls	Predispose patient to clot formation in lower extremities	Instruct patient in techniques of leg exercises and proper turning. Apply elastic stockings or intermittent pneumatic compression (IPC) devices. Administer anticoagulants as ordered by health care provider. Provide education regarding effects, side effects, and dietary considerations.
Integumentary System		
Decreased subcutaneous tissue and increased fragility of skin	Prone to pressure injuries and skin tears	Assess skin every 4 hours; pad all bony prominences during surgery. Turn or reposition at least every 2 hours.
Pulmonary System		
Decreased respiratory muscle strength and cough reflex (AORN, 2015)	Increased risk for atelectasis	Instruct patient in proper technique for coughing, deep breathing, and use of spirometer. Ensure adequate pain control to allow for participation in exercises.
Reduced range of movement in diaphragm	Residual capacity (volume of air left in lung after normal breath) increased, reducing amount of new air brought into lungs with each inspiration	When possible, have patient ambulate and sit in chair frequently.
Stiffened lung tissue and enlarged air spaces	Blood oxygenation reduced	Obtain baseline oxygen saturation; measure throughout perioperative period.
Gastrointestinal System		
Gastric emptying delayed	Increases risk for reflux and indigestion (AORN, 2015)	Position patient with head of bed elevated at least 45 degrees. Reduce size of meals in accordance with ordered diet.
Renal System		
Decreased renal function, with reduced blood flow to kidneys	Increased risk of shock when blood loss occurs; increased risk for fluid and electrolyte imbalance (AORN, 2015)	For patients hospitalized before surgery, determine baseline urinary output for 24 hours.
Reduced glomerular filtration rate and excretory times	Limited ability to eliminate drugs or toxic substances	Assess for adverse response to drugs.
Decreased bladder capacity	Increased risk for urgency, incontinence, and urinary tract infections (AORN, 2015). (Sensation of need to void often does not occur until bladder is filled.)	Instruct patient to notify nurse immediately when sensation of bladder fullness develops. Keep nurse call system and bedpan within easy reach. Toilet every 2 hours or more frequently if indicated.
Neurological System		
Sensory losses, including reduced tactile sense and increased pain tolerance	Decreased ability to respond to early warning signs of surgical complications	Inspect bony prominences for signs of pressure that patient is unable to sense. Orient patient to surrounding environment. Observe for nonverbal signs of pain.
Febrile response during surgery (AORN, 2015)	Increased risk of undiagnosed infection	Ensure careful, close monitoring of patient temperature; provide warm blankets; monitor heart function; warm intravenous fluids (AORN, 2015).
Decreased reaction time	Confusion and delirium after anesthesia; increased risk for falls	Allow adequate time to respond, process information, and perform tasks. Perform fall-risk screening and institute fall precautions. Screen for delirium with validated tools. Orient frequently to reality and surroundings.

TABLE 50.3 Physiological Factors that Place the Older Adult at Risk During Surgery—cont'd

Alterations	Risks	Nursing Implications
Metabolic System		
Lower basal metabolic rate	Reduced total oxygen consumption	Ensure adequate nutritional intake when diet is resumed but avoid intake of excess calories.
Reduced number of red blood cells and hemoglobin levels	Reduced ability to carry adequate oxygen to tissues	Administer necessary blood products as needed. Monitor blood test results and oxygen saturation.
Change in total amounts of body potassium and water volume	Greater risk for fluid or electrolyte imbalance	Monitor electrolyte levels and supplement as necessary. Provide cardiac monitoring (telemetry) as needed.

Association of PeriOperative Registered Nurses: *AORN position statement on care of the older adult in perioperative settings: position statement,* 2015. https://www.aorn.org/guidelines/clinical-resources/position-statements. Accessed July 18, 2018.

diminish, increasing the risk for postoperative atelectasis, pneumonia, and death. Obstructive sleep apnea (OSA), hypertension, coronary artery disease, diabetes mellitus, and heart failure are co-morbid conditions in the bariatric population. Patients who are obese often have difficulty resuming normal physical activity after surgery because of the pain and fatigue caused by surgery in addition to preexisting impaired physical mobility. This combination of factors increases the risk of developing venous thromboembolism (VTE). Obesity is a significant risk factor for wound infections, surgical blood loss, and a longer operation time (Tjeertes et al., 2015).

Excess weight placed on skin over bony prominences restricts blood flow and poses risks for pressure injuries to form on the operating table. Obesity also increases the risk of poor wound healing, wound infection, dehiscence, and evisceration because fatty tissue contains a poor blood supply, slowing the delivery of essential nutrients and antibodies needed for wound healing (see Chapter 48). In addition, surgeons often have difficulty closing surgical wounds because of the thick adipose layer.

Obstructive Sleep Apnea. Obstructive sleep apnea (OSA) is a chronic sleep disorder characterized by periodic episodes of narrowing or collapse of the upper airway (American Academy of Sleep Medicine, 2014). It occurs when muscles in the throat relax during sleep, causing soft tissue in the back of the throat to collapse and block the upper airway. A combination of structural and neuromuscular function, OSA results in pauses in breathing (apnea) that last at least 10 seconds during sleep. Most apneic episodes last between 10 and 30 seconds, but some may continue for 1 minute or longer, leading to significant oxygen desaturation. During an apnea episode, there is increasing negative intrathoracic pressure (down to −80 mm Hg), which makes it difficult for the heart to pump effectively against such a negative pressure; thus cardiac output decreases. In response to the oxygen desaturation, there is an arousal, which ends the apnea. The arousal is accompanied by a huge increase in sympathetic output, which causes a significant increase in blood pressure (American Academy of Sleep Medicine, 2014; Downey, 2018).

Patients with OSA often have co-morbid conditions such as asthma, atherosclerosis, myocardial infarction, heart failure, hypertension, atrial fibrillation, chronic kidney disease, and behavioral disorders, such as decreases in attention, vigilance, concentration, motor skills, and verbal and visuospatial memory (National Institute of Health, 2018). Some evidence suggests that the lack of sleep (for various reasons) may play a role in some older adults' mental decline a (National Institute of Health, 2018). The disorder hinders daily functioning because of chronic fatigue and sleepiness and adversely affects health and longevity. Patients who suffer from OSA develop numerous complications, including hypertension, heart disease, vascular disease,

neurological disease, and diabetes (Raveendran and Chung, 2015). Further, research suggests OSA is associated with insulin resistance, glucose tolerance, and type 2 diabetes independent of obesity (Kent et al., 2015).

Patients with OSA who are to undergo surgery present a significant risk. Receiving sedatives, opioid analgesics, and general anesthesia causes relaxation of the upper airway and may worsen OSA. The risk is higher when a patient is sedated and lying on his or her back. Patients have experienced severe apnea and hypoxemia, leading to death following surgical and diagnostic procedures under conscious sedation. Careful screening of patients at risk or symptomatic for OSA is essential before surgery (Raveendran and Chung, 2015). There is no evidence to suggest all surgical patients should be screened for OSA (US Preventive Services Task Force, 2017).

Immunosuppression. Patients with conditions that alter immune function (e.g., primary immune deficiency, acquired immunodeficiency syndrome [AIDS], cancer, bone marrow alterations, and organ transplants) are at an increased risk for developing infection after surgery. The risk for infection increases when patients receive radiation or chemotherapy for cancer treatment, take immunosuppressive medications to treat AIDS or prevent rejection after organ transplant, or require steroids to treat a variety of inflammatory or autoimmune conditions (Hannaman and Ertl, 2013). Radiation sometimes is given before surgery to reduce the size of a cancerous tumor so that it can be removed surgically. Ideally, a surgeon waits to perform surgery until 4 to 6 weeks after completion of radiation treatments because of the unavoidable effects that radiation has on normal tissue. Radiation thins the layers of the skin, destroys collagen, and impairs tissue perfusion. Otherwise, the patient may face serious wound-healing problems.

Fluid and Electrolyte Imbalance. The body responds to surgery as a form of trauma. Severe protein breakdown causes a negative nitrogen balance (see Chapter 45) and hyperglycemia. Both of these effects decrease tissue healing and increase the risk of infection. As a result of the adrenocortical stress response, the body retains sodium and water and loses potassium in the first 2 to 5 days after surgery. The severity of the stress response influences the degree of fluid and electrolyte imbalance. Extensive surgery results in a greater stress response. A patient who is hypovolemic before surgery or who has serious electrolyte alterations is at significant risk during and after surgery. For example, an excess or depletion of potassium increases the chance of dysrhythmias during or after surgery. The risk of fluid and electrolyte alterations is even greater in patients with preexisting diabetes mellitus, renal disease, or gastrointestinal (GI) or cardiovascular abnormalities (see Chapter 42).

Postoperative Nausea and Vomiting (PONV). The experience of having nausea and vomiting after surgery is uncomfortable and often immobilizing. PONV affects approximately 30% of patients in recovery rooms after surgery (Fetzer, 2015). It can lead to serious complications, including pulmonary aspiration, dehydration, and arrhythmias resulting from fluid and electrolyte imbalance. A patient who vomits frequently after surgery runs the risk of dehiscing surgical sutures. Patients predisposed to developing PONV are women, individuals with a history of PONV or motion sickness, nonsmoking status, and younger age. Anesthesia-related risk factors include the use of volatile anesthetics (e.g., nitrous oxide), duration of anesthesia, and perioperative opioid use. Certain types of surgery (e.g., abdominal procedures [cholecystectomies] and gynecological surgery) are also associated with PONV (Gan et al., 2014). Ambulatory surgery patients generally have less PONV. However, nausea and vomiting may occur after an ambulatory patient has left a surgical setting. This postdischarge nausea and/or vomiting (PDNV) may be particularly hazardous for ambulatory surgery patients because they no longer have immediate access to fast-onset intravenous antiemetic medications (Apfel et al., 2012). Screening for PONV is crucial. Patients with four or more risk factors have a higher incidence of PONV (Rothrock, 2019). Management of PONV begins before surgery.

Venous Thromboembolism. In 2008, the Centers for Medicare and Medicaid Services ruled that deep vein thrombosis (DVT) (clot formed in the deep veins) after total knee and hip surgery is a **never event** and refused to pay for hospital-acquired DVTs (CMS, 2010). If a patient develops a DVT after surgery, Medicare and some private insurance companies withhold payment to the hospital because DVTs are typically preventable. The Joint Commission (2017) has an updated set of accountability measures (i.e., quality measures that produce the greatest positive impact on patient outcomes when hospitals demonstrate improvement in them). One of the accountability measures is treatment and prevention of venous thromboembolism (VTE). Some VTEs are subclinical (without symptoms), whereas others present as sudden pulmonary embolus or symptomatic DVT. Patients most at risk for developing VTE are those who undergo surgical procedures with a general anesthetic and undergo a surgical time of more than 90 minutes, or 60 minutes if the surgery involves the pelvis or lower limb; acute surgical admissions with inflammatory or intraabdominal conditions; and those expected to have significant reduction in mobility after surgery. In addition, patients are at higher risk if they have one or more risk factors (Streiff et al., 2016):

- Active cancer or cancer treatment
- Age over 60 years
- Critical care admission
- Dehydration
- Known clotting disorders
- Obesity (body mass index [BMI] of 30 kg/m^2 or greater)

REFLECT NOW

A nurse conducts a preoperative assessment for an 85-year-old patient who is accompanied by a caregiver. The patient's caregiver assists the patient with ambulation and answers the nurse's questions.

A review of the patient's medical record reveals recent episodes of sleep apnea. What questions should the nurse ask to assess this patient's risks for surgical complications? Which risk factors place this patient at risk for surgical complications?

NURSING KNOWLEDGE BASE

Perioperative Communication

Continuity of care is pertinent when caring for surgical patients. Based on the delivery of care model utilized in the perioperative setting, some nurses may follow patients through the preoperative and intraoperative phases of surgery. In some instances, perioperative nurses follow patients through the postanesthesia care unit (PACU), assessing a patient's health status before surgery, identifying specific patient needs, teaching and counseling, preparing for the operating room (OR), and following a patient's recovery. However, different nurses and other health care providers also care for a patient during each phase of the surgical experience. A smooth communication "hand-off" between caregivers is needed to ensure continuity of care and reduce risk of medical errors (Benjamin et al., 2016). Transitions from one care provider to another place patients at risk for injuries, missed care, and errors in translating information. Nursing research shows that having a standardized checklist or protocol for hand-off communication between perioperative health care providers minimizes these risks (Scott et al., 2017). TJC National Patient Safety Goals address the importance of accurate patient identification and communication (TJC, 2020).

Glycemic Control and Infection Prevention

Evidence supports a relationship between wound and tissue infection and surgical patients' blood glucose levels. Poor control of blood glucose levels (specifically hyperglycemia) during and after surgery increases patients' risks for adverse outcomes, such as wound infection and mortality. Controlling blood sugars perioperatively reduces mortality in patients with or without diabetes who have general surgery and in patients who have cardiac surgery (van den Boom et al., 2018). Perioperative evaluation of patients coupled with appropriate insulin administration is a critical standard of care.

Pressure Injury Prevention

Patients who have surgery pose a unique challenge in pressure injury prevention (Shaw et al., 2014). Nursing research reveals that patients are at risk intraoperatively for pressure injuries as a result of intrinsic, extrinsic, and specific OR risk factors (EPUAP, NPIAP, PPPIA, 2019; Primiano et al., 2011):

Intrinsic risks (patient's tolerance to a pressure injury insult)—altered nutrition (albumin levels <3 g/dL), decreased mobility, older age, decreased mental status, infection, incontinence, impaired sensory perception, and co-morbidities such as diabetes, malnutrition, and weight (Kim et al., 2017; Saghaleini et al., 2018).

Extrinsic risks (variables that increase tissue susceptibility to sustain external pressure)—temperature, friction and shearing forces, and moisture.

OR risk factors—length of surgery, position on OR table, positioning devices used, warming devices, anesthetic agents, intraoperative hemodynamics, and length of time on the OR bed.

A preoperative assessment should include screening for these risk factors. Registered nurses assist in preventing pressure injuries intraoperatively by carefully positioning patients and using pressure-relieving surfaces. Positioning is a shared responsibility among the surgeon, the anesthesia provider, and OR nurses. The optimal position often involves a compromise between the best position for surgical access and the position a patient can tolerate (Welch, 2018). After surgery, perform a careful skin assessment and use appropriate pressure-reduction strategies (see Chapter 48).

CRITICAL THINKING

Successful critical thinking requires a synthesis of knowledge, experience, information gathered from patients, critical thinking attitudes,

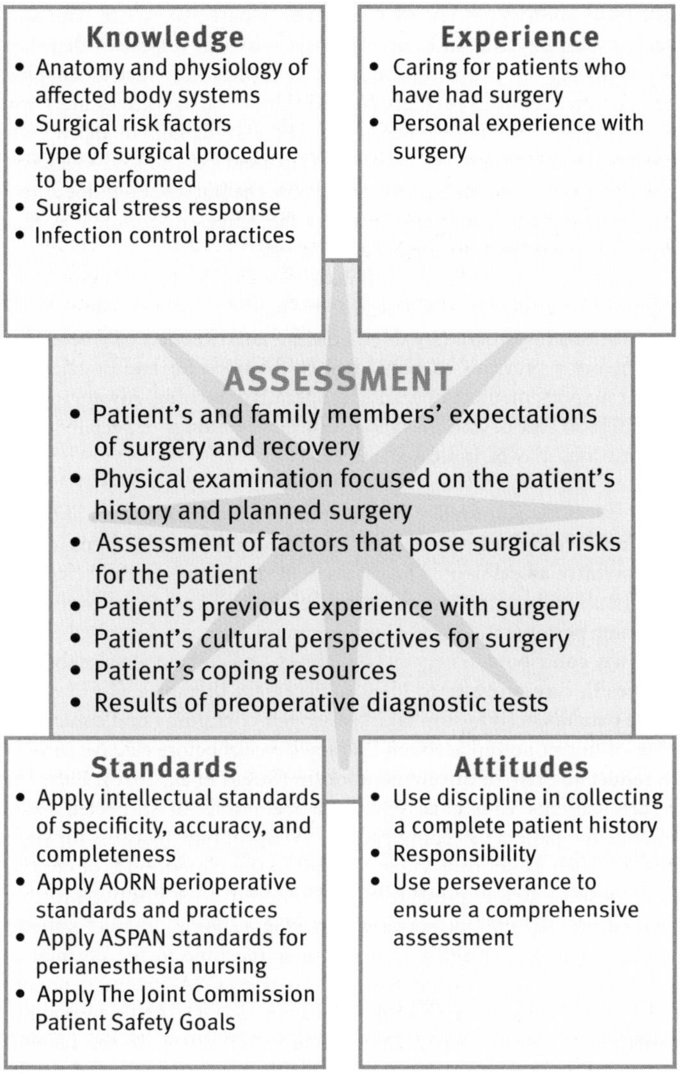

Knowledge
- Anatomy and physiology of affected body systems
- Surgical risk factors
- Type of surgical procedure to be performed
- Surgical stress response
- Infection control practices

Experience
- Caring for patients who have had surgery
- Personal experience with surgery

ASSESSMENT
- Patient's and family members' expectations of surgery and recovery
- Physical examination focused on the patient's history and planned surgery
- Assessment of factors that pose surgical risks for the patient
- Patient's previous experience with surgery
- Patient's cultural perspectives for surgery
- Patient's coping resources
- Results of preoperative diagnostic tests

Standards
- Apply intellectual standards of specificity, accuracy, and completeness
- Apply AORN perioperative standards and practices
- Apply ASPAN standards for perianesthesia nursing
- Apply The Joint Commission Patient Safety Goals

Attitudes
- Use discipline in collecting a complete patient history
- Responsibility
- Use perseverance to ensure a comprehensive assessment

FIG. 50.1 Critical thinking model for surgical patient assessment. *AORN,* Association of periOperative Registered Nurses; *ASPAN,* American Society of PeriAnesthesia Nurses.

and intellectual and professional standards. Clinical judgments require you to anticipate information, analyze the data, and make decisions regarding your patient's care. During assessment, consider all elements that build toward making an appropriate nursing diagnosis (Fig. 50.1).

When caring for a patient having surgery, integrate knowledge regarding the patient's specific clinical situation along with previous experiences in caring for surgical patients. Apply this knowledge using a patient-centered care approach, partnering with your patient to make clinical decisions. Using critical thinking attitudes (see Chapter 15) ensures that a plan of care is comprehensive and incorporates evidence-based principles for successful perioperative care. A key attitude for a perioperative nurse is responsibility (i.e., being responsible not only for standards of care but being a patient advocate as well). The use of professional perioperative standards developed by the Association of periOperative Registered Nurses (AORN) (http://www.aorn.org) and the American Society of PeriAnesthesia Nurses (ASPAN) (http://www.aspan.org/) provide valuable guidelines for perioperative management and evaluation of process and outcomes. TJC Hospital National Patient Safety Goals include two sets of recommendations for perioperative care: prevent infection and prevent mistakes in surgery (TJC, 2020). Always review these guidelines within the context of new

emerging evidence-based practice, agency policies, and the scope of practice of the state in which you practice.

REFLECT NOW

Think about a patient you cared for during his or her surgical experience. Develop a communication handoff for your patient that you would use to report to the nurse on the next shift.

PREOPERATIVE SURGICAL PHASE
❖ NURSING PROCESS

Apply the nursing process and use a critical thinking approach in your care of patients. The nursing process provides a clinical decision-making approach for you to develop and implement an individualized plan of care. Patients having surgery enter the health care setting in different levels of health. For example, a patient enters the hospital or ambulatory surgery center (ASC) on a predetermined day feeling relatively healthy and prepared to face elective surgery, while another person in a motor vehicle crash faces emergency surgery with no time to prepare. The ability to establish rapport and maintain a professional relationship with a patient and the patient's family is essential during the preoperative phase. Patients having surgery meet many health care personnel, including surgeons, nurse anesthetists, anesthesiologists, surgical technologists, and nurses. All play a role in a patient's care and recovery. Family members attempt to provide support through their presence but face many of the same stressors as the patient. As a nurse you need to form a caring relationship (see Chapter 7) and effectively communicate (see Chapter 24) with the patient and family to gain the patient's trust. This helps you to learn the depth of information needed to provide a patient-centered plan of care. Cultural sensitivity is equally important in developing a patient-centered plan of care reflecting the patient's physical, psychological, emotional, sociocultural, and spiritual well-being (see Chapter 9). You will learn to recognize a patient's degree of surgical risk, coordinate diagnostic tests, identify nursing diagnoses and nursing interventions, and establish outcomes in collaboration with patients and their families. It is a nurse's responsibility to communicate pertinent data and the plan of care to surgical team members.

Many hospitals have developed Enhanced Recovery After Surgery (ERAS) protocols. The protocols are interprofessional and based on published scientific evidence. Elements of an ERAS protocol might include minimally invasive surgical approaches instead of large incisions, management of fluids to seek fluid balance rather than large volumes of intravenous fluids, avoidance of or early removal of drains and tubes, early mobilization, and the serving of drinks and food the day of an operation (Ljungqvist et al., 2017). An ERAS protocol will include standards for preoperative and postoperative care.

◆ Assessment

During the assessment process, thoroughly assess each patient and critically analyze findings to ensure that you make patient-centered clinical decisions required for safe nursing care. The goal of the preoperative assessment is to identify a patient's normal preoperative function and the presence of any surgical risks and to recognize, prevent, and minimize possible postoperative complications. The extent of a nurse's assessment depends on the patient's condition, the surgical setting, the time the nurse has with a patient, and the urgency of a procedure. Ambulatory and same-day surgical programs offer challenges in gathering a complete assessment in a short time. In these settings, an interprofessional team approach is essential. Patients are admitted only hours before surgery; consequently, it is important for a nurse to organize and verify data obtained before surgery and implement a perioperative plan of care. This occurs both in ASCs and with patients who require a hospital stay.

Most surgical assessments begin before admission in the health care provider's office, preadmission clinic, anesthesia clinic, or by telephone. Some patients answer a self-report inventory before arriving at a center. Other times a health care provider performs a physical examination or orders laboratory tests. Nurses begin to teach, answer questions, and complete paperwork before surgery to streamline patient care on the day of surgery. When surgery is emergent with little time available, you prioritize an assessment based on the patient's presenting clinical condition and risk factors.

Through the Patient's Eyes. When possible it is important to determine a patient's expectations of surgery and recovery. Ask a patient what he or she hopes to gain as a result of surgery. Explore with questions such as "Tell me the type of surgery you are having in your own words" or "Do you understand the expected care and how long you will stay in the hospital after surgery? If not, what do you want to know?" or "Do you expect full pain relief or simply to have your pain reduced after surgery?" and "Do you expect to be independent immediately after surgery, or do you expect to be fully dependent on the nurse or your family?" These are only a few of the questions to ask to establish a plan of care that matches a patient's needs and expectations. Listen to the patient's explanation, be attentive, and explain expectations of surgery. Form a relationship with each patient to foster collaboration and shared decision making. Assessing patient expectations gives you a better understanding of the patient's health and health care needs.

Nursing History. A preoperative nursing history includes information similar to that described in Chapter 30. If a patient is unable to relay all of the necessary information, rely on family members (if appropriate) as resources. As with any admission to a health care agency, include information about advance directives. Ask if a patient has a durable power of attorney for health care or a living will (see Chapter 23) and include a copy in the patient's medical record. Often directives are modified before surgery but are reestablished after postoperative stabilization. To help ensure a thorough and accurate nursing assessment, electronic health records (EHRs) provide standardized documentation forms for data. Be sure to use all drop-down menus to most clearly portray a patient's history, but also be willing to enter full-text descriptions as needed.

Medical History. A review of a patient's medical history includes past illnesses and surgeries and the primary reason for seeking medical care. The medical history screens surgical candidates for major medical conditions that increase the risk of complications during or after surgery (Table 50.4). For example, a patient who has a history of heart failure is at risk for a further decline in cardiac function during and after surgery. The patient with heart failure in the preoperative period often requires beta-blocker medications, intravenous (IV) fluids infused at a slower rate, or administration of a diuretic after blood transfusions. Box 50.1 provides a list of assessment questions for a patient with a cardiac history. If a patient has surgical risks from medical conditions, surgery as an outpatient may be inadvisable, or special precautions will be necessary. In addition, the nurse asks about a family history of anesthetic complications such as malignant hyperthermia (an inherited disorder and life-threatening condition) that may occur during surgery.

Surgical History. A review of a patient's past experience with surgery reveals physical and potential psychological responses that may occur during the planned procedure. Complications such as anaphylaxis or malignant hyperthermia during previous surgeries alert you to the need for preventive measures and the availability of appropriate emergency equipment. For example, if a patient experienced an allergic reaction to latex during a previous surgery, the nurse should document the patient's history and ensure that a latex-free environment is provided for the patient during hospitalization.

A history of postoperative complications such as persistent vomiting or uncontrolled pain will lead to the selection of more appropriate medications (as ordered by the medical team). Reports of severe anxiety before a previous surgery identify the need for additional emotional support, medications, and preoperative teaching. Always inform the surgeon and/or anesthesiologist of these findings, especially when medications may be indicated.

Risk Factors. Knowledge of potential surgical risk factors and risk factors for complications (e.g., pressure injuries) provides focus for the preoperative assessment. The assessment data from careful screening of patients will contain information useful for necessary precautions in planning perioperative care. Consider any risk factors described earlier that may contribute to negative outcomes, and collaborate closely with the health care provider to identify necessary therapies. For example, some patients need to stop taking estrogen-containing oral contraceptives or hormone-replacement therapy 4 weeks before elective surgery to reduce the risk of thromboembolism (Streiff et al., 2016). Carefully screen patients who have signs and symptoms of suspected OSA. Include the patient's sleeping partner as appropriate to assess for signs of OSA such as snoring. Also, determine the patient's use of continuous positive airway pressure (CPAP), noninvasive positive-pressure ventilation (NIPPV), or apnea monitoring at home. Instruct patients who use CPAP or NIPPV to bring their machine to the hospital or surgery center. Many hospitals are now making OSA screening mandatory, using evidence-based tools such as the STOP-BANG sleep apnea assessment tool (Box 50.2) (Chung et al., 2013, 2016). Screen patients with simple questions regarding snoring, apnea during sleep, frequent arousals during sleep, morning headaches, daytime somnolence, and chronic fatigue (Ganzberg, 2016; Helvig et al., 2014).

Some patients need a detailed nutritional assessment to determine surgical risk. If a patient presents with signs of malnutrition, perform a nutritional screening using your agency's tool, or confer with a registered dietitian (see Chapter 45).

Medications. Review a patient's medications to determine if he or she is taking any medications that increase the risk for surgical complications (Table 50.5). Include all prescribed, OTC, and herbal medications in your assessment. Many medications interact unpredictably with anesthetic agents during surgery (Burchum and Rosenthal, 2019). Sometimes surgeons temporarily discontinue or adjust doses of a patient's prescription, over-the-counter (OTC) medications, and/or herbal supplements before surgery. Nurses in an outpatient setting should verify with surgeons which, if any, medications patients should take the morning of surgery. Often preprinted instruction sheets given to patients in physician offices contain this information. When working in an acute care setting, confirm with the surgeon all discontinued medications. If a patient is having inpatient surgery, all prescription medications taken before surgery are discontinued automatically after surgery unless reordered. It is important that as a patient moves through different areas (e.g., holding area to the OR), a complete list of medications is communicated accurately during hand-off report (TJC, 2020).

TABLE 50.4   Medical Conditions That Increase Risks of Surgery

Type of Condition	Reason for Risk
Bleeding disorders (thrombocytopenia, hemophilia)	Increases risk of hemorrhage during and after surgery.
Diabetes mellitus	Increases susceptibility to infection and impairs wound healing from altered glucose metabolism and associated circulatory impairment. Stress of surgery often results in hyperglycemia (Lewis et al., 2017).
Heart disease (recent myocardial infarction, dysrhythmias, heart failure) and peripheral vascular disease	Stress of surgery causes increased demands on myocardium to maintain cardiac output. General anesthetic agents depress cardiac function.
Hypertension	Increases risk for cardiovascular complications during anesthesia (e.g., stroke, inadequate tissue oxygenation).
Obstructive sleep apnea	Administration of opioids increases risk of airway obstruction after surgery. Patients desaturate as revealed by drop in oxygen saturation by pulse oximetry.
Upper respiratory infection	Increases risk of respiratory complications during anesthesia (e.g., pneumonia and spasm of laryngeal muscles).
Renal disease	Alters excretion of anesthetic drugs and their metabolites, increasing risk for acid-base imbalance and other complications.
Liver disease	Alters metabolism and elimination of drugs administered during surgery and impairs wound healing and clotting time because of alterations in protein metabolism.
Fever	Predisposes patient to fluid and electrolyte imbalances and sometimes indicates underlying infection.
Chronic respiratory disease (emphysema, bronchitis, asthma)	Reduces patient's means to compensate for acid-base alterations (see Chapter 42). Anesthetic agents reduce respiratory function, increasing risk for severe hypoventilation.
Immunological disorders (leukemia, acquired immunodeficiency syndrome [AIDS], bone marrow depression, and use of chemotherapeutic drugs or immunosuppressive agents)	Increases risk of infection and delayed wound healing after surgery.
Abuse of alcohol, opioid addiction	Alcohol abuse is associated with liver dysfunction and may interfere with the effects of anesthesia. Opioid addiction may result in health care and self-care neglect. Consequently, patients may have underlying diseases that may affect wound healing.
Chronic pain	Regular use of pain medications often results in higher tolerance. Increased doses of analgesics are sometimes necessary to achieve postoperative pain control.

Data from Mohabir PK: Preoperative evaluation, 2018, *Merck manual professional version*. https://www.merckmanuals.com/professional/special-subjects/care-of-the-surgical-patient/preoperative-evaluation. Last revised April 2018. Accessed August 3, 2018; and Lewis S, et al: *Medical-surgical nursing: assessment and management of clinical problems*, ed 10, St Louis, 2017, Elsevier.

BOX 50.1   Nursing Assessment Questions: Cardiac History

Nature of the Problem
- Do you have a history of heart attack, heart failure, angina (chest pain), irregular heartbeat, or valve disease?
- Which medications do you take?
- Are you taking any vitamins or other supplements?
- Have you had any recent medical testing or procedures on your heart (e.g., cardiac catheterization or echocardiogram)?
- Do you smoke cigarettes, including e-cigarettes? If so, how often and how many per day?

Signs and Symptoms
- Are you having any chest pain?
- How do you sleep at night (position, use of pillows, awakened with chest pain)?
- Do your feet swell?
- Are you short of breath, or do you have any difficulty breathing?

Onset and Duration
- How often do you have chest pain, when does it start, how long does it last, what alleviates it?

- When do your feet swell (all the time, end of the day, only after a busy day)?
- When do you become short of breath?

Severity
- On a scale of 0 to 10 (with 0 being no pain and 10 the worst pain), what number do you give your chest pain?
- Describe your usual activity level. Can you climb stairs; can you do housework?
- Do you exercise regularly? What exercise?

Self-Management and Culture
- Have you changed your activity level, sleep patterns, diet, or fluid intake recently?
- Are you taking any herbal or over-the-counter medications?

Through the Patient's Eyes
- How are you feeling about your upcoming surgery? Has it affected your symptoms?
- Are you currently having any additional stress?

BOX 50.2   The STOP-BANG Questionnaire

Height _____ cm /inches Weight _____ lb/kg
  Age _____
  Male/Female
  BMI _____
  Collar size of shirt: S, M, L, XL, or _____ cm /inches
  Neck circumference[a] _____ cm

1. **S**noring
   Do you *snore* loudly (louder than talking or loud enough to be heard through closed doors)?
   Yes No
2. **T**ired
   Do you often feel *tired*, fatigued, or sleepy during daytime?
   Yes No
3. **O**bserved
   Has anyone *observed* you stop breathing during your sleep?
   Yes No
4. Blood **P**ressure
   Do you have or are you being treated for high blood *pressure*?
   Yes No
5. **B**MI
   *B*MI more than 35 kg/m^2?
   Yes No
6. **A**ge
   *A*ge over 50 years old?
   Yes No
7. **N**eck circumference (measure with approved measuring tape)[a]
   *N*eck circumference greater than 40 cm?
   Yes No
8. **G**ender
   *G*ender male?
   Yes No

   Score of 4—High sensitivity of 88% for identifying severe obstructive sleep apnea (OSA)
   Score of 5 or more—High risk of OSA; a score of 6 is more specific

[a]Neck circumference is measured by staff.
BMI, Body mass index.
Modified from Chung F, et al: Predictive performance of the STOP-BANG score for identifying obstructive sleep apnea in obese patients, *Obes Surg* 23(12):2050, 2013; Chung F, et al: STOP-Bang questionnaire: a practical approach to screen for obstructive sleep apnea, *Chest* 149(3):631, 2016.

TABLE 50.5   Medications with Special Implications for the Surgical Patient

Drug Class	Effects During Surgery
Antibiotics	Potentiate (enhance action of) anesthetic agents. If taken within 2 weeks before surgery, aminoglycosides (gentamicin, neomycin, tobramycin) may cause mild respiratory depression from depressed neuromuscular transmission.
Antidysrhythmics	Medications (e.g., beta blockers) can reduce cardiac contractility and impair cardiac conduction during anesthesia.
Anticoagulants	Medications such as warfarin or aspirin alter normal clotting factors and thus increase risk of hemorrhaging. Discontinue at least 48 hours before surgery.
Anticonvulsants	Long-term use of certain anticonvulsants (e.g., phenytoin and phenobarbital) alters metabolism of anesthetic agents.
Antihypertensives	Medications such as beta blockers and calcium channel blockers interact with anesthetic agents to cause bradycardia, hypotension, and impaired circulation. They inhibit synthesis and storage of norepinephrine in sympathetic nerve endings.
Corticosteroids	With prolonged use, corticosteroids cause adrenal atrophy, reducing the ability of the body to withstand stress. Before and during surgery, dosages are often increased temporarily.
Insulin	A patient's insulin requirements fluctuate after surgery. For example, some patients need increased doses due to the stress response from surgery. Other patients need less insulin due to decreased nutritional intake following surgery.
Diuretics	Diuretics such as furosemide potentiate electrolyte imbalances (particularly potassium) after surgery.
Nonsteroidal antiinflammatory drugs (NSAIDs)	NSAIDs (e.g., ibuprofen) inhibit platelet aggregation and prolong bleeding time, increasing susceptibility to postoperative bleeding.
Herbal therapies: ginger, ginkgo, ginseng	These herbal therapies have the ability to affect platelet activity and increase susceptibility to postoperative bleeding. Ginseng increases hypoglycemia with insulin therapy.

Data from Kuwajerwala K: *Perioperative medication management,* Medscape, 2018. https://emedicine.medscape.com/article/284801-overview#a4. Last reviewed January 9, 2018. Accessed August 3, 2018.

Allergies. Allergies to medications, latex, and topical agents used to prepare the skin for surgery create significant risks for patients during surgery. An allergic response to any agent is potentially fatal, depending on severity. Latex allergies are on the rise, with 1% to 6% of the general population and 8% to 12% of the health care workforce sensitive to latex (OSHA, n.d.). Patients most at risk for a latex allergy include people with a genetic predisposition to latex allergy, children with spina bifida, patients with urogenital abnormalities or spinal cord injury (because of a long history of urinary catheter use), patients with a history of multiple surgeries, health care professionals, and workers who manufacture rubber products. Patients with an allergy to certain foods such as bananas, chestnuts, kiwifruit, avocados, potatoes, strawberries, nectarines, tomatoes, and wheat often have a cross-sensitivity to latex (Cleveland Clinic, 2017). Symptoms of a latex allergy vary in severity (e.g., contact dermatitis with redness, inflammation, and blisters; contact urticaria with pruritus, redness, and swelling; hay fever–like symptoms; and anaphylaxis). When you identify a patient allergy, provide an allergy identification band at the time of admission that remains on until discharge. List all allergies in the patient's medical record. It is also common to list allergies on the front of paper charts.

Smoking Habits. Screen all patients for a history of smoking, including cigarettes, cigars, electronic cigarettes, and pipes. This is usually included in the nursing health history. Use "pack-years" as a guide to determine the number of cigarette packs smoked per day and the number of years the patient has smoked. In addition, ask the patient about the use and frequency of other nicotine products such as snuff and chewing tobacco. Use this information to plan for aggressive pulmonary hygiene, including more frequent turning, deep breathing, coughing, and the use of incentive spirometry after surgery.

Alcohol Ingestion and Substance Use and Abuse. Habitual use of alcohol or illegal drugs and the misuse of prescription drugs predispose patients to adverse reactions to anesthetic agents. Some patients experience a cross-tolerance to anesthetic agents and analgesics, resulting in the need for higher-than-usual doses. Patients with a history of excessive alcohol ingestion are often malnourished, which delays wound healing. These patients are also at risk for liver disease, portal hypertension, and esophageal varices (which increase the risk of bleeding). A patient who habitually uses alcohol and is required to remain in the hospital longer than 24 hours is also at risk for acute alcohol withdrawal and its more severe form, delirium tremens (DTs).

It is important to assess all age-groups because there is a high prevalence of at-risk drinking and binge drinking (17% overall) in adults ages 18 years and older (CDC, 2018). It is common for patients to not disclose their use of alcohol or illegal drug use. Begin the assessment by asking the patient if he or she consumes wine, beer, whiskey, and other forms of alcohol. Assess the number of drinks the patient has during a typical day or week. Also ask about the use of illegal drugs and the use of prescription drugs, including the type, frequency, and method of delivery. Some health care facilities require the use of screening tools such as the Alcohol, Smoking and Substance Involvement Screening Test (ASSIST) to assess a patient's use of illegal drugs, smoking, and/or misuse of prescription drugs or the Alcohol Use Disorders Identification Test (AUDIT) to screen for alcohol use problems (World Health Organization, 2018; American Society of Addiction Medicine, 2019). Your findings will help in the planning of anesthetic and pain management. However, it is important postoperatively to consider opportunities to counsel those patients whose use of alcohol or illicit drugs is excessive.

Pregnancy. During preoperative assessment, routinely ask women of childbearing age who are scheduled for surgery about their last menstrual period and if it was "typical" for them. Also ask if they have had unprotected sex in the past month. Because many women do not know they are pregnant early in the first trimester, many institutions require a pregnancy test when a patient is scheduled for surgery. If a woman is pregnant, the perioperative plan of care addresses not one, but two patients: the mother and the developing fetus. A pregnant patient has surgery only on an emergent or urgent basis. Because all of a mother's major systems are affected during pregnancy, the risk for intraoperative complications increases. General anesthesia is administered with caution because of the increased risk of fetal death and preterm labor. Regional anesthesia is used in preference to general anesthesia when appropriate (Movasaghi et al., 2016). Psychological assessment of mother and family is also essential.

Perceptions and Knowledge Regarding Surgery. A patient's past experience with surgery influences potential physical and psychological responses to a procedure. Assess the patient's previous experiences with surgery as a foundation for anticipating his or her needs, providing teaching, addressing fears, and clarifying concerns. Ask him or her to discuss the previous type of surgery, level of discomfort, extent of disability, and overall level of care required. Address any complications that the patient experienced. Prior anesthesia records are a useful source of information if previous surgical problems occurred.

The surgical experience affects the family unit as a whole. Understanding a patient's and family's knowledge and expectations (following discharge) allows you to plan teaching and provide individualized emotional support measures. In many instances, patients fear surgery. Some fears are the result of past hospital experiences, warnings from friends and family, or lack of knowledge. Assess the patient's understanding of planned surgery, its implications, and planned postoperative activities. Ask questions, such as "Tell me what you think will happen before and after surgery" or "Explain what you know about surgery." Nurses face ethical dilemmas when patients are misinformed or unaware of the reason for surgery. Confer with the surgeon if a patient has an inaccurate perception or knowledge of the surgical procedure before the patient is sent to the surgical suite. Further, determine whether the health care provider explained routine preoperative and postoperative procedures, and assess the patient's readiness and willingness to learn. Reinforce the patient's knowledge of the surgical procedure and post-operative expectations.

Support Sources. Have your assessment include the identification of the patient's primary family caregiver or family support person. The patient usually cannot immediately assume the same level of physical activity enjoyed before surgery. With ambulatory surgery, patients and/or family caregivers assume responsibility for postoperative care immediately. The family caregiver is an important resource for a patient with physical limitations and provides the emotional support needed to motivate the patient to return to his or her previous state of health. Ask the family caregiver what type of support he or she provides. Is it sufficient to meet the patient's needs? What level of instruction or support is required?

Sometimes the family caregiver remembers preoperative and postoperative teaching better than the patient. Patients having ambulatory surgery will receive a postdischarge phone call to evaluate their recovery. Sometimes patients, especially older adults, are unable to hear or reach a phone after surgery. Ask if a family member will be staying with the patient to answer the phone. The nurse's responsibility is to fully prepare a patient and any family caregiver for patient self-care if the patient returns home. This includes providing information that allows the patient to anticipate any problems, know how to act, and be able to perform care measures (e.g., medication administration, dressing changes, exercises). Often a family member becomes the patient's coach, offering valuable support after surgery when a patient's participation in care is vital.

Occupation. Surgery often results in physical changes and restrictions that prevent a person from immediately returning to work. Assess the patient's occupational history to anticipate the possible effects of surgery on recovery, the time it will take to return to work, and eventual work performance. Explain postoperative restrictions set by the health care provider, such as lifting, walking, or climbing stairs, and the projected time frame for a patient to be able to return to work. When a patient is unable to return to a job, refer the patient to a social worker and/or occupational therapist for job-training programs or to seek economic assistance.

Preoperative Pain Assessment. Surgical manipulation of tissues, treatments, and positioning on the OR table contribute to postoperative pain. However, patients also often present preoperatively with painful conditions. Conduct a comprehensive pain assessment before surgery (see Chapter 44), including the character of any existing pain and the patient's and family's expectations for pain management after surgery. Ask patients to describe their perceived tolerance to pain, past experiences, and prior successful interventions.

Review of Emotional Health. Surgery is psychologically stressful and creates anxiety in patients and their families. Patients often feel powerless over their situation. Potential disruptions in lifestyle, a lengthy recovery period at home, and uncertainty about the long-term effects of surgery on a patient's life place stress on patients and their families. When a patient has a chronic illness, the family is either fearful that surgery will result in further disability or hopeful that it will improve the patient's lifestyle. To understand the effect of surgery on a patient's and family's emotional health, assess the patient's feelings about surgery, self-concept, body image, and coping resources.

It is difficult to assess a patient's feelings thoroughly when ambulatory surgery is scheduled because a nurse does not have much time to establish a therapeutic relationship with a patient. You can address these concerns initially with the patient during a home visit or on the telephone before surgery. In a hospital room, choose a private time for discussion after completing admitting procedures or diagnostic tests. Explain that it is normal to have fears and concerns. A patient's ability to share feelings partially depends on your willingness to listen, be supportive, and clarify misconceptions. Assure patients of their right to ask questions and seek information.

Self-Concept. Patients with a positive self-concept are more likely to approach surgical experiences with optimism. A person's personal and social identity coupled with a sense of competence in meeting one's own basic needs is a powerful resource for coping with the stress of surgery. Assess self-concept by asking patients to identify personal strengths and weaknesses (see Chapter 33). Patients who quickly criticize or scorn their own personal characteristics may have little self-regard or may be testing your opinion of their character. If the patient is testing your opinion of their character, focus on the facts and remain positive. Poor self-concept hinders the ability to adapt to the stress of surgery and may aggravate feelings of guilt or inadequacy.

Body Image. Surgery or surgical removal of any body part often leaves permanent scars, alteration in body function, or concern over mutilation. Change in or loss of body functions (e.g., with a colostomy or amputation) compounds a patient's fears. Assess patients' perceptions of anticipated body image alterations from surgery. Individuals respond differently, depending on their culture, self-concept, and self-esteem (see Chapter 33).

Some surgeries, such as removal of a breast, an ostomy, or removal of the prostate gland, may change the physical or psychological aspects of a patient's sexuality. In addition, some surgeries, such as a hernia repair, require patients to temporarily refrain from sexual intercourse until they return to normal physical activity. Encourage patients to express concerns about their sexuality. A patient facing even temporary sexual dysfunction requires understanding and support. Hold discussions about the patient's sexuality with his or her sexual partner so that the partner gains a shared understanding of how to cope with limitations in sexual function (see Chapter 34).

Coping Resources. Assessment of patients' feelings and self-concept reveals whether they have the ability to cope with the stress of surgery. Thus, ask patients about sources of stress in their lives, how they typically deal with stressful situations, and how stress affects their daily lives. Physiologically, stress causes activation of the endocrine system, resulting in the release of hormones and catecholamines, which increases blood pressure, heart rate, and respiration. Platelet aggregation also occurs, along with many other physiological responses. All patients will be affected physiologically by the stress response. If your patient has limited coping resources, your assessment findings will guide you in planning for stress management postoperatively by offering healthy coping strategies (see Chapters 32 and 37), initiating more frequent or comprehensive discussions about surgery, and involving social work or clergy as needed.

Cultural and Spiritual Factors. Culture is a system of beliefs and values developed over time and passed on through many generations (see Chapter 9). Each patient is unique in how he or she perceives and reacts to the surgical experience. Research shows that sometimes

---

BOX 50.3 CULTURAL ASPECTS OF CARE

Providing Culturally Sensitive Care for the Patient Having Surgery

Patients' culture and religion influence their health care beliefs (Douglas et al., 2014). The nurse's approach to perioperative care should respect patients' cultural values and involve partnering with the patient to provide a patient-centered care plan. The use of a wide variety of resources within a health care agency, in the literature, and from the Internet helps complement the data needed for nurses to provide culturally sensitive care.

Implications for Patient-Centered Care
- A cultural assessment for preoperative patients includes questions related to the patient's primary language, feelings regarding surgery and pain, pain management expectations, support system, and feelings toward self-care with postoperative implications (e.g., Does the patient relate to the concept of pain? Does the patient have feelings about gender of caregiver? Does the patient follow a custom of giving family members control over decisions? Does the patient have religious convictions that affect perioperative care, such as opposition to the administration of blood products?).
- Use sensitivity if a professional interpreter is needed to communicate with non–English-speaking patients because some patients may have difficulty sharing personal health information with people who are younger or of a specific gender.
- Use materials and teaching techniques that are culturally relevant and language-appropriate to communicate and assess the non–English-speaking patient for factors such as pain, general comfort, temperature, and need to void.
- Provide assessment tools and preoperative and postoperative educational materials in a variety of languages.

---

there is a discrepancy between the information provided before surgery and a patient's expectation, which highlights why nurses need to listen to patients to identify their expectations (Tocher, 2014). If you do not acknowledge and plan for cultural and spiritual differences in the perioperative plan of care, your patient may not achieve desired surgical outcomes (Box 50.3). To bridge cultural differences, the nurse explores and respects patients' beliefs as well as their meaning of illness, preferences, and needs. Understanding a patient's cultural and ethnic heritage helps the nurse care for a patient having surgery. Although it is important to recognize and plan for differences on the basis of culture, it is also necessary to recognize that members of the same culture are individuals and do not always hold these shared beliefs.

Physical Examination. Conduct a partial or complete physical examination, depending on the amount of time available and the patient's preoperative condition. Chapter 30 describes physical assessment techniques. Assessment focuses on a patient's medical history and on body systems that the surgery is likely to affect. While completing a nursing assessment, you validate existing information, reinforce basic preoperative teaching, and review standard discharge instructions. Individualized instruction occurs after all assessment data are collected.

General Survey. Observe a patient's gestures and body movements (gait, posture, purposeful movement), which may reflect decreased energy or weakness caused by illness. Height, body weight, and history of recent weight loss are important indicators of nutritional status and are used to calculate medication dosages. Preoperative vital signs, including pulse oximetry and blood pressure while sitting and standing, provide important baseline data with which to compare alterations

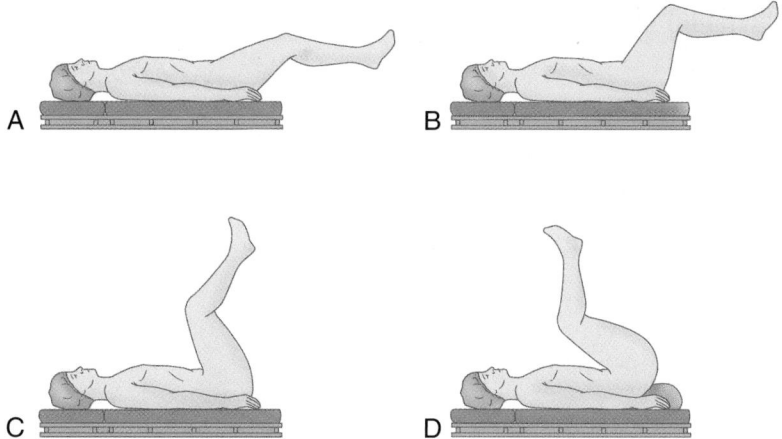

FIG. 50.2 Examples of patient positions requiring a lithotomy position during surgery. **A,** Low. **B,** Standard. **C,** High. **D,** Exaggerated. (From Rothrock J: *Alexander's care of the patient in surgery,* ed 16, St Louis, 2019, Mosby.)

that occur during and after surgery, including response to anesthetics and medications and fluid and electrolyte abnormalities (see Chapter 42). An elevated temperature is cause for concern. If a patient has an underlying infection, elective surgery is often postponed until the infection is treated or resolved. An elevated body temperature also alters drug metabolism and increases the risk for fluid and electrolyte changes. Notify the surgeon immediately if a patient has an elevated temperature.

Head and Neck. To determine if a patient is dehydrated, assess the patient's oral mucous membranes. Dehydration increases the risk for serious fluid and electrolyte imbalances during surgery. Inspect the area between the gums and cheek, the soft palate, and the nasal sinuses. Sinus drainage that is yellow or greenish may indicate respiratory or sinus infection. To rule out the presence of local or systemic infection, palpate the cervical lymph nodes and note any enlargement, which indicates systemic disease.

During the examination of the oral mucosa, identify any loose or capped teeth because they can become dislodged during endotracheal intubation. Note the presence of dentures, prosthetic devices, or piercings, so they can be removed before surgery, especially if the patient receives general anesthesia.

Integument. The overall condition of the skin reveals a patient's level of hydration. Carefully inspect the skin, especially over bony prominences such as the heels, elbows, sacrum, back of head, and scapula. In patients who are obese, separate the body folds to ensure that you examine the skin thoroughly. During surgery, patients often lie in a fixed position for several hours, placing them at increased risk for pressure injuries (see Chapter 48). Although physiological blood and lymphatic flow rates vary among patients, capillary pressures may increase to as much as 150 mm Hg during prolonged, unrelieved pressure without a position change. The normal pressure needed to keep capillaries open (10.5 to 22.5 mm Hg) was identified in classic research (Shore, 2000). When the intensity of pressure exerted on capillaries exceeds 10.5 to 22.5 mm Hg, ischemic injury to the skin can develop. Consider the type of surgery a patient will undergo and the position that is required on the OR table (Fig. 50.2) to identify areas at risk for pressure injury formation.

Multiple factors affect skin integrity during and after surgery. For example, chronic use of steroids increases a patient's susceptibility to skin tears. Older adults are at high risk for alteration in skin integrity from decrease in epidermis, positioning (pressure forces), and repositioning on the OR table (shearing forces).

Thorax and Lungs. Assess a patient's breathing pattern and chest excursion to detect presence of a decline in ventilation. When ventilation is reduced, a patient is at increased risk for respiratory complications (e.g., atelectasis) after surgery. Auscultation of breath sounds indicates whether the patient has pulmonary congestion or narrowing of airways, which can postpone a surgery. Breath sounds provide an important baseline for a patient's condition. Certain anesthetics potentially cause laryngeal muscle spasm. If you auscultate wheezing in the airways before surgery, a patient is at risk for further airway narrowing during surgery and after extubation (removal of the endotracheal tube). Notify the health care provider of any abnormalities noted during the assessment, especially if a decline in function is noted.

Heart and Vascular System. If a patient has a history of heart disease, assess the character of the apical pulse and listen to heart sounds. Assessment of peripheral pulses, capillary refill, and color and temperature of extremities is particularly important for all patients undergoing vascular or orthopedic surgery and for patients who will have constricting bandages or casts on an extremity after surgery. Screen a patient for causative factors of DVT formation as verified in coagulation laboratory tests (AORN, 2018a). If peripheral pulses are not palpable, use a Doppler instrument for assessment of their presence (McLendon and Attia, 2017). Acceptable capillary refill occurs in less than 2 seconds. Postoperative changes in circulatory status in a patient who had adequate circulation before surgery indicate impaired circulation.

Abdomen. Alterations in GI function after surgery often result in decreased or absent bowel sounds and abdominal distention. Assess the patient's usual abdominal anatomy for size, shape, symmetry, and presence of distention before surgery. Ask how often the patient has bowel movements, and inquire about the color and consistency of stools. Auscultate bowel sounds over all four abdominal quadrants.

Neurological Status. A surgical patient's level of consciousness changes as a result of anesthesia, sedatives, and complications that may develop during surgery. Preoperative assessment of baseline neurological status is important for all patients. The baseline neurological status helps with the assessment of ascent (awakening) from anesthesia. Patients should normally regain consciousness and return to normal preop states. However, it is also critical to assess neurological status to readily identify when patients develop delirium postoperatively. Delirium is an acute confusional state—not a degenerative process, but rather one linked with a specific medical condition that has caused changes to an individual's normal homeostasis and bodily function (Koutoukidis et al., 2017).

TABLE 50.6   Common Laboratory Tests for Surgical Patients

Test	Normal Values[a]	SIGNIFICANCE	
		Low	High
Complete Blood Count (CBC)			
Hemoglobin (Hgb)	Female: 12-16 g/dL; male: 14-18 g/dL	Anemia	Polycythemia (elevated red blood cell count)
Hematocrit (Hct)	Female: 36%-47%; male: 40%-52%	Fluid overload	Dehydration
Platelet count	150,000-400,000/mm³	Decreased clotting	Increased risk of blood clot
White blood cell count	5000-10,000/mm³	Decreased ability to fight infection	Infection
Blood Chemistry			
Sodium (Na)	136-145 mEq/L	Fluid overload	Dehydration
Potassium (K)	3.5-5.0 mEq/L	Cardiac rhythm irregularities	Cardiac rhythm irregularities
Chloride (Cl)	98-106 mEq/L	Follows shifts in sodium blood levels	Follows shifts in sodium blood levels
Carbon dioxide (CO₂)	23-30 mEq/L	Affects acid-base balance in blood	Affects acid-base balance in blood
Blood urea nitrogen (BUN)	10-20 mg/dL	Liver disease/fluid overload	Renal disease/dehydration
Glucose	74-106 mg/dL fasting	Insulin reaction, inadequate glucose intake	Diabetes mellitus and stress of surgery
Creatinine	0.5-1.1 mg/dL	Malnutrition	Renal disease
Coagulation Studies			
International Normalized Ratio (INR)	0.8-1.1	Risk of clot	Risk of bleeding
Prothrombin time (PT)	11-12.5 sec; 85%-100%	Risk of clot	Risk of bleeding
Partial thromboplastin time (PTT)	60-70 sec	Risk of clot	Risk of bleeding
Activated PTT	30-40 sec	Risk of clot	Excess heparin; risk of spontaneous bleeding (activated PTT)

[a]Normal ranges vary slightly among laboratories.
From Pagana KD et al.: *Mosby's diagnostic and laboratory test reference*, ed 14, St Louis, 2019, Elsevier.

Observe a patient's level of orientation, alertness, mood, and ease of speech, noting whether he or she answers questions appropriately and is able to recall recent and past events. Patients who have surgery for neurological disease (e.g., brain tumor or aneurysm) may demonstrate an impaired level of consciousness or altered behavior.

If a patient is scheduled for spinal or regional anesthesia, preoperative assessment of gross motor function and strength is important. Spinal anesthesia causes temporary paralysis of the lower extremities (see Chapter 44). Be aware of a patient entering surgery with weakness or impaired mobility of the lower extremities and communicate this to the perioperative team so that care providers do not become alarmed when full motor function does not return as the anesthetic wears off.

Diagnostic Screening. Patients often undergo diagnostic tests and procedures for preexisting abnormalities before surgery. Patients scheduled for elective or ambulatory surgery usually have tests done several days before surgery. Testing done the day of surgery is usually limited to tests designed to rule out or monitor potential problems, such as glucose monitoring for a patient with diabetes or an electrocardiogram (ECG) for patients with heart disease. If tests reveal severe problems, a surgeon or anesthesiologist will postpone surgery until the condition stabilizes. As a preoperative nurse you coordinate the completion of tests and verify that a patient is properly prepared. Be familiar with the purpose of diagnostic tests, know a patient's results, and alert a surgeon or anesthesiologist when findings are abnormal.

A patient's medical history, physical assessment findings, and surgical procedure determine the types of tests ordered. For example, a type and cross-match for blood are indicated before surgery for procedures in which blood loss is expected (e.g., hip replacements) in case a patient needs a blood transfusion during surgery. The surgeon designates the number of blood units to have available during surgery. Table 50.6 gives the purpose and normal values for common blood tests.

Maintenance of circulating blood volume is critical for any patient undergoing surgery and is accomplished with administration of whole blood or blood components. Patients undergoing elective surgery who will most likely need blood products will have a pre-transfusion type and screen sample taken 1 to 7 days before surgery (see agency policy) (Rothrock, 2019). This test ensures blood compatibility (if a transfusion is needed) and avoids antibodies that may emerge in response to exposure through transfusions or a patient's disease. Autotransfusion (i.e., the reinfusion of a patient's own blood intraoperatively) is more common today (Rothrock, 2019). During intraoperative autotransfusion (cell salvage), blood is collected as it is lost during the surgery and reinfused to the patient after it is filtered and washed. Predated (up to 1 month before surgery) autologous blood donation is in decreasing use (Rothrock, 2019).

REFLECT NOW

In preparing a preoperative patient for surgery, what are three questions you should ask a patient to identify the patient's religious and cultural preferences for surgery? If you have cared for a surgical patient, consider any specific patient behaviors that demonstrated religious and/or cultural practices.

BOX 50.4   Nursing Diagnostic Process

Fear Related to Insufficient Knowledge and Previous Surgical Experience

Assessment Activities	Assessment Findings
Ask patient to describe previous surgical experiences.	Apprehension over anesthesia and postoperative pain
Ask patient about understanding of preoperative education/preparation before admission.	Expresses feeling of dread, worry over complications that may result; unaware of preoperative testing
Observe patient's nonverbal behavior, including body movements.	Maintains poor eye contact, wrings hands when discussing surgery

◆ Nursing Diagnosis

Following assessment you group patterns of assessment findings to identify nursing diagnoses relevant for a surgical patient (Box 50.4). A patient with preexisting health problems is likely to have a variety of risk diagnoses. For example, a patient with type 2 diabetes who has fasting glucose levels exceeding 110 mg/dL is at risk for *Impaired Skin Integrity*. The nature of the surgery and assessment of the patient's health status provide assessment findings and risk factors for a number of nursing diagnoses. For example, because a patient will have a surgical incision and an intravenous (IV) infusion, there is a risk for developing infection at the surgical site, in the bloodstream (sepsis), or phlebitis (at the IV site). A diagnosis of *Risk for Infection* requires the nurse's attention from admission through recovery.

The related factors for problem-focused or negative diagnoses establish directions for nursing care that is provided during one or all surgical phases. For example, the diagnosis of *Impaired Mobility related to incisional pain* requires different interventions than the diagnosis *Impaired Mobility related to decreased muscle strength*. Preoperative nursing diagnoses allow nursing staff to take precautions and interventions so that care provided during the intraoperative and postoperative phases is consistent with the patient's needs.

Nursing diagnoses made before surgery may focus on the potential risks a patient may experience after surgery. Preventive care is essential to manage the surgical patient effectively. The following are common nursing diagnoses relevant to the patient having surgery:

- *Impaired Airway Clearance*
- *Anxiety*
- *Impaired Skin Integrity*
- *Risk for Infection*
- *Acute Pain*

◆ Planning

During the planning phase, synthesize information to establish a plan of care based on a patient's nursing diagnoses (see the Nursing Care Plan). Apply critical thinking in the selection of nursing interventions (Fig. 50.3). For example, apply knowledge of adult learning principles, standards for preoperative education (AORN, 2018a), and a patient's unique learning needs and anticipated needs after discharge to formulate a well-designed preoperative teaching plan for the diagnosis of *Anxiety*. Critical thinking ensures that a patient's plan of care integrates your knowledge, previous experiences, clinical reasoning, and established standards of practice. Previous experience in caring for surgical patients helps establish approaches to patient care (e.g., measures to prevent complications and how to anticipate and reduce a patient's

Knowledge
- Adult learning principles to apply when educating the patient and family
- Role other health care professionals may play in preoperative preparation
- Principles of communication in establishing trust
- Physiological risk factors for surgery

Experience
- Previous patient responses to planned preoperative care
- Personal experience with surgery

PLANNING
- Involve the patient and family in preoperative instruction
- Provide therapies aimed at minimizing the patient's fear or anxiety regarding surgery
- Plan therapies to reduce surgical risks
- Consult with other health care professionals

Standards
- Support the patient's autonomy and right to informed consent
- Apply AORN standards for preoperative teaching and practice
- Apply practice guidelines developed by agency

Attitudes
- Use creativity when preparing patients for outpatient surgery
- Speak with confidence when providing preoperative teaching

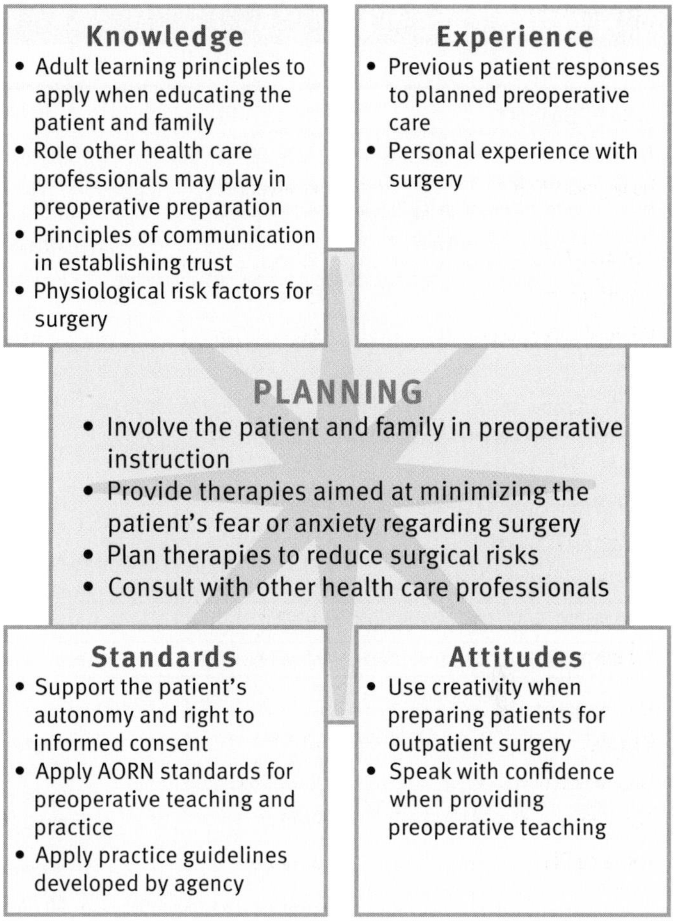

FIG. 50.3 Critical thinking model for surgical patient planning. *AORN*, Association of periOperative Registered Nurses.

anxiety). Use professional standards when selecting interventions for the nursing plan of care. These standards often use evidence-based guidelines for preferred nursing interventions.

Successful planning requires a patient-centered approach involving the patient and family to set realistic expectations for care. Early involvement of a patient and family caregiver when developing the surgical care plan minimizes surgical risks and postoperative complications and improves transition of care through discharge. A patient informed about the planned surgical experience is less likely to be fearful and is better able to participate in the postoperative recovery phase so that expected outcomes are met.

Goals and Outcomes. Establish goals and outcomes of care based on the individualized nursing diagnoses. Review and modify the plan during the intraoperative and postoperative periods. Outcomes established for each goal of care provide measurable evidence to gauge a patient's progress toward meeting stated goals. As an example, the goal "Patient will be able to perform postoperative exercises on the day of surgery" is measured through the following expected outcomes:

- Patient performs deep-breathing and coughing exercises on awakening from anesthesia.
- Patient performs postoperative leg exercises and early ambulation 12 hours after surgery.
- Patient performs incentive spirometry on return to patient care unit after surgery.
- Patient verbalizes rationale for early ambulation 24 hours after surgery.

◎ NURSING CARE PLAN

Anxiety

ASSESSMENT

Mr. Cooper is a 72-year-old patient scheduled for admission in 5 days for elective bowel resection to remove a cancerous tumor. You are the nurse in the ambulatory surgical center. During your initial encounter you note he is alert and oriented to person, place, and time. The patient has not had major surgery before. He lives at home with his wife, to whom he has been married 42 years.

Assessment Activities	*Assessment Findings[a]*
Ask Mr. Cooper what he understands about his surgical procedure.	He learned from his surgeon that he will have an incision down the middle of his abdomen that will take approximately 6 to 9 weeks to heal. Mr. Cooper states, "**I probably will need a colostomy; however, I am worried about how one works and what it will look like. Will I be able to take care of myself?**"
Ask Mr. Cooper about his knowledge of preoperative preparation and what he expects after surgery.	He correctly verbalizes understanding of medicines to take the morning of surgery and NPO status before surgery. Mr. Cooper indicated he is unsure about the length of time he will remain hospitalized, his diet after surgery, and plans for bowel elimination.
Assess Mr. Cooper's concerns about surgery.	He appears slightly anxious with reduced eye contact. His heart rate is 106 beats per minute and his blood pressure is 150/90 mm Hg (normal for patient 82 to 86 beats per minute, BP 130/78). He states, "This surgery will change my entire life. It is serious."

[a]**Assessment Findings** are shown in bold type.

NURSING DIAGNOSIS: Anxiety related to insufficient information about surgery

PLANNING

Goals	*Expected Outcomes (NOC)[b]*
	Anxiety Level
Mr. Cooper will exhibit reduced anxiety.	Patient will maintain eye contact during instructions.
	Patient will verbalize anxiety over change ostomy will have on body function.
	Knowledge: Treatment Procedures
Mr. Cooper will express understanding of expected postoperative care by the morning of surgery.	Mr. Cooper describes the importance of and demonstrates postoperative exercises by the morning of surgery.
	Mr. Cooper describes the need for a colostomy and progression of diet immediately after surgery.
Mr. Cooper will describe how ostomy functions and expectations regarding ostomy care by postoperative day two.	Mr. Cooper will explain location and expected output of colostomy.
	Patient will discuss plans for ostomy pouching and skin care by day two after surgery.

[b]Outcome classification labels from Moorhead S, et al: *Nursing Outcomes Classification (NOC)*, ed 6, St Louis, 2018, Elsevier.

INTERVENTIONS (NIC)[c]	RATIONALE
Anxiety Reduction	
Encourage verbalization of fears and concerns.	Minimizing apprehension over relevant concerns helps to relieve patient anxiety and allows for focusing instruction on those concerns.
Help patient identify specific aspects of surgery that cause him to be anxious.	
Refer patient to ostomy specialist in ambulatory care center to reinforce factual information about diagnosis and ostomy care.	Specialist plays an active role in helping patients perform self-care for their ostomy and adjust to it psychologically (Heideman, 2017).
Preoperative Teaching	
Provide Mr. Cooper, for home viewing, a compact disc (CD) program that explains a colostomy and the preoperative and postoperative routines to expect.	Preoperative education is effective in reducing patients' postoperative anxiety and improving their knowledge (Ramesh et al., 2017; Rothrock, 2019).
Make a follow-up call 24 hours before surgery to the patient encouraging him to ask questions and express concerns.	
Explain purpose and demonstrate to Mr. Cooper how to perform postoperative exercises.	Demonstration is an effective method to reinforce instruction (Tait et al., 2014).
Ostomy specialist will schedule visit morning of surgery to discuss with patient location and expected progress and output of colostomy, and plans for postop ostomy care.	Assists patient in having a realistic sense of postoperative condition and expectations for his involvement in care (Butcher et al., 2018)

[c]Intervention classification labels from Butcher HK, et al: *Nursing Interventions Classification (NIC)*, ed 7, St Louis, 2018, Elsevier.

◎ NURSING CARE PLAN—CONT'D

Anxiety

EVALUATION

Evaluation Activity	*Patient Response/Finding*	*Outcome Status*
Observe Mr. Cooper's nonverbal behavior and ask how he feels about surgery during instructional time.	Patient has numerous questions but maintains eye contact. At end of discussion states, "I am still a bit uneasy, but I think I am understanding more what to expect."	Patient maintains eye contact during instruction. Patient able to verbalize general concern. Requires ongoing discussion.
Ask Mr. Cooper to describe postoperative activities to expect.	He verbalizes understanding of purpose for postoperative exercises ("helps me to breath and be active") after surgery.	Mr. Cooper describes importance of exercises.
Observe Mr. Cooper demonstrate postoperative exercises.	He correctly demonstrates leg exercises and turning, coughing, and deep breathing (TCDB). Is having difficulty using incentive spirometer unassisted.	Mr. Cooper demonstrates leg exercises, turning, coughing and deep breathing. Needs further teaching and practice on incentive spirometer use.
Ostomy specialist asks Mr. Cooper to describe location and expected function of colostomy.	Patient describes area on abdomen where colostomy is to be located and type of stool that will be collected in ostomy pouch.	Mr. Cooper explains location and expected output of colostomy.

Setting Priorities. Use clinical judgment to prioritize nursing diagnoses and interventions based on the unique needs of each patient. Patients requiring emergent surgery often experience changes in their physiological status that require urgent reprioritizations. For example, if a patient's blood pressure begins to drop, hemodynamic stabilization becomes a priority over education and stress management. Ensure that the approach to each patient is thorough and reflects an understanding of the implications of a patient's age, physical and psychological health, educational level, cultural and religious practices, and stated and/or written wishes concerning advance medical directives.

Teamwork and Collaboration. For patients having surgery, the health care team needs to collaborate to ensure continuity of care. Preoperative planning ideally occurs days before admission to a hospital or surgical center. The collaboration between the health care provider's office, the surgical center, or hospital is crucial to prepare a patient for a procedure. Preoperative instruction gives patients time to think about their surgical experience, make necessary physical preparations (e.g., altering diet or discontinuing medication use), and ask questions about postoperative procedures. A patient having ambulatory surgery usually returns home on the day of surgery. Thus, well-planned preoperative care ensures that he or she is well informed and able to be an active participant during recovery. The family or significant others also play an active supportive role for a patient.

Collaboration among health care team members is very important when patients are admitted to a hospital for inpatient surgery. This is especially true for patients who have special problems (e.g., morbid obesity or advanced lung disease). Well-planned preoperative and postoperative care helps to ensure continuity of care during a patient's stay and after discharge. This means that nurses can anticipate expected interventions and the involvement of other professionals who will be taking part in the patient's care. The need for and implications for inpatient care are discussed with the patient and family before the surgery. Planning might include the use of an ERAS protocol. The postoperative plan of care for inpatients will focus on preventing postoperative complications but will also include interventions to inhibit exacerbations of co-morbid conditions. Postoperative care involves an interprofessional team whose members focus on patients' early recovery.

◆ Implementation

Preoperative nursing interventions provide patients (and families) with a complete understanding of the surgery and anticipated postoperative activities. During this time, you prepare patients physically and psychologically for surgical intervention and recovery.

Informed Consent. Except in emergencies, surgery cannot be performed legally or ethically until a patient fully understands a surgical procedure and all implications. Surgical procedures are not performed without documentation of a patient's informed consent in the medical record. In some instances, the patient's medical power of attorney may give consent if the patient is unable to do so. Persons with only general power of attorney cannot sign surgical consents. When a consent is obtained preoperatively, it must be done before a patient receives any form of sedation to ensure a clear level of consciousness at the time of signing. Chapter 23 discusses a nurse's responsibilities for informed consent. It is the surgeon's responsibility to explain the procedure, associated risks, benefits, alternatives, and possible complications before obtaining the patient's oral and documented informed consent (TJC, 2019). The patient also needs to know who will perform the procedure. To ensure that a patient understands the information about the surgery, TJC (2019). recommends that consent materials be written at a fifth-grade or lower reading level. After the patient or power of attorney signs the consent form, place it in the medical record. The record goes to the OR with the patient. If you have concerns about a patient's understanding of surgery, report these concerns to the operating surgeon or anesthesia provider before the patient goes to surgery (ACRP, 2017).

Privacy and Social Media. Although patients can now access their medical records electronically, confidentiality risks exist. Inappropriate discussions of a patient and any planned surgery in elevators, cafeterias, or social settings may end up being communicated "worldwide" (NCSBN, 2018). Nurses have the obligation to protect every patient's privacy by avoiding inappropriate discussions and not using social media to convey patient information. Posting patient information and photos on websites is prohibited; 26 state boards of nursing have taken disciplinary action against nurses who practice such behaviors (Rothrock, 2019), which are direct violations of federal and state patient privacy laws.

Health Promotion. Health promotion activities during the preoperative phase focus on health maintenance, patient safety, prevention of complications, and anticipation of the continued care needed after surgery.

Preoperative Teaching. Patient education is an important aspect of a patient's surgical experience (see Chapter 25). The topics and principles discussed depend on the type of surgery scheduled, whether a procedure is inpatient or outpatient, and the ability of a patient to attend to and learn the content provided. Providing patient education about pain reduces a patient's preoperative anxiety, which is frequently associated with postoperative pain (Chou et al., 2016). Education about the surgical experience increases patient satisfaction and knowledge, speeds up the recovery process, and facilitates a return to functioning (Lewis et al., 2017). Structured teaching throughout the perioperative period influences the following:

- *Ventilatory function*: Teaching improves the ability and willingness to deep breathe and cough effectively.
- *Physical functional capacity*: Teaching increases understanding and willingness to ambulate and resume activities of daily living.
- *Sense of well-being*: Patients who are prepared for surgery have less anxiety and report a greater sense of psychological well-being (Chou et al., 2016).
- *Length of hospital stay*: Being informed reduces a patient's length of hospital stay by preventing or minimizing complications.
- *Anxiety about pain and its management*: Patients who learn about pain and ways to relieve it before surgery are less anxious about it, ask for what they need, and require less analgesia after surgery (Chou et al., 2016).

The health care provider's office or hospital often provides preoperative information and instructions by telephone calls and home mailings. Instructions are available as preprinted teaching guidelines and checklists or in the form of videotapes or educational websites. The American College of Surgeons developed a patient education website titled *Surgical Patient Education Program,* which provides patient information and education materials on types of surgeries, health resources, insurance information, and even some home care skills training (American College of Surgeons, 2018). When a patient is scheduled for surgery (outpatient or inpatient), preadmission nurses call patients up to 1 week before the surgery to clarify questions and reinforce explanations (Rothrock, 2019). For example, they:

- Describe the time for a patient to arrive at the hospital or surgical center and the time of surgery (approximately).
- Explain the extent and purpose of food and fluid restrictions.
- Teach about physical preparation (e.g., bowel preparation, bathing or showering with antiseptic).
- Explain procedures performed in preanesthesia (holding area) just before transport to the OR (IV line insertion, preoperative medications).

Including family members in preoperative instruction is advisable. Often a family member is the coach for postoperative exercises when a patient returns from surgery. A family often has better retention of preoperative teaching and will be with the patient and able to help him or her in recovery. If anxious relatives do not understand routine postoperative events, it is likely that their anxiety heightens the patient's fear and concerns. Preoperative preparation of family members lessens anxiety and misunderstanding.

Reasons for Preoperative Instructions and Exercises. Patients are better prepared to participate in their recovery when they receive rationale for preoperative and postoperative procedures. Patients who undergo surgery need to learn how to promote a healthy recovery and prevent complications, which will allow them to return to a normal lifestyle as soon as possible. For example, a patient needs to know how recommended care activities (e.g., regular antibiotics, wound care) in the home will prevent wound infection, avoid wound-healing complications (e.g., activity restrictions prevent wound stress), and maintain a level of health (e.g., diet and progressive exercise allowed). Patients having surgery also need to know the signs of complications and when to call their surgeon.

Patients who have inpatient surgery need to additionally understand what is required to facilitate their recovery, including pain control, early ambulation, diet progression, wound care, and postoperative exercises (e.g., diaphragmatic breathing, incentive spirometry, coughing, turning, and leg exercises). Postoperative exercises and early ambulation help to prevent pulmonary and vascular complications and deconditioning (see Skill 50.1). Ideally instruction begins before surgery. After you explain each exercise, demonstrate it for the patient and use teach-back to confirm his or her understanding. Guide the patient through each exercise. Ask the patient to perform a return demonstration of the skill if possible, to reinforce it and increase the confidence in performing it.

Changes in the circulatory system, a patient's immobility during surgery, and a patient's underlying health condition create risks for development of DVT. Patients need to know which precautions to take after surgery to avoid DVT (e.g., leg exercises and use of compression hose or intermittent pneumatic compression [IPC] devices). Teach about the purposes and the specific nursing care associated with the devices (see Chapter 39).

Preoperative Routines. Explain the preoperative routines that a patient can expect. Knowing which tests and procedures are planned and why they are planned increases a patient's sense of control. Explain that an anesthesiologist will visit to complete a preanesthesia assessment either during the preoperative admission process or in the presurgical care unit of a hospital or surgical center.

Patients typically do not consume food or fluids by mouth for several hours before surgery to reduce the risk of vomiting and aspirating emesis during surgery. Instruct patients to eat and drink sufficient amounts during the week before surgery to ensure adequate fluid and nutrient intake. This is especially important for older adults living in long-term care settings, who often do not stay adequately hydrated. Recommend foods high in protein with sufficient amounts of carbohydrates, fat, and vitamins. Explain to patients and their families the importance of following oral intake instructions for food and liquids before surgery.

Surgical Procedure. After the surgeon explains the basic purpose of a surgical procedure and its steps, some patients may ask additional questions. First, clarify the information the patient discussed with the surgeon. Avoid using technical medical terms because this adds to a patient's confusion. Avoid saying anything that contradicts the surgeon's explanation. If a patient has little or no understanding about the surgery, notify the surgeon that the patient requires further explanation.

Time of Surgery. The scheduled operative time is only an anticipated time. Unanticipated delays occur for many reasons that often have nothing to do with the patient. Emphasize that the scheduled time is a rough estimate and that the actual time can be sooner or later. Make the family aware that delays occur for various reasons and do not necessarily indicate a problem. Communicate excessive delays when they do occur.

Postoperative Unit and Location of Family During Surgery and Recovery. Few patients are admitted to a hospital unit before surgery unless their case is emergent or a complication develops before the scheduled surgery. Even then it is common for patients to be assigned to a different room after surgery. When surgery is elective, patients and families will come to the surgical center admission area first. During the admission process, the patient and family will find out which patient care unit the patient most likely will be admitted to after surgery. Be sure to explain where the family can wait and where the surgeon will come to find family members after surgery. In many institutions, the circulating nurse gives periodic reports to the family in the waiting room for surgeries that are expected to be prolonged. Many hospitals use pagers to inform family through text messages about patient progress. If a patient will be taken to a special unit, it helps to orient the patient and family members to the environment of the unit before surgery.

Anticipated Postoperative Monitoring and Therapies. Inform a patient and family about routine postoperative monitoring and therapies (e.g., frequency of vital signs, IV therapy, dressings and drains, planned activity, and physical therapy). If they understand the frequency of anticipated monitoring and procedures, they are less apprehensive when nurses perform care activities. Try not to overprepare or underprepare a patient. It is easier to prepare a patient appropriately in elective cases when a surgeon has care guidelines such as an ERAS protocol for a specific procedure and you have adequate time for patient education. You cannot predict all of a patient's care requirements. Contradictions between your explanations and reality cause anxiety for a patient.

Sensory Preparation. Provide patients with information about the sensations typically experienced after surgery. Preparatory information helps them anticipate the steps of a procedure and thus form realistic images of the surgical experience. For example, warn that the OR is very bright and cold. Patients often undergo prewarming or are given warm blankets. A patient will have a cuff for a noninvasive blood pressure monitor placed around his or her arm. The monitor makes a hum and a beep, and the cuff tightens to take a reading. Informing a patient about these and other sensations in the OR reduces anxiety before the patient is anesthetized, which helps reduce the amount of anesthetic needed for induction. Postoperative sensations include blurred vision from ophthalmic ointment in the eyes, expected pain at the surgical site and in areas of the body affected by prolonged positioning, the tightness of dressings, dryness of the mouth, and the sensation of a sore throat resulting from an endotracheal tube (when one is inserted).

Postoperative Activity Resumption. The type of surgery determines how quickly patients can resume normal physical activity and regular eating habits. Explain what to expect after surgery. It is normal in most surgical cases for patients to progress their diet gradually. Many hospitals implement early mobility protocols to prevent hospital deconditioning. One example is the Go–Evaluate–Team Up–Unite–Promote (GETUP) program. It includes resources at the institution and how the nurse will implement a mobility program, evaluate the patient's capabilities (scale/tool/evaluation method), team up interprofessionally for progressive mobility, unite the patient and family members in mobility progression, and promote progress (Florida Hospital Association, 2018; Chua et al., 2017; Malarvizhi and Hemavathy, 2015). Some early ambulation protocols are more aggressive than others.

Pain-Relief Measures. Pain following surgery is one of a patient's most common fears. Even in local procedures (e.g., laparoscopy), air inflation into the abdomen causes significant discomfort in the area of surgery. The family is also concerned for the patient's comfort. Pain after surgery is expected. Inform the patient and family of the need to manage pain and the types of therapies likely to be used so that patients can resume activity quickly knowing they will receive pain relief (e.g., splinting, and relaxation exercises). Teach patients before surgery the type of pain to expect and how to use a pain scale, so they are prepared to rate their pain after surgery (see Chapter 44). Patient-controlled analgesia (PCA) may be ordered to provide patients with control over pain. Explain and demonstrate to a patient how to operate a PCA device and the

importance of administering medication as soon as pain becomes persistent (see Chapter 44). Patients who receive epidural analgesia need a thorough understanding of how it will affect their movement and sensation after surgery.

Some patients avoid taking pain-relief drugs after surgery for fear of the negative side effects or of becoming dependent on the drugs. Listen to their concerns and encourage patients to use analgesics as ordered. Unless pain is controlled, it is difficult for a patient to participate in postoperative therapy. Because of the well-publicized problem of opioid addiction, many patients are reluctant to take opioids even for short, appropriate time frames. There are states in the United States passing legislation that would create a "nonopioid directive" that patients can place in their medical files, formally notifying health care professionals they do not want to be prescribed or administered opioid medications (STATnews, 2017). When it is anticipated that patients will have severe pain postoperatively, have a serious discussion about how health care providers will gradually reduce the amount of opioids to use and switch to less addictive medication as patients progress.

Encourage patients to take pain medications at ordered intervals. Optimal pain management is based on patient assessment data throughout the perioperative experience and customized based on assessment findings and the surgical procedure involved, with follow-up evaluation and adjustments as needed.

Multimodal approaches to postoperative pain management vary depending on the patient, setting, and surgical procedure (Roger et al., 2016). Multimodal approaches include opioids and one or more additional pain-management methods, such as a peripheral nerve block, acetaminophen, gabapentin, nonsteroidal antiinflammatory drugs (NSAIDs), cyclooxygenase-2 (COX-2) inhibitors or ketamine (American Society of Anesthesiologists, 2018). When pain is not addressed regularly, it often becomes excruciating, and analgesics do not provide relief at the dose ordered. When educating patients, explain the length of time it takes for pain medications to take effect. Information from preoperative pain assessment is helpful when teaching about nonpharmacological pain-relief measures (such as positioning and splinting). Remember that pain is subjective, and you must accept patients' perception of pain.

Rest. Rest is essential for normal healing. Anxiety about surgery interferes with the ability to relax and sleep. Meet each patient's individual needs. If a patient is in the hospital, make the environment as quiet and comfortable as possible. The surgeon may order a sedative-hypnotic or antianxiety agent for the night before surgery. Sedative-hypnotics promote sleep. Antianxiety agents (e.g., alprazolam) act on the cerebral cortex and limbic system to relieve anxiety. The advantage of ambulatory surgery is that a patient can sleep at home or in a nearby hotel (for out-of-towners) the night before surgery.

Feelings Regarding Surgery. Some patients feel like part of an assembly line before surgery as a result of frequent staff visits and physical preparation for surgery. The patient has few opportunities to reflect on the experience. Recognize the patient as a unique individual. The patient and family need time to express feelings and concerns about surgery and to ask questions. The patient's level of anxiety influences the frequency of discussions. While delivering preoperative instruction, encourage expression of concerns, be patient, and listen attentively. The family may wish to discuss concerns without the patient present so that their fears do not frighten the patient and vice versa. Establishing a trusting and therapeutic relationship with a patient and family allows this process to happen.

Acute Care. Acute care activities in the preoperative phase focus on the preparation of a patient on the morning of surgery or before an emergent surgery.

Minimizing Risk for Surgical Wound Infection. A surgical site infection (SSI) is one of the National Quality Forum (NQF) incidents that hospitals report (NQF, 2015). As of 2008, the CMS (Centers for Medicaid and Medicare Services, 2018) no longer pays higher reimbursement for hospitalizations complicated by certain types of surgical site infections (e.g., mediastinitis after heart surgery, select orthopedic procedures) if they were not present on admission. Thus, there is great emphasis within hospitals on preventing the occurrence of SSIs. Antibiotics are sometimes ordered in the preoperative period. A reduction in wound infection rates occurs when an antibiotic is administered 60 minutes before the surgical incision is made and the antibiotics are stopped within 24 hours after surgery (Berríos-Torres et al., 2017). The surgeon orders a specific time before surgery for the patient to have an oral or IV antibiotic.

Preoperative care involves skin antisepsis (i.e., removing soil and transient microorganisms at the surgical site) to reduce the risk of a patient developing an SSI (Berríos-Torres et al., 2017). Routine components of skin antisepsis include preoperative bathing (showers or baths) and hair management, both of which reduce the number of microorganisms on the skin. Most patients bathe the evening before surgery or that morning. There is no one antiseptic agent found to be most effective (Berríos-Torres et al., 2017), but 2% chlorhexidine (CHG) in 70% alcohol is becoming the preferred antiseptic, with povidone iodine as an alternative when CHG is contraindicated (Kapadia et al., 2016; Poulin et al., 2014). Patients who have head and neck surgery typically shampoo the hair before surgery to reduce resident flora on the scalp.

The AORN (2018a) recommends that the nurse remove the hair at the surgical site only in select clinical situations. The current evidence supports leaving hair at the surgical site in place unless it interferes with exposure, closure, or dressing of the surgical site. When hair removal is required, clipping it is likely to result in less SSI than removal with a razor (AORN, 2018a). Use single-use clipper heads for each patient, and remove hair as close to the time of surgery as possible.

Maintaining Normal Fluid and Electrolyte Balance. A patient having surgery is vulnerable to fluid and electrolyte imbalance as a result of the stress of surgery, inadequate preoperative intake, and the potential for excessive fluid losses during surgery (see Chapter 42). The American Society of Anesthesiologists (ASA) has recommendations for fluid and food intake before nonemergent procedures requiring general and regional anesthesia or sedation/analgesia. These recommendations include fasting from intake of clear liquids for 2 or more hours, breast milk for 4 hours, formula and nonhuman milk for 6 hours, and a light meal of toast and clear liquids for 6 hours. A patient also cannot have any meat or fried foods 8 hours before surgery, unless explicitly specified by the anesthesiologist or surgeon (ASA, 2017). When a patient is hospitalized before surgery, remove all fluids and solid foods as ordered from the bedside and post a sign over the bed to alert personnel to fasting restrictions.

Despite the ASA standards, many surgeons still have patients maintain nothing by mouth after midnight. Ensure that you follow the health care provider's orders. During general anesthesia the muscles relax, and gastric contents can reflux into the esophagus. The anesthetic reduces the patient's gag reflex. Therefore, a patient is at risk for aspiration of food or fluids from the stomach into the lungs. The surgeon's orders will provide additional guidance for routine procedures (e.g., IV line placement and preoperative medications). Some patients are allowed to take specific medications (e.g., anticoagulants, cardiovascular medications, anticonvulsants, and antibiotics) with a sip of water as ordered by their health care providers. Allow patients time to rinse their mouths with water or mouthwash and brush their teeth immediately before surgery as long as they do not swallow water. Notify the surgeon and anesthesia provider if a patient eats or drinks during the fasting period.

If a patient cannot eat because of GI alterations or impairments in consciousness, the health care provider may order intravenous fluids. The health care provider assesses serum electrolyte levels to determine the type of IV fluids and electrolyte additives to administer before and during surgery. Patients with severe nutritional imbalances sometimes require supplements with concentrated protein and glucose such as total parenteral nutrition (see Chapter 45).

Preventing Bowel Incontinence and Contamination. Some patients receive a bowel preparation (e.g., a cathartic or enema) if the surgery involves the lower GI system. Manipulation of parts of the GI tract during surgery results in absence of peristalsis for 24 hours and sometimes longer. Enemas and cathartics (see Chapter 47) such as a polyethylene glycol electrolyte solution clean the GI tract to prevent intraoperative incontinence. An empty bowel reduces risk of injury to the intestines and minimizes contamination of the operative wound if colon surgery is planned or a part of the bowel is incised or opened accidentally. In addition, bowel cleansing reduces postoperative constipation. If a surgeon's order reads "give enemas until clear," this means that a nurse administers enemas until the enema return solution contains no solid fecal material. Too many enemas given over a short time can cause serious fluid and electrolyte imbalances (see Chapter 42). Most agencies limit the number of enemas (usually three) that a nurse may administer successively. Verify a patient's potassium level following bowel preparation. Diarrhea may cause hypokalemia.

Preparation On the Day of Surgery. You will commonly complete several routine procedures before releasing patients for surgery.

Hygiene. Basic hygiene measures provide additional comfort before surgery. If a patient is unwilling to take a complete bath, a partial bath is refreshing and removes irritating secretions or drainage from the skin. Provide a clean hospital gown as a patient cannot wear personal nightwear to the OR because it is restrictive and is a flammable hazard. When a patient is NPO for hours before surgery, his or her mouth is often very dry. Offer the patient nonalcohol-based mouthwash and toothpaste, again cautioning the patient not to swallow water.

Preparation of Hair and Removal of Cosmetics. During major surgery an anesthesiologist positions a patient's head to place an endotracheal tube into the airway (see Chapter 41). This involves manipulation of the hair and scalp. To avoid injury, ask the patient to remove hairpins or clips before leaving for surgery. Electrocautery is frequently used during surgery. Hairpins and clips can become an exit source for the electricity and cause burns. Remove hairpieces or wigs as well. Patients can braid long hair and wear disposable hats to contain hair before entering the OR.

During and after surgery, the anesthesia provider and nurse assess skin and mucous membranes to determine a patient's level of oxygenation, circulation, and fluid balance. A pulse oximeter is often applied to a finger to monitor oxygen saturation (see Chapter 30). Anesthesia providers also use end-tidal carbon dioxide, by way of capnography, to assess patients' physical status. When using a pulse oximeter, have patients remove all makeup (lipstick, powder, blush, nail polish) and at least one artificial fingernail to expose normal skin and nail color. Anything in or around the eye irritates or injures the eye during surgery. Have patients remove contact lenses, false eyelashes, and eye makeup. Give the patient's eyeglasses to the family immediately before the patient leaves for the OR. Document all valuables per agency policy.

Removal of Prostheses. It is easy for any type of prosthetic device to become lost or damaged during surgery. Have patients remove all removable prosthetics (e.g., artificial limbs, partial or complete dentures, artificial eyes, and hearing aids) for safekeeping just before leaving for surgery. If a patient has a brace or splint, check with the health care provider to determine whether it should remain in place. For many patients it is embarrassing to remove dentures, wigs, or other devices that enhance personal appearance. Offer privacy as a patient removes personal items. Patients are sometimes allowed to keep these until they reach the preoperative holding area. Place dentures in special containers labeled with the patient's name and other identification required by the agency for safekeeping to prevent loss or breakage. In many agencies, the nurse completes an inventory of all prosthetic devices or personal items and places them in a secured area. It is also common practice for nurses to give prostheses to family members. Document these actions in the appropriate portion of medical record per agency policy.

Safeguarding Valuables. If a patient has valuables, give them to family members or place in a secure designated location. Hospitals require patients to sign a release to free the facilities of responsibility for lost valuables. Prepare a list with a clear description of items, place a copy with a patient's medical record (see agency policy), and give a copy to a designated family member. Describe any jewelry, including color of stones or metal. For example, if the patient is wearing a silver ring with a red stone, document the ring as silver with a red stone and not as a ruby. There have been instances in which patients claim loss of a diamond, for example, when the actual stone was not a diamond. Patients are often reluctant to remove wedding rings or religious medals. A wedding band can be taped in place, but this is not the preferred practice. If there is a risk that the patient will experience swelling of the hand or fingers (mastectomy, hand surgery, fluid shifts), remove the band. Many hospitals allow patients to pin religious medals to their gowns, although the risk of loss increases. Remove other metal items such as piercings to reduce the risk of burns.

Preparing the Bowel and Bladder. Some patients receive an enema or cathartic agent the morning of surgery (see Chapter 47). If so, give at least 1 hour before a patient leaves for surgery, allowing time for him or her to defecate without rushing. Instruct a patient to urinate just before leaving for the OR and before giving preoperative medications. An empty bladder reduces discomfort and the risk of incontinence during surgery and makes abdominal organs more accessible to the surgeon. If a patient is unable to void, record this information on the preoperative checklist. The surgeon may order insertion of an indwelling catheter if the surgery is to be lengthy or the incision is in the lower abdomen (see Chapter 46).

Vital Signs. Monitor preoperative vital signs before surgery. The anesthesia provider uses these values as a baseline for intraoperative vital signs. If preoperative vital signs are abnormal, surgery is sometimes postponed. Notify the surgeon of any abnormalities before sending a patient to surgery. In addition, assess the patient for the presence and character of pain (see Chapter 44). Many patients have pain before surgery caused by the condition requiring surgery.

Prevention of Deep Vein Thrombosis—Antiembolism Devices. Preventing DVTs is a priority quality measure. The AORN (2018a) recommends that each health care organization implement a DVT prevention protocol. A patient's condition and type of surgery determine the preventive measures taken before surgery. For example, patients who have cardiac, GI, genitourinary (GU), gynecological (GYN), neurological, and orthopedic surgeries will likely have mechanical VTE prophylaxis applied the morning of surgery. This includes application of one of the following devices: antiembolism stockings (thigh or knee length), foot-impulse devices, or intermittent pneumatic compression (IPC devices: thigh or knee length) (Zhao et al., 2014; Kozek-Langenecker, 2018)). In addition, some patients receive pharmacological VTE prophylaxis, which includes medications such as low-molecular-weight heparin (LMWH) (Wan et al., 2015). The health care provider will screen patients carefully for the risk of bleeding before ordering pharmacological VTE prophylaxis.

When correctly sized and applied, antiembolism devices reduce the risk for DVT. Antiembolic stockings maintain compression of small veins and capillaries of the legs. The constant compression forces blood into larger vessels, thus promoting venous return and preventing venous stasis. The nurse attaches **intermittent pneumatic compression (IPC) stockings** to an air pump that inflates and deflates the stockings, allowing intermittent pressure sequentially from the ankle to the knee and alternating calves, mimicking normal venous return when walking (see Chapter 39). Foot-inflation devices simulate natural walking by compressing the plantar venous plexus (AORN, 2018a). Do not use antiembolism devices when patients have an allergy to the material (e.g., latex) or an unusual leg size or shape or a history of peripheral arterial disease, peripheral arterial bypass grafting, or peripheral neuropathy (Lim and Davies, 2014).

Administering Preoperative Medications. The increase in ambulatory surgeries has reduced the use of preoperative medications. However, the anesthesia provider or surgeon may order preanesthetic drugs ("on-call medications," "preops") to reduce patient anxiety, the amount of general anesthesia required, respiratory tract secretions, and the risk of nausea, vomiting, and possible aspiration. Typically, the nurse administers preoperative medications before a patient leaves for the OR. Complete all nursing care measures first. Preoperative drugs such as benzodiazepines, opioids, antiemetics, and anticholinergics usually cause dry mouth, drowsiness, and dizziness but do not induce sleep. To maintain patient safety, keep side rails in the up position, the bed in the low position, and the call light within easy reach. Instruct the patient to stay in bed until the surgical nursing assistant or transporter arrives. If the patient needs to get out of bed to void, explain the importance of using the call light to ask for assistance. A patient can easily fall, thinking nothing is wrong. Be sure that the patient has signed surgical consent before administering drugs that will alter consciousness.

Documentation and Hand-Off. Before a patient goes to the OR, an accurate medical record is essential to ensure safe and appropriate patient care. Check the contents of the medical record for the presence of ordered laboratory and imaging test results, accuracy and completeness of consent forms, and the preoperative checklist that agencies use as a tool to document all preoperative preparation activities. Carefully document surgical preparatory interventions and the patient's response to care. Once a patient is ready to go to the OR, a written (or electronic) record is inadequate to communicate information to the receiving health care team. The transfer of information about the patient from one health care provider to another requires an effective hand-off (AORN, 2018a). Box 50.5 lists critical elements for hand-offs from preoperative to intraoperative providers. The AORN (2018a) and TJC (2020) recommend that hand-off reports occur in person to ensure that the right patient receives the right surgery at the right surgical site.

Eliminating Wrong Site and Wrong Procedure Surgery. Because of errors made in the past with patients undergoing the wrong surgery or having surgery performed on the wrong site, TJC instituted Universal Protocol guidelines for preventing such mishaps. The Universal Protocol is part of TJC's ongoing National Patient Safety Goals (TJC, 2020). The preoperative-to-intraoperative hand-off described previously is an example of part of the protocol. Implement the Universal Protocol whenever an invasive surgical procedure is to be performed no matter the location (e.g., hospital, ASC, or health care provider office). The three principles of the protocol are (1) a preoperative verification that ensures all relevant documents (e.g., consent forms, allergies, medical history, physical assessment findings) and results of laboratory tests and diagnostic studies are available before the start of the procedure and that

BOX 50.5 Example of Elements of a Preoperative-to-Intraoperative Hand-Off Using SBAR Communication

Situation
- Name of patient, date of birth
- Name of operative procedure to be performed, including site and modifiers
- Pertinent documents (e.g., consent, test results) present and consistent

Background
- Elements of patient history pertinent to surgery
- Medical clearance
- Patient allergies and NPO status
- Patient's vital signs and pain level
- Medication profile and medications taken today; laboratory results; imaging results
- Code status of patient

Assessment
- Patient's current level of understanding of the surgery
- Special patient needs, risks, or precautions
- Pertinent cultural or emotional factors
- Anesthesia requests

Recommendations
- State whether the patient has been seen before surgery by a surgeon and anesthesia care provider.
- Determine if the patient is ready for surgery.
- Allow chance for all staff members to ask questions and voice concerns.

Adapted from Amato-Vealey EJ, et al: Hand-off communication: a requisite for patient safety, *AORN J* 88(5):766, 2008.

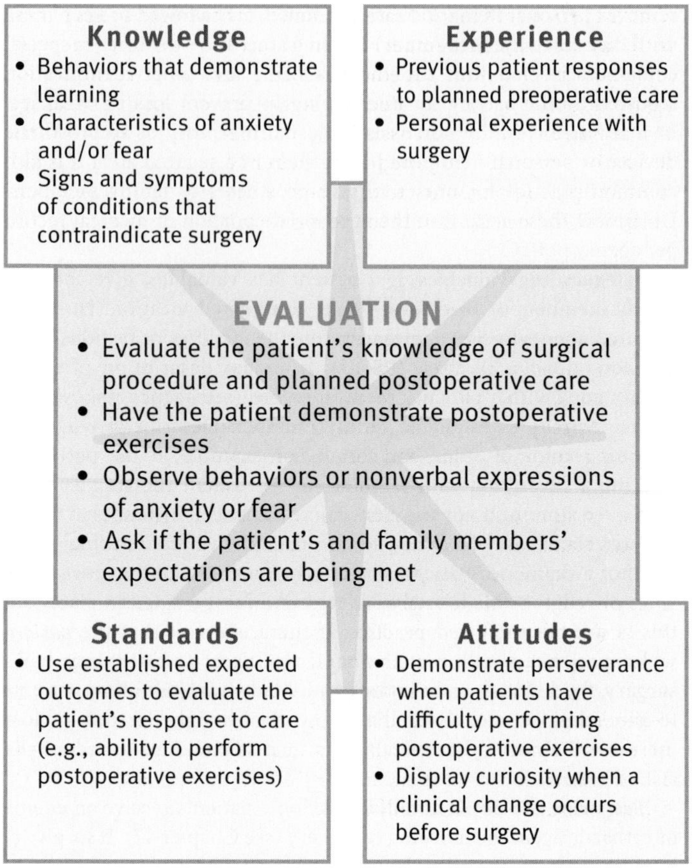

Knowledge
- Behaviors that demonstrate learning
- Characteristics of anxiety and/or fear
- Signs and symptoms of conditions that contraindicate surgery

Experience
- Previous patient responses to planned preoperative care
- Personal experience with surgery

EVALUATION
- Evaluate the patient's knowledge of surgical procedure and planned postoperative care
- Have the patient demonstrate postoperative exercises
- Observe behaviors or nonverbal expressions of anxiety or fear
- Ask if the patient's and family members' expectations are being met

Standards
- Use established expected outcomes to evaluate the patient's response to care (e.g., ability to perform postoperative exercises)

Attitudes
- Demonstrate perseverance when patients have difficulty performing postoperative exercises
- Display curiosity when a clinical change occurs before surgery

FIG. 50.4 Critical thinking model for surgical patient evaluation.

the type of surgery scheduled is consistent with the patient's expectations; (2) marking the operative site with indelible ink to mark left and right distinction, multiple structures (e.g., fingers), and levels of the spine; and (3) a "time-out" just before starting the procedure for final verification of the correct patient, procedure, site, and any implants (TJC, 2020). The marking and "time-out" most commonly occur in the holding area, just before the patient enters the OR. The individual who is performing the surgery and who is accountable for it must personally mark the site and involves the patient if possible (TJC, 2020). All members of the surgical/procedure team perform the time-out. This protocol includes the patient or a legally designated representative in the entire process. If the patient refuses a mark, document this on the procedure checklist.

QSEN Building Competency in Evidence-Based Practice You are a nurse in a surgical preoperative area. A patient asks, "After a previous surgery on my colon, I got an infection in the incision. What is the chance that I will get an infection or another complication after this surgery?" The patient verified that the previous surgery was uneventful but that within 48 hours after surgery the patient developed a fever of 103.6° F. The patient's question poses an important practice issue. Use the PICOT evidence-based practice framework and identify the question that will guide your inquiry of the evidence.

Answers to QSEN Activities can be found on the Evolve website.

◆ Evaluation

The nurse caring for a patient in the preoperative area evaluates initial patient outcomes (Fig. 50.4). Because limited time is available to evaluate outcomes before surgery, compare the patient's current status with expected outcomes to determine whether new or revised interventions and/or nursing diagnoses need to be implemented intraoperatively.

Through the Patient's Eyes. Evaluate whether the patient's expectations were met with respect to surgical preparation. For example, ask patients if they require additional information, if they desire to have their family members more involved, and if they have any unidentified needs. During evaluation, include a discussion of any misunderstandings so that patient concerns can be clarified. When patients have expectations about pain control, this is a good time to reinforce how it will be managed after surgery.

Patient Outcomes. Evaluate a patient's response to interventions designed for preoperative nursing diagnoses such as *Lack of Knowledge* and *Anxiety*. For example, ask the patient to describe the reason for postoperative exercises and the type of care activities to expect when he or she returns from surgery. Observe the patient's behaviors and discuss concerns to see if anxiety remains. Your evaluation is comprehensive to determine if further instruction or emotional support is needed after surgery. Interventions continue during and after surgery; thus the evaluation of many goals and outcomes does not occur until after surgery.

TRANSPORT TO THE OPERATING ROOM

Personnel in the OR notify the nursing unit or ambulatory surgery area when it is time for surgery. Inpatient facilities have transporters who bring stretchers to deliver patients to the preoperative care unit. In ambulatory care a patient simply walks into the preop suite if able and not medicated. A transporter or nurse in the holding area checks the patient's identification bracelet for two identifiers (name, birthday, or hospital number) (refer to institutional or agency policy) against the patient's medical record to ensure that the correct person is going to surgery. Because some patients receive preoperative sedatives, the nurses, assistive personnel, and transporter help the patient transfer from bed to stretcher to prevent falls. Provide the family an opportunity to visit before the patient is transported to the OR. Direct the family to the appropriate waiting area.

PREANESTHESIA CARE UNIT

In most hospitals, a patient enters a preanesthesia care unit (PCU) or presurgical care unit (PSCU) (sometimes called the *holding area*) outside the OR where preoperative preparations are completed. Nurses in the PCU are members of the OR staff and wear surgical scrub suits, hats, and footwear in accordance with infection control policies. In some ambulatory surgical settings, a perioperative primary nurse admits the patient, circulates during the operative procedure, and manages the patient's recovery and discharge.

If an IV catheter is not present already, a nurse or anesthesia provider inserts one into a vein to establish a route for fluid replacement, IV drugs, or blood products. The nurse also administers preoperative medications at this time. He or she monitors vital signs, including pulse oximetry. The anesthesia provider usually performs a patient assessment. Because of the preoperative medications, explain to the patient that he or she will begin to feel drowsy. The temperature in the PCU and adjacent OR suites is usually cool; therefore offer the patient an extra blanket or warming blanket. The patient will stay in the PCU only briefly.

INTRAOPERATIVE SURGICAL PHASE

Care of a patient intraoperatively requires careful preparation and knowledge of the events that occur during surgery. Another important feature of intraoperative care is safety of OR personnel. The OR environment poses unique risks resulting from the procedures followed. Members of the surgical team can suffer injury from skin sticks or cuts (e.g., needle or scalpel) or mucous membrane exposure (splashing of irrigated fluids) to contaminated body fluids. Proper use of personal protective equipment is critical. When nurses participate in laser surgical procedures, they use special safety precautions (e.g., use of laser protective eyewear or shields) to prevent injury to the eyes and skin.

NURSING ROLES DURING SURGERY

There are two traditional nursing roles in the OR: circulating nurse and scrub nurse (Fig. 50.5). The circulating nurse is an RN who does not scrub in and uses the nursing process in the management of patient care activities in the OR suite. The circulating nurse also manages patient positioning, antimicrobial skin preparation, medications, implants, placement and function of IPC devices, specimens, warming devices, and surgical counts of instruments and dressings (AORN, 2018a). The scrub nurse is either an RN or surgical technologist who is often certified (CST). The scrub nurse must have a thorough knowledge of each step of a surgical procedure and the ability to anticipate each instrument and supply needed by the surgeons (Rothrock, 2019). A circulating nurse and scrub nurse partner together to ensure patient safety by minimizing risk of error. The team also works together to ensure cost-efficient use of supplies.

A new role in the OR includes the RN first assistant (RNFA). This is an expanded role that requires formal academic education (AORN, 2018b). The RNFA collaborates with the surgeon by handling and cutting tissue, using instruments and medical devices, providing exposure of the surgical area and hemostasis, and suturing (Rothrock, 2019).

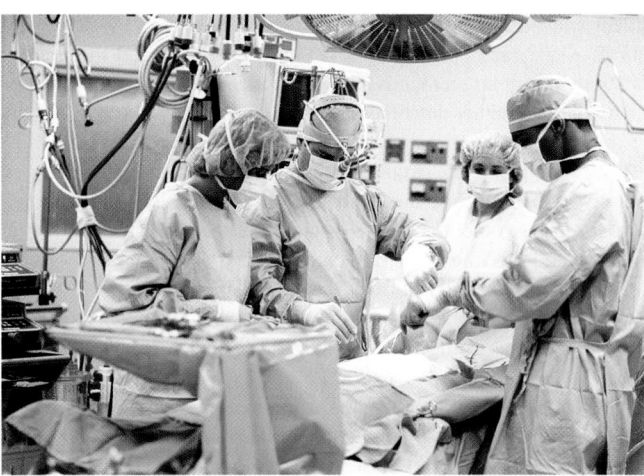

FIG. 50.5 Nurses in operating room (© 2011 Jupiterimages Corporation.)

❖ NURSING PROCESS

Apply the nursing process and use a critical thinking approach in your care of patients. The nursing process provides a clinical decision-making approach for you to develop and implement an individualized plan of care for intraoperative patients.

◆ Assessment

The circulating nurse in the OR thoroughly assesses the patient and critically analyzes findings to make patient-centered clinical decisions required for safe nursing care. Assessment focuses on a patient's immediate clinical status, skin integrity (over surgical site and dependent areas where patient will lie on operating table bed), and joint function (when unusual positions on the OR table are required). This allows the nurse to anticipate problems that predispose the patient to injury if he or she is positioned on the OR table incorrectly. Because patients are unable to speak for themselves while under general anesthesia, this assessment in the OR is very important for their safety. As the nurse, review the preoperative care plan to establish or revise the intraoperative care plan as indicated.

> **REFLECT NOW**
>
> One of the goals of preoperative nursing care is to prevent intraoperative and postoperative complications. Consider the surgical risk factors discussed in preoperative assessment and identify their relationship to potential complications that operating room nurses must prevent.

◆ Nursing Diagnosis

Review preoperative nursing diagnoses and modify them to individualize the care plan in the OR. The following are common nursing diagnoses relevant to the patient intraoperatively:

- *Impaired Airway Clearance*
- *Risk for Deep Vein Thrombosis*
- *Risk for Perioperative Positioning Injury*
- *Risk for Impaired Skin Integrity*
- *Risk for Latex Allergy*

◆ Planning

Goals and Outcomes. Patient-centered goals and outcomes of preoperative nursing diagnoses extend into the intraoperative phase. For example, a goal for the nursing diagnosis of *Impaired Airway Clearance* is "Airway will remain free of secretions." An expected outcome for this goal is: The patient will maintain a clear, open airway as evidenced by clear breath sounds, a respiratory rate of 12 to 20 breaths/minute, and the ability to effectively cough up secretions. How the patient responds during surgery will influence whether outcomes need to be adjusted.

Setting Priorities. The circulating nurse uses judgment to provide a safe operative experience for the patient. Ensuring an aseptic environment, conducting instrument and sponge counts according to policy, managing tissue and specimens correctly, and ensuring proper use of equipment and instruments are top priorities. If an unsafe practice occurs (e.g., break in sterility, missing sponge in wound), the circulating nurse is integral in ensuring the safety of the patient and operative personnel.

Teamwork and Collaboration. For optimal patient safety the preoperative health care team communicates assessment findings and patient problems via a formal hand-off with the surgical team to ensure a smooth transition in care (see Box 50.5). For example, alerting the operative team of a latex allergy or risk factors for complications during surgery (smoker) requires collaboration and timely communication among all team members.

◆ Implementation

A primary focus of intraoperative care is to prevent injury and complications related to anesthesia, surgery, positioning, and equipment use. The perioperative nurse is an advocate for the patient during surgery and always protects his or her dignity and rights.

Acute Care

Physical Preparation. A patient is usually still awake and notices health care providers in their surgical attire and masks when entering the OR. The staff members transfer a patient to the OR bed by being sure that the stretcher and bed are locked in place. Explain to the patient all the activities that will be performed before implementing the activities. Remember that a patient may be partially sedated as a result of medications; use caution. After safely securing the patient on the OR table with safety straps, the nurse applies monitoring devices such as continuous ECG electrodes, a pulse oximeter sensor, and blood pressure cuff. For ECG, place electrodes on the chest and extremities correctly to record electrical activity of the heart accurately. The anesthesia provider will use the cuff to monitor the patient's blood pressure. An electronic monitor in the OR will display the patient's heart rate, vital signs, and pulse oximetry continuously. Capnography is also used frequently to measure the patient's ongoing end-tidal carbon dioxide values. Now is also the time to apply antiembolism devices. The nurse also assists with the insertion of temperature probes via the bladder, esophagus, or rectum if required to continuously measure a patient's body temperature.

If a patient is to have a surgical procedure that uses a high-frequency electric current to heat biological tissue to cut or coagulate the tissue, a disposable or reusable grounding pad must be placed on the patient's skin. The grounding pad, adhered to the patient's skin away from the surgical site, is intended to safely return the electrical current from the patient back to the generator through a cord or cable. Correct placement of the pad prevents burns to the skin.

Intraoperative Warming. The unplanned occurrence of perioperative hypothermia is now minimized with the use of active intraoperative warming. Prevention of hypothermia (core temperature less than 36° C [96.8° F]) helps to reduce complications such as shivering, cardiac arrest, blood loss, SSI, pressure injuries, and mortality (Rightmyer and Singbartl, 2016). Evidence suggests that prewarming for a minimum of 30 minutes may reduce the occurrence of hypothermia (Rightmyer and Singbartl, 2016). The nurse in the OR applies warm cotton blankets, forced-air warmers, or circulating-water mattresses to patients. Forced-air warmers tend to be effective when used before surgery or intraoperatively.

Latex Sensitivity/Allergy. As the incidence and prevalence of latex sensitivity and allergy increase, the need for recognition of potential sources of latex is extremely critical. All medical supplies contain a label notifying the consumer of the latex content. The OR and PCU have many products that contain latex (e.g., gloves, IV tubing, syringes, and rubber stoppers on bottles and vials). It is also present in common objects such as adhesive tape, disposable electrodes, endotracheal tube cuffs, protective sheets, and ventilator equipment. Signs and symptoms of a latex reaction include local effects ranging from urticaria and flat or raised red patches to vesicular, scaling, or bleeding eruptions. Acute dermatitis is sometimes present. Rhinitis and/or rhinorrhea are other common reactions to mild and severe latex allergy. Immediate hypersensitivity reactions are life threatening, with the patient exhibiting focal or generalized urticaria and edema, bronchospasm, and mucus hypersecretion, all of which can compromise respiratory status. Vasodilation compounded by increased capillary permeability sometimes leads to circulatory collapse and eventual death. The draping of a patient during surgery blocks the ability to visualize the skin. Thus, be prepared to investigate any unexplained acute deterioration in a previously healthy patient for possible latex allergy.

A latex-free cart is available in an OR to create a latex-safe environment. All of the contents must be latex free. The Association of Surgical Technologists (AST) recommends that when facilities are not latex safe, nurses need to take steps to prepare an OR the night before to avoid the release of latex particles (AST, 2018). Any patient with a latex allergy should receive scheduling priority and be the first case in the morning. It is important to know that patients may develop anaphylaxis 30 to 60 minutes after being exposed to latex. Box 50.6 lists latex precautions.

Introduction of Anesthesia. The nature and extent of a patient's surgery and current physical status influence the type of anesthesia administered during surgery. Know the complications to anticipate after surgery for each type (Table 50.7).

General Anesthesia. Under general anesthesia a patient loses all sensation, consciousness, and reflexes, including gag and blink reflexes. The patient's muscles relax and the patient experiences amnesia. Amnesia is a protective measure that allows patients to forget any unpleasant events of the procedure. An anesthesia provider gives general anesthetics by IV infusion and inhalation routes through the three phases of anesthesia: induction, maintenance, and emergence. Surgery requiring general anesthesia involves major procedures with extensive tissue manipulation. During emergence, anesthetics are decreased, and the patient begins to awaken. Because of the short half-life of today's medications, emergence often occurs in the OR. The duration of anesthesia depends on the length of surgery.

Regional Anesthesia. Regional anesthesia results in loss of sensation in an area of the body by anesthetizing sensory pathways. This type of anesthesia is accomplished by injecting a local anesthetic along the pathway of a nerve from the spinal cord. A patient requires careful monitoring during and immediately after regional anesthesia for return of sensation and movement distal to the point of anesthetic injection. The circulating nurse protects the patient's limbs from injury until sensation returns. Serious complications such as respiratory paralysis occur if the level of anesthesia rises, moving upward in the spinal cord. Elevation of the upper body helps prevents respiratory paralysis. Some patients have a sudden fall in blood pressure, which results from extensive vasodilation caused by the anesthetic blocking sympathetic vasomotor nerves and pain and motor nerve fibers. Remember that grounding pad burns and other trauma can occur on the anesthetized part of the body without the patient being aware of the injury. It is necessary to observe frequently the position of the extremities and the condition of the skin.

Local Anesthesia. Local anesthesia involves loss of sensation at the desired site (e.g., a skin growth or the cornea of the eye) by inhibiting peripheral nerve conduction. It is commonly used in ambulatory surgery. A local can also be used in addition to general or regional anesthesia.

BOX 50.6 Latex Avoidance Precautions

- Health care workers can transmit the allergen by hand to patients after touching any object with latex. *Caution:* Keep the powder from the gloves away from patients because the powder acts as a carrier for the latex protein. Do not snap gloves on and off.
- Identify patients who are latex sensitive. The operating room (OR) needs to be labeled latex free to prevent personnel from bringing rubber products (e.g., wristbands, chart labels) into the room.
- Develop programs to educate health care workers in the care of latex-sensitive patients.

Recommendations for Patient Care (Patients with Latex Allergy or Latex Risk)

The Operating Room
- Notify the OR of patients who have potential latex allergies. Remove all latex products from the OR and bring a latex-free cart (if available) into the room.
- Use a latex-free reservoir bag, airways and endotracheal tubes, and laryngeal mask airways.
- Use a nonlatex anesthesia breathing circuit with plastic mask and bag.
- Place all monitoring devices and cords/tubes (oximeter, blood pressure, electrocardiograph wires) in stockinette and secure with tape to prevent direct skin contact. Rinse items sterilized in ethylene oxide before use. Residual ethylene oxide reacts and can cause an allergic response in a patient with a latex allergy.

Intravenous Line Preparation
- Use intravenous (IV) tubing without latex ports; use stopcocks if available.
- If unable to obtain IV tubing without latex ports, cover latex ports with tape.
- Cover all rubber injection ports on IV bags with tape and label as follows: *Do not inject or withdraw fluid through the latex port.* **NOTE:** *Pulmonary artery catheters (especially the balloon), central venous catheters, and arterial lines may contain latex components.*

Operating Room Patient Care
- Use nonlatex gloves. (*Caution:* Not all substitutes are equally impermeable to bloodborne pathogens; ensure that substitute gloves provide appropriate protection.)
- Use nonlatex tourniquets or nonlatex examination gloves or polyvinyl chloride tubing.
- Draw medication directly from opened multidose vials (remove stoppers) if medications are not available in ampules.
- The rubber allergen can possibly move from the plunger of a syringe into the medication, which sometimes causes an allergic reaction. The intensity of this reaction increases over time. Therefore, nurses draw up medications immediately before the beginning of the surgery or just before administration.
- Use latex-free or glass syringes.
- Use stopcocks to inject drugs rather than latex ports.
- Notify pharmacy and central supply that your patient is latex sensitive so these departments can use appropriate procedures when preparing medications and instruments. Also, notify radiology, respiratory therapy, housekeeping, food service, and postoperative care units so that they will take appropriate precautions to protect the patient.
- Place clear and readily visible signs on the doors of the OR to inform all who enter that the patient has a latex allergy.

Modified from *Perioperative Standards and Recommended Practices: AORN latex guideline,* Denver, 2018, AORN.

TABLE 50.7 Examples of Complications of Anesthesia

Type	Complications
General	Aspiration of vomitus, cardiac irregularities, decreased cardiac output, hypotension, hypothermia, hypoxemia, laryngospasm, malignant hyperthermia, nephrotoxicity, and respiratory depression
Regional: epidural, spinal and caudal blocks	Hypotension, hypothermia, injury to spinal cord, respiratory paralysis, spinal headache
Local	Hives, rash, anaphylaxis
Conscious sedation	Aspiration, decreased level of consciousness, hypoxemia, respiratory depression

The anesthetic agent (e.g., lidocaine) inhibits nerve conduction until the drug diffuses into the circulation. It is injected locally or applied topically. The patient experiences a loss in pain and touch sensation in the area of injection. Patients are at risk for having drug interactions and allergic effects. It is necessary to monitor patients continually during a local procedure. The frequency of observation and monitoring of patients is tailored to the patient, procedure, and the medications used (Kim and Kim, 2016).

Moderate (Conscious) Sedation. IV moderate sedation (i.e., conscious sedation) is used routinely for short-term surgical, diagnostic, and therapeutic procedures that do not require complete anesthesia but rather a depressed level of consciousness. A patient maintains spontaneous ventilation and a patent airway and requires no interventions during conscious sedation (Rothrock, 2019). In addition, the patient responds appropriately to physical (light touch) and verbal stimuli. The preferred sedative for conscious sedation is short-acting IV sedatives such as midazolam.

Advantages of conscious sedation include adequate sedation, reduction of fear and anxiety, amnesia, relief of pain and noxious stimuli, elevation of pain threshold, enhanced patient cooperation, stable vital signs, and rapid recovery. Nurses assisting with the administration of conscious sedation need to demonstrate competency in the care of these patients. Knowledge of anatomy, physiology, cardiac dysrhythmias, procedural complications, and pharmacological principles related to the administration of individual agents is essential. The nurse needs to assess, diagnose, and intervene in the event of unexpected reactions, such as an adverse reaction to a medication, and demonstrate skill in airway management and oxygen delivery. Resuscitation equipment must be readily available when using conscious sedation.

Positioning the Patient for Surgery. A patient will be placed on an operating room table in a position that offers access to the surgical site. Prevention of positioning injuries requires anticipation of the position and surgical approach to be used, the positioning equipment available to be used, and whether a patient has conditions causing risk for injury (AORN, 2018a). When possible, the position during surgery should be one that would be comfortable with the patient fully awake. Patients should be questioned about limited range of motion and their ability to lie comfortably in the expected position. If questions arise, the patient should be placed in the anticipated position as a trial before sedation or induction of anesthesia. If the operating table will be tilted either top to bottom, side to side, or moved into the sitting position (e.g., during breast reconstruction) during surgery, the anticipated position should be practiced before skin preparation and draping to make sure that supports and straps are secure and that the patient tolerates the position physiologically.

During general anesthesia, the nursing personnel and surgeon often wait to position a patient until the full stage of relaxation so that an injury is less likely to be caused by moving and lifting the patient's body parts. Ideally, a patient's position provides clear access to the operative site; sustains adequate circulatory and respiratory function; and ensures the patient's safety, comfort, and skin integrity. If a patient has conditions such as morbid obesity, malnourishment, existing pressure injuries, or chronic disease, special considerations are needed in positioning. It is important for the circulating nurse to assess circulatory, respiratory, integumentary, musculoskeletal, and neurological structures during surgery (AORN, 2018a).

An alert person maintains normal range of joint motion by pain and pressure receptors. If a joint is extended too far, pain stimuli provide a warning that muscle and joint strain is too great. In a patient who is anesthetized, normal defense mechanisms cannot guard against joint damage, muscle stretch, and strain. The muscles are so relaxed that it is relatively easy to place a patient in a position that the individual normally could not assume while awake. He or she often remains in a given position for several hours. Although it is sometimes necessary to place a patient in an unusual position, try to maintain correct alignment and protect skin from pressure, abrasion, and other injuries. Special mattresses, use of foam padding, and attachments to the OR table provide protection to extremities and bony prominences. Positioning should not impede normal movement of the diaphragm or interfere with circulation to body parts. If restraints are necessary, pad the skin to prevent trauma.

Documentation of Intraoperative Care. Throughout the surgical procedure, the circulating nurse keeps an accurate record of patient care activities and procedures performed by OR personnel (e.g., surgical count status, special equipment, IV and irrigation fluids, specimens, and medications). A standardized documentation format helps practitioners ensure continuity of information from the OR to the postanesthesia care unit (PACU) or recovery area (AORN, 2018a). The AORN recommends the use of verbal and standardized forms to transfer patient information between care providers.

◆ Evaluation

The circulating nurse conducts an ongoing evaluation to ensure that interventions such as patient position are implemented correctly during the intraoperative phase of surgery.

Through the Patient's Eyes. While a patient is undergoing surgery, it is important to keep the family informed. Pagers are used in some settings to text updates to family members. Hospitals vary on their policies for when and how often families are given updates of the patient's condition. Families expect an estimate of when surgery begins, how the surgery is progressing, and the length of time it will likely last. When you give an update to family members, ask if they have further questions or concerns and if their needs are being met.

Patient Outcomes. During surgery the anesthesia provider continuously monitors vital signs. The circulating nurse monitors and records intake and output (I&O), specimens obtained, medications and irrigations, type of dressing packing, and other treatments. Measurement of the patient's body temperature during and at completion of the surgery provides data to achieve the goal of keeping the patient normothermic. The circulating nurse will inspect the skin under the grounding pad and at areas where positioning exerts pressure.

▌ POSTOPERATIVE SURGICAL PHASE

There are three phases of anesthesia recovery. Phase I (immediate recovery) begins when a patient leaves the operating room (OR). It extends from the time a patient leaves the OR to the time he or she is stabilized in the PACU or ambulatory recovery area, meets discharge criteria, and is transferred to a nursing unit or other location. During phase I close monitoring is required; for the first 1 to 2 hours the focus is on assessing for the aftereffects of anesthesia, including airway clearance, cardiovascular complications, fluid management, temperature control, and neurological function. A patient's condition can change rapidly; assessments must be timely, knowledgeable, and accurate. When a patient has progressed beyond these elements of care, they can progress to the phase II level of care in which plans and care are provided to progress the patient home (ASPAN, 2018). This may be in the same physical location as phase I care, when a patient has had ambulatory surgery. Many PACUs provide blended levels of care, in which both levels of care are provided in the same location (ASPAN, 2018).

Phase III recovery (convalescence) focuses on providing ongoing care for patients who are hospitalized and require extended observation or intervention after transfer from phase I or phase II. Interventions are directed toward preparing the patient for self-care or care by family members. Phases of recovery are not locations but levels of care (ASPAN, 2018).

The type of anesthesia, nature of surgery, and a patient's previous condition determine the phases of recovery and the length of time spent on an acute care nursing unit. Typically, at the end of surgery the anesthesia provider and the circulating nurse accompany the patient to the PACU and provide a thorough hand-off report to the nursing staff.

IMMEDIATE POSTOPERATIVE RECOVERY (PHASE I)

When a PACU nurse receives a patient during hand-off, he or she obtains data from the surgical team to prepare for proper support of a patient's recovery status. This includes anticipating possible clinical problems based on assessment and being sure that special equipment needed for nursing care is available. Careful planning allows the nursing staff to consider placement of patients in the PACU. For example, patients who undergo spinal anesthesia are aware of their surroundings and benefit from being in a quieter part of the PACU, away from patients needing frequent monitoring. The nurse isolates patients with serious infections, such as tuberculosis, from other patients. Use Standard Precautions for infection control (see Chapter 28) for all patients.

When a patient is admitted to phase I recovery, personnel notify the nurses on the acute care nursing unit of his or her arrival. This allows the nursing staff to inform family members. Family members usually remain in the designated waiting area so that they are accessible when the surgeon arrives to explain the patient's condition. *It is the surgeon's responsibility to describe the patient's status, the results of surgery, and any complications that occurred.* The nurse is a valuable resource to the family for clarifying explanations if complications occur in the operative phase.

When a patient enters the PACU, the nurse and members of the surgical team discuss his or her status. A standardized approach or tool for "hand-off" communications helps to provide accurate information about a patient's care, treatment and services, current condition, and any recent or anticipated changes (Rothrock, 2019). The hand-off is interactive, interprofessional, and done at the patient's bedside, allowing for a communication exchange that gives caregivers the chance to dialogue and ask questions. The surgical team's report includes topics such as the type of anesthesia provided, vital sign trends, intraoperative medications, IV fluids, estimated blood and urine loss, and pertinent information about the surgical wound (e.g., dressings, tubes, drains) (Rothrock, 2019). The information obtained from hand-off report allows a recovery nurse to anticipate how quickly a patient should regain consciousness, any likely complications, and what his or her analgesic needs will be. A report on IV fluids or blood products administered during surgery from the anesthesia provider or perfusionist alerts the nurse to the patient's fluid and electrolyte balance. The surgeon or anesthesia provider often reports special concerns (e.g., whether the patient is at risk for hemorrhaging or infection) and whether there were complications during surgery such as excessive blood loss or cardiac irregularities. The circulating nurse also reports intraoperative patient positioning and condition of the skin. Frequently, this report takes place while PACU nurses are admitting the patient. The PACU nurse attaches the patient to monitoring equipment such as the noninvasive blood pressure monitor, ECG monitor, and pulse oximeter. Patients often receive some form of oxygen in this immediate recovery period.

After receiving hand-off communication from the OR, the PACU nurse conducts a complete systems assessment during the first few minutes of PACU care (Garrett, 2016) (Box 50.7). Patients will begin to gradually awaken while in the PACU. Try to arouse a patient by calling his or her name in a moderate tone of voice. If that is not successful, waken him or her by using touch or gently moving a body part. If painful stimulation is needed to arouse a patient, notify anesthesia immediately. Perform assessments at least every 15 minutes or more frequently, depending on the patient's condition and unit policy. This assessment continues until discharge from the PACU. Perform assessments quickly and thoroughly and target them to a patient's unique needs and type of surgery.

As patients awaken, they expectorate the oral airway, or the nurse asks the patient to expectorate the airway. The ability to do so signifies the return of a normal gag reflex. Before removing an artificial airway (or before the patient removes it), suction the back of the airway so that secretions are not retained. Be alert for nausea and vomiting, which may precipitate regurgitation. Avoid any rapid movement of the patient and keep his or her head elevated while lying on the side.

One of the greatest concerns is airway obstruction. A number of factors contribute to obstruction, including history of OSA; weak pharyngeal/laryngeal muscle tone from anesthetics; secretions in the pharynx, bronchial tree, or trachea; and laryngeal or subglottic edema. After anesthesia,

a patient's tongue causes the majority of airway obstructions. Ongoing assessment of airway patency is crucial even during phase III recovery. Patients remain in a side-lying position until airways are clear. Continue to assess respiratory status and breath sounds. Older patients, smokers, and patients with a history of respiratory disease are prone to developing complications such as atelectasis or pneumonia. Patients with OSA are often required to have continuous pulse oximetry while receiving IV opioids to detect oxygen desaturation quickly. Use of the Pasero Opioid-Induced Sedation Scale (POSS) in the PACU helps assess patients more accurately and meets the pain needs of the patient while preventing oversedation (Kobelt et al., 2014).

Normally a patient who received general anesthesia does not drink fluids in the PACU because of reduced peristalsis, risk of nausea and vomiting, and grogginess from general anesthesia. In the case of ambulatory surgery, once a patient awakens in the recovery area and feels no nausea, ice chips or clear liquids in small amounts will be given. For patients at high risk for the development of nausea and vomiting or those who must not vomit, the nurse administers a combination of antiemetics, as ordered by the surgeon, to block multiple receptors. A combination of antiemetic medications is often more effective than a single agent (Matsota et al., 2015). If a patient has an NG tube, keep it patent by irrigating it as ordered (see Chapter 47). Occlusion of an NG tube results in accumulation of gastric contents within the stomach, increasing risk of regurgitation and aspiration.

You will determine a patient's status and eventual readiness for discharge from the PACU based on vital sign stability compared with the preoperative data. Other outcomes for discharge include body temperature control, good ventilation and oxygenation status, orientation to surroundings, absence of complications, minimal pain and nausea, controlled wound drainage, adequate urine output, and fluid and electrolyte balance. Patients with more extensive surgery requiring anesthesia of longer duration usually recover more slowly. It is common for hospitals and ambulatory care centers to use objective scoring systems such as the Efficacy Safety Score to identify when patients are ready for discharge (Skraastad et al., 2017). Other standard tools include the modified Aldrete scoring system originally developed in 1970 (Aldrete, 1998) or the modified *postanesthesia recovery score* (PARS) and the DASAIM discharge assessment tool (Phillips et al., 2011). Health care providers use forms of both tools. Each assessment tool has criteria assessed at select time intervals (e.g., 5, 15, 30, 45, and 60 minutes) and on discharge from the PACU (see agency policy). A patient must receive a predetermined score before discharge from the PACU. If the patient's condition is still poor after 2 or 3 hours or if the stay lengthens, the surgeon may transfer him or her to an intensive care unit (ICU).

When a patient is discharged from the PACU and requires continued monitoring and care, another hand-off communication occurs at the patient's bedside between the PACU nurse and the nurse in the ambulatory care phase II area, acute nursing unit, or in an ICU. The nurses verify the patient's identification using two identifiers. The hand-off includes review of vital signs, the type of surgery and anesthesia performed, blood loss, level of consciousness, general physical condition, medications administered during surgery and in PACU, and the presence of IV lines, drainage tubes, and dressings. The PACU nurse's report helps the receiving nurse anticipate special patient needs and obtain necessary equipment. It is important to have uninterrupted time to review the recent pertinent events and ask questions. It is also important at this time for the patient's family members to be informed as soon as possible of the patient's transfer plan.

The PACU staff transport the patient to either the final recovery phase II area in an ambulatory setting or on a stretcher to an inpatient nursing unit. Staff members from the unit help to safely transfer the patient (see Chapter 38). The PACU nurse shows the receiving nurse the recovery room record and reviews the patient's condition and course of care. The PACU nurse also reviews the surgeon's orders that require attention. *Before*

BOX 50.7 Initial Postanesthesia Care Assessment: Parameters to Assess

Initial assessment in the PACU includes documentation of the following:

- Integration of data received at hand-off for transfer of care
- Vital signs
- Respiratory status—airway patency, breath sounds, type of artificial airway, mechanical ventilator settings, oxygen saturation, and end-tidal CO_2 values
- Intake and output
- Pain/sedation/comfort assessment (including psychoemotional status), presence of nausea or vomiting
- Neurological function: level of consciousness (may use Glasgow Coma scale), pupillary response (if indicated)
- Position of the patient
- Condition and color of skin, status of any suspected pressure areas
- Patient safety needs
- Neurovascular status: peripheral pulses and sensation of extremity or extremities
- Condition of surgical dressings or suture line, drains, tubes, receptacles
- Amount, appearance, and type of drainage
- Muscular response and strength/mobility
- Fluid therapy—location of intravenous (IV) lines, patency of IV lines, amount and type of solution (crystalloids or blood products) infused, next fluid to be administered
- Procedure-specific assessments, such as expected drainage amount, specific positioning aids for orthopedic surgery

Adapted from Rothrock JC: *Alexander's care of the patient in surgery,* ed 16, St, Louis, 2019, Elsevier.

the PACU nurse leaves the acute care area, the staff nurse assuming care for the patient takes a complete set of vital signs to compare with PACU findings. Minor vital sign variations normally occur after transporting the patient.

RECOVERY IN AMBULATORY SURGERY (PHASE II)

After patients stabilize and no longer require close monitoring, phase II recovery begins. This may occur in the same recovery area of the PACU for ambulatory patients or a different nearby location. With new anesthetic agents and minimally invasive surgical techniques, *fast-track surgery* is becoming more common, with patients experiencing a more rapid awakening in the OR, quicker recovery, and reduced morbidity (Nanavati and Prabhakar, 2014). Because of this, many ambulatory surgery patients can bypass phase I and immediately enter phase II in the recovery area.

In ambulatory surgery, phase II recovery is performed in a room equipped with medical recliner chairs, side tables, and foot rests. Kitchen facilities for preparing light snacks and beverages are usually located in the area, along with bathrooms. The phase II environment promotes a patient's and family's comfort and well-being until discharge. Nurses continue to monitor patients' vital signs and level of responsiveness but not at the same intensity as during phase I. In phase II recovery, you will initiate postoperative teaching with patients and family members (Box 50.8).

Patients are discharged to home following ambulatory surgery after they meet certain criteria, such as a designated score on the PARS assessment tool. Patients with known OSA or at high risk for the condition are not discharged from the recovery area to home until they are no longer at risk for postoperative respiratory depression, which may require a longer stay (ASA, 2014). Postoperative nausea and vomiting (PONV) sometimes occur once the patient is home, even if the symptoms were not present in the surgery center. Options for therapy include the transcutaneous AccuPoint electrical stimulation or the prophylactic use of drugs such as ondansetron, aprepitant, dolasetron, or a transdermal scopolamine patch (Rothrock, 2019).

Review written postoperative instructions and prescriptions with the patient and family caregiver before releasing the patient, and ensure that they verbalize understanding of these instructions. Always discharge the patient to a responsible adult who can drive the patient home.

RECOVERY OF INPATIENTS: POSTOPERATIVE RECOVERY AND CONVALESCENCE

Inpatients remain in the PACU until their condition stabilizes; they then return to the postoperative nursing unit for either continuing phase II or phase III convalescence. Nursing care focuses on returning the patient to a relatively functional level of wellness as soon as possible. The speed of recovery depends on the type or extent of surgery, risk factors, pain management, and postoperative complications.

❖ NURSING PROCESS

Apply the nursing process and use a critical thinking approach in your care of patients. The nursing process provides a clinical decision-making approach for you to develop and implement an individualized plan of care. Once a surgical patient is transferred to an acute care nursing unit, ongoing postoperative care is essential to support recovery.

◆ Assessment

During the assessment process, thoroughly assess each patient and critically analyze findings to ensure you make patient-centered clinical decisions required for safe postoperative nursing care. Apply critical thinking while you synthesize information from the preoperative nursing assessment, knowledge regarding the surgical procedure performed, and events occurring during surgery and phase I recovery. A variation from the patient's norm possibly indicates the onset of surgically related complications.

Before a patient arrives on the nursing unit, prepare the bed and room for his or her return if he or she is returning to the same nursing unit. The nurse is better prepared to care for the patient after surgery if the room is readied before the patient's return. A postoperative bedside unit includes the following:

1. Sphygmomanometer and/or automated noninvasive blood pressure monitor, stethoscope, and thermometer
2. Emesis basin
3. Incentive spirometer
4. Clean gown, washcloth, towel, and facial tissues
5. IV pole and infusion pump (if needed)
6. Suction equipment (if needed)
7. Oxygen equipment and oximetry monitor (if needed)
8. Extra pillows for positioning the patient comfortably
9. Bed pads to protect bed linen from drainage
10. Bed raised to stretcher height with bed linens pulled back and furniture moved to accommodate the stretcher and equipment (such as IV lines)

When a patient arrives on the acute care unit, monitor vital signs according to institution policy. Generally, you check vital signs every 15 minutes twice, every 30 minutes twice, hourly for 2 hours, and then every 4 hours or per orders. As the patient's condition stabilizes, the nurses usually assess the patient at least once a shift until discharge. Always base the frequency of assessment on a patient's current condition. *Do not assume that further monitoring is unnecessary if the patient appears normal during the initial assessment.* A patient's condition can change rapidly, especially during the postoperative period.

BOX 50.8 PATIENT TEACHING

Postoperative Instructions for an Ambulatory Surgical Patient

Objective
- Patient will describe signs and symptoms of postoperative problems to report to health care provider.

Teaching Strategies
- Give instruction sheet with contact information, including health care provider's telephone number, telephone number of surgery center, and follow-up appointment date and time. Provide an instruction sheet with clear, focused explanations.
- Allow patient and family to ask questions.
- Individualize standard instructions to patient's specific needs.
- Explain signs and symptoms of infection to family members.
- Explain name, dose, schedule, and purpose of medications and possible side effects. Provide printed drug information.
- Explain activity restrictions, diet progression, wound care guidelines, and the signs of any associated problems.

Evaluation
Use the principles of teach-back to evaluate patient/family caregiver learning:
- Patient explains when and how to call health care provider with problems.
- Patient recites date for follow-up appointment.
- Patient and family member describe signs and symptoms of infection.
- Patient verbalizes name of drug, dose, when to take, and common side effects.
- Patient demonstrates proper activity/movement and wound care.

Thoroughly document the initial nursing assessment findings. Enter patient data into the medical record on flow sheets, surgical assessment drop-down menus, or written progress notes. The initial findings provide a baseline for comparing postoperative changes.

Through the Patient's Eyes. When a patient initially returns to the acute care nursing unit, the family and patient have expectations of receiving prompt and attentive care. There is also the expectation that you will explain the patient's immediate status and the plan of care for the next few hours. Seeing the patient return from surgery is a relief in many ways, but if the patient has had complications or is not responding well, anxiety easily returns. As a patient stabilizes, it is important to assess the patient's and family's expectations for recovery and convalescence once he or she returns home. Be sure to review their expectations for management of pain and other symptoms. What do they expect from staff during the hospitalization? What are their expectations after the patient is discharged from the hospital? Who is the primary family caregiver and is he or she prepared to assume care at discharge? Make the patient and family partners in your assessment so that you can gather information necessary to develop a relevant plan of care. For example, ask the patient's caregivers to share their work schedules (if applicable) to determine whether the patient will have someone to provide transportation for follow-up appointments and outpatient rehabilitation (if prescribed), prepare meals, and assist with medication administration (if necessary).

Airway and Respiration. The priority in the care of a patient during phase III recovery is to maintain a patent airway. Assess airway patency, respiratory rate, rhythm, depth of ventilation, symmetry of chest wall movement, breath sounds, and color of mucous membranes and compare findings with data from the PACU. Be aware that certain anesthetic agents can still cause respiratory depression during this phase. A patient may present with snoring, little or no air movement on auscultation of the lungs, retraction of intercostal muscles, and decreased oxygen saturation. Be alert for shallow, slow breathing and a weak cough. If breathing is unusually shallow, place your hand near the patient's nose or mouth to feel exhaled air. Normal pulse oximetry values range between 92% and 100% saturation. Postoperative confusion is frequently secondary to hypoxia, especially in older adults. When a patient is responsive, assess his or her initial ability to use an incentive spirometer and note the volume achieved.

Circulation. The patient is at risk for cardiovascular complications resulting from actual or potential blood loss from the surgical site, side effects of anesthesia, electrolyte imbalances, and depression of normal circulatory-regulating mechanisms and ischemia. Careful assessment of heart rate and rhythm, along with blood pressure, reveals a patient's cardiovascular status. Compare vital signs from preoperative condition and phase I recovery with postoperative values during phase III. If a patient's blood pressure drops progressively with each check or if the heart rate changes or becomes irregular, notify the health care provider. An ECG rhythm strip of the heart is obtained after surgery, compared with preoperative ECG tracings, and placed in the medical record.

Assess circulatory perfusion by noting capillary refill, pulses, and the color and temperature of the nail beds and skin. If a patient had vascular surgery or has casts or constricting devices that may impair circulation, assess peripheral pulses and capillary refill distal to the site of surgery. For example, after surgery to the femoral artery, assess posterior tibial and dorsalis pedis pulses. In addition, compare pulses in the affected extremity with those in the unaffected extremity.

A common early circulatory problem is bleeding or hemorrhage. Blood loss may occur internally or externally through a drain or incision. Either type of hemorrhage results in a fall in blood pressure; elevated heart and respiratory rates; thready pulse; cool, clammy, pale skin; and restlessness.

Notify the surgeon if these changes occur. Maintain IV fluid infusion. Monitor the patient's vital signs every 15 minutes or more frequently until the patient's condition stabilizes. Continue oxygen therapy. The surgeon may consider medications or volume replacement and order blood counts and coagulation studies.

Temperature Control. The OR and recovery room environments are extremely cool. A patient's anesthetically depressed level of body function results in a lowering of metabolism and fall in body temperature. When patients begin to awaken more fully, they complain of feeling cold and uncomfortable. Older adults and pediatric patients are at higher risk for developing problems associated with postoperative hypothermia (temperature less than 36° C [96.8° F]). Also, closely assess the body temperature of other at-risk patients, including those of female gender, patients with burns, patients who received general anesthesia, patients who are cachexic or had low temperatures intraoperatively, and those whose surgery involved the use of cold irrigants (Rothrock, 2019).

In rare instances a genetic disorder known as malignant hyperthermia (MH), a life-threatening complication of anesthesia, develops. It is a hypermetabolic state occurring within skeletal muscle cells that become triggered by anesthesia. It results in an increase in intracellular calcium ion concentration. It is a potentially lethal condition that can occur in patients receiving various inhaled anesthetic agents and succinylcholine. The hyperthermic condition results in high carbon dioxide levels, metabolic and respiratory acidosis, increased oxygen consumption, production of heat, activation of the sympathetic nervous system, high serum potassium levels, and multiple organ dysfunction and failure. Early signs of malignant hyperthermia include tachypnea, tachycardia, heart arrhythmias, hyperkalemia, hypercarbia, and muscular rigidity. Later signs include elevated temperature, myoglobinuria, and multiple organ failure (AANA, 2018). In nearly all cases, the first signs and symptoms of MH occur in the operating room during induction of anesthesia; however, MH may also occur in the early postoperative period or after repeated exposures to anesthesia (Rosenberg et al., 2013; Sinha et al., 2017). Without prompt detection and treatment, it is potentially fatal.

Monitor temperature closely in the acute care area. Because an elevated temperature may be the first indication of an infection, assess the patient for a potential source of infection, including the IV site (if present), the surgical incision/wound, and the respiratory and urinary tracts. Notify the health care provider because further evaluation is often necessary.

Fluid and Electrolyte Balance. Because of the risk for fluid and electrolyte abnormalities after surgery, assess a patient's hydration status and monitor for signs of electrolyte alterations (see Chapter 42). Monitor and compare laboratory values with the patient's baseline. Maintain the patency of IV infusions. The patient's only source of fluid intake immediately after surgery is through IV catheters until the gag reflex and bowel sounds resume. Inspect the patient's catheter insertion site to ensure that the catheter is properly positioned within a vein, fluid flows freely, and the site is free of phlebitis or infiltration. Accurate recording of I&O assesses renal and circulatory function. Measure all sources of output, including urine, drainage from surgically placed drains, and gastric and wound drainage; note any insensible loss from diaphoresis. Assess daily weight for the first several days after surgery and compare with the preoperative weight. If the patient has a known cardiac history such as heart failure, continue daily weights. It is important to use a consistent scale, amount of clothing, and time of day to obtain accurate weight measurement.

Neurological Functions. After leaving the PACU a patient will still be drowsy. As anesthetic agents begin to metabolize, his or her reflexes return, muscle strength is regained, and a normal level of orientation returns. Monitor neurological status routinely by assessing whether the patient is oriented to self and the hospital and responds to questions appropriately. Assess pupil and gag reflexes, hand grips, and movement of extremities (see Chapter 30). If a patient had surgery involving part of the neurological system, conduct a more thorough neurological assessment. For example, if the patient had low-back surgery, assess leg movement, sensation, and strength.

Patients with regional anesthesia experience a return in motor function before tactile sensation returns. Typically, patients will have remained in the PACU until sensation and voluntary movement of the lower extremities return. Check the patient's sensation to touch (see Chapter 30). Knowing where regional anesthesia was introduced helps you check the distribution of the spinal nerves affected. Typically assess sensation by touching the patient bilaterally in the same area (e.g., lower arm on both sides or leg on both sides) and note where the patient feels touch. Test the sense of touch by using hand pressure or a gentle pinch of the skin. Extremity strength assessment continues to be important if a patient had spinal or epidural anesthesia.

Skin Integrity and Condition of the Wound. During recovery and acute postoperative care, assess the condition of the skin, noting pressure areas, rashes, petechiae, abrasions, or burns. A rash often indicates a drug sensitivity or allergy. Abrasions or petechiae sometimes result from a clotting disorder or inappropriate positioning or restraining that injures skin layers. Burns may indicate that an electrical cautery grounding pad was placed incorrectly on the patient's skin. Document burns or serious injury to the skin on an occurrence or adverse-event report according to agency policy (see Chapter 23). Note if the patient is complaining of any burning or pain in the eye, which could indicate a corneal abrasion.

After surgery, a patient may have only butterfly tape, skin staples, or even glue to close small wounds (see Chapter 48). Look at the incision carefully and notice any drainage or swelling. Most surgical wounds that are larger have dressings that protect the wound site and collect drainage. Observe the amount, color, odor, and consistency of drainage on dressings. It is most common to see serosanguineous drainage immediately after surgery. Estimate the amount of drainage by noting the number of saturated gauze sponges. If drainage appears on the outer surface of a dressing, another way of assessing it is to mark the outer perimeter of the drainage with tape or to mark and date it with the time noted. This way the nurse can easily note whether drainage is increasing (see Chapter 48). However, this is not the most accurate measure of volume of fluid lost. Reinforce the dressing as needed and call the surgeon if wound drainage is leaking through the dressing.

Many surgeons prefer to change surgical dressings the first time so that they can inspect the incisional area. This applies to both outpatients and inpatients. You have the opportunity on the acute care nursing unit to view and thoroughly assess and document the status of the incision/wound at the time of this initial dressing change. Assess whether wound edges are approximated and whether bleeding or drainage is present. It is also important to assess the patient's mobility level. If he or she is unable or unwilling to turn because of pain from the incisional area, pressure injury development is a concern. Institute the use of the Braden Scale or another assessment tool to determine a patient's risk of developing pressure injuries.

Metabolism. Research over the past decade shows that postoperative hyperglycemia (blood glucose greater than 180 mg/dL) is associated with surgical wound infection and longer hospital stays in surgical patients. Maintaining normoglycemia or a glucose level less than 150 mg/dL and reducing blood glucose variability are recommended as an evidence-based practice for safe and effective patient management (Sudhakaran and Surani, 2015). Nurses need to monitor blood glucose levels routinely based on surgeon order or hospital policy.

Genitourinary Function. Depending on the surgery, some patients do not regain voluntary control over urinary function for 6 to 8 hours after anesthesia. An epidural or spinal anesthetic often prevents a patient from feeling bladder fullness. Palpate the lower abdomen just above the symphysis pubis for bladder distention. Another option is to use a bladder scan or ultrasound to assess bladder volume. If the patient has a urinary catheter, there should be a continuous flow of urine of approximately 30 to 50 mL/hr in adults (see agency policy). Observe the color and odor of urine. Surgery involving parts of the urinary tract normally causes bloody urine for at least 12 to 24 hours, depending on the type of surgery. A urine output of less than 0.5 mL/kg/hr is reported to the surgeon or health care provider (Lewis et al., 2017).

Gastrointestinal Function. General anesthetics slow GI motility and often cause nausea. In addition, manipulation of the intestines during abdominal surgery further impairs peristalsis. Faint or absent bowel sounds are typical immediately after surgery. Normally patients who undergo abdominal or pelvic surgery have decreased peristalsis for at least 24 hours or longer (Rothrock, 2019). Paralytic ileus (i.e., loss of function of the intestine), which causes abdominal distention, is always possible after surgery. Auscultate bowel sounds in all four quadrants, noting faint or absent bowel sounds. Inspect the abdomen for distention caused by accumulation of gas. Ask whether a patient is passing flatus, an important sign indicating return of normal bowel function. The return of flatus is usually more indicative of normal bowel function return than the return of bowel sounds (Rothrock, 2019). If a nasogastric (NG) tube is in place for decompression, assess the patency of the tube and the color and amount of drainage (see Chapter 47).

Mobility. Postoperative mobility is necessary to promote respiratory, circulatory, and gastrointestinal function. Immobility may result in deconditioning and increase the patient's risk for hospital-acquired conditions (e.g., pressure injuries) and falls (Pashikanti and Von Ah, 2012). Current research concludes that the use of an early mobilization protocol improves outcomes for patients recovering from major surgery (Rupich et al., 2018). Assess the patient's range of motion, ability to move in the bed and sit on the side of the bed, gait, and balance. As a result of current research indicating improved outcomes in surgical patients, many hospitals have implemented early ambulation protocols to prevent hospital-acquired conditions. Thus, early ambulation protocols have become common practice on many surgical floors.

Comfort and Sleep. As patients awaken from general anesthesia, the sensation of pain becomes prominent. They perceive pain before regaining full consciousness. Acute incisional pain causes them to become restless and is often responsible for temporary changes in vital signs. It is difficult for patients to begin coughing and deep-breathing exercises when they experience incisional pain. The patient who had regional or local anesthesia usually does not experience pain initially because the incisional area is still anesthetized. Ongoing assessment of the patient's discomfort and the evaluation of pain-relief therapies (pharmacological and nonpharmacological) are essential throughout the postoperative course (Box 50.9). Use a pain scale for assessing postoperative pain, evaluating the response to analgesics, and objectively documenting pain severity (see Chapter 44). Using preoperative pain assessments as a baseline, evaluate the effectiveness of interventions throughout the patient's recovery.

Postoperatively, it is common for patients to experience sleep disturbances, often resulting from preoperative co-morbidity, type of anesthesia, severity of surgical trauma, postoperative pain, and environmental stress (Su and Wang, 2017). Some studies have shown that postoperative patients who experience sleep disorders are at higher risk for experiencing delirium, pain sensitivity, cardiovascular issues, and delayed recovery. In

BOX 50.9   EVIDENCE-BASED PRACTICE

Prevention of Acute Pain in the Postsurgical Patient

PICOT Question: In postoperative patients, how effective is preoperative education/pain management planning, compared to traditional/as-needed pain management approaches in controlling postoperative pain?

Evidence Summary

Evidence suggests postoperative pain is managed inadequately in more than 80% of patients in the United States. However, the type of surgery performed, analgesics/anesthetic interventions prescribed, and time elapsed after surgery influence postoperative pain (Gan, 2017). Correlation exists between poorly controlled acute postoperative pain and increased morbidity, functional and quality-of-life impairment, delayed recovery time, prolonged duration of opioid use, and higher health care costs (Gan, 2017). The presence and intensity of acute pain during the intraoperative and postoperative periods are predictive of the development of chronic pain. More effective analgesic/anesthetic measures in the perioperative period are needed to prevent the progression to persistent pain (Gan, 2017). Studies suggest local anesthetics and nonopioid analgesics are beneficial as preventive interventions (Gan, 2017).

The American Pain Society, the American Society of Anesthesiologists, and the American Society for Regional Anesthesia have endorsed pain management recommendations that are based on the principal that optimal management starts in the preoperative period with assessment of the patient and development of a patient-centered plan (Chou et al., 2016). Of the 32 recommendations, four of the recommendations impact nursing practice (Chou et al., 2016). The panel recommends:

- Individualized patient-centered and family-centered/caregiver plans reflecting and documenting the goals for postoperative management.
- Patient assessments in the preoperative phase for medical and psychiatric co-morbidities, medications, history of chronic pain, substance abuse, and previous postoperative treatment regimens and responses.
- The use of a validated pain assessment tool to track responses to postoperative pain treatments and adjust treatment plans accordingly.

- Multimodal analgesia, or the use of a variety of analgesic medications and techniques combined with nonpharmacological interventions, for the treatment of postoperative pain in children and adults.
- The use of cognitive behavioral modalities in adults as part of a multimodal approach.

Application to Nursing Practice

- Use patient-centered educational programs for patients and their families preoperatively. Educational modalities within the preoperative program could range from single episodes of face-to-face instruction to the provision of written materials, videos, audiotapes, or Web-based educational information for more intensive multicomponent preoperative interventions, including individualized and supervised exercise, education, and telephone calls.
- Conduct a comprehensive history and physical examination to develop an individually customized pain management plan through teamwork and collaboration with other members of the interprofessional team. The pain management plan is based on factors unique to the patient, such as the type of surgery or surgical site, the patient's previous experiences with surgery and postoperative treatment, medication allergies and intolerances, cognitive status, co-morbidities, preferences for treatment, and treatment goals.
- Pain assessment includes quantifying the intensity of pain. Pain assessments determine which interventions have been effective for the patient's pain, how the pain affects the patient's function, the type of pain (e.g., neuropathic, visceral, somatic, muscle spasms), and barriers to effective pain management, such as cultural or language differences, cognitive deficits, or patient misconceptions about pain management.
- A variety of analgesic medications and techniques that target different mechanisms of action may be combined with nonpharmacological interventions to offer more effective pain relief compared with single-modality interventions.
- Cognitive behavioral modalities are effective as adjunctive treatments in postoperative patients. These include guided imagery (i.e., relaxation), hypnosis, and music.

addition, noise that occurs in the hospital prevents patients from sleeping (DuBose and Hadi, 2016). Implement nonpharmacological and pharmacological measures (as prescribed) to promote a patient's postoperative sleep.

◆ Nursing Diagnosis

Determine the status of preoperative nursing diagnoses by clustering new postoperative assessment data. Then either revise or resolve preoperative diagnoses and identify relevant new diagnoses after surgery. A previously defined diagnosis such as *Risk for Impaired Skin Integrity* may continue as a postoperative problem, particularly if your assessment reveals continued risks such as reduced mobility or excess diaphoresis. It is common to identify new nursing diagnoses after surgery because of the risks or problems associated with it. Also consider the assessed needs of a patient's family when you identify nursing diagnoses. In the formulation of nursing diagnoses, be accurate in identifying a related factor (when appropriate). For example, *Impaired Mobility related to reduced lower-extremity strength* compared with *Impaired Mobility related to exercise intolerance* requires different nursing interventions. Potential nursing diagnoses for the postoperative patient include the following:

- *Impaired Airway Clearance*
- *Risk for Infection*
- *Impaired Mobility*
- *Impaired Skin Integrity*
- *Acute Pain*

◆ Planning

During the recovery phase, use current physical assessment data and analysis of the preoperative nursing history to plan the patient's care. The surgeon's postoperative orders and surgical team's report of the patient's operative condition also provide valuable data. In many institutions, early recovery after surgery (ERAS) protocols are being used, incorporating standard postoperative orders. Typical postoperative orders include:

- Frequency of vital signs monitoring and special assessments.
- Types of IV fluids and rates of infusion.
- Postoperative medications (especially those for pain and nausea).
- Resumption of preoperative medications as condition allows (some oral medications are converted to the IV route with appropriate dose adjustment).
- Fluids and food allowed by mouth.
- Level of activity that the patient can resume, including progressive mobility protocols.
- Measures to prevent deep vein thrombosis (e.g., sequential compression devices).
- Position that the patient is to maintain while in bed.
- I&O and daily weights.
- Laboratory tests and x-ray film studies.
- Special directions (e.g., surgical drains to suction, tube irrigations, dressing changes).

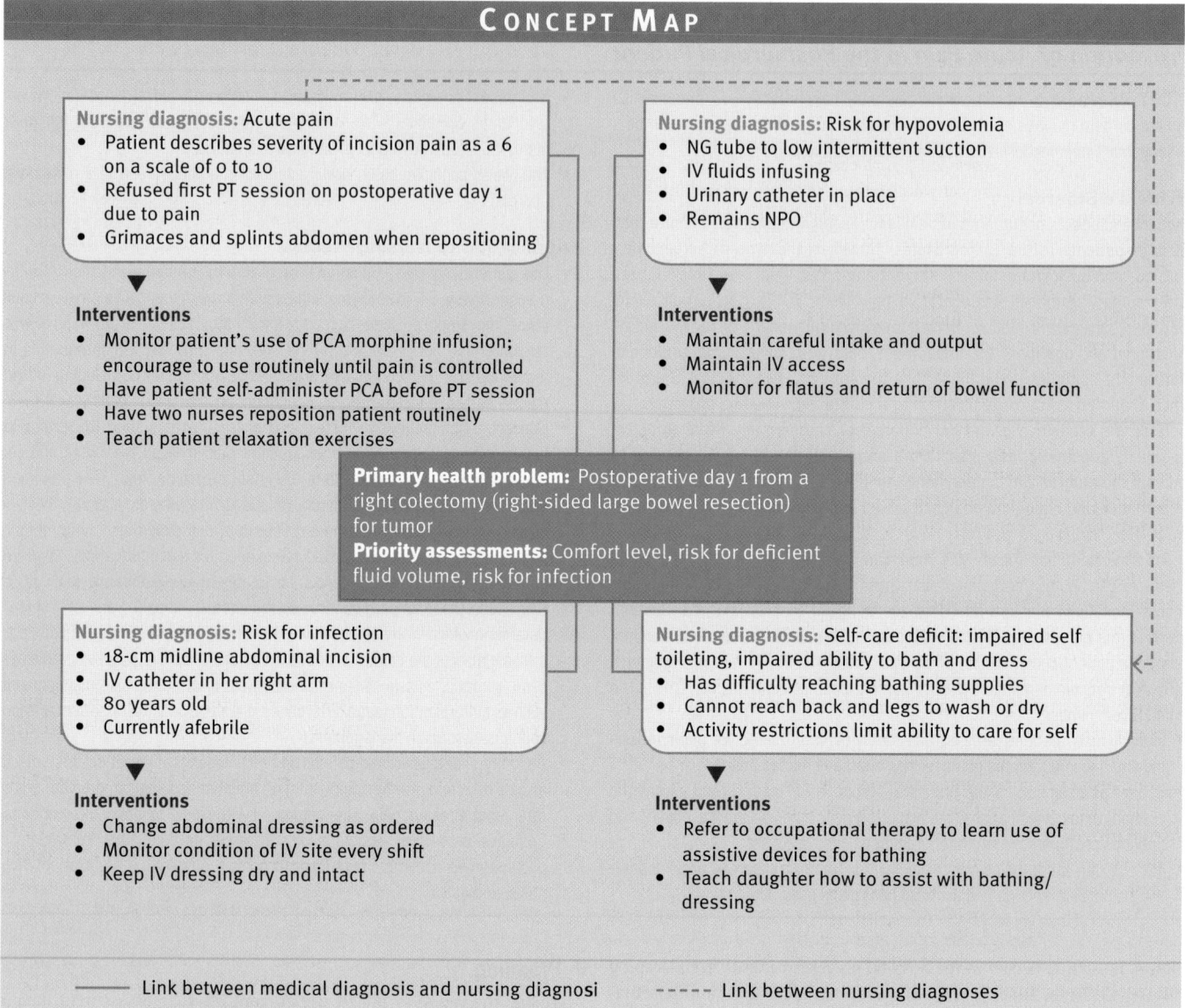

CONCEPT MAP

Nursing diagnosis: Acute pain
- Patient describes severity of incision pain as a 6 on a scale of 0 to 10
- Refused first PT session on postoperative day 1 due to pain
- Grimaces and splints abdomen when repositioning

▼

Interventions
- Monitor patient's use of PCA morphine infusion; encourage to use routinely until pain is controlled
- Have patient self-administer PCA before PT session
- Have two nurses reposition patient routinely
- Teach patient relaxation exercises

Nursing diagnosis: Risk for hypovolemia
- NG tube to low intermittent suction
- IV fluids infusing
- Urinary catheter in place
- Remains NPO

▼

Interventions
- Maintain careful intake and output
- Maintain IV access
- Monitor for flatus and return of bowel function

Primary health problem: Postoperative day 1 from a right colectomy (right-sided large bowel resection) for tumor
Priority assessments: Comfort level, risk for deficient fluid volume, risk for infection

Nursing diagnosis: Risk for infection
- 18-cm midline abdominal incision
- IV catheter in her right arm
- 80 years old
- Currently afebrile

▼

Interventions
- Change abdominal dressing as ordered
- Monitor condition of IV site every shift
- Keep IV dressing dry and intact

Nursing diagnosis: Self-care deficit: impaired self toileting, impaired ability to bath and dress
- Has difficulty reaching bathing supplies
- Cannot reach back and legs to wash or dry
- Activity restrictions limit ability to care for self

▼

Interventions
- Refer to occupational therapy to learn use of assistive devices for bathing
- Teach daughter how to assist with bathing/dressing

—— Link between medical diagnosis and nursing diagnosi   ----- Link between nursing diagnoses

FIG. 50.6 Concept map for Mr. Cooper. *IV,* Intravenous; *NG,* nasogastric; *PCA,* patient-controlled analgesia; *PT,* physical therapy.

Goals and Outcomes. Review nursing diagnoses when establishing goals, expected outcomes, and interventions for your patient. Measurable outcomes provide specific guidelines for determining a patient's progress toward recovery from surgery. For example, a patient recovering from knee replacement surgery with the diagnosis of *Impaired Mobility related to pain and lower-extremity weakness* has specific outcomes that include targeted ambulation (e.g., steps to take and distance down hallway), pain relief, and improved range of joint movement. After meeting each outcome, a patient ultimately achieves the goal of independent ambulation at a preoperative level or better. At times, goals and outcomes extend from the recovery period into the home setting. The nurse considers all goals of care established during the preoperative surgical phase that are still relevant. For example, a goal for the diagnosis of *Risk for Infection* would be "Patient will remain free of infection after surgery." Expected outcomes for this goal include:

- Patient's incision remains closed and intact.
- Patient's incision remains free of infectious drainage.
- Patient remains afebrile.

Setting Priorities. During the convalescent phase of recovery from general anesthesia, priorities for the first 24 hours include maintenance of respiratory, circulatory, and neurological status; wound management; pain control; and early mobility. Most surgeons are aggressive in increasing a patient's activity as soon as possible. If a patient is to be placed on an early mobility protocol, patients and families need to understand that the patient is not being rushed unnecessarily but that early mobility prevents hospital deconditioning. As a patient progresses, focus priorities on the advancement of patient activity (e.g., mobility, diet tolerance) to return the patient to preoperative functioning or better. A patient generally has multiple nursing diagnoses (Fig. 50.6). Reestablish priorities as the status of the patient's health problems change.

Teamwork and Collaboration. During Phase III recovery collaborate on the plan of care with respiratory therapy, physical therapy, occupational therapy, dietary, social work, home care, and others. Include family caregivers as much as possible, especially if they will be assuming care responsibilities in the home. The goal of an interprofessional approach to care is to help the patient return to the best possible level of functioning with a smooth transition to home, rehabilitation, or long-term care. Acute care settings often have a nurse or social worker in a case-manager role to coordinate interprofessional care so that the most appropriate resources are available to patients.

◆ **Implementation**

Acute Care. Primary causes for postoperative complications include impaired healing of the surgical wound, the effects of prolonged immobilization during surgery and recovery, and the influence of anesthesia and analgesics. If a patient has surgical risks before surgery, the likelihood of complications is greater (Box 50.10). Your aim is to direct postoperative nursing interventions at preventing complications so that the patient returns to the highest level of functioning possible. Failure of a patient to become actively involved in recovery adds to the risk of complications (Table 50.8). Virtually any body system can be affected. Consider the interrelationship of all systems and therapies provided.

Hospitals have instituted purposeful hourly rounds to improve nurse responsiveness and patient satisfaction. Purposeful rounds include the *4 Ps* (i.e., *p*ain, *p*otty, *p*ositioning, and *p*eriphery). Nursing staff ask patients about their pain and if they need to toilet, the patients are positioned for comfort, and an environmental check is done of the periphery to ensure that possessions such as a phone and call light are in reach (Mitchell et al., 2014). However, some patient care providers have expanded the *4 Ps* model to *7 Ps*, adding *p*lan, *p*ersonal needs, and *p*resence to the care model. The three additional activities in the *7 Ps* model include the patient's daily priorities and personal needs and the nurse's accessibility to the patient. The implementation of purposeful rounding improves patient safety by decreasing the occurrence of patient preventable events and proactively addresses problems before they occur (Daniels, 2016).

Maintaining Respiratory Function. To prevent respiratory complications, begin pulmonary interventions early. The benefits of thorough preoperative teaching are reached when patients can participate actively in postoperative exercises. When patients awaken from anesthesia, help them maintain a patent airway. Position the patient on one side with the face downward and the neck slightly extended to facilitate a forward movement of the tongue and the flow of mucus secretions out of the mouth. A small folded towel supports the head. Another positioning technique to promote a patent airway involves elevating the head of the bed slightly and extending the patient's neck slightly, with the head turned to the side. In the PACU, the nurse may need to perform a jaw-thrust maneuver and/or chin lift continuously to maintain the patient's airway. Never position a patient with arms over or across the chest because this reduces maximum chest expansion.

Place patients with known OSA or at risk for OSA in the lateral, prone, or upright position, never the supine position, throughout the perioperative period (Olson et al., 2018). Suction artificial airways and the oral cavity for secretions of mucus (see Chapter 41). Avoid continually eliciting the gag reflex, which might cause vomiting. The following interventions promote expansion of the lungs:

- Encourage diaphragmatic breathing exercises every hour while patients are awake.
- Administer CPAP or NIPPV to patients who use this modality at home (Olson et al., 2018).
- Instruct patients to use an incentive spirometer for maximum inspiration. The patient should try to reach the inspiratory target volume achieved before surgery on the spirometer.
- Encourage early ambulation. Walking causes patients to assume a position that does not restrict chest wall expansion and stimulates an increased respiratory rate. Ambulation increases peristalsis.
- Help patients who are restricted to bed to turn on their side every 1 to 2 hours while awake and to sit on the side of the bed when possible.

BOX 50.10 FOCUS ON OLDER ADULTS
Care of the Older Adult After Surgery

- Decreased cardiac reserve decreases cardiac output during physiological stress, which may result in a delay in recovery from tachycardia and the inability to tolerate fluid depletion (AORN, 2015).
- Preexisting medical conditions combined with reduction in physiological reserve are predictors for poor postoperative outcomes in older adults.
- During the perioperative period, assess for changes that occur as a result of infection, hemorrhage, alterations in blood pressure, and fluid/electrolyte abnormalities. Ongoing, focused assessments are necessary.
- Older patients are at greater risk for postoperative delirium associated with an acute onset. Reduced level of consciousness, reduced ability to maintain attention, perceptual disturbances, and memory impairment characterize the typical presentation (Meiner and Yeager,2019; AORN, 2015).
- Implement individualized measures to help the older adult achieve rest, sleep, and orientation in the postoperative period to reduce the risk of delirium development.
- Altered and unexpected drug responses are often related to different pharmacokinetics in the older adult. The possibility of high risk for adverse medication events with the administration of anesthetic agents and postoperative analgesics, especially narcotics, is likely (AORN, 2015). "Start low and go slow" is the guiding principle when medicating older adults because of their slow drug-clearance capability.

- Keep the patient comfortable. A patient who is comfortable can participate in deep breathing and coughing. Administer analgesics on time so that pain does not become severe.

The following measures promote removal of pulmonary secretions if they are present:

- Encourage coughing exercises every 1 to 2 hours while patients are awake, and maintain pain control to promote a deep, productive cough. *For patients who have had eye, intracranial, or spinal surgery, coughing may be contraindicated because of the potential increase in intraocular or intracranial pressure.*
- Provide oral hygiene to facilitate expectoration of mucus. The oral mucosa becomes dry when patients are NPO or placed on limited fluid intake.
- Initiate orotracheal or nasotracheal suction for patients who are too weak or unable to cough (see Chapter 41).
- Administer oxygen as ordered and monitor oxygen saturation with a pulse oximeter. Continue to monitor oxygen saturation for patients at risk for respiratory compromise from OSA (Olson et al., 2018). Administer oxygen to patients at risk for or diagnosed with OSA until they can maintain their baseline oxygen saturation while breathing room air.

Preventing Circulatory Complications. Some patients are at greater risk of venous stasis because of the nature of their surgery or medical history. The following interventions promote normal venous return and circulatory blood flow:

- Provide pain medications as prescribed and nonpharmacological therapies to ensure that patients ambulate early. Early ambulation promotes venous return and circulatory blood flow.
- Encourage patients to perform leg exercises at least every hour while awake. Exercise may be contraindicated in an extremity with a vascular repair or realignment of fractured bones and torn cartilage.
- Apply graded compression stockings or IPC devices as ordered by the health care provider. Remove the stockings or device at least once per shift. Perform a thorough reassessment of the skin of the lower extremities at this time.

TABLE 50.8   Postoperative Complications

Complication	Cause
Respiratory System	
Atelectasis: Collapse of alveoli with retained mucus secretions. Signs and symptoms include elevated respiratory rate, dyspnea, fever, crackles auscultated over involved lobes of lungs, and productive cough.	Inadequate lung expansion. Anesthesia, analgesia, and immobilized position prevent full lung expansion. There is greater risk in patients with upper abdominal surgery who have pain during inspiration and repress deep breathing.
Pneumonia: Inflammation of alveoli involving one or several lobes of lung. Development in lower dependent lobes of lung is common in patient who is immobilized after surgery. Signs and symptoms include fever, chills, productive cough, chest pain, purulent mucus, and dyspnea.	Poor lung expansion with retained secretions or aspirated secretions. Common resident bacterium in respiratory tract is *Diplococcus pneumoniae,* which causes most cases of pneumonia.
Hypoxemia: Inadequate concentration of oxygen in arterial blood. Signs and symptoms include restlessness, confusion, dyspnea, hypertension or hypotension, tachycardia or bradycardia, diaphoresis, and cyanosis.	Anesthetics and analgesics depress respirations. Increased retention of mucus with impaired ventilation occurs because of pain or poor positioning. Patients with obstructive sleep apnea are at increased risk for hypoxemia.
Pulmonary embolism: Embolus blocking pulmonary arterial blood flow to one or more lobes of lung. Signs and symptoms include dyspnea, sudden chest pain, cyanosis, tachycardia, and drop in blood pressure.	Same factors lead to formation of thrombus or embolus. Patients with preexisting circulatory or coagulation disorders and who are immobile are at risk.
Circulatory System	
Hemorrhage: Loss of large amount of blood externally or internally in short period of time. Signs and symptoms include hypotension, weak and rapid pulse, cool and clammy skin, rapid breathing, restlessness, and reduced urine output.	Slipping of suture or dislodged clot at incisional site. Patients with coagulation disorders are at greater risk.
Hypovolemic shock: Inadequate perfusion of tissues and cells from loss of circulatory fluid volume. Signs and symptoms are same as for hemorrhage.	Hemorrhage usually causes hypovolemic shock after surgery.
Thrombophlebitis: Inflammation of vein often accompanied by clot formation. Veins in legs are most commonly affected. Signs and symptoms include swelling and inflammation of involved site and aching or cramping pain. Vein feels hard, cordlike, and sensitive to touch.	Prolonged sitting or immobilization aggravates venous stasis. Trauma to vessel wall and hypercoagulability of blood increase risk of vessel inflammation.
Thrombus: Formation of clot attached to interior wall of a vein or artery, which can occlude the vessel lumen. Symptoms include localized tenderness along distribution of the venous system, swollen calf or thigh, calf swelling >3 cm (1.2 inches) compared to asymptomatic leg, pitting edema in symptomatic leg, and decrease in pulse below location of thrombus (if arterial).	Venous stasis (see discussion of thrombophlebitis) and vessel trauma. Venous injury is common after surgery of hips and legs, abdomen, pelvis, and major vessels. Patients with pelvic and abdominal cancer or traumatic injuries to the pelvis or lower extremities are at high risk for thrombus formation.
Embolus: Piece of thrombus that has dislodged and circulates in bloodstream until it lodges in another vessel (commonly lungs, heart, brain, or mesentery).	Thrombi form from increased coagulability of blood (e.g., polycythemia and use of birth-control pills containing estrogen).
Musculoskeletal System	
Hospital-associated deconditioning (HAD): Deficits in physical function secondary to immobilization during an acute hospitalization are collectively defined as hospital-associated deconditioning (HAD).	Older adults are particularly vulnerable. During an acute hospitalization, older adults spend approximately 83% of their hospital stay in bed and only 12% of their time in a chair. Prolonged immobility is associated with declines in muscle strength and muscle mass and with reduced cognitive function, muscle protein synthesis, and physical function (Falvey et al., 2015).
Gastrointestinal System	
Paralytic ileus: Nonmechanical obstruction of the bowel caused by physiological, neurogenic, or chemical imbalance associated with decreased peristalsis. Common in initial hours after abdominal surgery.	Handling of intestines during surgery leads to loss of peristalsis for a few hours to several days.
Abdominal distention: Retention of air within intestines and abdominal cavity during gastrointestinal surgery. Signs and symptoms include increased abdominal girth, patient complaints of fullness, and "gas pains."	Slowed peristalsis from anesthesia, bowel manipulation, or immobilization. During laparoscopic surgeries influx of air for procedure causes distention and pain up to shoulders.
Nausea and vomiting: Symptoms of improper gastric emptying or chemical stimulation of vomiting center. Patient complains of gagging or feeling full or sick to stomach.	Abdominal distention, fear, severe pain, medications, eating or drinking before peristalsis returns, and initiation of gag reflex.
Genitourinary System	
Urinary retention: Involuntary accumulation of urine in bladder as result of loss of muscle tone. Signs and symptoms include inability to void, restlessness, and bladder distention. It appears 6-8 hours after surgery.	Effects of anesthesia and narcotic analgesics. Local manipulation of tissues surrounding bladder and edema interfere with bladder tone. Poor positioning of patient impairs voiding reflexes.

TABLE 50.8   Postoperative Complications—cont'd

Complication	Cause
Urinary tract infection: Infection of the urinary tract as a result of bacterial or yeast contamination. Signs and symptoms include dysuria, itching, abdominal pain, possible fever, cloudy urine, presence of white blood cells, and leukocyte esterase positive on urinalysis.	Most frequently a result of catheterization of the bladder.
Integumentary System	
Wound infection: Invasion of deep or superficial wound tissues by pathogenic microorganisms; signs and symptoms include warm, red, and tender skin around incision; fever and chills; purulent material exiting from drains or from separated wound edges. Infection usually appears 3-6 days after surgery.	Infection is caused by poor aseptic technique or contaminated wound or surgical site before surgical exploration. For example, with a bowel perforation patient is at increased risk for a wound infection because of bacterial contamination from the large intestine.
Wound dehiscence: Separation of wound edges at suture line. Signs and symptoms include increased drainage and appearance of underlying tissues. This usually occurs 6-8 days after surgery.	Malnutrition, obesity, preoperative radiation to surgical site, old age, poor circulation to tissues, and unusual strain on suture line from coughing or positioning.
Wound evisceration: Protrusion of internal organs and tissues through incision. Incidence usually occurs 6-8 days after surgery.	See discussion of wound dehiscence. Patient with dehiscence is at risk for developing evisceration.
Skin breakdown: Result of pressure or shearing forces. Patients are at increased risk if alterations in nutrition and circulation are present, resulting in edema and delayed healing.	Prolonged periods on the operating room (OR) table and in the bed after surgery lead to pressure breakdown. Skin breakdown results from shearing during positioning on the OR table and improperly pulling patient up in bed.
Nervous System	
Intractable pain: Pain that is not amenable to analgesics and pain-alleviating interventions.	Intractable pain may be related to the wound or dressing, anxiety, or positioning.
Malignant hyperthermia: Severe hypermetabolic state and rigidity of the skeletal muscles caused by an increase in intracellular calcium ion concentration.	Rare genetic condition triggered with exposure to inhaled anesthetic agents and the depolarizing muscle relaxant succinylcholine.

- Encourage early ambulation. Most patients ambulate after surgery, depending on the severity of surgery and their conditions. Early ambulation protocols require patients to ambulate sometimes within 2 to 3 hours of having surgery (Resnick et al., 2016). The degree of activity allowed progresses as the patient's condition improves. Encourage ambulation even if a patient has an epidural catheter or PCA device.
- Before ambulation, assess the patient's vital signs at rest. Abnormalities such as hypotension or certain arrhythmias may contraindicate ambulation. If vital signs are at baseline, first help the patient sit on the side of the bed. A patient's complaint of dizziness is a sign of postural hypotension. A recheck of blood pressure determines whether ambulation is safe. Assist with ambulation by standing on the patient's strong side and making sure that he or she is able to walk steadily. Patients may be able to walk only a few feet the first few times out of bed. This usually improves each time. Assess a patient's tolerance to activity by periodically assessing how he or she responds to exercise. Using the baseline resting heart rate, compare it with the heart rate as the patient ambulates. Also note the heart rhythm. You can assess exercise tolerance by knowing the patient's maximum heart rate and then consider an appropriate target rate. One simple method to calculate a predicted maximum heart rate is by using this formula (AHA, 2015):

200 − Patient's age = Predicted maximum heart rate

The predicted maximum heart rate should then be multiplied by 50% to 85%, depending on the patient's condition and progress with exercise, to obtain a target rate.

Example: A 70-year-old patient has an average resting heart rate of 84 beats/min. The patient's predicted maximum heart rate equals:

220 − 70 = 150 beats/min

The patient's **target heart rate** will range from 50% to 85% of the maximum heart rate, or in this example:

75 to 128 beats/min

By comparing resting rate with the patient's actual rate during exercise, you can determine whether it is in a safe target range. Remember that a patient's acute surgical condition may not allow him or her to reach a target rate. *Confer with the patient's surgeon or physical therapist about a safe heart rate target.* Always ask patients how they feel during exercise and whether they note chest pain or shortness of breath.

- Avoid positioning patients in a manner that interrupts blood flow to extremities. Do not place pillows or rolled blankets under a patient's knees while in bed. Compression of the popliteal vessels can cause thrombi. When patients sit in chairs, elevate their legs on footstools. Never allow a patient to sit with one leg crossed over the other.
- Administer anticoagulant drugs as ordered. Patients at greatest risk for thrombus formation often receive prophylactic doses of anticoagulants such as LMWH (e.g., enoxaparin) or low-dose unfractionated heparin (LDUH) for anticoagulation.
- Promote adequate fluid intake orally or intravenously (IV). Adequate hydration prevents concentrated accumulation of formed blood elements such as platelets and red blood cells. When the plasma volume is low, these elements gather and form small clots within blood vessels.

Promoting Early Mobility. Many surgical postoperative protocols now include early mobility guidelines, which are designed to minimize or prevent hospital-acquired deconditioning (HAD) (see Chapter 39). Using early mobility protocols is associated with improved outcomes such as reduced deep vein thrombosis, reduced length of stay in patients with community-acquired pneumonia, and maintained or improved functional status from admission to discharge in the elderly and patients who undergo major surgery (Pashikanti and Von Ah, 2012). Explain to patients and family members how quickly patients will begin activities such as range-of-motion exercises, sitting on the side of the bed, and assisted ambulation, and the projected distance for walking independently. Activities will typically begin within 12 hours of a patient's return to the inpatient nursing unit. Also assure patients that appropriate mobility aids will be used and that assistance by nursing staff will ensure their safety (Pashikanti and Von Ah, 2012). There are patients who will not be able to initiate early mobility until their conditions have stabilized. Explain that it is normal for a patient to progress gradually in activity. If a patient tolerates activity, activity levels progress more quickly.

Achieving Rest and Comfort. Pain control is a priority to facilitate a patient's recovery. Without pain control, a patient will not move or ambulate as readily or as early or initiate coughing exercises after surgery. The anesthesia provider orders medications for pain management in the PACU. IV opioid analgesics such as morphine sulfate are the drugs of choice immediately postoperative. Advances have been made in the use of multimodal analgesia (more than one analgesic), which combines different drug classes delivered through various routes, including use of local anesthetics alone or in combination with other nerve blocks or therapies such as PCA. The goal is to enhance the efficacy of pain control while minimizing the side effects of each modality (Tan et al., 2015).

A patient's pain increases after surgery as the effects of anesthesia diminish. The patient becomes more aware of the surroundings and more perceptive of discomfort. The incisional area is only one source of pain. Irritation from drainage tubes, tight dressings, or casts and the muscular strains caused from positioning on the OR table also cause discomfort.

After assessing that a patient is in discomfort, check to be sure whether the ordered dose of analgesic is within the recommended range. Patients have the most surgical pain in the first 24 to 48 hours after surgery. IV PCA or epidural analgesia may be ordered. A PCA device delivers analgesic medications by IV or subcutaneous infusion. The PCA system allows patients to administer their own IV analgesics from a specially prepared pump (see Chapter 44). If patients gain a sense of control over their pain, they usually have fewer postoperative problems. Many patients receive regional analgesia, such as epidural analgesia, continuously throughout the recovery period, especially for thoracic and abdominal surgery. Studies show that continuous epidural analgesia provides superior pain relief in terms of less analgesic use, better postoperative pain relief (especially in the first 24 hours), less sedation, and faster return of GI function (Cummings et al., 2018; Hwang et al., 2018). Epidural techniques are especially useful in patients with OSA who are at increased risk of airway compromise and postoperative complications with the use of systemic opioids after surgery. Nonsteroidal antiinflammatory agents are an alternative to systemic opioids in patients with OSA (ASA, 2014). Monitor patients closely for side effects and educate them and family caregivers regarding the pain-management therapy and expected response.

As the patient begins to tolerate oral fluids, surgical protocols usually include changing pain medication from IV or epidural to oral administration. Do not overlook the importance of nonpharmacological interventions (see Chapter 44). Assess which care routines contribute to pain and use nonpharmacological measures to address this pain. An example is to lower the head of the bed and use a pillow for incisional splinting while turning a patient with recent abdominal surgery. Other methods to promote pain relief include positioning, back rubs, distraction, or imagery. Remember, *do not assume that a patient's pain is incisional.* When a patient without PCA or an epidural analgesic asks for pain medication, obtain orders to provide analgesics as often as allowed around-the-clock (ATC) in the first 24 to 48 hours after surgery to improve pain control. If pain medications are not relieving discomfort, notify the health care provider for additional orders. Nurses need to recognize potential complications of analgesics and know what to do if they occur.

Temperature Regulation. Unless intraoperative warming is used, patients are usually still cool when arriving in the surgical unit. Provide warmed blankets or heated air blankets if no other warming device is available. Increasing a patient's body temperature raises metabolism and improves circulatory and respiratory function.

Sometimes shivering is a side effect of certain anesthetic agents instead of hypothermia. Clonidine in small increments can decrease shivering as prescribed by the health care provider. When this happens, encourage your patient to use deep breathing and coughing to help to expel retained anesthetic gases.

If a patient develops signs or symptoms of malignant hyperthermia, recognize this as a potential emergency. Be prepared to administer dantrolene sodium as ordered by the health care provider (Malignant Hyperthermia Association of the United States, 2018). The medication is administered to prevent muscle stiffness and spasms caused by the rapid rise in body temperature and severe muscle contractions that accompany malignant hyperthermia.

Patients are at risk for infection after surgery for various reasons. If a patient becomes febrile, be aggressive in providing routine postoperative nursing interventions. For example, deep breathing and coughing, early ambulation, prompt removal of indwelling urinary catheter (if appropriate), and aseptic care of the surgical wound decrease the risk of postoperative infections. If a patient no longer requires intravenous fluids, prompt removal of IV catheters also reduces infection rates. Since microorganisms require time to incubate, infections are rare within the first 48 hours after surgery. If the health care provider suspects an infection, he or she orders wound and or blood cultures.

Maintaining Neurological Function. Deep breathing and coughing expel retained anesthetic gases and facilitate a patient's return to consciousness. Continue monitoring the patient's level of consciousness and responsiveness to questions. When patients are elderly, know the status of their renal function because delayed renal clearance of operatively administered anesthetic agents slows awakening. As a patient regains consciousness, orientation to the environment is important in maintaining the patient's mental status. Reorient the patient, explain that surgery is completed, and describe procedures and nursing measures.

Maintaining Fluid and Electrolyte Balance. Immediately after surgery, patients receive fluids only IV. It is important to maintain patency of IV infusions postoperatively (see Chapter 42). The nurse typically removes an IV catheter once a patient awakens after ambulatory surgery and can tolerate water without GI upset. A more seriously ill patient on a surgical unit requires IV fluids for a longer period to achieve hydration and electrolyte balance and sometimes to receive antibiotics. Some patients require blood products after surgery, depending on the amount of blood loss during surgery. A surgeon orders a prescribed solution and rate for each IV infusion. As a patient begins to take and tolerate oral fluids, the nurse decreases the IV rate as ordered by the surgeon. When patients no longer need a continuous IV infusion, the nurse will most likely saline lock the IV line (as ordered by the surgeon) to preserve the site for the administration of medications such as antibiotics or other types of intravenous therapy (see Chapter 42). In order to continuously monitor fluid status, measure contents of urinary catheter, NG tube, or wound drainage collection devices every 8 hours for output recording. Measure and empty wound drainage devices more often if drainage is excessive.

Promoting Normal Gastrointestinal Function and Adequate Nutrition. A patient likely begins to take ice chips or sips of fluids when arriving on an acute surgical care unit. If fluids are tolerated, the diet progresses with clear liquids next. Interventions for preventing GI complications promote the return of normal elimination and faster return of normal nutritional intake. It takes several days for a patient who has had GI surgery (e.g., a colon resection) to resume a normal diet. Normal peristalsis often does not return for 2 to 3 days. In contrast, the patient whose GI tract is unaffected directly by surgery can resume dietary intake after recovering from the effects of anesthesia. The following measures promote the return of normal elimination:

- Advance a patient's dietary intake gradually. Most surgeons rely on the return of flatus or bowel sounds to order a normal diet. Use patient assessment data to determine how quickly to advance the patient's diet. For example, provide clear liquids such as water, apple juice, broth, or tea after nausea subsides. Ingesting large amounts of fluids leads to distention and vomiting. If a patient tolerates liquids without nausea, advance the diet as ordered. Patients who had abdominal surgery are usually NPO the first 24 to 48 hours. As flatus and peristalsis return, provide clear liquids, followed by full liquids, a light diet of solid foods, and finally a patient's usual diet. Encourage intake of foods high in protein and vitamin C.
- Promote ambulation and exercise. Physical activity stimulates a return of peristalsis. A patient who has abdominal distention and "gas pain" may obtain relief when walking.
- Maintain an adequate fluid intake. Fluids keep fecal material soft for easy passage. Fruit juices and warm liquids are especially effective.
- Promote adequate food intake by stimulating a patient's appetite; remove sources of noxious odors and provide small servings of nonspicy foods.
- Avoid moving a patient suddenly to minimize nausea.
- Help the patient get into a comfortable position during mealtime. If possible, have him or her sit to minimize pressure on the abdomen.
- Provide frequent oral hygiene. Adequate hydration and cleaning of the oral cavity eliminate dryness and bad tastes.
- Administer fiber supplements, stool softeners, and rectal suppositories as ordered. If constipation or distention develops, the health care provider orders cathartics or enemas to stimulate peristalsis.
- Provide meals when the patient is rested and free from pain. Often a patient loses interest in eating if mealtime follows exhausting activities such as ambulation, coughing and deep-breathing exercises, or extensive dressing changes. When a patient has pain, the associated nausea often causes a loss of appetite.

Promoting Urinary Elimination. The depressant effects of anesthetics and analgesics impair the sensation of bladder fullness. A full bladder is painful and causes a patient awakening from surgery to be restless or agitated. Patients who have abdominal surgery or surgery of the urinary system often have indwelling catheters inserted until voluntary urination returns. Patients without a catheter need to void within 8 to 12 hours after surgery; otherwise it is sometimes necessary to insert a straight catheter. If a patient has an indwelling urinary catheter, the goal is to remove it as soon as possible because of the high risk for the development of a catheter-associated urinary tract infection (CAUTI). The Centers for Disease Control and Prevention (2016) recommend that in operative patients who have an indication for an indwelling catheter the catheter should be removed as soon as possible postoperatively, preferably within 24 hours, unless there are appropriate indications for continued use. The following measures promote normal urinary elimination (see Chapter 46):

- Help patients assume their normal position to void if possible.
- Check a patient frequently for the need to void when a catheter is not in place. The feeling of bladder fullness is often sudden, and you need to respond promptly when a patient calls for assistance.
- Assess for bladder distention. If a patient does not void within 8 to 12 hours of surgery or if bladder distention is present, you will insert a straight urinary catheter if you have an order from a health care provider. Continued difficulty in voiding sometimes requires an indwelling catheter, which increases the risk for a UTI. Although the evidence is inconclusive, some agencies use bladder ultrasound to assess bladder volume and assist in the decision to place a urinary catheter.

- Monitor I&O. If a patient has an indwelling catheter, expect an output of about 30 to 50 mL/hr. Another way to gauge adequacy of output is by determining a patient's weight. An accepted level of urinary output is at least 0.5 mL/kg/hr to 1 mL/kg/hr for adults (MDCalc, 2018; Lewis et al., 2017). If the urine is dark, concentrated, and low in volume, notify a health care provider. Patients easily become dehydrated as a result of fluid loss from surgical wounds and inadequate fluid intake. Measure I&O for several days after surgery until a patient achieves normal fluid intake and urinary output.

Skin and Wound Care. Wound healing is complicated by impaired circulation, inadequate nutrition and metabolic alterations (see Chapter 48). All of these factors can affect rate of healing and risk for infection. A wound also undergoes considerable physical stress on the suture line and wound bed. Strain on sutures from coughing, vomiting, distention, and movement of body parts can disrupt wound layers. Protecting a wound promotes healing. A critical time for wound healing is 24 to 72 hours after surgery, after which a seal is established. If infection of a clean surgical wound occurs, you will usually find symptoms of infection 4 to 5 days after surgery. Monitor surgical patients on an ongoing basis for fever, tenderness at a wound site, and presence of local drainage on dressings (i.e., yellow, green or brown, and odorous). A clean surgical wound usually does not regain strength against normal stress for 15 to 20 days after surgery.

Surgical dressings (if present) remain in place the first 24 hours after surgery to reduce the risk of infection. During this time, add an extra layer of gauze on top of the original dressing if drainage develops. After that, use aseptic technique during dressing changes and wound care (see Chapter 48). Time any dressing change to begin 5 to 30 minutes after giving a patient pain medication (depending on route—5 minutes IV, 30 minutes oral). Keep surgical drains patent so that accumulated secretions can escape from the wound bed.

Maintaining/Enhancing Self-Concept. The appearance of wounds, bulky dressings, drains, and tubes threatens a patient's self-concept. The effects of surgery, such as disfiguring scars, often create permanent changes in a patient's body image. If surgery leads to impairment in body function, a patient's role within the family can change significantly. Observe patients for behaviors reflecting alterations in self-concept (see Chapter 33). Some patients show revulsion toward their appearance by refusing to look at incisions, carefully covering dressings with bedclothes, or refusing to get out of bed because of tubes and devices. The fear of being unable to return to a functional family role causes some patients to avoid participation in the plan of care.

A family often plays an important role in efforts to improve a patient's self-concept. Explain the patient's appearance to the family and ways to avoid nonverbal expressions of revulsion or surprise. Encourage the family to accept the patient's needs and support his or her independence. The following measures help to maintain a patient's self-concept:

- Provide privacy during dressing changes or inspection of the wound. Keep room curtains closed around the bed and drape the patient to expose only the dressing or incisional area.
- Maintain the patient's hygiene. Wound drainage and antiseptic solutions from the surgical skin preparation dry on the surface of the skin, causing foul odor and skin irritation. A complete bath the first day after surgery renews the patient. Offer a clean gown and washcloth. Keep the patient's hair neatly combed and offer frequent oral hygiene every 2 hours while awake, especially if the patient is NPO.
- Prevent drainage devices from overflowing.
- Maintain a pleasant environment. Being in pleasant, comfortable surroundings heightens self-concept. Store or remove unused supplies. Keep the patient's bedside orderly and clean.
- Offer opportunities for the patient to discuss feelings about appearance. A patient who avoids looking at an incision possibly needs to

discuss fears or concerns. A patient having surgery for the first time is often more anxious than one who has had multiple surgeries. When a patient looks at an incision for the first time, make sure that the area is clean. Eventually he or she will be able to care for the incision site by applying simple dressings or bathing the affected area.

- Provide the family with opportunities to discuss ways to promote the patient's self-concept. Encouraging independence is sometimes difficult for a family member who has a strong desire to help the patient in any way. Family members are more able to be supportive during dressing changes when they know about the appearance of a wound or incision. Help family members know when it is appropriate to discuss future plans. This allows the patient and family to discuss realistic plans for a patient's return home.

Restorative and Continuing Care. In the postoperative period, the nurse, patient, and family collaborate to prepare the patient for discharge. Patients often must continue wound care, follow activity or diet restrictions, continue medication therapy, and observe for signs and symptoms of complications at home. Education for the preparation of patients to assume self-care is an ongoing process throughout hospitalization. It is important to provide specific, culturally appropriate, and accurate verbal and written discharge instructions to enhance the ability of patients to care for themselves at home (Marcus, 2014). Make education relevant. For example, if a patient has a limitation on what he or she can lift, understand the type of lifting normally done by the patient (e.g., picking up a small child or pet). Help patients anticipate how to apply restrictions at home.

Boston University School of Medicine developed a model for the hospital discharge process (National Academies of Science, 2014). The model involved development of 11 components for discharge instructions that formed a checklist, which has been adopted by the National Quality Forum. The 11 components include:

1. Make appointments for follow-up care.
2. Plan for the follow-up of results from pending tests.
3. Organize postdischarge services and equipment.
4. Identify the correct medications and plan for patient to obtain those medications.
5. Reconcile the discharge plan with national guidelines.
6. Teach a written discharge plan the patient can understand.
7. Educate the patient about diagnoses and medications.
8. Assess the degree of the patient's understanding of the plan.
9. Expedite transmission of the discharge summary to the primary care physician.
10. Provide telephone reinforcement.
11. Review appropriate steps for what to do if a problem arises.

Provide a wide variety of written educational materials for all patients after surgery. For example, offer materials with more pictures and illustrations for patients who do not speak English or have limited reading ability. Ensure that all materials are sensitive to various cultures and religions. Patients receive a copy of signed discharge instructions, and one copy remains in the medical or electronic record.

Surgical recovery is slowed if patients are deconditioned and then fail to exercise regularly. It is important to keep frail older adults active after surgery by offering assistive devices and referral to rehabilitation (AORN, 2015). A person is considered frail if he or she has three of the following:

unintentional weight loss, low physical activity, slowed motor performance, weakness, and fatigue or exercise intolerance. Aerobic exercise and physical resistance training sometimes improve patients' gait speed and ability to perform ADLs (Van Abbema et al., 2015). Collaborate with physical and occupational therapists in finding strategies to help patients adhere to recommended exercise and active ADL programs. Involve family caregivers in the patient's exercise program.

Some patients need home care assistance after discharge. For example, nurses make referrals to home care for skilled nursing requirements when patients need ongoing wound care, IV therapy, or drain management. In addition, patients who are more physically dependent often require assistance from assistive personnel to provide bathing and hygiene needs. The case coordinator or social worker at the hospital helps with discharge coordination. Encourage patients to show their discharge instructions to home care providers.

Other patients, especially older adults, sometimes require discharge to a rehabilitation or skilled nursing center after their hospital recovery. During their recovery, patients work to gain mobility and recovery of their independent living skills. In addition, nurses provide wound care and other specialized services. A case coordinator or social worker works with the patient, family, and nurse to coordinate transfer to the skilled nursing center.

◆ Evaluation

Through the Patient's Eyes. Consult with a patient and family to gather evaluation data and remember that evaluation is ongoing. Ask specific questions that evaluate patient expectations and perceptions during your hourly rounds. For example, you ask, "Is your pain being managed well?" "How well are you sleeping?" and "Is there anything I can do for you at this time?" Evaluate your patient's level of comfort and ensure that the patient understands all aspects of nursing care. Resolve any concerns or issues and answer the patient's and family caregiver's questions before discharge.

Patient Outcomes. Evaluate the effectiveness of care based on the patient-centered expected outcomes established after surgery for each nursing diagnosis. If a patient fails to progress as expected, revise his or her care plan based on evaluation findings and the patient's needs.

Make sure to evaluate for pain relief using a pain scale. Determine the efficacy of both pharmacological and nonpharmacological measures. Use appropriate evaluative measures; inspect the condition of a wound, monitor usage of the incentive spirometer, measure the distance or number of times that a patient can ambulate, and monitor the amount of fluid and food intake.

Part of an evaluation is to determine the extent to which the patient and family caregiver learn self-care measures. Use the teach-back method of patient education by having the patient restate information that you taught in his or her own words (Bastable, 2019). If a patient must perform any skill at home such as a dressing change or exercise, evaluate through return demonstration (see Chapter 25).

Many agencies call patients at home 24 hours after discharge to help evaluate patient outcomes. This allows for monitoring the progress of a patient's recovery and for identifying the development of complications. This also allows the nurse to evaluate and reinforce a patient's understanding of restrictions, wound care, medications, and necessary follow-up.

SAFETY GUIDELINES FOR NURSING SKILLS

Ensuring patient safety is an essential role of the professional nurse. To ensure patient safety, communicate clearly with the members of the health care team, assess and incorporate the patient's priorities of care and preferences, and use the best evidence when making decisions about the patient's care. When performing the skill in this chapter, remember the following points to ensure safe, individualized patient-centered care:

- Coughing and deep breathing are sometimes contraindicated after brain, spinal, head, neck, or eye surgery (prevents intracranial and intraocular pressure increases).
- Patients who are severely obese sometimes have more improved lung function and vital capacity in the reverse Trendelenburg or side-lying position.
- Report any signs of VTE such as pain, tenderness, redness, warmth, or swelling in the upper or lower extremities to the medical team immediately.

SKILL 50.1   TEACHING AND DEMONSTRATING POSTOPERATIVE EXERCISES

DELEGATION AND COLLABORATION

The skills of preoperative teaching cannot be delegated to assistive personnel (AP). AP can reinforce and help patients perform postoperative exercises. The nurse instructs the AP about:

- Any precautions or safety issues unique to the patient (e.g., fall risks, mobility limitations, bleeding precautions).
- Informing the nurse of any identified concerns (e.g., inability to perform exercise).

Equipment

- Pillow
- Incentive spirometer
- Preoperative education flow sheet
- Positive expiratory pressure (PEP) device
- Stethoscope

STEP	RATIONALE
ASSESSMENT	
1. Identify patient using at least two identifiers (e.g., name and birthday or name and medical record number) according to agency policy.	Ensures correct patient. Complies with The Joint Commission standards and improves patient safety (TJC, 2020).
2. Identify patient's cognitive level, language, and culture. If patient does not speak English or is deaf, have a professional interpreter available to assist you.	These factors may alter patient's ability to understand meaning of surgery and can affect postoperative healing if full understanding is not present.
3. Assess patient's/family caregiver's knowledge, experience, and health literacy.	Ensures patient/family caregiver has the capacity to obtain communicate, process, and understand basic health information (CDC, 2019).
4. Ask about previous experience with surgery and anesthesia; have patient clarify whether any undesirable outcomes occurred.	Information helps to prevent recurrent problems, particularly if the patient had problems with understanding instructions or plan of care.
5. Assess patient's understanding of the intended surgery and anesthesia. Ask patient to offer a description rather than asking a simple yes or no question (e.g., "Tell me what your surgery will involve"). Ask about patient's and family caregiver's expectations of surgery and care. Include questions concerning time frame for surgery and recovery, fears, cultural practices, and religious or spiritual beliefs.	Patients may have misconceptions and incomplete knowledge. Asking about fears, cultural practices, and religious or spiritual beliefs allows you to anticipate priorities of care and adapt teaching and support accordingly.
6. Assess patient's risk factors for postoperative respiratory complications (nursing history and ability to breathe deeply, cough). Check nursing history for patient's height and age.	General anesthesia predisposes patient to respiratory problems (Mills, 2018). Presence of underlying respiratory conditions or patient's inability to perform postoperative respiratory exercises increases the risk for pulmonary complications. Height and age are used to set incentive spirometer parameters.
7. Assess patient's anxiety related to surgery by noting responses and observing nonverbal behavior.	Directs you to provide additional emotional support, which may be needed to facilitate the patient's readiness to learn.
8. Assess family caregiver's ability and willingness to learn and support patient following surgery.	Family caregiver's presence after surgery is an important factor in patient recovery. Caregiver can coach patient through postoperative exercise, help with medication administration, and observe for postoperative complications.
9. Assess patient's medical record for type of surgery and approach.	The surgical procedure itself may require patients to limit activities postoperatively. Anticipating any limitations that might affect how patient can perform postoperative exercises allows you to adapt your instruction preoperatively.
PLANNING	
1. Perform hand hygiene. Prepare equipment and room for instructions and demonstrations.	Reduces transmission of microorganisms. A well-equipped room provides a conducive environment to learning.
2. Provide patient privacy	Maintaining privacy promotes patient dignity and respect.
3. Position the patient in a semi-Fowler's position or upright on the side of the bed as tolerated.	Appropriate positioning allows for increased participation in postoperative exercises and optimal comfort.
4. Plan teaching session for when the patient is not in pain.	Pain distracts patients from focusing on learning. Decreased pain promotes patient participation in the postoperative exercises.
5. Prepare health literacy–appropriate teaching materials. Provide instruction when family caregiver is present (if appropriate).	Promotes patient understanding of instructions. Family caregiver can be important resource for patient's recovery postoperatively.

Continued

| SKILL 50.1 | TEACHING AND DEMONSTRATING POSTOPERATIVE EXERCISES—cont'd | |

STEP	RATIONALE

IMPLEMENTATION

STEP	RATIONALE
1. Inform patient and family caregiver of date, time, and location of surgery; anticipated length of surgery; additional time in postanesthesia recovery area; and where to wait.	Accurate information helps reduce stress of uncertainty associated with surgery.
2. Encourage and answer questions patient and family caregiver ask.	Responding to patient and family caregiver questions helps to decrease anxiety and demonstrates your concern for them.
3. Instruct patient about preoperative bowel or skin preparations as needed in the home. Check medical orders and agency policies regarding number of preoperative showers and agent to be used for each shower (2% chlorhexidine gluconate is used most often). Following each preoperative shower, instruct patient to rinse the skin thoroughly and dry with a fresh clean, dry towel. Patient should don clean clothing.	Proper skin preparation is critical in preventing surgical site infections (SSIs). Rinsing skin removes residual antiseptic preparation that may cause skin irritation. After use, towels contain microorganisms that can grow in presence of moisture. Using fresh towel after each shower and donning clean clothing minimizes risk of reintroducing microorganisms to clean skin (AORN, 2018a; Berrios-Torres et al., 2017).
4. Instruct patient about extent and purpose of food and fluid restrictions for period specified by health care provider before surgery. For example, clear liquids may be ingested up to 2 hours before procedures requiring general anesthesia, regional anesthesia, or procedural sedation and analgesia. A light meal may be ingested for up to 6 hours before elective procedures requiring general anesthesia, regional anesthesia, or procedural sedation. (ASA, 2017).	During general anesthesia muscles relax, and gastric contents can reflux into esophagus, leading to aspiration. Anesthetic eliminates patient's ability to gag.
5. Describe perioperative routines (e.g., time-out procedure, operative site marking, insertion of IV catheter and therapy, urinary catheterization, hair clipping or removal, laboratory tests, transport to operating room [OR]).	Allows patient to anticipate and recognize routine procedures, reducing anxiety. Empowers patient with information about what the staff does to keep patient safe for operative process.
6. Describe planned effect of preoperative medications.	Provides information about what to expect, decreasing anxiety.
7. Review which routine medications patient needs to discontinue at home before surgery.	Some medications are discontinued before surgery to minimize effects that can cause surgical risks. For example, anticoagulants may increase bleeding and are usually discontinued several days before surgery. Insulin dosages are usually adjusted because of reduced intake of food before surgery.
8. Describe perioperative sensations and sounds to expect in holding area or OR (e.g., blood pressure cuff tightening, electrocardiogram [ECG] leads, cool room, and beep of monitors).	Misconceptions and concerns about perioperative sensations and sounds have been ranked high among preoperative patients for causing anxiety.
9. Describe pain-control methods to be used after surgery. Discuss what pain is acceptable; explain that patient will not be pain-free but that pain will be managed. Explain use of PCA (when appropriate).	Patients are fearful of postoperative pain. Explaining pain-management techniques reduces fear. This helps you understand what degree of pain the patient feels is acceptable, and allows you to educate the patient that although he or she will not be pain-free, the pain will be managed.
10. Describe what patient will experience after surgery (e.g., where patient will be upon awakening; that frequent vital signs will be taken; presence of dressing, catheters, drains, tubes; alternating pressure from sequential compression device; postoperative exercises; and the activity level to be expected).	Provides objective description of what patient can expect after surgery so that patient is prepared.
11. Explain any early mobility protocol; purpose and normal progression from sitting on side of bed to ambulation. Demonstrate how to sit on side of bed. Clarify that protocol starts early during recovery.	Full patient participation is essential for early ambulation to be successful.
12. Perform hand hygiene.	Reduces transmission of microorganisms.
13. Teach turning:	
a. Instruct patient on turning and sitting up (especially suited for abdominal and thoracic surgery):	Promotes circulation and ventilation.
(1) Have patient turn onto right side, assume supine position, and move to side of bed (in this case left side) if permitted by surgery. Instruct patient to move by bending knee and pressing heels against mattress to raise and move buttocks (see illustration). Top side rails on both sides of bed should be in upright position.	Positioning begins on side of bed so that turning to other side does not cause patient to roll toward edge of bed. Buttocks lift prevents shearing force against sheets. If patient's bed has a turn-assist feature, use it to help position him or her.
(2) Have patient splint incision with right hand or with right hand with pillow over incisional area; keep right leg straight and flex left knee up (see illustration); grab right side rail with left hand, pull toward right, and roll onto right side. Reverse process to turn to left side.	Supports incision and decreases discomfort while turning.
(3) Instruct patient to turn every 2 hours from side to side while awake. Often patient requires assistance with turning after surgery.	Reduces risk of vascular, pulmonary, and pressure injury complications.

CLINICAL DECISION: *Some patients, such as those who have had back surgery or vascular repair, are restricted from flexing their legs after surgery. Some patients are restricted from turning or may need help for positioning.*

STEP	RATIONALE

(4) To sit up on right side of bed, elevate head of bed and have patient turn onto right side. While lying on right side, patient pushes on mattress with left arm and swings feet over edge of bed with nurse's help. To sit up on left side of bed, reverse this process. Assess if patient feels dizzy while sitting up. Return to bed if dizziness occurs (see Chapter 38).

Sitting position lowers diaphragm to permit fuller lung expansion. Screening for dizziness detects orthostatic hypotension.

CLINICAL DECISION: *Caution patient to always use the nurse call system to ask for assistance when sitting on side of bed to reduce risk of a fall.*

14. Teach coughing and deep breathing:

Patient may hesitate to take deep breaths because of weakness or pain, resulting in secretions remaining in bases of lungs. Collection of secretions increases risk of pulmonary atelectasis and pneumonia. This is especially important for patients with a history of smoking, pneumonia, or chronic obstructive pulmonary disease (COPD) or patients who are confined to bed rest.

a. Assist patient to high-Fowler's position in bed with knees flexed, or have patient sit on side of bed or chair in upright position.

Sitting position facilitates diaphragmatic expansion.

b. Instruct patient to place palms of hands across from one another lightly along lower border of rib cage or upper abdomen (see illustration).

Allows patient to feel rise and fall of abdomen during deep breathing.

c. Have patient take slow, deep breaths, inhaling through nose. Explain that patient will feel normal downward movement of diaphragm during inspiration. Demonstrate as follows:

Helps to prevent hyperventilation or panting. Slow, deep breath allows for more complete lung expansion.

(1) Have patient avoid using chest and shoulder muscles while inhaling.

Increases unnecessary energy expenditure and does not promote full lung expansion.

(2) Have patient take slow, deep breath through the nose, hold for count of 3 seconds, and slowly exhale through mouth as if blowing out candle (pursed lips).

Resistance during exhalation helps to prevent alveolar collapse.

(3) Have patient repeat breathing exercise 3 to 5 times.

Repetition reinforces learning.

(4) Have patient take two slow, deep breaths, inhaling through nose and exhaling through pursed lips.

Deep breaths expand lungs fully to aid gas exchange and remove anesthetic agent so that patient regains consciousness (Lewis et al., 2017). Deep breaths also move air behind mucus to facilitate coughing.

(5) Have patient inhale deeply a third time and hold breath to count of 3. Cough fully for two to three consecutive coughs without inhaling between coughs.

Coughing prevents alveolar collapse and moves respiratory secretions to larger airways for expectoration (Lewis et al., 2017).

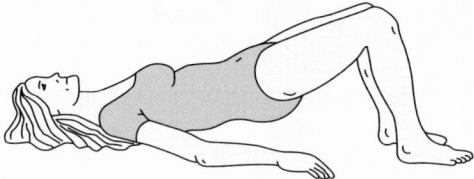

STEP 13a(1) Buttocks lift for moving to side of bed. (From Lowdermilk D, Perry SE: *Maternity and women's health care*, ed 9, St Louis, 2007, Mosby.)

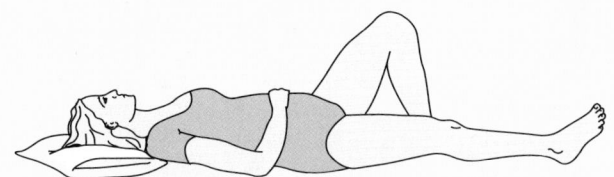

STEP 13a(2) Leg position when turning to right. (From Lowdermilk D, Perry SE: *Maternity and women's health care*, ed 9, St Louis, 2007, Mosby.)

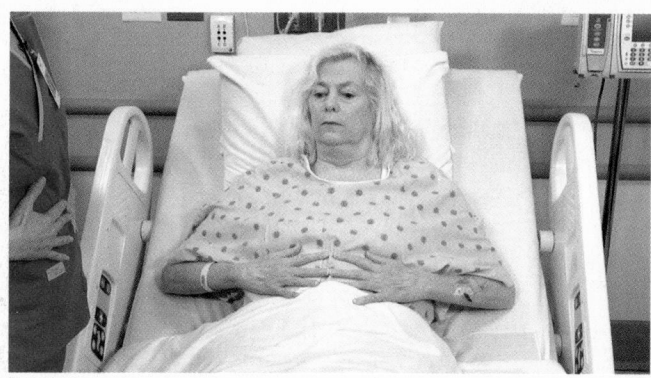

STEP 14b Deep-breathing exercise—placement of hands on upper abdomen during inhalation. (Copyright © Mosby's Clinical Skills: Essentials Collection.)

Continued

| SKILL 50.1 | TEACHING AND DEMONSTRATING POSTOPERATIVE EXERCISES—cont'd | |

STEP	RATIONALE
d. Caution patient against just clearing throat without deep breathing.	Clearing throat does not remove mucus from deeper airways.
e. Have patient practice several times. Instruct patient to perform turning, coughing, and deep breathing every 1 to 2 hours while awake (Lewis et al., 2017). Have family caregiver coach patient to exercise.	Allows for full chest expansion and increased perfusion of both lungs (Lewis et al., 2017). Decreases risk of postoperative pneumonia developing.
15. Teach use of an incentive spirometer	Provides visual aid of respiratory effort. Encourages deep breathing to loosen secretions in lung bases.
a. Explain purpose of incentive spirometer and how it works. Position patient in sitting position in chair or in reclining position with head of bed elevated at least 45 degrees.	Promotes cooperation. Facilitates diaphragm lowering and lung expansion.
b. Set targeted tidal volume on the incentive spirometer according to manufacturer directions. Explain that this is the volume level to be reached with each breath.	Establishes goal of volume level necessary for adequate lung expansion. Manufacturers determine target on basis of patient height and age.
c. Explain how to place mouthpiece of incentive spirometer so that lips completely cover mouthpiece. Have patient demonstrate until position is correct (see illustration).	Validates patient's understanding of instructions and evaluates psychomotor skills.
d. Instruct patient to exhale completely; then position mouthpiece so that lips completely cover it, and inhale slowly, maintaining constant flow through unit until reaching targeted tidal volume (see illustration).	Promotes complete inflation of lungs and minimizes atelectasis. Aiming toward target volume offers visual feedback of respiratory effort.
e. Once maximum inspiration is reached, have patient hold breath for 2 to 3 seconds and exhale slowly. Compare what patient achieves to set target.	Promotes alveolar inflation. Establishes measure of normal maximum breath by patient. Used to determine outcome postoperatively.

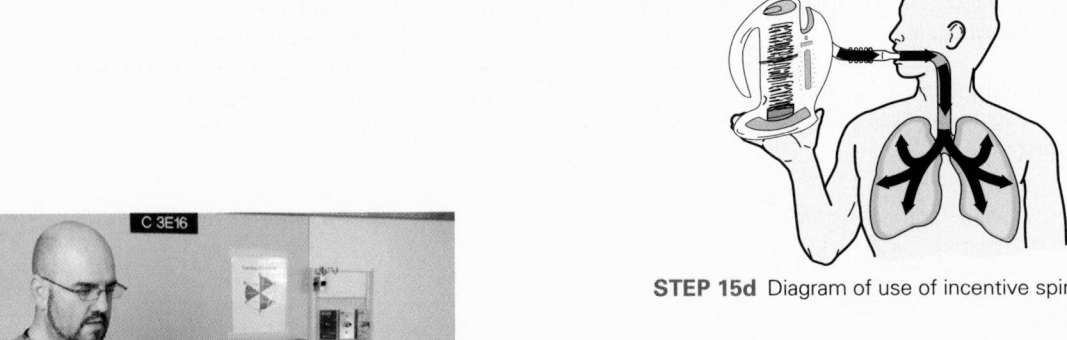

STEP 15d Diagram of use of incentive spirometer.

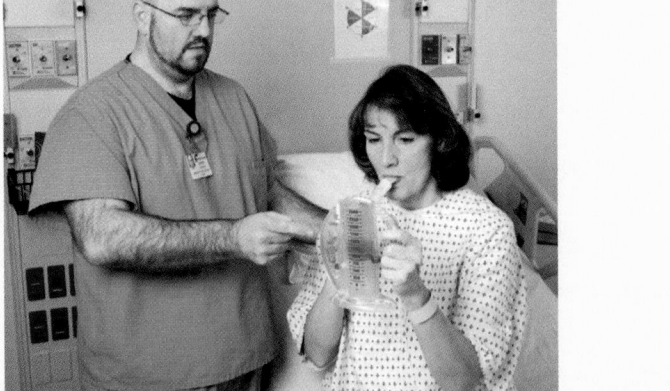

STEP 15c Patient demonstrates incentive spirometry.

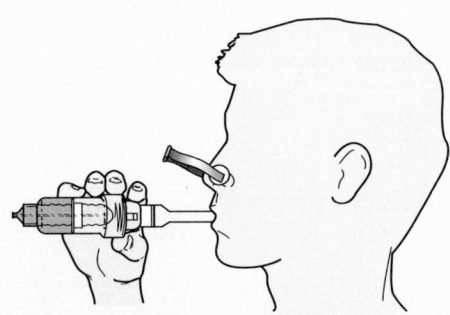

STEP 16b Diagram of use of positive expiratory pressure device.

STEP	RATIONALE
f. Instruct patient to breathe normally for short period between each of the 10 breaths taken on incentive spirometer. Repeat every hour while awake.	Prevents hyperventilation and fatigue.
16. Teach positive expiratory pressure (PEP) therapy:	
a. Explain purpose of PEP device and how it works. Set PEP device for setting ordered.	Promotes cooperation. Higher settings require more effort.
b. Instruct patient to assume semi-Fowler's or high-Fowler's position in bed or to sit in a chair. Place nose clip on patient's nose (see illustration).	Promotes optimum lung expansion and expectoration of mucus.
c. Have patient place lips around mouthpiece. Instruct patient to take full breath and exhale 2 or 3 times longer than inhalation. Repeat pattern for 10 to 20 breaths.	Ensures that patient does all breathing through mouth. Ensures that patient uses device properly.
d. Remove device from mouth and have patient take slow, deep breath and hold for 3 seconds.	Promotes lung expansion before coughing.
e. Instruct patient to exhale with a deep cough. Repeat exercise every 2 hours while awake.	Coughing promotes bronchial hygiene by increasing expectoration of secretions.
17. Teach controlled coughing:	Deep breaths expand lungs fully so that air moves behind mucus and facilitates effective coughing.
a. Explain importance of maintaining upright position in bed or chair; have patient lean slightly forward.	Position facilitates diaphragm excursion and enhances thorax and abdominal expansion.
b. Demonstrate coughing. Fold arms across abdomen and take a slow, deep breath, inhaling through the nose	Expands lungs.
c. To exhale: lean forward, pressing your arms against your abdomen. Cough 2 or 3 times without inhaling between coughs. Cough through a slightly open mouth (see illustration). Coughs should be short and sharp (Cleveland Clinic, 2017).	Clearing throat does not remove mucus from deeper airways. Full, forceful cough is most effective in removing mucus.
d. Breathe in again by "sniffing" slowly and gently through the nose.	Prevents mucus from moving back down airways.
e. Caution patient against just clearing throat instead of coughing deeply. Have patient rest a few minutes and repeat exercise	Clearing throat does not remove mucus from deeper airways.
f. If surgical incision is thoracic or abdominal, teach patient to place either hands or pillow over incisional area and place hands over pillow to splint incision (see illustration). During breathing and coughing exercises, press gently against incisional area for splinting and support.	Surgical incision cuts through muscles, tissues, and nerve endings. Deep-breathing and coughing exercises place additional stress on suture line and cause discomfort. Splinting incision with hands or pillow provides firm support and reduces incisional pulling and pain.
g. Instruct patient to cough 2 to 3 times every 2 hours while awake and to continue to practice coughing exercises, splinting imaginary incision (see illustration).	Deep coughing with splinting effectively expectorates mucus with minimal discomfort.
h. Instruct patient to examine sputum for consistency, odor, amount, and color changes and to notify a nurse if any changes are noted.	Sputum consistency, odor, amount, and color changes may indicate presence of pulmonary complication such as pneumonia.

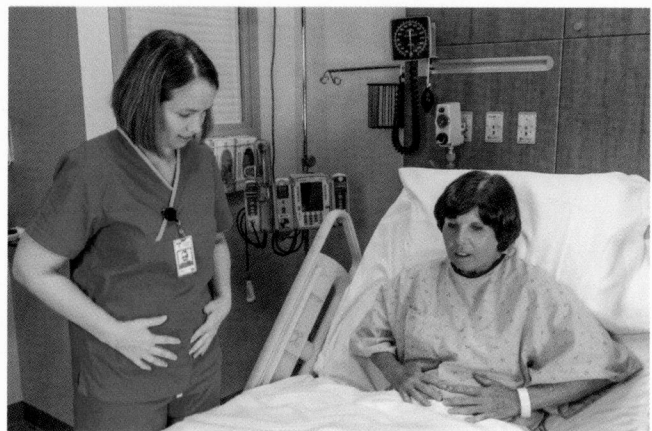

STEP 17c Controlled coughing with placement of hands on upper abdomen.

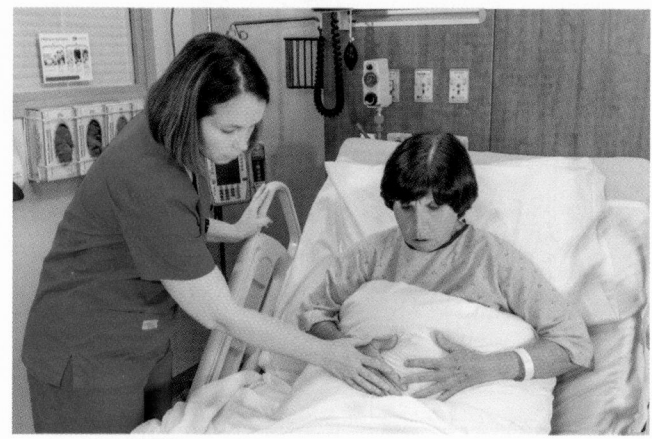

STEP 17f Techniques for splinting incisions.

Continued

SKILL 50.1	TEACHING AND DEMONSTRATING POSTOPERATIVE EXERCISES—cont'd

STEP	RATIONALE

18. Teach leg exercises:

CLINICAL DECISION: *Leg exercises are recommended for patients restricted to bed or during times when patients are ambulatory but resting in bed or in a chair. The ideal exercise to promote venous return and improve lung vital capacity is early mobility (see Chapter 38).*

STEP	RATIONALE
a. Instruct patient to perform leg exercises every 1 to 2 hours while awake: ankle rotation, dorsiflexion and plantar flexion, leg extension and flexion, and straight leg raises.	Leg exercises facilitate venous return from lower extremities and reduce risk of circulatory complications such as venous thromboembolism.
b. Position patient supine.	
c. Instruct patient to rotate each ankle in complete circle and draw imaginary circles with big toe 5 times (see illustration).	Promotes joint mobility.
d. Alternate dorsiflexion and plantar flexion while instructing patient to feel calf muscles tighten and relax (see illustration). Repeat 5 times.	Helps maintain joint mobility and promote venous return to prevent thrombus formation.
e. Perform quadriceps setting by tightening thigh and bringing knee down toward mattress and relaxing (see illustration). Repeat 5 times.	Quadriceps-setting exercises contract muscles of upper legs, maintain knee mobility, and improve venous return to heart.
f. Instruct patient to alternate raising legs straight up from bed surface. Leg should be kept straight (see illustration). Repeat 5 times.	Causes quadriceps muscle contraction and relaxation, which help promote venous return.
g. Explain to patient the expected progression of activity for early mobility and when it will begin.	Early mobility protocols usually advance from bedrest to sitting on side of bed to sitting in chair and progressive ambulation. (see Chapter 38).

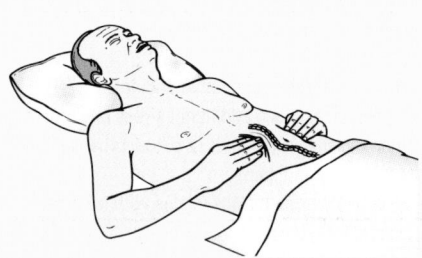
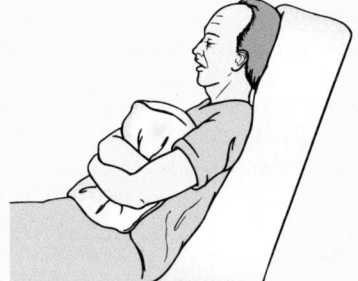
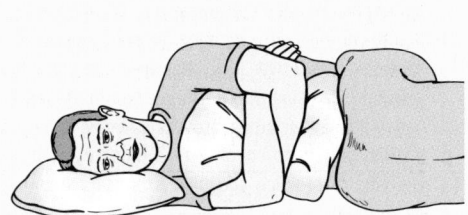

STEP 17g Patient splinting abdomen with pillow. (From Lewis S et al: *Medical-surgical nursing: assessment and management of clinical problems,* ed 9, St Louis, 2014, Mosby.)

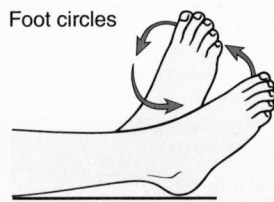

Foot circles

STEP 18c Foot circles. (From Lewis S, et al: *Medical-surgical nursing: assessment and management of clinical problems,* ed 9, St Louis, 2014, Mosby.)

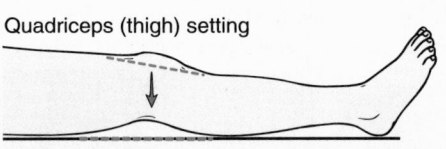

Quadriceps (thigh) setting

STEP 18e Quadriceps (thigh) setting. (From Lewis S, et al: *Medical-surgical nursing: assessment and management of clinical problems,* ed 9, St Louis, 2014, Mosby.)

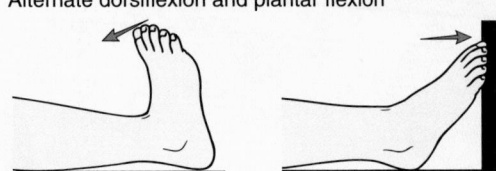

Alternate dorsiflexion and plantar flexion

STEP 18d Alternate dorsiflexion and plantar flexion. (From Lewis S, et al: *Medical-surgical nursing: assessment and management of clinical problems,* ed 9, St Louis, 2014, Mosby.)

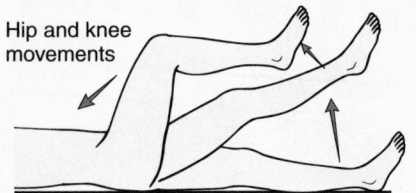

Hip and knee movements

STEP 18f Hip and leg lift. (From Lewis S, et al: *Medical-surgical nursing: assessment and management of clinical problems,* ed 9, St Louis, 2014, Mosby.)

STEP	RATIONALE
19. Have patient continue to practice exercises before surgery at least every 2 hours while awake. Teach patient to coordinate turning and leg exercises with diaphragmatic breathing and use of incentive spirometer.	Leg exercises stimulate circulation, which prevents venous stasis to help prevent formation of deep vein thrombosis (DVT). Coordinating exercises helps patient continuously work toward best outcomes for recovery.
20. Answer questions and verify patient's expectations of surgery. Coach expectations as needed.	Can reduce postoperative anxiety or anger.
21. Reinforce therapeutic coping strategies (e.g., meditation, calming conversation [Aust et al., 2016], listening to music).	Therapeutic coping strategies that self-distract patients reduce preoperative anxiety.
22. Help patient to a comfortable position.	Gives patient a sense of well-being.
23. Be sure nurse call system is in an accessible location within patient's reach.	Ensures patient can call for assistance if needed.
24. Raise side rails (as appropriate) and lower bed to lowest position.	Ensures patient safety.
25. After **completion** of preoperative teaching, appropriately dispose of supplies and equipment and perform hand hygiene.	Reduces transmission of microorganisms.

EVALUATION

1. If possible, observe patient demonstrating splinting, turning and sitting, deep breathing, use of incentive spirometer, PEP therapy, and leg exercises.	Validates patient's ability to correctly perform postoperative exercises and use devices.
2. Ask family member(s) to describe postoperative exercises patient is to perform.	Demonstrates learning.
2. Ask family caregiver to describe how he/she can coach patient with exercises at home before surgery.	Demonstrates understanding of role family member can play to support patient.
3. **Use Teach-Back:** "I want to be sure I explained what you need to know about the exercises we want you to perform after surgery. Tell me which exercises you will do and how to do them." Revise your instruction now or develop a plan for revised patient/family caregiver teaching if patient/family caregiver is not able to teach back correctly.	Determines patient's/family caregiver's level of understanding of instructional topic.

UNEXPECTED OUTCOMES AND RELATED INTERVENTIONS

1. Patient or caregiver identifies incorrect surgical procedure, site, date, or time of surgery.
   - Provide correct information verbally and in writing for patient and family caregiver.
2. Patient incorrectly performs/describes postoperative exercise(s).
   - Explain and demonstrate correct exercise technique.
   - Explain importance of the postoperative exercise as it pertains to patient recovery.
   - Instruct patient to repeat demonstration after clarification.

RECORDING AND REPORTING

- Document preoperative teaching on the appropriate form within the patient's medical record. There is often a preoperative education flow sheet or designated agency form where this information should be documented.
- Document evaluation of patient learning.
- Report patient's inability to identify procedure and site of surgery, as well as understanding of postoperative exercise(s) and teaching to health care provider.

HOME CARE CONSIDERATIONS

- Incorporate teaching of family members to help patient implement postoperative exercises at home. Be sure family has access to resources (e.g., dressing supplies, dietary food options) at home to support patient appropriately.

KEY POINTS

- Perioperative nursing includes the preoperative, intraoperative, and postoperative phases.
- The assessment of risk factors such as history of smoking, obesity, and obstructive sleep apnea allows a nurse to anticipate patient needs and the types of preparation required preoperatively to prevent intraoperative and postoperative complications.
- Malnutrition, diabetes, obesity, smoking, age, obstructive sleep apnea, and cardiac disorders increase patients' risks for perioperative complications.
- A nurse assesses a patient's potential psychological response by identifying the patient's previous experiences with surgery to anticipate his or her needs, providing teaching, addressing fears, and clarifying concerns
- A standard preoperative teaching plan includes instruction that influences maintenance of ventilatory function, physical functional capacity, and sense of well-being, as well as the reduction of patient anxiety and the patient's length of hospital stay.
- Postoperative exercises prevent pulmonary and vascular complications and deconditioning.
- An intraoperative assessment that focuses on a patient's immediate clinical status, skin integrity, and joint function allows the nurse to anticipate problems that predispose the patient to injury if he or she is not positioned on the OR table correctly.
- The primary differences between intraoperative phases are the level of monitoring and progressive change in focus from acute recovery to preparing patients for convalescence and recovery.
- Hand-off communication ensures that each patient receives the right surgery at the right surgical site by verifying the patient's situation (S) (the patient's problem and type of surgery), background (B) (history), assessment data (A), and recommendations (R) for the interventions that need to be implemented.
- Standardized protocols for hand-off communication between perioperative health care providers minimize surgical risks and promotes seamless transition between each surgical phase.
- Postoperative priorities include maintenance of a patent airway, circulatory and perfusion regulation, temperature control, pain control, fluid and electrolyte balance, and wound care.
- Postoperative patient education should be relevant and specific, culturally appropriate, and accurate to enhance the ability of patients to care for themselves at home.
- When caring for patients who had ambulatory surgery, prioritize education because of the limited time available, including involvement of the family or support system.

REFLECTIVE LEARNING

- Consider a postoperative patient who you cared for during your clinical rotation. Reflect on the priorities and outcomes that you set for the patient during your care. What nursing interventions were most successful in achieving the established outcomes for the patient?
- Reflect on a clinical situation when you provided discharge teaching for a patient following surgery. What were the major concerns of the patient and caregiver? How did you address their concerns?
- Discuss how you were aware of the cultural background and incorporated the cultural beliefs of your patient when you developed a preoperative teaching plan. What teaching strategies did you find most effective?

REVIEW QUESTIONS

1. The nurse prepares a patient with type 2 diabetes for a surgical procedure. The patient weighs 112.7 kg (248 lb) and is 5 feet, 2 inches in height. Which factors increase this patient's risk for surgical complications? (Select all that apply.)
   1. Obesity
   2. Prolonged bleeding time
   3. Delayed wound healing
   4. Ineffective vital capacity
   5. Immobility secondary to height

2. Which assessment questions should the nurse ask a preoperative patient preparing for surgery? (Select all that apply.)
   1. "Are you experiencing any pain?"
   2. "Do you exercise on a daily basis?"
   3. "When do you regularly take your medications?"
   4. "Do you have any medication allergies?"
   5. "Do you use drugs and/or tobacco products?"

3. Communication between a nurse caring for a patient in the preoperative holding area and the circulating nurse in the operating room (OR) can best be enhanced by which of the following? (Select all that apply.)
   1. Documenting assessment findings in the medical record
   2. Using a standardized SBAR tool
   3. Being responsive in using nonverbal communication techniques
   4. Giving specific information to a transport technician
   5. Listening to the OR nurse's questions

4. Which postoperative intervention best prevents atelectasis?
   1. Use of intermittent compression stockings
   2. Heel-toe flexion
   3. Use of the incentive spirometer
   4. Abdominal splinting when coughing

5. An 85-year-old patient returns to the inpatient surgical unit after leaving the PACU. Which of the following place the patient at risk during surgery? (Select all that apply.)
   1. Stiffened lung tissue
   2. Reduced diaphragmatic excursion
   3. Increased laryngeal reflexes
   4. Reduced blood flow to kidneys
   5. Increased cholinergic transmission

6. A postoperative patient experiences tachypnea during the first hour of recovery. Which nursing intervention is a priority?
   1. Elevate the head of the patient's bed.
   2. Give ordered oxygen through a mask at 4 L/min.
   3. Ask the patient to use an incentive spirometer.
   4. Position the patient on one side with the face down and the neck slightly extended so that the tongue falls forward.

7. Which is the best intervention the nurse should implement to promote bowel function?
   1. Early ambulation
   2. Deep-breathing exercises
   3. Repositioning on the left side
   4. Lowering the head of the patient's bed

8. Match the nursing interventions on the left with the complication to be prevented on the right. An intervention may apply to more than one complication.

Nursing Intervention	Complication
1. Offering glasses or hearing aid	a. Deep vein thrombosis
2. Early ambulation	b. Wound infection
3. Strict aseptic technique	c. Delirium

Nursing Intervention	Complication
4. Deep breathing exercise	**d.** Atelectasis
5. Hydration	

9. A nurse cares for a postoperative patient in the PACU. Upon assessment, the nurse finds the surgical dressing is saturated with serosanguineous drainage. Which interventions are a priority? (Select all that apply.)
1. Notify surgeon.
2. Maintain the intravenous fluid infusion.
3. Provide 2 L/min of oxygen via nasal cannula.
4. Monitor the patient's vital signs every 5 to 10 minutes.
5. Reinforce the dressing.

10. A patient who returned from surgery 3 hours ago following a kidney transplant is reporting pain at a 7 on a scale of 0 to 10. The nurse has tried repositioning with no improvement in the patient's pain report. Unmanaged surgical pain can lead to which of the following problems? (Select all that apply.)
1. Delayed ambulation
2. Reduced ventilation
3. Catheter-associated urinary tract infection
4. Retained pulmonary secretions
5. Reduced appetite

Answers: 1. 1, 3; **2.** 1, 4, 5; **3.** 2, 3; **4.** 3, 5; **5.** 1, 2, 4; **6.** 1; **7.** 1; **8.** 1 c, 2 a and c, 3 b, 4 d, 5 a and d; **9.** 1, 5; **10.** 1, 2, 4, 5.

Rationales for Review Questions can be found on the Evolve website.

REFERENCES

Aldrete JA: Modifications to the postanesthesia score for use in ambulatory surgery, *J Perianesth Nurs* 13(3):148, 1998.

American Association of Nurse Anesthetists (AANA): *Malignant hyperthermia crisis preparedness and treatment: position statement,* revised 2018. http://hhhwww.aana.com/docs/default-source/practice-aana-com-web-documents-(all)/malignant-hyperthermia-crisis-preparedness-and-treatment.pdf?sfvrsn=630049b1_8. .

American College of Surgeons: *Surgical patient education program: prepare for the best recovery,* updated 2018. https://www.facs.org/education/patient-education. Accessed August 3, 2018.

American Heart Association (AHA): *Target heart rates,* 2015. http://www.heart.org/HEARTORG/HealthyLiving/PhysicalActivity/Target-HeartRates_UCM_434341_Article.jsp?appName=MobileApp. Accessed March 4, 2019.

American Society of Addiction Medicine: *Screening and assessment tools,* 2019. https://www.asam.org/education/live-online-cme/fundamentals-program/additional-resources/screening-assessment-for-substance-use-disorders/screening-assessment-tools. Accessed February 6, 2019.

American Society of Anesthesiologists (ASA): Practice guidelines for the perioperative management of patients with obstructive sleep apnea: an updated report by the American Society of anesthesiologists Task force on perioperative management of patients with obstructive sleep apnea, *Anesthesiology* 120(2):268, 2014.

American Society of Anesthesiologists (ASA): Practice guidelines for preoperative fasting and the use of pharmacologic agents to reduce the risk of pulmonary aspiration: application to healthy patients undergoing elective procedures, *Anesthesiology* 126(3):376, 2017.

American Society of Anesthesiologists: *Multimodal approach to pain management reduces opioid use, prescriptions after joint replacement,* 2018. https://www.asahq.org/about-asa/newsroom/news-releases/2018/03/multimodal-approach-to-pain-management-reduces-opioid-use. Accessed February 13, 2019.

American Society of PeriAnesthesia Nurses (ASPAN): *Frequently asked questions,* 2018. http://www.aspan.org/Clinical-Practice/FAQs. Accessed March 13, 2018.

Apfel CC, et al.: Who is at risk for postdischarge nausea and vomiting after ambulatory surgery? *Anesthesiology* 117(3):475, 2012.

Association of Clinical Research Professionals (ACRP): *Should physicians be solely responsible for informed consent? One state thinks so,* 2017. https://www.acrp-net.org/2017/08/11/physicians-solely-responsible-informed-consent-one-state-thinks/. Accessed August 3, 2018.

Association of PeriOperative Registered Nurses (AORN): *AORN position statement on care of the older adult in perioperative settings,* 2015. https://www.aorn.org/guidelines/clinical-resources/position-statements. Accessed July 18, 2018.

Association of PeriOperative Registered Nurses (AORN): *Guidelines for perioperative practice,* Denver, 2018a, AORN.

Association of PeriOperative Registered Nurses (AORN): *AORN position statement on RN first assistants,* RNFA-Standards-of-Practice.pdf, 2018b. https://www.aorn.org/-/media/aorn/guidelines/position-statements/aorn_position_statement_rnfa.pdf. Accessed August 3, 2018.

Association of Surgical Technologists (AST): *Guidelines for best practices for the natural rubber latex allergic patient,* 2018. http://www.ast.org/uploadedFiles/Main_Site/Content/About_Us/Guideline_Latex_Allergy.pdf. Accessed August 3, 2018.

Aust H, et al.: Coping strategies in anxious surgical patients, *BMC Health Serv Res* 16:250, 2016.

Bastable SB: *Nurse as educator: principles of teaching and learning for nursing practice,* Burlington, MA, 2019, Jones and Bartlett Learning.

Benjamin MF, et al.: Using the Targeted Solutions Tool® to improve emergency department handoffs in a community hospital, *Jt Comm J Qual Patient Saf* 42(3):107–114, 2016.

Berríos-Torres SI, et al.: Centers for Disease Control and Prevention guidelines for the prevention of surgical site infection, *JAMA Surg* 152(8):784–791, 2017.

Burchum JR, Rosenthal LD: *Lehne's pharmacology for nursing care,* ed 10, St Louis, 2019, Elsevier.

Butcher HK, et al.: *Nursing interventions classification (NIC),* ed 7, St Louis, 2018, Elsevier.

Centers for Disease Control and Prevention (CDC): *Alcohol and public health: Fact sheets – binge drinking,* 2018. https://www.cdc.gov/alcohol/fact-sheets/binge-drinking.htm. Accessed July 1, 2018.

Centers for Disease Control and Prevention (CDC): *Guideline for prevention of catheter-associated urinary tract infections – 2009,* updated 2016. https://www.cdc.gov/infectioncontrol/guidelines/cauti/index.html. Accessed November 21, 2018.

Centers for Disease Control and Prevention (CDC): *What is health literacy,* 2019. https://www.cdc.gov/healthliteracy/learn/index.html. Accessed December 23, 2019.

Centers for Medicaid and Medicare Services: *Hospital-acquired condition reduction program (HACRP),* 2018. https://www.cms.gov/medicare/medicare-fee-for-service-payment/acuteinpatientpps/hac-reduction-program.html. Accessed July 30, 2018.

Centers for Medicaid and Medicare Services: *Adverse events in hospitals: public disclosure of information about events,* Washington, DC, 2010, Office of Inspector General. http://oig.hhs.gov/oei/reports/oei-06-09-00360.pdf. Accessed November 19, 2019.

Chou R, et al.: Guidelines on the management of postoperative pain, *J Pain* 17(2):131–157, 2016.

Chung F, et al.: STOP-Bang questionnaire: a practical approach to screen for obstructive sleep apnea, *Chest* 149(3):631, 2016.

Clinic C: *Coughing: controlled coughing: management and treatment,* 2017. https://my.clevelandclinic.org/health/diseases/8697-coughing-controlled-coughing/management-and-treatment. Accessed March 6, 2019.

Daniels JF: Purposeful and timely nursing rounds: a best practice implementation project, *JBI Database System Rev Implement Rep* 14(1):248, 2016.

Douglas MK, et al.: Guidelines for implementing culturally competent nursing care, *J Transcult Nurs* 25(2):109, 2014.

DuBose JR, Hadi K: Improving inpatient environments to support patient sleep, *Int J Qual Health Care* 28(5):540, 2016.

European Pressure Ulcer Advisory Panel (EPUAP) and National Pressure injury Advisory Panel (NPIAP), and Pan Pacific Pressure Injury Alliance: *Treatment of pressure ulcers/injuries: Clinical Practice Guideline. The International Guideline,* Emily Haesler (ED). EPUAP/NPIAP/PPPIA, 2019.

Falvey JR, et al.: Rethinking hospital-associated deconditioning: proposed paradigm shift, *Phys Ther* 95(9):1307, 2015.

Fetzer SJ: Postoperative nausea and vomiting. In Schick L, Windle PE, editors: *PeriAnesthesia nursing core curriculum: preprocedure, phase I and phase II PACU nursing,* ed 3, St Louis, 2015, Elsevier.

Florida Hospital Association: *Getup! Mobilizing patients to return to function more quickly,* 2018. http://www.f-ha.org/files/HIIN/GET-UP-Toolkit-Resource-Guide-2018.pdf. .

Gan TJ: Poorly controlled postoperative pain: prevalence, consequences, and prevention, *J Pain Res* 10:2287, 2017.

Ganzberg S: Obstrutive sleep apnea and office-based surgery, *Anesth Prog* 63(2):53, 2016.

Garrett JH: Effective perioperative communication to enhance patient care, *AORN J* 104(2):112, 2016.

Heideman BH: *Helping patients overcome ostomy challenges, Wound Care Advisor*, 2017. https://woundcareadvisor.com/helping-patients-overcome-ostomy-challenges-vol4-no3/. Accessed February 12, 2019.

Helvig A, et al.: Postoperative management of patients with obstructive sleep apnea: implications for the medical-surgical nurse, *Medsurg Nurs* 23(3):171, 2014.

Kim SE, Kim E: Local anesthesia with monitored anesthesia care for patients undergoing thyroidectomy: a case series, *Korean J Anesthesiol* 69(6):635, 2016.

Koutoukidis G, et al.: *Tabbner's Nursing care: theory and practice*, ed 7, Chatswood, Australia, 2017, Elsevier.

Kozek-Langenecker S, et al: European guideline on perioperative venous thromboembolism prophylaxis: surgery in the elderly, *Eur J Anaesthesiol* 35(2):116, 2018.

Lewis S, et al.: *Medical-surgical nursing: assessment and management of clinical problems*, ed 10, St Louis, 2017, Elsevier.

Lim CS, Davies AH: Graduated compression stockings, *CMAJ (Can Med Assoc J)* 186(10):e391, 2014.

Ljungqvist O, et al.: Enhanced recovery after surgery: a review, *JAMA Surg* 152(3):292, 2017.

Malarvizhi A, Hemavathy V: Knowledge on complications of immobility among the immobilized patients in selected wards at selected hospital, *J Nurs Health Sci* 4(2):2320, 2015.

Malignant Hyperthermia Association of the United States: *Dantrolene administration after an MH event*, 2018. https://www.mhaus.org/healthcare-professionals/mhaus-recommendations/dantrolene-administration-after-an-mh-event/. Accessed August 8, 2018.

Marcus C: Strategies for improving the quality of verbal patient and family education: a review of the literature and creation of the EDUCATE model, *Health Psychol Behav Med* 2(1):482, 2014.

Matsota P, et al.: Ondansetron-droperidol combination vs. ondansetron or droperidol monotherapy in the prevention of postoperative nausea and vomiting, *Arch Med Sci* 11(2):362, 2015.

McLendon K, Attia M: *Deep venous thrombosis (DVT) risk factors*, updated November 2017. In StatPearls [Internet], Treasure Island, FL, 2018, StatPearls Publishing. https://www.ncbi.nlm.nih.gov/books/NBK470215/.

MDCalc: *Urine output and fluid balance*, 2018. https://www.mdcalc.com/urine-output-fluid-balance.

Meiner SE, Yeager JJ: *Gerontologic nursing*, ed 6, St Louis, 2019, Elsevier.

Mills GH: Respiratory complications of anaesthesia, *Anaesthesia* 73(Suppl 1):25, 2018.

Mitchell MD, et al.: Hourly rounding to improve nursing responsiveness: a systematic review, *J Nurs Adm* 44(9):462, 2014.

Movasaghi G, et al.: Comparison between spinal and general anesthesia in percutaneous nephrolithotomy, *Int Anesth Res Soc* 123(35):207, 2016.

Nanavati AJ, Prabhakar S: Fast-track surgery: toward comprehensive peri-operative care, *Anesth Essays Res* 8(2):127, 2014.

National Academies of Science: *Facilitating patient understanding of discharge instructions: workshop summary*, Bethesda, MD, 2014, National Academies of Science. https://www.ncbi.nlm.nih.gov/books/NBK268650/. Accessed March 6, 2019.

National Council of State Boards of Nursing (NCSBN): *A nurse's guide to the use of social media*, 2018. https://www.ncsbn.org/NCSBN_SocialMedia.pdf. Accessed November 18, 2019.

National Quality Forum (NQF): *NQF-endorsed measures for surgical procedures: technical report*, 2015. https://www.qualityforum.org/Publications/2015/02/NQF-Endorsed_Measures_for_Surgical_Procedures.aspx . Accessed March 6, 2019.

Occupational Safety and Health Administration (OSHA): *Healthcare Wide Hazards: latex allergy*, n.d. https://www.osha.gov/SLTC/etools/hospital/hazards/latex/latex.html. Accessed March 6, 2019.

Olson E, et al: Postoperative management of adults with obstructive sleep apnea, *UpToDate*, updated June 15, 2018. https://www.uptodate.com/contents/postoperative-management-of-adults-with-obstructive-sleep-apnea#H2526407. Accessed August 8, 2018.

Pashikanti L, Von Ah D: Impact of early mobilization protocol on the medical-surgical inpatient population: an integrated review of literature, *Clin Nurse Spec* 26(2):87, 2012.

Phillips NM, et al.: Post-anaesthetic discharge scoring criteria: a systematic review, *JBI Libr Syst Rev* 9(41):1679, 2011.

Primiano M, et al.: Pressure ulcer prevalence and risk factors among prolonged surgical procedures in the OR, *AORN J* 94(6):555–566, 2011 Dec.

Resnick B, et al.: Feasibility and efficacy of function-focused care for orthopedic trauma patients, *J Trauma Nurs* 23(3):144, 2016.

Rightmyer J, Singbartl K: Preventing perioperative hypothermia, *Nursing* 46(9):57, 2016.

Roger C, et al.: Guidelines on the management of postoperative pain, *J Pain* 17(2):131, 2016.

Rosenberg H, et al: Malignant hyperthermia susceptibility, *GeneReviews*, updated January 31, 2013. https://www.ncbi.nlm.nih.gov/books/NBK1146/.

Rothrock JC: *Alexander's Care of the patient in surgery*, ed 16, St Louis, 2019, Elsevier.

Scott A, et al.: Understanding facilitators and barriers to care transitions: insights from Project ACHIEVE site visits, *Jt Comm J Qual Patient Saf* 43(9):433,2017.

Shore AC: Capillaroscopy and the measurement of capillary pressure, *Br J Clin Pharmacol* 50(6):501, 2000.

Sinha AK, et al.: Postoperative malignant hyperthermia- a medical emergency: a case report and review of literature, *J Clin Diagn Res* 11(4):1, 2017.

STATnews: No opioids, please: a growing movement lets patients refuse prescriptions, 2017. https://www.statnews.com/2017/03/19/opioid-prescription-refuse/

Streiff MB, et al.: Guidance for the treatment of deep vein thrombosis and pulmonary embolism, *J Thromb Thrombolysis* 41(1):32, 2016.

Su X, Wang DX: Improve postoperative sleep: what can we do? *Curr Opin Anaesthesiol* 31(1):83, 2017.

Sudhakaran S, Surani SR: Guidelines for perioperative management of the diabetic patient, *Surg Res Pract* 2015:284063, 2015. https://www.ncbi.nlm.nih.gov/pubmed/26078998.

Tait AR: Enhancing patient understanding of medical procedures: evaluation of an interactive multimedia program with in-line exercises, *Int J Med Inform* 83(5):376–384, 2014.

Tan M, et al.: Optimizing pain management to facilitate Enhanced Recovery after Surgery pathways, *Can J Anaesth* 62(2):203, 2015.

The Joint Commission (TJC): *2020 National Patient Safety Goals*, Oakbrook Terrace, IL, 2020, The Commission. https://www.jointcommission.org/en/standards/national-patient-safety-goals/. Accessed January 2, 2020.

The Joint Commission: *Comprehensive Accreditation and Certification manual, January 1, 2019*, Oakbrook Terrace, IL, 2019, The Commission.

The Joint Commission: *Joint Commission measures effective January 1, 2017*, 2017. https://www.jointcommission.org/joint_commission_measures_effective_january_1_2017/. Accessed 5 February 2019.

US Preventive Services Task Force: Recommendation statement: screening for obstructive sleep apnea in adults, *J Am Med Assoc* 317(4):407, 2017.

Van Abbema R, et al.: What type, or combination of exercise can improve preferred gait speed in older adults? A meta-analysis, *BMC Geriatr* 15:72, 2015.

van den Boom W, et al.: Effect of A1C and glucose on postoperative mortality in noncardiac and cardiac surgeries, *Diabetes Care* 41(4):782, 2018.

Wan B, et al.: Low-molecular-weight heparin and intermittent pneumatic compression for thromboprophylaxis in critical patients, *Exp Ther Med* 10(6):2331, 2015.

Welch MB: *Patient positioning for surgery and anesthesia in adults, UpToDate*, 2018. https://www.uptodate.com/contents/patient-positioning-for-surgery-and-anesthesia-in-adults. Accessed February 5, 2019.

World Health Organization (WHO): *The ASSIST Project - alcohol, smoking and substance involvement screening test*, 2018. https://www.who.int/substance_abuse/activities/assist/en/. Accessed December 20, 2018.

Zhao JM, et al.: Different types of intermittent pneumatic compression devices for preventing venous thromboembolism in patients after total hip replacement, *Cochrane Database Syst Rev* 12, 2014.

RESEARCH REFERENCES

American Academy of Sleep Medicine: *International classification of sleep disorders*, ed 3, Darien, IL, 2014, American Academy of Sleep Medicine.

Chua MJ, et al.: Early mobilisation after total hip or knee arthroplasty: a multicentre prospective observational study, *PLoS One* 12(6):e0179820, 2017.

Chung F, et al.: Predictive performance of the STOP-BANG score for identifying obstructive sleep apnea in obese patients, *Obes Surg* 23(12):2050, 2013.

Cummings KC, et al.: Epidural compared with non-epidural analgesia and cardiopulmonary complications after colectomy: a retrospective cohort study of 20,880 patients using a national quality database, *J Clin Anesth* 47(12), 2018.

Downey R: *Obstructive sleep apnea*, updated January 9, 2018, Medscape. https://emedicine.medscape.com/article/295807-overview#a2. Accessed July 8, 2018.

Fracol M, et al.: The surgical impact of e-cigarettes: a case report and review of the current literature, *Arch Plast Surg* 44(6):477, 2017.

Gan TJ, et al.: Consensus guidelines for the management of postoperative nausea and vomiting, *Anesth Analg* 118(1):85, 2014.

Hales CM, et al.: *Prevalence of obesity among adults and youth: United States, 2015–2016, NCHS Data Brief, No. 288*, Hyattsville, MD, 2017, National Center for Health Statistics.

Hannaman MJ, Ertl MJ: Patients with immunodeficiency, *Med Clin North Am* 97(6):1139, 2013.

Hwang BY, et al.: Comparison of patient-controlled epidural analgesia with patient-controlled intravenous analgesia for laparoscopic radical prostatectomy, *Korean J Pain* 31(3):191, 2018.

Kapadia BH, et al.: A randomized, clinical trial of preadmission chlorhexidine skin preparation for lower extremity total joint arthroplasty, *J Arthroplasty* 31(12):2856, 2016.

Kent BD, et al.: Insulin resistance, glucose intolerance and diabetes mellitus in obstructive sleep apnea, *J Thorac Dis* 7(8):1343, 2015.

Kim JM, et al.: Perioperative factors associated with pressure ulcer development after major surgery, *Korean J Anesthesiol* 71(1):48, 2017.

Kobelt P, et al.: Evaluation of a standardized sedation assessment for opioid administration in the post anesthesia care unit, *Pain Manag Nurs* 15(3):672, 2014.

Lin HS, et al.: Frailty and post-operative outcomes in older surgical patients: a systematic review, *BMC Geriatr* 16(1):157, 2016.

Linnaus ME, Ostlie DJ: Complications in common general pediatric surgery procedures, *Semin Pediatr Surg* 25(6):404, 2016.

Mistry PR, et al.: Prediction of surgical complications in the elderly: can we improve outcomes? *Asian J Urol* 4(1):44, 2017.

National Center for Health Statistics: Health, United States: *2016: with chartbook on long-term trends in health*, Hyattsville, MD, 2017, National Center for Health Statistics.

National Institute of Health (NIH): National, heart, lung, and blood Institute: *Sleep apnea*, 2018. https://www.nhlbi.nih.gov/health-topics/sleep-apnea. Accessed July 18, 2018.

Nicholas JA: Preoperative optimization and risk assessment, *Clin Geriatr Med* 30(2):207, 2014.

Poulin P, et al.: Preoperative skin antiseptics for preventing surgical site infections: what to do? *ORNAC J* 32(3):12–15, 2014, 24.

Ramesh C, et al.: Effect of preoperative education on postoperative outcomes among patients undergoing cardiac surgery: a systematic review and meta-analysis, *J Perianesth Nurs* 32(6):518, 2017.

Raveendran R, Chung F: Ambulatory anesthesia for patients with sleep apnea, *Dovepress* 2:143, 2015.

Rupich K, et al.: The benefits of implementing an early mobility protocol in postoperative neurosurgical spine patients, *Am J Nurs* 118(6):46, 2018.

Saghaleini SH, et al.: Pressure ulcer and nutrition, *Indian J Crit Care Med* 22(4):283, 2018.

Shaw LF, et al.: Incidence and predicted risk factors of pressure ulcers in surgical patients: experience at a medical center in Taipei, Taiwan, *BioMed Res Int* 416896, 2014, Published online 2014 Jun 26.

Skraastad E, et al.: Development and validation of the Efficacy Safety Score (ESS), a novel tool for postoperative patient management, *BMC Anesthesiol* 17:50, 2017.

Tjeertes E, et al.: Obesity –a risk factor for postoperative complications in general surgery? *BMC Anesthesiol* 15:112, 2015.

Tocher JM: Expectations and experiences of open abdominal aortic aneurysm repair patients: a mixed methods study, *J Clin Nurs* 23(3/4):421, 2014.

Wechter DG, et al.: *Smoking and surgery*, MedLinePlus, 2016. https://medlineplus.gov/ency/patientinstructions/000437.htm. Accessed July 8, 2018.

Weimann A, et al.: ESPEN guideline: clinical nutrition in surgery, *Clin Nutr* 36(3):623, 2017.

GLOSSARY

A

abduction Movement of a limb away from the body.

abrasion Scraping or rubbing away of epidermis; may result in localized bleeding and later weeping of serous fluid.

absorption Passage of drug molecules into the blood. Factors influencing drug absorption include route of administration, ability of the drug to dissolve, and conditions at the site of absorption.

acceptance Fifth stage of Kübler-Ross's stages of grief and dying. An individual comes to terms with a loss rather than submitting to resignation and hopelessness.

accessory muscles Muscles in the thoracic cage that assist with respiration.

accommodation Process of responding to the environment through new activity, thinking, and changing the existing schema or developing a new schema to deal with the new information. For example, a toddler whose parent consistently corrects him when he calls a horse a "doggie" accommodates and forms a new schema for horses.

accountability State of being answerable for one's actions—a nurse answers to himself or herself, the patient, the profession, the employing institution such as a hospital, and society for the effectiveness of nursing care performed.

accreditation Process whereby a professional association or nongovernmental agency grants recognition to a school or institution for demonstrated ability to meet predetermined criteria.

acculturation The process through which an individual or group transitions from one culture to develop the traits of another culture.

acne Inflammatory, papulopustular skin eruption, usually occurring on the face, neck, shoulders, and upper back.

acromegaly Chronic metabolic condition caused by overproduction of growth hormone and characterized by gradual, marked enlargement and elongation of bones of the face, jaw, and extremities.

active listening Listening attentively with the whole person—mind, body, and spirit. It includes listening for main and supportive ideas; acknowledging and responding; giving appropriate feedback; and paying attention to the other person's total communication, including the content, intent, and feelings expressed.

active range-of-motion (ROM) exercise Exercise to the joint by the patient while doing activities of daily living or during joint assessment.

active strategies of health promotion Activities that depend on the patient's motivation to adopt a specific health program.

active transport Movement of materials across the cell membrane by means of chemical activity that allows the cell to admit larger molecules than would otherwise be possible.

activities of daily living (ADLs) Activities usually performed in the course of a normal day in the patient's life such as eating, dressing, bathing, brushing the teeth, or grooming.

activity tolerance Type and amount of exercise or work that a person is able to perform without undue exertion or injury.

actual loss Loss of an object, person, body part or function, or emotion that is overt and easily identifiable.

acuity recording Mechanism by which entries describing patient care activities are made over a 24-hour period. The activities are then translated into a rating score, or acuity score, that allows for a comparison of patients who vary by severity of illness.

acute care Pattern of health care in which a patient is treated for an acute episode of illness, for the sequelae of an accident or other trauma, or during recovery from surgery.

acute illness Illness characterized by symptoms that are of relatively short duration, are usually severe, and affect the functioning of the patient in all dimensions.

adduction Movement of a limb toward the body.

adolescence Period in development between the onset of puberty and adulthood. It usually begins between 11 and 13 years of age.

adult day care center Facility for the supervised care of older adults; provides activities such as meals and socialization during specified day hours.

advanced practice registered nurse (APRN) Generally the most independently functioning nurse. An APRN has a master's degree in nursing; advanced education in pathophysiology, pharmacology, and physical assessment; and certification and expertise in a specialized area of practice.

advanced sleep phase syndrome Common in older adults; a disturbance in sleep manifested by early waking in the morning with an inability to get back to sleep. It is thought that this syndrome is caused by advancing of the circadian rhythm of the body.

adventitious sounds Abnormal lung sounds heard with auscultation.

adverse effect Harmful or unintended effect of a medication, diagnostic test, or therapeutic intervention.

adverse reaction Any harmful, unintended effect of a medication, diagnostic test, or therapeutic intervention.

advocacy Process whereby a nurse objectively provides patients with the information they need to make decisions and supports the patients in whatever decisions they make.

afebrile Without fever.

affective learning Acquisition of behaviors involved in expressing feelings about attitudes, appreciation, and values.

afterload Resistance to left ventricular ejection; the work the heart must overcome to fully eject blood from the left ventricle.

age-related macular degeneration Progressive disorder in which the macula (the specialized portion of the retina responsible for central vision) degenerates as a result of aging and loses its ability to function efficiently. First signs include blurring of reading matter, distortion or loss of central vision, sensitivity to glare, and distortion of objects.

agnostic Individual who believes that any ultimate reality is unknown or unknowable.

airborne precautions Safeguards designed to reduce the risk of transmission of infectious agents through the air that a person breathes.

alarm reaction Mobilization of the defense mechanisms of the body and mind to cope with a stressor; the initial stage of the general adaptation syndrome.

aldosterone Mineralocorticoid steroid hormone produced by the adrenal cortex with action in the renal tubule to regulate sodium and potassium balance in the blood.

allergic reaction Unfavorable physiological response to an allergen to which a person has previously been exposed and has developed antibodies.

alopecia Partial or complete loss of hair; baldness.

Alzheimer's disease Disease of the brain parenchyma that causes a gradual and progressive decline in cognitive functioning.

AMBULARM Device used for the patient who climbs out of bed unassisted and is in danger of falling. This device is worn on the leg and signals when the leg is in a dependent position such as over the side rail or on the floor.

amino acid Organic compound of one or more basic groups and one or more carboxyl groups. Amino acids are the building blocks that construct proteins and the end products of protein digestion.

anabolism Constructive metabolism characterized by conversion of simple substances into more complex compounds of living matter.

analgesic Relieving pain; drug that relieves pain.

analogies Resemblances made between things otherwise unlike.

anaphylactic reaction Hypersensitive condition induced by contact with certain antigens.

aneurysm Localized dilations of the wall of a blood vessel; usually caused by atherosclerosis, hypertension, or a congenital weakness in a vessel wall.

anger Second stage of Kübler-Ross's stages of grief and dying. During this stage an individual resists loss by expressing extreme displeasure, indignation, or hostility.

angiotensin Polypeptide occurring in the blood, causing vasoconstriction, increased blood pressure, and the release of aldosterone from the adrenal cortex.

anion gap Difference between the concentrations of serum cations and anions; determined by measuring the concentrations of sodium cations and chloride and bicarbonate anions.

anions Negatively charged electrolytes.

anthropometric measurements Body measures of height, weight, and skinfolds to evaluate muscle atrophy.

anthropometry Measurement of various body parts to determine nutritional and caloric status, muscular development, brain growth, and other parameters.

antibodies Immunoglobulins essential to the immune system that are produced by lymphoid tissue in response to bacteria, viruses, or other antigens.

anticipatory grief Grief response in which the person begins the grieving process before an actual loss.

antidiuretic hormone (ADH) Hormone that decreases the production of urine by increasing the resorption of water by the renal tubules. ADH is secreted by cells of the hypothalamus and stored in the posterior lobe of the pituitary gland.

antiembolic stockings Elasticized stockings that prevent formation of emboli and thrombi, especially after surgery or during bed rest.

antigen Substance, usually a protein, that causes the formation of an antibody and reacts specifically with that antibody.

antipyretic Substance or procedure that reduces fever.

anxiolytics Drugs used primarily to treat episodes of anxiety.

aphasia Abnormal neurological condition in which language function is defective or absent; related to injury to speech center in cerebral cortex, causing receptive or expressive aphasia.

apical pulse Heartbeat as listened to with the bell or diaphragm of a stethoscope placed on the apex of the heart.

apnea Absence of respirations for a period of time.

apothecary system System of measurement. The basic unit of weight is a grain. Weights derived from the grain are the gram, ounce, and pound. The basic measure for fluid is the minim. The fluidram, fluid ounce, pint, quart, and gallon are measures derived from the minim.

approximate To come close together, as in the edges of a wound.

arcus senilis Opaque ring, gray to white in color, that surrounds the periphery of the cornea. The condition is caused by deposits of fat granules in the cornea. Occurs primarily in older adults.

asepsis Absence of germs or microorganisms.

aseptic technique Any health care procedure in which added precautions are used to prevent contamination of a person, object, or area by microorganisms.

assault Unlawful threat to bring about harmful or offensive contact with another.

assertive communication Type of communication based on a philosophy of protecting individual rights and responsibilities. It includes the ability to be self-directive in acting to accomplish goals and advocate for others.

assessment First step of the nursing process. Activities required in the first step are data collection, validation, sorting, and documentation. The purpose is to gather information for health problem identification.

assimilation The process in which an individual adapts to the host's cultural values and no longer prefers the traditions, values, and beliefs of the culture of origin.

assisted living Residential living facilities in which each resident has his or her own room and shares dining and social activity areas.

associative play Form of play in which a group of children participates in similar or identical activities without formal organization, direction, interaction, or goals.

atelectasis Collapse of alveoli, preventing the normal respiratory exchange of oxygen and carbon dioxide.

atheist Individual who does not believe in the existence of God.

atherosclerosis Common arterial disorder characterized by yellowish plaques of cholesterol, lipids, and cellular debris in the inner layers of the walls of the large- and medium-size arteries.

atrioventricular (AV) node Part of the cardiac conduction system located on the floor of the right atrium; receives electrical impulses from the atrium and transmits them to the bundle of His.

atrophied Wasted or reduced size or physiological activity of a part of the body caused by disease or other influences.

attachment Initial psychosocial relationship that develops between parents and the neonate.

attentional set Mental state that allows the learner to focus on and comprehend a learning activity.

auditory Related to or experienced through hearing.

auscultation Method of physical examination; listening to the sounds produced by the body, usually with a stethoscope.

auscultatory gap Disappearance of sound when obtaining a blood pressure; typically occurs between the first and second Korotkoff sounds.

authority Right to act in areas in which an individual has been given and accepts responsibility.

autologous transfusion Procedure in which blood is removed from a donor and stored for a variable period before it is returned to the donor's own circulation.

autonomy Ability or tendency to function independently.

B

back-channeling Active listening technique that prompts a respondent to continue telling a story or describing a situation. Involves use of phrases such as "Go on," "Uh-huh," and "Tell me more."

bacteremia Presence of bacteria in the bloodstream.

bacteriuria Presence of bacteria in the urine.

balance Position in which the person's center of gravity is correctly positioned so that falling does not occur.

bandages Available in rolls of various widths and materials, including gauze, elasticized knit, elastic webbing, flannel, and muslin. Gauze bandages are lightweight and inexpensive, mold easily around contours of the body, and permit air circulation to underlying skin to prevent maceration. Elastic bandages conform well to body parts but can also be used to exert pressure over a body part.

bargaining Third stage of Kübler-Ross's stages of grief and dying. A person postpones the reality of a loss by attempting to make deals in a subtle or overt manner with others or with a higher being.

baridi Condition among the Bena people of Tanzania attributed to disrespectful behavior within the family or transgression of cultural taboos. The person experiences physical and psychological symptoms and is usually treated by a traditional healer, who has the person make a public admission or an apology or who treats the person with herbal remedies.

basal cell carcinoma Malignant epithelial cell tumor that begins as a papule and enlarges peripherally, developing a central crater that erodes, crusts, and bleeds. Metastasis is rare.

basal metabolic rate (BMR) Amount of energy used in a unit of time by a fasting, resting subject to maintain vital functions.

battery Legal term for touching another's body without consent.

bed boards Boards placed under the mattress of a bed that provide extra support to the mattress surface.

bed rest Placement of the patient in bed for therapeutic reasons for a prescribed period.

benchmarking Identifying best practices and comparing them with current organizational practices to improve performance. This process helps to support the claims of quality care delivery by the institution.

beneficence Doing good or actively promoting doing good; one of the four principles of the ethical theory of deontology.

benign breast disease (fibrocystic) Benign condition characterized by lumpy, painful breasts and sometimes nipple discharge. Symptoms are more apparent before the menstrual period. Known to be a risk factor for breast cancer.

bereavement Response to loss through death; a subjective experience that a person suffers after losing a person with whom there has been a significant relationship.

biases and prejudices Beliefs and attitudes associating negative permanent characteristics to people who are perceived as different from oneself.

bi-level positive airway pressure (Bi-PAP) Ventilatory support used to treat patients with obstructive sleep apnea, patients with congestive heart failure, and preterm infants with underdeveloped lungs.

bilineally Kinship that extends to both the mother's and father's sides of the family.

binders Bandages made of large pieces of material to fit specific body parts.

bioethics   Branch of ethics within the field of health care.

biological clock   Cyclical nature of body function. Functions controlled from within the body are synchronized with environmental factors; same meaning as biorhythm.

biological half-life   Time it takes for the body to lower the amount of unchanged medication by half.

biotransformation   Chemical changes that a substance undergoes in the body such as by the action of enzymes.

blanchable hyperemia   Redness of the skin caused by dilation of the superficial capillaries. When pressure is applied to the skin, the area blanches, or turns a lighter color.

body image   Peoples' subjective concept of their physical appearance.

body mechanics   Coordinated efforts of the musculoskeletal and nervous systems to maintain proper balance, posture, and body alignment.

bone resorption   Destruction of bone cells and release of calcium into the blood.

borborygmi   Audible abdominal sounds produced by hyperactive intestinal peristalsis.

botanica   Place that sells religious and herbal remedies.

bradycardia   Slower-than-normal heart rate; heart contracts fewer than 60 times/min.

bradypnea   Abnormally slow rate of breathing.

bronchospasm   Excessive and prolonged contraction of the smooth muscle of the bronchi and bronchioles, resulting in an acute narrowing and obstruction of the respiratory airway.

bruit   Abnormal sound or murmur heard while auscultating an organ, gland, or artery.

buccal   Of or pertaining to the inside of the cheek or the gum next to the cheek.

buccal cavity   Consists of the lips surrounding the opening of the mouth, the cheeks running along the side walls of the cavity, the tongue and its muscles, and the hard and soft palate.

buffer   Substance or group of substances that can absorb or release hydrogen ions to correct an acid-base imbalance.

bundle of His   Part of the cardiac conduction system that arises from the distal portion of the atrioventricular (AV) node and extends across the AV groove to the top of the intraventricular septum, where it divides into right and left bundle branches.

C

cachexia   Malnutrition marked by weakness and emaciation, usually associated with severe illness.

capitation   Payment mechanism in which a provider (e.g., health care network) receives a fixed amount of payment per enrollee.

capnography   Also known as end-tidal CO_2 monitoring, it provides instant information about how effectively CO_2 is eliminated by the pulmonary system, how effectively it is transported through the vascular system, and how effectively CO_2 is produced by cellular metabolism. Capnography is measured near the end of exhalation.

carbohydrates   Dietary classification of foods comprising sugars, starches, cellulose, and gum.

carbon monoxide   Colorless, odorless, poisonous gas produced by the combustion of carbon or organic fuels.

cardiac index   Adequacy of the cardiac output for an individual. It takes into account the body surface area (BSA) of the patient.

cardiac output (CO)   Volume of blood expelled by the ventricles of the heart, equal to the amount of blood ejected at each beat multiplied by the number of beats in the period of time used for computation (usually 1 minute).

cardiopulmonary rehabilitation   Actively assisting the patient with achieving and maintaining an optimal level of health through controlled physical exercise, nutritional counseling, relaxation and stress management techniques, prescribed medications and oxygen, and compliance.

cardiopulmonary resuscitation (CPR)   Basic emergency procedures for life support consisting of artificial respiration and manual external cardiac massage.

care   To feel concern for or interest in one who has sorrow or difficulties.

care bundle   A group of interventions related to a disease process or condition that when implemented together result in better patient outcomes than when the interventions are implemented individually.

caring   Universal phenomenon that influences the way we think, feel, and behave in relation to one another.

carriers   People or animals who harbor and spread an organism that causes disease in others but do not become ill themselves.

case management   Organized system for delivering health care to an individual patient or group of patients across an episode of illness and/or a continuum of care; includes assessment and development of a plan of care, coordination of all services, referral, and follow-up; usually assigned to one professional.

case management plan   Multidisciplinary model for documenting patient care that usually includes plans for problems, key interventions, and expected outcomes for patients with a specific disease or condition.

catabolism   Breakdown of body tissue into simpler substances.

cataplexy   Condition characterized by sudden muscular weakness and loss of muscle tone.

cataracts   Abnormal progressive condition of the lens of the eye characterized by loss of transparency.

cathartics   Drugs that act to promote bowel evacuation.

catheterization   Introduction of a catheter into a body cavity or organ to inject or remove fluid.

cations   Positively charged electrolytes.

center of gravity   Midpoint or center of the weight of a body or object.

centigrade   Denotes temperature scale in which 0° is the freezing point of water and 100° is the boiling point of water at sea level; also called Celsius.

cerumen   Yellowish or brownish waxy secretion produced by sweat glands in the external ear.

chancres   Skin lesions or venereal sores (usually primary syphilis) that begin at the site of infection as papules and develop into red, bloodless, painless ulcers with a scooped-out appearance.

change-of-shift report   Report that occurs between two scheduled nursing work shifts. Nurses communicate information about their assigned patients to nurses working on the next shift of duty.

channel   Method used in the teaching-learning process to present content: visual, auditory, taste, smell. In the communication process, a method used to transmit a message: visual, auditory, touch.

charting by exception (CBE)   Charting methodology in which data are entered only when there is an exception from that which is normal or expected; reduces time spent documenting in charting. It is a shorthand method for documenting normal findings and routine care.

chest percussion   Striking the chest wall with a cupped hand to promote mobilization and drainage of pulmonary secretions.

chest physiotherapy (CPT)   Group of therapies used to mobilize pulmonary secretions for expectoration.

chest tube   Catheter inserted through the thorax into the chest cavity for removing air or fluid; used after chest or heart surgery or pneumothorax.

Cheyne-Stokes respiration   Occurs when there is decreased blood flow or injury to the brainstem.

chronic illness   Illness that persists over a long time and affects physical, emotional, intellectual, social, and spiritual functioning.

circadian rhythm   Repetition of certain physiological phenomena within a 24-hour cycle.

circular transactional communication process   Communication model that enhances the linear communication by enabling the sender and receiver to view perceptions, attitudes, and potential reactions of others via a mental picture. This is a continuous and interactive activity.

circulating nurse   Assistant to the scrub nurse and surgeon whose role is to provide necessary supplies; dispose of soiled instruments and supplies; and keep an accurate count of instruments, needles, and sponges used.

civil law   Statutes concerned with protecting a person's rights.

climacteric   Physiological, developmental change that occurs in the male reproductive system between the ages of 45 and 60.

clinical criteria   Objective or subjective signs and symptoms, clusters of signs and symptoms, or risk factors.

clinical decision making   Problem-solving approach that nurses use to define patient problems and select appropriate treatment.

clinical-decision support systems   Computerized programs used within the health care setting to support decision making.

Clinical Information System (CIS) A computer-based system that collects, stores, and manipulates data to allow health care providers to make informed decisions about patient care.

closed-ended question Form of question that limits a respondent's answer to one or two words.

clubbing Bulging of the tissues at the nail base caused by insufficient oxygenation at the periphery, resulting from conditions such as chronic emphysema and congenital heart disease.

code of ethics Formal statement that delineates a profession's guidelines for ethical behavior. A code of ethics sets standards or expectations for the professional to achieve.

cognitive learning Acquisition of intellectual skills that encompass behaviors such as thinking, understanding, and evaluating.

collaborative interventions Therapies that require the knowledge, skill, and expertise of multiple health care professionals.

collaborative problem Physiological complication that requires the nurse to use nursing- and health care provider–prescribed interventions to maximize patient outcomes.

colloid osmotic pressure Abnormal condition of the kidney caused by the pressure of concentrations of large particles such as protein molecules that will pass through a membrane.

colon Portion of the large intestine from the cecum to the rectum.

colonization Presence and multiplication of microorganisms without tissue invasion or damage.

comforting Acts toward another individual that display both an emotional and physical calm. The use of touch, the establishment of presence, the therapeutic use of silence, and the skillful and gentle performance of a procedure are examples of comforting nursing measures.

common law One source for law that is created by judicial decisions as opposed to those created by legislative bodies (statutory law).

communicable disease Any disease that can be transmitted from one person or animal to another by direct or indirect contact or by vectors.

communication Ongoing, dynamic series of events that involves the transmission of meaning from sender to receiver.

community-based nursing Acute and chronic care of individuals and families to strengthen their capacity for self-care and promote independence in decision making.

community health nursing Nursing approach that combines knowledge from the public health sciences with professional nursing theories to safeguard and improve the health of populations in the community.

co-morbidity A chronic, long-term condition existing simultaneously with and usually independently of another medical condition.

compassion The feeling that arises when a person is confronted with another's suffering and feels motivated to relieve that suffering. Compassion shows kindness, caring, and a willingness to help others.

competence Specific range of skills necessary to perform a task.

complete bed bath Bath in which the entire body of a patient is washed in bed.

compress Soft pad of gauze or cloth used to apply heat, cold, or medications to the surface of a body part.

computer-based patient record Comprehensive computerized system used by all health care practitioners to permanently store information pertaining to a patient's health status, clinical problems, and functional abilities.

concentration Relative content of a component within a substance or solution.

concentration gradient Gradient that exists across a membrane, separating a high concentration of a particular ion from a low concentration of the same ion.

concept map Care-planning tool that assists in critical thinking and forming associations between a patient's nursing diagnoses and interventions.

confianza Trust.

confidentiality Act of keeping information private or secret; in health care the nurse shares information about a patient only with other nurses or health care providers who need to know private information about a patient to provide care for him or her; information can only be shared with the patient's consent.

conjunctivitis Highly contagious eye infection. The crusty drainage that collects on eyelid margins can easily spread from one eye to the other.

connectedness Having close spiritual relationships with oneself, others, and God or another spiritual being.

connotative meaning Shade or interpretation of the meaning of a word influenced by the thoughts, feelings, or ideas that people have about the word.

conscious sedation Administration of central nervous system–depressant drugs and/or analgesics to provide analgesia, relieve anxiety, and/or provide amnesia during surgical, diagnostic, or interventional procedures.

constipation Condition characterized by difficulty in passing stool or an infrequent passage of hard stool.

consultation Process in which the help of a specialist is sought to identify ways to handle problems in patient management or in planning and implementing programs.

Contact Precautions Safeguards designed to reduce the risk of transmission of epidemiologically important microorganisms by direct or indirect contact.

content The product and information obtained from the system.

continent urinary diversion (CUR) Surgical diversion of the drainage of urine from a diseased or dysfunctional bladder. Patient uses a catheter to drain the pouch.

continuous positive airway pressure (CPAP) Ventilatory support used to treat patients with obstructive sleep apnea, patients with congestive heart failure, and preterm infants with underdeveloped lungs.

convalescence Period of recovery after an illness, injury, or surgery.

coping Making an effort to manage psychological stress.

core temperature Temperature of deep structures of the body.

cough Sudden, audible expulsion of air from the lungs. The person breathes in, the glottis is partially closed, and the accessory muscles of expiration contract to expel the air forcibly.

counseling Problem-solving method used to help patients recognize and manage stress and enhance interpersonal relationships. It helps patients examine alternatives and decide which choices are most helpful and appropriate.

crackles Fine bubbling sounds heard on auscultation of the lung; produced by air entering distal airways and alveoli, which contain serous secretions.

crime Act that violates a law and that may include criminal intent.

criminal law Concerned with acts that threaten society but may involve only an individual.

crisis Transition for better or worse in the course of a disease, usually indicated by a marked change in the intensity of signs and symptoms.

crisis intervention Use of therapeutic techniques directed toward helping a patient resolve a particular and immediate problem.

critical pathways Tools used in managed care that incorporate the treatment interventions of caregivers from all disciplines who normally care for a patient. Designed for a specific care type, a pathway is used to manage the care of a patient throughout a projected length of stay.

critical period of development Specific phase or period when the presence of a function or reasoning has its greatest effect on a specific aspect of development.

critical thinking Active, purposeful, organized, cognitive process used to carefully examine one's thinking and the thinking of other individuals.

crutch gait Gait achieved by a person using crutches.

cue Information that a nurse acquires through hearing, visual observations, touch, and smell.

cultural and linguistic competence Set of congruent behaviors, attitudes, and policies that come together in a system or agency or among professionals that enables effective work in cross-cultural situations.

cultural assessment Systematic and comprehensive examination of the cultural care values, beliefs, and practices of individuals, families, and communities.

cultural awareness Gaining in-depth awareness of one's own background, stereotypes, biases, prejudices, and assumptions about other people.

cultural care accommodation or negotiation Adapting or negotiating with the patient/family to achieve beneficial or satisfying health outcomes.

cultural care preservation or maintenance Retaining and/or preserving relevant care values so that patients are able to maintain their well-being, recover from illness, or face handicaps and/or death.

cultural care repatterning or restructuring Reordering, changing, or greatly modifying a patient's/family's customs for a new, different, and beneficial health care pattern.

cultural competence Process in which the health care professional continually strives to achieve the ability and availability to work effectively with individuals, families, and communities.

cultural encounters Engaging in cross-cultural interactions; refining intercultural communication skills; gaining in-depth understanding of others and avoiding stereotypes; and managing cultural conflict.

cultural imposition Using one's own values and customs as an absolute guide in interpreting behaviors.

cultural knowledge Obtaining knowledge of other cultures; gaining sensitivity to, respect for, and appreciation of differences.

cultural pain Feeling that a patient has after a health care worker disregards the patient's valued way of life.

cultural respect Behavior that is respectful and responsive to the needs of the diverse patient.

cultural skills Communication, cultural assessment, and culturally competent care.

culturally congruent care Care that fits people's valued life patterns and sets of meanings generated from the people themselves. Sometimes this differs from the professionals' perspective on care.

culturally ignorant or blind Uneducated about other cultures.

culture Integrated patterns of human behavior that include the language, thoughts, communications, actions, customs, beliefs, values, and institutions of racial, ethnic, religious, or social groups.

culture-bound syndromes Illnesses restricted to a particular culture or group because of its psychosocial characteristics.

culture care theory Leininger's theory that emphasizes culturally congruent care.

culturological nursing assessment Systematic and comprehensive examination of the cultural care values, beliefs, and practices of individuals, families, and communities.

cutaneous stimulation Stimulation of a person's skin to prevent or reduce pain perception. A massage, warm bath, hot and cold therapies, and transcutaneous electrical nerve stimulation are some ways to reduce pain perception.

cyanosis Bluish discoloration of the skin and mucous membranes caused by an excess of deoxygenated hemoglobin in the blood or a structural defect in the hemoglobin molecule.

D

DAR (data, action, patient response) Format used in focus charting for recording patient information.

data analysis Logical examination of and professional judgment about patient assessment data; used in the diagnostic process to derive a nursing diagnosis.

data cluster Set of signs or symptoms that are grouped together in logical order.

database Store or bank of information, especially in a form that can be processed by computer.

debridement Removal of dead tissue from a wound.

decentralized management Organizational philosophy that brings decisions down to the level of the staff. Individuals best informed about a problem or issue participate in the decision-making process.

decision making Process involving critical appraisal of information that begins with recognizing a problem and ends with generating, testing, and evaluating a conclusion. Comes at the end of critical thinking.

deconditioning Physiological change following a period of inactivity, bed rest or sedentary lifestyle. It results in functional losses in such areas as mental status, degree of continence, and ability to accomplish activities of daily living.

defecation Passage of feces from the digestive tract through the rectum.

defendant Individual or organization against whom legal charges are brought in a court of law.

defining characteristics The observable assessment cues that cluster as manifestations of a problem-focused or health promotion nursing diagnosis.

dehiscence Separation of the edges of a wound, revealing underlying tissues.

dehydration Excessive loss of water from the body tissues accompanied by a disturbance of body electrolytes.

delegation Process of assigning another member of the health care team to be responsible for aspects of patient care (e.g., assigning nurse assistants to bathe a patient).

delirium Acute state of confusion that is potentially reversible and often has a physical cause.

dementia Generalized impairment of intellectual functioning that interferes with social and occupational functioning.

denial Unconscious refusal to admit an unacceptable idea.

denotative meaning Meaning of a word shared by individuals who use a common language. For example, the word *baseball* has the same meaning for all individuals who speak English, but the word *code* primarily denotes cardiac arrest to health care providers.

dental caries Abnormal destructive condition in a tooth caused by a complex interaction of food, especially starches and sugars, with bacteria that form dental plaque.

deontology Traditional theory of ethics that proposes to define actions as right or wrong based on the characteristics of fidelity to promises, truthfulness, and justice. The conventional use of ethical terms such as *justice, autonomy, beneficence,* and *nonmaleficence* constitutes the practice of deontology.

depression (1) Reduction in happiness and well-being that contributes to physical and social limitations and complicates the treatment of concomitant medical conditions. It is usually reversible with treatment. (2) Fourth stage of Kübler-Ross's stages of grief and dying. In this stage the person realizes the full impact and significance of the loss.

dermis Sensitive vascular layer of the skin directly below the epidermis; composed of collagenous and elastic fibrous connective tissues that give the dermis strength and elasticity.

determinants of health Many variables that influence the health status of individuals or communities.

detoxify To remove the toxic quality of a substance. The liver acts to detoxify chemicals in drug compounds.

development Qualitative or observable aspects of the progressive changes that one makes in adapting to the environment.

developmental crises Crises associated with normal and expected phases of growth and development (e.g., the response to menopause); same as maturational crises.

diabetic retinopathy Disorder of retinal blood vessels. Pathological changes secondary to increased pressure in the blood vessels of the retina result in decreased vision or vision loss caused by hemorrhage and macular edema.

diagnosis-related group (DRG) Classifications based on a hospitalized patient's primary and secondary medical diagnoses that are used as the basis for establishing Medicare reimbursement for patient care.

diagnostic process Mental steps (data clustering and analysis, problem identification) that follow assessment and lead directly to the formulation of a diagnosis.

diagnostic reasoning Process that enables an observer to assign meaning to and classify phenomena in clinical situations by integrating observations and critical thinking.

diaphoresis Secretion of sweat, especially profuse secretion associated with an elevated body temperature, physical exertion, or emotional stress.

diaphragmatic breathing Respiration in which the abdomen moves out while the diaphragm descends on inspiration.

diarrhea Increase in the number of stools and the passage of liquid, unformed feces.

diastolic Pertaining to diastole, or the blood pressure at the instant of maximum cardiac relaxation; the pressure of the blood in the arteries when the heart is filling

dietary reference intake (DRI) Information on each vitamin or mineral to reflect a range of minimum-to-maximum amounts that avert deficiency or toxicity.

diffusion Movement of molecules from an area of high concentration to one of lower concentration.

digestion Breakdown of nutrients by chewing, churning, mixing with fluid, and chemical reactions.

direct care interventions Treatments performed through interaction with the patient. For example, a patient may require medication administration, insertion of an intravenous infusion, or counseling during a time of grief.

discharge planning Activities directed toward identifying future proposed therapy and the need for additional resources before and after returning home.

discrimination Prejudicial outlook, action, or treatment.

disease Malfunctioning or maladaptation of biological or psychological processes.

disinfection Process of destroying all pathogenic organisms except spores.

disorganization and despair One of Bowlby's four phases of mourning in which an individual endlessly examines how and why the loss occurred.

distress Damaging stress; one of the two types of stress identified by Selye.

disuse osteoporosis Reductions in skeletal mass routinely accompanying immobility or paralysis.

diuresis Increased rate of formation and excretion of urine.

documentation Written entry into the patient's medical record of all pertinent information about him or her. These entries validate the patient's problems and care and exist as a legal record.

dominant culture Customs, values, beliefs, traditions, and social and religious views held by a group of people that prevail over another secondary culture.

dorsiflexion Flexion toward the back.

drainage evacuators Convenient portable units that connect to tubular drains lying within a wound bed and exert a safe, constant, low-pressure vacuum to remove and collect drainage.

Droplet Precautions Safeguards designed to reduce the risk of droplet transmission of infectious agents.

dysmenorrhea Painful menstruation.

dysphagia Difficulty swallowing; commonly associated with obstructive or motor disorders of the esophagus.

dyspnea Sensation of shortness of breath.

dysrhythmia Deviation from the normal pattern of the heartbeat.

dysuria Painful urination resulting from bacterial infection of the bladder and obstructive conditions of the urethra.

E

ecchymosis Discoloration of the skin or bruise caused by leakage of blood into subcutaneous tissues as a result of trauma to underlying tissues.

ectropion Eversion of the eyelid that exposes the conjunctival membrane and part of the eyeball.

edema Abnormal accumulation of fluid in interstitial spaces of tissues.

egocentric Developmental characteristic wherein a toddler is only able to assume the view of his or her own activities and needs.

electrocardiogram (ECG) Graphic record of the electrical activity of the myocardium.

electrolyte Element or compound that, when melted or dissolved in water or other solvent, dissociates into ions and can carry an electrical current.

electronic health record (EHR) An electronic record of patient health information generated whenever a patient accesses medical care in any health care delivery setting.

electronic infusion device Piece of medical equipment that delivers intravenous fluids at a prescribed rate through an intravenous catheter.

electronic medical record Part of the electronic health record that contains patient data gathered in a health care setting at a specific time and place.

embolism Abnormal condition in which a blood clot (embolus) travels through the bloodstream and becomes lodged in a blood vessel.

emerging adulthood The time from adolescence to the young adult when responsibilities of a stable job, marriage, and parenthood begin. It includes five features: the age of identity exploration, the age of instability, the age of self-focus, the age of feeling in between, and the age of possibilities.

emic world view The inside perspective of a cultural encounter.

emotional intelligence Assessment and communication technique used to better understand and perceive emotions of themselves. This assists in building a therapeutic relationship.

empathy Understanding and acceptance of a person's feelings and the ability to sense the person's private world.

empowered Gave legal authority to or enabled an individual or group; promoted self-actualization of an individual or group.

endogenous infections Infections produced within a cell or organism.

endorphins Hormones that act on the mind and produce a sense of well-being and reduction of pain.

endotracheal tube Short-term artificial airways to administer mechanical ventilation, relieve upper airway obstruction, protect against aspiration, or clear secretions.

enema Procedure involving introduction of a solution into the rectum for cleansing or therapeutic purposes.

enteral nutrition (EN) Provision of nutrients through the gastrointestinal tract when the patient cannot ingest, chew, or swallow food but can digest and absorb nutrients.

entropion Condition in which the eyelid turns inward toward the eye.

environment All of the many factors (e.g., physical and psychological) that influence or affect the life and survival of a person.

epidermis Outer layer of the skin that has several thin layers in different stages of maturation; shields and protects the underlying tissues from water loss, mechanical or chemical injury, and penetration by disease-causing microorganisms.

epidural infusion Type of nerve block anesthesia in which an anesthetic is intermittently or continuously injected into the lumbosacral region of the spinal cord.

erythema Redness or inflammation of the skin or mucous membranes that is a result of dilation and congestion of superficial capillaries; sunburn is an example.

eschar Thick layer of dead, dry tissue that covers a pressure injury or thermal burn. It

may be allowed to be sloughed off naturally, or it may need to be surgically removed.

ethical dilemma Dilemma existing when the right thing to do is not clear. Resolution requires the negotiation of differing values among those involved in the dilemma.

ethical principles Set of guidelines for the expectations of a profession and the standards of behavior for its members.

ethics Principles or standards that govern proper conduct.

ethics of care Delivery of health care based on ethical principles and standards of care.

ethnic/cultural identity Individuals identify consciously or unconsciously with those with whom they feel a common bond because of similar traditions, behaviors, values, and beliefs.

ethnicity Shared identity related to social and cultural heritage such as values, language, geographical space, and racial characteristics.

ethnocentrism Tendency to hold one's own way of life as superior to that of others.

ethnohistory Significant historical experiences of a particular group.

etic world view The outside perspective of a cultural encounter.

etiology Study of all factors that may be involved in the development of a disease.

eupnea Normal respirations that are quiet, effortless, and rhythmical.

eustress Stress that protects health; one of the two types of stress identified by Selye.

evaluation Determination of the extent to which established patient goals have been achieved.

evidence-based knowledge Knowledge that is derived from the integration of best research, clinical expertise, and patient values.

evidence-based practice Use of current best evidence from nursing research, clinical expertise, practice trends, and patient preferences to guide nursing decisions about care provided to patients.

evisceration Protrusion of visceral organs through a surgical wound.

exacerbations Increases in the gravity of a disease or disorder as marked by greater intensity in signs or symptoms.

excessive daytime sleepiness Extreme fatigue felt during the day. Signs of this include falling asleep at inappropriate times such as while eating, talking, or driving. May indicate a sleep disorder.

excoriation Injury to the surface of the skin caused by abrasion.

exhaustion stage Phase that occurs when the body can no longer resist the stress (i.e., when the energy necessary to maintain adaptation is depleted).

exogenous infection Infection originating outside an organ or part.

exostosis Abnormal benign growth on the surface of a bone.

expected outcomes Expected conditions of a patient at the end of therapy or a disease process, including the degree of wellness and the need for continuing care, medications, support, counseling, or education.

extended care facility   Institution devoted to providing medical, nursing, or custodial care for an individual over a prolonged period such as during the course of a chronic disease or the rehabilitation phase after an acute illness.

extension   Movement by certain joints that increases the angle between two adjoining bones.

extracellular fluid (ECF)   Portion of body fluids composed of the interstitial fluid and blood plasma.

exudate   Fluid, cells, or other substances that have been discharged from cells or blood vessels slowly through small pores or breaks in cell membranes.

F

face-saving   Way of speaking or acting that preserves dignity.

Fahrenheit   Denotes temperature scale in which 32° is the freezing point of water and 212° is the boiling point of water at sea level.

faith   Set of beliefs and a way of relating to self, others, and a Supreme Being.

fajita   Cotton binder used on a newborn's abdomen among Hispanics and Filipinos to prevent gas and umbilical hernia.

family   Group of interacting individuals composing a basic unit of society.

family as context   Nursing perspective in which the family is viewed as a unit of interacting members having attributes, functions, and goals separate from those of the individual family members.

family caregiving   A family process that occurs in response to an illness and encompasses multiple cognitive, behavioral, and interpersonal processes.

family diversity   The uniqueness of each family unit. For example, some families experience marriage for the first time and then have children in later life

family durability   A system of support and structure within a family that extends beyond the walls of the household.

family dynamics   The interactions between family members which is affected by a family's makeup (configuration), structure, function, problem-solving, and coping capacity.

family forms   Patterns of people considered by family members to be included in the family.

family function   Focuses on the processes used by the family to achieve its goals. Some processes include communication among family members, goal setting, conflict resolution, caregiving, nurturing, and use of internal and external resources.

family hardiness   Internal strengths and durability of the family unit; characterized by a sense of control over the outcome of life events and hardships, a view of change as beneficial and growth-producing, and an active rather than passive orientation in responding to stressful life events.

family health   Determined by the effectiveness of the family's structure, the processes that the family uses to meet its goals, and internal and external forces.

family as patient   Nursing approach that takes into consideration the effect of one intervention on all members of a family.

family resiliency   Family's ability to cope with expected and unexpected stressors.

family structure   Based on organization (i.e., ongoing membership) of the family and the pattern of relationships.

farmacia   Place to obtain prescribed medications.

febrile   Pertaining to or characterized by an elevated body temperature.

fecal immunochemical test (FIT)   A screening test for colon cancer. It detects occult blood in the stool and is not affected by medication or foods ingested.

fecal impaction   Accumulation of hardened fecal material in the rectum or sigmoid colon.

fecal incontinence   Inability to control passage of feces and gas from the anus.

fecal occult blood test (FOBT)   Measures microscopic amounts of blood in the feces.

feces   Waste or excrement from the gastrointestinal tract.

feedback   Process in which the output of a given system is returned to the system.

felony   Crime of a serious nature that carries a penalty of imprisonment or death.

feminist ethics   Ethical approach that focuses on the nature of relationships to guide participants in making difficult decisions, especially relationships in which power is unequal or in which a point of view has become ignored or invisible.

fever   Elevation in the hypothalamic set point so that body temperature is regulated at a higher level.

fictive   Nonblood kin; considered family in some collective cultures.

fidelity   Agreement to keep a promise.

fight-or-flight response   Total physiological response to stress that occurs during the alarm reaction stage of the general adaptation syndrome. Massive changes in all body systems prepare a human being to choose to flee or remain and fight the stressor.

filtration   Straining of fluid through a membrane.

fistula   Abnormal passage from an internal organ to the surface of the body or between two internal organs.

flashback   Recollection so strong that the individual thinks that he or she is actually experiencing the trauma again or seeing it unfold before his or her eyes.

flatus   Intestinal gas.

flora   Microorganisms that live on or within a body to compete with disease-producing microorganisms and provide a natural immunity against certain infections.

flow sheets   Documents on which frequent observations or specific measurements are recorded.

fluctuance   Soft, boggy feeling when tissue is palpated; usually a sign of tissue infection.

fluid volume deficit (FVD)   Fluid and electrolyte disorder caused by failure of bodily homeostatic mechanisms to regulate the

retention and excretion of body fluids. The condition is characterized by decreased output of urine, high specific gravity of urine, output of urine that is greater than the intake of fluid in the body, hemoconcentration, and increased serum levels of sodium.

fluid volume excess (FVE)   Fluid and electrolyte disorder characterized by an increase in fluid retention and edema, resulting from failure of bodily homeostatic mechanisms to regulate the retention and excretion of body fluids.

focus charting   Charting methodology for structuring progress notes according to the focus of the note (e.g., symptoms and nursing diagnosis). Each note includes data, actions, and patient response.

focused cultural assessment   Method of evaluating a patient's ethnohistory, biocultural history, social organization, and religious and spiritual beliefs to find issues that are most relevant to the problem at hand.

food poisoning   Toxic processes resulting from the ingestion of a food contaminated by toxic substances or bacteria-containing toxins.

food security   All members of a household have access to sufficient safe, nutritious food to maintain a healthy lifestyle.

foot boots   Soft, foot-shaped devices designed to reduce the risk of footdrop by maintaining the foot in dorsiflexion.

footdrop   Abnormal neuromuscular condition of the lower leg and foot characterized by an inability to dorsiflex, or evert, the foot.

friction   Effects of rubbing or the resistance that a moving body meets from the surface on which it moves; a force that occurs in a direction to oppose movement.

functional health illiteracy   Inability of an individual to obtain, interpret, and understand basic information about health.

functional health patterns   Method for organizing assessment data based on the level of patient function in specific areas (e.g., mobility).

functional nursing   Method of patient care delivery in which each staff member is assigned a task that is completed for all patients on the unit.

future orientation   Time dimension emphasized by dominant American culture. It is characterized by direct communication and is focused on task achievement, whereas past orientation communication is circular and indirect and is focused on group harmony.

G

gait   Manner or style of walking, including rhythm, cadence, and speed.

gastrostomy feeding tube   Insertion of a feeding tube through a stoma into the stomach to provide enteral nutrition.

general adaptation syndrome (GAS)   Generalized defense response of the body to stress; consists of three stages: alarm, resistance, and exhaustion.

general anesthesia   Intravenous or inhaled medications that cause the patient to lose all sensation and consciousness.

genomics Describes the study of all the genes in a person and interactions of those genes with one another and with that person's environment.

geriatrics Branch of health care dealing with the physiology and psychology of aging and the diagnosis and treatment of diseases affecting older adults.

gerontology Study of all aspects of the aging process and its consequences.

gingivae Gums of the mouth; mucous membrane with supporting fibrous tissue that overlies the crowns of unerupted teeth and encircles the necks of teeth that have erupted.

glaucoma Abnormal condition of elevated pressure within an eye caused by obstruction of the outflow of aqueous humor. If untreated, it often results in peripheral visual loss, decreased visual acuity with difficulty adapting to darkness, and a halo effect around lights.

globalization Worldwide scope or application.

glomerulus Cluster or collection of capillary vessels within the kidney involved in the initial formation of urine.

gluconeogenesis Formation of glucose or glycogen from substances that are not carbohydrates such as protein or lipid.

glucose Primary fuel for the body; needed to carry out major physiological functions.

glycogen Polysaccharide that is the major carbohydrate stored in animal cells.

glycogenesis Process for storing glucose in the form of glycogen in the liver.

goals Desired results of nursing actions set realistically by the nurse and patient as part of the planning stage of the nursing process.

Good Samaritan laws Legislation enacted in some states to protect health care professionals from liability in rendering emergency aid unless there is proven willful wrong or gross negligence.

graduated measuring container Receptacle for volume measurement.

granny midwives Amateur health practitioners that assist in labor and delivery.

granulation tissue Soft, pink, fleshy projections of tissue that form during the healing process in a wound not healing by primary intention.

graphic record Charting mechanism that allows for the recording of vital signs and weight in such a manner that caregivers can quickly note changes in the patient's status.

grief Form of sorrow involving the person's thoughts, feelings, and behaviors that occurs as a response to an actual or perceived loss.

grieving process Sequence of affective, cognitive, and physiological states through which the person responds to and finally accepts an irretrievable loss.

grounded Connection between the electric circuit and the ground, which becomes part of the circuit.

growth Measurable or quantitative aspect of an individual's increase in physical dimensions as a result of an increase in number of cells. Indicators of growth include changes in height, weight, and sexual characteristics.

guided imagery Method of pain control in which the patient creates a mental image, concentrates on that image, and gradually becomes less aware of pain.

gustatory Pertaining to the sense of taste.

H

halal Foods permissible for Muslims to eat.

hand rolls Rolls of cloth that keep the thumb slightly adducted and in opposition to the fingers.

hand-wrist splints Splints individually molded for the patient to maintain proper alignment of the thumb, slight adduction of the wrist, and slight dorsiflexion.

haram Foods prohibited by Muslim religious standards.

health Dynamic state in which individuals adapt to their internal and external environments so that there is a state of physical, emotional, intellectual, social, and spiritual well-being.

health belief model Conceptual framework that describes a person's health behavior as an expression of his or her health beliefs.

health beliefs Patient's personal beliefs about levels of wellness that can motivate or impede participation in changing risk factors, participating in care, and selecting care options.

health care–acquired infection Infection that was not present or incubating at the time of admission to a health care setting.

health care problems Any conditions or dysfunctions that the patient experiences as a result of illness or treatment of an illness.

health disparities Preventable differences in the burden of disease, injury, violence, or opportunities to achieve optimal health that are experienced by socially and economically disadvantaged populations.

health informatics Application of computer and information science in all basic and applied biomedical sciences to facilitate the acquisition, processing, interpretation, optimal use, and communication of health-related data.

health literacy Patients' reading and mathematics skills, comprehension, ability to make health-related decisions, and successful functioning as a consumer of health care.

health promotion Activities such as routine exercise and good nutrition that help patients maintain or enhance their present level of health and reduce their risk of developing certain diseases.

health promotion model Defines health as a positive, dynamic state, not merely the absence of disease. The health promotion model emphasizes well-being, personal fulfillment, and self-actualization rather than reaction to the threat of illness.

health status Description of health of an individual or community.

heat exhaustion Abnormal condition caused by depletion of body fluid and electrolytes resulting from exposure to intense heat or the inability to acclimatize to heat.

heat stroke Continued exposure to extreme heat that raises the core body temperature to 40.5° C (105° F) or higher.

hematemesis Vomiting of blood, indicating upper gastrointestinal bleeding.

hematoma Collection of blood trapped in the tissues of the skin or an organ.

hematuria Abnormal presence of blood in the urine.

hemolysis Breakdown of red blood cells and release of hemoglobin that may occur after administration of hypotonic intravenous solutions, causing swelling and rupture of erythrocytes.

hemoptysis Coughing up blood from the respiratory tract.

hemorrhoids Permanent dilation and engorgement of veins within the lining of the rectum.

hemostasis Termination of bleeding by mechanical or chemical means or the coagulation process of the body.

hemothorax Accumulation of blood and fluid in the pleural cavity between the parietal and visceral pleurae.

hernia Protrusion of an organ through an abnormal opening in the muscle wall of the cavity that surrounds it.

hilots Amateur health practitioners who assist in labor and delivery among Filipinos.

holistic Of or pertaining to the whole; considering all factors.

holistic health Comprehensive view of the person as a biopsychosocial and spiritual being.

home care Health service provided in the patient's place of residence to promote, maintain, or restore health or minimize the effects of illness and disability.

homeostasis State of relative constancy in the internal environment of the body; maintained naturally by physiological adaptive mechanisms.

hope Confident but uncertain expectation of achieving a future goal.

hospice System of family-centered care designed to help terminally ill people be comfortable and maintain a satisfactory lifestyle throughout the terminal phase of their illness.

Hoyer lift Mechanical device that uses a canvas sling to easily lift dependent patients for transfer.

humidification Process of adding water to gas.

humor Coping strategy based on an individual's cognitive appraisal of a stimulus that results in behavior such as smiling, laughing, or feelings of amusement that lessen emotional distress.

hydrocephalus Abnormal accumulation of cerebrospinal fluid in the ventricles of the brain.

hydrostatic pressure Pressure caused by a liquid.

hyperactive/overactive bladder Common bladder complaint that occurs more frequently with aging and includes the symptoms of urgency, frequency, nocturia, and urge incontinence.

hypercalcemia Greater-than-normal amount of calcium in the blood.

hypercapnia Greater-than-normal amounts of carbon dioxide in the blood; also called hypercarbia.

hyperextension Position of maximal extension of a joint.

hyperglycemia Elevated serum glucose levels.

hypertension Disorder characterized by an elevated blood pressure persistently exceeding 120/80 mm Hg.

hyperthermia Situation in which body temperature exceeds the set point.

hypertonic Situation in which one solution has a greater concentration of solute than another; therefore the first solution exerts greater osmotic pressure.

hypertonicity Excessive tension of the arterial walls or muscles.

hyperventilation Respiratory rate in excess of that required to maintain normal carbon dioxide levels in the body tissues.

hypnotics Class of drug that causes insensibility to pain and induces sleep.

hypostatic pneumonia Pneumonia that results from fluid accumulation as a result of inactivity.

hypotension Abnormal lowering of blood pressure that is inadequate for normal perfusion and oxygenation of tissues.

hypothermia Abnormal lowering of body temperature below 35° C, or 95° F, usually caused by prolonged exposure to cold.

hypotonic Situation in which one solution has a smaller concentration of solute than another; therefore the first solution exerts less osmotic pressure.

hypotonicity Reduced tension of the arterial walls or muscles.

hypoventilation Respiratory rate insufficient to prevent carbon dioxide retention.

hypovolemia Abnormally low circulating blood volume.

hypoxemia Arterial blood oxygen level less than 60 mm Hg; low oxygen level in the blood.

hypoxia Inadequate cellular oxygenation that may result from a deficiency in the delivery or use of oxygen at the cellular level.

I

identity Component of self-concept characterized by one's persisting consciousness of being oneself, separate and distinct from others.

idiosyncratic reaction Individual sensitivity to effects of a drug caused by inherited or other bodily constitution factors.

illness (1) Abnormal process in which any aspect of a person's functioning is diminished or impaired compared with his or her previous condition. (2) The personal, interpersonal, and cultural reaction to disease.

illness behavior Ways in which people monitor their bodies, define and interpret their symptoms, take remedial actions, and use the health care system.

illness prevention Health education programs or activities directed toward protecting patients from threats or potential threats to health and minimizing risk factors.

immobility Inability to move about freely; caused by any condition in which movement is impaired or therapeutically restricted.

immunity Quality of being insusceptible to or unaffected by a particular disease or condition.

immunization Process by which resistance to an infectious disease is induced or augmented.

implementation Initiation and completion of the nursing actions necessary to help the patient achieve health care goals.

impression management Ability to interpret others' behavior within their own context of meanings and behave in a culturally congruent way to achieve desired outcomes of communication.

incentive spirometry Method of encouraging voluntary deep breathing by providing visual feedback to patients of the inspiratory volume they have achieved.

incident rates Rate of new cases of a disease in a specified population over a defined period of time.

incident report Confidential document that describes any patient accident while the person is on the premises of a health care agency. (See occurrence report.)

independent practice association (IPA) Managed care organization that contracts with physicians or health care providers who usually are members of groups and whose practices include fee-for-service and capitated patients.

indirect care interventions Treatments performed away from the patient but on behalf of the patient or group of patients.

induration Hardening of a tissue, particularly the skin, because of edema or inflammation.

infection Invasion of the body by pathogenic microorganisms that reproduce and multiply.

inference (1) Judgment or interpretation of informational cues. (2) Taking one proposition as a given and guessing that another proposition follows.

infiltration Dislodging an intravenous catheter or needle from a vein into the subcutaneous space.

inflammation Protective response of body tissues to irritation or injury.

informed consent Process of obtaining permission from a patient to perform a specific test or procedure after describing all risks, side effects, and benefits.

infusion pump Device that delivers a measured amount of fluid over a period of time.

infusions Introduction of fluid into the vein, giving intravenous fluid over time.

inhalation Method of medication delivery through the patient's respiratory tract. The respiratory tract provides a large surface area for drug absorption. Inhalation can be through the nasal or oral route.

injections Parenteral administration of medication; four major sites of injection: subcutaneous, intramuscular, intravenous, and intradermal.

inpatient prospective payment system (IPPS) Payment mechanism for reimbursing hospitals for inpatient health care services in which a predetermined rate is set for treatment of specific illnesses.

input For the nursing process, the data or information that comes from a patient's assessment.

insensible water loss Water loss that is continuous and not perceived by the person.

insomnia Condition characterized by chronic inability to sleep or remain asleep through the night.

inspection Method of physical examination by which the patient is visually and systematically examined for appearance, structure, function, and behavior.

instillation To cause to enter drop by drop or very slowly.

institutional ethics committee Interdisciplinary committee that discusses and processes ethical dilemmas that arise within a health care institution.

instrumental activities of daily living (IADLs) Activities necessary for independence in society beyond eating, grooming, transferring, and toileting; include such skills as shopping, preparing meals, banking, and taking medications.

integrated delivery network (IDN) Set of providers and services organized to deliver a coordinated continuum of care to the population of patients served at a capitated cost.

interpersonal communication Exchange of information between two persons or among persons in a small group.

interstitial fluid Fluid that fills the spaces between most of the cells of the body and provides a substantial portion of the liquid environment of the body.

interview Organized, systematic conversation with the patient designed to obtain pertinent health-related subjective information.

intracellular fluid Liquid within the cell membrane.

intradermal (ID) Injection given between layers of the skin into the dermis. Injections are given at a 5- to 15-degree angle.

intramuscular (IM) Injections given into muscle tissue. The intramuscular route provides a fast rate of absorption that is related to the greater vascularity of the muscle. Injections are given at a 90-degree angle.

intraocular Method of medication delivery that involves inserting a medication disk similar to a contact lens into the patient's eye.

intrapersonal communication Communication that occurs within an individual (i.e., people "talk with themselves" silently or form an idea in their own mind).

intravascular fluid Fluid circulating within blood vessels of the body.

intravenous Injection directly into the bloodstream. Action of the drug begins immediately when given intravenously.

intravenous fat emulsions Soybean- or safflower oil–based solutions that are isotonic and may be infused with amino acid and dextrose solution through a central or peripheral line.

intubation Insertion of a breathing tube through the mouth or nose into the trachea to ensure a patent airway.

intuition Inner sensing that something is so.

irrigation Process of washing out a body cavity or wounded area with a stream of fluid.

ischemia Decreased blood supply to a body part such as skin tissue or to an organ such as the heart.

isolation Separation of a seriously ill patient from others to prevent the spread of an infection or protect the patient from irritating environmental factors.

isometric exercises Activities that involve muscle tension without muscle shortening, do not have any beneficial effect on preventing orthostatic hypotension but may improve activity tolerance.

isotonic Situation in which two solutions have the same concentration of solute; therefore both solutions exert the same osmotic pressure.

J

jaundice Yellow discoloration of the skin, mucous membranes, and sclera caused by greater-than-normal amounts of bilirubin in the blood.

jejunostomy tube Hollow tube inserted into the jejunum through the abdominal wall for administration of liquefied foods to patients who have a high risk of aspiration.

joint contracture Abnormality that may result in permanent condition of a joint; is characterized by flexion and fixation; and is caused by disuse, atrophy, and shortening of muscle fibers and surrounding joint tissues.

joints Connections between bones; classified according to structure and degree of mobility.

judgment Ability to form an opinion or draw sound conclusions.

justice Ethical standard of fairness.

K

Kardex Trade name for card-filing system that allows quick reference to the particular need of the patient for certain aspects of nursing care.

karma Asian Indian belief that attributes mental illness to past deeds in one's previous life.

knowing the patient An in-depth knowledge of the patient's patterns of responses; fosters skilled clinical decision making.

Korotkoff sound Sound heard during the taking of blood pressure using a sphygmomanometer and stethoscope.

Kussmaul respiration Increase in both rate and depth of respirations.

kyphosis Exaggeration of the posterior curvature of the thoracic spine.

L

la cuarentena Period of rest and restricted physical activity after childbirth that usually lasts 40 days.

laceration Torn, jagged wound.

language Code that conveys specific meaning as words are combined.

laryngospasm Sudden uncontrolled contraction of the laryngeal muscles, which in turn decreases airway size.

lateral violence Hostile, aggressive, and harmful verbal and nonverbal behavior by a nurse to another nurse via attitudes, actions, words,

or behaviors. This behavior includes criticizing, intimidations, blaming, fighting, public humiliation, isolating, withholding assistance, or undermining efforts in completing assignments. This leaves the nurse feeling bullied, inadequate and powerless.

law Rule, standard, or principle that states a fact or relationship between factors.

laxatives Drugs that act to promote bowel evacuation.

learning Acquisition of new knowledge and skills as a result of reinforcement, practice, and experience.

learning objective Written statement that describes the behavior that a teacher expects from an individual after a learning activity.

left-sided heart failure Abnormal condition characterized by impaired functioning of the left ventricle caused by elevated pressures and pulmonary congestion.

leukoplakia Thick, white patches observed on oral mucous membranes.

licensed practical nurse (LPN) Also known as the licensed vocational nurse (LVN) or in Canada, registered nurse's assistant (RNA); trained in basic nursing skills and the provision of direct patient care.

licensed vocational nurse (LVN) The LVN is the same as a licensed practical nurse (LPN), an individual trained in the United States in basic nursing techniques and direct patient care who practices under the supervision of a registered nurse. The LVN is licensed by a board after completing what is usually a 12-month educational program and passing a licensure examination. In Canada an LVN is called a certified nursing assistant.

lipids Compounds that are insoluble in water but soluble in organic solvents.

lipogenesis Process during which fatty acids are synthesized.

living wills Instruments by which a dying person makes wishes known.

local anesthesia Loss of sensation at the desired site of action.

logroll Maneuver used to turn a reclining patient from one side to the other or completely over without moving the spinal column out of alignment.

lordosis Increased lumbar curvature.

M

maceration Softening and breaking down of skin from prolonged exposure to moisture.

mal de ojo Evil eye.

malignant hyperthermia Autosomal-dominant trait characterized by often fatal hyperthermia in affected people exposed to certain anesthetic agents.

malpractice Injurious or unprofessional actions that harm another.

malpractice insurance Type of insurance to protect the health care professional. In case of a malpractice claim, the insurance pays the award to the plaintiff.

managed care Health care system in which there is administrative control over primary health care services. Redundant facilities and

services are eliminated, and costs are reduced. Preventive care and health education are emphasized.

Maslow's hierarchy of needs Model developed by Abraham Maslow that is used to explain human motivation.

matrilineal Kinship that is limited to only the mother's side.

maturation Genetically determined biological plan for growth and development. Physical growth and motor development are a function of maturation.

maturational loss Loss, usually of an aspect of self, resulting from the normal changes of growth and development.

Medicaid State medical assistance to people with low incomes, based on Title XIX of the Social Security Act. States receive matching federal funds to provide medical care and services to people meeting categorical and income requirements.

medical asepsis Procedures used to reduce the number of microorganisms and prevent their spread.

medical diagnosis Formal statement of the disease entity or illness made by the physician or health care provider.

medical record Patient's chart; a legal document.

Medicare Federally funded national health insurance program in the United States for people over 65 years of age. The program is administered in two parts. Part A provides basic protection against costs of medical, surgical, and psychiatric hospital care. Part B is a voluntary medical insurance program financed in part from federal funds and in part from premiums contributed by people enrolled in the program.

medication abuse Maladaptive pattern of recurrent medication use.

medication allergy Adverse reaction such as rash, chills, or gastrointestinal disturbances to a medication. Once a drug allergy occurs, the patient can no longer receive that particular medication.

medication dependence Maladaptive pattern of medication use in the following patterns: using excessive amounts of the medication, increased activities directed toward obtaining the medication, or withdrawal from professional or recreational activities.

medication error Any event that could cause or lead to a patient's receiving inappropriate drug therapy or failing to receive appropriate drug therapy.

medication interaction Response that occurs when one drug modifies the action of another drug. The interaction can potentiate or diminish the actions of another drug, or it may alter the way a drug is metabolized, absorbed, or excreted.

melanoma Group of malignant neoplasms, primarily of the skin, that are composed of melanocytes. Common in fair-skinned people having light-colored eyes and in those who have been sunburned.

melena Abnormal black, sticky stool containing digested blood that is indicative of gastrointestinal bleeding.

menarche Onset of a girl's first menstruation.

Ménière's disease Chronic disease of the inner ear characterized by recurrent episodes of vertigo; progressive sensorineural hearing loss, which may be bilateral; and tinnitus.

menopause Physiological cessation of ovulation and menstruation that typically occurs during middle adulthood in women.

message Information sent or expressed by sender in the communication process.

metabolic acidosis Abnormal condition of high hydrogen ion concentration in the extracellular fluid caused by either a primary increase in hydrogen ions or a decrease in bicarbonate.

metabolic alkalosis Abnormal condition characterized by the significant loss of acid from the body or increased levels of bicarbonate.

metabolism Aggregate of all chemical processes that take place in living organisms and result in growth, generation of energy, elimination of wastes, and other functions concerned with the distribution of nutrients in the blood after digestion.

metacommunication Dependent not only on what is said but also on the relationship to the other person involved in the interaction. It is a message that conveys the sender's attitude toward self and the message and the attitudes, feelings, and intentions toward the listener.

metastasize Spread of tumor cells to distant parts of the body from a primary site (e.g., lung, breast, or bowel).

metatheory An area of study that examines the relationships of various components that make up the knowledge of a discipline, including philosophical, theoretical, and empirical components that provide a broad overview of the discipline.

metered-dose inhaler (MDI) Device designed to deliver a measured dose of an inhalation drug.

metric system Logically organized decimal system of measurement; metric units can easily be converted and computed through simple multiplication and division. Each basic unit of measurement is organized into units of 10.

microorganisms Microscopic entities such as bacteria, viruses, and fungi that are capable of carrying on living processes.

micturition Urination; act of passing or expelling urine voluntarily through the urethra.

milliequivalent per liter (mEq/L) Number of grams of a specific electrolyte dissolved in 1 L of plasma.

mindfulness A moment-to-moment present awareness with an attitude of nonjudgment, acceptance, and openness. Mindfulness meditative practices are effective in reducing psychological and physical symptoms or perceptions of stress.

mind mapping Graphic approach to represent the connections between concepts and ideas (e.g., nursing diagnoses) that are related to a central subject (e.g., the patient's health problems).

minerals Inorganic elements essential to the body because of their role as catalysts in biochemical reactions.

minimum data set (MDS) Required by the Omnibus Budget Reconciliation Act of 1987, the MDS is a uniform data set established by the Department of Health and Human Services. It serves as the framework for any state-specified assessment instruments used to develop a written and comprehensive plan of care for newly admitted residents of nursing facilities.

minimum effective concentration (MEC) The plasma level of a medication below which the effect of the medication does not occur.

misdemeanor Lesser crime than a felony; the penalty is usually a fine or imprisonment for less than 1 year.

mobility Person's ability to move about freely.

moderate sedation/analgesia/conscious sedation Administration of central nervous system depressant drugs and/or analgesics to provide analgesia, relieve anxiety, and/or provide amnesia during surgical, diagnostic, or interventional procedures. Routinely used for diagnostic or therapeutic procedures that do not require complete anesthesia but simply a decreased level of consciousness.

monosaturated fatty acid Fatty acid in which some of the carbon atoms in the hydrocarbon chain are joined by double or triple bonds. Monounsaturated fatty acids have only one double or triple bond per molecule and are found as components of fats in such foods as fowls, almonds, pecans, cashew nuts, peanuts, and olive oil.

morals Personal conviction that something is absolutely right or wrong in all situations.

motivation Internal impulse that causes a person to take action.

motivational interviewing Interview technique used to identify patients' thoughts, beliefs, fears, and current health care behavior with the aim of helping them to identify improved self-care behaviors.

mourning Process of grieving.

murmurs Blowing or whooshing sounds created by changes in blood flow through the heart or abnormalities in valve closure.

muscle tone Normal state of balanced muscle tension.

myocardial contractility Measure of stretch of the cardiac muscle fiber. It can also affect stroke volume and cardiac output. Poor contraction decreases the amount of blood ejected by the ventricles during each contraction.

myocardial infarction Necrosis of a portion of cardiac muscle caused by obstruction in a coronary artery.

myocardial ischemia Condition that results when the supply of blood to the myocardium from the coronary arteries is insufficient to meet the oxygen demands of the organ.

N

NANDA International North American Nursing Diagnosis Association, organized in 1973. It formally identifies, develops, and classifies nursing diagnoses.

narcolepsy Syndrome involving sudden sleep attacks that a person cannot inhibit. Uncontrollable desire to sleep may occur several times during a day.

nasogastric (NG) tube Tube passed into the stomach through the nose to empty the stomach of its contents or deliver medication and/or nourishment.

nebulization Process of adding moisture to inspired air by adding water droplets.

necessary losses Losses that every person experiences.

necrotic Of or pertaining to the death of tissue in response to disease or injury.

negative health behaviors Practices actually or potentially harmful to health such as smoking, drug or alcohol abuse, poor diet, and refusal to take necessary medications.

negative nitrogen balance Condition occurring when the body excretes more nitrogen than it takes in.

negligence Careless act of omission or commission that results in injury to another.

neonate Stage of life from birth to 1 month of age.

nephrons Structural and functional units of the kidney containing renal glomeruli and tubules.

neurotransmitter Chemical that transfers the electrical impulse from the nerve fiber to the muscle fiber.

Never Events Serious incidents that are wholly preventable because guidance or safety recommendations that provide strong systemic protective barriers are available at a national level and should have been implemented by all health care providers.

nociceptors Somatic and visceral free nerve endings of thinly myelinated and unmyelinated fibers. They usually react to tissue injury but may also be excited by endogenous chemical substances.

nocturia Urination at night; can be a symptom of renal disease or may occur in persons who drink excessive amounts of fluids before bedtime.

nonblanchable hyperemia Redness of the skin caused by dilation of the superficial capillaries. The redness persists when pressure is applied to the area, indicating tissue damage.

noninvasive positive-pressure ventilation (NPPV) Used to prevent using invasive artificial airways (endotracheal [ET] tube or tracheostomy) in patients with acute respiratory failure, cardiogenic pulmonary edema, or exacerbation of chronic obstructive pulmonary disease. It has also been used following extubation of an ET tube.

nonmaleficence Fundamental ethical agreement to do no harm. Closely related to the ethical standard of beneficence.

nonrapid eye movement (NREM) sleep Sleep that occurs during the first four stages of normal sleep.

nonshivering thermogenesis Occurs primarily in neonates. Because neonates cannot shiver, a limited amount of vascular brown adipose tissue present at birth can be metabolized for heat production.

nonverbal communication Communication using expressions, gestures, body posture, and positioning rather than words.

normal sinus rhythm (NSR) The wave pattern on an electrocardiogram that indicates normal conduction of an electrical impulse through the myocardium.

numbing One of Bowlby's four phases of mourning. It is characterized by a lack of feeling or by feeling stunned by a loss; may last a few days or many weeks.

nurse-initiated interventions Response of the nurse to the patient's health care needs and nursing diagnoses. This type of intervention is an autonomous action based on scientific rationale that is executed to benefit the patient in a predicted way related to the nursing diagnosis and patient-centered goals.

Nurse Practice Acts Statutes enacted by the legislature of any of the states or the appropriate officers of the districts or possessions that describe and define the scope of nursing practice.

Nursing Clinical Information System (NCIS) A system that incorporates the principles of nursing informatics to support the work that nurses do by facilitating documentation of nursing process activities and offering resources for managing nursing care delivery.

nursing diagnosis Formal statement of an actual or potential health problem that nurses can legally and independently treat; the second step of the nursing process, during which the patient's actual and potential unhealthy responses to an illness or condition are identified.

nursing health history Data collected about a patient's present level of wellness, changes in life patterns, sociocultural role, and mental and emotional reactions to illness.

nursing intervention Any treatment based on clinical judgment and knowledge that a nurse performs to enhance patient outcomes.

Nursing Outcomes Classification A systematic organization of nurse-sensitive outcomes into groups or categories based upon similarities, dissimilarities, and relationships among the outcomes.

nursing process Systematic problem-solving method by which nurses individualize care for each patient. The five steps of the nursing process are assessment, diagnosis, planning, implementation, and evaluation.

nursing-sensitive outcomes Outcomes that are within the scope of nursing practice; consequences or effects of nursing interventions that result in changes in the patient's symptoms, functional status, safety, psychological distress, or costs.

nurturant Behavior that involves caring for or fostering the well-being of another individual.

nutrients Foods that contain elements necessary for body function, including water, carbohydrates, proteins, fats, vitamins, and minerals.

O

obesity Abnormal increase in the proportion of fat cells, mainly in the viscera and subcutaneous tissues of the body.

objective data Information that can be observed by others; free of feelings, perceptions, prejudices.

occurrence report Confidential document that describes any patient accident while the person is on the premises of a health care agency. (See incident report.)

olfactory Pertaining to the sense of smell.

oncotic pressure Total influence of the protein on the osmotic activity of plasma fluid.

open-ended question Form of question that prompts a respondent to answer in more than one or two words.

operating bed Table for surgery.

operating room (1) Room in a health care facility in which surgical procedures requiring anesthesia are performed. (2) Informal: a suite of rooms or an area in a health care facility in which patients are prepared for surgery, undergo surgical procedures, and recover from the anesthetic procedures required for the surgery.

ophthalmic Drugs given into the eye in the form of either eye drops or ointments.

ophthalmoscope Instrument used to illuminate the structures of the eye to examine the fundus, which includes the retina, choroid, optic nerve disc, macula, fovea centralis, and retinal vessels.

opioid Drug substance derived from opium or produced synthetically that alters perception of pain and that, with repeated use, may result in physical and psychological dependence (narcotic).

oral hygiene Condition or practice of maintaining the tissues and structures of the mouth.

orthopnea Abnormal condition in which a person must sit or stand to breathe comfortably.

orthostatic hypotension Abnormally low blood pressure occurring when a person stands.

osmolality Concentration or osmotic pressure of a solution expressed in osmoles or milliosmoles per kilogram of water.

osmolarity Osmotic pressure of a solution expressed in osmoles or milliosmoles per kilogram of the solution.

osmoreceptors Neurons in the hypothalamus that are sensitive to the fluid concentration in the blood plasma and regulate the secretion of antidiuretic hormone.

osmosis Movement of a pure solvent through a semipermeable membrane from a solution with a lower solute concentration to one with a higher solute concentration.

osmotic pressure Drawing power for water, which depends on the number of molecules in the solution.

osteoporosis Disorder characterized by abnormal rarefaction of bone, occurring most frequently in postmenopausal women, sedentary or immobilized individuals, and patients on long-term steroid therapy.

ostomy Surgical procedure in which an opening is made into the abdominal wall to allow the passage of intestinal contents from the bowel (colostomy) or urine from the bladder (urostomy).

other provider interventions Therapies that require the combined knowledge, skill, and expertise of multiple health care providers; also called *interdependent interventions*.

otoscope Instrument with a special ear speculum used to examine the deeper structures of the external and middle ear.

ototoxic Having a harmful effect on the eighth cranial (auditory) nerve or the organs of hearing and balance.

outcome Condition of a patient at the end of treatment, including the degree of wellness and the need for continuing care, medication, support, counseling, or education.

outliers Patients with extended lengths of stay beyond allowable inpatient days or costs.

outpatient Patient who has not been admitted to a hospital but receives treatments in a clinic or facility associated with the hospital.

output The product and information obtained from the system.

oxygen desaturation A decrease in oxygen concentration in the blood resulting from any condition that affects the exchange of carbon dioxide and oxygen.

oxygen saturation Amount of hemoglobin fully saturated with oxygen, given as a percent value.

oxygen therapy Procedure in which oxygen is administered to a patient to relieve or prevent hypoxia.

P

pain Subjective, unpleasant sensation caused by noxious stimulation of sensory nerve endings.

palliative care Level of care that is designed to relieve or reduce intensity of uncomfortable symptoms but not to produce a cure. Palliative care relies on comfort measures and use of alternative therapies to help individuals become more at peace during end of life.

pallor Unnatural paleness or absence of color in the skin.

palpation Method of physical examination whereby the fingers or hands of the examiner are applied to the patient's body to feel body parts underlying the skin.

palpitations Bounding or racing of the heart associated with normal emotions or a heart disorder.

Papanicolaou (Pap) smear Painless screening test for cervical cancer. Specimens are taken of squamous and columnar cells of the cervix.

parallel play Form of play among a group of children, primarily toddlers, in which each one engages in an independent activity that is similar to but not influenced by or shared with the others.

paralytic ileus Usually temporary paralysis of intestinal wall that may occur after abdominal surgery or peritoneal injury and that causes cessation of peristalsis; leads to abdominal distention and symptoms of obstruction.

parenteral administration Giving medication by a route other than the gastrointestinal tract.

parenteral nutrition (PN) Administration of a nutritional solution into the vascular system.

parteras Lay midwives.

partial bed bath Bath in which body parts that might cause the patient discomfort if left unbathed (i.e., face, hands, axillary areas, back, and perineum) are washed in bed.

passive range-of-motion (PROM) exercises Range of movement through which a joint is moved with assistance.

passive strategies of health promotion Activities that involve the patient as the recipient of actions by health care professionals.

pathogenicity Ability of a pathogenic agent to produce a disease.

pathogens Microorganisms capable of producing disease.

pathological fractures Fractures resulting from weakened bone tissue; frequently caused by osteoporosis or neoplasms.

patient-centered care Concept to improve work efficiency by changing the way that patient care is delivered.

patient- and family-centered care Model of nursing care in which mutual partnerships between the patient, family and health care team are formed to plan, implement and evaluate the nursing and health care delivered.

patient-controlled analgesia (PCA) Drug delivery system that allows patients to self-administer analgesic medications on demand.

patrilineal, patrilineally Kinship that is limited to only the father's side.

pay for performance Quality improvement program that rewards excellence through financial incentives to motivate change to achieve measurable improvements and improve patient care quality and safety.

perceived loss Loss that is less obvious to others. Although easily overlooked or misunderstood, a perceived loss results in the same grief process as an actual loss.

perception An individual's mental image or concept of elements in their environment, including information gained through the senses.

percussion Method of physical examination whereby the location, size, and density of a body part is determined by the tone obtained from the striking of short, sharp taps of the fingers.

perfusion (1) Passage of a fluid through a specific organ or an area of the body. (2) Therapeutic measure whereby a drug intended for an isolated part of the body is introduced via the bloodstream. (3) Relates to the ability of the cardiovascular system to pump oxygenated blood to the tissues and return deoxygenated blood to the lungs.

perineal care Procedure prescribed for cleaning the genital and anal areas as part of the daily bath or after various obstetrical and gynecological procedures.

perioperative nursing Refers to the role of the operating room nurse during the preoperative, intraoperative, and postoperative phases of surgery.

peripherally inserted central catheter (PICC) Alternative intravenous access when the patient requires intermediate-length venous access greater than 7 days to 3 months. Intravenous access is achieved by inserting a catheter into a central vein by way of a peripheral vein.

peristalsis Rhythmical contractions of the intestine that propel gastric contents through the length of the gastrointestinal tract.

peritonitis Inflammation of the peritoneum produced by bacteria or irritating substances introduced into the abdominal cavity by a penetrating wound or perforation of an organ in the gastrointestinal or reproductive tract.

PERRLA Acronym for "pupils equal, round, reactive to light, accommodation"; the acronym is recorded in the physical examination if eye and pupil assessments are normal.

personalismo Personalistic.

petechiae Tiny purple or red spots that appear on skin as minute hemorrhages within dermal layers.

pharmacokinetics Study of how drugs enter the body, reach their site of action, are metabolized, and exit from the body.

phlebitis Inflammation of a vein.

physician-initiated interventions Based on the physician's response to a medical diagnosis, the nurse responds to his or her written orders.

PIE note Problem-oriented medical record; the four interdisciplinary sections are the database, problem list, care plan, and progress notes.

placebos Dosage form that contains no pharmacologically active ingredients but may relieve pain through psychological effects.

plaintiff Individual who files formal charges against an individual or organization for a legal offense.

planning Process of designing interventions to achieve the goals and outcomes of health care delivery.

plantar flexion Toe-down motion of the foot at the ankle.

pleural friction rub Adventitious lung sound caused by inflamed parietal and visceral pleura rubbing together on inspiration.

pneumothorax Collection of air or gas in the pleural space.

point of maximal impulse (PMI) Point where the heartbeat can most easily be palpated through the chest wall. This is usually the fourth intercostal space at the midclavicular line.

point of view Way of looking at issues that reflects an individual's culture and societal influences.

poison Any substance that impairs health or destroys life when ingested, inhaled, or absorbed by the body in relatively small amounts.

poison control center One of a network of facilities that provides information regarding all aspects of poisoning or intoxication, maintains records of their occurrence, and refers patients to treatment centers.

polypharmacy Use of a number of different drugs by a patient who may have one or several health problems.

polyunsaturated fatty acid Fatty acid that has two or more carbon double bonds.

population Collection of individuals who have in common one or more personal or environmental characteristics.

positive health behaviors Activities related to maintaining, attaining, or regaining good health and preventing illness. Common positive health behaviors include immunizations, proper sleep patterns, adequate exercise, and nutrition.

postanesthesia care unit (PACU) Area adjoining the operating room to which surgical patients are taken while still under anesthesia.

postmortem care Care of a patient's body after death.

postural drainage Use of positioning along with percussion and vibration to drain secretions from specific segments of the lungs and bronchi into the trachea.

postural hypotension Abnormally low blood pressure occurring when an individual assumes the standing posture; also called orthostatic hypotension.

posture Position of the body in relation to the surrounding space.

power of attorney for health care Person designated by the patient to make health care decisions for the patient if the patient becomes unable to make his or her own decisions.

preadolescence Transitional developmental stage that occurs between childhood and adolescence.

preanesthesia care unit Area outside the operating room where preoperative preparations are completed.

preload Volume of blood in the ventricles at the end of diastole, immediately before ventricular contraction.

preoperative teaching Instruction regarding a patient's anticipated surgery and recovery that is given before surgery. Instruction includes, but is not limited to, dietary and activity restrictions, anticipated assessment activities, postoperative procedures, and pain-relief measures.

presbycusis Hearing loss associated with aging. It usually involves both a loss of hearing sensitivity and a reduction in the clarity of speech.

presbyopia Gradual decline in ability of the lens to accommodate or focus on close objects; reduces ability to see near objects clearly. This condition commonly develops with advancing age.

prescriptions Written directions for a therapeutic agent (e.g., medication, drugs).

presence Deep physical, psychological, and spiritual connection or engagement between a nurse and patient.

present time orientation Time dimension that focuses on what is happening here and now. Communication patterns are circular, and this time orientation is in conflict with the dominant organizational norm in health care that emphasizes punctuality and adherence to appointments.

pressure injury Inflammation, sore, or ulcer in the skin over a bony prominence.

presurgical care unit (PSCU) Area outside the operating room where preoperative preparations are completed.

preventive nursing actions Nursing actions directed toward preventing illness and promoting health to avoid the need for primary, secondary, or tertiary health care.

primary appraisal Evaluating an event for its personal meaning related to stress.

primary care First contact in a given episode of illness that leads to a decision regarding a course of action to resolve the health problem.

primary health care Combination of primary and public health care that is accessible to individuals and families in a community and provided at an affordable cost.

primary intention Primary union of the edges of a wound, progressing to complete scar formation without granulation.

primary nursing Method of nursing practice in which the patient's care is managed for the duration by one nurse who directs and coordinates other nurses and health care personnel. When on duty, the primary nurse cares for the patient directly.

primary prevention First contact in a given episode of illness that leads to a decision regarding a course of action to prevent worsening of the health problem.

problem-focused diagnosis A clinical judgment concerning an undesirable human response to a health condition/life process that exists in an individual, family or community.

problem identification One of the steps of the diagnostic process in which the patient's health care problem is recognized as a result of data analysis based on professional knowledge and experience.

problem-oriented medical record (POMR) Method of recording data about the health status of a patient that fosters a collaborative problem-solving approach by all members of the health care team.

problem solving Methodical, systematic approach to explore conditions and develop solutions, including analysis of data, determination of causative factors, and selection of appropriate actions to reverse or eliminate the problem.

productive cough Sudden expulsion of air from the lungs that effectively removes sputum from the respiratory tract and helps clear the airways.

professional standards review organization (PSRO) Focuses on evaluation of nursing care provided in a health care setting. The quality, effectiveness, and appropriateness of nursing care for the patient are the focus of evaluation.

prone Position of the patient lying face down.

proprioception Ability of the body to sense its position and movement in space.

prostaglandins Potent hormonelike substances that act in exceedingly low doses on target organs. They can be used to treat asthma and gastric hyperacidity.

proteins Any of a large group of naturally occurring, complex, organic nitrogenous compounds. Each is composed of large combinations of amino acids containing the elements carbon; hydrogen; nitrogen; oxygen; usually sulfur; and occasionally phosphorus, iron, iodine, or other essential constituents of living cells. Protein is the major source of building

material for muscles, blood, skin, hair, nails, and the internal organs.

proteinuria Presence in the urine of abnormally large quantities of protein, usually albumin. Persistent proteinuria is usually a sign of renal disease or renal complications of another disease, hypertension, or heart failure.

protocol Written and approved plan specifying the procedures to be followed during an assessment or in providing treatment.

pruritus Symptom of itching; an uncomfortable sensation leading to the urge to scratch.

psychomotor learning Acquisition of ability to perform motor skills.

ptosis Abnormal condition of one or both upper eyelids in which the eyelid droops; caused by weakness of the levator muscle or paralysis of the third cranial nerve.

puberty Developmental period of emotional and physical changes, including the development of secondary sex characteristics and the onset of menstruation and ejaculation.

public health nursing Nursing specialty that requires the nurse to care for the needs of populations or groups.

public communication Interaction of one individual with large groups of people.

pulmonary hygiene More frequent turning, deep breathing, coughing, use of incentive spirometry, and chest physical therapy (PT) if ordered.

pulse deficit Condition that exists when the radial pulse is less than the ventricular rate as auscultated at the apex or seen on an electrocardiogram. The condition indicates a lack of peripheral perfusion for some of the heart contractions.

pulse pressure Difference between the systolic and diastolic pressures, normally 30 to 40 mm Hg.

Purkinje network Complex network of muscle fibers that spread through the right and left ventricles of the heart and carry the impulses that contract those chambers almost simultaneously.

pursed-lip breathing Deep inspiration followed by prolonged expiration through pursed lips.

pyrexia Abnormal elevation of the temperature of the body above 37° C (98.6° F) because of disease; same as fever.

pyrogens Substances that cause a rise in body temperature, as in the case of bacterial toxins.

Q

QSEN The Quality and Safety in the Education of Nurses (QSEN) initiative is the commitment of nursing to the competencies outlined in the Institute of Medicine report related to nursing education. QSEN encompasses six competencies: patient-centered care, teamwork, collaboration, evidence-based practice, quality improvement, and safety.

quality improvement Monitoring and evaluation of processes and outcomes in health care or any other business to identify opportunities for improvement.

quality indicator Quantitative measure of an important aspect of care that determines

whether quality of service conforms to requirements or standards of care.

R

race Common biological characteristics shared by a group of people.

racial identity One's self-identification with one or more social groups in which a common heritage with a racial group is shared.

Ramadan Religious observance held during the ninth month of the Islamic calendar year. It involves fasting from sunrise to sunset.

range of motion (ROM) Range of movement of a joint from maximum extension to maximum flexion as measured in degrees of a circle.

rapid eye movement (REM) sleep Stage of sleep in which dreaming and rapid eye movements are prominent; important for mental restoration.

reaction Component of the pain experience that may include both physiological responses, as in the general adaptation syndrome, and behavioral responses.

reality orientation Therapeutic modality for restoring an individual's sense of the present.

receiver Person to whom message is sent during the communication process.

reception Neurophysiological components of the pain experience in which nervous system receptors receive painful stimuli and transmit them through peripheral nerves to the spinal cord and brain.

record Written form of communication that permanently documents information relevant to health care management.

recovery Period of time immediately following surgery when the patient is closely observed for effects of anesthesia, changes in vital signs, and bleeding. The recovery area is usually in the postanesthesia care unit.

referent Factor that motivates a person to communicate with another individual.

reflection Process of thinking back or recalling an event to discover the meaning and purpose of that event. Useful in critical thinking.

refractive error Defect in the ability of the lens of the eye to focus light such as occurs in nearsightedness and farsightedness.

regional anesthesia Loss of sensation in an area of the body supplied by sensory nerve pathways.

registered nurse (RN) In the United States a nurse who has completed a course of study at a state-approved, accredited school of nursing and has passed the National Council Licensure Examination (NCLEX-RN).

regression Return to an earlier developmental stage or behavior.

regulatory agencies Local, state, provincial, or national agencies that inspect and certify health care agencies as meeting specified standards. These agencies can also determine the amount of reimbursement for health care delivered.

rehabilitation Restoration of an individual to normal or near-normal function after a physical or mental illness, injury, or chemical addiction.

reinforcement Provision of a contingent response to a learner's behavior that increases the probability of recurrence of the behavior.

related factor Any condition or event that accompanies or is linked with the patient's health care problem.

relaxation Act of being relaxed or less tense.

reminiscence Recalling the past to assign new meaning to past experiences.

remissions Partial or complete disappearances of the clinical and subjective characteristics of chronic or malignant disease; remission may be spontaneous or the result of therapy.

renal calculi Calcium stones in the renal pelvis.

renin Proteolytic enzyme produced by and stored in the juxtaglomerular apparatus that surrounds each arteriole as it enters a glomerulus. The enzyme affects the blood pressure by catalyzing the change of angiotensinogen to angiotensin, a strong repressor.

reorganization Last phase of Bowlby's phases of mourning. During this phase, which sometimes requires a year or more, the person begins to accept unaccustomed roles, acquire new skills, and build new relationships.

report Transfer of information from the nurses on one shift to the nurses on the following shift. Report may also be given by one of the members of the nursing team to another health care provider (e.g., a physician or therapist).

reservoir Place where microorganisms survive, multiply, and await transfer to a susceptible host.

residual urine Volume of urine remaining in the bladder after a normal voiding; the bladder normally is almost completely empty after micturition.

resistance stage Third stage of the stress response, when the person attempts to adapt to the stressor. The body stabilizes; hormone levels stabilize; and heart rate, blood pressure, and cardiac output return to normal.

resource utilization group (RUG) Method of classification for health care reimbursement for long-term care facilities.

respeto Respectful.

respiration Exchange of oxygen and carbon dioxide during cellular metabolism.

respiratory acidosis Abnormal condition characterized by increased arterial carbon dioxide concentration, excess carbonic acid, and increased hydrogen ion concentration.

respiratory alkalosis Abnormal condition characterized by decreased arterial carbon dioxide concentration and hydrogen ion concentration.

respite care Short-term health services to dependent older adults either in their homes or in an institutional setting.

responsibility Carrying out duties associated with a particular role.

restorative care Health care settings and services in which patients who are recovering from illness or disability receive rehabilitation and supportive care.

restraint Device to aid in the immobilization of a patient or patient's extremity.

return demonstration Demonstration after the patient has first observed the teacher and then practiced the skill in mock or real situations.

rhonchi Abnormal lung sound auscultated when the patient's airways are obstructed with thick secretions.

right-sided heart failure Abnormal condition that results from impaired functioning of the right ventricle; characterized by venous congestion in the systemic circulation.

risk factor Any internal or external variable that makes a person or group more vulnerable to illness or an unhealthy event.

risk management Function of hospital or other health facility administration that is directed toward identification, evaluation, and correction of potential risks that could lead to injury of patients, staff members, or visitors and result in property loss or damage.

risk nursing diagnosis A clinical judgment concerning the vulnerability of an individual, family, group, or community for developing an undesirable human response to health conditions/life processes.

role performance Way in which a person views his or her ability to carry out significant roles.

root cause analysis Process of data collection and analysis that aids in finding the real cause of the problem and working on dealing with it rather than just dealing with its effects.

S

Sabbath From sundown on Friday to sundown on Saturday, this religious observance is a day of rest and worship for Jews and some Christian sects.

sandbags Sand-filled plastic tubes that can be shaped to body contours. They can immobilize an extremity or maintain body alignment.

saturated fatty acid Fatty acid in which each carbon in the chain has an attached hydrogen atom.

scientific method Codified sequence of steps used in the formulation, testing, evaluation, and reporting of scientific ideas.

scientific rationale Reason why a specific nursing action was chosen based on supporting literature.

scoliosis Lateral spinal curvature.

scope of nursing practice A professional definition of what a nurse is licensed to perform.

scrub nurse Registered nurse or operating room technician who assists surgeons during operations.

secondary appraisal Evaluating one's possible coping strategies when confronted with a stressor.

secondary intention Wound closure in which the edges are separated; granulation tissue develops to fill the gap; and, finally, epithelium grows in over the granulation, producing a larger scar than results with primary intention.

secondary prevention Level of preventive medicine that focuses on early diagnosis, use of referral services, and rapid initiation of treatment to stop the progress of disease processes.

sedatives Medications that produce a calming effect by decreasing functional activity, diminishing irritability, and allaying excitement.

segmentation Alternating contraction and relaxation of gastrointestinal mucosa.

self-concept Complex, dynamic integration of conscious and unconscious feelings, attitudes, and perceptions about one's identity, physical being, worth, and roles; how a person perceives and defines self.

self-esteem Feeling of self-worth characterized by feelings of achievement, adequacy, self-confidence, and usefulness.

self-transcendence Sense of authentically connecting to one's inner self.

sender Person who initiates interpersonal communication by conveying a message.

sensible water loss Loss of fluid from the body through the secretory activity of the sweat glands and the exhalation of humidified air from the lungs.

sensory deficits Defects in the function of one or more of the senses, resulting in visual, auditory, or olfactory impairments.

sensory deprivation State in which stimulation to one or more of the senses is lacking, resulting in impaired sensory perception.

sensory overload State in which stimulation to one or more of the senses is so excessive that the brain disregards or does not meaningfully respond to stimuli.

sequential compression stockings Plastic stockings attached to an air pump that inflates and deflates the stockings, applying intermittent pressure sequentially from the ankle to the knee.

serum half-life Time needed for excretion processes to lower the serum drug concentration by half.

sexual dysfunction Inability or difficulty in sexual functioning caused by physiological or psychological factors or both.

sexual identity How a person thinks about himself or herself sexually; it includes gender identity, gender role, and sexual orientation

sexual orientation Clear, persistent erotic preference for a person of one sex or the other.

sexuality "A function of the total personality … concerned with the biological, psychological, sociological, spiritual and culture variables of life …" (Sex Information and Education Council of the United States, 1980).

sexually transmitted infection Infectious process spread through sexual contact, including oral, genital, or anal sexual activity.

shear Force exerted against the skin while the skin remains stationary and the bony structures move.

side effect Any reaction or consequence that results from medication or therapy.

side rails Bars positioned along the sides of the length of the bed or stretcher to reduce the patient's risk of falling.

simpatia Friendly.

sinoatrial (SA) node Called the *pacemaker of the heart* because the origin of the normal heartbeat begins at the SA node. The SA node is in the right atrium next to the entrance of the superior vena cava.

situational crisis Unexpected crisis that arises suddenly in response to an external event or a conflict concerning a specific circumstance.

situational loss Loss of a person, thing, or quality resulting from a change in a life situation, including changes related to illness, body image, environment, and death.

sitz bath Bath in which only the hips or buttocks are immersed in fluid.

skilled nursing facility Institution or part of an institution that meets criteria for accreditation established by the sections of the Social Security Act that determine the basis for Medicaid and Medicare reimbursement for skilled nursing care, including rehabilitation and various medical and nursing procedures.

sleep State marked by reduced consciousness, diminished activity of the skeletal muscles, and depressed metabolism.

sleep apnea Cessation of breathing for a time during sleep.

sleep deprivation Condition resulting from a decrease in the amount, quality, and consistency of sleep.

SOAP note Progress note that focuses on a single patient problem and includes subjective and objective data, analysis, and planning; most often used in the problem-oriented medical record (POMR).

social determinants of health Factors that contribute to a person's current state of health. These factors may be biological, socioeconomic, psychosocial, behavioral, or social in nature.

socializing Interacting with friends or other people; communicating with others to form relationships and help people feel relaxed.

solute Substance dissolved in a solution.

solution Mixture of one or more substances dissolved in another substance. The molecules of each of the substances disperse homogeneously and do not change chemically. A solution may be a liquid, gas, or solid.

solvent Any liquid in which another substance can be dissolved.

source record Organization of a patient's chart so that each discipline (e.g., nursing, medicine, social work, or respiratory therapy) has a separate section in which to record data. Unlike POMR, the information is not organized by patient problems. The advantage of a source record is that caregivers can easily locate the proper section of the record in which to make entries.

sphygmomanometer Device for measuring the arterial blood pressure that consists of an arm or leg cuff with an air bladder connected to a tube, a bulb for pumping air into the bladder, and a gauge for indicating the amount of air pressure being exerted against the artery.

spiritual distress State of being out of harmony with a system of beliefs, a Supreme Being, or God.

spiritual well-being Individual's spirituality that enables a person to love, have faith and hope, seek meaning in life, and nurture relationships with others.

spirituality Spiritual dimension of a person, including the relationship with humanity, nature, and a Supreme Being.

standard of care Minimum level of care accepted to ensure high-quality care to patients. Standards of care define the types of therapies typically administered to patients with defined problems or needs.

Standard Precautions Guidelines recommended by the Centers for Disease Control and Prevention (CDC) to reduce risk of transmission of bloodborne and other pathogens in hospitals.

standardized care plans Written care plans used for groups of patients who have similar health care problems.

standing order Written and approved documents containing rules, policies, procedures, regulations, and orders for the conduct of patient care in various stipulated clinical settings.

statutory law Of or related to laws enacted by a legislative branch of the government.

stenosis Abnormal condition characterized by the constriction or narrowing of an opening or passageway in a body structure.

stereotypes Generalizations that are made about individuals without further assessment.

sterilization (1) Rendering a person unable to produce children; accomplished by surgical, chemical, or other means. (2) A technique for destroying microorganisms using heat, water, chemicals, or gases.

stoma Artificially created opening between a body cavity and the surface of the body (e.g., a colostomy formed from a portion of the colon pulled through the abdominal wall).

stress Physiological or psychological tension that threatens homeostasis or a person's psychological equilibrium.

stressor Any event, situation, or other stimulus encountered in a person's external or internal environment that necessitates change or adaptation by the person.

striae Streaks or linear scars that result from rapid development of tension in the skin.

stroke volume (SV) Amount of blood ejected by the ventricles with each contraction. It can be affected by the amount of blood in the left ventricle at the end of diastole (preload), the resistance to left ventricular ejection (afterload), and myocardial contractility.

subacute care Level of medical specialty care provided to patients who need a greater intensity of care than that provided in a skilled nursing facility but who do not require acute care.

subcultures Various ethnic, religious, and other groups with distinct characteristics from the dominant culture.

subcutaneous (sub-Q) Injection given into the connective tissue under the dermis. The subcutaneous tissue absorbs drugs more slowly than those injected into muscle. Injections are usually given at a 45-degree angle.

subjective data Information gathered from patient statements; the patient's feelings and perceptions. Not verifiable by another except by inference.

sublingual Route of medication administration in which the medication is placed underneath the patient's tongue.

Sunrise Model A model developed by Leininger that aids the health care practitioner in designing care decisions and actions in a culturally congruent fashion.

supine Position of the patient in which the patient is resting on his or her back.

suprainfection Secondary infection usually caused by an opportunistic pathogen.

suprapubic catheter Catheter surgically inserted through abdomen into bladder.

surfactant Chemical produced in the lungs to maintain the surface tension of the alveoli and keep them from collapsing.

surgical asepsis Procedures used to eliminate any microorganisms from an area. Also called *sterile technique.*

sympathy Concern, sorrow, or pity felt by the nurse for the patient. Sympathy is a subjective look at another person's world that prevents a clear perspective of all sides of the issues confronting that person.

synapse Region surrounding the point of contact between two neurons or between a neuron and an effector organ.

syncope Brief lapse in consciousness caused by transient cerebral hypoxia.

synergistic effect Effect resulting from two drugs acting synergistically. The effect of the two drugs combined is greater than the effect that would be expected if the individual effects of the two drugs acting alone were added together.

systolic Pertaining to or resulting from ventricular contraction.

T

tachycardia Rapid regular heart rate ranging between 100 and 150 beats/min.

tachypnea Abnormally rapid rate of breathing.

tactile Relating to the sense of touch.

tactile fremitus Tremulous vibration of the chest wall during breathing that is palpable on physical examination.

teaching Implementation method used to present correct principles, procedures, and techniques of health care; to inform patients about their health status; and to refer patients and family to appropriate health or social resources in the community.

team nursing Decentralized system in which the care of a patient is distributed among the members of a team. The charge nurse delegates authority to a team leader, who must be a professional nurse.

teratogens Chemical or physiological agents that may produce adverse effects in the embryo or fetus.

tertiary prevention Activities directed toward rehabilitation rather than diagnosis and treatment.

therapeutic communication Process in which the nurse consciously influences a patient or helps the patient to a better understanding through verbal and/or nonverbal communication.

therapeutic effect Desired benefit of a medication, treatment, or procedure.

therapeutic range   The safe therapeutic range is between the minimum effective concentration and the toxic concentration.

thermogenesis   The physiological process of heat production in the body.

thermoregulation   Internal control of body temperature.

threshold   Point at which a person first perceives a painful stimulus as being painful.

thrill   Continuous palpable sensation like the purring of a cat.

thrombus   Accumulation of platelets, fibrin, clotting factors, and the cellular elements of the blood attached to the interior wall of a vein or artery, sometimes occluding the lumen of the vessel.

tinnitus   Ringing heard in one or both ears.

tissue ischemia   Point at which tissues receive insufficient oxygen and perfusion.

tolerance   Point at which a person is not willing to accept pain of greater severity or duration.

tort   Act that causes injury for which the injured party can bring civil action.

total patient care   Nursing delivery of care model originally developed during Florence Nightingale's time. In the model a registered nurse (RN) is responsible for all aspects of care for one or more patients. The RN works directly with the patient, family, physician or health care provider, and health care team members. The model typically has a shift-based focus.

touch   To come in contact with another person, often conveying caring, emotional support, encouragement, or tenderness.

toxic effect   Effect of a medication that results in an adverse response.

tracheostomy   Procedure whereby a surgical incision is made into the trachea and a short artificial airway (a tracheostomy tube) is inserted.

transcendence   The belief that there is a force outside of and greater than the person that exists beyond the material world.

transcultural   Concept of care extending across cultures that distinguishes nursing from other health disciplines.

transcultural nursing   Distinct discipline developed by Leininger that focuses on the comparative study of cultures to understand similarities and differences among groups of people.

transcutaneous electrical nerve stimulation (TENS)   Technique in which a battery-powered device blocks pain impulses from reaching the spinal cord by delivering weak electrical impulses directly to the surface of the skin.

transdermal disk   Medication delivery device in which the medication is saturated on a waferlike disk, which is affixed to the patient's skin. This method ensures that the patient receives a continuous level of medication.

transfer report   Verbal exchange of information between caregivers when a patient is moved from one nursing unit or health care setting to another. The report includes information necessary to maintain a consistent level of care from one setting to another.

transformational leadership   A leadership style that focuses on change and innovation through effective communication and team building. Engagement, empowerment, and accountability are critical to team effectiveness.

transfusion reaction   Systemic response by the body to the administration of blood incompatible with that of the recipient.

trapeze bar   Metal triangular-shaped bar that can be suspended over a patient's bed from an overhanging frame; permits patients to move up and down in bed while in traction or some other encumbrance.

trimester   Referring to one of the three phases of pregnancy.

trochanter roll   Rolled towel support placed against the hips and upper leg to prevent external rotation of the legs.

trough   The lowest serum concentration of a medication before the next medication dose is administered.

turgor   Normal resiliency of the skin caused by the outward pressure of the cells and interstitial fluid.

U

unconscious/implicit bias   A bias that an individual is unaware of and that happens outside his or her control; it is influenced by personal background, cultural environment, and personal experiences.

unsaturated fatty acid   Fatty acid in which an unequal number of hydrogen atoms are attached and the carbon atoms attach to one another with a double bond.

ureterostomy   Diversion of urine away from a diseased or defective bladder through an artificial opening in the skin.

urge incontinence   A type of urinary incontinence that results from sudden, involuntary contraction of the muscles of the urinary bladder, resulting in an urge to urinate.

urinal   Receptacle for collecting urine.

urinary diversion   Surgical diversion of the drainage of urine such as a ureterostomy.

urinary incontinence   Inability to control urination.

urinary reflux   Abnormal, backward flow of urine.

urinary retention   Retention of urine in the bladder; condition frequently caused by a temporary loss of muscle function.

urine hat   Receptacle for collecting urine that fits toilet.

urometer   Device for measuring frequent and small amounts of urine from an indwelling urinary catheter system.

urosepsis   Organisms in the bloodstream.

utilitarianism   Ethic that proposes that the value of something is determined by its usefulness. The greatest good for the greatest number of people constitutes the guiding principle for action in a utilitarian model of ethics.

utilization review (UR) committees   Physician-supervised committees to review admissions, diagnostic testing, and treatments provided by physicians or health care providers to patients.

V

validation   Act of confirming, verifying, or corroborating the accuracy of assessment data or the appropriateness of the care plan.

Valsalva maneuver   Any forced expiratory effort against a closed airway such as when an individual holds his or her breath and tightens his or her muscles in a concerted, strenuous effort to move a heavy object or change positions in bed.

value   Personal belief about the worth of a given idea or behavior.

valvular heart disease   Acquired or congenital disorder of a cardiac valve characterized by stenosis and obstructed blood flow or valvular degeneration and regurgitation of blood.

variance   Unexpected event that occurs during patient care and that is different from CareMap predictions. Variances or exceptions are interventions or outcomes that are not achieved as anticipated. Variance may be positive or negative.

variant   Differing from a set standard.

vascular access devices   Catheters, cannulas, or infusion ports designed for long-term, repeated access to the vascular system.

vasoconstriction   Narrowing of the lumen of any blood vessel, especially the arterioles and the veins in the blood reservoirs of the skin and abdominal viscera.

vasodilation   Increase in the diameter of a blood vessel caused by inhibition of its vasoconstrictor nerves or stimulation of dilator nerves.

venipuncture   Technique in which a vein is punctured transcutaneously by a sharp rigid stylet (e.g., a butterfly needle), a cannula (e.g., an angiocatheter that contains a flexible plastic catheter), or a needle attached to a syringe.

ventilation   Respiratory process by which gases are moved into and out of the lungs.

verbal communication   Sending of messages from one individual to another or to a group of individuals through the spoken word.

vertigo   Sensation of dizziness or spinning.

vibration   Fine, shaking pressure applied by hands to the chest wall only during exhalation.

Virchow's triad   The three broad categories of factors that are thought to contribute to formation of a venous thrombosis: hypercoagulability, hemodynamic changes, and endothelial injury or dysfunction.

virulence   Ability of an organism to rapidly produce disease.

visual   Related to or experienced through vision.

vital signs   Temperature, pulse, respirations, and blood pressure.

vitamins   Organic compounds essential in small quantities for normal physiological and metabolic functioning of the body. With few exceptions, vitamins cannot be synthesized by the body and must be obtained from the diet or dietary supplements.

voiding   Process of urinating.

vulnerable populations   Collection of individuals who are more likely to develop health problems as a result of excess risks, limits in access to health care services, or being dependent on others for care.

W

wellness Dynamic state of health in which an individual progresses toward a higher level of functioning, achieving an optimum balance between internal and external environments.

wellness education Activities that teach people how to care for themselves in a healthy manner.

wellness nursing diagnosis Clinical judgment about an individual, group, or community in transition from a specific level of wellness to a higher level of wellness.

wheezes, wheezing Adventitious lung sounds caused by a severely narrowed bronchus.

work redesign Formal process used to analyze the work of a certain work group and change the actual structure of the jobs performed.

workplace violence The act or threat of violence, ranging from verbal abuse to physical assault, directed toward persons at work or on duty.

worldview Cognitive stance or perspective about phenomena characteristic of a particular cultural group.

wound culture Specimen collected from a wound to determine the specific organism that is causing an infectious process.

Y

yearning and searching Second phase of Bowlby's phases of mourning. It is characterized by emotional outbursts of tearful sobbing and acute distress.

Z

Z-track injection Technique for injecting irritating preparations into muscle without tracking residual medication through sensitive tissues.

INDEX

Note: Page numbers followed by *b* indicate boxes, *f* indicate illustrations, and *t* indicate tables

SPECIAL FEATURES